210839
S/7

GOODMAN and GILMAN's
The Pharmacological Basis
of Therapeutics

EDITORS

Alfred Goodman Gilman
M.D., Ph.D.

Professor and Chairman, Department of Pharmacology,
The University of Texas Health Science Center at Dallas,
Dallas, Texas

Louis S. Goodman
M.A., M.D., D.Sc.(Hon.)

Distinguished Professor of Pharmacology,
University of Utah College of Medicine,
Salt Lake City, Utah

Alfred Gilman
Ph.D., D.Sc.(Hon.)

Lecturer in Pharmacology,
Yale University School of Medicine,
New Haven, Connecticut;
Professor Emeritus of Pharmacology,
Albert Einstein College of Medicine of Yeshiva University,
Bronx, New York

ASSOCIATE EDITORS

Steven E. Mayer
M.S., Ph.D.

Professor of Medicine,
Division of Pharmacology,
University of California, San Diego,
School of Medicine, La Jolla, California

Kenneth L. Melmon
M.D.

Professor of Medicine and Pharmacology, and Chairman, Department of Medicine,
Stanford University School of Medicine,
Stanford, California

GOODMAN and GILMAN's
The Pharmacological Basis of Therapeutics

SIXTH EDITION

MACMILLAN PUBLISHING CO., INC.

New York

COLLIER MACMILLAN CANADA, INC.

Toronto

COLLIER MACMILLAN PUBLISHERS

London

MACMILLAN PUBLISHING CO., INC.
866 Third Avenue • New York, N.Y. 10022

COLLIER MACMILLAN CANADA, INC.

COLLIER MACMILLAN PUBLISHERS • London

Library of Congress catalog card number 80-19261
ISBN 0-02-344720-6
Baillière Tindall SBN 0 7020 08265

Printing: 5 6 7 8   Year: 3 4 5 6

The use of portions of the text of USP XX–NF XV is by permission of the USP Convention. The Convention is not responsible for any inaccuracy of quotation or for any false or misleading implication that may arise from separation of excerpts from the original context or by obsolescence resulting from publication of a supplement.

In this textbook, reference to proprietary names of drugs is ordinarily made only in chapter sections dealing with preparations. Such names are given in SMALL-CAP TYPE, usually immediately following the official or nonproprietary titles. Proprietary names of drugs also appear in the Index.

PREFACE TO THE SIXTH EDITION

THE first edition of this textbook, published nearly 40 years ago, was written when basic pharmacology was not fully accepted as a meaningful or relevant biomedical discipline. The appearance of that book did much to change the picture. An eminent pharmacologist, commenting on the first edition many years after its publication, stated that it provided a renaissance or perhaps more properly the *naissance* of the teaching and practice of pharmacology. The second edition, published in the mid-1950s, reflected the immense impact of the post–World War II burgeoning of biomedical research. Subsequent editions have been written as multiauthored works—a reflection of the enormous change in the content, stature, and function of pharmacology; its role in the biomedical sciences; and its impact on the clinical sciences and rational therapeutics. The Preface to the First Edition is reprinted herein, because it clearly states the three primary objectives that have guided the writing of all subsequent editions. Adherence to these objectives has encouraged widespread and successful use of *The Pharmacological Basis of Therapeutics* by both students and practitioners of medicine and other health professions, both in the United States and abroad.

While those familiar with previous editions of this textbook will immediately recognize the organization of the present volume, several major changes deserve emphasis. The section on general principles (Section I) has been expanded and divided into three chapters, including a new introductory treatise on "Principles of Therapeutics" (Chapter 3). Pharmacokinetic data have become available at an accelerating rate, and there is thus continued attention to the basic and applied aspects of this subject. Fundamental discussion is presented in Chapter 1, and a practical approach to the optimal utilization of this information is presented in a major new unit (Appendix II), which includes both explanatory text and readily utilized tables for a large number of important agents. Parallel advances have been made in the understanding of drug interactions. The basic mechanisms of clinically relevant interactions are analyzed for individual drugs, and an index of drug interactions has been prepared for ready reference (Appendix III).

Other major changes include a new chapter on "Neurohumoral Transmission and the Central Nervous System" (Chapter 12), presented as an introduction to the section that describes drugs that modify the functions of the CNS; this chapter serves as an important complement to its well-known predecessor on "Neurohumoral Transmission and the Autonomic Nervous System" (Chapter 4). An entire new section of the textbook (Section XVII) is concerned with toxicology. While detailed presentation of toxicological information is naturally left to more specialized books, familiarity with the basic tenets of this discipline has assumed increasing importance for the practicing physician. Emphasis is placed on principles and on description of the most commonly encountered metallic and nonmetallic environmental toxins.

Studies of receptors for neurotransmitters, autacoids, hormones, and drugs are yielding important insights into mechanisms of drug action as well as the pathophysiology of disease. Examples discussed in the text include receptors for agents that regulate the synthesis of cyclic AMP, the role of antibodies to nicotinic cholinergic receptors in the etiology of myasthenia gravis, inhibition of the biosynthesis of prostaglandins and related autacoids by a number of anti-inflammatory agents, the role of Na^+, K^+-ATPase in the mechanism of action of digitalis glycosides, and many others.

Newly approved drugs are of course fully discussed, as are many that are still in the developmental stage but show promise as future therapeutic agents. Drugs described for the first time in this sixth edition include the newer benzodiazepines, valproic acid and clonazepam for the treatment of seizure disorders, opioid agonist-antagonists (nalbuphine, buprenorphine, butorphanol), anti-inflammatory agents (sulindac, propionic acid derivatives), antihypertensive agents (minoxidil, captopril, prazosin, saralasin), adrenergic blocking agents (metoprolol, nadolol, timolol), antibiotics (amikacin, cefamandole, cefoxitin, ticarcillin), antineoplastic drugs (cisplatin, tamoxifen), and many others.

Despite the large number of new drugs and a wealth of new information on these and older agents, intense effort has been made to prevent undue expansion of the sixth edition. This has required extensive rewriting and condensation of less dynamic areas. Nearly one half of the chapters of this edition have been entirely rewritten; most of the remainder have been vigorously revised.

Many of the contributors to the fifth edition were able and anxious to participate in the current undertaking, and we are indebted for this loyalty. We are also pleased to welcome several outstanding new authors and two new associate editors. Virtually everyone who was invited to participate did so enthusiastically and with recognition of the effort necessary for the production of a cohesive and comprehensive textbook.

In addition to paying tribute to our collaborators, we gratefully acknowledge the advice and help received from scores of individuals, too numerous to mention by name. However, note should be made of the contribution of Drs. Sam K. Shimomura and Larry J. Davis, who reviewed all sections of the text on pharmaceutical preparations and dosages. Special thanks are also due to our editorial assistants—Wendy Deaner, Jane Rall, and Debra Lewis—who performed untold tasks with skill and outstanding good humor. The editors and authors also owe a great debt to Joan Carolyn Zulch, Editor-in-Chief, Medical Books Department, Macmillan Publishing Co., Inc. Twenty-five years of experience with this textbook have afforded her ample opportunity to refine her skills as an expert editor, a self-taught pharmacologist, and an able manipulator of the procrastinating spirit. Prefaces to previous editions of this textbook allowed the original authors and editors to pay tribute to their long-lasting friendship; this sentiment is reaffirmed. Special note can now also be made of rewarding and satisfying communication between generations.

ALFRED GOODMAN GILMAN
LOUIS S. GOODMAN
ALFRED GILMAN

PREFACE TO THE FIRST EDITION

THREE objectives have guided the writing of this book—the correlation of pharmacology with related medical sciences, the reinterpretation of the actions and uses of drugs from the viewpoint of important advances in medicine, and the placing of emphasis on the applications of pharmacodynamics to therapeutics.

Although pharmacology is a basic medical science in its own right, it borrows freely from and contributes generously to the subject matter and technics of many medical disciplines, clinical as well as preclinical. Therefore, the correlation of strictly pharmacological information with medicine as a whole is essential for a proper presentation of pharmacology to students and physicians. Furthermore, the reinterpretation of the actions and uses of well-established therapeutic agents in the light of recent advances in the medical sciences is as important a function of a modern textbook of pharmacology as is the description of new drugs. In many instances these new interpretations necessitate radical departures from accepted but outworn concepts of the actions of drugs. Lastly, the emphasis throughout the book, as indicated in its title, has been clinical. This is mandatory because medical students must be taught pharmacology from the standpoint of the actions and uses of drugs in the prevention and treatment of disease. To the student, pharmacological data per se are valueless unless he is able to apply his information in the practice of medicine. This book has also been written for the practicing physician, to whom it offers an opportunity to keep abreast of recent advances in therapeutics and to acquire the basic principles necessary for the rational use of drugs in his daily practice.

The criteria for the selection of bibliographic references require comment. It is obviously unwise, if not impossible, to document every fact included in the text. Preference has therefore been given to articles of a review nature, to the literature on new drugs, and to original contributions in controversial fields. In most instances, only the more recent investigations have been cited. In order to encourage free use of the bibliography, references are chiefly to the available literature in the English language.

The authors are greatly indebted to their many colleagues at the Yale University School of Medicine for their generous help and criticism. In particular they are deeply grateful to Professor Henry Gray Barbour, whose constant encouragement and advice have been invaluable.

LOUIS S. GOODMAN
ALFRED GILMAN

New Haven, Connecticut
November 20, 1940

CONTRIBUTORS

Baldessarini, Ross J., M.D., M.A.(Hon.). Professor of Psychiatry, Harvard Medical School; Associate Director, Mailman Laboratories for Psychiatric Research, McLean Division of Massachusetts General Hospital, Belmont, Massachusetts

Benet, Leslie Z., Ph.D. Professor and Chairman, Department of Pharmacy, School of Pharmacy, University of California, San Francisco, California

Bianchine, Joseph R., M.D., Ph.D. Professor and Chairman, Department of Pharmacology, and Professor of Medicine, Ohio State University, Columbus, Ohio

Bigger, J. Thomas, Jr., M.D. Professor of Medicine and Pharmacology, Columbia University College of Physicians and Surgeons, New York, New York

Blaschke, Terrence F., M.D. Chief, Division of Clinical Pharmacology, Stanford University School of Medicine, Stanford, California

Bloom, Floyd E., M.D. Professor, The Salk Institute, La Jolla, California

Calabresi, Paul, M.D. Professor and Chairman, Department of Medicine, Brown University; Physician-in-Chief, Roger Williams General Hospital, Providence, Rhode Island

Cohn, Victor H., Ph.D. Professor of Pharmacology, George Washington University School of Medicine, Washington, D. C.

Cooperman, Lee H., M.D. Professor of Anesthesiology, University of Pennsylvania School of Medicine, Philadelphia, Pennsylvania

Danford, Darla Erhard, M.P.H., D.Sc. Department of Nutrition, Harvard University School of Public Health, Boston, Massachusetts

Davis, Larry J., Pharm.D. Assistant Clinical Professor of Pharmacy and Associate Director, Drug Information Analysis Service, Division of Clinical Pharmacy, School of Pharmacy, University of California, San Francisco, California

Douglas, William W., M.D., Ch.B. Professor of Pharmacology, Yale University School of Medicine, New Haven, Connecticut

Finch, Clement A., M.D. Professor of Medicine, University of Washington School of Medicine, Seattle, Washington

Fingl, Edward, Ph.D. Professor of Pharmacology, University of Utah College of Medicine, Salt Lake City, Utah

Flower, Roderick J., Ph.D. Senior Scientist, Department of Prostaglandin Research, Wellcome Research Laboratories, Beckenham, Kent, United Kingdom

Franz, Donald N., M.S., Ph.D. Associate Professor of Pharmacology, University of Utah College of Medicine, Salt Lake City, Utah

Gilman, Alfred Goodman, M.D., Ph.D. Professor and Chairman, Department of Pharmacology, The University of Texas Health Science Center at Dallas, Dallas, Texas

Greene, Nicholas M., M.D. Professor of Anesthesiology, Yale University School of Medicine, New Haven, Connecticut

Harvey, Stewart C., Ph.D. Professor of Pharmacology, University of Utah College of Medicine, Salt Lake City, Utah

Haynes, Robert C., Jr., M.D., Ph.D. Professor of Pharmacology, University of Virginia School of Medicine, Charlottesville, Virginia

Hays, Richard M., M.D. Professor of Medicine and Director, Division of Nephrology, Albert Einstein College of Medicine of Yeshiva University, Bronx, New York

Hillman, Robert S., M.D. Professor of Medicine, University of Washington School of Medicine, Seattle, Washington

Hoffman, Brian F., M.D. David Hosack Professor of Pharmacology, Columbia University College of Physicians and Surgeons, New York, New York

Jaffe, Jerome H., M.D. Professor of Psychiatry, University of Connecticut School of Medicine, Farmington, Connecticut

Johnson, Eugene M., Jr., Ph.D. Associate Professor of Pharmacology, Washington University School of Medicine, St. Louis, Missouri

Klaassen, Curtis D., Ph.D. Professor of Pharmacology and Toxicology, University of Kansas School of Medicine, Kansas City, Kansas

Larner, Joseph, M.D., Ph.D. Alumni Professor and Chairman, Department of Pharmacology, University of Virginia School of Medicine, Charlottesville, Virginia

Levy, Robert I., M.D. Director, National Heart, Lung, and Blood Institute, National Institutes of Health, Bethesda, Maryland

Mandel, H. George, Ph.D. Professor and Chairman, Department of Pharmacology, George Washington University School of Medicine, Washington, D. C.

Mandell, Gerald L., M.D. Professor of Medicine and Director, Division of Infectious Diseases, University of Virginia School of Medicine, Charlottesville, Virginia

Marshall, Bryan E., M.D., F.R.C.P. Professor of Anesthesia, University of Pennsylvania School of Medicine, Philadelphia, Pennsylvania

Martin, William R., M.D. Professor and Chairman, Department of Pharmacology, University of Kentucky College of Medicine, Lexington, Kentucky

Mayer, Steven E., M.S., Ph.D. Professor of Medicine, Division of Pharmacology, University of California, San Diego, School of Medicine, La Jolla, California

Melmon, Kenneth L., M.D. Professor of Medicine and Pharmacology, and Chairman, Department of Medicine, Stanford University School of Medicine, Stanford, California

Moncada, Salvador, M.D., Ph.D. Head, Department of Prostaglandin Research, Wellcome Research Laboratories, Beckenham, Kent, United Kingdom

Mudge, Gilbert H., M.D. Professor of Medicine and Pharmacology, Dartmouth Medical School, Hanover, New Hampshire

Munro, Hamish N., M.B., Ch.B., D.Sc. Professor of Physiological Chemistry, Department of Nutrition and Food Science, Massachusetts Institute of Technology, Cambridge, Massachusetts

Murad, Ferid, M.D., Ph.D. Chief, Department of Medicine, Palo Alto Veterans Administration Hospital; Professor, Departments of Medicine and Pharmacology, Stanford University School of Medicine, Stanford, California

Needleman, Philip, Ph.D. Professor and Chairman, Department of Pharmacology, Washington University School of Medicine, St. Louis, Missouri

O'Reilly, Robert A., M.D. Clinical Professor of Medicine, Stanford University; Clinical Professor of Medicine, University of California, San Francisco; Chairman, Department of Medicine, Santa Clara Valley Medical Center, San Jose, California

Parks, Robert E., Jr., M.D., Ph.D. Professor of Medical Science, Brown University, Providence, Rhode Island

Pathak, Madhu A., M.Sc.(Tech), M.B., M.S., Ph.D. Senior Associate in Dermatology and Research Professor, Harvard Medical School and Massachusetts General Hospital, Boston, Massachusetts

Rall, Theodore W., Ph.D., D.Med.(Hon.). Professor of Pharmacology and Director, Neuroscience Program, University of Virginia School of Medicine, Charlottesville, Virginia

Ritchie, J. Murdoch, Ph.D., D.Sc., F.R.S. Eugene Higgins Professor of Pharmacology, Yale University School of Medicine, New Haven, Connecticut

Rollo, Ian M., Ph.D. Professor of Pharmacology and Therapeutics, University of Manitoba Faculty of Medicine, Winnipeg, Manitoba, Canada

Sande, Merle A., M.D. Professor and Chairman, Department of Medicine, San Francisco General Hospital, University of California School of Medicine, San Francisco, California

Schleifer, Leonard S., M.D., Ph.D. Resident, Department of Neurology, Cornell University Medical College, New York, New York

Sheiner, Lewis B., M.D.   Associate Professor of Laboratory Medicine and Medicine, University of California, San Francisco, California

Shimomura, Sam K., Pharm.D.   Associate Clinical Professor of Pharmacy and Vice-Chairman, University of California, Irvine/Long Beach Program, Division of Clinical Pharmacy, School of Pharmacy, University of California, San Francisco, California

Smith, Theodore C., M.D.   Professor of Anesthesia, University of Pennsylvania School of Medicine, Philadelphia, Pennsylvania

Swinyard, Ewart A., M.S., Ph.D.   Professor Emeritus of Pharmacology and Former Dean, College of Pharmacy; Professor Emeritus of Pharmacology, University of Utah College of Medicine, Salt Lake City, Utah

Taylor, Palmer, Ph.D.   Professor and Head, Division of Pharmacology, Department of Medicine, University of California, San Diego, School of Medicine, La Jolla, California

Vane, John R., D.Sc., F.R.S.   Group Research and Development Director, The Wellcome Foundation, Ltd., Beckenham, Kent, United Kingdom

Weiner, Norman, M.D.   Professor and Chairman, Department of Pharmacology, University of Colorado School of Medicine, Denver, Colorado

Wollman, Harry, M.D.   Robert Dunning Dripps Professor and Chairman, Department of Anesthesia, and Professor of Pharmacology, University of Pennsylvania School of Medicine, Philadelphia, Pennsylvania

CONTENTS

PREFACE TO THE SIXTH EDITION   v

PREFACE TO THE FIRST EDITION   vii

CONTRIBUTORS   viii

SECTION
I

General Principles

1. INTRODUCTION; THE DYNAMICS OF DRUG ABSORPTION, DISTRIBUTION, AND ELIMINATION   *Steven E. Mayer, Kenneth L. Melmon, and Alfred G. Gilman*   1

2. PHARMACODYNAMICS: MECHANISMS OF DRUG ACTION AND THE RELATIONSHIP BETWEEN DRUG CONCENTRATION AND EFFECT   *Alfred G. Gilman, Steven E. Mayer, and Kenneth L. Melmon*   28

3. PRINCIPLES OF THERAPEUTICS   *Kenneth L. Melmon, Alfred G. Gilman, and Steven E. Mayer*   40

SECTION
II

Drugs Acting at Synaptic and Neuroeffector Junctional Sites

4. NEUROHUMORAL TRANSMISSION AND THE AUTONOMIC NERVOUS SYSTEM   *Steven E. Mayer*   56

5. CHOLINERGIC AGONISTS   *Palmer Taylor*   91

6. ANTICHOLINESTERASE AGENTS   *Palmer Taylor*   100

7. ATROPINE, SCOPOLAMINE, AND RELATED ANTIMUSCARINIC DRUGS   *Norman Weiner*   120

8. NOREPINEPHRINE, EPINEPHRINE, AND THE SYMPATHOMIMETIC AMINES   *Norman Weiner*   138

9. DRUGS THAT INHIBIT ADRENERGIC NERVES AND BLOCK ADRENERGIC RECEPTORS   *Norman Weiner*   176

10. GANGLIONIC STIMULATING AND BLOCKING AGENTS   *Palmer Taylor*   211

11. NEUROMUSCULAR BLOCKING AGENTS   *Palmer Taylor*   220

SECTION

III

Drugs Acting on the Central Nervous System

12. NEUROHUMORAL TRANSMISSION AND THE CENTRAL NERVOUS SYSTEM
    Floyd E. Bloom 235

13. HISTORY AND PRINCIPLES OF ANESTHESIOLOGY
    Theodore C. Smith, Lee H. Cooperman, and Harry Wollman 258

14. GENERAL ANESTHETICS *Bryan E. Marshall and Harry Wollman* 276

15. LOCAL ANESTHETICS *J. Murdoch Ritchie and Nicholas M. Greene* 300

16. THE THERAPEUTIC GASES
    Theodore C. Smith, Lee H. Cooperman, and Harry Wollman 321
    Oxygen, Carbon Dioxide, Helium, and Water Vapor

17. HYPNOTICS AND SEDATIVES *Stewart C. Harvey* 339

18. THE ALIPHATIC ALCOHOLS *J. Murdoch Ritchie* 376

19. DRUGS AND THE TREATMENT OF PSYCHIATRIC DISORDERS *Ross J. Baldessarini* 391

20. DRUGS EFFECTIVE IN THE THERAPY OF THE EPILEPSIES
    Theodore W. Rall and Leonard S. Schleifer 448

21. DRUGS FOR PARKINSON'S DISEASE; CENTRALLY ACTING MUSCLE RELAXANTS
    Joseph R. Bianchine 475

22. OPIOID ANALGESICS AND ANTAGONISTS
    Jerome H. Jaffe and William R. Martin 494

23. DRUG ADDICTION AND DRUG ABUSE *Jerome H. Jaffe* 535

24. CENTRAL NERVOUS SYSTEM STIMULANTS *Donald N. Franz* 585
    Strychnine, Picrotoxin, Pentylenetetrazol, and Miscellaneous Agents (Doxapram, Ethamivan, Nikethamide, Methylphenidate)

25. CENTRAL NERVOUS SYSTEM STIMULANTS (*Continued*) *Theodore W. Rall* 592
    The Xanthines

SECTION

IV

Autacoids

INTRODUCTION *William W. Douglas* 608

26. HISTAMINE AND 5-HYDROXYTRYPTAMINE (SEROTONIN) AND THEIR ANTAGONISTS
    William W. Douglas 609

27. POLYPEPTIDES—ANGIOTENSIN, PLASMA KININS, AND OTHERS
    William W. Douglas 647

28. PROSTAGLANDINS, PROSTACYCLIN, AND THROMBOXANE A_2
    Salvador Moncada, Roderick J. Flower, and John R. Vane 668

SECTION
V

Drug Therapy of Inflammation

29. ANALGESIC–ANTIPYRETICS AND ANTI-INFLAMMATORY AGENTS; DRUGS EMPLOYED IN THE TREATMENT OF GOUT
Roderick J. Flower, Salvador Moncada, and John R. Vane   682

SECTION
VI

Cardiovascular Drugs

30. DIGITALIS AND ALLIED CARDIAC GLYCOSIDES
Brian F. Hoffman and J. Thomas Bigger, Jr.   729

31. ANTIARRHYTHMIC DRUGS   *J. Thomas Bigger, Jr., and Brian F. Hoffman*   761

32. ANTIHYPERTENSIVE AGENTS AND THE DRUG THERAPY OF HYPERTENSION
Terrence F. Blaschke and Kenneth L. Melmon   793

33. VASODILATORS AND THE TREATMENT OF ANGINA
Philip Needleman and Eugene M. Johnson, Jr.   819

34. DRUGS USED IN THE TREATMENT OF HYPERLIPOPROTEINEMIAS
Robert I. Levy   834

SECTION
VII

Water, Salts, and Ions

35. AGENTS AFFECTING VOLUME AND COMPOSITION OF BODY FLUIDS
Gilbert H. Mudge   848

SECTION
VIII

Drugs Affecting Renal Function and Electrolyte Metabolism

INTRODUCTION   *Gilbert H. Mudge*   885

36. DIURETICS AND OTHER AGENTS EMPLOYED IN THE MOBILIZATION OF EDEMA FLUID   *Gilbert H. Mudge*   892

37. AGENTS AFFECTING THE RENAL CONSERVATION OF WATER   *Richard M. Hays*   916

38. INHIBITORS OF TUBULAR TRANSPORT OF ORGANIC COMPOUNDS
Gilbert H. Mudge   929

SECTION
IX

Drugs Affecting Uterine Motility

39. OXYTOCIN, PROSTAGLANDINS, ERGOT ALKALOIDS, AND OTHER AGENTS
                          Theodore W. Rall and Leonard S. Schleifer   935

SECTION
X

Locally Acting Drugs

40. SURFACE-ACTING DRUGS   *Ewart A. Swinyard and Madhu A. Pathak*   951

41. ANTISEPTICS AND DISINFECTANTS; FUNGICIDES; ECTOPARASITICIDES
                                               Stewart C. Harvey   964

42. GASTRIC ANTACIDS AND DIGESTANTS   *Stewart C. Harvey*   988

43. LAXATIVES AND CATHARTICS   *Edward Fingl*   1002

SECTION
XI

Chemotherapy of Parasitic Diseases

44. DRUGS USED IN THE CHEMOTHERAPY OF HELMINTHIASIS   *Ian M. Rollo*   1013

45. DRUGS USED IN THE CHEMOTHERAPY OF MALARIA   *Ian M. Rollo*   1038

46. DRUGS USED IN THE CHEMOTHERAPY OF AMEBIASIS   *Ian M. Rollo*   1061

47. MISCELLANEOUS DRUGS USED IN THE TREATMENT OF PROTOZOAL INFECTIONS
                                                       Ian M. Rollo   1070

SECTION
XII

Chemotherapy of Microbial Diseases

48. ANTIMICROBIAL AGENTS   *Merle A. Sande and Gerald L. Mandell*   1080
     General Considerations

49. ANTIMICROBIAL AGENTS (*Continued*)   *Gerald L. Mandell and Merle A. Sande*   1106
     Sulfonamides, Trimethoprim-Sulfamethoxazole, and Urinary Tract Antiseptics

50. ANTIMICROBIAL AGENTS (*Continued*)   *Gerald L. Mandell and Merle A. Sande*   1126
     Penicillins and Cephalosporins

51. ANTIMICROBIAL AGENTS (*Continued*)   *Merle A. Sande and Gerald L. Mandell*   1162
     The Aminoglycosides

52. ANTIMICROBIAL AGENTS (*Continued*)   *Merle A. Sande and Gerald L. Mandell*   1181
     Tetracyclines and Chloramphenicol

53. ANTIMICROBIAL AGENTS (*Continued*)   *Gerald L. Mandell and Merle A. Sande*   1200
Drugs Used in the Chemotherapy of Tuberculosis and Leprosy

54. ANTIMICROBIAL AGENTS (*Continued*)   *Merle A. Sande and Gerald L. Mandell*   1222
Miscellaneous Antibacterial Agents; Antifungal and Antiviral Agents

SECTION

XIII

Chemotherapy of Neoplastic Diseases

INTRODUCTION   *Paul Calabresi and Robert E. Parks, Jr.*   1249

55. ANTIPROLIFERATIVE AGENTS AND DRUGS USED FOR IMMUNOSUPPRESSION
                                      Paul Calabresi and Robert E. Parks, Jr.   1256

SECTION

XIV

Drugs Acting on the Blood and the Blood-Forming Organs

56. DRUGS EFFECTIVE IN IRON-DEFICIENCY AND OTHER HYPOCHROMIC ANEMIAS
                                                              Clement A. Finch   1315

57. VITAMIN B$_{12}$, FOLIC ACID, AND THE TREATMENT OF MEGALOBLASTIC ANEMIAS
                                                            Robert S. Hillman   1331

58. ANTICOAGULANT, ANTITHROMBOTIC, AND THROMBOLYTIC DRUGS
                                                          Robert A. O'Reilly   1347

SECTION

XV

Hormones and Hormone Antagonists

INTRODUCTION   *Ferid Murad and Robert C. Haynes, Jr.*   1367

59. ADENOHYPOPHYSEAL HORMONES AND RELATED SUBSTANCES
                                      Ferid Murad and Robert C. Haynes, Jr.   1369

60. THYROID AND ANTITHYROID DRUGS   *Robert C. Haynes, Jr., and Ferid Murad*   1397

61. ESTROGENS AND PROGESTINS   *Ferid Murad and Robert C. Haynes, Jr.*   1420

62. ANDROGENS AND ANABOLIC STEROIDS *Ferid Murad and Robert C. Haynes, Jr.*   1448

63. ADRENOCORTICOTROPIC HORMONE; ADRENOCORTICAL STEROIDS AND THEIR
SYNTHETIC ANALOGS; INHIBITORS OF ADRENOCORTICAL STEROID BIOSYNTHESIS
                                      Robert C. Haynes, Jr., and Ferid Murad   1466

64. INSULIN AND ORAL HYPOGLYCEMIC DRUGS; GLUCAGON   *Joseph Larner*   1497

65. AGENTS AFFECTING CALCIFICATION: CALCIUM, PARATHYROID HORMONE, CALCI-
TONIN, VITAMIN D, AND OTHER COMPOUNDS
                                      Robert C. Haynes, Jr., and Ferid Murad   1524

SECTION
XVI

The Vitamins

INTRODUCTION   *Darla Erhard Danford and Hamish N. Munro*   1551

66. WATER-SOLUBLE VITAMINS   *Darla Erhard Danford and Hamish N. Munro*   1560
The Vitamin B Complex and Ascorbic Acid

67. FAT-SOLUBLE VITAMINS   *H. George Mandel and Victor H. Cohn*   1583
Vitamins A, K, and E

SECTION
XVII

Toxicology

68. PRINCIPLES OF TOXICOLOGY   *Curtis D. Klaassen*   1602

69. HEAVY METALS AND HEAVY-METAL ANTAGONISTS   *Curtis D. Klaassen*   1615

70. NONMETALLIC ENVIRONMENTAL TOXICANTS: AIR POLLUTANTS, SOLVENTS AND
VAPORS, AND PESTICIDES   *Curtis D. Klaassen*   1638

APPENDIX I. PRINCIPLES OF PRESCRIPTION ORDER WRITING AND PATIENT COM-
PLIANCE INSTRUCTION   *Ewart A. Swinyard*   1660

APPENDIX II. DESIGN AND OPTIMIZATION OF DOSAGE REGIMENS; PHARMACOKI-
NETIC DATA   *Leslie Z. Benet and Lewis B. Sheiner*   1675

APPENDIX III. DRUG INTERACTIONS   *Kenneth L. Melmon and Alfred G. Gilman*   1738

INDEX   1753

GOODMAN and GILMAN's
The Pharmacological Basis
of Therapeutics

SECTION

I

General Principles

INTRODUCTION; THE DYNAMICS OF DRUG ABSORPTION, DISTRIBUTION, AND ELIMINATION

Steven E. Mayer, Kenneth L. Melmon, and Alfred G. Gilman

In its entirety, *pharmacology* embraces the knowledge of the history, source, physical and chemical properties, compounding, biochemical and physiological effects, mechanisms of action, absorption, distribution, biotransformation and excretion, and therapeutic and other uses of drugs. Since a *drug* is broadly defined as any chemical agent that affects living processes, the subject of pharmacology is obviously quite extensive.

For the physician and the medical student, however, the scope of pharmacology is less expansive than indicated by the above definitions. The clinician is interested primarily in drugs that are useful in the prevention, diagnosis, and treatment of human disease, or in the prevention of pregnancy. Study of the pharmacology of these drugs can be reasonably limited to those aspects that provide the basis for their rational clinical use. Secondarily, the physician is also concerned with chemical agents that are not used in therapy but are commonly responsible for household and industrial poisoning as well as environmental pollution. Study of these substances is justifiably restricted to the general principles of prevention, recognition, and treatment of such toxicity or pollution. Finally, all physicians share in the responsibility to help resolve the continuing sociological problem of the abuse of drugs.

The basic pharmacological concepts summarized in this chapter and the two that follow apply to the characterization, evaluation, and comparison of all drugs. A clear understanding of these principles is essential for the subsequent study of the individual drugs. Many of these topics have been more extensively discussed in the textbooks by Goldstein and coworkers (1974), Levine (1978), and Melmon and Morrelli (1978).

A brief consideration of its major subject areas will further clarify how the study of pharmacology is best approached from the standpoint of the specific requirements and interests of the medical student and practitioner. At one time, it was essential for the physician to have a broad botanical knowledge, since he had to select the proper plants from which to prepare his own crude medicinal preparations. However, fewer drugs are now obtained from natural sources, and, more importantly, most of these are highly purified or standardized and differ little from synthetic chemicals. Hence, the interests of the modern clinician in *pharmacognosy* are correspondingly limited. Nevertheless, scientific curiosity should stimulate the physician to learn something of the *sources* of drugs, and this knowledge often proves practically useful as well as interesting. Knowledge of the *history* of drugs is of similar value.

The preparing, compounding, and dispensing of medicines at one time lay within the province of the physician, but this work is now delegated almost completely to the pharmacist. However, to write intelligent prescription orders, the physician must have some knowledge of the *physical and chemical*

1

properties of drugs and their available *dosage forms,* and he must have a basic familiarity with the *practice of pharmacy.* When the physician shirks his responsibility in this regard, he invariably fails to translate his knowledge of pharmacology and medicine into prescription orders and medication best suited for the individual patient. The details essential to the writing of correct prescription orders are summarized in Appendix I.

Pharmacokinetics deals with the *absorption, distribution, biotransformation,* and *excretion* of drugs. These factors, coupled with dosage, determine the concentration of a drug at its sites of action and, hence, the intensity of its effects as a function of time. Many basic principles of biochemistry and enzymology and the physical and chemical principles that govern the active and passive transfer and the distribution of substances across biological membranes are readily applied to the understanding of this important aspect of pharmacology.

The study of the biochemical and physiological *effects* of drugs and their *mechanisms of action* is termed *pharmacodynamics* (*see* Chapter 2). It is an experimental medical science that dates back only to the latter half of the nineteenth century. As a border science, pharmacodynamics borrows freely from both the subject matter and the experimental technics of physiology, biochemistry, cellular and molecular biology, microbiology, immunology, genetics, and pathology. It is unique mainly in that attention is focused on the characteristics of drugs. As the name implies, the subject is a dynamic one. The student who attempts merely to memorize the pharmacodynamic properties of drugs is foregoing one of the best opportunities for correlating the entire field of preclinical medicine. For example, the actions and effects of the saluretic agents can be fully understood only in terms of the basic principles of renal physiology and of the pathogenesis of edema. Conversely, no greater insight into normal and abnormal renal physiology can be gained than by the study of the pharmacodynamics of the saluretic agents.

Another ramification of pharmacodynamics is the correlation of the actions and effects of drugs with their chemical structures. Such *structure-activity relationships* are an integral link in the analysis of drug action, and exploitation of these relationships among established therapeutic agents has often led to the development of better drugs. However, the correlation of biological activity with chemical structure is usually of interest to the physician only when it provides the basis for summarizing other pharmacological information.

The physician is understandably interested mainly in the effects of drugs in man. This emphasis on *clinical pharmacology* is justified, since the effects of drugs are often characterized by significant interspecies variation, and since they may be further modified by disease. In addition, some drug effects, such as those on mood and behavior, can be adequately studied only in man. However, technical, legal, and ethical considerations limit pharmacological evaluation in man, and the choice of drugs must be based in part on their pharmacological evaluation in animals. Consequently, some knowledge of *animal pharmacology* and *comparative pharmacology* is helpful in deciding the extent to which claims for a drug based upon studies in animals can be reasonably extrapolated to man (*see* Chapter 3).

Pharmacotherapeutics deals with the use of drugs in the prevention and treatment of disease. Many drugs stimulate or depress biochemical or physiological function in man in a sufficiently reproducible manner to provide relief of symptoms or, ideally, to alter favorably the course of disease. Conversely, chemotherapeutic agents are useful in therapy because they have only minimal effects on man but can destroy or eliminate pathogenic cells or organisms.

Whether a drug is useful for therapy is crucially dependent upon its ability to produce its desired effects with only tolerable undesired effects. Thus, from the standpoint of the physician interested in the therapeutic uses of a drug, the *selectivity* of its effects is one of its most important characteristics. Drug therapy is rationally based upon the correlation of the actions and effects of drugs with the physiological, biochemical, microbiological, immunological, and behavioral aspects of disease. Pharmacodynamics provides one of the best opportunities for this correlation during the study of both the preclinical and the clinical medical sciences.

Toxicology is that aspect of pharmacology that deals with the adverse effects of drugs. It is concerned not only with drugs used in therapy but also with the many other chemicals that may be responsible for household, environmental, or industrial intoxication. The adverse effects of the pharmacological agents employed in therapy are properly considered an integral part of their total pharmacology. The toxic effects of other chemicals is such an extensive subject that the physician must usually confine his attention to the general principles applicable to the prevention, recognition, and treatment of drug poisonings of any cause.

▶ Pharmacokinetics

To produce its characteristic effects, a drug must be present in appropriate concentrations at its sites of action. Although obviously a function of the amount of drug administered, the concentrations attained also depend upon the extent and rate of its absorption, distribution, binding or localization in tissues, biotransformation, and excretion. These factors are depicted in Figure 1–1.

PHYSICOCHEMICAL FACTORS IN TRANSFER OF DRUGS ACROSS MEMBRANES

The absorption, distribution, biotransformation, and excretion of a drug all involve its passage across cell membranes. It is essential,

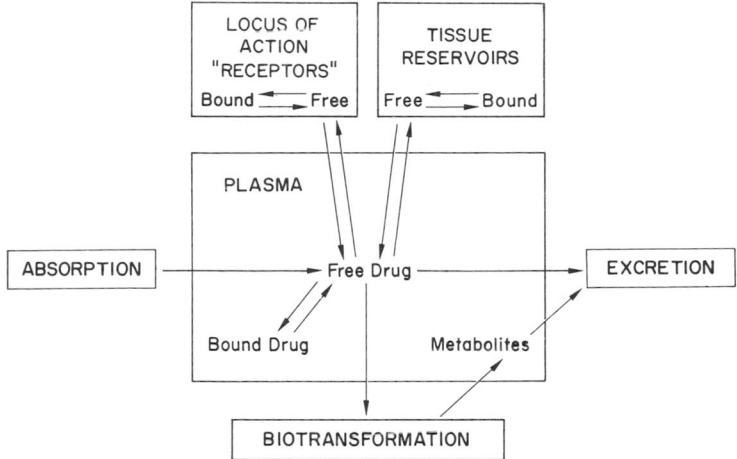

Figure 1-1. *Schematic representation of the interrelationship of the absorption, distribution, binding, biotransformation, and excretion of a drug and its concentration at its locus of action.*

Possible distribution and binding of metabolites are not depicted.

therefore, to consider the mechanisms by which drugs cross membranes and the physicochemical properties of molecules and membranes that influence this transfer. Important characteristics of a drug are its molecular size and shape, solubility at the site of its absorption, degree of ionization, and relative lipid solubility of its ionized and nonionized forms.

When a drug permeates a cell, it must obviously traverse the cellular plasma membrane. Other barriers to drug movement may be a single layer of cells (intestinal epithelium) or several layers of cells (skin). Despite these structural differences, the diffusion and transport of drugs across these various boundaries have many common characteristics, since drugs in general pass through cells rather than between them. The plasma membrane thus represents the common barrier.

Cell Membranes. The classical observations by Overton and by Collander and Bärlund led to the theory that the cell membrane was a thin layer of lipid-like material interspersed with minute water-filled channels. Subsequent studies suggested that the plasma membrane consisted of a lipid bilayer bound on both sides by protein, but this hypothesis has been broadened to a more dynamic model in which lipids and intrinsic and extrinsic proteins are viewed as being organized in a mosaic structure (*see* Symposium, 1972a). The intrinsic proteins are embedded or intercalated, in ordered or random arrangement, into a discontinuous lipid bilayer that forms the matrix of the mosaic. The intrinsic proteins

are globular but are oriented with their ionic and highly polar groups located largely on the membrane surfaces in contact with the extracellular and intracellular aqueous media, and with their nonpolar hydrophobic residues sequestered from contact with water in the membrane interior. Extrinsic proteins are bound to the exposed surfaces of the intrinsic proteins by electrostatic or hydrophobic interactions, but they are not involved in lipid-protein interactions that are critical to the membrane structure and its functions. Cell membranes are approximately 80 Å thick.

Passive Processes. Drugs cross membranes by either passive processes or by mechanisms involving the active participation of components of the membrane. In the former, the drug molecules penetrate by *passive diffusion* along a concentration gradient through aqueous channels in the membrane or by dissolving in the membrane. Such transfer is directly proportional to the magnitude of the concentration gradient across the membrane and the lipid:water partition coefficient of the drug. The greater the partition coefficient, the higher is the concentration of drug in the membrane and the faster is its diffusion. After a steady state is attained, the concentration of the free drug is the same on both sides of the membrane, if the drug is a nonelectrolyte. For ionic compounds, the steady-state concentrations will be dependent on differences in pH across the membrane, which may influence the state of ionization of the molecule on each side of the membrane, and on the electrochemical gradient for the ion. Passage through channels is called *filtration*, since it involves bulk flow of water as a result of a hydrostatic or osmotic difference across the membrane. The bulk flow of water carries with it any water-soluble molecule that is small enough to pass through the channels. Filtration is a common mechanism for transfer of many small, water-soluble, polar and nonpolar substances. The size of the membrane channels differs in the various body membranes. Capillary endothelial cells have large channels (40 Å), and molecules as large as albumin (molecular weight 67,000) may pass to a limited extent from the plasma to the extracellular fluid. In contrast, the channels in the red-cell membrane, the intestinal epithelium, and most cell membranes are about 4 Å in diameter and permit passage only of water, urea, and other small, water-soluble molecules. Such substances generally do not pass through channels in cell membranes if their molecular weights are greater than 100 to 200.

Most inorganic ions are sufficiently small to penetrate the channels in membranes, but their concentration gradient across the cell membrane is generally determined by the transmembrane potential (*e.g.*, chloride ion) or by active transport (*e.g.*, sodium and potassium ions).

Weak Electrolytes and Influence of pH. Most drugs are weak acids or bases and are present in solution as both the nonionized and ionized species. Since drugs generally are too large to pass through membrane channels, they must pass membrane barriers by diffusion through the lipid components of the membranes. The nonionized molecules are usually lipid soluble and can diffuse across the cell membrane. In contrast, the ionized fraction is usually unable to penetrate the lipid membrane because of its low lipid solubility.

The distribution of a weak electrolyte is usually determined by its pK_a and the pH gradient across the membrane. To illustrate the effect of pH on distribution of drugs, the partitioning of a weak acid ($pK_a = 4.4$) between plasma (pH = 7.4) and gastric juice (pH = 1.4) is depicted in Figure 1–2. It is assumed that the gastric mucosal membrane behaves as a simple lipid barrier that is permeable only to the lipid-soluble, nonionized form of the acid. The ratio of nonionized to ionized drug at each pH can be calculated from the Henderson-Hasselbalch equation. Thus, in plasma, the ratio of nonionized to ionized drug is 1:1000; in gastric juice, the ratio is 1:0.001. The total concentration ratio between the plasma and the gastric juice would therefore be 1000:1 if such a system came to a steady state. For a weak base with a pK_a of 4.4 ($BH^+ \rightleftharpoons B + H^+$), the ratio would be reversed. These considerations have obvious implications for the absorption and excretion of drugs, as will be discussed more specifically below. The establishment of concentration gradients of weak electrolytes across membranes with a pH gradient is a purely physical process and does not require an active transport system. All that is necessary is a membrane preferentially permeable to one form of the weak electrolyte and a pH gradient across the membrane. The establishment of the pH gradient is, however, an active process.

Bulk flow through *intercellular pores* is the major mechanism of passage of drugs across most capillary endothelial membranes, with the important exception of the central nervous system (CNS) (*see* below). These intercellular gaps are sufficiently large that diffusion across most capillaries is limited by blood flow and not by the lipid solubility of drugs or pH

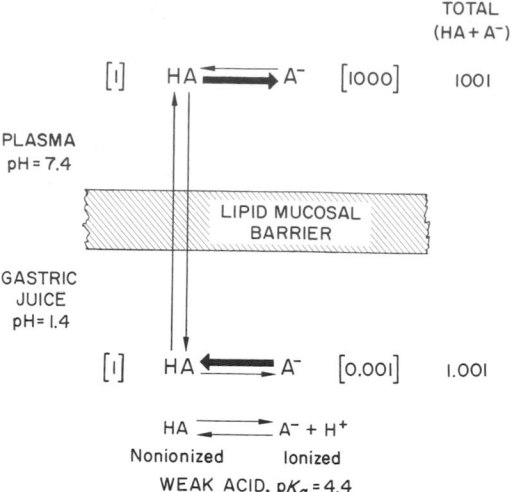

Figure 1–2. *Influence of pH on the distribution of a weak acid between plasma and gastric juice, separated by a lipid barrier.*

Only the nonionized moiety can readily penetrate the membrane; hence, it diffuses along its concentration gradient until, at steady state, its concentration is the same in both compartments. The degree of dissociation of the acid on each side depends on the pH of the plasma and gastric juice. The total concentration difference between the two sides is a direct function of the pH gradient across the membrane.

The values in brackets represent relative concentrations of the ionized and nonionized forms on each side of the membrane. The thick horizontal arrows point in the direction of the predominant form of the weak acid at the indicated pH.

gradients. This is an important factor in absorption of drugs after parenteral administration and in filtration across glomerular membranes in the kidney (*see* below). *Tight junctions* are characteristic of capillaries of the CNS and a variety of epithelia. Intercellular diffusion is consequently limited. *Pinocytosis*, the formation and movement of vesicles across cell membranes, has been implicated in drug absorption. However, the quantitative significance of pinocytosis is difficult to estimate and is controversial.

Carrier-Mediated Membrane Transport. Passive diffusion or bulk flow through water-filled pores is dominant in the absorption and, partly, in the excretion of drugs. Nevertheless, more active and selective mechanisms play important roles in pharmacokinetics. *Active transport* of some drugs occurs across neuronal membranes, the choroid plexus, renal tubular cells, and hepatocytes. The characteristics of active transport—selectivity, competitive inhibition by congeners, a requirement for energy, saturability, and movement against an electrochemical gradient—may play important roles in the mechanism of action of drugs that are subject to active transport or that interfere with the active transport of natural metabolites or neurotransmitters. The term *facilitated diffusion* describes a carrier-mediated transport process to which there is no input of energy, and movement of the substance in question thus cannot occur against an electrochemical gradient. Such mechanisms, which may also be highly selective for specific conformational structures of drugs, are necessary for the transport of endogenous compounds whose rate of movement across biological membranes by simple diffusion would otherwise be too slow.

ABSORPTION OF DRUGS

The manner in which drugs are absorbed has considerable importance. The rate of absorption affects the duration and intensity of drug action. Changes in this rate may therefore dictate the adjustment of the dose of a drug or the interval between doses in order to maintain a desired level of effect. The choice of the route of drug administration should be based on an understanding of the factors that influence absorption.

Factors That Modify Absorption. Many variables, in addition to the physicochemical factors discussed above, influence the absorption of drugs. Absorption, regardless of the site, is dependent upon drug *solubility.* Drugs given in aqueous solution are more rapidly absorbed than those given in oily solution, suspension, or solid form because they mix more readily with the aqueous phase at the absorptive site. For those given in solid form, the rate of *dissolution* may be the limiting factor in their absorption. Local conditions at the site of absorption alter solubility, particularly in the gastrointestinal tract. Aspirin, which is relatively insoluble in acidic gastric contents, is a common example of such a drug. The *concentration* of a drug influences its rate of absorption. Drugs ingested or injected in solutions of high concentration are absorbed more rapidly than are drugs in solutions of low concentration. The *circulation to the site of absorption* also affects drug absorption. Increased blood flow, brought about by massage or local application of heat, enhances absorption of a drug; decreased blood flow, produced by vasoconstrictor agents, shock, or other disease factors, can slow absorption. The area of the *absorbing surface* to which a drug is ex-

posed is one of the more important determinants of the rate of drug absorption. Drugs are absorbed very rapidly from large surface areas such as the pulmonary alveolar epithelium, the intestinal mucosa, or, in a few cases after extensive application, the skin. The absorbing surface is determined largely by the *route of administration.* Each of these factors separately or in conjunction with one another may have profound effects on the efficacy and toxicity of a drug.

Enteral (Oral) vs. Parenteral Administration. Often there is a choice of the route by which a therapeutic agent may be given, and a knowledge of the advantages and disadvantages of the different routes of administration is then of primary importance. Some characteristics of the major routes employed for systemic drug effect are compared in Table 1–1.

Oral ingestion is the most common method of drug administration. It is also the safest, most convenient, and most economical. Disadvantages to the oral route include emesis as a result of irritation to the gastrointestinal mucosa, destruction of some drugs by digestive enzymes or low gastric pH, irregularities in absorption or propulsion in the presence of food or other drugs, and necessity for cooperation on the part of the patient. In addition, drugs in the gastrointestinal tract may be metabolized by the enzymes of the mucosa, the intestinal flora, or the liver before they gain access to the general circulation.

The parenteral injection of drugs has certain distinct advantages over oral administration. In some instances, parenteral administration is essential for the drug to be absorbed in active form. Absorption is usually more rapid and more predictable than when a drug is given by mouth. The effective dose can therefore be more accurately selected. In emergency therapy, parenteral administration is particularly serviceable. If a patient is unconscious, uncooperative, or unable to retain anything given by mouth, parenteral therapy may become a necessity. The injection of drugs also has its disadvantages. Asepsis must be maintained to avoid infection, an intravascular injection may occur when it is not intended, pain may accompany the injection, and it is sometimes difficult for

Table 1–1. SOME CHARACTERISTICS OF COMMON ROUTES OF
DRUG ADMINISTRATION *

ROUTE	ABSORPTION PATTERN	SPECIAL UTILITY	LIMITATIONS AND PRECAUTIONS
Intravenous	Absorption circumvented Potentially immediate effects	Valuable for emergency use Permits titration of dosage Suitable for large volumes and for irritating substances, when diluted	Increased risk of adverse effects Must inject solutions *slowly*, as a rule Not suitable for oily solutions or insoluble substances
Subcutaneous	Prompt, from aqueous solution Slow and sustained, from repository preparations	Suitable for some insoluble suspensions and for implantation of solid pellets	Not suitable for large volumes Possible pain or necrosis from irritating substances
Intramuscular	Prompt, from aqueous solution Slow and sustained, from repository preparations	Suitable for moderate volumes, oily vehicles, and some irritating substances	Precluded during anticoagulant medication May interfere with interpretation of certain diagnostic tests (*e.g.*, creatine phosphokinase)
Oral ingestion	Variable; depends upon many factors (*see* text)	Most convenient and economical; usually more safe	Requires patient cooperation Absorption potentially erratic and incomplete for drugs that are poorly soluble, slowly absorbed, or unstable

* *See* text for more complete discussion and for other routes.

a patient to perform the injection himself if self-medication is a necessary procedure. Expense is another consideration.

Oral Ingestion. Absorption from the gastrointestinal tract is governed by factors that are generally applicable, such as surface area for absorption, blood flow to the site of absorption, the physical state of the drug, and its concentration at the site of absorption. In addition, since the first step in absorption, diffusion across the gastrointestinal epithelium, involves cells with tight intercellular junctions and small membrane pores, absorption is largely limited to nonionized species and is proportional to the lipid solubility of this form of the molecule. Furthermore, the large range of pH encountered in the gastrointestinal tract may affect the rate of absorption by altering the relative concentration of nonionized to ionized drug. The absorption of a lipid-soluble nonelectrolyte such as ethanol is very rapid, limited only by surface area and a few other factors (*e.g.*, presence of lipid-containing food). For very strong organic bases such as quaternary amines, the concentration of nonionized drug is so low that absorption by diffusion is negligible at any physiological pH. However, gastrointestinal pH is an important factor in absorption for weak organic acids and bases. Absorption will be maximal where ionization

is suppressed the most. Acids such as barbiturates and salicylates are more rapidly absorbed from the stomach, and bases such as ephedrine and quinine from the small intestine (*see* Figure 1–2). Furthermore, if the pH at the gastric mucosal surface is made more alkaline, as by antacids, the rate of absorption of acids should be reduced and that of bases increased.

However, these principles of drug absorption are modified by additional factors that are unique to the gastrointestinal tract. Gastric pH may affect drug solubility. The theorem of diffusion across lipid-containing membranes predicts that elevation of gastric pH should decrease the rate of absorption of aspirin (a weak acid), but an increase may actually be observed because the ionized species of this drug, which predominates with elevated pH, is more *soluble* in gastric juice than is the nonionized species. Microprecipitates of the latter may form on the mucosal surface, such that absorption is delayed until the drug redissolves. *Gastric emptying time* is another factor of importance. This is prolonged by antacids, thereby delaying the access of the gastric contents to the much larger *absorptive area* in the small intestine. Significant interactions of drugs occur as a consequence of such effects (*see* Chapter 3 and Appendix III).

Drugs that are destroyed by gastric juice or

that cause gastric irritation are sometimes administered in dosage forms with a coating that prevents dissolution in the acidic gastric contents. However, some *enteric-coated* preparations of a drug also may resist dissolution in the intestine, and very little of the drug may be absorbed.

Timed-Release Preparations. The rate of absorption of a drug administered as a tablet or other solid oral-dosage form is partly dependent upon its rate of dissolution in the gastrointestinal fluids. This factor is the basis for the so-called *timed-release, sustained-release,* or *prolonged-action* pharmaceutical preparations that are designed to produce slow, uniform absorption of the drug for 8 hours or longer. Potential advantages of such preparations are reduction in the frequency of administration of the drug as compared with conventional dosage forms, possibly with improved compliance by the patient, maintenance of a therapeutic effect overnight, and decreased incidence of undesired effects by elimination of the peaks in drug concentration that often occur after administration of other dosage forms.

Some timed-release preparations fulfill these theoretical expectations. Unfortunately, not all marketed preparations are reliable. The dissolution rate of some preparations in gastrointestinal fluid may be quite irregular because of technical problems associated with their manufacture or because of variations in gastrointestinal pH, gastric emptying, intestinal motility, and other physiological factors that influence drug absorption. Moreover, slow absorption from the gastrointestinal tract is often incomplete and erratic. In addition, each drug must be evaluated separately for its suitability as a timed-release preparation. Drugs given for a brief therapeutic effect should not be in the timed-release form. Conversely, timed-release preparations are not needed for drugs with an inherent long duration of effect. Also, timed-release preparations of some drugs might not be safe. Since the total dose of drug ingested at one time may be several times the dose of the conventional form of the drug, faulty release of the entire amount at once could lead to toxicity. Finally, failure of adequate release may compromise the therapeutic effect. It is thus incumbent on the physician who uses preparations of this type to establish a need for a timed-release preparation and also to assure himself of its uniformity, reliability, and safety. This is especially necessary since the timed-release formulations of different manufacturers may vary considerably from each other.

Sublingual Administration. Absorption from the oral mucosa has special significance for certain drugs, despite the fact that the surface area available is small. For example, nitroglycerin is effective when retained sublingually because it is nonionic and has a very high lipid solubility. The drug is also very *potent;* relatively few molecules need to be absorbed to produce the therapeutic effect. Since venous drainage from the mouth is to the superior vena cava, the drug is also protected from rapid inactivation by the liver. Drug absorbed from the stomach or intestines is delivered directly to the liver by the portal vein. In the case of nitroglycerin the rate of hepatic metabolism is sufficient to *prevent* the appearance of any active drug in the systemic circulation if the conventional tablet is swallowed.

Rectal Administration. The rectal route is often useful when oral ingestion is precluded by vomiting or when the patient is unconscious. In addition, the absorbed drug does not pass through the liver before entry into the systemic circulation. However, rectal absorption is often irregular and incomplete, and many drugs cause irritation of the rectal mucosa.

Parenteral Injection. The major routes of parenteral administration are intravenous, subcutaneous, and intramuscular. Absorption from subcutaneous and intramuscular sites occurs by simple diffusion along the gradient from drug depot to plasma. The rate is limited by the area of the absorbing capillary membranes and by the solubility of the substance in the interstitial fluid. Relatively large aqueous channels in the endothelial membrane account for the indiscriminate diffusion of molecules regardless of their lipid solubility. Larger molecules, such as proteins, slowly gain access to the circulation by way of lymphatic channels.

Intravenous. The factors concerned in absorption are circumvented by intravenous injection of drugs in aqueous solution, and the desired concentration of a drug in blood is obtained with an *accuracy* and *immediacy* not possible by any other procedure. In some instances, as in the induction of surgical anesthesia by a barbiturate, the dose of a drug is not predetermined but is adjusted to the response of the patient. Also, certain irritating solutions can be given only in this manner, for the blood vessel walls are relatively insensitive and the drug, if injected slowly, is greatly diluted by the blood.

As there are assets to the use of this route of administration, so are there liabilities. Unfavorable reactions are prone to occur, since high concentrations of drug may be attained rapidly in both plasma and tissues. Once the drug is injected there is no retreat. Repeated intravenous injections are dependent upon the ability to maintain a patent vein. Drugs in an oily vehicle or those that precipitate blood constituents or hemolyze erythrocytes should not be given by this route. *Intravenous injection must usually be performed slowly and with constant monitoring of the responses of the patient.*

Subcutaneous. Injection into a subcutaneous site is often utilized for the administration of drugs. It can be used only for drugs that are not irritating to tissue; otherwise, severe pain, necrosis, and slough may occur. The rate of absorption following subcutaneous injection of a drug is often sufficiently constant and slow to provide a sustained effect. Moreover, it may be varied intentionally. For example, the rate of absorption of a suspension of insoluble protamine insulin is slow compared with that of soluble insulin. The incorporation of a vasoconstrictor agent in a solution of a drug to be injected subcutaneously also retards absorption. Absorption of drugs implanted under the skin in a solid pellet form occurs slowly over a period of weeks or months; some hormones are effectively administered in this manner.

Intramuscular. Drugs in aqueous solution are rapidly absorbed after intramuscular injection. Very slow, constant absorption from the intramuscular site results if the drug is injected in solution in oil or suspended in various other repository vehicles. Penicillin is often administered in this manner. Substances too irritating to be injected subcutaneously may sometimes be given intramuscularly.

Intra-arterial. Occasionally a drug is injected directly into an artery to localize its effect in a particular tissue or organ. However, this practice usually has dubious therapeutic value. Diagnostic agents are sometimes administered by this route. Intra-arterial injection requires great care and should be reserved for experts.

Intrathecal. The blood-brain barrier and the blood–cerebrospinal fluid barrier often preclude or slow the entrance of drugs into the central nervous system (CNS). Therefore, when local and rapid effects of drugs on the meninges or cerebrospinal axis are desired, as in spinal anesthesia or acute CNS infections, drugs are sometimes injected directly into the spinal subarachnoid space.

Intraperitoneal. The peritoneal cavity offers a large absorbing surface from which drugs enter the circulation rapidly. Intraperitoneal injection is a common laboratory procedure, but it is seldom employed clinically. The dangers of infection and adhesions are too great to warrant the routine use of this route in man.

Pulmonary Absorption. Gaseous and volatile drugs may be inhaled and absorbed through the pulmonary epithelium and mucous membranes of the respiratory tract. Access to the circulation is rapid by this route, because the surface area is large. The principles governing absorption and excretion of the

anesthetic gases and vapors are discussed in Chapter 13.

In addition, solutions of drugs can be atomized and the fine droplets in air (aerosol) inhaled. Advantages are the almost instantaneous absorption of a drug into the blood, if this is desired, and, in the case of pulmonary disease, local application of the drug at the desired site of action. For example, epinephrine can be given in this manner for the treatment of bronchial asthma. The main disadvantages are poor ability to regulate the dose, cumbersomeness of the methods of administration, and the fact that many gaseous and volatile drugs produce irritation of the pulmonary epithelium.

Pulmonary absorption is an important route of entry of toxic environmental substances of varied composition and physical states (*see* Section XVII). Both local and systemic reactions to allergens may occur subsequent to inhalation; the lung is thus the target of action of numerous pharmacological agents (*see* Section IV).

Topical Application. *Mucous Membranes.* Drugs are applied to the mucous membranes of the conjunctiva, nasopharynx, oropharynx, vagina, colon, urethra, and urinary bladder primarily for their local effects. Occasionally, as in the application of antidiuretic hormone to the nasal mucosa, systemic absorption is the goal. Absorption through mucous membranes occurs readily. In fact, local anesthetics applied for local effect may sometimes be absorbed so rapidly that they produce systemic toxicity.

Skin. Few drugs readily penetrate the intact skin. Absorption of those that do is proportional to their lipid solubility since the epidermis behaves as a lipid barrier. The dermis, however, is freely permeable to many solutes; consequently, systemic absorption of drugs occurs much more readily through abraded or denuded skin. Inflammation and other conditions that increase cutaneous blood flow also enhance absorption. Toxic effects are sometimes produced by absorption through the skin of highly lipid-soluble substances (*e.g.,* a lipid-soluble insecticide in an organic solvent). Absorption through the skin can be enhanced by suspending the drug in an oily vehicle and rubbing the resulting preparation into the skin. This method of administration is known as *inunction.* Absorption through the skin is also increased by so-called occlusive dressings, which retain moisture and macerate the epidermis. (*See* Wepierre and Marty, 1979.)

Bioavailability. Pharmaceutical formulations of a drug are termed *chemically equivalent* if they meet the chemical and physical standards established by governmental or other regulatory agencies. They are said to be *biologically equivalent* if they yield similar concentrations of drug in blood and tissues, and they are designated *therapeutically equivalent* if they provide equal therapeutic benefit in clinical trial. Pharmaceutical preparations that are chemically equivalent but not biologically or therapeutically equivalent are said to differ in their *bioavailability*. Dosage forms of a drug from different manufacturers and even different lots of preparations from a single manufacturer sometimes differ in their bioavailability. Such differences are seen primarily among oral dosage forms of poorly soluble, slowly absorbed drugs. They result from differences in crystal form, particle size, or other physical characteristics of the drug that are not rigidly controlled in formulation and manufacture of the preparations. These factors affect disintegration of the dosage form and dissolution of the drug and, hence, rate and extent of drug absorption.

Biological nonequivalence of different drug preparations is a particularly acute problem because bioavailability of a preparation in man does not always correlate with laboratory tests of tablet dissolution or with tests of bioavailability in animals. Biological nonequivalence of practical importance has been detected among the preparations of a number of important drugs, including the cardiac glycoside digoxin and several antibiotics. Responsible drug manufacturers, interested medical and pharmaceutical scientists, and governmental agencies are cooperating to speed resolution of the problem by establishing tests for bioavailability of pharmaceutical preparations in man and by devising *in-vitro* tests for drug dissolution that have satisfactory predictive value. The significance of possible nonequivalence of drug preparations is further discussed in connection with drug nomenclature and the choice of drug name in prescription order writing (*see* Appendix I; Berliner *et al.*, 1974; American Pharmaceutical Association, 1978).

DISTRIBUTION OF DRUGS

After a drug is absorbed or injected into the bloodstream, it may be distributed into interstitial and cellular fluids. Patterns of drug distribution reflect certain physiological factors and physicochemical properties of drugs. An initial phase of distribution may be distinguished that reflects cardiac output and regional blood flow. Heart, liver, kidney, brain, and other highly perfused organs receive most of the drug during the first few minutes after absorption. Delivery of drug to muscle, most viscera, skin, and fat is slower, and these tissues may require several minutes to several hours before equilibration is attained. A second phase of drug distribution may therefore be distinguished; this is also limited by blood flow, and it involves a far larger fraction of the body mass than does the first phase. Superimposed on patterns of distribution of blood flow are factors that determine the rate at which drugs diffuse into tissues. Diffusion into the interstitial compartment occurs rapidly, because of the highly permeable nature of capillary endothelial membranes (except in brain). Lipid-insoluble drugs that permeate membranes poorly are restricted in their distribution and, hence, in their potential sites of action. Distribution may also be limited by drug binding to plasma protein, particularly albumin. An agent that is totally and strongly bound has no access to cellular sites of action, nor can it be metabolized and eliminated. Drugs may accumulate in tissues in higher concentrations than would be expected from diffusion equilibrium as a result of pH gradients, binding to intracellular constituents, or partitioning into fat.

Drug that has accumulated in a given tissue may serve as a reservoir that prolongs drug action in that same tissue or at a distant site reached through the circulation. An example that illustrates many of these factors is the use of the intravenous anesthetic thiopental. Thiopental is a highly lipid-soluble drug. Because blood flow to the brain is so high, the drug reaches its maximal concentration in brain within a minute after it is injected intravenously. After injection is concluded, the plasma concentration falls as thiopental diffuses into other tissues such as muscle. The concentration of the drug in brain follows that of the plasma, because there is little binding of the drug to brain constituents. Thus, onset of anesthesia is rapid, but so is its termination. Both are directly related to the concentration of the drug in brain. A third phase of distribution for this drug is due to the slow, blood flow–limited uptake by fat. With administration of successive doses of thiopental, accumulation of drug takes place in fat and other tissues that can store large amounts of the compound. These can become reservoirs for the maintenance of the plasma concentration, and, therefore, the brain concentration at or above the threshold required for anesthesia. Thus, a drug that is short acting because of rapid *redistribution* to sites at which the agent has no pharmacological action can become long acting when these storage sites are "filled" and termination of the drug's action becomes dependent on biotransformation and excretion. The absorption and distribution of drugs are also discussed in Appendix II (*see also* Benet, 1978).

Since the pH difference between intracellular and extracellular fluids is small (7.0 versus 7.4), this factor can result in only a relatively small concentration gradient of drug across the plasma membrane. Weak bases are concentrated slightly inside of cells, while the concentration of weak acids is slightly lower in the cells than in extracellular fluids. Lowering the pH of extracellular fluid increases the intracellular concentration of weak acids and decreases that of weak bases, provided that the intracellular pH does not also change and that the pH change does not simultaneously affect the binding, biotransformation, or excretion of the drug. Elevating the pH produces the opposite effects (*see* Figure 1–2).

Central Nervous System and Cerebrospinal Fluid. The distribution of drugs to the CNS from the blood stream is unique, mainly in that entry of drugs into the CNS extracellular space and cerebrospinal fluid is restricted. The restriction is similar to that across the gastrointestinal epithelium. Endothelial cells of the brain capillaries differ from their counterparts in most tissues by the absence of intercellular pores and pinocytotic vesicles. Tight junctions predominate, and aqueous bulk flow is thus severely restricted. This is not unique to the CNS capillaries (tight junctions appear in many muscle capillaries as well). It is likely that the unique arrangement of pericapillary glial cells also contributes to the slow diffusion of organic acids and bases into the CNS. The drug molecules probably must traverse not only endothelial but also perivascular cell membranes before reaching neurons or other drug target cells in the CNS. Cerebral blood flow is the only limitation to permeation of the CNS by highly lipid-soluble drugs. With increasing polarity the rate of diffusion of drugs into the CNS is proportional to the lipid solubility of the nonionized species (*see* Rall in the symposium edited by La Du *et al.,* 1971). Strongly ionized agents such as quaternary

amines or the penicillins are normally unable to enter the CNS from the circulation.

In addition, organic ions are extruded from the cerebrospinal fluid into blood at the choroid plexus by transport processes similar to those in the renal tubule. Lipid-soluble substances leave the brain by diffusion through the capillaries and the blood–choroid plexus boundary. Drugs and endogenous metabolites, regardless of lipid solubility and molecular size, also exit with bulk flow of the cerebrospinal fluid through the arachnoid villi.

The blood-brain barrier is adaptive in that exclusion of drugs and other foreign agents such as penicillin or *d*-tubocurarine protects the CNS against severely toxic effects. However, the barrier is neither absolute nor invariable. Very large doses of penicillin may produce seizures; meningeal or encephalitic inflammation increases the local permeability. Maneuvers to increase permeability of the blood-brain barrier are potentially important to enhance the efficacy of chemotherapeutic agents that are used to treat infections or tumors localized in the brain.

Drug Reservoirs. As mentioned, the body compartments in which a drug accumulates are potential reservoirs for the drug. If stored drug is in equilibrium with that in plasma and is released as the plasma concentration declines, a concentration of the drug in plasma and at its locus of action is sustained, and pharmacological effects of the drug are prolonged. However, if the reservoir for the drug fills rapidly, it so alters the distribution of the drug that larger quantities of the drug are required initially to provide a therapeutically effective concentration in the target organ.

Plasma Proteins. Many drugs are bound to plasma proteins, mostly to plasma albumin; binding to other plasma proteins generally occurs to a much smaller extent. The binding is usually reversible; covalent binding of reactive drugs such as alkylating agents occurs occasionally. The initial attraction that leads to binding is electrostatic, but this is reinforced by weaker forces, including hydrophobic bonds. Charge is thus not a major factor in the specificity and intensity of binding (*see* Koch-Weser and Sellers, 1976). The extent of the binding depends upon the particular drug. Some lipid-soluble organic acids, such as the penicillinase-resistant penicillins and the anticoagulant agent warfarin, are more than 90% bound to hydrophobic regions of the protein. Lipid-soluble organic bases may also be highly bound to albumin, but to different sites.

The fraction of total drug in plasma that is bound is determined by the drug concentration, its affinity for the binding sites, and the number of binding sites. Simple mass-action equations are used to describe the free and bound concentrations. At low concentrations of drug (less than the plasma protein–binding dissociation constant), the fraction bound is a function of the concentration of binding sites and the dissociation constant. At high drug concentrations (greater than the dissociation constant), the fraction bound is a function of the number of binding sites and the drug concentration. Statements that a given drug is $X\%$ bound are useless unless this additional information is also available; the usual implication is that therapeutic concentrations are being discussed.

Binding of a drug to plasma protein limits its concentration in tissues and at its locus of action, since only unbound drug is in equilibrium across membranes. Binding also limits glomerular filtration of the drug, since this process does not immediately change the concentration of free drug in the plasma (water is also filtered). However, plasma protein binding does *not* generally limit renal tubular secretion or biotransformation, since these processes lower the free drug concentration, and this is rapidly followed by dissociation of the drug-protein complex. If a drug is avidly transported or metabolized and its clearance, calculated on the basis of unbound drug, exceeds organ plasma flow, binding of the drug to plasma protein may be viewed as a transport mechanism that fosters drug elimination by delivering drug to sites for elimination.

Since binding of drugs to plasma albumin is rather nonselective, many drugs with similar physicochemical characteristics compete with each other and with endogenous substances for these binding sites. For example, displacement of unconjugated bilirubin from binding to albumin by the sulfonamides and other organic anions is known to increase the risk of bilirubin encephalopathy in the newborn, and drug toxicity has sometimes been attributed to similar competition between drugs for binding sites. Such interactions are often more complex than generally stated. Since drug displaced from plasma protein will redistribute into its full potential volume of distribution, the concentration of free drug in plasma and tissues after redistribution may be increased only slightly. The interaction may also involve altered elimination of the drug. Risk of adverse effect is greatest if

the displaced drug has a limited volume of distribution, if the competition extends to the drug bound in tissues, if elimination of the drug is also reduced, or if the displacing drug is administered in high dosage by rapid intravenous injection. Competition of drugs for plasma protein binding sites may also cause misinterpretation of measured serum concentrations of drugs.

Cellular Reservoirs. Many drugs accumulate in muscle and other cells in higher concentrations than in the extracellular fluids. If the intracellular concentration is high and if the binding is reversible, the tissue involved may represent a sizable drug reservoir, particularly if the tissue represents a large fraction of body mass. For example, during chronic administration of the antimalarial agent quinacrine, the concentration of the drug in liver may be several thousand times that in plasma. Accumulation in cells may be the result of active transport or, more commonly, binding. Tissue binding of drugs usually occurs with proteins, phospholipids, or nucleoproteins and is generally reversible.

Fat as a Reservoir. Many lipid-soluble drugs are stored by physical solution in the neutral fat. In obese persons, the fat content of the body may be as high as 50%, and even in starvation it constitutes 10% of body weight; hence, fat can serve as an important reservoir for lipid-soluble drugs. For example, as much as 70% of the highly lipid-soluble barbiturate thiopental may be present in body fat 3 hours after administration. However, fat is a rather stable reservoir because it has a relatively low blood flow.

Bone. The tetracycline antibiotics (and other divalent-metal-ion chelating agents) and heavy metals may accumulate in bone by adsorption onto the bone-crystal surface and eventual incorporation into the crystal lattice. Bone can become a reservoir for the slow release of toxic agents such as lead or radium into the blood. Their effects can thus persist long after exposure has ceased. Local destruction of the bone medulla may also lead to reduced blood flow and prolongation of the reservoir effect, since the toxic agent becomes sealed off from the circulation; this may further enhance the direct local damage to the bone. A vicious cycle results whereby the greater the exposure to the toxic agent the slower is its rate of elimination.

Transcellular Reservoirs. Drugs also cross epithelial cells and may accumulate in the transcellular fluids. The major transcellular reservoir is the gastrointestinal tract. Weak bases are passively concentrated in the stomach from the blood, because of the large pH differential between the two fluids, and some drugs are secreted in the bile in an active form or as a conjugate that can be hydrolyzed in the intestine. In these cases and when an orally administered drug is slowly absorbed, the gastrointestinal tract serves as a drug reservoir.

Other transcellular fluids, including *cerebrospinal fluid, aqueous humor, endolymph,* and *joint fluids,* do not generally accumulate significant total amounts of drugs.

Redistribution. Termination of drug effect is usually by biotransformation and excretion, but it may also result from redistribution of the drug from its site of action into other tissues or sites. Redistribution is a factor in terminating drug effect primarily when a highly lipid-soluble drug that acts on the brain or cardiovascular system is administered rapidly by intravenous injection or by inhalation. The factors involved in redistribution of drugs have been discussed above.

Placental Transfer of Drugs. A knowledge of the principles of transfer of drugs across the placenta is important, since drugs may cause congenital anomalies. Administered immediately prior to delivery, they may also have adverse effects upon the neonate. Drugs cross the placenta primarily by simple diffusion. Lipid-soluble, nonionized drugs readily enter the fetal blood from the maternal circulation. Penetration is least with drugs possessing a high degree of dissociation or low lipid solubility. The view that the placenta is a barrier to drugs is inaccurate. A more appropriate approximation is that the fetus is to at least some extent exposed to essentially all drugs taken by the mother (*see* Green *et al.,* 1979).

BIOTRANSFORMATION OF DRUGS

Many drugs are lipid-soluble, weak organic acids or bases that are not readily eliminated from the body. For example, after filtration at the renal glomerulus they are readily reabsorbed by diffusion through the renal tubular cells. To be excreted more rapidly, they must be transformed into more polar compounds. Drug metabolites usually are more polar and less lipid soluble than the parent molecule, and this enhances their excretion and reduces their volume of distribu-

tion. Biotransformation not only fosters drug elimination but also often results in inactivation of the compound. However, many drug metabolites have pharmacological activity. They may exert effects that are similar to or different from those of the parent molecule, and they may be responsible for important toxic effects that follow drug administration. Furthermore, advantage may sometimes be taken of drug-metabolizing enzymes by administration of an agent in an inactive form as a *prodrug.* This is necessary, for example, for purine or pyrimidine analogs used for cancer chemotherapy; in these cases the active chemical species, the nucleotide, is too polar to penetrate to intracellular sites of action, and drug is administered in the form of the purine or pyrimidine base or the corresponding nucleoside. If drug metabolites are active, termination of action takes place by further biotransformation or by excretion of the active metabolite in the urine. (For excellent summaries of drug biotransformation, *see* La Du *et al.,* 1971; Symposium, 1973b; Goldstein *et al.,* 1974; Lu, 1976; Lee *et al.,* 1977.)

Patterns of Biotransformation. The chemical reactions concerned in the biotransformation of drugs are classified as *nonsynthetic* and *synthetic.* The nonsynthetic reactions involve oxidation, reduction, or hydrolysis; they may result in activation, change in activity, or inactivation of the parent drug. The synthetic reactions, also called *conjugation reactions,* involve coupling between the drug or its metabolite and an endogenous substrate, usually a carbohydrate or an amino acid or a derivative of these, acetic acid, or inorganic sulfate.

Although many details of drug biotransformation are necessarily based upon observations in animals, the mechanisms in man are often similar. However, rates of the reactions in the various species are often quite different, and the patterns of biotransformation may be qualitatively different.

Various patterns of biotransformation, involving nonsynthetic and synthetic reactions and representing both activation and inactivation of drugs, are illustrated in Table 1–2. These reactions also emphasize that most drugs are converted concurrently or consecutively to multiple metabolites. The hepatic

Table 1-2. REPRESENTATIVE PATTERNS OF DRUG BIOTRANSFORMATION

Site of reaction: M = microsomal
N = nonmicrosomal

Type of reaction: 1 = conjugation
2 = oxidation
3 = reduction
4 = hydrolysis

microsomal enzyme systems are responsible for the biotransformation of the majority of drugs. Other tissues, including plasma, kidney, lung, and the gastrointestinal tract, also contribute to drug biotransformation.

The first reaction in Table 1-2, involving morphine, illustrates the common process of inactivation by glucuronide formation. The second series of reactions depicts the inactivation of the antiepileptic agent phenobarbital by oxidation. Subsequent conjugations of two types further facilitate excretion of the metabolite. The third reaction, oxidation of the antiepileptic agent trimethadione to the active metabolite dimethadione (DMO), demonstrates that oxidation need not inactivate a drug and that biotransformation does not always proceed to conjugation. DMO is not further metabolized but is slowly excreted in the urine. Oxidation may also result in conversion of an inactive drug to an active metabolite or the formation of a metabolite with qualitatively different activity than that of the parent drug, for example, the biotransformation of the antipyretic-analgesic phenacetin to a metabolite that causes methemoglobin formation. The fourth reaction sequence illustrates that a drug may be converted concurrently to active and inactive metabolites. The sedative-hypnotic chloral hydrate is both oxidized to inactive trichloroacetic acid and reduced to the active metabolite trichloroethanol, which is subsequently inactivated by conjugation. The time course of drug effect after administration of chloral hydrate

thus depends upon the relative rates of the three reactions. The fifth series of reactions involves the third general type of nonsynthetic reaction, hydrolysis. The neuromuscular blocking agent succinylcholine is hydrolyzed to succinylmonocholine, and this metabolite with weak activity is then further hydrolyzed to inactive choline. The final reaction sequence illustrates that conjugation, in this case, of 6-mercaptopurine to its ribonucleotide, occasionally results in activation of a drug.

Hepatic Microsomal Drug-Metabolizing Systems. The enzyme systems concerned in the biotransformation of many drugs are primarily located in the hepatic smooth endoplasmic reticulum. Fragments of this network are isolated by centrifugation of liver homogenates in the fraction generally called *microsomes.* These enzymes are present in other organs such as the kidney and gastrointestinal epithelium. Drugs absorbed from the intestine may thus be subject to the *first-pass effect.* This represents the combined action of gastrointestinal epithelial and hepatic drug-metabolizing enzymes, which may prevent the appearance of significant amounts of a drug in the circulation after oral administration (*see* Routledge and Shand, 1979).

Table 1-3. DRUG BIOTRANSFORMATION REACTIONS

I. *Oxidative Reactions* (Microsomal)

(1) N- and O-Dealkylation

$$RNHCH_2CH_3 \xrightarrow{[O]} RNH_2 + CH_3CHO$$

$$ROCH_3 \xrightarrow{[O]} ROH + CH_2O$$

(2) Side Chain (Aliphatic) and Aromatic Hydroxylation

$$RCH_2CH_3 \xrightarrow{[O]} R\overset{\displaystyle OH}{\underset{}{C}}HCH_3$$

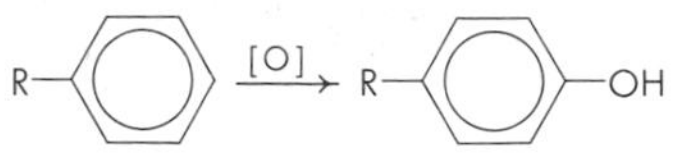

(3) N-Oxidation and N-Hydroxylation

$$(R)_3N \xrightarrow{[O]} R_3N{=}O$$

$$RNHR' \xrightarrow{[O]} R\overset{\displaystyle OH}{\underset{}{N}}R'$$

(4) Sulfoxide Formation

$$RSR' \xrightarrow{[O]} R\overset{\displaystyle O}{\underset{}{S}}R'$$

(5) Deamination of Amines

$$RCH_2NH_2 \xrightarrow{[O]} RCHO + NH_3$$

(6) Desulfuration

$$RSH \xrightarrow{[O]} ROH$$

II. *Glucuronide Synthesis* (Microsomal)

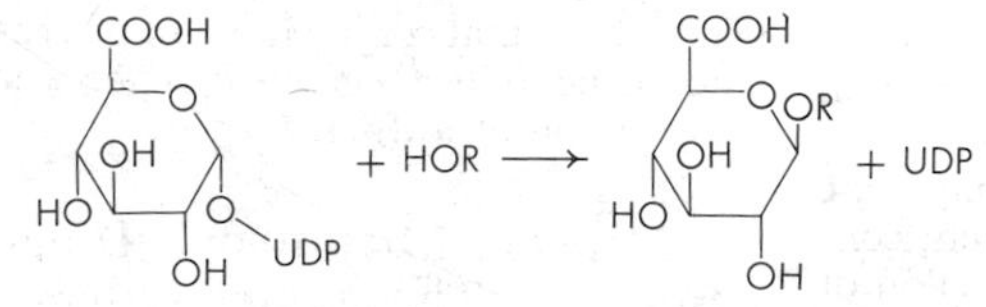

UDP–Glucuronic Acid

The endoplasmic reticulum resembles a canal system within the cell and may function also in intracellular transport. The reticulum consists of a membrane that bears small ribonucleoprotein particles, *ribosomes,* which cause the reticulum to have a rough surface. The rough-surfaced reticulum is the site of protein synthesis, including the synthesis of the smooth-surfaced reticulum that contains the enzymes that metabolize drugs.

The microsomal enzymes catalyze glucuronide conjugations and most of the oxidations of drugs (*see* Table 1–3). Reduction and hydrolysis of drugs are catalyzed by both microsomal and nonmicrosomal enzymes. Lipid solubility is an important, but not the only, requirement for a drug to be metabolized by the hepatic microsomes since this property favors the penetration of a drug into the endoplasmic reticulum and its binding with cytochrome P-450, a primary component of the oxidative enzyme system (Figure 1–3). Most endogenous metabolic intermediates are polar compounds and are not substrates. However, the microsomal enzymes do contribute to the biotransformation of fatty acids and steroid hormones and also conjugate bilirubin.

The hepatic microsomal enzyme systems are notable; not only do they participate in the biotransformation of many drugs but also

Table 1-3. DRUG BIOTRANSFORMATION REACTIONS (Continued)

III. *Other Conjugation Reactions*

(1) Acetylation

$$RNH_2 + CH_3\overset{\overset{\displaystyle O}{\|}}{C}SCoA \longrightarrow RNH\overset{\overset{\displaystyle O}{\|}}{C}CH_3 + CoA{-}SH$$

Acetyl CoA

(2) Conjugation with Glycine

$$RCOOH \longrightarrow R\overset{\overset{\displaystyle O}{\|}}{C}SCoA + NH_2CH_2COOH \longrightarrow R\overset{\overset{\displaystyle O}{\|}}{C}NHCH_2COOH + CoA{-}SH$$

(3) Conjugation with Sulfate

$$ROH + 3'\text{-phosphoadenosine } 5'\text{-phosphosulfate} \longrightarrow RO\overset{\overset{\displaystyle O}{\|}}{\underset{\underset{\displaystyle O}{\|}}{S}}OH + 3'\text{-phosphoadenosine } 5'\text{-phosphate}$$

(4) O-, S-, and N-Methylation

$$R{-}XH + S\text{-adenosylmethionine} \longrightarrow R{-}X{-}CH_3 + S\text{-adenosylhomocysteine}$$
$$(X = O, S, N)$$

IV. *Hydrolysis of Esters and Amides*

$$R\overset{\overset{\displaystyle O}{\|}}{C}OR' \longrightarrow RCOOH + R'OH$$

$$R\overset{\overset{\displaystyle O}{\|}}{C}NR' \longrightarrow RCOOH + R'NH_2$$

V. *Reduction*

(1) Azo Reduction

$$RN{=}NR' \longrightarrow RNH_2 + R'NH_2$$

(2) Nitro Reduction

$$RNO_2 \longrightarrow RNH_2$$

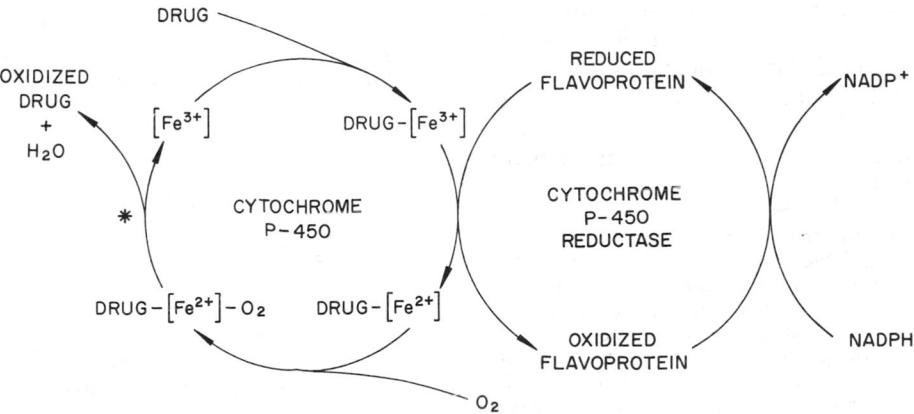

* Denotes contribution of a second electron and two hydrogen ions from NADH–flavoprotein–cytochrome b_5 or from NADPH–flavoprotein.

Figure 1-3. *Major components of the hepatic microsomal drug-metabolizing enzyme system.*

activity of these enzymes can be induced by many drugs and by chemicals encountered in the environment (*see* below). Both normal individual differences in microsomal enzyme activity and susceptibility to induction are genetically determined. Rates of biotransformation of drugs among individuals may vary sixfold or more.

The evolutionary development of drug-metabolizing systems is probably related to exposure of both vertebrates and invertebrates to toxic alkaloids in plants on which they have fed. Thus, drug metabolism has evolved as a means of protection against environmental toxins. However, the notion that biotransformation is equivalent to detoxication is incorrect, particularly with regard to drugs and man-made pollutants.

Oxidation. The hepatic endoplasmic reticulum contains an important group of oxidative enzymes called *mixed-function oxidases* or *monooxygenases* that require both reduced nicotinamide adenine dinucleotide phosphate (NADPH) and molecular oxygen. These enzymes are involved in the biotransformation of many drugs. Epoxide intermediates in these reactions are capable of covalent binding with macromolecules and may be responsible for tissue necrosis, carcinogenicity, and other toxic effects of drugs. The toxicity of several drugs (*e.g.,* acetaminophen, isoniazid, furosemide, methyldopa) appears to be due, at least in part, to the formation of such reactive nucleophils (*see* below and Figure 1–4).

The reactions catalyzed by the microsomal mixed-function oxidases include N- and O-dealkylation, aromatic ring and side chain hydroxylation, sulfoxide formation, N-oxidation, N-hydroxylation, deamination of primary and secondary amines, and the replacement of a sulfur by an oxygen atom (desulfuration). These reactions are depicted in Table 1–3.

The mixed-function oxidase system has not yet been fully characterized, since its components have not been purified in functional form. However, the electron-transport scheme is illustrated in Figure 1–3. The terminal oxidase is a hemoprotein (or group of proteins) designated cytochrome P-450, so named since it absorbs light at 450 nm when exposed to carbon monoxide. This property is also the basis for its analytical determination. Furthermore, carbon monoxide blocks the metabolism of many drugs by the system. The primary electron donor is NADPH;

the electron transfer involves a flavoprotein, cytochrome P-450 reductase. A phospholipid is essential for activity of the reconstituted system.

A drug substrate binds with oxidized cytochrome P-450 ([Fe^{3+}] in Figure 1–3). The resulting drug-cytochrome complex is reduced by the reductase, and the reduced complex then combines with molecular oxygen. A second electron and two hydrogen ions are acquired from the donor system, and the subsequent products are oxidized metabolite and water, with regeneration of the oxidized cytochrome P-450.

Interactions of substrates and inhibitors with oxidized cytochrome P-450 produce characteristic changes in the absorbance spectrum of the microsomes. These provide the basis for the designation of two types of drug binding sites or at least two types of cytochrome P-450 molecules. Clarification of the relationships between these spectral changes and the binding of drugs to the components of cytochrome P-450 and the interaction of binding sites is an area of active research.

The rate of drug biotransformation by the mixed-function oxidase system is determined by the concentration of cytochrome P-450, the proportions of the various forms of cytochrome P-450 and their affinities for the substrate, the concentration of cytochrome P-450 reductase, and the rate of reduction of the drug–cytochrome P-450 complex. Rate of biotransformation may also be influenced by competing endogenous and exogenous substrates. These many factors are responsible for the sometimes marked species, strain, and individual variations in drug metabolism by the microsomal system.

Glucuronide Synthesis. Glucuronides constitute the major proportion of metabolites of many phenols, alcohols, and carboxylic acids. Glucuronides are generally inactive and are rapidly secreted into the urine and bile by the transport mechanisms for anions. However, glucuronides eliminated in the bile may be subsequently hydrolyzed by intestinal or bacterial β-glucuronidase, and the liberated drug may be reabsorbed. This enterohepatic cycling may prolong the action of the drug.

Glucuronide formation is catalyzed by various microsomal glucuronyltransferases, with uridine diphosphate–glucuronic acid as the donor of glucuronic acid (Table 1–3). It is generated from glucose by enzymes in the cytosol. Glucuronide conjugation also occurs in the kidney and other tissues to a lesser extent.

Inhibition of Microsomal Drug Metabolism. Competitive inhibition between the many substrates for the microsomal enzymes is readily demonstrated *in vitro*. Such interactions are not usually of practical significance *in vivo*. This is not unexpected, since the inactivation of most drugs *in vivo* exhibits exponential (first-order) rather than linear (zero-order) kinetics; that is, the activity of drug-metabolizing enzymes is usually not rate limiting. Drug concentrations are commonly well below those necessary to saturate metabolizing enzymes, and competition between substrates is minimized under these conditions. An important corollary, however, is that significant mutual inhibition of drug metabolism is to be expected for drugs that normally exhibit zero-order inactivation kinetics. The best-established examples of inhibition of the metabolism of one drug by another during drug therapy do, in fact, involve phenytoin, dicumarol, and other drugs that, given alone, exhibit zero-order elimination.

Reduction in the rate of drug metabolism may also occur when biotransformation is so rapid that hepatic blood flow is the rate-limiting factor. Hepatic blood flow may decrease acutely after β-adrenergic blockade, and this can affect the rate of metabolism of drugs that are cleared from the plasma at very high rates (*e.g.*, lidocaine). Microsomal drug metabolism is inhibited by carbon monoxide and by hepatotoxic agents that destroy cytochrome P-450, interfere with hepatic metabolism, or chronically decrease hepatic blood flow.

In animals, a number of agents are impressive inhibitors of microsomal drug metabolism. Pretreatment with these compounds prolongs the effects of many other drugs by inhibition of their inactivation, or reduces the effects of those that are converted to active metabolites. The most extensively studied inhibitor is SKF 525A (β-diethylaminoethyl-2,2-diphenylpentanoate; proadifen). Inhibition of drug metabolism by SKF 525A and related agents may be simply competitive but often involves multiple mechanisms, including both competitive and noncompetitive interference with the binding of substrates to cytochrome P-450 and with the reduction of cytochrome P-450. These inhibitors may bind irreversibly with the enzyme, their metabolites may also be effective inhibitors, and most also cause induction of the microsomal system. In addition, such inhibitors may produce other pharmacological effects that contribute to drug interaction. Although not useful as therapeutic agents, they are valuable pharmacological tools for analysis of drug biotransformation and for characterization of the microsomal enzyme systems.

Induction of Microsomal Enzyme Activity. The activity of the microsomal enzymes can be increased by administration of certain drugs and by exposure to various chemicals in the environment; these inducers need not be substrates for the enzymes that are affected. The capacity of foreign compounds to induce microsomal drug metabolism is important for drug therapy and the transformation of environmental substances into highly toxic agents. That a drug can increase its own metabolism and that of other substrates has wide implications for chronic toxicity tests, crossover drug studies in animals and man, chronic drug therapy with single or multiple drugs, and the development of tolerance to drugs. (Chapter 3 and chapters on specific classes of drugs provide more information about the pharmacological and therapeutic aspects of induction of microsomal enzymes.)

In animals, the several hundred compounds known to stimulate the microsomal enzyme systems are loosely classified into two types, namely, those that resemble phenobarbital and those that are similar to the carcinogenic polycyclic hydrocarbons. Stimulation of the microsomal system by phenobarbital results in altered biotransformation of a wide variety of substrates. The increase in enzyme activity is attributed to induced synthesis of cytochrome P-450, cytochrome P-450 reductase, and other enzymes involved in drug metabolism, since the increase has typical latency, cannot be produced *in vitro*, is associated with proliferation of the endoplasmic reticulum, and can be prevented by inhibitors of nucleic acid and protein synthesis. Increased RNA polymerase activity and decreased microsomal ribonuclease activity have also been observed. Phenobarbital, but not all other inducers, also increases liver weight, hepatic blood flow, bile flow, and other hepatic proteins, including those thought to be important in the uptake of organic anions into the hepatocyte. Stimulation of the microsomal enzyme system by the polycyclic hydrocarbons is also attributed to induced protein synthesis, but the increase in drug metabolism is limited to relatively few substrates, does not result in an increase in cytochrome P-450 reductase, and is associated with the appearance of a qualitatively different terminal oxidase. Different receptors and different genes are thus probably involved in induction by these two classes of compounds. A widely used defoliant, trichlorophenoxyacetic acid (2,4,5-T), contains an inducer of this type as a contaminant, tetrachlorobenzo-*p*-dioxin. This compound can produce permanent induction of microsomal enzymes when submicrogram doses are given to experimental animals. This class of inducer can also accelerate the formation of reactive intermediates during metabolism of other drugs or of environmental chemicals.

Enzyme induction also occurs to a limited extent in kidney, gastrointestinal tract, adrenal, lung, placenta, skin, and pancreas. Upon removal of most inducing agents, the effects wane over a period of days or weeks, depending in part upon the time course for accumulation or elimination of the inducing agent.

Since chronic administration of a drug may stimulate its own metabolism and that of other agents, interactions may occur between drugs that are simultaneously administered. The concomitant administration of phenobarbital and warfarin results in lower plasma concentrations of warfarin and less anticoagulant effect than when the anticoagulant is administered alone. The desired therapeutic effect can be attained if dosage of the anticoagulant is increased. However, if the phenobarbital medication is stopped after the dosage of the anticoagulant has been adjusted, the plasma concentration and effect of warfarin increase, and severe bleeding may occur. Thus, during multiple-drug therapy involving an agent that stimulates drug metabolism, the effects of the other drugs must be carefully monitored, both when medication with the inducing agent is initiated and when it is discontinued.

Relationship of Drug Metabolism to Drug Toxicity. Reference has been made above to the formation of toxic metabolites as the result of microsomal oxidation of drugs. Microsomal oxidation can cause the formation of highly reactive compounds that normally have such a transient existence that they exert no biological action. Two examples of forma-

tion and inactivation of such substances are shown in Figure 1–4. As long as the terminal hydroxylation or conjugation keeps pace, accumulation of reactive intermediates does not occur. However, when induction occurs or when very large amounts of drug are present, oxidation by cytochrome P-450 is accelerated. Since glutathione is in limited supply in liver and kidney and can be depleted, the drug epoxide or quinone may reach a sufficient concentration to react with nucleophilic cell constituents. Hepatic or renal necrosis results. The discovery that the availability of glutathione determines the threshold for the toxic response has led to attempts to use thiols, for example, N-acetylcysteine, to treat poisoning by drugs such as acetaminophen.

Polycyclic hydrocarbons are potent inducers of microsomal metabolism and cause the accumulation of relatively small amounts of reactive intermediates that presumably intercalate into the DNA helix and initiate carcinogenesis. The experimental basis of this concept is well established; its clinical significance is not clear. It may be possible to evaluate the mutagenicity and carcinogenicity of drugs of this

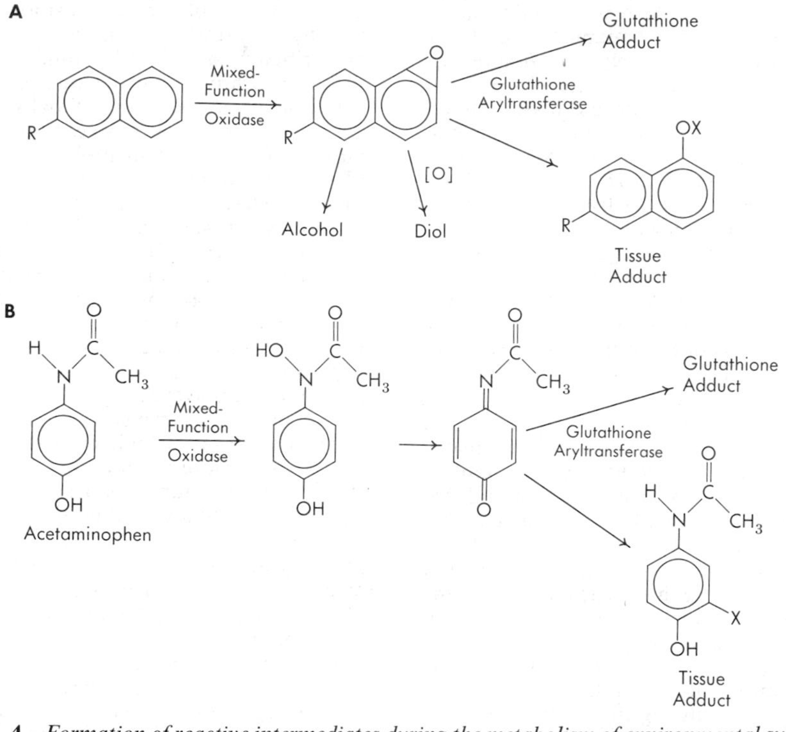

Figure 1–4. *Formation of reactive intermediates during the metabolism of environmental substances and drugs.*

A. A compound with an aromatic ring susceptible to hydroxylation may be metabolized to an arene oxide (epoxide) that can be converted spontaneously to the monoalcohol. The epoxide also can be converted enzymatically to a "diol" or can react with glutathione. The latter compound is eventually excreted as a mercapturic acid derivative. When concentrations of compounds such as glutathione are limiting, reaction can occur with macromolecular constituents of tissues.

B. Acetaminophen may be converted to a quinone type of reactive intermediate that is rapidly transformed to a mercapturate when the concentration of glutathione is not limiting. (The major route of acetaminophen metabolism is to an O-glucuronide.) *X* represents a tissue site of covalent reaction.

type that are used to treat very large populations, for example, those treated for *Schistosoma mansoni* infestation with polycyclic drugs such as lucanthone.

Drug Metabolism in the Fetus and Neonate. Activity of the hepatic microsomal enzyme systems is low in the neonate, particularly premature babies. Reduced conjugating activity contributes to the hyperbilirubinemia of the neonate and the risk of bilirubin encephalopathy. It is also the basis of the increased toxicity in the neonate of drugs such as chloramphenicol or certain opioid analgesics that are inactivated by glucuronide formation. Activity of nonmicrosomal enzymes involved in drug biotransformation is also reduced. The combination of a poorly developed blood-brain barrier, weak drug-metabolizing activity, and immature mechanisms for excretion combine to make the fetus and neonate very sensitive to toxic effects of drugs. Biotransformation capacity increases during the early months of postnatal life, although the pattern for different enzymes is variable.

Nonmicrosomal Drug Biotransformation. All conjugations other than glucuronide formation and some oxidation, reduction, and hydrolysis of drugs are catalyzed by nonmicrosomal enzymes. Such reactions contribute to the biotransformation of a number of common drugs, including aspirin and the sulfonamides. In addition, drugs that are only slowly metabolized may compete effectively with endogenous substrates. In certain such cases, as illustrated by the inhibition of xanthine oxidase by allopurinol, drug action and biotransformation are intimately related.

Nonmicrosomal biotransformation of drugs occurs primarily in the liver but also in plasma and other tissues. Although drug metabolism by the gastrointestinal tract and intestinal flora is usually minor relative to total drug elimination, biotransformation in the gastrointestinal tract sometimes contributes to what is superficially interpreted as poor oral absorption of a drug. Minor metabolites from the intestinal metabolism of a drug may contribute to drug toxicity. Intestinal hydrolysis of glucuronides secreted in the bile is an integral link in the enterohepatic cycling of drugs.

Individual variation in rates of drug bio-transformation is about the same for the nonmicrosomal enzymes as for the microsomal enzymes, namely, sixfold or greater. None of the nonmicrosomal enzymes involved in drug biotransformation is known to be inducible. Several, including pseudocholinesterase and the acetylating enzymes, exhibit genetic polymorphism. (*See* La Du *et al.*, 1971, for an excellent discussion of genetic modification of drug biotransformation.)

Conjugations. Inactivation of aromatic primary amines and hydrazines by conjugation with *acetic acid,* with acetyl coenzyme A as the acetyl donor, involves several N-acetyl transferases. These enzymes appear to represent the products of multiple genes, since genetic polymorphism (slow or fast acetylation by different individuals) is exhibited only to some substrates, including isoniazid, hydralazine, and many sulfonamides.

Aromatic carboxylic acids, such as salicylic acid, are often inactivated by conjugation with *glycine.* This reaction may exhibit zero-order kinetics when drug concentrations are high and first-order kinetics when they are lower. The kinetics of elimination of drugs metabolized by glycine conjugation thus appears to be highly variable, and adjustment of dosage may be very difficult.

Conjugation with *glutathione,* with subsequent formation of a mercapturate derivative, is not a quantitatively important route of biotransformation, but it contributes to inactivation of toxic epoxide intermediates produced by hydroxylation reactions (*see* discussion above and Figure 1–4).

Still other nonmicrosomal conjugations include *sulfate* conjugation of phenolic compounds, including steroids; *O-, S-,* and *N-methylation* of amines and phenols, including epinephrine and norepinephrine; and *ribonucleoside* and *ribonucleotide* formation, usually of analogs of the purines and pyrimidines to form active antimetabolites (*see* Figure 1–3).

Hydrolysis. Esters, such as procaine, are hydrolyzed by a variety of nonspecific esterases in liver, plasma, gastrointestinal tract, and other tissues. Hydrolysis of amides, such as lidocaine, occurs primarily in the liver. Peptidases in plasma, erythrocytes, and many other tissues are involved in the biotransformation of the biologically active polypeptides.

Oxidation. Some drugs are oxidized by a variety of flavoprotein enzymes in mitochondria and cytosol of the liver and other tissues. Examples include the oxidation of alcohols and aldehydes by *alcohol and aldehyde dehydrogenases,* the purine antimetabolite 6-mercaptopurine by *xanthine oxidase,* and drugs related to the catecholamines by *tyrosine hydroxylase* and *monoamine oxidase.*

Reduction. Microsomal and nonmicrosomal enzymes in the liver and other tissues can catalyze the reduction of nitro groups and the cleavage and reduction of the azo linkage. Examples include the nitro reduction of chloramphenicol and the azo reduction of PRONTOSIL. However, reduction of nitro and azo compounds *in vivo* is probably catalyzed mainly by the intestinal flora in the anaerobic environment of the gut (Scheline, 1973).

EXCRETION OF DRUGS

Drugs are eliminated from the body either unchanged or as metabolites. Excretory organs, the lung excluded, eliminate polar compounds more efficiently than substances with high lipid solubility. Lipid-soluble drugs are thus not readily eliminated until they are metabolized to more polar compounds.

The kidney is the most important organ for elimination of drugs and their metabolites. Substances excreted in the feces are mainly unabsorbed orally ingested drugs or metabolites excreted in the bile and not reabsorbed from the intestinal tract. Excretion of drugs in milk is important not because of the amounts eliminated but because the excreted drugs are potential sources of unwanted pharmacological effects in the nursing infant. Pulmonary excretion is important mainly for the elimination of anesthetic gases and vapors (*see* Chapter 13); occasionally, small quantities of other drugs or metabolites are excreted by this route.

Renal Excretion. Excretion of drugs and metabolites in the urine involves three processes: glomerular filtration, active tubular secretion, and passive tubular reabsorption.

The amount of drug entering the tubular lumen by *filtration* is dependent on its fractional plasma protein binding and glomerular filtration rate. In the proximal renal tubule, certain organic anions and cations are added to the glomerular filtrate by active, carrier-mediated tubular *secretion*. Many organic acids, such as penicillin, and metabolites, such as glucuronides, are transported by the system that secretes naturally occurring substances such as uric acid; organic bases, such as tetraethylammonium, are transported by a separate system that secretes choline, histamine, and other endogenous bases.

Both carrier systems are relatively nonselective, and organic ions of similar charge compete for transport. Both transport systems can also be bidirectional, and at least some drugs are both secreted and actively reabsorbed. However, transport of most ex-

ogenous ions is predominantly secretory. The outstanding example of the bidirectional tubular transport of an endogenous organic acid is uric acid. The characteristics of tubular transport systems for organic compounds are described in detail in Chapter 38.

In the proximal and distal tubules, the nonionized forms of weak acids and bases undergo net passive *reabsorption*. The concentration gradient for back diffusion is created by the reabsorption of water with sodium and other inorganic ions. Since the tubular cells are less permeable to the ionized forms of weak electrolytes, passive reabsorption of these substances is pH dependent. When the tubular urine is made more alkaline, weak acids are excreted more rapidly, primarily because they are more ionized and passive reabsorption is decreased. When the tubular urine is made more acid, the excretion of weak acids is reduced. Alkalinization and acidification of the urine have the opposite effects on the excretion of weak bases. In the treatment of drug poisoning, the excretion of some drugs can be hastened by appropriate alkalinization or acidification of the urine. Whether alteration of urine pH results in significant change in drug elimination depends upon the extent and persistence of the pH change and the contribution of pH-dependent passive reabsorption to total drug elimination. The effect is greatest for weak acids and bases with pK_a values in the range of urinary pH (5 to 8). However, alkalinization of urine can produce a fourfold to sixfold increase in excretion of a relatively strong acid such as salicylate when urinary pH is changed from 6.4 to 8.0. The fraction of nonionized drug would decrease from 1% to 0.04%.

Biliary and Fecal Excretion. Many metabolites of drugs formed in the liver are excreted into the intestinal tract in the *bile*. These metabolites may be excreted in the feces; more commonly, they are reabsorbed into the blood and ultimately excreted in the urine. Both organic anions, including glucuronides, and organic cations are actively transported into bile by carrier systems similar to those that transport these substances across the renal tubule. Both transport systems are nonselective, and ions of like charge may compete for transport. Steroids and related substances are transported into bile by a third carrier system. The effectiveness of the liver as an excretory organ for glucuronide conjugates is very much limited by their enzymatic hydrolysis after the bile is mixed with the contents of the small intestine.

Excretion by Other Routes. Excretion of drugs into *sweat, saliva,* and *tears* is quantitatively unimportant. Elimination by these routes is dependent mainly upon diffusion of the nonionized, lipid-soluble form of drugs through the epithelial cells of the glands and is pH dependent. Reabsorption of the nonionized drug from the primary secretion probably also occurs in the ducts of the glands, and active secretion of drugs across the ducts of the gland may also occur. Drugs excreted in the saliva enter the mouth, where they are usually swallowed. Their fate thereafter is the same as that of drugs taken orally. The concentration of some drugs in saliva parallels that in plasma. Saliva may therefore be a useful biological fluid in which to determine drug concentrations when it is difficult or inconvenient to obtain blood.

The same principles apply to excretion of drugs in *milk.* Since milk is more acidic than plasma, basic compounds may be slightly concentrated in this fluid, and the concentration of acidic compounds in milk is lower than in plasma. Nonelectrolytes, such as ethanol and urea, readily enter milk and reach the same concentration as in plasma, independent of the pH of the milk. (*See* summary of Plaa, in La Du *et al.,* 1971.)

Although excretion into *hair* and *skin* is also quantitively unimportant, sensitive methods of detection of toxic metals in these tissues have forensic significance. Arsenic in hair, detected 150 years after administration, has raised interesting questions about how Napoleon died, and by whose hand. Mozart's manic behavior during the preparation of his last major work, the *Requiem,* may have been due to mercury poisoning; traces of the metal have been found in his hair.

TIME COURSE OF DRUG EFFECT: PHARMACOKINETIC PRINCIPLES

Pharmacokinetic principles relate specifically to the variation with time of drug *concentration,* particularly in the blood, serum, or plasma as a result of *absorption, distribution,* and *elimination.* By extrapolation, they may be interpreted in terms of drug *effect.* Applied to therapy, pharmacokinetic principles aid in the selection and adjustment of drug dosage schedules and facilitate interpretation of measured serum concentrations of drugs. They are *not* a substitute for, but rather a supplement to, clinical monitoring and judgment. (Further information can be found in Appendix II; *see also* Gibaldi and Perrier, 1975; Melmon and Morrelli, 1978; Atkinson and Kushner, 1979.)

Basic Concepts. Pharmacokinetic principles have wide utility as a guide to therapy. These principles are useful, however, only if they are applied with appreciation of the assumptions upon which they are based. For example, the fundamental principles assume that the factors controlling drug elimination in the individual patient remain constant with time. Yet, drug elimination may change because of interaction with other drugs or following alterations in cardiovascular, renal, or hepatic function. Similarly, pharmacokinetic principles are most readily applied in terms of drug effect when effect is closely linked in time with drug concentration. However, the concentration-effect relationships for some drugs exhibit significant latency. These and other deviations from simple interpretation of kinetic patterns must be recognized, and modifications of the fundamental principles must be adopted for specific drugs and for the individual patient (*see* Melmon and Morrelli, 1978).

The fundamental pharmacokinetic principles are based upon the most elementary kinetic *model.* The body is considered a *single compartment. Distribution* of the drug within the compartment is assumed to be *relatively uniform, or of no practical consequence if not uniform,* and to occur *rapidly* relative to absorption and elimination. For this model, *volume of distribution* of a drug is that in which it would *appear* to be distributed during the steady state, if it existed throughout that volume at the same concentration as in plasma. If a drug is highly concentrated in tissues, its *apparent volume of distribution* (V_d) may be many times total body water. Thus:

$$V_d = \frac{\text{Total amount of drug in body}}{\text{Concentration of drug in plasma}}$$

Absorption and elimination of the drug are assumed to follow *exponential (first-order)* kinetics; that is, a constant *fraction* of drug present is eliminated per unit of time. Elimination of most drugs is exponential, since drug concentrations usually do not approach those required for saturation of the elimination process. In certain exceptional cases, the drug elimination processes may become saturated, and zero-order kinetics will result; that is, a constant *amount* of the drug present is eliminated per unit of time.

The rate of an *exponential process* may be expressed by its *rate constant k,* which expresses the *fractional change* per unit of time, or by its *half-time,* $t_{1/2}$, the time required for 50% completion of the process. The units of these two constants are time^{-1} and time, respectively. Both are independent of drug concentration (and dosage)—the hallmark of a first-order reaction. Simple calculations will reveal that the process is 93.75% complete after four half-times. A first-order rate constant and the half-time of the reaction are simply related ($kt_{1/2} = 0.693$) and may be interchanged accordingly. Total *body clearance* is the product of volume of distribution and elimination rate constant ($V_d k_e$) and expresses the volume of the V_d cleared per unit of time.

A *two-compartment model* of drug kinetics is more useful because it takes into account the phase of decreasing drug concentration that reflects the distribution of a drug from plasma into tissues (*see* Figure 1–5, *A*). As stated, this is ignored in the one-compartment model. However, if elimination of a drug is limited by blood flow to liver or kidney, as in congestive heart failure, the first phase may take on crucial significance. For further discussion, *see* Appendix II and Melmon and Morrelli (1978).

Single Doses. The time course of the plasma concentration of a hypothetical drug administered *intravenously* in a single dose is shown in Figure 1–5, *A*. As distribution of the drug occurs (the first phase in the two-compartment model), the concentration falls rapidly. *Following* this initial distribution phase, the kinetics of drug elimination is apparent. Since first-order elimination kinetics dictates that a constant *fraction* of drug is lost per unit of time, a plot of the log of drug concentration versus time is linear during this phase (absorption is complete). The half-time for drug elimination can be accurately determined from such a graph. Furthermore, extrapolation of the first-order elimination line to the drug-concentration axis (time = 0) yields an estimate of the drug concentration that would have obtained if distribution were instantaneous. Since the total amount of drug is known at this "zero-time" (the dose administered), the apparent volume of distribution can be calculated from the dose and the concentration obtained by extrapolation.

An *effect* of a single dose of a drug may be characterized by its *latency, time of peak effect, magnitude of peak effect,* and *duration.* The influence of dosage and rates of absorption and elimination on these parameters is also illustrated in Figure 1–5.

Differences in rate of absorption (Figure 1–5, *B*), particularly the large differences that result from administration of a drug by different routes or in different dosage forms, have a significant influence on all characteristics of the time course of drug concentration (and effect). When absorption is rapid relative to elimination, differences in rate of absorption are of less consequence, peak effect approaches that achieved after intravenous administration, and latency and time of peak effect are determined primarily by the rate of absorption.

As *dosage* is increased (Figure 1–5, *C*), latency is reduced and the peak effect is increased without change in the time of peak effect. Duration of effect is increased proportionately less than peak effect. Reduced *elimination* (Figure 1–5, *D*) results in the expected prolongation of drug effect. If the drug is rapidly absorbed, differences in rate of elimination have relatively minor influence on peak effect.

Repeated Doses. Since about four half-times are required for almost complete elimination of a drug, any dosage interval shorter than this must lead to *drug accumulation.* Provided that first-order kinetics continues to apply during repeated administration, drug accumulation continues until the rate of elimination equals the rate of drug administration. This follows from the principle that in first-order elimination the rate of elimination is proportional to dose; a constant *fraction* of the drug is eliminated per unit time. During repeated administration of a drug its concentration in plasma is characterized by the *time course* of accumulation, the *maximal*

Figure 1-5. *Fundamental pharmacokinetic relation-ships for single doses of drugs.*

A. A drug (500 mg) is administered *intravenously* to a 65-kg man, and plasma samples are obtained for determination of drug concentration. The concentration falls rapidly initially, as distribution occurs. First-order elimination kinetics follows. Extrapolation of this line indicates a hypothetical plasma concentration of 12 µg/ml at zero-time. The V_d is thus 500/0.012, or 41.7 l. This is indicative of distribution in total body water or drug sequestration at some nonplasma site. The half-time of drug elimination is estimated to be 3 hours.

B. Varied Absorption. Patterns to illustrate the influence of absorption (*a*) 100 times as rapid as, (*b*) ten times as rapid as, and (*c*) equal to elimination.

C. Varied Dosage. Patterns to illustrate the influence of a twofold difference in dosage (absorption ten times as rapid as elimination).

D. Varied Elimination. Patterns to illustrate the influence of a twofold difference in rate of elimination (lower curve, absorption:elimination = 10:1; upper curve, absorption:elimination = 10:0.5).

Graphs B, C, and D are based upon the elementary one-compartment model:

$$C_t = \frac{fD}{V_d}\left(\frac{k_a}{k_a - k_e}\right)[\exp(-k_e t) - \exp(-k_a t)]$$

where C_t = concentration of drug in plasma (mg/l) at time t, D = dose (mg), f = fractional absorption, V_d = volume of distribution (l), k_a = absorption rate constant (time^{-1}), and k_e = elimination rate constant (time^{-1}).

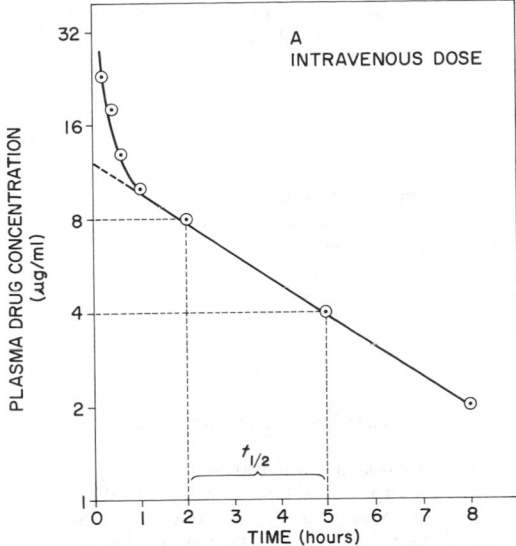

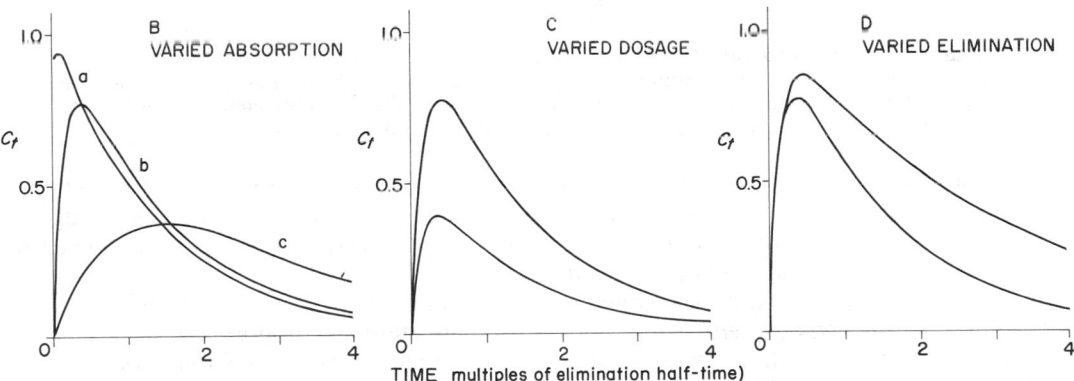

amount accumulated, and the *fluctuations* that result from the *dose interval* and the *half-time* of the drug (Figure 1–6).

When a drug is given repeatedly or continuously, the total body store increases exponentially to a plateau, with a half-time of increase that is equal to the elimination half-time for the agent (Figure 1–6). Thus, 50% of the maximal plateau level is achieved in one elimination half-time, 75% in two, 87.5% in three, and so forth. For practical purposes, maximal accumulation can be said to have occurred after about four half-times; at this time the rate of elimination is equal to that of administration.

The *average* total body store of drug at the plateau is a function of the maintenance dosage (dose/dosage interval) and the elimi-

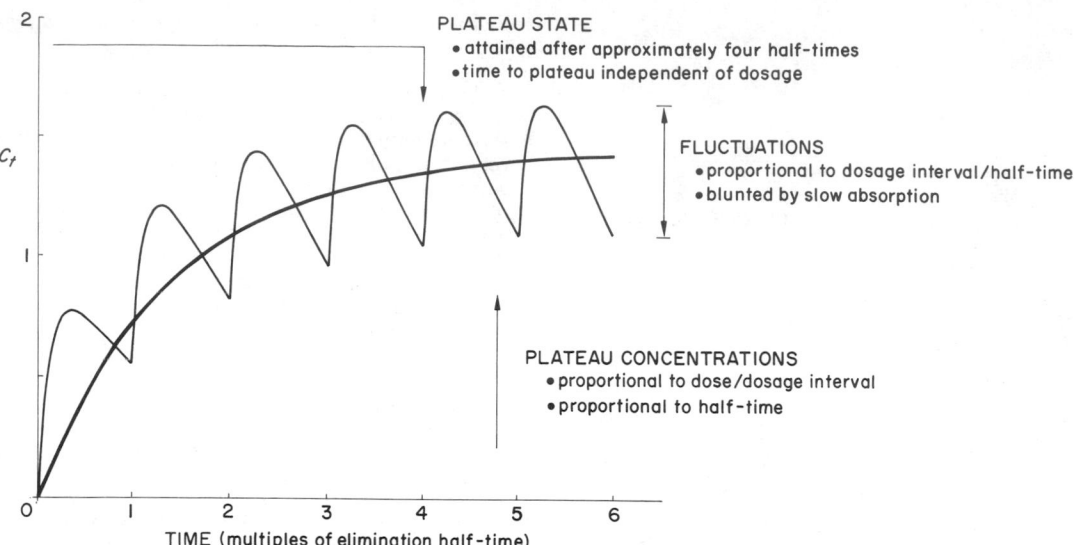

C_f

TIME (multiples of elimination half-time)

Within the figure:

PLATEAU STATE
• attained after approximately four half-times
• time to plateau independent of dosage

FLUCTUATIONS
• proportional to dosage interval/half-time
• blunted by slow absorption

PLATEAU CONCENTRATIONS
• proportional to dose/dosage interval
• proportional to half-time

Figure 1-6. *Fundamental pharmacokinetic relationships for repeated administration of drugs.*

Light line is the pattern of drug accumulation during repeated administration of a drug at intervals equal to its elimination half-time, when drug absorption is ten times as rapid as elimination. As the relative rate of absorption increases, the concentration maxima approach 2 and the minima approach 1 during the plateau state. Heavy line depicts the pattern during administration of equivalent dosage by continuous intravenous infusion. Curves are based upon the elementary one-compartment model.

Average concentration ($\bar{C}_p$) when the *plateau state* is attained during intermittent drug administration:

$$\bar{C}_p = \frac{fD}{V_d k_e T} = \frac{1.44\, t_{1/2} fD}{V_d T}$$

where $t_{1/2}$ = elimination half-time (time), T = dosage interval (time), and other symbols are as indicated in Figure 1–5. By substitution of infusion rate for D/T, the formula also provides the concentration maintained during the plateau state during continuous intravenous infusion. Note that both $t_{1/2}$ and dosage interval must be expressed in identical units of time.

nation half-time (Figure 1-6). These facts can be encompassed in an easily remembered statement: *the average total body store of drug at the plateau is approximately equal to 1.5 times (actually 1.44 times) the amount administered per half-time of elimination.* For example, if a drug has a half-time of 9 days and is administered once daily, it will accumulate to an average amount of 1.44 × 9, or 13 times that given daily (assuming complete absorption); more than one month will be required to achieve this result. These considerations apply equally well to continuous infusions of drugs—administration of an infinitely small dose at an infinitely small interval. If a drug is infused at 1 mg per minute and has a half-time of elimination of 60 minutes, it will accumulate to a total body store of approximately 90 mg. If the volume

of distribution of the drug is known, the calculated total body store of the drug can readily be expressed as a plasma concentration.

The fluctuations between doses during the plateau state are proportional to the ratio of the dosage interval and elimination half-time and are damped by slow absorption. When a rapidly absorbed drug is administered at intervals equal to its elimination half-time, the ratio of peak to minimal concentrations between doses approaches twofold. Half-doses at half-intervals will maintain the same average concentration with smaller fluctuations, an important achievement if the margin of safety of the drug is small.

Choice of Dosage Interval. Dosage interval should be selected primarily by consideration of the fluctuations in drug concentration that can be tolerated without excessive toxicity or loss of efficacy. On this basis, a dosage interval equal to or less than the elimination half-time is recommended for most drugs. However, longer intervals may be satisfactory if larger fluctuations can be tolerated, or if the drug is slowly absorbed. In addition, choice of dosage interval must sometimes be tempered by consideration of convenience for and compliance of the patient. For example, the penicillins in aqueous solution are often administered at intervals much greater than their half-times because a satisfactory effect can be achieved without toxicity despite the large fluctuations, and because the schedule is convenient for the patient.

Initial Loading Dose. When a drug is administered on a dosage schedule that is ultimately satisfactory for maintenance therapy, partial effect may occur promptly, but the full therapeutic and toxic effects of medication are necessarily delayed for the inevitable four elimination half-times. This may be a long time, indeed. If the therapeutic situation is not critical, such a dosage schedule may be preferred, since it minimizes the risk of excessive initial effect and permits adequate adjustment of dosage for the individual patient during the period of drug accumulation. If the desired full effect must be achieved more promptly, an initial so-called loading dose larger than the subsequent maintenance dose must be employed. It should be obvious, however, that if a dose larger than that required for maintenance is continued, accumulation and toxicity will result. If the dose given is only moderately greater than that required and if the elimination half-time is long, this toxicity may not become evident for an extended period of time. An estimated loading dose should be administered in divided fractions to permit at least some monitoring for efficacy and safety. Plateau concentrations during subsequent maintenance dosage are independent of the loading dose after the usual four half-times. Initial *total* loading dose (D^*), maintenance dosage (D/T; *e.g.,* 100 mg/8 hr or 300 mg/24 hr), and elimination half-time ($t_{1/2}$, in the same units of time) are related as follows: $D^* = 1.4\,t_{1/2}\,D/T$. Arguments for and against an initial loading dose are further discussed in connection with various

therapeutic agents, especially the cardiac glycosides, the antiarrhythmic drugs, and the oral anticoagulant agents (*see* Index).

Dose-Dependent Drug Elimination. Ethanol, aspirin, and phenytoin are examples of drugs that exhibit so-called dose-dependent elimination in the therapeutic range. As drug concentration (dosage) increases, elimination half-time and the time required to attain the plateau state also increase. In addition, plasma drug concentrations (and drug effects) during the plateau state increase disproportionately with increase in dosage. This pattern of deviation from first-order kinetics is expected if the concentration of the drug approaches that required for saturation of the elimination process. Further increases in dosage result in no further increase in the rate of elimination (zero-order kinetics). Similar deviation can occur if a metabolite of the drug inhibits its elimination. Saturation of carrier-mediated uptake of the drug by the liver and changes in fractional oral absorption or fractional plasma protein binding are the basis of other patterns of dose-dependent deviation from simple first-order kinetics.

Adjustment of Dosage Schedules for Impaired Elimination. To prevent excessive accumulation of a drug when its elimination is reduced in a patient with impaired renal, hepatic, or cardiovascular function, maintenance dosage (dose/dosage interval) must be reduced in proportion to the increase in elimination half-time. Whether the adjustment is accomplished by reducing the dose, increasing the dosage interval, or both depends upon the usual considerations of fluctuations and convenience. Since the therapeutic concentration desired has nothing to do with the rate of elimination, the initial loading dose need *not* be reduced for altered elimination *if the drug is rapidly absorbed,* but loading dose must be adjusted for altered volume of distribution. Plasma protein concentration and binding and other determinants of volume of distribution may be altered in renal, hepatic, and cardiovascular disease. In patients with reduced renal function, consideration must be given not only to drugs excreted unchanged in the urine but also to renal elimination of metabolites of drugs.

Adjustment of dosage schedules on the basis of pharmacokinetic principles, whether estimated by rule of thumb or by computer, is necessarily only an approximation; final adjustment must be made on the basis of the usual patient monitoring, including measurement of serum drug concentrations, if feasible. This important subject is discussed in more detail in Appendix II; *see also* Melmon and Morrelli (1978).

Adjustment of dosage schedules for patients with *impaired renal function* can be made precisely and with satisfactory results. Drug elimination by the kidney is correlated with endogenous creatinine clearance, serum creatinine concentration, and blood urea nitrogen concentration. These indices of renal function (listed in order of decreasing preference) provide an estimate of the necessary adjustment. Formulas, graphs, nomographs, and computer programs have been devised for adjustment of dosage schedules for individual drugs, including the cardiac glycosides and aminoglycoside antibiotics. The following simple formula, proposed by Giusti and Hayton (1973), appears to provide a suitable approximation of the adjustment for all drugs:

$$G = 1 - f\left(1 - \frac{C^r_{Cr}}{C_{Cr}}\right)$$

where G is the fraction of the usual maintenance dose that may be administered at usual dosage intervals, f is the fraction of the drug excreted unchanged in the urine in patients with normal renal function, C_{Cr} is normal endogenous creatinine clearance, and C^r_{Cr} is endogenous creatinine clearance measured in the patient or estimated from serum creatinine concentration. Alternatively, $1/G$ is the factor by which the dosage interval should be increased, if the choice is to administer usual doses of the drug at longer intervals. The formula does *not* include adjustment for possible changes in plasma protein binding or volume of distribution.

Adjustment of dosage schedules for patients with *imparied hepatic function* is difficult, since hepatic drug elimination is not consistently correlated with any of the routine hepatic function tests. In addition, CNS depressants and other drugs can precipitate encephalopathy in the cirrhotic patient for reasons other than excessive accumulation of the drug secondary to reduced drug elimination. The possibility of developing a simple test for hepatic drug-metabolizing activity that has predictive value for a variety of drugs is under active investigation. Monitoring of drug concentrations in serum is a more direct approach to adjusting dosage schedules for patients with liver disease, when such tests are available. When necessary, one must in essence determine the half-time of elimination for the patient in question and then apply the fundamental principles already discussed.

Monitoring of Drug Concentrations in Serum. Monitoring of drug concentrations in serum is particularly helpful in the use of drugs such as the antiepileptic agents, which are not readily monitored by direct clinical observation or other laboratory tests, and especially when these drugs are characterized by marked interpatient pharmacokinetic variation. This procedure is also a useful supplement to other monitoring in patients with impaired renal or hepatic function and whenever medication is unexpectedly ineffective or toxic. In addition, the patient's compliance may be improved merely by his knowing that drug concentrations are to be measured.

Serum drug concentrations are a reliable guide to therapy, however, only if the observations are interpreted in concert with other clinical information and with appropriate precautions. Serial measurements at selected intervals are always more useful than isolated determinations. Interpretation must include regard for the kinetic pattern for the particular drug, the interval between time of sampling and the last drug administration, and the plateau principle. Additional factors that must be considered include reliability of the analytical procedure, individual variation in serum concentrations associated with desired and undesired effects, possible active metabolites of the drug, factors that modify its concentration-effect relationship, concurrent medication, and possible drug tolerance. Finally, it must be recognized that the measured drug concentrations in serum, unless stated otherwise, represent both protein-bound and free drug. Potentially important differences in fractional binding of the drug are not detected by the usual measurements.

Studies with many drugs have shown that many apparent variations in drug potency among different species and different individuals are due primarily to variations in the rate of drug disposition. When dosage is adjusted so that equivalent serum concentrations are maintained, quantitative differences in response tend to disappear. This is obviously important for the establishment of optimal dosage for the individual patient.

General References

Goldstein, A.; Aronow, L.; and Kalman, S. M. *Principles of Drug Action: The Basis of Pharmacology,* 2nd ed. John Wiley & Sons, Inc., New York, **1974.**

Levine, R. R. *Pharmacology: Drug Actions and Reactions,* 2nd ed. Little, Brown & Co., Boston, **1978.**

Melmon, K. L., and Morrelli, H. F. (eds.). *Clinical Pharmacology: Basic Principles in Therapeutics,* 2nd ed. Macmillan Publishing Co., Inc., New York, **1978.**

Talalay, P. (ed.). *Drugs in Our Society.* The Johns Hopkins University Press, Baltimore, **1964.**

Historical Background

Holmstedt, B., and Liljestrand, G. (eds.). *Readings in Pharmacology.* Pergamon Press, Ltd., Oxford, **1963.**

Shuster, L. (ed.). *Readings in Pharmacology.* Little, Brown & Co., Boston, **1962.**

Absorption, Distribution, Biotransformation, and Excretion

Albert, A. Ionization, pH and biological activity. *Pharmacol. Rev.,* **1952,** *4,* 136–167.

American Pharmaceutical Association. *The Bioavailability of Drug Products,* cumulative ed. The Association, Washington, D. C., **1978.**

Berliner, R. W.; Clubb, L. E.; Doluisio, J. T.; Melmon, K. L.; Nados, A. S.; Oates, J. A.; Reigelmen, S.; Shideman, F. E.; Zelin, M.; and Robbins, F. C. *Drug Bioequivalence.* Office of Technological Assessment, U.S. Government Printing Office, Washington, D. C., **1974.**

Brodie, B. B., and Hogben, C. A. M. Some physiochemical factors in drug action. *J. Pharm. Pharmacol.,* **1957,** *9,* 345–380.

Conney, A. H. Pharmacological implications of microsomal enzyme induction. *Pharmacol. Rev.,* **1967,** *19,* 317–366. (379 references.)

Davson, H. The blood-brain barrier. In, *The Structure and Function of Nervous Tissue,* Vol. 4. (Bourne, G. H., ed.) Academic Press, Inc., New York, **1972,** pp. 321–445.

Green, T. P.; O'Dea, R. F.; and Mirkin, B. L. Determinants of drug disposition and effect in the fetus. *Annu. Rev. Pharmacol. Toxicol.,* **1979,** *19,* 285–322.

Hartiala, K. Metabolism of hormones, drugs, and other substances by the gut. *Physiol. Rev.,* **1973,** *53,* 496–534.

Koch-Weser, J., and Sellers, E. M. Binding of drugs to serum albumin. *N. Engl. J. Med.,* **1976,** *294,* 311–316, 526–531.

La Du, B. N.; Mandel, H. G.; and Way, E. L. (eds.). *Fundamentals of Drug Metabolism and Drug Disposition.* The Williams & Wilkins Co., Baltimore, **1971.**

Lee, D. H. K.; Falk, H. L.; Murphy, S. D.; and Geiger, S. R. (eds.). *Reactions to Environmental Agents. Handbook of Physiology,* Sect. 9. American Physiological Society, Bethesda, **1977.** (*See* especially Chapters 12 to 34 for absorption, distribution, and excretion of foreign agents.)

Lu, A. Y. H. Liver microsomal drug-metabolizing system: functional components and their properties. *Fed. Proc.,* **1976,** *35,* 2460–2463. (*See also* subsequent related articles, pp. 2464 and 2470.)

Reidenberg, M. M. *Renal Function and Drug Action.* W. B. Saunders Co., Philadelphia, **1971.**

Routledge, P. A., and Shand, D. G. Presystemic drug elimination. *Annu. Rev. Pharmacol. Toxicol.,* **1979,** *19,* 447–468.

Scheline, R. R. Metabolism of foreign compounds by gastrointestinal microorganisms. *Pharmacol. Rev.,* **1973,** *25,* 451–523.

Symposium. (Various authors.) Membrane structure and its biological applications. (Green, D. E., ed.) *Ann. N.Y. Acad. Sci.,* **1972a,** *195,* 1–519.

Symposium. (Various authors.) Pharmacogenetics. (Vesell, E. S., ed.) *Fed. Proc.,* **1972b,** *31,* 1253–1330.

Symposium. (Various authors.) Drug-protein binding. (Anton, A. H., and Solomon, H. M., eds.) *Ann. N.Y. Acad. Sci.,* **1973a,** *226,* 1–362.

Symposium. (Various authors.) Second international symposium on microsomes and drug oxidations. (Estabrook, R. W.; Gillette, J. R.; and Leibman, K. L.; eds.) *Drug Metab. Dispos.,* **1973b,** *1,* 1–487.

Tower, D. B., and Brady, R. O. (eds.). *Blood-Brain Barrier Systems. The Basic Neurosciences,* Vol. 1. *The Nervous System.* Raven Press, New York, **1975,** pp. 267–322.

Weissman, G., and Claiborne, R. (eds.). *Cell Membranes, Biochemistry, Cell Biology, and Pathology.* H. P. Publishing Co., New York, **1975.**

Wepierre, J., and Marty, J.-P. Percutaneous absorption of drugs. *Trends Pharmacol. Sci.,* **1979,** *1,* 23–26.

Pharmacokinetic Principles

Atkinson, A. J., Jr., and Kushner, W. Clinical pharmacokinetics. *Annu. Rev. Pharmacol. Toxicol.,* **1979,** *19,* 105–128.

Benet, L. Z. Biopharmaceutics as a basis for the design of drug products. In, *Drug Design,* Vol. IV. (Ariens, E. J., ed.) Academic Press, Inc., New York, **1973,** pp. 1–35.

———. Effect of route of administration and distribution on drug action. *J. Pharmacokinet. Biopharm.,* **1978,** *6,* 559–585.

Gibaldi, M., and Perrier, D. *Pharmacokinetics.* Marcel Dekker, Inc., New York, **1975.**

Giusti, D. L., and Hayton, W. L. Dosage regimen adjustments in renal impairment. *Drug Intell. Clin. Pharm.,* **1973,** *7,* 382–387.

Wagner, J. G. *Biopharmaceutics and Relevant Pharmacokinetics.* Drug Intelligence, Hamilton, Ill., **1971.**

2 PHARMACODYNAMICS: MECHANISMS OF DRUG ACTION AND THE RELATIONSHIP BETWEEN DRUG CONCENTRATION AND EFFECT

Alfred G. Gilman, Steven E. Mayer, and Kenneth L. Melmon

Pharmacodynamics may be defined as the study of the biochemical and physiological effects of drugs and their mechanisms of action. The latter aspect of the subject is perhaps the most fundamental challenge to the investigator of pharmacology, and information derived from such study is of basic utility to the clinician. The objectives of the analysis of drug action are identification of the primary action (as distinguished from description of resultant effects), delineation of the details of the chemical reaction between drug and cell, and characterization of the full action-effects sequence. Such a complete analysis provides a truly satisfactory basis for the rational therapeutic use of a drug on the one hand and for the design of new and superior chemical agents on the other.

MECHANISMS OF DRUG ACTION

While there are several types of exceptions, the effects of the preponderance of drugs result from their interaction with functional macromolecular components of the organism. Such interaction alters the function of the pertinent cellular component and thereby initiates the series of biochemical and physiological changes that are characteristic of the response to the drug. This concept—now almost obvious—had its origins in the experimental work of Ehrlich and Langley during the late nineteenth and early twentieth centuries. Ehrlich was struck by the high degree of chemical specificity for the antiparasitic and toxic effects of a variety of synthetic organic agents. Langley noted the ability of the South American arrow poison, curare, to inhibit chemically (nicotine) induced contraction of skeletal muscles; however, the tissue remained responsive to direct electrical stimulation. The terms *receptive substance* and, more simply, *receptor* were coined to denote the component of the organism with which the chemical agent was presumed to interact. There are fundamental corollaries to the statement that the receptor for a drug can be any functional macromolecular component of the organism. One is that a drug is potentially capable of altering the rate at which *any* bodily function proceeds; a second is that, by virtue of interactions with such receptors, drugs do not *create* effects but merely modulate rates of ongoing function. A simple pharmacological dictum thus states that a drug cannot impart a new function to a cell.

It must also be noted that one cannot, *a priori,* predict the result of interaction between a chemical agent and a macromolecule of interest. Functional changes may or may not follow; if effects are observed, they will result from either enhancement or inhibition of the unperturbed rate. Furthermore, as will be discussed below, a drug that has no direct action can cause functional change by competition for a binding site with another, active regulatory ligand of the receptor. Drugs are termed *agonists* when they cause effects as a result of direct alteration of the functional properties of the receptor with which they interact. Compounds that are themselves devoid of intrinsic pharmacological activity but cause effects by inhibition of the action of a specific agonist (*e.g.,* by competition for agonist binding sites) are designated as *antagonists.*

DRUG RECEPTORS

Chemical Properties. At least from a numerical standpoint, the proteins of the cell form the most important class of drug receptors. Obvious examples are the enzymes of crucial metabolic or regulatory pathways (*e.g.*, dihydrofolate reductase, acetylcholinesterase), but of equal interest are proteins involved in transport processes (*e.g.*, Na^+, K^+-ATPase) or those that serve structural roles (*e.g.*, tubulin). Specific binding properties of other cellular constituents can also be exploited. Thus, nucleic acids are important drug receptors, particularly for chemotherapeutic approaches to the control of malignancy; plant lectins show remarkable specificity for recognition of specific carbohydrate residues in polysaccharides and glycoproteins, although this has not been exploited therapeutically; drugs such as anesthetics interact with and alter the structure and function of the lipids of cellular membranes.

The binding of drugs to receptors, in various cases, involves all known types of interactions—ionic, hydrogen, van der Waals, and covalent. The last-named situation is frequently, but not necessarily, associated with a prolonged duration of drug action. Furthermore, noncovalent interactions of high affinity may appear to be essentially irreversible. In most interactions between drugs and receptors it is likely that bonds of multiple types are important and are formed between reactive groups on the drug and complementary, appropriately oriented regions of the receptor (*see* Goldstein *et al.*, 1974).

Functional Properties. The functional properties of the receptors that have been used as examples above are evident. In addition, however, there exist groups of cellular proteins whose normal function is to act as receptors for endogenous regulatory ligands—particularly hormones, neurotransmitters, and autacoids. The evolution of these systems has thus provided proteins whose collective functions are legion and that are regulated by the reversible binding of specific ligands. Much of pharmacology derives from attempts to understand and to exploit these crucial regulatory molecules, and they will be discussed throughout the text. Unfortunately, these interesting molecules are difficult to isolate and characterize because they are generally present in small quantities (thousands per cell) and many are integral components of plasma membranes. However, this location is crucial for the role that is served by these receptors—to sense extracellular regulatory signals and to translate them into intracellular physiological or metabolic events. While our detailed knowledge of such receptors remains somewhat limited, the rate of research is accelerating.

Examples of Membrane-Bound Receptor Systems of Physiological and Pharmacological Interest. The nicotinic cholinergic receptor is the best characterized of the membrane-bound proteins that serve as receptors for neurohormones, other regulatory ligands, and a multitude of drugs. It is relatively simple to prepare quantities of the homogeneous material, because of the availability of a rich source—the electric organs of certain eels and rays. The receptor *per se* appears to result from the association of several (three or more) subunits of molecular weight 40,000, which carry binding sites for cholinergic agonists and antagonists. There appears to be a common (or overlapping) site for these two classes of agents, which explains the competitive relationship between the action of such compounds as the agonist acetylcholine and the antagonist *d*-tubocurarine. The interaction of agonist ligands with the receptor results in changes in cation (Na^+) flux through the membrane as a result of a change in state of a specific *ionophore* or ion-conductance modulator. Evidence suggests that this ionophore is a protein that is distinct from the receptor, perhaps of molecular weight 43,000, and that the receptor and ionophore are strongly associated in the native membrane. Local anesthetics and certain toxins act as inhibitors of ion translocation, possibly by interacting directly with the ionophore protein. Further information on this important and interesting system will be found in Chapter 11 (*see also* Heidmann and Changeux, 1978).

Receptors for a number of hormones and autacoids function by regulation of the concentration of the intracellular second messenger, cyclic adenosine 3′,5′-monophosphate (cyclic AMP); this is accomplished by stimulation or inhibition of the activity of the membrane-bound enzyme adenylate cyclase (*see* Figure 4–7). A much studied but still relatively poorly characterized example of a receptor of this type is one that serves for the endogenous hormone epinephrine and for the neurotransmitter norepinephrine. It is also the site of action of exogenously administered agonists (*e.g.*, isoproterenol) and antagonists (*e.g.*, propranolol) of the β-adrenergic type (*see* Chapter 4). In this receptor-enzyme system, ligand binding sites (for hormone or drug) and enzyme catalytic sites are clearly on separate proteins, and the mechanism of interaction between the β-adrenergic receptor and adenylate cyclase is thus of considerable interest. An additional protein(s) appears to mediate this interaction, and its function is controlled by another essential regulatory ligand, guanosine triphosphate (GTP). Thus, receptor-mediated stimulation of cyclic AMP synthesis requires at least three proteins, the membrane, and two ligands—a β-adrenergic agonist and GTP. The mechanisms and significance of these reactions are discussed in several chapters in the text (*see* Index; *see also* Maguire *et al.*, 1977).

It is important to recognize that receptors of this type not only are the determinants of acute regulation of physiological and biochemical function but also are themselves subject to more chronic regulatory and homeostatic control. For example, continued stimulation of various types of cells with β-adrenergic agonists results in a state of *desensitization* (also referred to as *refractoriness* or *down regulation*), such that the effect that follows subsequent exposure to the same concentration of drug is diminished. This can become very important in therapeutic situations; an example is the repeated use of β-adrenergic bronchodilators such as isoproterenol for the treatment of asthma (*see* Chapter 8). There appear to be multiple mechanisms that are operative and that account for desensitization of different types. In some cases the signal from only a specific receptor becomes interrupted. This may involve alteration of the receptor within the membrane or, in some cases, the actual removal of the receptor from the membrane. In other situations, receptors for different hormones that, for example, may all stimulate the adenylate cyclase of a single cell become less effective; this type of regulation presumably is directed at some common point in the pathway distal to the receptor itself. *Hyperreactivity* or *supersensitivity* to receptor agonists is also frequently observed to follow reduction in the chronic level of receptor stimulation. Situations of this type can result from the long-term administration of antagonists such as propranolol (*see* Chapter 9). In at least some cases supersensitivity may result from the synthesis of additional receptors.

Drug-Receptor Interactions. As early as 1878, even before he coined the term *receptive substance,* Langley suggested that drug-cell combinations, and hence the actions and effects of drugs, were probably governed by the law of mass action. This view was extensively developed by A. J. Clark in the 1920s, and it remains the keystone of most theories of drug action. The many discrete relationships between chemical structure and biological activity and the competitive interaction of chemically similar drugs are, today, readily interpretable in these terms. Thus, drug-receptor kinetic theory borrows freely from that developed for ligand binding reactions and for enzyme action, and there is obvious coalescence when drug effect results from a direct interaction with an enzyme.

When one attempts to extend analysis of drug-receptor interactions beyond the initial reaction—the binding of drug to receptor— important questions arise as to the relationship between the concentration of drug-receptor complex and the magnitude of the effect that is observed. In the classical recep-

tor theory developed by Clark, it was assumed that drug effect is proportional to the fraction of receptors occupied by drug, and that maximal effect results when all receptors are occupied. While these assumptions are probably true in some cases, exceptions are common, particularly when the pathway leading from receptor to effect is complex (*e.g.,* drug-receptor interaction $\rightarrow \rightarrow$ alteration of cardiac contractility). However, the simplifying assumption serves as a useful point of departure.

Quantitative Descriptions of Drug Action. If one assumes that an agonist drug interacts reversibly with its receptor and that the resultant effect is proportional to the number of receptors occupied, the following reaction equation can be written:

$$\text{Drug } (D) + \text{Receptor } (R) \underset{k_2}{\overset{k_1}{\rightleftharpoons}} DR \longrightarrow \text{Effect}$$

This reaction sequence is analogous to the interaction of substrate with enzyme, and the magnitude of effect can be analyzed in a manner similar to that for enzymatic product formation.

The applicable equation is identical in form with the Michaelis-Menten equation:

$$\text{Effect} = \frac{\text{Maximal Effect } (D)}{K_D + (D)}$$

where $(D) = $ free drug concentration and K_D is the dissociation constant for the drug-receptor complex. This equation describes a simple rectangular hyperbola. There is no effect at $(D) = 0$; the effect is half-maximal when $(D) = K_D$, that is, when half of the receptors are occupied; the maximal effect is approached asymptotically as (D) increases above K_D (Figure 2–1, A). It is frequently convenient to plot the magnitude of effect versus log (D), since a wide range of drug concentrations is easily displayed and a portion of the curve is more linear. In this case, the result is the familiar sigmoidal log dose-effect curve (Figure 2–1, B).

Data analysis can be further facilitated if a linear form of the equation is written. This is obtained by taking the reciprocal of both sides of the expression and constructing the equivalent of a Lineweaver-Burk plot for enzyme kinetics:

$$\frac{1}{\text{Effect}} = \frac{K_D}{\text{Max. Effect } (D)} + \frac{1}{\text{Max. Effect}}$$

A plot of 1/Effect versus 1/(D) yields a straight line that intersects the Y-axis at 1/(Max. Effect) and that has a slope equal to K_D/(Max. Effect). Extrapolation of this line to the X-axis yields the value of the intercept, easily shown to be $-1/K_D$ (Figure 2–1, C). Thus, values for K_D and for the maximal effect can be readily calculated from such a plot. This representation is particularly useful for the analysis of drug antagonism.

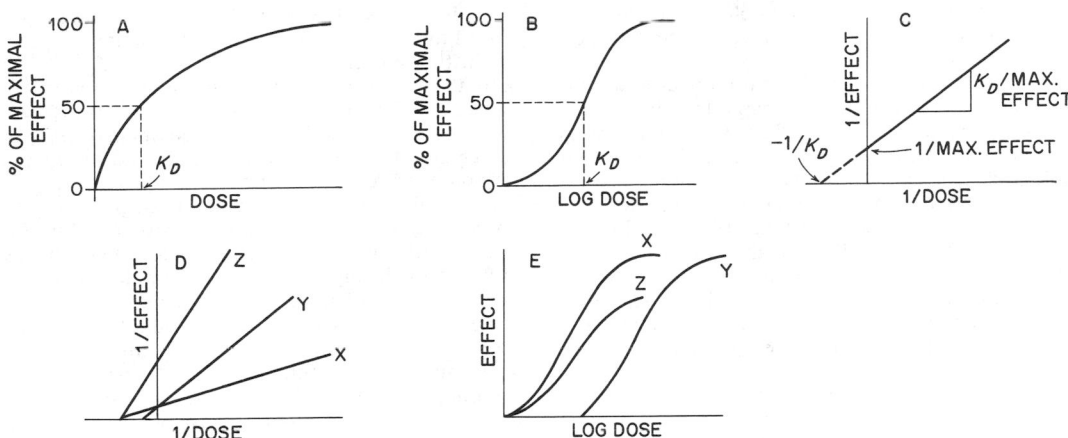

Figure 2-1. *Different representations of dose-effect curves.*

A. The ideal relationship between the concentration (dose) of a drug and the magnitude of response to it. When plotted on a linear scale of dose, a typical hyperbolic curve results.

B. A sigmoidal dose-effect curve results when the magnitude of effect observed is plotted versus the logarithm of the drug dose.

C. A double-reciprocal plot of the concentration dependence of drug effect (*see* text for explanation).

D and E. Representative double-reciprocal plots (*D*) and log dose-effect curves (*E*).

Curves X and Y. Two agonists with similar efficacy but differing in potency (X more potent than Y) *or* an agonist in the absence (X) and presence (Y) of a competitive antagonist.

Curves X and Z. Two agonists with similar potency but differing in efficacy (full agonist, X, and partial agonist, Z) *or* an agonist in the absence (X) and presence (Z) of a noncompetitive antagonist.

As stated above, certain drugs, termed antagonists, interact with the receptor or with other components of the effector mechanism to inhibit the action of an agonist, while initiating no effect themselves. If the inhibition can be overcome by increasing the concentration of the agonist, ultimately achieving the same maximal effect, the antagonist is said to be *surmountable* or *competitive*. This type of inhibition is commonly observed with antagonists that act reversibly at the receptor site. A somewhat similar situation will also result from reversible or irreversible interaction of the antagonist at other sites so that the affinity of the receptor for the agonist is altered. A conformational alteration of the receptor, with a reduction in affinity, could result from an action of an antagonist at a remote site. This is, however, more appropriately referred to as negative cooperativity than as competitive antagonism. Since the maximal effect can still be achieved if sufficient agonist is used, the double reciprocal plots of agonist alone versus agonist plus competitive antagonist *must* meet at the 1/Effect axis, where the concentration of agonist is infinite. The lines diverge at lower agonist concentrations; the apparent affinity of agonist for receptor is lowered (Figure 2–1, *D*). In the presence of a competitive antagonist, the log dose-effect curve for the agonist is shifted to the right (Figure 2–1, *E*). The maximal efficacy is unaltered, but the agonist appears to be less potent.

A noncompetitive antagonist *prevents* the agonist from producing any effect at a given receptor site.

This could result from irreversible interaction of the antagonist at any site to prevent binding of agonist. It would also follow reversible or irreversible interaction with any component of the system so as to prevent the successful initiation of effect following the binding of agonist. These results may be conceptualized as *removal* of receptor or response potential from the system. The maximal effect possible is reduced, but agonist can act normally at receptor-effector units not so influenced. The affinity of the agonist for the receptor and its potency are thus unaltered. The double reciprocal plot shows intersection of agonist and antagonist plus agonist lines on the 1/(D) axis at $-1/K_D$ (the affinity is unaltered). The maximal effect is different (Figure 2–1, *D*). Similarly, the log dose-effect curves show unaltered potency and reduced efficacy (Figure 2–1, *E*).

Antagonists may thus be classified as acting reversibly or irreversibly. If the antagonist binds at the active site for the agonist, reversible antagonists will be competitive and irreversible antagonist will be noncompetitive. If binding is elsewhere, however, these simple rules do not hold, and any combination is possible.

When two drugs bind to the same receptor, particularly if at the same site, why can one be an agonist and the other produce no effect—acting as an antagonist because of its presence? This question cannot be answered with precision, but fundamental differences in the physicochemical nature of the interaction must be operative. The following *model*, which can be stated in arbitrary physiological terms, may help to conceptualize a working answer to this question.

Consider a receptor (perhaps for a neurotransmitter) that itself constitutes *or* is capable of interacting with and regulating a specific channel for ions to permeate the plasma membrane. The ultimate physiological response of interest is a result of this change of ionic permeability. If this channel (receptor) can exist in two conformations that are in equilibrium (open, R_o, or closed, R_c) and the closed state predominates when no ligand for the receptor is present, the neurotransmitter or analogous drugs will affect the opening of the channel if it binds preferentially to (has greater affinity for) the open conformation.

$$R_c \rightleftharpoons R_o$$
$$\updownarrow \qquad \updownarrow$$
$$D \cdot R_c \rightleftharpoons D \cdot R_o$$

The *extent* to which the equilibrium $R_c \rightleftharpoons R_o$ is perturbed, and thus the magnitude of effect, is determined by the *relative* affinity of the drug for the two conformations (Figure 2–2). Thus, if a different but perhaps structurally analogous compound binds to the same site on R but with only slightly greater affinity for R_o than for R_c, the magnitude of effect observed may be less, despite the presence of maximally effective concentrations of the agent. A drug

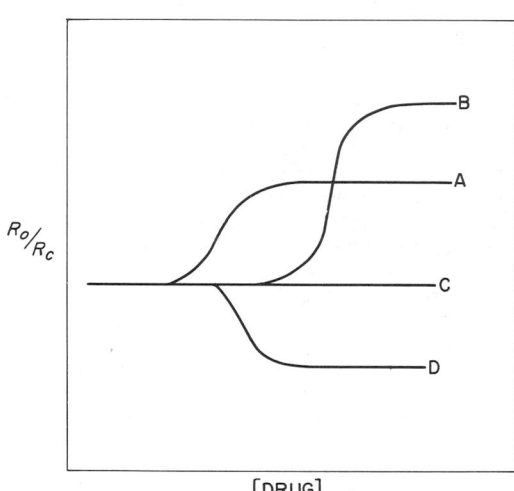

Figure 2-2. *Effects of drugs on the relative concentrations of two hypothetical forms of a receptor, R_o and R_c, that are in equilibrium* $(R_c \rightleftharpoons R_o)$.

Drugs A–D all bind to both forms of the receptor but with differing absolute and relative affinities. For drug A, affinity (K) for $R_o > R_c$, and binding affinity is relatively high; for drug B, K for $R_o \gg R_c$, but binding affinity is relatively poor; for drug C, K for $R_o = R_c$ (or K for $R_o = R_c = 0$); for drug D, K for $R_o < R_c$. (*See* text for additional explanation.)

that displays such intermediate effectiveness is referred to as a *partial agonist*. It then follows that an agent that has equal affinity for R_c and R_o will not alter the preexisting equilibrium; this compound will have no activity as an agonist but, when bound, will act as an antagonist because it impairs the ability of an agonist to alter the equilibrium and produce a response. (A drug with preferential affinity for R_c will actually inhibit the system, although if the *preexisting* equilibrium lies far in the direction of R_c this may be difficult to observe and the agent will be difficult to distinguish from the simple antagonist just described.) Finally, a partial agonist, when it binds to receptors but fails to produce a maximal response, will also act as an antagonist. A greater concentration of a full agonist will be required to produce a maximal effect because of the competitive effect of either a partial agonist or, of course, an antagonist.

It is obvious that something different from a simple receptor-occupancy theory has now been invoked, in that antagonists and partial agonists occupy receptors fully but do not produce maximal effects. It is thus useful to develop the concept of *intrinsic activity* or *efficacy* of drugs that act at the same receptor site but fail to produce equal effects. As a simple approximation, this concept can be quantified by the insertion of a drug-dependent rate constant in the initial equation:

$$D + R \underset{k_2}{\overset{k_1}{\rightleftharpoons}} DR \xrightarrow{k_3} \text{Effect}$$

For an antagonist, $k_3 = 0$.

It should be noted at this point that the use of the word *efficacy* can, at times, be confusing. While an antagonist has no efficacy in this sense as an initiator of an action-effects sequence, it may have great therapeutic efficacy when used as an antagonist.

Even if the molecular *action* of an agonist at a receptor site is proportional to its efficacy and to the number of receptor sites occupied, additional complications frequently make difficult the quantitative interpretation of the dose dependence of effect. This is particularly true when the drug-receptor interaction is but one event in a complex sequence of reactions ultimately resulting in an observable effect. For example, while occupancy of a certain number of receptors by agonist may initially lead to response, a later step in the pathway may become rate limiting at this stimulated level of function. Further receptor occupancy can then produce no additional effect. Analysis of situations of this type has led to the concept of *spare receptors* or *receptor reserve,* wherein a maximal effect can be achieved when a less-than-maximal fraction of receptors is occupied; in at least some such situations a certain number of receptors can be lost (*e.g.,* with an irreversible antagonist) without diminution of the maximal observable response. Conversely, if a drug is acting to inhibit a step in a reaction sequence, by interaction with its receptor, receptor occupancy will result in inhibition of the *ultimate effect* only when the step inhibited is or becomes the rate-limiting step. It may be necessary to occupy the majority of the receptors before any change in function is observed. In both this situation and in the case of "spare receptors," it should be apparent that the concentration of drug producing a half-maximal effect bears a complex relationship to the dissociation constant for the drug-receptor complex. When there are spare receptors, the concentration of drug required for a half-maximal effect is less than K_D, whereas the opposite holds when occupation of the initial fraction of receptors fails to cause a change in the function of interest (Figure 2–3).

Still other situations have required consideration of the possibilities that certain receptors may have multiple active sites or other drug binding (allosteric) sites. These sites may not act independently, and drug attachment at one point may alter the affinity for binding or reaction characteristics of agonists or antagonists at other locations. In this context one may note that the most detailed analysis of ligand binding reactions of this cooperative type has been possible with hemoglobin, a receptor for oxygen (if one is willing to accept oxygen as a drug), for the toxic gas carbon monoxide, and for experimental agents that can react with and alter the structure and function of variants of the protein molecule (e.g., hemoglobin S). It should be pointed out that different kinetic descriptions (or receptor theories) may be required when there are fundamental differences in the mechanism of drug action or in the structural and functional complexity of the responding system. Thus, these theories are not mutually exclusive, and

each may be true for individual situations. Further analysis of these models of receptor function may be found in the textbook by Goldstein and associates (1974). Analogous derivations for enzyme kinetics are detailed in texts such as those by Segel (1975) and White and colleagues (1978).

Structure-Activity Relationship. The affinity of a drug for a specific macromolecular component of the cell and its intrinsic activity are intimately related to its chemical structure. The relationship is frequently quite stringent, and relatively minor modifications in the drug molecule, particularly including such subtle changes as stereoisomerism, may result in major changes in pharmacological properties. Exploitation of structure-activity relationship has on many occasions led to the synthesis of valuable therapeutic agents. Since changes in molecular configuration need not alter all actions and effects of a drug equally, it is sometimes possible to develop a *congener* with a more favorable ratio of therapeutic to toxic effect or more acceptable secondary characteristics than those of the parent drug. In addition, effective therapeutic agents have been fashioned by developing structurally related competitive antagonists of other drugs or of endogenous substances known to be important in biochemical or physiological function.

Classification of Receptors and Drug Effects. Drug receptors have been identified and classified primarily on the basis of the effect or lack thereof of selective antagonists and by the relative potencies of representative agonists—the structure-activity relationship. For example, the effects of acetylcholine that are mimicked by the alkaloid muscarine and that are selectively antagonized by atropine are termed *muscarinic effects*. Other effects of acetycholine that are mimicked by nicotine and that are not readily antagonized by atropine but are selectively blocked by other agents (e.g., d-tubocurarine) are described as *nicotinic effects*. By *extension*, these two types of cholinergic effects are said to be mediated by muscarinic or nicotinic receptors. Such classification of receptors results in an internally consistent scheme that gives support to the view that two receptor types are involved. Although it contributes little to delineation of mechanism of drug action, such categorization does pro-

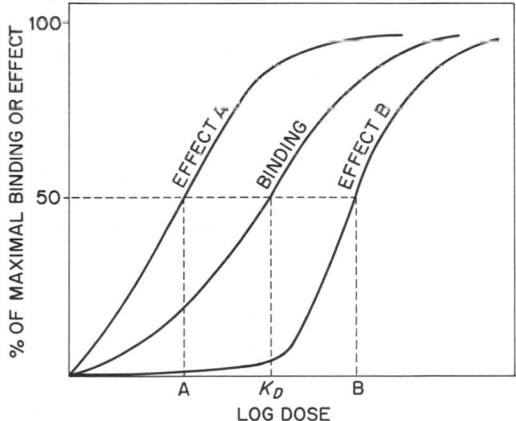

Figure 2–3. *Anomalous relationships between receptor occupation and response to a drug.*

The central curve, labeled *binding*, depicts the occupation of receptor by increasing concentrations of drug. Hypothetical dose-effect curve (*A*) is seen if maximal response results from less than maximal receptor occupation (spare receptors). Dose-effect curve (*B*) is seen if a significant fraction of receptors must be occupied before noticeable response to the drug occurs. The concentration of drug required to produce a half-maximal effect (*A* or *B*) thus bears a complex relationship to the dissociation constant of the drug-receptor complex (K_D).

vide a convenient basis for summarizing drug effects. If the effects and receptors in the various tissues have been classified, a statement that a drug activates a specified type of receptor is a succinct summary of its spectrum of effects and of the agents that will antagonize it. Similarly, a statement that a drug blocks a certain type of receptor specifies the agents that it will antagonize and at what sites.

The development, in the last decade, of high-specific-activity, radioactive ligands with great affinity and specificity for individual receptors has allowed the direct study of the drug-binding properties of individual receptors; this can proceed without the requirement for concurrent assessment of the change in function that normally follows occupation of a receptor by an appropriate agonist. There are significant benefits to this approach. Physiological and pathological alterations that influence the number or binding properties of individual receptors may be analyzed directly, without the need to infer their change from an alteration in the response that is observed. This is necessary, since the response may be many steps removed from the receptor, and change at any site in the pathway leading from receptor to ultimate effector will influence the response. Research of this type has led to some understanding of mechanisms of pathophysiology and therapeutic effects. For example, we now appreciate the neuromuscular disorder myasthenia gravis as an autoimmune disease wherein antibodies are directed toward the nicotinic cholinergic receptor. (*see* Chapters 6 and 11). Furthermore, ligand binding assays for many individual receptors are requisite for their purification and molecular characterization. Again, one may not be able to rely on the response that is characteristic of the drug-receptor complex for assay during receptor purification, since other components of the system necessary for the response may be lost. The ultimate goal of this type of research is to analyze the molecular events that are responsible for the interactions between the essential components of the system. Studies of this kind will allow a detailed definition of the differences between subtypes of receptors (*e.g.,* nicotinic and muscarinic) and an understanding of how receptors function and are regulated.

Significance of Receptor Subtypes. As described above, evolution has provided a diversity of receptors for a variety of *endogenous* regulators, and it is now clear that multiple subtypes of receptors exist for at least several of these molecules. In the case of acetylcholine, the existence of two major types of receptor—designated nicotinic and muscarinic—has been alluded to above. In addition, there are distinct differences in the ligand binding properties of the *nicotinic receptors* that are found in the ganglia of the autonomic nervous system versus those at the neuromuscular junction of the somatic nervous system. This difference is exploited for therapeutic benefit. Thus, antagonists that act preferentially at the nicotinic receptors in ganglia can be used to control blood pressure; they do not, happily, paralyze skeletal muscle. *d*-Tubocurarine and related agents constitute the converse example, and their ability to antagonize the action of acetylcholine is relatively well confined to the receptor sites at the neuromuscular junction. Other examples will be found in appropriate chapters. In particular, these include two types of receptor for histamine (H_1 and H_2) and a growing list of receptor subtypes for catecholamines (designated α_1, α_2, β_1, β_2). The utility of these observations and schemes of classification has been demonstrated by the recent development of a number of therapeutic agents that have selectivity for specific subtypes of receptors. This has allowed the clinician to utilize more fully the therapeutic efficacy of these compounds, while limiting the frequency of unwanted effects.

Cellular Sites of Drug Action. The general and major determinants of the primary site of drug action must be the localization of the specific receptors with which the drug interacts, their status and that of the entire receptor-effector system, and the concentration of drug to which the receptor is exposed. Localization of drug action is not necessarily dependent upon selective distribution of the drug. However, even if drug *action* is localized, the effects of the drug may be widespread and disseminated by a variety of secondary forces, chemical and physical.

If a drug acts by interaction with a relatively nonspecialized receptor, that is, a receptor that serves functions common to most cells, its effects will be widespread. If this is a vital function, the drug will be particularly dangerous to use. Nevertheless, such a drug may be clinically important. Digitalis glycosides are potent inhibitors of a fundamental and vital ion transport process, common to most cells. As such, they can cause widespread toxicity, and their margin of safety is dangerously low. Although their great utility is not to be denied, it would nevertheless be a boon to have a drug that accomplished the same therapeutic goal in a more selective way. Many similar examples could be cited, particularly in the area of cancer chemotherapy. Attempts have been made to restrict or direct the distribution of drugs by their attachment to soluble or insoluble carriers or by their encapsulation in liposomes. Another approach is the design of prodrugs that can be preferentially converted to the active species in only certain types of cells. These are areas of active investigation.

If a drug interacts with specialized receptors unique to specific types of differentiated cells, its effects are more specific. The hypothetical ideal drug would cause its therapeutic effect by virtue of such types of action. Side effects would be minimized, but toxicity might not be. If the differentiated function is a vital one, this type of drug could also be very dangerous. Some of the most lethal chemical agents known (*e.g.,* botulinus toxin) show such specificity and toxicity.

NONRECEPTOR-MEDIATED ACTIONS OF DRUGS

It must also be emphasized that several drugs do not act by virtue of combination with functional cellular components or receptors. Certain drugs may interact specifically with small molecules or ions that are normally or abnormally found in the body. The chelating agents, capable of forming strong bonds with a variety of metallic cations, are an excellent example, and chelators are available that show a remarkable degree of preference for specific ionic species—even among divalent cations. Thus, the affinity of ethylenediaminetetraacetate is ten orders of magnitude greater for Pb^{2+} than it is for Ba^{2+}, Sr^{2+}, or Mg^{2+}. A rather less specific but nonetheless often gratifying example is the therapeutic neutralization of gastric acid by a base (antacid).

Certain drugs that are structural analogs of normal biological constituents may be incorporated into cellular components and thereby alter their function. This has been termed a "counterfeit incorporation mechanism" (*see* Goldstein *et al.,* 1974), and has been particularly explored with analogs of pyrimidines and purines that can be incorporated into nucleic acids and that have clinical utility in cancer chemotherapy (*see* Chapter 55).

Additionally, there is a group of agents that act by more physicochemical mecha-nisms, some of which are poorly understood. A hint of this type of mechanism is provided by a lack of requirement for highly specific chemical structure. Stereoisomers of such drugs would not be expected to differ in their potency or efficacy. For example, certain relatively benign compounds, such as mannitol, can be administered in large quantities, sufficient to increase the osmolarity of various body fluids. Appropriate changes in the distribution of water result, and, depending on the agent and route of administration chosen, this effect can be exploited to promote diuresis, catharsis, expansion of circulating volume in the vascular compartment, or reduction of cerebral edema. The volatile general anesthetic agents interact with membranes to depress excitability. Their diversity of structure suggests a relatively nonspecific biophysical mechanism of action, and their individual potencies correlate well with the physical property of their oil:water partition coefficients.

RELATIONSHIP BETWEEN DOSE OF DRUG AND RESPONSE IN THE PATIENT

As discussed above, the relationship between drug concentration and the magnitude of the response that is observed may be complicated by numerous considerations, even where proximate responses to the agent are examined in simplified systems *in vitro.* However, under most such circumstances, dose-effect curves of the type shown in Figure 2–1 can be observed. When drugs are administered *in vivo,* however, there is no single characteristic relationship between intensity of drug effect and drug dosage. A dose-effect curve may be linear, concave upward, concave downward, or sigmoid. Moreover, if the observed effect is the composite of several effects of the drug, such as the change in blood pressure produced by a combination of cardiac, vascular, and reflex effects, the dose-effect curve need not be monotonic. However, a composite dose-effect curve can frequently be resolved into simple curves for each of its components; and simple dose-effect curves, whatever their precise shape, can be viewed as having four characteristic variables: potency, slope, maximal efficacy, and individual variation. These are

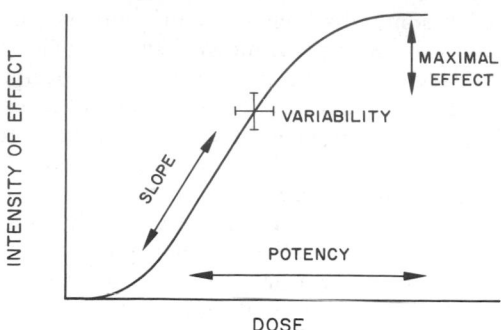

Figure 2–4. *The log dose-effect relationship.*

Representative log dose-effect curve, illustrating its four characterizing variables (*see* text for explanation).

illustrated in Figure 2–4 for the common sigmoid log dose-effect curve. As mentioned, the logarithmic transformation of dosage is often employed for the dose-effect relationship, because it permits display of a wide range of doses on a single graph and because it facilitates visual and mathematical comparisons between dose-effect curves for different drugs or for different responses to a single drug.

The characteristic variables of the dose-effect curve of Figure 2–4 of potency, maximal effect, and slope also characterize the drug-receptor interaction discussed above. However, as noted, the relationship between drug-receptor interaction and dose-effect curve is usually not simple, and it is compounded by the fourth factor—variation or *variance.* Nevertheless, appreciation of the general shape of the dose-effect curve for specific therapeutic agents is of considerable pragmatic significance.

Potency. The location of its dose-effect curve along the *dose axis* is an expression of the potency of a drug. Potency is influenced by the absorption, distribution, biotransformation, and excretion of a drug, as well as being determined by its inherent ability to combine with its receptors and the functional relationship between the receptor and the effector system. While knowledge of a drug's potency is obviously of paramount importance for decisions regarding drug dosage, potency *per se* is a relatively unimportant characteristic of a drug for clinical purposes. Thus, it makes little difference whether the

effective dose of a drug is 1 μg or 100 mg, as long as the drug can be administered conveniently. Potency is not necessarily correlated with any other characteristic of a drug, and there is no justification for the view that the more potent of two drugs is clinically superior. Low potency is a disadvantage only if the effective dose is so large that it is awkward to administer. Extremely potent drugs, particularly if they are volatile or are absorbed through the skin, may be hazardous and may require special handling.

For therapeutic applications, the potency of a drug is necessarily stated in *absolute* dosage units (25 μg, 10 mg/kg, etc.); for comparison of drugs, *relative potency,* the ratio of equieffective doses ($\frac{1}{10}$ ×, 5 ×, etc.), is a more convenient expression.

Maximal Efficacy. The maximal effect produced by a drug is referred to as its *maximal efficacy* or, simply, *efficacy.* Maximal efficacy of a drug may be determined by its inherent properties or those of the receptor-effector system and be reflected as a plateau in the dose-effect curve, but it may also be imposed by other factors. If the undesired effects of a drug limit its dosage, its efficacy will be correspondingly limited, even though it is inherently capable of producing a greater effect. Maximal efficacy of a drug is clearly one of its major characteristics. One of many important differences between morphine and aspirin is the difference in their maximal efficacy. The opioid provides relief of pain of nearly all intensities, whereas the salicylate is effective only against mild-to-moderate pain.

Efficacy and potency of a drug are not necessarily correlated, and these two characteristics of a drug should not be confused.

Slope. The slope of the dose-effect curve can be markedly influenced by the relationship between the receptor and the ultimate effector of the response as well as by the shape of the curve that describes the binding of the drug to the receptor. For example, if a drug must bind to most of the receptor molecules before a response is detected, the slope of dose-effect curve will be increased considerably (*see* Figure 2–3). While such phenomena are usually of little more than theoretical importance, they can have therapeutic significance. For example, a steep dose-effect curve for a CNS depressant implies that there is a small ratio between the dose that produces coma and that which causes mild sedation, and that excessive or inadequate effect may occur if the dose of the drug is not carefully adjusted. Nevertheless, many factors influence the margin of safety of a drug and the variability of its effects, and these characteristics of a drug are properly expressed by methods that summarize the contributions of all factors (see below).

Biological Variation. For our purposes, variation or *variance* can be defined as the appearance of differences in the magnitude of response among individuals in the same population given the same dose of drug. The more important factors that modify drug effect are discussed in Chapter 3. However, even when all known sources of variation are controlled or taken into account, drug effects are never identical in all patients, or even in a given patient on different occasions. A dose-effect curve applies only to a single

individual at one time or to the average individual. The intersecting brackets in Figure 2-4 indicate that biological variation of the dose-effect relationship can be visualized in either of two ways. The vertical bracket expresses the fact that a range of effects will be produced if a given dose of a drug is administered to a group of individuals; alternatively, the horizontal bracket expresses the fact that a range of doses is required to produce a specified intensity of effect in all individuals.

Dose-Percent Curve. The dose of a drug required to produce a specified effect in an individual is termed the *individual effective dose.* As defined, this is a *quantal* rather than a graded response, since the specified effect is either present or absent. Individual effective doses of most drugs are lognormally distributed, which means that the familiar *normal curve* of variation is obtained if the logarithms of the individual effective doses for a group of patients are expressed as a frequency distribution (Figure 2-5, A). A cumulative frequency distribution of individual

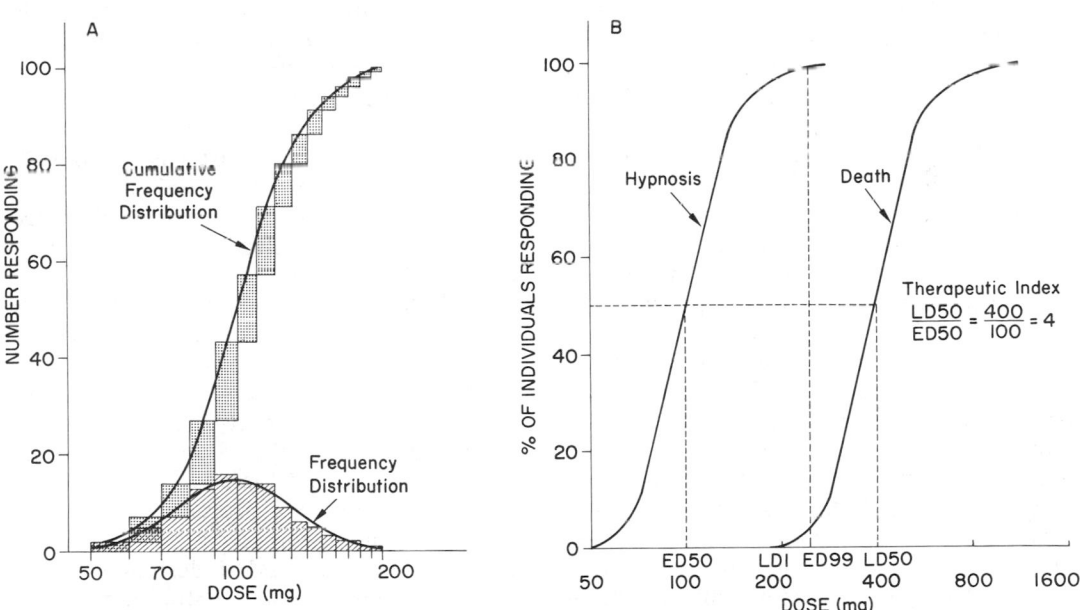

Figure 2-5. *Frequency distribution curves and quantal dose-effect curves.*

A. An experiment was performed on 100 subjects and the effective dose to produce a quantal response was determined for each individual. The number of subjects who required each dose is plotted, giving a lognormal frequency distribution (bars with diagonal lines). The stippled bars demonstrate that the normal frequency distribution, when summated, yields the cumulative frequency distribution—a sigmoidal curve that is a quantal dose-effect curve.

B. Quantal Dose-Effect Curves. Animals were injected with varying doses of a sedative-hypnotic, and the responses determined and plotted (*see* text for additional explanation).

effective doses, that is, the percentage of individuals that exhibit the effect plotted as a function of logarithm of dose, is known as a dose-percent curve or a quantal dose-effect curve. This is the integrated form of the normal frequency distribution. Although also a sigmoid curve, the dose-percent curve is an expression of individual variability for a single effect and has a slightly different meaning from the graded dose-effect curve discussed above. However, the graded dose-effect curve can be viewed similarly as representing the integral (summation) of a large number of quantal (molecular) responses.

The dose of a drug required to produce a specified intensity of effect in 50% of individuals is known as the *median effective dose* and is abbreviated ED50 (*not* ED_{50}) (Figure 2–5, *B*). If death is the end point, the median effective dose is termed the *median lethal dose* (LD50). The doses required to produce the stated effect in other percentages of the population are similarly expressed (ED20, LD90, etc.). Similar notations are also often used to refer to the dose of a drug required to produce a stated fraction of the maximal effect or a stated intensity of effect.

Population variation requires consideration of the significance of ED99 and LD1. If variation is marked, these doses may overlap even though the ED50 and LD50 differ by a wide margin (*see* below).

Terminology. Specific terms are used to refer to individuals who are unusually sensitive or unusually resistant to a drug, and to decribe those in whom a drug produces an unusual effect.

If a drug produces its usual effect at unexpectedly low dosage, the individual is said to be *hyperreactive* or *hypersensitive*. The latter term may, however, be confused with the pattern of effects associated with drug allergy. Hyperreactivity to a drug is usually termed *supersensitivity* only if the increased sensitivity is the result of denervation. If a drug produces its usual effect only at unusually large dosage, the individual is said to be *hyporeactive*. Decreased sensitivity is also described as *tolerance,* but this term has the connotation of hyporeactivity acquired as the result of prior exposure to the drug. Tolerance that develops rapidly after administration of only a few doses of a drug is termed *tachyphylaxis*. Reduced sensitivity should be described as *immunity* only if the acquired tolerance is the result of antibody formation.

An *unusual effect* of a drug, of whatever intensity and irrespective of dosage, that occurs in only a small percentage of individuals is often termed *idiosyncrasy*. However, this term is frequently considered a synonym for drug allergy and has so many other connotations that it perhaps should be abandoned. Unusual effects of drugs should simply be described as such or, when possible, by terms that refer to the underlying mechanism; they are often types of drug allergy or a consequence of genetic differences.

Selectivity. A drug is usually described by its most prominent effect or by the action thought to be the basis of that effect. However, such descriptions should not obscure the fact that *no drug produces only a single effect*. Morphine is correctly described as an analgesic, but it also suppresses cough and causes sedation, respiratory depression, constipation, bronchiolar constriction, release of histamine, antidiuresis, and a variety of other effects. A drug is adequately characterized only in terms of its full *spectrum of effects*. The relationship between the doses of a drug required to produce undesired and desired effects is termed its *therapeutic index, margin of safety,* or *selectivity*. Rarely is a drug sufficiently selective to be described as being *specific*. For therapeutic applications, selectivity of a drug is clearly one of its more important characteristics.

In clinical studies, drug selectivity is often expressed indirectly by summarizing the pattern and incidence of adverse effects produced by therapeutic doses of the drug and by indicating the proportion of patients who were forced to decrease drug dosage or discontinue medication because of adverse effects. These indirect procedures are often adequate, but comparison of dose-effect curves for desired and undesired effects is more consistently meaningful and is preferred whenever feasible (Figure 2–5, *B*).

In laboratory studies, therapeutic index is usually defined as the ratio between the median toxic dose and the median effective dose (TD50/ED50) or the median lethal dose and median effective dose (LD50/ED50). Because the ideal drug produces its desired effect in all patients without causing toxic effects in any, and because dose-percent curves need not be parallel, it can be logically argued that therapeutic index should be defined as the ratio between the minimal toxic dose and the maximal effective dose. However, minimal and maximal toxic and effective doses cannot be estimated with precision, particularly in the variable human population with which medical practice is concerned.

A drug does not have a single therapeutic index, but many. The margin of safety of aspirin for relief of headache is greater than its margin of safety for relief of arthritic pain, since the latter use requires larger dosage. Similarly, several therapeutic indices can be calculated for each desired effect. A synthetic opioid may cause less constipation than morphine and yet afford no advantage over the parent compound with regard to respiratory depression or sedation. Moreover, a drug may be selective within one context yet still be nonselective within another. The antihistamines are correctly described as selective antagonists of histamine, yet none of these drugs produces this selective peripheral effect without also causing significant central sedation. Finally, a drug may be correctly described as having an adequate margin of safety in most patients, but this description is meaningless for the patient who exhibits an unusual response to the drug. Penicillin is essentially nontoxic in the great majority of patients, yet it can cause death in those who have become allergic to it.

Albert, A. *The Selectivity of Drugs.* John Wiley & Sons, Inc., New York, **1975**.

Ariëns, E. J., and Beld, A. J. The receptor concept in evolution. *Biochem. Pharmacol.,* **1977,** *26,* 913–918.

Baxter, J. D., and Funder, J. W. Hormone receptors. *N. Engl. J. Med.,* **1979,** *301,* 1149–1161.

Clark, A. J. *The Mode of Action of Drugs on Cells.* E. Arnold & Co., London, **1933**.

Cuatrecasas, P. Membrane receptors. *Annu. Rev. Biochem.,* **1974,** *43,* 169–214.

Cuatrecasas, P., and Hollenberg, M. Membrane receptors and hormone action. *Adv. Protein Chem.,* **1976,** *30,* 251–451.

Dikstein, S. (ed.). *Fundamentals of Cell Pharmacology.* Charles C Thomas, Pub., Springfield, Ill., **1973**.

Featherstone, R. M. (ed.). *A Guide to Molecular Pharmacology-Toxicology,* Parts I–II. Marcel Dekker, Inc., New York, **1973**.

Goldstein, A.; Aronow, L.; and Kalman, S. M. *Principles of Drug Action: The Basis of Pharmacology,* 2nd ed. John Wiley & Sons, Inc., New York, **1974**.

Gringauz, A. *Drugs: How They Act and Why.* C. V. Mosby Co., St. Louis, **1978**.

Hansch, C. Enzyme study as a source of strategy in drug design. *Adv. Pharmacol. Chemother.,* **1975,** *13,* 45–81.

Heidmann, T., and Changeux, J.-P. Structural and functional properties of the acetylcholine receptor protein in its purified and membrane-bound states. *Annu. Rev. Biochem.,* **1978,** *47,* 317–357.

Iverson, L. L.; Iverson, S. D.; and Snyder, S. H. (eds.). *Principles of Receptor Research.* Plenum Press, New York, **1975**.

Kahn, C. R.; Megyesi, K.; Bar, R. S.; Eastman, R. C.; and Flier, J. S. New insights into the pathophysiology of disease states in man. *Ann. Intern. Med.,* **1977,** *86,* 205–219.

Klinge, E. (ed.). *Receptors and Cellular Pharmacology. Proceedings of the Sixth International Congress of Pharmacology,* Vol. 1. Pergamon Press, Ltd., Oxford, **1976**.

Korolkovas, A. *Essentials of Molecular Pharmacology.* John Wiley & Sons, Inc., New York, **1970**.

Levine, R. R. *Pharmacology: Drug Actions and Reactions,* 2nd ed. Little, Brown & Co., Boston, **1978**.

Maguire, M. E.; Ross, E. M.; and Gilman, A. G. β-Adrenergic receptor, ligand binding properties and the interaction with adenylyl cyclase. *Adv. Cyclic Nucleotide Res.,* **1977,** *8,* 1–83.

Porter, R., and O'Connor, M. (eds.). *Molecular Properties of Drug Receptors* (a Ciba Foundation symposium). J. & A. Churchill, Ltd., London, **1970**.

Rang, H. P. Receptor mechanisms: Fourth Gaddum Memorial Lecture, School of Pharmacy, University of London, January 1973. *Br. J. Pharmacol.,* **1973,** *48,* 475–495.

Segel, I. H. *Enzyme Kinetics.* John Wiley & Sons, Inc., New York, **1975**.

Smythies, J. R., and Bradley, R. J. (eds.). *Receptors in Pharmacology.* Marcel Dekker, Inc., New York, **1978**.

Van Rossum, J. M. (ed.). *Kinetics of Drug Action. Handbuch der Experimentellen Pharmakologie,* Vol. 47. Springer-Verlag, Berlin, **1977**.

White, A.; Handler, P.; Smith, E. L.; Hill, R. L.; and Lehman, I. R. *Principles of Biochemistry,* 6th ed. McGraw-Hill Book Co., New York, **1978**.

CHAPTER

3 PRINCIPLES OF THERAPEUTICS

*Kenneth L. Melmon, Alfred G. Gilman,
and Steven E. Mayer*

THERAPY AS A SCIENCE

Over a century ago Claude Bernard formalized criteria for gathering valid information in experimental medicine, but application of these criteria to therapeutics and to the process of making decisions about therapeutics has, until recently, been slow and inconsistent. At a time when the diagnostic aspects of medicine had become scientifically sophisticated, therapeutic decisions were often made on the basis of impressions and traditions. Historically, the absence of accurate data on the effects of drugs in man was in large part due to ethical standards of human experimentation. "Experimentation" in human beings was precluded, and it was not generally conceded that *every* treatment by any physician was and should be designed and in some sense recorded as an experiment.

Although there must always be ethical concern about experimentation in man, principles have been defined, and there are no longer ethical restraints on the gathering of either experimental or observational data on the efficacy and toxicity of drugs in *adults*. Furthermore, it should now be considered absolutely unethical to continue the *art* as opposed to the *science* of therapeutics on any patient who directly (the adult or child) or indirectly (the fetus) receives drugs for therapeutic purposes. Observational (nonexperimental) technics that can greatly add to our knowledge of the effects of drugs can be applied to all populations. The fact that such observational technics have largely been applied in an *ad-hoc,* nonsystematic fashion has led us to rely on a relative paucity of information about drugs. Therapeutics must now be dominated by objective evaluation of an adequate base of factual knowledge.

Conceptual Barriers to Therapeutics as a Science. The most important barrier that inhibited the development of therapeutics as a science seems to have been the belief that multiple variables in diseases and in the effects of drugs are uncontrollable. If this were true, the scientific method would not be applicable to the study of pharmacotherapy. Only recently has it been appreciated that clinical phenomena can be defined, described, and quantified with precision. Classification of diseases can be meaningful whether or not pathogenesis is known; analysis of measurements has become mathematically sound; experiments can be designed to yield valid conclusions about the pharmacological effects of drugs used for the treatment of patients. The approach to complex clinical data has been artfully discussed by Feinstein (1967; 1977a).

Another barrier to the realization of therapeutics as a science was overreliance on traditional *diagnostic labels* for disease. This encouraged the physician to think of a disease as a static rather than a dynamic entity, to view patients with the same "label" as a homogeneous rather than a heterogeneous population, and to consider a disease as an entity even when information about pathogenesis was not available. If diseases are not considered to be dynamic, "standard" therapies in "standard" doses will be the order of the day; decisions will be reflex in nature. Needed instead is an attitude that makes the physician responsible for recognition of and compensation for changes that occur in pathophysiology as the underlying process resolves or progresses. For example, the term *myocardial infarction* refers to localized destruction of myocardial cells caused by the interruption of the blood supply; however, decisions about therapy must take into account a variety of autonomic, hemodynamic, and electrophysiological variables that change as a function of time, as well as with the size of the infarction and its location. Furthermore, one often must focus on the presence of other diseases that could contribute to the infarction and that may require primary care separate from hemodynamic support (*e.g.*, management of the metabolic status of a patient with diabetes who has sustained a myocardial infarction). Failure to take all such variables into account while planning a therapeutic maneuver may result in ineffective therapy or toxicity. Differences in these variables among patients who are receiving the same therapy can account for different outcomes; conversely, if heterogeneous groups of patients receive alternative treatments, true differences in efficacy or toxicity between therapies may go unrecognized. A diagnosis or label of a disease or syndrome usually indicates a spectrum of possible causes and outcomes. Therapeutic experiments that fail to match groups for the known variables that affect prognosis yield uninterpretable data.

A third conceptual barrier was the incorrect notion that data derived empirically are useless because they are not generated by application of the scientific method. Empiricism is often defined as the practice of medicine founded on mere experience, without the aid of science or a knowledge of principles. The connotations of this definition are misleading; empirical observations need not be scientifically unsound. In fact, concepts of therapeutics have been greatly advanced by the astute clinical observer who makes careful and controlled observations on the outcome of a drug-induced clinical event. The results, even when the mechanisms of disease and their interactions with the effects of drugs are not understood, are nevertheless often crucial to appropriate therapeutic decisions. Often the initial suggestion that a drug may be efficacious in one condition arises from careful, empirical observations that are made while the drug is being used for another purpose. Recent examples of valid empirical observations that have resulted in new uses of drugs include the use of penicillamine to treat arthritis, lidocaine to treat cardiac arrhythmias, and propranolol to treat hypertension and angina. Conversely, empiricism *per se* often results in findings that are inadequate or invalid. For example, propranolol has been proposed for a large number of new uses; only a few of these have proved valid by controlled experimental or observational studies (Morrelli, 1973).

Clinical Trials. Application of the scientific method to experimental therapeutics is exemplified by a well-designed and well-executed clinical trial. To maximize the likelihood that useful information will result from the experiment, the objectives of the study must be defined, homogeneous populations of patients must be selected, appropriate control groups must be found, meaningful and sensitive indices of drug effects must be chosen for observation, and the observations must be converted into data and then into valid conclusions (Feinstein, 1977b). A number of excellent, critical summaries of the scientific requirements for clinical trials have been published (Hill, 1960, 1962). The *sine qua non* of any clinical trial is its controls. Many different types of controls may be used in a clinical trial, and the term *controlled study* is not synonymous with *randomized double-blind technic.* Selection of a proper control group is as critical to the eventual utility of an experiment as the selection of the experimental group. Feinstein (1977a) has written extensively about the difficulty and the importance of choosing controls for clinical trials. Although the randomized, double-blind controlled trial is the most effective design for distributing bias and unknown variables between the "treatment" and the "control" groups, it is not necessarily the optimal or applicable design for all studies. It may be impossible to use this design to study disorders that occur rarely, disorders in populations of patients that cannot, by regulation or ethics or both, be studied (*e.g.*, children, women of child-bearing age, the fetus, or some patients with psychiatric diseases), or the treatment of patients with a uniformly fatal disorder (*e.g.*, patients with rabies, where historical controls can be used).

There are several special considerations in the design of clinical trials if they are to be used to compare the relative effects of *alternative* therapies. (1) *Specific outcomes* of therapy that are clinically relevant and quantifiable must be measured. (2) The *accuracy of diagnosis* and the *severity of the disease* must be comparable in the groups being contrasted; otherwise, false-positive and false-negative errors may occur. (3) The *dosages* of the drugs must be chosen and individualized in a manner that allows relative efficacy to be compared at equivalent toxicities or allows relative toxicities to be compared at equivalent efficacies (Meffin *et al.,* 1977). (4) *Placebo effects,* which occur in a large percentage of patients, can confound many studies—particularly those that involve subjective responses; controls must take this into account (Beecher, 1959). Special designs, such as the "preference technic" (Jick *et al.*, 1966), may be required to evaluate the efficacy of drugs used for the relief of symptoms. In fact, subjective assessments that relate to the quality of life can be generated by the experimental subject and can be objectively tabulated and incorporated into evaluation of a therapy (Sheiner, 1979). (5) *Compliance* to the experimental regimens should be assessed *before* subjects are assigned to experimental or control groups. The drug-taking behavior of the subjects should be reassessed during the course of the trial. Noncompliance, even if randomly distributed between both groups, may cause falsely low estimates of the true potential benefits or toxicity of a particular treatment. (6) *Ethical considerations* may be major determinants of the types of controls that can be used and must be evaluated explicitly (Curran, 1979). For example, in therapeutic trials that involve life-threatening diseases, the use of a placebo is unethical, and new treatments must be compared with "standard" therapies. Depending upon such factors as the overall prognosis of the disease and the improvement in outcome or toxicity from the new treatment, very large numbers of subjects may be needed; otherwise, the possibility of a false-negative result is high (*i.e.,* no statistically significant differences between the two treatments will be found, even though differences actually exist) (Freiman *et al.,* 1978).

The results of clinical trials of new therapeutic agents or of old agents for new indications may have severe limitations in terms of what can be expected of drugs when they are used in an office practice. The selection of the patients for experimental trials usually eliminates those with coexisting diseases, and such trials usually assess the effect of only one or two drugs, not the many that might be given to or taken by the same patient under the care of a physician. Clinical trials are usually performed with relatively small numbers of patients for periods of time that may be shorter than are necessary in practice, and compliance may be better controlled than it can be in practice. All these factors, plus those that are described below (*see* section on Drug Development), lead to several inescapable conclusions:

1. If the result of a valid clinical trial of a drug is understood by the physician, he can only develop a hypothesis about what the drug might do to his patient, and he cannot be sure that what occurred in other patients will be seen in his own. In effect, the physician uses the results of a clinical trial to establish an experiment in his own patient. The detection of anticipated and unantici-

pated effects is the responsibility of the physician during his supervision of a therapeutic regimen.

2. If an anticipated effect of a drug does *not* occur in the patient, this does not mean that the effect cannot occur in that patient or in others. *Many factors in the individual patient may contribute to lack of efficacy of a drug.* They include, for example, misdiagnosis, poor compliance by the patient to the regimen, poor choice of dosage or dosage intervals, coincidental development of an undiagnosed separate illness that influences the outcome, the use of other agents that interact with primary drugs to nullify or alter their effects, undetected genetic or environmental variables that modify the disease or the pharmacological actions of the drug, or unknown therapy by another physician who is caring for the same patient. Such factors must be considered when a regimen is failing. More importantly, the physician should not attribute all success of a regimen to the therapy, and negative results in the course of an illness to the patient instead of to problems associated with therapy. Similarly, if an anticipated untoward or toxic effect is not seen in a particular patient, it can still occur in others. Physicians who use *only* their own experience with a drug to make decisions about its use unduly expose their patients to unjustifiable risk. For example, simply because a doctor has not seen a case of chloramphenicol-induced aplastic anemia in his own practice does not mean that such a disaster may not occur; the drug must still be used cautiously.

3. If an effect of a drug is not seen in a clinical trial, it may still be revealed in the setting of clinical practice. The necessity of determining whether an unanticipated change in the clinical course of a patient is or is not due to the drug(s) being used is one of the most important responsibilities of the physician. One half or more of both useful and adverse effects of drugs that were not recognized in the initial formal trials were subsequently found and reported by practicing physicians.

4. Rational therapy is therapy based on the use of the scientific method. It is no less crucial to have a scientific approach to the treatment of an individual patient than to use this approach when investigating drugs

in a research setting. In both instances, it is the patient who benefits.

INDIVIDUALIZATION OF DRUG THERAPY

As has been implied above, therapy as a science does not apply simply to the evaluation and testing of new, investigational drugs in animals and man. It applies with equal importance to the treatment of each patient as an individual. Therapists of every type have long recognized and acknowledged that individual patients show wide variability in response to the same drug or treatment modality. In recent years progress has been made in identifying the sources of variability (Smith and Rawlins, 1973; Rawlins, 1974). Important factors are presented in Figure 3-1; the basic principles that underlie these sources of variability have been presented in Chapters 1 and 2. The following discussion relates to the strategies that have been developed to minimize variability in the clinical setting. (*See also* Appendixes I to III; Sheiner *et al.*, 1975; Sheiner and Tozer, 1978.)

SOURCES OF VARIABILITY

After it has been determined that pharmacotherapy is necessary to modify the symptoms or outcome of a disease, the therapist is faced with two types of decisions: the first is qualitative (the initial choice to give or not to give a specific drug) and the second quantitative (the initial dosage regimen). Optimal treatment will result only when the physician is aware of the sources of variation in response to drugs and when the dosage regimen is designed on the basis of the best-available data about the diagnosis, severity and stage of the disease, presence of concurrent diseases or drug treatment, and *predefined goals* of acceptable efficacy and limits of acceptable toxicity. If objectively assessable expectations of drug therapy are not set before therapy is initiated, the patient is likely to be treated until he *obviously* responds in a grossly positive or grossly negative way before reconsideration of therapy will be likely.

In most clinical settings, the decision about the choice of drug is substantially influenced by the confidence the physician has in the accuracy of his diagnosis and estimates (both

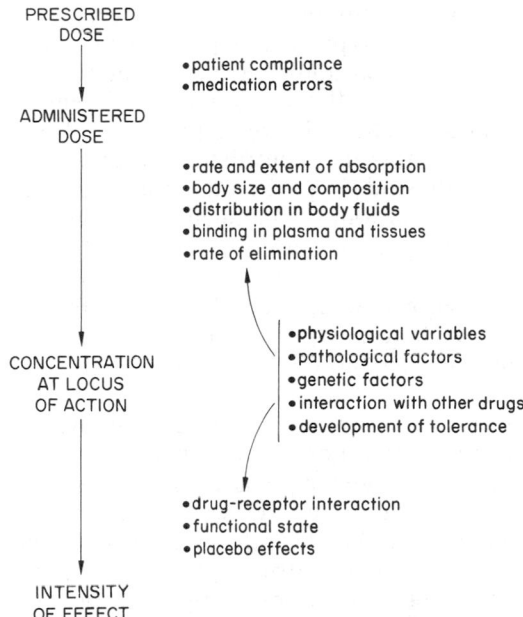

Figure 3-1. *Factors that determine the relationship between prescribed drug dosage and drug effect.* (Modified from Koch-Weser, 1972.)

clinical and laboratory) of the extent and severity of disease. However, there usually are insufficient data, either in the literature concerning the disease under treatment or from the clinical or laboratory profile of the patient, to indicate definitively the proper choice of drug (Peck, 1978). Based on the best-available information, the physician must decide on an initial drug from a group of reasonable alternatives. Subsequent adjustments should be based on whether the regimen is efficacious (*see* below) without adverse effects or at an acceptable level of toxicity.

VARIATION IN DISPOSITION OF A DRUG

After the choice of drug has been made, the next step is to choose an initial dosage regimen. Decisions must be made about the size of the first dose, the route of administration, the maintenance dose, and the interval between doses if more than one dose is necessary (*see* Chapter 1). Interpatient and intrapatient variation in disposition of a drug must be taken into account. For a given drug, there may be wide variation among individuals in its pharmacokinetic properties (absorption, distribution, metabolism, excretion, and binding to proteins in plasma). For some drugs, this variability may account for one half or more of the total variation in eventual response. The relative importance of the many factors that contribute to these differences depends in part on the drug itself and on its usual route of elimination. Drugs that are excreted primarily unchanged by the kidney tend to have smaller differences in disposition than do drugs that are inactivated by metabolism. Of drugs that are extensively metabolized, those with slower rates of clearance tend to have the largest variation in such rates between individuals. Studies in identical and nonidentical twins have revealed that genotype is a most important determinant of differences in the rates of metabolism (Vesell and Page, 1968; Vesell, 1979). For many drugs, physiological and pathological variations in organ function are major determinants of their rate of disposition. For example, the clearance of digoxin and gentamicin is related to the rate of glomerular filtration, whereas that of lidocaine and propranolol is primarily dependent on the rate of hepatic blood flow. The effect of disease states, especially those that involve the kidneys or liver, is to impair elimination and to increase the variability in the disposition of drugs. Disease may also affect responsiveness of tissues. In such settings, measurements of concentrations of drugs in biological fluids can be used to assist in the individualization of drug therapy (Koch-Weser, 1972).

The determination of concentrations of drug in, for example, plasma is particularly useful when certain well-defined criteria are fulfilled (Sheiner and Tozer, 1978). (1) There should be substantial *interpatient* variability in disposition of the drug (and small *intrapatient* variation). Otherwise, concentrations of drug in plasma could be predicted from dose alone. (2) It should be difficult to monitor intended or unintended effects of the drug. Whenever clinical effects or toxicity are easily measured (*e.g.*, the effect of a drug on blood pressure), such effects should be preferred in the decision to make any necessary adjustment of dosage of the drug. However, the effects of some drugs in certain settings are not easily monitored; for example, the hemodynamic changes caused by digitalis glycosides may be delayed and difficult to measure. Many drugs are used for *prophylaxis* of an uncommon or dangerous event; examples include anticonvulsants and antiarrhythmic agents. Some drugs (*e.g.*, antiarrhythmic agents) may also produce toxic effects that mimic symptoms or signs of the disease being treated, and titration of drug dosage may thus be aided by measurements of concentrations of the drug in blood. (3) The therapeutic index of the drug should be low, and its toxic effects should have the potential to increase morbidity. If this criterion is not met, patients could simply be given the largest dose known to be necessary to treat a disorder, as is commonly done with penicillin. However, if there is an overlap in the concentration-response relationship for desirable and undesirable effects of the drug, as is true for theophylline, determinations of concentration of drug in plasma may allow the dose to be optimized. All three of the above-described criteria must be met if the measurement of drug concentrations is to be of significant value in the adjustment of dosage. Knowledge of concentrations of drugs in plasma or urine is also particularly useful for detection of therapeutic failures that are due to lack of patient compliance with a medical regimen or for identification of patients with unexpected extremes in the rate of drug disposition.

The use of such measurements to assist the physician in achieving a desired concentration of drug in blood or plasma (*i.e.*, "targeting" the dose) is an example of the use of an *intermediate end point of therapy*. The concept of intermediate end points, including concentrations of drugs, as a guide to individualization of therapy can also be applied in other ways; one is to provide an indication for a change in the choice of drug therapy. Measurements of concentrations of drugs in plasma or preferably measurements of one or more pharmacological effects of the drug can provide an indication of probable lack of efficacy.

When measurements of the concentrations of drug in plasma are used, it must be remembered that they are almost always reported as the total concentration of drug, including both bound and unbound fractions. Changes in binding of the drug to plasma proteins, alterations of partitioning of the drug between tissues and plasma, and changes in responsiveness to the drug by the target tissue mean that quantitation of the concentration of drug in plasma is only useful as a guide, not as a sole determinant that automatically justifies change of the therapeutic regimen.

PHARMACODYNAMIC VARIABILITY

The availability of precise information about the pharmacokinetic properties of many drugs has contributed to understanding of the importance of differences in the responsiveness of target tissues to pharmacological agents. It is clear that considerable residual variation in response remains after the concentration of drug has been adjusted to the desired value; for some drugs this accounts for most of the total variation in the responsiveness of the individual. These observations have led to an increased interest in attempts to define and measure "sensitivity" to drugs in a clinical setting. Important progress has been made in understanding some of the determinants of sensitivity to drugs that act at specific receptors. For example, the number of receptors for insulin may be altered in diabetes (Flier *et al.*, 1979); responsiveness to adrenergic agonists (*e.g.*, isoproterenol or norepinephrine) may change because of disease (thyrotoxicosis) or because of the prior administration of either adrenergic agonists or antagonists (Lefkowitz, 1979); resistance to the antineoplastic agent methotrexate may occur because of gene amplification and subsequent synthesis of large quantities of the receptor for the cytotoxic action of this drug, dihydrofolate reductase (Schimke *et al.*, 1978). Receptors for drugs are not static components of the cell (*see* Chapter 2). They are in a dynamic state and are modulated by a variety of exogenous and endogenous factors that play a major role in the response to treatment.

OTHER FACTORS THAT AFFECT THERAPEUTIC OUTCOME

The variation in pharmacokinetic and pharmacodynamic parameters that accounts for much of the need to individualize therapy has been discussed. Other factors, listed in Figure 3–1, also should be considered as potential determinants of success or failure of

therapy. The following presentation serves as an introduction to these subjects, certain of which are also discussed elsewhere in the text.

Drug-Drug Interactions. Physicians face at least two difficult problems related to interactions between drugs. One is the acquisition of a perspective on the rapidly expanding body of information in this area. The other problem is to know whether a specific combination in a given patient has the potential to result in an interaction, and, if so, how to take advantage of the interaction if it leads to improvement in efficacy or how to avoid the consequences of an interaction if they are adverse.

A *potential drug interaction* refers to the possibility that one member of a class of drugs may alter the intensity of pharmacological effects of another drug given concurrently. The net result may be enhanced or diminished effects of one or both of the drugs, and this may be an intended or an unwanted or unexpected effect. Interactions may be either pharmacokinetic (alteration of the absorption, distribution, or disposition of one drug by another) or pharmacodynamic (*e.g.*, interactions between agonists and antagonists at drug receptors). Mechanisms are detailed in Appendix III.

Beneficial Drug-Drug Interactions. The concomitant use of two drugs is often essential to obtain a desired therapeutic objective. Examples abound, and the choice of drugs to be employed concurrently can be based on sound pharmacological principles. In the treatment of hypertension, a single drug is effective in only a modest percentage of patients. Moreover, tolerance to therapy is apt to occur due to compensatory reactions. The concurrent use of two drugs with different mechanisms of action can achieve a greater and more sustained reduction in blood pressure, particularly if one drug blocks some of the compensatory responses that result from the use of the other (*e.g.*, hydralazine plus propranolol). At the same time, the incidence of side effects may be reduced because each drug can be employed at a lower dosage than when used alone. In the treatment of heart failure, the concurrent use of a cardiac glycoside and a diuretic is often essential to achieve an adequate cardiac output and to maintain the patient in an edema-free state, especially if cardiac reserve is limited. Multiple-drug therapy is usual in cancer chemotherapy and for the treatment of certain infectious diseases. The goals in these cases are usually to improve efficacy and to delay the emergence of malignant cells or of microorganisms that are resistant to the effects of available drugs. Interactions between drugs are also frequently employed for the treatment of drug toxicity. This is most effective if a specific receptor blocking agent is available to counter the effects of a given agonist (*e.g.,* naloxone to treat opioid overdosage).

Alteration of the pharmacokinetic parameters of one drug by the administration of another may also be used for benefit. A familiar example is the administration of probenecid to inhibit the secretion of penicillin by the proximal tubule of the kidney. Drugs may be utilized to alter the pharmacokinetic profile of a toxicant (*see* Chapter 68).

The concomitant use of two or more drugs adds to the complexity of individualization of drug therapy. The dose of each drug should be adjusted to achieve optimal benefit. Thus, patient compliance is essential yet more difficult to achieve. To obviate the latter problem many fixed-dose drug combinations are marketed. The use of such combinations is advantageous only if the ratio of the fixed doses corresponds to the needs of the individual patient.

In the United States, a fixed-dose combination of drugs must be approved by the Food and Drug Administration (FDA) before it can be marketed, even though the individual drugs are available for concurrent use. To be approved, certain conditions must be met. The two drugs must act as synergists to achieve a better therapeutic response than either drug alone (*e.g.,* many antihypertensive drug combinations); or one drug must act to reduce the incidence of adverse effects caused by the other (*e.g.,* a diuretic that promotes the urinary excretion of potassium combined with a potassium-sparing diuretic).

Adverse Drug-Drug Interactions. These are also numerous, and the frequency of adverse interactions, as would be expected, increases with the number of drugs that a patient receives. The major mechanisms that lead to adverse interactions between drugs involve changes in the pharmacokinetic profile. Thus, one drug may interact with another to retard absorption, compete for binding sites on plasma proteins, alter metabolism by enzyme induction or inhibition, or change the rate of renal excretion.

Interactions can also occur at receptor sites. Interactions that are classified as adverse either compromise therapeutic efficacy, enhance toxicity, or both. It is thus incumbent upon the physician to be familiar with the basic principles of drug-drug interactions in planning a therapeutic regimen. Such reactions are discussed for individual drugs throughout this text and are summarized in Appendix III. (*See also* Cohen and Armstrong, 1974; Morrelli and Melmon, 1978; Hansten, 1979.)

Adverse drug interactions may frequently be avoided by appropriate modifications of dose, time, or route of administration, or by careful monitoring of the patient who is concurrently receiving drugs that may interact. Many drugs that have the potential to interact adversely must nevertheless be used in combination for optimal patient care (*e.g.,* K^+ loss due to diuretics may increase the toxicity of cardiac glycosides). Thus, the use of drugs that have the potential for adverse interactions is not necessarily contraindicated in certain clinical situations.

The frequency of significant beneficial or adverse drug interactions is unknown. Surveys that include data obtained *in vitro,* in animals, and in case reports tend to predict a frequency of interactions that is higher than actually occurs. While such reports have contributed to skepticism about the overall importance of drug interactions (Koch-Weser and Greenblatt, 1977), the physician must be alert for their occurrence. Recognition of beneficial effects and recognition and prevention of adverse drug interactions require a thorough knowledge of the intended and possible effects of drugs that are prescribed, a mental set to attribute unusual events to drugs rather than to disease, and adequate observation of the patient. Automated monitoring of prescription orders in the hospital or outpatient pharmacy may decrease the physician's need to memorize potential interactions. Nevertheless, knowledge of likely mechanisms of drug interactions is the only way the clinician can be prepared to analyze new findings systematically.

Placebo Effects. The net effect of drug therapy is the sum of the pharmacological effects of the drug and the nonspecific placebo effects associated with the therapeutic effort. Although identified specifically with administration of an inert substance in the guise of medication, *placebo effects are associated with the taking of any drug, active as well as inert.*

Placebo effects result from the physician-patient relationship, the significance of the therapeutic effort to the patient, and the mental "set" imparted by the therapeutic setting and by the physician. They vary significantly in different individuals and in any one patient at different times. Placebo effects are commonly manifest as alterations of mood, other subjective effects, and objective effects that are under autonomic or voluntary control. They may be favorable or unfavorable relative to the therapeutic objectives. Exploited to advantage, placebo effects can significantly supplement pharmacological effects and can represent the difference between success and failure of therapy. (*See* Bourne, 1978; Benson and McCallie, 1979.)

A placebo (in this context, better termed *dummy medication*) is an indispensable element of the controlled clinical trial. In contrast, a placebo has only a limited role in the routine practice of medicine. Although the inert medication may be an effective vehicle for a placebo effect, the physician-patient relationship is generally preferable. Relief or lack of relief of symptoms upon administration of a placebo is *not* a reliable basis for determining whether the symptoms have a "psychogenic" or "somatic" origin.

Tolerance. Tolerance may be acquired to the effects of many drugs, especially the opioids, barbiturates, and other CNS depressants. When this occurs, *cross-tolerance* may develop to the effects of pharmacologically related drugs, particularly those acting at the same receptor site, and drug dosage must be increased to maintain a given therapeutic effect. Since tolerance does not usually develop equally to all effects of a drug, the therapeutic index may decrease. However, there are also examples of the development of tolerance to the undesired effects of a drug and a resultant increase in its therapeutic index.

The mechanisms involved in the development of tolerance are only partially understood. In animals, tolerance often occurs as the result of induced synthesis of the hepatic microsomal enzymes concerned in drug biotransformation; the possible significance of this *drug-disposition* or *pharmacokinetic tolerance* during chronic medication in man is an area of continuing investigation. The most important factor in the development of tolerance to the opioids, barbiturates, and ethanol is some type of neuronal adaptation vaguely referred to as *cellular* or *pharmacodynamic tolerance.* Tachyphylaxis, such as that to histamine-releasing agents and to the sympathomimetic amines that act indirectly by releasing norepinephrine, has been attributed to depletion of available mediator, but other mechanisms may also contribute. The subject of tolerance is discussed in more detail in Chapter 23.

Genetic Factors. Genetic factors contribute to the normal variability of drug effects and are responsible for a number of striking quantitative and qualitative modifications of pharmacological activity. Many of these differences, such as the prolonged apnea in some patients after administration of usual doses of the neuromuscular blocking agent succinylcholine, have been traced to genetic influences on the enzymes involved in *drug biotransformation.* Other variations in drug effect, such as the greater incidence of drug-induced hemolytic anemia in non-Caucasians than in Caucasians, have been found to be related to genetic differences that modify the actions of drugs.

The objectives of *pharmacogenetics* include not only identification of differences in drug effects that have a genetic basis but also development of simple methods by which susceptible individuals can be recognized *before* the drug is administered.

APPROACH TO INDIVIDUALIZATION

It has been stated above that every therapeutic plan is and should be treated as an experiment. As such, most of the considerations that were specified above in the discussion of clinical trials must be applied to individual patients. Of utmost importance is the definition of specific goals of treatment and the means to assess whether these goals are being achieved successfully. Whenever possible, the objective end point should be related as closely as possible to the clinical goals of therapy (*e.g.,* suppression of an arrhythmia, shrinkage of a tumor, eradication of an infection). Many clinical goals are, however, difficult to assess (*e.g.,* the prevention of cardiovascular complications associated with hypertension and diabetes). In such cases it is necessary to set intermediate end points to therapy, such as a reduction in blood pressure or the concentration of glucose in plasma. These intermediate end points are based on demonstrated *or assumed* correlations with the ultimate clinical benefit. In many cases, such as normalization of the concentration of plasma glucose or reduction of the concentration of cholesterol in plasma by drugs, the intermediate goal is controversial.

Certain general considerations apply to the individualization of a drug regimen and the concept of intermediate end points. The initial choice of a drug can be made only after adequate clinical and laboratory assessment of the patient. The extent of this evaluation is itself dependent on many factors, including a cost-benefit analysis of diagnostic tests, and this must be based on the availability and specificity of alternative therapies (*e.g., see* Finnerty, 1975; Melby, 1975). The initial dosage regimen is determined by estimation, if possible, of the pharmacokinetic properties of the drug in the individual patient. The estimate must be based on an appreciation of the variables that are most likely to affect the disposition of the particular drug. These variables, among others, include age, body weight, renal and hepatic function, coexisting diseases such as congestive heart failure, or concurrent therapy with other drugs (*see* Figure 3–1). The value or utility of the regimen obviously needs to be assessed. The utility of a regimen can be defined as the benefit it produces plus the dangers of not treating the disease minus the sum of the adverse effects of therapy. Another common expression of the usefulness of a regimen is its ratio of risks to benefits (representing a balance between the efficacious and toxic effects of the drug). A definitive evaluation of the utility of a drug is not easy (Sheiner and Melmon, 1978). Some say it is not possible. Nevertheless, some sense of value of a regimen must be established in the minds of the physician and the patient. Knowledge of the usefulness of a given regimen may be a critical determinant of protracted compliance by the patient to a chronic regimen or logical discontinuation by the physician of a marginally efficacious and risky therapy.

DRUG REGULATION AND DEVELOPMENT

Drug Regulation

The history of drug regulation in the United States reflects the growing involvement by governments of most countries to assure the highest degree of efficacy and safety in marketed medicinal agents. The first act, the Federal Pure Food and Drug Act of 1906, was concerned only with the purity of drugs. There were no restrictions on sale nor obligations to establish efficacy and safety. However, few new drugs were marketed between 1908 and the advent of the sulfonamides in the mid 1930s, an era of therapeutic nihilism. The federal act was amended in 1938, following an epidemic of deaths that resulted from the marketing of a solution of sulfanilamide in diethylene glycol, an excellent but highly toxic solvent. The amended act, the enforcement of which was entrusted to the Food and Drug Administration (FDA), was primarily concerned with the labeling and safety of drugs. Toxicity studies were required, as well as approval of a new drug application (NDA), before a drug could be promoted and distributed. However, no proof of efficacy was required, and extravagant claims for therapeutic indications were commonly made. Drugs could go from the laboratory to clinical testing without approval by the FDA.

In this relatively relaxed atmosphere, research in basic and clinical pharmacology burgeoned in both industrial and academic laboratories. The result was a flow of new and effective drugs, called "wonder drugs" by the lay press, for the treatment of both infectious and organic disease. The risk-to-benefit ratio was seldom mentioned, but it emerged in dramatic fashion early in the 1960s. At that time thalidomide, a hypnotic with no obvious advantage over other drugs in its class, was introduced in the European market. After an appropriate period, it became apparent that the incidence of a relatively rare birth defect, phocomelia, was increasing. It soon reached epidemic proportion, and retrospective epidemiological research firmly established the causative agent to be thalidomide, taken early in the course of pregnancy. The reaction to the dramatic demonstration of the teratogenicity of a needless drug was worldwide. In the United States it resulted, in 1962, in the Harris-Kefauver Amendment to the Federal Pure Food and Drug Act.

The Harris-Kefauver Amendment is sound legislation. It requires extensive pharmacological and toxicological research before a drug can be tested in man. The data from such studies must be submitted in the form of an application for an investigational new drug (IND) and approved by the FDA before clinical studies can begin. Proof of efficacy is required, as is documentation of relative safety in terms of the risk-to-benefit ratio for the disease entity to be treated. Three extensive phases of clinical testing (*see* below) must be completed before a new drug application (NDA) can be submitted. Finally, proof of efficacy was required, retroactively, for all drugs marketed between 1938 and 1962.

The provisions of the amendment have greatly increased the time and the cost required to market a new drug. Moreover, although the law requires action on the part of the FDA within a period of 6 months, an NDA may be repeatedly returned to the applicant at 6-month intervals for additional basic or clinical research. The result has been a barrage of criticism from both the pharmaceutical industry and organized medicine, not of the law but of the rigid regulations imposed by the FDA in its enforcement. On the other hand, some consumer groups, with little appreciation of risk-to-benefit ratio, demand the recall of drugs that may play an important role in the therapeutic regimen of appropriately selected patients. In this climate, further amendments to the Federal Pure Food and Drug Act are being considered to speed the process of approval of an NDA without weakening, and hopefully even strengthening, requirements for safety and efficacy.

Drug Development

Except for concern about the so-called drug lag (Kennedy, 1978) and governmental interference with the practice of medicine, the average physician has not considered it to be important to understand the process of drug development. Yet an appreciation of this process is necessary if the therapist wishes to have the ability to estimate the risk-to-benefit ratio of a drug and to realize just when regulations can and cannot be relied upon for guarantees of efficacy and safety of a marketed product.

By the time an IND has been approved and a drug reaches the stage of testing in man, extensive evaluation of its pharmacokinetic, pharmacodynamic, and toxic properties have been performed in several species of animals and *in vitro*. As indicated above, the FDA issues regulations and guidelines that govern the type and extent of preclinical testing. Although the value of many requirements for preclinical testing is self-evident, such as those that screen for direct toxicity to organs and characterize dose-related effects, the value of others are controversial, particularly because of the well-known interspecies variation in the effects of drugs. Interestingly, although many of the preclinical tests have not been convincingly shown to predict effects that are eventually observed in man, the risk of cautious testing of a new drug in a normal person is surprisingly low.

Trials of drugs in man in the United States are generally conducted in phases, three of which must be completed before an NDA can be approved; these are outlined in Figure 3–2. Although assessment of risk is a major objective of such testing, this is far more difficult than is the determination of whether a drug is efficacious for a selected clinical condition (Temple *et al.*, 1979). Usually about 500 to 3000 carefully selected patients receive a new drug during phase-3 clinical trials. At most, only a few hundred are treated for more than 3 to 6 months, regardless of the likely duration of therapy that will be required in practice. Thus, the most profound and overt risks that occur almost immediately after the drug is given can be detected in a phase-3 study, if these occur more often than once per 100 administrations. Risks that are medically important but delayed or less frequent than 1 in 1000 administrations will not be revealed. However, to withhold a drug with important and proven efficacy until all of its untoward effects or unanticipated beneficial actions have been demonstrated is unconscionable. For instance, to detect an effect of a drug that occurs with a frequency of 1 in 50,000 administrations at a relative risk of 2 (*i.e.*, the

treated population would develop the event twice as frequently as it would appear spontaneously) within 1 year of giving the drug, requires the study of more than 1.5 million patients (Strom and Melmon, 1979). It is thus obvious that a number of unanticipated adverse and beneficial effects of drugs are only detectable after the drug is approved for distribution. The same can be more convincingly stated about most of the effects of drugs on children or the fetus, where premarketing experimental studies are restricted. It is for these reasons that many countries are considering the establishment of systematic methods for the surveillance of the effects of drugs after they have been approved for distribution (*see* Slone *et al.*, 1979; Strom and Melmon, 1980).

The problem of recognizing adverse effects during clinical trials is due not only to the limited number of studies but also to the selection of patients who are included. After marketing, the drug is used in patients with greater variations in their rates of absorption and elimination of drugs, in patients who have coexisting diseases, and so forth. Adverse reactions that may occur rarely or never in a carefully selected patient population, no matter how large, may be relatively frequent in the general population of patients (*e.g.*, *see* Naranjo *et al.*, 1979). Thus, while most physicians realize that it is medically and morally impractical to delay the release of a drug while awaiting the "definitive" information on all possible adverse effects, the limitations of available data at the time of release place an additional burden on the physician to be observant and critical in his use of new drugs and to consider the possibility of iatrogenic illness when undesirable reactions occur.

Before a drug can be marketed, an acceptable package insert must be prepared. This is a cooperative effort between the FDA and the pharmaceutical company. The insert usually contains basic pharmacological information, as well as essential clinical information in regard to approved indications, contraindications, precautions, warnings, adverse reactions, usual dosage, and available preparations. Advertising material cannot deviate from information contained in the insert.

The FDA is specifically prohibited from

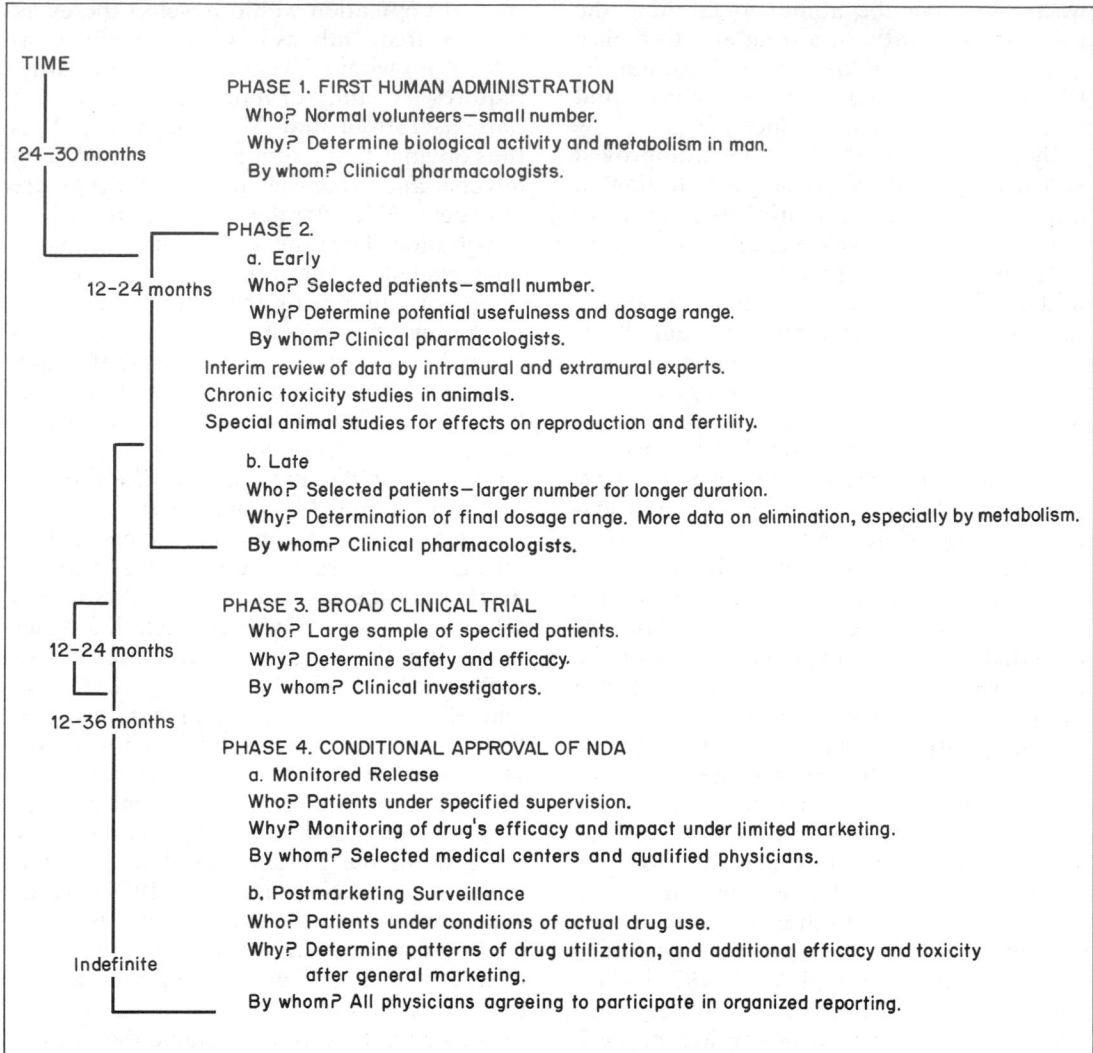

TIME

PHASE 1. FIRST HUMAN ADMINISTRATION
Who? Normal volunteers—small number.
Why? Determine biological activity and metabolism in man.
By whom? Clinical pharmacologists.

24–30 months

PHASE 2.
a. Early
Who? Selected patients—small number.
Why? Determine potential usefulness and dosage range.
By whom? Clinical pharmacologists.

12–24 months

Interim review of data by intramural and extramural experts.
Chronic toxicity studies in animals.
Special animal studies for effects on reproduction and fertility.

b. Late
Who? Selected patients—larger number for longer duration.
Why? Determination of final dosage range. More data on elimination, especially by metabolism.
By whom? Clinical pharmacologists.

PHASE 3. BROAD CLINICAL TRIAL
Who? Large sample of specified patients.
Why? Determine safety and efficacy.
By whom? Clinical investigators.

12–24 months

12–36 months

PHASE 4. CONDITIONAL APPROVAL OF NDA
a. Monitored Release
Who? Patients under specified supervision.
Why? Monitoring of drug's efficacy and impact under limited marketing.
By whom? Selected medical centers and qualified physicians.

b. Postmarketing Surveillance
Who? Patients under conditions of actual drug use.
Why? Determine patterns of drug utilization, and additional efficacy and toxicity after general marketing.
By whom? All physicians agreeing to participate in organized reporting.

Indefinite

Figure 3-2. *The phases of drug development in the United States.* (Modified from Melmon and Morrelli, 1978.)

modifying the practice of medicine. Yet, in modern society, the package insert imposes restraints on the individual physician. It is not within the scope of this textbook to discuss this problem further. Nevertheless, the physician should not ignore a well-conducted clinical investigation published in a well-respected archival journal that provides evidence for a new indication for an approved drug.

ADVERSE DRUG REACTIONS AND DRUG TOXICITY

Very few physicians believe that any drug, no matter how trivial its actions, is free of toxic effects. The use of the term *safe* in the 1938 amendments to the Federal Pure Food and Drug Act has led to unnecessary misunderstandings between the regulatory agencies, the medical profession, and consumers of drugs. Patients, to a much greater extent than physicians, do not understand the limitations of premarketing evaluation of risks, and the failure of the FDA to gather, systematically, useful information on the effects caused by drugs. The agency has had only limited success in cajoling the pharmaceutical industry into limited *postmarketing* studies. Generally, the public has had unwarranted confidence and expectations about the safety of drugs. More recently, the public has been told that thousands of patients are dying needlessly because of adverse effects of drugs. As is most often the case, the true situation lies somewhere between these two extremes, but precisely or even approximately where is unknown. For a review of the problems of defining, recognizing, classifying, and measuring the economic and human costs of adverse drug reactions, *see* Adverse Drug Reactions in the United States (1974) and Karch and Lasagna (1975).

As with drug interactions, classification of adverse effects of drugs according to information about their causes provides a framework for the transfer of principles to the clinical setting. Such classification appears in Chapter 68. In addition, the clinician obviously also needs to know the frequencies and types of untoward effects caused by each individual drug he prescribes; such information is presented throughout the text.

There is a danger that overemphasis of adverse drug reactions may cause physicians to lose sight of a most important aspect of therapy—the ratio of risks to benefits. Without consideration of this ratio it is impossible to establish the value of a drug. Procedures to estimate risk-to-benefit ratios for individuals (Pauker and Kassirer, 1975; Sheiner and Melmon, 1978) and for populations (Schoenbaum, 1978) have been tried but are not proven. A generally applicable method for the quantitation of utility will remain elusive until the rates of anticipated efficacy of a drug can be determined and until quantitative values can be placed on the state of health and on the probability of anticipated and unanticipated decreases in longevity, quality of life, and function (Sheiner and Melmon, 1978; Strom and Melmon, 1979). It must also be remembered that the physician and the patient may have very disparate opinions of these values.

GUIDE TO THE "THERAPEUTIC JUNGLE"

The flood of new drugs in recent years has provided many dramatic improvements in therapy, but it has also created a number of problems of equal magnitude. Not the least of these is the "therapeutic jungle," the term used to refer to the combination of the overwhelming number of drugs, the confusion over nomenclature, and the associated un-

certainty of the status of many of these drugs. A reduction in the marketing of close congeners and drug mixtures and an improvement in the quality of advertising are important ingredients in the remedy for the "therapeutic jungle." However, the physician can also contribute to the remedy by employing nonproprietary rather than proprietary names whenever appropriate, by using prototypes both as an instructional device and in clinical practice, by adopting a properly critical attitude toward new drugs, and by knowing and making use of reliable sources of pharmacological information. Most important, he should develop a "way of thinking about drugs" based upon pharmacological principles.

Drug Nomenclature. The existence of many names for each drug, even when reduced to a minimum, has led to a lamentable and confusing situation in drug nomenclature. In addition to its formal *chemical* name, a new drug is usually assigned a *code* name by the pharmaceutical manufacturer. If the drug appears promising, and the manufacturer wishes to place it on the market, a *United States Adopted Name* (USAN) is selected by the USAN Council, which is jointly sponsored by the American Medical Association, the American Pharmaceutical Association, and the United States Pharmacopeial Convention, Inc. This *nonproprietary* name is often referred to as the *generic* name. This term has become entrenched, but by definition it should be more properly reserved to designate a chemical or pharmacological class of drugs, such as sulfonamides or sympathomimetics. If the drug is eventually admitted to the U.S.P. (*see* below), the USAN becomes the *official* name. However, the nonproprietary name and the official name of an older drug may differ. Subsequently, the drug will also be assigned a *proprietary* name or *trademark* by the manufacturer. If the drug is marketed by more than one company, it may have several proprietary names. If mixtures of the drug with other agents are marketed, each such mixture may also have a separate proprietary name.

There is increasing worldwide adoption of the same name for each therapeutic substance. For newer drugs, the USAN is usually adopted for the nonproprietary name in other countries, but this is not true for older drugs. International agreement on drug names is mediated through the World Health Organization and the pertinent health agencies of the cooperating countries.

The nonproprietary or official name of a drug should be used whenever possible, and such a practice has been adopted in this textbook. The use of the nonproprietary name is clearly less confusing when the drug is available under multiple proprietary names, and when the nonproprietary name more readily identifies the drug with its pharmacological class. The best argument for the proprietary name is that it is frequently more easily pronounced and remembered as a result of advertising. For purposes of identification, proprietary names, designated by SMALL-CAP TYPE, appear throughout the text in chapter sections dealing with preparations as well as in the Index. This does not imply a complete listing of proprietary names, since the number for a single drug may be large and since proprietary names differ from country to country.

The question arises, however, whether the nonproprietary name or a proprietary name should be employed by the physician when he prescribes drugs. Use of the nonproprietary name, unless the source is designated, permits the pharmacist to dispense the preparation of any manufacturer, and this sometimes results in less expense for the patient. Based on a number of considerations, such as the frequency of use of a drug that is only available from a single manufacturer, the cost of filling a prescription, and the markup of the pharmacist, it appears as though the *overall savings* to society of prescribing the least expensive nonproprietary preparation is small, about 5% (*see* Trout and Lee, 1980). Of course, savings in individual situations can be very much greater. On the other hand, prescribing by nonproprietary name could result in the patient receiving a preparation of inferior quality or of uncertain bioavailability, and therapeutic failures due to decreased bioavailability do occur. On the urging of the Senate Subcommittee on Health, the FDA is currently attempting to establish standards for bioavailability and to compile information about the interchangeability of drug products (*see* Drug Bioequivalence: A Report of the Office of Technology Assessment, Drug Bioequivalence Study Panel,

1974). With the exception of drugs with known inconsistencies in bioavailability (Koch-Weser, 1974), nonproprietary names should be used when prescribing.

In practically all states with generic drug laws, a pharmacist may substitute a preparation that is presumably equivalent *unless* the physician indicates "no substitution" on the prescription. Likewise, if the nonproprietary name of a drug is employed, the physician has the privilege of indicating its source. In view of the discussion above on the individualization of drug therapy, it is understandable why a physician who has carefully adjusted the dose of a drug to a patient's individual requirements for chronic therapy may be reluctant to surrender control over the source of the drug that his patient receives.

Use of Prototypes. It is obviously crucial for the physician to be thoroughly familiar with the pharmacological properties of a drug before it is administered. It follows that the patient will benefit if the physician avoids the temptation to choose from many different drugs for the patient's regimen. A physician's needs for therapeutic agents can usually be satisfied by his thorough knowledge of one or two drugs in each therapeutic category. Inevitably, a small number of drugs can be used more effectively. When the clinical setting calls for a drug that the physician uses infrequently, he should feel obligated to learn about its effects, to use great caution in its administration, and to apply impeccable procedures in monitoring its effects.

For teaching purposes, as illustrated in this textbook, the confusion created by the welter of similar drugs is reduced by restricting major attention to prototypes in each pharmacological class. Focusing on the representative drugs results in better characterization of a class as a whole, and thereby permits sharper recognition of the occasional member that possesses unique properties. A teaching prototype is often the agent most likely to be employed in clinical use, but this is not always true. A particular drug may be retained as the prototype, even though a new congener is clinically superior, either because more is known about the older drug or because it is more illustrative for the entire class of agents.

Attitude toward New Drugs. A reasonable attitude toward new drugs is summarized by the adage that advises the physician to be "neither the first to use a new drug nor the last to discard the old." Only a minor fraction of the new drugs represents a significant therapeutic advance. The limitation of information about toxicity and efficacy at the time of release of a drug has been emphasized above, and this is particularly pertinent to comparisons with older agents in the same therapeutic class. Nevertheless, the important advances in therapeutics in the last 30 years emphasize the obligation to keep abreast of significant advances in pharmacotherapy.

SOURCES OF DRUG INFORMATION

The physician's need for objective, concise, and well-organized information on drugs is obvious. Among the available sources are textbooks of pharmacology and therapeutics, leading medical journals, drug compendia, professional seminars and meetings, and advertising. Despite this cornucopia of drug information, responsible medical spokesmen insist that most practicing physicians are unable to extract the objective and unbiased data required for the practice of rational therapeutics (*see* Task Force, 1969).

Depending on their aim and scope, *pharmacology textbooks* provide (in varying proportions) basic pharmacological principles, critical appraisal of useful categories of therapeutic agents, and detailed descriptions of individual drugs or prototypes that serve as standards of reference for assessing new drugs. In addition, pharmacodynamics and pathological physiology are correlated. For obvious reasons, textbooks cannot contain information on the most recently introduced drugs. Therapeutics is considered in virtually all textbooks of medicine, but often superficially.

The source of information described as most often used by physicians in an industry survey is the *Physicians' Desk Reference* (PDR). The brand-name manufacturers whose products appear support this book. No comparative data on efficacy, safety, or cost are included. The information is nearly identical to that contained in drug package inserts, which are largely based on the results of phase-3 testing.

AMA Drug Evaluations, compiled by the American Medical Association Department of Drugs, is free from some of these objections. Drugs are listed by therapeutic category and identified by both nonproprietary and proprietary names. The compendium includes information on uses, routes of administration, or dosages not always found in the package insert, recognizing that the physician's legitimate use of a drug for individual patients is not precluded by FDA-approved labeling limitations.

Industry promotion, in the form of direct-mail brochures, journal advertising, displays, professional courtesies, or the detail man, is intended to be persuasive rather than educational. The pharmaceutical industry cannot, should not, and indeed does not purport to be responsible for the education of physicians in the use of drugs.

Over 1500 medical journals are published regularly in the United States. However, of the 28 medical publications with circulations in excess of 70,000 copies, 25 are sent to physicians free of charge and paid for by the industry. Objective journals, which are not supported by drug manufacturers, include *Clinical Pharmacology and Therapeutics,* which is devoted primarily to the evaluation of the actions and effects of drugs in man. The *New England Journal of Medicine, Annals of Internal Medicine, Archives of Internal Medicine, British Medical Journal, Lancet,* and *Postgraduate Medicine* offer timely therapeutic reports and reviews. Four publications deserve special emphasis here because they exemplify effective attempts to provide objective drug information in easily assimilable form. These are *The Medical Letter, Clin-Alert, Rational Drug Therapy,* and *Drug Therapeutics: Concepts for Physicians. The Medical Letter* provides summaries of scientific reports and consultants' evaluations of the safety, efficacy, and rationale for use of a drug. *Clin-Alert* consists mainly of abstracts from the literature on drugs. *Rational Drug Therapy* presents a monthly review article on groups of drugs or on the management of specific conditions. *Drug Therapeutics* provides full review articles related to common problems in therapeutics.

The United States Pharmacopeia (U.S.P.)

and *The National Formulary* (N.F.) were recognized as "official compendia" by the Federal Pure Food and Drug Act of 1906. The approved therapeutic agents used in medical practice in the United States are described and defined with respect to source, chemistry, physical properties, tests for identity and purity, assay, storage, therapeutic dosage range, and class of use. The two official compendia are now published in a single volume; the current revision became official on July 1, 1980. U.S.P. XX includes 2314 monographs on drug substances and dosage forms; N.F. XV contains 196 monographs on pharmaceutical ingredients.

Benson, H., and McCallie, D. P. Angina pectoris and the placebo effect. *N. Engl. J. Med.,* 1979, *300,* 1424–1425.
Cohen, S. N., and others. A computer-based system for the study and control of drug interactions in hospitalized patients. In, *Drug Interactions.* (Morselli, P. L.; Garattini, S.; and Cohen, S. N.; eds.) Raven Press, New York, 1974, pp. 363–374.
Curran, W. J. Reasonableness and randomization in clinical trials: fundamental law and governmental regulation. *N. Engl. J. Med.,* 1979, *300,* 1273–1275.
Feinstein, A. R. Clinical biostatistics. XLI. Hard science, soft data and the challenges of choosing clinical variables in research. *Clin. Pharmacol. Ther.,* 1977a, *22,* 485–498.
Freiman, J. A.; Chalmers, T. C.; Smith, H.; and Kuebler, R. R. The importance of beta, the type II error and sample size in the design and interpretation of the randomized control trial. *N. Engl. J. Med.,* 1978, *299,* 690–694.
Jick, H.; Slone, D.; Dinan, B.; and Muench, H. Evaluation of drug efficacy by a preference technique. *N. Engl. J. Med.,* 1966, *275,* 1399–1403.
Kennedy, D. A calm look at "drug lag." *J.A.M.A.,* 1978, *239,* 423–426.
Lefkowitz, R. J. Direct binding studies of adrenergic receptors: biochemical, physiologic, and clinical implications. *Ann. Intern. Med.,* 1979, *91,* 450–458.
Meffin, P. J.; Winkle, R. A.; Blaschke, T. F.; Fitzgerald, J.; and Harrison, D. C. Response optimization of drug dosage: antiarrhythmic studies with tocainide. *Clin. Pharmacol. Ther.,* 1977, *22,* 42–57.
Naranjo, C. A.; Pontigo, E.; Valdenegro, C.; Gonzalez, G.; Ruiz, I.; and Bustio, U. Furosemide-induced adverse reactions in cirrhosis of the liver. *Clin. Pharmacol. Ther.,* 1979, *25,* 154–160.
Pauker, S. G., and Kassirer, J. P. Therapeutic decision making: a cost-benefit analysis. *N. Engl. J. Med.,* 1975, *293,* 229–234.
Schimke, R. T.; Kaufman, R. J.; Alt, F. W.; and Kellems, R. F. Gene amplification and drug resistance in cultured murine cells. *Science,* 1978, *202,* 1051–1055.
Schoenbaum, S. C. Vaccination for influenza—any alternatives? *N. Engl. J. Med.,* 1978, *298,* 621–622.
Sheiner, L. B.; Halkin, H.; Peck, C.; Rosenberg, B.; and Melmon, K. L. Improved computer-assisted digoxin therapy: a method using feedback of measured serum digoxin concentrations. *Ann. Intern. Med.,* 1975, *82,* 619–627.
Slone, D.; Shapiro, S.; Miettinen, O. S.; Finkle, W. D.; and Stolley, P. D. Drug evaluation after marketing. *Ann. Intern. Med.,* 1979, *90,* 257–261.
Temple, R. J.; Jones, J. K.; and Crout, J. R. Adverse effects of newly marketed drugs. *N. Engl. J. Med.,* 1979, *300,* 1046–1047.
Vesell, E. S., and Page, J. G. Genetic control of drug levels in man: phenylbutazone. *Science,* 1968, *159,* 1479–1480.

Monographs and Reviews
Adverse Drug Reactions in the United States: An Analysis of the Scope of the Problem and Recommendations for Future Approaches. Medicine in the Public Interest, Inc., Washington, D. C., 1974.
AMA Drug Evaluations, 3rd ed. PSG Publishing Co., Inc., Littleton, Mass., 1977.
Beecher, H. K. *Measurement of Subjective Responses: Quantitative Effects of Drugs.* Oxford University Press, New York, 1959.
Bourne, H. R. Rational use of placebo. In, *Clinical Pharmacology: Basic Principles in Therapeutics,* 2nd ed. (Melmon, K. L., and Morrelli, H. F., eds.) Macmillan Publishing Co., Inc., New York, 1978, pp. 1052–1062.
Cohen, S. N., and Armstrong, M. F. *Drug Interactions: A Handbook for Clinical Use.* The Williams & Wilkins Co., Baltimore, 1974.
Drug Bioequivalence: A Report of the Office of Technology Assessment, Drug Bioequivalence Study Panel. U.S. Government Printing Office, Washington, D. C., 1974.
Feinstein, A. R. *Clinical Judgment.* The Williams & Wilkins Co., Baltimore, 1967.
———. *Clinical Biostatistics.* C. V. Mosby Co., St. Louis, 1977b.
Finnerty, F. A. Extensive hypertension work-up: con. *J.A.M.A.,* 1975, *231,* 402–403.
Flier, J. S.; Kahn, C. R.; and Roth, J. Receptors, antireceptor antibodies and mechanisms of insulin resistance. *N. Engl. J. Med.,* 1979, *300,* 413–419.
Hansten, P. D. *Drug Interactions,* 4th ed. Lea & Febiger, Philadelphia, 1979.
Hill, A. B. *Controlled Clinical Trials: Conference of Council for International Organizations of Medical Sciences.* Blackwell Scientific Publications, Ltd., Oxford, 1960.
———. *Statistical Methods in Clinical and Preventive Medicine.* Oxford University Press, New York, 1962.
Karch, F. E., and Lasagna, L. Adverse drug reactions: a critical review. *J.A.M.A.,* 1975, *234,* 1236–1241.
Koch-Weser, J. Serum drug concentrations as therapeutic guides. *N. Engl. J. Med.,* 1972, *287,* 227–231.
———. Bioavailability of drugs. *N. Engl. J. Med.,* 1974, *291,* 233.
Koch-Weser, J., and Greenblatt, D. J. Drug interactions in clinical perspective. *Eur. J. Clin. Pharmacol.,* 1977, *11,* 405–408.
Melby, J. C. Extensive hypertension work-up: pro. *J.A.M.A.,* 1975, *231,* 399–401.
Melmon, K. L. Preventable drug reactions—causes and cures. *N. Engl. J. Med.,* 1971, *284,* 1361–1368.
Melmon, K. L.; Azarnoff, D. L.; Blaschke, T. F.; Goldberg, L. I.; Koch-Weser, J.; Nies, A. S.; Sheiner, L. B.; and Thompson, W. L. (eds.). *Drug Therapeutics: Concepts for Physicians.* Elsevier North-Holland, Inc., New York, 1979.
Melmon, K. L., and Morrelli, H. F. Drug reactions. In, *Clinical Pharmacology: Basic Principles in Therapeutics,* 2nd ed. (Melmon, K. L., and Morrelli, H. F., eds.) Macmillan Publishing Co., Inc., New York, 1978, pp. 951–981.
Morrelli, H. F. Propranolol. *Ann. Intern. Med.,* 1973, *78,* 913–917.
Morrelli, H. F., and Melmon, K. L. Drug interactions. In, *Clinical Pharmacology: Basic Principles in Therapeutics,* 2nd ed. (Melmon, K. L., and Morrelli, H. F., eds.) Macmillan Publishing Co., Inc., New York, 1978, pp. 982–1007.
Peck, C. C. Qualitative aspects of therapeutic decision making. In, *Clinical Pharmacology: Basic Principles in Therapeutics,* 2nd ed. (Melmon, K. L., and Morrelli,

H. F., eds.) Macmillan Publishing Co., Inc., New York, **1978**, pp. 1063–1083.

Rawlins, M. D. Variability in response to drugs. *Br. Med. J.,* **1974**, *4,* 91–94.

Sheiner, L. B. Clinical trials and the illusion of objectivity. In, *Drug Therapeutics: Concepts for Physicians.* (Melmon, K. L. *et al.,* eds.) Elsevier North-Holland, Inc., New York, **1979**, pp. 167–182.

Sheiner, L. B., and Melmon, K. L. The utility function of antihypertensive therapy. In, *Mild Hypertension: To Treat or Not to Treat.* (Perry, H. M., Jr., and Smith, W. M., eds.) *Ann. N.Y. Acad. Sci.,* **1978**, *304,* 112–122.

Sheiner, L. B., and Tozer, T. N. Clinical pharmacokinetics: the use of plasma concentrations of drugs. In, *Clinical Pharmacology: Basic Principles in Therapeutics,* 2nd ed. (Melmon, K. L., and Morrelli, H. F., eds.) Macmillan Publishing Co., Inc., New York, **1978**, pp. 71–109.

Smith, S. E., and Rawlins, M. D. *Variability in Human Drug Response.* Butterworths, London, **1973**.

Smith, W. M. Drug choice in disease states. In, *Clinical Pharmacology: Basic Principles in Therapeutics,* 2nd ed. (Melmon, K. L., and Morrelli, H. F., eds.) Macmillan Publishing Co., Inc., New York, **1978**, pp. 3–24.

Strom, B. L., and Melmon, K. L. Can post-marketing surveillance help to effect optimal drug therapy? *J.A.M.A.,* **1979**, *242,* 2420–2423.

———. Major challenges to post-marketing surveillance (PMS). *Kyoto International Conference on Drug Induced Sufferings.* **1980**.

Task Force on Prescription Drugs. *Final Report.* Department of Health, Education and Welfare, U.S. Government Printing Office, Washington, D. C., **1969**.

Trout, M. E., and Lee, A. M. Generic substitution: a boon or a bane to the physician and the consumer? In, *Drug Therapeutics: Concepts for Physicians.* (Melmon, K. L., ed.) Elsevier North-Holland, Inc., New York, **1980**.

The United States Pharmacopeia, 20th rev., and *The National Formulary,* 15th ed. (The United States Pharmacopeial Convention, Inc.) Mack Printing Co., Easton, Pa., **1980**.

Vesell, E. S. Pharmacogenetics—multiple interactions between genes and environment as determinants of drug response. *Am. J. Med.,* **1979**, *66,* 183–187.

Drugs Acting at Synaptic and Neuroeffector Junctional Sites

NEUROHUMORAL TRANSMISSION AND THE AUTONOMIC NERVOUS SYSTEM

Steven E. Mayer

The theory of *neurohumoral transmission* received direct experimental validation over half a century ago, and extensive investigation during the ensuing years has led to its general acceptance. The theory states that nerves transmit their impulses across most synapses and neuroeffector junctions by means of specific chemical agents known as *neurohumoral transmitters*. The actions of the so-called autonomic drugs that affect smooth muscle, cardiac muscle, and gland cells can be interpreted in terms of their mimicking or modifying the actions of the neurohumoral transmitters released by the autonomic fibers at either the ganglia or the effector cells.

Most of the general principles concerning the *physiology* and *pharmacology* of the peripheral autonomic nervous system and its effector organs apply with certain modifications to the neuromuscular junctions of skeletal muscle also, and in a more limited sense to the central nervous system (CNS) (*see* Chapter 12).

A clear understanding of the anatomy and physiology of the autonomic nervous system is essential to a study of the pharmacology of the *autonomic drugs*. The actions of an autonomic agent on various organs of the body can often be predicted if the responses to nerve impulses that reach the organs are known.

ANATOMY AND GENERAL FUNCTIONS OF THE AUTONOMIC NERVOUS SYSTEM

The autonomic nervous system is also called the visceral, vegetative, or involuntary nervous system. In the periphery, its representation consists of nerves, ganglia, and plexuses that provide the innervation to the heart, blood vessels, glands, other visceral organs, and smooth muscles. It is therefore widely distributed throughout the body and controls the so-called automatic, or vegetative, functions.

Differences between Autonomic and Somatic Nerves. A major difference between autonomic and somatic nerves is that of the structures innervated. The motor nerves of the involuntary system supply all structures of the body except skeletal muscle, which is innervated by somatic nerves. The most distal synaptic junctions in the autonomic reflex arc occur in ganglia that are entirely outside of the cerebrospinal axis, whereas the synapses of somatic nerves are entirely within the CNS. Autonomic nerves form extensive peripheral plexuses, whereas such networks are absent from the somatic system. The motor nerves to skeletal muscles are myelinated, whereas the postganglionic autonomic nerves are generally nonmyelinated. When the cerebrospinal nerves are interrupted, the skeletal muscles that they innervate are completely paralyzed and undergo atrophy, whereas smooth muscles and glands generally show some level of automatic activity independent of intact innervation. There are, however, certain similarities between these two nervous systems, as will be described later.

Visceral Afferent Fibers. The *afferent* fibers from visceral structures are the first link in the *reflex arcs of the autonomic system*. With certain exceptions, such as axon reflexes, most visceral reflexes are mediated through the CNS. The afferents are, for the most part, nonmyelinated fibers and are carried into the cerebrospinal axis by the vagus, pelvic, splanchnic, and other autonomic nerves. For example, about four fifths of the vagal nerve fibers are sensory. Other autonomic afferents from blood vessels in skeletal muscles and from certain integumental structures are carried in the somatic nerves. The cell bodies of visceral afferent fibers lie in the dorsal root ganglia of the spinal nerves and in the corresponding sensory ganglia of certain cranial nerves, such as the nodose ganglion of the vagus. The *efferent* link of the autonomic reflex arc is discussed in the sections that follow.

The autonomic afferent fibers are concerned with the mediation of visceral sensation (including pain and referred pain); with vasomotor, respiratory, and viscerosomatic reflexes; and with the regulation of interrelated visceral activities. A special example of an autonomic afferent system is that arising from the pressoreceptive endings in the carotid sinus and the aortic arch, and from the chemoreceptor cells in the carotid and aortic bodies; this system is important in the reflex control of blood pressure, heart rate, and respiration, and its afferent fibers pass in the glossopharyngeal and vagus nerves to the medulla.

There are no important physiological differences between visceral and somatic afferent fibers, and their responses to drugs do not differ significantly. The clinical importance of such fibers arises especially in connection with the relief of visceral pain by surgery or by local anesthetic block.

Central Autonomic Connections. There are probably no purely autonomic or somatic centers of integration, and extensive overlap occurs. Somatic responses are always accompanied by visceral responses and *vice versa*. Autonomic reflexes can be elicited at the level of the *spinal cord*. They are clearly demonstrable in the spinal animal, including man, and are manifested in sweating, blood pressure alterations, vasomotor responses to temperature changes, and reflex emptying of the urinary bladder, rectum, and seminal vesicles. Extensive central ramifications of the autonomic nervous system exist above the level of the spinal cord. The integration of the control of blood pressure and respiration in the *medulla oblongata* is well known, but there are even higher levels of integration of autonomic functions,

especially in the hypothalamus and cortex. The *hypothalamus* is the principal locus of integration of the entire autonomic system and is concerned in the regulation of body temperature, water balance, carbohydrate and fat metabolism, blood pressure, emotions, sleep, and sexual reflexes. Much information concerning central integration of autonomic functions has come not only from physiological experimentation but also from clinical investigation of such syndromes as diabetes insipidus, dystrophia adiposogenitalis, narcolepsy, hypothermia, hyperthermia, and diencephalic autonomic epilepsy. The hypothalamic nuclei that lie posteriorly and laterally are sympathetic in their main connections, and their stimulation results in massive discharge of the sympathoadrenal system. Parasympathetic functions are evidently integrated by the midline nuclei in the region of the tuber cinereum and by nuclei lying anteriorly. The supraoptic nuclei are involved in water metabolism through their connections with the posterior lobe of the hypophysis. This hypothalamiconeurohypophyseal system represents a centrally located autonomic mechanism that exerts its peripheral effects on the kidney by means of the antidiuretic hormone (ADH). *Thalamic* and *striatal* levels of autonomic representation have not been sufficiently investigated; however, the neostriatum is probably concerned in the regulation of certain vegetative functions, as indicated clinically by the autonomic disturbances accompanying lesions in this region. The *cortex* provides another suprasegmental level of integration for sympathetic and parasympathetic functions. It is also a locus for correlation between somatic and vegetative functions, both sensory and motor. The activities of the cardiovascular, gastrointestinal, and many other systems are partially regulated at this highest level. Of considerable theoretical and potentially therapeutic interest are attempts to control blood pressure and other autonomic functions through conditioning initiated at a level of conscious effort (Miller, 1978). Attention has also been focused on the importance of the *limbic* system, which includes the olfactory lobe, hippocampal formation, and the pyriform lobe, in the integration of emotional state with motor and visceral activities (*see* review by MacLean, 1970).

The actions of autonomic drugs on CNS transmission, although not fully understood, are often prominent and may at times overshadow the peripheral effects (*e.g.,* scopolamine, dextroamphetamine, di*iso*propyl phosphorofluoridate, etc.). Likewise, many centrally acting drugs may exert important visceral effects (*e.g.,* phenothiazines, barbiturates, morphine, pentylenetetrazol, etc.) (*see* Chapter 12).

Divisions of the Peripheral Autonomic System. On the efferent or motor side, the autonomic nervous system consists of two large divisions: (1) the *sympathetic* or *thoracolumbar* outflow and (2) the *parasympathetic* or *craniosacral* outflow. Only the briefest outline of those anatomical features necessary for an understanding of the actions of autonomic drugs will be given here.

The arrangement of the principal parts of the peripheral autonomic nervous system is presented schematically in Figure 4-1. As will be discussed subsequently, the neurohumoral transmitter of all preganglionic autonomic fibers, all postganglionic parasympathetic fibers, and a few postganglionic sympathetic fibers is *acetylcholine* (ACh); these so-called *cholinergic fibers* are depicted in *blue.* The *adrenergic fibers,* shown in *red,* comprise the majority of the postganglionic sympathetic fibers; here the transmitter is *norepinephrine (noradrenaline, levarterenol).* The transmitter of the *primary afferent fibers,* shown in *green,* has not been identified conclusively. The terms *cholinergic* and *adrenergic* were proposed originally by Dale to describe neurons that liberate ACh and norepinephrine (at that time, "sympathin"), respectively. Subsequently, Dale (1954) suggested the terms *cholinoceptive* and *adrenoceptive* to denote postjunctional sites that are acted upon by the respective transmitters.

Sympathetic Nervous System. The cells that give rise to the *preganglionic fibers* of this division lie mainly in the intermediolateral columns of the spinal cord and extend from the eighth cervical to the second or third lumbar segment. The axons from these cells are carried in the anterior nerve roots and synapse with neurons lying in sympathetic ganglia outside the cerebrospinal axis. The sympathetic ganglia comprise three groups—paravertebral, prevertebral, and terminal.

The *paravertebral sympathetic ganglia* consist of 22 pairs that lie on either side of the vertebral column to form the lateral chains. The ganglia are connected to each other by nerve trunks and to the spinal nerves by rami communicantes. The *white rami* are restricted to the segments of the thoracolumbar outflow; they carry the preganglionic myelinated fibers that issue from the spinal cord by way of the anterior spinal roots. The *gray rami* arise from the ganglia and carry postganglionic fibers back to the spinal nerves for distribution to sweat glands and pilomotor muscles, and to blood vessels of skeletal muscle and skin. The *prevertebral ganglia* lie in the abdomen and the pelvis near the ventral surface of the bony vertebral column, and consist mainly of the celiac (solar), superior mesenteric, aorticorenal, and inferior mesenteric ganglia. The *terminal ganglia* are few in number, lie near the organs that they innervate, and consist especially of those connected with the urinary bladder and rectum. In addition to the above ganglionic system, there are small *intermediate ganglia,* especially in the thoracolumbar region, that lie outside the conventional vertebral chain. They are variable in number and location, but are usually in close proximity to the communicating rami and to the anterior spinal nerve roots. Since they are not readily accessible to surgical resection, their continued presence after conventional types of sympathectomy may explain some of the poor results after surgery and the apparent return of autonomic functions.

Preganglionic fibers issuing from the spinal cord may synapse with the neurons of more than one sympathetic ganglion by means of collaterals issued en route. Their principal ganglia of termination need not correspond to the original level of issuance of the preganglionic fiber from the spinal cord. Many of the preganglionic fibers from the fifth to the last thoracic segment pass through the paravertebral ganglia and form the *splanchnic nerves.* Most of the splanchnic nerve fibers do not synapse until they reach the celiac ganglion.

Postganglionic fibers issuing from sympathetic ganglia reach all the visceral structures of the thorax, abdomen, head, and neck. The trunk and the limbs are supplied by means of sympathetic fibers in spinal nerves, as previously described. The prevertebral ganglia contain cell bodies the axons of which innervate the glands and the smooth muscles of the abdominal and the pelvic viscera. Many of the upper thoracic sympathetic fibers from the vertebral ganglia form *terminal plexuses,* such as the cardiac, esophageal, and pulmonary. The sympathetic distribution to the head and the neck (vasomotor, pupillodilator, secretory, and pilomotor) is by way of the cervical sympathetic chain and its three ganglia. All postganglionic fibers in this chain arise from cell bodies located in these three ganglia; all preganglionic fibers arise from the upper thoracic segments of the spinal cord, there being no sympathetic fibers that leave the CNS above the first thoracic level.

The *adrenal medulla* and other chromaffin tissue are embryologically and anatomically homologous to sympathetic ganglia, although the adrenal differs in that the principal catecholamine that is released in man and many other species is *epinephrine (adrenaline).* Secretory chromaffin cells originate from the same region of the neural crest as do the sympathetic ganglion cells and are innervated by typical preganglionic fibers.

Parasympathetic Nervous System. This system consists of three outflows of preganglionic fibers from the CNS and their postganglionic connections. The regions of central origin are the midbrain, the medulla oblongata, and the sacral part of the spinal cord. The *midbrain* or tectal outflow consists of fibers arising from the Edinger-Westphal nucleus of the *third* cranial nerve and going to the ciliary ganglion in the orbit. The *medullary* outflow comprises the parasympathetic components of the seventh, ninth, and tenth cranial nerves. The fibers in the *facial* nerve form the chorda tympani, which innervates the ganglia lying on the submaxillary and sublingual glands. They also form the greater superficial petrosal nerve, which innervates the sphenopalatine ganglion. The *glossopharyngeal* autonomic components innervate the otic ganglion. From the aforementioned peripheral ganglia, postganglionic parasympathetic fibers originate that supply the sphincter of the iris, the ciliary muscle, the salivary and lacrimal glands, and the mucous glands of the nose, mouth, and pharynx. These fibers also include vasodilator nerves to the organs mentioned. The *vagus* nerves arise in the medulla and contain preganglionic fibers, most of which do not synapse until they reach the many small ganglia lying directly on or in the viscera of the thorax and abdomen. In the intestinal wall, the vagal fibers terminate around ganglion cells in the plexuses of Auerbach and Meissner. The preganglionic fibers are thus very long and the postganglionic fibers quite short. The vagus nerve in addition carries a far greater number of afferent fibers (but apparently not pain fibers) from the viscera into the medulla; the cell bodies of these fibers lie mainly in the nodose ganglion. The *sacral* outflow consists of axons that arise from cells in the second, third, and fourth segments of the sacral cord and proceed as preganglionic fibers to form the pelvic nerves (nervi erigentes). They synapse in terminal ganglia lying near or within the bladder, rectum, and sexual organs. The vagal and sacral outflows provide motor, secretory, and vasodilator fibers to thoracic, abdominal, and pelvic organs, as indicated in Figure 4–1. The functions of these nerves are subsequently described.

Differences between Sympathetic and Parasympathetic Nerves. The *sympathetic system* is distributed to effectors throughout the body whereas the parasympathetic distribution is much more limited. Furthermore, the *sympathetic fibers* ramify to a much greater extent. A preganglionic sympathetic fiber may traverse a considerable distance of the sympathetic chain and pass through several ganglia before it finally synapses with a postganglionic neuron; also, its terminals make contact with a large number of postganglionic neurons. In some ganglia, the ratio of preganglionic axons to ganglion cells may be 1:20 or more. In this manner, a diffuse discharge of the sympathetic system is possible. In addition, there is an overlapping of synaptic innervation so that one ganglion cell is supplied by several preganglionic fibers.

The *parasympathetic system,* on the other hand, has its terminal ganglia very near to the organs innervated and thus is more discrete and limited in its discharge of impulses. In some organs, there appears to be a 1:1 relationship between the number of preganglionic and postganglionic fibers. On the other hand, the ratio of preganglionic vagal fibers to ganglion cells in Auerbach's plexus has been estimated as 1:8000. Hence, this distinction between the two systems does not apply to all sites.

Details of Innervation. The types and structures of nerve terminals within the CNS are described in Chapter 12. The axon of each somatic *motoneuron* divides into many branches, each of which innervates a single muscle fiber, so that more than 100 muscle fibers may be supplied by one motoneuron to form a *motor unit.* At each neuromuscular junction, or *motor endplate,* the axonal terminal loses its myelin sheath and forms a terminal arborization that lies in an invagination of the sarcoplasmic membrane. Mitochondria and a collection of synaptic vesicles are concentrated near the membrane.

The terminations of the *postganglionic autonomic fibers* at smooth muscle and gland cells show certain distinct differences from the foregoing pattern. In most autonomic effector organs, the innervation forms a rich plexus or terminal reticulum. The earlier literature has been reviewed critically by Hillarp (1959), according to whose interpretation, supported by subsequent histochemical and electron microscopic observations, the terminal reticulum is a triad. This consists of the final ramifications of the postganglionic sympathetic (adrenergic), parasympathetic (cholinergic), and visceral afferent fibers, all of which are enclosed within a frequently interrupted sheath of satellite or Schwann cells. At these interruptions, varicosities packed with vesicles are seen in the efferent fibers. Such varicosities occur repeatedly along the course of the ramifications of the axon, and, at these sites, there are no intervening structures between the varicosity and the cell that is so innervated. However, it is not certain whether every effector cell receives its own autonomic innervation in most organs. There is apparently wide variation in the distance between the nerve varicosities and smooth muscle fibers, ranging from 200 Å in the vas deferens to 10,000 Å in certain blood vessels. In some instances, nerve fibers appear actually to penetrate smooth muscle fibers (*see* review by Burnstock and Iwayama, 1971).

Between the smooth muscle fibers themselves, "protoplasmic bridges" have been described, which are believed to permit the conduction of impulses from cell to cell without the intervention of nervous elements. By such a mechanism, the direct actions of neurohumoral transmitters or drugs on a limited portion of the total cell population could be extended indirectly to large numbers of effector cells.

A structure long favored by physiologists as a relatively simple model for the study of synaptic transmission, the superior cervical *sympathetic ganglion* of the cat, has been shown to be extremely complex, both anatomically (Elfvin, 1963a, 1963b) and pharmacologically (Chapter 10). The preganglionic fibers lose their myelin sheaths, and divide repeatedly into a vast number of end fibers with diameters ranging from 0.1 to 0.3 μm; except at points of synaptic contact, they retain their satellite-cell sheaths. The vast majority of synapses are axodendritic. Apparently, a given axonal terminal may synapse with one or more dendritic processes at several points, as in the case of the innervation of smooth muscle described above. It is of interest that there are points of apparently intimate contact between neighboring ganglion cells that are dendrodendritic and dendrosomatic; the physiological significance of such contacts is not known. Additional elements of yet-unknown physiological significance that are present in varying numbers in sympathetic ganglia are small, catecholamine-containing chromaffin cells, some of which appear to make synaptic

Table 4-1. RESPONSES OF EFFECTOR ORGANS TO AUTONOMIC NERVE IMPULSES

EFFECTOR ORGANS	ADRENERGIC IMPULSES[1]		CHOLINERGIC IMPULSES[1]
	Receptor Type	Responses[2]	Responses[2]
Eye			
Radial muscle, iris	α	Contraction (mydriasis) + +	
Sphincter muscle, iris		———	Contraction (miosis) + + +
Ciliary muscle	β	Relaxation for far vision +	Contraction for near vision + + +
Heart			
S-A node	β_1	Increase in heart rate + +	Decrease in heart rate; vagal arrest + + +
Atria	β_1	Increase in contractility and conduction velocity + +	Decrease in contractility, and (usually) increase in conduction velocity + +
A-V node	β_1	Increase in automaticity and conduction velocity + +	Decrease in conduction velocity; A-V block + + +
His-Purkinje system	β_1	Increase in automaticity and conduction velocity + + +	Little effect
Ventricles	β_1	Increase in contractility, conduction velocity, automaticity, and rate of idioventricular pacemakers + + +	Slight decrease in contractility claimed by some
Arterioles			
Coronary	α,β_2	Constriction +; dilatation[3] + +	Dilatation ±
Skin and mucosa	α	Constriction + + +	Dilatation[4]
Skeletal muscle	α,β_2	Constriction + +; dilatation[3,5] + +	Dilatation[6] +
Cerebral	α	Constriction (slight)	Dilatation[4]
Pulmonary	α,β_2	Constriction +; dilatation[3]	Dilatation[4]
Abdominal viscera; renal	α,β_2	Constriction + + +; dilatation[5] +	———
Salivary glands	α	Constriction + + +	Dilatation + +
Veins (Systemic)	α,β_2	Constriction + +; dilatation + +	———
Lung			
Bronchial muscle	β_2	Relaxation +	Contraction + +
Bronchial glands	?	Inhibition (?)	Stimulation + + +
Stomach			
Motility and tone	α_2,β_2	Decrease (usually)[7] +	Increase + + +
Sphincters	α	Contraction (usually) +	Relaxation (usually) +
Secretion		Inhibition (?)	Stimulation + + +
Intestine			
Motility and tone	α_2,β_2	Decrease[7] +	Increase + + +
Sphincters	α	Contraction (usually) +	Relaxation (usually) +
Secretion		Inhibition (?)	Stimulation + +
Gallbladder and Ducts		Relaxation +	Contraction +
Kidney	β_2	Renin secretion + +	———
Urinary Bladder			
Detrusor	β	Relaxation (usually) +	Contraction + + +
Trigone and sphincter	α	Contraction + +	Relaxation + +
Ureter			
Motility and tone	α	Increase (usually)	Increase (?)
Uterus	α,β_2	Pregnant: contraction (α); nonpregnant: relaxation (β)	Variable[8]
Sex Organs, Male	α	Ejaculation + + +	Erection + + +
Skin			
Pilomotor muscles	α	Contraction + +	———
Sweat glands	α	Localized secretion[9] +	Generalized secretion + + +
Spleen Capsule	α,β_2	Contraction + + +; relaxation +	———
Adrenal Medulla		———	Secretion of epinephrine and norepinephrine

Table 4-1. RESPONSES OF EFFECTOR ORGANS TO AUTONOMIC NERVE IMPULSES (Continued)

| EFFECTOR ORGANS | ADRENERGIC IMPULSES[1] | | CHOLINERGIC IMPULSES[1] |
	Receptor Type	*Responses*[2]	*Responses*[2]
Liver	α,β_2	Glycogenolysis, gluconeogenesis[10] + + +	Glycogen synthesis +
Pancreas			
Acini	α	Decreased secretion +	Secretion + +
Islets (β cells)	α	Decreased secretion + + +	———
	β_2	Increased secretion +	———
Fat Cells	α,β_1	Lipolysis[10] + + +	———
Salivary Glands	α	Potassium and water secretion +	Potassium and water secretion + + +
	β	Amylase secretion +	
Lacrimal Glands		———	Secretion + + +
Nasopharyngeal Glands		———	Secretion + +
Pineal Gland	β	Melatonin synthesis	———

[1] The anatomical classes of adrenergic and cholinergic nerve fibers are described on page 57 and depicted in Figure 4–1 in red and blue, respectively. A long dash signifies no known functional innervation.

[2] Responses are designated 1 + to 3 + to provide an approximate indication of the importance of adrenergic and cholinergic nerve activity in the control of the various organs and functions listed.

[3] Dilatation predominates *in situ* due to metabolic autoregulatory phenomena.

[4] Cholinergic vasodilatation at these sites is of questionable physiological significance.

[5] Over the usual concentration range of physiologically released, circulating epinephrine, β-receptor response (vasodilatation) predominates in blood vessels of skeletal muscle and liver; α-receptor response (vasoconstriction), in blood vessels of other abdominal viscera. The renal and mesenteric vessels also contain specific dopaminergic receptors, activation of which causes dilatation, but their physiological significance has not been established (*see* review by Goldberg *et al.*, 1978).

[6] Sympathetic cholinergic system causes vasodilatation in skeletal muscle, but this is not involved in most physiological responses.

[7] It has been proposed that adrenergic fibers terminate at inhibitory β receptors on smooth muscle fibers, and at inhibitory α receptors on parasympathetic cholinergic (excitatory) ganglion cells of Auerbach's plexus.

[8] Depends on stage of menstrual cycle, amount of circulating estrogen and progesterone, and other factors.

[9] Palms of hands and some other sites ("adrenergic sweating").

[10] There is significant variation among species in the type of receptor that mediates certain metabolic responses.

contact with ganglion cells. Others are clustered predominantly around blood vessels (*see* Elfvin, 1971; Eränkö and Eränkö, 1971).

Responses of Effector Organs to Autonomic Nerve Impulses. A clear understanding of the response of the various effector organs to autonomic nerve impulses makes it possible to anticipate the actions of drugs that mimic or inhibit the actions of these nerves. In general, the sympathetic and parasympathetic systems are viewed as physiological antagonists. If one system inhibits a certain function, the other usually augments that function. Most viscera are innervated by both divisions of the autonomic nervous system, and the level of activity at any one moment represents the integration of influences of the two components. The action of one system is most easily demonstrated by surgical removal or drug-induced paralysis of the opposing system. However, despite the conventional concept of antagonism between the two portions of the autonomic nervous

system, their activities on specific structures may be either different and independent or integrated and interdependent. For example, the effects of sympathetic and parasympathetic stimulation of the heart and the iris follow a highly integrated pattern of antagonism (*see* Higgins *et al.*, 1973). Their actions on male sexual organs are complementary and are integrated to promote sexual function. The control of blood pressure is probably almost entirely due to sympathetic control of arteriolar resistance. The effects of stimulating the sympathetic (adrenergic) and parasympathetic (cholinergic) nerves to various organs, visceral structures, and effector cells are summarized in Table 4–1.

General Functions of the Autonomic Nervous System. The integrating action of the autonomic nervous system is of vital importance for the well-being of the organism. In general, the autonomic nervous system regulates the activities of structures that are not under voluntary control and that, as a rule, function below the level of consciousness. Thus, respiration, circulation, digestion, body temperature, metabolism, sweating, and the secretions of certain endocrine glands are regulated, in part or entirely, by the autonomic nervous system and its central connections. As Claude Bernard (1878–1879) and Cannon (1929, 1932) have emphasized, the constancy of the internal environment of the organism is to a large extent controlled by the vegetative, or autonomic, nervous system.

The sympathetic and parasympathetic systems have contrasting functions in regulating the internal environment. The *sympathetic system* and its associated adrenal medulla are not essential to life, and animals completely deprived of the sympathoadrenal system can continue a fairly normal existence within the sheltered confines of the laboratory. Under circumstances of stress, however, the lack of the sympathoadrenal functions becomes evident. Body temperature cannot be regulated when environmental temperature varies; the concentration of glucose in blood does not rise in response to urgent need; compensatory vascular responses to hemorrhage, oxygen want, excitement, and work are lacking; resistance to fatigue is lessened; sympathetic components of instinctive reactions to fright and danger are lost; pilomotor responses are absent; and other serious deficiencies in the protective forces of the body are discernible.

The *sympathetic system* is normally active at all times, the degree of activity varying from moment to moment and from organ to organ; in this manner, the finer adjustments to a constantly changing environment are accomplished. The *sympathoadrenal system* can also discharge as a unit. This occurs especially during rage and fright, under which circumstances sympathetically innervated structures over the entire body are affected simultaneously. The heart rate is accelerated; the blood pressure rises; red blood cells are poured into the circulation from the spleen (in certain species); the blood is shifted from the skin and splanchnic bed to the skeletal muscles; the concentration of blood glucose rises; the bronchioles and pupils dilate; and, on the whole, the organism is better prepared for "fight or flight." Many of these effects result primarily from, or are reinforced by, the actions of epinephrine, secreted by the adrenal medulla (*see* below).

The *parasympathetic system* is organized mainly for discrete and localized discharge and not for mass responses. It is concerned primarily with the functions of conservation and restoration of energy rather than with the expenditure of energy. It slows the heart rate, lowers the blood pressure, stimulates the gastrointestinal movements and secretions, aids absorption of nutrients, protects the retina from excessive light, and empties the urinary bladder and rectum. No useful purpose would be served in the body if the parasympathetic nerves all discharged at once.

NEUROHUMORAL TRANSMISSION

Nerve impulses elicit responses in smooth, cardiac, and skeletal muscles, exocrine glands, and postsynaptic neurons through liberation of specific chemical substances. The steps involved and the evidence for them will be outlined in some detail because the concept of chemical mediation of nerve impulses profoundly affects our knowledge of the mechanism of action of drugs at these sites.

HISTORICAL ASPECTS

The earliest concrete proposal of a neurohumoral mechanism was made shortly after the turn of the present century. Lewandowsky (1898) and Langley (1901) noted independently the similarity between the effects of injection of extracts of the adrenal gland and stimulation of sympathetic nerves. A few years later, in 1905, T. R. Elliott, while a student at Cambridge, England, extended these observations and postulated that sympathetic nerve impulses release minute amounts of an epinephrine-like substance in immediate contact with effector cells. He considered this substance to be the chemical step in the process of transmission. He also noted that long after sympathetic nerves had degenerated, the effector organs still responded characteristically to the hormone of the adrenal medulla. In 1905, Langley suggested that effector cells have excitatory and inhibitory "receptive substances," and that the response to epinephrine depended on which type of substance was present. In 1907, Dixon was so impressed by the correspondence between the effects of the alkaloid muscarine and the responses to vagal stimulation that he advanced the important idea that the vagus nerve liberated a muscarine-like substance that acted as a chemical transmitter of its impulses. In the same year, Reid Hunt announced his studies of acetylcholine (ACh) and other choline esters. In 1914, Dale thoroughly reinvestigated the pharmacological properties of ACh. He was so intrigued with the remarkable fidelity with which this drug reproduced the responses to stimulation of parasympathetic nerves that he introduced the term *parasympathomimetic* to characterize its effects. Dale also noted the brief duration of the action of this chemical and proposed that an esterase in the tissues rapidly splits ACh to acetic acid and choline, the latter being a much less potent compound.

The brilliant researches of Otto Loewi, begun in the winter of 1921, established the first real proof of the chemical mediation of nerve impulses by the peripheral release of specific chemical agents. Loewi's studies deserve description because the technic employed is basic to investigations in this field. He stimulated the vagus nerve of a perfused (donor) frog heart and allowed the perfusion fluid to come in contact with a second (recipient) frog heart used as a test object. A substance was liberated from the first organ that slowed the rate of the second. Loewi referred to this chemical substance as *Vagusstoff* ("vagus-substance"; parasympathin); subsequently, Loewi and Navratil (1926) presented evidence for its identification as *ACh*. Loewi also discovered that an accelerator substance similar to epinephrine was liberated into the perfusion fluid in summer, when the action of the sympathetic fibers in the frog's vagus, a mixed nerve, predominated over that of the inhibitory fibers. Loewi's discoveries were eventually confirmed and are now universally accepted. The essential features of the experiments are shown in Figure 4–2, which illustrates Bain's (1932) modification of Loewi's technic.

Evidence that the cardiac vagus-substance is also ACh in mammals was obtained in 1933 by Feldberg and Krayer. Many other investigations established quite conclusively that a chemical mediator, ACh, is instrumental in the transmission of parasympathetic impulses in mammals to other structures, including the iris, salivary glands, stomach, and small intestine.

In addition to its role as the neurohumoral transmitter of all postganglionic parasympathetic fibers and of a few postganglionic sympathetic fibers, such as those to the sweat glands and the sympathetic vasodilator fibers, ACh has been shown to have this transmitter function in three additional classes of nerves: (1) preganglionic fibers of both the sympathetic and the parasympathetic systems, (2) motor nerves to skeletal muscle, and (3) certain neurons within the CNS (*see* Feldberg, 1945, for early references). Subsequent evidence for this is discussed below.

Mention has already been made of Loewi's discovery of an accelerator substance released from frog hearts under certain conditions. In the same year, Cannon and Uridil (1921) reported that the liver, upon stimulation of the sympathetic hepatic nerves, released an epinephrine-like substance that in-

creased the blood pressure and the heart rate but did not dilate the pupil. Subsequent experiments, mainly by Cannon and coworkers, firmly established that this substance is the chemical mediator liberated by sympathetic nerve impulses at neuroeffector junctions. The mediator was originally called "sympathin" by Cannon in order to avoid premature implications regarding its chemical structure. The progressive steps by which Cannon and associates developed the concept of "sympathin" can be found in the monograph by Cannon and Rosenblueth (1937).

In many of its pharmacological and chemical properties, Cannon's "sympathin" closely resembled epinephrine, but the two substances differed in certain important respects. When epinephrine is injected into the body, it elicits both excitatory and inhibitory effects. Thus, it accelerates the rate of the heart but simultaneously dilates certain vascular beds while constricting others. In contrast, the excitatory effects of "sympathin" could be elicited separately. As early as 1910, Barger and Dale noted that the effects of sympathetic nerve stimulation were more closely reproduced by the injection of sympathomimetic primary amines than by that of epinephrine or other secondary amines. The possibility that demethylated epinephrine (*norepinephrine, levarterenol, noradrenaline*) might be "sympathin" had been repeatedly advanced by Z. M. Bacq and others, but definitive evidence for its role as the sympathetic nerve mediator was not obtained until specific chemical and biological assay methods were developed for the *quantitative* determination of small amounts of sympathomimetic amines in extracts of tissues and body fluids. Euler in 1946 found that the sympathomimetic substance in highly purified extracts of sympathetic nerves and effector organs bore

Figure 4–2. *Bain's modification of Loewi's technic for demonstrating the release of the vagus-substance upon stimulation of the cardiac nerve to the frog's heart.*

The donor heart (*D*) with nerves intact is perfused at constant pressure with a balanced salt solution. The perfusion fluid then passes to the isolated recipient heart (*R*). Cardiac contractions are recorded by means of writing levers; time (*T*), in 5-second intervals. The vagus fibers to the donor heart are stimulated (*S*) for 40 seconds, and the donor heart is quickly arrested. Slowing of the recipient heart is apparent within 15 seconds after arrest of the donor heart, and asystole occurs shortly thereafter. (After Bain, 1932. Courtesy of the *Quarterly Journal of Experimental Physiology and Cognate Medical Sciences* and Sir Edward Sharpey-Schafer's trustees.)

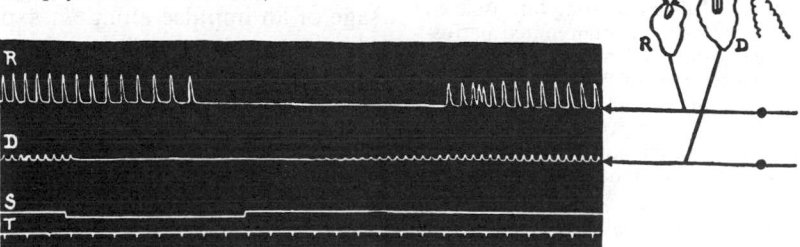

a strong resemblance to norepinephrine by all criteria used. He proposed that the sympathetic transmitter is norepinephrine. Numerous workers have confirmed and extended these observations, and all available evidence indicates that *norepinephrine* is the predominant sympathomimetic substance in postganglionic sympathetic nerves and is the adrenergic mediator liberated by their stimulation. (*See* review by Euler, 1972a.) Norepinephrine, its immediate precursor, dopamine, and epinephrine are also neurohumoral transmitters in the CNS. Their significance in the action of centrally acting drugs is discussed in Chapter 12.

EVIDENCE FOR NEUROHUMORAL TRANSMISSION

The concept of neurohumoral transmission was first developed primarily to explain observations relating to the transmission of impulses from postganglionic autonomic fibers to effector cells. The general lines of evidence in its support have included: (1) demonstration of the presence of a physiologically active compound, and of the enzymes necessary for its synthesis and breakdown, at appropriate sites; (2) recovery of the compound from the perfusate of an innervated structure during periods of nerve stimulation, but not (or in greatly reduced amounts) in the absence of stimulation; (3) demonstration that the compound, when administered appropriately, is capable of producing responses identical with those to nerve stimulation; and (4) demonstration that the responses to nerve stimulation and to the administered compound are modified in the same manner by various drugs. With the fulfillment of the foregoing criteria to varying degrees at several autonomic effector organs, the concept soon gained practically unanimous acceptance for these sites.

General acceptance of neurohumoral, rather than electrogenic, transmission at autonomic ganglia and the neuromuscular junction of skeletal muscle was withheld for a considerable period, chiefly for two reasons: (1) the extremely rapid time factors involved, in contrast to those at autonomic effector sites; and (2) discrepancies between the amount of the putative transmitter, ACh, recovered during nerve stimulation and that required to produce characteristic responses. Both objections have, for the most part, been answered satisfactorily through the development of modern technics of intracellular recording and microiontophoretic application of drugs, as will be described. The anatomical complexities and cellular barriers of the CNS are such that it is exceedingly difficult to stimulate isolated fiber tracts to, and recover uncontaminated perfusates from, selected groups of neurons. However, studies of individual neurons of the spinal cord and brain, particularly in the brilliant investigations of Eccles and his colleagues, have provided evidence of central neurohumoral transmission that has become increasingly convincing (*see* monographs by Eccles, 1964, 1973).

One important feature of junctional transmission that supports the concept of a neurohumoral mechanism is *the irreducible latent period between the arrival of an impulse at the axonal terminal and the appearance of the postjunctional potential.* Physiologists had long recognized a synaptic delay, sometimes as brief as a fraction of a millisecond, that could not be accounted for in terms of known conduction velocities in the presynaptic or postsynaptic neurons. However, there remained the possible explanation that conduction might be considerably slowed in the fine preterminal axonal branches. This limitation was overcome in an investigation of the giant synapse of the squid. Bullock and Hagiwara (1957) inserted fine-recording micropipettes into the presynaptic and postsynaptic fibers and simultaneously recorded from both following presynaptic stimulation. There was invariably a delay of 0.5 to 2.0 milliseconds, depending upon the temperature, between the arrival of the impulse at the presynaptic electrode and the recording of postsynaptic activity; furthermore, depolarization or hyperpolarization of either the presynaptic or the postsynaptic element induced no detectable change in the potential of the other (Hagiwara and Tasaki, 1958). These findings are consistent only with the chemical mediation of synaptic transmission and not with the direct spread of electrical current across the synapse.

In further support of neurohumoral transmission as a general phenomenon is the considerable indirect evidence indicating that most postsynaptic and postjunctional membranes are electrically inexcitable. *See* the reviews by Grundfest (1957) and Eccles (1964) for documentation and critical analysis.

There are instances where synaptic transmission undoubtedly does occur by the direct spread of current across the junction. Such electrotonic transmission of information across "gap junctions" occurs in the CNS (Schmitt *et al.*, 1976), and it might also have effects on synchronous firing of peripheral autonomic neurons.

STEPS INVOLVED IN NEUROHUMORAL TRANSMISSION

The sequence of events involved in neurohumoral transmission is of particular importance pharmacologically, since the actions of a great number of drugs, particularly those affecting the autonomic nervous system, can be related directly to the individual steps. In conformity with the usual convention, the term *conduction* will be reserved for the passage of an impulse along an axon or muscle fiber; *transmission* refers to the passage of an impulse across a synaptic or neuroeffector junction. With the exception of the local anesthetics, which are infiltrated in high concentrations in the immediate vicinity of nerve trunks, very few drugs modify axonal conduction in the doses employed therapeutically. Hence, this process will be described only briefly in order to introduce its role in triggering the first step in transmission.

Axonal Conduction. The most acceptable present hypothesis of conduction stems largely from the investigative work of Hodgkin and Huxley (1952).

At rest, the interior of the typical mammalian axon is approximately 70 mV negative to the exterior. The *resting potential* is essentially a *diffusion potential,* based chiefly on the 30- to 50-fold higher concentration of potassium ion in the axoplasm as compared with the extracellular fluid, and the relatively high permeability of the resting axonal membrane to potassium ions. Sodium and chloride ions are present in higher concentrations in the extracellular fluid than in the axoplasm, but their concentration gradients across the membrane are somewhat lower than that of potassium, and the axonal membrane at rest is considerably less permeable to these ions; hence their contribution to the resting potential is relatively minor. These ionic gradients are maintained by an energy-dependent active-transport or pump mechanism, which involves an adenosine triphosphatase (ATPase) activated by sodium at the inner and by potassium at the outer surface of the membrane (*see* Armstrong, 1974; Grundfest, 1975). At some sites, an electrogenic sodium pump may also contribute to the net resting potential (Castecls *et al.,* 1971).

In response to a stimulus above the threshold level, a nerve *action potential* (AP) or nerve impulse is initiated at a local region of the membrane. This is detectable first by a rapid deflection of the internal resting potential from its negative value toward zero, and continuing uninterruptedly to a positive overshoot. This local reversal of the membrane potential is due to a sudden, selective increase in the permeability of the membrane to *sodium* ions, which flow rapidly inward in the direction of their concentration gradient. Repolarization of the membrane follows immediately and results from the rapid replacement of this change by one of increased permeability to *potassium.* The transmembrane ionic currents produce local circuit currents around the axon. By such currents, adjacent inactive regions of the axon are activated, and excitation of the next excitable portion of the axonal membrane occurs. This brings about the propagation of the AP. The AP is therefore conducted without decrement along the axon. The region that has just been active remains momentarily in a refractory state. In myelinated fibers, permeability changes occur only at the nodes of Ranvier, thus causing a rapidly progressing type of jumping, or saltatory, conduction. The puffer fish poison, *tetrodotoxin,* is one of the few compounds that selectively block axonal conduction; it does so by preventing the increase in permeability to sodium ion associated with the rising phase of the AP (Kao, 1966). In contrast, *batrachotoxin,* an extremely potent steroidal alkaloid secreted by a South American frog, produces paralysis through a selective increase

in sodium permeability, which induces a persistent depolarization (Albuquerque *et al.,* 1973). The physiological and pharmacological aspects of axonal conduction have been reviewed in detail by Cole (1968) and Naharashi (1975).

Junctional Transmission. The arrival of the action potential (AP) at the axonal terminals initiates a series of events that effect the neurohumoral transmission of an excitatory or inhibitory impulse across the synapse or neuroeffector junction (*see* reviews by Eccles, 1964, 1973; Katz, 1966; Krnjević, 1974). These events, diagramed in Figure 4–3, are as follows:

1. *Release of the Transmitter.* The neurohumoral transmitters are probably synthesized in the region of the axonal terminals and stored there within the synaptic vesicles (*see* below), either in highly concentrated ionic form, as in the case of ACh, or as a readily dissociable complex or salt, as that of norepinephrine with adenosine triphosphate (ATP) and a specific protein. During the resting state, there is a continual, slow release of isolated quanta of the transmitter, ordinarily insufficient to cause initiation of a propagated impulse at the postjunctional site. However, this release of small amounts of transmitter produces electrical responses at the postjunctional membrane (miniature end-plate potentials, mepps) that are associated with the maintenance of physiological responsiveness of the effector organ (*see* Hall, 1972; Rang, 1975). The AP causes the synchronous release of several hundred quanta. The depolarization of the axonal terminal triggers this process; however, the intermediate steps are uncertain. One step is the influx of calcium ion, which enters the axonal cytoplasm and is believed to promote fusion of the vesicular and axoplasmic membranes. The contents of the vesicles are then discharged to the exterior by a process termed *exocytosis.* Other components of the vesicle, including enzymes and other proteins, are also discharged. Measurement of these components may provide useful information about the intensity and duration of prejunctional activity.

2. *Combination of the Transmitter with Postjunctional Receptors and Production of the Postjunctional Potential.* The transmitter diffuses across the synaptic or junctional

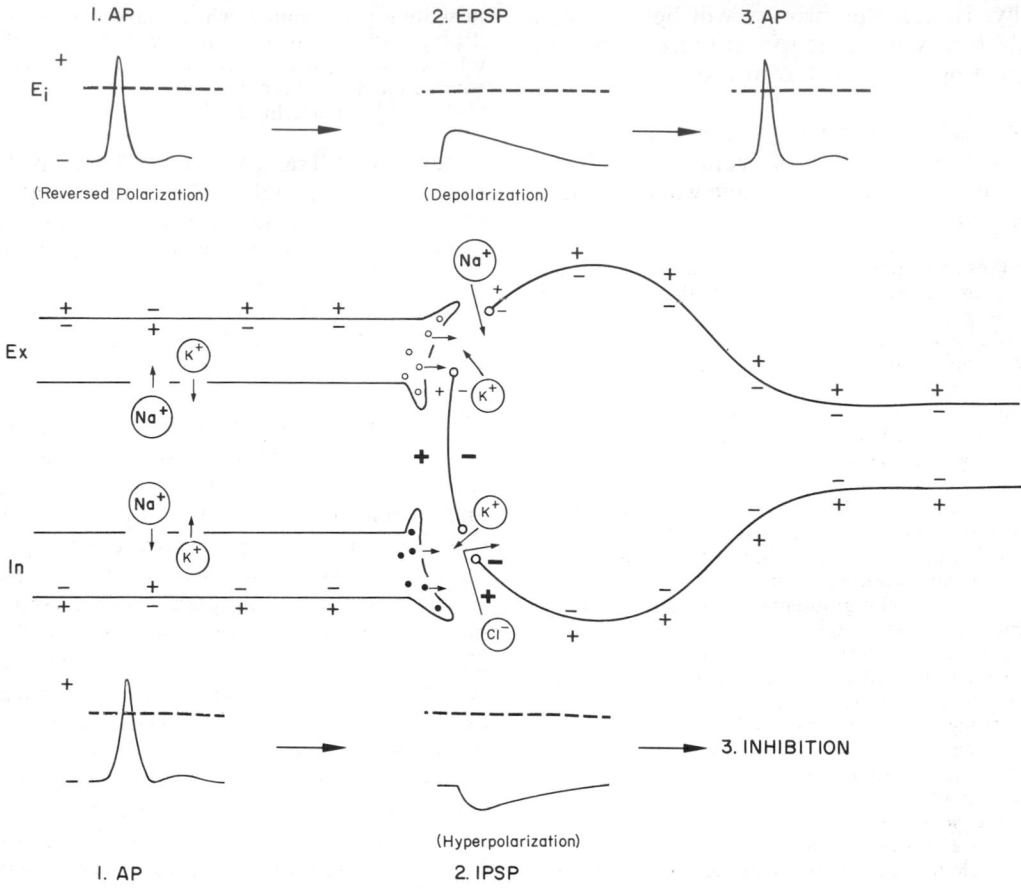

Figure 4-3. *Steps involved in excitatory* (Ex) *and inhibitory* (In) *neurohumoral transmission.*

1. The nerve action potential (AP), consisting in a self-propagated *reversal* of negativity (the internal potential, E_i, goes from a negative value, through zero potential, indicated by the broken line, to a positive value) of the axonal membrane, arrives at the presynaptic terminal and causes release of the excitatory (o) or inhibitory (●) transmitter.

2. Combination of the excitatory transmitter with postsynaptic receptors produces a localized depolarization, the excitatory postsynaptic potential (EPSP), through an increase in ionic permeability. The inhibitory transmitter causes a selective increase in permeability to the smaller ions (K^+ and Cl^-), resulting in a localized hyperpolarization, the inhibitory postsynaptic potential (IPSP).

3. The EPSP initiates a conducted AP in the postsynaptic neuron; this can, however, be prevented by the hyperpolarization induced by a concurrent IPSP.

The transmitter is dissipated by enzymatic destruction, by re-uptake into the presynaptic terminal or adjacent glial cells, or by diffusion. (Modified from Eccles, 1964, 1973; Katz, 1966; others.)

cleft, a distance of 100 to 500 Å, and combines with specialized macromolecular receptors on the postjunctional membrane; this results generally in a localized, nonpropagated increase in the ionic permeability, or conductance, of the membrane. With certain exceptions, noted below, either of two types of permeability change can occur: (1) a generalized increase in permeability to all types of ions, resulting in a localized depolarization of the membrane, that is, an *excitatory postsynaptic potential* (EPSP); or (2) a selective increase in permeability to only the smaller ions (*e.g.,* potassium and chloride), resulting in stabilization or actual hyperpolarization of the membrane, which constitutes an *inhibitory postsynaptic potential* (IPSP).

It should be emphasized that the potential

changes associated with the EPSP and IPSP at most sites are the results of passive flows of extracellular and intracellular ions down their concentration gradients. The changes in ionic permeability that cause these potential changes are specifically regulated by the specialized postjunctional receptors for the neurotransmitter that initiates the response (*see* Chapter 2 and the remainder of this section). Under normal conditions, these receptors may be highly localized on the effector-cell surface or distributed in an apparently random fashion.

3. *Initiation of Postjunctional Activity.* If an EPSP exceeds a certain threshold value, it initiates a propagated AP in a postsynaptic neuron or a muscle AP in most skeletal muscles or in cardiac muscle. In certain types of tonic skeletal muscle and in smooth muscle, in which propagated impulses do not occur, an EPSP initiates a localized contractile response; in gland cells, it initiates secretion. An IPSP will tend to oppose excitatory potentials initiated by other neuronal sources at the same time and site; whether a propagated impulse or other response ensues will depend on the algebraic sum of all these effects. In the CNS, and possibly at other sites, inhibition can also result from a relatively prolonged depolarizing action of a transmitter on presynaptic terminals, which in turn brings about a reduction in the amount of transmitter released by the terminals in response to nerve impulses (Eccles, 1964). This phenomenon of *presynaptic inhibition* has provided a tentative explanation of the mechanism of action of some centrally acting drugs.

4. *Destruction or Dissipation of the Transmitter.* When impulses can be transmitted across junctions at frequencies ranging from a few up to several hundred per second, it is obvious that there must be some efficient means of disposing of the transmitter following each impulse. At most cholinergic junctions, a highly specialized enzyme, *acetylcholinesterase* (AChE), is available for this function. It has been calculated that diffusion may account for termination of the action of ACh at some synapses. It is unlikely that any particular enzyme is directly involved in terminating the action of the adrenergic transmitter at the immediate receptor site in most organs; this is probably effected by a combination of re-uptake of most of the released norepinephrine by the axonal terminals, and simple diffusion (*see* Iversen, 1967, 1975; Moran, 1975; Cooper *et al.*, 1978).

5. *Nonelectrogenic Functions.* The continual, quantal release of neurotransmitters in amounts not sufficient to elicit a postjunctional response is probably important in the transjunctional control of neurotransmitter action. Not only the activity or synthesis of enzymes involved in the synthesis and inactivation of neurotransmitters but also the availability of receptors are probably controlled by *trophic* actions of neurotransmitters. This is especially well documented for the neuromuscular junction and neuroeffector junctions in the sympathetic nervous system (*see* Thesleff, 1970, 1973; Rang, 1975; Bullock *et al.*, 1977).

CHOLINERGIC TRANSMISSION

In close association with the neurotransmitter, acetylcholine (ACh), are two enzymes, *choline acetyltransferase* and *acetylcholinesterase* (AChE), which are involved in its synthesis and hydrolysis, respectively.

Choline Acetyltransferase (Choline Acetylase). This enzyme, a basic protein with a molecular weight of approximately 65,000, was first studied in cell-free extracts of the electric organ of the Amazonian electric eel, *Electrophorus electricus*. It has been partially purified from this and other sources by Nachmansohn and associates, who have played the major role in elucidating its properties (*see* Nachmansohn, 1959). Choline acetyltransferase catalyzes the final step in the synthesis of ACh—the acetylation of choline with acetyl coenzyme A (CoA) (*see* Hebb, 1972; Collier *et al.*, 1976; Rossier, 1977).

Acetyl CoA for this reaction is derived from pyruvate via the multistep pyruvate dehydrogenase reaction or is synthesized by acetate thiokinase, which catalyzes the reaction of acetate with ATP to form an enzyme-bound acyladenylate (acetyl AMP). In the presence of CoA, transacetylation and synthesis of acetyl CoA proceed.

Tremendous variations in choline acetyltransferase activity occur in mammalian nerve tissue. In general, high concentrations have been reported for peripheral cholinergic nerves (*e.g.*, ventral spinal roots, superior cervical ganglion) and thousandfold lower values are detected in afferent nerves (*e.g.*, dorsal spinal roots, optic nerve). Similar differences have been found by ultramicro determination of the concentrations of choline acetyltransferase in single cholinergic and noncholinergic neurons of autonomic ganglia (Buckley *et al.,* 1967). Various regions of the CNS also differ markedly in their ability to synthesize ACh (*see* Nachmansohn, 1959; Hebb, 1963). It is of interest that the human placenta, which is devoid of nervous tissue, also contains a high concentration of the enzyme (Kato, 1960).

Choline acetyltransferase, like other protein constituents of the neuron, is synthesized within the perikaryon and is then transported along the length of the axon to its terminal. The synaptic vesicles may be formed at the terminal, rather than in the perikaryon. In addition to the vesicles, the axonal terminals contain a large number of mitochondria, where acetyl CoA is synthesized as described. Choline is taken up from the extracellular fluid into the axoplasm by active transport. The final step in the synthesis probably occurs within the cytoplasm, following which most of the ACh is sequestered within the synaptic vesicles (*see* Potter, 1972). Moderately potent, selective inhibitors of choline acetyltransferase are available (Cavallito *et al.,* 1969). The storage and release of ACh are discussed below.

Acetylcholinesterase. For ACh to serve as the neurohumoral agent in peripheral junctional transmission, the ester must be removed or inactivated within the time limits imposed by the response characteristics of visceral neuroeffector junctions, motor endplates, and various types of neurons. These limits range from over a second to less than a millisecond. At the latter extreme, the mediator must be destroyed almost immediately—with "flashlike suddenness," as Dale has expressed it. Body fluids and tissues contain enzymes, first called *choline esterase,* that rapidly hydrolyze ACh to choline and acetic acid. The choline produced is pharmacologically weak in comparison with its acetylated precursor; for example, it possesses only 10^{-5} the vasodepressor potency of ACh. The general characteristics and distribution of acetylcholinesterase are discussed below; a more complete account of its molecular structure and its reactions with ACh and various inhibitors is presented in Chapter 6.

Acetylcholinesterase (AChE; also known as specific or true ChE) occurs in neurons, at the neuromuscular junction, and in certain other tissues (*see* below); it is responsible for the hydrolysis of ACh released in the process of cholinergic transmission. *Butyrocholinesterase* (BuChE; also known as cholinesterase, ChE, serum esterase, or pseudo-ChE) is present in various types of glial or satellite cells but only to a limited extent in neuronal elements of the

central and peripheral nervous systems, and in the plasma, liver, and other organs; its physiological function is unknown. Although both types of enzyme can hydrolyze ACh and certain other aliphatic and aromatic esters and as a group are inhibited selectively by physostigmine, they can be distinguished by several criteria.

The main reason for distinguishing between AChE and BuChE is that practically all the pharmacological effects of the anti-ChE agents (Chapter 6) are due to the inhibition of the AChE, with the consequent accumulation of endogenous ACh; inhibition of BuChE at most sites produces no apparent functional derangement.

AChE hydrolyzes ACh at a greater velocity than any other choline ester; it hydrolyzes acetyl-β-methylcholine (methacholine), but not benzoylcholine; and it is inhibited selectively by low concentrations of several *bis*-quaternary ammonium bases and by other agents. BuChE, on the other hand, exhibits a maximal velocity of hydrolysis with butyrylcholine as substrate; it hydrolyzes benzoylcholine, but not methacholine; and it is more sensitive than AChE to inhibition by a number of organophosphorus agents, such as di*iso*propyl phosphorofluoridate (DFP) and mipafox, and certain quaternary ammonium compounds (*see* Augustinsson, 1963).

It is possible to visualize, by histochemical technics, the sites of enzyme activity in relation to the various structural components of tissues and cells (*see* review by Koelle, 1975). Such studies have shown that neurons that give rise to the three categories of peripheral cholinergic fibers (postganglionic parasympathetic, preganglionic autonomic, somatic motor) contain relatively high concentrations of AChE throughout their entire length (dendrites, perikarya, axons). The concentrations in noncholinergic peripheral neurons (adrenergic, primary afferent) are, in general, considerably lower, but there are marked species variations. A small percentage of sympathetic ganglion cells in most species contains concentrations of AChE equivalent to those of their respective parasympathetic ganglion cells; evidence has been obtained that in the cat the former cells give rise to the cholinergic sympathetic fibers that innervate the sweat glands (Sjöqvist, 1963).

At the motor end-plates of skeletal muscle, most of the AChE is localized at the surface and infoldings of the postjunctional membrane, or subneural apparatus (Davis and Koelle, 1967; Couteaux, 1972). Accordingly, it is situated strategically for the rapid hydrolysis of ACh following the production of the end-plate potential (EPP). In skeletal muscle, there are several additional sites of AChE activity, such as the musculotendinous junction, for which no definite functional role can be assigned.

Storage and Release of Acetylcholine. In 1950, Fatt and Katz (1952) recorded at the motor end-plate of skeletal muscle and observed the random occurrence of small (approximately 0.1 to 3.0 mV) spontaneous depolarizations at a frequency of approximately one per second. The magnitude of these miniature end-plate potentials (mepps) is considerably below the threshold required to fire a muscle AP; that they are due to the release of ACh is indicated by their enhancement by neostigmine and their blockade by *d*-tubocurarine. This was the first evidence that ACh is stored in and released from motor-nerve endings in constant amounts or *quanta*. The morphological counterpart of this phenomenon was discovered shortly thereafter, in the form of synaptic vesicles noted in electron micrographs of nerve terminals by De Robertis and Bennett (1955). The storage and release of ACh have been investigated most extensively at motor end-plates; nevertheless, most of the principles discovered at this locus probably apply to other sites of cholinergic transmission as well, and in many respects to noncholinergic transmission (*see* reviews by Potter, 1972; Hubbard, 1973; Krnjević, 1974; Miyamoto, 1978).

When an AP arrives at the motor-nerve terminal, there is an explosive release of 100 or more quanta (or vesicles) of ACh, following a latent period of approximately 0.75 millisecond (Katz and Miledi, 1965). The intermediate steps appear to be as follows: the depolarization of the terminal permits the influx of calcium ions, which hypothetically then bind to sites bearing negative charges on the internal surface of the terminal axoplasmic membrane. This could facilitate fusion of axonal and vesicular membranes, resulting in the extrusion of the contents of the vesicles. The presence of calcium ions in the extracellular fluid is essential for the release of ACh elicited by the nerve impulse, and this effect is in turn antagonized by magnesium ions (*see* Douglas, 1968; Cooke *et al.*, 1973; Miyamoto, 1978).

While there is general agreement regarding certain steps involved in the storage and release of ACh, many of the details are still moot or unknown. Estimates of the ACh content of the synaptic vesicles range from 1000 to over 50,000 molecules per vesicle, and it has been calculated that a single motor-nerve terminal contains 300,000 or more vesicles. In addition, an uncertain but significant amount of ACh is present in the extravesicular cytoplasm. Mathematical treatment of the data obtained from postsynaptic recording at the motor end-plate during the continuous application of ACh to resting muscle has permitted estimation of the potential change induced by

a single molecule of ACh (3×10^{-7} V); from such calculations, it is evident that even the lower estimate of the ACh content per vesicle (1000 molecules) is sufficient to account for the magnitude of the mepps (Katz and Miledi, 1972).

In the superior cervical ganglion of the cat, approximately 85% of the total ACh content is stored in a releasable "depot" form, which is subdivided into more readily and less readily releasable reservoirs. The remaining 15% of the extractable ACh is in a "stationary" form and is perhaps located centrally to the axonal terminals. An additional "surplus" portion that may exceed the total depot ACh accumulates in the presence of an anti-ChE agent. The ganglion is able to support a remarkably high rate of ACh synthesis and release; when it is perfused with plasma and stimulated supramaximally at a frequency of 20 cycles per second, the ACh output during 1 hour is approximately six times the original content (Birks and MacIntosh, 1961).

The release of ACh by exocytosis through the prejunctional membrane is inhibited by toxin produced by *Clostridium botulinum*, one of the most potent toxins known. A small number of molecules of this toxin binds irreversibly to their sites of action, producing an essentially irreversible blockade of all cholinergic junctions (*see* Kao *et al.*, 1976). Death results from respiratory failure. Black widow spider toxin has a site of action similar to that of botulinus toxin, but with the opposite effect. Clumping of vesicles at the prejunctional membrane is associated with the release of excessive amounts of ACh (Frontali *et al.*, 1976; Pumplin and Reese, 1977).

Characteristics of Cholinergic Transmission at Various Sites. From the comparisons noted above, it is obvious that there are marked differences between various sites of cholinergic transmission with respect to general-architectural and fine-structural arrangements, the distributions of AChE, and the temporal factors involved in normal functioning. For example, in skeletal muscle the junctional sites occupy a small, discrete portion of the surface of the individual fibers and are relatively isolated from those of adjacent fibers; in the superior cervical ganglion, in contrast, approximately 100,000 ganglion cells are packed within a volume of a few cubic millimeters, and both the presynaptic and postsynaptic neuronal processes form complex networks. It is therefore to be expected that the specific features of cholinergic transmission will vary markedly at different sites.

1. *Skeletal Muscle.* In early studies, stimulation of a motor nerve resulted in the appearance of ACh in the output from perfused muscle; close intra-arterial injection of ACh produced muscular contraction similar to that elicited by stimulation of the

motor nerve. Later, it was demonstrated that the amount of ACh (10^{-17} mole) required to elicit an EPP following its microiontophoretic application to the motor end-plate of a rat diaphragm muscle fiber is equivalent to that recovered from each fiber following stimulation of the phrenic nerve (Krnjević and Miledi, 1958; Krnjević and Mitchell, 1961).

The combination of ACh with the receptors at the external surface of the postjunctional membrane induces an immediate, marked increase in permeability to Na^+ and K^+; it has been estimated that for each molecule of ACh that combines there is a flow of 50,000 cations across the postjunctional membrane (Katz and Miledi, 1972). This is the basis for the localized depolarizing EPP, which triggers the muscle AP, and the latter in turn leads to contraction. Further details concerning these events and their modification by neuromuscular blocking agents are presented in Chapter 11.

Following section and degeneration of the motor nerve to skeletal muscle or of the postganglionic fibers to autonomic effectors, there is a marked reduction in the threshold doses of the transmitters and of certain other drugs required to elicit a response, that is, *denervation supersensitivity* (Cannon and Rosenblueth, 1949). It has been shown that in skeletal muscle this change is accompanied by a spread of the cholinoceptive sites from the end-plate region to the adjacent portions of the sarcoplasmic membrane, which eventually involves practically its entirety (Axelsson and Thesleff, 1959).

The most important sources of material for study of both molecular and electrical postjunctional events have been the electric organs of the eel (*Electrophorus* species) and the electric elasmobranchs (*Torpedo, Raia* species) (*see* Colquhoun, 1975; Rang, 1975). A more detailed discussion is given in Chapter 11.

2. *Autonomic Effectors.*   In contrast to other cholinergically innervated cells (*i.e.,* skeletal muscle and neurons), smooth muscle and the cardiac conduction system (S-A node, atrium, A-V node, and the His-Purkinje system) normally exhibit intrinsic activity, both electrical and mechanical, that is modified but not initiated by nerve impulses. In the basal condition, smooth muscle and the cardiac conduction system exhibit spikes, or waves of increased membrane conduction, that are propagated from cell to cell at rates considerably slower than the AP of axons or skeletal muscle. The spikes are apparently initiated by rhythmic fluctuations in the membrane resting potential; in intestinal smooth muscle, the site of the pacemaker activity continually shifts, whereas in the heart it normally arises from the S-A node but can under certain circumstances arise from any part of the conduction system (*see* Chapter 31). As in skeletal muscle, the spike initiates a contraction.

The addition of ACh (10^{-7} to 10^{-6} M) to isolated intestinal muscle causes a fall in the resting potential (*i.e.,* the membrane potential becomes more positive) and an increase in the frequency of spike production, followed by a rise in tension. The primary action of ACh in initiating these effects is probably the partial depolarization of the cell membrane, brought about by an increase in sodium conductance; while there are changes in the conductances of potassium and

chloride also, their significance is uncertain (*see* review by Bolton, 1973). It is of interest, however, that ACh can also produce contraction of smooth muscle when the membrane has been completely depolarized by immersion in potassium-Ringer solution, provided calcium is present. Although the physiological significance of this observation is uncertain, there is increasing evidence that calcium ion fluxes across the muscle plasma membrane are affected by ACh and are directly involved in regulating the permeability of the membrane to sodium and in coupling membrane depolarization with contraction.

In the cardiac conduction system, particularly from the S-A to the A-V node, stimulation of the cholinergic innervation (of which the preganglionic fibers are in the vagus nerve) or the direct application of ACh causes inhibition, associated with hyperpolarization of the fiber membrane and a marked decrease in the rate of depolarization. These effects are due to a selective increase in permeability to potassium (Burgen and Terroux, 1953; Trautwein *et al.,* 1956; Lipsius and Vasalle, 1977). At the same time, the presence of a basal level of ACh may be essential for the maintenance of the transmembrane potential above a critical value of 60 mV (*see* Berne and Levy, 1972).

Although direct evidence is lacking, it is likely that, in those smooth muscle fibers where cholinergic impulses are inhibitory, ACh produces inhibition by the same mechanism as described above.

3. *Autonomic Ganglia.*   The evidence for cholinergic transmission in autonomic ganglia is similar to that obtained at the neuromuscular junction of skeletal muscle. When the perfusate from the isolated cat superior cervical ganglion is tested, ACh appears in the perfusion fluid after preganglionic but not after antidromic stimulation; it is not liberated spontaneously in significant amounts. The ganglion cells can be discharged by injecting very small amounts of ACh into the perfusion fluid or into the blood supply to the normally circulated ganglion (Feldberg and Gaddum, 1934; Emmelin and MacIntosh, 1956).

The capability of preganglionic impulses to discharge ganglion cells goes hand in hand with the capability of such impulses to release ACh into the perfusate. For example, when Locke's solution *without glucose* is perfused through a sympathetic ganglion, continued stimulation of the preganglionic nerve rapidly exhausts the mechanism of synaptic transmission, and the output of ACh from the ganglion simultaneously fails; both are restored at the same time when choline and glucose, lactate, or pyruvate are added to the perfusion fluid. When the Locke's solution lacks *calcium,* synaptic transmission and release of ACh by preganglionic nerve impulses fail at the same time; both are promptly and simultaneously restored by addition of calcium to the perfusion fluid. These effects of calcium are antagonized by *magnesium,* just as at the motor end-plate. After *preganglionic nerve section,* synaptic transmission and release of ACh by preganglionic impulses disappear together, at a time when axonal conduction is still unimpaired in the severed fiber.

Subsequent studies have disclosed that ganglionic transmission is a highly complex process, combining many of the features of transmission at the neuromuscular junctions of both skeletal and smooth muscle. Interneurons and additional transmitters may also be involved. An account of these events and their modification by drugs is presented in Chapter 10 (*see also* Purves and Lichtman, 1978).

Actions of Acetylcholine at Prejunctional Sites. Considerable attention has been focused on the possible involvement of *prejunctional cholinoceptive sites* in both cholinergic and noncholinergic transmission and in the actions of various drugs. The intra-arterial injection of ACh or an anti-ChE agent (physostigmine or neostigmine) produces both fasciculations (synchronous contractions of the skeletal muscle fibers of *entire motor units*) and antidromic APs that are conducted from the terminals of the motor nerves to the ventral spinal roots. Both effects are blocked by curare. These and related observations suggest that the compounds act at the prejunctional axonal terminals as well as at the postjunctional cholinoceptive sites. Several investigators, particularly Riker and associates (1957, 1969), have amplified and extended these observations (*see also* Chapter 11).

Cholinergic innervation of blood vessels may be prejunctional or directly on vascular smooth muscle. While the latter type of innervation is limited (*see* Uvnäs, 1954), *prejunctional cholinergic innervation* of sympathetic vasoconstrictor nerves appears likely (Steinsland *et al.,* 1973); such prejunctional cholinergic receptors represent a site of action of administered choline esters. The physiological role of this innervation is unclear, as is the presence of cholinergic receptors on most arterial and venous blood vessels in the absence of parasympathetic or cholinergic-sympathetic innervation. It is very unlikely that ACh plays a role as a circulating hormone analogous to that of epinephrine. The former compound is too rapidly hydrolyzed by local and circulating esterases.

Dilatation of blood vessels in response to administered choline esters could, therefore, involve several sites of action: prejunctional inhibitory synapses on sympathetic fibers, inhibitory neuroeffector junctions on smooth muscle, and cholinergic receptors on vascular smooth muscle cells that are not innervated. The last-named site of action probably contributes the most to the response of blood vessels to administered choline esters (*see* Chapter 5).

Participation of Acetylcholine in Transmission by Noncholinergic Neurons. Burn and Rand in 1959 introduced the concept of a *cholinergic link* in *adrenergic transmission.* According to this hypothesis, stimulation of *sympathetic fibers* results first in the release of ACh, which, in turn, causes the release of norepinephrine to act on the effector organs. The evidence to support this proposal includes the finding at several sites that, following a dose of atropine sufficient to block the direct effects of ACh on autonomic effector cells, injection of ACh produces sympathomimetic effects; if the animal is pretreated with reserpine to deplete adrenergic fibers of their norepinephrine content, the sympathomimetic response can no longer be obtained; but, when the sympathetic nerves of reserpine-treated animals are stimulated, ACh-like effects are produced; and finally, anti-ChE agents and other drugs modify the responses to stimulation of sympathetic nerves at cer-

tain sites in a manner consistent with the proposal. The concept is by no means generally accepted at present. There are observations at variance with the hypothesis (*e.g., see* Steinsland *et al.,* 1973), and there are more satisfactory explanations of the original observations. It is clear, however, that ACh can cause the release of norepinephrine by action at nicotinic receptors on cardiac sympathetic nerve endings (*see* Higgins *et al.,* 1973; Westfall, 1977).

ADRENERGIC TRANSMISSION

Under this general heading are included *norepinephrine,* the transmitter of most sympathetic postganglionic fibers and of certain tracts in the CNS, and *dopamine,* the predominant transmitter of the mammalian extrapyramidal system, as well as *epinephrine,* the major hormone of the adrenal medulla.

A tremendous amount of information has accumulated concerning catecholamines and related compounds during recent years. Two major reasons for this have been the application of new technics, especially radioisotopic labeling and histofluorescence localization of catecholamines, and indications of the importance of interactions between the endogenous catecholamines and many of the drugs now used in the treatment of hypertension, mental disorders, and a variety of other conditions. The details of these interactions and of the pharmacology of the sympathomimetic amines themselves will be found in subsequent chapters. (*See also* symposia edited by Acheson, 1966; Blaschko and Muscholl, 1972; Cotten, 1972; Usdin and Snyder, 1973; Usdin *et al.,* 1977.) The basic physiological, biochemical, and pharmacological features are presented briefly here.

Synthesis, Storage, and Release of Catecholamines. The *synthesis* of epinephrine from phenylalanine, by the steps shown in Figure 4–4, was proposed by Blaschko in 1939. This sequence has now been confirmed, and the enzymes involved have been identified and characterized. It is important to note that none of these enzymes is highly specific; consequently, many other endogenous substances as well as certain drugs are similarly acted upon at the various steps. For example, 5-hydroxytryptamine (5-HT, serotonin), tyramine, and histamine can be produced by L-aromatic amino acid decarboxylase (or dopa decarboxylase) (step 3) from their corresponding amino acids. Tyramine, in turn, can be oxidized (step 4) to octopamine, the phenol analog of norepinephrine; while octopamine is present only in small amounts in mammals, it is probably the major adrenergic transmitter in certain invertebrates (Barker *et al.,* 1972b). Dopa decarboxylase can also convert the drug methyldopa to α-methyldopamine, which, in turn, is converted by dopamine β-hydroxylase to the "false transmitter," α-methylnorepinephrine.

The relative velocities of each of these enzymatic steps in the body is of pharmacological significance. One approach to the treatment of hypertension has consisted in attempts to block the synthesis of norepinephrine by compounds that inhibit the various enzymes involved. This mode of attack can be expected to be fruitful only if the reaction involved is the *rate-limiting* one, for example, tyrosine hydroxylase (step 2) (Levitt *et al.,* 1965).

Unfortunately, inhibition of this enzyme is not of therapeutic benefit in controlling hypertension, perhaps because it is subject to several complex regulatory mechanisms. These include rapid feedback regulation by the end-product neurotransmitter, transsynaptic mechanisms that may inhibit (α-adrenergic) or activate (β-adrenergic) tyrosine hydroxylase, and perhaps presynaptic regulation by cholinergic nerves and other agents such as angiotensin and prostaglandins. Acute regulation probably involves

allosteric effectors that alter the affinity of the enzyme for cofactors, substrate, or end-product inhibitors. Long-term regulation may occur by other mechanisms. These appear to include alterations in the rate of synthesis of the enzyme and covalent modification of its structure (Almgren *et al.,* 1975; Baldessarini, 1975; Musacchio, 1975; Langer, 1977).

Current knowledge concerning the *cellular sites and mechanisms of synthesis, storage, and release* of catecholamines has been derived from studies of both adrenergically innervated organs and adrenal medullary tissue. Nearly all the *norepinephrine* content of the former is confined to the postganglionic sympathetic fibers; it disappears within a few days after section of the nerves. The small amount of residual catecholamine is largely *epinephrine,* which is presumably localized in chromaffin cells.

Understanding of the localization and function of adrenergic nerves has advanced rapidly because of the development of new technics. Formaldehyde-vapor histofluorescence studies have allowed visualization of a dense network of catecholamine-containing nerve fibers in smooth and cardiac muscle, blood vessels, and certain exocrine glands, which represents the postganglionic adrenergic component of the terminal reticular apparatus. Most of the catecholamine is present in frequently occurring vesicular swellings that are in close apposition to the muscle and gland cells (Carlsson *et al.,* 1962).

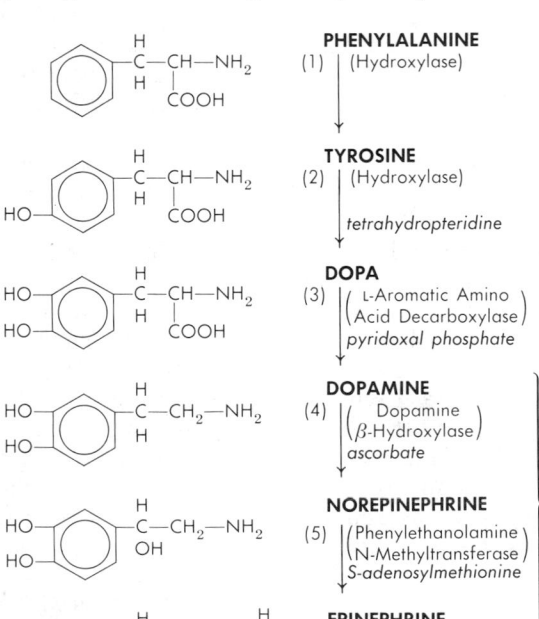

Intravesicular

Figure 4–4. *Steps in enzymatic synthesis of dopamine, norepinephrine, and epinephrine.*

The enzymes involved are shown in parentheses; essential cofactors, in italics.

The development of antibodies against enzymes that participate in the biosynthesis of catecholamines has allowed their visualization in tissues by sensitive immunofluorescence technics. Antibodies to dopamine-β-hydroxylase have been used to detect genetic differences in the biosynthesis of this enzyme and to measure its concentration in plasma as an estimate of adrenergic nerve activity (*see* below; *see also* Axelrod, 1972, 1973; Weinshilboum, 1978).

Another approach that is of considerable value for investigating the functions of adrenergic innervation has been the development of means of producing *immunosympathectomy* and *chemosympathectomy*. The former arose from observations that a protein, *nerve-growth factor,* present in various sources including salivary glands, produces a marked hypertrophy of sympathetic ganglia, both in tissue culture and in newborn animals. When an *antiserum* to the nerve-growth factor is injected into newborn animals under proper conditions, it suppresses the development of the peripheral sympathetic system (Levi-Montalcini and Angeletti, 1968). The same result can be obtained more simply in both newborn and adult animals by the administration of the chemosympathectomizing agent 6-hydroxydopamine. This compound is taken up selectively by adrenergic fibers and results in their destruction (Thoenen, 1972; Jonsson *et al.,* 1975).

The main features of the mechanisms of synthesis, storage, and release of catecholamines and their modifications by drugs are summarized in Figure 4–5. Osmophilic granules, 0.05 to 0.2 μm in diameter, have been isolated from the adrenal medulla, splenic nerves, and various regions of the CNS; they correspond to similar structures noted in electron micrographs of tissue sections (Bloom, 1973; Cooper *et al.,* 1978). The granules contain extremely high concentrations of catecholamines (approximately 21% dry weight) and ATP, in a molecular ratio of 4:1, as well as specific proteins or *chromogranins* and the enzyme dopamine β-hydroxylase (DBH). In the course of synthesis (Figure 4–4), the hydroxylation of tyrosine to dopa and the decarboxylation of dopa to dopamine (steps 2 and 3) take place in the cytoplasm. Dopamine then enters the granules, where it is converted to norepinephrine by DBH (step 4). In the adrenal medulla, most of the norepinephrine leaves the granules, is methylated in the cytoplasm to epinephrine (step 5), and then reenters a different group of intracellular granules, where it is stored until released. Thus, in the human adult, epinephrine accounts for approximately 80% of the catecholamines of the adrenal medulla, with norepinephrine mak-

ing up most of the remainder. (*See* reviews by Axelrod, 1963; Euler, 1972a; Stjärne, 1972; Rubin, 1974.)

It is likely that the enzymes that participate in the synthesis of norepinephrine are synthesized in the perikaryonal cell bodies of the adrenergic neurons and are then transported along the axons to their terminals. This can occur either slowly (1 to 3 mm per day) by bulk flow through axoplasm, as appears to be the case for tyrosine hydroxylase, or much more rapidly (1 to 10 mm per hour), as with dopamine β-hydroxylase. The microtubular system may participate in such rapid axonal transport and also in the formation and extrusion of the granules in which catecholamines are stored (*see* review by Kopin and Silberstein, 1972).

A major factor that controls the rate of synthesis of *epinephrine,* and hence the size of the store available for release from the adrenal medulla, is the level of glucocorticoids secreted by the adrenal cortex. The latter hormones are carried in high concentration, by the intra-adrenal portal vascular system, directly to the adrenal medullary chromaffin cells, where they induce the synthesis of phenylethanolamine-N-methyltransferase (Figure 4–4, step 5), the enzyme that methylates norepinephrine to epinephrine. Thus, any stress that persists sufficiently to invoke an enhanced secretion of corticotropin mobilizes the appropriate hormones of both the adrenal cortex (predominantly cortisol) and medulla (epinephrine) (see review by Wurtman *et al.,* 1972).

This remarkable relationship is present only in certain mammals, including man, where the adrenal chromaffin cells are enveloped entirely by steroid-secreting cortical cells. In the dogfish, for example, where the chromaffin cells and steroid-secreting cells are located in independent, noncontiguous glands, no epinephrine is formed (*see* review by Coupland, 1972).

In addition to its synthesis *de novo,* outlined above, there is a second major source of the norepinephrine of the terminal portions of the adrenergic fibers, namely, recapture by active transport of norepinephrine previously released to the extracellular fluid. This process, in fact, is probably the major one responsible for the termination of the effects of adrenergic impulses in most organs; the blood vessels apparently constitute an exception, where the immediate disposition of released norepinephrine is accomplished largely by a combination of enzymatic breakdown and diffusion (Spector *et al.,* 1972). In order to effect the re-uptake of norepinephrine and to maintain the concentration gradient of norepinephrine within the granules, at least two active transport systems are probably involved: one, across the axoplas-

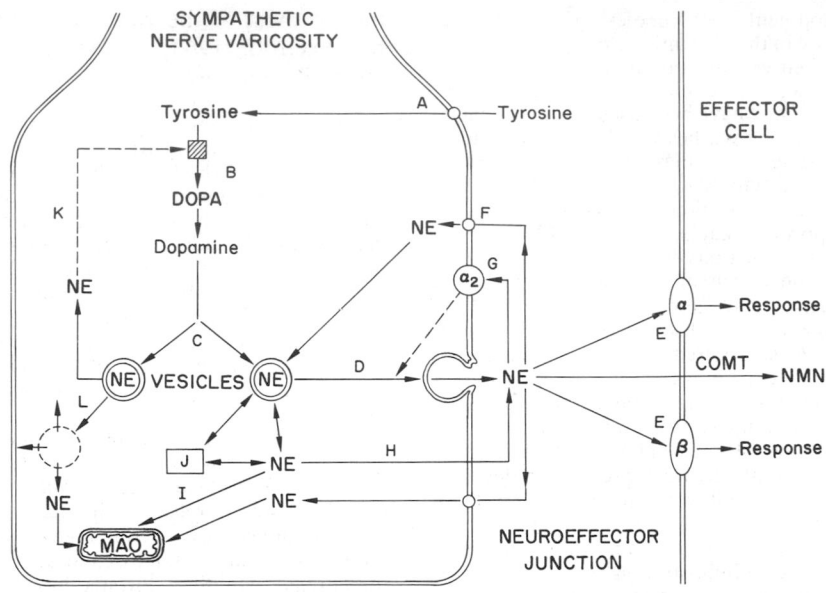

Figure 4–5. *Proposed sites of action of drugs on the synthesis, action, and fate of norepinephrine at sympathetic neuroeffector junctions.*

The events proposed to occur in this model of a sympathetic neuroeffector junction are as follows. Tyrosine is transported actively into the axoplasm (*A*) and is converted to dopa and then to dopamine by cytoplasmic enzymes (*B*). Dopamine is transported into the vesicles of the varicosity, where the synthesis and the storage of norepinephrine (NE) take place (*C*). An action potential causes an influx of Ca^{2+} into the nerve terminal (not shown), with subsequent fusion of the vesicle with the plasma membrane and exocytosis of NE (*D*). The transmitter then activates α and β receptors in the membrane of the postsynaptic cell (*E*). NE that penetrates into these cells is probably rapidly inactivated by catechol-O-methyltransferase (COMT) to normetanephrine (NMN). The most important mechanism for termination of the action of NE in the junctional space is by active re-uptake into the nerve and the storage vesicles (*F*). Norepinephrine in the synaptic cleft can also activate presynaptic (α_2) receptors (*G*), the result of which is to inhibit further exocytotic release of norepinephrine (dashed line).

NE can also be displaced from storage vesicles by sympathomimetic amines such as tyramine, which gain access to the nerve terminal by active uptake as in *F*. A portion of this NE diffuses out of the nerve (*H*) to react with receptors. Another portion of the NE released in this manner, or by spontaneous diffusion, is deaminated by mitochondrial monoamine oxidase (MAO) (*I*). Observations that only a fraction of the total NE content is available for release by either nerve stimulation or tyramine indicate that there are pools of the transmitter that are held in reserve (*J*).

The most important mechanism of regulation of NE synthesis involves the rate-limiting step, the hydroxylation of tyrosine. This regulation is complex but in part involves feedback inhibition by NE (*K*).

Sites of drug action in this scheme include:

1. Inhibition of MAO (*e.g.,* by pargyline) or COMT (no pharmacologically significant example of inhibitor).

2. Inhibition of plasma membrane uptake mechanism for NE (*F*) by tricyclic antidepressants or cocaine, making more NE available for binding to receptors.

3. Inhibition of vesicular storage of NE by reserpine and, in part, by guanethidine (*L*). The NE thereby released is normally inactivated by MAO. Guanethidine and bretylium also block coupling of the action potential to the release of NE.

4. Displacement of NE by indirectly acting sympathomimetic amines (*H*). Exocytosis of vesicular contents does not occur.

5. Direct interaction with adrenergic receptors by agonists and antagonists (*E, G*).

Anatomical elements are not drawn to scale. Mitochondria are about 0.25 μm in diameter and 0.75 μm long; vesicles, 0.05 μm; a nerve varicosity, 2 to 10 μm; the junctional space, 0.1 μm.

mic membrane from the extracellular fluid to the cytoplasm; and the other, from the cytoplasm into the storage granules.

The capacity of the adrenergic nerve terminal to store both the starting material for norepinephrine biosynthesis, tyrosine, and the neurotransmitter is exceptionally high. The active transport systems of the cellular and granular membranes may result in a 10,000-fold concentration of norepinephrine. Evidence for the former transport system is largely indirect and is based on the selective actions of various drugs, as discussed below.

Due to the relative ease of isolating pure preparations of granules, especially from the adrenal medulla, the second transport system has been characterized more fully. It can concentrate catecholamines against a 200-fold gradient across the granular membrane. The intragranular free norepinephrine is in equilibrium with a catecholamine-ATP-protein complex. This transport system requires ATP and magnesium ion, and it is blocked by very low concentrations (40 nM) of reserpine (Kirshner, 1962; Carlsson et al., 1963). The transport system across the axoplasmic membrane is blocked selectively by a number of other drugs, including *cocaine* and the *tricyclic antidepressants,* such as imipramine. Certain sympathomimetic drugs (*e.g., ephedrine, tyramine*) produce most of their effects indirectly, chiefly by displacing norepinephrine from the nerve-ending binding sites to the extracellular fluid, where the released endogenous transmitter then acts at the receptor sites of the effector cells. This action of so-called indirectly acting sympathomimetic amines is associated with the pharmacological phenomenon of *tachyphylaxis.* For example, repeated administration of tyramine results in rapidly decreasing effectiveness, whereas the effect of repeated administration of norepinephrine is not reduced and, in fact, reverses the tachyphylaxis to tyramine. One explanation of tachyphylaxis to tyramine and similarly acting sympathomimetic agents postulates that the pool of neurotransmitter available for displacement by these drugs is quite small relative to the total amount stored in the sympathetic nerve ending. Neurotransmitter release by displacement is not associated with the release of DBH and is thus not presumed to involve exocytosis.

The full sequence of steps by which the *nerve impulse* effects the *release of norepinephrine* from adrenergic fibers is not known. In the adrenal medulla, the triggering event is the liberation of ACh by the preganglionic fibers and its interaction with receptors on the chromaffin cells to produce a localized depolarization; a succeeding step is the entrance of calcium ions into these cells, which results in the extrusion by exocytosis of the granular contents (epinephrine, ATP, chromogranins, dopamine β-hydroxylase) to the extracellular fluid and hence into the circulation (Douglas, 1968; Kirshner, 1974). Calcium likewise appears to play an essential role in coupling the nerve impulse with the release of norepinephrine at adrenergic nerve terminals (Burn and Gibbons, 1965), as has been demonstrated also at cholinergic terminals. Evidence that exocytosis is the primary event in the release of norepinephrine from granules in adrenergic nerve terminals has recently become established. Enhanced activity of the sympathetic nervous system is accompanied by an increased concentration of both dopamine β-hydroxylase and chromogranins in the circulation. This should result only if the entire contents of the granule were released. Drugs can act at these steps either by promoting actively the release of norepinephrine (*e.g., guanethidine*), or by blocking this process (*e.g., bretylium*).

Adrenergic fibers can sustain the output of norepinephrine during prolonged periods of stimulation without exhausting their reserve supply, provided the mechanisms of synthesis and uptake of the transmitter are unimpaired. To meet increased needs for norepinephrine, regulatory mechanisms come into play that are directed at tyrosine hydroxylase (*see* above). However, the physiological response to prolonged or intense nerve stimulation may diminish before the stores of transmitter are exhausted. Transjunctional feedback regulatory mechanisms may inhibit tyrosine hydroxylase or cause the redistribution of transmitter between pools in the nerve ending. Postsynaptic sensitivity to the transmitter may also be regulated, either by alteration of the state or number of receptors or by changes in their ability to influence the activity of other components of the response system.

Termination of the Actions of Catecholamines. The actions of norepinephrine and epinephrine are terminated by (1) re-uptake into nerve terminals; (2) dilution by diffusion out of the junctional cleft; and (3) metabolic transformation. Two enzymes are important in the initial steps of metabolic transformation of catecholamines—monoamine oxidase (MAO) and catechol-O-methyltransferase (COMT) (*see* Axelrod, 1966; Kopin, 1972). However, in contrast to ACh, metabolic transformation is of relatively minor significance in terminating the actions of *endogenously* liberated neurotransmitter at sites other than blood vessels (Spector *et al.*, 1972). It was evident more than 30 years ago that a powerful enzymatic mechanism, such as that provided by AChE, was absent from the adrenergic nervous system, and Blaschko (1952) pointed out that the narrow spatial and temporal limitations of the action of ACh did not apply to adrenergic neuroeffector sites. Axelrod and colleagues demonstrated the significance of re-uptake into the sympathetic nerve ending (*see* reviews by Axelrod, 1966, 1973). Consistent with this are the observations that inhibitors of norepinephrine uptake by the nerve terminal (*e.g.*, cocaine, imipramine) potentiate the effects of the neurotransmitter; inhibitors of MAO and COMT have little effect. However, transmitter that is released *within* the nerve terminal is metabolized by MAO; COMT, particularly in the liver, is important to terminate the action of endogenous circulating and administered catecholamines.

Both MAO and COMT are widely distributed throughout the body, including the brain; the highest concentrations of each are in the liver and the kidney. However, there are distinct differences in their cytological locations; whereas MAO is associated chiefly with mitochondria, including those within the terminals of adrenergic fibers, COMT is confined largely to the cytoplasm and apparently has no selective association with adrenergic nerves. These factors are of importance both in determining the primary metabolic pathways followed by catecholamines in various circumstances and in explaining the effects of certain drugs. There are two different isozymes of MAO; MAO-A predominates in the intestinal mucosa and hepatocytes, while MAO-B is of greater importance in certain regions of the brain. Selective inhibitors of these two isozymes are being investigated (*see* Chapters 9 and 21).

Most of the epinephrine and norepinephrine that enters the circulation, from the adrenal medulla or from exogenous administration, or that is released rapidly from adrenergic fibers is first methylated by COMT to metanephrine or normetanephrine, respectively (Figure 4–6). Norepinephrine that is released slowly, either by drugs such as reserpine or by nerve impulses of low frequency, is probably initially deaminated by the MAO before it leaves the nerve ending to the corresponding aldehyde (not shown in Figure 4–6) and then converted rapidly at extraneuronal sites to 3,4-dihydroxymandelic acid. In either case, most of the metabolite resulting from attack by the initial enzyme is then converted by the other to the common product, 3-methoxy-4-hydroxymandelic acid, generally but incorrectly called "vanillylmandelic acid (VMA)," which constitutes the major metabolite of catecholamines excreted in the urine. The corresponding product of the metabolic degradation of dopamine, which contains no hydroxyl group in the side chain, is homovanillic acid (HVA). Other metabolic reactions are described in Figure 4–6. Normally in man the 24-hour urinary excretion of metabolites of endogenous catecholamines includes 2 to 4 mg of 3-methoxy-4-hydroxymandelic acid (representing in particular norepinephrine produced by adrenergic fibers and deaminated within them by MAO prior to release), 100 to 300 µg of normetanephrine (representing norepinephrine released by physiological stimulation of adrenergic fibers), and 100 to 200 µg of metanephrine (representing part of the epinephrine released by the adrenal medulla). In addition, 25 to 50 µg of norepinephrine and 2 to 5 µg of epinephrine also appear in the urine.

Inhibitors of MAO (*e.g., pargyline, nialamide*) can cause an increase in the level of norepinephrine in the brain and other tissues accompanied by a variety of pharmacological effects; however, some of the effects may be due to additional actions of these compounds (*see* below and Chapters 8 and 9). No striking pharmacological action can be attributed to the inhibition of COMT.

General Actions of Adrenergic Transmitters. The effects of norepinephrine released by adrenergic nerve impulses at various effector organs are listed in Table 4–1, and the actions of the catecholamines and other sympathomimetic agents are presented in detail in Chapter 8. Hence, it is necessary here to mention only the general principles relating to the role of the catecholamines as neurohumoral transmitters. Norepinephrine, epinephrine, and other catecholamines can cause either excitation or inhibition of *smooth muscle contraction,* depending on the site, the dose, and the catecholamine chosen. Norepinephrine is the most potent excitatory catecholamine and has correspondingly low activity as an inhibitor; *isoproterenol* exhibits the reverse pattern of activity. Epinephrine is relatively potent both as an excitor and as an inhibitor of smooth muscle contraction. On

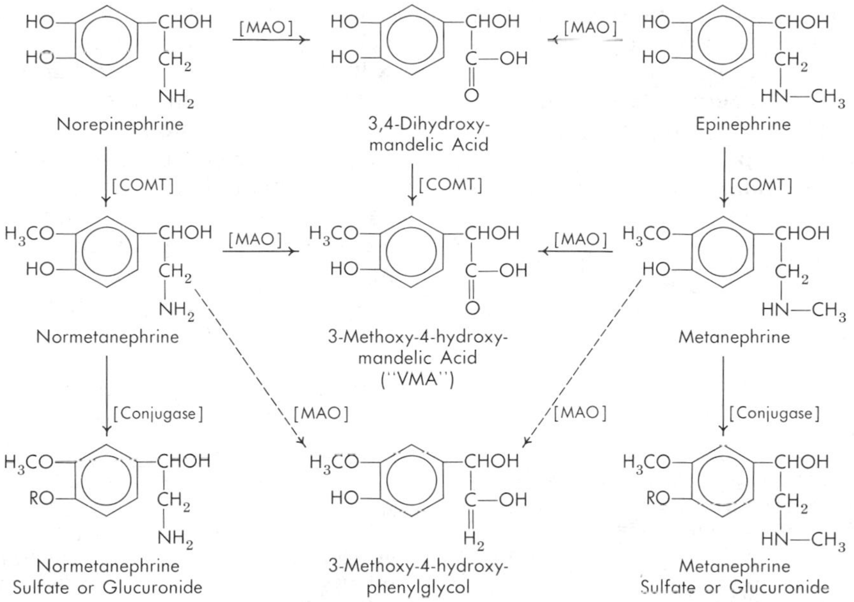

Figure 4-6. *Steps in the metabolic disposition of catecholamines.*

Both norepinephrine and epinephrine can initially be oxidatively deaminated by monoamine oxidase (MAO) to the corresponding aldehyde (not shown) and thence oxidized to 3,4-dihydroxy-mandelic acid; alternatively, they can first be methylated by catechol-O-methyltransferase (COMT) to normetanephrine and metanephrine, respectively. Most of the products of either type of reaction are then metabolized by the other enzyme to form the major excretory product, 3-methoxy-4-hydroxymandelic acid (frequently called vanillylmandelic acid ["VMA"]). Small amounts of normetanephrine and metanephrine are conjugated to the corresponding sulfates or glucuronides, and small portions of their initial aldehyde oxidation products are reduced to 3-methoxy-4-hydroxyphenylglycol (dashed arrows); the latter step occurs to a greater extent in the CNS. (Modified from Axelrod, 1966; others.)

the basis of such observations, Ahlquist (1948) proposed the terms α and β *receptors* for sites on smooth muscles where catecholamines produce excitatory and inhibitory responses, respectively. The gut is generally relaxed by catecholamines, but here the inhibitory response is mediated by both α and β receptors. Cardiac pacemakers and muscle respond to catecholamines and adrenergic impulses with an increase in rate and force of contraction (positive chronotropic and inotropic effects), but these have the pharmacological properties of β-adrenergic responses. Isoproterenol is thus the most potent agent in producing these effects. This classification of receptors has been corroborated by the findings that certain drugs (*e.g., phenoxybenzamine*) produce selective blockade of the effects of adrenergic nerve impulses and sympathomimetic agents at α-receptor sites, whereas others (*e.g., propranolol*) produce β-adrenergic blockade.

β Receptors can be subdivided into β_1 receptors (chiefly at cardiac sites) and β_2 receptors (elsewhere) on the basis of the relative selectivity of effects of both excitatory agents and antagonists (Lands *et al.*, 1967). The continuing development of highly selective drugs in these categories offers distinct therapeutic advantages (*see* Chapters 8 and 9; review by Moran, 1975).

There also appear to be two subtypes of α-adrenergic receptors (*see* Chapter 8). α_1 Receptors probably have a predominant postjunctional location and thus are responsible for the initiation of excitatory postsynaptic events. α_2 Receptors are at least in part located on presynaptic nerve terminals; activation of these receptors results in inhibition of the release of transmitter. Thus, α_2 receptors on adrenergic nerve terminals appear to mediate feedback inhibition of norepinephrine release (Figure 4–5), while such receptors on the cholinergic nerve terminals in the gastrointestinal tract are probably responsible for inhibitory effects of α-adrenergic agonists at this site. There is, however, insufficient evidence to permit classification of all prejunctional and all postjunctional α-adrenergic receptors as pharmacologically distinct, homogeneous groups (*see* Steppeler *et al.,* 1978).

In the smooth muscle of the guinea pig *vas deferens,* where adrenergic nerve impulses cause contraction by activation of α receptors, Burnstock and Holman (1961) have shown that effects at the muscle fiber membrane are quite similar to those produced by ACh on smooth muscles where the ester has an excitatory effect. Each adrenergic nerve impulse causes localized, partial depolarization; when the summation of successive responses attains a critical level of depolarization, a spike potential is induced; this is conducted over the adjacent muscle fibers and is followed by contraction. These effects are due primarily to an increase in Na^+ conductance (Magaribuchi *et al.,* 1971). Pyloric and ileocecal sphincters contain both α and β receptors, both of which mediate contraction (Reddy and Moran, 1968).

In contrast, in the guinea pig *taenia coli,* where the spontaneous rhythmic activity is inhibited by adrenergic nerve impulses through activation of both α and β receptors, the opposite effects are produced: suppression of spike discharges, abolition of conducted responses to electrical stimulation, and hyperpolarization. The basis for these effects is considerably more complex. The site of α-adrenergic action is most likely on the stimulatory cholinergic motoneurons that innervate the muscle, and the effect is to hyperpolarize the neuron and decrease its rate of firing. The β-receptor inhibitory component is exerted on the smooth muscle cell but is apparently not associated with any significant change in ionic conductance; it may be due to an increase in the binding of calcium to the cell membrane, which results in a stabilizing effect. The effects that result from the occupation of β-adrenergic receptors on smooth muscle cells are perhaps mediated by an increase in intracellular cyclic adenosine 3′,5′-monophosphate (cyclic AMP), as discussed below (*see* review by Bülbring, 1973).

In addition to the foregoing pharmacodynamic effects, epinephrine and its congeners produce an important group of *metabolic effects,* the manifestations of which include hyperglycemia, hyperlactacidemia, hyperlipemia, increased oxygen consumption, and hyperkalemia (*see* reviews by Himms-Hagen, 1967, 1972; Williamson, 1975; Mayer, 1978; Stull and Mayer, 1979). The key compound that is involved in the mediation of these effects, as well as those of a great number of other hormones, is *cyclic AMP,* as has been demonstrated in a brilliant series of investigations initiated by Sutherland, Rall, and their associates (*see* Robison *et al.,* 1971; Rall, 1972). Epinephrine enhances the accumulation of intracellular cyclic AMP by activating (via β receptors) a membrane-bound enzyme, adenylate cyclase, which catalyzes the conversion of ATP to cyclic AMP. Cyclic AMP then initiates a series of intracellular alterations, resulting in the characteristic metabolic effects of the catecholamines and participating in many of their pharmacodynamic effects as well.

The β receptors are particularly located in the plasma membranes with their catecholamine-binding sites oriented externally; the interaction of the receptor with adenylate cyclase requires at least one additional protein that binds guanine nucleotides (*see* Maguire *et al.,* 1977; Pfeuffer, 1977; Ross *et al.,* 1978). β-Adrenergic receptors have been quantified and characterized in many tissues by ligand-binding technics; progress is being made in the purification of this important protein.

Hyperglycemia induced by catecholamines and by glucagon is attributable in part to activation, via cyclic AMP, of hepatic *glycogen phosphorylase.* This enzyme converts glycogen to glucose-1-phosphate—the rate-limiting step in *glycogenolysis.* In addition, the action of cyclic AMP results in the inactivation of *glycogen synthase,* the enzyme that catalyzes the transfer of glycosyl units from UDP-glucose to glycogen. These two effects of cyclic AMP thus summate to increase the output of glucose from the liver.

The mechanism of action of cyclic AMP to produce these enzymatic changes is complex and is the result of the initiation of cascading series of protein phosphorylation reactions (Figure 4–7). Cyclic AMP interacts with its intracellular receptor, a *cyclic AMP–dependent protein kinase,* and causes the dissociation of this enzyme into activated catalytic subunits and regulatory subunits (the cyclic AMP–binding component). The activated protein kinase can phosphorylate a variety of proteins, ATP being used as a substrate. Thus, protein kinase phosphorylates glycogen synthase, and the result is *inactivation* of the enzyme by its conversion from a form that is independent (I) of a cofactor (glucose-6-phosphate) for activity to a form that is dependent (D) on the cofactor. Concurrently, the activated protein kinase phosphorylates and *activates* the enzyme *phosphorylase kinase.* Phosphorylase kinase is in fact another protein kinase, and it catalyzes the phosphorylation and *activation* of phosphorylase. In muscle, the phosphorylation of phosphorylase results in its conversion from the *b* form (dependent on 5′-AMP for activity) to the *a* (independent) form. In liver, a similar activation occurs, although *inactive* hepatic phosphorylase is only little affected by 5′-AMP. Since muscle does not contain glucose-6-phosphatase, an end product of glycogenolysis in muscle is lactate, and *hyperlactacidemia* results.

Similar types of reactions result in the activation of triglyceride lipase in adipose tissue, with resultant

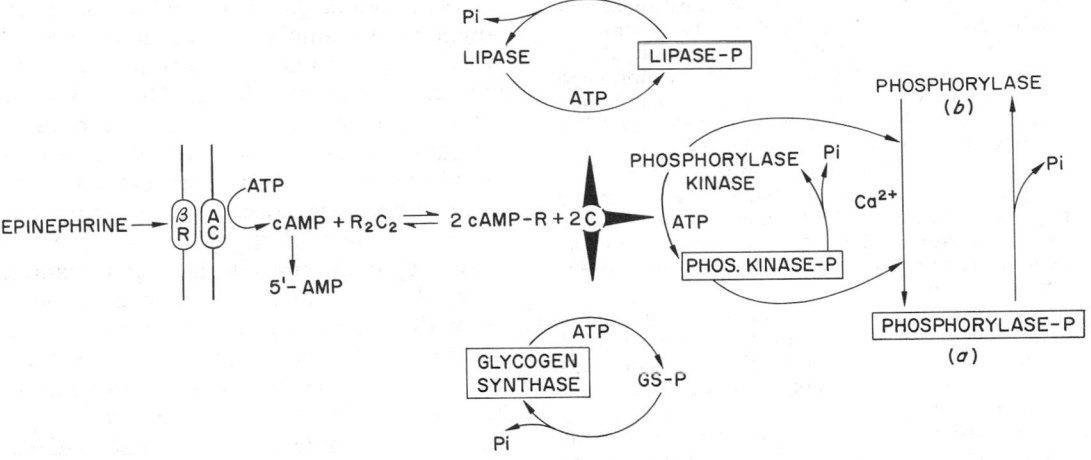

Figure 4-7. *Regulation of metabolism through β-adrenergic receptors.*

Cyclic adenosine 3′,5′-monophosphate (cyclic AMP, *cAMP*) is synthesized by adenylate cyclase (*AC*) at the inner face of the plasma membrane consequent to activation of β-adrenergic receptors (*βR*) by epinephrine or other β-adrenergic agonists. The intracellular receptor for cyclic AMP is a protein kinase (R_2C_2) that exists as a tetramer consisting of two regulatory (*R*) and two catalytic (*C*) subunits. Reaction with cyclic AMP causes dissociation and activation of the enzyme. The catalytic subunit phosphorylates a variety of proteins. The reactions shown in the figure are those that are most important ones for the regulation of glycogenolysis and lipolysis by the autonomic nervous system. Phosphorylation of triglyceride lipase and phosphorylase kinase increases enzyme activity. Phosphorylation of glycogen synthase, however, deactivates this enzyme. (The activated form of each enzyme is shown enclosed in a box.) Stimulation of glycogenolysis is thus the consequence of the concerted phosphorylation of two enzymes that have opposing actions. Removal of the hormonal stimulus is followed by rapid dephosphorylation of all the proteins by phosphoprotein phosphatases. The reactions shown represent a composite of the metabolic responses to epinephrine in skeletal muscle, heart, liver, and adipose tissue, but there are differences in the regulation of these reactions among these tissues.

hyperlipemia (Figure 4–7). This is a very important mechanism whereby catecholamines provide an increased supply of substrate for oxidative metabolism.

Hyperglycemia is also promoted by other catecholamine-induced mechanisms. *Gluconeogenesis* from lactate and amino acids is stimulated, via cyclic AMP, by catecholamines and glucagon. The mechanism of this action is less precisely understood. The critical reactions occur in mitochondria and involve the metabolic transformation of pyruvate to oxaloacetate to phosphoenolpyruvate. The latter is then converted to glucose by the action of several cytoplasmic enzymes. This is also an important action of glucocorticoids (*see* Chapter 63), by mechanisms not directly involving cyclic AMP.

Catecholamines have both an inhibitory effect on the secretion of insulin by the β cells of the pancreatic islets, via α receptors, and a cyclic AMP–mediated stimulatory effect, by means of β receptors. The inhibitory effect predominates strongly *in vivo*. Since insulin antagonizes many of the metabolic effects of catecholamines and glucagon, this inhibitory effect on the secretion of insulin reinforces the metabolic actions described above.

The catecholamine-induced efflux of potassium from the liver, following a transient influx, is probably mediated by cyclic AMP, as is the briefer outflow

of calcium. In the heart, catecholamines and glucagon increase the uptake of calcium.

The important question of a causal relationship between the accumulation of cyclic AMP induced by catecholamines and the pharmacodynamic actions of these agents at autonomic effector and synaptic sites remains a subject of extensive investigation. Most if not all the actions of catecholamines at β-receptor sites appear to require activation of adenylate cyclase and the consequent increase in the intracellular concentrations of cyclic AMP. This applies to inhibitory effects on smooth muscle, excitatory effects on the myocardium, secretory responses of exocrine glands, and quite possibly the action of norepinephrine as an inhibitory neurohumoral transmitter in the CNS.

The positive inotropic effect of catecholamines on the myocardium results from their interaction with β receptors and has been investigated extensively in an effort to determine whether it is causally related to the concurrent accumulation of cyclic AMP. Although there is an abundance of evidence on this matter, the interpretations remain somewhat equivocal. It is now clear that the positive inotropic response of the heart does not result from stimulated glycogenolysis. The phosphorylation of proteins important in the regulation of contraction may be the key, since the phosphorylation of a subunit of troponin appears to be a specific consequence of β-adrenergic stimulation (England, 1976; Brunton et al., 1979). Cyclic AMP may also mediate alterations in the permeability of the plasma membrane to Ca^{2+} and in Ca^{2+} transport by the sarcoplasmic reticulum. As pointed out by Sobel and Mayer (1973), the possibility cannot be excluded that catecholamines have actions on the myocardium, independent of cyclic AMP, that are involved in the inotropic response. While cyclic AMP appears to be necessary for the inotropic effect of catecholamines, its enhanced accumulation may not be sufficient to explain this response.

In some species, most notably the rat, the metabolic effects of catecholamines in liver are mediated through an α-adrenergic mechanism that is dependent on calcium and does not result in an increase in the concentration of cyclic AMP or the activation of cyclic AMP–dependent protein kinase. While rat hepatocytes contain functional β-adrenergic receptors, these do not appear to be quantitatively important in the overall metabolic response of liver to epinephrine or norepinephrine. For example, the increase in glycogenolysis and gluconeogenesis that follows stimulation of hepatocytes by catecholamines is unaffected by propranolol (which blocks the rise in cyclic AMP concentration induced by these agents) but is completely abolished by various α-adrenergic antagonists. Despite the fact that cyclic AMP–dependent protein kinase is not activated, *other* protein kinases are involved; the metabolic changes that occur appear to result from changes in the phosphorylation of target proteins that are similar to those that follow exposure of the livers of other species to β-adrenergic agonists (Garrison, 1978). Other metabolic sequences that appear to be regulated through the α-adrenergic pathway include ureagenesis and fatty acid synthesis. Moreover, some evidence suggests that carbohydrate metabolism in rat adipocytes can also be controlled by this mechanism. Neither the generality nor the importance of the α-adrenergic regulation of metabolism in other species has been established (*see* Exton, 1979, for a review).

RELATIONSHIP BETWEEN THE NERVOUS AND THE ENDOCRINE SYSTEMS

The concept that "humors" are secreted at certain sites to act elsewhere in the body can be traced back to Aristotle. In modern terms, the theory of neurohumoral transmission by its very designation implies at least a superficial resemblance between the nervous and the endocrine systems. Yet it should now be clear that the similarities extend considerably deeper, particularly with respect to the autonomic nervous system. In the regulation of homeostasis, the autonomic nervous system is responsible for rapid adjustments to changes in the total environment, which it

effects at both its ganglionic relays and postganglionic terminals by the liberation of chemical agents that act transiently at their immediate sites of release. The endocrine system, in contrast, regulates slower, more generalized adaptations by releasing its hormonal agents into the systemic circulation to act at distant, widespread sites over periods of hours or days. Both systems have major central representations in the hypothalamus, where they are integrated with each other and with subcortical, cortical, and spinal influences. Furthermore, there are structures that defy strict classification as belonging to the nervous system or to the endocrine system. One example is the *adrenal medulla.* Another is the *hypothalamiconeurohypophyseal tract,* which is analogous to the neurosecretory cells in certain invertebrates and fish (*see* reviews by Welsh, 1955; Scharrer, 1972). In fish, such cells exhibit both synaptic excitability and impulse conduction, as they presumably do in their mammalian counterpart. The neurohumoral theory may thus be said to provide a unitary concept of the evolution and functioning of the nervous and the endocrine systems, in which the differences are essentially only quantitative.

PHARMACOLOGICAL CONSIDERATIONS

In the foregoing sections, there are numerous references to the actions of drugs considered primarily as tools for the dissection and elucidation of physiological mechanisms. Here will be presented a classification of drugs that act upon the nervous system and its effector organs at some stage of neurohumoral transmission. In the immediately succeeding chapters, as well as elsewhere in the text, the systematic pharmacology of the important members of each of these classes is described.

Before proceeding with any classification of drugs, it is essential to emphasize an important general principle. The "first adage" of pharmacology is: "No drug has a single effect." Thus, a drug may be classified as an "anti-ChE agent," but this does not preclude its having direct effects at postsynaptic cholinoceptive sites or elsewhere. Likewise, iproniazid and other chemically related MAO inhibitors have also been shown to block the release of norepinephrine from adrenergic fibers; their therapeutic effect in the treatment of essential hypertension may be due to this blockade of release. Drugs are placed in a given class on the basis of what appears to be their primary or predominant action, but the decision must often be an arbitrary one. Additional effects or side effects constitute the major limitation to the usefulness of drugs as tools in the analysis of physiological and pharmacological mechanisms and in drug therapy. This problem has been and continues to be a serious one for agents acting on the autonomic nervous system. For example, ganglionic blocking agents, used in the treatment of hypertension, are badly compromised because of their lack of *selectivity* between sympathetic and parasympathetic ganglia. Nonselective β-adrenergic antagonists produce unwanted effects because they block hepatic and bronchial smooth-muscle β receptors. For these reasons both the pharmacologist and the clinician are constantly seeking drugs that have more selective effects, with respect to both mechanism and site.

Each step involved in neurohumoral transmission (Figure 4–3) represents a potential point of drug attack. This is depicted in the diagram of the adrenergic terminal and its postjunctional site, in Figure 4–5. Drugs that affect processes concerned in each step of transmission at both cholinergic and adrenergic junctions are summarized in Table 4–2, which lists representative agents that act by the mechanisms described below.

Interference with the Synthesis or Release of the Transmitter. *Cholinergic. Hemicholinium* (HC-3), a synthetic compound, blocks the transport system by which choline accumulates in the terminals of cholinergic fibers and thus it limits the synthesis of the ACh store available for release (Birks and MacIntosh, 1957). *Botulinus toxin* has been shown to prevent the release of ACh by all types of cholinergic fibers studied; fatality results from peripheral respiratory paralysis. Apparently, the toxin blocks release of vesicular ACh at the preterminal portion of the axon, but why this effect is confined to cholinergic fibers is not known.

Adrenergic. Several drugs in this category are discussed above as well as elsewhere (*see*

Index). *α-Methyltyrosine* blocks the synthesis of norepinephrine by inhibiting tyrosine hydroxylase, the enzyme representing the rate-limiting step. On the other hand, *methyldopa,* like dopa itself, is successively decarboxylated and hydroxylated in its side chain to form the putative "false neurotransmitter," *α-methylnorepinephrine.* The significance of these metabolic transformations of the drug is discussed in Chapter 32 (*see* review by Muscholl, 1972). *Bretylium* acts by preventing the release of norepinephrine by the nerve impulse.

Promotion of the Release of the Transmitter. *Cholinergic. Carbachol* (carbamylcholine) has been proposed to act in part by release of ACh at certain vascular smooth muscle neuroeffector junctions and in sympathetic ganglia (Renshaw *et al.,* 1938; Volle and Koelle, 1961). In addition, it acts directly at all postjunctional cholinergic receptors, as it does at the motor end-plate of skeletal muscle.

Adrenergic. Several drugs that promote the release of the adrenergic mediator have already been discussed. On the basis of the *rate* and the *duration* of the drug-induced release of norepinephrine from adrenergic terminals, one of two opposite effects can predominate. Thus, *tyramine, ephedrine, amphetamine,* and related drugs cause a relatively rapid, brief liberation of the transmitter and hence produce a sympathomimetic effect. On the other hand, *reserpine* and *guanethidine* bring about a slow, prolonged depletion of the transmitter, which is largely metabolized by MAO prior to its release; consequently, their sympathomimetic effects are slight, and their major effects are equivalent to adrenergic blockade. Reserpine and guanethidine also cause the release of 5-HT and possibly other, unidentified amines from central and peripheral sites, and many of their major effects may be based on this action.

Combination with Postjunctional Receptor Sites. *Cholinergic.* With the development of the theory of cholinergic transmission, the focus of attention was transferred from the nerve terminal to the postjunctional site as the probable locus of action of a large number of peripherally acting stimulating and

Table 4–2. TYPES OF ACTION OF REPRESENTATIVE DRUGS AT PERIPHERAL CHOLINERGIC AND ADRENERGIC SYNAPSES AND NEUROEFFECTOR JUNCTIONS

MECHANISM OF ACTION	SYSTEM	DRUGS	EFFECT
1. Interference with synthesis of transmitter	Cholinergic	Hemicholinium	Depletion of ACh
	Adrenergic	α-Methyltyrosine	Depletion of norepinephrine
2. Metabolic transformation by same pathway as precursor of transmitter	Adrenergic	Methyldopa	Displacement of norepinephrine by false transmitter (α-methylnorepinephrine)
3. Blockade of transport system of membrane of nerve terminal	Adrenergic	Cocaine, imipramine	Accumulation of norepinephrine at receptors
4. Blockade of transport system of storage granule membrane	Adrenergic	Reserpine	Destruction of norepinephrine by mitochondrial MAO, and depletion from adrenergic terminals
5. Displacement of transmitter from axonal terminal	Cholinergic	Carbachol	Cholinomimetic
	Adrenergic (rapid, brief)	Amphetamine, tyramine	Sympathomimetic
	Adrenergic (slow, prolonged)	Guanethidine	Depletion of norepinephrine from adrenergic terminal
6. Prevention of release of transmitter	Cholinergic	Botulinus toxin	Anticholinergic
	Adrenergic	Bretylium	Antiadrenergic
7. Mimicry of transmitter at postsynaptic receptor	Cholinergic Muscarinic Nicotinic	Methacholine Nicotine	Cholinomimetic Cholinomimetic
	Adrenergic Alpha Beta$_{1,2}$ Beta$_1$ Beta$_2$	Phenylephrine Isoproterenol Dobutamine Terbutaline	Sympathomimetic Nonselective β-adrenomimetic Selective cardiac stimulation Selective inhibition of smooth muscle contraction
8. Blockade of endogenous transmitter at postsynaptic receptor	Cholinergic Muscarinic Nicotinic	Atropine d-Tubocurarine, hexamethonium	Cholinergic blockade Cholinergic blockade
	Adrenergic Alpha Beta Beta$_1$	Phenoxybenzamine Propranolol Metoprolol	α-Adrenergic blockade β-Adrenergic blockade Selective adrenergic blockade (cardiac)
9. Inhibition of enzymatic breakdown of transmitter	Cholinergic	Anti-ChE agents (physostigmine, di*iso*propyl phosphorofluoridate [DFP])	Cholinomimetic
	Adrenergic	MAO inhibitors (pargyline, nialamide, tranylcypromine)	Accumulation of norepinephrine at certain sites; potentiation of tyramine

blocking drugs. This viewpoint has been of great value in the clarification and the classification of the effects of the majority of currently employed drugs in this category, and its application has led to the development of several new, more selectively acting compounds. Since ACh is the neurohumoral transmitter at various peripheral junctions, it can be assumed that the postjunctional cholinergic receptors all share certain common features. However, it has long been known that individual drugs vary with respect to their potency relative to that of ACh at different cholinoceptive sites. The various receptors must therefore have certain distinctive features, in addition to their common ones, based on specific chemical groupings or steric factors in their immediate vicinity. This constitutes the major basis of selectivity of drug action (see Figure 4-8). When a drug combines with a cholinergic receptor, it may produce one of two effects: the same effect as that of ACh (i.e., cholinomimetic); or no apparent direct effect but, by occupation of the receptor site, prevention of the action of endogenous ACh (i.e., cholinergic blockade). Many drugs produce both effects in sequence; nicotine is an outstanding example of such an agent.

The effects of the alkaloids *muscarine* and *nicotine* on cholinergic junctions provided the basis for Dale's classical differentiation of receptor types, which is still accurate for both the peripheral and central nervous systems. The parasympathomimetic effects of muscarine were well known at the turn of the cen-

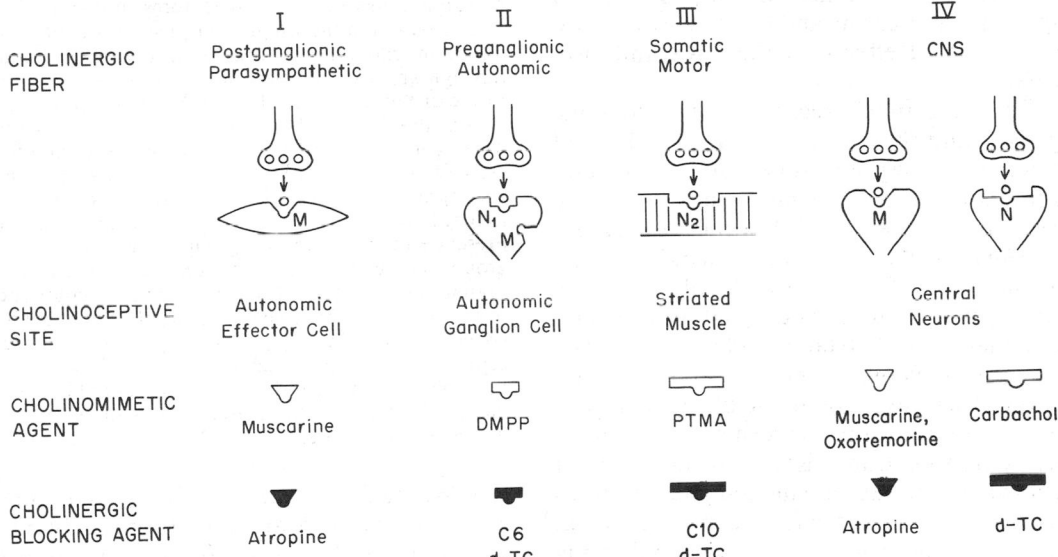

Figure 4-8. *Relative specificity of action of cholinomimetic and cholinergic blocking agents.*

Acetylcholine (ACh; depicted above as o), released by the nerve action potential from the four classes of cholinergic fibers (*I–IV*) or introduced from an exogenous source, can combine with the cholinoceptive sites of the corresponding postjunctional cells (*I–IV*) to produce its characteristic transmitter effects. The receptors of autonomic effector cells (*I*) are classified as *muscarinic* (*M*), and those of autonomic ganglion cells (*II*) and striated muscle (*III*) are classified as *nicotinic* (*N*). Although certain drugs act at nicotinic receptors on both *II* and *III* (e.g., *d*-tubocurarine, *d*-TC), others are more selective for *II* (e.g., hexamethonium, C6) or *III* (e.g., decamethonium, C10); hence, their designation here as N_1 and N_2, respectively. Cholinoceptive neurons of the CNS have predominantly either nicotinic (spinal cord) or muscarinic (thalamus, cerebral cortex) receptors.

Examples of drugs that act selectively to produce cholinomimetic effects at the foregoing cholinoceptive sites are muscarine (*I*), dimethylphenylpiperazinium (DMPP) (*II*), phenyltrimethylammonium (PTMA) (*III*), muscarine or oxotremorine (*IV-M*), and carbachol (*IV-N*). Cholinergic blocking agents also combine relatively selectively at such sites but have no important effects directly; their effects are due to blockade of the approach of endogenous ACh or exogenous cholinomimetic agents. Examples of drugs acting in this manner are atropine (*I*), hexamethonium (C6) (*II*), decamethonium (C10) (*III*), atropine (*IV-M*), and *d*-tubocurarine (*IV-N*).

Nicotine acts at nicotinic sites to produce stimulation in low doses, blockade in high doses.

tury and, in fact, prompted the early speculations by Dixon and Loewi concerning the possibility of neurohumoral transmission in the autonomic nervous system. By convention, the cholinomimetic effects of drugs and of ACh at *autonomic effector cells* are referred to as *muscarinic effects,* since the alkaloid activates these receptors. From the early work of Langley it is known that nicotine in low doses stimulates, and in higher doses paralyzes, autonomic ganglia; the same sequence was later shown to occur at the motor end-plates of certain types of skeletal muscle. The stimulation and then blockade of *autonomic ganglia* and the *end-plates of skeletal muscle,* as exhibited by ACh and various other drugs, are thus termed *nicotinic effects.* It must be emphasized that these effects by no means describe the full pharmacological spectra of muscarine and nicotine, which also have marked effects on the CNS and elsewhere.

The "nicotinic" receptors of autonomic ganglia and skeletal muscle are not identical since they respond differently to certain stimulating and blocking agents, as can be seen in Figure 4–8. *Dimethylphenylpiperazinium* (DMPP) and *phenyltrimethylammonium* (PTMA) are highly selective stimulants of autonomic ganglion cells and end-plates of skeletal muscle, respectively. *Tetraethylammonium* and *hexamethonium* are likewise selective ganglionic blocking agents. d-*Tubocurarine,* on the other hand, effectively blocks transmission at both motor end-plates and autonomic ganglia, although its action at the former site predominates, whereas *decamethonium,* a depolarizing agent, produces selective neuromuscular blockade. Some evidence suggests that the muscarinic receptors of smooth muscle may also be separable into more than one type (Burgen and Spero, 1968). The situation at autonomic ganglia is complicated further by the fact that the ganglion cells also have a secondary component of muscarinic receptors that have an unknown role in the physiology of ganglionic transmission (*see* Chapter 10).

Atropine selectively blocks all the muscarinic responses to injected ACh and related cholinomimetic drugs, whether they are excitatory, as in the intestine, or inhibitory, as in the heart. However, it is less effective in blocking responses to stimulation of certain postganglionic parasympathetic fibers. For example, although small doses of atropine prevent cardiac slowing or salivary secretion after nerve stimulation, even large doses will not abolish fully the responses of the smooth muscle of the intestine and urinary bladder to nerve impulses. A possible explanation is that such impulses are mediated in fact by purinergic, or ATP-releasing, fibers. Other belladonna alkaloids related to atropine and many synthetic compounds have similar blocking actions at cholinergic neuroeffector junctions.

With regard to the possible molecular basis for the difference between muscarinic and nicotinic receptors, it has been pointed out that ACh as well as numerous nicotinic and muscarinic activating and blocking drugs possess two features in common: a quaternary ammonium group or its equivalent; and an atom capable of forming a hydrogen bond, through an unshared pair of electrons, at an appropriate distance from the former. With the muscarinic agents, the distance between the two atoms is 4.3 to 4.4 Å, corresponding to that between the N^+ and the ester-O atom of ACh. For the nicotinic agents, the corresponding distance is 5.9 Å, which is equivalent to that between the N^+ and carbonyl-O of ACh. The presence of hydrophobic groups (*e.g.,* the methyl groups on the N^+ of ACh) is proposed to be involved both in the attraction of the drugs to the receptor and in the transition from activating to blocking activity (Beers and Reich, 1970). Thus, a picture of the receptors emerges that includes an anionic group, a nucleophilic group, and adjacent hydrophobic areas, not unlike that for the active centers of AChE, as discussed in Chapter 6.

Adrenergic. A vast number of synthetic compounds that bear structural resemblance to the naturally occurring catecholamines can combine at α- or β-adrenoceptive sites, or both, and produce sympathomimetic effects (*see* Chapter 8). *Phenylephrine* acts selectively at α-receptor sites, whereas *isoproterenol* exhibits selective action at β adrenoreceptors. Preferential stimulation of cardiac β_1 receptors follows the administration of *dobutamine* (*see* Tuttle and Mills, 1975; Sonnenblick *et al.,* 1979). *Terbutaline* is an example of a drug with relatively selective action on β_2 receptors; that is, it produces effective bronchodilatation with minimal effects on the heart. The main features of adrenergic blockade, including the selectivity of various blocking agents for α and β receptors, have been discussed. Here too, partial dissociation of effects at β_1 and β_2 adrenoreceptors has been achieved, as exemplified by the β_1-blocking agent *metoprolol*, which blocks the cardiac actions of catecholamines without causing an equivalent degree of antagonism at bronchioles. Several important drugs that promote the release of norepinephrine or deplete the transmitter resemble, in their effects, activators or blockers of postjunctional receptors (*e.g., tyramine* and *reserpine*, respectively). To date, there are relatively few examples of cholinomimetic drugs that have been demonstrated to act by comparable presynaptic mechanisms.

Interference with the Destruction of the Transmitter. *Cholinergic.* The *anti-ChE agents* (Chapter 6) constitute a large group of compounds, the primary action of which is inhibition of AChE, with the consequent accumulation and action of endogenous ACh at sites of cholinergic transmission.

Adrenergic. There appears to be no parallelism between the role of either COMT or MAO in terminating the action of the adrenergic transmitter and that of AChE in terminating the action of the cholinergic transmitter. The re-uptake of norepinephrine by the adrenergic nerve terminals is probably the major mechanism for terminating its transmitter action. Interference with this process has been proposed as the basis of the potentiating effect of *cocaine* on responses to adrenergic impulses and injected catecholamines; the antidepressant effect of *imipramine* and related drugs is perhaps due to a similar action at adrenergic synapses in the CNS. Inhibitors of COMT, such as pyrogallol and tropolone, produce only slight enhancement of the actions of catecholamines, whereas MAO inhibitors, such as *tranylcypromine*, potentiate the effects of tyramine but not of catecholamines. This action is important clinically. Patients who are being treated with MAO inhibitors may develop severe hypertensive episodes following the ingestion of foods rich in tyramine, such as certain cheeses, pickled herring, and certain red wines. This is because tyramine, which is normally metabolized by the MAO of the gut and the liver following absorption, now gains access to the systemic circulation and releases large amounts of norepinephrine from adrenergic nerve terminals. It may be possible to avoid such reaction by the use of selective inhibitors of MAO-B (*see* Chapter 9).

Central Neurohumoral Transmission. It is perhaps difficult for today's student to appreciate the impact that the concept of neurohumoral transmission has had on biomedical science. In the 1940s, the arguments that raged between the proponents of chemical transmission at synaptic sites (the "soup" men) and those who dismissed the thought and believed in electrical transmission (the "spark" men) can best be described as vitriolic. The latter accepted neurohumoral transmission at autonomic effector cells long before they did at ganglia and the neuromuscular junction. However, they finally struck their colors because of overwhelming evidence, largely provided by the use of drugs as research tools. The concept of neurohumoral transmission was quickly extended from the peripheral to the central nervous system. However, progress was slow for many years. Peripheral neurotransmitters are relatively few in number and can be studied in isolated structures in order to meet the rigid criteria that warrant the designation *neurotransmitter* without the reservation of *putative*. But with sophisticated technics, and again with the help of drugs as investigative tools, the role of specific neurotransmitters in central synaptic transmission has become firmly established. Interest in and knowledge of central neurohumors is now a burgeoning field, as described in the counterpart to this chapter, Chapter 12.

Ahlquist, R. P. A study of the adrenotropic receptors. *Am. J. Physiol.,* **1948,** *153,* 586–600.

Albuquerque, E. X.; Seyama, I.; and Narahashi, T. Characterization of batrachotoxin-induced depolarization of the squid giant axons. *J. Pharmacol. Exp. Ther.,* **1973,** *184,* 308–314.

Albuquerque, E. X.; Warnick, J. E.; Tasse, J. R.; and Sansone, F. M. Effects of vinblastine and colchicine on neural regulation of the fast and slow skeletal muscles of the rat. *Exp. Neurol.,* **1972,** *37,* 607–634.

Aurbach, G. D.; Fedak, S. A.; Woodward, C. J.; Palmer, J. S.; Hauser, D.; and Troxler, F. β-Adrenergic receptor: stereospecific interaction of iodinated β-blocking agent with high affinity site. *Science,* **1974,** *186,* 1223–1224.

Axelsson, J., and Thesleff, S. A study of supersensitivity in denervated mammalian skeletal muscle. *J. Physiol. (Lond.),* **1959,** *147,* 178–193.

Bain, W. A. Method of demonstrating humor transmission of effects of cardiac vagus stimulation in frog. *Q. J. Exp. Physiol.,* **1932,** *22,* 269–274.

Barger, G., and Dale, H. H. Chemical structure and sympathomimetic action of amines. *J. Physiol. (Lond.),* **1910,** *41,* 19–59.

Barker, D. L.; Molinoff, P. B.; and Kravitz, E. A. Octopamine in the lobster nervous system. *Nature* [*New Biol.*], **1972**, *236*, 61–63.

Bazemore, A. W.; Elliott, K. A. C.; and Florey, E. Isolation of factor I. *J. Neurochem.*, **1957**, *1*, 334–339.

Beers, W. H., and Reich, E. Structure and activity of acetylcholine. *Nature*, **1970**, *228*, 917–922.

Birks, R. I., and MacIntosh, F. C. Acetylcholine metabolism of a sympathetic ganglion. *Can. J. Biochem. Physiol.*, **1961**, *39*, 787–827.

Blaschko, H. The specific action of L-dopa decarboxylase. *J. Physiol.* (*Lond.*), **1939**, *96*, 50P–51P.

Brown, J. H.; Thompson, B. T.; and Mayer, S. E. Conversion of skeletal muscle glycogen synthase to multiple glucose 6-phosphate dependent forms by cyclic adenosine monophosphate dependent and independent protein kinases. *Biochemistry*, **1977**, *16*, 5501–5508.

Brunton, L. L.; Hayes, J. S.; and Mayer, S. E. Hormonally-specific phosphorylation of troponin I. *Nature*, **1979**, *280*, 78–80.

Buckley, G.; Consolo, S.; Giacobini, E.; and Sjöqvist, F. Cholinacetylase in innervated and denervated sympathetic ganglia and ganglion cells of the cat. *Acta Physiol. Scand.*, **1967**, *71*, 348–356.

Bullock, T. H., and Hagiwara, S. Intracellular recording from the giant synapse of the squid. *J. Gen. Physiol.*, **1957**, *40*, 565–577.

Burgen, A. S. V., and Spero, L. The action of acetylcholine and other drugs on the efflux of potassium and rubidium from smooth muscle of the guinea-pig intestine. *Br. J. Pharmacol.*, **1968**, *34*, 99–115.

Burgen, A. S. V., and Terroux, K. G. On the negative inotropic effects in the cat's auricle. *J. Physiol.* (*Lond.*), **1953**, *120*, 449–464.

Burn, J. H., and Gibbons, W. R. The release of noradrenaline from sympathetic fibres in relation to calcium concentrations. *J. Physiol.* (*Lond.*), **1965**, *181*, 214–223.

Burn, J. H., and Rand, M. J. Sympathetic postganglionic mechanism. *Nature*, **1959**, *184*, 163–165.

Burnstock, G., and Holman, M. E. The transmission of excitation from autonomic nerve to smooth muscle. *J. Physiol.* (*Lond.*), **1961**, *155*, 115–133.

Cannon, W. B., and Uridil, J. E. Studies on the conditions of activity in endocrine glands. VIII. Some effects on the denervated heart of stimulating the nerves of the liver. *Am. J. Physiol.*, **1921**, *58*, 353–354.

Carlsson, A.; Falck, B.; and Hillarp, N.-Å. Cellular localization of brain monoamines. *Acta Physiol. Scand.*, **1962**, *56*, Suppl. 196, 1–27.

Carlsson, A.; Hillarp, N.-Å.; and Waldeck, B. Analysis of the Mg++-ATP dependent storage mechanism in the amine granules of the adrenal medulla. *Acta Physiol. Scand.*, **1963**, *59*, Suppl. 215, 1–38.

Casteels, R.; Droogmans, G.; and Hendrickx, H. Electrogenic sodium pump in smooth muscle cells of the guinea-pig's taenia coli. *J. Physiol.* (*Lond.*), **1971**, *217*, 297–313.

Cavallito, C. J.; Yun, H. S.; Smith, J. C.; and Foldes, F. F. Choline acetyltransferase inhibitors. Configurational and electronic features of styrylpyridine analogs. *J. Med. Chem.*, **1969**, *12*, 134–138.

Chothia, C. Interaction of acetylcholine with different cholinergic nerve receptors. *Nature*, **1970**, *225*, 36–38.

Collier, B.; Barker, L. A.; and Mitlag, T. W. The release of acetylated choline by a sympathetic ganglion. *Mol. Pharmacol.*, **1976**, *12*, 340–344.

Cooke, J. D.; Okamoto, K.; and Quastel, D. M. J. The role of calcium in depolarization-secretion coupling at the motor nerve terminal. *J. Physiol.* (*Lond.*), **1973**, *228*, 459–497. (*See also* immediately preceding papers by same group on pages 377, 407, and 435.)

Dale, H. H. The action of certain esters and ethers of choline, and their relation to muscarine. *J. Pharmacol. Exp. Ther.*, **1914**, *6*, 147–190.

Dale, H. H.; Feldberg, W.; and Vogt, M. Release of acetylcholine at voluntary motor nerve endings. *J. Physiol.* (*Lond.*), **1936**, *86*, 353–380.

Davis, R., and Koelle, G. B. Electron microscopic localization of acetylcholinesterase and nonspecific cholinesterase at the neuromuscular junction by the gold-thiocholine and gold-thiolacetic acid methods. *J. Cell Biol.*, **1967**, *34*, 157–171.

De Robertis, E., and Bennett, H. S. Some features of the submicroscopic morphology of synapses in frog and earthworm. *J. Biophys. Biochem. Cytol.*, **1955**, *1*, 47–58.

Dixon, W. E. On the mode of action of drugs. *Med. Mag.* (*Lond.*), **1907**, *16*, 454–457.

Elfvin, L.-G. The ultrastructure of the superior cervical sympathetic ganglion of the cat. I. The structure of the ganglion cell processes as studied by serial sections. *J. Ultrastruct. Res.*, **1963a**, *8*, 403–440. II. The structure of the preganglionic end fibers and the synapses as studied by serial sections. *Ibid.*, **1963b**, *8*, 441–476.

———. Ultrastructural studies on the synaptology of the inferior mesenteric ganglion of the cat. *Ibid.*, **1971**, *37*, 411–425.

Elliott, T. R. The action of adrenalin. *J. Physiol.* (*Lond.*), **1905**, *32*, 401–467.

Emmelin, N., and MacIntosh, F. C. The release of acetylcholine from perfused sympathetic ganglia and skeletal muscles. *J. Physiol.* (*Lond.*), **1956**, *131*, 447–496.

England, P. J. Studies on the phosphorylation of the inhibitory subunit of troponin during modification of contraction in perfused rat heart. *Biochem. J.*, **1976**, *160*, 295–304.

Euler, U. S. von. Adrenaline and noradrenaline. Distribution and action. *Pharmacol. Rev.*, **1954**, *6*, 15–22.

Fatt, P., and Katz, B. Spontaneous subthreshold activity at motor nerve endings. *J. Physiol.* (*Lond.*), **1952**, *117*, 109–128.

Feldberg, W., and Gaddum, J. H. The chemical transmitter at synapses in a sympathetic ganglion. *J. Physiol.* (*Lond.*), **1934**, *81*, 305–319.

Feldberg, W., and Krayer, O. Das Auftreten eines azetylcholinartigen Stoffes in Herzvenenblut von Warmblütern bei Beizung der Nervi vagi. *Naunyn Schmiedebergs Arch. Exp. Pathol. Pharmakol.*, **1933**, *172*, 170–193.

Frontali, N.; Ceccarelli, B.; Gorio, A.; Mauro, A.; Siekevitz, P.; Tzeng, M.-C.; and Hurlburt, W. P. Purification from black widow spider venom of a protein factor causing depletion of synaptic vesicles at neuromuscular junction. *J. Cell Biol.*, **1976**, *68*, 462–479.

Garrison, J. C. The effects of glucagon, catecholamines, and the calcium ionophore A23187 on the phosphorylation of rat hepatocyte cytosolic proteins. *J. Biol. Chem.*, **1978**, *253*, 7091–7100.

Goldstein, M.; Fuxe, K.; and Hökfelt, T. Characterization and tissue localization of catecholamine synthesizing enzymes. *Pharmacol. Rev.*, **1972**, *24*, 293–309.

Gurin, S., and Delluva, A. The biological synthesis of radioactive adrenalin from phenylalanine. *J. Biol. Chem.*, **1947**, *170*, 545–550.

Hagiwara, S., and Tasaki, I. A study of the mechanism of impulse transmission across the giant synapse of the squid. *J. Physiol.* (*Lond.*), **1958**, *143*, 114–137.

Hartman, B. K., and Udenfriend, S. The application of immunological techniques to the study of enzymes regulating catecholamine synthesis and degradation. *Pharmacol. Rev.*, **1972**, *24*, 311–330.

Hayes, J. S.; Brunton, L. L.; Brown, J. H.; Reese, J. B.; and Mayer, S. E. Hormonally-specific expression of cardiac protein kinase activity. *Proc. Natl. Acad. Sci. U.S.A.*, **1979**, *76*, 1570–1574.

Hodgkin, A. L., and Huxley, A. F. A quantitative description of membrane current and its application to conduction and excitation in nerve. *J. Physiol.* (*Lond.*), **1952**, *117*, 500–544.

Holton, P. The liberation of adenosine triphosphate on antidromic stimulation of sensory nerves. *J. Physiol.* (*Lond.*), **1959**, *145*, 494–504.

Kao, I.; Drachman, D. B.; and Price, D. L. Botulinum toxin: mechanism of presynaptic action. *Science*, **1976**, *193*, 1256–1258.

Kato, J. Choline acetylase of human placenta. *J. Biochem.* (*Tokyo*), **1960**, *48*, 768–772.

Katz, B., and Miledi, R. The measurement of synaptic delay, and the time course of acetylcholine release at the neuromuscular junction. *Proc. R. Soc. Lond.* [*Biol.*], **1965**, *161*, 483–495.

———. The statistical nature of the acetylcholine potential and its molecular components. *J. Physiol.* (*Lond.*), **1972**, *224*, 665–699.

Kirshner, N. Uptake of catecholamines by a particulate fraction of the adrenal medulla. *J. Biol. Chem.*, **1962**, *237*, 2311–2317.

Koelle, G. B.; Davis, R.; Koelle, W. A.; Smyrl, E. G.; and Fine, A. V. The electron microscopic localization of acetylcholinesterase and pseudocholinesterase in autonomic ganglia. In, *Cholinergic Mechanisms.* (Waser, P. G., ed.) Raven Press, New York, **1975**, pp. 251–255.

Koelle, W. A., and Koelle, G. B. The localization of external or functional acetylcholinesterase at the synapses of autonomic ganglia. *J. Pharmacol. Exp. Ther.*, **1959**, *126*, 1–8.

Kravitz, E. A.; Slater, C. R.; Takahashi, K.; Bownds, M. D.; and Grossfeld, R. M. Excitatory transmission in vertebrates—glutamate as a potential neuromuscular transmitter compound. In, *Excitatory Synaptic Mechanisms.* (Andersen, P., and Jansen, J. K. S., eds.) Universitetsforlaget, Oslo, **1970**, pp. 85–93.

Krnjević, K., and Miledi, R. Acetylcholine in mammalian neuromuscular transmission. *Nature*, **1958**, *182*, 805–806.

Krnjević, K., and Mitchell, J. F. The release of acetylcholine in the isolated rat diaphragm. *J. Physiol.* (*Lond.*), **1961**, *155*, 246–262.

LaBrosse, E. H.; Axelrod, J.; Kopin, I. J.; and Kety, S. S. Metabolism of 7-H³-epinephrine-*d*-bitartrate in normal young men. *J. Clin. Invest.*, **1961**, *40*, 253–260.

Lands, A. M.; Arnold, A.; McAuliff, J. P.; Luduena, F. P.; and Brown, R. G., Jr. Differentiation of receptor systems activated by sympathomimetic amines. *Nature*, **1967**, *214*, 597–598.

Langley, J. N. Observations on the physiological action of extracts of the supra-renal bodies. *J. Physiol.* (*Lond.*), **1901**, *27*, 237–256.

Levin, E. Y.; Levenberg, B.; and Kaufman, S. The enzymatic conversion of 3,4-dihydroxyphenylethylamine to norepinephrine. *J. Biol. Chem.*, **1960**, *235*, 2080–2086.

Levitt, M.; Spector, S.; Sjoerdsma, A.; and Udenfriend, S. Elucidation of the rate-limiting step in norepinephrine biosynthesis in the perfused guinea pig heart. *J. Pharmacol. Exp. Ther.*, **1965**, *148*, 1–8.

Lewandowsky, M. Ueber eine Wirkung des Nebennierenextractes auf das Auge. *Zentralbl. Physiol.*, **1898**, *12*, 599–600.

Lipsius, S. L., and Vasalle, M. Effects of acetylcholine on potassium movements in the guinea-pig sinus node. *J. Pharmacol. Exp. Ther.*, **1977**, *201*, 669–677.

Loewi, O. Über humorale Übertragbarkeit der Herznervenwirkung. *Pflügers Arch. Gesamte Physiol.*, **1921**, *189*, 239–242.

Loewi, O., and Navratil, E. Über humorale Übertragbarkeit der Herznervenwirkung. X. Mitteilung. Über das Schicksal des Vagusstoff. *Pflügers Arch. Gesamte Physiol.*, **1926**, *214*, 678–688.

Longo, V. G. Acetylcholine, cholinergic drugs, and cortical electrical activity. *Experientia*, **1955**, *11*, 76–78.

Magaribuchi, T.; Ito, Y.; and Kuriyama, H. Effects of catecholamines on the guinea-pig vas deferens in various ionic environments. *Jpn. J. Physiol.*, **1971**, *21*, 691–708.

McIsaac, R. J., and Koelle, G. B. Comparison of the effects of inhibition of external, internal and total acetylcholinesterase upon ganglionic transmission. *J. Pharmacol. Exp. Ther.*, **1959**, *126*, 9–20.

Pfeuffer, T. GTP-binding proteins in membranes and the control of adenylate cyclase activity. *J. Biol. Chem.*, **1977**, *252*, 7224–7234.

Pumplin, D. W., and Reese, T. S. Action of brown widow spider venom and botulinum toxin on the frog neuromuscular junction examined with the freeze fracture technique. *J. Physiol.* (*Lond.*), **1977**, *273*, 444–457.

Reddy, V., and Moran, N. C. An evaluation of the adrenergic receptor types in isolated segments of the small intestine of the rabbit. *Arch. Int. Pharmacodyn. Ther.*, **1968**, *176*, 326–336.

Renshaw, R. R.; Green, D.; and Ziff, M. A basis for the acetylcholine action of choline derivatives. *J. Pharmacol. Exp. Ther.*, **1938**, *62*, 430–448.

Riker, W. F.; Roberts, J.; Standaert, F. G.; and Fujimoru, H. The motor nerve terminal as the primary focus for drug-induced facilitation of neuromuscular transmission. *J. Pharmacol. Exp. Ther.*, **1957**, *121*, 286–312.

Roach, P. J.; Takeda, Y.; and Larner, J. Rabbit skeletal muscle glycogen synthase: relation between phosphorylation state and kinetic properties. *J. Biol. Chem.*, **1976**, *251*, 1913–1919.

Ross, E. M.; Howlett, A. C.; Ferguson, K. M.; and Gilman, A. G. Reconstitution of hormone-sensitive adenylate cyclase activity with resolved components of the enzyme. *J. Biol. Chem.*, **1978**, *253*, 6401–6412.

Sjöqvist, F. Pharmacological analysis of acetylcholinesterase-rich ganglion cells in the lumbo-sacral sympathetic system of the cat. *Acta Physiol. Scand.*, **1963**, *157*, 352–362.

Soderling, T. R.; Jeff, M. F.; Hutson, N. J.; and Khatra, B.S. Regulation of glycogen synthase. *J. Biol. Chem.*, **1977**, *252*, 7517–7524.

Spector, S.; Tarver, J.; and Berkowitz, B. Effects of drugs and physiological factors in the disposition of catecholamines in blood vessels. *Pharmacol. Rev.*, **1972**, *24*, 191–202.

Steinsland, O. S.; Furchgott, R. F.; and Kirpekar, F. M. Inhibition of adrenergic neurotransmission by parasympathomimetics in the rabbit ear artery. *J. Pharmacol. Exp. Ther.*, **1973**, *184*, 346–356.

Steppeler, A.; Tanaka, T.; and Starke, K. A comparison of pre- and postsynaptic α-adrenergic effects of phenylephrine and tramazoline on blood vessels of the rabbit *in vivo*. *Naunyn Schmiedebergs Arch. Pharmacol.*, **1978**, *304*, 223–230.

Takeuchi, A., and Takeuchi, N. On the permeability of end-plate membrane during the action of transmitter. *J. Physiol.* (*Lond.*), **1960**, *154*, 52–67.

Thesleff, S. The cholinergic receptor in skeletal muscle. In, *Molecular Properties of Drug Receptors* (a Ciba Foundation symposium). (Porter, R., and O'Connor, M., eds.) J. & A. Churchill, Ltd., London, **1970**, pp. 33–39.

———. Functional properties of receptors in striated muscle. In, *Drug Receptors.* (Rang, H. P., ed.) University Park Press, Baltimore, **1973**, pp. 121–133.

Trautwein, W.; Kuffler, S. W.; and Edwards, C. Changes in membrane characteristics of heart muscle during inhibition. *J. Gen. Physiol.*, **1956**, *40*, 135–145.

Volle, R. L., and Koelle, G. B. The physiological role of acetylcholinesterase (AChE) in sympathetic ganglia. *J. Pharmacol. Exp. Ther.*, **1961**, *133*, 223–240.

Yamaguchi, N.; Champlain, J. de; and Nadeau, R. A. Regulation of norepinephrine release from cardiac sympathetic fibers by presynaptic α and β-receptors. *Circ. Res.*, **1977**, *41*, 108–116.

Monographs and Reviews

Acheson, G. H. (ed.). Second symposium on catecholamines. *Pharmacol. Rev.*, **1966**, *18*, Part 1, 1–803.

Almgren, O.; Carlsson, A.; and Engel, J. (eds.). *Regulation of Catecholamine Turnover. Chemical Tools in Catechola-*

mine Research, Vol. II. American Elsevier Publishing Co., Inc., New York, **1975,** pp. 3–310.

Armstrong, C. M. Ionic pores, gates and gating currents. *Q. Rev. Biophys.,* **1974,** *7,* 179–209.

Augustinsson, K.-B. Classification and comparative enzymology of the cholinesterases and methods for their determination. In, *Cholinesterases and Anticholinesterase Agents.* (Koelle, G. B., ed.) *Handbuch der Experimentellen Pharmakologie,* Vol. 15. Springer-Verlag, Berlin, **1963,** pp. 89–128.

Axelrod, J. The formation, metabolism, uptake and release of noradrenaline and adrenaline. In, *The Clinical Chemistry of Monoamines.* (Varley, H., and Gowenlock, A. H., eds.) Elsevier Publishing Co., Amsterdam, **1963,** pp. 5–18.

——. Methylation reactions in the formation and metabolism of catecholamines and other biogenic amines: the enzymatic conversion of norepinephrine (NE) to epinephrine (E). *Pharmacol. Rev.,* **1966,** *18,* 95–113.

——. Dopamine-β-hydroxylase: regulation of its synthesis and release from nerve terminals. *Ibid.,* **1972,** *24,* 233–243.

——. The fate of noradrenaline in the sympathetic neurone. *Harvey Lect.,* **1973,** *67,* 175–197.

Baldessarini, R. Release of catecholamines. In, *Handbook of Psychopharmacology,* Vol. 3. (Iversen, L. L.; Iversen, S. D.; and Snyder, S.; eds.) Plenum Press, New York, **1975,** pp. 37–137.

Bernard, C. *Leçons sur les phénomènes de la vie communs aux animaux et aux végétaux.* Baillière, Paris, **1878–1879.** (Two volumes.)

Berne, R. M., and Levy, M. N. *Cardiovascular Physiology,* 2nd ed. C. V. Mosby Co., St. Louis, **1972,** pp. 5–40.

Birks, R. I., and MacIntosh, F. C. Acetylcholine metabolism at nerve-endings. *Br. Med. Bull.,* **1957,** *13,* 157–161.

Blaschko, H. Amine oxidase and amine metabolism. *Pharmacol. Rev.,* **1952,** *4,* 415–458.

Blaschko, H., and Muscholl, E. (eds.). *Catecholamines. Handbuch der Experimentellen Pharmakologie,* Vol. 33. Springer-Verlag, Berlin, **1972.**

Bloom, F. E. Ultrastructural identification of catecholamine-containing central synaptic terminals. *J. Histochem. Cytochem.,* **1973,** *21,* 333–348.

Bolton, T. B. The permeability change produced by acetylcholine in smooth muscle. In, *Drug Receptors.* (Rang, H. P., ed.) University Park Press, Baltimore, **1973,** pp. 87–104.

Brodie, B. B.; Spector, S.; and Shore, P. A. Interactions of drugs with norepinephrine in the brain. *Pharmacol. Rev.,* **1959,** *11,* 548–564.

Bülbring, E. Actions of catecholamines on smooth muscle cell membrane. In, *Drug Receptors.* (Rang, H. P., ed.) University Park Press, Baltimore, **1973,** pp. 1–13.

Bullock, T. H.; Orkand, R.; and Grinnell, A. D. *Introduction to Nervous Systems.* W. H. Freeman & Co. Pub., San Francisco, **1977,** pp. 335–391.

Burnstock, G. Purinergic nerves. *Pharmacol. Rev.,* **1972,** *24,* 509–581.

Burnstock, G., and Iwayama, T. Fine-structural identification of autonomic nerves and their relation to smooth muscle. In, *Histochemistry of Nervous Transmission.* (Eränkö, O.) Elsevier Publishing Co., Amsterdam, **1971,** pp. 389–404.

Cannon, W. B. Organization for physiological homeostasis. *Physiol. Rev.,* **1929,** *9,* 399–431.

——. *The Wisdom of the Body.* W. W. Norton & Co., Inc., New York, **1932.**

Cannon, W. B., and Rosenblueth, A. *Autonomic Neuroeffector Systems.* The Macmillan Co., New York, **1937.**

——. *The Supersensitivity of Denervated Structures: A Law of Denervation.* The Macmillan Co., New York, **1949.**

Carlsson, A. The occurrence, distribution and physiological role of catecholamines in the nervous system. *Pharmacol. Rev.,* **1959,** *11,* 233–566.

Chagas, C., and Paes-de-Carvalho, A. (eds.). *Bioelectrogenesis: A Comparative Survey of Its Mechanisms, with Particular Emphasis on Electric Fishes.* Elsevier Publishing Co., Amsterdam, **1961.**

Cole, K. S. *Membranes, Ions and Impulses: A Chapter of Classical Biophysics.* University of California Press, Berkeley, **1968.**

Colquhoun, D. Mechanisms of action at the voluntary muscle endplate. *Annu. Rev. Pharmacol.,* **1975,** *15,* 307–326.

Cooper, J. R.; Bloom, F. E.; and Roth, R. H. *The Biochemical Basis of Neuropharmacology,* 3rd ed. Oxford University Press, New York, **1978.**

Cotten, M. deV. (ed.). Regulation of catecholamine metabolism in the sympathetic nervous system (N.Y. Heart Association Symposium). *Pharmacol. Rev.,* **1972,** *24,* 161–434.

Coupland, R. E. The chromaffin system. In, *Catecholamines.* (Blaschko, H., and Muscholl, E., eds.) *Handbuch der Experimentellen Pharmakologie,* Vol. 33. Springer-Verlag, Berlin, **1972,** pp. 16–45.

Couteaux, R. Structure and cytochemical characteristics of the neuromuscular junction. In, *Neuromuscular Blocking and Stimulating Agents,* Vol. 1. *International Encyclopedia of Pharmacology and Therapeutics,* Sect. 14. (Cheymol, J., ed.) Pergamon Press, Ltd., Oxford, **1972,** pp. 7–56.

Curtis, D. R., and Crawford, J. M. Central synaptic transmission—microelectrophoretic studies. *Annu. Rev. Pharmacol.,* **1969,** *9,* 209–240.

Dale, H. H. Chemical transmission of the effects of nerve impulses. *Br. Med. J.,* **1934,** *1,* 835–841.

——. The beginnings and the prospects of neurohumoral transmission. *Pharmacol. Rev.,* **1954,** *6,* 7–13.

Douglas, W. W. Stimulus-secretion coupling: the concept and clues from chromaffin and other cells (the First Gaddum Memorial Lecture, Cambridge, September 1967). *Br. J. Pharmacol.,* **1968,** *34,* 451–474.

Eccles, J. C. *The Physiology of Synapses.* Springer-Verlag, Berlin; Academic Press, Inc., New York, **1964.**

——. *The Understanding of the Brain.* McGraw-Hill Book Co., New York, **1973.**

Eränkö, O., and Eränkö, L. Small, intensely fluorescent granule-containing cells in the sympathetic ganglion of the rat. In, *Histochemistry of Nervous Transmission.* (Eränkö, O., ed.) Elsevier Publishing Co., Amsterdam, **1971,** pp. 39–51.

Euler, U. S. von. Synthesis, uptake and storage of catecholamines in adrenergic nerves. The effects of drugs. In, *Catecholamines.* (Blaschko, H., and Muscholl, E., eds.) *Handbuch der Experimentellen Pharmakologie,* Vol. 33. Springer-Verlag, Berlin, **1972a,** pp. 186–230.

——. Regulation of catecholamine metabolism in the sympathetic nervous system. *Pharmacol. Rev.,* **1972b,** *24,* 365–369.

Exton, J. H. Mechanisms involved in effects of catecholamines on liver carbohydrate metabolism. *Biochem. Pharmacol.,* **1979,** *28,* 2237–2240.

Feldberg, W. Present views on the mode of action of acetylcholine in the central nervous system. *Physiol. Rev.,* **1945,** *25,* 596–642.

Goldberg, L. I.; Volkman, P. H.; and Kohli, J. D. A comparison of the vascular dopamine receptor with other dopamine receptors. *Annu. Rev. Pharmacol. Toxicol.,* **1978,** *18,* 57–80.

Gray, E G. The fine structural characterization of different types of synapse. In, *Histochemistry of Nervous Transmission.* (Eränkö, O., ed.) Elsevier Publishing Co., Amsterdam, **1971,** pp. 149–160.

Grundfest, H. Electrical inexcitability of synapses and some consequences in the central nervous system. *Physiol. Rev.,* **1957,** *37,* 337–361.

——. Physiology of electrogenic excitable membranes. In, *The Nervous System,* Vol. 1. (Tower, D. B., ed.) Raven Press, New York, **1975,** pp. 153–164.

Hall, Z. W. Release of neurotransmitters and their interaction with receptors. *Annu. Rev. Biochem.,* **1972,** *41,* 925–947.

Hanin, I. (ed.). *Choline and Acetylcholine: Handbook of Chemical Assay Methods.* Raven Press, New York, **1974.**

Hebb, C. O. Formation, storage, and liberation of acetylcholine. In, *Cholinesterases and Anticholinesterase Agents.* (Koelle, G. B., ed.) *Handbuch der Experimentellen Pharmakologie,* Vol. 15. Springer-Verlag, Berlin, **1963,** pp. 56–88.

———. Biosynthesis of acetylcholine in nervous tissue. *Physiol. Rev.,* **1972,** *52,* 918–957.

Higgins, C. B.; Vatner, S. F.; and Braunwald, E. Parasympathetic control of the heart. *Pharmacol. Rev.,* **1973,** *19,* 119–155.

Hillarp, N.-Å. The construction and functional organization of the autonomic innervation apparatus. *Acta Physiol. Scand.,* **1959,** *46,* Suppl. 157, 1–39.

Himms-Hagen, J. Sympathetic regulation of metabolism. *Pharmacol. Rev.,* **1967,** *19,* 367–461.

———. Effects of catecholamines on metabolism. In, *Catecholamines.* (Blaschko, H., and Muscholl, E., eds.) *Handbuch der Experimentellen Pharmakologie,* Vol. 33. Springer-Verlag, Berlin, **1972,** pp. 363–462.

Hubbard, J. I. Microphysiology of vertebrate neuromuscular transmission. *Physiol. Rev.,* **1973,** *53,* 674–723.

Iversen, L. L. *The Uptake and Storage of Noradrenaline in Sympathetic Nerves.* Cambridge University Press, London, **1967.**

———. Uptake processes for biogenic amines. In, *Handbook of Psychopharmacology,* Vol. 3. (Iversen, L. L.; Iversen, S. D.; and Snyder, S.; eds.) Plenum Press, New York, **1975,** pp. 381–442.

Jonsson, G.; Malmfors, T.; and Sachs, C. (eds.). *6-Hydroxydopamine as a Denervation Tool in Catecholamine Research. Chemical Tools in Catecholamine Research,* Vol. I. American Elsevier Publishing Co., Inc., New York, **1975,** pp. 3–372.

Kao, C. Y. Tetrodotoxin, saxitoxin and their significance in the study of excitation phenomena. *Pharmacol. Rev.,* **1966,** *18,* 997–1049.

Katz, B. *Nerve, Muscle, and Synapse.* McGraw-Hill Book Co., New York, **1966.**

Kirshner, N. Function and organization of chromaffin vesicles. *Life Sci.,* **1974,** *14,* 1153–1167.

Koelle, G. B. Microanatomy and pharmacology of cholinergic synapses. In, *The Nervous System,* Vol. 1. (Tower, D. B., ed.) Raven Press, New York, **1975,** pp. 363–371.

Kopin, I. J. Metabolic degradation of catecholamines. The relative importance of different pathways under physiological conditions and after administration of drugs. In, *Catecholamines.* (Blaschko, H., and Muscholl, E., eds.) *Handbuch der Experimentellen Pharmakologie,* Vol. 33. Springer-Verlag, Berlin, **1972,** pp. 271–282.

Kopin, I. J., and Silberstein, S. D. Axons of sympathetic neurons: transport of enzymes *in vivo* and properties of axonal sprouts *in vitro. Pharmacol. Rev.,* **1972,** *24,* 245–254.

Krnjević, K. Chemical nature of synaptic transmission in vertebrates. *Physiol. Rev.,* **1974,** *54,* 418–540.

Langer, S. Z. Presynaptic regulation and their role in the regulation of transmitter release. *Br. J. Pharmacol.,* **1977,** *60,* 481–497.

Levi-Montalcini, R., and Angeletti, P. U. Nerve growth factor. *Physiol. Rev.,* **1968,** *48,* 534–569.

Lloyd, D. P. C. Cholinergy and adrenergy in the neural control of sweat glands. In, *Studies in Physiology.* (Curtis, D. R., and McIntyre, A. K., eds.) Springer-Verlag, New York, **1965,** pp. 169–178.

MacLean, P. D. The limbic brain in relation to the psychoses. In, *Physiological Correlates of Emotion.* (Black, P., ed.) Academic Press, Inc., New York, **1970,** pp. 130–146.

Maguire, M. M.; Ross, E. M.; and Gilman, A. G. β-Adrenergic receptor: ligand binding properties and the interaction with adenylyl cyclase. *Adv. Cyclic Nucleotide Res.,* **1977,** *8,* 2–83.

Mayer, S. E. Biochemical responses to *beta* adrenergic receptor activation. In, *Beta Adrenergic Blockade: A New Era in Cardiovascular Medicine.* (Braunwald, E., ed.) Excerpta Medica, Amsterdam, **1978,** pp. 25–37.

Michelson, M. J., and Zeimal, E. V. *Acetylcholine: An Approach to the Molecular Mechanism of Action.* Pergamon Press, Ltd., Oxford, **1973.**

Miller, N. E. Biofeedback and visceral learning. *Annu. Rev. Psychol.,* **1978,** *29,* 237–250.

Miyamoto, M. D. The actions of cholinergic drugs on motor nerve terminals. *Pharmacol. Rev.,* **1978,** *29,* 226–247.

Moran, N. C. Adrenergic receptors. In, *Adrenal Gland,* Vol. 6. Sect. 7., *Endocrinology. Handbook of Physiology.* (Blaschko, H.; Sayers, G.; and Smith, A. D.; eds.) American Physiological Society, Washington, D.C., **1975,** pp. 447–472.

Musacchio, J. M. Enzymes involved in biosynthesis and degradation by catecholamines. In, *Handbook of Psychopharmacology,* Vol. 3. (Iversen, L. L.; Iversen, S. D.; and Snyder, S.; eds.) Plenum Press, New York, **1975,** pp. 1–36.

Muscholl, E. Adrenergic false transmitters. In, *Catecholamines.* (Blaschko, H., and Muscholl, E., eds.) *Handbuch der Experimentellen Pharmakologie,* Vol. 33. Springer-Verlag, Berlin, **1972,** pp. 618–660.

Nachmansohn, D. *Chemical and Molecular Basis of Nerve Activity.* Academic Press, Inc., New York, **1959.**

———. The neuromuscular junction—the role of acetylcholine in excitable membranes. In, *The Structure and Function of Muscle,* 2nd ed., Vol. 3. (Bourne, G. H., ed.) Academic Press, Inc., New York, **1973,** pp. 31–116.

Naharashi, T. Neurotoxins: pharmacological dissection of ionic channels of nerve membranes. In, *The Nervous System,* Vol. 2. (Tower, D. B., ed.) Raven Press, New York, **1975,** pp. 101–110.

Potter, L. T. Synthesis, storage, and release of acetylcholine from nerve terminals. In, *The Structure and Function of Nervous Tissue,* Vol. 4. (Bourne, G. H., ed.) Academic Press, Inc., New York, **1972,** pp. 105–128.

Purves, D., and Lichtman, J. W. Formation and maintenance of synaptic connections in autonomic ganglia. *Physiol. Rev.,* **1978,** *58,* 821–857.

Rall, T. W. Role of adenosine 3′,5′-monophosphate (cyclic AMP) in actions of catecholamines. *Pharmacol. Rev.,* **1972,** *24,* 399–410.

Rall, T. W., and Gilman, A. G. (eds.). The role of cyclic AMP in the nervous system. *Neurosci. Res. Program Bull.,* **1970,** *8,* 221–323.

Rang, H. P. (ed.). *Drug Receptors.* University Park Press, Baltimore, **1973.**

———. Acetylcholine receptors. *Q. Rev. Biophys.,* **1975,** *7,* 283–397.

Riker, W. F., Jr., and Okamoto, M. Pharmacology of motor nerve terminals. *Annu. Rev. Pharmacol.,* **1969,** *9,* 173–208.

Robison, G. A.; Butcher, R. W.; and Sutherland, E. W. *Cyclic AMP.* Academic Press, Inc., New York, **1971.**

Rossier, J. Choline acetyltransferase: a review with special reference to its cellular and subcellular localization. *Int. Rev. Neurobiol.,* **1977,** *20,* 283–337.

Rothballer, A. B. The effects of catecholamines on the central nervous system. *Pharmacol. Rev.,* **1959,** *11,* 494–547.

Rubin, R. P. *Calcium and the Secretory Process.* Plenum Press, New York, **1974.**

Scharrer, B. Comparative aspects of neuroendocrine communication. *Gen. Comp. Endocrinol.,* **1972,** Suppl. 3, 515–517.

Schmitt, F. O.; Dev, P.; and Smith, B. H. Electrotonic processing of information by brain cells. *Science,* **1976,** *193,* 114–120.

Shepherd, J. T. Alteration in activity of vascular smooth

muscle by local modulation of adrenergic transmitter release. *Fed. Proc.,* **1978,** *37,* 179–221.

Sobel, B. E., and Mayer, S. E. Cyclic adenosine monophosphate and cardiac contractility. *Circ. Res.,* **1973,** *32,* 407–414.

Sonnenblick, E. H.; Frishman, W. H.; and LeJemtel, T. H. Dobutamine: a new synthetic cardioactive sympathetic amine. *N. Engl. J. Med.,* **1979,** *300,* 17–22.

Stjärne, L. The synthesis, uptake and storage of catecholamines in the adrenal medulla. The effects of drugs. In, *Catecholamines.* (Blaschko, H., and Muscholl, E., eds.) *Handbuch der Experimentellen Pharmakologie,* Vol. 33. Springer-Verlag, Berlin, **1972,** pp. 231–269.

Stull, J. T., and Mayer, S. E. Adrenergic and cholinergic mechanisms of modulation of myocardial contractility. In, *Heart,* Vol. 1. Sect. 2, *The Cardiovascular System. Handbook of Physiology.* (Berne, R. M., ed.) American Physiological Society, Bethesda, **1979,** pp. 741–774.

Thoenen, H. Surgical, immunological, and chemical sympathectomy. In, *Catecholamines.* (Blaschko, H., and Muscholl, E., eds.) *Handbuch der Experimentellen Pharmakologie,* Vol. 33. Springer-Verlag, Berlin, **1972,** pp. 813–844.

Tuttle, R. R., and Mills, J. Dobutamine: development of a new catecholamine to selectively increase cardiac contractility. *Circ. Res.,* **1975,** *36,* 185–196.

Usdin, E., and Snyder, S. (eds.). *Frontiers in Catecholamine Research.* Pergamon Press, Ltd., Oxford, **1973.**

Usdin, E.; Weiner, N.; and Youdim, M. B. H. (eds.). *Structure and Function of Monoamine Enzymes.* Marcel Dekker, Inc., New York, **1977.**

Uvnäs, B. Sympathetic dilator outflow. *Physiol. Rev.,* **1954,** *34,* 608–618.

Weiner, N.; Cloutier, G.; Bjur, R.; and Pfeffer, R. I. Modification of norepinephrine synthesis in intact tissue by drugs and during short-term adrenergic nerve stimulation. *Pharmacol. Rev.,* **1972,** *24,* 203–232.

Weinshilboum, R. M. Serum dopamine β-hydroxylase. *Pharmacol. Rev.,* **1978,** *30,* 133–166.

Welsh, J. H. Neurohormones. *Hormones (Lond.),* **1955,** *3,* 97–151.

Westfall, T. C. Local regulation of adrenergic neurotransmission. *Physiol. Rev.,* **1977,** *57,* 659–728.

Whittaker, V. P. Identification of acetylcholine and related esters of biological origin. In, *Cholinesterases and Anticholinesterase Agents.* (Koelle, G. B., ed.) *Handbuch der Experimentellen Pharmakologie,* Vol. 15. Springer-Verlag, Berlin, **1963,** pp. 1–39.

Williamson, J. R. Effects of epinephrine on glycogenolysis and myocardial contractility. In, *Adrenal Gland,* Vol. 6. Sect. 7, *Endocrinology. Handbook of Physiology.* (Blaschko, H.; Sayers, G.; and Smith, A. D.; eds.) American Physiological Society, Washington, D. C., **1975,** pp. 605–636.

Wolfe, B. B.; Harden, T. K.; and Molinoff, P. B. *In vitro* studies of β-adrenergic receptors. *Annu. Rev. Pharmacol. Toxicol.,* **1977,** *17,* 575–604.

Wurtman, R. J.; Pohorecky, L. A.; and Baliga, B. S. Adrenocortical control of the biosynthesis of epinephrine and proteins in the adrenal medulla. *Pharmacol. Rev.,* **1972,** *24,* 411–426.

CHAPTER
5 CHOLINERGIC AGONISTS

Palmer Taylor

Cholinergic agonists have as their primary action the excitation or inhibition of autonomic effector cells that are innervated by postganglionic parasympathetic nerves. When acting in this capacity, they may be referred to as *parasympathomimetic agents.* Additional actions are exerted on ganglia and on cells that do not receive extensive parasympathetic innervation but nevertheless possess cholinergic receptors. These drugs may be divided into two groups: (1) acetylcholine (ACh) and several synthetic choline esters and (2) the naturally occurring cholinomimetic alkaloids (particularly pilocarpine, muscarine, and arecoline) and their synthetic congeners. In addition, the anticholinesterase (anti-ChE) agents (Chapter 6) and the ganglionic stimulants (Chapter 10) have parasympathomimetic actions, but they also produce prominent effects at locations other than the postganglionic cholinergic effector site.

CHOLINE ESTERS

Acetylcholine (ACh) has had virtually no therapeutic applications because of its diffuseness of action and its rapid hydrolysis by both acetylcholinesterase (AChE) and plasma pseudocholinesterase. Consequently, numerous derivatives have been synthesized in attempts to obtain drugs with more selective and prolonged actions. Only the latter objective has met with much success.

History. ACh was first synthesized by Baeyer in 1867. Investigations culminating in its identification as a neurohumoral transmitter are described in Chapter 4.

Of several hundred synthetic choline derivatives investigated, only methacholine, carbachol, and bethanechol have had clinical application. The structures of these compounds are shown in Table 5–1. Although *methacholine,* the β-methyl analog of ACh, was studied by Hunt and Taveau as early as 1911, it was not until the systematic investigations of this compound by Simonart (1932) and Starr and associates (1933) that the drug received adequate

therapeutic trial. *Carbachol,* the carbamyl ester of choline, and *bethanechol,* its β-methyl analog, were synthesized in the early 1930s; their pharmacological actions were investigated by Molitor (1936) and others.

Mechanism of Action. The mechanisms of action of endogenous ACh at the postjunctional membranes of the effector cells and neurons that correspond to the four classes of cholinergic synapses are discussed in Chapter 4. By way of recapitulation, these are (1) autonomic effector sites, innervated by postganglionic parasympathetic fibers; (2) sympathetic and parasympathetic ganglion cells and the adrenal medulla, innervated by preganglionic autonomic fibers; (3) motor end-plates on skeletal muscle, innervated by somatic motor nerves; and (4) certain synapses within the central nervous system (CNS). When ACh is administered systemically, it has the potential to act at all of these sites; however, as a quaternary ammonium compound its penetration into the CNS is limited, and pseudocholinesterase reduces the concentrations of ACh that reach areas in the periphery with low blood flow.

Since muscarine was characterized originally as acting relatively selectively at *autonomic effector cells* to produce qualitatively the same effects as ACh, actions of ACh and related drugs at these sites are referred to as *muscarinic.* Accordingly, the *muscarinic,* or *parasympathomimetic,* actions of the drugs considered in this chapter are practically equivalent to the effects of postganglionic parasympathetic nerve impulses listed in Table 4–1 (page 60); the differences between the actions of the individual muscarinic agonists are largely quantitative, with limited selectivity for one organ system or another. It is now known that *muscarinic* receptors are also present to a variable degree on autonomic ganglion cells and on certain cortical and subcortical neurons, and hence the drugs of this class may have secondary effects at

91

Table 5-1. STRUCTURAL FORMULAS OF CHOLINE, ACETYLCHOLINE, AND CHOLINE ESTERS EMPLOYED CLINICALLY

Choline chloride	$(CH_3)_3\overset{+}{N}CH_2CH_2OH$	Cl^-
Acetylcholine chloride	$(CH_3)_3\overset{+}{N}CH_2CH_2O\overset{\overset{O}{\|\|}}{C}CH_3$	Cl^-
Methacholine chloride	$(CH_3)_3\overset{+}{N}CH_2\underset{CH_3}{CH}O\overset{\overset{O}{\|\|}}{C}CH_3$	Cl^-
Carbachol chloride	$(CH_3)_3\overset{+}{N}CH_2CH_2O\overset{\overset{O}{\|\|}}{C}NH_2$	Cl^-
Bethanechol chloride	$(CH_3)_3\overset{+}{N}CH_2\underset{CH_3}{CH}O\overset{\overset{O}{\|\|}}{C}NH_2$	Cl^-

these sites. All the actions of ACh and its congeners at muscarinic receptors can be blocked by *atropine* (*see* Chapter 7). The *nicotinic* actions of cholinergic agonists refer to their initial stimulation, and in high doses to subsequent blockade, of autonomic ganglion cells and the neuromuscular junction, actions comparable to those of nicotine.

Properties of Muscarinic Receptors. The muscarinic receptor has been quantified and characterized in various tissues in the periphery and in the CNS by analysis of binding isotherms for antagonists that interact with the putative receptor with high affinity (Snyder *et al.,* 1974; Birdsall and Hume, 1976; Birdsall *et al.,* 1978). Specificity of ligand binding to the receptor has been examined by study of competition by agonists, saturability, and stereospecificity of interaction. Specific binding is found in

tissues where muscarinic receptors are demonstrable pharmacologically. Unfortunately, our understanding of the events associated with activation of the receptor remains meager. Accumulation of cyclic guanosine 3′,5′-monophosphate (cyclic GMP) (George *et al.,* 1970), enhanced permeability of monovalent cations (Burgen and Spero, 1968), and increased turnover of phosphoinositol (Jafferji and Michell, 1976) have each been implicated in the sequence of steps that follows occupation of the receptor. Only stimulation of phosphoinositol turnover appears to be independent of Ca^{2+} and follows precisely the concentration dependence for occupation of the receptor by agonists (Birdsall and Hume, 1976), suggesting that it might be the most proximal of the three events.

Structure-Activity Relationship. The structure-activity relationship of cholinergic agonists has been described in detail (Simonart, 1932; Bebbington and Brimblecombe, 1965; Kosterlitz, 1967; Rand and Stafford, 1967). Attention is accorded here only to those drugs that are of therapeutic interest.

Acetyl-β-methylcholine (methacholine) differs from ACh chiefly in its greater duration and selectivity of action. Its action is more prolonged because it is hydrolyzed by AChE at a considerably slower rate than ACh and is almost totally resistant to hydrolysis by nonspecific cholinesterase or pseudocholinesterase. Its selectivity is manifested by a lack of significant nicotinic and a predominance of muscarinic actions, the latter being most marked on the cardiovascular system (Table 5–2).

Carbachol and *bethanechol,* which are unsubstituted carbamyl esters, are totally resistant to hydrolysis by either AChE or nonspecific cholinesterase; their half-lives are thus sufficiently long that they are distributed to areas of low blood flow. Bethanechol has mainly muscarinic actions, but both drugs act with some selectivity on the smooth muscle of the gastrointestinal tract and urinary bladder. Carbachol retains a high level of nicotinic activity, particularly on autonomic ganglia. It is likely that both its peripheral and its ganglionic actions are due, at least in part, to the release of endogenous ACh from the terminals of cholinergic fibers (*see* Chapter 4).

Table 5-2. SOME PHARMACOLOGICAL PROPERTIES OF CHOLINE ESTERS

CHOLINE ESTER	SUSCEPTIBILITY TO CHOLINESTERASES	Muscarinic				Antagonism by Atropine	Nicotinic
		Cardiovascular	Gastrointestinal	Urinary Bladder	Eye (topical)		
Acetylcholine	+ + +	+ +	+ +	+ +	+	+ + +	+ +
Methacholine	+	+ + +	+ +	+ +	+	+ + +	+
Carbachol	−	+	+ + +	+ + +	+ +	+	+ + +
Bethanechol	−	±	+ + +	+ + +	+ +	+ + +	−

PHARMACOLOGICAL PROPERTIES

Cardiovascular System. ACh has three primary effects upon the cardiovascular system: *vasodilatation,* a decrease in cardiac rate (the *negative chronotropic* effect), and a decrease in the force of cardiac contraction (the *negative inotropic* effect). The latter is particularly true of atrial muscle and is of lesser significance in the ventricle. However, certain of these above effects can be obscured by a number of factors, especially the release by ACh of catecholamines from both cardiac and extracardiac tissues and the dampening of the direct effects of ACh by baroreceptor and other reflexes.

Although ACh is rarely given systemically as a drug, its cardiac actions are of importance because of the involvement of cholinergic vagal impulses in the actions of the cardiac glycosides, antiarrhythmic agents, and many other drugs. The intravenous injection of a small (1 to 5 μg/kg) dose of ACh in an anesthetized animal produces an evanescent fall in blood pressure due to generalized vasodilatation, accompanied usually by reflex tachycardia. A considerably larger dose is required to elicit bradycardia or block of A-V nodal conduction from the direct action of ACh on the heart. If large doses of ACh are injected after the administration of atropine, an increase in blood pressure is observed due to stimulation of release of catecholamines from the adrenal medulla and activation of sympathetic ganglia. In *man,* intravenous infusions of ACh (20 to 60 mg per minute) produce little change other than vasodilatation and a slight fall in blood pressure, because of the rapid enzymatic hydrolysis of ACh and the efficient compensatory cardiovascular reflexes mediated through the caroticoaortic baroreceptors. When large doses (90 to 140 mg per minute) are administered intravenously, the complete pattern of bradycardia, hypotension, and the expected responses of other autonomic effectors is obtained.

ACh, when injected, produces *dilatation* of essentially *all vascular beds,* including the pulmonary (Aviado, 1965) and coronary (Levy and Zieske, 1969). However, it is unlikely that either parasympathetic vasodilator or sympathetic vasoconstrictor tone plays a major role in the regulation of coronary blood flow, in comparison with the effects of local oxygen tension and autoregulatory metabolic factors such as adenosine (Berne, 1974). The effect of choline esters to dilate vascular beds is due to the presence of muscarinic receptors at these sites, despite the lack of apparent cholinergic innervation of most vascular beds.

ACh has important actions on all types of specialized cardiac cells; the same is qualitatively true of vagal impulses, since cholinergic parasympathetic fibers are distributed extensively to the S-A and A-V nodes and the atrial muscle. Cholinergic innervation of the ventricular myocardium is sparse, and the axons terminate predominantly on specialized conduction tissue such as the Purkinje fibers (Kamijo and Koelle, 1955; Kent *et al.,* 1974; Priola, *et al.,* 1977).

In the *S-A node,* each normal cardiac impulse is initiated by the spontaneous depolarization of the pacemaker cells, due to a progressive fall in potassium conductance (*see* Chapter 31). At a critical level, the threshold potential, this depolarization initiates an action potential (AP). The AP is conducted over the course of the atrial muscle fibers to the A-V node and thence through the Purkinje system to the ventricular muscle. ACh slows the heart rate by decreasing the rate of spontaneous diastolic depolarization at the S-A node, thereby delaying the attainment of the threshold potential and the succeeding events in the cardiac cycle.

In *atrial muscle,* ACh decreases the strength of contraction. It also slows the rate of conduction of the AP and shortens the durations of the AP and the effective refractory period. The combination of these factors is the basis for the perpetuation or exacerbation by vagal impulses of atrial flutter or fibrillation arising at an ectopic focus. In contrast, primarily in the *A-V node* and to a much lesser extent in the *Purkinje conducting system,* ACh slows conduction but increases the refractory period. The decrement in A-V conduction is usually responsible for the complete heart block that may be observed when large quantities of cholinergic agonists are administered systemically. With an increase in vagal tone, such as is produced by the digitalis glycosides, the increased refractory period can contribute to the reduction in the frequency with which aberrant atrial impulses are transmitted to the ventricle, and thus decrease the ventricular rate during atrial flutter or fibrillation. The increased vagal tone also enhances electrical stability of the ventricles and reduces the incidence of spontaneous ventricular fibrillation (Kent *et al.,* 1974; Kent and Epstein, 1976). ACh normally decreases slightly the strength of contraction of the ventricle. This is particularly evident when contractility has been enhanced by adrenergic stimulation. The depressant effect is likely due in part to a decrease in release of norepinephrine and to a direct effect on the myocardium. At excessive concentrations, ACh may cause a positive inotropic effect, mainly through the local release of catecholamine (Buccino *et al.,* 1966). (*See also* Rand and Stafford, 1967; Higgins *et al.,* 1973; Levy, 1977.)

The effects produced in man by constant *intravenous* infusion of *methacholine* are identical with those obtained with ACh, but the effective dose is only about 0.5% as large. After a *subcutaneous* dose of 20 mg, a transient fall in blood pressure and a compensatory tachycardia occur. When methacholine is administered *orally,* doses 50 to 100 times as large as the effective subcutaneous dose must be employed before significant effects of this quaternary drug are observed; these are gradual in onset and mild in character. For example, after an oral dose of 1 g the blood pressure falls only moderately, the pulse rate slows, the typical flush appears, and the skin temperature of the extremities rises, indicative of vasodilatation. Methacholine administered parenterally can cause *cardiac arrhythmias,* such as various degrees of heart block including complete A-V dissociation. Cardiac arrhythmias caused by methacholine are particularly prone to occur in patients with hyperthyroidism.

In contrast to ACh and methacholine, the cardiovascular effects of *carbachol* and *bethanechol* ordinarily are less conspicuous following usual subcutaneous or oral doses that affect the gastrointestinal and urinary tracts; these generally consist only in a slight, transient fall in diastolic pressure accompanied by a mild reflex tachycardia.

Gastrointestinal System. All the compounds of this class are capable of producing increases in tone, amplitude of contractions, and peristaltic activity of the stomach and intestines, as well as enhanced secretory activity of the gastrointestinal tract. The enhanced motility may be accompanied by nausea, belching, vomiting, intestinal cramps, and defecation.

Urinary Tract. *Carbachol* and *bethanechol,* in contrast to ACh and methacholine, stimulate rather selectively the urinary tract as well as the gastrointestinal tract. The choline esters increase ureteral peristalsis, contract the detrusor muscle of the urinary bladder, increase the maximal voluntary voiding pressure, and decrease the capacity of the bladder. In addition, the trigone and external sphincter are relaxed. In animals with experimental lesions of the spinal cord or sacral roots, these drugs bring about satisfactory evacuation of the neurogenic bladder.

Miscellaneous Effect. ACh and its analogs stimulate secretion by all *glands* that receive parasympathetic innervation, including the lacrimal, tracheobronchial, salivary, digestive, and exocrine sweat glands. The effects on the *respiratory system,* in addition to increased tracheobronchial secretion, include bronchoconstriction and stimulation of the chemoreceptors of the carotid and aortic bodies. When instilled into the eye, they produce *miosis;* however, the resultant fall in the intraocular tension may be preceded by a temporary elevation due to an increase in the permeability of the blood–aqueous humor barrier and vasodilatation of small vessels.

The effects of ACh on *autonomic ganglia* and at the *neuromuscular junction* of skeletal muscle are described in Chapters 10 and 11, respectively. While the cholinergic agonists considered here can produce similar effects in isolated preparations, these are not significant with the doses employed clinically (with the possible exception of some responses to carbachol).

Synergisms and Antagonisms. ACh and methacholine are hydrolyzed by AChE, and their effects are markedly enhanced by the prior administration of anti-ChE agents. The latter drugs produce only additive effects with the stable analogs, carbachol and bethanechol.

The *muscarinic* actions of all the drugs of this class are blocked selectively by atropine, through competitive occupation of cholinergic receptor sites on the autonomic effector cells and on the secondary muscarinic receptors of autonomic ganglion cells. Epinephrine and other sympathomimetic amines likewise antagonize most of their muscarinic effects at sites where adrenergic and cholinergic impulses produce opposing effects (Table 4–1).

The *nicotinic* actions of ACh and its derivatives at autonomic ganglia are blocked by hexamethonium and related drugs; their actions at the neuromuscular junction of skeletal muscle are antagonized by *d*-tubocurarine and other competitive blocking agents.

Preparations, Routes of Administration, and Dosage. *Acetylcholine chloride* is used practically exclusively for compounding *acetylcholine chloride for ophthalmic solution* (MIOCHOL). The latter is available in vials for the extemporaneous preparation of a 1% solution in 5% mannitol.

Methacholine Chloride, U.S.P. (acetyl-β-methylcholine), is now rarely used clinically.

Bethanechol Chloride, U.S.P. (*carbamylmethylcholine chloride*; MYOTONACHOL, URECHOLINE, others), is available in tablets containing 5, 10, 25, or 50 mg and as an injection (5 mg/ml). It is used to stimulate contraction of the gastrointestinal tract and the urinary bladder. The *oral* dose for adults varies from 10 to 100 mg; the *subcutaneous* dose is 2.5 to 5.0 mg. The single dose may be given three to four times daily. *The drug should not be administered by the intramuscular or intravenous route.*

Carbachol, U.S.P. (*carbamylcholine chloride*), is used as *Carbachol Ophthalmic Solution*, U.S.P. (CARBACEL OPHTHALMIC, ISOPTO CARBACHOL), in concentrations of 0.75, 1.5, 2.25, and 3.0%. It is also available as *carbachol intraocular solution* (MIOSTAT INTRAOCULAR), a 0.01% solution that is used to produce miosis during ocular surgery. The solution (0.5 ml) is instilled into the anterior chamber.

Precautions, Toxicity, and Contraindications. Drugs of this class should be administered only by the *oral* or *subcutaneous* route for systemic effects; they are also used locally in the eye. If they are given intravenously or intramuscularly, their relative selectivity of action no longer holds, and the incidence and severity of toxic side effects are greatly increased. In order to *counteract* any serious toxic reactions to these drugs, *atropine sulfate* (0.5 to 1.0 mg) should be given intramuscularly or intravenously, and should be readily available. *Epinephrine* (0.1 to 1.0 mg, subcutaneously) is also of value in overcoming severe cardiovascular or bronchoconstrictor responses.

Among the major *contraindications* to the use of the choline esters are *asthma, hyperthyroidism, coronary insufficiency*, and *peptic ulcer*. As noted previously, their bronchoconstrictor action is liable to precipitate an asthmatic attack, and hyperthyroid patients may develop atrial fibrillation, particularly after methacholine. Hypotension induced by these agents can severely reduce coronary blood flow, especially if it is already compromised. The gastric acid secretion produced by the choline esters can aggravate the symptoms of peptic ulcer.

A number of *untoward clinical reactions* can follow the administration of *methacholine*, including nausea and vomiting, substernal pain or pressure, dyspnea, fainting, and transient complete heart block. Patients with hypertension may react to the drug with a precipitous fall in blood pressure. Overdosage may result in an alarming but transient syncopal reaction, with cardiac arrest and loss of consciousness. After *bethanechol*, untoward effects related to the cardiovascular system are less liable to occur. Undesirable effects may include flushing, sweating, epigastric distress, abdominal cramps, belching, a sensation of tightness in the urinary bladder, difficulty in visual accommodation, headache, and salivation.

THERAPEUTIC USES

Bethanechol is still used as a stimulant of the smooth muscle of the gastrointestinal tract and, particularly, the urinary bladder; *carbachol* is obsolete for these purposes because of its relatively larger component of nicotinic action at autonomic ganglia. The unpredictability of the intensity of response has virtually eliminated the use of *methacholine* as a vasodilator and cardiac vagomimetic agent.

Gastrointestinal Disorders. Bethanechol is of value in certain cases of *postoperative abdominal distention* and *gastric atony* or *stasis*. The oral route is preferred; the usual dose is 10 to 20 mg, three or four times daily. It may be necessary to insert a rectal tube to facilitate passage of flatus. The drug has likewise been used to advantage in certain patients with adynamic ileus secondary to toxic states. *Gastric atony and retention following bilateral vagotomy* for peptic ulcer are often satisfactorily relieved by bethanechol; in this condition, neostigmine is ineffective. Bethanechol is given by mouth with each main meal in cases without complete retention; when gastric retention is complete and nothing passes into the duodenum, the subcutaneous route is necessary because the drug is not adequately absorbed from the stomach. Bethanechol increases the volume and the acidity of secretion of the vagotomized stomach and hence should be given only with meals. Bethanechol is also of value in selected cases of *congenital megacolon*.

Urinary Bladder Disorders. Bethanechol may be useful in combating *urinary retention* when organic obstruction is absent, as in postoperative and postpartum retention and in certain cases of neurogenic bladder (Khanna, 1976; Finkbeiner *et al.*, 1977).

Catheterization, with its attendant risk of urinary tract infection, can thus be avoided. For *acute retention,* the drug is injected subcutaneously in the usual dose of 5 mg, which can be repeated after 15 to 30 minutes if necessary. The stomach should be empty at the time the drug is injected. In *chronic cases,* 10 mg of the drug may be given orally, three times daily, until voluntary or automatic voiding begins and then its administration is slowly withdrawn. Too large a dose will result in detrusor-sphincter dyssynergia; optimal dosage schedules must therefore be determined.

Opthalmological Uses. *Acetylcholine,* 1%, or *carbachol,* 0.01%, is used in cataract extractions and certain other surgical procedures on the anterior segment when it is desired to produce miosis rapidly; the action of acetylcholine is brief (Rizzuti, 1967). *Methacholine,* in concentrations up to 20%, in combination with neostigmine bromide, 5%, instilled intraconjunctivally at frequent intervals, has been recommended for the emergency treatment of acute attacks of *narrow-angle glaucoma.* For the chronic therapy of noncongestive, wide-angle glaucoma, *carbachol* (0.25 to 3.0%) has been employed. Carbachol will often reduce intraocular pressure in patients who have become resistant to pilocarpine or physostigmine.

Diagnostic Uses. If a patient is suspected of having poisoning due to atropine or other belladonna alkaloids, 10 to 30 mg of *methacholine* may be injected subcutaneously. The failure of appearance of the characteristic flush, sweating, lacrimation, rhinorrhea, salivation, and enhanced peristalsis is pathognomonic of *belladonna intoxication.* The specific antidote for this condition is *physostigmine* (*see* Chapter 6).

Methacholine and *bethanechol* have also been employed diagnostically in place of secretin as a test for *pancreatic enzymatic function;* by simultaneously stimulating secretion and constricting the ampullary mechanism, the drugs should normally cause an increase in the plasma amylase level. *Acetylcholine* has been employed as a transient vasodilator to improve visualization of hypovascular renal neoplasms.

CHOLINOMIMETIC NATURAL ALKALOIDS AND SYNTHETIC ANALOGS

The three major natural alkaloids in this group—*pilocarpine, muscarine,* and *arecoline*—have the same principal sites of action as the choline esters discussed above. Muscarine acts almost exclusively at *muscarinic* receptor sites, their classification as such being derived from this fact. Arecoline acts in addition at *nicotinic* receptors. Pilocarpine has a dominant muscarinic action, but it causes anomalous cardiovascular responses

and the sweat glands are particularly sensitive to the drug.

Although these naturally occurring alkaloids are of great value as pharmacological tools, present clinical use is largely restricted to the employment of pilocarpine as a miotic agent.

History and Sources. *Pilocarpine* is the chief alkaloid obtained from the leaflets of South American shrubs of the genus *Pilocarpus.* Although it was long known by the natives that the chewing of leaves of *Pilocarpus* plants caused salivation, the first experiments were apparently performed in 1874 by a Brazilian physician named Coutinhou. The alkaloid was isolated in 1875, and shortly thereafter the actions of pilocarpine on the pupil as well as on the sweat and salivary glands were described by Weber.

The poisonous effects of certain species of mushrooms have been known since ancient times, but it was not until Schmiedeberg isolated the alkaloid *muscarine* from *Amanita muscaria* that the properties of the drug could be systematically investigated. Schmiedeberg and Koppe published the first careful pharmacological study of muscarine in 1869. The role played by muscarine in the development of the neurohumoral theory has been recounted in Chapter 4.

Arecoline is the chief alkaloid of areca or betel nuts, the seeds of *Areca catechu.* The *betel nut* has been consumed as a euphoretic by the natives of the East Indies from early times in a masticatory mixture known as *betel* and composed of the nut, shell lime, and leaves of *Piper betle,* a climbing species of pepper.

Structure-Activity Relationship. The muscarinic alkaloids show marked differences as well as interesting relationships in structure (Table 5–3). *Arecoline* and *pilocarpine* are tertiary amines, but the former has been shown to be pharmacologically active chiefly in the protonated form (Burgen, 1965). *Muscarine,* a quaternary ammonium compound, has three asymmetric carbon atoms; all four pairs of enantiomorphs have been synthesized (Eugster *et al.,* 1958), including the naturally occurring L(+) form. *Oxotremorine* is a synthetic compound that is used as an investigative tool in the search for antiparkinsonism drugs and in other studies of the pharmacology of the CNS (Table 5–3). In the periphery, it acts as a potent muscarinic agonist. Its parkinsonism-like central effects include tremor, ataxia, and spasticity, which result apparently from activation of muscarinic receptors in the basal ganglia and elsewhere (Cho *et al.,* 1962). The chemistry and pharmacology of many natural and synthetic muscarinic compounds have been reviewed by Bebbington and Brimblecombe (1965) and Kosterlitz (1967).

PHARMACOLOGICAL PROPERTIES

Smooth Muscle. Pilocarpine, when applied locally to the *eye,* causes pupillary constriction, spasm of accommodation, and a transitory rise in intraocu-

Table 5-3. STRUCTURAL FORMULAS OF CHOLINOMIMETIC NATURAL
ALKALOIDS AND SYNTHETIC ANALOGS

Arecoline   Pilocarpine   Muscarine

Aceclidine   Oxotremorine

lar pressure, followed by a more persistent fall. Miosis lasts from several hours to a day, but fixation of the lens for near vision disappears in about 2 hours. The muscarinic alkaloids stimulate the smooth muscles of the *intestinal tract,* thereby increasing tone and motility; large doses cause marked spasm and tenesmus. The *bronchial musculature* is also stimulated; asthmatic patients uniformly respond to pilocarpine with a reduction in vital capacity, and a typical asthmatic attack may be precipitated. The tone and motility of the *ureters, urinary bladder, gallbladder,* and *biliary ducts* are also enhanced by pilocarpine and muscarine.

Exocrine Glands. Pilocarpine (10 to 15 mg, subcutaneously) causes marked diaphoresis in man; 2 to 3 liters of sweat may be secreted. Accompanying side effects may include hiccough, salivation, nausea, vomiting, weakness, and occasionally collapse. Muscarine and arecoline are also potent diaphoretic agents. The intradermal injection of a solution of pilocarpine or ACh in normally innervated skin causes local sweating and vasodilatation, which can be blocked by atropine. The salivary, lacrimal, gastric, pancreatic, and intestinal glands, and the mucous cells of the respiratory tract are also stimulated by these alkaloids. Normal saliva is hypotonic and is also unique in containing a larger amount of potassium than does the extracellular fluid from which it is derived; after pilocarpine, the composition of the saliva tends to approach that of an ultrafiltrate of the plasma (Dreisbach, 1961, 1963). The *gastric glands* are stimulated to secrete a juice rich in acid but especially abundant in pepsin and mucin, resembling that resulting from vagal stimulation.

Cardiovascular System. The most prominent cardiovascular effects following the intravenous injection of extremely small doses (0.01 to 0.03 µg/kg) of *muscarine* in various species are a marked fall in the blood pressure and a slowing or temporary cessation of the heart.

The actions of *pilocarpine* on the cardiovascular system are complex and defy satisfactory explanation. An intravenous injection of 0.1 mg/kg of pilocarpine produces a brief fall in blood pressure. However, if this is preceded by an appropriate dose

of a nicotinic blocking agent, pilocarpine produces a marked rise in pressure. Both the vasodepressor and pressor responses are prevented by atropine; the latter effect is also abolished by α-adrenergic blocking agents (Koppanyi, 1939; Levy and Ahlquist, 1962).

Central Nervous System. Pilocarpine, muscarine, and arecoline evoke a characteristic cortical arousal or activation response in cats following the intravenous injection of relatively small doses, similar to that produced by the injection of ACh or anti-ChE agents, or by electrical stimulation of the brain stem reticular formation. The arousal response to all these drugs is reduced or blocked by atropine and related agents (Rinaldi and Himwich, 1955a, 1955b). The spectrum of the known central actions of this group of drugs, ranging from those on individual neurons to the modification of complex behavioral processes, has been reviewed by Curtis and Crawford (1969) and Krnjević (1974).

Toxicology. Poisoning from pilocarpine, muscarine, or arecoline is characterized chiefly by exaggeration of their various parasympathomimetic effects, and resembles that produced by consumption of mushrooms of the genus *Inocybe* (*see* below). *Treatment* consists in the parenteral administration of atropine, and adequate measures to support the respiration and the circulation and to counteract pulmonary edema.

Preparations and Dosage. Official (U.S.P.) preparations of pilocarpine include ophthalmic solutions of both *Pilocarpine Hydrochloride* and *Pilocarpine Nitrate.* Pilocarpine hydrochloride solutions are sold under a variety of trade names in concentrations ranging from 0.25 to 10%, while the concentrations of pilocarpine nitrate solutions range from 0.5 to 6%. Combinations of pilocarpine with epinephrine or physostigmine are also available.

A drug-delivery system (OCUSERT) is available for achieving the sustained release of pilocarpine; it is placed in the cul-de-sac of the eyes. This is an elliptically shaped unit consisting of a pilocarpine-containing reservoir bounded by two layers of copolymer that control delivery of the drug. A relatively constant release of pilocarpine (20 or 40 μg per hour for the two dosage forms) is maintained for at least 7 days. Intraocular pressure may be effectively controlled without the stinging sensation and myopia experienced immediately after the application of pilocarpine solution. However, many patients find the foreign body uncomfortable and have difficulty with insertion of the device.

THERAPEUTIC USES

Pilocarpine is used in the treatment of *glaucoma*, where it is generally administered as a 0.5 to 4.0% aqueous solution. It can also be given in an ointment or as lamellae. The miotic action of pilocarpine is useful in overcoming the mydriasis produced by atropine; alternated with mydriatics, pilocarpine is employed to break adhesions between the iris and the lens.

Aceclidine (GLAUCOSTAT) is a synthetic compound that resembles arecoline (Table 5-3). In concentrations of 0.5 to 4.0%, it is approximately as effective as pilocarpine in reducing intraocular pressure in glaucoma, and it is a useful alternative for patients in whom the latter drug is unsatisfactory (Lieberman and Leopold, 1967; Romano, 1970). The drug is employed extensively in Europe but is not currently available in the United States.

MUSHROOM POISONING (MYCETISMUS)

Mushroom poisoning has been known for centuries. The Greek poet Euripides (fifth century B.C.) is said to have lost his wife and three children from this cause. In recent years the number of cases of mushroom poisoning has been increasing as the result of the current popularity of the consumption of wild mushrooms.

Although *Amanita muscaria* is the source from which *muscarine* has generally been isolated, its content of the alkaloid is so low (approximately 0.003%) that muscarine cannot be responsible for the major toxic effects. Much higher concentrations of muscarine are present in various species of *Inocybe* and *Clitocybe*. The symptoms of intoxication attributable to muscarine develop within 30 to 60 minutes of ingestion; they include salivation, lacrimation, nausea, vomiting, headache, visual disturbances, abdominal colic, diarrhea, bronchospasm, bradycardia, hypotension, and shock. Treatment with atropine (2 mg, parenterally) effectively blocks these effects.

Intoxication produced by *A. muscaria* and related species arises from the anticholinergic and hallucinogenic properties of a variety of isoxazole derivatives. Symptoms include irritability, restlessness, ataxia, hallucinations, and delirium. Treatment is mainly supportive; atropine is contraindicated, and sedatives are of questionable value (Becker *et al.*, 1976).

The most serious form of mycetismus is produced by *Galerina* species, *A. verna*, *A. virosa*, and *A. phalloides*, which are fairly common in both North America and Europe. These species account for 90% of all fatal cases. The principal toxins are the *phalloidins*, a group of cyclic heptapeptides that appear

to inhibit protein synthesis, and the *amanitins*, which inhibit RNA polymerase II and hence interfere with the synthesis of mRNA. The toxins disrupt hepatic cell membranes and the structure of the endoplasmic reticulum. Amanitin is also a directly acting nephrotoxin and causes tubular necrosis (Kedinger *et al.*, 1970; Becker *et al.*, 1976; Wieland and Faulstich, 1978). Symptoms are slow in onset, appearing 6 to 24 hours after ingestion; they include abdominal pain, hematuria, and diarrhea. Death usually results from hepatic or renal failure. Thioctic acid may be an effective antidote for the treatment of this type of mushroom poisoning (Becker *et al.*, 1976).

Baeyer, A. Ueber das Neurin. *Justus Liebigs Ann. Chem.,* **1867,** *142,* 322–326.

Becker, C. E.; Tong, T. G.; Boerner, U.; Roe, R. L.; Scott, R. A. T.; MacQuarrie, M. B.; and Bartter, F. Diagnosis and treatment of *Amanita phalloides*-type mushroom poisoning. *West. J. Med.,* **1976,** *125,* 100–109.

Birdsall, N. J. M.; Burgen, A. S. V.; and Hulme, E. C. The binding of agonists to brain muscarinic receptors. *Mol. Pharmacol.,* **1978,** *14,* 737.

Buccino, R. A.; Sonnenblick, E. H.; Cooper, T.; and Braunwald, E. Direct positive inotropic effect of acetylcholine on myocardium. Evidence for multiple cholinergic receptors in the heart. *Circ. Res.,* **1966,** *11,* 1097–1108.

Burgen, A. S. V. The role of ionic interaction at the muscarinic receptor. *Br. J. Pharmacol. Chemother.,* **1965,** *25,* 4–17.

Burgen, A. S. V., and Spero, L. The action of acetylcholine and other drugs on the efflux of potassium and rubidium from smooth muscle of guinea pig intestine. *Br. J. Pharmacol.,* **1968,** *34,* 99–115.

Cho, A. K.; Haslett, W. L.; and Jenden, D. J. The peripheral actions of oxotremorine, a metabolite of tremorine. *J. Pharmacol. Exp. Ther.,* **1962,** *138,* 249–257.

Dreisbach, R. H. Effect of pilocarpine on transfer of Ca^{45} and K^{42} to rat submaxillary gland and kidney. *J. Pharmacol. Exp. Ther.,* **1961,** *131,* 257–260.

———. Effect of parasympathetic stimulants on Ca^{45} transfer in rat parotid glands *in vitro. Am. J. Physiol.,* **1963,** *204,* 497–500.

Eugster, C. H.; Häfliger, F.; Denss, R.; and Girod, E. Die Spaltung von *d,l*-Muscarin in die optischen Antipoden. *Helv. Chim. Acta,* **1958,** *41,* 886–888.

George, W. J.; Polson, J. B.; O'Toole, A. G.; and Goldberg, N. D. Elevation of guanosine 3′,5′ cyclic phosphate in rat heart after perfusion with acetylcholine. *Proc. Natl. Acad. Sci. U.S.A.,* **1970,** *66,* 398–403.

Hollander, F. The secretion of gastric mucus and hydrochloric acid in response to pilocarpine: a review of the literature. *Gastroenterology,* **1944,** *2,* 201–211.

Hunt, R., and Taveau, R. DeM. The effects of a number of derivatives of choline and analogous compounds on the blood pressure. *U.S. Hyg. Lab. Bull.,* No. 73, Washington, D. C., **1911.**

Jafferji, S. S., and Michell, R. H. Muscarinic cholinergic stimulation of phosphoinositol turnover in longitudinal smooth muscle of guinea-pig ileum. *Biochem. J.,* **1976,** *154,* 63–67.

Kamijo, K., and Koelle, G. B. The histochemical localization of specific cholinesterase in the conduction system of beef heart. *J. Pharmacol. Exp. Ther.,* **1955,** *113,* 30.

Kedinger, C.; Gniazdowski, M.; Mandel, J. L., Jr.; Gissinger, F.; and Chambon, P. α-Amanitin: a specific inhibitor of one of two DNA-dependent RNA polymerase activities from calf thymus. *Biochem. Biophys. Res. Commun.,* **1970,** *38,* 165–171.

Kent, K. M., and Epstein, S. E. Neural basis for the genesis and control of arrhythmias associated with myocardial infarction. *Cardiology,* **1976,** *61,* 61–74.

Kent, K. M.; Epstein, S. E.; Cooper, T.; and Jacobowitz, D. M. Cholinergic innervation of the canine and human ventricular conducting system. *Circulation,* **1974,** *50,* 948–955.

Khanna, O. P. Disorders of micturition: neuropharmacologic basis and results of drug therapy. *Urology,* **1976,** *8,* 316–327.

Koppanyi, T. The hemodynamic effect of pilocarpine. *J. Pharmacol. Exp. Ther.,* **1939,** *66,* 19–20.

Levy, B., and Ahlquist, R. P. A study of sympathetic ganglionic stimulants. *J. Pharmacol. Exp. Ther.,* **1962,** *137,* 219–228.

Levy, M. N., and Zieske, H. Comparison of the cardiac effects of vagus nerve stimulation and acetylcholine infusions. *Am. J. Physiol.,* **1969,** *216,* 890–897.

Lieberman, T. W., and Leopold, I. H. The use of aceclydine in the treatment of glaucoma. *Am. J. Ophthalmol.,* **1967,** *64,* 405–415.

Light, R. U.; Bishop, C. C.; and Kendall, L. G. The response of the rabbit to pilocarpine administered into the cerebrospinal fluid. *J. Pharmacol. Exp. Ther.,* **1933,** *47,* 37–45.

Molitor, H. A comparative study of the effects of five choline compounds used in therapeutics: acetylcholine chloride, acetyl-beta-methycholine chloride, carbaminoyl choline, ethyl ether beta-methylcholine chloride, carbaminoyl beta-methylcholine chloride. *J. Pharmacol. Exp. Ther.,* **1936,** *58,* 337–360.

Priola, D. V.; Spurgeon, M. A.; and Geis, W. P. The intrinsic innervation of the canine heart: a functional study. *Circ. Res.,* **1977,** *40,* 5056.

Rinaldi, F., and Himwich, H. E. Alerting responses and actions of atropine and cholinergic drugs. *A.M.A. Arch. Neurol. Psychiatry,* **1955a,** *73,* 387–395.

———. Cholinergic mechanism involved in function of mesodiencephalic activating system. *Ibid.,* **1955b,** *73,* 396–402.

Rizzuti, A. B. Acetylcholine in surgery of the lens, iris and cornea. *Am. J. Ophthalmol.,* **1967,** *63,* 484–487.

Romano, J. H. Double-blind cross-over comparison of aceclidine and pilocarpine in open-angle glaucoma. *Br. J. Ophthalmol.,* **1970,** *54,* 510–521.

Simonart, A. On the action of certain derivatives of choline. *J. Pharmacol. Exp. Ther.,* **1932,** *46,* 157–193.

Starr, I., Jr.; Elsom, K. A.; Reisinger, J. A.; and Richards, A. N. Acetyl-β-methylcholin: action on normal persons with note on action of ethyl ether of β-methylcholin. *Am. J. Med. Sci.,* **1933,** *186,* 313–323.

Monographs and Reviews

Aviado, D. M. Acetylcholine and other parasympathomimetics. In, *The Lung Circulation.* Vol. 1, *Physiology and Pharmacology.* Pergamon Press, Ltd., Oxford, **1965,** pp. 329–341.

Bebbington, A., and Brimblecombe, R. W. Muscarinic receptors in the peripheral and central nervous systems. *Adv. Drug Res.,* **1965,** *2,* 143–172.

Berne, R. M. The coronary circulation. In, *The Mammalian Myocardium,* (Langer, G. A., and Brady, A. J., eds.) John Wiley & Sons, Inc., New York, **1974,** pp. 251–282.

Birdsall, N. J. M., and Hume, E. C. Biochemical studies on muscarinic acetylcholine receptors. *J. Neurochem.,* **1976,** *27,* 7–16.

Curtis, D. R., and Crawford, J. M. Central synaptic transmission—micro-electrophoretic studies. *Annu. Rev. Pharmacol.,* **1969,** *9,* 209–240.

Finkbeiner, A. E.; Bissada, N. K.; and Welch, L. T. Uropharmacology: choline esters and other parasympathomimetic drugs. *Urology,* **1977,** *10,* 83–89.

Higgins, C. B.; Vatner, S. F.; and Braunwald, E. Parasympathetic control of the heart. *Pharmacol. Rev.,* **1973,** *25,* 119–155.

Kosterlitz, H. W. Effects of choline esters on smooth muscle and secretions. In, *Physiological Pharmacology.* Vol. 3, *The Nervous System—Part C: Autonomic Nervous System Drugs.* (Root, W. S., and Hofmann, F. G., eds.) Academic Press, Inc., New York, **1967,** pp. 97–161.

Krnjević, K. Chemical nature of synaptic transmission in vertebrates. *Physiol. Rev.,* **1974,** *54,* 418–540.

Levy, M. N. Parasympathetic control of the heart. In, *Neural Regulation of the Heart.* (Randall, W. C., ed.) Oxford University Press, New York, **1977,** pp. 97–129.

Rand, M. J., and Stafford, A. Cardiovascular effects of choline esters. In, *Physiological Pharmacology.* Vol. 3, *The Nervous System—Part C: Autonomic Nervous System Drugs.* (Root, W. S., and Hofmann, F. G., eds.) Academic Press, Inc., New York, **1967,** pp. 1–95.

Schmiedeberg, O., and Koppe, R. *Das Muscarin, das giftige Alkaloid des Fliegenpilzes.* F. C. W. Vogel, Leipzig, **1869.**

Snyder, S. H.; Chang, K. J.; Kuhar, M. J.; and Yamamura, H. I. Biochemical identification of the mammalian muscarinic cholinergic receptor. *Fed. Proc.,* **1974,** *34,* 1915–1921.

Wieland, T., and Faulstich, H. Amatoxins, phallotoxins, phallolysin and antamanide: the biologically active components of poisonous *Amanita* mushrooms. *CRC Crit. Rev. Biochem.,* **1978,** *5,* 185–260.

CHAPTER

6 ANTICHOLINESTERASE AGENTS

Palmer Taylor

The function of acetylcholinesterase (AChE) in terminating the action of acetylcholine (ACh) at the junctions of the various cholinergic nerve endings with their effector organs or postsynaptic sites is considered in Chapter 4. Drugs that inhibit AChE are called *anticholinesterase* (anti-ChE) agents. They cause ACh to accumulate at cholinergic receptor sites and thus are potentially capable of producing effects equivalent to excessive stimulation of cholinergic receptors throughout the central and peripheral nervous systems. In view of the widespread distribution of cholinergic neurons, it is not surprising that the anti-ChE agents as a group have received more extensive application as toxic agents, in the form of agricultural insecticides and potential chemical-warfare "nerve gases," than as therapeutic agents. Nevertheless, there are members of this class of compounds that are clinically useful.

Prior to World War II, only the "reversible" anti-ChE agents were generally known, of which *physostigmine (eserine)* is the outstanding example. Shortly before and during World War II, a comparatively new class of highly toxic chemicals, the *organophosphates*, was developed chiefly by Schrader, of I.G. Farbenindustrie, first as agricultural insecticides and later as potential chemical-warfare agents. The extreme toxicity of these compounds was found to be due to their "irreversible" inactivation of AChE, thereby exerting long-lasting inhibitory activity. Since the pharmacological actions of both classes of anti-ChE agents are qualitatively similar, they will be discussed as a group. Certain effects of anti-ChE agents and their interactions with other drugs at autonomic ganglia and the neuromuscular junction are described in Chapters 10 and 11.

History. *Physostigmine,* also called *eserine,* is an alkaloid obtained from the Calabar or ordeal bean, the dried ripe seed of *Physostigma venenosum* Bal-

four, a perennial plant in tropical West Africa. The Calabar bean, also called Esére nut, chop nut, or bean of Etu Esére, was once used by native tribes of West Africa as an "ordeal poison" in trials for witchcraft.

The Calabar bean was brought to England in 1840 by Daniell, a British medical officer stationed in Calabar, and early investigations of its pharmacological properties were conducted by Christioson (1855), Fraser (1863), and Argyll-Robertson (1863). A pure alkaloid was isolated by Jobst and Hesse in 1864 and named *physostigmine;* the following year, Vee and Leven obtained the same alkaloid, which they named *eserine.* The first therapeutic use of the drug was in 1877 by Laqueur, in the treatment of glaucoma, one of its few clinical uses today. M. and M. Polonovski (1923) and Stedman and Barger (1925) elucidated the chemical structure of physostigmine, and its synthesis was accomplished by Julian and Pikl in 1935. Interesting accounts of the history of physostigmine have been presented by Rodin (1947), Karczmar (1970), and Holmstedt (1972).

As a result of the basic research of Stedman (1929a, 1929b) and associates in elucidating the chemical basis of the activity of physostigmine, Aeschlimann and Reinert (1931) systematically investigated a series of substituted phenyl esters of alkyl carbamic acids. *Neostigmine,* a most promising member of this series, was introduced into therapeutics in 1931 for its stimulant action on the intestinal tract. It was reported independently by Remen (1932) and Walker (1935) to be effective in the symptomatic therapy of myasthenia gravis.

It is remarkable that the first account of the synthesis of a highly potent compound of the *organophosphorus anti-ChE* series, *tetraethylpyrophosphate* (TEPP), was published by Clermont in 1854, 10 years prior to the isolation of physostigmine. More remarkable still, as Holmstedt (1963) has pointed out, is the fact that the investigator survived to report on the compound's taste; a few drops of the pure compound placed on the tongue would be expected to prove rapidly fatal. Modern investigations of the organophosphorus compounds, and the first hint of their toxicity, date from the 1932 publication of Lange and Krueger on the synthesis of dimethyl and diethyl phosphorofluoridates. The authors' statement that inhalation of the vapors of these compounds caused a persistent choking sensation and blurred vision apparently was instrumental in leading Schrader to explore this class for insecticidal activity.

During the synthesis and investigation of approximately 2000 compounds, Schrader (1952) defined the structural requirements for insecticidal (and, as learned subsequently, for anti-ChE) activity (*see* below). One compound in this early series, *parathion,* later became the most widely employed insecticide of this class. Prior to and during World War II, the efforts of Schrader's group were directed toward the development of chemical-warfare agents. The synthesis of several compounds of much greater toxicity than parathion, such as *sarin, soman,* and *tabun,* resulted but were kept secret by the German government. It is estimated that over 10,000 tons of the last-mentioned agent was manufactured at one German plant for this purpose. Investigators in the Allied countries also followed Lange and Krueger's lead in the search for potentially toxic compounds; di*iso*propyl phosphorofluoridate (DFP), synthesized by McCombie and Saunders (1946), was the organophosphorus compound studied most extensively by British and American scientists. It has been estimated that over 50,000 organophosphorus compounds have been synthesized and screened for insecticidal potency, of which over 3 dozen have been produced commercially (Chadwick, 1963).

In the 1950s, a series of heterocyclic, aromatic, and naphthyl *carbamates* was synthesized and found to have a high degree of selective toxicity against insects and to be potent anti-ChE agents (Gysin, 1954). Among those currently employed as insecticides are 1-naphthyl N-methylcarbamate (carbaryl; SEVIN) and 2-isopropoxyphenyl N-methylcarbamate (BAYGON) (*see* Fukuto, 1972; Murphy, 1980).

Structure of Acetylcholinesterase. Although early studies led to the isolation in pure form of an AChE from the eel, *Electrophorus electricus* (Leuzinger *et al.,* 1968), it is now evident that the native form of the enzyme is a more complex structure. The basic unit is tetrameric and is composed of equivalent subunits of 80,000 molecular weight, each of which contains an active center. Usually three tetrameric units are linked through disulfide bonds to a filament (50 × 2 nm) in an arrangement analogous to three flowers connected to a stalk (Dudai *et al.,* 1973; Cartaud *et al.,* 1975). Mild treatment with protease gives rise to the 320,000-molecular-weight tetramer with full retention of catalytic activity. The filamentous unit, which appears to serve only a structural role, is collagen-like in composition (Lwebuga-Mukasa *et al.,* 1976; Rosenberry and Richardson, 1977). The composition of AChE, along with studies of its removal from the synapse by collagenase, demonstrate that the enzyme is located in the outer basal lamina (basement membrane) rather than the postsynaptic membrane. A similar situation applies to AChE in skeletal muscle, where the elongated form of the enzyme is found specifically in junctional regions (Hall, 1973).

The active center of AChE consists of a negative subsite, which attracts the quaternary group of choline through both coulombic and hydrophobic forces, and an esteratic subsite, where nucleophilic attack occurs on the acyl carbon of the substrate (Figure 6–1, *I*). The catalytic mechanism resembles that of other serine esterases, where a serine hydroxyl group is rendered highly nucleophilic through a charge-relay system involving the close apposition of an imidazole group and, presumably, a carboxyl group on the enzyme. During enzymatic attack on

the ester, a tetrahedral intermediate is formed that collapses to an acetyl enzyme conjugate with the concomitant release of choline. The acetyl enzyme is labile to hydrolysis, which results in the formation of acetate and active enzyme (*see* Froede and Wilson, 1971; Rosenberry, 1975). AChE is one of the most efficient enzymes known and has the capacity to hydrolyze 3×10^5 ACh molecules per molecule of enzyme per minute; this is equivalent to a turnover time of 150 microseconds.

Mechanism of Action of AChE Inhibitors. The mechanisms of action of compounds that typify the three classes of anti-ChE agents are also shown in Figure 6–1 (*II, III, IV*).

Quaternary compounds inhibit the enzyme reversibly by combining either at the active center or at a site spatially removed from the active center called the peripheral anionic site (Mooser and Sigman, 1974; Taylor and Lappi, 1975). The potent reversible inhibitor, *edrophonium,* binds selectively to the active center. The complex is stabilized by interaction of the quaternary nitrogen at the anionic subsite and by hydrogen bonding (Wilson and Quan, 1958) (Figure 6–1, *II*). Edrophonium has a brief duration of action owing to the reversibility of its binding to AChE and rapid elimination by the kidneys following systemic administration.

Drugs such as *physostigmine* and *neostigmine* that have a carbamyl ester linkage are hydrolyzed by AChE, but much more slowly than is ACh (Goldstein and Hamlisch, 1952; Myers, 1956; Wilson *et al.,* 1960). Both the quaternary amine, neostigmine, and the tertiary amine, physostigmine, exist as cations, which contributes to their association with the active center. By serving as alternate substrates (Figure 6–1, *III*), the alcohol moiety is cleaved, giving rise to the carbamylated enzyme. In contrast to the acetyl enzyme, methylcarbamyl AChE or dimethylcarbamyl AChE is far more stable ($t_{1/2}$ for hydrolysis of the dimethylcarbamyl enzyme is 15 to 30 minutes) (Wilson and Harrison, 1961). Sequestration of the enzyme in its carbamylated form thus precludes the enzyme-catalyzed hydrolysis of ACh for extended periods of time. *In vivo,* the duration of inhibition by the carbamylating agents is 3 to 4 hours.

The *organophosphorus inhibitors,* such as DFP, serve as true hemisubstrates, since the resultant phosphorylated or phosphonylated enzyme is extremely stable (Figure 6–1, *IV*). Reaction occurs at the esteratic site and is enhanced by the geometry of the tetrahedral phosphates, which resemble the transition state for acetyl ester hydrolysis. Certain quaternary organophosphorus compounds (*e.g.,* echothiophate) interact with both the esteratic and anionic subsites in the active center to produce a stable complex; this contributes to the high potency of these agents (*see* Burgen and Hobbiger, 1951; Holmstedt, 1963). If the alkyl groups in the phosphorylated enzyme are ethyl or methyl, a significant degree of spontaneous regeneration of active enzyme requires several hours. Secondary (as in DFP) or

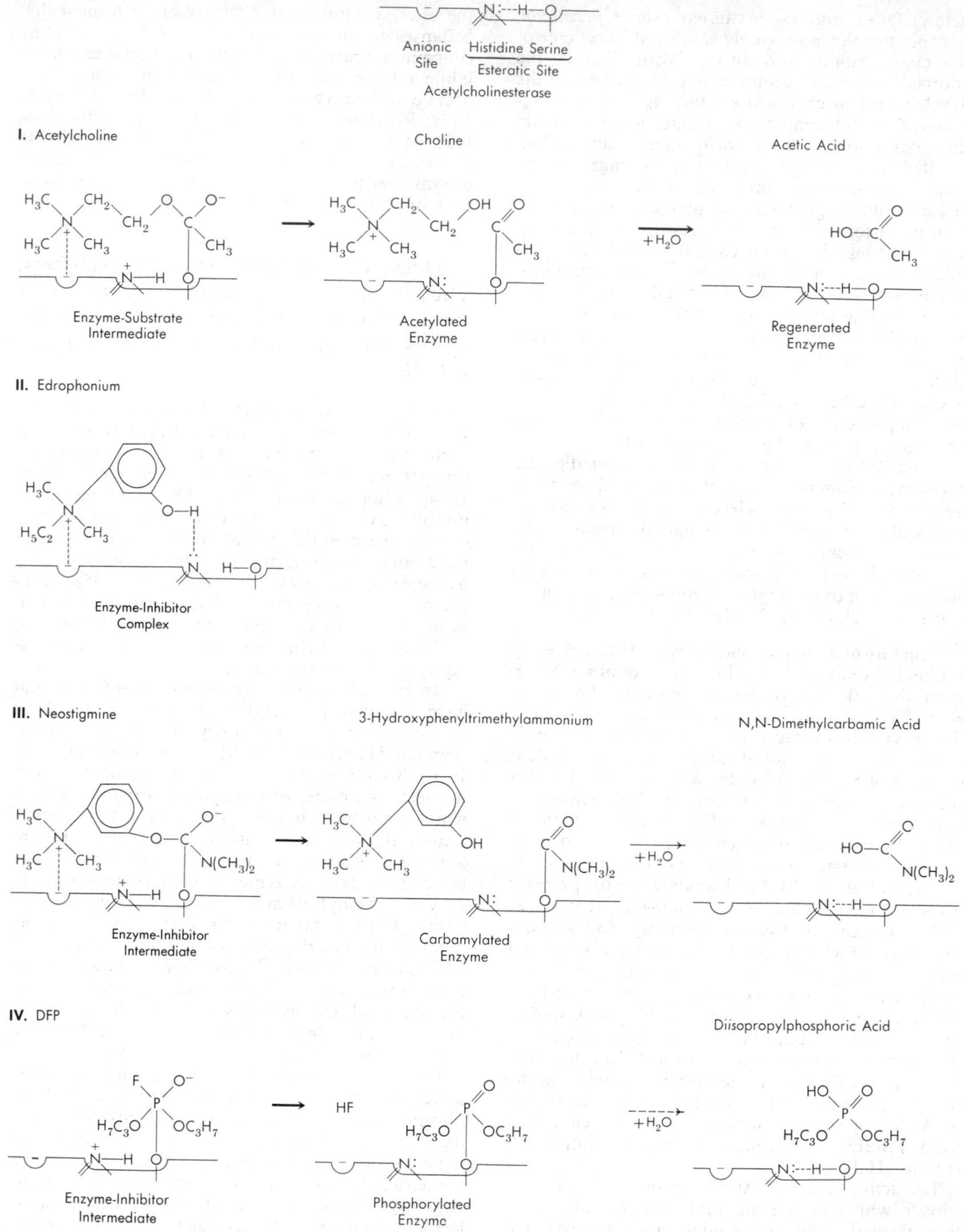

Figure 6-1. *Steps involved in the hydrolysis of acetylcholine (ACh) by acetylcholinesterase (AChE)* (I), *and in the inhibition of AChE by reversible* (II), *carbamyl ester* (III), *and organophosphorus* (IV) *agents.*

Heavy, light, and dashed arrows represent extremely rapid, intermediate, and extremely slow or insignificant reaction velocities, respectively. *See* text and references for description. Structures of the inhibitors appear in Tables 6-1 and 6-2.

tertiary alkyl groups enhance the stability of the phosphorylated enzyme, and significant regeneration of active enzyme is not observed. Hence, the return of AChE activity depends on synthesis of new enzyme. The stability of the phosphorylated enzyme is further enhanced through "aging," which results from the loss of one of the alkyl groups (see Figure 6-2; Aldridge, 1976; Hobbiger, 1976).

The methanesulfonyl group also serves as a hemisubstrate by forming a conjugate with the serine hydroxyl group on AChE. Like the phosphorylated enzyme, methanesulfonyl AChE is resistant to hydrolytic reactivation (Kitz and Wilson, 1963).

From the foregoing account, it is apparent that the terms "reversible" and "irreversible," as applied to the carbamyl ester and organophosphorus anti-ChE agents, respectively, reflect only quantitative temporal differences, and that both classes of drugs react covalently with the enzyme in essentially the same manner as does ACh.

Action at Effector Organs. The characteristic pharmacological effects of the anti-ChE agents are due primarily to the prevention of hydrolysis of ACh by AChE at sites of cholinergic transmission. Transmitter thus accumulates, and the action of ACh that is liberated by cholinergic impulses or that leaks from the nerve ending is enhanced. With most of the organophosphorus agents, such as DFP, virtually all the acute effects of moderate doses are attributable to this action. For example, the characteristic miosis that follows local application of DFP to the eye is not observed after chronic postganglionic denervation of the eye because there is no effective source of endogenous ACh. The consequences of enhanced concentrations of ACh at motor end-plates are unique to this site and are discussed below.

Among the classical anti-ChE agents, physostigmine, a tertiary amine, exerts a minimum of effects that are not related to inhibition of AChE. The quaternary ammonium anti-ChE compounds all have additional direct actions at some cholinergic receptor sites, either as agonists or antagonists. For example, the effects of neostigmine on the spinal cord and neuromuscular junction are based on a combination of its anti-ChE activity and direct cholinergic stimulation.

Chemistry and Structure-Activity Relationship. The structure-activity relationship of anti-ChE drugs has been reviewed extensively for the "reversible" inhibitors (Long, 1963), the organophosphorus

agents (Holmstedt, 1963), and both classes of compounds (Karczmar, 1967a; Usdin, 1970). Only those agents that are of general therapeutic or toxicological interest will be considered here.

"Reversible" Carbamate Inhibitors. Drugs of this class that are of therapeutic interest are shown in Table 6-1. After the structure of physostigmine was established, Stedman (1929a, 1929b) and associates undertook a systematic investigation of a number of related synthetic compounds. They concluded that the essential moiety of the physostigmine molecule was the methyl carbamate of a basically substituted simple phenol (right of the dash line in Table 6-1). The quaternary ammonium derivative, *neostigmine,* is a compound of greater stability and equal or greater potency. *Pyridostigmine* is a close congener that is also employed in the treatment of myasthenia gravis. The simple analogs of neostigmine that lack the carbamyl group, such as *edrophonium,* are less potent and much shorter-acting anti-ChE agents.

An increase in anti-ChE potency and duration of action can result from the linking of two quaternary ammonium nuclei by a chain of appropriate structure and length. One such example is the miotic agent *demecarium,* which consists of two neostigmine molecules connected at their carbamate nitrogen atoms by a series of ten methylene groups. The second quaternary group confers additional stability to the interaction on the enzyme surface since negative subsites peripheral to the active center have been identified on AChE. Another class of *bis*-quaternary compounds is represented by *ambenonium,* used in the treatment of myasthenia gravis. Ambenonium does not react covalently with AChE but binds noncovalently with a high affinity. In addition to its potent anti-ChE activity, this drug has a variety of actions at both the prejunctional and postjunctional membranes of the skeletal muscle motor end-plate (Karczmar, 1967b; Hobbiger, 1976).

The insecticide *carbaryl,* which is extensively used in garden products, inhibits ChE in a fashion identical to other carbamylating inhibitors. The signs and symptoms of poisoning closely resemble those of the organophosphates (Murphy, 1980). Carbaryl has a particularly low toxicity from dermal absorption. Its structure is as follows:

Carbaryl

Organophosphorus Inhibitors. The general formula for this class of cholinesterase inhibitors is presented in Table 6-2. A great variety of substituents is possible: R_1 and R_2 may be alkyl, alkoxy, aryloxy, amido, mercaptan, or other groups, and X may represent a halide, cyanide, thiocyanate, phenoxy, thiophenoxy, phosphate, or carboxylate group. A useful chemical classification of the compounds in this class that are of particular pharmacological or toxicological interest has been developed by Holmstedt (1963), upon which the listing in Table 6-2 is

Table 6–1. REPRESENTATIVE "REVERSIBLE" ANTICHOLINESTERASE AGENTS EMPLOYED CLINICALLY

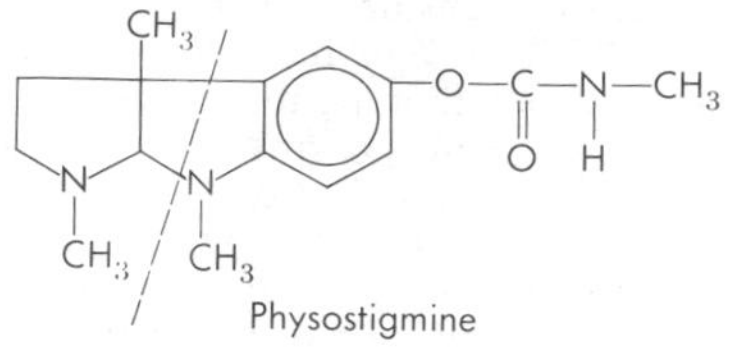

Physostigmine

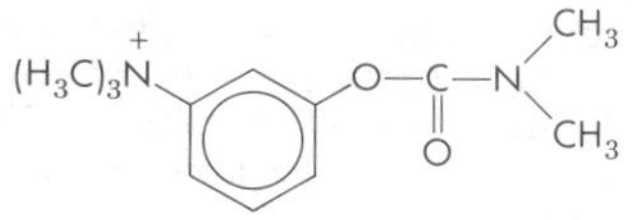

Neostigmine

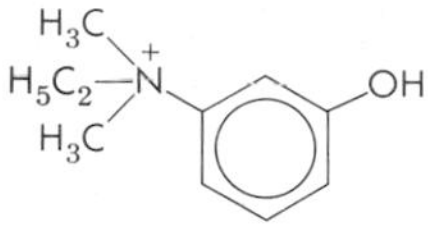

Edrophonium

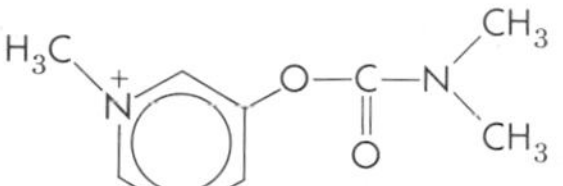

Pyridostigmine

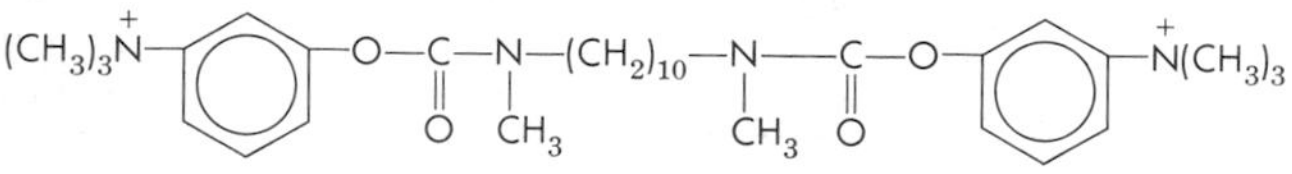

Demecarium

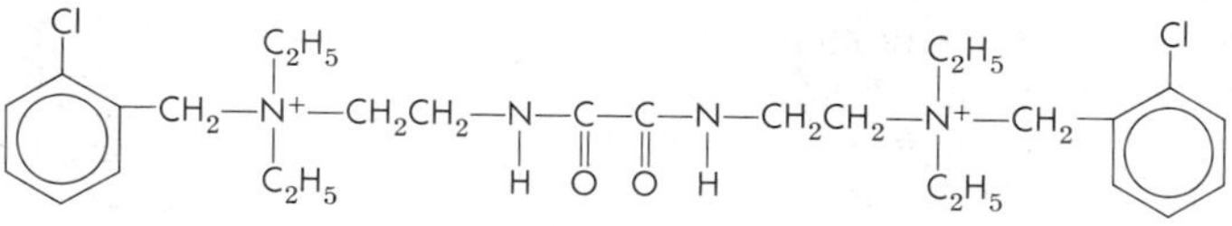

Ambenonium

based. Extensive compilations of the organophosphorus compounds and their toxicity may be found in the publications of Frear (1969) and Gaines (1969).

Diisopropyl phosphorofluoridate (DFP) is perhaps the best-known and most extensively studied compound of this general class, as the result both of its early development and toxicological evaluation during World War II and of certain of its properties that render it particularly valuable as an investigative tool. The latter include the virtually irreversible inactivation that it produces by alkylphosphorylation of AChE and certain other esterases; its high lipid solubility, resulting in penetration into the central nervous system (CNS); and its relative specificity.

The "nerve gases," *tabun, sarin,* and *soman,* are among the most potent synthetic toxic agents known; they are lethal to laboratory animals in submilligram doses.

Parathion was synthesized by Schrader in 1944. Because of its low volatility and stability in aqueous solution, it became widely used as an insecticide. It continues to be used extensively in agriculture, but less hazardous compounds have become popular, particularly for home and garden use. Early studies demonstrated that parathion, purified from its contaminants, was inactive in inhibiting AChE *in vitro* and that *paraoxon* was the active metabolite. The conversion is carried out predominantly in liver (DuBois *et al.,* 1949) by the mixed-function oxygenases in the endoplasmic reticulum (Neal, 1967). Other tissues also have some capacity for such conversion. Parathion has probably been responsible for more cases of accidental poisoning and death than

any other organophosphorus compound. The trade names and the code names that have been employed to designate the compound include NIRAN, E-605, COMPOUND 3422, AAT, ETILON, FOLIDOL, and SNP. (*See* Gosselin *et al.,* 1976, for listings of many pesticides and their trade names and synonyms.)

Some insecticides such as *malathion* can be detoxified by hydrolysis of the carboxyl ester linkage by plasma carboxylesterases. The detoxication reaction is much more rapid in mammals and birds than in insects, giving rise to a desirable degree of selective toxicity (*see* Murphy, 1980). However, its use is not without risk when protective measures are inadequate. *TEPP* has been used as an insecticide. A tetramide derivative of the same structural class, *OMPA,* is practically devoid of anti-ChE activity; but, like parathion, it is metabolized to an extremely active product, probably the N oxide or the isomeric hydroxymethyl compound. Apparently a similar transformation takes place in plants.

Among the quaternary ammonium organophosphorus compounds (group E, Table 6–2), only *echothiophate* is useful clinically. It is relatively resistant to spontaneous hydrolysis and can thus be stored for several weeks in aqueous solution.

PHARMACOLOGICAL PROPERTIES

Generally the pharmacological properties of anti-ChE agents can be predicted merely by knowing those loci where ACh is released physiologically by nerve impulses and the

Table 6–2. CHEMICAL CLASSIFICATION OF REPRESENTATIVE ORGANOPHOSPHORUS COMPOUNDS OF PARTICULAR PHARMACOLOGICAL OR TOXICOLOGICAL INTEREST *

General formula (Schrader, 1952):

$$\begin{array}{c} R_1 \\ \diagdown \\ P \\ \diagup \diagdown \\ R_2 \quad X \end{array} \quad = O$$

Group A, X = halogen, cyanide, or thiocyanate; group B, X = alkyl, alkoxy, or aryloxy; group C, thiol- or thionophosphorus compounds; group D, pyrophosphates and similar compounds; group E, quaternary ammonium compounds

GROUP	STRUCTURAL FORMULA	COMMON, CHEMICAL, AND OTHER NAMES	COMMENTS
A	$i\text{-}C_3H_7O$, $i\text{-}C_3H_7O$, O, F (P center)	DFP Diisopropyl phosphorofluoridate	Potent, irreversible inactivator
	$(CH_3)_2N$, C_2H_5O, O, CN (P center)	Tabun Ethyl N-dimethylphosphoramido-cyanidate	Extremely toxic "nerve gas"
	$i\text{-}C_3H_7O$, CH_3, O, F (P center)	Sarin (GB) Isopropyl methylphosphono-fluoridate	Extremely toxic "nerve gas"
	$(CH_3)_3CCHO$ with CH_3, CH_3, O, F (P center)	Soman Pinacolyl methylphosphono-fluoridate	Extremely toxic "nerve gas"
B	C_2H_5O, C_2H_5O, O, $O\text{-}$(phenyl)$\text{-}NO_2$ (P center)	Paraoxon, Mintacol, E 600 Diethyl 4-nitrophenyl phosphate	Active metabolite of parathion
C	C_2H_5O, C_2H_5O, S, $O\text{-}$(phenyl)$\text{-}NO_2$ (P center)	Parathion (see list of trade names in text) Diethyl O-(4-nitrophenyl) phosphorothioate	Widely employed agricultural insecticide, resulting in numerous cases of accidental poisoning
	C_2H_5O, (phenyl), S, $O\text{-}$(phenyl)$\text{-}NO_2$ (P center)	EPN O-Ethyl O-(4-nitrophenyl) phenylphosphonothioate	Widely employed agricultural insecticide
	CH_3O, CH_3O, S, $S\text{-}CHCOOC_2H_5$ / $CH_2COOC_2H_5$ (P center)	Malathion O,O-Dimethyl S-(1,2-dicarb-ethoxyethyl) phosphorodi-thioate	Widely employed insecticide of greater safety than parathion or EPN because of rapid detoxication by higher organisms
D	C_2H_5O, C_2H_5O, O—P—O, OC_2H_5, OC_2H_5 (pyrophosphate)	TEPP Tetraethyl pyrophosphate	Early insecticide
	$(CH_3)_2N$, $(CH_3)_2N$, O—P—O, $N(CH_3)_2$, $N(CH_3)_2$ (pyrophosphate)	OMPA, Schradan Octamethyl pyrophosphoramide	Insecticide; inactive in vitro, but metabolized by animals and plants to potent anti-ChE agent
E	C_2H_5O, C_2H_5O, O, $SCH_2CH_2N^+(CH_3)_3$, I^- (P center)	Echothiophate, Phospholine, 217MI Diethoxyphosphinylthiocholine iodide	Extremely potent choline derivative; employed in treatment of glaucoma; relatively stable in aqueous solution

* After Holmstedt, 1959, 1963. See also Usdin, 1970; Hobbiger, 1976.

responses of the corresponding effector organs to the chemical mediator (*see* Chapter 4). While this is true in the main, the diverse locations of cholinergic synapses increase the complexity of the response. Potentially, the anti-ChE agents can produce all the following effects: (1) stimulation of muscarinic receptor responses at autonomic effector organs; (2) stimulation, followed by depression or paralysis, of all autonomic ganglia and skeletal muscle (nicotinic actions); and (3) stimulation, with subsequent depression, of cholinergic receptor sites (primarily muscarinic) in the CNS. Following toxic or lethal doses of anti-ChE agents, most of these effects can actually be noted (*see* below). However, with smaller doses, particularly those employed therapeutically, several modifying factors are significant. The response of effector organs also depends on whether they receive cholinergic nerve impulses continuously or phasically. Moreover, little is known concerning the relative degree to which the drugs inactivate AChE in various tissues *in vivo*. Compounds such as parathion become more toxic when distributed systemically, owing to conversion to the active form, paraoxon. In general, compounds containing a quaternary ammonium group do not penetrate cell membranes readily; hence, anti-ChE agents in this category are absorbed poorly from the gastrointestinal tract and are excluded by the blood-brain barrier from exerting significant action on the CNS after moderate doses. On the other hand, such compounds act relatively selectively at the neuromuscular junctions of skeletal muscle, exerting their action both as anti-ChE agents and as direct agonists. They have comparatively less effect at autonomic effector sites; their ganglionic actions are generally intermediate. In contrast, the more lipid-soluble agents, such as tertiary amines and most organophosphorus compounds, are well absorbed after oral administration and have ubiquitous effects at both peripheral and central cholinergic receptor sites. The lipid-soluble organophosphates are also well absorbed through the skin.

The actions of anti-ChE agents on autonomic effector cells and on cortical and subcortical sites in the CNS, where the receptors are largely of the muscarinic type, are blocked by *atropine*. Likewise, atropine blocks some of the excitatory actions of anti-ChE agents on autonomic ganglia, since such agents also activate muscarinic receptors of the ganglion cells, in addition to nicotinic receptors normally involved in ganglionic synaptic transmission (*see* Chapter 10).

The main actions of anti-ChE agents that are of therapeutic importance are concerned with the *eye,* the *intestine,* and the *skeletal neuromuscular junction;* most of the other actions are of toxicological interest.

Eye.   When applied locally to the conjunctiva, anti-ChE agents cause conjunctival hyperemia and constriction of the sphincter of the iris (miosis) and ciliary muscle (spasm of accommodation and focusing to near vision). Miosis is apparent in a few minutes, becomes maximal in 0.5 hour, and lasts for several hours to days. Although the pupil may be "pinpoint" in size, it generally contracts further when exposed to light. The spasm of accommodation is more transient and generally disappears considerably before termination of the miosis. Intraocular pressure usually falls concomitantly, as the result of facilitation of outflow of the aqueous. humor; the reduction in tension is likely to be particularly marked in eyes in which the pressure is elevated. However, in some cases anti-ChE agents may cause a transient increase in intraocular pressure due to dilatation and engorgement of the finer blood vessels and to increased permeability of the blood–aqueous humor barrier. (A more complete account is given below in the discussion of glaucoma.)

Gastrointestinal Tract.   While the actions of various anti-ChE agents on the gastrointestinal tract are nearly identical, *neostigmine* has been studied most extensively in this regard. In man, neostigmine enhances *gastric* contractions and increases the secretion of gastric acid from the parietal cells. The drug tends to counteract the inhibition of gastric tone and motility induced by atropine, and enhances the stimulatory effect of morphine. After bilateral vagotomy, the gastric motor effects of neostigmine are greatly reduced. The lower portion of the *esophagus* is stimulated by neostigmine; in patients with marked achalasia and dilatation of the esophagus, the drug can cause a salutary increase in tone and peristalsis.

Neostigmine augments the motor activity

of the *small and large bowel;* the colon is particularly stimulated. Atony is overcome or prevented, propulsive waves are increased in amplitude and frequency, and transport is thus promoted. The total effect of anti-ChE agents on intestinal motility probably represents a combination of actions at the ganglion cells of Auerbach's plexus and at the muscle fibers, as a result of the preservation of ACh released by the cholinergic preganglionic and postganglionic fibers, respectively.

Skeletal Neuromuscular Junction. Most of the effects of potent anti-ChE drugs on muscle fibers can be adequately explained on the basis of their inhibition of AChE at neuromuscular junctions. However, there is good evidence for an accessory component of *direct action* of neostigmine and other quaternary ammonium anti-ChE agents on skeletal muscle. For example, the intra-arterial injection of neostigmine into chronically denervated muscle, or into normally innervated muscle in which essentially all the AChE has been inactivated by prior administration of DFP, evokes an immediate contraction, whereas physostigmine does not (Riker and Wescoe, 1946).

Normally, a single nerve impulse in a terminal motor-axon branch liberates enough ACh to produce a localized depolarization, the end-plate potential, of sufficient magnitude to initiate a propagated muscle action potential. The ACh released is rapidly hydrolyzed by AChE, such that the lifetime of free ACh within the synapse ($\sim$200 microseconds) is shorter than the decay of the end-plate potential or the refractory period of the muscle (Colquhoun, 1979). Therefore, each motor impulse gives rise to a single wave of depolarization. After inhibition of AChE the residence time of ACh in the synapse increases, allowing for rebinding of transmitter to receptors. A prolongation of the decay of the end-plate potential is observed (about threefold) due to successive stimulation at neighboring receptors. Quanta released by individual nerve impulses are no longer isolated. This destroys the synchrony between end-plate depolarization and the development of the action potential. Consequently, asynchronous excitation and fibrillation of muscle fibers are observed. When ACh persists in the synapse, it may also act

on the axon terminal, resulting in antidromic firing of the motoneuron; this contributes to fasciculations, which involve the entire motor unit. With sufficient inhibition of AChE, depolarization of the end-plate predominates and blockade due to depolarization ensues (*see* Chapter 11). Thus, a small dose of physostigmine or neostigmine may increase the skeletal muscle contraction produced by a single maximal nerve stimulus, but larger doses or repetitive nerve stimulation at a rapid rate results in depression or block.

The anti-ChE agents act as "decurarizing" drugs and will reverse the antagonism of competitive neuromuscular blocking agents. Neostigmine is not effective against the skeletal muscle paralysis caused by decamethonium, succinylcholine, or benzoquinonium, since these agents also produce neuromuscular blockade by sustained depolarization or desensitization of the motor end-plate (*see* Chapter 11).

Actions at Other Sites. *Secretory glands* that are innervated by postganglionic cholinergic fibers include the bronchial, lacrimal, sweat, salivary, gastric (antral G cells and parietal cells), intestinal, and acinar pancreatic glands; low doses of anti-ChE agents cause, in general, augmentation of their secretory responses to nerve stimulation, and higher doses produce an increase in the resting rate of secretion.

Smooth muscle fibers of the bronchioles and ureters are contracted by these drugs, and the ureters may show increased peristaltic activity.

The *cardiovascular actions* of anti-ChE agents are extremely complex, since they reflect both ganglionic and postganglionic effects of accumulated ACh on the heart and blood vessels. The predominant effect on the *heart* from the peripheral action of accumulated ACh is bradycardia, resulting in a fall in cardiac output.

The effective refractory period of cardiac muscle fibers is shortened, and the refractory period and conduction time of the conducting tissue are increased. The *blood vessels* are in general dilated, although the coronary and pulmonary circulation may show the opposite response. The sum of the foregoing effects should result in hypotension, but at the ganglionic level ACh has first an excitatory and at higher concentrations an inhibitory action. Hence, the excitatory action on the parasympathetic ganglion cells would tend to reinforce the above effects, whereas the opposite sequence would result from the action of ACh on sympathetic ganglion cells. Excitation followed by inhibition is also produced by ACh at the medullary vasomotor and cardiac centers. All these effects are complicated further by the hypoxemia resulting from the bronchoconstrictor and other actions of accumulated ACh on the respiratory system; this would reinforce both sympathetic tone and ACh-induced discharge of epinephrine from the adrenal medulla. Hence, it is not surprising that a wide variety of hemodynamic effects has been reported following anti-ChE agents, depending on the drug, dose, route of administration, species, and other factors.

At *autonomic ganglia,* as indicated above, low concentrations of ACh or of anti-ChE agents cause spontaneous firing of the ganglion cells in response to submaximal preganglionic stimulation. This effect results from the activation of *muscarinic* receptors. The ganglionic blockade from higher concentrations of anti-ChE drugs apparently results from persistent depolarization of the cell membrane induced at the *nicotinic* receptors, which masks the preceding excitatory effect (Dolivo and Koelle, 1970; *see also* Chapter 10).

The effects of anti-ChE drugs on the CNS are likewise characterized by stimulation or facilitation at various sites, succeeded by inhibition or paralysis at higher concentrations. In the EEG, for example, the initial characteristic change noted is desynchronization, or the appearance of waves of low voltage and high frequency, probably reflecting stimulation of the ascending reticular activating system. The respiratory and other subcortical centers likewise show stimulation after low doses and depression with higher or toxic doses. Hypoxemia is probably a major factor in CNS depression that appears after large doses of anti-ChE agents. The stimulant effects are antagonized by atropine, although not as completely as are the muscarinic effects at peripheral autonomic effector sites.

Absorption, Fate, and Excretion. *Physostigmine* is readily absorbed from the gastrointestinal tract, subcutaneous tissues, and mucous membranes. The conjunctival instillation of solutions of the drug may result in systemic effects if measures (*e.g.,* pressure on inner canthus) are not taken to prevent absorption from the nasal mucosa. The alkaloid

is largely destroyed in the body, mainly by hydrolytic cleavage at the ester linkage by cholinesterases; renal excretion plays only a minor role in its disposal. In man, a 1-mg dose of physostigmine injected subcutaneously is largely destroyed in 2 hours.

Neostigmine and related quaternary ammonium drugs are absorbed poorly after oral administration, such that much larger doses are needed than by the parenteral route. Whereas the effective parenteral dose of neostigmine in man is 0.5 to 2.0 mg, the equivalent oral dose may be 30 mg or more. Large oral doses may prove toxic if intestinal absorption is enhanced for any reason. Neostigmine is destroyed by plasma esterases, and the quaternary alcohol and parent compound are excreted in the urine. Pyridostigmine and its quaternary alcohol are also the predominant entities found in urine after administration of this drug to man (Somani *et al.,* 1972; Cohan *et al.,* 1976; Appendix II).

The commonly encountered *organophosphorus anti-ChE agents* are, with certain exceptions (*e.g.,* echothiophate), highly lipid-soluble liquids; many have high vapor pressures at ordinary temperatures. The less volatile agents that are commonly employed as agricultural insecticides (*e.g.,* parathion, malathion) are generally dispersed as aerosols or as dusts consisting of the organophosphorus compound adsorbed to an inert, finely particulate material. Consequently, the compounds are rapidly and effectively *absorbed* by practically all routes, including the gastrointestinal tract, as well as through the skin and mucous membranes following contact with the liquid form, and by the lungs after inhalation of the vapors, dusts, or aerosols.

Following their absorption, most organophosphorus compounds are *excreted* almost entirely as hydrolysis products in the urine. However, *oxidative enzymes* are also involved in the metabolism of the organophosphorus compounds.

The organophosphorus anti-ChE agents are hydrolyzed in the body by a group of enzymes known as "phosphorylphosphatases." They are widely distributed throughout plasma and the various tissues and can hydrolyze a large number of organophosphorus compounds (*e.g.,* DFP, tabun, sarin, paraoxon, TEPP) by splitting the anhydride-like P—F (or P—CN) or ester bond. The enzymes are not inhibited by organophosphorus compounds, presumably because the phosphorylated active site reacts rapidly with water to regenerate the free form, in contrast to its high stability in the case of the cholinesterases. It has been suggested that acquired resistance of insects to certain insecticides of this class results from the adaptive development of such enzymes (*see* review by Mounter, 1963). Malathion and other organophosphorus compounds containing carboxylesters undergo hydrolysis at these ester linkages. This reaction is catalyzed by plasma esterases that can be inhibited by organophosphorus compounds. Thus, the toxicity from exposure to two organophosphorus insecticides may be supra-additive (Su *et al.*, 1971; Murphy, 1980).

TOXICOLOGY

The toxicological aspects of the anti-ChE agents are of practical importance to the physician. In addition to numerous cases of accidental intoxication from the use and manufacture of organophosphorus compounds as agricultural insecticides, these agents have been employed frequently for homicidal and suicidal purposes, largely because of their accessibility. Occupational exposure is most common by the dermal and pulmonary routes, while oral ingestion is most common in cases of nonoccupational poisoning. In addition, chronic exposure to several organophosphorus compounds, in particular triarylphosphates, can produce a peculiar neuropathy characterized by demyelination and axonal degeneration; these effects are apparently not due to inhibition of AChE or other cholinesterases. It is common practice to screen for this toxicity in the evaluation of the safety of new insecticides.

Acute Intoxication. The effects of acute intoxication by anti-ChE agents are manifested by muscarinic and nicotinic signs and symptoms and, except for compounds of extremely low lipid solubility, by signs referable to the CNS. Effects may be *localized* or *generalized.* Local effects are due to the action of vapors or aerosols at their site of contact with the eyes or respiratory tract, or to the local absorption after liquid contamination of the skin or mucous membranes, including those of the gastrointestinal tract. General effects rapidly follow systemic absorption by any route; they appear most rapidly after inhalation of vapors or aerosols, where severe effects are present within a few minutes. In contrast, after gastrointestinal and percutaneous absorption, the onset of symptoms is delayed. The *duration* of effects is determined largely by the properties of the compound: its lipid solubility, whether it must be activated, the stability of the organophosphorus-AChE bond, and whether "aging" of the phosphorylated enzyme has occurred.

After *local exposure* to vapors or aerosols or after their *inhalation,* ocular and respiratory effects generally appear first. Ocular effects include marked miosis, ocular pain, conjunctival congestion, ciliary spasm, and brow ache, along with watery nasal discharge; respiratory effects consist in "tightness" in the chest and wheezing respiration, due to the combination of bronchoconstriction and increased bronchial secretion. Gastrointestinal symptoms occur earliest after *ingestion,* and include anorexia, nausea and vomiting, abdominal cramps, and diarrhea. With *percutaneous absorption* of liquid, localized sweating and muscular fasciculation in the immediate vicinity are generally the earliest manifestations.

Additional *muscarinic* effects after systemic absorption include those discussed under pharmacological properties; severe intoxication is manifested by extreme salivation, involuntary defecation and urination, sweating, lacrimation, bradycardia, and hypotension.

Nicotinic actions at the *neuromuscular junctions* of skeletal muscle usually consist in fatigability and generalized weakness, involuntary twitchings, scattered fasciculations, and eventually severe weakness and paralysis; undoubtedly a central component of action contributes to some of these effects. The most serious consequence of the neuromuscular actions is paralysis of the respiratory muscles.

The broad spectrum of effects on the CNS include confusion, ataxia, slurred speech, loss of reflexes, Cheyne-Stokes respiration, generalized convulsions, coma, and central respiratory paralysis. Actions on the vasomotor and other cardiovascular centers in the medulla oblongata further complicate the hemodynamic pattern and lead to hypotension.

The *time of death* after a single acute exposure may range from less than 5 minutes to nearly 24 hours, depending upon the dose, route, agent, and other factors. The *cause of death* is primarily *respiratory failure,* usually accompanied by a secondary *cardiovascular* component. Muscarinic, nicotinic, and central actions all contribute to respiratory embarrassment; they include laryngospasm, bronchoconstriction, increased tracheobronchial and salivary secretion, compromised voluntary control of the diaphragm and intercostal muscles, and central respiratory depression. Although the blood pressure may fall to alarmingly low levels and cardiac irregularities intervene, these effects probably result as much from hypoxemia as from the specific actions mentioned, since they are often reversed by the establishment of adequate pulmonary ventilation.

Diagnosis and Treatment. The *diagnosis* of severe, acute anti-ChE intoxication is readily made from the history of exposure and the characteristic signs and symptoms. In suspected cases of milder acute or chronic intoxication, determination of the ChE activities in erythrocytes and plasma will generally establish the diagnosis. Although these values vary considerably in the normal population, they will usually be depressed well below the normal range before any symptoms due to systemic anti-ChE intoxication are evident. Such figures do not reflect with any accuracy the activities of the corresponding enzymes in the tissues, the depression of which is the basis of the toxic effects.

Treatment is both specific and highly effective. *Atropine* in sufficient dosage (*see* below) effectively antagonizes the actions at muscarinic receptor sites, including the increased tracheobronchial and salivary secretion, the bronchoconstriction, the autonomic ganglionic stimulation, and to a moderate extent the central actions. Larger doses are required to get appreciable concentrations of atropine into the CNS. Atropine is virtually without effect against the peripheral neuromuscular activation and subsequent paralysis. The last-mentioned action of the anti-ChE agents as well as all other peripheral effects can be reversed by *pralidoxime,* a cholinesterase reactivator that is discussed in detail below.

In moderate or severe anti-ChE intoxication, the recommended adult dose of pralidoxime is 1 g, injected intravenously within not less than 2 minutes. If weakness is not relieved or if it recurs after 20 minutes, the dose may be repeated. Early treatment is very important to assure that the oxime reaches the phosphorylated AChE while the latter can still be reactivated.

In addition, certain general supportive measures may be necessary. These include (1) termination of exposure, by removal of the patient or application of a gas mask if the atmosphere is contaminated, copious washing of contaminated skin or mucous membranes with water, or gastric lavage; (2) maintenance of a patent airway; (3) artificial respiration, if required; (4) administration of oxygen; (5) alleviation of persistent convulsions by trimethadione (1 g, intravenously every 15 minutes, to a maximum of 5 g) or sodium thiopental (2.5% solution, intravenously); and (6) treatment of shock (*see* Grob, 1963a; Wills, 1970).

Atropine should be given in very large doses. Following an initial injection of 2 to 4 mg, given intravenously if possible, otherwise intramuscularly, the 2-mg dose should be repeated every 3 to 10 minutes until muscarinic symptoms disappear, and also if they reappear. As much as 50 mg may be required the first day. A mild degree of atropine block should then be maintained, by the oral administration of 1 or 2 mg at intervals of several hours, as long as symptoms are in evidence. Whereas the AChE *reactivators* represent a major advance in the therapy of anti-ChE intoxication (*see* below), their use must be supplemented by the administration of atropine as described.

Cholinesterase Reactivators.
While the phosphorylated esteratic site of AChE undergoes hydrolytic regeneration at a slow or negligible rate (Figure 6–2, upper reaction),

Wilson (1951) found that nucleophilic agents such as hydroxylamine (H_2NOH), hydroxamic acids ($RCONHOH$), and oximes ($RCH{=}NOH$), reactivate the enzyme more rapidly than does spontaneous hydrolysis. He reasoned that selective reactivation could be achieved by a site-directed nucleophil, wherein interaction of a quaternary nitrogen with the negative subsite of the active center would place the nucleophil in close apposition to the phosphorus. This goal was achieved to a remarkable degree by Wilson and Ginsberg (1955) with pyridine-2-aldoxime methyl chloride (2-PAM, 2-formyl-1-methylpyridinium chloride oxime, *pralidoxime;* Figure 6–2); reactivation with this compound occurs at a million times the rate of that with hydroxylamine. Certain *bis*-quaternary oximes were subsequently shown to be even more potent as reactivators; an example is *obidoxime chloride* (Hobbiger and Vojvodić, 1966), the structure of which follows:

Obidoxime

With these two agents the oxime is oriented proximally to exert a nucleophilic attack on the phosphorus; the oxime-phosphonate is then split off, leaving the regenerated enzyme (Figure 6–2, lower reaction) (Wilson, 1959).

The velocity of reactivation of phosphorylated AChE by pralidoxime varies with the nature of the phosphoryl group, and in general follows the same sequence as the order for spontaneous hydrolytic reactivation, that is, dimethylphosphoryl-AChE > diethylphosphoryl-AChE > di*iso*propylphosphoryl-AChE, and so forth. Moreover, phosphorylated AChE can undergo a fairly rapid process of "aging," so that within the course of minutes or hours it becomes completely resistant to the reactivators. The "aging" is probably due to the loss of one alkyl or alkoxy group, leaving a much more stable monoalkyl- or monoalkoxy-phosphoryl-AChE (Fleisher and Harris, 1965) (*see* Figure 6–2). Phosphonates containing tertiary alkoxy groups are more prone to "aging" than are the secondary or primary congeners (Aldridge, 1976). The oximes are not effective in antagonizing the toxicity of the carbamyl ester inhibitors, and, since pralidoxime itself has weak anti-ChE activity, *they are contraindicated in the*

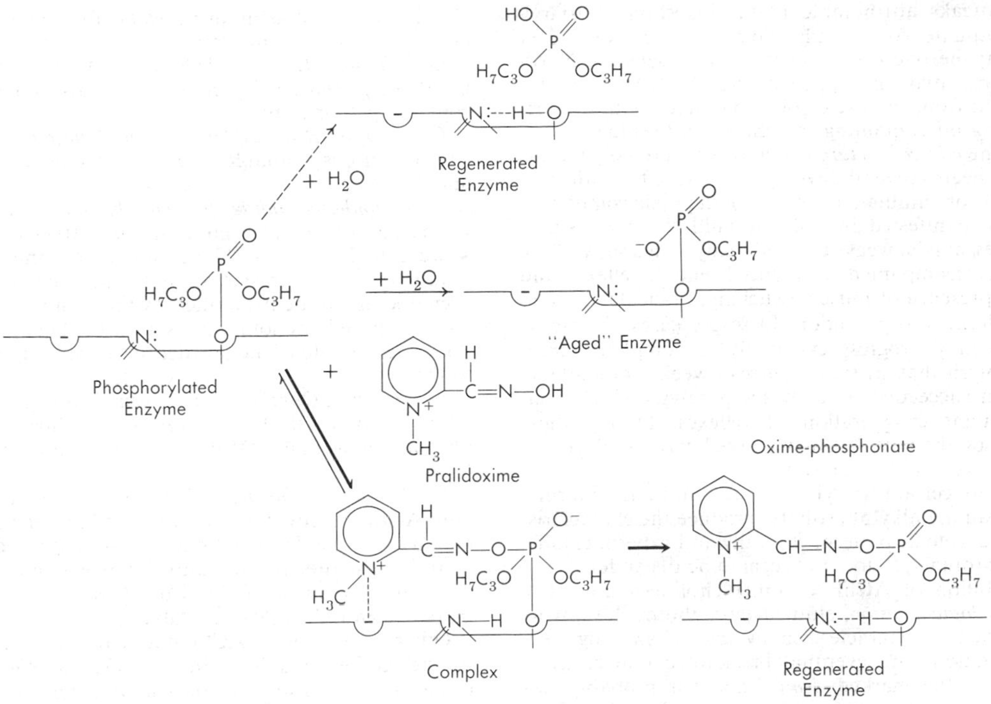

Figure 6-2. *Reactivation of alkylphosphorylated acetylcholinesterase (AChE).*

Following alkylphosphorylation of AChE by DFP (at left), spontaneous hydrolytic reactivation occurs at an insignificant rate (upper reaction), as indicated by the dashed arrow. "Aging" is the loss of one of the isopropoxy residues that occurs more rapidly than spontaneous hydrolysis; the product is very resistant to regeneration by pralidoxime. Pralidoxime (in lower reaction) combines with the anionic site by electrostatic attraction of its quaternary N atom, which orients the nucleophilic oxime group to react with the electrophilic P atom; the oxime-phosphonate is split off, leaving the regenerated enzyme. (Modified from Wilson, 1959; Froede and Wilson, 1971; Aldridge and Reiner, 1972.)

treatment of overdosage with neostigmine or physo stigmine or poisoning with carbaryl (O'Brien, 1969).

Pharmacology, Toxicology, and Disposition. The reactivating action of oximes and hydroxamic acids *in vivo* is most marked at the skeletal neuromuscular junction. Following a dose of an organophosphorus compound that produces total blockade of transmission, the intravenous injection of an oxime can restore the response to stimulation of the motor nerve within a few minutes. Antidotal effects are less striking at autonomic effector sites and insignificant in the CNS.

High doses of pralidoxime and related compounds can in themselves cause neuromuscular blockade and other effects, including inhibition of AChE; such actions are minimal at the doses recommended for clini-

cal use, 1 to 2 g intravenously. If pralidoxime is injected intravenously more rapidly than the recommended rate of 500 mg per minute, it can cause mild weakness, blurred vision, diplopia, dizziness, headache, nausea, and tachycardia.

The oximes as a group are largely metabolized by the liver, and the breakdown products are excreted by the kidney.

Chronic Neurotoxicity of Organophosphorus Compounds. Certain fluorine-containing alkylorganophosphorus anti-ChE agents (*e.g.,* DFP, mipafox) have in common with a number of triarylphosphates, of which triorthocresylphosphate (TOCP) is the classical example, the property of inducing a peculiar type of delayed neurotoxicity. This syndrome first received widespread attention following the demonstration that TOCP, an adulterant of Jamaica ginger, was responsible for an outbreak of thousands of cases of paralysis that occurred in the southern United States during prohibition. Several similar outbreaks attributable to the ingestion of triaryl-phosphate compounds have been recorded since then; the one occurring in 1959 in Meknes, North Africa, involving approximately 10,000 people, resulted from the use of olive oil mixed with a lubricating oil containing triorthocresylphosphate.

The *clinical picture* is that of a severe polyneuritis that begins several days after exposure to a sufficient single or cumulative amount of the toxic compound. It is manifested initially by mild sensory disturbances, ataxia, weakness, and ready fatigability of the legs, accompanied by reduced tendon reflexes and the presence of muscle twitching, fasciculation, and tenderness to palpation. In severe cases, the weakness may progress eventually to complete flaccid paralysis that, over the course of weeks or months, is often succeeded by a spastic paralysis with a concomitant exaggeration of reflexes. During these phases, the muscles show marked wasting. Recovery may require 2 or more years.

Only certain triarylphosphates and only fluorine-containing alkylphosphates produce the characteristic neurotoxic pattern, clinically and experimentally. Accordingly, it does not seem to be dependent upon inhibition of AChE or other cholinesterases. The *pathological lesion*, studied most thoroughly in the chicken, is characterized by *axonal* swelling, segmentation, and eventual breakdown into granular debris; the marked *demyelination* is probably secondary to the aforementioned axonal changes. Neither the biochemical basis nor any specific therapy for the neurotoxic syndrome is known (*see* Aldridge et al., 1969; Usdin, 1970). Experimental myopathies that result in generalized necrotic lesions and changes in end-plate cytostructure are also found after chronic treatment with organophosphates (Laskowski and Dettbarn, 1977).

PREPARATIONS

The compounds described here are those commonly used as anti-ChE drugs and cholinesterase reactivators in the United States. *Conventional dosages* and *routes of administration* are given in the discussion of therapeutic applications of these agents (*see* below).

Physostigmine, U.S.P. (*eserine*), *Physostigmine Salicylate*, U.S.P., and *Physostigmine Sulfate*, U.S.P., are available as crystalline powders for compounding oral and parenteral preparations in suitable dosage forms. Physostigmine salicylate (ANTILIRIUM) injection contains 2-mg amounts in 2-ml ampuls. *Physostigmine Sulfate Ophthalmic Ointment*, U.S.P. (0.25%), and *Physostigmine Salicylate Ophthalmic Solution*, U.S.P. (0.25% and 0.5%), are also available.

Neostigmine Bromide, U.S.P. (PROSTIGMIN), is available for *oral* use in 15-mg tablets. *Neostigmine Methylsulfate*, U.S.P. (PROSTIGMIN METHYLSULFATE), is marketed for *parenteral* injection in sterile solution in ampuls and vials containing 0.25, 0.5, or 1.0 mg/ml.

Ambenonium Chloride, U.S.P. (MYTELASE), is available for *oral* use in 10-mg tablets.

Pyridostigmine Bromide, U.S.P. (MESTINON), is available for *oral* use in 60-mg tablets, in 180-mg sustained-release tablets, and in a syrup that contains

12 mg/ml, as well as in an *injectable* form that contains 5 mg/ml in 2-ml ampuls.

Edrophonium Chloride, U.S.P. (TENSILON), is marketed for *parenteral* injection in ampuls and vials containing 10 mg/ml.

Demecarium Bromide Ophthalmic Solution, U.S.P. (HUMORSOL), is available in concentrations of 0.125 and 0.25%.

Echothiophate Iodide for Ophthalmic Solution, U.S.P. (ECHODIDE, PHOSPHOLINE), is marketed as a powder in 3.0-, 6.25-, 12.5-, and 25-mg amounts. Solutions of appropriate strength must be freshly prepared in a diluent supplied by the manufacturer. Once prepared, the solution is stable for about a year if kept refrigerated. The powder must not be applied to the eye.

Isoflurophate Ophthalmic Ointment, U.S.P. (FLORO-PRYL), contains 0.025% isoflurophate (di*iso*propyl phosphorofluoridate, DFP) in a suitable anhydrous base.

Pralidoxime Chloride, U.S.P. (PROTOPAM), is the only AChE reactivator currently available for general use in the United States. It is dispensed in ampuls in sterile, 1-g amounts for extemporaneous solution in 20 ml of sterile distilled water. It is also marketed in official 500-mg tablets.

Other reactivators of AChE not currently available in the United States include *obidoxime chloride* (TOXOGONIN), its analog *trimedoxime*, and *diacetyl monoxime*. *Obidoxime* is more potent than pralidoxime; the recommended dose is 3 to 6 mg/kg, injected intravenously over 5 to 10 minutes. The dose of *diacetyl monoxime* is 1 to 2 g, injected intravenously at a rate of 200 mg per minute; unlike pralidoxime or obidoxime, it penetrates the blood-brain barrier and reactivates AChE in the CNS. Both drugs can also be repeated in the same doses after 20 minutes.

THERAPEUTIC USES

Although anti-ChE agents have been recommended for the treatment of a wide variety of conditions, their superiority to other drugs and widespread acceptability have been established mainly in four areas: *atony of the smooth muscle of the intestinal tract and urinary bladder, glaucoma, myasthenia gravis,* and *termination of the effects of competitive neuromuscular blocking drugs*. In these conditions, certain anti-ChE agents can be recommended as the drugs of choice; other classes of drugs may sometimes be indicated as adjuncts or in preference to the anti-ChE agents. *Physostigmine* is also useful in the treatment of *atropine intoxication* (*see* below) and of poisoning with *phenothiazines* and *tricyclic antidepressants* (Chapter 19). *Edrophonium* can be used for terminating attacks of *paroxysmal supraventricular tachycardia*.

Paralytic Ileus and Atony of the Urinary Bladder. In the treatment of both these conditions, *neostigmine* is generally the most satisfactory of the anti-ChE agents. The direct parasympathomimetic agents, discussed in Chapter 5, are employed for the same purposes.

Neostigmine is used for the relief of *abdominal distention* from a variety of medical and surgical causes. The usual subcutaneous dose of neostigmine methylsulfate for postoperative paralytic ileus is 0.5 to 1.0 mg. Peristaltic activity commences in 10 to 30 minutes after parenteral administration, whereas 2 to 4 hours is required after oral administration of neostigmine bromide (15 mg). A rectal tube should be inserted to facilitate expulsion of gas, and it may be necessary to assist evacuation with a small low enema. The drug should not be used when there is mechanical obstruction of the intestine or urinary bladder, when peritonitis is present, or when the viability of the bowel is doubtful. Other supportive measures are not to be neglected, including intubation and suction as well as appropriate therapy with fluids and electrolytes. Indeed, neostigmine and other drugs are to be viewed mainly as adjuvant agents in the treatment of distention. The drug is not likely to be helpful in relieving atony of the stomach or upper gastrointestinal tract after vagotomy.

When neostigmine is employed for the treatment of atony of the detrusor muscle of the *urinary bladder,* postoperative dysuria is relieved and the time interval between operation and spontaneous urination is shortened. The drug is used in the same dose and manner as in the management of paralytic ileus.

Glaucoma. Glaucoma is a disease complex characterized chiefly by an increase in intraocular pressure that, if sufficiently high and persistent, leads to damage to the optic disc at the juncture of the optic nerve and the retina; this can cause irreversible blindness. Of the three types—primary, secondary, and congenital—anti-ChE agents are of great value in the management of the primary as well as of certain categories of the secondary type (*e.g.,* aphakic glaucoma, following cataract extraction); the congenital type rarely responds to therapy other than surgical treatment. Primary glaucoma is subdivided into narrow-angle (acute congestive) and wide-angle (chronic simple) types, based on the configuration of the angle of the anterior chamber where reabsorption of the aqueous humor occurs. Anti-ChE agents produce a fall in intraocular pressure in both types of primary glaucoma, chiefly by lowering the resistance to outflow of the aqueous humor. Effects on the volumes of the various intraocular vascular beds (*e.g.,* those of the iris, ciliary body, etc.) and on the rate of secretion of the aqueous humor into the posterior chamber may contribute secondarily to the lowering of pressure, or conversely may produce a rise in pressure preceding the fall. In narrow-angle glaucoma, the aqueous outflow is facilitated by the freeing of the entrance to the trabecular space at the canal of Schlemm from blockade by the iris, as the result of the drug-induced contraction of the sphincter muscle of the iris.

In wide-angle, or chronic simple, glaucoma, there is no physical obstruction to the entry to the trabecu-lae; rather, the trabeculae, which are a meshwork of pores of small diameter, lose their patency. In this circumstance, contraction of the sphincter muscle of the iris and the ciliary muscle enhances tone and alignment of the trabecular network to improve resorption and outflow of aqueous humor through the network to the canal of Schlemm (*see* reviews by Watson, 1972; Schwartz, 1978).

The foregoing distinctions are of great importance for therapy, since the roles of miotic drugs, including the anti-ChE agents, are quite different in the management of the two types of primary glaucoma. Acute congestive (narrow-angle) glaucoma is nearly always a medical emergency in which the drugs are essential in controlling the acute attack, but the long-range management is usually based predominantly on surgery (*e.g.,* peripheral or complete iridectomy). Chronic simple (wide-angle) glaucoma, on the other hand, has a gradual, insidious onset and is not generally amenable to surgical improvement; in this type, control of intraocular pressure is usually dependent upon drug therapy on a permanent basis.

Acute congestive glaucoma may be precipitated by the injudicious use of a mydriatic agent in patients over 40, or by a variety of factors that can cause pupillary dilatation or engorgement of intraocular vessels. The cardinal signs and symptoms include marked ocular inflammation, a semidilated pupil, severe pain, and nausea. Every effort must be made to reduce the intraocular pressure to the normal level and maintain it there for the duration of the attack. In general, an anti-ChE agent is instilled in the conjunctival sac in combination with a parasympathomimetic agent for greatest effectiveness. One such combination that is frequently employed is a solution of *physostigmine salicylate,* 1%, plus *pilocarpine nitrate,* 4%. This combination should be instilled six times at 10-minute intervals, then three times at 30-minute intervals, and thereafter as required. *Adjunctive therapy* should include the intravenous administration of a carbonic anhydrase inhibitor, such as *acetazolamide,* to reduce the secretion of aqueous humor, or of an osmotic agent, such as *mannitol* or *glycerol,* to induce intraocular dehydration. The long-acting organophosphorus compounds are not indicated in narrow-angle glaucoma because of vascular engorgement and an increase in the angle block.

Chronic simple glaucoma and *secondary glaucoma* require careful consideration of the needs of the individual patient in selecting the drug or combination of drugs to be employed. The choices available include (1) parasympathomimetic agents (*e.g.,* pilocarpine nitrate, 0.5 to 4%; *see* Chapter 5); (2) anti-ChE agents that are short acting (*e.g.,* physostigmine salicylate, 0.02 to 1%) and long acting (demecarium bromide, 0.125 to 0.25%; echothiophate, 0.03 to 0.25%; isoflurophate, 0.005 to 0.2%); and, paradoxically, (3) sympathomimetic agents (*e.g.,* epinephrine, 1 to 2%; phenylephrine, 10%; *see* Chapter 8). Drugs of the last-mentioned class are often most effective when used in combination with AChE inhibitors or cholinergic agonists. They reduce intraocular pressure by decreasing secretion of aqueous humor, and they prevent engorgement of small blood vessels. *Timolol,* a β-adrenergic antagonist, has also been found to be effective in reducing intraocular pressure (*see* Chapter 9). Timolol does not cause pupillary constriction but appears to act by reducing the production of aqueous humor (Boger *et al.,* 1978). Timolol is long acting, and administration is at 12-hour intervals. Although its chronic use has yet to be fully assessed, this may avoid the side effects of the long-acting inhibitors of AChE (Katz, 1978). Despite the convenience of less frequent administration and the high potency of long-acting anti-ChE agents, their use entails a greater risk of development of lenticular opacities and untoward autonomic effects.

Of the organophosphorus agents, *DFP* has the longest duration of action and is extremely potent when applied locally; solutions in peanut or sesame oil require instillation from once daily to once weekly, and may control intraocular pressure in severe cases that are resistant to other drugs. The oily vehicle is unpleasant to most patients. Consequently, DFP has largely been replaced by echothiophate.

Anti-ChE agents have been employed locally in the treatment of a variety of other ophthalmological conditions, including accommodative esotropia in children and myasthenia gravis confined to the extraocular and eyelid muscles, and, in alternation with a mydriatic drug such as atropine, for the breaking of adhesions between the iris and the lens or cornea. (For a complete account of the use of anti-ChE agents in ocular therapy, *see* Havener, 1978.)

Untoward Effects. Treatment of glaucoma with potent, long-acting anti-ChE agents (including demecarium, echothiophate, and isoflurophate) for 6 months or longer carries a high risk of the development of a specific type of *cataract,* which begins as anterior subcapsular vacuoles (Axelsson and Holmberg, 1966; de Roetth, 1966; Shaffer and Hetherington, 1966). Although formation of spontaneous cataracts is quite common within comparable age groups, the incidence of lenticular opacities under such circumstances can be as high as 50%; the hazard is apparently increased in proportion to the strength of the solution, frequency of instillation, duration of therapy, and age of the patient. The underlying mechanism remains elusive (*see* Laties, 1969).

Most of the studies that have implicated the long-acting anti-ChE agents in the formation of cataracts have been retrospective and uncontrolled. The reported incidence of cataracts attributable to such drugs may thus be distorted by selection of patients with more severe glaucoma; nevertheless, cataractogenesis should be considered when therapeutic decisions are made. Long-acting anti-ChE agents are, of course, not indicated when glaucoma can be controlled by parasympathomimetic drugs, physostigmine, or other agents. Since glaucoma leads to irreversible blindness if not adequately controlled, the long-acting cholinesterase inhibitors retain their therapeutic importance in situations where other agents are inadequate (Havener, 1978).

Treatment with *pilocarpine* (4%), alone or in combination with *physostigmine* (0.2%), one to five times daily, was found to entail no higher incidence of the development of lenticular opacities than appeared spontaneously in untreated patients in comparable age groups (Axelsson, 1969). At present, it seems clear that pilocarpine and other shorter-acting miotic drugs should be employed as long as they provide adequate control of intraocular tension. If they fail to do so, the hazards of cataract development must be balanced against those of increased intraocular pressure before resorting to the use of the potent, long-acting anti-ChE agents. When such drugs are used, patients should be examined for the appearance of lenticular opacities at intervals of 6 months or less.

Miscellaneous ocular side effects that may occur following local instillation of anti-ChE agents are headache, brow pain, blurred vision, phacodinesis, pericorneal injection, congestive iritis, various allergic reactions, and, rarely, retinal detachment. When anti-ChE drugs are instilled intraconjunctivally at frequent intervals, sufficient absorption may occur to produce various systemic effects, which result from inhibition of tissue AChE and plasma pseudo-ChE. Hence, cholinergic autonomic function will be augmented and the neuromuscular blockade produced by succinylcholine will be enhanced and prolonged (*see* Chapter 11.) Individuals with vagotonia and allergies are at particular risk. Systemic absorption of the drug can be minimized by digital compression of the inner canthus of the eye during and for a short period following its instillation.

Myasthenia Gravis. Myasthenia gravis is a neuromuscular disease characterized by weakness and marked fatigability of skeletal muscle (*see* Grob, 1963b; Drachman, 1978); exacerbations and partial remissions occur frequently. Its clinical manifestations were described before the turn of the century (Jolly, 1895; Campbell and Bramwell, 1900). Jolly noted the similarity between the symptoms of myasthenia gravis and curare poisoning in animals and suggested that *physostigmine,* an agent then known to antagonize curare, might be of therapeutic value. Forty years elapsed before his suggestion was given systematic trial (Walker, 1934). Remen (1932) and Walker (1935) independently showed *neostigmine* to be useful in the management of the disease, and, although *pyridostigmine* is also frequently employed today, neostigmine remains a standard for comparison of new agents.

The defect in myasthenia gravis is in synaptic transmission at the neuromuscular junction. When a motor nerve of a normal subject is stimulated at 25 Hz, electrical and mechanical responses are well sustained. A suitable margin of safety exists for maintenance of neuromuscular transmission. Initial responses in the myasthenic patient may be normal, but they diminish rapidly, which explains the difficulty experienced by the patient in maintaining voluntary muscle activity for more than brief periods. When the patient is given an appropriate dose of neostigmine, the response to tetanic stimulation is improved, along with symptomatic improvement in muscle strength. The same dose of neostigmine in control subjects leads to a *reduced* response to tetanic stimulation, accompanied by fasciculations, local weakness, and repetitive action potentials in response to a single stimulus (Grob, 1963b). Elmqvist and coworkers (1964) observed that the amplitude of miniature end-plate potentials was reduced in patients with myasthenia gravis and, since they were unable to demonstrate a reduction of receptor sensitivity, postulated that the change was due to a reduction in the number of ACh molecules per quantum. The relative importance of prejunctional and postjunctional defects was a matter of considerable debate until Patrick and Lindstrom (1973) found that rabbits immunized with the nicotinic receptor purified from electric eels slowly developed muscular weakness and respiratory difficulties that resembled the symptoms of myasthenia gravis. The rabbits also exhibited decremental responses following repetitive nerve stimulation, enhanced sensitivity to curare, and symptomatic and electrophysiological improvement of neuromuscular transmission following administration of anti-ChE agents. Although this *experimental allergic myasthenia gravis* and the naturally occurring disease differ somewhat, particularly in the marked acute phase of the experimental condition, this critical development of an animal model prompted intense investigation into whether the natural disease represented an autoimmune injury directed toward the ACh receptor. Antireceptor antibody was soon identified in patients with myasthenia gravis (Almon *et al.,* 1974). Receptor-binding antibody has been detected in sera of 87% of patients with myasthenia gravis, although the clinical status of the patients does not correlate precisely with the antibody titer (Lindstrom *et al.,* 1976). Passive transfer of antibody, by use of an immunoglobulin fraction prepared from myasthenic patients, produces the myasthenic syndrome in recipient animals (Toyka *et al.,* 1975). By use of the snake α-neurotoxins that were also essential for the purification and characterization of the isolated nicotinic receptor from eel (*see* Chapter 11), Fambrough and associates (1973) were able to detect a 70 to 90% reduction in the number of receptors per end-plate in myasthenic patients. This finding provided crucial support for the hypothesis that a decrease in receptors in the postsynaptic membrane accounts for the defects of the disease.

The picture that ultimately emerges is that myasthenia gravis is caused by an autoimmune response to the ACh receptor at the postjunctional end-plate. Antibodies, which are also present in plasma, reduce the number of receptors detectable either by toxin-binding assays or by electrophysiological measurements of ACh sensitivity (Drachman, 1978). In these patients, immune complexes have been detected at the postsynaptic membrane, along with marked ultrastructural abnormalities in the synaptic cleft (Engel *et al.,* 1977). The latter appear to be a consequence of the destructive autoimmune reaction.

Diagnosis. Although the diagnosis can usually be made from the history, signs, and symptoms, its differentiation from certain neurasthenic, infectious, endocrine, neoplastic, and degenerative neuromuscular diseases may sometimes be difficult. However, myasthenia gravis is the only condition in which the aforementioned deficiencies can be improved dramatically by anti-ChE medication. The *edrophonium test* is performed by injecting intravenously 2 mg of edrophonium chloride, followed 45 seconds later by an additional 8 mg if the first dose is without effect; a positive response consists in brief improvement in strength, unaccompanied by lingual fasciculation

(which generally occurs in nonmyasthenic patients).

An excessive dose of an anti-ChE drug results in a *cholinergic crisis.* The condition is characterized by weakness resulting from excessive depolarization of the motor end-plate; other features result from overstimulation of muscarinic receptors. The weakness resulting from depolarization block may closely resemble *myasthenic weakness,* which is due to insufficient anti-ChE medication. The distinction is of obvious practical importance, since the former is treated by withholding, and the latter by administering, the anti-ChE agent. When the edrophonium test is performed cautiously, limiting the dose to 1 or 2 mg, and with facilities for respiratory resuscitation immediately available, a further decrease in strength indicates cholinergic crisis, while improvement signifies myasthenic weakness. *Atropine sulfate,* 0.6 mg or more intravenously, should be given immediately if a severe muscarinic reaction ensues (for complete details, *see* Osserman and Genkins, 1966; Osserman *et al.,* 1972).

If the patient suspected of having myasthenia gravis exhibits minimal symptoms at the time of examination, a provocative test can be performed by injecting intravenously 0.1 to 0.5 mg of *d*-tubocurarine chloride. A positive response consists in the rapid precipitation of the characteristic weakness and associated symptoms; it should be reversed by the immediate intravenous injection of 2.0 mg of neostigmine methylsulfate. The *d*-tubocurarine test is a potentially hazardous procedure; it should be performed only with an anesthesiologist present and with facilities for respiratory and cardiovascular resuscitation immediately at hand. A regional curare test involving intra-arterial injection into one limb has been developed, which carries less risk (Horowitz *et al.,* 1976).

Treatment. Neostigmine, pyridostigmine, and *ambenonium* are the standard anti-ChE drugs used in the symptomatic treatment of myasthenia gravis. All can increase the response of myasthenic muscle to repetitive nerve impulses, primarily by the preservation of endogenous ACh; receptors over a greater cross-sectional area of the end-plate are then presumably exposed to concentrations of ACh that are sufficient for stimulation. In a normal end-plate, the density of receptors is sufficient so that recruitment of additional receptors is not necessary.

When the diagnosis of myasthenia gravis has been established, the optimal single oral dose of an anti-ChE agent can be determined by either of two empirical methods involving oral or intravenous titration.

In the oral test, baseline recordings are made of grip strength, vital capacity, and a number of signs and symptoms that reflect the strength of various muscle groups. The patient is then given an oral dose of neostigmine (7.5 mg), pyridostigmine (30 mg), or ambenonium (2.5 mg). The improvement in muscle strength and changes in other signs and symptoms are noted at frequent intervals until there is a return to the basal state. After an hour or longer in the basal state, the drug is given again with the dose increased to one and one-half times the initial amount, and the same observations are repeated. This sequence is continued, with increasing increments of one half the initial dose, until the optimal response is obtained. The result can be confirmed by the *edrophonium test*. If the dose of the longer-acting anti-ChE agent was insufficient, a further improvement in muscle strength will result. If the dose was adequate or excessive, no further change or a reduction in muscle strength will be evident. The optimal single oral dose may range from the initial doses given above to more than ten times these amounts.

Alternatively, the optimal dose can be determined by an intravenous titration test, as described in detail by Osserman and associates (1972). This involves recording of the same parameters as above, before and following the intravenous injection of successive, small increments of neostigmine (0.125 mg) or pyridostigmine (0.5 mg), at intervals of a few minutes. Prior to injection of the anti-ChE agent, the patient is given an intravenous injection of 0.4 to 0.6 mg of atropine to prevent muscarinic side effects. When the optimal total intravenous dose has been established, and confirmed by the edrophonium test, the optimal single oral dose is estimated as approximately 30 times that amount.

The duration of action of these drugs is such that the interval between oral doses required to maintain a reasonably even level of strength is usually 2 to 4 hours for neostigmine and 3 to 6 hours for pyridostigmine or ambenonium. However, the amount required may vary from day to day, and physical or emotional stress, intercurrent infections, and menstruation usually necessitate an increase in the frequency or size of the dose. In addition, unpredictable exacerbations and remissions of the myasthenic state may require adjustment of the dosage upward or downward. Although all patients with myasthenia gravis should be seen by a physician at regular intervals, most can be taught to modify their dosage regimens according to their changing requirements. *Pyridostigmine* is available in sustained-release tablets containing a total of 180 mg, of which 60 mg is released immediately and 120 mg over several hours; this preparation should be limited to use at bedtime and is of value in maintaining patients for 6- to 8-hour periods. Muscarinic cardiovascular and gastrointestinal side effects of anti-ChE agents can generally be controlled by atropine or other anticholinergic drugs (Chapter 7); in most patients, tolerance is developed eventually to the muscarinic effects, so that anticholinergic medication can be suspended. A number of drugs, including curariform agents and certain antibiotics and general anesthetics, interfere with neuromuscular transmission; their administration to patients with myasthenia gravis is hazardous without proper adjustment of anti-ChE dosage and other appropriate precautions. Parenteral administration of the standard anti-ChE agents is sometimes required in desperately ill myasthenic patients who do not respond adequately to oral medication; the subcutaneous, intramuscular, or intravenous route may be used.

In cases where administration of anti-ChE agents at optimal doses is not sufficient to enable near-normal motor activity, other therapeutic measures must be considered. Controlled studies reveal that *corticosteroids* promote clinical improvement in a high percentage of patients (Engel, 1976; Howard *et al.,* 1976; Mann *et al.,* 1976). However, when treatment with steroids is continued over a prolonged period, a high incidence of undesirable side effects may result (*see* Chapter 63). Gradual lowering of maintenance doses and alternate-day regimens are used as means for minimizing side effects (Seybold and Drachman, 1974; Howard *et al.,* 1976). In addition, initiation of steroid treatment augments muscle weakness; however, as the patient improves with continued administration of steroids, doses of anti-ChE drugs can be reduced (Drachman, 1978). The immunosuppressive activity of corticosteroids is likely of primary importance, since antireceptor activity is diminished in circulating lymphocytes following such treatment (Abramsky *et al.,* 1975).

Thymectomy should be considered in myasthenia associated with a thymoma or when the disease is not adequately controlled by anti-ChE agents. An improved prognosis following thymectomy is likely, and apparent remissions have been observed in some cases (Buckingham *et al.,* 1976). However, the relative risks and benefits of the surgical procedure versus anti-ChE and corticosteroid treatment requires careful assessment in each case (McQuillen and Leone, 1977). Since the thymus contains myoid cells, it has been suggested that the disease arises in this tissue (*see* Drachman, 1978); however, the thymus is not required for perpetuation of the condition.

In keeping with the presumed autoimmune etiology of myasthenia gravis, *plasmapheresis* has been performed with beneficial results in patients who have remained disabled despite thymectomy and treatment with steroids and anti-ChE agents (Dau *et al.,* 1977). Improvement in muscle strength correlates with the reduction of the titer of antibody directed against the cholinergic nicotinic receptor. The use of immunosuppressive agents such as azathioprine is also being explored.

Intoxication by Anticholinergic Drugs. Many of the peripheral and central effects of poisoning by atropine and related antimuscarinic drugs (Chapter 7) can be reversed by intravenous injection of physostigmine. Many other drugs, such as the phenothiazines, antihistamines, tricyclic antidepressants, and benzoquinamide, have central, as well as peripheral, anticholinergic activity, and *physostigmine salicylate* may be useful in reversing the central anticholinergic syndrome produced by overdosage or an unusual reaction to these drugs (Rumack, 1973; Aquilonius, 1977). An initial intravenous dose of 0.5 to 2 mg of physostigmine is indicated, with additional increments given as necessary. Physostigmine, a tertiary amine, crosses the blood-brain barrier in contrast to the quaternary anti-AChE drugs. The use of anti-ChE agents to reverse the effects of competitive neuromuscular blocking agents is discussed in Chapter 11.

Abramsky, O.; Aharonov, A.; Teitelbaum, D.; and Fuchs, S.   Myasthenia gravis and the acetylcholine receptor: effect of steroids in the clinical course and cellular immune response to acetylcholine receptor. *Arch. Neurol.,* **1975,** *32,* 684–687.

Aeschlimann, J. A., and Reinert, M.   Pharmacological

action of some analogues of physostigmine. *J. Pharmacol. Exp. Ther.,* **1931,** *43,* 413–444.

Aldridge, W. N.; Barnes, J. M.; and Johnson, M. K. Studies on delayed neurotoxicity produced by some organophosphorus compounds. *Ann. N.Y. Acad. Sci.,* **1969,** *160,* 314–322.

Almon, R. R.; Andrew, C. G.; and Appel, S. H. Serum globulin in myasthenia gravis: inhibition of α-bungarotoxin binding to acetylcholine receptors. *Science,* **1974,** *186,* 55–57.

Argyll-Robertson, D. The Calabar bean as a new agent in ophthalmic practice. *Edinb. Med. J.,* **1863,** *8,* 815–820.

Axelsson, U. Glaucoma miotic therapy and cataract. *Acta Ophthalmol. (Kbh.),* **1969,** Suppl. 102, 1–37.

Axelsson, U., and Holmberg, A. The frequency of cataract after miotic therapy. *Acta Ophthalmol. (Kbh.),* **1966,** *44,* 421–429.

Boger, W.; Steinert, R.; Puliafito, C.; and Pavah-Langston, D. Clinical trial comparing timolol ophthalmic solution in patients with open angle glaucoma. *Am. J. Ophthalmol.,* **1978,** *86,* 8–18.

Buckingham, J. M.; Howard, F. M.; Bernatz, P. E.; Payne, W. S.; Harrison, E. G.; O'Brien, P. C.; and Weiland, L. H. The value of thymectomy in myasthenia gravis. *Ann. Surg.,* **1976,** *184,* 543–548.

Burgen, A. S. V., and Hobbiger, F. The inhibition of cholinesterases by alkylphosphates and alkylphenolphosphates. *Br. J. Pharmacol. Chemother.,* **1951,** *6,* 593–605.

Campbell, H., and Bramwell, E. Myasthenia gravis. *Brain,* **1900,** *23,* 277–336.

Cartaud, J.; Reiger, F.; Bon, S.; and Massoulie, J. Fine structure of electric eel acetylcholinesterase. *Brain Res.,* **1975,** *88,* 127–130.

Christioson, R. On the properties of the ordeal bean of Old Calabar. *Mon. J. Med. (Lond.),* **1855,** *20,* 193–204.

Clermont, P. de. Chimie organique—note sur la préparation de quelques éthers. *C. R. Acad. Sci. [D] (Paris),* **1854,** *39,* 338–341.

Cohan, S. L.; Pohlmann, J. L. W.; Mikszewki, J.; and O'Doherty, D. S. The pharmacokinetics of pyridostigmine. *Neurology (Minneap.),* **1976,** *26,* 536–539.

Dau, P. C.; Lindstrom, J. M.; Cassel, C. K.; Denys, E. H.; Shev, F. E.; and Spitler, L. E. Plasmapheresis and immunosuppressive drug therapy in myasthenia gravis. *N. Engl. J. Med.,* **1977,** *297,* 1134–1140.

de Roeth, A., Jr. Lenticular opacities in glaucoma patients receiving echothiophate iodide therapy. *J.A.M.A.,* **1966,** *195,* 664–666.

Dolivo, M., and Koelle, G. B. Properties of nicotinic and muscarinic receptors in isolated rat ganglia. *Experientia,* **1970,** *26,* 679.

DuBois, K. P.; Doull, J.; Salerno, P. R.; and Coon, J. M. Studies on the toxicity and mechanisms of action of *p*-nitrophenyl diethyl thiono phosphate (parathion). *J. Pharmacol. Exp. Ther.,* **1949,** *95,* 79–91.

Dudai, Y.; Herzberg, M.; and Silman, I. Molecular structures of acetylcholinesterase from electric organ tissue of the electric eel. *Proc. Natl. Acad. Sci. U.S.A.,* **1973,** *70,* 2473–2476.

Elmqvist, D.; Hoffman, W. W.; Kugelberg, J.; and Quastel, D. M. J. An electrophysiological investigation of neuromuscular transmission in myasthenia gravis. *J. Physiol. (Lond.),* **1964,** *174,* 417–434.

Engel, A. G.; Lambert, E. H.; and Howard, F. M., Jr. Immune complexes (IgG and C3) at the motor endplate in myasthenia gravis. *Mayo Clin. Proc.,* **1977,** *52,* 267–280.

Engel, W. K. Myasthenia gravis: corticosteroids and anticholinesterases. *Ann. N.Y. Acad. Sci.,* **1976,** *274,* 623–630.

Fambrough, D. M.; Drachman, D. B.; and Satyamurti, S. Neuromuscular junction in myasthenia gravis; decreased acetylcholine receptors. *Science,* **1973,** *182,* 293–295.

Fleisher, J. H., and Harris, L. W. Dealkylation as a mechanism for aging of cholinesterase after poisoning with

pinacolyl methylphosphonofluoridate. *Biochem. Pharmacol.,* **1965,** *14,* 641–650.

Fraser, T. R. On the characters, actions and therapeutical uses of the ordeal bean of Calabar (*Physostigma venenosum,* Balfour). *Edinb. Med. J.,* **1863,** *9,* 36–56, 123–132, 235–248.

Gaines, T. B. Acute toxicity of pesticides. *Toxicol. Appl. Pharmacol.,* **1969,** *14,* 515–534.

Goldstein, A., and Hamlisch, R. E. Properties and behavior of purified human plasma cholinesterase. IV. Enzymatic destruction of the inhibitors prostigmine and physostigmine. *Arch. Biochem. Biophys.,* **1952,** *35,* 12–22.

Gysin, H. Über einige neue Insektizide. *Chimia,* **1954,** *8,* 205–210, 221–228.

Hall, Z. W. Multiple forms of acetylcholinesterase and their distribution in endplate and non-endplate regions of rat diaphragm muscle. *J. Neurobiol.,* **1973,** *4,* 343–361.

Hobbiger, F., and Vojvodić, V. The reactivating and antidotal actions of N,N′-trimethylenebis(pyridinium-4-aldoxime) (TMB-4) and N,N′-oxydimethylenebis(pyridinium-4-aldoxime) (toxogenin) with particular reference to their effect on phosphorylated acetylcholinesterase in brain. *Biochem. Pharmacol.,* **1966,** *15,* 1677–1690.

Horowitz, S. H.; Genkins, G.; and Kornfeld, P. Electrophysiologic diagnosis of myasthenia gravis and the regional curare test. *Neurology (Minneap.),* **1976,** *26,* 410–417.

Howard, F. M., Jr.; Duane, D. D.; Lambert, E. H.; and Daube, J. R. Alternate-day prednisolone: preliminary report of a double-blind controlled study. *Ann. N.Y. Acad. Sci.,* **1976,** *274,* 596–607.

Jolly, F. Pseudoparalysis myasthenica. *Neurol. Zentralbl.,* **1895,** *14,* 34.

Julian, P. L., and Pikl, J. Studies in indole series. V. Complete synthesis of physostigmine (eserine). *J. Am. Chem. Soc.,* **1935,** *57,* 755–757.

Kitz, R., and Wilson, I. B. Acceleration of the rate of reaction of methanesulfonyl fluoride and acetylcholinesterase by substituted ammonium ions. *J. Biol. Chem.,* **1963,** *238,* 745–748.

Lange, W., and Krueger, G. von. Über Ester der Mono fluorphosphorsäure. *Ber. Dtsch. Chem. Ges.,* **1932,** *65,* 1598–1601.

Laqueur, L. Ueber Atropin und Physostigmin in ihre Wirkung auf den intraocularen Druck: Ein Beitrag zur Therapie des Glaucoms. *Albrecht von Graefes Arch. Klin. Ophthalmol.,* **1877,** *23,* 149–176.

Laties, A. M. Localization in cornea and lens of topically-applied irreversible cholinesterase inhibitors. *Am. J. Ophthalmol.,* **1969,** *68,* 848–857.

Leuzinger, W.; Baker, A. L.; and Cauvin, E. Acetylcholinesterase. II. Crystallization, absorption spectra, isoionic point. *Proc. Natl. Acad. Sci. U.S.A.,* **1968,** *59,* 620–623.

Lindstrom, J. M.; Seybold, M. E.; Lennon, V. A.; Whittingham, S.; and Duane, D. D. Antibody to acetylcholine receptor in myasthenia gravis: prevalance, clinical correlates and diagnostic value. *Neurology (Minneap.),* **1976,** *26,* 1054–1059.

Lwebuga-Mukasa, J. S.; Lappi, S.; and Taylor, P. Molecular forms of acetylcholinesterase from *Torpedo californica:* their relationship to synaptic membranes. *Biochemistry,* **1976,** *15,* 1425–1434.

McCombie, H., and Saunders, B. C. Alkyl fluorophosphonates: preparation and physiological properties. *Nature,* **1946,** *157,* 287–289.

McQuillen, M. P., and Leone, M. G. A treatment carol: thymectomy revisited in the corticosteroid era. *Neurology (Minneap.),* **1977,** *27,* 1103–1106.

Mann, J. D.; Johns, T. R.; Campa, J. F.; and Muller, W. H. Long term prednisolone followed by thymectomy in myasthenia gravis. *Ann. N.Y. Acad. Sci.,* **1976,** *274,* 608–622.

Mooser, G., and Sigman, D. S. Ligand binding properties

of acetylcholinesterase determined with fluorescent probes. *Biochemistry,* **1974,** *13,* 2299–2307.

Myers, D. K. Studies on cholinesterase. 10. Return of cholinesterase activity in the rat after inhibition by carbamoyl fluorides. *Biochem. J.,* **1956,** *62,* 556–563.

Neal, R. A. Studies on the metabolism of diethyl 4-nitrophenyl phosphorothionate (parathion) *in vitro. Biochem. J.,* **1967,** *103,* 183–191.

O'Brien, R. D. Phosphorylation and carbamylation of cholinesterase. *Ann. N.Y. Acad. Sci.,* **1969,** *160,* 204–214.

Osserman, K. E., and Genkins, G. Critical reappraisal of the use of edrophonium (TENSILON) chloride tests in myasthenia gravis and significance of clinical classification. *Ann. N.Y. Acad. Sci.,* **1966,** *135,* 312–326.

Patrick, J. L., and Lindstrom, J. Autoimmune response to acetylcholine receptor. *Science,* **1973,** *180,* 871–872.

Polonovski, M., and Polonovski, M. Etúde sur les alcaloïdes de la fève de Calabar (XI). Quelques hypothèses sur la constitution de l'ésérine. *Bull. Soc. Chim. Fr.,* **1923,** *33,* 1117–1131.

Remen, L. Zur Pathogenese und Therapie der Myasthenia gravis pseudoparalytic. *Dtsch. Z. NervHeilk.,* **1932,** *128,* 66–78.

Riker, W. F., Jr., and Wescoe, W. C. The direct action of prostigmine on skeletal muscle: its relationship to the choline esters. *J. Pharmacol. Exp. Ther.,* **1946,** *88,* 58–66.

Rodin, F. H. Eserine: its history in the practice of ophthalmology (physostigmine): *Physostigma venenosum* (Balfour): (Calabar bean). *Am. J. Ophthalmol.,* **1947,** *30,* 19–28.

Rosenberry, T. L., and Richardson, J. M. Structure of 18S and 14S acetylcholinesterase. Identification of collagenlike subunits that are linked by disulfide bonds to catalytic subunits. *Biochemistry,* **1977,** *16,* 3550–3558.

Rumack, B. H. Anticholinergic poisoning: treatment with physostigmine. *Pediatrics,* **1973,** *52,* 449–451.

Seybold, M. E., and Drachman, D. B. Gradually increasing doses of prednisolone in myasthenia gravis: reducing the hazards of treatment. *N. Engl. J. Med.,* **1974,** *290,* 81–84.

Shaffer, R. N., and Hetherington, J., Jr. Anticholinesterase drugs and cataracts. *Am. J. Ophthalmol.,* **1966,** *62,* 613–618.

Somani, S. M.; Roberts, J. B.; and Wilson, A. Pyridostigmine metabolism in man. *Clin. Pharmacol. Ther.,* **1972,** *13,* 393–399.

Stedman, E. III. Studies on the relationship between chemical constitution and physiological action. Part II. The miotic activity of urethanes derived from the isomeric hydroxybenzyldimethylamines. *Biochem. J.,* **1929a,** *23,* 17–24.

———. Chemical constitution and miotic action. *Am. J. Physiol.,* **1929b,** *90,* 528–529.

Stedman, E., and Barger, G. Physostigmine (eserine). Part III. *J. Chem. Soc.,* **1925,** *127,* 247–258.

Su, M.; Kinoshita, F. K.; Frawley, F. P.; and DuBois, K. P. Comparative inhibition of aliesterases and cholinesterases in rats fed eighteen organophosphorus insecticides. *Toxicol. Appl. Pharmacol.,* **1971,** *20,* 241–249.

Taylor, P., and Lappi, S. Interaction of fluorescent probes with acetylcholinesterase. The site and specificity of propidium binding. *Biochemistry,* **1975,** *14,* 1989–1997.

Toyka, K. V.; Drachman, D. B.; Pestronk, A.; and Kao, I. Myasthenia gravis: passive transfer from man to mouse. *Science,* **1975,** *190,* 397–399.

Walker, M. B. Treatment of myasthenia gravis with physostigmine. *Lancet,* **1934,** *1,* 1200–1201.

———. Case showing effect of prostigmine on myasthenia gravis. *Proc. R. Soc. Med.,* **1935,** *28,* 759–761.

Wilson, I. B. Acetylcholinesterase. XI. Reversibility of tetraethyl pyrophosphate inhibition. *J. Biol. Chem.,* **1951,** *190,* 111–117.

Wilson, I. B., and Ginsburg, S. A powerful reactivator of

alkyl phosphate–inhibited acetylcholinesterase. *Biochim. Biophys. Acta,* **1955,** *18,* 168–170.

Wilson, I. B., and Harrison, M. A. Turnover number of acetylcholinesterase. *J. Biol. Chem.,* **1961,** *236,* 2292–2295.

Wilson, I. B.; Hatch, M. A.; and Ginsburg, S. Carbamylation of acetylcholinesterase. *J. Biol. Chem.,* **1960,** *235,* 2312–2315.

Wilson, I. B., and Quan, C. Acetylcholinesterase: studies on molecular complementariness. *Arch. Biochem. Biophys.,* **1958,** *73,* 131–143.

Monographs and Reviews

Aldridge, W. N. Survey of major points of interest about reactions of cholinesterases. *Croat. Chem. Acta,* **1976,** *47,* 225–233.

Aldridge, W. N., and Reiner, E. Enzyme inhibitors as substrates. *Front. Biol.,* **1972,** *26,* 3–328.

Aquilonius, S.-M. Physostigmine in the treatment of drug overdose. In, *Cholinergic Mechanisms and Psychopharmacology,* Vol. 24. (Jenden, D. J., ed.) Plenum Press, New York, **1977,** pp. 817–825.

Chadwick, L. E. Actions on insects and other invertebrates. In, *Cholinesterases and Anticholinesterase Agents.* (Koelle, G. B., ed.) *Handbuch der Experimentellen Pharmakologie,* Vol. 15. Springer-Verlag, Berlin, **1963,** pp. 741–798.

Colquhoun, D. The link between drug binding and response: theories and observations. In, *The Receptors: A Comprehensive Treatise,* Vol. I. (O'Brien, R. D., ed.) Plenum Press, New York, **1979,** pp. 93–142.

Drachman, D. H. Myasthenia gravis. *N. Engl. J. Med.,* **1978,** *298,* 136–142, 186–193.

Frear, D. E. H. *Pesticide Index,* 4th ed. College Science Publishers, State College, Pa., **1969.**

Froede, H. C., and Wilson, I. B. Acetylcholinesterase. In, *The Enzymes,* Vol. 5. (Boyer, P. D., ed.) Academic Press, Inc., New York, **1971,** pp. 87–114.

Fukuto, T. R. Metabolism of carbamate insecticides. *Drug Metab. Rev.,* **1972,** *1,* 117–151.

Gosselin, R. E.; Hodge, H. C.; Smith, R. P.; and Gleason, M. N. *Clinical Toxicology of Commercial Products,* 4th ed. The Williams & Wilkins Co., Baltimore, **1976.**

Grob, D. Anticholinesterase intoxication in man and its treatment. In, *Cholinesterases and Anticholinesterase Agents.* (Koelle, G. B., ed.) *Handbuch der Experimentellen Pharmakologie,* Vol. 15. Springer-Verlag, Berlin, **1963a,** pp. 989–1027.

———. Therapy of myasthenia gravis. *Ibid.,* **1963b,** pp. 1028–1050.

Havener, W. H. *Ocular Pharmacology,* 4th ed. C. V. Mosby Co., St. Louis, **1978,** pp. 318–335.

Hobbiger, F. Reactivation of phosphorylated acetylcholinesterase. In, *Cholinesterases and Anticholinesterase Agents.* (Koelle, G. B., ed.) *Handbuch der Experimentellen Pharmakologie,* Vol. 15. Springer-Verlag, Berlin, **1963,** pp. 921–988.

———. Pharmacology of anticholinesterase drugs. In, *Neuromuscular Junction.* (Zaimis, E., ed.) *Handbuch der Experimentellen Pharmakologie,* Vol. 42. Springer-Verlag, Berlin, **1976,** pp. 487–581.

Holmstedt, B. Pharmacology of organophosphorus cholinesterase inhibitors. *Pharmacol. Rev.,* **1959,** *11,* 567–688. (764 references.)

———. Structure-activity relationships of the organophosphorus anticholinesterase agents. In, *Cholinesterases and Anticholinesterase Agents.* (Koelle, G. B., ed.) *Handbuch der Experimentellen Pharmakologie,* Vol. 15. Springer-Verlag, Berlin, **1963,** pp. 428–485.

———. The ordeal bean of Old Calabar: the pageant of *Physostigma venenosum* in medicine. In, *Plants in the Development of Modern Medicine.* (Swain, T., ed.) Harvard University Press, Cambridge, **1972,** pp. 303–360.

Karczmar, A. G. Pharmacologic, toxicologic, and therapeutic properties of anticholinesterase agents. In, *Physiological Pharmacology*. Vol. 3, *The Nervous System Part C: Autonomic Nervous System Drugs*. (Root, W. S., and Hofmann, F. G., eds.) Academic Press, Inc., New York, **1967a**, pp. 163–322.

———. Multiple mechanisms of action of drugs at the neuromyal junction as studied in the light of the phenomenon of "reversal." *Laval Med.*, **1967b**, *38*, 465–480.

———. History of the research with anticholinesterase agents. In, *Anticholinesterase Agents*, Vol. 1. *International Encyclopedia of Pharmacology and Therapeutics*, Sect. 13. (Karczmar, A. G., ed.) Pergamon Press, Ltd., Oxford, **1970**, pp. 1–44.

Katz, I.   Beta-blockers and the eye: an overview. *Ann. Ophthalmol.*, **1978**, *10*, 847–850.

Laskowski, M. B., and Dettbarn, W. D.   The pharmacology of experimental myopathies. *Annu. Rev. Pharmacol. Toxicol.*, **1977**, *17*, 387–409.

Long, J. P.   Structure-activity relationships of the reversible anticholinesterase agents. In, *Cholinesterases and Anticholinesterase Agents*. (Koelle, G. B., ed.) *Handbuch der Experimentellen Pharmakologie*, Vol. 15. Springer-Verlag, Berlin, **1963**, pp. 374–427.

Mounter, L. A.   Metabolism of organophosphorus anticholinesterase agents. In, *Cholinesterases and Anticholinesterase Agents*. (Koelle, G. B., ed.) *Handbuch der Experimentellen Pharmakologie*, Vol. 15. Springer-Verlag, Berlin, **1963**, pp. 486–504.

Murphy, S. D.   Pesticides. In, *Casarett and Doull's Toxicology: The Basic Science of Poisons*, 2nd ed. (Doull, J.; Klaassen, C. D.; and Amdur, M. O.; eds.) Macmillan Publishing Co., Inc., New York, **1980**, pp. 357–408.

Osserman, K. E.; Foldes, F. F.; and Genkins, G.   Myasthenia gravis. In, *Neuromuscular Blocking and Stimulating Agents*, Vol. 11. *International Encyclopedia of Pharmacology and Therapeutics*, Sect. 14. (Cheymol, J., ed.) Pergamon Press, Ltd., Oxford, **1972**, pp. 561–618.

Rosenberry, T. L.   Acetylcholinesterase. *Adv. Enzymol.*, **1975**, *43*, 103–213.

Schrader, G.   *Die Entwicklung neuer Insektizide auf Grundlage von Organischen Fluor- und Phosphorverbindungen*. Monographie No. 62, Verlag Chemie, Weinheim, **1952**.

Schwartz, B.   The glaucomas. *New Engl. J. Med.*, **1978**, *290*, 182–186.

Usdin, E.   Reactions of cholinesterases with substrates inhibitors and reactivators. In, *Anticholinesterase Agents*, Vol. 1. *International Encyclopedia of Pharmacology and Therapeutics*, Sect. 13. (Karczmar, A. G., ed.) Pergamon Press, Ltd., Oxford, **1970**, pp. 47–354.

Watson, P. G. (ed.).   Glaucoma. *Br. J. Ophthalmol.*, **1972**, *56*, 145–318.

Wills, J. H.   Toxicity of anticholinesterases and treatment of poisoning. In, *Anticholinesterase Agents*, Vol. 1. *International Encyclopedia of Pharmacology and Therapeutics*, Sect. 13. (Karczmar, A. G., ed.) Pergamon Press, Ltd., Oxford, **1970**, pp. 355–471.

Wilson, I. B.   Molecular complementarity and antidotes for alkyl phosphate poisoning. *Fed. Proc.*, **1959**, *18*, 752–758.

CHAPTER

7 ATROPINE, SCOPOLAMINE, AND RELATED ANTIMUSCARINIC DRUGS

Norman Weiner

The drugs described in this chapter inhibit the actions of acetylcholine (ACh) on autonomic effectors innervated by postganglionic cholinergic nerves as well as on smooth muscles that lack cholinergic innervation; that is, they antagonize the muscarinic actions of ACh. They are therefore known as *antimuscarinic* or *muscarinic cholinergic blocking* agents. Because the main actions of all members of this class of drugs are qualitatively similar to those of the best-known member, atropine, the terms *atropinic* and *atropinelike* are also appropriately used.

In general, antimuscarinic agents have little effect on the actions of ACh at nicotinic receptor sites. Thus, at autonomic ganglia, where transmission normally involves an action of ACh on nicotinic receptors, atropine produces partial block only at relatively high doses. At the neuromuscular junction, where the receptors are principally or exclusively nicotinic, extremely high doses of atropine or related drugs are required to cause any degree of blockade. However, quaternary ammonium analogs of atropine and related drugs generally exhibit varying degrees of nicotinic blocking activity and, consequently, are more likely to interfere with ganglionic or neuromuscular transmission in doses of the same magnitude as those that produce muscarinic block. In the central nervous system (CNS), cholinergic transmission appears to be predominantly nicotinic in the spinal cord and both muscarinic and nicotinic at subcortical and cortical levels in the brain (Brimblecombe, 1974). Accordingly, many or most of the CNS effects of atropine-like drugs at ordinary doses are probably attributable to their central anticholinergic actions. At high or toxic doses, the central effects of atropine and related drugs consist, in general, of stimulation followed by depression; these are probably due to a combination of antimuscarinic and other actions. There is an increased release and turnover of ACh in the CNS associated with the administration of antimuscarinic drugs; this may result in the activation of nicotinic receptors in the brain and contribute to the central effects of this class of drugs (Weiner, 1974). Since quaternary compounds penetrate the blood-brain barrier poorly, antimuscarinic drugs of this type show little in the way of central effects.

Parasympathetic neuroeffector junctions in different organs are not equally sensitive to the antimuscarinic agents. However, the relative sensitivity of various parasympathetically innervated organs to blockade by atropinic agents varies little among the drugs. Small doses depress salivary and bronchial secretion and sweating. With larger doses, the pupil dilates, accommodation of the eye is inhibited, and vagal effects on the heart are blocked so that the heart rate is increased. Larger doses inhibit the parasympathetic control of the urinary bladder and gastrointestinal tract, thus inhibiting micturition and decreasing the tone and motility of the gut. Still larger doses are required to inhibit gastric secretion and motility. Since only the primary phase of gastric secretion is controlled by the vagus, the remaining hormonally controlled secretion remains unaffected. Thus, doses of any antimuscarinic drug that reduce the tone and motility of the stomach and the duodenum and depress gastric secretion also invariably affect salivary secretion, ocular accommodation, and micturition. The drugs produce the functional equivalent of resection or paralysis of postganglionic cholinergic nerves.

The actions and effects of the antimuscarinic agents usually differ only quantitatively from those of atropine, which is considered in detail as the prototype of the group. The properties of other antimuscarinic drugs are discussed in terms of their differences from those of atropine.

History. The naturally occurring antimuscarinic drugs are the alkaloids of the belladonna plants. The most important of these are *atropine* and *scopolamine*. Preparations of belladonna were known to the ancient Hindus and have been used by physicians for many centuries. During the time of the Roman Empire and in the Middle Ages the deadly nightshade plant was frequently used to produce obscure and often prolonged poisoning. This prompted Linné to name the shrub *Atropa belladonna,* after Atropos, the oldest of the Three Fates, who cuts the thread of life.

Accurate study of the actions of belladonna dates from the isolation of atropine in pure form by Mein in 1831. In 1867, Bezold and Bloebaum showed that atropine blocks the cardiac effects of vagal stimulation, and 5 years later Heidenhain found that it prevents salivary secretion due to stimulation of the chorda tympani. These fundamental observations were quickly followed by many others, and today there is an extensive and secure body of experimental and clinical information on the pharmacological actions of the belladonna alkaloids. Many semisynthetic congeners of the belladonna alkaloids, usually quaternary ammonium derivatives, and a large number of synthetic antimuscarinic compounds have been prepared, primarily with the still-unrealized objective of depressing gastric secretion without undesired antimuscarinic effects on other organs. These drugs have few advantages over the naturally occurring alkaloids and their derivatives.

ATROPINE, SCOPOLAMINE, AND RELATED BELLADONNA ALKALOIDS

Sources and Members. The belladonna drugs are widely distributed in nature, especially in the Solanaceae plants. *Atropa belladonna,* the deadly nightshade, yields mainly the alkaloid *atropine* (*dl-hyoscyamine*). The same alkaloid is found in *Datura stramonium,* known as Jamestown or Jimson weed,

stinkweed, thorn-apple, and devil's apple. The alkaloid *scopolamine* (*hyoscine*) is found chiefly in the shrub *Hyoscyamus niger* (henbane) and *Scopolia carniolica*. The official preparations of belladonna act chiefly by virtue of their content of atropine.

Chemistry. These alkaloids are organic esters formed by combination of an aromatic acid, *tropic acid,* and complex organic bases, either *tropine* (tropanol) or *scopine*. Scopine differs from tropine only in having an oxygen bridge between the carbon atoms designated as 6 and 7 in the structural formulas in Table 7-1. Homatropine is a semisynthetic compound produced by combining the base tropine with mandelic acid. *Methylatropine nitrate, methscopolamine bromide,* and *homatropine methylbromide* are the corresponding quaternary ammonium derivatives, modified by the addition of a second methyl group to the nitrogen.

Structure-Activity Relationship. The intact ester of tropine and tropic acid is essential for the antimuscarinic action of atropine, since neither the free acid nor the base exhibits significant antimuscarinic activity. The presence of a free OH group in the acid portion of the ester is also important. Substitution of other aromatic acids for tropic acid modifies but does not necessarily abolish the antimuscarinic activity. When given parenterally, quaternary ammonium derivatives of atropine and scopolamine are, in general, more potent than their parent compounds in both antimuscarinic and ganglionic blocking activity, and lack CNS activity because of poor penetration into the brain. Given orally, they are poorly and unreliably absorbed, as are other quaternary ammonium compounds.

There is an asymmetrical carbon atom in tropic and mandelic acids (boldface **C** in the formulas in Table 7-1). Scopolamine is *l*-hyoscine and is much more active than *d*-hyoscine. Atropine is racemized during extraction and consists of a mixture of equal parts of *d*- and *l*-hyoscyamine, but the antimuscarinic activity is almost wholly due to the naturally occurring *l* form. *l*-Hyoscyamine is thus twice as potent as atropine in its antimuscarinic activity. In central activity, *l*-hyoscyamine is 8 to 50 times as potent as the *d* isomer.

Table 7-1. STRUCTURAL FORMULAS OF ATROPINE, SCOPOLAMINE, AND HOMATROPINE

Atropine   Scopolamine   Homatropine

Mechanism of Action. The major action of the antimuscarinic agents is a *competitive* antagonism of the actions of ACh and other muscarinic agonists. The antagonism can therefore be overcome by increasing sufficiently the concentration of ACh at receptor sites of the effector organ. The receptors affected are those of peripheral structures that are either stimulated or inhibited by muscarine, that is, exocrine glands and smooth and cardiac muscle. Responses to postganglionic cholinergic nerve stimulation are also inhibited by antimuscarinic drugs, but less readily than are responses to injected choline esters. The difference may be due to release of ACh by cholinergic nerve terminals so close to receptors that very high concentrations of the neurotransmitter gain access to the receptors in the synaptic cleft. In addition, diffusion and other factors may limit the concentration of antagonist that can be attained at these receptor sites.

Interaction of Atropine and Related Drugs with Muscarinic Receptors. Much evidence supports the notion that atropine and related compounds compete with muscarinic agonists for identical binding sites on muscarinic receptors (Brimblecombe, 1974; Yamamura and Snyder, 1974; Hulme *et al.,* 1978). Based on an extensive study of the affinities of agonists and antagonists for muscarinic receptors in membranes prepared from rat cerebral cortex, Burgen and coworkers have proposed that there are two major populations of binding sites with different affinities for agonists and a third minor population with an extremely high affinity for muscarinic agonists (*see* Birdsall *et al.,* 1978a). In contrast, only one type of binding site for muscarinic antagonists could be demonstrated in these preparations (Hulme *et al.,* 1978). The low-affinity agonist binding site and the antagonist binding site closely resemble the muscarinic binding site that has been studied by ligand binding technics in peripheral smooth muscle (guinea pig ileum) (Yamamura and Snyder, 1974). Birdsall and associates (1978b) proposed that there may be only a single muscarinic binding site in cerebral cortex, which is identical to that in peripheral smooth muscle. In the periphery, this binding site is presumably coupled to effector systems that mediate the contractile response. As a consequence of the energy expended in this coupling reaction, the affinity constant for ligand binding to the receptor is thought to be less for the coupled than for the uncoupled receptor. In contrast, affinity constants for antagonists are proposed to be the same for all populations of receptors, since antagonists produce no alteration in the effector system. According to this hypothesis, only a fraction of the receptors in the cerebral cortex are coupled to effector systems, accounting for the heterogeneity of affinities for the binding of agonists (Birdsall *et al.,* 1978b, 1979).

Selectivity of Antagonism. Atropine is a highly selective antagonist of muscarinic agents at the corresponding receptors of smooth and cardiac muscle and exocrine gland cells. This antagonism is so selective that atropine blockade of the actions of a noncholinomimetic drug has been taken as evidence that the drug acts indirectly either through release of ACh or by some other cholinergic mechanism. For example, the stimulant action of 5-hydroxytryptamine (5-HT) on guinea pig ileum has been attributed to activation of intramural cholinergic neurons because it is blocked by atropine. However, atropine and other antimuscarinic agents are no exceptions to the general rule that selectivity of antagonism is rarely absolute and is usually lost when high doses are used. Conclusions based on selectivity of antagonism by atropine are therefore acceptable only when they are supported by more direct evidence. Under appropriate experimental conditions and usually in higher doses than are needed to antagonize ACh, atropine may block or reduce responses to histamine, 5-HT, and norepinephrine. Atropine is moderately active in relieving histamine-induced bronchoconstriction in man and experimental animals. It also antagonizes the action of 5-HT on rat uterus, the respiratory tract smooth muscle of guinea pig and cat, guinea pig atria, and the aneural smooth muscle of chick amnion, where 5-HT is presumed to act directly. Atropine in very large doses depresses contraction of the cat nictitating membrane induced by norepinephrine. In all cases, the antagonism of other types of agonists is less complete than that of ACh.

PHARMACOLOGICAL PROPERTIES

Atropine and scopolamine differ quantitatively in antimuscarinic actions. Scopolamine has a more potent action on the iris, ciliary body, and certain secretory (salivary, bronchial, and sweat) glands, but atropine is the more potent on heart, intestine, and bronchial muscle, and has a more prolonged action. Atropine does not depress the CNS in doses that are used clinically and, therefore, is given in preference to scopolamine for most purposes. Where some central depressant effect is no disadvantage or is desired, as in preanesthetic medication, scopolamine is frequently administered.

Central Nervous System. *Atropine* stimulates the medulla and higher cerebral centers. In doses used clinically (0.5 to 1.0 mg), this effect is usually confined to mild vagal excitation. The rate and occasionally the depth of breathing are increased, but this effect is probably the result of bronchiolar dilatation and the subsequent increase in physiological "dead space." With toxic doses of atropine, central excitation becomes more prominent, leading to restlessness, irritability, disorientation, hallucinations, or delirium (*see* the discussion of atropine poisoning). With still larger doses, stimulation is followed by depression, coma ensues, and medullary paralysis causes death. Even moderate doses of atropine may depress certain central motor mechanisms controlling muscle tone and movement, as seen in the salutary effect on the tremor and rigidity of parkinsonism (*see* Chapter 21 and Therapeutic Uses, below).

Scopolamine in therapeutic doses normally causes drowsiness, euphoria, amnesia, fatigue, and dreamless sleep with a reduction in rapid-eye-movement (REM) sleep. These effects are sometimes sought when scopolamine is used as an adjunct to anesthetic agents or for preanesthetic medication. However, the same doses of scopolamine occasionally cause excitement, restlessness, hallucinations, or delirium, especially in the presence of severe pain. These excitatory effects, which resemble the central effects of toxic doses of atropine, occur regularly after large doses of scopolamine.

Central Antimuscarinic Action. Doses of atropine required to inhibit peripheral responses to choline esters or anticholinesterase (anti-ChE) agents produce almost no detectable central effects; large doses are required. This may reflect difficulty of penetration of the drug into the CNS. Physostigmine is able to reverse the atropine-induced depression of the hypothalamus and reticular activating system in animals and the central effects of atropine poisoning in man. In animals, atropine antagonizes the action of ACh applied locally to the cerebral cortex and spinal cord. However, atropine also depresses the effects of noncholinergic stimuli, indicating that the drug has central actions other than blocking cholinergic synapses. (*See* Krnjević, 1969, 1974.)

EEG. Atropine promptly restores to normal the increased EEG activity due to isoflurophate (di*iso*propyl phosphorofluoridate, DFP). Given alone, it reduces the voltage and frequency of the *alpha* rhythm and consistently shifts the EEG rhythm to slow activity, a pattern typical of the EEG in drowsiness. Both atropine and scopolamine also depress the EEG arousal response to photostimulation (Ostfeld and Arguete, 1962). In experimental animals, atropine and particularly scopolamine antagonize EEG activation by hypothalamic or reticular formation stimulation and by several drugs, including sympathomimetic agents. In therapeutic doses, atropine reduced abnormal EEG waves in about one half of a group of patients with *grand mal* epilepsy (Grob *et al.,* 1947). It has also been reported to reduce spike-and-dome paroxysms in certain cases of *petit mal* epilepsy. Atropine or scopolamine disrupts several behavioral responses in experimental animals at the same time as the EEG is altered. Although in many cases physostigmine promptly and simultaneously restores both to normal, the correlation between EEG and behavioral changes has not been established. (*See* Longo, 1966.)

Antitremor Activity. The belladonna alkaloids and related antimuscarinic agents have long been used in parkinsonism. A central antimuscarinic mechanism is likely, since physostigmine reverses the beneficial effects of atropinic drugs and aggravates the symptoms in untreated patients (Duvoisin, 1967). The salutary effect of levodopa in parkinsonism has led to considerable insight into the relations between cholinergic and dopaminergic mechanisms in this disease (*see* Chapter 21).

Vestibular Function. Scopolamine is effective in preventing motion sickness. This action is probably either on the cortex or more peripherally on the maculae of the utricle and saccule.

Eye. The atropinic drugs block the responses of the sphincter muscle of the iris and the ciliary muscle of the lens to cholinergic stimulation (Table 7–4, page 134). Thus, they dilate the pupil (*mydriasis*) and paralyze accommodation (*cycloplegia*). The wide pupillary dilatation results in photophobia; the lens is fixed for far vision, near objects are blurred, and sometimes micropsia occurs. The normal pupillary reflex constriction to light or upon convergence of the eyes is abolished. These effects can occur after either local or systemic administration of the alkaloids. However, conventional systemic doses of atropine (0.6 mg) have little ocular effect, in contrast to equal doses of scopolamine, which cause definite mydriasis and loss of accommodation. Locally applied atropine or scopolamine produces ocular effects of considerable duration; accommodation and pupillary reflexes may not fully recover for 7 to 12 days. The atropinic mydriatics differ from the sympathomimetic agents in that the latter cause pupillary dilatation without loss of accommodation. Pilocarpine, choline esters, physostigmine, and DFP in sufficient concentrations can reverse the ocular effects of atropinic drugs at least partially and constrict the pupil.

Atropinic drugs when administered systemically have little effect on *intraocular pressure* except in patients with narrow-angle glaucoma, where the pressure may occasionally rise dangerously. This effect is because the iris, crowded back into the angle of the anterior chamber of the eye, interferes with drainage of aqueous humor. The drugs may precipitate a first attack in unrecognized cases of this rare condition. In patients with wide-angle glaucoma, a significant rise in pressure is unusual. Atropinic drugs can generally be used safely in this latter condition, particularly if the patient is also adequately treated with an appropriate miotic agent.

Respiratory Tract. The belladonna alkaloids inhibit secretions of the nose, mouth, pharynx, and bronchi, and thus dry the mucous membranes of the respiratory tract. This action is especially marked if there is excessive secretion, and is the basis for the use of atropine and scopolamine in preanesthetic medication. The smooth muscles of bronchi and bronchioles are relaxed, with a resulting slight widening of the airway, which decreases airway resistance but increases the volume of residual air. The increase in "dead space" due to bronchiolar dilatation may be the basis of the respiratory stimulation produced by atropine. Atropine is more potent than scopolamine as a bronchodilator. It is particularly effective against bronchoconstriction produced by parasympathomimetic drugs such as methacholine and anti-ChE agents, but it is also moderately active in histamine-induced experimental asthma in both animals and man. However, atropine is less effective than epinephrine or isoproterenol as a bronchial relaxant, even against bronchoconstriction from electrical stimulation of the vagus. The role of cholinergic factors in the causation of bronchial asthmatic attacks remains to be elucidated.

Atropine and scopolamine reduce the occurrence of laryngospasm during general anesthesia. This appears to be due to depression of respiratory tract secretions that can precipitate reflex laryngospasm, caused by contraction of the laryngeal skeletal muscle, which is not blocked by atropine.

Cardiovascular System. *Heart.* The main effect of atropine on the heart is to alter *rate*. With average clinical doses (0.4 to 0.6 mg), the rate often decreases, presumably due to central vagal stimulation, which occurs prior to the onset of peripheral muscarinic cholinergic blockade. A similar effect may be seen with low doses of atropine that do not produce peripheral antimuscarinic effects. The slowing is rarely marked, about 4 to 8 beats per minute, and is usually absent after rapid intravenous injection. There are no accompanying changes in blood pressure or cardiac output. Larger doses cause progressively increasing tachycardia by blocking vagal effects on the S-A nodal pacemaker. The resting heart rate is increased by about 35 to 40 beats per minute in young men given 2 mg intramuscularly; the maximal heart rate (*e.g.*, in response to exercise) is not altered by atropine. The influence of atropine is most noticeable in healthy young adults, in whom vagal tone is considerable. In infancy and old age, even large doses of atropine may fail to accelerate the heart. Atropine often causes cardiac arrhythmias, but without significant cardiovascular symptoms. Atrial arrhythmias and atrioventricular dissociation occur, the former most commonly in children given small doses that slow the heart, the latter usually in adults after small or large doses (Dauchot and Gravenstein, 1971; Hayes *et al.*, 1971).

With low doses of scopolamine (0.1 or 0.2 mg) the cardiac slowing is greater than with atropine. With higher doses, cardioacceleration occurs initially, but it is short lived and is followed within 30 minutes either by a return to the normal rate or by bradycardia. Thus, after a short initial period, doses of scopolamine that produce ocular effects do not accelerate cardiac rate. With atropine, ocular effects are accompanied by tachycardia.

Adequate doses of atropine can abolish many types of reflex vagal cardiac slowing or asystole, for example, from inhalation of irritant vapors, stimulation of the carotid sinus, pressure on the eyeballs, peritoneal stimulation, central stimulation of vagal nuclei, or the normal afferent impulses causing respiratory arrhythmia. It also prevents or abruptly abolishes bradycardia or asystole from injection of choline esters, anti-ChE agents, or other parasympathomimetic drugs, as well as cardiac arrest from electrical stimulation of the vagus.

The removal of vagal influence on the heart by atropine may also cause changes in *conduction*. A-V conduction time is decreased, even when heart rate is kept constant by atrial pacing, and the P-R interval is shortened. In certain cases of partial heart block, in which vagal activity is an etiological factor, atropine may lessen the degree of block. In some patients with complete heart block, the idioventricular rate may be accelerated by atropine; in others it is stabilized. Atropine may improve the clinical condition of patients with early myocardial infarction by relieving severe sinus or nodal bradycardia or A-V block (*see* Adgey *et al.*, 1968; and below). In contrast, toxic doses and, occasionally, a large therapeutic dose of atropine may cause A-V block and nodal rhythm.

Circulation. Atropine, in clincal doses, completely counteracts the peripheral vasodilatation and sharp fall in blood pressure caused by choline esters. In contrast, when given alone, its effect on blood vessels and blood pressure is neither striking nor constant. This is expected, because most vascular beds probably lack significant cholinergic innervation and the cholinergic sympathetic vasodilator fibers to vessels supplying skeletal muscle do not appear to be involved to any important extent in the normal regulation of tone.

Toxic amounts of atropine usually, and therapeutic doses occasionally, dilate cutaneous blood vessels, especially those in the blush area (*atropine flush*). The mechanism of this anomalous vascular response is unknown. It may be a compensatory reaction permitting the radiation of heat to offset the atropine-induced rise in temperature. On the other hand, it may represent a direct vasodilator action unrelated to cholinergic blockade. The scarlet appearance of the flushed skin, coupled with fever, has caused atropine intoxication to be mistakenly diagnosed as scarlet fever.

Gastrointestinal Tract. Interest in the actions of antimuscarinic drugs on the stomach and intestine has led to their use as antispasmodic agents for gastrointestinal disorders and in the treatment of peptic ulcer. Although atropine can completely abolish the effects of ACh (and other parasympathomimetic drugs) on the gastrointestinal tract, it inhibits only incompletely the effects of vagal impulses. This difference is particularly striking in the effects of atropine on motility of the gut. The cause is not known; it appears likely that it may be due to the involvement of gastrointestinal hormones or neurohumoral transmitters other than ACh and norepinephrine.

Secretion. Salivary secretion is particularly sensitive to inhibition by antimuscarinic agents, which can completely abolish the copious, watery, parasympathetically induced secretion. The mouth becomes dry, and swallowing and talking become difficult.

Gastric secretion is reduced in volume and total acid content. However, this reduction is notable only when relatively large doses are given to experimental animals. Gastric secretion in *man* is not greatly altered by conventional doses of the belladonna drugs; to be effective, doses must usually be given (1 mg or more) that invariably cause dry mouth, increase in heart rate, ocular disturbances, and other side effects. Secretion during both psychic and gastric phases is reduced

but not abolished. Volume is usually reduced, but the concentration of acid is not necessarily lowered. The intestinal phase of gastric secretion may be somewhat inhibited. Full doses of atropine diminish and may completely abolish the interdigestive (fasting) secretion of acid; this action is less prominent in patients with peptic ulcers. The duration of the effect of atropine on gastric secretion is brief when compared with that on salivary glands. Secretion induced by histamine, alcohol, or caffeine is reduced but not abolished by the doses of atropine tested in man.

The gastric cells that secrete mucin and enzymes are more directly under vagal influence than are the acid-secreting cells, and full doses of atropine may decrease the concentration of these organic constituents. Atropine completely blocks the copious secretion of gastric juice, rich in both acid and proteolytic enzymes, elicited by injection of choline esters (methacholine and carbachol) or pilocarpine. (*See* Code, 1951.)

Atropine reduces the loss of plasma proteins from the everted gastric mucosal pouch of vagally denervated dogs. The increased shedding of plasma proteins across the gastric mucosa produced by either histamine or ACh is also substantially inhibited by atropine, whereas that produced by ethanol is not affected (Davenport and Kauffman, 1975; Kauffman and Davenport, 1975). These results are of interest, since it has been reported that prolonged oral administration of antimuscarinic agents such as propantheline or atropine is efficacious in the management of Menétrier's disease, which is associated with giant hypertrophy of the gastric mucosa, peripheral edema, and excessive loss of protein from the stomach (Smith and Powell, 1978).

Atropine has little effect on the secretion of *pancreatic juice, bile,* or *succus entericus;* these processes are largely under hormonal rather than vagal control.

Motility. The belladonna alkaloids have marked effects on motility of the gastrointestinal tract, since the parasympathetic nerves almost exclusively supply the extrinsic nervous motor control of the gut; sympathetic nerve impulses play a relatively small part in the physiological regulation of tone and motility. The parasympathetic nerves enhance both tone and motility, and relax sphincters, thereby favoring the passage of chyme through the gut. However, the intestine has a complex system of intramural nerve plexuses that are mainly responsible for motility, and impulses from the CNS only modify the effects of the intrinsic reflexes. The terminal neurons of the intramural plexuses are cholinergic, and the effects of their activity can be blocked by atropine. However, atropine-resistant tone and movements of the gut are also observed.

Both in normal subjects and in patients with gastrointestinal disease, full therapeutic doses of atropine produce definite and prolonged inhibitory effects on the motor activity of the stomach, duodenum, jejunum, ileum, and colon, characterized by a decrease in tone and in amplitude and frequency of peristaltic contractions. It should be noted that the doses needed to produce inhibition are more than enough to depress salivary secretion and usually produce ocular and cardiac effects. Excessive motility and hypertonus (as produced by morphine, insulin hypoglycemia, parasympathomimetic drugs, and certain emotional stimuli) are readily inhibited by appropriate doses of atropine, and more normal motor activity is usually restored.

Atropine abolishes or prevents the excess motor activity of the gastrointestinal tract induced by parasympathomimetic drugs and anti-ChE agents. In moderate doses, the alkaloids do not block responses to other directly acting stimulants, such as histamine and vasopressin, that do not act on ACh receptors. However, responses to drugs acting through the intramural plexuses, such as nicotine, morphine, and 5-HT, are inhibited.

Other Smooth Muscle. *Urinary Tract.* Intravenous urographic studies in man indicate that atropine (1.2 mg, intravenously) dilates the pelves, calyces, ureters, and bladder, and increases the visibility of the kidneys. Atropine decreases the normal tone and amplitude of contractions of the *ureter* and *bladder*, and often eliminates drug-induced enhancement of ureteral tone.
Biliary Tract. Atropine exerts a mild antispasmodic action on the gallbladder and bile ducts in man. However, this is not sufficient to overcome or prevent the marked spasm and increase in biliary duct pressure induced by opioids. Both nitrites and theophylline are more effective than atropine in this respect. Atropine has no consistent effect on the choledochal sphincter mechanism in man. Emptying of the human gallbladder in response to a fat meal is delayed by prior administration of atropine. There is little basis for the use of atropine alone as a biliary antispasmodic.
Uterus. Atropine has negligible effects on the

human uterus. Given to women in labor to cause amnesia, scopolamine does not alter or interfere with uterine contractions or increase the duration of labor; although the drug crosses the placental barrier, the fetus is apparently not adversely affected, and the respiration of the newborn is not depressed.

Secretory Glands. Small doses of atropine or scopolamine inhibit the activity of *sweat glands,* despite the vasodilatation the drugs may cause in some skin areas. The skin becomes hot and dry; sweating may be depressed enough to raise the body temperature, but only notably so after toxic doses. Atropine more readily blocks sweating induced by injected muscarinic agents than it does thermoregulatory sweating. The anhidrotic action of atropine and stimulation of sweating by muscarinic agents appeared for many years to be a pharmacological anomaly, as the sweat glands are supplied only by nerves that are anatomically sympathetic. However, these fibers are, in fact, mainly cholinergic. The alkaloids also inhibit, although not strikingly, the *lacrimal glands.*

Body Temperature. The rise in body temperature due to the belladonna alkaloids is usually significant only after large doses. Nevertheless, in infants and small children moderate doses induce "atropine fever." In atropine poisoning in infants, the temperature may reach 43° C or higher. Suppression of sweating is doubtless a considerable factor in the production of the fever, especially when the environmental temperature is high, but other mechanisms may be important when large doses are taken. It has been suggested that atropine may exert a central effect on temperature regulation; however, animals that do not sweat, such as the dog, do not exhibit fever after atropine.

Absorption, Fate, and Excretion. The belladonna alkaloids are absorbed rapidly from the gastrointestinal tract. They also enter the circulation when applied locally to the mucosal surfaces of the body. Only limited absorption occurs from the intact skin. The total absorption of quaternary ammonium derivatives of the alkaloids after an oral dose is only about 10 to 25% (Levine, 1959; Jonkman *et al.*, 1977); nevertheless, some of these compounds, applied locally to the eye, can cause mydriasis and cycloplegia. Atropine disappears rapidly from the blood and is distributed throughout the entire body. Most is excreted in the urine within the first 12 hours, in part unchanged. Only about 1% of an oral dose of scopolamine is eliminated as such in the urine. Traces of atropine are found in various secretions, including milk.

Some species of animals, especially certain rodents and marsupials, tolerate large doses of belladonna alkaloids. This is commonly seen in some varieties of rabbit, which show no toxic effects when fed on a diet of belladonna leaves. The resistance of these rabbits is genetically determined and depends on the presence of an enzyme, *atropine esterase,* found in the blood and liver.

Poisoning by Belladonna Alkaloids. The deliberate or accidental ingestion of belladonna alkaloids or other classes of drugs with atropinic properties is a major cause of poisonings. Many H_1-histaminergic blocking agents, phenothiazines, and tricyclic antidepressants have antimuscarinic activity and, in sufficient dosage, may produce syndromes that include features of atropine intoxication. Infants and young children are especially susceptible to the toxic effects of atropinic drugs (Unna *et al.,* 1950; Rumack, 1973). Indeed, many cases of intoxication in children have resulted from conjunctival instillation of atropinic drugs, systemic absorption occurring either from the nasal mucosa after the drug has traversed the nasolacrimal duct or from the intestinal tract if it is swallowed. Delirium or toxic psychoses, without undue peripheral manifestations, have been reported in adults after instillation of atropine eyedrops. Poisoning also occurs from overdoses of the many "over-the-counter" sleeping medicines containing scopolamine, and from purposeful ingestion, for hallucinatory effects, of nonprescription remedies for asthma that contain belladonna. Serious intoxication may occur in children who ingest berries or seeds containing belladonna alkaloids. Reports of stramonium poisoning due to tea made from Jimson weed seeds date as far back as 1676 in the United States and are described in early editions of this textbook.

Shein and Smith (1978) have quantified the antimuscarinic activity of a series of tricyclic antidepressants. Agents such as imipramine, nortriptyline, protriptyline, and amitriptyline are approximately $1/20$ to $1/80$ as potent as atropine in inhibiting the effects of ACh on the guinea pig ileum. However, since these drugs are administered in therapeutic doses considerably higher than the effective dose of atropine, antimuscarinic effects are often observed clinically (*see* Chapter 19). Treatment of intoxication by tricyclic antidepressants may thus require the administration of physostigmine (*see* below; Rumack, 1973; Aquilonius, 1978).

Fatalities from intoxication with atropine and scopolamine are rare, but they sometimes occur in children, in whom 10 mg or less may be lethal. Idiosyncratic reactions are more common with scopolamine

than with atropine, and ordinary therapeutic doses sometimes cause alarming effects. Homatropine methylbromide is well tolerated in doses much larger than those used for therapy and is only about $1/50$ as toxic as atropine. Table 7-2 shows the doses of atropine giving undesirable responses or symptoms of overdosage.

Symptoms and Signs. These develop promptly after ingestion of the drug. The mouth becomes dry and burns; swallowing and talking are difficult or impossible, and there is marked thirst. The vision is blurred, and photophobia is prominent. The skin is hot, dry, and flushed. A rash may appear, especially over the face, neck, and upper part of the trunk; desquamation may follow. An atropine rash is more likely to occur in children. The body temperature rises, especially in infants. The pulse is weak and very rapid, but in infants and old people tachycardia may not be pronounced. Palpitation is prominent, and the blood pressure may be elevated. Urinary urgency and difficulty in micturition are sometimes noted. Abdominal distention may develop, especially in infants.

The patient is restless, excited, and confused, and exhibits weakness, giddiness, and muscular incoordination. Gait and speech are disturbed. Nausea and vomiting sometimes occur. The behavior and mental symptoms may suggest an acute organic psychosis. Memory is disturbed, orientation is faulty, hallucinations (especially visual) are common, the sensorium is clouded, and mania and delirium are not unusual (*see* Ketchum *et al.,* 1973). The diagnosis of an acute schizophrenic episode or alcoholic delirium has been mistakenly made, and some patients have been committed to psychiatric institutions for observation and diagnosis. The syndrome often lasts 48 hours or longer and may be punctuated by convulsions. Depression and circulatory collapse occur only in cases of severe intoxication; the blood pressure declines, respiration becomes inadequate, and death due to respiratory failure follows after a period of

Table 7-2. EFFECTS OF ATROPINE IN RELATION TO DOSAGE

DOSE	EFFECTS
0.5 mg	Slight cardiac slowing; some dryness of mouth; inhibition of sweating
1.0 mg	Definite dryness of mouth; thirst; acceleration of heart, sometimes preceded by slowing; mild dilatation of pupil
2.0 mg	Rapid heart rate; palpitation; marked dryness of mouth; dilated pupils; some blurring of near vision
5.0 mg	All the above symptoms marked; speech disturbed; difficulty in swallowing; restlessness and fatigue; headache; dry, hot skin; difficulty in micturition; reduced intestinal peristalsis
10.0 mg and more	Above symptoms more marked; pulse rapid and weak; iris practically obliterated; vision very blurred; skin flushed, hot, dry, and scarlet; ataxia, restlessness, and excitement; hallucinations and delirium; coma

paralysis and coma (*see* Shader and Greenblatt, 1972).

Diagnosis. Careful analysis of the symptoms readily indicates widespread paralysis of organs innervated by parasympathetic nerves. This should immediately arouse suspicion of belladonna poisoning. Particularly significant are the dry mucous membranes, widely dilated and unresponsive pupils, tachycardia, cutaneous flush, and fever. However, the mental symptoms may distract attention from the obvious peripheral autonomic signs. *Any patient with an acute onset of bizarre mental and neurological symptoms should be suspected of poisoning by drugs, including atropinic drugs.* A history of prior belladonna medication may help to confirm the diagnosis. If belladonna poisoning is still doubtful, subcutaneous injection of 1 mg of the anti-ChE agent physostigmine may be diagnostic. If the typical salivation, sweating, and intestinal hyperactivity do not occur, belladonna intoxication is almost certain.

Treatment. When the poison has been taken orally, gastric lavage and other measures to limit intestinal absorption should be initiated without delay. *Physostigmine,* long overlooked as a possible antidote to atropine poisoning, is the rational therapy. For example, the slow intravenous injection of 1 to 4 mg of physostigmine (0.5 to 1.0 mg in children) rapidly abolishes the delirium and coma caused by large doses of atropine. Since physostigmine is metabolized rapidly, the patient may again lapse into coma within 1 to 2 hours, and repeated doses may be needed (*see* Forrer and Miller, 1958; Ketchum *et al.,* 1973; Rumack, 1973). If marked excitement is present and more specific treatment is not available, diazepam is most suitable for sedation and for control of convulsions. Large doses should be avoided because the central depressant action may coincide with the depression occurring late in belladonna poisoning. Phenothiazines should not be used because their antimuscarinic action is likely to intensify toxicity. Artificial respiration may be necessary. Ice bags and alcohol sponges help to reduce fever, especially in children.

Preparations, Dosage, and Routes of Administration. *Belladonna Tincture,* U.S.P., is a widely used preparation that consists of an aqueous-alcoholic extract of belladonna leaves. The adult dose is 0.6 to 1.0 ml, which contains approximately 0.2 to 0.3 mg, respectively, of the alkaloids of the leaf (mainly atropine). *Belladonna Extract,* U.S.P., may be given in tablets; the dose is 15 mg, equivalent to approximately 0.2 mg of atropine. *Belladonna Leaf,* U.S.P., is used for the preparation of the tincture and extract. *Atropine,* U.S.P., is the main alkaloid of belladonna as the free base. The readily soluble salt, *Atropine Sulfate,* U.S.P., is official as a powder, in tablet form, as an injectable solution, and as an ophthalmic solution and ointment. The average adult dose of atropine sulfate is 0.5 mg. It is usually given orally, but may be injected subcutaneously or intravenously. *Scopolamine* (*l*-hyoscine) is marketed as the readily soluble salt, *Scopolamine Hydrobromide,* U.S.P. (*hyoscine hydrobromide*). The adult oral or parenteral dose is 0.6 mg.

SYNTHETIC AND SEMISYNTHETIC SUBSTITUTES FOR BELLADONNA ALKALOIDS

The lack of selectivity of the belladonna alkaloids for those parasympathetic functions that might profitably be blocked in various diseases, particularly of the gastrointestinal tract, has led to intensive efforts to discover antimuscarinic drugs with more selective effects. Success has been limited, and the available agents are not wholly satisfactory. Although there are minor variations, the sequence of block in various organ systems is very similar for all antimuscarinic drugs now used clinically.

The main differences in pharmacological properties are seen with those compounds having a quaternary ammonium structure. These drugs are poorly and unreliably absorbed after oral administration, and valid comparisons of their potencies with those of the belladonna alkaloids can be made only after parenteral administration (Jonkman *et al.,* 1977). Penetration of the conjunctiva is also poor, so that most quaternary ammonium compounds are of little value in ophthalmology. Central effects are generally lacking, because these agents do not readily pass the blood-brain barrier. The quaternary ammonium compounds usually have a somewhat more prolonged action; little is known of the fate and excretion of most of these agents. The ratio of ganglionic blocking to antimuscarinic activity is greater for compounds with the quaternary ammonium structure because of their greater potency at nicotinic receptors; some of the side effects seen after high doses are due to ganglionic blockade. Thus, impotence and postural hypotension can occur in patients who are given these drugs. Poisoning with quaternary ammonium compounds may also cause a curariform neuromuscular block, leading to respiratory paralysis. Thus, toxic doses of these agents produce the usual manifestations of antimuscarinic poisoning with additional effects of ganglionic and, rarely, neuromuscular block, but usually without significant CNS involvement.

There is a clinical impression that the quaternary ammonium compounds have a relatively greater effect on gastrointestinal activity and that the doses necessary to treat gastrointestinal disorders are, consequently, somewhat more readily tolerated; this has been attributed to the additional element of ganglionic block. These drugs, like atropine, do not appear to produce adequate control of gastric secretion or gastrointestinal motility at doses that are devoid of significant side effects due to muscarinic blockade at other sites (Ivey, 1975a). However, there is a more recent suggestion that propantheline, taken orally, significantly reduces secretion of gastric acid stimulated by food to the same extent at low doses (15 mg per day) as when larger amounts are given (45 mg per day); only the higher dose caused pronounced side effects (Feldman *et al.*, 1977).

The pharmacological properties of the drugs discussed below differ little from those of other agents in the same general category and range between those of atropine and those of oxyphenonium and methantheline, the quaternary ammonium compounds with the greatest ratio of ganglionic blocking to antimuscarinic activity. The names, chemical structures, dosage forms, and usual clinical doses of these and other drugs of the same class are given in Table 7–3.

Homatropine. This drug (Table 7–1) has about one tenth the potency of atropine. It is used solely as a topical *mydriatic* and *cycloplegic* in the form of 2 to 5% *Homatropine Hydrobromide Ophthalmic Solution,* U.S.P., or of the unofficial hydrochloride, for which purposes it is preferable to atropine in many cases because of its rapid onset and short duration of action (Table 7–4). Accommodation is usually normal within 24 hours, but a briefer cycloplegia can be obtained by a 1% solution, often used in combination with a sympathomimetic drug (*e.g.,* ephedrine). Homatropine does not usually cause complete cycloplegia in children. Some conjunctival vasodilatation occurs after instillation of the drug.

Quaternary Ammonium Derivatives of Belladonna Alkaloids

Methscopolamine Bromide. *Methscopolamine Bromide,* U.S.P. (PAMINE) lacks the central actions of scopolamine. It is less potent than atropine and is poorly absorbed; however, its action is more prolonged, the usual oral dose (2.5 mg) acting for 8 hours. Its limited use has been chiefly in gastrointestinal diseases. The drug is available in 2.5-mg tablets.

Homatropine Methylbromide. Used mainly to treat gastrointestinal disorders and sometimes for preanesthetic medication, *Homatropine Methylbromide,* U.S.P., is less potent than atropine in antimuscarinic activity (oral dose, 10 mg), but it is four times more potent as a ganglionic blocking agent. It is available in 10-mg tablets (RU-SPAS, SED-TENS SE).

Representative Synthetic Quaternary Ammonium Compounds

Methantheline. *Methantheline Bromide,* U.S.P. (BANTHINE), is a synthetic quaternary ammonium compound (Table 7–3) that differs from atropine in having a particularly high ratio of ganglionic blocking to antimuscarinic activity. High doses may cause impotence, an effect rarely produced by purely antimuscarinic drugs and indicative of ganglionic block. Toxic doses may paralyze respiration by neuromuscular block. CNS manifestations of restlessness, euphoria, fatigue, or, very rarely, acute psychotic episodes may appear in occasional patients. Gastrointestinal effects of methantheline appear to be relatively greater than those of atropine, and many clinicians have the impression that the doses of methantheline used in the treatment of gastrointestinal disorders cause fewer antimuscarinic side effects than does atropine. The action is somewhat more prolonged than that of atropine, the effects of a therapeutic dose lasting 6 hours. An additional toxic manifestation unrelated to the blocking actions is the occasional appearance of skin rashes, including exfoliative dermatitis.

Propantheline. Closely related chemically to methantheline, *Propantheline Bromide,* U.S.P. (PRO-BANTHINE) (Table 7–3), has similar properties but is two to five times more potent. It is one of the most widely used of the synthetic antimuscarinic drugs. Very high doses block the skeletal neuromuscular junction. The usual clinical dose (15 mg) acts for about 6 hours. Propantheline bromide, administered orally, slows gastric emptying in man (Hurwitz *et al.,* 1977). The significance of this pharmacological action of propantheline and other atropine-like compounds in the management of peptic ulcer has not been clarified.

Synthetic Tertiary-Amine Antimuscarinic Compounds

These tertiary amines are, in general, well absorbed after oral administration, and some (*e.g.,* cyclopentolate and tropicamide) are useful in ophthalmology. Their pharmacological properties are very similar to those of atropine.

Tertiary Amines with Antispasmodic Properties

Dicyclomine Hydrochloride, U.S.P. (BENTYL, others), and *thiphenamil hydrochloride* (TROCINATE) (Table 7–3) decrease spasm of the gastrointestinal tract, biliary tract, ureter, and uterus without producing characteristic atropinic effects on the salivary, sweat, or gastrointestinal glands, the eye, or the cardiovascular system, except in large doses. Their major action is purported to be a nonspecific direct relaxant action on smooth muscle rather than a competitive antagonism of ACh. Thiphenamil is chemically related to the local anesthetics and has local anesthetic activity. Clinical use of these drugs has been disappointing.

Table 7-3. REPRESENTATIVE SYNTHETIC ANTIMUSCARINIC DRUGS [1]

DRUG, DOSAGE FORM, AND USUAL SINGLE DOSE [2]	CHEMICAL STRUCTURE
Quaternary Ammonium Compounds Anisotropine methylbromide VALPIN Tablets: 50 mg 50 mg	
Clidinium Bromide, U.S.P. QUARZAN Capsules: 2.5 and 5 mg 2.5 to 5 mg	
Diphemanil Methylsulfate, U.S.P. PRANTAL [3] Tablets: 100 mg 100 to 200 mg	
Glycopyrrolate, U.S.P. ROBINUL [4] Tablets: 1 and 2 mg 1 to 2 mg	
Hexocyclium methylsulfate TRAL [3] Tablets: 25 mg 25 mg	
Isopropamide Iodide, U.S.P. DARBID Tablets: 5 mg 5 mg [5]	

Table 7–3. REPRESENTATIVE SYNTHETIC ANTIMUSCARINIC DRUGS [1] (Continued)

DRUG, DOSAGE FORM, AND USUAL SINGLE DOSE [2]	CHEMICAL STRUCTURE
Quaternary Ammonium Compounds (*Cont.*) Mepenzolate Bromide, U.S.P. CANTIL Tablets: 25 mg Liquid: 5 mg/ml 25 to 50 mg	
Methantheline Bromide, U.S.P. BANTHINE [4] Tablets: 50 mg 50 to 100 mg	
Oxyphenonium bromide ANTRENYL Tablets: 5 mg 5 to 10 mg	
Propantheline Bromide, U.S.P. PRO-BANTHINE [4] Tablets: 7.5 and 15 mg 15 mg	
Tridihexethyl Chloride, U.S.P. PATHILON [3,4] Tablets: 25 mg 25 to 50 mg	
Tertiary-Amine Compounds Methixene hydrochloride TREST Tablets: 1 mg 1 to 2 mg	

[1] Antimuscarinic agents employed primarily for their effects on the CNS are discussed in Chapter 21.

[2] Most of the drugs are given four times daily, before meals and at bedtime. Dosage should be adjusted for the individual patient until either the desired effect is achieved or intolerable side effects occur. Treatment of elderly persons may be initiated with lower-than-usual doses.

[3] Also available as a sustained-release tablet.

[4] Also available in a solution or as a powder for dissolution for injection.

Table 7–3. REPRESENTATIVE SYNTHETIC ANTIMUSCARINIC DRUGS [1] (Continued)

DRUG, DOSAGE FORM, AND USUAL SINGLE DOSE [2]	CHEMICAL STRUCTURE
Tertiary-Amine Compounds (Cont.) Oxyphencyclimine Hydrochloride, U.S.P. DARICON Tablets: 10 mg 5 to 10 mg [5]	
Piperidolate Hydrochloride, U.S.P. DACTIL Tablets: 50 mg 50 mg	
Tertiary-Amine Compounds with Antispasmodic Properties Dicyclomine Hydrochloride, U.S.P. [6] BENTYL, and others Capsules: 10 mg Tablets: 20 mg Syrup: 2 mg/ml 10 to 20 mg	
Thiphenamil hydrochloride [6] TROCINATE Tablets: 100 and 400 mg 400 mg	
Tertiary-Amine Compounds Used Primarily as Mydriatic Agents Cyclopentolate Hydrochloride, U.S.P. CYCLOGYL Ophthalmic solution: 0.5, 1.0, and 2.0%	
Tropicamide, U.S.P. MYDRIACYL Ophthalmic solution: 0.5 and 1%	

[5] Administration twice a day is recommended.
[6] It is claimed that these drugs also relax smooth muscle directly.

THERAPEUTIC USES OF ANTIMUSCARINIC DRUGS

The belladonna alkaloids have been employed in a wide variety of clinical conditions, predominantly to inhibit effects of parasympathetic nervous system activity. However, the lack of selectivity of the antimuscarinic agents makes it difficult to obtain desired therapeutic responses without concomitant side effects. The latter usually are not serious but are sufficiently disturbing to the patient to limit sharply the dosage tolerated and therefore the usefulness of these agents, particularly for chronic administration. In addition, the efficacy of atropine-like drugs for several gastrointestinal disorders, their major use, is marginal. Fortunately, an H_2-receptor blocker, cimetidine, is now available as an alternative for the treatment of ulcer disease.

Certain of the synthetic belladonna substitutes are used much more extensively than are the natural alkaloids in a number of clinical conditions. However, there are few situations in which this preference is supported by evidence.

Gastrointestinal Tract. Antimuscarinic agents have been widely employed in the management of peptic ulcer. Although these drugs can reduce the secretion of gastric acid and gastric motility, the doses required to produce these effects are usually associated with pronounced side effects, such as dryness of the mouth, loss of visual accommodation, photophobia, and difficulty in urination. As a consequence, patient compliance in the long-term management of symptoms of peptic ulcer with these drugs is poor. Although Feldman and coworkers (1977) reported that propantheline can inhibit the secretion of gastric acid (stimulated by food) in doses that produce minimal side effects, most investigators have concluded that antimuscarinic agents, even when administered in relatively high doses, are not unequivocally efficacious in the management of patients with peptic ulcer (Ivey, 1975a).

If an antimuscarinic drug is to be used, the official belladonna tincture is the most economical and is readily titrated to what can be considered the patient's optimal dose. A relatively high dose is less troublesome if taken at bedtime, so that peak side effects as well as inhibition of gastric secretion occur during sleep. The introduction of *cimetidine,* a histamine H_2-receptor blocking agent, has resulted in marked improvement in the short-term treatment of peptic ulcer (*see* Chapter 26). Most patients with this disease will also respond well to appropriate doses of antacids, which may be given alone or in conjunction with cimetidine if necessary. It is thus difficult to describe a useful role for antimuscarinic agents in the treatment of peptic ulcer.

The belladonna alkaloids and their synthetic substitutes have been employed and recommended in a wide variety of conditions known or supposed to involve increased tone ("*spasticity*") or motility of the gastrointestinal tract. These agents can reduce tone and motility when administered in maximal tolerated doses, and they might be expected to have a real effect if the condition in question is in fact due to excessive smooth muscle contraction, a point that is often in doubt. Although antimuscarinic agents are commonly used in the management of irritable colon syndrome, there is no convincing evidence that these drugs are effective in this condition. A difficulty in evaluation of the efficacy of any treatment for the management of irritable colon syndrome is the observation that placebo medication has been found to be effective in over 35% of patients with this condition (Ivey, 1975b).

The intestinal hypermotility and increased frequency of stools associated with administration of two antihypertensive agents, guanethidine and reserpine, are frequently well controlled by atropine-like drugs. Similarly, diarrhea sometimes associated with irritative conditions of the lower bowel, such as mild *dysenteries* and *diverticulitis,* may respond to such therapy. In these conditions, both the frequency of bowel movements and the associated abdominal cramps may be reduced or fully controlled. However, more severe conditions such as *salmonella dysenteries, ulcerative colitis,* and *regional enteritis* respond poorly.

The belladonna alkaloids and synthetic substitutes are very effective in reducing *excessive salivation,* such as that associated with heavy-metal poisoning or parkinsonism; indeed, the dosage must be adjusted carefully to avoid reducing secretion to the point where dry mouth is troublesome. Although these agents are rarely effective alone in relieving *biliary colic,* they are commonly administered with morphine or another opioid. Antimuscarinic agents can reduce the volume and tryptic activity of pancreatic secretion, perhaps largely secondary to retarded entry of acid gastric contents into the duodenum and thus delayed release of secretin. Several agents, particularly methantheline and propantheline, have been tried in the treatment of *acute pancreatitis;* however, evidence for their efficacy in this condition remains entirely unconvincing.

Uses in Ophthalmology. Effects limited to the eye are obtained by local administration of an antimuscarinic drug to produce mydriasis and cycloplegia. Cycloplegia is not attainable without mydriasis and requires higher concentrations or more prolonged application of a given agent. Mydriasis is often necessary for thorough examination of the retina and optic disc and in the therapy of *acute iritis, iridocyclitis,* and *keratitis.* The belladonna mydriatics may be alternated with miotics for breaking or preventing the development of adhesions between the iris and the lens. Complete cycloplegia may be necessary in the treatment of *iridocyclitis* and *choroiditis,* following cataract surgery, and for accurate *measurement of* *refractive errors.* In instances where complete cycloplegia is required, agents such as atropine or scopolamine, which are more effective, are preferred to drugs such as cyclopentolate and tropicamide. Details of the drugs commonly used and the duration of action of the usual solutions are given in Table 7–4. One or 2 drops of an aqueous solution, often containing a surface-active agent to facilitate penetration, is instilled into the conjunctival sac and repeated as necessary to produce the desired intensity and duration of effect. The values given vary with the frequency and duration of contact with the solution and with individual susceptibility. Although the effect of a single drop of a solution of atropine on healthy eyes is very prolonged, in acute inflammation two or three instillations a day may be required to maintain a full effect. Atropine occasionally causes local irritation of the eye, and in susceptible persons it may produce swelling of the eyelids and conjunctivitis. With continued use, the conjunctivitis may become chronic. Therapy with antihistaminic agents may control the atropine conjunctivitis, or therapy may be continued with another agent (*e.g.,* scopolamine).

Shorter-acting substitutes for atropine or scopolamine are used when prolonged mydriasis and cycloplegia are not required or may pose a hazard to the patient. The standard agents for this purpose are homatropine, cyclopentolate, and tropicamide. Of these homatropine has the longest action but may not provide adequate cycloplegia even with 5% solutions. Where mydriasis alone is desired, the weaker solutions of cyclopentolate or tropicamide may be used, if necessary in combination with a sympathomimetic drug such as phenylephrine. Psychotic reactions, behavioral disturbances, and convulsions have appeared after ophthalmic use of cyclopentolate.

It is of great importance to recognize patients who are predisposed to narrow-angle glaucoma. The ophthalmic use of any of the antimuscarinic drugs may increase intraocular pressure in eyes with a narrow angle between iris and cornea, precipitating an attack of *acute glaucoma* with the potential hazard of ensuing blindness, particularly if mydriasis is prolonged. Atropine and scopolamine are therefore particularly dangerous. Systemic use of the antimuscarinic agents can also precipitate glaucoma in such predisposed patients. In wide-angle glaucoma the drugs generally do not cause dangerous elevation of intraocular pressure, particularly if the patient is treated soon afterward with locally applied miotics. Although narrow-angle glaucoma is a very rare condition, the use of drugs with antimuscarinic properties is not; careful ophthalmological evaluation, including examination with tonometer and gonioscope, should be undertaken to detect the possible presence of a narrow-angle anterior chamber before starting therapy with these agents, particularly if therapy is to be intensive or prolonged. Mydriasis due to the shorter-acting agents may be counteracted by local application of pilocarpine (1 to 4%); mydriasis from atropine and scopolamine is usually only partly counteracted, even by physostigmine (0.25%) or isoflurophate (0.1%).

The photophobia associated with mydriasis may require that the patient wear dark glasses. Although absorption into the blood stream from the conjunctival sac is minimal, systemic toxicity can occur from an antimuscarinic agent that reaches more absorptive mucosal surfaces by way of the nasolacrimal duct. This danger should be minimized by pressure on the inner canthus of the eye for a few minutes after each instillation. This precaution is particularly important in small children, who are highly susceptible to the toxic effects of belladonna alkaloids.

Respiratory Tract. Atropine and other belladonna alkaloids and substitutes reduce secretion in both the upper and the lower respiratory tract, and they are common constituents of proprietary "cold" tablets. This effect in the nasopharynx may provide some symptomatic relief of *acute rhinitis* associated with *coryza* or *hay fever,* but such therapy does not affect the natural course of the condition. It is probable that the contribution of antihistamines employed in "cold" mixtures is also primarily due to their antimuscarinic properties, except in conditions with an allergic basis.

The belladonna alkaloids can induce bronchial dilatation and were formerly in common use as a

Table 7–4.   MYDRIATIC AND CYCLOPLEGIC PROPERTIES OF ANTIMUSCARINIC AGENTS

DRUG	STRENGTH OF SOLUTION * (*percent*)	MYDRIASIS Maximal (*minutes*)	MYDRIASIS Recovery † (*days*)	PARALYSIS OF ACCOMMODATION Maximal (*hours*)	PARALYSIS OF ACCOMMODATION Recovery ‡ (*days*)
Atropine sulfate	1.0	30–40	7–10	1–3	7–12
Scopolamine hydrobromide	0.5	20–30	3–7	½–1	5–7
Homatropine hydrobromide	1.0 §	40–60	1–3	½–1	1–3
Cyclopentolate hydrochloride	0.5–1.0	30–60	1	½–1	1
Tropicamide	0.5–1.0 ‖	20–40	¼	½	< ¼

* One instillation of 1 drop of solution.
† To within 1 mm of original pupillary diameter.
‡ To within 2 diopters of original accommodative power; ability to read fine print is possible by the third day after instillation of atropine or scopolamine and by 6 hours after homatropine.
§ Full mydriasis and loss of accommodation require instillation of a 5% solution.
‖ Adequate loss of accommodation lasting about 30 minutes requires instillation of a 1% solution.

remedy for bronchial asthma. They appear to have beneficial effects when there is obstruction of the airway associated with chronic bronchitis. *Ipratropium bromide,* a congener of methylatroprine that is currently available only for experimental use in the United States, is an effective bronchodilator when administered by inhalation in doses of 40 to 80 μg (Poppius and Salorinne, 1973). In this dose, ipratropium appears to be as effective as the β_2-adrenergic agonist albuterol (200 μg, by inhalation) in relieving airway obstruction in patients with chronic bronchitis. In contrast, albuterol is much more effective in cases of bronchial asthma (Petrie and Palmer, 1975). Ipratropium, administered by aerosol, produces a significant increase in forced expiratory volume (FEV_1) without significantly affecting the viscosity or volume of sputum. It appears to cause fewer systemic side effects than do β-adrenergic agonists used in the treatment of obstructive pulmonary disease and may become a useful agent for the management of selected patients with such afflictions (Symposium, 1975; May and Palmer, 1977).

When administered systemically, antimuscarinic agents may reduce the volume of bronchial secretion, which can result in decreased fluidity and subsequent inspissation of the residual secretion. This viscid material is difficult to remove from the respiratory tree, and its presence can dangerously obstruct airflow and predispose to infection. Because of the effect on bronchial secretion, repeated administration of any antimuscarinic drug to a patient with chronic lung disease is considered by some authorities to be potentially hazardous.

Cardiovascular System. Aside from inhibition of certain reflexes during anesthesia and surgery, the cardiovascular effects of the belladonna alkaloids have limited clinical application, and the synthetic substitutes are little used in this field. Atropine is a specific antidote for the cardiovascular collapse that may result from the injudicious administration of a choline ester.

Atropine may be of value in the *initial* treatment of carefully selected patients with *acute myocardial infarction* in whom excessive vagal tone causes sinus or nodal bradycardia accompanied by a falling blood pressure and a low cardiac output, or a high-grade A-V block resulting in ectopic ventricular tachyarrhythmia (*see* Thomas and Woodgate, 1966; Adgey *et al.,* 1968). Administered intravenously, small doses of atropine (0.2 to 0.4 mg) may restore a normal heart rate and increase the blood pressure to an adequate level within a few minutes. However, there are very substantial risks in this therapeutic maneuver. If the drug accelerates heart rate without improving coronary perfusion, myocardial ischemia will be even more pronounced. Uncontrollable tachyarrhythmias, including ventricular tachycardia and fibrillation, may result (*see* Richman, 1974). Repeated doses of atropine must therefore be avoided. Bradycardia, if persistent, should be controlled by the insertion of a pacemaker as soon as possible.

Atropine is occasionally useful in reducing the severe bradycardia and syncope associated with a *hyperactive carotid sinus reflex.* It has little effect on most ventricular rhythms. In some patients atropine may eliminate ventricular premature contractions associated with a very slow atrial rate. It may also reduce the degree of A-V block when increased vagal tone is a major factor in the conduction defect. Atropine is occasionally useful in the diagnosis of *anomalous A-V conduction* (Wolff-Parkinson-White syndrome) by restoring the QRS complex to normal duration.

Central Nervous System. For many years the belladonna alkaloids and subsequently the tertiary-amine synthetic substitutes were the only agents helpful in the treatment of *parkinsonism.* Levodopa is now the treatment of choice, but concurrent therapy with the synthetic antimuscarinic agents may be required (*see* Chapter 21). Synthetic agents such as benztropine are also useful in the treatment of parkinsonism-like symptoms induced by phenothiazines or butyrophenones (*see* Chapter 19).

The belladonna alkaloids were among the first drugs to be used in the prevention of *motion sickness.* Scopolamine is the most effective prophylactic agent for short (4- to 6-hour) exposures to severe motion, and probably for periods up to several days. Oral doses of 0.1 mg protect 75% of susceptible persons, and do not affect vision and rarely cause dryness of the mouth. Intramuscular injection of 0.2 mg controls symptoms of most seasick individuals; sedation is the major disadvantage. (*See* Brand and Whittingham, 1970.) The superiority of scopolamine is more apparent the more susceptible the subject and the more severe the stress. The drug is not recommended for nausea and vomiting due to most other causes. All agents used to combat motion sickness should be given *prophylactically;* they are much less effective after severe nausea or vomiting has developed. (For further discussion of motion sickness, *see* Chapter 26.)

The sedation, tranquilization, and amnesia produced by scopolamine are useful in a variety of circumstances, including *labor.* In this situation it is almost always combined with agents that produce analgesia or sedation. Given alone in the presence of pain or severe anxiety, scopolamine may induce outbursts of uncontrolled behavior.

Uses in Anesthesia. The belladonna alkaloids are often used prior to the administration of a general anesthetic agent, mainly to inhibit excessive salivation and secretions of the respiratory tract; their concomitant bronchodilator action is also of value. The increasing use of relatively nonirritating anesthetics lessens the importance of antimuscarinic agents for this purpose. Scopolamine may contribute to tranquilization and amnesia. Atropine is commonly given with neostigmine to counteract its parasympathomimetic effects when the latter agent is used to end curarization after surgery. Serious cardiac arrhythmias have occasionally occurred, perhaps due to the combination of initial central vagal stimulation by atropine and the cholinomimetic effect of neostigmine.

Genitourinary Tract. Atropine has often been given with an opioid in the treatment of *renal colic* in the hope that it will relax the ureteral smooth muscle; however, as in biliary colic, it probably does not make a major contribution to the relief of pain. The belladonna alkaloids and several synthetic substitutes can lower intravesicular pressure, increase capacity, and reduce the frequency of urinary bladder contractions by antagonizing the parasympathetic control of this organ. The block is less complete than in many other organs, but it has been taken as a basis for the use of such agents in *enuresis* in children, particularly when a progressive increase in bladder capacity is the objective, to reduce urinary frequency in spastic paraplegia, and to increase the capacity of the bladder in conditions in which irritation has led to hypertonicity. However, it has not been established that antimuscarinic drugs make a major contribution to the treatment of any of these conditions. Tricyclic antidepressants are used to manage enuresis; it is possible that at least a component of the efficacy of this approach is due to the atropine-like properties of this class of drugs.

Anticholinesterase and Mushroom Poisoning. The use of atropine in large doses for the treatment of poisoning by anti-ChE organophosphorus insecticides is discussed in detail in Chapter 6. Atropine may also be used to antagonize the parasympathomimetic effects of neostigmine or other anti-ChE agents administered in the treatment of myasthenia gravis. It does not interfere with the salutary effects at the skeletal neuromuscular junction, and is particularly useful early in therapy, before tolerance to muscarinic side effects has developed.

Atropine is a specific antidote for the so-called *rapid type* of *mushroom poisoning* due to the cholinomimetic alkaloid muscarine, found in *Amanita muscaria* and a few other fungi. Atropine is of no value in the *delayed type* of mushroom poisoning due to the toxins of *A. phalloides* and certain other species of the same genus. (*See* Chapter 5.)

Adgey, A. A. J.; Geddes, J. S.; Mulholland, H. C.; Keegan, D. A. J.; and Pantridge, J. F. Incidence, significance, and management of early bradyarrhythmia complicating acute myocardial infarction. *Lancet,* **1968,** *2,* 1097–1101.
Aquilonius, S.-M. Physostigmine in the treatment of drug overdose. In, *Cholinergic Mechanisms and Psychopharmacology,* Vol. 24. (Jenden, D. J., ed.) Plenum Press, New York, **1978,** pp. 817–825.
Birdsall, N. J. M.; Burgen, A. S. V.; and Hulme, E. C. The binding of agonists to brain muscarinic receptors. *Mol. Pharmacol.,* **1978a,** *14,* 723–736.
———. Correlation between the binding properties and pharmacological responses of muscarinic receptors. In, *Cholinergic Mechanisms and Psychopharmacology,* Vol. 24. (Jenden, D. J., ed.) Plenum Press, New York, **1978b,** pp. 25–33.
———. Multiple classes of muscarinic receptor binding sites in the brain. In, *Receptors,* Vol. 1. (Jacob, J., ed.) *Advances in Pharmacology and Therapeutics: Proceedings of the Seventh International Congress of Pharmacology.* Pergamon Press, Ltd., Oxford, **1979,** pp. 73–80.
Brand, J. J., and Whittingham, P. Intramuscular hyoscine in control of motion sickness. *Lancet,* **1970,** *2,* 232–234.
Dauchot, P., and Gravenstein, J. S. Effects of atropine on the electrocardiogram in different age groups. *Clin. Pharmacol. Ther.,* **1971,** *12,* 274–280.

Davenport, H. W., and Kauffman, G. L. Plasma shedding by the canine oxyntic and pyloric glandular mucosa induced by topical action of acetylcholine. *Gastroenterology,* **1975,** *69,* 190–197.
Duvoisin, R. C. Cholinergic-anticholinergic antagonism in parkinsonism. *Arch. Neurol.,* **1967,** *17,* 124–136.
Feldman, M.; Richardson, C. T.; Peterson, W. L.; Walsh, J. H.; and Fordtran, J. S. Effect of low-dose propantheline on food-stimulated gastric acid secretion. *N. Engl. J. Med.,* **1977,** *297,* 1427–1430.
Forrer, G. R., and Miller, J. J. Atropine coma: a somatic therapy in psychiatry. *Am. J. Psychiatry,* **1958,** *115,* 455–458.
Grob, D.; Harvey, A. M.; Langworthy, O. R.; and Lilienthal, J. L., Jr. The administration of di-isopropyl-fluorophosphate (DFP) to man. III. Effect on the central nervous system with special reference to the electrical activity of the brain. *Bull. Johns Hopkins Hosp.,* **1947,** *81,* 257–266.
Hayes, A. H., Jr.; Copelan, H. W.; and Ketchum, J. S. Effects of large intramuscular doses of atropine on cardiac rhythm. *Clin. Pharmacol. Ther.,* **1971,** *12,* 482–486.
Hulme, E. C.; Birdsall, N. J. M.; Burgen, A. S. V.; and Mehta, P. The binding of antagonists to brain muscarinic receptors. *Mol. Pharmacol.,* **1978,** *14,* 737–750.
Hurwitz, A.; Robinson, R. G.; and Herrin, W. F. Prolongation of gastric emptying by oral propantheline. *Clin. Pharmacol. Ther.,* **1977,** *22,* 206–210.
Ivey, K. J. Anticholinergics: do they work in peptic ulcer? *Gastroenterology,* **1975a,** *68,* 154–166.
———. Are anticholinergics of use in the irritable colon syndrome? *Ibid.,* **1975b,** *68,* 1300–1307.
Jonkman, J. H. G.; Van Bork, L. E.; Wijsbeek, J.; De Zeeuw, R. A.; and Orie, N. G. M. Variations in the bioavailability of thiazinamium methylsulfate. *Clin. Pharmacol. Ther.,* **1977,** *21,* 457–463.
Kauffman, G. L., and Davenport, H. W. Effect of atropine in reducing plasma protein shedding by the canine oxyntic glandular mucosa induced by topical irrigation with histamine or cobra venom. *Gastroenterology,* **1975,** *69,* 198–199.
Ketchum, J. S.; Sidell, F. R.; Crowell, E. B., Jr.; Aghajanian, G. K.; and Hayes, A. H., Jr. Atropine, scopolamine, and ditran: comparative pharmacology and antagonists in man. *Psychopharmacologia,* **1973,** *28,* 121–145.
Levine, R. M. The intestinal absorption of the quaternary derivatives of atropine and scopolamine. *Arch. Int. Pharmacodyn. Ther.,* **1959,** *121,* 146–149.
May, C. S., and Palmer, K. N. V. Effect of aerosol ipratropium bromide (Sch 1000) on sputum viscosity and volume in chronic bronchitis. *Br. J. Clin. Pharmacol.,* **1977,** *4,* 491–492.
Ostfeld, A. M., and Arguete, A. Central nervous system effects of hyoscine in man. *J. Pharmacol. Exp. Ther.,* **1962,** *137,* 133–139.
Petrie, G. R., and Palmer, K. N. V. Comparison of aerosol ipratropium bromide and salbutamol in chronic bronchitis and asthma. *Br. Med. J.,* **1975,** *1,* 430–432.
Poppius, H., and Salorinne, Y. Comparative trial of a new anticholinergic bronchodilator, Sch 1000, and salbutamol in chronic bronchitis. *Br. Med. J.,* **1973,** *4,* 134–136.
Richman, S. Adverse effect of atropine during myocardial infarction. Enhancement of ischemia following intravenously administered atropine. *J.A.M.A.,* **1974,** *228,* 1414–1416.
Rumack, B. H. Anticholinergic poisoning: treatment with physostigmine. *Pediatrics,* **1973,** *52,* 449–451.
Shein, K., and Smith, S. E. Structure-activity relationships for the anticholinoceptor action of tricyclic antidepressants. *Br. J. Pharmacol.,* **1978,** *62,* 567–571.
Smith, R. L., and Powell, D. W. Prolonged treatment of Menétrièr's disease with an oral anticholinergic drug. *Gastroenterology,* **1978,** *74,* 903–906.
Thomas, M., and Woodgate, D. Effect of atropine on

bradycardia and hypotension in acute myocardial infarction. *Br. Heart J.,* **1966,** *28,* 409–413.

Unna, K. R.; Glaser, K.; Lipton, E.; and Patterson, P. R. Dosage of drugs in infants and children. I. Atropine. *Pediatrics,* **1950,** *6,* 197–207.

Yamamura, H. I., and Snyder, S. H. Muscarinic cholinergic receptor binding in the longitudinal muscle of the guinea pig ileum with (^{3}H) quinuclidinyl benzilate. *Mol. Pharmacol.,* **1974,** *10,* 861–867.

Monographs and Reviews

Brimblecombe, R. W. *Drug Actions on Cholinergic Systems.* University Park Press, Baltimore, **1974.**

Code, C. F. The inhibition of gastric secretion: a review. *Pharmacol. Rev.,* **1951,** *3,* 59–106. (336 references.)

de Wied, D., and de Jong, W. Drug effects and hypothalamic–anterior pituitary function. *Annu. Rev. Pharmacol.,* **1974,** *14,* 389–412.

Goldstein, A.; Aronow, L.; and Kalman, S. M. *Principles of Drug Action: The Basis of Pharmacology,* 2nd ed. John Wiley & Sons, Inc., New York, **1974,** p. 111.

Krnjević, K. Central cholinergic pathways. *Fed. Proc.,* **1969,** *28,* 113–120. (64 references.)

———. Chemical nature of synaptic transmission in vertebrates. *Physiol. Rev.,* **1974,** *54,* 418–540.

Longo, V. G. Behavioral and electroencephalographic effects of atropine and related compounds. *Pharmacol. Rev.,* **1966,** *18,* 965–996. (184 references.)

Shader, R. I., and Greenblatt, D. J. Belladonna alkaloids and synthetic anticholinergics: uses and toxicity. In, *Psychiatric Complications of Medical Drugs.* (Shader, R. I., ed.) Raven Press, New York, **1972,** pp. 103–147.

Symposium. (Various authors.) The place of parasympatholytic drugs in the management of chronic obstructive airways disease. (Hoffbrand, B. I., ed.) *Postgrad. Med. J.,* **1975,** *51,* Suppl. 7, pp. 1–161.

Toman, J. E. P., and Davis, J. P. The effects of drugs upon the electrical activity of the brain. *Pharmacol. Rev.,* **1949,** *1,* 425–492. (349 references.)

Weiner, N. Neurotransmitter systems in the central nervous system. In, *Drugs and the Developing Brain.* (Vernadakis, A., and Weiner, N., eds.) Plenum Press, New York, **1974,** pp. 105–131.

CHAPTER

8 NOREPINEPHRINE, EPINEPHRINE, AND THE SYMPATHOMIMETIC AMINES

Norman Weiner

The sympathetic nervous system is vitally involved in the homeostatic regulation of a wide variety of central and peripheral functions, among which are heart rate, force of cardiac contraction, vasomotor tone, blood pressure, bronchial airway tone, carbohydrate and fatty acid metabolism, psychomotor activity, affect, and appetite. Stimulation of the sympathetic nervous system normally occurs in response to physical activity, psychological stress, generalized allergic reactions, and other situations in which the organism is provoked. Because of the diverse functions that are mediated or modified by the sympathetic nervous system, agents that mimic or alter its activity are useful in the treatment of several clinical disorders, including hypertension, shock, cardiac failure and arrhythmias, asthma, allergy, and anaphylaxis.

The host of physiological and metabolic responses that follows stimulation of sympathetic nerves in mammals is usually mediated by the neurotransmitter, norepinephrine. As part of the response to stress, the adrenal medulla is also stimulated, resulting in elevation of the concentrations of epinephrine and norepinephrine in the circulation. The actions of these two catecholamines are very similar at some sites but differ significantly at others. For example, both compounds stimulate the myocardium; however, epinephrine dilates blood vessels to skeletal muscle, whereas norepinephrine has a minimal constricting effect on them. Dopamine is a third, naturally occurring catecholamine. While it is found predominantly in the basal ganglia of the central nervous system (CNS), dopaminergic nerve endings and specific receptors for this catecholamine have been identified elsewhere in the CNS and in the periphery. The role of the catecholamines in the CNS is detailed in Chapter 12 and elsewhere. As might be expected, sympathomimetic amines—naturally occurring catecholamines and drugs that mimic their actions—comprise one of the more extensively studied groups of pharmacological agents.

Most of the actions of such compounds can be classified into six broad types: (1) a *peripheral excitatory action* on certain types of smooth muscle, such as those in blood vessels supplying skin and mucous membranes, and on gland cells, such as those in salivary and sweat glands; (2) a *peripheral inhibitory action* on certain other types of smooth muscle, such as those in the wall of the gut, in the bronchial tree, and in blood vessels supplying skeletal muscle; (3) a *cardiac excitatory action,* responsible for an increase in heart rate and force of contraction; (4) *metabolic actions,* such as an increase in rate of glycogenolysis in liver and muscle, and liberation of free fatty acids from adipose tissue; (5) *endocrine actions,* such as modulation of the secretion of insulin, renin, and pituitary hormones; and (6) *CNS actions,* such as respiratory stimulation and, with some of the drugs, an increase in wakefulness, psychomotor activity, and a reduction in appetite. All sympathomimetic drugs do not show each of the above types of action to the same degree. However, many of the differences in their effects are only quantitative, and description of the effects of each compound would be unnecessarily repetitive. Therefore, the pharmacological properties of these drugs as a class are described in detail for the prototypical agent, *epinephrine.*

History. The pressor effect of suprarenal extracts was first shown by Oliver and Schäfer in 1895. The active principle was named epinephrine by Abel in 1899 and synthesized independently by Stolz and Dakin (*see* Hartung, 1931). The development of our knowledge of epinephrine and norepinephrine as neurohumoral transmitters is outlined in Chapter 4. Barger and Dale (1910) studied the pharmacological activity of a large series of synthetic amines related to epinephrine and termed their action *sympathomimetic.* This important study determined the basic structural requirements for activity and indicated that the sympathomimetic amines had qualitatively similar effects but that there were considerable quantitative differences. When it was found that cocaine or chronic denervation of effector organs reduced their responses to ephedrine and tyramine but enhanced the effects of epinephrine (Tainter and Chang, 1927; Burn and Tainter, 1931), it became clear that the differences between sympathomimetic amines were not simply quantitative. It was then suggested that epinephrine acted directly on the effector cell while ephedrine and tyramine had an indirect effect by acting on the nerve endings. The discovery that reserpine depletes tissues of norepinephrine, first made by Bertler and coworkers (1956), was followed by evidence that tyramine does not act on tissues from animals that have been treated with reserpine (Carlsson *et al.*, 1957). Burn and Rand (1958), confirming these observations, concluded that some sympathomimetic amines act by releasing endogenous norepinephrine. Many subsequent investigations have been directed toward clarifying this mechanism (*see* below).

Sites and Mechanism of Action.   α- *and β-Adrenergic Receptors or Adrenoceptors.*   In 1948, Ahlquist conducted a systematic examination of the effects of epinephrine, norepinephrine, and isoproterenol on a variety of target tissues. He observed in particular that the rank order of potency of these compounds depended on the target organ examined. Analysis of the data led him to propose that differences in the actions of these catecholamines could be explained by the presence of two distinct, differentially sensitive receptors for the catecholamines, and these were denoted as α and β. More recently, the development of even more selective agonists and antagonists that act at adrenergic receptors has allowed their subclassification. Lands and coworkers (1967a, 1967b) categorized β receptors as either β_1 or β_2; β_1-adrenergic receptors predominate in cardiac tissues, while β_2 receptors are present primarily in smooth muscle and gland cells. However, different tissues may possess both β_1 and β_2 receptors in varying proportions (*see* Minneman *et al.*, 1979). α Receptors also appear to be heterogeneous. Those designated α_1 predominate at postsynaptic effector sites of smooth muscle and gland cells; α_2 receptors, which are proposed to exist on nerve terminals, are believed to mediate the presynaptic feedback inhibition of neural release of norepinephrine and, perhaps, ace-

tylcholine. Activation of such α_2 receptors on cholinergic nerve terminals may contribute to the inhibition of intestinal activity caused by α-adrenergic agonists. α_2 Receptors may also be present on postsynaptic cells in several tissues, including the cerebral cortex, platelets, uterus, and parotid gland. Many of the adrenergic receptors in the CNS and those that mediate certain metabolic responses to catecholamines have not been definitively classified at the present time (*see* Furchgott, 1972; Cubeddu *et al.*, 1974b; Starke, 1977).

The relative sensitivities of these adrenergic receptors to epinephrine, norepinephrine, and isoproterenol, the three major catecholamines, are as follows: (1) at α_1 receptors, epinephrine is equal to or more potent than norepinephrine, which in turn is much more potent than isoproterenol; (2) at α_2 receptors, epinephrine is either more or less potent than norepinephrine, depending on the tissue, and isoproterenol is ineffective; (3) at β_1 receptors, isoproterenol is more potent than epinephrine, which is equipotent with norepinephrine; (4) at β_2 receptors, isoproterenol is equal to or more potent than epinephrine, which is much more potent than norepinephrine. Drugs that activate or block these receptors more selectively are detailed in this and the next chapter. Particularly notable has been the development of β_1- and β_2-adrenergic agonists and of β_1 antagonists. The distributions of these receptors and the responses that occur when they are activated are detailed in Table 4–1 (page 60).

In general, the effect of activation of α_1 receptors in smooth muscle is excitatory while that of β_2 receptors at such sites is inhibitory, although this is not an absolute rule. In other tissues, β-adrenergic receptors can mediate stimulatory effects (*see* Table 4–1). Thus, activation of β receptors results in stimulation of various secretions (*e.g.*, that of insulin), and the stimulatory effects of catecholamines on the heart are mediated by β_1 receptors.

Catecholamines inhibit propulsive contractions and reduce the tone of most intestinal smooth muscle; these effects appear to be mediated by both α- and β-adrenergic receptors. Activation of β receptors located on smooth muscle cells results in their relaxation. α Receptors appear to inhibit gastrointestinal motility by a presynaptic action. Thus, activation of α receptors on cholinergic nerve terminals within the intestinal wall is associated with inhibition of the release of acetylcholine. For this reason the presence of both an α- and a β-blocking agent is required to prevent completely the inhibitory effect of epinephrine on the intestine (Ahlquist and Levy, 1959).

An important factor in the response of an organ to sympathomimetic amines is the proportion and density of α and β receptors in the tissue. Norepinephrine has little effect on bronchial air flow because the receptors in bronchial smooth muscle appear to be largely of the β_2 type. In contrast, isoproterenol and epinephrine are potent bronchodilators. Cutaneous blood vessels possess α receptors almost exclusively; thus, norepinephrine and epinephrine cause marked constriction of such vessels, while isoproterenol has little effect. The smooth muscle of blood vessels supplying skeletal muscles has both β_2 receptors, the activation of which by low concentrations of epinephrine causes vasodilatation, and α receptors that allow epinephrine to constrict these vessels. In this tissue the threshold concentration of epinephrine for activation of β_2 receptors is lower, but when both types of receptors are activated the response to α receptors predominates.

Release of Stored Norepinephrine. Many sympathomimetic drugs, such as *amphetamine* and *ephedrine*, exert a large fraction of their effects by releasing norepinephrine from storage sites in the sympathetic nerves to the effector organ. The responses they elicit are therefore similar to those of norepinephrine but are slower in onset and generally longer lasting than those of a single equipressor dose of norepinephrine. They also exhibit tachyphylaxis; that is, repeated injections or continuous infusions of these indirectly acting drugs become less effective as the releasable stores of norepinephrine are depleted. Many sympathomimetic drugs owe only part of their effect to norepinephrine release and also act directly on adrenergic receptors. These agents are generally called mixed-acting sympathomimetic amines (*see* below).

Role of Sympathomimetic Amines in the Modulation of Neural Release of Norepineph-

rine. α-Adrenergic agonists are able to inhibit profoundly the release of norepinephrine by neurons (Haggendahl, 1970; Starke, 1971; Enero *et al.*, 1972; Cubeddu and Weiner, 1975a). Conversely, when the sympathetic nerve to a tissue is stimulated in the presence of an α-adrenergic antagonist, there is a marked increase in the amount of norepinephrine released per nerve impulse (Brown and Gillespie, 1957; DePotter *et al.*, 1971). The inhibitory effect of norepinephrine on its release from noradrenergic nerve terminals appears to be mediated by α receptors that are pharmacologically distinct from the classical α_1 postsynaptic receptor. As mentioned, these receptors have been designated α_2 and are presumed to be located on presynaptic nerve terminals (Starke, 1972). There is also evidence that α_2 receptors may occur postsynaptically. Certain drugs, such as nordefrin (α-methylnorepinephrine) and clonidine, are more potent agonists at α_2 than at α_1 receptors, and, at appropriate concentrations, they preferentially inhibit the release of norepinephrine. A major component of the antihypertensive effect of these agents may rely on this action, predominantly at central sites (*see* Chapter 32; Starke and Altmann, 1973; Berthelsen and Pettinger, 1977). Phenylephrine and methoxamine, in contrast, activate postsynaptic α_1 receptors at much lower concentrations than are required to inhibit the release of transmitter (Starke *et al.*, 1975; Langer, 1977; Starke, 1977). Agonists that stimulate β-adrenergic receptors appear to enhance the release of norepinephrine from neurons (Farnebo and Hamberger, 1974; Adler-Graschinsky and Langer, 1975; Dixon *et al.*, 1979). However, these effects are modest when compared with the powerful inhibitory effects of α agonists, and it is not clear that this β-adrenergic regulatory mechanism operates *in vivo* under normal circumstances (Dixon *et al.*, 1979).

Reflex Effects. The ultimate response of a target organ to sympathomimetic amines is determined not only by the direct effects of the agent but also by the reflex homeostatic adjustments of the organism. One of the most striking effects of many sympathomimetic amines is a rise in arterial blood pressure due to stimulation of α receptors in vascular beds. This elicits compensatory reflexes through the caroticoaortic baroreceptor system, resulting in a diminution of overall sympathetic tone that tends to lessen the effect of the sympathomimetic drugs and is accompanied by an increase in vagal tone that slows the heart. This compensatory mechanism is of special importance for drugs having little β-receptor activity and, therefore, little direct cardioaccelerator action. To cite a clinical application, phenylephrine, a drug with negligible β-receptor activity, can be used to treat paroxysmal atrial or nodal tachycardia because it raises blood pressure and thereby reflexly lessens sympathetic cardioaccelerator tone and increases parasympathetic cardiodecelerator tone, the combined effects of which may be enough to end the episode of tachycardia.

Mechanism of Direct Action on Sympathetic Effectors. Catecholamines act directly on sympathetic effector cells by binding to receptors located in cellular plasma membranes. Sympathomimetic drugs influence biochemical reactions as well as functional responses in virtually all tissues they affect, and the relation between these effects has been extensively studied. Production of cyclic adenosine 3',5'-monophosphate (cyclic AMP) by stimulation of adenylate cyclase has had particular attention as a possible step linking β-receptor activation to both functional and metabolic changes. This subject is discussed in Chapters 2 and 4.

The relationship of electrical phenomena, ion fluxes, and changes of tension in smooth muscle has been extensively studied without the establishment of a general pattern. The ionic movements differ between α- and β-receptor activation, and probably between smooth muscles. Visceral smooth muscle contractions are generally associated with slow waves of partial depolarization, in some muscles with superimposed action potentials that travel for some distance along adjacent cells. Contractions due to α-receptor stimulation are accompanied in some muscles by graded depolarization only; in others, there is a concomitant appearance or increased frequency of superimposed action potentials. The ionic mechanisms associated with these changes are also discussed in Chapter 4. In muscles inhibited by β-receptor stimulation the membrane becomes hyperpolarized and action potentials disappear or are less frequent. These changes are not consistently accompanied by potassium movement. The relationship of hyperpolarization to sodium movement is in dispute, and entry of calcium has been proposed as a component of the complex ionic mechanism. (*See* Somlyo and Somlyo, 1968; Daniel *et al.*, 1970; Marshall, 1973.) Although the effects of epinephrine appear to be related to changes in *transmembrane*

potentials, neither its excitatory nor inhibitory actions can depend entirely on the electrical changes. Isolated smooth muscle preparations, depolarized by being bathed in a solution with a high potassium content, can still be stimulated or inhibited by epinephrine; the muscle contraction due to epinephrine is reduced to about half by such depolarization. Both α- and β-adrenergic blocking agents have their usual effects on epinephrine-induced actions on depolarized muscles. These observations do not necessarily exclude a mechanism of action involving ionic movements; in depolarized preparations epinephrine increases the permeability of the cell membrane to ions, and does not cause contraction in the absence of calcium. Observations on the rabbit stomach, where hyperpolarization instead of depolarization accompanies contraction due to epinephrine, also indicate that broad generalizations should not be made about the nature and importance of electrical changes (*see* Furchgott, 1960; Schild, 1960).

Refractoriness to Catecholamines. Chronic exposure of catecholamine-sensitive cells and tissues to adrenergic agonists causes a diminution in their capacity to respond to such agents. This phenomenon is variously termed refractoriness, desensitization, down regulation, or tachyphylaxis. While descriptions of such adaptive changes are common in a variety of experimental and clinical situations, mechanisms are only partially understood. They have been studied extensively in cells that synthesize cyclic AMP in response to β-adrenergic agonists. Following the constant application of isoproterenol or similar agents to such cells, the capacity to synthesize cyclic AMP may be markedly reduced within a few hours. There is evidence for multiple points of regulation. The number of receptors detectable by radioactive ligand binding assays may be reduced (perhaps because of their internalization), triggered in some way by the agonist. Under other circumstances the interaction between the receptor and adenylate cyclase or the catalytic activity of the enzyme itself may be impaired (*see* Lefkowitz and Williams, 1978; Perkins *et al.*, 1978). Regulation of this type is not unique to adrenergic receptors; rather, it is the rule in most neural and endocrine systems.

Chemistry and Structure-Activity Relationship of Sympathomimetic Amines. β-Phenylethylamine (Table 8–1) can be viewed as the parent compound of the sympathomimetic amines, consisting of a benzene ring and an ethylamine side chain. The structure permits substitutions to be made on the aromatic ring, the α- and β-carbon atoms, and the terminal amino group, to yield a great variety of compounds with sympathomimetic activity. Norepinephrine, epinephrine, dopamine, and isoproterenol have OH groups substituted in the 3 and 4 positions of the benzene ring. Since *o*-dihydroxybenzene is also known as *catechol,* sympathomimetic amines with these OH substitutions in the aromatic ring are termed *catecholamines.*

The structure-activity relationship (SAR) of sympathomimetic drugs has been studied extensively since the classical investigations of Barger and Dale (1910). The pressor effects have been investigated

Table 8-1. CHEMICAL STRUCTURES AND MAIN CLINICAL USES OF IMPORTANT SYMPATHOMIMETIC DRUGS †

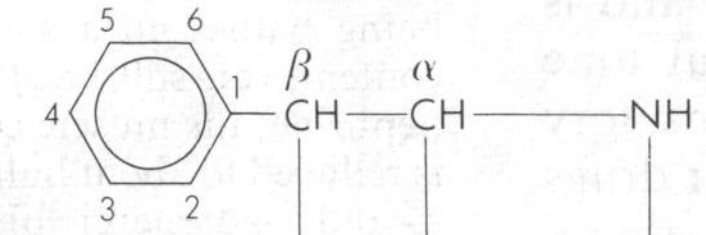

Prototype formula (ring positions 5, 6, 4, 1, 3, 2):
β CH — α CH — NH

Drug	Ring substituent	β	α	N	α Receptor (A N P V)	β Receptor (B C)	CNS,0
Phenylethylamine		H	H	H			
Epinephrine	3-OH,4-OH	OH	H	CH$_3$	A, P,V	B,C	
Norepinephrine	3-OH,4-OH	OH	H	H	P		
Epinine	3-OH,4-OH	H	H	CH$_3$			
Dopamine	3-OH,4-OH	H	H	H	P		
Dobutamine	3-OH,4-OH	H	H	1 *		C	
Nordefrin	3-OH,4-OH	OH	CH$_3$	H	V		
Ethylnorepinephrine	3-OH,4-OH	OH	CH$_2$CH$_3$	H		B	
Isoproterenol	3-OH,4-OH	OH	H	CH(CH$_3$)$_2$		B,C	
Protokylol	3-OH,4-OH	OH	H	2 *		B	
Isoetharine	3-OH,4-OH	OH	CH$_2$CH$_3$	CH(CH$_3$)$_2$		B	
Metaproterenol	3-OH,5-OH	OH	H	CH(CH$_3$)$_2$		B	
Terbutaline	3-OH,5-OH	OH	H	C(CH$_3$)$_3$		B	
Metaraminol	3-OH	OH	CH$_3$	H	P		
Phenylephrine	3-OH	OH	H	CH$_3$	N,P		
Tyramine	4-OH	H	H	H			
Hydroxyamphetamine	4-OH	H	CH$_3$	H	N,P	C	
Methoxyphenamine	2-OCH$_3$	H	CH$_3$	CH$_3$		B	
Methoxamine	2-OCH$_3$,5-OCH$_3$	OH	CH$_3$	H	P		
Albuterol	3-CH$_2$OH,4-OH	OH	H	C(CH$_3$)$_3$		B	
Amphetamine		H	CH$_3$	H			CNS,0
Methamphetamine		H	CH$_3$	CH$_3$	P		CNS,0
Benzphetamine		H	CH$_3$	3 *			0
Ephedrine		OH	CH$_3$	CH$_3$	N,P	B,C	
Phenylpropanolamine		OH	CH$_3$	H	N		
Mephentermine		H	4 *	CH$_3$	N,P		
Phentermine		H	4 *	H			0
Chlorphentermine	4-Cl	H	4 *	H			0
Fenfluramine	3-CF$_3$	H	CH$_3$	C$_2$H$_5$			0
Tuaminoheptane	CH$_3$(CH$_2$)$_3$	H	CH$_3$	H	N		
Propylhexedrine	5 *	H	CH$_3$	CH$_3$	N		
Diethylpropion	6 *						0
Phenmetrazine	7 *						0
Phendimetrazine	8 *						0

Substituent structures:

1. $-$CH$-$(CH$_2$)$_2-$[phenyl]$-$OH, with CH$_3$
2. $-$CH$-$CH$_2-$[benzodioxole ring], with CH$_3$
3. CH$_3$, $-$N, $-$CH$_2-$[phenyl]
4. CH$_3$, $-$C$-$, CH$_3$
5. [cyclohexane ring]
6. 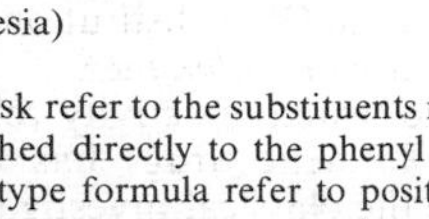 $-$C$-$CH$-$N$-$C$_2$H$_5$, O CH$_3$ C$_2$H$_5$
7. O$-$CH$_2$, $-$CH, CH$_2$, CH$-$NH, CH$_3$
8. O$-$CH$_2$, $-$CH, CH$_2$, CH$-$N, CH$_3$ CH$_3$

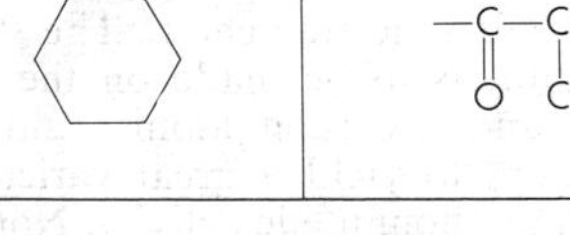

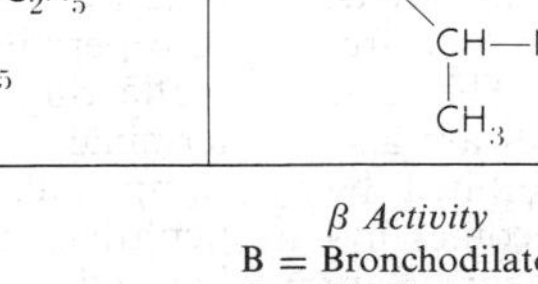

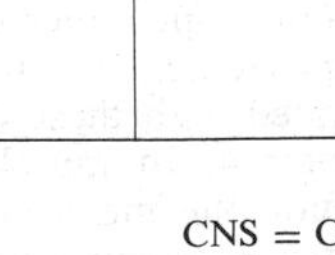

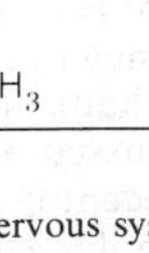

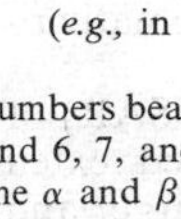

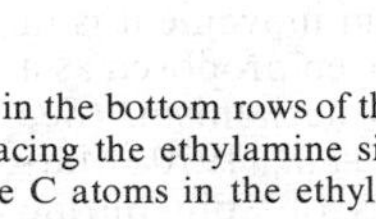

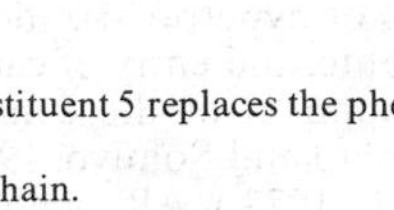

α Activity
A = Allergic reactions (includes β action)
N = Nasal decongestion
P = Pressor (may include β action)
V = Other local vasoconstriction (e.g., in local anesthesia)

β Activity
B = Bronchodilator
C = Cardiac

CNS = Central nervous system
0 = Anorectic

* Numbers bearing an asterisk refer to the substituents numbered in the bottom rows of the table; substituent 5 replaces the phenyl ring, and 6, 7, and 8 are attached directly to the phenyl ring, replacing the ethylamine side chain.

† The α and β in the prototype formula refer to positions of the C atoms in the ethylamine side chain.

more than other properties of the drugs. However, the pressor responses are the resultant of many effects on a complex system and involve many interacting factors that preclude their exact interpretation. Most directly acting sympathomimetic drugs influence both α and β receptors, but the ratio of the α and β activity varies tremendously between drugs in a continuous spectrum from an almost pure α activity (phenylephrine) to an almost pure β activity (isoproterenol). Since α activity on vascular beds raises the blood pressure and β activity on vascular beds lowers the blood pressure, it is virtually impossible to determine SAR from measurements of blood pressure alone unless one class of receptors has been blocked by a selective adrenergic blocking agent. There is a similarly wide spectrum in the ratio between direct action on adrenergic receptors and indirect effects through the release of norepinephrine. The SAR of directly acting agents is best studied in isolated systems where norepinephrine stores have been depleted by denervation or by drugs such as reserpine (Trendelenburg *et al.,* 1962; Trendelenburg, 1972). Among the sympathomimetic amines, only the β-hydroxylated catecholamines do not release norepinephrine to any significant degree. Despite the multiplicity of the sites of action of sympathomimetic amines, several generalizations can be made, as presented below.

Separation of Aromatic Ring and Amino Group. By far the greatest sympathomimetic activity occurs when two carbon atoms separate the ring from the amino group. This rule applies with few exceptions to all types of action.

Substitution on the Amino Group. The effects of amino substitution are most readily seen in the actions of catecholamines on α and β receptors. Increase in the size of the alkyl substituent increases β-receptor activity. Norepinephrine has, in general, rather feeble β_2 activity; this is greatly increased in epinephrine with the addition of a methyl group, and both β_1 and β_2 activity are maximal in isoproterenol with an isopropyl substituent. A notable exception is phenylephrine, which has a N-methyl substituent but is a pure α agonist. Selective β_2-receptor stimulants require a large amino substituent, but depend on other substitutions for their selectivity for β_2 rather than for β_1 receptors. α-Receptor activity is also modified by alkyl substitution on the amino group. In general, the less the substitution on the amino group the greater is the selectivity for α activity, although N-methylation increases the potency of primary amines. Thus, α activity is maximal in epinephrine, less in norepinephrine, and almost absent in isoproterenol.

Substitution on the Aromatic Nucleus. Maximal α and β activity depends on the presence of OH groups in the 3 and 4 positions. When one or both of these groups are absent, without other aromatic substitution, the overall potency is reduced. Phenylephrine is thus less potent than epinephrine on both α and β receptors, with β activity almost completely absent. Hydroxy groups in the 3 and 5 positions confer β_2-receptor selectivity on compounds with large amino substituents. Thus, metaproterenol, terbutaline, and other similar compounds relax the bronchial musculature in patients with asthma without

causing significant tachycardia. The response to noncatecholamines is in part determined by their capacity to release norepinephrine from sites of storage. These agents thus cause mostly effects that are mediated by α and β_1 receptors, since norepinephrine is a weak β_2 agonist.

Since substitution of polar groups on the phenylethylamine structure makes the resultant compounds less lipophilic, unsubstituted or alkyl-substituted compounds cross the blood-brain barrier more readily and have more central activity. Thus, ephedrine, amphetamine, and methamphetamine exhibit considerable CNS activity. In addition, the absence of polar hydroxyl groups results in a loss of direct peripheral sympathomimetic activity. A dose of 50 mg of ephedrine elicits central effects without inordinate cardiovascular effects.

Catecholamines have only a brief duration of action and are ineffective after oral administration because they are rapidly inactivated in the intestinal mucosa and in the liver before reaching the systemic circulation (*see* Chapter 4). Absence of one or both OH substituents, particularly the 3-OH group, increases the oral effectiveness and the duration of action of many of these compounds, especially if they also possess an α-methyl group.

Groups other than OH have been substituted on the aromatic ring. In general, potency on α receptors is reduced and β-receptor activity is minimal; the compounds may even block β receptors. For example, methoxamine, with methoxy substituents on positions 2 and 5, has highly selective α-stimulating activity and in large doses blocks β receptors. Albuterol, a selective β_2-receptor stimulant, has a CH_2OH substituent on position 3 and is an important exception to the general rule of low β activity.

Substitution on the α-Carbon Atom. This substitution blocks oxidation by monoamine oxidase (MAO), thus greatly prolonging the duration of action of noncatecholamines, the detoxication of which depends largely on breakdown by MAO since they are unaffected by catechol-O-methyltransferase (COMT). The duration of action of nordefrin (α-methylnorepinephrine) is not prolonged, whereas the duration of action of noncatecholamines with an α-methyl group, such as ephedrine or amphetamine, is measured in hours rather than in minutes. Since intraneuronal MAO is an important enzyme for degradation of phenylethylamines that lack an α-methyl substituent, compounds with such a group persist in the nerve terminal and are more likely to release norepinephrine from sites of storage. Agents such as metaraminol thus exhibit a greater degree of indirect sympathomimetic activity (*see* below).

Substitution on the β-Carbon Atom. Substitution of an OH group on the β carbon generally decreases central stimulant action, largely because of the lower lipid solubility of such compounds. However, such substitution greatly enhances agonistic activity, both at α and β receptors. Thus, ephedrine is less potent than methamphetamine as a central stimulant, but it is more powerful in dilating bronchioles and increasing blood pressure and heart rate. Similarly epinine is less potent than epinephrine on both α and β receptors.

Absence of the Benzene Ring. CNS stimulant

activity is reduced without a corresponding decrease in α and β activity when the benzene ring is replaced by an appropriate aliphatic chain (e.g., tuaminoheptane, methylhexaneamine), by a saturated ring (e.g., cyclopentamine, propylhexedrine), or by a different unsaturated ring (e.g., naphazoline; Table 8–2). Naphazoline, in fact, is a powerful α-receptor stimulant, but it differs from other sympathomimetic amines in that it depresses instead of stimulates the CNS. Two other imidazolines, clonidine (Chapter 32) and oxymetazoline, exhibit preferential effects on α_2 receptors.

The proportion of α to β activity varies with the compound; however, in general these amines have rather more marked α than β activity. Consequently, many of them are used primarily as nasal decongestants because of their vasoconstrictor properties.

Optical Isomerism. Substitution on either α or β carbon yields optical isomers. Levorotatory substitution on the β carbon confers the greater peripheral activity, so that the naturally occurring *l*-epinephrine and *l*-norepinephrine are ten or more times as potent as their unnatural *d* isomers. Dextrorotatory substitution on the α carbon generally provides a more potent compound than the *l* isomer in central stimulant activity. *d*-Amphetamine is more potent than *l*-amphetamine in central but not peripheral activity.

I. Catecholamines

EPINEPHRINE

PHARMACOLOGICAL PROPERTIES

In general, the responses to epinephrine resemble the effects of stimulation of adrenergic nerves. However, they are not identical due to differences between epinephrine and the adrenergic mediator, norepinephrine, in their properties as α- and β-receptor agonists. Most of the responses listed in Table 4–1 (page 60) are seen after injection of epinephrine in man, although the occurrence of sweating, piloerection, and mydriasis depends on the physiological state of the subject. Particularly prominent are the actions on the heart and the vascular and other smooth muscle. So enormous is the literature

on almost every aspect of the many changes in bodily function caused by epinephrine that this discussion is limited largely to the actions of the drug in man and refers to the more abundant results in animals when studies in man are limited.

Blood Pressure. Epinephrine is one of the most potent vasopressor drugs known. Given rapidly *intravenously* it evokes a characteristic effect on blood pressure, which rises rapidly to a peak that is proportional to the dose. The increase in systolic pressure is greater than in diastolic pressure, so that the pulse pressure increases. The mean pressure then falls below normal before returning to the control level. Repeated doses of epinephrine continue to have the same pressor effect, in sharp contrast to amines that owe a major part of their effect to release of norepinephrine.

The mechanism of the rise in blood pressure due to epinephrine is threefold: a direct myocardial stimulation that increases the strength of ventricular contraction (positive inotropic action), an increased heart rate (positive chronotropic action), and, most important, vasoconstriction in many vascular beds, especially in the precapillary resistance vessels of skin, mucosa, and kidney, along with marked constriction of the veins. The pulse rate, at first accelerated, may be slowed markedly at the height of the rise by compensatory vagal discharge. This bradycardia is absent if the effects of vagal discharge are blocked by atropine. Minute doses of epinephrine (0.1 μg/kg) may cause the blood pressure to fall. The depressor effect of small doses and the biphasic response to larger doses are due to greater sensitivity to epinephrine of vasodilator β_2 receptors than of constrictor α receptors.

The effects are somewhat different when

Table 8–2. CHEMICAL STRUCTURES OF IMIDAZOLINE DERIVATIVES

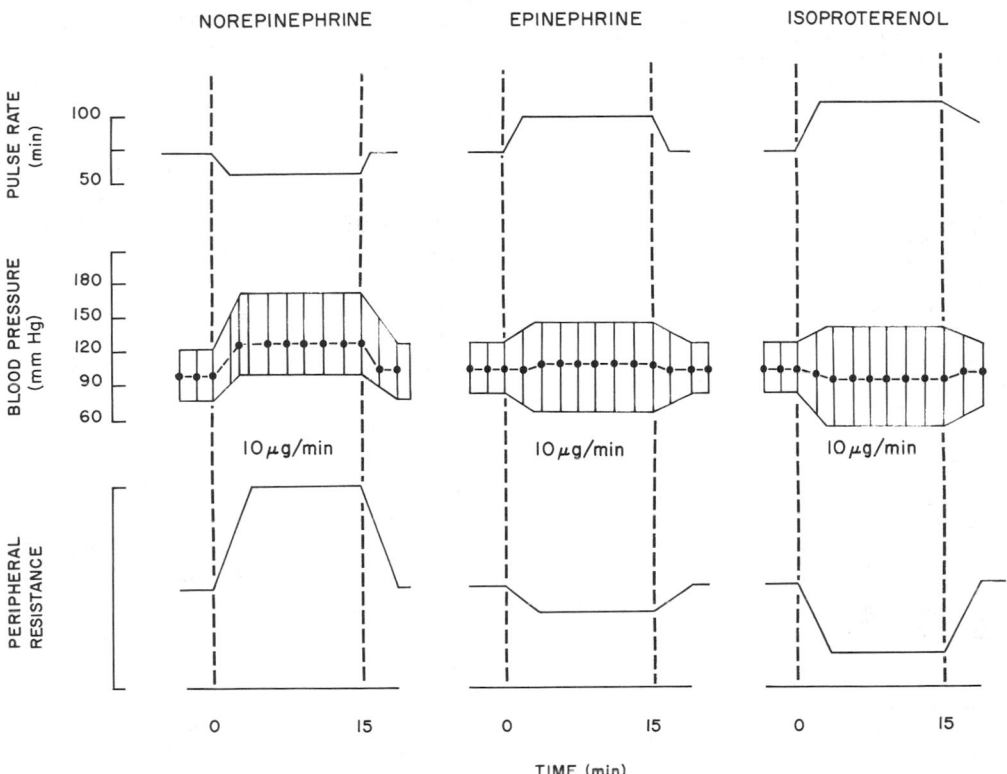

NOREPINEPHRINE   EPINEPHRINE   ISOPROTERENOL

Figure 8-1. *The effects of intravenous infusion of norepinephrine, epinephrine, and isoproterenol in man.* (After Allwood, Cobbold, and Ginsburg, 1963. Courtesy of the *British Medical Bulletin.*)

the drug is given by slow *intravenous infusion* or by *subcutaneous injection*. Absorption of epinephrine after subcutaneous injection is slow due to the drug's local vasoconstrictor action; the effects of doses as large as 0.5 to 1.5 mg can be duplicated by intravenous infusion at a rate of 10 to 30 μg per minute. There is a moderate increase in systolic pressure due to increased cardiac contractile force and a rise in cardiac output (Figure 8-1). Peripheral resistance decreases, due to the dominant action on β_2 receptors of vessels in skeletal muscle, where blood flow is enhanced, often doubled, after a subcutaneous dose of 0.5 to 1.0 mg; as a consequence, diastolic pressure usually falls. Since the mean blood pressure is not, as a rule, greatly elevated, compensatory reflexes do not antagonize appreciably the direct cardiac actions. Occasionally there is no change or even a slight rise in peripheral resistance and diastolic pressure, depending upon the ratio of α to β responses in the various vascular beds, which in turn are dependent on the dose administered. Heart rate, cardiac output,

stroke volume, and left ventricular work per beat are increased due to direct cardiac stimulation and to increased venous return to the heart, which is reflected by an increase in right atrial pressure. The details of the effects of intravenous infusion of epinephrine, norepinephrine, and isoproterenol in man are compared in Table 8-3 and Figure 8-1.

Vascular Effects. The chief vascular action of epinephrine is exerted on the smaller arterioles and precapillary sphincters, although veins and large arteries also respond to the drug. Various vascular beds react differently (*see* Table 4-1, page 60).

Injected epinephrine markedly reduces *cutaneous blood flow,* constricting precapillary vessels and subpapillary venules. However, skin pallor due to cutaneous vasoconstriction during "flight-or-fight" reactions is mainly due to increased sympathetic discharge rather than to released epinephrine. Cutaneous vasoconstriction accounts for a marked decrease in blood flow in the hands and feet. The "aftercongestion" of mucosae

Table 8–3. COMPARISON OF THE EFFECTS OF INTRAVENOUS INFUSION OF EPINEPHRINE AND NOREPINEPHRINE IN MAN *

	EPINEPH-RINE	NOREPINEPH-RINE
Cardiac		
Heart rate	+	− †
Stroke volume	+ +	+ +
Cardiac output	+ + +	0, −
Arrhythmias	+ + + +	+ + + +
Coronary blood flow	+ +	+ +
Blood Pressure		
Systolic arterial	+ + +	+ + +
Mean arterial	+	+ +
Diastolic arterial	+,0,−	+ +
Mean pulmonary	+ +	+ +
Peripheral Circulation		
Total peripheral resistance	−	+ +
Cerebral blood flow	+	0, −
Muscle blood flow	+ + +	0, −
Cutaneous blood flow	− −	− −
Renal blood flow	−	−
Splanchnic blood flow	+ + +	0, +
Metabolic Effects		
Oxygen consumption	+ +	0, +
Blood glucose	+ + +	0, +
Blood lactic acid	+ + +	0, +
Eosinopenic response	+	0
Central Nervous System		
Respiration	+	+
Subjective sensations	+	+

* 0.1 to 0.4 μg/kg/min

+ = increase;   0 = no change;   − = decrease;   † = after atropine, +

(After Goldenberg, Aranow, Smith, and Faber, 1950. Courtesy of *Archives of Internal Medicine*.)

following the vasoconstriction from locally applied epinephrine is probably due to changes in vascular reactivity as a result of tissue hypoxia rather than to β-receptor activity of the drug on mucosal vessels.

Blood flow to *skeletal muscles* is increased by therapeutic doses in man. Epinephrine infused intravenously in man at the rate of 30 μg per minute causes a very large but transient increase in blood flow, followed by a fall to about double the resting flow. This is due to a powerful β_2-receptor vasodilator action followed by a partially counterbalancing vasoconstrictor action on the α receptors that are also present in this vascular bed. If an α-adrenergic blocking agent is given, the pronounced vasodilatation in muscle due to epinephrine is sustained; after β-blocking agents, only vasoconstriction occurs. These vascular effects are independent of cardiac or central reflex effects and occur also in sympathectomized limbs.

The effect of epinephrine on *cerebral circulation* is related to systemic blood pressure. In usual therapeutic doses, the drug has no significant constrictor action on cerebral arterioles; moreover, autoregulatory mechanisms tend to limit the increase in cerebral blood flow due to increased blood pressure. In man, intravenous infusion of pressor doses (20 to 70 μg per minute) increases both cerebral blood flow and oxygen uptake without altering cerebrovascular resistance (King *et al.*, 1952).

Intravenous infusion of 0.1 μg/kg per minute in man markedly increases *hepatic blood flow* and decreases *splanchnic vascular resistance,* concomitantly with a large increase in hepatic glucose output and in the consumption of oxygen as measured in the splanchnic vascular bed (*see* Bearn *et al.*, 1951; Greenway and Stark, 1971).

The effects of epinephrine on *renal function* are variable, but the *renal vascular changes* in man are clear (Smythe *et al.*, 1952; Gombos *et al.*, 1962). Doses of epinephrine (3 to 23 μg per minute, intravenously) that have little effect on mean arterial pressure consistently increase renal vascular resistance and reduce renal blood flow by as much as 40%. All segments of the renal vascular bed contribute to the increased resistance. Since the glomerular filtration rate is only slightly and variably altered, the filtration fraction is consistently increased. Excretion of sodium, potassium, and chloride is decreased; urine volume may be increased, decreased, or unchanged. Maximal tubular reabsorptive and excretory capacities are unchanged. The secretion of renin is increased as a consequence of a direct action of epinephrine on β receptors in the juxtaglomerular apparatus.

Arterial and venous *pulmonary pressures* are raised. Although direct pulmonary vasoconstriction can be shown under suitable conditions, redistribution of blood from the systemic to the pulmonary circulation, due to constriction of the more powerful musculature in the systemic great veins, doubtless plays an important part in the increase in pulmonary pressure. Overdosage of epinephrine may cause death by pulmonary edema precipitated by elevated pulmonary capillary filtration pressure.

Coronary blood flow is enhanced by epinephrine or by cardiac sympathetic stimulation in man as well as in animals. The increased flow occurs even with doses that do not increase the aortic blood pressure and is the net result of three factors. The first is the increase in mechanical compression of the coronary vessels due to more forcible contraction of the surrounding myocardium, tending to reduce coronary flow; however, an opposite effect results from the increased duration of diastole. The increased flow during diastole is further enhanced if aortic blood pressure is elevated by epinephrine, and, as a consequence, there may be an increase in total coronary flow because of this effect. The second factor is the direct action of the drug on coronary vessels, which have both α and β receptors; in man this is predominantly constrictor via α receptors (Anderson *et al.,* 1972). The effect of direct action normally is of little importance compared to the overriding influence of the third factor, a metabolic dilator effect consequent upon the increased strength of contraction, and due to locally produced metabolites (such as adenosine) resulting from a relative myocardial hypoxia. (*See* Gregg and Fisher, 1963; Dempsey and Cooper, 1972.)

An exception to the effects of increased sympathetic activity on coronary blood flow is seen clinically in patients with Prinzmetal's variant angina. Such patients apparently are supersensitive to the vasoconstrictor α component of sympathetic nerve discharge and can experience angina at rest even though their vascular bed may be relatively free of atherosclerotic lesions. The decrease in coronary blood flow may be sufficiently great and prolonged to cause myocardial infarction (*see* Chapter 33).

Cardiac Effects. Epinephrine is a powerful cardiac stimulant. It acts directly on β_1 receptors of the myocardium and of the cells of the pacemaker and conducting tissues. This stimulation is independent of alterations in cardiac function secondary to increased venous return and other peripheral vascular effects. The heart rate increases and the rhythm is often altered. Cardiac systole is shorter and more powerful, cardiac output is enhanced, and the work of the heart and its oxygen consumption are markedly increased. Cardiac efficiency (work done relative to oxygen consumption) is lessened. The direct actions of epinephrine uncomplicated by

secondary effects can be most readily observed in isolated cardiac preparations from animals. Examples are responses of the isolated papillary muscle of the cat, where the actions include increases in contractile force, accelerated rate of rise of isometric tension, increased excitability, enhanced oxygen consumption, acceleration of the rate of spontaneous beating, and induction of automaticity in quiescent muscles.

In accelerating the heart within the physiological range, epinephrine shortens systole more than diastole so that the duration of diastole per minute is increased. Epinephrine speeds the heart by accelerating the slow depolarization of S-A cells that takes place during diastole, that is, during phase 4 of microelectrode recordings. Thus, the transmembrane potential of the pacemaker cells falls more rapidly to the threshold level at which sodium conductance suddenly increases and initiates the action potential. The amplitude of the action potential and the maximal rate of depolarization (phase 0) are also increased. A shift in the location of the pacemaker in the S-A node often occurs, indicating the activation of latent pacemaker cells. In Purkinje fibers, epinephrine accelerates diastolic depolarization and further facilitates activation of latent pacemaker cells. These changes do not occur in atrial and ventricular muscle fibers, where epinephrine has little effect on the stable, phase-4 resting potential after repolarization. Some effects of epinephrine on cardiac tissues are largely secondary to the increase in heart rate, and are small or inconsistent in preparations where the heart rate is kept constant. For example, the effect of epinephrine on repolarization of atrium, Purkinje fibers, or ventricle is small if the heart rate is unchanged. When the heart rate is increased, the duration of the action potential is consistently shortened, and the refractory period is correspondingly decreased. Similarly, acceleration of the heart rate plays an important part in increasing the conduction velocity in the bundle of His, Purkinje fibers, and ventricle. Thus, the drug shortens the refractory period of atrial and ventricular muscle and speeds A-V conduction. It also decreases the grade of A-V block occurring as a result of disease, drugs, or vagal stimulation.

Conduction through the Purkinje system depends on the level of membrane potential at the time of excitation. Excessive reduction of this potential results in conduction disturbances, ranging from slowed conduction to complete inexcitability. Epinephrine increases the membrane potential and improves conduction in canine Purkinje fibers that have been excessively depolarized. Since circumstances favoring such excessive depolarization are common in diseased hearts, this mechanism has been proposed to account for the salutary effects of epinephrine in various human arrhythmias—as, for example, in patients with complete heart block until more definitive measures can be instituted (Singer *et al.,* 1967). If large doses of epinephrine are given, premature ventricular systoles occur and may herald more serious ventricular arrhythmias. This is rarely seen with conventional doses in man, but ventricular extrasystoles, tachycardia, or even fibrillation may be precipitated by release of endogenous epinephrine when the heart has been sensitized to this action of epinephrine by certain anesthetics or in cases of myocardial infarction. The mechanism of induction of these cardiac arrhythmias is not clear. During anesthesia, some of the arrhythmias, such as ventricular tachycardia, may not be due to the emergence of ventricular pacemakers but to the effect of epinephrine in modifying impulse conduction through areas of cardiac tissue in which conduction has been depressed by the anesthetic agent, thus permitting irregular reentry of delayed impulses to unaffected areas of the conduction system and contractile tissue (*see* Dresel *et al.,* 1960).

The refractory period of the human A-V node is normally shortened by epinephrine, but may be prolonged indirectly by doses that slow the heart through reflex vagal discharge, an effect reversed by atropine. Supraventricular arrhythmias are apt to occur from the combination of epinephrine and cholinergic stimulation. Depression of sinus rate and A-V conduction by vagal discharge probably plays a part in epinephrine-induced ventricular arrhythmias, since various drugs that block the vagal effect confer some protection. The cardiac arrest occasionally caused by vagal discharge due to pressure on the eyeball or carotid sinus can be abolished by epinephrine, which induces or accelerates impulse formation in the ventricles. The action of epinephrine in enhancing cardiac automaticity and its action in causing arrhythmias are effectively antagonized by β-blocking agents such as propranolol. However, α-adrenergic blocking agents such as phenoxybenzamine protect against epinephrine-induced cardiac irregularities during anesthesia; protection is due in part to prevention of the rise in blood pressure (which sensitizes the myocardium to epinephrine-induced ectopic rhythms). This leaves in doubt whether the arrhythmic action is entirely on β receptors or partly on α receptors in addition. There appear to be α receptors in at least some regions of the heart, since the α-receptor stimulant phenylephrine and, during β-receptor block, epinephrine prolong the refractory period and strengthen contractions of isolated atria; these effects are antagonized by α-blocking agents (Benfey and Varma, 1967).

Cardiac arrhythmias have been recorded in man after accidental intravenous administration of conventional subcutaneous doses of epinephrine. Systolic and diastolic pressures rise alarmingly, sometimes as high as $400/300$ mm Hg for a short time; cerebrovascular hemorrhage has occurred from this error. Venous pressure rises, hyperventilation occurs (occasionally preceded by a brief period of apnea), pallor and palpitation are prominent, and heart rate is accelerated after a transient bradycardia. Ventricular premature systoles usually appear within the first minute after injection, frequently followed by multifocal ventricular tachycardia (prefibrillation rhythm). As the effects on the ventricle subside 1 or 2 minutes after their appearance, a marked atrial tachycardia ensues, occasionally associated with A-V block.

In the human *ECG,* epinephrine decreases the amplitude of the T wave in all leads in normal persons. In animals given relatively larger doses, additional effects are seen on the T wave and S-T segment. After being decreased in amplitude, the T wave may become biphasic and the S-T segment deviates either above or below the isoelectric line before abnormal ventricular deflections appear. Such S-T segment changes are similar to the downward deviation found in patients with *angina pectoris* during spontaneous or epinephrine-induced attacks of pain. These electrical changes have therefore been attributed to myocardial hypoxia.

Effects on Smooth Muscles. The effects of epinephrine on the smooth muscles of different organs and systems depend upon the type of adrenergic receptor in the muscle (Table 4–1, page 60). Gastrointestinal smooth muscle is, in general, relaxed by epinephrine. Intestinal tone and the frequency and amplitude of spontaneous contractions are reduced. The stomach is usually relaxed and the pyloric and ileocecal sphincters are contracted, but these effects depend upon the preexisting tone of the muscle. If tone is already high, epinephrine causes relaxation; if low, contraction. Epinephrine contracts the *splenic capsule* and reduces the size of the spleen in some species but not in man.

The responses of *uterine muscle* to epinephrine vary with species, phase of the sexual cycle, state of gestation, and the dose given. Epinephrine contracts strips of pregnant or nonpregnant human uterus *in vitro* in any effective concentration by interaction with α receptors. The effects of epinephrine on the human uterus *in situ,* however, differ. During the last month of pregnancy and at parturition, epinephrine inhibits uterine tone and contractions; this effect is of no clinical value because it is brief and accompanied by cardiovascular effects. However, other more selective β_2-receptor stimulants, such as albuterol or terbutaline, have been used successfully to delay premature labor. (*See* Bieniarz *et al.,* 1972; Liggins and Vaughan, 1973; Wallace *et al.,* 1978.)

Epinephrine relaxes the detrussor muscle of the *bladder* as a result of activation of β receptors and contracts the trigone and sphincter muscles due to its α-agonistic activity. This can result in hesitancy in urination and may contribute to retention of urine in the bladder.

Respiratory Effects. Epinephrine stimulates respiration, but this effect is brief and has no clinical value. Given intravenously to animals or man, epinephrine may cause a brief period of apnea before stimulation is seen. The apnea is probably due in part to a transient reflex inhibition of the respiratory center through the baroreceptor mechanism and in part to direct inhibition of the center.

Epinephrine can affect respiration more significantly by its peripheral actions, particularly by relaxing bronchial muscle. It has a powerful bronchodilator action, most evident when bronchial muscle is contracted due to disease, as in bronchial asthma, or in response to drugs or various autacoids. In such situations, epinephrine has a striking therapeutic effect as a physiological antagonist to the constrictor influences since it is not limited to specific competitive antagonism such as occurs with antihistaminic drugs against histamine-induced bronchoconstriction. Epinephrine also alters respiration by its α-receptor action in both normal and asthmatic persons; it increases vital capacity by relieving congestion of the bronchial mucosa and, when its action is limited as much as possible to the pulmonary vascular bed by administration as an aerosol, by constricting pulmonary vessels. Its effect in asthma may be due in part to an additional action shown by Assem and Schild (1969), namely, inhibition of antigen-induced release of histamine; this action is shared by selective β_2-receptor stimulants (*see* Chapter 26).

Epinephrine increases respiratory rate and tidal volume, and thereby reduces alveolar carbon dioxide content in normal subjects. However, inordinately large doses in man may cause death by interference with gaseous exchange due to development of pulmonary edema. Administration of a rapidly acting α-blocking agent or intermittent positive-pressure respiration (to increase intra-alveolar pressure) may be lifesaving.

Effects on Central Nervous System. Epinephrine in conventional therapeutic doses is not a powerful CNS stimulant. This is largely due to the inability of this rather polar compound to enter the CNS. While the drug may cause restlessness, apprehension, headache, and tremor in many persons, these effects may in part be secondary to the profound cardiorespiratory and peripheral metabolic effects of the catecholamine.

In animals, small intravenous doses cause arousal from natural sleep and large doses cause stupor, emesis, exaggerated knee jerks, spasticity, and even convulsions. In patients with Parkinson's disease, epinephrine increases rigidity and tremor, but the locus and mechanism of action are unclear.

Metabolic Effects. Epinephrine has a number of important influences on metabolic processes. Epinephrine elevates the concentrations of *glucose* and *lactate* in blood by mechanisms described in Chapter 4. *Insulin secretion* is inhibited via α receptors and is enhanced by activation of β receptors; the predominant effect seen with epinephrine is inhibition. Epinephrine also decreases the uptake of glucose by peripheral tissues, at least in part because of its effects on the secretion of insulin. Glycosuria rarely occurs. The effect of epinephrine to stimulate glycogenolysis in most tissues and in most species involves β receptors (*see* Chapter 4).

Epinephrine raises the concentration of *free fatty acids* in blood by activation of triglyceride lipase, which accelerates the breakdown of triglycerides to form free fatty acids and glycerol. Fat is deposited in muscle and liver, probably due to the increased amount of free fatty acid in the blood. This lipolytic action also appears to be mediated by cyclic AMP via β_1-adrenergic receptors. Infusions of epinephrine generally increase plasma cholesterol, phospholipid, and low-density lipoproteins. It has been speculated that the increased incidence of atherosclerosis and coronary artery disease associated with chronic stress may be due, at least in part, to the metabolic consequences of sympathetic nerve stimulation. The *calorigenic action* of epinephrine (increase in metabolism) is reflected in man by an increase of 20 to 30% in oxygen consumption after conventional doses. Studies in animals have shown that this effect, although composite, is mainly due to enhanced breakdown of triglycerides in brown adipose tissue, providing an increase in oxidizable substrate. (*See* Himms-Hagen, 1967, 1972; Porte and Robertson, 1973; Chapter 4.)

Epinephrine produces a transient rise in the concentration of *potassium* in plasma, mainly due to release of the ion from the liver. This hyperkalemia is followed by a more prolonged fall in plasma potassium. During these changes hepatic potassium rapidly enters the blood and is taken up by muscle; subsequently the pool of potassium in muscle falls during the period of hypokalemia and is transferred to the liver. The concentration of *inorganic phosphate* in plasma is decreased by epinephrine.

Miscellaneous Effects. Epinephrine reduces circulating *plasma volume* by loss of protein-free fluid to the extracellular space, thereby increasing *erythrocyte* and *plasma protein concentrations.* However, conventional doses of epinephrine in man do not significantly alter plasma volume or packed red-cell volume under normal conditions, although such doses are reported to have variable effects in shock, hemorrhage, hypotension, and anesthesia. Epinephrine increases *total leukocyte count* but causes *eosinopenia.* Epinephrine has long been known to accelerate blood coagulation in animals and man, an effect probably due to increased activity of factor V (Forwell and Ingram, 1957).

The effects of epinephrine on *secretory glands* are not marked; in most glands secretion is usually inhibited, partly due to reduced blood flow caused by vasoconstriction. Epinephrine stimulates *lacrimation* and a scanty mucous secretion from salivary glands. *Sweating* and *pilomotor activity* are not seen after systemic administration of epinephrine, but occur after intradermal injection of very dilute solutions of either epinephrine or norepinephrine. Such effects are inhibited by α-blocking agents.

Mydriasis is readily seen during physiological sympathetic stimulation but not when epinephrine is instilled into the conjunctival sac of normal eyes. However, epinephrine usually lowers *intraocular pressure* from normal levels and in wide-angle glaucoma; the mechanism is not clear, but both reduced production of aqueous humor due to vasoconstriction and enhanced outflow probably occur (*see* Grant, 1969). Paradoxically, β-adrenergic antagonists also reduce intraocular pressure and are useful in the treatment of glaucoma (*see* Chapter 9).

Although epinephrine does not directly excite *skeletal muscle,* it facilitates neuromuscular transmission. The mechanism of this effect is not clear. It also acts directly on the muscle cell, a β-receptor action that prolongs the active state of white, fast-contracting fibers and shortens the active state of red, slow-contracting fibers. Epinephrine temporarily abolishes fatigue due to prolonged rapid stimulation of the motor nerve (*see* Bowman and Nott, 1969). Given intra-arterially in patients with myasthenia gravis, epinephrine causes a real increase in motor power of the injected limb for 30 minutes or more. Given orally, ephedrine and amphetamine have this same effect; although these two drugs have been used clinically in this condition, the improvement in muscle strength does not approach that seen after neostigmine. Skeletal muscles of hypocalcemic patients are hypersensitive to epinephrine, which causes immediate local tetany upon intra-arterial injection; the mechanism of this action is not known.

Large or repeated doses of epinephrine or other sympathomimetic amines given to experimental animals lead to *damage to arterial walls and myocar-dium,* so severe as to cause the appearance of necrotic areas, indistinguishable in the heart from myocardial infarcts. The mechanism of this injury is not yet clear, but verapamil (which inhibits entry of calcium into the myocardial cell), propranolol, phentolamine, dipyridamole, indomethacin, or aspirin gives substantial protection against the damage. Similar lesions occur in many patients with pheochromocytoma or after prolonged infusions of norepinephrine (*see* Vliet *et al.,* 1966).

Absorption, Fate, and Excretion. *Absorption.* Epinephrine does not reach pharmacologically active concentrations in the body after oral administration because it is rapidly conjugated and oxidized in the gastrointestinal mucosa and liver. Absorption from subcutaneous tissues occurs slowly because of local vasoconstriction; heat and massage hasten the rate. Absorption is more rapid after intramuscular than after subcutaneous injection. When relatively concentrated solutions (1%) are nebulized and inhaled, the actions of the drug are largely restricted to the respiratory tract; although systemic reactions may occur from such inhalation, they are usually mild unless large amounts are used.

Fate and Excretion. Epinephrine is rapidly inactivated in the body despite its stability in the blood. The liver, which is rich in both of the enzymes responsible for destruction of circulating epinephrine, is an important, although not essential, tissue in the degradation process. While only small amounts appear in the urine of normal persons, the urine of patients with pheochromocytoma contains large amounts of epinephrine and norepinephrine.

The greater part of a dose of epinephrine injected into man is accounted for by excretion of metabolites in the urine. Most of the injected drug is first metabolized by COMT and MAO, as already described (*see* Figure 4–6, page 77). Congeners of epinephrine are metabolized by the same enzyme systems; amines lacking the 3-OH group are unaffected by COMT, and their disposal depends upon MAO or other enzymes, mostly in the liver. Destruction of these amines is generally slower than that of epinephrine, and inhibition of MAO by a variety of drugs may prolong their action in the body. (*See* Sharman, 1973.) Amines with an α-methyl substituent are resistant to deamination by MAO.

Preparations, Dosage, and Routes of Administration. Many preparations of epinephrine are available. Epinephrine is the official U.S.P. term; adrenaline, the B.P. term.

Epinephrine, U.S.P., is the *l* isomer of β-(3,4,-dihydroxyphenyl)-α-methylaminoethanol (*see* Table 8-1). It is only very slightly soluble in water but forms water-soluble salts with acids. It is unstable in alkaline solution and on exposure to air or light, turning pink from oxidation to adrenochrome and then brown from formation of polymers. Epinephrine may be given by injection, usually subcutaneously, inhaled as an aerosol, or applied locally to mucous membranes or abraded surfaces, as an aqueous solution, ointment, or suppository.

Epinephrine Injection, U.S.P., is a 1:1000 sterile solution of epinephrine hydrochloride in distilled water for parenteral injection, and is available in 1-ml ampuls and 30-ml vials. The usual adult dose given *subcutaneously* ranges from 0.1 to 0.5 ml (0.1 to 0.5 mg). The *intravenous* route is used cautiously if an immediate and reliable effect is mandatory. If the solution is given by vein, it must be adequately diluted and injected *very slowly.* The dose is seldom as much as 0.25 mg. *Intracardiac* injection is occasionally used for attempted resuscitation in emergencies. An unofficial aqueous 1:200 suspension of crystalline epinephrine (SUS-PHRINE) has a prolonged duration of action because of its low solubility. Injected subcutaneously the initial adult dose is 0.1 ml, and the maximum is 0.3 ml, repeated no sooner than after 4 hours. *Epinephrine suspensions must never be injected intravenously.*

Epinephrine Inhalation, U.S.P., is a nonsterile 1% aqueous solution of epinephrine hydrochloride for oral (not nasal) inhalation, either from a nebulizer or from an intermittent positive-pressure breathing apparatus. It is used to relieve bronchial constriction and is available in 7.5-ml vials. *Every precaution must be taken not to confuse this 1:100 solution with the 1:1000 solution designed for parenteral administration.* Injection of the 1:100 solution has caused death.

Epinephrine Nasal Solution, U.S.P., is a 1:1000 preparation of epinephrine hydrochloride identical with *epinephrine injection* except that it is not sterile. It is generally used in preparing more dilute solutions (1:50,000 to 1:2000) for sprays to constrict vessels of mucosa or abraded skin. *Epinephrine Bitartrate,* U.S.P., is available as an official *ophthalmic* solution in concentrations of 0.25, 0.5, 1.0, and 2% of epinephrine base, and as an official pressurized *aerosol* (MEDIHALER-EPI) delivering measured doses of 0.3 mg (0.16 mg of epinephrine base) for oral inhalation.

Toxicity, Side Effects, and Contraindications.

Epinephrine may cause disturbing reactions, such as *fear, anxiety, tenseness, restlessness, throbbing headache, tremor, weakness, dizziness, pallor, respiratory difficulty,* and *palpitation.* The effects rapidly subside with rest, quiet, recumbency, and reassurance, but the patient is often alarmed.

Hyperthyroid and hypertensive individuals are particularly susceptible to the untoward and pressor responses to epinephrine. In psychoneurotic individuals, existing symptoms are often markedly aggravated by the administration of epinephrine.

More serious accidents consist in *cerebral hemorrhage* and *cardiac arrhythmias.* The use of large doses or the accidental rapid *intravenous* injection of epinephrine may result in cerebral hemorrhage from the sharp rise in blood pressure. Subarachnoid hemorrhage and hemiplegia have occurred even after a subcutaneous dose of 0.5 ml of the 1:1000 U.S.P. injection. Rapidly acting vasodilators such as the nitrites or sodium nitroprusside can counteract the marked pressor effects of large doses of epinephrine; α-blocking agents may also be of use.

Ventricular arrhythmias may follow the administration of epinephrine. If ventricular fibrillation develops, it is usually fatal unless immediate remedial measures are employed; fibrillation is particularly likely to occur if the drug is used unwisely during anesthesia, especially with halogenated hydrocarbon anesthetics, or in individuals with organic heart disease. Patients with long-standing bronchial asthma and a significant degree of emphysema, who have reached the age in which degenerative heart disease is prevalent, must be given epinephrine only with considerable caution. In patients suffering from shock, the drug may accentuate the underlying disorder. Anginal pain is readily induced by epinephrine in patients with angina pectoris.

Therapeutic Uses. Epinephrine has a wide variety of clinical uses in medicine and surgery. In general, these are based on the actions of the drug on blood vessels, heart, and bronchial muscle. The most common uses of epinephrine are to relieve respiratory distress due to *bronchospasm,* to provide rapid relief of *hypersensitivity reactions* to drugs and other allergens, and to *prolong the action of infiltration anesthetics.* Its cardiac effects may be of use in restoring cardiac rhythm in patients with *cardiac arrest* due to various causes. It is also used as a *topical hemostatic* on bleeding surfaces. The therapeutic uses of epinephrine are further discussed later in this chapter, together with those of other sympathomimetic drugs.

NOREPINEPHRINE (LEVARTERENOL)

Norepinephrine (levarterenol, *l*-noradrenaline, *l*-β-[3,4-dihydroxyphenyl]-α-aminoethanol) is the chemical mediator liberated by mammalian postganglionic adrenergic nerves. It differs from epinephrine only by lacking the methyl substitution in the amino group (see Table 8–1). As with epinephrine, the d isomer has pharmacological properties similar to those of the l form, but it is much less active. Norepinephrine constitutes 10 to 20% of the catecholamine content of human adrenal medulla and as much as 97% in some pheochromocytomas. The history of its discovery and its role as a neurohumoral mediator are discussed in Chapter 4.

Pharmacological Actions. The pharmacological actions of norepinephrine and epinephrine have been extensively compared *in vivo* and *in vitro* (see Table 8–3). Both drugs are direct agonists on effector cells, and their actions differ mainly in the ratio of their effectiveness in stimulating α and β_2 receptors. Both are approximately equipotent in stimulating β_1 (cardiac) receptors. Norepinephrine is a potent agonist at α receptors and has little action on β_2 receptors; however, it is somewhat less potent than epinephrine on the α receptors of most organs.

Cardiovascular Effects. The cardiovascular effects of intravenous infusion of 10 μg of norepinephrine per minute in man are shown in Figure 8–1. Systolic and diastolic pressures and usually pulse pressure are increased. Cardiac output is unchanged or decreased, and the total peripheral resistance is raised. Compensatory vagal reflex activity slows the heart, overcoming the direct cardioaccelerator action, and the stroke volume is thus increased. The peripheral vascular resistance increases in most vascular beds, and the blood flow is reduced through kidney, liver, and usually skeletal muscle. A marked venoconstriction contributes to the increased resistance. Glomerular filtration rate is maintained unless the decrease in renal blood flow is quite marked. Norepinephrine constricts mesenteric vessels and reduces splanchnic and hepatic blood flow in man. Coronary flow is substantially increased, probably due to both indirectly induced coronary dilatation, as with epinephrine, and elevated blood pressure. (However, see page 147.) Unlike epinephrine, small doses of norepinephrine do not cause vasodilatation or lower blood pressure, since the blood vessels of skeletal muscle are constricted instead of dilated; α-block-

ing agents therefore abolish the pressor effects but do not cause significant reversal. The circulating blood volume is reduced by loss of protein-free fluid to the extracellular space, probably due to postcapillary vasoconstriction. The usual ECG change is sinus bradycardia due to a reflex increase in vagal tone, with or without prolongation of the P-R interval. Nodal rhythm, A-V dissociation, bigeminal rhythm, ventricular tachycardia, and fibrillation have also been observed.

Other Effects. Other responses to norepinephrine are not prominent in man. The drug causes hyperglycemia and other metabolic effects similar to those produced by epinephrine, but these are observed only when larger doses are given. Respiratory minute volume is slightly increased. Effects on the CNS are somewhat less prominent than those of epinephrine. Intradermal injection of suitable doses in man causes sweating that is not blocked by atropine. Increased frequency of contraction of the pregnant human uterus has been observed, but the effects on the other smooth muscles are slight.

Absorption, Fate, and Excretion. Norepinephrine, like epinephrine, is ineffective when given orally and is absorbed poorly from sites of subcutaneous injection. It is rapidly inactivated in the body by the same enzymes that methylate and oxidatively deaminate epinephrine (see above). Only 4 to 16% of an administered dose is excreted unchanged in the urine. Negligible amounts are normally found in the urine, but as much as 15 mg per day may be excreted by persons with pheochromocytoma.

Preparations, Dosage, and Route of Administration. *Norepinephrine Bitartrate,* U.S.P. (LEVOPHED BITARTRATE), is the water-soluble, crystalline monohydrate salt. Like epinephrine, it is readily oxidized. *Norepinephrine Bitartrate Injection,* U.S.P., is a 0.2% sterile solution of the bitartrate, equivalent to 0.1% of norepinephrine base. It is usually given by *intravenous infusion,* as a solution containing 4μg/ml of norepinephrine base, obtained by diluting 4 ml of the official injection in 1000 ml of 5% dextrose. After the cardiovascular response to a test dose of 0.1 to 0.2 μg/kg of body weight is observed, the infusion is adjusted to obtain the desired pressor response. Normally the infusion of 2 to 4 μg of base per minute (0.5 to 1.0 ml per minute) is adequate. The pressor response to the drug can be readily controlled since it disappears within 1 or 2 minutes after the infusion is stopped. In patients in whom intravenous infusion of large volumes of fluid is undesirable, less dilute solutions may be used cautiously. Oral administration is ineffective.

Toxicity, Side Effects, and Precautions. The untoward effects of norepinephrine are similar to those of epinephrine, but they are usually less pronounced and less frequent. Anxiety, respiratory difficulty, awareness of the slow, forceful heart beat, and transient headache are the most common effects. Overdoses or conventional doses in hypersensitive persons (*e.g.*, hyperthyroid patients) cause severe hypertension with violent headache, photophobia, stabbing retrosternal and pharyngeal pain, pallor, intense sweating, and vomiting. The risk of cardiac arrhythmias contraindicates the use of the drug during anesthesia with agents that sensitize the automatic tissue of the heart.

Care must be taken that *necrosis* and *sloughing* do not occur at the site of intravenous injection, due to extravasation of the drug. The infusion should be made high in the limb, preferably through a long plastic cannula extending centrally, and the site of infusion should be changed at least every 12 hours. Impaired circulation at injection sites, with or without extravasation of norepinephrine, may be relieved by hot packs and infiltration of the area with phentolamine or a local anesthetic. Norepinephrine infusions should never be left unattended. Blood pressure must be determined at least every 15 minutes during the infusion and more frequently during initial adjustment of the rate. Blood pressure should not be raised to more than normotensive levels. Reduced blood flow to vital areas is a constant danger in the use of norepinephrine. The drug should not be used in pregnant women because of its contractile action on the pregnant uterus.

Therapeutic Uses and Status. Norepinephrine has only limited therapeutic value. The therapeutic use of norepinephrine and of other sympathomimetic amines in hypotension due to shock is discussed later in this chapter.

ISOPROTERENOL

Isoproterenol (isopropylarterenol, isopropylnorepinephrine, isoprenaline, isopropylnoradrenaline, *dl*-β-[3,4-dihydroxyphenyl]-α-isopropylaminoethanol) (Table 8–1) is the most active of the sympathomimetic amines

that act almost exclusively on β receptors by virtue of their N-alkyl substitution. First studied by Konzett (1940), it has since been the subject of extensive animal and clinical research.

Pharmacological Actions. Isoproterenol has a powerful action on all β receptors and almost no action on α receptors. Its main actions, therefore, are on the heart, the smooth muscle of bronchi, skeletal muscle vasculature, and the alimentary tract. In addition, it exerts prominent metabolic effects in adipose tissue, skeletal muscle, and, in some species, liver. The *l* isomer is much more potent than is the *d* isomer. The major cardiovascular effects of isoproterenol, epinephrine, and norepinephrine in man are compared in Figure 8–1.

Cardiovascular System. Intravenous infusion of isoproterenol in man lowers peripheral vascular resistance, mainly in skeletal muscle but also in renal and mesenteric vascular beds, and diastolic pressure falls. Cardiac output is raised by an increase in the venous return to the heart, combined with the positive inotropic and chronotropic actions of the drug. With usual doses of isoproterenol in man, the increase in cardiac output is generally enough to maintain or raise the systolic pressure, although the mean pressure is reduced. Renal blood flow is decreased in normotensive subjects but is markedly increased in patients in cardiogenic or septicemic shock. Pulmonary arterial pressure is unchanged. Larger doses cause a striking fall in mean blood pressure.

Smooth Muscle. Isoproterenol relaxes almost all varieties of smooth muscle when the tone is high, but this action is most pronounced on bronchial and gastrointestinal smooth muscle. It prevents or relieves bronchoconstriction due to drugs and bronchial asthma in man, but tolerance to this effect develops with overuse of the drug. Its effect in asthma may be due in part to an additional action to inhibit antigen-induced release of histamine (Assem and Schild, 1969); this action is shared by selective β_2-receptor stimulants. The drug decreases the tone and motility of intestinal musculature and inhibits uterine motility even when epinephrine causes contraction.

Metabolic and Central Nervous System Actions. In man, isoproterenol causes less hyperglycemia than does epinephrine, but it is as effective as epinephrine in releasing *free fatty acids.* Insulin secretion is stimulated both by glucose and by direct β-adrenergic activation of pancreatic islet cells. The *calorigenic* actions of isoproterenol and epinephrine are similar. Like epinephrine, isoproterenol can cause central excitation, but this is not significant with doses used clinically.

Absorption, Fate, and Excretion. Isoproterenol is readily absorbed when given parenterally or as an aerosol. Absorption of sublingual or oral doses is unreliable. It is metabolized primarily in the liver and other tissues by COMT. Isoproterenol is a relatively poor substrate for MAO and is not taken up by sympathetic neurons to the same extent as are epinephrine and norepinephrine. The duration of action of isoproterenol may therefore be longer than is that of epinephrine, but it is still brief.

Preparations, Dosage, and Routes of Administration. *Isoproterenol Hydrochloride,* U.S.P. (ISUPREL), is a white, water-soluble powder; it is oxidized on exposure to air or alkali. *Isoproterenol Hydrochloride Inhalation,* U.S.P., is available as a 0.25% aerosol (ISUPREL MISTOMETER, NORISODRINE AEROTROL) and as solutions (0.5 and 1%). A usual dose to relieve bronchoconstriction in asthma is 0.5 ml of the 0.5% solution. This is diluted to approximately 2.5 ml with water or isotonic saline solution and is given as a mist over 10 to 20 minutes. The drug is also available as *Isoproterenol Hydrochloride Injection,* U.S.P., containing 200 μg/ml. Sublingual and oral preparations of isoproterenol are unreliable, and their use is not recommended.

Toxicity and Side Effects. The acute toxicity of isoproterenol is much less than that of epinephrine. Palpitation, tachycardia, headache, and flushing of the skin are common; anginal pain, nausea, tremor, dizziness, weakness, and sweating are less frequent. Cardiac arrhythmias can occur readily, although they are not usually serious. Large or repeated doses in animals may lead to myocardial necrosis, as with epinephrine, or to cardiac arrest when the heart is subjected to an increased work load (Lockett, 1965).

Overdosage of isoproterenol administered by inhalation can be fatal, presumably as a result of the induction of ventricular arrhythmias. Approximately 10 years ago, an isoproterenol nebulizer containing five times the usual concentration of the drug was introduced for use in England and Wales for the management of intractable asthma. This nebulizer provided approximately 0.4 mg of isoproterenol per inhalation. During the time when this preparation was popular in the United Kingdom, there was a considerable increase in mortality among asthmatics. A similar increase was not seen in other countries where such preparations were not available. This unfortunate experience serves to illustrate dramatically the hazards of excessive doses of β-adrenergic agonists (Stolley, 1972).

Therapeutic Uses. Isoproterenol is employed clinically only as a *bronchodilator* in respiratory disorders and as a *cardiac stimulant* in heart block, cardiogenic shock after myocardial infarction, and septicemic shock. Its use in these conditions and its value in relation to other sympathomimetic agents are discussed later in this chapter.

PROTOKYLOL

Protokylol hydrochloride (VENTAIRE) is a derivative of isoproterenol (*see* Table 8-1). The larger, nonpolar substituent on the amine endows this drug with more favorable pharmacokinetic properties. It is more reliably absorbed from the gastrointestinal tract than is isoproterenol and can be given orally. Following this route of administration, bronchodilatation becomes manifest within 30 to 90 minutes and persists for 3 to 4 hours. Its cardiovascular effects and other pharmacological properties are similar to those of isoproterenol. The usual oral dose of protokylol hydrochloride is 2 to 4 mg four times daily.

ETHYLNOREPINEPHRINE

Ethylnorepinephrine Hydrochloride, U.S.P. (BRONKEPHRINE), is primarily a β-adrenergic agonist, despite the fact that it is a primary amine (Table 8-1). Its actions are similar to those of isoproterenol, although it is less potent. The drug is administered intramuscularly or subcutaneously; it is available in a solution for injection that contains 2 mg/ml, and the usual dose is 1 to 2 mg.

DOPAMINE

Dopamine (3,4-dihydroxyphenylethylamine) (Table 8-1) is the immediate metabolic precursor of norepinephrine and epinephrine; it is a central neurotransmitter (Chapters 12 and 21) and possesses important intrinsic pharmacological properties. Dopamine is a substrate for both MAO and COMT and thus is ineffective when administered orally.

Cardiovascular Effects. Dopamine exerts a positive inotropic effect on the myocardium, acting as an agonist at β_1 receptors. In addition, it has the capacity to release norepinephrine from nerve terminals, and this also contributes to its effects on the heart. Tachycardia is less prominent during infusions of dopamine than of isoproterenol. Dopamine appears to increase systolic and pulse pressure and has either no effect on or slightly increases diastolic blood pressure. Total peripheral resistance is usually unchanged when low or intermediate therapeutic doses are given. This is probably due to the ability of dopamine to reduce regional arterial resistance in the mesentery and the kidney, while producing minor increases in other vascular beds. The effect of dopamine on the renal vasculature appears to be mediated by a specific dopaminergic receptor. In relatively low doses, infusion of dopamine is associated with an increase in glomerular filtration rate, renal blood flow, and sodium excretion. As a consequence, dopamine is especially useful in the management of cardiogenic, traumatic, or hypovolemic shock, where major increases in sympathetic activity may particularly compromise renal function. Since dopamine is a potent sympathomimetic agent, its use in life-threatening states of shock must be carefully monitored, and particular attention must be paid to avoidance of elevated blood pressure or reduction in renal function as a consequence of renal vasoconstriction. This may occur during administration of high doses of dopamine as a consequence of its stimulatory effect at α receptors. Many aspects of the pharmacology of dopamine have been reviewed by Goldberg (1972).

Other Effects. Although there are specific dopaminergic receptors in the CNS, injected dopamine usually has no central effects because it does not readily cross the blood-brain barrier (*see* Chapters 12, 19, and 21).

Preparations, Dosage, and Route of Administration. *Dopamine hydrochloride* (INTROPIN) is a water-soluble, light-sensitive, white crystalline powder, marketed in solution in 5-ml ampuls containing 40 mg/ml of the drug. It is used only by the intravenous route. The contents of the ampul must be diluted in 250 or 500 ml of an appropriate sterile solution (0.9% sodium chloride or 5% dextrose), to yield a final concentration of 800 or 400 μg/ml. The drug is administered at a rate of 5 μg/kg per minute initially, and this rate may be increased gradually up to 20 to 50 μg/kg per minute as the clinical situation dictates. During the infusion, all patients require intermittent evaluation of blood volume and frequent assessment of myocardial function, perfusion of vital organs, and the production of urine. Reduction in urine flow, tachycardia, and the development of arrhythmias may be indications to slow or terminate the infusion. The duration of action of dopamine is quite brief, and hence the rate of administration can be used to control the intensity of effect.

Precautions, Adverse Reactions, and Contraindications. Before dopamine is administered to patients in shock, hypovolemia should be corrected by transfusion of whole blood, plasma, or appropriate fluids. The patient must be monitored as indicated above. Untoward effects due to overdosage are generally attributable to excessive sympathomimetic activity (although this may also be the response to worsening shock). Nausea, vomiting, tachycardia, anginal pain, arrhythmias, headache, hypertension, and vasoconstriction may be encountered during infusion of dopamine. Since the drug has an extremely short half-life in plasma, these effects usually disappear quickly if the infusion is slowed or interrupted. Rarely, the use of a short-acting α-blocking agent such as phentolamine may be required. Extravasation of large amounts of dopamine during infusion may cause ischemic necrosis and sloughing. Rarely, gangrene of the fingers or toes has followed the prolonged infusion of the drug. If this is threatened, local infiltration of the region with phentolamine should be instituted.

Dopamine should be avoided or used at a much reduced dosage (one tenth or less) if the patient has received an inhibitor of MAO. Careful adjustment of dosage is also necessary for the patient who is taking tricyclic antidepressants.

Therapeutic Uses. Dopamine is useful in the treatment of some types of shock. It is particularly beneficial for patients with oliguria and with low or normal peripheral vascular resistance. The drug is also of value in the treatment of cardiogenic and bacteremic shock, as well as profound hypotension following removal of pheochromocytoma (from patients who were inadequately treated with adrenergic blocking agents prior to surgery). In all such situations the prognosis is more favorable when therapy is instituted early and especially before the rate of urine flow is seriously decreased (below 0.3 ml per minute). The management of shock is more fully discussed later in this chapter. Dopamine may also be of value in the treatment of *chronic refractory congestive heart failure* (*see* Goldberg, 1974).

DOBUTAMINE

Dobutamine resembles dopamine chemically but possesses a bulky aromatic substituent on the amino group (Table 8–1). Despite the absence of a β-OH group, dobutamine is a directly acting agent with selectivity for β_1 receptors; its indirect actions are slight (Sonnenblick *et al.*, 1979).

Cardiovascular Effects. Dobutamine appears to be relatively more effective in enhancing the contractile force of the heart than in increasing heart rate (Tuttle and Mills, 1975; Tuttle *et al.*, 1976). The drug acts directly on β_1 receptors to produce its inotropic effect. While dobutamine enhances the automaticity of the sinus node in man, this action is not as prominent as that produced by isoproterenol. Dobutamine does not appear to affect atrial conduction velocity in man, although it does augment conduction velocity through the A-V node. There is little or no effect on ventricular impulse conduction. In contrast to dopamine, dobutamine does not have an effect on the dopaminergic receptors in the renal vasculature and, therefore, does not produce renal vasodilatation (Goldberg *et al.*, 1977).

In animals, dobutamine, administered at a rate of 2.5 to 15 μg/kg per minute, increases cardiac contractility and cardiac output. Total peripheral resistance is not much affected. The heart rate increases only modestly when the rate of administration of dobutamine is maintained at less than 20 μg/kg per minute. After administration of β-blocking agents, infusion of dobutamine fails to increase cardiac output, but total peripheral resistance increases, suggesting that dobutamine does have modest direct effects on α receptors in the vasculature. Reflex tachycardia associated with isoproterenol-induced hypotension cannot explain the greater chronotropic effect of isoproterenol as compared with dobutamine, since neither vagotomy nor agents that interfere with the function of sympathetic neurons eliminate the difference in the chronotropic effects of the two drugs.

Route of Administration, Dosage, and Preparations. Dobutamine is not effective when given orally, and, since its half-life in plasma is approxi-mately 2 minutes, it must be administered by continuous intravenous infusion. The usual dose is 2.5 to 10 μg/kg per minute. The drug is rapidly metabolized in the liver to inactive conjugates with glucuronic acid and to 3-0-methyldobutamine.

Dobutamine hydrochloride (DOBUTREX) is supplied in 20-ml vials that contain 250 mg of the drug. The compound is dissolved in 10 ml of sterile water or 5% dextrose solution, and this solution is then further diluted to at least 50 ml for use.

Toxicity and Precautions. Since the electrophysiological effects caused by dobutamine are not markedly different from those of isoproterenol or dopamine, serious arrhythmias may be expected; however, it appears that the incidence is lower (Sonnenblick *et al.*, 1979). Nevertheless, because dobutamine enhances A-V conduction, the drug should be used with considerable caution or avoided in individuals with atrial fibrillation. In approximately 5 to 10% of patients, dobutamine may produce a marked increase in heart rate or systolic pressure. These effects can be rapidly reversed by reduction in the rate of administration of the drug. Less frequent side effects include nausea, headache, palpitations, shortness of breath, and anginal pain. Infusions of the drug have been performed for as long as 3 days.

Therapeutic Uses. Dobutamine causes a dose-related improvement in cardiac output in patients with congestive heart failure. Infusions at rates ranging from 2.5 to 15 μg/kg per minute produce progressive increases in cardiac output and decreases in pulmonary wedge pressure, indicative of a reduction in diastolic filling pressure in the left ventricle. Urine output and sodium excretion are increased, presumably secondarily to the improvement in cardiovascular status. Dobutamine appears to be particularly useful in patients who have undergone procedures involving cardiopulmonary bypass. Even greater beneficial effects are obtained under these circumstances when sodium nitroprusside is administered concomitantly with dobutamine.

Dobutamine appears to have advantages over other catecholamines for the improvement of myocardial function in heart failure. Since the effects of dobutamine on heart rate and systolic pressure are minimal in comparison to the other catecholamines, the oxygen demands of the myocardium are increased to a lesser degree. Increased contractility and reduction in left ventricular filling pressure in the failing heart should augment the gradient for diastolic coronary blood flow. The reduction in heart size also reduces wall tension at any given level of systolic pressure, and this tends to reduce oxygen demand. These favorable effects on myocardial perfusion are less likely to occur in the absence of cardiac failure. As a consequence, the use of dobutamine has been recommended for patients with acute myocardial infarction when congestive heart failure is superimposed (particularly if peripheral vascular resistance and heart rate are high). If cardiogenic shock and severe hypotension are also present, coronary perfusion may be compromised and, under these circumstances, a vasopressor or expansion of plasma volume may also be required. Such procedures should be instituted only if pulmonary arterial and pulmonary wedge pressures can be monitored. Dobutamine, as well as other inotropic agents, is contraindicated in patients with marked obstruction to cardiac ejection, such as in idiopathic hypertrophic subaortic stenosis.

II. Noncatecholamines

Until slightly more than 2 decades ago, it was presumed that all sympathomimetic amines produced their effects by acting directly on adrenergic receptors. However, some observations were not compatible with this notion. For example, following chronic postganglionic adrenergic denervation, the effects of epinephrine and norepinephrine on target organs were found to be potentiated, whereas those of tyramine and many other noncatechol sympathomimetic amines were found to be reduced or abolished. Similarly, after animals or isolated organs were treated with cocaine in concentrations sufficient to block the uptake of catecholamines into the adrenergic nerve terminal, the effects of norepinephrine and epinephrine were potentiated, whereas the actions of tyramine were inhibited. In 1958, Burn and Rand reported that the effects of tyramine were markedly reduced if it was tested on isolated organs prepared from animals treated with reserpine; again, there was no impairment of the effects of either norepinephrine or epinephrine. Since reserpine was known to deplete profoundly tissue stores of catecholamines, Burn and Rand proposed that tyramine was not interacting directly with α-adrenergic receptors to produce its pharmacological actions. They argued instead that tyramine and related amines acted indirectly, following uptake into the adrenergic nerve terminal, by stoichiometric displacement of norepinephrine from storage sites in the synaptic vesicles or from extravesicular binding sites. Norepinephrine could then exit from the adrenergic

nerve terminal, traverse the synaptic cleft, and interact with receptors to produce the sympathomimetic effects. Following chronic postganglionic adrenergic denervation, adrenergic nerve terminals degenerate, which explains the lack of effect of tyramine under this condition. In the presence of cocaine, the high-affinity neuronal transport system for catecholamines and certain congeners is inhibited, and tyramine and related amines are unable to enter the adrenergic nerve terminal. In this manner cocaine inhibits the actions of indirectly acting sympathomimetic amines, while potentiating the effects of directly acting agents that are normally removed from the synaptic cleft by this transport system (see Chapter 4).

A wide variety of sympathomimetic amines were then investigated with regard to their ability to act either directly upon adrenergic receptors or indirectly via release of neurotransmitter (Trendelenburg, 1972). The most common experimental procedure is to compare the dose-response curve of the amine on a particular target tissue before and after treatment with reserpine. Such studies revealed that the actions of compounds such as norepinephrine, epinephrine, isoproterenol, and phenylephrine were essentially unaffected after treatment with reserpine; however, responses of peripheral tissues to agents such as tyramine, phenylethylamine, and amphetamine were abolished. Most agents exhibited some degree of residual sympathomimetic activity after the administration of reserpine, but higher doses of these amines were required to produce comparable effects. The first group of drugs is classified as directly acting sympathomimetic amines, since they activate adrenergic receptors directly; the second group of agents is termed indirectly acting amines, since they act only by releasing norepinephrine from presynaptic stores; and the group of compounds that exhibits residual but lower activity following treatment with reserpine is classified as mixed-acting sympathomimetic amines—that is, they have both direct and indirect actions.

It has not been possible to categorize all sympathomimetic amines precisely, because of variability of the pattern observed between different tissues and species. This is particularly true of the agents with mixed actions. Nevertheless, some generalizations can be stated (Trendelenburg *et al.*, 1962; Trendelenburg, 1972).

Phenylethylamines that lack both hydroxyl groups on the ring and the β-hydroxyl group on the side chain act almost exclusively indirectly. Agents that lack hydroxyl groups on the aromatic ring but possess a β-hydroxyl group (*e.g.*, ephedrine) have the capacity to act both directly and indirectly to produce sympathomimetic effects. Similarly, phenylethylamines that possess the catechol structure but lack the β-hydroxyl group, such as dopamine, exhibit mixed actions, although the effects tend to be primarily indirect. Phenylethylamines with both a *meta*-hydroxyl group on the aromatic ring and a β-hydroxyl group, such as phenylephrine, tend to be primarily directly acting, although they are less potent than β-hydroxylated catecholamines. Other aspects of the SAR of the indirectly acting sympathomimetic amines are discussed above.

There is some controversy over whether nonpolar sympathomimetic amines exert their actions in the CNS by a direct, indirect, or mixed action. If catecholamines in the CNS are severely depleted by reserpine, the actions of amphetamine are not abolished (Smith, 1963). However, the effects of amphetamine are markedly reduced when animals are treated with α-methyltyrosine, an inhibitor of norepinephrine synthesis (Rech, 1964; Moore *et al.*, 1970). It has been suggested that newly synthesized norepinephrine may be much more crucial to the function of adrenergic neurons in the CNS and that amphetamine may act indirectly by releasing a pool of newly synthesized catecholamines that is not depleted by reserpine.

Since the actions of norepinephrine are more marked on α and β_1 receptors than on β_2 receptors, many noncatecholamines that release norepinephrine have predominantly α-receptor-mediated and cardiac effects. However, many noncatecholamines with both direct and indirect effects on adrenergic receptors show powerful β_2-agonistic activity and are widely used clinically for the effects that result. Thus, ephedrine, although dependent upon norepinephrine release for some of its effect, relieves bronchospasm by its action on β_2 receptors in bronchial muscle, an effect virtually absent with norepinephrine. It must also be recalled that some noncatecholamines, for example, phenylephrine, act primarily and directly on effector cells. It is therefore impossible to predict precisely the characteristic effects of noncatecholamines simply on the basis that they all provoke the release of at least some norepinephrine.

With few exceptions the actions and effects of noncatecholamines, except those on the CNS, fit within the framework of α- and β-receptor activity as listed in Table 4-1 (page 60), and, therefore, only the main differences in their properties will be presented. The additional CNS effects, most prominent with sympathomimetic amines lacking substituents on the benzene ring, have been most extensively studied with amphetamine and, consequently, are discussed in detail in relation to the properties and clinical uses of that drug.

False-Transmitter Concept. As indicated above, indirectly acting amines are taken up into adrenergic nerve terminals and storage vesicles, where they presumably replace norepinephrine in the storage complex. Phenylethylamines that lack a β-hydroxyl group are retained there poorly, but β-hydroxylated phenylethylamines and compounds that subsequently become hydroxylated in the synaptic vesicle by dopamine-β-hydroxylase are retained in the synaptic vesicle for relatively long periods of time (Musacchio *et al.*, 1965; Kopin, 1968). Such substances can produce a persistent diminution in the content of norepinephrine at functionally critical sites in the adrenergic nerve terminal. When the nerve is stimulated, the content of a relatively constant number of synaptic vesicles is presumably released by exocytosis. If these vesicles contain a considerable proportion of phenylethylamines that are much less potent than norepinephrine, activation of postsynaptic adrenergic receptors will be diminished.

This hypothesis, known as the *false-transmitter concept,* is a possible explanation for the hypotensive effect that results from the administration of inhibitors of MAO. Phenylethylamines are normally synthesized in the gastrointestinal tract as a result of the action of bacterial tyrosine decarboxylase. The tyramine that is formed in this fashion is usually oxidatively deaminated in the gastrointestinal tract and the liver, and the amine does not reach the systemic circulation in significant concentrations. However, when an MAO inhibitor is administered, tyramine may be absorbed systemically. It is transported into the adrenergic nerve terminal, where its catabolism is again prevented because of the inhibition of MAO at this site; it is then β-hydroxylated to octopamine and stored in the vesicles in this form. As a consequence, there is gradual displacement of norepinephrine, and stimulation results in the release of a relatively small amount of norepinephrine along with a fraction of octopamine. The latter amine has relatively little ability to activate either α- or β-adrenergic receptors. There is thus a functional impairment of sympathetic nerve transmission following chronic administration of MAO inhibitors.

Despite such functional impairment, patients who have received MAO inhibitors may experience severe hypertensive crises if they ingest cheese, beer, or red wine. These and related foods, which are produced by a fermentation process, contain a large quantity of tyramine and, to a lesser degree, other phenylethylamines. When gastrointestinal and hepatic MAO is inhibited, the large quantity of tyramine that is ingested is absorbed rapidly and reaches the systemic circulation in high concentration. A massive and precipitous release of norepinephrine can result, with consequent hypertension that can be sufficiently severe to cause myocardial infarction or a cerebrovascular accident. Hypertensive crises may not be a danger when selective inhibitors of monoamine oxidase-B (MAO-B) are administered. In man, a considerable fraction of the MAO in the gastrointestinal tract appears to be of the A type (Houslay and Tipton, 1976). Thus, during therapy with a selective MAO-B inhibitor, there remains, in the gastrointestinal tract and liver, sufficient MAO-A to deaminate tyramine. Inhibitors of MAO-B may thus find considerable use in the treatment of disorders of the CNS such as depression and Parkinson's disease (Riederer *et al.,* 1978; *see* Chapters 19 and 21).

The false-transmitter concept can also be invoked to explain the hypotension that often follows infusions of metaraminol. Metaraminol possesses both direct and indirect sympathomimetic actions and has been infused for many hours for the maintenance of blood pressure in individuals who are severely hypotensive. When the infusion is terminated, patients may relapse into a severe hypotensive state, despite correction of the factors responsible for their shock. Presumably, the maintenance of adequate blood pressure at this time is largely dependent upon intrinsic sympathomimetic activity. However, a considerable fraction of the norepinephrine in the nerve terminal may have been replaced by metaraminol, and the release of this less potent sympathomimetic amine, along with norepinephrine, is apparently insufficient to produce adequate vasoconstriction. To manage this problem, patients can be given an infusion of norepinephrine for a period of time sufficient to allow replenishment of the stores of the neurotransmitter.

Absorption, Distribution, and Fate of Noncatecholamines.

In contrast to the catecholamines, most of the noncatecholamines that are used clinically are effective when given orally and many act for long periods. These properties are due in part to resistance to the inactivating enzymes of liver and other tissues and in part to the fact that relatively large amounts are given. Phenylisopropylamines, the most commonly used noncatecholamines, become localized in tissues soon after their administration; and, in contrast to catecholamines, which cross the blood-brain barrier with difficulty, they are found in high concentration in brain and cerebrospinal fluid. This accounts in part for their relatively powerful CNS activity. Although several pathways, including p-hydroxylation, N-demethylation, deamination, and conjugation in the liver, take part in their disposal, a substantial fraction of these drugs is excreted in the urine unchanged. Urinary excretion of amphetamine and many other noncatecholamines is greatly influenced by urinary pH. Since the pK_a of amphetamine is 9.9, the percentage of nonionized drug increases in alkaline urine, and the drug is readily reabsorbed by the renal tubules; at pH 8.0 only 2 to 3% is excreted. If the urine is acidic, urinary excretion may be as much as 80% (Beckett and Rowland, 1965). The effects of amphetamine are greatly prolonged in patients with alkaline urine, and acidification of the urine by the administration of ammonium chloride is a logical procedure in the treatment of amphetamine poisoning. A large number of noncatecholamines have pK_a values between 9.0 and 10.3 (Vree *et al.,* 1969), and similar striking effects of urinary pH can be expected.

Patients treated with MAO inhibitors should not take noncatecholamines or ingest foods that contain tyramine (*see* above). Even sympathomimetic drugs that are resistant to MAO (*e.g.,* amphetamine and ephedrine) should not be administered to such individuals, since these drugs provoke the release of norepinephrine, and the actions of the neurotransmitter can be potentiated by MAO inhibitors in this circumstance (Smith, 1966).

AMPHETAMINE

Amphetamine, racemic β-phenylisopropylamine (Table 8–1), has powerful CNS stimulant actions in addition to the peripheral α and β actions common to indirectly acting sympathomimetic drugs. Unlike epinephrine, it is effective after oral administration and its effects last for several hours.

History. The pressor effects of amphetamine were first described by Piness and associates (1930). Alles (1933) observed its bronchodilator, respiratory stimulant, and analeptic actions and, comparing it with epinephrine, found its cardiovascular effects to be of much longer duration but its potency to be much lower. The central stimulant effects of amphetamine were first used clinically by Prinzmetal and Bloomberg (1935) to treat narcolepsy and have since been employed in a variety of conditions, including obesity, fatigue, parkinsonism, and poisoning by CNS depressants.

PHARMACOLOGICAL PROPERTIES

Cardiovascular Responses. In man and animals, amphetamine given orally raises both systolic and diastolic blood pressures. Heart rate is often reflexly slowed; with large doses, cardiac arrhythmias may occur. Cardiac output is not enhanced by therapeutic doses, and cerebral blood flow is little changed. The *l* isomer is slightly more potent than the *d* isomer in its cardiovascular actions.

Other Smooth Muscles. In general, smooth muscles respond to amphetamine as they do to other sympathomimetics. Bronchial muscle is relaxed, but the effect is not sufficiently marked to be of therapeutic value. The contractile effect on the urinary bladder sphincter is particularly marked, and has been used in treating enuresis and incontinence. Pain and difficulty in micturition occasionally occur. The gastrointestinal effects of amphetamine are unpredictable. If enteric activity is pronounced, amphetamine may cause relaxation and delay the movement of intestinal contents; if the gut is already relaxed, the opposite effect may be seen. The response of the human uterus varies, but usually there is an increase in tone.

Central Nervous System. Amphetamine is one of the most potent sympathomimetic amines with respect to stimulation of the CNS. It stimulates the medullary respiratory center, lessens the degree of central depression caused by various drugs, and produces other signs of stimulation of the CNS. Animals given sufficient doses of amphetamine show tremor, restlessness, increased motor activity, agitation, and sleeplessness; these effects are thought to be due to cortical stimulation and possibly to stimulation of the reticular activating system. In contrast, the drug can obtund the maximal electroshock seizure discharge and prolong the ensuing period of depression; these properties may be related to the usefulness of amphetamine in certain cases of epilepsy. In elicitation of CNS excitatory effects, the *d* isomer (dextroamphetamine) is three to four times as potent as the *l* isomer.

In man, the marked *analeptic* action is exemplified by the fact that anesthesia produced by 0.5 g of amobarbital sodium given intravenously can be greatly lessened by 10 to 30 mg of amphetamine injected intravenously. The *psychic* effects depend on the dose and the mental state and personality of the individual. The main results of an oral dose of 10 to 30 mg are as follows: wakefulness, alertness, and a decreased sense of fatigue; elevation of mood, with increased initiative, self-confidence, and ability to concentrate; often elation and euphoria; increase in motor and speech activity. Performance of only simple mental tasks is improved; and, although more work may be accomplished, the number of errors is not necessarily decreased. Physical performance, for example, in athletes, is improved, and the drug is abused for this purpose. These effects are not invariable, and may be reversed by overdosage or repeated usage. Prolonged use or large doses are nearly always followed by mental depression and fatigue. Many individuals given amphetamine experience headache, palpitation, dizziness, vasomotor disturbances, agitation, confusion, dysphoria, apprehension, delirium, or fatigue. (*See* review by Weiss and Laties, 1962.)

Fatigue and Sleep. Prevention and reversal of fatigue by amphetamine have been studied extensively in the laboratory, in military field studies, and in athletics. In general, the duration of adequate performance is prolonged before fatigue appears and the effects of fatigue are at least partly reversed. The most striking improvement due to amphetamine appears to occur when performance has been reduced by fatigue and lack of sleep. Such improvement may be partly due to alteration of unfavorable attitudes toward the task. However, amphetamine reduces the frequency of attention lapses that impair performance after prolonged sleep deprivation, and thus improves execution of tasks requiring sustained attention. Rapid-eye-movement (REM) sleep is reduced to about 10%, less than half the normal proportion of total sleeping time. The need for sleep may be postponed, but it obviously cannot be indefinitely avoided. When the drug is discontinued after long use, total sleep increases, and REM sleep appears more rapidly than usual and is unduly prolonged. The pattern of sleep may take as long as 2 months to return to normal. (*See* reviews by Weiss and Laties, 1962; Oswald, 1968.)

Analgesia. Amphetamine and some other sympathomimetic amines have a small analgesic effect in man and experimental animals. However, this is not sufficiently pronounced to be useful therapeutically.

EEG. In general, amphetamine accelerates and

desynchronizes the EEG. It causes a shift of the resting EEG toward the higher frequencies in man, but to a smaller degree than that occurring during attention. It reduces the amplitude and the duration of the large delta waves that are present during sleep after prolonged insomnia and in narcolepsy. In some children with petit mal and typical 3-per-second spike-and-dome dysrhythmia, amphetamine may abolish both the seizures and the abnormal EEG discharges; this may be due, in part, to an effect on alertness and activity. In children with behavioral disorders and abnormal EEG (6-cycle-per-second rhythm), amphetamine may improve behavior with or without altering the EEG. (*See* review by Toman and Davis, 1949.)

Spinal Cord, Reticular Formation, and Respiratory Center. Amphetamine facilitates monosynaptic and polysynaptic transmission in the spinal cord. In common with ephedrine, it enhances excitatory activity, promotes righting movements and postural activity, and speeds the recovery of responses in spinal, decerebrate, and decorticate animals. Amphetamine can reverse the depressant effect of barbiturates on the reticular formation, and it lowers the threshold for arousal by electrical stimulation of this region (Bradley and Key, 1958).

The *respiratory center* is stimulated by amphetamine in animals, and the rate and depth of respiration are increased. In normal man, usual doses of the drug do not appreciably increase respiratory rate or minute volume. Nevertheless, when respiration is depressed by centrally acting drugs, amphetamine may stimulate respiration.

Depression of Appetite. Amphetamine and similar drugs have been widely used in the treatment of obesity, although the wisdom of this use is at best questionable. Weight loss in obese humans treated with amphetamine is almost entirely due to reduced food intake and only in small measure to increased metabolism. The site of action is probably in the lateral hypothalamic feeding center; injection of amphetamine into this area, but not into the ventromedial satiety center, suppresses food intake (*see* Blundell and Leshem, 1973). In man, some drug-induced loss of acuity of smell and taste has been described, and increased physical activity may also contribute to the loss of weight. In dogs, the effect is powerful and may lead to complete starvation if amphetamine is given each day 1 hour before the daily meal. The effect is much less in man, and tolerance to acceptable doses develops rapidly. The effect is insufficient to reduce weight continuously in obese individuals without dietary restriction. Amphetamine has little effect in reducing food intake in those persons whose overeating is impelled by psychological factors.

Mechanisms of Action in the CNS. Amphetamine appears to exert most or all of its effects in the CNS by releasing biogenic amines from their storage sites in the nerve terminals. The alerting effect of amphetamine, its anorectic effect, and at least a component of its locomotor-stimulating action are presumably mediated by release of norepinephrine from central noradrenergic neurons. These effects can be prevented by treatment of the animal with α-methyltyrosine, an inhibitor of tyrosine hydroxylase and, therefore, of catecholamine synthesis. Some aspects of locomotor activity and the stereotyped behavior induced by amphetamine are probably a consequence of the release of dopamine from dopaminergic nerve terminals, particularly in the neostriatum. Higher doses are required to produce these behavioral effects, and this is correlated with the need for higher concentrations of amphetamine to release dopamine from brain slices or synaptosomes *in vitro*. With still higher doses of amphetamine, disturbances of perception and overt psychotic behavior occur. These effects may be due to release of 5-hydroxytryptamine (5-HT) from tryptaminergic neurons and of dopamine in the mesolimbic system. In addition, amphetamine may exert direct agonistic effects on central receptors for 5-HT (*see* Weiner, 1972).

Metabolic Effects. Although large doses of amphetamine markedly increase oxygen consumption in animals, conventional therapeutic doses cause either no change, a small fall, or a modest rise (10 to 15%) in the metabolic rate in man. Some patients show a slight increase in body temperature. The apparent calorigenic action may be due to restlessness caused by the drug. Amphetamine increases the plasma concentration of free fatty acids but, in contrast to epinephrine, does not modify carbohydrate utilization or increase the concentration of blood glucose or lactate, and the respiratory quotient is unaltered.

Preparations, Route of Administration, and Dosage. *Amphetamine Sulfate,* U.S.P. (BENZEDRINE), is a white, water-soluble powder, available in 5- and 10-mg tablets and 15-mg slow-release capsules. The *d* isomer is available as *Dextroamphetamine Phosphate,* U.S.P., in 5-mg tablets; and as *Dextroamphetamine Sulfate,* U.S.P. (DEXEDRINE), in 5- and 10-mg tablets, in an official elixir (1 mg/ml), and in 5-, 10-, and 15-mg slow-release capsules.

With the usual oral dose of 2.5 to 5.0 mg of dextroamphetamine, the effects appear within ½ to 1 hour. The patient's sensitivity should first be tested with a dose of 2.5 mg. For chronic medication the usual dosage is 5 mg, two or three times daily. The last dose is generally given not later than 4 P.M., to avoid insomnia. The amphetamines are schedule-II drugs under federal regulations (*see* Appendix I).

Toxicity and Side Effects. The *acute toxic effects* of amphetamine are usually extensions of its therapeutic actions and, as a rule, result from overdosage. The *central effects* commonly include restlessness, dizziness, tremor, hyperactive reflexes, talkativeness, tenseness, irritability, weakness, insomnia, fever, and sometimes euphoria. Confusion, assaultiveness, increased libido, anxiety, delirium, paranoid hallucinations, panic states, and suicidal or homicidal tendencies occur, especially in mentally ill patients. However, these psychotic effects can be elicited in any individual if sufficient quantities of amphetamine are ingested for a prolonged period. Fatigue and depression usually follow the central stimulation. *Cardiovascular effects* are common and include headache, chilliness, pallor or flushing, palpitation, cardiac arrhythmias, anginal pain, hypertension or hypotension, and circulatory collapse. Excessive sweating occurs. Symptoms referable to the *gastrointestinal system* include dry mouth, metallic taste, anorexia, nausea, vomiting, diarrhea, and abdominal cramps. Fatal poisoning usually terminates in convulsions and coma, and cerebral hemorrhages are the main pathological finding.

The *toxic dose* of amphetamine varies widely. Toxic manifestations occasionally occur as an idiosyncrasy after as little as 2 mg, but are rare with doses of less than 15 mg. Severe reactions have occurred with 30 mg, yet doses of 400 to 500 mg are not uniformly fatal. Larger doses can be tolerated after chronic use of the drug.

Treatment of acute amphetamine intoxication should include acidification of the urine by administration of ammonium chloride. Excretion of amphetamine is negligible in alkaline urine and is vastly increased in acidic urine. Chlorpromazine is effective treatment for the CNS symptoms, and additionally its α-receptor blocking action reduces the elevated blood pressure; a nitrite or a rapidly acting α-receptor blocking agent may also be required if hypertension is marked.

Chronic intoxication with amphetamine causes symptoms similar to those of acute overdosage, but abnormal mental conditions are more common. Weight loss may be marked, and occasionally dermatitis occurs. A psychotic reaction with vivid hallucinations and paranoid delusions, often mistaken for schizophrenia, is the most common serious effect. Recovery is usually rapid after withdrawal of the drug, but occasionally the condition becomes chronic. In these persons amphetamine may act as a precipitating factor hastening the onset of an incipient schizophrenia (*see* Angrist and Gershon, 1972).

Precautions and Contraindications. The abuse of amphetamine by the laity as a means of overcoming sleepiness and of increasing energy and alertness should be discouraged. The drug should be used only under medical supervision. The additional *contraindications* and *precautions* in the use of amphetamine are generally similar to those described above for epinephrine. Its use is inadvisable in patients with anorexia, insomnia, asthenia, psychopathic personality, or a history of homicidal or suicidal tendencies.

Dependence and Tolerance. Psychological dependence often occurs when amphetamine or dextroamphetamine is used chronically, as discussed in Chapter 23. *Tolerance* almost invariably develops to the anorexigenic effect of amphetamines, and is often seen also in the need for increasing doses to maintain improvement of mood in psychiatric patients. A period without the drug usually restores the patient's sensitivity. Tolerance is striking in individuals who are dependent on the drug, and a daily intake of 1700 mg without apparent ill effects has been reported. Development of tolerance is not invariable, and cases of narcolepsy have been treated for years without requiring an increase in the initially effective dose.

Therapeutic Uses. Amphetamine and dextroamphetamine are used chiefly for their CNS effects. They have been largely supplanted by other sympathomimetic agents for their peripheral effects. Dextroamphetamine, with greater CNS action and less peripheral action, is generally preferred to amphetamine; it is used in obesity, narcolepsy, hyperkinetic syndrome in children (minimal brain damage), parkinsonism, behavior disorders, and absence seizures. These uses are discussed later in this chapter.

METHAMPHETAMINE

Methamphetamine is closely related chemically to amphetamine and ephedrine (Table 8–1). Its *pharmacological actions* are similar to those of amphetamine, but it exhibits a different ratio between central and peripheral actions. Small doses have prominent central stimulant effects without significant peripheral actions; somewhat larger doses produce a sustained rise in systolic and diastolic blood pressure, due in man mainly to cardiac stimulation. Cardiac output is increased, although the heart rate may be reflexly slowed. Venous constriction causes peripheral venous pressure to increase. These factors tend to increase the venous return and, therefore, the cardiac output. Pulmonary arterial pressure is raised, probably secondary to increased cardiac output. Renal blood flow is also enhanced. Although moderate doses stimulate cardiac contraction, excessive doses depress the myocardium. (*See* Aviado, 1959, 1970; Eckstein and Abboud, 1962.)

Preparations, Route of Administration, and Dosage. *Methamphetamine hydrochloride* (DESOXYN, FETAMIN) is the *d* isomer. It is available in tablets containing 2.5 or 5 mg and in sustained-release tablets containing 5, 10, or 15 mg. The usual oral dose for central effects varies from 2.5 mg daily to 5 mg three times daily.

Methamphetamine is a schedule-II drug under federal regulations (*see* Appendix I).

Therapeutic Uses. Methamphetamine is principally used for its *central effects,* which are more pronounced than those of amphetamine and are accompanied by less prominent peripheral actions. These uses are discussed below in the section of this chapter on therapeutic uses.

EPHEDRINE

Ephedrine occurs naturally in various plants. It was used in China for at least 2000 years before being introduced into Western medicine in 1924 (*see* Chen and Schmidt, 1930). Prepared synthetically in 1927, it has since been used extensively for clinical conditions in which either peripheral or CNS actions of sympathomimetic drugs are desired. Its central actions are less pronounced than those of the amphetamines. Ephedrine stimulates both α and β receptors and has clinical uses related to both types of action. The drug owes part of its peripheral action to release of norepinephrine, but it also has direct effects on receptors and exhibits substantial effects in reserpine-treated animals and man (Krogsgaard, 1956). Tachyphylaxis develops to its peripheral actions, and rapidly repeated doses become less effective, probably as a result of the depletion of norepinephrine stores.

Since ephedrine contains two asymmetrical carbon atoms, four compounds are possible. Only *l*-ephedrine and racemic ephedrine are commonly used clinically; their pharmacological properties and uses are essentially similar. The structure of ephedrine is depicted in Table 8–1.

Pharmacological Actions. Ephedrine differs from epinephrine mainly in its efficacy after oral administration, its much longer duration of action, its more pronounced central actions, and its much lower potency. *Cardiovascular effects* of ephedrine are in many ways similar to those of epinephrine, but they persist about ten times as long. The drug elevates the systolic and usually also the diastolic pressure in man, and pulse pressure increases. Pressor responses are due partly to vasoconstriction but mainly to cardiac stimulation, provided venous return is adequate. The heart rate may not be altered, but it increases if vagal reflexes are blocked. The force of myocardial contraction and cardiac output are augmented by the drug; the renal and splanchnic blood flows are decreased whereas the coronary, cerebral, and muscle blood flows are increased.

Bronchial muscle relaxation is less prominent but more sustained with ephedrine than with epinephrine. Consequently, ephedrine is of value only in milder cases of acute asthma and in chronic cases that need continued medication. *Mydriasis* occurs after local application of the drug to the eye. Reflexes to light are not abolished, accommodation is unaffected, and intraocular pressure is unchanged. Ephedrine and other sympathomimetics are of little use as mydriatics in the presence of inflammation. The drug is less effective in individuals who have heavily pigmented irides than in those in whom the iris is light colored. Other smooth muscles are generally affected by ephedrine in the same manner as by epinephrine. However, the activity of the human *uterus* is usually reduced by ephedrine, regardless of the effect of epinephrine, and thus this agent has been used to relieve the pain of dysmenorrhea. Ephedrine is less effective than epinephrine in elevating the concentration of *glucose* in the *blood.* The *CNS effects* of ephedrine are similar to those of amphetamine but are considerably less marked.

Preparations, Routes of Administration, and Dosage. *Ephedrine Sulfate,* U.S.P., is the *l* isomer. It is available in 25- and 50-mg tablets and capsules and in a 4-mg/ml syrup; the oral dose varies from 15 to 50 mg. For continued medication, small doses are given at 3- to 4-hour intervals. Sterile solutions (25 and 50 mg/ml) are available; in hypotensive states, 15 to 50 mg may be given subcutaneously or, if a rapid response is necessary, 20 mg can be injected intravenously. Solutions of 1 and 3% in water are available for nasal mucosal decongestion, and aqueous solutions of 0.1% are applied to the eye to produce mydriasis.

Toxic Reactions. These are similar to the untoward reactions observed after epinephrine, with additional reactions referable to the CNS effects of ephedrine. Insomnia is common with continued medication, but it is readily counteracted by sedatives if necessary. *Precautions* in the use of ephedrine are similar to those outlined for epinephrine and the amphetamines.

Therapeutic Uses. The main clinical applications of ephedrine are in *bronchospasm,* in *Stokes-Adams syndrome,* as a *nasal decongestant,* as a *mydriatic,* and in certain *allergic disorders.* The drug has also been employed as a *pressor* agent, particularly during spinal anesthesia, and for its central stimulant action in *narcolepsy.* These uses are discussed below in the section of this chapter on therapeutic uses.

MEPHENTERMINE

Mephentermine is N-methyl-ω-phenyl-*tertiary*-butylamine (Table 8–1). It is one of several pressor agents currently used in various hypotensive conditions. Its duration of action is prolonged, pressor effects lasting 30 to 60 minutes after subcutaneous and up to 4 hours after intramuscular doses. Its peripheral actions and effects appear to be similar to those of methamphetamine, but its central actions are relatively feeble. Mephentermine acts both directly and by release of endogenous norepinephrine. Cardiac contraction is enhanced, and cardiac output and systolic and diastolic pressures are usually increased. The change in heart rate is variable, depending on the degree of vagal tone; large doses can depress the heart. The pressor response involves both increased cardiac output and peripheral vasoconstriction. In some cases the net vascular effect may be vasodilatation, which appears not to involve β receptors (Caldwell and Goldberg, 1970). Coronary blood flow is increased, forearm blood flow is reduced, and venous tone is increased. Marked mucosal vasoconstriction can be produced by local application of the drug. CNS effects may occur with large doses of mephentermine. These include drowsiness, weeping, incoherence, and convulsions, and rapidly disappear on withdrawal of the drug. (For references, *see* Aviado, 1959, 1970; Eckstein and Abboud, 1962; Zaimis, 1968.)

Preparations, Routes of Administration, and Dosage. *Mephentermine Sulfate,* U.S.P. (WYAMINE), is available in sterile solution (15 and 30 mg/ml) for parenteral injection. Given *intramuscularly* the dose is usually 10 to 30 mg. Slow *intravenous infusions* are also given, the rate being varied to produce the desired pressor effect.

Therapeutic Uses. Mephentermine is mainly used as a pressor agent in various *hypotensive states,* as discussed below in the section of this chapter on therapeutic uses.

HYDROXYAMPHETAMINE

Hydroxyamphetamine, synthesized in Germany in 1913, came into clinical use only after reinvestigation 2 decades later (Alles, 1933). Its chemical structure differs from that of amphetamine only by the addition of a 4-OH group (*see* Table 8–1).

In many respects the actions of hydroxyamphetamine resemble those of ephedrine, with the exception that the drug almost entirely lacks CNS stimulant activity. The duration of action after oral or subcutaneous administration is from 90 to 120 minutes; after intravenous injection, 20 to 30 minutes. While the drug has been employed for the treatment of hypotensive states and to maintain an adequate ventricular rate in the Stokes-Adams syndrome, the only current use of hydroxyamphetamine in the United States is as a mydriatic. *Hydroxyamphetamine Hydrobromide,* U.S.P. (PAREDRINE), is available as a 1% ophthalmic solution.

METARAMINOL

Metaraminol, 3-hydroxyphenylisopropanolamine (Table 8–1), is used almost exclusively for the treatment of hypotensive states. It has both direct and indirect actions and its overall effects are similar to those of norepinephrine, but it is much less potent and has a more prolonged action. It lacks CNS stimulant effects. Metaraminol is absorbed after oral administration; however, for equal effects, oral doses must be five or six times greater than doses given intramuscularly or intravenously. The pressor effect of an intramuscular dose of 5 mg lasts for about 1½ hours.

Cardiovascular Actions. The cardiovascular actions in man are reflected in a sustained rise in systolic and diastolic pressures, almost entirely due to vasoconstriction and usually accompanied by a marked reflex bradycardia. Occasionally sinus arrhythmia also occurs. In normotensive subjects, cardiac output is unchanged or may decrease slightly, but the force of myocardial contraction is enhanced. Cardiac output increases strikingly when slowing of the heart is prevented by atropine. Increased cardiac output may play a larger role in patients with hypotension and shock, in which conditions the drug increases cardiac output as well as peripheral resistance. Metaraminol increases venous tone and decreases renal and cerebral blood flows, the latter even when blood pressure is raised as much as 40%. In dogs, limb and splanchnic blood flows are also decreased and coronary blood flow is increased, but these effects have not yet been confirmed in man. Pulmonary vasoconstriction occurs in man, and the pulmonary blood pressure is elevated by the drug even when cardiac output is reduced. (*See* Aviado, 1959, 1970; Eckstein and Abboud, 1962; Zaimis, 1968.)

Preparations, Routes of Administration, and Dosage. *Metaraminol Bitartrate,* U.S.P. (ARAMINE), is available in 1-ml ampuls and 10-ml vials as a sterile solution (10 mg/ml) for intramuscular injection, usually in a dose of 2 to 10 mg, or, after suitable dilution, for intravenous infusion. The rate of administration is regulated according to the individual's response to the drug. Subcutaneous injections should be avoided since tissue sloughing may occur.

Therapeutic Uses. The principal use of metaraminol is as a pressor agent in certain *hypotensive states,* the treatment of which is discussed below in the section of this chapter on therapeutic uses.

PHENYLEPHRINE

Phenylephrine differs chemically from epinephrine only in lacking an OH in the 4 position on the benzene ring (Table 8–1). It was first studied by Barger and Dale (1910), but was not used clinically until years later when it was found to have greater potency than other monohydroxyl derivatives. Phenylephrine is a powerful postsynaptic α-receptor stimulant with little effect on the β receptors of the heart. A direct action on receptors accounts for the greater part of its effects, only a small part being due to its ability to release norepinephrine. Central stimulant action is minimal.

Cardiovascular Actions. The predominant actions of phenylephrine are on the *cardiovascular system.* Intravenous, subcutaneous, or oral administration causes a rise in systolic and diastolic pressures in man and other species. Responses are more sustained than those to epinephrine, lasting 20 minutes after intravenous and as long as 50 minutes after subcutaneous injection. Accompanying the pressor response to phenylephrine is a marked reflex bradycardia that can be blocked by atropine; after atropine, large doses of the drug increase the heart rate only slightly. In man, cardiac output is slightly decreased and peripheral resistance is considerably increased. Circulation time is slightly prolonged, and venous pressure is slightly increased; venous constriction is not marked. Most vascular beds are constricted, and renal, splanchnic, cutaneous, and limb blood flows are reduced but coronary blood flow is increased. Pulmonary vessels are constricted, and pulmonary arterial pressure is raised. The drug is a powerful vasoconstric-

tor, with properties very similar to those of norepinephrine but almost completely lacking the chronotropic and inotropic actions on the heart. Cardiac irregularities are seen only very rarely even with large doses, and the reflex slowing is sufficient to permit use of the drug to end attacks of paroxysmal atrial tachycardia. (*See* Aviado, 1959, 1970; Eckstein and Abboud, 1962.)

Preparations, Routes of Administration, and Dosage. *Phenylephrine Hydrochloride,* U.S.P. (ISOPHRIN, NEO-SYNEPHRINE), is the *l* isomer. It is available as a sterile solution (10 mg/ml) for parenteral use, an elixir (1 mg/ml), various nasal (0.125, 0.25, 0.5, and 1.0%) and ophthalmic (2.5 and 10%) solutions, and a viscous ophthalmic solution (10%). For children, the weaker solutions should be used because of the possibility of toxic effects. Roughly equipressor doses are 0.8 mg intravenously, 5 mg subcutaneously or intramuscularly, and 250 mg orally. However, absorption after oral administration is unreliable. For treatment of hypotension during spinal anesthesia, the usual dose is 5 to 10 mg, administered intramuscularly. The rate of intravenous infusion in hypotensive states should be regulated according to the patient's response.

Therapeutic Uses. Phenylephrine is used mainly as a *nasal decongestant,* a pressor agent in *hypotensive states,* a *mydriatic,* a local vasoconstrictor (0.005%) in solutions of local anesthetics, and in the relief of *paroxysmal atrial tachycardia.* These uses are discussed below in the section of this chapter on therapeutic uses.

METHOXAMINE

Methoxamine is β-hydroxy-β-(2,5-dimethoxyphenyl) isopropylamine (Table 8–1). Its pharmacological properties are almost exclusively those characteristic of α-receptor stimulation, since it acts directly at these sites. Its pharmacological actions are thus similar to those of phenylephrine. The outstanding effect is an increase in blood pressure due entirely to vasoconstriction. The drug has virtually no stimulant action on the heart and lacks β-receptor action on smooth muscle. It causes little or no CNS stimulation.

Cardiovascular Actions. Methoxamine, given intravenously or intramuscularly in man, causes a rise in systolic and diastolic blood pressures that persists for 60 to 90 minutes. The pressor effect is due almost exclusively to an increase in peripheral resistance. Cardiac output is decreased or unchanged. Renal blood flow is reduced in man to a greater extent than after equipressor doses of norepinephrine or metaraminol. Cerebral, splanchnic, and limb blood flows are reduced in dogs, and coronary blood flow is unchanged; whether the effects are similar in man is not known. In man, the venous pressure increases, but the constrictor action on forearm veins is feeble. Methoxamine has no significant stimulant action on the heart, and does not increase the ventricular rate in patients with heart block. Reflex bradycardia is prominent, and, therefore, the drug is used clinically to relieve attacks of paroxysmal atrial tachycardia. When the vagal effects are blocked by atropine, methoxamine often slows the heart slightly. This is probably due to a direct action on α receptors. Injection of the drug into the artery leading to the sinus node slows the heart, an effect blocked by phentolamine (James *et al.*, 1968). Methoxamine does not appear to precipitate cardiac arrhythmias. In contrast to epinephrine, methoxamine prolongs ventricular muscle action potentials and refractory period and slows A-V conduction (Gilbert *et al.*, 1958). Tachyphylaxis to the drug occurs in experimental animals, but has not been reported in man. (*See* Aviado, 1959, 1970; Eckstein and Abboud, 1962; Zaimis, 1968.)

In man, pressor doses of methoxamine cause pilomotor stimulation and often a desire to micturate. Occasionally tingling of the extremities and a feeling of coldness follow intravenous injection of the drug.

Preparations, Routes of Administration, and Dosage. *Methoxamine Hydrochloride,* U.S.P. (VASOXYL), is available as a solution (10 or 20 mg/ml) for intramuscular injection. The dose varies from 10 to 20 mg. Intravenous injections of 3 to 5 mg may also be given with the precautions properly accorded to intravenous injections of sympathomimetic amines.

Therapeutic Uses. Methoxamine is almost solely used as a pressor agent in *hypotensive states* and to end attacks of *paroxysmal atrial tachycardia.* These conditions are discussed below in the section of this chapter on therapeutic uses.

METHOXYPHENAMINE

Methoxyphenamine, β-(o-methoxyphenyl) isopropylmethylamine, differs from methamphetamine only in having a methoxy substituent in the 2 position on the benzene ring (Table 8–1), but its pharmacological properties differ greatly. Its main sympathomimetic action is on β receptors of smooth muscle. By this action, the drug causes *bronchodilatation,* its usual clinical use. Its bronchodilator effect is greater than that of ephedrine, and the accompanying cardiovascular effects are considerably less. The α-receptor and central stimulant actions of the drug are minimal. Methoxyphenamine also exhibits weak antihistaminic properties.

Preparations, Route of Administration, and Dosage. *Methoxyphenamine Hydrochloride,* U.S.P. (ORTHOXINE), is marketed in 100-mg tablets and in a syrup (10 mg/ml). The usual oral dose is 50 to 100 mg, repeated every 3 or 4 hours if necessary.

Therapeutic Uses. Methoxyphenamine is used mainly in mild cases of *asthma* and other *allergic conditions,* as discussed below.

SELECTIVE β_2-ADRENERGIC STIMULANTS

The considerable incidence and intensity of untoward effects of isoproterenol, when administered either parenterally or by inhalation for the treatment of bronchoconstrictive disease, have caused investigators to conduct an intensive search for more specific β_2-adrenergic agonists. *Metaproterenol* and *terbutaline,* two such compounds, have already been introduced into therapy in the United States and elsewhere. *Albuterol* (*salbutamol*) is in clinical use in Canada and Europe. Other β_2 agonists that are currently under investigation include *carbuterol, rimiterol, salmefamol, fenoterol, soterenol, tretoquinol,* and *quinterenol* (Webb-Johnson and Andrews, 1977). While most of these compounds are not catecholamines, a few do possess a catechol nucleus in their structure. The structures of metoproterenol, terbutaline, and albuterol are shown in Table 8–1. Because of their relative specificity for β_2 receptors, these drugs relax smooth muscle of the bronchi, uterus, and vascular supply to skeletal muscle, but generally have much less stimulant action on the heart than does isoproterenol. Thus, in asthmatic patients albuterol and isoproterenol are approximately equipotent as bronchodilators when given by aerosol, whereas ten times the dose of albuterol is required to cause equal cardioacceleration. Metaproterenol is somewhat less selective than albuterol for β_2 receptors. Nevertheless, cardiac stimulation is sufficiently limited to give the drug a considerable therapeutic advantage over isoproterenol.

METAPROTERENOL

Metaproterenol is quite similar to isoproterenol chemically, except that the two hydroxyl groups are attached at the meta positions on the benzene ring rather than at the meta and para positions. As a consequence, metaproterenol is resistant to methylation by COMT. It is effective when administered orally and has a somewhat longer duration of action than does isoproterenol.

Pharmacological Properties. Metaproterenol is primarily a β_2-adrenergic agonist. When administered by inhalation, it has relatively little effect on the β_1 receptors of the heart. Following either oral administration or inhalation of metaproterenol, there is an increase in 1-second forced expiratory volume (FEV$_1$) and in the maximal rate of forced expiratory flow (FEF), and a decrease in airway resistance. With a single oral dose of 20 mg of the drug, significant improvement in airway function is demonstrable for up to 4 hours. After administration of the drug by inhalation, improved respiratory function is apparent for a more variable period of time, ranging from 1 to 5 hours. There is some suggestion that tolerance develops after repeated administration of metaproterenol. This is manifested primarily as a shortened duration of action of the drug. A similar phenomenon is seen with ephedrine.

Approximately 40% of metaproterenol is absorbed after oral administration. The drug is excreted in the urine primarily as conjugates with glucuronic acid.

Preparations, Routes of Administration, and Dosage. *Metaproterenol sulfate* (ALUPENT, METAPREL) is available for oral inhalation as a micronized powder. The metered-dose inhaler contains 225 mg of the drug, and approximately 0.65 mg is nebulized per dose. Administration is generally performed by 2 or 3 deep inhalations, and this may be repeated at 4-hour intervals; the total daily dose should not exceed 12 inhalations. The drug is also available in 20-mg tablets. The usual adult dose is 20 mg, taken three or four times a day. A syrup (10 mg/5 ml) is suitable for use in children. The usual dose in children who are 6 to 9 years of age or who weigh less than 27 kg is 5 ml, given three or four times a day. Children over 9 years of age or who weigh over 27 kg may receive 10 ml three or four times a day.

Toxicity and Precautions. Adverse reactions are generally those expected from sympathomimetic stimulation and include tachycardia, hypertension, nervousness, tremor, palpitations, nausea, and vomiting. The drug should be used with special caution in patients with hypertension, coronary artery disease, congestive heart failure, hyperthyroidism, or diabetes.

Therapeutic Uses. Metaproterenol is useful as a *bronchodilator* in the treatment of bronchial asthma and for reversible bronchospasm associated with bronchitis or emphysema. When administered by inhalation, it is approximately as effective as isoproterenol and its duration of action is considerably longer. When administered orally, it is at least as effective as ephedrine.

TERBUTALINE

Terbutaline sulfate is a synthetic sympathomimetic agent that is administered orally and subcutaneously for the treatment of reversible obstruction of the airway. It is a relatively selective β_2 agonist. Like metaproterenol, terbutaline is not a catechol and is not methylated by COMT.

Pharmacological Properties. Terbutaline, given orally in a dose of 5 mg to patients with asthma, produces bronchodilatation after about 1 hour that lasts for approximately 7 hours. There is a significant increase in pulmonary function, as demonstrated by an increase of 15% or more in FEV$_1$ and FEF. When the drug is administered subcutaneously, the improvement in pulmonary function occurs in approximately 5 minutes and persists for up to 4 hours. However, the selectivity of this agent for β_2 receptors is much less apparent when the drug is administered by this route, and cardiovascular effects similar to those caused by isoproterenol may be expected.

Side effects associated with the administration of terbutaline are generally those produced by other sympathomimetic agents. Nervousness and muscle tremors are common; other effects include headache, tachycardia, palpitations, drowsiness, nausea, vomiting, and sweating. These reactions are usually mild, and their frequency appears to diminish with continued therapy. The precautions to be observed are the same as those for other sympathomimetic drugs.

Preparations, Routes of Administration, and Dosage. *Terbutaline Sulfate*, U.S.P. (BRETHINE, BRICANYL), may be administered either subcutaneously or orally. The usual subcutaneous dose is 0.25 mg. If significant clinical improvement does not occur in 15 to 30 minutes, a second dose may be administered. A total dose of 0.5 mg should not be exceeded within a 4-hour period. The usual oral dose of terbutaline is 5 mg, administered at intervals of approximately 6 hours three times a day. If side effects are notable, the dose may be reduced to 2.5 mg three times daily. Terbutaline is available in tablets containing either 2.5 or 5 mg of the drug and as an injection containing 1 mg/ml.

Therapeutic Uses. Terbutaline is an effective *bronchodilator* when administered orally and is useful in the management of asthma and other bronchospastic diseases. Like metaproterenol and other relatively selective β_2 agonists, terbutaline appears to possess modest therapeutic advantages over less selective bronchodilators such as ephedrine.

Terbutaline, metaproterenol, and albuterol have been used successfully by continuous intravenous infusion to *delay delivery in premature labor.* Side effects are more prominent with the large doses required and include nervousness, tremor, headache, nausea and vomiting, hypotension, and maternal and fetal tachycardia (*see* Liggins and Vaughan, 1973; Wallace *et al.*, 1978).

OTHER β_2 AGONISTS

Albuterol, available in Canada and Europe as *salbutamol,* may be administered either by inhalation or orally. The usual oral dose is 2 to 4 mg, given three or four times a day. Its pharmacological properties are similar to those of terbutaline. When inhaled, its peak effect occurs in 30 to 40 minutes, and effects are detectable for 3 to 6 hours.

Isoetharine is available for the treatment of bronchospastic disease as a solution for nebulization (BRONKOSOL) or in a metered-dose, pressurized inhaler as the mesylate (BRONKOMETER). It is purported to produce fewer cardiac side effects than does either epinephrine or isoproterenol, as is claimed for all of the agents in this group.

MISCELLANEOUS SYMPATHO-MIMETIC DRUGS

Several sympathomimetic drugs are used primarily as vasoconstrictors for local application to the nasal mucous membrane or the eye. Their structures are depicted in Tables 8–1 and 8–2. They vary from simple aliphatic amines to complex imidazoline derivatives Their nonproprietary and trade names as well as available preparations are as follows: *Propylhexedrine,* U.S.P. (BENZEDREX), nasal inhaler (250 mg); *Tuaminoheptane Sulfate,* U.S.P. (TUAMINE), nasal inhaler (325 mg); *Naphazoline Hydrochloride,* U.S.P. (PRIVINE), 0.05% nebulizer or 0.1% nasal solution and 0.02 to 0.1% ophthalmic solution; *Tetrahydrozoline Hydrochloride,* U.S.P., 0.05 and 0.1% nasal solutions (TYZINE) and 0.05% ophthalmic solution (VISINE); *Oxymetazoline Hydrochloride,* U.S.P. (AFRIN), 0.025 and 0.05% nasal solution; *Xylometazoline Hydrochloride,* U.S.P. (OTRIVIN), 0.05 and 0.1% nasal solutions.

Phenylpropanolamine Hydrochloride, U.S.P. (PROPADRINE), shares the pharmacological properties of ephedrine and is approximately equal in potency except that it causes less CNS stimulation. The drug is available in 25- and 50-mg capsules and in an elixir (4 mg/ml). It is also the ingredient of numerous proprietary mixtures that are marketed for the oral treatment of nasal and sinus congestion, usually in combination with an antihistaminic drug.

THERAPEUTIC USES OF SYM-PATHOMIMETIC DRUGS

The success that has attended efforts to develop therapeutic agents that can influence adrenergic receptors selectively and the variety of vital functions that are regulated by the sympathetic nervous system have resulted in a class of drugs that have a large number of important therapeutic uses.

Use of Vascular Effects. *Control of Hemorrhage.* The vasoconstrictor action of epinephrine may control superficial hemorrhage from skin and mucous membranes when the drug is applied topically as a spray or on cotton or gauze pledgets. It is effective only against bleeding from arterioles and capillaries and does not control venous oozing or hemorrhage from larger vessels.

Decongestion of Mucous Membranes. Sympathomimetic amines with α-receptor action cause marked vasoconstriction and blanching when applied to nasal and pharyngeal mucosal surfaces. They are therefore useful in the treatment of mucosal congestion accompanying *hay fever, allergic rhinitis, acute coryza, sinusitis,* and other respiratory conditions. The short duration of action of many of the amines, such as epinephrine, limits their value in shrinking the nasal mucosa when applied topically, and longer-acting congeners are more commonly used in these conditions. Some of the sympathomimetic amines more widely used topically for nasal decongestion are indicated as *N* in Table 8–1. All have the disadvantage that their use may be followed by "aftercongestion" and that prolonged use often results in chronic rhinitis. Some (*e.g.*, naphazoline) also irritate the nasal mucosa, causing a brief but sharp stinging sensation when first applied. Sufficient absorption of any of the imidazoline derivatives (Table 8–2) may cause CNS depression, leading to coma and marked reduction in body temperature, especially in infants. These drugs should not be used in young children.

Epinephrine is used in many surgical procedures on the nose, throat, and larynx, to shrink the mucosa and improve visualization by limiting hemorrhage. Since epinephrine is relatively nonirritating, it is especially suitable for use in treatment of congestion of the conjunctiva.

The efficacy of locally applied sympathomimetic vasoconstrictors in shrinking the nasal mucosa has led to the use of amines that may have this effect when given orally. Since the vessels of the nasal mucosa have not been shown to be more sensitive than most other vessels to sympathomimetic drugs, doses of orally administered sympathomimetics large enough to afford relief from nasal congestion will be expected to constrict other vascular beds and to raise the blood pressure. Ephedrine and pseudoephedrine have been given orally as nasal decongestants; their effects on nasal congestion due to colds are not of much consequence, but *allergic rhinitis* often responds well. While they do not raise blood pressure to any marked extent in doses that have this decongestant effect, they redistribute blood flow and cause cardiac stimulation. Several oral preparations promoted for the relief of colds and other upper respiratory conditions contain a sympathomimetic amine in combination with a variety of other agents (*e.g.,* antihistamines, antimuscarinic drugs, antipyretic-analgesics, caffeine, antitussives). There is no convincing evidence that such concoctions provide other than the symptomatic relief that is likely due to the presence of the aspirin-like drug.

Use with Local Anesthetics. Epinephrine is widely used to retard the absorption of local anesthetics. Other sympathomimetic amines are of value in preventing the fall in blood pressure that may accompany spinal anesthesia (*see* Chapter 15).

Hypotension. Sympathomimetic amines with predominant α-receptor activity can be used to relieve hypotension in various conditions, such as that associated with spinal anesthesia or due to overdosage of an antihypertensive agent. However, hypotension *per se* is not a sufficient reason to use pressor agents. There should be evidence that the hypotension is the cause of inadequate perfusion of vital organs before treatment with such drugs is initiated, and other maneuvers may be safer and more effective. For example, hypotension during spinal anesthesia may be managed by attention to fluid volumes and tilting of the patient. Sympathomimetic amines must be used very cautiously in patients under general anesthesia, since halogenated hydrocarbons sensitize the heart to the arrhythmic action of catecholamines and related drugs.

Administration of sympathomimetic agents for their pressor effect may be a useful *emergency measure* until other therapy can be instituted in certain hypotensive states (*e.g.,* in acute hemorrhage). Sympathomimetics may be used to raise the blood pressure and sustain the coronary and cerebral circulation until measures can be taken to restore an adequate circulating blood volume. However, this therapy must be regarded as only a temporary expedient that can obscure the extent of blood volume replacement required and can in itself cause loss of fluid from the vascular compartment. Vasopressor therapy can thus increase the risk of further circulatory deterioration.

The release of large amounts of catecholamines during operation on patients with *pheochromocytoma* can lead to a considerable decrease in the circulating blood volume, and the blood pressure may drop precipitously as soon as the tumor has been removed. Infusion of norepinephrine has been used to sustain the blood pressure postoperatively, but adequate fluid-volume replacement appears to be more rational therapy. Alternatively, the loss of circulating volume can be largely prevented and the postoperative fall in pressure much reduced or eliminated by inhibiting the vasoconstriction due to released catecholamines with an α-adrenergic blocking agent (*see* Chapter 9).

The blood pressure of patients with *orthostatic hypotension* due to various factors, including neurological diseases such as syringomyelia and tabes dorsalis, may be supported by treatment orally with ephedrine or other long-acting pressor sympathomimetic agents. However, responses are highly variable and control of the blood pressure in these conditions remains a very difficult problem.

Shock. Shock is a clinical state in which there is inadequate perfusion of tissues. The management of shock and the prognosis are determined by the pathogenesis of the syndrome. For example, hypovolemic shock due to the loss of fluid from either the vascular or extravascular compartments is treated by replacement of blood, plasma, or water and electrolytes, as appropriate. Adequate delivery of oxygen and the restoration of circulating blood volume, in addition to correction of the factors that resulted in hypovolemia, are generally sufficient to treat hypovolemic shock. Although these maneuvers are not likely to be adequate for other forms of shock, they are no less important in the treatment of the syndrome no matter what the cause.

Cardiogenic shock as a consequence of myocardial infarction is a vexing problem; there is no standard, accepted treatment, and the prognosis is poor no matter what the therapy. Replacement of fluid to restore circulatory volume is essential, but judicious administration is mandatory and the consequences must be monitored by measurement of either central venous pressure or pulmonary arterial wedge pressure. Blood pressure must be adequate to restore perfusion of vital organs, including the heart, but the pressure should not be so high as to place undue demands for oxygen on an already severely compromised myocardium; the output of urine must be assessed as an index of renal perfusion, especially if α-adrenergic agonists are employed to restore blood pressure. Dopamine appears to be particularly appropriate for this purpose, because of its ability to produce vasoconstriction while maintaining flow through the renal and mesenteric vascular beds. Dobutamine has been recommended because of its positive inotropic effects that are accompanied by modest peripheral vasoconstriction. Isoproterenol has also been employed. Improvement of cardiac performance and cardiac output can lead to a rise in blood pressure and improved perfusion of tissues. Glucagon has also been employed in cardiogenic shock, and it can increase the strength of cardiac contraction by a mechanism that does not involve β-adrenergic receptors. Unfortunately there are no convincing data that support the use of one drug in preference to another in this condition.

Under exceptional circumstances peripheral vasoconstrictors may be required to maintain an adequate blood pressure. Infusions of norepinephrine, metaraminol, and mephentermine, as well as epinephrine, have been employed for this purpose. As was discussed above, care must be taken to avoid an excessive increase in blood pressure, since the advantages of improving coronary perfusion may be more than offset by the increased demands placed on the myocardium; circulation to the kidneys and other vital organs may also be compromised. It is well to remember that, except in neurogenic shock and shock associated with spinal anesthesia, reflex vasoconstriction mediated by the sympathetic nervous system is probably already intense, and vasoconstrictors may only further compromise blood flow.

Because of the intense vasoconstriction associated with most forms of shock, several investigators have recommended the use of either α-adrenergic antagonists or vasodilators in the management of this condition. Such agents are likely to improve blood flow to tissues if a minimally effective blood pressure can be maintained. In addition, the reduction of afterload and preload on the heart reduces cardiac work and the myocardial requirement for oxygen at any given cardiac output. Rapidly acting vasodilator agents such as sodium nitroprusside appear to be superior to α-blocking agents in this circumstance, in part because of the ease of moment-to-moment control of the action of the drug (see Chapter 33).

The hemodynamic abnormalities of septic shock are treated in a manner similar to that for cardiogenic shock, at least insofar as one can apply the same principles of adequate oxygenation, tissue perfusion, and circulating volume, as well as maintenance of a respectable, but not excessive, blood pressure and correction of electrolyte or acid-base imbalance. Administration of appropriate antibiotics is of course indicated. Claims have also been made for the value of administration of large doses of adrenocorticosteroids and other agents that may reduce the elaboration of the vasoactive substances that are mediators of this syndrome. There is no convincing evidence of the efficacy of such treatment (see Reichgott and Melmon, 1975).

Use of Reflex Cardiac Effects of Pressor Drugs. Attacks of *paroxysmal atrial* or *nodal tachycardia* may be ended by reflex vagal discharge caused by pressor responses to phenylephrine or methoxamine, drugs without significant cardiac excitatory action. The dose, given slowly intravenously, should not raise the blood pressure above 160 mm Hg; for phenylephrine, the dose may be 0.15 to 0.8 mg; for methoxamine, 3 to 5 mg. A short-acting anticholinesterase agent such as edrophonium may be safer for this purpose (see Chapter 6).

Use of Cardiac Effects. *Cardiac Arrest and Heart Block with Syncopal Seizures.* Syncope in *Stokes-Adams syndrome,* generally occurring at the transition from partial to complete A-V block, may be due to ventricular standstill or to prefibrillatory rhythm leading to ventricular fibrillation. Epinephrine and isoproterenol are of value in prophylaxis and symptomatic treatment of the attacks, but physical measures should be applied first in the acute attack. Circulation may sometimes be restored by a precordial blow followed by external cardiac compression or, if readily at hand, by an electrical pacemaker or defibrillator. Next, cardiac puncture with or without intracardiac injection of epinephrine may be effective and, as a last resort, thoracotomy and manual cardiac massage may rarely be required. To restore the intrinsic cardiac rhythm once some circulation has been established, intravenous infusion of epinephrine or isoproterenol may be necessary. These catecholamines are likely to precipitate ventricular fibrillation if injudiciously used in patients with prefibrillatory rhythm, and, therefore, extreme care

should be taken in their *intravenous* administration. When the indications are less urgent, repeated subcutaneous injections of epinephrine or intramuscular injections of epinephrine in oil may give the desired results. Epinephrine has been used to maintain an adequate ventricular rate (30 to 40 beats or more per minute) for as long as a week, but other sympathomimetic amines are more suitable for prolonged and prophylactic treatment. Ephedrine and hydroxyamphetamine are both orally effective and longer acting. Either can prevent recurrence of syncopal attacks. *However, drug therapy is a temporary measure only to be used until an electrical pacemaker can be fitted to supply optimal and reliable ventricular regulation.*

The problem of reviving patients apparently dead from *drowning, electrocution,* or *anesthetic accidents* is not substantially different from that of the syncope in Stokes-Adams syndrome, and the same principles apply. In all cases of cardiac arrest, adequate artificial ventilation is crucial. Anesthetic cardiac accidents may be due either to asystole or to ventricular fibrillation. Since the heart is sensitized to the arrhythmic action of epinephrine by many anesthetics, the drug may convert asystole to ventricular fibrillation. Physical measures, especially the use of an electrical pacemaker are obviously more appropriate. Electrical countershock is indicated in ventricular fibrillation. Although the use of epinephrine in anesthetic accidents is theoretically inadvisable in cardiac arrest or after defibrillation, many patients have recovered when the drug has been administered. It is impossible to decide whether recovery is due to the drug, to mechanical stimulation of the myocardium by the needle prick, or to other procedures simultaneously applied. In patients who do not respond to other measures, it is not unreasonable to resort to the cardiac excitatory action of epinephrine. (See Bellet, 1960; Zoll and Linenthal, 1963.)

Uses in Allergic Disorders. *Bronchial Asthma.* Epinephrine, isoproterenol, and the newer selective β_2-receptor stimulants are the mainstay of the symptomatic treatment of respiratory distress due to bronchospasm. Relief is due to the β_2-receptor action that relaxes smooth muscle; with epinephrine, a contributory factor may be an α-receptor action that constricts bronchial mucosal vessels, thereby reducing congestion and edema. Acute asthmatic attacks are usually relieved within 3 to 5 minutes after subcutaneous injection of 0.2 to 0.5 mg of epinephrine or after oral inhalation of a 1% solution of epinephrine, a 0.5 or 1% solution of isoproterenol, or 0.65 mg of metaproterenol from a metered-dose inhaler. The decrease in vital capacity and the increase in residual air characteristic of these attacks are rapidly corrected, and maximal breathing capacity and velocity of expiration increase.

Whatever the drug or route of administration, the smallest dose affording relief should be used. Inhalations of isoproterenol or epinephrine may have to be repeated at intervals of 2 or 3 minutes, and subcutaneous injections of epinephrine at 15- to 20-minute intervals until relief of acute attacks is obtained. If symptoms recur, massage of the site of injection may give relief by enhancing absorption of the drug. With the longer-acting β_2-receptor stimulants such as terbutaline, 1 or 2 inhalations are often sufficient and repetition is unnecessary for 4 hours.

Complete refractoriness to epinephrine and isoproterenol is not uncommon after protracted therapy in severe cases and in status asthmaticus, especially when bronchospasm is associated with the presence of viscid mucus plugs in the bronchi. Epinephrine reduces bronchial secretion and may make these plugs more viscid and difficult to dislodge. Measures to facilitate removal of mucus plugs are important in these cases and include expectorants and increased hydration of the patient to liquefy the plugs, and mechanical removal of retained secretion by bronchoscopic suction. Suitable chemotherapy is used to combat respiratory infection when this common precipitating cause is present.

In cases of *refractory asthma,* intravenous administration of aminophylline is sometimes useful, but administration of adrenocorticosteroids is often required to interrupt the severe asthmatic cycle. Because of the serious side effects of prolonged use of such steroids (*see* Chapter 63), their administration should be discontinued as early as practicable; fortunately, such discontinuation is possible in virtually all cases. Susceptibility to small doses of epinephrine and other sympathomimetic amines is usually restored once repeated and progressive bronchial relaxation has been achieved. For prolonged relief from bronchospasm, usually in chronic asthma, *epinephrine in oil* is sometimes used, and a dose of 1 ml may permit a night's sleep free from attacks. The longer-acting oral sympathomimetics with prominent β-receptor action are more commonly used to prevent attacks. Metaproterenol (20 mg) or terbutaline (5 mg), administered every 6 hours, is perhaps more useful for this purpose. Ephedrine (20 to 50 mg), given at 4-hour intervals, is also an effective prophylactic. The use of methylxanthines such as aminophylline in asthma is discussed in Chapter 25.

Miscellaneous Allergic Disorders. Epinephrine is the drug of choice to relieve the symptoms of acute hypersensitivity reactions to drugs (*e.g.,* penicillin) and of other acute allergic reactions. A subcutaneous injection of epinephrine rapidly relieves itching, urticaria, and swelling of lips, eyelids, and tongue, and the drug may be lifesaving when edema of the glottis threatens suffocation. Only epinephrine is administered to relieve these acute reactions since it acts particularly rapidly; however, ephedrine, having a more prolonged action, can be used for the continued treatment of allergic disorders, such as hay fever. When skin tests are performed for hypersensitivity to various foods, drugs, pollens, or other allergens, epinephrine should always be at hand to control acute untoward reactions. If chronic medication with ephedrine is being used for allergic conditions, the drug should not be given for at least 12 hours before sensitivity tests are made; otherwise, positive reactions may be prevented. When conjunctival tests for serum or drug hypersensitivity are made, epinephrine solution instilled into the eye readily controls the local discomfort of positive reactions.

Ophthalmic Uses. Local application of various sympathomimetic amines to the conjunctiva is used to dilate the pupil, mainly to permit adequate examination of the fundus. The mydriatic effect of these drugs, notably ephedrine (0.1%), hydroxyamphetamine (1%), and phenylephrine (1 to 2%), lasts for only a few hours. The sympathomimetics have the additional advantage that they do not cause cycloplegia and usually do not increase intraocular pressure. Sympathomimetic mydriatics are also used to reduce the incidence of posterior synechiae in uveitis, and epinephrine (0.25 to 2%) or phenylephrine (10%) is used to treat wide angle glaucoma, reducing the intraocular pressure by their local vasoconstrictor action, which decreases production of aqueous humor.

Use of Central Effects. Apart from a series of drugs used only as anorectics (*see* below), the main sympathomimetics used for central effects are ephedrine, amphetamine, dextroamphetamine, methamphetamine, and mephentermine. Of these, dextroamphetamine and methamphetamine are most widely employed. The peripheral actions of ephedrine, mephentermine, and, to a lesser extent, amphetamine are disproportionately great, and central effects cannot be obtained without side effects from the peripheral actions.

Narcolepsy. Ephedrine, amphetamine, methamphetamine, and dextroamphetamine have been used to treat narcoleptic patients. The amphetamines largely prevent attacks of sleep in nearly all patients, and cataplexy is often much improved. The usual dose of dextroamphetamine varies from 5 to 60 mg daily, in divided portions, the last dose being taken not later than 4 P.M. so that the nocturnal sleep is not prevented. Tolerance does not appear to develop to these agents in the treatment of narcolepsy.

Parkinsonism. Dextroamphetamine partially alleviates various symptoms of parkinsonism, but it has been superseded by levodopa and other antiparkinsonism drugs. If levodopa cannot be tolerated, dextroamphetamine can be given as an adjuvant to the other drugs. It has little effect on tremor, but decreases rigidity in many patients and frequently relieves oculogyric crises. The drug brings about a better sleep cycle, a subjective improvement in muscle strength and rigidity, and elevates the mood, a most important objective in the treatment of the patients. The total daily dose varies from 10 to 50 mg or more. In certain other diseases of the extrapyramidal system, such as *spasmodic torticollis* and spasmodic movements of a limb, dextroamphetamine may relieve symptoms.

Obesity and Weight Reduction. Whatever the etiology of obesity, a factor common to all cases is necessarily an intake of amounts of food that supply more energy than the body uses. Of the two possible measures to correct this imbalance, attempts to reduce food intake have been more popular in Western civilization. Persistent dietary restraint has proven both essential and difficult to achieve, and various sympathomimetic and related drugs that depress appetite have been used to make a low-calorie diet more tolerable. These appetite depressants are of no value without an accompanying stringent dietary regimen, and it has been regularly demonstrated that, without consistent supervision, no prescribed regimen of drug or diet is predictably successful. Several factors have a part in determining this unsatisfactory situation. In many patients the etiology of obesity is psychological, and compulsive overeating is difficult to eradicate even with psychiatric help. The central stimulant and anorectic effects of most of these drugs have proven inseparable. This compromises their use in the latter part of the day; given after 4 P.M., they interfere with sleep at night. Since much of the overeating takes place in the evening, their value is obviously limited. The anorectic agents are often given with a soporific to overcome this difficulty, but without conspicuous success. In addition, tolerance develops within a few weeks and increased dosage is limited both by the peripheral actions that these drugs exert and by such symptoms of central stimulation as nervousness and irritability. Even during the early period of administration, peripheral effects, although seldom pronounced, are rarely completely absent.

None of the drugs used in obesity has proven superior to dextroamphetamine or methamphetamine, either in effectiveness or in lack of peripheral side effects. However, certain other agents have not so far presented a significant problem of drug abuse and, therefore, are preferable. Regulations are currently under consideration in the United States to interdict the prescribing of amphetamines for weight reduction. In contrast to other amphetamine derivatives, fenfluramine (Table 8–1) causes drowsiness and does not interfere with REM sleep. The preparations are as follows: *benzphetamine hydrochloride* (DIDREX), 25- and 50-mg tablets; *chlorphentermine hydrochloride* (PRE-SATE), 65-mg slow-release tablets; *Diethylpropion Hydrochloride,* U.S.P. (TENUATE, TEPANIL), 25-mg tablets and 75-mg slow-release tablets; *fenfluramine hydrochloride* (PONDIMIN), 20-mg tablets; *phendimetrazine tartrate* (PLEGINE), 35-mg tablets; *Phenmetrazine Hydrochloride,* U.S.P. (PRELUDIN), 25-mg tablets and 50- and 75-mg slow-release tablets; *phentermine hydrochloride* (IONAMIN, WILPO), 8-, 15-, and 30-mg slow-release capsules. The usual dose is one tablet three times a day, but the effect of a single dose should first be tested; a single slow-release dose should be taken at least 12 hours before bedtime.

Psychogenic Disorders. Amphetamines have been used in mild mental disorders such as mood disturbances, chronic nervous exhaustion, and psychoneuroses. In most conditions they have been superseded by other psychoactive drugs (*see* Chapter 19).

Hyperkinetic Syndrome. The amphetamines have a dramatic effect in calming a high proportion of abnormally hyperactive children. Restlessness, distractibility, and impulsive behavior are reduced, attention span is lengthened, and behavior becomes more tolerable to parents and teachers. Concomitant psychotherapy and parent counseling are necessary. Long-term drug therapy is essential; withdrawal leads to deterioration of performance. However, since the demands of school aggravate the condition, the drug can often be stopped during vacations. The usual dose of dextroamphetamine is 5 to 10 mg three times daily. Tolerance to this effect does not appear to develop. Side effects include insomnia, headache, irritability, depression, periods of excessive crying,

and gastrointestinal cramps, but these do not often require discontinuation of the drug. Continued use of dextroamphetamine depresses growth in these children by reducing appetite; a rebound weight gain occurs when the drug is stopped. Methylphenidate, which is equally effective, may cause less inhibition of growth. There is evidence that the long-term use of these stimulant drugs does not lead to subsequent abuse of the drug. It is alarming that the number of hyperkinetic children is estimated at 5%. A careful assessment of the condition must be made before therapy is begun. (*See* Sroufe and Stewart, 1973; Chapters 19 and 24.)

The mechanism of action of amphetamine in children with the hyperkinetic syndrome is probably related to the effect of the drug on CNS neurotransmitters (*see* Weiner, 1972; Snyder, 1973). It is not difficult to correlate the alerting and attention-span effects of the drug with its central actions, but the calming effect seems paradoxical.

Epilepsy. In *grand mal,* dextroamphetamine may be a valuable adjunct to phenobarbital, counteracting the ataxia and drowsiness produced by the barbiturate and thus allowing effective amounts to be given. It is also useful in *absence seizures* (petit mal) to counteract the sedative effect of trimethadione if this is troublesome. In some cases of petit mal, dextroamphetamine, either alone or in conjunction with an oxazolidinedione or succinimide, may prevent the attacks and restore the EEG to normal.

Miscellaneous Uses. Ephedrine and amphetamine have been reported to prevent *syncopal reactions* of the vagal or vasodepressor type due to abnormal sensitivity of the carotid sinuses. Ephedrine, amphetamine, and other sympathomimetics have been used with variable success to treat *urinary incontinence* and *nocturnal enuresis.* The benefit may be due partly to central effects of the drugs and partly to contraction of the vesical sphincter. Terbutaline or other selective β_2 agonists may be useful to delay delivery in *premature labor.*

Ablad, B.; Carlsson, E.; and Ek, L. Pharmacological studies of two new cardioselective adrenergic beta-receptor antagonists. *Life Sci.,* **1973,** *12,* Pt. I, 107–119.

Adler-Graschinsky, E., and Langer, S. Z. Possible role of a beta-adrenoceptor in the regulation of noradrenaline release by nerve stimulation through a positive feed-back mechanism. *Br. J. Pharmacol.,* **1975,** *53,* 43–50.

Ahlquist, R. P. A study of adrenotropic receptors. *Am. J. Physiol.,* **1948,** *153,* 586–600.

Ahlquist, R. P., and Levy, B. Adrenergic receptive mechanism of canine ileum. *J. Pharmacol. Exp. Ther.,* **1959,** *127,* 146–149.

Alles, G. A. The comparative physiological actions of *dl-β*-phenylisopropylamines. I. Pressor effect and toxicity, *J. Pharmacol. Exp. Ther.,* **1933,** *47,* 339–354.

Alles, G. A., and Prinzmetal, M. The comparative physiological actions of *dl-β*-phenylisopropylamines. II. Bronchial effect. *J. Pharmacol. Exp. Ther.,* **1933,** *48,* 161–174.

Anderson, R.; Holmberg, S.; Svedmyr, N.; and Åberg, G. Adrenergic α- and β-receptors in coronary vessels in man: an *in vitro* study. *Acta Med. Scand.,* **1972,** *191,* 241–244.

Assem, E. S. K., and Schild, H. O. Inhibition by sympathomimetic amines of histamine release induced by antigen in passively sensitized human lung. *Nature*, **1969**, *224*, 1028–1029.

Barger, G., and Dale, H. H. Chemical structure and sympathomimetic action of amines. *J. Physiol. (Lond.)*, **1910**, *41*, 19–59.

Bearn, A. G.; Billing, B.; and Sherlock, S. The effect of adrenaline and noradrenaline on hepatic blood flow and splanchnic carbohydrate metabolism in man. *J. Physiol. (Lond.)*, **1951**, *115*, 430–441.

Beckett, A. H., and Rowland, M. Urinary excretion kinetics of amphetamine in man. *J. Pharm. Pharmacol.*, **1965**, *17*, 628–639.

Benfey, B. G., and Varma, D. R. Interactions of sympathomimetic drugs, propranolol and phentolamine, on atrial refractory period and contractility. *Br. J. Pharmacol. Chemother.*, **1967**, *30*, 603–611.

Bertler, A.; Carlsson, A.; and Rosengren, E. Release by reserpine of catecholamines from rabbit hearts. *Naturwissenschaften*, **1956**, *43*, 521.

Bieniarz, J.; Motew, M.; and Scommegna, A. Uterine and cardiovascular effects of ritodrine in premature labor. *Obstet. Gynecol.*, **1972**, *40*, 65–73.

Blundell, J. E., and Leshem, M. B. Dissociation of the anorexic effects of fenfluramine and amphetamine following intrahypothalamic injection. *Br. J. Pharmacol.*, **1973**, *47*, 183–185.

Bradley, P. B., and Key, B. J. The effect of drugs on arousal responses produced by electrical stimulation of the reticular formation of the brain. *Electroencephalogr. Clin. Neurophysiol.*, **1958**, *10*, 97–110.

Brown, G. L., and Gillespie, J. S. The output of sympathetic transmitter from the spleen of the cat. *J. Physiol. (Lond.)*, **1957**, *138*, 81–102.

Burn, J. H., and Rand, M. J. The action of sympathomimetic amines in animals treated with reserpine. *J. Physiol. (Lond.)*, **1958**, *144*, 314–336.

Burn, J. H., and Tainter, M. L. An analysis of the effect of cocaine on the actions of adrenaline and tyramine. *J. Physiol. (Lond.)*, **1931**, *71*, 169–193.

Caldwell, R. W., and Goldberg, L. I. An evaluation of the vasodilation produced by mephentermine and certain other sympathomimetic amines. *J. Pharmacol. Exp. Ther.*, **1970**, *172*, 297–309.

Caliva, F. S.; Eich, R.; Taylor, H. L.; and Lyons, R. H. Some cardiovascular effects of phenyl-2-butyl-norsupifren hydrochloride (ARLIDIN). *Am. J. Med. Sci.*, **1959**, *238*, 174–179.

Carlsson, A.; Rosengren, E.; Bertler, A.; and Nilsson, J. Effect of reserpine on the metabolism of catecholamines. In, *Psychotropic Drugs*. (Garattini, S., and Ghetti, V., eds.) Elsevier Publishing Co., Amsterdam, **1957**.

Choo-Kang, Y. F. J.; Parker, S. S.; and Grant, I. W. B. Response of asthmatics to isoprenaline and salbutamol aerosols administered by intermittent positive-pressure ventilation. *Br. Med. J.*, **1970**, *4*, 465–468.

Cubeddu, L. X.; Barnes, E.; Langer, S. Z.; and Weiner, N. Release of norepinephrine and dopamine-β-hydroxylase by nerve stimulation. I. Role of neuronal and extraneuronal uptake and of alpha presynaptic receptors. *J. Pharmacol. Exp. Ther.*, **1974a**, *190*, 431–450.

Cubeddu, L. X.; Langer, S. Z.; and Weiner, N. The relationships between alpha receptor block, inhibition of norepinephrine uptake and the release and metabolism of ³H-norepinephrine. *J. Pharmacol. Exp. Ther.*, **1974b**, *188*, 368–385.

Cubeddu, L. X., and Weiner, N. Release of norepinephrine and dopamine-β-hydroxylase by nerve stimulation. III. Effects of norepinephrine depletion on the alpha presynaptic regulation of release. *J. Pharmacol. Exp. Ther.*, **1975a**, *192*, 1–14.

——————. Release of norepinephrine and dopamine-β-hydroxylase by nerve stimulation. IV. An evaluation of a role for cyclic adenosine monophosphate. *Ibid.*, **1975b**, *193*, 105–127.

DePotter, W. P.; Chubb, I. W.; Put, A.; and De Schaepdryver, A. F. Facilitation of the release of noradrenaline and dopamine-β-hydroxylase at low stimulation frequencies by α-blocking agents. *Arch. Int. Pharmacodyn. Ther.*, **1971**, *193*, 191–197.

Dixon, W. R.; Mosimann, W. F.; and Weiner, N. The role of presynaptic feedback mechanisms in regulation of norepinephrine release by nerve stimulation. *J. Pharmacol. Exp. Ther.*, **1979**, *209*, 196–204.

Dresel, P. E.; MacCannell, K. L.; and Nickerson, M. Cardiac arrhythmias induced by minimal doses of epinephrine in cyclopropane-anesthetized dogs. *Circ. Res.*, **1960**, *8*, 948–955.

Enero, M. A.; Langer, S. Z.; Rothlin, R. P.; and Stefano, F. J. E. Role of the alpha-adrenergic receptor in regulating noradrenaline overflow by nerve stimulation. *Br. J. Pharmacol.*, **1972**, *44*, 672–688.

Farnebo, L.-O., and Hamberger, B. Influence of α- and β-adrenoceptors on the release of noradrenaline from field stimulated atria and cerebral cortex slices. *J. Pharm. Pharmacol.*, **1974**, *26*, 644–646.

Forwell, G. D., and Ingram, G. I. C. The effect of adrenaline infusion on human blood coagulation. *J. Physiol. (Lond.)*, **1957**, *135*, 371–383.

Furchgott, R. F. Receptors for sympathomimetic amines. In, *Adrenergic Mechanisms* (a Ciba Foundation symposium). (Vane, J. R.; Wolstenholme, G. E. W.; and O'Connor, M.; eds.) Little Brown & Co., Boston; J. & A. Churchill, Ltd., London, **1960**, pp. 246–252.

Gilbert, J. L.; Lange, G.; Polevoy, I.; and Brooks, C. McC. Effects of vasoconstrictor agents on cardiac irritability. *J. Pharmacol. Exp. Ther.*, **1958**, *123*, 9–15.

Goldberg, L. I. Dopamine—clinical uses of an endogenous catecholamine. *N. Engl. J. Med.*, **1974**, *291*, 707–710.

Goldenberg, M.; Aranow, H., Jr.; Smith, A. A.; and Faber, M. Pheochromocytoma and essential hypertensive vascular disease. *Arch. Intern. Med.*, **1950**, *86*, 823–836.

Gombos, E. A.; Hulet, W. H.; Bopp, P.; Goldring, W.; Baldwin, D. S.; and Chasis, H. Reactivity of renal and systemic circulations to vasoconstrictor agents in normotensive and hypertensive subjects. *J. Clin. Invest.*, **1962**, *41*, 203–217.

Grunfeld, C.; Grollman, A. P.; and Rosen, O. M. Structure-activity relationships of adrenergic compounds on the adenylate cyclase of frog erythrocytes. *Mol. Pharmacol.*, **1974**, *10*, 605–614.

Haggendahl, J. Some further aspects on the release of the adrenergic transmitter. In, *Bayer Symposium II. New Aspects of Storage and Release Mechanisms of Catecholamines*. (Schumann, H. J., and Kroneberg, G., eds.) Springer-Verlag, Berlin, **1970**, pp. 100–109.

Hartung, W. H. Epinephrine and related compounds: influence of structure on physiologic activity. *Chem. Rev.*, **1931**, *9*, 389–465.

James, T. N.; Bear, E. S.; Lang, K. F.; and Green, E. W. Evidence for adrenergic alpha receptor depressant activity in the heart. *Am. J. Physiol.*, **1968**, *215*, 1366–1375.

King, B. D.; Sokoloff, L.; and Wechsler, R. L. The effects of l-epinephrine and l-norepinephrine upon cerebral circulation and metabolism in man. *J. Clin. Invest.*, **1952**, *31*, 273–279.

Konzett, H. Neue broncholytisch hochwirksame Körper der Adrenalinreihe. *Naunyn Schmiedebergs Arch. Exp. Pharmakol. Pathol.*, **1940**, *197*, 27–40.

Krogsgaard, A. R. The effect of intravenously injected reserpine on blood pressure, renal function and sodium excretion. *Acta Med. Scand.*, **1956**, *154*, 41–51.

Lands, A. M.; Arnold, A.; McAuliff, J. P.; Luduena, F. P.; and Brown, T. G., Jr. Differentiation of receptor systems activated by sympathomimetic amines. *Nature*, **1967a**, *214*, 597–598.

Lands, A. M.; Luduena, F. P.; and Buzzo, H. J. Differentiation of receptors responsive to isoproterenol. *Life Sci.,* **1967b,** *6,* 2241–2249.

Lefkowitz, R. J., and Williams, L. T. Molecular mechanisms of activation and desensitization of adenylate cyclase coupled β-adrenergic receptors. *Adv. Cyclic Nucleotide Res.,* **1978,** *9,* 1–18.

Levy, B., and Wilkenfeld, B. E. An analysis of selective beta receptor blockade. *Eur. J. Pharmacol.,* **1969,** *5,* 227–234.

Liggins, G. C., and Vaughan, G. S. Intravenous infusion of salbutamol in the management of premature labour. *J. Obstet. Gynaecol. Br. Commonw.,* **1973,** *80,* 29–33.

Lockett, M. Dangerous effects of isoprenaline in myocardial failure. *Lancet,* **1965,** *2,* 104–106.

Manley, E. S., and Lawson, J. W. Effect of beta adrenergic receptor blockade on skeletal muscle vasodilatation produced by isoxsuprine and nylidrin. *Arch. Int. Pharmacodyn. Ther.,* **1968,** *175,* 239–250.

Minneman, K. P.; Hegstrand, L. R.; and Molinoff, P. B. Simultaneous determination of beta-1 and beta-2 adrenergic receptors in tissues containing both receptor subtypes. *Mol. Pharmacol.,* **1979,** *15,* 286–298.

Moore, K. E.; Carr, L. A.; and Dominic, J. A. Functional significance of amphetamine-induced release of brain catecholamines. In, *Amphetamines and Related Compounds.* (Costa, E., and Garattini, S., eds.) Raven Press, New York, **1970,** pp. 371–384.

Musacchio, J. M.; Kopin, I. J.; and Weise, V. K. Subcellular distribution of some sympathomimetic amines and their β-hydroxylated derivatives in the rat heart. *J. Pharmacol. Exp. Ther.,* **1965,** *148,* 22–28.

Oliver, G., and Schäfer, E. A. The physiological effects of extracts from the suprarenal capsules. *J. Physiol. (Lond.),* **1895,** *18,* 230–276.

Perkins, J. P.; Johnson, G. L.; and Harden, T. K. Drug-induced modification of the responsiveness of adenylate cyclase to hormones. *Adv. Cyclic Nucleotide Res.,* **1978,** *9,* 19–31.

Piness, G.; Miller, H.; and Alles, G. A. Clinical observations on phenylaminoethanol sulphate. *J.A.M.A.,* **1930,** *94,* 790–791.

Prinzmetal, M., and Bloomberg, W. The use of BENZEDRINE for the treatment of narcolepsy. *J.A.M.A.,* **1935,** *105,* 2051–2054.

Rech, R. H. Antagonism of reserpine behavioral depression by *d*-amphetamine. *J. Pharmacol. Exp. Ther.,* **1964,** *146,* 369–376.

Reichgott, M. J., and Melmon, K. L. The role of corticosteroids in the treatment of shock. In, *Steroid Therapy.* (Azarnoff, D. L., ed.) W. B. Saunders Co., Philadelphia, **1975,** pp. 118–133.

Riederer, P.; Youdim, M. B. H.; Birkmayer, W.; and Jellinger, K. Monoamine oxidase activity during (−)-deprenil therapy: human brain postmortem studies. *Adv. Biochem. Psychopharmacol.,* **1978,** *19,* 377–382.

Schild, H. O. Effect of adrenaline on depolarized smooth muscle. In, *Adrenergic Mechanisms* (a Ciba Foundation symposium). (Vane, J. R.; Wolstenholme, G. E. W.; and O'Connor, M.; eds.) Little, Brown & Co., Boston; J. & A. Churchill, Ltd., London, **1960,** pp. 288–292.

Singer, D. H.; Lazzara, R.; and Hoffman, B. F. Interrelationships between automaticity and conduction in Purkinje fibers. *Circ. Res.,* **1967,** *21,* 537–558.

Smith, C. B. Enhancement by reserpine and α-methyl-dopa of the effects of *d*-amphetamine upon the locomotor activity of mice. *J. Pharmacol. Exp. Ther.,* **1963,** *142,* 343–350.

———. The role of monoaminoxidase in the intraneuronal metabolism of norepinephrine released by indirectly-acting sympathomimetic amines or by adrenergic nerve stimulation. *Ibid,* **1966,** *151,* 207–220.

Smythe, C. McC.; Nickel, J. F.; and Bradley, S. E. The effect of epinephrine (USP), *l*-epinephrine and *l*-norepinephrine on glomerular filtration rate, renal plasma flow

and the urinary excretion of sodium, potassium and water in normal man. *J. Clin. Invest.,* **1952,** *31,* 499–506.

Snyder, S. H. How amphetamine acts in minimal brain dysfunction. *Ann. N.Y. Acad. Sci.,* **1973,** *205,* 310–320.

Sonnenblick, E. H.; Frishman, W. H.; and LeJemtel, T. H. Dobutamine: a new synthetic cardioactive sympathetic amine. *N. Engl. J. Med.,* **1979,** *300,* 17–22.

Spoerel, W. E.; Seleny, F. L.; and Williamson, R. D. Shock caused by continuous infusion of metaraminol bitartrate (ARAMINE). *Can. Med. Assoc. J.,* **1964,** *90,* 349–353.

Starke, K. Influence of alpha receptor stimulants on noradrenaline release. *Naturwissenschaften,* **1971,** *58,* 420.

———. Alpha-sympathomimetic inhibition of adrenergic and cholinergic transmission in the rabbit heart. *Naunyn Schmiedebergs Arch. Pharmakol.,* **1972,** *274,* 18–45.

Starke, K., and Altmann, K. P. Inhibition of adrenergic neurotransmission by clonidine: an action on prejunctional α-receptors. *Neuropharmacology,* **1973,** *12,* 339–347.

Starke, K.; Endo, T.; and Taube, H. D. Relative pre- and postsynaptic potencies of alpha adrenoceptor agonists in the rabbit pulmonary artery. *Naunyn Schmiedebergs Arch. Pharmacol.,* **1975,** *291,* 55–78.

Stolley, P. D. Asthma mortality—why the United States was spared an epidemic of deaths due to asthma. *Am. Rev. Respir. Dis.,* **1972,** *105,* 883–890.

Tainter, M. L., and Chang, D. K. The antagonism of the pressor action of tyramine by cocaine. *J. Pharmacol. Exp. Ther.,* **1927,** *30,* 193–207.

Tolbert, M. E. M.; Butcher, F. R.; and Fain, J. N. Lack of correlation between catecholamine effects of cyclic adenosine 3′:5′-monophosphate and gluconeogenesis in isolated rat liver cells. *J. Biol. Chem.,* **1973,** *248,* 5686–5692.

Trendelenburg, U.; Muskus, A.; Fleming, W. W.; and de la Sierra, B. G. A. Modification by reserpine of the action of sympathomimetic amines in spinal cats: a classification of sympathomimetic amines. *J. Pharmacol. Exp. Ther.,* **1962,** *138,* 170–180.

Tuttle, R. R.; Hillman, C. C.; and Toomey, R. E. Differential β adrenergic sensitivity of atrial and ventricular tissue assessed by chronotropic, inotropic, and cyclic AMP responses to isoprenaline and dobutamine. *Cardiovasc. Res.,* **1976,** *10,* 452–458.

Tuttle, R. R., and Mills, J. Dobutamine: development of a new catecholamine to selectively increase cardiac contractility. *Circ. Res.,* **1975,** *36,* 185–196.

Vliet, P. D. V.; Burchell, H. B.; and Titus, J. L. Focal myocarditis associated with pheochromocytoma. *N. Engl. J. Med.,* **1966,** *274,* 1102–1108.

Vree, T. B.; Muskens, A. T. J. M.; and van Rossum, J. M. Some physicochemical properties of amphetamine and related drugs. *J. Pharm. Pharmacol.,* **1969,** *21,* 774–775.

Wallace, R. L.; Caldwell, D. L.; Ansbacher, R.; and Otterson, W. N. Inhibition of premature labor by terbutaline. *Obstet. Gynecol.,* **1978,** *51,* 387–392.

Webb-Johnson, D. C., and Andrews, J. L. Bronchodilator therapy. *N. Engl. J. Med.,* **1977,** *297,* 476–482.

Wolfe, J. D.; Tashkin, D. P.; Calvarese, B.; and Simmons, M. Bronchodilator effects of terbutaline and aminophylline alone and in combination in asthmatic patients. *N. Engl. J. Med.,* **1978,** *298,* 363–367.

Yamaguchi, N.; DeChamplain, J.; and Nadeau, R. A. Regulation of norepinephrine release from cardiac sympathetic fibers in the dog by presynaptic alpha and beta receptors. *Circ. Res.,* **1977,** *41,* 108–117.

Monographs and Reviews

Allwood, M. J.; Cobbold, A. F.; and Ginsburg, J. Peripheral vascular effects of noradrenaline, isopropylnoradrenaline and dopamine. *Br. Med. Bull.,* **1963,** *19,* 132–136.

Angrist, B. M., and Gershon, S. Psychiatric sequelae of amphetamine use. In, *Psychiatric Complications of Medical Drugs.* (Shader, R. I. ed.) Raven Press, New York, **1972,** pp. 175–199.

Aviado, D. M., Jr. Cardiovascular effects of some commonly used pressor amines. *Anesthesiology,* **1959,** *20,* 71–97. (228 references.)

———. *Sympathomimetic Drugs.* Charles C Thomas, Pub., Springfield, Ill., **1970.**

Bellet, S. Mechanism and treatment of A-V heart block and Adams-Stokes syndrome. *Prog. Cardiovasc. Dis.,* **1960,** *2,* 691–705.

Berthelsen, S., and Pettinger, W. A. A functional basis for classification of α-adrenergic receptors. *Life Sci.,* **1977,** *21,* 595–606.

Bowman, W. C., and Nott, M. W. Actions of sympathomimetic amines and their antagonists on skeletal muscle. *Pharmacol. Rev.,* **1969,** *21,* 27–72.

Chen, K. K., and Schmidt, C. F. Ephedrine and related substances. *Medicine (Baltimore),* **1930,** *9,* 1–117.

Daniel, E. E.; Paton, D. M.; Taylor, G. S.; and Hodgson, B. J. Adrenergic receptors for catecholamine effects on tissue electrolytes. *Fed. Proc.,* **1970,** *29,* 1410–1425.

Dempsey, P. J., and Cooper, T. Pharmacology of the coronary circulation. *Annu. Rev. Pharmacol.,* **1972,** *12,* 99–110.

Eckstein, J. W., and Abboud, F. M. Circulatory effects of sympathomimetic amines. *Am. Heart J.,* **1962,** *63,* 119–135.

Furchgott, R. F. The classification of adrenoceptors (adrenergic receptors). An evaluation from the standpoint of receptor theory. In, *Catecholamines.* (Blaschko, H., and Muscholl, E., eds.) *Handbuch der Experimentellen Pharmakologie,* Vol. 33. Springer-Verlag, Berlin, **1972,** pp. 283–335.

Furness, J. B., and Burnstock, G. Role of circulating catecholamines in the gastrointestinal tract. In, *Adrenal Gland,* Vol. 6. Sect. 7, *Endocrinology. Handbook of Physiology.* (Blaschko, H.; Sayers, G.; and Smith A. D.; eds.) American Physiological Society, Washington, D. C., **1975,** pp. 515–536.

Goldberg, L. I. Cardiovascular and renal actions of dopamine: potential clinical applications. *Pharmacol. Rev.,* **1972,** *24,* 1–29.

Goldberg, L. I.; Hsieh, Y.-Y.; and Resnekov, L. Newer catecholamines for treatment of heart failure and shock; an update on dopamine and a first look at dobutamine. *Prog. Cardiovasc. Dis.,* **1977,** *19,* 327–340.

Grant, W. M. Action of drugs on movement of ocular fluids. *Annu. Rev. Pharmacol.,* **1969,** *9,* 85–94.

Greenway, C. V., and Stark, R. D. Hepatic vascular bed. *Physiol. Rev.,* **1971,** *51,* 23–65.

Gregg, D. E., and Fisher, L. C. Blood supply to the heart. In, *Circulation,* Vol. 2. Sect. 2, *The Cardiovascular System. Handbook of Physiology.* (Hamilton, W. F., ed.) American Physiological Society, Washington, D. C., **1963,** pp. 1517–1584.

Himms-Hagen, J. Sympathetic regulation of metabolism. *Pharmacol. Rev.,* **1967,** *19,* 367–461.

———. Effects of catecholamines on metabolism. In, *Catecholamines.* (Blaschko, H., and Muscholl, E., eds.)

Handbuch der Experimentellen Pharmakologie, Vol. 33. Springer-Verlag, Berlin, **1972,** pp. 363–462.

Houslay, M. D., and Tipton, K. F. Multiple forms of monoamine oxidase; fact and artefact. *Life Sci.,* **1976,** *19,* 467–478.

Kopin, I. J. False adrenergic transmitters. *Annu. Rev. Pharmacol.,* **1968,** *8,* 377–394.

Langer, S. Z. Presynaptic receptors and their role in the regulation of transmitter release. *Br. J. Pharmacol.,* **1977,** *60,* 481–497.

Marshall, J. M. Effects of catecholamines on the smooth muscle of the female reproductive tract. *Annu. Rev. Pharmacol.,* **1973,** *13,* 19–32.

Oswald, I. Drugs and sleep. *Pharmacol. Rev.,* **1968,** *20,* 273–303. (134 references.)

Porte, D., Jr., and Robertson, R. P. Control of insulin secretion by catecholamines, stress, and the sympathetic nervous system. *Fed. Proc.,* **1973,** *32,* 1792–1796.

Sharman, D. F. The catabolism of catecholamines: recent studies. *Br. Med. Bull.,* **1973,** *29,* 110–115.

Somlyo, A. P., and Somlyo, A. V. Vascular smooth muscles. I. Normal structure, pathology, biochemistry and biophysics. *Pharmacol. Rev.,* **1968,** *20,* 197–272.

Sroufe, L. A., and Stewart, M. A. Treating problem children with stimulant drugs. *N. Engl. J. Med.,* **1973,** *289,* 407–413.

Starke, K. Regulation of noradrenaline release by presynaptic receptor systems. *Rev. Physiol. Biochem. Pharmacol.,* **1977,** *77,* 1–124.

Toman, J. E. P., and Davis, J. P. The effects of drugs upon the electrical activity of the brain. *Pharmacol. Rev.,* **1949,** *1,* 425–492.

Trendelenburg, U. Factors influencing the concentration of catecholamines at the receptors. In, *Catecholamines.* (Blaschko, H., and Muscholl, E., eds.) *Handbuch der Experimentellen Pharmakologie,* Vol. 33. Springer-Verlag, Berlin, **1972,** pp. 726–761.

Weiner, N. Regulation of norepinephrine synthesis. *Annu. Rev. Pharmacol.,* **1970,** *10,* 273–290.

———. Pharmacology of central nervous system stimulants. In, *Drug Abuse: Proceedings of the International Conference.* (Zarafonetis, C. J. D., ed.) Lea & Febiger, Philadelphia, **1972,** pp. 243–251.

———. The role of cyclic nucleotides in the regulation of neurotransmitter release from adrenergic neurons by neuromodulators. In, *Essays in Neurochemistry and Neuropharmacology,* Vol. 4. (Youdim, M. B. H.; Lovenberg, W.; Sharman, D. F.; and Lagnado, J. R.; eds.) John Wiley & Sons, Inc., New York, **1980,** pp. 69–124.

Weiss, B., and Laties, V. G. Enhancement of human performance by caffeine and the amphetamines. *Pharmacol. Rev.,* **1962,** *14,* 1–36. (118 references.)

Zaimis, E. Vasopressor drugs and catecholamines. *Anesthesiology,* **1968,** *29,* 732–762. (162 references.)

Zoll, P. M., and Linenthal, A. J. A program for Stokes-Adams disease and cardiac arrest. *Circulation,* **1963,** *27,* 1–4.

9 DRUGS THAT INHIBIT ADRENERGIC NERVES AND BLOCK ADRENERGIC RECEPTORS

Norman Weiner

Many substances of diverse structure and mechanism of action interfere with the function of the sympathetic nervous system. Several such drugs are extremely valuable in clinical medicine, particularly for the control of hypertension and cardiac disorders.

Certain drugs, termed *adrenergic neuron blocking agents,* interfere with the release of norepinephrine consequent to nerve stimulation. They may produce this effect by inhibition of the synthesis, storage, or release of the neurotransmitter. Irrespective of the precise mechanism, the consequence of these effects is a reduction in the amount of norepinephrine released by each nerve impulse. Such agents do not interfere significantly with the actions of circulating or exogenous catecholamines or other sympathomimetic amines that act directly on postsynaptic adrenergic receptors. Since the physiology and pharmacology of peripheral adrenergic neurons that innervate different organs are quite similar, drugs that interfere with adrenergic neuronal function affect all peripheral adrenergic neurons in a similar manner. A subgroup of this class of agents, of which clonidine and methyldopa are members, inhibits sympathetic nervous activity by reducing impulse traffic from sympathetic centers in the brain that modulate the activity of peripheral sympathetic neurons.

Other drugs, *adrenergic receptor blocking agents,* inhibit the ability of the neurotransmitter or other sympathomimetic amines to interact effectively with their receptors. Since the pharmacological sensitivities of adrenergic receptors vary considerably, these agents may interfere selectively with the different responses that are normally mediated by the sympathetic nervous system. For example, selective blockers of β_1-adrenergic receptors antagonize the actions of epinephrine and norepinephrine on the heart but do not block vasoconstrictor responses mediated by α receptors.

A knowledge of autonomic physiology and the sites of action of drugs that interfere with sympathetic function is essential for understanding of the pharmacology and clinical uses of these important classes of drugs. The appropriate background is presented in Chapters 4 and 8.

Side Effects Common to Agents That Interfere with the Function of Sympathetic Neurons. The sympathetic nervous system is intimately involved in the modulation of a host of homeostatic mechanisms. Interference with its functions impairs the capacity of the organism to generate appropriate physiological responses that are required to react to adverse or provocative environmental inputs. As a consequence, a number of effects that are associated with the administration of such blocking agents are predictable. Since many of the side effects caused by these drugs are common to all agents that interfere with sympathetic function, they can be discussed collectively. Exceptions will be mentioned at this point and explained in more detail in the discussion of the individual drugs.

Postural Hypotension. Hypotension, and particularly postural hypotension, is a common effect of agents that interfere with sympathetic function. The sympathetic nervous system is critically involved in the regulation of blood pressure, particularly by modulation of vasomotor tone and cardiac rate and contractility. Venous tone is under the control of the sympathetic nervous system, and, if this regulation is impaired, blood pools in the capacitance vessels when the erect position is assumed. Thus, postural hypotension is particularly troublesome in individuals with minimal sympathetic nervous system function. Postural hypotension is especially common with adrenergic neuron blocking agents such as guanethidine and methyldopa and with α-adrenergic blocking agents.

Sedation or Depression. Agents that interfere with adrenergic function in the central nervous system (CNS) frequently cause sedation or depression. Locomotor activity, alertness, and affect appear to be importantly regulated by central noradrenergic neurons (*see* Chapter 12). Agents that interfere with peripheral adrenergic function and that are sufficiently lipophilic to enter the CNS may therefore be expected to produce behavioral effects. Drugs of this type include reserpine, methyldopa, phenoxybenzamine, and clonidine. The effects of guanethidine on the CNS are minimal, since this very polar compound does not gain access to central adrenergic neurons to any significant degree.

Monoamine oxidase (MAO) inhibitors, which interfere with peripheral sympathetic nervous system function, enhance affect and stimulate psychomotor activity by a central mechanism; several factors appear to contribute. The rates of synthesis and release of catecholamines appear to be considerably greater in the CNS than in the periphery. It is likely that inhibition of the metabolism of catecholamines is more significant when their rate of turnover is more rapid. Furthermore, interference with peripheral adrenergic activity by MAO inhibitors is hypothesized to be due to the accumulation of false neurotransmitters derived from dietary amines such as tyramine (*see* Chapter 8); penetration of tyramine into the CNS is not nearly as rapid as it is into peripheral adrenergic neurons.

Increased Gastrointestinal Motility and Diarrhea. Sympathomimetic agents inhibit gastrointestinal function by two mechanisms. β-Adrenergic agonists cause relaxation of intestinal smooth muscle directly; α agonists act presynaptically to inhibit the release of neurotransmitter from cholinergic neurons in the intestinal wall (Chapter 8; Furness and Burnstock, 1975). Thus, it is to be expected that agents that interfere with sympathetic function would increase gastrointestinal motility and cause diarrhea. These side effects are seen particularly with drugs such as reserpine, methyldopa, and guanethidine.

Impaired Ability to Ejaculate. Contraction of the vas deferens and other accessory reproductive organs is mediated by the sympathetic nervous system, and agents that interfere with sympathetic function will thus inhibit ejaculation. This problem is most frequent when the more powerful adrenergic neuron blocking agents, such as guanethidine and methyldopa, are administered.

Increased Blood Volume and Sodium Retention. Hypotension can cause a reduction of renal blood flow. If the rate of glomerular filtration is reduced, more complete reabsorption of sodium and water can occur, and there will be an increase in the volume of blood and extracellular fluid. These effects tend to negate the reduction in blood pressure and may account for the tolerance to their hypotensive effect that sometimes develops. Retention of sodium is particularly prominent with the more powerful hypotensive agents, such as guanethidine and methyldopa. This side effect accounts for one of the attributes of the concomitant use of a diuretic agent in the treatment of hypertension (*see* Chapters 32 and 36).

Nasal Stuffiness. This is an annoying side effect that is common to agents that block either adrenergic neurons or α receptors. It is due to vasodilatation in the mucous membranes of the nasopharynx.

Extrapyramidal Symptoms. Symptoms of akinesia, rigidity, and tremor, characteristic of Parkinson's disease, are commonly caused by agents that enter the CNS and interfere with sympathetic nervous function by a presynaptic mechanism. These alterations are presumably due to inhibitory effects on dopaminergic neurons. Reserpine and methyldopa commonly produce such side effects.

Side Effects Limited to α-Adrenergic Blocking Agents. Agents that interfere with sympathetic function by blockade of α receptors cause most of the side effects listed above, with the exception of extrapyramidal symptoms. In addition, reflex tachycardia is an important side effect of such drugs. Postural hypotension with reflex stimulation of the sympathetic nervous system results in tachycardia and increased myocardial contractility, effects mediated by β receptors and not blocked by α-adrenergic antagonists. In addition, many α blocking agents that act at postsynaptic (α_1) receptors also inhibit presynaptic (α_2) receptors; this results in enhanced output of norepinephrine per nerve impulse and presumably intensifies the effects of reflex sympathetic stimulation on the heart. Phentolamine and phenoxybenzamine produce this presynaptic effect, whereas prazosin is relatively ineffective in blocking presynaptic α_2 receptors. Prazosin is thus less likely to cause reflex tachycardia.

Side Effects Limited to β-Adrenergic Blocking Agents. The side effects common to β-adrenergic blocking agents are largely restricted to the cardiovascular and respiratory systems and to alterations of metabolism. Bradycardia and reduced cardiac output are important changes, particularly when the contractility of the myocardium is already impaired; congestive heart failure may be precipitated. Sensitivity to insulin and oral hypoglycemic drugs is also associated with the administration of β blockers, since glycogenolysis in muscle and, in some species, in liver is mediated by β receptors. Bronchoconstriction is a common side effect of β_2-blocking drugs and nonselective β-adrenergic antagonists, particularly in patients with pulmonary disease.

Epinephrine, which is secreted by the adrenal medulla, is an important physiological bronchodilator. The release of catecholamines from the adrenal medulla is not greatly affected by the usual doses of adrenergic neuron blocking agents. Thus, drugs that interfere with the function of the sympathetic nervous system by a presynaptic mechanism but do not affect secretion of epinephrine by the adrenal medulla do not interfere to any significant extent with the compensatory mechanisms that are evoked by bronchoconstriction or hypoglycemia.

I. α-Adrenergic Blocking Agents

α-Adrenergic blocking agents bind selectively to the α class of adrenergic receptors and thereby interfere with the capacity of sympathomimetic amines to initiate actions at these sites. Phenoxybenzamine and dibenamine bind covalently to the α receptor and produce an irreversible and insurmountable type of blockade. Phentolamine, tolazoline, and prazosin bind reversibly and antagonize the actions of sympathomimetic amines competitively.

There are prominent differences in the relative abilities of α-adrenergic blocking agents to antagonize the effects of sympathomimetic amines at the two subtypes of α receptors. Phenoxybenzamine is approximately 100-fold more potent in blocking α_1 (postsynaptic) receptors than α_2 receptors that modulate neural release of transmitter (presumed presynaptic receptors). Prazosin is also a highly selective α_1-blocking agent, while phentolamine is only three to five times more potent in inhibiting α_1- than α_2-adrenergic receptors. In contrast, yohimbine is a selective α_2 blocker and has been shown to prevent the antihypertensive effects of clonidine (Starke *et al.*, 1975; Langer, 1977).

PHENOXYBENZAMINE AND RELATED HALOALKYLAMINES

Phenoxybenzamine and *dibenamine* are haloalkylamines with a relatively specific capability to interact with and block α-adrenergic receptors; they have no α-adrenergic agonistic activity (Nickerson and Goodman, 1947). Phenoxybenzamine is the compound most commonly used at the present time and the only member of the series that has been

studied extensively in man. It is six to ten times as potent as dibenamine and is somewhat better absorbed after oral administration.

Chemistry. Dibenamine is N,N-dibenzyl-β-chloroethylamine, and phenoxybenzamine differs from it only in the replacement of one benzyl group by a phenoxyisopropyl moiety. Their structural formulas are as follows:

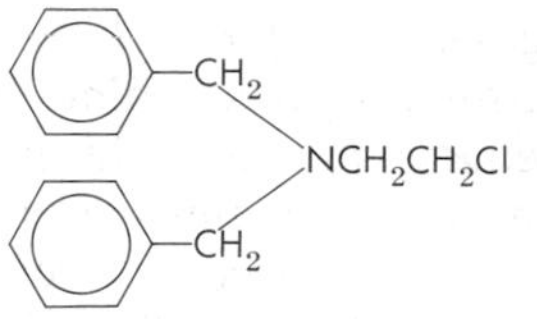

Dibenamine

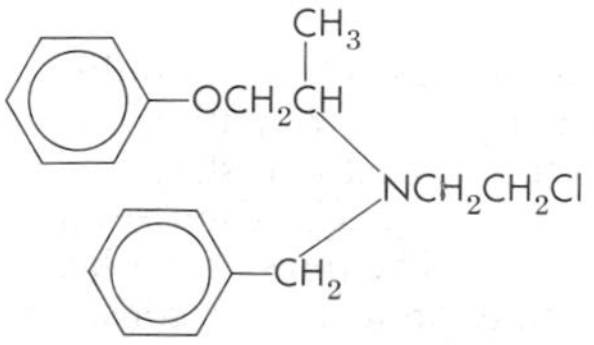

Phenoxybenzamine

The haloalkylamine adrenergic blocking agents are closely related chemically to the nitrogen mustards; like the latter, the tertiary amine cyclizes to form a reactive ethylenimonium intermediate (Chapter 55). The molecular configuration directly responsible for blockade is probably a highly reactive carbonium ion formed when the three-membered ring breaks. The relatively slow onset of action, even after intravenous administration, is probably due to the time required for the formation of these reactive intermediates, which can then alkylate various biological materials. It is presumed that the arylalkyl amine moiety of the molecule is responsible for the relative specificity of action of these agents, since the reactive intermediate can presumably react with sulfhydryl, amino, and hydroxy groups on many macromolecules. The major structural requirements for production of the characteristic nonequilibrium blockade have been reviewed by Nickerson and Gump (1949) and Graham (1962).

Locus and Mechanism of Action. α-Adrenergic blockade is due to a direct action of these drugs on α receptors and is independent of any effects on adrenergic neurons or on the basic response mechanisms of effector cells. β-Adrenergic receptors are not affected by conventional doses of any α-blocking agent in current use.

The presence of a catecholamine or an α-adrenergic blocking agent of the competitive type during development of blockade by a haloalkylamine can decrease the degree of block attained (Nickerson and Gump, 1949; Furchgott, 1954). This appears to involve a competition for the same population of receptors, and indicates that the initial binding of the haloalkylamine to its site of action is due to the same relatively weak forces (ionic, hydrogen bond, etc.) involved in the actions of most agonists and of adrenergic blocking agents of most other chemical classes (competitive antagonists). After blockade by a haloalkylamine has fully developed, it is unaffected by exposure to another drug capable of interacting with the same receptors. This stage is referred to as *nonequilibrium blockade* and is the result of formation of a stable covalent bond between the antagonist and the receptor (Nickerson, 1957).

While it was anticipated that a radioactive haloalkylamine could be used to label the α-adrenergic receptor selectively to facilitate its identification and purification, this has not been possible because of reaction of such compounds with many other macromolecules. However, more selective (although noncovalently binding) radioactive ligands such as (^{3}H)dihydroergocryptine have been used successfully to quantify and characterize α-adrenergic receptors in various tissues (Newman *et al.*, 1978; Tsai and Lefkowitz, 1978).

In addition to producing postsynaptic α-adrenergic blockade, the haloalkylamines, and to varying degrees other classes of α-blocking agents, exert important effects on the metabolism of catecholamines. Phenoxybenzamine increases the rate of turnover of norepinephrine in the periphery, which is associated with increased tyrosine hydroxylase activity. In intact animals, these effects are probably predominantly due to increased sympathetic nerve activity, a reflex response to α-adrenergic blockade, since the effect can be inhibited by ganglionic blocking agents (Mueller *et al.*, 1970). Phenoxybenzamine and other α-blocking agents also increase the amount of neurotransmitter released by each nerve impulse. This appears to be due to blockade of presynaptic α_2 receptors, which mediate a negative feedback mechanism that inhibits the release of norepinephrine (Potter *et al.*, 1971; Cubeddu *et al.*, 1974b; Langer, 1977; Starke, 1977; Weiner, 1980). There is a parallel increase in the output of both norepinephrine and dopamine β-hydroxylase, implicating the facilitation of exocytosis in the mechanism (Cubeddu *et al.*, 1974b).

Phenoxybenzamine and many congeners inhibit the uptake of catecholamines into both adrenergic nerve terminals and extraneuronal tissues (Cubeddu *et al.*, 1974a). The ratios of effectiveness against these two processes vary considerably among members of the series (Iversen *et al.*, 1972).

PHARMACOLOGICAL PROPERTIES

Phenoxybenzamine and dibenamine effectively inhibit responses that are mediated by α-adrenergic agonists. Thus, α-receptor-mediated excitatory responses of smooth muscle and exocrine glands are antagonized (Table 4–1, page 60). While the *actions* of all

sympathomimetic agents that stimulate α receptors are inhibited essentially to the same extent, the *net effects* of different sympathomimetic amines on a complex parameter such as blood pressure may be antagonized to very different degrees because of different effects of these agonists on other receptors. For example, a dose of phenoxybenzamine that completely eliminates the pressor response to epinephrine or converts it to a depressor response may produce only a partial inhibition of the pressor response to norepinephrine. Epinephrine produces both vasoconstriction and vasodilatation, and moderate inhibition of the former may allow the latter to predominate; norepinephrine, on the other hand, has very little vasodilator action, and all of the residual constriction is manifested in the pressor response. It should also be noted that the effects of any blocking agent are highly dependent on the level of activity of the system on which it acts. Thus, the vasodilatation induced by phenoxybenzamine may vary markedly in different vascular beds, depending on their degree of adrenergic vasomotor tone, and may vary over a wide range in a single vascular bed, depending on its physiological state (*see* Nickerson and Hollenberg, 1967).

Blockade by most haloalkylamines develops relatively slowly, and the peak effect is usually not attained in less than an hour after intravenous administration. The blockade produced by a single dose of dibenamine or phenoxybenzamine disappears with a half-life of roughly 24 hours in intact laboratory animals and man. Demonstrable effects thus persist for at least 3 or 4 days, and the effects of daily administration are cumulative for nearly a week.

Many tissues appear to contain receptors in excess of the number required for a full response to most agonists ("spare receptors"), and a considerable proportion can be inactivated irreversibly before the tissue is incapable of a maximal response (*see* Chapter 2). With increasing doses of the blocking agent, the dose-response curve for an agonist is shifted progressively to the right as the number of available receptors is reduced. When the number of functional receptors is reduced to the degree that the original maximal response is no longer attainable with a full agonist, the dose-response curve does not shift further to the right; additional receptor blockade now causes a depression of the maximal response. The reduction in maximal response then is proportional to the further irreversible blockade of the remaining receptors. Many aspects of the general pharmacology of the haloalkylamines are reviewed by Graham (1962), Nickerson and Hollenberg (1967), and Furchgott (1972).

In addition to the blockade of α-adrenergic receptors, the haloalkylamines can inhibit responses to 5-hydroxytryptamine (5-HT, serotonin), histamine, and acetylcholine (ACh). Blockade of these other types of agonists has the same general pharmacological characteristics as does the adrenergic blockade. Although nonequilibrium blockade of responses to histamine and 5-HT requires the same basic chemical configuration as does α-adrenergic blocking activity and the same intermediate transformations are probably involved, potency with respect to these properties varies considerably. For example, dibenamine has relatively low antihistaminic activity, whereas phenoxybenzamine is as potent in this regard as many of the antihistamines now employed clinically. Effective blockade of responses to ACh usually requires relatively high doses of haloalkylamine.

Cardiovascular System. *Blood Pressure.* The usual blocking dose of phenoxybenzamine (1.0 mg/kg in man) or of dibenamine infused slowly intravenously into healthy, recumbent, normovolemic subjects causes little change in systemic blood pressure, although the diastolic pressure tends to fall somewhat. However, a sharp drop may occur in any situation involving compensatory sympathetic vasoconstriction, such as upright posture or hypovolemia. Thus, a prominent effect of the blockade is *postural hypotension.* In addition, impairment of compensatory vasoconstriction sensitizes to the hypotensive effects of a variety of agents and conditions that tend to produce vasodilatation, including hypercapnia, anesthetic agents, and analgesics such as morphine and meperidine. Rapid injection of a haloalkylamine can cause a precipitous fall in blood pressure, which probably involves factors other than α-adrenergic blockade.
Blood Flows. Phenoxybenzamine produces a prominent and progressive increase in cardiac output and decrease in total peripheral resistance in normal recumbent subjects. However, the changes in blood flow and resistance induced in specific vascular beds vary widely with the conditions under which the blocking agent is administered. In general, the greater the degree of adrenergic vasomotor tone in a vascular bed, the more pronounced is the relaxant effect of the haloalkylamines (*see* Nickerson and Hollenberg, 1967). Cerebral and coronary resistances are not significantly altered by α-adrenergic blockade *per se.* Cerebral flow is little affected unless the blood pressure is greatly reduced, and coronary flow increases in parallel with reflex cardiac stimulation. Phenoxybenzamine increases resting blood flow in muscle and, in a cool environment, enhances cutaneous blood flow. However, sympathetic vasoconstriction exerts little restraint on muscle blood flow during exercise or on cutaneous blood flow in a warm environment, and under these conditions α blockade produces little change. Splanchnic and renal blood flows are not altered remarkably in the normovolemic subject at rest; however, in the presence of the increased adrenergic vasoconstrictor tone induced by circumstances such as hypovolemia or the infusion of norepinephrine, phenoxybenzamine increases flow to a major degree in both these areas. In the kidney, perfusion of the outer cortex is most markedly affected. Pulmonary arteries and veins are also relaxed; however, because of a greater systemic vasodilatation, blood volume in the pulmonary circuit is usually decreased.

Other important effects of haloalkylamines, and of other agents that inhibit sympathetic vasoconstriction, are diversion of a higher percentage of the total blood flow through channels that exchange metabolites effectively with tissue cells ("nutrient channels"), and movement of fluid from the interstitial to the vascular compartment, the result of differential effects on precapillary and postcapillary resistance vessels (Nickerson and Hollenberg, 1967; Hollenberg and Nickerson, 1970).
Responses to Adrenergic Stimuli. Pressor responses to epinephrine and other sympathomimetic amines are blocked or reversed by phenoxybenzamine and dibenamine (Figure 9–1). A reduction in the pressor response without reversal is usually seen when the capacity for adrenergic vasodilatation is limited by any factor, for example, the sympathomimetic amine used (norepinephrine,

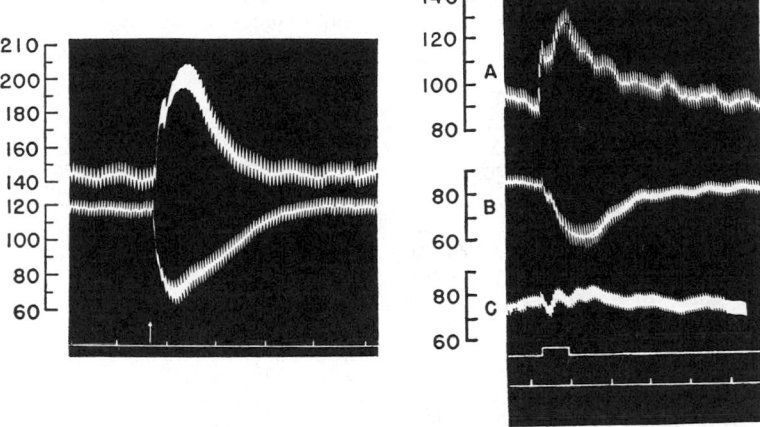

Figure 9-1. *Effect of dibenamine on blood pressure responses of anesthetized cat.*

Left. Responses to a small dose of epinephrine. Upper record before and lower record after intravenous administration of dibenamine (15 mg/kg). The arrow indicates intravenous injections of epinephrine (2.5 μg/kg). The pressor response is converted to depressor by selective blockade of the vasoconstrictor (α-receptor) action of epinephrine, which allows expression of the concurrent vasodilator (β₂-receptor) action. Ordinate, blood pressure in mm Hg; abscissa, time in minutes.

Right. Responses to splanchnic nerve stimulation. *A* before and *B* after dibenamine; *C* after dibenamine and removal of adrenal glands. Ordinate, blood pressure in mm Hg; abscissa, time in minutes. Period of stimulation is indicated by upward deflection of signal line. The initial sharp component of the pressor response in tracing A is due to the local effect of norepinephrine released from sympathetic nerve endings in splanchnic vessels. The subsequent slower component of the rise is predominantly due to catecholamines released from the adrenal medulla. In tracing B each of the two components of the original pressor response is reversed. The initial rapid fall is small. The second, slower component of the reversal represents the vasodilator response to circulating catecholamines, predominantly the effect of epinephrine. After removal of the adrenal glands, only the local (splanchnic) component of the response remains. (After Nickerson and Goodman, 1947. Courtesy of the *Journal of Pharmacology and Experimental Therapeutics.*)

phenylephrine, or other agents with minimal β₂-adrenergic agonistic activity) or the preparation employed (*e.g.*, pithed animals, where vasodilatation is already near maximal).

Many effects induced directly or indirectly by stimulation of α-adrenergic receptors of vascular smooth muscle are prevented by the haloalkylamines. These include the lethal effects of epinephrine and many other sympathomimetic amines, the changes in erythrocyte and leukocyte counts induced by fright or struggle, and the pulmonary lesions resulting from exposure to oxygen at high pressure. Similarly, a number of secondary pathological effects of infused epinephrine or norepinephrine, including pulmonary edema, reduction in plasma volume, accumulation of pericardial fluid, adrenocortical necrosis, and changes in hepatic cells, are effectively blocked.

Cardiac Effects. The chronotropic and inotropic effects of epinephrine, norepinephrine, and direct or reflex sympathetic nerve stimulation on the mammalian myocardium are not inhibited by the haloalkylamines or by other α-adrenergic blocking agents (Nickerson and Chan, 1961). Indeed, the tachycardia in intact animals is usually exaggerated because the pressor response is prevented and reflex vagal stimulation is minimized. Phenoxybenzamine and dibenamine induce reflex tachycardia; this is a characteristic component of the response to peripheral vasodilatation and may be accentuated by enhanced release of norepinephrine and decreased inactivation of the amine due to inhibition of neuronal and extraneuronal uptake mechanisms.

In both laboratory animals and man, haloalkylamines effectively inhibit cardiac arrhythmias that involve catecholamines in their genesis, with or without specific sensitization of the myocardium by drugs such as halogenated anesthetics. Both inhibition of the adrenergic pressor response and a direct blocking effect on the heart are involved, but it is not known if the latter is related to the small component of α-adrenergic receptors that is present in the myocardium. However, arrhythmias following acute coronary artery occlusion or precipitated by hypothermia are not inhibited.

Metabolic Effects. The receptors involved in metabolic responses to catecholamines are predominantly β, but important α-adrenergic actions also participate. The effects of phenoxybenzamine *in vivo* appear particularly complex, primarily because many of the measured responses are composite. For example, agents such as epinephrine stimulate hepatic glycogenolysis (β, in some species) and inhibit insulin secretion (α). However, there is also a weaker β-adrenergic stimulatory effect on insulin secretion. In the presence of phenoxybenzamine, the inhibitory action of epinephrine on insulin secretion is blocked, and the response to β-receptor stimulation and the direct effect of glucose are revealed. The subsequent rise in insulin concentration may facilitate glucose uptake to the extent that hyperglycemia (from glycogenolysis) is obscured. The result is an *apparent* block of the glycogenolytic effect of epinephrine by phenoxybenzamine when, in fact, this is not the case. Phenoxybenzamine does not specifically antagonize the effects of catecholamines on glycogenolysis in muscle, nor does it inhibit catecholamine-augmented lipolysis. In some species, however (*e.g.*, rat), phenoxybenzamine can block the effect of catecholamines on hepatic glycogenolysis. Under some circumstances α-adrenergic blockade can considerably *increase* norepinephrine-induced lipolysis in human adipose tissue. (*See* Himms-Hagen, 1967; Symposium, 1970.)

Central Nervous System. Interest in possible physiological functions of catecholamines in the CNS has led to many studies of the central effects of α-adrenergic blocking agents (*see* Chapter 12).

Dibenamine, phenoxybenzamine, and congeners can stimulate the CNS to cause nausea, vomiting, hyperventilation, motor excitability, and even convulsions, particularly when a relatively large dose is rapidly injected intravenously. In man, a characteristic loss of time perception may occur. These effects develop and terminate much more rapidly than does the blockade, and hydrolysis products of the active agents, which do not block α receptors, are also effective CNS stimulants. Mild-to-moderate sedation commonly results from the slow intravenous infusion of the usual blocking dose of phenoxybenzamine in man, and fatigue and lethargy may accompany oral medication. This sedation is very similar to that produced by drugs that appear to activate central α receptors (*e.g.*, clonidine).

Other Effects. Phenoxybenzamine and dibenamine effectively antagonize the wide variety of responses to endogenous and exogenous sympathomimetic amines that are mediated by α-adrenergic receptors. Stimulation of the radial fibers of the iris is readily blocked, and miosis is a prominent component of the response to phenoxybenzamine by man, but accommodation is not significantly affected. Contractions of the nictitating membrane, retractor penis, arrector pili, and the uterus of several species are inhibited. Motility of the nonpregnant human uterus *in situ* is reduced and stimulation by norepinephrine is prevented (Wansbrough *et al.*, 1968). Estrogen-induced tubal block of ovum transport is inhibited in rabbits, and it is of interest that the circular fibers of the human tubal isthmus have a particularly dense adrenergic innervation (Owman *et al.*, 1967). However, phenoxybenzamine and estrogen have very similar central effects in inhibiting the secretion of luteinizing hormone (LH) in ovariectomized monkeys (Bhattacharya *et al.*, 1972). Salivary secretion of water and electrolytes evoked by cervical sympathetic nerve stimulation or injected sympathomimetic drugs is blocked. The volume and enzyme content of pancreatic exocrine secretion are increased by α- and decreased by β-adrenergic blockade. The limited adrenergic sweating observed in man, particularly of the hands and axillae, is also blocked.

Inasmuch as the predominantly inhibitory effects of sympathomimetic agents on the gastrointestinal tract are mediated by α as well as by β receptors, combined α- and β-adrenergic blockade is usually required to inhibit completely relaxation by epinephrine or norepinephrine. A very limited overall effect of α-adrenergic blockade on gastrointestinal function is indicated by the fact that dibenamine and phenoxybenzamine do not appreciably alter the rate of passage of barium sulfate through the human gastrointestinal tract.

Absorption, Fate, and Excretion. Haloalkylamine adrenergic blocking agents are effective when administered by all routes, but injection should be only intravenously because of their irritant properties. Absorption from the gastrointestinal tract is incomplete and somewhat capricious; 20 to 30% of orally administered phenoxybenzamine appears to be absorbed in active form.

Phenoxybenzamine has a high lipid solubility at body pH, and accumulation in fat may occur after large doses. The metabolic fate of these highly unstable agents is poorly understood. Over 50% of the radioactivity of intravenously administered phenoxybenzamine is excreted in 12 hours and over 80% in 24 hours, but small amounts remain in various tissues for at least a week.

Preparations, Routes of Administration, and Dosage. *Phenoxybenzamine Hydrochloride*, U.S.P. (DIBENZYLINE), is available for *oral* use in 10-mg capsules; ampuls for intravenous use (100 mg of the drug in 2 ml) are available for investigational purposes. The oral dose usually varies between 20 and 60 mg per day, and full dosage should be approached incrementally. When administered *intravenously,* phenoxybenzamine must be well diluted and infused slowly. Most commonly a dose of 1.0 mg/kg is diluted in 250 to 500 ml of 5% glucose or 0.9% sodium chloride solution and infused over a period of at least 1 hour.

Toxicity, Side Effects, and Precautions. Untoward effects of phenoxybenzamine are largely due to the blockade of α-adrenergic receptors. Loss of vasomotor control can result in postural hypotension and reflex tachycardia in ambulatory patients, or a sharp fall in blood pressure in those who are hypovolemic. The postural hypotension and palpitation may disappear despite continued blockade, but can reappear under conditions that promote vasodilatation, such as exercise, eating a large meal, or consuming alcohol. Because of the danger of severe hypotension when the drug is administered in the presence of hypovolemia, intravenous administration must be slow, the patient must be kept under constant observation, and blood or an appropriate plasma-volume expander must be on hand to correct any deficit revealed by the hemodynamic response. Inhibition of compensatory vasoconstriction also exaggerates the depressor effects of opioids and other agents that act directly to relax vascular smooth muscle. Other results of α-receptor blockade include miosis, nasal stuffiness, and inhibition of ejaculation. Effects not clearly related to blockade are local tissue irritation, sedation, and a generalized feeling of weakness and tiredness. Local irritation is probably involved in the nausea and occasional vomiting that may follow large oral doses, particularly if administered on an empty stomach.

Therapeutic Uses. The clinical uses of haloalkylamines are discussed below, along with those of other α-adrenergic blocking agents.

PHENTOLAMINE AND TOLAZOLINE

Tolazoline (2-benzyl-2-imidazoline) was first reported in the pharmacological literature as a vasodepressor agent with effects similar to those of histamine. Its α-adrenergic blocking action was noted only during subsequent investigations. *Phentolamine* was introduced later, with particular attention to its α-adrenergic blocking activity.

Chemistry. The 2-substituted imidazolines have a wide range of pharmacological actions, including adrenergic blocking, sympathomimetic, antihypertensive, antihistaminic, histamine-like, and cholinomimetic; slight changes in structure may make one or another of these properties dominant. At the present time, members of the series are marketed for each of the first four properties listed. The structural formulas of *phentolamine* and *tolazoline* are as follows:

Phentolamine

Tolazoline

PHARMACOLOGICAL PROPERTIES

Phentolamine and *tolazoline* produce a moderately effective competitive α-adrenergic blockade that is relatively transient. Responses to 5-HT are also inhibited. These substances have important actions on cardiac and smooth muscle that may be divided into three classes: (1) "sympathomimetic," including cardiac stimulation; (2) "parasympathomimetic," including stimulation of the gastrointestinal tract that is blocked by atropine; and (3) "histamine-like," including stimulation of gastric secretion and peripheral vasodilatation (*see* Nickerson, 1949). Phentolamine is a considerably more potent α-adrenergic blocking agent than is tolazoline, and its other effects are somewhat less prominent.

The usual clinical doses of tolazoline produce very little α-adrenergic blockade, and the block produced by doses of phentolamine that are tolerated by man is far from complete. Tolazoline or phentolamine given intravenously produces vasodilatation and cardiac stimulation; the blood pressure response varies with the relative contributions of the two effects. Phentolamine usually causes a fall in pressure, but the net effect of tolazoline commonly is pressor. Both agents can decrease peripheral resistance and increase venous capacity. The dilatation is predominantly due to a *direct action on vascular smooth muscle* in the dose range now usually employed in man (Taylor *et al.,* 1965). However, high doses of phentolamine can produce a hemodynamic picture characteristic of α-adrenergic blockade (Moyer and Caplovitz, 1953); at this dose level side effects are severe. Pulmonary arterial pressure and vascular resistance are usually reduced by tolazoline or phentolamine. The acute response is variable, but is of considerable magnitude in some patients with elevated pulmonary pressures; significant chronic reductions have not been achieved. A paradoxical increase in pulmonary resistance has been reported, and it has been suggested that these drugs may have a direct vasoconstrictor action that is usually masked (*see* Yoran and Glassman, 1973). Many imidazoline derivatives are partial α-adrenergic agonists. Clonidine, a potent agonist at both α_1 and α_2 receptors, is also an imidazoline derivative.

Therapeutic doses of phentolamine and tolazoline cause cardiac stimulation that is more than just a reflex response to peripheral vasodilatation, and this can be associated with cardiac arrhythmias in both laboratory animals and man (Das and Parratt, 1971). Enhanced neural release of norepinephrine due to presynaptic α_2 blockade may contribute to these effects.

Phentolamine and tolazoline can block many responses that involve α-adrenergic receptors. However, the intrinsic eye muscles are relatively resistant, and in intact laboratory animals and man tolazoline may cause mydriasis rather than miosis. The imidazoline blocking agents stimulate salivary, lacrimal, respiratory tract, and pancreatic secretion, and tolazoline can cause profuse sweating in man. This may be due to a direct action of the drug on muscarinic cholinergic receptors. Tolazoline has been reported to induce secretion from denervated salivary glands. Phentolamine and tolazoline produce hyperperistalsis and diarrhea in laboratory animals and man, effects that are blocked by atropine. Abdominal discomfort is a very common side effect of phentolamine administration. Phentolamine and tolazoline stimulate gastric secretion of both acid and pepsin.

Absorption, Fate, and Excretion. *Tolazoline* is well absorbed after both parenteral and oral administration. However, it is considerably less effective when given orally because rapid renal excretion prevents accumulation of adequate concentrations during the slow absorption from the gastrointestinal tract. It is largely excreted unchanged by the organic-base transport system of the renal tubules. Little is known about the fate of *phentolamine* in the body. It is not more than 20% as active after oral as after parenteral administration, and only 10% of an injected dose is recovered in the urine in active form.

Toxicity, Side Effects, and Precautions. The most disturbing clinical side effects of phentolamine and tolazoline are attributable to cardiac and gastrointestinal stimulation. Both drugs can cause alarming tachycardia, cardiac arrhythmias, and anginal pain, most frequently after parenteral administration. Tolazoline has been implicated as a precipitating factor in myocardial infarction and occasionally may produce severe hypertension. Gastrointestinal stimulation may result in abdominal pain, nausea, vomiting, diarrhea, and exacerbation of peptic ulcer. Effective doses of tolazoline quite frequently produce piloerection, chilliness, and apprehension. The imidazoline blocking agents should be used with caution in patients with gastritis, peptic ulcer, or coronary artery disease.

Preparations, Routes of Administration, and Dosage. *Phentolamine Mesylate,* U.S.P. (REGITINE MESYLATE), is marketed for parenteral use in sterile ampuls containing 5 mg. The standard dose that has been employed in the diagnosis of pheochromocytoma in adults is 5 mg, given intravenously. However, it is more prudent to initiate testing with lower doses, particularly if suspicion is high that the patient does indeed have a pheochromocytoma. *Phentolamine Hydrochloride,* U.S.P. (REGITINE), is available for oral use in tablets containing 50 mg.

Tolazoline Hydrochloride, U.S.P. (PRISCOLINE), is marketed for oral use in tablets containing 25 mg, in long-acting tablets containing 80 mg, and for injection in 10-ml multiple-dose vials (25 mg/ml). The most commonly employed oral dosage is 25 mg four to six times a day, although considerably larger doses are required to produce significant α-adrenergic blockade. Alternatively, 80 mg (long-acting preparation) can be given every 12 hours. A full parenteral dose is 50 to 200 mg, given intravenously, intramuscularly, or subcutaneously. However, tolazoline is infrequently administered parenterally except for investigational purposes.

Therapeutic Uses. Clinical applications of the adrenergic blocking and vasodilating actions of phentolamine and tolazoline are discussed with those of other α-adrenergic blocking agents later in this chapter (*see also* Chapters 32 and 33).

PRAZOSIN

Prazosin is a recently developed antihypertensive agent that appears to exert its vasodilator action through blockade of postsynaptic α_1 receptors. Administration of prazosin causes reversal of pressor responses to epinephrine, and it blocks pressor responses to norepinephrine. Prazosin appears to be a rather selective α_1-blocking agent. It probably has little effect on α_2 receptors, and prazosin thus does not cause enhanced neural release of norepinephrine. This may explain the relatively modest degree of tachycardia associated with the administration of this α-adrenergic antagonist. Prazosin reduces vascular tone in both resistance and capacitance vessels. This is associated with a reduction in venous return and cardiac output. The hemodynamic effects associated with prazosin, namely, decreased arterial pressure, reduction in arterial and venous tone, and relatively little change in cardiac output, heart rate, or right atrial pressure, are similar to the hemodynamic consequences of directly acting vasodilators, such as sodium nitroprusside (Graham and Pettinger, 1979). Additional information about prazosin is presented in Chapter 32.

ERGOT ALKALOIDS

The ergot alkaloids were the first adrenergic blocking agents to be discovered, and most aspects of their general pharmacology were disclosed by the classical studies of Dale (1906).

Ergot alkaloids exhibit a complex variety of important pharmacological properties. Most notably, these agents act as partial agonists or antagonists at α-adrenergic, tryptaminergic, and dopaminergic receptors (Berde and Stürmer, 1978; *see* Table 39–2). Distinctions among individual members of this family of compounds are apparently due to the differences in the potencies of the individual compounds at various receptors and the manner in which each interacts with different receptors.

Chemistry. Details of the chemistry of the ergot alkaloids are presented in Chapter 39. However, certain aspects are significant for the present discussion of α-adrenergic blockade. Compounds of the *ergonovine* type, which lack a polypeptide side chain, have no adrenergic blocking activity. Of the natural ergot preparations, "ergotoxine" has the greatest α-adrenergic blocking potency. It was studied for almost 40 years before it was shown to be a mixture of three alkaloids—*ergocornine, ergocristine,* and *ergocryptine;* fortunately, these have very similar pharmacological properties. Dihydrogenation of the lysergic acid nucleus increases α-adrenergic blocking activity and decreases, but does not eliminate, the ability to stimulate smooth muscle by an action on tryptaminergic receptors.

PHARMACOLOGICAL PROPERTIES

Both the natural and the dihydrogenated peptide alkaloids produce *α-adrenergic blockade*. This is relatively persistent for a competitive antagonist, but it is of much shorter duration than that produced by a haloalkylamine. These drugs also are effective antagonists of 5-HT. Although the hydrogenated ergot alkaloids are among the most potent α-adrenergic blocking agents known, side effects prevent the administration of doses that could produce more than minimal blockade in man.

The most important effects of all the ergot alkaloids are due to actions on the CNS and direct stimulation of smooth muscle. The latter occurs in many different organs (*see* Chapter 39), and even dihydroergotoxine has been observed to produce spastic contractions of the intestine in man.

The peptide ergot alkaloids can reverse the pressor response to epinephrine to depressor (α-adrenergic blockade), but they can also convert the depressor response to isoproterenol to pressor. The latter effect appears to be due to an increase in cardiac output in the presence of a vascular bed already constricted by the alkaloid. All the *natural ergot alkaloids* cause a significant rise in blood pressure as a result of peripheral vasoconstriction, which is more pronounced in postcapillary than in precapillary vessels (Mellander and Nordenfelt, 1970). Although hydrogenation reduces this action, dihydroergotamine is still an effective vasoconstrictor, and a residual constrictor action of dihydroergotoxine is also demonstrable. Ergotamine, and probably all other ergot alkaloids,

can produce coronary vasoconstriction, often with associated ischemic changes in the ECG and anginal pain in patients with coronary artery disease. *Dihydroergotoxine* produces only limited vasoconstriction, and its overall effects include peripheral vasodilatation and a fall in arterial pressure. These effects are predominantly due to central depression of vasomotor nerve activity (Barcroft *et al.,* 1951). The ergot alkaloids usually induce bradycardia even when the blood pressure is not increased. This is predominantly due to increased vagal activity, but a central reduction in sympathetic tone and direct myocardial depression may also be involved.

The natural and hydrogenated ergot alkaloids all inhibit epinephrine-induced hepatic glycogenolysis and hyperglycemia more effectively than do other α-adrenergic blocking agents. This is not correlated with the blockade of cardiovascular or other smooth muscle responses, and may not be a specific α-receptor effect. Glycogenolysis in skeletal muscle and the consequent lactacidemia are not similarly inhibited.

Several aspects of the pharmacology of the ergot alkaloids are discussed in more detail by Rothlin (1947), Nickerson (1949), and Nickerson and Hollenberg (1967), and in a volume edited by Berde and Schild (1978).

Toxicity and Side Effects. The dose of dihydroergotoxine in man is strictly limited by the production of nausea and vomiting. Prolonged or excessive administration of any of the natural peptide ergot alkaloids can cause vascular insufficiency and gangrene of the extremities. This is particularly likely to occur in the presence of preexisting vascular pathology or infection. In severe cases, prompt vasodilatation is essential. There have been no comparative studies on the treatment of this sporadic condition, but a direct-acting drug such as *nitroprusside* appears to be most effective (Carliner *et al.,* 1974). Toxic effects of the ergot alkaloids are described in more detail in Chapter 39.

Therapeutic Uses and Preparations. The primary uses of ergot alkaloids are to stimulate contraction of the uterus post partum and to relieve the pain of migraine. These and other applications are described in Chapter 39; the effect of bromocriptine on the secretion of prolactin, of which advantage is taken clinically, is described in Chapter 59. The various preparations of ergot alkaloids are listed in Chapter 39.

OTHER α-ADRENERGIC BLOCKING AGENTS

Natural and synthetic compounds of several other chemical classes exhibit α-adrenergic blocking activity. A number of these are discussed in the reviews of Bovet and Bovet-Nitti (1948) and Nickerson (1949). *Chlorpromazine, haloperidol,* and many other neuroleptic drugs produce significant α blockade in both laboratory animals and man. Chlorpromazine has also been reported to prolong and, under appropriate conditions, enhance the pressor response to norepinephrine, possibly as a result of the capability of this compound to block neuronal re-uptake of the neurotransmitter. Haloperidol also inhibits dopamine-induced renal vasodilatation, which is not affected by the common α- or β-adrenergic blocking agents. (*See* Webster, 1965; Yeh *et al.,* 1969; Goldberg, 1972.)

Benzodioxans. Many members of this series, which was first described over 40 years ago by Fourneau and Bovet, produce a relatively transient, competitive α-adrenergic blockade. Some compounds, such as *piperoxan,* inhibit responses to circulating catecholamines much more effectively than those to adrenergic nerve activity. *Dibozane* is a later addition to the series. The benzodioxans have many and varied actions in addition to adrenergic blockade (*see* reviews by Bovet and Bovet-Nitti, 1948; Nickerson, 1949).

Yohimbine. Yohimbine is an indolealkylamine alkaloid with a chemical similarity to reserpine. Yohimbine and a diastereoisomer, *corynanthine,* and a derivative, *ethyl yohimbine,* produce competitive α-adrenergic blockade of limited duration. Yohimbine also blocks peripheral 5-HT receptors. It has little direct effect on smooth muscle, but readily penetrates the CNS and produces a complex pattern of responses in doses lower than required to produce peripheral α-adrenergic blockade. These include antidiuresis, due to release of antidiuretic hormone (ADH), and a general picture of central excitation, including elevations of blood pressure and heart rate, increased motor activity, irritability, and tremor in both unanesthetized laboratory animals and man. Sweating, nausea, and vomiting are also common after parenteral administration in man (Garfield *et al.,* 1967). Yohimbine has been reported to be a relatively selective inhibitor of α_2-adrenergic receptors. It enhances neural release of norepinephrine at concentrations less than those required to block postsynaptic α_1 receptors. This may account for some of the effects of this drug, which resemble those of sympathomimetic agents (Starke, 1977).

Azapetine. Azapetine (6-allyl-6,7-dihydro-5H-dibenz[c,e]azepine) has blocking and direct vasodilating actions that are qualitatively and quantitatively very similar to those of tolazoline. Most smooth muscle responses mediated by α-adrenergic receptors are blocked about equally. Azapetine tends to lower the blood pressure more than does tolazoline, probably because it causes less cardiac stimulation. (*See* review by Nickerson and Hollenberg, 1967.)

THERAPEUTIC USES OF α-ADRENERGIC BLOCKING AGENTS

α-Adrenergic blockade has been employed or suggested as therapy in a wide variety of conditions, but it has few well-established uses. Quite possibly the clinical application of these drugs will always be severely limited by the fact that efferent sympathetic pathways operating through α-adrenergic receptors are critical to the cardiovascular reflexes that allow man to function as a biped, and it is often difficult to balance the therapeutic benefits of blockade against the disadvantages of disrupting this essential regulatory function.

Cardiovascular Uses. *Hypertension.* Several drugs currently used in the treatment of essential hypertension act by inhibiting sympathetic vasoconstrictor tone. However, with the exception of prazosin, results with α-adrenergic blocking agents in this condition have been disappointing. An important factor is that β receptors are unaffected, and reflex tachycardia and palpitation are added to the other side effects associated with inhibition of sympathetic vasoconstriction. The usefulness of prazosin in hypertension may in part be due to its lack of potency in inhibiting presynaptic α receptors. Small doses of phenoxybenzamine have been found useful in patients who have developed resistance to adrenergic neuron blocking drugs on the basis of vascular supersensitivity to catecholamines (Sandler *et al.,* 1968). Phenoxybenzamine and phentolamine have also been used successfully to control acute hypertensive episodes due to sympathomimetics, and to certain foods and drugs in the presence of MAO inhibition. The treatment of hypertension is discussed in Chapter 32.

Pheochromocytoma. Many pharmacological tests for the diagnosis of pheochromocytoma have been employed in the past, including provocative tests with histamine, methacholine, and glucagon, as well as blocking tests with phentolamine and other drugs. Determinations of the amounts of catecholamines and their metabolites, particularly vanillylmandelic acid, metanephrine, and normetanephrine in urine and catecholamines in plasma, are now generally accepted as the most reliable methods of diagnosis (*see* Wolf *et al.,* 1970). While the pharmacological tests are now much less helpful, there are times when the use of phentolamine and histamine can aid greatly in establishing the diagnosis. A few patients with symptoms and signs that are very suggestive of pheochromocytoma will not have abnormal concentrations of catecholamines or their metabolites in plasma or urine, despite the presence of the tumor. The patient can be treated with phentolamine prior to the performance of a histamine challenge test. Protection is thus secured from life-threatening hypertension or arrhythmias caused by catecholamines. However, high concentrations of catecholamines may be detected in plasma just after the histamine is administered or in urine collected for 2 hours after the test (Melmon, 1980).

Adrenergic blocking agents are useful in the *preoperative management* of patients with pheochromocytoma, for their *prolonged treatment* if the tumor is malignant or otherwise not amenable to surgery, and to prevent paroxysmal hypertension during *operative manipulation* of the tumor. Oral phenoxybenzamine is the preferred drug in the first two of these situations. The stable, persistent blockade may allow improvement in the general cardiovascular status of the patient prior to operation, and it permits expansion of the blood volume, which may be severely reduced as a result of the excessive adrenergic vasoconstriction. Patients with inoperable tumors have been adequately controlled with phenoxybenzamine for many years (*see* Engelman and Sjoerdsma, 1964). Propranolol is also frequently employed in these patients in order to antagonize the β_1-receptor-mediated effects of catecholamines on the heart. In the preoperative management of pheochromocytoma, phenoxybenzamine can be administered orally, starting with daily doses of 50 mg. If the patient has evidence of catecholamine-induced myocarditis or myocardiopathy, such treatment can be continued for weeks. The drug is given for shorter periods if cardiovascular and metabolic abnormalities are corrected quickly. In the operative period, phenoxybenzamine (1 mg/kg) given intravenously 36 hours and again approximately 12 hours prior to surgery provides reasonable protection against both pressor episodes and cardiac arrhythmias. During the operation, 2 to 5 mg of phentolamine can also be given intravenously to block effects of large amounts of catecholamines that may be released suddenly. If preoperative treatment is effective, removal of the tumor should not precipitate a period of hypotension. The judicious use of small doses of propranolol or special anesthetic procedures may be necessary to prevent arrhythmias (*see* Ross *et al.*, 1967; Crout and Brown, 1969). Preoperative treatment with α-methyltyrosine, an inhibitor of catecholamine synthesis, may be preferred if the patient is sensitive to adrenergic blocking agents.

Shock. Largely because of preoccupation with low blood pressure as a criterion of shock, vasopressor agents have been used extensively in its treatment. However, vasoconstriction is a prominent feature of shock *per se,* and there is little evidence that its accentuation by drugs is beneficial, as long as a minimally acceptable blood pressure can be maintained (*see* Chapter 8). Indeed, hyperactivity of the sympathetic nervous system or infusion of a vasoconstrictor such as norepinephrine can accentuate the development of shock initiated by hemorrhage, trauma, or infection, and can itself induce lethal shock in both laboratory animals and man.

Many agents that induce vasodilatation by inhibiting sympathetic vasoconstriction or by directly relaxing vascular smooth muscle improve the survival rate of experimental animals subjected to various shock-inducing procedures. Protection can be attributed to at least three distinct cardiovascular effects: (1) increased cardiac output and total blood flow; (2) local redistribution of blood flow so that a larger percentage passes through channels that readily exchange metabolites with tissue cells, presumably true capillaries; and (3) reversal of the vasoconstriction-induced shift of fluid from the vascular to the interstitial compartment. Two other effects of α-blocking agents such as phentolamine can make important contributions to the practical clinical management of this condition: (1) The fall in blood pressure induced when it is administered in the presence of hypovole-

mia provides a quick and reliable indication of the adequacy of intravascular fluid–volume replacement, a point often difficult to determine even with careful monitoring of the central venous pressure. (2) The shift of blood from the pulmonary to the systemic vascular bed associated with blockade of sympathetic vasomotor tone allows administration of larger volumes of fluid more rapidly than would otherwise be possible, particularly in patients with some myocardial inadequacy. It should be emphasized that any drug therapy in shock is secondary to fully adequate replacement of intravascular fluid volume with blood or other appropriate fluids. *Phentolamine or phenoxybenzamine should not be given unless the central venous pressure has been elevated by fluid administration without an adequate circulatory response;* inhibition of vasoconstrictor reflexes makes the circulation highly vulnerable to hypovolemia. In addition, the blocking agent must be administered slowly and suitable fluids must be immediately available for use if a sharp drop in blood pressure indicates that replacement has in fact been inadequate. (*See* Nickerson, 1962; Hardaway, 1968.) Direct vasodilators are also being used to treat shock, particularly that associated with myocardial failure (*see* Chapter 33).

Peripheral Vascular Disease. Many α-adrenergic blocking drugs, direct-acting vasodilators (*see also* Chapter 33), and drugs with mixed actions are promoted for the treatment of inadequacies of blood flow, particularly to the skin and muscles of the extremities. Ischemia in these areas arises from a variety of pathological processes, but morphological changes that limit flow in relatively large vessels are commonly involved. In general, the results of drug therapy in this broad group of diseases have been disappointing, and vasoactive drugs should not be given precedence over conservative medical management or surgery, where the latter is indicated and possible. Although there are many reports of the efficacy of α-adrenergic blocking agents and of other vasodilators in *intermittent claudication,* there is no convincing evidence that any agent or procedure can increase skeletal muscle blood flow beyond the level produced by exercise to the limit of tolerance. Such exercise is also generally accepted as the most effective mechanism for improving the collateral circulation to ischemic muscle.

The most favorable clinical responses to α-adrenergic blockade are in conditions with a large component of adrenergic vasoconstriction, such as *Raynaud's syndrome* and *acrocyanosis.* These are less common and threatening than occlusive arterial disease, but even here drug therapy is probably secondary to other measures. Phenoxybenzamine and tolazoline have been observed to relieve vasospasm and reduce sensitivity to cold in Raynaud's syndrome. Satisfactory results are obtained in most cases with oral doses that produce only a relatively low level of adrenergic blockade (Friend and Edwards, 1954; Gifford, 1971). Vasospasm induced by an exogenous sympathomimetic is readily antagonized, and local infiltration with 2.5 to 5.0 mg of phentolamine or addition of the drug to the intravenous solution effectively prevents the severe local vasoconstriction and skin necrosis that can be associated with infusion of a vasoconstrictor such as norepinephrine, particularly if there is some extravasation.

Other Cardiovascular Uses. High spinal cord transection commonly leads to autonomic hyperreflexia with paroxysmal elevations in blood pressure from both cutaneous and visceral stimuli, particularly those from the urinary bladder. It has been reported that these pressor episodes and the associated signs and symptoms can be well controlled by relatively small oral doses of phenoxybenzamine (Sizemore and Winternitz, 1970).

Any inadequacy of cardiac output, particularly of relatively acute onset, can cause an increase in sympathetic vasomotor tone, which increases peripheral resistance and decreases venous compliance. Because the constriction is greater in the systemic bed, blood is shifted to the pulmonary circuit, and increased pulmonary blood volume and pressure can cause *pulmonary congestion and edema.* It has been repeatedly shown that block of sympathetic vasoconstriction can rapidly reverse these processes and decrease myocardial work and pulmonary congestion. α-Adrenergic blockade has been shown to be beneficial in heart failure with pulmonary edema (*see* Majid *et al.,* 1971), and in acute myocardial infarction where pain can accentuate the vasoconstriction (Kelly *et al.,* 1973). Other vasodilator drugs such as nitroprusside (*see* Chapter 33) are also effective.

II. β-Adrenergic Blocking Agents

β-Adrenergic blocking agents have received major attention in the last decade because of their utility in the management of cardiovascular disorders, including hypertension, angina pectoris, and cardiac arrhythmias.

The first drug shown to produce a selective blockade of β-adrenergic receptors was *dichloroisoproterenol* (DCI) (Powell and Slater, 1958). Studies with DCI made a substantial contribution to the understanding of effects mediated by β receptors, but it was not used in man, largely because it has a prominent β-receptor stimulant action; that is, it is a partial agonist. *Propranolol* was the first β-adrenergic antagonist to come into wide clinical use, and it remains the most important of these compounds. It is a highly potent, nonselective β-adrenergic blocking agent with no intrinsic sympathomimetic activity. However, because of its ability to block β receptors in bronchial smooth muscle and skeletal muscle, propranolol interferes with bronchodilatation produced by epinephrine and other sympathomimetic amines and with glycogenolysis, which ordinarily occurs during hypoglycemia. Thus, the

drug is usually not used in individuals with bronchial asthma and must be used cautiously in diabetics who are receiving insulin or oral hypoglycemic agents. As a consequence, there has been a search for β-adrenergic blocking agents that are cardioselective (*see* Karow *et al.,* 1971), and a number of drugs have now been developed that exhibit some degree of specificity for β₁-adrenergic receptors. *Practolol* was the first such agent, and it was widely employed in Europe and elsewhere for the treatment of hypertension. However, disturbing toxicities that involved epithelial structures in particular were noted after long-term use of the drug.

Among the relatively *nonselective β-adrenergic blocking agents* that are either available in the United States or under clinical investigation are propranolol, alprenolol, nadolol, oxprenolol, penbutolol, pindolol, sotalol, and timolol. Propranolol and nadolol are currently available for systemic use in the United States. *Selective β₁-adrenergic blocking agents* that have either been introduced into therapy or are under investigation include *metoprolol, atenolol, acebutolol,* and *tolamolol.* It is important to remember that the selectivity of the β₁ blockers is not absolute; larger doses of these compounds will inhibit all β-adrenergic receptors (*see* Prichard, 1978). Propranolol and metoprolol will be discussed as prototypes of nonselective and cardioselective β₁-adrenergic blocking agents, respectively.

Butoxamine is a somewhat selective β₂-adrenergic antagonist. It blocks β₂-vasodilator and other smooth muscle inhibitory effects of isoproterenol, but relatively little antagonism of the cardiac effects is observed in anesthetized animals; in unanesthetized dogs, however, it blocks the chronotropic action (Levy, 1966; Burns *et al.,* 1967).

Chemistry. Most of the more effective β-adrenergic blocking agents can be considered to be derivatives of the β-receptor agonist isoproterenol. The structural formulas of DCI and of the β-adrenergic blocking agents that are available for general use in the United States are as follows:

Dichloroisoproterenol (DCI)

OH CH$_3$

—OCH$_2$—C—CH$_2$NHCH

H CH$_3$

Propranolol

HO
H
H
HO

OH CH$_3$

OCH$_2$—C—CH$_2$NHC—CH$_3$

H CH$_3$

Nadolol

OH CH$_3$

OCH$_2$—C—CH$_2$NHC—CH$_3$

H CH$_3$

Timolol

CH$_3$OCH$_2$CH$_2$—

OH CH$_3$

—OCH$_2$—C—CH$_2$NHCH

H CH$_3$

Metoprolol

The structural similarity between β-receptor agonists and antagonists is closer than in the case of drugs acting at α receptors. The side chain with an isopropyl or bulkier substituent on the amine appears to favor interaction with β receptors. The nature of substituents on the aromatic ring determines whether the effect will be predominantly activation or blockade. These substituents also affect cardioselectivity. The aliphatic hydroxyl appears to be essential for activity. It gives the molecule optical activity, and the levorotatory forms of both β-adrenergic agonists and antagonists are much more potent than the dextrorotatory forms. This difference is useful in distinguishing the effects of β-receptor blockade from those of other pharmacological actions of the molecule; for example, the *d* isomer of propranolol has less than 1% of the potency of the *l* isomer of propranolol in blocking β-adrenergic receptors, but the two are equipotent as local anesthetics (Barrett and Cullum, 1968).

PHARMACOLOGICAL PROPERTIES

As in the case of the α-adrenergic blocking agents, much of the pharmacology of β-adrenergic blockade can be deduced from a knowledge of the functions subserved by the involved receptors (Table 4–1, page 60) and the physiological or pathological conditions under which they are activated. Thus, β-receptor blockade has little effect on the normal heart with the subject at complete rest, but may have profound effects when sympathetic control of the heart is high, as during exer-

cise. The overall response to a β-adrenergic blocking agent may also be modified by other properties of the drug in question. β-Receptor stimulation ("intrinsic sympathomimetic activity") is an important part of the response to certain β-adrenergic antagonists, such as practolol, pindolol, acebutolol, alprenolol, and oxprenolol (Prichard, 1978). Some of these drugs also have direct actions on cell membranes, which are commonly described as membrane stabilizing, local anesthetic, and quinidine-like. The local anesthetic potency of propranolol is about equal to that of lidocaine, while oxprenolol is about half as potent; sotalol, timolol, atenolol, tolamolol, and pindolol are almost devoid of this property.

In isolated atria, propranolol and oxprenolol decrease spontaneous frequency, maximal driving frequency, and contractility, and increase electrical threshold. They also increase A-V conduction time and decrease the spontaneous rate of depolarization of ectopic pacemakers in intact hearts. Resting membrane potential and repolarization are not greatly affected by propranolol, but the height and rate of rise of the action potential are reduced because the drug decreases the inward sodium current (Tarr *et al.*, 1973). These quinidine-like effects are associated with generalized depression of myocardial function, which can cause death with large doses. It has been suggested that β-adrenergic blocking agents without membrane-stabilizing activity are less likely than propranolol to precipitate heart failure. However, direct myocardial depression requires doses much higher than those necessary for β-adrenergic blockade, and it appears that block of sympathetic stimulation is by far the most important factor in the occasional precipitation of heart failure in a patient with an inadequate cardiac reserve. The quinidine-like effects of β-adrenergic blocking drugs appear to contribute little to the treatment of cardiac arrhythmias; effective concentrations of propranolol in blood are below those that cause much membrane stabilization, and β blockers without this property are also effective antiarrhythmic agents (*see* Black and Prichard, 1973; Shand, 1975).

Binding Studies with Labeled β-Adrenergic Antagonists. β-Adrenergic receptors have been identified and characterized in many tissues with the use of highly potent and selective β-adrenergic blocking agents that are labeled with a radioisotope of high specific activity, such as (^{125}I)iodohydroxybenzylpindolol (Aurbach *et al.*, 1974) or (^{3}H)dihydroalprenolol (Williams *et al.*, 1976). Such studies have allowed determination of the molecular properties of the receptor and have increased the knowledge about its mechanism of interaction with adenylate cyclase (*see* Maguire *et al.*, 1977; Ross *et al.*, 1978). Furthermore, the affinities of various agents for β$_1$ and β$_2$ receptors can be determined with precision

(Minneman *et al.*, 1979a). Thus, metoprolol and practolol exhibit the greatest (10- to 20-fold) degree of selectivity for β_1 receptors, while atenolol is about threefold more potent in binding to β_1- than to β_2-adrenergic receptors; propranolol, pindolol, sotalol, and timolol have equal affinity for both subtypes. The relative proportions of β_1 and β_2 receptors in a tissue can also be determined by ligand binding technics (Minneman *et al.*, 1979b). For example, in rat tissues, the proportion of β_1 to β_2 receptors is about 4:1 in heart and cerebral cortex and about 1:5 in lung and cerebellum.

NONSELECTIVE β-ADRENERGIC BLOCKING AGENTS: PROPRANOLOL

As mentioned, propranolol is a nonselective β-adrenergic blocking agent that is used widely for the treatment of hypertension, the prophylaxis of angina pectoris, and the control of certain types of cardiac arrhythmias. It blocks both β_1 and β_2 receptors competitively and does not exhibit any intrinsic agonistic properties.

Cardiovascular System. The most important effects of β-adrenergic blocking drugs are on the cardiovascular system, predominantly due to actions on the heart. Propranolol decreases heart rate and cardiac output, prolongs mechanical systole, and slightly decreases blood pressure in resting subjects (Robin *et al.*, 1967; Helfant *et al.*, 1971). The effects on cardiac output and heart rate are more dramatic during exercise. Peripheral resistance is increased as a result of compensatory sympathetic reflexes, and blood flow to all tissues except the brain is reduced (Nies *et al.*, 1973). The major effects of propranolol on the heart are absent in animals in which norepinephrine stores have been depleted (Shanks, 1966).

The cardiac effects of β-adrenergic blockade are often reflected in changes in sodium excretion. The normal diurnal pattern is reversed, as in patients with moderate myocardial inadequacy, and there is a slow adjustment to a new steady state with increased total body sodium and extracellular fluid volume. These effects are most obvious in patients with some preexisting myocardial inadequacy. In some patients with severe heart disease, β-adrenergic blockade can cause progressive accumulation of sodium and water, edema, and frank congestive heart failure (Epstein and Braunwald, 1966). These effects on sodium excretion probably result from intrarenal hemodynamic changes that are part of the adjustment to the decreased cardiac output (Nies *et al.*, 1971). The magnitude of the effect appears to parallel the dependence of the heart on adrenergic stimulation to maintain adequate function. Occasionally a β-adrenergic blocking agent, particularly when given intravenously, can precipitate acute heart failure.

The effect of β-adrenergic blockade on the heart is more marked under conditions of increased demand and sympathetic tone. The cardiac response to fluid load is reduced, as is the tachycardia associated with exercise, nitrite hypotension, or the Valsalva maneuver (Black and Prichard, 1973). Ventricular dimensions and contractility are little affected in normal, supine, resting subjects, but the decreases in end-diastolic and end-systolic ventricular size and the increase in myocardial contractility associated with exercise are reduced. In patients with occlusive coronary artery disease, propranolol can cause significant increases in ventricular end-diastolic volumes and pressures, and in the tension-time index; it can also cause or increase ventricular asynergy (*see* Robin *et al.*, 1967; Helfant *et al.*, 1971). Maximal exercise tolerance is considerably decreased in normal individuals, but can be increased in patients with angina pectoris (Sowton *et al.*, 1971).

Total coronary blood flow and myocardial oxygen consumption are also decreased as a result of reductions of heart rate, ventricular systolic pressure, and contractility (Wolfson and Gorlin, 1969). The reduction is predominantly in subepicardial blood flow, which leads to a relative redistribution of flow (Gross and Winbury, 1973). A similar internal shunting after β-adrenergic blockade allows blood flow to ischemic areas of the heart to be altered less than that to other regions (Pitt and Craven, 1970). While prolongation of systolic ejection and dilatation of the ventricle caused by propranolol tend to increase oxygen requirements, the oxygen-sparing effects predominate (*see* Chapter 33).

In appropriate doses, all β-adrenergic blocking drugs reduce the chronotropic and inotropic effects of cardiac sympathetic nerve activity and of circulating β-receptor agonists.

Stimulation by other agents, including calcium, barium, methylxanthines, and digitalis, is little affected. The relative effectiveness of various β-adrenergic antagonists against circulating compared to locally released catecholamines is not entirely clear, but it appears that propranolol blocks the two types of stimuli about equally (Ledsome et al., 1974).

Blood Pressure. Propranolol is an effective antihypertensive agent. Chronic treatment of hypertensive patients with a β-adrenergic blocking agent results in a slowly developing reduction in blood pressure. Propranolol is particularly useful clinically in combination with vasodilators that act directly on the vasculature. The reflex tachycardia that is a prominent feature of the response to the latter drugs is effectively blocked by the β-adrenergic antagonist (*see* Chapter 32).

Several mechanisms have been proposed for the efficacy of propranolol in the management of hypertension, and more than one mechanism may contribute to this effect. Reduction in cardiac output occurs rather promptly after administration of propranolol. However, the hypotensive effects of propranolol do not usually appear as rapidly. β-Adrenergic agonists are known to increase modestly the release of norepinephrine from adrenergic nerve terminals (Adler-Graschinsky and Langer, 1975; Starke, 1977; Dixon et al., 1979); propranolol blocks this effect, and such impairment of the release of norepinephrine following sympathetic nerve stimulation might contribute to the antihypertensive effects of the drug.

The release of renin from the juxtaglomerular apparatus is stimulated by β_2-adrenergic agonists, and this effect is blocked by drugs such as propranolol (*see* Ganong, 1973). They also reduce, but do not completely block, the increase in plasma renin activity induced by sodium deprivation (Michelakis and McAllister, 1972). Buhler and associates (1972) observed that the antihypertensive effect of propranolol, administered in relatively modest doses, is much more prominent in individuals with elevated plasma renin activity than in those in whom this value is relatively low. It has thus been proposed that propranolol may exert at least a portion of its antihypertensive effect by inhibiting the secretion of renin by the kidney. However, hypertensive patients who have low activity of renin in plasma do respond to propranolol if larger doses are employed (Zacharias et al., 1972; Oates et al., 1977). Furthermore, some β-blocking agents reduce blood pressure but do not inhibit the secretion of renin significantly. Thus, Weber and colleagues (1974) have concluded that the antihypertensive effects of β blockers are not mediated by a reduction in plasma renin (*see also* Stokes et al., 1974).

Esler and coworkers (1977) have suggested that hypertensive patients who respond to propranolol can be classified into two groups. Those who exhibit hypotensive responses when the concentration of propranolol in plasma is relatively low (3 to 30 ng/ml) tend to have high activity of renin in plasma and elevated concentrations of circulating catecholamines. Many of the remaining subjects respond when the concentration of propranolol in plasma is in the range of 30 to 100 ng/ml.

Effect on Vascular Responses to Drugs. Propranolol and other nonselective β-adrenergic blocking drugs inhibit the vasodepressor and vasodilator effects of isoproterenol, and augment the pressor effect of epinephrine. Pressor responses to norepinephrine may be slightly decreased because its cardiac actions are blocked, but those to phenylephrine are unchanged. These effects are entirely predictable from a knowledge of the relative activities of different sympathomimetics on vascular α and β receptors. Vasodilatation due to histamine, ACh, and nitroglycerin is unaffected. β-Adrenergic blockade does not inhibit renal vasodilatation induced by dopamine, although the limited responses to isoproterenol in this vascular bed and to dopamine in the femoral vasculature are eliminated (McNay and Goldberg, 1966).

Effects on Cardiac Rhythm and Automaticity. Propranolol reduces sinus rate, decreases the spontaneous rate of depolarization of ectopic pacemakers, and slows conduction in the atria and in the A-V node. Large doses of propranolol appear to exert a quinidine-like effect on the myocardium, which might contribute to the antiarrhythmic effect of this drug. However, the β-adrenergic blocking activity of propranolol appears to be its major mechanism of action (Shand, 1975). The utility of propranolol in the management of cardiac arrhythmias is discussed in Chapter 31.

Central Nervous System. Propranolol readily penetrates into the brain, but it has few, if any, effects that can be clearly attributed to blockade of β-adrenergic receptors in the CNS. While there has been speculation that central actions of propranolol might contribute to its antihypertensive effects, there is no convincing evidence.

Metabolic Effects. β-Adrenergic blocking agents can considerably modify carbohydrate and fat metabolism, although many species and tissue variations as well as composite effects confuse this complex field (*see* reviews by Himms-Hagen, 1967, and several articles in Symposium, 1970). Most of the effects of catecholamines on carbohydrate and fat metabolism are mediated by β receptors and changes in adenylate cyclase activity, with resultant production of cyclic adenosine 3′,5′-monophosphate (cyclic AMP). Adrenergic blocking agents that inhibit metabolic responses act on this sequence of events. In man, propranolol inhibits the rise in plasma free fatty acids induced by sympathomimetic amines or by enhanced sympathetic nervous system activity. It also effectively and selectively inhibits the lipolytic action of catecholamines on isolated adipose tissue of several species. The actions of adrenergic blocking agents on carbohydrate metabolism are more complicated. The hyperglycemic response to epinephrine is reduced by β-adrenergic blocking drugs in most species and by α blockers in only a few. The effects of the latter agents also involve actions on insulin secretion (*see* above). Glycogenolysis in heart and skeletal muscle is inhibited by β- and not by α-adrenergic blocking drugs. The effects on hepatic glycogenolysis are dependent on the species (*see* Chapter 4). The release of insulin by isoproterenol is blocked by propranolol, but apparently not by practolol (Loubatieres *et al.*, 1971). Propranolol does not affect plasma glucose or insulin concentrations in normal individuals, or the rate or magnitude of the fall of plasma glucose after insulin, but it does slow the subsequent recovery of glucose concentration and prevents the usual rebound of plasma glycerol. These effects are presumably due to inhibition of the glycogenolytic and lipolytic actions of endogenous catecholamines released in response to hypoglycemia. Consequently, β-adrenergic blocking agents must be used with caution in patients prone to hypoglycemia and particularly in diabetics treated with insulin. Many aspects of the adrenergic control of insulin secretion have been reviewed by Porte and Robertson (1973).

Other Effects. Propranolol blocks the action of sympathomimetic amines on β-adrenergic receptors in many structures. However, when administered in the absence of a specific agonist, the most important response to β blockade outside of the cardiovascular system is that of the bronchi and bronchioles. Adrenergic bronchodilatation is mediated by β_2 receptors, but the presence of significant intrinsic adrenergic bronchodilator activity was not demonstrated before the clinical availability of β-adrenergic blocking agents. Propranolol consistently increases airway resistance. This effect is small and of no clinical significance in normal individuals, but it can be marked and potentially dangerous in asthmatics (*see* Nicolaescu *et al.*, 1972). Because bronchodilatation is a β_2-adrenergic response, selective β_1 blockers such as metoprolol are much less likely than propranolol to induce bronchoconstriction, and they have been used in asthmatic patients with minimal effects on airway resistance (*see* Formgren, 1972).

β-Adrenergic blocking agents antagonize relaxation of the uterus by catecholamines, but they have no effect under conditions in which the response is excitatory (Tothill, 1967). Propranolol increases the activity of the human uterus, more in the nonpregnant than in the pregnant state (Wansbrough *et al.*, 1968). β-Receptor blockade inhibits the action of epinephrine that prevents local edema formation in response to the injection of a variety of irritants in the rat paw (*see* Green, 1972), and both propranolol and practolol block the "antianaphylactic" effect of catecholamines on antigen-induced histamine release from sensitized lung (Assem and Schild, 1971). Circulating eosinophils increase in man during the administration of propranolol, and the reduction characteristically induced by epinephrine is blocked (Koch-Weser, 1968).

The effects of β-adrenergic blocking agents on skeletal neuromuscular transmission are variable, and appear to be unrelated to either β-adrenergic blockade or local anesthetic activity (Wislicki, 1969). Drugs that block β-adrenergic receptors antagonize epinephrine-induced tremor in man, and large doses of propranolol can reduce tremorine-induced tremor in laboratory animals. However, propranolol is not consistently effective in controlling essential tremor or the tremor of parkinsonism (Gilligan *et al.*, 1972). It is likely that the antitremor effect is peripheral.

Absorption, Fate, and Excretion. Propranolol is almost completely absorbed following oral administration. However, much of the administered drug is metabolized by the liver during its first passage through the portal circulation, and only up to about one third reaches the systemic circulation. In addition, there is considerable interindividual variation in the degree of presystemic hepatic elimination of propranolol, and this contributes to the great variability (up to 20-fold) in plasma concentrations found after oral administration of comparable doses to patients. The degree of hepatic extraction of propranolol is less as the dose is increased, suggesting that a saturable mechanism is involved (Evans *et al.,* 1973b). Furthermore, somewhat less of the drug is removed during the first circulation through the liver after repeated administration than after the initial dose, which accounts for a gradual increase in the half-life of the drug after chronic oral administration (about 4 hours) compared with the half-life of the initial oral dose (about 3 hours) (Shand *et al.,* 1970; Shand, 1975).

Propranolol is bound to plasma proteins to the extent of 90 to 95% (Evans *et al.,* 1973a). This may also contribute to variability in the concentration of the drug in plasma and the relative unreliability of total plasma concentration as a guide to therapeutic efficacy.

Propranolol is virtually completely metabolized before excretion in the urine (Hayes and Cooper, 1971). One of the products of hepatic metabolism is 4-hydroxypropranolol, which appears to exhibit β-adrenergic blocking activity comparable to that of the parent compound (Fitzgerald and O'Donnell, 1971). However, the half-life of 4-hydroxypropranolol is short, and it probably contributes relatively little to the therapeutic effect of the drug. Other metabolic products that have been identified in the urine include naphthoxylactic acid, isopropylamine, and propranolol glycol. A considerable fraction of the metabolites of propranolol is apparently glucuronide conjugates (Shand, 1975; Oates *et al.,* 1977).

Preparations, Routes of Administration, and Dosage. *Propranolol Hydrochloride,* U.S.P. (INDERAL), is available in tablets containing 10, 20, 40, or 80 mg for oral administration, and in 1-ml ampuls containing 1.0 mg for intravenous use.

In the management of hypertension, propranolol is administered orally. The initial dose is usually 40 mg, given twice daily. The dose is increased gradually to a level of 160 to 480 mg per day. When the doses are large, the drug can often be taken once daily. In the treatment of angina pectoris or for the control of arrhythmias, doses of 40 to 320 mg per day may be employed. As in the treatment of hypertension, the initial doses should be low and increased gradually until either therapeutic benefit or toxicity is noted. Propranolol may be administered intravenously for the management of life-threatening arrhythmias. Under these circumstances the usual dose is 1 to 3 mg, administered slowly and with careful and frequent measurement of blood pressure, ECG, and cardiac function. If an adequate response is not obtained, a second dose may be given after a few minutes. In the event of overdosage, atropine should be administered to counteract the bradycardia, and cardiac glycosides and diuretics should be given in the event of cardiac failure. Vasopressors may be required to counteract a profound fall in blood pressure.

Toxicity, Side Effects, and Precautions. The major dangers of therapy with propranolol or other β-adrenergic blocking drugs are related to the blockade *per se.* Serious cardiac depression is uncommon, but heart failure may develop suddenly or slowly, usually in patients whose hearts are severely compromised by disease or by other drugs (*e.g.,* anesthetics). Acute failure is rare with oral administration. Propranolol should be given with caution to any patient with inadequate myocardial function, but it may be beneficial if the patient has severe hypertension or a treatable arrhythmia or if excessive sinus rate contributes significantly to the inadequacy. The inotropic action of digitalis is not prevented by propranolol, but both drugs depress A-V conduction. Propranolol can cause A-V dissociation and cardiac arrest in patients with preexisting partial heart block due to digitalis or other factors.

Administration of propranolol, and presumably any β-adrenergic blocking agent, renders patients susceptible to a withdrawal syndrome that may be due to supersensitivity of β-adrenergic receptors (due, hypothetically, to adaptive changes in receptor number). Some patients may experience a severe exacerbation of anginal attacks, and myocardial infarction has occurred. Patients being treated for hypertension may have a life-threatening rebound of blood pressure to levels that can exceed pretreatment values. Such problems appear within hours to 1 to 2 days after the drug is abruptly discontinued. Some patients develop premonitory signs and symptoms, such as nervousness, sweating, and tachycardia. If therapy is to be stopped, it should be done gradually. If the patient discontinues his own medication, treatment should be reinstituted promptly and, if there is evidence of difficulty, in the hospital.

Another important danger from β-adrenergic blockade is an increase in airway resistance, which can be life threatening in asthmatics. Asthma is a contraindication to the use of propranolol. The effectiveness of epinephrine in the treatment of acute allergic reactions may be reduced in patients who receive propranolol chronically. Cardio-selective (β_1) adrenergic antagonists will probably replace propranolol for use in asthmatics and other patients with a history of severe allergy. However, none of the compounds developed thus far is sufficiently selective to be considered safe in patients with obstructive airway disease. They should not be administered to such individuals unless the therapist is prepared to counter unwanted bronchoconstriction.

Propranolol augments the hypoglycemic action of insulin by reducing the compensatory effect of sympathoadrenal activation, and masks the tachycardia that is an important sign of developing hypoglycemia. Consequently, any patient susceptible to episodes of hypoglycemia who is also taking propranolol must be taught to respond to subtle signs of hypoglycemia. If possible, propranolol should not be given to diabetic patients who are being treated with insulin or oral hypoglycemic agents.

Side effects of propranolol that are not extensions of the desired pharmacological action are usually not serious and frequently disappear during continued drug administration. Nausea, vomiting, mild diarrhea, and constipation have been reported. CNS effects are not common, but many have been observed, including hallucinations, nightmares, insomnia, lassitude, dizziness, and depression (*see* Greenblatt and Shader, 1972). In double-blind studies, many of these CNS complaints occurred with equal frequency during administration of a placebo. Rash, fever, and purpura probably reflect an allergic response; they are infrequent but require discontinuation of the drug. Unwanted effects of propranolol have been reviewed by Greenblatt and Koch-Weser (1973).

Therapeutic Uses. Propranolol can be especially useful in the management of hypertension. In general, the drug is combined with a diuretic agent. It is also frequently used as an adjunct to treatment with a vasodilator in order to minimize reflex tachycardia and compensatory increases in cardiac output (*see* Chapter 32). Propranolol is indicated for the management of both supraventricular and ventricular arrhythmias. It seems to be especially valuable in the management

of arrhythmias associated with digitalis intoxication (*see* Chapter 31). Propranolol has proven efficacious in the prophylaxis of angina pectoris; this subject is discussed in Chapter 33.

Propranolol is also used in *hypertrophic obstructive cardiomyopathies*. In these conditions forceful contraction of the myocardium along a ventricular outflow tract can greatly increase outflow resistance, particularly during exercise. β-Adrenergic blockade may have little effect when the patient is at rest, but it has been shown to improve hemodynamic parameters considerably during exercise, and relatively long-term treatment has been reported to be beneficial (*see* Shand *et al.*, 1971). Propranolol is sometimes useful in the management of tachycardia and arrhythmias in patients with *pheochromocytoma*. However, it is less important than α-adrenergic blockade in this condition and should not be given except in the presence of the latter. When used alone, β-adrenergic blocking drugs can cause a dangerous increase in blood pressure. Similarly, they can accentuate vasospasm in conditions such as Raynaud's syndrome.

β-Adrenergic blockade has been shown to have palliative value in a variety of conditions that involve adrenergic signs and symptoms. In *hyperthyroidism* propranolol decreases heart rate, cardiac output, and tremor; the drug provides rapid, dramatic improvement in thyroid crises (*see* Malcolm, 1972; Chapter 60). A central mechanism of action has been suggested to explain the beneficial effects of propranolol in various *anxiety states*, but peripheral block of symptoms such as palpitation and tremor, which tend to reinforce the anxiety, appears to be the most likely mechanism (*see* Bonn *et al.*, 1972).

During investigation of the use of propranolol for the prevention of angina pectoris, it was observed that one patient who also suffered from migraine headaches had a decreased frequency of attacks (Rabkin *et al.*, 1966). Subsequent well-controlled studies have demonstrated that propranolol is an effective agent for the *prophylaxis of migraine* (Weber and Reinmuth, 1972). The pathophysiology of migraine is complex and incompletely understood, and the mechanism of action of propranolol to prevent such headaches is unknown (*see* Chapter 39). Propranolol has *not* been demonstrated to be an effective agent for the management of the symptoms of an acute attack. The dose of propranolol for the prophylaxis of migraine must be determined for each patient. The usual procedure is to begin with 40 mg per day in divided doses. If no effect is observed, this is gradually increased to a maximal dose of 240 mg per day. If there is no benefit in 4 to 6 weeks, therapy with propranolol is gradually discontinued.

Recent studies have suggested that mortality after myocardial infarction may be reduced by the administration of β-adrenergic blocking agents. Mortality in patients less than 65 years old was reduced by nearly 50% during the first year after infarction by the administration of alprenolol (Andersen *et al.*, 1979). Similar trials of propranolol and metoprolol are currently underway.

NADOLOL

Nadolol is a nonselective β-adrenergic blocking agent that has recently been approved for clinical use in the United States. It is essentially devoid of agonist or local anesthetic activity and is nearly as potent as propranolol. The unique aspect of the pharmacology of nadolol is that the compound is not metabolized, and it is primarily excreted unchanged in the urine. The half-life is relatively long (20 to 24 hours), and the drug can thus be administered once daily (*see* Symposium, 1979).

Nadolol (CORGARD) is available for oral administration in 40-, 80-, and 120-mg tablets. The usual initial dose for the treatment of hypertension or for angina pectoris is 40 mg, given once daily. The dosage is increased gradually in increments of 40 to 80 mg and with recognition of the fact that several days must pass before steady-state concentrations of the drug are achieved in plasma. The usual daily maintenance dose for angina is 80 to 240 mg; for hypertension, the usual range is 80 to 320 mg. Adjustment of dosage is necessary in patients with impaired renal function. The major adverse reactions that follow administration of nadolol appear to be the same as those described above for propranolol.

TIMOLOL

Timolol is a nonselective β-adrenergic antagonist without demonstrable local anesthetic properties and with minimal agonist activity. It is five to ten times more potent than propranolol as a β-adrenergic blocking agent (Scriabine *et al.*, 1973). Its duration of action after oral administration of 4 mg is approximately 4 hours. Clinical studies suggest that it is a highly effective antihypertensive agent.

Timolol maleate (TIMOPTIC) has been approved for use in the United States as an ophthalmic preparation for the treatment of chronic wide-angle glaucoma, aphakic glaucoma, and secondary glaucoma. β-Adrenergic blocking agents have been shown to lower intraocular pressure, presumably by reducing the production of aqueous humor; however, the exact mechanism of this effect is unclear. Timolol does not change the size of the pupil nor the tone of the ciliary body, and it does not interfere with vision. The drug is administered as eyedrops, and solutions of 0.25 and 0.5% are available. The recommended dosage is 1 drop of 0.25% timolol solution in each eye twice a day. The duration of the beneficial effect of timolol is in excess of 7 hours. Although mild ocular irritation is noted occasionally, the side effects with this agent are minimal; patients may rarely complain of blurred vision. Systemic absorption of the drug can occur, leading to slowing of the heart, and the drug should be used with caution in individuals with asthma, heart block, or heart failure.

In a comparative study of timolol and pilocarpine in the management of wide-angle glaucoma, Boger and associates (1978) demonstrated that these agents reduce intraocular pressure to an equal degree. Preparations of timolol were better accepted by the patients, since there was no evidence of miosis and spasm of accommodation. In this study, tolerance to the effect of timolol did not develop over a period of 10 weeks.

OTHER NONSELECTIVE β-ADRENERGIC BLOCKING AGENTS

Several other β-adrenergic antagonists are being investigated for clinical utility; none of these is currently available in the United States. Some of their pertinent properties are summarized in Table 9–1, as are those of propranolol, nadolol, timolol, and the cardioselective β₁-adrenergic antagonists.

CARDIOSELECTIVE (β₁) ADRENERGIC BLOCKING AGENTS: METOPROLOL

Metoprolol is a relatively selective β_1-adrenergic antagonist that is devoid of agonistic activity. Metoprolol effectively inhibits the inotropic and chronotropic responses to isoproterenol; its potency in this regard is similar to that of propranolol. In contrast, to inhibit the vasodilator response to isoproterenol, the dose of metoprolol must be 50 to 100 times that of propranolol. This relative β_1 selectivity of metoprolol is the basis for its potential therapeutic advantage over less selective agents (Ablad *et al.*, 1973). Other, investigational cardioselective (β_1) adrenergic blocking agents are listed in Table 9–1.

When beagle dogs received metoprolol (0.4 mg/kg, intravenously) prior to infusions of epinephrine (0.5 µg/kg per minute), minimal changes in mean aortic blood pressure and only a moderate increase in peripheral resistance were observed. In contrast, when propranolol was administered to these animals (0.2 mg/kg, intravenously), a subsequent intravenous infusion of epinephrine caused a marked increase in mean aortic blood pressure and peripheral resistance. These results suggest that propranolol effectively blocks the peripheral vasodilator (β_2) effect of epinephrine, allowing the expression of the α-adrenergic agonistic properties of the catecholamine. The consequent increases in total peripheral resistance and blood pressure are marked because of the blockade of the partially offsetting β_2 response. In contrast, metoprolol does not substantially inhibit the peripheral vasodilator effect of epinephrine. Thus, the increases in peripheral resistance and blood pressure produced by activation of α receptors are mitigated considerably by vasodilatation (Ablad *et al.*, 1974).

Absorption, Distribution, and Excretion. Metoprolol is efficiently and rapidly absorbed from the gastrointestinal tract. However, metoprolol, like propranolol, is subject to first-pass metabolism in the liver, and, in

Table 9-1.   PHARMACOLOGICAL CHARACTERISTICS OF β-ADRENERGIC RECEPTOR BLOCKING AGENTS *

COMPOUND	POTENCY AS β BLOCKER (PROPRANOLOL = 1.0)	LOCAL ANESTHETIC ACTIVITY	INTRINSIC SYMPATHOMIMETIC ACTIVITY	HALF-LIFE IN PLASMA (HOURS) †
I. Nonselective ($\beta_1 + \beta_2$) Adrenergic Blocking Agents				
Alprenolol	0.3–1	+	+ +	2–3
Bunolol	50	0	0	6
Nadolol	0.5	0	0	20
Oxprenolol	0.5–1	+	+ +	1–2
Penbutolol	5–10	+	0	26 ‡
Pindolol	5–10	±	+ +	3–4
Propranolol	1	+ +	0	3–5
Sotalol	0.3	0	0	5–12
Timolol	5–10	0	±	4–5
II. Cardioselective (β_1) Adrenergic Blocking Agents				
Acebutolol	0.3	+	+	3–4
Atenolol	1	0	0	6–8
Metoprolol	0.5–2	±	0	3–4
Practolol	0.3	0	+ +	5–10
Tolamolol	0.3–1	±	0	3–6

   * Based on data in Waal-Manning, 1976; Brogden *et al.,* 1977; McDevitt, 1977; Benson *et al.,* 1978; Prichard, 1978; Scriabine, 1979. *See also* Appendix II.

   † The duration of effect, in general, is considerably longer than might be expected from the plasma $t_{1/2}$.

   ‡ Plasma $t_{1/2}$ of slow phase of disposition. A rapid phase ($t_{1/2}$, 1 to 2 hours) is also demonstrable.

man, only about 40% of the drug reaches the systemic circulation. Peak concentrations in plasma are achieved after 90 minutes (*see* Brogden *et al.,* 1977). Metoprolol has a relatively short half-life in the plasma, averaging about 3 hours. The drug is extensively metabolized in the body, and 10% or less of the drug is excreted unchanged. The metabolites of metoprolol, which include hydroxylated and O-demethylated compounds, appear to lack significant pharmacological activity.

Toxicity, Side Effects, and Precautions. Metoprolol causes some reduction in forced expiratory volume (FEV_1) in asthmatic patients, but the effect is less than that produced by propranolol when the drugs are administered in doses that cause equal degrees of β_1-adrenergic blockade. In contrast to propranolol, metoprolol does not significantly inhibit the bronchodilatation induced by isoproterenol. However, exacerbation of respiratory symptoms has occurred in asthmatic patients who have received relatively high doses of metoprolol. Such individuals should probably not be treated with metoprolol unless bronchoconstriction is controlled simultaneously with a β_2-adrenergic agonist or other antiasthmatic drug (Brogden *et al.,* 1977).

Metoprolol reduces plasma renin activity in hypertensive patients and in normal subjects and inhibits the rise in the plasma renin activity normally induced by cardiovascular stress, such as prolonged standing. There is some evidence that metoprolol may impair glucose tolerance in diabetic patients and perhaps in normal individuals, implying that the β-receptor-mediated release of insulin is to some degree inhibited by this drug. Should hypoglycemia occur in a diabetic patient, metoprolol, like propranolol, can mask some of the signs because of inhibition of the associated reflex tachycardia.

The most common side effects associated with the administration of metoprolol are fatigue, headache, dizziness, and insomnia. These effects are generally not sufficiently severe to require cessation of treatment.

As with all β-adrenergic antagonists, metoprolol should not be used if there is a risk of congestive heart failure unless the patient is monitored closely; the administration of digitalis may be necessary. Similarly, the drug must be used with caution in individuals with disturbances of cardiac conduction.

Preparations, Route of Administration, and Dosage. *Metoprolol tartrate* (LOPRESSOR) is administered orally. The initial dose is 50 mg twice daily, and the dose may be gradually increased to a maximum of 450 mg per day, depending upon the response. Metoprolol is available in 50- and 100-mg tablets.

Therapeutic Uses. Metoprolol is an effective antihypertensive agent, and its efficacy appears to be comparable to that of propranolol in the management of mild or moderate disease. Metoprolol is frequently administered in combination with other antihypertensive drugs (*see* Chapter 32). Although it is logical to assume that metoprolol should be effective in the management of cardiac arrhythmias and angina pectoris, data are not yet available.

LABETALOL

Labetalol is an antihypertensive agent with unique pharmacological properties; it exhibits both α- and β-adrenergic blocking activity (Brittain and Levy, 1976; Richards and Prichard, 1978). It is also able to inhibit the re-uptake of norepinephrine into nerve terminals. The structural formula of labetalol is as follows:

Labetalol

Labetalol is approximately one tenth as potent as phentolamine in its ability to block α receptors, and it is approximately one third as potent as propranolol in blocking β receptors. Labetalol possesses no intrinsic sympathomimetic activity. In low doses, its pharmacological effects resemble those of propranolol. In higher doses, its actions are similar to those of adrenergic neuron blocking drugs.

Labetalol is well absorbed when administered orally. Like propranolol, a considerable fraction of the drug is metabolized in the first circulation through the liver. Its half-life in plasma is approximately 5 hours, and about 5% of the drug is excreted in the urine unchanged (Martin *et al.*, 1976).

Labetalol is a potent hypotensive agent (Prichard and Boakes, 1976). It has been used successfully to treat essential hypertension, the hypertension and other cardiovascular effects associated with pheochromocytoma, and the hypertensive response during abrupt withdrawal of clonidine (Rosei *et al.*, 1976). Postural hypotension occurs in a small fraction of patients.

III. Centrally Acting Agents That Interfere with Adrenergic Neuronal Function

The activity of the peripheral sympathetic nervous system is regulated by the CNS in a complex manner that remains incompletely understood. Psychic factors can profoundly affect sympathetic activity, suggesting that the cortex is involved in this process. Regions of the brain stem such as the hypothalamus and nucleus tractus solitarius also are critically involved in central sympathetic regulation of cardiovascular activity and blood pressure. Neurons in these regions of the brain stem that are *themselves* adrenergic are involved in regulation of peripheral sympathetic activity, but the nature and mechanism of this control are unclear (*see* below).

Clonidine and *methyldopa* are two useful antihypertensive agents that act by inhibiting the outflow of sympathetic neural traffic from the CNS. While their pharmacological properties are primarily presented in Chapter 32, brief descriptions of these drugs follow to facilitate comparison with other agents that interfere with the function of the sympathetic nervous system.

CLONIDINE

Clonidine is an antihypertensive agent that, paradoxically, possesses primarily α-adrenergic agonistic properties (*see* Chapter 32). However, clonidine owes its antihypertensive effect to a predominant action on the CNS, where it apparently produces a decrease in the sympathetic outflow from the brain.

The major pharmacological actions of clonidine appear to be related to its capacity to stimulate both central and peripheral α_1- and α_2-adrenergic receptors. Shortly after the parenteral administration of clonidine, an elevation in blood pressure is observed. This appears to be the result of direct interaction of the drug with peripheral α_1 (postsynaptic) receptors, resulting in a transient vasoconstriction. Within a short period of time, the hypotensive effect of clonidine becomes apparent, presumably as a result of a direct α-agonistic effect in the CNS.

The exact site at which clonidine exerts this central effect is not precisely known. It appears to inhibit central sympathetic outflow by acting upon α receptors in the lower brain stem region, possibly in the nucleus tractus solitarius (Haeusler, 1973a, 1973b, 1974). This region of the brain is rich in cell bodies and nerve terminals that contain epinephrine or norepinephrine (Van der Gugten *et al.*, 1976). Lesion of this region is associated with a fulminating hypertensive response (Doba and Reis, 1973). Conversely, electrical stimulation of this region is associated with a reduction in blood pressure (De Jong *et al.*, 1975). However, the actions of clonidine on blood pressure may be mediated in the lower brain stem, in the spinal cord, or at several levels in the cerebrospinal axis.

Clonidine has been shown to exhibit potent agonistic activity on α_2 (presynaptic) receptors. As a consequence, neural release of norepinephrine is inhibited by the drug. This could lead to a reduction of central sympathetic neuronal activity, which might then be responsible for the reduced peripheral sympathetic outflow. Since the effect of clonidine on blood pressure can be inhibited by yohimbine, which is primarily an α_2 antagonist, it is conceivable that clonidine inhibits adrenergic neuronal activity by an α_2 presynaptic mechanism (Starke and Altmann, 1973). Conversely, activation of α_1 (postsynaptic) receptors in certain nuclei in the brain stem may be associated with inhibition of central sympathetic outflow (Haeusler, 1974).

METHYLDOPA

It is now generally accepted that methyldopa exerts its antihypertensive effect by a central mechanism (Porter *et al.*, 1977; *see* Chapter 32). The drug enters the CNS quite readily, and it is then decarboxylated to α-methyldopamine and β-hydroxylated to α-methylnorepinephrine in central adrenergic neurons. The α-methylnorepinephrine that is released from such neurons is a potent agonist at α receptors in the CNS and, in some manner, perhaps analogous to that of clonidine, inhibits central sympathetic outflow. α-Methylnorepinephrine, like clonidine, is a more potent stimulator at presynaptic (α_2) receptors than at postsynaptic receptors (Starke, 1977).

IV. Adrenergic Neuron Blocking Agents

Interference with chemical mediation at postganglionic adrenergic nerve endings can occur by several mechanisms, including depletion of the stores of mediator and direct prevention of its release. However, many drugs in this class appear to act by more than one mechanism, and the contribution of each to a given effect is often unclear. It is particularly difficult to assess the contribution of reduced norepinephrine content to inhibition of the function of adrenergic neurons. In some cases block occurs only after extensive depletion; in others, with only minor changes in total content. In the latter instance the assumption has often been made that a crucial "pool" or "compartment" of transmitter

has been depleted. However, it is likely in such cases that the blockade of the adrenergic neuron is unrelated to the depletion of norepinephrine.

GUANETHIDINE

Guanethidine may be considered representative of drugs that depress the function of postganglionic adrenergic nerves. Guanethidine and related compounds, such as bretylium (*see* below), have a strongly basic moiety such as the guanidine grouping or a quaternary nitrogen. The structural formula of guanethidine is as follows:

Guanethidine

Locus and Mechanism of Action. The major effect of guanethidine is inhibition of responses to stimulation of sympathetic nerves and to indirectly acting sympathomimetic amines (*e.g.*, tyramine, amphetamine). The site of this inhibition is clearly presynaptic and, during chronic administration of guanethidine, it is due to impaired release of neurotransmitter from peripheral adrenergic neurons.

Guanethidine has considerable local anesthetic activity, but concentrations that prevent responses to adrenergic nerve stimulation do not block conduction along adrenergic axons. Essentially complete inhibition of responses to adrenergic nerve activity can develop very rapidly, and this change precedes any detectable alteration in tissue stores of catecholamines, which subsequently decline slowly. Chronic administration of guanethidine can, however, greatly reduce tissue concentrations of norepinephrine, and the depletion persists for several days after the drug has been discontinued.

Guanethidine is taken up by and stored in adrenergic nerves, and this accumulation is essential for its action. Uptake involves the same mechanism responsible for the nerve membrane transport of norepinephrine, and the uptake and subsequent action of guanethidine can be inhibited by sympathomimetic amines, phenoxybenzamine, cocaine, phenothiazines, and tricyclic antidepressants. Guanethidine apparently accumulates in and displaces norepinephrine from intraneuronal storage granules, and is itself released by nerve stimulation. Thus, it fits the definition of a "false transmitter," but this mechanism appears not to be responsible for its effects. Guanethidine can also be released by reserpine, amphetamine, and tyramine; while release by the latter two drugs is associated with a decreased response, it is not clear whether the granule-bound or some other pool of guanethidine with which it is in equilibrium is primarily responsible for the nerve block. (*See* Boura and Green, 1965; Mitchell and Oates, 1970; Kirpekar and Furchgott, 1972; Shand *et al.,* 1973.)

A considerable part of the norepinephrine released from adrenergic nerve terminals by guanethidine is first deaminated by intraneuronal MAO. The percentage is less than that deaminated during release by reserpine, but more than with tyramine. However, sufficient amounts of unchanged norepinephrine are released initially to produce sympathomimetic effects, including hypertension, contraction of the nictitating membrane, piloerection, and cardiac stimulation. Guanethidine directly depresses the myocardium previously depleted of catecholamines. In addition to its indirect effects, guanethidine has been shown to produce vasodilatation in animals pretreated with reserpine; this is at least partly prevented by β-adrenergic blockade, which suggests a direct action on β-adrenergic receptors.

Chronic administration of guanethidine produces a supersensitivity of effector cells that is very similar to that due to sympathetic postganglionic denervation. It reaches a maximum in 10 to 14 days, is greater for norepinephrine than for epinephrine, and can be explained by chronic absence of released mediator (Emmelin and Engström, 1961). Guanethidine can also cause an acute increase in the sensitivity of tissues to catecholamines. This could involve a "presynaptic" component due to competition for the amine transport mechanism at the nerve membrane, but it is at least partly due to an action unrelated to adrenergic nerves (Maxwell, 1965).

PHARMACOLOGICAL PROPERTIES

The most important effects of guanethidine are attributable to reduction of re-

sponses to sympathetic nerve activation because of diminution in the release of transmitter. Thus, in contrast to adrenergic blocking agents, responses mediated by α- and β-adrenergic receptors are suppressed about equally. Guanethidine usually causes a roughly parallel shift to the right of frequency-response curves for stimulation of adrenergic nerves, but with some preferential block of responses to low frequencies. The concentration of catecholamines in the adrenal medulla is not lowered by guanethidine, and responses that involve the release of amines from this site may be unaffected or even augmented. Similarly, concentrations of catecholamines in the CNS are not altered by guanethidine, since this polar drug does not penetrate the blood-brain barrier in sufficient concentrations to exert prominent CNS effects.

Cardiovascular System. Rapid intravenous injection of guanethidine produces a characteristic triphasic response. There is an initial rapid fall in blood pressure associated with increased cardiac output and decreased peripheral resistance; the latter is probably due to a transient direct action of the drug on resistance vessels. The fall in blood pressure is followed by hypertension, which may persist for several hours and is much accentuated by prior ganglionic blockade or spinal cord section. Infusion of the doses employed in man causes a definite, but relatively small and transient increase in blood pressure.

In both laboratory animals and man, the initial changes are followed by a progressive fall in both systemic and pulmonary arterial pressures that may last for several days. This period of hypotension is usually associated with bradycardia, decreased pulse pressure, and decreased cardiac output. Systolic pressure in the erect position is most markedly reduced, and changes in supine blood pressure are often small. Peripheral resistance is not usually decreased, but the absence of a consistently increased peripheral resistance in the presence of decreased transmural pressure indicates some relaxation of peripheral arterioles. At least under resting conditions the distribution of blood flow is not greatly affected, although the hepatosplanchnic and renal beds may receive a smaller percentage of the cardiac output after guanethidine.

During chronic administration of guanethidine, the cardiac output may return toward or to normal, probably as a result of the sodium and water retention and increased blood volume induced by guanethidine. The heart rate is usually decreased for the duration of the antihypertensive response. The effect of guanethidine on plasma renin activity has received little attention, but it appears to cause a decrease, as do most other drugs and procedures that decrease stimulation at β_2-adrenergic receptors in the kidney (Stokes et al., 1970).

Guanethidine inhibits cardiovascular reflexes such as those elicited by bilateral carotid artery occlusion in laboratory animals or by the Valsalva maneuver or cold pressor test in man. Blockade may be incomplete with the doses usually employed in man. However, a significant antihypertensive effect is always associated with some impairment of cardiovascular adjustments, and postural and exercise hypotension are common. (See review by Sannerstedt and Conway, 1970.)

Other Effects. Guanethidine has been studied primarily for its cardiovascular effects. However, it has been shown to produce a generalized depression of responses to sympathetic nerve stimulation and augmentation of responses to catecholamines in both in-vivo and in-vitro experiments on a large number of tissues and organs.

Guanethidine and most other adrenergic neuron blocking drugs increase *gastrointestinal motility* and can cause diarrhea. This is commonly attributed to parasympathetic predominance after blockade of adrenergic fibers, but it is not well correlated with such blockade; for example, reserpine causes relatively more and bethanidine relatively less diarrhea than does guanethidine. The effect of guanethidine on gastrointestinal motility has been roughly correlated with release of intestinal 5-HT (Cass and Spriggs, 1961), but this mechanism is not fully established. It has also been suggested that altered histamine metabolism may be involved (LeBlanc et al., 1972). The *salt and water retention* commonly seen in hypertensive patients treated with guanethidine can probably be accounted for by hemodynamic effects, but the drug has been shown to stimulate sodium transport in frog skin and a renal tubular effect in man has not been ruled out.

Absorption, Fate, and Excretion. Under the usual conditions of chronic oral administration, absorption of guanethidine can vary from 3 to about 30%; it appears to be relatively constant in a given patient. However, differences in absorption account for only part of the wide variation in dose required for a satisfactory antihypertensive effect. Guanethidine is rapidly cleared by the kidney, but small amounts may remain in the body for as long as 14 days; retention probably involves both specific (adrenergic nerves) and nonspecific tissue uptake. Almost all the guanethidine that enters the circulation in man is accounted for by renal excretion of the parent compound and of two more polar and much less active metabolites. Metabolism appears to be by hepatic microsomal enzymes, and the percentage metabolized is considerably higher after oral than after parenteral administration. (See McMartin and Simpson, 1971.)

Preparations, Routes of Administration, and Dosage. *Guanethidine Sulfate,* U.S.P. (ISMELIN), is available in 10- and 25-mg tablets for oral administration. The usual daily dose is 25 to 50 mg, but it varies widely; because of its long duration of action, a single daily dose is satisfactory. The starting dose for ambulatory patients is usually 10 mg, and this may be increased at intervals of about 1 week until the desired effects are obtained or unacceptable side effects supervene. Carefully supervised patients in the hospital may receive a somewhat higher initial dose, and it may be increased more rapidly.

Toxicity, Side Effects, and Precautions. The effects of guanethidine are cumulative over extended periods. Adverse effects can appear or progress for many days or even weeks after an increase in dosage, and may not subside for several days after complete cessation of therapy. The therapeutic effect of guanethidine can be antagonized by tricyclic antidepressants (Mitchell et al., 1970), and a similar antagonism has been reported with chlorpromazine. If high doses of guanethidine are administered to overcome such antagonism, subsequent withdrawal of, for example, a tricyclic antidepressant can lead to profound hypotension and shock if the dose of guanethidine is not adjusted appropriately beforehand. Sensitization by guanethidine to some sympathomimetics found in "cold remedies" can result in hypertensive crises.

The most important complication of guanethidine therapy is *postural hypotension;* it is most prominent shortly after arising from sleep and may be accentuated by hot weather, alcohol, or exercise. Hypotensive episodes may be associated with symptoms of cerebral and myocardial ischemia. It is important that both standing and supine blood pressures be considered in adjusting dosage. A generalized subjective "weakness" is common; it is partially but not entirely attributable to postural hypotension. Fluid retention occurs and can lead to edema and resistance to the antihypertensive effect if a diuretic is not given concurrently. Guanethidine can also decrease myocardial competence by decreasing adrenergic nerve effects, and this plus fluid accumulation can lead to frank heart failure in patients with limited cardiac reserve. Some tendency to diarrhea is associated with guanethidine therapy in a high percentage of cases, but this can often be controlled by relatively small doses of an anticholinergic agent, paregoric, or a kaolin-pectin preparation. Guanethidine can cause severe hypertensive reactions in patients with pheochromocytoma.

Therapeutic Uses. The only major use of guanethidine is in the treatment of *hypertension.* This subject is discussed in Chapter 32. It also effectively controls the pressor episodes associated with the hyperreflexia of high spinal cord lesions. Local application of guanethidine has received limited trial in the treatment of *glaucoma,* sometimes in combination with epinephrine (Roth, 1973), and to produce a partial Horner's syndrome in cases of *abnormal eyelid retraction* (Gay *et al.,* 1967).

BRETYLIUM

Choline 2,6-xylyl ether (TM10) was the first of many strongly basic compounds shown to inhibit responses to adrenergic nerve stimulation without impairing responses to exogenous catecholamines; interest in this type of specific blockade of adrenergic nerves led to the study of many congeners, of which *bretylium* was the first to be used in man.

Discovered in the late 1950s, bretylium was first regarded as a potentially useful antihypertensive agent. Its development was greatly hampered, however, because of its poor and unpredictable absorption after oral administration. More recently, bretylium has been demonstrated to be an effective antiarrhythmic agent, and it is now available for use in the United States for that purpose. Only the effects of bretylium on the function of the adrenergic neuron will be discussed here; other pharmacological properties of this drug are described in Chapter 31.

Bretylium, like guanethidine, inhibits the release of norepinephrine from adrenergic nerve endings. Autoradiographic studies have shown that the drug is concentrated in adrenergic nerve terminals, and it

appears to exert a selective local anesthetic effect at that site. As with many compounds that affect sympathetic neurons, bretylium exerts multiple effects on the metabolism of norepinephrine. Acute, parenteral administration of bretylium may be associated with sympathomimetic effects as a result of the capacity of this agent to release norepinephrine from nerve terminals. Subsequently, bretylium blocks the release of norepinephrine associated with nerve stimulation. Bretylium has also been reported to inhibit the uptake of norepinephrine and epinephrine into adrenergic nerve endings. As a consequence of this cocaine-like action, bretylium is able to potentiate the actions of circulating catecholamines (Haeusler *et al.,* 1969).

Bretylium and guanethidine produce very similar early inhibition of responses to adrenergic nerve stimulation and to amphetamine and other indirectly acting sympathomimetics, although the action of bretylium is more readily antagonized by such drugs. Agents that block the amine transport mechanism at adrenergic nerve-terminal membranes, such as imipramine, inhibit the action of both guanethidine and bretylium (Toda, 1972). In contrast to guanethidine, a single blocking dose of bretylium produces little reduction of the concentrations of catecholamines in tissues. Only large, repeated doses produce depletion. Bretylium can cause an initial increase in tissue catecholamines, antagonize the depleting action of guanethidine, and delay the release of norepinephrine during nerve degeneration. The initial "sympathomimetic" effects of bretylium are less prominent and more transient than those of guanethidine. Like guanethidine, bretylium does not block release of catecholamines from the adrenal medulla, and responses of effector cells to circulating catecholamines may be much increased. The pharmacology of bretylium has been discussed by Boura and Green (1965).

BETHANIDINE, DEBRISOQUIN

A large number of compounds within the general guanethidine-bretylium spectrum of activity have been synthesized and tested. The most successful from a therapeutic standpoint have combined a very basic guanidine or amidine moiety, similar to that in guanethidine, with an aromatic ring constituent, as in bretylium. Two of these compounds, *bethanidine* (1-benzyl-2,3-dimethylguanidine) and *debrisoquin* (3,4-dihydro-2[1H]-isoquinolinecarboxamidine), have proven to be useful antihypertensive drugs. Their hemodynamic effects are essentially the same as those of guanethidine or bretylium, and the reduction in blood pressure has a large postural component. In other respects their pharmacological properties appear to be similar to those of bretylium. Compared to guanethidine, their durations of action are much shorter, they produce lesser sympathomimetic effects when injected intravenously, and they cause considerably less depletion of norepinephrine stores. (*See* Moe *et al.,* 1964; Boura and Green, 1965.) In occasional patients the shorter duration of action of bethanidine and debrisoquin or the lesser tendency to produce diarrhea may be a significant advantage, but in general they have the same role as guanethidine in antihypertensive therapy. These compounds are not available for general use in the United States.

RESERPINE

History. Descriptions of the use of extracts of plants resembling rauwolfia may be traced back to ancient Hindu ayurvedic writings. They were used in primitive Hindu medicine for a variety of diseases, including snakebite (because of the resemblance of the root to a snake), hypertension, insomnia, and insanity.

Rauwolfia serpentina (Benth) is a climbing shrub of the Apocynaceae family, indigenous to India and neighboring countries. A French botanist, Plumier, in 1703 named the plant *Rauwolfia serpentina* in honor of Dr. Leonhard Rauwolf of Augsburg, a sixteenth century botanist who never saw the plant or even knew of its existence. Therapeutic applications of the whole root for the treatment of psychoses and hypertension were described in an Indian medical journal in 1931 by Sen and Bose. Little attention was paid to this finding until 1955, when Vakil wrote the first report of its antihypertensive effect in a Western medical journal.

In 1954, Kline reported that rauwolfia or reserpine was helpful in the treatment of psychotic patients. Subsequent discovery of the ability of rauwolfia alkaloids and related compounds to release biogenic amines from storage sites in the body initiated a great number of investigations directed at elucidating the interactions between these amines and reserpine.

Chemistry. There are a number of rauwolfia alkaloids with complex structures. The structure of reserpine is as follows:

Reserpine

Locus and Mechanism of Action. Reserpine depletes stores of catecholamines and 5-HT in many organs, including the brain and adrenal medulla, and most of its pharmacological effects have been attributed to this action. Depletion is slower and less complete in the adrenal medulla than in other tissues.

Reduced concentrations of catecholamines can be measured within an hour after administration of reserpine, and depletion is maximal by 24 hours. Most of the catecholamine is deaminated intraneuronally, and pharmacological effects of the released mediator are minimal unless MAO has been inhibited. The doses used in most laboratory experiments reduce tissue catecholamines to negligible levels. Major impairment of adrenergic nerve function usually begins at levels below 30% of normal, and is roughly related to the degree of depletion below that value. Tissue catecholamines are restored slowly; consequently, repeated doses have a cumulative action when administered even at intervals of up to a week or longer. Chronic administration of reserpine in doses of less than 1.0 mg per day produces a marked depletion of the norepinephrine content of the human myocardium (Chidsey *et al.*, 1963).

Depletion of catecholamines by reserpine is at least partially dependent on nerve activity and can be reduced by spinal cord section or ganglionic blockade. Studies with labeled drug indicate that reserpine itself is not released by nerve activity even in the period up to 18 hours after administration when some of the drug is reversibly bound; all reserpine remaining in tissues after 24 to 30 hours is firmly bound and may persist for many days (Norn and Shore, 1971).

It is clear that reserpine interferes with intracellular storage of catecholamines, but the amounts of reserpine in tissues are much too small to assume a stoichiometric displacement. Reserpine antagonizes the uptake of norepinephrine by isolated chromaffin granules, apparently by inhibiting the ATP-Mg^{2+}–dependent uptake mechanism of the granule membrane. This may be irreversible, because it appears that restoration of normal intraneuronal stores of norepinephrine is dependent on transport of new storage vesicles down the axon (Häggendal and Dahlström, 1972).

Inhibition of reserpine-induced depletion of catecholamines by MAO inhibitors has been attributed to an increased intracellular concentration of free amine. The decrease in norepinephrine synthesis induced by reserpine may be due to block of dopamine uptake into storage granules that contain the enzyme dopamine β-hydroxylase. Furthermore, the increased concentration of free catecholamine presumably feeds back to inhibit tyrosine hydroxylase, since norepinephrine competes with the pterin cofactor for the enzyme (Pfeffer *et al.*, 1975). On the other hand, the compensatory increased firing of adrenergic nerves after reserpine and other drugs that inhibit their effects causes an acute increase in tyrosine hydroxylase activity, and chronic administration of reserpine is associated with increased tissue activity of the enzyme and an increased turnover rate of norepinephrine. (*See* Weiner, 1970; Weiner *et al.*, 1978.)

Supersensitivity to catecholamines is observed following chronic administration of reserpine. The site of change is presumably postjunctional and may be due to alterations of the adrenergic receptors. Such adaptive change is usual following chronic deprivation of transmitter. It has also been suggested that an increased availability of calcium in effector cells may be involved (Carrier and Jurevics, 1973).

A number of observations suggest that reserpine has other actions. Reserpine administered intra-arterially produces peripheral vasodilatation in both normal and sympathectomized human extremities. It directly depresses several parameters of myocardial function (Nayler, 1962), and chronic administration of small doses has been reported to produce morphological changes in the myocardium. Release of gastrin via a central vagal mechanism appears to be involved in the increased gastric acid secretion induced by reserpine (Emås and Fyrö, 1965). The drug can produce a variety of endocrine changes in experimental animals (see Gaunt et al., 1963); this may be due to depletion of dopamine and perhaps other biogenic amines in the median eminence that are involved in regulation of the secretion of pituitary hormones.

Pharmacological Properties. After a transient sympathomimetic effect, seen only after parenteral administration of relatively large doses, reserpine causes a slowly developing fall in blood pressure frequently associated with bradycardia. In recumbent subjects, the reduction in blood pressure may involve a decrease in peripheral resistance; this is most marked in the skin, and cutaneous blood flow may be increased. However, the antihypertensive effect of chronic administration of reserpine is usually associated with a reduced cardiac output (Cohen et al., 1968). Pressor responses, such as those induced by carotid artery occlusion or stimulation of the central end of the cut vagus nerve, are effectively inhibited by the doses of reserpine commonly employed in experimental animals. Most observations in man indicate that cardiovascular reflexes are only partially inhibited, probably because of the small doses administered. However, reflex responses of veins can be comparably depressed by guanethidine and reserpine, and the two drugs appear to have a similar potential to decrease cardiac output and produce postural hypotension at equivalent levels of inhibition of efferent nerve function. Responses to indirectly acting sympathomimetic amines are potentiated during the initial phase of reserpine action, but later they are depressed. (See reviews by Alper et al., 1963; Sannerstedt and Conway, 1970.)

Reserpine acts centrally to produce characteristic sedation and a state of indifference to environmental stimuli. These central effects resemble those of the phenothiazines (Chapter 19), but they are not identical. It is assumed that these changes are due to depletion of stores of catecholamines and 5-HT in the brain. Following prolonged administration of high doses, extrapyramidal effects are noted.

Preparations, Routes of Administration, and Dosage. The oral antihypertensive dose of reserpine ranges from 0.1 to 1.0 mg daily, usually taken in two or three divided doses. Higher doses are now rarely employed because of increased side effects. It requires up to 3 weeks for the full antihypertensive effect to develop. Reserpine is now used only rarely in psychiatric patients for its behavioral effects.

The rauwolfia fractions, alkaloids, and derivatives are available in a large variety of preparations. Two that are official are the whole root, *Rauwolfia Serpentina*, U.S.P., and the purified alkaloid, *Reserpine*, U.S.P. Rauwolfia serpentina (RAUDIXIN, others) is available in tablets containing 50 or 100 mg. Orally, 200 to 300 mg of powdered whole root is equivalent to 0.5 mg of reserpine. Reserpine (SANDRIL, SERPASIL) is available in tablets that contain 0.1, 0.25, 0.5, or 1 mg; in capsules that contain 0.5 mg; as an elixir (0.2 mg/4 ml); or as an injection (2.5 mg/ml) in 2 ml-ampuls and 10-ml vials.

Toxicity, Side Effects, and Precautions. Untoward responses to reserpine are predominantly referable to the CNS and the gastrointestinal tract, and have resulted in a progressive reduction in the doses employed in the treatment of hypertension. The mild sedative effect of small doses may be desirable in some apprehensive patients. However, even doses as small as 0.25 mg per day can produce a considerable incidence of nightmares and psychic depression (Quetsch et al., 1959), sometimes severe enough to require hospitalization or to end in suicide. *Reserpine should not be administered to patients with a history of depressive episodes,* and it should be discontinued if suggestive signs or symptoms develop. Extrapyramidal disturbances rarely occur with the usual antihypertensive dose. Reserpine commonly increases gastrointestinal tone and motility, with abdominal cramps and diarrhea. Single doses of 0.25 mg or more quite consistently increase gastric acid secretion. The secretory effects of chronic administration and their relation to reports of gastrointestinal ulceration and hemorrhage are less clear-cut, but reserpine probably should not be given to patients with a history of peptic ulcer and it should be discontinued if signs or symptoms of peptic ulceration appear. Reserpine quite commonly causes weight gain.

Hypotensive episodes are rare with doses of less than 1 mg of reserpine per day, but patients may be sensitized to this reaction following a cerebrovascular accident. Vascular side effects include flushing and nasal congestion; these are usually of minor importance, but the latter may occasionally cause serious respiratory problems in infants born of mothers receiving reserpine. Reserpine has been reported to produce cardiovascular lability during anesthesia, but careful studies have failed to substantiate this, and it does not appear necessary to discontinue the drug prior to anesthesia and surgery (Munson and Jenicek, 1962).

In a retrospective study in the United States, subsequently confirmed in the United Kingdom and Finland, it was found that the long-term administration of reserpine as an antihypertensive drug in women was associated with over a threefold increase in the incidence of *carcinoma of the breast* (*see* Boston Collaborative Drug Surveillance Program, 1974; Editorial, 1974). However, considerable controversy ensued over the statistical validity of this conclusion. It remains uncertain if the chronic administration of reserpine is associated with an increased incidence of any type of malignancy.

Therapeutic Uses. The only important application of the cardiovascular effects of reserpine is in the treatment of *hypertension;* this subject is discussed in Chapter 32. Because of the severity of the dose-related side effects of reserpine, the drug is administered in low doses and is used only in conjunction with other types of antihypertensive agents.

SPECIFIC INHIBITORS OF CATECHOLAMINE SYNTHESIS

Much of the work on adrenergic neuron blocking drugs has assumed a cause-and-effect relationship between depletion of norepinephrine stores and failure of nerve function. Consequently, it appeared that inhibition of norepinephrine synthesis would represent the ultimate mechanism of adrenergic neuron blockade. Inhibitors of each step of the biosynthesis have been studied, but major depletion occurs only

with drugs that act on the rate-limiting step, the hydroxylation of tyrosine. Of these inhibitors, α-methyltyrosine (α-MT) is the most thoroughly studied and one of the most effective. The pattern of effects produced by α-MT differs considerably from that of the classical adrenergic neuron blocking drugs. Almost complete depletion of norepinephrine stores in brain and peripheral tissues in laboratory animals by α-MT does not lower blood pressure, and only limited signs of sympathetic inadequacy have been reported; responses to both tyramine and norepinephrine are depressed (Spector *et al.*, 1965). Conversely, it has been reported that a single intravenous dose of α-MT can considerably inhibit the reduction in hindlimb perfusion induced by sympathetic nerve stimulation at a time when the norepinephrine content of arterial walls is unaltered (Redisch *et al.*, 1969). Norepinephrine synthesis has been decreased by about 70% in man by α-MT; this produces considerable improvement in patients with pheochromocytoma, but has little effect on the blood pressure of those with essential hypertension (Engelman *et al.*, 1968).

MONOAMINE OXIDASE INHIBITORS

Monoamine oxidase (MAO) inhibitors were introduced into therapy for the treatment of depression in 1957. Paradoxically, these agents, which inhibit the oxidative deamination of norepinephrine, were found to cause hypotension. However, because of their toxicity and the occurrence of dangerous interactions between MAO inhibitors and certain other drugs and foods, they are now used only occasionally as antidepressants (*see* Chapter 19); they currently have little or no place in the management of hypertension.

The effects of MAO inhibitors on blood pressure are attributed to the accumulation of false transmitters (impotent phenylethylamines) in peripheral adrenergic neurons, and they thus appear to act as adrenergic neuron blocking agents. The false-transmitter concept and the action of MAO inhibitors are discussed in Chapter 8, as is the etiology of the hypertensive crisis that can follow the ingestion of foods that contain tyramine by patients taking these drugs.

There has, however, been a resurgence of interest in MAO inhibitors as possible therapeutic agents following the discovery that there are isozymes of MAO and that these isozymes have different substrate specificities and can be inhibited selectively (Sandler and Youdim, 1972). Physical separation of isozymes of MAO has been achieved; there is evidence to suggest that the active site of the isozymes is identical and that the different properties of the enzymes are related to the lipid environment in which they are situated (Tipton, 1975; Houslay and Tipton, 1976).

Clorgyline, closely related structurally to pargyline, was found to be a rather selective inhibitor of MAO type A (MAO-A) (Johnston, 1968). A chemically similar compound, *deprenyl,* was found to be selectively effective against MAO type B (MAO-B) (Knoll, 1976). Pargyline exhibits somewhat greater inhibitory activity against MAO-B, but its selectivity is not great. MAO A preferentially deaminates physiological substrates such as 5-HT, norepinephrine, epinephrine, metanephrine, and normetanephrine. It also deaminates other β-hydroxylated phenylethylamines, such as octopamine. Preferential substrates for MAO-B include benzylamine, tryptamine, 5-O-methyltryptamine, and phenylethylamine. Tyramine, dopamine, and 3-O-methyltyramine are metabolized by both isozymes to similar degrees (Houslay and Tipton, 1976).

It was originally proposed that MAO-A is localized in neuronal tissue, whereas MAO-B is extraneuronal; however, this generalization is not entirely correct. Rat liver and brain contain approximately equal proportions of the two isozymes. Rat superior cervical ganglion and spleen contain almost entirely MAO-A. The intestine contains approximately 70% MAO-A. Of particular interest is the observation that human platelets and striatum contain MAO-B. Thus, administration of deprenyl (10 mg per day) inhibits MAO-B in brain by greater than 90% and appears to have a beneficial effect in patients with Parkinson's disease (Riederer et al., 1978; see also Chapter 21). This agent is purported not to produce the "beer, cheese, and wine" type of hypertensive crisis, since MAO-A, which is present in liver and gastrointestinal tract, is not inhibited. Tyramine, which is absorbed from the gastrointestinal tract, can still be effectively metabolized in individuals treated with deprenyl.

DRUGS THAT DESTROY ADRENERGIC NERVE FIBERS

Interest in 6-hydroxydopamine (6-OHDA) was first aroused by the observation that it caused a prolonged decrease in the catecholamine content of the heart (Porter et al., 1963). This effect was subsequently shown to be due to destruction of sympathetic nerve endings. Most peripheral sympathetic nerves are affected by adequate doses, but there are some quantitative differences in sensitivity. The adrenal medulla and peripheral cholinergic neurons are unaffected. 6-OHDA does not damage peripheral adrenergic nerve-cell bodies or proximal axons in adult animals, and regeneration of the terminal usually occurs completely. In newborn animals the entire adrenergic neuron may be destroyed and a permanent sympathectomy produced. This is usually more complete than that produced by antisera against the nerve-growth factor (immunosympathectomy) (see Levi-Montalcini and Angeletti, 1966).

The action of 6-OHDA on peripheral adrenergic nerves is dependent on its accumulation by the nerve-membrane amine pump and can be prevented by drugs such as desipramine that block this process. Although 6-OHDA is taken up by intraneuronal storage granules, this step appears not to be necessary for nerve damage because the drug is fully effective in animals pretreated with reserpine.

Morphological changes in adrenergic nerve endings have been detected as early as 1 hour after administration of 6-OHDA, and subsequent events are similar to those following nerve section. The first responses to 6-OHDA administration are sympathomimetic, due to the release of endogenous norepinephrine. Later effects are very similar to those due to guanethidine or surgical sympathectomy.

6-OHDA does not penetrate the CNS from the blood stream, but it can act on central neurons after local or intraventricular administration. Central neurons containing either norepinephrine or dopamine are affected; the former are usually considered to be the more susceptible. However, there may be only a small differential in the amounts required to damage monoaminergic neurons and to affect all other cellular elements (Poirier et al., 1972). In contrast to peripheral neurons, many cell bodies in the CNS are damaged and little regeneration occurs.

6-OHDA has been evaluated for possible therapeutic use in the treatment of glaucoma. Subconjunctival injection of the drug results in destruction of noradrenergic neurons that innervate the anterior structures of the eye, resulting in long-lasting reduction in intraocular pressure. Unfortunately, the beneficial effect persists for only 3 to 4 months and dissipates as the adrenergic nerve terminals regenerate. Repeated injections of the neurotoxin are thus required. Subsequent injections tend to cause inflammation and fibrosis, and the treatment becomes progressively less satisfactory.

The pharmacology of 6-OHDA has been reviewed by Thoenen and Tranzer (1973) and Kostrzewa and Jacobowitz (1974).

Ablad, B.; Carlsson, B.; Carlsson, E.; Dahlof, C.; Ek, L.; and Hultberg, E. Cardiac effects of β-adrenergic antagonists. *Adv. Cardiol.,* **1974,** *12,* 290–302.

Ablad, B.; Carlsson, E.; and Ek, L. Pharmacological studies of two new cardioselective adrenergic beta-receptor antagonists. *Life Sci.,* **1973,** *12,* Pt. I, 107–119.

Adler-Graschinsky, E., and Langer, S. Z. Possible role of a beta-adrenoceptor in the regulation of noradrenaline release by nerve stimulation through a positive feed-back mechanism. *Br. J. Pharmacol.,* **1975,** *53,* 43–50.

Andersen, M. P.; Frederiksen, J.; Jürgensen, H. J.; Pedersen, F.; Bechsgaard, P.; Hansen, D. A.; Nielsen, B.; Pedersen-Bjergaard, O.; and Rasmussen, S. L. Effects of alprenolol on mortality among patients with definite or suspected acute myocardial infarction. *Lancet,* **1979,** *2,* 865–867.

Assem, E. S. K., and Schild, H. O. Antagonism by β-adrenoceptor blocking agents of the antianaphylactic effect of isoprenaline. *Br. J. Pharmacol.,* **1971,** *42,* 620–630.

Aurbach, G. D.; Fedak, S. A.; Woodard, C. J.; Palmer, J. W.; Hauser, D.; and Troxler, F. Beta-adrenergic receptor: stereospecific interaction of iodinated beta-blocking agent with high affinity site. *Science,* **1974,** *185,* 1223–1224.

Barcroft, H.; Konzett, H.; and Swan, H. J. C. Observations on the action of the hydrogenated alkaloids of the ergotoxine group on the circulation in man. *J. Physiol. (Lond.),* **1951,** *112,* 273–291.

Barrett, A. M., and Cullum, V. A. The biological properties of the optical isomers of propranolol and their effects on cardiac arrhythmias. *Br. J. Pharmacol.,* **1968,** *34,* 43–55.

Benson, M. K.; Berrill, W. T.; Cruickshank, J. M.; and Sterling, G. S. A comparison of four β-adrenoceptor antagonists in patients with asthma. *Br. J. Clin. Pharmacol.,* **1978,** *5,* 415–419.

Bhattacharya, A. N.; Dierschke, D. J.; Yamaji, T.; and

Knobil, E.   The pharmacologic blockade of the circhoral mode of LH secretion in the ovariectomized rhesus monkey. *Endocrinology,* **1972,** *90,* 778–786.

Boger, W. P., III; Steinert, R. F.; Puliafito, C. A.; and Pavan-Langston, D.   Clinical trial comparing timolol ophthalmic solution to pilocarpine in open-angle glaucoma. *Am. J. Ophthalmol.,* **1978,** *86,* 8–18.

Bonn, J. A.; Turner, P.; and Hicks, D. C.   Beta-adrenergic receptor blockade with practolol in treatment of anxiety. *Lancet,* **1972,** *1,* 814–815.

Boston Collaborative Drug Surveillance Program.   Reserpine and breast cancer. *Lancet,* **1974,** *2,* 669–671.

Brittain, R. T., and Levy, G. P.   A review of the animal pharmacology of labetalol, a combined alpha and beta adrenoceptor blocking drug. *Br. J. Clin. Pharmacol.,* **1976,** *3,* 681–694.

Brogden, R. N.; Heel, R. C.; Speight, T. M.; and Avery, G. S.   Metoprolol: a review of its pharmacological properties and therapeutic efficacy in hypertension. *Drugs,* **1977,** *14,* 321–348.

Buhler, F. R.; Laragh, J. H.; Baer, L.; Vaughn, D. E.; and Brunner, H. R.   Propranolol inhibition of renin secretion. *N. Engl. J. Med.,* **1972,** *287,* 1209–1214.

Burns, J. J.; Salvador, R. A.; and Lemberger, L.   Metabolic blockade by methoxamine and its analogs. *Ann. N.Y. Acad. Sci.,* **1967,** *139,* 833–840.

Carliner, N. H.; Denune, D. P.; Finch, C. S., Jr.; and Goldberg, L. I.   Sodium nitroprusside treatment of ergotamine-induced peripheral ischemia. *J.A.M.A.,* **1974,** *227,* 308–309.

Carrier, O., Jr., and Jurevics, H. A.   The role of calcium in "nonspecific" supersensitivity of vascular muscle. *J. Pharmacol. Exp. Ther.,* **1973,** *184,* 81–94.

Cass, R., and Spriggs, T. L. B.   Tissue amine levels and sympathetic blockade after guanethidine and bretylium. *Br. J. Pharmacol. Chemother.,* **1961,** *17,* 442–450.

Chidsey, C. A.; Braunwald, E.; Morrow, A. G.; and Mason, D. T.   Myocardial norepinephrine concentration in man. Effects of reserpine and of congestive heart failure. *N. Engl. J. Med.,* **1963,** *269,* 653–658.

Cohen, S. I.; Young, M. W.; Lau, S. H.; Haft, J. I.; and Damato, A. N.   Effects of reserpine therapy on cardiac output and atrioventricular conduction during rest and controlled heart rates in patients with essential hypertension. *Circulation,* **1968,** *37,* 738–746.

Crout, J. R., and Brown, B. R., Jr.   Anesthetic management of pheochromocytoma: the value of phenoxybenzamine and methoxyflurane. *Anesthesiology,* **1969,** *30,* 29–36.

Cubeddu, L. X.; Barnes, E.; Langer, S. Z.; and Weiner, N.   Release of norepinephrine and dopamine-β-hydroxylase by nerve stimulation. I. Role of neuronal and extraneuronal uptake and of alpha presynaptic receptors. *J. Pharmacol. Exp. Ther.,* **1974a,** *190,* 431–450.

Cubeddu, L. X.; Langer, S. Z.; and Weiner, N.   The relationships between alpha receptor block, inhibition of norepinephrine uptake and the release and metabolism of ^{3}H-norepinephrine. *J. Pharmacol. Exp. Ther.,* **1974b,** *188,* 368–385.

Das, P. K., and Parratt, J. R.   Myocardial and haemodynamic effects of phentolamine. *Br. J. Pharmacol.,* **1971,** *41,* 437–444.

De Jong, W.; Zandberg, P.; and Bohus, B.   Central inhibitory noradrenergic cardiovascular control. *Prog. Brain Res.,* **1975,** *42,* 285–298.

Dixon, W. R.; Mosimann, W. F.; and Weiner, N.   The role of presynaptic feedback mechanisms in regulation of norepinephrine release by nerve stimulation. *J. Pharmacol. Exp. Ther.,* **1979,** *209,* 196–204.

Doba, N., and Reis, D. J.   Acute fulminating neurogenic hypertension produced by brainstem lesions in the rat. *Circ. Res.,* **1973,** *32,* 584–593.

Editorial.   Rauwolfia derivatives and cancer. *Lancet,* **1974,** *2,* 701–702.

Emås, S., and Fyrö, B.   Vagal release of gastrin in cats following reserpine. *Acta Physiol. Scand.,* **1965,** *63,* 358–369.

Emmelin, N., and Engström, J.   Supersensitivity of salivary glands following treatment with bretylium or guanethidine. *Br. J. Pharmacol. Chemother.,* **1961,** *16,* 315–319.

Engelman, K.; Horwitz, D.; Jéquier, E.; and Sjoerdsma, A.   Biochemical and pharmacologic effects of α-methyltyrosine in man. *J. Clin. Invest.,* **1968,** *47,* 577–594.

Engelman, K., and Sjoerdsma, A.   Chronic medical therapy for pheochromocytoma: a report of four cases. *Ann. Intern. Med.,* **1964,** *61,* 229–241.

Epstein, S. E., and Braunwald, E.   The effect of β-adrenergic blockade on patterns of urinary sodium excretion: studies in normal subjects and in patients with heart disease. *Ann. Intern. Med.,* **1966,** *65,* 20–27.

Esler, M.; Zweifler, A.; Randall, O.; and DeQuattro, V.   Pathophysiologic and pharmacokinetic determinants of the antihypertensive response to propranolol. *Clin. Pharmacol. Ther.,* **1977,** *22,* 299–308.

Evans, G. H.; Nies, A. S.; and Shand, D. G.   The disposition of propranolol. III. Decreased half-life and volume of distribution as a result of plasma binding in man, monkey, dog and rat. *J. Pharmacol. Exp. Ther.,* **1973a,** *186,* 114–122.

Evans, G. H.; Wilkinson, G. R.; and Shand, D. G.   The disposition of propranolol. IV. A dominant role for tissue uptake in the dose-dependent extraction of propranolol by the perfused rat liver. *J. Pharmacol. Exp. Ther.,* **1973b,** *186,* 447–454.

Fitzgerald, J. D., and O'Donnell, S. R.   Pharmacology of 4-hydroxypropranolol, a metabolite of propranolol. *Br. J. Pharmacol.,* **1971,** *43,* 222–235.

Formgren, H.   Practolol in the treatment of tachyarrhythmias in patients with bronchial asthma. *Am. Heart J.,* **1972,** *84,* 710–712.

Friend, D. G., and Edwards, E. A.   Use of DIBENZYLINE as a vasodilator in patients with severe digital ischemia. *Arch. Intern. Med.,* **1954,** *93,* 928–937.

Furchgott, R. F.   Dibenamine blockade in strips of rabbit aorta and its use in differentiating receptors. *J. Pharmacol. Exp. Ther.,* **1954,** *111,* 265–284.

Garfield, S. L.; Gershon, S.; Sletten, I.; Sundland, D. M.; and Ballou, S.   Chemically induced anxiety. *Int. J. Neuropsychiatry,* **1967,** *3,* 426–433.

Gay, A. J.; Salmon, M. L.; and Wolkstein, M. A.   Topical sympatholytic therapy for pathologic lid retraction. *Arch. Ophthalmol.,* **1967,** *77,* 341–344.

Gifford, R. W., Jr.   The arteriospastic diseases: clinical significance and management. *Cardiovasc. Clin.,* **1971,** *3,* No. 1, 128–139.

Gilligan, B. S.; Veale, J. L.; and Wodak, J.   Propranolol in the treatment of tremor. *Med. J. Aust.,* **1972,** *1,* 320–322.

Graham, R. M., and Pettinger, W. A.   Drug therapy: prazosin. *N. Engl. J. Med.,* **1979,** *300,* 232–236.

Green, K. L.   The anti-inflammatory effect of catecholamines in the peritoneal cavity and hind paw of the mouse. *Br. J. Pharmacol.,* **1972,** *45,* 322–332.

Gross, G. J., and Winbury, M. M.   Beta adrenergic blockade on intramyocardial distribution of coronary blood flow. *J. Pharmacol. Exp. Ther.,* **1973,** *187,* 451–464.

Haeusler, G.   Activation of the central pathway of the baroreceptor reflex, a possible mechanism of the hypotensive action of clonidine. *Naunyn Schmiedebergs Arch. Pharmacol.,* **1973a,** *278,* 231–246.

————.   Further similarities between the action of clonidine and a central activation of the depressor baroreceptor reflex. *Ibid.,* **1973b,** *285,* 1–14.

————.   Clonidine-induced inhibition of sympathetic nerve activity: no indication for a central presynaptic or an indirect sympathomimetic mode of action. *Ibid.,* **1974,** *286,* 97–111.

Haeusler, G.; Haefly, W.; and Huerlimann, A.   On the

mechanism of the adrenergic nerve blocking action of bretylium. *Naunyn Schmiedebergs Arch. Pharmakol.,* **1969,** *265,* 260–277.

Häggendal, J., and Dahlström, A. The recovery of the capacity for uptake-retention of [³H] noradrenaline in rat adrenergic nerves after reserpine. *J. Pharm. Pharmacol.,* **1972,** *24,* 565–574.

Hayes, A., and Cooper, R. G. Studies on the absorption, distribution and excretion of propranolol in rat, dog and monkey. *J. Pharmacol. Exp. Ther.,* **1971,** *176,* 302–311.

Helfant, R. H.; Herman, M. V.; and Gorlin, R. Abnormalities of left ventricular contraction induced by beta adrenergic blockade. *Circulation,* **1971,** *43,* 641–647.

Hollenberg, N. K., and Nickerson, M. Changes in pre- and postcapillary resistance in pathogenesis of hemorrhagic shock. *Am. J. Physiol.,* **1970,** *219,* 1483–1489.

Iversen, L. L.; Salt, P. J.; and Wilson, H. A. Inhibition of catecholamine uptake in the isolated rat heart by haloalkylamines related to phenoxybenzamine. *Br. J. Pharmacol.,* **1972,** *46,* 647–657.

Johnston, J. P. Some observations upon a new inhibitor of monoamine oxidase in brain tissue. *Biochem. Pharmacol.,* **1968,** *17,* 1285–1297.

Kelly, D. T.; Delgado, C. E.; Taylor, D. R.; Pitt, B.; and Ross, R. S. Use of phentolamine in acute myocardial infarction associated with hypertension and left ventricular failure. *Circulation,* **1973,** *47,* 729–735.

Kirpekar, S. M., and Furchgott, R. F. Interaction of tyramine and guanethidine in the spleen of the cat. *J. Pharmacol. Exp. Ther.,* **1972,** *180,* 38–46.

Knoll, J. Analysis of the pharmacological effects of selective monoamine oxidase inhibitors. In, *Monoamine Oxidase and Its Inhibition* (a Ciba Foundation symposium). (Wolstenholme, G. E. W., and Knight, J., eds.) Elsevier Publishing Co., Amsterdam, **1976,** pp. 135–162.

Koch-Weser, J. Beta adrenergic blockade and circulating eosinophils. *Arch. Intern. Med.,* **1968,** *121,* 255–258.

LeBlanc, J.; Côté, J.; Doré, F.; and Rousseau, S. Effects of guanethidine and related compounds on histamine excretion. *Can. J. Physiol. Pharmacol.,* **1972,** *50,* 539–544.

Ledsome, J. R.; Kellett, R. P.; and Burkhart, S. M. The ability of propranolol to antagonize induced changes in heart rate. *J. Pharmacol. Exp. Ther.,* **1974,** *188,* 198–206.

Levy, B. The adrenergic blocking activity of N-*tert*-butylmethoxamine (butoxamine). *J. Pharmacol. Exp. Ther.,* **1966,** *151,* 413–422.

Loubatieres, A.; Mariani, M. M.; Sorel, G.; and Savi, L. The action of β-adrenergic blocking and stimulating agents on insulin secretion. Characterization of the type of β receptor. *Diabetologia,* **1971,** *7,* 127–132.

McDevitt, R. G. The assessment of β-adrenoceptor blocking drugs in man. *Br. J. Clin. Pharmacol.,* **1977,** *4,* 413–425.

McMartin, C., and Simpson, P. The absorption and metabolism of guanethidine in hypertensive patients requiring different doses of the drug. *Clin. Pharmacol. Ther.,* **1971,** *12,* 73–77.

McNay, J. L., and Goldberg, L. I. Comparison of the effects of dopamine, isoproterenol, norepinephrine, and bradykinin on canine renal and femoral blood flow. *J. Pharmacol. Exp. Ther.,* **1966,** *151,* 23–31.

Majid, P. A.; Sharma, B.; and Taylor, S. H. Phentolamine for vasodilator treatment of severe heart-failure. *Lancet,* **1971,** *2,* 719–724.

Martin, L. E.; Hopkins, R.; and Bland, R. Metabolism of labetalol by animals and man. *Br. J. Clin. Pharmacol.,* **1976,** *3,* Suppl., 695–710.

Maxwell, R. A. Concerning the mode of action of guanethidine and some derivatives in augmenting the vasomotor action of adrenergic amines in vascular tissues of the rabbit. *J. Pharmacol. Exp. Ther.,* **1965,** *148,* 320–328.

Mellander, S., and Nordenfelt, I. Comparative effects of dihydroergotamine and noradrenaline on resistance, ex-

change and capacitance functions in the peripheral circulation. *Clin. Sci.,* **1970,** *39,* 183–201.

Michelakis, A. M., and McAllister, R. G. The effect of chronic adrenergic receptor blockade on plasma renin activity in man. *J. Clin. Endocrinol. Metab.,* **1972,** *34,* 386–394.

Minneman, K. P.; Hegstrand, L. R.; and Molinoff, P. B. The pharmacological specificity of beta-1 and beta-2 adrenergic receptors in rat heart and lung *in vitro. Mol. Pharmacol.,* **1979a,** *15,* 21–33.

————. Simultaneous determination of beta-1 and beta-2 adrenergic receptors in tissues containing both receptor subtypes. *Ibid.,* **1979b,** *15,* 34–46.

Mitchell, J. R.; Cavanaugh, J. H.; Arias, L.; and Oates, J. A. Guanethidine and related agents. III. Antagonism by drugs which inhibit the norepinephrine pump in man. *J. Clin. Invest.,* **1970,** *49,* 1596–1604.

Mitchell, J. R., and Oates, J. A. Guanethidine and related agents. I. Mechanism of the selective blockade of adrenergic neurons and its antagonism by drugs. *J. Pharmacol. Exp. Ther.,* **1970,** *172,* 100–107.

Moe, R. A.; Bates, H. M.; Palkoski, Z. M.; and Banziger, R. Cardiovascular effects of 3,4-dihydro-2(1H) isoquinoline carboxamidine (DECLINAX). *Curr. Ther. Res.,* **1964,** *6,* 299–318.

Moyer, J. H., and Caplovitz, C. The clinical results of oral and parenteral administration of 2-(N′-*p*-tolyl-N′-*m*-hydroxyphenylaminomethyl) imidazoline hydrochloride (REGITINE) in the treatment of hypertension and an evaluation of cerebral hemodynamics. *Am. Heart J.,* **1953,** *45,* 602–610.

Mueller, R. A.; Thoenen, H.; and Axelrod, J. Inhibition of neuronally induced tyrosine hydroxylase by nicotinic receptor blockade. *Eur. J. Pharmacol.,* **1970,** *10,* 51–56.

Munson, W. M., and Jenicek, J. A. Effect of anesthetic agents on patients receiving reserpine therapy. *Anesthesiology,* **1962,** *23,* 741–746.

Nayler, W. G. A direct effect of reserpine on ventricular contractility. *J. Pharmacol. Exp. Ther.,* **1962,** *139,* 222–229.

Newman, K. D.; Williams, L. T.; Bishopric, N. H.; and Lefkowitz, R. J. Identification of α-adrenergic receptors in human platelets by (³H)dihydroergocryptine binding. *J. Clin. Invest.,* **1978,** *61,* 395–402.

Nickerson, M., and Chan, G. C.-M. Blockade of responses of isolated myocardium to epinephrine. *J. Pharmacol. Exp. Ther.,* **1961,** *133,* 186–191.

Nickerson, M., and Goodman, L. S. Pharmacological properties of a new adrenergic blocking agent: N,N-dibenzyl-β-chloroethylamine (dibenamine). *J. Pharmacol. Exp. Ther.,* **1947,** *89,* 167–185.

Nickerson, M., and Gump, W. S. The chemical basis for adrenergic blocking activity in compounds related to dibenamine. *J. Pharmacol. Exp. Ther.,* **1949,** *97,* 25–47.

Nicolaescu, V.; Manicatide, M.; and Stroescu, V. β-Adrenergic blockade with practolol in acetylcholine-sensitive asthma patients. *Respiration,* **1972,** *29,* 139–154.

Nies, A. S.; Evans, G. H.; and Shand, D. G. Regional hemodynamic effects of beta-adrenergic blockade with propranolol in the unanesthetized primate. *Am. Heart J.,* **1973,** *85,* 97–102.

Nies, A. S.; McNeil, J. S.; and Schrier, R. W. Mechanism of increased sodium reabsorption during propranolol administration. *Circulation,* **1971,** *44,* 596–604.

Norn, S., and Shore, P. A. Failure to affect tissue reserpine concentrations by alteration of adrenergic nerve activity. *Biochem. Pharmacol.,* **1971,** *20,* 2133–2135.

Owman, C.; Rosengren, E.; and Sjöberg, N.-O. Adrenergic innervation of the human female reproductive organs: a histochemical and chemical investigation. *Obstet. Gynecol.,* **1967,** *30,* 763–773.

Pfeffer, R. I.; Mosimann, W. F.; and Weiner, N. Time course of the effect of reserpine administration on tyrosine hydroxylase activity in adrenal glands and vasa deferentia. *J. Pharmacol. Exp. Ther.,* **1975,** *193,* 533–548.

Pitt, B., and Craven, P. Effect of propranolol on regional myocardial blood flow in acute ischaemia. *Cardiovasc. Res.,* **1970,** *4,* 176–179.

Poirier, L. J.; Langelier, P.; Roberge, A.; Boucher, R.; and Kitsikis, A. Non-specific histopathological changes induced by the intracerebral injection of 6-hydroxydopamine (6-OH-DA). *J. Neurol. Sci.,* **1972,** *16,* 401–416.

Porter, C. C.; Totaro, J. A.; and Stone, C. A. Effect of 6-hydroxydopamine and some other compounds on the concentration of norepinephrine in the hearts of mice. *J. Pharmacol. Exp. Ther.,* **1963,** *140,* 308–316.

Potter, W. P. de; Chubb, I. W.; Put, A.; and Schaepdryver, A. F. de. Facilitation of the release of noradrenaline and dopamine-β-hydroxylase at low stimulation frequencies by α-blocking agents. *Arch. Int. Pharmacodyn. Ther.,* **1971,** *193,* 191–197.

Powell, C. E., and Slater, I. H. Blocking of inhibitory adrenergic receptors by a dichloro analog of isoproterenol. *J. Pharmacol. Exp. Ther.,* **1958,** *122,* 480–488.

Prichard, B. N. C., and Boakes, A. J. Labetalol in long term treatment of hypertension. *Br. J. Clin. Pharmacol.,* **1976,** *3,* 743–750.

Quetsch, R. M.; Achor, R. W. P.; Litin, E. M.; and Faucett, R. L. Depressive reactions in hypertensive patients: a comparison of those treated with rauwolfia and those receiving no specific antihypertensive treatment. *Circulation,* **1959,** *19,* 366–375.

Rabkin, R.; Stables, D. P.; Levin, N. W.; and Suzman, M. M. The prophylactic value of propranolol in angina pectoris. *Am. J. Cardiol.,* **1966,** *18,* 370–380.

Redisch, W.; Terry, E. N.; Rouen, L. R.; and Clauss, R. H. Effects of alpha-methyl-tyrosine upon catecholamine levels in arterial tissue and plasma and upon peripheral blood flow measurements in the anesthetized dog. *J. Cardiovasc. Surg.,* **1969,** *10,* 291–298.

Richards, D. A., and Prichard, B. N. C. Concurrent antagonism of isoproterenol and norepinephrine after labetalol. *Clin. Pharmacol. Ther.,* **1978,** *23,* 253–258.

Riederer, P.; Youdim, M. B. H.; Birkmayer, W.; and Jellinger, K. Monoamine oxidase activity during (−)-deprenil therapy: human brain postmortem studies. In, *Advances in Biochemical Psychopharmacology,* Vol. 19. (Roberts, P. J.; Woodruff, G. N.; and Iversen, L. L.; eds.) Raven Press, New York, **1978,** pp. 377–382.

Robin, E.; Cowan, C.; Puri, P.; Ganguly, S.; DeBoyrie, E.; Martinez, M.; Stock, T.; and Bing, R. J. A comparative study of nitroglycerin and propranolol. *Circulation,* **1967,** *36,* 175–186.

Rosei, E. A.; Brown, J. J.; Lever, A. F.; Robertson, A. S.; Robertson, J. I. S.; and Trust, P. M. Treatment of phaeochromocytoma and of clonidine withdrawal hypertension with labetalol. *Br. J. Clin. Pharmacol.,* **1976,** *3,* 809–815.

Ross, E. J.; Prichard, B. N. C.; Kaufman, L.; Robertson, A. I. G.; and Harries, B. J. Preoperative and operative management of patients with phaeochromocytoma. *Br. Med. J.,* **1967,** *1,* 191–198.

Ross, E. M.; Howlett, A. C.; Ferguson, K. M.; and Gilman, A. G. Reconstitution of hormone-sensitive adenylate cyclase activity with resolved components of the enzyme. *J. Biol. Chem.,* **1978,** *253,* 6401–6412.

Roth, J. A. Guanethidine and adrenaline used in combination in chronic simple glaucoma. *Br. J. Ophthalmol.,* **1973,** *57,* 507–510.

Sandler, G.; Leishman, A. W. D.; and Humberstone, P. M. Guanethidine-resistant hypertension. *Circulation,* **1968,** *38,* 542–551.

Scriabine, A. β-Adrenoceptor blocking drugs in hypertension. *Annu. Rev. Pharmacol. Toxicol.,* **1979,** *19,* 269–284.

Scriabine, A.; Torchiana, M. L.; Stavorski, J. M.; Ludden, C. T.; Minsker, D. H.; and Stone, C. A. Some cardiovascular effects of timolol, a new beta adrenergic blocking agent. *Arch. Int. Pharmacodyn. Ther.,* **1973,** *205,* 76–93.

Sen, G., and Bose, K. C. *Rauwolfia serpentina,* a new Indian drug for insanity and high blood pressure. *Indian Med. World,* **1931,** *2,* 194–201.

Shand, D. G.; Morgan, D. H.; and Oates, J. A. The release of guanethidine and bethanidine by splenic nerve stimulation: a quantitative evaluation showing dissociation from adrenergic blockade. *J. Pharmacol. Exp. Ther.,* **1973,** *184,* 73–80.

Shand, D. G.; Nuckolls, E. M.; and Oates, J. A. Plasma propranolol levels in adults with observations in four children. *Clin. Pharmacol. Ther.,* **1970,** *11,* 112–120.

Shand, D. G.; Sell, C. G.; and Oates, J. A. Hypertrophic obstructive cardiomyopathy in an infant—propranolol therapy for three years. *N. Engl. J. Med.,* **1971,** *285,* 843–844.

Shanks, R. G. The pharmacology of beta sympathetic blockade. *Am. J. Cardiol.,* **1966,** *18,* 308–316.

Sizemore, G. W., and Winternitz, W. W. Autonomic hyper-reflexia—suppression with alpha-adrenergic blocking agents. *N. Engl. J. Med.,* **1970,** *282,* 795.

Sowton, E.; Smithen, C.; Leaver, D.; and Barr, I. Effect of practolol on exercise tolerance in patients with angina pectoris. *Am. J. Med.,* **1971,** *51,* 63–70.

Spector, S.; Sjoersdma, A.; and Udenfriend, S. Blockade of endogenous norepinephrine synthesis by α-methyl-tyrosine, an inhibitor of tyrosine hydroxylase. *J. Pharmacol. Exp. Ther.,* **1965,** *147,* 86–95.

Starke, K., and Altmann, K. P. Inhibition of adrenergic neurotransmission by clonidine: an action on prejunctional α-receptors. *Neuropharmacology,* **1973,** *12,* 339–347.

Starke, K.; Borowski, E.; and Endo, T. Preferential blockade of presynaptic alpha receptors by yohimbine. *Eur. J. Pharmacol.,* **1975,** *34,* 385–388.

Stokes, G. S.; Goldsmith, R. F.; Starr, L. M.; Gentle, J. L.; Mani, M. K.; and Stewart, J. H. Plasma renin activity in human hypertension. *Circ. Res.,* **1970,** *27,* Suppl. 2, II-207–II-214.

Stokes, G. S.; Weber, M. A.; and Thornell, I. R. β-Blockers and plasma renin activity in hypertension. *Br. Med. J.,* **1974,** *1,* 60–62.

Tarr, M.; Luckstead, E. F.; Jurewicz, P. A.; and Haas, H. G. Effect of propranolol on the fast inward sodium current in frog atrial muscle. *J. Pharmacol. Exp. Ther.,* **1973,** *184,* 599–610.

Taylor, S. H.; Sutherland, G. R.; MacKenzie, G. J.; Staunton, H. P.; and Donald, K. W. The circulatory effects of phentolamine in man with particular respect to changes in forearm blood flow. *Clin. Sci.,* **1965,** *28,* 265–284.

Toda, N. Interactions of bretylium and drugs that inhibit the neuronal membrane transport of norepinephrine in isolated rabbit atria and aortae. *J. Pharmacol. Exp. Ther.,* **1972,** *181,* 318–327.

Tothill, A. Investigation of adrenaline reversal in the rat uterus by the induction of resistance to isoprenaline. *Br. J. Pharmacol. Chemother.,* **1967,** *29,* 291–301.

Tsai, B. S., and Lefkowitz, R. J. (^{3}H)Dihydroergocryptine binding to alpha adrenergic receptors in canine aortic membranes. *J. Pharmacol. Exp. Ther.,* **1978,** *204,* 606–614.

Van der Gugten, J.; Palkovits, M.; Wijnen, H. L. J. M.; and Versteeg, D. H. G. The regional distribution of adrenaline in the rat brain. *Brain Res.,* **1976,** *107,* 171–175.

Waal-Manning, H. J. Which beta-blocker? *Drugs,* **1976,** *12,* 412–441.

Wansbrough, H.; Nakanishi, H.; and Wood, C. The effect of adrenergic receptor blocking drugs on the human uterus. *J. Obstet. Gynaecol. Br. Commonw.,* **1968,** *75,* 189–198.

Weber, M. A.; Stokes, G. S.; and Gain, J. M. Comparison of the effect of renin release of beta adrenergic antagonists with differing properties. *J. Clin. Invest.,* **1974,** *54,* 1413–1419.

Weber, R. G., and Reinmuth, O. M. The treatment of migraine with propranolol. *Neurology (Minneap.)*, **1972**, *22*, 366–369.

Webster, R. A. The antiadrenaline activity of some phenothiazine derivatives. *Br. J. Pharmacol. Chemother.*, **1965**, *25*, 566–576.

Weiner, N.; Lee, F.-L.; Dreyer, E.; and Barnes, E. The activation of tyrosine hydroxylase in noradrenergic neurons during acute nerve stimulation. *Life Sci.*, **1978**, *22*, 1197–1216.

Williams, L. T.; Snyderman, R.; and Lefkowitz, R. J. Identification of β-adrenergic receptors in human lymphocytes by (−)(^{3}H)alprenolol binding. *J. Clin. Invest.*, **1976**, *57*, 149–155.

Wislicki, L. Excitatory and depressant effects of β-adrenoceptor blocking agents on skeletal muscle. *Arch. Int. Pharmacodyn. Ther.*, **1969**, *182*, 310–317.

Wolfson, S., and Gorlin, R. Cardiovascular pharmacology of propranolol in man. *Circulation*, **1969**, *40*, 501–511.

Yeh, B. K.; McNay, J. L.; and Goldberg, L. I. Attenuation of dopamine renal and mesenteric vasodilatation by haloperidol: evidence for a specific dopamine receptor. *J. Pharmacol. Exp. Ther.*, **1969**, *168*, 303–309.

Yoran, C., and Glassman, E. The paradoxic effect of tolazoline hydrochloride on pulmonary hypertension of mitral stenosis. *Chest*, **1973**, *63*, 843–846.

Zacharias, F. J.; Cowen, K. J.; Priest, J.; Vickers, J.; and Wall, B. G. Propranolol in hypertension. A study of long-term therapy, 1964–1970. *Am. Heart J.*, **1972**, *83*, 755–761.

Monographs and Reviews

Alper, M. H.; Flacke, W.; and Krayer, O. Pharmacology of reserpine and its implications for anesthesia. *Anesthesiology*, **1963**, *24*, 524–542.

Bein, H. J. The pharmacology of rauwolfia. *Pharmacol. Rev.*, **1956**, *8*, 435–483.

Berde, B., and Schild, H. O. (eds.). *Ergot Alkaloids and Related Compounds. Handbuch der Experimentellen Pharmakologie*, Vol. 49. Springer-Verlag, Berlin, **1978**.

Berde, B., and Stürmer, E. Introduction to the pharmacology of ergot alkaloids and related compounds as a basis of their therapeutic application. In, *Ergot Alkaloids and Related Compounds.* (Berde, B., and Schild, H. O., eds.) *Handbuch der Experimentellen Pharmakologie*, Vol. 49. Springer-Verlag, Berlin, **1978**, pp. 1–28.

Black, J. W., and Prichard, B. N. C. Activation and blockade of β adrenoceptors in common cardiac disorders. *Br. Med. Bull.*, **1973**, *29*, 163–167.

Boura, A. L. A., and Green, A. F. Adrenergic neurone blocking agents. *Annu. Rev. Pharmacol.*, **1965**, *5*, 183–212.

Bovet, D., and Bovet-Nitti, F. *Médicaments du Système Nerveaux Végétatif.* S. Karger, Basel, **1948**.

Dale, H. H. On some physiological actions of ergot. *J. Physiol. (Lond.)*, **1906**, *34*, 163–206.

Furchgott, R. F. The classification of adrenoceptors (adrenergic receptors). An evaluation from the standpoint of receptor theory. In, *Catecholamines.* (Blaschko, H., and Muscholl, E., eds.) *Handbuch der Experimentellen Pharmakologie*, Vol. 33. Springer-Verlag, Berlin, **1972**, pp. 283–335.

Furness, J. B., and Burnstock, G. Role of circulating catecholamines in the gastrointestinal tract. In, *Adrenal Gland*, Vol. 6. Sect. 7, *Endocrinology. Handbook of Physiology.* (Blaschko, H.; Sayers, G.; and Smith, A. D.; eds.) American Physiological Society, Washington, D. C., **1975**, pp. 515–536.

Furst, C. I. The biochemistry of guanethidine. *Adv. Drug Res.*, **1967**, *4*, 133–161.

Ganong, W. F. Biogenic amines, sympathetic nerves, and renin secretion. *Fed. Proc.*, **1973**, *32*, 1782–1784.

Gaunt, R.; Chart, J. J.; and Renzi, A. A. Interactions of drugs with endocrines. *Annu. Rev. Pharmacol.*, **1963**, *3*, 109–128.

Goldberg, L. I. Cardiovascular and renal actions of dopamine: potential clinical applications. *Pharmacol. Rev.*, **1972**, *24*, 1–29.

Graham, J. D. P. 2-Halogenoalkylamines. *Prog. Med. Chem.*, **1962**, *2*, 132–175.

Greenblatt, D. J., and Koch-Weser, J. Adverse reactions to propranolol in hospitalized medical patients: a report from the Boston Collaborative Drug Surveillance Program. *Am. Heart J.*, **1973**, *86*, 478–484.

Greenblatt, D. J., and Shader, R. I. On the psychopharmacology of beta adrenergic blockade. *Curr. Ther. Res.*, **1972**, *14*, 615–625.

Hardaway, R. M., III. *Clinical Management of Shock.* Charles C Thomas, Pub., Springfield, Ill., **1968**.

Himms-Hagen, J. Sympathetic regulation of metabolism. *Pharmacol. Rev.*, **1967**, *19*, 367–461.

Houslay, M. D., and Tipton, K. F. Multiple forms of monoamine oxidase: fact and artefact. *Life Sci.*, **1976**, *19*, 467–478.

Karow, A. M., Jr.; Riley, M. W.; and Ahlquist, R. P. Pharmacology of clinically useful beta-adrenergic blocking drugs. *Fortschr. Arzneimittforsch.*, **1971**, *15*, 103–122.

Koch-Weser, J. Drug therapy: bretylium. *N. Engl. J. Med.*, **1979**, *300*, 473–477.

Kostrzewa, R. M., and Jacobowitz, D. M. Pharmacological actions of 6-hydroxydopamine. *Pharmacol. Rev.*, **1974**, *26*, 199–288.

Langer, S. Z. Presynaptic receptors and their role in the regulation of transmitter release. *Br. J. Pharmacol.*, **1977**, *60*, 481–497.

Levi-Montalcini, R., and Angeletti, P. U. Immunosympathectomy. *Pharmacol. Rev.*, **1966**, *18*, 619–628.

Levy, B., and Wilkenfeld, B. E. Selective interactions with beta adrenergic receptors. *Fed. Proc.*, **1970**, *29*, 1362–1364.

Maguire, M. M.; Ross, E. M.; and Gilman, A. G. β-Adrenergic receptor: ligand binding properties and the interaction with adenylyl cyclase. *Adv. Cyclic Nucleotide Res.*, **1977**, *8*, 2–83.

Malcolm, J. Adrenergic beta receptor inhibition and hyperthyroidism. *Acta Cardiol.*, **1972**, Suppl. 15, 307–326.

Marley, E., and Stephenson, J. D. Central actions of catecholamines. In, *Catecholamines.* (Blaschko, H., and Muscholl, E., eds.) *Handbuch der Experimentellen Pharmakologie*, Vol. 33. Springer-Verlag, Berlin, **1972**, pp. 463–537.

Melmon, K. L. The adrenal medulla. In, *Textbook of Endocrinology*, 6th ed. (Williams, R. H., ed.) W. B. Saunders Co., Philadelphia, **1980**.

Nickerson, M. The pharmacology of adrenergic blockade. *Pharmacol. Rev.*, **1949**, *1*, 27–101.

———. Nonequilibrium drug antagonism. *Pharmacol. Rev.*, **1957**, *9*, 246–259.

———. Drug therapy of shock. In, *Shock: Pathogenesis and Therapy* (a Ciba Foundation symposium). (Bock, D. K., ed.) Springer-Verlag, Berlin, **1962**, pp. 356–370.

Nickerson, M., and Hollenberg, N. K. Blockade of α-adrenergic receptors. In, *Physiological Pharmacology.* Vol. 4, *The Nervous System—Part D: Autonomic Nervous System Drugs.* (Root, W. S., and Hofmann, F. G., eds.) Academic Press, Inc., New York, **1967**, pp. 243–305.

Oates, J. A.; Conolly, M. E.; Prichard, B. N. C.; Shand, D. G.; and Schapel, G. The clinical pharmacology of antihypertensive drugs. In, *Antihypertensive Agents.* (Gross, F., ed.) *Handbuch der Experimentellen Pharmakologie*, Vol. 39. Springer-Verlag, Berlin, **1977**, pp. 571–632.

Porte, D., Jr., and Robertson, R. P. Control of insulin secretion by catecholamines, stress, and the sympathetic nervous system. *Fed. Proc.*, **1973**, *32*, 1792–1796.

Porter, C. C.; Torchiana, M. L.; and Stone, C. A. False

transmitters as antihypertensive agents. In, *Antihypertensive Agents.* (Gross, F., ed.) *Handbuch der Experimentellen Pharmakologie,* Vol. 39. Springer-Verlag, Berlin, **1977,** pp. 263–297.

Prichard, B. N. C.   β-Adrenergic receptor blockade in hypertension, past, present and future. *Br. J. Clin. Pharmacol.,* **1978,** *5,* 379–399.

Rothlin, E.   The pharmacology of the natural and dihydrogenated alkaloids of ergot. *Bull. Schweiz. Akad. Med. Wiss.* **1947,** *2,* 249–273.

Sandler, M., and Youdim, M. B. H.   Multiple forms of MAO: functional significance. *Pharmacol. Rev.,* **1972,** *24,* 331–348.

Sannerstedt, R., and Conway, J.   Hemodynamic and vascular responses to antihypertensive treatment with adrenergic blocking agents: a review. *Am. Heart J.,* **1970,** *79,* 122–127.

Schmitt, H.   The pharmacology of clonidine and related products. In, *Antihypertensive Agents.* (Gross, F., ed.) *Handbuch der Experimentellen Pharmakologie,* Vol. 39. Springer-Verlag, Berlin, **1977,** pp. 299–396.

Shand, D. G.   Drug therapy: propranolol. *N. Engl. J. Med.,* **1975,** *293,* 280–284.

Starke, K.   Regulation of noradrenaline release by presynaptic receptor systems. *Rev. Physiol. Biochem. Pharmacol.,* **1977,** *77,* 1–124.

Symposium. (Various authors.)   Adrenergic receptors mediating metabolic responses. *Fed. Proc.,* **1970,** *29,* 1350–1429.

Symposium. (Various authors.)   Interrelationship of angina pectoris and hypertension. *Br. J. Clin. Pharmacol.,* **1979,** *7,* Suppl. 2, 157S–267S.

Thoenen, H., and Tranzer, J. P.   The pharmacology of 6-hydroxydopamine. *Annu. Rev. Pharmacol.,* **1973,** *13,* 169–180.

Tipton, K. F.   Monoamine oxidase. In, *Adrenal Gland,* Vol. 6. Sect. 7, *Endocrinology. Handbook of Physiology.* (Blaschko, H.; Sayers, G.; and Smith, A. D.; eds.) American Physiological Society, Washington, D. C., **1975,** pp. 677–697.

Weiner, N.   Regulation of norepinephrine biosynthesis. *Annu. Rev. Pharmacol.,* **1970,** *10,* 273–290.

———.   The role of cyclic nucleotides in the regulation of neurotransmitter release from adrenergic neurons by neuromodulators. In, *Essays in Neurochemistry and Neuropharmacology,* Vol. 4. (Youdim, M. B. H.; Lovenberg, W.; Sharman, D. F.; and Lagnado, J. R.; eds.) John Wiley & Sons, Inc., New York. **1980,** pp. 69–124.

Wolf, R. L.; Mendlowitz, M.; and Fruchter, A.   Diagnosis and treatment of pheochromocytoma. *Mt. Sinai J. Med. N.Y.,* **1970,** *37,* 549–567.

CHAPTER

10 GANGLIONIC STIMULATING AND BLOCKING AGENTS

Palmer Taylor

The pharmacology of ganglionic transmission is based largely on modifications of the availability or action of the primary neurotransmitter, acetylcholine (ACh). Accordingly, the passage of impulses in autonomic ganglia can be influenced by drugs that (1) interfere with the storage or synthesis of the transmitter (*e.g.*, hemicholinium), (2) prevent the liberation of ACh from the preganglionic nerve endings (*e.g.*, botulinus toxin, local anesthetics), (3) inactivate ganglionic cholinesterases (*e.g.*, physostigmine, DFP), and (4) either mimic or prevent the interactions between ACh and its ganglionic (nicotinic) cholinergic receptor sites.

Neurotransmission in autonomic ganglia has long been recognized to be a far more complex process than that described by a single neurotransmitter-receptor system, and intracellular recordings reveal at least four different changes in potential that can be elicited by stimulation of the preganglionic nerve (Eccles and Libet, 1961; Nishi and Koketsu, 1968; Weight *et al.*, 1979). The *primary pathway* involves the depolarization of postsynaptic sites by ACh. The receptors are classified as nicotinic, and the pathway is sensitive to classical non-depolarizing blocking agents such as *hexamethonium*. Activation of this primary pathway gives rise to an initial *excitatory postsynaptic potential* (EPSP). This depolarizing event has a latency of about 1 millisecond and a duration of 10 to 20 milliseconds.

An *action potential* is generated in the postganglionic neuron when the initial EPSP attains a critical amplitude. In mammalian sympathetic ganglia *in vivo*, it may be necessary for multiple synapses to be activated before transmission is effective. The initial EPSP (and the initial depolarization that can be evoked experimentally by iontophoretic application of ACh to the postganglionic neuron) can be attributed to increases in the conductances of sodium and potassium. Since this event is rapid, it is necessary to envision a tightly coupled relationship between occupation of the receptor and activation of the channel that gives rise to the enhanced conductance. In this sense, the mechanism of generation of the initial EPSP parallels that seen at the neuromuscular junction (*see* Chapter 11).

The *secondary pathways* are insensitive to blockade by hexamethonium and its analogs and involve the transmission of both *excitatory* and *inhibitory* impulses. Both the *inhibitory postsynaptic potential* (IPSP) and the *late excitatory postsynaptic potential* (late EPSP) are of lower amplitude and of far longer duration. In the mammalian superior cervical ganglion, the IPSP has a latency of 35 milliseconds and a duration of several seconds; the late EPSP has a latency of several hundred milliseconds and an equally long duration.

The late EPSP can be preferentially generated with agonists that act selectively on muscarinic receptors; this potential is not blocked by hexamethonium, but it is sensitive to blockade by atropine (Koketsu, 1969; Libet, 1970). Thus, the delayed depolarization described by the late EPSP appears to be mediated by muscarinic receptors. In contrast to the initial EPSP, there is an *increase* in membrane resistance during the late EPSP that is attributed to a decrease in potassium conductance (Weight and Votava, 1970; Weight *et al.*, 1979). It is likely that the late EPSP serves to facilitate transmission of impulses through the primary pathway, since an enhanced resistance can increase the amplitude of convergent fast EPSPs and hence increase the efficiency of transmission across ganglionic synapses.

Like the late EPSP, the IPSP is unaffected by the classical ganglionic blocking agents but, in many systems, is sensitive to blockade by atropine. Substantial electrophysiological and morphological evidence has accumulated to suggest that one or several catecholamines participate in the generation of the IPSP. Dopamine and norepinephrine cause hyperpolarization of ganglia, and both the IPSP and the catecholamine-induced hyperpolarization are blocked by α-adrenergic antagonists. Since the IPSP is sensitive in most systems to blockade by *both* atropine and α-adrenergic antagonists, ACh that is released at the preganglionic terminal may act on a catecholamine-containing interneuron to stimulate the release of dopamine or norepinephrine; the catecholamine, in turn, produces hyperpolarization (an IPSP) of the ganglion cell (Eccles and Libet, 1961; Libet, 1970). Morphological studies indicate that catecholamine-containing cells are present in ganglia. These include the dopamine- or norepinephrine-containing small, intensely fluorescent (SIF) cells and adrenergic nerve terminals. The precise role played by the SIF cells remains to be established (Libet, 1977; Eranko, 1978). Stimulation of adrenergic fibers has been shown to inhibit transmission in parasympathetic ganglia of the bladder (de Groat and Saum, 1972). The electrogenic mechanism of the IPSP has yet to be resolved.

In addition, a *late, slow* EPSP has been observed in amphibian ganglia (Weight *et al.,* 1979). Although the transmitter responsible for this potential is unknown, the late, slow EPSP also facilitates transmission of the initial EPSP.

Stimulation of preganglionic nerve fibers increases the content of cyclic adenosine $3',5'$-monophosphate (cyclic AMP) and cyclic guanosine $3',5'$-monophosphate (cyclic GMP) in sympathetic ganglia. These changes in the concentrations of cyclic nucleotides result from activation of postsynaptic muscarinic receptors (McAfee *et al.,* 1971, Weight *et al.,* 1974). Catecholamines cause only an increase in the concentration of cyclic AMP. However, other procedures that affect the generation or availability of cyclic nucleotides in ganglia do not cause the changes in permeability or potential that would be expected if the cyclic nucleotides served as obligatory mediators of the electrophysiological responses (Gallagher and Shinnick-Gallagher, 1977; Quenzer *et al.,* 1979; Weight *et al.,* 1979). Thus, the role of cyclic nucleotides in the regulation of the slow changes in potential remains to be established.

Other synaptic mediators appear to influence ganglionic transmission, but their precise sites of action remain to be ascertained. Furthermore, the relative importance of the secondary pathways and even the nature of the modulating transmitters appear to differ among individual ganglia and between parasympathetic and sympathetic ganglia. It should be emphasized that the secondary synaptic events serve to modulate the initial EPSP. Conventional ganglionic blocking agents can inhibit ganglionic transmission completely; the same cannot be said for muscarinic antagonists or α-adrenergic agonists (*see* Volle, 1969; Weight *et al.,* 1979).

Drugs that stimulate cholinergic receptor sites on autonomic ganglia can be grouped into two major categories. The first group consists of drugs with nicotinic specificity, including *nicotine* itself. Their excitatory effects on ganglia are rapid in onset, are blocked by non-depolarizing ganglionic blocking agents, and mimic *the initial EPSP.* The second group is composed of drugs such as *muscarine* and *methacholine,* and, in part, the *anticholinesterase* (anti-ChE) *agents.* Their excitatory effects on ganglia are de-

layed in onset, blocked by atropine-like drugs, and mimic *the late EPSP.*

Ganglionic blocking agents impair transmission by actions at the primary nicotinic receptor and also may be classified into two groups. The *first group* includes those drugs that initially stimulate the ganglia by an ACh-like action and then block because of a persistent depolarization (*e.g.,* nicotine); prolonged application of nicotine results in desensitization of the cholinergic receptor site and continued blockade. (*See* reviews by Volle, 1969; Haefely, 1972.) The blockade of autonomic ganglia produced by the *second group* of blocking drugs, of which *hexamethonium* can be regarded as a prototype, does not involve prior ganglionic stimulation or changes in the ganglionic potentials. Such agents impair transmission by competing with ACh for ganglionic cholinergic receptor sites and, in a manner analogous to the blockade of transmission at the neuromuscular junction by curare, prevent the development of the postsynaptic depolarization (initial EPSP). Some evidence indicates that these drugs may also block the channel that is associated with the activated receptor. Compounds in this group have no effect on nerve conduction or on the release of transmitter substance from the nerve terminals. It is this class of conventional ganglionic blocking agents that is employed in therapy (*see* below).

GANGLIONIC STIMULATING DRUGS

Although the ganglionic stimulating drugs have no essential therapeutic uses, they are of considerable interest as experimental tools.

History. Two natural alkaloids, nicotine and lobeline, owe much of their pharmacological activity to their actions at autonomic ganglia. *Nicotine* (Table 10–1) was first isolated from leaves of tobacco, *Nicotiana tabacum,* by Posselt and Reiman in 1828, and Orfila initiated the first pharmacological studies of the alkaloid in 1843.

Langley and Dickinson (1889) painted the superior cervical ganglion of rabbits with nicotine and demonstrated that its site of action was the ganglion, rather than the preganglionic or postganglionic nerve fiber. *Lobelia* (Indian tobacco) is obtained from the dried leaves and tops of an herb, *Lobelia inflata.* *Lobeline* (α-lobeline) (Table 10–1) is the chief constituent of lobelia and was first obtained in crystalline form by Wieland in 1915. Lobeline has many

Table 10-1. GANGLIONIC STIMULANTS

Nicotine

Lobeline

Tetramethylammonium

1,1-Dimethyl-4-phenylpiperazinium

of the same actions in the body as nicotine but is less potent.

A number of synthetic compounds also have prominent actions at ganglionic receptor sites. The actions of the *onium compounds,* of which *tetramethylammonium* (TMA) is the simplest prototype, were explored in considerable detail in the last half of the nineteenth century and in the early decades of the twentieth century. The structure-activity relationship of the onium compounds has been reviewed by Ing (1956). In 1951, Chen and coworkers described the ganglionic stimulating properties of *1,1-dimethyl-4-phenylpiperazinium (DMPP) iodide,* a relatively specific ganglionic stimulant.

NICOTINE

Nicotine has no therapeutic application. However, its high toxicity and presence in tobacco give nicotine a considerable measure of medical importance. The chronic effects of nicotine and the untoward effects of the chronic use of *tobacco* are considered in Chapter 23.

Chemistry. *Nicotine* is one of the few natural liquid alkaloids. It is a colorless, volatile base ($pK_a = 8.5$) that turns brown and acquires the odor of tobacco on exposure to air. The alkaloid is readily soluble in water and forms water-soluble salts. The *d* and *l* forms of nicotine appear to have the same potency.

Pharmacological Actions. The complex and often unpredictable changes that occur in the body after administration of nicotine are due not only to its actions on a variety of neuroeffector and chemosen-

sitive sites but also to the fact that the alkaloid has both stimulant and depressant phases of action. The ultimate response of any one structure or system represents the summation of the several different and opposing effects of nicotine. For example, the drug can increase the heart rate by excitation of sympathetic or paralysis of parasympathetic cardiac ganglia, and it can slow the heart rate by paralysis of sympathetic or stimulation of parasympathetic cardiac ganglia. In addition, the effects of the drug on the chemoreceptors of the carotid and aortic bodies and on medullary centers influence heart rate, as do also the cardiovascular compensatory reflexes resulting from changes in blood pressure caused by nicotine. Finally, nicotine causes a discharge of epinephrine from the adrenal medulla, and this hormone accelerates cardiac rate and raises blood pressure.

Peripheral Nervous System. The major action of nicotine consists initially in transient stimulation and subsequently in a more persistent depression of all autonomic ganglia. Small doses of nicotine stimulate the ganglion cells directly and facilitate the transmission of impulses. When larger doses of the drug are applied, the initial stimulation is followed very quickly by a blockade of transmission. Whereas stimulation of the ganglion cells coincides with their depolarization, depression of transmission by adequate doses of nicotine occurs both during the depolarization and after it has subsided (Ginsborg and Guerrero, 1964). Nicotine also possesses a biphasic action on the adrenal medulla; small doses evoke the discharge of catecholamines, and larger doses prevent their release in response to splanchnic nerve stimulation.

Nicotine also causes the release of catecholamines in a number of isolated organs. This action results in a sympathomimetic response to nicotine that is blocked by drugs known to prevent the effects of catecholamines (*see* Burn *et al.,* 1959; Ferry, 1963).

The effects of nicotine on the neuromuscular junction are similar to those on ganglia. However, with the exception of avian and denervated mammalian muscle, the stimulant phase is largely obscured by the rapidly developing paralysis. In the latter stage, nicotine also produces neuromuscular blockade due to receptor desensitization. In contrast to autonomic ganglia, where lobeline causes depolarization and acts like nicotine, the end-plate of skeletal muscle fibers is blocked but not depolarized by lobeline.

Nicotine, like ACh, is known to stimulate a number of sensory receptors. These include mechanoreceptors that respond to stretch or pressure of the skin, mesentery, tongue, lung, and stomach; chemoreceptors of the carotid body; thermal receptors of the skin and tongue; and pain receptors. Prior administration of hexamethonium prevents the stimulation of the sensory receptors by nicotine, but has little effect, if any, on the activation of the sensory receptors by physiological stimuli. The explanation of these observations is controversial (Douglas and Gray, 1953; Armette and Ritchie, 1961).

Central Nervous System. Nicotine markedly stimulates the central nervous system (CNS). Appropriate doses produce *tremors* in both man and laboratory animals; with somewhat larger doses, the tremor is followed by *convulsions*. The *excitation of respiration* is a particularly prominent action of nicotine; although large doses act directly on the medulla oblongata, smaller doses augment respiration reflexly by excitation of the chemoreceptors of the carotid and aortic bodies, as first demonstrated by Heymans and coworkers (1931). Stimulation of the CNS is followed by depression, and death results from failure of respiration due to both central paralysis and peripheral blockade of muscles of respiration.

Nicotine and lobeline cause *vomiting* by a complex of central and peripheral actions. The central component of the vomiting response is due to stimulation of the emetic chemoreceptor trigger zone in the area postrema of the medulla oblongata (Laffan and Borison, 1957). In addition, nicotine activates a number of vagal and spinal afferent nerves that form the sensory input of the reflex pathways involved in the act of vomiting.

Nicotine exerts an *antidiuretic action* as the result of stimulation of the hypothalamiconeurohypophyseal system with the consequent release of antidiuretic hormone (ADH).

Cardiovascular System. When administered intravenously to the dog, nicotine characteristically produces an increase in heart rate and blood pressure. The latter is usually a more sustained response. In general, the cardiovascular responses to nicotine are due to stimulation of sympathetic ganglia and the adrenal medulla, together with the discharge of catecholamines from sympathetic nerve endings and chromaffin tissues of various organs (Gebber, 1969). Also contributing to the sympathomimetic response to nicotine is the activation of chemoreceptors of the aortic and carotid bodies, which reflexly results in *vasoconstriction, tachycardia,* and *elevated blood pressure.*

Gastrointestinal Tract. In contrast to the cardiovascular actions of nicotine, the effects of the drug on the gastrointestinal tract are due largely to parasympathetic stimulation. The combined activation of parasympathetic ganglia and cholinergic nerve endings results in increased tone and motor activity of the bowel. Nausea, vomiting, and occasionally diarrhea are observed following systemic absorption of nicotine.

Exocrine Glands. Nicotine causes an initial stimulation of salivary and bronchial secretions that is followed by inhibition. Salivation caused by smoking is reflexly produced by the irritant smoke rather than by a systemic effect of nicotine.

Absorption, Fate, and Excretion. Nicotine is readily absorbed from the respiratory tract, buccal mucous membranes, and skin. Severe poisoning has resulted from percutaneous absorption. Being a relatively strong base, its absorption from the stomach is minimal unless intragastric pH is raised (Ivey and Triggs, 1978). Intestinal absorption is far more efficient.

Approximately 80 to 90% of nicotine is altered in the body, mainly in the liver but also in the kidney and lung. A significant fraction of inhaled nicotine is metabolized by the lung (Turner *et al.,* 1975). The major metabolites of nicotine are conitine and nicotine-1'-N-oxide, which are formed respectively from oxidation of the α carbon and N-oxidation of the pyrrolidine ring. The half-life of nicotine following inhalation or parenteral administration is 30 to 60 minutes. Both nicotine and its metabolites are rapidly eliminated by the kidney (Russell and Feyerabend, 1978). The rate of urinary excretion of nicotine is dependent upon the pH of the urine; excretion diminishes when the urine is alkaline. Nicotine is also excreted in the *milk* of lactating women who smoke. The milk of heavy smokers may contain 0.5 mg per liter.

Acute Nicotine Poisoning. Poisoning from nicotine may occur from accidental ingestion of insecticide sprays in which nicotine is present as the effective agent or in children from ingestion of tobacco products. The acutely fatal dose of nicotine for an adult is probably about 60 mg of the base. Smoking tobacco usually contains 1 to 2% nicotine. When smoked, cigarettes currently manufactured in the United States deliver 0.05 to 2.5 mg of nicotine each (*see* Chapter 23). Apparently the gastric absorption of nicotine from tobacco taken by mouth is delayed because of slowed gastric emptying, so that vomiting caused by the central effect of the initially absorbed fraction removes much of the tobacco remaining in the stomach.

The onset of symptoms of acute, severe nicotine poisoning is rapid; they include nausea, salivation, abdominal pain, vomiting, diarrhea, cold sweat, headache, dizziness, disturbed hearing and vision, mental confusion, and marked weakness. Faintness and prostration ensue; the blood pressure falls; breathing is difficult; the pulse is weak, rapid, and irregular; and collapse may be followed by terminal convulsions. Death may result within a few minutes from respiratory failure caused by paralysis of the muscles of respiration.

Therapy. Vomiting should be induced with syrup of ipecac, or gastric lavage should be performed in order to remove the nicotine. Alkaline solutions should be avoided. A slurry of activated charcoal is then passed through the tube and left in the stomach. Artificial respiration with oxygen should be instituted if needed and continued for as long as necessary. Other necessary therapy may include treatment of shock.

OTHER GANGLIONIC STIMULANTS

Stimulation of ganglia by TMA or DMPP differs from that produced by nicotine in that the initial stimulation is not followed by a dominant blocking action. Demonstration of ganglionic blockade caused by DMPP or TMA requires large intra-arterial doses or application of the drug *in vitro*. Their stimulatory action for the most part mimics the initial EPSP and is blocked by hexamethonium. Part of the facilitation of transmission may, however, be due to a muscarinic action. DMPP is about three times more potent than nicotine.

Parasympathomimetic drugs (muscarine, pilocarpine, and the synthetic choline esters) can also stimulate ganglia; however, their effects are usually obscured by stimulation of peripheral neuroeffector sites.

GANGLIONIC MODULATORS

In addition to the ganglionic stimulating agents related to the ACh-AChE system, *gamma-aminobutyric acid, substance P, 5-hydroxytryptamine,* and *angiotensin II* modify neurotransmission in certain ganglia or in the adrenal medulla. Since the actions of these substances are not antagonized by either hexamethonium or atropine, noncholinergic ganglionic receptors are involved. 5-Hydroxytryptamine initially stimulates and then depresses transmission in parasympathetic ganglia in the bladder (Saum and de Groat, 1973); in ganglia of the myenteric plexus, it is stimulatory and produces a slow EPSP (Wood and Mayer, 1979).

Catecholamines have mixed excitatory and inhibitory actions on sympathetic ganglia. *Isoproterenol* causes depolarization of the ganglion cells and facilitates transmission of impulses in both curare- and atropine-sensitive cholinergic pathways. In isolated ganglia, isoproterenol can depress transmission. The excitatory actions of isoproterenol are prevented by β-adrenergic blocking compounds. *Norepinephrine, epinephrine,* and *dopamine* usually cause a depression of transmission and hyperpolarization of the ganglion cells. Catecholamines also depress the release of transmitter, and this action may contribute to ganglionic blockade (Christ and Nishi, 1971; Haefely, 1972). When these inhibitory effects are prevented by α-adrenergic blocking compounds, norepinephrine and epinephrine display the excitatory actions of isoproterenol.

GANGLIONIC BLOCKING DRUGS

In contrast to nicotine and related compounds, a number of drugs block transmission in autonomic ganglia without producing any preceding or concomitant change in the membrane potentials of ganglion cells. In general, they do not modify the conduction of impulses in preganglionic or postganglionic fibers and do not prevent release of ACh by preganglionic impulses. They produce ganglionic blockade by occupying receptor sites and by stabilizing the postsynaptic membranes against the actions of ACh liberated from presynaptic nerve endings.

The chemical diversity of compounds sharing this action on autonomic ganglia is illustrated in Table 10–2. The structure-activity relationship of these compounds has been extensively analyzed and reviewed (Paton and Zaimis, 1952; Ing, 1956).

HEXAMETHONIUM AND RELATED DRUGS

History and Structure-Activity Relationship. Although Marshall (1913) and Burn and Dale (1915) first described the "nicotine paralyzing" action of *tetraethylammonium* (TEA) on ganglia, and other

Table 10–2. NON-DEPOLARIZING GANGLIONIC BLOCKING AGENTS

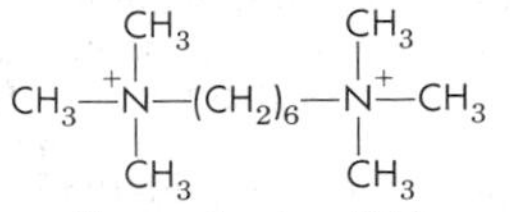

Hexamethonium (C6)

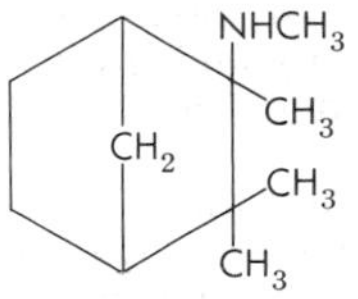

Mecamylamine

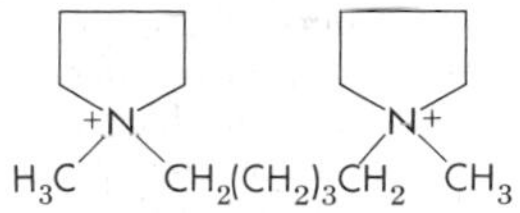

Pentolinium

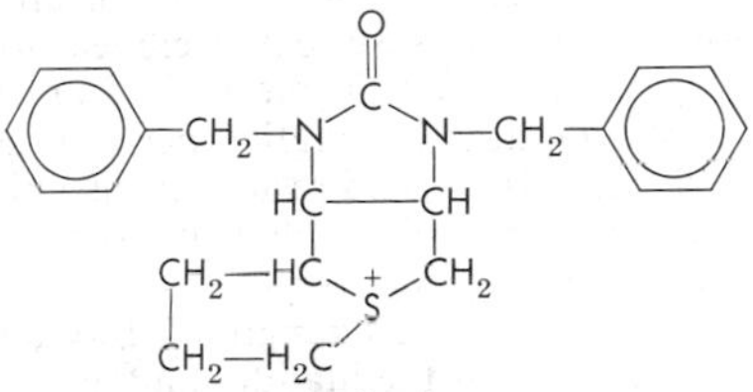

Trimethaphan

investigators had reported certain additional pharmacological properties, TEA was largely overlooked until Acheson and Moe (1946) and Acheson and Pereira (1946) published their definitive analyses of the effects of the ion on the cardiovascular system and autonomic ganglia. They also proposed the use of TEA for the treatment of hypertension. The *bis*-quaternary ammonium salts were developed and studied independently by Barlow and Ing (1948) and Paton and Zaimis (1949, 1952). These agents were found to be more potent and to have a longer duration of action.

The prototypical ganglionic blocking drug in this series, *hexamethonium* (C6), has a bridge of six methylene groups between the two quaternary nitrogen atoms (Table 10–2). C6 and its congener C5 are competitive blocking agents at the ganglia, with minimal neuromuscular and muscarinic blocking activity. Subsequently, several series of *bis*-quaternary ammonium compounds were investigated for ganglionic blocking activity, and some drugs so discovered have been employed clinically, including *pentolinium, chlorisondamine,* and *trimethidinium.* Pentolinium has a longer duration of action than hexamethonium and was widely used to produce controlled hypotension in anesthesia after Enderby's initial favorable report in 1954. Triethylsulfonium salts, like the quaternary and *bis*-quaternary ammonium ions, possess ganglionic blocking actions. This knowledge led to the development of other sulfonium ganglionic blocking agents and culminated in the synthesis of *trimethaphan* (Randall *et al.*, 1949) (Table 10–2).

The synthesis of secondary amines with ganglionic blocking activity represented somewhat of a departure in the chemistry of these agents. The pharmacological properties of *mecamylamine* (Table 10–2) were first reported in the mid-1950s, and the drug was soon thereafter introduced into therapy (Stone *et al.*, 1956). Its antagonism of acetylcholine has both a competitive and noncompetitive component. *Pempidine,* a tertiary amine with similar properties, was introduced shortly after mecamylamine.

Pharmacological Properties. Nearly all of the physiological alterations observed after the administration of hexamethonium and related drugs can be attributed to the blockade of transmission in autonomic ganglia by the mechanisms already considered. Since all members of this group of drugs exhibit essentially the same pharmacological activity, their actions *in vivo* can be discussed together.

The alteration of physiological processes attending ganglionic blockade can be anticipated with reasonable accuracy by a careful inspection of Figure 4–1 (facing page 58) and by knowing which division of the autonomic nervous system exercises dominant control of various organs (Table 10–3). For example, blockade of sympathetic ganglia interrupts adrenergic control of arterioles and results in vasodilatation, improved peripheral blood flow in some vascular beds, and a fall in blood pressure.

In addition, generalized ganglionic blockade may result also in atony of the bladder and gastrointestinal tract, cycloplegia, xerostomia, diminished perspiration, and, by abolishing circulatory reflex pathways, postural hypotension. Many of these changes represent the generally undesirable features of ganglionic blockade, which limit the therapeutic efficacy of ganglionic blocking agents.

Cardiovascular System. The importance of existing sympathetic tone in determining the degree to which blood pressure is lowered by ganglionic blockade is illustrated by the fact that blood pressure may be decreased only minimally in recumbent normotensive subjects but may fall markedly in sitting or standing subjects. As originally noted by Organe and coworkers (1949), *postural hypotension* occurs and may cause syncope. Postural hypotension per-

sists longer than recumbent hypotension and is a major problem in ambulatory patients receiving ganglionic blocking drugs; it is relieved to some extent by muscular activity and completely by recumbency, and tends to become less prominent after continued medication. Sympathetically mediated vasomotor reflexes are inhibited, and the cold pressor response is reduced. The drugs induce a hypotensive response even in sympathectomized patients, probably because there are ganglionic vasoconstrictor pathways not removed by surgery.

Changes in *cardiac rate* following ganglionic blockade depend largely on existing vagal tone. In man, mild tachycardia usually accompanies the hypotension, a sign that indicates fairly complete ganglionic blockade. However, a decrease may occur if the heart rate is initially high.

Cardiac output is often reduced by ganglionic blocking drugs in patients with normal cardiac function, probably as a consequence of diminished venous return resulting from venous dilatation and peripheral pooling of the blood. In patients with cardiac failure, ganglionic blockade frequently results in increased cardiac output due to a reduction in peripheral resistance and to decreased right-heart pressure resulting from a decrease in venous return. In hypertensive subjects, cardiac output, stroke volume, and left ventricular work are diminished.

Although *total systemic vascular resistance* is decreased in patients who receive ganglionic blocking agents, the changes in *blood flow* and *vascular resistance* of individual vascular beds are variable. The *skin temperature* is elevated mostly in the hands and feet, and blood flow to the limbs may increase. The retinal and choroidal vessels dilate. Reduction of *cerebral blood flow* is small unless mean systemic blood pressure falls below 50 to 60 mm Hg (Miletick and Ivankovich, 1978). *Skeletal muscle blood flow* is unaltered, and *splanchnic blood flow* decreases following ganglionic blockade. Trimethaphan appears to cause some vasodilatation by a direct mechanism (Wang *et al.*, 1977).

The *renal effects* of ganglionic blockade in normotensive subjects include a decrease in glomerular filtration rate and renal blood flow and an increase in renal vascular resistance.

Gastrointestinal Tract. The volume and the acidity of *gastric secretions* are generally decreased by the

Table 10–3. USUAL PREDOMINANCE OF SYMPATHETIC (ADRENERGIC) OR PARASYMPATHETIC (CHOLINERGIC) TONE AT VARIOUS EFFECTOR SITES, WITH CONSEQUENT EFFECTS OF AUTONOMIC GANGLIONIC BLOCKADE

SITE	PREDOMINANT TONE	EFFECT OF GANGLIONIC BLOCKADE
Arterioles	Sympathetic (adrenergic)	Vasodilatation; increased peripheral flow; hypotension
Veins	Sympathetic (adrenergic)	Dilatation; pooling of blood; decreased venous return; decreased cardiac output
Heart	Parasympathetic (cholinergic)	Tachycardia
Iris	Parasympathetic (cholinergic)	Mydriasis
Ciliary muscle	Parasympathetic (cholinergic)	Cycloplegia
Gastrointestinal tract	Parasympathetic (cholinergic)	Reduced tone and motility; constipation
Urinary bladder	Parasympathetic (cholinergic)	Urinary retention
Salivary glands	Parasympathetic (cholinergic)	Xerostomia
Sweat glands	Sympathetic (cholinergic)	Anhidrosis

ganglionic blocking agents. The secretory response to insulin-induced hypoglycemia is diminished, as is the increase in *pancreatic secretions* stimulated by the consumption of a test meal of milk. *Salivary secretion* is also diminished. The *tone* and *motility* of the gastrointestinal tract in man are reduced, and propulsive movements of the small intestine may be completely blocked.

Other Effects. Ganglionic blockade causes partial or total impairment of the voiding contractions of the *urinary bladder,* with a resultant increase in vesical capacity. This is due to blockade of parasympathetic ganglia along the efferent pathways of the spinal reflex concerned with micturition, so that bladder distention causes no urge to void. Moderate dosage in some subjects may result in incomplete emptying of the bladder and a large residual urine. In the male, both penile erection and ejaculation are impaired. Ganglionic blockade causes incomplete *mydriasis* and partial loss of *accommodation* as a result of impaired transmission in the ciliary ganglion. *Sweating* is reduced.

Untoward Responses and Severe Reactions. Among the milder untoward responses observed are visual disturbances (such as mydriasis and difficulty in accommodation), dry mouth, conjunctival suffusion, urinary hesitancy, decreased potentia, subjective chilliness, moderate constipation, occasional diarrhea, abdominal discomfort, anorexia, heartburn, nausea, eructation and bitter taste, and the signs and symptoms of syncope caused by postural hypotension. These side effects tend to become less pronounced as administration of the drug is continued.

More severe reactions include *marked hypotension, constipation, paralytic ileus, urinary retention,* and *cycloplegia.* Syncope may occur without warning. Unlike the quaternary ammonium ganglionic blocking agents, which do not readily reach the CNS, large doses of *mecamylamine* can produce *prominent central effects,* resulting in tremors, mental confusion, seizures, mania, or depression.

Absorption, Fate, and Excretion. The absorption of quaternary ammonium compounds from the enteric tract is incomplete and unpredictable. This is due both to the limited ability of quaternary ammonium ions to penetrate cell membranes and to the depression of propulsive movements of the stomach and small intestine. Gastric emptying time may be so delayed that two or three doses may be retained in the stomach; the gastric contents may then suddenly enter the duodenum, and the absorption of the accumulated toxic amounts of drug can cause severe hypotension and collapse. Although the absorption of mecamylamine is less erratic, a danger exists of reduced bowel activity leading to frank paralytic ileus.

After absorption, the quaternary ammonium blocking agents are confined primarily to the extracellular space. Penetration of the blood-brain barrier is limited. Most of a parenteral dose is excreted unchanged by the kidney. Mecamylamine is not confined to the extracellular space; high concentrations accumulate in the liver and kidney. Meca-

mylamine is excreted slowly by the kidney in unchanged form and is a relatively long-acting ganglionic blocking agent.

Preparations, Routes of Administration, and Dosage. Of the numerous ganglionic blocking agents that have appeared on the therapeutic scene, only *mecamylamine* and *trimethaphan* are currently official in the United States. *Pempidine, pentolinium,* and *chlorisodamine* are still used to a limited extent in Europe.

Mecamylamine Hydrochloride, U.S.P. (INVERSINE), is available for oral administration in tablets containing 2.5 and 10 mg of the drug. The usual initial dose is 2.5 mg, given twice daily.

Trimethaphan Camsylate, U.S.P. (ARFONAD), is available as an injection, in 10-ml ampuls containing 50 mg/ml. It possesses a short duration of action and may be given by intravenous drip. When administered in this manner, a 0.1% solution in 5% dextrose is employed.

THERAPEUTIC USES

Historically the major therapeutic use of the ganglionic blocking agents has been in the management of *hypertensive cardiovascular disease.* However, these drugs have been supplanted by superior agents for the treatment of *chronic hypertension.* Some physicians still use ganglionic blocking agents in the emergency treatment of *hypertensive crises* (*see* Chapter 32). In this situation, trimethaphan is infused intravenously at a rate of 0.3 to 3 mg per minute. Abrupt reduction of blood pressure or reduction below the normal range is particularly dangerous in individuals with coronary or cerebrovascular insufficiency. Infusions should be terminated gradually while the blood pressure is monitored. Since trimethaphan can stimulate the release of histamine, it should be used with caution in patients with a history of allergy (Larson, 1964).

Trimethaphan is also employed in the management of *autonomic hyperreflexia.* This syndrome is typically seen in patients with injuries of the upper spinal cord and results from a massive sympathetic discharge. A common stimulus for such discharge is distention of the bladder; it is often associated with catheterization or irrigation of the bladder, cystoscopy, or transurethral resection. Since normal central inhibition of the reflex is lacking in such patients, the spinal reflex is dominant. It can be controlled successfully with ganglionic blocking agents (Texter *et al.,* 1976; Basta *et al.,* 1977).

An additional therapeutic use of the ganglionic blocking agents is in the production of *controlled hypotension;* a reduction in blood pressure during surgery may be sought deliberately to minimize hemorrhage in the operative field, to reduce blood loss in various orthopedic procedures, and to facilitate surgery on blood vessels (Leigh, 1975; Salem, 1978).

Acheson, G. H., and Moe, G. K. The action of tetraethylammonium ion on the mammalian circulation. *J. Pharmacol. Exp. Ther.,* **1946,** *87,* 220–236.
Acheson, G. H., and Pereira, S. A. The blocking effect of

tetraethylammonium ion on the superior cervical ganglion of the cat. *J. Pharmacol. Exp. Ther.*, **1946**, *87*, 273–280.

Armette, C. J., and Ritchie, J. M. The action of acetylcholine and some related substances on conduction in mammalian non-myelinated nerve fibers. *J. Physiol. (Lond.)*, **1961**, *155*, 372–384.

Barlow, R. B., and Ing, H. R. Curare-like action of polymethylene bis-quaternary ammonium salts. *Br. J. Pharmacol. Chemother.*, **1948**, *3*, 298–304.

Basta, J. W.; Nlejadlik, K.; and Pallares, V. Autonomic hyperflexia: intraoperative control with pentolinium tartrate. *Br. J. Anaesth.*, **1977**, *49*, 1087–1090.

Burn, J. H., and Dale, H. H. The action of certain quaternary ammonium bases. *J. Pharmacol. Exp. Ther.*, **1915**, *6*, 417–438.

Burn, J. H.; Leach, E. H.; Rand, M. J.; and Thompson, J. W. Peripheral effects of nicotine and acetylcholine resembling those of sympathetic stimulation. *J. Physiol. (Lond.)*, **1959**, *148*, 332–352.

Chen, G.; Portman, R.; and Wickel, A. Pharmacology of 1,1-dimethyl-4-phenylpiperazinium iodide, a ganglion-stimulating agent. *J. Pharmacol. Exp. Ther.*, **1951**, *103*, 330–336.

Christ, D. D., and Nishi, S. Site of adrenaline blockade in the superior cervical ganglion of the rabbit. *J. Physiol. (Lond.)*, **1971**, *213*, 107–117.

de Groat, W. C., and Saum, W. R. Sympathetic inhibition of the urinary bladder and of pelvic ganglionic transmission in the cat. *J. Physiol. (Lond.)*, **1972**, *220*, 297–314.

Douglas, W. W., and Gray, J. A. B. The excitant action of acetylcholine and other substances on cutaneous sensory pathways and its prevention by hexamethonium and *d*-tubocurarine. *J. Physiol. (Lond.)*, **1953**, *119*, 118–128.

Eccles, R. M., and Libet, B. Origin and blockade of the synaptic responses of curarized sympathetic ganglia. *J. Physiol. (Lond.)*, **1961**, *157*, 484–503.

Enderby, G. E. H. Pentolinium tartrate in controlled hypotension. *Lancet*, **1954**, *2*, 1097.

Ferry, C. B. The sympathomimetic effect of acetylcholine on the spleen of the cat. *J. Physiol. (Lond.)*, **1963**, *167*, 487–504.

Gallagher, J. P., and Shinnick-Gallagher, P. Cyclic nucleotides injected intracellularly into rat superior cervical ganglion cells. *Science*, **1977**, *198*, 851–852.

Gebber, G. L. Neurogenic basis for the rise in blood pressure evoked by nicotine in the cat. *J. Pharmacol. Exp. Ther.*, **1969**, *166*, 255–269.

Ginsborg, B. L., and Guerrero, S. On the action of depolarizing drugs on sympathetic ganglion cells of the frog. *J. Physiol. (Lond.)*, **1964**, *172*, 189–206.

Heymans, C.; Bouckaert, J. J.; and Dautrebande, I. Sinus carotidien et réflexes respiratoires. III. Sensibilité des sinus carotidiens aux substances chimiques. Action stimulante respiratoire réflexe du sulfure de sodium, du cyanure de potassium, de la nicotine et de la lobéline. *Arch. Int. Pharmacodyn. Ther.*, **1931**, *40*, 54–91.

Ivey, K. J., and Triggs, E. J. Absorption of nicotine by the human stomach and its effect on gastric ion fluxes and potential difference. *Am. J. Dig. Dis.*, **1978**, *23*, 809–814.

Laffan, R. J., and Borison, H. L. Emetic action of nicotine and lobeline. *J. Pharmacol. Exp. Ther.*, **1957**, *121*, 468–476.

Langley, J. N., and Dickinson, W. L. On the local paralysis of peripheral ganglia, and on the connexion of different classes of nerve fibers with them. *Proc. R. Soc. Lond. [Biol.]*, **1889**, *46*, 423–431.

McAfee, D. A.; Schunderet, M.; and Greengard, P. Adenosine 3′,5′-monophosphate in nervous tissue: increase associated with synaptic transmission. *Science*, **1971**, *171*, 1156–1158.

Marshall, C. R. Studies on the pharmaceutical action of

tetra-alkyl-ammonium compounds. *Trans. R. Soc. Edinb.*, **1913**, *1*, 17–40.

Nishi, S., and Koketsu, K. Early and late after-discharges of amphibian sympathetic ganglion cells. *J. Neurophysiol.*, **1968**, *31*, 109–121.

Organe, G.; Paton, W. D. M.; and Zaimis, E. J. Preliminary trials of bistrimethylammonium decane and pentane diiodide (C_{10} and C_5) in man. *Lancet*, **1949**, *1*, 21–23.

Paton, W. D. M., and Zaimis, E. J. The pharmacological actions of polymethylene bistrimethylammonium salts. *Br. J. Pharmacol. Chemother.*, **1949**, *4*, 381–400.

Quenzer, L.; Yahn, D.; Alkadhi, K.; and Volle, R. L. Transmission blockade and stimulation of ganglionic adenylate cyclase by catecholamines. *J. Pharmacol. Exp. Ther.*, **1979**, *208*, 31–36.

Randall, L. O.; Peterson, W. G.; and Lehmann, G. The ganglionic blocking action of thiophanium derivatives. *J. Pharmacol. Exp. Ther.*, **1949**, *97*, 48–57.

Saum, W. P., and de Groat, W. C. The actions of 5-hydroxytryptamine on the urinary bladder and on vesical autonomic ganglia in the cat. *J. Pharmacol. Exp. Ther.*, **1973**, *185*, 70–82.

Stone, C. A.; Torchiana, M. L.; Navarro, A.; and Beyer, K. H. Ganglionic blocking properties of 3-methylamino-isocamphane hydrochloride (mecamylamine): a secondary amine. *J. Pharmacol. Exp. Ther.*, **1956**, *117*, 169–183.

Texter, J. H.; Reece, R. W.; and Hranowsky, N. Pentolinium in the management of hyperreflexia. *J. Urol.*, **1976**, *116*, 350–352.

Turner, D. M.; Armitage, A. K.; Briant, R. H.; and Dollery, C. T. Metabolism of nicotine by the isolated perfused dog lung. *Xenobiotica*, **1975**, *5*, 539–551.

Wang, H. H.; Liu, L. M. P.; and Katz, R. L. A comparison of the cardiovascular effects of sodium nitroprusside and trimethaphan. *Anesthesiology*, **1977**, *46*, 40–48.

Weight, F. F.; Petzold, G.; and Greengard, P. Guanosine 3′5′-monophosphate in sympathetic ganglia: increase associated with synaptic transmission. *Science*, **1974**, *186*, 942–944.

Weight, F. F., and Votava, J. Slow synaptic excitation in sympathetic ganglion cells; evidence for synaptic inactivation of potassium conductance. *Science*, **1970**, *170*, 755–758.

Wood, J. D., and Mayer, C. J. Serotonergic activation of tonic-type enteric neurons in guinea pig small bowel. *J. Neurophysiol.*, **1979**, *42*, 582–593.

Monographs and Reviews

Eranko, O. Small intensely fluorescent (SIF) cells and nervous transmission in sympathetic ganglia. *Annu. Rev. Pharmacol. Toxicol.*, **1978**, *18*, 417–430.

Haefely, W. Electrophysiology of the adrenergic neuron. In, *Catecholamines.* (Blaschko, H., and Muscholl, E., eds.) *Handbuch der Experimentellen Pharmakologie*, Vol. 33. Springer-Verlag, Berlin, **1972**, pp. 661–725.

Ing, H. R. Structure-action relationships of hypotensive drugs. In, *Hypotensive Drugs.* (Harrington, M., ed.) Pergamon Press, Ltd., Oxford, **1956**, pp. 7–22.

Koketsu, K. Cholinergic synaptic potentials and the underlying ionic mechanisms. *Fed. Proc.*, **1969**, *28*, 101–112.

Larson, A. G. Deliberate hypotension. *Anesthesiology*, **1964**, *25*, 682–706.

Leigh, J. M. The history of controlled hypotension. *Br. J. Anaesth.*, **1975**, *47*, 745–749.

Libet, B. Generation of slow inhibitory and excitatory postsynaptic potentials. *Fed. Proc.*, **1970**, *29*, 1945–1956.

———. The role SIF cells play in ganglionic transmission. *Adv. Biochem. Psychopharmacol.*, **1977**, *16*, 541–546.

Miletick, D. J., and Ivankovich, A. D. Cardiovascular effects of ganglionic blocking drugs. *Int. Anesthesiol. Clin.*, **1978**, *16*, 151–170.

Paton, W. D. M., and Zaimis, E. J. The methonium compounds. *Pharmacol. Rev.,* **1952,** *4,* 219–253. (187 references.)

Russell, M. A. H., and Feyerabend, C. Cigarette smoking: a dependence on high nicotine level boli. *Drug Metab. Rev.,* **1978,** *8,* 29–57.

Salem, M. R. Therapeutic uses of ganglionic blocking drugs. *Int. Anesthesiol. Clin.,* **1978,** *16,* 171–200.

Volle, R. L. Ganglionic transmission. *Annu. Rev. Pharmacol.,* **1969,** *9,* 135–146.

Weight, F. F.; Schulman, J. A.; Smith, P. A.; and Busis, N. A. Long-lasting synaptic potentials and the modulation of synaptic transmission. *Fed. Proc.,* **1979,** *38,* 2084–2094.

CHAPTER

11 NEUROMUSCULAR BLOCKING AGENTS

Palmer Taylor

Several drugs employed clinically have as their major action the interruption of transmission of the nerve impulse at the skeletal neuromuscular junction. On the basis of distinct electrophysiological differences in their mechanism of action, they are classified either as *competitive* (*stabilizing*) agents, of which curare is the classical example, or as *depolarizing* agents, such as succinylcholine.

History, Sources, and Chemistry. *Curare* is a generic term for various South American arrow poisons. The drug has a long and romantic history. It has been employed for centuries by the Indians along the Amazon and Orinoco Rivers and in other parts of the continent for killing wild animals used for food; death results from paralysis of skeletal muscles. The technic of preparation of curare was long shrouded in mystery and was entrusted only to tribal witch doctors. Soon after the discovery of the American continent, Sir Walter Raleigh and other early explorers and botanists became interested in curare, and late in the sixteenth century samples of the native preparations were brought to Europe for examination and investigation. Following the pioneering work of the scientist-explorer von Humboldt, in 1805, the *botanical sources* of curare quite early became the object of much field search. The curares from eastern Amazonia contain various species of *Strychnos* as their chief ingedient. It is noteworthy that most of the South American species of *Strychnos* examined contain chiefly quaternary, neuromuscular blocking alkaloids, whereas the Asiatic, African, and Australian species nearly all contain tertiary, strychnine-like alkaloids. Certain species of *Chondrodendron* also yield curare. Research on curare was greatly accelerated by the work of Gill (1940), who, after prolonged and intimate study of the native methods of preparing curare, brought to the United States a sufficient amount of the authentic drug prepared from *C. tomentosum* to permit chemical and pharmacological investigations.

The modern clinical use of curare probably dates from 1932, when West employed highly purified fractions in patients with tetanus and spastic disorders. In 1940, Bennett introduced the drug as an adjuvant in the pentylenetetrazol shock treatment of psychiatric disorders. The first trial of curare for promoting muscular relaxation in general anesthesia was reported by Griffith and Johnson (1942). The advantage of obtaining the desired degree of muscular relaxation without the use of dangerously high concentrations of anesthetic became recognized over the next decade. The achievement of muscle relaxation during abdominal surgery or tracheal intubation thus emerged as the chief therapeutic use of curare.

The fascinating history of curare, the reports of early travelers, and the complex problems of botanical source, nomenclature, and chemical identification of the curare alkaloids have been presented in extensive reviews (*see* McIntyre, 1947, 1972; Bovet, 1972; and *previous editions* of this textbook).

The essential structure of *d-tubocurarine* was established by King (1935). One of the nitrogen atoms was later found to constitute a tertiary amine (Everett *et al.,* 1970; Codding and James, 1973; Table 11–1). A synthetic derivative *metocurine* (formerly called *dimethyl d-tubocurarine*), contains three additional methyl groups, one of which quaternizes the tertiary nitrogen; the other two form methyl ethers at the phenolic hydroxyl groups. This compound possesses about three times the potency of *d*-tubocurarine in man.

The most potent of all curare alkaloids are the *toxiferines*, obtained from *Strychnos toxifera* (*see* Waser, 1972). A semisynthetic derivative, *alcuronium chloride* (*diallylbisnortoxiferin*), is employed clinically in Europe (Table 11–1).

The seeds of the trees and shrubs of the genus *Erythrina*, widely distributed in tropical and subtropical areas, contain substances with curare-like activity. A hydrogenated derivative, *dihydro-β-erythroidine*, of the parent alkaloid, *erythroidine*, has been studied most carefully and subjected to clinical trial.

Gallamine (Table 11–1) is one of a series of synthetic substitutes for curare described by Bovet and coworkers in 1949 (*see* review by Bovet, 1972). Exploration of the structure-activity relationship of the plant alkaloids led to the development of the *polymethylene bis-trimethylammonium series* (referred to herein by the generic term *methonium compounds*) simultaneously and independently by Barlow and Ing (1948) and Paton and Zaimis (1949 *et seq.*). The most potent agent was found when the chain contained ten carbon atoms (*decamethonium* [*C10*], Table 11–1). The member of the series containing six carbon atoms in the chain, *hexamethonium* (*C6*), was found to be particularly effective as a ganglionic blocking agent (*see* Chapter 10).

The use of curarized animals by Hunt and Taveau in 1906 in experiments on *succinylcholine* (Table 11–1) prevented them from observing the neuromuscular blocking activity of the drug, and this property went unrecognized for more than 40 years. In 1949, the curariform action of the compound was

**Table 11-1.   STRUCTURAL FORMULAS OF MAJOR NEUROMUSCULAR
BLOCKING AGENTS**

COMPETITIVE AGENTS

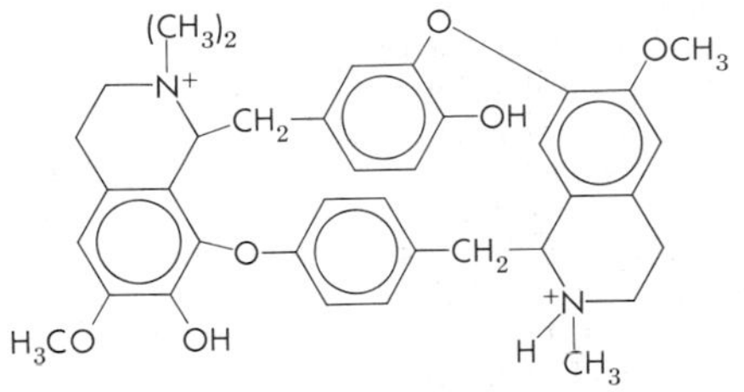

d-Tubocurarine

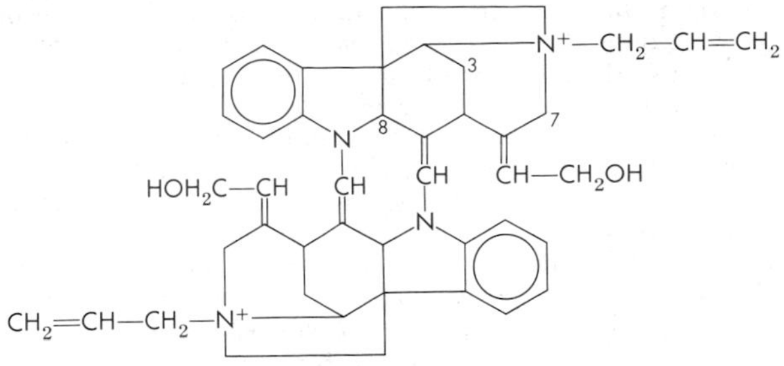

Alcuronium

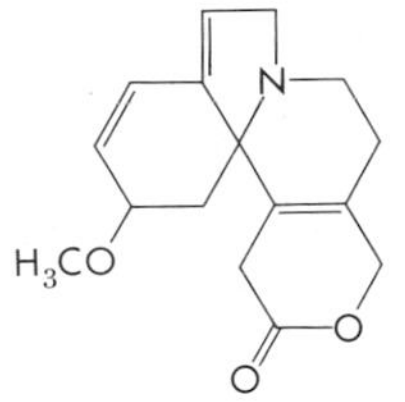

β-Erythroidine

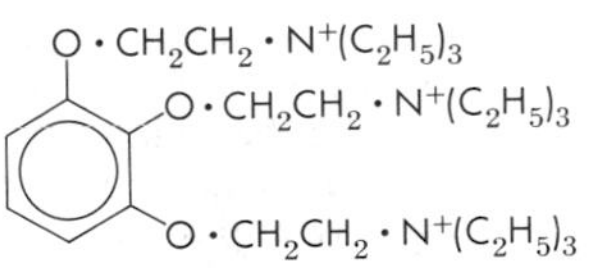

Gallamine

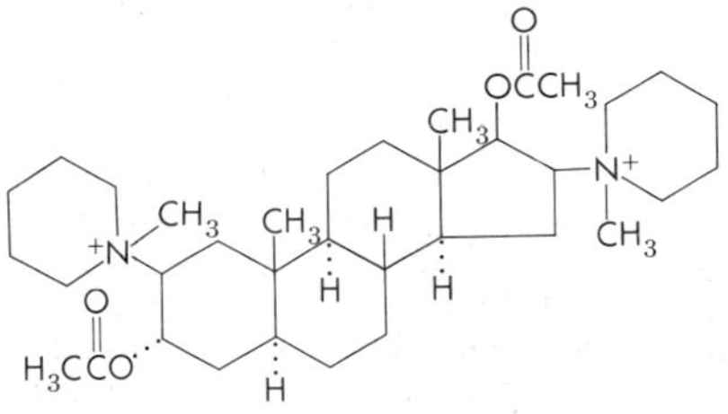

Pancuronium

DEPOLARIZING AGENTS

Decamethonium

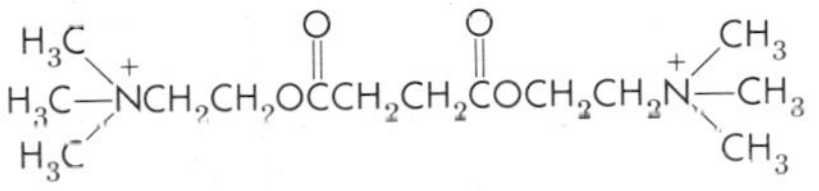

Succinylcholine

COMBINED ACTION

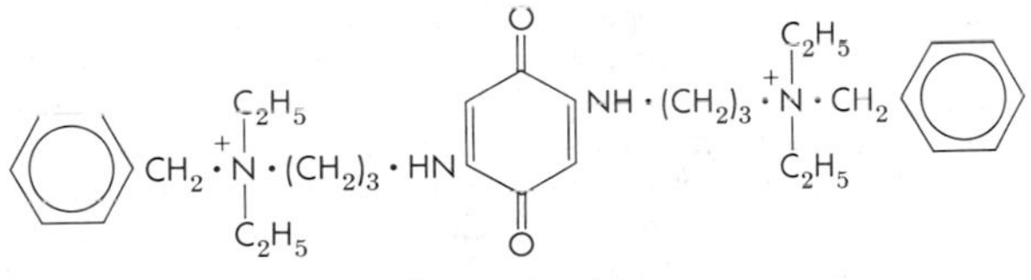

Benzoquinonium

described independently by workers in Italy, Great Britain, and the United States, and its clinical application soon followed.

Benzoquinonium is a synthetic neuromuscular blocking agent obtained by quaternization of a compound originally synthesized as a potential antibacterial substance (Table 11–1). It combines certain features of both the competitive and depolarizing agents, and in addition has considerable anticholinesterase (anti-ChE) activity (Hoppe, 1950).

Pancuronium is a member of a series of *bis*-quaternary ammonium steroids that were synthesized in 1964. Extensive pharmacological and clinical studies have shown that it is approximately five times as potent as *d*-tubocurarine as a competitive neuromuscular blocking agent, with minimal cardiovascu-

lar and little or no histamine-releasing or hormonal actions (Buckett *et al.,* 1968; Speight and Avery, 1972). *Fazadinium* was developed recently in Great Britain as a competitive blocking agent. Its extensive metabolism by the liver makes it unique among this class of drugs.

Structure-Activity Relationship.   The first attempts to analyze the structure-activity relationship of drugs were made in the field of neuromuscular blocking agents (*see* Crum Brown and Fraser, 1868, 1869), although neither the structure of the active ingredients of curare nor the role of acetylcholine (ACh) in neuromuscular transmission was then known.

For both theoretical and practical reasons, the

structural features that distinguish *competitive* from *depolarizing* neuromuscular blocking agents have received particular attention. Although exceptions can be cited, a few useful generalizations can be made about the differences in structure between these two groups of agents. The *competitive* or *stabilizing* agents are for the most part relatively bulky, rigid molecules (*e.g.*, *d*-tubocurarine, the toxiferines, *β*-erythroidine, gallamine, pancuronium), whereas the *depolarizing* agents (*e.g.*, decamethonium, succinylcholine) generally have a more flexible structure that enables free bond rotation (*see* Table 11–1; Bovet, 1972; Cheymol and Bourillet, 1972; Waser, 1972). While the distance between quaternary groups in the flexible depolarizing agents can vary up to the limit of the maximal bond distance (1.45 nm for decamethonium), the distance for the rigid competitive blockers is usually 1.0 ± 0.1 nm. The *tris*-quaternary compound gallamine, the tertiary amine *β*-erythroidine, and fazadinium, in which the cationic charge is delocalized, represent exceptions to this generalization. The crystal structure of *d*-tubocurarine has been elucidated (Sobell *et al.*, 1972), and the internitrogen distance is 1.03 nm. Moreover, all the polar groups reside on one of its surfaces. *l*-Tubocurarine, which is 20- to 60-fold less potent than the *d* isomer, has an equivalent internitrogen distance but does not have the polar groups confined to one surface.

The functional relationship of curare to ACh focuses attention on the role of quaternary ammonium groups. Many well-known drugs (atropine, quinine, strychnine, etc.) show a marked increase in neuromuscular blocking potency when their nitrogen atom is quaternized. On the other hand, many nonquaternary ammonium compounds block the neuromuscular junction (quinine, nicotine, erythroidine derivatives, etc.). The neuromuscular blocking activity of *β*-erythroidine and dihydro-*β*-erythroidine is actually abolished by quaternization of the nitrogen. Other atoms can substitute for cationic quaternary nitrogen; thus, neuromuscular blocking activity has been reported for sulfonium, phosphonium, arsonium, stibonium, iodinium, platinum, and osmium compounds.

The *bis*-quaternary ammonium structure of most of the compounds in Table 11–1 suggests that electrostatic or coulombic association occurs between the two ionized cationic centers of the drug and certain anionic groups of the receptor site; for example, replacement of one quaternary moiety of decamethonium by a primary amine group results in a considerable loss of potency, which is likely a consequence of increased hydration of the cation (Barlow *et al.*, 1955). The quaternary moiety ensures that the cationic charge is maintained in a minimally hydrated environment.

With a further increase in the length of the polymethylene chain of the *methonium compounds* beyond C10, a second peak has been found for potency of depolarizing neuromuscular blockade at C14 to C18, representing a distance between the quaternary ammonium groups of approximately 2.0 nm (Barlow and Zoller, 1964; Khromov-Borisov and Michelson, 1966).

Cholinergic Receptor Site. The concept of the nicotinic cholinergic receptor, with which ACh combines to initiate the end-plate potential (EPP), is introduced in Chapter 4. By taking advantage of specialized evolutionary events related to cholinergic neurotransmission, it has been possible in recent years to isolate and characterize the cholinergic nicotinic receptor. These accomplishments represent landmarks in the development of molecular pharmacology. The electric organs from the aquatic species of *Electrophorus* and, especially, *Torpedo* provide rich sources of receptor. The electric organ is derived embryologically from myoid tissue; however, in contrast to skeletal muscle, a significant fraction of the surface of the membrane is excitable and contains cholinergic receptor (Bennett, 1970). In vertebrate skeletal muscle, motor end-plates occupy 0.1% or less of the cell surface. The discovery of seemingly irreversible antagonism of neuromuscular transmission by an *α* toxin from venoms of the krait, *Bungarus multicinctus,* or varieties of the cobra, *Naja naja* (Chang and Lee, 1963), offered a suitable marker for identification of the receptor. The *α* toxins are peptides of around 8000 molecular weight that can be isolated and labeled with radioisotopes. The interaction of *α* toxins with the receptor was initially applied to an assay for identification of the isolated cholinergic receptor *in vitro* by Changeux and colleagues in 1970. The *α* toxins have extremely high affinities and slow rates of dissociation from the receptor, yet the interaction is noncovalent. *In situ* and *in vitro* their behavior resembles that expected for a high-affinity antagonist.

Parallel studies employing a site-directed, irreversible sulfhydryl-labeling reagent, *maleimidobenzyl trimethylammonium,* identified a 40,000-dalton peptide in the preparations containing receptor, the labeling of which is protected by agonists (Karlin, 1969). This peptide also predominates in preparations that were subsequently purified by use of the *α*-toxin assay (Karlin and Cowburn, 1973). Thus, two separate approaches, which rely on distinctly different aspects of receptor specificity, identify the same protein (or peptide therefrom) as the nicotinic cholinergic receptor. Further evidence that the isolated protein was the receptor came from immunological studies (Patrick and Lindstrom, 1973), since initial attempts at reconstitution of receptor function in isolated membranes met with only marginal success. More recently, several of the expected properties of receptor function have been reconstituted by the addition of soluble receptor to phospholipid vesicles. The immunological approach has continued to yield critical information on the location and disposition of the receptor in the membrane. Furthermore, immunization of experimental animals with purified receptor results in the production of antibody that reacts with endogenous nicotinic receptor and a syndrome that in many ways resembles the human disease, *myasthenia gravis* (*see* Chapter 6).

The *α* toxins, with their high affinity and selectivity for the receptor, were initially employed to facilitate its isolation. Their additional value as markers for examination of the biosynthesis, location, and turnover of the receptor is also now clear (Heidmann and Changeux, 1978; Patrick *et al.*, 1978; Fambrough, 1979).

Despite its relative paucity in muscle, the nicotinic receptor has also been isolated from mammalian skeletal muscle; it has virtually the same biochemical properties as does the receptor of electric fish (Dolly and Barnard, 1977; Froehner *et al.*, 1977). Subcellular fractions that bind α toxins have been extracted from brain (Wang *et al.*, 1978) and a cultured pheochromocytoma (Patrick and Stallcup, 1977). In the latter cells, the ACh receptor that mediates changes in ion permeability is distinct from the α-neurotoxin binding entity. This is not totally unexpected, since the nicotinic receptor of cells that originate from the neural crest (which gives rise to autonomic ganglia) has a different pharmacological specificity than does the receptor of the neuromuscular junction (*see* Chapter 10). Thus, α toxins may be specific markers only for nicotinic receptors whose embryonic origin is skeletal muscle.

The isolated receptor is an asymmetrical (14 nm $\times$ 8 nm) molecule of 250,000 daltons. It is composed of multiple subunits of 40,000 to 69,000 daltons, with two α-toxin and one or two agonist-antagonist binding sites per receptor molecule (Heidmann and Changeux, 1978). The agonist-antagonist recognition site is on the 40,000-dalton peptide, and the functional role played by the other peptides remains unknown. Measurement of the number of receptors per unit area and the membrane conductance have demonstrated that rates of ion translocation are sufficiently rapid (5×10^7 ions per second) to require movement through an open channel, rather than by a rotating carrier of ions (Karlin, 1973). Moreover, agonist-mediated changes in ion permeability (inward movement of sodium and outward movement of potassium) apparently can occur through a single class of channels (Dionne *et al.*, 1978). Thus, the agonist binding site appears to be intimately coupled with an ion channel; binding of agonist results in a rapid conformational change that opens the channel.

In junctional areas the receptor is present in high densities ($10,000/\mu m^2$) (Cartaud *et al.*, 1978); there is a tendency for localization at the tips of the postsynaptic folds (Fertuck and Salpeter, 1976). The protein spans the membrane, as expected if a channel mechanism prevails, with an additional 3- to 4-nm extension at the extracellular face (Figure 11–1). On the extracellular surface, a cavity exists within the receptor molecule that collects electron-dense stain. Thus, the view perpendicular to the membrane surface is of closely packed rosette-like structures, 8 nm in diameter (*see* Potter and Smith, 1977; Ross *et al.*, 1977).

PHARMACOLOGICAL PROPERTIES

Skeletal Muscle. The peripheral locus of the paralytic action of curare was first adequately described by Bernard (1856, 1857). His classical experiments on the localization, as described below, are still instructively performed with the purified alkaloid, d-tubocurarine, by students in the pharmacological laboratory.

If the hindleg of a pithed frog is ligatured in a manner that deprives the limb of its circulation but allows the sciatic nerve to remain free, the injection of curare into the ventral lymph sac produces typical effects in all parts of the frog except in the ligatured limb. In this unpoisoned leg, electrical stimulation of the sciatic nerve produces typical muscular contraction, whereas the opposite poisoned extremity is unresponsive to nerve stimulation. Furthermore, afferent stimulation of the sciatic nerve of the poisoned limb elicits crossed-reflex responses in the unpoisoned extremity. It is thus clear that curare, in producing the observed effects, does not act centrally (spinal cord) or on peripheral nerve, but must reach skeletal muscle in order to exert its effect. Further localization of the action to the neuromuscular junction is accomplished by showing that the curarized muscle is electrically excitable when stimulated directly and that the sciatic nerve, when soaked in a solution of curare, is still capable of carrying impulses.

Mechanism of Action. The cellular locus and mechanism of action of d-tubocurarine and other *competitive* neuromuscular blocking agents have been well defined by modern technics, including microiontophoretic application of drugs and intracellular recording. In brief, d-tubocurarine combines with the cholinergic receptor sites at the postjunctional membrane and thereby blocks competitively the transmitter action of ACh. When the drug is applied directly to the end-plate of a single isolated muscle fiber under microscopic control, the muscle cell becomes insensitive to motor-nerve impulses and to directly applied ACh; however, the end-plate region and the remainder of the muscle fiber membrane retain their normal sensitivity to the application of potassium ions, and the muscle fiber still responds to direct electrical stimulation.

Before further analysis of the action of antagonists at the neuromuscular junction, it is important to consider certain details of receptor activation. The steps involved in the release of ACh by the nerve action potential (AP), the development of miniature end-plate potentials (mepps), their summation to form a postjunctional end-plate potential (EPP), the triggering of the muscle AP, and contraction have been described in Chapter 4. In the last decade electrophysiological experimentation has revealed the electrical event associated with the opening and closing of the individual receptor channels associated with activation by agonist. This was achieved by statistical analysis of membrane potential or con-

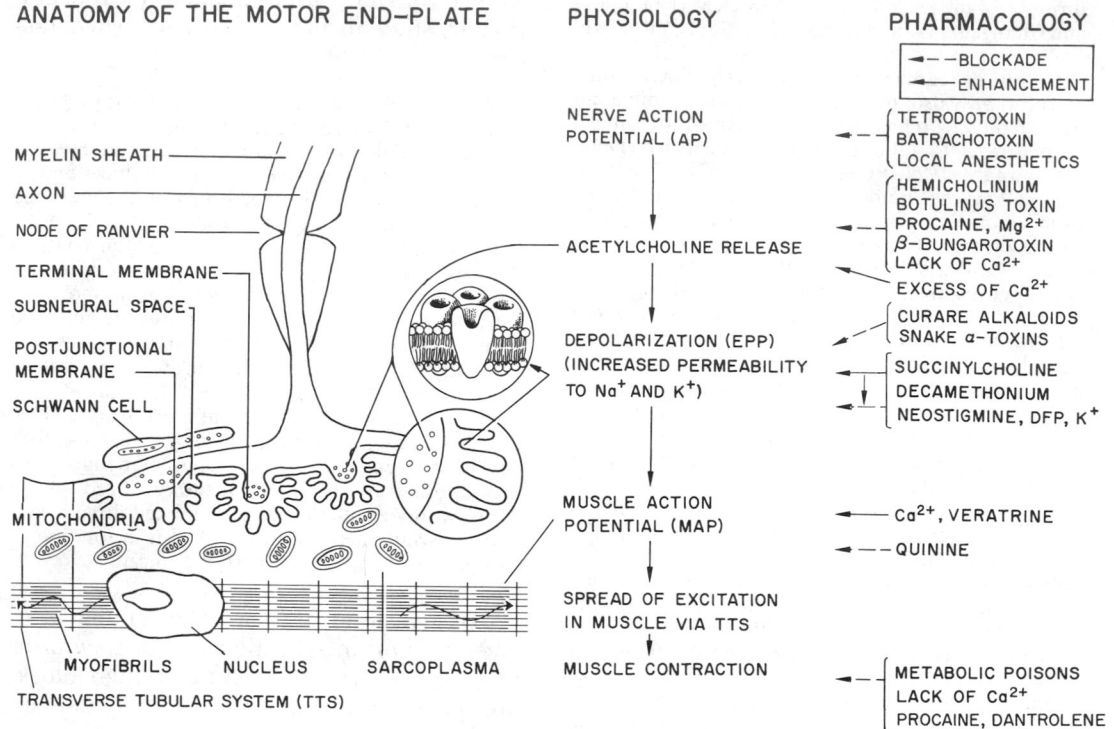

Figure 11-1. *Sites of action of agents at the neuromuscular junction and adjacent structures.*

The anatomy of the motor end-plate, shown at the left, and the sequence of events from liberation of acetylcholine (ACh) by the nerve action potential (AP) to contraction of the muscle fiber, indicated in the middle column, are described in some detail in Chapter 4. The modification of these processes by various agents is shown on the right; the dashed arrows indicate inhibition or block; the solid arrows, enhancement or activation. The circled inserts are an enlargement of the indicated structures. The highest magnification depicts the receptor in the bilayer of the postsynaptic membrane (Ross *et al.*, 1977). (Modified from Waser, 1958.)

ductance fluctuations during continuous administration of agonist (Katz and Miledi, 1972; Anderson and Stevens, 1973) and, more recently, by direct recording from a single receptor channel with a suction electrode on denervated skeletal muscle (Neher and Sakmann, 1976). The fundamental event elicited by agonist is an "all-or-none" opening and closing of channels, which gives rise to a square-wave pulse with an average open-channel conductance of ~30 picoSiemens and a duration that is exponentially distributed around a time of about 1 millisecond. The duration of channel opening is far more dependent on the nature of the agonist than is the value of the open-channel conductance (Colquhoun, 1979).

The influence of increasing concentrations of the competitive antagonist, *d*-tubocurarine, is progressively to diminish the amplitude and shorten the duration of the EPP. The amplitude of the EPP may fall to below 70% of its initial value before it is insufficient to initiate the propagated muscle AP. Analysis of the antagonism of *d*-tubocurarine on single-channel events shows that it reduces the frequency of channel-opening events but does not af-

fect the conductance or duration of opening for a single channel (Katz and Miledi, 1973). This behavior is precisely that expected for a competitive antagonist. The rates of onset and offset of antagonism by curare are slower than those of ACh because of the tendency of curare to rebind to successive receptors before exit from the synapse by diffusion (Armstrong and Lester, 1979).

The duration of the end-plate current (or EPP) parallels the lifetime for channel closing. Since the former event is a consequence of multiple quanta of ACh interacting with receptors during nerve stimulation, individual ACh molecules released presynaptically do not successively rebind to receptors to activate multiple channels before hydrolysis by acetylcholinesterase (AChE). The concentration of unbound ACh diminishes more rapidly than does the decay of the end-plate current.

If anti-ChE drugs are present, the EPP (or end-plate current) is prolonged, which is indicative of rebinding of transmitter to neighboring receptors before removal from the synapse (Magee and Terrar, 1975). It is then not surprising that anti-ChE agents and *d*-tubocurarine are competitive, since increasing the duration of action of ACh in the synapse should favor occupation of the receptor by transmitter relative to *d*-tubocurarine. *d*-Tubocurarine also partially prevents the prolongation of the EPP by the anti-AChE compounds (Fatt and Katz, 1951; Mageby and Terrar, 1975). This is, in part, a consequence of longer diffusion distances between unoccupied receptors and a diminished probability of agonist rebinding to neighboring receptors when antagonist is present.

The *depolarizing agents,* such as *succinylcholine* and *decamethonium,* act by a different mechanism. Their initial action is to depolarize the membrane in the same manner as ACh; however, since they persist at the neuromuscular junction, the depolarization is longer lasting. This results in a brief period of repetitive excitation, which may be manifested by transient muscular fasciculation. This phase is followed by block of neuromuscular transmission. The details of the sequence of excitation and depression vary with different species and muscles in the same species, so that the dominance of repetitive excitation, contracture, or block will differ. In man, the sequence of repetitive excitation (fasciculations) followed by block

of transmission and neuromuscular paralysis is observed; however, even this sequence is influenced by such factors as the identity of the anesthetic agent used concurrently and the type of muscle. Depolarization blockade exhibits several distinct differences from that produced by *d*-tubocurarine and related drugs; these are listed in Table 11-2.

A partial explanation of these distinctive features of neuromuscular blockade by the depolarizing agents was provided by the discovery by Burns and Paton (1951) that, in contrast to the stabilizing action of *d*-tubocurarine on the motor end-plate, decamethonium produces an immediate and persistent depolarization of both the end-plate and the immediately adjacent area of the sarcoplasmic membrane in the gracilis muscle of the cat. Much the same result is obtained with high, paralyzing doses of ACh in the presence of an anti-ChE agent. Thus, it was assumed that neuromuscular blockade was due to the inability of the depolarized area just beyond the end-plate to initiate propagated muscle APs in response to the continued depolarization of the end-plate itself. However, this proposal was inadequate to explain several subsequent observations, particularly the persistence of neuromuscular blockade considerably beyond the period of depolarization of the end-plate (*see* below).

Many of the characteristics of depolarizing blocking agents listed in Table 11-2 apply only to man

Table 11-2. COMPARISON OF COMPETITIVE (*d*-TUBOCURARINE) AND DEPOLARIZING (DECAMETHONIUM) BLOCKING AGENTS *

	d-TUBOCURARINE	DECAMETHONIUM (C10)
Effect of *d*-tubocurarine chloride administered previously	Additive	Antagonistic
Effect of decamethonium administered previously	No effect, or antagonistic	Some tachyphylaxis; usually no cumulative effect
Effect of anti-ChE agents on block	Reversal of block	No antagonism
Effect on motor end-plate	Elevated threshold to ACh; no depolarization	Partial, persisting depolarization
Initial excitatory effect on striated muscle	None	Transient fasciculations
Character of muscle response to indirect tetanic stimulation during *partial* block	Poorly sustained contraction	Well-sustained contraction
Effect of KCl or of a tetanus on block	Transient reversal of the block	No antagonism
Effect of current applied to end-plate region:		
—cathodal	Lessens paralysis	Intensifies paralysis
—anodal	Intensifies paralysis	Lessens paralysis
Effect of lowering muscle temperature on block	Antagonism and shortening of effect	Amplification and prolongation of effect
Effect on denervated mammalian muscle	Transient fibrillation	Contracture
Effect on avian muscle	Flaccid paralysis	Contracture, spastic to flaccid paralysis
Mammalian species sensitivity	Rat > Mouse > Rabbit > Cat	Cat > Rabbit > Monkey > Mouse > Rat
Muscle selectivity (cat)	$\frac{\text{Activity in cat}}{\text{Activity in rat}} \doteq 0.5$	$\frac{\text{Activity in cat}}{\text{Activity in rat}} \doteq 200$
	Paralyzes respiratory ("red") muscles more than limb ("white") muscles	Paralyzes respiratory muscles less than limb muscles

* Based on data in Paton and Zaimis, 1949, 1952; Zaimis, 1976; Zaimis and Head, 1976.

and to the twitch ("white") muscles of the cat. In all muscles investigated in the monkey, dog, rabbit, and rat, and in the slowly contracting soleus muscle of the cat, decamethonium and succinylcholine produce a type of blockade that combines certain features of both the depolarizing and the competitive agents described above and that has some characteristics not associated with either; this type of action has been termed a "dual" mechanism by Zaimis (1953, 1959, 1976). In such cases, the depolarizing agents produce initially the characteristic fasciculations and potentiation of the maximal twitch; this response is potentiated by anti-ChE agents. However, following the onset of blockade, there is a poorly sustained response to tetanic stimulation of the motor nerve, intensification of the block by *d*-tubocurarine, and antagonism by anti-ChE agents.

The dual action of the depolarizing blocking agents is also seen in intracellular recordings of membrane potential; when agonist is applied continuously, the initial depolarization is followed by a gradual repolarization (Thesleff, 1955, 1958; Elmqvist and Thesleff, 1962). The second phase, repolarization, resembles receptor desensitization (Katz and Thesleff, 1957).

In man, most of the early evidence indicated that decamethonium and succinylcholine produced a depolarization blockade, wherein anti-ChE drugs potentiate depolarization and tetanic stimulation gives rise to a well-sustained contraction. However, behavior characteristic of a dual type of blockade has also been frequently reported under clinical circumstances. Here, with increasing concentrations of succinylcholine and in time, the block converts from a depolarizing to a non-depolarizing type, termed phase-I and phase-II block (Churchill-Davidson and Katz, 1966; Katz, 1973). Zaimis (1976) has observed that the pattern of neuromuscular blockade produced by depolarizing drugs in anesthetized patients has changed in recent years. Prolonged apnea and slow recovery are now observed more frequently, and the characteristics of depolarization blockade are less evident following prolonged administration of succinylcholine or decamethonium. Zaimis has suggested that the general anesthetic employed may be an important factor, with fluorinated hydrocarbons predisposing the system to non-depolarization blockade (*see also* Fogdall and Miller, 1975). Thus, the anesthetic may induce some change in the postsynaptic membrane so that different features of neuromuscular blockade are accentuated.

Although fasciculations may result from stimulation of the prejunctional motor-nerve terminal by the depolarizing agent, giving rise to stimulation of the motor unit in an antidromic fashion (Riker, 1975), the primary site of blockade of neuromuscular transmission is the postjunctional membrane (Katz and Miledi, 1965; Standaert and Adams, 1965; Auerbach and Betz, 1971).

Depolarizing agents produce channel opening, which can be measured by the statistical analysis of fluctuation of EPPs. The probability of channel opening associated with the binding of drug to the receptor is less with decamethonium than with ACh or carbamylcholine (Katz and Miledi, 1973). The diminished probability of channel opening would serve to classify decamethonium as a partial agonist that acts on the postsynaptic membrane. Higher concentrations of decamethonium also interfere with ion translocation by blocking the channel directly (Adams and Sakmann, 1978).

Many ions, drugs, and toxins block neuromuscular transmission by other mechanisms, such as interference with the synthesis or release of ACh (*see* Chapter 4); but these agents are not employed clinically for this purpose. The sites of action and interrelationship of some of them are indicated in Figure 11-1.

Sequence and Characteristics of Paralysis. *Animals* poisoned by *d-tubocurarine* or other *competitive blocking agents* first exhibit motor weakness, and ultimately the muscles become totally flaccid and inexcitable through their motor innervation. Small, rapidly moving muscles such as those of the fingers, toes, jaw, eyes, and ears are involved before those of the limbs, neck, and trunk. Ultimately the intercostal muscles and finally the diaphragm are paralyzed, and respiration then ceases. Death is caused by hypoxia secondary to peripheral respiratory paralysis. Terminal asphyxial convulsions may appear, but these are mild because of the muscular paralysis. Life can be saved by artificial respiration, particularly because the duration of action of *d*-tubocurarine is relatively brief. Recovery of muscles usually occurs in the reverse order to that of their paralysis, and thus the diaphragm is ordinarily the first to regain function. The action of *d*-tubocurarine is entirely reversible so that recovery is eventually complete.

When an appropriate dose of *d*-tubocurarine (10 to 15 mg) is injected *intravenously in man,* the onset of effects is very rapid. Slight dizziness and a sensation of warmth are first experienced. Difficulty in focusing and weakness in the jaw muscles are then observed, and difficulty in speech and ptosis soon follow. Ptosis, strabismus, diplopia, dysarthria, and dysphagia are indicative of the early involvement of the small muscles of the head and neck. Relaxation of the small muscles of the middle ear improves acuity of hearing for low tones. The limbs feel heavy and are difficult to move. Respiratory movements become more diaphragmatic as the intercostal muscles are involved. Despite adequate artificially controlled respiration, "shortness of breath" is experienced. The accumulation of unswallowed saliva in the pharynx causes the sensation of choking. Head movement soon becomes impossible, and ultimately the ability to move the limbs and trunk is lost. Throughout the stage of complete muscular paralysis, consciousness and sensorium remain entirely undisturbed (*see* below). The experience is definitely unpleasant.

The *small motor-nerve system* in mammals innervates the intrafusal fibers of muscle spindles; when the intrafusal fibers shorten, afferent volleys are discharged from the activated spindles and initiate spinal reflexes that enhance skeletal muscle tone. *d*-Tubocurarine has also been shown to block the responses of intrafusal fibers to small motor-nerve stimulation and to ACh. (*See* Hunt and Kuffler, 1950; Smith, 1963.)

Prior to causing paralysis, the *depolarizing agents* decamethonium and succinylcholine evoke transient muscular fasciculations, observed especially over the chest and abdomen; however, these are less common in the anesthetized patient. As the paralytic effect progresses, the neck, arm, and leg muscles are involved at a time when there is only slight weakness of facial, masticatory, lingual, pharyngeal, and laryngeal muscles; at this stage, respiratory muscular weakness is not pronounced and vital capacity is reduced only 25%.

With the exception of succinylcholine, the foregoing effects of the neuromuscular blocking agents become apparent within a few minutes after the intravenous administration of the usual clinical dose and persist over the course of 30 to 60 minutes.

After a single intravenous dose of 10 to 30 mg of *succinylcholine,* muscular fasciculation ensues briefly; then relaxation occurs within 1 minute, becomes maximal within 2 minutes, and disappears as a rule within 5 minutes. Transient apnea usually occurs at the time of maximal effect. Muscular relaxation of longer duration can be achieved by repeated injections at appropriate intervals or by continuous intravenous infusion. Even after discontinuance of an infusion, the effects of the drug usually disappear rapidly because of its rapid hydrolysis by the pseudocholinesterase of the plasma and liver. The degree of muscular relaxation can usually be altered within 30 to 60 seconds by a change in the rate of infusion. Muscle soreness may follow the administration of succinylcholine. The duration of action of succinylcholine can be greatly enhanced and the initial muscular fasciculation practically abolished by the prior administration of *hexafluorenium bromide,* 0.4 mg/kg, intravenously, a drug that has the combined actions of inhibition of pseudocholinesterase and mild, competitive

neuromuscular blockade (Torda *et al.,* 1967).

During prolonged depolarization, muscle cells may lose significant quantities of K^+ and gain Na^+, Cl^-, and Ca^{2+}. In patients in whom there has been extensive injury to soft tissues, the efflux of K^+ following continued administration of succinylcholine can be life threatening.

Central Nervous System. *d*-Tubocurarine and other quaternary neuromuscular blocking agents are virtually devoid of central effects following the intravenous administration of ordinary clinical doses because of their inability to penetrate effectively the blood-brain barrier.

The most decisive experiment performed to settle the problem whether curare significantly affects central functions in the dose range employed clinically is that of Smith and associates (1947). Smith (an anesthesiologist) permitted himself to receive intravenously two and one-half times the amount of *d*-tubocurarine necessary for paralysis of all skeletal muscles. Adequate respiratory exchange was maintained by artificial respiration with oxygen. Included among the various functions continuously or repeatedly examined were the EEG, sensorium, pain threshold, mentation and memory, vision, smell and hearing, neurological signs, ECG, pulse rate, respiration, and blood pressure. At no time was there any evidence of lapse of consciousness, impairment of memory, clouding of sensorium, analgesia, disturbance of special senses, or alteration in the resting EEG or its response to pattern vision. No evidence of central respiratory or vasomotor stimulation was observed. It was concluded that *d*-tubocurarine given intravenously even in large doses has no significant central stimulant, depressant, or analgesic effect in man, and that its sole action of value in anesthesia is the peripheral paralytic effect on skeletal muscle.

Autonomic Ganglia. Although the nicotinic receptors of autonomic ganglion cells have certain features in common with those at the motor end-plate, the two types are not identical, as discussed above and in Chapter 4. Hence, neuromuscular blocking agents vary with respect to their relative potencies in producing ganglionic blockade. Just as at the motor end-plate, ganglionic blockade by *d*-tubocurarine and other stabilizing drugs is antagonized effectively by anti-ChE agents, such as neostigmine; however, in ganglia, the antagonism is reinforced by the additional action of endogenous ACh at the muscarinic receptors of the ganglion cells, as described in Chapters 6 and 10.

At the doses of d-tubocurarine employed clinically, some degree of blockade is probably produced, both at autonomic ganglia and at the adrenal medulla, which results in a fall in blood pressure and tachycardia. Gallamine in doses used clinically blocks selectively the cardiac vagus nerve, but whether this occurs at the ganglionic or at a more peripheral site is uncertain; this action results in sinus tachycardia and occasionally in cardiac arrhythmias and hypertension. Pancuronium, metocurine, and alcuronium have less marked ganglionic effects at common clinical doses. The maintenance of cardiovascular reflex responses is usually desired during anesthesia.

Of the *depolarizing agents,* decamethonium rarely causes effects attributable to ganglionic blockade; although instances of bradycardia, tachycardia, and even cardiac arrest have been reported, it is difficult to dissociate such occurrences from the actions of the anesthetic agent or other circumstances. Cardiovascular effects that are probably due to the successive stimulation of vagal ganglia (manifested by bradycardia) and of sympathetic ganglia (resulting in hypertension and tachycardia) are more frequently associated with the administration of succinylcholine. With extremely high doses, ganglionic blockade may ensue (*see* Foldes, 1966; Dijl, 1972).

Histamine Release. Following the demonstration by Alam and coworkers (1939) that histamine is released from muscle by the intra-arterial injection of curare in dogs, Comroe and Dripps (1946) discovered that d-tubocurarine produced typical histamine-like wheals when injected intracutaneously or intra-arterially in man. They suggested that certain clinical responses to d-tubocurarine (bronchospasm, hypotension, excessive bronchial and salivary secretion) might be caused by the release of histamine, and that antihistaminic drugs might be used to advantage to overcome such effects. Subsequently, many workers verified and extended these findings and conclusions. The decreased coagulability of the blood that has been noted after d-tubocurarine is probably due to the concomitant release of heparin from the mast cells. Metocurine and succinylcholine also cause histamine release, but to a lesser extent (Savarese *et al.,* 1977). Deca-

methonium, pancuronium, alcuronium, and gallamine apparently release detectable amounts of histamine only when administered in excessive dosage.

Cardiovascular System. The rapid intravenous injection of large doses of d-tubocurarine in man may cause a rapid and severe fall in blood pressure. The major causes of the hypotension are peripheral vasodilatation from the release of histamine and sympathetic ganglionic blockade. Additional factors are diminished venous return due to loss of skeletal muscle tone, diminished respiratory excursion, and the consequences of intermittent positive pressure in the airway for the purpose of restoring the adequacy of respiration. Pancuronium is unique in that rapid injection can increase blood pressure, possibly because of ganglionic stimulation.

The cardiovascular and certain other side effects of *benzoquinonium* are due primarily to its anti-ChE activity. They include bradycardia, hypotension, and possible circulatory collapse. Atropine is an effective prophylactic measure; epinephrine is useful in cases of syncope.

Miscellaneous Actions. Ganglionic blockade is chiefly responsible for the decreased tone and motility of the gastrointestinal tract. Decamethonium and succinylcholine exhibit muscarinic actions, but only in extremely high doses; the latter drug may cause an increase in intraocular tension. The depolarizing agents can release potassium rapidly from intracellular sites; this may be a factor in the production of prolonged apnea that has been noted in patients who receive these drugs while in electrolyte imbalance (Dripps, 1953, 1976). Such alterations in the distribution of potassium may be particularly important in patients with congestive heart failure who are receiving digitalis or diuretics. Caution should be used or depolarizing blocking agents should be avoided in patients with extensive soft-tissue trauma or burns. Neonates may have an enhanced sensitivity to competitive neuromuscular blocking agents and some resistance to depolarizing drugs (Smith, 1976).

Synergisms and Antagonisms. The interactions between the competitive and depolarizing neuromuscular blocking agents have already been considered. From a clinical viewpoint, the most important pharmacological interactions of these drugs are with certain *general anesthetics,* certain *antibiotics,* and *anti-ChE compounds.*

Ether exerts a stabilizing effect on the postjunctional membrane and, therefore, acts synergistically with the *competitive blocking agents,* including benzoquinonium. Consequently, when such blocking drugs are employed for muscular relaxation as adjuncts to ether anesthesia, their doses should be reduced to a range of one third to one half the standard doses employed. *Halothane, cyclopropane, fluroxene, methoxyflurane,* and *enflurane* likewise act synergistically with the competitive blocking agents, but to a lesser extent (*see* Foldes, 1966).

Streptomycin in sufficiently high doses was shown by Brazil and Corrado (1957) to produce neuromuscular blockade in much the same manner as do magnesium ions, by inhibition of ACh release from the preganglionic terminal (through competition with calcium ions) and to a lesser extent by stabilization of the postjunctional membrane. The blockade is antagonized by calcium salts, but only inconsistently by anti-ChE agents (Galindo, 1972). This action is shared to varying degrees by other aminoglycosides (*see* Chapter 51). The *tetracycline antibiotics* can also produce neuromuscular block, possibly by chelation of calcium ions; Ca^{2+} will also reverse their block. Additional antibiotics that have neuromuscular blocking action, through unidentified mechanisms, include the *polypeptides* (*polymyxins A and B, colistin*), *clindamycin*, and *lincomycin*. (*See* review by Pittinger and Adamson, 1972.) Accordingly, when neuromuscular blocking agents are to be administered to patients who are receiving any of these antibiotics, special consideration should be given to the dose and to the judicious use of a calcium salt as an antagonist if recovery of spontaneous respiration is delayed.

Since the anti-ChE agents neostigmine and edrophonium preserve endogenous ACh and also act directly on the neuromuscular junction, they can be employed in the treatment of overdosage with *d*-tubocurarine or other competitive blocking agents. Similarly, upon completion of the surgical procedure many anesthesiologists employ neostigmine to reverse and decrease the duration of competitive neuromuscular blockade (Dripps, 1976). The anti-ChE agents, however, are synergistic with the depolarizing blocking agents, particularly in their initial phase of action. Thus, the distinction in the type of neuromuscular blocking agent must be clear.

Epinephrine and *norepinephrine* exert an anticurare effect, probably by increasing the amount of ACh released at the nerve terminal (*see* Bowman and Nott, 1969).

Miscellaneous drugs that may have significant interactions with either competitive or depolarizing neuromuscular blocking agents include *trimethaphan, opioid analgesics, procaine, lidocaine, quinidine, phenelzine, propranolol, magnesium salts, corticosteroids, digitalis glycosides, chloroquine*, and *diuretics* (*see* Maclagan, 1976; Zaimis, 1976; Argov and Mastaglia, 1979; Hansten, 1979).

Toxicology. Poisoning from the neuromuscular blocking agents is almost always the result of overdosage. The important untoward responses are *prolonged apnea, cardiovascular collapse*, and those resulting from *histamine release*.

Failure of respiration to become adequate in the postoperative period may not always be due directly to the drug. An obstruction of the airway, decreased arterial carbon dioxide tension secondary to hyperventilation during the operative procedure, or the neuromuscular depressant effect of excessive amounts of neostigmine used to reverse the action of the competitive blocking drugs are also causes of the failure to resume adequate ventilation. Directly related factors may also include alterations in body temperature (an increased temperature potentiating the competitive drugs, and a decreased temperature exerting the same effect on the action of the depolarizing substances); electrolyte imbalance, particularly of potassium; decreased plasma cholinesterase (*e.g.*, congenital deficiency or liver disease, resulting in reduction in the rate of destruction of succinylcholine); the presence of latent myasthenia gravis or of malignant disease such as oat-cell carcinoma of the bronchus (myasthenic syndrome); reduced blood flow to skeletal muscles causing delayed removal of the blocking drugs; decreased elimination of the relaxants secondary to reduced renal function; and interactions with any of the drugs noted above. Great care should be taken when administering muscle relaxants to dehydrated or desperately ill patients.

A severe rapid rise in temperature has occurred occasionally in patients receiving *halothane* and *succinylcholine*, and more rarely with other combinations of general anesthetics and neuromuscular blocking agents. This condition, known as *malignant hyperthermia*, has a familial tendency. The inducing agent causes widespread muscular rigidity and enhanced heat production by muscle. The hyperthermia may be fatal, and steps should be taken to dissipate heat quickly. Subsequent muscle damage is usually evident. Malignant hyperthermia should be treated by rapid cooling, inhalation of 100% oxygen, and control of the acidosis that is generally present. Procainamide, procaine, or dantrolene, administered intravenously, antagonize the release of or the effect of calcium; these agents are partially effective (Dijl, 1972; Gordon *et al.*, 1973; Symposium, 1978).

Treatment of respiratory paralysis should be by positive-pressure artificial respiration with oxygen and maintenance of a patent airway until the complete recovery of normal respiration is assured. With the competitive blocking agents, this may be hastened by the administration of neostigmine methylsulfate

(1 to 3 mg, intravenously, combined with 0.6 to 1.2 mg of atropine sulfate) or edrophonium (10 mg, intravenously, repeated as required).

Neostigmine antagonizes only the skeletal muscular blocking action of the competitive blocking agents, and it may aggravate such side effects as hypotension or bronchospasm. In such circumstances, sympathomimetic amines may be given to support the blood pressure. The position of the patient should be such as to favor the return of venous blood from the flaccid musculature. Antihistamines are definitely beneficial to counteract the responses that follow the release of histamine, provided they are administered before the neuromuscular blocking agent.

Absorption, Fate, and Excretion. Quaternary ammonium neuromuscular blocking agents are very poorly and irregularly absorbed from the gastrointestinal tract. *d*-Tubocurarine is inactive after oral administration, unless huge doses are ingested; this fact was well known to the South American Indians, who ate with impunity the flesh of game killed with curare-poisoned arrows. Absorption is quite adequate from intramuscular sites.

When a single moderate dose of *d-tubocurarine* is injected intravenously, the action begins to wear off in about 20 minutes, yet some residual effect is still discernible after 2 to 4 hours or more. However, when a second dose is given as late as 24 hours after a first, less drug is needed for an equivalent degree of paralysis. The brief duration of paralysis following the initial dose is probably due chiefly to redistribution of the drug; when repeated doses are administered, the tissues become saturated and factors of degradation and excretion then directly influence intensity and duration of action. In man, about one third of an administered dose of *d*-tubocurarine is excreted in the urine over a period of several hours, independent of dose and parenteral route of injection; smaller quantities appear in the bile, and a variable amount is metabolized (Crankshaw and Cohen, 1975). The slow redistribution is responsible for the decline of plasma concentrations after a single dose even in cases of renal failure (Maclagan, 1976). In patients with renal insufficiency, accumulation may occur follow-

ing multiple doses (Gibaldi *et al.,* 1972). For practical purposes, no significant amount of *d*-tubocurarine crosses the placenta late in pregnancy to reach the fetus.

Distribution and elimination of *metocurine* are similar to those of *d*-tubocurarine, as is its duration of action (Savarese *et al.,* 1977). *Pancuronium* is partially hydroxylated in the liver but also has a similar duration of action (Agoston *et al.,* 1977). *Gallamine* and *decamethonium* are almost entirely excreted by the kidney, with no apparent metabolic degradation. Approximately 75% of an injected dose of *benzoquinonium* is excreted unchanged.

The extremely brief duration of action of *succinylcholine* is due largely to its rapid hydrolysis by the pseudocholinesterase of liver and plasma. The initial metabolite, *succinylmonocholine,* has a much weaker, predominantly competitive type of neuromuscular blocking action. Among the occasional patients who exhibit prolonged apnea following the administration of succinylcholine, a considerable number have an atypical plasma cholinesterase or a deficiency of the enzyme, due to a genetic factor, hepatic disease, or a nutritional disturbance; however, in some the enzymatic activity in plasma has been normal (Kalow and Gunn, 1957; Kalow, 1965).

Preparations, Routes of Administration, and Dosage. Neuromuscular blocking agents are administered parenterally and nearly always *intravenously.* Detailed information on *dosage* can be found in anesthesiology textbooks (*see* Feldman, 1978; Vickers *et al.,* 1978). *The neuromuscular blocking agents are potentially hazardous drugs. Consequently, they should be administered to patients only by anesthesiologists and other clinicians who have had extensive training in their use and in a setting where facilities for respiratory and cardiovascular resuscitation are immediately at hand.*

Tubocurarine Chloride, U.S.P. (*d-tubocurarine chloride;* TUBARINE, others), is marketed as a sterile solution containing 3 or 15 mg/ml. The solution containing 15 mg/ml should always be diluted before injection. The use of *d*-tubocurarine to produce muscular relaxation for surgical purposes may be cited as an example of one dose schedule employed. In conjunction with usual preanesthetic medication and light surgical anesthesia, 6 to 9 mg of the drug may be given as a single intravenous injection in adults. One half of this dose may be given after 3 to 5 minutes, if necessary, and small supplements employed later, as required. If *ether* is used, only one third the recommended dose should be given; with certain other general anesthetics, intermediate doses should be employed.

Metocurine Iodide, U.S.P. (*dimethyl tubocurarine iodide;* METUBINE IODIDE), is available as a solution containing 2 mg/ml. Since this drug is two to three times as potent as *d*-tubocurarine in man, the doses employed are only one third those of the parent alkaloid.

Gallamine Triethiodide, U.S.P. (FLAXEDIL), is available as a sterile solution containing 20 or 100 mg/ml. For muscular relaxation in conjunction with surgical anesthesia, gallamine triethiodide is usually injected intravenously in a dose not exceeding 1.0 mg/kg of body weight, and an additional amount (0.5 to 1.0 mg/kg) may be given after 40 to 50 minutes, if necessary.

Succinylcholine Chloride, U.S.P. (ANECTINE, QUELICIN, SUCOSTRIN, SUX-CERT), is marketed as a sterile powder (0.5 and 1.0 g) and as a sterile solution containing 20, 50, or 100 mg/ml. For brief surgical procedures in adults, the usual intravenous dose is 20 mg, but the optimal dose varies considerably (10 to 30 mg or more). The drug is given by intravenous drip infusion for more prolonged procedures, in order to obtain sustained muscular relaxation; the dose varies widely from patient to patient (0.5 to 5.0 mg or more per minute), and must be highly individualized. Moment-to-moment control of relaxation can be obtained by careful attention to the rate of infusion and the response of the patient.

Hexafluorenium Bromide, U.S.P. (MYLAXEN; hexamethylenebis [9-fluorenyldimethylammonium]), is a selective inhibitor of plasma cholinesterase with mild competitive neuromuscular blocking potency. It is given to prolong the blocking action of *succinylcholine* and to minimize the fasciculation that occurs prior to neuromuscular block with this agent. The drug is available in a solution in 10-ml vials (20 mg/ml). Following an intravenous dose of hexafluorenium of 0.4 mg/kg (not to exceed a total dose of 36 mg), the initial dose of succinylcholine is 0.2 mg/kg, intravenously (not to exceed a total dose of 18 mg), which causes muscular relaxation for 20 to 30 minutes.

Decamethonium Bromide, U.S.P. (SYNCURINE), is marketed as a sterile solution containing 1 mg/ml. The initial intravenous dose in adults varies from 0.5 to 3.0 mg, injected at the rate of 0.5 to 1.0 mg per minute. Supplements may be injected at 10- to 30-minute intervals, if required.

Pancuronium bromide (PAVULON) is available in solutions containing 1 or 2 mg/ml. The usual intravenous dose is 0.04 to 0.10 mg/kg.

Alcuronium chloride (*diallylbisnortoxiferin chloride;* ALLOFERIN) is provided in ampuls containing 5 mg/ml; the recommended intravenous dose is 10 to 15 mg. The drug is not yet marketed in the United States.

Fazadinium bromide is employed in Europe as a rapidly acting competitive blocking agent. It is unique among the neuromuscular blocking agents in

that the decline of plasma concentrations is primarily due to reduction of the diazo linkage in the liver (Brittain and Tyers, 1973). The agent may have a distinct advantage in short surgical or diagnostic procedures or in patients whose renal function is compromised. The agent has yet to be marketed or tested extensively in the United States.

Measurement of Neuromuscular Blockade in Man. Assessment of neuromuscular block is usually performed by stimulation of the ulnar nerve. Responses are monitored from compound action potentials or muscle tension developed in the adductor pollicis muscle. Responses to repetitive or tetanic stimulae are most useful for evaluation of blockade of transmission since individual measurements of twitch tension must be related to control values obtained prior to the administration of drugs. Thus, stimulus schedules such as the "train of four" or responses to tetanic stimulation are preferred procedures (Waud and Waud, 1972; Ali and Savarese, 1976).

THERAPEUTIC USES

The main clinical use of the neuromuscular blocking agents is as an *adjuvant in surgical anesthesia* to obtain relaxation of skeletal muscle, particularly of the abdominal wall, so that operative manipulations are facilitated. With muscular relaxation no longer dependent upon the depth of general anesthesia, a much lighter level of anesthesia suffices. This situation is of obvious advantage since the risk of respiratory and cardiovascular depression is minimized. Moreover, the postanesthetic recovery period is reduced. Muscle relaxation is also of value in various orthopedic procedures, such as the correction of dislocations and the alignment of fractures. Neuromuscular blocking agents are often employed to facilitate intubation with an endotracheal tube and have been used to facilitate laryngoscopy, bronchoscopy, and esophagoscopy in combination with a general anesthetic.

Use to Prevent Trauma in Electroshock Therapy. Electroconvulsive therapy of psychiatric disorders is occasionally complicated by trauma to the patient; the grand mal seizures induced may cause dislocations or fractures. Inasmuch as the muscular component of the convulsion is not essential for benefit from the procedure, various means have been tried to minimize overt motor manifestations of the seizure. Among these is the use of neuromuscular blocking agents and thiopental. The combination of the blocking drug, the anesthetic agent, and postictal depression usually results in respiratory depression or temporary apnea. An endotracheal tube and oxygen should always be available, and the previously described precautions must be rigidly observed. An oropharyngeal airway should be inserted as soon as the jaw muscles relax (after the seizure) and provision made to prevent aspiration of mucus and saliva. Since the introduction of curare for this purpose in 1940, practically all the neuromuscular blocking agents have been similarly employed. Succinylcholine is now most often used because of the brevity of its effect.

Miscellaneous Uses. *d*-Tubocurarine has been sporadically employed for its "lissive" action in the symptomatic therapy of a variety of *spastic disorders,* but the results have been disappointing. Curare has had sporadic clinical trial for the symptomatic control of muscular spasms in *acute convulsive states,* such as *tetanus, status epilepticus, convulsant drug intoxication,* and *other convulsions* (*e.g.,* following the bite of the *black widow spider*); its major limitation in such conditions is the narrow margin between the dose that affords relief and that which produces respiratory paralysis.

Diagnostic Uses. Curare can be employed diagnostically for the *detection of pain due to nerve-root compression* masked by painful spasm of muscles involved in protective splinting. The use of *d*-tubocurarine to assist in the *diagnosis of myasthenia gravis* and its potential hazards are presented in Chapter 6.

Adams, P. R., and Sakmann, B. Decamethonium both blocks and opens end plate channels. *Proc. Natl. Acad. Sci. U.S.A.,* **1978,** *75,* 2994–2998.

Agoston, S.; Crul, J. F.; Kersten, U. W.; and Scaf, A. H. J. Relationship of serum concentration of pancuronium to its neuromuscular activity in man. *Anesthesiology,* **1977,** *15,* 509–512.

Alam, M.; Anrep, G. V.; Barsoum, G. S.; Talaat, M.; and Wieninger, E. Liberation of histamine from the skeletal muscle by curare. *J. Physiol. (Lond.),* **1939,** *95,* 148–158.

Ali, H. H., and Savarese, J. J. Monitoring of neuromuscular function. *Anesthesiology,* **1976,** *14,* 216–249.

Anderson, C. R., and Stevens, C. F. Voltage clamp analysis of acetylcholine produced current fluctuations at the frog neuromuscular junction. *J. Physiol. (Lond.),* **1973,** *235,* 655–672.

Armstrong, D. L., and Lester, H. A. The kinetics of tubocurarine action and restricted diffusion within the synaptic cleft. *J. Physiol. (Lond.),* **1979,** *294,* 365–386.

Auerbach, A., and Betz, W. Does curare affect transmitter release? *J. Physiol. (Lond.),* **1971,** *213,* 691–705.

Barlow, R. B.; Blaschko, H.; Himms, J. M.; and Trendelenburg, U. Observations on Ω-amino-polymethylene trimethylammonium compounds. *Br. J. Pharmacol. Chemother.,* **1955,** *10,* 116–123.

Barlow, R. B., and Ing, H. R. Curare-like action of polymethylene *bis*-quaternary ammonium salts. *Br. J. Pharmacol. Chemother.,* **1948,** *3,* 298–304.

Barlow, R. B., and Zoller, A. Some effects of long chain polymethylene bis-onium salts on junctional transmission in the peripheral nervous system. *Br. J. Pharmacol. Chemother.,* **1964,** *23,* 131–150.

Bennett, A. E. Preventing traumatic complications in convulsive shock therapy by curare. *J.A.M.A.,* **1940,** *114,* 322–324.

Bernard, C. Analyse physiologique des propriétés des systèmes musculaire et nerveux au moyer du curare. *C. R. Acad. Sci. (Paris),* **1856,** *43,* 825–829.

Brazil, O. V., and Corrado, A. P. The curariform action of

streptomycin. *J. Pharmacol. Exp. Ther.,* **1957,** *120,* 452–459.

Brittain, R. T., and Tyers, M. B. The pharmacology of AH 8165: a rapid-acting, short-lasting competitive neuromuscular blocking drug. *Br. J. Anaesth.,* **1973,** *45,* 837–843.

Buckett, W. R.; Marjoribanks, C. E. B.; Marwick, F. A.; and Morton, M. B. The pharmacology of pancuronium bromide (Org. NA97), a new potent steroidal neuromuscular blocking agent. *Br. J. Pharmacol. Chemother.,* **1968,** *32,* 671–682.

Burns, B. D., and Paton, W. D. M. Depolarization of the motor end-plate by decamethonium and acetylcholine. *J. Physiol. (Lond.),* **1951,** *115,* 41–73.

Cartaud, J.; Benedetti, E. C.; Sobel, A.; and Changeux, J.-P. A morphological study of the cholinergic receptor protein from *Torpedo marmorata* in its membrane environment and in its detergent extracted form. *J. Cell Sci.,* **1978,** *29,* 313–325.

Chang, C. C., and Lee, C. Y. Isolation of neurotoxins from the venom of *Bungarus multicinctus* and their modes of neuromuscular blocking action. *Arch. Int. Pharmacodyn. Ther.,* **1963,** *144,* 241–257.

Changeux, J.-P.; Kasai, M.; and Lee, C. Y. Use of a snake venom toxin to characterize the cholinergic receptor protein. *Proc. Natl. Acad. Sci. U.S.A.,* **1970,** *67,* 1241–1247.

Churchill-Davidson, H. C., and Katz, P. L. Dual, phase II, or desensitization block? *Anesthesiology,* **1966,** *33,* 536–538.

Codding, P. W., and James, M. N. G. The crystal and molecular structure of a potent neuromuscular blocking agent: *d*-tubocurarine dichloride pentahydrate. *Acta Crystallogr.,* **1973,** *29B,* 935–954.

Comroe, J. H., Jr., and Dripps, R. D. The histamine-like action of curare and tubocurarine injected intracutaneously and intra-arterially in man. *Anesthesiology,* **1946,** *7,* 260–262.

Crum Brown, A., and Fraser, T. R. On the connection between chemical constitution and physiological action. Part I. On the physiological action of the salts of the ammonium bases, derived from strychnia, brucia, thebaia, codeia, morphia, and nicotia. *Trans. R. Soc. Edinb.,* **1868,** *25,* 151–203.

————. Part II. On the physiological action of the ammonium bases derived from atropia and conia. *Ibid.,* **1869,** *25,* 693–739.

Dionne, V. E.; Steinbach, J. H.; and Stevens, C. F. An analysis of the dose-response relationship at voltage-clamped frog neuromuscular junctions. *J. Physiol. (Lond.),* **1978,** *281,* 421–444.

Dolly, J. O., and Barnard, E. A. Purification and characterization of an acetylcholine receptor from mammalian skeletal muscle. *Biochemistry,* **1977,** *16,* 5053–5060.

Dripps, R. D. Abnormal respiratory responses to various "curare" drugs during surgical anesthesia: incidence, etiology and treatment. *Ann. Surg.,* **1953,** *137,* 145–155.

Everett, A. J.; Lowe, L. A.; and Wilkinson, S. Revision of the structure of (+)-tubocurarine chloride and (+)-chondrocurine. *Chem. Commun.,* **1970,** *16,* 1020–1021.

Fatt, P., and Katz, B. An analysis of the end-plate potential recorded with an intra-cellular electrode. *J. Physiol. (Lond.),* **1951,** *115,* 320–369.

Fertuck, H. C., and Salpeter, M. M. Quantitation of junctional and extrajunctional acetylcholine receptors by electron microscope autoradiography after ^{125}I-α-bungarotoxin binding at mouse neuromuscular junctions. *J. Cell Biol.,* **1976,** *69,* 144–158.

Fogdall, R. P., and Miller, R. D. Neuromuscular effects of enflurane, alone and combined with *d*-tubocurarine, pancuronium and succinylcholine in man. *Anesthesiology,* **1975,** *42,* 173–178.

Froehner, S. C.; Reiness, C. G.; and Hall, Z. W. Subunit structure of the acetylcholine receptor from denervated rat skeletal muscle. *J. Biol. Chem.,* **1977,** *252,* 8589–8596.

Galindo, A. The role of prejunctional effects in myoneural transmission. *Anesthesiology,* **1972,** *36,* 598–608.

Gibaldi, M.; Levy, G.; and Hayton, W. L. Tubocurarine and renal failure. *Br. J. Anaesth.,* **1972,** *44,* 163–165.

Griffith, H. R., and Johnson, G. E. The use of curare in general anesthesia. *Anesthesiology,* **1942,** *3,* 418–420.

Hoppe, J. O. A pharmacological investigation of 2,5-*bis*-(3-diethylaminopropylamino) benzoquinone-*bis*-benzylchloride (WIN 2747): a new curarimimetic drug. *J. Pharmacol. Exp. Ther.,* **1950,** *100,* 333–345.

Hunt, R., and Taveau, R. M. On the physiological action of certain choline derivatives and new methods for detecting choline. *Br. Med. J.,* **1906,** *2,* 1788–1791.

Kalow, W., and Gunn, D. R. The relation between dose of succinylcholine and duration of apnea in man. *J. Pharmacol. Exp. Ther.,* **1957,** *120,* 203–214.

Karlin, A., and Cowburn, D. W. The affinity-labeling of partially purified acetylcholine receptor from electric tissue of *Electrophorus. Proc. Natl. Acad. Sci. U.S.A.,* **1973,** *70,* 3636–3640.

Katz, B., and Miledi, R. Propagation of electric activity in motor nerve terminals. *Proc. R. Soc. Lond. [Biol.],* **1965,** *161,* 453–482.

———. The statistical nature of the acetylcholine potential and its molecular components. *J. Physiol. (Lond.),* **1972,** *224,* 665–699.

———. The characteristics of "end plate noise" produced by different depolarizing drugs. *Ibid.,* **1973,** *231,* 549–574.

Katz, B., and Thesleff, S. A study of "desensitization" produced by acetylcholine at the motor end-plate. *J. Physiol. (Lond.),* **1957,** *138,* 63–80.

Katz, R. L. Electromyographic and mechanical effects of suxamethonium and tubocurarine on twitch, tetanic and post-tetanic responses. *Br. J. Anaesth.,* **1973,** *45,* 849–859.

King, H. Curare alkaloids. I. Tubocurarine. *J. Chem. Soc.,* **1935,** 1381–1389.

Mageby, K., and Terrar, D. A. Factors affecting the time course of decay of end-plate currents: a possible cooperative action of acetylcholine on receptors at the frog neuromuscular junction. *J. Physiol. (Lond.),* **1975,** *244,* 467–482.

Neher, E., and Sakmann, B. Single channel currents recorded from the membrane of denervated frog muscle fibres. *Nature,* **1976,** *260,* 799–800.

Paton, W. D. M., and Zaimis, E. J. The pharmacological actions of polymethylene bistrimethylammonium salts. *Br. J. Pharmacol. Chemother.,* **1949,** *4,* 381–400.

Patrick, J., and Lindstrom, J. Auto-immune response to acetylcholine receptor. *Science,* **1973,** *180,* 871–872.

Patrick, J., and Stallcup, B. α-Bungarotoxin binding and cholinergic receptor function on a rat sympathetic nerve line. *J. Biol. Chem.,* **1977,** *252,* 8629–8633.

Potter, L., and Smith, D. S. Postsynaptic membranes in the electric tissue of *Narcine.* I. Organization and innervation of electric cells. *Tissue Cell,* **1977,** *9,* 585–602.

Ross, M. J.; Klymkowsky, M. W.; Agard, D. A.; and Stroud, R. M. Structural studies of a membrane-bound acetylcholine receptor from *Torpedo californica. J. Mol. Biol.,* **1977,** *116,* 635–659.

Savarese, J. J.; Ali, H. H.; and Antonio, R. P. The clinical pharmacology of metocurine. *Anesthesiology,* **1977,** *47,* 277–284.

Smith, S. M.; Brown, H. O.; Toman, J. E. P.; and Goodman, L. S. The lack of cerebral effects of *d*-tubocurarine. *Anesthesiology,* **1947,** *8,* 1–14.

Sobell, H. M.; Sokore, T. D.; Tavale, S. S.; Canepa, F. G.; Pauling, P.; and Petcher, T. J. Stereochemistry of a curare alkaloid: O,O′,N-trimethyl-*d*-tubocurarine. *Proc. Natl. Acad. Sci. U.S.A.,* **1972,** *69,* 2212–2215.

Standaert, F. G., and Adams, J. E. The actions of succinylcholine on the mammalian motor nerve terminal. *J. Pharmacol. Exp. Ther.,* **1965,** *149,* 113–123.

Thesleff, S. The mode of neuromuscular block caused by

acetylcholine, nicotine, decamethonium and succinylcholine. *Acta Physiol. Scand.,* **1955,** *34,* 218–231.

———. A study of the interaction between neuromuscular blocking agents and acetylcholine at the mammalian motor end-plate. *Acta Anaesthesiol. Scand.,* **1958,** *2,* 69–79.

Torda, T. A. G.; Foldes, F. F.; Bailey, M. B.; Klonymus, D. H.; and Kuwabara, S. The interactions of neuromuscular blocking agents in man: the role of hexafluorenium. *Anesthesiology,* **1967,** *28,* 1010–1019.

Wang, G.; Molinaro, S.; and Schmidt, J. O. Ligand responses of the α-bungarotoxin binding sites from skeletal muscle and the optic lobe of the chick. *J. Biol. Chem.,* **1978,** *253,* 8507–8512.

Waud, B. E., and Waud, D. R. The relation between the response to "train of four" stimulation and receptor occlusion during competitive neuromuscular block. *Anesthesiology,* **1972,** *37,* 413–416.

West, R. Curare in man. *Proc. R. Soc. Med.,* **1932,** *25,* 1107–1116.

Zaimis, E. J. Motor end-plate differences as a determining factor in the mode of action of neuromuscular blocking substances. *J. Physiol. (Lond.),* **1953,** *122,* 238–251.

Monographs and Reviews

Argov, Z., and Mastaglia, F. L. Disorders of neuromuscular transmission caused by drugs. *N. Engl. J. Med.,* **1979,** *301,* 409–413.

Bennett, M. V. L. Comparative physiology: electric organs. *Annu. Rev. Physiol.,* **1970,** *32,* 471–528.

Bernard, C. *Leçons sur les effets des substances toxiques et médicamenteuses.* J.-B. Baillière et Fils, Paris, **1857.**

Bovet, D. Synthetic inhibitors of neuromuscular transmission, chemical structures and structure activity relationships. In, *Neuromuscular Blocking and Stimulating Agents,* Vol 1. *International Encyclopedia of Pharmacology and Therapeutics,* Sect. 14. (Cheymol, J., ed.) Pergamon Press, Ltd., Oxford, **1972,** pp. 243–294.

Bowman, W. C., and Nott, M. W. Actions of sympathomimetic amines and their antagonists on skeletal muscle. *Pharmacol. Rev.,* **1969,** *21,* 27–72. (385 references.)

Cheymol, J., and Bourillet, F. Inhibitors of post-synaptic receptors. In, *Neuromuscular Blocking and Stimulating Agents,* Vol. 1. *International Encyclopedia of Pharmacology and Therapeutics,* Sect. 14. (Cheymol, J., ed.) Pergamon Press, Ltd., Oxford, **1972,** pp. 297–356.

Colquhoun, D. The link between drug binding and response: theories and observations. In, *The Receptors: A Comprehensive Treatise.* (O'Brien, R. D., ed.) Plenum Press, New York, **1979,** pp. 93–142.

Crankshaw, D. P., and Cohen, E. N. Uptake, distribution and elimination of skeletal muscle relaxants. In, *Muscle Relaxants.* (Katz, R., ed.) Excerpta Medica, Amsterdam, **1975,** pp. 125–141.

Dijl, W., van. Neuromuscular blocking agents. In, *Side Effects of Drugs,* Vol. 7. (Meyler, L., and Herxheimer, A., eds.) Excerpta Medica, Amsterdam, **1972,** pp. 209–223.

Dripps, R. D. The clinician looks at neuromuscular blocking drugs. In, *Neuromuscular Junction.* (Zaimis, E., ed.) Springer-Verlag, Berlin, **1976,** pp. 583–592.

Elmqvist, D., and Thesleff, S. Ideas regarding receptor desensitization at the motor end plate. *Rev. Can. Biol.,* **1962,** *21,* 220–234.

Fambrough, D. Control of acetylcholine receptors in skeletal muscle. *Physiol. Rev.,* **1979,** *59,* 165–227.

Feldman, S. Neuromuscular blocking drugs. In, *A Practice of Anaesthesia,* 4th ed. (Churchill-Davidson, H. C., and Wylie, W. D., eds.) W. B. Saunders Co., Philadelphia, **1978,** pp. 865–911.

Foldes, F. F. (ed.). *Muscle Relaxants.* F. A. Davis Co., Philadelphia, **1966.**

Gill, R. C. *White Waters and Black Magic.* Henry Holt & Co., New York, **1940.**

Gordon, R. A.; Britt, B. A.; and Kalow, E. (eds.). *International Symposium on Malignant Hyperthermia.* Charles C Thomas, Pub., Springfield, Ill., **1973.**

Hansten, P. D. *Drug Interactions,* 4th ed. Lea & Febiger, Philadelphia, **1979.**

Heidmann, T., and Changeux, J.-P. Structural and functional properties of the acetylcholine receptor protein in its purified and membrane bound states. *Annu. Rev. Biochem.,* **1978,** *47,* 317–357.

Hunt, C. C., and Kuffler, S. W. Pharmacology of the neuromuscular junction. *Pharmacol. Rev.,* **1950,** *2,* 96–120.

Kalow, W. Genetic factors in relation to drugs. *Annu. Rev. Pharmacol.,* **1965,** *5,* 9–26.

Karlin, A. Chemical modification of the active site of the acetylcholine receptor. *J. Gen. Physiol.,* **1969,** *54,* 245S–264S.

———. Molecular interactions of the acetylcholine receptor. *Fed. Proc.,* **1973,** *32,* 1847–1853.

Khromov-Borisov, N. V., and Michelson, M. J. The mutual disposition of cholinoceptors of locomotor muscles, and the changes in their disposition in the course of evolution. *Pharmacol. Rev.,* **1966,** *18,* 1051–1090.

McIntyre, A. R. *Curare: Its History, Nature, and Clinical Use.* University of Chicago Press, Chicago, **1947.**

———. History of curare. In, *Neuromuscular Blocking and Stimulating Agents,* Vol. 1. *International Encyclopedia of Pharmacology and Therapeutics,* Sect. 14. (Cheymol, J., ed.) Pergamon Press, Ltd., Oxford, **1972,** pp. 187–203.

Maclagan, J. Competitive neuromuscular blocking drugs. In, *Neuromuscular Junction.* (Zaimis, E., ed.) Springer-Verlag, Berlin, **1976,** pp. 421–474.

Paton, W. D. M., and Zaimis, E. J. The methonium compounds. *Pharmacol. Rev.,* **1952,** *4,* 219–253.

Patrick, J.; Heinemann, S.; and Schubert, D. Biology of cultured nerve and muscle. *Annu. Rev. Neurosci.,* **1978,** *1,* 417–443.

Pittinger, C., and Adamson, R. Antibiotic blockade of neuromuscular function. *Annu. Rev. Pharmacol.,* **1972,** *12,* 169–184.

Riker, W. F. Prejunctional effects of neuromuscular blocking and facilitatory drugs. In, *Muscle Relaxants.* (Katz, R., ed.) Excerpta Medica, Amsterdam, **1975,** pp. 59–102.

Smith, C. M. Neuromuscular pharmacology: drugs and muscle spindles. *Annu. Rev. Pharmacol.,* **1963,** *3,* 223–242.

Smith, S. C. Neuromuscular blocking drugs in man. In, *Neuromuscular Junction.* (Zaimis, E., ed.) Springer-Verlag, Berlin, **1976,** pp. 593–660.

Speight, T. M., and Avery, G. S. Pancuronium bromide: a review of its pharmacological properties and clinical application. *Drugs,* **1972,** *4,* 163–226.

Symposium. (Various authors.) *Second International Symposium on Malignant Hyperthermia.* (Aldrete, A., and Britt, B. A., eds.) Grune & Stratton, Inc., New York, **1978,** pp. 1–560.

Vickers, M. D.; Wood-Smith, F. G.; and Stewart, H. C. *Drugs in Anaesthetic Practice.* Butterworths, London, **1978.**

Waser, P. G. Chemistry and pharmacology of natural curare compounds. In, *Neuromuscular Blocking and Stimulating Agents,* Vol. 1. *International Encyclopedia of Pharmacology and Therapeutics,* Sect. 14. (Cheymol, J., ed.) Pergamon Press, Ltd., Oxford, **1972,** pp. 205–239.

Zaimis, E. The neuromuscular junction: area of uncertainty. In, *Neuromuscular Junction.* (Zaimis, E., ed.) Springer-Verlag, Berlin, **1976,** pp. 1–18.

Zaimis, E., and Head, S. Depolarizing neuromuscular blocking drugs. In, *Neuromuscular Junction.* (Zaimis, E., ed.) Springer-Verlag, Berlin, **1976,** pp. 365–420.

Zaimis, E. J. Mechanisms of neuromuscular blockade. In, *Curare and Curare-like Agents.* (Bovet, D.; Bovet-Nitti, F.; and Marini-Bettòlo, G. B.; eds.) Elsevier Publishing Co., Amsterdam, **1959,** pp. 191–203.

Drugs Acting on the Central Nervous System

CHAPTER

12 NEUROHUMORAL TRANSMISSION AND THE CENTRAL NERVOUS SYSTEM

Floyd E. Bloom

Drugs that act upon the central nervous system (CNS) influence the lives of everyone, everyday. These agents are invaluable therapeutically because they can produce specific physiological and psychological effects. Without general anesthetics, modern surgery would be impossible. Drugs that affect the CNS may selectively relieve pain or fever, suppress disorders of movement, or prevent epileptic seizures. They may induce sleep or arousal, reduce the desire to eat, or allay the tendency to vomit. They may be used to treat anxiety, mania, depression, or schizophrenia without altering consciousness. The brain also responds secondarily to drugs that are used to treat diseases of peripheral organs.

The nonmedical, self-use of CNS drugs is widely practiced. Socially acceptable stimulants and antianxiety agents produce stability, relief, and even pleasure for many. However, the excessive use of these and other drugs can also adversely affect lives when an individual becomes addicted or because of toxic side effects that may include lethal overdosage.

The unique quality of drugs that affect the nervous system and behavior places pharmacologists who study the CNS in the midst of one of the ultimate scientific challenges— the attempt to understand the cellular and molecular basis for the enormously complex and varied functions of the human brain. In this effort, pharmacologists have two major goals: to use drugs to dissect the cellular and molecular mechanisms that operate in the normal CNS and to develop appropriate drugs to correct pathophysiological events in the abnormal CNS.

Approaches to the elucidation of the sites and mechanisms of action of CNS drugs demand fundamental understanding of the cellular and molecular biology of the brain. Although knowledge of the anatomy, physiology, and chemistry of the nervous system is far from complete, the acceleration of interdisciplinary research on the CNS has allowed remarkable progress over the past decade. This chapter develops guidelines and fundamental principles for the comprehensive analysis of drugs that affect the CNS.

ORGANIZATIONAL PRINCIPLES OF THE BRAIN

The brain is an assembly of interrelated systems that regulate activity within and between each other in a dynamic, complex fashion. Its largest anatomical divisions provide a superficial classification of the distribution of brain functions.

MACROFUNCTIONS OF BRAIN REGIONS

Cerebral Cortex. The two cerebral hemispheres constitute the largest division of the brain. Regions of the cortex are classified in several ways: (1) by the modality of information processed (*e.g.*, sensory, including somatosensory, visual, auditory, and olfactory, as well as motor and associational); (2) by anatomical position (frontal, temporal, parietal, and occipital); and (3) by the geometrical relationship between cell types in the major cortical layers (so-called cytoarchitectonic classifications). Presently, emphasis on cortical structure is focused upon the rather regular columnar organization of cells within vertically oriented cylinders at right angles to the cortical surface. These vertical arrays, each of which contains slightly more than 100 neurons in their most elemental form, may constitute the basic modules of the cortex for processing information. Individual columns can be assembled into large ensembles of hundreds to thousands of neurons by functional association with adjacent vertical arrays or with functionally related units in other areas of the cortex. Mountcastle and Edelman (1978) view these ensembles as "interconnected . . . nested distributed systems" and suggest that the associations are rapidly modifiable as information is processed. The 50 billion neurons of the human cortex provide an astronomical number of recombinant possibilities for such processing. Cortical areas termed association areas receive and somehow process information that is relayed to the primary cortical sensory regions, producing the still-unexplained higher cortical functions such as abstract thought, memory, and consciousness.

The cerebral cortices also provide for supervisory integration of the autonomic nervous system, and they may integrate somatic and vegetative functions, including those of the cardiovascular and gastrointestinal systems. For example, the control of blood pressure and of gastric motility may be susceptible to conscious feedback control in human beings (Miller, 1978).

Limbic System. This region, which consists of the *hippocampus, amygdaloid complex, septum, hypothalamus, olfactory* and *pyriform lobes, basal ganglia,* and parts of the *thalamus,* is sometimes called the visceral brain. These structures lie beneath the cortical mantle and act in a complex, concerted manner to integrate emotional state with motor and visceral activities.

Parts of the limbic system also participate individually in functions that are capable of more precise definition. Thus, the basal ganglia or neostriatum (the *caudate nucleus, putamen, globus pallidus,* and *lentiform nucleus*) form an essential segment of the *extrapyramidal motor system.* This system complements the function of the pyramidal (or voluntary) motor system; damage to the extrapyramidal system results in inhibition of voluntary movements and the appearance of disorders characterized by involuntary movements, such as the tremors and rigidity of Parkinson's disease or the uncontrollable limb movements of Huntington's chorea. Similarly, the hippocampus may be crucial to the formation of recent memory, since this function is lost in patients with extensive bilateral damage to the hippocampus.

The *thalamus* lies in the center of the brain, beneath the cortex and basal ganglia and above the hypothalamus. The neurons of the thalamus are arranged into distinct clusters, or nuclei, which are either paired or midline structures. These nuclei act as relays between the incoming sensory pathways and the cortex, between the discrete regions of the thalamus and hypothalamus, and between the basal ganglia and the association regions of the cerebral cortex. The thalamic nuclei and the basal ganglia both exert regulatory control over visceral functions; for example, aphagia and adipsia, as well as general sensory neglect, have been observed to follow damage to the corpus striatum (Ungerstedt, 1971).

The *hypothalamus* is the principal integrating region for the entire autonomic nervous system, and it regulates among other functions, body temperature, water balance, intermediary metabolism, blood pressure, sexual and circadian cycles, secretion of the adenohypophysis, sleep, and emotion. Recent advances in the cytophysiological and chemical dissection of the hypothalamus have clarified the connections and possible functions of individual hypothalamic nuclei (Guillemin, 1978).

Midbrain and Brain Stem. The *mesencephalon, pons,* and *medulla oblongata* connect the cerebral hemispheres and thalamus-hypothalamus to the spinal cord. These "bridge portions" of the CNS contain most of the nuclei of the cranial nerves, as well as the major inflow and outflow tracts from the cortices and spinal cord. It is within these regions that the *reticular activating system* is found, which is an important but incompletely characterized region of gray matter linking peripheral sensory and motor events with higher levels of nervous integration. The major monoamine-containing neurons of the brain are found within this zone. These regions together represent the points of central integration for coordination of essential reflexive acts such as swallowing and vomiting and those that involve the cardiovascular and respiratory systems; these areas also include the primary receptive regions for most visceral afferent sensory information. The reticular activating system is essential for the regulation of sleep and wakefulness, as well as for coordination of gaze and eye tracking movements. The fiber systems projecting from the reticular formation have been called "nonspecific" because the targets to which these fibers project are considerably more diffuse in distribution than are the connections from many other neurons (*e.g.*, specific thalamocortical projections). However, the reticular systems may innervate targets in a coherent, functional manner even though their targets are widely distributed (*see* Symposium, 1979b).

Cerebellum. This small and highly organized cortical region arises from the posterior pons behind the cerebral hemispheres. Although it is also highly laminated and redundant in its detailed cytological organization, the lobules and folia of the cerebellum project onto specific deep cerebellar nuclei, which in turn make relatively selective projections to the motor cortex (by way of the thalamus) and to the brain stem nuclei concerned with vestibular (position-stabilization) function. The cerebellum is generally regarded as playing an important role in the maintenance of appropriate body posture in space. In addition to maintaining the proper tone of antigravity musculature and providing continuous feedback during volitional movements of the trunk and extremities, the cerebellum may also regulate heart rate, possibly to maintain blood flow despite changes in posture.

Spinal Cord. The cord extends from the caudal end of the medulla oblongata to the lower lumbar vertebrae. Within this mass of nerve cells and tracts, the sensory information from skin, muscles, joints, and viscera is locally coordinated with motoneurons and with primary sensory relay cells to project to and receive signals from higher levels. The spinal cord is divided into anatomical segments (cervical, thoracic, lumbar, and sacral) that correspond to divisions of the peripheral nerves and spinal column. Ascending and descending tracts of the spinal cord are located within the white matter at the perimeter of the cord, while intersegmental connections and synaptic contacts are concentrated within the H-shaped internal mass of gray matter. Within the H, sensory information flows into the dorsal portion, and motor outflow exits from the ventral portion. The preganglionic neurons of the autonomic nervous system are found in the intermediolateral columns of the gray matter, approximately at the external boundary of the middle of the H of the gray matter. Autonomic reflexes (*e.g.*, changes in skin vasculature with alteration of temperature) can easily be elicited within local segments of the cord, as shown by the maintenance of these reflexes after the cord is severed (Rothlin and Berde, 1953).

MICROANATOMY OF THE BRAIN

Cellular Organization of the Brain. Present understanding of the cellular organization of the CNS depends upon two separate concepts of interconnections between neurons (Szentagothai and Arbib, 1974; Rakic, 1975). In the first, *long-hierarchical* neuronal organizations are stressed, while in the second, *short-* or *local-circuit* organizations are emphasized. In the primary sensory and motor pathways, the transmission of information is highly sequential, and interconnected neurons are related to each other in a hierarchical fashion. Primary receptors (in the retina, middle ear, olfactory epithelium, tongue, or skin) transmit first to primary relay cells and then to the primary sensory fields of the cerebral cortex. For motor output systems, the reverse sequence holds, descending from the motor cortex to the final

common output of the spinal motoneuron. The essential feature of the hierarchical scheme of CNS organization is that destruction of any link incapacitates the system. Despite moderate search, no neurotransmitter has yet been identified for any of the major links in any sensory or motor pathway, except for the final junction between motoneuron and muscle, where acetylcholine (ACh) is, of course, the transmitter.

In the local-circuit neuron concept of organization, attention is focused on neurons whose connections are mainly established within the immediate vicinity of their location. Such local-circuit neurons are frequently small and may have very few processes. They are thought to regulate the flow of information through their small spatial domain, and they may do this *without* the necessity for the generation of action potentials, which permit the long-distance transmission between hierarchically connected neurons. The neurotransmitter for some local-circuit neurons has been identified as either gamma aminobutyrate (GABA) or glycine.

Evidence also suggests that a third organizational scheme may be useful in attempting to understand certain neuronal systems of the pons and brain stem that contain one of the monoamines—that is, norepinephrine (NE), dopamine (DA), or 5-hydroxytryptamine (5-HT). These neurons extend multiple-branched connections to many target cells, almost all of which lie outside of the brain region in which the neurons are located. In no case do these monoamine-containing cells appear to be sequential elements within any known hierarchical system; rather, they appear to be special local-circuit neurons whose spatial domains are one to two orders of magnitude larger than the classical intraregional interneurons. For example, norepinephrine-containing neurons of the locus ceruleus project from pons to cerebellum, spinal cord, thalamus, and several cortical zones, but the function of these target regions is not obviously disrupted when the adrenergic fibers are destroyed experimentally, indicating their divergent but nonhierarchical structure. These systems could mediate linkages between regions that may require temporary integration. Many other long projecting systems that arise from the midbrain could also fit into this organizational scheme, which is neither hierarchical nor strictly local circuit. The neurotransmitter is not yet known for most of these types of internuncial connections.

Cell Biology of Neurons. Morphological properties of central neurons have been very useful for the description of their functional characteristics. Neurons are classified in many different ways, including designation according to function (sensory, motor, or interneuron), the identity of the transmitter they synthesize, and location. Microscopic analysis focuses on their general shape, and, in particular, the number of extensions from the cell body. Most neurons have one axon, which carries signals from the cell of origin to other cells. Other processes extend from the nerve cell to receive synaptic contacts from other neurons; these processes, called dendrites, may branch in extremely complex patterns. Neurons exhibit the cytological characteristics of highly active secretory cells: large nuclei; large amounts of smooth and rough endoplasmic reticulum; and frequent clusters of specialized smooth endoplasmic reticulum (Golgi apparatus), where secretory products of the cell are packaged into organelles bound with membrane for transport out of the cell (Figure 12–1). The synaptic vesicles that are characteristic of distal axons are not easily observed within the neuronal cell body; larger vesicles seen in the Golgi zone may thus form the synaptic vesicles after transport to the nerve terminals. Neurons and their cellular extensions are rich in microtubules—elongated tubules of approximately 24-nm diameter. Their functions may be to support the elongated axons and dendrites and to assist in the reciprocal transport of essential macromolecules and organelles between the cell body and the axon or dendrites.

Synaptic Relationships. Synaptic arrangements in the CNS fall into a wide variety of morphological and functional forms that are specific for the cells involved. Specific synaptic connections that have one origin will tend to form contacts upon particular surface zones of their target cells in a mosaic arrangement that may reflect the underlying distribution of chemical receptors. Electron microscopic observations of target neurons reveal two major structural details as characteristic of the site presumed to be the active zone of contact. The presynaptic structure is enriched in small vesicles; their shape, size, and chemical properties vary with the identity of the neurotransmitter. Each vesicle probably contains several thousand molecules of transmitter, a number that approaches the lower estimate of transmitter molecules in a "quantum," the elemental package responsible for miniature postsynaptic potentials (see Chapter 4). In addition, the presynaptic and postsynaptic membranes exhibit a specialized attachment site, termed the *synaptolemma* by Bodian (1972).

Many spatial arrangements are possible within synaptic relationships (Figure 12–1). The most common arrangement, typical of the hierarchical pathways, is the axodendritic or axosomatic arrangement in which the axons of the cell of origin make their functional contact with the dendrites or cell body of the target. In other cases, functional contacts may occur between the adjacent cell bodies (somasomatic) or between overlapping dendrites (dendrodendritic). The latter is typical of some of the monoaminergic neurons within their nuclei of origin. Many local-circuit neurons do not possess distinct axons and yet enter into synaptic relationships through modified dendrites, sometimes termed *telodendrites;* these modified dendrites can be either the presynaptic or the postsynaptic element. Another relatively frequent arrangement, particularly within the spinal cord, is the serial axoaxonic relationship in which the axon of an interneuron ends upon the terminal of a long-distance neuron as that terminal contacts a dendrite in the dorsal horn. Many presynaptic axons contain enlargements along their length that show collections of typical synaptic vesicles, often without a specialized synaptolemma. It is not yet clear if sites with specialized synaptolemma also act as specific sites of release of transmitter; "nonspecialized" axonal enlargements (or *boutons en passage*) could also be sites of some other function. Neurons of the peripheral autonomic nervous system do not exhibit specialized synaptolemma at the point of their contact with glandular or smooth muscle cells, where transmitter is certainly released; they do, however, exhibit typical axodendritic, dendrodendritic, and somasomatic contacts within autonomic ganglia.

The bioelectric properties of neurons and junctions in the CNS generally follow the outlines and details already described for the peripheral autonomic nervous system (see Chapter 4), except that a much more varied range of intercellular mechanisms has been discerned in CNS. Although not yet fully clarified, some description of these various forms of presumptive exchange of information appears below.

IDENTIFICATION OF CENTRAL TRANSMITTERS

To provide rigorous scientific proof that one chemical substance is the transmitter for a given central synaptic connection, criteria have been established by analogy with those that were utilized to demonstrate that ACh and NE were the predominant transmitters of the autonomic nervous system (see Chapter 4).

1. *The transmitter must be shown to be present in the presynaptic terminals of the synapse and in the neurons from which those presynaptic terminals arise.* Extensions of this criterion involve the demonstration that the presynaptic neuron synthesizes and catabolizes the transmitter substance, rather than simply storing it after accumulation from a nonneural source. Microscopic cytochemistry

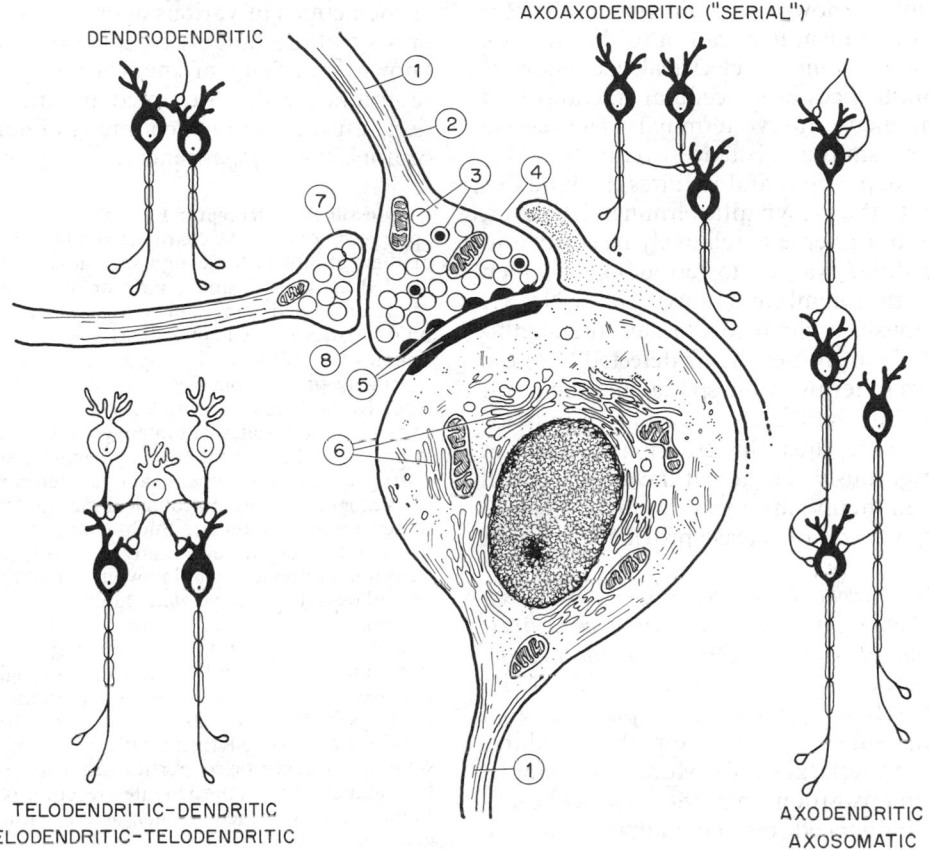

Figure 12-1. *Drug-sensitive sites in synaptic transmission.*

Schematic view of the drug-sensitive sites in some prototypical synaptic complexes. In the center, a postsynaptic neuron receives a somatic synapse (shown greatly oversized) from an axonic terminal; an axoaxonic terminal is shown in contact with this presynaptic nerve terminal. Drug-sensitive sites include: (*1*) microtubules responsible for orthograde and retrograde transport of macromolecules between the neuronal cell body and distal processes; (*2*) electrically conductive membranes; (*3*) sites for the storage and synthesis of transmitters; (*4*) sites for the active uptake of some transmitters into nerve terminals or glia; (*5*) sites for the release of transmitter and sites (receptors) to generate responses; (*6*) cytoplasmic organelles and postsynaptic membranes for maintenance of synaptic activity and for long-term mediation of altered physiological states; and (*7*) presynaptic receptors on adjacent presynaptic processes and (*8*) on nerve terminals (autoreceptors). Around the central neuron are schematic illustrations of the more common synaptic relationships in the CNS. (Modified from Bodian, 1972, and Cooper *et al.*, 1978.)

(Bloom, 1970, 1975; Hokfelt *et al.*, 1978b) and subcellular fractionation and analysis of brain tissue are particularly useful to evaluate this criterion in the CNS. These technics are often combined with the production of surgical or chemical lesions of presynaptic neurons or their tracts to demonstrate that the lesion causes the disappearance of the alleged transmitter from the target region.

2. *The transmitter must be released from the presynaptic nerve concomitantly with presyn-* *aptic nerve activity.* This criterion is generally evaluated by electrical stimulation of the nerve pathway *in vivo* and collection of the transmitter in an enriched extracellular fluid within the synaptic target area (Nieoullon *et al.*, 1977). However, devices for collection such as push-pull cannulae are still hundreds of times larger than individual synapses, and the sensitivity of the methods for detection of transmitters requires that collection extend for periods that are thousands of times longer

than most known synaptic potentials. Release of transmitter can also be studied *in vitro* by ionic or electrical activation of thin brain slices or subcellular fractions that are enriched in nerve terminals. The release of all transmitter substances so far studied is voltage dependent and requires the influx of Ca^{2+} into the presynaptic terminal. However, transmitter release is relatively insensitive to extracellular Na^+ or to tetrodotoxin, which blocks transmembrane movement of Na^+. It is obviously difficult to evaluate the significance of transmitter that is detected by these technics in terms of the spatial and temporal characteristics of transmission at an individual synapse. Thus, this criterion has not yet been rigorously satisfied at the cellular level, although many instances of more general documentation of release provide significant clues.

3. *The effects of the alleged substance, when applied experimentally to the target cells, must be identical to the effects of stimulating the presynaptic pathway.* This criterion can be met loosely by qualitative comparisons (*e.g.*, both the substance and the pathway inhibit or excite the target cell). More convincing is the demonstration that the ionic conductances influenced by the pathway are the same as those affected by the candidate transmitter. More specifically, the equilibrium value of the synaptic potential and that to which the cell is driven by the alleged transmitter should be identical. These tests require intracellular recording for long periods of time, and this is difficult to achieve, particularly for many of the smaller or deeply placed target neurons of the brain. Alternatively, the criterion can be satisfied less rigorously by demonstration of pharmacological identity of receptors. In general, pharmacological antagonism of the pathway's actions and those of the candidate transmitter should be achieved by similar doses of the same drug. To be convincing, the antagonistic drug should not affect responses of the target neurons to other unrelated pathways or to chemically distinct transmitter candidates. Actions that are qualitatively identical to those that follow stimulation of the pathway should also be observed when synthetic agonists that mimic the transmitter are tested. Pharmacological characterization

of the actions of various agonists and antagonists will presumably be consistent with the known specificity of the various classes of receptors for the presumed natural agonist (*e.g.*, muscarinic or nicotinic cholinergic receptors, β_1- or β_2-adrenergic receptors, etc.).

Assessment of Receptor Properties. Central synaptic receptors may be characterized by examination of their ability to bind high-specific-activity radiolabeled agonists or antagonists or of the ability of other unlabeled compounds to compete for such binding sites (*see* Chapter 2; Maguire *et al.*, 1977; Simon and Hiller, 1978; Snyder *et al.*, 1978). The specificity of such binding must be evaluated with care. Radioligand binding assays can be used to quantify binding sites within a region, to follow their appearance throughout the phylogenetic scale and during brain development, and to determine how physiological or pharmacological manipulation regulates receptor number. Such characterization of the opiate receptor eventually contributed to the detection of previously unknown peptide transmitter candidates—the *enkephalins* and *endorphins* (*see* below).

The properties of the cellular response to the transmitter can be studied electrophysiologically by the use of *microiontophoresis* (combination of recordings from single cells and highly localized drug administration) (*see* Krnjevic, 1974; Bloom, 1975). In some cases, receptor properties can also be studied biochemically when the activated receptor is coupled to an enzymatic reaction, such as the synthesis of a cyclic nucleotide.

With limitations, these methods can provide quantitative information on the adaptive self-regulation of receptors for a neurotransmitter that follows pharmacological or pathological perturbations (*e.g.*, denervation supersensitivity, drug-induced subsensitivity, etc.). Drug-receptor interactions should be considered to be constantly modifiable relationships. Postsynaptic receptivity on CNS neurons is continuously regulated in terms of the number of receptive sites and the threshold required for generation of a response. Receptor number is often dependent upon the concentration of agonist to which the target cell is exposed. Thus, chronic excess of agonist can lead to a reduced number of receptors (desensitization or down-regulation) and consequently to subsensitivity or tolerance to the transmitter. A deficit of transmitter can lead to increased numbers of receptors and supersensitivity of the system (Kahn, 1976; Schwartz *et al.*, 1978; Sulser *et al.*, 1978). These adaptive processes become especially important when drugs are used to treat chronic illness of the CNS. *With prolonged periods of exposure to drug, the actual mechanisms underlying the therapeutic effect may differ strikingly from those that operate when the agent is first introduced into the system.* Similar adaptive modifications of neuronal systems can also occur at presynaptic sites, such as those concerned with transmitter synthesis, storage, re-uptake, and release (*see* Mandell, 1973). These adaptive changes frustrate attempts to interpret the effects of behaviorally active drugs in terms of specific neurotransmitters (*see* Iversen and Iversen, 1975).

NEUROTRANSMITTERS, NEURO-HORMONES, AND NEUROMODU-LATORS: CONTRASTING PRINCIPLES OF NEURONAL REGULATION

Neurotransmitters. Until recently, relatively few known substances were considered to be candidates as synaptic transmitters in the CNS. All transmitters were originally thought to operate in a monolithic fashion, leading either to excitation or inhibition by causing rapid changes in the ionic conductivity of the membrane and consequent shifts in the membrane potential as the target cell approaches the equilibrium potential for those ions.

Over the past decade, experiments on the peripheral and central nervous systems have indicated that chemical communication across synapses and other neuroeffector junctions can also operate through mechanisms other than the archetypical rapid increases in postsynaptic membrane conductances. So-called slow synaptic potentials were encountered in photoreceptors and sympathetic ganglia in which the polarization of the membrane was changed through inactivation of finite resting conductances (*i.e.,* a "leaky" resting membrane). Shortly thereafter, studies on central synaptic mechanisms detected similar slow potential changes attributable to noradrenergic β receptors or to muscarinic cholinergic receptors; these responses appear to depend upon changes in polarization that are accompanied by *decreased* membrane conductances, although the molecular mechanisms accounting for these changes are still unknown. Considerable evidence has been presented that favors the view that such synaptic events may be mediated through the postsynaptic generation of cyclic nucleotides (*see* below; *see also* Bloom, 1975, and Greengard, 1978). Regardless of the mechanisms that underlie such synaptic operations, their temporal and biophysical characteristics differ substantially from the rapid onset-offset type of effect previously thought to describe all synaptic events. These differences have thus raised the issue of whether substances that produce slow synaptic effects should be described with the same term—*neurotransmitter*. Some of the alternate terms deserve brief survey with regard to mechanisms of drug action.

Neurohormones. Peptide-secreting cells of the hypothalamicohypophyseal circuits were originally described as neurosecretory cells, a form of neuron that was both fish and fowl, receiving synaptic information from other central neurons yet secreting their transmitter in a hormone-like fashion into the circulation (Scharrer, 1969). The transmitter of such neurons was termed a *neurohormone*, that is, a hormone arising from a neuron. However, this term has lost most of its original meaning because these hypothalamic neurons may also synapse with neurons in the brain stem and spinal cord (Barker, 1977; Swanson, 1977); cytochemical evidence would indicate that transmission at these sites is also mediated by the same substance that is secreted as a hormone in the posterior pituitary (oxytocin, antidiuretic hormone). Thus, the designation of hormone relates to the site of release at the pituitary and does not necessarily describe all of the actions of the peptide.

Neuromodulators. Florey (1967) employed the term *modulator* to describe substances that can influence neuronal activity differently than do neurotransmitters. In the context of this definition, the distinctive feature of a modulator is that it originates from cellular and nonsynaptic sites, yet influences the excitability of nerve cells. Florey specifically designated substances such as CO_2 and ammonia, arising from active neurons or glia, as potential modulators through nonsynaptic actions. Similarly, circulating steroid hormones (Zigmond, 1975), locally released adenosine (Burnstock, 1975; McIlwain, 1977), and prostaglandins (Symposium, 1971; Horrobin, 1978) might all now be regarded as modulators. If a modulator is to be defined simply on the basis of its nonsynaptic origin, then substances that are released at junctional sites could not be so designated.

The term *neuromodulator* has also been employed in a different way to distinguish neural substances that influence the general level of neuronal excitability without altering the membrane potential. This special type of effect was first ascribed to the actions of substance P in the spinal cord (*see* Nicoll, 1978), and similar definitions of modulation have recently been reactivated from studies of the effects of thyrotropin-releasing hormone (TRH) (Nicoll, 1978) and enkephalins on spinal neurons (Zieglgansberger and Bayerl, 1976; Barker *et al.,* 1978). In the latter cases, the modulator function is described as one that does not directly alter neuronal membrane potential or ionic conductances but, nevertheless, does alter the ability of other neurotransmitters to elicit such changes.

Neuromediators. Substances that participate in the elicitation of the postsynaptic response to a transmitter or a modulator fall under this heading. The clearest examples of such mediation are provided by the involvement of cyclic adenosine 3′,5′-monophosphate (cyclic AMP), and perhaps of cyclic guanosine 3′,5′-monophosphate (cyclic GMP), as second messengers at specific sites of synaptic transmission (Bloom, 1975; Greengard, 1978). However, there are technical difficulties in the demonstration that a change in the concentration of cyclic nucleotides occurs prior to the generation of the synaptic potential and that this change in concentration is both necessary and sufficient for the generation of the synaptic potential; this forces the more conservative position that, while cyclic nucleotides are likely to be involved in synaptic events at these sites, additional precise quantitative data are needed for secure proof of mediation. It is possible that the changes in the concentration of cyclic nucleotides that can be observed under certain conditions supplement and enhance the generation of the synaptic potentials. Activation of cyclic nucleotide-dependent protein phosphorylation reactions (*see* Chapter 4) could alter properties of membrane proteins that are known to be substrates in these reactions (Greengard, 1978). These possibilities are pertinent to the action of the central catecholaminergic circuits described below.

The criteria for identification of synaptic transmitters rely heavily on the demonstrations that a substance contained in a neuron is secreted by that neuron to transmit infor-

mation to its postsynaptic target. Given this level of functional description and a definite effect of neuron A on its target cell B, a substance found in neuron A, secreted from neuron A, and producing the effect of A on B would then operationally be the transmitter from A to B. Within this broad definition, substances may act to transmit their information in a variety of ways, many of which are only now beginning to be characterized as to mechanisms. In some cases, transmitters may produce minimal effects on bioelectric properties, yet activate or inactivate biochemical mechanisms necessary for responses to other circuits. Alternatively, the action of a transmitter may vary with the context of ongoing synaptic events— enhancing excitations or inhibitions, rather than operating to impose direct excitation or inhibition. Each chemical substance that fits within the broad definition of a transmitter may, therefore, require operational definition within the spatial and temporal domains in which a specific cell-cell circuit is defined. Those same properties may or may not be generalized to other cells that are contacted by the same presynaptic neurons, with the differences in operation related to differences in the postsynaptic receptor and the mechanisms by which the activated receptor produces its effect (Bloom, 1975).

ACTIONS OF DRUGS IN THE CNS

Specificity and Nonspecificity of CNS Drug Action. The effect of a drug is considered to be specific when it affects an identifiable molecular mechanism unique to target cells that bear receptors for the drug. Conversely, a drug is regarded as nonspecific when it produces effects on many different target cells and acts by diverse molecular mechanisms. This terminology thus distinguishes *broad* actions at many levels of the CNS through effects on specific molecular mechanisms (*e.g.,* atropine blockade of muscarinic receptors) from nonspecific actions. This separation is often a property of the dose-response relationship of the drug and the cell or mechanisms under scrutiny. Even a drug that is highly selective when tested at a low concentration may exhibit nonspecific actions at substantially higher doses. (For example, many specific antagonists of β-adrenergic receptors can also cause local anesthesia at high concentrations; similar nonspecific effects may be seen with tricyclic antidepressants at doses one to two orders of magnitude higher than those required to cause selective changes in rates of transmitter uptake or release.) Conversely, even generally acting drugs may not act equally on all levels of the CNS. For example, sedatives, hypnotics, or general anesthetics would have very limited utility if central neurons that control the respiratory and cardiovascular systems were not less sensitive to their actions. Drugs with specific actions may produce nonspecific effects when the dose and route of administration initially produce high tissue concentrations; their specificity of action becomes apparent only later, when the concentrations fall.

As the number of putative neurotransmitters has increased and as technics have evolved for the analysis of the actions of drugs upon specific target neurons, the list of drugs that have been regarded as having general actions has become considerably shorter. Thus, more and more drugs exhibit actions that can be related to specific mechanisms. For example, the effects of the broadly acting stimulants strychnine and picrotoxin can now be attributed to interference with inhibitory actions that are mediated at receptors for glycine and GABA, respectively (Curtis *et al.,* 1971); similarly, barbiturates have been found to have relatively selective effects on synaptic mechanisms (MacDonald and Barker, 1978). Drugs whose mechanisms currently appear to be general or nonspecific are classed according to whether they produce behavioral depression or stimulation, while specifically acting CNS drugs can be classed more definitively according to their locus of action or specific therapeutic usefulness.

General (Nonspecific) CNS Depressants. This category includes the anesthetic gases and vapors, the aliphatic alcohols, and some hypnotic-sedative drugs. These agents share the ability to depress excitable tissue at all levels of the CNS by stabilization of neuronal membranes, leading to a decrease in amount of transmitter released by the nerve impulse, as well as to general depression of postsynaptic responsiveness and ion movement.

General (Nonspecific) CNS Stimulants. The drugs that remain in this category are pentylenetetrazol and related agents that are capable of powerful excitation of the CNS and the methylxanthines, which have a much weaker stimulant action. Stimulation may be accomplished by one of two general mechanisms: by blockade of inhibition or by direct neuronal excitation (which may involve increased transmitter release, more prolonged transmitter action, labilization of the postsynaptic membrane, or a decrease in synaptic recovery time).

Drugs That Selectively Modify CNS Function. The agents in this group *may* cause either depression or excitation. In some instances, a drug may produce both effects simultaneously on different systems. Some agents in this category have little effect upon the level of excitability in doses that are used therapeutically. The principal classes of these CNS drugs are the following: anticonvulsants, antiparkinsonism drugs, narcotic and nonnarcotic analgesics, appetite suppressants, antiemetics, analgesic-antipyretics, certain stimulants, neuroleptics (antidepressants and antimanic and antipsychotic agents), hypnotics, sedatives, and tranquilizers.

Although selectivity of action may be remarkable, a drug usually affects several CNS functions to varying degrees. When only one constellation of effects is wanted in a therapeutic situation, the remaining effects of the drug are regarded as limitations in selectivity, *i.e.,* unwanted or side effects.

The specificity of a drug's action is frequently overestimated. This is partly due to the fact that the drug is identified with the effect that is implied by the class name. For example, levodopa, atropine and other muscarinic antagonists, and some antihistamines are all antiparkinsonism drugs, yet all have substantial additional effects that are therapeutically useful. However, since all centrally acting drugs are more or less selective, it will be profitable to consider some of the probable bases for their selectivity; such considerations are inseparable from discussion of the mechanisms of their action.

Factors That Affect the Intensity and Duration of the Effects of Drugs on the CNS. Apart from the exceptional instances in which drugs are introduced directly into the CNS, the concentration of the agent in the blood after oral or parenteral administration obviously has great bearing on the concentration in the CNS. However, this relationship is often not as simple as for peripheral structures.

Although not anatomically defined, the *blood-brain barrier* represents an important boundary between the peripheral and central nervous systems in the form of a permeability barrier to the passive diffusion of substances from the blood stream into various regions of the CNS. Evidence of the barrier is provided by the greatly diminished rate of access of chemicals from plasma to the brain (*see* Chapter 1). This phenomenon is much less prominent in the hypothalamus and in several small specialized organs lining the third and fourth ventricles of the brain: the median eminence, area postrema, pineal gland, subfornical organ, and subcommissural organ. While severe limitations are imposed upon the diffusion of macromolecules, selective barriers to permeation also exist for small charged molecules such as neurotransmitters, their precursors and metabolites, and some drugs. These diffusional barriers are at present best conceived as a combination of the partition of solute across the vasculature (which governs passage by definable properties such as molecular weight, charge, and lipophilicity) and the presence or absence of energy-dependent transport systems. Active transport of certain agents may occur across the barrier in either direction. For example, amino acids are actively transported into brain by stereospecific systems in which groups of amino acids compete for uptake sites (Wurtman and Fernstrom, 1974). The diffusional barriers retard the movement of substances from brain to blood as well as from blood to brain, but the brain clears metabolites of transmitters into the cerebrospinal fluid by excretion through the acid transport system of the choroid plexus (*see* Wood, 1979). Substances that can rarely gain access to the brain from the blood stream can often reach the brain after injection directly into the cerebrospinal fluid.

Other factors may also influence the *duration* of a drug's effect. Where the action of a drug is to reduce storage of a transmitter substance, the onset of the effect may be delayed; however, the drug may have a prolonged effect that persists after it has disappeared from the CNS. For example, reserpine reduces stores of catecholamines and 5-HT in the central and peripheral nervous systems. The full biochemical and behavioral effect of this drug appears only after many hours but is apparent for a considerable time after reserpine has been eliminated from the body; yet long-term therapy with reserpine may result in transmitter stores that are only slightly reduced. Covalent or high-affinity binding of a drug to a receptor can also, of course, produce a prolonged effect.

General Characteristics of CNS Drugs. Combinations of centrally acting drugs are frequently administered to therapeutic advantage (*e.g.*, an anticholinergic drug and levodopa for Parkinson's disease). However, other combinations of drugs may be detrimental, because of potentially dangerous additive effects, or mutually antagonistic, because of interactions between their central effects.

The effect of a CNS drug is additive with the physiological state and with the effects of other depressant and stimulant drugs. For example, anesthetics are less effective in a hyperexcitable subject than in a normal patient; the converse is true with respect to the effects of stimulants. In general, depressant effects of drugs from all categories are additive (*e.g.*, the fatal combination of barbiturates or benzodiazepines with ethanol), as are the effects of stimulants. Therefore, respiration depressed by morphine is further impaired by depressant drugs, while stimulant drugs can augment the excitatory effects of morphine to produce vomiting and convulsions.

Antagonism between depressants and stimulants is variable. Some instances of true pharmacological antagonism among CNS drugs are known; for example, opioid antagonists are very selective in blocking the effects of opioid analgesics, and trimethadione (an anticonvulsant) completely blocks the convulsions produced by pentylenetetrazol over a wide dosage range. However, the antagonism exhibited between two CNS drugs is usually physiological in nature. Thus, an individual who has received one drug cannot be returned entirely to normal by another. However, remarkable antagonism between depressants and stimulants (*e.g.*, haloperidol and amphetamine) may be noted with respect to certain functions.

The selective effects of drugs on specific neurotransmitter systems may be additive or competitive. This potential for drug interaction must be considered whenever such drugs are administered concurrently. The prolonged duration of action of certain agents may necessitate a drug-free period before therapy with other drugs can be started in order to avoid such interactions. An excitatory effect on some functions is commonly observed with low concentrations of some depressant drugs due either to depression of inhibitory systems or to a transient increase in the release of excitatory transmitters. Examples are the "stage of excitement" during induction of general anesthesia and the "stimulant" effects of alcohol. The excitatory phase occurs only with low concentrations of the depressant; uniform depression ensues with increasing drug concentration. The excitatory effects can be minimized, when appropriate, by pretreatment with a depressant drug that is devoid of such effects (*e.g.*, benzodiazepines in preanesthetic medication). Acute, excessive stimulation of the cerebrospinal axis is normally followed by depression (amphetamine, strychnine), which is in part the consequence of neuronal fatigue and exhaustion of metabolites and stores of transmitters. This postictal depression is additive with the effects of depressant drugs. Acute, drug-induced depression is not, as a rule, followed by stimulation. However, chronic drug-induced sedation or depression is followed by prolonged hyperexcitability upon abrupt withdrawal of medication (barbiturates, alcohol). This type of hyperexcitability can be effectively controlled by the same or another depressant drug (*see* Chapter 23).

Organization of CNS-Drug Interactions. The structural and functional properties of neurons provide a means to specify the possible sites at which drugs could interact specifically or generally in the CNS (Figure 12–1). In this scheme, drugs that affect neuronal energy metabolism, maintenance of membrane integrity, or transmembrane ionic equilibria would be generally acting compounds. Similarly general in action would be drugs that affect the two-way intracellular transport systems (*e.g.*, colchicine). These general effects can still exhibit differ-

ent dose-response or time-response relationships among different neurons based, for example, on such neuronal properties as rate of firing, dependence of discharge on external stimuli or internal pacemaker, resting ionic fluxes, or axon length. In contrast, when drug actions can be related to specific aspects of the metabolism, release, or function of a neurotransmitter, the site, specificity, and mechanism of action of a drug can be defined by systematic studies of dose-response and time-response relationships. From such data the most sensitive, rapid, or persistent neuronal event can be identified.

Transmitter-dependent actions of drugs can be organized conveniently into *presynaptic* and *postsynaptic* categories. The presynaptic category includes all of the events in the perikaryon and nerve terminal that result in transmitter synthesis (including the acquisition of adequate substrates and cofactors), storage, release, re-uptake, and catabolism. Transmitter concentrations can be lowered by blockade of synthesis or storage or both. Otherwise, the amount released per impulse is relatively unalterable, but effects that follow release may be enhanced by inhibition of re-uptake or by blockade of catabolic enzymes. The transmitter that is released at a synapse can also exert actions upon the terminal from which it was released by interaction with receptors at these sites (termed *autoreceptors*). Activation of presynaptic autoreceptors can slow the rate of discharge of transmitter and thereby provide a feedback mechanism that controls the concentration of transmitter in the synaptic cleft (*see* Carlsson, 1975; Chapters 4 and 8).

The postsynaptic category includes all of the events that follow release of the transmitter in the vicinity of the postsynaptic receptor—in particular, the molecular mechanisms by which occupation of the receptor by the transmitter produces changes in the properties of the membrane of the postsynaptic cell (shifts in membrane potential) as well as more enduring biochemical actions (changes in intracellular cyclic nucleotides, protein kinase activity, and related substrate proteins). Direct postsynaptic effects of drugs generally require relatively high affinity for the receptors or resistance to metabolic degradation. Each of these presynaptic or postsynaptic actions is potentially highly specific and can be envisioned as being restricted to a single, chemically defined subset of CNS cells.

CENTRAL NEUROTRANSMITTERS

In examining the effects of drugs on the CNS with reference to the neurotransmitters for specific circuits, attention should be devoted to the general organizational principles of neurons. The view that synapses represent drug-modifiable control points within neuronal networks thus requires the explicit delineation of the sites at which given neurotransmitters may operate and the degree of specificity or generality by which such sites may be affected. One principle that underlies the following summaries of individual transmitter substances is the chemical-specificity hypothesis of Dale (1935), which holds that a given neuron releases the same transmitter substance at every one of its synaptic terminals. Although there have been indications that some neurons may contain more than one transmitter substance (Hokfelt *et al.,* 1978a), Dale's principle remains generally valid. This principle could also be taken to mean that a transmitter produces the same functional effect (hyperpolarization, depolarization) wherever it is released (functional specificity), but this latter corollary has *not* yet been established. Table 12-1 provides an overview of the pharmacological properties of those amino acid and monoamine transmitters that have been most fully studied in the CNS.

Amino Acids. The CNS contains uniquely high concentrations of certain amino acids, notably glutamate and gamma aminobutyrate (GABA); these amino acids are extremely potent in their ability to alter neuronal discharge. However, many physiologists were extremely reluctant to accept these simple substances as central neurotransmitters. This reluctance was based in part on conceptual problems of how to discriminate amino acids acting as transmitters from the same compounds as precursors for protein synthesis. The ubiquitous distribution of amino acids within the brain also posed problems in relating release to activity of a single neuronal circuit. Other important arguments against amino acids as transmitters

were that they produced prompt, powerful, and readily reversible but redundant effects on every neuron tested; the dicarboxylic amino acids produced excitation, and the monocarboxylic ω-amino acids (*e.g.,* GABA, glycine, β-alanine, taurine) produced qualitatively similar inhibitions (Kelly and Beart, 1975). This redundancy of effect was taken as further support of a nonspecific action on neuronal discharge, and this view was seemingly supported by the early observations that iontophoretic application of amino acids produced excitations or inhibitions that differed from those produced by activation of relevant synapses. Research was also hampered by the facts that selective antagonists of the amino acids were not available and there were no cytochemical methods that could visualize such junctions. In the last 15 years most of these conceptual arguments have proven to be unjustified and the evidence is quite strong that certain amino acids, especially GABA and glycine, are central transmitters.

GABA was identified as a unique chemical constituent of brain in 1950, but its potency as a CNS depressant was not immediately recognized. In the crustacean stretch receptor, GABA mimicked the actions of stimulation of the inhibitory nerve, and picrotoxin antagonized both the effects of applied GABA and stimulation of the inhibitory nerve. In the crusteacean, work by Kravitz and coworkers (1963) demonstrated that GABA was the only inhibitory amino acid found exclusively in the inhibitory nerve and that the inhibitory potency of extracts of this nerve were accounted for by their content of GABA. Release of GABA was then correlated with the frequency of nerve stimulation. Intracellular recordings from the muscle indicated that the inhibitory nerve and GABA produced identical increases of Cl^- conductance in the muscle. These observations thus fully satisfy the criteria for identification of a transmitter (*see* Otsuka, 1973).

These same physiological and pharmacological properties were later found to be useful models in tests of a role for GABA in the CNS. Evidence strongly supports the idea that GABA mediates the inhibitory actions of local interneurons in the brain regions rostral to the spinal cord, and that GABA may also mediate presynaptic inhibition within the spinal cord (*see* Otsuka, 1973; Ryall, 1975). Presumptive GABA-ergic inhibitory synapses have been demonstrated most clearly between cerebellar Purkinje neurons and their targets in Deiter's nucleus; between small interneurons and the major output cells of cerebellar cortex, olfactory bulb, cuneate nucleus, hippocampus, and the lateral septal nucleus; and between the vestibular nucleus and the trochlear motoneurons. GABA may also mediate the effects of inhibitory neurons within the cerebral cortex (*see* Kelly and Beart, 1975). The existence of a GABA-ergic pathway from caudate nucleus to substantia nigra is supported by neurochemical and cytochemical evidence (Kelly and Beart, 1975). Presumptive GABA-ergic neurons and nerve terminals have been localized with immunocytochemical methods that visualize glutamic acid decarboxylase (Ribak *et al.*, 1978). The reaction catalyzed by this pyridoxal phosphate–requiring enzyme provides the major source of GABA. The most useful drugs for confirmation of GABA-ergic mediation have been *bicuculline* (Curtis *et al.*, 1971) and *picrotoxin* (Obata *et al.*, 1970); however, many convulsants whose actions were previously unexplained (including penicillin and pentylenetetrazol) may also act as selective antagonists of GABA (MacDonald and Barker, 1978). Useful therapeutic effects have not yet been obtained by the use of agents that mimic GABA (such as muscimol), that inhibit the active re-uptake of the transmitter (2,4-diaminobutyrate, nipecotic acid, and guvacine; *see* Johnston, 1978), or that alter the rate of synthesis or degradation of GABA (such as aminooxyacetic acid; *see* Iversen, 1978). Picrotoxin and bicuculline appear to antagonize the actions of GABA; however, while bicuculline is able to compete with GABA for putative receptor binding sites, picrotoxin cannot (Iversen, 1978). The benzodiazepines may either simulate or antagonize the actions of GABA on the CNS.

Glycine was not found to be a particularly potent agent when its inhibitory effects were first evaluated by the iontophoretic technic in spinal cord. However, Werman and associates (1968) have assembled neurochemical and electrophysiological evidence that strongly supports a role for glycine as the inhibitory transmitter between spinal interneurons and motoneurons.

Glycine is the most abundant amino acid with inhibitory activity found in the ventral-quadrant gray matter of the spinal cord, and concentrations of glycine drop in proportion to the degeneration of ventral-quadrant interneurons following transient ischemia of the cord. Glycine has also been localized to spinal interneurons by electron-microscopic autoradiography. It is concentrated in nerve terminals that can be discriminated from those that accumulate GABA (Iversen, 1978). The hyperpolarization of motoneurons produced by iontophoretic application of glycine is relatively transient but approaches the equilibrium potential for the indirectly activated inhibitory postsynaptic potential; however, tests with GABA also indicate similar electrophysiological effects and a similar increase in Cl⁻ conductance. The major evidence that favors glycine as the mediator of intraspinal postsynaptic inhibition is the selective antagonism of its effects by strychnine. Strychnine does not usually antagonize responses to GABA (*see* Ryall, 1975), but it is able to inhibit the hyperpolarizing responses to β-alanine, another naturally occurring amino acid (Nicoll, 1978). Glycine also appears to be the most likely transmitter for inhibitory interneurons in the reticular formation but not in the cuneate nucleus. Except for experiments with strychnine, there has been little pharmacological manipulation of neurons that release glycine. Aspects of the synthesis or degradation of glycine that are unique to the CNS are not appreciated.

Glutamate and *aspartate* are found in very high concentrations in brain, and both of these amino acids have extremely powerful excitatory effects on neurons in virtually every region of the CNS. However, the widespread distribution of these two dicarboxylic acids in the CNS and their roles in intermediary metabolism have tended to obscure the action that they might have as transmitters.

While a strong circumstantial case can be built for glutamate as the transmitter at the neuromuscular junction of insect muscle (Usherwood and Machili, 1968), efforts to support either glutamate or aspartate as excitatory transmitters in the mammalian CNS have been hampered by the unavailability of a convincingly selective receptor antagonist. Evidence for selective, high-affinity re-uptake systems for glutamate and aspartate favors a transmitter role, as does the correlation of the concentrations of glutamate and aspartate with microdissections of brain regions following selective lesions (Nadler *et al.*, 1978). Glutamic acid diethylester (GDEE) may selectively suppress effects of glutamate on thalamic neurons without suppressing responses to either ACh or aspartate (McLennan, 1975). However, pathways sensitive to blockade with GDEE have not been found. At present, the best that can be said for the possible transmitter roles of glutamate and aspartate in the CNS is the absence of data that disqualify them (McLennan, 1975). Glutamate and a rigid analog, kainic acid, have been employed as neurotoxins to produce lesions in neuronal cell bodies while selectively sparing axons in the vicinity (Coyle *et al.*, 1977); these effects may depend upon the existence of postsynaptic receptors for glutamate, but all neurons are not equally susceptible to the toxic action.

Acetylcholine. After it was established that ACh is the transmitter at neuromuscular and parasympathetic neuroeffector junctions, as well as at the major synapse of autonomic ganglia (*see* Chapter 4), the amine began to receive considerable attention as a potential central neurotransmitter. Based on the finding of an irregular distribution within the regions of the CNS and the observation that peripheral cholinergic drugs could produce marked behavioral effects after central administration, many were willing to consider that ACh might be "the" central neurotransmitter. In the late 1950s Eccles and colleagues demonstrated the recurrent excitation of spinal Renshaw neurons to be sensitive to nicotinic cholinergic antagonists; these cells were also found to be cholinoceptive. Such observations were consistent with the chemical and functional specificity of Dale's hypothesis that all branches of a neuron released the same transmitter substance and, in this case, produced similar

Table 12-1. OVERVIEW OF THE PHARMACOLOGY OF AMINO ACID AND MONOAMINE TRANSMITTERS IN THE CENTRAL NERVOUS SYSTEM

TRANSMITTER	ANATOMY-CYTOLOGY	PRESYNAPTIC PHARMACOLOGY			POSTSYNAPTIC PHARMACOLOGY			
		Synthesis	Storage	Re-uptake	Agonists	Antagonists	Receptor Mechanisms	Catabolism
GABA	Supraspinal interneurons	—	—	2-Hydroxy-GABA, guvacine, and nipecotic acid inhibit	Muscimol, β-alanine, taurine	Bicuculline, picrotoxin	Increases Cl⁻ conductance; hyperpolarizes	Blocked with aminooxyacetic acid
Glycine	Spinal interneurons	—	—	—	Taurine (?), β-alanine (?)	Strychnine	Increases Cl⁻ conductance; hyperpolarizes	—
Glutamate; aspartate	Interneurons at all levels	—	—	—	Homocysteic acid, kainic acid	Glutamate diethylester (?)	Increases Na⁺ and cation conductances; depolarizes	—
Acetylcholine	All levels; probable long and short connections	Hemicholinium blocks	—	Choline uptake can be enhanced with loading	Muscarine	Quinuclidinyl benzoate, atropine, scopolamine	Excitatory	Cholinesterase inhibitors block
	Motoneuron–Renshaw cell				Nicotine	Dihydro-β-erythroidine	Excitatory	
Dopamine	All levels; short, medium, and long connections	α-Methyltyrosine inhibits; levodopa enhances	Tetrabenazine, reserpine, α-methyl-m-tyrosine inhibit; amphetamine releases; γ-hydroxybutyrate inhibits release	Benztropine, amitriptyline inhibit; 6-hydroxydopamine accumulates and is toxic	Apomorphine, bromocryptine	Haloperidol, phenothiazines	Associated with cyclic AMP at certain sites; probably inhibitory	Monoamine oxidase inhibitors block

					Agonists	Antagonists		
Norepinephrine	All levels; long axons from pons and brain stem	Same as for dopamine; FLA-63 * and diethyldithiocarbamate inhibit dopamine β-hydroxylase	Reserpine, tetrabenazine, α-methyl-m-tyrosine inhibit; amphetamine releases	Desipramine inhibits; 6-hydroxydopamine accumulates and is toxic	α:Clonidine	Phenoxybenzamine, phentolamine, piperoxan	—	Same as for dopamine
					β:Isoproterenol	Propranolol, others	Associated with cyclic AMP; generally inhibitory	
Epinephrine	Midbrain and brain stem to diencephalon	Same as for norepinephrine	Probably same as for norepinephrine	—	Probably same as for norepinephrine	Probably same as for norepinephrine	—	Probably same as for dopamine
5-Hydroxytryptamine	Midbrain and pons to all levels	p-Chlorophenylalanine blocks; tryptophan may increase	Reserpine, tetrabenazine inhibit	Clomipramine and fluoxetine inhibit; 5,7-dihydroxytryptamine accumulates and is toxic	LSD	—	—	Same as for dopamine

* FLA-63 is bis-(1-methyl-4-homopiperazinyl-thiocarbonyl) disulfide.

types of postsynaptic action (*see* Eccles, 1964). Although the ability of ACh to elicit neuronal discharge has subsequently been replicated on scores of CNS cells (*see* review by Krnjević, 1974), the spinal Renshaw cell remains the best if not the sole example of a central cholinergic nicotinic junction.

In most regions of the CNS, the effects of ACh, assessed either by iontophoresis (Krnjević, 1974) or by radioligand receptor-displacement assays (Kuhar, 1978), would appear to be generated by interaction with a mixture of nicotinic and muscarinic receptors. The precise cytological distribution of these receptors within any target region remains unclear. Several sets of presumptive cholinergic pathways have been proposed in addition to that of the motoneuron-Renshaw cell. These include the following: medial septal nucleus to dentate gyrus and subiculum of hippocampus habenula to interpeduncular nucleus; cortical interneurons to cortical pyramidal neurons; and thalamus, putamen, and caudate to neurons in the caudate. The thalamic-striatal circuit may be partially antagonized by iontophoretic administration of atropine, and many of the iontophoretic actions of ACh on a host of identified test cells are also reversed by muscarinic antagonists, including those on the cerebrocortical and the hippocampal pyramidal neurons (Stone, 1972). However, the major support for the cholinergic nature of these proposed pathways is the loss of ACh and the enzyme responsible for its synthesis (choline acetyltransferase) that follows lesions of the presumed cells of origin. Furthermore, maps may be constructed of neurons and fibers that stain cytochemically for specific acetylcholinesterase activity (Lewis and Shute, 1978).

Thus, while ACh has long been the subject of intense investigation as a CNS transmitter, compelling evidence has been accumulated for only a few sites. A major impediment has been the lack of an adequate anatomical method for mapping cholinergic tracts; this would facilitate the challenge of target neurons with cholinergic agonists, and with cholinergic antagonists during experimental activation of such pathways. However, the present data are fully in keeping with the possibility that both interregional and intraregional circuits may have ACh as their transmitter. When administered to man and animals, both cholinergic and anticholinergic drugs cause marked behavioral effects (*see* Chapters 6 and 7; Iversen and Iversen, 1975).

Catecholamines. The brain contains separate neuronal systems that utilize three different catecholamines—*dopamine, norepinephrine,* and *epinephrine.* Each system is anatomically distinct and presumably serves separate functional roles. There has been extensive investigation of these systems with a variety of technics, and a wealth of descriptive details is thus available for each (*see*

Moore and Bloom, 1978, 1979; Symposium, 1979a).

Dopamine. Although originally regarded only as a precursor of norepinephrine, assays of distinct regions of the CNS eventually revealed that the distributions of dopamine and norepinephrine are markedly different. In fact, more than half of the CNS content of catecholamine is dopamine, and extremely high amounts are found in the basal ganglia (especially the caudate nucleus), the nucleus accumbens, the olfactory tubercle, the central nucleus of the amygdala, the median eminence, and restricted fields of the frontal cortex. Due to the availability of histochemical methods that can reveal all the catecholamines (formaldehyde- or glyoxylic acid–induced fluorescence; Dahlstrom and Fuxe, 1964) or immunohistochemical methods for enzymes that synthesize individual catecholamines (Hokfelt *et al.,* 1978b), the anatomical connections of the dopamine-containing neurons are known with some precision, at least for the rodent brain. These studies indicate that there are three major morphological classes of dopaminergic neurons: (1) ultrashort neurons within the amacrine cells of the retina and periglomerular cells of the olfactory bulb; (2) intermediate-length neurons within the tuberobasal ventral hypothalamus that innervate the median eminence and intermediate lobe of the pituitary, incertohypothalamic neurons that connect the dorsal and posterior hypothalamus with the lateral septal nuclei, and small series of neurons within the perimeter of the dorsal motor nucleus of the vagus, the nucleus of the solitary tract, and the periaqueductal gray matter; and (3) long projections between the major dopamine-containing nuclei in the substantia nigra and ventral tegmentum and their targets in the striatum, in the limbic zones of the cerebral cortex, and in other major regions of the limbic system except the hippocampus (*see* Moore and Bloom, 1978). At the cellular level, the nature of the actions of dopamine remains somewhat controversial. While most iontophoretic studies indicate that inhibition is the predominant action, studies of the effects of electrical stimulation on transmembrane properties of the target neurons in the striatum suggest that there are depolarizing effects; however, these latter observations are open to substantial criticism (Siggins, 1978). Responses of striatal neurons to iontophoretic tests are compatible with the view that a dopamine-sensitive adenylate cyclase in the striatum may be related to synaptic function. Many, but not all, classes of antipsychotic drugs have been shown to antagonize the ability of dopamine to activate this adenylate cyclase (*see* Chapter 19). In other tests these antipsychotic drugs may also affect the electrically stimulated release of dopamine from brain slices, increase rates of synthesis of dopamine, and produce effects related to other neurotransmitters. Although acute treatment of experimental animals with antipsychotic agents can inhibit the effect of dopamine on its target neurons and effect an acute secondary increase in the synthesis of dopamine, chronic treatment results either in loss of this antagonism or in greatly diminished rates of metabolism of dopamine. The molecular mechanism responsible for the therapeutic effect is therefore not known (Symposium, 1977). Moreover, recent work suggests that CNS receptors for dopamine may be subclassified into those that affect adenylate cyclase and those that do not (Kebabian, 1978).

Norepinephrine. Relatively large amounts of norepinephrine occur within the hypothalamus and in certain zones of the limbic system, such as the central nucleus of the amygdala and the dentate gyrus of the hippocampus, but this catecholamine is also present in significant but lower amounts in most brain regions. Detailed mapping studies indicate that most noradrenergic neurons arise either in the locus ceruleus of the pons or in neurons of the lateral tegmental portion of the reticular formation. From these neurons, multiple branched axons innervate specific target cells in a large number of cortical, subcortical, and spinomedullary fields.

Examination of the effects of iontophoretic application of norepinephrine and of stimulation of the locus ceruleus indicates that the predominant acute effect of norepinephrine is inhibitory. This is mediated by β-adrenergic receptors and results in hyperpolarization of the postsynaptic membrane, accompanied by an increase in the passive resistance of the membrane. These actions are relatively slower in onset and longer in duration than are effects of inhibitory amino acids (Siggins *et al.*, 1971a, 1971b), and they can be simulated by iontophoretic application of cyclic AMP on cerebellar Purkinje cells, hippocampal pyramidal cells, and cerebrocortical pyramidal cells (*see* Bloom, 1975). These results support those of Rall and coworkers that demonstrate a β-adrenergic-sensitive adenylate cyclase system in cerebellar slices (*see* Rall, 1972). In some brain regions the effects of norepinephrine on adenylate cyclase may involve both α- and β-adrenergic receptors (*see* Bloom, 1975).

Depending on the species and brain region examined, *adenosine* can markedly potentiate the effects of norepinephrine and other biogenic amines on the synthesis of cyclic AMP. While the methylxanthines potentiate the effects of norepinephrine, cyclic AMP, and stimulation of the locus ceruleus on cerebellar Purkinje cells, they *antagonize* the ability of adenosine to activate adenylate cyclase or to inhibit the discharge of cells that are targets for norepinephrine (*see* Chapter 25; Sattin and Rall, 1970; Bloom, 1975; Stone and Taylor, 1977). Antipsychotic drugs, especially phenothiazines, also have effects upon the norepinephrine-activated adenylate cyclase in certain cortical areas (Sulser *et al.*, 1978). Tricyclic antidepressants influence binding of α-receptor ligands (U'Prichard *et al.*, 1978) as well as their better-known ability to inhibit the re-uptake of norepinephrine. Although the latter action potentiates the effects of norepinephrine acutely, chronic treatment with these drugs can result in desensitization of noradrenergic receptors (Sulser *et al.*, 1978; Wolfe *et al.*, 1978).

Examination of the effects of lesions of noradrenergic pathways and of parenterally injected drugs has suggested a long list of physiological events that are regulated by norepinephrine. These include feeding, sleeping, memory, learning, and attention. Because the neurophysiological bases of these functions are not well understood, details of the involvement of norepinephrine in the multiple circuits that underlie such behaviors remain to be elucidated.

Epinephrine. Neurons in the CNS that contain epinephrine were recognized only recently following the development of sensitive enzymatic assays for phenylethanolamine-N-methyltransferase (*see* Chapter 4) and immunocytochemical staining technics for the enzyme (Hokfelt *et al.*, 1974). Epinephrine-containing neurons are found in the medullary reticular formation and make relatively restricted connections to a few pontine and diencephalic nuclei, eventually coursing as far rostrally as the paraventricular nucleus of the dorsal midline thalamus (Hokfelt *et al.*, 1974). The physiological properties of these connections have not been studied as yet, but in locus ceruleus, which receives such adrenergic innervation, the effects are inhibitory (Cedarbaum and Aghajanian, 1976).

5-Hydroxytryptamine. Following the chemical determination that a biogenic substance found both in serum ("serotonin") and in gut ("enteramine") was 5-HT, assays for this substance revealed its presence in brain (Brodie and Shore, 1957). Since that time, studies of 5-HT have had a pivotal role in the neuropharmacology of the CNS. Fluorescence and other cytochemical methods have been used to trace the central anatomy of 5-HT-containing neurons in several species (*see* Azmitia, 1978). Tryptaminergic neurons are localized to some nine nuclei lying in or adjacent to the midline (raphe) regions of the pons and upper brain stem, corresponding to well-defined nuclear ensembles (Dahlstrom and Fuxe, 1964).

More precise localization is made by study of losses of 5-HT in selected regions of brain after individual raphe-nuclei lesions are produced electrolytically or chemically (with the indolamine-specific neurotoxins 5,6- or 5,7-dihydroxytryptamine; Baumgarten *et al.*, 1976) and through the use of orthograde and retrograde tracing technics (Azmitia, 1978). The more rostral raphe nuclei appear to innervate forebrain regions, while the more caudal raphe nuclei project within the brain stem and spinal cord. The median raphe nucleus contributes a major portion of the tryptaminergic innervation of the limbic system, and the dorsal raphe nucleus contributes a major portion of similar innervation of cortical regions and the neostriatum.

In the mammalian CNS, cells receiving cytochemically demonstrable tryptaminergic input, such as the suprachiasmatic nucleus, ventrolateral geniculate body, and amygdala, exhibit a uniform and dense investment of reactive terminals. Recordings obtained from such neurons show uniform inhibition after stimulation of the raphe neurons, and this effect is mimicked by iontophoretic application of 5-HT (Aghajanian and Wang, 1978).

Of the many different drugs that are antagonists of 5-HT in various peripheral structures, such as autonomic ganglia or smooth muscle (*see* Chapter 26), none seems to act as an antagonist of 5-HT at any proven tryptaminergic synapse within the CNS (Aghajanian and Wang, 1978). This result is remarkable since much speculation on the function of 5-HT in the CNS was predicted on knowledge of the hallucinogenic properties of lysergic acid diethylamide (LSD) and its ability to antagonize the actions of 5-HT on smooth muscle. Although LSD, in high concentration, does block the action of 5-HT at peripheral tryptaminergic receptors, it mimics 5-HT in the CNS, especially on 5-HT-containing neurons (Aghajanian and Wang, 1978). LSD and some of the other peripheral antagonists of 5-HT can inhibit responses to 5-HT applied by microiontophoresis to randomly encountered cells in various regions of the CNS. However, none of these cells has been proven to be a physiological target for a tryptaminergic neuron. It has been hypothesized that altered function of tryptaminergic pathways is a factor in various mental illnesses and CNS dysfunctions, including schizophrenia, the affective disorders, infantile autism, and minimal brain dysfunction, as well as the mental defects accompanying phenylketonuria and Down's syndrome (*see* Symposium, 1974). Drug treatments of animals and correlations of 5-HT metabolism with experimental manipulations have provided some indications that 5-HT-containing neurons may also be involved in other, simpler functions, such as regulation of temperature, neuroendocrine control (regulation of release of hypophysiotropic hormones), and activity of the extrapyramidal system (*see* Symposium, 1974). These proposals of behavioral functions of such highly divergent and overlapping long-axon systems are subject to the limitations mentioned above for the catecholamines. Many different classes of centrally active drugs can affect physiological or biochemical parameters of various tryptaminergic neuronal systems by influencing direct responses to 5-HT or its uptake, synthesis, storage, release, or catabolism. The list includes hallucinogens such as LSD, N,N-dimethyltryptamine (DMT), and other congeners of the biogenic amine, mescaline, reserpine, chlorpromazine, tricyclic antidepressants, monoamine oxidase inhibitors, amphetamines (particularly the chloroamphetamines), lithium, morphine, methylxanthines, and ethyl alcohol. Since almost all of these drugs have been demonstrated to have effects on catecholamine-containing and other chemically defined neurons, the functional importance of the effects on mechanisms that involve 5-HT is difficult to interpret.

LSD is among the most interesting of the compounds that interact with 5-HT. It reduces turnover of 5-HT in the brain, and it inhibits the firing of raphe neurons (*see* Aghajanian, 1972; Freedman and Halaris, 1978). In iontophoretic tests, LSD and 5-HT are both potent inhibitors of the firing of raphe (5-HT) neurons, but LSD and other hallucinogens are far less potent depressants than is 5-HT on neurons that receive innervation from the raphe. The inhibitory effect of LSD on raphe neurons offers a plausible explanation of the drug's hallucinogenic effects, namely, that they result from depression of activity in a system that tonically inhibits visual and other sensory inputs. However, typical LSD-induced behavior is still seen in animals with raphe nuclei destroyed or after blockade of the synthesis of 5-HT by *p*-chlorophenylalanine. Other evidence against this explanation of LSD-induced hallucinations is the potentiation of LSD by administration of the precursor of 5-HT, 5-hydroxytryptophan. In addition, one LSD-like behavioral response in rats (poor habituation to sensory stimulation) is replicated by electrical stimulation of raphe nuclei (*see* Freedman and Halaris, 1978).

Histamine. For many years, histamine and antihistamines that are active in the periphery have been known to produce significant effects on animal behavior. Only relatively recently, however, has evidence accumulated to suggest that histamine might be a central neurotransmitter.

Efforts to document the presence of histamine within neurons are hampered by lack of an effective cytochemical method and by the presence of mast cells, which have rich stores of histamine, in the CNS. However, only about half of the brain content of histamine can be released by drugs such as compound 48/80 or polymyxin B, which are effective in liberating the amine from mast-cell granules; the histamine that remains can be localized by subcellular fractionation technics to fractions of brain homogenates rich in nerve terminals. The histamine content has been shown to vary irregularly from one hypothalamic nucleus to another, which is suggestive of a neuron-specific distribution. Furthermore, lesions of the lateral hypothalamus result in a depletion of histidine decarboxylase activity on the side of the lesion. The time course of disappearance parallels that expected for postlesion nerve-fiber degeneration (Schwartz, 1975). Unlike the monoamines and amino acid transmitters, there does not appear to be an active re-uptake process for histamine to conserve transmitter after its release. In fact, no direct evidence has been obtained for histamine release *in vivo* or *in vitro* associated with neuronal activity.

Histamine can activate adenylate cyclase in some brain regions of some species (*see* Rall, 1972; Greengard, 1978), and this action can also be potentiated by adenosine. In brain regions with high contents of histamine, such as hypothalamus and reticular formation, the effects of iontophoretically applied histamine are inhibitory; in some cases, these effects can be simulated by application of cyclic AMP and potentiated by inhibitors of cyclic nucleotide phosphodiesterase (*see* Bloom, 1975). Cyclic AMP may serve as a second messenger to mediate the actions of histamine in the CNS. The functions of presumptive histaminergic neural systems remain uncertain.

Peptides. The discovery of several endogenous peptides in brain that elicit striking effects on the activity of neural systems has produced considerable excitement among those who are interested in the functions of the CNS (*see* Guillemin, 1978; Iversen *et al.*, 1978). Technics for rapid determination of the amino acid sequences of such peptides and for their synthesis in large quantities have greatly facilitated progress. The peptide's physiological effects can then be studied, and its localization can be probed by radioimmunoassay and by immunocytochemical procedures.

An imposing catalog of previously unknown neuropeptides has accumulated. In addition, certain peptides previously thought to be restricted to the gut or to endocrine glands have also been found in the CNS. Study of the effects of these peptides in brain may provide answers to the larger question of the relationship between multiple roles for a given substance in widely different locations. Relatively detailed maps are now available for neurons that show immunoreactivity to antisera prepared against *luteinizing hormone–releasing hormone* (LHRH) (Hoffman *et al.*, 1978), *somatostatin* (Hokfelt *et al.*, 1976, 1978b), *substance P* (Cuello and Kanazawa, 1978), *enkephalin* (Sar *et al.*, 1978), *endorphins* (Bloom *et al.*, 1978), and *oxytocin* and *vasopressin* (Swanson, 1977; Defendini and Zimmerman, 1978). Less detailed maps and assay data indicate that peptides such as *vasoactive intestinal polypeptide* (Hokfelt *et al.*, 1978b), *gastrin* and *cholecystokinin* (Hokfelt *et al.*, 1978b), *thyrotropin-releasing hormone* (TRH) (Hokfelt *et al.*, 1974), and angiotensin (Chapter 27) may also be found in various neurons.

Although each peptide is obviously unique, the current research effort is epitomized by the numerous experiments on the *endorphins* and *enkephalins*. This family of previously unrecognized neuropeptides was detected, isolated, and eventually identified on the basis of their ability to react with receptors that mediate responses to morphine and other opioids. Following the demonstration of a high-affinity binding site in synaptic membranes with selectivity for opioids (*see* Kosterlitz *et al.*, 1977), Hughes, Kosterlitz and their colleagues in Aberdeen demonstrated that brain extracts contained two substances that competed with radiolabeled opioids for such sites. These materials, which also showed opioid-like activity *in vitro*, were both identified as pentapeptides; they share a common N-terminal tetrapeptide sequence (Tyr-Gly-Gly-Phe-X) and differ only in the C-terminal position, which is either methionine or leucine. The peptides were named *enkephalins* and are referred to as met^5-enkephalin

and leu^5-enkephalin (Hughes *et al.*, 1975). Of great interest, the entire structure of met^5-enkephalin is contained within the 91–amino acid sequence of the pituitary hormone β-lipotropin (β-LPH), which was isolated and sequenced by Li and associates (1966). β-LPH shows no opioid activity *per se*.

Almost immediately after these studies, other groups reported isolation, purification, chemical structures, and synthesis of three additional endogenous peptides with opioid-like activity (*endorphins*): α-endorphin (β-LPH 61-76), γ-endorphin (β-LPH 61-77), and β-endorphin (β-LPH 61-91) (*see* Chapters 22 and 59).

By the use of immunocytochemical technics, the brain, pituitary, and gastrointestinal tract have each been found to contain enkephalin and β-endorphin, but a single cell does not contain both substances (Bloom *et al.*, 1978). Iontophoretic application of enkephalins and β-endorphin suggests that neurons throughout the CNS can be depressed by these peptides; such effects are qualitatively identical to those of opioid agonists and can be selectively antagonized with the opioid antagonist naloxone (Zieglgansberger *et al.*, 1978). Behavioral tests indicate that β-endorphin is a potent analgesic in animals and man. Analgesia induced by brain stimulation in man releases β-endorphin into the cerebrospinal fluid. Animals made dependent on morphine show cross-tolerance to the effects of endorphin (Tseng *et al.*, 1976). Although the role of these peptides in central and peripheral neural function is far from clear, their possible involvement in abnormal behavioral states seems likely.

PERSPECTIVES FOR FUTURE DEVELOPMENT

Concepts of the relationship between the actions of a drug and the functions of specific brain systems have progressed through three phases, particularly in the relatively brief history of psychopharmacology (Mandell, 1973). In the first phase, drug-induced changes in function were correlated directly with changes in the concentrations of neurotransmitters or their metabolites. An exemplary anomaly revealed at this stage was the relationship between the behavioral depression that follows administration of reserpine and the decreased storage of 5-HT (and also norepinephrine and dopamine) in the brain (Brodie and Shore, 1957). The time course of the change in behavior coincides initially with alterations in the content of biogenic amines; however, when the analysis is extended past the first 48 hours, it becomes clear that the concentrations of amines remain depressed while behavior returns toward normal.

A second phase of investigation began

with demonstrations that many drugs with potent behavioral actions (*e.g.*, LSD, amphetamine, tricyclic antidepressants, antipsychotics) produced relatively minor changes in the concentrations of transmitter. Attempts were thus made to relate the effects of drugs to alterations in the dynamics of neuronal metabolism, from which it was hoped that information about changes in neuronal activity could be inferred. For example, estimates have been made of the turnover rates of neurotransmitters (*see* Costa and Meek, 1974), and single-unit electrophysiological recordings have also been employed as indices of the effects of drugs on the functional activity of chemically characterized neuronal systems. This approach suffers from at least two problems that are also shared by experiments that rely on assessment of concentrations of transmitters. (1) Neurochemical experiments proceed on a time scale of minutes to hours, while neuronal events occur in milliseconds or seconds; changes that are measured may therefore be quite removed from those that occur at the primary site of action. (2) Neurotransmitters that have not yet been identified obviously cannot be measured. Because of these and other limitations, it is entirely possible for changes to occur after a drug treatment that are correctly correlated, perhaps even selectively, with aspects of the metabolism or action of one or more transmitter substances, and yet the two effects—that on function and that on specific neuronal systems—may not be causally related.

Current efforts in CNS pharmacology are also in a third phase that focuses on the adaptive changes imposed on the nervous system by chronic treatment with drugs. Thus, for example, the therapeutic effects of lithium or of tricyclic antidepressants require periods of treatment of 1 to 2 weeks before therapeutic results are evident (*see* Chapter 19; Bunney *et al.*, 1977). While the metabolic changes and functional effects that are observed during acute treatment were assumed to continue, it has become clear that they do not persist and are replaced by changes that may in fact be opposite to those seen acutely. For example, tricyclic antidepressants, when given acutely, potentiate the cellular and behavioral effects of norepinephrine by inhibition of its re-uptake. It has

been inferred that depression results from a deficiency of catecholamine and that tricyclic antidepressants are effective by increasing the amounts of catecholamine at the postsynaptic receptor. However, in animals treated chronically with desmethylimipramine, sensitivity of β-adrenergic receptors is decreased, even though presynaptic re-uptake of norepinephrine remains fully inhibited (Sulser *et al.*, 1978; Wolfe *et al.*, 1978). Bunney has proposed that the therapeutic effect of lithium in manic-depressive psychosis could be related to a general stabilization of such adaptive responses of receptors (Bunney *et al.*, 1977).

Future efforts to provide explanations for drug-induced neurological changes will undoubtedly continue to focus on synaptic transmitters and their mechanisms. As more transmitter substances are characterized and more synaptic circuits and mechanisms of transmission are defined, it may be useful to consider three general properties by which neuronal circuits can be described and to employ them in efforts to correlate the molecular actions of drugs with the neurological and behavioral effects that result. A *spatial domain* describes those areas of the brain or of peripheral receptive fields that feed signals to a given cell and those areas to which that cell sends its signals. A *temporal domain* describes the duration of the effects of a cell on its targets. A *functional domain* describes the molecular mechanisms by which the cell influences its targets. Within these three domains, neurons can be defined in terms of their transmitters, receptors, and functional location, as well as in the more classical categories of sensory, motor, or interneuronal. All of these properties must be borne in mind simultaneously in the attempt to develop comprehensive explanations of the acute and chronic effects of drugs.

Aghajanian, G. K. LSD and CNS transmission. *Annu. Rev. Pharmacol.*, **1972**, *12*, 157–168.

Barker, J. L.; Neale, J. H.; Smith, T. G.; and MacDonald, R. L. Opiate peptide modulation of amino acid responses suggests novel form of neuronal communication. *Science*, **1978**, *199*, 1451–1453.

Bloom, F.; Battenberg, E.; Rossier, J.; Ling, N.; and Guillemin, R. Neurons containing β-endorphin in rat brain exist separately from those containing enkephalin: immunocytochemical studies. *Proc. Natl. Acad. Sci. U.S.A.*, **1978**, *75*, 1591–1595.

Brodie, B. B., and Shore, P. A. A concept for a role of

serotonin and norepinephrine as chemical mediators in the brain. *Ann. N.Y. Acad. Sci.*, **1957**, *66*, 631–642.

Bunney, W. E., Jr.; Post, R. M.; Anderson, A. E.; and Kopanda, R. T. A neuronal receptor sensitivity mechanism in affective illness (a review of evidence). *Commun. Psychopharmacol.*, **1977**, *1*, 393–405.

Cedarbaum, J. M., and Aghajanian, G. K. Noradrenergic neurons of the locus coeruleus: inhibition by epinephrine and activation by the alpha antagonist piperoxan. *Brain Res.*, **1976**, *112*, 413–419.

Coyle, J. T.; Schwarcz, R.; Bennet, J. P.; and Campochiaro, P. Clinical, neuropathologic and pharmacologic aspects of Huntington's disease: correlates with a new animal model. *Prog. Neuro-psychopharmacol.*, **1977**, *1*, 13–30.

Cuello, A. C., and Kanazawa, I. The distribution of substance P immunoreactive fibers in the rat central nervous system. *J. Comp. Neurol.*, **1978**, *178*, 129–156.

Curtis, D. R.; Duggan, A. W.; Felix, D.; Johnston, G. A. R.; and McLennan, H. Antagonism between bicuculline and GABA in the cat brain. *Brain Res.*, **1971**, *33*, 57–73.

Dahlstrom, A., and Fuxe, K. Evidence for the existence of monoamine-containing neurons in the central nervous system. I. Demonstration of monoamines in the cell bodies of brain stem neurons. *Acta Physiol. Scand.,* **1964**, *232*, Suppl. 62, 1–55.

Hoffman, G. E.; Knigge, K. M.; Moynihan, J. A.; Melnyk, V.; and Arimura, A. Neuronal fields containing luteinizing hormone releasing hormone (LHRH) in mouse brain. *Neuroscience*, **1978**, *3*, 219–232.

Hokfelt, T.; Elde, R.; Johansson, O.; Luft, R.; Nilsson, G.; and Arimura, A. Immunohistochemical evidence for separate populations of somatostatin-containing and substance P–containing primary afferent neurons in the rat. *Neuroscience*, **1976**, *1*, 131–136.

Hokfelt, T.; Fuxe, K.; Goldstein, M.; and Johansson, O. Immunohistochemical evidence for the existence of adrenaline neurons in the rat brain. *Brain Res.,* **1974**, *66*, 235–251.

Hokfelt, T.; Ljungdahl, A.; Steinbusch, H.; Verhofstad, A.; Nilsson, G.; Pernow, B.; and Goldstein, M. Immunohistochemical evidence of substance P–like immunoreactivity in some 5-hydroxytryptamine-containing neurons in the central nervous system. *Neuroscience*, **1978a**, *3*, 517–538.

Hughes, J. W.; Smith, T.; Kosterlitz, H.; Fothergill, L.; Morgan, B.; and Morris, H. Identification of two related pentapeptides from the brain with potent opiate agonist activity. *Nature*, **1975**, *255*, 577–579.

Kebabian, J. W. Multiple classes of dopamine receptors in mammalian central nervous system: the involvement of dopamine-sensitive adenyl cyclase. *Life Sci.*, **1978**, *23*, 479–484.

Kravitz, E. A.; Kuffler, S. W.; and Potter, D. D. Gamma-aminobutyric acid and other blocking compounds in Crustacea. Their relative concentrations in separated motor and inhibitory axons. *J. Neurophysiol.*, **1963**, *26*, 739–751.

Li, C. H.; Barnafi, L.; Chretien, M.; and Chung, D. Isolation and amino-acid sequence of β-LPH from sheep pituitary glands. *Nature*, **1966**, *208*, 1093–1094.

MacDonald, R. L., and Barker, J. L. Specific antagonism of GABA-mediated postsynaptic inhibition in cultured mammalian spinal cord neurons: a common mode of convulsant action. *Neurology (Minneap.)*, **1978**, *28*, 325–330.

Mandell, A. J. Redundant macromolecular mechanisms in central synaptic regulation. In, *New Concepts in Neurotransmitter Regulation.* (Mandell, A. J., ed.) Plenum Press, New York, **1973**, pp. 259–277.

Nadler, J. V.; White, W. F.; Vaca, K. W.; Perry, B. W.; and Cotman, C. W. Biochemical correlates of transmission mediated by glutamate and aspartate. *J. Neurochem.,* **1978**, *31*, 147–155.

Nieoullon, A.; Cheramy, A.; and Glowinski, J. An adaptation of the push-pull cannula method to study the *in vivo* release of ^{3}H-dopamine synthesized from ^{3}H-tyrosine in the cat caudate nucleus: effects of various physical and pharmacological treatments. *J. Neurochem.,* **1977**, *28*, 819–828.

Obata, K.; Takeda, K.; and Shinozaki, H. Further study on pharmacological properties of the cerebellar inhibition of Deiters neurones. *Exp. Brain Res.,* **1970**, *11*, 327–342.

Otsuka, M. Gamma aminobutyric acid and some other transmitter candidates in the nervous system. In, *Pharmacology and the Future of Man: Proceedings of the Fifth International Congress on Pharmacology*, Vol. 4. (Acheson, G. H., and Bloom, F. E., eds.) S. Karger, Basel, **1973**, pp. 186–201.

Ribak, C. E.; Vaughan, J. E.; and Saito, K. Immunocytochemical localization of glutamic acid decarboxylase in neuronal somata following colchicine inhibition of axonal transport. *Brain Res.*, **1978**, *140*, 315–332.

Sar, M.; Stumpf, W. E.; Miller, R. J.; Chang, K. J.; and Cuatrecasas, P. Immunohistochemical localization of enkephalin in rat brain and spinal cord. *J. Comp. Neurol.,* **1978**, *182*, 17–38.

Sattin, A., and Rall, T. W. The effect of adenosine and adenine nucleotides on the adenosine 3′,5′-phosphate content of guinea pig cerebral cortex slices. *Mol. Pharmacol.*, **1970**, *6*, 13–23.

Siggins, G. R.; Hoffer, B. J.; Oliver, A. P.; and Bloom, F. E. Activation of a central noradrenergic projection to cerebellum. *Nature*, **1971a**, *233*, 481–483.

Siggins, G. R.; Oliver, A. P.; Hoffer, B. J.; and Bloom, F. E. Cyclic adenosine monophosphate and norepinephrine: effects on transmembrane properties of cerebellar Purkinje cells. *Science*, **1971b**, *171*, 192.

Stone, T. W. Cholinergic mechanisms in the rat somatosensory cerebral cortex. *J. Physiol. (Lond.)*, **1972**, *225*, 485–499.

Stone, T. W., and Taylor, D. A. An electrophysiological demonstration of a synergistic interaction between norepinephrine and adenosine in rat cerebral cortex. *J. Physiol. (Lond.)*, **1977**, *266*, 523–543.

Swanson, L. Immunohistochemical evidence for a neurophysin-containing autonomic pathway arising in the paraventricular nucleus of the hypothalamus. *Brain Res.,* **1977**, *128*, 346–351.

Tseng, L. F.; Loh, H. H.; and Li, C. H. Beta endorphin: cross tolerance to and cross physical dependence on morphine. *Proc. Natl. Acad. Sci. U.S.A.*, **1976**, *73*, 4187–4189.

Ungerstedt, U. Adipsia and aphagia after 6-hydroxydopamine induced degeneration of the nigro-striatal dopamine system. *Acta Physiol. Scand.*, **1971**, *367*, Suppl., 95–122.

U'Prichard, D. C.; Greenberg, D. A.; Sheehan, P. P.; and Snyder, S. H. Tricyclic antidepressants: therapeutic properties and affinity for alpha-noradrenergic receptor binding sites in the brain. *Science*, **1978**, *199*, 197–198.

Usherwood, P. N. R., and Machili, P. Pharmacological properties of excitatory neuromuscular synapses in the locust. *J. Exp. Biol.*, **1968**, *49*, 341–361.

Werman, R.; Davidoff, R. A.; and Aprison, M. H. Inhibitory action of glycine on spinal neurons in the cat. *J. Neurophysiol.*, **1968**, *31*, 81–95.

Wolfe, B. B.; Harden, T. K.; Sporn, J. R.; and Molinoff, P. B. Presynaptic modulation of beta adrenergic receptors in cerebral cortex after treatment with antidepressants. *J. Pharmacol. Exp. Ther.*, **1978**, *207*, 446–457.

Zieglgansberger, W., and Bayerl, H. The mechanism of inhibition of neuronal activity by opiates in the spinal cord of cat. *Brain Res.*, **1976**, *115*, 111–128.

Monographs and Reviews

Aghajanian, G. K., and Wang, R. Y. Physiology and pharmacology of central serotonergic neurons. In, *Psy-*

chopharmacology—A Generation of Progress. (Lipton, M. A.; DiMascio, A.; and Killam, K. F.; eds.) Raven Press, New York, **1978**, pp. 171–184.

Azmitia, E. C. The serotonin-producing neurons of the midbrain median and dorsal raphe nuclei. In, *Handbook of Psychopharmacology,* Sect. II, Vol. 9. (Iversen, L. L.; Iversen, S. D.; and Snyder, S. H.; eds.) Plenum Press, New York, **1978**, pp. 233–314.

Barker, J. L. Physiological roles of peptides in the nervous system. In, *Peptides in Neurobiology.* (Gainer, H., ed.) Plenum Press, New York, **1977**, pp. 295–344.

Baumgarten, H. G.; Bjorklund, A.; Lachenmayer, L.; and Nobin, A. Evaluation of the effects of 5,7-dihyroxytryptamine on serotonin and catecholamine neurons in the rat CNS. *Acta Physiol. Scand.,* **1976**, *391,* Suppl., 3–19.

Bloom, F. E. Localization of neurotransmitters by electron microscopy. *Res. Publ. Assoc. Res. Nerv. Ment. Dis.,* **1970**, *50,* 25–57.

———. The role of cyclic nucleotides in central synaptic function. *Rev. Physiol. Biochem. Pharmacol.,* **1975**, *74,* 1–103.

Bodian, D. Neuron junctions: a revolutionary decade. *Anat. Rec.,* **1972**, *174,* 73–82.

Burnstock, G. Purinergic transmission. In, *Handbook of Psychopharmacology,* Sect. I, Vol. 5. (Iversen, L. L.; Iversen, S. D.; and Snyder, S. H.; eds.) Plenum Press, New York, **1975**, pp. 131–194.

Carlsson, A. Autoreceptors. In, *Pre- and Postsynaptic Receptors.* (Usdin, E., and Bunney, W. E., Jr., eds.) Marcel Dekker, Inc., New York, **1975**, pp. 49–65.

Cooper, J. R.; Bloom, F. E.; and Roth, R. H. *The Biochemical Basis of Neuropharmacology,* 3rd ed. Oxford University Press, New York, **1978**.

Costa, E., and Meek, J. L. Regulation of biosynthesis of catecholamines and serotonin in the CNS. *Annu. Rev. Pharmacol.,* **1974**, *14,* 491–512.

Dale, H. H. Pharmacology and nerve endings. *Proc. R. Soc. Med.,* **1935**, *28,* 319–332.

Defendini, R., and Zimmerman, E. A. The magnocellular neurosecretory system of the mammalian hypothalamus. In, *The Hypothalamus.* (Reichlin, S.; Baldessarini, R. J.; and Martin, J. B.; eds.) Raven Press, New York, **1978**, pp. 137–152.

Eccles, J. C. *The Physiology of Synapses.* Academic Press, Inc., New York, **1964**.

Florey, E. Neurotransmitters and modulators in the animal kingdom. *Fed. Proc.,* **1967**, *26,* 1164–1176.

Freedman, D. X., and Halaris, A. Monoamines and the biochemical mode of action of LSD at synapses. In, *Psychopharmacology—A Generation of Progress.* (Lipton, M. A.; DiMascio, A.; and Killam, K. F.; eds.) Raven Press, New York, **1978**, pp. 347–360.

Greengard, P. *Cyclic Nucleotides, Phosphorylated Proteins, and Neuronal Function: Distinguished Lecture Series of the Society of General Physiologists,* Vol. 1. Raven Press, New York, **1978**.

Guillemin, R. Peptides in the brain: the new endocrinology of the neuron. *Science,* **1978**, *202,* 390–402.

Hokfelt, T., and others. Aminergic and peptidergic pathways in the nervous system with special reference to the hypothalamus. In, *The Hypothalamus.* (Reichlin, S.; Baldessarini, R. J.; and Martin, J. B.; eds.) Raven Press, New York, **1978b**, pp. 69–136.

Horrobin, D. F. *Prostaglandins: Physiology, Pharmacology and Clinical Significance.* Eden Press, Montreal, **1978**.

Iversen, L. L. Biochemical psychopharmacology of GABA. In, *Psychopharmacology—A Generation of Progress.* (Lipton, M. A.; DiMascio, A.; and Killam, K. F.; eds.) Raven Press, New York, **1978**, pp. 25–38.

Iversen, L. L.; Nicoll, R. A.; and Vale, W. W. Neurobiology of peptides. *Neurosci. Res. Program Bull.,* **1978**, *16,* 214–370.

Iversen, S. D., and Iversen, L. L. *Behavioral Pharmacology.* Oxford University Press, New York, **1975**.

Johnston, G. A. R. Neuropharmacology of amino acid inhibitory transmitters. *Annu. Rev. Pharmacol. Toxicol.,* **1978**, *18,* 269–289.

Jones, E. G., and Hartman, B. K. Recent advances in neuroanatomical methodology. *Annu. Rev. Neurosci.,* **1978**, *1,* 215–298.

Kahn, C. R. Membrane receptors for hormones and neurotransmitters. *J. Cell Biol.,* **1976**, *60,* 261–286.

Kelly, J. S., and Beart, P. M. Amino acid receptors in CNS. II. GABA in supraspinal regions. In, *Handbook of Psychopharmacology,* Sect. I, Vol. 4. (Iversen, L. L.; Iversen, S. D.; and Snyder, S. H.; eds.) Plenum Press, New York, **1975**, pp. 129–209.

Kosterlitz, H. W.; Hughes, J.; Lord, J. A. H.; and Waterfield, A. A. *Enkephalins, Endorphins, and Opiate Receptors,* Vol. 2. Society for Neuroscience, Bethesda, **1977**, pp. 291–307.

Krnjević, K. Chemical nature of synaptic transmission in vertebrates. *Physiol. Rev.,* **1974**, *54,* 419–540.

Kuhar, M. J. Central cholinergic pathways: physiologic and pharmacologic aspects. In, *Psychopharmacology—A Generation of Progress.* (Lipton, M. A.; DiMascio, A.; and Killam, K. F.; eds.) Raven Press, New York, **1978**, pp. 199–204.

Lewis, P. R., and Shute, C. C. D. Cholinergic pathways in CNS. In, *Handbook of Psychopharmacology,* Sect. I, Vol. 9. (Iversen, L. L.; Iversen, S. D.; and Snyder, S. H.; eds.) Plenum Press, New York, **1978**, pp. 315–356.

Maguire, M. E.; Ross, E. M.; and Gilman, A. G. Beta adrenergic receptor: ligand binding properties and the interaction with adenylyl cyclase. *Adv. Cyclic Nucleotide Res.,* **1977**, *8,* 1–83.

McIlwain, H. Extended roles in the brain for second-messenger systems. *Neuroscience,* **1977**, *2,* 357–372.

McLennan, H. Excitatory amino acid receptors in the central nervous system. In, *Handbook of Psychopharmacology,* Sect. I, Vol. 4. (Iversen, L. L.; Iversen, S. D.; and Snyder, S. H.; eds.) Plenum Press, New York, **1975**, pp. 211–228.

Miller, N. E. Biofeedback and visceral learning. *Annu. Rev. Psychol.,* **1978**, *29,* 237–250.

Moore, R. Y., and Bloom, F. E. Central catecholamine neuron systems: anatomy and physiology of the dopamine systems. *Annu. Rev. Neurosci.,* **1978**, *1,* 129–169.

———. Central catecholamine neuron systems: anatomy and physiology. *Ibid.,* **1979**, *2,* 113–168.

Mountcastle, V. B., and Edelman, G. M. An organizing principle for cerebral function: the unit module and the distributed system. In, *The Mindful Brain.* (Edelman, G. M., and Mountcastle, V. B., eds.) The MIT Press, Cambridge, Mass., **1978**, pp. 7–50.

Nicoll, R. A. Physiological studies on amino acids and peptides as prospective transmitters in the CNS. In, *Psychopharmacology—A Generation of Progress.* (Lipton, M. A.; DiMascio, A.; Killam, K. F.; eds.) Raven Press, New York, **1978**, pp. 103–118.

Rakic, P. Local circuit neurons. *Neurosci. Res. Program Bull.,* **1975**, *13,* 293–446.

Rall, T. W. Role of adenosine 3′-5′-monophosphate (cyclic AMP) in actions of catecholamines. *Pharmacol. Rev.,* **1972**, *24,* 399–409.

Rothlin, E., and Berde, B. The structural and functional principles of the autonomic nervous system. *Aerztl. Monatsschr.,* **1953**, *5,* 865–905.

Ryall, R. W. Amino acid receptors in CNS. I. GABA and glycine in spinal cord. In, *Handbook of Psychopharmacology,* Sect. I, Vol. 4. (Iversen, L. L.; Iversen, S. D.; and Snyder, S. H.; eds.) Plenum Press, New York, **1975**, pp. 83–128.

Scharrer, B. Neurohumors and neurohormones: definitions and terminology. *J. Neurovisc. Relat.,* **1969**, *9,* Suppl., 1–20.

Schmitt, F. O., and Worden, F. G. (eds.). *The Neurosci-*

ences: A Fourth Study Program. The MIT Press, Cambridge, Mass., **1979.**

Schwartz, J. C. Histamine as a transmitter in brain. *Life Sci.,* **1975,** *17,* 503–513.

Schwartz, J. C.; Costenin, J.; Martres, M. P.; Protais, P.; and Baudry, M. Modulation of receptor mechanisms in the CNS: hyper- and hyposensitivity to catecholamines. *Neuropharmacology,* **1978,** *17,* 665–685.

Siggins, G. R. Electrophysiological role of dopamine in striatum: excitatory or inhibitory? In, *Psychopharmacology—A Generation of Progress.* (Lipton, M. A.; DiMascio, A.; and Killam, K. F.; eds.) Raven Press, New York, **1978,** pp. 143–158.

Simon, E. J., and Hiller, J. M. The opiate receptors. *Annu. Rev. Pharmacol. Toxicol.,* **1978,** *18,* 371–394.

Snyder, S. H.; U'Prichard, D. C.; and Greenberg, D. A. Neurotransmitter receptor binding in the brain. In, *Psychopharmacology—A Generation of Progress.* (Lipton, M. A.; DiMascio, A.; and Killam, K. F.; eds.) Raven Press, New York, **1978,** pp. 361–370.

Sulser, F.; Vetulani, J.; and Mobley, P. L. Mode of action of antidepressant drugs. *Biochem. Pharmacol.,* **1978,** *27,* 257–261.

Symposium. (Various authors.) Prostaglandins. (Ramwell, P., and Shaw, J., eds.) *Ann. N.Y. Acad. Sci.,* **1971,** *180,* 5–568.

Symposium. (Various authors.) Serotonin—new vistas: histochemistry and pharmacology. (Costa, E.; Gessa, G. L.; and Sandler, M.; eds.) *Adv. Biochem. Psychopharmacol.,* **1974,** *10,* 1–329.

Symposium. (Various authors.) Nonstriatal dopaminergic neurons. (Costa, E., and Gessa, G. L., eds.) *Adv. Biochem. Psychopharmacol.,* **1977,** *16,* 1–686.

Symposium. (Various authors.) The endorphins. (Costa, E., and Trabucchi, M., eds.) *Adv. Biochem. Psychopharmacol.,* **1978,** *18,* 1–366.

Symposium. (Various authors.) *Catecholamines—Basic and Clinical Frontiers: Proceedings of the Fourth International Catecholamine Symposium.* (Usdin, E., ed.) Pergamon Press, Ltd., Oxford, **1979a.**

Symposium. (Various authors.) *Reticular Formation—Revisited.* (Hobson, J. A., ed.) Raven Press, New York, **1979b.**

Szentagothai, J., and Arbib, M. A. Conceptual models of neural organization. *Neurosci. Res. Program Bull.,* **1974,** *12,* 310–510.

Werman, R. Amino acids as central transmitters. In, *Neurotransmitters: Proceedings of the Association for Research in Nervous and Mental Disease,* Vol. 50. (Kopin, I. J., ed.) The Williams & Wilkins Co., Baltimore, **1972,** pp. 147–180.

Wood, J. W. (ed.). *Neurobiology of the Cerebrospinal Fluid.* Plenum Press, New York, **1979.**

Wurtman, R. J., and Fernstrom, J. D. Nutrition and the brain. In, *The Neurosciences: A Third Study Program.* (Schmitt, F. O., and Worden, F G., eds.) The MIT Press, Cambridge, Mass., **1974,** pp. 685–694.

Zieglgansberger, W.; Siggins, G. R.; French, E.; and Bloom, F. E. Effects of opioids on single units. In, *Characteristics and Function of Opioids.* (Van Ree, J., and Terenius, L., eds.) Elsevier Publishing Co., Amsterdam, **1978,** pp. 75–86.

Zigmond, R. E. Binding, metabolism, and action of steroid hormones in the central nervous system. In, *Handbook of Psychopharmacology,* Sect. I, Vol. 5. (Iversen, L. L.; Iversen, S. D.; and Snyder, S. H.; eds.) Plenum Press, New York, **1975,** pp. 239–328.

13 HISTORY AND PRINCIPLES OF ANESTHESIOLOGY

Theodore C. Smith, Lee H. Cooperman, and Harry Wollman

I. History of Surgical Anesthesia

Anesthesia before 1846. Surgical procedures were uncommon before 1846. Understanding of the pathophysiology of disease and of the rationale for its treatment by surgery was rudimentary. Aseptic technic and the prevention of wound infection were almost unknown. In addition, the lack of satisfactory anesthesia was a major deterrent. Because of all these factors few operations were attempted and mortality was frequent. Typically, surgery was of an emergency nature—for example, amputation of a limb for open fracture, cystotomy for bladder stone, or drainage of an abscess. Fine dissection and careful technic were not possible in patients for whom relief of pain was inadequate.

Some means of attempting to relieve surgical pain were available and, in fact, had been used since ancient times (Davison, 1965). Drugs like alcohol, hashish, and opium derivatives, taken by mouth, provided some consolation. Physical methods for the production of analgesia, such as packing a limb in ice or making it ischemic with a tourniquet, were occasionally used. Unconsciousness induced by a blow to the head or by strangulation did provide relief from pain, although at a high cost. However, the most common method used to achieve a relatively quiet surgical field was simple restraint of the patient by force. It is no wonder that surgery was looked upon as a last resort.

Sad to say, the analgesic properties of both nitrous oxide and diethyl ether had been known to a few for years, but the agents were not utilized for medical purposes (Keys, 1963). Nitrous oxide was synthesized by Priestley in 1776, and both he and Humphry Davy some 20 years later commented upon its anesthetic properties (Faulconer and Keys, 1965). Davy in fact suggested that ". . . it may probably be used with advantage during surgical operations in which no great effusion of blood takes place." Another 20 years passed before Michael Faraday wrote that the inhalation of diethyl ether produced effects similar to those of nitrous oxide. However, except for their inhalation in carnival exhibitions or to produce "highs" at "ether frolics," these drugs were not used in man until the mid-nineteenth century.

Green (1971) has presented an analysis of the reasons for the introduction of anesthesia in the 1840s. The time was then right, since concern for the well-being of one's fellows, a humanitarian attitude, was more prevalent than it had been in the previous century. "So long as witches were being burned in Salem, anesthesia could not be discovered 20 miles away in Boston." While humanitarian concern extended to the relief of pain, chemistry and medicine had simultaneously advanced to such an extent that a chemically pure drug could be prepared and then used with some degree of safety. There was, too, growth of the inquisitive spirit—a search for improvement of man's lot.

Public Demonstration of Ether Anesthesia. Dentists were instrumental in the introduction of both diethyl ether and nitrous oxide. They, even more than physicians, came into daily contact with persons complaining of pain; often, as a by-product of their work, they produced pain. It was at a stage show that Horace Wells, a dentist, noted that one of the participants, while under the influence of nitrous oxide, injured himself yet felt no pain. The next day Wells, while breathing nitrous oxide, had one of his own teeth extracted, painlessly, by a colleague. Shortly thereafter, in 1845, Wells attempted to demonstrate his discovery at the Massachusetts General Hospital in Boston. Unfortunately the patient cried out during the operation, and the demonstration was deemed a failure.

William T. G. Morton, a Boston dentist (and medical student), was familiar with the use of nitrous oxide from a previous association with Horace Wells. Morton learned of ether's anesthetic effects, thought it more promising, and practiced with it on animals and then on himself. Finally, he asked permission to demonstrate the drug's use, publically, as a surgical anesthetic.

The story of this classical demonstration in 1846 has been retold countless times. The operating room ("ether dome") at the Massachusetts General Hospital remains as a memorial to the first public demonstration of surgical anesthesia. In the gallery of this room skeptical spectators gathered, for the news had spread that a second-year medical student had developed a method for abolishing surgical pain. The patient, Gilbert Abbott, was brought in and Dr. Warren, the surgeon, waited in formal morning clothes. Operating gowns, masks, gloves, surgical asepsis, and the bacterial origin of infection were entirely unknown at that time. Everyone was ready and waiting, including the strong men to hold down the struggling patient, but Morton did not appear. Fifteen minutes passed, and the surgeon, becoming impatient, took his scalpel and turning to the gallery said, "As Dr. Morton has not arrived, I presume he is otherwise engaged." While the audience smiled and the patient cringed, the surgeon turned to make his incision. Just then Morton entered, his tardiness being due to the necessity for completing an apparatus with which to administer the ether. Warren stepped back, and pointing to the man strapped to the operating table said, "Well, sir, your patient is ready." Surrounded by a silent and unsympathetic audience, Morton went quietly to work. After a few minutes of ether inhalation, the patient was unconscious, whereupon Morton looked up and said, "Dr. Warren, *your* patient is ready." The operation was begun. The patient showed no sign of pain, yet he was alive and breathing. The strong men were not needed. When the operation was completed, Dr. Warren turned to the astonished audience and made the famous statement, "Gentlemen, this is no humbug." Dr. Henry J. Bigelow, an eminent surgeon attending the demonstration, remarked, "I have seen something today that will go around the world."

Following initial disbelief, news of the successful demonstration spread rapidly. Within a month, ether was in use in other cities of the United States and had been given in Great Britain as well. Its use was soon established as legitimate medical therapy.

The lives of those involved in the introduction of surgical anesthesia did not have so salubrious an outcome. Morton initially tried to patent the use of ether to produce anesthesia and, when this failed, patented instead his device for its administration. Considerable wrangling ensued as to who was the legitimate discoverer of anesthesia. Never receiving what he felt to be his due, Morton died an embittered man.

Charles Jackson, Morton's chemistry teacher at Harvard, also claimed priority in the discovery; it was he who had suggested that Morton use pure sulfuric ether. Jackson became insane, a fate that also befell Horace Wells, the man who had failed in the public demonstration of nitrous oxide anesthesia. Crawford Long, a physician in rural Georgia, had used ether anesthesia since 1842 but neglected to publish his experiences. He survived and prospered, but Morton rightfully receives credit for the introduction of surgical anesthesia. A monument erected by the citizens of Boston over the grave of Dr. Morton in Mt. Auburn Cemetery near Boston bears the following inscription written by Dr. Jacob Bigelow:

WILLIAM T. G. MORTON
Inventor and Revealer of Anaesthetic Inhalation.
Before Whom, in All Time, Surgery Was Agony.
By Whom Pain in Surgery Was Averted and Annulled.
Since Whom Science Has Control of Pain.

Anesthesia after 1846. Although it is rarely used today, ether was the ideal "first" anesthetic. Chemically, it is readily made in pure form. It is relatively easy to administer, since it is a liquid at room temperature but is readily vaporized. Ether is potent, unlike nitrous oxide, and thus a few volumes percent can produce anesthesia without diluting the oxygen in room air to hypoxic levels. It supports both respiration and circulation, crucial properties at a time when human physiology was not understood well

enough for assisted respiration and circulation to be possible. And ether is not toxic to vital organs.

The next anesthetic to receive wide use was chloroform. Introduced by the Scottish obstetrician James Simpson in 1847, it became quite popular, perhaps because of its more pleasant odor. Other than this and its nonflammability, there was little to recommend it (Sykes, 1960). The drug is a hepatotoxin and a severe cardiovascular depressant. Despite the relatively high incidence of intraoperative and postoperative death associated with the use of chloroform, it was championed, especially in Great Britain, for nearly 100 years (Duncum, 1947). Because of the danger and difficulty in administering chloroform, distinguished British physicians early became interested in anesthetics and their administration, a trend that was evident in the United States only 100 years later.

The course of anesthesiology in the United States, after the initial burst of enthusiasm, was one of slow change and limited progress (Vandam, 1973). Furthermore, despite the relative comfort that the surgical patient experienced, the amount and scope of surgery increased only slightly in the 1840s and 1850s (Greene, 1979). The incidence of mortality was little changed, for postoperative infection was still a serious problem. Only with the introduction of aseptic technics 20 years after the discovery of anesthesia did surgery come into its own.

Other Anesthetic Agents. Nitrous oxide fell into disuse after the apparent failure in Boston in 1845. It was reintroduced in 1863 into American dental and surgical practice, largely through the efforts of a showman, entrepreneur, and partially trained physician, Gardner Q. Colton. In 1868, the administration of nitrous oxide with oxygen was described by Edmond Andrews, a Chicago surgeon, and soon thereafter the two gases became available in steel cylinders, greatly increasing their practicality (Thomas, 1975). Nitrous oxide is still widely used today.

The anesthetic properties of cyclopropane were accidentally discovered in 1929 when chemists were analyzing impurities in an isomer, propylene (Lucas, 1961). After extensive clinical trial at the University of Wisconsin, the drug was introduced into practice; cyclopropane was perhaps the most widely used general anesthetic for the next 30 years. However, with the prominent risk of explosion in the operating room brought about by the increasing use of electronic equipment, the need for a safe, nonflammable anesthetic increased, and several groups pursued the search. Efforts by the British Research Council and by chemists at Imperial Chemical Industries were rewarded by the development of halothane, a nonflammable anesthetic. It was introduced into clinical practice in 1956, and has since become the most widely used, potent general anesthetic. Most of the newer agents, which are halogenated hydrocarbons and ethers, are modeled after halothane.

The skeletal muscle relaxants (neuromuscular blocking agents) were also discovered and their pharmacological properties demonstrated long before their introduction into clinical practice (McIntyre, 1959; Bennett, 1967). Curare, in crude form, had long been used by South American Indians as a poison on their arrow tips (*see* Chapter 11). Its first clinical use was in spastic disorders, where it could decrease muscle tone without embarrassing respiration excessively. It was then used to modify the violent muscle contractions associated with convulsive therapy of psychiatric disorders. Finally, in the 1940s, anesthesiologists used curare to provide the muscular relaxation that previously could be obtained only with deep levels of general anesthesia. Over the next half-dozen years several synthetic substitutes were made and used clinically. It is difficult to overemphasize the importance of muscle relaxants in anesthetic practice. Their use permits adequate conditions for surgery with light levels of general anesthesia; cardiovascular depression is thus minimized, and the patient awakens promptly when the anesthetic is discontinued.

Although the desirability of an intravenous anesthetic agent must have been apparent to physicians early in the twentieth century, the drugs at hand were few and unsatisfactory. The situation changed dramatically in 1935, when Lundy demonstrated the clinical usefulness of thiopental, a rapidly acting thiobarbiturate. It was originally considered useful as a sole anesthetic agent, but the heroic doses required resulted in serious depression of the circulatory, respiratory, and nervous systems. Thiopental has, however, been enthusiastically accepted as an agent for the rapid induction of general anesthesia. Other barbiturates (*e.g.,* thiamylal and methohexital) are also used for this purpose, but they are less popular.

Various combinations of tranquilizers and narcotic drugs have been used recently as anesthetic agents, usually in combination with nitrous oxide. The term *neurolept anesthesia* is applied to such technics. A similar state, dissociative anesthesia, is often produced with the drug ketamine (*see* Chapter 14). However convenient these agents may be to use, their side effects have limited their clinical usefulness to special situations.

II. Principles of the Administration of General Anesthetics

UPTAKE AND DISTRIBUTION OF INHALATIONAL ANESTHETICS

A firm understanding of general anesthesia requires appreciation of the pharmacokinetics of drugs that are inhaled. During general anesthesia produced with an inhalational agent, the depth of anesthesia varies directly with the tension of anesthetic agent in the brain, and the rates of induction and recovery depend upon the rate of change of tension in this tissue. The terms *tension* and *partial pressure* are used interchangea-bly. The tension of anesthetic agent in the brain is always approaching the tension in arterial blood. The factors that determine the tension of anesthetic gas in the arterial blood and in the brain can be considered under four headings: (1) concentration of the anesthetic agent in inspired gas, (2) pulmonary ventilation delivering the anesthetic to the lungs, (3) transfer of the gas from the alveoli to the blood flowing through the lungs, and (4) loss of the agent from the arterial blood to all the tissues of the body. (*See* Kety, 1950, 1951.)

CONCENTRATION OF THE ANESTHETIC AGENT IN INSPIRED GAS

The concentration of an individual gas in a mixture of gases is proportional to its tension, and one often refers to them interchangeably when speaking of the inspired gases.

When a constant tension of anesthetic gas is inhaled, the tension in arterial blood approaches that of the agent in the inspired mixture, in the manner shown in Figure 13–1 for several different anesthetics. (The tension of the inspired vapor or gas is commonly called the "inspired tension.") For drugs such as nitrous oxide, the arterial tension reaches 90% of the inspired tension in about 20 minutes. When methoxyflurane is administered, the approach to a steady state is much slower, and 90% of the inspired tension would be reached in arterial blood only after many hours. This difference is determined by the physical properties of the two agents (*see* below).

In practice the inspired tension is rarely constant. An anesthetizing concentration of some agents may irritate the airway of an awake or lightly anesthetized patient, so that the inspired concentration must be increased slowly. In other cases, where the vapor is not irritating, the speed of induction may be increased by giving the inhalational anesthetics in concentrations greater than those ultimately desired. Anesthetic tensions are thus produced in blood and tissues sooner than would be possible if maintenance concentrations were used for induction. As anesthesia proceeds, the inspired concentration of anesthetic is reduced to a level suitable for the maintenance of anesthesia.

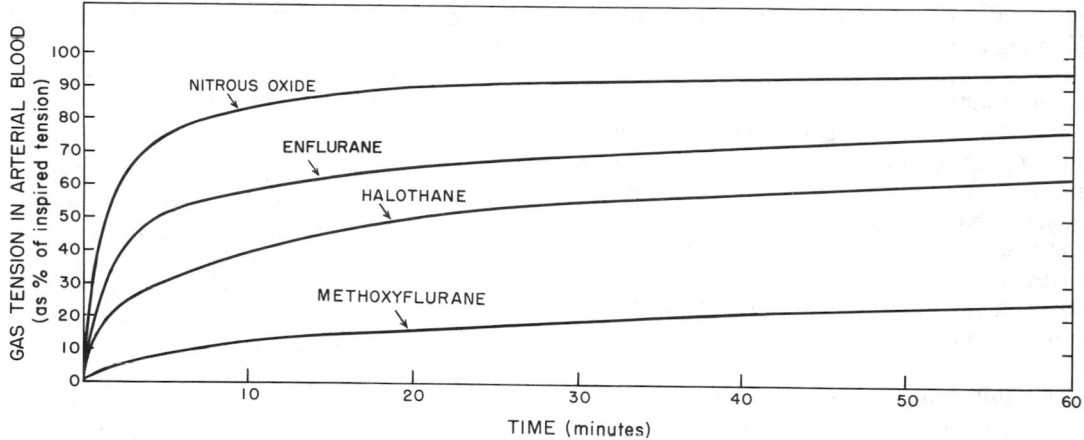

Figure 13–1. *The tensions of anesthetic gases in arterial blood.*

The curves demonstrate how arterial blood tension of the anesthetics increases toward the inspired tension. The increase in partial pressure is rapid for the relatively insoluble gases, and slower for those that are more soluble in blood. For the first comprehensive theoretical analysis of the shape of uptake curves, *see* Kety (1950, 1951). For an early experimental approach to the uptake of anesthetic gases, *see* Haggard (1924).

The course of events is illustrated here for an idealized situation, where the inhaled concentration remains constant, and pulmonary ventilation and cardiac output and its regional distribution remain constant at normal values. In fact, as anesthesia deepens, alveolar ventilation and cardiac output fall, and distribution of regional circulation and agent solubility are variably altered. These and other factors can result in up to 11% difference between predicted and actual concentration (Cowles *et al.,* 1972). Alinear analyses have been proposed that take these factors into consideration (Smith *et al.,* 1972; Munson *et al.,* 1973).

PULMONARY VENTILATION

Each inspiration delivers some anesthetic gas to the lung. If the respiratory minute ventilation is great, the tension of the anesthetic in alveoli increases quickly, as does its tension in arterial blood. Thus, the partial pressure of anesthetic gas in blood can be increased by overventilation during induction. This can be achieved by stimulation of respiration with carbon dioxide or by mechanical control of this function. Conversely, decreased ventilation (resulting, for instance, from respiratory depression by premedication or an anesthetic agent) can lead to a slower rate of change of arterial gas tension.

The effects of the rate of respiration to slow or speed induction are transient for gases such as nitrous oxide that have low solubility in blood and tissues and thus equilibrate quickly. However, the volume of respiration exerts a more significant and prolonged effect on the rate of uptake of more soluble and slowly equilibrating drugs such

as methoxyflurane. (For further discussion, *see* Eger, 1964.)

TRANSFER OF ANESTHETIC GASES FROM ALVEOLI TO BLOOD

The normal alveolar membrane poses no barrier to the transfer of anesthetic gases in both directions. Although the diffusion of anesthetic gases may be normal, certain situations can occur during clinical anesthesia that impede the efficient transfer of gases into blood flowing through the lung. One of these is maldistribution of alveolar ventilation such as may occur in pulmonary emphysema. There is then a lower tension of anesthetic gas in the poorly ventilated alveoli, and thus a lower anesthetic tension in the blood draining them. The contribution of this blood to the arterial pool results in slowing of the rate of change of tension of the anesthetic in arterial blood. Mismatch of ventilation and perfusion in the lung also produces a difference between alveolar and arterial tensions of anesthetic gases. This, too, results in slowing of the rate of induction of, or recovery from, anesthesia (*see* Eger and Severinghaus, 1964).

In the absence of ventilation-perfusion disturbances, three factors determine how rapidly anesthetics pass from the inspired gases to blood. These are (1) the solubility of the agent in blood, (2) the rate of blood flow through the lung, and (3) the partial pressures of the agent in arterial and mixed venous blood.

Solubility of the Agent in Blood. This is usually expressed as the blood:gas partition coefficient, or λ, which represents the ratio of anesthetic concentration in blood to anesthetic concentration in a gas phase when the two are in equilibrium (*i.e.,* when the partial pressure is equal in both phases). The blood:gas partition coefficient is as high as 12 for very soluble agents such as methoxyflurane and as low as 0.47 for relatively insoluble anesthetics such as nitrous oxide. *The more soluble an anesthetic is in blood, the more of it must be dissolved in blood to raise its partial pressure there appreciably. Therefore, the blood tension of soluble agents rises slowly. The potential reservoir for relatively insoluble gases is small and can be filled more quickly. Therefore, their tension in blood can increase more rapidly.*

The blood:gas partition coefficients for the commonly used anesthetic agents are given in Table 14–1 (page 277). The feature of the curves in Figure 13–1 that is largely determined by the blood solubility of the agents is the height and sharpness of the bend, or "knee," in the uptake curve. The more soluble the agent (*i.e.,* the higher the λ), the lower and less sharp is the "knee" of the curve, and the slower is the approach of blood tension to that of the inhaled gases.

Rate of Pulmonary Blood Flow. The pulmonary blood flow (*i.e.,* the cardiac output) affects the rate at which anesthetics pass from the alveolar gases into the arterial blood. An increase in pulmonary blood flow slows the initial portion of the arterial tension curve; but the latter part of the curve tends to catch up, with the overall result that there is little change in the total time required for complete equilibration. (For the reasons why this should be so, *see* Kety, 1950, 1951; Mapleson, 1963; Mapleson, in the text by Papper and Kitz, 1963; Eger, 1964.)

Partial Pressures in Arterial and Mixed Venous Blood. After taking up anesthetic gas in the lung, the blood circulates to the tissues, and anesthetic gas is transferred from the blood to all tissues of the body. Blood cannot approach equilibrium with inhaled gas tension until this process, which tends to decrease the blood tension, is nearly complete. The mixed venous blood returning to the lungs has more anesthetic gas in it with each passage through the body. After a few minutes of anesthesia the difference between arterial (or alveolar) and mixed venous gas tension decreases continuously. Since the rate of diffusion across the pulmonary membrane is proportional to the difference between alveolar and mixed venous gas tensions, the volume of gas transferred to arterial blood during each minute decreases as time passes. Thus, arterial tension rises more slowly in the final portion of the curves in Figure 13–1.

LOSS OF ANESTHETIC GASES FROM
ARTERIAL BLOOD TO TISSUES

When the inhalational agents are delivered by arterial blood to the tissues, the tension rises in tissues to approach that in arterial blood. The rate at which a gas passes into tissues depends on (1) the solubility of the gas in the tissues, (2) the rate at which the gas is delivered to the tissues (*i.e.,* the blood flow to the various areas of the body), and (3) the partial pressures of the gas in arterial blood and tissues. Note that these three factors affecting transfer of the gas from blood to tissue are similar to the three that affect transfer of the anesthetic from lung to blood (*see* above).

Solubility of Gas in Tissues. This is expressed as a tissue:blood partition coefficient, a concept analogous to the blood:gas partition coefficient previously discussed. With most anesthetic agents, the tissue:blood partition is near unity for many of the body's lean tissues; that is, these agents are equally soluble in lean tissue and blood. An anesthetic concentration in blood or tissue is the product of partial pressure and solubility. Thus, the concentration of most anesthetics in lean tissues, such as the gray matter of brain, approaches that in blood as tissue tension builds up toward arterial blood tension. On the other hand, the tissue:blood coefficient for all anesthetics is large for fatty tissues. Their concentration in the fatty tissue is much greater than that in blood at the time of equilibrium (when tissue tension equals blood tension).

Tissue solubility is of importance in determining the slope of the final portion, or "tail," of the gas tension curves (Figure 13–1). High tissue solubility, especially high fat solubility, tends to depress the rate of rise of the "tail" of the curve.

Tissue Blood Flow. The higher the blood flow to a tissue, the faster is the delivery of the anesthetic agent, and the more rapidly will its tension and concentration rise in that area. Thus, the concentration of an inert gas in brain approaches that in arterial blood more rapidly when cerebral blood flow is high, and more slowly when cerebral blood flow decreases. It has been suggested that anesthetic induction and emergence can be speeded by allowing the patient to inhale some carbon dioxide. This agent, by increasing ventilation, accelerates the rise in the arterial tension curve (*see* above). In addition, by dilating cerebral vessels, carbon dioxide increases cerebral blood flow and thus hastens the rate at which brain tension of the anesthetic changes. Since brain tension of the anesthetic is the important factor for anesthesia, this procedure results in more rapid induction or emergence but *not* in more profound anesthesia.

Only tissues with high rates of blood flow will exhibit rapid rises in concentration of anesthetic, and only high-flow areas take up significant amounts of the agent during the early stages of anesthesia. Since blood flow to adipose tissue is very limited, anesthetic gases will be delivered to, and taken up by, fatty tissues so slowly that these tissues contain a significant amount of anesthetic agent only after a considerable time has elapsed.

Partial Pressures in Arterial Blood and Tissues. As the tissues take up anesthetic agent, the partial pressure of the gas in tissues increases toward that of the arterial blood. Since the rate at which gas diffuses from arterial blood to tissues varies with the partial-pressure difference between them, tissue concentration changes rapidly in the early minutes of anesthesia; however, as the tissue tension comes closer to the arterial tension, the tissue uptake of gas slows.

In *summary,* during the administration of an anesthetic, its tension in blood rises toward that in the inspired gas, at first rapidly, then more slowly. Tissue tensions increase concomitantly, approaching the arterial tension. The partial pressure increases most rapidly in tissues with high rates of blood flow, and lags considerably in areas where blood flow is lower.

ELIMINATION OF INHALATIONAL ANESTHETICS

The major factors that affect rate of elimination of the anesthetics are the same as those that are important in the uptake phase: pulmonary ventilation, blood flow, and solubility in blood and tissue. However, the administration of anesthesia is usually completed before arterial tension has reached inspired tension, and long before tissues of low blood flow or high gas solubility have reached inspired tension. As ventilation with anesthetic-free gas washes out the lungs, the arterial blood tension declines first, followed by that in the tissues. An example of tissue concentrations during 60 minutes of nitrous oxide inhalation and 45 minutes of washout is shown in Figure 13–2 (*see* Cowles *et al.,* 1968). Soon after elimination begins, the tension in lung and blood has fallen to very low (nonanesthetic) levels. Because of the high blood flow to brain, its tension of anesthetic gas decreases rapidly, accounting for the rapid awakening from anesthesia noted with relatively insoluble agents such as nitrous oxide. The agent persists for a longer time in tissues with lower blood flow such as muscle, and for yet longer times in fat where blood flow is very low, and from which the agent is therefore very slowly released.

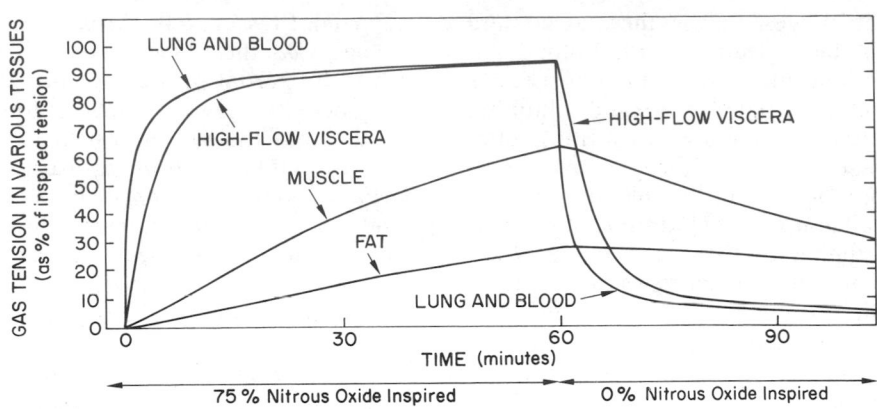

Figure 13-2. *Tissue tensions of an anesthetic gas during uptake and elimination.*

The curves demonstrate how tissue tensions of nitrous oxide approach the inspired tension during a 60-minute anesthetic uptake phase and a subsequent 45-minute elimination phase. The high-blood-flow viscera include brain, heart, and kidney. Liver and intestine have lower blood flows, and their tensions would lie between those of the high-blood-flow viscera and muscle. (Modified from Cowles, Borgstedt, and Gillies, 1968.)

OTHER ROUTES OF ELIMINATION
OF ANESTHETICS

The anesthetic gases are metabolized in the body to a variable extent. With most agents this is small. However, up to 15% of halothane and 70% of methoxyflurane are metabolized to various intermediate compounds, and in some cases to ionized halogens (*see* Chapter 14; Cohen, 1971). The bulk of metabolism of anesthetics occurs after clinical anesthesia has been discontinued, and is greatest for the more fat-soluble drugs (Berman *et al.*, 1973). The importance of the metabolism of anesthetic agents is not in the termination of their action; rather, metabolites of anesthetics may be responsible for certain of their toxic effects or aftereffects.

Additional small losses of anesthetic gases from the body occur by diffusion across skin and mucous membranes, and by means of urinary excretion of the agent or its breakdown products (Stoelting and Eger, 1969; Cohen, 1971).

MINOR EFFECTS

Minor pharmacokinetic effects distinguish the uptake, distribution, and elimination of soluble gases, such as nitrous oxide, from those of insoluble gases, such as nitrogen or helium.

Concentration Effect and Second-Gas Effect. The *concentration effect* may be defined as follows: when higher concentrations of an anesthetic gas are inhaled, arterial tension increases at a slightly greater rate than it would have if a lesser concentration of the anesthetic had been inhaled (*see* Eger, 1963). Consider a patient who is inhaling 75% nitrous oxide and 25% oxygen. Although nitrous oxide is relatively insoluble, when the inhaled concentration is high, the rate of uptake of the gas by blood and tissues may be as great as 1 liter per minute during the early

minutes of anesthesia. As this volume of gas disappears from the lung, fresh gases are literally sucked into the lung from the breathing circuit to replace the volume taken up. The rate at which the inspired gas mixture is delivered to the lung is then 1 liter per minute greater than the minute ventilation would have provided without this effect. Therefore, the rate of rise of the arterial tension curve for nitrous oxide is increased during induction of anesthesia. However, if only 10% nitrous oxide is inhaled, the body's uptake of approximately 150 ml per minute results in no significant change in the rate of gas delivery to the lung, and there is little or no acceleration of the arterial tension.

The simultaneous presence of two anesthetic gases in the lung can introduce a closely related phenomenon known as the *second-gas effect.* An illustration may be taken in which 75% nitrous oxide and 1% halothane are administered together with 24% oxygen. The same disappearance of 1 liter per minute of nitrous oxide from the lung into the body takes place, and the rate at which 1% halothane is delivered to the alveoli becomes 1 liter per minute greater than the minute ventilation would otherwise have provided. As a result, the arterial tension of halothane rises a little more rapidly in the presence of nitrous oxide. (*See* Epstein *et al.*, 1964.)

Diffusion Hypoxia. The reverse of the concentration effect can occur after the anesthetic has been discontinued, and will be illustrated for nitrous oxide. The elimination of nitrous oxide from blood to lung may proceed at a rate as great as the uptake. The additional gas added to the alveoli dilutes the available oxygen, and reduces alveolar oxygen concentration. The phenomenon is known as *diffusion hypoxia* (*see* Fink, 1955). It is seen in the early minutes following the end of a nitrous oxide administration, if the patient is breathing air. The hypoxia is usually mild, and is rarely a clinical threat. It can be prevented by oxygen inhalation for a few minutes at the end of the anesthetic administration.

Although *diffusion hypoxia* can theoretically occur after the withdrawal of any anesthetic agent, its magnitude is insignificant unless high concentrations of a soluble agent such as nitrous oxide have been inhaled for some time. Under these circumstances a considerable volume of inert gas has been dissolved in the body (up to 30 liters), and much of it is eliminated through the lungs in the first few minutes after its administration is discontinued. When lower concentrations of an agent (*e.g.*, 2% halothane) are inhaled, even after a long time only a few liters will have been taken up in the body. When administration is discontinued, the elimination of 100 ml per minute or less of halothane is not sufficient to dilute the alveolar oxygen to hypoxic levels.

Intertissue Diffusion. During the approach to equilibrium, the gas being inhaled may be present at different partial pressures in adjacent tissues, the partial pressure being higher in the areas with greater flow and in those where the gas is less soluble. The anesthetic will diffuse into the areas where its tension is lower. The rates of diffusion are such that tissue tensions are not much affected in areas with high blood flow and areas where the gas is relatively insoluble. However, tissue concentrations can be significantly changed by diffusion in areas where flow rates are low and gas solubility is high, as in adipose tissue (*see* Eger, 1973).

ADMINISTRATION OF INHALATIONAL ANESTHETICS

ANESTHETIC MACHINES

With these devices, the anesthesiologist is able to deliver measured quantities of anesthetic gases and oxygen through accurate flowmeters, and with the use of special vaporizers it is possible to add the vapor of volatile anesthetic liquids to the gas stream. Tanks of oxygen and anesthetic gases are attached to the machine by fittings that are pin-indexed, so that a tank cannot be mounted in the wrong slot (*see* Epstein and Hunter, 1968).

Vaporizers. Liquid anesthetic agents can be vaporized in several ways (*see* Hill, 1968). They may be slowly dripped into the gas mixture. They may be vaporized by a gas stream that passes over the surface of the liquid, or past a wick saturated with the liquid. Some vaporizers can deliver a precisely known concentration of anesthetic vapor. Bimetalic valves incorporated in these vaporizers keep the output concentration constant over a range of room temperature, by altering the ratio of through flow to by-pass flow of gases. A gas may also be passed through the liquid, as in the modern, precise, "saturation-type" vaporizers such as the copper kettle. In these devices, gas bubbles pass through a liquid anesthetic in such a way that saturation of the gas bubbles with the liquid agent is complete. Equilibration occurs within the vaporizer, the amount of liquid volatilized by the gas depending only upon the vapor pressure, which, in turn, is determined by

the particular liquid and its temperature. Since vaporization of liquids tends to cool them, some vaporizers are made of materials that conduct heat well, and are thermally connected to the anesthesia machine, which provides a large heat reservoir. As a result, the temperature inside a copper kettle tends to remain constant, even when liquids are vaporized rapidly. The decrease in vapor pressure that occurs when temperature declines is thus minimized (Morris and Feldman, 1958).

As the vapor pressures of many liquid anesthetics are several hundred millimeters Hg at room temperature (*see* Table 14–1, page 277), saturation vaporizers can deliver far more than is necessary or desirable. Therefore, the outflow of gases from the vaporizer is diluted with additional flows of oxygen or nitrous oxide to attain the desired anesthetic concentrations.

BREATHING CIRCUITS

The gases and vapors are delivered into a system of wide-bore tubes with valves, a distensible bag that provides a reservoir for the gases, and usually an absorber for expired carbon dioxide. Gases are administered to the patient by means of a face mask or endotracheal tube. Two types of gas delivery systems are illustrated in Figure 13–3.

Valves. These may be one-way valves, which can act as non-rebreathing valves or can ensure that the gases are unidirectionally circulated in a *circle system*. They may be demand valves, which ensure that fresh gas can flow into the system only during inspiration and only in amounts required by the patient; or they may be pop-off valves, which permit the escape of excess gases from the circuit but do not allow entry of room air (*see* Foregger, 1959).

Reservoir Bag. In the absence of a demand valve, there must be a reservoir of gas from which the patient can inhale. This is usually provided by a distensible bag that partially empties during inhalation and refills during exhalation. In non-rebreathing systems, the bag refills with fresh gases from the flowmeters. In rebreathing systems, it refills not only with fresh gas, but also with exhaled gases after they have passed through a carbon dioxide absorber. The bag also provides a means for the assistance or control of respiration by the anesthesiologist, who can compress the bag and thus force gas into the patient's lungs. When pressure on the bag is released, the lungs empty and the bag refills.

Carbon Dioxide Absorption or Elimination. In systems where rebreathing is permitted, one must provide for elimination of the exhaled carbon dioxide (*see* Gates and Adriani, 1962; Brown *et al.*, 1964). For this purpose, a canister of carbon dioxide-absorbing material can be included in the breathing circuit. This material is a basic substance, such as soda lime, that reacts with carbonic acid formed by carbon dioxide and water. As a result of the reaction, a carbonate and water are produced and heat is generated (*see* Bracken and Cox, 1968).

Another way in which carbon dioxide can be

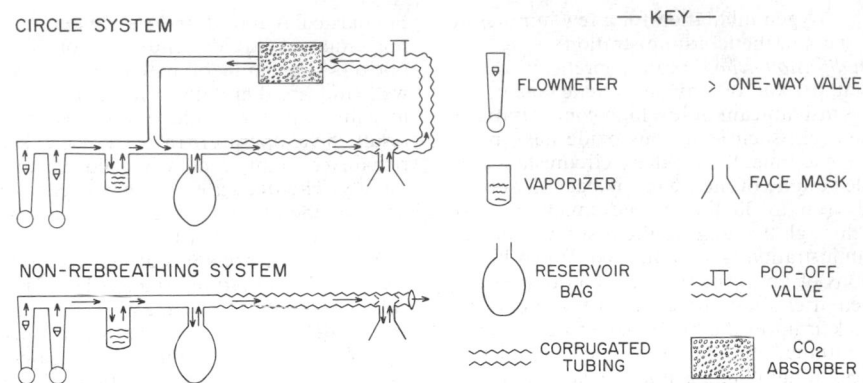

Figure 13-3. *Systems used for delivering inhalational anesthetics.*

Two breathing circuits are shown; they are made up of similar components arranged in slightly different ways.

Circle System. Gases are delivered through flowmeters and past the vaporizer, and then circulate in one direction around the circle. If large amounts of fresh gas are added, the excess is eliminated through the one-way, pop-off valve. If, on the other hand, rebreathing of the exhaled gases takes place, only small amounts of fresh gases are added from the machine to replace the oxygen used by the patient in metabolism and the anesthetic gases taken up by the patient. In this case, no gas flows out through the pop-off valve, and the exhaled carbon dioxide is absorbed chemically. (For a discussion of optimal placement of the various components of circle systems, *see* Eger and Ethans, 1968.)

Non-rebreathing System. Gases are delivered through flowmeters and past the vaporizer, as in the circle system. They then pass to the reservoir bag and the patient. All exhaled gases escape through the one-way exhalation valve, and carbon dioxide absorption is unnecessary. Fresh gases must be delivered at a rate sufficient to supply the patient's minute ventilation.

If the one-way valve between the bag and the face mask is eliminated, this system becomes the popular Magill circuit, and the amount of rebreathing that takes place then depends on the flow rate of the gases (*see* Mapleson, 1954).

eliminated from an anesthetic system is by washout with high flows of fresh gases, the carbon dioxide being carried out in the overflow of other gases. The higher the flow rate, the greater is the overflow and the more complete the elimination of carbon dioxide (*see* Mapleson, 1954; Adriani, 1960; Brown *et al.,* 1964). In *non-rebreathing systems,* all the exhaled carbon dioxide is eliminated from the system by means of the non-rebreathing valve.

Information on Exact Concentrations. The concentrations of anesthetics and oxygen being inhaled by the patient are identical to those being delivered by the machine only in non-rebreathing circuits. In these circuits, if the anesthesiologist has accurate flowmeters for gases and a dependable vaporizer for liquids, he can determine what concentrations of anesthetics and oxygen are being delivered to the patient. However, in systems where rebreathing occurs, the situation is considerably different. Denitrogenation of the patient dilutes the gases in the system; humidification of the gases in the system lowers their concentrations somewhat; oxygen is lost from the system as the patient utilizes it for metabolic requirements; and anesthetic gases are taken up by the patient at a changing rate. At the same time, small amounts of oxygen and anesthetic are added to the circuit. It is apparent that in a low-flow system, the inhaled gases are a mixture with a composition

that is difficult to estimate. As the flow rates increase, the characteristics of the system become less like the low-flow and more like the non-rebreathing system, and the inhaled gas concentrations approach the concentrations being delivered from the flowmeters and the vaporizer. Nitrous oxide is most frequently delivered in high-flow systems; the anesthesiologist is then assured of at least 20% inhaled oxygen and very nearly 80% inhaled concentration of this rather weak anesthetic gas (*see* Smith, 1966).

Gas, Heat, and Water Exchange in Anesthesia Systems. Three liters of nitrogen may be eliminated from the lung and from tissues in the first hour of anesthesia if a nitrous oxide–oxygen mixture is inspired. This nitrogen must be exhausted from the breathing circuit if high concentrations of both oxygen and nitrous oxide are desired. Unlike carbon dioxide, it cannot be absorbed, but it can be eliminated by non-rebreathing circuits or diluted and vented through a pop-off valve.

Water vapor and the heat to vaporize it are provided under normal conditions by the nasal turbinates. However, during anesthesia, the machine delivers dry gas that has been chilled by its expansion from compressed gas cylinders, and the patient inspires it through oropharyngeal or endotracheal tubes that bypass the nasal turbinates; cooling and drying of the tracheobronchial mucosa thus occur.

While the heat and water loss may be tolerable in a normal patient for a short operation, the small, the elderly, and those who lose a great deal of heat and water when a large mass of tissue is exposed during long procedures benefit from the conservation of water and heat. This may be provided by the use of low-flow or closed systems or by warming and humidifying inspired gases. Such measures are often undertaken in pediatric anesthesia.

DOSAGE AND POTENCY OF GENERAL ANESTHETICS

General anesthetics are among the most dangerous drugs approved for general use, in that the margin of safety in their use is small. Therapeutic indices range from about two to four. That is, the dose that produces circulatory arrest may be only two to four times that which produces adequate anesthesia. Thus, accurate methods are required for choosing the dose of an anesthetic and for evaluating the depth of anesthesia.

When a tablet is swallowed or a solution injected into a muscle, the dose is described in terms of the mass of drug that is administered. However, when a drug is inhaled as a gas or vapor, a very large fraction of it is exhaled within the next 1 or 2 seconds. Moreover, since it is the brain and not the lung that is the site of action of inhalational anesthetics, the agent must partition between the alveolar gas and the blood and then again between the blood and the brain cells before exerting its action. It is difficult to specify the concentration in the brain of experimental animals and impossible to measure it in man. Yet the need to specify a dose to conduct pharmacological and physiological studies and for the administration of general anesthesia is inescapable. Anesthesiologists have therefore accepted a measure of potency of inhalational agents known as MAC, which stands for *minimum alveolar concentration* of anesthetic at 1 atmosphere that produces immobility in 50% of patients or animals exposed to a noxious stimulus (Eger *et al.*, 1965). The rationale for using the concentration in the alveoli rather than that in the brain to measure a dose is based on the following considerations: concentration in the lung can be easily, frequently, and accurately measured; at steady state, the partial pressure of anesthetic in the lung and the partial pressure in the brain are equal;

and relatively high blood flow to the brain causes rapid transport of blood-borne agents to the brain and thus rapid equilibration between blood and brain.

Among the characteristics of MAC that recommend it as a measure of anesthetic dose and potency are that MAC is invariant with a variety of noxious stimuli from tail clamping to abdominal incision; that variability within individuals of a given species is small; that sex, height, weight, and duration of anesthesia do not alter MAC (although temperature and age do); and, finally, that doses of anesthetic agents appear to be additive (*i.e.*, one half of a MAC of one drug plus one half of a MAC of another drug will cause immobility following noxious stimulation in 50% of individuals tested) (Cullen *et al.*, 1969; Millar *et al.*, 1969).

The slopes of the dose-response curves for inhalational anesthetics are steep. Thus, although only 50% of individuals may fail to respond to stimulation at 1.0 MAC, more than 99% are unresponsive at a dose of 1.1 MAC. The latter concentration is, therefore, the surgically useful dose of each anesthetic if it is used without supplementation. Modern anesthesiologists tend to provide "light" anesthesia with concentrations of inhaled anesthetic of 0.9 to 1.1 MAC, in combination with judicious use of adjuvant drugs.

MAC represents only a single point on the dose-response curve for the production of anesthesia. Doubling the concentration of an anesthetic may produce more or less than a doubling of the intensity of another effect (*e.g.*, decrease in blood pressure), depending on the slope of the dose-response curve of that drug for that effect.

DEPTH OF ANESTHESIA

SIGNS AND STAGES OF ANESTHESIA

Between 1847 and 1858, John Snow described certain signs that helped him determine the depth of anesthesia in patients receiving chloroform or ether. These included the onset of rhythmic, automatic breathing and the loss of winking in response to touching the conjunctiva as surgical anesthesia was reached, and the gradual disappearance of intercostal muscle activity and cessation of eyeball movement as anesthesia was deepened. In 1920, Guedel, using these and other signs, outlined four stages of general anesthesia, dividing the third stage, that of surgical anesthesia, into four planes. Guedel's observations related primarily to ether, a substance with such great solubility in blood that the onset and progressive deepening of anesthesia were predictably slow. Opportunity is thus afforded the anesthesiologist to watch the unfolding of a series of changes involving respiration, muscle tone, and reflex activity. The somewhat arbitrary division is as follows: I—stage of analgesia; II—stage of delirium; III—stage of surgical anesthesia; IV—stage of medullary depression.

I. *Stage of Analgesia.* The first stage begins with the administration of the anesthetic and lasts until consciousness is lost. Artusio (1954, 1955) demonstrated that certain major operations requiring minimal muscular relaxation can be completed during the analgesia characterizing this stage.

II. *Stage of Delirium.* This stage extends from the loss of consciousness to the beginning of surgical anesthesia. Excitement and involuntary activity may be minimal or marked. Under the latter circumstance, the patient may laugh, shout, sing, and thrash about. The jaw becomes set, skeletal muscular tone increases, and breathing is irregular. Incontinence of urine and feces may occur, as may retching or vomiting. The pupils may dilate. Hypertension and tachycardia may be marked. Anesthesiologists try to reduce the duration and the intensity of this stage to the minimum.

III. *Stage of Surgical Anesthesia.* The third stage extends from the end of the second stage until cessation of spontaneous respiration occurs. The transition to stage III occurs when the excitement and the respiratory irregularity of stage II disappear. The third stage can be divided into four planes, numbered from 1 to 4, in order of increasing depth of anesthesia. The major differences in physical signs in the various planes relate to the character of the *respiration,* the character of the *eyeball movements,* the presence or absence of certain *reflexes,* and the size of the *pupils* (Gillespie, 1943).

IV. *Stage of Medullary Depression.* This stage starts as soon as the weakened respiration of plane 4 ceases, and it ends with failure of the circulation.

These signs and stages are partly recognizable during administration of many other general anesthetics, although they are often obscured by effects of modern anesthetics that differ from those of ether. Halothane causes hypotension more readily than does ether. Nitrous oxide is incapable of producing muscular relaxation; thus, neuromuscular blocking agents play an important role during anesthesia with nitrous oxide. The accompanying paralysis of respiration associated with neuromuscular blockade deprives the anesthesiologist of much information about depth of anesthesia, as does controlled ventilation, which is commonly used in modern anesthetic technics. Complete muscular paralysis eliminates all the skeletal muscular indices of depth, such as eyeball movement, changes in respiration, tightness of the jaw, and ability to phonate, swallow, move, or close the glottis. Eye signs may be obscured by the intense pupillary constriction that accompanies administration of narcotic analgesics. Other preanesthetic medications may obscure still other signs of the depth of anesthesia, and rapid induction of anesthesia with thiopental virtually eliminates the stage of excitement. Cullen and coworkers (1972) demonstrated that no single one of the major signs described by Guedel correlated satisfactorily with the measured alveolar concentrations of anesthetic during prolonged stable states.

A PRACTICAL APPROACH TO EVALUATING DEPTH OF ANESTHESIA

The following approach is useful for almost any general anesthetic. If the eyelids blink when the eyelashes are stroked, if the patient is swallowing, if respiration is irregular in rate and depth, and if one knows that not a great deal of anesthetic has been administered, surgical anesthesia is *not* present.

Loss of the eyelash reflex and the development of rhythmic respiration indicate the beginning of surgical anesthesia. If the skin incision is made at once, indications of "light" anesthesia may include an increase in respiratory rate or a rise in arterial blood pressure. Jaw muscles may become tight, and even if the mouth can be opened an oral airway may not be tolerated; an attempt to insert it may produce gagging, coughing, vomiting, or laryngospasm.

As anesthesia deepens, these responses are reduced in degree or abolished altogether. With most of the general anesthetics, an increase in depth brings progressive reduction in respiratory tidal volume. Tracheal tug may become evident as accessory muscles of respiration come into play. Diaphragmatic activity becomes jerky or snapping in character, and the lower chest is pulled in as the diaphragm descends. When the potent halogenated agents are used, arterial blood pressure tends to vary directly with the depth of anesthesia, and hypotension can be used as an index of dosage. Suggestions that anesthesia is becoming "lighter" are the formation of tears, apnea following peritoneal stimulation, increasing resistance to inflation of the lungs, and the return of those indices of light anesthesia listed above.

Severe respiratory depression or cessation of breathing (excluding breath-holding seen during early phases of anesthesia) and marked hypotension or asystole must be regarded as evidence of deep anesthesia unless other causes, for example, the effect of muscle relaxants, blood loss, and hypoxia, or the influence of vagal reflexes, can explain these findings.

Thus, common sense and experience, combined with constant observation of the patient's responses to anesthetic drugs and to stimuli, permit the successful estimation of depth of anesthesia.

The Electroencephalogram as an Index of Depth of General Anesthesia. In 1937, Gibbs and associates suggested that the EEG be used as a measure of the depth of anesthesia during surgical operations. Since that time a number of workers have classified the EEG changes produced by the inhalational agents and barbiturates (*see* Faulconer and Bickford, 1960; Clark and Rosner, 1973; Rosner and Clark, 1973a).

Use of the EEG as the sole index of anesthetic depth may be unreliable, since many factors influence the activity of the central nervous system (CNS). Hypoxia, hypoglycemia, hypothermia, and inadequate cerebral circulation can markedly alter the EEG at a time when anesthetic concentration remains constant (Marshall *et al.*, 1965). Furthermore, although EEG changes produced by a given agent may correlate with brain concentration, they also vary widely when different anesthetics are compared. (For a detailed examination of this subject, the reader should consult Clark and Rosner, 1973; Rosner and Clark, 1973a; McDowall, 1976.)

Muscular Relaxation. In the absence of neuromuscular blocking drugs, suppression of spinal reflex activity is the major mechanism by which general anesthetics produce muscle relaxation (Ngai *et al.*, 1965). Thus, in both animals (de Jong and Robles, 1968; de Jong *et al.*, 1968) and man (de Jong *et al.*, 1967) there is an excellent correlation between anesthetic concentration, suppression of spinal reflex activity, and muscular relaxation. Observation of muscle tone can thus serve as an index of the depth of anesthesia. It should be stressed that the concentration required to produce muscle relaxation in the aged, debilitated patient is far less than that necessary in the robust young man.

PREANESTHETIC MEDICATION

Preanesthetic medication should decrease anxiety without producing excessive drowsiness, facilitate a smooth, rapid induction without prolonging emergence, provide amnesia for the perioperative period while maintaining cooperation prior to loss of consciousness, relieve preoperative and postoperative pain if it is present, and minimize some of the undesirable side effects of anesthetic agents, notably salivation, bradycardia, and postanesthetic vomiting (Shearer, 1960, 1961). The accomplishment of these multiple purposes usually requires the concomitant use of two or three drugs. The most commonly employed classes include hypnotics, tranquilizers, opioids, antiemetics, and anticholinergics.

The wide variety of preanesthetic regimens in current use testifies to the lack of agreement on optimal combinations. Comparisons are difficult for a number of reasons. Many of the drugs produce nearly indistinguishable effects (Elliot *et al.*, 1969). Premedication may produce differing results depending on the operative procedure; the choice of anesthetic drugs and technic; and the patient's disease, age, sex, physical status, and current drug therapy. The more ill, the more elderly, the less robust and active the patient, the greater are the effects exerted by sedatives, tranquilizers, and analgesics.

HYPNOTICS

While drowsiness does not imply loss of all anxiety, most drugs in use for preanesthetic medication have some of both effects. The important classes of hypnotics include barbiturates and nonbarbiturate sedatives and antihistamines (*see* Chapter 17).

Barbiturates. *Pentobarbital* and *secobarbital* are the barbituric acid derivatives used most frequently to provide sedation and relieve apprehension before operation. They may be administered orally or intramuscularly to adults in doses of 100 to 200 mg, and to infants and children in doses of 3 to 5 mg/kg of body weight. These drugs have minimal depressant action on respiration and circulation and rarely produce nausea or vomiting (*see* Andersen and Gravenstein, 1966). Patients receiving barbiturates for preanesthetic medication usually awaken more promptly from a general anesthetic than if an opioid analgesic had been given, but the incidence of emergence excitement tends to be higher, presumably because of greater awareness of pain. Tolerance to the usually administered doses of barbiturates is observed in patients who have been taking many kinds of drugs, including other barbiturates, alcohol, and even aspirin and some anticoagulants.

Antihistamines. Sedation is a variable side effect of this group of drugs. *Hydroxyzine,* 50 to 150 mg intramuscularly, has found wide usage. It exhibits many minor benefits, such as bronchodilatory, antisialogogic, antiemetic, antiarrhythmic, and ataractic effects. It produces minimal circulatory and respiratory depression (Andersen and Gravenstein, 1966; Lauria *et al.*, 1968) and does not prolong anesthesia (Kim and Dobkin, 1973).

TRANQUILIZERS (ANTIANXIETY AGENTS)

Just as sedatives have some ataractic action, so do tranquilizers produce some sedation. The major groups include benzodiazepines, phenothiazines, and butyrophenones (*see* Chapters 17 and 19).

Benzodiazepines. The members of this class of drugs are used extensively for preanesthetic medication. They provide amnesia in 60% of patients after doses that produce only mild sedation (Frumin *et al.*, 1976; Pandit *et al.*, 1976). The amnesic effect is especially likely when the benzodiazepines are combined with scopolamine (Clarke *et al.*, 1970; Dundee and Haslett, 1970). Benzodiazepines can raise the threshold for CNS toxicity of local anesthetics (de Jong and Heavner, 1973). *Diazepam* in doses of 5 to 10 mg has been most widely used. It is active orally but is less predictable after intramuscular injection because low solubility slows uptake (Hillestad *et al.*, 1974). It has little effect on respiration unless loss of consciousness is produced by overdosage. It does not potentiate respiratory depression produced by opioids (Aukburg *et al.*, 1976). *Lorazepam* may be given intramuscularly and appears to produce amnesia frequently (Fragen and Caldwell, 1976).

Phenothiazines. Many different phenothiazine derivatives and other tranquilizers have been recommended for preanesthetic medication. These substances were suggested because of sedative, antiarrhythmic, antihistaminic, and antiemetic properties. They are sometimes combined in reduced dosage with a barbiturate or an opioid for greater sedation. Prolongation of postanesthetic sleep and greater respiratory depression are probable, and decrease in blood pressure is possible (*see* Dobkin *et al.*, 1962; Hoffman and Smith, 1970). The value of phenothiazines in premedication must be carefully weighed against their side effects. Phenothiazines commonly used in premedication include *promazine, promethazine,* and *propiomazine,* all in intramuscular dosage of 20 to 50 mg. (For a comparative study of 16 different phenothiazines and a useful bibliography, *see* Dundee *et al.*, 1965.)

Butyrophenones. The usual dose for premedication is 2.5 to 5 mg of droperidol, which provides 6 to 12 hours of ataraxia (*see* Downes *et al.*, 1967; Edmonds-Seal and Prys-Roberts, 1970). Some antiemetic activity can be expected, and there is reasonable cardiovascular stability, despite slight α-adrenergic blocking activity. Both restlessness and extrapyramidal dyskinesia can occur, especially in children; these effects may be countered by the administration of atropine.

OPIOIDS

Surgical pain is often severe, and even minor preoperative pain is deleterious to smooth induction of anesthesia. Therefore, when analgesics are used in premedication, only strong opioids have proven adequate. The major difference among opioids that governs the choice for premedication is duration of activity (*see* Chapter 22).

Morphine. Morphine in doses of 8 to 12 mg intramuscularly is frequently used prior to operation. If pain is present before operation, morphine is one of the drugs of choice. It is the pain-relieving property that in all probability minimizes the incidence of restlessness or excitation during emergence from general anesthesia. The drug is useful also for depressing the cough reflex. Preanesthetic medication with an opioid reduces the amount of general anesthetic required by 10 to 20% (Saidman and Eger, 1964; Munson *et al.*, 1965).

Unfortunately, morphine may have undesirable side effects. It often prolongs the awakening from general anesthesia since its clinical effects persist for 4 to 6 hours. Its stimulant effect on smooth muscle may cause spasm of the bile duct or of the ureters; colicky pain, often relieved by atropine but always abolished by naloxone, may result from this effect on smooth muscle. Wheezing may develop in patients with asthma. Constipation and urinary retention may be annoying. Nausea and vomiting are not uncommon. A vagotonic effect may be evidenced by bradycardia (Marta *et al.*, 1973). Hypotension can occur after the use of morphine or other opioid analgesics. The respiratory depressant action of morphine may increase intracranial pressure through retention of carbon dioxide and subsequent cerebral vasodilatation. While this can be undesirable in patients in whom intracranial pressure is already elevated, the effect can be abolished through adequate pulmonary ventilation. The respiratory and circulatory effects of opioids have been reviewed by Eckenhoff and Oech (1960), and differences among opioids have been considered by Loan and coworkers (1969) and Morrison and associates (1969).

Meperidine. This drug in 50- to 100-mg doses intramuscularly is used for preanesthetic medication, but it shares all the disadvantages of morphine, including depression of blood pressure, cardiac output, and respiration. Tachycardia occasionally occurs, posing a problem in differential diagnosis. Respiratory depression lasts 2 to 3 hours (Downes *et al.*, 1967).

Fentanyl. This synthetic opioid is useful in some cases because of its short duration of action, 1 to 2 hours (*see* Downes *et al.*, 1967). The usual dose is 0.05 to 0.10 mg intramuscularly.

ANTIEMETICS

Often the sequelae of prophylactic antiemetics (notably hypotension) are as disturbing and frequent as emetic episodes. However, if a drug is otherwise useful in a given instance, its antiemetic effect is an additional welcome benefit. *Droperidol* and *hydroxyzine* are sometimes useful for their antiemetic effects. *Benzquinamide* is a mild tranquilizer with some respiratory stimulant activity, probably via peripheral chemoreceptors. It is also a mild vasopressor and hence does not share some of the drawbacks of other antiemetics (Klein *et al.*, 1970; Mull and Smith, 1974). *Other drugs* that provide an antiemetic effect following intramuscular administration include scopolamine, 0.4 to 0.6 mg; cyclizine, 50 mg; trimethobenzamide, 200 mg; and a variety of phenothiazines.

ANTICHOLINERGIC DRUGS

The excessive respiratory tract secretions seen during open-drop administration of ether suggested the use of an anticholinergic drug prior to anesthetization. With the advent of less irritating anesthetic agents, secretions have become less of a problem. The emphasis has now shifted to the desire to counteract the vagal effects that may frequently occur during anesthesia. Thus, atropine or a similar substance continues to be given by most anesthesiologists (Eger, 1962; *see* Chapter 7).

Atropine. Atropine produces oral dryness and blurred vision within 10 to 15 minutes after intramuscular injection of the standard 0.4- to 0.6-mg dose. The vagal blocking action of such an amount may not be sufficient to prevent parasympathetically induced cardiovascular effects such as hypotension and bradycardia that result from increase in ocular pressure, visceral traction, manipulation of the carotid sinus, or injection of multiple doses of succinylcholine. However, the intravenous injection of an additional dose of atropine often promptly restores the cardiac rate and the arterial pressure toward normal. Small doses may have a cardiac-slowing effect (Dauchot and Gravenstein, 1971).

Atropine is not contraindicated in patients with glaucoma. Increased intraocular pressure does not result from the doses recommended (*see* Schwartz *et al.*, 1957). Some have advised that anticholinergic premedication be omitted in patients with asthma. However, inspissation of respiratory secretions has not proven to be a problem when the drugs are used in asthmatics. Their use in febrile patients may be unwise, since they depress the mechanism of heat loss by sweating.

Scopolamine. Scopolamine is usually given intramuscularly, in a dose of 0.4 to 0.6 mg. It is superior to atropine as an antisialogogue but is less effective in preventing reflex bradycardia during general anesthesia, particularly in children (Freeman and Bachman, 1959). The sedative effect of scopolamine is more marked than that of atropine (*see* Domino and Corssen, 1967); occasionally, however, patients become restless or disoriented after scopolamine, and the incidence of emergence excitement appears greater after its administration (Eckenhoff *et al.*, 1961). The combination of scopolamine with a barbiturate is subjectively more unpleasant than scopolamine plus a narcotic analgesic, or atropine with a barbiturate or an opioid analgesic (*see* Stephen *et al.*, 1969).

Glycopyrrolate. This longer-acting quaternary amine produces less sedation than scopolamine but is a more effective antisialogogue than atropine. It is also more effective in blocking the secretion of gastric acid (Taylor *et al.*, 1970; Salem *et al.*, 1976).

MOLECULAR MECHANISM OF ACTION OF GENERAL ANESTHETICS

Despite a considerable effort to formulate unitary hypotheses of the mechanism of action of general anesthetics, there is as yet no single theory that is generally accepted. Direct correlation between molecular events that are affected by anesthetics and the physiological effects that result from these actions is difficult. It is important to understand that many of the hypotheses that have been offered are only descriptive of the effects of anesthetics on specific biochemical and biological systems. While it is certain that these agents can affect a variety of processes, a basic theory must explain the relationship between the biochemical and physiological effects of anesthetics and their primary action.

Most theories of anesthesia are based on the physicochemical characteristics of the anesthetic drugs. These proposals rely heavily on the correlation between the potency of an anesthetic agent and the solubility of the drug in oil, first demonstrated by Meyer (1899, 1901) and Overton (1901). The precise nature of this correlation is demonstrated in Figure 13–4, where the MAC value for a number of anesthetics is plotted versus the olive oil:gas partition coefficient at 37° C. Interpretation of this fundamental result is thought to be crucial to the understanding of the action of anesthetics. It should be noted that other properties of molecules are also correlated with their potency as anesthetics. These include the ability to reduce surface tension (Traube, 1904; Clements and Wilson, 1962) and the ability to induce the formation of clathrates of water (ordered, crystal-like structures) (Miller, 1961; Pauling, 1961). However, such molecular properties are closely related to the fundamental physical forces that determine hydrophobicity.

The physical force that promotes the high relative solubility of molecules in oil compared to water is the so-called hydrophobic interaction. Molecules such as potent anesthetics that cannot form a significant number of hydrogen bonds and that are nonpolar distribute to sites in which they are removed from the aqueous environment. For this reason and because of the correlation of lipophilicity with anesthetic potency, it has been concluded that the primary site of action of anesthetics is either the lipid matrix of the biological membrane or hydrophobic regions of specific receptor proteins. Anesthetics can bind to proteins, presumably to hydrophobic sites. However, the absence of a satisfactory structure-activity relationship for anesthetic agents suggests that they do not produce their effects by specific interaction with a receptor protein. Thus, the most attractive possibility is that the primary action of anesthetics is exerted on the lipid matrix of the biological membrane.

Anesthesia in experimental animals can be reversed by the application of moderate pressure (~100 atmospheres) (Miller *et al.*, 1973). One interpretation of this observation is that a large change of volume may be crucially associated with the fundamental action of anesthetics. Phospholipids in artificial (model) membranes undergo a change of state as temperature is increased—the so-called gel-liquid crystalline transition of the phospholipid matrix. The temperature at which this occurs is dependent on the identity of the phospholipid, and the change in state is associated with an increase in the molar volume of the lipid. If anesthetics are present, the transition

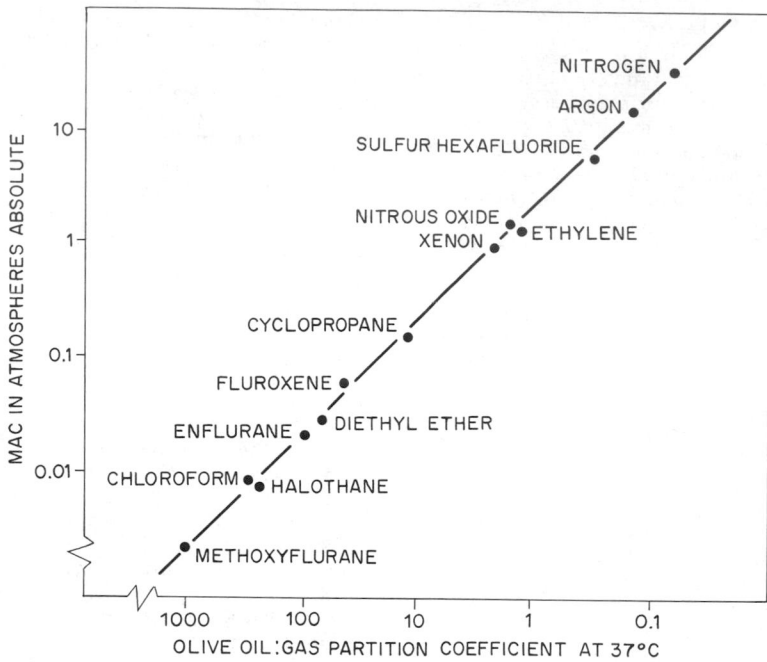

Figure 13-4. *The correlation of anesthetic potency with olive oil:gas partition coefficient.*

The correlation is shown for a number of general anesthetic agents and other inert gases not usually used for anesthesia. Note the log scales and the excellent correlation over a very wide range of fat solubilities and potencies (*see* Paton, 1974). (Modified from Eger, Lundgren, Miller, and Stevens, 1969; Miller, Paton, Smith, and Smith, 1972.)

from the gel to the liquid crystalline state of the phospholipids is more likely to happen; that is, it occurs at lower temperatures (Trudell *et al.,* 1973b). It is possible to rationalize the effect of pressure to reverse anesthesia based on such considerations. Furthermore, anesthetics broaden the melting curve for the gel-liquid crystalline transition (as if water melted between 0° and 5° C), indicative of a reduction in the number of phospholipid molecules that interact cooperatively at any time. The application of physical technics, such as nuclear-magnetic resonance and electron-spin resonance, indicates that anesthetics cause a local disordering of the lipid matrix (Trudell *et al.,* 1973a; Trudell and Hubbell, 1976). Because anesthetics appear to decrease the number of molecules of phospholipid that alternate *simultaneously* between the gel and liquid crystalline states, these drugs reduce the magnitude of fluctuations of volume that probably occur in dynamic biological membranes (Mountcastle *et al.,* 1978). It is hypothesized that such fluctuations are sufficiently large to be important in the regulation of the structural state of membrane-bound proteins (*e.g.,* their state of aggregation) and, therefore, of their functional properties (*see* Halsey, 1974). As inhibitors of such fluctuations, anesthetics could readily influence the fluxes of ions, which are crucial determinants of neuronal excitability, or other functions of membranes that are determined by the proteins that function in the milieu of a dynamic lipid matrix.

While many features of such hypotheses are conjectural, they are attractive and represent recent advances toward understanding of this interesting subject.

Adam, N. Effects of general anesthetics on memory functions in man. *J. Comp. Physiol. Psychol.,* **1973,** *38,* 294–305.

Adriani, J. Disposal of carbon dioxide from devices used for inhalational anesthesia. *Anesthesiology,* **1960,** *21,* 742–748.

Allison, Z. C., and Nunn, J. F. Effects of general anaesthetics on microtubules. *Lancet,* **1968,** *2,* 1326–1329.

Andersen, T. W., and Gravenstein, J. S. Cardiovascular effects of sedative doses of pentobarbital and hydroxyzine. *Anesthesiology,* **1966,** *27,* 272–278.

Artusio, J. J., Jr. Di-ethyl ether analgesia: detailed description of the first stage of ether anesthesia in man. *J. Pharmacol. Exp. Ther.,* **1954,** *111,* 343–398.

———. Ether analgesia during major surgery. *J.A.M.A.,* **1955,** *157,* 33–36.

Aukburg, S. J.; Miller, J.; and Smith, T. C. Interaction between meperidine and diazepam on the ventilatory response to carbon dioxide. *Clin. Res.,* **1976,** *24,* 506a.

Bancroft, W. S., and Richter, G. H. The chemistry of anesthesia. *J. Phys. Chem.,* **1931,** *35,* 215–268.

Bennett, A. E. How "Indian arrow poison" curare became a useful drug. *Anesthesiology,* **1967,** *28,* 446–451.

Berman, M. L.; Lowe, H. J.; Bochantin, J.; and Hagler, K. Uptake and elimination of methoxyflurane as influenced by enzyme induction in the rat. *Anesthesiology,* **1973,** *38,* 352–357.

Bernard, C. *Leçons sur les anésthesiques et sur l'asphyxie.* Baillière et fils, Paris, **1875.**

Bracken, A., and Cox, L. A. Apparatus for carbon dioxide absorption. *Br. J. Anaesth.,* **1968,** *40,* 660–665.

Brown, E. S.; Seniff, A. M.; and Elam, J. O. Carbon dioxide elimination in semi-closed systems. *Anesthesiology,* **1964,** *25,* 31–36.

Bruce, D., and Christiansen, R. Morphologic changes in the giant amoeba *Chaos chaos* induced by halothane and ether. *Exp. Cell Res.,* **1965,** *40,* 544–553.

Clarke, P. R. F.; Eccersley, P. S.; Frisby, J. P.; and Thornton, J. A. The amnesic effect of diazepam (valium). *Br. J. Anaesth.,* **1970,** *42,* 690–697.

Clements, J. A., and Wilson, K. M. The affinity of narcotic agents for interfacial films. *Proc. Natl. Acad. Sci. U.S.A.,* **1962,** *48,* 1008–1014.

Cowles, A. L.; Borgstedt, H. H.; and Gillies, A. J. Uptake and distribution of inhalation anesthetic agents in clinical practice. *Anesth. Analg. (Cleve.),* **1968,** *47,* 404–414.

———. The uptake and distribution of four inhalation anesthetics in dogs. *Anesthesiology,* **1972,** *36,* 558–570.

Cullen, D. J., and others. Clinical signs of anesthesia. *Anesthesiology,* **1972,** *36,* 21–36.

Cullen, S. C.; Eger, E. I., ii; Cullen, B. F.; and Gregory, P. Observations on the anesthetic effect and the combination of xenon and halothane. *Anesthesiology,* **1969,** *31,* 305–309.

Darbinjan, T. M.; Golovchinsky, V. B.; and Plehotkina, S. I. The effects of anesthetics on reticular and cortical activity. *Anesthesiology,* **1971,** *34,* 219–229.

Dauchot, P., and Gravenstein, J. S. Effects of atropine on the electrocardiogram in different age groups. *Clin. Pharmacol. Ther.,* **1971,** *12,* 274–280.

de Jong, R. H.; Freund, F. G.; Robles, R.; and Morikawa, K. I. Anesthetic potency determined by depression of synaptic transmission. *Anesthesiology,* **1968,** *29,* 1139–1144.

de Jong, R. H., and Heavner, J. E. Diazepam and lidocaine-induced cardiovascular changes. *Anesthesiology,* **1973,** *39,* 633–638.

de Jong, R. H.; Hershey, W. N.; and Wagman, I. H. Measurement of a spinal reflex (H-reflex) during general anesthesia in man: association between reflex depression and muscular relaxation. *Anesthesiology,* **1967,** *28,* 382–389.

de Jong, R. H., and Robles, R. Monosynaptic transmission in the cat's spinal cord: a quantitative measure of anesthetic dose. *Anesthesiology,* **1968,** *29,* 887–891.

de Jong, R. H., and Wagman, I. H. Block of afferent impulses in the dorsal horn of monkey. A possible mechanism of anesthesia. *Exp. Neurol.,* **1968,** *20,* 352–358.

Dobkin, A. B.; Israel, J. S.; and Criswick, V. G. Prolongation of thiopental anaesthesia with hydroxyzine, SA 97, thiethylperazine, and thioridazine. *Can. Anaesth. Soc. J.,* **1962,** *9,* 342–346.

Domino, E. F., and Corssen, G. Central and peripheral effects of muscarinic cholinergic blocking agents in man. *Anesthesiology,* **1967,** *28,* 568–574.

Downes, J. J.; Kemp, R. V. F.; and Lambertsen, C. J. The magnitude and duration of respiratory depression due to fentanyl and meperidine in man. *J. Pharmacol. Exp. Ther.,* **1967,** *158,* 416–423.

Dundee, J. W., and Haslett, W. H. K. The benzodiazepines. *Br. J. Anaesth.,* **1970,** *42,* 217–234.

Dundee, J. W.; Moore, J.; Love, W. J.; Nicholl, R. M.; and Clarke, R. S. J. Studies of drugs given before anesthesia. VI. The phenothiazine derivatives. *Br. J. Anaesth.,* **1965,** *37,* 332–353.

Eckenhoff, J. E.; Kneale, D. H.; and Dripps, R. D. The incidence and etiology of postanesthetic excitement. *Anesthesiology,* **1961,** *22,* 667–673.

Edmonds-Seal, J., and Prys-Roberts, C. Pharmacology of drugs used in neuroleptanalgesia. *Br. J. Anaesth.,* **1970,** *42,* 207–216.

Eger, E. I., ii. Effect of inspired anesthetic concentration on the rate of rise of alveolar concentration. *Anesthesiology,* **1963,** *24,* 153–157.

———. Respiratory and circulatory factors in uptake and distribution of volatile anaesthetic agents. *Br. J. Anaesth.,* **1964,** *36,* 155–171.

———. Intertissue diffusion of anesthetics. *Anesthesiology,* **1973,** *38,* 201.

Eger, E. I., ii, and Ethans, C. T. The effects of inflow, overflow, and valve placement on economy of the circle system. *Anesthesiology,* **1968,** *29,* 93–100.

Eger, E. I., ii; Lundgren, C.; Miller, S. F.; and Stevens, W. C. Anesthetic potencies of sulfur hexafluoride, carbon tetrafluoride, chloroform and ethrane in dogs: correlation with the hydrate and lipid theories of anesthetic action. *Anesthesiology,* **1969,** *30,* 129–135.

Eger, E. I., ii; Saidman, L. J.; and Brandstater, B. Minimum alveolar anesthetic concentration, a standard of anesthetic potency. *Anesthesiology,* **1965,** *26,* 756–763.

Eger, E. I., ii, and Severinghaus, J. W. Effect of uneven pulmonary distribution of blood and gas on induction with inhalation anesthetics. *Anesthesiology,* **1964,** *25,* 620–626.

Elliot, H. W.; Fisher, C. W.; de Lappe, A.; Davis, K.; and Botnik, E. Propiomazine, pentobarbital, hydroxyzine, and placebo: double-blind comparison of sedative effects. *Anesthesiology,* **1969,** *31,* 233–236.

Epstein, H. G., and Hunter, A. R. Anaesthetic apparatus: a pictorial review of the development of the modern anaesthetic machine. *Br. J. Anaesth.,* **1968,** *40,* 636–647.

Epstein, R. M.; Rackow, H.; Salanitre, E.; and Wolf, G. Influence of the concentration effect on the uptake of anesthetic mixtures: the second gas effect. *Anesthesiology,* **1964,** *25,* 364–371.

Finck, A. D.; Ngai, S. H.; and Berkowitz, B. A. Antagonism of general anesthesia by naloxone in the rat. *Anesthesiology,* **1977,** *46,* 241–245.

Fink, B. R. Diffusion anoxia. *Anesthesiology,* **1955,** *16,* 511–519.

Foregger, R. The classification and performance of respiratory valves. *Anesthesiology,* **1959,** *20,* 296–308.

Fragen, R. J., and Caldwell, N. Lorazepam premedication. *Anesth. Analg. (Cleve.),* **1976,** *55,* 792–796.

Freeman, A., and Bachman, L. Pediatric anesthesia: an evaluation of preoperative medication. *Anesth. Analg. (Cleve.),* **1959,** *38,* 429–432.

Frumin, M. J.; Herckar, V. R.; and Jarvik, M. E. Amnesic action of diazepam and scopolamine in man. *Anesthesiology,* **1976,** *45,* 406–412.

Gates, G., and Adriani, J. Disposal of carbon dioxide from apparatus used for inhalational anesthesia. *Anesthesiology,* **1962,** *23,* 148–149.

Gibbs, F. A.; Gibbs, E. L.; and Lennox, W. G. Effect on the electroencephalogram of certain drugs which influence nervous activity. *Arch. Intern. Med.,* **1937,** *60,* 154–166.

Gillespie, N. A. The signs of anaesthesia. *Curr. Res. Anesth. Analg.,* **1943,** *22,* 275–282.

Greene, N. M. A consideration of factors in the discovery of anesthesia and their effects on its development. *Anesthesiology,* **1971,** *35,* 515–522.

———. Anesthesia and the development of surgery (1846–1896). *Anesth. Analg. (Cleve.),* **1979,** *58,* 5–12.

Haggard, H. W. Absorption, distribution, and elimination of ethyl ether. *J. Biol. Chem.,* **1924,** *59,* 737–802.

Halsey, M. J. Mechanisms of general anesthesia. In, *Anesthetic Uptake and Action.* (Eger, E. I., ii, ed.) The Williams & Wilkins Co., Baltimore, **1974,** pp. 45–76.

Hill, D. W. The design and calibration of vaporizers for volatile anaesthetic agents. *Br. J. Anaesth.,* **1968,** *40,* 648–659.

Hillestad, L.; Hansen, T.; Melsom, H.; and Driveness, A. Diazepam metabolism in normal man. *Clin. Pharmacol. Ther.,* **1974,** *16,* 479–489.

Hoffman, J. C., and Smith, T. C. The respiratory effects of meperidine and propiomazine in man. *Anesthesiology,* **1970,** *32,* 325–331.

Kety, S. S. The physiological and physical factors governing the uptake of anesthetic gases by the body. *Anesthesiology,* **1950,** *11,* 517–526.

Kim, D., and Dobkin, A. B. Effect of premedication on duration of anaesthesia with halogenated vapours: chloroform, trichloroethylene, halothane, methoxyflurane, enflurane (ETHRANE) and isoflurane (FORANE). *Can. Anaesth. Soc. J.,* **1973,** *20,* 479–493.

Klein, R. L.; Graves, C. L.; Kim, Y.; and Blatnick, R. Inhibition of apomorphine-induced vomiting by benzquinamide. *Clin. Pharmacol. Ther.,* **1970,** *11,* 530–537.

Lauria, J. I.; Markello, R.; and King, B. D. Circulatory and respiratory effects of hydroxyzine in volunteers and geriatric patients. *Anesth. Analg. (Cleve.),* **1968,** *47,* 378–382.

Loan, W. B.; Morrison, J. D.; Dundee, J. W.; Clarke, R. S. J.; Hamilton, R. C.; and Brown, S. S. Studies of drugs given before anaesthesia. XVII. The natural and semi-synthetic opiates. *Br. J. Anaesth.,* **1969,** *41,* 57–63.

Lucas, G. H. The discovery of cyclopropane. *Anesth. Analg. (Cleve.),* **1961,** *40,* 15–27.

McDowall, D. G. Monitoring the brain. *Anesthesiology,* **1976,** *45,* 117–134.

McIntyre, A. R. Historical background, early use and development of muscle relaxants. *Anesthesiology,* **1959,** *20,* 409–415.

Mapleson, W. W. The elimination of rebreathing in various semi-closed anaesthesia systems. *Br. J. Anaesth.,* **1954,** *26,* 323–332.

———. An electric analogue for uptake and exchange of inert gases and other agents. *J. Appl. Physiol.,* **1963,** *18,* 197–204.

Marshall, M.; Longley, B. P.; and Stanton, W. H. Electroencephalography in anaesthetic practice. *Br. J. Anaesth.,* **1965,** *37,* 845–857.

Marta, J. A.; Davis, H. S.; and Eisele, J. H. Vagomimetic effects of morphine and INNOVAR in man. *Anesth. Analg. (Cleve.),* **1973,** *52,* 817–821.

Meyer, H. H. Zur Theorie de Alkoholnarkose. I. Mitt. Welche Eigenschaft der Anästhetika bedingt ihre narkotische Wirkung? *Arch. Exp. Pathol. Pharmakol.,* **1899,** *42,* 109.

———. Zur Theorie der Alkoholnarkose. III. Mitt. Der Einfluss wechselnder Temperatur auf Wirkungsstärke und Teilungskoeffizient der Narkotika. *Ibid.,* **1901,** *46,* 338.

Millar, R. D.; Wahrenbrock, E. A.; Schroeder, C. F.; Knipstein, T. W.; Eger, E. I., II; and Buechel, D. R. Ethylene-halothane anesthesia: addition or synergism? *Anesthesiology,* **1969,** *31,* 301–304.

Miller, K. W.; Paton, W. D. M.; Smith, E. B.; and Smith, R. A. Physicochemical approaches to the mode of action of general anesthetics. *Anesthesiology,* **1972,** *36,* 339–351.

Miller, K. W.; Paton, W. D. M.; Smith, R. A.; and Smith, E. B. The pressure reversal of general anesthesia and the critical volume hypothesis. *Mol. Pharmacol.,* **1973,** *9,* 131–143.

Miller, S. L. A theory of gaseous anesthetics. *Proc. Natl. Acad. Sci. U.S.A.,* **1961,** *47,* 1515–1524.

Morris, L. E., and Feldman, S. A. Considerations in design and function of anesthetic vaporizers. *Anesthesiology,* **1958,** *19,* 642–649.

Morrison, J. D.; Loan, W. B.; Dundee, J. W.; McDowell, S. A.; and Brown, S. S. Studies of drugs given before anaesthesia. XVIII. The synthetic opiates. *Br. J. Anaesth.,* **1969,** *41,* 987–993.

Mountcastle, D. B.; Biltonen, R. L.; and Halsey, M. J. Effect of anesthetics and pressure on the thermotropic behavior of multilamellar dipalmitoylphosphatidyl choline liposomes. *Proc. Natl. Acad. Sci. U.S.A.,* **1978,** *75,* 4906–4910.

Mull, T. D., and Smith, T. C. Comparison of the ventilatory effects of two antiemetics, benzquinamide and prochlorperazine. *Anesthesiology,* **1974,** *40,* 581–587.

Munson, E. S.; Eger, E. I., II; and Bowers, D. L. Effects of anesthetic-depressed ventilation and cardiac output on anesthetic uptake: a computer nonlinear simulation. *Anesthesiology,* **1973,** *38,* 251–259.

Munson, E. S.; Saidman, L. J.; and Eger, E. I., II. Effect of nitrous oxide and morphine on the minimum alveolar concentration of fluroxene. *Anesthesiology,* **1965,** *26,* 134–139.

Ngai, S. H.; Hanks, E. C.; and Farhie, S. E. Effects of anesthetics on neuromuscular transmission and somatic reflexes. *Anesthesiology,* **1965,** *26,* 162–167.

Overton, E. *Studien über die Narkose zugleich ein Beitrag zur allgemeinen Pharmakologie.* G. Fischer, Jena, **1901.**

Pandit, S. K.; Heisterkamp, D. V.; and Cohen, P. J. Further studies of the anti-recall effect of lorazepam. *Anesthesiology,* **1976,** *45,* 495–500.

Pauling, L. A molecular theory of general anesthesia. *Science,* **1961,** *134,* 15–21.

Quastel, J. H. Metabolic activity of neurons. *Ann. N.Y. Acad. Sci.,* **1963,** *109,* 436–450.

Rosner, B. S., and Clark, D. L. Neurophysiologic effects of general anesthetics. II. Sequential regional actions in the brain. *Anesthesiology,* **1973a,** *39,* 59–81.

Saidman, L. J., and Eger, E. I., II. Effect of nitrous oxide and of narcotic premedication on the alveolar concentration of halothane required for anesthesia. *Anesthesiology,* **1964,** *25,* 302–306.

Salem, M. R.; Wong, A. Y.; Mani, M.; Bennett, E. J.; and Toyama, T. Premedicant drugs and gastric juice pH and volume in pediatric patients. *Anesthesiology,* **1976,** *44,* 216–219.

Schwartz, H.; deRoetth, A., Jr.; and Papper, E. M. Preanesthetic use of atropine and scopolamine in patients with glaucoma. *J.A.M.A.,* **1957,** *165,* 144–146.

Seifritz, W. The effects of various anesthetic agents on protoplasm. *Anesthesiology,* **1950,** *11,* 24–32.

Smith, N. T.; Zwart, A.; and Beneken, J. E. W. Interaction between the circulatory effects and the uptake and distribution of halothane: use of a multiple model. *Anesthesiology,* **1972,** *37,* 47–58.

Smith, T. C. Nitrous oxide and low inflow circle systems. *Anesthesiology,* **1966,** *27,* 266–271.

Stephen, G. W.; Banner, M. P.; Wollman, H.; and Smith, T. C. Respiratory pharmacology of mixtures of scopolamine with secobarbital and with fentanyl. *Anesthesiology,* **1969,** *31,* 237–242.

Stoelting, R. K., and Eger, E. I., II. Percutaneous loss of nitrous oxide, cyclopropane, ether and halothane in man. *Anesthesiology,* **1969,** *30,* 278–289.

Taylor, W. J. R.; Llewellyn-Thomas, E.; and Sellers, E. A. A comparative evaluation of intramuscular atropine, dicyclomine, and glycopyrrolate using healthy medical students as volunteer subjects. *Int. Z. Klin. Pharmakol. Ther. Toxikol.,* **1970,** *3,* 358–364.

Torri, G.; Damia, G.; Fabiani, M. L.; and Frova, G. Uptake and elimination of enflurane in man: a comparative study between enflurane and halothane. *Br. J. Anaesth.,* **1972,** *44,* 789–794.

Traube, J. Theorie der Osmose und Narkose. *Arch. Ges. Physiol.,* **1904,** *105,* 541–559.

Trudell, J. R. A unitary theory of anesthesia based on lateral phase separations in nerve membranes. *Anesthesiology,* **1977,** *46,* 5–10.

Trudell, J. R., and Hubbell, W. L. Localization of molecular halothane in phospholipid bilayer model nerve membranes. *Anesthesiology,* **1976,** *44,* 202.

Trudell, J. R.; Hubbell, W. L.; and Cohen, E. N. The effect of two inhalation anesthetics on the order of spin-labeled phospholipid vesicles. *Biochim. Biophys. Acta,* **1973a,** *291,* 321–327.

———. Pressure reversal of inhalation anesthetic-induced

disorder in spin-labeled phospholipid vesicles. *Ibid.*, **1973b**, *291*, 328–334.

Vandam, L. D. Early American anesthetists—the origins of professionalism in anesthesia. *Anesthesiology*, **1973**, *38*, 264–274.

Warburg, O. The enzyme problem and biological oxidations. *Bull. Johns Hopkins Hosp.*, **1930**, *46*, 341–358.

Winterstein, H. *Die Narkose*, 2nd ed. Springer-Verlag, Berlin, **1926**.

Monographs and Reviews

Brazier, M. A. B. *The Neurophysiological Background for Anesthesia*. Charles C Thomas, Pub., Springfield, Ill., **1972**.

Clark, D. L., and Rosner, B. S. Neurophysiologic effects of general anesthetics. I. The electroencephalogram and sensory evoked responses in man. *Anesthesiology*, **1973**, *38*, 564–582.

Cohen, E. N. Metabolism of the volatile anesthetics. *Anesthesiology*, **1971**, *35*, 193–202.

Davison, M. H. A. *The Evolution of Anesthesia*. The Williams & Wilkins Co., Baltimore, **1965**.

Duncum, B. M. *The Development of Inhalation Anesthesia*. Oxford University Press, New York, **1947**.

Eckenhoff, J. E., and Oech, S. R. The effects of narcotics and antagonists upon respiration and circulation in man. *Clin. Pharmacol. Ther.*, **1960**, *1*, 483–524. (262 references.)

Eger, E. I., II. Atropine, scopolamine, and related compounds. *Anesthesiology*, **1962**, *23*, 365–383.

Eyring, H.; Woodbury, J. W.; and D'Arrigo, J. S. A molecular mechanism of general anesthesia. (Editorial.) *Anesthesiology*, **1973**, *38*, 415–424.

Faulconer, A., Jr., and Bickford, R. G. *Electroencephalography in Anesthesiology*. Charles C Thomas, Pub., Springfield, Ill., **1960**.

Faulconer, A., and Keys, T. E. (eds.). *Foundations of Anesthesiology*. Charles C Thomas, Pub., Springfield, Ill., **1965**.

Guedel, A. E. *Inhalation Anesthesia: A Fundamental Guide*, 2nd ed. The Macmillan Co., New York, **1951**.

Halsey, M. J.; Millar, R. A.; and Sutton, J. A. (eds.). *Molecular Mechanisms in General Anaesthesia*. Churchill-Livingstone, Ltd., London, **1974**.

Kaufman, R. D. Biophysical mechanisms of anesthetic action: historical perspective and review of current concepts. *Anesthesiology*, **1977**, *46*, 49–62.

Kety, S. S. The theory and applications of the exchange of inert gas at the lungs and tissues. *Pharmacol. Rev.*, **1951**, *3*, 1–41. (133 references.)

Keys, T. E. *The History of Surgical Anesthesia*. Dover Publications, Inc., New York, **1963**.

Papper, E. M., and Kitz, R. J. (eds.). *Uptake and Distribution of Anesthetic Agents*. McGraw-Hill Book Co., New York, **1963**.

Paton, W. D. M. Unconventional unanaesthetic molecules. In, *Molecular Mechanisms in General Anaesthesia*. (Halsey, M. J.; Millar, R. A.; and Sutton, J. A.; eds.) Churchill-Livingstone, Ltd., London, **1974**, pp. 48–64.

Richards, C. D. The action of general anaesthetics on synaptic transmission within the central nervous system. In, *Molecular Mechanisms in General Anaesthesia*. (Halsey, M. J.; Millar, R. A.; and Sutton, J. A.; eds.) Churchill-Livingstone, Ltd., London, **1974**, pp. 99–111.

Rosner, B. S., and Clark, D. L. Neurophysiologic effects of general anesthetics. II. Sequential regional actions in the brain. *Anesthesiology*, **1973b**, *39*, 59–81.

Roth, S. H. Physical mechanisms of anesthesia. *Annu. Rev. Pharmacol. Toxicol.*, **1979**, *19*, 159–178.

Shearer, W. M. The evolution of premedication. *Br. J. Anaesth.*, **1960**, *32*, 554–562; **1961**, *33*, 219–225.

Snow, J. *The Inhalation of the Vapour of Ether in Surgical Operations*. John Churchill, London, **1847**.

Sykes, W. S. *Essays on the First Hundred Years of Anesthesia*. E. & S. Livingstone, Edinburgh, **1960**.

Thomas, K. B. *The Development of Anaesthetic Apparatus*. Blackwell Scientific Publications, Oxford, **1975**.

14 GENERAL ANESTHETICS

Bryan E. Marshall and Harry Wollman

The state of general anesthesia is a drug-induced absence of perception of all sensations. Depths of anesthesia appropriate for the conduct of surgical procedures can be achieved with a wide variety of drugs, either alone or, more often, in combinations. General anesthetics can be administered by a variety of routes, but intravenous or inhalational administration is preferred, because the effective dose and the time course of action are more predictable when these technics are used. In this chapter the inhalational general anesthetic agents are described in some detail. The intravenous agents, including the barbiturates, opioids, and neuroleptics, are discussed in detail elsewhere (*see* Index) and, therefore, only their use for anesthesia will be presented here.

I. Inhalational Anesthetics

An ideal inhalational general anesthetic agent would be characterized by: (1) rapid and pleasant induction of, and recovery from, anesthesia; (2) rapid changes in the depth of anesthesia; (3) adequate relaxation of skeletal muscles; (4) a wide margin of safety; and (5) the absence of toxic effects or other adverse properties in normal doses. However, the availability of ultrashort-acting barbiturates, potent opioid analgesics with short durations of action, and specific muscle relaxants has reduced the necessity for the first three properties. The margin of safety and incidence of adverse effects are, therefore, the principal factors that now determine the acceptability of a general anesthetic agent.

The inhalational general anesthetic agents in current use are nitrous oxide, halothane, enflurane, and methoxyflurane; isoflurane is likely to become available soon in the United States. The inorganic compound nitrous oxide (N_2O) is a gas at normal ambient temperature and pressure, whereas the other four agents are volatile organic liquids (Table 14–1). None of these agents possesses all of the ideal properties. Certain generalizations are appropriate concerning the relative potency and the properties that result from their physical and chemical characteristics.

Potency. A standard of comparison for potency of general anesthetic agents has been elusive, and the introduction of the concept of *minimum alveolar concentration* (MAC; *see* Chapter 13) by Eger and associates (1965) provided an important and practical definition. The values of MAC in Table 14–1 demonstrate both the wide range of relative potencies and the greater potencies of the volatile agents compared to nitrous oxide. A dose of 1 MAC will prevent movement in response to surgical incision in 50% of subjects; doses that span the approximate range of 0.5 to 2 MAC are necessary for adequate anesthesia in individual subjects. A dose of less than 1 MAC may also be effective when requirements are reduced by disease or the presence of other drugs.

Vaporization. Volatile anesthetics are administered by flowing a carrier gas mixture (usually rich in oxygen) through a chamber that promotes the vaporization of the liquid compound. The greater the vapor pressure of the agent at room temperature, the greater is the volume of vapor that will emerge from the vaporizer mixed with the carrier gas. The saturated vapor pressures for the volatile anesthetics shown in the second column of Table 14–1 indicate that concentrations far exceeding 1 MAC are easily obtained. For example, the saturated vapor pressure of halothane is 243 torr, and, therefore, a carrier gas may emerge from the vaporizer with a concentration of approximately 30% (assuming the atmospheric pressure is 760 torr). This mixture must then be diluted with fresh

Table 14-1. PROPERTIES OF INHALATIONAL ANESTHETIC AGENTS

ANESTHETIC	MAC * (%)	VAPOR PRESSURE (torr at 20° C)	BLOOD:GAS PARTITION COEFFICIENT (at 37° C)	OIL:GAS PARTITION COEFFICIENT (at 37° C)
Methoxyflurane	0.16	22.5	12.0	970
Halothane	0.75	243	2.3	224
Enflurane	1.68	175	1.9	98
Isoflurane	1.40	250	1.4	99
Nitrous oxide	105 †	Gas	0.47	1.4

* MAC = minimum alveolar concentration (see text for further definition).
† A value of MAC greater than 100% means that hyperbaric conditions would be required to reach 1 MAC.

carrier gas, not containing halothane, to reduce the concentration respired by the patient to the range that is required for maintenance of anesthesia (0.3 to 1.5%). Precise design of vaporizers and careful metering of the anesthetic dose are necessary to avoid overdosage. In contrast, for nitrous oxide, not even 1 MAC can be administered at normal barometric pressures.

Induction of Anesthesia. None of the agents listed in Table 14-1 is irritating to breathe, and their odors are not unpleasant. The ease with which anesthesia may be induced depends, therefore, on the potency and the blood:gas partition coefficient; the former expresses what tension or partial pressure is necessary in the brain for anesthesia, and the latter is a measure of the quantity of vapor that must be transferred to the blood from the alveolar gas in order to achieve a given tension (see Chapter 13). The product of MAC and blood:gas partition coefficient is a guide to the relative dose of each agent. Compared to methoxyflurane or halothane, the achievement of the same depth of anesthesia with enflurane requires that 50% more anesthetic be absorbed; the similar use of nitrous oxide necessitates more than a 25-fold increase.

The fourth column in Table 14-1 lists the oil:gas partition coefficients. The greater the value, the more slowly the agent equilibrates in the fatty tissues and, conversely, the longer the period of elimination after discontinuation of the anesthetic.

Most of what follows in this chapter concerns the pharmacological properties of anesthetic drugs. Their influences on the lungs, heart, and circulation, as well as the less apparent actions on other organ systems, are

side effects that always accompany general anesthesia; accurate knowledge of these properties is required for safe management of the patient. Although inhalational anesthetics in current use are relatively inert and nontoxic, some are more prone than others to be metabolized. Certain of these metabolic products are now believed to determine the toxicity that follows the use of these drugs.

HALOTHANE

Chemistry and Physical Properties. Halothane, U.S.P. (FLUOTHANE), is 2-bromo-2-chloro-1,1,1-trifluoroethane (Table 14-2). It is supplied for anesthesia in amber-colored bottles, and its stability is further enhanced by the addition of 0.01% thymol. Soda lime does not accelerate the decomposition of halothane. Mixtures of halothane with air or oxygen are not explosive. Partition coefficients and the MAC value for halothane are listed in Table 14-1.

All metals tested (silver, brass, copper, stainless steel, magnesium, aluminum, bronze, and tin) except nickel and titanium are tarnished or corroded by halothane. The compound interacts with rubber and some plastics, but not with polyethylene.

The solubility of halothane in rubber can theoret-

Table 14-2. STRUCTURES OF VOLATILE GENERAL ANESTHETIC AGENTS *

* Note the varying halogen substitutions and that all of the agents, except halothane, are ethers. While isoflurane and enflurane are isomers, there are some important differences in their pharmacological properties (see text).

ically slow the induction of and the emergence from anesthesia as a consequence of the uptake or release of the anesthetic from the rubber elements in the anesthesia circuit when low-flow technics are used.

PHARMACOLOGICAL PROPERTIES

General Characteristics. Halothane is a potent anesthetic agent with properties that allow a smooth and rather rapid loss of consciousness that progresses to anesthesia with abolition of responses to painful stimulation. In practice, the rapidity, convenience, and pleasantness associated with the intravenous administration of thiopental are usually preferred for induction of anesthesia; halothane is then introduced for maintenance of anesthesia during the surgical procedure. The circumstances and requirements of the surgical procedure determine whether the patient is allowed to breathe spontaneously or is ventilated manually or mechanically; whether the trachea is intubated; and whether additional drugs, such as muscle relaxants or analgesics, are administered.

The clinical popularity of halothane is based primarily on the ease with which depth of anesthesia can be changed, the rapid awakening when its administration is stopped, and the relatively low incidence of toxic effects associated with its use. However, the margin of safety of halothane is not wide; circulatory depression with profound reduction of arterial blood pressure is readily produced.

The classical signs of depth of anesthesia summarized by Gillespie (1943) for ether anesthesia were based on changes in the pupil size, eye movements, respiratory pattern, and other actions that depend on certain properties peculiar to that agent (*e.g.*, sympathetic activation, respiratory stimulation, and slow induction). With halothane anesthesia, the pupils remain small because the sympathetic nervous system is not stimulated, respiration is depressed early, and induction is quite rapid. The signs of depth of anesthesia of most practical value are, therefore, the blood pressure, which is progressively depressed, and the response to surgical stimulation (*e.g.*, pulse rate, blood pressure, movement, or even awakening). The concentration of anesthetic agent that is necessary in the inspired gas mixture for induction of anesthesia must be appropriately reduced as

the alveolar concentration increases during maintenance if progressive increase in depth of anesthesia and decrease in blood pressure are to be avoided.

Circulation. Administration of halothane is characterized by a dose-dependent reduction of arterial blood pressure (Deutsch *et al.*, 1962), accompanied by reduction in cardiac output and stroke volume, as well as evidence of substantial alterations in the distribution of blood flow to various organs.

An important concept advanced by Price (1961) is that the hemodynamic changes observed with anesthetic agents depend on a balance between the pharmacological actions of the agent and the sympathoadrenal responsiveness of the recipient. The administration of some agents, such as ether, cyclopropane, and fluroxene (all seldom used or now unavailable), is associated with evidence of enhanced sympathetic activity and increased concentrations of both norepinephrine and epinephrine in the circulation. With these agents, cardiovascular depression can be readily demonstrated only in isolated organs or when the sympathoadrenal system is inactivated; in the intact animal, blood pressure is well maintained until the stage of anesthesia is deep.

With halothane and the other commonly used volatile agents, anesthesia is not associated with increased sympathoadrenal activity; concentrations of catecholamines in blood do not increase (Millar and Morris, 1961a; Perry *et al.*, 1974), and cardiovascular depression is evident. However, at clinical depths of anesthesia, sympathoadrenal response to stimulation is not abolished by halothane. An appropriate stimulus, for example, increased carbon dioxide tension or surgical stimulation, may cause an active sympathetic response with increases of blood pressure, heart rate, and concentrations of catecholamines in plasma (Price *et al.*, 1960).

Baroreceptor Control. Baroreceptors in the aorta and carotid sinus are the principal sensory organs for the afferent limb of baroreceptor reflexes. A decrease of blood pressure induces decreased discharge via afferent nerve fibers to the brain stem and release of inhibition of the vasomotor center with increased sympathoadrenal output to the effector sites; increased cardiac output and heart rate and vasoconstriction in various organs result.

Early work on this system demonstrated that halothane influenced the afferent discharge by "resetting" the baroreceptors to respond around a lower "set point" (Biscoe and Millar, 1964), depressed the vasomotor response of the brain stem (Price *et al.*, 1960), and reduced the sympathetic outflow that results (Alper *et al.*, 1969). However, the observed changes were small, and other investigations of the entire baroreceptor system led to the conclusion that the action of halothane on its central neural components accounted for only part of the depression of baroreceptor response (Epstein *et al.*, 1968).

Thus, in cross-circulation experiments with separate perfusion of the head from the rest of the body, Wang and associates (1968) demonstrated that administration of halothane to the head induced less hypotension than did administration to the rest of the body. In addition, there is little effect of halothane on the response of preganglionic sympathetic neurons to stimulation of baroreceptors (Skovsted *et al.*, 1969). It is concluded that the predominant actions of halothane are at the effector sites in the heart that control cardiac rate and/or contractility. Bagshaw and Cox (1977) demonstrated that baroreceptor adjustments of total peripheral resistance are well maintained during anesthesia with halothane.

Organ Blood Flow. Halothane influences the blood flow to every organ. In the skin and cerebral circulation, flow may increase as the vessels dilate. However, the cerebrovascular bed, as well as the renal and splanchnic circulations, loses some of its ability to autoregulate flow, and perfusion of these tissues decreases if blood pressure falls excessively. The coronary circulation remains responsive to myocardial needs for oxygen; vasodilatation occurs in poorly ventilated areas of the lung because of inhibition of pulmonary vasoconstriction that normally occurs in response to hypoxia.

In an individual patient, blood flow to each of these organs can be influenced by pH and carbon dioxide tension, posture, temperature, age, disease, and the administration of other drugs. It is, therefore, not surprising that conflicting results have been reported. However, there is agreement that, despite the differences from organ to organ, the total peripheral vascular resistance changes very little when hypotension occurs with halothane (Eger *et al.*, 1970; Sonntag *et al.*, 1978). Dilatation in one organ bed is offset by reduced flow in another, and, thus, the primary cause of hypotension is not generalized peripheral vasodilatation.

Heart. When anesthesia is induced by inspiration of halothane at concentrations necessary for surgery (0.8 to 1.2%), cardiac output is reduced by 20 to 50% from the level characteristic of the awake state (Marshall *et al.*, 1969). Both increased concentration of halothane and reduced arterial carbon dioxide tension (hyperventilation) accentuate the reduction (Prys-Roberts *et al.*, 1968).

It was suggested by Price (1960) that hypotension with halothane was due to depression of myocardial contractility, and study of preparations of heart muscle *in vitro* has repeatedly demonstrated such a dose-dependent depression (Sugai *et al.*, 1968). Confirmation in the clinical setting has been more difficult. For example, in man after some 2 to 5 hours of constant halothane anesthesia, all of the cardiovascular changes (*i.e.*, hypotension, depressed cardiac output, and bradycardia) tend to return toward normal; this has been attributed to sympathetic activation with time (Eger *et al.*, 1970). Nevertheless, there is general agreement that myocardial contractility is reduced during halothane anesthesia in man (Sonntag *et al.*, 1978). Animal studies have established that autoregulation of coronary flow remains intact and that any reduction of flow that is observed reflects the reduced oxygen consumption and work of the heart. No deficiency in supply of metabolic substrates to the myocardium is detectable in the normal heart, and there is no evidence of anaerobic metabolism. Merin and associates (1977) have concluded that interference with myocardial metabolism does not account for changes in contractility. While the mechanism of this depression of contractility is thus unclear, it can be reversed experimentally by administration of Ca^{2+}. It is suggested from the studies of Price (1974) and Shimosato and Yasuda (1978) that halothane may interfere with the availability of Ca^{2+} in the sarcoplasm. This hypothesis remains to be confirmed.

Thus, hypotension during halothane anesthesia results from two main effects. First, there is a direct depression of the myocardium and decreased cardiac output and, second, the normal baroreceptor-mediated tachycardia in response to hypotension is reduced.

Cardiac Rhythm. The heart rate is slowed

during anesthesia with halothane. This is, in part, reversible by atropine and is due to reduction of cardiac sympathetic activity with consequent vagal predominance. However, direct slowing of the S-A nodal discharge *in vitro* was observed by Reynolds and associates (1970), and atropine does not alter this effect. There appears to be both a reduction of the rate of phase-4 depolarization, which is normally responsible for the automaticity of pacemaker tissue, and an increased threshold for the generation of an action potential. During halothane anesthesia in man, vagal activity is further enhanced by manipulation of the airway. Sinus bradycardia, wandering pacemaker, or junctional rhythms are not uncommon at this time, but they are generally benign.

Tachyarrhythmias may also occur in the presence of halothane. Some of these may be of the reentrant type (*see* Chapter 31). Since halothane slows the conduction of impulses and also probably increases refractory periods in conducting tissue, it creates the conditions necessary for reentry, a unidirectional block with slow retrograde conduction (Atlee and Rusy, 1977).

Halothane may also increase the automaticity of the myocardium; this effect is exaggerated by adrenergic agonists and leads to propagated impulses from ectopic sites within the atria or ventricles (Zink *et al.*, 1975). Increased secretion of endogenous epinephrine may result from stimulation during surgery, if anesthesia is insufficient, or from increased arterial tension of carbon dioxide, if ventilation is inadequate. Alternatively, exogenously administered epinephrine may initiate the arrhythmia. Tachyarrhythmias are unlikely if, in the presence of halothane anesthesia, ventilation is adequate and epinephrine is used in concentrations of 1:100,000 or less and the dose in adults does not exceed 0.1 mg in 10 minutes or 0.3 mg in 1 hour (Katz *et al.*, 1962).

While all of the above-mentioned arrhythmias are generally benign in patients with a healthy myocardium, they may not be so in the presence of cardiac disease, hypoxia, acidosis, or electrolyte abnormalities.

Respiration. If the patient anesthetized with halothane is allowed to breathe spontaneously, an increased partial pressure of carbon dioxide in the arterial blood is common and is indicative of ventilatory depression; there is also an increased difference between the partial pressure of oxygen in the alveolar gas and in the arterial blood, indicating less efficient exchange of gas. Halothane thus influences both ventilatory control and the efficiency of oxygen transfer. To compensate for these effects, ventilation is frequently assisted or controlled by manual or mechanical means, and the concentration of oxygen that is inspired is increased.

Ventilatory Control. Characteristically, respirations are rapid and shallow during halothane anesthesia. Minute volume is reduced, and arterial carbon dioxide tension is increased to approximately 50 torr. Halothane causes a dose-related reduction in the ventilatory response to carbon dioxide (Munson *et al.*, 1966). While the precise effects of the anesthetic on the function of central and peripheral chemoreceptors are uncertain, the changes in the ventilatory response to carbon dioxide and the altered pattern of breathing caused by halothane are probably predominantly mediated at central sites of action (Ngai *et al.*, 1965).

In the awake state, the total ventilatory response to carbon dioxide is altered little by denervation of peripheral chemoreceptors. Therefore, despite evidence from Biscoe and Millar (1964) that halothane depresses the activity of the carbon dioxide–stimulated carotid body, it seems unlikely that this effect can be responsible for the ventilatory depression that is observed.

In contrast, the carotid bodies are the only chemoreceptors responsible for increased ventilation in response to arterial hypoxemia. This is abolished by denervation and by halothane (Hirshman *et al.*, 1977). It follows that adequacy of oxygenation during anesthesia cannot be assessed by observing ventilatory exchange. However, halothane depresses responsiveness to carbon dioxide even when the blood is hyperoxic.

The above considerations lead to the conclusion that depression of respiratory sensitivity to carbon dioxide by halothane results from a central action on the respiratory centers themselves. This view is further supported by investigations of factors that determine the rapid and shallow pattern of ventilation that accompanies halothane anesthesia. Some evidence of minor changes in sensitivity of pulmonary stretch receptors has been adduced by Coleridge and associates (1968), but, in general, the phasic activity of the vagal afferents is unchanged by halothane, and the essential sites of action are in the brain stem.

Pulmonary Oxygen Transfer. Efficient transfer of oxygen from the alveolar gas to hemoglobin in the alveolar capillary red blood cell depends on a proper balance between alveolar ventilation and perfusion. This balance is importantly controlled by the effects of gravity and various structural mechanical factors, and fine adjustments are provided by changes in the tone of the smooth muscle of bronchial airways and pulmonary vessels. All of these may be altered during halothane anesthesia. The influence of gravity obviously differs when the patient is in the horizontal position, particularly when ventilation is achieved by intermittent positive pressure. Halothane changes the relative movements of the rib cage and diaphragm (Tusiewicz *et al.*, 1977), alters lung volume (Laws, 1968), dilates bronchial smooth muscle (a useful property in asthmatic patients) (Coon and Kampine, 1975), depresses mucociliary flow (Forbes, 1976), and inhibits pulmonary vascular constriction in the presence of hypoxia (Bjertnaes *et al.*, 1976). The outcome is more or less impairment of oxygen exchange (Marshall and Wyche, 1972), with evidence of an increased fraction of blood to which no oxygen is added as it traverses the lungs (pulmonary shunt) and increased mismatching of ventilation and perfusion (Landmark *et al.*, 1977).

Nervous System. Electrical activity of the cerebral cortex recorded by a frontooccipital EEG shows progressive replacement of fast, low voltage activity by slow waves of greater amplitude as halothane anesthesia is deepened. Surgical stimulation may reverse this pattern, and such arousal reactions may be associated with recall of intraoperative events by patients, as in a dream (Bimar and Bellville, 1977). This sequence resembles arousal of the brain by activation of the brain stem reticular formation, but reticular neuronal activity is depressed by halothane (Shimoji *et al.*, 1977).

Cerebral vessels dilate during halothane anesthesia, cerebral blood flow increases unless blood pressure falls excessively (Wollman *et al.*, 1964), autoregulation is impaired (Miletich *et al.*, 1976), and cerebrospinal fluid pressure increases (Lassen and Christensen, 1976). The delivery of oxygen and substrates to the brain appears to be adequate, and there is no indication that halothane anesthesia interferes with energy metabolism in the brain unless excessive doses are employed (Smith and Wollman, 1972; Michenfelder and Theye, 1975).

Recovery of mental function after even brief anesthesia with halothane is not complete for several hours (Korttila *et al.*, 1977), but this phenomenon probably contributes little to the more prolonged impairment of psychological performance that has been reported after major surgery. Shivering during recovery is common and probably represents both a response to heat loss and an ill-defined expression of neurological recovery.

Muscle. Relaxation of skeletal muscle is desirable or necessary for many surgical procedures. Anesthesia with halothane causes some relaxation by central depression; in addition, the duration and magnitude of the muscular relaxation induced by competitive skeletal muscle relaxants such as *d*-tubocurarine or pancuronium are markedly increased (Katz and Gissen, 1967). The mechanism of this effect is not known but appears to be based on increased sensitivity of the endplate to the action of the competitive neuromuscular blocking agents.

Rarely, induction of anesthesia with halothane or any of the other halogenated inhalational anesthetics triggers a peculiar, uncontrolled hypermetabolic reaction in skeletal muscle of susceptible patients. The resultant syndrome of *malignant hyperpyrexia* is characterized by a rapid rise in body temperature and a massive increase in oxygen consumption; death may result. While this effect is probably dependent on a preexisting defect in muscle, it is a dramatic exaggeration of halothane's ability to interfere with calcium movement in muscle (Aldrete and Britt, 1978).

Uterine smooth muscle is relaxed by halothane. This effect is of sufficient magnitude to allow manipulation of the fetus (version) during the prenatal period. Inhibition of natural or induced uterine contractions by halothane during parturition may prolong the process of delivery, as well as increase blood loss. Thus, other agents or technics may be preferred for the relief of obstetrical pain.

Kidney. Anesthesia with halothane at a level of about 1 MAC causes dose-dependent reductions of renal blood flow and the rate of glomerular filtration to approximately 40% and 50% of normal, respectively (Mazze *et al.*, 1963). These effects can be attenuated or abolished by preoperative hydration (Barry *et al.*, 1964), and few effects are demonstrable in the absence of hypotension. Halothane does not interfere greatly with autoregulation of renal blood flow nor, in the normotensive state, with the distribution of flow between the renal cortex and medulla (Leighton and Bruce, 1975). Anesthesia is normally accompanied by the production of a small volume of concentrated urine. While some effects on tubular transport and endocrine regulation of the kidney have been noted, the changes in urine volume are probably secondary to circulatory responses and reduced glomerular filtration (Deutsch *et al.*, 1966).

In an occasional elderly patient, retention of water postoperatively results in hyponatremia, reduced serum osmolality, and mental confusion. There is no direct evidence that halothane anesthesia is responsible for this syndrome of inappropriate secretion of antidiuretic hormone. The renal effects of halothane anesthesia are rapidly reversed, and there is no evidence of postoperative renal impairment.

Liver. Hepatic function is depressed by halothane. The extent of this depression is similar to that produced by other inhalational anesthetics, and it is rapidly reversed when administration of halothane is stopped.

Splanchnic and, therefore, hepatic blood flow is reduced by halothane as a passive consequence of reduced perfusion pressure, but there is no evidence of ischemic dysfunction (Epstein *et al.*, 1966; Larson *et al.*, 1974).

Hepatitis. Hepatitis that occurs in the postoperative period is most often due to transmission of hepatitis virus (*e.g.*, in transfused blood), involvement of the liver by disease processes, or damage by known hepatotoxic drugs. However, a retrospective analysis of the records of more than 850,000 administrations of anesthetics suggested a small incidence of hepatic necrosis in which the above etiological factors did not appear to be present (Summary of the National Halothane Study, 1966).

Typically, some 2 to 5 days after anesthesia and surgery, a fever develops, accompanied by anorexia, nausea, and vomiting. Occasionally, a rash occurs and analysis of blood reveals eosinophilia and biochemical abnormalities characteristic of hepatitis. There may be a progression to hepatic failure, and death occurs in about 50% of these patients. The incidence of the syndrome is low, approximately 1 in 10,000 anesthetic administrations. Since it is seen most often after repeated administrations of halothane over a short period of time, the term *halothane hepatitis* is used. However, it should be emphasized that halothane is by far the most common general anesthetic agent in use, and the adjusted rate of occurrence is not statistically different for halothane than for any other general anesthetic agent. Thus, the conclusion that halothane should not be given repeatedly, and particularly not when the previous administration was followed by the signs or symptoms of the syndrome, probably applies equally to all the other potent inhalational agents in current use.

A possible basis for the above-described syndrome has been provided by the observation that halothane and all other general anesthetic agents are metabolized, at least to some extent (*see* below). Chemically reactive or immunogenic products may result. An excess of a toxic product or of a metabolite capable of inducing an immune response may lead to hepatitis. While evidence that such reactions occur has been obtained in both animals and man, this has only been observed in extraordinary circumstances (Sipes and Brown, 1976; Williams *et al.*, 1977).

Biotransformation. Approximately 60 to 80% of absorbed halothane is eliminated unchanged in the exhaled gas in the first 24 hours after its administration, and smaller amounts continue to be exhaled for several days or even weeks. Of the fraction not exhaled, approximately 15% undergoes biotransformation, and the rest is eliminated unchanged by other routes.

The mixed-function oxidase or cytochrome P-450 system in the endoplasmic reticulum of the hepatocyte is responsible for this metabolism. Chloride and bromide ions are removed from halothane but only a small amount of fluoride (the bond energy for C-F is nearly twice that for C-Br or C-Cl). It has been suggested that the concentrations of circulating bromide may be sufficient to cause changes in mood or intellectual function in the postoperative period (Johnstone *et al.*, 1975). The urine contains organic fluorine-containing compounds, mostly trifluoroacetic acid (Rehder *et al.*, 1967; Sakai and Takaori, 1978). Induction of microsomal enzymes may follow exposure to various drugs, including halothane, and metabolic breakdown may thereby be increased (Cohen, 1971). In addition, hypoxia or other abnormal circumstances related to disease may alter the metabolic pathways and result in the production of unusually toxic substances.

Several studies have suggested that occupational exposure to an environment containing halothane or other anesthetic agents for a prolonged period may result in an increased incidence of miscarriage of pregnancy (Vessey, 1978). While this has not yet been confirmed, effective steps to reduce environmental contamination are relatively simple and have already been instituted in most operating rooms; this seems prudent, indeed.

Evaluation. *Disadvantages and Limitations.* General anesthesia for surgery requires sleep, analgesia, suppression of visceral reflexes, and, to a variable extent, muscle relaxation; only the first is completely obtained with halothane. Analgesia must often be accomplished by the use of opiates or nitrous oxide, muscular relaxation is enhanced by specific relaxant drugs, and visceral reflexes are managed with other drugs as appropriate (*e.g.*, atropine for bradycardia or local anesthesia to obtund responses to visceral traction). Hypoxemia, hypotension, and transient arrhythmias may occur and sometimes require modification of the anesthetic technic; respiratory depression usually necessitates supplemental ventilation.

Advantages and Uses. Halothane has a moderately high potency and a moderately low blood:gas partition coefficient. Induction of and recovery from anesthesia are, therefore, not prolonged. Halothane is nonflammable. The larynx is not irritated, bronchospasm is uncommon, and, thus, induction is smooth. Nevertheless, thiopental is most commonly injected to induce sleep prior to the administration of halothane. Halothane is compatible with soda lime and may be used with oxygen to provide maximal oxygenation or combined with other gas mixtures such as nitrous oxide and oxygen. Its potential for inducing hypotension is sometimes utilized deliberately to reduce blood loss under carefully controlled conditions. Uterine relaxation can be valuable during version or extraction of a fetus.

Status. Halothane has enjoyed wide popularity for 20 years, and it is utilized for the entire range of surgical procedures. Its administration is associated with an excellent safety record (Summary of National Halothane Study, 1966). Appropriate equipment is available for precise administration of this agent in all situations. The introduction of enflurane and the availability of a variety of intravenous agents have somewhat reduced the use of halothane, but it remains the current standard for comparison.

ENFLURANE

Chemistry and Physical Properties. *Enflurane*, U.S.P. (ETHRANE), is 2-chloro-1,1,2-trifluoroethyl difluoromethyl ether. It is a clear, colorless, nonflammable liquid with a mild, sweet odor. It is extremely stable chemically and does not contain a preservative. It does not attack aluminum, tin, brass, iron, or copper. The partition coefficients and the MAC value for enflurane are listed in Table 14–1. Enflurane is soluble in rubber (partition coefficient = 74), and this may prolong induction and recovery somewhat, as described for halothane.

PHARMACOLOGICAL PROPERTIES

General Characteristics. The physical properties of enflurane assure that induction of and emergence from anesthesia and adjustment of anesthetic depth during maintenance can be smooth and moderately rapid. Technics of administration are very similar to those for halothane. Induction of anesthesia to depths appropriate for surgery may be achieved in less than 10 minutes when approximately 4% enflurane is inhaled. A short-acting barbiturate is usually infused intravenously to render the patient unconscious. As with any inhalational agent, the alveolar concentration approaches the inspired concentration with time, and the latter must be progressively reduced. Anesthesia is maintained with inspired concentrations of 1.5 to 3% enflurane.

There is mild stimulation of salivation and tracheobronchial secretions, but these are not usually troublesome, and the preoperative use of muscarinic antagonists is not routinely required. Laryngeal and pharyngeal reflexes are obtunded early, and excitement during induction is seldom observed.

The pupils remain small, and eye movements are not prominent; respiration is depressed, and ventilatory assistance is usually required; and, as with halothane, the most useful signs of depth of anesthesia are changes in arterial blood pressure, pulse rate, or movement in response to surgical stimulation.

Circulation. Arterial blood pressure decreases progressively as the depth of anesthesia increases with enflurane, to about the same degree as it does with halothane. Studies of the effects of the agent on the baroreceptor responses and preganglionic sympathetic activity are also similar (Skovsted and Price, 1972); there is evidence of reduced adrenergic activity, and there is no increase in the concentration of circulating catecholamines (Göthert and Wendt, 1977).

In-vitro preparations of myocardium show dose-dependent, reversible depression of contractility (Shimosato et al., 1969), similar to that caused by halothane at equivalent doses. In the intact animal, Merin and associates (1976) have demonstrated that depression of myocardial work is paralleled by diminished consumption of oxygen by the heart. There is no evidence of myocardial hypoxia.

No major differences between the potent volatile anesthetic agents have been observed with regard to their effects on blood flow to vital organs. There are, however, small differences. Bradycardia does not usually occur during anesthesia with enflurane; the pulse rate remains constant. Cardiac output is not decreased as much as with halothane (Marshall et al., 1971), at least at concentrations below 1.5 MAC, and the decreased blood pressure is due, in part, to decreased peripheral vascular resistance. In response to surgical stimulation or hypercarbia, cardiovascular depression may be reversed and blood pressure and cardiac output return toward preanesthetic levels. Administration of the β-adrenergic antagonist propranolol exaggerates hypotension induced by enflurane (Horan et al., 1977); this is also observed with other anesthetic agents. Doses of general anesthetics are, therefore, often reduced for patients who are receiving such drugs.

Cardiac Rhythm. In addition to the absence of bradycardia with enflurane, there is also a reduced tendency to arrhythmias. Enflurane does not interfere with impulse conduction in the heart to the same extent as does halothane (Atlee and Rusy, 1977), and the heart is not as sensitized to catecholamines (Johnston et al., 1976). Hypercarbia or the use of epinephrine for hemostasis or prolongation of the action of local anesthetic agents seldom promotes cardiac arrhythmias in patients receiving enflurane. However, it is prudent not to exceed the concentration and dosage of epinephrine that are advised with the use of halothane (*see* above).

Respiration. Enflurane causes increasing respiratory depression as its concentration is increased. At the level of 1 MAC, the arterial tension of carbon dioxide is greater than with other anesthetics, and depression of the responses to both hypoxia and hypercarbia are greater than with halothane (Hirshman et al., 1977). Curiously, and in contrast to halothane, tachypnea is less common. Assisted or controlled ventilation is usually employed; nevertheless, in order to reduce the incidence of central nervous system (CNS) seizure activity (*see* below), hyperventilation should be avoided. As with all inhalational agents, pulmonary exchange of oxygen may become less efficient during anesthesia, and inspired oxygen concentrations of 35% or more are given to avoid hypoxemia, especially in the elderly. Enflurane causes bronchodilatation and usually inhibits bronchoconstriction.

Nervous System. The occurrence of tonic-clonic muscle activity in a small proportion of subjects was noted early in the clinical use of enflurane (Virtue et al., 1966). Subsequently it was demonstrated that a characteristic EEG pattern may emerge when higher concentrations of enflurane are used or when there is hypocarbia. A high-voltage, fast-frequency (14- to 18-Hz) pattern progresses to spike-dome complexes; these alternate with periods of electrical silence or frank seizure activity with motor movements. Jerking or twitching of the muscles of the jaw, face, neck, or limbs may be seen. There is no evidence of anaerobic metabolism in the brain during the seizure (Wollman *et al.*, 1969) and, postoperatively, no unusual impairment of mental function. Furthermore, the seizures are of short duration, are self-limited, and may be prevented by avoiding deep anesthesia and/or hyperventilation. This excitatory action of enflurane is not thought to be of special concern, but the drug should be avoided in patients with seizure foci.

The other effects of enflurane on the CNS are similar to those of halothane. Cerebral oxygen consumption is reduced. Cerebral blood flow is increased when perfusion pressure remains constant, since vasodilatation occurs, and intracranial pressure is also increased. As the blood pressure declines, cerebral blood flow is at first maintained and then decreases if low values of pressure are reached.

Muscle. Skeletal muscle relaxation increases with the depth of anesthesia and is greater than that produced by halothane (Fogdall and Miller, 1975). Relaxation may be sufficient for abdominal surgery. Competitive skeletal muscle relaxants are more effective in the presence of enflurane (Waud, 1977), and the administration of small doses of these agents allows the use of lighter stages of anesthesia. The muscle relaxant activity of enflurane is caused by actions in the CNS and at the postjunctional membrane of the neuromuscular junction; it is not reversed by neostigmine.

Uterine muscle is relaxed by enflurane, and increased blood loss may occur during parturition, cesarean section, or therapeutic abortion.

Kidney. Reductions of renal blood flow, glomerular filtration rate, and urine volume during anesthesia with enflurane are similar to those that occur with equivalent depths of anesthesia from halothane; they are reversed rapidly when the anesthetic is discontinued.

Fluoride is a metabolite of enflurane (Mazze *et al.*, 1977; Sakai and Takaori, 1978); however, despite circulating concentrations (up to 20 μM) that far exceed those derived from halothane, concentrations of fluoride do not reach the threshold for renal toxicity (>40 μM). Even when there is renal failure in animals, plasma concentrations of fluoride decline rapidly after enflurane is discontinued, probably due to entry of the anion into bone. It is probable that anesthesia with enflurane is safe in patients with renal disease as long as the depth and duration are not excessive.

Liver and Gastrointestinal Tract. Evidence of hepatic impairment has been obtained during and after surgical anesthesia with enflurane. However, postanesthetic impairment is not apparent in volunteers and the hepatic effects of enflurane are rapidly reversed. Hepatic necrosis associated with repeated administration of enflurane has been reported, and another anesthetic agent should be selected if sensitivity is suspected from a previous administration of the drug (*see* above).

No unusual effects on the gastrointestinal tract have been reported. Splanchnic blood flow is reduced in proportion to perfusion pressure, but delivery of oxygen is not compromised. Nausea and vomiting occur in the postoperative period in perhaps 3 to 15% of patients, but to a lesser extent than with halothane or methoxyflurane.

Biotransformation. About 80% of the enflurane that is administered can be recovered unchanged in the expired gas. Of the remainder, some 2 to 5% is metabolized in the liver. This quantity is small because the presence of fluorine and chlorine, the absence of bromine, and the incorporation of an ether bond in the molecule increase its stability. In addition, the oil:gas partition coefficient is less than that of other halogenated anesthetic agents. For this reason, enflurane leaves the fatty tissues more rapidly in the postoperative period and is available for degradation for a relatively brief time. Biotransformation may be increased if hepatic enzymes are induced. The metabolic products that have been identified include difluoromethoxydifluoroacetic acid and fluoride ion. The significance of circulating fluoride with regard to renal function is discussed above.

Evaluation. *Disadvantages and Limitations.* Deep anesthesia with enflurane is associated with respiratory and circulatory depression. Seizure activity may occur when concentrations of enflurane are relatively high, especially when there is hypocarbia. This agent should be avoided when patients have preexisting abnormalities in the EEG or history of a seizure disorder. Uterine relaxation caused by enflurane provides a relative contraindication to the use of deep levels of enflurane anesthesia during labor.

Advantages. Enflurane allows rapid, smooth adjustments of the depth of anesthesia with little change in pulse or respiratory rate. While arrhythmias, postoperative shivering, nausea, and vomiting occur, they do so to a lesser extent than with halothane or methoxyflurane. Relaxation of skeletal muscle is often adequate for surgery, and interactions with competitive muscle relaxants allow smaller doses of enflurane to be used. If epinephrine is used parenterally with the same precautions as are described for halothane, arrhythmias are even less likely to occur than with the latter agent.

Status. Enflurane was introduced into general clinical use in 1973. It was utilized initially mainly as a substitute to avoid repeated administration of halothane, but it is now employed quite widely whenever an inhalational anesthetic agent is desired. Halothane is the more commonly utilized drug, but awareness of enflurane is still increasing. As more is learned, the differences between the two agents seem less striking.

METHOXYFLURANE

Chemistry and Physical Properties. *Methoxyflurane,* U.S.P. (PENTHRANE), is 2,2-dichloro-1,1-difluoroethyl methyl ether (Table 14–2). It is a clear, colorless liquid with a sweet, fruity odor. To retard decomposition, it is supplied in opaque bottles containing 0.01% butylated hydroxytoluene. It is stable in the presence of soda lime and is nonflammable and nonexplosive in air or oxygen in anesthetic concentrations. Physical properties of methoxyflurane and its MAC value are listed in Table 14–1; it is very soluble in rubber (partition coefficient = 635).

PHARMACOLOGICAL PROPERTIES

General Characteristics. Methoxyflurane is the most potent of the inhalational agents. Because of its low vapor pressure at room temperature, the maximal inspired concentration that can be obtained is only 3%. Because of extreme solubility in rubber, as much as 30% of the administered drug may be absorbed by components of an anesthetic circuit, thus reducing the concentration available. Furthermore, the unusually large blood:gas partition coefficient reduces still further the alveolar and hence the arterial tension of the drug early in administration. Nevertheless, since the MAC is only 0.16%, induction of anesthesia with methoxyflurane can be accomplished with inhaled concentrations of 2 to 3%. Induction is slow, requires perhaps 20 to 30 minutes, and is often associated with a stage of excitement. Overdosage is obviously unusual at this stage. For these reasons and because it is desirable to minimize the total dose, methoxyflurane is usually administered after anesthesia has been induced by the intravenous administration of a rapidly acting barbiturate. The inspired concentration of methoxyflurane that is required for maintenance of anesthesia is between 0.2% and 0.8%, and muscle relaxants are used as required. As with all inhalational agents, the administered concentration must be reduced as time passes, to maintain a constant depth of anesthesia. This may be estimated by evaluation of the extent of respiratory and circulatory depression, particularly as reflected in response to surgical stimulation.

The extraordinarily great solubility of methoxyflurane in lipid results in its accumulation in fatty tissue. Slow diffusion from these sites accounts for the prolonged and sometimes restless, albeit pain-free, recovery period.

Circulation. Cardiovascular depression with methoxyflurane is generally similar to that produced by halothane (Walker *et al.,* 1962). Systemic arterial blood pressure, pulse rate, and cardiac output are decreased progressively with increasing depth of anesthesia. Total peripheral vascular resistance is not changed, and, as with halothane, the primary effect appears to be decreased myocardial contractility (Shimosato and Etsten, 1969). Myocardial consumption of oxygen and coronary blood flow decrease, but there is no evidence of hypoxia.

Anesthesia with this agent is not accompanied by stimulation of the sympathetic nervous system, and concentrations of circulating catecholamines do not increase (Millar and Morris, 1961b). Cardiac arrhythmias are not frequent, but sinus bradycardia is the most common; it is responsive to atropine (Reynolds et al., 1970). If anesthesia is profound, A-V nodal rhythm may occur. If the sympathetic nervous system is activated by hypercarbia or by tracheal or surgical stimulation in the presence of an inadequate depth of anesthesia, ventricular arrhythmias may occasionally appear. The myocardium is sensitized to the action of injected epinephrine, but less so than with halothane. Arrhythmias can be avoided by observation of the same precautions.

Respiration. Ventilatory depression, as measured by the arterial tension of carbon dioxide, the response to increased carbon dioxide, or the response to hypoxia, is proportional to the depth of anesthesia and is slightly less than that observed with halothane (Larson et al., 1969). When spontaneous respiration is allowed, changes in ventilatory minute volume can be useful as a sign of depth of anesthesia. Methoxyflurane is not irritating to the respiratory tract. Secretions are not stimulated (hence premedication with atropine is not necessary), and bronchoconstriction does not occur (Coon and Kampine, 1975).

Muscle. Relaxation of skeletal muscles can be marked at deeper levels of anesthesia with methoxyflurane. The action appears to be a combination of central (Ngai and Hanks, 1962) and peripheral (Waud and Waud, 1975) effects and is additive with the action of the competitive neuromuscular blocking agents. However, the latter drugs are usually used to achieve relaxation of skeletal muscle so that the dose of methoxyflurane can be minimized.

Methoxyflurane does not relax the uterus and in normal doses has little effect on uterine contractions during labor. Its use in obstetrical practice, particularly during the first stage of labor, is thus of value.

Nervous System. As anesthesia is established with methoxyflurane, the fast, low-amplitude pattern that is characteristic of the EEG of the awake subject is progressively replaced by slower waves of greater amplitude. As with other agents, attempts to regulate the administration of methoxyflurane automatically based on changes in the EEG wave form have met with only limited success thus far.

Dilatation of cerebral vessels occurs and results in increased cerebral blood flow and increased intracranial pressure; cerebral consumption of oxygen is decreased (Lassen and Christensen, 1976).

Liver and Gastrointestinal Tract. Depression of hepatic function occurs as it does with other agents and is rapidly reversible. There is no evidence of direct hepatic toxicity, although postoperative hepatic necrosis has been reported, as with other halogenated anesthetics (see above).

Nausea or vomiting may occur in the postoperative period. The incidence is less than 20% and varies with the surgical procedure, premedication, and other factors.

Kidney. Renal blood flow, glomerular filtration rate, and urine flow are reduced, as they are with halothane. However, in the postoperative period, high-output renal failure may occur under certain circumstances. Crandell and associates (1966) first drew attention to this association, but 5 years passed before the cause-and-effect nature of the relationship was established by Mazze and coworkers (1971). All patients who receive methoxyflurane have concentrations of circulating fluoride as a result of biotransformation of the anesthetic. When the administration of methoxyflurane exceeds the equivalent of a dose of 1 MAC for more than 2 hours, the concentration of fluoride in plasma may exceed $40 \mu M$, and direct damage to the renal tubules occurs. The toxic syndrome is characterized by an inability to concentrate the urine, even in response to vasopressin (Cousins and Mazze, 1973). The resulting polyuria may result in dehydration, hypernatremia, and azotemia. Recovery is usual, but it may take a year; mortality rates in such patients have been reported to be as high as 20%.

It is this complication that has curtailed the use of methoxyflurane. To avoid renal toxicity, the dose and duration must be limited. Justification of its use in the first stage of labor is based on intermittent administration of the agent immediately preceding each uterine contraction.

Biotransformation. Methoxyflurane is metabolized to a greater extent than any other inhalational agent (Sakai and Takaori, 1978). As much as 50 to 70% of the absorbed dose is metabolized in the liver to free fluoride, oxalic acid, difluoromethoxyacetic acid, and dichloroacetic acid. The first two substances, particularly fluoride, cause renal damage.

Two characteristics of methoxyflurane are responsible for this occurrence. The molecule, despite the ether bond, is more susceptible to metabolism than are the other halogenated methyl ethyl ethers. Probably of greater importance is the great propensity of methoxyflurane to diffuse into fatty tissues. The drug is released slowly from this reservoir and becomes available for biotransformation for many days. The peak concentration of free fluoride in the plasma is found on the second to fourth postanesthetic day. There is considerable variation in the concentration of fluoride that is achieved. It is greater in obese subjects, in the elderly, and after induction of hepatic microsomal enzymes by drugs such as phenobarbital or phenytoin.

Evaluation. *Disadvantages and Limitations.* The potential renal toxicity of this agent dictates that it should not be used to achieve profound anesthesia nor for prolonged periods of time. Contraindications to its use include the presence of renal disease or the concomitant administration of drugs that induce hepatic enzymes or that are nephrotoxic. Respiratory and circulatory depression can be profound. Induction, maintenance, and adjustment of the depth of anesthesia are slow compared to halothane or enflurane.

Advantages and Uses. This agent was quite widely used for all types of anesthesia following its introduction into clinical practice in 1960. It is nonflammable, and it provides profound analgesia and good relaxation of skeletal muscles. Uterine contractions are not inhibited. Postoperative nausea and vomiting are not troublesome. It was initially thought that the low vapor pressure and delayed response to changes in the inspired concentration would provide a valuable increase in the margin of safety. The advent of precision vaporizers and appropriate technics of administration have lessened the need for such considerations.

Status. As a result of its renal toxicity, the use of methoxyflurane as a general anesthetic is limited. It is valued mainly for its analgesic potency during the first stage of labor, where small doses administered discontinuously do not result in sufficient accumulation of methoxyflurane or its metabolites to produce observable renal toxicity.

ISOFLURANE

Isoflurane (FORANE) is 1-chloro-2,2,2-trifluoroethyl difluoromethyl ether (Table 14–2). It is a volatile anesthetic with the physical properties summarized in Table 14–1. These values are similar to those of enflurane, since the two compounds are isomers. Induction of and recovery from anesthesia with isoflurane are slightly more rapid than with enflurane.

Myocardial function is well maintained with isoflurane (Perry *et al.*, 1974), and, in this respect, it is unlike all of the preceding halogenated agents. Blood pressure decreases with dose, but mainly as a result of dilatation of peripheral vessels. Cardiac output may increase markedly in response to hypercarbia. Cardiac arrhythmias are uncommon, and the heart is not sensitized to the actions of epinephrine (Johnston *et al.*, 1976).

Respiratory depression is more profound with isoflurane than with halothane, but this is characterized by decreasing tidal volume without change in respiratory rate (Hirshman *et al.*, 1977).

Skeletal muscle relaxation is adequate for many types of surgery; if a competitive neuromuscular blocking agent is required, its dose can be markedly reduced. There is less evidence of excitation of the CNS than there is with enflurane.

The properties of this general anesthetic agent are, therefore, attractive. However, in 1976, Corbett reported an increased incidence of hepatic neoplasm in mice repeatedly anesthetized with isoflurane, and the drug was withdrawn from clinical studies. A recent and more carefully controlled study has not confirmed Corbett's conclusions (Eger *et al.*, 1978). It thus seems probable that studies will resume and that this potentially useful general anesthetic agent may become available.

NITROUS OXIDE

Chemistry and Physical Properties. *Nitrous Oxide,* U.S.P. (dinitrogen monoxide; N_2O), is a colorless gas without appreciable odor or taste. It is the only inorganic gas that is practical for clinical anesthesia. It is marketed in steel cylinders as a colorless liquid under pressure and in equilibrium with its gas phase. The vapor pressure at room temperature is approximately 50 atmospheres. As it is released from the cylinder, some of the liquid nitrous oxide returns to the gaseous state; the pressure in the tank thus remains nearly constant until all the liquid has evaporated. The heat required for its vaporization is obtained from the walls of the cylinder and surrounding air, with the result that the tank becomes cold to the touch and may accumulate a deposit of frost. Nitrous oxide is heavier than air. Although nitrous oxide is not flammable, it supports combustion as actively as does oxygen when it is present in proper concentration with a flammable anesthetic. Fatal explosions have occurred with ether–nitrous oxide mixtures.

Nitrous oxide has relatively low solubility in blood, the blood:gas partition ratio at 37° C being 0.47. The drug is carried in the blood in physical solution only. Other properties are listed in Table 14 1.

PHARMACOLOGICAL PROPERTIES

General Characteristics. Since Colton administered nitrous oxide in 1844, it has passed through periods of greater or lesser popularity. It is currently used as an adjuvant during most procedures in which general anesthesia is employed.

Nitrous oxide can cause surgical anesthesia predictably only when administered under hyperbaric conditions. Paul Bert demonstrated this in 1879 by the use of 85% nitrous oxide in oxygen at 1.2 atmospheres in a pressure chamber. The MAC value is 105%, but there is considerable variability among individuals. Analgesia equivalent to that produced by morphine follows the inspiration of 20% nitrous oxide; some patients lose consciousness when breathing 30% nitrous oxide in oxygen, and most will become unconscious with 80%.

Nitrous oxide has been used as the sole anesthetic agent at inspired concentrations up to 80% and even beyond. In this situation the danger of hypoxia is obvious. The avoidance of hypoxic organ damage and the maintenance of satisfactory anesthesia for any but the briefest of procedures require maneuvering between very narrow limits, and this should no longer be attempted.

Another technic for the administration of nitrous oxide that has enjoyed considerable success includes induction of sleep by the intravenous administration of thiopental, accomplishment of skeletal muscle relaxation with neuromuscular blocking agents, and hyperventilation to reduce the arterial tension of carbon dioxide to approximately 25 torr. It has been suggested that the total muscle paralysis and the absence of respiratory drive augment the analgesia provided by nitrous oxide. Conditions for surgery are excellent, organ functions are depressed minimally, and recovery is rapid. However, there have been several reports of recall by patients of events that occurred during this type of "anesthesia." The subjects are immobilized and unable to communicate and their unconsciousness cannot be assured without appropriate supplementation with potent inhalational agents or intravenous drugs such as morphine.

The value of nitrous oxide is as an adjuvant. In the presence of 70% nitrous oxide in oxygen, the concentration of potent inhalational agents can be reduced. Reductions of MAC values in these circumstances are from 0.75% to 0.29% for halothane and from 1.68% to 0.6% for enflurane. Smaller doses of the halogenated agents, combined with some nitrous oxide, result in less respiratory and circulatory depression and more rapid recovery.

The uptake and distribution of nitrous oxide are influenced in relatively unique ways by its physical properties (Eger, 1974). A normal adult breathing 70% nitrous oxide will achieve 90% equilibration in about 15 minutes. During this time, approximately 10 liters of nitrous oxide will have been absorbed from the alveolar gas into the body. This volume change is more than ten times that which occurs during the inhalation of 1% halothane. This large uptake of gas has two effects, called the second-gas effect and the concentration effect (*see* Chapter 13). As nitrous oxide is removed from the alveoli, some additional fresh gas must flow in from the airways; this augments the ventilatory volume and increases the delivery of all the gases to the alveoli. This is the second-gas effect. At the same time, the flow of nitrous oxide into the blood stream reduces somewhat the total gas volume, so that the remaining gases are concentrated; this is the concentration effect. Clinically, the second-gas and concentration effects are useful during induction of anesthesia, since they increase the rapidity of uptake of a potent inhalational agent and also increase the alveolar concentration of oxygen, thus minimizing hypoxia. The reverse process occurs when the administration of nitrous oxide is discontinued (*see* Chapter 13). If air is abruptly substituted, the exchange of nitrous oxide from tissue and blood to alveolar gas results in a transient substantial decrease in the alveolar tension and, hence, the arterial tension of oxygen. This has been labeled *diffusional hypoxia* and can be a cause of postoperative hypoxemia, particularly when there also is respiratory depression following prolonged hyperventilation. Diffusional hypoxia has a limited time span, and adverse effects can be avoided by the administration of supplemental oxygen during the early recovery period.

Nitrous oxide exchanges with nitrogen whenever a nitrous oxide–containing mixture of gases is administered to a patient who had previously been breathing air. Since the blood:gas partition coefficient for nitrous oxide is 34 times that for nitrogen, a great deal more nitrous oxide is available for exchange. As a result, when nitrous oxide is administered, pockets of trapped gas in the body will expand as nitrogen leaves and is replaced by larger amounts of nitrous oxide (*see* Chapter 13). Such pockets may be found in an occluded middle ear, a pneumothorax, loops of intestine, lung, or renal cysts. Even air within the skull following a pneumoencephalogram is subject to expansion. This can result in large increases in pressure and volume, and nitrous oxide is thus best avoided in these circumstances.

Circulation. Nitrous oxide is generally employed as only one of several agents for general anesthesia. The potent inhalational agents have such marked effects on the cardiovascular system that the subtle influence of nitrous oxide may be easily overlooked.

When nitrous oxide is added to halothane in combined concentrations that do not alter the depth of anesthesia, the pupils dilate and the concentration of circulating norepinephrine increases. Under these conditions, arterial blood pressure, total peripheral vascular resistance, and cardiac output all rise

(Hornbein *et al.,* 1969; Smith *et al.,* 1970). Nitrous oxide depresses myocardial contractility *in vitro* but increases the responsiveness of vascular smooth muscle to epinephrine. The net effect of supplementation of halothane with nitrous oxide is a substantial reduction in the amount of halothane required to maintain anesthesia and, thus, less hypotension.

Supplementation of enflurane anesthesia with 70% nitrous oxide results in reduction of the concentration of enflurane that is required and in similar, but less marked, activation of the sympathetic nervous system. When combined with narcotics, nitrous oxide causes only further circulatory depression.

Respiration. The effects of nitrous oxide on ventilatory drive are generally small. Slight or no depression of the response to carbon dioxide has been reported with 50% nitrous oxide; however, when nitrous oxide is added to other anesthetic agents, further depression is unequivocal (Hornbein *et al.,* 1969). The response to hypoxia is reduced when 50% nitrous oxide is given alone (Yacoub *et al.,* 1976).

The relatively nonspecific changes in respiratory function that may result in an increased difference between alveolar and arterial oxygen tension during general anesthesia reemphasize the importance of augmentation of the tension of inspired oxygen. A concentration of not less than 30% oxygen is wise, and, therefore, not more than 70% nitrous oxide should be employed.

Effects on Other Organs. Like other anesthetic agents, nitrous oxide provides analgesia, unconsciousness, and depression of reflexes. It does not exert toxic effects on the CNS. Cerebral blood flow remains responsive to carbon dioxide, and autoregulation continues as perfusion pressure changes in the presence of 70% nitrous oxide (Wollman *et al.,* 1965).

Skeletal muscle does not relax in the presence of 80% nitrous oxide, and blood flow to muscle does not change. Unlike the halogenated general anesthetics, nitrous oxide is most unlikely to contribute to the production of malignant hyperpyrexia.

The liver, kidneys, and gastrointestinal

tract show no marked effects of nitrous oxide, and there is no evidence of toxicity (Larson et al., 1974). Nausea or vomiting occurs postoperatively in approximately 15% of patients.

Following very prolonged administration of nitrous oxide, there is evidence of interference with production of both leukocytes and red blood cells by bone marrow (Lassen et al., 1956). These effects do not occur within the time frame of clinical surgery (Amess et al., 1978). While long-term inhalation of nitrous oxide has been utilized to treat pain and discomfort, its value is limited. Of more practical concern is the effect of long-term, low-dose exposure of operating room personnel to the gas. As with halothane, there is little definitive evidence of adverse effects. However, with simple procedures to prevent contamination, the atmosphere of an operating room should not contain more than 50 ppm of nitrous oxide.

Biotransformation. Nitrous oxide is rapidly and predominantly eliminated as such in the expired gas, and a little diffuses out through the skin. Sufficiently precise methods have not been utilized to determine to what extent biotransformation may occur.

Evaluation. *Disadvantages.* Nitrous oxide is a weak agent, and attempts to provide adequate anesthesia may be accompanied by hypoxia if it is used alone. Transient postanesthetic hypoxia may also occur as large volumes of nitrous oxide are exhaled. Air pockets in closed spaces may expand in the abdomen, chest, and skull. Nausea or vomiting occurs to a minor degree postoperatively.

Advantages. Nitrous oxide is a nonflammable, nonirritating, and powerful analgesic agent; there is very rapid onset of and recovery from its effects. Its principal use is as a supplement to other specific and/or potent agents, and this allows the use of smaller doses of the latter and reduces the likelihood of complications.

Status. As a sole agent, nitrous oxide is used intermittently to provide analgesia for dental procedures and during the first stage of parturition. In combination with other drugs, nitrous oxide is given to the majority of patients who require general anesthesia.

DIETHYL ETHER (ETHER), ETHYL CHLORIDE, VINYL ETHER, FLUROXENE, CYCLOPROPANE, AND ETHYLENE

These six agents are chemically and physically dissimilar, but they have in common one property that renders them practically obsolete. They are all flammable and/or explosive at concentrations necessary for anesthesia, particularly in oxygen-enriched mixtures.

The use of diverse types of electrical equipment in the operating room resulted in the implementation of cumbersome and expensive procedures to prevent ignition of flammable gas mixtures. The search for nonflammable general anesthetic agents was a principal stimulus that led to the successful development of the halogenated agents described in this chapter.

In the past, diethyl ether and cyclopropane were of such significance as general anesthetic agents that, in some areas and for variable periods of time, they were relied on as the sole drugs for the production of anesthesia for all types of surgery. However, compared to the nonflammable halogenated drugs available today, flammable agents do not possess enough desirable properties to justify their use. Anesthesia with diethyl ether is characterized by prolonged induction and emergence, and a high incidence of postanesthetic nausea or vomiting. Anesthesia with cyclopropane is frequently associated with cardiac arrhythmias, and recovery is often associated with nausea or vomiting and sometimes hypotension. Ethylene has an unpleasant smell and only slightly greater potency than nitrous oxide.

There were thought to be certain redeeming features of anesthesia with diethyl ether, cyclopropane, or fluroxene. Their use is accompanied by increased concentrations of circulating catecholamines and evidence of sympathoadrenal activity. The cardiovascular system is stimulated and cardiac output and blood pressure are often maintained at or above normal values. This feature was once valued for patients with cardiac disease or hypotension following trauma, hemorrhage, and so forth. It is now recognized that these conditions require specific treatment and that sympathoadrenal stimulation from an anesthetic may add to the cardiac burden and hasten deterioration. Further information on these agents can be found in the *fifth* and *previous editions* of this textbook.

TRICHLOROETHYLENE AND CHLOROFORM

These two agents represent the older and now less useful halogenated compounds. They were popular in the past but are no longer used. Trichloroethylene offers no special advantages. It decomposes to form neurotoxins in the presence of hot soda lime and thus cannot be used in most breathing circuits. At adequate depths of anesthesia it produces bradycardia and tachypnea with shallow respirations and thus is useful only when supplemented with other drugs. Chloroform is hepatotoxic and nephrotoxic.

Even with current technics for precise administration, its toxicity exceeds that of other agents. Cardiac arrhythmias are not infrequent with either of these drugs and, particularly with chloroform, can lead to cardiac arrest.

II. Intravenous Anesthetics

The requirements for general anesthesia and surgery may necessitate the administration of several intravenous drugs with different actions to ensure hypnosis, analgesia, relaxation, and control of visceral reflex responses. While the use of intravenous drugs thus adds flexibility, it also increases the complexity. The relatively short duration of action of many inhalational agents is not an attribute of most nonvolatile compounds.

In this section the special properties of barbiturates and other agents that have special utility in surgical procedures will be discussed. More detailed discussions of each class of drug and their uses in other circumstances are presented elsewhere (*see* Index).

BARBITURATES

Barbiturates with a duration of action appropriate to the requirements of surgery became available with the introduction of thiopental by Lundy in 1935. Its use during general anesthesia continues greatly to exceed that of any other barbiturate.

Chemistry and Preparations. *Thiopental Sodium,* U.S.P. (PENTOTHAL), is supplied for clinical use as the water-soluble sodium salt (*Thiopental Sodium for Injection,* U.S.P.). Included with each gram of thiopental sodium is 60 mg of sodium carbonate. Solutions of the mixture are thus strongly alkaline (pH 11). After injection into the blood stream, the sodium carbonate is neutralized and the thiopental is converted in large part into its acidic, nonionized form. It does not precipitate in the blood because it is rapidly diluted and strongly bound to plasma proteins, especially albumin. When thiopental sodium is dissolved in *Sterile Water for Injection,* U.S.P., a 2.8% solution is isotonic; concentrations less than 2% may cause hemolysis.

Other ultrashort-acting barbiturates include *Methohexital,* U.S.P. (BREVITAL), which is supplied for use as *Methohexital Sodium for Injection,* U.S.P. The pH of its aqueous solutions is 11. Thiamylal (SURITAL) is available as *Thiamylal Sodium for Injection,* U.S.P.

PHARMACOLOGICAL PROPERTIES

Pharmacokinetics. Following a single intravenous anesthetic dose of thiopental sodium, unconsciousness occurs after 10 to 20 seconds (the time required for the drug to circulate from the arm to the brain). The depth of anesthesia may increase for up to 40 seconds and then decreases progressively until consciousness returns in 20 to 30 minutes. This sequence reflects the changes in concentration of thiopental at its sites of action in the brain and is a consequence of the initial distribution of the drug to the brain, followed by its subsequent redistribution to other tissues. This is discussed fully in Chapters 1 and 17. At the time of awakening, the plasma concentration may be 10% of the peak value. When all tissues contain sufficient quantities of thiopental, redistribution does not result in such a precipitous drop of the concentrations in plasma, and the duration of action is prolonged. When too great a total quantity of thiopental is administered, recovery may require many hours.

Thiopental is metabolized slowly in the liver and, while this may involve only a fraction of the circulating drug, it has been shown by Saidman and Eger (1966) to be a significant factor in limiting the duration of anesthesia. For methohexital, metabolic degradation may be of even greater importance. Other factors, such as the binding of thiopental by plasma proteins, change in the nonionized fraction of the drug following changes in blood pH, or changes in the distribution of blood flow, may also influence the depth of anesthesia.

General Anesthetic Action. Neurophysiologic investigations in animals and man suggest that general anesthesia with thiopental results from suppression of the reticular activating system in the brain stem. With small doses of thiopental, excitatory responses may be observed, suggesting release from higher control as inhibitory regions are depressed first. The signs of anesthesia are not particularly characteristic; pupils are of small or normal size, eyeballs are fixed and usually central, eyelash and tendon reflexes are diminished, and respiration and circulation are somewhat depressed. However, thiopental and other barbiturates are poor analgesics and may even increase the sensitivity to pain when administered in inadequate amounts (Dundee, 1960). In these circumstances, evidence of sympathetic response becomes manifest with tachycardia, dilated pupils, tears, sweating, tachypnea, increased blood pressure, and movement or vocalization in response to surgery.

Respiration. Unlike some of the inhalational anesthetics, thiopental is not irritating to the respiratory tract, and yet coughing, laryngospasm, and even bronchospasm occur with some frequency. The basis of these reactions is unknown; they disappear as a deeper phase of anesthesia is established. The presence of saliva, the insertion of an airway, or partial obstruction by soft tissues may trigger one or all of these responses. Moderate doses of thiopental do not depress these airway reflexes.

Thiopental produces a dose-related depression of respiration that can be profound. Both the response to carbon dioxide and the response to hypoxia are reduced or even abolished (Hirshman *et al.*, 1975). Following a dose of thiopental sufficient to cause sleep, tidal volume is decreased, and, despite a small increase of respiratory rate, the minute volume is reduced; the arterial tension of carbon dioxide rises slightly. Larger doses of thiopental cause more profound changes, and respiration is maintained only by movements of the diaphragm. Surgical manipulations provide a stimulus to respiration and, within limits, can offset the respiratory depression.

Circulation. Direct exposure of heart muscle to thiopental and other barbiturates *in vitro* causes inhibition of myocardial contractility (Altura and Altura, 1975), and the tone of vascular smooth muscle is generally decreased *in vitro. In vivo*, following the administration of an anesthetic dose of thiopental to a normal adult, the arterial blood pressure decreases only *transiently* and then returns essentially to normal. Cardiac output is usually decreased somewhat, but total peripheral vascular resistance is unchanged or increased. Blood flow to the skin and brain is decreased, but that to other organs remains essentially normal.

However, in the presence of hemorrhage or other form of hypovolemia, circulatory instability, sepsis, toxemia, or shock, the administration of a "normal" dose of thiopental may result in hypotension, circulatory collapse, and cardiac arrest. In such patients, thiopental or any other general anesthetic agent should be used very cautiously.

The baroreceptor system appears unaffected, but there is a reduction of sympathetic nerve activity. Concentrations of catecholamines in plasma are not increased, and the heart is not sensitized to epinephrine. Arrhythmias are uncommon except in the presence of hypercarbia or arterial hypoxemia.

Cerebral blood flow and cerebral metabolic rate are reduced with thiopental and other barbiturates. There is a marked reduction of intracranial pressure, and this effect is utilized clinically in anesthesia for neurosurgery or in other circumstances when elevated intracranial pressures are expected (Shapiro, 1975). When prolonged effects on cerebral blood flow, metabolic rate, and intracranial pressure are desired, a longer-acting barbiturate (*e.g.*, pentobarbital) is more appropriate.

Other Organs. Relaxation of skeletal muscle is transient and occurs only at the onset of anesthesia. When procedures require additional relaxation of skeletal muscle, other agents must be used in addition. Thiopental has little effect on uterine contractions, but it does cross the placenta and depresses the fetus. The functions of liver and kidney are depressed only with large doses, and then only transiently.

Clinical Use. Thiopental sodium is administered intravenously. It may be injected either as a single bolus, intermittently, or as a continuous infusion. The latter technic has had some popularity, and fixed mixtures of several drugs (*e.g.*, thiopental, an opioid analgesic, and a muscle relaxant) have been infused to obtain full surgical anesthesia. However, this approach is to be deplored, for it eliminates the one principal advantage of intravenous anesthesia—the ability to choose drugs with very specific actions and to titrate doses to suit the response of the patient. In addition, the use of a continuous infusion increases the likelihood of overdosage, with a subsequent prolonged recovery period.

For single or intermittent injections of thiopental sodium, the concentration employed should not exceed 2.5% in aqueous solution. Solutions of thiopental are irritating and painful if deposited extravascularly, and the effective dose then cannot be precisely determined; injections are, therefore, most safely made into the side port of a flowing intravenous infusion of saline solution or 5% dextrose in water.

If concentrations greater than 2.5% are injected extravascularly, the pain may be severe and tissue necrosis can occur. Of even greater concern are the results of inadvertent intra-arterial injection of concentrated solutions of thiopental. The arterial endothelium and deeper layers are immediately damaged and endarteritis follows, often with thrombosis exacerbated by arteriolar spasm as norepinephrine is released (Brown et al., 1968). Vascular ischemia and even gangrene may result. Because damage to the arterial wall is instantaneous, the aim of treatment is to reduce the response and hence limit the lesion. If the infusion needle is still in situ, 5 to 10 ml of 1% procaine may serve to reduce the pain and the arteriospasm. Heparin may inhibit thrombosis, and a regional block of the sympathetic nerves may also induce arterial dilatation. Permanent and serious sequelae have not been reported to follow intra-arterial injection of 2.5% solutions of thiopental and do not occur with 1% solutions of methohexital.

For induction of anesthesia in an adult patient, the usual procedure is to inject a 50-mg test dose moderately rapidly, observe the response, and then inject an additional 100 to 200 mg over 20 seconds. In a muscular, robust individual, as much as 500 mg may occasionally be necessary to induce general anesthesia. If the dose is injected too slowly, a stage of excitement may be encountered that can result in dislodgment of the needle. Such excitatory movements are more common with methohexital. Conversely, if too much drug is injected too rapidly, profound anesthesia may supervene with apnea and hypotension. The usual response after a correctly chosen dose is for the patient to experience a faint taste of garlic, followed by a suppressed yawn and then the smooth, rapid appearance of sleep. There is an initial and transient period of relaxation, which may be appropriate for very short procedures such as correction of a dislocation, and the airway may become impaired by the infolding of soft tissues around the tongue and pharynx.

After this point the drugs to be used for maintenance of anesthesia can be administered. Most commonly, these will be an inhalational agent with or without nitrous oxide, opioid analgesics, or muscle relaxants. For short procedures that are not especially painful, intermittent doses of thiopental combined with nitrous oxide are satisfactory, particularly if an analgesic was given preoperatively. A total dose of 1 g of thiopental should not generally be exceeded if prolonged recovery is to be avoided. The larger the initial dose of thiopental that is required, the larger the supplementary doses must be, even in patients of the same size. Patients who require a large initial dose of thiopental will awaken despite plasma concentrations that would normally cause sleep. This phenomenon is termed acute tolerance, and, while its nature is obscure, it is important in its effects on total drug dosage (Dundee et al., 1956).

Recovery following thiopental should be characterized by smooth, rapid awakening to consciousness. However, if there is postoperative pain, restlessness may become evident and analgesics should be given (an antianalgesic effect of thiopental at low circulating concentrations may be partially responsible). There is often shivering postoperatively as heat is generated to restore body temperature that has decreased during anesthesia and surgery. Postural hypotension may be encountered, and patients should not be moved too hurriedly.

Evaluation. *Disadvantages.* Most of the complications associated with the use of thiopental are minor and can be avoided or minimized by judicious use of the drug. Extravenous or intra-arterial injection should be uncommon and, if concentrations no greater than 2.5% are used, are unlikely to cause serious damage. Cough, laryngospasm, and bronchospasm can be serious in certain patients, such as those with elevated intracranial pressure, pharyngeal infections, unstable aneurysms, or asthma. In each such case, adequate anesthesia should be ensured prior to stimulation of the airway.

Overdosage can occur if the specific requirements for each patient are not estimated correctly. The result is hypotension, respiratory depression, and/or prolongation of awakening. There is no effective agent to antagonize the actions of the barbiturates. Hexobarbital and methohexital both cause a higher incidence of motor movements during induction of anesthesia.

The presence of *variegate porphyria* (South African) or *acute intermittent porphyria* constitutes an absolute contraindication to the use of barbiturates. In these two forms of porphyria, thiopental or other barbiturates may precipitate a widespread demyelination of peripheral and cranial nerves and disseminated lesions throughout the CNS, resulting in pain, weakness, and paralysis that may be life threatening (Dean, 1971). Other types of porphyria do not contraindicate the use of barbiturates; this has been a point of confusion.

Advantages. The outstanding advantages of thiopental are rapid, pleasant induction of anesthesia and fast recovery therefrom, with little postanesthetic excitement or vomiting. The use of methohexital is associated with even more rapid recovery of consciousness. These drugs may be given to induce anesthesia prior to administration of a more potent agent, or they can be used alone to provide anesthesia for short procedures that are associated with little pain. They are useful to promote light sleep during regional local anesthesia and for quieting excitement or controlling convulsions.

Status. The ultrashort-acting barbiturates have an important place in the practice of anesthesiology. Thiopental sodium remains the standard for comparison. General anesthesia is most often initiated by an injection of thiopental to induce sleep prior to administration of the more potent agents that are necessary for the surgical procedure.

OPIOID ANALGESICS

The detailed pharmacology of the opioids is discussed in Chapter 22. Morphine, meperidine, fentanyl, or other analgesics are frequently employed as supplements during general anesthesia with inhalational or intravenous agents. For this purpose, intravenous doses of 1 to 2 mg of morphine, 10 to 25 mg of meperidine, and 0.05 to 0.1 mg of fentanyl are approximately equivalent and may provide analgesia for about 90, 45, and 30 minutes, respectively. Respiratory depression, mild decreases in blood pressure, some delay in awakening, and an appreciable incidence of postoperative nausea or vomiting accompany the use of these drugs.

In some situations, very large doses of morphine have been infused to obtain anesthesia. Morphine has been given slowly intravenously in doses of 1 to 3 mg/kg over 15 to 20 minutes to induce analgesia and unconsciousness. Respiratory depression is severe, and ventilation must be mechanically controlled, often for extended periods of time. The addition of nitrous oxide adds further to the anesthesia, and administration of competitive skeletal muscle relaxants provides good conditions for surgery. It is perhaps unexpected that the cardiovascular system is not severely depressed with such large doses of morphine. Lowenstein and associates (1969) showed that patients with normal cardiac function experienced no significant changes, while an increase in cardiac output and stroke volume and a decrease in total peripheral resistance often occur in those with cardiac disease. Blood flow to organs is maintained. For example, autoregulation of the cerebral circulation is unimpaired even at the higher dose range (3 mg/kg); similarly, renal function is well maintained.

The morphine–nitrous oxide technic has been utilized quite widely for cardiac surgery. Despite the large doses of morphine, some patients are evidently not sufficiently anesthetized and may become hypertensive during surgery; postoperative recall of events as a terrifying dream or psychosis may also occur. The addition of nitrous oxide provides a greater depth of anesthesia but nullifies the stimulatory effects of morphine on the circulation of those with cardiac disease (Stoelting and Gibbs, 1973).

Status. Opioid analgesics are widely used to provide relief from pain during general anesthesia of all types. Judicious use of these agents intravenously can provide analgesia of rapid onset and appropriate duration; smaller doses of general anesthetics are then required.

When large doses of morphine are employed to provide general anesthesia, reversal of its effects with naloxone is unsatisfactory, and it is usually necessary to ventilate patients mechanically for an additional 12 to 24 hours. The technic has fallen from favor for this reason.

NEUROLEPTIC-OPIOID COMBINATIONS

Neuroleptic compounds, such as the butyrophenone derivative *droperidol* (INAPSINE), produce a state of quiescence with reduced motor activity, reduced anxiety, and indifference to the surroundings. Sleep is not necessarily induced, and patients are responsive to commands. In addition to inducing neurolepsis, droperidol has adrenergic blocking, antiemetic, antifibrillatory, and anticonvulsant actions, and it enhances the effects of other CNS depressants.

When a potent narcotic analgesic such as fentanyl citrate is combined with droperidol, a state of neurolept analgesia is established, during which a variety of diagnostic or minor surgical procedures can be accomplished; these include bronchoscopy, radiological studies, burn dressings, cystoscopy, and the like. Neurolept analgesia can be converted to neurolept anesthesia by the concurrent administration of 65% nitrous oxide in oxygen.

Clinical Use. Droperidol and fentanyl citrate may be used alone or together, the dose of each being adjusted individually, but most often a precompounded mixture (INNOVAR) is used. Each milliliter of this preparation contains 0.05 mg of fentanyl citrate and 2.5 mg of droperidol.

A useful technic for adults is to mix a dose of 0.1 ml/kg of INNOVAR in 250 ml of 5% dextrose in water and to infuse this solution intravenously over a period of 5 to 10 minutes. If the rate of infusion is too slow, delirium and excitement may occur, sometimes with laryngospasm. If the rate is too rapid, spasm of the chest wall may supervene, and respiratory exchange can become impossible, even by artificial means. This untoward response is easily managed by the intravenous administration of a rapidly acting neuromuscular blocking agent, such as succinylcholine. Normally, after approximately 3 to 4 minutes, the recipient appears to fall asleep and may cease to breathe, except on command. Should an endotracheal tube be required to ensure adequate ventilation, a smaller dose of the combination will suffice if the larynx and trachea are anesthetized by the topical application of a local anesthetic.

Circulatory effects of neurolept anesthesia are not generally marked. Droperidol has a slight α-adrenergic blocking action that results in moderate hypotension. A parasympathomimetic effect of fentanyl accounts for bradycardia; administration of atropine will prevent this. Cerebral blood flow and cerebral metabolism are reduced, and there may be marked reduction of elevated intracranial pressure, provided that the arterial tension of carbon dioxide does not increase when respiration is depressed. Care should be taken to avoid abrupt changes in posture, since severe hypotension may be precipitated. Other than bradycardia, cardiac arrhythmias are rare, and the heart is not sensitized to the effects of epinephrine.

In contrast to the circulatory effects, respiratory depression is marked (Dunbar et al., 1967). Assisted or controlled ventilation is necessary, and respiration of an oxygen-enriched gas mixture is desirable.

Droperidol has a prolonged duration of action (3 to 6 hours), whereas fentanyl exerts its analgesic effect for only about 30 minutes. Following induction of neurolept anesthesia, supplementary doses of fentanyl alone (1 μg/kg) are injected at intervals of approximately 20 minutes. Indications for additional doses include evidence of sympathetic activity with increasing pulse rate and blood pressure, sweating, and limb movements.

Recovery. Consciousness is recovered rapidly after the administration of nitrous oxide is stopped, but patients remain free of pain and drowsy, although arousable. Nausea or vomiting occurs in 5 to 10% of patients; confusion and a depressed mental state may become apparent.

Respiratory depression may persist into the postoperative period and can last for 3 to 4 hours (Harper et al., 1976). The opioid antagonist naloxone can reverse this respiratory depression, but it will also abolish the analgesia. A less abrupt procedure is to support ventilation until spontaneous respiration is adequate.

A side effect of droperidol is the occurrence of extrapyramidal muscle movements. Approximately 1% of patients receiving droperidol exhibit this side effect, which is sometimes delayed for 12 hours after the termination of anesthesia. The movements are self-limited and can be controlled with atropine or benztropine. Neurolept analgesia should not be used for patients with Parkinson's disease.

Status. Neurolept analgesia and neurolept anesthesia are safe and simple procedures, although induction of these states is slow. Circulatory changes are minimal unless the patient is hypovolemic or subjected to postural changes. Respiratory depression is severe but predictable. This is a useful technic in the elderly or the seriously ill or debilitated.

When neuromuscular blocking agents are also used, adequate conditions can be provided for all types of surgery, but the technic is generally not preferred over the use of potent inhalational agents for most types of major surgery. It has specialized uses for certain diagnostic procedures and for some types of peripheral operations.

TRANQUILIZERS

The benzodiazepine *diazepam* (Chapters 17 and 19) produces sedation, relaxation of skeletal muscle, and amnesia and is an anticonvulsant. There is a 1- to 2-minute delay before the effects of diazepam become apparent during intravenous infusion, and the dose required to induce anesthesia is quite variable (0.2 to 1.5 mg/kg). Because of these two features, it is important that the injection be slow and that the infusion rate not exceed 10 mg per minute if excessive dosage is to be avoided. A dose of 0.6 mg/kg given intravenously to an adult will usually result in

a sequence of drowsiness, amnesia, and finally unconsciousness with light anesthesia.

The tidal volume decreases and respiratory rate increases, but ventilation is generally little altered; diazepam can, however, augment the respiratory depressant effect of opioid analgesics. The cardiovascular system is also little altered. Pulse rate may increase without change in cardiac output or blood pressure (Dalen et al., 1969).

Diazepam, U.S.P. (VALIUM), is insoluble in water and is supplied for injection dissolved in a mixture of organic solvents. It develops a cloudy appearance in water and should not be diluted, and the solution is incompatible with many other drugs. It should be injected intravenously into the side port of an intravenous infusion to minimize a burning sensation and the possibility of venous thrombosis.

Status. Diazepam can be used when sedation is required for a minor procedure or during regional local anesthesia. Alternatively, diazepam may be substituted for thiopental for induction of anesthesia when it is desirable to minimize cardiovascular effects. Diazepam is most useful preoperatively to reduce anxiety and to reduce the requirement for potent anesthetic agents, and as an adjuvant during and after surgery.

DISSOCIATIVE ANESTHESIA

Some arylcycloalkylamines may induce a state of sedation, immobility, amnesia, and marked analgesia. The name *dissociative anesthesia* is derived from the strong feeling of dissociation from the environment that is experienced by the subject to whom such an agent is administered. This condition is similar to neurolept analgesia but results from the administration of a single drug (Winters et al., 1972).

Phencyclidine was the first drug used for this purpose, but the frequent occurrence of unpleasant hallucinations and psychological problems soon led to its abandonment. These effects are much less frequent with *Ketamine Hydrochloride,* U.S.P. (2-[o-chlorophenyl]-2-[methylamino] cyclohexanone hydrochloride; KETAJECT, KETALAR).

Ketamine hydrochloride is supplied as an acidic solution for intravenous or intramuscular use in ampuls containing 10 or 50 mg of ketamine base per milliliter.

Clinical Use. For the induction of dissociative anesthesia in an adult, ketamine hydrochloride is administered in a dose of 1 to 2 mg/kg over a period of about 1 minute. (A similar induction follows the intramuscular injection of 4 to 6 mg/kg.) A sensation of dissociation is noticed within 15 seconds, and unconsciousness becomes apparent within another 30 seconds. Intense analgesia and amnesia are established rapidly. Following a single dose, unconsciousness lasts for 10 to 15 minutes and analgesia persists for some 40 minutes; amnesia may be evident for a period of 1 to 2 hours following the initial injection. If anesthesia of longer duration is necessary, supplementary doses of about one third or one half of the initial amount may be administered.

Muscular relaxation is poor, muscle tone may be

increased, purposeless movements sometimes occur, and occasionally violent and irrational responses to stimuli are observed. A soothing and quiet environment is necessary for success with this technic.

Hypoxic or hypercarbic stimulation of respiration is not seriously affected following usual doses of ketamine (Hirshman *et al.*, 1975). Pharyngeal and laryngeal reflexes are retained, and, while the cough reflex is depressed, airway obstruction does not normally occur. Airway resistance is in fact decreased, and bronchospasm may be abolished (Bovill *et al.*, 1971). Arterial blood pressure increases by as much as 25%, and cardiac output and rate increase. When myocardial tissue is exposed to ketamine *in vitro*, depression of contractility occurs. The stimulation observed *in vivo* is attributed to increased sympathetic activity. Concentrations of norepinephrine in the circulation are increased. Cerebral blood flow, metabolic rate, and intracranial pressure are augmented (Lassen and Christensen, 1976), as is intraocular pressure.

Recovery. Unlike the conventional intravenous agents, ketamine does not act primarily on the reticular activating system in the brain stem; rather, it acts on the cortex and the limbic system (Winters *et al.*, 1972). Perhaps this is the reason that recovery after ketamine has some unusual features. Awakening often requires several hours and is not infrequently characterized by disagreeable dreams and even hallucinations. Sometimes these unpleasant occurrences may recur days or weeks later. Almost half of adults over the age of 30 years exhibit delirium or excitement, or experience visual disturbances. The incidence of such adverse psychological experiences is greatly reduced in children and young adults. It is thought that the incidence of such unpleasant effects can be lowered by the prior administration of morphine and scopolamine and by the substitution of diazepam or thiopental for the last dose of ketamine.

Status. Ketamine hydrochloride is not indicated for patients with hypertension or psychiatric disorders. Intraocular pressure is increased with ketamine and, therefore, its use is not advisable for many types of eye surgery. It can be employed for induction of anesthesia, or, in combination with nitrous oxide, to produce adequate general anesthesia.

Ketamine is especially useful in children for the management of minor surgical or diagnostic procedures or for repeated procedures that require intense analgesia, such as changing burn dressings. When the burns involve the face and neck, the maintenance of an unobstructed airway with ketamine makes it a valuable agent.

Alper, M. H.; Fleisch, J. H.; and Flacke, W. The effects of halothane on the response of cardiac sympathetic ganglia on various stimulants. *Anesthesiology*, **1969**, *31*, 429–436.

Altura, B. T., and Altura, B. M. Barbiturates and aortic and venous smooth-muscle function. *Anesthesiology*, **1975**, *43*, 432–444.

Amess, J. A. L.; Burman, J. F.; Rees, G. M.; Nancekievill, D. G.; and Mollin, D. L. Megaloblastic hemopoiesis in patients receiving nitrous oxide. *Lancet*, **1978**, *2*, 339–341.

Atlee, J. L., and Rusy, B. F. Atrioventricular conduction times and atrioventricular nodal conductivity during enflurane anesthesia in dogs. *Anesthesiology*, **1977**, *47*, 498–503.

Bagshaw, R. J., and Cox, R. H. Baroreceptor control of regional haemodynamics during halothane anaesthesia in the dog. *Br. J. Anaesth.*, **1977**, *49*, 535–544.

Barry, K. G.; Mazze, R. I.; and Schwartz, F. D. Prevention of surgical oliguria and renal-hemodynamic suppression by sustained hydration. *N. Engl. J. Med.*, **1964**, *270*, 1371–1377.

Benumof, J., and Wahrenbrock, E. A. Local effects of anesthetic on regional hypoxic pulmonary vasoconstriction. *Anesthesiology*, **1975**, *43*, 525–532.

Bimar, J., and Bellville, J. W. Arousal reaction during anesthesia in man. *Anesthesiology*, **1977**, *47*, 449–454.

Biscoe, T. J., and Millar, R. A. Effects of inhalation anaesthetics on carotid body chemoreceptor activity. *Br. J. Anaesth.*, **1968**, *40*, 2–12.

Bjertnaes, L. J.; Hauge, A.; Nakken, K. F.; and Bredeson, J. E. Hypoxic pulmonary vasoconstriction: inhibition due to anaesthesia. *Acta Physiol. Scand.*, **1976**, *96*, 283–289.

Bovill, J. G.; Clarke, R. S. J.; Davis, E. A.; and Dundee, J. W. Some cardiovascular effects of ketamine in man. *Br. J. Pharmacol.*, **1971**, *41*, 411P–412P.

Brown, S. S.; Lyons, S. M.; and Dundee, J. W. Intra-arterial barbiturates: a study of some factors leading to intravascular thrombosis. *Br. J. Anaesth.*, **1968**, *40*, 13–19.

Coleridge, H. M.; Coleridge, J. C. G.; Luck, J. C.; and Norman, J. The effect of four volatile anaesthetic agents in the impulse activity of two types of pulmonary receptor. *Br. J. Anaesth.*, **1968**, *40*, 484–492.

Coon, R. L., and Kampine, J. P. Hypocapnic bronchoconstriction and inhalation anesthetics. *Anesthesiology*, **1975**, *43*, 635–641.

Corbett, T. H. Cancer and congenital anomalies associated with anesthetics. *Ann. N.Y. Acad. Sci.*, **1976**, *271*, 58–66.

Cousins, M. J., and Mazze, R. I. Methoxyflurane nephrotoxicity: a study of dose-response in man. *J.A.M.A.*, **1973**, *225*, 1611–1616.

Crandell, W. B.; Pappas, S. G.; and MacDonald, A. Nephrotoxicity associated with methoxyflurane anesthesia. *Anesthesiology*, **1966**, *27*, 591–607.

Dalen, J. E.; Evans, G. L.; Banas, J. S., Jr.; Brooks, H. L.; Paraskos, J. A.; and Dexter, L. The hemodynamic and respiratory effects of diazepam (VALIUM). *Anesthesiology*, **1969**, *30*, 259–263.

Dean, G. *Porphyrias: A Story of Inheritance and Environment*, 2nd ed. Pitman, London, **1971**.

Deutsch, S.; Goldberg, M.; Stephens, G. M.; and Wu, W. H. Effects of halothane anesthesia on renal function in normal man. *Anesthesiology*, **1966**, *27*, 793–804.

Deutsch, S.; Linde, H. W.; Dripps, R. D.; and Price, H. L. Circulatory and respiratory actions of halothane in normal man. *Anesthesiology*, **1962**, *23*, 631–638.

Dunbar, B. S.; Ovassapian, A.; Dripps, R. D.; and Smith, T. C. The respiratory response to carbon dioxide during INNOVAR–nitrous oxide anaesthesia in man. *Br. J. Anaesth.*, **1967**, *39*, 861–866.

Dundee, J. W. Alterations in response to somatic pain associated with anaesthesia. II. The effect of thiopentone and pentobarbitone. *Br. J. Anaesth.*, **1960**, *32*, 407–414.

Dundee, J. W.; Price, H. L.; and Dripps, R. D. Acute tolerance to thiopentone in man. *Br. J. Anaesth.*, **1956**, *28*, 344–352.

Eger, E. I., II; Saidman, L. J.; and Brandstater, B. Minimum alveolar anesthetic concentration: a standard of anesthetic potency. *Anesthesiology*, **1965**, *26*, 756–763.

Eger, E. I., II; Smith, N. T.; Stoelting, R. K.; Cullen, D. J.; Kadis, L. B.; and Whitcher, C. E. Cardiovascular effects of halothane in man. *Anesthesiology*, **1970**, *32*, 396–409.

Eger, E. I., II; White, A.; Brown, C.; Biava, C.; Corbett, T.; and Steven, W. A test of carcinogenicity of enflurane, halothane and nitrous oxide in mice. (Abstract.) *American Society of Anesthesiology Scientific Papers, 1978, 295–296.

Epstein, R. M.; Deutsch, S.; Cooperman, L. H.; Clement, A. J.; and Price, H. L. Splanchnic circulation during halothane anesthesia and hypercapnia in normal man. *Anesthesiology,* 1966, 27, 654–661.

Epstein, R. A.; Wang, H.; and Bartelstone, H. J. The effects of halothane on circulatory reflexes of the dog. *Anesthesiology,* 1968, 29, 867–876.

Fogdall, R. P., and Miller, R. D. Neuromuscular effects of enflurane alone and combined with *d*-tubocurarine, pancuronium, and succinylcholine in man. *Anesthesiology,* 1975, 42, 173–178.

Forbes, A. R. Halothane depresses mucociliary flow in the trachea. *Anesthesiology,* 1976, 45, 59–63.

Gillespie, N. A. The signs of anesthesia. *Anesth. Analg. (Cleve.),* 1943, 22, 275–282.

Göthert, M., and Wendt, J. Inhibition of adrenal medullary catecholamine secretion by enflurane. I. Investigations *in vivo. Anesthesiology,* 1977, 46, 400–403.

Harper, M. H.; Hickey, R. F.; Cromwell, T. H.; and Linwood, S. The magnitude and duration of respiratory depression produced by fentanyl and fentanyl plus droperidol in man. *J. Pharmacol. Exp. Ther.,* 1976, 199, 464–468.

Hirshman, C. A.; McCullough, R. E.; Cohen, P. J.; and Weil, J. V.ᐟ Hypoxic ventilatory drive in dogs during thiopental, ketamine or pentobarbital anesthesia. *Anesthesiology,* 1975, 43, 628–634.

———. Depression of hypoxic ventilatory response by halothane, enflurane and isoflurane in dogs. *Br. J. Anaesth.,* 1977, 49, 957–963.

Horan, B. F.; Prys-Roberts, C.; Hamilton, W. K.; and Roberts, J. G. Haemodynamic responses to enflurane anaesthesia and hypovolaemia in the dog and their modification by propranolol. *Br. J. Anaesth.,* 1977, 49, 1189–1197.

Hornbein, T. F.; Martin, W. E.; Bonica, J. J.; Freund, F. G.; and Parmentier, P. Nitrous oxide effects on the circulatory and ventilatory responses to halothane. *Anesthesiology,* 1969, 31, 250–260.

Johnston, R. R.; Eger, E. I., ii; and Wilson, C. A comparative interaction of epinephrine with enflurane, isoflurane and halothane in man. *Anesth. Analg. (Cleve.),* 1976, 55, 709–712.

Johnstone, R. E.; Kennell, E. M.; Behar, M. G.; Brummond, W.; Ebersole, R. C.; and Shaw, L. M. Increased serum bromide concentration after halothane anesthesia in man. *Anesthesiology,* 1975, 42, 598–601.

Katz, R. L., and Gissen, A. J. Neuromuscular and electromyographic effects of halothane and its interaction with *d*-tubocurarine in man. *Anesthesiology,* 1967, 28, 564–567.

Katz, R. L.; Matteo, R. S.; and Papper, E. M. The injection of epinephrine during general anesthesia. II. Halothane. *Anesthesiology,* 1962, 23, 597–600.

Korttila, V.; Tammisto, T.; Ertama, P.; Pfaffli, P.; Blomgren, E.; and Hakkinen, S. Recovery, psychomotor skills and simulated driving after brief inhalational anesthesia with halothane or enflurane combined with nitrous oxide and oxygen. *Anesthesiology,* 1977, 46, 20–27.

Landmark, S. J.; Knopp, T. J.; Rehder, K.; and Sessler, A. D. Regional pulmonary perfusion and V/Q in awake and anesthetized-paralyzed man. *J. Appl. Physiol.,* 1977, 43, 993–1000.

Larson, C. P.; Eger, E. I., ii; Maullem, M.; Buechel, D. R.; Munson, E. S.; and Eisele, J. H. The effects of diethyl ether and methoxyflurane on ventilation. II. A comparative study in man. *Anesthesiology,* 1969, 30, 174–184.

Larson, C. P.; Mazze, R. I.; and Cooperman, L. H. Effects of anesthetics on cerebral, renal and splanchnic circulations: recent developments. *Anesthesiology,* 1974, 41, 169–181.

Lassen, H. C. A.; Henriksen, E.; Neukirch, F.; and Kristensen, H. S. Treatment of tetanus: severe bone-marrow

depression after prolonged nitrous-oxide anaesthesia. *Lancet,* 1956, 1, 527–530.

Lassen, N. A., and Christensen, M. S. Physiology of cerebral blood flow. *Br. J. Anaesth.,* 1976, 48, 719–734.

Laws, A. K. Effects of induction of anaesthesia and muscle paralysis on functional residual capacity of the lungs. *Can. Anaesth. Soc. J.,* 1968, 15, 325–331.

Leighton, K., and Bruce, C. Distribution of kidney blood flow: a comparison of methoxyflurane and halothane effects as measured by heated thermocouple. *Can. Anaesth. Soc. J.,* 1975, 22, 125–137.

Lowenstein, E.; Hallowell, P.; Levine, F. H.; Daggett, W. M.; Austen, W. G.; and Laver, M. B. Cardiovascular response to large doses of intravenous morphine in man. *N. Engl. J. Med.,* 1969, 281, 1389–1393.

Lundy, J. S. Intravenous anesthesia: preliminary report of the use of two new thiobarbiturates. *Proc. Staff Meet. Mayo Clin.,* 1935, 10, 536–543.

Marshall, B. E.; Cohen, P. J.; Klingenmaier, C. H.; and Aukburg, S. Pulmonary venous admixture before, during and after halothane:oxygen anesthesia in man. *J. Appl. Physiol.,* 1969, 27, 653–657.

Marshall, B. E.; Cohen, P. J.; Klingenmaier, C. H.; Neigh, J. L.; and Pender, J. W. Some pulmonary and cardiovascular effects of enflurane (ETHRANE) anaesthesia with varying $PaCO_2$ in man. *Br. J. Anaesth.,* 1971, 43, 996–1002.

Mazze, R. I.; Calverley, R. K.; and Smith, N. T. Inorganic fluoride nephrotoxicity: prolonged enflurane and halothane anesthesia in volunteers. *Anesthesiology,* 1977, 46, 265–271.

Mazze, R. I.; Schwartz, F. D.; Slocum, H. C.; and Barry, K. G. Renal function during anesthesia and surgery. I. The effects of halothane anesthesia. *Anesthesiology,* 1963, 24, 279–284.

Mazze, R. I.; Shue, G. L.; and Jackson, S. H. Renal dysfunction associated with methoxyflurane anesthesia. *J.A.M.A.,* 1971, 216, 278–288.

Merin, R. G.; Kumazawa, T.; and Luka, N. L. Enflurane depresses myocardial function, perfusion and metabolism in the dog. *Anesthesiology,* 1976, 45, 501–507.

Merin, R. G.; Verdouw, P. D.; and de Jong, J. W. Dose-dependent depression of cardiac function and metabolism by halothane in swine (*Sus scrofa*). *Anesthesiology,* 1977, 46, 417–423.

Michenfelder, J. D., and Theye, R. A. *In vivo* toxic effects of halothane on canine cerebral metabolic pathways. *Am. J. Physiol.,* 1975, 229, 1050–1055.

Miletich, D. J.; Ivankovich, A. D.; Albrecht, R. F.; Reimann, C. R.; Rosenberg, R.; and McKissic, E. D. Absence of autoregulation of cerebral blood flow during halothane and enflurane anesthesia. *Anesth. Analg. (Cleve.),* 1976, 55, 100–109.

Millar, R. A., and Morris, M. E. Sympatho-adrenal responses during general anesthesia in the dog and man. *Can. Anaesth. Soc. J.,* 1961a, 8, 356–386.

———. A study of methoxyflurane anesthesia. *Ibid.,* 1961b, 8, 210–215.

Munson, E. S.; Larson, C. P., Jr.; Babad, A. A.; Regan, M. J.; Buechel, D. R.; and Eger, E. I., ii. The effects of halothane, fluroxene, and cyclopropane on ventilation: a comparative study in man. *Anesthesiology,* 1966, 27, 716–728.

Ngai, S. H., and Hanks, E. C. Effect of methoxyflurane on electromyogram, neuromuscular transmission and spinal reflexes. *Anesthesiology,* 1962, 23, 158–159.

Ngai, S. H.; Katz, R. L.; and Farhie, S. E. Respiratory effects of trichloroethylene, halothane, and methoxyflurane in the cat. *J. Pharmacol. Exp. Ther.,* 1965, 148, 123–130.

Perry, L. B.; VanDyke, R. A.; and Theye, R. A. Sympathoadrenal and hemodynamic effects of isoflurane, halothane, and cyclopropane in dogs. *Anesthesiology,* 1974, 40, 465–470.

Price, H. L. General anesthesia and circulatory homeostasis. *Physiol. Rev.,* **1960**, *40,* 187–218.

———. Circulatory action of general anesthetic agents and the homeostatic roles of epinephrine and norepinephrine in man. *Clin. Pharmacol. Ther.,* **1961**, *2,* 163–176.

———. Calcium reverses myocardial depression caused by halothane. *Anesthesiology,* **1974**, *41,* 576–579.

Price, H. L.; Lurie, A. A.; Black, G. W.; Sechzer, P. H.; Linde, H. W.; and Price, M. L. Modification by general anesthetics (cyclopropane and halothane) of circulatory and sympathoadrenal responses to respiratory acidosis. *Ann. Surg.,* **1960**, *152,* 1071–1077.

Prys-Roberts, C.; Kelman, G. R.; Greenbaum, R.; Kain, M. L.; and Bay, J. Hemodynamic and alveolar-arterial PO_2 differences at varying $PaCO_2$ in anesthetized man. *J. Appl. Physiol.,* **1968**, *25,* 80–87.

Rehder, K.; Forbes, J.; Alter, H.; Hessler, O.; and Stier, A. Halothane biotransformation in man: a quantitative study. *Anesthesiology,* **1967**, *28,* 711–715.

Reynolds, A. K.; Chiz, J. F.; and Pasquet, A. F. Halothane and methoxyflurane. A comparison of their effects on cardiac pacemaker fibers. *Anesthesiology,* **1970**, *33,* 602–610.

Saidman, L. J., and Eger, E. I., II. The effect of thiopental metabolism on duration of anesthesia. *Anesthesiology,* **1966**, *27,* 118–126.

Sakai, T., and Takaori, M. Biodegradation of halothane, enflurane, and methoxyflurane. *Br. J. Anaesth.,* **1978**, *50,* 785–791.

Shapiro, H. M. Intracranial hypertension: therapeutic and anesthetic considerations. *Anesthesiology,* **1975**, *43,* 445–471.

Shimoji, K.; Matsuki, M.; Shimizu, H.; Maruyama, Y.; and Aida, S. Dishabituation of mesencephalic reticular neurons by anesthetics. *Anesthesiology,* **1977**, *47,* 349–352.

Shimosato, S., and Etsten, B. E. Effect of anesthetic drugs on the heart: a critical review of myocardial contractility and its relationship to hemodynamics. *Clin. Anesth.,* **1969**, *3,* 17–72.

Shimosato, S.; Sugai, N.; Iwatsuki, N.; and Etsten, B. E. The effect of ETHRANE on cardiac muscle mechanics. *Anesthesiology,* **1969**, *30,* 513–518.

Shimosato, S., and Yasuda, I. Cardiac performance during prolonged halothane anaesthesia in the cat. *Br. J. Anaesth.,* **1978**, *50,* 215–219.

Sipes, I. G., and Brown, B. R. An animal model of hepatotoxicity associated with halothane anesthesia. *Anesthesiology,* **1976**, *45,* 622–628.

Skovsted, P., and Price, H. L. The effects of ETHRANE on arterial pressure, preganglionic sympathetic activity and barostatic reflexes. *Anesthesiology,* **1972**, *36,* 257–262.

Skovsted, P.; Price, M. L.; and Price, H. L. The effects of halothane on arterial pressure, preganglionic sympathetic activity, and barostatic reflexes. *Anesthesiology,* **1969**, *31,* 507–514.

Smith, A. L., and Wollman, H. Cerebral blood flow and metabolism. Effect of anesthetic drugs and techniques. *Anesthesiology,* **1972**, *36,* 378–400.

Smith, N. T.; Calverley, R. K.; Prys-Roberts, C.; Eger, E. I., II; and Jones, C. W. Impact of nitrous oxide on the circulation during enflurane anesthesia in man. *Anesthesiology,* **1978**, *48,* 345–349.

Smith, N. T.; Eger, E. I., II; Stoelting, R. K.; Whayne, T. F.; Cullen, D.; and Kadis, L. B. The cardiovascular and sympathomimetic responses to the addition of nitrous oxide to halothane in man. *Anesthesiology,* **1970**, *32,* 410–421.

Sonntag, H.; Donath, U.; Hillebrand, W.; Merin, R. G.; and Radke, J. Left ventricular function in conscious man and during halothane anesthesia. *Anesthesiology,* **1978**, *48,* 320–324.

Stoelting, R. K., and Gibbs, P. S. Hemodynamic effects of morphine and morphine–nitrous oxide in valvular heart

disease and coronary artery disease. *Anesthesiology,* **1973**, *38,* 45–52.

Sugai, N.; Shimosato, S.; and Etsten, B. E. Effect of halothane on force-velocity relations and dynamic stiffness of isolated heart muscle. *Anesthesiology,* **1968**, *29,* 267–274.

Summary of the National Halothane Study. *J.A.M.A.,* **1966**, *197,* 775–788.

Tusiewicz, K.; Bryan, A. C.; and Froese, A. B. Contributions of changing rib cage-diaphragm interactions to the ventilatory depression of halothane anesthesia. *Anesthesiology,* **1977**, *47,* 327–337.

Vessey, M. P. Epidemiological studies of the occupational hazards of anaesthesia—a review. *Anaesthesia,* **1978**, *33,* 430–438.

Virtue, R. W.; Lund, L. O.; Phelps, M., Jr.; Vogel, J. H. K.; Beckwitt, H.; and Heron, M. Difluoromethyl 1,1,2-trifluoro-2-chloroethyl ether as an anaesthetic agent: results with dogs, and a preliminary note on observations with man. *Can. Anaesth. Soc. J.,* **1966**, *13,* 233–241.

Walker, J. A.; Eggers, G. W. N.; and Allen, C. R. Cardiovascular effects of methoxyflurane anesthesia in man. *Anesthesiology,* **1962**, *23,* 639–642.

Wang, H.; Epstein, R. A.; Markee, S. J.; and Bartelstone, H. J. The effects of halothane on peripheral and central vasomotor control mechanisms of the dog. *Anesthesiology,* **1968**, *29,* 877–886.

Waud, B. E., and Waud, D. R. Comparison of the effects of general anesthetics on the end-plate of skeletal muscle. *Anesthesiology,* **1975**, *43,* 540–547.

Williams, B. D.; White, N.; Amlot, P. L.; Slaney, J.; and Toseland, P. A. Circulating immune complexes after repeated halothane anaesthesia. *Br. Med. J.,* **1977**, *2,* 159–162.

Winters, W. D.; Ferrer-Allado, T.; and Guzman-Flores, C. The cataleptic state induced by ketamine: a review of the neuropharmacology of anesthesia. *Neuropharmacology,* **1972**, *11,* 303–315.

Wollman, H.; Alexander, S. C.; Cohen, P. J.; Chase, P. E.; Melman, E.; and Behar, M. G. Cerebral circulation of man during halothane anesthesia: effects of hypocarbia and *d*-tubocurarine. *Anesthesiology,* **1964**, *25,* 180–184.

Wollman, H.; Alexander, S. C.; Cohen, P. J.; Smith, T. C.; Chase, P. E.; and van der Molen, R. A. Cerebral circulation during general anesthesia and hyperventilation in man. Thiopental induction to nitrous oxide and *d*-tubocurarine. *Anesthesiology,* **1965**, *26,* 329–334.

Wollman, H.; Smith, A. L.; Neigh, J. L.; and Hoffman, J. C. Cerebral blood flow and oxygen consumption in man during electroencephalographic seizure patterns associated with ETHRANE anesthesia. In, *Cerebral Blood Flow.* (Brock, M., and Fieschi, C., eds.) Springer-Verlag, Berlin, **1969**, pp. 246–248.

Yacoub, O.; Doell, D.; Kryger, M. H.; and Anthonisen, N. R. Depression of hypoxic ventilatory response by nitrous oxide. *Anesthesiology,* **1976**, *45,* 385–389.

Zink, J.; Sasyniuk, B. I.; and Dresel, P. E. Halothane-epinephrine-induced cardiac arrhythmias and the role of heart rate. *Anesthesiology,* **1975**, *43,* 548–555.

Monographs and Reviews

Aldrete, J. A., and Britt, B. A. (eds.). *Malignant Hyperthermia.* Grune & Stratton, Inc., New York, **1978**.

Cohen, E. N. Metabolism of the volatile anesthetics. *Anesthesiology,* **1971**, *35,* 193–202.

Eger, E. I., II. *Anesthetic Uptake and Action.* The Williams & Wilkins Co., Baltimore, **1974**.

Marshall, B. E., and Wyche, M. Q. Hypoxemia during and after anesthesia. *Anesthesiology,* **1972**, *37,* 178–209.

Waud, B. E. Neuromuscular blocking agents. In, *Current Problems in Anesthesia and Critical Care Medicine,* Vol. 4. (Brunner, E. A., ed.) Year Book Medical Publishers, Inc., Chicago, **1977**, pp. 5–47.

CHAPTER

15 LOCAL ANESTHETICS

J. Murdoch Ritchie and Nicholas M. Greene

GENERAL PHARMACOLOGY OF LOCAL ANESTHETICS

Local anesthetics are drugs that block nerve conduction when applied locally to nerve tissue in appropriate concentrations. They act on any part of the nervous system and on every type of nerve fiber. For example, when they are applied to the motor cortex impulse transmission from that area stops, and when they are injected into the skin they prevent the initiation and the transmission of sensory impulses. A local anesthetic in contact with a nerve trunk can cause both sensory and motor paralysis in the area innervated. Many kinds of compounds interfere with conduction, but they often permanently damage the nerve cells. The great practical advantage of the local anesthetics is that their action is reversible; their use is followed by complete recovery in nerve function with no evidence of structural damage to nerve fibers or cells.

Since ionic mechanisms of excitability are similar in nerve and muscle, it is not surprising that these agents also can have prominent actions on all types of muscular tissue.

History. The first local anesthetic to be discovered was cocaine, an alkaloid contained in large amounts (0.6 to 1.8%) in the leaves of *Erythroxylon coca,* a shrub growing in the Andes Mountains 1000 to 3000 m above sea level. Nearly 9 million kilograms of these leaves are consumed annually by about 2 million inhabitants of the highlands of Peru, who chew or suck the leaves for the sake of the cocaine. For many centuries it has played an important role in the social and political life of these people because of the sense of well-being it produces.

The pure alkaloid was first isolated by Niemann, a pupil of Wöhler, who noted that it had a bitter taste and produced a peculiar effect on the tongue, making it numb and almost devoid of sensation. Von Anrep in 1880 studied its pharmacological actions and observed that the skin became insensitive to the prick of a pin when cocaine was infiltrated subcutaneously. He recommended that the alkaloid be used clinically as a local anesthetic. His suggestion, how-ever, was not acted upon, and credit for the introduction of cocaine into clinical use as a local anesthetic is usually given to two young Viennese physicians, Sigmund Freud and Karl Koller. In 1884, Freud made a general study of the physiological effects of cocaine. He was particularly impressed by the central actions of the drug and used it to wean one of his colleagues from morphine. He was successful in this attempt, but at the cost of producing one of the first-known cocaine addicts of modern times. Koller quickly appreciated that the anesthetizing properties of cocaine had great practical importance and soon introduced cocaine into ophthalmology as a local anesthetic.

The acceptance of cocaine as a local anesthetic was immediate, and in this way the history of local anesthesia differs sharply from that of general anesthesia. Other investigators rapidly extended Koller's initial observation. Within a short time, Hall in 1884 introduced local anesthesia into dentistry, and the next year Halsted, by demonstrating that cocaine could stop transmission in nerve trunks, laid the foundation for nerve block anesthesia in surgery. Corning in 1885 produced spinal anesthesia in dogs, but several years passed before his technic was employed in clinical surgery.

A chemical search for synthetic substitutes for cocaine started in 1892 with the work of Einhorn and his colleagues. This resulted in 1905 in the synthesis of procaine, which is still a prototype for local anesthetic drugs.

Properties Desirable in Local Anesthetics. A good local anesthetic should combine several properties. It should not be irritating to the tissue to which it is applied, nor should it cause any permanent damage to nerve structure; most local anesthetics in common use fulfill these requirements. Its systemic toxicity should be low because it is eventually absorbed from its site of application. Therefore, the therapeutic index is an important factor in evaluating the efficacy and safety of local anesthetic agents. Since this can vary greatly among local anesthetics, there is a constant search for new, more effective, and safer agents. The ideal local anesthetic must be effective regardless of whether it is injected into the tissue or whether it is applied locally to mucous membranes. It is usually important that the time required for the onset of anesthesia should be as short as possible. Furthermore, the action must last long enough to allow time for the contemplated surgery, yet not so long as to entail an extended period of recovery. There are many agents that satisfy this latter requirement. Occasionally, a local anesthetic action lasting for days or even weeks or months is desirable, for example, in the control of chronic pain. Unfortunately, the available compounds employed for anesthesia of such long duration have high local toxicity. Neurolysis with slough and necrosis of surrounding tissues occurs, and partial or complete transverse injury of the spinal cord with permanent paralysis may result if such a reaction occurs in the vicinity of the cord.

GENERAL PROPERTIES

The local anesthetics have many actions in common, and before discussing the pharmacology of the individual members these general properties will be considered.

Chemistry and Structure-Activity Relationship. Table 15-1 shows that the structures of most of the useful local anesthetics contain hydrophilic and hydrophobic domains that are usually separated by an intermediate alkyl chain. The hydrophilic group is usually a tertiary amine, but it may also be a secondary amine; the hydrophobic domain is an aromatic residue. In almost all cases linkage to the aromatic group is of the ester or amide type, and the nature of this bond is a determinant of certain of the pharmacological properties of these agents. The ester link is important because this bond is readily hydrolyzed during metabolic degradation and inactivation in the body. Procaine is typical of local anesthetics with the esteratic link. The molecule can be divided into three main portions: the aromatic acid (para-aminobenzoic), the alcohol (ethanol), and the tertiary amino group (diethylamino) (see Table 15-1). Changes in any part of the molecule alter the anesthetic potency and the toxicity of the compound, an observation that provides the basis for the vast number of available local anesthetics. Increasing the length of the alcohol group leads to a greater anesthetic potency. It also leads to an increase in toxicity so that compounds with an ethyl ester, such as procaine, exhibit the least toxicity. The length of the two

terminal groups on the tertiary amino nitrogen is similarly important. The structure-activity relationship and the physicochemical properties of local anesthetics have been reviewed by Büchi and Perlia (1971).

Mechanism of Action. Local anesthetics prevent both the generation and the conduction of the nerve impulse. Their main site of action is the cell membrane, and there is seemingly little direct action of physiological importance on the axoplasm. The work of Hodgkin, Huxley, and their colleagues has led to a better understanding of the nature of the nerve impulse, and it is now relatively easy to explain, at least partially, the action of local anesthetics within the framework of the ionic theory of nervous activity.

Local anesthetics and other classes of agents (e.g., alcohols and barbiturates) block conduction by decreasing or preventing the large *transient* increase in the permeability of the membrane to sodium ions that is produced by a slight depolarization of the membrane (see Ritchie, 1975; Strichartz, 1976). As the anesthetic action progressively develops in a nerve, the threshold for electrical excitability gradually increases and the safety factor for conduction decreases; when this action is sufficiently well developed, block of conduction is produced.

Raising the calcium concentration in the medium bathing a nerve tends to relieve the conduction block produced by local anesthetics. This relief occurs because calcium alters the surface potential on the membrane,

Table 15-1. STRUCTURAL FORMULAS OF SELECTED LOCAL ANESTHETICS

* Chloroprocaine has a chlorine atom in position 2 of the aromatic moiety of procaine.
† Bupivacaine has a butyl group in place of the N-methyl substituent of mepivacaine.

and hence the transmembrane electrical field. This, in turn, reduces the degree of inactivation of the sodium channels and the affinity of the latter for the local anesthetic molecules (*see* Hille, 1977).

The local anesthetics also reduce the permeability of *resting* nerve to potassium as well as to sodium ions. This accounts for the observation that the block in conduction is not accompanied by any large or consistent change in the resting potential (Straub, 1956).

Quaternary analogs of local anesthetics block conduction when applied internally to perfused giant axons of squid, but they are relatively ineffective when applied externally. These observations, together with others on the effects of varying pH on the potency of related tertiary amines, suggest that the site at which local anesthetics act, at least in their charged form, is accessible only from the inner surface of the membrane (Narahashi and Frazier, 1971). Local anesthetics applied externally must therefore first cross the membrane, in the uncharged form, before they can exert a blocking action. Furthermore, several studies show that the binding of the charged form of the local anesthetic to the receptor is voltage dependent, in a way that suggests that the receptor is about halfway down the sodium channel (Strichartz, 1973; Hille, 1977).

The exact mechanism whereby a local anesthetic influences the permeability of the membrane is at present unknown, but it is interesting that the relative anesthetic potency of a series of compounds exactly parallels their effectiveness in increasing the surface pressure of monomolecular films of lipids (*see* Skou, 1961). On the basis of this work, Shanes (1958) suggested that local anesthetics achieve block by increasing the surface pressure of the lipid layer that constitutes the nerve membrane, thereby closing the pores through which ions move. This would cause a general decrease in the resting permeability and would also limit the increase in sodium permeability, the fundamental change necessary for the generation of the action potential. In contrast, Metcalfe and Burgen (1968) have suggested that local anesthetics affect permeability by increasing the degree of disorder of the membrane. The partial reversal of local anesthetic block by high external pressure (Kendig and Cohen, 1977) is consistent with this latter view. However, at least one mechanism of action of local anesthetics involves their combination with a specific receptor site within the sodium channel, hence physically blocking it (Narahashi and Frazier, 1971; Ritchie, 1975; Strichartz, 1976; Hille, 1977).

Differential Sensitivity of Nerve Fibers to Local Anesthetics. As a general rule, small nerve fibers seem to be more susceptible to the action of local anesthetics than are large fibers. This was clearly established for the myelinated A fibers by Gasser and Erlanger (1929), who showed that when cocaine is applied to a cutaneous nerve the γ waves (from small cutaneous afferent fibers) are the first and the α waves (from large fibers) the last to disappear. The smallest mammalian nerve fibers are nonmyelinated and, on the whole, are blocked more readily than the myelinated fibers. However, the spectrum of sensitivity of the nonmyelinated fibers overlaps that of the myelinated fibers to some extent. Thus, some myelinated A delta fibers are blocked earlier, and with lower concentrations of anesthetic, than are most of the C fibers (Nathan and Sears, 1961). The sensitivity to local anesthetics is not determined by fiber size alone, therefore, but also by the anatomical fiber type. This is not surprising in view of the great difference between the physiological mode of conduction in the myelinated fibers, in which conduction is saltatory, and that of the nonmyelinated fibers, in which it is continuous. Still other factors as yet unknown may determine the susceptibility of a fiber to a local anesthetic. For example, it is not known whether myelinated autonomic B fibers and myelinated A fibers of the same diameter differ in sensitivity. Although there is general agreement on the differential *rate* of blockade produced by local anesthetics in fibers of different sizes, there is some question whether a similar differential effect obtains after sufficient time has been allowed for full equilibration of the local anesthetic with the tissue. Indeed, Franz and Perry (1974) found that *absolute* differential blockade occurred only when the length of nerve exposed to the anesthetic was limited to a few millimeters.

The sensitivity of a fiber to local anesthetics does not seem to depend on whether it is sensory or motor, in spite of a widespread belief to the contrary. The misconception seems to have arisen in the following way. When a local anesthetic is applied to a muscle-nerve trunk, which contains both sensory and motor fibers, the contractions elicited reflexly, by jerking a tendon, for example, are blocked before those elicited by electrical stimulation of the nerve. This led to the belief that an appropriate concentration of anesthetic could block completely the sensory fibers without abolishing the conduction of impulses in motor fibers. In 1957, however, Matthews and Rushworth made the first direct comparison of the relative sensitivity of muscle proprioceptive afferent and muscle efferent fibers, both of which are of the same large diameter. These investigators found that the two types of fibers were *equally* sensitive. However, the smaller γ *motor* fibers supplying the muscle spindles were much more rapidly blocked by the local anesthetic, and it is this preferential blockade of the smaller motor fibers, rather than the sensory fibers, that leads to the preferential loss of the muscle reflexes. Franz and Perry (1974) suggest that differential block cannot result from differences in minimal concentrations necessary to block axons of different diameters. Rather, it results from differences in the critical lengths of axons that must be exposed to the anesthetic, smaller axons having shorter critical lengths because of their smaller internodal distances. In the early stages of development of anesthetic action, small discrete lengths of the most accessible portions of the nerve trunk are the first to be exposed to the anesthetic as it diffuses inward along various intrafascicular routes. Smaller fibers with their shorter critical lengths are thus blocked more quickly by anesthetic solutions than are larger fibers; the same reasoning accounts for their slower recovery when the process is reversed.

The differential sensitivity to block exhibited by fibers of varying sizes is of great practical importance and may explain why there is a definite order in which the sensory functions of a nerve are affected by local anesthetics. Fortunately for the patient, the sensation of pain is usually the first modality to disappear, and it is followed in turn by the sensations of cold, warmth, touch, and deep pressure, although there is great individual variation. Gasser and Erlanger (1929) were impressed by the fact that, when pressure was applied to a nerve, the resulting anesthesia appeared in a sequence roughly *opposite* to that observed after block by anesthetic drugs; that is, pain was the last sensation to disappear and touch the first. They suggested that touch is mediated by the largest sensory fibers in a nerve, pain by the smallest sensory fibers, and temperature by fibers of intermediate diameters. Although open to certain criticisms (Douglas and Ritchie, 1962), this suggestion has been extremely useful in the analysis of sensory function.

Effect of pH. The local anesthetics in the form of the unprotonated amine tend to be only slightly soluble. Therefore, they are generally marketed in the form of their water-soluble salts, usually the hydrochlorides. Inasmuch as the local anesthetics are weak bases, these salt solutions are quite acidic, a condition that fortunately increases the stability of the local anesthetic and any accompanying vasoconstrictor substance. A

small amount of unprotonated amine must, however, always be present, and it is in this form that the drug can penetrate the tissues and produce an anesthetic action.

Numerous investigations in which anesthetics were applied to isolated nerve trunks or to the cornea, where the buffering capacity of the tissue fluids is limited, have shown that the addition of base to local anesthetic solutions enhances activity. However, alkaline solutions of the drugs are not more effective clinically. The explanation probably is that, under conditions usually encountered in clinical use, the pH of the local anesthetic is rapidly brought to that of the extracellular fluids, regardless of the pH of the solution in which it is injected.

All the commonly used local anesthetics contain a tertiary (or secondary) nitrogen atom and, therefore, can exist either as the uncharged tertiary (or secondary) amine or as the positively charged substituted ammonium cation, depending on the dissociation constant (pK_a) of the compound and the pH of the solution. The ionization of a typical local anesthetic may be depicted as follows:

$$\begin{array}{c} R_1 \\ | \\ R_2\!-\!\overset{+}{N}H \\ | \\ R_3 \end{array} \rightleftharpoons \begin{array}{c} R_1 \\ | \\ R_2\!-\!N \\ | \\ R_3 \end{array} + H^+$$

The pK_a of any typical local anesthetic in common use lies between 8.0 and 9.0, so that only 5 to 20% will be in the form of the unprotonated amine at the pH of the tissues. This fraction, although small, is important because the drug usually has to diffuse through connective tissue and other cellular membranes to reach its site of action, and it is generally agreed that it can do so only in the form of the uncharged amine. There is still a difference of opinion as to which form is active once the anesthetic has reached the nerve. It has been suggested that the form of the molecule active in nerve fibers is the cation. This conclusion has been supported by the results of experiments on anesthetized mammalian nonmyelinated fibers (Ritchie and Greengard, 1966) in which conduction could be blocked or unblocked merely by setting the pH of the bathing medium at pH 7.2 or pH 9.6, respectively, without altering the amount of anesthetic present. When the pH is low, and conduction is blocked, most of the anesthetic must be in its cationic form. This seems to indicate that the cation is the molecular form that combines with some receptor in the membrane to prevent the generation of an action potential. Furthermore, the *major* role of the cation has been clearly demonstrated by Narahashi and colleagues using quaternary analogs of the amine local anesthetics (Narahashi and Frazier, 1968). However, it is now evident that both molecular forms possess anesthetic activity (Hille, 1977; Mrose and Ritchie, 1978; Ritchie, 1979).

Frequency Dependence and Use Dependence. The degree of block produced by a given concentration of local anesthetic depends markedly on how much and how recently the nerve has been stimulated. Thus, a resting nerve is much less sensitive to a local anesthetic than one that has been recently and repetitively stimulated: the higher the frequency of preceding stimulation, the greater is the degree of block obtained to a test shock. These frequency- and use-dependent effects of local anesthetics occur because the local anesthetic molecule in its quaternary form gains access to the receptor only when the "gates" at the inner face of the sodium channel are open and because the affinity of the local anesthetic for the receptor in the sodium channel is voltage dependent (*see* Strichartz, 1973; Courtney, 1975; Hille, 1977; Courtney *et al.*, 1978; Ritchie, 1979). Local anesthetics exhibit these properties to different extents, depending, for example, on their pK_a and lipid solubility. An anesthetic that blocked high-frequency sensory discharge while permitting passage of low-frequency motor discharge would clearly be valuable clinically.

Prolongation of Action by Vasoconstrictors. The duration of action of a local anesthetic is proportional to the time during which it is in actual contact with nervous tissues. Consequently, procedures that maintain the localization of the drug at the nerve greatly prolong the period of anesthesia. Cocaine itself constricts blood vessels, probably by potentiating the action of norepinephrine (*see* Chapters 4 and 8); therefore, it prevents its own absorption. Braun in 1903 demonstrated that the addition of epinephrine to local anesthetic solutions greatly prolongs and intensifies their action. In clinical practice, therefore, the solution of a local anesthetic usually also contains epinephrine (1 part in 200,000), norepinephrine (1 part in 100,000), or a suitable synthetic congener, for example, phenylephrine. In general, the concentration of such constrictor agents should be kept at the minimal effective level. The epinephrine performs a dual service. By decreasing the rate of absorption, epinephrine not only localizes the anesthetic at the desired site but also allows the rate at which it is destroyed in the body to keep pace with the rate at which it is absorbed into the circulation. This reduces its systemic toxicity.

Some of the vasoconstrictor agent may be absorbed systemically, occasionally to an extent sufficient to cause untoward reactions, such as restlessness, an increase in heart rate, palpitation, and chest pain. When a paste of cocaine and epinephrine is applied to mucous membranes during plastic surgical procedures, the systemic effects may be life threatening. In such circumstances, the use of α- or β-adrenergic antagonists should be considered to counter the most prominent untoward manifestations of adrenergic stimulation. There may also be a delay in wound healing, tissue edema, or necrosis after local anesthesia. These effects seem to occur in part because sympathomimetic amines produce an increase in the oxygen consumption of the tissue, and this, together with the vasoconstriction, leads to hypoxia and local tissue damage. This is a particularly serious problem when local anesthetics are used in surgery on the digits, hands, or feet. Prolonged constriction of major arteries in the presence of limited collateral circulation can produce irreversible hypoxic damage and gangrene. In addition, the local anesthetics themselves may interfere with the reparative processes of wound healing.

Pharmacological Actions. In addition to blocking conduction in nerve axons in the peripheral nervous system, local anesthetics interfere with the function of all organs in which conduction or transmission of impulses occurs. Thus, they have important effects on the central nervous system (CNS), the autonomic ganglia, the neuromuscular junction, and all forms of muscle fiber (for review, *see* de Jong, 1977).

Central Nervous System. Following absorption, all nitrogenous local anesthetics may cause stimulation of the CNS, producing restlessness and tremor that may proceed to clonic convulsions. In general, the more potent the anesthetic the more readily convulsions may be produced. Alterations of

CNS activity are thus predictable from the local anesthetic agent in question and the blood concentration achieved. Central stimulation is followed by depression, and death is usually due to respiratory failure. It is possible to protect animals from several lethal doses of a local anesthetic by the use of artificial respiration.

Frank and Sanders (1963) have suggested that the apparent stimulation and the subsequent depression produced by applying local anesthetics to the CNS are both, in fact, due solely to *depression* of neuronal activity. The apparent stimulation is due perhaps to a selective depression of inhibitory neurons. The evidence for this hypothesis is that, when procaine is applied to the cortical neurons in isolated slabs of cerebral cortex, only depression of the directly evoked electrical responses is obtained. Depression of activity is also the only effect that procaine produces in monosynaptic and polysynaptic spinal reflexes (Taverner, 1960). This depressant action also accounts for the findings in laboratory animals that local anesthetics can produce a condition indistinguishable from general anesthesia when given after subanesthetic doses of a general anesthetic. It would also account for the suppressive effects of local anesthetics against convulsions produced by electric shock and by pentylenetetrazol (Tanaka, 1955).

Rapid systemic administration of local anesthetics, or large doses of the more toxic agents administered locally, may produce death with only transient or no signs of CNS stimulation. Under these conditions the concentration of the drug probably rises so rapidly that all neurons are depressed simultaneously. Alternatively, the function of critical centers that control respiration and vasomotor tone may be impaired quickly, depriving neurons that are involved in apparently stimulatory effects of local anesthetics of oxygen and glucose.

The support of respiration is the essential feature of treatment in the late stage of intoxication. While the barbiturates are capable of arresting convulsions resulting from toxic doses of local anesthetics, a near-anesthetic dose of barbiturate is required. The usual clinical dose merely provides psychic sedation and affords little protection. Diazepam is the drug of choice for both the prevention and the arrest of convulsions.

All the local anesthetics stimulate the CNS. For example, although drowsiness is the most frequent complaint, lidocaine may produce euphoria and muscle twitching at a blood concentration of 5 μg/ml. Cocaine seems to be unique in that it has a particularly powerful action on the cortex. This property of cocaine and its potential for abuse are discussed in Chapter 23. The synthetic local anesthetics, in contrast, are less stimulating to the higher cerebral centers and are not abused.

Neuromuscular Junction and Ganglionic Synapse. Local anesthetics also affect transmission at the neuromuscular junction. Close intra-arterial injection of 0.2 mg of procaine into the cat's tibialis anterior muscle reduces twitches and tetanic responses evoked by maximal motor-nerve volleys, and the response of the muscle to injected acetylcholine. The muscle, however, responds normally to direct electrical stimulation (Harvey, 1939). Other work suggests that procaine also diminishes the release of acetylcholine by the motor-nerve endings (*see* de Jong, 1977). Similar effects are obtained when procaine is added to the fluid perfusing an autonomic ganglion. The effects of procaine and physostigmine are antagonistic, and those of procaine and curare additive. The postsynaptic action of procaine, however, differs from that of curare in that the end-plate current is much prolonged by local anesthetics and has a multicomponent time course of decay (*see* Ruff, 1977). Local anesthetics do not interfere with transmission by simply competing with acetylcholine for the receptor. Rather, studies of the effect of these drugs on miniature end-plate currents and acetylcholine-induced end-plate currents suggest that a complex of transmitter, receptor, and local anesthetic is formed that seems to have negligible conductance (Ruff, 1977).

Cardiovascular System. Following systemic absorption, local anesthetics act on the cardiovascular system. The primary site of action is the myocardium, where decreases in electrical excitability, conduction rate, and force of contraction occur. In addition, most local anesthetics cause arteriolar dilatation. The cardiovascular effects are usually seen only after high systemic concentrations are attained. However, on rare occasion small amounts of anesthetic employed for simple infiltration anesthesia will cause cardiovascular collapse and death. The exact mechanism is unknown, but it probably results from cardiac arrest due to either an action on the pacemaker or the sudden onset of ventricular fibrillation. Such a reaction may follow inadvertent intravascular administration of the agent. Both the ionized and the nonionized forms of the local anesthetic may be important for these effects. It has been suggested that the effects on threshold and conduction time depend on the presence of the local anesthetic cations in the extracellular medium; on the other hand, the effect on strength of myocardial contractions depends exclusively on the presence of the nonionized form, presumably indicating that this is an intracellular action (Baird and Hardman, 1961).

Studies on isolated atrial and ventricular muscle reveal that procaine resembles quinidine in its cardiac action in that it increases the effective refractory period, raises the threshold for stimulation, and prolongs conduction time. These cardiac actions of procaine, and the accompanying characteristic changes in the ECG, would be of therapeutic interest were it not for the rapid metabolic destruction of the compound and the propensity of procaine and other local anesthetics to cause central stimulation. Therefore, studies of procaine congeners were undertaken to find a compound that possessed the quinidine-like action on the heart but not the other undesirable properties. The result was the introduction of procainamide; the cardiac actions of this agent are fully discussed in Chapter 31.

Smooth Muscle. The local anesthetics depress contractions in strips of isolated intestine and in the intact bowel (*see* Zipf and Dittmann, 1971). On the isolated intestine, there is little correlation between anesthetic potency and antispasmodic efficacy, and this spasmolytic action, which can antagonize the contractions produced by a variety of chemical agents, seems to be caused by a direct depression of smooth muscle.

Spinal and epidural anesthesia, as well as instillation of local anesthetics into the peritoneal cavity, cause sympathetic nervous system paralysis that can result in increased tone of gastrointestinal musculature. Most local anesthetics may increase the resting tone and decrease the contractions of isolated human uterine muscle; however, uterine contractions are seldom depressed during intrapartum regional anesthesia (de Jong, 1977).

Hypersensitivity to Local Anesthetics. Rare individuals exhibit a hypersensitivity to local anesthetics. This may manifest itself as an allergic dermatitis, a typical asthmatic attack, or a fatal anaphylactic reaction (*see* de Jong, 1977). Hypersensitivity seems to occur most prominently in response to local anesthetics of the *ester type* and frequently extends to chemically related compounds. For example, individuals sensitive to procaine may also react to structurally similar compounds (*e.g.,* tetracaine). Agents of the amide type are essentially free of this prob-

lem, and substitution of such a compound to avoid group specificity is usually possible. Certain antihistamines are occasionally used as local anesthetics for individuals who have become hypersensitive to all the conventional agents. These antihistamines presumably have the general structural features necessary for local anesthetic activity without sharing the specific antigenic determinants of the conventional drugs.

Fate of Local Anesthetics. The metabolic fate of local anesthetics is of great practical importance because their toxicity depends largely on the balance between their rate of absorption and their rate of destruction. As noted above, the rate of absorption of anesthetic agents can be reduced considerably by the incorporation of a vasoconstrictor agent in the anesthetic solution. However, the rate at which they are destroyed varies greatly, and this is a major factor in determining the safety of a particular anesthetic agent. Furthermore, binding of the anesthetic to tissues reduces the amount that appears in the systemic circulation and, consequently, reduces toxicity. For example, in intravenous regional anesthesia of an extremity, about half of the original anesthetic dose is still tissue bound 30 minutes after release of the tourniquet (de Jong, 1977). Many of the common local anesthetics (*e.g.,* procaine and tetracaine) are esters, and their toxicity is usually lost as the result of hydrolysis, which occurs in both the liver and the plasma. Animals with experimentally produced hepatic damage are much more susceptible to the toxic actions of local anesthetics, so that the extensive use of a local anesthetic in patients with severe hepatic damage should be avoided. However, the ester type of local anesthetic is degraded not only by liver esterase but also by a plasma esterase, probably plasma cholinesterase. Metabolic degradation by the plasma esterase is particularly important in man, whose plasma can hydrolyze local anesthetics of the ester type 4 to 20 times faster than can the plasma of any other animal (Foldes *et al.,* 1956). Indeed, Brodie and coworkers (1948) have shown that in man the hydrolysis of procaine occurs mainly in the plasma and only to a small extent in the liver. Since spinal fluid contains little or no esterase, anesthesia produced by the intrathecal injection of an anesthetic agent will persist until the local anesthetic agent has been absorbed into the blood.

The metabolism of the amide-linked local anesthetics is more complex (see Hansson, 1971). Lidocaine is degraded by hepatic microsomes, the initial reactions involving N-dealkylation and subsequent hydrolysis. The general features of the metabolism of mepivacaine and prilocaine are probably similar.

Those anesthetic agents that are slowly destroyed by·the liver are in small part eliminated in the urine.

COCAINE

Source. Cocaine occurs in the leaves of *Erythroxylon coca* and other species of *Erythroxylon,* trees indigenous to Peru and Bolivia, where the leaves have been used for centuries by the natives to increase endurance and promote a sense of well-being.

Chemistry. Cocaine is benzoylmethylecgonine. Ecgonine is an amino alcohol base closely related to tropine, the amino alcohol in atropine. Cocaine is thus an ester of benzoic acid and a nitrogen-containing base. It has the fundamental structure previously described for the synthetic local anesthetics (see Table 15–1).

Pharmacological Actions. The most important action of cocaine clinically is its ability to block the initiation or conduction of the nerve impulse following local application. Its most striking systemic effect is stimulation of the CNS. In addition, cocaine has numerous important side actions.

Central Nervous System. Cocaine stimulates the CNS generally. In man, this is manifested first in a feeling of well-being and euphoria; sometimes dysphoria may result. These effects may be accompanied by garrulousness, restlessness, and excitement. After small amounts of cocaine, motor activity is well coordinated; however, as the dose is increased, tremors and eventually clonic-tonic convulsions may result from stimulation of lower motor centers and enhancement of cord reflexes. The vasomotor and vomiting centers may also share in the stimulation, and emesis may result. Central stimulation is soon followed by depression. Eventually the vital medullary centers are depressed, and death results from respiratory failure. The cerebral actions of cocaine and the subject of *cocaine abuse* are discussed in Chapter 23.

Cardiovascular System. Small doses of cocaine given systemically may slow the heart as a result of central vagal stimulation, but after moderate doses the heart rate is increased. The increased cardiac rate probably results from increased central sympathetic stimulation as well as from the peripheral effects of cocaine on the sympathetic nervous system, as discussed below. Although the blood pressure may finally fall, there is at first a prominent rise in blood pressure due to sympathetically mediated tachycardia and vasoconstriction. A large intravenous dose of cocaine may cause immediate death from cardiac failure due to a direct toxic action on the heart muscle.

Skeletal Muscle. There is no evidence that cocaine increases the intrinsic strength of muscular contraction. The relief of fatigue by cocaine seems to result from central stimulation, which masks the sensation of fatigue.

Body Temperature. Cocaine is markedly pyrogenic. The increased muscular activity attending stimulation by cocaine augments heat production; vasoconstriction decreases heat loss. Also, there is reason to believe that cocaine has a direct action on the heat-regulating centers, for the onset of cocaine fever is often heralded by a chill, which indicates that the body is adjusting its temperature to a higher level. Cocaine pyrexia is often a striking feature of cocaine poisoning and can easily be elicited in animals by sublethal doses.

Sympathetic Nervous System. Cocaine potentiates both the excitatory and the inhibitory responses of sympathetically innervated organs to norepinephrine, and sympathetic nerve stimulation and, to a lesser degree, to epinephrine. Cocaine potentiation was first observed by Frölich and Loewi in 1910, and many explanations have been offered to account for the phenomenon. It now seems well established that cocaine blocks the uptake of catecholamines at adrenergic nerve endings; this uptake process is primarily responsible for terminating the actions of both adrenergic impulses and circulating catecholamines (see Chapter 4).

Cocaine is the only local anesthetic that is known to interfere with the uptake of norepinephrine by the adrenergic nerve terminals and, therefore, is the only local anesthetic to produce sensitization to catecholamines. This provides a plausible explanation of why cocaine, unlike other local anesthetics, produces vasoconstriction and mydriasis. The peripheral component of the cardioacceleration produced by cocaine is probably of similar origin.

Local Anesthetic Actions. The most important local action of cocaine is its ability to block nerve conduction when brought into direct contact with nerve tissue. Cocaine was once used extensively in ophthalmological procedures, but it causes sloughing of the corneal epithelium. Because of this, and because of its potential for abuse, cocaine is now restricted to topical use, especially in the upper respiratory passages. Even this use may be accompanied by severe toxicity.

Absorption, Fate, and Excretion. Cocaine is absorbed from all sites of application, including mucous membranes and the gastrointestinal mucosa. Absorption is enhanced in the presence of inflammation, and systemic effects of the drug may thereby be markedly increased. For example, such may occur if cocaine is used in cystography when the urinary bladder is inflamed.

After absorption, cocaine is degraded by plasma esterases (Van Dyke *et al.,* 1976) and, at least in some animals, by hepatic enzymes (see de Jong, 1977). A little may be excreted unchanged in the urine (Lemberger and Rubin, 1976; de Jong, 1977). The half-life of cocaine in the plasma after oral or nasal administration is approximately 1 hour (Van Dyke *et al.,* 1978).

Tolerance, Abuse, and Acute Poisoning. Cocaine is a powerful cerebrocortical stimulant and is often abused for this effect. Overdosage may lead to acute poisoning. The effects and treatment of poisoning and the misuse of cocaine are discussed in Chapter 23.

Preparations and Dosage. *Cocaine,* U.S.P., and *Cocaine Hydrochloride,* U.S.P., are the official preparations of the alkaloid. The alkaloidal base is freely soluble in organic solvents; the hydrochloride salt, in water. Cocaine is not prepared to be used internally or injected. Solutions employed clinically for surface anesthesia vary from 1.0 to 10% depending on the mucosa being anesthetized. Epinephrine is usually incorporated in these solutions. Occasionally, dry cocaine powder is moistened with epinephrine solution to form so-called cocaine mud for use on the nasal mucosa. In view of the dangerous potentiative interaction between cocaine and catecholamines, this practice is to be condemned.

Cocaine, because of its addicting potency, is included among the drugs controlled by the federal drug-abuse regulations (*see* Appendix I).

PROCAINE

Procaine was synthesized by Einhorn in 1905 and introduced under the trade name NOVOCAIN. It is still a useful local anesthetic. The chemical structure of procaine has already been discussed.

Pharmacological Actions. The pharmacological actions that procaine shares with other local anesthetic drugs have been presented. However, one property unique to procaine and some related drugs deserves brief consideration.

Procaine-Sulfonamide Antagonism. Procaine and many other ester-type local anesthetics are hydrolyzed in the body to produce para-aminobenzoic acid, which inhibits the action of sulfonamides. This fact is occasionally of practical importance. Procaine and its congeners also interfere with the chemical determination of sulfonamide concentration in biological fluids.

Absorption, Fate, and Excretion. Procaine is readily absorbed following parenteral administration and thus does not long remain at the site of injection. In order to retard absorption, vasoconstrictor drugs may be added to procaine solutions. Following absorption, procaine, like the other ester-type drugs, is rapidly hydrolyzed, mostly in the circulation, by an esterase, presumably plasma cholinesterase.

Preparations. *Procaine Hydrochloride,* U.S.P. (NOVOCAIN, others), occurs as a white crystalline powder that is freely soluble in water. It is available as an official injection. Market preparations include the following: ampuls or vials of a 0.5, 1, 2, or 10% solution without epinephrine, or 1 or 2% solution with epinephrine in a concentration of 1:50,000 to 1:100,000, for infiltration and nerve block; 5 to 20% solution in ampuls, for spinal anesthesia; ampuls of sterile procaine hydrochloride crystals (50 to 500 mg), for spinal anesthesia; 0.1 or 0.2% procaine hydrochloride in isotonic sodium chloride solution, for intravenous infusion.

Clinical Uses. Procaine has a variety of clinical uses as a local anesthetic. It also has two special uses.

Procaine and the Aging Process. Systemic administration of procaine has been claimed to delay the aging process or alter favorably the course of the common chronic diseases of middle or later life. A critical review of the extensive literature (Ostfeld *et al.,* 1977) fails to substantiate this claim.

Procaine Salts of Other Drugs. Procaine can form poorly soluble salts or conjugate with other drugs and prolong their action. This property is unrelated to the ability of procaine to produce local anesthesia. For example, after the intramuscular injection of procaine penicillin G, the antibiotic is absorbed very slowly so that detectable concentrations of penicillin exist in the blood and urine for prolonged periods, as discussed in more detail in Chapter 50. The possibility of allergy to procaine must be considered when hypersensitivity to such preparations occurs.

LIDOCAINE

Lidocaine, introduced in 1948, is one of the most widely used local anesthetics. Its chemical structure is shown in Table 15–1.

Pharmacological Actions. The pharmacological actions that lidocaine shares with other local anesthetic drugs have been presented. Lidocaine produces more prompt, more intense, longer-lasting, and more extensive anesthesia than does an equal concentration of procaine. Unlike procaine it is an aminoethylamide. It is an agent of choice, therefore, in individuals sensitive to ester-type local anesthetics.

Absorption, Fate, and Excretion. Lidocaine is relatively quickly absorbed after parenteral administration and from the gastrointestinal tract (*see* Boyes *et al.,* 1971; Hansson, 1971; Keenaghan and Boyes, 1972). Although it is effective when used without any vasoconstrictor, in the presence of epinephrine the rate of absorption and the toxicity are thereby decreased and the duration of action is prolonged. Lidocaine is metabolized in the liver by the microsomal mixed-function oxidases by dealkylation to monoethylglycine and xylidide. The latter compound retains significant local anesthetic and toxic activity. In man about 75% of xylidide is excreted in the urine as the further metabolite, 4-hydroxy-2,6-dimethylaniline (Keenaghan and Boyes, 1972).

Toxicity. In experimental animals, overdosage of lidocaine produces death from ventricular fibrillation or cardiac arrest; procaine, on the other hand, tends to depress respiration rather than the circulation (de Jong, 1971). A notable side effect of lidocaine is sleepiness. There is also a high incidence of dizziness, which may be caused by a metabolite rather than by lidocaine itself (Boyes *et al.,* 1971).

Preparations. *Lidocaine Hydrochloride,* U.S.P. (*lignocaine;* XYLOCAINE, others), is very soluble in water and alcohol. The official preparations include injections and a cream, ointment, jelly, topical solution, and topical aerosol. Market preparations (0.5 to 4.0%), available in ampuls, vials, or prefilled syringes with and without epinephrine (1:100,000 to 1:200,000), are suitable for infiltration (0.5%), block (1 to 2%), and topical mucosal anesthesia (1 to 2%). Other preparations include ointments (2.5 to 5%), a jelly (2%), a cream (3%), and topical solutions (2 and 4%).

Clinical Uses. Lidocaine has a variety of clinical uses as a local anesthetic. In addition, lidocaine is used intravenously as an antiarrhythmic agent, as described in Chapter 31.

OTHER SYNTHETIC LOCAL ANESTHETICS

The number of synthetic local anesthetics is so large that it is impractical to consider all of them. Therefore, discussion will be limited mainly to those that are official in the U.S.P.

Some local anesthetic agents are too toxic to be given by injection. Their use is restricted to topical application to the eye, the mucous membranes, or the skin. Many local anesthetics are suitable, however, for infiltration or injection to produce nerve block; some of them are also useful for topical application. The main categories of local anesthetics are given below; the agents are listed in alphabetical order.

LOCAL ANESTHETICS SUITABLE FOR INJECTION

Bupivacaine hydrochloride (MARCAINE) is an amide type of local anesthetic; its structure is identical to that of mepivacaine except that a butyl group replaces the methyl substituent on the amino nitrogen. It is a potent agent capable of producing prolonged analgesia. Its mean duration of action is greater than that of tetracaine, while the toxicity of the two compounds is similar. Bupivacaine hydrochloride is available in solutions for injection (0.25, 0.5, and 0.75%) with or without epinephrine (1:200,000).

Chloroprocaine Hydrochloride, U.S.P. (NESACAINE), is a halogenated derivative of procaine, the pharmacological properties of which it shares almost completely. Its anesthetic potency is at least twice as great as that of procaine, and its toxicity is lower. Chloroprocaine hydrochloride is available in solutions for injection (1.0, 2.0, and 3.0%).

Dibucaine Hydrochloride, U.S.P. (*cinchocaine;* NUPERCAINE, others), is a quinoline derivative. It is one of the most potent, most toxic, and longest acting of the commonly employed local anesthetics. It is about 15 times as potent and as toxic as procaine, and its anesthetic action lasts about three times as

long. Dibucaine hydrochloride is infrequently used either topically or by injection.

Etidocaine hydrochloride (DURANEST) is a long-acting derivative of lidocaine. The time required for induction of anesthesia with etidocaine is about the same as that for lidocaine, but its analgesic action lasts two to three times longer (*see* de Jong, 1977). It is not employed for spinal anesthesia, but is useful for epidural and for all types of infiltration and regional anesthesia. It usually blocks motor before sensory fibers because of frequency dependence (*see* above). Etidocaine hydrochloride is marketed in solutions for injection (0.5 and 1.0%) with or without epinephrine (1:200,000) and in a 1.5% solution with epinephrine (1:200,000).

Mepivacaine Hydrochloride, U.S.P. (CARBOCAINE), is a local anesthetic of the amide type (*see* Table 15–1). Its pharmacological properties are somewhat similar to those of lidocaine, which it resembles chemically. Its action is more rapid in onset and somewhat more prolonged than that of lidocaine. It has been employed for all types of infiltration and regional nerve block anesthesia as well as for spinal anesthesia. Mepivacaine hydrochloride is marketed in solutions for injection (1.0, 1.5, 2.0, and 3.0% without, and 2% with, levonordefrin as a vasoconstrictor).

Prilocaine Hydrochloride, U.S.P. (CITANEST), is a local anesthetic of the amide type. Its pharmacological properties resemble those of lidocaine. Its onset and duration of action are longer than those of lidocaine. Like lidocaine, it may produce sleepiness. A unique toxic aftereffect is *methemoglobinemia,* and its use is declining for this reason. It has been employed for all types of infiltration and regional nerve block anesthesia as well as for spinal anesthesia. Prilocaine hydrochloride is marketed in solutions for injection (1.0, 2.0, and 3.0%).

Tetracaine Hydrochloride, U.S.P. (AMETHOCAINE, PONTOCAINE), is a derivative of para-aminobenzoic acid (*see* Table 15–1). It is about ten times more toxic and more active than procaine after intravenous injection. For topical anesthesia of the eye, a 0.5% solution or ointment is used; for the mucous membranes of the nose and throat, a 2.0% solution. For spinal anesthesia, a total dose of 10 to 20 mg is adequate. Tetracaine has been rather extensively employed for continuous caudal anesthesia, but its onset of action at this site is very slow. The initial dose usually consists of 30 ml of a 0.25% solution. The effects are longer lasting than those of procaine. Tetracaine hydrochloride is available in solutions and in ampuls containing the dry salt. An official ophthalmic solution of tetracaine and an official ophthalmic ointment of 0.5% tetracaine base in white petrolatum are also marketed.

LOCAL ANESTHETICS LARGELY RESTRICTED TO OPHTHALMOLOGICAL USE

While certain of the agents described above can be used in the eye, the following local anesthetic agents are largely restricted to the production of corneal anesthesia. Their main advantage over the prototype, cocaine, is that they produce little or no mydriasis or corneal injury.

Benoxinate Hydrochloride, U.S.P. (DORSACAINE), is a benzoic acid ester related to procaine. It is an effective surface anesthetic agent that is useful in ophthalmology. A single instillation of 1 or 2 drops of a 0.4% solution produces within 60 seconds a sufficient degree of anesthesia to permit tonometry. It is marketed as a 0.4% solution.

Proparacaine Hydrochloride, U.S.P. (ALCAINE, OPHTHAINE, OPHTHETIC), is a benzoate ester, but it is chemically distinct from procaine, benoxinate, and tetracaine. This difference in chemical structure may explain the lack of cross-sensitization between proparacaine and other local anesthetic agents. It is about as potent as tetracaine. Unlike some topical anesthetics, proparacaine hydrochloride produces little or no initial irritation. It is available in a 0.5% official ophthalmic solution for topical application.

Local Anesthetics Used Mainly to Anesthetize the Less Delicate Mucous Membranes and the Skin

Some anesthetics are either too irritating or too ineffective to be applied to the eye. However, they are useful as topical anesthetic agents on the skin and the less delicate mucous membranes. These preparations are effective in the symptomatic relief of anal and genital pruritus, ivy poisoning, and numerous other acute and chronic dermatoses.

Cyclomethycaine Sulfate, U.S.P. (SURFACAINE), acts on damaged or diseased skin and on the mucosa of the rectum and genitourinary system, but it is relatively ineffective on the mucous membranes of the mouth, nose, bronchi, and eye. The compound is marketed as a cream (0.5%), an ointment (1.0%), a jelly for urethral application (0.75%), and suppositories containing 10 mg.

Dimethisoquin Hydrochloride, U.S.P. (QUOTANE), is an active surface anesthetic that is not of the benzoate ester type. The high anesthetic potency of dimethisoquin makes it of unique value as an antipruritic for the relief of itching and pain associated with various dermatological lesions. The compound appears to be less sensitizing when applied topically than antipruritic ointments containing antihistaminic drugs, but isolated cases of contact dermatitis have been reported. Dimethisoquin is marketed as an ointment (0.5%) and lotion (0.5%).

Dyclonine Hydrochloride, U.S.P. (DYCLONE), has a rapid onset of action and a duration of effect comparable to that of procaine. It is absorbed through the skin and mucous membranes. The compound is used as a 0.5 to 1.0% solution for topical anesthesia in otolaryngology.

Hexylcaine Hydrochloride, U.S.P. (CYCLAINE), was previously used for infiltration, spinal, topical, and nerve block anesthesia. It is about twice as potent as procaine. Hexylcaine hydrochloride is available for topical application as a 5% solution and for injection as a 1% solution.

Pramoxine Hydrochloride, U.S.P. (TRONOTHANE), is a surface anesthetic agent that is not of the benzoate ester type. Its distinct chemical structure is likely to minimize the danger of cross-sensitivity reactions in patients allergic to other local anesthetics. Pramoxine produces satisfactory surface anesthesia and is reasonably well tolerated on the skin and less delicate mucous membranes. It is too irritating to be used on the eye or in the nose. Official preparations are available for topical application as a 1% cream or jelly.

Anesthetics of Low Solubility

Some local anesthetics are poorly soluble in water and, consequently, too slowly absorbed to be toxic. They can be applied directly to wounds and ulcerated surfaces where they remain localized for long periods of time, which accounts for their sustained anesthetic action. Chemically, they are esters of para-aminobenzoic acid that lack the terminal tertiary or secondary amino group possessed by the previously described local anesthetics. The most important members of the series are *Benzocaine,* U.S.P. (*ethyl aminobenzoate;* ANESTHESIN), and *Butamben,* U.S.P. (*butyl aminobenzoate;* BUTESIN). Benzocaine is identical to procaine structurally, except that it lacks the terminal diethylamino group. They may be applied as dusting powders, undiluted or diluted with sterile talc. They are soluble in oil and may be incorporated in oily solutions, ointments, and suppositories.

Some salts of the tertiary amino group of local anesthetics are very insoluble. For example, the hydroiodide salt of tetracaine may produce anesthesia of 45-hours' duration when sprinkled in a surgical wound (Cherney, 1963).

Tetrodotoxin and Saxitoxin

These toxins are two of the most potent poisons known, the minimal lethal dose of each in the mouse being about 8 μg/kg. Both toxins are responsible for outbreaks of fatal poisoning in man. Tetrodotoxin is found in the gonads and other tissues of some fish of the order Tetraodontiformes (to which the Japanese *fugu,* or puffer fish, belongs); it also occurs in the skin of some newts of the family Salamandridae. Saxitoxin, and possibly some related toxins, are elaborated by the dinoflagellates *Gonyaulax catenella* and *Gonyaulax tamerensis,* and are retained in the tissues of clams and other shellfish that eat these organisms. Given the right conditions of temperature and light the *Gonyaulax* may multiply so rapidly as to discolor the ocean—hence the term *red tide.* Shellfish feeding on *Gonyaulax* at this time become extremely toxic to man and are responsible for the periodic outbreaks of *paralytic shellfish poisoning* (see Kao, 1966, 1972).

Although the toxins are chemically different from each other, their *mechanism of action* seems identical (see Narahashi, 1972). Both toxins, in nanomolar concentrations, specifically block the sodium channels in the membranes of excitable cells. As a result, the sodium currents are inhibited and the action potential is blocked. Blockade of vasomotor nerves, together with a relaxation of vascular smooth muscle, seems to be responsible for the hypotension that is characteristic of tetrodotoxin poisoning (Kao, 1972). Both toxins cause death by paralysis of the respiratory muscles. The *treatment* of severe cases of poisoning therefore requires artificial ventilation. Early gastric lavage and therapy to support the blood pressure are also indicated. If the patient survives paralytic shellfish poisoning for 24 hours, the prognosis is good (*see* Ogura, 1971; Schantz, 1971).

Apart from toxicological considerations, there are two other reasons for current interest in these toxins. First, since the toxins are much more specific and potent than the local anesthetics described above, they might serve as prototypes for new chemical classes of local anesthetics. Indeed, in animal experiments a combination of saxitoxin and a local anesthetic produces nerve block of longer duration than does either agent alone (Adams *et al.*, 1976). Second, they are important in the analysis of the molecular basis of the action potential. Experiments with radioactively labeled toxins have been used to determine the density of sodium channels in a variety of nerves (*see* Ritchie, 1979).

CLINICAL USES OF LOCAL ANESTHETICS

Local anesthesia is the loss of sensation without the loss of consciousness, and central control of vital functions is not impaired. A major advantage, therefore, is that the physiological trespass associated with general anesthesia is avoided. Local anesthetics are not, however, devoid of the potential to produce deleterious side effects. The choice of a local anesthetic and the technic of its use are the determinants of such toxicity.

The following discussion concerns the pharmacological and physiological consequences of the use of local anesthetics; these are evaluated in terms of the potential advantages and disadvantages of local anesthetics under clinical conditions. Technics for the administration of local anesthetics are described in detail elsewhere (Moore, 1965; Bromage, 1978).

SURFACE ANESTHESIA

Anesthesia of mucous membranes of the nose, mouth, throat, tracheobronchial tree, esophagus, and genitourinary tract can be produced by direct application of aqueous solutions of salts of many local anesthetics. Cocaine (4 to 10%), tetracaine (1 to 2%), and lidocaine (2 to 4%) are most often used. Procaine and mepivacaine are ineffective; they penetrate mucous membranes too poorly. Cocaine has the unique advantage of producing vasoconstriction as well as anesthesia. The shrinking of mucous membranes decreases operative bleeding while improving surgical visualization. Comparable vasoconstriction can be achieved with other local anesthetics by the addition of a low concentration of a vasoconstrictor such as phenylephrine (0.005%). Phenylephrine should not be added to solutions of cocaine. Epinephrine, topically applied, has no significant local effect. It penetrates mucous membranes too poorly. Maximal safe total dosages for topical anesthesia in a healthy 70-kg adult are 200 mg for cocaine and lidocaine and 60 mg for tetracaine.

Peak anesthetic effect following topical application of cocaine or lidocaine occurs within 2 to 5 minutes (3 to 8 minutes with tetracaine), and anesthesia lasts for 30 to 45 minutes (30 to 60 minutes with tetracaine). Anesthesia is entirely superficial; it does not extend to submucosal structures. This technic does not alleviate pain or discomfort from pressure or distortion of adjacent structures. Topical anesthesia of the respiratory tract also inhibits ciliary action, a matter of possible concern in patients with excessive tracheobronchial secretions.

Local anesthetics are rapidly absorbed into the circulation following topical application to mucous membranes. Such topical anesthesia thus always carries the risk of systemic toxic reactions. Absorption is particularly rapid when local anesthetics are applied to the tracheobronchial tree. Concentrations in blood after instillation of effective local anesthetics into the airway are nearly the same as those that follow intravenous injection of the drug. Blood concentrations are lower and peak values are reached more slowly when a given amount of topical anesthetic is applied over a longer period of time. When topical anesthetics are applied to the mouth, nose, or throat, the patient should be cautioned to expectorate the excess solution of the anesthetic to avoid excessive absorption. Surface anesthetics for the skin and cornea have been described above.

INFILTRATION ANESTHESIA

Infiltration anesthesia consists in injection of a solution of local anesthetic directly into the tissue to be incised or mechanically stimulated. Infiltration anesthesia can be so superficial as to include only the skin. It can also include deeper structures, including intra-abdominal organs when these, too, are infiltrated.

The duration of infiltration anesthesia (or any other regional anesthetic technic except topical anesthesia) can be approximately doubled by the addition of epinephrine (1:200,000; 5 µg/ml) to the solution. By decreasing the rate of absorption of drug into the blood stream, epinephrine also decreases peak concentrations of local anesthetics in blood and the rate at which these are achieved. The likelihood of adverse systemic reactions is thereby proportionately decreased. Epinephrine-containing solutions should not, however, be injected into tissues supplied by end arteries, for example, fingers and toes, ears, the nose, and the penis. To do so may result in gangrene. For the same reason, epinephrine should be avoided in solutions injected intracutaneously. Since epinephrine is also absorbed into the circulation, it should not be used in patients in whom adrenergic stimulation is undesirable, especially those with ventricular arrhythmias, hypertension, or hyperthyroidism. Epinephrine is contraindicated during the administration of anesthetics, such as cyclopropane, that markedly increase ventricular excitability. Epinephrine can be used cautiously during the administration of halothane; maximal doses are 10 ml of a 1:100,000 solution in 10 minutes, or 30 ml per hour in a healthy 70-kg adult. Epinephrine is often not used in combination with an exceptionally long-acting local anesthetic (*e.g.,* bupivacaine) because of the possibility of inordinate prolongation of anesthesia (24 hours or more). Long duration of local anesthetic action may be advantageous during prolonged operations or as a means for providing relief of postoperative pain. Long duration may, however, prove disadvantageous in ambulatory patients because of concurrent loss of motor function and possible hazards associated with prolonged loss of cutaneous sensation.

The local anesthetics most frequently used for infiltration anesthesia are lidocaine and procaine. When used without epinephrine, up to 7 mg/kg of 0.5 to 1.0% lidocaine solution or 10 mg/kg of 0.5 to 1.0% procaine solution can be used for infiltration anesthesia in healthy individuals. Doses must be decreased in patients who are at risk of untoward effects. The duration of anesthesia is 45 to 60 minutes with either agent. When epinephrine is added, the amount of lidocaine or procaine that is used can be increased by one third.

The advantage of infiltration anesthesia and other regional anesthetic technics is that it is possible to provide good anesthesia without disruption of normal bodily functions. The chief disadvantage of infiltration anesthesia is that relatively large amounts of drug must be used to anesthetize relatively small areas. This is no problem with minor surgery. When major surgery is performed, however, the amount of local anesthetic that is required may make systemic toxic reactions likely. Whereas intra-abdominal procedures are technically feasible under infiltration anesthesia, substantially better operating conditions are more readily and safely achieved with lesser amounts of local anesthetic administered by other regional technics.

FIELD BLOCK ANESTHESIA

Field block anesthesia is produced by subcutaneous injection of a solution of local anesthetic in such a manner as to interrupt nerve transmission proximal to the site to be anesthetized. For example, subcutaneous infiltration of the proximal portion of volar surface of the forearm results in an extensive area of cutaneous anesthesia that starts 2 to 3 cm distal to the site of injection. The same principle can be applied with particular benefit to the scalp, the anterior abdominal wall, and the lower extremity.

The drugs used and the concentrations and doses recommended are the same as for infiltration anesthesia. The advantage of field block anesthesia is that less drug can be used to provide a greater area of anesthesia than when infiltration anesthesia is used. Knowledge of the relevant neuroanatomy is obviously essential for successful field block anesthesia.

NERVE BLOCK ANESTHESIA

Injection of a solution of a local anesthetic into or about individual peripheral nerves or nerve plexuses produces even greater areas of anesthesia with a smaller amount of drug than do the technics described above. Blockade of mixed peripheral nerves

and nerve plexuses also usually anesthetizes somatic motor nerves, a matter of importance in certain types of surgery. The areas of sensory and motor denervation usually start several centimeters distal to the site of injection. Particularly useful are blocks of the brachial plexus for procedures on the upper extremity distal to insertion of the deltoid, intercostal nerve blocks for anesthesia and relaxation of the anterior abdominal wall, cervical plexus block for surgery of the neck, sciatic and femoral nerve blocks for surgery distal to the knee, blocks of individual nerves at the wrist and at the ankle or blocks of individual nerves such as the median or ulnar at the elbow, and blocks of sensory cranial nerves.

The onset of sensory anesthesia following injection about a peripheral nerve depends on the pK_a of the anesthetic, that is, the amount that exists in the unprotonated form at a tissue pH of 7.4. The onset of action of lidocaine occurs in about 3 minutes; 35% of lidocaine is in the basic form at this pH. Onset of action of bupivacaine requires about 15 minutes; only 5 to 10% of bupivacaine is not protonated at pH 7.4. Latency is also determined by the need for diffusion of the agent from its site of injection to its site of action. Diffusion is more important in determining rapidity of onset when nerve plexuses are blocked than when single nerves are anesthetized. The latency of the anesthetic effect of lidocaine injected about the ulnar nerve is 3 minutes, but this value is nearly 15 minutes when the drug is injected about the brachial plexus. The latency of bupivacaine is over 20 minutes in brachial plexus block. In practice, local anesthetics such as lidocaine, which act rapidly but relatively briefly, are often combined with an anesthetic such as bupivacaine, which, although slow in onset, has a long duration of action.

Duration of nerve block anesthesia depends upon the physical characteristics of the local anesthetic used. Especially important are lipid solubility and protein binding. In general, local anesthetics can be divided into three categories: those such as procaine with a short duration of action (20 to 45 minutes) following anesthetization of a mixed peripheral nerve; those with an intermediate duration of action (60 to 120 minutes), such as lidocaine, mepivacaine, and prilocaine; and those with a long duration of action (400 to 450 minutes), such as tetracaine, bupivacaine, and etidocaine. Duration of nerve block anesthesia can be extended by increasing the amount of drug injected. However, this is of relatively limited value because the possibility of systemic toxic reactions is increased more than is the duration of action of the drug. Increasing the volume of anesthetic injected also increases the likelihood of spread of the solution to nearby structures that one may not wish to affect. Duration of action is more safely prolonged by the addition of epinephrine.

The types of nerve fibers that are blocked when a local anesthetic is injected about a mixed peripheral nerve depend upon the concentration of drug used, nerve-fiber size, and internodal distance. Frequency and pattern of nerve-impulse transmission also determine the types of nerves that are affected (*see* above), as exemplified by the propensity of etidocaine to produce block of somatic motor nerves more readily than block of somatic sensory fibers (Bromage *et al.,* 1974).

Pharmacological factors that determine latency, duration of action, and sensitivity of nerve fibers to the effects of local anesthetics are to be distinguished from anatomical factors, which are similarly important. A mixed peripheral nerve or nerve trunk consists of individual nerves surrounded by an investing epineurium. The vascular supply is usually centrally located. When a local anesthetic is deposited about a peripheral nerve, it diffuses from the outer surface toward the core along a concentration gradient (Winnie *et al.*, 1977). Consequently, nerves located in the outer mantle of the mixed nerve are blocked first. These fibers are usually distributed to more proximal anatomical structures than are those situated near the core of the mixed nerve. If the volume and concentration of local anesthetic solution deposited about the nerve are adequate, the local anesthetic will eventually diffuse inwardly in amounts adequate to block even the most centrally located fibers. Lesser amounts of drug will block only nerves in the mantle and smaller and more sensitive central fibers. Furthermore, since uptake of local anesthetics usually occurs primarily in the core of a mixed nerve or nerve trunk where the vascular supply is located, the duration of blockade of centrally located nerves is shorter than that of more peripherally situated fibers. The sequence of onset of block and recovery from block of sympathetic, sensory, and motor fibers in mixed peripheral nerves depends, therefore, as much upon the anatomical location of the fibers within the mixed nerve as upon their sensitivity to local anesthetics.

Which local anesthetic is to be used for a nerve block, as well as the amount and concentration to be used, depends upon which nerves or plexuses are to be blocked, the types of fibers to be blocked, the duration of anesthesia required, and the size and physical status of the patient. Procaine (0.5 to 2.0% solution) and lidocaine (1.0 to 2.0% solution) can be used in the amounts recommended above under Infiltration Anesthesia. Mepivacaine (up to 7 mg/kg of a 1.0 to 3.0% solution) provides anesthesia that lasts about as long as that from lidocaine. Bupivacaine (0.25 to 0.75% solution) can be used in amounts up to 3 mg/kg when long duration of action is required. Tetracaine (up to 1.5 mg/kg of a 0.1 to 0.2% solution) also produces anesthesia of long duration. Chloroprocaine (1 to 2% solution) is especially useful when short duration of effect is desired; up to 20 mg/kg may be injected because chloroprocaine is so rapidly hydrolyzed by plasma cholinesterase. As with other regional anesthetic technics, addition of 1:200,000 epinephrine prolongs duration and allows the use of greater amounts of local anesthetic.

Peak concentrations of local anesthetics in blood and the potential for systemic reactions depend upon the amount injected, the physical characteristics of the local anesthetic, and whether epinephrine is used. They also are determined by the rate of blood flow to the site of injection. This is of particular importance in nerve block anesthesia. Peak concentrations of lidocaine in blood following injection of 400 mg for intercostal nerve blocks average 7 μg/ml; the same amount of lidocaine used for block of the brachial plexus results in peak concentrations in blood of approximately 3 μg/ml (Covino and Vas-

sallo, 1976). The amounts of local anesthetic that can be safely injected as outlined in the preceding paragraph must, therefore, be adjusted according to the anatomical site of the nerve(s) to be blocked. Multiple nerve blocks (*e.g.*, intercostal block) require reduction in the amount of anesthetic that can be safely given because the surface area for absorption is increased. Nerve blocks in richly vascular areas must also be performed with less drug.

Successful nerve blocks are impossible without thorough knowledge of neuroanatomy. Armed with such knowledge, however, the expert anesthesiologist can predictably block any nerve by using one of two technics. He can place the needle for injection in the same fascial compartment in which the nerve to be blocked lies and then inject a relatively large volume of anesthetic solution. Diffusion of the solution is restricted by anatomical boundaries, and an effective concentration can thus be delivered to the nerve. This technic is frequently used, for example, in blocks of the brachial plexus via the axillary approach. It is essential when nonsensory nerves are to be blocked, for example, in paravertebral sympathetic or splanchnic nerve blocks. Alternatively, the anesthesiologist can assure himself that the tip of the needle lies immediately adjacent to the nerve to be blocked. Smaller amounts of local anesthetic need then be injected because of reliance on accurate placement of the drug. Assurance that the tip of the needle lies immediately adjacent to the nerve requires that a paresthesia be elicited, and the most accurate placement is ensured when a paresthesia is produced by injection of the anesthetic solution. This degree of precision is essential when the nerve to be blocked, for example, the sciatic, does not lie in a well-defined anatomical compartment. Even when nerves that do lie in anatomical compartments are to be blocked, elicitation of paresthesias substantially enhances the likelihood of producing successful anesthesia. Reliance on paresthesias also decreases the amount of anesthetic that need be injected. There is no convincing evidence that deliberate production of paresthesias, including those that occur upon injection, is associated with development of postanesthetic traumatic neuritis.

INTRAVENOUS REGIONAL ANESTHESIA

Intravenous regional anesthesia consists in the injection of local anesthetic solution into a vein of an extremity previously exsanguinated with a Esmarch bandage and kept exsanguinated by a pneumatic tourniquet placed on the upper part of the extremity and inflated above arterial pressure. Lidocaine (1.5 mg/kg of 0.5% solution) is frequently used for intravenous regional anesthesia of the upper extremity. Onset of anesthesia occurs in 2 to 3 minutes. At the end of surgery when the tourniquet is released, approximately 15 to 30% of the lidocaine injected into the isolated extremity enters the systemic circulation. Peak concentrations in blood, reached within 4 to 5 minutes, are less than those observed following brachial plexus or lumbar epidural block.

Intravenous regional anesthesia is not as effective in the lower as it is in the upper extremity. In the latter case it is used for operations at the level of or distal to the elbow. Intravenous regional anesthesia cannot be used when fractures or other tender lesions exist in the extremity because of pain produced by exsanguination with the Esmarch bandage. The safety of intravenous regional anesthesia depends upon maintenance of pressure in the tourniquet adequate to occlude arterial flow at all times.

SPINAL ANESTHESIA

Spinal anesthesia is produced by injection of a local anesthetic into the lumbar subarachnoid space below the termination of the cord (second lumbar vertebra). Spread of the agent within the subarachnoid space and, thus, the level of anesthesia are controlled by the injection of solutions that are heavier or lighter than cerebrospinal fluid; the patient is then placed in the head-up or head-down position. Addition of 10% glucose solution to that of the local anesthetic produces a solution that is heavier than cerebrospinal fluid (hyperbaric spinal anesthesia). With the patient in the head-down position the glucose–local anesthetic solution then ascends in the subarachnoid space. The height that it achieves is determined by the volume of solution injected and the degree of tilt of the patient. Hyperbaric solutions remain in the distal subarachnoid space when injected with the patient sitting or in the head-up position. Hypobaric spinal anesthesia is produced by addition of sterile distilled water to the solution of local anesthetic. These mixtures are used less frequently than are hyperbaric solutions.

The concentration of local anesthetic in cerebrospinal fluid decreases rapidly after injection as the drug is bound to tissue and absorbed into the vascular system. Furthermore, within 10 to 15 minutes a hyperbaric solution becomes isobaric. At this point changes in position of the patient no longer affect distribution of the local anesthetic within the subarachnoid space. The level of anesthesia becomes "fixed."

Local anesthetics within the subarachnoid space act on superficial layers of the spinal cord, but their primary site of anesthetic action is on nerve fibers. Because the concentration of local anesthetic in spinal fluid decreases as a function of distance from the site of injection and because different types of nerve fibers differ in their sensitivity to the effects of local anesthetics, zones of differential anesthesia develop. Since preganglionic sympathetic fibers are blocked by concentrations of local anesthetics that are inadequate to affect somatic sensory or motor fibers, the level of sympathetic denervation during hyperbaric spinal anesthesia extends an average of two spinal segments cephalad to the level that is unresponsive to painful stimuli. On the other hand, since somatic motor fibers are more resistant to the action of local anesthetics than are somatic sensory fibers, the level of motor blockade is an average of two spinal segments below the level made unresponsive to painful stimuli during hyperbaric spinal anesthesia.

The goal of spinal anesthesia is to block somatic sensory and motor fibers. The accompanying sympathetic denervation, however, alters physiological responses. Blood concentrations of local anesthetics during spinal anesthesia are relatively low and play no role in altering physiological responses. The amount of drug that is injected is too low, and the rate of absorption is too slow. The physiological effects of spinal anesthesia are those of sympathetic blockade, and the safe practice of spinal anesthesia requires comprehension of its consequences (Greene, 1958).

Cardiovascular Consequences of Sympathetic Blockade in Spinal Anesthesia. The most cephalad preganglionic sympathetic fibers arise from the spinal cord at the level of the first thoracic segment. Because of the two-segment zone of differential sympathetic block, sympathetic denervation is complete when sensory anesthesia is obtained at the third thoracic segmental level. Since the physiological responses to spinal anesthesia depend upon the level of sympathetic denervation, the consequences of spinal anesthesia with sensory loss to midcervical levels are essentially the same as those associated with sensory effects that extend only to the third thoracic segmental level. Furthermore, sympathetic denervation by spinal anesthesia involves preganglionic fibers, and each preganglionic fiber ascends and descends in the paravertebral chain to synapse with up to 18 postganglionic fibers, which are then distributed peripherally in a nonsegmental manner. Thus, blockade of sympathetic fibers at, for example, the fourth thoracic segmental level is associated with diffuse peripheral responses that extend three or four segments above the peripheral sensory area that is innervated by fibers arising at the fourth thoracic segmental level.

Even low segmental levels of sensory spinal anesthesia are usually associated with some degree of sympathetic blockade. The most distal preganglionic sympathetic fibers arise from the spinal cord at the second lumbar segmental level. Spinal anesthetic solutions are usually injected between the third and fourth lumbar vertebrae. Turbulence associated with injection, together with subsequent diffusion of the local anesthetic in spinal fluid, almost invariably results in sympathetic blockade at the second lumbar segmental level, even when sensory denervation involves only low lumbar or sacral roots.

The most important consequence of the sympathetic blockade of spinal anesthesia is alteration of cardiovascular function. Arteries and arterioles dilate in sympathetically denervated areas; total peripheral vascular resistance and mean arterial blood pressure thus decrease. Reduction in blood pressure due to peripheral vasodilatation during spinal anesthesia is, however, not proportional to the extent of the sympathetic block. Compensatory vasoconstriction occurs in areas where sympathetic innervation is intact. This increases regional vascular resistance and tends to restore blood pressure. Compensatory vasoconstriction occurs mainly in the upper extremities. It does not involve the cerebral vasculature. However, even with total sympathetic blockade the decrease in total peripheral resistance averages no more than 12 to 14% in normal individuals. The change is relatively small because the smooth muscles of arteries and (especially) arterioles retain a certain degree of autonomous tone, and they do not dilate maximally. Furthermore, sympathetic arteriolar tone is relatively low in the recumbent, normovolemic individual. Because the decrease in total peripheral resistance is relatively minor in normal individuals, even with total sympathetic blockade during spinal anesthesia, severe arterial hypotension is not brought about by changes in the arterial side of the circulation.

The postarteriolar circulation is also altered by the sympathetic denervation associated with spinal anesthesia. Spontaneous vasomotion consisting in rhythmic contraction and relaxation of precapillary sphincters ceases. Arteriovenous metarteriolar thoroughfare channels dilate. Arterial hydrostatic pressures are more directly transmitted to postarteriolar channels. As a result, there are changes in the route, volume, and velocity of postarteriolar and capillary blood flow. Whether these result in an increase or a decrease in tissue blood flow and oxygenation depends on the degree of autonomous tone maintained by denervated postarteriolar vascular structures, as well as on changes in effective perfusion pressure, that is, the difference between arteriolar and venular pressures. The former varies so greatly from one organ to another that it becomes impossible to make generalizations about whether tissue blood flow increases or decreases during spinal anesthesia.

The most important cardiovascular responses to spinal anesthesia are those that result from changes in the venous side of the circulation. Sympathetic tone to veins and venules is lost during spinal anesthesia to the same extent as is that to arteries and arterioles. Unlike arteries and arterioles, however, denervated veins and venules retain little autonomous tone. They can dilate maximally, and the extent to which they do is determined by intraluminal hydrostatic pressure. As they increase their capacity, they sequester within them a greater percentage of the blood volume, and venous return to the heart decreases. This can cause an appreciable fall in cardiac output and blood pressure.

The safety of spinal anesthesia thus depends upon maintenance of an adequate venous return to the heart. This is best accomplished by elevation of sympathetically blocked areas above the level of the right atrium. The slight (10° to 15°) head-down position is appropriate. In normal individuals in the slight head-down position, cardiac output remains normal even during total preganglionic sympathetic blockade. The head-up position, on the other hand, is associated with severe decreases in cardiac output and profound arterial hypotension. Cardiac arrest may occur. The head-up position should, of course, be used to restrict spread of hyperbaric anesthetic solutions in the subarachnoid space; however, if the level of anesthesia becomes unexpectedly high or if severe hypotension develops, the patient must unhesitatingly and immediately be placed in the head-down position. The resulting level of anesthesia may be embarrassingly high, but the patient will survive. Because adequate venous return is essential to the safe management of patients during spinal anesthesia, this form of anesthesia is contraindicated in the presence of hypovolemia from any cause.

Treatment of arterial hypotension during spinal anesthesia should, as a general rule, be initiated if systolic blood pressure falls by approximately 25% of normal *resting* levels. The patient is placed in the slight head-down position and oxygen is administered. Vasopressors are of some value but should not be relied upon exclusively. When used, vasopressors should be given intravenously in small doses. α-Adrenergic agonists, such as methoxamine and phenylephrine, are best avoided. The increase in peripheral vascular resistance produced by such agents may so increase afterload that the myocardium, already suffering from a decrease in preload, may fail acutely. Vasopressors that act solely by virtue of their positive inotropic effects are also of limited value in the absence of an adequate venous return. The most satisfactory vasopressors are those that decrease venous compliance. While no vasopressor acts solely on the venous circulation, agents such as mephentermine and ephedrine have desirable effects. They also have moderate positive inotropic effects, yet do not produce severe and undesirable increases in peripheral vascular resistance. Hypotension during spinal anesthesia may also be treated by the rapid intravenous infusion of balanced salt solutions, sometimes in amounts as great as 1.5 to 2 liters or more. While hypovolemia must be treated during spinal anesthesia (or any other type of anesthesia), the administration of large volumes of intravenous fluids to normovolemic patients rendered hypotensive by sympathetic blockade during spinal anesthesia may be questioned. Cardiac output is restored by rapid infusion of balanced salt solutions to the extent that venous return is increased, but the increase is accomplished by hemodilution, not by increasing the ouput of blood with a normal content of oxygen. Use of large volumes of intravenous fluids in this way also sharply increases the incidence of postoperative urinary retention and the need for catheterization.

Spinal anesthesia is, in the absence of parasympatholytic premedication, characterized by a decrease in pulse rate. The bradycardia is due to a combination of two factors: preganglionic blockade of cardiac accelerator fibers (first through fourth thoracic spinal segments), and responses of intrinsic stretch receptors in the right side of the heart that mediate chronotropic responses to changes in central venous and right atrial pressure. The role of intrinsic stretch receptors in regulation of heart rate during spinal anesthesia to midthoracic levels is illustrated by the effects of changes in posture on heart rate after the local anesthetic is fixed and changes in the level of anesthesia are no longer possible: lowering the patient's head increases pulse rate as venous return and right atrial pressure increase, while elevation of the head decreases pulse rate as venous return and right atrial pressure decrease.

Coronary blood flow decreases during spinal anesthesia in proportion to the decrease in mean aortic pressure. Myocardial work, however, also decreases. Myocardial oxygen requirements decrease because of the decrease in afterload, the decrease in preload, and the bradycardia. In normal individuals the decrease in the myocardial requirement for oxygen slightly exceeds the decrease in oxygen supply (coronary flow); the myocardium is thus relatively hyperfused. It is not known if the same relationship holds true in patients with coronary artery disease.

Cerebrovascular autoregulatory mechanisms maintain cerebral circulation at normal levels even though arterial hypotension may develop during spinal anesthesia. Only when mean aortic pressure decreases to the range of 55 to 60 torr does cerebral blood flow begin to diminish. The level of blood pressure at which cerebrovascular autoregulation is no longer able to compensate for decreases in arterial perfusion pressure is greater in hypertensive than in normotensive patients. Thus, hypotension should be treated sooner in hypertensive patients than in normal subjects.

Renovascular autoregulation also compensates for changes in arterial blood pressure over a wide range. When arterial hypotension is severe enough to diminish renal blood flow, glomerular filtration and urinary output decrease, but circulation remains adequate to maintain the viability of glomerular and tubular cells. The oliguria is transient and disappears as the effects of the spinal anesthetic wear off and blood pressure returns to normal.

Respiratory Complications. Pulmonary ventilation is little affected by spinal anesthesia. Even levels of sensory denervation high enough to include lower cervical dermatomes are associated with normal tensions of carbon dioxide and oxygen in arterial blood. The phrenic nerves remain unaffected during such high levels of anesthesia because of the existence of the two-segment zone of differential motor blockade mentioned above. The diaphragm compensates for intercostal paralysis, particularly since relaxation of the anterior abdominal wall associated with intercostal paralysis decreases resistance to descent of the diaphragm during inhalation. Diaphragmatic excursions during high spinal anesthesia may be impaired, however, in obese patients, in patients with ascites, in pregnant women at term, or in other situations in which intra-abdominal pressure may be increased, including use of the extreme head-down or Trendelenburg position.

While respiratory tidal volume and maximal inspiratory capacity are unaffected by high spinal anesthesia, forced expiration is impaired because of paralysis of the abdominal musculature. Patients with high spinal anesthesia are unable to cough normally. High spinal anesthesia may therefore be hazardous in patients with excessive tracheobronchial secretions.

Respiratory arrest, while rare, can occur during spinal anesthesia. Its most frequent cause is ischemic paralysis of the medullary respiratory centers associated with profound decreases in cardiac output and arterial blood pressure. Only a small percentage of such incidents is due to phrenic nerve paralysis during lumbar spinal anesthesia. Apnea is also not due to ascent of the local anesthetic in cerebrospinal fluid with direct depression of chemotactic respiratory neurons in the brain stem. Concentrations of local anesthetic in cisternal spinal fluid during high spinal anesthesia are inadequate to produce pharmacological effects; they are even lower in ventricular cerebrospinal fluid and have no effect on either vasomotor or respiratory nuclei in the medulla.

The fundamental importance of inadequate cerebral perfusion as the primary cause of apnea during spinal anesthesia is demonstrated by the observation that respiratory arrest almost always immediately precedes or follows cardiac arrest. Furthermore, prompt restoration of cardiac output by appropriate means will result in immediate restoration of ventilation. This would not occur if the apnea were due to phrenic nerve paralysis or to direct depression of the respiratory centers.

The incidence, magnitude, and type of postoperative respiratory complications are the same after spinal anesthesia (or other forms of regional anesthesia) as after general anesthesia for the same operative procedure. Postoperative respiratory complications are related to age, sex, smoking habits, use of narcotics, quality of intraoperative and postoperative ventilatory care, preexisting pulmonary disease, and, above all, the anatomical site and nature of the surgery. When these factors are taken into consideration, postoperative respiratory complications are not related to the type of anesthesia. Regional anesthesia, including spinal anesthesia, provides no advantage for the avoidance of pulmonary complications in the postoperative period.

Hepatic Function. Hepatic function is unaffected by spinal anesthesia, even in the presence of hypotension. Postoperative hepatic function is principally determined by the type and nature of the surgery performed. The magnitude and duration of postoperative hepatic dysfunction are the same following spinal or other forms of regional anesthesia as they are following similar operations performed under commonly used general anesthetics. The same holds true for patients with preexisting hepatic disease. Spinal and other forms of regional anesthesia confer no special benefits in patients with liver disease.

Neurological Complications. Residual neurological deficits associated with spinal anesthesia are so rare in modern practice that, if they do occur, aggressive and complete diagnostic tests must be undertaken immediately to assure that they are not due to other causes. The majority of neurological disorders that follow spinal anesthesia are coincidental manifestations of other pathology, ranging from tumors of the cord and demyelinating diseases to malpositioning of the patient with pressure-induced neuropathy of peripheral nerves. When neurological deficits do occur that are directly ascribable to spinal anesthesia, they may present themselves either immediately or they may develop days or a week or more after the procedure. Neurological complications with acute onset may be due to the unwitting injection of a toxic substance, most often alcohol or a detergent or antiseptic solution; this may result in chemical transection of the cord. The deficits may also be due to the injection of a local anesthetic with histotoxic properties or to the injection of an excessive concentration of a local anesthetic that normally does not cause histotoxicity. Tetracaine, procaine, and lidocaine are devoid of neurotoxicity. When neurological complications follow the use of these local anesthetics, they are, in the absence of chemical contamination of the solution, the result of injection in such a manner as to expose nerve roots and the spinal cord to excessive concentrations of the drug. They are not due to "allergic" responses to the agent.

Another cause of the immediate appearance of neurological deficits following spinal anesthesia is traumatic damage to a nerve root incurred during performance of the lumbar puncture. This characteristically involves a single nerve root. Nerve damage during lumbar puncture usually occurs when the needle is directed so far laterally that it impinges on a nerve root at its point of exit from the subarachnoid space through the dura—the point at which a nerve is sufficiently fixed to be susceptible to direct trauma. Such damage to a nerve root in the cauda equina is rare.

Neurological sequelae of spinal anesthesia that are delayed in onset are usually the result of chronic arachnoiditis; this is produced by the inadvertent injection of materials (lint, talc, etc.) or chemicals that initiate a chronic inflammatory response. Avoidance of this type of reaction depends upon meticulous attention to details of technic during administration of the drug and the use of equipment that is chemically uncontaminated as well as sterile.

Spinal anesthesia is commonly regarded as contraindicated in patients with preexisting disease of the spinal cord. The assumption is that abnormal neural tissue is more susceptible to the histotoxic effects of local anesthetics. No experimental evidence exists to support this hypothesis. It is, nonetheless, prudent to avoid spinal anesthesia in patients with progressive diseases of the spinal cord, since worsening of the disease may be blamed on the anesthetic agent or the procedure. There is no reason, however, to avoid spinal anesthesia in patients with peripheral neuropathies or with diseases or conditions that affect intracranial portions of the CNS. Indeed, the latter category of patients may benefit from the use of spinal anesthesia instead of general anesthesia, provided there is no associated increase in intracranial pressure.

Headaches may follow any lumbar puncture, whether for diagnostic or anesthetic purpose. Characteristically postural in nature, these disappear when the patient is supine. The incidence of such headaches is related to the size of the needle used and to the age and sex of the patient. When 25-gauge needles are used, the incidence of headaches after spinal anesthesia is 1% or less (even in obstetrical patients, who constitute the most susceptible group). Spinal needles larger than 22-gauge should be avoided. Severe headaches may be accompanied by temporary palsy of the abducens nerve, with resulting diploplia. Headaches with meningismus indicate irritation, and the cause must be carefully evaluated.

Dosage and Duration of Anesthesia. Dosages of local anesthetics used for spinal anesthesia vary according to the volume of the subarachnoid space (*i.e.,* the height of the patient), the segmental level of anesthesia desired, and the duration of anesthesia required. Since all local anesthetics carry with them the potential for production of neurotoxic responses if used in excessively high concentrations, the amounts used in spinal anesthesia should be adjusted to avoid concentrations in spinal fluid in excess of those needed to produce anesthesia. Tetra-caine should not be injected in concentrations exceeding 0.5%; injected concentrations of lidocaine and procaine should not exceed 5%. When high thoracic levels of anesthesia are sought, 16 mg of tetracaine, 125 mg of lidocaine, or 200 mg of procaine may be used. The duration of anesthesia averages approximately 1.75 hours with this dose of tetracaine during high thoracic spinal anesthesia, about 60 minutes with lidocaine, and 45 to 60 minutes with procaine. Slightly longer duration may be achieved with 18 mg of tetracaine, 150 mg of lidocaine, or 250 mg of procaine; these doses should not be exceeded regardless of the height of anesthesia desired. At the opposite extreme, 4 to 6 mg of tetracaine, 25 to 50 mg of lidocaine, and 50 to 75 mg of procaine are appropriate doses when anesthesia of low lumbar and sacral roots is desired. Intermediate doses are indicated for intermediate segmental levels of anesthesia.

The duration of spinal anesthesia with a given dose of local anesthetic to a given segmental level of anesthesia is prolonged in elderly patients because of decreased rates of vascular absorption. Duration of any spinal anesthetic may be safely extended by 75 to 100% by addition of epinephrine to the solution of local anesthetic. The amount of epinephrine used ranges from 0.1 to 0.5 mg, depending upon the level of anesthesia.

Evaluation of Spinal Anesthesia. Modern spinal anesthesia is a safe and effective technic. Its value is greatest during surgery involving the lower abdomen, the extremities, or the perineum. It is often combined with intravenous medication to provide sedation and amnesia. With low spinal anesthesia the potential for physiological trespass is less than that associated with general anesthesia. The same does not apply for high spinal anesthesia. The sympathetic blockade that accompanies levels of spinal anesthesia adequate for mid or upper abdominal surgery is so extensive that equally satisfactory and safer operating conditions are usually achieved by the administration of a general anesthetic and a neuromuscular blocking agent. Low spinal anesthesia and high spinal anesthesia are, in physiological terms, totally different technics. One is frequently indicated, the other only rarely.

EPIDURAL ANESTHESIA

Injection of a solution of local anesthetic into the epidural space is a popular form of regional anesthesia. When injected into the lumbar, or less frequently, the thoracic area, the anesthetic acts in two places. It diffuses across the dura into the subarachnoid space, where it acts on nerve roots and the spinal cord much as it does when injected directly into the subarachnoid space during spinal anesthesia. The drug also diffuses into the paravertebral area through the intervertebral foramina, producing, in essence, multiple paravertebral nerve blocks. The former is the more important site of action. When local anesthetics are injected into the epidural space via the caudal canal (caudal anesthesia), the anesthetic acts less by diffusing across the dura and more by blocking nerves as they pass through the epidural space; diffusion through sacral foramina also plays an important role.

The choice of drugs to be used during epidural anesthesia is dictated primarily by the duration of anesthesia desired. Particularly popular are bupivacaine, when long duration is sought, and lidocaine, when a shorter-acting agent is indicated. Chloroprocaine is useful when very short duration of action is required. The duration of action of lidocaine is frequently prolonged (and its systemic toxicity decreased) by addition of epinephrine (1:200,000). Duration of anesthesia is also frequently extended by serial injections through a catheter placed in the epidural space.

The volumes of local anesthetic injected during epidural anesthesia are determined principally by the segmental level of anesthesia required. The larger the volume, the greater is the spread within the epidural space and the more extensive the area of anesthesia. The volume of anesthetic needed to achieve a given level of anesthesia may be decreased in older patients because the patency of intervertebral foramina is decreased and less anesthetic diffuses into the paravertebral area.

Concentrations of local anesthetic used are determined by the types of nerve fibers to be blocked. The lowest concentrations are used when only sympathetic fibers are to be blocked. The highest concentrations are used when sympathetic, somatic sensory, and somatic motor blockade are required. Intermediate concentrations allow somatic sensory anesthesia without muscle relaxation. The total amounts of drug that can be safely injected at one time are approximately the same as those mentioned above in the section on Nerve Block Anesthesia and the section on Infiltration Anesthesia. The technic of epidural anesthesia and the volumes, concentrations, and types of drugs used are described in detail by Bromage (1978).

Responses to lumbar epidural anesthesia, the most frequently employed form of epidural anesthesia, are in many ways similar to those that follow spinal anesthesia. This is not unexpected in view of the subarachnoid site of action of local anesthetics placed in the epidural space. There are, however, distinguishing features. One is in the zones of differential blockade associated with the two technics. There is no zone of differential sympathetic blockade with epidural anesthesia, and the level of sympathetic denervation is thus the same as the level of sensory denervation. On the other hand, the zone of differential motor blockade is four to five spinal segments with epidural anesthesia, whereas it is only two segments with spinal anesthesia.

Another significant difference between epidural and spinal anesthesia is that drugs used by the epidural technic are injected in amounts sufficient to produce high concentrations in blood following absorption. Peak concentrations of lidocaine in blood following injection of 400 mg (without epinephrine) into the lumbar epidural space average 3 to 4 μg/ml. The same amount of lidocaine injected into the caudal epidural space results in slightly higher values. Addition of epinephrine (1:200,000) to the lidocaine decreases peak concentrations in blood by about 25%. Peak concentrations of bupivacaine in

blood after the lumbar epidural injection of 150 mg average 1.0 μg/ml. These concentrations are a function of the total dose of drug rather than the concentration or volume of solution following epidural or other forms of regional anesthesia, except for spinal anesthesia (Covino and Vassallo, 1976).

Because epidural anesthesia is not associated with the zone of differential sympathetic blockade that is observed during spinal anesthesia, it might be assumed that cardiovascular responses to epidural anesthesia would be less prominent. In practice, this is not the case; this potential advantage of epidural anesthesia is offset by the cardiovascular responses to the high concentration of anesthetic in blood that is achieved during epidural anesthesia. This is most apparent when, as is often the case, epinephrine is added to the epidural injection. The resulting concentration of epinephrine in blood is sufficient to produce significant β-adrenergic stimulation. As a consequence, peripheral vasodilatation is so pronounced that blood pressure decreases, even though cardiac output increases due to the positive inotropic and chronotropic effects of epinephrine. The result is peripheral hyperperfusion and hypotension. Differences in cardiovascular responses to equal levels of spinal and epidural anesthesia are also observed when a local anesthetic such as lidocaine is used without epinephrine. The direct effects of the high concentration of lidocaine on peripheral smooth muscle and the effects of the agent on the heart may become significant. The magnitude of the differences in responses to equal sensory levels of spinal and epidural anesthesia varies, however, with the local anesthetic used for the epidural injection (assuming no epinephrine is used). Local anesthetics such as bupivacaine, which are highly lipid soluble, are distributed less into the circulation than are less lipid-soluble agents such as lidocaine.

High concentrations of local anesthetics in blood during epidural anesthesia are of special importance when this technic is used to control pain during labor and delivery. Local anesthetics cross the placenta, enter the fetal circulation, and may cause depression of the neonate (Scanlon et al., 1974). The extent to which they do so is determined by dosage, the level of protein binding in both maternal and fetal blood (Tucker, et al., 1970), placental blood flow, and solubility of the agent in fetal tissue. The persistence of abnormal neonatal neurobehavioral activity for 24 or even 48 hours after delivery may be related to placental transfer of local anesthetics during labor and delivery and to the relative inability of the neonate to metabolize the drugs, particularly those of the amide type. These potential hazards to the neonate can be offset to some extent by use of local anesthetics (e.g., bupivacaine) that are less distributed into the circulation. Such lipid-soluble agents are long acting. Furthermore, since control of the segmental level of anesthesia is in part determined by the duration of action of the agent when a serial-injection catheter technic is used, the anesthesiologist loses some control of the level of anesthesia.

The greater zone of differential motor blockade that results with epidural anesthesia means that this procedure has less effect on pulmonary ventilation than does an equal sensory level of spinal anesthesia.

This potential benefit is offset, however, during abdominal operations, because higher sensory levels of epidural anesthesia must be achieved to obtain the same degree of surgical relaxation of abdominal muscles that is produced by spinal anesthesia.

Adams, H. J.; Blair, M. R.; and Takman, B. H. The local anesthetic activity of saxitoxin alone and with vasoconstrictor and local anesthetic agents. *Arch. Int. Pharmacodyn. Ther.,* **1976,** *224,* 275–282.

Baird, W. M., and Hardman, H. F. An analysis of the effect of pH, procaine cation, nonionized procaine and procaine ethylchloride cation upon cardiac conduction time, stimulation threshold, amplitude of contraction and the relationship of these parameters to antiarrhythmic activity. *J. Pharmacol. Exp. Ther.,* **1961,** *132,* 382–391.

Boyes, R. N.; Scott, D. B.; Jebson, P. J.; Godman, M. J.; and Julian, D. G. Pharmacokinetics of lidocaine in man. *Clin. Pharmacol. Ther.,* **1971,** *12,* 105 116.

Brodie, B. B.; Lief, P. A.; and Poet, R. The fate of procaine in man following its intravenous administration and methods for the estimation of procaine and diethylaminoethanol. *J. Pharmacol. Exp. Ther.,* **1948,** *94,* 359–366.

Bromage, P. R.; Datta, S.; and Dunford, L. A. An evaluation of etidocaine in epidural analgesia for obstetrics. *Can. Anaesth. Soc. J.,* **1974,** *21,* 535–545.

Cherney, L. S. Tetracaine hydroiodide: a long-lasting local anesthetic agent for the relief of pain. *Anesth. Analg. (Cleve.),* **1963,** *42,* 477–481.

Courtney, K. R. Mechanism of frequency-dependent inhibition of sodium currents in frog myelinated nerve by the lidocaine derivative GEA 968. *J. Pharmacol. Exp. Ther.,* **1975,** *195,* 225–236.

Courtney, K. R.; Kendig, J. J.; and Cohen, E. N. Frequency-dependent conduction block: the role of nerve impulse pattern in local anesthetic potency. *Anesthesiology,* **1978,** *48,* 111–117.

Douglas, W. W., and Ritchie, J. M. Mammalian nonmyelinated nerve fibers. *Physiol. Rev.,* **1962,** *42,* 297–334.

Foldes, F. F.; Colavincenzo, J. W.; and Birch, J. H. Epidural anesthesia: a reappraisal. *Anesth. Analg. (Cleve.),* **1956,** *35,* 33–47.

Frank, G. B., and Sanders, H. D. A proposed common mechanism of action for general and local anesthetics in the central nervous system. *Br. J. Pharmacol. Chemother.,* **1963,** *21,* 1–9.

Franz, D. N., and Perry, R. S. Mechanisms for differential block among single myelinated and non-myelinated axons by procaine. *J. Physiol. (Lond.),* **1974,** *236,* 193–210.

Gasser, H. S., and Erlanger, J. The role of fiber size in the establishment of a nerve block by pressure or cocaine. *Am. J. Physiol.,* **1929,** *88,* 581–591.

Harvey, A. M. The actions of procaine on neuromuscular transmission. *Bull. Johns Hopkins Hosp.,* **1939,** *65,* 223–238.

Hille, B. Local anesthetics: hydrophilic and hydrophobic pathways for the drug-receptor reaction. *J. Gen. Physiol.,* **1977,** *69,* 497–515.

Keenaghan, J. B., and Boyes, R. N. The tissue distribution, metabolism and excretion of lidocaine in rats, guinea pigs, dogs and man. *J. Pharmacol. Exp. Ther.,* **1972,** *180,* 454–463.

Kendig, J., and Cohen, E. N. Pressure antagonism to nerve conduction block by anesthetic agents. *Anesthesiology,* **1977,** *47,* 6–10.

Matthews, P. B. C., and Rushworth, G. The relative sensitivity of muscle nerve fibres to procaine. *J. Physiol. (Lond.),* **1957,** *135,* 263–269.

Metcalfe, J. C., and Burgen, A. S. V. Relaxation of anaesthetics in the presence of cyto-membranes. *Nature,* **1968,** *220,* 587–588.

Mrose, H., and Ritchie, J. M. Local anesthetics: do benzocaine and lidocaine act at the same site? *J. Gen. Physiol.,* **1978,** *71,* 223–225.

Narahashi, T., and Frazier, D. T. Site of action and active form of local anesthetics in nerve fibers. *Fed. Proc.,* **1968,** *27,* 408.

Nathan, P. W., and Sears, T. A. Some factors concerned in differential nerve block by local anaesthetics. *J. Physiol. (Lond.),* **1961,** *157,* 565–580.

Ruff, R. L. A quantitative analysis of local anaesthetic alteration of miniature end-plate currents and end-plate current fluctuations. *J. Physiol. (Lond.),* **1977,** *264,* 89–124.

Scanlon, J. W.; Brown, W. U., Jr.; Weiss, J. B.; and Alper, M. H. Neurobehavioral responses of newborn infants after maternal epidural anesthesia. *Anesthesiology,* **1974,** *40,* 121–128.

Skou, J. C. The effect of drugs on cell membranes with special reference to local anaesthetics. *J. Pharm. Pharmacol.,* **1961,** *13,* 204–217.

Straub, R. Effects of local anesthetics on resting potential of myelinated nerve fibres. *Experientia,* **1956,** *12,* 182–187.

Strichartz, G. R. The inhibition of sodium currents in myelinated nerve by quaternary derivatives of lidocaine. *J. Gen. Physiol.,* **1973,** *62,* 37–57.

Tanaka, K. Anticonvulsant properties of procaine, cocaine, adiphenine and related structures. *Proc. Soc. Exp. Biol. Med.,* **1955,** *90,* 192–195.

Taverner, D. The action of local anaesthetics on the spinal cord of the cat. *Br. J. Pharmacol. Chemother.,* **1960,** *15,* 201–206.

Tucker, G. T.; Boyes, R. N.; Bridenbaugh, P. O.; and Moore, D. C. Binding of anilide-type local anesthetics in human plasma. II. Implications *in vivo,* with special reference to transplacental distribution. *Anesthesiology,* **1970,** *35,* 304 314.

Van Dyke, C.; Barash, P. G.; Jatlow, P.; and Byck, R. Cocaine: plasma concentrations after intranasal application in man. *Science,* **1976,** *191,* 859–861.

Van Dyke, C.; Jatlow, P.; Ungerer, J.; Barash, P. G.; and Byck, R. Oral cocaine: plasma concentrations and central effects. *Science,* **1978,** *200,* 211–213.

Winnie, A. P.; Tay, C. H.; Patel, K. P.; Ramanmurthy, S.; and Durrani, Z. Pharmacokinetics of local anesthetics during plexus blocks. *Anesth. Analg. (Cleve.),* **1977,** *56,* 852–861.

Monographs and Reviews

Bromage, P. R. *Epidural Analgesia.* W. B. Saunders Co., Philadelphia, **1978.**

Büchi, J., and Perlia, X. Structure-activity relations and physicochemical properties of local anesthetics. In, *Local Anesthetics,* Vol. 1. *International Encyclopedia of Pharmacology and Therapeutics,* Sect. 8. (Lechat, P., ed.) Pergamon Press, Ltd., Oxford, **1971,** pp. 39–130.

Covino, B. G., and Vassallo, H. G. *Local Anesthetics: Mechanisms of Action and Clinical Use.* Grune & Stratton, Inc., New York, **1976.**

de Jong, R. H. *Local Anesthetics.* Charles C Thomas, Pub., Springfield, Ill., **1977.**

Greene, N. M. *Physiology of Spinal Anesthesia.* The Williams & Wilkins Co., Baltimore, **1958;** reprinted by Robert E. Krieger Publishing Co., Huntington, N.Y., **1976.**

Hansson, E. Absorption, distribution, metabolism and excretion of local anesthetics. In, *Local Anesthetics,* Vol. 1. *International Encyclopedia of Pharmacology and Therapeutics,* Sect. 8. (Lechat, P., ed.) Pergamon Press, Ltd., Oxford, **1971,** pp. 239–260.

Kao, C. Y. Tetrodotoxin, saxitoxin and their significance in the study of excitation phenomena. *Pharmacol. Rev.,* **1966,** *18,* 997–1049.

———. Pharmacology of tetrodotoxin and saxitoxin. *Fed. Proc.,* **1972,** *31,* 1117–1123.

Lemberger, L., and Rubin, A. *Physiologic Disposition of*

Drugs of Abuse. Spectrum Publications, Inc., New York, **1976.**

Moore, D. C. *Regional Block.* Charles C Thomas, Pub., Springfield, Ill., **1965.**

Narahashi, T. Mechanism of action of tetrodotoxin and saxitoxin on excitable membranes. *Fed. Proc.,* **1972,** *31,* 1124–1132.

Narahashi, T., and Frazier, D. T. Site of action and active form of local anesthetics. *Neurosci. Res.,* **1971,** *4,* 65–99.

Ogura, Y. Fugu (puffer-fish) poisoning and the pharmacology of crystalline tetrodotoxin poisoning. In, *Neuropoisons: Their Pathophysiological Actions.* Vol. 1, *Poisons of Animal Origin.* (Simpson, L. L., ed.) Plenum Press, New York, **1971,** pp. 139–156.

Ostfeld, A.; Smith, C. M.; and Stotsky, B. A. The systemic use of procaine in the treatment of the elderly: a review. *J. Am. Geriatr. Soc.,* **1977,** *25,* 1–19.

Ritchie, J. M. Mechanism of action of local anesthetic agents and biotoxins. *Br. J. Anaesth.,* **1975,** *74,* 191–198.

———. A pharmacological approach to the structure of sodium channels in myelinated axons. *Annu. Rev. Neurosci.,* **1979,** *2,* 341–362.

Ritchie, J. M., and Greengard, P. On the mode of action of local anesthetics. *Annu. Rev. Pharmacol.,* **1966,** *6,* 405–430.

Schantz, E. J. Paralytic shellfish poisoning and saxitoxin. In, *Neuropoisons: Their Pathophysiological Actions.* Vol. 1, *Poisons of Animal Origin.* (Simpson, L. L., ed.) Plenum Press, New York, **1971,** pp. 159–168.

Shanes, A. M. Electrochemical aspects of physiological and pharmacological action in excitable cells. *Pharmacol. Rev.,* **1958,** *10,* 59–273.

Strichartz, G. Molecular mechanisms of nerve block by local anesthetics. *Anesthesiology,* **1976,** *45,* 421–441.

Zipf, H. F., and Dittmann, E. C. General pharmacological effects of local anesthetics. In, *Local Anesthetics,* Vol. 1. *International Encyclopedia of Pharmacology and Therapeutics,* Sect. 8. (Lechat, P., ed.) Pergamon Press, Ltd., Oxford, **1971,** pp. 191–238.

16 THE THERAPEUTIC GASES

Oxygen, Carbon Dioxide, Helium, and Water Vapor

*Theodore C. Smith, Lee H. Cooperman,
and Harry Wollman*

The therapeutic gases discussed in this chapter, most notably oxygen, are obviously not uniquely relevant to the central nervous system. They are placed in Section III primarily for proximity to the general anesthetic agents, many of which are also administered by inhalation.

OXYGEN

The importance of oxygen, water, and food to the animal organism is fundamental. Of these three basic essentials for the maintenance of life, the deprivation of oxygen leads to death most rapidly. Therapy with oxygen is useful or necessary for life in several diseases and intoxications that interfere with normal oxygenation of the blood or tissues. In addition, pure oxygen administered at ambient pressures greater than 1 atmosphere has both unique applications as a therapeutic agent and multiple toxic effects.

History. Soon after Priestley's discovery of oxygen in 1772 and Lavoisier's elucidation of its role in respiration, oxygen therapy was introduced in England by Beddoes. His publication in 1794, entitled "Considerations on the Medicinal Use and Production of Factitious Airs," can be considered the beginning of inhalational therapy (*see* Leigh, 1974a). Beddoes, overcome with enthusiasm for his project, treated all kinds of diseases with oxygen. They included such diverse conditions as scrofula, leprosy, and paralysis. Such indiscriminate therapeutic applications naturally led to many failures, and Beddoes died a disconsolate man. It is interesting to note that Beddoes' collaborator was James Watt, engineer and inventor of the steam engine, and his assistant was Sir Humphry Davy. When Beddoes' experiments proved disappointing, Davy left the laboratory in order to pursue his own investigations on the properties of nitrous oxide. Davy's contribution to the history of anesthesia is mentioned in Chapter 13.

It was only following such pioneer investigations as those of Haldane, Hill, Barcroft, Krogh, L. J. Henderson, and Y. Henderson that oxygen therapy was placed upon a sound physiological basis (*see* Sackner, 1974).

OXYGEN DEPRIVATION

Etiology of Hypoxia. *Hypoxia* is a broad term used to designate deprivation of oxygen regardless of etiology or site. Since hypoxia can arise from a variety of causes, and because methods of treatment are closely allied to etiology, a classification of the types of hypoxia is useful. One can consider five categories of hypoxia:

1. *Inadequate Oxygen Content of Inspired Gas.* In this situation, the oxygen tension in the pulmonary alveoli is below normal. This may be due to low inspired concentration of oxygen at normal ambient pressure, such as occurs when inert gases are present in greater-than-normal concentration. Alternatively, it may be caused by low ambient pressure, such as occurs at high altitude.

2. *Inadequate Delivery of Inspired Gas to the Lungs.* In this category, inspired gas has normal oxygen tension but is not delivered to the lungs in adequate amounts. This may be due to respiratory tract obstruction, to muscular weakness induced by disease (*e.g.,* myasthenia gravis) or by drugs (*e.g.,* neuromuscular blocking agents), or to lack of respiratory drive because of central nervous sytem (CNS) disease or the effect of central respiratory depressant drugs (*e.g.,* opioids and barbiturates).

3. *Inadequate Oxygenation of Blood Due to Abnormal Pulmonary Gas Exchange.* In the presence of a normal tension of oxygen in the inspired air and adequate ventilation, a defect in pulmonary function prevents the normal oxygenation of blood. The defect in pulmonary function may be a diffusion block,

321

due to thickening of the alveolar-capillary membrane. It may be caused by venous-arterial (right-to-left) shunts. It may also reflect a functional inequality of ventilation and perfusion in the lung, such as occurs in most acute and chronic pulmonary diseases.

4. *Inadequate Transport of Oxygen by the Circulation.* The delivery of adequate inspired oxygen to normally ventilated and perfused alveoli results in normal arterial oxygen tension. However, the arterial blood may fail to deliver sufficient oxygen to the tissues. This can be caused by low cardiac output, as in shock, or by maldistribution of the cardiac output, such as occurs following thrombosis or vasospasm. Another cause may be low oxygen-carrying capacity of the blood due to anemia or abnormal hemoglobin structure or function (carboxyhemoglobin; 2,3-diphosphoglycerate [2,3-DPG] deficiency) (*see* Desforges, 1976).

5. *Inadequate or Excessive Utilization by Tissues.* In this situation, tissues are unable to extract and utilize enough oxygen from the normally oxygenated blood that is delivered. This may be due to abnormally high metabolic demand (*e.g.,* thyrotoxicosis, hyperpyrexia) or to malfunctioning cellular enzyme systems (*e.g.,* cyanide poisoning, uncoupling of oxidative phosphorylation) (*see* Robin, 1977).

Actually, a combination of several kinds of hypoxia may exist and the dangers are then far greater. For instance, an organ with low blood flow due to atherosclerotic changes can sustain serious damage if the oxygen tension of its arterial supply should decrease only slightly.

Effects of Hypoxia. The signs and symptoms of hypoxia are varied and widespread. They are most clearly seen in the individual who is subjected to inadequate oxygenation of the blood acutely or subacutely, as with inhalation of low oxygen mixtures, respiratory depression, or respiratory obstruction. The picture differs in the patient acclimatized to hypoxic conditions; this complex subject cannot be considered here (*see* Lahiri, 1977). Nor will comment be made on the greater resistance to hypoxia manifested by the newborn of most species (*see* Mott, 1961).

The changes produced by hypoxia include alterations in the transport of oxygen in blood, which sometimes produce cyanosis. In addition, respiratory, cardiovascular, and CNS changes occur, as well as effects on individual organs and tissues and on metabolism. All these effects are discussed below.

Oxygen Saturation and Tension of Oxygen in Blood. The oxygen saturation, or content, of blood is related to its oxygen tension (P_{O_2}), as illustrated by the oxygen-hemoglobin dissociation curve (Figure 16–1) (*see* Severinghaus, 1966). The oxygen tension of the blood *and* the oxygen saturation of the circulating hemoglobin are both reduced when: (1) the partial pressure of oxygen in the inspired air is lowered, (2) the amount of oxygen delivered to the alveoli per minute is below physiological requirements, or (3) the exchange of oxygen from alveoli to blood is inadequate. The resulting reduction of *both* oxygen *tension* and *content* of the blood contrasts with other situations where blood P_{O_2} is normal but oxygen content is low, such as occurs in anemia.

Cyanosis. This is an unreliable guide to the arterial oxygen saturation. Cyanosis appears when about 5 g/dl of reduced hemoglobin is present in arterial blood. This figure represents an oxygen saturation of 67% when a normal amount of hemoglobin (15 g/dl) is present. However, when anemia lowers the hemoglobin to 10 g/dl, then cyanosis does not appear until the arterial blood saturation has decreased to 50%. Furthermore, the ability to recognize cyanosis clinically is extremely variable (Comroe and Botelho, 1947).

Respiration. Hypoxia stimulates both rate and depth of respiration reflexly through the chemoreceptors of the carotid and aortic bodies. Although moderate reductions in oxygen saturation fail to increase the respiratory minute volume markedly, the inhalation of gas mixtures containing 7% or less of oxygen nearly doubles the pulmonary ventilation. Furthermore, the respiratory response to carbon dioxide is considerably enhanced when the P_{O_2} of arterial blood is lowered (*see* Weil and Zwillich, 1976). It is important to realize that, as a result of the hyperpnea induced by hypoxia, there is a fall in arterial carbon dioxide tension (P_{CO_2}). Some of the physiological changes observed in hypoxic persons may be partly due to this mild hypocarbia. With decrease in the normal carbon

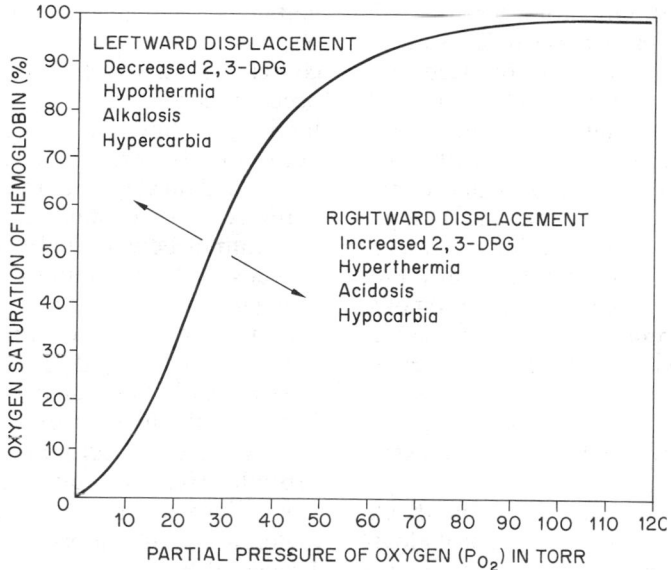

Figure 16-1. *The oxygen-hemoglobin dissociaton curve.*

Saturation of normal hemoglobin with oxygen is determined by the partial pressure of oxygen (P_{O_2}) and is modified by a number of other factors. The most important of these are certain phosphate compounds, temperature, and pH. Molecular CO_2 has a small effect opposite in direction to that of the hydrogen ions that result from hydration and dissociation of CO_2. A leftward shift of the curve limits the availability of oxygen, since a lower P_{O_2} is required to remove the same fraction of hemoglobin-bound oxygen. A rightward shift increases the supply of oxygen available to tissues. Different hemoglobins may have different dissociation curves. For example, the curve for fetal hemoglobin is above and to the left of normal. 2,3-DPG is 2,3-diphosphoglycerate. (Based on data in Arturson *et al.,* 1974.)

dioxide central respiratory drive, the increase in ventilation due to hypoxia at the peripheral chemoreceptors is somewhat self-limiting.

Normal individuals breathing low concentrations of oxygen fail to experience dyspnea because hypoxia and dyspnea are not necessarily associated. Dyspnea occurs when the respiratory minute volume approaches the maximal breathing capacity. In the normal individual, with a maximal breathing capacity of 160 liters per minute, an extreme degree of hypoxia does not provide sufficient stimulus for the minute ventilation to reach levels associated with dyspnea. On the other hand, if the maximal breathing capacity is reduced to 15 to 30 liters per minute by pulmonary abnormalities, any slight respiratory stimulation might raise the minute volume sufficiently to cause dyspnea. There are many stimuli to respiration in addition to hypoxia, for example, acidosis, hypercarbia, and activation of stretch receptors originating in the lungs. Thus, the indication for

oxygen therapy is not dyspnea but hypoxia or the threat of severe hypoxemia. When oxygen is given to a patient who has both hypoxia and dyspnea, therapy should not be stopped if oxygen fails to relieve the dyspnea (*see* Comroe and Dripps, 1950).

Cardiovascular System. The cardiac output increases with hypoxia, largely due to autoregulatory vasodilatation of the coronary and cerebral vasculature (*see* Cohen *et al.,* 1967; Kravec *et al.,* 1972). However, hypoxia leads to pulmonary vasoconstriction and thus pulmonary hypertension (*see* Zapol *et al.,* 1977). This response is an exaggeration of the pulmonary arterial vasomotion that matches regional perfusion to regional ventilation in the normal lung (*see* Haab *et al.,* 1969).

Acute hypoxia results in an increase in *heart rate,* probably mediated through some mechanism other than the carotid and aortic chemoreceptors (Daly and Scott, 1958; Krasney and Koehler, 1977). In normal individuals exposed to reduced oxygen tensions in the inspired air, the increase in pulse rate varies with the oxygen saturation of arterial blood, reaching about a 30% increase at 70% saturation. Tachycardia is such a consistent response to hypoxia that a reduction in heart rate of 10 beats per minute within a few minutes after the initiation of oxygen therapy has been taken as presumptive evidence that acute hypoxia existed (Comroe and Dripps, 1950). Continuing hypoxia, however, can result in a decrease in heart rate toward normal values, and the prolonged inhalation of 4 to 5% oxygen can produce circulatory failure.

The *blood pressure* increases in normal individuals subjected experimentally to acute hypoxia, but significant increases are not observed unless the inhaled oxygen concentration is below 10%.

Central Nervous System. Hypoxia affects the CNS both functionally and morphologically. An acute reduction of the arterial oxygen saturation to 85% ($P_{O_2} = 50$ torr) decreases mental effectiveness, visual acuity, emotional stability, and finer muscular coordination. Further reduction to 75% saturation ($P_{O_2} = 40$ torr) leads to faulty judgment, analgesia, and considerable impairment of muscular coordination. If the arterial oxygen saturation is reduced below 65% ($P_{O_2} = 32$ torr), unconsciousness and a progressive, descending depression of the CNS supervene (*see* Anderson *et al.*, 1946; Flynn *et al.*, 1977). Finally, circulatory failure occurs. Because hypoxia is so pernicious and reduces acuity of sensation and judgment, a person inhaling a low oxygen mixture may lose consciousness before realizing that any changes have taken place.

Under certain conditions the inhalation of carbon dioxide may offer some protection to the hypoxic brain, for three reasons. First, it counteracts the respiratory alkalosis produced when hypoxia induces hyperpnea, thus moving the oxygen dissociation curve to the right and making more oxygen available to tissues. Second, it increases the ventilation, resulting in more rapid delivery of oxygen to alveoli and therefore in a higher arterial P_{O_2}. Third, it tends to dilate cerebral vessels and increase blood flow to the brain (*see* Pierce *et al.*, 1962).

The manifestations of cerebral hypoxia produced by acute arrest of the cerebral circulation are sudden and dramatic. Changes in the EEG include the appearance of high-voltage slow waves (delta waves), which occur within seconds, as does the loss of consciousness. The first histological changes occur in cortical gray matter and some thalamic cells after 3 or 4 minutes of circulatory occlusion; the cerebellum is more resistant to hypoxic damage, and the brain stem and cord are most resistant. Full return of function cannot be expected if circulatory arrest exceeds 3 to 5 minutes, and irreversible damage and death may be expected if the cerebral circulation remains static for longer periods (*see* Plum, 1973; Safar *et al.*, 1978).

Individual Organs and Tissues. The brain is usually the first organ to manifest hypoxic damage; the myocardium is also highly susceptible. Hypoxic injury to other organs is slower in onset, but can occur as a result of generalized circulatory insufficiency. Cerebrovascular responses and compensatory vasomotor reflexes combine to deflect an inordinately large proportion of the cardiac output from visceral channels to organs such as the brain and heart. Under these circumstances, hypoxic damage to the liver and kidney as well as other organs can be demonstrated. The effect of oxygen lack on the eye is loss of visual acuity, which is manifested most noticeably by the abrupt development of a sensation of brightening following restoration of the normal supply of oxygen. Muscle is capable of sustaining an oxygen debt for periods of several hours by means of anaerobic metabolism.

Metabolism. Oxygen consumption and carbon dioxide production by the whole body and by various organs do not change measurably until extremes of hypoxia are reached. However, there are changes in carbohydrate metabolism associated with a shift from aerobic to anaerobic metabolic pathways. Those changes most frequently observed are hyperglycemia and increased production of lactic acid, with an increase in the lactate:pyruvate ratio in blood and metabolic acidosis. A summary of the metabolic effects of hypoxia has been provided by Cohen (1972).

ADMINISTRATION OF OXYGEN

Normally the inspired air contains 20.9% oxygen. At a barometric pressure of 760 torr this represents a partial pressure or tension of oxygen in the inspired air of 159 torr. However, oxygen uptake and dilution with water vapor and carbon dioxide reduce the P_{O_2} in the alveoli to about 100 torr. There is a small tension gradient between alveolar gas and arterial blood, resulting in a normal arterial P_{O_2} of about 90 torr (96% saturation). The inhalation of oxygen at 1 or more atmospheres of ambient pressure raises the arterial P_{O_2} to many times its normal value. This change is naturally followed by physiological adjustments, and under some circumstances by functional disturbances of the tissues exposed to these high oxygen tensions (*see* Lambertsen, 1965).

Effect on Blood Gases. *Oxygen.* Arterial blood carries oxygen in two forms. Most is normally bound to hemoglobin, as described by the sigmoid curve in Figure 16–1; a smaller amount is free in solution. The amount of oxygen carried in each way depends on the P_{O_2}. When fully saturated with oxygen, each gram of hemoglobin binds 1.3 volumes % of oxygen. At 37° C, 0.003 volume % of oxygen is dissolved in blood per torr of partial pressure of oxygen. These facts permit calculation of arterial content of oxygen from arterial P_{O_2} (*see* Table 16–1). Inspiration of oxygen at a variety of ambient pressures and concentrations may produce the same arterial P_{O_2}, as suggested by the examples in the right-hand column of Table 16–1. The oxygen utilized by tissue usually comes from hemoglobin; however, if sufficient oxygen is dissolved (due to very high P_{O_2}, as in a hyperbaric chamber), all the oxygen utilized by tissue may be supplied by dissolved oxygen.

Carbon Dioxide. One of the ways in which carbon dioxide is carried by blood is in the form of bicarbonate. This mechanism of carbon dioxide transfer operates more readily when a hydrogen ion acceptor is made available, as occurs in the capillaries when oxyhemoglobin is converted to deoxyhemoglobin, a stronger base and therefore a better hydrogen ion acceptor. When large amounts of oxygen are carried in simple solution, the amount of physically dissolved oxygen may be sufficient to satisfy the requirements of tissue (*see* Table 16–1). Little or no oxygen is then extracted from oxyhemoglobin, and deoxyhemoglobin is not formed. Carbon dioxide is then carried away from tissues less efficiently, and the P_{CO_2} of the tissues rises by several torr (*see* Lambertsen *et al.,* 1953).

Nitrogen. Normally, the blood is in equilibrium with alveolar air, which contains close to 80% nitrogen. As a result, several liters of this inert gas are in solution in body fluids and are present in body cavities. When pure oxygen is inhaled, the partial pressure of nitrogen in the alveoli falls rapidly. Nitrogen diffuses from the tissues to be eliminated by the lungs. Most of the nitrogen of the body can be exhaled in this manner within a few hours. The effects of this absence of "inert gas" from the body are discussed in the section on Untoward Effects of Oxygen Inhalation, as well as under Therapeutic Uses.

Respiration. The immediate effect of the inhalation of 100% oxygen by normal subjects is a mild respiratory depression, presumably due to withdrawal of tonic impulses from the chemoreceptors. After a few minutes the situation becomes far more complex, and there is no general agreement on the effects of steady-state concentrations of 100% oxygen on respiration (Lambertsen, 1966).

Cardiovascular System. There is a slight decrease in the heart rate of normal subjects inhaling pure oxygen. Cardiac output is reduced by 8 to 20%, which may be caused in part by oxygen-induced myocardial depression. There is little change in blood pressure. The inhalation of oxygen also affects blood flow to some important vascular beds. Coronary blood flow in the dog is reduced by the administration of oxygen. Cerebral blood flow is decreased slightly. Some attribute this to the mild hypocarbia attending oxygen inhalation. Whether oxygen itself has any direct effect on cerebral vessels is not yet clear. In the pulmonary vascular bed, high tensions of oxygen cause dilatation and reduced pulmonary arterial pressure. Oxygen inhalation appears to relax the pulmonary vasculature in hypoxic animals and man, and in persons with pulmonary hypertension. (*See* Fishman, 1961; Aviado, 1965; Stark *et al.,* 1973.)

Metabolism. When 100% oxygen is inhaled by man, changes are not detectable in oxygen consumption, carbon dioxide pro-

Table 16-1. THE CARRIAGE AND TRANSFER OF OXYGEN IN BLOOD *

ARTERIAL OXYGEN TENSION (torr)	ARTERIAL OXYGEN CONTENT (vol %)			MIXED VENOUS OXYGEN CONTENT (vol %)			MIXED VENOUS OXYGEN TENSION (torr)	EXAMPLES
	Dissolved	Bound to Hemoglobin	Total	Dissolved	Bound to Hemoglobin	Total		
30	0.1	10.9	11.0	0.06	5.9	6.0	20	Individual at high altitude or with respiratory failure breathing air
90	0.3	19.2	19.5	0.12	14.4	14.5	41	Normal man breathing air; patient with respiratory failure breathing oxygen
300	0.9	19.5	20.4	0.12	15.3	15.4	44	Anesthesia with 50% O_2—50% N_2O; individual at high altitude breathing oxygen
600	1.8	19.6	21.4	0.14	16.3	16.4	49	Normal man breathing oxygen
1800	5.4	19.6	25.0	0.45	19.6	20.1	150	Normal man breathing hyperbaric oxygen

* The table illustrates the carriage and transfer of oxygen in blood under a variety of circumstances. As arterial oxygen tension increases, so does the amount of dissolved oxygen, which is directly proportional to the P_{O_2}. As oxygen tension increases, oxygen bound to hemoglobin rises to, but does not exceed, 19.6 volumes % (100% saturation of hemoglobin at 15 g/dl). Increasing the oxygen tension by increasing inspired concentration, pressure, or both increases the amount of dissolved oxygen, which can be used by tissues. This is a small fraction of the total demand at normal oxygen tension, but at elevated ambient pressures (in hyperbaric facilities) dissolved oxygen may supply a large part or all of the requirement for oxygen.

The figures in this table are approximations based on the assumptions of 15 g/dl of hemoglobin, 5 volumes % of oxygen extraction by the whole body, constant cardiac output, and the ventilatory changes usually observed under the circumstances illustrated. When severe anemia is present, arterial oxygen tensions are little affected, but arterial content of oxygen is lower. Oxygen extraction continues, and, therefore, mixed venous blood has a considerably lower oxygen content and oxygen tension.

duction, respiratory quotient, or glucose utilization.

UNTOWARD EFFECTS OF OXYGEN INHALATION

The administration of oxygen, particularly at more than 1 atmosphere of pressure, can cause undesirable effects. However, none of these should interdict the use of high partial pressures of oxygen when they are indicated.

Pulmonary Atelectasis. When the alveoli of the lungs are filled predominantly with oxygen, subsequent airway obstruction may result in complete absorption of the gas with consequent alveolar collapse. Similarly, if a body cavity is filled with oxygen and subsequently its access to the atmosphere becomes obstructed, complete absorption of the gas can cause discomforting symptoms. For example, occlusion of the Eustachian tubes may lead to retraction of the eardrums, and obstruction of the paranasal sinuses may produce a "vacuum-type" headache.

Oxygen Apnea. In several situations the response of the respiratory centers to carbon dioxide may be so depressed that respiration is maintained largely by the activity of the carotid and aortic chemoreceptors. This phenomenon may attend cerebral injuries involving the respiratory centers, barbiturate intoxication, or long periods of exposure to hypercarbia or hypoxia (*e.g.*, chronic pulmonary disease). In these instances, the administration of oxygen may cause apnea by the removal of the chemoreceptor drive to respiration. The occurrence of oxygen apnea is not a contraindication to, but rather a convincing indication of the need for, the administration of oxygen. It is better to have the patient well oxygenated with controlled artificial respiration than to have him poorly oxygenated from breathing spontaneously, but inadequately, in response to a hypoxic drive from the chemoreceptor mechanism. Fortunately, in many cases it is possible to administer carefully controlled concentrations of oxygen sufficient to increase arterial oxygenation, but not great enough to cause apnea; the patient must be monitored constantly and the conditions controlled stringently.

Retrolental Fibroplasia. Retrolental fibroplasia occurs in some premature infants who have been exposed to high concentrations of oxygen at birth. Retinal changes begin to appear between the third and sixth week of life. These may regress entirely or may progress through retinal detachment to blindness. The incidence of this disease has been greatly reduced in recent years by administering oxygen only to those infants who require it and only for as long as it is required, and by limiting the inspired oxygen concentration to 35 to 40% when possible. However, the infant who is cyanotic despite inhalation of 40% oxygen should be exposed to higher concentrations; this can be done without increasing the danger of retrolental fibroplasia, for it is the *arterial* P_{O_2} and not the *inspired* P_{O_2} that is the crucial determinant of this disease. Retinal damage can also occur in adults following inhalation of 100% oxygen at greater-than-atmospheric pressures. This is particularly liable to occur in those patients whose retinal circulation has been previously compromised, for example, by retinal detachment (*see* Nichols and Lambertsen, 1969; Flynn *et al.*, 1977; Kushner *et al.*, 1977).

Oxygen Poisoning. *Effects on the Respiratory Tract.* The inhalation, at atmospheric pressure, of 80% oxygen for more than about 12 hours can cause a symptom complex mainly referable to irritation of the respiratory tract. Normal subjects exposed to these tensions of oxygen in the inspired air manifest a progressive decrease in vital capacity, coughing, nasal stuffiness, sore throat, and substernal distress, followed by tracheobronchitis and later by the development of pulmonary congestion, transudation, exudation, or atelectasis (*see* Clark and Lambertsen, 1971).

This syndrome is not experienced by subjects breathing 50% oxygen, nor by those breathing 100% oxygen at ½ atmosphere for 24 hours or longer. Thus, it is clear that the important factor in the causation of this symptom complex is the P_{O_2} and *not* the concentration of oxygen in the inhaled gas (*see* Winter and Smith, 1972). The onset and progression of signs and symptoms are more rapid at greater inspired P_{O_2}. When inspired P_{O_2} becomes greater than 2 atmospheres,

CNS toxicity is the first symptom to appear (Lambertsen, 1965). Figure 16–2 shows a comparison of the times of onset of pulmonary and CNS symptoms of oxygen toxicity.

In addition, breathing of oxygen depresses the mucociliary transport mechanism of the respiratory tract, with subsequent inhibition of the tracheal flow of mucus. This effect can be demonstrated after several hours of inhalation of oxygen and is influenced by both duration and degree of the hypoxia for which the patient is being treated. Inhibition of mucociliary transport impairs the host's pulmonary defenses (see Wanner, 1977).

Effects on the Central Nervous System. When pure oxygen is inhaled at pressures greater than 2 atmospheres, a characteristic syndrome is observed. Signs and symptoms include muscular twitching, nausea, vertigo, mood changes, paresthesias, and, finally, loss of consciousness and generalized convulsions. The appearance of this syndrome is related both to the length of exposure and to the ambient P_{O_2}. The symptoms may appear in persons at rest in less than 2 hours at 3 atmospheres, in ½ hour at 4 atmospheres, and in a few minutes at 6 atmospheres of oxygen. However, wide individual variations are observed in the susceptibility to oxygen poisoning. The latent period before oxygen toxicity appears is decreased by physical exertion and by inhalation of carbon dioxide. CNS toxicity produced by high pressures of oxygen appears to be reversible with decrease in the inspired P_{O_2}. Following a period of postictal depression, recovery of normal function is complete and relatively rapid.

Although the mechanism of this type of oxygen poisoning is not known, it may be related to the presence of free radicals containing oxygen, possible damage to cellular membranes by lipid peroxidation, and the oxidation of vital tissue components, including glutathione, ascorbic acid, and enzymes. Some protection against the oxygen toxicity syndrome is offered by the administration of gamma-amino-butyric acid, succinate, chelating agents, certain anesthetics, and tromethamine (*tris*-[hydroxymethyl] aminomethane). The mechanisms by which these agents offer protection are as numerous and conjectural as the possible mechanisms of CNS oxygen toxicity itself. (For detailed discussion, *see* Clark, 1974; Fridovich, 1975; Wolfe and DeVries, 1975.)

PREPARATIONS

Official U.S.P. preparations of oxygen are of a specified purity. Oxygen is marketed in a compressed

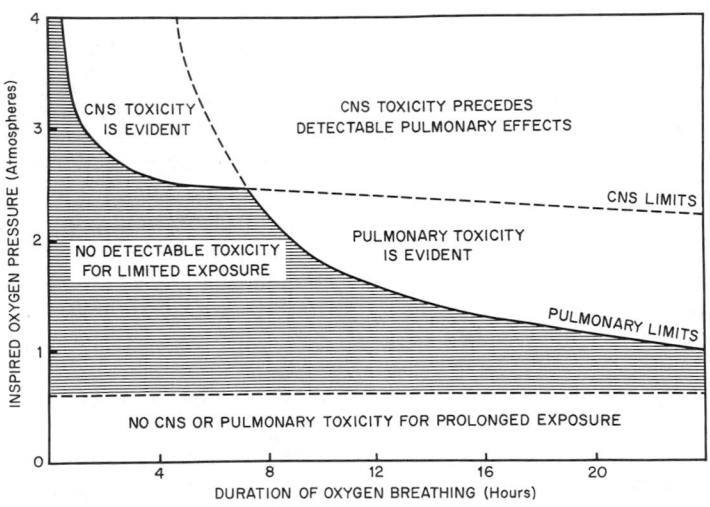

Figure 16–2. *Oxygen-toxicity limits in man.*

The two areas most affected are the CNS and the lungs. The occurrence of toxicity depends upon both the inspired oxygen pressure (P_{O_2}) and the duration of exposure. The safe duration of exposure becomes shorter as the inspired P_{O_2} increases. Below ½ atmosphere of inspired oxygen, indefinite exposure appears to be safe; between ½ and approximately 2 atmospheres, pulmonary toxicity occurs after prolonged exposures but CNS effects are not detectable; above 2 atmospheres, CNS toxicity appears before pulmonary effects are detectable. (Drawn from suggestions and analysis by C. J. Lambertsen, Institute for Environmental Medicine, University of Pennsylvania.)

form in steel cylinders fitted with reducing valves for delivery of the gas. They are usually color coded (green in the United States), and those for use on anesthetic machines are pin indexed.

METHODS OF ADMINISTRATION

The various methods for the administration of oxygen will be discussed only briefly. They have been reviewed by Barach (1962), Leigh (1974b), and Young and Crocker (1976).

Nasal Cannulas. A simple device for the administration of oxygen is a soft rubber or plastic catheter, which is inserted into a nostril, but not far enough to traverse the nasopharynx and enter the esophagus. Short, paired catheters that just extend into both nares are called nasal prongs. Humidified oxygen is passed through these tubes, and the rate of flow largely determines the concentration that enters the alveoli. It is rare that more than 50% oxygen can be introduced into the lungs by this means (Gibson et al., 1976). The nasal cannula causes minimal discomfort for the patient, and permits him freedom of movement while allowing attending personnel easier access to the patient.

Face Masks. Another, more effective method for the administration of oxygen is a face mask. Such masks may be equipped with a system of valves to permit elimination of carbon dioxide and dilution of the inspired oxygen with ambient air, if this is desired. It is possible to administer nearly 100% oxygen with a tightly fitted face mask and reservoir bag. The procedure is economical and efficient, and the transparent plastic devices are well accepted by patients. Masks are almost essential for use at high altitudes, in aviation, and in pressure chambers. Furthermore, they make possible the use of assisted or controlled ventilation, which can be of value in the treatment of pulmonary edema, asthma, and certain chronic pulmonary diseases. A device similar to the mask is the mouthpiece used in conjunction with a nose clip, but this is less comfortable and is not suitable for the depressed patient, who cannot maintain an airtight seal with this device.

Other Routes. Oxygen tents and hoods that fit over the patient's head in a fairly airtight manner are used occasionally. They are comfortable for the patient but restrict access of attendants. Oxygen must be delivered to them at relatively high flow rates. Administration of oxygen through an endotracheal tube or a tracheostomy in conjunction with mechanical ventilation is used for the seriously ill.

In a few cases where patients have been in the final stages of respiratory failure due to pulmonary disease, extracorporeal oxygenation has been used. A heart-lung machine oxygenates part of the patient's blood flow during this procedure. The hope was that several hours or, at the most, several days of such mechanical support would permit sufficient pulmonary improvement to make further extracorporeal support unnecessary; results have been disappointing (see Zapol et al., 1977).

THERAPEUTIC USES

Haldane stated years ago that *hypoxia not only stops the machine but wrecks the machinery.* The treatment of hypoxia is obviously a medical emergency, and, therefore, all therapeutic measures for its relief should be marshaled. Since the primary objective is the correction of the basic defect responsible for the deficiency, and since the causes of hypoxia are diverse, the therapeutic measures for its relief are numerous and varied. The administration of oxygen frequently does not correct the basic defect. Rather, oxygen is employed as a stopgap until more fundamental measures can be instituted or become effective, or occasionally because specific therapy for the underlying disease is unavailable. In this capacity the administration of oxygen can be lifesaving. The alert therapist does not wait until the signs and symptoms of severe hypoxia are evident but administers the gas in anticipation of its need.

As discussed above, the indication for oxygen therapy is not dyspnea but hypoxia. When oxygen is given to a patient who has both hypoxia and dyspnea, therapy should not be stopped if oxygen fails to relieve the dyspnea.

The therapeutic uses of oxygen are conveniently considered under the headings used above to classify the etiology of hypoxia.

Inadequate Oxygen Content of Inspired Gas. When there is a deficiency of oxygen in the atmosphere, for example, at high altitudes, the administration of supplemental oxygen will assure an adequate P_{O_2} in the alveoli. Above an altitude of 3.7 km (12,000 ft), where barometric pressure is below 500 torr, it is necessary to administer supplemental oxygen; above 10.1 km (33,000 ft), even 100% oxygen will not maintain normal alveolar P_{O_2}.

Inadequate Delivery of Inspired Gas to the Lungs. Inadequate oxygenation of the normal lung does not always call for therapy with oxygen. Rather, the basic cause of the hypoxia should be removed. For example, obstruction of the airway can often be corrected by mechanical means; insufficiency of the respiratory muscles or respiratory depression calls for artificial ventilation. However, there are circumstances under which oxygen therapy can be of great value. For instance, when obstruction to breathing is due to bronchoconstriction that proves difficult to overcome, hypoxia can be relieved when oxygen is administered by mask.

Inadequate Oxygenation of Blood Due to Abnormal Pulmonary Gas Exchange. This constitutes the chief indication for oxygen (*see* Pontoppidan *et al.,* 1973; Hedley-Whyte *et al.,* 1976; Sykes *et al.,* 1976). This is especially true when hypoxia is the result of poor diffusion of gases across the alveolar-capillary membrane or of inequality of ventilation and perfusion.

Diffusion Barriers. Oxygen diffuses less readily through the alveolar-capillary membrane than does carbon dioxide. Therefore, in situations where a diffusion barrier exists in the lung, the P_{O_2} of blood may fall considerably while the P_{CO_2} rises little. Oxygen will diffuse poorly across the alveolar-capillary membrane when anatomical changes occur, as in pulmonary fibrosis, or when the membrane is temporarily thickened, as in pulmonary edema. In such situations, oxygen inhalation is of great value in overcoming the diffusion barrier, and adequate arterial oxygenation can usually be obtained with only a small increase in inspired oxygen concentration. Pure diffusion block is rare, and other pulmonary defects in association with it are usually of greater functional importance.

Ventilation-Perfusion Inequalities. When some alveoli are poorly ventilated, the oxygenation of blood flowing past them is decreased. This blood will mix with well-oxygenated blood coming from more normal areas of lung, and the resulting mixed arterial blood will be intermediate in its content of oxygen. If the ventilation-perfusion defect is serious enough to produce significant desaturation of the arterial blood, therapy with oxygen is indicated. This treatment increases the P_{O_2} of gas in all alveoli, and some reversal of hypoxemia can be expected.

Venous-Arterial Shunts. A small amount of right-to-left shunting of blood is normal from Thebesian and pleural veins. Abnormal degrees of shunting may be due to congenital anatomical defects, or they may be acquired, as in patients with atelectasis or pneumonia. Since the shunted blood is never exposed to respiratory gases, administration of oxygen cannot increase its saturation. The increase in oxygen content of blood draining normal oxygen-containing alveoli is small, as it represents mostly dissolved oxygen (*see* Table 16–1). When this blood mixes with partially unsaturated blood, the resulting arterial pool may still be inadequately oxygenated. Thus, some improvement can be obtained by administering oxygen in the presence of right-to-left shunting; however, if the defect is great, arterial blood saturation may not be returned completely to normal.

Mixed Defects in Pulmonary Function. In most disease states, more than one factor contributes to the production of hypoxemia. For example, in *pneumonia* there is a diffusion defect. Atelectasis is present in some areas of the lung, and there is also a ventilation-perfusion defect. Finally, tachypnea and shallow respiration result in less effective alveolar ventilation. In this disease, as in many others, oxygen administration compensates for some of the abnormalities better than for others. It may overcome the diffusion barrier completely and successfully treat the ventilation-perfusion defect, but may only partially compensate for the shunting of blood past atelectatic alveoli. The inefficient ventilatory pattern usually improves with relief of the hypoxia. Oxygen

obviously does not remove the basic cause of the disease; improvement is symptomatic.

In the treatment of *pulmonary edema,* the administration of oxygen by mask or endotracheal tube with controlled or assisted ventilation can be of value. Particular benefit derives from the increased intrapulmonary pressure that is transmitted to the great veins, thereby retarding the flow of blood into the right heart.

Inadequate Transport of Oxygen by the Circulation. Oxygen is useful in certain types of circulatory disorders, in which it provides a valuable adjunct to more fundamental therapy.

Hemoglobin Deficiency. The administration of oxygen is of importance in the treatment of *carbon monoxide poisoning,* because it accelerates the conversion of carboxyhemoglobin to oxyhemoglobin. In addition, the breathing of pure oxygen leads to increased transport of this gas in solution in the plasma, and in this manner tissue hypoxia is partially relieved (*see* Chapter 70). Similarly, oxygen inhalation can also be of value in anemia.

Circulatory Deficiency. Oxygen has been used effectively in certain instances of generalized circulatory deficiency, including cardiac decompensation and shock. In *cardiac decompensation* the oxygen saturation of the blood may be reduced due to pulmonary edema. In addition, there is tissue hypoxia associated with circulatory inadequacy. Oxygen therapy often results in the relief of cyanosis and a slowing of the pulse rate. Although treatment should be directed primarily toward improving cardiac function, oxygen affords temporary relief due to better oxygenation of the myocardium.

Oxygen administration is of limited value in the therapy of the tissue hypoxia present during *shock.* Nevertheless, oxygen is often administered to patients with peripheral circulatory failure for whatever benefit can be gained from the increase in blood P_{O_2} and the additional oxygen carried in solution.

Oxygen may also be of some value in cases of localized circulatory deficiency, such as occurs in *coronary occlusion.* The higher P_{O_2} and oxygen content of the circulating blood may aid in the delivery of oxygen to hypoxic areas of the myocardium. Improvement is frequently noted, with relief of pain and restlessness, improvement of circulation, and relief of cyanosis. Oxygen inhalation may also be of value in some instances of *cerebrovascular accidents,* permitting better oxygenation of marginally hypoxic areas of the brain.

Miscellaneous Uses of Oxygen. A unique although uncommon use of oxygen is in the treatment of *abdominal distention.* In such conditions as intestinal obstruction, ileus, or postoperative distention, the gas accumulating in the bowel consists largely of nitrogen. Very little of this nitrogen will dissolve in blood, for it has already been exposed in the lungs to an atmosphere containing 80% nitrogen. If, however, 100% oxygen is breathed and the partial pressure of nitrogen in the alveoli falls, nitrogen diffuses out of the blood into the exhaled gases. As the nitrogen content of the blood decreases, the gas in the intestine diffuses into the circulation and is eliminated through the lungs. For similar reasons, inhalation of 100% oxygen has also been suggested for treatment of *spontaneous pneumothorax* and *air embolism.*

Oxygen inhalation is also used by workers in *pressurized spaces,* to decrease the inhaled nitrogen concentration and thus to lessen the likelihood of *caisson disease,* or bends, to shorten the required decompression time, and to minimize nitrogen narcosis. Under these conditions one must be careful not to exceed the time and concentration limits for avoidance of oxygen toxicity.

Finally, in *anesthesia,* oxygen is a common diluent for the gaseous and volatile anesthetic agents. The anesthetized patient may inhale up to 98% oxygen when 2% halothane is being administered in a nonrebreathing system, or as little as 20% oxygen when 80% nitrous oxide is given.

HYPERBARIC OXYGEN THERAPY

Although most uses of oxygen do not require more than 1 atmosphere of the gas, there are some conditions where administration of greater tensions may be desirable.

The administration of more than 1 atmosphere of oxygen as a therapeutic measure had its beginnings in the high-pressure experiments of Paul Bert in 1878. In recent decades serious studies of the effects of high-pressure oxygen by investigators such as Behnke, Boerema, and Lambertsen have provided some basis for the use of "hyperbaric oxygen" in clinical medicine.

Hyperbaric oxygenation is accomplished in pressure chambers. These range in size from those designed for a few small experimental animals, through those large enough for a man, up to chambers that accommodate an entire operating suite. Since it is neither practical nor economical to fill the larger chambers with oxygen, they may be brought to ambient pressures of more than 1 atmosphere with compressed air. The patients then inhale oxygen at these ambient pressures through a face mask or mouthpiece.

There are many practical difficulties associated with this type of treatment. The facilities and their proper maintenance and operation are expensive; there is a fire hazard in the enclosed space of the chamber; oxygen toxicity and nitrogen narcosis are distinct possibilities; and decompression sickness can occur in patients or attendants (*see* Committee on Hyperbaric Oxygenation, 1966). However, many potential uses for this method of therapy have been explored. Presently its use is justified in a few situations (*see* Trapp *et al.,* 1974; Davis and Hunt, 1977).

Gas Emboli and Bubbles. Hyperbaric oxygenation can be useful in the treatment of decompression sickness. It can also provide immediate relief of symptoms in situations where gas emboli in the vascular tree can be compressed by high pressures, such as diving accidents and postcardiopulmonary-bypass gas emboli. During slow decompression these bubbles, which become filled with oxygen, are gradually absorbed.

Anaerobic Infections. Intermittent treatment with hyperbaric oxygen may be of value in the treatment of infections produced by *Clostridium perfringens,* the anaerobic bacillus causing *gas gangrene.* The increased tissue oxygen pressure achieved inhibits growth and production of toxin by these bacteria. Antibiotics and other supportive therapy are still necessary. Results are less satisfactory in the treatment of *tetanus* with hyperbaric oxygen, as the toxin may already be bound to neural tissue, and, although the microorganism is killed or prevented from multiplying, irreversible damage may have occurred (*see* Alfery and Rauscher, 1979).

Hyperbaric oxygen may prove to be useful in the treatment of other anaerobic infections and for some cases of chronic, refractory osteomyelitis (*see* Medical Letter, 1979).

Carbon Monoxide Poisoning. The use of 2 atmospheres of oxygen will result in faster conversion of carboxyhemoglobin to oxyhemoglobin than will 100% oxygen at sea level. Little practical benefit is gained by increasing pressure much further. One treatment with 2 atmospheres of oxygen for 30 to 90 minutes is usually sufficient even for patients who are comatose. The greatest difficulty encountered in the use of this therapy is the problem of rapidly transporting the patient to a hyperbaric chamber. The use of 1 atmosphere of oxygen during transport is recommended and may make hyperbaric treatment unnecessary (*see* Chapter 70).

Circulatory Disturbances. If the blood flow to a tissue is decreased due to disease such as atherosclerosis, its P_{O_2} might be maintained near normal by increasing the P_{O_2} and oxygen content of its arterial blood. The increase in arterial and venous blood oxygenation produced by inhaling 3 atmospheres of oxygen is shown in Table 16–1. The *diffusion* of significant amounts of oxygen *through the skin* into blood and deeper tissues only begins at pressure above 10 atmospheres.

With the hope of improving tissue oxygenation by raising the arterial blood P_{O_2}, hyperbaric oxygen has been used as a therapeutic measure in such *local circulatory disturbances* as stroke, peripheral arterial insufficiency, and compromised skin grafts. The possibility of oxygen toxicity makes continuous therapy dangerous, and, therefore, intermittent treatments are used. The efficacy of this method of therapy in these diseases depends on the presence of some circulation to the tissues, that is, only partial occlusion of vessels or the existence of collateral channels for those that are blocked. This application of hyperbaric oxygen has had minimal success.

CARBON DIOXIDE

It was not until the end of the eighteenth century that Priestley discovered this gas and Lavoisier described its role in respiration. A century later Miesher demonstrated its effects on the respiration of man. The gas is of paramount importance in the regulation of many vital functions, and small changes in P_{CO_2} in the body have marked physiological effects.

TRANSFER AND ELIMINATION OF CARBON DIOXIDE

Several hundred milliliters per minute of carbon dioxide are produced by the body's metabolism at rest, and up to ten times that much during heavy exercise. The gas diffuses readily from the cells that produce it into the blood stream, where it is carried partly as bicarbonate ion, partly in chemical combination with hemoglobin and plasma proteins, and also in solution at a partial pressure of about 47 torr in mixed venous blood. It is transported to the lung, where it is normally exhaled at the same rate at which it is produced, leaving a partial pressure of about 40 torr in the alveoli and in the arterial blood.

The P_{CO_2} of air is a fraction of 1 torr. When 4% carbon dioxide is inhaled, the P_{CO_2} of inspired gas rises to about 30 torr. This increases the alveolar P_{CO_2}, decreases the gradient for its transfer from mixed venous blood to alveoli, and temporarily slows its elimination by the lung. However, as carbon dioxide accumulates, the tissue and blood P_{CO_2} rises, and a new steady state is reached in which carbon dioxide tensions are greater than normal. The difference in P_{CO_2} between mixed venous blood and alveoli is reestablished, ventilation is increased, and the minute volume of carbon dioxide produced by metabolic processes can again be exhaled through the lungs. When 8% carbon dioxide is inhaled, the P_{CO_2} of inspired gas is about 60 torr, which is *higher* than the blood and tissue tensions. Carbon dioxide is thus *taken up* by the body for a period of time. As the gas is both taken up and produced by the body, tissue and blood tensions increase to levels high enough again to provide a gradient from mixed venous blood to the alveoli. With the reestablished gradient and increased ventilation, elimination of carbon dioxide can again occur at the same rate as its metabolic production.

Under some circumstances, for example, with certain anesthetic technics (*see* Chapter 13), deliberate hyperventilation is carried out, resulting in a rate of carbon dioxide elimination that exceeds the rate of its production. The body's stores of carbon dioxide become depleted, and the arterial P_{CO_2} may decrease to 25 torr or less. Some of the effects of hypocarbia are discussed below.

When carbon dioxide is inhaled, or when alveolar ventilation is decreased, the P_{CO_2} in arterial blood rises and its pH falls. This decrease in pH is referred to as *respiratory acidosis.* When overventilation lowers the P_{CO_2} of blood, the pH rises and *respiratory alkalosis* is present. As carbon dioxide can freely diffuse into and out of cells, the changes in blood P_{CO_2} and pH are soon reflected by intracellular changes of P_{CO_2} and pH (*see* Chapter 35).

EFFECTS OF CARBON DIOXIDE

Alterations of P_{CO_2} and pH have widespread effects in the body. Here a description will be given of the important effects of carbon dioxide on respiration, circulation, and the CNS. (For a more complete discussion of these and other effects, *see* Nahas and Schaefer, 1974; Nunn, 1977.)

Respiration. Carbon dioxide is a potent stimulus to respiration. The inhalation of 2% carbon dioxide produces a measurable increase in both rate and depth of ventilation. Ten percent carbon dioxide can produce respiratory volumes of 75 liters per minute in normal individuals. The inhalation of even higher concentrations produces little additional increase in ventilation. Respiratory stimulation begins in seconds following the inhalation of even low concentrations of carbon dioxide, and maximal stimulation by the inhaled carbon dioxide is usually attained in less than 5 minutes (*see* Lourenco, 1976). The respiratory effects of carbon dioxide inhalation disappear within a few minutes after its withdrawal.

There are at least two *sites* where carbon dioxide acts to stimulate respiration. Respiratory integration areas in the brain stem are acted upon by impulses from medullary chemoreceptors and from peripheral arterial chemoreceptors. The mechanism by which carbon dioxide acts on these receptors particularly involves the decrease in pH produced by the gas (*see* Mitchell and Berger, 1975; Neff and Talmage, 1978).

Circulation. The circulatory effects of carbon dioxide are the result of its direct local effects and its centrally mediated effects on the autonomic nervous system. The direct effect of carbon dioxide on the *heart* results from pH changes and produces diminished contractile force and slowing of the rate of contraction (*see* Ng *et al.,* 1967). The cardiac rhythm is usually not affected. The direct effect on systemic *blood vessels* results in vasodilatation.

The autonomic effects of carbon dioxide result in widespread activation of the *sympathetic nervous system* with an increase in concentrations of epinephrine and norepinephrine in plasma (*see* Sechzer *et al.,* 1960; Hamilton *et al.,* 1966). The response is mediated by various subcortical centers in the hypothalamus, brain stem reticular formation, and medulla. These areas can be locally excited by carbon dioxide, but they also receive afferents from the carotid and aortic chemoreceptors that are sensitive to changes in carbon dioxide in the blood. The results of sympathetic nervous system activation are, in general, opposite to the local effects of carbon dioxide. The sympathetic effects consist in increase in the force and rate of cardiac contraction and constriction of many vascular beds.

The total circulatory response to carbon dioxide, therefore, is determined by the balance of the opposing effects on local tissues and on the sympathetic nervous sytem effects. The overall effects of carbon dioxide inhalation in normal man are increase in cardiac output and heart rate, elevation of systolic and diastolic blood pressures, and increase in pulse pressure (*see* Blackburn *et al.,* 1972; Cullen and Eger, 1974). There is a *decrease* in total peripheral resistance when carbon dioxide is breathed. The local vasodilating effects of carbon dioxide appear to exert more of an influence than do the sympathetically mediated vasoconstrictor effects. In the heart, the marked increase in cardiac output reflects a predominance of the sympathetic over the local effects. When carbon dioxide is breathed by an individual whose vasomotor impulses are blocked, for example, by spinal anesthesia or extensive sympathectomy, the peripheral action of carbon dioxide predominates and the blood pressure falls.

Cardiac arrhythmias due to inhalation of carbon dioxide are rare, even when arterial P_{CO_2} reaches 80 torr (Sechzer *et al.*, 1960). However, when the arrhythmia threshold is decreased by factors such as the inhalation of some of the halogenated anesthetics, carbon dioxide is more likely to produce cardiac arrhythmias.

The cerebral circulation, which does not have functionally important sympathetic innervation, undergoes significant dilatation when carbon dioxide is inhaled (*see* Kety and Schmidt, 1948). To a lesser extent carbon dioxide produces coronary vasodilatation (Rowe, 1974; Neill and Hattenhauer, 1975).

Following the termination of carbon dioxide inhalation, a mild fall in blood pressure is noted in awake man, along with tachycardia (Dripps and Comroe, 1947; Sechzer *et al.*, 1960).

The circulatory effects of lower-than-normal tensions of carbon dioxide may be observed during voluntary or mechanical hyperventilation. They consist in vascular dilatation in muscle and vasoconstriction in skin, intestine, brain, and kidney. Blood pressure is reduced; cardiac output, oxygen consumption, and heart rate are increased (*see* Kety and Schmidt, 1946; McGregor *et al.*, 1962; Rowe *et al.*, 1962; Zwillich *et al.*, 1976). The mechanisms through which these changes are effected are complex. Part of the changes may be attributed to hypocarbia and part to the mechanical effects of hyperventilation or the increased airway pressure caused by mechanical ventilation (*see* Prys-Roberts *et al.*, 1967).

Central Nervous System. The inhalation of low concentrations of carbon dioxide depresses the excitability of the cerebral cortex and increases the threshold for the production of seizures by drugs or electroshock. It also increases the cutaneous pain threshold through a central action. This central depression is of importance in the therapeutic application of the gas, for carbon dioxide can cause further depression of an already depressed brain. However, when high concentrations of carbon dioxide (25 to 30%) are breathed, subcortical areas that have cortical projections are activated. This activation overcomes the depressant effect of carbon dioxide on the cortex. The increased cortical excitability that results can progress to convulsions. The inhalation of even higher concentrations of carbon dioxide (about 50%) produces marked cortical and subcortical depression of a type similar to that produced by anesthetic agents. The effects of carbon dioxide inhalation on the EEG depend on the concentration of the gas that is inhaled. When low concentrations are inhaled and cortical depression is present, EEG waves of increased frequency appear. The inhalation of 30% carbon dioxide produces intermittent high-voltage bursts in the EEG, coinciding with clinical seizure activity. An anesthetic concentration of carbon dioxide (50%) causes flattening of the EEG. A decrease in P_{CO_2} below normal values results in the appearance of high-voltage slow waves (theta and delta), particularly in the frontal leads (*see* Woodbury and Karler, in Symposium, 1960).

Untoward Effects of Carbon Dioxide Inhalation. The normal subject inhaling concentrations of carbon dioxide up to 5 or 6% experiences the sensation of increased respiration, but rarely experiences dyspnea. Some notice an acidic taste, as carbon dioxide forms carbonic acid in the presence of water. The inhalation of higher concentrations, up to about 10%, produces dyspnea, headache, dizziness, sweating, restlessness, paresthesias, and a general feeling of discomfort. Higher concentrations result in pronounced discomfort. The CNS effects of very high concentrations of carbon dioxide are described above. As with oxygen poisoning, the CNS toxicity of carbon dioxide is a reversible phenomenon.

Following the abrupt withdrawal of inhaled concentrations of carbon dioxide above 5%, a few subjects experience headache or dizziness. These symptoms can be avoided by slowly decreasing the inhaled concentration rather than withdrawing it suddenly.

Untoward circulatory effects of carbon dioxide include marked elevation of blood pressure, tachycardia, and possible arrhythmias. Acidosis resulting from high concentrations of carbon dioxide renders effector organs less sensitive to the effects of catecholamines; this is usually undesirable.

CHEMISTRY AND PREPARATIONS

Carbon dioxide is approximately one and one-half times as dense as air. *Carbon Dioxide*, U.S.P., is of a specified purity. It is marketed in metal cylinders compressed to 58 atmospheres, under which condition it exists as a liquid, vaporizing as it is delivered from the cylinder. For medicinal purposes, carbon dioxide is usually administered in combination with oxygen, and cylinders containing the two gases in varying proportions are available. Since carbon dioxide solidifies at approximately $-78°$ C, it can also be obtained in solid form (dry ice).

METHODS OF ADMINISTRATION

Carbon dioxide is frequently administered by means of a tight-fitting face mask, the gas being supplied from a cylinder containing a mixture of 5 to 10% carbon dioxide in oxygen. It is also possible to deliver 100% carbon dioxide from a cylinder through a tube held a few inches above the patient's face. Carbon dioxide, being heavier than air, falls over the patient's face and is inhaled, diluted with room air. Although this technic requires little equipment, it does not allow one to know the inhaled concentration of carbon dioxide.

Another method of administration of carbon dioxide is the rebreathing technic, where the supply of carbon dioxide comes from the patient's exhaled gases, which are rebreathed, for example, from a paper bag. Since the inspired oxygen concentration falls as the inhaled carbon dioxide concentration rises, this should not be continued for longer than a few minutes.

THERAPEUTIC USES

Inhalation of carbon dioxide has been suggested as a means of therapy in many commonly encountered situations, but for most of these there are other treatments available that are more effective and offer fewer disadvantages.

Respiratory Depression, Asphyxia, and Coma. The usefulness of carbon dioxide in stimulating depressed respiration is very limited. When respiratory minute volume is reduced, the excretion of carbon dioxide is impaired and the tension of this gas in blood and tissues rises. Thus, there is already an elevated P_{CO_2}. A further elevation of the tension by the administration of carbon dioxide may not increase ventilation and will only worsen the respiratory acidosis. Elevation of P_{CO_2} may also further depress the neurons of the respiratory centers. Reliance should be placed on mechanical support of the respiration plus the administration of oxygen.

Carbon Monoxide Poisoning. The inhalation of 5 to 7% carbon dioxide in oxygen has been used in the treatment of carbon monoxide poisoning, as carbon dioxide increases both the ventilatory exchange and the rate of dissociation of carbon monoxide from carboxyhemoglobin. A disadvantage is the production of serious acidosis when the respiratory acidosis produced by carbon dioxide is added to the metabolic acidosis already present in cases of severe carbon monoxide poisoning.

Uses in Anesthesia. Carbon dioxide inhalation can increase the speed of induction and emergence from anesthesia by increasing minute ventilation (*see* Chapter 13), but respiratory acidosis occurs. Hyperventilation with its attendant respiratory alkalosis has some uses in anesthesia. It increases the apparent depth of anesthesia. By constricting the cerebral vessels, it decreases brain size slightly and may facilitate the performance of neurosurgical operations.

Uses in Research and Diagnosis. Carbon dioxide inhalation has been of value in the study of the control of respiration and of cerebral blood flow, and carbon dioxide–sensitivity curves have been used to investigate the effects of drugs on respiration and cerebral blood flow. Hyperventilation to lower P_{CO_2} is of use for diagnostic purposes in eliciting the characteristic EEG pattern of absence seizures, but other methods are also used, such as photostimulation or induced sleep.

Miscellaneous Uses. Inhalation of carbon dioxide is one of many suggested treatments for *hiccoughs,* and it has been successful in some cases. Carbon dioxide inhalation may terminate seizures in patients with *status petit mal.* The gas must be mixed with oxygen for use in certain types of pump oxygenators to maintain a normal P_{CO_2} in blood.

HELIUM

Helium is an inert gas; its limited medical applications are due exclusively to physical properties. The low density of helium (specific gravity = 0.14) is the basis for its use when respiration is embarrassed by an obstruction of an airway that produces turbu-

lence. The low aqueous solubility of helium (one half that of nitrogen) makes it useful for divers and others who work in environments with high ambient pressure and as a volume tracer in tests of pulmonary function. However, the high velocity of acoustic transmission in helium (1300 m per second) and the increased heat transfer that results from its high thermal conductivity create problems from distortion of the voice and from hypothermia.

History and Preparations. Helium was identified spectroscopically in the sun's atmosphere in 1868, as α radiation from uranium ore in 1895, and as a component in natural gas in 1905. The United States maintains a supply of helium from wells in Louisiana and Texas, presently the sole commercial source. Helium is recovered after liquefaction of natural gas and is marketed in compressed form in steel cylinders. *Helium,* U.S.P., consists of not less than 95% helium, the remainder being mostly nitrogen. Various mixtures with oxygen are also available.

Methods of Administration. The apparatus that is used to breathe helium is chosen largely on the basis of the specific application. In saturation diving applications, individuals are placed in a closed environment consisting largely of helium. In pulmonary function testing, one breath of helium may be inhaled or it may be breathed from closed spirometers by way of a mask or mouthpiece. Because so little helium dissolves in the body, only oxygen need be added and carbon dioxide absorbed. For intermittent positive pressure breathing, a non-rebreathing circuit is commonly employed with either a mask or endotracheal tube.

Applications. The use of helium is theoretically helpful in patients with an obstruction of the upper tracheobronchial tree that causes turbulent flow of gas. Beneficial results have not been conclusively documented in generalized obstruction, but patients may improve temporarily (Chan-Yeung *et al.,* 1976). The main uses of helium are for physiological investigations and diagnostic tests and for the prevention of nitrogen narcosis and decompression sickness in hyperbaric atmospheres.

Respiratory Obstruction. During normal breathing, gas flow is laminar in airways that are smaller than 3 to 5 mm in diameter, and the energy required to produce flow is more dependent on the viscosity than on the density of the gas. The kinematic viscosity of helium is several times that of oxygen. However, when there is laryngeal or tracheal obstruction and turbulent flow of gas, the energy required for flow is inversely related to the *density* of the gas. If obstruction is significant and the work of breathing air or oxygen is very high, mixtures of helium and oxygen may be respired more easily and result in greater washout of carbon dioxide. However, such mixtures are always less effective than is 100% oxygen in raising the P_{O_2} in blood.

Careful clinical trials of mixtures of helium and oxygen administered by intermittent positive-pressure technics have demonstrated that there is a slight reduction in P_{CO_2}, but this is probably due to a physical artifact (*see* Smith and Weiner, 1977).

The use of increased pressure or the maintenance of a greater tidal volume with oxygen alone has the same effect. When helium mixtures are administered, the patient's high-pitched, distorted voice is most noticeable. This dramatic change probably accounts for some of the belief that mixtures of helium and oxygen are beneficial in chronic lung disease.

Diagnostic Uses. Helium is useful in pulmonary function testing because it is nearly as insoluble as hydrogen but is not flammable. If a bolus of helium is introduced into a spirometer circuit, a small amount is taken up by the patient. Its dilution following mixing within the lungs and spirometer is used in calculations of diffusing capacity and functional residual capacity of the lungs.

Hyperbaric Applications. The production of oxygen toxicity at 2 atmospheres and of nitrogen narcosis at 5 atmospheres limits the barometric pressure at which man can function in a mixture of these gases (Brauer and Way, 1970). Furthermore, under high pressure, significant amounts of nitrogen dissolve in blood and, particularly, in lipid. If decompression is rapid, nitrogen will effervesce from body stores and produce gas emboli in joints, the CNS, and blood; the results are excruciating pain, chronic disability, and even death. This decompression sickness, also known as "the bends" or caisson disease, can be avoided by slow decompression, which permits the dissolved nitrogen to diffuse gradually into the blood and be eliminated by the lungs. Because helium is one third as soluble in lipid as nitrogen and because it has little demonstrable narcotic effect up to 30 atmospheres (Brauer and Way, 1970), respiration of mixtures of helium and oxygen permit deeper diving and safer, quicker decompression. Furthermore, helium's low density reduces the work of breathing required at very high pressures. In some undersea missions, subjects have lived in a helium-oxygen atmosphere. Problems encountered included garbled, distorted speech, increased loss of body heat, and gas emboli at the junction of skin and subcutaneous fat or of body fat and blood vessels. The latter is due to the phenomenon of isobaric counterdiffusion of nitrogen and helium (Lambertsen and Idicula, 1975).

WATER VAPOR

Because of extensive hydrogen bonding, water is a liquid with a large heat of vaporization, a high specific heat, and considerable ability to dissolve or disperse a wide variety of other compounds. Water in aerosolized form is used to carry drugs into the respiratory tract for topical effect (*e.g.,* in asthma or bronchitis) or for rapid absorption and systemic effect. Inhalation and exhalation of water vapor normally take place with every breath, and inhalation of supplemental amounts of water vapor can be an important therapeutic procedure.

Inspired air is warmed to body temperature and humidified to saturation by the time it reaches the larynx or upper trachea. While deeper rapid breathing may move the boundary of saturation deeper into the chest, the air-conditioning function of the nasal turbinates and upper airway still provides the bulk of humidification. Normal man can tolerate a temporary shift in the site of humidification to the tracheobronchial tree during endotracheal anesthesia (Knudsen *et al.,* 1973) or the chronic shift that results from tracheostomy if no additional stress is placed on the airways. More than 50 mg of water may be needed for each liter of inspired dry gas to saturate it at body temperature. Failure of humidification is deleterious to mucociliary transport because of increased viscosity of secretions, decreased ciliary activity, and increased loss of heat (Chalon *et al.,* 1972; Déry, 1973; Forbes, 1973).

Uses of Inspired Water Vapor. The proper amount of water vapor in an environment contributes to maintenance of comfort. Excessively dry or humid atmospheres may produce symptoms, especially in patients with chronic nasal and upper airway disease. The inhalation of a cold or warm aerosol may be soothing in acute inflammation (laryngitis and croup). Water vapor is particularly therapeutic for patients whose airways are chronically intubated (as in respiratory care units); it decreases crusting of respiratory mucosa, liquefies thick secretions, promotes mucociliary clearance, helps supply body water in the presence of a deficit, and tends to conserve body heat by limiting evaporation in the airway. Water vapor may be used to deliver drugs such as bronchodilators, mucolytics, hydroscopics, steroids, and antibiotics to the respiratory tract (Pierce and Saltzman, 1974).

Methods of Administration. Inspired water may be provided as vapor from humidifiers or as vapor and particulate water from aerosol generators (nebulizers). Either may provide water warmed to body temperature or cooled below room temperature, as occasionally desired in laryngitis. The water used may be locally prepared distilled water, commercially prepared sterile distilled water, or various solutions, most commonly 0.45% or 0.9% (isotonic) sodium chloride (*see* Mercer, 1973; Egan, 1977).

The amount of water provided by humidifiers is limited to a maximum that is determined by the temperature of the gas. At room temperature (20° C), air that is saturated with water vapor contains 20 mg of water per liter at a partial pressure of 17.5 torr. At body temperature, 100% relative humidity is equivalent to a water content of 53 mg per liter and a pressure of 47 torr.

While the content of water vapor in inspired gas is limited to a maximum set by temperature, additional water may be administered by dispersing small droplets with mechanical, pneumatic, or ultrasonic aerosol generators. The size of the aerosol particles may be varied from less than 1 μm to more than 100 μm, thus permitting some control over the disposition of the aerosol. Particles larger than 50 μm tend to settle rapidly or coalesce, forming the rain familiar in oxygen tents and steam hoods. Particles of 10 to 20 μm are governed largely by inertia and tend to impact on the walls of conduits at bends. The turbulence created by the turbinate bones of the nose, the glottis, and the carina tend to remove all of these particles in the upper airway and trachea. Particles of 5 to 10 μm are more stable, but inertia and Brownian movement cause them to impact on the walls of the airways, so that many of these particles are deposited in medium-sized and small bronchi. Particles of 1 to 5 μm may penetrate all the way to the alveolar exchange surface. Particles of less than 1 μm are so aerodynamically stable that the bulk of such inhaled particles may be completely exhaled in the subsequent breath. They are neither heavy enough to impact on the airways nor light enough to diffuse from alveolar ducts to alveoli during the course of one breath.

Untoward Effects. Potential problems include thermal damage from overheated inspired gas, water overload from deposition of particles in the tracheobronchial tree, and bronchoconstriction from direct irritation of the bronchi by the droplets. This bronchoconstriction may be blocked by anesthesia with halothane or by isoproterenol, administered topically or systemically (Cheney and Butler, 1968; Waltemath and Bergman, 1973). Thermal damage is due not only to the temperature of the gas but also to the delivery of 580 calories per gram of steam upon condensation. Chronic inhalation of an aerosol mist may result in the net absorption of 300 to 500 ml of water a day by adult patients and disproportionately more (relative to weight) by children and infants.

Anderson, D. P.; Allen, W. J.; Barcroft, H.; Edholm, O. G.; and Manning, G. W.   Circulatory changes during fainting and coma caused by oxygen lack. *J. Physiol. (Lond.)*, **1946**, *104*, 426–434.

Arturson, G.; Garby, L.; Robert, M.; and Zaar, B.   The oxygen dissociation curve of normal human blood with special reference to the influence of physiological effector ligands. *Scand. J. Clin. Lab. Invest.*, **1974**, *34*, 9–13.

Barach, A. L.   Historical background. In, Symposium—inhalational therapy. *Anesthesiology*, **1962**, *23*, 407–421.

Barcroft, J.   Anoxaemia. *Lancet*, **1920**, *2*, 485–489.

Behnke, A. R., Jr.; Johnson, F. S.; Poppen, J. R.; and Motley, E. P.   The effect of oxygen on man at pressures from 1 to 4 atmospheres. *Am. J. Physiol.*, **1935**, *110*, 565–572.

Blackburn, J. P.; Conway, C. M.; Leigh, J. M.; Lindop, M. J.; and Reitan, J. A. $PaCO_2$ and the pre-ejection period: the $PaCO_2$/inotropy response curve. *Anesthesiology*, **1972**, *37*, 268–276.

Boerema, I.; Meyne, N. G.; Brummelkamp, W. K.; Bouma, S.; Mensch, M. H.; Kamermans, F.; Stern Hanf, M.; and Van Aalderen, W.   Life without blood. *J. Cardiovasc. Surg. (Torino)*, **1960**, *1*, 133–146.

Brauer, R. W., and Way, R. O.   Relative narcotic potencies of hydrogen, helium, nitrogen and their mixtures. *J. Appl. Physiol.*, **1970**, *29*, 23–31.

Chalon, J.; Lowe, D. A.; and Malebranche, J.   The effects of dry anesthetic gases on tracheobronchial ciliated epithelium. *Anesthesiology*, **1972**, *37*, 338–343.

Chan-Yeung, M.; Abboud, R.; Ming, S. T.; and Mac-Lean, L.   Effect of helium on maximum expiratory flow in patients with asthma before and during induced bronchoconstriction. *Am. Rev. Respir. Dis.*, **1976**, *113*, 434–443.

Cheney, F. W., and Butler, J.   The effects of ultrasonically produced aerosols on airway resistance in man. *Anesthesiology*, **1968**, *29*, 1099–1106.

Clark, J. M.   The toxicity of oxygen. *Am. Rev. Respir. Dis.*, **1974**, *110*, Suppl., 40–50.

Cohen, P. J.; Alexander, S. C.; Smith, T. C.; Reivich, M.; and Wollman, H.   Effects of hypoxia and normocarbia on cerebral blood flow and metabolism in conscious man. *J. Appl. Physiol.*, **1967**, *23*, 183–189.

Comroe, J. H., Jr., and Botelho, S.   The unreliability of cyanosis in the recognition of arterial anoxemia. *Am. J. Med. Sci.*, **1947**, *214*, 1–6.

Cullen, D. J., and Eger, E. I., II.   Cardiovascular effects of CO_2 in man. *Anesthesiology*, **1974**, *41*, 345–349.

Daly, M. B., and Scott, M. J.   The effects of stimulation of the carotid body chemoreceptors on heart rate in the dog. *J. Physiol. (Lond.)*, **1958**, *144*, 148–166.

Déry, R.   The evolution of heat and moisture in the respiratory tract during anesthesia with non-rebreathing system. *Can. Anaesth. Soc. J.*, **1973**, *20*, 296–309.

Desforges, J. F.   Hemoglobin—a working molecule. *N. Engl. J. Med.*, **1976**, *295*, 164–165.

Dripps, R. D., and Comroe, J. H., Jr.   The respiratory and circulatory response of normal man to inhalation of 7.6 and 10.4 per cent CO_2 with a comparison of the maximal ventilation produced by severe muscular exercise, inhalation of CO_2 and maximal voluntary hyperventilation. *Am. J. Physiol.*, **1947**, *149*, 43–51.

Flynn, J. T.; O'Grady, G. E.; Herrera, J.; Kushner, B. J.; Cantolino, S.; and Milam, W.   Retrolental fibroplasia. I. Clinical observations. *Arch. Ophthalmol.*, **1977**, *95*, 217–223.

Forbes, A. R.   Humidification and mucus flow in the intubated trachea. *Br. J. Anaesth.*, **1973**, *45*, 874–878.

Fridovich, I.   Superoxide dismutase. *Annu. Rev. Biochem.*, **1975**, *44*, 147–159.

Gibson, R. L.; Comer, P. B.; Beckman, R. W.; and McGraw, C. P.   Actual tracheal oxygen concentrations with commonly used oxygen equipment. *Anesthesiology*, **1976**, *44*, 71–73.

Haab, P.; Held, D. R.; Ernst, H.; and Farhi, L. E.   Ventilation-perfusion relationships during high altitude adaptation. *J. Appl. Physiol.*, **1969**, *26*, 77–81.

Haldane, J. S.; Meakins, J. C.; and Priestley, J. C.   The effects of shallow breathing. *J. Physiol. (Lond.)*, **1919**, *52*, 433–453.

Haldane, J. S., and Priestley, J. G.   The regulation of the lung-ventilation. *J. Physiol. (Lond.)*, **1905**, *32*, 225–266.

Hamilton, J. T.; Hersey, L. W.; and Twiss, J. L.   The role of the adrenal medulla in the blood pressure response to carbon dioxide following hexamethonium. *Arch. Int. Pharmacodyn. Ther.*, **1966**, *160*, 29–43.

Henderson, Y., and Haggard, H. W.   The treatment of carbon monoxide asphyxia by means of oxygen plus carbon dioxide inhalation. *J.A.M.A.*, **1922**, *79*, 1137–1145.

Kety, S. S., and Schmidt, C. F.   The effect of active and passive hyperventilation on cerebral blood flow, blood oxygen consumption, cardiac output, and blood pressure of normal young men. *J. Clin. Invest.*, **1946**, *25*, 107–119.

———.   The effects of altered arterial tension of carbon dioxide and oxygen on cerebral blood flow and cerebral oxygen consumption of normal young men. *Ibid.*, **1948**, *27*, 484–492.

Knudsen, J.; Lomholt, N.; and Wisborg, K.   Postoperative pulmonary complications using dry and humidified anesthetic gases. *Br. J. Anaesth.*, **1973**, *45*, 363–368.

Krasney, J. A., and Koehler, R. C.   Influence of arterial hypoxia on cardiac and coronary dynamics in the conscious sinoaortic-denervated dog. *J. Appl. Physiol.*, **1977**, *43*, 1012–1018.

Kravec, T. F.; Eggers, G. W. N., Jr.; and Kettel, L. J.   Influence of patient age on forearm and systemic vascular response to hypoxaemia. *Clin. Sci.*, **1972**, *42*, 555–565.

Krogh, M.   Diffusion of gases through the lungs of man. *J. Physiol. (Lond.)*, **1915**, *49*, 271–300.

Kushner, B. J.; Essner, D.; Cohen, I. J.; and Flynn, J. T.   Retrolental fibroplasia. II. Pathologic correlation. *Arch. Ophthalmol.*, **1977**, *95*, 29–38.

Lambertsen, C. J.; Ewing, J. H.; Kough, R. H.; Gould, R.; and Stroud, M. W.   Oxygen toxicity. Arterial and internal jugular blood gas composition in man during inhalation of air, 100% O_2 and 2% CO_2 in O_2 at 3.5 atmospheres ambient pressure. *J. Appl. Physiol.*, **1955**, *8*, 255–263.

Lambertsen, C. J., and Idicula, J. A. A new gas lesion syndrome in man induced by "isobaric gas counter diffusion." *J. Appl. Physiol.,* 1975, *39,* 434–443.

Lambertsen, C. J.; Kough, R. H.; Cooper, D. Y.; Emmel, G. L.; Loeschcke, H. H.; and Schmidt, C. F. Oxygen toxicity. Effects in man of oxygen inhalation at 1 and 3.5 atmospheres upon blood gas transport, cerebral circulation and cerebral metabolism. *J. Appl. Physiol.,* 1953, *5,* 471–486.

Lambertsen, C. J., and Wendel, H. An alveolar P_{CO_2} control system: its use to magnify respiratory depression by meperidine. *J. Appl. Physiol.,* 1960, *15,* 43–48.

Leigh, J. M. Early treatment with oxygen: the pneumatic institute and the panaceal literature of the nineteenth century. *Anaesthesia,* 1974a, *29,* 194–208.

————. Evolution of oxygen therapy apparatus. *Ibid.,*1974b, *29,* 462–485.

Lourenco, R. V. Clinical methods for the study of regulation of ventilation. *Chest,* 1976, *70,* 109–195.

McGregor, M.; Donevan, R. E.; and Anderson, N. M. Influence of carbon dioxide and hyperventilation on cardiac output in man. *J. Appl. Physiol.,* 1962, *17,* 933–937.

Medical Letter. Hyperbaric oxygen therapy. 1979, *20,* 51–52.

Mott, J. C. The ability of young mammals to withstand total oxygen lack. *Br. Med. Bull.,* 1961, *17,* 144–147.

Neff, T. A., and Talmage, P. Neuromuscular and chemical control of breathing. *Chest,* 1978, *73,* 247–308.

Neill, W. A., and Hattenhauer, M. Impairment of myocardial O_2 supply due to hyperventilation. *Circulation,* 1975, *52,* 854–858.

Ng, M. L.; Levy, M. N.; and Zieske, H. A. Effects of changes of pH and of carbon dioxide tension on left ventricular performance. *Am. J. Physiol.,* 1967, *213,* 115–120.

Nichols, C. W., and Lambertsen, C. J. Effects of high oxygen pressures on the eye. *Med. Prog.,* 1969, *281,* 25–30.

Pierce, E. C., Jr.; Lambertsen, C. J.; Strong, M. J.; Alexander, S. C.; and Steele, D. Blood P_{CO_2} and brain oxygenation at reduced ambient pressure. *J. Appl. Physiol.,* 1962, *17,* 899–908.

Plum, F. The clinical problem: how much anoxia-ischemia damages the brain? *Arch. Neurol.,* 1973, *29,* 359–360.

Prys-Roberts, C.; Kelman, G. R.; Greenbaum, R.; and Robinson, R. H. Circulatory influences of artificial ventilation during nitrous oxide anesthesia in man. II. Results: the relative influences of mean intrathoracic pressure and arterial carbon dioxide tension. *Br. J. Anaesth.,* 1967, *39,* 533–547.

Raymond, K.; Weiskopf, R. B.; Halsey, G. J.; Goldfien, A.; Eger, E. I., II; and Severinghaus, J. W. Possible mechanism for the antiarrhythmic effect of helium in anesthetized dogs. *Science,* 1972, *176,* 1250–1252.

Robin, E. D. Dysoxia—abnormal tissue oxygen utilization. *Arch. Intern. Med.,* 1977, *137,* 905–910.

Rowe, G. G. Responses of the coronary circulation to physiologic changes and pharmacologic agents. *Anesthesiology,* 1974, *41,* 182–196.

Rowe, G. G.; Castillo, C. A.; and Crumpton, G. W. Effects of hyperventilation on systemic and coronary hemodynamics. *Am. Heart J.,* 1962, *63,* 67–77.

Sackner, M. A. A history of oxygen usage in chronic obstructive pulmonary disease. *Am. Rev. Respir. Dis.,* 1974, *110,* Suppl., 25–34.

Safar, P.; Bleyaert, A.; Nemoto, E. M.; Moossy, J.; and Snyder, J. V. Resuscitation after global brain ischemia-anoxia. *Crit. Care Med.,* 1978, *6,* 215–227.

Sechzer, P. H.; Egbert, L. D.; Linde, H. W.; Cooper, D. Y.; Dripps, R. D.; and Price, H. L. Effect of CO_2 inhalation on arterial pressure, ECG, and plasma catecholamines and 17-OH corticosteroids in normal man. *J. Appl. Physiol.,* 1960, *15,* 454–458.

Severinghaus, J. W. Blood gas calculator. *J. Appl. Physiol.,* 1966, *21,* 1108–1116.

Smith, T. C., and Weiner, S. Helium: rational treatment in respiratory therapy? *Resp. Care,* 1977, *22,* 417.

Stark, R. D.; Finnegan, P.; and Bishop, J. M. Long-term domiciliary oxygen in chronic bronchitis with pulmonary hypertension. *Br. Med. J.,* 1973, *3,* 467–470.

Waltemath, C. L., and Bergman, N. A. Increased respiratory resistance provoked by endotracheal administration of aerosols. *Am. Rev. Respir. Dis.,* 1973, *108,* 520–525.

————. Effect of histamine and halothane on increased respiratory resistance provoked by aerosols. *Anesthesiology,* 1974, *41,* 473–476.

Weil, J. V., and Zwillich, C. W. Assessment of ventilatory response to hypoxia: methods and interpretations. *Chest,* 1976, *70,* Suppl. 1, 124–128.

Wolfe, W. G., and DeVries, W. C. Oxygen toxicity. *Annu. Rev. Med.,* 1975, *26,* 203–217.

Zapol, W. M., and Snider, M. T. Pulmonary hypertension in severe acute respiratory failure. *N. Engl. J. Med.,* 1977, *296,* 476–480.

Zapol, W. M.; Snider, M. T.; and Schneider, R. C. Extracorporeal membrane oxygenation for acute respiratory failure. *Anesthesiology,* 1977, *46,* 272–285.

Zwillich, C. W.; Pierson, D. J.; Creagh, E. M.; and Weil, J. V. Effects of hypocapnia and hypocapnic alkalosis on cardiovascular function. *J. Appl. Physiol.,* 1976, *40,* 333–337.

Monographs and Reviews

Alfery, D. D., and Rauscher, L. A. Tetanus: a review. *Crit. Care Med.,* 1979, *7,* 176–181.

Aviado, D. M. *The Lung Circulation,* Vols. 1 and 2. Pergamon Press, Ltd., Oxford, 1965.

Barcroft, J. *The Respiratory Function of the Blood.* Cambridge University Press, Cambridge, Vol. I, 1925; Vol. II, 1928.

Berne, R. M. Regulation of coronary blood flow. *Physiol. Rev.,* 1964, *44,* 1–29.

Bert, P. *Barometric Pressure: Researches in Experimental Physiology.* (Hitchcock, M. A., and Hitchcock, F. A., transls.) College Book Co., Columbus, Ohio, 1943.

Clark, J. M., and Lambertsen, C. J. Pulmonary oxygen toxicity: a review. *Pharmacol. Rev.,* 1971, *23,* 37–133.

Cohen, P. J. The metabolic function of oxygen and biochemical lesions of hypoxia. *Anesthesiology,* 1972, *37,* 148–177.

Committee on Hyperbaric Oxygenation (eds.). *Fundamentals of Hyperbaric Medicine.* National Academy of Sciences–National Research Council, Washington, D. C., 1966.

Comroe, J. H., Jr., and Dripps, R. D. *The Physiological Basis for Oxygen Therapy.* Charles C Thomas, Pub., Springfield, Ill., 1950.

Davis, J. C., and Hunt, T. K. (eds.). *Hyperbaric Oxygen Therapy.* Undersea Medical Society, Bethesda, 1977.

Egan, D. F. *Fundamentals of Respiratory Therapy,* 3rd ed. C. V. Mosby Co., St. Louis, 1977.

Fishman, A. P. Respiratory gases in the regulation of the pulmonary circulation. *Physiol. Rev.,* 1961, *41,* 214–280.

Flynn, J. T.; O'Grady, G. E.; Herrera, J.; Kushner, B. J.; Cantolino, S.; and Milam, W. Retrolental fibroplasia. I. Clinical observations. *Arch. Ophthalmol.,* 1977, *95,* 217–223.

Grant, W. J. *Medical Gases: Their Properties and Uses.* Year Book Medical Publishers, Inc., Chicago, 1978.

Haldane, J. S., and Priestley, J. G. *Respiration.* The Clarendon Press, Oxford, 1935.

Hedley-Whyte, J.; Burgess, G. E.; Feeley, T. W.; and Miller, M. G. *Applied Physiology of Respiratory Care.* Little, Brown & Co., Boston, 1976.

Henderson, Y. *Adventures in Respiration: Modes of Asphyxiation and Methods of Resuscitation.* The Williams & Wilkins Co., Baltimore, 1938.

Hill, L. *Caisson Sickness* (an international medical monograph). Edward Arnold & Co., London, **1912.**

Kuntz, I. E., and Zipp, A. Water in biological systems. *N. Engl. J. Med.,* **1977,** *297,* 262–266.

Lahiri, S. Physiological responses and adaptations to high altitude. *Int. Rev. Physiol.,* **1977,** *15,* 217–251.

Lambertsen, C. J. Effects of oxygen at high partial pressure. In, *Respiration,* Vol. 2. Sect. 3, *Handbook of Physiology.* (Fenn, W. O., and Rahn, H., eds.) American Physiological Society, Washington, D. C., **1965,** pp. 1027–1040.

———. Physiological effects of oxygen inhalation at high partial pressures. In, *Fundamentals of Hyperbaric Medicine.* (Committee on Hyperbaric Oxygenation, eds.) National Academy of Sciences–National Research Council, Washington, D. C., **1966,** pp. 12–20.

Mercer, T. T. Production and characterization of aerosols. *Arch. Intern. Med.,* **1973,** *131,* 39–46.

Mitchell, R. A. Cerebrospinal fluid and the regulation of respiration. In, *Advances in Respiratory Physiology.* (Caro, C. G., ed.) The Williams & Wilkins Co., Baltimore, **1966,** pp. 1–47.

Mitchell, R. A., and Berger, A. J. Neural regulation of respiration. *Am. Rev. Respir. Dis.,* **1975,** *111,* 206–224.

Nahas, G., and Schaefer, K. E. *Carbon Dioxide and Metabolic Regulation.* Springer-Verlag, New York, **1974.**

Nichols, C. W., and Lambertsen, C. J. Effects of oxygen upon ophthalmic structures. In, *Underwater Physiology.* (Lambertsen, C. J., ed.) Academic Press, Inc., New York, **1971,** pp. 57–66.

Nunn, J. F. Carbon dioxide. In, *Applied Respiratory Physiology,* 2nd ed. Butterworths, London, **1977,** pp. 334–374.

Pierce, A. K., and Saltzman, H. A. The scientific basis of respiratory therapy (the Sugarloaf Conference). *Am. Rev. Respir. Dis.,* **1974,** *110,* Pt. 2, 1–204.

Pontoppidan, H.; Geffin, B.; and Lowenstein, E. *Acute Respiratory Failure in the Adult.* Little, Brown & Co., Boston, **1973.**

Sykes, M. K.; McNicol, M. W.; and Campbell, E. J. M. *Respiratory Failure.* Blackwell Scientific Publications, Oxford, **1976.**

Symposium. (Various authors.) Carbon dioxide. (Eckenhoff, J. E., ed.) *Anesthesiology,* **1960,** *21,* 585–766.

Trapp, W. G.; Banister, E. W.; Davison, A. J.; and Trapp, P. A. *Proceedings of the Fifth International Hyperbaric Conference,* Vols. I and II. Price Printing, Ltd., Canada, **1974.**

Wanner, A. Clinical aspects of mucociliary transport. *Am. Rev. Respir. Dis.,* **1977,** *116,* 73–125.

Winter, P. M., and Smith, G. The toxicity of oxygen. *Anesthesiology,* **1972,** *37,* 210–241.

Young, J. A., and Crocker, D. *Principles and Practice of Inhalation Therapy.* Year Book Medical Publishers, Inc., Chicago, **1976.**

CHAPTER

17 HYPNOTICS AND SEDATIVES

Stewart C. Harvey

The principal use of sedative-hypnotic drugs is to produce drowsiness and promote sleep. The application of the term *sedative* to this group is somewhat misleading. It dates from the era when the sedative-hypnotic compounds were the only drugs (apart from alcohol, opiates, and belladonna) that could be used to calm anxious and disturbed patients. With the proliferation of psychopharmacological agents, the drugs traditionally described as "sedative-hypnotics" have come to play a lesser role in daytime sedation. This role will be discussed in connection with the pharmacotherapy of anxiety in Chapter 19. In the present chapter, the hypnotic properties and uses of these drugs are emphasized.

A *sedative* drug decreases activity, moderates excitement, and calms the recipient. A *hypnotic* drug produces drowsiness and facilitates the onset and maintenance of a state of sleep that resembles natural sleep in its electroencephalographic characteristics and from which the recipient may be easily aroused; the effect is sometimes called hypnosis, but the sleep induced by hypnotic drugs does not resemble that artificially induced passive state of suggestibility also called hypnosis. Sedation, pharmacological hypnosis, and general anesthesia are usually regarded as only increasing depths of a continuum of central nervous system (CNS) depression. Indeed, most sedative or hypnotic drugs, when used in high doses, can induce general anesthesia. One important exception, however, is the benzodiazepines.

Since sedative-hypnotic drugs usually have the capability of producing widespread depression of the CNS, it is not surprising to find that CNS functions, in addition to the state of wakefulness, are usually depressed by these drugs. Thus, various sedative-hypnotic drugs are employed as antiepileptic agents (Chapter 20), muscle relaxants (Chapter 21), and antianxiety drugs (Chapter 19); some may also be used to produce amnesia or general anesthesia (Chapter 14). It is not certain whether the effects of these drugs on wakefulness and anxiety are truly distinct, and their separation in this textbook may represent an artificial division.

Throughout the world, more prescriptions are written for sedative-hypnotic-antianxiety drugs than for any other class of drugs. In the United States in 1976, there were 128 million such prescriptions, of which 27 million (about one billion doses) were for hypnotic effects.

History. Since antiquity, potions have been used to induce sleep. History and folklore have provided accounts of both sinister and romantic uses of laudanum, alcoholic beverages, and various herbals to produce stupor, during which intrigue, adultery, or magical transformation could take place. Potions were also used for sedation and hypnosis, but they were too unpredictable to bequeath to modern medicine. The first agent to be specifically introduced as a sedative and soon thereafter as a hypnotic was bromide (1853, 1864). Only four more sedative-hypnotic drugs (chloral hydrate, paraldehyde, urethan, and sulfonal) were in use before 1900. Barbital was introduced in 1903 and phenobarbital in 1912. Their success spawned the synthesis and testing of over 2500 barbiturates, of which approximately 50 were distributed commercially. The barbiturates held the stage so dominantly that less than a dozen other sedative-hypnotics were successfully marketed before 1960, and several popular old drugs slipped into oblivion. The introduction of chlordiazepoxide in 1961 began an era in which the inferior barbiturates and other hypnotics were expected to become obsolete, but the medical profession has been reluctant to abandon the older sedative-hypnotics. However, in the United States, the number of prescriptions written annually for benzodiazepine sedative-hypnotic-antianxiety drugs is about 100 million. Meanwhile, a few non-benzodiazepine agents continue to appear and command careful examination.

BENZODIAZEPINES

While there are many similarities among the benzodiazepines, they are difficult to characterize as a class. However, it is usually assumed that they all exert the same qualitative actions and have the same mechanism(s) of action, even though there are quantitative differences in their pharmacodynamic spectra. Both hypnotic and nonhypnotic benzodiazepines will be described in this chapter to illustrate the general properties of the group and the important differences between individual agents; only those benzodiazepines used primarily for hypnosis will be discussed in detail (*see also* Chapter 19).

Chemistry. Over 2000 benzodiazepines have been synthesized, and more than 100 have been tested for hypnotic and other activities. The basic structure for most benzodiazepines is shown below, as are those of flurazepam and triazolam. The structures of other commonly used benzodiazepines appear in Chapter 19.

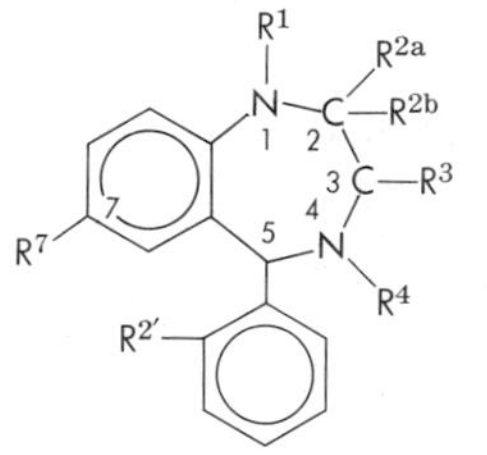

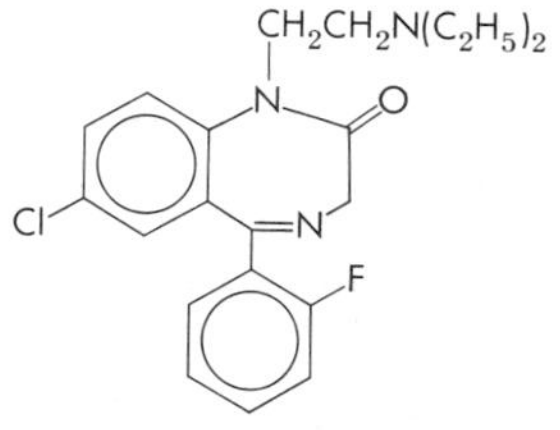

Flurazepam

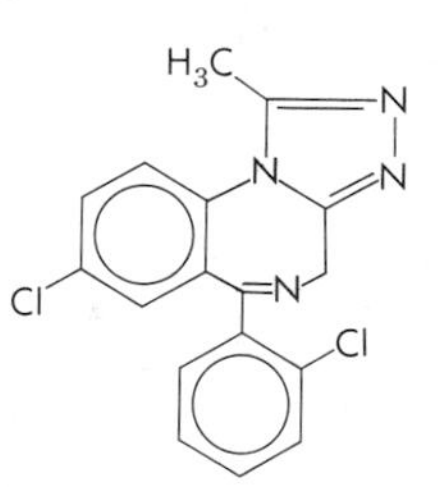

Triazolam

The 1,4-benzodiazepine structure is only the fused-ring portion in which key positions are numbered. However, all the important CNS-depressant benzodiazepines contain a 5-aryl or 5-cyclohexenyl substituent, so that the term benzodiazepine has come to mean the 5-aryl-1,4-benzodiazepines. Other than the apparent requirement for the 5-aryl group, the structure-activity relationship is not stringent. At the 7 position, electron-withdrawing groups enhance and electron-releasing and large groups suppress activity. Substituents elsewhere in this aromatic ring have a negative effect. The chemical nature of substituents at positions 1 to 3 varies widely. A low electron density at the 4 nitrogen is common among all useful or promising benzodiazepines. A 2' (or ortho) substituent on 5 phenyl is not essential, but electron-withdrawing groups enhance potency; substituents elsewhere on this ring decrease activity. Study of the structure-activity relationship thus far has failed to explain the different pharmacological spectra of the various benzodiazepines, except that the 7-nitro group enhances anticonvulsant potency. The chemistry and structure-activity relationship have been reviewed by Sternbach (1973) and Greenblatt and Shader (1974b).

PHARMACOLOGICAL PROPERTIES

The effects of the benzodiazepines virtually all result from actions of these drugs on the CNS, even when lethal doses are taken. In man and other mammals, the most prominent of these effects are sedation, hypnosis, decreased anxiety, muscle relaxation, and anticonvulsant activity. One benzodiazepine, alprazolam, may have antidepressant activity. Only two effects of these drugs appear to result from actions on peripheral tissues: coronary vasodilatation, seen after intravenous administration of therapeutic doses of certain benzodiazepines, and neuromuscular blockade, seen with very high doses. High concentrations of benzodiazepines *in vitro* can impair conduction in nerves, depress smooth and striated muscle, and kill certain bacteria and schistosomes.

Central Nervous System. While the benzodiazepines affect activity at all levels of the neuraxis, some structures are affected to a much greater extent than are others. In addition, some effects of the drugs are indirect. The benzodiazepines are not general neuronal depressants, as are the barbiturates, ethanol, various other sedative-hypnotic drugs, and general anesthetics. All of the benzodiazepines have the same pharmacological profile, except for the anticonvulsant and possibly analgesic effects of certain members. Nevertheless, there are wide differences in selectivity among the drugs, and the clinical usefulness of individual benzodiazepines thus varies considerably. While some of these differences are described below, detailed discussion may be found in the monographs and reviews listed in the bibliography.

The pharmacological profile for a given drug varies markedly from species to species. In some species, the subject may become alert before there is evidence of CNS depression. For example, the 7-nitrobenzodiazepines induce hyperactivity in mice, rats, and monkeys, but not in most other species; flurazepam causes convulsions only in cats. Interestingly, muscle relaxation in cats and anticonvulsant activity against pentylenetetrazol in mice correlate better with the sedative, antianxiety, and hypnotic properties in man than do the actions to suppress motor activity, induce sleep, and release suppressed behavior in experimental animals.

In man, as the dose of a benzodiazepine is increased, sedation progresses to hypnosis and hypnosis to stupor, as expected of a general CNS depressant. Clinical literature often refers to the "anesthetic" effects and uses of certain benzodiazepines, but the drugs do not cause a true general anesthesia, since awareness usually persists and relaxation sufficient to allow surgery cannot be achieved. However, retrograde amnesia may occur, which creates the illusion of previous anesthesia. For true surgical anesthesia, benzodiazepines must be combined with other CNS-depressant drugs. Similarly in some experimental animals, righting reflexes or certain other CNS functions are not abolished until lethal or nearly lethal doses of benzodiazepines are given. In contrast, the barbiturates can cause anesthesia.

Like probably all sedative-hypnotic drugs, "preanesthetic" doses of benzodiazepines impair recent memory and interfere with the establishment of the memory trace. Hence they cause retrograde amnesia for events that occur while therapeutic concentrations of the drug are present.

The question whether the so-called antianxiety actions of benzodiazepines are the same as or different from the sedative and hypnotic actions has not been resolved. In various experimental models of aggressive behavior in animals, benzodiazepines and meprobamate, but not barbiturates or phenothiazines, can selectively diminish aggressiveness without causing impairment of neurological function or decrease in general activity. The so-called antianxiety benzodiazepines have a greater effect than do others in most tests of the antiaggressive effects. However, in colonies of muricidal rats and mice, benzodiazepines, but not barbiturates, actually *increase* mortality. Thus, the benzodiazepines are said to have an effect to diminish defensive aggressiveness but to augment or not affect offensive (attack) aggressiveness. These effects on either defensive or attack aggressiveness appear to represent selective actions on the CNS.

Shuttle avoidance behavior, discriminative fear conditioning, and conflict behavior in operant conditioning studies possibly provide better models for "anxiety" than does so-called defensive aggressiveness. Rats, cats, monkeys, and pigeons have been tested in various ways designed to produce conflict between positively reinforced (rewarded) or approach behavior and negatively reinforced (punished) behavior. Benzodiazepines with prominent antianxiety activity and meprobamate increase the suppressed (punished) behavior, even when given in doses that decrease rewarded behavior. They also suppress conditioned avoidance behavior and restore behavior averted by bitter taste or brain stimulation. The release of previously suppressed behavior, which is greater for antianxiety than for hypnotic benzodiazepines, has been called the disinhibitory effect. However, these drugs also increase frequency of response in partial reinforcement schedules, in which there is no aversive stimulation; this effect is often attributed to so-called nonspecific arousal (*see* Tye *et al.,* 1977). The effect of benzodiazepines on conflict behavior is prevented by prior treatment with bicuculline (*see* Chapter 12) or thiosemicarbazide. Phenothiazines and other antipsychotic drugs do not act selectively on such behavior; the effects of barbiturates vary with species. High doses of any of these drugs will suppress both punished and rewarded behavior. These findings indicate that the effects of benzodiazepines on such behavior cannot be attributed to general depression of the CNS.

Studies on tolerance in animals are often cited to support the belief that disinhibitory effects of benzodiazepines are separate from their general depressant effects. Thus, tolerance to the ability of the drug to decrease general activity and impair locomotor performance occurs very rapidly and can be detected even after a single dose of a benzodiazepine (Christensen, 1973). After several days of treatment, tolerance to the depressant effects of benzodiazepines on rewarded or neutral behavior also occurs; this is not, however, observed with the disinhibitory effects. In fact, the disinhibitory effects of the drugs are augmented by the development of tolerance to their depressant effects. There is also tolerance to the effects of benzodiazepines on the turnover of brain norepinephrine but not to the effects on 5-hydroxytryptamine (5-HT) (*see* below). In man, tolerance to both the hypnotic and antianxiety effects can occur, but quantitative data are not available to ascertain which develops more easily.

Some benzodiazepines induce muscle hypotonia without interfering with normal locomotion. They also decrease decerebrate rigidity in cats and rigidity in patients with cerebral palsy. They increase the patellar reflex. In cats, muscle relaxation is effected in doses that are two (flurazepam) to four (clonazepam) orders of magnitude less than those that abolish the righting reflex. Diazepam is ten times more selective than meprobamate. However, this remarkable degree of selectivity is not seen in man; clonazepam in nonsedative doses does cause muscle relaxation in man, but diazepam and most other benzodiazepines do not. Tolerance occurs to both the muscle relaxant and ataxic effects of these drugs.

Experimentally, benzodiazepines inhibit seizure activity induced by either pentylenetetrazol or picrotoxin, but strychnine- and maximal electroshock-induced seizures are suppressed only with doses that also severely impair locomotor activity. Flunitrazepam, triazolam, clonazepam, bromazepam, and nitrazepam are more selective anticonvulsants than are other benzodiazepines. Benzodiazepines also suppress photic seizures in baboons and ethanol-withdrawal seizures in man. The site of anticonvulsant action is not at the seizure focus; rather, the drugs prevent the subcortical spread of seizure activity. Tolerance to the anticonvulsant effects develops more rapidly than it does to the sedative-hypnotic effects.

Only diazepam is selectively analgesic in mice. In man, it causes a transient analgesia after intravenous administration. No analgesic effect in man has been reported for other benzodiazepines. Various interactions with the effects of different analgesics have been observed in experimental animals. Their clinical significance remains to be clarified. Unlike the barbiturates, benzodiazepines do not cause hyperalgesia.

Effects on EEG and Sleep Stages. The effects of benzodiazepines on the waking EEG resemble those of other sedative-hypnotic drugs. Alpha activity is decreased, and there is an increase in low-voltage, fast activity, especially beta activity. The shift in activity occurs more in the frontal and rolandic areas than elsewhere in the brain; unlike the effect of barbiturates, there is little or no posterior spread. The benzodiazepines reduce the amplitude of cortical somatosensory-evoked potentials in the human EEG; the latency of the early peak is shortened and that of the late peak prolonged. This effect and the shift to beta activity appear to correlate with the antianxiety effects. Benzodiazepines resemble barbiturates in that tolerance occurs to the effects on the EEG.

Interest in and understanding of the stages of sleep have increased greatly in recent years. Some characteristics of these stages are summarized in Table 17–1. The effects of benzodiazepines on the stages of sleep have been studied in over 80 investigations. An

excellent compilation of findings and discussion of 66 of these may be found in the review by Kay and associates (1976) (*see also* Greenblatt and Shader, 1974b; Mendelson *et al.,* 1977). From these studies it may be concluded that, with a few important exceptions, the benzodiazepines are all rather similar in their effects on the important sleep parameters. However, a few studies suggest that high doses of some benzodiazepines produce effects that are qualitatively different from those that are seen after low doses. Most studies have been on normal subjects. It appears that insomniacs and patients with various psychiatric disorders may respond differently than do normal individuals. Unfortunately, not enough research has been conducted on those subjects for whom hypnotics are mostly intended—those with insomnia of various etiologies.

Most benzodiazepines decrease sleep latency, especially when first used, and diminish the number of awakenings and the time spent in stage 0 (a stage of wakefulness). They have been shown to increase the awakening threshold (Itil, 1976). Time in stage 1 (descending drowsiness) is usually decreased by flurazepam, lorazepam, nitrazepam, and temazepam, but it is increased by chlordiazepoxide, diazepam, and oxazepam. Time spent in stage 2 (which is the major fraction of non-rapid-eye-movement [REM] sleep) is increased by all benzodiazepines. Benzodiazepines prominently decrease the time spent in slow-wave sleep (SWS; stages 3 and 4); usually both stages 3 and 4 are shortened, but in neurotic patients or those with endogenous depression temazepam has been found to prolong stage 3 and shorten stage 4. The shortening of stage-4 sleep does not decrease the total number of delta waves during a night because they are transferred to stage 2 (Feinberg *et al.,* 1977). The decrease in stage-4 sleep is accompanied by a reduction in night terrors and nightmares; however, if the decrease is marked, these phenomena may be shifted to the waking hours ("daymares").

Much attention has been paid to the effects on REM sleep. All benzodiazepines increase REM latency (time from onset of spindle sleep to the first REM burst), except that flurazepam has been reported to shorten latency in some insomniac neurotic or psychotic individuals. The frequency of eyeball movement during REM sleep is decreased. The time spent in REM sleep is usually shortened. However, REM sleep may not be shortened when lower doses of flurazepam, clobazam, or perhaps other benzodiazepines are used, even though substantial shortening of SWS and prolongation of stage-2 sleep may occur. Triazolam diminishes REM sleep in the early hours, but the lost time is made up later in the sleep time; it is not known if this is the result of acute tolerance or rapid elimination of the drug. Even with benzodiazepines that cause a substantial reduction in total time spent in REM sleep, the number of cycles

**Table 17–1. ELECTROENCEPHALOGRAPHIC AND OTHER CHARACTERISTICS
OF THE STAGES OF SLEEP**

STAGE *	EEG WAVE ACTIVITY †	EYEBALL ACTIVITY	EFFECT OF DEPRIVATION	OTHER OBSERVATIONS
0 (Awake) Eyes open Eyes closed	 Beta Alpha	Irregular, except slowly rolling when drowsy	—	Insomniacs have longer stages 0 and 1 than normal subjects
1 ("Descending" sleep; dozing)	Alpha Beta Theta	Slight, but bursts of rolling movement	Prevents all following sleep stages; no selective deprivation	
2 (Unequivocal sleep)	Theta Spindles K complexes	Slight rolling movements; occasional REM ‡	Prevents following stages	Subject easily aroused; sensory stimuli evoke K complexes
Slow-Wave Sleep (SWS, Deep Sleep) — 3 (Deep-sleep transition)	Theta Delta Spindles K complexes	Slight	Prevents stage 4	Subject hard to arouse; K complexes are hard to evoke
4 ("Cerebral" sleep)	Delta	Slight	Suicidal ideation and day terrors Rebound excessive; SWS begins on first night of restored sleep and may last for weeks	Subject very hard to arouse; K complexes cannot be evoked Night terrors and somnambulism occur in this stage Insomniacs have normal SWS
REM sleep ‡ (REMS)	Mixed frequency but no spindles or K complexes	Considerable; darting, irregular, in bursts (REM) ‡·§	Anxiety, overeating, behavioral disturbances, decreased concentration and learning, hypersexuality, decreased seizure threshold	Stage of recallable dreaming; 74% of dreams occur in REMS Dreams are more vivid, sexual, and bizarre than in non-REMS; nightmares usually occur during REMS In the male, REMS frequently begins with an erection

* Order of sleep stages is 0, 1, 2, 3, 4, REMS, 1, 2, 3, 4, REMS, etc.; stage 0 may also be repeated, especially in insomniacs. A complete cycle takes approximately 90 minutes. Narcoleptics may bypass any or all of stages 1 to 4. In young adults, the percentage of total sleep time spent in the various stages is as follows: stage 0, 1 to 2%; stage 1, 3 to 6%; stage 2, 40 to 52%; stage 3, 5 to 8%; stage 4, 10 to 19%; REMs, 23 to 34%.

† Alpha is high-amplitude, sinusoidal activity of 8 to 14 cycles per second (cps); beta is low amplitude, 15 to 35 cps; delta is high amplitude (>75 μvolt), 0.5 to 3 cps; theta is low amplitude, 4 to 7 cps; spindles are bursts (each, 0.5-second duration) of high amplitude, 12 to 15 cps; K complex is a high-amplitude negative wave followed by a positive wave, with spindles sometimes superimposed.

‡ REM stands for rapid eyeball movement.

§ REM activity is expressed as "density," *i.e.,* number of movements per epoch.

of REM sleep is usually increased, mostly late in the sleep time. Various benzodiazepines may actually increase time in REM sleep and fast activity during REM sleep in depressed schizophrenics and other psychotics, patients with endogenous depression or neuroses, unspecified insomnias, and persons who alternately work during the day or night. Nitrazepam often increases REM sleep.

Benzodiazepines do not appear to lessen the relaxation of neck muscles that occurs at the onset of REM sleep. They diminish the magnitude of the bursts of tachycardia that occur during REM sleep and the fluctuations in skin resistance that occur in both stage-2 and REM sleep; the effect is greater in normal than in neurotic subjects (Monti *et al.*, 1975). Tolerance rapidly develops to the effects on skin resistance. Flunitrazepam increases the sexual and aggressive content of dreams during REM sleep (Gaillard and Phelippeau, 1976).

Despite the shortening of stage-4 and REM sleep, the net effect of administration of benzodiazepines is an increase in total sleep time. The effect is greatest in subjects with the shortest-baseline total sleep time, for whom sleep time may triple, and least (or even insignificant) in those who normally enjoy a long sleep time (Dement *et al.,* 1973). In addition, despite the increase in the number of REM cycles, the number of shifts to lighter sleep stages (1 and 0) and the amount of body movement are diminished. The nocturnal peaks in the concentration of growth hormone in plasma and the concentrations of prolactin and luteinizing hormone are not affected by flurazepam or nitrazepam.

Use of benzodiazepines imparts a sense of deep or refreshing sleep, but it is uncertain to which effect on sleep parameters this can be attributed. Many workers believe it is the result of the diminution in REM sleep, but some hold it to be also the result of the suppression of SWS. Itil (1976) states that the decrease in REM sleep correlates with increased sleep comfort and decreased restlessness and wakefulness, in contrast to natural sleep, in which the sense of deep sleep usually correlates with the amount of SWS. The extent of increase in fast beta activity may correlate with hangover and a sense of having had a non-refreshing sleep.

During chronic nocturnal use of benzodiazepines the effects on the various stages of sleep usually decline within a few nights but do not disappear. Tolerance is more pronounced to the effects on the REM-sleep than to the non-REM-sleep parameters. During chronic use the number of dreams may double, although dreams usually are less bizarre (Oswald *et al.,* 1973). If after 3 to 4 weeks of nightly use of a benzodiazepine the drug is discontinued, there may be a considerable rebound in the amount and density of REM sleep. Withdrawal from clorazepate, lorazepam, or nitrazepam causes a rebound decrease in REM-sleep latency and an increase in REM-sleep time that may last for a long period. With flurazepam and triazolam, the rebound in REM sleep appears to be slight or negligible. During the period of such rebound the number of dreams per night is about the same as before the drug was taken, but their bizarre character may increase. There is also usually a rebound in SWS, which may exceed the rebound in REM sleep. Withdrawal of flurazepam causes only a slight rebound. However, after flunitrazepam, SWS may remain depressed for several weeks, gradually returning to the baseline condition without rebound. Usually there is a rebound increase in total wake time, which may be especially evident with triazolam (Kales *et al.,* 1978); total wake time is not changed after withdrawal of flurazepam (Kales *et al.,* 1977).

Sites and Mechanism of CNS Actions. The benzodiazepines selectively act on polysyn-aptic and not monosynaptic neuronal pathways throughout the CNS. The action is mainly that of presynaptic inhibition, although at some sites, such as in the cuneate nucleus, there may be postsynaptic inhibition; whether inhibition is presynaptic or postsynaptic, it simulates that of gamma-aminobutyric acid (GABA). Polysynaptic responses may be diminished or augmented, according to whether synaptic inhibition subserves an inhibitory or facilitatory function in the integrated response.

The effects of the benzodiazepines on the midbrain reticular formation are of special interest because of the importance of this region for the maintenance of wakefulness. The mesoencephalic reticular formation is quite sensitive, and effects are noted at tenfold lower concentrations of the drugs than are required to influence spinal neurons. The benzodiazepines decrease both the spontaneous activity and the response to afferent sensory input. In man, somatosensory-evoked potentials, thought to be modulated by the midbrain reticular formation, are diminished in amplitude, and the latency of the early potential is prolonged (Saletu *et al.,* 1972).

The effects on the medullary and forebrain hypnogenic areas require elucidation. The effects on the REM-sleep loci are also poorly known, but the lack of an action on the frequency of ponto-geniculo-occipital (PGO) spike discharge suggests that the benzodiazepines lack prominent effects on the caudal locus ceruleus, where the discharges originate. However, in the cat, the mutiple-unit activity in the midbrain reticular formation following PGO spikes is suppressed by benzodiazepines (Tsuchiya and Fukushima, 1977), but the locus for this action may be in the median forebrain bundle (*see* Haefely *et al.,* 1975). PGO spiking precedes bursts of rapid eyeball movement during REM sleep, and the suppression of the midbrain afterdischarge may be a manifestation of the negative effects of benzodiazepines on REM sleep.

The threshold for behavioral arousal and vascular constriction caused by electrical stimulation of the hypothalamus is diminished by doses of benzodiazepines that cause no general neurological impairment. Various autonomic responses that can be elicited by electrical stimulation at more than one site in the hypothalamus can be suppressed by benzodiazepines only when the stimulation is applied to certain of these sites (*see* Chinn and Barnes, 1978). This suggests that benzodiazepines do not directly inhibit neuronal activity in the primary autonomic centers but do remove facilitatory influences.

There has been lively interest in the effects of

benzodiazepines on the limbic system and hypothalamic and motor cortical connections. The drugs affect neuronal activity in the *hippocampus* quite selectively. Tsuchiya and Kitigawa (1976) reported that hippocampal potentials evoked by stimulation in the amygdala, ventromedial hypothalamus, and cortical gray matter (but not the septum) were facilitated. The preoptic region was moderately depressed selectively, but the reticular area was not.

Seizures elicited by repetitive stimulation of the amygdala are prevented by both diazepam and phenobarbital (Wise and Chinerman, 1974). The drugs prevent the spread of a seizure rather than suppress the afterdischarge, although phenobarbital but not diazepam does elevate the threshold for afterdischarge. In hippocampal pyramidal cells that are recurrently inhibited by stimulation of the fimbria or alveus, inhibition is prolonged by direct application of benzodiazepines (Wolf and Haas, 1977).

The *muscle relaxant effects* of benzodiazepines probably can be explained by actions mostly at supraspinal loci. The effect of stimulation in the medullary reticular formation on spinal neurons is suppressed by small doses of these drugs; the tonic facilitatory influence on spinal gamma neurons is diminished, and gamma rigidity is thus attenuated (*see* Schallek *et al.*, 1972). In the spinal cord, somewhat higher doses of benzodiazepines enhance presynaptic but not postsynaptic inhibition and thus inhibit polysynaptic reflexes.

Benzodiazepine-induced ataxia possibly results from actions in the cerebellum. Benzodiazepines decrease the firing rate of Purkinje cells (Haefely *et al.*, 1975; Critchett and Lippa, 1978). High doses of drug may cause a "burst-suppression" type of firing; that is, long periods of inactivity are interrupted by brief bursts of activity.

The *mechanism of action* of the benzodiazepines appears to be in some way related to the metabolism or action of GABA. Wherever GABA causes either presynaptic or postsynaptic inhibition, the benzodiazepines elicit a similar effect. Their actions are blocked by bicuculline and picrotoxin, which are antagonists of GABA. However, the benzodiazepines are not truly GABA-mimetic, because they are inactive when GABA has been depleted. Furthermore, their ability to compete with GABA for putative receptor binding sites correlates poorly with their effects in man (Snyder and Enna, 1975). Inhibitors of GABA synthesis, such as thiosemicarbazone, prevent the effects of benzodiazepines, and inhibitors of GABA degradation, such as aminoxyacetic acid, augment them. Therefore, benzodiazepines appear to act indirectly. The simulation of the effects of GABA by benzodiazepines may be due to an action of the drugs to antago-

nize a protein that inhibits the binding of GABA to its receptor (Costa *et al.*, 1978; Guidotti *et al.*, 1978). The dissociation constants of the benzodiazepine-protein complex are in the range of 10 to 100 nM, which is also about that for the stereospecific binding sites for benzodiazepines in rat and human brain. The dissociation constants for various drugs correlate strongly with their human muscle relaxant and antianxiety activities (Baestrup *et al.*, 1977; Möhler and Okada, 1978; Speth *et al.*, 1978).

The mechanisms of the paradoxical excitement that is sometimes caused by benzodiazepines and of the convulsant effect of overdosage in some animals are unknown, but it is of interest that Peričić and associates (1977) found that certain benzodiazepines inhibit the synthesis of GABA. This inhibition apparently occurs only in certain parts of the brain, which might explain the unevenness of depressant effects of the drugs throughout the CNS. One convulsant benzodiazepine is an antagonist of GABA. Unevenness in the effects at various GABA-sensitive loci and differences among the pharmacological spectra of the sundry benzodiazepines might also be attributed to differences in their actions on cyclic nucleotide phosphodiesterases. Some of the benzodiazepines strongly inhibit this activity; the inhibition is not uniform throughout the brain. Alteration of cyclic nucleotide concentrations might affect the release and postsynaptic effects of not only GABA but also other neurotransmitters as well.

In preparations of synaptic membranes from the brain stem and spinal cord, benzodiazepines can bind to sites that also have high affinity for strychnine. Their relative affinities for such sites correlate moderately well with certain pharmacological properties. Since strychnine is thought to act as an antagonist at receptors for glycine (*see* Chapter 12), it has been proposed that some actions of benzodiazepines may result from their interaction with such receptors (*see* Snyder *et al.*, 1977). However, the binding affinities are much too low to account for the pharmacological actions of the benzodiazepines, the drugs do not have a selective action to block effects of strychnine, and they have not been observed to interact with glycine at any site. It is noteworthy that bicuculline, but not strychnine, antagonizes the postsynaptic depressant effects of benzodiazepines on medullary neurons that respond to both glycine and GABA (Dray and Straughan, 1976). The roles of GABA and glycine in the action of benzodiazepines have been reviewed by Costa and coworkers (1975), Bloom (1977), and Haefely (1977), and in a symposium (1978).

The benzodiazepines affect the brain content and turnover of various neurotransmitters, but these effects probably result from the GABA-like actions of the drugs. The benzodiazepines decrease the turnover of norepinephrine throughout the brain; they decrease that of dopamine in some regions and increase it in others. The turnover of 5-HT is also decreased, especially in the mesencephalon and rhombencephalon.

Tolerance to the effects of benzodiazepines on the turnover of norepinephrine, but not 5-HT, occurs with repetitive exposure to the drugs (*see* Stein *et al.*, 1973). This has suggested that experimental antianxiety effects, to which tolerance does not occur, are mediated by tryptaminergic nerves and that depressant effects, to which tolerance does occur, are mediated by noradrenergic nerves. There is no evidence that ataxia or the actions on polysynaptic reflexes, to which tolerance occurs, involve noradrenergic nerves. The details of the effects of benzodiazepines on brain monoamines may be found in the monographs edited by Garattini and associates (1973) and Costa and Greengard (1975).

Administration of a benzodiazepine results in an increased content of acetylcholine in certain parts of the brain (Consolo *et al.*, 1975; Sethy, 1978). Davies and Polc (1978) have reported that a water-soluble benzodiazepine can antagonize the actions of acetylcholine on the Renshaw cell without affecting the dorsal root potential; this is the only known example of a selective interaction of a benzodiazepine with a transmitter other than GABA.

Respiration. The benzodiazepines have only slight effects on respiration. Hypnotic doses of triazolam and flurazepam are without effect in normal subjects. Preanesthetic doses of diazepam and flurazepam slightly depress alveolar ventilation and cause respiratory acidosis (Rao *et al.*, 1973; Clarke and Lyons, 1977). The effect appears to result from a decrease in the hypoxic and not the hypercapneic drive, since the response to CO_2 is unaffected (Lakshminarayan *et al.*, 1976). The rate of expiratory flow is depressed only under hypoxic conditions (Gabel *et al.*, 1976). Large doses of lorazepam do, however, moderately depress the response to CO_2 (Elliott *et al.*, 1971; Gasser *et al.*, 1975).

Despite the innocuousness of the respiratory effects in normal persons, nitrazepam, diazepam (in doses used in endoscopy), and perhaps other benzodiazepines decrease alveolar ventilation and P_{O_2}, increase P_{CO_2}, and may cause CO_2 narcosis in patients with chronic obstructive pulmonary disease (Clark *et al.*, 1971; Rao *et al.*, 1973). Furthermore, diazepam can cause apnea during anesthesia and also when given with opioids. Despite the occasional adverse interaction with opioids, the benzodiazepines do not alter the effect of meperidine on the response to CO_2 (*see* Greenblatt and Shader, 1974b). It is noteworthy that in scores of cases of intoxi-

cation involving benzodiazepines the only patients who required respiratory assistance were those who had also taken another CNS-depressant drug, especially alcohol (*see* Greenblatt *et al.*, 1977).

Cardiovascular System. The cardiovascular effects of benzodiazepines are minor, except in severe intoxication. The effects are not alike among all members of the group. Hypnotic doses of triazolam and flurazepam do not affect cardiovascular functions in man (Knapp *et al.*, 1977). So-called anesthetic doses of diazepam and lorazepam moderately decrease left ventricular stroke work, stroke volume, and cardiac output and consequently decrease systolic blood pressure and reflexly increase systemic peripheral resistance and heart rate (Elliott *et al.*, 1971; Rao *et al.*, 1973). Coronary flow is increased (Ikram *et al.*, 1973); this has been shown in dogs to be a direct effect on the coronary vasculature. Bromazepam diminishes systolic and diastolic blood pressures about equally, without significantly changing heart rate; myocardial oxygen demand is reduced, and efficiency is increased (Pozenel *et al.*, 1977). Flunitrazepam decreases blood pressure and cardiac work and reflexly increases heart rate by a vasodilator action that appears mainly to decrease afterload (Seitz *et al.*, 1977). The cardiovascular effects of benzodiazepines have been reviewed by Greenblatt and Shader (1974b).

Gastrointestinal Tract. Several benzodiazepines are employed in combinations with other types of drugs that supposedly improve a variety of "anxiety-related" gastrointestinal disorders (*see* Greenblatt and Shader, 1974b). There is no experimental evidence that benzodiazepines have significant direct gastrointestinal actions.

Pharmacokinetics. Benzodiazepines used for their hypnotic effects are usually administered orally. Some are absorbed within 0.5 to 1 hour, while others take longer than 6 hours; the differences may reflect, in part, the properties of the tablets (*e.g.*, rate of disintegration) rather than pharmacokinetic differences in the compounds. Bioavailability is relatively consistent with some preparations and erratic with others. When administered by the intramuscular route, the water-soluble benzodiazepines are predictably well absorbed, a feature important in the effectiveness of certain benzodiazepines in the emergency treatment of *status epilepticus* and some other types of seizures.

All benzodiazepines bind to human plasma albumin. The extent of binding varies from probably only a few percent with flurazepam to nearly 99% with diazepam. The binding site is stereospecific, at least for oxazepam. Binding correlates strongly with lipid solubility. It is not known to what extent benzodiazepines may interact with other protein-bound drugs, but the paucity of documented adverse interactions suggests that the competition is clinically insignificant.

The plasma concentrations of most benzodiazepines exhibit kinetic patterns that are consistent with two-compartment models (*see* Chapter 1 and Appendix II), but three-compartment models appear to be more appropriate for the highly lipid-soluble compounds. There is a fast uptake into the gray matter of the brain, followed by a slower phase of redistribution into the white matter and adipose tissue. In man, this slower phase of distribution lasts from 11 minutes to 12 hours, depending on the compound. Once redistribution is achieved, the volumes of distribution are quite large, especially for the lipid-soluble benzodiazepines. Benzodiazepines cross the placental barrier and are also secreted into human milk.

The pharmacokinetics of diazepam, nitrazepam, bromazepam, and perhaps others is complicated by apparent enterohepatic circulation. During the early distribution phase, there is probably considerable biliary secretion of drug; hours later, there is a surge in the plasma concentration as drug is reabsorbed, and pharmacological effects result. Food enhances this late return of diazepam into the plasma (Linnoila *et al.*, 1975). The presence of drug or metabolites in feces after intravenous administration also suggests that there is hepatic secretion into bile.

The biotransformations of the benzodiazepines differ from most drugs that contain phenyl or benzo groups in that the benzodiazepines are resistant to hydroxylation at these sites. Trace amounts of a phenolic metabolite have been found only with oxazepam. The only metabolism that involves the benzo ring is reduction of nitro substituents and acetylation of the resulting amines. With these exceptions, metabolic attack occurs only on the 1,4-diazepine moiety. Nevertheless, biotransformations of this ring produce numerous metabolites. For example, medazepam yields at least 11 nonconjugated metabolites, of which two result from rupture of the ring. The major type of conjugate is glucuronide; traces of sulfates have been found with some benzodiazepines. Acetamides are the predominant conjugated metabolites of the 7-nitro compounds. Many of the nonconjugated metabolites of benzodiazepines themselves have biological activity; medazepam yields at least five active metabolites (including diazepam, temazepam, and oxazepam). The accumulation of active metabolites complicates the clinical pharmacology and pharmacokinetics of certain benzodiazepines.

Most biotransformations appear to take place in the liver. However, Mahon and co-workers (1977) have demonstrated a very rapid biotransformation of flurazepam by the small intestine in man. This metabolism may be so rapid that, when small doses are given, only the metabolite appears in the circulation. However, the small intestine usually plays a minor role in the metabolism of most benzodiazepines.

The rate at which benzodiazepines are eliminated is slower in elderly than in young persons. The half-lives of some benzodiazepines are increased in patients with cirrhosis and viral hepatitis.

Evidence obtained *in vitro* and *in vivo* indicates that benzodiazepines are biotransformed by the microsomal drug-metabolizing system. However, the benzodiazepines usually do not induce the synthesis of these enzymes significantly. In man, the induction of the metabolism of other substances has been negligible in all studies thus far. Although it is generally believed that benzodiazepines do not induce their own metabolism, chlordiazepoxide, diazepam, and flurazepam appear to do so (*e.g., see* Linnoila *et al.*, 1975). During the repetitive administration of flurazepam the "steady-state" concentrations in plasma may fall to negligible levels and the elimination half-life of the desamino metabolite also decreases (Hasegawa and Matsubara, 1975).

Further details about the elimination of benzodiazepines are given only for those that are used primarily for hypnosis. The bioavailability of flurazepam varies betwen 30 and 60%. After a single oral dose of 30 mg, the plasma concentration rises to a peak of 1 to 2 ng/ml at 1 hour and falls rapidly with a half-life of about 3 hours. About 70% of flurazepam is converted to metabolites during its first pass through the intestine and liver. There are at least six nonconjugated metabolites of the drug, of which five are more potent in various activities than is flurazepam. Clinically, the desamino (group at position 1 converted to HOC_2H_4–) and desalkyl (group at position 1 removed) metabolites are of major significance. Not only are they an order of magnitude more potent than is flurazepam in animal tests, but also they reach higher concentrations in plasma than does flurazepam. After a 30-mg dose of flurazepam, the peak concentration (at 1 to 3 hours) of the desalkyl metabolite is 0.5 to 1.8 ng/ml and that of the desamino compounds is 6 to 8 ng/ml. The elimination half-life of the desamino compound is 10 to 20 hours and that of the desalkyl metabolite is 1 day (Hasegawa and Matsubara, 1975) or longer (*see* Breimer, 1977). Therefore, with daily administration, these metabolites accumulate to rather high concentrations over a period of several days to a few weeks. Since pharmacological activity is attributable to these metabolites, a few days of daily administration are required for the onset of the full effect of flurazepam, and residual effects ("hangover") are common. Less than 0.2% of flurazepam is excreted unchanged; 30 to 55% of the drug is converted to the desamino metabolite.

Following oral administration, the absorption of nitrazepam ranges from 50 to 95%. In fasting subjects, an oral dose of 10 mg may provide a peak concentration of about 70 to 100 ng/ml in 0.5 to 5 hours. Once absorbed, the drug is bound to plasma albumin to the extent of 87%. There is a distribution phase, which lasts 2 to 3 hours, following which there is a slight rise in concentration before the final elimination phase. The elimination half-life ranges from 18 to 34 hours; the drug thus accumulates during nightly repetitive administration. Of five nonconjugated metabolites, only one has significant biological activity. The major metabolic pathway is reduction of the 7-nitro group to the amine, followed by acetylation.

Triazolam has an average absorption half-time of less than 10 minutes. One milligram will yield a peak concentration of about 9 ng/ml. The pharmacokinetics appears to fit the one-compartment model. The plasma half-life has been reported to be about 4.5 hours (Metzler *et al.,* 1977), but unpublished data suggest that it may be as short as 2.7 hours. The principal unconjugated metabolite is the 1-hydroxymethyl derivative, which has a hypnotic potency in man nearly equal to that of triazolam.

The pharmacokinetics of flunitrazepam is not well defined. The elimination half-life is probably about 15 hours. This implies that there is accumulation of drug during daily administration. The 7-amino derivative is the principal unconjugated metabolite.

The elimination half-lives of antianxiety drugs sometimes used as hypnotics are given in Table 17–2 (*see also* Appendix II).

The pharmacokinetics and biotransformations of benzodiazepines have been reviewed by Randall and Kappell (1973), Greenblatt and Shader (1974b), and Breimer (1977).

Untoward Effects. At the time of peak concentration in plasma, hypnotic doses of benzodiazepines can be expected to cause varying degrees of light-headedness, lassitude, increased reaction time, motor incoordination, ataxia, impairment of mental and psychomotor functions, disorganization of thought, confusion, dysarthria, retrograde amnesia, dry mouth, and a bitter taste. Cognition appears to be affected less than motor performance. All of these effects greatly impair driving skills. When the drug is given before the intended time of sleep, they may not even be noticed, but the persistence of these effects during the waking hours is adverse. *Interaction with ethanol* may be especially serious. The persistence of objective side effects is generally predictable from a knowledge of the pharmacokinetics, but that of the subjective effects may not be. The residual effects of a single dose are more prominent after diazepam, lorazepam, and nitrazepam than after flurazepam and triazolam. During repeated administration, the effects of nitrazepam may persist for nearly 20 hours and those of flurazepam for over 10 hours; they may persist even longer if alcohol is ingested concurrently (Mendelson *et al.,* 1976). The effects of flunitrazepam may last for 10 to 24 hours, and effects of triazolam on mood possibly last as long as 16 hours (Veldkamp *et al.,* 1974), which is inconsistent with its reputed short half-life. Central-depressant adverse effects increase with age.

Other relatively common side effects of benzodiazepines are weakness, headache, blurred vision, vertigo, nausea and vomiting, epigastric distress, and diarrhea; joint pains, chest pains, and incontinence may occur in a few percent or less of recipients.

The possible adverse effects of alterations in the sleep pattern will be discussed at the end of this chapter.

Adverse Psychological Effects. Benzodiazepines may cause paradoxical effects. Nitrazepam frequently and flurazepam occasionally increase the incidence of nightmares, especially during the first week of use. Flura-zepam occasionally causes garrulousness, anxiety, irritability, tachycardia, and sweating. In one case, euphoria, restlessness, insomnia, hallucinations, and hypomanic behavior, which lasted several days, occurred after the administration of flurazepam. Similar behavior has resulted after use of chlordiazepoxide. Anticonvulsant benzodiazepines sometimes induce motor stimulation and precipitate grand mal seizures. Antianxiety benzodiazepines have been reported to release bizarre uninhibited behavior in some users with low levels of anxiety; hostility and rage may occur in others. Paranoia, depression, and suicidal ideation occasionally accompany the use of antianxiety benzodiazepines. However, it is not possible to decide if these effects are a consequence of a primary emotional disorder, are the result of potentiation of the disorder by the drugs, or are caused primarily by the benzodiazepines.

Although benzodiazepines have a reputation for causing only a low rate of *abuse* and *dependence,* the possibility of this adverse complication of chronic use must not be overlooked. The overwhelming preponderance of reported cases involve benzodiazepines used to treat anxiety, often in combination with other abused drugs. High doses and prolonged periods of use appear to be necessary. A few cases of dependence upon flurazepam, nitrazepam, and flunitrazepam have been reported. In some of these, the patients had previously abused other drugs, including antianxiety benzodiazepines (*e.g., see* Misra, 1975). Whether dependence can occur with a single nightly therapeutic dose of a short-acting hypnotic benzodiazepine over an extended period remains to be determined, but some tolerance has been reported under these conditions (*e.g., see* Kales *et al.,* 1977). Tolerance to benzodiazepines confers cross-tolerance to methaqualone, barbiturates, and, to some extent, ethanol. It is recommended that the drug be discontinued at the first sign of an increase in the dose required. Withdrawal signs and symptoms include depression, anxiety, and agitation, as well as abnormalities of sleep and dreams. Acute psychosis and delirium may follow withdrawal of benzodiazepines with antianxiety activity; convulsions may be precipitated during withdrawal of those with anticonvul-

sant activity. Habituation and dependence upon benzodiazepines have been reviewed by Greenblatt and Shader (1974b) and Allgulander (1978).

The potential for adverse effects on the elimination of CO_2 in persons with obstructive pulmonary disease has been discussed above.

A wide variety of allergic, hepatotoxic, and hematologic reactions to antianxiety benzodiazepines has been reported (*see* Greenblatt and Shader, 1974b), but the incidence is quite low. Hypnotic benzodiazepines can be expected to cause similar reactions.

Only diazepam has hitherto been reported to be teratogenic, causing cleft lip and palate in man (Safra and Oakley, 1975) and mice (Miller and Becker, 1975), but it is advisable to withhold any benzodiazepine during pregnancy, especially during the first trimester. Large doses taken just prior to or during labor may cause hypothermia, hypotonia, and mild respiratory depression in the neonate. Abuse by the pregnant mother can result in a withdrawal syndrome in the newborn infant.

Except for additive effects with other CNS-depressant drugs, most frequently ethanol and valproate, reports of clinically important drug interactions between benzodiazepines and other drugs have been rare and unconfirmed. Ethanol increases both the absorption of benzodiazepines and the CNS depression (*see* Ascione, 1978). Valproate and benzodiazepines in combination may cause psychotic episodes.

THERAPEUTIC USES

The use of the benzodiazepines as hypnotics is discussed at the end of this chapter; there is also some discussion of their employment as sedatives. Other uses of benzodiazepines are as antianxiety agents (Chapter 19), anticonvulsants (Chapter 20), muscle relaxants (Chapter 21), for preanesthetic medication (Chapter 13), and in anesthesia (Chapter 14).

Preparations and Dosage. The aqueous solubility of benzodiazepines ranges from less than 1/10,000 (chlordiazepoxide, lorazepam, oxazepam) to 1/2 (flurazepam hydrochloride). Solubilities in lipid are generally low; however, because of the generally low aqueous solubilities, lipid : water partition coefficients are usually high. The official names, trade names, preparations, and sedative and hypnotic doses of these agents are given in Table 17–2.

BARBITURATES

The barbiturates have enjoyed a long period of extensive use as sedative-hypnotic drugs; however, except for a few specialized uses, they have been largely replaced by the

Table 17-2.   HALF-LIVES, DOSAGE FORMS, AND ORAL DOSES OF SEDATIVE-HYPNOTIC DRUGS

DRUG CLASSES, NONPROPRIETARY NAMES, AND TRADE NAMES	HALF-LIFE (hr)	DOSAGE FORMS [1] (mg or mg/vol)	ADULT ORAL DOSE [2] (mg)	
			Sedative	Hypnotic
Benzodiazepines				
Bromazepam [3] (LECTOPAM)	8–19	—	6–12, 3–4×d [4]	24(?)
Chlordiazepoxide (LIBRITABS)	7–28	T:5,10,25	5–10, 2–3×d	25
Chlordiazepoxide·HCl (LIBRIUM)	7–28	C:5,10,25	5–20, 3–4×d	25
Diazepam (VALIUM)	20–90	T:2,5,10	2–10, 2–4×d	10
Flunitrazepam [3] (ROHYPNOL)	10–20	—	—	1–2
Flurazepam·HCl (DALMANE)	24–100 [5]	C:15,30	—	15–30
Lorazepam (ATIVAN)	10–20	T:0.5,1,2	0.5–1, 2–3×d	2–4
Nitrazepam [3] (MOGADON)	18–34	—	—	5–10
Oxazepam (SERAX)	3–21	C:10,15,30; T:15	10–15, 3–4×d	10–30
Oxazolam [3] (SERENAL)	~4.5 [6]	—	—	—
Prazepam (VERSTRAN)	24–200 [5]	T:10	10–20, 2–3×d	10–20
Temazepam [3] (CEREPAX, LEVANXOL)	—	—	—	10–30
Triazolam [3] (HALCION)	2.7–4.5(?)	T:0.25,0.5,1	0.25–0.5, 2–3×d	0.5–1
Barbiturates				
Amobarbital (AMYTAL)	8–42	E:44/5; T:15,30,50,100	22–50, 2–3×d	100–200
Amobarbital Na (AMYTAL SODIUM)	8–42	C:65,200	—	65–200
Aprobarbital (ALURATE)	—	E:40/5	40–80, 3×d	40–160
Butabarbital Na (BUTISOL SODIUM)	34–42	E:30/5; C,T:15,30,50,100	7.5–60, 3–4×d	100–200
Butalbital (SANDOPTAL)	—	M. C,T:50	50–100, 3–4×d	100–200
Hexobarbital (SOMBULEX)	2.7–7	T:250	—	250–500
Pentobarbital (NEMBUTAL)	15–48	E:18.2/5	20, 3–4×d	90–180
Pentobarbital Na (NEMBUTAL SODIUM)	15–48	C:50,100	30, 2–4×d	100
Phenobarbital (various trade names)	24–140	E:7.5/5, 20/5; T:15,30,60,100	15–30, 2–3×d	100–200
Phenobarbital Na (various trade names)	24–140	T:15,30,60,100	15–30, 2–3×d	100–200
Secobarbital (SECONAL)	19–34	E:22/5	30–50, 3–4×d	100
Secobarbital Na (SECONAL SODIUM)	19–34	C:50,100	30–50, 3–4×d	100
Talbutal (LOTUSATE)	—	T:30,50,120	30, 2–3×d	120
Miscellaneous				
Chloral Betaine (BETA-CHLOR)	4–9.5 [5]	T:870(=500 hydrate)	—	870–1000
Chloral Hydrate (various trade names)	4–9.5 [5]	C:250,500; S:250/5,500/5,800/5	250, 3×d	500–2000
Ethchlorvynol (PLACIDYL)	10–25 [7]	C:100,500,750	100–200, 2–3×d	500–1000
Ethinamate (VALMID)	—	C,T:500		500–1000

Table 17-2. HALF-LIVES, DOSAGE FORMS, AND ORAL DOSES OF SEDATIVE-HYPNOTIC DRUGS (Continued)

DRUG CLASSES, NONPROPRIETARY NAMES, AND TRADE NAMES	HALF-LIFE (hr)	DOSAGE FORMS [1] $(mg \ or \ mg/vol)$	ADULT ORAL DOSE [2] (mg)	
			Sedative	Hypnotic
Glutethimide (DORIDEN)	5–22	C:500; T:125,250,500	125–250, 1–3×d	250–500
Meprobamate (EQUANIL, MILTOWN)	6–17	ERC:200,400; T:200,400,600	400, 3–4×d or 400–800ERC, 1–2×d	800
Methaqualone (QUAALUDE, SOPOR)	10–42	T:75,150,300	75, 3–4×d	150–300
Methaqualone·HCl (PAREST, SOMNAFAC)	10–42	C:200,400	100, 4×d	200–400
Methyprylon (NOLUDAR)	—	C:300; T:50,200	50–100, 3–4×d	200–400
Paraldehyde	—	C:1000; L:30	5–10 ml [2]	10–30 ml [2]
Triclofos Na (TRICLOS)	4–9.5 [5]	S:500/5; T:750	—	1500
L-Tryptophan [3]	—	—	—	1000–5000

[1] T = tablet; C = capsule; S = syrup; L = liquid; E = elixir; ERC = extended-release capsule; M = marketed only in mixtures. For solid dosage forms, number is milligrams per unit dose; for liquid forms, number is milligrams per unit dose, volume in milliliters.

[2] For parenteral, rectal, or pediatric doses, see U.S.P. or manufacturer's literature.

[3] Not yet available in the United States. All other agents are listed in the U.S.P. except aprobarbital, chloral betaine, lorazepam, prazepam, and triclofos.

[4] Dose, number per day.

[5] Half-life of the active metabolite to which the effects can be mainly attributed.

[6] Limited data; range is undoubtedly much wider.

[7] For acute use, half-life of distribution phase (1 to 3 hours) may be more appropriate.

somewhat safer benzodiazepines. A more detailed description of the barbiturates can be found in the *fifth edition* of this textbook.

Chemistry. Barbituric acid is 2,4,6-trioxohexahydropyrimidine. The compound lacks central-depressant activity, but the presence of alkyl or aryl groups at position 5 confers sedative-hypnotic and sometimes other activities. The general structural formula for the barbiturates and the structures of those compounds available in the United States are shown in Table 17-3.

The carbonyl group at position 2 takes on acidic character because of lactam ("keto")-lactim ("enol") tautomerization favored by its location between the two electronegative amido nitrogens. The lactim form is favored in alkaline solution, and salts result. The barbituric acid derivatives do not dissolve readily in water, although they are quite soluble in nonpolar solvents, a feature that they share with many other organic compounds that depress the CNS. The sodium salts of barbiturates dissolve in water, forming alkaline and often unstable solutions.

Barbiturates in which the oxygen at C2 is replaced by sulfur are called *thiobarbiturates.* Although only those compounds having a barbituric acid ring (oxygen at C2) are properly called *barbiturates,* it has become common practice to refer to both groups of compounds as barbiturates and to distinguish between them, when necessary, by using the terms *thiobarbiturates* and *oxybarbiturates.* Thiobarbiturates are more lipid soluble than the corresponding oxybarbiturates.

In general, structural changes that increase lipid solubility decrease duration of action, decrease la-

Table 17-3. BARBITURATES AVAILABLE CURRENTLY IN THE UNITED STATES: NAMES AND STRUCTURES

GENERAL FORMULA:

BARBITURATE	R_{5a}	R_{5b}
Amobarbital	ethyl	isopentyl
Aprobarbital	allyl	isopropyl
Barbital	ethyl	ethyl
Butabarbital	ethyl	sec-butyl
Butalbital	allyl	isobutyl
Hexobarbital *	methyl	1-cyclohexen-1-yl
Mephobarbital *	ethyl	phenyl
Metharbital *	ethyl	ethyl
Methohexital *	allyl	1-methyl-2-pentynyl
Pentobarbital	ethyl	1-methylbutyl
Phenobarbital	ethyl	phenyl
Secobarbital	allyl	1-methylbutyl
Talbutal	allyl	sec-butyl
Thiamylal †	allyl	1-methylbutyl
Thiopental †	ethyl	1-methylbutyl

* R_3 = H, except in hexobarbital, mephobarbital, metharbital, and methohexital, where it is replaced by CH_3.

† O, except in thiamylal and thiopental, where it is replaced by S.

tency to onset of activity, accelerate metabolic degradation, and often increase hypnotic potency. Thus, large aliphatic groups at C5 confer greater activity than do methyl groups, but the compounds have a shorter duration of action; however, groups larger than seven carbons tend to have convulsant activity. Introduction of polar groups, such as ether, keto, hydroxyl, amino, or carboxyl groups, into alkyl side chains decreases lipid solubility and abolishes hypnotic activity. Methylation of the 1-N atom increases lipid solubility and shortens duration of action, although demethylation to a longer-acting metabolite may occur. Lipid solubility also favors interaction with hydrophobic regions in proteins. It correlates roughly with binding to plasma protein and cytochrome P-450 and closely with binding to NADH–cytochrome c oxidoreductase.

PHARMACOLOGICAL PROPERTIES

The barbiturates reversibly depress the activity of all excitable tissues. Not all tissues are affected at the same dose or concentration; the CNS is exquisitely sensitive, and, when barbiturates are given in sedative or hypnotic doses, there is very little effect on skeletal, cardiac, or smooth muscle. Even in anesthetic concentrations, direct effects on peripheral excitable tissues are weak and do not create difficulties if the duration of anesthesia is not prolonged. However, if depression is extended, as in acute barbiturate intoxication, serious deficits in cardiovascular and other peripheral functions occur.

Central Nervous System. The barbiturates can produce all degrees of depression of the CNS, ranging from mild sedation to general anesthesia. The use of barbiturates for general anesthesia is discussed in Chapter 14. Certain barbiturates, particularly those containing a 5-phenyl substituent (phenobarbital, mephobarbital) have selective anticonvulsant activity; in doses that have only minor effects on the reticular system, they elevate the threshold for the initiation of afterdischarges, shorten the period of afterdischarge, and suppress the spread of seizures. The anticonvulsant uses are discussed in Chapter 20. There is an old belief that barbiturates, especially phenobarbital, have useful antianxiety properties and also exert effects on certain psychosomatic disorders, but evidence is equivocal at best, and the antianxiety properties are certainly not equivalent to those thought to be exerted by benzodiazepines. The barbiturates may have euphoriant effects, which, when maximal, are comparable to those of morphine (McClane and Martin, 1976).

Except for the anticonvulsant activities of phenobarbital and its congeners, the barbiturates possess a low degree of selectivity and therapeutic index. Thus, it is not possible to achieve a desired effect without evidences of general depression of the CNS. However, there is one function, namely, pain perception and reaction, that is relatively unimpaired until the moment of unconsciousness. Indeed, in small doses, the barbiturates are *hyperalgesic* and increase the reaction to painful stimuli. Hence they cannot be relied upon to produce sedation or sleep in the pres-

ence of even moderate pain. Although barbiturates have been claimed to enhance analgesia from other drugs, a sound clinical assessment of their contribution to the efficacy of various combinations of analgesic drugs remains to be made. Barbiturates are said to antagonize analgesics in experimental animals, but Geller and associates (1977) found no such interaction.

In some individuals and in some circumstances, such as in the presence of pain, barbiturates cause overt excitement instead of sedation. The fact that such paradoxical excitement occurs with other CNS depressants suggests that it may result from depression of inhibitory centers. As with ethanol, the degree and quality of excitement are variable, depending on both personality and environment.

Effects on EEG. In small intravenous doses or after oral ingestion, barbiturates decrease low-frequency electrical activity determined by electroencephalography and increase the low-voltage, fast activity (15 to 35 Hz). Fast activity from the frontal cortex spreads to the parietal and occipital cortex and recedes in the reverse order as the effect of the drug wanes. The early high-frequency response resembles that from electrical arousal of the reticular formation, and the threshold for EEG arousal may be transiently lowered; however, the hippocampal component of the arousal response is missing, and true arousal does not occur.

Activation of the EEG is accompanied by clouding of consciousness and, occasionally, euphoria. As the dose is increased, large-amplitude, random slow waves (5 to 12 Hz) similar to those in sleep appear, and consciousness is lost, although the patient may continue to respond to strong, painful stimuli. These slow waves usually occur in spindle-shaped bursts; they differ from normal sleep spindles in spectra and topographic distribution. The spindle pacemaker resides in the thalamus. There is greater thalamicocortical coherence than in normal sleep. The EEG is very stable in this and subsequent stages.

A further increase in dose causes the wave frequency to decrease to 1 to 3 Hz. Limbic neuronal firing rates become depressed. Mild-to-moderate noxious stimuli now fail to evoke responses. With still higher doses the amplitudes of the waves diminish, and there are occasional brief periods of electrical silence, but EEG coherence among the limbic structures persists even during such burst suppression. Major surgical procedures can be undertaken at this time. The periods of electrical silence become longer as depression becomes more severe, and eventually all electrical activity disappears. The EEG patterns are grossly similar to those produced by gaseous and volatile anesthetic agents (Chapter 14); however, there are minor differences, particularly during induction.

The effects of barbiturates on the resting EEG and evoked responses have been reviewed by Clark and Rosner (1973) and Rosner and Clark (1973).

Effects on Stages of Sleep. Hypnotic doses of barbiturates always alter the stages of sleep, and they do so in a dose-dependent manner. They decrease sleep latency, slightly increase delta bursts and fast-EEG activity during sleep, decrease the number of stage shifts to stages 0 and 1 (number of awakenings), and decrease body movement. Stages 3 and 4 (slow-wave sleep, SWS) are generally shortened considerably, except in some patients with anxiety and in barbiturate addicts. Furthermore, phenobarbital sometimes increases stage-4 sleep in healthy persons and may also increase total SWS in enuretic and somnambulistic persons. Thiopental has also been reported to increase stage-4 sleep. The latent period before REM sleep is prolonged, and total time spent in REM sleep, the number of REM cycles, and REM activity are diminished; with the short-acting barbiturates, these effects occur primarily during the first third of the night and are compensated for in the last third. The nocturnal peaks of plasma growth hormone concentration are increased after single and repetitive administration, but those of adrenocorticoids are decreased. It is of interest that administration of barbiturates during the day may decrease REM sleep at night (Feinberg *et al.,* 1974).

During repetitive nightly administration, some tolerance to the effects on sleep occurs within a few days, and the effect on total sleep time may be reduced by as much as 50% after two weeks of use (*see* Kales *et al.,* 1977). In all of nine studies reviewed by Kay and associates (1976), discontinuation led to rebound increases in all the parameters reported to be decreased by barbiturates. There may be an increase in REM sleep even if there was no reduction of this phenomenon during the time of drug administration (Kales *et al.,* 1970a). A rebound decrease in stage-2 sleep is said also to occur. However, Kales and coworkers (1970a, 1977) did not observe a rebound in stage-4 or total sleep time after cessation of nightly administration of 100 mg of secobarbital, and Feinberg and associates (1974) did not find a rebound in REM sleep parameters after repetitive use of amobarbital, phenobarbital, or secobarbital.

The effects of barbiturates on sleep have been reviewed by Kay and associates (1976) and Mendelson and coworkers (1977).

Tolerance. Both pharmacodynamic (functional) and pharmacokinetic tolerance to barbiturates can occur. The former contributes more to the decreased effect than does the latter. Indeed, after a single dose of barbiturate, the plasma concentration upon awakening may be higher than when sleep ensued. After a second dose, a higher level is required to reestablish sleep than with the first dose. Acute tolerance thus appears to occur substantially earlier than does induction of microsomal enzymes. With chronic administration of gradually increasing doses, pharmacodynamic tolerance continues to develop over a period of weeks to months, depending upon the dosage schedule, whereas pharmacokinetic tolerance reaches its peak in a few days. Tolerance to the effects on mood, sedation, and hypnosis occurs more readily and is greater than that to the anticonvulsant and lethal effects; thus, as tolerance increases, the therapeutic index decreases. When tolerance becomes maximal, the effective dose of a barbiturate may be increased by as much as six times; this is twofold to threefold greater than can be accounted for by enhanced metabolic disposition.

Supervised chronic sedation for weeks to months

with therapeutic doses of secobarbital or pentobarbital causes a negligible degree of tolerance (*see* Wikler, 1976), and it might be concluded that once-a-day use of recommended hypnotic doses would be unlikely to cause tolerance. However, tolerance to the effects on sleep stages may occur or the chronic disruption of the normal sleep pattern may in itself make sleep less satisfying; the result is that the patient may increase his dosage in an attempt to improve his sleep and therein enhance the probability or degree of tolerance.

Caldwell and Sever (1974) state that pharmacodynamic tolerance is negligible with barbiturates with short half-lives, but this is critically dependent on the dosage regimen. The degree of tolerance is determined by the time-averaged extent of depression of the CNS. When short- and long-acting barbiturates are administered such that the duration of CNS depression is equivalent, the degrees of tolerance are the same.

Since pharmacodynamic tolerance may be viewed as a homeostatic excitatory feedback response to depression, it is not surprising that signs and symptoms of withdrawal resemble exaggerations of the functions originally depressed and that cross-tolerance occurs to other similar depressants of the CNS. Thus, tolerance to barbiturates confers tolerance to all general CNS-depressant drugs, such as meprobamate, glutethimide, methaqualone, and general anesthetics. There may even be cross-tolerance to the pharmacodynamically dissimilar opioids and phencyclidine, only a part of which is due to induction of hepatic enzymes. There is some evidence of cross-tolerance to the antianxiety and hypnotic effects of benzodiazepines, but not to the muscle relaxant effects. The syndrome of withdrawal from barbiturates is discussed in Chapter 23.

Abuse and Dependence. Like other CNS-depressant drugs, barbiturates are abused, and some individuals develop a dependence upon them. Dependence upon and tolerance to barbiturates are closely related, the former generating the drug-seeking behavior that leads to increased usage and consequent higher level of tolerance. The liabilities of various barbiturates to produce dependence appear to be equal when based on equivalent cumulated exposure to their depressant effects.

The severity of the abstinence syndrome relates to the degree of tolerance and hence to the extent, duration, and continuity of abuse prior to withdrawal. It is also dependent upon the rate of elimination of the drug; slow elimination allows time for the CNS to diminish its compensatory excitatory response more nearly in phase with the diminution in drug-induced depression. Persons dependent upon various barbiturates may be withdrawn more smoothly if long-acting phenobarbital is substituted for a shorter-acting drug prior to withdrawal.

The discontinuation of barbiturate medication in epileptics may result in status epilepticus, even when the patient has been using the long-acting phenobarbital in relatively small daily doses. Neither phenytoin nor chlorpromazine will prevent seizures caused by withdrawal from barbiturates; barbiturates themselves are indicated to suppress them.

Various aspects of tolerance, physical dependence, and abuse of barbiturates are discussed in the proceedings of the conference edited by Thompson and Unna (1976), by Oswald (1976) and Allgulander (1978), and in Chapter 23.

Sites and Mechanism of Actions on the CNS. In experimental animals, nonanesthetic doses of the depressant barbiturates have been shown to depress monosynaptic responses only transiently, but they delay synaptic recovery and, at some synapses, decrease postsynaptic resistance. Polysynaptic responses are affected to a somewhat greater extent. When paired stimuli are tested, barbiturates decrease facilitation and enhance inhibition. The depression at most sensitive synapses probably results from a presynaptic effect to decrease transmitter release, but postsynaptic inhibition has also been demonstrated at membranes upon which GABA but not glycine has an inhibitory action. Occasionally, barbiturates may alter the GABA inversion potential (Ransom and Barker, 1976). The inhibitory actions at synapses confer a particular efficacy against repetitive activity in a number of CNS pathways; small doses of certain barbiturates may have almost no effect on the initial impulse in a train, yet greatly depress the responses to the subsequent impulses. Posttetanic potentiation is not affected.

Although only a few studies have directly compared the actions of barbiturates and GABA, it appears that low doses of barbiturates either have a GABA-like action (*e.g., see* Polc and Haefely, 1976) or enhance the effects of GABA (Nicoll, 1978). Examination of the effects of stereoisomers of pentobarbital on cultured spinal neurons suggests that the S(−) isomer is predominantly responsible for these effects; the R(+) isomer produces excitatory responses (Huang and Barker, 1980). Experimental elevation of GABA concentration in the brain lengthens the time of sleep induced by barbiturates and lowering the concentration shortens it (Tzeng and Ho, 1977). The mechanism of these GABA-like effects is not clear. Cutler and associates (1974) and Sutton and Simmonds (1974) adduced evidence that nonaromatic barbiturates acutely inhibit a neuronal uptake system for GABA. Some barbiturates also appeared to cause the release of GABA. However, Ticku and Olsen (1978) could not confirm these findings; instead, they found that barbiturates competed with dihydropicrotoxinin at a site thought to be a GABA receptor-modulated ionophore.

The above-cited GABA-like effects of barbiturates suggest similarities with the benzodiazepines. Among these are their effects on the reticulohypothalamic systems that regulate hippocampal activity (Tsuchiya and Kitigawa, 1976), their effects on amygdaloid seizures (Wise and Chinerman, 1974), and their inhibition of the turnover of dopamine, norepinephrine, and 5-HT. One distinct difference between barbiturates and benzodiazepines is that the margin of selectivity is quite small with the former but not the latter; that is, with barbiturates only a slight elevation in dose produces nonselective depression in addition to selective synaptic depression. Thus, the segmental component of a somatovisceral reflex studied by Schlosser and associates (1975) was suppressed by phenobarbital almost as readily as was the suprasegmental response. Responses to various excitatory transmitters are also nonselectively inhibited by higher doses of barbiturates.

The GABA-like effects do not preclude the possibility of selective interactions with other neurotransmitter systems. Barbiturates may selectively abolish noradrenergic excitation but not inhibition at various synapses. Concentrations that produce anesthesia decrease the release and turnover of acetylcholine (Sundwall, 1973; Richter and Waller, 1977), which may be the result of nonselective neuronal depression. However, when there is tolerance to barbiturates, there is also supersensitivity to the actions of pilocarpine on the CNS (Wahlström and Eckwall, 1976). Hemicholinium-3 prevents and reverses tolerance to barbiturates. A role for acetylcholine in the development of tolerance is thus suggested.

Very high concentrations of barbiturates interfere with calcium entry into rat brain synaptosomes, prevent stimulus-secretion coupling in mouse forebrain, suppress the calcium spike in giant squid synapses and decrease the calcium-sensitive sodium activation parameter, and release calcium from neuronal mitochondria, resulting in increased membrane permeability and intracellular sodium. It is not clear if these effects have any relevance to the CNS-depressant actions of the drugs.

During barbiturate-induced anesthesia, there is approximately a 50% decrease in oxygen utilization by the brain and an increase in glycogen and high-energy phosphate content, probably secondary to the decrease in neuronal activity. This is thought to be the basis for the prevention of cerebral edema by barbiturate and its protection against cerebral infarction during cerebral ischemia and head injury (*see* Smith, 1977).

Peripheral Nervous Structures. Barbiturates selectively depress transmission in *sympathetic ganglia* in concentrations that have no detectable effect on nerve conduction, neuroeffector junctions, or cardiovascular or other smooth muscle. The effect is not presynaptic, although higher doses may diminish transmitter release. The response of the ganglion cells to both preganglionic stimulation and choline esters is diminished. The ganglion cells are not depolarized, and they remain responsive to potassium chloride. The ganglionic depressant action is sufficiently pronounced to be of clinical interest; it may account, at least in part, for the fall in blood pressure produced by intravenous oxybarbiturates and by severe barbiturate intoxication.

At *skeletal neuromuscular junctions,* the twitch response to a single electrical shock applied to the motor nerve may be augmented by subanesthetic concentrations of barbiturates. In toxic doses, barbiturates increase transmitter release and reduce the sensitivity of the postsynaptic membrane to the depolarizing effect of acetylcholine and decamethonium. The transient inward sodium conductance is decreased, but the outward sodium current is increased (Seyama and Narahashi, 1975). The neuromuscular blocking effects of both *d*-tubocurarine and decamethonium are enhanced during barbiturate anesthesia.

Transmission at *autonomic neuroeffector junctions* is also depressed by barbiturates, but the effects are of relatively little significance.

Respiration. Barbiturates depress both the respiratory drive and the mechanisms responsible for the rhythmic character of respiration; however, low doses of barbiturate occasionally enhance the response to CO_2 slightly. The neurogenic drive is diminished by hypnotic doses, but usually no more so than during natural sleep. *Neurogenic drive is essentially eliminated by a dose three times greater than that normally used to induce sleep.* Such doses also suppress the hypoxic and chemoreceptor drives; the hypoxic drive is affected by lower doses than is the chemoreceptor drive, but some function nevertheless persists after doses that obliterate the response to CO_2. Thus, with increasing depth of depression of the CNS, the dominant respiratory drive shifts to the carotid and aortic bodies. Eventually, if the dose is increased still further, the powerful hypoxic drive also fails. However, the margin between the lighter planes of surgical anesthesia and dangerous respiratory depression is sufficient to permit the ultrashort-acting barbiturates to be used, with suitable precautions, as anesthetic agents.

The barbiturates only slightly depress protective reflexes until the degree of intoxication is sufficient to produce severe respiratory depression. In animals, the cough reflex is depressed only by doses that seriously embarrass respiration, and, in this respect, the barbiturates differ from opioids and other antitussives that may exert a selective effect on cough reflexes. Coughing, sneezing, hiccoughing, and laryngospasm may occur when barbiturates are employed as intravenous anesthetic agents. Indeed, laryngospasm is one of the chief respiratory complications of barbiturate anesthesia.

Cardiovascular System. When given orally in sedative or hypnotic doses, the barbiturates do not produce significant overt cardiovascular effects, except for a slight decrease in blood pressure and heart rate such as occurs in normal sleep. During thiopental anesthesia, there is usually either no change or a fall in mean arterial pressure, the latter being more pronounced in hypertensive patients. Hypotension is caused, in part, by partial inhibition of ganglionic transmission. Histamine release occurs, but it is rarely of clinical consequence. However, when there is congestive heart failure or hypovolemic shock and reflexes are already operating maximally, barbiturates can cause an exaggerated fall in blood pressure. Because barbiturates impair reflex cardiovascular adjustments to inflation of the lung, positive-pressure respiration should be used cautiously and only when necessary to maintain adequate pulmonary ventilation in patients who are anesthetized or intoxicated with a barbiturate.

Apart from changes in blood pressure the following cardiovascular changes have often been noted when thiopental and other intravenous thiobarbiturates are administered after conventional preanesthetic medication: a decrease in cardiac output; considerable decrease in renal plasma flow; an increase in total calculated peripheral resistance, which develops only over a period of time and is probably partly compensatory to decreased cardiac output and partly central in origin; an increase or no change in heart rate; a decrease in myocardial utilization of free fatty acids; a decrease in intrathoracic blood volume; an increase in blood flow and volume in the extremities; a decrease or no change in the central, right atrial, and peripheral venous pressures; and a decrease in cerebral blood flow, with a marked fall in cerebrospinal fluid pressure. Cardiac arrhythmias are observed only rarely in man (but frequently in animals) and do not result from sensitization of the myocardium to catecholamines. In general, the effects of thiopental anesthesia on the cardiovascular system are benign in comparison with those of other (volatile) anesthetic agents and do not constitute a hazard in normal clinical practice. Direct depression of cardiac contractility occurs only when doses several times those required to cause anesthesia are administered. This probably contributes to the cardiovascular depression that accompanies acute barbiturate poisoning, as does depression of vascular smooth muscle. Both cardiac glycosides and β-adrenergic agonists can overcome the myocardial depressant effect.

Gastrointestinal Tract. The oxybarbiturates tend to decrease the tonus of the gastrointestinal musculature and the amplitude of rhythmic contractions. The locus of action is partly peripheral and partly central, depending on the dose. Hypnotic doses of amobarbital reduce the motility of the sigmoid colon in fasted human subjects; a similar effect occurs during physiological sleep. On emergence from barbiturate-induced sleep, there may be a period of intestinal and colonic hypermotility. A hypnotic dose does not significantly delay gastric emptying in man. Gastric secretions may be somewhat depressed by barbiturates. The relief of various gastrointestinal symptoms by sedative doses is probably largely due to the central-depressant action.

Liver. The best-known effects of barbiturates on the liver are those on the microsomal drug-metabolizing system (*see* Chapter 1), about which there is now an extensive literature.

The barbiturates combine with cytochrome P-450 and thus competitively interfere with the biotransformations of a number of substrates of this enzyme, which include other drugs as well as endogenous substrates, such as steroids. Thus, adverse drug interactions and potential endocrine imbalance can result from such inhibition. The other substrates may reciprocally inhibit barbiturate biotransformations. The nature of the inhibition is not simple, however, because barbiturates do not inhibit the biotransformations of all drugs that are substrates of the microsomal enzyme system. The barbiturates themselves do not necessarily have to be oxidized by the enzyme system in order to inhibit the biotransformations of other drugs. Various barbiturates differ in their affinity for cytochrome P-450. Barbiturates also inhibit NADH–cytochrome c oxidoreductase, but it is not clear to what extent this effect contributes to the overall inhibition of the system.

The barbiturates cause a marked increase in the

enzyme, protein, and lipid content of the hepatic smooth endoplasmic reticulum. Their capacity to induce the synthesis of these components correlates with the plasma half-life of the drug but is unrelated to its metabolism by the enzyme system, since barbital is an effective inducer. Not only is the rate of metabolism of a number of drugs increased but also that of steroid hormones, cholesterol, bile salts, certain other endogenous substrates, and vitamin K and possibly vitamin D. Glucuronyl transferase activity is increased. Not all microsomal biotransformations of drugs and endogenous substrates are affected to the same degree, but a convenient rule of thumb is that, at maximal induction in man, the rates are approximately doubled. The inducing effect is not limited to the microsomal enzymes; for example, there is an increase in δ-aminolevulinic acid (ALA) synthetase, a mitochondrial enzyme, and aldehyde dehydrogenase, a cytoplasmic enzyme, and in the rate of conjugation of sulfobromophthalein with glutathione. The effect of barbiturates on ALA synthetase represents an action on feedback control of porphyrin synthesis, which provides heme for the induced cytochrome P-450. Excessive activation of the enzyme is associated with exacerbation of porphyria (see below). Barbiturates may also increase the rate of synthesis of certain proteins, such as the Y and Z proteins, which are believed to regulate the entry of anionic compounds into hepatic cells.

The induction of the microsomal enzymes can be responsible for a host of adverse drug interactions. The capacity of barbiturates to increase the synthesis of porphyrins may be responsible for one of the more bizarre and dangerous side effects of the drugs. In patients suffering from acute intermittent porphyria, the drugs may precipitate a severe attack, possibly culminating in paralysis and death.

The effect of the barbiturates that are themselves metabolized by hepatic endoplasmic reticulum to increase the rate of their own metabolism accounts for part of the tolerance to the drugs. Many sedative-hypnotics, various anesthetics, and ethanol also are metabolized by and/or induce the microsomal enzymes, and cross-tolerance can occur on this basis. A number of other drugs, chlorinated hydrocarbon insecticides, lipid-rich foods, and certain food additives can also induce the microsomal enzymes, but only under exceptional circumstances have they been shown to increase the rate of elimination of barbiturates significantly in man.

Choleresis results from treatment with phenobarbital but not other barbiturates. Both bile salt–dependent flow and bile salt–independent flow are increased by barbiturates in persons with cholestasis (see Sharp and Mirkin, 1972; Stiehl et al., 1973). Biliary excretion of phospholipids, sulfobromophthalein, indocyanine green, rose bengal, and various drugs is also increased. The increase in bile salt secretion probably affects the absorption of various drugs and foodstuffs. Nevertheless, during chronic administration of phenobarbital, the biliary fluxes of phospholipids, bile acids, and cholesterol were found to be unaltered in normal subjects (Ginsberg and Garnick, 1977). Phenobarbital decreases the hepatic uptake of choline. In man, barbiturates induce a *deficiency* of steroid Δ^4-5α-reductase (Kappas *et al.,* 1977).

Genitourinary Tract. In hypnotic doses, barbiturates do not significantly impair uterine activity during labor. Full anesthetic doses decrease the force and frequency of uterine contractions. More important in the use of barbiturates during labor is their respiratory depressant effect on the infant, since the placenta offers no significant barrier to their passage. Hypnotic doses do not affect the urinary bladder or ureter, but anesthetic doses may cause some depression of contraction.

Kidney. In the concentrations required to produce deep anesthesia, the barbiturates exert direct effects on renal tubular transport mechanisms. The maximal rate of secretion of *p*-aminohippurate may be depressed by as much as 15 to 25%. Pentobarbital also appears to depress the reabsorptive processes for sodium and glucose by a direct action on tubular cells. However, the direct effects may be overshadowed, at least in part, by the reflex vasoconstriction and decreased renal plasma flow consequent to systemic hypotension, and also by stimulation of the secretion of antidiuretic hormone (ADH). The net effect is a decrease in urine flow. The effect on electrolyte excretion varies, depending on the previous condition of the subject. The administration of a hypnotic dose of secobarbital to subjects undergoing maximal water diuresis is usually followed by a slight reduction in urine flow; this is attributable to a hemodynamic action rather than to the release of ADH, since there is no corresponding increase in the osmolarity of the urine. Severe oliguria or anuria may occur in acute barbiturate poisoning, largely as a result of the marked hypotension.

Pharmacokinetics. *Absorption and Routes of Administration.* For hypnotic use, the barbiturates are usually administered orally. The intravenous route is usually employed for the management of convulsive emergencies or for general anesthesia; the rectal route is used occasionally in infants. Intramuscular injection is avoided, because the alkalinity of soluble preparations causes pain and necrosis at the site of injection.

By the oral route, the rate-limiting step in absorption from the empty stomach is that of dissolution and dispersal of the drug in the gastrointestinal contents. Absorption takes place mainly from the intestine, despite the favorable pH partition in the stomach. The sodium salts are more rapidly absorbed than are the free acids because of rapid dissolution. Absorption is faster when barbiturates are well diluted than when taken without water because the drug is dispersed over a large surface area and remains in solution. Food in the stomach decreases the rate of absorption but not the bioavailability.

Distribution. Barbiturates are bound to plasma albumin to various extents. Lipid solubility is the primary determinant of binding; thus, approximately 80% of thiopental but only 5% of barbital is bound. Weak acids, such as aspirin and warfarin, can displace barbiturates from albumin. The concentration of drug in cerebrospinal fluid equals that of unbound barbiturate in plasma. Barbiturates partition into fat in proportion to their lipid solubility.

Highly lipid-soluble barbiturates, such as thiopental, methohexital, thiamylal, thiohexital, and hexobarbital, undergo a rapid, flow-limited uptake into the most vascular areas of the brain, going first into the gray matter. Maximal uptake occurs within 30 seconds, and sleep may be induced within a few circulation times. Within 30 minutes there is then a redistribution into the less vascular areas of the brain and to other tissues; as little as 10% of the peak amount remains in the gray matter. The ultrashort duration of action is the result of this rapid distribution phase. For such drugs, there is no correlation between duration of action and elimination half-life. The highly vascular kidney, liver, and heart equilibrate almost as fast as does the brain, so that maximal tissue concentrations of thiopental, for example, occur within 1 minute to a few minutes after intravenous administration. Fifteen to 30 minutes is required for equilibration of resting muscle and skin, and more than an hour in the poorly vascular fat. The less lipid-soluble oxybarbiturates equilibrate much more slowly, since uptake is more limited by permeability and less by flow. Cerebral uptake is slower, and as long as 20 minutes may be required for sleep to occur after intravenous administration of barbital or phenobarbital. Barbiturates also distribute to fetal blood, and concentrations approach those in maternal plasma. When a steady state is reached, the highest concentrations of drug in nonadipose tissue occur in the liver and kidney; the concentrations are greater in fat.

Elimination. All barbiturates are filtered by the renal glomerulus in proportion to the concentration of the unbound drug in plasma. Barbiturates with a high lipid:water partition coefficient not only are largely bound and consequently poorly filtered but are also readily reabsorbed from the lumen of the tubule. The burden of elimination is thus put on the drug-metabolizing systems. While a few barbiturates with low lipid:water partition coefficients (*e.g.,* barbital, aprobarbital, and phenobarbital) are largely excreted unchanged in the urine, this occurs slowly. Only 20% of an oral hypnotic dose of barbital is eliminated in the urine of normal adults in the first 24 hours. Traces of barbital may be detected in the urine as long as 8 to 12 days after administration. Phenobarbital and aprobarbital are also eliminated slowly, over a period of several days. Renal excretion can be significantly increased by osmotic diuresis. Alkalinization of the urine also hastens excretion because of the shift toward increased ionization of a weak organic acid.

When renal function is impaired, barbiturates that depend upon the kidney for elimination may cause severe CNS and cardiovascular depression and thereby may further diminish renal function.

Small amounts of barbiturates are secreted into milk after a single dose, but the concentration in milk may approach that in plasma during repetitive administration of long-acting barbiturates. Barbiturates are also secreted into saliva, which may be used to monitor the concentration in plasma; for phenobarbital and amobarbital the plasma concentration is approximately three times that of saliva.

The oxybarbiturates are metabolized only in the liver; thiobarbiturates are also biotransformed to a small extent in kidney, brain, and perhaps other tissues. The products are usually inactive, but demethylation of N-methyl congeners yields active products; thus, mephobarbital and methabarbital give rise to phenobarbital and barbital, respectively. The metabolites are invariably more polar than the parent compounds and hence are excreted more rapidly.

Barbiturates are transformed by oxidation of radicals at C5 to alcohols, ketones, phenols, or carboxylic acids, which may appear in the urine as such or as glucuronic acid conjugates. Other biotransformations include N-hydroxylation (*see* Tang *et al.,* 1977), N-dealkylation of N-alkylbarbiturates to active metabolites, desulfuration of thiobarbiturates to oxybarbiturates, and opening of the barbituric acid ring. Side chain oxidation is the most important biotransformation responsible for the termination of biological activity. The biotransformations of the barbiturates have been reviewed by Freudenthal and Carroll (1973).

At one time, barbiturates were classified as long-, intermediate-, short-, and ultrashort-acting drugs. The discovery that the elimination half-lives did not conform to the apparent duration of action has led to the virtual abandonment of this classification. However, a more serviceable classification has not been forthcoming, and it is still useful to distinguish among barbiturates in terms of the duration of their major effects. However, it is important to know that absorption and redistribution are critical determinants of the time of onset and duration of anesthetic and hypnotic effects of ultrashort- and short-acting barbiturates; the rate of elimination determines the time course of residual effects and accumulation of the drug during repetitive use.

The data on half-lives in Table 17–2 show that, among the barbiturates used for hypnosis in the United States, only hexobarbital appears to have an elimination half-life that is sufficiently short for virtually complete elimination to occur in 24 hours. *All other barbiturates will accumulate during repetitive administration unless appropriate adjustments in dosage are made. Furthermore, the persistence of the drug in plasma during the day favors the development of tolerance and abuse.* There is, however, a defect in the application of all present pharmacokinetic data to the clinical situation, in that the half-lives are based on assays that determine both the $R(+)$ and $S(-)$ enantiomers, yet the enantiomers have different half-lives as well as effects.

Half-lives are affected by various factors. With drugs that are metabolized, repetitive use shortens the half-life; for example, that of butabarbital is shortened by 20 to 25% during chronic administration of a single dose per day. Metabolic elimination is more rapid among young people than in the elderly and infants; in children, the half-life of phenobarbital is about half but in infants is two to five times that of the adult. Half-lives are increased during pregnancy, partly because of increased binding to plasma protein.

The effect of hepatic disease on the half-life is variable. Changes in intrinsic hepatic clearance, blood flow, and plasma protein binding are important factors. Chronic liver disease increases the half-life of biotransformable barbiturates in some but not all patients (*see* Breimer, 1977). Cirrhosis increases both the half-life of certain barbiturates and the sensitivity of the patient to the CNS-depressant effects of the drugs. Because many alternative drugs are available, there seems to be little reason to use barbiturates in a patient with cirrhosis. If they must be employed, small doses should be tested. Barbiturates or other hypnotics should not be administered to patients showing premonitory signs of hepatic coma. The pharmacokinetics of barbiturates and the effects of hepatic and renal diseases have been reviewed by Breimer (1977).

Untoward Effects. *Aftereffects.* Drowsiness may last for only a few hours after a hypnotic dose of barbiturate, but residual depression of the CNS (hangover) is sometimes frankly evident the following day. Even in the absence of overt evidence of residual depression, subtle distortions of mood and impairment of judgment and fine motor skills may be demonstrable. For example, a 200-mg dose of secobarbital has been shown to impair performance of driving or flying skills for 10 to 22 hours. However, impairment by recommended hypnotic doses may not be as prevalent as commonly thought. When 100 mg of secobarbital is given, negative residual effects on performance were observed in only 3 of 16 tests; aftereffects were more common with 200-mg doses (Bixler *et al.,* 1975). Findings with butabarbital and secobarbital were similar. Nevertheless, users should be emphatically warned about piloting aircraft, driving automobiles, and operating dangerous machinery and also about potential deterioration of intellectual performance during the day following hypnotic use. Residual effects may also take the form of vertigo, nausea, vomiting, or diarrhea, especially in neurotic persons.

The aftereffects of barbiturates may sometimes be manifested as overt excitement. The user may awaken slightly intoxicated and feel euphoric and energetic; later, as the demands of his daytime activities challenge his possibly impaired faculties, he may display irritability and temper. It is not certain whether excitatory aftereffects are caused by persistence of the excitatory R(+) enantiomer or to withdrawal symptoms resulting from acute tolerance. Aftereffects such as nightmares and night terrors may be caused by deprivation of REM and/or stage-4 sleep, especially after several nights of use.

Paradoxical Excitement. In some persons, barbiturates repeatedly produce excitement rather than depression, and the patient may appear to be inebriated. This type of idiosyncracy is relatively common among geriatric and debilitated patients and occurs most frequently with phenobarbital and N-methylbarbiturates.

Pain. Rarely, the use of barbiturates results in localized or diffuse myalgic, neuralgic, or arthritic pain, especially in psychoneurotic patients with insomnia. The pain may occur in paroxysms, is most intense in the early morning hours, and is most frequently located in the neck, shoulder girdle, and upper limbs. Symptoms may last for days after the drug is discontinued. Like other nonanalgesic hypnotic drugs, barbiturates may cause restlessness, excitement, and even delirium when given in the presence of pain.

Hypersensitivity. Allergic reactions occur especially in persons who tend to have asthma, urticaria, angioedema, and similar conditions. Hypersensitivity reactions in this category include localized swellings, particularly of the eyelids, cheeks, or lips and erythematous dermatitis. Rarely, exfoliative dermatitis may be caused by phenobarbital and can prove fatal; the skin eruption may be associated with fever, delirium, and marked degenerative changes in the liver and other parenchymatous organs.

Drug Interactions. Barbiturates combine with other CNS depressants to cause severe depression; ethanol is the most frequent offender, and interactions with antihistamines are also common. Isoniazid, methylphenidate, and monoamine oxidase inhibitors also increase the CNS-depressant effects.

The greatest number of drug interactions results from induction of hepatic microsomal enzymes. There is significant acceleration of the disappearance of corticosteroids, oral anticoagulants, digitoxin, doxycycline, oral contraceptives, phenytoin, sulfadimethoxine, testosterone, tricyclic antidepressants, and zoxazolamine. In experimental animals, the metabolism of vitamins D and K are accelerated, and deficiencies in the coagulation factors II and VIII have also been shown. This finding may be pertinent to reported instances of coagulation defects in neonates whose mothers were taking phenobarbital. Elderly patients may have low concentrations of calcium in plasma as the probable result of accelerated elimination of vitamin D (Young *et al.,* 1977); barbiturates increase the incidence of fractures, probably in part because of an increased number of falls. Hepatic enzyme induction lowers endogenous steroid hormone concentrations, which may cause endocrine disturbances. Barbiturates also induce the hepatic generation of toxic metabolites of chlorocarbon anesthetics and carbon tetrachloride and consequently promote lipid peroxidation, which facilitates the periportal necrosis of the liver caused by these agents.

Barbiturates competitively inhibit the metabolism of certain other drugs. The most important interaction of this type is with tricyclic antidepressants.

Although barbiturates compete with other weak acids for binding to plasma albumin, the only clinically important displacement is that of thyroxine. The absorptions of dicumarol and griseofulvin are decreased by barbiturates, especially phenobarbital.

Other Untoward Effects. Because barbiturates enhance porphyrin synthesis, they are absolutely contraindicated in patients with acute intermittent porphyria or porphyria variegata. In hypnotic doses, the effects of barbiturates on the control of respiration are minor; however, in the presence of pulmonary insufficiency, serious respiratory depression may occur and the drugs are thus contraindicated. Rapid intravenous injection of a barbiturate may cause cardiovascular collapse before anesthesia ensues, so that the CNS signs of depth of anesthesia may fail to give an adequate warning of impending toxicity. Blood pressure can fall to shock levels; even slow intravenous injection of barbiturates often produces apnea and occasionally laryngospasm, coughing, and other respiratory difficulties.

BARBITURATE POISONING

In part because of the ready availability and pro-miscuous use of barbiturates, poisoning with these drugs is a major clinical problem; death occurs in 0.5 to 12% of cases. Most of the cases are the result of deliberate attempts at suicide, but some are from accidental poisonings in children or in drug abusers. A widely held concept is that poisoning often is the result of "drug automatism." This behavior relates to the patient who fails to fall asleep after the first or second dose of a hypnotic, becomes confused, and unwittingly ingests an overdose; on recovery, there is no memory of having taken the additional doses. The extent of poisoning from confusion during self-administration is controversial. Aitken and Proud-foot (1969) could attribute no more than 2 cases out of 994 to automatism; they believe the failure to recall suicidal intent is the result of psychogenic defense mechanisms, a conclusion also reached by Dorpat (1974). Nevertheless, Jansson (1961), after investigating 488 cases of intoxication, estimated that approximately one fourth of the cases were classi-fiable as "drug automatism"; a higher percentage of these individuals had cerebral lesions than did the patients with suicidal intent, and they were thus probably more disposed to confusional states during mild intoxication.

The *lethal dose* of barbiturate varies with many factors and cannot be stated with certainty. Severe poisoning is likely to occur when more than ten times the full hypnotic dose has been ingested at once. The barbiturates with short half-lives and high lipid sol-ubility are more potent and more toxic than the more polar, long-acting compounds, such as phenobarbi-tal and barbital. The potentially fatal dose of pheno-barbital is 6 to 10 g, whereas that of amobarbital, secobarbital, or pentobarbital is 2 to 3 g. The lowest concentration of drug in plasma associated with lethal overdosage has been 6 mg/dl for phenobarbi-tal and barbital but only 1 mg/dl for shorter-acting agents such as amobarbital and pentobarbital; if alcohol or other depressant drugs are also present, the concentrations that can cause death are lower. The finding of a high concentration in blood of necropsy does not in itself constitute *prima-facie* evidence of death from barbiturate poisoning. Pa-tients with much higher blood concentrations than those mentioned above have recovered satisfactorily. Bailey and Jatlow (1975) reported a case in which the plasma concentration of barbital was 120 mg/dl—the highest ever recorded; the patient recovered without hemodialysis. The highest blood concentration of phenobarbital from which a patient has recovered is 29 mg/dl. Patients who ingest fatal amounts of the long-acting agents more frequently die in the hospital, whereas those who are poisoned by barbiturates with shorter half-lives are more fre-quently found dead. This would suggest that poison-ing with the short-acting agents is somewhat more dangerous, since the measures that are available for the treatment of acute barbiturate intoxication are most effective if they are instituted before serious depression of the respiratory and cardiovascular systems has developed.

Individuals who are disposed toward self-destruction are likely to have a bountiful supply of CNS depressants on hand, and a barbiturate may not be the only intoxicant. Ingestion of these drugs may follow the consumption of large quantities of alcohol. Physical examination alone is rarely suffi-cient to differentiate poisoning by the various agents and, particularly, by mixtures of CNS depressants. Ultimately, the diagnosis depends on the chemical identification of the compounds in body fluids.

The *signs and symptoms* of barbiturate poisoning are referable especially to the CNS and the cardio-vascular system. Moderate intoxication resembles alcoholic inebriation. In severe intoxication, the pa-tient is comatose, and the level of reflex activity conforms in a general way to the intensity of the central depression. The deep reflexes may persist for some time despite coexistent coma. The Babinski sign is often positive. The EEG may be of the burst-suppression type with brief periods of electrical si-lence. The pupils may be constricted and react to light, but late in the course of barbiturate poisoning hypoxic paralytic dilatation may appear. Respiration is affected early. Breathing may be either slow, or rapid and shallow; Cheyne-Stokes rhythm may be present. Superficial observation of respiration may be misleading with regard to actual minute volume and to the degree of respiratory acidosis and cerebral hypoxia; arterial P_{CO_2} and P_{O_2} must be determined. Eventually, blood pressure falls due to the direct effect of the drug and of hypoxia on medullary vasomotor centers with consequent arteriolar and venous dilatation; depression of cardiac contractility, sympathetic ganglia, and vascular smooth muscle also contribute. The patient thus develops shock, with a weak and rapid pulse, cold and sweaty skin, a rise in the hematocrit, and renal ischemia. Hypo-thermia, sometimes with temperatures as low as 32° C, often occurs. Pulmonary complications (atelectasis, edema, and bronchopneumonia) and renal failure are likely to be the fatal complications of severe barbiturate poisoning.

Not uncommonly, patients suffering from acute barbiturate intoxication develop necrosis of sweat glands and bullous cutaneous lesions, which are not due to hypersensitivity or hypothermia. These lesions heal slowly, sometimes requiring many weeks.

The optimal *treatment* of acute barbiturate intoxi-cation is based upon general supportive measures and, often, the use of dialysis or hemoperfusion. A highly organized intensive care unit, prepared for around-the-clock effort with continuous monitoring of the patient, can reduce the mortality rate to less than 2%. Formerly, when CNS stimulants were used in attempts to antagonize barbiturates, mortality rates were as high as 40%. The present treatment is applicable in most respects for poisoning by any CNS depressant.

The depth of coma and adequacy of ventilation are first evaluated. If fewer than 24 hours have elapsed since ingestion, gastric lavage should be considered, even though little barbiturate is usually recovered from the stomach after 4 hours. Lavage or emesis should be attempted only after precautions have been taken to avoid aspiration. Apomorphine-induced emesis evacuates the stomach more rapidly and reliably than does ipecac. Adsorption of barbiturate in the stomach with activated charcoal has been widely used. However, its effectiveness with acidic drugs has been questioned and its inherent toxicity may be significant. After lavage, a saline cathartic should be administered and repeated every 1 to 2 hours as long as bowel sounds are present.

Close and constant attention must be given to the maintenance of a patent airway and to the prevention of hypostatic pneumonia. Oxygen should be administered by a nasal catheter or by a catheter through the pharyngeal airway. Measures to prevent or treat atelectasis should be taken. Blood P_{CO_2} and pH should be monitored, and mechanical ventilation should be initiated when indicated. Fever or roentgenographic evidence of pneumonia calls for appropriate therapy.

Measures should be taken to prevent further loss of body heat, but it is not universally agreed that it is necessary to restore the body temperature to normal.

In severe acute barbiturate intoxication, circulatory collapse is a major threat. Often the patient is admitted to the hospital with severe hypotension or shock. The hypovolemic, vascular, and cardiodepressant factors are evaluated. Dehydration is often severe. Hypovolemia must be corrected, and, if necessary, the blood pressure can be supported with dopamine. Some authorities advocate the use of digitalis if central venous pressure is elevated subsequent to the use of intravenous fluids and there is no diuresis.

Renal failure consequent to shock and hypoxia accounts for perhaps one sixth of the deaths. Such failure also contributes to delayed elimination of long-acting barbiturates. Therefore, parameters of renal function and changes in the concentration of drug in plasma are assessed frequently. Anuria and uremia may ensue, even after the patient has recovered consciousness.

Should renal failure occur, the most effective method of disposing of the poison is hemodialysis or hemoperfusion. Elimination of the drug is achieved very much faster by these procedures than by endogenous mechanisms. Hemodialysis is more effective in removing long-acting than short-acting compounds because there is less protein binding of the former. More effective extraction of the lipid-soluble, short-acting barbiturates can be achieved by the use of a lipid-containing dialysate or by hemoperfusion through activated charcoal or ion-exchange resins. Perfusion through the lipid-adsorptive resin, AMBERLITE XAD-4, has been reported to clear the blood in 2.5 to 10 hours (Rosenbaum et al., 1976). Peritoneal dialysis is only 25% as rapid as hemodialysis in removing barbiturates from the body. If renal and cardiac function are satisfactory and the patient is hydrated, forced diuresis and alkalinization of the urine will significantly hasten the excretion of some but not all barbiturates. The likelihood of success is increased if the drug is only partly bound to plasma protein, has a relatively low pK_a, and is relatively slowly reabsorbed. These are characteristics of the long-acting barbiturates. It is desirable to achieve a diuresis of 8 to 14 liters per day. Because of elevated ADH levels, hypotonic solutions are usually less effective than osmotic or high-ceiling diuretics. When diuresis of this magnitude is achieved, it is absolutely necessary to maintain water and electrolyte balance. Even though forced diuresis and alkalinization can increase the renal clearance of pentobarbital by as much as 15 times, the total rate of detoxication is increased by only 15 to 25%, since little of this drug is usually excreted in the urine. In contrast, the rates of detoxication of barbital, phenobarbital, apobarbital, and allobarbital—barbiturates for which renal excretion is a significant fraction of total elimination—are increased 30 to 180%; this can shorten the duration of coma substantially.

Various aspects of acute intoxication with barbiturates and its management are discussed in reviews by Mann and Sandberg (1970), Matthew, (1971), Robinson and coworkers (1971), and Spear and Protass (1973).

THERAPEUTIC USES

The use of barbiturates as sedative-hypnotic drugs is justifiably on the decline because they lack specificity of effect in the CNS, they have a lower therapeutic index than do the benzodiazepines, tolerance occurs more frequently than with benzodiazepines, the liability for abuse is greater, and there is a considerable number of drug interactions.

CNS Uses. The use of barbiturates as hypnotics is included in the general discussion on page 369. Barbiturates may be used in large doses in the management of acute maniacal states, delirium, and certain psychoneurotic disorders, although they are being superseded by newer agents.

The era when barbiturates (particularly phenobarbital) were virtually the only drugs recommended for daytime sedation has long passed, and they have largely been replaced by benzodiazepines and other compounds. However, they are still available as "sedatives" in a host of inefficacious combinations for the treatment of functional gastrointestinal disorders, hypertension, asthma, and coronary artery disease. They are also included in analgesic combinations, possibly counterproductively. Although they may effectively decrease hyperactivity in hyperthyroidism, benzodiazepines are preferred. The barbiturates still have valid uses as sedatives to decrease restlessness during illnesses in children such as colic, whooping cough, pylorospasm, and nausea and vomiting of functional origin, to suppress excitement of various abnormal origins, and to decrease apprehension preparatory to minor medical and dental procedures.

Barbiturates are sometimes used to antagonize unwanted CNS-stimulant effects of various drugs, such as ephedrine, dextroamphetamine, and theophylline; butabarbital and phenobarbital are most commonly used for such purposes. In these uses, they are probably superior to benzodiazepines.

Barbiturates are still used for their rapid onset of action in the *emergency treatment* of *convulsions,* such as occur in tetanus, eclampsia, status epilepticus, cerebral hemorrhage, and poisoning by convulsant drugs; however, benzodiazepines are generally superior in these uses. Some representative dose ranges for intravenous administration are as follows: phenobarbital sodium, 0.15 to 0.3 g; pentobarbital sodium, 0.3 to 0.5 g; amobarbital sodium, 0.4 to 0.8 g; thiopental sodium, 0.1 to 0.2 g. The injection should be made slowly, with the usual precautions necessary for intravenous administration. Phenobarbital sodium is frequently used because of its anticonvulsant efficacy; however, even when administered intravenously, 15 minutes or more may be required for it to attain peak concentrations in the brain. Thus, the practice of continuing to administer phenobarbital until convulsions stop results in brain concentrations that continue to rise and may eventually exceed that required to control the seizures. The subsequent barbiturate-induced depression may summate with postictal depression. Administration of phenobarbital requires restraint and patience until the anticonvulsant effect develops before deciding whether a second dose is necessary. While the rapidity of onset of the ultrashort- and short-acting barbiturates would seem to have appeal, these drugs have a low ratio of anticonvulsant to hypnotic action. Diazepam offers many advantages for the emergency treatment of certain convulsive disorders, particularly for *status epilepticus*. The use of phenobarbital, mephobarbital, and methabarbital in the symptomatic therapy of epilepsy is also discussed in Chapter 20.

The barbiturates are being replaced by benzodiazepines for preanesthetic medication and basal anesthesia. The ultrashort-acting agents continue to be employed as intravenous anesthetics (Chapter 14). Short- and ultrashort-acting barbiturates are occasionally used as adjuncts to other agents in the production of obstetrical anesthesia. Although several studies have failed to affirm gross depression of respiration in the neonate at birth, evaluation of the effects on the fetus and neonate is difficult; it is prudent to avoid the use of barbiturates in obstetrics.

The barbiturates are employed as diagnostic and therapeutic aids in psychiatry, in *narcoanalysis* and *narcotherapy*. They are used to activate latent abnormalities in the EEG. In low concentrations, amobarbital has been administered directly into the carotid artery as a means of identifying the dominant cerebral hemisphere for speech prior to neurosurgery.

Anesthetic doses of barbiturates attenuate cerebral edema resulting from surgery, head injury, or cerebral ischemia, and they decrease infarct size and increase survival (*see* Smith, 1977). The death rate from head injuries among juveniles and adults has been reported to be reduced by 80% and 50%, respectively. General anesthetics do not provide protection; CNS depression alone cannot, therefore, explain the protective effect.

Hepatic Metabolic Uses. Because hepatic glucuronyl transferase and the bilirubin-binding Y protein are increased by the barbiturates, phenobarbital has been successfully used to treat *hyperbilirubinemia* and *kernicterus* in the neonate (*see* Stern *et al.,* 1970); complete failure of this treatment can probably be attributed to premature discontinuation of the drug. The nondepressant barbiturate phetharbital (N-phenylbarbital) works equally well. Phenobarbital may improve the hepatic transport of bilirubin in patients with hemolytic jaundice (Perona *et al.,* 1973). The effect of phenobarbital on bile salt metabolism and excretion has been employed in the treatment of selected cases of *cholestasis* (*see* Sharp and Mirkin, 1972; Linarelli *et al.,* 1973; Stiehl *et al.,* 1973). Phenobarbital has not proven to be of value in the dissolution of cholesterol gallstones.

Preparations and Dosage. Barbiturates are marketed in a vast array of preparations. In the United States, phenobarbital is an ingredient in more than 80 proprietary remedies, which are best ignored in favor of nonproprietary preparations. Special slow-release forms are pointless and potentially dangerous in view of the long half-lives of most barbiturates, and they are disadvantageous in hypnotic use.

Oxybarbiturates are poorly soluble in cold water but are soluble in alcohol and hot water. Aqueous solutions are acidic. The sodium salts are freely soluble in water, and their solutions are quite alkaline.

The hypnotic and sedative doses of the barbiturates are listed in Table 17-2.

CHLORAL DERIVATIVES

The pharmacology and uses of the chloral derivatives that are employed clinically are essentially the same, because they are all converted in the body to the same active intermediate. Therefore, what is said below about *chloral hydrate* applies equally well to *chloral betaine* and *triclofos sodium*, unless otherwise indicated.

Chemistry. *Chloral* is 2,2,2-trichloroacetaldehyde, an unstable, disagreeable oil that does not lend itself well to pharmaceutical formulations. Therefore, it was introduced into medicine in the form of its hydrate, formed by adding one molecule of water to the carbonyl group. The formula of chloral hydrate is $CCl_3CH(OH)_2$.

Chloral can form hemiacetals of the general formula $CCl_3CH(OH)(OR)$, of which *chloral alcoholate, chloral betaine, α-chloralose,* and *dichloralphenazone* are examples. They generate chloral hydrate *in vivo*. Their metabolite, *trichloroethanol* (CCl_3CH_2OH), is an excellent hypnotic, but it is not conveniently used as such, owing to its physical and irritant properties; instead, it is used as the monosodium salt of the phosphate ester, *triclofos sodium*, $CCl_3CH_2OPO_3H^- \cdot Na^+$.

Local Actions. Chloral hydrate is quite irritating to the skin and mucous membranes. Gastrointestinal side effects are particularly likely to occur if the drug is insufficiently diluted or if it is taken on an empty stomach. Chloral betaine and triclofos generate some chloral in the stomach and hence cause some gastrointestinal irritation. They lack the disagreeable taste of chloral hydrate.

Systemic Actions. Like the barbiturates, chloral hydrate has little analgesic activity, and excitement or delirium may be initiated by pain. It is effective against experimentally induced convulsions produced by strychnine, pentylenetetrazol, and electroshock and has been used in the treatment of eclampsia and tetanus; however, the ratio of anticonvulsant to sedative effects is low, and diazepam, clonazepam, or barbiturates are preferable in the treatment of acute convulsive disorders. The margin of safety is too narrow to permit the drug to be used as a general anesthetic agent.

During the first week of use of chloral hydrate, there is a decrease in the sleep latency and the number of awakenings, a slight variable decrease in total sleep time, and a slight decrease in slow-wave sleep. In only one of seven studies in which the dose ranged between 0.5 and 1.5 g was REM sleep suppressed (*see* Kay *et al.*, 1976). Similarly, 1 g of triclofos has a negligible effect on sleep stages; however, 500 mg of α-chloralose decreases REM sleep but increases stage-4 or slow-wave sleep. During repetitive nightly use, the effects on sleep supposedly disappear within 2 weeks (Kales *et al.*, 1970a, 1970b); however, Hartmann (1976) has reported that total sleep time and REM latency remain elevated, even though the number of awakenings is increased. After discontinuation of the drug, a significant rebound in REM sleep does not occur (Hartmann and Cravens, 1973).

In therapeutic doses, chloral hydrate has little effect on respiration and blood pressure. Toxic doses produce severe respiratory depression and hypotension. In large doses, chloral hydrate depresses cardiac contractility and shortens the refractory period, as do many hydrocarbon anesthetics. Untoward cardiac effects may occur when toxic doses are administered, especially to patients with heart disease; however, there is no evidence of deleterious effects on the heart from the continued use of the compound in therapeutic doses.

The pharmacological properties of *trichloroethanol* closely resemble those of chloral hydrate. Clinically, trichloroethanol is at least as effective as chloral hydrate, is approximately equipotent to chloral hydrate as a central depressant, and is as effective as a hypnotic. In the body, chloral hydrate is very rapidly reduced to trichloroethanol with a half-time of a few minutes, and significant amounts of chloral hydrate have not been detected in the blood after its oral administration; therefore, it is generally believed that the central depressant effects are caused by trichloroethanol.

Distribution and Fate. Chloral hydrate and trichloroethanol are sufficiently lipid soluble to permeate plasma membranes and enter cells throughout the body. Chloral hydrate has been detected in cerebrospinal fluid, milk, and fetal blood. Dichloralphenazone and the more water-soluble derivatives, chloral betaine and triclofos, are rapidly hydrolyzed to chloral hydrate and trichloroethanol, respectively, after which they are comparably distributed.

Chloral hydrate is reduced to trichloroethanol, apparently largely by alcohol dehydrogenase in the liver. Ethanol accelerates the reduction, because its own oxidation provides NADH to drive the reduction of chloral hydrate. Chloral inhibits alcohol dehydrogenase. A small but variable amount of chloral hydrate and a larger fraction of trichloroethanol are oxidized to trichloroacetic acid, mainly in the smooth endoplasmic reticulum of the liver and kidney. Trichloroethanol is mainly conjugated with glucuronic acid, and the product (urochloralic acid) is excreted mostly into the urine and to a limited extent into the bile. The plasma half-life of trichloroethanol ranges from 4 to 12 hours. The pharmacokinetics of chloral hydrate and trichloroethanol have been reviewed by Breimer (1977).

Untoward Effects. The irritant actions of chloral hydrate give rise to an unpleasant taste, epigastric distress, nausea, occasional vomiting, and flatulence. Gastric necrosis has occurred after intoxicating doses. Undesirable CNS effects include light-headedness, malaise, ataxia, and nightmares. "Hangover" may also occur, although it is less common than with most barbiturates and some benzodiazepines. The tendency of hypnotics to cause persistent effects in the elderly is less pronounced with chloral hydrate than with agents that are metabolized by the hepatic microsomal enzyme system.

Rarely, patients exhibit *idiosyncratic reactions* to chloral hydrate. Occasionally, a patient becomes somnambulistic after receiving the drug, and may be disoriented and incoherent and show paranoid behavior. *Allergic reactions* include erythema, scarlatiniform exanthems, urticaria, and eczematoid dermatitis. The eruption usually begins on the face or back and spreads to the neck, chest, and arms; it may be followed by desquamation or exfoliation. The dermatitis may appear within several hours or as long as 10 days after ingestion of the drug. Eosinophilia and leukopenia may also occur. Chloral hydrate is contraindicated in patients with marked hepatic or renal impairment, and it should perhaps be avoided in patients with severe cardiac disease. Toxic doses may depress myocardial contractility as well as cause ventricular and supraventricular tachyarrhythmias (*see* Gustafson *et al.*, 1977). If gastritis is present, the drug should not be given orally but may be administered in olive oil as a retention enema.

Chloral hydrate appears to both inhibit and enhance the metabolism of some drugs in man. It may respectively potentiate or antagonize oral anticoagulants (*see* Udall, 1975, and Breimer, 1977, for references); the clinical significance is in dispute. Chloral hydrate accelerates the biotransformation of amitriptyline. The final effect on the action of other drugs may be complicated by the fact that trichloroacetic acid formed by the metabolism of chloral hydrate displaces acidic drugs from plasma-protein binding sites, thus temporarily increasing their plasma concentrations in spite of shortening the half-lives. Since many drugs are acidic and are protein bound, there may be a considerable potential for adverse interactions. Malach and Berman (1975) have confirmed that the combination of chloral hydrate and furosemide in some persons may cause vasodilatation and flushing, tachycardia, hypotension or hypertension, and sweating, which they attribute to displacement of thyroxine from binding proteins. At present, chloral derivatives probably should be avoided in patients with intermittent porphyria. An exacerbation by chloral hydrate of the metabolic defect in an infant with a tyrosinemia-like syndrome has been reported (Watts *et al.*, 1975). The subject of microsomal enzyme induction and displacement of protein-bound drugs by chloral derivatives has been reviewed by Greenblatt and Shader (1972).

A study by Sellers and associates (1972) is sometimes cited to dispute the popular belief that chloral hydrate and ethanol in combination (the "Mickey Finn") are not supra-additive. However, the dose of chloral hydrate chosen for the study was only marginally hypnotic, and the dose of alcohol probably did not yield a blood concentration much above 30 mg/dl; a pronounced depressant effect with higher doses cannot be ruled out. Experimental studies in several species have confirmed the existence of an interaction between these drugs. Its basis is presumed to be mutual inhibition of the metabolism of the other agent, in addition to the combined depressant effect of the two drugs.

Acute Intoxication. The toxic oral dose of chloral hydrate for adults is approximately 10 g, although death has been reported from as little as 4 g and individuals have survived after ingesting as much as 30 g. Poisoning by chloral hydrate resembles acute barbiturate intoxication, and the same supportive treatment is indicated. Gastric irritation may result in initial vomiting and even gastric necrosis. Pinpoint pupils may be seen, as in morphine poisoning. If the patient survives, icterus due to hepatic damage and albuminuria from renal irritation may appear. Treatment is the same as that for intoxication with other CNS depressants (*see* Barbiturate Poisoning, page 359); hemodialysis is effective (Stalker *et al.,* 1978).

Abuse and Chronic Intoxication. The habitual use of chloral hydrate may result in the development of tolerance, physical dependence, and addiction. Chloral addicts may take enormous doses of the drug. The chloral habit is similar to alcohol addiction, and sudden withdrawal may result in delirium and seizures with a high frequency of death, when untreated. The chloral habitué may suddenly exhibit what was formerly termed a "break in tolerance," and death may occur, either as a result of an overdose or a failure of the detoxication mechanism due to hepatic damage. In patients suffering from chronic intoxication, gastritis is common and skin eruptions may develop. Parenchymatous renal injury may also occur.

Dosage and Preparations. The dosage and preparations of *chloral hydrate* are listed in Table 17-2. Only brief comment is made here. The often-recommended dose of 0.5 to 1 g has only a slight effect on sleep, at best. Many individuals require as much as 2 g of chloral hydrate. To minimize irritation, solutions of the drug should be taken well diluted with water or milk. It is too irritating to be given parenterally. *Chloral betaine* is more palatable and less irritating than chloral hydrate. A dose of 870 mg is equivalent to 500 mg of chloral hydrate. A dose of *triclofos sodium* of 1.5 g will yield a blood concentration of trichloroethanol approximately equal to that from 900 mg of chloral hydrate.

ETHCHLORVYNOL

Ethchlorvynol is a sedative-hypnotic drug with a rapid onset and short duration of action. It has the following structure:

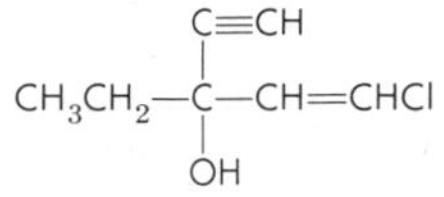

$$CH_3CH_2-\underset{\underset{OH}{|}}{\overset{\overset{C\equiv CH}{|}}{C}}-CH=CHCl$$

Ethchlorvynol

CNS Effects. Ethchlorvynol has anticonvulsant and muscle relaxant properties as well as sedative-hypnotic activity. Although the drug is said to produce less initial excitement than do the barbiturates, valid clinical confirmation is needed. The EEG pattern following ethchlorvynol resembles that seen after barbiturates. Ethchlorvynol administered to two subjects for 2 weeks decreased sleep latency, wake time, REM sleep, and stage-4 time and increased stage-2 and total sleep time (Kripke *et al.,* 1978); after withdrawal, rebound occurred in sleep latency and REM latency, wake time, and time spent in stage 2, but not in REM sleep or stage-4 sleep. If ethchlorvynol is taken along with ethanol, an exaggerated hypnotic effect may occur.

Absorption and Fate. Oral ethchlorvynol acts within 15 to 30 minutes. The maximal concentration in blood is attained in 1 to 1.5 hours. The apparent volume of distribution is about 4 liters per kilogram. The drug passes the placental barrier. Two-compartment kinetics is manifested, with a distribution half-life of about 1 to 3 hours and an elimination half-life of 10 to 25 hours (from data of Cummins *et al.,* 1971). After intoxicating doses, dose-dependent rates of elimination may be seen. Approximately 90% of the drug is destroyed in the liver.

Side Effects, Intoxication, and Abuse. The most common side effects caused by ethchlorvynol are mintlike aftertaste, dizziness, nausea, vomiting, hypotension, and facial numbness. In persons in whom absorption is especially rapid, giddiness and ataxia frequently occur; these effects can be controlled by giving the drug with food. Mild "hangover" is also relatively common. An occasional patient responds with profound hypnosis, muscular weakness, and syncope unrelated to marked hypotension. Positional nystagmus or diplopia may occur, especially after overdoses. Idiosyncratic responses range from mild stimulation to marked excitement and hysteria. Ethchlorvynol should not be used with antidepressants, because delirium may result. Hypersensitivity reactions include urticaria, rare but sometimes fatal thrombocytopenia, and occasionally cholestatic jaundice. Because of a reported effect to suppress the anticipated response to dicumarol, the drug should be used cautiously in combination with drugs metabolized by the liver, and it is contraindicated in intermittent porphyria. Pulmonary edema may follow intravenous injection (*see* Glauser *et al.,* 1976) and may even occur after large oral doses.

The therapeutic index of ethchlorvynol is probably about the same as that of barbiturates with an intermediate duration of action. Acute intoxication is characterized by prolonged deep coma, severe respiratory depression, hypotension, bradycardia, and hypothermia. Death has occurred with a blood concentration of 14 mg/dl. The lethal dose usually ranges from 10 to 25 g, but death has followed a dose of 2.5 g (ethanol was also present), and one patient survived 50 g (with intensive care) after a coma lasting 7 days. Treatment is similar to that for acute barbiturate intoxication. Substantial amounts of ethchlorvynol have been recovered from the stomach by lavage as late as 5 hours after ingestion. Hemodialysis clears the blood at least three times faster than does forced diuresis or peritoneal dialysis, but is still inadequate; dialysis against oil is more effective (Welch *et al.*, 1972).

Chronic abuse of ethchlorvynol results in tolerance and physical dependence. Abusers may take up to 4 g of drug per day. Usually they show signs of intoxication, such as incoordination, tremors, ataxia, slurred speech, confusion, asthenia, hyperreflexia, nystagmus, diplopia, and sometimes toxic amblyopia, dichromatism, scotoma, and reversible peripheral or optic neuritis. Withdrawal symptoms may resemble delirium tremens and are sometimes suggestive of a schizophrenic reaction. They are especially severe in elderly patients.

Preparations and Dosage. These are listed in Table 17–2. A dose of 770 mg of ethchlorvynol is approximately equivalent to 100 mg of secobarbital.

GLUTETHIMIDE

Glutethimide is 3-ethyl-3-phenyl-2,6-piperidine-dione and is similar to methyprylon (*see* below). Their structures are as follows:

Glutethimide   Methyprylon

Glutethimide has little to recommend its continued use as a sedative-hypnotic drug. Its addiction liability and the severity of withdrawal symptoms are equal to those of the barbiturates, and certain features of acute intoxication make its treatment more difficult.

Pharmacological Actions. The pharmacology of glutethimide is like that of barbiturates in that it can induce hypnosis without selective analgesic, antitussive, or anticonvulsant actions. It is also similar in its effects on the EEG pattern and in its suppression of REM sleep. Glutethimide differs from barbiturates, however, in that doses that affect REM sleep do not alter the number of awakenings per night or the total sleep time (Kales *et al.*, 1970a, 1970c). It also differs

in that a dose of 125 mg confers protection against motion sickness for 3 or 4 hours. The drug exhibits pronounced anticholinergic activity, which is most prominent in the iris but which also is manifested by inhibition of salivary secretion and intestinal motility.

Absorption and Fate. Glutethimide is quite erratically absorbed from the gastrointestinal tract. The drug has a high lipid:water partition coefficient, so that following intravenous injection it quickly penetrates the brain and then redistributes in the same manner as does thiopental. It passes the placental barrier and is probably also excreted into milk. About 50% of the drug is bound to plasma proteins. Less than 2% of a usual dose is excreted into the urine unchanged, and most of the drug is metabolized in the liver; its half-life ranges from 5 to 22 hours. Glutethimide is a racemate; the *d* isomer is converted to 4-hydroxy-2-ethyl-2-phenylglutarimide, and the *l* isomer to 2-(*l*-hydroxyethyl)-2-phenylglutarimide. The 4-hydroxy metabolite is active in animals but does not contribute to the effects of single therapeutic doses in man (Crow *et al.*, 1977); it may contribute to intoxication (Hansen *et al.*, 1975). Both hydroxylated metabolites are converted to glucuronides, which enter the enterohepatic circulation; their excretion into the urine is quite slow. Approximately 2% of the *d* isomer is converted to the active metabolite, α-phenyl-α-ethyl glutaconimide. Recently identified metabolites include 4-hydroxyphenyl, 3-methoxy-4-hydroxyphenyl, and other phenyl oxidation products, as well as α-phenyl-γ-butyrolactone. The biological disposition of glutethimide has been discussed by Curry and coworkers (1971).

Glutethimide stimulates the hepatic microsomal enzyme system. The half-life of vitamin D$_3$ may be decreased by about 50%, and the rate of excretion of 6β-hydroxycortisol is increased by about eightfold. The effects of warfarin may be diminished (Udall, 1975). However, glutethimide inhibits the conversion of corticosterone to 18-hydroxycorticosterone. It decreases bilirubin turnover but increases its clearance (Blaschke *et al.*, 1974). In animals, glutethimide increases δ-ALA synthetase activity and the metabolism of barbiturates and other drugs, and it probably also does so in man. Glutethimide is contraindicated for patients with intermittent porphyria.

Adverse Effects. With therapeutic doses, toxic side effects are rare and consist in "hangover," excitement, blurring of vision, gastric irritation, headache, and, infrequently, skin rashes, including exfoliative dermatitis. Thrombocytopenia, aplastic anemia, and leukopenia may also occur.

Acute Intoxication. Intoxication may be caused by overdoses of glutethimide or by a combination of glutethimide and other CNS depressants. The symptoms of acute intoxication are similar to those of barbiturate poisoning. Respiratory depression is usually less severe than with barbiturate intoxication, but circulatory failure is at least equally severe. The antimuscarinic actions cause xerostomia, ileus, atony of the urinary bladder, and long-lasting mydriasis and hyperpyrexia, which may persist for hours after the patient regains consciousness. In some cases of glutethimide poisoning, occasional bouts of tonic muscular spasms, twitching, and even convulsions occur. Patients also tend to show cyclic variations in the level of intoxication (see Myers and Stockard, 1975). A dose of 5 g is sufficient to produce severe intoxication. The lethal dose is between 10 and 20 g; plasma concentrations associated with lethality range from 2 to 80 μg/ml. In acute intoxication, the plasma half-life may exceed 100 hours but averages about 40 hours; hemodialysis shortens the half-life to about 14 hours. The fall in the plasma concentration of the drug may be followed by increased absorption from the intestinal tract, resulting in a rapid, secondary rise in the blood concentration following the initial dialysis. When hydrogel-coated charcoal is used, elimination is greatly accelerated (see Vale et al., 1975).

Chronic Use and Abuse. Excessive use of glutethimide leads to tolerance and psychic and physical dependence. The abstinence syndrome includes tremulousness, nausea, tachycardia, fever, tonic muscle spasms, and generalized convulsions. The same symptoms occasionally occur in patients who have been taking glutethimide regularly in moderate doses (0.5 to 3 g daily) even when there is no evidence of abstention, and also in patients being treated for acute intoxication who have no previous history of drug abuse. In the latter case, tonic muscular spasms and, infrequently, generalized convulsions are seen. Catatonia and dyskinesias may be observed after abusers are withdrawn from a combination of glutethimide and an antihistamine (Good, 1976). Chronic use may cause osteomalacia.

Preparations and Dosage. These are listed in Table 17–2. The hypnotic dose may be repeated, if necessary, but not less than 4 hours before arising. Considering the lack of any specific utility of glutethimide and the complications of treatment of its acute or chronic abuse, it is difficult to justify the continued use of this agent.

METHYPRYLON

Methyprylon is 3,3-diethyl-5-methyl-2,4-piperidinedione. Its structure is shown with that of glutethimide on page 364.

Much still remains to be learned about the pharmacology and toxicology of methyprylon. In a dose of 300 mg, its hypnotic effect is indistinguishable from that of 200 mg of secobarbital, but it is not as effective as the benzodiazpine triazolam. This dose also suppresses REM sleep as much as does 100 mg of pentobarbital.

Approximately 97% of methyprylon appears to be metabolized. The metabolites are partly conjugated to glucuronides. Only 60% of the free metabolites and glucuronides is recoverable from urine. The plasma half-life is 4 hours, but it is longer in acute intoxication (see Pancorbo et al., 1977). Methyprylon stimulates the hepatic microsomal enzyme system and δ-ALA synthetase; it should probably be avoided in patients with intermittent porphyria.

Untoward effects of methyprylon are not frequent, but include "hangover," nausea, vomiting, epigastric distress, diarrhea, esophagitis, headache, and rash. Neutropenia and thrombocytopenia of unproven origin have been reported in persons taking methyprylon. An idiosyncratic excitement occasionally occurs.

Acute intoxication resembles that caused by barbiturates, and the general principles of management are the same. Hypotension, shock, and pulmonary edema are more conspicuous features than is respiratory depression. Hemodialysis is an effective component of treatment. Peritoneal dialysis may also be effective; at pH 7.4, methyprylon is quite water soluble, which facilitates dialysis. The lethal dose is unknown; death has occurred after ingestion of 6 g, but recovery has occurred after 27 g. Coma may last for up to 5 days.

Habituation, tolerance, physical dependence, and addiction can occur. The abstinence syndrome is like that of the barbiturates and includes insomnia, confusion, hallucinations, and convulsions.

The dosage and preparations are shown in Table 17–2.

MEPROBAMATE

Meprobamate is a *bis*-carbamate ester with the following structural formula:

Meprobamate

Although it was synthesized as a potential muscle relaxant, its psychopharmacological properties became of greater interest, and it was introduced for use as an antianxiety agent in 1955. There was a phenomenal and immediate acceptance of meprobamate, and there developed both a medical and popular craze for the drug. Despite the emergence of the benzodiazcpines, meprobamate is still widely used.

Neuropharmacological Properties. In the usual clinical doses in man, meprobamate is often difficult to distinguish from a placebo on the one hand and an intermediate-acting barbiturate on the other. In higher doses in man and laboratory animals, its properties might be characterized as being somewhere between those of the barbiturates and the benzodiazepines.

Although meprobamate can cause widespread depression of the CNS, it does so unevenly; there is considerable selectivity in its influence on various CNS functions, and it does not cause anesthesia.

Meprobamate can depress polysynaptic reflexes in the spinal cord without affecting monosynaptic reflexes, and it is more selective than barbiturates in this respect. This effect is thought to contribute to its muscle relaxant properties, although suprasegmental loci of action cannot be discounted. With clinical doses in man, the muscle relaxant effects are negligible, although there may be some decrease in spasm as a result of a lessening of anxiety. The N-isopropyl derivative, *carisoprodol* (Chapter 21), has more prominent muscle relaxant activity. Although the drug has been reported to have a slight hyperalgesic action (Kantor *et al.*, 1973), it appears to have a mild analgesic effect when there is musculoskeletal pain (Gilbert and Koepke, 1973), and it enhances the analgesic effects of other drugs.

As an anticonvulsant, meprobamate resembles trimethadione. It antagonizes pentylenetetrazol and raises the electroshock seizure threshold in laboratory animals but does not prevent seizures from maximal electroshock. In man, meprobamate suppresses absence seizures, but it may aggravate grand mal and myoclonic epilepsy. Grand mal convulsions frequently occur as the result of abrupt withdrawal from chronic use of large doses.

Aggressive animals become tame and docile when given doses of meprobamate that cause negligible impairment of locomotor and general activity. Behavior patterns that have been previously suppressed by punishment are restored ("released") by meprobamate. The drug inhibits a variety of responses to hypothalamic stimulation and shortens electrical afterdischarges in the limbic system; it also suppresses amygdalohippocampal-evoked potentials in doses that do not affect the arousal response evoked by stimulation of the reticular formation of the brain stem. Despite these selective experimental effects, which are usually thought to correlate with antianxiety effects in man, clinical proof of efficacy as a selective antianxiety agent is lacking. In their review of the clinical literature, Greenblatt and Shader (1971) stated, "In only five of 26 studies was meprobamate clearly shown to be more effective than a placebo in psychoneurotic patients, and in only one of ten studies was meprobamate clearly more useful than a barbiturate."

Doses of meprobamate above 1600 mg increase the amount and amplitude of fast activity in the human EEG. The augmentation is more selective for certain frequencies than with barbiturates. Meprobamate differs from both barbiturates and benzodiazepines in that there is little activation of the EEG in the frontal lobe. Usual clinical doses do not affect the EEG. Only two studies have been made on the effect of meprobamate on the stages of sleep (*see* Kay *et al.*, 1976). In one, the drug decreased stage-1 sleep and increased the time spent in stage-2 and REM sleep without affecting slow-wave sleep.

Absorption, Fate, and Excretion. Meprobamate is well absorbed when administered orally; when tablets are taken, peak concentrations are reached in plasma in 1 to 3 hours. During chronic administration of sedative doses, concentrations in blood usually range between 5 and 20 μg/ml. There is little binding to plasma proteins. Eighty to 92% of the drug is metabolized in the liver, mainly to a side chain hydroxy derivative and a glucuronide; the remainder is excreted unchanged in the urine. The half-life of a single dose in plasma ranges from 6 to 17 hours, but it has been reported to be as long as 24 to 48 hours during chronic administration; the kinetics of elimination may be dependent on the dose. Meprobamate can induce some hepatic microsomal enzymes. It is not clear whether the drug induces the

enzymes responsible for its own metabolism (*see* Meyer and Straughn, 1977).

Adverse Effects and Intoxication. The major unwanted effects of sedative doses of meprobamate are drowsiness and ataxia. According to the findings of Kornetsky (1958; but *see* McNair, 1973), a single dose of 400 mg has little effect on the performance of psychometric tests; however, there is considerable impairment of learning and motor coordination and prolongation of reaction time when doses of 1600 mg are given.

Hypotension may occur in response to meprobamate. Allergic reactions have been reported in from 0.2 to 3.4% of different series of patients and appear most frequently in those with a history of dermatological or allergic conditions. Urticaria or an erythematous rash is the most common manifestation. Acute nonthrombocytopenic purpura has also been reported, and angioedema and bronchospasm have occurred occasionally.

Study of the effects of the concurrent administration of meprobamate and ethanol have yielded conflicting data (*see* Forney and Hughes, 1968; Carpenter, 1975). Tricyclic antidepressants and monoamine oxidase (MAO) inhibitors increase the CNS-depressant effects of meprobamate. It is prudent to assume that the CNS-depressant effect of any drug will be exaggerated by therapeutic doses of meprobamate.

Within a year of the introduction of meprobamate into medicine, abuse was reported, and this soon became a major problem; it has continued despite a substantial decrease in the clinical use of the drug. After chronic medication with doses usually in excess of 2.4 g a day for several weeks, abrupt discontinuation evokes a withdrawal syndrome usually characterized by anxiety, insomnia, tremors, gastrointestinal disturbances, and, frequently, hallucinations; grand mal–like convulsions occur in about 10% of cases. Allgulander (1978) reported 40% of drug habitués with serious withdrawal syndromes had been using meprobamate, a considerably higher percentage than had been taking barbiturates. Mild symptoms sometimes occur after withdrawal from chronic doses of as low as 1.6 g a day.

Meprobamate overdosage continues to contribute appreciably to hospital admissions (Allen *et al.*, 1977). Moderate overdosage, which results in blood concentrations in the range of 30 to 100 μg/ml, may cause vertigo, ataxia, slurred speech, impaired stance, stupor, or light coma. Ingestions that result in concentrations of 100 to 200 μg/ml cause coma, hypotension, respiratory depression, shock, pulmonary edema, and heart failure. Although a single dose of 12 g has been fatal, lethal doses usually exceed 40 g. The principles of the management of intoxication are essentially those described for barbiturate intoxication (*see* above). Hemodialysis or hemoperfusion is indicated only if brain stem functions are inadequate. Hemoperfusion with AMBERLITE XAD-4 resin or charcoal may be superior to hemodialysis, but more data are needed. Elimination can be considerably enhanced by diuresis promoted by the administration of saline and furosemide.

Conflicting reports have appeared on the effects of exposure of the fetus to meprobamate; it is recommended that meprobamate not be taken during pregnancy, especially during the first trimester.

Induction of hepatic microsomal enzymes by meprobamate may result in exacerbation of intermittent porphyria and may also be the cause of various drug interactions. The elimination of warfarin, estrogens, and oral contraceptives is increased by large doses of meprobamate, but interactions appear to be slight when usual doses are taken.

Therapeutic Uses.   Even though the antianxiety effects of meprobamate are equivocal, several million prescriptions are written each year for this indication and for the closely allied purpose of daytime sedation. Meprobamate is also used as a hypnotic agent in the treatment of insomnia. It has especially been advocated for hypnotic use in geriatric patients, for whom it has been reported to be as effective as flurazepam and flunitrazepam (Keston and Brocklehurst, 1974; Brocklehurst *et al.*, 1978), more predictable than chloral hydrate, and subject to fewer dosage problems than barbiturates and probably flurazepam. The sedative and hypnotic doses are listed in Table 17–2.

METHAQUALONE

The 2,3-disubstituted quinazolines possess hypnotic activity. Of these, only methaqualone is marketed. It has the following structure:

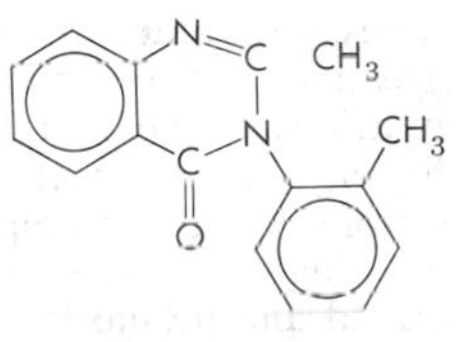

Methaqualone

Pharmacodynamics.   In addition to sedative-hypnotic properties, methaqualone possesses anticonvulsant, antispasmodic, local anesthetic, and weak antihistaminic properties. In high doses, it selectively depresses polysynaptic pathways in the spinal cord. The drug has antitussive activity comparable to that of codeine; although it lacks analgesic activity, it enhances analgesia from codeine. Methaqualone may also possess tranquilizing properties, but it is not clear that these are distinct from its sedative effects; evaluations from drug abusers suggest that they may be distinct (*see* below). Tolerance occurs to the depressant, anticonvulsant, and behavioral effects. In anesthetic doses, methaqualone exerts a myocardial depressant action that is the principal cause of hypotension.

Reports of the effects of methaqualone on the stages of sleep are contradictory (*see* review by Kay *et al.*, 1976). If there is an effect on stage-4 and REM sleep, it is one of suppression, except that low doses (150 mg) have been reported to cause an increase in REM activity. Effects on stage 2 are variable; sleep latency may decrease.

Absorption and Fate.   In man, 99% of methaqualone is absorbed in 2 hours. In the plasma, 70 to 90% is bound to albumin. More than 99% of the drug is metabolized by the hepatic microsomal system, and 4'-hydroxymethaqualone and the N'-oxide are the major primary metabolites. At least eight other hydroxyl metabolites are formed; these are mainly conjugated and excreted in the urine, but the 4-hydroxy metabolite is excreted into bile. The pharmacokinetics is that of a two-compartment system, with a distribution half-life of less than 1 hour and an elimination half-life of 10 to 40 hours (Delong *et al.*, 1976). A moderate degree of hepatic microsomal enzyme induction occurs. 17-Ketosteroid concentrations in the plasma are increased.

Side Effects, Intoxication, and Dependence.   During sedation with methaqualone, fatigue and occasionally dizziness and torpor may occur. With hypnotic doses, there may be transient paresthesias preceding the onset of sleep. Persisting paresthesias and other signs of peripheral neuropathy that last for months to years may also occur (*e.g., see* Marks, 1974; Hoaken, 1975). Occasionally, restlessness and anxiety are observed instead of sedation and sleep. Excessive dreaming and somnambulism also sometimes occur. "Hangover" is frequent. Other side effects include xerostomia, anorexia, nausea, vomiting, diarrhea, epigastric discomfort, sweating, bromidrosis, urticaria, and exanthems. Rarely, aplastic anemia has developed, but the relationship to methaqualone has not been proven. Severe CNS depression may occur when methaqualone is taken in combination with ethanol or other CNS depressants. Methaqualone increases the effects of MAO inhibitors and tricyclic antidepressants. In combination with phenothiazines and tricyclic antidepressants, it may cause epistaxis and menstrual irregularities (*see* Marriott, 1976). Methaqualone does not appear to interact significantly with warfarin. It has been used without difficulty in patients with intermittent porphyria.

Mild overdosage usually causes excessive central depression much like that from barbiturates, but restlessness and excitement sometimes result instead. With severe overdosage, delirium, pyramidal signs (such as hypertonicity, hyperreflexia, and myoclonus), and frank convulsions may occur. Myoclonic episodes and amnesia have been reported, in one case with a dose as low as 400 mg. During coma, cardiovascular and respiratory depression are less severe than with barbiturates. Coma has been noted after 2.4 g and death after 8 g. Most fatalities occur in persons who have also ingested ethanol. Treatment is primarily supportive. While hemodialysis and peritoneal dialysis are poorly effective, theoretical considerations suggest that hemoperfusion through activated charcoal, oil, or cation-exchange resins might be of value.

Methaqualone has come to be widely abused. The unexpectedly explosive pace with which methaqualone was incorporated into the drug culture stems from a popular view among abusers that it has aphrodisiac activity and that it promotes unreserved interpersonal relations. Drug culturists contend also that it causes a dissociative "high" achieved without the drowsiness caused by barbiturates; in fact, many abusers liken the effects of methaqualone to those of heroin. Abusers employ doses of 75 mg to 2 g a day, with an average of about 725 mg. Severe grand mal convulsions may occur after abrupt withdrawal from such high doses.

The biochemistry, experimental and clinical pharmacology, and toxicity of methaqualone have been reviewed by Brown and Goenechea (1973).

Dosage and Preparations. These are listed in Table 17-2. Capsules of the hydrochloride have a very rapid dissolution rate, and the onset of action is quite prompt with this dosage form.

PARALDEHYDE

Paraldehyde is a polymer of acetaldehyde, but it is perhaps best regarded as a polyether of cyclic structure, as follows:

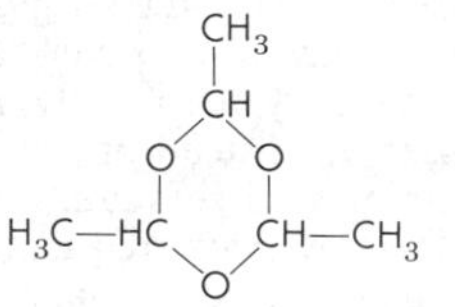

Paraldehyde

Because of some limited virtues and despite its disadvantages, paraldehyde has managed to survive a century of use; it deserves to be retired.

Pharmacological Actions. Paraldehyde is a rapidly acting hypnotic; after a therapeutic oral dose, sleep usually ensues in 10 to 15 minutes. The drug does not possess analgesic properties, and it may produce excitement or delirium in the presence of pain. In large doses, it is effective against all types of convulsions and against delirium.

Paraldehyde has little effect on respiration and blood pressure in ordinary therapeutic doses. In large doses, it produces respiratory depression and hypotension.

Pharmacokinetics. Oral paraldehyde is rapidly absorbed. With hypnotic doses, 70 to 80% is metabolized in the liver, most of the remainder is exhaled, and a small amount is excreted in urine. In hepatic insufficiency, the rate of elimination is slowed, and the proportion excreted in the expired air is increased. It is believed that paraldehyde is depolymerized to acetaldehyde in the liver and then oxidized by aldehyde dehydrogenase to acetic acid, which is ultimately metabolized to carbon dioxide and water.

The drug readily crosses the placental barrier. Some delay in onset of respiratory movements has been observed in the neonate following its administration to the mother during labor.

Untoward Effects and Poisoning. Paraldehyde has a strong aromatic odor and a disagreeable taste. Orally, it is irritating to the throat and stomach, and intramuscularly or subcutaneously it may cause necrosis and also nerve injury. Intravenously it may cause cyanosis, cough, and hypotension.

Adverse effects and intoxication with paraldehyde are uncommon only because its use has been essentially restricted to hospitalized or institutionalized patients. The lethal dose is difficult to ascertain; death has occurred from 25 g, but one person has survived 150 g. According to one estimate, the minimal lethal blood level is about 50 mg/dl.

Patients poisoned by paraldehyde commonly exhibit very rapid, labored respiratory movements, possibly due to the injurious effect of paraldehyde or its decomposition products on the lungs and possibly, in some cases, due to acidosis. Acidosis, bleeding gastritis, muscular irritability, azotemia, oliguria, albuminuria, leukocytosis, fatty changes in the liver and kidney with toxic hepatitis and nephrosis, pulmonary hemorrhages and edema, and dilatation of the right ventricle have all been observed in cases of severe acute or chronic paraldehyde poisoning.

Chronic paraldehyde intoxication results in *tolerance* and *dependence*. The paraldehyde addict may become acquainted with the drug when it is used in the treatment of alcoholism and then, surprisingly in view of its disagreeable taste and odor, prefer it to alcohol. Paraldehyde addiction resembles alcoholism, and sudden withdrawal may result in delirium tremens and vivid hallucinations.

Some paraldehyde habitués suffer from metabolic acidosis of unknown etiology, but it is in excess of that consequent to the oxidation of paraldehyde-derived acetaldehyde.

Therapeutic Uses. Paraldehyde has been used chiefly for the treatment of abstinence phenomena and other psychiatric states characterized by excitement; for the emergency treatment of convulsive episodes arising from tetanus, eclampsia, status epilepticus, and poisoning by convulsive drugs; and for basal and obstetrical anesthesia. Its most persisting use has been in the treatment of delirium tremens. Advocates point out that it may be administered more easily—as a retention enema—to restrained, difficult-to-manage patients (including children) than are intravenous or oral CNS depressants or anticonvulsants.

Dosage and Preparations. The hypnotic dose is shown in Table 17-2. When given rectally as a retention enema, the drug is usually added to 2 volumes of olive oil. In no case should paraldehyde be taken from old, partially empty containers, since an appreciable proportion of the drug may have been oxidized to acetic acid and other decomposition products; these products have been implicated as contributing factors in several intoxications. It is best stored away from light in 2- or 5-ml amber ampuls, which can be opened freshly and the unused contents discarded. Since paraldehyde reacts rapidly with certain plastics, it should be measured with glass syringes.

MISCELLANEOUS SEDATIVE-HYPNOTIC DRUGS

Ethinamate and Mebutamate. *Ethinamate* is a urethane with the following structure:

Ethinamate

It has a rapid onset and a short duration of action. Its effect on REM sleep is unknown. Ethinamate is inactivated at least partly by the liver, by hydroxylation of the cyclohexyl ring; the product is conjugated and excreted as the glucuronide. Side effects of ethinamate include nausea, occasional vomiting, and infrequently rash. Idiosyncratic excitement may be noted, especially in children. Fever and thrombocytopenia occur rarely. The lethal dose is unknown; death has resulted from the ingestion of 15 g, but there has been recovery after 28 g. Chronic use of larger-than-recommended doses may lead to psychic and physical dependence. The abstinence syndrome is similar to that for the barbiturates. It is often stated that 500 mg is equivalent to 100 mg of secobarbital, but some studies have found this dose to be little better than a placebo.

The urethane *mebutamate,* for which antihypertensive effects have been claimed, has hypnotic properties. It suppresses REM sleep, but no rebound occurs; stage-4 sleep is increased.

Monoureides. The monoureides in general are short-acting sedative-hypnotics with a low therapeutic index. Consequently, they are very little used. *Carbromal* (bromodiethylacetylurea) and *bromisovalum* (α-bromoisovalerylurea) are obsolete monoureides that are still available; they both release bromide ion and can thus cause bromide poisoning. In intoxication, shock-lung and an intravascular coagulation defect may occur. *Capuride,* available in Europe, appears to have a more favorable therapeutic index.

Bromides. Bromides have an exceedingly slow onset and offset of action and hence were used only as sedatives and anticonvulsants, for which they are now obsolete. The reader is referred to *previous editions* of this textbook for details of the action and toxicity of bromide ion.

Others. *Clomethiazole* (chlormethiazole) is a sedative–muscle relaxant–anticonvulsant drug used outside the United States, especially for the management of withdrawal from ethanol. Given alone, its effects on respiration are slight, and the therapeutic index is high. However, deaths from adverse interaction with ethanol are relatively frequent.

Benzoctamine is used outside the United States as an antianxiety agent; it appears to be an excellent hypnotic drug. In therapeutic doses it has negligible effects on respiration and may even improve it in chronic obstructive pulmonary disease and asthma. Consequently, it may be of particular value as a hypnotic in persons with respiratory disorders.

Etomidate is a short-acting hypnotic drug of recent origin that is widely used outside the United States. It appears to have GABA-like effects. In anesthetic doses it has negligible effects on the respiratory and cardiovascular systems and hence is advocated as an intravenous anesthetic; however, myoclonus, especially in response to pain, is sometimes troublesome.

L-*Tryptophan* in doses of 1 to 5 g may diminish sleep latency and prolong stage-2 sleep; 5-hydroxytryptophan in doses of 100 to 200 mg has similar effects. REM sleep may be suppressed. Hypnosis presumably is the result of an increase in brain 5-HT. There is presently a considerable interest in the effects of these substances for the treatment of various dyskinesias and depression.

Various *β-adrenergic receptor blocking drugs* are under active investigation as hypnotics. Oxprenolol and alprenolol may be more active than propranolol. The hypnotic effects are said to be markedly enhanced in combination with L-tryptophan.

Antihistamines and Nonprescription Hypnotics. Diphenhydramine, doxylamine, methapyrilene, promethazine, and pyrilamine have all been used as hypnotics. Methapyrilene, formerly included in virtually all nonprescription sleep aids in the United States, was removed from these products in 1979 because of its possible carcinogenic properties. Outside of the United States, diphenhydramine is marketed in combination with methaqualone, and it has undergone trials in the United States. A dose of 1 mg/kg in children reduces sleep latency and wake time but does not differ from a placebo in its effects on restlessness and nightmares; in adults, 50 mg of diphenhydramine can be distinguished from a placebo. Among other potentially hypnotic ingredients in such products are the antihistamine pyrilamine and the antimuscarinic drug scopolamine or its amine oxide. Scopolamine markedly increases REM-sleep latency and diminishes REM activity at first, but tolerance occurs after two or three nights, and rebound occurs after discontinuation of use (Sagalés *et al.,* 1977). The third most common component of nonprescription hypnotic mixtures is sodium salicylamide. A dose of 1.3 g has a slight sedative effect; the dose included in nonprescription products is 200 to 380 mg. Aspirin or sodium salicylate in amounts of 25 to 228 mg is included in a few mixtures. It is most dubious whether any of the salicylates contribute to hypnosis in these products. Certain nonprescription mixtures exert appreciable side effects, yet statistically they cannot be distinguished from a placebo as sedative-antianxiety drugs (Rickels and Hesbacher, 1973); other products, however, can (Wolff, 1974).

MANAGEMENT OF INSOMNIA

Few clinical disorders have been more casually and carelessly treated than insomnia. Insomnia has many causes, and an accurate differential diagnosis is required before treatment should be considered. Prescription of a hypnotic without regard to the underlying disturbance subjects the patient to the risk of abuse, may mask the signs and symptoms of a pernicious pathology, and may dangerously exacerbate an unrecognized sleep apnea. Furthermore, nonhypnotic drugs may be superior to hypnotic drugs when there is a specific cause of the insomnia. For example, dextroamphetamine or similar drugs may improve sleep in some hyperkinetic patients and those with Parkinson's disease; other examples include antidepressants for those with endogenous depression (10 days or more of treatment may be required), phenothiazines or haloperidol for psychotics (after a latency), phenytoin when there are paroxysmal nightmares, dextroamphetamine or appropriate anticonvulsants when there is sleep epilepsy or myoclonus, analgesics when sleep is impaired by (even subliminal) pain, insulin in improperly managed diabetes, antithyroid drugs or β-adrenergic antagonists in hyperthyroidism, metoclopramide or bethanechol in nocturnal gastroesophageal reflux, cimetidine in peptic ulcer, and so forth.

Even when no specific pathological etiology can be identified, insomnia may nevertheless relate to identifiable causes, such as ingestion of food or coffee near bedtime, various drugs, a defective mattress or pillow, or a host of other factors known to many. Only when specific causes cannot be eliminated or compensated for should a nonspecific, hypnotic drug be considered.

Nature does not compel man to sleep 8 hours a day, and many persons function well on much less sleep. Sometimes simple assurance of this fact is sufficient to improve sleep or at least to decrease the concern about nocturnal sleeplessness. A relaxing activity before bedtime is often efficacious.

When a hypnotic is to be used, various considerations determine the choice. Because of both temporal and personality factors, choices differ according to whether the problem with sleep is short term (situational), such as jet lag or sleeping in an unfamiliar place, or chronic. The problems of drug accumulation, alteration of sleep pattern, tolerance, and abuse potential are of much greater concern in long-term than in transient situational use.

The choice of drug differs according to whether the patient has difficulty only in falling asleep or also in remaining asleep. In the former situation, a drug with only a very short duration of action is desirable. Unfortunately, in the United States, there is not presently available an oral-dosage form of a drug with a suitably short half-life. Triazolam and oxazolam appear to have nearly ideal half-lives and are likely to become drugs of first choice when they are made available. Triazolam is also released from its dosage form and absorbed rapidly, so that both pharmacokinetic and biopharmaceutical factors favor its use. Since the average sleep latency among insomniacs is less than an hour and may be more nearly 30 minutes, the latency can, at best, be shortened by only 20 to 30 minutes. The saving usually does not amount to an appreciable amount of sleep. Consequently, the most important role of the physician may be to convince the patient that a short period of wakefulness is less serious than are the potential complications of dependence on hypnotics.

For persons who may need an effect of drug throughout sleep, hypnotic drugs with half-lives of 4 to 8 hours should be preferred to those with shorter half-lives, but the risk of appreciable residual effects, tolerance, drug interactions, and abnormalities in sleep patterns is increased. Triazolam, oxazolam, and flunitrazepam may be good choices. Hexobarbital and chloral derivatives have suitable half-lives, but their use creates other problems. Flurazepam generates active metabolites of very long half-life, but empirically it has become an acceptable hypnotic drug for inducing sleep of long duration. The long half-lives of the metabolites may explain the absence of significant rebound, since withdrawal is automatically very gradual. Since most persons who have difficulty falling asleep also need all-night coverage, hypnotic drugs with half-lives in the 4- to 8-hour range probably have the greatest all-around serviceability. These patients are usually anxious, so that the antianxiety properties of the benzodiazepines may be particularly helpful to them.

Subjects who suffer from early-morning awakening, often with a feeling of panic, are frequently depressives for whom psychotherapy and antidepressants should be considered.

When sleep apnea interrupts sleep, hypnotics without respiratory depressant properties are indicated. Thus, triazolam and flurazepam are suitable, but nitrazepam may not be. Even diphenhydramine may be considered.

It is relevant to consider alterations in sleep pattern, both during use and after withdrawal of a drug. Since night terrors and somnambulism most frequently occur during stage 4 of sleep, drugs that shorten or lighten this stage may be indicated. However, caution is in order, since, with some hypnotics, rebound effects on stage 4 may be quite severe or protracted. Furthermore, strong suppression of stage 4 may cause the emergence of day terrors or of suicidal ideation. Similarly, nightmares that normally occur during REM sleep may transfer to stage 2. Nocturnal enuresis may be prevented by drugs that suppress REM sleep. Suppression of REM sleep may also improve endogenous depression (*see* Greenberg and Pearlman, 1974).

For chronic hypnotic therapy, continual nightly medication should be avoided; after a good night's sleep, the drug should be discontinued for 2 to 3 days, thus minimizing tolerance and the likelihood of abuse, cumulative effects of disruption of sleep patterns, hepatic enzyme induction, and drug accumulation. Both tolerance and rebound effects generate anxiety and mislead the user to believe that higher and more frequent doses are necessary, with the result that a vicious cycle of increasing use and tolerance and continuing disruption of normal sleep patterns occurs. In this situation, abuse and dependence are increasingly more likely to develop. It is important to emphasize the potential for dependence to the patient; he should also be educated about the effects of disruption of the normal sleep pattern. Family counseling may be important. It is of utmost importance to proceed cautiously with a patient who has a history of any kind of drug abuse. After a period of continual use of a hypnotic, withdrawal should be gradual.

Except when specific drug therapy or nonpharmacological interventions are indicated, *benzodiazepines should be considered to be the hypnotic drugs of choice,* since they have better therapeutic indices, fewer drug interactions, less effect on respiration, and probably lower abuse liability than do the barbiturates and the other prescription hypnotic drugs available in the United States. This applies even to the venerable chloral derivatives; were they to be used to the same extent as barbiturates, they would prove to have most of the shortcomings. Similarly, the benzodiazepines are the preferred sedatives.

Insomnia and its treatment have been reviewed by Kales and associates (1974; 1975), Johns (1975), and Hartmann (1977).

Aitken, R. C. B., and Proudfoot, A. T. Barbiturate automatism—myth or malady? *Postgrad. Med. J.,* **1969,** *45,* 612–616.
Allen, M. D.; Greenblatt, D. J.; and Noel, B. Meprobamate overdosage: a continuing problem. *Clin. Toxicol.,* **1977,** *11,* 501–515.
Baestrup, C.; Albrechtsen, R.; and Squires, R. F. High densities of benzodiazepine receptors in human cortical areas. *Nature,* **1977,** *269,* 702–704.
Bailey, D. N., and Jatlow, P. I. Barbital overdose and abuse. A new problem. *Am. J. Clin. Pathol.,* **1975,** *64,* 291–296.
Bekersky, I.; Maggio, A. C.; Mattaliano, V., Jr.; Boxenbaum, H. G.; Maynard, D. E.; Cohn, P. D.; and Kaplan, S. A. Influence of phenobarbital on the disposition of clonazepam and antipyrine in the dog. *J. Pharmacokinet. Biopharm.,* **1977,** *5,* 507–512.
Blaschke, T. F.; Berk, P. D.; Rodkey, F. L.; Scharschmidt, B. F.; Collison, H. A.; and Waggoner, J. G. Drugs and the liver. I. Effects of glutethimide and phenobarbital on hepatic bilirubin clearance, plasma bilirubin turnover, and carbon monoxide production in man. *Biochem. Pharmacol.,* **1974,** *23,* 2795–2806.
Brocklehurst, J. C.; Carty, M. H.; and Skorecki, J. The use of a kymograph in a comparative trial of flunitrazepam and meprobamate in elderly patients. *Curr. Med. Res. Opin.,* **1978,** *5,* 663–668.
Brown, S. S., and Goenechea, S. Methaqualone: metabolic, kinetic, and clinical pharmacologic observations *Clin. Pharmacol. Ther.,* **1973,** *14,* 314–324.
Caldwell, J., and Sever, P. S. The biochemical pharmacology of abused drugs. II. Alcohol and barbiturates. *Clin. Pharmacol. Ther.,* **1974,** *16,* 737–749.
Carpenter, J. A. (ed.). Drug interactions: the effects of alcohol and meprobamate applied singly and jointly in human subjects. *J. Stud. Alcohol,* **1975,** *7,* Suppl., 1–193.
Chinn, C., and Barnes, C. D. Comparative effects of propranolol and diazepam on hypothalamically-evoked sympathetic responses. *Pharmacologist,* **1978,** *20,* 207.
Chou, D. T., and Wang, S. C. Unit activity of amygdala and hippocampal neurons: effects of morphine and benzodiazepines. *Brain Res.,* **1977,** *126,* 427–440.
Christensen, J. D. Tolerance development with chlordiazepoxide in relation to the plasma levels of the parent compound and its main metabolites in mice. *Acta Pharmacol. Toxicol. (Kbh.),* **1973,** *33,* 262–272.
Clark, T. J. H.; Collins, J. V.; and Tong, D. Respiratory depression caused by nitrazepam in patients with respiratory failure. *Lancet,* **1971,** *2,* 737–738.
Clarke, R. S. J., and Lyons, S. M. Diazepam and flunitrazepam as induction agents for cardiac surgical operations. *Acta Anaesthesiol. Scand.,* **1977,** *21,* 282–292.
Consolo, S.; Garattini, S.; and Ladinski, H. Action of the benzodiazepines on the cholinergic system. In, *Mechanism of Action of Benzodiazepines.* (Costa, E., and Greengard, P., eds.) Raven Press, New York, **1975,** pp. 63–80.
Critchett, D. J., and Lippa, A. S. Evidence for the GABA-ergic properties of benzodiazepines: effects of iontophoretically applied flurazepam on cerebellar Purkinje cells. *Fed. Proc.,* **1978,** *37,* 347.
Crow, J. W.; Lain, P.; Bochner, F.; Shoeman, D. W.; and Azarnoff, D. L. Glutethimide and 4-OH glutethimide:

pharmacokinetics and effect on performance in man. *Clin. Pharmacol. Ther.,* **1977,** *22,* 458–464.

Cummins, L. M.; Martin, Y. C.; and Scherfling, E. E. Serum and urine levels of ethchlorovynol in man. *J. Pharm. Sci.,* **1971,** *60,* 261–263.

Curry, S. H.; Riddall, D.; Gordon, J. S.; Simpson, P.; Binns, T. B.; Rondel, R. K.; and McMartin, C. Disposition of glutethimide in man. *Clin. Pharmacol. Ther.,* **1971,** *12,* 849–857.

Cutler, R. W. P.; Markowitz, D.; and Dudzinsky, D. S. The effect of barbiturates on [³H]GABA transport in rat cerebral cortex slices. *Brain Res.,* **1974,** *81,* 189–197.

Davies, J., and Polc, P. Effect of a water soluble benzodiazepine on the responses of spinal neurones to acetylcholine and excitatory amino acid analogs. *Neuropharmacology,* **1978,** *17,* 217–220.

Delong, A. F.; Smyth, R. D.; Polk, A.; Nayak, R. K.; and Reavey-Cantwell, N. H. Blood levels of methaqualone in man following chronic therapeutic doses. *Arch. Int. Pharmacodyn. Ther.,* **1976,** *222,* 322–331.

Dement, W. C.; Zarcone, V. P.; Hoddes, E.; Smythe, H.; and Carskadon, M. Sleep laboratory and clinical studies with flurazepam. In, *The Benzodiazepines.* (Garattini, S.; Mussini, E.; and Randall, L. O.; eds.) Raven Press, New York, **1973,** pp. 599–611.

Dorpat, T. L. Drug automatism, barbiturate poisoning, and suicide behavior. *Arch. Gen. Psychiatry,* **1974,** *31,* 216–220.

Dray, A., and Straughan, D. W. Benzodiazepines: GABA and glycine receptors on single neurons in the rat medulla. *J. Pharm. Pharmacol.,* **1976,** *28,* 314–315.

Elliott, H. W.; Nomof, N.; Navarro, G.; Reulius, H. W.; Knowles, J. A.; and Comer, W. H. Central nervous system and cardiovascular effects of lorazepam in man. *Clin. Pharmacol. Ther.,* **1971,** *12,* 468–481.

Feinberg, I.; Fein, G.; Walker, J. M.; Price, L. J.; Floyd, T. C.; and March, J. D. Flurazepam effects on slow-wave sleep: stage 4 suppressed but number of delta waves constant. *Science,* **1977,** *198,* 847–848.

Feinberg, I.; Hibi, S.; Cavness, C.; and March, J. Absence of REM rebound after barbiturate withdrawal. *Science,* **1974,** *185,* 534–535.

Gabel, R. A.; Irving, S. P.; and Weiskopf, R. B. Depression of human ventilatory response to hypoxia by diazepam and by meperidine-diazepam. *Fed. Proc.,* **1976,** *35,* 728.

Gaillard, J.-M., and Phelippeau, M. Benzodiazepine-induced modifications of dream content: the effect of flunitrazepam. *Neuropsychobiology,* **1976,** *2,* 37–44.

Gasser, J. C.; Kaufman, R. D.; and Bellville, J. W. Respiratory effects of lorazepam, pentobarbital, and pentazocine. *Clin. Pharmacol. Ther.,* **1975,** *18,* 170–174.

Geller, E. B.; Durlofsky, L.; Harakal, C.; Cowan, A.; and Adler, M. W. Pentobarbital does not influence the antinociceptive effects of morphine in naive or morphine-tolerant rats. *Pharmacologist,* **1977,** *19,* 142.

Gilbert, M. M., and Koepke, H. H. Relief of musculoskeletal and psychopathological symptoms with meprobamate and aspirin: a controlled study. *Curr. Ther. Res.,* **1973,** *15,* 820–832.

Ginsberg, R. L., and Garnick, M. B. Effect of phenobarbital on biliary lipid metabolism in normal man. *Gastroenterology,* **1977,** *72,* 1221–1227.

Glauser, F. L.; Smith, W. R.; Caldwell, A.; Hoshiko, M.; Dolan, G. S.; Baer, H.; and Olsher, N. Ethchlorvynol (PLACIDYL)-induced pulmonary edema. *Ann. Intern. Med.,* **1976,** *84,* 46–48.

Good, M. I. Catatonialike symptomatology and withdrawal dyskinesias. *Am. J. Psychiatry,* **1976,** *133,* 1454–1456.

Greenberg, R., and Pearlman, C. Cutting the REM nerve: an approach to the adaptive role of REM sleep. *Perspect. Biol. Med.,* **1974,** *17,* 513–521.

Greenblatt, D. J.; Allen, M. D.; Noel, B. J.; and Shader, R. I. Acute overdosage with benzodiazepine derivatives. *Clin. Pharmacol. Ther.,* **1977,** *4,* 497–514.

Gustafson, A.; Svensson, S.-E.; and Ugander, L. Cardiac arrhythmias in chloral hydrate poisoning. *Acta Med. Scand.,* **1977,** *201,* 227–230.

Haefely, W.; Kulcsár, A.; Möhler, H.; Pieri, L.; Polc, P.; and Schaffner, R. Possible involvement of GABA in the central actions of benzodiazepines. In, *Mechanism of Action of Benzodiazepines.* (Costa, E., and Greengard, P., eds.) Raven Press, New York, **1975,** pp. 131–151.

Hansen, A. R.; Kennedy, K. A.; Ambre, J. J.; and Fischer, L. J. Glutethimide poisoning. A metabolite contributes to morbidity and mortality. *N. Engl. J. Med.,* **1975,** *292,* 250–252.

Hartmann, E. Long-term administration of psychotropic drugs: effects on human sleep. In, *Pharmacology of Sleep.* (Williams, R. L., and Karacan, I., eds.) John Wiley & Sons, Inc., New York, **1976,** pp. 211–223.

Hartmann, E., and Cravens, J. The effects of long term administration of psychotropic drugs on human sleep. V. The effects of chloral hydrate. *Psychopharmacologia,* **1973,** *33,* 219–232.

Hasegawa, M., and Matsubara, I. Metabolic fates of flurazepam. I. Gas chromatographic determination of flurazepam and its metabolites in human urine and blood using electron capture detector. *Chem. Pharm. Bull. (Tokyo),* **1975,** *23,* 1826–1833.

Hindmarch, I. A repeated dose comparison of three benzodiazepine derivatives (nitrazepam, flurazepam and flunitrazepam) on subjective appraisals of sleep and measures of psychomotor performance the morning following night-time medication. *Acta Psychiatr. Scand.,* **1977,** *56,* 373–381.

Hoaken, P. C. S. Adverse effect of methaqualone. *Can. Med. Assoc. J.,* **1975,** *112,* 685.

Huang, L. M., and Barker, J. L. Pentobarbital: stereospecific actions of ($+$) and ($-$) isomers revealed on cultured mammalian neurons. *Science,* **1980,** *207,* 195–197.

Ikram, H.; Rubin, A. P.; and Jewkes, R. F. Effect of diazepam on myocardial blood flow of patients with and without coronary artery disease. *Br. Heart J.,* **1973,** *35,* 626–630.

Itil, T. M. Discrimination between some hypnotic and anxiolytic drugs by computer-analyzed sleep. In, *Pharmacology of Sleep.* (Williams, R. L., and Karacan, I., eds.) John Wiley & Sons, Inc., New York, **1976,** pp. 225–238.

Jansson, B. Drug automatism as a cause of pseudosuicide. *Postgrad. Med.,* **1961,** *30,* A34–A40.

Kales, A.; Allen, C.; Scharf, M. B.; and Kales, J. D. Hypnotic drugs and their effectiveness. All-night studies of insomniac subjects. *Arch. Gen. Psychiatry,* **1970a,** *23,* 226–232.

Kales, A.; Bixler, E. O.; Kales, J. D.; and Scharf, M. B. Comparative effectiveness of nine hypnotic drugs: sleep laboratory studies. *J. Clin. Pharmacol.,* **1977,** *17,* 207–213.

Kales, A.; Kales, J. D.; Scharf, M. B.; and Tan, T.-L. Hypnotics and altered sleep patterns. II. All-night EEG studies of chloral hydrate, flurazepam and methaqualone. *Arch. Gen. Psychiatry,* **1970b,** *23,* 219–225.

Kales, A.; Preston, T. A.; Tan, T.-L.; and Allen, C. Hypnotics and altered sleep-dream patterns. I. All-night EEG studies of glutethimide, methaprylon, and pentobarbital. *Arch. Gen. Psychiatry,* **1970c,** *23,* 211–218.

Kales, A.; Scharf, M. B.; and Kales, J. D. Rebound insomnia: a new clinical syndrome. *Science,* **1978,** *201,* 1039–1040.

Kantor, T. G.; Laska, E.; and Streem, A. An apparent algesic effect of meprobamate. *J. Clin. Pharmacol.,* **1973,** *13,* 152–159.

Kappas, A.; Bradlow, H. L.; Bickers, D. R.; and Alvares, A. P. Induction of a deficiency of steroid Δ^4-5α-reductase activity in liver by a porphyrinogenic drug. *J. Clin. Invest.,* **1977,** *59,* 159–164.

Keston, M., and Brocklehurst, J. C. Flurazepam and meprobamate: a clinical trial. *Age Ageing,* **1974,** *3,* 54–58.

Knapp, R.; Remen, D.; Linsenmeyer, G.; and Boyd, E. An evaluation of the cardiopulmonary safety and efficacy of triazolam, flurazepam, and placebo as oral hypnotic agents. *Clin. Pharmacol. Ther.*, **1977**, *21*, 107–108.

Kornetsky, C. Effects of meprobamate, phenobarbital and dextroamphetamine on reaction time and learning in man. *J. Pharmacol. Exp. Ther.*, **1958**, *123*, 216–219.

Kripke, D. F.; Lavie, P.; and Hernandez, J. Polygraphic evaluation of ethchlorvynol (14 days). *Psychopharmacology*, **1978**, *56*, 221–223.

Lakshminarayan, S.; Sahn, S. A.; Hudson, L. D.; and Weil, J. V. Effect of diazepam on ventilatory responses. *Clin. Pharmacol. Ther.*, **1976**, *20*, 178–183.

Linarelli, L. G.; Hengstenberg, F. H.; and Drash, A. L. Effect of phenobarbital on hyperlipemia in patients with intrahepatic and extrahepatic cholestasis. *J. Pediatr.*, **1973**, *83*, 291–298.

Linnoila, M.; Korttila, M.; and Mattila, M. J. Effect of food and repeated injections on serum diazepam levels. *Acta Pharmacol. Toxicol. (Kbh.)*, **1975**, *36*, 181–186.

McClane, T. K., and Martin, W. R. Subjective and physiologic effects of morphine, pentobarbital, and meprobamate. *Clin. Pharmacol. Ther.*, **1976**, *20*, 192–198.

McNair, D. M. Antianxiety drugs and human performance. *Arch. Gen. Psychiatry*, **1973**, *29*, 611–617.

Mahon, W. A.; Inaba, T.; and Stone, R. M. Metabolism of flurazepam by the small intestine. *Clin. Pharmacol. Ther.*, **1977**, *22*, 228–233.

Malach, M., and Berman, N. Furosemide and chloral hydrate. Adverse drug reaction. *J.A.M.A.*, **1975**, *232*, 638–639.

Marks, P. Methaqualone and peripheral neuropathy. *Practitioner*, **1974**, *212*, 721–722.

Marriott, P. F. Methaqualone with psychotropic drugs: adverse interaction. *Med. J. Aust.*, **1976**, *1*, 412.

Mendelson, W. B.; Goodwin, D. W.; Hill, S. Y.; and Reichman, J. D. The morning after: residual EEG effects of triazolam and flurazepam alone and in combination with alcohol. *Curr. Ther. Res.*, **1976**, *19*, 155–163.

Metzler, C. M.; Ko, H.; Royer, M. E.; Veldkamp, W.; and Linet, O. I. Bioavailability and pharmacokinetics of orally administered triazolam in normal subjects. *Clin. Pharmacol. Ther.*, **1977**, *21*, 111–112.

Meyer, M. C., and Straughn, A. B. Meprobamate. Bioavailability monograph. *J. Am. Pharm. Assoc.*, **1977**, *17*, 173–176.

Miller, R. P., and Becker, B. A. Teratogenicity of oral diazepam and diphenylhydantoin in mice. *Toxicol. Appl. Pharmacol.*, **1975**, *32*, 53–61.

Misra, P. C. Nitrazepam (MOGADON) dependence. *Br. J. Psychiatry*, **1975**, *126*, 81–82.

Möhler, H., and Okada, T. Biochemical identification of the site of action of benzodiazepines in human brain by ^{3}H-diazepam binding. *Life Sci.*, **1978**, *22*, 985–996.

Monti, J. M.; Altier, H.; Prando, M.; and Gil, J. L. The actions of flunitrazepam (ROHYPNOL) on heart and respiratory rates and skin potential fluctuations during the sleep cycle in normal volunteers and neurotic patients with insomnia. *Psychopharmacologia*, **1975**, *43*, 187–190.

Myers, R. R., and Stockard, J. J. Neurologic and electroencephalographic correlates in glutethimide intoxication. *Clin. Pharmacol. Ther.*, **1975**, *17*, 212–220.

Nicoll, R. A. Pentobarbital: differential postsynaptic actions on sympathetic ganglion cells. *Science*, **1978**, *199*, 451–452.

Oswald, I.; Lewis, S. A.; Tagney, J.; Firth, H.; and Haider, I. Benzodiazepines and human sleep. In, *The Benzodiazepines.* (Garattini, S.; Mussini, E.; and Randall, L. O.; eds.) Raven Press, New York, **1973**, pp. 613–625.

Pancorbo, A. S.; Palagi, P. A.; Piecoro, J. J.; and Wilson, H. D. Hemodialysis in methyprylon overdose. Some pharmacokinetic considerations. *J.A.M.A.*, **1977**, *237*, 470–471.

Peričić, D.; Walters, J. R.; and Chase, T. N. Effect of diazepam and pentobarbital on aminooxyacetic acid-induced accumulation of GABA. *J. Neurochem.*, **1977**, *29*, 839–846.

Perona, G.; Corrocher, R.; Frezza, M.; Falezza, G. C.; Cellerino, R.; Tiribelli, C.; Fusaro, A.; and DeSandre, G. Phenobarbitone sensitivity of jaundice in haemolytic patients. *Br. J. Haematol.*, **1973**, *25*, 723–736.

Polc, P., and Haefely, W. Effects of two benzodiazepines, phenobarbitone, and baclofen on synaptic transmission in the cat cuneate nucleus. *Naunyn Schmiedebergs Arch. Pharmacol.*, **1976**, *294*, 121–131.

Pozenel, H.; Bückert, A.; and Amrein, R. The antihypertensive effect of LEXOTAN (bromazepine)—a new benzodiazepine derivative. *Int. J. Clin. Pharmacol. Biopharm.*, **1977**, *15*, 31–39.

Ransom, B. R., and Barker, J. L. Pentobarbital selectively enhances GABA-mediated post-synaptic inhibition in tissue cultured mouse spinal neurons. *Brain Res.*, **1976**, *114*, 530–535.

Rao, S.; Sherbaniuk, R. W.; Prasad, K.; Lee, S. J. K.; and Sproule, B. J. Cardiopulmonary effects of diazepam. *Clin. Pharmacol. Ther.*, **1973**, *14*, 182–189.

Reeves, R. L. Comparison of triazolam, flurazepam, and placebo as hypnotics in geriatric patients with insomnia. *J. Clin. Pharmacol.*, **1977**, *17*, 319–323.

Report, Boston Collaborative Drug Surveillance Program. Clinical depression of the central nervous system due to diazepam and chlordiazepoxide in relation to cigarette smoking and age. *N. Engl. J. Med.*, **1973**, *288*, 277–280.

Richter, J., and Waller, M. B. Effects of pentobarbital on the regulation of acetylcholine content and release in different regions of rat brain. *Biochem. Pharmacol.*, **1977**, *26*, 609–615.

Rickels, K., and Hesbacher, P. T. Over-the-counter daytime sedatives. A controlled study. *J.A.M.A.*, **1973**, *223*, 29–33.

Rosenbaum, J. L.; Kramer, M. S.; and Raja, R. Resin hemoperfusion for acute drug intoxication. *Arch. Intern. Med.*, **1976**, *136*, 263–266.

Safra, M. J., and Oakley, G. P., Jr. Association between cleft lip with or without cleft palate and prenatal exposure to diazepam. *Lancet*, **1975**, *2*, 478–480.

Sagalés, T.; Erill, S.; and Domino, E. F. Effects of repeated doses of scopolamine on the electroencephalographic stages of sleep in normal volunteers. *Clin. Pharmacol. Ther.*, **1977**, *18*, 727–732.

Saletu, B.; Saletu, M.; and Ital, T. Effect of minor and major tranquilizers on somatosensory evoked potentials. *Psychopharmacologia*, **1972**, *24*, 347–358.

Schlosser, W.; Franco, S.; and Sigg, E. B. Differential attenuation of somatovisceral reflexes by diazepam, phenobarbital and diphenylhydantoin. *Neuropharmacology*, **1975**, *14*, 525–531.

Seitz, W.; Hempelman, G.; and Piepenbrock, S. Zur kardiovaskulären Wirkung von Flunitrazepam (ROHYPNOL, Ro-5-4200). *Anaesthesist*, **1977**, *26*, 249–256.

Sellers, E. M.; Carr, G.; Bernstein, J. G.; Sellers, S.; and Koch-Weser, J. Interaction of chloral hydrate and ethanol in man. II. Hemodynamics and performance. *Clin. Pharmacol. Ther.*, **1972**, *13*, 50–58.

Sethy, V. H. Effects of hypnotic and anxiolytic agents on regional concentrations of acetylcholine in rat brain. *Naunyn Schmiedebergs Arch. Pharmacol.*, **1978**, *301*, 157–161.

Seyama, I., and Narahashi, T. Mechanism of blockade of neuromuscular transmission by pentobarbital. *J. Pharmacol. Exp. Ther.*, **1975**, *192*, 95–104.

Sharp, H. L., and Mirkin, B. L. Effect of phenobarbital on hyperbilirubinemia, bile acid metabolism, and microsomal enzyme activity in chronic intrahepatic cholestasis of childhood. *J. Pediatr.*, **1972**, *81*, 116–126.

Smith, A., and Rawlins, M. D. Benzodiazepines. *Br. Med. J.*, **1977**, *2*, 447.

Smith, A. R. Barbiturate protection in cerebral hypoxia. *Anesthesiology*, **1977**, *47*, 285–293.

Snyder, S. H.; Enna, S. J.; and Young, A. B. Brain mechanisms associated with therapeutic actions of benzodiazepines: focus on neurotransmitters. *Am. J. Psychiatry,* **1977,** *134,* 662–665.

Speth, R. C.; Wastek, G. J.; Johnson, P. C.; and Yamamura, H. I. Benzodiazepine binding in human brain: characterization using [³H]flunitrazepam. *Life Sci.,* **1978,** *22,* 859–866.

Stalker, N. E.; Gambertoglio, J. G.; Fukumitsu, C. J.; Naughton, J. L.; and Benet, L. Z. Acute massive chloral hydrate intoxication treated with hemodialysis: a clinical pharmacokinetic analysis. *J. Clin. Pharmacol.,* **1978,** *18,* 136–142.

Stein, L.; Wise, C. D.; and Berger, B. D. Antianxiety action of benzodiazepines: decrease in activity of serotonin neurons in the punishment system. In, *The Benzodiazepines.* (Garattini, S.; Mussini, E.; and Randall, L. O.; eds.) Raven Press, New York, **1973,** pp. 299–326.

Stern, L.; Khanna, N. N.; Levy, G.; and Yaffe, S. J. Effect of phenobarbital on hyperbilirubinemia and glucuronide formation in newborns. *Am. J. Dis. Child.,* **1970,** *120,* 26–31.

Stiehl, A.; Thaler, M.; and Amirand, W. H. Effects of phenobarbital on bile salt metabolism in cholestasis due to intrahepatic bile duct hyplasia. *Pediatrics,* **1973,** *51,* 992–997.

Sundwall, A. Effect of pentobarbital on the turnover of acetylcholine in brain nerve terminals *in vivo. Brain Res.,* **1973,** *62,* 531–536.

Sutton, I., and Simmonds, M. A. Effects of acute and chronic pentobarbitone on the γ-aminobutyric acid system in rat brain. *Biochem. Pharmacol.,* **1974,** *23,* 1801–1808.

Tang, B. K.; Inaba, T.; and Kalow, W. N-Hydroxylation of pentobarbital in man. *Drug Metab. Dispos.,* **1977,** *5,* 71–74.

Ticku, M. K., and Olsen, R. W. Interaction of barbiturates with dihydropicrotoxinin binding sites related to the GABA receptor–ionophore system. *Life Sci.,* **1978,** *22,* 1643–1651.

Tsuchiya, T. Effects of 1,4-benzodiazepines with a long side chain in position 1 on the evoked potentials recorded in the limbic system and hypothalamus. *Neuropharmacology,* **1977,** *16,* 259–266.

Tsuchiya, T., and Fukushima, H. Effects of benzodiazepines on PGO firings and multiple unit activity in the midbrain reticular formation in cat. *Electroencephalogr. Clin. Neurophysiol.,* **1977,** *43,* 700–706.

Tsuchiya, T., and Kitigawa, S. Effects of benzodiazepines and pentobarbital on the evoked potentials in the cat brain. *Jpn. J. Pharmacol.,* **1976,** *26,* 411–418.

Tye, N. C.; Sahgal, A.; and Iverson, S. D. Benzodiazepines and discrimination behavior: dissociation of response and sensory factors. *Psychopharmacology,* **1977,** *52,* 191–194.

Tzeng, S., and Ho, I. K. Effect of acute and continuous pentobarbital administration on the gamma-aminobutyric acid system. *Biochem. Pharmacol.,* **1977,** *26,* 699–704.

Udall, J. A. Clinical implications of warfarin interactions with five sedatives. *Am. J. Cardiol.,* **1975,** *35,* 67–69.

Vale, J. A.; Rees, A. J.; Widdop, B.; and Goulding, R. Use of charcoal hemoperfusion in the management of severely poisoned patients. *Br. Med. J.,* **1975,** *1,* 5–9.

Veldkamp, W.; Straw, R. N.; Metzler, C. M.; and Demissianos, H. V. Efficacy and residual effect evaluation of a new hypnotic, triazolam. *J. Clin. Pharmacol.,* **1974,** *14,* 102–111.

Wahlström, G., and Eckwall, T. Tolerance to hexobarbital and supersensitivity to pilocarpine after chronic barbital treatment in the rat. *Eur. J. Pharmacol.,* **1976,** *38,* 123–129.

Watts, R. W. E.; Chalmers, R. A.; Liberman, M. M.; and Lawson, A. M. Some biochemical effects of chloral hydrate in an infant with a tyrosinemia-like syndrome. *Pediatr. Res.,* **1975,** *9,* 875–878.

Welch, L. T.; Bower, J. D.; Ott, C. E.; and Hume, A. S. Oil

dialysis for ethchlorvynol intoxication. *Clin. Pharmacol. Ther.,* **1972,** *13,* 745–749.

Wise, R. A., and Chinerman, J. Effects of diazepam and phenobarbital on electrically-induced amygdaloid seizures and seizure development. *Exp. Neurol.,* **1974,** *45,* 355–363.

Wolf, P., and Haas, H. L. Effects of diazepines and barbiturates on hippocampal recurrent inhibition. *Naunyn Schmiedebergs Arch. Pharmacol.,* **1977,** *299,* 211–218.

Wolff, B. B. Evaluation of hypnotics in outpatients with insomnia using a questionnaire and a self-rating technique. *Clin. Pharmacol. Ther.,* **1974,** *15,* 130–140.

Young, R. E.; Ramsay, L. E.; and Murray, T. S. Barbiturates and serum calcium in the elderly. *Postgrad. Med.,* **1977,** *53,* 212–215.

Monographs and Reviews

Allgulander, C. Dependence on sedative and hypnotic drugs. *Acta Psychiatr. Scand.,* **1978,** Suppl. 270, 1–120.

Ascione, F. J. Benzodiazepines with alcohol. *Drug Ther.,* **1978,** *9,* 58–71.

Bixler, E. O.; Scharf, M. B.; Leo, L. A.; and Kales, A. Hypnotic drugs and performance. A review of theoretical and methodological considerations. In, *Hypnotics: Methods of Development and Evaluation.* (Kagan, F.; Harwood, T.; Rickels, K.; Rudzik, A. D.; and Sorer, H.; eds.) Spectrum Publications, Inc., New York, **1975,** pp. 175–194.

Bloom, F. E. Neural mechanisms of benzodiazepine actions. *Am. J. Psychiatry,* **1977,** *134,* 669–672.

Breimer, D. D. Clinical pharmacokinetics of hypnotics. *Clin. Pharmacokinet.,* **1977,** *2,* 93–109.

Browne, T. R. Clonazepam. A review of a new anticonvulsant drug. *Arch. Neurol.,* **1976,** *33,* 326–332.

Clark, D. L., and Rosner, B. S. Neurophysiologic effects of general anesthetics. I. The electroencephalogram and sensory evoked responses in man. *Anesthesiology,* **1973,** *38,* 564–582. (114 references.)

Costa, E., and Greengard, P. (eds.). *Mechanism of Action of Benzodiazepines.* Raven Press, New York, **1975.**

Costa, E.; Guidotti, A.; Mao, C. C.; and Suria, A. New concepts on the mechanism of action of benzodiazepines. *Life Sci.,* **1975,** *17,* 167–186. (59 references.)

Costa, E.; Guidotti, A.; and Toffano, G. Molecular mechanisms mediating the action of diazepam on GABA receptors. *Br. J. Psychiatry,* **1978,** *133,* 239–248.

Dundee, J. W., and Haslett, W. H. K. The benzodiazepines: a review of their actions and uses relative to anaesthetic practice. *Br. J. Anaesth.,* **1970,** *42,* 217–234.

Dundee, J. W., and Keilty, S. R. Diazepam. *Int. Anesthesiol. Clin.,* **1969,** *7,* 91–121.

Forney, R. B., and Hughes, F. W. *Combined Effects of Alcohol and Other Drugs.* Charles C Thomas, Pub., Springfield, Ill., **1968.**

Freudenthal, R. I., and Carroll, F. I. Metabolism of certain commonly used barbiturates. *Drug Metab. Rev.,* **1973,** *2,* 265–278. (42 references.)

Garattini, S.; Mussini, E.; and Randall, L. O. (eds.). *The Benzodiazepines.* Raven Press, New York, **1973.**

Greenblatt, D. J., and Shader, R. I. Meprobamate: a study of irrational drug use. *Am. J. Psychiatry,* **1971,** *127,* 1297–1303. (72 references.)

———. The clinical choice of sedative-hypnotics. *Ann. Intern. Med.,* **1972,** *77,* 91–100. (138 references.)

———. Benzodiazepines. *N. Engl. J. Med.,* **1974a,** *291,* 1011–1015, 1239–1243. (34 references.)

———. *Benzodiazepines in Clinical Practice.* Raven Press, New York, **1974b.**

Greenblatt, D. J.; Shader, R. I.; and Koch-Weser, J. Flurazepam hydrochloride. *Clin. Pharmacol. Ther.,* **1975a,** *17,* 1–14.

———. Flurazepam hydrochloride, a benzodiazepine hypnotic. *Ann. Intern. Med.,* **1975b,** *83,* 237–241.

Guidotti, A.; Toffano, G.; and Costa, E. An endogenous

protein modulates the affinity of GABA and benzodiazepine receptors in rat brain. *Nature,* **1978,** *275,* 553–555.

Haefely, W. E. Synaptic pharmacology of barbiturates and benzodiazepines. *Agents Actions,* **1977,** *7,* 353–359.

Hartmann, E. Drugs for insomnia. *Ration. Drug Ther.,* **1977,** *11,* No. 12, 1–5.

Johns, M. W. Sleep and hypnotic drugs. *Drugs,* **1975,** *9,* 448–478. (95 references.)

Kagan, F.; Harwood, T.; Rickels, K.; Rudzik, A. D.; and Sorer, H. (eds.). *Hypnotics: Methods of Development and Evaluation.* Spectrum Publications, Inc., New York, **1975.**

Kales, A.; Kales, J.; and Bixler, E. O. Insomnia: an approach to management and treatment. *Psychiatr. Ann.,* **1974,** *4,* 28–44.

Kales, A.; Kales, J.; Bixler, E. O.; and Martin, E. Common shortcomings in the evaluation and treatment of insomnia. In, *Hypnotics: Methods of Development and Evaluation.* (Kagan, F.; Harwood, T.; Rickels, K.; Rudzik, A. D.; and Sorer, H.; eds.) Spectrum Publications, Inc., New York, **1975,** pp. 29–40.

Kay, D. C.; Blackburn, A. B.; Buckingham, J. A.; and Karacan, I. Human pharmacology of sleep. In, *Pharmacology of Sleep.* (Williams, R. L., and Karacan, I., eds.) John Wiley & Sons, Inc., New York, **1976,** pp. 83–210. (294 references.)

Mann, J. B., and Sandberg, D. H. Therapy of sedative overdosage. *Pediatr. Clin. North Am.,* **1970,** *17,* 617–628.

Matthew, H. (ed.). *Acute Barbiturate Poisoning.* Excerpta Medica, Amsterdam, **1971.**

Mendelson, W. B.; Gillin, J. C.; and Wyatt, R. J. *Human Sleep and Its Disorders.* Plenum Press, New York, **1977.**

Oswald, I. Dependence upon hypnotic and sedative drugs. In, *Contemporary Psychiatry: Selected Reviews from the British Journal of Hospital Medicine.* (Silverstone, T., and Barraclough, B., eds.) Headey Brothers, Ltd., Asford, **1976,** pp. 272–277.

Randall, L. O., and Kappell, B. Pharmacological activity of some benzodiazepines and their metabolites. In, *The Benzodiazepines.* (Garattini, S.; Mussini, E.; and Randall, L. O.; eds.) Raven Press, New York, **1973,** pp. 27–51. (38 references.)

Randall, L. O.; Schallek, W.; Sternbach, L. H.; and Ning, R. Y. Chemistry and pharmacology of the 1,4-benzodiazepines. In, *Psychopharmacological Agents.* (Gordon, M., ed.) Academic Press, Inc., New York, **1974,** pp. 175–281.

Robinson, R. R.; Gunnels, J. C., Jr.; and Clapp, J. R. Treatment of acute barbiturate intoxication. *Mod. Treat.,* **1971,** *8,* 561–579.

Rosner, B. S., and Clark, D. L. Neurophysiologic effects of general anesthestics. II. Sequential regional actions in the brain. *Anesthesiology,* **1973,** *39,* 59–81. (181 references.)

Rudzik, A. D.; Hester, J. B.; Tang, A. H.; Straw, R. N.; and Friis, W. Triazolobenzodiazepines, a new class of central nervous system–depressant compounds. In, *The Benzodiazepines.* (Garattini, S.; Mussini, E.; and Randall, L. O.; eds.) Raven Press, New York, **1973,** pp. 285–297.

Schallek, W.; Schlosser, W.; and Randall, L. O. Recent developments in the pharmacology of the benzodiazepines. *Adv. Pharmacol. Chemother.,* **1972,** *10,* 119–183.

Snyder, S. H., and Enna, S. J. The role of central glycine receptors in the pharmacological actions of benzodiazepines. In, *Mechanism of Action of Benzodiazepines.* (Costa, E., and Greengard, P., eds.) Raven Press, New York, **1975,** pp. 81–91.

Solomon, F.; White, C. C.; Parron, D. L.; and Mendelson, W. B. Sleeping pills, insomnia and medical practice. *N. Engl. J. Med.,* **1979,** *300,* 803–808.

Spear, P. W., and Protass, L. M. Barbiturate poisoning—an endemic disease. Five years' experience in a municipal hospital. *Med. Clin. North Am.,* **1973,** *57,* 1471–1479.

Sternbach, L. H. Chemistry of 1,4-benzodiazepines and some aspects of the structure-activity relationship. In, *The Benzodiazepines.* (Garattini, S.; Mussini, E.; and Randall, L. O.; eds.) Raven Press, New York, **1973,** pp. 1–26.

Symposium. (Various authors.) Oxazepam update. (Ayd, F. J., Jr., ed.) *Dis. Nerv. Syst.,* **1975,** *36,* No. 5, Sect. 2, 1–32.

Symposium. (Various authors.) Central action of benzodiazepines. *Br. J. Psychiatry,* **1978,** *133,* 231–268.

Thompson, T., and Unna, K. R. (eds.). *Predicting Dependence Liability of Stimulant and Depressant Drugs.* University Park Press, Baltimore, **1976.**

Wikler, A. Review of research on sedative drug dependence at the addiction research center and University of Kentucky. In, *Predicting Dependence Liability of Stimulant and Depressant Drugs.* (Thompson, T., and Unna, K. R., eds.) University Park Press, Baltimore, **1976,** pp. 147–163.

Zbinden, G., and Randall, L. O. Pharmacology of benzodiazepines: laboratory and clinical correlations. *Adv. Pharmacol.,* **1967,** *5,* 213–291.

18 THE ALIPHATIC ALCOHOLS

J. Murdoch Ritchie

ETHYL ALCOHOL

Alcoholic beverages have been used since the dawn of history, and the opinions and traditions of the past often cloud the discussion of this subject. The oldest alcoholic drinks were fermented beverages of relatively low alcohol content, that is, the beers and wines. When the Arabs introduced the then recent technic of distilling into Europe in the Middle Ages, the alchemists believed that alcohol was the long-sought elixir of life. Alcohol was therefore held to be a remedy for practically all diseases, as indicated by the term *whisky* (Gaelic: *usquebaugh,* meaning "water of life"). It is now recognized that the therapeutic value of alcohol is much more limited than its social value.

PHARMACOLOGICAL PROPERTIES

Local Actions. Alcohol injures cells by precipitating and dehydrating protoplasm, and can therefore act as an astringent. It is also an irritant to denuded surfaces and to mucosae. The more concentrated the alcohol, the more pronounced are its effects.

Skin. Alcohol cools the skin by evaporation, and so alcohol sponges are commonly used in fever. Alcohol rubbed on the skin produces mild redness and burning, and it is therefore employed as a counterirritant and rubefacient. It is often used in bedridden patients to prevent bedsores and decubitus ulcers, for it hardens and cleans the skin and helps to prevent sweating.

Mucous Membranes. The irritant action of alcohol is particularly marked on mucosae. High concentrations may produce considerable inflammation of the gastric mucosa, for example.

Subcutaneous Tissues. Alcohol injected hypodermically causes considerable pain followed by anesthesia. If the injection is made close to nerves, neuritis and nerve degeneration may occur. Injections in or near nerves are deliberately used to cause anesthesia of protracted or even permanent character in the treatment of severe pain, for example, in *tic douloureux.*

Action on Bacteria. The bactericidal action of alcohol is discussed in Chapter 41.

Peripheral Nerves. Alcohol blocks conduction in peripheral nerve by decreasing the maximal values of both the sodium and the potassium conductances. The resting potential usually becomes slightly less negative. While it is tempting to ascribe the central effects of alcohol to its ability to block nervous conduction, the concentrations required for peripheral blockade (about 5 to 10%) are greatly in excess of those needed to produce the central effects (*see* Wallgren and Barry, 1970; Israel *et al.,* 1971).

Central Nervous System. The central nervous system (CNS) is more markedly affected by alcohol than any other system of the body. The question whether alcohol is a "stimulant" has long been debated. Laymen in particular view alcoholic drinks as stimulating. However, there seems little doubt that alcohol, like other general anesthetics, is a primary and continuous depressant of the CNS. The apparent stimulation results from the unrestrained activity of various parts of the brain that have been freed from inhibition as a result of the depression of inhibitory control mechanisms.

Electrophysiological studies suggest that alcohol, like other general anesthetics, exerts its first depressant action upon those parts of the brain involved in the most highly integrated functions. The polysynaptic structures of the reticular activating system and certain cortical sites are particularly susceptible (Himwich and Callison, 1972). The cortex is thus released from its integrating control. As a result, the various processes related to thought occur in a jumbled, disorganized fashion and the smooth operation of motor processes becomes disrupted. The first mental processes to be affected are those that depend on training and previous experience and that usually make for sobriety and self-restraint. The finer grades of discrimination, memory, concentration, and insight are dulled and then lost. Confidence abounds, the personality becomes expansive and vivacious, and speech may become eloquent and occasionally brilliant. Mood swings are uncontrolled and emotional outbursts frequent.

These psychic changes are accompanied by sensory and motor disturbances. For example, spinal reflexes are at first enhanced because they have been freed from central inhibitions; as intoxication becomes more advanced, however, this first phase of enhanced reflex activity is succeeded by a general impairment of nervous function and a condition of general anesthesia ultimately prevails.

Carefully performed experiments have shown that, in general, alcohol increases neither mental nor physical abilities. Although the individual often firmly believes that his performance is greatly improved, psychometric tests involving typewriting, target practice, and complicated mental problems indicate that efficiency is, in fact, decreased. Tasks requiring less skill, thought, and attention are less markedly affected, especially if they are mechanical in nature (*see* Wallgren and Barry, 1970). However, alcohol may cause some improvement in performance in *special* circumstances; for example, if a person's mental inhibitions prevent him from carrying out a task at which he is normally skilled, *moderate* amounts of alcohol, by relieving the inhibitions, may allow him to function more effectively.

In general, the effects of alcohol on the CNS are proportional to the concentration of alcohol in the blood (*see* Maling, 1970). However, the effects are more marked when the concentration is rising than when it is falling. If the rate of absorption of alcohol from the gastrointestinal tract is rapid, a relatively high blood concentration may result from the ingestion of quite a small amount of alcohol. The same applies if the fraction of the cardiac output delivered to tissues such as muscle is low compared to brain; an effect on the CNS is then rapidly obtained. However, redistribution of the alcohol soon occurs and the effects, as a result, are relatively brief.

Alcohol differs from the volatile general anesthetics in that over 90% of it is oxidized in the body and relatively little is excreted unchanged. The rate of oxidation is low, with the result that general anesthesia from alcohol lasts much longer than does that from conventional inhalational anesthetics. There is little margin between the full surgical anesthetic dose and that which is dangerous to respiration. For these reasons alcohol is not employed as a general anesthetic. It is still occasionally used as an analgesic and hypnotic, but much more so by the laity than by the medical profession. The ingestion of 60 ml of 95% alcohol raises the pain threshold approximately 35 to 40%, but it does not alter other sensory perceptions. Like morphine, alcohol also causes euphoria, and it changes the patient's reaction to pain from one of concern to one of relative detachment. The neurological and physiological effects of alcohol have been reviewed by Trémolières (1970), Wallgren and Barry (1970), Kissin and Begleiter (1971, 1972, 1974), Gross (1977), and in a report by the U.S. Department of Health, Education, and Welfare (1978).

Chronic excessive ingestion of ethanol is directly associated with serious neurological and mental disorders (*e.g.*, brain damage, memory loss, sleep disturbances, and psychoses). In addition, nutritional and vitamin deficiencies, incident to the poor food intake or the faulty gastrointestinal function of the alcoholic (*see* Hillman, 1974), seem to cause many neuropsychiatric syndromes that are common in alcoholics, such as Wernicke's encephalopathy, Korsakoff's psychosis, polyneuritis, and nicotinic acid deficiency encephalopathy (*see* Wallgren and Barry, 1970; Turner *et al.*, 1977; Chapter 66).

Respiration. Moderate amounts of alcohol in man may stimulate or depress respiration; the ventilatory response to carbon dioxide is, however, always depressed (Johnstone and Reier, 1973). Large amounts (sufficient to produce a blood concentration of 400 mg/dl or more) produce dangerous or lethal depression of respiration.

EEG. Alcohol produces a slowing of the alpha rhythm of the brain, and this effect becomes particularly prominent as intoxication develops. Chronic alcoholics, however, show no consistent, permanent pathological changes in rhythm (Begleiter and Platz, 1972; Turner *et al.*, 1977).

Anticonvulsant Action. In laboratory animals, alcohol can effectively *suppress convulsions* induced by pentylenetetrazol and by electroshock (McQuarrie and Fingl, 1958; Workman *et al.*, 1958), but only in amounts that cause general depression of the CNS. The anticonvulsant action is followed by a period of hyperexcitability that lasts from 12 hours (after a single dose) to several days (after cessation of chronic administration). This is presumably one reason why alcohol may precipitate convulsions in man and why some advocate that it not be ingested by patients with epilepsy.

Brain Metabolism. Many attempts have been

made to find a metabolic basis for the effects of ethanol on the CNS, but these have not had much success. Thus, any effect of alcohol on tissue respiration in the whole animal or *in vitro* is slight or absent. Effects that are seen appear to be secondary to the functional changes produced by alcohol in the neurons (*see* Wallgren, 1971).

Cardiovascular System. The *immediate* effects of alcohol on the circulation are relatively minor (Wallgren and Barry, 1970; Zsotér and Sellers, 1977). The blood pressure, cardiac output, and force of myocardial contraction do not change significantly after a moderate amount of alcohol. The pulse rate may increase, but this is usually due to muscular activity or reflex stimulation. The cardiovascular depression that is observed in acute severe alcoholic intoxication is due mainly to central vasomotor factors and to the respiratory depression. A direct depression of the heart by alcohol has been observed following its acute administration to experimental animals; both myocardial contractility and working efficiency may be adversely affected by a blood concentration as low as 100 mg/dl (Wallgren and Barry, 1970).

Recent studies make it clear that chronic excessive use of alcohol has a deleterious effect on the heart (*see* Myerson, 1971; Burch and Giles, 1974; Regan *et al.*, 1977). Electron microscopic observations reveal characteristic intracellular lesions in the myocardium, associated with congestive heart failure; prognosis for return of muscle function is guarded. Other cardiovascular abnormalities occasionally observed in chronic heavy drinkers are largely the result of malnutrition and vitamin deficiency (*see* Hillman, 1974). The precise role of alcohol in the etiology of alcoholic cardiomyopathy is unclear (Turner *et al.*, 1977).

Alcohol in moderate doses causes vasodilatation, especially of the cutaneous vessels, and produces a warm and flushed skin. The vasodilatation is most likely the result of central vasomotor depression, because the direct action of alcohol on blood vessels is insignificant. The widespread belief that the coronary arteries are dilated and that the coronary blood flow is increased by moderate doses of alcohol is unsupported by acceptable laboratory or clinical evidence. Although alcohol compares favorably with nitroglyc-

erin in its ability to prevent anginal pain in patients with coronary arteriosclerosis subjected to a standard exercise test, it does not prevent the characteristic changes in the RS-T segments and the T waves of the ECG that are associated with myocardial ischemia, implying that alcohol does not improve oxygenation of cardiac muscle. This suggests that any salutary response to alcohol observed in angina pectoris is probably due to its central depressant properties (*see* Wallgren and Barry, 1970). Alcohol administered to human subjects in doses sufficient to produce facial vasodilatation and mild inebriation causes no change in cerebral blood flow, cerebral metabolism, or cerebral vascular resistance. A plasma concentration associated with severe alcoholic intoxication (300 mg/dl) does indeed markedly increase mean cerebral blood flow and diminish cerebrovascular resistance. However, cerebral oxygen uptake is much reduced (*see* Wallgren, 1971). There is no rational basis, therefore, for the use of alcohol as a vasodilator in patients with cerebrovascular disease. Furthermore, several studies (*see* Klatsky *et al.*, 1977) indicate that regular use of large amounts of alcohol results in a higher-than-normal blood pressure. Alcohol may thus be a risk factor for hypertension.

Plasma Lipoproteins. In contrast to the potential deleterious effects of alcohol on the cardiovascular system described above, several studies show a clear negative correlation between chronic ingestion of ethanol and the incidence of coronary heart disease. This protective effect may occur because ethanol increases the concentration of α- or high-density lipoproteins and decreases that of β- or low-density lipoproteins in plasma (Yano *et al.*, 1977). Apparently the lower the concentration of high-density lipoprotein in blood, the greater is the risk of coronary heart disease (Gordon *et al.*, 1977; *see* Chapter 34).

Skeletal Muscle. The total amount of work accomplished by an individual under the influence of small doses of alcohol may increase. This is chiefly the result of the central action of the alcohol, for although alcohol is a readily available source of energy for muscular work and, in addition, may improve the circulation in muscle, the increased performance is largely due to a lessened appreciation of fatigue. Large doses of alcohol cause CNS depression and thereby decrease the amount of muscular work accomplished. Such doses also directly damage the muscle (Song and Rubin, 1972), causing an alcoholic skeletal myopathy similar in many respects to the alcoholic cardiomyopathy (*see* Myerson, 1971; Perkoff, 1971). There is a marked increase in the activity of creatine phosphokinase in plasma, indicative of muscle damage, and striking ultrastructural changes in the muscle.

Body Temperature. After ingestion of alcohol, there is a feeling of warmth because alcohol enhances cutaneous and gastric blood flow. Increased sweating may also occur. Heat is therefore lost more rapidly, and the internal temperature consequently falls. With large amounts of alcohol, the central temperature-regulating mechanism itself becomes depressed and the fall in body temperature may become pronounced. The action of alcohol in lowering body temperature is naturally greater when the environmental temperature is low, or when the mechanisms for dissipating heat are disturbed, as during fever. Although moderate amounts of ethanol (0.2 to 1 g/kg) may have beneficial effects during exposure to cold, heavy intoxication is clearly dangerous if the conservation of body heat is essential (*see* Wallgren and Barry, 1970). Those experienced in polar exploration are well acquainted with the dangers of this temptation.

Gastrointestinal Tract. The effects of various concentrations and types of alcoholic beverages on the gastrointestinal motor and secretory functions are influenced by a number of factors. Among these are the state of the digestive processes, the presence or absence of gastrointestinal disease, the amount and type of food present, the degree of tolerance for alcohol, accompanying psychological factors, and so forth.

Gastric secretions, like salivary secretions, are usually stimulated *psychically* by alcohol, especially if the individual likes it. The gastric juice produced in this way is rich in acid and normal in pepsin content. Alcohol may also *reflexly* stimulate the secretion of salivary and gastric juice by exciting sensory endings in the buccal and gastric mucosae. Finally, alcohol may evoke gastric secretion through a more *direct* action on the stomach, possibly involving the release of gastrin (Cooke, 1975). Alcohol is a very effective stimulus for gastric acid secretion, and, clearly, the drinking of alcoholic beverages is inadvisable in patients with peptic ulcer.

The presence in the stomach of alcohol in concentrations of about 10% results in a gastric secretion rich in acid, but it is poor in pepsin unless psychic secretion is also elicited. However, although the pepsin content is decreased, there is no interference with peptic digestion, and gastric motility is not reduced. As the concentration of alcohol in ingested beverages is raised above about 20%, gastric secretion tends to be inhibited and peptic activity is depressed. Malt liquors and wine cause a similar inhibition even though the alcohol concentrations are relatively low, because they contain colloidal substances, tannins, and organic acids. Strong alcoholic drinks, of 40% concentration and over, are quite irritating to the mucosa and cause congestive hyperemia and inflammation, with an accompanying loss of plasma protein into the gastrointestinal lumen (Chowdhury *et al.*, 1977). In such high concentrations alcohol produces an erosive gastritis (*see* Leevy *et al.*, 1971; Lorber *et al.*, 1974). This may explain why one out of three heavy drinkers suffers from chronic gastritis. The presence of food in the stomach tends to lessen irritation because it decreases the concentration of alcohol by dilution and the concentration of hydrogen ions by its buffering action. Further protection against excessive irritation is afforded by the stomach itself, which responds to the presence of alcohol by secreting mucus that both protects the mucosa and dilutes the alcohol. Aspirin, in the presence of hydrochloric acid, can produce severe gastric damage and brisk gastric bleeding in dogs (Davenport, 1969). This effect is much enhanced by alcohol, and it is caused by an impairment of the mucosal barrier to back diffusion of intraluminal hydrogen ions into the mucosa (Smith *et al.*, 1971). Microscopic examination of the gastrointestinal tract indicates that ethanol damages both the gastric mucosa (Eastwood and Kirchner, 1974) and the intestinal mucosa (Baraona *et al.*, 1974).

The habitual use of immoderate amounts of alcohol may lead to constipation, due probably to an inadequate food intake and an insufficient bulk residue. On the other hand, diarrhea may occur, as a result of the irritant action of certain flavoring oils; in the chronic inebriate, however, it may signify vitamin deficiency or a reduction in intestinal absorption of Na$^+$ and water (Mekhjian and May, 1977). Alcohol taken in moderate amounts does not significantly influence the motor activity of the colon, but taken to the point of intoxication it results in virtual cessation of gastrointestinal secretory and motor functions. Absorption is delayed, and pylorospasm and vomiting may occur independently of any reflex due to local irritation.

Alcohol contributes to the production of lesions of the esophagus and duodenum and is also an etiological factor in acute and chronic pancreatitis (Pirola and Lieber, 1974; Turner et al., 1977). The pancreatitis appears to occur because ethanol produces not only increased secretion but also an obstruction of the pancreatic duct (see Wallgren and Barry, 1970), perhaps as a result of increased plasma concentrations of secretin that have been observed to follow the ingestion of alcohol by normal human subjects (Straus et al., 1975). A spectrum of problems can follow, ranging from the formation of inflammatory cysts and pseudocysts to frank pancreatic insufficiency, with inadequate production of bicarbonate and malabsorption of dietary fat and the fat-soluble vitamins (A, D, E, and K). Early signs and symptoms of this problem can be very subtle and difficult to diagnose.

Liver. Acute alcoholic intoxication in man is probably not associated with any great change in hepatic function. Alcohol increases the rate at which isolated liver slices synthesize fat. This enhanced lipid anabolism seems to be caused by the increased NADH:NAD ratio that results from the oxidation of alcohol. This *direct* effect on the liver would therefore provide a plausible biochemical basis for the finding that alcohol promotes the hepatic accumulation of fat in animals. However, alcohol may also promote the accumulation of fat in the liver *indirectly*, for it causes the mobilization of fat from peripheral tissues. Even after the ingestion of relatively small amounts of alcohol, accumulation of fat in the liver of normal individuals can be demonstrated (see Feinman and Lieber, 1974). While protein synthesis can be inhibited acutely by the ingestion of alcohol,

its prolonged use results in the accumulation of protein in the liver (Baraona and Lieber, 1977). The prognostic implications of the accumulation of fat and protein may at first be benign, but, eventually, these processes become irreversible and can proceed to various stages of hepatic disease that are characteristic of the cirrhosis that is seen in many chronic alcoholics (see Lieber, 1978). Although malnutrition and vitamin deficiency may contribute to these conditions in man (Scheig, 1970; Galambos, 1972; Feinman and Lieber, 1974), experiments in baboons make it clear that these effects are directly caused by ethanol and do not depend upon a dietary inadequacy (Lieber et al., 1975; Lieber, 1978).

There seems no doubt that the *continued* use of *large* amounts of alcohol has serious effects on gastrointestinal and hepatic functions. The crucial problem centers about the occasional use of moderate amounts of alcoholic beverages. It seems that relatively small amounts (between 3 and 6 oz of whisky per day) are not necessarily deleterious. If one enjoys alcohol, it may even affect digestion favorably if taken with meals. The influence of alcohol in the digestive tract has been extensively reviewed by Wallgren and Barry (1970).

Teratogenic Effects. Although suspected for centuries, the *fetal alcohol syndrome* has only recently been fully described. The abnormality, which occurs with a frequency of 4 to 7 per 1000 live births (see Clarren and Smith, 1978), consists in CNS dysfunction (such as low IQ and microcephaly), slowness in growth, a characteristic cluster of facial abnormalities (such as short palpebral fissures, hypoplastic upper lip, and short nose), and a variable set of major and minor malformations. These features may be due, at least in part, to a direct action of ethanol to inhibit embryonic cellular proliferation early in gestation (Brown et al., 1979). Ethanol seems to be the most frequent cause of teratogenically induced mental deficiency that is known in the Western world; even moderate drinking of alcohol is clearly contraindicated during pregnancy.

Longevity and Heredity. Heavy drinkers have a shorter length of life on the average than do abstainers (*see* Schmidt and de Lint, 1973; report by U.S. Department of Health, Education, and Welfare, 1978). However, there appears to be little or no difference in the life expectancy of abstainers as compared to *temperate* drinkers. Existing evidence does not support the claim that alcoholism injures human germ cells. The number of miscarriages tends to be higher in alcoholic women. This is mainly because they are prone to have a larger number of children, and the number of miscarriages increases as the number of conceptions increases. Likewise, the higher infant mortality in alcoholic families is largely due to neglect of the neonate as well as the mother during her pregnancy.

Sexual Functions. It is a popular notion that alcohol is an aphrodisiac; indeed, aggressive sexual behavior is often seen after alcohol, usually as a result of a loss of inhibition and restraint. Shakespeare, however, realized that inebriation interferes with coitus. In *Macbeth,* for example, the following conversation occurs (Act 2, scene 3):

MACDUFF: What three things does drink especially provoke?
PORTER: Marry, sir, nose-painting, sleep, and urine. Lechery, sir, it provokes, and unprovokes; it provokes the desire, but it takes away the performance. . . .

The experiments of Gantt (1952) on the effects of alcohol on the sexual reflexes of normal dogs support the observations of Shakespeare; in neurotic dogs, alcohol has some therapeutic value. Objective measurements of penile tumescence and vaginal pressure show that ethanol significantly decreases sexual responsiveness in both men and women (Wilson, 1977).

In man, chronic ingestion of alcohol may lead to impotence, sterility, and gynecomastia. This feminization in alcoholic men has a dual origin. First, alcohol-induced hepatic injury leads to a hyperestrogenization and a reduced rate of production of testosterone; second, by increasing the activity of the enzymes of the hepatic endoplasmic reticulum, ethanol markedly increases the rate of metabolic inactivation of testosterone (Van Thiel and Lester, 1976; Turner *et al.,* 1977).

Alcohol and Cancer. Compared to the general population, heavy drinkers show markedly excessive mortality from cancers of the mouth, pharynx, larynx, esophagus, liver, and lung (*see* report by U.S. Department of Health, Education, and Welfare, 1978). It is unclear whether this is necessarily a direct effect of ethanol, or if it results from the alcohol acting in cooperation with some other factors, such as smoking or contaminants in food or alcoholic beverages.

Kidney. That alcohol exerts a *diuretic effect* has been established by a number of investigators and by most consumers. Although the large amounts of fluid ordinarily ingested with alcoholic beverages undoubtedly contribute to the increased urine flow, alcohol in itself can be demonstrated to produce a marked diuretic response in man by virtue of a decrease in renal tubular reabsorption of water. Considerable evidence indicates that alcohol causes this diuresis by acting on the supraopticoneurohypophyseal system to inhibit the secretion of antidiuretic hormone. The diuretic effect is roughly proportional to the blood alcohol concentration and occurs when the concentration is rising but not when it is stationary or falling (*see* Wallgren and Barry, 1970). Indeed, alcohol in repeated doses may have an antidiuretic effect (Beard and Knott, 1971).

Although the kidneys of habitual heavy drinkers may not be normal, this cannot necessarily be attributed to alcohol as such. With the possible exception of some individuals with arteriosclerotic nephritis, the ingestion of varying amounts of alcohol has no deleterious action on renal function either in normal subjects or in patients with acute or chronic nephritis.

Endocrine Glands. Relatively large doses of alcohol stimulate the release of adrenocortical hormones by promoting the secretion of corticotropin (*see* Stokes, 1971).

Alcohol, even in moderate doses, produces a prompt increase in urinary excretion of epinephrine, norepinephrine, and their metabolites. This is associated with inhibition of the uptake of catecholamines into cells, leading to a decrease in the catecholamine content of the adrenal medulla and the CNS; 5-hydroxytryptamine is also released from the CNS (Feldstein, 1971). The increased concentration of circulating catecholamines might be partly responsible for the transient hyperglycemia, the pupillary dilatation, and the slight rise in blood pressure that often occur during the early stages of intoxication. It has been suggested that the altered CNS distribution of biogenic amines, particularly 5-hydroxytryptamine, mediates both the sleep and the tolerance associated with alcohol ingestion (*see* Truitt, 1973). Furthermore, the biogenic amines have been implicated in ethanol addiction: opioid-like alkaloids are supposedly formed in the brain by a condensation between biogenic amines and acetaldehyde, a metabolite of ethanol (*see* Myers, 1978; Collins *et al.,* 1979).

Blood. Alcohol produces a number of hematologic effects (*see* Lindenbaum, 1974). Some, such as sideroblastic and megaloblastic anemias, occur only if malnutrition coexists; alcohol also seemingly acts as a weak folate antagonist in man. Other effects, such as thrombocytopenia and vacuolization of the precursors of red and white cells, occur even when the diet is adequate and seem to result from a direct depressant action of alcohol on the bone marrow. There is also a depression of leukocyte migration into inflamed areas, which may partly account for the poor resistance of alcoholics to infection.

Interaction with Other Drugs. The impairment of muscular coordination and of judgment that is associated with ingestion of a moderate amount of alcohol (sufficient to produce a blood concentration of up to

50 mg/dl) may be very much enhanced in a person who has also taken sedatives, hypnotics, anticonvulsants, antidepressants, tranquilizers, or analgesic agents such as propoxyphene or opioids. *Psychopharmacological agents are now so widely used that it is important for the physician to warn patients given such medication of the enhanced effects of alcohol and of the consequent increased danger of driving an automobile after drinking alcohol.*

Unusual side effects may occur when alcohol is taken in association with other drugs. For example, patients treated with oral hypoglycemic agents may experience unpleasant symptoms similar to those experienced by patients who take disulfiram after the ingestion of alcohol (*see* below). The combination of alcohol and an oral hypoglycemic agent may also cause unpredictable fluctuations of plasma glucose concentrations, apparently because of an additive hypoglycemic effect of alcohol and because chronic consumption of ethanol can decrease the half-life of tolbutamide. Alcohol may also interfere with the therapeutic actions of a wide variety of drugs, for example, the coumarin type of anticoagulant, by enhancement of their metabolism. The possible relationships between such interactions and the metabolism of alcohol by the hepatic microsomal oxidase system is discussed below (page 383). As mentioned above, the irritant effect of alcohol on the gastric mucosa may be responsible for increased bleeding when salicylates are taken concurrently. An excellent compendium of references to such interactions has been prepared by Polacsek and coworkers (1972). (*See also* Kissin, 1974; Pirola, 1978.)

Absorption, Fate, and Excretion. *Absorption.* Alcohol is rapidly absorbed from the stomach, small intestine, and colon. Vaporized alcohol can be absorbed through the lungs, and fatal intoxication has occurred as a result of its inhalation. It can also be absorbed from subcutaneous sites; however, if the concentration is excessive the astringent action of alcohol prevails, with the result that the local blood supply is effectively shut off and, in consequence, absorption is limited. Absorption of alcohol through the human skin is negligible.

Many factors modify the absorption of alcohol from the *stomach*. At first absorption is rapid, but then it decreases to a very slow rate although the gastric concentration is still high. If the emptying of the stomach is delayed, for example, by pylorospasm due to high concentrations of alcohol, the subsequent absorption of alcohol from the intestine will also be delayed. The volume, character, and dilution of the alcoholic beverage, the presence of food, the period of time taken to ingest the drink, and individual peculiarities are major influences on the rate at which the stomach empties. Depending on these factors, complete absorption may require from 2 to 6 hours or more. With increasing concentration of ingested alcohol, absorption is facilitated until concentrations are reached that impede absorption. Most foods in the stomach tend to retard absorption, milk being especially efficacious. Beer exerts a retarding action, like that of food.

Absorption from the *small intestine* is extremely rapid and complete, and it is largely independent of the presence of food in the stomach or intestine. Some carbohydrates have actually been noted to augment the rate of intestinal absorption of ethanol (Broitman et al., 1976). The rapidity of absorption of alcohol from the small intestine is probably the reason why patients who have undergone gastrectomy may complain that they become intoxicated by amounts of alcohol that would have been innocuous prior to the operation (Muehlberger, 1958). Indeed, the time of gastric emptying and, consequently, of the onset of the phase of extremely rapid intestinal absorption may well be the prime factor that determines the wide variety of rates of absorption of ingested alcohol that are seen in different individuals and under different conditions.

Distribution in the Body. After absorption, alcohol is fairly uniformly distributed throughout all tissues and all fluids of the body. The plasma concentration is somewhat higher than that in erythrocytes. The placenta is permeable to alcohol; thus, alcohol gains free access to the fetal circulation. Inasmuch as alcohol affects primarily the CNS, much attention has been focused on the concentration in the brain, where, as a result of a large blood supply, the concentration of alcohol quickly approaches that of the blood.

The amount of alcohol in brains of persons dying of alcoholic intoxication varies from 300 to 600 mg/100 g. Alcohol is also present in cerebrospinal fluid, at a concentration lower than that in the blood when the blood concentration is rising and higher when the blood concentration is falling.

Metabolism. Ninety to 98% of the alcohol that enters the body is completely oxidized. The metabolism of alcohol differs from that of most substances in that the rate of oxidation is constant with time, and it is little increased by raising the concentration in the blood (zero-order kinetics). The amount of alcohol oxidized per unit of time is roughly proportional to body weight and probably to liver weight. In the adult, the *average* rate at which alcohol can be metabolized is about 10 ml per hour. Thus, the alcohol in about 120 ml (4 oz) of whisky or 1.2 liters of beer would require 5 to 6 hours to be oxidized by a person of average size. The relatively slow and constant rate of metabolism places a definite limit on the amount of alcohol that can be consumed over a given period of time without an individual becoming drunk due to an accumulation of alcohol. Direct determination in man indicates that the *maximal* daily metabolism of alcohol is about 450 ml (*see* Kalant, 1971; *see also* Appendix II). Various dietary, hormonal, and pharmacological factors can alter the metabolism of alcohol. For example, starvation lowers and insulin increases the rate of oxidation of alcohol. However, such effects are slight and probably have little significance in the treatment of acute alcoholic intoxication (*see* Stokes, 1971).

The initial oxidation of alcohol occurs chiefly in the liver, and the rate of metabolism is considerably reduced in hepatectomized animals. The primary step is the oxidation of alcohol to acetaldehyde by *alcohol dehydrogenase,* which is a zinc-containing enzyme of molecular weight about 80,000 that utilizes NAD as the hydrogen acceptor (*see* Wartburg, 1971). The acetaldehyde is converted to acetyl coenzyme A, which is then oxidized through the citric acid cycle or utilized in the various anabolic reactions involved in the synthesis of cholesterol, fatty acids, and other tissue constituents. Many metabolic changes accompany or follow the metabolism of alcohol. Some changes, such as the increased production of lactate and fatty acid, the hyperuricemia, and, possibly, the decreases in the hepatic citric acid cycle activity and in fatty acid oxidation, seem to be a direct consequence of the increased NADH:NAD ratio produced by the oxidation of the alcohol (*see* Lieber *et al.,* 1975). The causes of a variety of other metabolic changes, including a decrease in urinary excretion of uric acid and an enhanced urinary loss of magnesium, calcium, and zinc, are obscure (Flink, 1971).

Alcohol can also be metabolized to acetaldehyde by another system of enzymes, namely, the microsomal mixed-function oxidases that occur in the smooth endoplasmic reticulum of the liver. The extent to which this system metabolizes ethanol in man is probably very small, but it provides one basis for the known interactions between ethanol and the host of other drugs also metabolized by this system (*see* Teschke *et al.,* 1977; Pirola, 1978). For example, ethanol first decreases and then increases the activity of the enzymes of the hepatic endoplasmic reticulum. Rubin and Lieber (1968) have suggested that this dual effect might explain why chronic alcoholics when inebriated are less resistant than normal individuals to barbiturates, but are more resistant when sober.

Alcohol as a Food. Alcohol is a ready, albeit expensive, source of energy that is utilized more rapidly than most foods because it is quickly absorbed from the gastrointestinal tract and requires no preliminary digestion. The energy released per gram of ethyl alcohol is approximately 7 kcal. Some alcoholic beverages also contain protein and carbohydrate; for example, beer contains about 500 kcal per liter, only half of which is provided by its alcohol content. In contrast, distilled spirits contain no such foodstuffs, and their calories are derived purely from alcohol. Moreover, they contain no vitamins. Many of the diseases of chronic alcoholics occur because they may supply one half or more of their daily caloric requirements by drinking alcohol, and frequently continue to do so for many years. As a result, they may neglect to eat other foods that would balance their diet, and vitamin and other dietary deficiencies develop.

Excretion. Normally about 2% of ingested alcohol escapes oxidation; under special circumstances, such as when large doses of alcohol have been consumed, this value may be as high as 10%. Although small amounts of alcohol can be detected in sweat, tears, bile, gastric juice, saliva, and other secretions, most of the alcohol that escapes oxidation is excreted through the kidneys and lungs. Simple arithmetic explains why attempts to hasten significantly the emergence from intoxication by the use of diuretics or agents inducing hyperpnea are doomed to failure. At most, the concentration in the urine is slightly greater than, and the concentration in the alveolar air only 0.05%, that of the blood. A severely intoxicated individual with a blood alcohol concentration of 300 mg/dl therefore could lose at most about 3 g of alcohol per liter of urine and about 0.2 g per 100 liters of expired air.

Tolerance and Addiction to Alcohol. The repeated use of alcohol results in the development of tolerance, so that larger doses must be taken in order to produce characteristic effects. However, the degree of tolerance is not as marked as for morphine and nicotine. Tolerance and addiction to alcohol are discussed in Chapter 23.

Acute Alcoholic Intoxication. The characteristic signs and symptoms of alcoholic intoxication are well known. Nevertheless, the erroneous diagnosis of drunkenness is often made in patients who appear inebriated, but who have not ingested alcohol. Diabetic coma, for example, may be mistaken for severe alcoholic intoxication. Drug intoxications, cardiovascular accidents, and fractured skulls seem to be common causes for the diagnostic errors (*see* Morgan and Cagan, 1974). The odor of the breath, which is *not* due to any alcohol vapor but to impurities in the alcoholic beverages or to other causes, is a notoriously unreliable guide and may often be seriously misleading. For medicolegal purposes, the concentration of alcohol in the blood, exhaled air, or urine should be determined.

In severe acute alcoholic intoxication the patient is stuporous or comatose. The skin is cold and clammy, the body temperature is low, respirations are slow and noisy, the pupils may be normal or dilated, and the heart rate is accelerated. If this condition persists for 8 or 10 hours, hypostatic pneumonia or increased intracranial pressure may ensue. Death is rare unless unconsciousness continues for many hours or trauma, infection, or the concurrent ingestion of other CNS depressants complicates the case. Recovery is jeopardized if deep coma persists for over 12 hours.

Treatment. The patient should be kept warm. The stomach may be lavaged, but care must be taken to prevent pulmonary aspiration of the return flow. Analeptics such as pentylenetetrazol or caffeine have no value. If significant respiratory depression is present, steps should be taken to protect the airway from aspiration and to provide ventilatory assistance if indicated. Increased intracranial pressure due to cerebral edema is treated by the usual medical measures, such as hypertonic mannitol solution intravenously, spinal fluid drainage, and so forth. Since ethanol is so freely miscible in water, it lends itself ideally to removal by hemodialysis (*see* Morgan and Cagan, 1974). In general, the therapy of the type of acute alcoholic intoxication where the patient is somnolent or comatose does not differ significantly from that of acute central depression caused by conventional general anesthetics or hypnotics. Reference should be made to the treatment of acute barbiturate intoxication for further measures (*see* Chapter 17).

Acute alcoholic intoxication is not always associated with coma. Usually therapy is not required, and it is sufficient for the patient to wait while his tissues metabolize the ingested alcohol at the characteristic constant rate until sobriety ensues. However, in some individuals the release of central inhibitory control of thought and action may lead to a condition that is characterized by nausea, vomiting, restlessness, hyperexcitability, and hyperactivity often of an extremely violent nature. Sedatives and hypnotics such as paraldehyde, chloral hydrate, and barbiturates have been extensively employed to quiet such a patient. Great care must be taken, however, when sedatives are used to treat a patient who has already treated himself to an excessive amount of a CNS depressant, namely, alcohol; physical restraints are safer. Phenothiazines are sometimes used to treat violent patients (Morgan and Cagan, 1974), and have been employed both to relieve the nausea and to produce relaxation and control of the patient's excessive motor activity without causing any dangerous increase in the degree of central depression. The subject of acute alcoholic intoxication has been extensively reviewed by various authors (*e.g.,* Newman, 1941; Morgan and Cagan, 1974).

Concentration of Alcohol in Body Fluids in Relation to Alcoholic Intoxication. It is generally agreed that threshold effects (such as an increased reaction time, diminished fine motor control, and an impaired critical faculty) appear when the concentration of alcohol in the blood is 20 to 30 mg/dl; and more than 50% of persons are grossly intoxicated when the concentration is 150 mg/dl. The average concentration in fatal cases is about 400 mg/dl (Committee on Medicolegal Problems, 1968).

The determination of alcohol in body fluids is often important for medicolegal purposes to establish how much alcohol was ingested. Methods of determining the concentration of alcohol are given by the Committee on Medicolegal Problems (1968) and by Harger (1974). The concentration of alcohol in the blood may be determined directly. Alternatively it can be estimated from the concentration either in expired air, which is about 0.05% that in the blood or, less frequently, in the urine, which is about 130% that in the blood.

Diagnosis of Intoxication. All but a few states have passed laws embodying the recommendations of the National Safety Council and the American Medical Association concerning the driving of motor vehicles by persons who are drunk. If the defendant's blood has a concentration of alcohol of 100 mg/dl or over, he should be considered as being under the influence of intoxicating beverages; if 50 mg/dl or under, not under the influence; if between 50 and 100 mg/dl, this fact must be considered only with other competent positive evidence with regard to the guilt or innocence of the defendant. The importance of such legislation is emphasized by the fact that the average person with a blood alcohol concentration of 100 or 150 mg/dl is 7 or 25 times, respectively, more likely to have a fatal accident than the driver with no alcohol in his blood (*see* reports by U.S. Department of Health, Education, and Welfare, 1974, 1978).

The problem of the *intoxicated pedestrian* must also be recognized because negligence on the part of inebriated pedestrians may be an important factor in traffic accidents. For example, about one third of the pedestrians killed in highway accidents have blood alcohol concentrations of 100 mg/dl or more (*see* reports by U.S. Department of Health, Education, and Welfare, 1974, 1978). Alcohol is also involved in 35% of general aviation crashes (*see* report by U.S. Department of Transportation, 1968). In addition, alcohol is a factor in a large number of *violent deaths* unassociated with traffic accidents. For example, studies in typical communities in the United States revealed that alcohol was a contributing or responsible factor in about 50% of violent deaths (*see* Tinklenberg, 1973).

From the medicolegal point of view the major factor in judging the degree of intoxication is the concentration of alcohol in the blood. The individual, on the other hand, is often concerned more with the *quantity* of alcohol he can safely drink. Unfortunately for him this is not a simple question because many factors, such as his weight and the rate of absorption from the gastrointestinal tract, determine the concentration of alcohol in the blood produced by the ingestion of a given amount of alcohol (*see* Wallgren and Barry, 1970). On the average, ingestion of 44 g of alcohol taken as whisky (4 oz) or martini cocktail (5.5 oz) on an empty stomach results in a maximal blood concentration of 67 to 92 mg/dl; after a mixed meal, 30 to 53 mg/dl. Ingestion of the same amount of alcohol taken as conventional-strength beer (1.2 liters) on an empty stomach results in a maximal blood concentration of 41 to 49 mg/dl; after a mixed meal, 23 to 29 mg/dl. After gastrointestinal absorption is complete, the concentration in the blood at any time after ingestion can be estimated from the volume of distribution of the alcohol, which averages 0.54 liter/kg, and the rate of metabolism, which is about 120 mg/kg per hour (*see* Appendix II; Committee on Medicolegal Problems, 1968).

Contraindications. Contraindications to the use of alcohol largely follow from toxicological considerations. Patients with hepatic disease should not use alcohol, and gastrointestinal ulcers are also contraindications. Alcohol should be avoided by patients with alcoholic skeletal or cardiac myopathy. Clearly, it should be taken only in great moderation, or not at all, by pregnant women, and alcohol should be forbidden absolutely to patients who were once addicted to it (*see* Chapter 23). In general, the use of alcohol in the presence of any particular disease is a matter that the physician and patient must decide in each individual case.

Preparations. Alcohol is currently, and whisky, brandy, and sherry wine were formerly, official preparations. *Alcohol*, U.S.P. (*ethanol, ethyl alcohol*), contains not less than 94.9% by volume of C_2H_5OH. *Diluted Alcohol*, N.F., contains about 49% C_2H_5OH by volume (about 41.5% by weight); it is thus nearly equivalent to 100-proof alcohol, which in the United States contains 50% C_2H_5OH by volume. *Whisky* (whiskey) and *brandy* are alcoholic liquids obtained by distillation of fermented mash and wholly or partly malted cereal grains, and the fermented juice of sound ripe grapes, respectively. They contain about 50% of C_2H_5OH by volume. *Sherry wine*, obtained by fermenting the juice of sound ripe grapes and fortifying it with brandy, contains approximately 20% of C_2H_5OH by volume. In addition, numerous other alcoholic beverages are commercially obtainable. *Rubbing Alcohol*, U.S.P., contains about 70% (by volume) of ethanol, the remainder being acetone, methyl isobutyl ketone, coal tar colors, perfume oils, and water.

The relationship between chemical structure and pharmacological and toxicological action in a large number of aliphatic alcohols is reviewed by Derache (1970).

Therapeutic Uses of Alcohol. Alcohol and alcoholic beverages are widely used by the laity for numerous ailments, and the proper delineation of their legitimate uses in medicine is sometimes difficult (*see* Leake and Silverman, 1966).

External. Alcohol is an excellent *solvent* for many drugs and is frequently employed for medicinal mixtures as a vehicle. Alcohol is a solvent for the *toxicodendrol* causing ivy poisoning; early and thorough washing of the affected parts with alcohol may abort or lessen the severity of the dermatitis. In *phenol skin burns* alcohol should be used immediately as a wash if castor oil is not available; it is not to be employed for gastric lavage, however, when phenol has been swallowed. Alcohol *cools* the skin when it is allowed to evaporate, and alcohol sponges are therefore used to treat fever. It is also *rubefacient* and is included in liniments. Alcohol (50 to 70% by volume) is employed as a rubbing agent on the skin of bedridden patients in order to prevent *decubitus ulcers*. It is also used to *decrease sweating*, and is an ingredient of many anhidrotic and astringent lotions. Ethyl alcohol still remains the most popular *skin disinfectant* (*see* Chapter 41).

Alimentary Tract. Alcoholic beverages, if enjoyed by the patient, may be given before meals as a *stomachic* to improve appetite and digestion, especially in convalescent and debilitated or elderly patients (Turner *et al.*, 1977).

Injection for Relief of Pain. Dehydrated alcohol may be injected in the close proximity of nerves or sympathetic ganglia for the relief of the long-lasting pain that occurs in *trigeminal neuralgia, inoperable carcinoma,* and other conditions. Epidural, subarachnoid, and lumbar paravertebral injections of alcohol have also been employed in appropriate circumstances. For example, lumbar paravertebral injections of alcohol may destroy sympathetic ganglia and thereby produce vasodilatation, relieve pain, and promote healing of lesions in patients with vascular disease of the lower extremities.

Systemic Uses. Alcohol acts as a *hypnotic* and *antipyretic,* and is widely employed for these purposes by lay persons. Alcoholic beverages are sometimes valuable during convalescence as rapidly assimilable sources of energy or as remedies for insomnia. Although sometimes used for this purpose, alcohol is ineffective in causing vasodilatation in persons with peripheral vascular disease or coronary artery disease; any benefits that may be noted from the ingestion of alcoholic beverages in such patients are probably due to a central depressant action rather than to an increase in peripheral or coronary blood flow.

For generations alcoholic beverages have been used to check impending *"head colds."* Perhaps the greatest therapeutic advantage of such therapy is to make the patient drowsy and sleepy so that he stays in bed, whereas otherwise he would be ambulant to the detriment of at least his associates. Hamburger (1936) humorously advised the following therapy, culled from an old English book, to be instituted at the first inkling of a cold, namely, to hang one's hat on the bedpost, drink from a bottle of good whisky until two hats appear, and then get into bed and stay there.

METHYL ALCOHOL

Methyl alcohol (CH$_3$OH), also called *methanol, wood alcohol,* and *Columbian spirit,* is the simplest of the alcohols. The pharmacology, biochemistry, toxicology, and clinical aspects of methyl alcohol have been extensively reviewed by Koivusalo (1970) and Morgan and Cagan (1974). It is widely employed industrially as a solvent. It is also used as an adulterant to "denature," and thereby make unfit to drink, the ethyl alcohol that is used for cleaning purposes, paint removal, and a variety of other uses. Such alcohol, being tax free, is considerably less expensive than more conventional alcoholic beverages and, unless denatured, offers considerable temptation to the derelict. Methyl alcohol is purely of toxicological interest. Poisoning results from its ingestion as a substitute for, or as an adulterant of, ethyl alcohol. For example, 6% of all blindness in the United States Armed Forces during World War II was caused by methanol (Greear, 1950). Serious or fatal poisoning can also occur from industrial exposure.

Fate in the Body. After absorption, methyl alcohol is widely distributed in body tissues. While small amounts of the alcohol are then excreted in the urine and in the expired air, methyl alcohol is largely oxidized in the body to formaldehyde and formic acid. Animals differ in their ability to oxidize methanol to formic acid and to oxidize formic acid itself. In the rabbit only 1% is excreted as formic acid in the urine, compared with 20% in the dog; an intermediate value is obtained in man.

The oxidation of methanol, like that of ethanol, proceeds independently of the concentration in the blood. The rate, however, is only one seventh that of ethanol, so that complete oxidation and excretion of methyl alcohol usually require several days. Oxidation occurs mainly in the liver and kidney.

Relation of Methanol to Ethanol Oxidation. Although experiments with isolated rat tissue slices have emphasized the importance of catalase in the oxidation of methanol, it is still generally agreed that in man alcohol dehydrogenase is involved in the first step of oxidation (*see* Cooper and Kini, 1962; Koivusalo, 1970). The fact that it is this same enzyme that is responsible for the oxidation of ethyl alcohol is presumably the explanation for the finding *in vitro* that ethanol very considerably depresses the rate of oxidation of methanol. The common biochemical pathway of oxidation of both alcohols also accounts for the clinical observations that simultaneous administration of ethanol may ameliorate the toxic sequelae of methanol poisoning (*see* Koivusalo, 1970). This is because the products of oxidation of methanol are toxic rather than methanol itself, and, therefore, the degree of poisoning is minimized if the rate of oxidation of methanol is reduced as much as possible.

Methyl Alcohol Poisoning. Poisoning due to methyl alcohol results from a combination of the following: (1) a minor factor of CNS depression, similar to that produced by ethyl alcohol; (2) a major factor of acidosis due to the production of formic acid (Clay *et al.,* 1975); and (3) a specific toxicity of the oxidation products of methanol (probably formaldehyde) for the retinal cells.

Symptoms. Methanol is less inebriating than ethanol; indeed, inebriation is not a prominent symptom of methanol intoxication unless a very large amount is consumed or ethanol is also ingested. An asymptomatic latent period of 8 to 36 hours may precede the onset of symptoms; if ethanol is simultaneously imbibed in sufficient amount, methanol poisoning may be considerably delayed, or, on occasion, even averted. In such cases ethanol intoxication is prominent, and methanol ingestion may not be suspected.

Symptoms and *signs* of methanol poisoning consist in headache, vertigo, vomiting, severe upper abdominal pain, back pain, dyspnea, motor restlessness, cold clammy extremities, blurring of vision, hyperemia of the optic disc, and, occasionally, diarrhea. Blood pressure is usually unaffected. The pulse is slow in severely ill patients, and bradycardia constitutes a grave prognostic sign. The visual disturbance can proceed to blindness, and the pupils then do not react to light. Restlessness and delirium may be marked. Despite the severe acidosis, Kussmaul respiration is not common. Coma can develop with amazing rapidity in relatively asymptomatic subjects. In moribund patients the respiration is slow, shallow, gasping, and "fish mouth" in type. Death may be sudden, or it may occur only after many hours of coma. Death occurs in inspiratory apnea, with terminal opisthotonos and convulsions.

Laboratory findings include evidence of severe acidosis, methanol and formic acid in blood and urine, moderate ketonemia, normal serum sodium and potassium concentrations, albuminuria, and slight or moderate acetonuria. The ketonemia and acetonuria are mild in comparison with the severity of the acidosis. Cerebral blood flow and cerebral oxygen consumption are both markedly reduced during methanol poisoning. Serum amylase is elevated as a result of pancreatitis; indeed, pancreatic injury probably accounts for the violent epigastric pain. Cerebrospinal fluid pressure is often elevated.

Death from methanol is nearly always preceded by blindness. As little as 4 ml of methanol has caused blindness, and ingestion of 80 to 150 ml is usually fatal. The formaldehyde is probably the cause of the selective injury to the retinal cells (*see* Koivusalo, 1970).

Treatment and Prognosis. The cardinal feature of methanol poisoning is the acidosis, and the correction of acidosis is the keystone of proper therapy if the patient is to survive. It is also believed that the prognosis with respect to salvage of vision is directly dependent on the rapidity and the completeness of the correction of the acidosis. However, acidosis itself is not the cause of the ocular disturbances, because these phenomena are not observed in other types of acidosis. Indeed, retinal changes may occur in methanol poisoning despite seemingly adequate therapy with alkali. All the available evidence is consistent with the idea that blindness is induced by an intermediary product of methanol metabolism, probably formaldehyde, the effect of which is *enhanced* by acidosis (Mardones, 1963). Because of the slow oxidation of methanol the risk of recurrence of acidosis after a period of successful treatment is great, and hence close observation and proper therapy should be continued for several days to prevent sudden relapse and death. The metabolic acidosis is treated with alkali (*see* Chapter 35); hypokalemia from alkali therapy may require administration of potassium salts. In general, water and electrolyte balance and nutrition must be maintained. The use of hemodialysis or peritoneal dialysis will hasten the removal of methanol from the body (Wenzl *et al.,* 1968; Koivusalo, 1970). The patient should be kept warm and his eyes protected from strong light.

The administration of ethanol is recommended on the basis that it retards the oxidation of methanol, as explained above, and is a specific measure for the prevention of blindness that may otherwise follow. Ethanol administration may also be a lifesaving procedure if alkali therapy must be postponed for any reason. Neurological damage, giving rise to a permanent motor dysfunction, may follow methanol poisoning; the rigidity and hypokinesis may be relieved by levodopa (Guggenheim *et al.,* 1971).

DISULFIRAM

History. *Tetraethylthiuram disulfide* (*disulfiram*) was used in the rubber industry as an antioxidant.

Workers exposed to disulfiram developed a hypersensitivity to ethanol. Two Danish physicians, who had taken disulfiram in the course of an investigation of its potential anthelmintic usefulness and who became ill at a cocktail party, were quick to realize that the disulfiram had altered their response to alcohol. They then initiated a series of pharmacological and clinical studies that provided the basis for the use of disulfiram as an adjunct in the treatment of chronic alcoholism. Similar sensitization is produced by various congeners of disulfiram, industrial exposure to cyanamide, eating the fungus *Coprinus atramentarius,* the hypoglycemic sulfonylureas, metronidazole, and the ingestion of *animal charcoal* (*see* Kitson, 1977).

Mechanism of Action. Disulfiram, given by itself, is a relatively nontoxic substance, and few untoward effects are observed when it is administered alone in reasonable doses in animals or man. However, disulfiram markedly alters the intermediary metabolism of alcohol. When ethanol is given to an animal or to an individual previously treated with disulfiram, the blood acetaldehyde concentration rises five to ten times higher than in an untreated animal or individual. This effect is accompanied by marked signs and symptoms, known as the *acetaldehyde syndrome.* Within about 5 to 10 minutes the face feels hot, and soon afterwards it is flushed and scarlet in appearance. As the vasodilatation spreads over the whole body, intense throbbing is felt in the head and neck, and a pulsating headache may develop. Respiratory difficulties, nausea, copious vomiting, sweating, thirst, chest pain, considerable hypotension, orthostatic syncope, marked uneasiness, weakness, vertigo, blurred vision, and confusion are observed. The facial flush is replaced by pallor, and the blood pressure may fall to shock level. As little as 7 ml of alcohol will cause mild symptoms in sensitive persons, and the effect, once elicited, lasts between 30 minutes (in mild cases) and several hours (in severe cases). After the symptoms wear off, the patient is exhausted and may sleep for several hours, after which he is well again.

Most of the signs and symptoms observed after the ingestion of disulfiram plus alcohol are attributable to the resulting increase in the concentration of acetaldehyde in the body. They can, in fact, be produced in normal humans by the intravenous injection of acetaldehyde. Acetaldehyde is produced as a result of the initial oxidation of ethanol by the alcohol dehydrogenase of the liver. It does not accumulate in the tissues because it is further oxidized almost as soon as it is formed, most likely primarily by the enzyme aldehyde dehydrogenase. In the presence of disulfiram, however, the concentration of acetaldehyde rises because disulfiram seems to compete with NAD for the active centers of the enzyme aldehyde dehydrogenase and thereby reduces the rate of oxidation of the acetaldehyde. Diethyldithiocarbamate, a major metabolite of disulfiram, also inhibits alcohol dehydrogenase. This would account for the increased concentration of ethanol in blood sometimes reported during treatment with disulfiram. Some aspects of the disulfiram-ethanol reaction, however, are still obscure. For example, *hypo*tension is characteristic of the disulfiram-ethanol reaction, whereas injection of acetaldehyde into animals usually causes *hyper*tension (*see* Kitson, 1977). The hypotension could result from the known inhibition by diethyl-dithiocarbamate of dopamine β-hydroxylase, with a consequent reduction of norepinephrine synthesis in sympathetic nerve terminals (*see* Morgan and Cagan, 1974; Kitson, 1977).

Absorption, Fate, and Excretion. Disulfiram is rapidly and completely absorbed from the human gastrointestinal tract. However, a period of 12 hours is required for its full action, perhaps because, being highly soluble in lipid, it is initially localized in fat. Elimination is relatively slow, and about one fifth still remains in the body at the end of a week. The greater part of the absorbed drug is oxidized, probably chiefly in the liver, and excreted in the urine as the sulfate, partly free and partly esterified.

Toxic Reactions and Contraindications. Disulfiram by itself is largely, but not completely, innocuous. It may cause acneform eruptions, allergic dermatitis, urticaria, lassitude, fatigue, tremor, restlessness, reduced sexual potency, headache, dizziness, a garlic-like or metallic taste, and mild gastrointestinal disturbances. In contrast to these relatively mild effects, however, alarming reactions may result from the ingestion of even small amounts of alcohol in persons being treated with disulfiram. Marked respiratory depression, cardiovascular collapse, cardiac arrhythmias, myocardial infarction, acute congestive heart failure, unconsciousness, convulsions, and sudden and unexplained fatalities have occurred. Obviously the use of disulfiram as a therapeutic agent is not without danger, and it should be attempted only under careful medical and nursing supervision. The patient must be warned that, as long as he is taking disulfiram, the ingestion of alcohol in any form will make him sick and may endanger his life. He must learn to avoid disguised forms of alcohol, such as sauces, fermented vinegar, cough syrups, and even aftershave lotions and backrubs.

Chemistry and Preparation. The chemical structure of disulfiram is as follows:

$$H_5C_2 \diagdown N-C-S-S-C-N \diagup C_2H_5$$
$$H_5C_2 \diagup \quad \underset{S}{\|} \quad \quad \underset{S}{\|} \quad \diagdown C_2H_5$$

Disulfiram

The drug, which is almost insoluble in water, forms chelates with certain metals, especially iron and copper. *Disulfiram,* U.S.P. (ANTABUSE), is available in the form of oral, scored tablets that contain 250 or 500 mg of the drug.

Administration and Dosage. Disulfiram should be administered only by a physician, and therapy is usually commenced in the hospital. The maintenance dose is about 0.5 g per day, although sometimes it may have to be reduced to 0.25 g or less if unpleasant side effects appear. The daily dose should be taken in the morning, the time when the resolve

not to drink may be strongest. Sensitization to alcohol may last for as long as 6 to 12 days after the ingestion of disulfiram because of its slow rate of elimination.

Therapeutic Use. The only therapeutic use of disulfiram is in the treatment of *chronic alcoholism.* Disulfiram is not a cure for alcoholism, but merely affords the volunteer a crutch by which the sincere desire to stop drinking can be fortified. The rationale for its use is that the patient knows that if he is to avoid the devastating experience of the "acetaldehyde syndrome" he cannot drink for at least 3 or 4 days after taking disulfiram. The subject is further discussed in Chapter 23, which deals with the therapy of drug abuse.

Baraona, E., and Lieber, C. S. Effects of ethanol on hepatic protein synthesis and secretion. In, *Currents in Alcoholism.* (Seixas, F. A., ed.) Grune & Stratton, Inc., New York, **1977**, pp. 33–46.

Baraona, E.; Pirola, R.; and Lieber, C. S. Small intestinal damage and changes in cell population produced by ethanol ingestion in the rat. *Gastroenterology,* **1974,** *66,* 226–234.

Broitman, S. A.; Gottlieb, L. S.; and Vitale, J. J. Augmentation of ethanol absorption by mono- and disaccharides. *Gastroenterology,* **1976,** *70,* 1101–1107.

Brown, N. A.; Goulding, E. H.; and Fabro, S. Ethanol embryotoxicity: direct effects on mammalian embryos *in vitro. Science,* **1979,** *206,* 573–575.

Chowdhury, A. R.; Malmud, L. S.; and Dinoso, V. P. Gastrointestinal plasma protein loss during ethanol ingestion. *Gastroenterology,* **1977,** *72,* 37–40.

Clarren, S. K., and Smith, D. W. The fetal alcohol syndrome. *N. Engl. J. Med.,* **1978,** *298,* 1063–1067.

Clay, K. L.; Murphy, R. C.; and Watkins, W. D. Experimental methanol toxicity in the primate: analysis of metabolic acidosis. *Toxicol. Appl. Pharmacol.,* **1975,** *34,* 49–61.

Collins, M. A.; Num, W. P.; Borge, G. F.; Teas, G.; and Goldfarb, C. Dopamine-related tetrahydroisoquinolines: significant urinary excretion by alcoholics after alcohol consumption. *Science,* **1979,** *208,* 1184–1186.

Cooke, A. Gastrin release by ethanol. *Gastroenterology,* **1975,** *68,* 192–193.

Cooper, J. R., and Kini, M. M. Biochemical aspects of methanol poisoning. *Biochem. Pharmacol.,* **1962,** *11,* 405–416.

Davenport, H. W. Gastric mucosal hemorrhage in dogs. Effects of acid, aspirin, and alcohol. *Gastroenterology,* **1969,** *56,* 439–449.

Eastwood, G. L., and Kirchner, J. P. Changes in the fine structure of mouse gastric epithelium produced by ethanol and urea. *Gastroenterology,* **1974,** *67,* 71–84.

Gantt, W. H. Effect of alcohol on the sexual reflexes of normal and neurotic male dogs. *Psychosom. Med.,* **1952,** *14,* 174–181.

Gordon, T.; Castelli, W. P.; Hjortland, M. C.; Kannel, W. B.; and Dawber, T. R. High density lipoprotein as a protective factor against coronary heart disease. *Am. J. Med.,* **1977,** *62,* 707–714.

Greear, J. N. The causes of blindness. In, *Blindness: Modern Approaches to the Unseen Environment.* (Zahl, P. A., ed.) Princeton University Press, Princeton, N.J., **1950.**

Guggenheim, M. A.; Couch, J. R.; and Weinberger, W. Motor dysfunction as a permanent complication of methanol ingestion. *Arch. Neurol.,* **1971,** *24,* 550–554.

Hamburger, L. P. Some minor ailments: their importance in the medical curriculum. *Yale J. Biol. Med.,* **1936,** *8,* 365–386.

Johnstone, R. E., and Reier, C. E. Acute respiratory effects of ethanol in man. *Clin. Pharmacol. Ther.*, **1973,** *11,* 501–508.

Klatsky, A. L.; Friedman, G. D.; Siegelaub, A. B.; and Gerard, M. J. Alcohol consumption and blood pressure. Kaiser-Permanente multiphasic health examination data. *N. Engl. J. Med.,* **1977,** *296,* 1194–1200.

McQuarrie, D. G., and Fingl, E. Effects of single doses and chronic administration of ethanol on experimental seizures in mice. *J. Pharmacol. Exp. Ther.,* **1958,** *124,* 264–271.

Mekhjian, H. S., and May, E. S. Acute and chronic effects of ethanol on fluid transport in the human small intestine. *Gastroenterology,* **1977,** *72,* 1280–1286.

Muehlberger, C. W. The physiological action of alcohol. *J.A.M.A.,* **1958,** *167,* 1842–1845.

Rubin, E., and Lieber, C. S. Hepatic microsomal enzymes in man and rat: induction and inhibition by ethanol. *Science,* **1968,** *162,* 690–691.

Scheig, R. Effects of ethanol on the liver. *Am. J. Clin. Nutr.,* **1970,** *23,* 467–473.

Schmidt, W., and de Lint, J. Causes of death of alcoholics. *J. Stud. Alcohol,* **1973,** *33,* 171–185.

Smith, B. M.; Skillman, J. J.; Edwards, B. G.; and Silen, W. Permeability of the human gastric mucosa. Alteration by acetylsalicylic acid and ethanol. *N. Engl. J. Med.,* **1971,** *285,* 716–721.

Song, S. K., and Rubin, E. Ethanol produces muscle damage in human volunteers. *Science,* **1972,** *175,* 327–328.

Straus, E.; Urbach, H.-J.; and Yalow, R. S. Alcohol-stimulated secretion of immunoreactive secretin. *N. Engl. J. Med.,* **1975,** *293,* 1031–1032.

Teschke, R.; Matsuzaki, S.; Ohnishi, K.; Hasamura, Y.; and Lieber, C. S. Metabolism of alcohol at high concentrations: role and biochemical nature of the hepatic microsomal oxidizing system. In, *Alcohol Intoxication and Withdrawal IIIa.* (Gross, M. M., ed.) Vol. 85A, *Advances in Experimental Medicine and Biology.* Plenum Press, New York, **1977,** pp. 257–280.

Van Thiel, D. H., and Lester, R. Sex and alcohol: a second peek. *N. Engl. J. Med.,* **1976,** *295,* 835–836.

Wenzl, J. E.; Mills, S. D.; and McCall, J. T. Methanol poisoning in an infant. Successful treatment with peritoneal dialysis. *Am. J. Dis. Child.,* **1968,** *116,* 445–447.

Wilson, G. T. Alcohol and human sexual behavior. *Behav. Res. Ther.,* **1977,** *15,* 239–252.

Workman, R. L., Jr.; Swinyard, E. A.; Rigby, O. F.; and Swinyard, C. A. Correlation between anticonvulsant activity and plasma concentration of ethanol. *J. Am. Pharm. Assoc.,* **1958,** *47,* 769–772.

Yano, K.; Rhoads, G. G.; and Kagan, A. Coffee, alcohol and risk of coronary heart disease among Japanese men living in Hawaii. *N. Engl. J. Med.,* **1977,** *297,* 405–409.

Zsotér, T. T., and Sellers, E. M. Effect of alcohol on cardiovascular reflexes. *J. Stud. Alcohol,* **1977,** *38,* 1–10.

Monographs and Reviews

Beard, J. O., and Knott, D. H. The effect of alcohol on fluid and electrolyte metabolism. In, *The Biology of Alcoholism.* Vol. 1, *Biochemistry.* (Kissin, B., and Begleiter, H., eds.) Plenum Press, New York, **1971,** pp. 353–376.

Begleiter, H., and Platz, A. The effects of alcohol on the central nervous system in humans. In, *The Biology of Alcoholism.* Vol. 2, *Physiology and Behavior.* (Kissin, B., and Begleiter, H., eds.) Plenum Press, New York, **1972,** pp. 293–343.

Burch, G. E., and Giles, T. D. Alcoholic cardiomyopathy. In, *The Biology of Alcoholism.* Vol. 3, *Clinical Pathology.* (Kissin, B., and Begleiter, H., eds.) Plenum Press, New York, **1974,** pp. 435–460.

Committee on Medicolegal Problems. *Alcohol and the Impaired Driver: A Manual on the Medicolegal Aspects of Chemical Tests for Intoxication,* American Medical Association, Chicago, **1968.**

Derache, R. Toxicology, pharmacology and metabolism of higher alcohols. In, *Alcohols and Derivatives.* (Trémolières, J., ed.) Vol. 2, *International Encyclopedia of Pharmacology and Therapeutics,* Sect. 20. Pergamon Press, Ltd., Oxford, **1970,** pp. 507–522.

Feinman, L., and Lieber, C. S. Liver disease in alcoholism. In, *The Biology of Alcoholism.* Vol. 3, *Clinical Pathology.* (Kissin, B., and Begleiter, H., eds.) Plenum Press, New York, **1974,** pp. 303–338.

Feldstein, A. Effect of ethanol on neurohumoral amine metabolism. In, *The Biology of Alcoholism.* Vol. 1, *Biochemistry.* (Kissin, B., and Begleiter, H., eds.) Plenum Press, New York, **1971,** pp. 127–159.

Flink, E. B. Mineral metabolism in alcoholism. In, *The Biology of Alcoholism.* Vol. 1, *Biochemistry.* (Kissin, B., and Begleiter, H., eds.) Plenum Press, New York, **1971,** pp. 377–395.

Galambos, J. T. Alcoholic hepatitis: its therapy and prognosis. *Prog. Liver Dis.,* **1972,** *4,* 567–588.

Gross, M. M. (ed.). *Alcohol Intoxication and Withdrawal.* Vols. A and B, *Advances in Experimental Medicine and Biology.* Plenum Press, New York, **1977.**

Harger, R. H. Recently published analytical methods for determining alcohol in body materials. Alcohol countermeasures literature review. *Report to Department of Transportation (DOT-HS-031-3-722).* National Technical Information Service, Springfield, Va., **1974.**

Hillman, R. W. Alcoholism and malnutrition. In, *The Biology of Alcoholism.* Vol. 3, *Clinical Pathology.* (Kissin, B., and Begleiter, H., eds.) Plenum Press, New York, **1974,** pp. 513–586.

Himwich, H. E., and Callison, D. A. The effects of alcohol on evoked potentials of various parts of the central nervous system of the cat. In, *The Biology of Alcoholism.* Vol. 2, *Physiology and Behavior.* (Kissin, B., and Begleiter, H., eds.) Plenum Press, New York, **1972,** pp. 67–84.

Israel, Y.; Rosenmann, E.; Hein, S.; Colombo, G.; and Canessa-Fischer, M. Effects of alcohol on the nerve cell. In, *Biological Basis of Alcoholism.* (Israel, Y., and Mardones, J., eds.) John Wiley & Sons, Inc., New York, **1971,** pp. 53–72.

Kalant, H. Absorption, diffusion, distribution, and elimination of ethanol: effects on biological membranes. In, *The Biology of Alcoholism.* Vol. 1, *Biochemistry.* (Kissin, B., and Begleiter, H., eds.) Plenum Press, New York, **1971,** pp. 1–62.

Kissin, B. Interactions of ethyl alcohol and other drugs. In, *The Biology of Alcoholism.* Vol. 3, *Clinical Pathology.* (Kissin, B., and Begleiter, H., eds.) Plenum Press, New York, **1974,** pp. 109–161.

Kissin, B., and Begleiter, H. (eds.). *The Biology of Alcoholism.* Vol 1, *Biochemistry.* Plenum Press, New York, **1971.**

———. *Ibid.* Vol. 2, *Physiology and Behavior.* Plenum Press, New York, **1972.**

———. *Ibid.* Vol. 3, *Clinical Pathology.* Plenum Press, New York, **1974.**

Kitson, T. M. The disulfiram-ethanol reaction. *J. Stud. Alcohol,* **1977,** *38,* 96–113.

Koivusalo, M. Methanol. In, *Alcohols and Derivatives.* (Trémolières, J., ed.) Vol. 2, *International Encyclopedia of Pharmacology and Therapeutics,* Sect. 20. Pergamon Press, Ltd., Oxford, **1970,** pp. 465–505.

Leake, C. D., and Silverman, M. *Alcoholic Beverages in Clinical Medicine.* Year Book Medical Publishers, Inc., Chicago, **1966.**

Leevy, C. M.; Tanribilir, A. K.; and Smith, F. Biochemistry of gastrointestinal and liver disease in alcoholism. In, *The Biology of Alcoholism.* Vol. 1, *Biochemistry.* (Kissin, B., and Begleiter, H., eds.) Plenum Press, New York, **1971,** pp. 307–325.

Lieber, C. S. Pathogenesis and early diagnosis of alcoholic liver injury. *N. Engl. J. Med.,* **1978,** *298,* 888–893.

Lieber, C. S.; Teschke, R.; Hasumura, Y.; and Decarli, L. M. Differences in hepatic and metabolic changes after acute and chronic alcohol consumption. *Fed. Proc.,* **1975,** *34,* 2060–2074.

Lindenbaum, J. Hematologic effects of alcohol. In, *The Biology of Alcoholism.* Vol. 3, *Clinical Pathology.* (Kissin, B., and Begleiter, H., eds.) Plenum Press, New York, **1974,** pp. 461–480.

Lorber, S. H.; Dinoso, V. P., Jr.; and Chey, W. Y. Diseases of the gastrointestinal tract. In, *The Biology of Alcoholism.* Vol. 3, *Clinical Pathology.* (Kissin, B., and Begleiter, H., eds.) Plenum Press, New York, **1974,** pp. 339–357.

Maling, H. M. Toxicology of single doses of ethyl alcohol. In, *Alcohols and Derivatives.* (Trémolières, J., ed.) Vol. 2, *International Encyclopedia of Pharmacology and Therapeutics,* Sect. 20. Pergamon Press, Ltd., Oxford, **1970,** pp. 277–299.

Mardones, J. The alcohols. In, *Physiological Pharmacology,* Vol. 1. (Root, W. S., and Hofmann, F. G., eds.) Academic Press, Inc., New York, **1963.**

Mendelson, J. H., and Mello, N. K. Biologic concomitants of alcoholism. *N. Engl. J. Med.,* **1979,** *301,* 912–921.

Morgan, R., and Cagan, E. J. Acute alcohol intoxication, the disulfiram reaction, and methyl alcohol intoxication. In, *The Biology of Alcoholism.* Vol. 3, *Clinical Pathology.* (Kissin, B., and Begleiter, H., eds.) Plenum Press, New York, **1974,** pp. 163–189.

Myers, R. D. Psychopharmacology of alcohol. *Annu. Rev. Pharmacol. Toxicol.,* **1978,** *18,* 125–144.

Myerson, R. M. Effects of alcohol on cardiac and muscular function. In, *Biological Basis of Alcoholism.* (Israel, Y., and Mardones, J., eds.) John Wiley & Sons, Inc., New York, **1971,** pp. 183–208.

Newman, H. W. *Acute Alcoholic Intoxication: A Critical Review.* Stanford University Press, Stanford, Calif., **1941.**

Perkoff, G. T. Alcoholic myopathy. *Annu. Rev. Med.,* **1971,** *5,* 125–132.

Pirola, R. C. *Drug Metabolism and Alcohol.* University Park Press, Baltimore, **1978.**

Pirola, R. C., and Lieber, C. S. Acute and chronic pancreatitis. In, *The Biology of Alcoholism.* Vol. 3, *Clinical Pathology.* (Kissin, B., and Begleiter, H., eds.) Plenum Press, New York, **1974,** pp. 359–402.

Polacsek, E.; Barnes, T.; Turner, N.; Hall, R.; and

Weise, C. *Interaction of Alcohol and Other Drugs.* Addiction Research Foundation, Toronto, **1972.**

Regan, T. J.; Ettinger, P. O.; Haider, B.; Ahmed, S. S.; Oldewurtel, H. A.; and Lyons, M. M. The role of ethanol in cardiac disease. *Annu. Rev. Med.,* **1977,** *28,* 393–409.

Stokes, P. E. Alcohol-endocrine relationships. In, *The Biology of Alcoholism.* Vol. 1, *Biochemistry.* (Kissin, B., and Begleiter, H., eds.) Plenum Press, New York, **1971,** pp. 397–436.

Tinklenberg, J. R. Alcohol and violence. In, *Alcoholism. Progress in Research and Treatment.* (Bourne, P. G., and Fox, R., eds.) Academic Press, Inc., New York, **1973,** pp. 195–210.

Trémolières, J. (ed.). *Alcohols and Derivatives.* Vols. 1 and 2, *International Encyclopedia of Pharmacology and Therapeutics,* Sect. 20. Pergamon Press, Ltd., Oxford, **1970.**

Truitt, E. B. A biogenic amine hypothesis for alcohol tolerance. *Ann. N.Y. Acad. Sci.,* **1973,** *215,* 177–182.

Turner, T. B.; Mezey, E.; and Kimball, A. W. Measurement of alcohol-related effects in man: chronic effects in relation to levels of alcohol consumption. *Johns Hopkins Med. J.,* **1977,** *5,* 235–248, 273–286.

U.S. Department of Health, Education, and Welfare. *Alcohol and Health.* (Second and Third Special Reports to the Congress from the Secretary of Health, Education, and Welfare.) The Department, Washington, D. C., **1974, 1978.**

U.S. Department of Transportation. *Alcohol and Highway Safety.* (A Report to the Congress from the Secretary of Transportation.) The Department, Washington, D. C., **1968.**

Wallgren, H. Effect of ethanol on intracellular respiration and cerebral function. In, *The Biology of Alcoholism.* Vol. 1, *Biochemistry.* (Kissin, B., and Begleiter, H., eds.) Plenum Press, New York, **1971,** pp. 103–125.

Wallgren, H., and Barry, H., III. *Actions of Alcohol,* Vols. I and II. American Elsevier Publishing Co., Inc., New York, **1970.**

Wartburg, J. P. von. The metabolism of alcohol in normals and alcoholics: enzymes. In, *The Biology of Alcoholism.* Vol. 1, *Biochemistry.* (Kissin, B., and Begleiter, H., eds.) Plenum Press, New York, **1971,** pp. 63–102.

CHAPTER

19 DRUGS AND THE TREATMENT OF PSYCHIATRIC DISORDERS

Ross J. Baldessarini

The use of drugs with well-demonstrated efficacy in psychiatric disorders has become widespread since the mid-1950s. Today, 20% of the prescriptions written in the United States are for medications intended to affect mental processes, namely, to sedate, stimulate, or otherwise change mood, thinking, or behavior. This practice reflects both the very high frequency of primary emotional disorders and the nearly inevitable emotional, psychological, and social reactions of persons with primarily medical illnesses. In addition, a large number of drugs used for other purposes also modify emotions and cognition either as part of their usual actions or as toxic effects of overdosage.

In this chapter, agents used primarily for the treatment of psychiatric disorders are discussed. Other drugs may so alter the function of the central nervous system (CNS) as to warrant their designation as *psychotoxic.* These include useful substances with particular abuse liability (*e.g.,* opioids, sedatives); agents without established therapeutic use, including many natural products that have arisen from popular or folk practices (*e.g.,* alcohol, coffee, tobacco, marihuana, methylated aromatic amine hallucinogens, lysergic acid diethylamide); and agents with accepted medical indications that can produce psychiatric side effects (*e.g.,* antihypertensives, cocaine, sedatives, stimulants, steroids, cardiac glycosides). Discussion of these agents is beyond the scope of this chapter, and the reader is referred to other sections dealing with CNS drugs and their potential behavioral toxicity. (*See* especially Chapter 23 and specialized reviews by Efron *et al.,* 1967; Shader, 1972; Usdin and Efron, 1972; Schultes, 1978.) Drugs used in the treatment of psychiatric disorders as well as psychotoxic agents are often collectively called *psychoactive* or *psychotropic.* Over 1500 compounds classified primarily as psychotropic agents have been described (Usdin and Efron, 1972; Usdin, 1978a).

In the presentation of each drug group, a prototypical agent is sometimes used to exemplify the characteristics of the class. Important differences from the prototype are discussed when appropriate. An attempt is also made to define the characteristics of treatable conditions and to indicate how drugs are used in psychiatric patients. Although several alternative schemes exist, the psychotherapeutic agents described in this chapter are placed into three major categories. *Antipsychotic* or *neuroleptic* drugs are those used to treat the most severe psychiatric illnesses, the psychoses; they have beneficial effects on mood and thought but carry the risk of producing neurotoxic effects that mimic neurological diseases. *Mood-stabilizing* drugs (notably, lithium salts) and *antidepressants* (mood-elevating agents) are those used to treat affective disorders. *Antianxiety-sedative* agents, particularly the benzodiazepines, are those used for the drug therapy of anxiety states.

The use of drugs in the treatment of psychiatric disorders is complicated by uncertainties and inaccuracies of diagnosis characteristic of clinical psychiatry. However, psychiatric diagnosis continues to gain objectivity, coherence, and reliability. The association between specific clinical syndromes and predictable responses to psychotropic drugs has supported the impressive recent progress in this area. Testable hypotheses about possible biological bases of severe psychiatric illnesses have been stimulated by knowledge of the mechanisms of action of psychotropic agents, assisted by the emergence of a medical discipline commonly known as *biological psychiatry.* Although there is sometimes disagreement among psychiatrists concerning diagnosis and the indications for various treatments, these uncertainties do not invalidate the many salutary effects of drugs on mental symptoms. The diagnostic terminology and criteria currently employed in the United States is well described in the *Diagnostic and Statistical Manual of Mental Disorders* of the American Psychiatric Association (1968, 1979).

History. Modification of behavior, mood, and emotion by drugs has always been a favorite indulgence of mankind. The use of psychoactive drugs evolved along two related paths. The first was in the use of drugs to modify normal behavior and to produce altered states of feeling for religious, ceremonial, or recreational purposes. The second was to alleviate mental ailments. A fascinating account of the early history and characteristics of many psychoactive compounds is presented by Lewin (1924). More modern reviews are those of Efron and associates (1967), Caldwell (1978), and Schultes (1978). In 1845, Moreau proposed that hashish intoxication provided a model psychosis useful in the study of insanity. Three decades later, Freud presented his study of cocaine and suggested its potential uses in pharmacotherapy. Soon thereafter, Kraepelin founded the first laboratory of clinical psychopharmacology in Dorpat, where he evaluated psychological effects of drugs in man. In 1931, Sen and Bose published the first report of the use of *Rauwolfia serpentina* in the treatment of insanity. Insulin shock, pentylenetetrazol-induced convulsions, and electroconvulsive therapy followed in 1933, 1934, and 1937, respectively, and treatment of both depression and schizophrenia thus became available. Amphetamine was the first synthetic drug to provide a model psychosis. In 1943, Hofmann purposefully ingested a minute amount of lysergic acid diethylamide (LSD) to experience its psychic effects. His report of the high potency of LSD made the concept that a toxic metabolic product might be the cause of mental illness more popular. Accounts of this and other early experiments in psychopharmacology have been presented by the original participants (*see* Ayd and Blackwell, 1970).

The first report on the treatment of mania with *lithium* was that of Cade (1949). This discovery was slow in gaining general acceptance by the medical community. In 1950, *chlorpromazine* was synthesized in France. The recognition of the unique effects of chlorpromazine by Laborit (1952) and its use in psychiatric patients by Delay and Deniker (1952) marked the beginnings of modern psychopharmacology. The history of this revolutionary era in psychiatric therapy is recounted by Ayd and Blackwell (1970), Swazey (1974), and Caldwell (1978). The term *tranquilizer* was introduced in the early 1950s by Yonkman to characterize the psychic effect of reserpine. Despite its popularity, this ambiguous and misleading term is not used in this chapter.

The report on *meprobamate* by Berger (1954) marked the beginning of investigations of modern sedatives with useful antianxiety properties. An antitubercular drug, *iproniazid,* was introduced in the early 1950s and was soon recognized as a monoamine oxidase inhibitor and antidepressant (Crane, 1959); in 1958, Kuhn recognized the antidepressant effect of *imipramine. Chlordiazepoxide,* the first of the antianxiety benzodiazepines, was developed by Sternbach in 1957. In the following year Janssen discovered the antipsychotic properties of *haloperidol,* a butyrophenone, and thus still another class of antipsychotic agents became available.

During the 1960s there was a rapid expansion of psychopharmacological research, and many new theories of psychoactive drug effects were introduced. The clinical efficacy of many of these agents was firmly established during this decade.

In recent years, emphasis has centered on biogenic amines in the CNS, their probable mediation of many effects of psychotropic drugs, and their possible causal involvement in mental illness. In addition, much attention is now being paid to the liabilities of treatment with psychotherapeutic drugs, especially their limited efficacy in severe or chronic mental illnesses, their risk of serious toxic effects, and the limitations of screening methods used to develop new agents, most of which offer few advantages over drugs available for nearly 2 decades. A balanced view of their advantages and disadvantages is beginning to emerge. While not nearly the curative "wonder drugs" they promised to be initially, antipsychotic and antidepressant agents used to treat the most severe mental illnesses have had a remarkable impact on psychiatric practice and theory—an impact that can legitimately be called revolutionary.

Nosology. The various classes of psychotherapeutic agents are fairly selective in their ability to modify the symptoms of mental illnesses. The optimal use of such drugs thus requires experience in the differential diagnosis of psychiatric conditions. A few salient aspects of psychiatric nosology are summarized briefly, and some further information is provided in the discussion of the specific classes of drugs.

A most important distinction is made between the *psychoses* and the less severe conditions usually called the *neuroses* (or psychoneuroses). The psychoses are the most severe psychiatric diseases, in which there is not only a marked impairment of behavior but also a serious inability to think coherently, to comprehend reality, or to gain insight into the abnormality; these conditions often include *delusions* and *hallucinations.* The psychotic disorders include *organic* conditions (notably, *delirium* and *dementia*), which are typically associated with definable toxic, metabolic, or neuropathologic changes and are characterized by confusion, disorientation, and memory disturbances as well as behavioral disorganization, and *idiopathic* (or "functional") disorders, for which underlying causes remain completely obscure. The latter are characterized by the retention of orientation and memory in the presence of severely disordered emotion, thought, and behavior, except in unusually severe stuporous states sometimes encountered in these illnesses. Those primary disorders characterized by abnormal emotion or *mood* (disorders of *affect* with depression, dysphoria, or elation or mania) are called *manic-depressive* disorders (Winokur *et al.,* 1969). These may ("bipolar" illnesses) or may not ("unipolar" illnesses) include periods of elation or excitement alternating with severe depression and autonomic changes, notably insomnia, anorexia, and diurnal alterations in mood or activity. In addition, depression can occur as a milder or neurotic disorder or as a symptom associated with other psychiatric or medical illnesses. The idiopathic psychoses characterized mainly by disordered thinking and emotional withdrawal and often associated with paranoid delusions and auditory hallucinations are called *schizophrenia,* which can vary in severity and present a variety of specific symptom clusters. In addition, there are disorders marked by more or less isolated delusions; these may represent a separate category of illness called "paranoid state" or *paranoia.*

Antipsychotic drugs exert beneficial effects in virtually all classes of psychotic illness, and, contrary to a common misconception, are *not* selective for schizophrenia. Moreover, antidepressant drugs that are especially beneficial in manic-depressive disease or in very severe depression can also exert useful effects on less severe depressive syndromes and on conditions that are not obviously depressive in nature (*e.g.,* enuresis, persistent pain, panic attacks). Thus, in general, psychotropic drugs are not disease specific; they provide clinical benefit for specific syndromes or complexes of symptoms.

The less pervasive psychiatric disorders are the *neuroses.* While the ability to comprehend reality is retained, suffering and disability are sometimes very severe. Neuroses may be acute and transient or, more commonly, persistent or recurrent. They involve abnormal symptoms or patterns of behavior, generally believed to be associated with *anxiety.* Neurotic symptoms may include mood changes (anxiety, panic, depression) or limited abnormalities of thought (obsessions, irrational fears) or of behavior (rituals or compulsions, pseudoneurological or "hysterical" conversion signs). In such disorders, drugs may have some beneficial effects for short periods. The drugs particularly modify associated anxiety and depression.

Other so-called characterological disorders may or may not respond to medical intervention; these conditions include characteristic personality styles (*e.g.,* paranoid, withdrawn, psychopathic, hypochondriacal) or behavior patterns (*e.g.,* abuse of alcohol or other substances, socially deviant or perverse behavior) that may run counter to societal expectations. Typically, drugs are not effective in such chronic conditions except when episodes of anxiety or depression occur or in cases of withdrawal from addicting substances (*see* Chapter 23).

Biological Hypotheses in Mental Illness. The introduction of relatively effective and selective drugs for the management of schizophrenic and manic-depressive patients in the 1950s encouraged formulation of biological concepts of the pathogenesis of these mental illnesses. This was followed by increased understanding of the actions of psychopharmacological agents. In addition, other agents were discovered that mimic some of the symptoms of severe mental illnesses. These include the induction of paranoid states by the abuse of amphetamines, the induction of hallucinations and altered emotional states by synthetic agents such as LSD or by natural products that can be formed in mammalian tissues (notably, N,N-dimethyltryptamine), and the occasional production of depression by antihypertensive agents (notably, reserpine and methyldopa) that alter the metabolism of biogenic amines in the CNS.

The leading hypothesis to arise from such considerations was based on data that indicated that antidepressants enhance the biological activity of monoamine neurotransmitters in the CNS and that antiadrenergic compounds can induce depression. It was then reasonable to speculate that a deficiency of amine neurotransmission in the CNS might be causative of depression or that an excess could result in mania. Further, since antipsychotic agents antagonize the actions of dopamine as a neurotransmitter in the forebrain, it has been proposed that there may be a state of functional overactivity of dopamine in the limbic system or cortex in schizophrenia or mania. Alternatively, an endogenous psychotomimetic compound might be produced either uniquely or in excessive quantities in psychotic patients. This "pharmacocentric" approach to the construction of hypotheses is appealing in its seeming rationality, and it has gained abundant support from studies of the actions of antipsychotic and antidepressant drugs over the past 3 decades. In turn, the plausibility of such biological hypotheses has encouraged interest in genetic and family studies, as well as in clinical and biochemical studies. Despite extensive efforts, the attempts to document metabolic changes in human subjects predicted by these hypotheses have not, on balance, provided consistent or compelling corroboration. Simultaneously, genetic studies have provided evidence that inheritance can account for only a *portion* of the causation of mental illnesses, leaving room for environmental and psychological hypotheses. Thus, the hopes of the 1950s and 1960s for the discovery of clearly defined, genetically determined inborn errors of metabolism to explain psychiatric disease have not been realized.

Moreover, there is a growing realization that there may be an oversimplification in the attempt to formulate hypotheses about the causes of mental illness from the tenets of psychopharmacology. Thus, it was commonly hoped that knowledge of the mechanisms of action of antipsychotic or antidepressant drugs would point the way to the discovery of underlying pathophysiological changes in schizophrenia or manic-depressive illness that are functionally opposite to the effects of the drugs. This has not proven to be the case.

The antipsychotic, antimanic, and antidepressant drugs have effects on cortical, limbic, hypothalamic, and brain stem mechanisms that are of fundamental importance for the regulation of arousal, consciousness, affect, and autonomic functions. It is entirely possible that physiological and pharmacological modification of these brain regions might have important behavioral consequences and useful clinical effects regardless of the fundamental nature or cause of the mental disorder in question. Moreover, the relatively poor temporal correlations between the known effects of most psychotropic drugs, which for the most part occur rapidly, and their clinical effects suggest that secondary or even more indirect changes brought about by the drugs may mediate their clinical actions.

Even if the most generous interpretations of the actions of psychotropic drugs could be taken to provide insights into the clinical pathophysiology or the etiology of mental illnesses, many other serious problems remain. They include biological heterogeneity, even within groups of the most carefully diagnosed patients. In addition, the already discussed lack of disease specificity of psychotropic drugs tends to minimize the chances of finding a discrete metabolic correlate for a specific disease. Finally, the technical problems associated with attempts to study metabolic changes in or the post-mortem chemistry of the human CNS are awesome. Among these are artifacts introduced by drug treatment itself.

Nevertheless, the efforts of the past 3 decades have not been without reward. Thus, the introduction of pharmacologically oriented hypotheses concerning biological bases of the serious mental illnesses has encouraged rational research in psychiatry. These efforts have led to marked improvements in clinical investigative technics, fostered improved methods of differential diagnosis, and encouraged difficult and sophisticated genetic and family studies (such as natural "cross-fostering" experiments among adopted children as a method of separating genetic and environmental influences). In short, psychiatry has drawn closer to the mainstream of modern medicine. Much of the research in this complex field has been reviewed critically elsewhere, starting with the masterful critique by Kety in 1959. (More recent articles on research in schizophrenia and manic-depressive illness are listed under Monographs and Reviews at the end of this chapter.)

In *summary,* the available information does not permit a conclusion as to whether crucial, discrete biological lesions are the basis of the most severe mental illnesses (other than certain deliria and dementias). Moreover, it is not necessary to presume that such a basis is operative in order to provide effective drug treatment for psychiatric patients with medications. Furthermore, it would be clinical folly to underestimate the importance of psychological and social factors in the manifestations of mental illnesses or to overlook psychological aspects of the conduct of biological therapies (Baldessarini, 1977b).

Animal Experiments and Psychopharmacology. Because the essential characteristics of human mental disease cannot be reproduced in animals, studies of etiology and treatment are greatly hampered. In man, psychiatric illness can manifest itself by disturbances in interpersonal relationships and communication. Internal conflict, anxiety, and depression are often revealed only through verbalization. Social structure and communication in subhuman animals are so rudimentary as to make the human achievements in this area unique. The intellectual superiority of man over even the highest other primates is so great as to make comparison of respective psychopathology exceedingly difficult.

Although the study of animal behavior has not yet yielded much information concerning the mode of action of drugs in abnormal human behavior, such studies have led to screening procedures for the selection of drugs in the treatment of mental illness. The usefulness of many compounds in the treatment of psychiatric disorders was discovered fortuitously in patients receiving them for other purposes. However, many psychiatrically useful phenothiazines and drugs such as haloperidol, chlordiazepoxide, and others were discovered by means of animal screening technics. Once a therapeutically useful drug has been found, its properties in animal tests can be ascertained and new compounds with similar actions can be synthesized. The chance of discovering a unique therapeutic agent with this method is small, but variations in efficacy and toxicity may be found.

Clinical Evaluation of Psychotropic Drugs. Although there are problems in the evaluation of the efficacy of any drug, the difficulties in evaluating psychoactive drugs are particularly severe. Assessment of change and improvement in psychiatric illness has never been easy. The most striking example of this problem is found in literature concerning the efficacy of psychotherapy. Although psychotherapy seems to have salutary effects in individual patients, no study has demonstrated this in a scientifically acceptable way. The problem should be simpler in the evaluation of pharmacotherapy, for here one presumes that the agent is uniform and administered to all patients in the same way. Unfortunately, results are still frequently equivocal. The criteria for evaluation of the efficacy of drugs in clinical trials are presented in Chapter 3. Detailed reviews of the principles and problems in establishing the efficacy and safety of psychotropic drugs are available (Levine *et al.,* 1971; Baldessarini, 1977b; Hardesty and Burdock, 1978).

The discussions of psychotropic drugs in the following sections place major emphasis on the results of carefully controlled studies whenever these are available. Unfortunately, in many areas controlled studies have never been done. Since the literature is so vast, reference is often made to review articles. As with all classes of drugs, the prudent physician will employ only a limited number of proven agents and become thoroughly familiar with their use.

I. Drugs Used in the Treatment of Psychoses

Several classes of drugs are effective in the symptomatic treatment of psychoses. They are most appropriately used in the therapy of schizophrenia, organic psychoses, and the manic phase of manic-depressive illness. Their occasional use may be indicated in depression or in severe anxiety. These classes include compounds such as the phenothiazines, the structurally similar thioxanthenes, and the dibenzodiazepines and dibenzoxazepines; butyrophenones (phenylbutylpiperidines) and the newer diphenylbutylpiperidines; indolones and other heterocyclic compounds; and the rauwolfia alkaloids and related synthetic heterocyclic amine-depleting agents. Since these many chemically dissimilar drugs share many pharmacological properties, information about their pharmacology and clinical uses will be presented for the group as a whole. Particular attention will be paid to chlorpromazine, the oldest representative of the phenothiazine-thioxanthene class of drugs, and haloperidol, the original butyrophenone and representative of several related and rapidly expanding classes of aromatic butylpiperidine derivatives.

The use of these antipsychotic agents is extremely widespread, as is evident from the fact that several hundreds of millions of patients have been treated with them since their introduction in the 1950s. While the antipsychotic drugs have had a revolutionary, beneficial impact on medical and psychiatric practice, their liabilities, especially their almost relentless association with extrapyramidal neurological effects, must also be emphasized (see Crane, 1973; Marsden et al., 1975; Gardos and Cole, 1976). The antipsychotic effects of these drugs appear to be unique; in the present chapter, they will be referred to as antipsychotic or neuroleptic agents.

PHENOTHIAZINES AND OTHER ANTIPSYCHOTIC AGENTS

The phenothiazines as a class, and especially chlorpromazine, the prototype, are among the most widely used drugs in medical practice. Chlorpromazine and the many other related agents that have been devel-

oped in the last 3 decades are primarily employed in the management of patients with serious psychiatric illnesses. In addition, many members of the group have other clinically useful properties, including antiemetic, antinausea, and antihistaminic effects and the ability to potentiate analgesics, sedatives, and general anesthetics; many of these actions are discussed elsewhere in this text (see Index). At the present time, there are more than 30 phenothiazine drugs that are used in psychiatric conditions and still others that are primarily intended for other uses.

History. The history of the antipsychotic agents is especially well summarized by Swazey (1974) and Caldwell (1978). Historical precedence should be given to the introduction of lithium salts for mania in 1949 (see below, page 431), and even earlier to the description of hypotensive and sedating properties of *Rauwolfia* plant extracts in the Indian medical literature (Sen and Bose, 1931). Plant products have been a part of Hindu medicine since ancient times, but there was little interest in their systematic use in Western psychiatry until the 1950s. In the early 1950s, some encouraging results were obtained with carefully prepared natural extracts of *Rauwolfia* (Kline, 1958) and then with pure *reserpine*, which was isolated, characterized, and synthesized by Woodward. While reserpine and related compounds that share its ability to deplete monoamines from their vesicular storage sites in neurons do exert useful antipsychotic effects, these are relatively weak and are often associated with severe side effects, including profound hypotension, excessive salivation, diarrhea, and sedation. Thus, the clinical utility of reserpine is now primarily as an antihypertensive agent (see Chapters 9 and 32).

Phenothiazine compounds were synthesized in Europe in the late nineteenth century as part of the development of aniline dyes such as methylene blue. The history of these dyestuffs is intimately related to the early development by Ehrlich and others of the theory of specific drug-tissue interactions—a cornerstone of pharmacology. Ehrlich even suggested in the 1890s that methylene blue might be used to treat psychoses. In the late 1930s a derivative of phenothiazine, promethazine, was prepared by Charpentier and was found to have antihistaminic properties and a strong sedative effect. Attempts to treat agitation in psychiatric patients with promethazine and other antihistamines followed in the period 1940–1950, but without much success.

Meanwhile, the ability of promethazine to cause a marked prolongation of barbiturate sleeping time in rodents was discovered, and during 1949–1952 the French surgeon Laborit introduced the drug into clinical anesthesia as a potentiating agent (Laborit et al., 1952). This work prompted a search for other phenothiazine derivatives with anesthesia-potentiating actions as well as greater central activities, and in 1949–1950 Charpentier synthesized chlorpromazine. Soon thereafter, Laborit and colleagues described the ability of this compound to potentiate anesthetics and produce "artificial hibernation." They noted that chlorpromazine by itself did not cause a loss of consciousness but produced only a tendency to sleep and a marked lack of interest in what was going on. These central actions became known as *ataractic* or *neuroleptic* soon thereafter.

Courvoisier and associates (1953) described an amazingly large number of actions manifested by chlorpromazine. These included gangliolytic, adrenolytic, antifibrillatory, antiedematous, antipyretic, antishock, anticonvulsant, and antiemetic properties. In addition, chlorpromazine was found to enhance the activity of a number of analgesic and central depressant drugs.

The first report on the treatment of mental illness by chlorpromazine alone is often credited to Delay and Deniker (1952). However, colleagues of Laborit, Colonel Paraire and other psychiatrists at the Parisian military hospital of Val-de-Grace, first reported the beneficial effects of this agent in a manic patient at a meeting in February, 1952. Even earlier (December, 1951), Sigwald had treated a paranoid woman with the new drug. Not until March, 1952, did Delay and Deniker begin their often-quoted early work with chlorpromazine. They were convinced that chlorpromazine achieved more than symptomatic relief of agitation or anxiety and that it could have an ameliorative effect upon psychotic processes with quite diverse symptomatology. In 1954, Lehmann and Hanrahan reported, for the first time in the Western Hemisphere, the use of chlorpromazine in the treatment of psychomotor excitement and manic states. Subsequently, the drug was released for marketing in the United States. It was first employed clinically as an antiemetic, but it was also noted that it produced sedation, relaxation, and hypothermia. In addition, it was considered promising as a potentiating agent for a variety of other centrally acting drugs. Clinical studies soon revealed that the most important use of chlorpromazine was in the treatment of psychotic states, and it has since been used primarily for psychiatric purposes.

In the years that followed, a large number of structural analogs of chlorpromazine and other more novel compounds were prepared, tested on animal behavior, and reached clinical trial or application. Particularly important in this regard was the research of Janssen, who worked in the late 1950s in Belgium with a series of derivatives of normeperidine in the hope of developing an improved analgesic agent. He found that propiophenones had analgesic effects, but that the addition of one methylene group to produce a butyrophenone led either to quite unexpected neuroleptic effects in animals or to a mixture of analgesic and neuroleptic effects. Modification of the butyrophenone structure led to virtually pure neuroleptic activity with potency seen previously only with some piperazine phenothiazines or thioxanthenes. The first of these new substances to be made available for clinical use in psychiatry was haloperidol (1958).

Chemistry and Structure-Activity Relationship. This topic has been reviewed by Zirkle and Kaiser (1970) and, more recently, by Biel and coworkers

(1978). Phenothiazine has a three-ring structure in which two benzene rings are linked by a sulfur and a nitrogen atom (*see* Table 19–1, page 408). If the nitrogen at position 10 is replaced by a carbon atom with a double bond to the side chain, the compound becomes a thioxanthene. Other modifications of the middle ring have included substitution of a nitrogen atom for the sulfur in position 5 and a carbon atom for the nitrogen at position 10 to yield the still-experimental *acridanes,* such as chlomocran.

Substitutions of interest in the phenothiazine nucleus are at positions 2 and 10. Substitution of an electron-withdrawing group at position 2 (but not positions 3 or 4) increases the efficacy of phenothiazines and other tricyclic congeners, possibly by biasing the position of their side chains toward the substituted lateral ring—a conformation that seems to favor superimposition on the structure of catecholamines.

The nature of the substituent at position 10 also influences pharmacological activity. As can be seen in Table 19–1 (page 408), the phenothiazines and thioxanthenes can be divided into groups on the basis of substitution at this site. The group with an *aliphatic* side chain includes chlorpromazine and triflupromazine among the phenothiazines; these compounds are relatively low in potency (but *not* in clinical efficacy). The second group, with similar or somewhat greater potency, contains a *piperidine* moiety in the side chain; it includes thioridazine, mesoridazine, and piperacetazine. There appears to be a lower incidence of extrapyramidal side effects with this substitution, at least in the case of thioridazine, possibly due to increased central antimuscarinic activity. The most potent phenothiazine and thioxanthene antipsychotic compounds are those of the third group, which have a *piperazine* (or piperazinyl) group; fluphenazine is an example. Use of these potent compounds entails a much greater risk of inducing acute extrapyramidal effects but less tendency to produce sedation or autonomic side effects such as hypotension, unless unusually large doses are employed. At least two piperazine phenothiazines have been esterified with long-chain fatty acids (enanthic [heptanoic] or decanoic) to produce slowly absorbed and hydrolyzed, long-acting, lipophilic prodrugs; fluphenazine enanthate and decanoate are the only such derivatives currently available in the United States.

The thioxanthenes are similarly available with aliphatic and piperazine substituents; piperidines are not available. The analog of chlorpromazine among the thioxanthenes is chlorprothixene. The piperazine-substituted thioxanthenes include clopenthixol, flupentixol, and thiothixene; they are all highly potent and effective antipsychotic agents, although to date only thiothixene is available in the United States. Since thioxanthenes have an olefinic double bond between the central-ring carbon atom at position 10 and the side chain, geometric isomers exist; the *cis* (or α) isomers are the more active, perhaps again by facilitating superimposability of structure upon that of dopamine or other catecholamines. This concept of superimposability of the structures of tricyclic antipsychotic compounds and dopamine is supported by stereochemical models and computations, as well as by some limited crystallographic data (Feinberg and Snyder, 1975).

All of the phenothiazines and thioxanthenes used in psychiatry have three carbon atoms interposed between position 10 of the central ring and the first amino nitrogen atom of the side chain at this position; in addition, the amine is always tertiary. This structure of neuroleptic compounds contrasts with that of antihistaminic phenothiazines (*e.g.*, promethazine) or strongly anticholinergic phenothiazines (*e.g.*, ethopropazine, diethazine), which have only two carbon atoms separating the amino group from position 10 of the central ring; addition of a fourth carbon atom similarly results in a reduction or loss of neuroleptic activity. When one or two of the methyl or other substituents of the tertiary amino group of the side chain are removed (as can occur in the natural metabolism of chlorpromazine), there is an increasing loss of activity; in addition, increasing the size of amino N-alkyl substituents leads to a reduction of activity.

The structure-activity relationship has also been studied in some detail for a large number of butyrophenones and their congeners. About 20 of these compounds have been prepared and characterized; many have been used in clinical trials, for the most part in Europe. The largest group of butyrophenones includes substituted piperidine compounds that are analogs of haloperidol. Among these is spiroperidol, one of the most potent neuroleptics yet discovered. In addition, there are several investigational piperazine-substituted butyrophenones and a short-acting tetrahydropyridine derivative, droperidol, which is used almost exclusively in anesthesia.

More recently a second and closely related family of interesting drugs has been developed, the *diphenylbutylpiperidines*. These compounds include fluspirilene, penfluridol, and pimozide, all of which are under active clinical study. These agents are both extraordinarily potent and very long acting (several days to a week or more) after *oral* administration, unlike any other type of neuroleptic agent. Further discussion of the structure-activity relationship of the butyrophenones and diphenylbutylpiperidines can be found in the review articles cited above.

Several other classes of heterocyclic compounds have neuroleptic or antipsychotic effects, but too few are available or sufficiently well characterized to permit conclusions regarding structure-activity relationship. These include a small number of *indole* compounds (notably, molindone and oxypertine) and several piperazine-substituted tricyclic compounds with various seven-membered central rings. These latter agents bear some resemblance to the imipramine-like antidepressant drugs and include *dibenzoxazepines* (notably, loxapine, a typical neuroleptic) and *dibenzodiazepines* (notably, clozapine, a most interesting antipsychotic agent that seems to have little neurological toxicity and minimal central antidopaminergic activity; unfortunately bone-marrow toxicity may preclude its clinical use).

Other heterocyclic compounds include butaclamol, a pentacyclic compound with active (dextrorotatory) and inactive enantiomeric forms that have been useful in characterization of the stereochemistry of the sites of action of neuroleptic agents. Sulpiride is a drug with several similarities to clozapine, except that it is not strongly anticholinergic and it has not been reported to be toxic to the bone marrow. This agent may produce mild extrapyramidal effects, and it has at least some antipsychotic efficacy. The availability of drugs such as clozapine, sulpiride, and, to some extent, thioridazine is encouraging, since they represent at least partial exceptions to the formerly almost-inevitable association of neurotoxic with antipsychotic effects.

PHARMACOLOGICAL PROPERTIES

The antipsychotic drugs share many pharmacological effects and therapeutic applications. Chlorpromazine is commonly taken as a prototype for the group. Many antipsychotic drugs, and especially chlorpromazine and other agents of low potency, have sedative effects. These are especially conspicuous early in treatment, although tolerance to this effect is typical; sedation may not be noticeable when very agitated psychotic patients are treated. Antipsychotic drugs also have well-demonstrated antianxiety effects. However, this class of agents is not generally used for such a purpose, largely because of their neurological and autonomic side effects.

The term *neuroleptic* was introduced by Delay and Deniker in the early 1950s and was based on their observation of the effects of chlorpromazine and reserpine in psychiatric patients. By the use of this term, they intended to contrast the effects of the new agents with those of classical CNS depressants such as the general anesthetics, sedatives and hypnotics, and opioids. As described, the neuroleptic syndrome consisted in suppression of spontaneous movements and complex behavior, while spinal reflexes and unconditioned nociceptive-avoidance behaviors remained intact. In man, the neuroleptic drugs cause a striking lack of initiative, disinterest in the environment, little display of emotion, and a limited range of affect. Initially, there might be some slowness in response to external stimuli and drowsiness. However, subjects are easily aroused, capable of giving appropriate answers to direct questions, and seem to have their intellectual functions intact; there is no ataxia, incoordination, or dysarthria. Psychotic patients become less agitated and restless, and withdrawn or autistic patients sometimes become more responsive and communicative. Aggressive and impulsive behavior diminishes. Gradually (usually over a period of days), psychotic symptoms of hallucinations, delusions, and disorganized or incoherent thinking tend to disappear. In addition, early clinical reports of the effects of chlorpromazine described neurological effects, including bradykinesia, mild rigidity, some tremor, and occasional subjective restlessness (akathisia), that resemble those of postencephalitic or idiopathic Parkinson's disease. Indeed, some clinicians believed that the neurological and antipsychotic actions were inevitably, and perhaps causally, associated and even advocated their provocation as a test of effectiveness of the drug.

While the original use of the term *neuroleptic* appears to have encompassed the whole unique syndrome just described, and to this day is commonly used as a synonym for *antipsychotic* in Europe, there is now a tendency to use the term *neuroleptic* to emphasize the more neurological aspects of the syndrome (*i.e.,* the extrapyramidal, parkinsonian aspects) and to consider these effects as nonessential or even undesirable. The description of drugs such as clozapine that are clearly antipsychotic and have little extrapyramidal action has reinforced this trend. At the present time, virtually all of the drugs with antipsychotic activity that are available in the United States also have effects on movement and posture and can thus be called neuroleptic. However, the more general and hopeful term *antipsychotic* is commonly used and may be preferable.

General Psychophysiological and Behavioral Effects. In animals and in man, the most prominent observable effects of typical neuroleptic agents are strikingly similar. In low doses, operant behavior is reduced but spinal reflexes are unchanged. Exploratory behavior is diminished, and responses to a variety of stimuli are fewer, slower, and smaller, although the ability to discriminate stimuli is retained. Conditioned avoidance behaviors are selectively inhibited, while unconditioned escape or avoidance responses are not. The highly reinforcing self-stimulation of the animal brain (typically with electrodes placed in the monoamine-rich median forebrain bundle) is blocked, although the capacity to press the stimulation-inducing lever is not lost. Behavioral activation, stimulated environmentally or pharmacologically, is blocked. Feeding is inhibited. Most neuroleptics block the emesis and aggression induced by apomorphine—a dopaminergic agonist. In high doses, most neuroleptic agents induce characteristic cataleptic immobility that allows the animal to be placed in abnormal postures that persist. Muscle tone is altered, and ptosis is typical. The animal appears to be indifferent to most stimuli, although it continues to withdraw from those that are noxious or painful. Many learned tasks can still be performed if sufficient stimulation and motivation are provided. Even very high doses of most neuroleptics do not induce coma, and the lethal dose is extraordinarily high. Many of these effects are well summarized by Fielding and Lal (1978).

Effects on Motor Activity. Nearly all of the neuroleptic agents used in psychiatry can diminish spontaneous motor activity in every species of animal studied, including man. However, one of the more disturbing side effects of chlorpromazine, *akathisia,* is manifested by a marked increase in motor activity (page 407). The cataleptic immobility of animals treated with phenothiazines, described above, resembles the *catatonia* seen in some schizophrenics and in a variety of metabolic and neurological disorders affecting the CNS. In man, catatonic signs, along with other features of schizophrenia, are sometimes relieved by antipsychotic agents. However, rigidity and bradykinesia, which can mimic catatonia, can be induced in patients, especially by large doses of the more potent neuroleptic agents, and reversed by removal of the drug or the addition of an antiparkinsonian agent (*see* Fielding and Lal, 1978; Janssen and Van Bever, 1978).

Chlorpromazine causes skeletal muscular relaxation in some types of spastic conditions. Since it has little effect at spinal levels, actions on motor activity must be mediated at a higher level, perhaps in the basal ganglia. The drug does not produce blockade of the neuromuscular junction.

Phenothiazines and other antipsychotic drugs often produce parkinsonism and other extrapyramidal effects. Theories concerning the mechanisms underlying these extrapyramidal reactions, as well as descriptions of their clinical presentations and management, are given below.

Effects on Sleep. The effect of antipsychotic drugs on sleep patterns is not consistent, but they tend to normalize sleep disturbances characteristic of many psychoses. The ability to prolong and enhance the effect of opioid and hypnotic drugs appears to parallel the sedative potency of the particular agent. The more potent neuroleptic agents that do not cause drowsiness also do not enhance hypnosis produced by other drugs.

Effects on Conditioned Responses. Courvoisier and colleagues (1953) found that chlorpromazine impairs the ability of animals to make a conditioned avoidance response to a learned sensory cue that signals the onset of punishing shock avoidable by moving to a safe place in an experimental box. Under the influence of small doses of the drug, animals ignore the warning signal but still attempt to escape once the shock is applied. General CNS depressants affect both avoidance (the conditioned response) and escape (the unconditioned response) to approximately the same extent. Cook and Weidley (1957) confirmed and extended these observations on chlorpromazine, and showed that barbiturates and meprobamate affect the conditioned as well as the unconditioned responses to about the same extent, and only in doses that produce ataxia or hypnosis. Since then, many variations on the conditioned avoidance paradigm have been developed, utilizing operant conditioning technics in which the avoidance behavior requires bar pressing, which can be evaluated quantitatively and automatically (Fielding and Lal, 1978). Passive avoidance behavior, requiring immobility, is also suppressed by neuroleptic drugs, in contrast to what might be expected in the case of drugs that suppress locomotion nonspecifically (Iwahara *et al.*, 1968).

Since correlations between antipsychotic effectiveness and conditioned avoidance tests are quite good for many types of neuroleptic agents, they have, as mentioned, become the basis for screening procedures in pharmaceutical psychopharmacology laboratories. Despite their empirical utility and quantitative characteristics, effects on conditioned avoidance do not provide important models or insights into the basis of antipsychotic effects in man. For example, the effects of neuroleptic drugs on conditioned avoidance are subject to tolerance and are blocked by anticholinergic agents, while their clinical antipsychotic actions are not. Moreover, the extraordinarily close correlation between the potencies of drugs in conditioned avoidance tests and their ability to block the behavioral effects of dopaminergic agonists such as amphetamine or apomorphine suggests that such avoidance tests may be specifically *selective* for drugs with extrapyramidal and other neurological effects. The inability of the atypical and more selective antipsychotic drugs, such as clozapine and sulpiride, to antagonize dopamine agonists or to block conditioned avoidance responses in animal behavioral tests also supports this interpretation. (*See* Barchas *et al.,*1978; Fielding and Lal, 1978; Janssen and Van Bever, 1978.)

Effects on Complex Behavior. Antipsychotic drugs impair vigilance in human subjects performing a variety of tasks, such as continuous pursuit-rotor and tapping-speed tests. The drugs produce relatively little impairment of digit-symbol substitution, a test of intellectual functioning. On the other hand, secobarbital causes greater impairment in performance in digit-symbol substitution than in continuous performance and other vigilance tests. In normal subjects, neuroleptic agents of low potency may inhibit the performance of complex intellectual tasks such as story writing, but such experiments are difficult to design and interpret.

Effects on Specific Areas of the Nervous System. The effects of antipsychotic drugs are apparent at all levels in the nervous system. Although the actions underlying the antipsychotic and many of the neurological effects of antipsychotic drugs remain unknown, theories based on their ability to antagonize the actions of dopamine as a neurotransmitter in the basal ganglia and limbic portions of the forebrain have become most prominent and are supported by a large body of data.

Cortex. Since psychosis involves a disorder of higher functions and thought processes, cortical effects of antipsychotic drugs are of great interest. However, there is little information available about specific effects on the cortex that shed light on the mechanisms of action of antipsychotic drugs. On the other hand, there is an abundance of data concerning cortical or scalp recordings of the EEG in animals and man.

EEG. When neuroleptic drugs are given to animals, there is slowing and a decrease in the variability of frequencies (*synchronization*) and a decrease in arousal-induced changes in the EEG; these effects are reversed by dopaminergic agonists, which also tend to induce arousal and desynchronization of the EEG (Longo, 1978). Similarly, when chlorpromazine is administered to man, there is a slowing of the EEG pattern, with an increase in the occurrence of theta waves and, to a lesser degree, delta waves, a decrease in alpha waves and fast-beta activity, and some increase in burst activity and spiking (Fink, 1969; Itil, 1978). The increased synchronization is accompanied by an increase in voltage. There is also a reduction of the arousing effects of sensory stimuli (*e.g.,* blocking of alpha rhythm). Many studies have been conducted on the effects of antipsychotic drugs on sensory-evoked EEG potentials. These have usually suggested either decreases in amplitudes and increases in latencies or a tendency toward "normalization" of aberrant responses, perhaps especially in patients who respond favorably to treatment (Shagass and Straumanis, 1978).

Seizure Threshold. Many neuroleptic drugs can lower the seizure threshold and induce discharge patterns in the EEG that are associated with epileptic seizure disorders. Aliphatic phenothiazines with low potency (particularly chlorpromazine) seem particularly able to do this, while the more potent neuroleptic piperazine phenothiazines and thioxanthenes (notably, fluphenazine and thiothixene) seem least likely to have this effect (Itil, 1978). The butyrophenones have variable and unpredictable effects on seizure activity; molindone may have the least activity of this type among neuroleptic agents. Overt seizures associated with the administration of antipsychotic drugs are more likely to be seen in patients who have either a history of epilepsy or a condition that predisposes to seizures. Neuroleptic agents, especially low-potency phenothiazines and thioxanthenes, should be used with *extreme caution,* if at all, in untreated epileptic patients and in patients undergoing withdrawal from central depressants such as alcohol or barbiturates. Antipsychotic drugs, especially the piperazines, can be used safely in epileptics if moderate doses are attained gradually and if concomitant anticonvulsant drug therapy is maintained (*see* Chapter 20).

Basal Ganglia. Because the extrapyramidal effects of nearly all of the available antipsychotic drugs are prominent, a great deal of interest has centered on the actions of these drugs in the basal ganglia, notably the caudate nucleus, putamen, globus pallidus, and allied nuclei, which are believed to play a crucial role in the control of posture and the involuntary (extrapyramidal) aspects of movement. Current understanding of the role of a deficiency of dopamine in this region in the pathogenesis of Parkinson's disease, the modest success of levodopa in treating this disease, and the striking resemblance between the clinical manifestations of Parkinson's disease and the neurological effects of neuroleptic drugs have all focused attention on the possible role of a deficiency of dopamine activity in neuroleptic-induced extrapyramidal effects.

The suggestion that interference with the transmitter function of dopamine in the mammalian forebrain might contribute to the neurological and possibly also the antipsychotic effects of the neuroleptic drugs was first made by European pharmacologists in the early 1960s. This hypothesis arose largely from the observation that neuroleptic drugs consistently increased the concentrations of the metabolites of dopamine, but had variable effects on the metabolism of other neurotransmitters (Carlsson and Lindqvist, 1963). The importance of dopamine was also strongly supported by early histochemical studies of amine-containing neurons in the mammalian brain, which indicated a preferential distribution of dopamine-containing fibers between midbrain and the basal ganglia (notably, the nigroneostriatal tract), and within the hypothalamus (*see* Chapters 12 and 21). More recently, neuroanatomists have come to appreciate the existence of other dopamine-containing projections from midbrain tegmental nuclei to forebrain regions associated with the limbic system, as well as to temporal and prefrontal cerebral cortical areas closely interlinked with the limbic system. A somewhat simplistic, but attractive, concept arose: many extrapyramidal neurological effects of the antipsychotic drugs might be mediated by antidopaminergic effects in the basal ganglia. Their antipsychotic effects might be mediated by antagonism of dopaminergic neurotransmission in the limbic, mesocortical, and hypothalamic systems.

A compelling body of data has now accumulated to support the theory that antagonism of dopamine-mediated synaptic neurotransmission is an important action of neuroleptic drugs (Baldessarini, 1977a; Carlsson, 1978; Creese *et al.,* 1978; Baldessarini and Tarsy, 1979). Thus, antipsychotic drugs with neuroleptic actions, but not their inactive congeners, increase the rate of production of dopamine metabolites (notably, 3-methoxytyramine and dihydroxyphenylacetic and homovanillic acids), the rate of conversion of the precursor amino acid tyrosine to dopamine and its metabolites (Sedvall, 1975), and the rate of firing of putative dopamine-containing cells in the midbrain (Bunney *et al.,* 1973). These effects have usually been interpreted to represent secondary or compensatory responses of plastic and adaptive neuronal systems attempting to maintain homeostasis in the face of what is assumed to be a primary interruption of synaptic transmission at dopaminergic terminals in the caudate nucleus and other areas of the forebrain.

Evidence that a crucial primary event may be the blockade of postsynaptic dopamine receptor sites includes the observations that small doses of neuroleptic drugs block behavioral or neuroendocrine effects of dopaminergic agonists. Examples are stereotypical gnawing behavior in the rat induced by apomorphine, possibly by a direct dopaminergic effect on the caudate nucleus; locomotor excitement induced by the injection of dopamine or apomorphine into the limbic terminals, such as the nucleus accumbens septi; and the effect of apomorphine or levodopa to inhibit secretion of prolactin, believed to be mediated by hypothalamic or pituitary receptors for dopamine. Notably, atypical antipsychotic drugs such as clozapine and pimozide are characterized by their very weak actions or inactivity in such tests.

More direct evidence of receptor blockade by neuroleptic drugs has been provided by their antagonism of a selective dopamine-sensitive adenylate cyclase system in homogenates of caudate or limbic tissue (Clement-Cormier *et al.,* 1974; Greengard, 1978) and their interference with electrophysiological responses to dopamine or apomorphine applied iontophoretically to receptive cells in the caudate nucleus. This latter blockade can be overcome by what is presumably circumvention of the receptor sites on the cell surface by the iontophoresis of analogs of cyclic adenosine 3',5'-monophosphate (cyclic AMP) (Siggins *et al.,* 1976). A more recent development is the application of radioligand binding assays that use homogenates or membrane fractions from mammalian caudate tissue as a source of receptors and low concentrations of tritiated neuroleptic drugs (particularly haloperidol and the very potent compound spiroperidol) or dopaminergic agonists (dopamine itself or apomorphine) as ligands (*see* Creese *et al.,* 1978; Snyder *et al.,* 1978). Pharmacological evidence supports the concept that the binding of these ligands to brain tissue represents, at least partially, an interaction with a dopaminergic receptor site. Questions remain about the validity of the assumptions involved in these technics. However, the correlation is generally excellent between the potency *in vitro* of antipsychotic drugs of *all types* to interfere with the binding of these ligands and esti-

mates of their clinical potency or of their ability to block the effects of dopaminergic agonists in animals (Baldessarini, 1977a; Creese *et al.,* 1978). Analogs and isomers of the antipsychotic drugs that are inactive clinically lack the ability to compete for relevant ligand binding sites.

Together, these findings strongly support the theory that antipsychotic drugs interfere with the actions of dopamine as a synaptic neurotransmitter in the brain. At the same time, they do not prove that antidopaminergic effects are either necessary or sufficient to account for the diverse extrapyramidal effects of the neuroleptic drugs, let alone their antipsychotic actions.

Limbic System. Dopaminergic projections from the midbrain terminate on several septal nuclei, the olfactory tubercle, the amygdala, and other structures within the temporal and prefrontal lobes of the cerebrum. In view of the dopamine hypothesis just reviewed with respect to the extrapyramidal aspects of the actions of neuroleptic drugs, it is not surprising that much attention has also been given to the mesolimbic system as a possible site of mediation of at least some of the antipsychotic effects of these agents. Speculations about the pathophysiology of the idiopathic psychoses such as schizophrenia have centered around the limbic area for many years. These have been given some indirect encouragement by repeated "natural experiments" that have associated psychotic mental phenomena with lesions of the temporal lobe and other portions of the limbic system (*see* Baldessarini, 1977a; Barchas *et al.,* 1978).

Many of the behavioral, neurophysiological, biochemical, and pharmacological findings about the dopaminergic system of the basal ganglia have been extended to mesolimbic and mesocortical tissue as well. Since there are a number of differences in the extrapyramidal and antipsychotic actions of the neuroleptic drugs, there have been many attempts to define differences in the regulation of dopaminergic systems in the various regions of the brain to account for these differences. They include the observations that many of the acute extrapyramidal effects of the neuroleptic drugs tend to diminish or to disappear over a period of weeks or a few months and that some of these effects are very sensitive to concurrent administration of anticholinergic, antiparkinsonism drugs; neither observation is true of the antipsychotic effects. A most encouraging early finding was that, while anticholinergic agents block the increase in turnover of dopamine induced by neuroleptic agents in the basal ganglia, they seem not to do so in limbic areas containing dopaminergic terminals (Carlsson, 1978). There are other findings that also support the impression that not all dopaminergic systems are similar, either functionally or in their manner of regulation or response to drugs (*see* Bunney and Aghajanian, 1978; Moore and Kelly, 1978; Sulser and Robinson, 1978). For example, the development of *tolerance* to the effect of antipsychotic drugs to enhance the turnover of dopamine may not be as prominent in limbic as in extrapyramidal areas. However, there is even more evidence that many of the effects of antipsychotic drugs are similar in both regions. Thus, the regional similarities are particularly striking in the case of *in-vitro* tests of dopamine receptor blockade, such as inhibition of dopamine-sensitive adenylate cyclase (Clement-Cormier *et al.,* 1974) and the competition for binding of ligands purported to interact with receptors for dopamine (Creese *et al.,* 1978). For further discussions of this topic, *see* Carlsson (1978) and other references already cited.

Hypothalamus. In addition to neurological and antipsychotic effects that appear to be mediated in part by antidopaminergic actions of the neuroleptic drugs, there are endocrine changes that have been related to effects of these agents on the hypothalamus or pituitary that might involve dopamine. Prominent among these is the ability of most neuroleptic drugs to increase the rate of secretion of prolactin in man.

The effect of neuroleptic agents on prolactin secretion may be due to a blockade of the tuberoinfundibular dopaminergic system that projects from the arcuate nucleus of the hypothalamus to the median eminence or to a direct antagonistic action at dopaminergic receptors localized on cells of the anterior pituitary. The existence of dopaminergic receptors in the pituitary itself, as well as morphological evidence of an intimate relationship between dopamine-containing neurosecretory terminals in the median eminence and the small blood vessels of the hypophyseal portal system, has encouraged speculation that dopamine itself may be the elusive prolactin release-inhibiting hormone known to exist in the hypothalamus (*see* Reichlin and Boyd, 1978; Chapter 59).

Correlations between the potencies of neuroleptic drugs to stimulate prolactin secretion and to cause behavioral effects are excellent in both animals and man. They prevail for many classes of drugs (Meltzer *et al.,* 1978; Sachar, 1978). There are, however, a few discrepancies. The effects of neuroleptic drugs on prolactin secretion tend to occur at lower doses than do their antipsychotic effects; this may reflect their action outside the blood-brain barrier in the inferior hypothalamus or in the pituitary gland. There is no tolerance to the effect of antipsychotic drugs on prolactin, even after years of treatment. However, the effect is rapidly reversible when the drugs are discontinued (Overall, 1978). It seems likely that this effect of antipsychotic agents is responsible for the breast engorgement and galactorrhea that is sometimes associated with their use, even in male patients.

The effects of neuroleptics on other hypothalamic neuroendocrine functions are much less well characterized, although they do inhibit the release of growth hormone (Martin *et al.,* 1978) and chlorpromazine may reduce the secretion of corticotropin-regulatory hormone in response to certain stresses (Frohman, 1972). In addition to neuroendocrine effects, it is likely that the other autonomic effects of some antipsychotic drugs may be mediated by the hypothalamus. An important example is the *poikilothermic effect* of chlorpromazine, which is sometimes used to facilitate the induction of surgical hypothermia.

Brain Stem. Chlorpromazine can depress brain stem functions. Ordinarily clinical doses of the phenothiazines have little effect upon *respiration.* In human subjects, slight depression of respiratory minute and tidal volumes has been reported following a single intravenous or intramuscular injection (Dobkin *et al.,* 1954). *Vasomotor reflexes* mediated by either the hypothalamus or the brain stem are depressed by relatively low doses of chlorpromazine. This effect might occur at many points in the reflex pathway, and the net result is a centrally mediated fall in blood pressure. Even when there is acute overdosage with suicidal intent, the phenothiazines usually do not cause life-threatening coma or suppression of vital functions; this contributes importantly to their safety.

Chemoreceptor Trigger Zone (CTZ). Most neuroleptic agents have a marked protective action against the nausea- and emesis-inducing effects of apomorphine and certain ergot alkaloids, all of which can interact with central dopaminergic receptors in the CTZ of the medulla. The antiemetic effect of most neuroleptics occurs with very low doses. However, thioridazine, uniquely, has no clinical efficacy as an antiemetic in man. Drugs or other stimuli that cause emesis by an action on the nodose ganglion or locally on the gastrointestinal tract are not antagonized by antipsychotic drugs, but potent piperazines and butyrophenones are sometimes effective against nausea due to vestibular stimulation. Several antipsychotic agents have become especially popular for the treatment of nausea and vomiting (*see* below).

Spinal Cord. Disagreement exists concerning the effects of chlorpromazine upon spinal reflexes; certain investigators claim that chlorpromazine has little or no effect upon such reflexes, while others claim depression of one or another. For the antipsychotic drugs as a group, the current consensus is that depressant actions on the spinal cord are minor, if present at all, and contribute little to the actions of these drugs.

Peripheral Nerves. Chlorpromazine is a potent

local anesthetic, but the drug has never been used for this purpose. Indeed, most of the antipsychotic drugs and even their clinically ineffective congeners exert local anesthetic or so-called membrane-stabilizing effects, especially at high concentrations (typically above 10 μM); these have little to do with the important actions of the drugs (Seeman, 1972; *see also* Creese *et al.*, 1978).

Autonomic Nervous System. Since various antipsychotic agents have peripheral cholinergic blocking activity, α-adrenergic blocking actions, and adrenergic activity (secondary to the block of neuronal re-uptake of amines), their effects on the autonomic nervous system are complex and unpredictable. Antihistaminic and antitryptaminergic effects of these agents further complicate the picture.

Chlorpromazine does have significant α-adrenergic antagonistic activity and can either block or reverse the pressor effects of epinephrine. Based on the extent of antagonism of the effects of norepinephrine *in vivo* and competition for binding sites with radioligands believed to be selective for α-adrenergic receptors, the relative potencies of several antipsychotic drugs as α-adrenergic antagonists can be ranked as follows: relatively strong (piperacetazine > droperidol > triflupromazine > chlorpromazine); moderate (thioridazine > fluphenazine > haloperidol); relatively weak (trifluperazine > clozapine $\gg$ pimozide). Since piperazines and haloperidol are used in low doses to produce antipsychotic effects, it follows that they should show little antiadrenergic activity in patients; indeed, this seems to be true (*see* Creese *et al.*, 1978; Janssen and Van Bever, 1978; Snyder *et al.*, 1978).

The cholinergic blocking effects of antipsychotic drugs are relatively weak, but the blurring of vision commonly experienced with chlorpromazine may be due to an anticholinergic action on the ciliary muscle. Chlorpromazine regularly produces a miosis in man, which can be due to α-adrenergic blockade. Other phenothiazines can cause mydriasis, and this is especially likely to occur with thioridazine, which is the most potent muscarinic antagonist of the group. Chlorpromazine has intermediate antimuscarinic potency and can cause constipation and decreased gastric secretion and motility. Doses of 1 to 3 mg/kg can block the effects of physostigmine on intestinal tone and peristalsis, presumably as a result of cholinergic blockade. Decreased sweating and salivation are probably additional manifestations of the anticholinergic effects of the phenothiazines. Urinary retention is rare, but can occur in males with prostatism. Anticholinergic effects are least frequently caused by piperazines and other potent neuroleptics, including haloperidol (*see* Snyder *et al.*, 1978). The anticholinergic status of clozapine remains controversial. It is very potent in several tests *in vitro* but does not seem to be active *in vivo* (*see* Carlsson, 1978).

The phenothiazines inhibit ejaculation without interfering with erection. Thioridazine produces this effect with some regularity, and there are thus problems in its acceptance by male patients. Attribution of this effect to adrenergic blockade is logical but unsubstantiated inasmuch as thioridazine is less potent than chlorpromazine in its antiadrenergic effects.

For further discussion of the autonomic pharmacology of the phenothiazines, the exhaustive monographs by Gordon (1967, 1974) should be consulted. Reviews by Sigg (1968), Klein and Davis (1969), and Shader and DiMascio (1970) also describe the autonomic side effects of numerous psychotropic drugs.

Endocrine System. The effects of neuroleptic drugs on hypothalamic regulatory hormones result in profound changes in the endocrine system, as mentioned above with respect to increased secretion of prolactin. Chlorpromazine can also reduce urinary concentrations of gonadotropins, as well as those of estrogens and progestins. As a result of these derangements, galactorrhea and gynecomastia can occur. Amenorrhea is also seen with chlorpromazine, but this is relatively infrequent. In animals, the drug can block ovulation, suppress the estrous cycle, cause infertility and pseudopregnancy, and maintain an endometrial decidual reaction. Inhibition of secretion of gonadotropin also can result in decreased testicular weight.

Since antipsychotic drugs are used chronically and thus cause prolonged elevations of concentrations of prolactin, there has been concern over a possible increased risk of carcinoma of the breast. To date, there is no evidence that the use of antipsychotic agents entails this risk (Brugmans *et al.*, 1973; Schyve *et al.*, 1978). Nevertheless, neuroleptic and other agents that stimulate the secretion of prolactin should be avoided in patients with established cases of carcinoma of the breast.

Nonreproductive endocrinological functions are also affected. Chlorpromazine may cause a decrease in the secretion of adrenocorticosteroids as a result of diminished release of corticotropin. It interferes with the secretion of pituitary growth hormone, an effect utilized for a while in the treatment of acromegaly (Kolodny *et al.*, 1971). Neuroleptics are in fact poor therapy for acromegaly (Dimond *et al.*, 1973), and there is no evidence that they retard growth or development of children. In addition, chlorpromazine can decrease the secretion of neurohypophyseal hormones. Weight gain and an increase in appetite occur with all phenothiazines but not with haloperidol. Chlorpromazine may also impair glucose tolerance and insulin release to a clinically appreciable degree in some prediabetic patients (Erle *et al.*, 1977). Peripheral edema occurs in 1 to 3% of patients and may be of endocrine origin.

Kidney. Chlorpromazine may have weak diuretic effects in animals and man, due either to a depressant action upon the secretion of antidiuretic hormone (ADH) or to inhibition of reabsorption of water and electrolytes by a direct action on the renal tubule, or both. The slight fall in blood pressure that occurs with chlorpromazine is not associated with any significant change in glomerular filtration rate; indeed, there is a tendency toward an increase in renal blood flow.

Cardiovascular System. The actions of chlorpromazine on the cardiovascular system are complex because the drug produces direct effects on the heart and blood vessels, and also indirect ones through actions on CNS and autonomic reflexes. In normal man, the intravenous administration of chlorpromazine causes *orthostatic hypotension,* due to a combination of central actions and peripheral α-adrenergic blockade, and reflex *tachycardia.* Oral therapy causes mild hypotension, systolic blood pressure being affected more than diastolic. Tolerance develops to the hypotensive effect, so that after several weeks of chronic administration the pressures return toward normal (Sakalis *et al.,* 1972). However, some degree of orthostatic hypotension may persist indefinitely. The orthostatic hypotension occurs more frequently with chlorpromazine and thioridazine, and less so with piperazine derivatives, haloperidol, loxapine, and molindone. Chlorpromazine also has a direct depressant action on the heart; cat papillary muscle shows a negative inotropic response to relatively low concentrations of chlorpromazine. The drug has a vasodilating action due to both its effects on the autonomic nervous system and a direct action on blood vessels. An increase in coronary blood flow may result from administration of the drug.

Chlorpromazine has an antiarrhythmic effect upon the heart, which may be due either to a quinidine-like action or to a local anesthetic effect. ECG changes include prolongation of the Q-T and P-R intervals, blunting of T waves, and S-T segment depression. Thioridazine, in particular, causes a high incidence of T wave changes. Cardiotoxicity of a more severe nature has been reported in young patients (Alexander and Nino, 1969). These effects are less common when the more potent antipsychotic agents are administered.

Liver. Aside from the hypersensitivity reactions occasionally seen after administration of the antipsychotic drugs, such as an obstructive form of jaundice (*see* below), these agents have no characteristic hepatic effects. The drugs may be used in patients with hepatic disease, but caution is advisable. Since their metabolism may be delayed or modified, they may compromise an already diseased liver.

Miscellaneous Biochemical Effects. There are a number of reports of interactions of antipsychotic drugs with central neurohumors other than dopamine that may contribute to their antipsychotic effects or other actions (*see* Carlsson, 1978). For example, many neuroleptics enhance the turnover of acetylcholine, especially in the basal ganglia. This effect may be secondary to the blockade of dopamine receptors on cholinergic neurons. In addition, as already discussed above, there is an inverse relationship between antimuscarinic potency of antipsychotic drugs in the brain and the likelihood of extrapyramidal effects (Snyder *et al.,* 1978). There is also a suggestion that β-adrenergic blockade may contribute to central actions of neuroleptic agents (Sulser and Robinson, 1978), and speculation that other amines (*e.g.,* 5-hydroxytryptamine [5-HT]), amino acids (gamma-aminobutyric acid, GABA), or peptides (substance P, endorphins) that are known to affect dopamine neurons may also provide likely sites of action of some antipsychotic agents (*see* Carlsson, 1978). Although chlorpromazine and a few other low-potency phenothiazines have mild antag-

onistic actions at receptors for histamine and 5-HT, these affects are not shared by all antipsychotic drugs and are unlikely to contribute in an important way to their major actions.

Absorption, Fate, and Excretion. The study of the pharmacokinetics and metabolism of the antipsychotic drugs is one of the most active aspects of their evaluation. At the present time few conclusions with clinical relevance can be drawn. This situation is due in part to limitations of the laboratory technics involved, the complex metabolism of some antipsychotic agents, and, very importantly, the many frustrations inherent in diagnosis and objective evaluation of clinical change in psychotic patients.

A few generalizations can be made. Most antipsychotic drugs tend to have erratic and unpredictable patterns of absorption, particularly with oral administration and even when liquid preparations are used. Parenteral (intramuscular) administration can increase the availability of active drug by four to ten times. The drugs are highly lipophilic, highly membrane or protein bound, and accumulate in the brain, lung, and other tissues with a high blood supply. Antipsychotic agents enter the fetal circulation quite easily. It is virtually impossible (and, fortunately, usually not necessary) to remove these agents by dialysis.

The pharmacokinetics of all antipsychotic drugs follows a multiphasic pattern. The usually stated elimination half-lives with respect to total concentrations in plasma are typically 10 to 20 hours. The biological effects of single doses usually persist for at least 24 hours; this encourages the common current practice of giving the entire daily dose at one time, once the patient has accommodated to the initial side effects of the drug. Elimination from the plasma may be more rapid than from sites of high lipid content and binding, notably in the CNS. Direct pharmacokinetic studies on this issue are few and inconclusive. Nevertheless, metabolites of some agents have been detected in the urine for as long as several months after the drug has been discontinued. Slow removal of drug may contribute to the typically slow rate of exacerbation of psychosis after stopping drug treatment, and this complicates evaluation of psychotic patients who have been on antipsychotic therapy.

The main routes of metabolism of the antipsychotic drugs are by oxidative processes mediated largely by hepatic microsomal and other drug-metabolizing enzymes. Conjugation with glucuronic acid is a very prominent route of metabolism. Hydrophilic metabolites of these drugs are excreted in the urine and, to some extent, in the bile. Most oxidized metabolites of antipsychotic drugs are also biologically *inactive,* but a few are not (notably, 7-hydroxychlorpromazine and mesoridazine) and may contribute to the biological activity of the parent substance, as well as complicate the problem of correlating assays of drug in blood with clinical effects. A bioassay that detects active metabolites that can compete for binding of a radioligand may help to simplify this problem (*see* Creese *et al.,* 1978). The less potent antipsychotic drugs may induce their own hepatic metabolism or conjugation, since concentrations of chlorpromazine and other phenothiazines in blood are lower after several weeks of treatment with the same dosage; it is also possible that alterations of gastrointestinal motility are partially responsible. Age is an important determinant of the rate of metabolism and excretion of antipsychotic drugs. The fetus, the infant, and the elderly have diminished capacity to metabolize and eliminate these agents (Morselli, 1977).

The pharmacokinetics of antipsychotic drugs has been reviewed by Cooper and associates (1976), Morselli (1977), Hollister (1978a), May and Van Putten (1978), and Baldessarini (1979a).

Detailed comments on the pharmacokinetics can be offered for only a few agents that have been well studied. Chlorpromazine is preeminent in this regard, not only because the drug has been in use for decades, but also because it is employed in large doses and relatively high concentrations of drug and metabolites are thus available for assay. Unfortunately, its extraordinarily complex metabolism limits its usefulness as a model agent (*see* May and Van Putten, 1978). The absorption of tablets of chlorpromazine is very erratic, although the bioavailability seems to be increased somewhat by the use of liquid concentrates, as is true for many of the antipsychotic agents. However, these preparations tend to be expensive and inconvenient to use. Peak concentrations in plasma are attained in about 2 to 4 hours. Intramuscular administration of the drug avoids much of the first-pass metabolism in the liver (and possibly also the gut) and provides measurable concentrations in plasma within 15 to 30 minutes; bioavailability is increased up to tenfold. The gastrointestinal absorption of chlorpromazine is modified unpredictably by food and is decreased by orally administered colloidal antacids and by anticholinergic drugs such as certain of the antiparkinsonian agents that are often given with neuroleptics to ameliorate their extrapyramidal effects (Rivera-Calimlin *et al.,* 1973). Chlorpromazine and other antipsychotic agents bind significantly to membranes and to plasma albumin. Concentrations of the drug in brain can be up to ten times those in the blood, and the apparent volume of distribution of the drug is high (about 20 liters per kilogram). Elimination of the drug from plasma includes a rapid ($t_{1/2}$ about 2 hours) and a slower ($t_{1/2}$ about 30 hours) phase, but markedly variable values have been reported; the half-life of elimination from human brain is unknown. The rate of elimination and of metabolism of chlorpromazine and other antipsychotic drugs decreases with advancing age, and smaller doses of the drug must be used in elderly patients.

Attempts to correlate plasma concentrations of chlorpromazine or of its metabolites with clinical responses have not been especially successful (*see* Cooper *et al.,* 1976; May and Van Putten, 1978). They indicate that wide variations (at least tenfold) in plasma concentrations occur among individuals. These are not eliminated by controlling the dose, timing, and prior exposure to the drug, suggesting that individual genetic determinants may be responsible. Although it appears that plasma concentrations of chlorpromazine below 30 ng/ml are not likely to produce an adequate antipsychotic response and that levels above 750 ng/ml are likely to be associated with unacceptable toxicity (Rivera-Calimlin *et al.,* 1973), it is not yet possible to state the concentrations in plasma that are likely to be associated with optimal clinical responses.

There may be as many as 10 or 12 metabolites of chlorpromazine that occur in man in *appreciable* quantities (Morselli, 1977). The most important metabolites, quantitatively, are nor$_2$-chlorpromazine (doubly demethylated), chlorophenothiazine (removal of entire side chain), methoxy and hydroxy products, and glucuronide conjugates of the hydroxylated compounds. In the urine, 7-hydroxylated and dealkylated (nor$_2$) metabolites and their conjugates predominate.

There is less information about other antipsychotic drugs. Thioridazine has been studied relatively well (Buyze *et al.,* 1973; Gottschalk *et al.,* 1975). Its pharmacokinetics and metabolism are similar to those of chlorpromazine, but the strong anticholinergic action of thioridazine on the gut can modify its own absorption. Major metabolites include sulfoxy products at ring-position 5 (inactive) or at the substituent at position 2 (including the *active* metabolite, mesoridazine). Demethylation of the piperidine ring is very rapid, but the activity of this metabolite is unknown. The thioxanthenes are similar to chlorpromazine, except that metabolism to sulfoxides is common and ring-hydroxylated products are uncommon. Piperazine derivatives of the phenothiazines and thioxanthenes are also handled much like chlorpromazine, although metabolism of the piperidine ring itself occurs. Haloperidol and other butyrophenones are metabolized by an N-dealkylation reaction; the resultant fragments can be conjugated with glucuronic acid, and it is believed that all of the metabolites of haloperidol are inactive (Forsman and Öhman, 1974).

Tolerance and Physical Dependence. The antipsychotic drugs are not addicting, as the term is defined in Chapter 23. However, some degree of physical dependence may occur. There are reports of muscular discomfort and difficulty in sleeping that develop several days after abrupt discontinuation. EEG changes upon sudden withdrawal have not been detected. Monkeys given the human equivalent of nearly 600 mg of chlorpromazine daily for over a month showed no obvious withdrawal symptoms when the drug was discontinued.

Tolerance develops to the sedative effects of chlorpromazine and other phenothiazines. This takes place over a period of days or weeks, and has been demonstrated by a variety of objective tests. Tolerance to various antipsychotic drugs and cross-tolerance among the agents are also demonstrable in behavioral and biochemical experiments in animals, particularly those directed toward evaluation of the blockade of dopaminergic receptors in the basal ganglia (see Baldessarini and Tarsy, 1979). This form of tolerance may be less prominent in limbic areas of forebrain. One correlate of tolerance in forebrain dopaminergic systems is the development of *disuse supersensitivity* of those systems, possibly mediated by changes in the receptors for the neurotransmitter. This mechanism may underlie the clinical phenomenon of *withdrawal-emergent dyskinesias* (the development of choreoathetosis on abrupt discontinuation of antipsychotic agents, especially following prolonged use of high doses of potent agents) (Jacobson *et al.,* 1974). Although there may be cross-tolerance among neuroleptic drugs for some effects, clinical problems occur in making rapid changes from high doses of one type of agent to another; hypotension, other autonomic effects, and acute extrapyramidal reactions often result.

Preparations, Routes of Administration, and Dosage. Since there are a large number of agents with known neuroleptic or antipsychotic effects, Table 19-1 summarizes only those that are currently marketed in the United States. A few available agents are excluded that are now known to have inferior antipsychotic effects or that are no longer commonly used in psychiatric patients. These include butaperazine (REPOISE), carphenazine (PROKETAZINE), mepazine (PACATAL), promazine (SPARINE), reserpine and other rauwolfia alkaloids, and thiopropazate (DARTAL). Prochlorperazine (COMPAZINE) has questionable utility as an antipsychotic agent and produces acute extrapyramidal reactions frequently; it is thus not commonly employed in psychiatry, although it is used as an antiemetic. One agent that is deserving of specific comment is thiethylperazine (TORECAN), which is currently marketed only as an antiemetic, although it is a potent dopaminergic antagonist with many neuroleptic-like properties; it is an efficacious antipsychotic agent (Rotrosen *et al.,* 1978). The United States has been particularly slow to accept many psychotropic agents that are in common use in Europe.

Toxic Reactions and Side Effects. The antipsychotic drugs have a high therapeutic index and are remarkably safe agents. Furthermore, most phenothiazines have a relatively flat dose-response curve, so that they can be used over a wide range of dosages. Although occasional deaths from overdosage have been reported, this is a rare event if the patient is given even minimal medical care and if an overdosage is not complicated by the concurrent ingestion of alcohol or other drugs. Based on animal data, the therapeutic index is lowest for thioridazine (20) and chlorpromazine (200) and is in excess of 1000 for the more potent agents (Janssen and Van Bever, 1978). Adult patients have survived doses of chlorpromazine up to 10,000 mg, and deaths due to haloperidol appear to be unknown.

Side effects are often extensions of the many pharmacological actions of the drugs, which have already been discussed. The most important are those on the *CNS, cardiovascular system, autonomic nervous system,* and *endocrine functions.* The *extrapyramidal effects,* which are of great importance, are discussed in detail below (see also Shader and DiMascio, 1970). Other dangerous effects are agranulocytosis and pigmentary degeneration of the retina, both of which are extremely rare (see below).

Therapeutic doses of phenothiazines may cause faintness, palpitation, nasal stuffiness, dry mouth, and some slight constipation. The patient may complain of being cold, drowsy, or weak. The most troublesome side effect is *orthostatic hypotension,* which may result in syncope. A fall in blood pressure is most likely to occur from administration of the phenothiazines with aliphatic side chains. Congeners of the piperazine type, as well as other potent neuroleptic agents, produce less hypotension and may be used when this side effect is to be avoided. A mild elevation of temperature may be seen during the first few days, particularly if the drug is given parenterally. On the other hand, hypothermia can occur and may be due both to the action on the heat-regulating center and to direct peripheral vasodilatation. Sensitivity and adaptation to changes of environmental temperature are impaired so that fatal hyperthermia and heat stroke are possible complications.

Neurological Side Effects of Neuroleptic Drugs. A variety of neurological syndromes, involving particularly the extrapyramidal system, occur following the use of almost all antipsychotic drugs. These reactions are particularly prominent during treatment with the piperazine group of phenothiazine drugs and with haloperidol. There is less likelihood of acute extrapyramidal side effects with thioridazine and with several other agents (notably, clozapine and sulpiride) that are not available in the United States. Neurological effects associated with antipsychotic drugs are described in detail by the American College of Neuropsychopharmacology Task Force (1973), Marsden and associates (1975), and Baldessarini (1979b).

There are probably five varieties of extrapyramidal syndromes associated with the use of antipsychotic drugs. Three of these usually appear concomitantly with the administration of the drug, and two are late-appearing syndromes that occur following prolonged treatment for many months or years. The clinical features of these five syndromes and guidelines for their management are summarized in Table 19-2.

A *parkinsonian syndrome* that may be indistinguishable from idiopathic parkinsonism may develop during administration of antipsychotic drugs. Its incidence varies with different agents (Table 19-1), and in some patients it may not be seen at all. Clinically, there is a generalized slowing of volitional movement (akinesia) with mask facies and a reduction in arm movements. The most noticeable signs are *rigidity* and *tremor at rest,* especially involving the upper extremities. "Pill-rolling" movements may be seen. Parkinsonian side effects may be mistaken for depression since the flat facial expression and retarded movements resemble signs of depression.

Another extrapyramidal effect seen during antipsychotic drug therapy is *akathisia.* This term refers to the compelling need of the patient to be in constant movement rather than to any specific movement pattern. The patient feels that he must get up and walk or continuously move about, and he may be unable to keep this under control. Akathisia can be mistaken for agitation in psychotic patients; the distinction is critical, since agitation might be appropriately treated with an increase in dosage. Parenteral administration of benztropine sometimes allows a differential diagnosis between the two conditions, inasmuch as psychotic agitation will not respond to this drug; however, in most cases, the clinical response is equivocal. Due to the frequently unsatisfactory response of akathisia to antiparkinsonian or other drugs, treatment typically requires reduction of antipsychotic drug dosage.

Acute dystonic reactions are occasionally seen with the initiation of antipsychotic drug therapy. Facial grimacing and torticollis can occur and may be associated with oculogyric crisis. These syndromes may be mistaken for hysterical reaction or seizures, but they respond dramatically to parenteral administration of anticholinergic antiparkinsonian drugs. Once again, the differential diagnosis is important.

Tardive dyskinesia is a late-appearing neurological syndrome associated with antipsychotic drug use. It occurs more frequently in older patients, and an incidence that averages about 10 to 20% has been reported in chronically institutionalized patients. It may be more common in females and those with a history of prior brain damage. Its incidence with specific drug groups is not known, but it has been associated with every class of neuroleptic agents in common clinical use. The incidence appears to be very low with the experimental antipsychotic agents clozapine and sulpiride. Tardive dyskinesia is characterized by stereotyped involuntary movements consisting in sucking and smacking of the lips, lateral jaw movements, and fly-catching dartings of the tongue. There may be choreiform and purposeless, quick movements of the extremities. All these movements disappear during sleep, as they do in parkinsonism. Although the tardive dyskinesias may be masked by large doses of antipsychotic drugs, this form of treatment is considered dangerous and is only employed in very compelling circumstances, such as severely incapacitating dyskinesia, particularly with continuing psychosis. Symptoms may persist indefinitely after discontinuation of the medication, although sometimes tardive dyskinesias will disappear with time. This is perhaps more likely to occur in younger patients. Antiparkinsonian drugs typically exacerbate tardive dyskinesias and other forms of choreoathetosis, such as in Huntington's disease, and no adequate therapy has as yet been devised. Experimental treatments include the use of large amounts (several grams a day) of choline or phosphatidylcholine (lecithin) to attempt to increase the availability of acetylcholine in the brain (Growdon *et al.,* 1978; *see* Chapter 66).

A rare movement disorder that can appear late in

Table 19-1. SELECTED ANTIPSYCHOTIC DRUGS: CHEMICAL STRUCTURES, DOSES, SIDE EFFECTS, AND DOSAGE FORMS

Phenothiazines

Ring numbering: positions 1,2,3,4 and 5 (S), 6,7,8,9, 10 (N), with R_1 on N (position 10) and R_2 at position 2.

NONPROPRIETARY NAME / TRADE NAME	R_1	R_2	DOSE — Antipsychotic Dose Range—Daily Dosage, Usual (mg)	Extreme* (mg)	Single Intramuscular Dose† (mg)	Sedative Effects	Extrapyramidal Effects	Hypotensive Effects	DOSAGE FORMS — Oral (T = tablet (mg), C = capsule (mg), S = syrup, E = elixir, C = concentrate)	Injection (A = ampul, V = vial, S = syringe)
Chlorpromazine Hydrochloride, U.S.P. THORAZINE	—(CH$_2$)$_3$—N(CH$_3$)$_2$	—Cl	300–800	25–2000	25–50	+++	++	I.M. +++ Oral ++	(T)10,25,50 100,200 (C)sustained release; 30,75,150, 200,300 (S)10 mg/5 ml (C)30 mg/ml, 100 mg/ml ‡	(A)25 mg/ml, 50 mg/2 ml (V)25 mg/ml in 10 ml
Triflupromazine Hydrochloride, U.S.P. VESPRIN	—(CH$_2$)$_3$—N(CH$_3$)$_2$	—CF$_3$	100–150	50–300	20–50	++	+++	++	(T)10,25,50 ‡	(V)i0 mg/ml in 10 ml; 20 mg/ml (S)10 mg/ml
Mesoridazine Besylate, U.S.P. SERENTIL	—(CH$_2$)$_2$— (2-methylpiperidine, N—CH$_3$)	—SCH$_3$ (S=O)	75–300	25–400	25				(T)10,25 50,100 (C)25 mg/ml	(A)25 mg/ml
Piperacetazine, U.S.P. QUIDE	—(CH$_2$)$_3$—N (piperidine, 4-(CH$_2$)$_2$OH)	—COCH$_3$	20–160	5–200					(T)10,25	

Drug	R	Dose						Preparations		
Thioridazine Hydrochloride, U.S.P. (MELLARIL) — side chain $-(CH_2)_2-$ with N–CH$_3$ ring	$-SCH_3$	200–600	50–800		+++	+	++	(T)10,15,25,50, 100,150, 200	(C)30 mg/ml 100 mg/ml	
Acetophenazine Maleate, U.S.P. (TINDAL) — $-(CH_2)_3-N$ $N-(CH_2)_2-OH$	$-COCH_3$	60–120	20–600		++	++	+	(T)20		
Fluphenazine Hydrochloride, U.S.P. / Fluphenazine Enanthate, U.S.P. / Fluphenazine decanoate (PERMITIL and PROLIXIN (HYDROCHLORIDES) (PROLIXIN ENANTHATE and DECANOATE)) — $-(CH_2)_3-N$ $N-(CH_2)_2-OH$	$-CF_3$	2.5–20	1–30	1.25–2.5 (decanoate or enanthate: 25–50 every 1–3 weeks)	+	+++	+	(T)0.25,1, 2.5,5,10 (T)sustained release; 1	(C)5 mg/ml (E)0.5 mg/ml	(V)2.5 mg/ml in 10 ml Enanthate and decanoate: (S)25 mg/ml (V)25 mg/ml in 5 ml
Perphenazine, U.S.P. (TRILAFON) — $-(CH_2)_3-N$ $N-(CH_2)_2-OH$	$-Cl$	8–32	4–64	5–10	–+	+++	+	(T)2,4,8,16 (T)sustained release; 8	(C)16 mg/5 ml (A)5 mg/ml	
Trifluoperazine Hydrochloride, U.S.P. (STELAZINE) — $-(CH_2)_3-N$ $N-CH_3$	$-CF_3$	6–20	2–60	1–2	+	+++	+	(T)1,2.5,10	(C)10 mg/ml	(V)2 mg/ml in 10 ml

* Extreme dosage ranges are occasionally exceeded cautiously and only when other appropriate measures have failed.

† Except for the enanthate and decanoate forms of fluphenazine, dosage can be given intramuscularly up to every 6 hours for agitated patients.

‡ Chlorpromazine, U.S.P., is available as the free base in rectal suppositories in 25- and 100-mg sizes; the hydrochloride is also available in nonproprietary preparations. Thiothixene, U.S.P., is available as the free base in 1-, 2-, 5-, and 10-mg capsules. Triflupromazine, U.S.P., is available as the free base in oral suspension, *equivalent to* 50 mg of the hydrochloride per 5 ml.

409

Table 19-1. SELECTED ANTIPSYCHOTIC DRUGS: CHEMICAL STRUCTURES, DOSES, SIDE EFFECTS, AND DOSAGE FORMS (Continued)

NONPROPRIETARY NAME	TRADE NAME	DOSE			SIDE EFFECTS			DOSAGE FORMS	
		Antipsychotic Dose Range—Daily Dosage		Single Intramuscular Dose † (mg)	Sedative Effects	Extra-pyramidal Effects	Hypotensive Effects	Oral T = tablet (mg) C = capsule (mg) S = syrup E = elixir C = concentrate	Injection A = ampul V = vial S = syringe
		Usual (mg)	Extreme * (mg)						

Thioxanthenes

R₁, R₂ structure (thioxanthene nucleus, positions 1–10)

		R_2	Usual (mg)	Extreme (mg)	IM	Sedative	Extrapyramidal	Hypotensive	Oral	Injection
Chlorprothixene, U.S.P. $R_1 = CH-(CH_2)_2-N(CH_3)_2$	TARACTAN	$-Cl$	50–400	30–600	25–50	+++	++	++	(T)10,25,50,100 (C)100 mg/5 ml	(A)25 mg/2 ml
Thiothixene Hydrochloride, U.S.P. $R_1 = CH(CH_2)_2-N$ (piperazine) $N-CH_3$	NAVANE	$-SO_2N(CH_3)_2$	6–30	6–60	2–6	+ to ++	++	++	(C)1,2,5,10,20 ‡ (C)5 mg/ml	(A)4 mg/2 ml

Other Heterocyclic Compounds

			Usual	Extreme	IM	Sedative	Extrapyramidal	Hypotensive	Oral	Injection
Haloperidol, U.S.P.	HALDOL		6–20	2–100	2.5–5	+	+++	+	(T)0.5,1,2,5,10 (C)2 mg/ml	(A)5 mg/ml, as the lactate (V)5 mg/ml, as the lactate, in 10 ml

Loxapine succinate DAXOLIN, LOXITANE	60–100	20–250	+	++	+	(C)5,10, 25,50	(C)25 mg/ml, as the hydrochloride
Molindone hydrochloride LIDONE, MOBAN	50–225	15–400	++	+	0	(T)5,10,25 (C)5,10,25	

* Extreme dosage ranges are occasionally exceeded cautiously and only when other appropriate measures have failed.

† Except for the enanthate and decanoate forms of fluphenazine, dosage can be given intramuscularly up to every 6 hours for agitated patients.

‡ Chlorpromazine, U.S.P., is available as the free base in rectal suppositories in 25- and 100-mg sizes; the hydrochloride is also available in nonproprietary preparations. Thiothixene, U.S.P., is available as the free base in 1-, 2-, 5-, and 10-mg capsules. Triflupromazine, U.S.P., is available as the free base in oral suspension, *equivalent to* 50 mg of the hydrochloride per 5 ml.

Table 19-2. NEUROLOGICAL EFFECTS OF NEUROLEPTIC DRUGS

REACTION	FEATURES	TIME OF MAXIMAL RISK	PROPOSED MECHANISM	TREATMENT
Acute dystonia	Spasm of muscles of tongue, face, neck, back; may mimic seizures; *not* hysteria	1 to 5 days	Unknown	Many treatments can alter, but effects of antiparkinsonian agents are diagnostic and curative *
Parkinsonism	Bradykinesia, rigidity, variable tremor, mask facies, shuffling gait	5 to 30 days	Antagonism of dopamine	Antiparkinsonian agents helpful †
Akathisia	Motor restlessness; *not* anxiety or "agitation"	5 to 60 days	Unknown	Reduce dose or change drug; antiparkinsonian agents † or benzodiazepines may help
Tardive dyskinesia	Oral-facial dyskinesia; widespread choreoathetosis	After months or years of treatment (worse on withdrawal)	Excess function of dopamine hypothesized	Prevention crucial; treatment unsatisfactory
Perioral tremor ("rabbit" syndrome)	Perioral tremor (may be a late variant of parkinsonism)	After months or years of treatment	Unknown	Antiparkinsonian agents often help †

   * Many drugs have been claimed to be helpful for acute dystonia. Among the most commonly employed treatments are diphenhydramine hydrochloride, 25 or 50 mg intramuscularly, or benztropine mesylate, 1 or 2 mg intramuscularly or slowly intravenously, followed by oral medication with the same agent for a period of days to perhaps several weeks thereafter.
   † For details regarding the use of oral antiparkinsonian agents, *see* the text and Chapter 21.

treatment of chronically ill patients with antipsychotic agents is *perioral tremor,* sometimes referred to as the "rabbit" syndrome (Jus *et al.,* 1974) due to the peculiar movements that characterize this condition. While sometimes categorized with other tardive (late or slowly evolving) dyskinesias, this term is usually reserved for choreoathetotic reactions. The "rabbit" syndrome, in fact, shares many features with parkinsonism, since the tremor has a frequency of about 5 to 7 Hz and there is a favorable response to anticholinergic agents.

Histological examination of brains of patients who had signs of tardive dyskinesia or of brains of animals exposed to high doses of neuroleptic agents for prolonged periods have not revealed a clear or consistent lesion. Moreover, the pathophysiology of tardive dyskinesia remains obscure, although it is hypothesized that compensatory increases in the function of dopamine as a neurotransmitter in the basal ganglia may be involved. This idea is supported by comparison of therapeutic responses in patients with Parkinson's disease to those with tardive dyskinesia or other choreoathetotic dyskinesias such as Huntington's disease. Thus, antidopaminergic drugs tend to ameliorate tardive dyskinesia, while dopaminergic agonists worsen the condition; antimuscarinic agents tend to worsen tardive dyskinesia, and cholinergic agents sometimes help. In addition, there are now abundant data to support the concept

of *disuse supersensitivity* of dopaminergic systems in the animal brain. Since supersensitivity to dopaminergic agonists tends not to persist for more than a few weeks after exposure to antagonists of the transmitter, this phenomenon is most likely to play a role in those variants of tardive dyskinesia that resolve rapidly; these are usually referred to as *withdrawal-emergent dyskinesias.* The theoretical and clinical aspects of this complex and troublesome problem have been reviewed in detail elsewhere (Baldessarini and Tarsy, 1978, 1979).

It is important to prevent the neurological syndromes that complicate the use of antipsychotic drugs. Certain therapeutic guidelines should be followed. Thus, the routine use of antiparkinsonian agents in an attempt to *avoid* early extrapyramidal reactions is usually unnecessary. Furthermore, this adds complexity, anticholinergic and other side effects, and expense to the treatment regimen. The use of antiparkinsonian agents should be reserved for cases of *overt* extrapyramidal reactions that respond favorably to such intervention. The early extrapyramidal reactions are most likely to be encountered with the high-potency piperazine and butyrophenone neuroleptics and are least likely with thioridazine, among currently available drugs. In addition, since tolerance to these early extrapyramidal effects commonly occurs after several weeks or months, the need for antiparkinsonian agents will ordinarily diminish with time; their doses should be adjusted accordingly. Most of the available antiparkinsonian agents, including amantadine, have been used successfully in the management of antipsychotic drug-induced extrapyramidal reactions; however, levodopa is almost never employed, since this entails a high risk of inducing agitation and worsening psychosis (*see* Chapter 21). The thoughtful and conservative use of antipsychotic drugs in patients with chronic or frequently recurrent psychotic disorders can reduce the risk of tardive dyskinesia. Although reduction of the dose of an antipsychotic agent is the best way to minimize its neurological side effects, this may not be practical in a patient with uncontrollable psychotic illness. The best preventive practice is to use minimally effective doses of antipsychotic drugs for long-term therapy and to discontinue treatment as soon as it seems reasonable to do so or if a satisfactory response cannot be obtained.

Jaundice. Jaundice was observed in patients shortly after the introduction of chlorpromazine into medical practice and was the cause for some alarm. The incidence of this complication is very low and has been on the decrease since the 1960s. This is presumably due to improved quality of the products or to a shift in popularity toward more potent agents, which tend to have less systemic toxicity than do the low-potency phenothiazines. Commonly occurring during the second to fourth week of therapy, the jaundice is characterized by bile in the urine and abnormally high levels of alkaline phosphatase associated with high concentrations of bilirubin in plasma. It is generally mild, with the plasma bilirubin rarely rising higher than 15 mg/100 ml; the direct bilirubin is higher than the indirect. Fever, anorexia, and hepatic tenderness are usually not present but may be prodromal symptoms of impending jaundice. Despite the presence of jaundice, patients rarely complain of pruritus.

The jaundice is of the obstructive type. Biopsy specimens show centralobular cholestasis, with little or no parenchymatous damage and with mild inflammatory response. The presence of inspissated bile in the hepatic canaliculi may be caused by an increase in viscosity of the bile, precipitation of its macromolecular components, or periductal edema.

There is general agreement that the jaundice following phenothiazine administration is a manifestation of hypersensitivity. Eosinophilic infiltration of the liver as well as eosinophilia are frequently present. There is prompt recurrence of jaundice when the patient is again given the same drug, and there is no correlation between the dose administered and the appearance of jaundice. Ayd (1962) has indicated that desensitization to chlorpromazine may occur with repeated administration in individuals exhibiting jaundice. If jaundice is not observed within the first month of treatment with a phenothiazine, the chance of its later occurrence decreases with time. Since there is always the possibility of shifting a patient from one drug to another without the recurrence of a hypersensitivity reaction, it is felt by some investigators that therapy should be carefully continued in cases of jaundice when the psychiatric disorder calls for uninterrupted drug therapy.

Blood Dyscrasias. Leukocytosis, leukopenia, and eosinophilia occur with phenothiazine medication. It is difficult to determine whether a leukopenia occurring during the administration of a phenothiazine is a forewarning of impending agranulocytosis. This serious but rare complication occurs in not more than 1 in 10,000 patients receiving chlorpromazine or other low-potency agents, particularly in high doses; it usually appears within the first 8 to 12 weeks of treatment (DuComb and Baldessarini, 1977). Since the onset of blood dyscrasia may be sudden, the appearance of an apparent upper respiratory infection in a patient being treated with an antipsychotic drug should be followed immediately by a complete blood count.

Skin Reactions. Dermatological reactions to the phenothiazines are common. Urticaria or dermatitis occurs in about 5% of patients receiving chlorpromazine. Three types of skin disorders are associated with the use of phenothiazines. The first is a hypersensitivity reaction that may be urticarial, maculopapular, petechial, or edematous. It usually occurs between the first and eighth week of treatment. The skin clears following discontinuation of the drug and may remain so even if drug therapy is reinstituted. Secondly, contact dermatitis may occur in personnel who handle chlorpromazine, and there may be a certain degree of cross-sensitivity to the other phenothiazines. Thirdly, photosensitivity occurs, the reaction resembling that seen with severe sunburn. This complication may be prevented simply by keeping the patient well covered. An effective sunscreen preparation containing para-aminobenzoic acid should be prescribed for outpatients during the summer.

Abnormal pigmentation induced by long-term administration of phenothiazines in high doses to chronic schizophrenics has been reported, but it is very rare with current practices. Patients showing this effect have generally received any of a number of phenothiazines, but chlorpromazine is the drug most commonly implicated. The reaction manifests itself as a gray-blue pigmentation in regions exposed to the sun. The dermis contains deposits of melanin located throughout the depth of the corium. Ultraviolet light with wavelengths above 3200 Å seems to be primarily responsible for the effects.

Epithelial keratopathy is often observed in patients on long-term therapy with chlorpromazine, and opacities in the cornea and in the lens of the eye have also been noted. In very extreme cases the deposits in the lens may result in impairment of vision. Active treatment of this condition (*e.g.*, with penicillamine) has not been especially helpful, and the deposits tend to disappear spontaneously, although slowly, following discontinuation of the low-potency drug usually implicated. Pigmentary retinopathy, which has been reported particularly following the use of high doses of thioridazine, may be a closely related toxic effect of the phenothiazines (Zelickson and Zeller, 1964; Prien *et al.*, 1970); thus far it has been reported only with doses of thioridazine in excess of 1000 mg per day. A maximal daily dose of 800 mg is therefore currently recommended.

Metabolic Effects. Chlorpromazine raises plasma

cholesterol concentrations consistently and significantly (Clark *et al.,* 1967). It is not known if other antipsychotic drugs have this effect or if they share the previously mentioned impairment of glucose tolerance occasionally associated with chlorpromazine (Erle *et al.,* 1977).

Interactions with Other Drugs. The phenothiazines with low potency and the thioxanthenes markedly affect the actions of a number of other drugs, and cognizance must be taken of this fact. Chlorpromazine was originally introduced to potentiate central depressants, and it and some of its congeners have continued to be used for this purpose, especially in anesthesiology. In addition, such drugs can strongly potentiate sedatives and analgesics prescribed for medical purposes, as well as nonprescription sedatives and hypnotics, antihistamines, and cold remedies. Patients should also be warned to expect enhancement of the effects of alcohol. Chlorpromazine clearly increases the miotic and sedative effects of morphine and is believed also to increase its analgesic actions. Furthermore, the drug markedly increases the respiratory depression produced by meperidine and can be expected to have similar effects when administered concurrently with other opioid analgesics. As should be clear from the discussion of the actions of neuroleptic drugs, they inhibit the actions of direct dopaminergic agonists and of levodopa.

Other interactive effects can be manifest on the cardiovascular system. Chlorpromazine and some other antipsychotic drugs, in common with most tricyclic antidepressants, may block the antihypertensive effects of guanethidine. The mechanism appears to involve blockade of uptake of guanethidine into sympathetic nerves. The more potent antipsychotic agents, especially molindone, seem to be much less likely to cause this effect. On the other hand, the phenothiazines can promote hypotension, possibly due to their α-adrenergic blocking properties. Thus, the interaction between phenothiazines and antihypertensives can be quite unpredictable.

Cardiac depressant effects have been ascribed to thioridazine, and its relatively strong anticholinergic action can cause tachycardia. In addition, this antipsychotic agent may partially nullify the inotropic effect of digitalis by its quinidine-like action that can cause myocardial depression, decreased efficiency of repolarization, and increased risk of tachyarrhythmias. The antimuscarinic action of thioridazine can also enhance the peripheral and central effects (confusion, delirium) of other anticholinergic agents, such as the tricyclic antidepressants.

Agents such as phenobarbital and other sedatives that induce microsomal drug-metabolizing enzymes

can enhance the metabolism of antipsychotic agents (Loga *et al.,* 1975); this effect may sometimes have significant clinical consequences.

DRUG TREATMENT OF PSYCHOSES

The antipsychotic drugs do not seem to show particular specificity for the diagnostic type of psychosis to be treated. They are clearly effective in acute psychoses of unknown etiology, including mania, paranoid states, and acute exacerbations of schizophrenia, although most controlled clinical data exist for the acute and chronic phases of schizophrenia. In addition, antipsychotic drugs are used empirically in many other disorders, whether idiopathic or organic, in which psychotic symptoms and severe agitation are prominent. Unfortunately, for disorders other than schizophrenia and mania, there have been but few controlled comparisons with a placebo or sedatives, and reliable guidelines to dosage are meager.

The fact that phenothiazines and other neuroleptic agents are indeed antipsychotic was very slow to gain acceptance, particularly by physicians in the United States. However, many scientifically rigorous clinical trials have established beyond reasonable doubt that these agents are effective and that they are superior to agents such as the barbiturates or the benzodiazepines, or to alternative types of treatment such as electroconvulsive shock. The "target" symptoms for which the neuroleptic agents seem to be especially effective include tension, hyperactivity, combativeness, hostility, negativism, hallucinations, acute delusions, insomnia, poor self-care, anorexia, and sometimes withdrawal and seclusiveness; less likely is improvement in insight, judgment, memory, and orientation. The most favorable prognosis is for patients with relatively acute illnesses of brief duration who had relatively healthy personalities prior to the illness.

Despite the great success of the antipsychotic drugs, their use alone does not constitute optimal care of psychotic patients. The acute care, protection, and support of acutely psychotic patients, as well as mastery of technics employed in their long-term care and rehabilitation, continue to be important medical skills. Many detailed reviews of the clinical use of antipsychotic drugs are available (May, 1968; Klein and Davis, 1969; Baldessarini, 1977b; Davis and Garver, 1978; Hollister, 1978a).

In order to assess changes in the patient's condition, an accurate evaluation of his mental and physical status at the start of therapy is necessary. Treatment goals should then be defined. Although rating scales for symptom complexes are available (*see* Levine *et al.*, 1971), the physician can define treatable symptoms on the basis of clinical examinations or simple scales.

No one drug or combination of drugs has a selective effect on a particular symptom complex in groups of schizophrenic patients, although individual patients appear to do better with one agent than another; this can only be determined by trial and error. Since compliance with medication schedules can be poor on both inpatient and outpatient services, it is important to simplify the treatment regimen and to try to ensure that the patient is receiving the drug. In cases of severe and dangerous noncompliance, the patient can be treated with injections of fluphenazine decanoate or enanthate, long-acting preparations. Since delusional paranoid patients frequently believe that the medicine is "poison," this group is particularly appropriate for the administration of long-acting injectable preparations.

Since the choice of a drug cannot be made on the basis of anticipated therapeutic effect, the *selection* of a particular medication for treatment often depends on side effects. If a patient has responded well to a drug in the past, it should probably be used again. If the patient has a history of cardiovascular disease or stroke and the threat from hypotension is serious, a potent neuroleptic should be used in the smallest dose that is effective (*see* Table 19–1). If because of age, medical condition, or disease factors there is a marked risk of development of extrapyramidal symptoms, thioridazine should be considered, although small doses of potent antipsychotic drugs may be safer in the elderly. If the patient would be seriously discomforted by interference with ejaculation or if there are serious risks of cardiovascular or other autonomic toxicity, thioridazine should be avoided. If sedative effects are undesirable, a potent agent is preferable. If the patient has compromised hepatic function or if there is a potential threat of jaundice, haloperidol is probably a safe choice, although other high-potency agents may also be used. Choice can also be conditioned by the physician's experience in the use of a particular drug, a factor that can outweigh all others. Skill in the use of these drugs also depends on selection of an adequate dosage, knowledge of what to expect, and judgment as to when to stop therapy or change drugs.

Some patients do not respond satisfactorily to antipsychotic drug treatment, and many chronically disorganized schizophrenic patients, while helped during periods of acute exacerbation of their disease, may show highly unsatisfactory responses between the more acute phases of illness. Since the individual nonresponder cannot be identified beforehand with certainty, the physician must accept the fact that there is a small subgroup of patients who do poorly or even become worse on medication, at least during some phases of their illness. If a patient does not improve after a course of adequate treatment and if he fails to respond to another drug given in adequate dosage, therapy should be discontinued and the diagnosis reevaluated.

The *time course of response* to antipsychotic drugs is such that 3 weeks or more is required to demonstrate positive effects in hospitalized schizophrenics. Full effect may require 6 weeks to 6 months. In contrast, improvement of some acutely psychotic patients can be seen within 48 hours. A few inconclusive reports have suggested that parenteral administration of an antipsychotic drug at the start of an acute psychosis may be particularly efficacious. However, it is not clear to what extent nonspecific sedative effects may contribute to early changes in such patients (Anderson and Kuehnle, 1974).

After the initial response of the patient, drugs are frequently used in conjunction with other psychological and supportive treatments. Although there is no clear statistical evidence that formal psychotherapy greatly affects prognosis (Grinspoon *et al.*, 1968; May, 1968; Feinsilver and Gunderson, 1972; Hogarty and Ulrich, 1977), psychotherapy and other treatments are believed to assist the patient in adjusting to his environment.

There is no convincing evidence that combinations of antipsychotic drugs offer any advantage. A combination of an antipsychotic drug and an antidepressant may be useful in some cases, especially in depressed psychotic patients or in cases of agitated depression. However, the suggestion that a tricyclic antidepressant can reduce apathy and withdrawal in schizophrenia is not proven.

The *duration of treatment* has received a great deal of attention. In a review of 22 controlled prospective studies involving nearly 3200 schizophrenic patients, Davis (1975) noted that the mean overall relapse rate was 56% for those patients who were withdrawn from antipsychotic drugs and given a placebo, compared to only 15% of those who continued on proper drug therapy. It is sometimes found, at least for short periods (weeks or a few months), that dosage in chronic cases can be lowered to 100 to 300 mg of chlorpromazine (or its equivalent) per day without signs of relapse, although the average lowest effective dose for long-term maintenance treatment in schizophrenia is still not known (Davis and Garver, 1978). Intermittent therapy can be useful, particularly in reducing the incidence of side effects. Effective maintenance with monthly injections of a fluphenazine ester has been reported (Hirsch *et al.*, 1973).

Optimal dosage of antipsychotic drugs is difficult to determine because of the variable dose-response curves and the difficulties in defining an end point of therapeutic response. In the treatment of acute psychoses, one should increase the dose of antipsychotic drug as rapidly as feasible, over a few days at most, to achieve control of symptoms. The dose is then adjusted during the next several weeks as the patient's condition warrants. Parenteral medication is often indicated for acutely agitated patients. Small doses (25 to 50 mg of chlorpromazine, 5 mg of haloperidol, or comparable doses of another agent) are given *intramuscularly* (and almost never by other routes); these can be repeated as frequently as hourly to obtain the desired response. One must, of course, remain alert for hypotension or acute dystonic reactions, which are especially likely with such treatment. The desired effect may be delayed for several hours. Some antipsychotic drugs, including fluphenazine, other piperazines, and haloperidol, have been given in doses of several hundred milligrams a day orally without disaster, although there is no convincing evidence that such high doses of potent agents achieve superior results (Quitkin *et al.*, 1974). After an initial period of stabilization, regimens based on a single daily dose are efficacious and safe; they may also allow some degree of selection of the time at which unwanted effects occur so as to minimize the patient's discomfort.

Table 19–1 (page 408) gives usual and extreme ranges of dosage for antipsychotic drugs employed in the United States. These ranges are only guidelines, and they have been established, for the most part, in the treatment of schizophrenic patients. Higher doses have been used, but must still be considered experimental. While acutely disturbed inpatients may require higher doses of an antipsychotic drug than do more stable outpatients, the concept that a low-maintenance dose will suffice during follow-up care of a partially recovered or chronic psychotic patient is poorly substantiated. The minimal effective dose to achieve clear antipsychotic effects seems to be approximately 300 to 400 mg of chlorpromazine daily or the equivalent amount of another agent (Davis and Garver, 1978). Careful observation of the patient's changing response is the best guide to appropriate dosage.

The treatment of *organic mental syndromes* (*i.e.*, delirium or dementia) is another accepted use of the antipsychotic drugs. They may be administered temporarily, while a specific and correctable structural, infectious, metabolic, or toxic cause is vigorously sought. They are used chronically when no correctable cause can be found. Once again, there are no drugs of choice or clearly established dosage guidelines (*see* Prien, 1973). In patients with acute "brain syndromes" without likelihood of seizures, frequent small doses (perhaps 2 to 6 mg) of a piperazine or haloperidol may be effective in controlling agitation. Agents with low potency should be avoided because of their greater tendency to produce sedation, hypotension, and seizures. The potent antipsychotic drugs are much less likely to cause excitement or additional confusion, as is common when barbiturates or other sedatives are given to such patients. This is also true for demented patients in whom use of small doses of potent antipsychotic drugs can be very helpful.

The use of antipsychotic drugs in *mania* and *depression* has met with some success. Haloperidol and chlorpromazine are both effective in the treatment of mania and are often used concomitantly with the institution of lithium therapy (*see* below). In fact, it is often impractical to attempt to manage a manic patient with lithium alone during the first week of illness, when the antipsychotic drugs are usually required. There is no controlled study to date of possible long-term preventive effects of antipsychotic

drugs in manic-depressive illness. The treatment of depression with phenothiazines is more controversial. Controlled studies have demonstrated the efficacy of several antipsychotic drugs in some depressed patients, especially those with striking agitation or psychotic delusions (*see* Overall *et al.*, 1964; Baldessarini, 1977b).

Anxiety is considered by some to be an indication for the use of antipsychotic drugs. In view of the wide range of disturbing and serious side effects, the use of these drugs for such a purpose is inappropriate. However, for patients who have crippling anxiety that does not respond to sedative-antianxiety drugs, a brief trial of an antipsychotic agent might be warranted. (An antidepressant drug could be appropriate if, for example, panic attacks are present.) The long-term utility of antipsychotic drugs for the treatment of anxiety is not established, nor is it known at what rate tolerance to their antianxiety effects may occur. Patients who require or demand medication for anxiety for prolonged periods require careful medical and psychiatric evaluation. The physician should recall that the risk of tardive dyskinesia is *not* clearly related to the dose of antipsychotic drugs (Baldessarini and Tarsy, 1978). Thus, their use for prolonged periods, even in relatively small doses, can be expected to carry such a risk.

The status of the drug treatment of *childhood psychosis* and other behavioral disorders of children is confused by diagnostic inconsistencies and a paucity of controlled studies. Neuroleptics can benefit children with disorders that are characterized by some of the same features that occur in adult psychoses. Low doses of the more potent agents seem to be preferred in an attempt to avoid interference with daytime activities or performance in school (Campbell, 1975). Due to the wide range of behavioral disorders of children that are sometimes called psychoses, one can expect a proportion of children so treated to respond unfavorably to these agents. In evaluating the behavioral disorders of children, it is important to consider the syndrome of "minimal brain dysfunction" or "hyperactivity"; this responds poorly to antipsychotic agents but uniquely well to certain stimulant drugs, especially dextroamphetamine and methylphenidate (*see* De La Cruz *et al.*, 1973). Information on dosages of antipsychotic drugs for children is very limited, as is the number of drugs currently approved in the United States for use in preadolescents (*see* Anders and Ciaranello, 1977). Most relevant experience is with chlorpromazine, for which the recommended daily doses are approximately 2 mg/kg of body weight. A suggested limit is 200 mg per day (orally) for preadolescents, 40 mg per day (intramuscularly) for children under 5 years of age or 23 kg of body weight, and 75 mg per day (intramuscularly) under age 12 years or 45 kg. Usual daily doses for other agents are: triflupromazine, 0.2 mg/kg; thioridazine, 0.5 to 3 mg/kg; chlorprothixene, 10 to 100 mg (over the age of 6); trifluoperazine and thiothixene, 1 to 15 mg and 1 to 30 mg for children over age 6 and 12 years, respectively. Haloperidol, utilized to treat the rare syndrome of Gilles de la Tourette in children and adolescents (Shapiro *et al.*, 1973), is recommended at doses of 2 to 16 mg per day in children over 12 years of age.

For patients at the other end of the age spectrum, poor tolerance of the side effects of the antipsychotic drugs often limits the doses of drugs that can be given. One should proceed cautiously, using small, divided doses, with the expectation that the very elderly will require doses that are one half or less of those needed for young adults (*see* Baldessarini, 1977b; Prien and Cole, 1978).

MISCELLANEOUS MEDICAL USES FOR ANTIPSYCHOTIC DRUGS

Neuroleptic drugs have a variety of uses in addition to the treatment of psychiatric patients. Predominant among these are the treatment of nausea and vomiting (for which some antihistamines are also effective; Table 19-3), alcoholic hallucinosis, certain neuropsychiatric diseases marked by movement disorders (notably, Gilles de la Tourette's syndrome and Huntington's disease), and, occasionally,

intractable hiccough and pruritus (for which trimeprazine is recommended).

Nausea and Vomiting. Chlorpromazine, in relatively low, nonsedative doses, can prevent vomiting of certain etiologies. The potent and selective antiemetic action of the drug has found useful clinical application in a number of disorders characterized by vomiting, such as uremia, gastroenteritis, carcinomatosis, radiation sickness, and emesis caused by a number of drugs including estrogens, the tetracyclines, opioid analgesics, agents used in the chemotherapy of malignancy, and disulfiram. Chlorpromazine has also been used in nausea and vomiting of pregnancy, but pregnant patients should not be given the drug for this purpose (*see* Morselli, 1977; Goldberg and DiMascio, 1978). Chlorpromazine does not appear to control motion sickness. Although prochlorperazine is a very potent antiemetic agent, it produces a very high incidence of dystonias, especially when given intramuscularly, and hence should

Table 19-3. PHENOTHIAZINES USED IN THE TREATMENT OF NAUSEA AND VOMITING

NONPROPRIETARY NAME AND TRADE NAME	ROUTE, DOSAGE FORM, AND ADULT DOSE		
	Oral T = tablet S = syrup C = concentrate SC = sustained-release capsule	*Suppository*	*Intramuscular* A = ampul S = syringe
Chlorpromazine (THORAZINE) Base, U.S.P. Hydrochloride, U.S.P.	*	25,100 mg	*
(Dosage)	10–25 mg every 4–6 hr	25–100 mg every 6–8 hr	25–50 mg every 2–4 hr
Perphenazine, U.S.P. (TRILAFON)	*		*
(Dosage)	8–16 mg/day		5 mg
Prochlorperazine (COMPAZINE) Base, U.S.P. Edisylate, U.S.P. Maleate, U.S.P.	(S)5 mg/ml (C)10 mg/ml (T)5,10,25 mg (SC)10,15,30,75 mg	2.5,5,25 mg	(A)5 mg/ml (1 or 10 ml) (S)5 mg/ml (2 ml)
(Dosage)	5–10 mg, 3–4 times/day 10 mg, 2 times/day (SC)	25 mg twice a day	5–10 mg every 3–4 hr (up to 40 mg/day)
Promethazine Hydrochloride, U.S.P. (PHENERGAN)	(T)12.5,25,50 mg (S)6.25,25 mg/5 ml	12.5,25,50 mg	25,50 mg/ml
(Dosage)	12.5–25 mg every 4–6 hr	12.5–25 mg every 4–6 hr	12.5–25 mg every 4–6 hr
Thiethylperazine maleate (TORECAN MALEATE)	(T)10 mg	10 mg	(A)10 mg/2 ml
(Dosage)	10–30 mg/day	10–30 mg/day	20 mg, 1–3 times/day
Triflupromazine Hydrochloride, U.S.P. (VESPRIN)	*		*
(Dosage)	20–30 mg/day		5–15 mg every 4–6 hr (up to 60 mg/day)

* Dosage forms provided in Table 19-1.

be used with caution. The same precautions should be observed in the use of phenothiazines for nausea and vomiting as with the use of potent analgesics in the treatment of pain, because they may mask diagnostic symptoms in acute surgical conditions or neurological syndromes. Not all the phenothiazines are equally effective as antiemetics, and thioridazine is a notable exception to the general rule that most neuroleptic agents have antiemetic effects. It should be remembered that this action of most antipsychotic agents may thwart attempts to induce emesis pharmacologically (*e.g.,* with apomorphine) in the management of cases of acute drug overdosage. The preparations and dosages of phenothiazines that are effective in the treatment of nausea and vomiting are listed in Table 19–3. Surprisingly, nausea is occasionally seen as a side effect of antipsychotic drugs.

Hiccough. An interesting use of chlorpromazine is in the control of *intractable hiccough.* The mechanism of action in this disorder is unknown.

Withdrawal Syndromes. Antipsychotic drugs are *not* useful in the management of withdrawal from opioids, and their use in the management of withdrawal from barbiturates and other nonbarbiturate sedatives is *contraindicated,* due to the high risk of seizures. This risk also precludes the use of neuroleptics during withdrawal from alcohol. However, they can be employed safely and effectively in certain psychoses associated with chronic alcoholism—especially the syndrome known as *alcoholic hallucinosis (see* Freedman *et al.,* 1975).

Other Neuropsychiatric Disorders. Antipsychotic drugs are useful in the management of several rare syndromes with psychiatric features that are also characterized by movement disorders. These include, in particular, Gilles de la Tourette's syndrome (marked by tics, other involuntary movements, grunts, and vocalizations that are frequently obscene) (*see* Van Woert *et al.,* 1976) and Huntington's disease (marked by severe and progressive choreoathetosis, psychiatric symptoms, and a clear genetic basis) (*see* Chase, 1976). Haloperidol is currently regarded as the drug of choice for these conditions.

II. Drugs Used in the Treatment of Disorders of Mood

Affective disorders—*mania* and *depression*—are characterized by changes in mood as the primary symptom. Either of these two extremes of mood may be accompanied by psychosis with disordered thought and delusional perceptions. Psychosis may have, as a secondary symptom, a change in mood, and it is this overlap that causes much confusion in diagnosis. Severe mood changes without psychosis frequently occur and are often accompanied by *anxiety (see* below). The deci-

sion to use an antidepressant drug rather than an antipsychotic agent, for example, may rest on such factors as predominant symptomatology, family and personal history, and precise information on the onset and course of the current episode of the disease.

Mania, characterized by elation (often tinged with dysphoria), hyperactivity, and uncontrollable thought and speech, is treated with both antipsychotic drugs and lithium carbonate. *Depression,* characterized by feelings of intense sadness or pessimistic worry, agitation, self-deprecation, physical changes (including insomnia, anorexia, and loss of drive, enthusiasm, and libido), and mental slowing, can be treated with the tricyclic antidepressant drugs, the monoamine oxidase inhibitors, some antipsychotic agents, lithium carbonate, and electroconvulsive shock treatment (ECT). There is no obvious chemical similarity between the various therapeutic modalities, but there are striking similarities in their effects on brain amines. However, the importance of amine metabolism in their mechanisms of action, much less in the biology of the mood disorders, remains undefined (*see* Baldessarini, 1975; van Praag, 1978). Problems of selection of treatment, as well as the decision to treat affective disorders, are discussed below.

TRICYCLIC ANTIDEPRESSANTS

Imipramine (a dibenzazepine derivative), *amitriptyline* (a dibenzocycloheptadiene derivative), and other closely related compounds are the drugs currently most widely used for the treatment of depression. Because of their structure (*see* below), they are often referred to as the tricyclic antidepressants. Their efficacy in alleviating depression has been well established.

History. In the late nineteenth century, Thiele and Holzinger synthesized iminodibenzyl and described its chemical characteristics in detail. The pharmacological properties were not investigated until the late 1940s, when Häfliger and Schindler synthesized a series of more than 40 derivatives of iminodibenzyl for possible uses as antihistamines, sedatives, analgesics, and antiparkinsonian drugs. One of these was *imipramine,* a dibenzazepine compound, which differs from the phenothiazines only by replacement of the sulfur with an ethylene linkage to produce a seven-membered central ring. Following screening in animals, a few compounds, including imipramine, were selected on the basis of sedative or hypnotic properties for therapeutic trial.

During clinical investigation of these phenothiazine analogs, Kuhn (1958) found quite fortuitously that, unlike the phenothiazines, imipramine was relatively ineffective in quieting agitated psychotic patients. Instead, it apparently bestowed remarkable benefit upon certain depressed patients. Subsequently, Kuhn administered imipramine to approximately 50 patients suffering from a variety of depressive syndromes and concluded that it was most useful in "endogenous" depressions characterized by regression and inactivity, whereas patients with hyperactive, agitated, and anxious depressions were made worse by the drug. Since then, further evidence for the effectiveness of this compound has accumulated (*see* Klein and Davis, 1969).

The search for chemically related compounds has yielded, to date, six tricyclic compounds that are in common clinical use in the United States. In addition to the dibenzazepines, *imipramine* and its secondary-amine congener (and major metabolite) *desipramine*, there are *amitriptyline* and its N-demethylated product *nortriptyline* (dibenzocycloheptadienes), as well as *doxepin* (a dibenzoxepine) and *protriptyline* (a dibenzocycloheptatriene). There is little evidence that there are important differences in the efficacy of these agents.

Chemistry and Structure-Activity Relationship. The structures of the tricyclic antidepressant compounds are given in Table 19-4. Although dibenzazepines seem to be similar to the phenothiazines chemically, the ethylene group of imipramine's middle ring imparts dissimilar stereochemical properties and prevents conjugation among the rings, as occurs with the phenothiazines. The demethylated congener of imipramine, the secondary amine desipramine, has similar activity to that of imipramine as an antidepressant, although there are some pharmacological dissimilarities as discussed below. It was suggested that desipramine might be not only *an* active metabolite of imipramine but also *the* active drug, although this has been almost impossible to prove with *in-vivo* experiments. It is now certain that desipramine is no more effective or rapidly acting

than imipramine. The same generalizations can be made from the comparison between amitriptyline and nortriptyline. The latter pair are the structural homologs of the thioxanthenes among the antipsychotic drugs (*c.f.*, Tables 19-4 and 19-1); however, unlike the thioxanthenes, they do not occur as geometric isomers since there is no center of asymmetry. Geometric isomers of doxepin do exist; both are active and are included in available products. The 3-chloro analog of imipramine (the homolog of chlorpromazine), called clomipramine, is quite sedative and is in common clinical use in Europe as an antidepressant. In further contrast to the phenothiazines, compounds with only two carbon atoms separating the amino nitrogen of the side chain from the central ring retain some activity. Except for these few facts, the structure-activity relationship of the tricyclic antidepressants remains poorly understood. The chemistry and structure-activity relationship of a variety of experimental antidepressant agents are discussed in more detail by Kaiser and Zirkle (1970) and Usdin (1978a, 1978b).

PHARMACOLOGICAL PROPERTIES

Central Nervous System. One might expect an effective antidepressant drug to have a stimulating or mood-elevating effect when given to a normal subject. Although this may occur with the monoamine oxidase (MAO) inhibitors, it is not true of the tricyclic antidepressants.

If a dose of 100 mg of imipramine is given to a normal subject, he feels sleepy and tends to be quieter, his blood pressure falls slightly, and he feels light-headed. Often unpleasant anticholinergic effects (dry mouth and blurred vision) appear. There is little, if any, change in pupillary size. Gait may become unsteady, and the subject feels tired and clumsy. These drug effects are usually perceived as unpleasant, and cause a feeling of "unhappiness" and an *increase* in anxiety.

Table 19-4.   TRICYCLIC ANTIDEPRESSANTS

Imipramine — $CH_2CH_2CH_2N(CH_3)_2$

Amitriptyline — $CHCH_2CH_2N(CH_3)_2$

Doxepin — $CHCH_2CH_2N(CH_3)_2$

Desipramine — $CH_2CH_2CH_2NHCH_3$

Nortriptyline — $CHCH_2CH_2NHCH_3$

Protriptyline — $CH_2CH_2CH_2NHCH_3$

There may be a deterioration in tests of performance (DiMascio *et al.*, 1964). These acute drug effects thus resemble those seen with certain phenothiazines.

Repeated administration for several days may lead to accentuation of these symptoms and, in addition, to difficulty in concentrating and thinking, comparable to that experienced during the course of similar treatment with chlorpromazine (Grunthal, 1958). Imipramine seems to produce greater impairment of cognitive and affective processes and lesser reduction in physical movement than does chlorpromazine.

In contrast, if the drug is given over a period of time to depressed patients, an elevation of mood occurs. *About 2 to 3 weeks must pass before the therapeutic effects of the drug are evident.* For this reason, the tricyclic antidepressants are not prescribed on an "as-needed" basis. The explanation of the slow onset of effects remains a matter of conjecture.

The manner in which imipramine relieves the signs and symptoms of depression is not clear. Its effect has been described as a dulling of depressive ideation rather than as euphoric stimulation. However, reports of manic excitement as well as of euphoria and insomnia indicate that imipramine does have a stimulant action under certain circumstances (Bunney *et al.*, 1972). Hallucinations, excitement, and confusion, which occur in a small percentage of patients receiving antidepressants (Lehmann *et al.*, 1958; Baldessarini and Willmuth, 1968), may represent central anticholinergic effects (*see* below; Granacher and Baldessarini, 1975).

Effects on Sleep. The tricyclic antidepressants occasionally have been used as hypnotics because of their sedative property. Although this effect may be useful in the initial therapy of a depressed patient who is not sleeping well, their general use for hypnosis is not recommended. In adequate doses they cause hangover and are not as effective as a conventional hypnotic. The drugs decrease the number of awakenings, increase stage-4 sleep, and markedly decrease time in rapid-eye-movement (REM) sleep. Amitriptyline and the investigational agent clomipramine appear to be especially sedative, while the secondary-amine antidepressants are less so.

EEG Effects. EEG studies in animals and man have revealed many complex effects, some of which change with the dose. Low doses of tricyclic antidepressants tend to have synchronizing effects that resemble those of sedatives or the phenothiazines; sometimes, particularly with amitriptyline, alpha rhythm is suppressed. High doses tend to produce stimulation and arousal and can induce seizure activity (*see* Itil, 1978; Longo, 1978).

Effects on Animal Behavior. Despite its clinical antidepressant effects, imipramine produces depression of spontaneous motor activity in laboratory animals. It impairs both acquisition and performance of conditioned avoidance responses. In all these tests, it is far less potent than chlorpromazine, although it bears some similarities to diazepam. Effects on hexobarbital- or alcohol-induced sedation are unpredictable; ataxia and mild hypothermia are usual.

Although imipramine decreases spontaneous motor activity in animals, it is also capable of stimulating a great variety of behavior patterns. Blockade of the reserpine-induced sedative or "depressive" patterns in animals is a characteristic of all the tricyclic antidepressants. The latter drugs must be given before the reserpine because an intact CNS store of amines must be present for this blocking effect to become evident. Since reserpine depletes the brain of both 5-HT and norepinephrine, it is not clear which amine, if not both, is important for this action. Although this interaction has been favored as a screening test for antidepressant agents and has helped to provide support for the "amine hypothesis" of affective disorders, the relationship between these animal tests and clinical depression is tenuous. Other effects in animals have been described that seem to represent stimulant-like activity. These include potentiation of adrenergic agonists, notably amphetamine, methylphenidate, and levodopa, and augmentation of some operant behaviors, food-reward reinforced behavior, and self-stimulation of the brain. Aggressive behavior induced by hypothalamic lesions can also be increased, as can shock-induced aggression in rodents after prolonged treatment with imipramine (*see* Lowe *et al.*, 1978). Many of these behavioral effects seem to be related to potentiation of amine-mediated (particularly noradrenergic) synaptic transmission in the CNS.

Actions on Brain Amines. Tricyclic antidepressants potentiate the action of biogenic amines in the CNS by blockade of their major means of physiological inactivation—re-uptake at nerve terminals. However, there is increasing doubt that this is either a necessary or sufficient explanation of the antidepressant action of these drugs. Similar doubts concerning the role of altered amine metabolism in the pathophysiology of manic-depressive illness have already been discussed above (*see* page 393). This reservation concerning the actions of antidepressants is supported by the observation that several antidepressants are unable to potentiate the effects of biogenic amines. Moreover, other agents that are potent inhibitors of the transport of norepinephrine, notably amphetamine and cocaine, are poor antidepressants, despite the fact that they have stimulant and even euphoriant effects in some persons.

Related hypotheses have emphasized the interactions of antidepressants with other CNS amines, particularly 5-hydroxytryptamine (5-HT, serotonin) and acetylcholine. Since some antidepressants (amitriptyline, imipramine, and especially clomipramine) block the uptake of 5-HT, this CNS neurohumor may be involved in the effects of certain antidepressants (*see* van Praag, 1978). Nevertheless, the physiological importance of re-uptake of 5-HT versus its enzymatic deamination by MAO is uncertain, and many effective antidepressants have little apparent interaction with tryptaminergic neurons. It has also been suggested that the potent antimuscarinic action of many tricyclic antidepressants may contribute to their major effects. The idea has received some clinical support from the observation that the cholinesterase inhibitor physostigmine may aggravate depression and have antimanic effects (Janowsky *et al.,* 1974). However, the anticholinergic activity of the antidepressants correlates poorly with their main effects (Snyder and Yamamura, 1977), and other strongly antimuscarinic compounds, such as atropine, scopolamine, and many anticholinergic antiparkinsonian agents, are not effective antidepressants.

Despite many shortcomings of the concept that antidepressant drugs alter amine-mediated neurotransmission in the CNS, this point of view has dominated the field for 2 decades. At the present time, a few apparently valid generalizations can be made. Thus, all tricyclic antidepressants in current use in the United States block the neuronal transport (uptake) of norepinephrine, 5-HT, or both. Accordingly, they potentiate the effects of directly acting sympathomimetic amines, whether they are released endogenously or administered systemically. They block the effects of indirectly acting amines, such as tyramine, which presumably must be taken up by sympathetic neurons to cause the release of norepinephrine (*see* Chapter 8). Clomipramine is a rather selective blocker of 5-HT transport and causes a decreased turnover of the amine in the tryptaminergic-containing neurons of the midbrain raphe nuclei. In turn, their firing rate is de-

creased. In contrast, the demethylated antidepressants are thought to be much more selective in blocking the uptake of norepinephrine, and, accordingly, reduce its turnover and the firing rate of adrenergic neurons in the locus ceruleus (*see* Svenssen and Usdin, 1978). These effects appear to represent integrated responses to the *increased* availability of neurotransmitters, and are the obverse of the effects of antipsychotic drugs (dopamine *antagonists*) to enhance firing rates and turnover of neurotransmitter in dopaminergic neurons (*see* above).

There are additional interactions between antidepressants and amine neurotransmitters that are less completely understood. These include apparent α-adrenergic antagonistic actions (U'Pritchard *et al.,* 1978), a gradually increasing release of norepinephrine (apparent increase in quantum released per nerve impulse) that may be related to presynaptic α-adrenergic autoreceptors (Crews and Smith, 1978), neurophysiologically defined stabilizing effects on norepinephrine-containing cells of the locus ceruleus (*see* Chapter 12) (Svenssen and Usdin, 1978), and a gradually evolving increased sensitivity of forebrain neurons to 5-HT (DeMontigny and Aghajanian, 1978). In addition, prolonged enhancement of the availability of norepinephrine due to inhibition of transport of the neurotransmitter may cause desensitization of β-adrenergic systems, perhaps as a result of reduction of the number of available receptors (*see* Sulser and Robinson, 1978). It remains to be determined if slowly evolving changes in receptor number or sensitivity or the activity of central noradrenergic systems can help to account for the typically prolonged onset of the clinical effects of antidepressant drugs.

Autonomic Nervous System. In contrast to the weak anticholinergic effects of the phenothiazines, the anticholinergic responses to therapeutic doses of the tricyclic antidepressants are prominent. These are manifested in blurred vision, dry mouth, constipation, and urinary retention. Amitriptyline seems to cause the highest incidence of these effects, while desipramine has relatively less anticholinergic effect in man (Blackwell *et al.,* 1978). Tachycardia is frequent and may in part be an adrenergic effect caused by the blockade of norepinephrine re-uptake in the heart. Since the autonomic changes that accompany depression may include some of these symptoms, the determination of what is a true autonomic side effect of a tricyclic antidepressant must rest on a careful physical examination and history obtained before the initiation of drug therapy.

Cardiovascular System.   Tricyclic antidepressants have marked effects on the cardiovascular system even in therapeutic doses (*see* Raisfeld, 1972; Jefferson, 1975). Imipramine lowers the blood pressure in anesthetized dogs and obtunds various cardiovascular reflexes, including the carotid occlusion reflex, the Bezold-Jarisch reflex, and postural responses. There is an increased tendency for arrhythmias to develop in patients on tricyclic drugs, and there have been several reports of unexpected deaths (Williams and Sherter, 1971; Moir *et al.,* 1972). These adverse reactions may be related to the blockade of amine re-uptake by these drugs and the resultant high concentrations of norepinephrine in cardiac tissue. Orthostatic hypotension is commonly observed with therapeutic doses. Myocardial infarction and the precipitation of congestive heart failure during the course of treatment have been attributed to imipramine administration. Tachycardia is a common finding. The most prominent ECG change observed following the use of imipramine consists in inversion or flattening of the T waves. Direct, quinidine-like myocardial depressant effects of imipramine (and, presumably, of its congeners) can be prominent in human subjects (Bigger *et al.,* 1977). One should be wary of potentially dangerous enhancement of the effects of other cardiac depressant drugs by tricyclic antidepressants.

Since the tricyclic antidepressants can cause orthostatic hypotension, produce arrhythmias, and interact in deleterious ways with other drugs (*see* below), great caution must be observed in their use in patients with cardiac disease. Unfortunately, since many depressed patients fall in an age group where cardiac problems are common and coexistence of depressive illness and cardiovascular disease is frequent, the physician is faced with a dilemma. This can be resolved by consideration of the usual self-limited time course of depressions, treatment of associated anxiety and sleep disorders with other medication (*see* below), and use of electroconvulsive therapy (ECT) in serious depressions.

Respiration.   Imipramine in clinically useful doses produces little effect on respiration. Respiratory depression has been observed following poisoning with imipramine and with amitriptyline (*see* below).

Absorption, Distribution, Fate, and Excretion.   Imipramine and other tricyclic antidepressant agents are well absorbed after oral administration. While they are usually initially used in divided doses, their relatively long half-lives and rather wide range of tolerated concentrations permit a gradual transition toward a single daily dose given at bedtime. This is most safely done for doses up to the equivalent of 150 mg of imipramine. High doses of these strongly anticholinergic agents can slow gastrointestinal activity and gastric emptying time, resulting in slower or erratic absorption of these and other drugs taken concomitantly; this can complicate the management of acute overdosage. Concentrations in plasma typically peak within 2 to 8 hours, but this can be delayed for over 12 hours. Intramuscular administration of tricyclic antidepressants can be performed under unusual circumstances, particularly with severely depressed, anorexic patients who may refuse oral medication. The pharmacokinetics of these agents is discussed by Morselli (1977) and Hollister (1978a); *see also* Appendix II.

Once absorbed, these lipophilic drugs are widely distributed; their pharmacokinetic properties are similar to those of the phenothiazines. They are strongly bound to plasma protein and to the constituents of tissues. The latter fact accounts for their large volumes of apparent distribution, which are typically 10 to 50 liters per kilogram. Toxic effects of these drugs can be expected when their concentrations in plasma rise above 1 μg/ml and can occur at even half this value. These concentrations are just a few times greater than those associated with therapeutic effects—100 to 300 ng/ml.

The tricyclic antidepressants are oxidized by hepatic microsomal enzymes, followed by conjugation with glucuronic acid. The major route of metabolism of imipramine is to the active drug desipramine; inactivation of either compound occurs largely by oxidation to 2-hydroxy metabolites and conjugation with glucuronic acid. In contrast, amitriptyline (while mainly demethylated to nortriptyline) and nortriptyline undergo preferential oxidation at the 10 position, followed by glucuronidation; the 10-hydroxy metabolites may have some biological activity. While the demethylated metabolites of both imipramine and amitriptyline clearly possess antidepressant activity, it is not known if this accounts for most or all of the activity of the parent drugs. It is clear that these demethylated products can accumulate in concentrations approaching, or even exceeding, those of their precursors. Doxepin also appears to be converted to an active metabolite, nordoxepin, by N-demethylation (Ziegler *et al.*, 1978).

There is marked variation among subjects (up to 50-fold) in the ratio of methylated to demethylated molecules following administration of imipramine or amitriptyline in man (Nagy and Johansson, 1975). This variation, as well as that of the concentrations of the drug in blood, appears to be characteristic of the individual and is presumably under genetic control (Alexanderson and Sjöqvist, 1971). The question of possible correlations between concentrations of tricyclic antidepressants in blood and clinical response or toxicity is under active investigation. (For reviews, *see* Åsberg, 1974, 1976; Lader, 1974; Cooper *et al.*, 1976; Glassman *et al.*, 1977; Glassman and Perel, 1978; Baldessarini, 1979a.) While conclusions remain rather tentative, concentrations between 50 and 300 ng/ml or, more narrowly, between 100 and 200 ng/ml have been suggested to correlate best with clinically satisfactory antidepressant responses. When the plasma concentration of imipramine, amitriptyline, or doxepin is determined, it is customary to report the results for the sum of the parent compound and the demethylated metabolite.

The inactivation and elimination of tricyclic antidepressants occur over a period of several days, and half-lives range from about 10 to 20 hours for imipramine to an extreme of about 80 hours for protriptyline; the other agents have intermediate values (*see* Appendix II). It follows that most tricyclic antidepressants should be inactivated and excreted within a week after termination of treatment, with notable exceptions being ordinary doses of protriptyline and overdosage with the other agents (Spiker and Biggs, 1976). Indeed, cardiac arrhythmias have been reported for 10 days or more following the acute phase of intoxication with large doses of drugs such as amitriptyline (Rasmussen, 1966; Vohra and Burrows, 1974). Tricyclic antidepressants are not removed effectively by any available dialysis technic.

Tolerance and Physical Dependence. Tolerance to the anticholinergic effects, such as dry mouth, constipation, blurred vision, and tachycardia, tends to develop with continued use of imipramine. Orthostatic hypotension similar to that seen with the phenothiazines may occur initially, but tolerance to this effect is acquired. Occasional patients will show physical or psychic dependence on the tricyclic antidepressants (Shatan, 1966). A withdrawal syndrome consisting in malaise, chills, coryza, and muscle aching has been reported to follow abrupt discontinuation of high doses of imipramine. Despite these occasional problems, it is important to emphasize that tricyclic antidepressants have frequently been used for prolonged periods (years) by patients with severe recurring depression (so-called unipolar manic-depressive illness) without evidence of tolerance to their desirable effects (*see* Davis, 1976).

Preparations, Routes of Administration, and Dosage. These are presented in Table 19-5. A further consideration of dosage and the use of antidepressant drugs appears below.

Toxic Reactions and Side Effects. Significant toxic effects of tricyclic antidepressant drugs are relatively common, and estimates of prevalence have run as high as 5% (Boston Collaborative Drug Surveillance Program, 1972). Most of these reactions involve antimuscarinic effects of the drugs and cerebral toxicity, but cardiac toxicity also represents a serious problem. The tricyclic antidepressants can be placed in the following approximate rank order of antimuscarinic potency: amitriptyline > imipramine > doxepin = nortriptyline > desipramine = protriptyline (Richelson and Diventz-Romero, 1977; Snyder and Yamamura, 1977; *see also* Blackwell *et al.*, 1978). Clinical consequences of this effect include dry mouth and a sour or metallic taste, epigastric distress, constipation, dizziness, tachycardia, palpitations, blurred vision, and urinary retention. Special precautions should be taken in men with pros-

Table 19-5. ANTIDEPRESSANT DRUGS: PREPARATIONS, DOSAGE FORMS, AND DOSES

NONPROPRIETARY NAME	TRADE NAMES	DOSAGE FORMS *	USUAL DAILY DOSE (*mg*)	EXTREME DAILY DOSE (*mg*) †
Tricyclics				
Imipramine Hydrochloride, U.S.P. ‡	IMAVATE, JANIMINE, PRESAMINE, SK-PRAMINE, TOFRANIL	(T)10,25,50 mg (A)25 mg/2 ml	100–200	30–300
Desipramine Hydrochloride, U.S.P.	NORPRAMIN, PERTOFRANE	(C)25,50 mg (T)25,50,75, 100,150 mg	100–200	25–300
Amitriptyline Hydrochloride, U.S.P. ‡	AMITRIL, ELAVIL, ENDEP	(T)10,25,50,75, 100,150 mg (V)10 mg/ml in 10 ml	75–200	50–300
Nortriptyline Hydrochloride, U.S.P.	AVENTYL HYDROCHLORIDE, PAMELOR	(C)10,25 mg (S)10 mg/5 ml	75–150 §	20–150
Doxepin Hydrochloride, U.S.P.	ADAPIN, SINEQUAN	(C)10,25,50,75, 100,150 mg (S)10 mg/ml	75–150	25–300
Protriptyline Hydrochloride, U.S.P.	VIVACTYL	(T)5,10 mg	15–40	10–60
Monoamine Oxidase Inhibitors				
Isocarboxazid, U.S.P.	MARPLAN	(T)10 mg	10–30	10–30
Phenelzine Sulfate, U.S.P.	NARDIL	(T)15 mg	15–30	15–90
Tranylcypromine Sulfate, U.S.P.	PARNATE	(T)10 mg	20–30	10–30

* T = tablet; C = capsule; V = vial for intramuscular injection; A = ampul for intramuscular injection; S = oral solution or concentrate.

† Extreme doses are for very young and very elderly patients at the low end and for hospital use in severe or treatment-resistant depression at the high end. In addition, due to the long biological half-life of MAO inhibition, small doses of MAO inhibitors are used after several days to weeks of treatment.

‡ Imipramine is also available as the pamoate (TOFRANIL-PM) in capsules containing 75, 100, 125, or 150 mg of the drug, but its advantages over the hydrochloride are not established. Amitriptyline hydrochloride is also available mixed with fixed doses of perphenazine in tablets containing 2/10, 4/10, 2/25, 4/25, or 4/50 mg of perphenazine/amitriptyline (ETRAFON, TRIAVIL) and mixed with chlordiazepoxide in tablets containing 5/12.5 or 10/25 mg of chlordiazepoxide/amitriptyline (LIMBITROL).

§ Although the recommended maximal daily dose is 100 mg, recent evidence indicates that many patients have relatively low concentrations in plasma and inferior clinical responses unless doses exceed 100 mg, while a few may have an excessive amount at doses above 150 mg/day (Åsberg, 1976).

tatic hypertrophy. Paradoxically, excessive sweating is a fairly common complaint; the mechanism of this response is not known. Weakness and fatigue are attributable to central effects of the drug and may resemble those seen with the phenothiazines. There are marked individual differences in the type and the frequency of these side effects, and they may be related to concentrations of active drug in plasma. Older patients tend to suffer more from dizziness, postural hypotension, constipation, delayed micturition, edema, and muscle tremors. Very rarely, amitriptyline may cause inappropriate secretion of ADH.

Another undesirable effect of imipramine (and of all forms of treatment of depression) is a transition in certain patients from depression to hypomanic or *manic excitement*. This striking feature of so-called bipolar manic-depressive illness is sometimes referred to as the "switch process" and has been studied in detail by Bunney and associates (1972). In addition to manic reactions to tricyclic antidepressants, delirium is common. These may be seen in approximately 10% of treated patients (and in over 30% of patients over age 50) (Davies *et al.*, 1971). These common drug-related problems are still frequently overlooked or misinterpreted as being part of the primary illness, particularly in the elderly. Small doses of physostigmine may aid in the diagnosis in some cases (*see* Granacher and Baldessarini, 1975). Among the CNS problems associated with tricyclic antidepressants, extrapyramidal reactions are rare, although *tremor* is not unusual. A fine tremor occurs in about 10%

of those receiving a tricyclic agent, although the prevalence of this effect is also much higher in elderly patients, particularly when high doses of drug are administered. Tremor may respond to small doses of propranolol. It is important to clarify the problem of the therapy of the various CNS-based toxic or psychiatric reactions to tricyclic antidepressants. *Antipsychotic drugs* are to be *avoided,* except for the management of manic reactions or severe agitation. They may exacerbate toxic confusional states, rather than help them. In any of these reactions, whether manic or toxic-organic, the best first step is to *stop the antidepressant.* Physostigmine may be effective in some cases, and, if sedation is urgently required, small doses of diazepam may be considered.

Although *loss of accommodation* is a common ophthalmological side effect of any strongly anticholinergic agent, including tricyclic antidepressants, the precipitation of *glaucoma,* while frequently mentioned, is actually a rare event. The risk is probably highest in elderly patients with the narrow-angle type of glaucoma. They require emergency treatment with a miotic agent if an attack is precipitated. Tricyclic antidepressants can still be used in patients with glaucoma, provided that pilocarpine eyedrops or an equivalent medication is continued (Nouri and Cuendet, 1971). The most rational choice of an antidepressant in such a case would be desipramine, due to its relatively low anticholinergic potency and moderate half-life.

Various types of *cardiovascular difficulties* have already been described above; these are also discussed by Raisfeld (1972), Moir and associates (1973), Vohra and Burrows (1974), Jefferson (1975), and Burrows and coworkers (1976). In one series, sudden deaths among cardiac patients receiving tricyclic antidepressants were four times more frequent than in those who were not so treated (Moir *et al.,* 1973). Patients at risk for ventricular arrhythmias may be especially vulnerable to the intrusion of ectopic ventricular contractions during the prolonged myocardial repolarization time that is induced by the tricyclic drugs. There is also a suspicion that antidepressant drugs may contribute to cardiomyopathies and to the worsening of congestive heart failure in some cases (Raisfeld, 1972).

Hypotension is frequent with antidepressants and may add further to the risk of ischemic damage to the heart or brain in vulnerable individuals. Dihydroergotamine (10 mg per day) has been used safely to treat such hypotension (Bojanovsky and Tolle, 1974). Although clinical studies of the relative risk of cardiac toxicity among antidepressants are few and inconclusive, and animal studies may not be pertinent, the current impression is that amitriptyline, protriptyline, and perhaps imipramine may be more dangerous than doxepin or mianserin in depressed patients with cardiac disease (*see* Burrows *et al.,* 1976; Hollister, 1978b). The cardiotoxic effects of tricyclic antidepressants produce especially dangerous complications following acute overdosage.

Miscellaneous toxic effects of tricyclic antidepressants include jaundice, agranulocytosis, and rashes, but these are very infrequent. Weight gain has been described; while its mechanism is obscure, increased appetite and caloric intake are usually implicated. Delay of orgasm and *orgasmic impotence* have been described in men and women. The safety of antidepressants during pregnancy and lactation or in the treatment of young children is not well established. Evidence concerning the possibility of *teratogenic effects* of the tricyclic agents is mixed but unconvincing (*see* Goldberg and DiMascio, 1978). Nevertheless, the possibility of toxic effects on fetal tissue remains unresolved (Morselli, 1977). For severe depression during pregnancy and lactation, ECT may be a relatively safe and effective alternative. Antidepressants are generally not recommended for use in children, although small doses of imipramine are used for the treatment of enuresis in those over 6 years of age. Children seem to be especially vulnerable to cardiotoxic and seizure-inducing effects of high doses of tricyclic compounds (Morselli, 1977), and deaths have occurred in children after accidental or deliberate overdosage with only a few hundred milligrams of drug.

Acute poisoning with tricyclic antidepressants is occurring with increasing frequency and, unlike acute overdosage with antipsychotic drugs, is life threatening. Unfortunately, most of the drugs used in the treatment of severe disorders of mood (tricyclic agents, MAO inhibitors, and lithium salts) are potentially lethal in doses that are readily available to patients with a high risk of suicide. While the margin of safety for the tricyclic antidepressants is not accurately known for man, deaths have been reported with doses of approximately 2000 mg of imipramine (or the equivalent of another drug), and severe intoxication can be expected at doses above 1000 mg. As a general rule, *it is unwise to dispense more than a week's supply of an antidepressant to an acutely depressed patient.*

The presenting of symptoms and the course of events in acute poisoning due to a tricyclic antidepressant is often complex (Noble and Matthew, 1969). A typical pattern is a brief phase of excitement and restlessness, sometimes with myoclonus, grand mal seizures, or dystonia, followed by rapid development of coma, often with depressed respiration, hypoxia, depressed reflexes, hypothermia, hypotension, and striking evidence of anticholinergic effects, with mydriasis, flushed dry skin and dry mucosae, decreased bowel sounds, urinary retention, and tachycardia. At this crucial stage the patient must be treated in an intensive care unit that allows constant cardiac monitoring and defibrillation and resuscitation when necessary. The most urgent needs are to support vital functions. Gastric lavage is sometimes used early in treatment, but this is best done only with a cuffed endotracheal tube safely in place. Although dialysis and diuresis are useless in such cases, administration of activated charcoal to adsorb the drug in the gut has some demonstrated utility (Crome *et al.,* 1977). The comatose phase disappears gradually, usually over 1 to 3 days, depending on the severity of the poisoning. A period of excitement and delirium is then very typical, again with prominent anticholinergic signs. Even when this phase of delirious intoxication has passed, the risk of life-threatening cardiac arrhythmias continues for at least several days, requiring close medical supervision and continued cardiac monitoring.

The efficacy and safety of various pharmacological interventions to counter tricyclic poisoning remain unsettled. Although physostigmine salicylate can sometimes produce dramatic effects to alleviate many of the antimuscarinic, cardiotoxic, and neurotoxic features of this syndrome (*see* Granacher and Baldessarini, 1975), indications for the use of this approach are not entirely clear. The major difficulty involves the toxicity of physostigmine itself, and seizures may result, particularly when large doses are given very rapidly (Baldessarini and Gelenberg, 1979). Its safety and efficacy seem to be greater in cases of mild intoxication, characterized by confusion and delirium but with stable vital functions and the absence of coma. Physostigmine is the only reversible anticholinesterase with appreciable capability to cross the blood-brain barrier to exert central actions. The usual dose is between 0.5 and 2 mg, given intramuscularly or by *slow* intravenous injection; the injection is then repeated as often as required by clinical signs. Typically, doses can be given

every 30 to 90 minutes due to the short half-life of this agent. (For further details on the use of physostigmine, *see* Granacher and Baldessarini, 1975.) Cardiac toxicity and hypotension in such poisonings can be especially difficult to manage. The heart is usually hyperactive, with supraventricular tachycardia and a high cardiac output, but the arteriovenous pressure differential is decreased. The QRS complex of the ECG is moderately responsive to tricyclic antidepressants, and in acute overdosage it is typically prolonged to over 100 milliseconds. Generally, cardiac glycosides and depressants such as quinidine or procainamide are contraindicated, but phenytoin has been given safely and may simultaneously be useful to suppress the convulsive seizures that are often present. In addition, propranolol has been recommended (*see* Vohra and Burrows, 1974). Diazepam has been used to control seizures and myoclonic and dystonic features of tricyclic antidepressant poisoning. Aside from the problems of management created by the specific effects of tricyclic antidepressants, very serious hypoxia, hypertension or hypotension, and metabolic acidosis may have to be treated. In the presence of high concentrations of tricyclic antidepressants, the effects of α-adrenergic agonists, used as pressor agents, may be inhibited, and maintenance of intravascular volume may be difficult to achieve.

Interactions with Other Drugs. The tricyclic antidepressants are involved in several clinically important drug interactions. The binding of tricyclic antidepressants to plasma albumin can be reduced by competition with phenytoin, phenylbutazone, aspirin, aminopyrine, scopolamine, and phenothiazines (*see* Morselli, 1977). Other interactions that may also potentiate the effects of tricyclic drugs can result from interference with their metabolism in the liver. This effect has been associated with neuroleptic drugs, methylphenidate, and certain steroids, including oral contraceptives (*see* Morselli, 1977). In the opposite direction, barbiturates and certain other sedatives can increase the hepatic metabolism of the antidepressants by inducing microsomal enzyme systems, and the concurrent administration of these drugs should probably be avoided; benzodiazepines do not seem to have this effect (Gram *et al.,* 1973).

Antidepressants potentiate the effects of alcohol, and probably other sedatives (Seppälä *et al.,* 1975). The anticholinergic activity of tricyclic antidepressants makes it important to monitor the results if the drugs must be used simultaneously with antiparkinsonian agents, antipsychotic drugs (especially thioridazine), or other compounds with antimuscarinic activity. The tricyclic antidepressants have prominent and potentially dangerous potentiative interactions with biogenic amines, such as norepinephrine, which normally are removed from their site of action by neuronal uptake. Presumably by a similar mechanism, the action of adrenergic neuron blocking agents such as guanethidine is prevented by the tricyclic antidepressants. This effect may be somewhat less noticeable with doxepin, which is a less potent blocker of re-uptake of norepinephrine by sympathetic neurons.

Tricyclic agents can also block the centrally mediated antihypertensive action of clonidine. A particularly severe, but rare, interaction has been noted following the concurrent administration of an MAO inhibitor and a tricyclic antidepressant. The resultant syndrome can include severe CNS toxicity, marked by hyperpyrexia, convulsions, and coma. Although this reaction is rare and the two classes of antidepressant agents have been combined safely (*see* Goldberg and Thornton, 1978), this use should be contraindicated, since the interaction has a potentially catastrophic outcome. There is no evidence that treatment with tricyclic agents plus MAO inhibitors is more efficacious than a tricyclic antidepressant alone. Tricyclic antidepressants can be used safely during ECT.

Therapeutic Uses. The use of tricyclic antidepressants in depressed patients is discussed below (*see* page 434). While several other possible indications for these drugs have been suggested, only *enuresis* in children over 6 years of age has been accepted as a possible use for imipramine (and only in doses up to 2.5 mg/kg, or 50 mg total, daily); the efficacy of such treatment is not completely settled (*see* Medical Letter, 1974; Stewart, 1975). Other areas of suggested use that remain investigational include certain syndromes that may mimic depression, overlap diagnostically with depression, or be accompanied by or complicated by secondary depression. These include *alcoholism* and the neuroses, especially *phobic-anxiety syndromes* (Klein *et al.*, 1978) and some cases of *obsessive-compulsive neurosis*. The latter is notoriously difficult to treat by any method, and it remains unclear if the occasional benefit

seemingly provided by antidepressant drugs reflects an action on the primary disorder or on secondary depression that frequently accompanies it. *Chronic pain, neuralgias,* and *migraine* are other syndromes that may belong in the same category and that sometimes respond favorably to tricyclic agents or to other treatments used for depression.

MONOAMINE OXIDASE (MAO) INHIBITORS

The MAO inhibitors comprise a rather heterogeneous group of drugs that have in common the ability to block oxidative deamination of naturally occurring monoamines. However, the relationship between MAO inhibition and some of the ancillary therapeutic actions of these drugs is not firmly established. These drugs have numerous other effects, many of which are still poorly understood. For example, they lower blood pressure and were at one time used to treat hypertension. Their use in psychiatry has also become very limited as the tricyclic antidepressants have come to dominate the treatment of depression and allied conditions. Thus, MAO inhibitors are used when tricyclic antidepressants give an unsatisfactory result and when ECT is inappropriate or refused. In addition, it has been repeatedly suggested, with some scientific support (*see* Robinson *et al.*, 1978), that whereas severe depression may not be the most favorable indication for these agents, certain neurotic illnesses with depressive features, and also with anxiety and phobias, may respond especially favorably. However, the record of success of MAO inhibitors in controlled trials in comparison with tricyclic antidepressants or ECT is not good (*see* Klein and Davis, 1969). One possible determinant of their poor efficacy in severe depression may be the use of insufficient dosage (Robinson *et al.*, 1978). Moreover, the complex, sometimes severe, and often unpredictable interactions between MAO inhibitors and many drugs and food-derived amines, as well as their tendency to damage the hepatic parenchyma, have made their medical use difficult and hazardous.

History. In 1951, *isoniazid* and its isopropyl derivative, *iproniazid,* were developed for the treatment of tuberculosis. It was soon found that iproniazid had mood-elevating effects in tuberculous patients. In 1952, Delay and collaborators investigated the action of isoniazid in the treatment of depressed states and Zeller and coworkers found that iproniazid, in contrast to isoniazid, was capable of inhibiting the enzyme MAO. In 1957, following investigations by Kline and colleagues and by Crane, it was applied in psychiatry for the treatment of depressed patients. MAO inhibitors had an important impact on the development of modern biological psychiatry. (For reviews of this topic, *see* Weil-Malherbe, 1967; Baldessarini, 1975, 1977b.)

Because of toxicity, there has been a great deal of flux in the introduction and withdrawal of MAO inhibitors. Drugs no longer available include *iproniazid, pheniprazine, etryptamine,* and *nialamide.* *Tranylcypromine* was withdrawn from the market during 1964, but again became available for use in patients under close medical observation. At present, the MAO inhibitors available for use in depression are *isocarboxazid, phenelzine,* and *tranylcypromine.*

Chemistry and Structure-Activity Relationship. The first MAO inhibitors to be used in the treatment of depression were hydrazide derivatives of hydrazine, a highly hepatotoxic substance. Subsequently, compounds unrelated to hydrazine were found to be very potent MAO inhibitors. Several of these agents were structurally related to amphetamine and were synthesized in an attempt to enhance central stimulant properties. Cyclization of the side chain of amphetamine resulted in the nonhydrazide MAO inhibitor *tranylcypromine.* Details of the structure-activity relationship and the chemistry of these agents can be found elsewhere (*see* Kaiser and Zirkle, 1970; Biel *et al.,* 1978). Structures of the MAO inhibitors currently available in the United States for psychiatric patients are as follows:

Tranylcypromine

Phenelzine

Isocarboxazid

PHARMACOLOGICAL PROPERTIES

MAO inhibitors exert their effects mainly on organ systems influenced by sympathomimetic amines and 5-HT. These agents inhibit not only MAO but other enzymes as well (*see* Costa and Sandler, 1972), and *they interfere with the hepatic metabolism of many drugs.* In addition, they are believed to exert effects not directly related to enzyme inhibition. MAO is a flavin-containing enzyme that is localized in mitochondrial membranes, whether in nerve terminals or the liver. It is biochemically dissimilar to other nonspecific amine oxidases found, for example, in plasma. It is closely linked functionally with an aldehyde reductase in all tissues, but the products of these reactions can be carboxylic acids *or* alcohols, depending on the substrate and the tissue. MAO is important in regulating the metabolic degradation of catecholamines and 5-HT in neural or target tissues, and hepatic MAO has a crucial defensive role in inactivating circulating monoamines or those, such as tyramine, that originate in the gut and are absorbed into the portal circulation (*see* Baldessarini and Fischer, 1978). It appears that MAO exists in at least two forms with dissimilar substrate preferences and differential sensitivity to selective inhibitors (*clorgyline* versus MAO-A and *deprenyl* versus MAO-B); this might offer therapeutic advantages when it is desirable to potentiate certain amines selectively. (Extensive discussions of this and other aspects of MAO and its inhibitors are provided in the monograph edited by Costa and Sandler, 1972; *see also* Chapters 4, 8, 9, 12, and 21.)

The hydrazines isocarboxazid and phenelzine (and the nonhydrazine antihypertensive agent pargyline) bind irreversibly to MAO. In the clinical setting, maximal inhibition is usually achieved within a few days, although the antidepressant effect of these drugs may be delayed for 2 or 3 weeks. Since new enzyme molecules must be synthesized to restore amine metabolism to normal, it takes up to 2 weeks for the effect to be reversed. Enzyme inhibition by tranylcypromine, unlike that produced by the hydrazines or pargyline, is reversed much more rapidly, since this drug is not irreversibly bound to the enzyme. In addition, tranylcypromine has a more rapid onset of action. The enzyme-inhibitory effects of these drugs can be evaluated in human subjects by assay of urinary amines and their deaminated metabolites, sometimes after a test dose of an amine (Levine and Sjoerdsma, 1963), or by direct assay of MAO activity in conveniently biopsied tissues, such as skin or jejunum, or, more commonly, in blood platelets. The platelet technic is currently favored as a means of monitoring the actions of MAO inhibitors and has led to the impression that favorable clinical responses are likely to occur when platelet MAO is inhibited by at least 70% (Robinson *et al.,* 1978).

The capacity of MAO inhibitors to act as antidepressants has most often been assumed to reflect the increased availability of one or more monoamines in the CNS or sympathetic nervous system, although this assumption has been difficult to prove. One problem with this hypothesis is that the acute biochemical and pharmacological actions of MAO inhibitors precede the palliative effects in psychiatric illnesses by as long as 2 or more weeks. Reasons for this delay of therapeutic effects remain unexplained.

Effects on Sleep and the EEG. MAO inhibitors are among the most effective suppressors of REM sleep that are known. This effect has been used therapeutically in the treatment of narcolepsy (Wyatt *et al.,* 1971). Moreover, when they are effective in the treatment of depression, MAO inhibitors correct the accompanying disorder of sleep, whether it is an increase or decrease of sleep time. In man, the effects of the MAO inhibitors upon the EEG are slight. Tranylcypromine does, however, have stimulant-like effects on the EEG.

Animal Behavior. The administration of single doses of an MAO inhibitor produces either minor changes in the behavior of animals or none at all, even when biochemical studies reveal marked alteration in the activity of the enzymes in the brain and significant elevations of concentrations of dopamine, norepinephrine, and 5-HT in the brain. However, when these drugs are combined with other agents, marked effects upon behavior and CNS function may be seen. Thus, in animals pretreated with MAO inhibitors, reserpine and tetrabenazine produce excitement rather than sedation, hexobarbital sleeping time is prolonged, and the actions of many other CNS depressants and stimulants may be augmented.

Cardiovascular System. MAO inhibitors lower blood pressure and provide symptomatic relief in angina pectoris. Their use as antihypertensive agents, now obsolete, is described in *previous editions* of this textbook (*see also* Chapters 8 and 9).

Absorption, Fate, and Excretion. All the currently employed MAO inhibitors are readily absorbed when given by mouth. They are never given parenterally. These drugs produce maximal inhibition of MAO in biopsy samples from man within 5 to 10 days. There is little information on their pharmacokinetics. However, their biological activity is prolonged due to the characteristics of their interaction with the enzyme.

The hydrazide MAO inhibitors are thought to be cleaved, with resultant liberation of active products. They are inactivated primarily by acetylation. About one half the population in the United States and Europe (and more in other populations, such as Eskimos and certain Orientals) are "slow acetylators" of the hydrazine-type drugs, including phenelzine, and this may explain the exaggerated effects observed in some patients given conventional doses of phenelzine (Vesell, 1972).

Toxic Reactions and Side Effects. Toxic reactions from *overdosage* may occur in a matter of hours despite the long delay in onset of a therapeutic response. Reported effects of overdosage include agitation, hallucinations, hyperreflexia, hyperpyrexia, and convulsions. Both hypotension and hypertension have been reported. Treatment of such intoxication presents a problem. Sympathomimetic amines and barbiturates should be used with extreme caution. Conservative treatment aimed at maintaining normal temperature, respiration, blood pressure, and proper fluid and electrolyte balance has often been successful. Since the inhibition of the enzyme is irreversible, late toxic effects may appear. Patients with known overdosage of MAO inhibitors should be observed in the hospital for at least a week after the poisoning.

The potential toxic effects of the MAO inhibitors are greater and more serious than those of any other group of psychotherapeutic agents. The most dangerous are those involving the liver, the brain, and the cardiovascular system. Hepatotoxicity does not seem to be related to dosage or duration of therapy, and the incidence with currently used MAO inhibitors is low. Nevertheless, when it does occur, it can be serious because the hydrazide compounds cause cellular damage to the hepatic parenchyma. This problem has led to discontinuation of the use of several MAO inhibitors.

Excessive central stimulation consisting in tremors, insomnia, and hyperhidrosis may occur and might be considered extensions of the pharmacological effects. Agitation and hypomanic behavior may also occur, and on rare occasions hallucinations and confusion are observed. *Convulsions* have also been reported. Peripheral *neuropathy* following the use of hydrazides may possibly be related to a pyridoxine deficiency.

Orthostatic hypotension occurs with the use of all the MAO inhibitors currently employed. The immediate condition readily yields to recumbency, but the dose may have to be reduced or the medication withdrawn.

A variety of other less serious side effects have been reported, including dizziness and vertigo (perhaps related to orthostatic hypotension), headache, inhibition of ejaculation, difficulty in urination, weakness, fatigue, dry mouth, blurred vision, and skin rashes. Constipation is common, but the cause is not known.

Interactions with Other Drugs. The paucity of grossly observable signs following the administration of MAO inhibitors is deceptive, for major changes have occurred in the body's capacity to handle endogenous or exogenous biogenic amines and to respond normally to a wide spectrum of pharmacological agents. When MAO is inhibited, biogenic amines are not deaminated but remain active and produce behavioral and pharmacodynamic effects.

Because of their interference with various enzymes, the MAO inhibitors prolong and intensify the effects of other drugs and interfere with the metabolism of various naturally occurring substances. There is considerable evidence that administration of *precursors of biogenic amines* may cause marked effects when administered following MAO inhibitors. Thus, the administration of levodopa or 5-hydroxytryptophan increases the concentrations of catecholamines or 5-HT in brain, respectively, and produces signs of central excitation in animals. The concurrent administration of levodopa and an MAO inhibitor to patients can be expected to produce agitation and hypertension.

The actions of *sympathomimetic amines* are potentiated following the use of MAO inhibitors. The effect is greater with indirectly acting amines (*e.g.,* amphetamine and tyramine) than with directly acting amines, which are potentiated in man to a greater degree by the tricyclic antidepressants. Since administered catecholamines are largely inactivated by catechol-O-methyltransferase and by neuronal reuptake, the MAO inhibitors have less effect in prolonging and intensifying their action. On the other hand, inasmuch as certain sympathomimetic amines such as amphetamine and tyramine act peripherally, primarily by releasing the stores of catecholamines in nerve endings, and since the concentration of amines is raised by MAO inhibitors, profound potentiation of effects such as pressor responses may be expected (*see* below).

MAO inhibitors also interfere with detoxication mechanisms for certain other drugs. They prolong and intensify the effects of central depressant agents, such as general anesthetics, sedatives, antihistamines, alcohol, and potent analgesics; of anticholinergic agents, particularly those used in the treatment of parkinsonism; and of antidepressant agents, especially imipramine and amitriptyline. A serious *hyperpyrexic* reaction occurs after the concomitant use of *meperidine.* This reaction may be mediated by the release of 5-HT, since it does not occur in experimental animals if they are pretreated with inhibitors of 5-HT synthesis.

Hypertensive crisis is a most serious toxic effect of MAO inhibitors related to drug interaction. Hypertensive crises were noted to be associated with the ingestion of cheese in patients receiving MAO inhibitors, particularly tranylcypromine and phenelzine but also other agents in this class. Acting on the suggestion of an alert pharmacist, Blackwell suggested that certain cheeses might contain a pressor amine or substance capable of liberating stored catecholamines (*see* Ayd and Blackwell, 1970). *Tyramine* was soon implicated as the culpable substance. The average meal of natural or aged cheeses contains enough tyramine to provoke a marked rise in blood pressure and other cardiovascular changes. Presumably as a result of hepatic MAO inhibition, tyramine and other monoamines in food or produced by bacteria in the gut escape oxidative deamination in the liver and release catecholamines that are present in supranormal amounts in nerve endings and the adrenal medulla. Other foods implicated in this syndrome include beer, wine, pickled herring, snails, chicken liver, yeast, large quantities of coffee citrus fruits, canned figs, broad beans (which contain dopa), and chocolate and cream or their products. Realistically, since more than 10 mg of tyramine seems to be required to produce significant hypertension, the most dangerous foods are aged cheeses and yeast products used as food supplements (*see* Marley and Blackwell, 1970; Baldessarini, 1977b). Patients being treated with MAO inhibitors and their families should be given a list of foods to be avoided and a general warning about the use of *any* medication by the patient without permission. Care must even be exercised here, since certain depressed patients have used such a list as a compilation of potential suicidal agents.

In certain instances, intracranial bleeding has occurred, and death has sometimes followed. Headache is a common symptom, and fever frequently accompanies the hypertensive episode. Narcotics should never be used for such headaches, and blood pressure should be evaluated immediately when a patient taking an MAO inhibitor reports a severe throbbing headache. There is a clinical similarity of the hypertensive syndrome to that seen in pheochromocytoma. Such episodes may also be encountered when MAO inhibitors are used with sympathomimetic amines, methyldopa, dopamine, and tryptophan. Acute increases in blood pressure can also follow the initial doses of reserpine and adrenergic neuron blocking agents such as guanethidine when these are given concurrently with an MAO inhibitor. It should be noted that tranylcypromine can cause a reaction if administered when the effect of phenelzine is still present. Switching a patient from one MAO inhibitor to another or to a tricyclic antidepressant requires that a rest period of 2 weeks intervenes.

Treatment of the hypertensive crisis is directed at lowering the blood pressure. For this purpose a short-acting α-adrenergic blocking agent (*e.g.*, phentolamine, 2 to 5 mg, intravenously) is recommended. In an emergency, chlorpromazine (50 to 100 mg, intramuscularly) can be used if phentolamine is not at hand; chlorpromazine can even be given to patients to use orally (100 mg) if an intense headache develops and medical help is not available. Fever may be reduced by external cooling.

The actual incidence of serious side effects is very difficult to determine. It has been estimated that by 1970 3.5 million patients had used tranylcypromine and, of these, 50 persons sustained cerebrovascular accidents and 15 died. Coincidental presence of nondrug-induced pathology probably plays an important role. There is no evidence that the relative incidence of hypertensive crises is any greater with tranylcypromine than with the other agents in this class, but the absolute number of patients treated with the latter drugs is considerably smaller. However, tranylcypromine is not recommended for use in patients over 60 years of age, or in those with cardiac disease or hypertension or at risk of stroke; it is questionable whether *any* MAO inhibitor should be used by patients in these categories.

Therapeutic Uses. The MAO inhibitors have been used primarily in the treatment of *depression* and certain *phobic-anxiety states.* Their possible use in *narcolepsy* is mentioned above; since the specific indication for their use is not yet clear and their toxicity relatively great, they have been reserved mainly for patients refractory to other treatments. They were at one time employed in the therapy of hypertension. The use of MAO inhibitors in psychiatry is discussed below, with other drug treatments for disorders of mood (page 435).

LITHIUM SALTS

Lithium salts were introduced into psychiatry in 1949 for the treatment of mania. However, they were not accepted in the United States for this use until 1970, in part due to reluctance of American physicians to accept the safety of this treatment. This was the result of reports of severe intoxication with lithium chloride from its use as a sodium substitute. In addition, lack of commercial interest in this inexpensive, unpatentable mineral meant that research to establish its efficacy in manic-depressive illness was carried out without industrial support. Nevertheless, the clinical research supporting the efficacy and safety of lithium salts for mania and for the prevention of recurrent attacks of manic-depressive illness is now highly impressive. Many details of the pharmacology and uses of lithium salts in psychiatry and medicine are reviewed elsewhere (Baldessarini and Lipinski, 1975; Johnson, 1975; Johnson and Johnson, 1978).

History. Lithium urate is quite soluble, and, accordingly, lithium salts were used as a treatment of gout in the nineteenth century. The bromide of lithium was employed in that era as a sedative and anticonvulsant as well. Thereafter, lithium salts were little used until the late 1940s, when lithium chloride was employed as a salt substitute for cardiac and other chronically ill patients. This ill-advised usage led to several reports of severe intoxication and death and to considerable notoriety concerning lithium salts within the medical profession. Cade in Australia, while looking for toxic nitrogenous substances in the urine of mental patients for testing in guinea pigs, administered lithium salts to the animals in an attempt to increase the solubility of urates. Lithium carbonate made the animals lethargic, and, in an inductive leap, Cade gave lithium carbonate to several agitated or manic psychiatric patients. In 1949, he reported that this treatment seemed to have a specific effect in mania. For a more detailed account of the early development of lithium salts in psychiatric therapeutics, *see* Schou (1957, 1968, 1969) and Ayd and Blackwell (1970).

Chemistry. Lithium is the lightest of the alkali metals (group Ia); the salts of this monovalent cation share some characteristics with those of sodium and potassium, but not others. It is readily assayed in biological fluids by flame-photometric and atomic-absorption spectrophotometric methods. Traces of lithium ion occur in animal tissues, but it has no known physiological role. It is very abundant in many alkaline mineral-spring waters. Lithium carbonate is the salt in therapeutic use in the United States.

PHARMACOLOGICAL PROPERTIES

Therapeutic concentrations of lithium have almost no discernable psychotropic effects in normal man. It is not a sedative, depressant, or euphoriant, and this characteristic differentiates lithium from all other psychotropic agents. The general biology and pharmacology of the lithium ion have been reviewed in detail by Shou (1957). The mechanism of action of lithium as a mood-stabilizing agent remains unknown, although

effects on biological membranes are suspected.

A most important characteristic of the lithium ion is that it has a relatively small gradient of distribution across biological membranes, unlike sodium and potassium; while it can replace sodium in supporting a single action potential in a nerve cell, it is not an adequate "substrate" for the sodium pump and it cannot, therefore, maintain membrane potentials. It is uncertain if important interactions occur between lithium (at therapeutic concentrations of about 1 mEq per liter) and the transport of other monovalent or divalent cations by nerve cells.

Central Nervous System. In addition to speculations about altered distribution of ions in the CNS, much attention has centered on the effects of low concentrations of lithium ion on the metabolism of the biogenic monoamines that have been implicated in the pathophysiology of mood disorders. In animal brain tissue, lithium ion at concentrations of 1 to 10 mEq per liter inhibits the depolarization-provoked and calcium-dependent release of norepinephrine and dopamine, but *not* 5-HT, from nerve terminals. It may also slightly alter the re-uptake and presynaptic storage of catecholamines in directions consistent with increased inactivation of the amines. The ion has little effect on catecholamine-sensitive adenylate cyclase activity or on the binding of ligands to putative adrenergic receptors in brain tissue, although there is some evidence that lithium can inhibit the effects of receptor blocking agents to cause supersensitivity in such systems (Pert *et al.,* 1978). Lithium has been noted to modify hormonal responses mediated by adenylate cyclase in other tissues (*see* below). The effects of lithium on the distribution of sodium, calcium, and magnesium and on glucose metabolism have all been suggested to contribute to the antimanic or mood-stabilizing effects of the ion, but none of these hypotheses has been substantiated (*see* Baldessarini and Lipinski, 1975; Johnson and Johnson, 1978).

When given to manic patients who characteristically sleep very little, lithium corrects the sleep disorder as the mania abates. However, there are no well-established primary effects of lithium salts on sleep, except for some suppression of REM phases. Treatment with lithium also produces high-voltage slow waves in the human EEG, sometimes with superimposed fast-beta activity. Changes similar to those associated with ECT are occasionally observed and can include marked degrees of epileptiform discharge, even in subjects without a prior history of a seizure disorder (*see* Itil, 1978).

Absorption, Distribution, and Excretion. Lithium ions are readily and almost completely absorbed from the gastrointestinal tract. Complete absorption occurs in about 8 hours, with peak concentrations in plasma occurring 2 to 4 hours after an oral dose. The ion is initially distributed in the extracellular fluid and then gradually accumulated in various tissues to different degrees. The concentration gradients across cellular membranes are much smaller than those for sodium and potassium. The final volume of distribution is equal to that of total body water. Passage through the blood-brain barrier is slow, but when a steady state is achieved the concentration of lithium in the cerebrospinal fluid is about 40% of the concentration in plasma. There is no evidence of the ion binding to plasma proteins.

Approximately 95% of a single dose of lithium is eliminated in the urine. About one third to two thirds of an acute dose is excreted during a 6- to 12-hour initial phase of excretion, followed by a slow excretion over the next 10 to 14 days. With repeated administration, lithium excretion increases during the first 5 to 6 days until equilibrium is reached between ingestion and excretion. When therapy with lithium is stopped, there is a rapid phase of renal excretion followed by a slow 10- to 14-day phase. Since 80% of the filtered lithium is reabsorbed by the renal tubules, lithium clearance by the kidney is about 20% of that for creatinine, ranging between 15 and 30 ml per minute. This is somewhat lower in elderly patients (10 to 15 ml per minute) and higher in young persons. Sodium loading produces a small enhancement of lithium excretion, but *sodium depletion* promotes a clinically important degree of *retention of lithium.*

Because of the *low therapeutic index* for the lithium ion (as low as 2 or 3), concentrations in plasma or serum must be determined to facilitate the safe use of the drug. This must be done daily in the treatment of acutely manic patients. Indeed, the risks of such early treatment are sufficiently great that it may be wiser to postpone treatment with lithium until some degree of behavioral control and metabolic stability have been attained with antipsychotic drugs. Although the concentration of lithium in blood is usually measured at a trough of the oscillations that result from repetitive administration, the peaks can be two or three times higher than the steady-state concentration. When the peaks are reached, intoxication may result. (This can occur even when concentrations in morning samples of plasma are in the acceptable range of 1 mEq per liter.) Because of the very low margin of safety of the lithium ion and because of its short half-life during initial distribution, *divided daily doses must be used in man* (at least until experimental long-acting preparations are perfected).

While the pharmacokinetics of lithium tends to vary considerably between subjects, it is relatively stable, with time, in the individual patient (Baldessarini and Stephens, 1970). However, well-established regimens can be complicated by occasional periods of sodium loss, such as may occur with an intercurrent medical illness or with excessive sweating; hence, all patients should have plasma concentrations checked at least occasionally. The relatively stable and characteristic pharmacokinetics of the lithium ion in single patients makes it possible to predict dosage requirements of an individual based on the results of administration of a single test dose of lithium carbonate, followed by a single plasma assay 24 hours later (Cooper and Simpson, 1978).

Most of the renal tubular reabsorption of the lithium ion seems to occur in the proximal tubule. Nevertheless, its retention can be increased by any diuretic that leads to sodium depletion (*e.g.*, furosemide, ethacrynic acid, and thiazides) (Himmelhoch *et al.*, 1977; Jefferson and Greist, 1979). Renal excretion can be increased somewhat by the administration of osmotic diuretics, acetazolamide, or aminophylline, although this is of little help in the management of lithium-induced toxicity. Triamterene may increase excretion of lithium, suggesting that some reabsorption of the ion may occur in the distal nephron; however, spironolactone does not increase the excretion of lithium.

Less than 1% of ingested lithium leaves the human body in the feces, and 4 to 5% is excreted in the sweat. Lithium is secreted in saliva in concentrations about twice those in plasma, and this fluid has been used experimentally to monitor lithium concentrations. Since the ion is also secreted in human milk, women should not breast-feed infants; otherwise, lithium intoxication of the child may occur.

Preparations, Route of Administration, and Dosage. Preparations currently used in the United States are 300-mg tablets or capsules of Li_2CO_3. These include ESKALITH (capsules), LITHANE (tablets), LITHONATE (capsules), LITHOTABS (tablets), and nonproprietary preparations. In Europe and elsewhere different quantities are sometimes prepared (*e.g.*, a 250-mg tablet), and salts other than the carbonate have been used, including a liquid solution of the citrate. The carbonate salt is favored for tablets and capsules because it is relatively less hygroscopic and less irritating to the gut than other salts, especially the chloride. Parenteral administration is never employed. Long-acting, "once-a-day" tablets are under investigation.

Unlike most other drugs, the lithium ion is not prescribed merely by dose. Instead, due to the very low therapeutic index of this agent, determination of the concentration of the drug in blood is crucial, and lithium cannot be used safely in patients who cannot have regular determinations of its concentration in plasma or serum. The concentration that is currently considered to be optimal is between 0.8 and 1.5 mEq per liter; the range of 1.0 to 1.5 mEq per liter is favored for treatment of manic or hypomanic patients; somewhat lower values (0.8 to 1.0 mEq per liter) are considered adequate and safer for long-term use for prevention of recurrent manic-depressive illness. These concentrations refer to blood samples obtained at 10 $\pm$ 2 hours after the last oral dose of the day. The recommended concentration is often attained by doses of 900 to 1500 mg per day in outpatients and 1200 to 2700 mg per day in hospitalized manic patients; the optimal dose tends to be larger in younger and heavier patients.

Toxic Reactions and Side Effects. Lithium therapy is initially associated with a transient increase in the excretion of 17-hydroxycorticosteroids, sodium, potassium, and water. This effect is usually not sustained beyond 24 hours. In the subsequent 4 to 5 days of lithium therapy, the excretion of potassium becomes normal, sodium is retained, and, in some cases, pretibial edema forms. Sodium retention has been associated with increased aldosterone secretion and responds to administration of spironolactone. Edema and sodium retention frequently disappear spontaneously after several days.

A small number of lithium-treated patients develop a benign, diffuse, nontender thyroid enlargement, suggestive of compromised thyroid function. In patients treated with lithium, thyroid ^{131}I uptake is increased, plasma protein-bound iodine and free thyroxine tend to be slightly low, and thyroid-stimulating hormone (TSH) secretion may be slightly elevated. However, patients usually remain euthyroid and obvious hypothyroidism is rare. In rats, the ion inhibits thyrotropin activation of thyroid adenylate cyclase, and inhibitory effects of lithium have been noted on the synthesis of cyclic AMP in several

other situations (Baldessarini and Lipinski, 1975; Forrest, 1975). It is unknown if there is a cause-and-effect relationship between this action of lithium and any of its subsequent effects. In patients who develop goiter, discontinuation of lithium or treatment with thyroid hormone results in shrinkage of the gland.

Polydipsia and polyuria occur in patients treated with lithium, occasionally to a disturbing degree. Several cases of acquired nephrogenic diabetes insipidus have been reported in patients maintained at therapeutic plasma concentrations of the ion. The polyuria disappears with termination of lithium therapy. The mechanism of this effect may involve inhibition of the action of ADH on renal adenylate cyclase, resulting in decreased ADH stimulation of renal reabsorption of water. However, there is also evidence that lithium may exert an action at a step beyond cyclic AMP synthesis to alter both thyroid and renal function. While there is thus uncertainty of the precise site of action of the cation, its effectiveness in blocking the renal response to ADH has aroused interest in its therapeutic usefulness in the treatment of the syndrome of inappropriate secretion of ADH (White and Fetner, 1975).

The lithium ion also has a weak action on carbohydrate metabolism that resembles somewhat that of insulin. In intact rats, lithium causes an increase in skeletal muscle glycogen accompanied by severe depletion of glycogen from the liver. The mechanisms of action of insulin and lithium probably differ inasmuch as maximal amounts of the two agents produce additive effects on glucose metabolism in the isolated rat diaphragm (Haugaard *et al.*, 1974).

The prolonged use of lithium causes a benign and reversible depression of the T wave of the ECG, an effect not related to depletion of sodium or potassium (Demers and Heninger, 1971).

Lithium causes EEG changes characterized by diffuse slowing, widened frequency spectrum, and potentiation with disorganization of background rhythm. There are conflicting reports with regard to lithium and convulsive disorders. Seizures have been reported in nonepileptic patients with plasma lithium concentrations in the therapeutic range (Baldessarini and Stephens, 1970).

An increase in circulating leukocytes occurs during the chronic use of lithium and is reversed within 1 week after termination of treatment.

Allergic reactions such as dermatitis and allergic vasculitis can occur with lithium administration.

The occurrence of toxicity is related to the plasma lithium concentration and its rate of rise following administration. Acute intoxication is characterized by vomiting, profuse diarrhea, ataxia, coma, and convulsions. Symptoms of milder toxicity that are most likely to occur at the absorptive peak of lithium include nausea, vomiting, abdominal pain, diarrhea, sedation, and fine tremor. The more serious effects involve the nervous system and consist in mental confusion, hyperreflexia, gross tremor, dysarthria, seizures, and cranial-nerve and focal neurological signs, progressing to coma and death (Saron and Gaind, 1973). Other toxic effects are cardiac arrhythmias, hypotension, and albuminuria. In pregnancy, concomitant use of natriuretics and low-sodium diets is the most common cause of maternal and neonatal lithium intoxication (Goldfield and Weinstein, 1973), and during post-partum diuresis one can anticipate potentially toxic retention of lithium by the mother. The use of lithium in pregnancy has been associated with neonatal goiter, CNS depression, hypotonia, and cardiac murmur. All these conditions reverse with time. More ominously, however, recent epidemiological data suggest that the use of lithium in early pregnancy may be associated with a severalfold increase in the incidence of cardiovascular anomalies of the newborn (especially Ebstein's malformation) (see Goldberg and DiMascio, 1978). For these reasons, the safety of lithium salts in pregnancy is at least uncertain, and such use is not recommended.

Examination of renal biopsies from patients exposed to lithium carbonate for periods ranging from less than one to several years has revealed degenerative changes and inflammatory responses in the kidney. These include swelling, deformation, and apparent destruction of the nephron. Since attempts to demonstrate significant losses of glomerular or tubular renal function have not been convincing, the significance of these observations remains in doubt. Renal function should be evaluated at least semiannually in patients receiving chronic therapy with lithium (see Jefferson and Greist, 1979).

Treatment of Lithium Intoxication. Since there is no specific antidote for lithium intoxication, treatment is supportive. If renal function is adequate, excretion can be accelerated slightly with osmotic diuresis and intravenous sodium bicarbonate solution. Dialysis is probably the most effective means of removing the ion from the body and should be considered in severe poisonings. When the concentration of lithium in plasma is lowered by dialysis or other means, recovery is still slow. This suggests that the intracellular concentration of lithium may be the prime determinant of the appearance of clinical toxicity.

Interactions with Other Drugs. Interactions between lithium and diuretics have been discussed above. Compensation should also be made for abnormal sodium loss, such as that caused by increased sweating or diarrhea. Lithium decreases the pressor response to norepinephrine in man. Thiazide diuretics may correct the nephrogenic diabetes insipidus caused by lithium (see Chapter 37). Lithium is often used in conjunction with antipsychotic and antidepressant drugs. Several case reports have suggested a risk of increased CNS toxicity of lithium when it is combined with haloperidol; this is, however, at variance with more than a decade of experience with this combination in Europe (see Tupin and Schuller, 1978). The antipsychotic drugs may block the nausea, which can be a sign of lithium toxicity. Urinary retention due to the anticholinergic effects of the tricyclic antidepressants can become particularly uncomfortable in the presence of a lithium-induced diuresis. There is, however, no absolute contraindication to the concurrent use of lithium and other psychotropic drugs.

Therapeutic Uses. The use of lithium in *manic-depressive illness* is discussed below.

Lithium treatment is ideally conducted only in patients with normal sodium intake and with normal cardiac and renal function. Very occasionally, patients with severe systemic illnesses can be treated with lithium, provided there are sufficiently compelling indications. Its use in medically healthy *adults or adolescents* for *acute mania* or the prevention of *recurrences of bipolar manic-depressive illness* are the only indications currently approved in the United States. In addition, based on compelling evidence of efficacy (see Davis, 1976), it is also sometimes used as an alternative to tricyclic antidepressants in severe recurrent depression (unipolar manic-depressive illness).

Lithium salts have also been tried, with very mixed results, to treat acute depression and a variety of disorders characterized by a recurrent or episodic course. These include premenstrual tension, drug-abuse syndromes including alcoholism, episodic aggression or anger, irregularity of food intake (notably in anorexia nervosa and the Klein-Levin syndrome with hypersomnia and hyperphagia), periodic catatonia (Gjessing's syndrome), and a variety of other neurotic, psychotic, or other behavioral disorders. In addition, lithium has undergone limited evaluation in several neurological disorders (especially Huntington's chorea and tardive dyskinesia), has been tried as an antithyroid agent, and has been used in the syndrome of inappropriate secretion of ADH. These trials have all had mixed results, and they have not led to generally accepted treatments for any of the conditions listed (see Schou, 1978).

DRUG TREATMENT OF DISORDERS OF MOOD

Disorders of mood (*affective* disorders) are extremely common in general medical practice, as well as in psychiatry. The severity of these conditions covers an extraordinarily broad range, from normal grief reactions to death of a loved one, to severe, incapacitating, and frequently fatal psychosis. The lifetime risk of suicide in primary depression and manic-depressive illness is about 15%. Clearly, not all of the grief, misery, and disappointments of the human condition are indications for medical treatment, and affective disorders have a very high rate of spontaneous remission, provided that sufficient time passes. The antidepressant agents or lithium salts are thus generally reserved for the more severe and incapacitating disorders of mood, and the most satisfactory results tend to occur in patients who have the more severe illnesses. The data from clinical research in support of the efficacy of antidepressant agents and of lithium are now overwhelming (*see* Klein and Davis, 1969; Klerman, 1972; Glassman and Perel, 1973; Morris and Beck, 1974; Baldessarini, 1977b). Nevertheless, many shortcomings and problems continue to be associated with all drugs used to treat affective disorders. In addition to less-than-dramatic efficacy in some cases, virtually all of the drugs used to treat disorders of mood are potentially lethal when acute overdosage occurs and can cause an appreciable degree of less severe morbidity even with careful clinical use.

Despite their recognized limitations, the antidepressants and lithium carbonate have a well-established and important place in medical practice. Currently the tricyclic agents are the most widely used antidepressants. They are all apparently similar in efficacy for depression, provided that adequate doses are used for a sufficient period of time. Effective doses, calculated in terms of imipramine or its equivalent of a similar drug, are currently estimated to exceed 100 mg per day, and doses above 200 mg per day are best reserved for severely ill inpatients. Since the onset of action of all antidepressant drugs is delayed for up to 2 or 3 weeks, a trial of treatment with an adequate dose cannot be judged a failure for at least 1 month.

Secondary considerations govern the selection of a specific antidepressant. If some sedation seems desirable early in treatment, amitriptyline or doxepin is usually selected. If anticholinergic side effects are to be avoided, desipramine may be a rational choice. Prior success with a specific agent is an additional consideration. The tertiary-amine tricyclic antidepressants are highly effective and commonly used; however, if they fail to produce satisfactory results, it is probably best to change to a secondary amine and to increase the dose. This advice is based on research that indicates a complex biphasic relationship between the concentration of drug in blood and the clinical response for the *de*methylated tricyclic agents (*see* Baldessarini, 1979a).

Disappointing responses to antidepressant therapy usually result from the use of inadequate doses (*see* Kline, 1974) or too short a therapeutic trial (*see* Klerman, 1978). Unless a patient is very debilitated or unusually sensitive to the side effects of a tricyclic antidepressant, it is best to begin treatment with about 50 mg per day and to increase the dose rapidly to the equivalent of 150 mg per day or more of imipramine. For severely ill hospitalized patients, the dose can be raised to the range of 200 to 300 mg per day, although little added benefit and much more toxicity are likely to result. It is also wise to avoid single doses above 150 mg in outpatients. Due to the high rate of relapse within the first year following recovery from an acute, severe depressive illness, treatment is usually continued for at least several months (*see* Hollister, 1978b; Klerman, 1978; Mandel and Klerman, 1978). In this phase of treatment, doses below 100 mg per day of imipramine or its equivalent are less likely to be effective, and, as an approximate guideline, 100 to 150 mg per day for 3 to 6 months can be tried. Some physicians have attempted to discontinue treatment gradually over several months, in accordance with the clinical response observed. In addition to this approach to the management of the post-recovery phase of acute depression, there is increasing evidence that the prolonged use of a tricyclic agent can have important ameliorative or preventive effects on recurrent depression (unipolar manic-depressive illness). This treatment can be considered as an alternative to the use of lithium carbonate to prevent recurrent depression (*see* Davis, 1976; Klerman, 1978; Mandel and Klerman, 1978).

While acute mania is a primary indication for the use of lithium carbonate, it is, in actual practice, an inferior agent for the management of severe manic attacks. These episodes represent a serious medical problem and require urgent hospitalization for the protection and careful medical management of the patient. While a few mildly hypomanic patients can be managed successfully as outpatients with lithium alone, it is more common to begin treatment of severely manic patients with large doses of an antipsychotic drug (the type selected makes little difference). As the intake of food and fluids becomes stable and the patient becomes more cooperative over 5 to 10 days, lithium can be introduced gradually and safely. While the long-term benefits of antipsychotic drugs in bipolar disorders of mood have yet to be proven, the preventive effects of lithium carbonate have become its most compelling clinical indication. This is most clear with bipolar affective disorders, but lithium is probably also efficacious in the prevention of the emergence of recurrent depression (*see* Davis, 1976; Klerman, 1978). Tricyclic antidepressants are usually contraindicated in bipolar illness, except to treat acute depressive phases, because of their tendency to provoke a "switch" to mania or hypomania (Bunney *et al.,* 1972). In view of the very low therapeutic index for lithium salts, as well as recent suggestions that they may lead to degenerative changes in the kidney (*see* above), it is important to be circumspect when advising a patient or family to embark on a prolonged regimen involving lithium. Factors that enter into this decision include the severity of the illness, the frequency of recurrence, and the probable reliability of the patient.

Other forms of treatment of depression have not been well established or are no longer regularly employed, with the important exception of ECT, which remains the most rapid and effective treatment for severe acute depression and is sometimes lifesaving for acutely suicidal patients (*see* Avery and Winokur, 1977; Freeman *et al.,* 1978). The MAO inhibitors are generally inferior to other forms of treatment in severe depression, based on controlled trials, although tranylcypromine may be about as effective as the tricyclic agents (*see* Klein and Davis, 1969). Doses of phenelzine that inhibit MAO activity in platelets by more than 75 or 80% are probably effective (Robinson *et al.,* 1978). Evidence in support of the efficacy of isocarboxazid is poor, and this agent can be considered virtually obsolete (*see* Hollister, 1978a). Despite the favorable results obtained with tranylcypromine and with doses of phenelzine above 60 mg per day, the toxicity of the former (*see* above) and the impracticality of MAO assays for most practitioners limit their clinical application. Nevertheless, MAO inhibitors are sometimes tried when a vigorous trial of a tricyclic antidepressant (*e.g.,* 200 to 300 mg daily of imipramine or its equivalent for 4 weeks) has been unsatisfactory and when ECT is refused. In addition, MAO inhibitors may have selective benefits for conditions other than ordinary depression, including neurotic illnesses marked by phobias and anxiety as well as dysphoria (Tyrer *et al.,* 1973). Thus, the indications for the MAO inhibitors are few and must be weighed against their potential toxicity and their complex interactions with many other drugs. Stimulants, with or without added sedatives, are an outmoded treatment for severe psychiatric depression; not only are they ineffective compared to a placebo, but they actually worsen dysphoria and agitation in some patients (*see* Klein and Davis, 1969; Mandel and Klerman, 1978).

III. Drugs Used in the Treatment of Anxiety

Sedatives with useful antianxiety effects are consistently among the most commonly prescribed drugs. The appropriate generic term for this group of agents remains uncertain, although there is some reason to suspect that terms such as *antianxiety agents, anxiolytics,* and *tranquilizers* represent to some extent wishful thinking and the impact of advertising. With the possible exception of the benzodiazepines (and some of the antihistamines or anticholinergics), most drugs used to treat anxiety are either sedatives or at least have many properties in common with traditional sedatives, such as the barbiturates. Even the benzodiazepines share some of these properties, particularly when high doses are given. The wide diversity of compounds used to treat anxiety greatly complicates attempts to make generalizations about them. Many of these drugs are discussed in other chapters of this text (*see* Chapters 17, 18, 20, 21, 23, and 26). This section covers only a limited group of agents that are commonly used to treat anxiety and mild dysphoria, and only this use is emphasized. Since the benzodiazepines now dominate this field, they are given the most attention; the

other agents are mentioned only briefly. More extensive reviews of the pharmacology of these drugs, particularly the benzodiazepines, are available (*see* Ludwig and Potterfield, 1971; Garattini *et al.,* 1973; Greenblatt and Shader, 1974; Baldessarini, 1977b; Chapter 17).

History. Man has sought chemical agents to modify the effects of stress and the feelings of discomfort, tension, anxiety, and dysphoria throughout recorded history. Many of these efforts have led to the development of agents that are often classed as sedatives, and the single most widely used of these is one of the oldest—*ethanol.* In the last century, *bromide* salts and the *barbiturates* were introduced into medical practice as sedatives, along with compounds similar in effect to alcohol, including *paraldehyde* and *chloral hydrate.* By the 1930s it became apparent that bromides had cumulative toxic effects on the CNS, and their use in medical practice waned, although the availability of bromides in nonprescription preparations, remarkably, still continues. Throughout the early decades of this century, the barbiturates continued to be the dominant antianxiety agents in medical practice; however, by the 1950s, there was great concern with their propensity to induce tolerance, sometimes followed by physical dependence and potentially lethal reactions during withdrawal. These problems strongly colored professional and popular attitudes about sedatives, encouraged the search for safer agents, and appear to contribute to the use of new terms that emphasize their dissimilarities from the barbiturates and related sedatives. Some of this effort led to studies of derivatives of aliphatic polyalcohols; one of these, mephenesin, the *o*-methyl-phenyl derivative of propanetriol, was found to have putative muscle relaxant and sedative properties, but was impractically short acting. Its chemical modifications led directly to the introduction of the *propanediol carbamates* (*meprobamate* and congeners) in the early 1950s, along with a variety of other analogs of barbiturates or derivatives of higher alcohols.

Throughout the 1950s, despite enormous popularity of some of these compounds for daytime sedation or for hypnotic effects, an increasing awareness developed that they shared many of the undesirable properties of barbiturates. These included an unclear separation between their useful antianxiety effects and excessive sedation and an impressive propensity to cause physical dependence and severe acute intoxication on overdosage. This set the scene for the discovery of *chlordiazepoxide* in the late 1950s and the introduction of more than a dozen *benzodiazepine* congeners since that time. This class of sedatives has come to dominate the market and medical practice; in recent years, chlordiazepoxide and diazepam have been among the frontrunners in terms of numbers of prescriptions written for all drugs used in medical practice, accounting for perhaps 75% of approximately 100 million prescriptions for all sedatives annually in the United States alone, at a cost of about 500 million dollars.

BENZODIAZEPINE COMPOUNDS

Six benzodiazepine derivatives are presently available for the treatment of anxiety. In their order of introduction, they are *chlordiazepoxide, diazepam, oxazepam, clorazepate, lorazepam,* and *prazepam*. Although commonly used for treating anxiety, they share other therapeutic indications; these are discussed elsewhere (*see* Index).

History. Compounds of this type were initially synthesized in the 1930s. The first successful benzodiazepine, *chlordiazepoxide,* was developed by Sternbach's group at the Roche Laboratories in the late 1950s. Tests in animals indicated that chlordiazepoxide had interesting muscle relaxant, antistrychnine, and spinal reflex-blocking properties. It also produced "taming" of a number of species of animals in doses much lower than those producing ataxia or measurable hypnosis. This "taming" effect in monkeys led to the clinical trial of the drug in man for the determination of antianxiety effects. (For further details, *see* Garattini *et al.,* 1973.)

Chemistry and Structure-Activity Relationship. Over 2000 benzodiazepines have been synthesized. The structure-activity relationship of this group has been reviewed by Sternbach (1973). Chlordiazepoxide was the first compound introduced for clinical use, but several useful congeners have been developed. The structures of the six benzodiazepines that are available for treatment of anxiety are shown in Table 19-6.

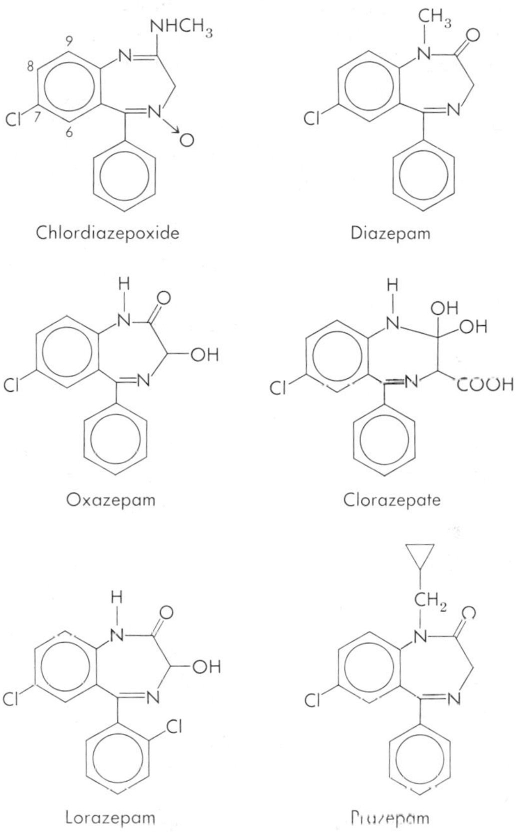

PHARMACOLOGICAL PROPERTIES

Chlordiazepoxide and diazepam can be considered prototypical drugs for their class. They have achieved wide use as antianxiety agents but have other therapeutic applications as well.

Central Nervous System. *Behavioral and Neurophysiological Effects.* The effects of the benzodiazepines in the relief of anxiety can readily be demonstrated in experimental animals. In conflict punishment procedures, benzodiazepines greatly reduce the suppressive effects of punishment. Positive effects in this experimental model are not seen with antidepressants and antipsychotics. The behavioral effects of antianxiety agents are extensively reviewed by Sepinwall and Cook (1978).

Difficulties in evaluating the therapeutic efficacy of psychotropic drugs in man are particularly great in the case of the antianxiety drugs, owing largely to the contribution

Table 19-6. BENZODIAZEPINES FOR THE TREATMENT OF ANXIETY

Chlordiazepoxide

Diazepam

Oxazepam

Clorazepate

Lorazepam

Prazepam

of nonpharmacological factors to the treatment of anxiety; disparate results have thus been obtained. Many studies have shown that chlordiazepoxide and its congeners are more effective than a placebo in the treatment of varied groups of anxious neurotic patients. However, negative results have also been reported (*see* Klein and Davis, 1969). The clinical popularity of these drugs apparently is the result of a combination of their pharmacological actions, their relative safety, and an extraordinary demand for agents of this type by both doctors and patients.

In common with barbiturates, chlordiazepoxide blocks EEG arousal from stimulation of the brain stem reticular formation. Central depressant actions of diazepam and other benzodiazepines on spinal reflexes occur and are in part mediated by the brain stem reticular system. Like meprobamate and the barbiturates, chlordiazepoxide depresses the duration of electrical afterdischarge in the limbic system, including the septal region, the amygdala, the hippocampus, and the hypothalamus. These and other limbic and autonomic effects are the focus of particular theoretical interest at the present time, as are observations of potentiation of the effects of GABA or other inhibitory transmitters in the CNS by the benzodiazepines (*see* Bloom, 1977; Iversen, 1978; Tallman *et al.*, 1980; Chapter 17).

Effects on Sleep. Benzodiazepines can be used effectively as hypnotics in conjunction with their use as antianxiety drugs. They seem to have only mild effects to suppress REM periods, but they do have a tendency to suppress the deeper phases of sleep, especially stage 4 (while *increasing* total sleep time). The significance of this is not known, but diazepam has been used in the treatment of "night terrors" that arise out of stage-4 sleep.

EEG Effects. The benzodiazepines cause an increase in fast-beta activity with an increase in amplitude of the EEG. This is a pattern similar to that of meprobamate and other sedatives. Virtually all benzodiazepines increase *seizure threshold* and are anticonvulsant. Diazepam is used clinically for this purpose, especially in status epilepticus (*see* Chapter 20).

Cardiovascular and Respiratory Systems. Considerable attention must be paid to the cardiovascular effects of the benzodiazepines since they are used so widely in cardiac patients. Diazepam, in an intravenous dose of 5 to 10 mg, causes a slight decrease in respiration, blood pressure, and left ventricular stroke work. Increase in heart rate and decrease in cardiac output can also occur. The effects are minimal, and it is unlikely that there is significant depression of cardiovascular function when the benzodiazepines are given in usual therapeutic doses by the oral route.

Skeletal Muscle. Diazepam is widely used as a muscle relaxant, although controlled studies rarely show any advantage of any benzodiazepine over either placebo or aspirin. Some muscle relaxation occurs after administration of any of the CNS depressants, and there seems to be no particular advantage to any one of them when given by the oral route. (*See* Chapter 21.)

Absorption, Fate, and Excretion. Chlordiazepoxide, oxazepam, and several other benzodiazepines are absorbed relatively slowly following oral administration, and peak concentrations in plasma may not be attained for several hours. In contrast, diazepam is one of the most rapidly absorbed benzodiazepines, reaching peak concentrations in about an hour in adults, but as quickly as 15 to 30 minutes in children. This rapidity of uptake, even after oral administration, may largely account for the euphoriant or intoxicating effect of large doses of diazepam that contributes to its popularity as a "street drug." Most of the benzodiazepines are bound to plasma protein to a great extent (85 to 95%)—a factor that limits the efficacy of dialysis in the treatment of acute poisonings. The apparent volumes of distribution for most benzodiazepines are high—about 1 to 3 liters per kilogram. Secondary peaks in the plasma concentration have been described for several benzodiazepines, for example, at 6 to 12 hours after an oral dose of diazepam. These are most likely due to enterohepatic recirculation (*see* Morselli, 1977).

The pharmacokinetic parameters that have been reported for these agents may be somewhat misleading for several reasons. Assay technics have not all been of high specificity, and active metabolites can markedly alter the actual biological half-life (*e.g.*, the formation of nordiazepam from diazepam and even from chlordiazepoxide can extend biological half-life by twofold or threefold). The actual kinetics for some benzodiazepines is quite complex and is not easily analyzed by traditional models. Thus, the usually stated half-life for the elimination phase of the drug does not adequately depict the kinetics of the early distributive phase, which can be very important clinically. For example, the distributive (alpha) half-life of diazepam is about 2.5 hours, while the elimination (beta) half-time is about 1.5 days initially and even longer after prolonged treatment. Moreover, while correlations between plasma concentrations of benzodiazepines and clinical effects are imperfect (*see* Gottschalk, 1978), it is apparent that concentrations in plasma that border on twice the values usually considered to be effective are associated with undesirable degrees of sedation (*see* Morselli, 1977). For this reason, the benzodiazepines are *not* effectively or safely given once a day, despite their relatively long elimination half-lives; doses should be divided in two to four portions for the treatment of daytime anxiety.

With the probable exception of oxazepam and lorazepam, which are primarily conjugated with glucuronic acid to form inactive metabolites, the benzodiazepines used for anxiety are typically converted to active metabolites. Most of these are products of hepatic microsomal enzymatic activity, which leads to N-dealkylated or otherwise-oxidized products. In addition, clorazepate, which is probably inert as such, is converted nonenzymatically in gastric acid to an active metabolite, desmethyldiazepam or *nordiazepam,* which is also an active metabolite of chlordiazepoxide and diazepam. The benzodiazepines as a class tend to have minimal pharmacokinetic interactions with other drugs, with the exception of the MAO inhibitors. The *premature neonate* and the *elderly* may have half-lives for diazepam that are three or four times longer than those of young adults, children, or even full-term neonates. In addition, severe hepatic disease can increase the half-life of diazepam by a factor of two to five. Since formation of glucuronide is not restricted to hepatic microsomes, oxazepam and lorazepam may be safer agents for those with severely impaired hepatic function; they may also be safer for elderly patients, if only because of their relatively short duration of action. Most of the benzodiazepines are excreted almost entirely in the urine and in the form of oxidized and glucuronide-conjugated metabolites.

Information on the pharmacokinetic properties and metabolism of the benzodiazepines is described by Garattini and associates (1973), Greenblatt and Shader (1974), Morselli (1977), Gottschalk (1978), and Hollister (1978a); *see also* Appendix II.

Tolerance and Physical Dependence. High doses of benzodiazepines must be given for long periods of time and then abruptly withdrawn before marked withdrawal symptoms, including seizures, appear (*see* Allquander, 1978). Habituation can occur; however, because of the long half-lives and conversion to active metabolites, *withdrawal symptoms* after chronic use may not appear for a week after abrupt discontinuation of the drug. In most instances after usual doses, there is no withdrawal syndrome.

Toxic Reactions and Side Effects. The expected side effects of CNS depressants of drowsiness and ataxia are extensions of the pharmacological actions of these drugs. With diazepam, antianxiety effects can be expected at blood concentrations of 400 to 600 ng/ml, while some sedative effects and psychomotor impairment begin at concentrations just over 300 to 400 ng/ml, and gross CNS intoxication can be expected at concentrations over 900 to 1000 ng/ml (*see* Morselli, 1977). Therapeutic concentrations of chlordiazepoxide approximate 700 to 1000 ng/ml.

An *increase* in hostility and irritability, as well as vivid or disturbing dreams, is often reported as possible effects of the benzodiazepines, with the possible exception of oxazepam. Equally paradoxical is an *increase* in anxiety. Such a response is especially likely to occur in patients who feel threatened by being dulled by the sedative effects of antianxiety agents. Both psychoses and sudden suicidal impulses have occasionally been reported in patients receiving high doses of benzodiazepines, although their significance is obscure in many cases. On the other hand, one of the most common causes of reversible *confusional states in the elderly* is surely the *overuse of sedatives* of all kinds, including what would ordinarily be referred to as "small" doses of benzodiazepines.

In general, the clinical toxicity of the benzodiazepines is low. Weight gain, which may be the result of renewed appetite, occurs in some patients. Many of the side effects reported for these drugs so overlap with symptoms of anxiety that unless a careful history is taken one is hard put to ascribe these effects to the drug. Among the other toxic reactions seen with chlordiazepoxide are skin rash, nausea, headache, impairment of sexual function, vertigo, and light-headedness. Agranulocytosis has also been reported rarely. Menstrual irregularities have been noted, and women may fail to ovulate while taking benzodiazepines.

Overdosage with the benzodiazepines is frequent, but serious sequelae are rare unless other drugs or ethanol are also administered. A few deaths have been reported at doses greater than 700 mg of diazepam or chlordiazepoxide. The striking advantage of this group of drugs is the remarkable margin of safety. Treatment for overdosage is purely supportive of respiratory and cardiovascular function.

The question of teratogenic effects of benzodiazepines or other toxic effects on the fetus is controversial (*see* Safra and Oakley, 1975; Morselli, 1977; Goldberg and DiMascio, 1978). The most persistent, but unproven, suggestion has been that there may be a small increase in the risk of midline cleft deformities of the lip or palate, although these remain well below the overall risk of birth defects (about 2% in the general population) and are correctable by surgery. It is clear that benzodiazepines depress CNS function in the neonate, and especially in the premature newborn. Concentrations of these drugs in umbilical cord blood may exceed those in the maternal circulation; as mentioned, the fetus and newborn are much less able to metabolize benzodiazepines than are adults.

Interactions with Other Drugs. These are infrequent with the benzodiazepines, and, except for an additive effect with other CNS depressants, they are usually not significant. Heavy cigarette smoking may decrease the effectiveness of usual doses of these drugs. The ability of benzodiazepines to induce the hepatic metabolism of other agents is much smaller than that of many other sedatives, especially the barbiturates.

Preparations, Routes of Administration, and Dosage. These are presented in Table 19–7.

Therapeutic Uses. The benzodiazepines are used in the treatment of *anxiety* (*see* below). In addition, chlordiazepoxide has been widely employed in the treatment of *alcohol withdrawal syndromes* (*see* Chapter 23). The substitution of an antianxiety agent for alcohol in chronic alcoholism is a common practice, but this does not appear significantly to reduce alcohol intake or in any way to be an effective treatment of alcoholism. Other uses are as premedication in *anesthesia,* and in *obstetrics* during labor (*see* Chapters 13 and 14).

Table 19-7. BENZODIAZEPINES USED FOR ANXIETY: PREPARATIONS, DOSAGE FORMS, AND DOSES

NONPROPRIETARY NAME	TRADE NAMES	DOSAGE FORMS * (*mg*)	USUAL DAILY DOSE (*mg*) †	EXTREME DAILY DOSES (*mg*)
Chlordiazepoxide, U.S.P.	LIBRITABS	(T)5,10,25	15–60	10–100
Chlordiazepoxide Hydrochloride, U.S.P. §	LIBRIUM, A-POXIDE, SK-LYGEN	(T)5,10,25 (C)5,10,25 (A)100/2 ml	15–60 50–100(i.v. per dose)	10–100 300(i.v.)
Clorazepate dipotassium ‡	TRANXENE	(C)3.75,7.5,15	30	7.5–90
Clorazepate monopotassium	AZENE	(C)3.25,6.5,13	13–52	6.5–78
Diazepam, U.S.P. §	VALIUM	(T)2,5,10 (A)10/2 ml (V)50/10 ml (S)10/2 ml	4–40 2–20(i.v. per dose)	2–40 30(i.v.)
Lorazepam	ATIVAN	(T)0.5,1,2	2–6	1–10
Oxazepam, U.S.P.	SERAX	(C)10,15,30 (T)15	30–60	30–120
Prazepam	VERSTRAN	(T)10	20–40	10–60

* T = tablet; C = capsule; A = ampul; V = vial; S = syringe.

† The daily doses are given as total milligrams per day, assuming doses are divided into two to four portions per day. All doses are for adults or adolescents. For children 6 to 12 years of age, chlordiazepoxide may be given in divided daily doses of 10 to 30 mg. Diazepam may be given in divided daily doses of 3 to 10 mg to children over 6 months of age. For younger children, consult the manufacturer's instructions.

‡ Chlorazepate dipotassium is also available as slow-release tablets (TRANXENE-SD), containing either 11.5 or 22.5 mg, to be taken once daily.

§ Parenteral preparations are available only for chlordiazepoxide hydrochloride and diazepam; intramuscular administration is not advisable; for details concerning intravenous use, *see* the manufacturer's instructions.

Diazepam has also been employed as a skeletal muscle relaxant. It has been used successfully in the treatment of *tetanus* in the intravenous dose of 2 to 20 mg at intervals of 2 to 8 hours. In conventional doses it has been claimed, but not proven, to relieve the muscular spasticity of *upper motoneuron* disorders. On the other hand, there is evidence from controlled studies that diazepam is effective in relieving spasticity and athetosis in patients with *cerebral palsy*. The use of diazepam in *cardioversion* is well documented. Diazepam is also employed in the management of *seizure disorders* and a number of other medical, neurological, and surgical conditions, about which there is further information in Chapters 17 and 20.

OTHER SEDATIVES USED FOR ANXIETY

Many other classes of drugs that act on the CNS have been used in the past for daytime sedation and the treatment of anxiety. Many of these uses are now virtually obsolete. They include that of the propanediol carbamates (notably, *meprobamate*), the barbiturates (which still have medical uses and are discussed in Chapter 17), many other pharmacologically similar nonbarbiturates, and yet another group of drugs that are sometimes called "sedative-autonomic" agents; the last-named group includes certain antihistamines and anticholinergic agents, some of which are included in nonprescription and prescription sedatives. Many of the dosage forms and usual doses of these are provided in Table 17-2 (page 350), and others are discussed elsewhere (*see* Chapter 26). The demise of most of these agents in modern psychiatric practice is due to the many problems associated with the use of traditional sedatives; these particularly include their tendency to cause unwanted degrees of sedation or frank intoxication and their liability to produce tolerance, physical dependence, and severe withdrawal reactions. However, it is worth noting that some of these agents are relatively safe and have rarely been abused. These include some of the "sedative-autonomic" agents, such as *diphenhydramine*, which is still used occasionally, especially in pediatric practice.

DRUG TREATMENT OF ANXIETY

Anxiety is not only a cardinal symptom of many psychiatric disorders but also an almost-inevitable component of many medical and surgical conditions. Indeed, it is a universal human emotion, closely allied with appropriate fear, and often serving psychobiologically adaptive purposes. A most important clinical generalization is that anxiety is rather infrequently a "disease" in itself, although in truth the anxiety associated with many of the psychoneurotic disorders often seems to have an incomprehensible life of its own, not readily explained by biological or psychoanalytical investigation. On the other hand, anxiety is often associated with medical or psychiatric problems that can readily be diagnosed and effectively treated. Sometimes, despite a thoughtful evaluation of a patient, no treatable primary illness is found, or, if one is found and treated, it may be desirable to deal directly with the anxiety at the same time. In such situations, antianxiety medications are frequently and appropriately used.

Currently, the most useful drugs seem to be the benzodiazepines. The specific drug chosen seems to make little difference, although the older agents, because of their long tenure, have been more thoroughly investigated. In patients with impaired hepatic function or in the elderly, oxazepam is currently favored; since lorazepam has similar characteristics, it may be a suitable alternative. Only chlordiazepoxide and diazepam have been used extensively in children.

Clinical experience strongly indicates that the most favorable responses to the benzodiazepines are obtained in situations that involve relatively acute anxiety reactions in medical or psychiatric patients who have either modifiable primary illnesses or primary anxiety neuroses. However, this group of anxious patients also has a high response rate to placebo and is the group most likely to undergo spontaneous improvement. Antianxiety drugs are also used in the management of more persistent or recurrent anxiety associated with the neuroses; guidelines for their appropriate use are less clear in these situations. Although there is a great deal of concern about the potential for habituation and abuse of sedatives, recent studies have suggested that physicians tend to be conservative and may even *undertreat* patients with anxiety. They may either withhold drug unless symptoms or dysfunction are severe or interrupt treatment within a few weeks, causing a high proportion of relapses (*see* Rickels *et al.,* 1978). However, patients with very long-lasting or persistent patterns of dissatisfaction or insecurity or those who have diagnosable character disorders (*see* American Psychiatric Association, 1968, 1979) may be particularly difficult to treat successfully with antianxiety agents. They may be at higher risk of a gradual escalation of dose, physical dependence, or impulsive overdosing. Nevertheless, the few data available suggest that such abuses are relatively infrequent or, when one considers the millions of patients using such drugs, even rare (*see* Frazier, 1978).

Other agents have been tried experimentally in anxiety. β-Adrenergic antagonists have been used in an attempt to block the peripheral autonomic manifestations of anxiety, but controlled trials are few and generally do not show better results than those obtained with the benzodiazepines (*see* Frazier, 1978). Other methods of treatment, including psychotherapy and behavioral technics, are discussed by Frazier (1978). There are important, nonpharmacological factors that bear on the use and effects of antianxiety drugs. Discussions of the nonspecific and placebo aspects of such treatment are provided by Wolf (1959), Rickels (1968), Baldessarini (1977b), and Rickels and associates (1978). The general topic of the evaluation and treatment of anxiety is well reviewed by Cole and Davis (1975), Frazier (1978), and Rickels and associates (1978); aspects of the abuse of sedatives are reviewed by Muller (1972) and Frazier (1978). Useful guidelines for the safe and rational use of sedatives in general practice are provided by an American Medical Association Committee (1974). The current status of some of the effective sedative-antianxiety agents as federally *controlled substances* is reviewed in Appendix I.

Alexander, C. S., and Nino, A. Cardiovascular complications in young patients taking psychotropic drugs. *Am. Heart J.,* **1969,** *78,* 757–769.

Alexanderson, B., and Sjöqvist, F. Individual differences in the pharmacokinetics of monomethylated tricyclic antidepressants: role of genetic and environmental factors and clinical importance. *Ann. N.Y. Acad. Sci.,* **1971,** *179,* 739–751.

American College of Neuropsychopharmacology Task Force. Drug therapy: neurological syndromes associated with antipsychotic-drug use. *N. Engl. J. Med.,* **1973,** *289,* 20–23.

American Medical Association Committee on Alcoholism and Drug Dependence. Barbiturates and barbiturate-like drugs. Considerations in their medical use. *J.A.M.A.,* **1974,** *230,* 1440–1441.

Anderson, W. H., and Kuehnle, J. C. Strategies for the treatment of acute psychosis. *J.A.M.A.,* **1974,** *229,* 1884–1889.

Avery, D., and Winokur, G. The efficacy of electroconvulsive therapy and antidepressants in depression. *Biol. Psychiatry,* **1977,** *12,* 507–523.

Ayd, F. J., Jr. A critical appraisal of chlordiazepoxide. *J. Neuropsychiatr.,* **1962,** *3,* 177–180.

Baldessarini, R. J. Schizophrenia. *N. Engl. J. Med.,* **1977a,** *297,* 988–995.

Baldessarini, R. J., and Gelenberg, A. J. Use of physostigmine in antidepressant-induced intoxication. *Am. J. Psychiatry,* **1979,** *136,* 1608–1609.

Baldessarini, R. J., and Stephens, J. H. Clinical pharmacology and toxicology of lithium salts. *Arch. Gen. Psychiatry,* **1970,** *22,* 72–77.

Baldessarini, R. J., and Willmuth, R. L. Psychotic reactions during amitriptyline therapy. *Can. Psychiatr. Assoc. J.,* **1968,** *13,* 571–573.

Berger, F. M. The pharmacological properties of 2-methyl-2-*n*-propyl-1,3 propanediol dicarbamate (MILTOWN), a new interneuronal blocking agent. *J. Pharmacol. Exp. Ther.,* **1954,** *112,* 413–423.

Bigger, J. T.; Giardina, E. G.; and Perel, J. J. Cardiac antiarrhythmic effects of imipramine hydrochloride. *N. Engl. J. Med.,* **1977,** *296,* 206–208.

Blackwell, B.; Stefopoulos, A.; and Enders, P. Anticholinergic activity of two tricyclic antidepressants. *Am. J. Psychiatry,* **1978,** *135,* 722–724.

Bloom, F. E. Neural mechanisms of benzodiazepine actions. *Am. J. Psychiatry,* **1977,** *134,* 669–672.

Bojanovsky, J., and Tölle, R. Dihydroergotamin gegen die Kreislaufwirkungen der Thymoleptika. *Dtsch. Med. Wochenschr.,* **1974,** *99,* 1064–1065.

Boston Collaborative Drug Surveillance Program. Adverse reactions to tricyclic-antidepressant drugs. *Lancet,* **1972,** *1,* 529–530.

Brugmans, J.; Verbruggen, F.; Dom, J.; and Schuermans, V. Prolactin, phenothiazines and admission to mental hospital, and carcinoma of the breast. *Lancet,* **1973,** *2,* 502–503.

Bunney, B. S., and Aghajanian, G. K. Mesolimbic and mesocortical dopaminergic systems: physiology and pharmacology. In, *Psychopharmacology: A Generation of Progress.* (Lipton, M. A.; DiMascio, A.; and Killam, K. F.; eds.) Raven Press, New York, **1978,** pp. 159–169.

Bunney, B. S.; Walters, J. R.; Roth, R. H.; and Aghajanian, G. K. Dopaminergic neurons: effect of antipsychotic drugs and amphetamine on single cell activity. *J. Pharmacol. Exp. Ther.,* **1973,** *185,* 560–571.

Bunney, W. E., Jr.; Murphy, D. L.; and Goodwin, F. K. The "switch process" in manic-depressive illness. *Arch. Gen. Psychiatry,* **1972,** *27,* 295–302.

Burrows, G. D.; Vohra, J.; Hunt, D.; Sloman, J. G.; Soggins, B. A.; and Davies, B. Cardiac effects of different tricyclic antidepressant drugs. *Br. J. Psychiatry,* **1976,** *129,* 335–341.

Buyze, G.; Egberts, P.; Muuse, R.; and Poslavsky, A. Blood levels of thioridazine and some of its metabolites in psychiatric patients. *Psychiatr. Neurol. Neurochir.,* **1973,** *76,* 229–239.

Cade, J. F. J. Lithium salts in the treatment of psychotic excitement. *Med. J. Aust.,* **1949,** *2,* 349–352.

Campbell, M. Psychopharmacology in childhood psychosis. *Int. J. Ment. Health,* **1975,** *4,* 238–254.

Carlsson, A. Mechanism of action of neuroleptic drugs. In, *Psychopharmacology: A Generation of Progress.* (Lipton, M. A.; DiMascio, A.; and Killam, K. F.; eds.) Raven Press, New York, **1978,** pp. 1057–1070.

Carlsson, A., and Lindqvist, M. Effect of chlorpromazine and haloperidol on formation of 3-methoxytyramine and normetanephrine in mouse brain. *Acta Pharmacol. Toxicol.* (*Kbh.*), **1963,** *20,* 140–144.

Carpenter, W. T., Jr.; Strauss, J. S.; and Bartko, J. J. Flexible system for the diagnosis of schizophrenia: report from the WHO international pilot study of schizophrenia. *Science,* **1973,** *182,* 1275–1277.

Clark, M. L.; Ray, T. S.; Paredes, A.; Ragland, R. E.; Costilee, J. P.; Smith, C. W.; and Wolf, S. Chlorpromazine in women with chronic schizophrenia: the effects on cholesterol levels and cholesterol-behavioral relationships. *Psychosom. Med.,* **1967,** *29,* 634–642.

Clement-Cormier, Y. C.; Kebabian, J. W.; Petzold, G. L.; and Greengard, P. Dopamine-sensitive adenylate cyclase in mammalian brain: a possible site of action of antipsychotic drugs. *Proc. Natl. Acad. Sci. U.S.A.,* **1974,** *71,* 1113–1117.

Cook, L., and Weidley, E. Behavioral effects of some psychopharmacological agents. *Ann. N.Y. Acad. Sci.,* **1957,** *66,* 740–752.

Cooper, T. B., and Simpson, G. M. Kinetics of lithium and clinical response. In, *Psychopharmacology: A Generation of Progress.* (Lipton, M. A.; DiMascio, A.; and Killam, K. F.; eds.) Raven Press, New York, **1978,** pp. 923–931.

Courvoisier, S.; Fournel, J.; Ducrot, R.; Kolsky, M.; and Koetschet, P. Propiétés pharmacodynamiques du chlorhydrate de chloro-3(dimethylamino-3'propyl)-10 phenothiazine (4560 RP). *Arch. Int. Pharmacodyn. Ther.,* **1953,** *92,* 305–361.

Crane, G. E. Iproniazid (MARSILID) phosphate, a therapeutic agent for mental disorders and debilitating disease. *Psychiatr. Res. Rep.,* **1959,** *8,* 142–152.

————. Clinical psychopharmacology in its 20th year. *Science,* **1973,** *181,* 124–128.

Creese, I.; Burt, D.; and Snyder, S. H. Biochemical actions of neuroleptic drugs: focus on dopamine receptor. In,

Handbook of Psychopharmacology, Vol. 10. (Iversen, L. L.; Iversen, S. D.; and Snyder, S. H.; eds.) Plenum Press, New York, **1978,** pp. 37–89.

Crews, F. T., and Smith, C. B. Presynaptic alpha-receptor subsensitivity after long-term antidepressant treatment. *Science,* **1978,** *202,* 322–324.

Crome, P.; Dawling, S.; and Braithwaite, R. A. Effect of activated charcoal on absorption of nortriptyline. *Lancet,* **1977,** *2,* 1203–1205.

Davies, R. K.; Tucker, G. J.; Harrow, M.; and Detre, T. P. Confusional episodes and antidepressant medication. *Am. J. Psychiatry,* **1971,** *128,* 127.

Delay, J., and Deniker, P. Trente-huit cas de psychoses traitées par la cure prolongée et continue de 4560 RP. Le Congrès des Al. et Neurol. de Langue Fr. In, *Compte rendu du Congrès.* Masson et Cie, Paris, **1952.**

Demers, R. G., and Heninger, G. R. Electrocardiographic T-wave changes during lithium carbonate treatment. *J.A.M.A.,* **1971,** *218,* 381–386.

DeMontigny, C., and Aghajanian, G. K. Tricyclic antidepressants: long-term treatment increases responsivity of rat forebrain neurons to serotonin. *Science,* **1978,** *202,* 1303–1305.

DiMascio, A.; Heninger, G.; and Klerman, G. L. Psychopharmacology of imipramine and desipramine: a comparative study of their effects in normal males. *Psychopharmacologia,* **1964,** *5,* 361–371.

Dimond, R. C.; Brammer, S. R.; Atkinson, R. L., Jr.; Howard, W. J.; and Earll, J. M. Chlorpromazine treatment and growth hormone secretory responses in acromegaly. *J. Clin. Endocrinol. Metab.,* **1973,** *36,* 1189–1195.

Dobkin, A. B.; Gilbert, R. G. B.; and Lamoureu, L. Physiological effects of chlorpromazine. *Anaesthesia,* **1954,** *9,* 157–174.

DuComb, L., and Baldessarini, R. J. Timing and risk of bone marrow depression by psychotropic drugs. *Am. J. Psychiatry,* **1977,** *134,* 1294–1295.

Erle, G.; Basso, M.; Federspil, G.; Sicolo, N.; and Scandellari, C. Effect of chlorpromazine on blood glucose and plasma insulin in man. *Eur. J. Clin. Pharmacol.,* **1977,** *11,* 15–18.

Feinberg, A. P., and Snyder, S. H. Phenothiazine drugs: structure activity relationships explained by a conformation that mimics dopamine. *Proc. Natl. Acad. Sci. U.S.A.,* **1975,** *72,* 1899–1903.

Feinsilver, D., and Gunderson, J. Psychotherapy for schizophrenics—is it indicated? *Schizophr. Bull.,* **1972,** *6,* 11–23.

Forrest, J. J., Jr. Lithium inhibition of cAMP-mediated hormones: a caution. *N. Engl. J. Med.,* **1975,** *292,* 423–424.

Forsman, A., and Öhman, R. On the pharmacokinetics of haloperidol. *Nord. Psykiatr. Tidskr.,* **1974,** *28,* 441–448.

Freeman, C. P.; Basson, J. V.; and Crighton, A. Double-blind controlled trial of electroconvulsive therapy (ECT) and simulated ECT in depressive illness. *Lancet,* **1978,** *1,* 738–740.

Frohman, L. A. Clinical neuropharmacology of hypothalamic releasing factors. *N. Engl. J. Med.,* **1972,** *286,* 1391–1398.

Gardos, G., and Cole, J. O. Maintenance antipsychotic therapy: is the cure worse than the disease? *Am. J. Psychiatry,* **1976,** *133,* 32–36.

Glassman, A. H.; Perel, J. M.; Shostak, M.; Kantor, S. J.; and Fleiss, J. L. Clinical implications of imipramine plasma levels for depressive illness. *Arch. Gen. Psychiatry,* **1977,** *34,* 197–204.

Goldberg, R. B., and Thornton, W. E. Combined tricyclic-MAOI therapy for refractory depression: a review with guidelines for appropriate usage. *J. Clin. Pharmacol.,* **1978,** *18,* 143–147.

Goldfield, M. D., and Weinstein, M. R. Lithium carbonate in obstetrics: guidelines for clinical use. *Am. J. Obstet. Gynecol.,* **1973,** *116,* 15–22.

Gottschalk, L. A. Pharmacokinetics of the minor tranquilizers and clinical response. In, *Psychopharmacology. A Generation of Progress.* (Lipton, M. A.; DiMascio, A.; and Killam, K. F.; eds.) Raven Press, New York, **1978,** pp. 975–985.

Gottschalk, L. A.; Biener, R.; Noble, E.; Birch, H.; Wilbert, D.; and Heizer, J. Thioridazine plasma levels and clinical response. *Compr. Psychiatry,* **1975,** *16,* 323–337.

Gram, L. F.; Christiansen, J.; and Overo, K. F. Pharmacokinetic interaction between tricyclic antidepressants and other psychopharmaca. *Acta Psychiatr. Scand. [Suppl.],* **1973,** *243,* 52–53.

Granacher, R. P., and Baldessarini, R. J. Physostigmine in the acute anticholinergic syndrome associated with antidepressant and antiparkinson drugs. *Arch. Gen. Psychiatry,* **1975,** *32,* 375–380.

Grinspoon, L.; Ewalt, J. R.; and Shader, R. Psychotherapy and pharmacotherapy in chronic schizophrenia. *Am. J. Psychiatry,* **1968,** *124,* 1645–1652.

Growdon, J. H.; Gelenberg, A. J.; Doller, J.; Hirsch, M. J.; and Wurtman, R. J. Lecithin can suppress tardive dyskinesia. *N. Engl. J. Med.,* **1978,** *298,* 1029–1030.

Grunthal, E. Untersuchungen über die besondere psychologische Wirkung des Thymolepticums TOFRANIL. *Psychiatr.-Neurol. Wochenschr.,* **1958,** *136,* 402–408.

Hardesty, A. S., and Burdock, E. I. Quantitative clinical evaluation in psychopharmacology. In, *Psychopharmacology: A Generation of Progress.* (Lipton, M. A.; DiMascio, A.; and Killam, K. F.; eds.) Raven Press, New York, **1978,** pp. 871–878.

Haugaard, E. S.; Mickel, R.; and Haugaard, N. Actions of lithium ions and insulin on glucose utilization, glycogen synthesis and glycogen synthase in the isolated rat diaphragm. *Biochem. Pharmacol.,* **1974,** *23,* 1675–1685.

Himmelhoch, J. M.; Poust, R. I.; and Mallinger, A. G. Adjustment of lithium dose during lithium-chlorothiazide therapy. *Clin. Pharmacol. Ther.,* **1977,** *22,* 225–227.

Hirsch, S. R.; Gaind, R.; Rohde, P. D.; Stevens, B. C.; and Wing, J. K. Outpatient maintenance of chronic schizophrenic patients with long-acting fluphenazine: double blind placebo trial. *Br. Med. J.,* **1973,** *1,* 633–637.

Hogarty, G. E., and Ulrich, R. F. Temporal effects of drug and placebo in delaying relapse in schizophrenic outpatients. *Arch. Gen. Psychiatry,* **1977,** *34,* 297–301.

Iwahara, S.; Iwasaki, T.; and Hasegawa, Y. Effects of chlorpromazine and homofenazine on a passive avoidance response in rats. *Psychopharmacologia,* **1968,** *13,* 320–331.

Jacobson, G.; Baldessarini, R. J.; and Manschreck, T. Tardive and withdrawal dyskinesia associated with haloperidol. *Am. J. Psychiatry,* **1974,** *131,* 910–913.

Janowsky, D. S.; El-Yousef, M. K.; Davis, J. M. Acetylcholine and depression. *Psychosom. Med.,* **1974,** *36,* 248–257.

Jus, K.; Jus, A.; Gautier, J.; Villeneuve, A.; Pires, P.; Pineau, R.; and Villeneuve, R. Studies of the actions of certain pharmacological agents on tardive dyskinesia and on the rabbit syndrome. *Int. J. Clin. Pharmacol.,* **1974,** *9,* 138–145.

Klein, D. F.; Zitrin, C. M.; and Woerner, M. Antidepressants, anxiety, panic, and phobia. In, *Psychopharmacology: A Generation of Progress.* (Lipton, M. A.; DiMascio, A.; and Killam, K. F.; eds.) Raven Press, New York, **1978,** pp. 1401–1410.

Klerman, G. L. Drug therapy of clinical depressions. *J. Psychiatr. Res.,* **1972,** *9,* 253–270.

Kline, N. S. Clinical experience with iproniazid (MARSILID). *J. Clin. Exp. Psychopathol.,* **1958,** *19,* Suppl., 72–78.

———. Antidepressant medications: a more effective use by general practitioners, family physicians, internists and others. *J.A.M.A.,* **1974,** *227,* 1158–1160.

Kolodny, H. D.; Sherman, L.; Singh, A.; Kim, S.; and

Benjamin, F. Acromegaly treated with chlorpromazine. *N. Engl. J. Med.,* **1971,** *284,* 819–822.

Kuhn, R. The treatment of depressive states with G22355 (imipramine hydrochloride). *Am. J. Psychiatry,* **1958,** *115,* 459–464.

Laborit, H.; Huguenard, P.; and Alluaume, R. Un nouveau stabilisateur vegetatif, le 4560 RP. *Presse Méd.,* **1952,** *60,* 206–208.

Lehmann, H. E.; Cahn, C. H.; and de Vertouil, R. L. The treatment of depressive conditions with imipramine (G22355). *Can. Psychiatr. Assoc. J.,* **1958,** *3,* 155–164.

Lehmann, H. E., and Hanrahan, G. E. Chlorpromazine, a new inhibiting agent for psychomotor excitement and manic states. *Arch. Neurol. Psychiatry,* **1954,** *71,* 227–257.

Levine, R. J., and Sjoerdsma, A. Estimation of monoamine oxidase activity in man: techniques and applications. *Ann. N.Y. Acad. Sci.,* **1963,** *107,* 966–974.

Loga, S.; Curry, S.; and Lader, M. Interactions of orphenadrine and phenobarbitone with chlorpromazine: plasma concentrations and effects in man. *Br. J. Clin. Pharmacol.,* **1975,** *2,* 197–208.

Mandel, M. R., and Klerman, G. L. Clinical use of antidepressants, stimulants, tricyclics and monoamine oxidase inhibitors. In, *Principles of Psychopharmacology,* 2nd ed. (Clark, W. G., and del Guidice, J., eds.) Academic Press, Inc., New York, **1978,** pp. 537–551.

Medical Letter. Imipramine for enuresis. **1974,** *16,* 22–24.

Meltzer, H. Y.; Goode, D. J.; and Fang, V. S. The effect of psychotropic drugs on endocrine function. In, *Psychopharmacology: A Generation of Progress.* (Lipton, M. A.; DiMascio, A.; and Killam, K. F.; eds.) Raven Press, New York, **1978,** pp. 509–529.

Moir, D. C.; Cornwell, W. B.; Dingwall-Fordyce, I.; Crooks, J.; O'Malley, K.; Turnbull, M. J.; and Weir, R. D. Cardiotoxicity of amitriptyline. *Lancet,* **1972,** *2,* 561–564.

Moir, D. C.; Dingwall-Fordyce, I.; and Weir, R. D. A follow-up study of cardiac patients receiving amitriptyline. *Eur. J. Clin. Pharmacol.,* **1973,** *6,* 98–101.

Moore, K. E., and Kelly, P. H. Biochemical pharmacology of mesolimbic and mesocortical dopaminergic neurons. In, *Psychopharmacology: A Generation of Progress.* (Lipton, M. A.; DiMascio, A.; and Killam, K. F.; eds.) Raven Press, New York, **1978,** pp. 221–234.

Nagy, A., and Johansson, R. Plasma levels of imipramine and desipramine in man after different routes of administration. *Naunyn Schmiedebergs Arch. Pharmacol.,* **1975,** *290,* 145–160.

Noble, J., and Matthew, H. Acute poisoning by tricyclic antidepressants: clinical features and management of 100 patients. *Clin. Toxicol.,* **1969,** *2,* 403–421.

Nouri, A., and Cuendet, J. F. Atteintes oculaires au coures des traitements aux thymoleptiques. *Schweiz. Med. Wochenschr.,* **1971,** *101,* 1178.

Overall, J. E. Prior psychiatric treatment and the development of breast cancer. *Arch. Gen. Psychiatry,* **1978,** *35,* 898–899.

Overall, J. E.; Hollister, L. E.; Meyer, F.; Kimball, I.; and Shelton, J. Imipramine and thioridazine in depressed and schizophrenic patients. *J.A.M.A.,* **1964,** *189,* 93–96.

Pert, A.; Rosenblatt, J. E.; Sivit, C.; Pert, C. B.; and Bunney, W. E., Jr. Long-term treatment with lithium prevents the development of dopamine receptor supersensitivity. *Science,* **1978,** *201,* 171–173.

Prien, R. F.; Delong, S. L.; Cole, J. O.; and Levine, J. Ocular changes occurring with prolonged high dose chlorpromazine therapy. *Arch. Gen. Psychiatry,* **1970,** *23,* 464–468.

Quitkin, F.; Rifkin, A.; and Klein, D. F. Very high dosage vs. standard dosage fluphenazine in schizophrenia. *Arch. Gen. Psychiatry,* **1974,** *32,* 1276–1281.

Raisfeld, I. H. Cardiovascular complications of antidepressant therapy: interactions at the adrenergic neuron. *Am. Heart J.,* **1972,** *83,* 129–133.

Rasmussen, J. Poisoning with amitriptyline. *Dan. Med. Bull.,* **1966,** *16,* 201–203.

Richelson, E., and Diventz-Romero, S. Blockade by psychotropic drugs on muscarinic acetylcholine receptor in cultured nerve cells. *Biol. Psychiatry,* **1977,** *12,* 771–785.

Rivera-Calimlin, L.; Casteneda, L.; and Lasagna, L. Effects of mode of management on plasma chlorpromazine in psychiatric patients. *Clin. Pharmacol. Ther.,* **1973,** *14,* 978–986.

Rotrosen, J.; Angrist, B. M.; Gershon, S.; Aronson, M.; Gruen, P.; Sachar, E.; Denning, R. K.; Matthysse, S.; Stanley, M.; and Wilk, S. Thiethylperazine. *Arch. Gen. Psychiatry,* **1978,** *35,* 1112–1118.

Sachar, E. J. Neuroendocrine responses to psychotropic drugs. In, *Psychopharmacology: A Generation of Progress.* (Lipton, M. A.; DiMascio, A.; and Killam, K. F.; eds.) Raven Press, New York, **1978,** pp. 499–507.

Safra, M. J., and Oakley, G. P., Jr. Association between cleft lip with or without cleft palate and prenatal exposure to diazepam. *Lancet,* **1975,** *2,* 478–480.

Sakalis, G.; Curry, S. H.; Mould, G. P.; and Lader, M. H. Physiologic and clinical effects of chlorpromazine and their relationship to plasma level. *Clin. Pharmacol. Ther.,* **1972,** *13,* 931–946.

Saron, B. M., and Gaind, R. Lithium. *Clin. Toxicol.,* **1973,** *6,* 257–269.

Schou, M. Lithium in psychiatric therapy and prophylaxis. *J. Psychiatr. Res.,* **1968,** *6,* 67–95.

Sedvall, G. Receptor feedback and dopamine turnover in CNS. In, *Handbook of Psychopharmacology,* Vol. 6. (Iversen, L. L.; Iversen, S. D.; and Snyder, S. H.; eds.) Plenum Press, New York, **1975,** pp. 127–177.

Sen, G., and Bose, K. C. *Rauwolfia serpentina,* a new Indian drug for insanity and high blood pressure. *Indian Med. World,* **1931,** *2,* 194–201.

Seppalä, T.; Linniola, M.; Elonen, E.; Mattita, M. J.; and Mäki, M. Effect of tricyclic antidepressants and alcohol on psychomotor skills related to driving. *Clin. Pharmacol. Ther.,* **1975,** *17,* 515–522.

Shagass, C., and Straumanis, J. J. Drugs and human sensory evoked potentials. In, *Psychopharmacology: A Generation of Progress.* (Lipton, M. A.; DiMascio, A.; and Killam, K. F.; eds.) Raven Press, New York, **1978,** pp. 699–709.

Shapiro, A. K.; Shapiro, E.; and Wayne, H. L. Treatment of Tourette's syndrome with haloperidol. Review of 34 cases. *Arch. Gen. Psychiatry,* **1973,** *28,* 92–97.

Shatan, C. Withdrawal symptoms after abrupt termination of imipramine. *Can. Psychiatr. Assoc. J.,* **1966,** *2,* 150–157.

Snyder, S. H.; U'Pritchard, D.; and Greenberg, D. A. Neurotransmitter receptor finding in the brain. In, *Psychopharmacology: A Generation of Progress.* (Lipton, M. A.; DiMascio, A.; and Killam, K. F.; eds.) Raven Press. New York, **1978,** pp. 361–370.

Snyder, S. H., and Yamamura, H. Antidepressants and the muscarinic acetylcholine receptor. *Arch. Gen. Psychiatry,* **1977,** *34,* 236–239.

Spiker, D. G., and Biggs, J. T. Tricyclic antidepressants: prolonged plasma levels after overdose. *J.A.M.A.,* **1976,** *236,* 1711–1712.

Stewart, M. Treatment of bedwetting. *J.A.M.A.,* **1975,** *232,* 181–183.

Sulser, F., and Robinson, S. E. Clinical implications of pharmacological differences among antipsychotic drugs. In, *Psychopharmacology: A Generation of Progress.* (Lipton, M. A.; DiMascio, A.; and Killam, K. F.; eds.) Raven Press, New York, **1978,** pp. 943–954.

Svenssen, T. H., and Usdin, T. Feedback inhibition of brain noradrenaline neurons by tricyclic antidepressants: α-receptor mediation. *Science,* **1978,** *202,* 1089–1091.

Tupin, J. P., and Schuller, A. B. Lithium and haloperidol incompatibility reviewed. *Psychiatr. J. Univ. Ottawa,* **1978,** *3,* 245–251.

Tyrer, P.; Candy, J.; and Kelly, D. A study of the clinical effects of phenelzine and placebo in the treatment of phobic anxiety. *Psychopharmacologia,* **1973,** *32,* 237–254.

U'Pritchard, D. C.; Greenberg, D. A.; Sheehan, P. P.; and Snyder, S. H. Tricyclic antidepressants: therapeutic properties and affinity for alpha-noradrenergic receptor binding sites in the brain. *Science,* **1978,** *199,* 197–198.

Vohra, J., and Burrows, G. D. Cardiovascular complications of tricyclic antidepressant overdosage. *Drugs,* **1974,** *8,* 432–437.

White, M. G., and Fetner, C. D. Treatment of the syndrome of inappropriate secretion of antidiuretic hormone with lithium carbonate. *N. Engl. J. Med.,* **1975,** *292,* 390–392.

Williams, R. B., and Sherter, C. Cardiac complications of tricyclic antidepressant therapy. *Ann. Intern. Med.,* **1971,** *74,* 395–398.

Zelickson, A. S., and Zeller, H. C. A new and unusual reaction to chlorpromazine. *J.A.M.A.,* **1964,** *188,* 394–396.

Ziegler, V. E.; Biggs, J. T.; and Wylie, L. T. Doxepin kinetics. *Clin. Pharmacol. Ther.,* **1978,** *23,* 573–579.

Monographs and Reviews

Allquander, C. Dependence on sedative and hypnotic drugs. *Acta Psychiatr. Scand.* [*Suppl.*], **1978,** *270,* 1–120.

American Pharmaceutical Association Scientific Review Subpanel on Psychotherapeutic Drugs. *Evaluation of Drug Interactions.* The Association, Washington, D. C., **1973.**

American Psychiatric Association. *Diagnostic and Statistical Manual of Mental Disorders,* Vols. II and III. The Association, Washington, D. C., **1968** and **1979.**

Anders, T. F., and Ciaranello, R. Psychopharmacology of childhood disorders. In, *Psychopharmacology: From Theory to Practice.* (Barchas, J. D.; Berger, P. A.; Ciaranello, R.; and Elliott, G. R.; eds.) Oxford University Press, New York, **1977,** pp. 407–447.

Åsberg, M. Individualization of treatment with tricyclic compounds. *Med. Clin. North Am.,* **1974,** *58,* 1083–1091.

————. Treatment of depression with tricyclic drugs: pharmacokinetic and pharmacodynamic aspects. *Pharmakopsychiatrie,* **1976,** *9,* 18–26.

Ayd, F. J., Jr., and Blackwell, B. (eds.). *Discoveries in Biological Psychiatry.* J. B. Lippincott Co., Philadelphia, **1970.**

Baldessarini, R. J. The basis for amine hypotheses in affective disorders: a critical evaluation. *Arch. Gen. Psychiatry,* **1975,** *32,* 1087–1093.

————. *Chemotherapy in Psychiatry.* Harvard University Press, Cambridge, Mass., **1977b.**

————. Mood drugs. *D.M.,* **1977c,** *11,* 1–65.

————. Status of psychotropic drug blood level assays and other biochemical measurements in clinical practice. *Am. J. Psychiatry,* **1979a,** *136,* 1177–1180.

————. The "neuroleptic" antipsychotic drugs. 1. Mechanisms of action. *Postgrad. Med.,* **1979b,** *65,* 108–111, 114–119. 2. Neurologic side effects. *Ibid.,* **1979b,** *65,* 123–128.

Baldessarini, R. J., and Fischer, J. E. Trace amines and alternative neurotransmitters in the central nervous system. *Biochem. Pharmacol.,* **1978,** *27,* 621–626.

Baldessarini, R. J., and Lipinski, J. G. Lithium salts: 1970–1975. *Ann. Intern. Med.,* **1975,** *83,* 527–533.

Baldessarini, R. J., and Tarsy, D. Tardive dyskinesia. In, *Psychopharmacology: A Generation of Progress.* (Lipton, M. A.; DiMascio, A.; and Killam, K. F.; eds.) Raven Press, New York, **1978,** pp. 993–1004.

————. Relationship of the actions of neuroleptic drugs to the pathophysiology of tardive dyskinesia. *Int. Rev. Neurobiol.,* **1979,** *21,* 1–45.

Barchas, J. D.; Berger, P. A.; Ciaranello, R. D.; and Elliott, G. R. (eds.). *Psychopharmacology: From Theory to Practice.* Oxford University Press, New York, **1977.**

Barchas, J. D.; Berger, P. A.; Matthysse, S.; and Wyatt, R. J. The biochemistry of affective disorders and schizo-

phrenia. In, *Principles of Psychopharmacology,* 2nd ed. (Clark, W. G., and del Guidice, J., eds.) Academic Press, Inc., New York, **1978,** pp. 105–132.

Biel, J. H.; Bopp, B.; and Mitchell, B. D. Chemistry and structure-activity relationships of psychotropic drugs. In, *Principles of Psychopharmacology,* 2nd ed. (Clark, W. G., and del Guidice, J., eds.) Academic Press, Inc., New York, **1978,** pp. 140–168.

Bradley, P. B. Phenothiazine derivatives. *Pharmacol. Physicians,* **1963,** *1,* 417–477.

Caldwell, A. E. History of psychopharmacology. In, *Principles of Psychopharmacology,* 2nd ed. (Clark, W. G., and del Guidice, J., eds.) Academic Press, Inc., New York, **1978,** pp. 9–40.

Chase, T. N. Rational approaches to the pharmacotherapy of chorea. In, *The Basal Ganglia.* Association for Research in Nervous and Mental Disease Publications, Vol. 55. (Yahr, M. D., ed.) Raven Press, New York, **1976,** pp. 337–350.

Clark, W. G., and del Guidice, J. (eds.). *Principles of Psychopharmacology,* 2nd ed. Academic Press, Inc., New York, **1978.**

Cole, J. O., and Davis, J. M. Minor tranquilizers, sedatives, and hypnotics. In, *Comprehensive Textbook of Psychiatry,* 2nd ed. (Freedman, A. M.; Kaplan, H. I.; and Sadock, B. J.; eds.) The Williams & Wilkins Co., Baltimore, **1975,** pp. 1956–1968.

Conney, A. H. Pharmacological implications of microsomal enzyme induction. *Pharmacol. Rev.,* **1967,** *19,* 317–366.

Cooper, J. R.; Bloom, F. E.; and Roth, R. H. *The Biochemical Basis of Neuropharmacology,* 3rd ed. Oxford University Press, New York, **1978.**

Cooper, T. B.; Simpson, G. M.; and Lee, H. J. Thymoleptic and neuroleptic drug plasma levels in psychiatry: current status. *Int. Rev. Neurobiol.,* **1976,** *19,* 269–309.

Costa, E., and Sandler, M. (eds.). *Monoamine Oxidases—New Vistas. Advances in Biochemical Psychopharmacology,* Vol. 5. Raven Press, New York, **1972.**

Davis, J. M. Overview: maintenance therapy in psychiatry. I. Schizophrenia. *Am. J. Psychiatry,* **1975,** *132,* 1237–1245.

————. Overview: maintenance therapy in psychiatry. II. Affective disorders. *Ibid.,* **1976,** *133,* 1–13.

Davis, J. M., and Garver, D. L. Neuroleptics: clinical use in psychiatry. In, *Handbook of Psychopharmacology,* Vol. 10. (Iversen, L. L.; Iversen, S. D.; and Snyder, S. H.; eds.) Plenum Press, New York, **1978,** pp. 129–164.

De La Cruz, F. F.; Fox, B. H.; and Roberts, R. H. (eds.). Minimal brain dysfunction. *Ann. N.Y. Acad. Sci.,* **1973,** *205,* 1–396.

Efron, D. H.; Holmstedt, B.; and Kline, N. S. (eds.). *Ethnopharmacologic Search for Psychoactive Drugs.* Public Health Service Publication No. 67–1645, U.S. Government Printing Office, Washington, D. C., **1967.**

Feighner, J. P.; Robins, E.; Guze, S.; Woodruff, R. A., Jr.; Winokur, G.; and Munoz, R. Diagnostic criteria for use in psychiatric research. *Arch. Gen. Psychiatry,* **1972,** *26,* 57–63.

Fielding, S., and Lal, H. Behavioral actions of neuroleptics. In, *Handbook of Psychopharmacology,* Vol. 10. (Iversen, L. L.; Iversen, S. D.; and Snyder, S. H.; eds.) Plenum Press, New York, **1978,** pp. 91–128.

Fink, M. EEG and human psychopharmacology. *Annu. Rev. Pharmacol.,* **1969,** *9,* 241–258.

Frazier, S. H. (ed.). The anxious patient. *McLean Hosp. J.,* **1978,** *3,* 1–64.

Freedman, A. M.; Kaplan, H. I.; and Sadock, B. J. (eds.). *Comprehensive Textbook of Psychiatry,* 2nd ed. The Williams & Wilkins Co., Baltimore, **1975.**

Garattini, S.; Mussini, E.; and Randall, L. O. (eds.). *The Benzodiazepines.* Raven Press, New York, **1973.**

Glassman, A. H., and Perel, J. M. The clinical pharmacology of imipramine. *Arch. Gen. Psychiatry,* **1973,** *28,* 649–653.

——. Tricyclic blood levels and clinical outcome: a review of the art. In, *Psychopharmacology: A Generation of Progress.* (Lipton, M. A.; DiMascio, A.; and Killam, K. F.; eds.) Raven Press, New York, **1978,** pp. 917–921.

Goldberg, H. L., and DiMascio, A. Psychotropic drugs in pregnancy. In, *Psychopharmacology: A Generation of Progress.* (Lipton, M. A.; DiMascio, A.; and Killam, K. F.; eds.) Raven Press, New York, **1978,** pp. 1047–1055.

Gordon, M. *Psychopharmacological Agents,* Vols. II and III. Academic Press, Inc., New York, **1967** and **1974.**

Greenblatt, D. J., and Shader, R. I. *Benzodiazepines in Medical Practice.* Raven Press, New York, **1974.**

Greengard, P. *Cyclic Nucleotides, Phosphorylated Proteins, and Neuronal Function.* Raven Press, New York, **1978,** pp. 25–37.

Hollister, L. E. *Clinical Pharmacology of Psychotherapeutic Agents.* Churchill-Livingstone, Ltd., New York, **1978a.**

——. Tricyclic antidepressants. *N. Engl. J. Med.,* **1978b,** *299,* 1106–1109, 1168–1172.

Irwin, S. Psychoactive drug evaluation. In, *Search for New Drugs.* (Rubin, A. A., ed.) Marcel Dekker, Inc., New York, **1972,** pp. 201–232.

Itil, T. M. Effects of psychotropic drugs on qualitatively and quantitatively analyzed human EEG. In, *Principles of Psychopharmacology,* 2nd ed. (Clark, W. G., and del Guidice, J., eds.) Academic Press, Inc., New York, **1978,** pp. 261–277.

Iversen, L. L. Biochemical psychopharmacology of GABA. In, *Psychopharmacology: A Generation of Progress.* (Lipton, M. A.; DiMascio, A.; and Killam, K. F.; eds.) Raven Press, New York, **1978,** pp. 25–38.

Iversen, L. L.; Iversen, S. D.; and Snyder, S. H. (eds.). *Handbook of Psychopharmacology,* 14 vols. Plenum Press, New York, **1976–1978.**

Janssen, P. A. Butyrophenones and diphenylbutyl-piperidines. In, *Psychopharmacological Agents,* Vol. 3. (Gordon, M., ed.) Academic Press, Inc., New York, **1974,** pp. 128–158.

Janssen, P. A., and Van Bever, W. F. Preclinical psycho-pharmacology of neuroleptics. In, *Principles of Psycho-pharmacology,* 2nd ed. (Clark, W. G., and del Guidice, J., eds.) Academic Press, Inc., New York, **1978,** pp. 279–295.

Jefferson, J. W. A review of the cardiovascular effects and toxicity of tricyclic antidepressants. *Psychosom. Med.,* **1975,** *37,* 160–179.

Jefferson, J. W., and Greist, J. H. Lithium and the kidney. *Semin. Psychiatry,* **1979,** 81–104.

Johnson, F. N. (ed.). *Lithium Research and Therapy.* Academic Press, Inc., New York, **1975.**

Johnson, F. N., and Johnson, S. *Lithium in Medical Practice.* University Park Press, Baltimore, **1978.**

Kaiser, G., and Zirkle, C. L. Antidepressant drugs. In, *Medicinal Chemistry,* 2nd ed. (Burger, A., ed.) John Wiley & Sons, Inc., New York, **1970,** pp. 1470–1497.

Kaufman, J. S. Drug interactions involving psychotherapeutic agents. In, *Drug Treatment of Mental Disorders.* (Simpson, L. L., ed.) Raven Press, New York, **1976,** pp. 289–309.

Kety, S. S. Biochemical theories of schizophrenia. *Science,* **1959,** *29,* 1528–1532, 1590–1596.

Kety, S. S., and Matthysse, S. (eds.). Prospects for research on schizophrenia. *Neurosci. Res. Program Bull.,* **1972,** *10,* 370–507.

Killam, K. E. Pharmacology of the reticular formation. In, *Psychopharmacology: A Review of Progress, 1957–1967.* (Efron, D. H., ed.) U.S. Government Printing Office, Washington, D. C., **1968,** pp. 411–445.

Klein, D. F., and Davis, J. M. *Diagnosis and Drug Treatment of Psychiatric Disorders.* The Williams & Wilkins Co., Baltimore, **1969.**

Klerman, G. L. Long-term treatment of affective disorders. In, *Psychopharmacology: A Generation of Progress.* (Lipton, M. A.; DiMascio, A.; and Killam, K. F.; eds.) Raven Press, New York, **1978,** pp. 1303–1311.

Lader, M. Plasma concentrations of tricyclic antidepressive drugs. *Br. J. Clin. Pharmacol.,* **1974,** *1,* 281–283.

Levine, J.; Schiele, B. C.; and Bouthilet, L. (eds.). *Principles and Problems in Establishing the Efficacy of Psychotropic Agents.* Public Health Service Publication No. 2138, U.S. Government Printing Office, Washington, D. C., **1971.**

Lewin, L. *Phantastica, Narcotic and Stimulating Drugs; Their Use and Abuse.* Berlin, **1924;** English translation, London, **1931;** E. P. Dutton & Co., New York, **1931.**

Lipton, M. A.; DiMascio, A.; and Killam, K. F. (eds.). *Psychopharmacology: A Generation of Progress.* Raven Press, New York, **1978.**

Longo, V. G. Effects of psychotropic drugs on the EEG of animals. In, *Principles of Psychopharmacology,* 2nd ed. (Clark, W. G., and del Guidice, J., eds.) Academic Press, Inc., New York, **1978,** pp. 247–260.

Lowe, M. C.; Horita, A.; Gelenberg, A. J.; and Klerman, G. L. Preclinical pharmacology of antidepressants. In, *Principles of Psychopharmacology,* 2nd ed. (Clark, W. G., and del Guidice, J., eds.) Academic Press, Inc., New York, **1978,** pp. 311–323.

Ludwig, B. J., and Potterfield, J. R. The pharmacology of propanediol carbamates. *Adv. Pharmacol. Chemother.,* **1971,** *9,* 173–240.

Marley, E., and Blackwell, B. Interactions of monoamine oxidase inhibitors, amines, and foodstuffs. *Adv. Pharmacol. Chemother.,* **1970,** *8,* 185–239.

Marsden, C. D.; Tarsy, D.; and Baldessarini, R. J. Spontaneous and drug-induced movement disorders in psychiatric patients. In, *Psychiatric Aspects of Neurologic Disease.* (Benson, D. F., and Blumer, D., eds.) Grune & Stratton, Inc., New York, **1975,** pp. 219–265.

Martin, J. B.; Brazeau, P.; Tannenbaum, G. S.; Willoughby, J. O.; Epelbaum, J.; Terry, L. C.; and Durand, D. Neuroendocrine organization of growth hormone regulation. In, *The Hypothalamus.* Association for Research in Nervous and Mental Disease Publications, Vol. 56. (Reichlin, S.; Baldessarini, R. J.; and Martin, J. B.; eds.) Raven Press, New York, **1978,** pp. 329–357.

Matthysse, S., and Lipinski, J. F. Biochemical aspects of schizophrenia. *Annu. Rev. Med.,* **1975,** *26,* 551–565.

Matthysse, S., and Sugarman, J. Neurotransmitter theories of schizophrenia. In, *Handbook of Psychopharmacology,* Vol. 10. (Iversen, L. L.; Iversen, S. D.; and Snyder, S. H.; eds.) Plenum Press, New York, **1978,** pp. 211–242.

May, P. R. A. *Treatment of Schizophrenia: A Comparative Study of Five Treatment Methods.* Science House, New York, **1968.**

May, P. R. A., and Van Putten, T. Plasma levels of chlorpromazine in schizophrenia: a critical review of the literature. *Arch. Gen. Psychiatry,* **1978,** *35,* 1081–1087.

Meltzer, H. Y., and Stahl, S. M. The dopamine hypothesis of schizophrenia: a review. *Schizophr. Bull.,* **1976,** *2,* 19–76.

Morris, J. B., and Beck, A. T. The efficacy of antidepressant drugs. *Arch. Gen. Psychiatry,* **1974,** *30,* 667–674.

Morselli, P. L. Psychotropic drugs. In, *Drug Disposition during Development.* (Morselli, P. L., ed.) Spectrum Publications, Inc., New York, **1977,** pp. 431–474.

Muller, C. The overmedicated society: forces in the marketplace for medical care. *Science,* **1972,** *176,* 488–492.

Murphy, D. L.; Campbell, I.; and Costa, J. L. Current status of the indoleamine hypothesis of the affective disorders. In, *Psychopharmacology: A Generation of Progress.* (Lipton, M. A.; DiMascio, A.; and Killam, K. F.; eds.) Raven Press, New York, **1978,** pp. 1235–1248.

Pope, H. G., and Lipinski, J. F. Diagnosis in schizophrenia and manic-depressive illness. *Arch. Gen. Psychiatry,* **1978,** *35,* 811–828.

Praag, H. M. van. Amine hypotheses of affective disorders. In, *Handbook of Psychopharmacology,* Vol. 13. (Iversen, L. L.; Iversen, S. D.; and Snyder, S. H.; eds.) Plenum Press, New York, **1978,** pp. 187–297.

Prien, R. F. Chemotherapy in chronic organic brain syndrome—a review of the literature. *Psychopharmacol. Bull.*, **1973**, *9*, 5–20.

Prien, R. F., and Cole, J. O. The use of psychopharmacological drugs in the aged. In, *Principles of Psychopharmacology*, 2nd ed. (Clark, W. G., and del Guidice, J., eds.) Academic Press, Inc., New York, **1978**, pp. 593–605.

Reichlin, S., and Boyd, A. E., III. Neural control of prolactin secretion in man. *Psychoneuroendocrinology*, **1978**, *3*, 113–130.

Rickels, K. *Non-Specific Factors in Drug Therapy.* Charles C Thomas, Pub., Springfield, Ill., **1968**.

Rickels, K.; Downing, R. W.; and Winokur, A. Antianxiety drugs: clinical use in psychiatry. In, *Handbook of Psychopharmacology*, Vol. 13. (Iversen, L. L.; Iversen, S. D.; and Snyder, S. H.; eds.) Plenum Press, New York, **1978**, pp. 395–430.

Robinson, D. S.; Nies, A.; Ravaris, C. L.; Ives, J. O.; and Bartlett, D. Clinical psychopharmacology of phenelzine: MAO activity and clinical response. In, *Psychopharmacology: A Generation of Progress.* (Lipton, M. A.; DiMascio, A.; and Killam, K. F.; eds.) Raven Press, New York, **1978**, 961–973.

Schildkraut, J. J. The catecholamine hypothesis of affective disorders: a review of the supporting evidence. *Am. J. Psychiatry*, **1965**, *122*, 509–522.

———. Current status of the catecholamine hypothesis of the affective disorders. In, *Psychopharmacology: A Generation of Progress.* (Lipton, M. A.; DiMascio, A.; and Killam, K. F.; eds.) Raven Press, New York, **1978**, pp. 1223–1234.

Schou, M. Biology and pharmacology of the lithium ion. *Pharmacol. Rev.*, **1957**, *9*, 17–58.

———. The biology and pharmacology of lithium: a bibliography. *Psychopharmacol. Bull.*, **1969**, *5*, 33–62.

———. The range of clinical uses of lithium. In, *Lithium in Medical Practice.* (Johnson, F. N., and Johnson, S., eds.) University Park Press, Baltimore, **1978**, pp. 21–39.

Schultes, R. E. Ethnopharmacological significance of psychotropic drugs of vegetal origin. In, *Principles of Psychopharmacology*, 2nd ed. (Clark, W. G., and del Guidice, J., eds.) Academic Press, Inc., New York, **1978**, pp. 41–70.

Schyve, P. M.; Smithline, F.; and Meltzer, H. Y. Neuroleptic-induced prolactin level elevation and breast cancer: an emerging issue. *Arch. Gen. Psychiatry*, **1978**, *35*, 1291–1301.

Seeman, P. The membrane actions of anesthetics and tranquilizers. *Pharmacol. Rev.*, **1972**, *24*, 583–655.

Sepinwall, J., and Cook, L. Behavioral pharmacology of antianxiety drugs. In, *Handbook of Psychopharmacology*, Vol. 13. (Iversen, L. L.; Iversen, S. D.; and Snyder, S. H.; eds.) Plenum Press, New York, **1978**, pp. 345–393.

Shader, R. J. (ed.). *Psychiatric Complications of Medical Drugs.* Raven Press, New York, **1972**.

———. (ed.). *Manual of Psychiatric Therapeutics: Practical Psychopharmacology and Psychiatry.* Little, Brown & Co., Boston, **1975**.

Shader, R. I., and DiMascio, A. *Psychotropic Drug Side Effects: Chemical and Theoretical Perspectives.* The Williams & Wilkins Co., Baltimore, **1970**.

Shore, P. A., and Giachetti, A. Reserpine: basic and clinical pharmacology. In, *Handbook of Psychopharmacology*, Vol. 10. (Iversen, L. L.; Iversen, S. D.; and Snyder, S. H.; eds.) Plenum Press, New York, **1978**, pp. 197–219.

Sigg, E. B. Autonomic side-effects induced by psychotherapeutic agents. In, *Psychopharmacology: A Review of Progress, 1957–1967.* (Efron, D. H.; Cole, J. O.; Levine, J.; and Wittenborn, J. R.; eds.) U.S. Government Printing Office, Washington, D. C., **1968**, pp. 581–588.

Siggins, G. R.; Hoffer, B. J.; Bloom, F. E.; and Ungerstedt, U. Cytochemical and electrophysiological studies of dopamine in the caudate nucleus. In, *The Basal Ganglia.* Association for Research in Nervous and Mental Disease Publications, Vol. 55. (Yahr, M., ed.) Raven Press, New York, **1976**, pp. 227–248.

Spitzer, R. L.; Fleiss, J. L.; and Endicott, J. Problems in classification: reliability and validity. In, *Psychopharmacology: A Generation of Progress.* (Lipton, M. A.; DiMascio, A.; and Killam, K. F.; eds.) Raven Press, New York, **1978**, pp. 857–869.

Sternbach, L. H. Chemistry of 1,5-benzodiazepines and some aspects of the structure-activity relationship. In, *The Benzodiazepines.* (Garattini, S.; Mussini, E.; and Randall, L. O.; eds.) Raven Press, New York, **1973**, pp. 1–26.

Swazey, J. P. *Chlorpromazine in Psychiatry: A Study in Therapeutic Innovation.* M.I.T. Press, Cambridge, Mass., **1974**.

Tallman, J. F.; Paul, S. M.; Skolnick, P.; and Gallager, D. W. Receptors for the age of anxiety: pharmacology of the benzodiazepines. *Science*, **1980**, *207*, 274–281.

Usdin, E. Classification of psychotropic drugs. In, *Principles of Psychopharmacology*, 2nd ed. (Clark, W. G., and del Guidice, J., eds.) Academic Press, Inc., New York, **1978a**, pp. 193–246.

———. (ed.). Symposium on the plasma level monitoring of tricyclic antidepressants. *Comm. Psychopharmacol.*, **1978b**, *2*, 371–456.

Usdin, E., and Efron, D. H. *Psychotropic Drugs and Related Compounds*, 2nd ed. Public Health Service Publication No. 72-9074, U.S. Government Printing Office, Washington, D. C., **1972**.

Van Woert, M. H.; Jutkowitz, R.; Rosenbaum, D.; and Bowers, M. B., Jr. Gilles de la Tourette's syndrome: biochemical approaches. In, *The Basal Ganglia.* Association for Research in Nervous and Mental Disease Publications, Vol. 55. (Yahr, M. D., ed.) Raven Press, New York, **1976**, pp. 459–465.

Vesell, E. S. Pharmacogenetics. *N. Engl. J. Med.*, **1972**, *287*, 904–909.

Weil-Malherbe, H. The biochemistry of the functional psychoses. *Adv. Enzymol.*, **1967**, *29*, 479–553.

Winokur, G.; Clayton, P. J.; and Reich, T. *Manic-Depressive Illness.* C. V. Mosby Co., St. Louis, **1969**.

Wolf, S. The pharmacology of placebos. *Pharmacol. Rev.*, **1959**, *11*, 689–704.

Wyatt, R. J.; Termini, B. A.; and Davis, J. M. Biochemical and sleep studies of schizophrenia. *Schizophr. Bull.*, **1971**, *4*, 10–66.

Zirkle, C. L., and Kaiser, C. Antipsychotic drugs. In, *Medicinal Chemistry*, 2nd ed. (Berger, A., ed.) John Wiley & Sons, Inc., New York, **1970**, pp. 1410–1469.

20 DRUGS EFFECTIVE IN THE THERAPY OF THE EPILEPSIES

Theodore W. Rall and Leonard S. Schleifer

GENERAL CONSIDERATIONS

Classification of Epileptic Seizures. The term *epilepsies* is a collective designation for a group of chronic central nervous system (CNS) disorders having in common the occurrence of sudden and transitory episodes (seizures) of abnormal phenomena of motor (convulsion), sensory, autonomic, or psychic origin. The seizures are nearly always correlated with abnormal and excessive EEG discharges.

The prevalence of epilepsy is between 3 and 6 per 1000 population (Hauser, 1978). The term *primary* or *idiopathic epilepsy* denotes those cases where no cause for the seizures can be identified. *Secondary* or *symptomatic epilepsy* designates the disorder when such factors as trauma, neoplasm, infection, developmental abnormalities, cerebrovascular disease, or various metabolic conditions contribute to the etiology.

For purposes of drug treatment, it is more useful to classify patients according to the type of seizure they experience. A simplified form of the International Classification of Epileptic Seizures (Gastaut, 1970), based on the clinical manifestations of the attacks and the pattern of the EEG, is presented in Table 20–1. Accurate diagnosis is essential, since pharmacotherapy is selective for a particular type of seizure (*see* below). A more complete description of the various types of seizures has been provided by Aird and Woodbury (1974).

Nature and Mechanisms of Seizures. Almost a century ago John Hughlings Jackson, the father of modern concepts of epilepsy, proposed that seizures were caused by "occasional, sudden, excessive, rapid and local discharges of gray matter," and that a generalized convulsion resulted when normal brain tissue was invaded by the seizure activity initiated in the abnormal focus. In the intervening years little has been added to Jackson's concepts except for the electrical proof of their correctness. The EEG amply demonstrates that seizures are in fact electrical explosions of the brain and serves as the basic method of modern differential diagnosis of the epilepsies (Gibbs and Gibbs, 1954, 1964).

Both clinical and EEG observations suggest that seizure activity in most patients with epilepsy has a focal or at least a relatively localized origin (*see* Pedley, 1978). However, there is as yet no definitive explanation of the cause of high-frequency and synchronous firing in a seizure focus. Local biochemical changes, ischemia, and loss of vulnerable small-cell inhibitory systems are among the possible mechanisms. The pathological origins of such foci include congenital defects, head trauma and hypoxia at birth, inflammatory vascular changes subsequent to infectious illnesses of childhood, concussion or depressed skull fracture, abscess, neoplasm, and vascular occlusion of whatever etiology. Although these different lesions have somewhat different predilections for various brain areas, the type of chronic stable focus appears to be similar, and the type of seizure pattern shown by the patient seems more related to the anatomical connections of the focus than to the original etiology.

An abnormal feature of the neuron engaged in seizure activity is the "paroxysmal depolarizing shift" (PDS), often associated with high-frequency bursts of action potentials, loss of inhibitory post-synaptic potentials, and synchronous discharge of other cells of the same columnar group; the PDS correlates well with the familiar, bizarre seizure wave of the gross-surface EEG. Neurons in a chronic-seizure focus exhibit a kind of denervation sensitivity with regard to excitatory stimuli, and may also be relatively lacking in inhibitory input. A factor that may be important in synchronizing cortical neuronal aggregates is the phenomenon termed *backfiring* (*see* Pedley, 1978). In this situation the action potential is initiated ectopically in the axon and then propagates into the cell body. For example, axons of thalamocortical relay cells that project into a cortical epileptic focus can be excited nonsynaptically by substances released in the region of axonal processes—possibly potassium or glutamate. The antidromic firing of a single thalamic relay cell can

Table 20-1. CLASSIFICATION OF EPILEPTIC SEIZURES *

SEIZURE TYPE †		CHARACTERISTICS
I. *Partial Seizures* (Focal Seizures)	A. Partial seizures with elementary symptomatology (*cortical focal*)	Various manifestations, generally without impairment of consciousness, including convulsions confined to a single limb or muscle group (*Jacksonian motor epilepsy*), specific and localized sensory disturbances (*Jacksonian sensory epilepsy*), and other limited signs and symptoms depending upon the particular cortical area producing the abnormal discharge
	B. Partial seizures with complex symptomatology (*temporal lobe, psychomotor*)	Attacks of confused behavior, generally with impairment of consciousness, with a wide variety of clinical manifestations, associated with bizarre generalized EEG activity during the seizure but with evidence of anterior temporal lobe focal abnormalities even in the interseizure period in many cases
	C. Partial seizures secondarily generalized	
II. *Generalized Seizures* (Bilateral, Symmetrical Seizures)	A. Absences (*petit mal*)	Brief and abrupt loss of consciousness associated with high-voltage, bilaterally synchronous, 3-per-second spike-and-wave pattern in the EEG, usually with some symmetrical clonic motor activity varying from eyelid blinking to jerking of the entire body, sometimes with no motor activity
	B. Bilateral massive epileptic myoclonus	Isolated clonic jerks associated with brief bursts of multiple spikes in the EEG
	C. Infantile spasms	Progressive disorder in infants with motor spasms or other convulsive signs, bizarre diffuse changes in the interseizure EEG (hypsarhythmia), and progressive mental deterioration
	D. Clonic seizures	In young children, rhythmic clonic contractions of all muscles, loss of consciousness, and marked autonomic manifestations
	E. Tonic seizures	In young children, opisthotonus, loss of consciousness, and marked autonomic manifestations
	F. Tonic-clonic seizures (*grand mal*)	Major convulsions, usually a sequence of maximal tonic spasm of all body musculature followed by synchronous clonic jerking and a prolonged depression of all central functions
	G. Atonic seizures	Loss of postural tone, with sagging of the head or falling
	H. Akinetic seizures	Impairment of consciousness and complete relaxation of all musculature, secondary to excessive inhibitory discharge

* Modified from the International Classification of Epileptic Seizures (Gastaut, 1970).

† Some classifications include unilateral seizures as a distinct category. Additional seizure types are presently unclassified due to incomplete data.

influence large numbers of cortical cells and could represent a powerful mechanism for recurrent excitation.

Various experimental models have been used by investigators to study the nature and mechanisms of seizures (see Symposium, 1972b). Application of alumina cream to the motor cortex of the monkey creates an epileptogenic focus that causes chronically recurring, spontaneous seizures of focal onset; this experimental model resembles human focal epilepsy in many ways (see Ward, in Symposium, 1969, 1972b). In such models and also in man, anatomical and neurophysiological studies suggest that "epileptic" neurons are responsible for initiating seizure discharges. Although many cases of human focal epilepsy are associated with areas of local glial scarring similar to the lesions produced in the vicinity of instillation of alumina cream, some patients with focal epilepsy have no demonstrable pathological changes (see Pedley, 1978). Further, it has been repeatedly shown that independent secondary epileptic foci develop in areas that are richly innervated by efferents from a primary lesion produced by alumina cream (see Wilder, in Symposium, 1972b). These secondary foci persist after the surgical removal of the primary focus and are not associated with any consistent changes in histological characteristics.

A more recent and potentially very useful experimental model for human focal epilepsy is that produced in a variety of animal species by a procedure termed kindling (see Symposium, 1976). This involves delivery of brief, localized trains of electrical stimuli to various areas of the brain at widely spaced intervals, optimally of about 24 hours. With time, progressively longer and more intense periods of afterdischarge are produced at sites both near to and remote from the point of stimulation. Ultimately, motor seizures, characterized by loss of balance and generalized clonic jerking (myoclonus), can be regularly elicited even when many months have elapsed between stimulations. Although spontaneous, chronically recurring seizures are not produced, "kindled" animals are much more sensitive to a variety of convulsive stimuli, both chemical and sensory. As in the model produced by application of alumina cream, histologically normal, secondary epileptic foci are found that persist after destruction of the original site of stimulation, and interictal, spontaneous focal discharges can be detected. Kindling may account in part for the delay between hypoxic or traumatic insult to the CNS and the onset of overt seizures, as well as for the sometimes-progressive character of human epilepsy.

Other experimental models utilize animals that are genetically susceptible to convulsive seizures precipitated by appropriate sensory stimuli (see Symposium, 1972b). These include audiogenic seizures in certain strains of mice and seizures elicited by intermittent photic stimulation, prevalent in a specific group of baboons. While these may be appropriate models for cases of evoked epilepsy in man, they may be more significant for calling attention to inherited factors that are suspected to play a role in the genesis of human epilepsy.

A seizure focus in man may remain quiescent over long periods of time, discharging only intermittently as revealed by EEG analysis, and may cause no signs or symptoms. The spread of convulsive activity to neighboring normal cells is presumably restrained by normal inhibitory mechanisms. However, physiological changes that cannot in themselves cause seizures may trigger the focus or facilitate spread of abnormal electrical activity to normal tissue. Among such factors are changes in blood glucose concentration, blood gas tensions, plasma pH, and total osmotic pressure and electrolyte composition of extracellular fluid; endocrine changes, fatigue, emotional stress, and nutritional deficiencies may also contribute. Many factors can interact to precipitate seizures in a brain predisposed by injury or inherited defect, and the physician should not be perplexed when some patients with seemingly identical seizure patterns respond quite differently to drug therapy.

Given a seizure focus and suitable precipitating circumstances, the abnormal activity may, as mentioned, spread to normal brain tissue. If the spread is sufficiently extensive, the entire brain is activated and a tonic-clonic convulsion with unconsciousness ensues. If the spread is localized, the seizure produces signs and symptoms characteristic of the anatomical focus. More distant areas and centers may be driven indirectly without themselves participating in the production of high-frequency seizure discharges, but with disruption of their normal function. For example, a driving focus is suggested by the characteristic dysrhythmia of the cortical EEG (3-per-second spike and wave) and the associated unconsciousness of absence seizures, which disappear as abruptly as they began with no evidence of cortical postseizure fatigue.

Once initiated, a seizure is undoubtedly maintained by reentry of excitatory impulses in a closed feedback pathway that need not include the original seizure focus. Contributing to the self-limitation and eventual abrupt collapse of the seizure are the elevated threshold and prolonged refractoriness that result from hyperactivity, and also inhibition from pathways external to the seizure loop. Metabolic factors, such as accumulation of carbon dioxide and adenosine and depletion of oxygen and high-energy phosphate intermediates, may also contribute to self-limitation of seizure discharge.

Mechanisms of Action of Antiepileptic Agents. There are two general ways in which drugs might abolish or attenuate seizures: effects on pathologically altered neurons of seizure foci to prevent or reduce their excessive discharge, and effects that would reduce the spread of excitation from seizure foci and prevent detonation and disruption of function of normal aggregates of neurons. Most, if not all, antiepileptic agents that are presently available act at least in part by the second mechanism, since all modify the ability of the brain to respond to various seizure-evoking stimuli. A variety of neuro-physiological effects of such drugs have been noted, including reduction of Na^+ or Ca^{2+} fluxes, potentiation of presynaptic or post-synaptic inhibition, reduction of posttetanic potentiation (PTP), and reduction of evoked responses in various monosynaptic or poly-synaptic pathways. However, it must be admitted that mechanisms of action of anti-epileptic agents are only poorly understood. All of these effects generally embarrass normal functions of the brain, leading to undesired side effects. Investigators frequently fail to define those neurophysiological effects that might be prominent at therapeutic concentrations or those that are not characteristic of local anesthetics or sedatives. Useful antiepileptic agents may be capable of causing some mixture of mutually reinforcing actions that permits therapeutic responses without undue disruption of normal function. With these general considerations in mind, the more plausible hypotheses of the action of antiepileptic agents will be discussed in the sections that deal with the individual drugs.

Chemical Structure and Antiepileptic Selectivity. The useful antiepileptic agents belong to several chemical classes, and experimental compounds are even more diverse in structure (*see* Krall *et al.*, 1978b). Most of the drugs introduced before 1965 are closely related in structure to phenobarbital, the oldest member of this therapeutic class. These include the hydantoins, the deoxybarbiturates, the oxazolidinediones, and the succinimides. The agents introduced after 1965 include benzodiazepines (*clonazepam*), an iminostilbene (*carbamazepine*), and a branched-chain carboxylic acid (*valproic acid*). The structure-activity relationships of these and other classes of compounds are summarized by Close and Spielman (1961), Murray and Kier (1977), Popp (1977), and Vida and Gerry (1977).

The laboratory screening tests for potential anti-epileptic drugs have relied heavily on the capacity to modify the effects of maximal electric shock (inhibition of tonic hindlimb extension) and to elevate the dose of pentylenetetrazol required to precipitate tonic-clonic convulsions; this emphasis persists today after about 40 years of investigation (*see* Krall *et al.*, 1978a). While the former test usually predicts activity against generalized tonic-clonic and cortical focal convulsions and the latter against absence seizures, there are a number of important exceptions to this generalization. In addition, some agents that can modify convulsions produced by maximal electric shock without appreciable effect on the threshold dose of pentylenetetrazol have been found to suppress absence seizures and to exacerbate tonic-clonic

convulsions in patients (*see* Fromm *et al.*, 1978). These and other observations indicate the need for continued development of model systems for the detection and evaluation of potential therapeutic agents.

Therapeutic Aspects. The ideal antiepileptic drug would obviously suppress all seizures without causing any unwanted effects. Unfortunately, the drugs used currently not only fail to control seizure activity in some patients, but they frequently cause side effects that range in severity from minimal impairment of the CNS to death from aplastic anemia. The physician who treats patients with epilepsy is thus faced with the task of selecting the appropriate drug or combination of drugs that best controls seizures in an individual patient at an acceptable level of untoward effects. It is generally held that complete control of seizures can be achieved in up to 50% of patients and possibly another 25% can be improved significantly (*see* Meinardi *et al.*, 1977). The *degree of success* is largely dependent on the type of seizure and the extent of associated neurological abnormalities (*see* below).

For the purposes of drug therapy the classification of seizures given above may be further condensed. *Absence* (petit mal) seizures respond well to one group of drugs, and *generalized tonic-clonic* (grand mal) and *cortical focal* convulsions are usually adequately controlled by another. *Temporal lobe* (psychomotor) seizures tend to be refractory to therapy and respond only to some of the agents in the second group. *Infantile* myoclonus and the types of epilepsy that occur in *young children* represent a group for which therapy is generally unsatisfactory. Multiple-drug therapy is often required, since two or more seizure types may occur in the same patient. Generalized tonic-clonic seizures are common in patients with other minor types of attack, since the grand mal convulsion is essentially the invasion of the entire brain by convulsive activity restrained to limited foci and pathways in all other lesser seizure types.

The general principles of the drug therapy of the epilepsies are summarized below, following discussion of the individual agents. Details of diagnosis and therapy can be found in the monographs and reviews listed at the end of the chapter.

Plasma Concentrations of Antiepileptic Drugs. Measurement of drug concentrations in plasma greatly facilitates antiepileptic medication, especially multiple-drug therapy (Symposium, 1972a; Aird and Woodbury, 1974). However, the physician must recognize that recommended concentrations are only guidelines for therapy. Thus, for some drugs clinical effects correlate well with their concentrations in plasma, but for others the correlation is extremely poor. Contributing to this problem is the variability that has been noted in the chemical analysis of certain compounds, and a concerted effort is being made to make these measurements more reliable (*see* Symposium, 1978b). Another difficulty is that the values determined usually represent total concentrations in plasma. Many antiepileptic drugs are highly bound to plasma proteins; the concentration of free drug is only a small fraction of the total and may be variable. Plasma drug concentrations recommended for maintenance antiepileptic therapy, as well as other pharmacokinetic characteristics essential for interpretation of measured concentrations and for devising drug dosage schedules, are discussed with the individual agents and in Appendix II. The value of monitoring plasma concentrations of the antiepileptic agents is discussed further at the end of the chapter.

HYDANTOINS

PHENYTOIN (DIPHENYLHYDANTOIN)

Phenytoin (diphenylhydantoin) is a primary drug for all types of epilepsy except absence seizures. It has been more thoroughly studied in the laboratory and clinic than any other antiepileptic agent.

History. Phenytoin was first synthesized in 1908 by Biltz, but its anticonvulsant activity was not discovered until 1938 (Merritt and Putnam, 1938a). In contrast to the earlier accidental discovery of the anticonvulsant properties of bromide and phenobarbital, phenytoin was the product of a search among nonsedative structural relatives of phenobarbital for agents capable of suppressing electroshock convulsions in laboratory animals. It was introduced for the symptomatic treatment of epilepsy in the same year (Merritt and Putnam, 1938b). The discovery of phenytoin was a signal advance. Since this agent is not a sedative in ordinary doses, it established that antiepileptics need not impair consciousness; and since, unlike phenobarbital, the drug is effective in some cases of temporal lobe epilepsy, it encouraged the search for basic differences between the various convulsive disorders and for drugs with selective anticonvulsant action.

Structure-Activity Relationship. Phenytoin has the following structural formula:

Phenytoin

A 5-phenyl or other aromatic substituent appears essential for activity against clinical generalized tonic-clonic seizures and for abolition of the maximal electroshock seizure pattern in laboratory animals. Alkyl substituents in position 5 contribute to sedation, a property absent in phenytoin. The 5 carbon permits asymmetry, as in mephenytoin, but there appears to be little difference in activity between isomers. (*See* Toman and Goodman, 1948; Close and Spielman, 1961; Vida and Gerry, 1977.)

Pharmacological Effects. *Central Nervous System.* Phenytoin exerts antiepileptic activity without causing general depression of the CNS. In toxic doses it may produce excitatory signs and at lethal levels a type of decerebrate rigidity. The most easily demonstrated properties of phenytoin are its ability to limit the development of maximal seizure activity and to reduce the spread of the seizure process from an active focus. Both features are undoubtedly related to its clinical usefulness. Phenytoin can induce complete remission of generalized tonic-clonic and certain other partial seizures but does not completely eliminate the sensory aura or other prodromal signs.

The anticonvulsant properties of phenytoin have been reviewed by Toman and Goodman (1948) and Woodbury (Symposium, 1969). Unlike phenobarbital, phenytoin does not elevate the threshold for seizures induced by injection of such convulsant drugs as strychnine, picrotoxin, or pentylenetetrazol. It also has only limited ability to elevate threshold for electroshock seizures. Phenytoin does, however, restore abnormally increased excitability toward normal.

Probably the most significant effect of phenytoin is its ability to modify the pattern of maximal electroshock seizures. The characteristic tonic phase can be abolished completely, but the residual clonic seizure may be exaggerated and prolonged. The drug produces similar alterations in the convulsions of psychiatric patients undergoing electroconvulsive therapy (Toman *et al.,* 1947) and in maximal seizures induced in animals by picrotoxin and pentylenetetrazol. This seizure-modifying action is observed also with other typical antiepileptics effective against generalized tonic-clonic seizures.

In various species, as revealed by a variety of stimulation-recording technics, the ability of phenytoin to reduce the duration of afterdischarge and to limit the spread of seizure activity is more prominent than its effect on threshold for stimulation. Moreover, elevation of threshold is relatively selective for the cerebral cortex and hippocampus. Morrell and coworkers (1959) noted that phenytoin was superior to phenobarbital in blocking cortical spread of focal seizure activity but inferior to the barbiturate in suppressing focal activity. They considered these differences significant to their clinical efficacy. In addition, concentrations of phenytoin within the therapeutic range have been found to reduce cortical potentials evoked by delivery of paired stimuli to thalamic nuclei (Englander *et al.,* 1977). This effect was noted over a range of pulse intervals without appreciable change in the threshold for stimulation.

An *excitatory* effect on the cerebellum, to activate inhibitory pathways that extend to the cerebral cortex, has been suggested to contribute to the anticonvulsant effect of phenytoin. Halpern and Julien (1972) and Julien and Halpern (1972) noted that reduction of seizure activity in a cortical epileptogenic focus by the drug was associated with increased cerebellar Purkinje-cell discharge. After cerebellectomy, cortical focal seizure activity increased and phenytoin was less effective. While chronic electrical stimulation of the cerebellum has been used in the treatment of intractable epilepsy (*see* Symposium, 1978a), the results have been inconclusive (Van Buren *et al.,* 1978). The effects of cerebellar stimulation on thalamocortical excitability can be distinguished qualitatively and quantitatively from those of phenytoin (Englander *et al.,* 1977; Johnson *et al.,* 1979). Thus, the participation of cerebellar excitation in the antiepileptic action of phenytoin remains to be established. The effects of the drug in developing animals are also of interest. In the early postnatal period, phenytoin has predominantly excitatory effects on the CNS (Vernadakis and Woodbury, 1969, and in Symposium, 1969). These excitatory effects become less prominent and the anticonvulsant effects more consistent as the animal develops, in parallel with maturation of postsynaptic inhibitory systems.

Phenytoin reduces PTP of synaptic transmission in the spinal cord and stellate ganglion of the cat (Esplin, 1957). Since PTP could facilitate the spread of seizure activity emanating from foci that discharge periodically, this action of phenytoin has long been considered crucial in its therapeutic effect. However, the doses used in the animal studies were high, and it is difficult to estimate the extent to which suppression of PTP is involved in the antiepileptic effects of the drug.

Mechanism of Action. A stabilizing effect of phenytoin is apparent on all neuronal membranes, including those of peripheral nerves, and probably on all excitable as well as nonexcitable membranes (*see* Woodbury, in Symposium, 1969; *see also* Chapter 31). There is considerable evidence that this effect, as well as those on PTP and synaptic transmission, result directly or indirectly from effects on the movement of ions across cell membranes. In a variety of systems, phenytoin has been observed to decrease resting fluxes of sodium ions as well as sodium currents that flow during action potentials or chemically induced depolarizations (*see* Ayala and Johnston, 1977). In addition, influx of calcium ion during depolarization is decreased, either independently or as a consequence of reduced intracellular concentration of sodium. Phenytoin can also delay the activation of outward potassium current during an action potential, leading to an increased refractory period and a decrease in repetitive firing (*see* Ayala and Johnston, 1977). Although these ionic effects can usually be distinguished both quantitatively and qualitatively from those produced by local anesthetics, they seldom have been demonstrated at concentrations of phenytoin at or below 10 μM, the maximal plasma concentration of free drug that usually can be tolerated during therapy.

Absorption, Distribution, Biotransformation, and Excretion.

The pharmacokinetic characteristics of phenytoin are markedly influenced by its limited aqueous solubility and its dose-dependent elimination. Its inactivation by the hepatic microsomal enzyme system is susceptible to inhibition by other drugs.

Phenytoin is a weak acid with a pK_a of about 8.3; its aqueous solubility is limited, even in the intestine. Upon intramuscular injection, the drug precipitates at the injection site and is slowly absorbed, as if it had been administered in a repository preparation.

Absorption of phenytoin after oral ingestion is slow, sometimes variable, and occasionally incomplete. Significant differences in bioavailability of oral pharmaceutical preparations have been detected (Melikian *et al.,* 1977). Peak concentration after a single dose may occur in plasma as early as 2 hours or as late as 6 hours. Slow absorption during chronic medication blunts the fluctuations of drug concentration between doses.

Phenytoin is extensively (about 90%) bound to plasma proteins, mainly albumin (Booker and Darcey, 1973). A greater fraction remains unbound in the neonate, in patients with hypoalbuminemia, and in uremic patients (Reidenberg *et al.,* 1971). The drug is widely distributed in all tissues. Fractional binding in tissues, including brain, is about the same as in plasma. Thus, its apparent volume of distribution is about 64% of body weight, but would be about seven times larger if calculated on the basis of unbound drug. Concentration in the cerebrospinal fluid (CSF) is equal to the unbound fraction in plasma.

Approximately 2% of phenytoin is excreted unchanged in the urine. The remainder is metabolized primarily by the hepatic microsomal enzymes. The major metabolite, the parahydroxyphenyl derivative, is inactive. It accounts for 60 to 70% of a single dose of the drug and a somewhat smaller fraction during chronic medication. It is excreted initially in the bile and subsequently in the urine, in large part as the glucuronide. Other apparently inactive metabolites include the dihydroxy catechol and its 3-methoxy derivative, and the dihydrodiol. At plasma concentrations below 10 μg/ml, elimination is exponential (first order); plasma half-time averages about 24 hours but varies at least fourfold. At higher concentrations, dose-dependent elimination is apparent; plasma half-time increases with concentration (dose), perhaps because the hydroxylation reaction approaches saturation or is inhibited by the metabolites. A genetically determined limitation in ability to metabolize phenytoin has been detected (Kutt *et al.,* 1964). (*See* Dill *et al.,* 1956; Arnold and Gerber, 1970; Chang *et al.,* 1970, 1972; Symposium, 1972a; Glazko, 1973.)

Toxicity. The toxic effects of phenytoin depend upon the route and duration of exposure as well as dosage. When it is administered intravenously at an excessive rate in the emergency treatment of cardiac arrhythmias or status epilepticus, the most notable toxic signs are *cardiovascular collapse* and/or *CNS depression.* Acute overdosage by the oral route features primarily signs referable to the cerebellum and vestibular system. Toxic effects associated with chronic medication are also primarily dose-related *cerebellar-vestibular effects* but include *other CNS effects, behavioral changes, increased frequency of seizures, gastrointestinal symptoms, gingival hyperplasia, osteomalacia,* and *megaloblastic anemia. Hirsutism* is an annoying untoward effect in young females. These phenomena can usually be made bearable by proper adjustment of dosage and do not usually interfere with therapy. Serious adverse effects, including those on the skin, bone marrow, and liver, are probably manifestations of *drug allergy.* Although rare, they necessitate withdrawal of the drug.

The toxicity of phenytoin has been extensively reviewed in a symposium (1972a).

Central nervous system toxicity is the most consistent effect of phenytoin overdosage. *Nystagmus, ataxia, diplopia,* and *vertigo* and other cerebellar-vestibular effects are common. *Blurred vision, mydri-*

asis, and *hyperactive tendon reflexes* also occur. *Behavioral* effects include *hyperactivity, silliness, confusion, dullness, drowsiness,* and *hallucinations. Peripheral neuropathy,* sometimes with absent tendon reflexes, has been reported in 7 to 30% of patients, particularly the elderly, who have received the drug in high dosage for many years. The relationship to cyanocobalamin metabolism remains uncertain (*see* Symposium, 1972a). Cerebellar Purkinje cells exhibit damage following high doses of phenytoin only in the presence of concurrent hypoxia (Dam, 1972; Symposium, 1972a).

Gingival hyperplasia occurs in about 20% of all patients during chronic therapy and is probably the most common manifestation of phenytoin toxicity in children and young adolescents. The overgrowth of tissue appears to involve altered collagen metabolism (Symposium, 1972a; Hassell *et al.,* 1976). Toothless portions of the gums are not affected. The condition does not necessarily require withdrawal of medication, and it can be minimized by good oral hygiene.

Gastrointestinal disturbances, including *nausea, vomiting, epigastric pain,* and *anorexia,* can be reduced by taking the drug with meals or in more frequent divided doses.

A variety of *endocrine* effects have been reported. Inhibition of release of *antidiuretic hormone* (ADH) has been observed in patients with inappropriate ADH secretion. *Hyperglycemia* and *glycosuria* appear to be due to inhibition of insulin secretion (Kiser *et al.,* 1970; Levin *et al.,* 1970). *Osteomalacia,* with hypocalcemia and elevated alkaline phosphatase activity, has been attributed to both altered metabolism of vitamin D and inhibition of intestinal absorption of calcium (Symposium, 1972a). This condition is relatively resistant to vitamin D administration.

Hypersensitivity reactions include *morbilliform rash* in 2 to 5% of patients and occasionally more serious skin reactions, including *Stevens-Johnson syndrome. Systemic lupus erythematosus* and potentially fatal *hepatic necrosis* have been reported rarely. *Hematological* reactions include *neutropenia, leukopenia, thrombocytopenia, agranulocytosis,* and *aplastic anemia. Megaloblastic anemia* has been attributed to altered folate absorption but probably also involves altered folate metabolism (Symposium, 1972a). It is rare and responds to administration of folic acid. Similar effects have been reported during medication with phenobarbital, primidone, and mephenytoin. *Lymphadenopathy,* resembling Hodgkin's disease and malignant lymphoma, is associated with reduced immunoglobulin A (IgA) production (Sorrell *et al.,* 1971). *Hypoprothrombinemia* and *hemorrhage* have occurred in the newborn of mothers who received phenytoin during pregnancy; vitamin K is effective treatment or prophylaxis.

Preparations, Routes of Administration, and Dosage. *Phenytoin Sodium,* U.S.P. (*diphenylhydantoin sodium;* DILANTIN), is available as 30- and 100-mg capsules for oral use, and as a sterile solution of 50 mg/ml, with a special solvent, for parenteral use. Preparations of *Phenytoin,* U.S.P., include 50-mg tablets and oral suspensions containing 30 mg/5 ml or 125 mg/5 ml. There are significant differences in bioavailability among various preparations of phenytoin, and patients should thus be treated with the drug product of a single manufacturer (*see* Melikian *et al.,* 1977).

Choice and adjustment of the dosage of phenytoin and interpretation of measured concentrations of the drug in plasma must be dominated by recognition of the dose-dependent kinetics of elimination of the drug. As dosage is increased, plasma half-life and the time required to attain the plateau state increase. Plasma drug concentration increases disproportionately as dosage is increased. Several investigators have attempted to provide methods for prediction of the plasma concentration obtained with a given regimen. The dose-dependent elimination of phenytoin can be described in terms of a Michaelis-Menten model. Unfortunately, the kinetic constants vary widely between individuals, and nomograms are thus of limited usefulness. Alternatively, data from an individual patient can be used to determine the kinetic parameters for that subject (*see* Mullen, 1978; Appendix II).

Initial daily dosage for adults is 3 to 4 mg/kg (100 mg, twice daily). Dosage is subsequently increased, preferably with monitoring of plasma concentration, as needed for control of seizures or as limited by toxicity. Increments in dosage may be made at 1-week intervals at low dosage but at 2-week intervals when dosage exceeds 300 mg daily. Doses greater than 500 mg daily are rarely tolerated if taken regularly. Because of its relatively long half-life and slow absorption, a single daily dose is often satisfactory for adults, but gastric intolerance may dictate divided dosage. Divided dosage is recommended for children (4 to 7 mg/kg per day). If loading dosage is deemed necessary, 600 to 1000 mg, in divided portions over 8 to 12 hours, will provide effective plasma concentrations within 24 hours in most patients.

Intravenous administration of phenytoin should not exceed 50 mg per minute. A slower rate is preferred, especially in elderly patients. Intramuscular administration is not recommended.

Plasma Drug Concentrations. A good correlation is usually observed between the total concentration of phenytoin in plasma and the clinical effect. Thus, control of seizures is generally obtained with concentrations above 10 μg/ml, while toxic effects such as nystagmus develop around 20 μg/ml. Ataxia is apparent at 30 μg/ml and lethargy at about 40 μg/ml.

The degree of protein binding of phenytoin and, therefore, the concentration of drug that is free in plasma at any given total concentration vary from patient to patient. Such factors can confuse interpretation of measured concentrations of the drug. In a series of 25 patients studied by Booker and Darcey (1973), clinical signs of toxicity correlated far better with the concentration of unbound phenytoin than with that of the total.

Drug Interactions. Well-documented *increase* in the concentration of phenytoin in plasma, by inhibition of its inactivation, has occurred during concurrent administration of *chloramphenicol, dicumarol, disulfiram, isoniazid,* or certain *sulfonamides.* Less well-documented or variable increase has been reported for a variety of other drugs. Inhibition of inactivation of phenytoin should be suspected for other agents that are also hydroxylated by the microsomal enzyme system. *Sulfisoxazole, phenylbutazone,* and possibly *salicylates* can *increase* effective concentrations of phenytoin by competing for plasma-protein binding sites.

A well-documented *decrease* in phenytoin concentration is caused by *carbamazepine,* which may enhance the metabolism of phenytoin. Conversely, the concentration of carbamazepine may be reduced by phenytoin. There is some evidence that chronic administration of *folate* can decrease the effectiveness of phenytoin either by inhibiting drug absorption or by a direct antagonism of the central antiepileptic effects of phenytoin.

Interaction between phenytoin and *phenobarbital* is variable. Phenobarbital may increase the biotransformation of phenytoin, by induction of the hepatic microsomal enzyme system, but may also decrease its inactivation, apparently by competitive inhibition. In addition, phenobarbital may reduce the oral absorption of phenytoin. Conversely, the phenobarbital concentration is sometimes increased by phenytoin. *Ethanol* has similar opposing effects on the inactivation of phenytoin.

Phenytoin has been demonstrated to enhance the metabolism of *corticosteroids.* The suggested mechanism for this effect is an induction of metabolizing enzymes, although phenytoin is only a weak inducer of the hepatic microsomal enzyme system in man.

Therapeutic Uses. *Epilepsy.* Phenytoin is one of the more widely used antiepileptic agents, and it is effective in most forms of epilepsy except absence seizures. The use of phenytoin and other agents in the therapy of epilepsies is discussed further at the end of the chapter.

Other Uses. Phenytoin has been used with variable results for the treatment of *disturbed nonepileptic psychotic patients.* A favorable response is more likely when there is initially an abnormal EEG, especially when the abnormality is of a paroxysmal type that suggests that an underlying seizure mechanism is disrupting normal behavior. Some cases of *trigeminal and related neuralgias* respond well to phenytoin, but carbamazepine is the preferred agent. The use of phenytoin in the treatment of *cardiac arrhythmias* is discussed in Chapter 31.

OTHER HYDANTOINS

Mephenytoin. *Mephenytoin,* U.S.P. (MESANTOIN), 3-methyl-5,5-phenylethylhydantoin, is N-demethylated to NIRVANOL (Butler, 1953). This metabolite was employed clinically in the 1920s but was abandoned because of a high incidence of serious toxicity. The metabolite probably accounts, at least in part, for the therapeutic benefit and toxicity of chronic medication with mephenytoin.

Pharmacological Effects. Mephenytoin is active in most anticonvulsant tests in animals (Toman *et al.,* 1947; Goodman *et al.,* 1948; Brown *et al.,* 1953). Like phenytoin, it inhibits PTP. Unlike phenytoin, it antagonizes pentylenetetrazol, elevates seizure threshold, and is a sedative. Also unlike phenytoin, mephenytoin is rapidly absorbed after oral administraton. Its N-demethylation and the subsequent inactivation of the metabolite by hydroxylation are catalyzed by the hepatic microsomal enzymes.

Therapeutic Uses and Toxicity. Mephenytoin was introduced in 1945 for the treatment of epilepsy (*see* Loscalzo, 1952). Its antiepileptic spectrum is the same as that of phenytoin, and it may exacerbate absence seizures. Very limited pharmacokinetic information is available (Plaa and Hine, 1960). A half-life of 144 hours in patients previously unexposed to the drug has been reported (*see* Troupin *et al.,* 1976). Although sometimes dramatically superior to phenytoin therapeutically (Lennox and Lennox, 1960), this advantage is offset by its toxicity. Mephenytoin causes significantly less ataxia, gingival hyperplasia, gastric distress, and hirsutism than does phenytoin and less sedation than does phenobarbital. However, serious toxicity is common. These adverse effects include morbilliform rash (in 10% of patients), fever, lymphadenopathy, leukopenia, pancytopenia, agranulocytosis, hepatotoxicity, periarteritis nodosa, and lupus erythematosus. Death attributed to aplastic anemia has occurred. Acute overdosage results in coma.

Well-controlled studies of the usefulness of mephenytoin in epilepsy have not been performed. However, a recent retrospective study suggests it is useful in the prevention of focal seizures and that effective concentrations in plasma may approximate 25 to 40 μg/ml (*see* Troupin *et al.,* 1976). When mephenytoin is used, it is generally concurrently with other agents, in the lowest dose possible, and only in patients who fail to respond to or do not tolerate safer agents. Because of its sedative effects, mephenytoin is more rationally employed concurrently with phenytoin than with phenobarbital or primidone.

Preparations and Dosage. Typical daily dosage is 300 to 600 mg in adults and 100 to 400 mg in children. The drug is available in 100-mg tablets.

Ethotoin. *Ethotoin* (PEGANONE) is 3-ethyl-5-phenylhydantoin. Introduced by Schwade and co-workers (1956), it appeared to be of some value in the treatment of temporal lobe as well as generalized tonic-clonic seizures and to be relatively free of the typical adverse effects of phenytoin. However, because of its low efficacy, it is employed only occasionally, mostly as an adjunct to other agents, in the therapy of generalized tonic-clonic seizures. The usual daily dose for adults is 2 to 3 g. Ethotoin is available in 250- and 500-mg tablets.

Skin rash, gastrointestinal distress, and drowsiness are the common adverse effects of ethotoin. Lymphadenopathy has also been reported. Metabolites, produced by the hepatic microsomal enzymes, include the N-dealkyl and parahydroxyphenyl derivatives.

ANTICONVULSANT BARBITURATES

The pharmacology of the barbiturates as a class is considered in Chapter 17; discussion in this chapter is limited to the three barbiturates employed for therapy of the epilepsies.

PHENOBARBITAL

Phenobarbital was the first effective organic antiepileptic agent (Hauptmann, 1912). It has relatively low toxicity, is inexpensive, and is still one of the more effective and widely used drugs for this purpose.

Structure-Activity Relationship. The structural formula of phenobarbital is shown in Table 17–3 (page 351). The structure-activity relationship of the barbiturates has been studied extensively and summarized by Vida and Gerry (1977). Maximal anticonvulsant activity is obtained when one substituent at position 5 is a phenyl group. The 5,5-diphenyl derivative has less anticonvulsant potency than phenobarbital but is virtually devoid of hypnotic activity. By contrast, 5,5-dibenzyl barbituric acid causes convulsions.

Anticonvulsant Properties. Most barbiturates have anticonvulsant properties. However, the capacity of some of these agents, such as phenobarbital, to exert maximal anticonvulsant action at doses below those required for hypnosis determines their clinical utility as antiepileptics. Phenobarbital is active in most anticonvulsant tests in animals but is relatively nonselective. It limits the spread of seizure activity and also elevates seizure threshold. Some of its actions in animal models and screening tests are discussed above.

The ability of some barbiturates to be selective anticonvulsants suggests that different mechanisms of action are involved in the anticonvulsant and hypnotic effects. Unfortunately, most electrophysiological studies have failed to distinguish between anticonvulsant and hypnotic barbiturates. Recently, Macdonald and Barker (1979a) examined the electrophysiological effects of various barbiturates in dissociated cell cultures of mammalian spinal cord neurons. Barbiturates that display clinical anticonvulsant activity only at hypnotic doses exerted a gamma-aminobutyric acid (GABA)–like effect and caused an augmentation of the postsynaptic inhibitory responses to GABA. In contrast, the useful anticonvulsant barbiturates, such as phenobarbital and mephobarbital, failed to exhibit GABA-like effects at concentrations where augmentation of postsynaptic responses to GABA was observed. These observations suggest that the ability of anticonvulsants to reduce the spread of seizures may depend on the potentiation of inhibitory pathways that are recruited during discharge of epileptogenic foci; sedation, on the other hand, may be a consequence of more generalized stimulation of receptors for GABA.

Absorption, Distribution, Biotransformation, and Excretion. Oral absorption of phenobarbital is complete but somewhat slow; peak concentrations in plasma occur several hours after a single dose. It is 40 to 60% bound to plasma proteins and bound to a similar extent in tissues, including brain. The volume of distribution is approximately 0.9 liter per kilogram. Up to 25% of phenobarbital is eliminated by pH-dependent renal excretion; the remainder is inactivated by the hepatic microsomal enzymes. The major metabolite, the parahydroxyphenyl derivative, is inactive and is excreted in the urine partly as the sulfate conjugate (Butler, 1956). The plasma half-life of phenobarbital is about 90 hours in adults and somewhat shorter and more variable in children.

Toxicity. The adverse effects of phenobarbital have been reviewed by Browning and Maynert (Symposium, 1972a). *Sedation,* the most frequent undesired effect of phenobarbital, is apparent to some extent in all patients upon initiation of therapy, but tolerance develops during chronic medication. *Nystagmus* and *ataxia* occur at excessive dosage. Phenobarbital sometimes produces *irritability* and *hyperactivity* in children and *confusion* in the elderly.

Scarlatiniform or *morbilliform rash,* possibly with other manifestations of drug allergy, occurs in 1 to 2% of patients. Fatal *exfoliative dermatitis* is rare. *Hypoprothrombinemia* with hemorrhage has been observed in the newborn of mothers who have received phenobarbital during pregnancy; vitamin K is effective for treatment or prophylaxis. *Megaloblastic anemia* that responds to folate and *osteomalacia* that responds to high doses of vitamin D occur during chronic phenobarbital therapy of epilepsy, as they do during phenytoin medication. Other adverse effects of phenobarbital are discussed in Chapter 17.

Preparations, Routes of Administration, and Dosage. *Phenobarbital,* U.S.P., and *Phenobarbital Sodium,* U.S.P., are available in a variety of dosage forms for oral and parenteral use. The usual daily dose for *adults* is 1 to 5 mg/kg (60 to 200 mg). Since plasma half-time averages 90 hours, weeks are required to attain the plateau state. Double dosage for the initial 4 days provides an effective plasma drug concentration more promptly, but sedation will be prominent. The usual initial daily dose for *children* is 3 to 6 mg/kg, in two divided portions. Dosage is subsequently increased or adjusted, as required for control of seizures or as limited by toxicity.

Plasma Drug Concentrations. During chronic medication in adults, plasma concentration of phenobarbital averages 10 μg/ml per daily dose of 1 mg/kg; in children, the value is 5 to 7 μg/ml per 1 mg/kg. Although higher concentrations are frequently maintained, particularly in institutionalized patients with refractory seizures, plasma concentrations of 10 to 25 μg/ml are usually recommended for control of epilepsy; 15 μg/ml is the minimum for prophylaxis against febrile convulsions. Whether tolerance develops to the antiepileptic effects of phenobarbital is uncertain.

The relationship between plasma concentration of phenobarbital and adverse effects varies with the development of tolerance. Sedation, nystagmus, and ataxia are usually absent at concentrations below 30 μg/ml during chronic medication, but adverse effects may be apparent for several days at lower concentrations when therapy is initiated or whenever dosage is increased. Concentrations greater than 60 μg/ml may be associated with marked intoxication in the nontolerant individual.

Since significant behavioral toxicity may be present despite the absence of overt signs of toxicity, the tendency to maintain patients, particularly children, on excessively high doses of phenobarbital should be resisted. Plasma phenobarbital concentration should be increased above 30 to 40 μg/ml only if the increment is adequately tolerated and only if it contributes significantly to seizure control. (*See* Svensmark and Buchthal, 1963; Buchthal *et al.,* 1968; Buchthal and Svensmark, 1971; Symposium, 1972a.)

Drug Interactions. Interactions between phenobarbital and other drugs usually involve induction of the hepatic microsomal enzyme system by phenobarbital (*see* Chapters 1 and 17). The variable interaction with phenytoin has been discussed previously (page 455). Concentrations of phenobarbital in plasma may be elevated by as much as 40% during concurrent administration of valproic acid (*see* below).

Therapeutic Uses. Phenobarbital is an effective agent for *generalized tonic-clonic* (grand mal) and *cortical focal seizures.* Its efficacy, low toxicity, and low cost make it a primary agent for these types of epilepsy, particularly in children. The use of phenobarbital in the therapy of the epilepsies is discussed further at the end of the chapter.

OTHER BARBITURATES

Mephobarbital. *Mephobarbital,* U.S.P. (MEBARAL), is N-methylphenobarbital. It is N-demethylated by the hepatic microsomal enzymes, and most of its activity during chronic medication can be attributed to the accumulation of phenobarbital produced by this conversion. Consequently, the pharmacological properties, toxicity, and clinical uses of mephobarbital are the same as those for phenobarbital. However, oral absorption of mephobarbital is usually incomplete, and its dose is approximately twice that of phenobarbital. The plasma concentration of phenobarbital provides a guide to adjustment of mephobarbital dosage.

Metharbital. *Metharbital,* U.S.P. (GEMONIL), is N-methylbarbital. It is N-demethylated by the hepatic microsomal enzymes to barbital, which is excreted unchanged in the urine. Most of the activity of metharbital during chronic medication is probably attributable to the metabolite. Metharbital has greater sedative and less antiepileptic activity than does phenobarbital. It has been reported to be effective for infantile myoclonic spasms (Perlstein, 1950, 1957). The initial dosage for infants and small children is 50 mg, one to three times daily; for adults, 100 mg, two to three times daily.

DEOXYBARBITURATES

PRIMIDONE

Primidone is an effective agent for treatment of all types of epilepsy except absence seizures.

Chemistry. Primidone may be viewed as a congener of phenobarbital in which the carbonyl oxygen of the urea moiety is replaced by two hydrogen atoms:

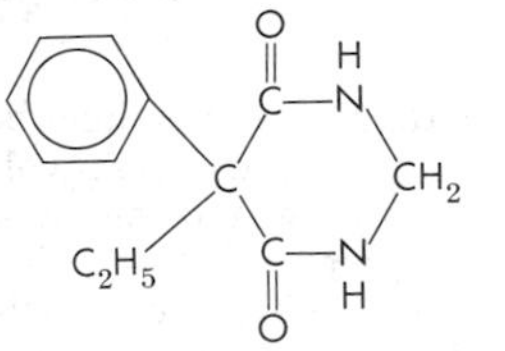

Primidone

Anticonvulsant Effects. Primidone resembles phenobarbital in many laboratory anticonvulsant effects, but it is rather more selective in modifying electroshock seizure pattern in animals and man (Bogue and Carrington, 1953; Goodman *et al.*, 1953). The anticonvulsant effects of administered primidone in animals are attributed to both the parent drug and its active metabolites (Symposium, 1972a).

Absorption, Distribution, Biotransformation, and Excretion. Primidone is rapidly and almost completely absorbed after oral administration, although individual variability can be great. Peak concentrations in plasma are usually observed approximately 3 hours after ingestion. The plasma half-time of primidone is about 8 hours; in children, about 40% of the drug is excreted unchanged in the urine.

Primidone is converted to two active metabolites, phenobarbital and phenylethylmalonamide (PEMA). Primidone and PEMA are bound to plasma proteins to only a small extent, whereas about half of phenobarbital is so bound. The half-life of PEMA in plasma is 24 to 48 hours; both it and phenobarbital (plasma half-life: 48 to 120 hours) accumulate during chronic medication. The appearance of phenobarbital in plasma may be delayed several days upon initiation of therapy with primidone.

Toxicity. The toxicity of primidone has been reviewed by Booker (Symposium, 1972a). The more common complaints are *sedation, vertigo, dizziness, nausea, vomiting, ataxia, diplopia,* and *nystagmus.* There may also be an *acute feeling of intoxication* immediately following administration of primidone. This occurs before there is any significant metabolism of the drug. The relationship of adverse effects to dosage is complex, since they result from both the parent drug and its two active metabolites and since tolerance develops during chronic medication. Side effects are occasionally quite severe when therapy is initiated.

Serious adverse effects are relatively uncommon, but *maculopapular* and *morbilliform rash, leukopenia, thrombocytopenia, systemic lupus erythematosus,* as well as *lymphadenopathy* have been reported. Acute *psychotic reactions,* usually in patients with temporal lobe epilepsy, have also occurred. *Hemorrhagic disease* in the neonate, *megaloblastic anemia,* and *osteomalacia* similar to those discussed previously in connection with phenytoin and phenobarbital have also been described.

Preparations and Dosage. *Primidone,* U.S.P. (MYSOLINE), is available as 50- and 250-mg tablets and as an oral suspension (250 mg/5 ml). The usual daily dose for adults is 500 to 1500 mg given in divided doses; for children, 5 to 20 mg/kg. Therapy should be initiated at lower dosage and increased gradually. Lower dosage may be possible or necessary when the drug is used concurrently with phenytoin.

Plasma Drug Concentrations. During chronic medication, the plasma concentration of phenobarbital generated by biotransformation of primidone averages 2 to 4 μg/ml per mg/kg daily dose of primidone. The plasma concentration of primidone fluctuates significantly between doses but averages about 0.5 to 1 μg/ml per daily dose of 1 mg/kg of primidone. The plasma concentration of the active metabolite PEMA is usually intermediate between those of primidone and phenobarbital. Dosage of primidone may be adjusted primarily with reference to the concentration of phenobarbital, as outlined previously for administered phenobarbital, and secondarily with reference to the concentration of the parent drug. Concentrations of primidone greater than 10 μg/ml are usually associated with significant ataxia and lethargy. A disproportionately high primidone:phenobarbital concentration ratio during chronic medication usually implies that medication has not been taken regularly. The relationship of plasma concentration of PEMA to efficacy and toxicity has not been established. (*See* Booker and Gallagher and Baumel, in Symposium, 1972a.)

Drug Interactions. *Phenytoin* has been reported to *increase* the conversion of primidone to phenobarbital. *Isoniazid* has been demonstrated in one patient to *decrease* the conversion of primidone to phenobarbital and PEMA. Other drug interactions to be anticipated are those for phenobarbital.

Therapeutic Uses. Clinical antiepileptic efficacy of primidone was first reported by Handley and Stewart (1952). It is useful against *generalized tonic-clonic, cortical focal,* and *temporal lobe epilepsy.* It may be effective alone in patients refractory to other medications but is more effective when used concurrently with phenytoin. Its use in combination with phenobarbital is illogical. Primidone is ineffective against absence seizures but sometimes useful against myoclonic seizures in young children. The therapeutic use of primidone and other antiepileptic agents is discussed further at the end of the chapter.

IMINOSTILBENES

CARBAMAZEPINE

Carbamazepine was approved in the United States for use as an antiepileptic agent in 1974. It has been employed since the 1960s for the treatment of trigeminal neuralgia (Blom, 1963).

Chemistry. Carbamazepine is related chemically to the tricyclic antidepressants. It is a derivative of iminostilbene with a carbamyl group at the 5 position; this moiety is essential for potent antiepileptic activity. The structural formula of carbamazepine is as follows:

Carbamazepine

There is considerable overlap of the three-dimensional structures of phenytoin and carbamazepine (*see* Julien and Hollister, in Symposium, 1975).

Anticonvulsant Effects. The anticonvulsant effects of carbamazepine in animals resemble those of phenytoin. At therapeutic concentrations, carbamazepine can inhibit maximal electroshock seizures, abolish focal brain discharges induced by locally applied penicillin, and suppress seizure activity caused by similarly applied alumina cream. In addition, it is more effective than phenytoin in raising the threshold for minimal electroshock seizures and in blocking seizures in response to pentylenetetrazol. However, Krupp (1969) reported that carbamazepine has only a slight inhibitory effect on PTP in the spinal cord of the cat. The electrophysiological and biochemical actions responsible for the anticonvulsant effects of carbamazepine are unknown.

Absorption, Distribution, Biotransformation, and Excretion. Carbamazepine is absorbed rapidly after oral administration, but with considerable individual variability. Peak concentrations in plasma are observed 2 to 6 hours after oral ingestion, and binding to plasma proteins occurs to the extent of about 80%. Carbamazepine is metabolized to the 10,11-epoxide, and this compound also has anticonvulsant activity. The half-life of the parent compound in plasma after chronic administration is between 13 and 17 hours. Because of autoinduction of drug metabolism, this is shorter than that in individuals who have received only a single dose. The half-life of the 10,11-epoxide is probably shorter than that of the parent compound, ranging from 5 to 8 hours.

Less than 1% of carbamazepine is recovered in the urine as the parent compound or the epoxide. There is further metabolism to carbamazepine-10,11-dihydroxide and subsequent conjugation with glucuronic acid.

Toxicity. The more frequent untoward effects of carbamazepine include *diplopia, blurred vision, drowsiness, dizziness, nausea, vomiting,* and *ataxia.* A wide variety of other CNS, gastrointestinal, cardiovascular, and dermatological effects have also been reported. Other adverse effects and precautions are similar to those for the tricyclic antidepressants. Some tolerance develops to the untoward effects of carbamazepine, and they can be minimized by gradual increase in dosage and adjustment of maintenance dosage.

Carbamazepine has caused deaths from *aplastic anemia* and from its *cardiovascular effects;* nevertheless, it is a valuable drug (Livingston *et al.,* 1974). Serious adverse effects, in addition to bone-marrow depression, include *leukopenia, thrombocytopenic purpura, hepatocellular* and *cholestatic jaundice, acute oliguria* with *hypertension, thrombophlebitis, left ventricular failure,* and *cardiovascular collapse. Skin rash,* often with other manifestations of drug allergy, is said to occur in 3% of patients. *Stevens-Johnson syndrome, exfoliative dermatitis, photosensitivity, altered skin pigmentation,* and *systemic lupus erythematosus* have been reported.

Preparations and Dosage. *Carbamazepine,* U.S.P. (TEGRETOL), is available in 200-mg tablets for oral administration. Therapy for *epilepsy* is usually started at a dosage of 200 mg, taken twice daily to minimize side effects. Dosage is then increased gradually to 600 to 1200 mg per day for adults and 20 to 30 mg/kg for children. The short half-life of carbamazepine often necessitates dosage intervals of 6 to 8 hours to minimize fluctuations in plasma concentrations.

Therapy for *trigeminal neuralgia* is generally started at a dose of 200 mg per day; dosage may be increased gradually, as needed, to a level of 1200 mg per day if this is tolerated.

Plasma Drug Concentrations. There is no simple relationship between the dose of carbamazepine and concentrations of the drug in plasma (*see* Morselli, in Symposium, 1975). Therapeutic concentrations are reported to be 6 to 8 μg/ml, although there is considerable variation. Side effects referable to the CNS are frequent at concentrations of 8.5 to 10 μg/ml.

Drug Interactions. There are apparently few interactions between carbamazepine and other drugs. Phenobarbital is said to increase the metabolism of carbamazepine; the biotransformation of phenytoin may be enhanced by carbamazepine.

Therapeutic Uses. *Epilepsy.* Carbamazepine is useful in patients with *temporal lobe epilepsy,* whether the condition occurs alone or in combination with *generalized tonic-clonic seizures. When it is employed, renal, hepatic, and bone-marrow function must be monitored;* such hematological evaluation may have contributed to the lack of recent reports of fatal aplastic anemia associated with the use of carbamazepine. The therapeutic use of carbamazepine is discussed further at the end of the chapter.

Neuralgia. Carbamazepine was introduced by Blom in the early 1960s and is now the primary agent for treatment of *trigeminal* and *glossopharyngeal neuralgias* (*see* Crill, 1973). It is also effective for *lightning tabetic pain.* Carbamazepine is *not* an analgesic and should *not* be employed for relief of other types of pain.

Most patients with neuralgia are benefited initially, but only 70% obtain continuing relief. Adverse effects have required discontinuation of medication in 5 to 20% of patients. Concurrent medication with phenytoin may be useful when carbamazepine alone is not satisfactory.

SUCCINIMIDES

ETHOSUXIMIDE

The succinimides evolved from a systematic search for effective agents less toxic than the oxazolidinediones for the treatment of absence seizures. Ethosuximide is a primary agent for this type of epilepsy.

Structure-Activity Relationship. Ethosuximide has the following structural formula:

$$C_2H_5 \quad \overset{H_2}{\underset{\quad}{C}} $$

Ethosuximide

The structure-activity relationship of the succinimides is in accord with that for other anticonvulsant classes (Chen *et al.,* 1963). Methsuximide and phensuximide have phenyl substituents and are more active against maximal electroshock seizures.

Ethosuximide, with alkyl substituents, is the most active against seizures induced by pentylenetetrazol and is the most selective for clinical absence seizures.

Anticonvulsant Properties. The anticonvulsant spectrum of ethosuximide in animals resembles that of trimethadione. The most prominent characteristic of both drugs is protection against the convulsant action of pentylenetetrazol. Ethosuximide also elevates threshold for electroshock seizures, but it abolishes the tonic extensor component of maximal electroshock seizures only in anesthetic doses. In addition, it blocks spiking activity in both the primary and secondary foci and the associated clonic seizure activity produced by the local application of cobalt to the frontal cortex of the rat.

A shortcoming of many of the early electrophysiological studies of the effects of ethosuximide was the failure to correlate effects with concentrations of the drug in plasma. Several recent studies have addressed this issue. Englander and colleagues (1977) demonstrated that ethosuximide, at concentrations in the recommended therapeutic range, had a characteristic effect on thalamocortical excitation when compared to phenytoin. At short intervals of paired stimuli, ethosuximide had little effect on the cortical response and actually lowered the threshold for stimulation. With pulse intervals greater than 200 milliseconds, ethosuximide markedly decreased cortical responses and elevated the threshold for stimulation. Frequency-dependent effects were not observed for phenytoin.

Guberman and colleagues (1975) studied the effects of ethosuximide and phenytoin in acute penicillin-induced epilepsy in the cat. Epileptic bursts in the EEG, often resembling the spike-and-wave pattern of absence seizures, were reduced more effectively by ethosuximide than by phenytoin. Furthermore, there was a good correlation between the concentration of ethosuximide in plasma and effect, and concentrations were similar to those associated with therapeutic effects in patients with absence seizures.

Absorption, Distribution, Biotransformation, and Excretion. The extent of absorption of ethosuximide from the gastrointestinal tract is unknown. Peak concentrations occur in plasma in 1 to 7 hours after a single oral dose. Ethosuximide is not significantly bound to plasma proteins; during chronic medication, the concentration in the CSF is similar to that in plasma. In animals, it is relatively evenly distributed in all tissues and does not accumulate in fat.

In man, 20% of the drug is excreted unchanged in the urine. The remainder is metabolized by hepatic microsomal enzymes. The major metabolite, the hydroxyethyl derivative, accounts for about 40% of administered drug, is inactive, and is excreted as such and as the glucuronide in the urine. Other metabolites include the corresponding ketone derivative and an open-ring succinamic acid compound. The plasma half-time of ethosuximide averages about 30 hours in children and 60 hours in adults (*see* Symposium, 1972a).

Toxicity. The toxicity of ethosuximide has been reviewed by Buchanan (Symposium, 1972a). The most common dose-related side effects are *gastrointestinal* complaints (*nausea, vomiting,* and *anorexia*) and *CNS* effects (*drowsiness, lethargy, euphoria, dizziness, headache,* and *hiccough*). Some tolerance to these effects develops. *Parkinson-like symptoms* and *photophobia* have also been reported. *Restlessness, agitation, anxiety, aggressiveness, inability to concentrate,* and other behavioral effects have occurred primarily in patients with a prior history of psychiatric disturbance.

Urticaria and other skin reactions, including *Stevens-Johnson syndrome*, as well as *systemic lupus erythematosus, eosinophilia, leukopenia, thrombocytopenia, pancytopenia,* and *aplastic anemia* have also been attributed to the drug. The leukopenia may be transient, despite continuation of the drug, but several deaths have resulted from bone-marrow depression. Renal or hepatic toxicity has not been reported.

Preparations and Dosage. *Ethosuximide*, U.S.P. (ZARONTIN), is available for oral administration as 250-mg capsules and as a syrup (250 mg/5 ml). An initial daily dose of 250 mg in children and 500 mg in adults is increased by 250-mg increments at weekly intervals until seizures are adequately controlled or toxicity intervenes. Usual maintenance dosage is 20 to 40 mg/kg. Increased caution is required if daily dosage exceeds 1500 mg in adults or 750 to 1000 mg in children.

Plasma Drug Concentrations. During chronic medication in children, the plasma concentration of ethosuximide averages 2 to 4 μg/ml per daily dose of 1 mg/kg. However, because of variation, concentrations in plasma cannot be predicted accurately. The plateau state is attained in 4 to 6 days. A plasma concentration of 40 to 100 μg/ml is required for satisfactory control of absence seizures in most patients (*see* Browne *et al.,* 1975). However, some patients may be completely controlled at lower concentrations, and others are incompletely controlled at higher concentrations. A relationship between plasma concentration and adverse effects has not been established. Concentrations as high as 160 μg/ml have been tolerated without excessive toxicity. (*See* Symposium, 1972a.)

Drug Interactions. Interactions between ethosuximide and other drugs have not been reported. Increased toxicity should be anticipated with other drugs having similar dose-related adverse effects.

Therapeutic Uses. Ethosuximide is more effective than trimethadione against *absence seizures* (Vossen, 1958; Zimmerman and Burgemeister, 1958; Symposium, 1972a) and has a lower risk of serious adverse effects; it is an important therapeutic agent for this type of epilepsy. The use of ethosuximide and the other antiepileptic agents is discussed further at the end of the chapter.

OTHER SUCCINIMIDES

Methsuximide. Methsuximide, N,2-dimethyl-2-phenylsuccinimide, was introduced by Zimmerman (1956) for the therapy of absence seizures. Ethosuximide subsequently proved more effective. Methsuximide, particularly when given concurrently with other drugs, may also be useful in the treatment of temporal lobe epilepsy. Adverse gastrointestinal and central effects are similar in pattern to those of ethosuximide. Severe depression, skin rash, fever, periorbital edema, leukopenia, aplastic anemia, nephropathy, and hepatotoxicity have also been reported.

Methsuximide, U.S.P. (CELONTIN), is available as 150- and 300-mg capsules. Medication is initiated with 300 mg, given daily. The usual daily dose for adults is 600 to 1200 mg. Patients receiving higher doses, especially in multiple-drug therapy, should be carefully monitored.

Methsuximide is rapidly absorbed and metabolized (Symposium, 1972a). It is not bound significantly to plasma proteins, and less than 1% is excreted unchanged in the urine. Metabolism by the hepatic microsomal enzymes in the dog yields N-demethyl and parahydroxyphenyl derivatives and their glucuronides (Dudley *et al.,* 1974). The N-demethyl metabolite has been implicated in the production of delayed coma after acute overdosage of methsuximide (Karch, 1973) and has been detected in much higher concentration than the parent drug in the plasma of patients during chronic administration of methsuximide (Strong *et al.,* 1974). Inadequate study of this active metabolite limits the value of the meager pharmacokinetic information on methsuximide.

Phensuximide. The first succinimide introduced for the therapy of absence seizures (Zimmerman, 1951) was phensuximide, N-methyl-2-phenylsuccinimide. Low efficacy has relegated it to secondary

status. Adverse gastrointestinal and central effects are similar to those for ethosuximide. A dreamlike state, skin rash, fever, granulocytopenia, leukopenia, and reversible nephropathy have also been reported.

Phensuximide, U.S.P. (MILONTIN), is available as 250- and 500-mg capsules and as a suspension containing 300 mg/5 ml. The usual daily dose for adults is 2 to 4 g. Phensuximide is rapidly absorbed and converted to the N-demethyl metabolite, an active species; renal excretion of unchanged drug is negligible. The parent drug is not bound to plasma proteins (Porter *et al.,* 1977).

VALPROIC ACID

Valproic acid is the latest antiepileptic drug to be approved for use in the United States. The antiepileptic properties of valproate were discovered serendipitously when it was used as a vehicle for other compounds that were being screened for antiepileptic activity (Meunier *et al.,* 1963).

Chemistry. Valproic acid (*n*-dipropylacetic acid) is a simple branched-chain carboxylic acid; its structural formula is as follows:

$$CH_3CH_2CH_2 \diagdown \atop CH_3CH_2CH_2 \diagup CHCOOH$$

Valproic Acid

Certain other branched-chain carboxylic acids with fewer or the same number of carbon atoms have potencies similar to that of valproic acid in antagonizing pentylenetetrazol-induced convulsions. However, straight-chain acids and *n*-dibutylacetic acid have little or no activity. The primary amide of valproic acid has been reported to be about twice as potent as the parent compound (*see* Murray and Kier, 1977).

Pharmacological Effects. Valproic acid has antiepileptic activity against a variety of types of seizures while causing only minimal sedation and other CNS side effects. It prevents pentylenetetrazol-induced seizures in mice with a potency greater than that of ethosuximide but less than that of phenobarbital. It also eliminates hindlimb extension in mice subjected to maximal electroshock but only at relatively high doses. These results suggest that valproate would be more useful in absence than in generalized tonic-clonic seizures (*see* Pinder *et al.,* 1977; Bruni and Wilder, 1979). While the drug is also effective in a variety of other model systems considered useful for predicting efficacy in absence seizures, it also reduces the frequency and severity of spontaneous seizures in monkeys rendered epileptic by implantation of alumina cream (Lockard *et al.,* 1977). Furthermore, valproate can prevent induced convulsions in kindled rats (Tanaka and Lange, 1975; Wada, 1977) and, at lower doses, can prevent the establishment of the kindling phenomenon in cats (Leviel and Naquet, 1977).

The mechanism of action of valproate is unknown, although several investigators have proposed a possible interaction with the metabolism of GABA in the brain (*see* Pinder *et al.,* 1977; Bruni and Wilder, 1979). It has been suggested that selective increases in concentrations of GABA in synaptic regions may be promoted by inhibition of GABA transaminase or succinic semialdehyde dehydrogenase, inhibition of re-uptake by glial cells and nerve endings, or some combination of these actions. One observation that supports this notion is that valproate blocks the convulsant effects of GABA antagonists (picrotoxin and bicuculline) at doses similar to or lower than those required to block pentylenetetrazol-induced seizures (Frey and Löscher, 1976). On the other hand, valproate augments the GABA-mediated postsynaptic inhibition of cultured spinal neurons without influencing the time course of the response (Macdonald and Bergey, 1979). This suggests a postsynaptic site of action.

Absorption, Distribution, Biotransformation, and Excretion.

Valproic acid is rapidly and almost completely absorbed after oral administration. Peak concentrations in plasma are observed in 1 to 4 hours, although this can be delayed for several hours if the drug is ingested with meals.

Binding of valproate to plasma proteins varies between 80 and 94% in healthy subjects and in patients with epilepsy. Its volume of distribution is consistent with equilibration mainly in the extracellular space (Klotz and Antonin, 1977). Concentrations of valproate in CSF are about 10% of the value in plasma, suggesting equilibration between the CSF and the free valproate in the blood.

After a single dose of valproic acid, unchanged drug is not found in the urine in significant amounts. More than 70% is present as various metabolites, mainly the glucuronide conjugate of 2-propylglutaric acid (Ferrandes and Eymard, 1977). There is some excretion of valproate in the feces. The half-life of valproate in epileptic patients is approximately 15 hours (*see* Appendix II).

Toxicity. The incidence of toxicity associated with the use of valproic acid is remarkably low compared to other antiepileptic drugs. The most common side effects are gastrointestinal symptoms; these include anorexia, nausea, and vomiting in about 16% of patients (*see* Simon and Penry, 1975). Effects on the CNS, such as sedation, ataxia, and incoordination, occur very infrequently. There have been several reports that suggest a link between the administration of valproic acid and hepatotoxicity. Willmore and colleagues (1978) noted that 4 of 25 patients who had valproic acid added to their anticonvulsant regimen showed biochemical evidence of hepatic injury. Suchy and coworkers (1979) described fatal hepatotoxicity in two children receiving the drug; it was the sole medication in one of the children. *In toto,* approximately 20 deaths have been reported that were secondary to liver failure and associated with the administration of valproic acid. It is recommended that tests of hepatic function be performed prior to and every 2 months after initiation of such therapy.

Preparation and Dosage. *Valproic acid* (DEPAKENE) is available in 250-mg capsules and in a syrup containing 250 mg/5 ml of the sodium salt. The usual daily doses are 1000 to 3000 mg in adults and 30 to 60 mg/kg in children (*see* Medical Letter, 1979); dosage is usually started at a lower level, and divided doses are given.

Plasma Drug Concentrations. The concentration of valproate in plasma that appears to be associated with therapeutic effects is approximately 50 to 100 µg/ml (Appendix II). However, the correlation between this concentration and efficacy is poor; the short half-life of the drug and a variable degree of protein binding probably contribute to this problem (Wulff *et al.,* 1977).

Drug Interactions. There is well-documented interaction between valproate and phenobarbital. Concentrations of phenobarbital in plasma rise by as much as 40% when valproate is given concurrently. The underlying mechanism is unknown, although inhibition of hepatic enzymes has been suggested (*see* Bruni and Wilder, 1979).

Jeavons and colleagues (1977) noted that 5 of 12 patients who received valproate and clonazepam concurrently developed *absence status epilepticus.* However, a similar interaction between these two drugs was not observed by Wilder and associates (1978). Concentrations of phenytoin in plasma may be altered when patients receive valproate and phenytoin concurrently, but the changes have been inconsistent; the concentrations of valproate, however, do seem to be lower during administration of such regimens (see Pinder et al., 1977).

Therapeutic Uses. The therapeutic uses of valproic acid in epilepsy have recently been reviewed (see Simon and Penry, 1975; Pinder et al., 1977; Bruni and Wilder, 1979). The drug is particularly effective in absence seizures, both simple and complex; this is the only current indication for the administration of valproate in the United States. The drug has also been shown to be effective in a variety of other types of epilepsy, including myoclonic and grand mal seizures; it is less effective in controlling partial seizures. The therapeutic uses of valproate in epilepsy are discussed further at the end of this chapter.

OXAZOLIDINEDIONES

TRIMETHADIONE

Although no longer the clinical agent of choice, trimethadione has been extensively studied in the laboratory and clinic, and, in this regard, it may still be considered the prototype for agents useful against absence seizures.

History. The demonstration by Perlstein and the confirmation by many others of the selectivity of trimethadione in the treatment of absence seizures was an important advance in the therapy of the epilepsies (Lennox, 1945; Goodman et al., 1946; Perlstein and Andelman, 1946; Richards and Perlstein, 1946). It provided the first clear indication that drugs could be selective for the various types of epilepsy and spurred research on the basic physiological mechanism of the absence seizures, which previously had been refractory to therapy. Moreover, it provided a new pharmacological tool for such investigations. In addition, it reemphasized the value of a systematic search for new anticonvulsants by means of laboratory tests (Everett and Richards, 1944; Goodman et al., 1946).

Structure-Activity Relationship. Trimethadione has the structural formula as shown.

Trimethadione

The oxazolidinediones contain the structural common denominator typical of many other classes of antiepileptic agents. The alkyl substituents on the carbon in position 5 appear important for the selectivity of the oxazolidinediones both as antagonists of pentylenetetrazol in animals and as clinically useful agents in the therapy of absence seizures. The same is true for the succinimides. The structure-activity relationship for these compounds has been reviewed by Toman and Goodman (1948), Close and Spielman (1961), and Chen and coworkers (1963).

Pharmacological Effects. The outstanding anticonvulsant property of trimethadione in laboratory animals is its protective effect against pentylenetetrazol seizures, in which property it differs markedly from phenytoin (Everett and Richards, 1944; Toman and Goodman, 1948). Conversely, it is far inferior to phenytoin in its ability to modify the maximal electroshock seizure pattern.

Dimethadione, the N-demethyl metabolite of trimethadione, is active and resembles the parent drug in most respects. In general, compared with the parent drug, the metabolite is more potent (Withrow et al., 1968).

Unlike typical antiepileptic barbiturates and hydantoins, trimethadione fails to modify the maximal seizure pattern in psychiatric patients undergoing electroconvulsive therapy, even in doses well above the accepted level for suppression of clinical absence seizures (Toman et al., 1947). Neurophysiological studies have also identified significant differences between the effects of trimethadione and phenytoin. Schallek and Kuehn (1963) observed that trimethadione considerably elevates the threshold for seizure discharge by repetitive stimulation of the central lateral nucleus of the thalamus of the cat, in doses lower than required for other areas and in contrast to the lack of effect of phenytoin on the thalamus. Morrell and associates (1959) noted that trimethadione depressed the projection of seizure activity from cortical foci to thalamus while leaving cortical spread relatively unaffected. Phenytoin produces the opposite effect. Although trimethadione also elevates the cortical seizure threshold (Delgado and Mihailović, 1956), some thalamic nuclei are particularly sensitive to the drug. Since the thalamocortical system appears particularly important in the genesis of absence seizures, the relatively selective effect of trimethadione on thalamic nuclei could account for its clinical efficacy against this type of epilepsy.

Trimethadione also markedly decreases spinal cord transmission during repetitive stimulation without modifying transmission of single impulses, and it antagonizes the effects of pentylenetetrazol on the spinal cord (Esplin and Curto, 1957; Woodbury and Esplin, 1959). Unlike phenytoin, trimethadione has no effect on PTP in the spinal cord or stellate ganglia.

Absorption, Distribution, Biotransformation, and Excretion. Trimethadione is rapidly absorbed from the gastrointestinal tract; the peak plasma concentration after a single dose occurs in 0.5 to 2 hours (Frey and Schulz, 1970). It is not bound significantly to plasma proteins and is uniformly distributed in tissues; its apparent volume of distribution is 60% of body weight. Trimethadione is largely demethylated by the hepatic microsomal enzymes to the active metabolite dimethadione (Butler *et al.,* 1965). Dimethadione is not further metabolized but is excreted unchanged in the urine with a half-time of 6 to 13 days. During chronic medication, the metabolite accumulates and is responsible for the major activity of the medication. (*See* Symposium, 1972a.)

Toxicity. The most common undesired effects of trimethadione are *sedation* and *hemeralopia* (blurring of vision in bright light or glare effect). The latter appears to be an effect upon the neural layers of the retina rather than on the photochemical process (Sloan and Gilger, 1947). Hemeralopia does not usually require discontinuation of medication and can be overcome by the use of tinted glasses. Children are not as susceptible as adults. Drowsiness tends to diminish with continued medication. Trimethadione may also precipitate generalized *tonic-clonic seizures* in some patients with absence seizures associated with grand mal.

Less common but more serious untoward effects include *exfoliative dermatitis* and other *skin rashes, blood dyscrasias, hepatitis,* and *nephrosis.* Fatalities have been reported. Moderate *neutropenia* is not uncommon (incidence as high as 20%); fulminating *pancytopenia* and *aplastic anemia* have occurred. *Lupus erythematosus* and *lymphadenopathy* have been observed. A *myasthenic syndrome* has also been reported (Booker *et al.,* 1968). (*See* Gallagher, in Symposium, 1972a.)

Preparations and Dosage. *Trimethadione,* U.S.P. (TRIDIONE), is available for oral use as 300-mg capsules, 150-mg sweetened tablets, and a flavored solution (40 mg/ml). The usual daily dose is 900 to 2100 mg for adults and 20 to 60 mg/kg (300 to 900 mg) for children. However, larger doses are sometimes necessary, and dosage is individualized for each patient to provide maximal efficacy with minimal side effects. Although commonly administered in divided doses, once-daily medication may be satisfactory.

Plasma Drug Concentrations. During chronic medication, plasma concentration of trimethadione averages 0.6 μg/ml per daily dose of 1 mg/kg, with moderate fluctuations between doses. Plasma concentrations of the active metabolite dimethadione are 20 times higher (12 μg/ml per 1 mg/kg) and provide the guide for adjustment of dosage. Several weeks are required to attain the plateau state when therapy is initiated and when dosage is changed. A disproportionately high trimethadione:dimethadione concentration ratio usually implies that the patient has not been taking medication regularly. The plasma concentration of dimethadione must usually be maintained above 700 μg/ml for control of seizures. The relationship between plasma concentration and adverse effects has not been established. (*See* Jensen, 1962; Chamberlin *et al.,* 1965; Symposium, 1972a.)

Drug Interactions. Interactions between trimethadione and other drugs have not been reported.

Therapeutic Uses. Trimethadione is employed only in the treatment of *absence seizures,* and usually only in patients who are inadequately controlled by or do not tolerate other agents. Because of its potential for serious toxicity, treatment with trimethadione necessitates close medical supervision of the patient, especially during the initial year of therapy. The therapeutic use of trimethadione and other agents in the treatment of absence seizures is discussed further at the end of the chapter.

PARAMETHADIONE

Paramethadione was first reported to be clinically useful for *absence seizures* by Davis and Lennox (1947). It differs from trimethadione only in the replacement of one of the methyl groups on the carbon in the 5 position by an ethyl substituent. Its pharmacological properties, therapeutic uses, dosage, and toxicity are similar to those of trimethadione.

Paramethadione, U.S.P. (PARADIONE), is available as 150- and 300-mg capsules and in a flavored solution (300 mg/ml).

Although the undesired effects of paramethadione and trimethadione are similar, the reported incidence of serious adverse effects may be less for paramethadione (Lennox and Lennox, 1960). More importantly perhaps, individuals who do not tolerate one of the oxazolidinediones may tolerate the other.

Paramethadione is N-demethylated by the hepatic microsomal enzymes to an active metabolite that is slowly excreted in the urine (Butler and Waddell, 1955). The metabolite accumulates during chronic medication and is probably responsible for most of the anticonvulsant activity of the parent drug, as dimethadione is for trimethadione.

BENZODIAZEPINES

The benzodiazepines are employed clinically primarily as sedative-antianxiety drugs; their pharmacology is presented in detail in Chapters 17 and 19. Discussion in this chapter is limited to consideration of their usefulness in the therapy of the epilepsies. A large number of benzodiazepines have broad antiepileptic properties, but only clonazepam has received approval for chronic treatment of certain types of seizures. Diazepam is extremely valuable for the management of *status epilepticus*.

Chemistry. The structure of diazepam is shown in Table 19–6 (page 437); that of clonazepam is as follows:

Clonazepam

Although superficially unrelated, the benzodiazepines and the other antiepileptic agents have a similar steric configuration (Camerman and Camerman, 1970). The structure-activity relationship for the anticonvulsant effect of the benzodiazepines has been summarized by Popp (1977).

Anticonvulsant Properties. In animals, prevention of pentylenetetrazol-induced seizures by the benzodiazepines is much more prominent than their modification of the maximal electroshock seizure pattern (Swinyard and Castellion, 1966; Millichap, 1969). In experimental models of epilepsy, they suppress the spread of seizure activity produced by epileptogenic foci in the cortex, thalamus, and limbic structures but do not abolish the abnormal discharge of the focus (*see* Browne and Penry, 1973; Symposium, 1973). In low dosage, the benzodiazepines suppress polysynaptic activity in the spinal cord and decrease neuronal activity in the mesencephalic reticular system. Clonazepam

appears to be more potent than diazepam in various experimental seizures.

Benzodiazepines facilitate a variety of GABA-mediated synaptic systems, involving both presynaptic and postsynaptic inhibition (*see* Haefely *et al.*, 1979). In cultured spinal cord neurons, diazepam augments the increase in chloride conductance produced by GABA, but not that produced by glycine, without influencing the time course of the response to GABA (Macdonald and Barker, 1979b). Based on these data and on the ability of benzodiazepines to increase the apparent affinity of GABA for binding sites in preparations of brain membranes, it has been proposed that benzodiazepines somehow increase the potency or effectiveness of this inhibitory neurotransmitter (*see* Guidotti *et al.*, 1979). Even though the available data indicate that regulation of the function of receptors for GABA may be quite complex, it appears that the antiepileptic actions of benzodiazepines, barbiturates, and valproate may in part involve similar mechanisms.

Absorption, Distribution, Biotransformation, and Excretion. Clonazepam is well absorbed after oral administration, and concentrations in plasma are usually maximal within 2 to 4 hours (*see* Pinder *et al.*, 1976). After intravenous administration, both clonazepam and diazepam are redistributed in a manner typical of that for highly lipid-soluble agents (*see* Chapter 1). Central effects develop promptly but wane rapidly as the drugs move to other tissues. About 50% of the clonazepam in the circulation is bound to plasma proteins (*see* Browne, 1978).

Clonazepam is metabolized principally by reduction of the nitro group to produce the inactive 7-amino derivative; hydroxylated derivatives are minor metabolites. Less than 1% of the drug can be recovered unchanged in the urine, and the remainder is excreted as conjugated and unconjugated metabolites. The plasma half-life is about 1 to 2 days.

The major metabolite of diazepam, the N-demethyl derivative, is biologically active; other active metabolites include a ring-hydroxylated derivative and oxazepam, which is both demethylated and hydroxylated. Both the parent drug and the demethylated metabolite have a plasma half-life of 1 to 2 days or longer.

Toxicity. The acute toxicity of clonazepam is low relative to usual clinical dosage. Oral ingestion of as much as 60 mg (small child) or 100 mg (adult) has occurred without permanent sequelae (*see* Pinder *et al.,* 1976); therapy consisted in gastric lavage and supportive measures. *Cardiovascular* and *respiratory depression* may occur after *intravenous* administration of diazepam or clonazepam, particularly if other anticonvulsants or central depressants have been administered previously (*see* Greenblatt and Koch-Weser, 1973).

The principal side effect of chronic oral medication with clonazepam is the syndrome of drowsiness, somnolence, fatigue, and lethargy. This occurs in about 50% of patients initially, but tends to subside with continued administration. While these symptoms can usually be kept to tolerable levels by reduction in the dosage or the rate at which it is increased, they sometimes force discontinuation of the drug. *Muscular incoordination* and *ataxia* are common but less frequent side effects, followed by *hypotonia, dysarthria,* and *dizziness. Behavioral disturbances,* especially in children, can be very troublesome; these include aggression, hyperactivity, irritability, and difficulty in concentration. Both anorexia and hyperphagia have been reported. *Increased salivary* and *bronchial secretions* may cause difficulties in children. *Seizures* are sometimes exacerbated (*see* Browne, 1978), and *status epilepticus* may be precipitated if the drug is discontinued abruptly. Other aspects of the toxicity of the benzodiazepines are discussed in Chapters 17 and 19.

Preparations, Routes of Administration, and Dosage. *Clonazepam* (CLONOPIN) is available as 0.5-, 1-, and 2-mg tablets. The initial dose for adults is 1.5 mg per day, and for children it is 0.01 to 0.03 mg/kg per day. The dose-dependent side effects are reduced if two or three divided doses are given each day. Dosage may be increased every 3 to 7 days by 0.25 to 0.5 mg per day in children and 0.5 mg per day in adults. The maximal recommended dosage is 20 mg per day for adults and 0.2 mg/kg per day for children. The concentration of clonazepam in plasma produced by a given dose cannot be predicted accurately.

Diazepam, U.S.P. (VALIUM), is available as 2-, 5-, and 10-mg tablets and in solution (5 mg/ml) for injection. The solvent for the commercial parenteral preparation is a propylene glycol–ethanol–water mixture. If this solution is diluted, precipitation may occur. It may be possible to dilute the preparation with aqueous solutions in glass containers (Morris, 1978). For *status epilepticus,* diazepam is administered *slowly* and intravenously. The usual dose for adults and older children is 5 to 10 mg, as required; this may be repeated at intervals of 10 to 15 minutes, up to a maximal dose of 30 mg. If necessary, this regimen can be repeated in 2 to 4 hours, but no more than 100 mg should be administered in a 24-hour period.

Plasma Drug Concentrations. Effective concentrations of clonazepam in plasma range from 5 to 70 ng/ml. However, a similar range of concentrations is observed in patients who have a poor therapeutic response or various side effects (*see* Browne, 1978). Thus, neither clear-cut minimal therapeutic concentrations nor usually toxic concentrations can be stated.

Drug Interactions. Significant drug interactions with clonazepam have not been reported (*see* Pinder *et al.,* 1976). However, it must be remembered that diazepam and other benzodiazepines are known to potentiate the action of CNS depressant drugs such as ethanol.

Therapeutic Uses. Clonazepam is useful in the therapy of absence seizures as well as myoclonic seizures in children. Diazepam is the agent of choice for the treatment of *status epilepticus;* it is not useful as an oral agent for the treatment of seizure disorders. These applications are discussed further at the end of the chapter. Other uses of the benzodiazepines are described primarily in Chapters 17 and 19.

OTHER ANTIEPILEPTIC AGENTS

Phenacemide. Phenacemide (phenylacetylurea) is the straight-chain analog of 5-phenylhydantoin. It was introduced by Gibbs and coworkers (1949). Even if its efficacy remained unchallenged, its clinical value and use would be severely limited by its potential for serious toxicity. Phenacemide should be used only in the therapy of temporal lobe epilepsy refractory to other agents, in association with other drugs, and only if adequate supervision and monitoring are possible. Periodic assessment of hepatic, renal, and bone-marrow function is mandatory. The patient and his family must be alerted to the possible hazards of the drug.

Phenacemide, U.S.P. (PHENURONE), is available as 500-mg tablets. Usual daily dosage in adults has varied from 1.5 to 5 g. Phenacemide is almost completely absorbed from the gastrointestinal tract. Biotransformation by hepatic microsomal enzymes includes inactivation by *p*-hydroxylation of the phenyl substituent; ring closure to form a hydantoin does not occur. Unchanged drug is not excreted in the urine (Everett and Richards, 1952). Plasma concentrations associated with efficacy and safety have not been established.

Serious *adverse effects* of phenacemide severely limit its use and often necessitate withdrawal of the drug. As summarized by Tyler and King (1951), behavioral effects may occur in 17% of patients and include personality changes, aggressive behavior, paranoid and depressive reactions, and acute psychosis. Other adverse effects include gastrointestinal symptoms (8%), skin rash (5%), drowsiness (4%), aplastic anemia (2%), hepatitis (2%), and occasional nephritis. Deaths from aplastic anemia have occurred.

Acetazolamide. Acetazolamide, the prototype for the carbonic anhydrase inhibitors, is discussed with the saluretic agents in Chapter 36. It has anticonvulsant properties in animals and is sometimes an effective antiepileptic agent, particularly against absence seizures. However, its usefulness is limited by the rapid development of tolerance. (*See* Lombroso and Forsythe, 1960; Millichap, 1971.) *Acetazolamide,* U.S.P. (DIAMOX), is available as 125- and 250-mg tablets and as a solution (500 mg per vial) for parenteral use.

Acetazolamide is rapidly absorbed from the gastrointestinal tract, is highly bound to plasma proteins, and is eliminated unchanged in the urine. Adverse effects are minimal when it is employed in moderate dosage for limited periods. Drowsiness and paresthesias may occur at high doses and during prolonged medication. Skin rash and other allergic reactions are not common.

The anticonvulsant properties of the carbonic anhydrase inhibitors resemble those of carbon dioxide. In animals, they abolish the tonic extensor component of maximal electroshock convulsions, elevate seizure threshold, and protect against audiogenic seizures and those produced by withdrawal from high concentrations of carbon dioxide. In the spinal cord, monosynaptic pathways are selectively depressed without effect on synaptic recovery or PTP. Threshold for stimulation of the diencephalon is also increased. These effects may result from inhibition of glial-cell carbonic anhydrase, with subsequent accumulation of carbon dioxide and reduced flux of sodium into neurons. (*See* Woodbury and Kemp, 1970.)

GENERAL PRINCIPLES AND CHOICE OF DRUGS FOR THE THERAPY OF THE EPILEPSIES

Accurate evaluation of the type of seizure is essential for the rational pharmacotherapy of epilepsy. This requires a thorough examination of the patient, including the EEG. Epilepsy is a chronic condition, and long-term treatment is the rule; patients with conditions that might be mistaken for epilepsy (*e.g.,* withdrawal from chronic use of a sedative-hypnotic agent) or those who have experienced a single seizure precipitated by a reversible abnormality (*e.g.,* hypoglycemia)

should not be treated continuously (*see* Solomon and Plum, 1976). Furthermore, an attempt should be made to ascertain the cause of the epilepsy with the hope of discovering a correctable lesion, either structural or metabolic. This is more likely in the very young patient or when the first seizure appears during adulthood.

Once the decision has been made to use drugs to control the seizures, and this is often the case even if a specific etiology is found, medication is selected to "fit the fit." The goal of therapy is to keep the patient free of seizures without interfering with normal function.

Even when it is anticipated that multiple-drug therapy will be required, *medication is initiated with a single drug. Initial dosage* is usually that expected to provide a plasma drug concentration during the plateau state at least in the lower portion of the range associated with clinical efficacy. However, to minimize dose-related adverse effects, therapy with some drugs is initiated at reduced dosage, and the clinically effective amount is attained gradually. Loading dosage is employed only if the urgency for control of seizures exceeds the risk of adverse effects during the initial therapy.

The results of the initial medication should be assessed with appropriate regard for the time required to attain the plateau state, the usual variability of incidence of seizures, and the anticipation that some tolerance usually develops to the sedative and other minor adverse effects of these drugs. Dosage is increased at appropriate intervals, as required for control of seizures or as limited by toxicity, and such adjustment is preferably assisted by monitoring of drug concentrations in plasma.

If a single drug fails to provide adequate control of seizures in maximal tolerated dosage, *another drug should be substituted or a second drug may be added.* The choice between these alternatives is usually determined by consideration of the adverse effects of the drug in the individual patient. Unless serious adverse effects of the drug dictate otherwise, *dosage should always be reduced gradually* when a drug is being discontinued, to minimize the risk of precipitating status epilepticus. No drug should be discarded as useless unless obvious toxicity or monitoring of drug concentrations in plasma indicates that the patient has actually been taking the medication as prescribed.

Essential to optimal management of epilepsy is the *filling-out of a seizure chart* by the patient or a relative; *frequent visits to the physician or seizure clinic,* particularly in the early period of treatment, since hematological and other possible somatic side effects require consideration of change in medication; and *long-term follow-up,* including repetition of EEG and neurological examination. Most crucial for successful management is *regularity of medication.*

Common *causes of failure* of antiepileptic medication are improper diagnosis of the type of seizure, incorrect choice of drug, inadequate or excessive dosage, too frequent changes in medication without regard for the time required for transition between plateau states, failure to utilize fully the advantages of multiple-drug medication, inattention to ancillary aspects of therapy, and poor compliance by the patient. Poor compliance may take the form of erratic medication, with only partial control of seizures; consistent failure to take medication, with failure ever to attain adequate drug concentration; or excessive medication, with needless toxicity. Poor compliance sometimes persists despite the best efforts of the physician, but it can usually be corrected. Similarly, failure of therapy because of inattention to recommendations about diet, rest, avoidance of alcohol, and similar ancillary factors can usually be prevented.

Measurement of *plasma drug concentration* at appropriate intervals greatly facilitates the *initial adjustment* of dosage for individual differences in drug elimination and the *subsequent adjustment* of dosage to minimize dose-related adverse effects without sacrifice of seizure control. If control of seizures is less than complete, monitoring can assist in the choice between adjusting dosage of the existing medication, substituting an alternative drug, or adding a second drug. Periodic monitoring during *maintenance therapy* can detect failure of the patient to take the medication as prescribed; for the patient with infrequent seizures and apparent control, periodic monitoring can provide assurance that seizure control is, in fact, being maintained. Knowledge of plasma drug concentration can be especially helpful during *multiple-drug therapy.* If toxicity occurs, monitoring helps to identify the particular drug responsible, and, if pharmacokinetic drug interaction occurs, it can guide readjustment of dosage. In general, monitoring of drug concentrations in plasma during antiepileptic therapy is likely to be an aid whenever therapy is less than satisfactory or whenever it is associated with toxicity or an unexpected or atypical clinical response.

Duration of Therapy. In an attempt to provide guidelines for withdrawal of anticonvulsant drugs,

Holowach and coworkers (1972) studied the effects of withdrawing treatment from 148 children who had been free of seizures for 4 years. One quarter of the children had a recurrence of seizures during the next 5 to 12 years. Most of these were children who had focal seizures. The recurrence rates were lowest in children who had only grand mal (8%) or absence (12%) seizures.

Other studies have suggested that the rate of recurrence for adults is around 40% (*see* Meinardi *et al.,* 1977). A history of a single recent seizure may interfere with employment or the right to have a driver's license; these are important considerations in adult patients.

If a decision to withdraw antiepileptic drugs is made, such withdrawal should be done gradually over a period of months. The risk of *status epilepticus* is great with abrupt cessation of therapy.

Generalized Tonic-Clonic (Grand Mal) and Cortical Focal Seizures. Phenytoin and phenobarbital are the principal agents used to treat generalized tonic-clonic seizures. Phenobarbital is generally the agent of choice in children under the age of 5, while phenytoin is usually used first for older children and adults. Concurrent administration of the two drugs is often advantageous. Their differing side effects permit full dosage of each and, therefore, a relatively greater common anticonvulsant effect. The combined use is also of value because the full effect of phenytoin alone may leave a residuum of focal seizures, aura or prodromata, or a subclinical focal EEG dysrhythmia. This residuum can be prevented by concurrent use of phenobarbital. Conversely, the combined use of the two drugs is advantageous in mixed generalized tonic-clonic and temporal lobe seizures because phenobarbital alone is usually ineffective against the latter component.

Carbamazepine is also useful in the treatment of generalized tonic-clonic seizures, although it is generally considered to be more toxic than phenobarbital or phenytoin. A recent double-blind study of a small number of patients demonstrated that carbamazepine is as effective as phenytoin in the treatment of generalized tonic-clonic and focal seizures (Kosteljanetz *et al.,* 1979). Although valproic acid has not yet been approved for use in the United States in the treatment of generalized tonic-clonic seizures, clinical experience has suggested that it is an effective agent for such patients (*see* Bruni and Wilder, 1979).

Primidone alone may be effective in patients who are refractory to phenytoin and phenobarbital. However, it is more commonly employed concurrently with phenytoin. Since it is metabolized in part to phenobarbital, primidone is logically a substitute for, not a supplement to, phenobarbital. Mephenytoin is sometimes dramatically superior to phenytoin, but the advantage is offset by the greater risk of serious toxicity. Cortical focal seizures usually respond to the agents employed for generalized tonic-clonic seizures.

Absence (Petit Mal) Seizures. Trimethadione was the first agent of selective benefit against absence seizures in children (Lennox, 1945; Richards and Perlstein, 1946). As a result, its reputation has somewhat exceeded its true worth. Ethosuximide is more effective and has a lower risk of serious toxicity. Complete control of absence seizures can be attained in about 50% of patients, and significant reduction in seizure frequency is achieved in another 25%.

Numerous controlled studies have demonstrated the effectiveness of valproic acid in absence seizures. It may be possible to achieve a 75% reduction in the frequency of such seizures in approximately two thirds of patients by administration of this drug (Simon and Penry, 1975; Pinder et al., 1977). Some investigators suggest that valproate might offer the advantage of preventing the emergence of tonic-clonic seizures without the need for additional therapy.

Clonazepan is also effective in the treatment of absence seizures, particularly those with a myoclonic component. However, because tolerance may develop to the antiepileptic effects, other agents are generally preferred.

Phenytoin, phenobarbital, and primidone are ineffective against absence seizures and may increase their frequency, but medication with one of these agents is often required as additional therapy against the emergence of generalized tonic-clonic seizures (Livingston et al., 1965).

Partial Seizures with Complex Symptomatology. The treatment of partial seizures with complex symptomatology (psychomotor or temporal lobe seizures) is generally less effective than is that of generalized or absence seizures. Essential to appropriate therapy is differentiation between absence seizures and partial seizures with complex symptomatology. The latter are characterized by an aura, a longer duration, and postictal confusion (see Dreifuss, in Symposium, 1975). The agents used to treat absence seizures are generally ineffective for partial seizures with complex symptomatology.

The agents effective for generalized tonic-clonic seizures are also employed for control of partial seizures with complex symptomatology. Phenytoin is often the preferred drug, particularly if there are associated tonic-clonic seizures. Primidone is generally used in preference to phenobarbital, although both are employed. Carbamazepine is also a very useful agent in the treatment of complex partial seizures and may be effective in cases that are refractory to other agents. Its use has been limited by fear of hematological side effects. Some investigators maintain that the risks of cautious treatment with carbamazepine are very low and consider it to be a drug of first choice (see Parsonage, in Symposium, 1975).

Febrile Convulsions. Two to four percent of children experience a convulsion associated with a febrile illness. About 33% of these children will have another febrile convulsion, and 2 to 3% become epileptic in later years. This is a sixfold increase in risk compared to the general population.

The treatment, if any, of febrile seizures is controversial (see Fishman, 1979). Several alternatives have been proposed, including no treatment, regular treatment with phenobarbital, or initiation of phenobarbital at the onset of a febrile illness. The latter course of action is doomed to failure because of the pharmacokinetic properties of phenobarbital. It takes several days to reach effective concentrations in blood, and the use of a sufficient loading dose results in toxic effects.

One approach to the problem of febrile seizures is to institute chronic therapy in those children who are at greatest risk for a recurrence of seizures. This includes children who have their first seizure before 18 months of age, those who have significant neurological abnormalities, and those in whom the seizures last more than 15 minutes or are complex in nature (see Fishman, 1979). Phenobarbital is the drug of choice. If the child has experienced no seizures for 30 months and is otherwise normal, therapy is usually discontinued.

Seizures in Infants and Young Children. Infantile myoclonic spasms with hypsarhythmia are refractory to the usual antiepileptic agents; corticotropin or the adrenocorticosteroids are the agents of choice. The earlier the diagnosis is established and treatment initiated, the more successful is therapy. Clonazepam may be a useful adjunct, but tolerance often develops.

Primidone may be effective against myoclonic, akinetic, and atonic seizures in young children. Clonazepam is also a useful agent in such cases.

Phenytoin is relatively ineffective and may produce restlessness and hyperactivity when employed in young children (Laurance, 1970). Phenobarbital is the drug of choice for generalized tonic-clonic seizures in children under 5 years of age.

Posttraumatic Epilepsy. Head injuries can predispose to the development of epilepsy; with penetrating wounds the risk may be as high as 30 to 40%. There is some clinical evidence to suggest that prophylactic therapy may be effective in preventing the development of a seizure disorder in such cases. This would be consistent with the kindling model of epilepsy, discussed above. The agents effective for treatment of focal seizures and generalized tonic-clonic convulsions are employed.

Status Epilepticus and Other Convulsive Emergencies. Status epilepticus is a neurological emergency; untreated it may be fatal. In addition to specific drug therapy, supportive care is essential. Attention must be paid to electrolyte abnormalities, cardiac arrhythmias, dehydration, hypoglycemia, and the possibility of hypotensive shock. Diazepam, administered intravenously, is the agent of choice for control of status epilepticus; the dosage is discussed above. It is effective in 80 to 90% of cases, largely independent of seizure type or etiology. Phenobarbital or phenytoin may also be employed intravenously. The latter agent must be administered at a rate less than 50 mg per minute, and even more slowly in elderly patients, to minimize the risk of central and cardiovascular toxicity. Whatever agent is employed, equipment for maintenance of an airway and for mechanical support of ventilation must be immediately available. After seizures are controlled, appropriate chronic antiepileptic therapy should be initiated.

Convulsive emergencies associated with *drug poisoning* and *drug-induced seizures* in previously nonepileptic patients during medication with agents such as the local anesthetics may also be controlled by diazepam and phenobarbital or another barbiturate. The control of *drug-withdrawal seizures* associated with abuse of alcohol, barbiturates, or related sedative-hypnotics is discussed in Chapter 23.

Antiepileptic Therapy and Pregnancy. Children of epileptic mothers who received anticonvulsant medication during the early months of pregnancy have an increased incidence of a variety of birth defects. Evidence is greatest for therapy with phenobarbital, phenytoin, or trimethadione, and there is suggestive evidence of a similar relationship for other antiepileptic agents. Retrospective studies suggest that a specific set of fetal abnormalities is associated with maternal use of trimethadione; the incidence of this *fetal trimethadione syndrome* may be very high (German *et al.,* 1970; Zackai *et al.,* 1975). A *fetal hydantoin syndrome* has also been described (Hanson and Smith, 1975).

Most (> 90%) *epileptic mothers treated with antiepileptic drugs bear normal children.* In addition, epilepsy itself probably carries a risk of fetal defects, and abrupt discontinuation of medication incurs a definite risk of status epilepticus and its hazards for the fetus and mother. For these reasons, antiepileptic medication should *not* be discontinued in pregnant epileptic women for whom the medication is necessary for the prevention of major seizures. However, depending upon the frequency and severity of seizures in the *individual patient,* cautious reduction of dosage to a minimum may be feasible and advisable, particularly in the first trimester. Therapeutic abortion should be considered when trimethadione has been used during pregnancy. Folic acid deficiency, if present, should be corrected. (*See* Fedrick, 1973; Lowe, 1973; Monson *et al.,* 1973.)

The newborn of mothers who received phenobarbital, primidone, or phenytoin during pregnancy may also develop a deficiency of vitamin K–dependent clotting factors, and serious hemorrhage may occur during the first 24 hours of life. Bleeding can be prevented by administration of vitamin K.

Arnold, K., and Gerber, N. The rate of decline of diphenylhydantoin in human plasma. *Clin. Pharmacol. Ther.,* **1970,** *11,* 121–134.

Blom, S. Tic douloureux treated with new anticonvulsant. *Arch. Neurol.,* **1963,** *9,* 285–290.

Bogue, J. Y., and Carrington, H. C. The evaluation of "MYSOLINE"—a new anticonvulsant drug. *Br. J. Pharmacol.,* **1953,** *8,* 230–236.

Booker, H. E.; Chun, R. W. M.; and Sanguino, M. Myasthenic syndrome associated with trimethadione. *Neurology (Minneap.),* **1968,** *18,* 274.

Booker, H. E., and Darcey, B. Serum concentrations of free diphenylhydantoin and their relationship to clinical intoxication. *Epilepsia,* **1973,** *14,* 177–184.

Brown, W. C.; Schiffman, D. O.; Swinyard, E. A.; and Goodman, L. S. Comparative assay of antiepileptic drugs by "psychomotor" seizure test and minimal electroshock threshold test. *J. Pharmacol. Exp. Ther.,* **1953,** *107,* 273–283.

Browne, T. R. Clonazepam. *N. Engl. J. Med.,* **1978,** *299,* 812–816.

Browne, T. R.; Dreifuss, F. E.; Dyken, P. R.; Goode, D. J.; Penry, J. K.; Porter, R. J.; White, B. G.; and White, P. T. Ethosuximide in the treatment of absence (petit mal) seizures. *Neurology (Minneap.),* **1975,** *25,* 515–524.

Browne, T. R., and Penry, J. K. Benzodiazepines in the treatment of epilepsy: a review. *Epilepsia,* **1973,** *14,* 277–310.

Bruni, J., and Wilder, B. J. Valproic acid. *Arch. Neurol.,* **1979,** *36,* 393–398.

Buchthal, F., and Svensmark, O. Serum concentrations of diphenylhydantoin (phenytoin) and phenobarbital and their relation to therapeutic and toxic effects. *Psychiatr. Neurol. Neurochir.,* **1971,** *74,* 117–136.

Buchthal, F.; Svensmark, O.; and Simonsen, H. Relation of EEG and seizures to phenobarbital in serum. *Arch. Neurol.,* **1968,** *19,* 567–572.

Butler, T. C. Quantitative studies of the physiological disposition of 3-methyl-5-ethyl-5-phenyl hydantoin (MESANTOIN) and 5-ethyl-5-phenyl hydantoin (NIRVANOL). *J. Pharmacol. Exp. Ther.,* **1953,** *109,* 340–345.

————. The metabolic hydroxylation of phenobarbital. *Ibid.,* **1956,** *116,* 326–336.

Butler, T. C., and Waddell, W. J. A pharmacological comparison of the optical isomers of 5-ethyl-5-methyl-2,4-oxazolidinedione and of 3,5-dimethyl-5-ethyl-2,4-oxazolidinedione (paramethadione, PARADIONE). *J. Pharmacol. Exp. Ther.,* **1955,** *113,* 238–240.

Butler, T. C.; Waddell, W. J.; and Poole, D. T. Demethylation of trimethadione and metharbital by rat liver microsomal enzymes: substrate concentration-yield relationships and competition between substrates. *Biochem. Pharmacol.,* **1965,** *14,* 937–942.

Camerman, A., and Camerman, M. Diphenylhydantoin and diazepam. Molecular structure similarities and steric basis of anticonvulsant activity. *Science,* **1970,** *168,* 1457–1458.

Chamberlin, H. R.; Waddell, W. J.; and Butler, T. C. A study of the product of demethylation of trimethadione in the control of petit mal epilepsy. *Neurology (Minneap.),* **1965,** *15,* 449–454.

Chang, T.; Okerholm, R. A.; and Glazko, A. J. Identification of 5-(3,4-dihydroxyphenyl)-5-phenylhydantoin: a metabolite of 5,5-diphenylhydantoin (DILANTIN) in rat urine. *Anal. Letters,* **1972,** *5,* 195–202.

Chang, T.; Savory, A.; and Glazko, A. J. A new metabolite of 5,5-diphenylhydantoin (DILANTIN). *Biochem. Biophys. Res. Commun.,* **1970,** *38,* 444–449.

Chen, G.; Weston, J. K.; and Bratton, A. C., Jr. Anticonvulsant activity and toxicity of phensuximide, methsuximide and ethosuximide. *Epilepsia,* **1963,** *4,* 66–76.

Crill, W. E. Carbamazepine. *Ann. Intern. Med.,* **1973,** *79,* 844–847.

Dam, M. The density and ultrastructure of the Purkinje cells following diphenylhydantoin treatment in animals and man. *Acta Neurol. Scand.,* **1972,** *48,* Suppl. 49, 1–65.

Davis, J. P., and Lennox, W. G. The effect of trimethyloxazolidine dione and dimethyl ethyloxazolidine dione on seizures and on the blood. *Proc. Assoc. Res. Nerv. Ment. Dis.,* **1947,** *36,* 423–436.

Delgado, J. M. R., and Mihailović, L.   Use of intracerebral electrodes to evaluate drugs that act on the central nervous system. *Ann. N.Y. Acad. Sci.,* **1956,** *64,* 644–666.

Dill, W. A.; Kazenko, A.; Wolf, L. M.; and Glazko, A. J.   Studies on 5,5-diphenylhydantoin (DILANTIN) in animals and man. *J. Pharmacol. Exp. Ther.,* **1956,** *118,* 270–279.

Dreifuss, F. E.   Use of anticonvulsant drugs. *J.A.M.A.,* **1979,** *241,* 607–609.

Dudley, K. H.; Bius, D. L.; and Waldrop, C. D.   Urinary metabolites of N-methyl-α-methyl-α-phenylsuccinimide (methsuximide) in the dog. *Drug Metab. Dispos.,* **1974,** *2,* 113–122.

Englander, R. N.; Johnson, R. N.; Brickley, J. J.; and Hanna, G. R.   Effects of antiepileptic drugs on thalamocortical excitability. *Neurology (Minneap.),* **1977,** *27,* 1134–1139.

Esplin, D. W.   Effects of diphenylhydantoin on synaptic transmission in cat spinal cord and stellate ganglion. *J. Pharmacol. Exp. Ther.,* **1957,** *120,* 301–323.

Esplin, D. W., and Curto, E. M.   Effects of trimethadione on synaptic transmission in the spinal cord; antagonism of trimethadione and pentylenetetrazol. *J. Pharmacol. Exp. Ther.,* **1957,** *121,* 457–467.

Everett, G. M., and Richards, R. K.   Comparative anticonvulsive action of 3,5,5-trimethyloxazolidine-2,4-dione (TRIDIONE), DILANTIN and phenobarbital. *J. Pharmacol. Exp. Ther.,* **1944,** *81,* 402–407.

————.   Pharmacological studies of phenacetylurea (PHENURONE), an anticonvulsant drug. *Ibid.,* **1952,** *106,* 303–313.

Fedrick, J.   Epilepsy and pregnancy: a report from the Oxford Record Linkage Study. *Br. Med. J.,* **1973,** *2,* 442–448.

Ferrandes, B., and Eymard, P.   Metabolism of valproate sodium in rabbit, rat, dog, and man. *Epilepsia,* **1977,** *18,* 169–182.

Fishman, M. A.   Febrile seizures: the treatment controversy. *J. Pediatr.,* **1979,** *94,* 174–184.

Frey, H.-H., and Löscher, W.   Di-n-propylacetic acid—a profile of anticonvulsant activity in mice. *Arzneim. Forsch.,* **1976,** *26,* 299–301.

Frey, H.-H., and Schulz, R.   Time course of the demethylation of trimethadione. *Acta Pharmacol. Toxicol. (Kbh.),* **1970,** *28,* 477–483.

Fromm, G. H.; Wessel, H. B.; Glass, J. D.; Alvin, J. D.; and Van Horn, G.   Imipramine in absence and myoclonic-astatic seizures. *Neurology (Minneap.),* **1978,** *28,* 953–957.

Gastaut, H.   Clinical and electroencephalographical classification of epileptic seizures. *Epilepsia,* **1970,** *11,* 102–113.

German, J.; Kowal, A.; and Ehlers, K. H.   Trimethadione and human teratogenesis. *Teratology,* **1970,** *3,* 349–362.

Gibbs, F. A.; Everett, G. M.; and Richards, R. K.   PHENURONE in epilepsy. *Dis. Nerv. Syst.,* **1949,** *10,* 47–49.

Glazko, A. J.   Diphenylhydantoin metabolism: a prospective review. *Drug Metab. Dispos.,* **1973,** *1,* 711–714.

Goodman, L. S.; Swinyard, E. A.; Brown, W. C.; Schiffman, D. O.; Grewal, M. S.; and Bliss, E. L.   Anticonvulsant properties of 5-phenyl-5-ethyl-hexahydropyrimidine-4,6-dione (MYSOLINE), a new antiepileptic. *J. Pharmacol. Exp. Ther.,* **1953,** *108,* 428–436.

Goodman, L. S.; Toman, J. E. P.; and Swinyard, E. A.   The anticonvulsant properties of TRIDIONE: laboratory and clinical investigations. *Am. J. Med.,* **1946,** *1,* 213–228.

————.   Anticonvulsant properties of 5,5-phenyl thienyl hydantoin in comparison with DILANTIN and MESANTOIN. *Proc. Soc. Exp. Biol. Med.,* **1948,** *68,* 584–587.

Greenblatt, D. J., and Koch-Weser, J.   Adverse reactions to intravenous diazepam: a report from the Boston Collaborative Drug Surveillance Program. *Am. J. Med. Sci.,* **1973,** *266,* 261–266.

Guberman, A.; Gloor, P.; and Sherwin, A. L.   Response of

generalized penicillin epilepsy in the cat to ethosuximide and diphenylhydantoin. *Neurology (Minneap.),* **1975,** *25,* 758–764.

Halpern, L. M., and Julien, R. M.   Augmentation of cerebellar Purkinje cell discharge rate after diphenylhydantoin. *Epilepsia,* **1972,** *13,* 377–385.

Handley, R., and Stewart, A. S. R.   MYSOLINE: a new drug in the treatment of epilepsy. *Lancet,* **1952,** *1,* 742–744.

Hanson, J. W., and Smith, D. W.   The fetal hydantoin syndrome. *J. Pediatr.,* **1975,** *87,* 285–290.

Hassell, T. M.; Page, R. C.; Narayanan, A. S.; and Cooper, C. G.   Diphenylhydantoin (DILANTIN) gingival hyperplasia: drug-induced abnormality of connective tissue. *Proc. Natl. Acad. Sci. U.S.A.,* **1976,** *73,* 2909–2912.

Hauptmann, A.   LUMINAL bei Epilepsie. *Munch. Med. Wochenschr.,* **1912,** *59,* 1907–1909.

Hauser, W. A.   Epidemiology of epilepsy. *Adv. Neurol.,* **1978,** *19,* 313–339.

Holowach, J.; Thurston, D. L.; and O'Leary, J.   Prognosis in childhood epilepsy: follow-up study of 148 cases in which therapy has been suspended after prolonged anticonvulsant control. *N. Engl. J. Med.,* **1972,** *286,* 169–174.

Jeavons, P. M.; Clark, J. E.; and Maheshwari, M. C.   Treatment of generalized epilepsies of childhood and adolescence with sodium valproate (EPILIM). *Dev. Med. Child Neurol.,* **1977,** *19,* 9–25.

Jensen, B. N.   Trimethadione in serum of patients with petit mal epilepsy. *Dan. Med. Bull.,* **1962,** *9,* 74–79.

Johnson, R. N.; Charlton, J. D.; Englander, R. N.; Brickley, J. J.; Nowack, W. J.; and Hanna, G. R.   Cerebellar stimulation: regional effects on a thalamocortical system. *Epilepsia,* **1979,** *20,* 247–254.

Julien, R. M., and Halpern, L. M.   Effects of diphenylhydantoin and other antiepileptic drugs on epileptiform activity and Purkinje cell discharge rates. *Epilepsia,* **1972,** *13,* 387–400.

Karch, S. B.   Methsuximide overdose: delayed onset of profound coma. *J.A.M.A.,* **1973,** *223,* 1463–1465.

Kiser, J. S.; Vargas-Cordon, M.; Brendel, K.; and Bressler, R.   The in vitro inhibition of insulin secretion by diphenylhydantoin. *J. Clin. Invest.,* **1970,** *49,* 1942–1948.

Klotz, U., and Antonin, K. H.   Pharmacokinetics and bioavailability of sodium valproate. *Clin. Pharmacol. Ther.,* **1977,** *21,* 736–743.

Kosteljanetz, M.; Christiansen, J.; Dan, A. M.; Hansen, B. S.; Lyon, B. B.; Pedersen, H.; and Dam, M.   Carbamazepine *vs.* phenytoin. *Arch. Neurol.,* **1979,** *36,* 22–24.

Krall, R. L.; Penry, J. K.; Kupferberg, H. J.; and Swinyard, E. A.   Antiepileptic drug development. I. History and a program for progress. *Epilepsia,* **1978a,** *19,* 393–408.

Krall, R. L.; Penry, J. K.; White, B. G.; Kupferberg, H. J.; and Swinyard, E. A.   Antiepileptic drug development. II. Anticonvulsant drug screening. *Epilepsia,* **1978b,** *19,* 409–428.

Krupp, P.   The effect of TEGRETOL on some elementary neuronal mechanisms. *Headache,* **1969,** *9,* 42–46.

Kutt, H.; Wolk, M.; Scherman, R.; and McDowell, F.   Insufficient parahydroxylation as a cause of diphenylhydantoin toxicity. *Neurology (Minneap.),* **1964,** *14,* 542–548.

Laurance, B. M.   Idiopathic epilepsy. *Practitioner,* **1970,** *205,* 331–332.

Lennox, W. G.   The petit mal epilepsies: their treatment with TRIDIONE. *J.A.M.A.,* **1945,** *129,* 1069–1073.

Leviel, V., and Naquet, R.   A study of the action of valproic acid on the kindling effect. *Epilepsia,* **1977,** *18,* 229–234.

Levin, S. R.; Booker, J., Jr.; Smith, D. F.; and Grodsky, G. M.   Inhibition of insulin secretion by diphenylhydantoin in the isolated perfused pancreas. *J. Clin. Endocrinol. Metab.,* **1970,** *30,* 400–401.

Livingston, S.; Pauli, L. L.; and German, W.   Carbamazepine (TEGRETOL) in epilepsy. Nine year follow-up study with special emphasis on untoward reactions. *Dis. Nerv. Syst.,* **1974,** *35,* 103–107.

Livingston, S.; Torres, I.; Pauli, L. L.; and Rider, R. V.

Petit mal epilepsy: results of a prolonged follow-up study of 117 patients. *J.A.M.A.*, **1965**, *194*, 227–232.

Lockard, J. S.; Levy, R. H.; Congdon, W. C.; DuCharme, L. L.; and Patel, I. H. Efficacy testing of valproic acid compared to ethosuximide in monkey model. II. Seizure, EEG, and diurnal variations. *Epilepsia*, **1977**, *18*, 205–224.

Lombroso, C. T., and Forsythe, I. A long term follow-up of acetazolamide (DIAMOX) in the treatment of epilepsy. *Epilepsia*, **1960**, *1*, 493–500.

Loscalzo, A. E. MESANTOIN in the control of epilepsy. *Neurology (Minneap.)*, **1952**, *2*, 403–411.

Löscher, W. Rapid determination of valproate sodium in serum by gas-liquid chromatography. *Epilepsia*, **1977**, *18*, 225–227.

Lowe, C. R. Congenital malformations among infants born to epileptic women. *Lancet*, **1973**, *1*, 9–10.

Macdonald, R. L., and Barker, J. L. Anticonvulsant and anesthetic barbiturates: different postsynaptic actions in cultured mammalian neurons. *Neurology (Minneap.)*, **1979a**, *29*, 432–447.

———. Enhancement of GABA-mediated postsynaptic inhibition in cultured mammalian spinal cord neurons: a common mode of anticonvulsant action. *Brain Res.*, **1979b**, *167*, 323–336.

Macdonald, R. L., and Bergey, G. K. Valproic acid augments GABA-mediated postsynaptic inhibition in cultured mammalian neurons. *Brain Res.*, **1979**, *170*, 558–562.

Medical Letter. Drugs for epilepsy. **1979**, *21*, 25–28.

Melikian, A. P.; Straughn, A. B.; Slywka, G. W. A.; Whyatt, P. L.; and Meyer, M. C. Bioavailability of 11 phenytoin products. *J. Pharmacokinet. Biopharm.*, **1977**, *5*, 133–146.

Merritt, H. H., and Putnam, T. J. A new series of anticonvulsant drugs tested by experiments on animals. *Arch. Neurol. Psychiatry*, **1938a**, *39*, 1003–1015.

———. Sodium diphenyl hydantoinate in treatment of convulsive disorders. *J.A.M.A.*, **1938b**, *111*, 1068–1073.

Meunier, G.; Carraz, G.; Neunier, Y.; Eymard, P.; and Aimard, M. Propriétés pharmacodynamiques de l'acide n-dipropylacétique. *Therapie*, **1963**, *18*, 435–438.

Millichap, J. G. Relation of laboratory evaluation to clinical effectiveness of antiepileptic drugs. *Epilepsia*, **1969**, *10*, 315–328.

———. Drug therapy and management of the child with epilepsy. *Drug Ther.*, **1971**, *1*, No. 10, 15–29.

Monson, R. R.; Rosenberg, L.; Hartz, S. C.; Shapiro, S.; Heinonen, O. P.; and Sloane, D. Diphenylhydantoin and selected congenital malformations. *N. Engl. J. Med.*, **1973**, *289*, 1049–1052.

Morrell, F.; Bradley, W.; and Ptashne, M. Effects of drugs on discharge characteristics of chronic epileptogenic lesions. *Neurology (Minneap.)*, **1959**, *9*, 492–498.

Morris, M. E. Compatibility and stability of diazepam injection following dilution with intravenous fluids. *Am. J. Hosp. Pharm.*, **1978**, *35*, 669–672.

Mullen, P. W. Optimal phenytoin therapy: a new technique for individualizing dosage. *Clin. Pharmacol. Ther.*, **1978**, *23*, 228–232.

Pedley, T. A. The pathophysiology of focal epilepsy: neurophysiological considerations. *Ann. Neurol.*, **1978**, *3*, 2–9.

Perlstein, M. A. GEMONAL (5,5-diethyl 1-methyl barbituric acid): a new drug for convulsive and related disorders. *Pediatrics*, **1950**, *5*, 448–451.

———. Metharbital (GEMONIL) in myoclonic spasms of infancy and related disorders. *Am. J. Dis. Child.*, **1957**, *93*, 425–429.

Perlstein, M. A., and Andelman, M. B. TRIDIONE: its use in convulsive and related disorders. *J. Pediatr.*, **1946**, *29*, 20–40.

Plaa, G. L., and Hine, C. H. Hydantoin and barbiturate blood levels observed in epileptics. *Arch. Int. Pharmacodyn. Ther.*, **1960**, *78*, 375–382.

Porter, R. J.; Penry, J. K.; Lacy, J. R.; Newmark, M. E.; and Kupferberg, H. J. The clinical efficacy and pharmacokinetics of phensuximide and methsuximide. *Neurology (Minneap.)*, **1977**, *27*, 375–376.

Reidenberg, M. M.; Odar-Cedarlöf, I.; von Bahr, C.; Borgå, O.; and Sjöqvist, F. Protein binding of diphenylhydantoin and desmethylimipramine in plasma from patients with poor renal function. *N. Engl. J. Med.*, **1971**, *285*, 264–267.

Richards, R. K., and Perlstein, M. A. TRIDIONE, a new drug for the treatment of convulsive and related disorders. *Arch. Neurol. Psychiatry*, **1946**, *55*, 164–165.

Schallek, W., and Kuehn, A. Effects of trimethadione, diphenylhydantoin, and chlordiazepoxide on afterdischarges in brain of cat. *Proc. Soc. Exp. Biol. Med.*, **1963**, *112*, 813–817.

Schwade, E. D.; Richards, R. K.; and Everett, G. M. PEGANONE, a new antiepileptic drug. *Dis. Nerv. Syst.*, **1956**, *17*, 155–158.

Simon, D., and Penry, J. K. Sodium di-*n*-propylacetate (DPA) in the treatment of epilepsy. *Epilepsia*, **1975**, *16*, 549–573.

Sloan, L. L., and Gilger, A. P. Visual effects of TRIDIONE. *Am. J. Ophthalmol.*, **1947**, *30*, 1387–1405.

Sorrell, T. C.; Forbes, I. J.; Burness, F. R.; and Rischbieth, R. H. C. Depression of immunological function in patients treated with phenytoin sodium (sodium diphenylhydantoin). *Lancet*, **1971**, *2*, 1233–1235.

Strong, J. M.; Abe, T.; Gibbs, E. L.; and Atkinson, A. J., Jr. Plasma levels of methsuximide and N-desmethylmethsuximide during methsuximide therapy. *Neurology (Minneap.)*, **1974**, *24*, 250–255.

Suchy, F. J.; Balistreri, W. F.; Buchino, J. J.; Sondheimer, J. M.; Bates, S. R.; Kearns, G. L.; Stull, J. D.; and Bove, K. E. Acute hepatic failure associated with the use of sodium valproate. *N. Engl. J. Med.*, **1979**, *300*, 962–966.

Svensmark, O., and Buchthal, F. Accumulation of phenobarbital in man. *Epilepsia*, **1963**, *4*, 199–206.

Swinyard, E. A., and Castellion, A. W. Anticonvulsant properties of some benzodiazepines. *J. Pharmacol. Exp. Ther.*, **1966**, *151*, 369–375.

Tanaka, T., and Lange, H. L'effet d'embrasement (kindling effect) par stimulation amygdalienne chez le chat at le rat. *Rev. Electroencephalogr. Neurophysiol. Clin.*, **1975**, *5*, 41–44.

Toman, J. E. P.; Loewe, S.; and Goodman, L. S. Physiology and therapy of convulsive disorders. I. Effect of anticonvulsant drugs on electroshock seizures in man. *Arch. Neurol. Psychiatry*, **1947**, *58*, 312–324.

Toman, J. E. P., and Sabelli, H. C. Comparative neuronal mechanisms. *Epilepsia*, **1969**, *10*, 179–192.

Troupin, A. S.; Ojemann, L. M.; and Dodrill, C. B. Mephenytoin: a reappraisal. *Epilepsia*, **1976**, *17*, 403–414.

Tyler, M. W., and King, E. Q. Phenacemide in treatment of epilepsy. *J.A.M.A.*, **1951**, *147*, 17–21.

Van Buren, J. M.; Wood, J. H.; Oakley, J.; and Hambrecht, F. Preliminary evaluation of cerebellar stimulation by double-blind stimulation and biological criteria in the treatment of epilepsy. *J. Neurosurg.*, **1978**, *48*, 407–416.

Vernadakis, A., and Woodbury, D. M. The developing animal as a model. *Epilepsia*, **1969**, *10*, 163–178.

Vossen, R. On the anticonvulsant effect of succinimides. *Dtsch. Med. Wochenschr.*, **1958**, *83*, 1227–1230.

Wada, J. A. Pharmacological prophylaxis in the kindling model of epilepsy. *Arch. Neurol.*, **1977**, *34*, 389–395.

Wilder, B. J.; Willmore, L. J.; and Bruni, J. Valproic acid: interaction with other anticonvulsant drugs. *Neurology (Minneap.)*, **1978**, *28*, 892–896.

Willmore, L. J.; Wilder, B. J.; Bruni, J.; and Villarreal, H. J. Effect of valproic acid on hepatic function. *Neurology (Minneap.)*, **1978**, *28*, 961–964.

Withrow, C. D.; Stout, R. J.; Barton, L. J.; Beacham, W. S.; and Woodbury, D. M. Anticonvulsant effects of 5,5-dimethyl-2,4-oxazolidinedione (DMO). *J. Pharmacol. Exp. Ther.*, **1968**, *161*, 335–341.

Wulff, K.; Flachs, H.; Würtz-Jørgensen, A.; and Gram, L. Clinical pharmacological aspects of valproate sodium. *Epilepsia,* **1977,** *18,* 149–157.

Zackai, E. H.; Mellman, W. J.; Neiderer, B.; and Hanson, J. W. The fetal trimethadione syndrome. *J. Pediatr.,* **1975,** *87,* 280–284.

Zimmerman, F. T. Use of methylphenylsuccinimide in treatment of petit mal epilepsy. *A.M.A. Arch. Neurol. Psychiatry,* **1951,** *66,* 156–162.

———. Evaluation of N-α,α-methylphenyl succinimide in the treatment of petit mal epilepsy. *N.Y. State J. Med.,* **1956,** *56,* 1460–1465.

Zimmerman, F. T., and Burgemeister, B. B. A new drug for petit mal epilepsy. *Neurology (Minneap.),* **1958,** *8,* 769–775.

Monographs and Reviews

Aird, R. B., and Woodbury, D. M. *Management of Epilepsy.* Charles C Thomas, Pub., Springfield, Ill., **1974.**

Ayala, G. F., and Johnston, D. The influences of phenytoin on the fundamental electrical properties of simple neural systems. *Epilepsia,* **1977,** *18,* 299–307.

Close, W. J., and Spielman, M. A. Anticonvulsant drugs. In, *Medicinal Chemistry,* Vol. 5. (Hartung, W. H., ed.) John Wiley & Sons, Inc., New York, **1961.**

Gibbs, F. A., and Gibbs, E. L. *Atlas of Electroencephalography,* Vols. 2 and 3. Addison-Wesley Press, Reading, Mass., **1954** and **1964.**

Guidotti, A.; Toffano, G.; Baraldi, M.; Schwartz, J. P.; and Costa, E. A molecular mechanism for facilitation of GABA receptor function by benzodiazepines. In, *GABA-Neurotransmitters.* (Larsen-Krogsgaard, P.; Scheel-Kruger, J.; and Kofod, H.; eds.) Academic Press, Inc., New York, **1979,** pp. 406–415.

Haefely, W.; Pole, P.; Schaffner, R.; Keller, H. H.; Pieri, L.; and Möhler, H. Facilitation of GABA-ergic transmission by drugs. In, *GABA-Neurotransmitters.* (Larsen-Krogsgaard, P.; Scheel-Kruger, J.; and Kofod, H.; eds.) Academic Press, Inc., New York, **1979,** pp. 357–375.

Lennox, W. G., and Lennox, M. A. *Epilepsy and Related Disorders.* Little, Brown & Co., Boston, **1960.** (Two volumes, 1128 references.)

Meinardi, H.; van Heycop ten Ham, M. W.; Meijer, J. W. A.; and Bongers, E. Long-term control of seizures. In, *Epilepsy: The Eighth International Symposium.* (Penry, J. K., ed.) Raven Press, New York, **1977,** pp. 17–26.

Murray, W. J., and Kier, L. B. Noncyclic anticonvulsants. In, *Anticonvulsants.* (Vida, J. A., ed.) Academic Press, Inc., New York, **1977,** pp. 578–616.

Pinder, R. M.; Brogden, R. N.; Speight, T. M.; and Avery, G. S. Clonazepam: a review of its pharmacological properties and therapeutic efficacy in epilepsy. *Drugs,* **1976,** *12,* 321–361.

———. Sodium valproate: a review of its pharmacological properties and therapeutic efficacy in epilepsy. *Ibid.,* **1977,** *13,* 81–123.

Popp, F. P. Other heterocyclic drugs. In, *Anticonvulsants.* (Vida, J. A., ed.) Academic Press, Inc., New York, **1977,** pp. 331–548.

Solomon, G. E., and Plum, F. *Clinical Management of Seizures: A Guide for the Physician.* W. B. Saunders Co., Philadelphia, **1976.**

Symposium. (Various authors.) *Basic Mechanisms of the Epilepsies.* (Jasper, H. H.; Ward, A. A., Jr.; and Pope, A.; eds.) Little, Brown & Co., Boston, **1969.**

Symposium. (Various authors.) *Antiepileptic Drugs.* (Woodbury, D. M.; Penry, J. K.; and Schmidt, R. P.; eds.) Raven Press, New York, **1972a.**

Symposium. (Various authors.) *Experimental Models of Epilepsy: A Manual for the Laboratory Worker.* (Purpura, D. P.; Penry, J. K.; Tower, D.; Woodbury, D. M.; and Walter, R.; eds.) Raven Press, New York, **1972b.**

Symposium. (Various authors.) *The Benzodiazepines.* (Garattini, S.; Mussini, E.; and Randall, L. O.; eds.) Raven Press, New York, **1973.**

Symposium. (Various authors.) *Advances in Neurology,* Vol. 11. (Penry, J. K., and Daly, D. D., eds.) Raven Press, New York, **1975.**

Symposium. (Various authors.) *Kindling.* (Wada, J., and Ross, R. T., eds.) Raven Press, New York, **1976.**

Symposium. (Various authors.) *Cerebellar Stimulation in Man.* (Cooper, I. S., ed.) Raven Press, New York, **1978a.**

Symposium. (Various authors.) *Antiepileptic Drugs: Quantitative Analysis and Interpretation.* (Pippinger, C. E.; Penry, J. K.; and Kutt, H.; eds.) Raven Press, New York, **1978b.**

Toman, J. E. P., and Goodman, L. S. Anticonvulsants. *Physiol. Rev.,* **1948,** *28,* 409–432. (216 references.)

Vida, J. A., and Gerry, E. H. Cyclic ureides. In, *Anticonvulsants.* (Vida, J. A., ed.) Academic Press, Inc., New York, **1977,** pp. 152–284.

Woodbury, D. M., and Esplin, D. W. Neuropharmacology and neurochemistry of anticonvulsant drugs. *Proc. Assoc. Res. Nerv. Ment. Dis.,* **1959,** *37,* 24–56.

Woodbury, D. M., and Kemp, J. W. Some possible mechanisms of action of antiepileptic drugs. *Pharmakopsychiat. Neuropsychopharmakol.,* **1970,** *3,* 201–226.

CHAPTER

21 DRUGS FOR PARKINSON'S DISEASE; CENTRALLY ACTING MUSCLE RELAXANTS

Joseph R. Bianchine

Drugs described in this chapter have in common the ability to improve skeletal muscle function by primary actions on the central nervous system (CNS). These drugs fall into two distinct categories on the basis of their sites of action within the CNS, their pharmacological properties, and their therapeutic uses. The first group acts primarily on the basal ganglia; its members exert either dopaminergic or anticholinergic effects, and they are useful for the treatment of Parkinson's disease and related disorders. *Levodopa* is the prototype of central dopaminergic drugs, while *trihexyphenidyl* is the prototypical central anticholinergic agent. The second group of drugs, the centrally acting skeletal muscle relaxants, depress with varying degrees of selectivity certain neuronal systems that control muscle tone. Members of this group are used for treating acute and chronic muscle spasm, tetanus, and certain types of poorly defined low back pain.

Research on basic and clinical aspects of Parkinson's disease and the success of its treatment have advanced rapidly during the past 15 years. Consequently, the major emphasis of this chapter is placed on drugs that are effective in this condition. Similar advances have not been made in the development of effective skeletal muscle relaxants.

I. Drugs for Parkinson's Disease

Parkinsonism: Clinical Overview. Parkinson's disease, first described by James Parkinson in 1817 as *paralysis agitans,* is a prevalent, serious neurological disease. It afflicts more than one-half million persons in the United States alone. A parkinsonism-like syndrome may arise from several causes (Barbeau, 1976; Pearce, 1978). The most common documented etiologies are cerebral atherosclerosis, viral encephalitis, and the

untoward effects of certain drugs. Drugs that produce parkinsonism have in common the capacity to prevent the action of dopamine in the basal ganglia of the brain (Calne *et al.,* 1979). For example, antipsychotic drugs such as the phenothiazines and butyrophenones block postsynaptic receptors for dopamine and cause extrapyramidal symptoms that resemble parkinsonism, especially in older patients (*see* Chapter 19). In contrast, reserpine produces a parkinsonism-like syndrome by depleting dopamine available for release by the presynaptic neuron. Progressive supranuclear palsy, olivopontocerebellar degeneration, Shy-Drager syndrome, carbon monoxide poisoning, manganese poisoning, and Wilson's disease commonly are associated with certain symptoms that are characteristic of Parkinson's disease. However, in these rare disorders, parkinsonism is only one aspect of a more widespread cerebral disorder. With the exception of manganese poisoning, dopaminergic drugs induce little improvement in these conditions.

Parkinson's disease, independent of specific etiology, usually appears insidiously in the latter decades of life and produces a slowly increasing disability in movement (Yahr, 1975; Pearce, 1978). The disease is usually characterized by four major clinical features: tremor, bradykinesia, rigidity, and a disturbance of posture (Bianchine, 1976).

Tremor results from rhythmically alternating, "pill-rolling" contractions (three to five per second) of a muscle group and its antagonist. Distal muscles are more commonly involved than proximal ones. Tremor can be present during rest, often disappears on purposeful movement (or during sleep), and usually increases remarkably with anxiety or stress. Tremor is commonly superimposed on the hypertonicity of mutually antagonistic groups of skeletal muscles. Initiation of movements becomes increasingly difficult, ponderous, and extremely inefficient and fatiguing.

Bradykinesia is characterized by three components—marked poverty of spontaneous movement, loss of normal associated movements, and slow initiation of all voluntary movements. The "masked" facial expression in parkinsonism classically demonstrates all these features.

Rigidity is due to increased muscle tone; a "cogwheel" or "ratchet" resistance to passive movement of an extremity characterizes this feature.

A *postural defect* appears late in the progression of the disease. The patient is unable to maintain an upright position of the trunk while standing or walking. Consequently, a progressively stooped position is assumed and a festinating gait may occur.

In advanced stages of parkinsonism, loss of motor function causes a variety of other signs and symptoms, such as impairment of postural reflexes, reduced blinking, micrographia, microphonia, and impaired ocular convergence. Autonomic symptoms of sialorrhea and seborrhea are also common.

Parkinsonism: A Striatal Dopamine-Deficiency Syndrome.

A prominent feature of the basal ganglia is their conspicuously high concentration of two neurotransmitters, dopamine and acetylcholine (*see* Lloyd, 1978). A simplistic, but useful, neurochemical model of the functions of the basal ganglia suggests that the striatal tracts, important for the smooth control of voluntary movements, normally contain balanced dopaminergic (inhibitory) and cholinergic (excitatory) components (*see* Calne, 1978a). It is now clear that any imbalance in these individual systems produces specific disorders of movement. For example, the hyperkinetic locomotion and the behavior that are characteristic of Huntington's chorea may be the result of excessive dopaminergic activity in the basal ganglia (Bernheimer *et al.*, 1973; Klawans *et al.*, 1977). In contrast, there is a marked deficiency in the dopaminergic component of the basal ganglia in parkinsonism. This relative deficiency of dopamine results in the signs and symptoms noted above (Yahr, 1975). Consequently, the theoretical goal of the treatment of parkinsonism is to balance striatal activity by reducing cholinergic activity or enhancing dopaminergic function with centrally acting anticholinergic and dopaminergic drugs, respectively. Often, these two classes of drugs are combined effectively.

The understanding that parkinsonism is a syndrome of dopamine deficiency and the discovery of levodopa as an important drug for the treatment of the disease were the logical culmination of a series of related basic and clinical observations (*see* review by

Hornykiewicz, 1973a). The first may have been the clinical finding that reserpine could induce a parkinsonism-like syndrome as a dose-dependent side effect. Reserpine was later shown to release and thereby deplete stores of 5-hydroxytryptamine (5-HT) and catecholamines in the brain. Subsequently, Carlsson and coworkers (1957) found that the akinesia and sedation produced by reserpine in mice could be reversed by the administration of dopa but not of 5-hydroxytryptophan, the precursor of 5-HT. The relevant clinical observation that the phenothiazines also may induce symptoms of parkinsonism provided another clue that helped focus on the basal ganglia as a site of action for this important class of drugs. The presence of dopamine in the brain, first reported by Montagu (1957), was confirmed by Carlsson and coworkers, who also showed depletion of the putative neurotransmitter by reserpine and its replenishment by dopa (Carlsson *et al.*, 1958).

Measurements of regional concentrations of dopamine in human brains provided the basic link between laboratory studies and clinical applications. Bertler and Rosengren (1959) and Carlsson (1959) found that about 80% of the dopamine in the human brain is concentrated in the basal ganglia, mostly in the caudate nucleus and putamen (corpus striatum). The pivotal discovery by Ehringer and Hornykiewicz (1960) that there is a marked deficiency of striatal dopamine (10% or less of normal) in the basal ganglia of patients with parkinsonism furnished the crucial evidence. The degree of deficiency correlated with the loss of melanin-containing neurons in the pars compacta of the substantia nigra, the most consistent pathological finding of parkinsonism. Since dopamine does not pass the blood-brain barrier when administered systemically, it has no therapeutic effect in parkinsonism. However, levodopa, the immediate metabolic precursor of dopamine, does permeate into striatal tissue, where it is decarboxylated to dopamine.

Initial clinical trials with small intravenous doses of D,L-dopa provided encouraging results, but the drug caused prominent adverse reactions. Cotzias and associates (1967) first clearly demonstrated that small, gradual increments in oral dosage minimized unwanted effects of D,L-dopa. These clinical studies demonstrated the value of replenishment of depleted stores of dopamine in parkinsonism and fulfilled the prediction made by the basic scientists in the previous decade. The clinical findings were quickly confirmed and extended in a number of trials with the active isomer, levodopa, which proved more effective than the racemic mixture. Several symposia and extensive reviews on the use of levodopa in parkinsonism have been published (*see* Marks, 1974; Stern, 1975; Sweet and McDowell, 1975; Yahr, 1975; Bianchine, 1976; Symposium, 1977; Yahr, 1978; Calne *et al.*, 1979). The introduction of levodopa has been critically important not only for the care of the majority of patients with Parkinson's disease but also because it provided the first outstanding example of the successful therapeutic application of biochemically derived information to a chronic degenerative neurological disorder. The very reasonable expectation is that similar neurochemical approaches will soon lead to advances in therapy of other debilitating diseases of the nervous system (Klawans, 1977; Lord et al., 1977; Rinne, 1978; Calne et al., 1979).

LEVODOPA

The introduction of levodopa, L-3,4-dihydroxyphenylalanine, for the treatment of Parkinson's disease was followed by prompt and enthusiastic recognition of its remarkable therapeutic action in the majority of cases. The more recent introduction of "potentiators" of levodopa (dopa decarboxylase inhibitors) has further augmented the clinical value of this drug.

Chemistry. Levodopa is formed from L-tyrosine as an intermediary in the enzymatic synthesis of catecholamines. Dopamine is synthesized directly from levodopa by a cytoplasmic enzyme, aromatic L-amino acid decarboxylase. The structures of levodopa and dopamine are shown in Figure 21–1 (page 479).

There is an active search underway to find specific and useful analogs of dopamine for the treatment of Parkinson's disease (see Goldberg et al., 1978). Two such classes of dopaminergic agonists, the aporphines and the ergolines, are described briefly below. Structural similarities between dopamine and prototypes of these classes of dopaminergic agonists are shown in Figure 21–2 (page 484). As expected, these agonists share many pharmacological properties with levodopa.

PHARMACOLOGICAL PROPERTIES

The main effects of levodopa are produced by the product of its decarboxylation, dopamine; levodopa, as such, is practically inert pharmacologically. Since about 95% of orally administered levodopa is rapidly decarboxylated in the periphery to dopamine, which does not penetrate the blood-brain barrier, large doses must be taken to allow sufficient accumulation of levodopa in the brain, where its decarboxylation raises the central dopamine concentration. Tolerance to the necessarily large dosage is achieved only by gradual upward titration of the dose over a period of weeks until a maximal clinical response is obtained or until the emergence of unacceptable side effects.

Approximately 75% of patients with parkinsonism respond at least reasonably well to levodopa. Therapeutic response in some patients is seemingly "miraculous," especially at the outset. Essentially all signs and symptoms of parkinsonism can respond to the administration of levodopa.

Central Nervous System. The pharmacological effects of levodopa on muscle tone and movement are not seen in normal individuals. Bradykinesia and rigidity usually respond more quickly and consistently than does tremor, but a significant reduction in tremor is often obtained with continued therapy. Amelioration of these primary neurological symptoms is accompanied by similar improvements in overall functional ability. Secondary motor manifestations such as disturbances in posture, gait, associated movements, facial expression, speech, handwriting, swallowing, and respiration are also proportionately improved.

Psychic Effects. In most patients, levodopa at least partially relieves the changes in mood that are characteristic of Parkinson's disease. Early in therapy, feelings of apathy are generally replaced by increased vigor and a sense of well-being. The result is described as a general alerting response characterized by apparent improvement in mental function and an increased interest in self, surroundings, and family. However, a significant number of patients develop serious behavioral side effects, as discussed below.

Cardiovascular System. Peripheral decarboxylation of levodopa markedly increases the concentration of dopamine in blood. Dopamine is a pharmacologically active catecholamine with prominent effects on α- and β-adrenergic receptors, although its potency is much less than that of epinephrine, norepinephrine, or isoproterenol (Goldberg et al., 1978). The reluctance of early investigators to test the effects of high doses of levodopa for parkinsonism rested largely on the expectation of potentially toxic cardiovascular effects, particularly hypertension and cardiac dysrhythmias. Contrary to such expectation, therapeutic doses of levodopa frequently cause only modest and asymptomatic *orthostatic hypotension;* tolerance to this effect develops within a few weeks of chronic treatment. The mechanism by which levodopa produces hypotension is not fully understood.

Therapeutic doses of levodopa produce *cardiac stimulation* by an action of dopamine on β-adrenergic receptors. Transient tachycardia and other cardiac arrhythmias may occur in some patients, and myocardial contractility may be increased for several hours after a large dose of levodopa, especially early in therapy. Tolerance to these effects also develops after several weeks of chronic treatment. The cardiac effects of levodopa mediated by dopamine are usually blocked by β-adrenergic antagonists such as propranolol.

Metabolic and Endocrine Effects. The tuberoinfundibular neurons of the hypothalamus comprise a major central dopaminergic system. These neurons play an important and as yet incompletely defined role in the modulation of hypothalamic-pituitary function (*see* Chapter 59). Dopamine inhibits the secretion of prolactin in man; it acts directly on the relevant cells of the adenohypophysis and may also stimulate the release of a prolactin inhibitory factor. Thus, levodopa and other dopaminergic agonists decrease the secretion of prolactin, while dopaminergic antagonists have an opposite effect. However, studies suggest that hypothalamic regulation of the adenohypophysis may be abnormal in Parkinson's disease (Langston and Forno, 1978). Consequently, the release of growth hormone that is noted in response to the administration of levodopa in normal subjects (*see* Chapter 59) is minimal or absent when levodopa is administered to patients with Parkinson's disease (Eddy *et al.*, 1971). A hypothalamic defect in the regulation of growth hormone might explain why earlier predictions of the production of acromegaly in patients receiving levodopa have proven to be false (Sirtori *et al.*, 1972). Inhibition of prolactin secretion is useful in a variety of clinical situations. Levodopa or dopaminergic agonists are often efficacious in the syndromes of Chiari-Frommel and Forbes-Albright, as well as in puerperal and nonpuerperal galactorrhea and amenorrhea-galactorrhea (*see* Bianchine *et al.*, 1978).

Mechanism of Action. Since abundant evidence suggests that parkinsonism is a syndrome of deficiency of striatal dopamine, it follows that the immediate metabolic precursor of dopamine, levodopa, would act by replenishing these depleted stores. Evidence in favor of this mechanism includes a positive correlation between the symptoms of Parkinson's disease and loss of nigrostriatal neurons. Furthermore, the brains of patients with Parkinson's disease who had been on high doses of levodopa until death contain concentrations of dopamine in the striatum that are five to eight times higher than those in untreated patients and that appear to be correlated with their clinical response to the drug. These findings indicate that dopamine storage capacity of the terminals of the nigrostriatal fibers is not completely lost in patients with parkinsonism. The striatal concentration of aromatic L-amino acid decarboxylase, the enzyme that converts levodopa to dopamine, is markedly reduced in parkinsonism, but sufficient enzymatic activity remains to account for the replenishment of dopamine following the administration of levodopa (*see* Hornykiewicz, 1973a, 1973b).

The actions of dopamine in the basal ganglia have been studied at the molecular level, and it has been shown that the transmitter causes a substantial accumulation of cyclic adenosine 3′,5′-monophosphate (cyclic AMP) in the corpus striatum by activation of the dopamine-sensitive adenylate cyclase that is present at this site (Kebabian and Saavedra, 1976; Philipson and Horn, 1976; Shibuya, 1979). While the significance of this finding remains unclear, it is hypothesized that cyclic AMP is the intracellular mediator of the actions of dopamine in the basal ganglia (*see* Chapters 12 and 19). Other crucial questions, such as how dopamine modulates striatal output and the cause of the degeneration of the striatal nerve cells in Parkinson's disease, remain unanswered (Calne *et al.*, 1979).

No matter how attractive, it now seems clear that the above proposed mechanism of action is much too simplistic. Actually, there have been few attempts to test this hypothesis by correlating individual clinical features of parkinsonism with regional striatal concentrations of neurotransmitters or their metabolites (Calne, 1977). However, one such study by Lloyd (1978) clearly indicates that the problem is truly multifaceted and no simple correlation is possible. One difficulty with attempts to correlate functional, anatomical, and pharmacological parameters is directly related to the diffuse nature of the nigrostriatal tracts. Factors such as the clinical impact of striatal denervation hypersensitivity, the role of dopamine-sensitive adenylate cyclase, the effect of other locally important neurotransmitters (GABA, 5-HT), and the possibility that certain metabolites of levodopa may have pharmacological activity (Sourkes, 1971; Sandler *et al.*, 1973) complicate our understanding of the action of levodopa in man.

Absorption, Distribution, Fate, and Excretion. Levodopa is rapidly absorbed from the small bowel by an active transport system for aromatic amino acids. Concentrations of the drug in plasma usually peak between 0.5 and 2 hours after an oral dose. The half-life in plasma is short—only 1 to 3 hours. The rate of absorption of levodopa is greatly dependent upon the rate of gastric emptying, the pH of gastric juice, and the length of time the drug is exposed to the degradative enzymes of the gastric mucosa and intestinal flora. For example, sluggish gastric emptying (caused either by intrinsic factors or by anticholinergic drugs), hyperacidity of gastric juice, and competition for absorption sites in the small bowel by amino acids each may interfere with the bioavailability of levodopa (Bianchine and Shaw, 1976).

More than 95% of levodopa is decarboxylated in the periphery by the widely distributed extracerebral aromatic L-amino acid decarboxylase. The drug is extensively decarboxylated in its first passage through the liver, which is rich in decarboxylase, so that relatively little unchanged drug reaches the cerebral circulation and probably less than 1% penetrates into the CNS. Inhibition of peripheral decarboxylase markedly increases the fraction of administered levodopa that remains unmetabolized and available to cross the blood-brain barrier.

The principal metabolic pathways for levodopa are depicted in Figure 21-1. A small amount is methylated to 3-O-methyldopa, which accumulates in the CNS due to its long half-life. Most is converted to dopamine, small amounts of which in turn are metabolized to norepinephrine and epinephrine. Biotransformation of dopamine proceeds rapidly to yield the principal excretion products, 3,4-dihydroxyphenylacetic acid (DOPAC) and 3-methoxy-4-hydroxyphenylacetic acid (homovanillic acid, HVA). At least 30 metabolites of levodopa have been identified (Goodall and Alton, 1969). Several of these have powerful pharmacological effects that contribute to the spectrum of toxicity. Some evidence indicates that the metabolism of levodopa may be accelerated during prolonged therapy, possibly due to enzyme induction.

Metabolites of dopamine are rapidly excreted in the urine; about 80% of a radioactively labeled dose is recovered within 24 hours. The principal metabolites, DOPAC and HVA, account for up to 50% of the administered dose. These metabolites, as well as small amounts of levodopa and dopamine, also appear in the cerebrospinal fluid. Negligible amounts are found in the feces. After prolonged therapy with levodopa, the ratio of DOPAC to HVA excreted may increase, probably reflecting a depletion of methyl donors necessary for metabolism by cate-

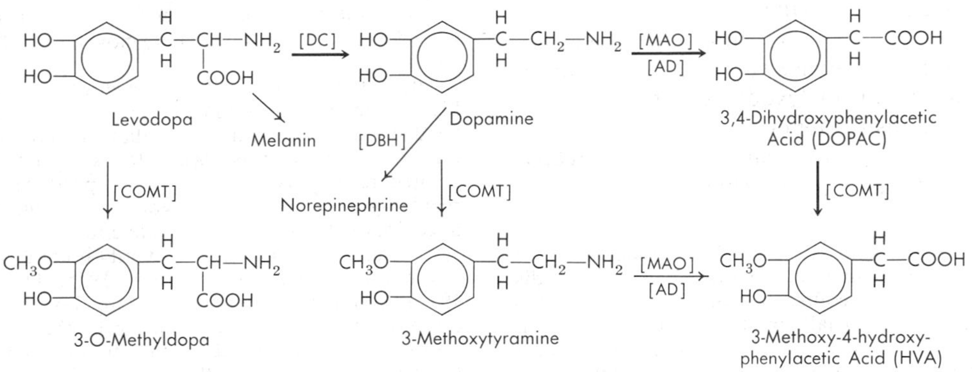

Figure 21-1. *Important catabolic pathways of levodopa* (L-*dopa*).

Major pathways are shown by heavy arrows; minor pathways, by light arrows. *AD,* aldehyde dehydrogenase; *COMT,* catechol-O-methyltransferase; *DBH,* dopamine β-hydroxylase; *DC,* aromatic L-amino acid decarboxylase; *MAO,* monoamine oxidase. (For biosynthetic pathway, *see* Figure 4-4, page 72.)

chol-O-methyl transferase; it is estimated that about three fourths of dietary methionine is utilized for the metabolism of large therapeutic doses of levodopa.

Side Effects and Toxicity. Careful and judicious administration of levodopa to an informed and cooperative patient is essential to optimize the ratio of benefit to toxicity (Duvoisin, 1977; Marsden and Parkes, 1977; Marx, 1979). The majority of patients with Parkinson's disease who are treated with levodopa experience side effects. Their intensity and type vary greatly at different stages of therapy. Although many are relatively innocuous, others are troublesome and necessitate reduction in dosage or complete withdrawal of the drug. Side effects are generally dose dependent and reversible. Elderly patients and those with postencephalitic parkinsonism are especially intolerant of large doses.

The most common side effects *early* in therapy with levodopa are nausea and vomiting. Cardiac arrhythmias occur in some patients, especially those with preexisting disturbances in cardiac conduction. The majority of patients on *long-term* therapy develop abnormal involuntary movements, which vary considerably in pattern and severity and often limit the tolerated dosage of levodopa. Psychiatric disturbances are produced by levodopa in a significant proportion of patients and frequently limit the dose that can be tolerated. All side effects are reversible and can generally be controlled by a reduction in dosage.

Because of these potential side effects, it is important to exercise very special care in the administration of levodopa to patients with coronary insufficiency, cardiac arrhythmias, occlusive cerebrovascular disease, affective disorders, or major psychoses.

Gastrointestinal. About 80% of patients experience anorexia, nausea, vomiting, or epigastric distress early in the course of treatment with levodopa. This is caused partially by stimulation of the medullary emetic center and is most likely to occur if dosage is increased too rapidly, if individual doses are too large, or if the drug is taken without food. Anorexia may result in transient weight loss in some patients. These symptoms are controlled by concurrent administration of food (which decreases the peak concentration of levodopa in plasma) or by

lowering of the dosage administered. Although certain phenothiazines are highly effective antiemetic drugs, they should not be used for the control of nausea in this situation, since they interfere with the action of dopamine at striatal receptor sites. Gastrointestinal side effects tend to disappear with continuing therapy as tolerance develops. Bleeding and perforation of peptic ulcers have been reported in a few patients.

Hypotension. About 30% of patients develop slight orthostatic hypotension early in therapy. It is usually asymptomatic, but some patients experience dizziness and, rarely, syncope. Careful regulation of dosage is necessary in such individuals, and the usual measures for controlling orthostatic hypotension should be employed. Despite continuation of therapy, blood pressure tends to return to values that obtained prior to treatment. The mechanism that underlies this effect remains unclear.

Cardiac Irregularities. Cardiac arrhythmias are not uncommon in the older-age group of patients with Parkinson's disease; consequently, a direct association between the development of an arrhythmia and therapy with levodopa is difficult to establish. However, the β-adrenergic action of dopamine on the heart, as well as direct β-adrenergic receptor stimulation by other catecholamine metabolites of the drug, presents a potentially serious side effect of levodopa. Fortunately, the incidence of arrhythmias is low. Sinus tachycardia, atrial and ventricular extrasystoles, atrial flutter and fibrillation, and ventricular tachycardia have been reported. These cardiac arrhythmias, which are more likely to occur in patients with coronary artery disease, can usually be controlled by the administration of propranolol.

Abnormal Involuntary Movements. These movements appear in approximately 50% of patients within 2 to 4 months after the initiation of treatment with levodopa. Unfortunately, they often coincide temporally with what would otherwise be optimal improvement. They appear with increasing frequency as drug administration continues and are directly related to the dose of the drug and to the degree of clinical improvement. About 80% of patients on full therapeutic doses for a year or longer will develop some abnormal movements (Yahr, 1978).

The abnormal involuntary movements are variable in type and include faciolingual tics, grimacing, head bobbing, and various oscillatory and rocking movements of the arms, legs, or trunk. Rarely, exaggerated respiratory movements can produce an irregular gasping pattern or hyperventilation. Tolerance does not develop to this side effect; in fact, the symptoms tend to increase in severity if the dosage is not reduced (Stern, 1975; Yahr, 1975; Duvoisin, 1977). Although such movements are abolished by a decrease in the dose of levodopa or by the administration of pyridoxine, it is unfortunate that both these maneuvers reduce the therapeutic efficacy of levodopa as well. Therefore, the physician must carefully titrate the dose and time of administration of levodopa to maximize the therapeutic benefit while minimizing side effects. These abnormal involuntary movements are the most important side effect of levodopa that limit the dose that can be given. No satisfactory means, pharmacological or otherwise, have yet been found to antagonize this side effect selectively.

Behavioral Disturbances. The population with parkinsonism is aged, and individuals often have impairment of memory or judgment or even dementia. Furthermore, patients often experience isolation and loss of social esteem because of their disease. In this setting, the central stimulant effect of levodopa can result in hallucinations, paranoia, mania, insomnia, anxiety, nightmares, and emotional depression (Yahr, 1978). The actions of levodopa on the hypothalamus may cause renewed sexual interest, and this can cause additional behavioral changes.

Serious behavioral disturbances occur in about 15% of patients who receive levodopa and usually require reduction of dosage or, for some, complete withdrawal of the drug (Malitz, 1972). One of the more common disturbances resembles an organic brain syndrome and is characterized by confusion, sometimes progressing to frank delirium. Although the mental depression of many patients is often improved by levodopa, some appear to develop a more severe depression, which in a few cases has led to suicidal gestures. Tricyclic antidepressant drugs have been helpful in some cases. Fully developed psychotic reactions with paranoid delusions or hallucinations are most likely to occur in patients with a history of mental disorder, organic brain syndrome including dementia, or postencephalitic parkinsonism (Sacks *et al.*, 1972). A few patients develop classical symptoms of hypomania, one manifestation of which may be inappropriate or excessive sexual behavior (Goodwin *et al.*, 1971).

Abnormalities of Laboratory Tests. Urinary metabolites of levodopa cause false-positive tests for ketoacidosis by the dip-stick test; they also color the urine red, then black, on exposure to air or alkali.

Interactions with Other Drugs. Decarboxylation of levodopa to dopamine is catalyzed by the pyridoxine-dependent enzyme L-amino acid decarboxylase, and doses of *pyridoxine* that are only modestly in excess of the recommended dietary allowance enhance the extracerebral metabolism of levodopa at this step. Less levodopa is then available for conversion to dopamine in the basal ganglia. Consequently, when administered with levodopa, pyridoxine may completely reverse its therapeutic effect or promptly reduce its toxic side effects, depending on the clinical circumstances. Patients should be aware that pyridoxine is present in many *multivitamin preparations* in amounts in excess of 5 mg. A multivitamin preparation that does not contain pyridoxine is available. It is important to note that, when levodopa is coadministered with an inhibitor of L-amino acid decarboxy-

lase, the interactive antagonistic effect of pyridoxine is lost (Yahr, 1975).

Antipsychotic drugs, such as *phenothiazines, butyrophenones,* and *reserpine,* can produce a parkinsonism-like syndrome. Reserpine acts by depleting stores of central dopamine, while the other agents block receptors for dopamine. Since these drugs nullify the therapeutic effects of levodopa, they are contraindicated. This possible etiological drug factor should be considered in every newly diagnosed case of parkinsonism. If the exposure to these antipsychotic drugs was short, it is likely that their prompt withdrawal alone will cause disappearance of symptoms of parkinsonism. As previously mentioned, the phenothiazines should not be used to combat the emetic effect of levodopa (Stern, 1975).

Nonspecific monoamine oxidase inhibitors, such as *phenelzine* and *isocarboxazid,* interfere with inactivation of dopamine, norepinephrine, and other catecholamines. Hence, they exaggerate, unpredictably, the central effects of levodopa and its catecholamine metabolites. Hypertensive crisis and hyperpyrexia are very real and dangerous sequelae of concurrent administration of two such drugs. A monoamine oxidase inhibitor should be withdrawn at least 14 days prior to the administration of levodopa. It is interesting to note that a selective inhibitor of monoamine oxidase B is now under investigation as a drug for Parkinson's disease (*see* below).

Anticholinergic drugs, such as *trihexyphenidyl, benztropine, procyclidine,* and others, act synergistically with levodopa to improve certain symptoms of parkinsonism, especially tremor. However, large doses of anticholinergic drugs can slow gastric emptying sufficiently to cause a delay in the absorption of levodopa by the small bowel. This effect can be so pronounced as to detract from the therapeutic benefit of levodopa (Bianchine and Sunyapridakul, 1973; Stern, 1975).

Preparations and Dosage. *Levodopa,* U.S.P. (BENDOPA, DOPAR, LARODOPA, others), is available for oral use as tablets or capsules containing 100, 250, or 500 mg of the drug.

The optimal maintenance dosage of levodopa is determined by careful titration in each patient. The usual initial dose is 0.5 to 1 g daily, divided into three or four equal portions. The total daily dosage is then gradually increased by increments of 100 to 750 mg, every 3 to 7 days. The rate of increase in dosage is determined primarily by the patient's tolerance to nausea and vomiting. Significant objective improvement may appear during the second or third week as the daily dosage reaches 2 to 3 g. Further benefit accrues gradually with increasing dosage, even after the dose is stabilized at an apparently optimal level. Good therapeutic responses are not reached in some patients for as long as 1 to 6 months. Therefore, levodopa should not be considered ineffective until full doses have been administered for such periods. In general, younger patients with less severe symptoms derive greater benefit than do severely debilitated, elderly patients in whom maximal tolerated doses are often limited by side effects. The usual daily maintenance dose ranges from 3 to 8 g, taken in at least four divided doses. More frequent administration of smaller doses may reduce side effects and yield better results.

INHIBITORS OF AROMATIC L-AMINO ACID DECARBOXYLASE

Concurrent administration of levodopa with an inhibitor of aromatic L-amino acid (dopa) decarboxylase that is unable to penetrate into the CNS readily diminishes the decarboxylation of levodopa in peripheral tissues. Such reduction allows a greater proportion of levodopa to reach the desired receptor sites in the nigrostriatum.

Several studies describe the pharmacokinetics of levodopa administered either alone or in combination with an inhibitor of the decarboxylase. Concentrations of levodopa in plasma are higher and the half-life is longer after concurrent administration of a decarboxylase inhibitor and levodopa than when levodopa is given alone (Bianchine and Shaw, 1976). At present, *carbidopa* is the only such inhibitor that is clinically available in the United States, and it is supplied in combination with levodopa in a fixed ratio of 1 to 10 by weight. *Benserazide* has similar properties and is marketed in Europe and Canada (Palfreyman *et al.*, 1978). Carbidopa has the following structure:

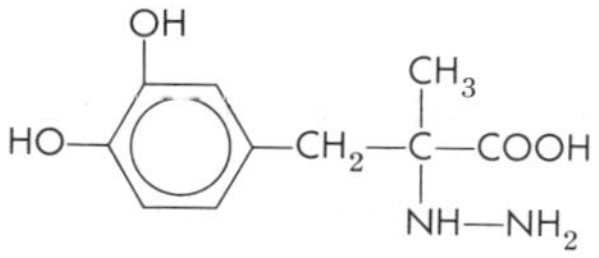

Carbidopa

Several clinical studies have clearly demonstrated distinct advantages of combined therapy with a decarboxylase inhibitor and levodopa. These may be summarized as follows: (1) The optimally effective dose of levodopa can be reduced by about 75%, inasmuch as a much larger proportion of levodopa enters the brain. (2) Nausea and vomiting from stimulation of receptors for dopamine in the medullary emetic center are largely eliminated. Likewise, the cardiac side effects are diminished or prevented. (3) Effective dosage of levodopa can be achieved much more quickly during initial therapy since the necessity to develop tolerance to the peripheral effects of dopamine is minimized. (4) Antagonism of the therapeutic efficacy of levodopa by pyridoxine is avoided. (5) The frequency and intensity of diurnal variations in control of symptoms by levodopa are reduced, presumably by avoidance of large fluctuations of the concentration of dopamine in the CNS. The number of divided doses per day may often be reduced without loss of control. (6) The percentage of patients who are improved and the degree of improvement appear to be somewhat greater than with dopa alone (Stern, 1975; Yahr, 1978).

However, some of the problems of therapy with levodopa are not resolved by the concomitant use of peripheral decarboxylase inhibitors. Abnormal involuntary movements not only occur with the same frequency but also tend to develop earlier in therapy and may be more severe. Adverse mental effects also occur with about the same frequency but appear earlier in the course of therapy.

Untoward Effects. In recommended doses the peripheral decarboxylase inhibitors that are currently employed are essentially devoid of pharmacological activity when administered alone, and toxic effects have not been observed (Chase and Watanabe, 1972; Papavasiliou *et al.*, 1972). However, when administered in combination with levodopa, carbidopa generally will enhance, quantitatively, the pharmacological action of levodopa. In this sense, the side effects of carbidopa when administered with levodopa are those associated with enhancement of the effects of levodopa.

Preparations and Dosage. Carbidopa is available in scored tablets that contain 10 mg of the drug in combination with 100 mg of levodopa (SINEMET 10/100) or that contain 25 mg of carbidopa and 250 mg of levodopa (SINEMET 25/250). Physicians can obtain carbidopa as a single agent (LODOSYN) upon request of the manufacturer.

Generally, therapy is initiated with 400 mg of levodopa (40 mg of carbidopa) daily in divided doses. If a greater therapeutic effect is needed, the dose of the combination can be increased progressively to a daily maximum of about 2000 mg of levodopa (200 mg of carbidopa). For patients treated previously with levodopa alone, dosage with levodopa must be withheld overnight (8 hours) before starting the combination of levodopa and carbidopa. As a first approximation, the total daily dosage of levodopa must be reduced by approximately 75%.

AMANTADINE

Amantadine, introduced as an antiviral agent for the prophylaxis of A_2 influenza (see Chapter 54), was unexpectedly found to cause symptomatic improvement of patients with parkinsonism (Schwab et al., 1972). This drug probably acts by releasing dopamine from intact dopaminergic terminals that remain in the nigrostriatum of patients with Parkinson's disease. Because of this facilitated release of dopamine, it appears that the therapeutic efficacy of amantadine is enhanced by the concurrent administration of levodopa. However, patients receiving near-maximal benefit from levodopa generally experience little additional improvement from amantadine.

Many studies confirm that amantadine is clearly less efficacious than levodopa but slightly more so than the anticholinergic drugs (Parkes et al., 1970; Mawdsley et al., 1972). Amantadine acts maximally within a few days but usually loses a portion of its efficacy in 6 to 8 weeks of continuous treatment. Consequently, many physicians use amantadine episodically for short (2- to 3-week) intervals whenever the patient requires additional therapeutic assistance.

Amantadine is readily absorbed from the gastrointestinal tract and has a relatively long duration of action. It is excreted unchanged in the urine and, therefore, can accumulate in the body when renal function is inadequate.

Mechanism of Action. Amantadine was observed to release dopamine from peripheral neuronal storage sites of animals who have received infusions of the transmitters; this peripheral effect suggested that amantadine might exert a similar action on the residual, intact dopaminergic terminals in the striatum of patients with parkinsonism. Amantadine causes release of dopamine from central neurons and facilitates its release by nerve impulses. Release of dopamine by amantadine may also occur from central sites other than nigrostriatal neurons.

Untoward Effects. Compared to levodopa or anticholinergic agents, amantadine is relatively free of side effects. They are generally mild, often transient, and always reversible. Their incidence and severity

increase markedly when the daily dosage exceeds 200 mg. Hallucinations, confusion, and nightmares are more common when the drug is administered concurrently with anticholinergic agents or when the patient has an underlying psychiatric disorder. Insomnia, dizziness, lethargy, drowsiness, and slurred speech have also been reported. Nausea, vomiting, anorexia, and constipation occur infrequently (Forssman et al., 1972).

Long-term use of amantadine may result in the appearance of livido reticularis in the lower extremities. Although this complication is often cosmetically unacceptable, it merely reflects the local release of catecholamines with resultant vasoconstriction (Pearce et al., 1974).

Preparations and Dosage. Amantadine Hydrochloride, U.S.P. (SYMMETREL), is available as 100-mg capsules and in a syrup containing 50 mg/5 ml. The usual dose is 100 mg, given twice daily.

APORPHINES

Apomorphine, commonly used as an emetic in the management of oral drug overdosage, was the first dopaminergic agonist reported to have beneficial effects in Parkinson's disease. Because of renal damage associated with the chronic administration of large doses of apomorphine, Cotzias and associates (1976) shifted their investigations to N-propylnoraporphine, an analog of apormorphine. This compound and others of this type remain under investigation.

ERGOLINES

Several ergot derivatives demonstrate dopaminergic activity in animal models of parkinsonism and mimic the neuroendocrinological effects of dopamine on the secretion of prolactin and growth hormone (see Chapter 39). These derivatives include lergotrile, lisuride, and bromocriptine (Calne, 1977); the last-named compound has been studied most thoroughly and hence logically serves as a prototype for the ergolines. Its structure is shown in Figure 21–2. Bromocriptine is available for clinical use in the United States for the short-term management of galactorrhea; its use for the treatment of hyperprolactinemia and acromegaly is considered experimental (see Chapter 59). Bromocriptine and other dopaminergic agonists of this type are being investigated actively for their possible utility in the treatment of Parkinson's disease (Calne, 1978b; Goldstein et al., 1978; Keller and Daprada, 1979; Lieberman et al., 1979).

In man, bromocriptine is rapidly absorbed, and concentrations of the drug usually peak in plasma within 2 hours; therapeutic concentrations for the treatment of Parkinson's disease persist three to four times longer than do those of levodopa (given without a decarboxylase inhibitor). Unfortunately, the dosage of bromocriptine required to control parkinsonism (20 to 150 mg daily) is approximately ten times larger than that required to suppress galactorrhea, and this quantity of the drug is very expensive.

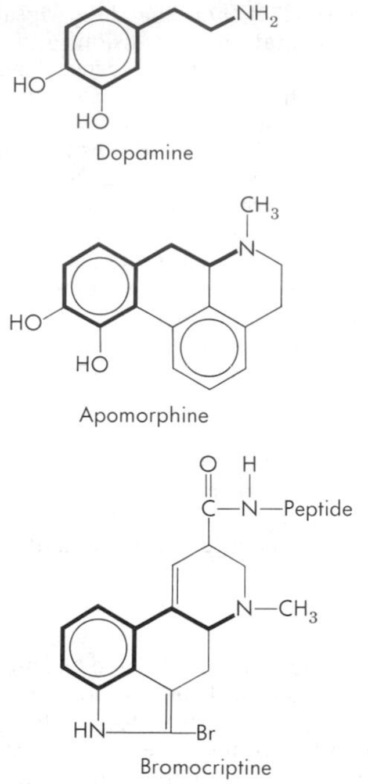

Figure 21–2. *Structural similarities (heavy lines) between dopamine, apomorphine, and bromocriptine.*

Efforts are thus being made to develop less complex and hence less costly ergoline analogs; an example is lergotrile, which does not contain the amide substituent present in bromocriptine. While studies with lergotrile in parkinsonism demonstrate pharmacological properties very similar to those of bromocriptine, clinical investigation with lergotrile has been halted because of hepatotoxicity. An active search for safer derivatives continues. An alternative approach has been to supplement regimens that rely on levodopa with small doses of bromocriptine. While clinical investigation of bromocriptine in parkinsonism is limited, a few observations appear established: (1) Patients with parkinsonism who experience excessive "on-off" phenomenon (*see* below) or who are not reasonably controlled with levodopa (or by the combination of levodopa and carbidopa) may be managed more smoothly when bromocriptine is added to the therapeutic regimen. This may be the main clinical value of bromocriptine. (2) In many patients with Parkinson's disease, high doses of bromocriptine (50 to 100 mg) elicit therapeutic responses that are equivalent to those obtained with levodopa. (3) Optimal clinical results may be achieved by a combination of submaximal doses of bromocriptine and levodopa (Calne, 1977; Godwin-Austen and Smith, 1977; Lieberman *et al.*, 1979). (4) Visual and auditory hallucinations are more frequent with bromocriptine than with levodopa. (5) Symptomatic hypotension and cutaneous *livido reticularis* are far more common with bromocriptine than with levodopa. (6) Bromocriptine induces less dyskinesia than does levodopa. (7) Similar to levodopa, bromocriptine induces a nonspecific arousal of the CNS that may be effective in treating patients who are comatose because of hepatic encephalopathy (Morgan *et al.*, 1977).

DEPRENYL

There are two isoenzymes that oxidize monoamines. Monoamine oxidase A (MAO-A) inactivates monoamines of intestinal origin, while the isoenzyme MAO-B predominates in certain regions of the CNS (*see* Chapter 9). Deprenyl (phenylisopropyl-N-methylpropinylamine) is a highly selective inhibitor of MAO-B (Birkmayer *et al.*, 1977; Knoll, 1978; Rinne *et al.*, 1978; Yahr, 1978). In striking contrast to the known nonspecific MAO inhibitors (*e.g.*, phenelzine and isocarboxazid), deprenyl does not result in profound and potentially lethal potentiation of the effects of catecholamines when administered concurrently with a centrally effective amine. For example, a patient receiving deprenyl may eat cheeses (that contain tyramine) or take levodopa without danger (Knoll, 1978). However, administration of deprenyl inhibits the intracerebral metabolic degradation of dopamine. The resultant preservation of dopamine in the basal ganglia appears to maximize the therapeutic efficacy of levodopa. Consequently, when deprenyl is added to the therapeutic regimen, the dose of levodopa can be reduced without loss of therapeutic benefit. Preliminary clinical trials with this compound are encouraging. Deprenyl is not generally available in the United States.

ANTICHOLINERGIC DRUGS

Anticholinergic agents were the most effective drugs for treatment of Parkinson's disease for more than a century. However, the introduction of levodopa and, more recently, the availability of decarboxylase inhibitors such as carbidopa have relegated anticholinergics to a supportive role in the treatment of the disorder. Nonetheless, the anticholinergic drugs are still very useful for patients with minimal symptoms, for those unable to tolerate levodopa because of side effects or contraindications, and for those who are not benefited by levodopa. Furthermore, more than half the patients who derive therapeutic benefit from levodopa experience further amelioration of symptoms after supplemental treatment with an anticholinergic drug. These drugs are also useful to alleviate the parkinsonism-like syndrome induced by antipsychotic drugs.

The deficiency of dopamine in the striatum of patients with parkinsonism intensifies the excitatory effects of the cholinergic system within the striatum. Anticholinergics aid such patients by blunting this component of the nigrostriatal pathway (Calne, 1978a).

PHARMACOLOGICAL PROPERTIES

Trihexyphenidyl, the prototype of this group of drugs, qualitatively resembles the belladonna alkaloids in its pharmacological actions and side effects (*see* Chapter 7). The drug favorably influences the tremor that is characteristic of parkinsonism. It is less effective in improving rigidity and bradykinesia. Among the secondary symptoms of parkinsonism, the anticholinergic agents improve excessive sialorrhea by inhibiting salivary secretion. Although the peripheral anticholinergic actions of the synthetic compounds selected for use in Parkinson's disease are less prominent than are those of the natural antimuscarinic alkaloids such as atropine, side effects of cycloplegia, constipation, and urinary retention may become troublesome, especially for the aged patient (Cunningham *et al.,* 1949).

Side effects referable to the CNS, such as mental confusion, delirium, somnolence, and hallucinations, may also limit the utility of these drugs. Although there are essentially no pharmacological differences among the anticholinergic agents commonly used in parkinsonism, certain patients clearly appear to tolerate one preparation better than another.

The anticholinergic drugs used for the treatment of Parkinson's disease are listed in Table 21–1, as are certain antihistamines. The antihistamines listed in Table 21–1 are structurally related to diphenhydramine, possess some central anticholinergic properties, and are well tolerated, especially by elderly patients. While these antihistamines produce fewer side effects, they are not as efficacious as are the anticholinergic agents. Their sedative effect may be helpful in certain patients.

Preparations and Dosage. Patients should be started at the lower end of the range of daily dosage listed in Table 21–1, and this should be divided into two or three equal portions. Dosage should then be gradually increased until there is maximal improvement or, more likely, until the onset of intolerable side effects. It is especially important to tailor the medication to achieve the optimal balance between control of the disabling symptoms and the adverse reactions to the drugs. The optimal dose of a given drug for a particular individual cannot be stated. In general, elderly patients are less able to tolerate large doses of the drugs than are young patients. The drugs with prominent peripheral anticholinergic effects must be used with great caution in individuals suffering from narrow-angle glaucoma or urinary retention secondary to disorders of the prostate.

THERAPEUTIC USES OF DRUGS FOR PARKINSON'S DISEASE

Many aspects of the clinical use of levodopa, the combination of levodopa and carbidopa, and other dopaminergic drugs have been described in the preceding pages. The relative importance of these drugs is still not certain. Most neurologists agree that the combination of levodopa with the decarboxylase inhibitor is now the most effective preparation available in the United States for treatment of Parkinson's disease (Medical Letter, 1979). Some neurologists suggest that since dopaminergic drugs are limited in the duration of their effectiveness (and this limit is not altered by the decarboxylase inhibitor), these drugs should be reserved for the more severe stages of parkinsonism (Fahn and Calne, 1978). Consequently, it is not uncommon for physicians to initiate treatment for mild parkinsonism with anticholinergic agents. Levodopa may be added when the disease progresses moderately. When the symptoms become serious, the combination of levodopa and carbidopa is substituted for levodopa. Other neurologists use the combination preparation earlier in the course of the disease instead of using levodopa alone.

Yahr (1975) distinguished two phases of treatment with levodopa. There is an initial induction phase that lasts several weeks and a subsequent, long-term maintenance phase. During the induction phase, the daily dosage of levodopa is increased slowly to minimize the likelihood of side effects such as insomnia, nausea, and anorexia. *One critical factor in successful therapy during this phase is the careful and slow titration of dosage for each patient.* This point can hardly be overemphasized. Too rapid an increase in dosage generally results in a therapeutic failure because of side effects and toxicity. The full benefits of treatment with levodopa become apparent in the maintenance phase; this level of improvement generally lasts for about 2 years. However, careful monitoring of the patient and judicious modification of all the therapeutic measures are required to maintain a desirable response. Attempts to eradicate every

Table 21-1. MISCELLANEOUS DRUGS FOR PARKINSONISM

DRUG CLASS, NONPROPRIETARY NAME, AND TRADE NAME	CHEMICAL STRUCTURE	DOSAGE FORMS *	RANGE OF AVERAGE DAILY DOSE
Anticholinergic Agents			
Benztropine Mesylate, U.S.P. (COGENTIN)		T:0.5,1,2 mg I:2 mg/2 ml	1–6 mg
Trihexyphenidyl Hydrochloride, U.S.P. (ARTANE, others)		T:2,5 mg C(S):5 mg E:2 mg/5 ml	1–10 mg
Procyclidine Hydrochloride, U.S.P. (KEMADRIN)		T:2,5 mg	6–20 mg
Cycrimine Hydrochloride, U.S.P. (PAGITANE)		T:1.25,2.5 mg	3.75–15 mg
Biperiden Hydrochloride, U.S.P. (AKINETON)		T:2 mg I:5 mg/ml †	2–10 mg
Ethopropazine Hydrochloride, U.S.P. ‡ (PARSIDOL)		T:10,50,100 mg	50–600 mg
Antihistamines			
Diphenhydramine Hydrochloride, U.S.P. (BENADRYL, others)	*See* Chapter 26	C,T:25,50 mg E,S:12.5 mg/5 ml I:10 mg/ml, 50 mg/ml	100–200 mg

Table 21-1. MISCELLANEOUS DRUGS FOR PARKINSONISM (Continued)

DRUG CLASS, NONPROPRIETARY NAME, AND TRADE NAME	CHEMICAL STRUCTURE	DOSAGE FORMS *	RANGE OF AVERAGE DAILY DOSE
Chlorphenoxamine Hydrochloride, U.S.P. (PHENOXENE)		T:50 mg	150–400 mg
Orphenadrine hydrochloride (DISIPAL)		T:50 mg	50–250 mg

* T = tablet; I = injection; C(S) = sustained-release capsule; E = elixir; C = capsule; S = syrup.
† As Biperiden Lactate, U.S.P.
‡ Ethopropazine is a phenothiazine with significant anticholinergic activity.

vestige of symptoms of parkinsonism with levodopa usually require doses that cause unacceptable side effects. Two major limiting factors of long-term therapy with levodopa are the development of abnormal involuntary movements and the "on-off" phenomenon. It is not clear why both these undesirable effects are so delayed in appearance. Day-to-day and even within-the-day variations in the severity of symptoms have always been among the most characteristic features of parkinsonism. Treatment with levodopa has greatly increased their complexity and importance. Marsden and Parkes (1977) state that the swings from "on" and "off" periods essentially represent a marked change from mobility to relative immobility. These fluctuations may occur many times a day and often with startling rapidity. "On" periods are usually associated with high or rising concentrations of levodopa in plasma, whereas "off" periods often correlate with low or falling values.

It is not necessary to discontinue previous anticholinergic medication upon initiation of treatment with levodopa, although the dose of the former drug may need reduction. There is ample evidence that the judicious combination of levodopa and anticholinergic drugs may be beneficial.

Effects of Long-Term Treatment. The result of the initial therapy (1 or 2 years) is usually more impressive than the therapeutic benefit derived from long-term treatment (more than 3 years). Sweet and McDowell (1975) reviewed the outcome of 100 patients 5 years after starting levodopa. The adjusted death rate among patients receiving levodopa was less than that reported before the drug was available. However, the average "functional" status of the patients approaches pretreatment levels after 5 years despite remarkable improvement, particularly between 0.5 and 2 years of therapy. Yahr (1975) postulated that this slow loss of efficacy reflects advancement of the underlying disease (slow but progressive

loss of neurons), rather than a specific loss of the effect of levodopa *per se*. Abnormal involuntary movements, rapid oscillations in motor performance ("on-off" phenomena), and postural instability are the major adverse effects of long-term treatment with levodopa or with the combination of levodopa and carbidopa (Granérus, 1978). Thus, while levodopa does not cure Parkinson's disease, it does provide symptomatic relief for a long time and remains the most effective treatment available for this illness. It makes possible a more self-sufficient existence for a longer time than was possible before the drug became available (Joseph *et al.*, 1978).

Drug-Induced Parkinsonism. Parkinsonism, acute dyskinesia, and dystonias that are induced by the phenothiazines and other antipsychotic agents usually respond readily to low doses of anticholinergic drugs. There is some controversy over whether anticholinergic agents should be administered routinely upon the initiation of chronic treatment with antipsychotic drugs in an attempt to prevent or delay the appearance of these symptoms of parkinsonism (*see* Chapter 19).

Miscellaneous Uses of Drugs for Parkinson's Disease. The efficacy of levodopa in Parkinson's disease has prompted clinical trials of the drug for a number of other neurological conditions characterized by disordered extrapyramidal function, such as torsion dystonia, cerebral palsy, and progressive supranuclear palsy. The results have been unimpressive. Administration of levodopa may provoke a nonspecific "awakening" of patients in hepatic coma (Morgan *et al.*, 1977) or coma associated with encephalitis or Reye's syndrome (Chandra, 1978). Levodopa has not been found to be useful for the treatment of any psychiatric disorder; in fact, the drug tends to exacerbate latent or active psychotic states, both organic and functional. In addition, dopaminergic agents are not useful in controlling or reversing the extrapyramidal side effects induced by antipsychotic drugs such as the phenothiazines and butyrophenones, since the latter agents presumably block the activation of dopaminergic receptors.

II. Centrally Acting Muscle Relaxants

Drugs used to relieve spasticity of skeletal muscle should reduce excessive muscle tone. In contrast to the neuromuscular blocking drugs, which act primarily at the neuromuscular junction, most of the skeletal muscle relaxants described in this section act on the CNS; dantrolene, an exception, acts directly on skeletal muscle.

Spasticity of skeletal muscle develops when there is an abnormal increase in resistance to passive movement of a muscle group and is due to an augmented tonic stretch reflex; other proprioceptive reflexes may also be hyperactive. Spasticity occurs in a wide variety of neurological conditions and is highly variable in its etiology and presentation. Several different synaptic loci within a spinal segment may significantly alter the condition (*e.g.*, α and γ motoneurons, primary afferent fiber terminals, and interneurons). Importantly, spasticity requires a finite time to develop following initiation of neural injury and is highly variable in severity during various stages of recovery from injury or the progression of disease. Factors such as neural plasticity, axonal sprouting, and development of denervation hypersensitivity affect the specific nature of the condition. Consequently, it is impossible to explain all the abnormalities of the reflexes of spastic patients with a single neurophysiological hypothesis. Similarly, it is unreasonable to expect that muscular spasticity of diverse etiologies will respond effectively to a drug directed toward a particular aspect of the function of nerve or skeletal muscle.

MEPHENESIN

Although little used clinically at present, mephenesin is the oldest and probably the most extensively studied skeletal muscle relaxant. The pharmacological actions of many newer relaxants are, in general, qualitatively similar to those of mephenesin. It is a prototype for the drugs that produce relaxation of skeletal muscle by a central action with relatively little sedation. Smith (1965) and Davidoff (1978) have reviewed in depth the pharmacological actions of drugs that possess muscle relaxant activity.

All types of experimental hypertonia and hyperreflexia, such as produced by decerebration or by spinal or supraspinal lesions, are diminished by mephenesin. Specifically, mephenesin depresses transmission through a number of spinal and supraspinal polysynaptic pathways. Both facilitation and inhibition of muscle stretch reflexes resulting from stimulation of appropriate areas in the reticular formation are depressed by mephenesin. On the other hand, the central polysynaptic pathways concerned with arousal elicited by stimulation of the midbrain reticular formation are little affected by the drug. In the intact animal, actions of mephenesin at both spinal and supraspinal sites apparently contribute to the muscular relaxation. Mephenesin prolongs synaptic recovery time and reduces repetitive discharges of interneurons. Such effects may underlie the selectivity of the drug for certain tonically active systems controlling muscle tone.

The mechanism of action of mephenesin and other centrally acting muscle relaxants is poorly understood. Neuronal conduction, neuromuscular transmission, and muscle excitability are not depressed except by nearly lethal doses. A prominent effect of muscle relaxants is to depress spinal polysynaptic reflexes perferentially over monosynaptic reflexes. This effect of mephenesin was recognized early and is exhibited by the other muscle relaxants; hence, they are characterized as *interneuronal blocking agents*. However, this characterization is both unrevealing as to mechanism and imprecise, because depression is not restricted to interneurons (Davidoff, 1978). Furthermore, certain agents that do not produce muscular relaxation also show some preferential depression of polysynaptic reflexes; therefore, this effect is not an identifying characteristic of the class (Domino, 1956; Longo, 1961; Esplin, 1963; Smith, 1965).

The centrally acting muscle relaxants that are similar to mephenesin in their pharmacological effects include *carisoprodol, chlorphenesin carbamate, chlorzoxazone, metaxalone, methocarbamol,* and *orphenadrine*. Their chemical structures, trade names, and dosages are summarized in Table 21–2. There are no well-controlled studies in which the relative safety and efficacy of these compounds are compared. As a result, selection of one of these preparations over another remains highly empirical and subjective.

Three clinically useful, centrally active skeletal muscle relaxants appear to differ from mephenesin in their mode of action; they are the benzodiazepines, baclofen, and cyclobenzaprine.

BENZODIAZEPINES

This group of drugs is discussed in detail in Chapters 17 and 19. Only selected aspects of their muscle relaxant action will be presented here. Diazepam and other benzodiazepines are widely used as skeletal muscle relaxants for a variety of spastic states. These agents may be useful in painful spasms of flexor muscles. Benzodiazepines appear to have a more selective action on reticular neuronal mechanisms that control muscle tone than on spinal interneuronal activity, whereas mephenesin-like drugs exhibit no such selectivity (Tseng and Wang, 1971). The molecular mechanism underlying these observations remains unclear (Verrier *et al.,* 1975; Calne, 1976). Sedation may limit the efficacy of diazepam as a muscle relaxant. The dosages and preparations of the benzodiazepines are described in Chapter 17.

BACLOFEN

A derivative of the putative neurotransmitter gamma-aminobutyric acid (GABA), baclofen (β-[4-chlorophenyl]GABA) was recently released in the

Table 21-2. CENTRALLY ACTING MUSCLE RELAXANTS CURRENTLY AVAILABLE

NONPROPRIETARY NAME AND TRADE NAME	CHEMICAL STRUCTURE	DOSAGE FORMS *	SINGLE DOSE
Baclofen (LIORESAL)	Cl—⬡—CHCH$_2$COOH / CH$_2$NH$_2$	T:10 mg	5–20 mg
Carisoprodol (RELA, SOMA)	CH$_2$CH$_2$CH$_3$ / H$_2$NCOOCH$_2$CCH$_2$OOCNHCH(CH$_3$)$_2$ / CH$_3$	T:350 mg	350 mg
Chlorphenesin carbamate (MAOLATE)	Cl—⬡—OCH$_2$CHCH$_2$OOCNH$_2$ (OH)	T:400 mg	800 mg
Chlorzoxazone (PARAFLEX)	Cl-benzoxazolone structure	T:250 mg	250–750 mg
Cyclobenzaprine Hydrochloride, U.S.P. (FLEXERIL)	·HCl, HCCH$_2$CH$_2$N(CH$_3$)$_2$	T:10 mg	10 mg
Mephenesin	CH$_3$ / ⬡—OCH$_2$CHCH$_2$OH (OH)	T:500 mg	1–2 g
Metaxalone (SKELAXIN)	H$_3$C— ... —OCH$_2$ oxazolidinone — H$_3$C	T:400 mg	800 mg
Methocarbamol, U.S.P. (ROBAXIN, others)	OCH$_3$ / ⬡—OCH$_2$CH—CH$_2$OOCNH$_2$ (OH)	T:500,750 mg / I:100 mg/ml	1–2 g, oral / 1–3 g, i.v., slowly
Orphenadrine Citrate, U.S.P. (NORFLEX, others)	*See* Table 21–1	T:100 mg / I:30 mg/ml	100 mg, oral / 60 mg, i.m. or i.v.

* T = tablet; I = injection.

United States for the treatment of spasticity in patients with multiple sclerosis. It may be of some value in patients with spasticity due to spinal cord injury or disease. Because it is an obvious analog of GABA, an initial postulate was that baclofen activated receptors for the transmitter in the spinal cord. To the contrary, since baclofen hyperpolarizes primary afferent fiber terminals whereas GABA depolarizes them, it appears that the inhibitory action of baclofen in spasticity is not related to its GABA-like structure (Davidoff and Sears, 1974; Calne, 1976; Fukuda *et al.,* 1977; Potashner, 1978). The drug is absorbed rapidly after oral administration and has a half-life in plasma of about 3 to 4 hours. It is largely excreted unchanged by the kidney. The use of baclofen may be limited by its adverse effects, which include drowsiness, insomnia, dizziness, weakness, and mental confusion. Sudden withdrawal of baclofen after chronic administration may cause auditory and visual hallucinations, anxiety, and tachycardia. Coma, respiratory depression, and seizures have been reported following significant overdosage. The threshold for initiation of seizures may be lowered in patients with epilepsy.

Baclofen is variably effective in the treatment of spasticity caused by multiple sclerosis or other diseases of the spinal cord. Similar to other muscle relaxants, it may impair the ability of the patient to walk or stand. It is not recommended for the management of the spasticity in rheumatic disorders, stroke, cerebral palsy, or the muscular rigidity of parkinsonism (Davidoff, 1978).

Preparation and Dosage. The available preparation of baclofen is listed in Table 21-2. Determination of optimal dosage in individual patients requires careful titration. Treatment is initiated with an oral dose of 5 mg, given three times daily, and after 3 days the individual dose is increased to 10 mg. The maximal dosage is 20 mg, four times daily. Abrupt withdrawal of the drug should be avoided. Baclofen should be administered cautiously and in decreased dosage to patients with impaired renal function.

CYCLOBENZAPRINE

Closely related to the tricyclic antidepressants both structurally and pharmacologically (Table 21-2), cyclobenzaprine is difficult to categorize in comparison with other available skeletal muscle relaxants (Ashby *et al.*, 1972). It is clear that this drug acts neither at the neuromuscular junction nor directly on skeletal muscle. Few data are available that suggest a mechanism by which this drug modifies muscle spasm. In a 2-week, crossover study Bercel (1977) compared cyclobenzaprine with placebo in the management of patients with osteoarthritis and posterior neck or low back pain; the drug was minimally more effective than placebo. Clinical studies comparing this agent with other muscle relaxants are in progress.

In keeping with its structural similarity to the tricyclic antidepressants, cyclobenzaprine has side effects in common with that group of drugs. These are anticholinergic in nature and include drowsiness, dry mouth and mucous membranes, tachycardia, blurred vision, and paresthesias. Administration within 2 weeks of treatment with MAO inhibitors is contraindicated. The drug should be avoided in patients with cardiac arrhythmias or heart block because of the known cardiotoxic action of the tricyclic antidepressants. The usual dose of cyclobenzaprine is 10 mg orally, given three times daily.

DANTROLENE

Dantrolene is unique, in comparison to the muscle relaxants listed in Table 21-2, in that it exerts its effects by direct actions on skeletal muscle (Snyder *et al.*, 1967; Van Winkle, 1976; Davidoff, 1978). Dantrolene has the following chemical structure:

Dantrolene

Pharmacological Properties. Dantrolene reduces contraction of skeletal muscle by a direct action on excitation–contraction coupling, perhaps by decreasing the amount of calcium released from the sarcoplasmic reticulum (Van Winkle, 1976). Although the drug produces some CNS depressant effects, it does not impair polysynaptic reflexes preferentially as do the centrally acting muscle relaxants. Dantrolene diminishes the force of electrically induced twitches in man without altering muscle action potentials, and it reduces reflex more than voluntary contraction (Herman *et al.*, 1972). Dantrolene does not affect neuromuscular transmission, nor does it change the electrical properties of skeletal muscle membranes (Davidoff, 1978).

In patients with upper motoneuron lesions, spasticity is generally diminished by treatment with dantrolene, and functional capacity is often improved. Unfortunately, the drug also tends to cause a generalized muscle weakness that negates functional improvement.

Dantrolene is also effective in alleviating the signs of malignant hyperthermia in susceptible animals and in patients. This rare, genetically determined syndrome is usually precipitated by the administration of neuromuscular blocking agents and inhalational anesthetics during surgery (*see* Chapter 11). Contraction of skeletal muscle apparently occurs as a result of excessive release of calcium from the sarcoplasmic reticulum.

Absorption of dantrolene from the gastrointestinal tract is slow and incomplete but sufficiently consistent to provide dose-related concentrations in plasma. The mean half-life of the drug in adults is about 9 hours after a 100-mg dose. It is slowly metabolized by the liver, and the 5-hydroxy and acetamido metabolites are excreted with unchanged drug in the urine.

Untoward Effects and Precautions. Dantrolene has a serious potential to cause hepatotoxicity. Fatal hepatitis has been reported in approximately 0.1 to 0.2% of patients treated with the drug for 60 days or longer. Symptomatic hepatitis may occur in 0.5% of patients treated with dantrolene for more than 60 days, while chemical abnormalities of hepatic function are noted in up to 1%. In view of this potential for hepatic injury, chronic administration of dantrolene should be halted if clear benefits are not evident within 45 days, and hepatic function should be monitored. The most common major side effect of dantrolene is weakness, which is probably an extension of its effect on skeletal muscle. Although weakness may be transient or mild, its persistence in some ambulatory patients may compromise therapeutic benefit. Euphoria, light-headedness, dizziness, drowsiness, and fatigue often occur early in treatment, but these side effects are generally transient; nevertheless, patients should be cautioned against driving or participating in hazardous occupations. Although the diarrhea that occurs in some patients can usually be controlled by a more gradual increase in dosage, it may necessitate withdrawal of the drug.

Preparations and Dosage. *Dantrolene sodium* (DANTRIUM) is available for oral use in capsules containing 25, 50, 75, or 100 mg of the drug and in a suspension (5 mg/ml). The starting dose of 25 mg once a day is gradually increased weekly by increments of 50 to 100 mg per day to a maximal dose of 400 mg daily, given in four divided doses. For children, the recommended starting dose of 1 mg/kg once a day is gradually increased to a maximum of 3 mg/kg four times a day, but not to exceed 400 mg daily. Dantrolene is also available for intravenous administration in vials containing 20 mg of the drug.

Therapeutic Uses. Dantrolene can relieve spasticity, but the weakness it produces may handicap the patient more than the spasticity it relieves. Dantrolene provides significant and sustained reduction of spasticity and improves functional capacity for the majority of paraplegic and hemiplegic patients; clonus, mass-reflex movements, and abnormal resistance to passive stretch are reduced. About one half of patients with athetoid cerebral palsy or multiple sclerosis are also sufficiently improved to warrant continued treatment. In general, patients whose functional rehabilitation is retarded by spasticity appear to gain most from the drug. Tolerance to its therapeutic effect does not appear. (*See* Chyatte and Basmajian, 1973; Chyatte *et al.*, 1973; Gelenberg and Poskanzer, 1973; Mayer *et al.*, 1973; Symposium, 1974; Davidoff, 1978.)

Dantrolene should be administered intravenously as soon as the syndrome of malignant hyperthermia is recognized; the initial dose is 1 mg/kg, and this may be repeated as necessary to a total of 10 mg/kg. Supportive measures are also important. These include discontinuation of anesthetics, administration of oxygen, management of acidosis and fever, and attention to urine output and water and electrolyte balance. Oral administration of dantrolene (1 to 2 mg/kg four times a day) may be necessary for 1 to 3 days to prevent recurrence of the condition.

THERAPEUTIC STATUS

Currently, there is no completely satisfactory form of therapy for alleviation of skeletal muscle spasticity (Davidoff, 1978). While several of the drugs presently available to the clinician are capable of providing variable relief of spasticity in given circumstances, troublesome muscle weakness, adverse effects on gait, and a variety of other side effects minimize their overall usefulness. These drugs may temporarily abate some of the symptoms of cerebral palsy, but they have a minor role in the overall management of this disorder. Muscle relaxants are of little value in Parkinson's disease or in other dysfunctions resulting from diseases of the brain. Muscle relaxants administered intravenously have established value in treating acute muscle spasms associated with trauma and inflammation and are also beneficial in producing muscle relaxation for certain orthopedic manipulations.

Many agents with muscle relaxant properties produce notable sedation in ordinary oral doses. Such agents enjoy particularly wide use in the treatment of muscle tension and pains associated with anxiety states and psychosomatic disorders. Favorable reports of the effects of such drugs for the conditions mentioned are numerous; however, whether the benefits are attributable to the sedative effect of the drugs or to a placebo effect have not been determined critically.

Anderson, R. J., and Raines, A. Suppression of decerebrate rigidity by phenytoin and chlorpromazine. *Neurology (Minneap.)*, **1976**, *26*, 858–862.

Ashby, P.; Burke, D.; and Rao, S. Assessment of cyclobenzaprine in the treatment of spasticity. *J. Neurol. Neurosurg. Psychiatry*, **1972**, *35*, 599–605.

Barbeau, A. Parkinson's disease: etiologic considerations. *Res. Publ. Assoc. Res. Nerv. Ment. Dis.*, **1976**, *55*, 281–292.

Bercel, N. A. Cyclobenzaprine in the treatment of skeletal muscle spasm in osteoarthritis of the cervical and lumbar spine. *Curr. Ther. Res.*, **1977**, *22*, 462–468.

Berger, F. M., and Bradley, W. The pharmacological properties of α:β-dihydroxy-γ-(2-methylphenoxy)-propane (MYANESIN). *Br. J. Pharmacol. Chemother.*, **1946**, *1*, 265–272.

Bernheimer, H.; Birkmayer, W.; and Hornykiewicz, O. Brain dopamine and the syndromes of Parkinson and Huntington: clinical, morphological and neurochemical correlations. *J. Neurol. Sci.*, **1973**, *20*, 415–455.

Bertler, A., and Rosengren, E. Occurrence and distribution of dopamine in brain and other tissues. *Experientia*, **1959**, *15*, 10–11.

Bianchine, J. R., and Shaw, G. M. Clinical pharmacokinetics of levodopa in Parkinson's disease. *Clin. Pharmacokinet.*, **1976**, *1*, 313–358.

Bianchine, J. R.; Shaw, G. M.; Greenwald, J. E.; and Dandalides, S. M. Clinical aspects of dopamine agonists and antagonists. *Fed. Proc.*, **1978**, *37*, 2434–2439.

Bianchine, J. R., and Sunyapridakul, L. Individualization of levodopa therapy. *Med. Clin. North Am.*, **1974**, *58*, 1071–1081.

Birkmayer, W.; Riederer, P.; Ambrozi, L.; and Youdim, M. B. H. Implications of combined treatment with "MODAPAR" and L-deprenyl in Parkinson's disease. *Lancet*, **1977**, *1*, 439–440.

Burke, D. J. An approach to the treatment of spasticity. *Drugs*, **1975**, *10*, 112–120.

Calne, D. B. The pharmacology of spasticity. In, *Clinical Neuropharmacology.* (Klawans, H. L., ed.) Raven Press, New York, **1976**, pp. 137–145.

————. Developments in the pharmacology and therapeutics of parkinsonism. *Ann. Neurol.*, **1977**, *1*, 111–119.

————. Parkinsonism, clinical and neuropharmacologic aspects. *Postgrad. Med.*, **1978a**, *64*, 82–88.

————. Role of ergot derivatives in the treatment of parkinsonism. *Fed. Proc.*, **1978b**, *37*, 2207–2209.

Carlsson, A. The occurrence, distribution, and physiological role of catecholamines in the nervous system. *Pharmacol. Rev.*, **1959**, *11*, 490–493.

————. Biochemical implications of dopa-induced actions on the central nervous system, with particular reference to abnormal movements. In, *L-Dopa and Parkinsonism.* (Barbeau, A., and McDowell, F. H., eds.) F. A. Davis Co., Philadelphia, **1970**, pp. 205–213.

Carlsson, A.; Lindqvist, M.; and Magnusson, T. 3,4-Dihydroxyphenylalanine and 5-hydroxytryptophan as reserpine antagonists. *Nature*, **1957**, *180*, 1200.

Carlsson, A.; Lindqvist, M.; Magnusson, T.; and Waldeck, B. On the presence of 3-hydroxytyramine in brain. *Science*, **1958**, *127*, 471.

Chandra, B. Treatment of disturbances of consciousness caused by measles encephalitis with levodopa. *Eur. Neurol.*, **1978**, *17*, 265–270.

Chase, T. N., and Watanabe, A. M. Methyldopahydrazine as an adjunct to L-dopa therapy in parkinsonism. *Neurology (Minneap.)*, **1972**, *22*, 384–392.

Chyatte, S. B., and Basmajian, J. V. Dantrolene sodium: long-term effects in severe spasticity. *Arch. Phys. Med. Rehabil.*, **1973**, *54*, 311–315.

Chyatte, S. B.; Birdsong, J. H.; and Roberson, D. L. Dantrolene sodium in athetoid cerebral palsy. *Arch. Phys. Med. Rehabil.*, **1973**, *54*, 365–368.

Cotzias, G. C.; Papavasiliou, P. S.; Tolosa, E. S.; Mendez, J. S.; and Bell-Midura, M. Treatment of parkinsonism with aporphines: possible role of growth hormone. *N. Engl. J. Med.*, **1976**, *294*, 567–572.

Cotzias, G. C.; Van Woert, M. H.; and Schiffer, L. M. Aromatic amino acids and modification of parkinsonism. *N. Engl. J. Med.*, **1967**, *276*, 374–379.

Cunningham, R. W.; Harned, B. K.; Clark, M. C.;

Cosgrove, R. R.; Daugherty, N. S.; Hine, C. H.; Vessey, R. E.; and Yuda, N. N. The pharmacology of 3-(N-piperidyl)-1-phenyl-1-cyclohexyl-1-propranol HCl (ARTANE) and related compounds: new antispasmodic agents. *J. Pharmacol. Exp. Ther.,* **1949,** *96,* 151–165.

Davidoff, R. A., and Sears, E. S. The effects of lioresal on synaptic activity in the isolated spinal cord. *Neurology (Minneap.),* **1974,** *24,* 957–963.

Duvoisin, R. C. Problems in the treatment of parkinsonism. *Adv. Exp. Med. Biol.,* **1977,** *90,* 131–155.

Eddy, R. L.; Jones, A. L.; Chakmakjian, Z. H.; and Silverthorne, M. C. Effect of levodopa (L-dopa) on human hypophyseal trophic hormone release. *J. Clin. Endocrinol. Metab.,* **1971,** *33,* 709–712.

Ehringer, H., and Hornykiewicz, O. Verteilung von Noradrenalin und Dopamin (3-hydroxytyramin) im Gehirn des Menschen und ihr Verhalten bei Erkrankungen des extrapyramidalen Systems. *Klin. Wochenschr.,* **1960,** *38,* 1236–1239.

Ellis, K. O., and Carpenter, J. F. Studies on the mechanism of action of dantrolene sodium, a skeletal muscle relaxant. *Naunyn Schmiedebergs Arch. Pharmacol.,* **1972,** *275,* 83–94.

———. Mechanism of control of skeletal-muscle contraction by dantrolene sodium. *Arch. Phys. Med. Rehabil.,* **1974,** *55,* 362–369.

Esplin, D. W. Criteria for assessing effects of depressant drugs on spinal cord synaptic transmission, with examples of drug selectivity. *Arch. Int. Pharmacodyn. Ther.,* **1963,** *143,* 479–497.

Fahn, S., and Calne, D. B. Considerations in the management of parkinsonism. *Neurology (Minneap.),* **1978,** *28,* 5–7.

Forssman, B.; Kihlstrand, S.; and Larsson, L. E. Amantadine therapy in parkinsonism. *Acta Neurol. Scand.,* **1972,** *48,* 1–18.

Fukuda, T.; Kudo, Y.; and Ono, H. Effects of β-(p-chlorophenyl)-GABA (baclofen) on spinal synaptic activity. *Eur. J. Pharmacol.,* **1977,** *44,* 17–24.

Gelenberg, A. J., and Poskanzer, D. C. The effect of dantrolene sodium on spasticity in multiple sclerosis. *Neurology (Minneap.),* **1973,** *23,* 1313–1315.

Godwin-Austen, R. B., and Smith, N. J. Comparison of the effects of bromocriptine and levodopa in Parkinson's disease. *J. Neurol. Neurosurg. Psychiatry,* **1977,** *40,* 479–482.

Goldberg, L. I.; Volkman, P. H.; and Kohli, J. D. A comparison of the vascular dopamine receptor with other dopamine receptors. *Annu. Rev. Pharmacol. Toxicol.,* **1978,** *18,* 57–79.

Goldstein, M.; Lieberman, A.; Battista, A. F.; Lew, J. Y.; and Matsumoto, Y. Experimental and clinical studies on bromocriptine in the parkinsonian syndrome. *Acta Endocrinol. (Kbh.),* **1978,** *88,* Suppl. 216, 57–66.

Goodall, M. C., and Alton, H. Dopamine (3-hydroxytyramine) metabolism in parkinsonism. *J. Clin. Invest.,* **1969,** *48,* 2300–2308.

Goodwin, F. K.; Murphy, D. L.; Brodie, H. K. H.; and Bunney, W. E. Levodopa: alterations in behavior. *Clin. Pharmacol. Ther.,* **1971,** *12,* 383–396.

Granérus, A. K. Factors influencing the occurrence of "on-off" symptoms during long-term treatment with L-dopa. *Acta Med. Scand.,* **1978,** *203,* 75–81.

Greengard, P., and Kebabian, J. W. Role of cyclic AMP in synaptic transmission in the mammalian peripheral nervous system. *Fed. Proc.,* **1974,** *33,* 1059–1067.

Herman, R.; Mayer, N.; and Mecomber, S. A. Clinical pharmaco-physiology of dantrolene sodium. *Am. J. Phys. Med.,* **1972,** *51,* 296–311.

Hornykiewicz, O. Dopamine in the basal ganglia. *Br. Med. Bull.,* **1973b,** *29,* 172–178.

Hutt, C. S.; Snider, S. R.; and Fahn, S. Interaction between bromocriptine and levodopa; biochemical basis for an improved treatment for parkinsonism. *Neurology (Minneap.),* **1977,** *27,* 503–510.

Joseph, C.; Chassan, J. B.; and Koch, M. L. Levodopa in Parkinson's disease. *Ann. Neurol.,* **1978,** *3,* 116–118.

Kebabian, J. W., and Saavedra, J. M. Dopamine-sensitive adenylate cyclase occurs in a region of substantia nigra containing dopaminergic dendrites. *Science,* **1976,** *193,* 683–685.

Keller, H. H., and Daprada, M. Central dopamine agonistic activity and microsomal biotransformation of lisuride, lergotrile and bromocriptine. *Life Sci.,* **1979,** *24,* 1211–1222.

Klawans, H. L.; Goetz, C.; Nausieda, P. A.; and Weiner, W. J. Recent advances in the biochemical pharmacology of extrapyramidal movement disorders. *Adv. Exp. Med. Biol.,* **1977,** *90,* 21–47.

Knoll, J. The possible mechanisms of action of (−) deprenyl in Parkinson's disease. *J. Neural Transm.,* **1978,** *43,* 177–198.

Langston, J. W., and Forno, L. S. The hypothalamus in Parkinson's disease. *Ann. Neurol.,* **1978,** *3,* 129–133.

Lieberman, A.; Kupersmith, M.; Estey, E.; and Goldstein, M. Treatment of Parkinson's disease with bromocriptine. *N. Engl. J. Med.,* **1976,** *295,* 1400–1404.

Lieberman, A. N.; Kupersmith, M.; Gopinathan, G.; Estey, E.; Goodgold, A.; and Goldstein, M. Bromocriptine in Parkinson's disease: further studies. *Neurology (Minneap.),* **1979,** *29,* 363–369.

Lloyd, K. G. Neurochemical compensation in Parkinson's disease. In, *Parkinson's Disease, Concepts and Prospects.* (Lakke, J. P. W. F.; Korf, J.; and Wesseling, H.; eds.) Excerpta Medical, Amsterdam, **1978,** pp. 61–72.

Longo, V. G. Effects of mephenesin on the repetitive discharge of spinal cord interneurones. *Arch. Int. Pharmacodyn. Ther.,* **1961,** *132,* 222–236.

Lord, J. A. H.; Waterfield, A. A.; Hughes, J.; and Kosterlitz, H. W. Endogenous opioid peptides: multiple agonists and receptors. *Nature,* **1977,** *267,* 495–499.

Mars, H. Modification of levodopa effect by systemic decarboxylase inhibition. *Arch. Neurol.,* **1973,** *28,* 91–95.

Marsden, C. D., and Parkes, J. D. Success and problems of long-term levodopa therapy in Parkinson's disease. *Lancet,* **1977,** *1,* 345–349.

Marx, J. L. Parkinson's disease: search for better therapies. *Science,* **1979,** *203,* 737–738.

Mawdsley, C.; Williams, I. R.; Pullar, I. A.; Davidson, D. L.; and Kinloch, N.E. Treatment of parkinsonism by amantadine and levodopa. *Clin. Pharmacol. Ther.,* **1972,** *13,* 575–583.

Mayer, N.; Mecomber, S. A.; and Herman, R. Treatment of spasticity with dantrolene sodium. *Am. J. Phys. Med.,* **1973,** *52,* 18–29.

Medical Letter. Drugs for parkinsonism. **1979,** *21,* 37–38.

Montagu, K. A. Catechol compounds in rat tissues and in brains of different animals. *Nature,* **1957,** *180,* 244–245.

Morgan, M. Y.; Jakobovits, A.; Elithorn, A.; James, I. M.; and Sherlock, S. Successful use of bromocriptine in the treatment of a patient with chronic portasystemic encephalopathy. *N. Engl. J. Med.,* **1977,** *296,* 793–794.

Palfreyman, M. G.; Danzin, C.; Bey, P.; Jung, M. J.; Riberbeau-Gayon, G.; Aubry, M.; Vevert, J. P.; and Sjoerdsma, A. Difluoromethyl dopa, a new enzyme-activated irreversible inhibitor of aromatic L-amino acid decarboxylase. *J. Neurochem.,* **1978,** *31,* 927–932.

Papavasiliou, P. S.; Cotzias, G. C.; Duby, S. E.; Steck, A. J.; Fehling, C.; and Bell, M. A. Levodopa in parkinsonism; potentiation of central effects with a peripheral inhibitor. *N. Engl. J. Med.,* **1972,** *285,* 8–14.

Parkes, J. D.; Zilkha, K. J.; Calver, D. M.; and Knill-Jones, R. P. Controlled trial of amantadine hydrochloride in Parkinson's disease. *Lancet,* **1970,** *1,* 259–262.

Pearce, J. M. S. Aetiology and natural history of Parkinson's disease. *Br. Med. J.,* **1978,** *2,* 1664–1666.

Pearce, L. A.; Waterbury, L. D.; and Green, H. D. Amantadine hydrochloride: alteration in peripheral circulation. *Neurology (Minneap.)*, **1974**, *24*, 46–48.

Philipson, O. T., and Horn, A. S. Substantia nigra of the rat contains a dopamine adenylate cyclase. *Nature*, **1976**, *261*, 418–420.

Phillis, J. W. Is β-(4-chlorophenyl)-GABA a specific antagonist of substance P on cerebral cortical neurons? *Experientia*, **1976**, *32*, 593–594.

Potashner, S. J. Baclofen: effects on amino acid release. *Can. J. Physiol. Pharmacol.*, **1978**, *56*, 150–154.

Putney, J. W., Jr., and Bianchi, C. P. Site of action of dantrolene in frog sartorius muscle. *J. Pharmacol. Exp. Ther.*, **1974**, *189*, 202–212.

Rinne, U. K. Recent advances in research on parkinsonism. *Acta Neurol. Scand.*, **1978**, *57*, Suppl. 67, 77–113.

Rinne, U. K.; Sonninen, V.; and Surtola, T. Treatment of Parkinson's disease with ʟ-dopa and decarboxylase inhibitor. *Z. Neurol.*, **1972**, *202*, 1–20.

Rinne, U. K.; Surtola, T.; and Sonninen, V. ʟ-Deprenyl treatment of "on-off" phenomena in Parkinson's disease. *J. Neural Transm.*, **1978**, *43*, 253–262.

Roszkowski, A. P. A pharmacological comparison of therapeutically useful centrally acting skeletal muscle relaxants. *J. Pharmacol. Exp. Ther.*, **1960**, *129*, 75–81.

Sacks, O. W.; Kohl, M. S.; Messeloff, C. R.; and Schartz, W. F. Effects of levodopa in parkinsonian patients with dementia. *Neurology (Minneap.)*, **1972**, *22*, 516–519.

Sandler, M.; Carter, S. B.; Hunter, K. R.; and Stern, G. M. Tetrahydroisoquinoline alkaloids; *in vivo* metabolites of ʟ-dopa in man. *Nature*, **1973**, *241*, 439–443.

Sandler, M., and Ruthven, C. R. J. The biosynthesis and metabolism of the catecholamines. *Prog. Med. Chem.*, **1969**, *6*, 200–210.

Schwab, R. S.; Poskanzer, D. C.; England, A. C.; and Young, R. R. Amantadine in Parkinson's disease. Review of more than two years' experience. *J.A.M.A.*, **1972**, *222*, 792–795.

Shibuya, M. Dopamine-sensitive adenylate cyclase activity in the striatum in Parkinson's disease. *J. Neural Transm.*, **1979**, *44*, 297–302.

Sirtori, C. R.; Bolme, P.; and Azarnoff, D. L. Metabolic responses to acute and chronic ʟ-dopa administration in patients with parkinsonism. *N. Engl. J. Med.*, **1972**, *287*, 729–733.

Snyder, H. R., Jr.; Davis, C. S.; Bickerton, R. K.; and Halliday, R. P. 1-[(5-Arylfurfurylidene)amino]hydantoins. A new class of muscle relaxants. *J. Med. Pharm. Chem.*, **1967**, *10*, 807–810.

Sourkes, R. L. Possible new metabolites mediating actions of ʟ-dopa. *Nature*, **1971**, *229*, 413–414.

Tseng, T. C., and Wang, S. C. Locus of action of centrally acting muscle relaxants, diazepam and tybamate. *J. Pharmacol. Exp. Ther.*, **1971**, *178*, 350–360.

Van Winkle, W. B. Calcium release from skeletal muscle sarcoplasmic reticulum: site of action of dantrolene sodium? *Science*, **1976**, *193*, 1130–1131.

Verrier, M.; MacLeod, S.; and Ashby, P. The effects of diazepam on presynaptic inhibition in patients with complete and incomplete spinal cord lesions. *Can. J. Neurol. Sci.*, **1975**, *2*, 179–184.

Von Voigtlander, P. F., and Moore, K. E. Dopamine: release from the brain *in vivo* by amantadine. *Science*, **1971**, *174*, 408–410.

Yahr, M. D. Overview of present day treatment of Parkinson's disease. *J. Neural Transm.*, **1978**, *43*, 227–238.

Monographs and Reviews

Berger, F. M. Spinal cord depressant drugs. *Pharmacol. Rev.*, **1949**, *1*, 243–278. (136 references.)

Bernheimer, H.; Birkmayer, W.; Hornykiewicz, O.; Jellinger, K.; and Seitelberger, F. Brain dopamine and the syndromes of Parkinson and Huntington. *J. Neurol. Sci.*, **1973**, *20*, 415–455. (115 references.)

Bianchine, J. R. Drug therapy of parkinsonism. *N. Engl. J. Med.*, **1976**, *295*, 814–818.

Bianchine, J. R., and Sunyapridakul, L. Interactions between levodopa and other drugs: significance in the treatment of Parkinson's disease. *Drugs*, **1973**, *6*, 364–388. (118 references.)

Calne, D. B.; Kebabian, J.; Silbergeld, E.; and Evarts, E. Advances in the neuropharmacology of parkinsonism. *Ann. Intern. Med.*, **1979**, *90*, 219–229.

Davidoff, R. A. Pharmacology of spasticity. *Neurology (Minneap.)*, **1978**, *28*, 46–51.

Domino, E. F. The correlation between animal testing procedures and clinical effectiveness of centrally acting muscle relaxants of the mephenesin type. *Ann. N.Y. Acad. Sci.*, **1956**, *64*, 705–729. (177 references.)

Hornykiewicz, O. Parkinson's disease: from brain homogenate to treatment. *Fed. Proc.*, **1973a**, *32*, 183–190.

Malitz, S. (ed.). *ʟ-Dopa and Behavior.* Raven Press, New York, **1972**.

Marks, J. (ed.). *The Treatment of Parkinsonism with ʟ-Dopa.* American Elsevier Publishing Co., New York, **1974**.

Smith, C. M. Relaxants of skeletal muscle. In, *Physiological Pharmacology.* Vol. 2, *The Nervous System—Part B: Central Nervous System Drugs.* (Root, W. S., and Hofmann, F. G., eds.) Academic Press, Inc., New York, **1965**, pp. 2–96. (459 references.)

Stern, G. (ed.). *The Clinical Uses of Levodopa.* University Park Press, Baltimore, **1975**.

Sweet, R. D., and McDowell, F. H. Five years' treatment of Parkinson's disease with levodopa: therapeutic results and survival of 100 patients. *Ann. Intern. Med.*, **1975**, *83*, 456–463.

Symposium. (Various authors.) Spasticity—its etiology, physiology and the pharmacology of a new agent. *Arch. Phys. Med. Rehabil.*, **1974**, *55*, 331–392.

Symposium. (Various authors.) *Parkinson's Disease: Concepts and Prospects.* (Lakke, J. P. W. F.; Korf, J.; and Wesseling, H.; eds.) Excerpta Medica, Amsterdam, **1977**.

Yahr, M. D. Levodopa. *Ann. Intern. Med.*, **1975**, *83*, 677–682.

22 OPIOID ANALGESICS AND ANTAGONISTS

Jerome H. Jaffe and William R. Martin

This chapter presents the pharmacological properties of the opioids (opioid agonists) and the opioid antagonists. The term *opioid* is used here to designate a group of drugs that are, to varying degrees, opium- or morphine-like in their properties. The opioids are employed primarily as analgesics, but they have many other pharmacological effects as well. Opioids interact with what appear to be several closely related receptors, and they share some of the properties of certain peptides, the *enkephalins* and the *endorphins,* which probably are present in the nervous system of all vertebrates.

History. Although the psychological effects of opium may have been known to the ancient Sumerians, the first undisputed reference to poppy juice is found in the writings of Theophrastus in the third century B.C. The word *opium* itself is derived from the Greek name for juice, the drug being obtained from the juice of the poppy, *Papaver somniferum.* Arabian physicians were well versed in the uses of opium; Arabian traders introduced the drug to the Orient, where it was employed mainly for the control of dysenteries. Paracelsus (1493–1541) is credited with repopularizing the use of opium in Europe; it had fallen into disfavor because of its toxicity. By the middle of the sixteenth century, the uses of opium that are still valid were fairly well understood, and, in 1680, Sydenham wrote, "Among the remedies which it has pleased Almighty God to give to man to relieve his sufferings, none is so universal and so efficacious as opium."

In the eighteenth century opium smoking became popular in the Orient. At that time the use of opiates for their subjective effects was considerably more acceptable than it is at present. In Europe, the ready availability of opium led to some degree of overuse, but the problem of opium eating never became as prevalent or as socially destructive as the abuse of alcohol.

Opium contains more than 20 distinct alkaloids. In 1803, Sertürner isolated and described an opium alkaloid that he named morphine, after Morpheus, the Greek god of dreams. The discovery of other alkaloids in opium quickly followed that of morphine (codeine by Robiquet in 1832, papaverine by Merck in 1848). By the middle of the nineteenth century the use of pure alkaloids rather than crude opium preparations began to spread throughout the medical world.

The invention of the hypodermic needle and the parenteral use of morphine tended to produce a more severe variety of compulsive drug use. In the United States, the extent of the opioid-use problem was accentuated by the influx of opium-smoking Chinese laborers, the widespread use of morphine among wounded Civil War soldiers, and the unrestricted availability of opium that prevailed until the early years of this century. The history of opium and its alkaloids and the problems of addiction are described by Terry and Pellens (1928) and by Musto (1973).

The problem of addiction to opioids stimulated a search for potent analgesics that would be free of the potential to produce addiction. In 1915, Pohl observed that N-allylnorcodeine prevented or abolished morphine- and heroin-induced respiratory depression. More than 25 years elapsed before Unna as well as Hart and McCawley independently described the more pronounced morphine-antagonizing properties of nalorphine. The clinical significance of this antagonistic effect was not explored until 1951, when Eckenhoff and coworkers reported the use of nalorphine as an antidote for morphine poisoning in man. By this time chemists had synthesized a number of entities that were chemically quite distinct from morphine but produced almost the same pattern of pharmacological effects, including addiction. In 1953, Wikler and associates demonstrated that nalorphine would precipitate acute abstinence syndromes in postaddicts who had received opioids for brief periods, and that in the majority of nonaddicted subjects large doses of nalorphine produced dysphoria and anxiety rather than euphoria. Shortly thereafter, Lasagna and Beecher noted that, although nalorphine antagonized the analgesic effects of morphine, it was, nevertheless, an effective analgesic when given to patients with postoperative pain. The dysphoric side effects produced by nalorphine make it unsuitable for clinical use as an analgesic; however, since the low abuse potential of nalorphine had already been observed, the report of its analgesic effects raised the hope that other narcotic antagonists might be free of these dysphoric effects and still have analgesic activity. The search for useful compounds led to the discovery of new drugs, such as the relatively pure antagonist *naloxone* and compounds with mixed actions (*e.g., pentazocine, butorphanol,* and *buprenorphine*). Such agents not only have enlarged the range of available therapeutic entities but also, in conjunction with the subsequent discovery of receptors for opioids and endogenous peptides that bind to these receptors, have helped to change our views about the actions of the opioids.

By 1967, researchers had concluded that the complex interactions among morphine-like drugs, antagonists, and what were then called mixed agonist-antagonists could best be explained by postulating the existence of more than one type of receptor for the opioids and related drugs (Martin, 1967). Following a methodological approach developed by Goldstein and coworkers, investigators in several laboratories (Pert and Snyder, 1973; Simon *et al.,* 1973; Terenius, 1973) independently reported the discovery of saturable, stereospecific binding sites or receptors for opioid drugs in the mammalian nervous system. Shortly thereafter, Hughes and Kosterlitz and their coworkers described the isolation from pig brain of two pentapeptides that exhibited morphine-like actions on the guinea pig ileum—actions that were specifically antagonized by naloxone (*see* Hughes *et al.,* 1975). Within the same year, Goldstein and colleagues reported the presence of a peptide-like substance in the bovine pituitary gland with opioid activity (Cox *et al.,* 1975; Teschemacher *et al.,* 1975). This substance proved to be a polypeptide with 31 amino acid residues; it, too, exhibited opioid-like actions that were antagonized by naloxone. Hughes and coworkers named the pentapeptides leucine- (leu-) and methionine- (met-) *enkephalin.* The larger peptide was designated *β-endorphin.* These recent developments have been reviewed by Goldstein (1976), Kosterlitz and Hughes (1978), Miller and Cuatrecasas (1978a, 1979), Simon and Hiller (1978), and Terenius (1978).

Terminology. The term *opiate* was once used to designate drugs derived from opium—morphine, codeine, and the many semisynthetic congeners of morphine. Soon after the development of totally synthetic entities with morphine-like actions, the word *opioid* was introduced to refer in a generic sense to all drugs, natural and synthetic, with morphine-like actions. Some writers continued to use the term *opiate* in a generic sense, and in such contexts *opiate* and *opioid* are interchangeable. With the advent of drugs that bind to some receptors for opioids but do not share all of the actions of morphine, the word *opioid* required redefinition. In this chapter the term *opioid* is retained as a generic designation for all exogenous substances that bind specifically to any of several subspecies of opioid receptors and produce some agonist actions. Drugs that meet this definition may or may not have a pharmacological profile similar to that of morphine. Some may bind to subspecies of receptors in a pattern that differs from that of morphine, and, although they can be displaced from these receptors by the antagonist *naloxone,* their pharmacological actions may be distinct from those of morphine. Some substances,

like naloxone, appear to bind to receptors for opioids but initiate little agonistic action; they are designated here as *opioid antagonists.* There are still other compounds that in some situations appear to have both agonistic and antagonistic effects, depending on the dose, the species, and the test situation.

There is, at present, no entirely satisfactory classification of the opioids and the antagonists that have been studied. In this chapter these substances have been divided into three groups: opioid agonists (morphine and morphine-like opioids), opioid antagonists, and opioids with mixed actions; the last-named category includes the agonist-antagonists. Further discussion of receptor subtypes is found in the section on Opioid Antagonists and Agonist-Antagonists.

The term *narcotic* was obsolete long before the discovery of endogenous opioid-like ligands and receptors for these substances. Derived from the Greek word for stupor and at one time applied to any drug that induced sleep, it was, for a number of years, used to refer to morphine-like strong analgesics. With the development of mixed agonist-antagonists, some of which do not suppress morphine-like physical dependence, and with the increasing use of the term in a legal context to refer to any substance that can cause dependence, the term *narcotic* is no longer useful in a pharmacological context. However, it is not likely to disappear soon.

MORPHINE AND CHEMICALLY RELATED OPIOIDS

There are now many compounds that produce analgesia and other effects similar to those produced by morphine. Some of these may have some special properties, but none has proven to be clinically superior in relieving pain. Morphine remains the standard against which new analgesics are measured. Although morphine can be synthesized in the laboratory, it is still obtained from opium.

Source and Composition of Opium. Opium is obtained from the milky exudate of the incised unripe seed capsules of the poppy plant, *Papaver somniferum.* Once indigenous to Asia Minor, the plant is now grown legally and illegally in many parts of the world. The milky juice is dried in the air and forms a brownish, gummy mass. This is further dried and powdered to make the official powdered opium, containing a number of alkaloids. Only a few—morphine, codeine, and papaverine—have clinical usefulness. The alkaloids constitute about

25% by weight of opium and can be divided into two distinct chemical classes, *phenanthrenes* and *benzylisoquinolines.*

The principal phenanthrenes are morphine (10% of opium), codeine (0.5%), and thebaine (0.2%). The principal benzylisoquinolines are papaverine (1.0%), which is a smooth muscle relaxant (*see* Chapter 33), and noscapine (6.0%).

Chemistry of Morphine and Related Opioids. The structure of morphine, originally proposed by Gulland and Robinson in 1925, is as follows:

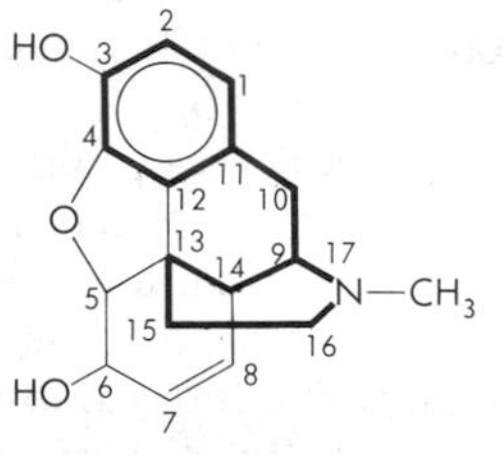

Morphine

Although morphine can be synthesized in the laboratory with great difficulty, many semisynthetic derivatives are made by relatively simple modifications of the morphine or thebaine molecule. *Codeine* is methylmorphine, the methyl substitution being on the phenolic OH. *Thebaine* differs from morphine only in that both OH groups are methylated and that there are two double bonds in the ring ($\Delta^{6,7}$, $\Delta^{8,14}$). It has little analgesic action and produces seizures at a relatively low dosage. However, thebaine is a precursor of several important 14-OH compounds, such as *oxycodone* and *naloxone.* Certain derivatives of thebaine are more than 1000 times as potent as morphine (*e.g., etorphine*). *Diacetylmorphine,* or *heroin,* is made from morphine by the acetylation of both the phenolic and the alcoholic OH groups. *Apomorphine,* which can also be prepared from morphine, is a potent emetic and dopaminergic agonist (*see* Chapter 21). *Hydromorphone, oxymorphone, hydrocodone,* and *oxycodone* are also made by modifying the morphine molecule. The structural relationship between morphine and some of its surrogates and antagonists is shown in Table 22-1.

Structure-Activity Relationship of the Opioids. In addition to morphine, codeine, and the semisynthetic derivatives of the natural opium alkaloids, there are a number of other structurally distinct chemical classes of drugs with pharmacological actions similar to those of morphine. These diverse groups share the capacity to produce analgesia, respiratory depression, gastrointestinal spasm, and morphine-like physical dependence. Toxic doses produce convulsions, and the analgesic, gastrointestinal, depressant, and convulsant effects can be antagonized by naloxone and related antagonists. Clinically useful compounds include the morphinans, benzomorphans, methadones, phenylpiperidines, and propionanilides. In addition, *thiambutene* and *benzimidazole* derivatives possess morphine-like activity (for references, *see* Braenden *et al.,* 1955). Although the flat two-

Table 22-1. STRUCTURES OF OPIOIDS AND OPIOID ANTAGONISTS CHEMICALLY RELATED TO MORPHINE

NONPROPRIETARY NAME	CHEMICAL RADICALS AND POSITIONS			OTHER CHANGES †
	3 *	6 *	17 *	
Morphine	—OH	—OH	—CH_3	—
Heroin	—$OCOCH_3$	—$OCOCH_3$	—CH_3	—
Hydromorphone	—OH	=O	—CH_3	(1)
Oxymorphone	—OH	=O	—CH_3	(1),(2)
Levorphanol	—OH	—H	—CH_3	(1),(3)
Codeine	—OCH_3	—OH	—CH_3	—
Hydrocodone	—OCH_3	=O	—CH_3	(1)
Oxycodone	—OCH_3	=O	—CH_3	(1),(2)
Nalorphine	—OH	—OH	—$CH_2CH{=}CH_2$	—
Naloxone	—OH	=O	—$CH_2CH{=}CH_2$	(1),(2)
Naltrexone	—OH	=O	—CH_2—◁	(1),(2)
Buprenorphine	—OH	—OCH_3	—CH_2—◁	(1),(2),(4)
Butorphanol	—OH	—H	—CH_2—◇	(2),(3)
Nalbuphine	—OH	—OH	—CH_2—◇	(1),(2)

* The numbers 3, 6, and 17 refer to positions in the morphine molecule, as shown above.

† Other changes in the morphine molecule are as follows:
  (1) Single instead of double bond between C7 and C8.
  (2) OH added to C14.
  (3) No oxygen between C4 and C5.
  (4) *Endo*etheno bridge between C6 and C14; 1-hydroxy-1,2,2-trimethylpropyl substitution on C7.

dimensional representations of these chemically diverse compounds appear to be quite different, molecular models show certain common characteristics; these are indicated by the heavy lines in the structure of morphine shown above. Among the important properties of the opioids that can be altered by structural modification are their affinity for various subspecies of receptors for opioids, agonistic versus antagonistic activity, lipid solubility, resistance to metabolic breakdown, and binding to albumin in plasma. Structure-activity relationships among the exogenous opioids and opioid antagonists have been reviewed by Lewis and coworkers (1971) and Barnett and associates (1978).

The discovery of endogenous ligands (enkephalins and endorphins) with high affinities for opioid receptors has added new dimensions to the study of structure-activity relationships of opioid agonists and to the concept of the diversity of opioid receptors (for structures, *see* below under Mechanism of Action). The enkephalins and endorphins share the pharmacological properties of the agonistic opioid alkaloids. The enkephalins have a very brief duration of action due to rapid hydrolysis by peptidases. Their pharmacological properties can only be demonstrated *in vitro* or by intracerebral injection, and their binding characteristics can only be determined with accuracy in the presence of protease inhibitors. However, due to their relatively simple structure, modern technics have led to the synthesis of scores of congeners, many of which are stable, share the binding characteristics and pharmacological actions of opioid alkaloids (including the capacity to induce tolerance and cause addiction), cross the blood-brain barrier, and are active by all routes of administration including oral. Activity is retained and the half-life is prolonged when D-amino acids are substituted in the 2 or 5 (or both) positions of leu-enkephalin. D-ala[2]-D-leu[5]-enkephalin is remarkable in this respect. Substitution in the 1, 3, or 4 position reduces activity. For recent developments in this area, *see* Miller and Cuatrecasas (1978b), Chang and Cuatrecasas (1979), and Chang and coworkers (1979).

The clinical applicability of the synthetic enkephalins remains to be determined. The synthesis of an enkephalin with a high affinity for an opioid receptor at a specific site would be a notable achievement.

PHARMACOLOGICAL PROPERTIES

Morphine and related opioids produce their major effects on the central nervous system (CNS) and the bowel. The effects are remarkably diverse and include analgesia, drowsiness, changes in mood, respiratory depression, decreased gastrointestinal motility, nausea, vomiting, and alterations of the endocrine and autonomic nervous systems.

The older literature on opium alkaloids has been reviewed by Reynolds and Randall (1957), Winter (1965), and Martin (1967). For more recent reviews and references, *see* Kosterlitz and associates (1973), Braude and colleagues (1974), Martin and Sloan (1977), and Adler and associates (1978).

Mechanism of Action. Opioids act as agonists, interacting with stereospecific and saturable binding sites or receptors in the brain and other tissues. These binding sites are widely but unevenly distributed throughout the CNS. They are present in highest concentration in the limbic system (frontal and temporal cortex, amygdala, and hippocampus), thalamus, striatum, hypothalamus, midbrain, and spinal cord (Snyder *et al.*, 1974; Simon and Hiller, 1978). The affinity of many, but not all, opioid analgesics for the binding sites correlates well with their potency as analgesics. Since many factors determine the fraction of an administered dose that reaches the receptors, this is a remarkable finding.

The opioid receptors appear to be the normal sites of action of several endogenous ligands. Two pentapeptides, methionine-enkephalin (met-enkephalin) (Tyr-Gly-Gly-Phe-Met) and leucine-enkephalin (leu-enkaphalin) (Tyr-Gly-Gly-Phe-Leu), and several larger polypeptides have been isolated from brain and other tissues; they interact with receptors for opioids and produce patterns of effects similar but not always identical to those seen with the opioid drugs. The amino acid sequence of met-enkephalin is identical to sequence 61 to 65 in the pituitary hormone β-lipotropin (β-LPH), a protein with 91 amino acid residues. The larger polypeptides that bind to receptors for opioids are also identical to portions of β-LPH. The carboxy terminus (β-LPH 61-91), which is now designated β-*endorphin*, is the most potent of the endogenous opioid-like substances isolated thus far. Other sequences with opioid activity are α-endorphin (β-LPH 61-76) and γ-endorphin (β-LPH 61-77) (*see* Figure 59-2; *see also* Simon and Hiller, 1978; Terenius, 1978; Beaumont and Hughes, 1979). A nonpeptide endogenous substance has been reported to cross-react with morphine-specific antibodies and is distributed throughout the brain in a pattern distinct from that of the enkephalins or β-endorphin (Gintzler *et al.,* 1978).

The binding sites or receptors for opioids are found particularly in synaptosomal fractions of brain. The enkephalins are located in neurons and their processes, and their distribution correlates well with that of the receptors. Endogenous opioid-like peptides are present particularly in areas of the CNS that are presumed to be related to the perception of pain (laminae I and II of the spinal cord, spinal trigeminal nucleus, periaqueductal gray, periventricular gray, and medullary raphe nuclei); to movement, mood, and behavior (globus pallidus, stria terminalis, locus ceruleus); and to the regulation of neuroendocrinological functions (median eminence). They are also found in cells whose functions relate to the motility of the bowel (nerve plexuses and exocrine glands of the stomach and intestine). Enkephalins are believed to be contained in short interneurons. Sectioning of the spinal cord does not reduce the content of enkephalin in the cord below the level of the lesion, and the concentrations are unaltered by section of the dorsal roots. In contrast, β-endorphin is found principally in the pars intermedia and pars distalis of the pituitary gland and in the hypothalamus. However, some of the neurons that contain β-endorphin have axons that ascend and descend; certain of these axons have terminals in the central gray matter, an area that appears to play a major role in modulation of pain and where there is also a high concentration of enkephalins (see Snyder, 1978; Terenius, 1978; Beaumont and Hughes, 1979).

The enkephalins and β-endorphin appear to belong to two functionally and anatomically distinct systems and to function as neurotransmitters, modulators of neurotransmission, or neurohormones. Because of the location of β-endorphin in the hypothalamus and the pituitary and its relatively longer duration of action, it is viewed as a probable neurohormone. The wider distribution of enkephalins, their very rapid destruction, their location in synaptosomes, and the observation that their release following depolarization of brain or intestinal tissues is calcium dependent suggest that they function as neurotransmitters or modulators of synaptic function. It is assumed that exogenous opioids (morphine-like drugs and opioids with mixed actions) produce their effects by mimicking the actions of the endogenous ligands. However, since there appear to be several subspecies of receptors, there is also the possiblity that exogenous opioids may have actions on some receptors that, in a given species, are not strongly activated by its own endogenous ligands—at least those discovered to date. For example, in certain species, exogenous opioids cause excitation and seizures. In general, however, when β-endorphin is injected into animals or man, the effects are similar to those of morphine. Tolerance to and physical dependence on exogenously administered met-enkephalin and β-endorphin have been demonstrated, as has cross-tolerance between these peptides and exogenous opioids (see Snyder, 1978; Terenius, 1978).

The β-endorphin that is found in the pituitary is produced by the cleavage of a protein that is synthesized in cells within the hypothalamus, probably in the arcuate nucleus. Because this protein is the prohormone for both ACTH and β-LPH (which, in turn, contains β-endorphin), it is sometimes referred to as pro-opiocortin (see Chapter 59). ACTH and β-LPH or β-endorphin (or both) are stored in the same cells. In the rat, stress and other manipulations that result in secretion of ACTH also cause release of equimolar quantities of β-endorphin (see Guillemin, 1978). However, in studies of human subjects, β-endorphin is not normally detectable in plasma; injection of antidiuretic hormone, which produces a sharp increase in the circulating concentration of ACTH, causes an increase in the concentration of β-LPH in plasma, but not in that of β-endorphin (Suda et al., 1978). Enkephalins are not formed from β-endorphin; they are synthesized in brain tissue by proteolysis of a distinct precursor. The role of endogenous opioid-like peptides in normal human physiology, in addictive states, and in psychiatric disorders remains unknown (see Guillemin, 1978; Snyder, 1978; Terenius, 1978; Verebey et al., 1978; Beaumont and Hughes, 1979).

Cellular and Biochemical Aspects of the Actions of Opioids. The binding of an exogenous opioid agonist or an endogenous ligand to its receptor initiates the events that ultimately produce the effects that are observed. Opioid agonists as well as the endogenous opioid-like peptides decrease the activity of adenylate cyclase in specialized cultures of cells derived from the nervous system. This effect is antagonized by naloxone. When exposed to morphine for several days, the cells become "tolerant" to this effect, and adenylate cyclase activity and concentrations of cyclic AMP return to baseline values. When morphine is removed, there is an enhanced activity of adenylate cyclase, and excessive quantities of cyclic adenosine 3',5'-monophosphate (cyclic AMP) accumulate (Sharma et al., 1975).

Such cell cultures represent an important system for the study of the actions of opioids. While there is no doubt that receptors for opioids can, at least under certain circumstances, regulate the activity of adenylate cyclase, there is little information on whether changes in the concentration of cyclic AMP in neurons have anything to do with the primary actions of the opioids or their endogenous counterparts. The effects of opioids on cyclic AMP in the brain appear to depend on the preparation, the area of the brain studied, and the concentration of calcium ion. Opioids appear to produce a selective and naloxone-reversible inhibition of adenylate cyclase activity in slices prepared from at least certain regions of the CNS (see Simon and Hiller, 1978).

The affinity of opioids for receptors *in vitro* is related to the concentration of Na^+, but not to that of other monovalent cations. Elevation of $[Na^+]$ reduces the affinity of binding of agonists, while increasing that of antagonists (Snyder, 1978). The physiological significance of these observations is not apparent.

Since opioids can alter the release of a number of neurotransmitters, they may influence some mechanism that is fundamental to neuronal function. The transmembrane transport of Ca^{2+} may be such a process. Administration of morphine produces a depletion of Ca^{2+} in the brain (and within synaptosomes prepared therefrom) and prevents uptake of Ca^{2+} into brain slices and synaptosomes. Calcium ion antagonizes the analgesia produced by morphine (see Way, 1978). Opioids also appear to suppress the activation by calcium of a membrane-bound protein kinase that is involved in the phosphorylation of other membrane proteins (Clouet *et al.*, 1978; Schulman and Greengard, 1978).

It has been postulated that enkephalin-containing interneurons exert their actions on presynaptic neural processes, with resultant alterations in the rate of release of other transmitters. In the CNS, opioids and endogenous opioid-like peptides inhibit the release of acetylcholine, norepinephrine, and substance P and alter the release of dopamine (*see* Snyder, 1978; Terenius, 1978; Beaumont and Hughes, 1979).

Central Nervous System. In man, morphine produces *analgesia, drowsiness, changes in mood,* and *mental clouding.* A significant feature of the analgesia is that it occurs without loss of consciousness. When therapeutic doses of morphine are given to patients with pain, they report that the pain is less intense, less discomforting, or entirely gone. Drowsiness occurs commonly both in volunteers and in patients with clinical pain. The extremities feel heavy and the body warm, the face (especially the nose) may itch, and the mouth becomes dry. In addition to relief of distress, some patients experience euphoria. If the external situation is favorable, sleep may ensue.

When morphine in the same dose is given to a presumably normal, pain-free individual, the experience is not always pleasant. Nausea is common, and vomiting may also occur. Feelings of drowsiness and inability to concentrate, difficulty in mentation, apathy, lessened physical activity, reduced visual acuity, and lethargy may ensue. In postaddict volunteers, mental clouding is less prominent than in normal subjects, and the euphoria is more pronounced.

As the dose is increased, subjective effects become more pronounced; there is increased drowsiness that leads to sleep; in individuals who experience euphoria, the euphoric effect is accentuated; patients with severe pain that is not adequately relieved by smaller doses of morphine are usually relieved by larger doses (15 to 20 mg). The incidence of nausea and vomiting is also increased, and respiratory depression, the major toxic effect of morphine-like drugs, may become pronounced; but even large doses are not anticonvulsant and do not cause slurred speech or significant motor incoordination.

Analgesia. The relief of pain by morphine and its surrogates is relatively selective, in that other sensory modalities (touch, vibration, vision, hearing, etc.) are not obtunded. Patients frequently report that the pain is still present but that they feel more comfortable (*see* below). Continuous dull pain is relieved more effectively than sharp intermittent pain, but with sufficient amounts of morphine it is possible to relieve even the severe pain associated with renal or biliary colic.

The selectivity of opioid-induced analgesia is greater than that of many other drugs that act on the CNS. Thus, the inhalation of nitrous oxide (20 to 40 volumes %), while producing analgesia that is approximately equivalent to 15 mg of morphine, also produces an overall impairment of consciousness, marked drowsiness, alterations in judgment, impairment of immediate and delayed memory, and nausea. Similarly, low concentrations of ether, high doses of barbiturates, or gross intoxication with alcohol produce significant analgesia, but only in association with sedation and impairment of motor coordination, intellectual acuity, emotional control, and judgment. For a given degree of analgesia, the mental clouding produced by therapeutic doses of morphine is considerably less pronounced and of a qualitatively different character; morphine and related drugs rarely produce the garrulous, silly, and emotionally labile behavior frequently seen during intoxication with alcohol or a barbiturate. The characteristics of the subjective effects produced by narcotic analgesics have been extensively studied in patients and nonaddict volunteers by Beecher, Keats, Lasagna, and their coworkers (*see* Beecher, 1959; Smith *et al.*, 1962), while the comparative effects of morphine, barbiturates, and other drugs in postaddicts have been studied at the Addiction Research Center, Lexington, Kentucky (*see* Wikler, 1958; Hill *et al.*, 1963).

Any meaningful discussion of the action of analgesic agents must include some distinction between *pain as a specific sensation,* subserved by distinct neurophysiological structures, and *pain as suffering* (the original sensation plus the reactions evoked by the sensation). There is general agreement that all types of painful experiences, whether produced with experimental technics or occurring clinically as a result of pathology, include both the *original sensation* and the *reaction to that sensation* (*see* Sternbach, 1978).

The effects of analgesics on both experimentally produced and pathological pain have been carefully studied in man. The latter type of pain cannot be terminated at will, and the meaning of the sensation and the distress it engenders are markedly affected by the individual's previous experiences and current expectations. In experimentally produced pain, measurements of the effects of morphine on *pain threshold* have not always been consistent; some workers find that analgesics reliably elevate the threshold (*see* Gracely *et al.*, 1979), while many others do not obtain consistent changes. By contrast, moderate doses of morphine are quite effective in relieving clinical pain and increasing the capacity to *tolerate* experimentally induced pain (*see* Smith *et al.*, 1968; Wolff *et al.*, 1969). Opioids obtund the response to painful stimuli at several loci in the brain. Not only is the sensation of pain altered by opioid analgesics, but the affective response is changed as well. This latter effect is best assessed by asking patients with clinical pain about the degree of relief produced by the drug administered. When pain does not evoke its usual responses (anxiety, fear, panic, and suffering), *a patient's ability to tolerate the pain may be markedly increased even when the capacity to perceive the sensation is relatively unaltered* (*see* Beecher, 1959; Sternbach, 1978).

Mechanisms and Sites of Opioid-Induced Analgesia. Opioid-induced analgesia is due to actions at several sites within the CNS and involves several systems of neurotransmitters. The opioids do not alter the threshold or responsivity of afferent nerve endings to noxious stimulation, nor do they impair the conduction of the nerve impulse along peripheral nerves. The presence of receptors for opioids in laminae I and II (substantia gelatinosa) of the spinal cord and in the spinal nucleus of the trigeminal nerve in the brain stem is consistent with the view that noxious stimuli can be altered and diminished at this first level of sensory integration. In patients with complete transection of the spinal cord, morphine depresses nociceptive withdrawal reflexes below the level of the lesion, an effect that also can be demonstrated in other species. The patellar reflexes are relatively unaffected (*see* Wikler, 1958; Domino, 1968; Kerr and Wilson, 1978).

It is postulated that the exogenous opioids or endogenous enkephalins alter the central release of neurotransmitters from afferent nerves sensitive to noxious stimuli. The activity elicited in lamina V of the spinal cord by noxious stimulation is suppressed by the microinjection of opioids into the substantia gelatinosa. The distribution of substance P in areas involved in the modulation of pain and the inhibition of its release by opioid drugs suggest that it might be an excitatory transmitter or neuromodulator of noxious afferent input.

Afferent nerves and the enkephalin-containing interneurons are also affected by the input from descending tracts from supraspinal structures and perhaps by circulating β-endorphin. In both animals and man, electrical stimulation of various parts of the brain, most reliably the periaqueductal gray, the dorsal raphe nuclei, and the periventricular gray, produces a profound and relatively selective analgesia. The analgesia outlasts the period of stimulation by periods varying from seconds to hours; it is largely reversible by naloxone. A similar pattern of analgesia can be produced by microinjection of opioids or opioid-like peptides into the same regions. Cross-tolerance develops between analgesia produced by electrical stimulation of the brain and microinjection of opioids into the brain (or to systemically administered opioids).

Analgesia produced by stimulation of the periaqueductal gray appears to involve the release of endogenous peptides, which, in turn, influences other ascending and descending fiber tracts involved in the modulation of pain impulses and in the subjective response to pain. Microinjection of opioids also activates these fiber tracts. The descending tracts exert an inhibitory influence on spinal interneurons that modulate the effects of incoming noxious sensory stimuli. It is likely that a major descending inhibitory tract consists of tryptaminergic neurons, since procedures that deplete 5-hydroxytryptamine (5-HT) or that interrupt tryptaminergic pathways abolish analgesia produced by stimulation of the periaqueductal gray and dorsal raphe nuclei. Stimulation of the periaqueductal gray also increases turnover of 5-HT in higher levels of the brain, suggesting that some ascending tracts may also be tryptaminergic (*see* Akil *et al.*, 1978; Cannon *et al.*, 1978; Beaumont and Hughes, 1979).

There are other sites, such as the hypothalamus, where stimulation produces analgesia and where tryptaminergic fibers do not seem to be involved to the same degree. Stimulation of the periaqueductal gray may also result in antidromic stimulation of β-endorphin-containing nerve fibers located in the hypothalamus, and the analgesia that outlasts the stimulation may be due to release of β-endorphin (Hosobuchi *et al.*, 1979). Most of the sites where stimulation produces analgesia appear to be parts of extralemniscal pathways linked to limbic structures and seem to be related to the affective component of the responses to noxious stimuli (Van Ree, 1977).

Analgesia can also be induced by electrical or mechanical stimulation of peripheral nerves at specific points (acupuncture). Since this analgesia can be antagonized by naloxone, it probably involves endogenous opioid-like peptides (Pomeranz and Chiu, 1976). Similar evidence suggests that the analgesic response to a placebo also involves the release of endogenous peptides, but that the analgesia induced by hypnosis does not.

Mechanism of Other CNS Effects. High doses of opioids can produce *muscular rigidity* in man, and both opioids and endogenous peptides cause catelepsy, circling, and stereotypical behavior in rats and other animals. These effects are probably related to actions at opioid receptors in the substantia nigra and striatum, and involve interactions with both dopaminergic and GABAergic neurons (Moroni *et al.*, 1979). Chronic administration of dopaminergic antagonists (*e.g.*, haloperidol, pimozide) or lithium increases the concentration of met-enkephalin in the striatum (*see* Beaumont and Hughes, 1979).

The mechanisms by which opioids produce *tranquility, euphoria,* and other alterations of mood remain unsettled. The *locus ceruleus* contains both noradrenergic neurons and high concentrations of opioid receptors and is postulated to play a critical role in feelings of alarm, panic, fear, and anxiety. Activity in locus ceruleus is inhibited by α-adrenergic agonists and by both exogenous opioids and endogenous opioid-like peptides (Korf *et al.,* 1974; Svensson *et al.,* 1975; Young *et al.,* 1977). The role of the locus ceruleus in opioid withdrawal is discussed in Chapter 23.

Effects on the Hypothalamus. Morphine decreases the response of the hypothalamus to afferent stimulation, but does not significantly alter its response to direct electrical stimulation. In many species, opioids alter the equilibrium point of the hypothalamic heat-regulatory mechanisms so that an animal will maintain a lower body temperature. Thus, in the dog, morphine initiates a period of panting that gradually subsides as the temperature decreases; the panting reappears if attempts are made to raise body temperature to the pre-morphine level. In man, body temperature falls slightly after single therapeutic doses of morphine, although it appears to be increased by chronic high dosage. In the cat and other animals in which morphine causes excitement and mania, body temperature is increased.

Effects on Pituitary Hormones. In animals, opioids stimulate the release of ACTH, an effect that is blocked by naloxone and to which tolerance develops. In patients who are undergoing surgery, however, opioids inhibit the stress-induced release of ACTH. During chronic administration of morphine or methadone, concentrations of cortisol in plasma are within the normal range, but they rise sharply after the drug is withdrawn.

In man, opioids and opioid-like peptides suppress the secretion of luteinizing hormone (LH) and thyrotropin, and enhance the release of prolactin and, in some cases, growth hormone. The suppression of the secretion of LH leads to a substantial decrease in the concentration of testosterone in plasma; only partial tolerance develops to this effect. Depending on the dose and the degree of tolerance, males maintained on methadone exhibit decreased sexual drive, as well as decreased motility of sperm and volume of ejaculate.

The endogenous opioid-like peptides may play a role in the normal regulation of the secretion of several pituitary hormones, since the administration of naloxone increases concentrations of LH and follicle-stimulating hormone (FSH) in plasma and depresses those of prolactin and growth hormone (Bruni *et al.,* 1977). The mechanisms involved are unclear, but a likely possibility is an alteration of the release of neurotransmitters (*e.g.,* dopamine) that ordinarily regulate the secretion of pituitary hormone releasing factors and release-inhibiting factors (*see* Chapter 59; Fishman, 1978; Beaumont and Hughes, 1979). Morphine and other opioids have been regarded as stimulators of the release of antidiuretic hormone; however, the oliguria that follows the administration of opioids may represent a direct renal or a hemodynamic effect.

EEG. In man, single therapeutic doses of opioids produce a shift toward increased voltage and lower frequencies in the EEG, such as occurs in natural sleep or after very low doses of barbiturates. In postaddicts, single doses of morphine suppress the rapid-eye-movement (REM) or "paradoxical sleep" phase of the EEG; slow-wave sleep is also reduced, while light sleep and waking time are increased. With repeated administration, some tolerance develops to these effects; whether they are also seen with other opioids such as methadone is not clear (*see* Martin and Kay, 1977).

Pupil. Morphine and many of its surrogates cause constriction of the pupil in man. Miosis is due to an excitatory action on the autonomic segment of the nucleus of the oculomotor nerve in the dog (Lee and Wang, 1975), and the same mechanism may be presumed in man. Following toxic doses of opioids, *the miosis is marked and pinpoint pupils are pathognomonic;* however, marked mydriasis occurs when asphyxia intervenes. Tolerance to the miotic effect of morphine is not prominent, and the morphine or heroin addict continues to have constricted pupils.

The pupillary effects of morphine vary with the species. Cats (excited by morphine) and monkeys (sedated by morphine) show mydriasis. Therapeutic doses of morphine increase accommodative power and lower intraocular tension in both normal and glaucomatous eyes.

Excitatory Effects. Extremely high doses of morphine and its surrogates produce convulsions. The mechanism is unclear, and different opioids may produce different patterns of seizures. Supraspinal structures are more sensitive to the convulsant effect than is the spinal cord, since convulsant doses produce seizures above the level of a cord transection but not below it. With most opioids, convulsant effects are seen only at dose levels far in excess of those required to produce profound analgesia. However, with some agents convulsant effects may occur at doses only moderately higher than those required for analgesia. The convulsant effect of opioids can be reversed by naloxone, but the dose required varies considerably among the various agents. In some instances, metabolites may have more convulsant activity than the parent drug, as is the case with meperidine. The seizures may not involve the same receptors that are responsible for opioid-induced analgesia. When seizures are induced by the microinjection of opioids, they are elicited more reproducibly in areas of the brain that are not involved in the production of analgesia (Gilbert and Martin, 1975; Frenk *et al.,* 1978).

In some species, relatively low doses of morphine produce gross excitation and hyperthermia. In the cat, for example suitable doses produce not only analgesia but also a state in which the animal is continually restless, seems frightened, and cowers and scrambles to avoid being handled. Larger doses lead to seizures and death. These effects can be antagonized by naloxone and prevented by phenytoin, and do not occur after lesions in the caudal hypothalamus. Following high doses of opioids, mice show increased locomotor activity. Animals stimulated rather than sedated by morphine include pigs, cows, sheep, goats, lions, tigers, bears, and horses.

Respiration. Morphine is a primary and continuous depressant of respiration, at least in part by virtue of a direct effect on the brain stem respiratory centers. The respiratory depression is discernible even with doses too small to disturb consciousness, and increases progressively as the dose is increased. In man, death from morphine poisoning is nearly always due to respiratory arrest. Therapeutic doses of morphine in man depress all phases of respiratory activity (rate, minute volume, and tidal exchange). The diminished respiratory volume is due primarily to a slower rate of breathing, and with toxic amounts the rate may fall to 3 or 4 per minute. Morphine and related opioids may also produce irregular and periodic breathing; in man, this is often seen even after therapeutic doses.

Maximal respiratory depression occurs within approximately 7 minutes after intravenous administration of morphine, but may not be seen for as long as 30 minutes after intramuscular administration or as long as 90 minutes following subcutaneous administration. The sensitivity of the respiratory center begins to return toward normal within 2 to 3 hours; however, respiratory minute volume is still considerably below normal for as long as 4 to 5 hours following therapeutic doses.

The *mechanism* of respiratory depression by morphine involves a reduction in the responsiveness of the brain stem respiratory centers to increases in carbon dioxide tension (P_{CO_2}). Opioids also depress the pontine and medullary centers involved in regulating respiratory rhythmicity and the responsiveness of medullary respiratory centers to electrical stimulation (*see* Pentiah *et al.,* 1966; Flórez *et al.,* 1968).

The influence of various afferent stimuli on the respiratory center is not affected to the same degree. Hypoxic stimulation of the chemoreceptors may still be effective when the respiratory center shows decreased responsiveness to CO_2. When the main stimulus to respiration is hypoxia, the inhalation of high tensions of O_2 may produce apnea. In addition to a marked depression of the automatic regulation of respiration, voluntary control of respiration may also be altered. After large doses of morphine or synthetic analogs, patients will breathe if instructed to do so, but without such instruction they may remain relatively apneic.

Within minutes after an intravenous therapeutic dose of morphine, there is a decrease in minute volume, followed by an increase in CO_2 in the blood and alveolar gas. As CO_2 accumulates, it again drives the respiratory center to a degree dictated by the opioid. Thus, respiratory rate and sometimes even minute volume can be unreliable indicators of the degree of respiratory depression. Natural sleep also produces a decrease in the sensitivity of the medullary center to CO_2, and the effects of morphine and sleep are additive.

Effects of Other Opioids. In equianalgesic doses, respiration in man is depressed by parenteral codeine and morphine to about the same degree (120 mg of codeine, 10 mg of morphine), but death as a result of codeine overdosage is rare. Numerous studies have compared morphine with other opioids with respect to their ratios of analgesic to respiratory depressant activities. It is clear that all the opioids are capable of producing respiratory depression, and most studies have found that, when equianalgesic doses are used, the degree of respiratory depression observed is not significantly different from that seen with morphine (*see* Eckenhoff and Oech, 1960).

Morphine and related opioids also depress the *cough reflex,* at least in part by a direct effect on a cough center in the medulla (Chakravarty *et al.,* 1956). There is, however, no obligatory relationship between depression of respiration and depression of coughing, and effective antitussive agents are available that do not depress respiration (*see* below).

Nauseant and Emetic Effects. Nausea and vomiting produced by morphine and its derivatives are unpleasant side effects caused by direct stimulation of the chemoreceptor trigger zone (CTZ) for emesis, in the area postrema of the medulla. Apomorphine, a dopaminergic agonist, also causes vomiting by stimulation of the CTZ. The emetic effect of morphine is counteracted by some phenothiazine derivatives, particularly those with a potent dopamine-blocking action (*see* Chapter 19). Certain individuals never vomit after morphine, whereas others do so each time the drug is administered.

Nausea and vomiting are relatively uncommon in recumbent patients given therapeutic doses of morphine, but nausea occurs in approximately 40% and vomiting in 15% of ambulatory patients given 15 mg of the drug subcutaneously. This suggests that a vestibular component is also operative. Indeed, it has been shown that the nauseant and emetic effects of morphine in man are markedly enhanced by vestibular stimulation, and that morphine and related synthetic analgesics produce an increase in vestibular sensitivity (Gutner *et al.,* 1952). Drugs that are useful in motion sickness are sometimes helpful in reducing opioid-induced nausea in ambulatory patients.

After a therapeutic dose of morphine, subsequent doses are unlikely to produce vomiting; other emetics are also ineffective after morphine. All clinically useful opioids produce some degree of nausea and vomiting. Careful, controlled clinical studies usually demonstrate that in equianalgesic dosage the incidence of such side effects is not significantly lower than that seen with morphine. Although the opioid antagonists do not prevent or relieve emesis induced by apomorphine, patients treated therapeutically with such antagonists (*see* Chapter 23) rarely vomit, even after huge doses of morphine or heroin.

Cardiovascular System. In the supine patient, therapeutic doses of morphine or synthetic opioids have no major effect on blood pressure or cardiac rate and rhythm. Despite obvious respiratory depression from doses that cause toxicity, the blood pressure is usually maintained until relatively late in the course of intoxication, and falls largely as a result of hypoxia. Thus, artificial respiration or administration of oxygen may cause the blood pressure to rise despite the persisting medullary depression. Morphine and related opioid agonists dilate resistance and capacitance vessels and thereby decrease the capacity of the cardiovascular system to respond to gravitational shifts; therefore, when supine patients assume the head-up position, orthostatic hypotension and fainting may occur. The *peripheral arteriolar and venous dilatation* produced by morphine involves several mechanisms. Morphine and most opioids provoke the release of *histamine,* which sometimes plays a large role in the hypotension; vasodilatation is usually only partially blocked by histamine-receptor (H_1) blocking agents (*see* Eckenhoff and Oech, 1960). Morphine also induces arteriolar dilatation by a central suppression of adrenergic tone and blunts the reflex vasoconstriction caused by increased P_{CO_2} (Zelis *et al.,* 1977).

Effects on the myocardium are not significant in normal man; the cardiac rate is either unaffected or slightly increased, and there is no consistent effect on cardiac output. The ECG is not altered. In patients with coronary artery disease but no acute medical problems, 8 mg of morphine intravenously produces a decrease in oxygen consumption, left ventricular end-diastolic pressure, and cardiac work; effects on cardiac index are inconsistent (Alderman *et al.,* 1972; Popio *et al.,* 1978). In patients with acute myocardial infarction, the cardiovascular responses to morphine are generally similar (Lee *et al.,* 1976); they may, however, be more variable than in normal subjects, and the magnitude of changes (*e.g.,* the decrease in blood pressure) may be more pronounced (Thomas *et al.,* 1965).

Very large doses of morphine can be used to provide anesthesia, particularly during cardiac surgery (*see* Chapter 14). The depressant effects of most anesthetics on cardiac performance are thus avoided.

Morphine and related agents should be used with caution in patients who have a decreased blood volume since they are prone to develop hypotension. Morphine should be used with great care in patients with cor pulmonale, since deaths following ordinary therapeutic doses have been reported. The concurrent use of certain phenothiazines may increase the risk of morphine-induced hypotension.

Cerebral circulation is not directly affected by therapeutic doses of morphine. However, respiratory depression and CO_2 retention result in cerebral vasodilatation and an increase in cerebrospinal fluid pressure; the pressure increase does not occur when P_{CO_2} is maintained at normal levels by artificial ventilation.

Gastrointestinal Tract. The use of opium for relief of diarrhea and dysentery preceded by many centuries its employment for analgesia. The observed effects of morphine and related drugs on the bowel may vary widely, depending on the species, the dose, and the experimental technics. Therefore, the present discussion will concentrate on the effects observed in man.

Stomach. Morphine and related drugs cause some decrease in the secretion of hydrochloric acid; this can be overcome by chemical or psychic stimulation. A more pronounced effect is the decrease in motility associated with an increase in the tone of the antral portion of the stomach. There is also an increase in the tone of the first part of the duodenum, which often makes therapeutic intubation exceedingly difficult, delays the passage of the gastric contents through the duodenum for as much as 12 hours, and retards the absorption of drugs that are administered orally. This delay accounts for about one half of the total gastrointestinal delay, which is the basis of constipation produced by morphine.

Small Intestine. Both biliary and pancreatic secretions are diminished by morphine, and digestion of food in the small intestine is delayed. There is an increase in resting tone, and periodic spasms are observed. The amplitude of the nonpropulsive type of rhythmic, segmental contractions is usually enhanced, but *propulsive contractions are markedly decreased.* The upper part of the small intestine, particularly the duodenum, is affected more than the ileum. A period of relative atony may follow the hypertonicity. Water is more completely absorbed from the chyme because of the delayed passage of the bowel contents, and the viscosity of the chyme is thereby increased. The tone of the ileocecal valve is enhanced. Large doses of atropine may counteract, in part, the gastrointestinal responses to morphine, but resection of the extrinsic nerves and ganglionic blocking agents do not do so. The actions of morphine on the small intestine are thought to cause about one fourth of the total constipating effect of the alkaloid. (*See* Chapman *et al.,* 1950; Vaughan Williams and Streeten, 1950; Daniel *et al.,* 1959.)

Large Intestine. Propulsive peristaltic waves in the colon are diminished or abolished after morphine, and tone is increased to the point of spasm. The resulting delay in the passage of the contents causes considerable desiccation of the feces, which, in turn, retards its advance through the colon. The amplitude of the nonpropulsive type of rhythmic contractions of the colon is usually enhanced. The tone of the anal sphincter is greatly augmented, and this, combined with inattention to the normal sensory stimuli for the defecation reflex due to the central actions of the drug, further contributes to morphine-induced constipation. The actions of morphine on the large intestine combine to contribute about one fourth of the entire constipating effect.

Atropine partially antagonizes the spasmogenic action on the human colon, but it has little effect on the decreased propulsive activity produced by morphine.

Whereas the intestinal responses to opium and morphine are unpleasant side effects when the drugs are given for analgesia, they can be desirable therapeutic objectives in themselves, especially in patients with exhausting diarrhea or dysentery. In patients with chronic ulcerative colitis, opioids may stimulate colonic motility, and the use of opioids during acute episodes of the disease sometimes leads to a toxic dilatation of the colon (Garrett *et al.,* 1967). Codeine and all the morphine surrogates produce qualitatively similar effects on the motility of the bowel. There are, however, quantitative differences, and not all opioid analgesics are useful in the treatment of diarrheas.

Mechanism of Action on the Bowel. Neither the administration of ganglionic blocking agents nor the removal of the extrinsic innervation of the bowel prevents the characteristic actions of morphine and its surrogates in the unanesthetized animal. Morphine has many effects on the myenteric plexus of the intestine, including actions on cholinergic, tryptaminergic, and enkephalinergic receptors (*see* Burks, 1976). However, its constipating and antidiarrheal actions may not be due entirely to local actions on the intestine. Injection of minute quantities of morphine into the cerebral ventricles inhibits gastrointestinal propulsive activity, an effect abolished by intraventricular administration of opioid antagonists (Parolaro *et al.,* 1977) or by vagotomy (Stewart *et al.,* 1978). Although some tolerance develops to the effects of opioids on gastrointestinal motility, patients who take opioids chronically remain constipated.

Biliary Tract. Therapeutic doses of morphine, codeine, and other morphine surrogates can cause a marked increase in pressure in the biliary tract. For example, after the subcutaneous injection of 10 mg of morphine sulfate the pressure in the common bile duct rises from the normal of less than 20 mm of water to a level of 200 to 300 mm. The response begins within 5 minutes after injection, reaches its peak in 15 minutes, and persists for 2 hours or more. Symptoms often accompany the increased pressure and vary from epigastric distress to typical biliary colic.

Some patients with biliary colic may experience exacerbation and not relief of pain when given these drugs. Furthermore, an occasional individual complains of pain in the epigastrium or right hypochondrium after morphine, probably due to duodenal or biliary tract spasm. Spasm of the biliary tract produced by morphine is evident roentgenographically as well as manometrically, and a sharp constriction becomes apparent at the lower end of the common bile duct (sphincter of Oddi). This spasm prevents emptying and thus causes the intraductal pressure to rise, and is probably responsible for the elevations of plasma amylase and lipase that are sometimes found after patients have been given morphine. Such elevations may persist for 24 hours after therapeutic doses and may confuse the diagnosis of intra-abdominal pathology, especially when acute pancreatitis is one of the diseases under consideration. Biliary spasm is not, however, a consistent effect of therapeutic doses of morphine, and some patients show no changes in bile duct size or pressure. Atropine only partially prevents morphine-induced biliary spasm, but opioid antagonists prevent or relieve it. Nitroglycerin (0.6 mg) administered sublingually also decreases the elevated intrabiliary pressure. Some analgesics such as meperidine, phenoperidine, and pentazocine seem to produce less pronounced increases in biliary pressure (Economou and Ward-McQuaid, 1971).

Other Smooth Muscle. *Ureter and Urinary Bladder.* Therapeutic doses of morphine increase the tone and amplitude of contractions of the *ureter,* especially of the lower third. The response of the ureters in man to opioids is quite variable. When the antidiuretic effects of the drugs are prominent and urine flow decreases, the ureter may become quiescent.

The tone of the detrusor muscle of the *urinary bladder* is augmented by morphine; this sometimes causes urinary urgency. The tone of the vesical sphincter is also enhanced by morphine; this effect may make urination difficult, and catheterization is sometimes required following therapeutic doses of morphine. In addition, the central effects of these drugs may make the patient inattentive to the stimuli arising in the bladder and may play a role in morphine-induced urinary retention.

Uterus. Studies of the effects of therapeutic doses of morphine in women suggest that labor may be somewhat prolonged (*see* Campbell *et al.,* 1961). The mechanism involved is not clear; however, it has been noted that, if the uterus is made hyperactive by oxytocics, morphine tends to restore tone, frequency, and amplitude of contractions to normal. In addition, the central effects of morphine may affect the degree to which the parturient is able to cooperate in the delivery. Neonatal mortality may thus be increased by the injudicious use of opioids during labor as a result of these factors and the high sensitivity of the neonate to the respiratory depressant effect of these drugs.

Bronchial Musculature. Although large doses of morphine and meperidine produce constriction of the bronchi, this effect is rarely seen after therapeutic doses in man. The possible role of morphine-induced bronchoconstriction in the aggravation of asthma is discussed below.

Skin. In man, therapeutic doses of morphine cause cutaneous blood vessels to dilate. The skin of the face, neck, and upper thorax frequently becomes flushed and warm. These changes in cutaneous circulation may, in part, be due to the release of histamine and may be responsible for the *pruritus* and the *sweating* that commonly follow the administration of morphine. Histamine release probably accounts for the urticaria commonly seen at the site of injection.

Tolerance, Physical Dependence, and Liability for Abuse. The development of tolerance and physical dependence with repeated use is a characteristic feature of all the opioid drugs, and the possibility of developing psychological dependence on the effects of these drugs is one of the major limitations of their clinical use. It is important to emphasize that the overall liability for abuse of an agent is not established by any one single factor; rather, it is a composite based on a number of factors. These include: (1) the capacity of the drug to produce the kind of physical dependence in which drug withdrawal causes sufficient distress to bring about drug-seeking behavior; (2) its ability to suppress withdrawal symptoms caused by withdrawal of other agents; (3) the degree to which it induces euphoria similar to that produced by morphine and other opioids; (4) the patterns of toxicity that occur when the dose is increased beyond the usual therapeutic range; and (5) physical characteristics of the drug, such as water solubility, that may determine whether it is likely to be abused by the parenteral route. There is evidence to suggest that the overall abuse liability of some of the analgesics related to the opioid antagonists is lower than that of morphine. The implications of the differences in abuse potential for the choice of agents in therapy are discussed below, and the subject of compulsive drug use is elaborated in detail in Chapter 23.

Absorption, Distribution, Fate, and Excretion. *Absorption.* The opioids are readily absorbed from the gastrointestinal tract; they are also absorbed from the nasal mucosa and the lung (as when heroin is used as snuff or opium is smoked), and after subcutaneous or intramuscular injection. With most opioids, including morphine, the effect of a given dose is less after oral than after parenteral administration, due to significant first-pass metabolism in the liver. The shape of the time-effect curve also varies with the route of administration, so that the duration of action is often somewhat longer with the oral route. Such differences in time-effect curves are illustrated in Figure 22-1.

When morphine and most of its congeners are given intravenously, they act promptly. However, the more lipid-soluble compounds have a somewhat more rapid onset of action after subcutaneous administration due to differences in the rate of absorption. The durations of action show relatively little variation (*see* Table 22-2).

Distribution and Fate. When therapeutic concentrations of morphine are present in plasma, about one third of the drug is protein bound. Free morphine rapidly leaves the blood and accumulates in parenchymatous tissues, such as the kidney, lung, liver, and spleen. Skeletal muscle has a somewhat lower level of morphine, but because of its mass it accounts for the major fraction of the drug in the body. Morphine does not persist in tissues, and 24 hours after the last dose tissue concentrations are quite low.

Although the primary site of action of morphine is in the CNS, in the adult only small quantities pass the blood-brain barrier. Compared to other opioids such as codeine, heroin, and methadone, morphine crosses the blood-brain barrier at a considerably lower rate (*see* Oldendorf *et al.,* 1972). Transport of opioids by the choroid plexus has been noted, but its significance remains uncertain.

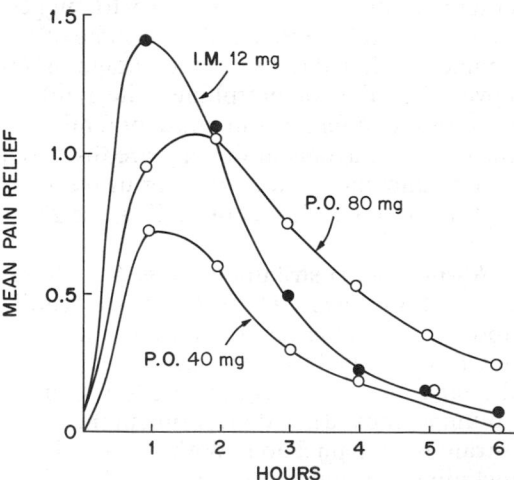

Figure 22-1. *Time-effect curves for oral* (P.O.) *and intramuscular* (I.M.) *morphine.*

Changes in pain relief in cancer patients are shown on an arbitrary scale after drug administration. (After Houde, Wallenstein, and Beaver, 1965. Courtesy of Academic Press, Inc.)

The major pathway for the detoxication of morphine is conjugation with glucuronic acid, and after the intravenous administration of morphine the concentrations of free morphine in tissues decline progressively while those of conjugated morphine (morphine-3-monoglucuronide) increase and then decline more slowly. In young adults, the half-life of morphine in plasma is about 2.5 to 3 hours (Brunk and Delle, 1974; Stanski *et al.,* 1978). This value may be longer in older patients. For many opioids, N-demethylation occurs in several mammalian species including man, but in the case of morphine it does not appear to be a major pathway in man.

Excretion. Small amounts of free morphine and larger amounts of conjugated morphine are found in the urine, and these account for most of the administered drug. Although traces of morphine are detectable in the urine for well over 48 hours, 90% of the total excretion takes place during the first day. The major route of elimination of the metabolites is by glomerular filtration. About 7 to 10% of administered morphine eventually appears in the feces, and this comes almost exclusively from the bile as conjugated morphine. Enterohepatic circulation of morphine and morphine glucuronide occurs, which probably accounts for the presence of small amounts of morphine in the urine for several days after the last dose.

Codeine, in contrast to morphine, is approximately two thirds as effective orally as parenterally, both as an analgesic and as a respiratory depressant. Very few opioids have so high an oral-parenteral potency ratio; also in this group is oxycodone. Their greater oral efficacy is due to less first-pass metabolism in the liver, presumably due to the presence of a methoxy group in position 3, the principal site of metabolism of morphine. Once absorbed, codeine is metabolized by the liver and excreted chiefly in the urine, largely in inactive forms. A small fraction (approximately 10%) of administered codeine is demethylated to form morphine, and both free and conjugated morphine can be found in the urine after therapeutic doses of codeine. Codeine has an exceptionally low affinity for the opioid receptor, and the analgesic effect of codeine may be due to its conversion to morphine. The half-life of codeine in plasma is 2.5 to 3 hours (Findlay *et al.,* 1978).

Heroin (diacetylmorphine) is rapidly hydrolyzed to monoacetylmorphine (MAM), which, in turn, is hydrolyzed to morphine. In the adult, the blood-brain barrier tends to impede entry of morphine into the brain; the barrier is considerably less effective

Table 22-2. A COMPARISON OF OPIOID ANALGESICS WITH RESPECT TO DOSAGE, DURATION OF ACTION, WITHDRAWAL SYMPTOMS, AND DISTINGUISHING FEATURES

NONPROPRIETARY NAME	TRADE NAME	DOSE * (mg)	DURATION OF ACTION * (hours)	WITHDRAWAL SYMPTOMS	DISTIN-GUISHING FEATURES ▲
Morphine		10	4–5	*see* text	*see* text
Heroin (diacetyl-morphine)		3 (2–8)	3–4	like morphine	2
Hydromorphone (dihydromorphinone)	DILAUDID	1.5	4–5	like morphine	
Oxymorphone (dihydro-hydroxymorphinone)	NUMORPHAN	1.0–1.5	4–5	like morphine	
Metopon (methyldihydro-morphinone)		3.5	4–5	like morphine	3
Codeine		120 (10–30)	(4–6)	*see* text	*see* text
Hydrocodone (dihydro-codeinone)	HYCODAN †	(5–10)	(4–8)	between morphine and codeine	4,7
Dihydrocodeine	PARACODIN †	60	4–5	between morphine and codeine	
Oxycodone (dihydro-hydroxycodeinone)	PERCODAN †	10–15 (3–5)	4–5 (4–5)	close to morphine	7
Pholcodine (β-morph-olinylethylmorphine)	ETHNINE, PHOLDINE	(10–15)	(4–5)	much less than codeine	3,4,5
Levorphanol	LEVO-DROMORAN	2–3	4–5	like morphine	7
Methadone	DOLOPHINE, etc.	7.5–10	3–5	*see* text	6,8
Dextromoramide	PALFIUM	5–7.5	4–5	like methadone	3,6,8
Dipipanone	PIPADONE	20–25	4–5	like methadone	3,6,8,9
Phenadoxone	HEPTALGIN, etc.	10–20	1–3	less than mor-phine	3,9
Meperidine	DEMEROL, etc.	80–100	2–4	*see* text	1,7
Alphaprodine	NISENTIL	25–35	1–2	like meperidine	1,7
Anileridine	LERITINE	25–30	2–4	like meperidine	1,7

* *Dose* shown is the amount given *subcutaneously* that produces approximately the same analgesic effects as 10 mg of morphine administered subcutaneously. The figures in *parentheses* are the *doses* and the *duration* of action for *oral, antitussive* doses; they are not necessarily equieffective doses. *Duration of action* shown is for *subcutaneous* administration; after *intravenous* administration, peak effects are somewhat more pronounced but overall effects are of shorter duration. The doses and durations shown in this table are based primarily on papers reviewed by Eddy and coworkers (1957), Reynolds and Randall (1957), Murphree (1962), and Lasagna (1964), and are augmented by more recent studies of newer drugs.

▲ 1 = causes little or no constipation; 2 = manufacture or importation into the United States illegal; 3 = not available in the United States; 4 = by tradition used mainly as an antitussive; 5 = little or no analgesic or euphorigenic activity; 6 = may exhibit cumulative effects on repeated dosage; 7 = retains fair degree of efficacy when given orally; 8 = retains most of its analgesic efficacy when given orally; 9 = marked irritation at injection sites.

† These opioids are marketed in the United States only in combination with additional ingredients.

against heroin and MAM since both are more lipid soluble than morphine. Most of the current evidence suggests that morphine and MAM are responsible for the pharmacological actions of heroin. Heroin is mainly excreted in the urine largely as free and conjugated morphine.

The absorption, fate, and distribution of morphine-like drugs have been reviewed by Way and Adler (1960, 1962), Way, (1968), and Misra (1978).

Idiosyncrasy, Variations in Response, and Precautions. Morphine and related opioids produce a wide spectrum of unwanted effects, such as nausea, vomiting, dizziness, mental clouding, dysphoria, constipation, and increased pressure in the biliary tract. These occur so commonly that they cannot

be considered idiosyncratic, even though there are many patients who do not experience such effects. Rarely, a patient may develop a delirium. *Increased sensitivity* to pain after the analgesia has worn off may also occur.

Allergic phenomena occur with opioid analgesics, but they are not common. They are usually manifested as urticaria and other types of skin rashes; contact dermatitis in nurses and pharmaceutical workers has been reported. Wheals at the site of injection of morphine, codeine, and related drugs are probably caused by the release of histamine. Anaphylactoid reactions have been reported after intravenous codeine and morphine, but such reactions are quite rare; however, it has been suggested, but not proven, that they are responsible for some of the sudden deaths, episodes of pulmonary edema, and other complications that occur among addicts who use heroin intravenously (Challenor *et al.,* 1973).

A number of factors may alter the sensitivity to opiate analgesics, including the integrity of the blood-brain barrier. For example, when morphine is administered to the mother prior to delivery, the newborn infant may exhibit respiratory depression even though the drug produced no significant depression in the mother (*see* Way *et al.,* 1965). Since the blood-brain barrier does not play as prominent a role in limiting the access of all opioids to the CNS, some, such as meperidine, produce relatively less respiratory depression in the newborn. After the neonatal period, there is little change in analgesic response to opioids until late in life. In patients over 60 years old there seems to be both a decrease in sensitivity to pain and an increased analgesic response to opioids (Bellville *et al.,* 1971).

The patient with severe pain may tolerate larger doses of morphine (three to four therapeutic doses over a period of a few hours) but may exhibit subjective and respiratory depression should the pain suddenly subside. *Illnesses* of various types may increase or decrease the sensitivity to morphine and related drugs. Patients with *myxedema* and *multiple sclerosis* are more sensitive to the depressant effects, whereas *hyperthyroid* patients seem more tolerant; controlled studies, however, are lacking. All the opioid analgesics are metabolized by the liver, and the drugs should be used with caution in patients with hepatic disease, since cumulative effects may occur. Because the metabolic pathways for some synthetic opioids are different from those for morphine, it is possible that some might be safer than others in such patients (*see* Way and Adler, 1962; Misra, 1978).

Patients with *reduced blood volume* are considerably more susceptible to the hypotensive effects of morphine and related drugs, and these agents must be employed cautiously in patients with any type of hemorrhage. The respiratory depressant effects of morphine and the related capacity to elevate intracranial pressure may be markedly exaggerated in the presence of head injury or of an already elevated cerebrospinal fluid pressure produced by trauma. Therefore, while *head injury per se* does not constitute an absolute contraindication to the use of opioids, the possibility of exaggerated depression of respiration must be considered. Furthermore, since opioids produce mental clouding and side effects such as miosis and vomiting, which are important signs in following the clinical course of patients with head injuries, the advisability of their use must be carefully weighed. In patients with *prostatic hypertrophy,* morphine may precipitate acute urinary retention, requiring repeated catheterization.

Morphine and related opioids must be used with great caution in any situation in which there is decreased respiratory reserve, such as *emphysema, kyphoscoliosis,* or even severe *obesity.* In patients with chronic *cor pulmonale,* death has occurred following therapeutic doses of morphine. Although many patients with such conditions seem to be functioning within normal limits, they are already utilizing compensatory mechanisms, such as increased respiratory rate. Many have chronically elevated levels of plasma CO_2, and may be less sensitive to the stimulating actions of CO_2. The further imposition of the depressant effects of opioids can be disastrous.

Opioids can precipitate attacks of *asthma* in anesthetized patients, but the risk does not seem to be high. There is general agreement, however, that during an asthmatic attack morphine and related drugs should be avoided. All opioid analgesics depress the respiratory center, release histamine, depress the cough reflex, and tend to dry secretions. Giving such agents to asthmatic patients, in whom the airway resistance may be many times greater than normal, invites disaster by producing a decrease in respiratory drive without a corresponding decrease in airway resistance.

Interactions with Other Drugs. The depressant effects of some opioids may be exaggerated and prolonged by phenothiazines, monoamine oxidase inhibitors, and tricyclic antidepressants; the mechanisms of these supra-additive effects are not fully understood, but may involve alterations in the rate of metabolic transformation of the opioid or alterations in neurotransmitters involved in the actions of opioids. Some, but not all, phenothiazines reduce the amount of narcotic required to produce a given level of analgesia. However, the respiratory depressant effects seem also to be enhanced, the degree of sedation is increased, and the hypotensive effects of phenothiazines become an additional complication. *Some phenothiazine derivatives enhance the sedative effects, but at the same time seem to be antianalgesic* and increase the amount of opioid required to produce satisfactory relief from pain (Moore and Dundee, 1961). Small doses of amphetamine increase the effects of morphine substantially (Forrest *et al.,* 1977), as does the antihistamine hydroxyzine, when given intramuscularly (Beaver and Feise, 1976).

Preparations, Routes of Administration, and Dosage of Opium and Its Alkaloids. *Powdered Opium,* U.S.P., is a light-brown powder. The official morphine content of opium is 10.0 to 10.5% by weight. Thus, a dose of 60 mg taken orally is equivalent to 6 mg of morphine. PANTOPON is the proprietary name of a commonly used preparation of purified opium alkaloids. It is available as an injection. *Opium Tincture,* U.S.P. (*laudanum, deodorized opium tincture*), is a hydroalcoholic solution containing 10% of opium (1.0% of morphine). The average adult dose is 0.6 to 1.5 ml (equivalent to 6 to 15 mg of morphine), taken orally. *Opium (gum opium)* is still official in the U.S.P.; the dose is the same as for the powder. These preparations are infrequently employed. *Paregoric,* U.S.P. (*camphorated opium tincture*), is a hydroalcoholic preparation in which there is also benzoic acid, camphor, and anise oil. The usual adult dose is 5 to 10 ml, which corresponds to 2 to 4 mg of morphine. Paregoric represents a needlessly complex therapeutic survival of a former day.

Morphine. Morphine is available as the alkaloidal base, but it is prescribed only in the form of its water-soluble salts. The two most common salts are *Morphine Sulfate,* U.S.P., and *morphine hydrochloride.* The salts are bitter, white powders that are quite soluble in water and exhibit characteristic alkaloidal incompatibilities. Solutions of morphine salts are not irritating on injection. *Morphine Sulfate Injection,* U.S.P., is a sterile aqueous solution for parenteral use, and usually contains 8, 10, or 15 mg in 1 ml.

Hypodermically, 10 mg/70 kg of body weight is generally considered to be an optimal initial dose of morphine and provides satisfactory analgesia in approximately 70% of patients with moderate-to-severe pain (*e.g.,* postoperative pain) with only a moderate incidence of side effects. Subsequent doses may be higher or lower, depending on the analgesic response and the side effects produced. The average *oral* adult dose of morphine is often stated as 8 to 20 mg. However, controlled studies have shown that oral administration is only about one sixth to one fifteenth as effective as parenteral administration (depending on whether *peak* or *total analgesia* is measured).

Occasionally morphine sulfate is given *intravenously,* and it has been employed by this route for the control of severe postoperative pain and restlessness, for preoperative medication in emergencies, for minor surgical procedures when general anesthesia is not indicated, for severe cardiac pain, for severe biliary and renal colic, and for pulmonary edema. The usual dose is 2.5 to 15 mg. Maximal respiratory depression is manifest within 10 minutes.

The dose of opiates for *infants and children* is 0.1 to 0.2 mg/kg, injected subcutaneously or intramuscularly.

Codeine. Codeine is available as the free alkaloidal base (*Codeine,* U.S.P.) and in the form of its water-soluble salts. The most common salts of codeine are *Codeine Sulfate,* U.S.P., and *Codeine Phos-*

phate, U.S.P. Both are available as official tablets containing 15, 30, or 60 mg of the drug. *Codeine Phosphate Injection,* U.S.P., contains 15, 30, or 60 mg/ml of the salt. Codeine phosphate has the advantage of being much more soluble in water than is the sulfate. Also available is *Terpin Hydrate and Codeine Elixir,* U.S.P., used mainly for cough and containing 10 mg in a 5-ml dose.

Although a dose of 120 mg of codeine, administered subcutaneously, produces analgesia equivalent to that resulting from 10 mg of morphine, the former drug has few advantages over morphine when used parenterally. However, codeine has a high oral-parenteral potency ratio; in terms of total analgesia, codeine is about 60% as potent when given orally as when injected intramuscularly. In this respect it has definite advantages over morphine. Orally, a dose of 30 mg of codeine is approximately equianalgesic with 325 to 600 mg of aspirin; when these two drugs are combined, the analgesic effect equals or sometimes exceeds that of 60 mg of codeine. The variability of the analgesic response at this dosage level is considerable (*see* Beaver, 1966; Cooper and Beaver, 1976; Moertel, 1976; Bloomfield *et al.,* 1977). The effects of 15 mg of codeine orally can be demonstrated by objective technics to reduce the frequency of pathological cough, and progressively greater cough suppression is seen as the dose is increased up to 60 mg (Sevelius *et al.,* 1971). The abuse liability of codeine is much lower than that of morphine, as discussed more fully in Chapter 23.

Apomorphine. Apomorphine, U.S.P., a dopaminergic agonist, is obtained by exposure of morphine to strong mineral acids. Its analgesic properties are diminished, but it retains the capacity to stimulate the medullary CTZ and to produce a combination of CNS excitation and depression. It has been used therapeutically for the production of emesis; the usual dose is 5 mg, given subcutaneously.

Etorphine hydrochloride (M-99; IMMOBILON) is an analog of thebaine used exclusively for immobilizing large animals. In man, it is 400 times as potent as morphine in producing subjective effects and suppressing opioid withdrawal. Its duration of action is relatively short (Jasinski *et al.,* 1975). Poisoning with etorphine should be treated in the same way as morphine poisoning.

Other Semisynthetic Morphine and Codeine Derivatives. There are many drugs that can substitute for morphine and codeine. Their names, doses, and special characteristics are shown in Table 22–2.

Hydromorphone Hydrochloride, U.S.P. (DILAUDID), is available in 1-, 2-, 3-, and 4-mg tablets; in ampuls containing 1, 2, 3, and 4 mg; and as 3-mg rectal suppositories.

Hydrocodone Bitartrate, U.S.P., is used in combination with other ingredients in a variety of proprietary antitussive and analgesic-antipyretic mixtures (*e.g.,* HYCODAN). Similarly, *oxycodone* is available only as an ingredient in analgesic and antitussive mixtures. Oxycodone is about as potent as morphine and is 10 to 12 times more potent than codeine. Like codeine, it retains about 50% of its efficacy when given orally. *Oxymorphone Hydrochloride,* U.S.P. (NUMORPHAN), is available as an injection containing 1 mg/ml and in 5-mg rectal suppositories.

Acute Opioid Poisoning

Acute opioid poisoning may result from clinical overdosage, accidental overdosage in addicts, or attempts at suicide. Occasionally, a delayed type of poisoning may occur from the injection of an opioid into chilled skin areas or in patients with low blood pressure and shock. The drug is not fully absorbed, and, therefore, a subsequent dose may be given. When normal circulation is established, an excessive amount may suddenly be absorbed. Because tolerance to the opioids develops so rapidly, and because there is great individual variation in sensitivity, it is difficult to state the exact amount of any opioid that is toxic or lethal to man. Recent experiences with methadone indicate that in nontolerant individuals serious toxicity may follow the oral ingestion of 40 to 60 mg. Older literature suggests that, in the case of morphine, a normal, pain-free adult is not likely to die after oral doses of less than 120 mg, or to have serious toxicity with less than 30 mg parenterally.

Symptoms and Diagnosis. By the time he is seen by the physician, the patient who has taken an overdose of an opioid is usually asleep or stuporous. If a large overdose has been taken, he cannot be aroused and may be in a *profound coma*. The *respiratory rate* is quite low (sometimes only 2 to 4 per minute), and *cyanosis* may be present. As the respiratory exchange becomes poorer, *blood pressure*, at first maintained near normal, falls progressively. If adequate oxygenation is restored early, the blood pressure will improve; if hypoxia persists untreated, however, there may be capillary damage, and measures to combat *shock* may then be required. The *pupils* are symmetrical and pinpoint in size; however, if hypoxia is severe, they may be dilated. *Urine formation* is depressed. *Body temperature* falls, and the skin becomes cold and clammy. The *skeletal muscles* are flaccid, the jaw is relaxed, and the tongue may fall back and block the airway. Frank convulsions may occasionally be noted in infants and children. When death occurs, it is nearly always due to respiratory failure. Sometimes, even if respiration is restored, death may still occur as a result of complications, such as pneumonia or shock, that develop during the period of coma. *Pulmonary edema* is commonly seen with opioid poisoning. It is probably not due to contaminants or to anaphylactoid reactions, and has been observed following toxic doses of morphine, methadone, propoxyphene, and uncontaminated heroin.

The triad of *coma, pinpoint pupils,* and *depressed respiration* strongly suggests opioid poisoning. Since deliberate or accidental overdosage is common among addicts, the finding of needle marks suggestive of addiction further supports the diagnosis. Mixed poisonings, however, are not uncommon. In such cases, other agents such as a barbiturate or alcohol may also be contributing to the clinical picture. Chemical examination of the urine and gastric contents for opioids and other CNS depressants may help to clarify the diagnosis, but the results usually become available too late to influence treatment.

Treatment. The first step is to establish a patent airway and ventilate the patient. Opioid antagonists such as naloxone can produce dramatic reversal of the severe respiratory depression (*see* below), and the use of naloxone is now the treatment of choice. The safest approach is the administration of small intravenous doses (*e.g.,* 0.4 mg of naloxone); this dose may be repeated after 2 to 3 minutes. For children, the initial dose is 0.01 mg/kg. If no effect is seen after two or three such doses, one can reasonably question the accuracy of the diagnosis. Pulmonary edema sometimes associated with opioid overdosage may be countered by positive-pressure respiration. Grand mal seizures, occasionally seen as part of the toxic syndrome with meperidine and propoxyphene, are ameliorated by treatment with naloxone.

Opioid antagonists, such as nalorphine and levallorphan, that also have agonistic actions should be used with care since they may further embarrass respiration that has been depressed by alcohol, barbiturates, or related CNS depressants. Since naloxone has no direct respiratory depressant action, it is the drug of choice. The presence of alcohol or a barbiturate does not prevent the salutary effect of an antagonist, and in cases of mixed intoxications the situation will be improved largely due to antagonism of the respiratory depressant effects of the opioid. However, there is an emerging body of data that suggest that naloxone and naltrexone may also antagonize some of the depressant actions of sedative-hypnotics (*see* below). Although opioid antagonists also counteract the sedative effects of morphine, one need not attempt to restore the patient to full consciousness. The duration of action of antagonists is usually shorter than that of many opioids; hence, the patient must be carefully watched, lest he slip back into coma. This is particularly important when the overdosage is due to methadone or *l*-acetylmethadol. The depressant effects of these drugs may persist for 24 to 72 hours, and fatalities have occurred as a result of premature discontinuation of treatment with an antagonist drug.

The use of an opioid antagonist to treat acute

poisoning in an addict should be undertaken with care, since the antagonist may precipitate a severe withdrawal syndrome that cannot be readily suppressed during the period of action of the antagonist. In some situations, this withdrawal syndrome can be more life threatening than the respiratory depression itself.

These principles are appropriate in treating acute poisoning with any of the opioid agonists. Toxicity due to overdose of pentazocine and opioids with mixed actions can be alleviated by high doses of naloxone, which, unlike nalorphine, antagonizes the agonistic effects of these agents. The pharmacological actions of opioid antagonists are discussed in more detail below.

THERAPEUTIC USES

Sir William Osler referred to morphine as "God's own medicine." The years since Osler have seen the introduction of scores of synthetic and semisynthetic agents that are equal to morphine in their ability to produce analgesia; undoubtedly the search for better analgesics will continue. For the present, however, the opioids retain their very special place in the treatment of pain.

General Principles. When opioid analgesics are administered for the relief of pain, cough, or diarrhea, only symptomatic treatment is being provided and the underlying pathology remains. The physician must constantly weigh the benefits of this relief against its costs and risks to the patient. Such costs and risks are frequently quite different, depending upon whether the symptom is a manifestation of an acute or a chronic disease.

In acute problems, opioids may obscure the symptoms or the progress of the disease. However, because relief of pain can also facilitate history taking and examination, there are times when the skillful use of opioids may even aid in diagnosis.

The problems that arise in the *treatment of chronic conditions* involve more complex considerations. Repeated daily administration will eventually produce some tolerance to the therapeutic effects of the drug, and some degree of physical dependence as well. The degree will depend on the particular drug, the frequency of administration, and the quantity administered. The risk of developing psychological dependency is always present. Thus, a decision to relieve any chronic symptom, especially pain, by the parenteral administration of an opioid may be shortsighted and can be a disservice to the patient. Measures other than drugs should be employed to relieve chronic pain when they are effective and available. To cite but one example, cutaneous stimulation or stimulation of the dorsal columns may be of some value in alleviating chronic pain. The general principles to be observed in order to mimimize the incidence of medical addiction are discussed in Chapter 23.

In the usual doses, opioids relieve suffering by altering the emotional component of the painful experience as well as by producing analgesia. The physician who views his patient as a whole person responding to a physically and emotionally stressful illness, who realizes the importance of his own relationship to the patient, and who utilizes this relationship to provide psychological support will need to prescribe considerably less opioid than a physician who cannot offer this kind of support. In addition to emotional support, the physician should also take into account the substantial variability in both the capacity to tolerate pain and the response to opioids. Some patients may require considerably more than the average dose of a drug to experience any relief from pain; others, perhaps because of more rapid metabolic disposition, may require a drug at shorter intervals. Some clinicians, out of an exaggerated concern for the possibility of inducing addiction, tend to prescribe initial doses of opioids that are too low or too infrequent to alleviate pain, and then respond to the patient's continued complaints with an even more exaggerated concern about dependence, despite the high probability that the request for more drug is only the expected consequence of the inadequate dosage prescribed (*see* Marks and Sachar, 1973). It is useful to remember that the typical dose of 10 mg of morphine relieves postoperative pain in only two thirds of patients.

Pain. *The Selection of a Drug.* The differences between morphine and its surrogates have been considerably overestimated (*see* Table 22–2). In equianalgesic doses, most of these drugs produce approximately the same incidence and degree of unwanted side effects. Nevertheless, there are some patients who may have side effects with one agent and not with another. Some drugs have shorter durations of action, others are particularly efficacious when given by mouth, and a few are considered to have a lower risk for producing opioid dependence. The availability of a wide range of agents provides for therapeutic flexibility. When pain is not too severe, codeine, oxycodone, or hydrocodone orally will often provide very satisfactory relief, especially when given with a nonopioid analgesic such as aspirin. Combination of an opioid with a small dose of amphetamine may augment analgesia while reducing the sedative effects. When the pain is associated with biliary spasm, meperidine may produce less increase in the spasm than will an equianalgesic dose of morphine. When the pain is likely to be of short duration (e.g., diagnostic procedures, cystoscopy, orthopedic manipulation, etc.), a drug with a shorter duration of action, such as meperidine or alphaprodine, might be preferable to morphine or methadone.

The Pain of Terminal Illness. Although they are not requisite or even desirable in all cases of terminal cancer, the euphoria, tranquility, and relief of pain afforded by the wise use of opioids are a blessing to the patient and his family. Some degree of physical dependence and tolerance develops whenever an opioid is given in therapeutic dosage several times a day over a prolonged period. In patients with painful terminal illnesses such considerations should not in any way prevent the physician from fulfilling his primary obligation to ease the patient's discomfort. The physician should not wait until the pain becomes agonizing; *no patient should ever wish for death because of his physician's reluctance to use adequate amounts of effective opioids.* Such patients, while they may be physically dependent, are not considered "addicts" even though they may need large doses on a regular basis; in states that require the reporting of addicts, patients with terminal illnesses are not reportable. The use of parenteral opioids should be reserved until nonopioid drugs or other measures no longer give adequate relief. Then codeine or a comparable effective oral drug should be employed together with nonopioid analgesics and the doses increased until pain can no longer be controlled without the more effective parenteral preparations.

Some clinicians who are experienced in the management of terminal illness now recommend that opioids be administered not on demand, but at sufficiently short, fixed intervals so that pain is continually under control and patients do not dread its return. There has been a renewed interest in analgesic mixtures. "Brompton's mixture" (which originated in Brompton Hospital in England) is now used in a generic sense to designate an alcoholic solution containing an opioid (usually morphine or heroin) and either cocaine and/or a phenothiazine. There are no controlled studies that demonstrate special efficacy for oral heroin. Amphetamines have demonstrable mood-elevating and analgesic effects and enhance opioid-induced analgesia; similar effects might be expected from cocaine. However, not all terminal patients require the euphoriant effects of cocaine or amphetamine and some experience side effects. Routine use of such agents seems to be losing popularity. Since phenothiazines would be expected to antagonize the effects of cocaine or amphetamine, the combination of drugs in a single mixture seems illogical (Twycross, 1977). Clinicians who have administered "Brompton's mixture" have observed that the development of tolerance is not rapid and analgesia can be maintained for many months.

When opioids and other analgesics are no longer satisfactory, nerve block by injections of alcohol, chordotomy, or other types of neurosurgical intervention such as neurostimulation may be required if the nature of the lesion permits.

Postoperative Pain. Opioid analgesics are commonly employed to control pain and discomfort in the immediate postoperative period, but they should be considered two-edged swords. If used indiscriminately, they may obscure the outcome of surgery and the course of recovery, and prevent the early recognition of complications. They may also decrease the effectiveness of coughing, decrease respiratory ventilation, predispose to pneumonia, reduce bowel motility, and cause urinary retention. On the other hand, the reduction of pain associated with movements of the chest can increase the patient's ability to breathe deeply and to cough voluntarily, and can also facilitate early ambulation. When pain is not too severe, oral codeine or oxycodone with aspirin often provides adequate analgesia without the side effects associated with the use of usual doses of morphine. When there is inflammation or pain from uterine muscle, 600 mg of aspirin may provide more analgesia than 60 mg of codeine (*see* Cooper and Beaver, 1976; Bloomfield *et al.,* 1977).

Headache. Headache is often a recurrent problem, sometimes reflecting emotional disturbances, and opioid analgesics, with the possible exception of codeine, should not be employed unless all other measures have failed. Even then, considerable care should be employed to minimize psychological dependence and addiction.

Obstetrical Analgesia. The use of morphine and its synthetic surrogates in obstetrical analgesia is a highly specialized field requiring experience and sound judgment to ensure safety. For any given agent, three factors must be considered: efficacy in relieving pain, effect on the progress of labor, and effect on the fetus. All the available, fully effective opioids are powerful respiratory depressants, and the fetus seems more susceptible to their respiratory depressant effects than does the mother. In equianalgesic doses, morphine and methadone appear somewhat more depressant to the fetus than are meperidine and closely related drugs (*see* Eddy *et al.,* 1957; Campbell *et al.,* 1961). The pharmacological basis for this difference has been discussed above. The differences are sufficient to justify the selection of meperidine-like drugs in preference to morphine for obstetrical use. Regardless of the specific opioid analgesic that is selected, opioid-induced respiratory depression in the newborn can be immediately reversed by a small dose of naloxone injected into the umbilical vein.

Sedation and Sleep. Whenever possible, drugs other than opioids should be prescribed for sedation, tranquilization, or sleep. When sleeplessness is due to *pain* or *cough,* opioids are often necessary, and when properly used they foster rest and thus conserve the patient's strength. Although long years of use have demonstrated the value of opioids as pre-anesthetic medication, controlled clinical studies suggest that preanesthetic medication with a sedative or an antianxiety agent is just as effective in reducing preoperative apprehension and does not cause vomiting. The routine use of opioids in pain-free patients is difficult to justify on the basis of available evidence.

Cough. The opioids remain among the most effective agents for suppressing cough. This antitussive effect can be demonstrated experimentally against the coughing induced by electrical stimulation of the medulla or by chemical or mechanical irritation of the respiratory tract. The dose of any given opioid required to suppress cough induced by these technics seems to be lower than that required for analgesia. A 15-mg oral dose of codeine, although ineffective for analgesia, produces a demonstrable antitussive effect, and higher doses of codeine produce even more suppression of chronic cough. Interestingly, the degree of relief reported by patients does not necessarily correlate with actual reduction in the frequency of coughing (Sevelius et al., 1971), and it has been suggested that the usual doses of opioids produce their major effect on the patient's subjective reactions to the cough, rather than on the frequency and intensity of coughing.

Considerable progress has been made in separating analgesic actions from antitussive activity, and there are now a number of effective nonopioid, non-addictive antitussives available for clinical use (see below).

Dyspnea. Certain forms of dyspnea may be markedly relieved by morphine. This is especially true of the dyspnea of acute left ventricular failure and pulmonary edema, in which the response to intravenous morphine may be dramatic. The mechanism underlying this relief is still not clear. It may involve an alteration of the patient's reaction to impaired respiratory function and an indirect reduction of the work of the heart due to reduced fear and apprehension. However, it is more probable that the major benefit is due to cardiovascular effects such as decreased peripheral resistance and an increased capacity of the peripheral and splanchnic vascular compartments (see Vasko et al., 1966; Vismara et al., 1976). Opioids are contraindicated in pulmonary edema due to respiratory irritants unless severe pain is also present; contradictions to their use in asthma have already been discussed.

Constipating Effects. The opioids remain the most effective agents for causing constipation or treating diarrhea. Mild constipation and a drier stool are often desirable after ileostomy or colostomy, and the constipating action is especially valuable in treating exhausting diarrhea and dysenteries due to a number of causes. As in the case for cough, it requires considerably less morphine to affect the gut than to produce analgesia. Traditionally, opium preparations (opium tincture, 0.5 to 1.0 ml; paregoric, 4 ml) rather than the pure alkaloids are used; the morphine content of these doses cannot provide significant analgesia (especially by the oral route),

but such dosage is, nevertheless, effective treatment for diarrhea. Synthetic opioids also produce a decrease in bowel motility; several of these, such as diphenoxylate, loperamide, and difenoxin, are used exclusively for this purpose (see below).

Special Anesthesia. High doses of morphine or other opioids have been used as the primary anesthetic agents in certain surgical procedures. Although respiration is so depressed that physical assistance is required, the patient retains consciousness (see Chapter 14).

LEVORPHANOL AND CONGENERS

Levorphanol is the only commercially available opioid agonist of the morphinan series. The d isomer (dextrorphan) is relatively devoid of analgesic action and makes little contribution to the activity of the racemate (racemorphan). The structure of levorphanol is indicated in Table 22-1.

The pharmacological effects of levorphanol in all species including man closely parallel those of morphine (for references, see Reynolds and Randall, 1957). However, clinical reports suggest that it produces less nausea and vomiting. The nonanalgesic isomer dextrorphan possesses considerable antitussive activity (see below). Levorphanol is promptly absorbed from subcutaneous sites. Although it is less effective when given orally, its oral-parenteral potency ratio is considerably better than that of morphine. The average dose, 2 to 3 mg subcutaneously, is approximately equianalgesic with 10 mg of morphine. Maximal analgesia occurs 60 to 90 minutes after subcutaneous injection. Clinical studies of levorphanol have been reviewed by Eddy and coworkers (1957) and Lasagna (1964); its absorption, fate, and excretion have been reviewed by Way and Adler (1962) and Misra (1978). The drug is available as Levorphanol Tartrate, U.S.P. (LEVO-DROMORAN), in tablets containing 2 mg and as an injection containing 2 mg/ml.

MEPERIDINE AND CONGENERS

History. Meperidine is a synthetic, analgesic drug introduced by Eisleb and Schaumann in 1939. Originally studied as an atropine-like agent, it was soon discovered to have considerable analgesic activity. Although it exhibits some of the pharmacological effects of morphine in man, it is chemically quite dissimilar. Meperidine is an effective and widely used analgesic agent.

Chemistry. The structural formulas of meperidine, a phenylpiperidine, and some of its congeners are shown in Table 22-3.

PHARMACOLOGICAL PROPERTIES

Meperidine, like other opioids, binds to opioid receptors and exerts its chief pharmacological actions on the CNS and the neural elements in the bowel.

Table 22-3. CHEMICAL STRUCTURES OF PHENYLPIPERIDINE ANALGESICS

COMPOUND	R_1	R_3
Meperidine	CH_3	$-COCH_2CH_3$ (C=O)
Alphaprodine	$-CH_3$	$-OCCH_2CH_3$ (C=O)
Anileridine	$-CH_2CH_2-\bigcirc-NH_2$	$-COCH_2CH_3$ (C=O)
Diphenoxylate	$-CH_2CH_2C-CN$ (with two phenyl groups)	$-COCH_2CH_3$ (C=O)
Fentanyl	$-CH_2CH_2-\bigcirc$	$-N-C-CH_2CH_3$ (C=O) †

* R_2 = H, except in alphaprodine, where R_2 = CH_3.
† The sole *para* substitution on the piperidine ring is as shown.

Central Nervous System. Meperidine produces a pattern of effects similar to those described for morphine.

Analgesia. In patients or experimental subjects, the analgesic effects of meperidine are detectable about 15 minutes after oral administration, reach a peak in about 2 hours, and subside gradually over several hours. The onset of analgesic effect is faster (within 10 minutes) after subcutaneous or intramuscular administration and reaches a peak in about 1 hour. In clinical use, the duration of action is shorter than that of morphine, being approximately 2 to 4 hours. This necessitates a shorter interval between injections for the relief of continuing pain. The peak analgesic effect corresponds closely to peak concentrations in plasma.

In general, 80 to 100 mg of meperidine given parenterally is approximately equivalent to 10 mg of morphine. Since neither morphine nor meperidine in these doses produces satisfactory analgesia in all patients in all situations, there are times when larger doses are appropriate. In terms of total analgesic effect, meperidine is less than one half as effective when given by mouth as when given parenterally (*see* review by Lasagna, 1964).

Sedation, Euphoria, and Excitation. In equianalgesic doses, meperidine produces as much sedation as does morphine, and as much euphoria (10 to 20% of patients). A few patients may experience dysphoria. Meperidine differs from morphine in that toxic doses sometimes cause CNS excitation, characterized by tremors, muscle twitches, and seizures (*see* below).

Respiration. In equianalgesic doses, meperidine depresses respiration to the same degree as does morphine. Peak respiratory depression is observed within 1 hour after intramuscular administration, and after usual therapeutic doses there is a return toward normal starting at about 2 hours, although minute volume is usually measurably depressed for as long as 4 hours (Lambertsen *et al.,* 1961). The respiratory depression produced by meperidine can be antagonized by naloxone, nalorphine, and related opioid antagonists.

Miscellaneous Effects on the Nervous System. After systemic administration, meperidine may obtund or abolish the corneal reflex. Like other opioids, meperidine causes pupillary constriction. It has considerable local anesthetic activity but is somewhat irritating when applied locally. Meperidine appears to increase the sensitivity of the labyrinthine apparatus in human subjects (Gutner *et al.,* 1952), a fact that may partially explain the higher incidence of dizziness, nausea, and vomiting encountered when the drug is given to ambulatory patients; it lacks anticonvulsant activity. Meperidine has effects on the secretion of pituitary hormones similar to those of morphine.

EEG. Upon continued administration of large doses at short intervals, slow waves appear in the EEG after a few days, and then become progressively slower and of greater amplitude. The slow waves persist even after tolerance has developed to the drug. The EEG changes differ from those observed after morphine in that abnormal slow-wave activity occurs only when morphine is administered more rapidly than tolerance develops. The meperidine-induced alterations persist for about 48 hours after withdrawal of the drug, after which time the EEG record slowly returns to its original character. Large doses of meperidine regularly produce EEG evidence of convulsive activity in animals.

Cardiovascular System. In therapeutic doses, meperidine has no significant untoward effects on the cardiovascular system, particularly when patients are recumbent; myocardial contractility is not depressed, and the ECG is unaltered. Ambulatory patients given meperidine may experience syncope associated with a fall in blood pressure, but symptoms rapidly clear if the recumbent position is assumed. After the intravenous administration of meperidine, there is an increase in peripheral blood flow and a decrease in peripheral arterial and venous resistance, effects that are not blocked by prior oral administration of antihistamines. The mechanisms involved may be similar to those described above for morphine. Intramuscular administration of meperidine does not significantly affect heart rate, but intravenous administration frequently produces an increased rate that is sometimes alarming. As with morphine, respiratory depression is responsible for an accumulation of CO_2, which, in turn, produces cerebrovascular dilatation, increase in cerebral blood flow, and elevation of cerebrospinal fluid pressure (*see* Eckenhoff and Oech, 1960).

Smooth Muscle. Meperidine has a spasmogenic effect on certain smooth muscles, similar to that observed with other opioids.

Gastrointestinal Tract. The effects of meperidine are qualitatively similar to those of morphine. However, clinical observations indicate that it does not cause as much constipation when given over prolonged periods of time; this may be related to its shorter duration of action, which permits periods of normal function, or to a more favorable ratio of analgesic to gastrointestinal effects. After equianalgesic doses, the spasm in the biliary tract, as well as the rise in pressure in the common bile duct, induced by meperidine is less than that caused by morphine but greater than that by codeine.

Uterus. The intact uterus of nonpregnant women is usually mildly stimulated by meperidine. Late in pregnancy, the drug does not significantly alter the activity of the normally contracting uterus, but appears to increase the tone and the frequency and intensity of contraction in the uterus made hyperactive by oxytocics. Administered prior to an oxytocic, meperidine does not exert any antioxytocic effect. Therapeutic doses given during labor appear neither to delay the birth process nor to alter the rhythmic uterine contractions (*see* Eddy *et al.,* 1957). The drug does not interfere with normal post-partum contraction or involution of the uterus, and it does not increase the incidence of post-partum hemorrhage.

Absorption, Fate, and Excretion. Meperidine is absorbed by all routes of administration. While peak concentrations in plasma are usually observed between the first and second hour after oral administration, only about 50% of the drug escapes first-pass metabolism to enter the circulation (Mather and Tucker, 1976).

Meperidine is metabolized chiefly in the liver. After intravenous administration, the rapid decline of the concentration in plasma due to distribution is followed by a slower phase with a half-time of about 3 hours. In patients with cirrhosis, the half-life is increased to 6 hours (Klotz *et al.,* 1974). Approximately 60% of meperidine in plasma is protein bound. Heavy drinkers of alcohol have an increased apparent volume of distribution that leads to concentrations in plasma that are initially lower than would be found in nondrinkers. Older patients have higher concentrations in plasma and decreased binding to plasma proteins, both of which may account for their increased response to therapeutic doses (Mather *et al.*, 1975).

In man, meperidine is hydrolyzed to meperidinic acid, which, in turn, is partially conjugated. Meperidine is also N-demethylated to normeperidine, which may then be hydrolyzed to normeperidinic acid and subsequently conjugated. About one third of administered meperidine can be accounted for in the urine as N-demethylated derivatives; the clinical significance of the formation of normeperidine is discussed further under toxicity. Very little meperidine is excreted unchanged (*see* Way and Adler, 1962; Way, 1968; Misra, 1978).

Preparations, Routes of Administration, and Dosage. Trade names for meperidine include DEMEROL and PETHADOL. The international nonproprietary name is *pethidine. Meperidine Hydrochloride, U.S.P., Meperidine Hydrochloride Injection, U.S.P., Meperidine Hydrochloride Tablets, U.S.P.*, and *Meperidine Hydrochloride Syrup, U.S.P.*, are the official preparations. The drug is available for oral use in 50- and 100-mg tablets, and as a syrup containing 50 mg/5 ml; for parenteral use it is available in unit dosage forms and in multiple-dose vials containing 50, 75, or 100 mg/ml. It is usually given orally or intramuscularly. Intravenous use increases the incidence and severity of untoward effects, and subcutaneous or intramuscular administration causes local irritation and tissue induration; frequent repetition may lead to severe fibrosis of muscle tissue (*see* Johnson *et al.*, 1976). The dose varies with the clinical situation. Most patients with moderate-to-severe pain are relieved by 100 mg parenterally. The effectiveness of the drug by the oral route is not reduced to the same degree as is that of morphine, but its oral-parenteral potency ratio is lower than that of codeine. Doses for infants and children may be calculated on a weight basis.

Congeners of meperidine are also available in the United States; only those that are official are described here. *Alphaprodine Hydrochloride, U.S.P.* (NISENTIL), is available in 1-ml ampuls containing 40 or 60 mg/ml, and in 10-ml multiple-dose vials containing 60 mg/ml. *Anileridine Hydrochloride, U.S.P.* (LERITINE), is available as 25-mg tablets. *Anileridine Injection, U.S.P.*, is marketed for parenteral administration in ampuls and multiple-dose vials containing 25 mg/ml of anileridine phosphate. Doses, durations of action, and distinguishing pharmacological features of alphaprodine and anileridine are shown in Table 22–2.

Untoward Effects, Precautions, and Contraindications. The pattern and overall incidence of untoward effects that follow the use of meperidine are similar to those observed after equianalgesic doses of morphine, except that constipation and urinary retention are less common. Patients who experience nausea and vomiting with morphine may not do so with meperidine; the converse may also be true. As with other opioids, tolerance develops to some of these effects. The contraindications are the same as for other opioids. In patients or addicts who are tolerant to the depressant effects of meperidine, large doses repeated at short intervals produce tremors, muscle twitches, dilated pupils, hyperactive reflexes, and convulsions.

Normeperidine, a metabolite of meperidine, differs from meperidine in having greater excitant and less depressant effect. When toxic doses of meperidine are given parenterally, the rate of absorption exceeds the rate of formation of normeperidine, and the picture is primarily one of CNS depression. When toxic doses of meperidine are given orally, the rate of absorption does not exceed the capacity of the liver to convert meperidine to normeperidine. Hence the ratio of normeperidine to meperidine increases, producing a picture of mixed stupor and convulsions; a similar syndrome may also be seen in patients with renal failure, in whom concentrations of normeperidine may be abnormally high (Szeto *et al.*, 1977). Opioid antagonists block the convulsant effect of normeperidine in the mouse (Gilbert and Martin, 1975).

Interaction with Other Drugs. There have been reports of severe reactions following the administration of meperidine to patients being treated with monoamine oxidase (MAO) inhibitors. These consisted in excitation, delirium, hyperpyrexia, and convulsions or severe respiratory depression. Chlorpromazine increases the respiratory depressant effects of meperidine (Lambertsen *et al.*, 1961), as may tricyclic antidepressants; this is not true of diazepam. Concurrent administration of drugs such as promethazine or chlorpromazine may also greatly enhance meperidine-induced sedation. As with morphine, concomitant administration of *amphetamine* has been reported to enhance the analgesic effects of meperidine and its congeners.

Tolerance, Physical Dependence, and Liability for Abuse. In situations where they are administered chronically, the duration of action of meperidine is considerably shorter than that of morphine, and continuous depression of the CNS is attained only when the drug is used at less than 4-hour intervals. This may account for the slower development of tolerance to meperidine. Tolerance to the excitatory effects of meperidine does not seem to develop even after prolonged use of high doses. When patients who have become tolerant to the respiratory depressant effects of meperidine are given high doses at frequent intervals, excitatory effects, including hallucinations and seizures, may occur (*see* above; Chapter 23).

The pattern of withdrawal symptoms after abrupt discontinuation of meperidine differs somewhat from that after morphine in that there are fewer autonomic effects and the symptoms develop more rapidly and are of shorter duration. It should be emphasized that the degree of physical dependence that a drug induces is only one factor in determining its abuse liability (*see* above). Actually, the need to use a drug repeatedly at short intervals can be viewed as a factor favoring the reinforcement of drug-seeking behavior. Some congeners of meperidine can produce a marked degree of physical dependence, and withdrawal symptoms following abrupt discontinuation result in a severe morphine-like withdrawal syndrome. The abuse potential of the clinically available meperidine congeners is similar to that of meperidine.

THERAPEUTIC USES

The major use of meperidine is for analgesia. Unlike morphine and its congeners, meperidine is not useful for the treatment of cough and diarrhea.

Analgesia. Meperidine can be used in any situation where an opioid analgesic is required. However, there are a number of clinical conditions in which its lesser spasmogenic effects or its better oral efficacy make meperidine preferable to morphine. For example, in equianalgesic doses meperidine has less spasmogenic effect on the biliary tract than does morphine. On the other hand, in bronchoscopy the relative lack of antitussive activity of meperidine makes it less valuable. Because of concern about drug dependence, many clinicians prescribe doses of meperidine that are too low or too infrequent, thereby causing unnecessary suffering. This is discussed above, in the section on therapeutic uses of morphine.

Meperidine crosses the placental barrier and even in reasonable analgesic doses causes a significant increase in the percentage of babies who show delayed respiration, decreased respiratory minute volume, or decreased oxygen saturation, or who require resuscitation (*see* review by Eddy *et al.*, 1957). Concentrations of meperidine in cord blood at birth may be higher than those in maternal blood (Morgan *et al.*, 1978). However, meperidine produces less respiratory depression in the newborn than does an equianalgesic dose of morphine or methadone (*see* above).

OTHER CONGENERS OF MEPERIDINE

Diphenoxylate. Diphenoxylate is a meperidine congener that has a definite constipating effect in

man. While it has been proposed as a maintenance drug in the treatment of opioid dependence, its only recognized use is in the treatment of diarrhea. Although single doses in the therapeutic range (*see* below) produce little or no morphine-like subjective effects, at high doses (40 to 60 mg) the drug shows typical opioid activity, including euphoria, suppression of morphine abstinence, and a morphine-like physical dependence after chronic administration. Diphenoxylate is unusual in that even its salts are virtually insoluble in aqueous solution, thus obviating the possibility of abuse by the parenteral route. *Diphenoxylate Hydrochloride*, U.S.P., *Diphenoxylate Hydrochloride and Atropine Sulfate Oral Solution*, U.S.P., and *Diphenoxylate Hydrochloride and Atropine Sulfate Tablets*, U.S.P., are the official preparations. In the combination (LOMOTIL, others), each tablet or 5 ml contains 2.5 mg of diphenoxylate and 25 μg of atropine sulfate. The recommended daily dosage for treatment of *diarrhea* in adults is 20 mg, in divided doses. It is a schedule-V narcotic (*see* Appendix I). *Difenoxin* (diphenoxylic acid) is one of the metabolites of diphenoxylate; it has actions similar to those of the parent compound.

Loperamide. Loperamide, like diphenoxylate, is a piperidine derivative (4-[*p*-chlorophenyl]-4-hydroxy-N,N-dimethyl-α,α-diphenyl-1-piperidinebutyramide). It slows gastrointestinal motility by effects on the circular and longitudinal muscles of the intestine. It binds to opioid receptors in brain homogenates and intestinal strips; its constipating action is probably due, at least in part, to actions at these receptors. In controlling chronic diarrhea, the drug is as effective as diphenoxylate. In clinical studies, the most common side effect is abdominal cramps. Little tolerance develops to its constipating effect (Galambos *et al.*, 1976).

In human volunteers taking large doses, concentrations of loperamide in plasma peak about 4 hours after ingestion; this long latency may be due to inhibition of gastrointestinal motility (Weintraub *et al.*, 1977). The apparent elimination half-time is 7 to 14 hours. Loperamide is not well absorbed after oral administration and, in addition, apparently does not penetrate well into the brain (Stahl *et al.*, 1977); these properties contribute to the selectivity of its action. A large proportion of the drug is excreted in the feces.

Despite the finding that the drug does not readily enter the CNS, high doses of loperamide do suppress withdrawal symptoms in morphine-dependent monkeys. However, the drug is unlikely to be abused parenterally because of its low solubility, and large doses of loperamide (18 to 54 mg) given to human volunteers do not elicit pleasurable effects typical of opioids. Its overall potential for abuse is probably lower than that of diphenoxylate. The drug is available as *loperamide hydrochloride* (IMODIUM) in 2-mg capsules. The usual dosage is 4 to 8 mg per day; the daily dose should not exceed 16 mg.

Ethoheptazine. Ethoheptazine (1-methyl-4-carbethoxy-4-phenylhexamethyleneimine) is structurally related to meperidine. The abuse potential is extremely low, but its efficacy as an analgesic is not impressive. *Ethoheptazine citrate* (ZACTANE) is available as tablets containing 75 mg, and as tablets containing 75 mg in combination with 325 mg of aspirin (ZACTIRIN).

FENTANYL

Fentanyl is a synthetic opioid related to the phenylpiperidines (Table 22–3). As an analgesic it is estimated to be 80 times as potent as morphine. Its respiratory depressant effect is of shorter duration than that of meperidine; its analgesic and euphoric effects are antagonized by opioid antagonists, but are not significantly prolonged or intensified by *droperidol,* a neuroleptic agent with which it is usually combined for use as an intravenous anesthetic (*see* Chapter 14). The subjective effects of the combination depend on the relative proportions of the two agents. High doses of fentanyl produce marked muscular rigidity, possibly as a result of the effects of opioids on dopaminergic transmission in the striatum; this effect can be antagonized by naloxone. Fentanyl is usually used only for anesthesia. It is available as *Fentanyl Citrate,* U.S.P., and *Fentanyl Citrate Injection,* U.S.P. (SUBLIMAZE), containing 50 μg of fentanyl citrate per milliliter in 2- and 5-ml ampuls.

METHADONE AND CONGENERS

Methadone was synthesized by German chemists and came into clinical use at the end of World War II. The pharmacological properties of methadone are qualitatively similar to those of morphine.

Chemistry.   Methadone has the following structural formula:

Methadone

In spite of the fact that the two-dimensional structure of methadone does not remotely resemble that of morphine, steric factors force the molecule to simulate the pseudopiperidine ring configuration that appears to be essential for opioid activity. The analgesic activity of the racemate is almost entirely the result of its content of *l*-methadone, which is 8 to 50 times more potent than the *d* isomer (depending upon the species and analgesic test employed). *d*-Methadone also lacks significant respiratory depressant action and addiction liability, but it does possess antitussive activity.

A large number of structural isomers and congeners of methadone have been compared pharmac-

ologically with methadone and morphine (*see* Braenden *et al.,* 1955). As analgesics, these drugs have no demonstrable superiority over the parent compound. The dose, durations of action, and other effects of the congeners are compared to those of other opioid analgesics in Table 22–2.

Pharmacological Actions.   The pharmacological actions of single doses of methadone are qualitatively identical to those of morphine. The outstanding properties of methadone are its effective analgesic activity, its efficacy by the oral route, its extended duration of action in suppressing withdrawal symptoms in physically dependent individuals, and its tendency to show persistent effects with repeated administration.

Central Nervous System.   After parenteral administration in man, a single dose of methadone is an effective analgesic, equal in potency and duration of action to morphine. Single doses of methadone may be slightly less hypnotic than comparable doses of morphine; however, upon repeated administration, marked sedative effects are seen in some patients (Martin *et al.,* 1973a). Methadone produces respiratory depression, miosis, antitussive effects, and effects on the secretion of pituitary hormones that are qualitatively similar to those of morphine.

Smooth Muscle.   Methadone, like morphine, increases intestinal tone, diminishes the amplitude of contractions, and produces a marked decrease in propulsive activity; it is constipating and causes biliary tract spasm. After therapeutic doses, the ureters become quiescent, perhaps because of the antidiuretic effect. The uterus at term is not significantly affected.

Absorption, Fate, and Excretion.   Appreciable concentrations of methadone can be found in the plasma within 10 minutes after its subcutaneous injection. It is also well absorbed from the gastrointestinal tract and can be detected in plasma within 30 minutes after oral ingestion; it reaches peak concentrations at about 4 hours. After therapeutic doses, about 85% of methadone is bound to plasma proteins; only a fraction enters the brain. Peak concentrations occur in the brain within 1 or 2 hours after subcutaneous or intramuscular administration, and this correlates well with the intensity and duration of analgesia. Methadone appears to be firmly bound to protein in various tissues, including brain. Some of its effects after repeated administration are due to its gradual accumulation in tissues. When administration is discontinued, low concentrations are maintained in plasma by slow release from extravascular binding sites (Dole and Kreek, 1973; Harte *et al.,* 1976).

Methadone undergoes extensive biotransformation in the liver. The major metabolites, the results of N-demethylation and cyclization to form pyrrolidines and pyrroline, are excreted in the urine and the bile along with small amounts of unchanged drug. The amount of methadone excreted in the urine is increased when the urine is acidified. In nontolerant subjects the mean apparent half-life of methadone after a single dose is approximately 15 hours (Inturrisi and Verebey, 1972). After chronic administration, the apparent half-life is 22 hours (Verebey *et al.,* 1975).

The use of methadone in the treatment of compulsive heroin users has revived interest in other methadone congeners, such as α-*dl*- and *l*-acetylmethadol (methadyl acetate). In subjects physically dependent on α-*dl*-acetylmethadol, opioid withdrawal symptoms are not perceived for 72 to 96 hours after the last oral dose, and subjects are entirely comfortable when given a single dose of the drug as infrequently as every 72 hours (Fraser and Isbell, 1952; Jaffe *et al.,* 1972; Ling *et al.,* 1978). The relatively slow onset and protracted duration of action of this drug, which is probably inactive, are thought to be due in part to its conversion to active metabolites (noracetylmethadol, dinoracetylmethadol, and normethadol) that are slowly further metabolized or excreted (*see* Misra, 1978).

Preparations, Routes of Administration, and Dosage. *Methadone Hydrochloride,* U.S.P., is a bitter white powder, soluble in water and ethanol. Trade names of methadone include DOLOPHINE and WESTADONE. All conventional routes of administration may be used, but subcutaneous administration may cause local irritation. *Methadone Hydrochloride Tablets,* U.S.P., are available for oral use in 5- and 10-mg amounts. *Methadone Hydrochloride Injection,* U.S.P., is available in single ampuls and multiple-dose vials containing 10 mg/ml. The *oral analgesic dose* for adults is 5 to 15 mg, depending on the severity of the pain and the response of the patient; the initial parenteral dose is usually 5 to 10 mg.

In the United States, special controls on methadone have been enacted in an effort to prevent its unregulated large-scale use in the treatment of opioid addiction. Specialized dosage forms used in opioid addiction include tablets containing 2.5, 5, 10, or 40 mg of the drug.

Side Effects, Toxicity, Drug Interactions, and Precautions. Side effects caused by methadone are similar to those caused by morphine. The principal danger of overdosage is diminished pulmonary ventilation. The conditions that alter sensitivity to methadone are similar to those outlined for morphine, and the therapy of acute methadone intoxication is the same as for morphine. During chronic administration there may be excessive sweating, lymphocytosis, and increased concentrations of prolactin, albumin, and globulins in the plasma. Rifampin accelerates the metabolism of methadone and has been observed to precipitate withdrawal symptoms. Tricyclic antidepressants and diazepam inhibit the metabolism of methadone in rats (*see* Kreek, 1978).

Tolerance, Physical Dependence, and Liability for Abuse. The abuse liability of methadone and its congeners in man has been thoroughly assessed. Volunteer postaddicts who received subcutaneous or oral methadone daily developed partial *tolerance* to the nauseant, anorectic, miotic, sedative, respiratory depressant, and cardiovascular effects of methadone. Tolerance develops more slowly to methadone than to morphine in some patients, especially with respect to the depressant effects. However, this may be related in part to cumulative effects of the drug or its metabolites. Sedation with concomitant slowing of the EEG occurs during experimental addiction (Martin *et al.,* 1973a). Tolerance to the constipating effect of methadone does not develop as fully as does tolerance to other effects. The behavior of the addicts who use methadone parenterally is strikingly similar to that of the morphine addict, but many former heroin users treated with oral methadone show virtually no overt behavioral effects (*see* Chapter 23).

Development of physical dependence during the chronic administration of methadone can be demonstrated by drug withdrawal or by administration of an opioid antagonist. Subcutaneous administration of 10 to 20 mg of methadone in former opioid addicts produces definite euphoria, equal in duration to that caused by morphine. On the basis of definitive studies, the overall abuse potential of methadone is rated comparable to that of morphine (Martin *et al.,* 1973a).

Therapeutic Uses. The primary uses of methadone are relief of pain, treatment of opioid abstinence syndromes, and treatment of heroin users. It is not widely used as an antiperistaltic agent, but it is an effective antitussive. It should be employed with extreme caution, if at all, in labor.

Analgesia. The onset of analgesia occurs 10 to 20 minutes following parenteral administration and 30 to 60 minutes after oral medication. The duration of action of single doses is essentially the same as that of morphine. With repeated usage, some cumulative effects are seen, so that either lower dosage or longer intervals between doses become possible. *In contrast to morphine, methadone and many of its congeners retain a considerable degree of their effectiveness when given orally.* In terms of total analgesic effects, methadone given orally is about 50% as effective as the same dose administered intramuscularly; however, the oral-parenteral potency ratio is considerably lower when peak analgesic effect is considered (Beaver *et al.,* 1967). In equianalgesic doses, the pattern and incidence of untoward effects caused by methadone and morphine are similar.

PROPOXYPHENE

Of the four stereoisomers, only the alpha racemate, known as *propoxyphene,* has analgesic activity. Its analgesic effect resides in the dextrorotatory isomer, *d*-propoxyphene (dextropropoxyphene). However, levopropoxyphene seems to have some antitussive activity. As can be seen from the following formula, propoxyphene is related structurally to methadone.

Propoxyphene

Pharmacological Actions. Propoxyphene binds to opioid receptors and produces analgesia and other CNS effects that are qualitatively similar to those seen with codeine and other opioids. It has no significant antipyretic or anti-inflammatory effects. It is likely that at equianalgesic doses the incidence of side effects such as nausea, anorexia, constipation, abdominal pain, and drowsiness would be similar to those of codeine.

There is some question about the minimal dosage required to relieve pain in clinical situations. Most studies have reported that 32 mg of propoxyphene is no better than a placebo; higher doses produce analgesia somewhat more reliably. Beaver (1966) estimated that it requires 90 to 120 mg of propoxyphene hydrochloride administered orally to equal the analgesic effects of 60 mg of codeine, a dose that usually produces about as much analgesia as 600 mg of aspirin. The statement that, at the usual clinical dosage, propoxyphene or codeine is no more effective than aspirin is probably true, but it can be misleading. The analgesic effectiveness of aspirin in relieving moderate pain, especially where there is inflammation, has been repeatedly demonstrated; it is about one fifth to one tenth as potent as codeine, depending on the clinical situation. Since 30 to 60 mg of codeine given orally sometimes produces no more analgesia than placebo (*see* Cooper and Beaver, 1976; Bloomfield *et al.,* 1977), it is not surprising that 32 mg of the less potent propoxyphene hydrochloride is often of marginal value. Higher doses of either propoxyphene or codeine would probably yield more analgesia, although the inci-

dence of side effects is also greater. Furthermore, combinations of propoxyphene and aspirin (like combinations of codeine and aspirin) afford a higher level of analgesia than does either agent given alone (*see* Lasagna, 1964; Beaver, 1966; Moertel, 1976).

Absorption, Fate, and Excretion. Propoxyphene is absorbed after oral or parenteral administration. After oral administration the water-soluble hydrochloride appears to be absorbed somewhat more rapidly than the relatively water-insoluble napsylate. However, differences in peak plasma concentrations between the two preparations are small. Concentrations in plasma reach their highest values at about 2 hours, then slowly decrease. The mean half-life of propoxyphene following oral administration is approximately 12 hours (Wolen *et al.,* 1975). With repeated oral administration every 6 hours, plasma concentrations increase, reaching a steady state after 1 to 2 days. There is great variability between subjects in terms of the plasma concentrations that are achieved; metabolism of propoxyphene may be more rapid in smokers. In man, the major route of metabolism is N-demethylation to yield norpropoxyphene, which is then slowly excreted in the urine (McMahon *et al.,* 1971; *see also* Misra, 1978).

Toxicity. In the usual therapeutic doses propoxyphene produces no significant effects on the cardiovascular system. Given orally, it is approximately one third as potent as orally administered codeine in depressing respiration (Bellville and Seed, 1968). Moderately toxic doses usually produce CNS and respiratory depression, but with still larger doses the clinical picture may be complicated by convulsions in addition to respiratory depression. Delusions, hallucinations, and confusion have also been noted following the ingestion of toxic doses, and deaths due to propoxyphene overdosage are often accompanied by pulmonary edema. Respiratory depressant effects are significantly enhanced when alcohol or sedative-hypnotic agents are ingested concurrently, and deaths have occurred when excessive quantities of propoxyphene have been taken in conjunction with such agents. Naloxone reverses the toxic effects of propoxyphene, but the effects of other antagonists such as nalorphine seem to be more variable.

Liability for Abuse. Very large doses (800 mg of the hydrochloride or 1200 mg of the napsylate per day) reduce the intensity of the morphine withdrawal syndrome somewhat less effectively than do 1500-mg doses of codeine. Maximal tolerated doses are equivalent to daily doses of 20 to 25 mg of morphine, given subcutaneously, or 10 mg of methadone. It does not appear to be longer acting than morphine in suppressing withdrawal (Jasinski *et al.,* 1977). For most would-be abusers, use of higher doses of propoxyphene is prevented by untoward side effects and the occurrence of toxic psychoses. When very large doses are used in morphine-tolerant addicts, some respiratory depression is seen, suggesting that there is not a high degree of cross-tolerance between propoxyphene and morphine. Abrupt discontinuation of chronically administered propoxyphene hydrochloride (up to 800 mg per day, given for almost 2 months) results in mild abstinence phenomena, and large oral doses (300 to 600 mg) produce subjective effects that are considered pleasurable by postaddicts. Administered intravenously, it is recognized as an opioid; however, the drug is quite irritating when administered either intravenously or subcutaneously, so that abuse by these routes results in severe damage to veins and soft tissues, which limits the time the drug can be used parenterally.

Although propoxyphene has less potential for abuse than codeine, the incidence of abuse (corrected for the number of equianalgesic doses) has been approximately the same as with codeine. Further, some patients who have consumed very large overdoses of propoxyphene (about 1 g or more) have died. For these reasons, propoxyphene has been placed in schedule IV of the Controlled Substances Act in the United States (*see* Appendix I).

Preparations, Route of Administration, Dosage, and Therapeutic Uses. Although it has been used experimentally for the suppression of withdrawal symptoms in cases of opioid addiction (*see* Jasinski *et al.*, 1977), the only recognized use of propoxyphene is for the treatment of mild-to-moderate pain that is not adequately relieved by aspirin. When appropriate doses are selected, combinations of aspirin and propoxyphene can be as effective as the combination of codeine and aspirin. However, the latter combination is considerably less costly; inasmuch as the situations calling for analgesics of this type are commonly chronic conditions, the factor of cost cannot be discounted. The current wide popularity of propoxyphene in clinical situations in which codeine was once used seems to be largely a result of unrealistic overconcern about the addictive potential of codeine.

The drug is available as *Propoxyphene Hydrochloride*, U.S.P. (DARVON, DOLENE, others), and as *Propoxyphene Napsylate*, U.S.P. (DARVON-N). Capsules of the hydrochloride contain 32 or 65 mg; tablets of the napsylate contain 100 mg (equivalent to 65 mg of the hydrochloride), and a suspension is available at concentrations of 10 mg/ml. Combinations of propoxyphene with aspirin or acetaminophen are also marketed in a variety of dosage forms.

OPIOID ANTAGONISTS AND AGONIST-ANTAGONISTS

The concept of antagonism of the actions of opioids is relatively complex. There are probably several subspecies of opioid receptor, each with its own set of affinities for exogenous drugs and endogenous ligands and each apparently mediating different effects when activated. There is no theoretical reason to expect that any substance would have identical activities at these various binding sites. Among the opioids already studied, there are compounds that appear to exhibit saturable, stereospecific binding at one subtype of receptor while exerting little agonistic activity; yet they can bind and exert strong agonistic actions at another. *Naloxone* comes closest to being a relatively pure competitive antagonist; however, it, too, varies considerably in its capacity to antagonize the agonistic actions of other substances at different subspecies of receptor.

On the basis of pharmacological actions in man and experimental animals, Martin and coworkers (Martin *et al.*, 1976; Gilbert and Martin, 1977) have postulated the existence of three subspecies of opioid receptors, designated μ, κ, and σ. Within this framework, the μ receptor is involved in the production of supraspinal analgesia, respiratory depression, euphoria, and physical dependence. Some drugs may also have activity at κ receptors, which, when activated, induce spinal analgesia, miosis, and sedation. The action of κ-receptor agonists on respiratory function has not been studied in depth. However, the κ agonists nalorphine and pentazocine do cause a modest degree of respiratory depression. The drug *ethylketocyclazocine* appears to be a selective κ-receptor agonist and acts at spinal and supraspinal sites. To what extent supraspinal sites are involved in its analgesic activity in man is not known. Activation of σ receptors causes dysphoria and hallucinations, as well as respiratory and vasomotor stimulatory effects. Since all of the actions of known opioids cannot be explained within this model, it is possible that other subspecies of receptors will be identified. A receptor distinct from the μ receptor and designated δ has been described in the mouse vas deferens (Lord *et al.*, 1977); its relationship to the κ and σ receptors is still unclear. Most opioids and opioid antagonists appear to have different affinities for the different receptors.

The drugs discussed in the previous sections are thought to exert their agonistic actions primarily at the μ receptor, and to a lesser degree at the κ receptor. The drugs to be discussed in this section presumably bind to the μ receptor and can therefore compete with other substances for these sites, but either they exert no actions (*i.e.*, they are *competitive antagonists* at the μ receptor) or they exert only limited actions (*i.e.*, they are *partial agonists* at the μ receptor). Drugs such as nalorphine and cyclazocine, which are competitive antagonists at the μ receptor (and block the effects of morphine-like drugs), exert agonistic actions at the κ and σ receptors. The term *agonist-antagonist* has evolved to describe this complex pattern of actions. As mentioned, there are a few drugs that appear to act as partial agonists at one receptor type or another. Such drugs exhibit a ceiling effect. They can substitute for a morphine-like drug (μ-receptor agonist) when there are low levels of physical dependence, but they precipitate signs and symptoms of abstinence in subjects who are dependent on high levels of a morphine-like agonist. While they are primarily μ-receptor agonists, they can under certain circumstances reduce total agonistic activity by displacement of a stronger agonist.

The concepts of multiple types of receptors for opioids and of partial agonists remain only inferences from pharmacological experiments. However, some of the observations that are explained by these constructs are described below.

Drugs such as nalorphine and cyclazocine prevent or reverse most of the effects of morphine-like opioids, but in the absence of opioids they produce analgesia, cause constriction of the pupil, depress respiration, and induce a type of physical dependence; these effects are clearly similar to those of morphine and related opioid agonists. However, they also differ from morphine-like agonists in several respects. Among these are the following: (1) some antagonists (*e.g.*, nalorphine, cyclazocine) produce psychotomimetic and other subjective effects that are qualitatively distinct from those produced by morphine; (2) antagonists of the nalorphine type produce a form of physical dependence that results in a withdrawal syndrome that is qualitatively distinct from that seen after withdrawal of morphine; (3) the antagonists pentazocine, cyclazocine, and nalorphine produce a type of analgesia in experimental animals that differs from that of morphine—they clearly interrupt nociceptive input in the spinal cord, while morphine also acts at supraspinal loci in producing analgesia; (4) study of the interactions between morphine and nalorphine give rise to a biphasic curve, in which lower doses of nalorphine antagonize the effects of morphine while larger doses produce a lesser degree of antagonism; (5) when various opioids and synthetic analogs of met-enkephalin and leu-enkephalin are tested in two distinct bioassay preparations (guinea pig ileum and mouse vas deferens) and in binding studies *in vitro*, their potency ratios in the two preparations vary widely, as does the amount of naloxone required to antagonize their effects.

There are several reasons to believe that certain drugs that bind to opioid receptors (*e.g.*, nalorphine, propiram, and buprenorphine) act as *partial agonists*. Their dose-response curves exhibit a ceiling effect, in which their maximal effect is less than that produced by a strong agonist such as morphine. Furthermore, partial agonists will precipitate withdrawal in subjects who are dependent on a high level of a strong agonist but substitute for the agonist at lower levels of dependency. The actions of some prototypical opioids and antagonists at postulated receptors are listed in Table 22–4.

Chemistry and Structure-Activity Relationship. Relatively minor changes in the structure of an opioid can convert a drug that is primarily an agonist into one with antagonistic actions at one or more of the receptor subtypes. The most common such substitution is that of a larger moiety (*e.g.*, an allyl or methylcyclopropyl group) for the N-methyl group on an opioid such as codeine, morphine, or levorphanol. Such substitutions sometimes produce congeners that are relatively pure antagonists, such as naloxone, but more often produce drugs that are agonist-antagonists. Some agonist-antagonists have profiles of action that are distinctly different from those of morphine and seem to exert their actions primarily at μ or σ receptors. The close structural similarities

Table 22–4. SUMMARY OF THE ACTIONS OF PROTOTYPICAL AGONISTS, ANTAGONISTS, AND AGONIST-ANTAGONISTS AT HYPOTHETICAL SUBTYPES OF OPIOID RECEPTOR

COMPOUND	RECEPTOR TYPES [*]		
	μ	κ	σ
Morphine	Ag [†]	Ag	—
Naloxone [‡]	Ant	Ant	Ant
Pentazocine	Ant	Ag	Ag
Nalorphine	Ant	pAg	Ag
Buprenorphine	pAg	—	
Propiram	pAg	—	
N-allyl-normetazocine	Ant		Ag

[*] The μ receptor is thought to mediate supraspinal analgesia, respiratory depression, euphoria, and physical dependence; the κ receptor, spinal analgesia, miosis, and sedation; the σ receptor, dysphoria, hallucinations, and respiratory and vasomotor stimulation. *See* text for further explanation.

[†] Ag = agonist; Ant = competitive antagonist; pAg = partial agonist; the absence of an entry means that the compound has not yet been fully studied; — = no significant action.

[‡] Naloxone is more potent in antagonizing the effects of μ agonists than κ or σ agonists and is thus thought to have the highest affinity for the μ receptor.

between agonists and antagonists related to morphine are illustrated in Table 22–1. The chemistry and the structure-activity relationship of the opioid antagonists have been reviewed by Archer and associates (1973) and Harris (1974). For recent references, *see* Barnett and coworkers (1978).

PHARMACOLOGICAL PROPERTIES

The pharmacological actions of opioid antagonists and agonist-antagonists depend upon whether another opioid-like substance has been administered previously and the degree to which physical dependence has developed to that substance.

Effects in the Absence of Opioid Drugs. *Naloxone* is almost devoid of agonistic effects. In man, subcutaneous doses up to 12 mg produce no discernible subjective effects, and 24 mg causes only slight drowsiness. *Naltrexone* also appears to be a relatively pure antagonist, but with higher oral efficacy and a longer duration of action (Martin *et al.*, 1973b; Verebey *et al.*, 1976).

The subjective effects of *nalorphine* in man depend largely upon the dose, the subject, and the situation. In patients with postoperative pain, a dose of 10 to 15 mg of nalorphine is about as effective as 10 mg of morphine in producing analgesia. While most patients relax and become drowsy, a significant percentage experience unpleasant reactions that range from anxiety, "crazy feelings," and vivid, disturbing, "unreal" daydreams to frank hallucinatory phenomena, usually visual. Other side effects include difficulty in focusing the eyes, sweating, nausea, and the feeling of being groggy or drunk and of being sleepy but unable to sleep. These dysphoric and psychotomimetic effects appear more frequently as the dose is increased, but there is not a consistent increase in analgesia. Postaddicts report that the effects of low doses of nalorphine are more like those of short-acting barbiturates or alcohol than those of morphine. The dysphoric effects can be antagonized by large doses of naloxone.

Nalorphine produces some degree of respiratory depression and certain autonomic effects, such as lowering of body temperature and miosis. In contrast to morphine, the respiratory depression produced by nalorphine does not increase as the dose is raised. For example, a dose of 75 mg does not produce significantly greater respiratory depression than is seen with 10 to 20 mg. Nalorphine might thus be considered to have only antagonistic actions at the μ receptor, but significant agonistic actions at the κ and σ receptors. It requires a considerably higher dose of naloxone to antagonize the effects of nalorphine than those of morphine.

Although high doses of antagonists might be expected to alter the actions of *endogenous* opioid-like peptides, the detectable effects are both subtle and limited. This remains a paradox. While in man naloxone alters the analgesia induced by placebos and acupuncture, it does not decrease tolerance for experimentally induced pain (Grevert and Goldstein, 1978). The effects of both naloxone and naltrexone on mood are minimal (Gritz et al., 1976; Verebey et al., 1976). Oral doses of more than 1 g of naloxone have been administered without producing any major subjective or physiological effects (Zaks et al., 1971). Naloxone may increase concentrations of LH and FSH in plasma and decrease those of prolactin and GH, consistent with the hypothesis that endogenous opioid-like substances play a role in regulation of pituitary function (Bruni et al., 1977).

Antagonistic Actions. Small doses (0.4 to 0.8 mg) of *naloxone* given intramuscularly or intravenously in man prevent or promptly reverse the effects of morphine-like opioid agonists. In patients with respiratory depression, there is an increase in respiratory rate within 1 or 2 minutes. Sedative effects are reversed, and blood pressure, if depressed, returns to normal. One milligram of naloxone intravenously completely blocks the effects of 25 mg of heroin (Zaks et al., 1971). Antagonistic effects last from 1 to 4 hours, depending on the dose of naloxone. It can also reverse the psychotomimetic and dysphoric effects of agonist-antagonists such as pentazocine, but higher doses (10 to 15 mg) are required. Antagonism of opioid effects by naloxone is often accompanied by "over-

shoot" phenomena; for example, respiratory rate depressed by opioids transiently becomes higher than that prior to the period of depression. This "overshoot" is probably related to the "unmasking" of acute physical dependence (*see* below).

Although the antagonistic effects of opioid antagonists are seen most dramatically in the presence of opioid agonists and agonist-antagonists, antagonism of the analgesic and respiratory depressant effects on nonopioids in both animals and man has been reported. In rats, naloxone antagonizes the analgesia produced by nitrous oxide. In the spinal dog, naltrexone antagonizes some of the depressant effects of pentobarbital (Gilbert and Martin, 1977). Antagonism of depressant actions of diazepam by naloxone has also been reported in man. Pure opioid antagonists such as naloxone, which produce no respiratory depression themselves, may thus have significant advantages in situations where the etiology of the respiratory depression is not clear.

Nalorphine also prevents or abolishes opioid-induced CNS and gastrointestinal effects, with certain minor exceptions. The antagonism of severe opioid-induced respiratory depression is seen within 1 or 2 minutes after the intravenous injection of 5 to 10 mg of nalorphine and lasts 1 to 4 hours. Patients may not show complete reversal of sedative effects.

The degree of opioid antagonism observed depends not only on the dose of the antagonist but also on which opioid has been given and the degree to which physical dependence has developed. Thus, 10 mg of nalorphine does not antagonize the relatively mild respiratory depression produced by 10 mg of morphine, perhaps because its antagonistic effects at the μ receptor are counterbalanced by its own weak respiratory depressant activity. However, smaller doses of nalorphine antagonize the severe depression produced by 70 mg of morphine. In patients who are physically dependent, very small doses (2 to 5 mg) of nalorphine or small doses of naloxone may be sufficient not only to antagonize respiratory depression but also to precipitate withdrawal phenomena. In such individuals, large doses of opioid antagonists can produce severe withdrawal symptoms.

Effects in Physical Dependence. In subjects who are dependent on morphine-like opioids, small subcutaneous doses of naloxone (0.5 mg) precipitate a moderate-to-severe withdrawal syndrome that is very similar to that seen after abrupt withdrawal of opioids, except that the syndrome appears within minutes after administration and subsides in about 2 hours. The severity and duration of the syndrome are related to the dose of the antagonist and the degree and type of dependence. Higher doses of naloxone will precipitate withdrawal from pentazocine, butorphanol, or nalbuphine.

Naloxone produces "overshoot" phenomena suggestive of early acute physical dependence 24 hours after a single large dose of morphine, and it precipitates withdrawal symptoms 5 days after a single 40-mg dose of methadone (Nutt and Jasinski, 1974). Antagonists of the nalorphine type do not precipitate withdrawal symptoms after chronic use of pentazocine, but do precipitate a morphine type of withdrawal syndrome following use of propiram.

Tolerance, Physical Dependence, and Liability for Abuse. Tolerance develops to the agonistic but not to the antagonistic effects of opioid agonist-antagonists and partial agonists. Tolerance to the subjective effects, including the dysphoric and the psychotomimetic responses to both nalorphine and cyclazocine, has been demonstrated in man; cross-tolerance between these agents has also been shown (see Martin, 1967). However, even in subjects highly tolerant to the dysphoric, sedative, and motor effects of cyclazocine, a small (4-mg) dose continues to prevent the euphoric, miotic, respiratory depressant, and physical dependence-producing properties of morphine and heroin.

Even after prolonged administration of high doses, discontinuation of naloxone is not followed by any recognizable withdrawal syndrome, and the withdrawal of naltrexone, another relatively pure antagonist, produces very few signs and symptoms. However, after chronic administration of high dosage, abrupt discontinuation of either nalorphine or cyclazocine causes a characteristic withdrawal syndrome that is similar for both drugs. One early sign is repeated brief episodes of a sensation that is described by some subjects as "electric shocks to the head" and by others as light-headedness or fainting spells. It does not appear to be a convulsive phenomenon, and consciousness is not lost. Later signs and symptoms include lacrimation, rhinorrhea, yawning, chills, diarrhea, fever, and loss of appetite and body weight. Although the intensity of these withdrawal signs and symptoms in the nalorphine withdrawal syndrome is generally less than comparable manifestations of the morphine withdrawal syndrome, a more striking contrast is the absence of "craving" or drug-seeking behavior. Drug-seeking behavior is present in the syndromes that characterize withdrawal from pentazocine, butorphanol, or nalbuphine, which have characteristics of both the nalorphine- and the morphine-type withdrawal syndromes (see below).

Since nalorphine, cyclazocine, and naloxone (1) do not support physical dependence of the mor-

phine type, (2) are viewed by postaddicts as either neutral or unpleasant drugs in terms of their subjective effects, and (3) do not produce a variety of physical dependence that leads to drug-seeking behavior, they are considered to have little or no potential for abuse (for references, see Martin, 1967; Jasinski et al., 1971; Jasinski, 1973).

Absorption, Fate, and Excretion. The effects of naloxone are seen almost immediately after its intravenous administration. The drug is metabolized in the liver, primarily by conjugation with glucuronic acid; other metabolites are produced in small amounts (Weinstein et al., 1974). Following parenteral administration, the duration of action of naloxone is about 1 to 4 hours; its half-life in plasma is about 1 hour (see Misra, 1978). The drug is absorbed after oral administration, but it is metabolized so rapidly in its first passage through the liver that it is only one fiftieth as potent as when given parenterally (see Nutt and Jasinski, 1974). Oral doses of more than 1 g are almost completely metabolized in less than 24 hours.

Like naloxone, nalorphine is much more effective after parenteral than oral administration, probably because of rapid biotransformation in the liver (mainly conjugation with glucuronic acid). After parenteral administration of nalorphine, the onset of action is prompt, but the half-life is short. The onset and duration of action of levallorphan are similar to those of nalorphine.

Unlike naloxone, cyclazocine and naltrexone, both of which have cyclopropylmethyl substitutions on the nitrogen, retain much of their efficacy by the oral route, and their durations of action are longer, approaching 24 hours after moderate oral doses (see Martin et al., 1973b). In the treatment of patients addicted to opioids, naltrexone is used in large oral doses (over 100 mg) to prevent the euphorigenic effects of opioids. After such doses, peak concentrations in plasma are reached within 1 to 2 hours and then slowly decline with a half-life of 10 hours; this value does not change after chronic use. In man, naltrexone is metabolized to 6-naltrexol, which is a weak antagonist and has a longer half-life. Naltrexone is much more potent than naloxone, and 100-mg oral doses produce concentrations in tissues sufficient to block for 48 hours the effects of 25 mg of heroin (taken intravenously) (see Verebey et al., 1976).

Preparations and Route of Administration. Naloxone Hydrochloride Injection, U.S.P. (NARCAN), is available in 1-ml ampuls at a concentration of 0.4 mg/ml. It is the drug of choice in most situations where an opioid antagonistic effect is required. An injectable preparation for use in neonates (NARCAN NEONATAL) contains 0.02 mg/ml in 2-ml ampuls. Nalorphine Hydrochloride Injection, U.S.P. (NAL-

LINE), is available for pediatric use in 1-ml ampuls containing 0.2 mg. It is also available in 1-, 2-, and 10-ml ampuls containing 5 mg/ml. The dose is highly dependent on the clinical situation. *Levallorphan Tartrate Injection,* U.S.P. (LORFAN), is available in a concentration of 1 mg/ml. It is approximately ten times as potent as nalorphine, and its therapeutic indications are virtually identical. *Naltrexone* and *cyclazocine* are available only for investigational use.

Therapeutic Uses. Opioid antagonists are used in the treatment of opioid-induced respiratory depression. They are also used in the diagnosis of physical dependence on opioids and as therapeutic agents in the treatment of compulsive users of opioids, as discussed in Chapter 23. Agonist-antagonists are also used as analgesics (*see* below).

Treatment of Opioid Overdosage. The dramatic effects of opioid antagonists in reversing opioid-induced respiratory depression in the adult have already been discussed. Opioid antagonists have also been effectively employed to decrease neonatal respiratory depression secondary to the administration of opioids to the mother. When employed for this purpose, the antagonist may be given either to the mother shortly before delivery (preferable) or to the infant by way of the umbilical vein following delivery. The usual dose of naloxone is 0.4 or 0.8 mg for the mother; in the neonate, the initial dose is 10 μg/kg. There is overwhelming evidence that all known opioids, even in reasonable therapeutic doses (*e.g.,* 10 mg of morphine, 100 mg of meperidine), produce a significant increase in the incidence of depression of respiration in the neonate compared to deliveries in which no general anesthetic or opioid is used. This increased depression is not great; however, even if the use of opioid antagonists results in only a slight decrease in the incidence of such respiratory depression, their routine use would still appear justified whenever opioids are administered during labor (*see* review by Eddy *et al.,* 1957). Antagonists with agonistic actions should not be used.

Analgesia. Pure opioid antagonists are of no value as analgesics; several agonist-antagonists are now in clinical use and are discussed separately, below.

PENTAZOCINE

Pentazocine is one of the many compounds synthesized as part of a deliberate effort to develop an effective analgesic with little or no abuse potential. A benzomorphan derivative, pentazocine has both agonistic actions and weak opioid antagonistic activity. The pharmacology of pentazocine has been reviewed by Brogden and associates (1973).

Chemistry. Pentazocine, a white powder soluble in acidic aqueous solutions, has the following structural formula:

Pentazocine

The analgesic and respiratory depressant activity of the racemate is due mainly to the *l* isomer.

Pharmacological Actions. Pentazocine exerts its major effects on the CNS and smooth muscle. The pattern of *CNS effects* is generally similar to that of the opioids, including analgesia, sedation, and respiratory depression. A dose of approximately 20 mg, administered parenterally, produces the same degree of respiratory depression as does a 10-mg dose of morphine. Increasing the dose of pentazocine beyond 30 mg does not ordinarily produce proportionate increases in respiratory depression (Engineer and Jennett, 1972). However, at doses of 60 to 90 mg, nalorphine-like dysphoric and psychotomimetic effects may occur that can be antagonized by naloxone but not by nalorphine.

The effects of low doses of pentazocine on the *gastrointestinal tract* are qualitatively similar to those of the opioids; relatively small intramuscular doses (15 mg) significantly decrease gastric emptying time. However, higher doses (30 to 45 mg) increase the transit time through the intestinal tract and produce less elevation of biliary pressure than equianalgesic doses of morphine (Economou and Ward-McQuaid, 1971).

The *cardiovascular responses* to pentazocine differ from those seen with the morphine-like opioids, in that high doses cause an increase in blood pressure and heart rate. In normal subjects, pentazocine causes a decrease in effective renal plasma flow but no decrease in glomerular filtration rate (Sigman and Elwood, 1967). In patients with coronary artery disease, pentazocine (intravenously) elevates mean aortic pressure, left ventricular end-diastolic pressure, and mean pulmonary artery pressure, and causes an increase in cardiac work (Alderman *et al.,* 1972; Lee *et al.,* 1976). Pentazocine produces a rise in the concentrations of catecholamines in plasma; this may account for its effects on blood pressure (Tammisto *et al.,* 1971).

The effects of pentazocine on *uterine contractility* do not appear to differ from those of meperidine. Pentazocine also has weak opioid antagonistic activity (approximately one fiftieth as potent as nalorphine). It does not antagonize the respiratory depression produced by morphine; however, when given to patients who have been receiving opioids on a regular basis, it may precipitate opioid withdrawal symptoms (Beaver *et al.,* 1966). In patients tolerant to opioids, pentazocine reduces the analgesia produced by morphine, even when clear-cut withdrawal symptoms are not produced. Pentazocine is presumed to exert its agonistic actions at the κ and σ receptors.

Absorption, Fate, and Excretion. Pentazocine is well absorbed from the gastrointestinal tract and from subcutaneous and intramuscular sites. Concentrations in plasma coincide closely with the onset, duration, and intensity of analgesia; peak values occur 15 minutes to 1 hour after intramuscular administration and 1 to 3 hours after oral administration. The half-life in plasma is 2 to 3 hours (Berkowitz *et al.,* 1969). First-pass metabolism in the liver is extensive, and somewhat less than 20% of pentazocine enters the systemic circulation (Ehrnebo *et al.,* 1977).

Although some free pentazocine is excreted in the urine, the action of the drug is terminated largely by biotransformation in the liver; the metabolites, products of the oxidation of the terminal methyl groups and glucuronide conjugates, are excreted by the kidney. There is considerable variability between individuals in terms of rate of pentazocine metabolism, and this may account for the variability of analgesic response (*see* Brogden *et al.,* 1973). Pentazocine passes the placental barrier but to a lesser extent than does meperidine (Beckett and Taylor, 1967).

Preparations, Routes of Administration, and Dosage. *Pentazocine Lactate Injection,* U.S.P. (TALWIN), is available in 1-, 1.5-, and 2-ml ampuls and 10-ml multiple-dose vials, each milliliter containing an amount equivalent to 30 mg of the base. *Pentazocine Hydrochloride Tablets,* U.S.P., for oral use contain 50 mg of the base. It is included under schedule IV of the Controlled Substances Act (*see* Appendix I). In terms of analgesic effect, a 30- to 50-mg dose given parenterally is approximately equivalent to 10 mg of morphine. An oral dose of about 50 mg of pentazocine results in analgesia equivalent to that produced by 60 mg of codeine. In terms of peak effect, pentazocine is approximately one fourth as potent orally as parenterally; in terms of total analgesic effect, one third as potent. (*See* Beaver *et al.,* 1966, 1968; Kantor *et al.,* 1966.)

Side Effects, Toxicity, and Precautions. Side effects from pentazocine differ somewhat from those of opioids. The most commonly reported effect is sedation, followed by sweating, and dizziness or lightheadedness; nausea also occurs, but vomiting is less common than with morphine. Nalorphine-like psychotomimetic effects such as anxiety, nightmares, weird thoughts, and hallucinations have been reported. These are not common with doses in the therapeutic range but are seen with increasing frequency with doses above 60 mg. The clinical picture of overdosage has not been well defined. High doses produce marked respiratory depression associated with increased blood pressure and tachycardia. The respiratory depression is antagonized by naloxone. Pentazocine is irritating when administered subcutaneously or intramuscularly. Repeated injections over long periods may cause extensive fibrosis of subcutaneous and muscular tissue (Johnson *et al.,* 1976). Patients who have been receiving opioids on a regular basis may experience withdrawal symptoms when given pentazocine. After an opioid-free interval of 1

to 2 days, it is usually possible to administer pentazocine without producing such withdrawal effects.

Tolerance, Physical Dependence, and Liability for Abuse. With frequent and repeated use, tolerance develops to the analgesic and subjective effects of pentazocine; however, it is not clear if the rate of development of this tolerance is comparable to that seen with morphine-like opioids or is the same for all effects of the drug. When given intravenously or subcutaneously to postaddicts, pentazocine (40 mg) produces essentially morphine-like effects; when the dose is increased to 60 mg, the effects begin to resemble the nervousness and loss of energy produced by nalorphine. In contrast to morphine and other opioids, pentazocine does not prevent or ameliorate the morphine withdrawal syndrome when substituted in subjects physically dependent on morphine. Instead, when high doses of pentazocine are given to such subjects, its antagonistic actions, although weak, precipitate withdrawal symptoms.

After chronic administration (60 to 90 mg every 4 hours), postaddicts develop physical dependence that can be demonstrated by abrupt withdrawal or precipitated by naloxone but not by nalorphine. The withdrawal syndrome after chronic doses of more than 500 mg per day is similar in some respects to that seen after withdrawal of nalorphine, but it also has some of the characteristics of morphine withdrawal, including abdominal cramps, anxiety, chills, elevated temperature, vomiting, lacrimation, and sweating. Although milder in intensity, the syndrome is associated with drug-seeking behavior; that is, subjects request additional medicine to alleviate the withdrawal syndrome (Jasinski *et al.,* 1970).

On the basis of early testing, pentazocine was not believed to have a significant potential for abuse, and it was released for general use subject to no special controls. Many physicians believed that the drug had no abuse potential at all and permitted unlimited refilling of prescriptions and self-administration of the parenteral preparation by ambulatory patients. Subsequently, cases of compulsive self-administration primarily of *parenteral* pentazocine were reported. The availability of the oral preparation, greater appreciation of its potential for abuse, and more supervision by physicians and pharmacists have reduced the tendency to prescribe the parenteral form of pentazocine. Despite the absence of legal controls, pentazocine was not misused by heroin addicts to any significant extent until 1977, when the combination of pentazocine (usually extracted from the oral tablet) and the antihistamine pyribenzamine, used intravenously, became popular in the addict subculture of several large urban areas. Pentazocine was then included under schedule IV of the Controlled Substances Act. The contribution of pyribenzamine to the reinforcing effects of the combination remains uncertain. Clearly pentazocine should be used with prudence. When it is necessary to relieve pentazocine withdrawal symptoms, the predominant opinion is that this should be done with gradual reduction of pentazocine itself, rather than by substitution of low doses of methadone. A syndrome of withdrawal from pentazocine has also been observed in neonates.

Therapeutic Uses. Pentazocine is used primarily as an analgesic. Because it may be employed in situations where there is chronic severe pain or where the risk of drug dependence is higher than average (e.g., individuals with past histories of alcoholism or excessive self-administration of drugs), it is likely that cases of dependence will continue to develop. Because abuse patterns appear to be less likely to develop with oral administration, this route should be used whenever possible. The problem will remain one in which the physician must choose among a number of unattractive alternatives—inadequate relief of pain, risk of dependence on pentazocine, or risk of dependence on an opioid of higher abuse potential. Pentazocine may have advantages when it is important to minimize the risk of compulsive drug use. Other mixed agonist-antagonists now available may cause fewer side effects.

BUTORPHANOL

Butorphanol is a morphinan congener with a profile of actions similar to those of pentazocine. It has recently become available for clinical use in the United States. The structural formula of butorphanol is shown in Table 22–1.

Pharmacological Actions and Side Effects. In postoperative patients, a parenteral dose of 2 to 3 mg of butorphanol produces analgesia and respiratory depression approximately equal to that produced by 10 mg of morphine or 80 mg of meperidine; the onset, peak, and duration of action are similar to those that follow the administration of morphine (see Gilbert et al., 1976). Like pentazocine and other drugs whose actions are hypothesized to be exerted primarily on κ and σ receptors, the increase in respiratory depression is much less pronounced as the dose is increased than it is with morphine and other μ-receptor agonists (Nagashima et al., 1976). Also like pentazocine, analgesic doses of butorphanol produce an increase in pulmonary arterial pressure and in the work of the heart; systemic arterial pressure is slightly decreased (Popio et al., 1978).

The major side effects of butorphanol are drowsiness, weakness, sweating, feelings of floating, and nausea. While the incidence of psychotomimetic side effects is lower than that with equianalgesic doses of pentazocine, they are qualitatively similar (see above).

Tolerance, Physical Dependence, and Liability for Abuse. Single doses of butorphanol cause subjective effects that resemble those produced by cyclazocine, pentazocine, and nalorphine, rather than those by morphine. In subjects who are dependent on 60 mg of morphine per day, butorphanol neither suppresses nor precipitates a withdrawal syndrome. Postaddicts stabilized on 12 mg of butorphanol four times a day complain of drowsiness, constipation, difficulty in urinating, and inability to sleep. The drug is identified much more frequently as a barbiturate than as an opioid, and postaddicts express indifference or mild dislike for it. After chronic administration of butorphanol, the administration of 4 mg of naloxone

or abrupt withdrawal of the drug produces a withdrawal syndrome characterized by discomfort and requests for medicine for relief. The peak intensity of withdrawal symptoms occurs 48 hours after discontinuation and is not as severe as that seen with equianalgesic doses of morphine; it resembles the syndrome that follows the use of cyclazocine and is largely over by the eighth day. It is not clear if butorphanol will be any less subject to abuse than pentazocine. As with the latter drug, oral preparations will probably cause fewer problems than the parenteral preparation.

Therapeutic Uses, Route of Administration, Dosage, and Preparations. Since butorphanol is available only in parenteral form, it is better suited for the relief of acute rather than chronic pain. Because of its side effects on the heart, it is less useful than morphine or meperidine in patients with congestive heart failure or myocardial infarction. The usual dose is between 1 and 4 mg of the tartrate, given intramuscularly, intravenously, or subcutaneously; this may be repeated every 3 to 4 hours. *Butorphanol tartrate* (STADOL) is available in 1-ml vials containing 1 mg and in 1-, 2-, and 10-ml vials at a concentration of 2 mg/ml. The drug is not currently listed in any schedule of the Controlled Substances Act.

NALBUPHINE

Pharmacological Actions and Side Effects. Nalbuphine is structurally related to both naloxone and oxymorphine (see Table 22–1). It produces analgesia and weak antagonist effects, hypothetically by actions at μ receptors. An intramuscular dose of 10 mg causes analgesia equivalent to that which follows the administration of 10 mg of morphine; the onset and duration of both analgesic and subjective effects are similar to those of morphine (Jasinski and Mansky, 1972; Beaver and Feise, 1978). Nalbuphine depresses respiration as much as do equianalgesic doses of morphine; however, nalbuphine exhibits a ceiling effect, such that increases in dosage beyond 30 mg produce no further respiratory depression. In contrast to pentazocine and butorphanol, 10 mg of nalbuphine given to patients with stable coronary artery disease does not produce an increase in cardiac index, pulmonary arterial pressure, or cardiac work, and systemic blood pressure is not significantly altered (Romagnoli and Keats, 1978). Its gastrointestinal effects are probably similar to those of pentazocine. Nalbuphine produces few side effects at doses of 10 mg or less; sedation, sweating, and headache are the most common. Side effects resemble those of nalorphine at much higher doses (70 mg) (dysphoria, racing thoughts, and distortions of body image). Nalbuphine is metabolized in the liver and has a half-life in plasma of about 5 hours.

Tolerance, Physical Dependence, and Liability for Abuse. Postaddicts "like" the effects of single (8-mg) doses of nalbuphine as much as they do those of morphine. When the dose of nalbuphine is increased to 72 mg, the degree of "liking" and euphoria is increased only slightly, and sedative as well as nalorphine-like side effects (racing thoughts, sensory distortion) begin to occur. High doses of nalbuphine are more likely to be identified as a barbiturate than as an opiate.

In subjects dependent on low doses of morphine (60 mg per day), nalbuphine precipitates an abstinence syndrome. As an antagonist, it is one fourth as potent as nalorphine (Jasinski and Mansky, 1972). During the first week of chronic administration, experimental subjects are relaxed and enjoy the drugged feeling; they usually identify nalbuphine as morphine-like, but occasionally as a barbiturate or an amphetamine. After 7 days (daily dose of 142 mg), subjects begin to complain of headache, difficulty in concentration, strange thoughts and dreams, irritability, and depression. Although complaints persist, some subjects continue to tolerate these effects; in these subjects, the administration of 4 mg of naloxone (but not 30 mg of nalorphine) produces an abstinence syndrome. Subjects describe this as morphine-like withdrawal and demand drugs for relief. The syndrome is similar in intensity to that seen with pentazocine, and symptoms are greatly diminished by the seventh day. The potential for abuse of nalbuphine is probably similar to that of pentazocine.

Therapeutic Uses, Route of Administration, Dosage, and Preparations. Nalbuphine can be used to produce analgesia in a variety of painful syndromes. However, because it is an agonist-antagonist, administration to patients who have been receiving morphine-like opioids may create difficulties unless a brief drug-free interval is interposed. *Nalbuphine hydrochloride* (NUBAIN) is supplied as an injectable solution for intramuscular, subcutaneous, or intravenous use in 1- and 2-ml ampuls and 10-ml multiple-dose vials that contain 10 mg/ml.

BUPRENORPHINE

Buprenorphine is a semisynthetic, highly lipophilic opioid derived from thebaine (Table 22–1). It is 25 to 50 times more potent than morphine.

Pharmacological Actions and Side Effects. Buprenorphine produces analgesia and other CNS effects that are qualitatively similar to those of morphine. About 0.4 mg of buprenorphine is equianalgesic with 10 mg of morphine given intramuscularly. While the duration of analgesia may be somewhat longer than with morphine, the subjective and respiratory depressant effects are unequivocally slower in onset and last longer than those of morphine. Peak miosis occurs about 6 hours after intramuscular injection, while maximal respiratory depression is observed at about 3 hours.

In receptor binding studies, buprenorphine behaves like an antagonist (judged by the effect of Na$^+$ on affinity). In abstinent, morphine-dependent dogs, buprenorphine suppresses signs of withdrawal, while in stabilized opioid-dependent dogs, it precipitates withdrawal. Depending on dose, buprenorphine may cause symptoms of abstinence in patients who have been receiving morphine-like drugs (μ-receptor agonists) for several weeks (Houde, 1979). Although

respiratory depression has not been a major problem in clinical trials, the respiratory depressant actions of buprenorphine are not readily reversed, even by high doses of naloxone (4 to 16 mg). It is not clear whether respiratory depression exhibits a ceiling, as is seen with nalbuphine and pentazocine. Cardiovascular effects appear to be similar to those of morphine. Side effects are similar to those of other opioids and include sedation, nausea, vomiting, dizziness, sweating, and headache.

Buprenorphine is relatively well absorbed by most routes, including the sublingual; 0.4 to 0.8 mg of the drug administered sublingually produces satisfactory analgesia in postoperative patients. Concentrations in blood peak 2 hours after oral ingestion and persist for more than a day. Both N-dealkylated and conjugated metabolites are detected in the urine, but most of the drug is excreted unchanged in the feces. About 96% of the circulating drug is bound to protein.

Tolerance, Physical Dependence, and Liability for Abuse. In postaddicts, subcutaneous doses of buprenorphine ranging from 0.2 to 2 mg produce typical morphine-like effects, including euphoria and pupillary constriction. Miosis is detectable for 72 hours, as is a subtle feeling of lethargy.

During chronic administration of 8 mg of buprenorphine per day, subjects identify the drug as morphine-like and "like" the effects as much as comparable subjects receiving 120 mg of morphine daily. In these subjects, naloxone, in doses sufficient to produce severe withdrawal in addicts who are dependent on morphine, pentazocine, or butorphanol, does not precipitate a withdrawal syndrome; at the same time, the subjective and physiological effects of subcutaneous morphine (in doses of up to 120 mg) are prevented or markedly attenuated. This attenuation or "blockade" persists for more than 30 hours after the last dose of buprenorphine.

When discontinued, a withdrawal syndrome develops that is delayed in onset (some subjects report symptoms after the second to third day; others not until the fifteenth day), consists in typical morphine-like withdrawal signs and symptoms, and persists for about 1 to 2 weeks. Subjects describe the intensity as mild to moderate, but they demand drugs for relief. Overall, the potential for abuse of buprenorphine is probably less than that of morphine (Jasinski *et al.,* 1978).

Therapeutic Uses, Route of Administration, and Dosage. *Buprenorphine* (TEMGESIC) may be used as an analgesic; its use as a maintenance drug for opioid-dependent subjects has also been proposed. Buprenorphine is available for parenteral use as the hydrochloride in 1- and 2-ml ampuls containing 0.3 mg/ml. The usual dose is 0.3 to 0.6 mg, given every 6 to 8 hours.

NONOPIOID ANTITUSSIVES

Cough is a useful physiological mechanism serving to clear the respiratory passages of foreign material and excess secretions. It should not be suppressed indiscriminately. There are, however, many situations in which cough does not serve any useful purpose but may, instead, only annoy the patient or prevent rest and sleep. In such situations the physician should use a drug that will reduce the frequency or intensity of the coughing. The cough reflex is complex, involving the central and peripheral nervous systems as well as the smooth muscle of the bronchial tree. It has been suggested that irritation of the bronchial mucosa causes bronchoconstriction, which, in turn, stimulates cough receptors (which probably represent a specialized type of stretch receptor) located in tracheobronchial passages (*see* Salem and Aviado, 1970). Afferent conduction from these receptors is via fibers in the vagus nerve; central components of the reflex probably involve several mechanisms or centers that are distinct from the mechanisms involved in the regulation of respiration.

The drugs that can affect this complex mechanism directly or indirectly are quite diverse. For example, drugs that cause bronchodilation could alter the initiation of coughing without having any significant central effects; other drugs might act primarily on the central or the peripheral nervous system components of the cough reflex. The literature on antitussives has been exhaustively reviewed by Eddy and associates (1969) and by Salem and Aviado (1970). This section describes a few of the many drugs that have been in clinical use and that are believed to act on the nervous system in modifying cough.

A number of drugs are known to reduce cough as a result of their central actions, although the exact mechanisms are still not entirely clear. Included among them are the opioid analgesics discussed above (codeine, hydrocodone, and hydromorphone are the opioids most commonly used to prevent cough) as well as a number of nonopioid agents. In selecting a specific agent for a particular patient, *the advantages of a low abuse potential per se should not be overvalued.* It is true that opioid addicts who cannot obtain their drug of choice, and occasionally adolescents seeking new experiences, often turn to cough preparations containing opioids or to paregoric; however, despite the extensive use and ready availability of such

preparations, the number of persons dependent on them is exceedingly small. Nonopioid antitussives having no significant liability for abuse would seem to be most advantageous in treating *chronic cough* or in treating individuals who seem *psychologically predisposed* to drug dependence; nevertheless, in the overwhelming majority of situations requiring a cough suppressant, liability for abuse need not be a major consideration.

Much more significant considerations are the *antitussive efficacy against pathological cough* and the *incidence of side effects.* Most of the nonopioid agents now offered as antitussives are effective against cough induced by a variety of experimental technics. Some of these technics are able to distinguish 30 mg of codeine from a placebo, but their validity for predicting clinical efficacy is still open to question.

Dextromethorphan. *Dextromethorphan* (*d*-3-methoxy-N-methylmorphinan) is the *d* isomer of the codeine analog of levorphanol; however, unlike the *l* isomer, it has no analgesic or addictive properties. The drug acts centrally to elevate the threshold for coughing. Its effectiveness in patients with pathological cough has been demonstrated in controlled studies, where it was found to be about the equal of codeine. Unlike codeine, it rarely produces drowsiness or gastrointestinal disturbances. In therapeutic dosage the drug does not inhibit ciliary activity. Its toxicity is quite low, but extremely high doses may produce CNS depression.

Dextromethorphan Hydrobromide, U.S.P., is available as a syrup containing 15 mg/5 ml. The average adult dose is 15 to 30 mg, three to four times daily; however, as is the case with codeine, higher doses are often required. *Terpin Hydrate and Dextromethorphan Hydrobromide Elixir,* U.S.P., containing 10 mg/5 ml, is also available. The drug is generally marketed for "over-the-counter" sale in syrups and lozenges, or in combinations with an antihistamine for prescription orders under multiple brand names in many countries throughout the world.

Levopropoxyphene Napsylate, U.S.P. (NOVRAD), in doses of 50 to 100 mg orally appears to suppress cough to about the same degree as does 30 mg of dextromethorphan. Unlike dextropropoxyphene, levopropoxyphene has little or no analgesic activity. It is available in 100-mg capsules and as a suspension containing 50 mg/ml.

Noscapine is a naturally occurring opium alkaloid of the benzylisoquinoline group; except for its antitussive effect, it has no significant actions on the CNS in doses within the therapeutic range. In dogs, the drug is a potent releaser of histamine, and large doses cause bronchoconstriction and transient hypotension. Toxic doses produce convulsions in animals. The average adult dose is 15 to 30 mg, three or four times daily, but single doses of 60 mg have been used. It is the primary ingredient in several proprietary mixtures.

Other drugs that have been used as centrally acting antitussives include *carbetapentane, caramiphen,* and *diphenhydramine.* Each is a member of a distinct pharmacological class unrelated to the opioids; in general their toxicity is low, but controlled clinical studies are still insufficient to determine whether they merit consideration as alternatives to more thoroughly studied agents.

Benzonatate, U.S.P. (TESSALON), is a long-chain polyglycol derivative chemically related to procaine and believed to exert its antitussive action on stretch or cough receptors in the lung, as well as by a central mechanism. It has been administered by all routes; the oral dose is about 100 mg, but higher doses have been used.

Akil, A.; Watson, S. J.; Holman, R. B.; and Barchas, J. D. Parallels between the neuromodulator mechanisms of stimulation analgesia and morphine analgesia. In, *Factors Affecting the Action of Narcotics.* (Adler, M. L.; Manara, L.; and Samanin, R.; eds.) Raven Press, New York, **1978,** pp. 565–578.

Alderman, E. L.; Barry, W. H.; Graham, A. F.; and Harrison, D. C. Hemodynamic effects of morphine and pentazocine differ in cardiac patients. *N. Engl. J. Med.,* **1972,** *287,* 623–627.

Beaver, W. T., and Feise, G. Comparison of the analgesic effects of morphine, hydroxyzine, and their combination in patients with postoperative pain. In, *Advances in Pain Research and Therapy,* Vol. 1. (Bonica, J. J., and Albe-Fessard, D., eds.) Raven Press, New York, **1976,** pp. 553–557.

———. A comparison of the analgesic effect of intramuscular nalbuphine and morphine in patients with postoperative pain. *J. Pharmacol. Exp. Ther.,* **1978,** *204,* 487–496.

Beaver, W. T.; Wallenstein, S. L.; Houde, R. W.; and Rogers, A. A comparison of the analgesic effects of pentazocine and morphine in patients with cancer. *Clin. Pharmacol. Ther.,* **1966,** *7,* 740–751.

———. A clinical comparison of the analgesic effects of methadone and morphine administered intramuscularly, and of orally and parenterally administered methadone. *Ibid.,* **1967,** *8,* 415–426.

———. A clinical comparison of the effects of oral and intramuscular administration of analgesics: pentazocine and phenazocine. *Ibid.,* **1968,** *9,* 582–597.

Beckett, A. H., and Taylor, J. F. Blood concentrations of pethidine and pentazocine in mother and infant at time of birth. *J. Pharm. Pharmacol.,* **1967,** *19,* Suppl., 50s–52s.

Bellville, J. W., and Forrest, W. H., Jr. Respiratory and subjective effects of *d-* and *l-*pentazocine. *Clin. Pharmacol. Ther.,* **1968,** *9,* 142–151.

Bellville, J. W.; Forrest, W. H., Jr.; Miller, E.; and Brown, B. W. Influence of age on pain relief from analgesics. *J.A.M.A.,* **1971,** *217,* 1835–1841.

Bellville, J. W., and Seed, J. C. A comparison of the respiratory depressant effects of dextropropoxyphene and codeine in man. *Clin. Pharmacol. Ther.,* **1968,** *9,* 428–434.

Berkowitz, B. A.; Asling, J. H.; Shnider, S. M.; and Way, E. L. Relationship of pentazocine plasma levels to pharmacological activity in man. *Clin. Pharmacol. Ther.,* **1969,** *10,* 320–328.

Bloomfield, S. S.; Barden, T. P.; and Mitchell, J. Naproxen, aspirin and codeine in postpartum uterine pain. *Clin. Pharmacol. Ther.,* **1977,** *21,* 414–421.

Bruni, J. F.; Van Vugt, D.; Marshall, S.; and Meites, J. Effects of naloxone, morphine and methionine enkephalin on serum prolactin, luteinizing hormone, follicle stimulating hormone, thyroid stimulating hormone and growth hormone. *Life Sci.,* **1977,** *21,* 461–466.

Brunk, S. F., and Delle, M. Morphine metabolism in man. *Clin. Pharmacol. Ther.,* **1974,** *16,* 51–57.

Campbell, C.; Phillips, O. C.; and Frazier, T. M. Analgesia during labor: a comparison of pentobarbital, meperidine, and morphine. *Obstet. Gynecol.,* **1961,** *17,* 714–718.

Chakravarty, N. K.; Matallana, A.; Jensen, R.; and Borison, H. L. Central effects of antitussive drugs on cough and respiration. *J. Pharmacol. Exp. Ther.,* **1956,** *117,* 127–135.

Challenor, Y. B.; Richter, R. W.; Brunn, B.; and Pearson, J. Nontraumatic plexitis and heroin addiction. *J.A.M.A.,* **1973,** *225,* 958–961.

Chang, K.-J.; Cooper, B. R.; Hazum, E.; and Cuatrecasas, P. Multiple opiate receptors: different regional distribution in the brain and differential binding of opiates and opioid peptides. *Mol. Pharmacol.,* **1979,** *16,* 91–104.

Chang, K.-J., and Cuatrecasas, P. Multiple opiate receptors. *J. Biol. Chem.,* **1979,** *254,* 2610–2618.

Chapman, W. P.; Rowlands, E. N.; and Jones, C. M. Multiple-balloon kymographic recording of the comparative action of DEMEROL, morphine and placebos on the motility of the upper small intestine in man. *N. Engl. J. Med.,* **1950,** *243,* 171–177.

Clouet, D. H.; O'Callaghan, J. P.; and Williams, N. Inhibition of calcium-stimulated protein kinase activity in striatal synaptic membranes by opioids. In, *Characteristics and Function of Opioids.* (Ree, J. van, and Terenius, L., eds.) Elsevier/North Holland Biomedical Press, New York, **1978,** pp. 351–352.

Cooper, S. A., and Beaver, W. T. A model to evaluate mild analgesics in oral surgery outpatients. *Clin. Pharmacol. Ther.,* **1976,** *20,* 241–250.

Cox, B. M.; Opheim, K.; Teschemacher, H.; and Goldstein, A. A peptide-like substance from pituitary that acts like morphine. 2. Purification and properties. *Life Sci.,* **1975,** *16,* 1777–1782.

Daniel, E. E.; Sutherland, W. H.; Bogoch, A.; (and Kent, J. T. [tech. asst.]). Effects of morphine and other drugs on the motility of the terminal ileum. *Gastroenterology,* **1959,** *36,* 510–523.

Dole, V. P., and Kreek, M. J. Methadone plasma level: sustained by a reservoir of drug in tissue. *Proc. Natl. Acad. Sci. U.S.A.,* **1973,** *70,* 10.

Economou, G., and Ward-McQuaid, J. N. A cross-over comparison of the effect of morphine, pethidine, pentazocine, and phenazocine on biliary pressure. *Gut,* **1971,** *12,* 218–221.

Ehrnebo, M.; Boréus, L.; and Lönroth, U. Bioavailability and first-pass metabolism of oral pentazocine in man. *Clin. Pharmacol. Ther.,* **1977,** *22,* 888–892.

Engineer, S., and Jennett, S. Respiratory depression following single and repeated doses of pentazocine and pethidine. *Br. J. Anaesth.,* **1972,** *44,* 795–801.

Findlay, J. W. A.; Jones, E. C.; Butz, R. F.; and Welch, R. M. Plasma codeine and morphine concentrations after therapeutic oral doses of codeine-containing analgesics. *Clin. Pharmacol. Ther.,* **1978,** *24,* 60–68.

Flórez, J.; McCarthy, L. E.; and Borison, H. L. A comparative study in the cat of the respiratory effects of morphine injected intravenously and into the cerebrospinal fluid. *J. Pharmacol. Exp. Ther.,* **1968,** *163,* 448–455.

Forrest, W. H., Jr.; Brown, B. W., Jr.; Brown, C. R.; Defalque, R.; Gold, M.; Gordon, H. E.; James, K. E.; Katz, J.; Mahler, D. L.; Schroff, P.; and Teutsch, G. Dextroamphetamine with morphine for the treatment of postoperative pain. *N. Engl. J. Med.,* **1977,** *296,* 712–715.

Fraser, H. F., and Isbell, H. Actions and addiction liabilities of alpha-acetylmethadols in man. *J. Pharmacol. Exp. Ther.,* **1952,** *105,* 458–465.

Frenk, H.; McCarty, B. C.; and Liebeskind, J. C. Different brain areas mediate the analgesic and epileptic properties of enkephalin. *Science,* **1978,** *200,* 335–337.

Galambos, J. T.; Hersh, T.; Schroder, S.; and Wenger, J. Loperamide: a new antidiarrheal agent in the treatment of chronic diarrhea. *Gastroenterology,* **1976,** *70,* 1026–1029.

Garrett, J. M.; Sauer, W. G.; and Moertel, C. G. Colonic motility in ulcerative colitis after opiate administration. *Gastroenterology,* **1967,** *53,* 93–100.

Gilbert, M. S.; Hanover, R. M.; Moylan, B. S.; and Caruso, F. S. Intramuscular butorphanol and meperidine in postoperative pain. *Clin. Pharmacol. Ther.,* **1976,** *20,* 359–364.

Gilbert, P. E., and Martin, W. R. Antagonism of the convulsant effects of heroin, *d*-propoxyphene, meperidine, normeperidine and thebaine by naloxone in mice. *J. Pharmacol. Exp. Ther.,* **1975,** *192,* 538–541.

———. The effect of morphine- and nalorphine-like drugs in the non-dependent, morphine-dependent and cyclazocine-dependent chronic spinal dog. *Ibid.,* **1976,** *198,* 66–83.

———. Antagonism of the effects of pentobarbital in the chronic spinal dog by naltrexone. *Life Sci.,* **1977,** *20,* 1401–1406.

Gintzler, A. R.; Gershon, M. D.; and Spector, S. A nonpeptide morphine-like compound: immunocytochemical localization in the mouse brain. *Science,* **1978,** *199,* 447–448.

Gracely, R. H.; Dubner, R.; and McGrath, P. A. Narcotic analgesia: fentanyl reduces the intensity but not the unpleasantness of painful tooth pulp sensations. *Science,* **1979,** *203,* 1261–1263.

Grevert, P., and Goldstein, A. Endorphins: naloxone fails to alter experimental pain or mood in humans. *Science,* **1978,** *199,* 1093–1095.

Gritz, E. R.; Shiffman, S. M.; Jarvik, M. E.; Schlesinger, J.; and Charuvastra, V. C. Naltrexone: physiological and psychological effects of single doses. *Clin. Pharmacol. Ther.,* **1976,** *19,* 773–776.

Gutner, L. B.; Gould, W. J.; and Batterman, R. C. The effects of potent analgesics upon vestibular function. *J. Clin. Invest.,* **1952,** *31,* 259–266.

Harte, E. H.; Gutjahr, C. L.; and Kreek, M. J. Long-term persistence of *d,l*-methadone in tissues. *Clin. Res.,* **1976,** *24,* 623A.

Hill, H. E.; Haertzen, C. A.; Wolbach, A. B., Jr.; and Miner, E. J. The Addiction Research Center Inventory: standardization of scales which evaluate subjective effects of morphine, amphetamine, pentobarbital, alcohol, LSD-25, pyrahexyl and chlorpromazine. *Psychopharmacologia,* **1963,** *4,* 167–205.

Hosobuchi, Y.; Rossier, J.; Bloom, F. E.; and Guillemin, R. Stimulation of human periaqueductal gray for pain relief increases immunoreactive β-endorphin in ventricular fluid. *Science,* **1979,** *203,* 279–281.

Houde, R. W. Analgesic effectiveness of the narcotic agonist-antagonists. *Br. J. Clin. Pharmacol.,* **1979,** *1,* Suppl. 3, 297s–308s.

Houde, R. W.; Wallenstein, S. L.; and Beaver, W. T. Clinical measurement of pain. In, *Analgetics.* (deStevens, G., ed.) Academic Press, Inc., New York, **1965,** pp. 75–122.

Hughes, J. W.; Smith, T.; Kosterlitz, H.; Fothergill, L.; Morgan, B.; and Morris, H. Identification of two related pentapeptides from the brain with potent opiate agonist activity. *Nature,* **1975,** *255,* 577–579.

Inturrisi, C. E., and Verebey, K. Disposition of methadone in man after single oral dose. *Clin. Pharmacol. Ther.,* **1972,** *13,* 923–930.

Jaffe, J. H.; Senay, E. C.; Schuster, C. R.; Renault, P. R.; Smith, B.; and DiMenza, S. Methadyl acetate vs methadone. A double blind study of heroin users. *J.A.M.A.,* **1972,** *222,* 437–442.

Jasinski, D. R. Effects in man of partial morphine agonists. In, *Agonist and Antagonist Actions of Narcotic Analgesic Drugs.* (Kosterlitz, H. W.; Collier, H. O. J.; and Villarreal, J. E.; eds.) University Park Press, Baltimore, **1973,** pp. 94–103.

Jasinski, D. R.; Griffith, J. D.; and Carr, C. B. Etorphine in man. I. Subjective effects and suppression of morphine abstinence. *Clin. Pharmacol. Ther.,* **1975,** *17,* 267–272.

Jasinski, D. R., and Mansky, P. A. Evaluation of nalbuphine for abuse potential. *Clin. Pharmacol. Ther.,* **1972,** *13,* 78–90.

Jasinski, D. R.; Martin, W. R.; and Hoeldtke, R. D. Effects of short- and long-term administration of pentazocine in man. *Clin. Pharmacol. Ther.,* **1970,** *11,* 385–403.

———. Studies of the dependence-producing properties of GPA-1657, profadol, and propiram in man. *Ibid.,* **1971,** *12,* 613–649.

Jasinski, D. R.; Pevnick, J. S.; Clark, S. C.; and Griffith, J. D. Therapeutic usefulness of propoxyphene napsylate in narcotic addiction. *Arch. Gen. Psychiatry,* **1977,** *34,* 227–233.

Jasinski, D. R.; Pevnick, J. S.; and Griffith, J. D. Human pharmacology and abuse potential of the analgesic buprenorphine. *Arch. Gen. Psychiatry,* **1978,** *35,* 501–516.

Johnson, K. R.; Hsueh, W. A.; Glusman, S. M.; and Arnett, F. C. Fibrous myopathy. A rheumatic complication of drug abuse. *Arthritis Rheum.,* **1976,** *19,* 923–926.

Kantor, T. G.; Sunshine, A.; Laska, E.; Meisner, M.; and Hopper, M. Oral analgesic studies: pentazocine hydrochloride, codeine, aspirin, and placebo and their influence on response to placebo. *Clin. Pharmacol. Ther.,* **1966,** *7,* 447–454.

Klotz, U.; McHorse, T. S.; Wilkinson, G. R.; and Schenker, S. The effect of cirrhosis on the disposition and elimination of meperidine in man. *Clin. Pharmacol. Ther.,* **1974,** *16,* 667–675.

Korf, J.; Bunney, B. S.; and Agajanian, G. K. Noradrenergic neurons: morphine inhibition of spontaneous activity. *Eur. J. Pharmacol.,* **1974,** *25,* 165–169.

Kreek, M. J. Effects of drugs and alcohol on opiate disposition and action. In, *Factors Affecting the Action of Narcotics.* (Adler, M. W.; Manara, L.; and Samanin, R.; eds.) Raven Press, New York, **1978,** pp. 717–739.

Lambertsen, C. J.; Wendel, H.; and Longenhagen, J. B. The separate and combined respiratory effects of chlorpromazine and meperidine in normal men controlled at 46 mm Hg alveolar pCO_2. *J. Pharmacol. Exp. Ther.,* **1961,** *131,* 381–393.

Lee, G.; DeMaria, A.; Amsterdam, E. A.; Realyvasquez, E.; Angel, J.; Morrison, S.; and Mason, D. T. Comparative effects of morphine, meperidine and pentazocine on cardiocirculatory dynamics in patients with acute myocardial infarction. *Am. J. Med.,* **1976,** *60,* 949–955.

Lee, H. K., and Wang, S. C. Mechanism of morphine induced miosis in the dog. *J. Pharmacol. Exp. Ther.,* **1975,** *192,* 415–431.

Ling, W.; Klett, C. J.; and Gillis, R. D. A cooperative clinical study of methadyl acetate. *Arch. Gen. Psychiatry,* **1978,** *35,* 345–353.

Lord, J.; Waterfield, A. A.; Hughes, J.; and Kosterlitz, H. W. Endogenous opioid peptides: multiple agonists and receptors. *Nature,* **1977,** *267,* 495–499.

McMahon, R. E.; Ridolfo, A. S.; Culp, H. W.; Wolen, R. L.; and Marshall, F. J. The fate of radiocarbon-labeled propoxyphene in rat, dog, and human. *Toxicol. Appl. Pharmacol.,* **1971,** *19,* 427–444.

Marks, R. M., and Sachar, E. J. Undertreatment of medical inpatients with narcotic analgesics. *Ann. Intern. Med.,* **1973,** *78,* 173–181.

Martin, W. R.; Eades, C. G.; Thompson, J. A.; Huppler,

R. E.; and Gilbert, P. E. The effects of morphine- and nalorphine-like drugs in the non-dependent and morphine-dependent chronic spinal dog. *J. Pharmacol. Exp. Ther.,* **1976,** *197,* 517–532.

Martin, W. R.; Jasinski, D. R.; Haertzen, C. A.; Kay, D. C.; Jones, B. E.; Mansky, P. A.; and Carpenter, R. W. Methadone—a reevaluation. *Arch. Gen. Psychiatry,* **1973a,** *28,* 286–295.

Martin, W. R.; Jasinski, D. R.; and Mansky, P. A. Naltrexone, an antagonist for the treatment of heroin dependence. *Arch. Gen. Psychiatry,* **1973b,** *28,* 784–791.

Mather, L. E., and Tucker, G. T. Systemic availability of orally administered meperidine. *Clin. Pharmacol. Ther.,* **1976,** *20,* 535–540.

Mather, L. E.; Tucker, G. T.; Pflug, A. E.; Lindop, M. J.; and Wilkerson, C. Meperidine kinetics in man. *Clin. Pharmacol. Ther.,* **1975,** *17,* 21–30.

Miller, R. J., and Cuatrecasas, P. The enkephalins. Peptides with morphine-like activity. *Naturwissenschaften,* **1978b,** *65,* 507–514.

Moertel, C. G. Relief of pain with oral medications. *Aust. N.Z. J. Med.,* **1976,** *6,* Suppl. 1, 1–8.

Moore, J., and Dundee, J. W. Alterations in response to somatic pain associated with anaesthesia. VII. The effect of nine phenothiazine derivatives. *Br. J. Anaesth.,* **1961,** *33,* 422–431.

Morgan, D.; Moore, G.; Thomas, J.; and Triggs, E. Disposition of meperidine in pregnancy. *Clin. Pharmacol. Ther.,* **1978,** *23,* 288–295.

Moroni, F.; Peralta, E.; Cheney, D. L.; and Costa, E. On the regulation of gamma-aminobutyric acid neurons in caudatus, pallidus, and nigra: effects of opioids and dopamine agonists. *J. Pharmacol. Exp. Ther.,* **1979,** *208,* 190–194.

Nagashima, H.; Karamanian, A.; Malovany, R.; Rodnay, P.; Ang, M.; Koerner, S.; and Folder, F. F. Respiratory and circulatory effects of intravenous butorphanol and morphine. *Clin. Pharmacol. Ther.,* **1976,** *19,* 738–745.

Nutt, J. G., and Jasinski, D. R. Methadone-naloxone mixtures for use in methadone maintenance programs. I. An evaluation in man of their pharmacological feasibility. II. Demonstration of acute physical dependence. *Clin. Pharmacol. Ther.,* **1974,** *15,* 156–166.

Oldendorf, W. H.; Hyman, S.; Braun, L.; and Oldendorf, S. Z. Blood-brain barrier penetration of morphine, codeine, heroin, and methadone after carotid injection. *Science,* **1972,** *178,* 984–986.

Parolaro, D.; Sala, M.; and Gori, E. Effect of intracerebroventricular administration of morphine upon intestinal motility in rat and its antagonism with naloxone. *Eur. J. Pharmacol.,* **1977,** *46,* 329–338.

Pentiah, P.; Reilly, F.; and Borison, H. L. Interactions of morphine sulfate and sodium salicylate on respiration in cats. *J. Pharmacol. Exp. Ther.,* **1966,** *154,* 110–118.

Pert, C. B., and Snyder, S. H. Opiate receptor: its demonstration in nervous tissue. *Science,* **1973,** *179,* 1011–1014.

Pomeranz, B., and Chiu, D. Naloxone blockade of acupuncture analgesia: endorphin implicated. *Life Sci.,* **1976,** *19,* 1757–1762.

Popio, K. A.; Jackson, D. H.; Ross, A. M.; Schreiner, B. F.; and Yu, P. N. Hemodynamic and respiratory depressant effects of morphine and butorphanol. *Clin. Pharmacol. Ther.,* **1978,** *23,* 281–287.

Romagnoli, A., and Keats, A. S. Comparative hemodynamic effects of nalbuphine and morphine in patients with coronary artery disease. *Cardiovasc. Dis.: Bull. Texas Heart Inst.,* **1978,** *5,* 19–24.

Schulman, H., and Greengard, P. Calcium-dependent protein phosphorylation system in membranes from various tissues, and its activation by the "calcium-dependent regulator". *Proc. Natl. Acad. Sci. U.S.A.,* **1978,** *75,* 5432–5436.

Sevelius, H.; McCoy, J. F.; and Colmore, J. P. Dose

response to codeine in patients with chronic cough. *Clin. Pharmacol. Ther.,* **1971,** *12,* 449–455.

Sharma, S. K.; Klee, W. A.; and Nirenberg, M. Dual regulation of adenylate cyclase accounts for narcotic dependence and tolerance. *Proc. Natl. Acad. Sci. U.S.A.,* **1975,** *72,* 3092–3096.

Sigman, E. M., and Elwood, C. M. Effect of intramuscular pentazocine on renal hemodynamics in normal human subjects. *Anesth. Analg. (Cleve.),* **1967,** *46,* 57–60.

Simon, E. J.; Hiller, J. M.; and Edelman, I. Stereospecific binding of the potent narcotic analgesic ^{3}H etorphine to rat-brain homogenate. *Proc. Natl. Acad. Sci. U.S.A.,* **1973,** *70,* 1947–1949.

Smith, G. M.; Lowenstein, E.; Hubbard, J. H.; and Beecher, H. K. Experimental pain produced by the submaximum effort tourniquet technique: further evidence of validity. *J. Pharmacol. Exp. Ther.,* **1968,** *163,* 468–474.

Smith, G. M.; Semke, C. W.; and Beecher, H. K. Objective evidence of mental effects of heroin, morphine and placebo in normal subjects. *J. Pharmacol. Exp. Ther.,* **1962,** *136,* 53–58.

Snyder, S. H.; Pert, C. B.; and Pasternak, G. W. The opiate receptor. *Ann. Intern. Med.,* **1974,** *81,* 534–540.

Stahl, K. D.; Van Bever, W.; Janssen, P.; and Simon, E. J. Receptor affinity and pharmacological potency of a series of narcotic analgesic, antidiarrheal and neuroleptic drugs. *Eur. J. Pharmacol.,* **1977,** *46,* 199–205.

Stanski, D. R.; Greenblatt, D. J.; and Lowenstein, E. Kinetics of intravenous and intramuscular morphine. *Clin. Pharmacol. Ther.,* **1978,** *24,* 52–59.

Stewart, J. J.; Weisbrodt, N. W.; and Burks, T. F. Central and peripheral actions of morphine on intestinal transit. *J. Pharmacol. Exp. Ther.,* **1978,** *205,* 547–555.

Suda, T.; Liotta, A. S.; and Krieger, D. T. β-Endorphin is not detectable in plasma from normal human subjects. *Science,* **1978,** *202,* 221–223.

Svenson, T. H.; Bunney, B. S.; and Agajanian, G. K. Inhibition of both noradrenergic and serotonergic neurons in brain by the alpha-adrenergic agonist clonidine. *Brain Res.,* **1975,** *92,* 291–306.

Szeto, H. H.; Inturrisi, C. E.; Houde, R.; Saal, S.; Cheigh, J.; and Reidenberg, M. M. Accumulation of normeperidine, an active metabolite of meperidine in patients with renal failure or cancer. *Ann. Intern. Med.,* **1977,** *86,* 738–741.

Tammisto, T.; Jaattela, A.; Nikki, P.; and Takki, S. Effect of pentazocine and pethidine on plasma catecholamine levels. *Ann. Clin. Res.,* **1971,** *3,* 22–29.

Terenius, L. Stereospecific interaction between narcotic analgesics and a synaptic plasma membrane fraction of rat cerebral cortex. *Acta Pharmacol. Toxicol. (Kbh.),* **1973,** *32,* 317–320.

Teschemacher, H.; Opheim, K. E.; Cox, B. M.; and Goldstein, A. A peptide-like substance from pituitary that acts like morphine. I. Isolation. *Life Sci.,* **1975,** *16,* 1771–1776.

Thomas, M.; Malmcrona, R.; Fillmore, S.; and Shillingford, J. Haemodynamic effects of morphine in patients with acute myocardial infarction. *Br. Heart J.,* **1965,** *27,* 863–875.

Twycross, R. Value of cocaine in opiate-containing elixirs. *Br. Med. J.,* **1977,** *2,* 1348.

Van Ree, J. M. Multiple brain sites involved in morphine antinociception. *J. Pharm. Pharmacol.,* **1977,** *29,* 765–767.

Vasko, J. S.; Henney, R. P.; Oldham, H. N.; Brawley, R. K.; and Morrow, A. G. Mechanisms of action of morphine in the treatment of experimental pulmonary edema. *Am. J. Cardiol.,* **1966,** *18,* 876–883.

Vaughan Williams, E. M., and Streeten, D. H. P. The action of morphine, pethidine, and AMIDONE upon the intestinal motility of conscious dogs. *Br. J. Pharmacol. Chemother.,* **1950,** *5,* 584–603.

Verebey, K.; Volavka, J.; and Clouet, D. Endorphins in psychiatry. *Arch. Gen. Psychiatry*, **1978**, *35*, 877–888.

Verebey, K.; Volavka, J.; Mule, S.; and Resnick, R. Methadone in man: pharmacokinetic and excretion studies in acute and chronic treatment. *Clin. Pharmacol. Ther.*, **1975**, *18*, 180–190.

———. Naltrexone: disposition, metabolism, and effects after acute and chronic dosing. *Ibid.*, **1976**, *20*, 315–328.

Vismara, L. A.; Leamon, D. M.; and Zelis, R. The effects of morphine on venous tone in patients with acute pulmonary edema. *Circulation*, **1976**, *54*, 335–337.

Way, W. L.; Costley, E. C.; and Way, E. L. Respiratory sensitivity of the newborn infant to meperidine and morphine. *Clin. Pharmacol. Ther.*, **1965**, *6*, 454–461.

Weinstein, S. H.; Pfeffer, M.; and Schor, J. Metabolism and pharmacokinetics of naloxone. In, *Narcotic Antagonists.* (Braude, M. C.; Harris, L. S.; May, E. L.; Smith, J. P.; and Villarreal, J. E.; eds.) Raven Press, New York, **1974**, pp. 525–535.

Weintraub, H. S.; Killinger, J. M.; Keykants, J.; Kanzler, M.; and Jaffe, J. H. Studies on the elimination rate of loperamide in man after administration of increasing oral doses of IMODIUM. *Curr. Ther. Res.*, **1977**, *21*, 867–876.

Wolen, R. L.; Ziege, E. A.; and Gruber, C. M. Determination of propoxyphene and norpropoxyphene by chemical ionization mass fragmentation. *Clin. Pharmacol. Ther.*, **1975**, *17*, 15–20.

Wolff, B. B.; Kantor, T. G.; Jarvik, M. F.; and Laska, E. Response of experimental pain to analgesic drugs. III. Codeine, aspirin, secobarbital, and placebo. *Clin. Pharmacol. Ther.*, **1969**, *10*, 217–228.

Young, W. S.; Bird, S. J.; and Kuhar, M. J. Iontophoresis of methionine-enkephalin in the locus coeruleus area. *Brain Res.*, **1977**, *129*, 366–370.

Zaks, A.; Jones, T.; Fink, M.; and Freedman, A. Treatment of opiate dependence with high dose oral naloxone. *J.A.M.A.*, **1971**, *215*, 2108–2110.

Zelis, R.; Flaim, S. F.; and Eisele, J. H. Effects of morphine on reflex arteriolar constriction induced in man by hypercapnia. *Clin. Pharmacol. Ther.*, **1977**, *22*, 172–178.

Monographs and Reviews

Adler, M. W.; Manara, L.; and Samanin, R. (eds.). *Factors Affecting the Action of Narcotics.* Raven Press, New York, **1978**.

Archer, S.; Albertson, N. F.; and Pierson, A. K. Structure-activity relationships in the opioid antagonists. In, *Agonist and Antagonist Actions of Narcotic Analgesic Drugs.* (Kosterlitz, H. W.; Collier, H. O. J.; and Villarreal, J. E.; eds.) University Park Press, Baltimore, **1973**, pp. 25–29.

Barnett, G.; Trsic, M.; and Willette, R. E. (eds.). *QuaSAR: Quantitative Structure Activity Relationships of Analgesics, Narcotic Antagonists, and Hallucinogens.* National Institute on Drug Abuse Research Monograph No. 22, U.S. Government Printing Office, Washington, D. C., **1978**.

Beaumont, A., and Hughes, J. Biology of opioid peptides. *Annu. Rev. Pharmacol. Toxicol.*, **1979**, *19*, 245–267.

Beaver, W. T. Mild analgesics, a review of their clinical pharmacology (Part II). *Am. J. Med. Sci.*, **1966**, *251*, 576–599.

Beecher, H. K. *The Measurement of Subjective Responses: Quantitative Effects of Drugs.* Oxford University Press, New York, **1959**.

Braenden, O. J.; Eddy, N. B.; and Halbach, H. Synthetic substances with morphine-like effect. Relationship between chemical structure and analgesic action. *Bull. WHO*, **1955**, *13*, 937–998.

Braude, M. C.; Harris, L. S.; May, E. L.; Smith, J. P.; and Villarreal, J. E. (eds.). *Narcotic Antagonists.* Raven Press, New York, **1974**.

Brogden, R. N.; Speight, T. M.; and Avery, G. S. Pentazo-cine: a review of its pharmacological properties, therapeutic efficacy and dependence liability. *Drugs*, **1973**, *5*, 6 91. (181 references.)

Burks, T. F. Gastrointestinal pharmacology. *Annu. Rev. Pharmacol. Toxicol.*, **1976**, *16*, 15–31.

Cannon, J. T.; Liebeskind, J. C.; and Frenk, H. Neural and neurochemical mechanisms of pain inhibition. In, *The Psychology of Pain.* (Sternbach, R. A., ed.) Raven Press, New York, **1978**, pp. 27–47.

Domino, E. F. Effects of narcotic analgesics on sensory input, activating system and motor output. *Res. Publ. Assoc. Res. Nerv. Ment. Dis.*, **1968**, *46*, 117–149.

Eckenhoff, J. E., and Oech, S. R. The effects of narcotics and antagonists upon respiration and circulation in man. *Clin. Pharmacol. Ther.*, **1960**, *1*, 483–524. (262 references.)

Eddy, N. B.; Friebel, H.; Hohn, K.; and Halbach, H. Codeine and its alternates for pain and cough relief. *Bull. WHO*, **1969**, *40*, 639–719.

Eddy, N. B.; Halbach, H.; and Braenden, O. J. Synthetic substances with morphine-like effect. Clinical experience: potency, side-effects, addiction liability. *Bull. WHO*, **1957**, *17*, 569–863.

Fishman, J. The opiates and the endocrine system. In, *The Bases of Addiction.* (Fishman, J., ed.) Dahlem Konferenzen. Abakon Verlagsgesellschaft, Berlin, **1978**, pp. 257–279.

Goldstein, A. Opioid peptides (endorphins) in pituitary and brain. *Science*, **1976**, *193*, 1081–1086.

Guillemin, R. Peptides in the brain: the new endocrinology of the neuron. *Science*, **1978**, *202*, 390–402.

Harris, L. S. Narcotic antagonists: structure-activity relationships. In, *Narcotic Antagonists.* (Braude, M. C.; Harris, L. S.; May, E. L.; Smith, J. P.; and Villarreal, J. E.; eds.) Raven Press, New York, **1974**, pp. 13–20. (51 references.)

Kerr, F. W. L., and Wilson, P. R. Pain. *Annu. Rev. Neurosci.*, **1978**, *1*, 83–102.

Kosterlitz, H. W.; Collier, H. O. J.; and Villarreal, J. E. (eds.). *Agonist and Antagonist Actions of Narcotic Analgesic Drugs.* University Park Press, Baltimore, **1973**.

Kosterlitz, H. W., and Hughes, J. Development of the concepts of opiate receptors and their ligands. *Adv. Biochem. Psychopharmacol.*, **1978**, *18*, 31–44.

Kosterlitz, H. W., and Waterfield, A. A. *In vitro* models in the study of structure-activity relationships of narcotic analgesics. *Annu. Rev. Pharmacol. Toxicol.*, **1975**, *15*, 29–47.

Lasagna, L. The clinical evaluation of morphine and its substitutes as analgesics. *Pharmacol. Rev.*, **1964**, *16*, 47–83.

Lewis, J. W.; Bentley, K. W.; and Cowan, A. Narcotic analgesics and antagonists. *Annu. Rev. Pharmacol. Toxicol.*, **1971**, *11*, 241–270. (305 references.)

Martin, W. R. Opioid antagonists. *Pharmacol. Rev.*, **1967**, *19*, 463–521. (373 references.)

Martin, W. R., and Kay, D. C. Effects of opioid analgesics and antagonists on the EEG. In, *Handbook of Electroencephalography and Clinical Neurophysiology*, Vol. 7, Pt. C. (Longo, V. G., ed.) Elsevier Publishing Co., Amsterdam, **1977**, pp. 97–109.

Martin, W. R., and Sloan, J. W. Neuropharmacology and neurochemistry of subjective effects, analgesia, tolerance, and dependence produced by narcotic analgesics. In, *Handbook of Experimental Pharmacology.* Vol. 45/I, *Drug Addiction I: Morphine, Sedative/Hypnotic and Alcohol Dependence.* (Martin, W. R., ed.) Springer-Verlag, Berlin, **1977**, pp. 43–158. (750 references.)

Miller, R. J., and Cuatrecasas, P. Enkephalins and endorphins. *Vitam. Horm.*, **1978a**, *36*, 297–382.

———. Neurobiology and neuropharmacology of the enkephalins. *Adv. Biochem. Psychopharmacol.*, **1979**, *20*, 187–225.

Misra, A. L. Metabolism of opiates. In, *Factors Affecting the Action of Narcotics.* (Adler, M. L.; Manara, L.; and

Samanin, R.; eds.) Raven Press, New York, **1978**, pp. 297–343.

Murphree, H. B.   Clinical pharmacology of potent analgesics. *Clin. Pharmacol. Ther.,* **1962,** *3,* 473–504.

Musto, D. F.   *The American Disease.* Yale University Press, New Haven, **1973.**

Reynolds, A. K., and Randall, L. O.   *Morphine and Allied Drugs.* University of Toronto Press, Toronto, **1957.** (More than 1600 references.)

Salem, H., and Aviado, D. M. (eds.).   *Antitussive Agents,* Vols. 1, 2, and 3. *International Encyclopedia of Pharmacology and Therapeutics,* Sect. 27. Pergamon Press, Ltd., Oxford, **1970.**

Simon, E. J., and Hiller, J. M.   The opiate receptors. *Annu. Rev. Pharmacol. Toxicol.,* **1978,** *18,* 371–394.

Snyder, S. H.   The opiate receptor and morphine-like peptides in the brain. *Am. J. Psychiatry,* **1978,** *135,* 645–652.

Sternbach, R. A. (ed.).   *The Psychology of Pain.* Raven Press, New York, **1978.**

Terenius, L.   Endogenous peptides and analgesia. *Annu. Rev. Pharmacol. Toxicol.,* **1978,** *18,* 189–204.

Terry, C. E., and Pellens, M.   *The Opium Problem.* Bureau of Social Hygiene, Inc., New York, **1928.**

Way, E. L.   Distribution and metabolism of morphine and its surrogates. *Res. Publ. Assoc. Res. Nerv. Ment. Dis.,* **1968,** *46,* 13–31.

———.   Common and selective mechanisms in drug dependence. In, *The Bases of Addiction.* (Fishman, J., ed.) Dahlem Konferenzen. Abakon Verlagsgesellschaft, Berlin, **1978,** pp. 333–352.

Way, E. L., and Adler, T. K.   The pharmacologic implications of the fate of morphine and its surrogates. *Pharmacol. Rev.,* **1960,** *12,* 383–446.

———.   *The Biological Disposition of Morphine and Its Surrogates.* World Health Organization, Geneva, **1962.**

Wikler, A.   *Mechanisms of Action of Opiates and Opiate Antagonists: A Review of Their Mechanisms of Action in Relation to Clinical Problems.* Public Health Monograph No. 52, U.S. Government Printing Office, Washington, D. C., **1958.** (195 references.)

Winter, C. A.   The physiology and pharmacology of pain and its relief. In, *Analgetics.* Vol. 5, *Medicinal Chemistry.* (deStevens, G., ed.) Academic Press, Inc., New York, **1965,** pp. 10–74. (283 references.)

Yaksh, T. L., and Rudy, T. A.   Narcotic analgesics: CNS sites and mechanisms of action as revealed by intracerebral injection techniques. *Pain,* **1978,** *4,* 299–359.

23 DRUG ADDICTION AND DRUG ABUSE

Jerome H. Jaffe

As far back as recorded history, every society has used drugs that produce effects on mood, thought, and feeling. Moreover, there were always a few individuals who digressed from custom with respect to the time, the amount, and the situation in which these drugs were to be used. Thus, both the nonmedical use of drugs and the problem of drug abuse are as old as civilization itself.

Problems of Terminology. *Drug abuse* refers to the use, usually by self-administration, of any drug in a manner that deviates from the approved medical or social patterns within a given culture. The term conveys the notion of social disapproval, and it is not necessarily descriptive of any particular pattern of drug use or its potential adverse consequences.

Since this definition is largely a social one, it is not surprising that for any particular drug there is a great variation in what is considered abuse, not only from culture to culture but also from time to time and from one situation to another within the same culture. For example, in Western society, chronic intoxication with alcohol is usually considered drug abuse, yet on certain occasions gross intoxication with alcohol is not. The use of medically prescribed barbiturates to induce sleep is permissible, but the self-administration of the same amount of barbiturates to induce euphoria in a social situation would be abuse. The use of medically prescribed opioid analgesics for the relief of pain is quite proper; however, the self-administration of the same drugs, in the same dosages, for relief of depression or tension or to induce euphoria is considered flagrant abuse. Temporal variations are common. For example, 2 decades ago the use of psychedelic (hallucinogenic, psychotomimetic) compounds such as lysergic acid diethylamide (LSD) was a practice limited to a few college students and research workers in the United States; it was not illegal, and there was no social condemnation of the users. By the mid-1960s, experimentation with psychedelic drugs was widespread among both college and high school students; the use of these drugs had become equivalent to abuse; and the possession, manufacture, or sale of such drugs had been made a criminal offense under federal law.

Nonmedical drug use is a less pejorative term but is so general that it encompasses behaviors ranging from the occasional use of alcohol to compulsive use of opioids, and includes behaviors that may or may not be associated with any adverse effects. Nonmedical drug use may consist in *experimental use* of a drug on one or a few occasions, because of curiosity about its effects, or in order to conform to the expectations of peer groups. It may involve the *casual* or *"recreational" use* of modest amounts of a drug for its pleasurable effects, or *circumstantial use,* in which certain drug effects are sought because they are helpful in particular circumstances, as when students or truck drivers take amphetamines to alleviate fatigue. These various forms of nonmedical use may then lead to more *intensive patterns* of use in terms of frequency or amount and, in some cases, to patterns of *dependence* or *compulsive drug use.*

Compulsive Drug Use. One of the hazards in the use of drugs to alter mood and feeling is that some individuals eventually develop a dependence on the drug; they have diminished flexibility in terms of their behavior toward a particular drug. They continue to take it in the absence of medical indications, often despite adverse social and medical consequences, and they behave as if the effects of the drugs are needed for continued well-being. The intensity of this "need" or dependence may vary from a mild desire to a "craving" or "compulsion" to use the drug, and, when the availability of the drug is uncertain, they may exhibit a preoccupation with its procurement. In extreme forms, the behavior exhibits the characteristics of a chronic relapsing disorder. Since *intense reliance* on the effects of self-administered drugs *per se* is generally a deviation from approved and expected patterns of use, the terms *compulsive drug use* and *compulsive abuse* are often interchangeable. However, there are often striking inconsistencies in the way the terms *drug dependence* and *drug abuse* are employed.

Until recently in Western society, the attitude toward the use of tobacco was so permissive that even chronic, heavy, compulsive use damaging to the user's health, and over which he may have little control, was rarely thought of as compulsive abuse or dependence. This overly permissive attitude toward tobacco is changing. Compulsive smoking is increasingly thought of as a form of behavior that is appropriately grouped with other drug dependencies (*see* Surgeon General, 1979).

Dependence on a drug *per se* is not necessarily cause for concern. If the substance used has low toxicity and is relatively inexpensive (*e.g.,* caffeine), a drug-using behavior may meet the criteria for dependence but may not constitute a significant medical or social problem. More commonly, however, compulsive use of drugs is usually detrimental both to the user and to the society of which he is a part. However, detrimental effects can be determined only after an evaluation of the pattern of use by a given individual and a consideration of the available alternatives. For example, if the only alternative to the use of opioids is the compulsive use of alcohol, there are many who would take the view that opioid dependence is far less destructive to the individual and society, and that some provision should be made to permit that particular individual to use opioid drugs.

Compulsive drug use is commonly, but not necessarily, associated with the development of tolerance and physical dependence. *Tolerance* has developed when, after repeated administration, a given dose of a drug produces a decreased effect or, conversely, when increasingly larger doses must be administered to obtain the effects observed with the original dose. *Physical dependence* refers to an altered physiological state produced by the repeated administration of a drug, which necessitates the continued administration of the drug to prevent the appearance of a stereotypical syndrome, *the withdrawal or abstinence syndrome,* characteristic for the particular drug. The theoretical bases for the phenomena of tolerance and physical dependence are discussed below.

Addiction. It is possible to describe all known patterns of drug use without employing the terms *addict* or *addiction.* In many respects this would be advantageous, for the term *addiction,* like the term *abuse,* has been used in so many ways that it can no longer be employed without further qualification or elaboration. However, since it is not likely that the term will be dropped from the language, it is appropriate to make an effort to delimit its meaning. The definition used here is somewhat arbitrary, and it is not necessarily identical with other definitions of addic-

tion or drug dependence (*see* National Commission, 1973; World Health Organization, 1973). In this chapter, the term *addiction* will be used to mean *a behavioral pattern of drug use, characterized by overwhelming involvement with the use of a drug (compulsive use), the securing of its supply, and a high tendency to relapse after withdrawal.* Addiction is thus viewed as an extreme on a continuum of involvement with drug use and refers in a *quantitative* rather than a *qualitative* sense to the degree to which drug use pervades the total life activity of the user and to the range of circumstances in which drug use controls his behavior. In most instances it will not be possible to state with precision at what point compulsive use should be considered addiction. Anyone who is addicted would be considered drug dependent within the WHO definitions, but *within the set of definitions used here the term* addiction *cannot be used interchangeably with* physical dependence. *It is possible to be physically dependent on drugs without being addicted and, in some special circumstances, to be addicted without being physically dependent* (*see* below).

Risks of Nonmedical Drug Use. The risk of becoming dependent is only one of a number of hazards related to the nonmedical use of drugs. The particular hazards vary considerably and depend on the drug, the dose, the route of administration, the setting in which it is used, and the psychological state and drug-related experiences of the user. Certain risks are not limited to more intensive drug-use patterns, but may be associated with experimental, recreational, or circumstantial use as well. For example, if the dose is excessive, even the first experience with a drug may produce serious toxicity, and even occasional parenteral drug use can cause infections if hygienic precautions are inadequate. Other risks may be entirely unrelated to the pharmacological actions of the drugs used. In many societies certain forms of nonmedical drug use may lead to social ostracism or criminal prosecution. However, in this chapter the emphasis will be on the pharmacological and biochemical aspects of nonmedical drug use.

GENESIS OF DRUG USE AND DEPENDENCE

Whether the use of a drug is socially acceptable or subject to extreme disapproval, multiple factors determine who will experiment with the drug and experience its effects; other factors determine who will continue to use it casually or recreationally; and still other factors decide who will progress from casual to intensive or compulsive use.

Experimentation is largely a matter of availability, curiosity, the attitude and drug-using behavior of one's friends, the social acceptability of a given form of drug use, the risks believed to be associated with experimental use, and the tendency of the individual to respect social norms. Sometimes, drug experimentation may involve the use of substances that produce unpleasant effects. The host of materials ingested over the centuries for supposed aphrodisiac effects bears witness to this. However, from the thousands of substances that have been self-administered over the years, only a few have become staples in mankind's pharmacopoeia of drugs for nonmedical use; of these, still fewer give rise to serious problems of dependence. A full exploration of the interactions between man, environment, and drugs is beyond the scope of this chapter. (*See* Brecher, 1972; National Commission, 1973; World Health Organization, 1974.)

The emphasis here will be on the interactions of man and drug, and on those aspects of the interaction that are relevant to clinical situations and to the development of dependence.

Drugs as Reinforcers. Man's tendency to take drugs is shared with other mammals. Laboratory animals quickly learn to self-administer most of the drugs commonly used for nonmedical purposes, including opioids, barbiturates, alcohol, anesthetic gases, local anesthetics, volatile solvents, central nervous system (CNS) stimulants, phencyclidine, nicotine, and caffeine. Whether an animal will self-administer a drug depends on a number of factors, including the properties of the drug itself, the route of administration, the size of the individual dose, the amount of work required to obtain a dose and the time between the work and the drug administration (schedule of reinforcement), the presence of other drugs, and the kinds of drugs the animal has been given previously (*see* Schuster and Thompson, 1969; Kalant *et al.,* 1978; Woods, 1978). When given continuous access, animals show patterns of self-administration that are strikingly similar to those exhibited by human users of the same drug. Such observations suggest that preexisting psychopathology is not a requisite for initial or even continued drug taking, and that drugs themselves are powerful reinforcers, even in the absence of physical dependence.

Some drugs (*e.g.,* chlorpromazine) are never self-administered; they appear instead to have aversive properties, and animals learn to avoid maneuvers that result in small injections of such drugs. On the other hand, animals will press a lever more than four thousand times to get a single injection of cocaine, and when given free access, they immediately begin self-administering high daily doses that may produce severe toxic effects and induce self-mutilating behavior. With stimulants such as amphetamine and cocaine, periods of self-imposed abstinence alternate with periods of drug administration; generally the animals die of toxic effects and inanition after a period of several weeks of continuous use. If saline solution is substituted for cocaine or amphetamine, there is a burst of rapid lever pressing for several hours, then abruptly all responding ceases and is not resumed. In contrast, animals self-administering morphine gradually raise the daily dose over a period of weeks, then self-administer the drug at a steady rate that avoids both gross toxicity and withdrawal symptoms. When saline solution is substituted for morphine, however, the animal continues to press the lever (except during the peak of withdrawal) and does so at a slow but steady rate over a period of weeks (*see* Thompson and Pickens, 1970; Woods, 1978).

Tolerance and Physical Dependence. In addition to the primary reinforcing effects, when drugs are used chronically other factors come into play that profoundly affect the pattern of use and the likelihood that the drug use will be continued. Among these are the capacities of some substances, but not others, to produce *tolerance* and/or *physical dependence.* These phenomena, as previously defined, are often assumed to be inextricably linked to each other and to the problem of compulsive drug use. Neither of these assumptions is valid. Tolerance and physical dependence develop not only with opioids, alcohol, and hypnotics but also after chronic administration of a wide variety of drugs that are not self-administered by animals or used compulsively by man. Such drugs include anticholinergics, chlorpromazine, imipramine, and cyclazocine, a synthetic opioid antagonist (*see* Chapter 22). Nor does physical dependence invariably occur in every situation where tolerance develops. Tolerance is a very general phenomenon observed with a host of substances and involves many independent mechanisms.

In addition to *innate* tolerance to various classes of drugs, it is possible to distinguish three varieties of *acquired* pharmacological tolerance: dispositional, pharmacodynamic, and behavioral. Drug *disposi-*

tional tolerance results from changes in the pharmacokinetic properties of the agent in the organism, such that reduced concentrations are present at the sites of drug action. The most common mechanism is an increased rate of metabolism. Dispositional tolerance has relatively little effect on the peak intensity of action and does not usually result in more than a threefold decrease in sensitivity. *Pharmacodynamic tolerance* results from adaptive changes within affected systems, such that the response is reduced in the presence of the same concentration of the drug. *Behavioral tolerance* has been defined as a change in the response to a drug due to behavioral mechanisms (Dews, 1977). When a reduced effect of a drug on behavior is used as the measure of tolerance, it is a consistent finding that tolerance develops more rapidly and to a greater degree when the effect of the drug has a behavioral "cost" to the organism (*i.e.,* when it impairs its capacity to earn a reward or to avoid punishment) than when it does not. Thus, rats tested daily on a moving belt under the influence of alcohol develop more tolerance to the ataxic effects than rats receiving the same dose after the test, and both groups develop tolerance more rapidly than rats given an even larger dose of alcohol without daily testing. Similar relationships between behavioral conditions and the development of tolerance have been observed with opioids, marihuana, and amphetamines. Behavioral tolerance must ultimately be understood in pharmacodynamic terms. In any given situation, several types of tolerance and more than one mechanism may operate concurrently (*see* Kalant *et al.,* 1971; Martin and Sloan, 1977a; Smith, 1977; Kalant, 1978; Siegel, 1978).

Tolerance to Opioids.

Tolerance does not develop uniformly to all the actions of opioid drugs. There may be complete tolerance to some actions, while responses to others are unaltered. Tolerance to opioids is characterized by a shortened duration and decreased intensity of the analgesic, euphorigenic, sedative, and other CNS depressant effects as well as by a marked elevation in the average lethal dose. While animals that are tolerant to opioids may metabolize them somewhat more rapidly, most of the tolerance seen with opioids is due to adaptation of cells in the nervous system to the drug's action.

Although tolerance itself does not necessarily affect the likelihood of continued use, it can affect patterns of use by increasing the amount of drug that must be taken to produce a given effect (*e.g.,* euphoria). The use of increased amounts may in turn enhance the risk of toxic effects or produce other problems if the drug is expensive or obtained illicitly.

Tolerance to opioid drugs can develop with remarkable rapidity. In the dog, considerable recovery from behavioral depression occurs during the course of a continuous 8-hour infusion of morphine (acute tolerance). Although such rapid changes do not occur in man (Elliot *et al.,* 1971), former morphine addicts can attain a dosage of 500 mg of morphine per day within 10 days. However, even with prolonged administration of opioids to experimental animals, there appears to be little tolerance to the facilitatory effect of such drugs on electrical self-stimulation of the brain or to their capacity to serve as discriminative stimuli (*see* Kornetsky *et al.,* 1979). Associative processes akin to learning may be involved in the interactions between tolerance to opioids and the conditions under which they are given, as well as in certain forms of long-lasting residual tolerance. Furthermore, animals and man previously dependent on opioids become physically dependent more rapidly on reexposure, and drugs that inhibit the synthesis of proteins interfere with memory as well as with the development of tolerance to opioids (*see* Siegel, 1978). Since most theories attempt to account for both tolerance and physical dependence within a single model, further consideration of tolerance is included below in the discussion of physical dependence.

Tolerance to Alcohol, Barbiturates, and Related Hypnotics.

Animals made tolerant to barbiturates or alcohol show significantly less sedation and ataxia than do nontolerant animals at the same blood concentrations. However, as the blood concentrations are increased, there is progressively less difference between tolerant and nontolerant animals in the degree of CNS depression and, in contrast to the tolerance seen with opioids, animals tolerant to alcohol or barbiturates show only modest elevation of the lethal blood concentration. If the use of the CNS depressant has produced only ataxia and has been insufficient to depress respiration to some degree, there is little or no tolerance to the respiratory depressant and lethal effects of the drug. It appears that only those systems that have been challenged or altered by the agent become tolerant to its effects (Okamoto *et al.,* 1978).

In the case of short-acting barbiturates (*e.g.,* pentobarbital), alcohol, and a number of nonbarbiturate hypnotics (glutethimide, meprobamate, etc.), a more rapid enzymatic degradation of the drug can also be demonstrated in tolerant animals. Thus, in the same animal two independent mechanisms, *pharmacodynamic* tolerance and *dispositional* tolerance, contribute to the decreased duration and intensity of the response to a given dose of drug. Both modes of adaptation are relevant to clinical problems. Dispositional tolerance, however, does not seem closely related to the phenomena of physical dependence and pharmacodynamic tolerance; changes in the rate of enzymatic degradation of barbiturates can be induced by pretreatment with substances that do not in themselves produce CNS depression or pharmacodynamic tolerance.

With this group of drugs, as with the opioids, tolerance does not directly increase the probability of continued or compulsive use. However, tolerance to toxic effects may not develop in parallel with tolerance to CNS depression and, in the case of alcohol particularly, the consumption of more drug in order to obtain CNS effects may increase the likelihood of direct drug-induced organ damage (see Lieber, 1972). Furthermore, the shortened duration of action may increase the frequency of drug taking, thereby increasing the number of times that drug-taking behavior will be reinforced.

Some aspects of tolerance to general CNS depressants develop with surprising rapidity. Thus, in man, when the blood concentration is falling after administration of a large dose of alcohol, the signs and symptoms of intoxication disappear at a concentration that was associated with gross intoxication when the blood level was rising. This apparently rapid or *acute* CNS tolerance has also been observed repeatedly in animals with pentobarbital, thiopental, paraldehyde, and trichloroethanol, and the degree of tolerance that develops (as measured by the blood concentration of the drug when signs of ataxia disappear) seems directly related to the depth of the CNS depression that was produced by the drug. It is not clear whether the mechanisms underlying acute tolerance are related to those involved in the tolerance that develops over longer periods. The subject of tolerance to alcohol and related general CNS depressants has been reviewed by Kalant and associates (1971) and Smith (1977). Tolerance to CNS sympathomimetics, nicotine, cannabinoids, and psychedelics is also discussed under clinical characteristics of their abuse.

Physical Dependence. Physical dependence has been studied after chronic administration of opioids, general depressants of the CNS (alcohol, barbiturates, and related hypnotics), amphetamines, cannabinoids, nicotine, and opioid antagonists. The withdrawal symptoms associated with many of these classes of agents are characterized by rebound effects in those same physiological systems that were modified initially by the drug (*rebound hyperexcitability*). For example, general depressants elevate the seizure threshold, but spontaneous seizures are seen during withdrawal; morphine depresses the flexor and crossed extensor spinal reflexes, but these same polysynaptic reflexes are

hyperexcitable during morphine withdrawal. Amphetamines alleviate fatigue, suppress appetite, and elevate mood; amphetamine withdrawal is characterized by lack of energy, hyperphagia, and depression. Nicotine tends to suppress anger and produce an alerting pattern in the EEG; irritability and drowsiness are common complaints following abrupt cessation in heavy smokers. It is not certain whether all the complex patterns of symptoms seen during withdrawal from opioids or general depressants should be considered rebound effects, nor whether such a generalization is applicable to the stereotypical, distinct syndromes observed after abrupt withdrawal of drugs such as chlorpromazine, imipramine, and cyclazocine.

Time Required. The time required to produce physical dependence on any drug depends on a number of factors, but the most important seem to be the degree to which function in the CNS is altered by the drug and the continuity of this alteration. However, whether a withdrawal syndrome is clinically observable depends on (1) the criteria for withdrawal symptoms, (2) the sensitivity of technics used to detect withdrawal phenomena, and (3) the rate at which the drug is removed from its site of action.

Patients who have received therapeutic doses of morphine several times a day for 1 to 2 weeks will have only mild symptoms that may not be recognized as withdrawal symptomatology when the drug is stopped; symptoms are even less pronounced when the opioid is one that is slowly eliminated (such as methadone). However, if the drug is not simply discontinued but an opioid antagonist (naloxone) is used to induce withdrawal, it is possible to demonstrate withdrawal symptoms in man after therapeutic doses of morphine, methadone, or heroin given four times per day for as short a period as 2 to 3 days. In former heroin addicts naloxone precipitates mild withdrawal symptoms 1 week after a single 40-mg dose of methadone, indicating the presence of an otherwise-subclinical level of physical dependence. In short, the phenomenon of opioid physical dependence is initiated by the first dose, and this rapid development has important clinical implications (*see* below).

The time required to produce physical dependence with general CNS depressants is likewise short; when rapidly metabolized drugs are used, the earliest signs of rebound excitability can be detected after surprisingly brief periods of CNS depression. Using the threshold for seizures in mice as a measure, McQuarrie and Fingl (1958) were able to demonstrate that a single large dose of alcohol produces an elevation of the seizure threshold that is followed by a period of subnormal threshold. After 3 days of chronic exposure to ethanol, mice develop marked physical dependence, with spontaneous seizures upon abrupt withdrawal (Goldstein, 1973). In cats, evidence of withdrawal hyperexcitability can be demonstrated after as little as 26 hours of deep pentobarbital intoxication. In man, it may require weeks of *mild intoxication* with short-acting barbiturates to produce clinically significant physical dependence, but 10% of patients who were kept *deeply intoxicated* (semicomatose) for 16 to 20 hours per day, for 10 to 12 days, became so physically dependent that they developed seizures and delirium on abrupt withdrawal (Alexander, 1951). If rebound changes in the EEG or insomnia are used as criteria, only 1 or 2 weeks of ordinary dosage at night is enough to induce low levels of physical dependence on CNS depressants (Kales *et al.*, 1974, 1978).

In contrast to the short-acting drugs, abrupt discontinuation of long-acting opioids, such as methadone or acetylmethadol, produces withdrawal symptoms that are slow in onset and generally less severe. Conversely, when methadone is displaced from its receptors by an antagonist, a severe withdrawal syndrome ensues. It is as if a great deal of latent hyperexcitability is explosively released rather than gradually dissipated over a period of time. Thus, it is necessary to distinguish between the degree of *latent* hyperexcitability and the amount manifested when the drug is stopped. The same principle holds for the general depressants of the CNS (Boisse and Okamoto, 1978). Continuous action on neural pathways theoretically produces a greater degree of physical dependence. However, such factors as tissue binding or slow metabolism may result in a very slow reversal of the process, a slower onset of withdrawal phenomena, and a generally less severe clinical syndrome.

These observations suggest that the adaptational processes that eventually produce grossly observable withdrawal symptoms, at least with opioids and general CNS depressants, actually begin with the first dose. This has obvious implications not only for the problem of deciding just when physical dependence is present but also for the problem of determining the causes of compulsive abuse. It is quite conceivable that individuals who use short-acting drugs to induce euphoria or reduce tensions can perceive an exacerbation of these same tensions (rebound effects) as the drug effects wane. Such increases in tension might then contribute to the motivation to repeat the use of the drug, and the alleviation of withdrawal phenomena might increase the effectiveness of the drug as a reinforcer of drug-using behavior. Similar subtle post-drug-use effects are also seen with amphetamines and possibly with nicotine.

The relationship between compulsive drug use and physical dependence is variable and complex. For example, some degree of physical dependence develops in medical patients who receive opioids regularly for more than a few days. The overwhelming majority of such patients do not exhibit drug-seeking behavior and do not become compulsive users. Even those who administer such drugs to themselves for brief periods discontinue the drug when the medical condition is relieved. A large proportion of the young men who served in the United States Army in Vietnam used heroin, and about half of this group became physically dependent. Nevertheless, a substantial percentage simply stopped their heroin use before their return to the United States, and many did so without benefit of any special treatment (*see* Robins, 1974).

It is probable that at least some degree of physical dependence on CNS depressants (including alcohol) develops after relatively brief periods of continuous use, yet the majority of individuals are able to tolerate minor withdrawal phenomena and do not become compulsive drug users.

Thus, although some compulsive users attribute their drug problems entirely to "getting hooked" (either iatrogenically or out of ignorance in the course of using drugs illicitly), physical dependence is currently viewed not so much as a direct cause of compulsive use but as one of several factors that contribute to its development and to the tendency to relapse after withdrawal (*see* below).

Degree of Physical Dependence and Locus of Changes. Although it is possible to demonstrate changes in the biochemical and physiological properties of tissues (*e.g.*, brain, intestine) in dependent animals (*see* Herz and Schulz, 1978; Johnson *et al.*, 1978), the degree of physical dependence is still measured by the severity of the withdrawal syndrome produced either by abrupt withdrawal or by use of drug antagonists. In man, there appears to be an upper limit to the degree of physical dependence on opioids. This upper limit seems to be a negative exponential function of total daily dose, so that increasing the daily dose in man beyond the equivalent of 500 mg of morphine does not significantly increase the severity of the withdrawal syndrome. Since the abrupt withdrawal of hypnotics or alcohol after high dosage produces seizures and delirium that can be fatal in man and animals, it is difficult to establish an upper limit of physical dependence on these agents.

In view of the distribution and widespread effects of endogenous opioid-like substances (*see* Chapters 12 and 22), it is not surprising that adaptive changes to the administration of exogenous opioids and withdrawal phenomena can be demonstrated throughout the autonomic and central nervous systems. Withdrawal hyperexcitability is observed in decerebrate animals, in the spinal cord of man, and in animals after cord transection. With local administration, the spinal cord or other structures can be made "dependent" on opioids with minimal involvement of the rest of the CNS (*see* Yaksh *et al.,* 1977). Recent studies suggest an important role for a noradrenergic center in the brain stem—the locus ceruleus. Opioids suppress activity in the locus ceruleus, an effect that is reversed by naloxone. Clonidine, an antihypertensive agent, also inhibits activity in these neurons, apparently by agonistic actions at α_2-adrenergic receptors (Korf *et al.,* 1974; Aghajanian, 1978); clonidine also suppresses the signs and symptoms of withdrawal from opioids in rats and man (Tseng *et al.,* 1975; Paalzow, 1978) and produces analgesia in rats. Tolerance develops to this analgesic effect, and there is cross-tolerance to morphine (Paalzow, 1978). It is postulated that some of the affective and physiological aspects of the opioid withdrawal syndrome are due to hyperactivity in the locus ceruleus or to increased sensitivity (supersensitivity) of structures that are innervated by neurons of the locus ceruleus (*see* Gold *et al.,* 1978).

It is now quite clear that changes occur throughout the *entire* neuraxis during the development of physical dependence on CNS depressants, including, probably, alcohol (*see* Smith, 1977; Rosenberg and Okamoto, 1978).

Cross-Dependence.

The ability of one drug to suppress the manifestations of physical dependence produced by another and to maintain the physically dependent state is referred to as *cross-dependence.* Cross-dependence may be partial or complete, and the degree is more closely related to pharmacological effects than to chemical similarities.

In general, any potent morphine-like opioid will show cross-dependence with other opioids. Partial cross-dependence is also seen between alcohol and barbiturates, whereby in man alcohol can very substantially but not completely suppress the symptoms of barbiturate withdrawal (Fraser *et al.,* 1957).

Animal studies show a high degree of cross-dependence among general CNS depressants; most sedative-hypnotics (*e.g.,* paraldehyde, chloral hydrate, meprobamate, benzodiazepines, etc.) will show a reasonable degree of cross-dependence with each other and with alcohol and barbiturates. There is also some cross-dependence between barbiturates and volatile anesthetics. Clinical reports are consistent with these findings, although there are few well-controlled studies.

If a long-acting drug such as methadone is substituted over several days for morphine, abrupt discontinuation produces a withdrawal syndrome characteristic of the long-acting drug rather than that of morphine. This aspect of cross-dependence has important clinical implications, since the withdrawal symptoms that occur with drugs with longer half-lives (methadone, phenobarbital, chlordiazepoxide) are generally less severe but more protracted. This phenomenon is the basis for the *substitution treatment* of physical dependence for both opioids and CNS depressants.

In animals, there is cross-tolerance and cross-dependence between opioid drugs and endogenous opioid-like peptides. There is, however, little cross-tolerance and cross-dependence between drugs that act on different species of opioid receptors (*see* Chapter 22). Animals tolerant to ketocyclazocine (a κ agonist) are not tolerant to morphine, and ketocyclazocine does not suppress the opioid withdrawal syndrome (*see* Woods and Carney, 1977). The implications of these findings for the clinical use of newer analgesics, such as nalbuphine, butorphanol, and buprenorphine, are still unclear.

Theories of Physical Dependence. Most theories postulate some form of CNS counteradaptation to the agonistic actions of the drugs. Counteradaptation results in the development of a "latent hyperexcitability" in neural systems affected by the drugs, which becomes manifest in the form of rebound or overshoot phenomena when the drugs are stopped or, in the case of opioids, when they are displaced from the receptor by an antagonist. The theories differ largely in the level of explanation or in the mechanisms proposed to account for the counteradaptive changes; most involve models that account for the observation that physical dependence is generally accompanied by tolerance and that the two phenomena develop and decay at about the same rate.

Martin (1968) has proposed a homeostatic and redundancy model in which tolerance is due to the opening of redundant pathways within the CNS when the primary pathway is blocked by the action of the drug. With drug withdrawal, activity in the primary pathway is restored, which in combination with continuing activity in the redundant pathway results in a rebound hyperexcitability of the pathways once depressed by the drug. While developed largely to account for opioid physical dependence, this theory is applicable to other drugs as well. Others have speculated that decreased neural activity in any functional system results in a "disuse supersensitivity" analogous to the denervation supersensitivity that develops in peripheral autonomic structures. The supersensitivity is thought to begin as soon as input is reduced and to account for decreased drug effect (tolerance); abrupt withdrawal of the drug or its displacement by an antagonist restores input to supersensitive elements, producing a "rebound" hyperactivity in the very systems that were depressed by the drug (*see* Jaffe and Sharpless, 1968). This model does not require that the drug be present on the ultimate neuronal receptor itself. Supersensitivity to various neurotransmitters has been demonstrated after chronic administration of opioids, ethanol, or other drugs to experimental animals (*see* Castellani *et al.,* 1978; Herz and Schulz, 1978; Johnson *et al.,* 1978).

A related theory postulates that alterations in neural input cause an increase in the number of receptors, which, in turn, may be "active" or "silent." An increase in receptors for neurotransmitters would account for tolerance, and the rebound effects occur when drug withdrawal restores normal neurotransmitter activity to a system with excess receptors (*see* Collier, 1966). It has not been possible to demonstrate changes in the affinity or number of opioid receptors or in concentrations of endogenous opioid-like peptides in animals who are dependent on such drugs (*see* Simon and Hiller, 1978).

Enzyme induction theories postulate that drugs that cause dependence inhibit an enzyme that synthesizes a product important for cell activity (*e.g.,* a neurotransmitter), and that the level of the enzyme itself is regulated by its product, the neurotransmitter. The initial drug effect is a result of the decrease in transmitter concentration, but this decrease also leads to increased synthesis of the enzyme and a new steady-state level that restores transmitter concentration, resulting in tolerance; when the drug is withdrawn there is excess enzyme, which then causes excess synthesis of transmitter, and this produces rebound effects until the enzyme activity falls to a new steady state (*see* Goldstein and Goldstein, 1968; Shuster, 1971). These theories are applicable to both opioid and CNS-depressant types of physical dependence.

There appears to be at least one biochemical system that reacts in this way. Opioids and endogenous opioid-like peptides inhibit adenylate cyclase activity in certain cultured neuronal cells. After a few days of incubation with such compounds, adenylate cyclase activity and concentrations of cyclic adenosine 3′,5′-monophosphate (cyclic AMP) return to control values, despite the continued presence of the opioids (tolerance). When the opioids are removed or naloxone is added to the medium, there is a rebound increase in adenylate cyclase activity that results in a sharp increase in the intracellular concentration of the cyclic nucleotide (Sharma *et al.,* 1975).

Specific neurotransmitters are believed to play an important role in the development of tolerance and physical dependence. Depletion of 5-hydroxytryptamine (5-HT) appears to interfere with the development of tolerance to both opioids and ethanol (*see* Frankel *et al.,* 1978; Way, 1978), while depletion of norepinephrine is reported to interfere with the development of tolerance (but not physical dependence) to barbiturates (Tabakoff *et al.,* 1978). Depletion of catecholamines aggravates the alcohol withdrawal syndrome, and drugs that induce cross-dependence or that raise concentrations of gamma-aminobutyric acid (GABA) in brain have an ameliorative effect (*see* Goldstein, 1973, 1979).

At present no single model can account for all the complex phenomena that are seen with the many classes of drugs that produce tolerance and physical dependence. It is likely that multiple mechanisms are involved and that each model may reflect a facet of truth. For additional references, *see* Martin and Sloan (1977a), Smith (1977), and several reviews in Fishman (1978).

Learning, Conditioning, and Relapse. Within the framework of learning theory, drug use, whether casual or compulsive, can be viewed as behavior that is maintained by its consequences; consequences that strengthen a behavior pattern are reinforcers. Drugs may reinforce the antecedent drug-taking behavior by inducing pleasurable effects (positive reinforcement) or by terminating some aversive or unpleasant situation (negative reinforcement), as when a drug alleviates pain or anxiety. Secondary or social reinforcement entirely independent of pharmacological effects may also play a role, as is the case when drug use results in special status, membership in a desired group, or the approval of friends. Sometimes social reinforcement maintains experimental behavior until the individual comes to appreciate the primary drug effect or becomes tolerant to some initial aversive effects of the particular drug. This seems to be the case with many young people who do not like the initial effects of tobacco or who perceive nothing pleasurable about the initial effects of smoking marihuana. Although it is not as widely appreciated, many naive individuals find the effects of an initial dose of heroin, with its associated nausea and vomiting, somewhat unpleasant; however, social reinforcement may maintain the behavior until tolerance develops to these effects.

The development of physical dependence gives rise to the possibility of another variety of reinforcement; each time drug use alleviates withdrawal distress the antecedent drug-using behavior is further reinforced. Even when tolerance attenuates the initial reinforcing effects, drugs that induce physical dependence create a regularly recurring sense of distress that is immediately eliminated by another dose of the drug. During the withdrawal state, drug use can simultaneously alleviate distress and produce euphoria, a particularly powerful reinforcement (*see* Wikler, 1975).

It is uncertain to what extent euphorigenic effects of drugs continue to contribute to their reinforcing effects once tolerance develops. After as little as 5 days of self-administration of alcohol or heroin in a laboratory setting, alcoholic or heroin addicts show more depression, dysphoria, and anxiety than a sense of well-being. In the case of opioids, however, there is a brief period immediately after each dose when mood is elevated (Meyer and Mirin, 1979). The latter finding is consistent with studies in animals, which show little or no tolerance to the opioid-induced lowering of thresholds for electrical self-stimulation of the brain or to the capacity of the drugs to serve as discriminative cues (*see* Kornetsky *et al.,* 1979).

A *protracted opioid abstinence syndrome,* characterized by physiological and psychological abnormalities, commonly follows the acute syndrome due to withdrawal of opioids, and this condition can persist for weeks. Since the subjective sense of not being quite normal is immediately relieved by very small doses of opioid drugs, the protracted abstinence syndrome may predispose to relapse by creating a prolonged period of increased vulnerability, during which the effects of opioids are especially reinforcing (*see* Cushman and Dole, 1973; Martin *et al.,* 1973). Such a protracted state may also exist following withdrawal of other drugs that cause dependence.

In both animals and man, drug effects, withdrawal phenomena, and relief of withdrawal symptoms by drugs can be conditioned to environmental stimuli (*see* Wikler, 1973, 1975; O'Brien *et al.,* 1977). Such conditioning helps to explain how the rituals and circumstances surrounding drug use can act as secondary reinforcers, and how the mere taking of an inert pill or the use of a needle and syringe containing no drug can evoke the feelings (including relief of withdrawal symptoms) previously produced when the pill or syringe contained an active substance. The observation that withdrawal distress can become conditioned to the environment in which it occurs may underlie reports that former opioid addicts may experience sensations very similar to withdrawal symptoms, including an intensified craving for drugs, when they return to an environment where drugs are available. Alcoholics may have similar experiences, particularly when they are exposed to the sight and smell of alcohol (Ludwig *et al.,* 1974). The conditions that elicit the most severe withdrawal and the most intense "craving" for opioids are those associated with the availability and use of the drug, rather than those associated with withdrawal (*e.g.,* being offered some heroin by a friend or watching someone else use the drug) (O'Brien *et al.,* 1977; Meyer and Mirin, 1979). Anecdotal reports suggest that these are also the circumstances that increase craving in recently abstinent alcoholics and cigarette smokers.

Vulnerability. In man, drugs may produce effects experienced as pleasurable, novel, or tension reducing, but these effects are not such powerful reinforcers that repetitive drug use is inevitable. Much research has centered on why some individuals stop after experimentation, others continue drug use but do not become dependent, and still others become compulsive drug users.

Individuals who later become regular users of socially disapproved drugs tend to be more impulsive, more rebellious with respect to social norms, and less tolerant of frustration, but they do not fall into any single diagnostic category. To date, no clearly recognized addictive personality or constellation of traits has been identified that is equally applicable to all varieties of compulsive drug users. Indeed, given the different pharmacological effects of various drugs, it would be surprising if all compulsive drug users were similar.

There are many factors that could contribute to increased vulnerability to continued or compulsive drug use. Some individuals may experience a more intense response to the initial reinforcing properties of the drugs, such as a more intense euphoria or a more profound reduction of unpleasant feelings of anger, depression, or anxiety. Such intense reactions, in turn, could be due to differences in sensitivity to drug effects or to initially higher levels of distress. Thus, for some, drug use may be viewed as self-treatment for internal distress. Although the agent selected or the pattern of use may sometimes run counter to social norms, for some individuals the alternative may be a state of tension that may be felt to be intolerable. On the other hand, the contributory factors may be entirely social, as in the case of young people who continue to smoke cigarettes (despite some initial unpleasant reactions) more to conform to the pressures from friends than because of an especially intense need for the pharmacological effects of nicotine. Still other possibilities include differences in intensity of adverse effects of the drugs or in the intensity of withdrawal phenomena as experienced by different users (*see* above).

Efforts to delineate the factors that contribute to vulnerability have included studies of the personalities and family structures of different types of drug users, and the role of peer groups, social factors, and economic conditions in generating tension and frustration. In some cases, constitutional and genetic factors have been identified that might be responsible either for abnormal states of tension or for unusually positive or negative responses to drug use or drug withdrawal (*see* Goodwin, 1979). But it would appear that for any given pattern of continued drug use the outcome is the result of an interaction between social, biological, and environmental factors. (*See* Platt and Labate, 1976; Jaffe, 1977; Jessor, 1978; Dupont *et al.*, 1979.)

Sociological Factors. Social factors have a major influence on which individuals have access to various drugs, and social attitudes determine which drugs are acceptable for casual or "recreational" use, which may be used for relief of tension, and which are prohibited. In addition, the nature of a society often determines the kinds of tensions induced in its members, as well as the kinds of behaviors that are viewed as socially acceptable. Thus, until recently in Western cultures the pressures to perform sexually and aggressively were greater for males than for females, while the pressures against use of opioids or alcohol were greater for females than for males. In general, when the use of a drug is widely accepted, the number of users tends to be large and their personal characteristics are quite diverse, including the characteristics of the small proportion who become compulsive users. When a particular form of drug use meets with severe disapproval, those who use it despite such sanctions tend to be very different from the average person in society in terms of attitudes and emotional adjustment even before use. Consequently, a high proportion may become intensive or compulsive users, sometimes leading to the conclusion that the particular drug is "more addicting" than those drugs used by larger and more diverse populations. Drugs may indeed differ in the degree to which they induce dependence, but the ratio of experimenters to addicts is not always a valid measure of the liability of a drug to cause dependence.

The acceptability of a drug may increase or decrease with time in a fadlike fashion. Sometimes the use of a drug may become identified with acceptance

of the values of particular groups within a society, and individuals may participate in drug-using behavior as a way of symbolizing their group affiliation. Membership, even in highly deviant groups, may in turn represent an attempted solution to problems of personal identity, since some groups have elaborate sets of behavioral norms.

Chronic drug use may establish a complex equilibrium among family members, and abstinence on the part of the user, with its attendant changes in behavior and role, can also induce tension in other members of the family. Relapse to drugs or alcohol sometimes restores the previous pathological equilibrium. Cultural attitudes toward addicts and alcoholics and the legal or medical complications of drug use further increase the drug user's difficulties in obtaining realistic gratifications (alternative reinforcers) and simultaneously foster his return to an environment (the local bar or group of heroin addicts) where he is accepted, where the drug is available, and where its use is acceptable and has been repeatedly reinforced.

CLINICAL CHARACTERISTICS

Most of the pharmacological agents commonly used for subjective purposes (excluding caffeine) can be placed into eight major classes, as follows: (1) opioids, (2) general CNS depressants, (3) CNS sympathomimetics (including cocaine), (4) nicotine and tobacco, (5) cannabinoids, (6) psychedelics (hallucinogens, psychotomimetics, psychotogens), (7) arylcyclohexylamines (*e.g.,* phencyclidine), and (8) inhalants (*e.g.,* nitrous oxide, ethyl ether, volatile solvents). Although the agents within each class have many actions in common, there are also differences, and the classification is offered merely for its didactic convenience.

Opioids

Incidence and Patterns of Use. In the late 1960s the use of heroin increased considerably, in both the United States and Great Britain. Some of the reasons for the increase include changes in social attitudes toward drug use and toward established social norms in general, increased availability of drugs, and the substantial increase in the adolescent population (a result of the sharp increase in births following World War II), with its associated social changes. In the United States, heroin use, once centered in large urban areas, has spread to smaller communities. Members of racial and ethnic groups from lower socioeconomic strata continue to be overrepresented, but the use of heroin is now observed with greater frequency among more affluent members of society. A survey taken in 1977 indicated that 2 to 3% of young adults (age 18 to 25) had tried heroin at some time in their lives. During the period of peak prevalence (1970–1973), there were probably more than 500,000 heroin addicts in the United States.

In the United States there are three basic patterns of opioid use and dependence. One involves individuals whose drug use begins in the context of medical treatment and who obtain their initial supplies through medical channels. This group constitutes a very small percentage of the addicted population. Another pattern begins with experimental or "recreational" drug use, progresses to more intensive use, and involves primarily adolescents and young adults, with males far outnumbering females. Most of these users are introduced to the drug by other users. This is true both of the initial contact and of those subsequent contacts leading to relapse after periods of withdrawal. The way in which drug use spreads from one friend to another in epidemic fashion has been well documented (Hughes *et al.,* 1972). A third pattern involves users who begin in one or another of the preceding ways but later switch to oral opioids (methadone) obtained from organized treatment programs.

A user's first experience with opioids is often quite unpleasant, with nausea and vomiting as the outstanding features. Some may not try again for days or weeks; others, however, discover a new world of inner satisfaction with the first dose and make a conscious decision to continue to use the drug as frequently as their finances will permit. Some may struggle with the impulse to use it again and may do so only intermittently for many months or years before becoming regular users; some may never become compulsive users. Although there are no statistics to support the notion, the most common pattern may be to try the drug once or twice and then, with awareness of the dangers, to avoid it thereafter. Despite the medical and legal risks, where group values support opioid use and relatively pure drugs are easily available, a very high percentage of users may become physically dependent. In 1971, about 42% of United States Army enlisted men in Vietnam used opioids at least once, and about half of these users reported that at some time during their year in Vietnam they were physically dependent (*see* Robins, 1974).

The incidence of opioid addiction among physicians, nurses, and those in the related health professions is many times higher than in any group with comparable educational background. Most physician-addicts state that they first took the drug to overcome fatigue, depression, or to alleviate some bodily ailment, and few indicate that they were seeking thrills; the original motive, however, has little effect on the pattern and the consequences of the addiction that later develops. These are often related more to chance factors, such as whether they are prosecuted by enforcement agencies for their drug use. Considering the frequency with which opioid analgesics are used in clinical medicine, addiction as a complication of medical treatment is quite uncommon. When it does occur, the pattern it follows depends on both the emotional adjustment of the patient prior to involvement with opioids and the source of the drug. Those individuals who continue to obtain it from physicians usually avoid many of the problems associated with illicit drugs. Those who must obtain drugs from illicit traffic encounter the same problems that are faced by heroin users. The personality characteristics of physician-addicts, and probably those of "medical" addicts in general, are distinct from those of the urban heroin addict.

Rapid intravenous injection of an opioid produces a warm flushing of the skin and sensations in the lower abdomen described by addicts as similar in intensity and quality to sexual orgasm; this lasts for about 45 seconds and is known as a "rush," "kick," or "thrill." Although heroin is the most commonly used illicit opioid, it has few special pharmacological properties that account for its popularity. Given subcutaneously, even experienced users cannot reliably distinguish heroin from morphine. This is understandable, since heroin is rapidly converted into morphine in the body. When these two drugs are given intravenously, addicts are better able to distinguish between them, probably because of the greater lipid solubility of heroin in comparison to morphine. This results in a higher rate of crossing the blood-brain barrier, and effects on the CNS are thus produced rapidly (Oldendorf, 1978). In the brain, heroin is rapidly deacetylated to 6-monoacetyl morphine and then to morphine. In this sense, heroin carries morphine rapidly into the brain. On a weight basis, heroin is about two and one-half times as potent as morphine as an analgesic, but, given subcutaneously, it does not produce more euphoria or greater physical dependence (Martin and Fraser, 1961).

Symptoms and Effects of Compulsive Use. The behavior, social adjustment, and medical problems observed among opioid users and addicts are surprisingly varied. Experience with thousands of patients maintained on high daily doses of methadone for periods of more than 10 years has shown no direct injurious effects (Kreek, 1973, 1979; Wilmarth and Goldstein, 1974). Good health and productive work are thus not incompatible with regular use of opioids. However, it is now clear that the behavior of the individual prior to opioid use and the purposes and patterns of use play a large role in determining the social and physiological consequences.

In England, where chronic opioid users may still obtain pure heroin from legitimate medical sources at no cost, the patterns of social adjustment are extremely varied. The majority of opioid users in Britain are young people who were introduced to drug use by friends, began out of curiosity, and continue because of the euphoric effects. The preferred route of administration is intravenous. The patterns of adjustment among the patients receiving treatment at London clinics are similar to those observed in the United States. Four major patterns have been noted: (1) "stables"—patients who are legitimately employed, do not engage in criminal activity, do not associate with other addicts, and do not buy extra heroin illicitly; (2) "junkies"—patients who are the opposite of the stable patients in these respects; (3) "loners"—patients who are on welfare rather than engaging in crime, do not associate with other addicts, but do use a wide variety of drugs not prescribed by the clinic; and (4) "two-worlders"— patients who are employed but associate with other addicts, buy extra drugs, and engage in criminal activities. The disorganized behavior and criminality of the "junkies" and the organized behavior of the "stables" antedate the addiction (Stimson, 1973). Despite the legal source of drugs, those receiving heroin at London clinics had a high incidence of infections (due to neglect of hygienic procedures or to shared needles) and a surprisingly high mortality rate, ranging from 2 to 6% per year (Stimson, 1973). A follow-up study of young heroin addicts treated at London clinics revealed that 7 years later only 48% were still using opioids (43% obtained drugs from the clinics), 32% were abstinent and not abusing other drugs, and 12% were dead (Stimson et al., 1978).

Similar variations in patterns of behavior, social adjustment, and impaired health have been noted among heroin addicts in the United States despite the exclusively illegal sources of their drugs. Undoubtedly, the high cost and impurities of illicit drugs in the United States exact their toll. Many females earn their drug money through prostitution, and there is a high incidence of venereal disease among female heroin addicts. The average annual death rate among young-adult heroin addicts is several times higher than that for nonaddicts of similar age and ethnic backgrounds. In the younger group, much of this increase is due to fatal opioid overdosage that is usually an accidental outcome of the dangerous fluctuations in the purity of illicit heroin or to combinations of opioids with alcohol or other CNS depressants. Another frequent cause of sudden death has been termed an "anaphylactoid reaction," which probably results from the intravenous injection of a drug containing certain impurities. The suicide rate among adult addicts is likewise consid-

erably higher than that of the general population, and a surprisingly high percentage die violent deaths at the hands of others. The medical complications common among drug users include infections (e.g., septicemia, endocarditis, hepatitis, tetanus, and pulmonary, cerebral, and subcutaneous abscesses) due to shared needles and unhygienic procedures, foreign-body emboli, granulomata due to injection of contaminants, and a variety of neurological, musculoskeletal, and other lesions that may be due to hypersensitivity reactions. The medical problems associated with opioid use have been reviewed by Sapira (1968) and Thornton and Thornton (1974).

The health and social adjustment of patients maintained on oral methadone are equally varied. Many hold jobs, raise children, commit no crimes, and use no socially disapproved drugs. Yet other patients continue to commit crimes, do not obtain employment, and use other drugs or excessive amounts of alcohol. A substantial number experience significant depression (Weissman et al., 1976). The mortality rate among patients in maintenance programs is higher than that among others of comparable age and socioeconomic status, but the general consensus is that the high rate is not related to the effects of oral methadone per se, but directly or indirectly to problems that antedated methadone use or to the excessive use of alcohol and other drugs.

Opioids reduce pain, aggression, and sexual drives, and their use, therefore, is unlikely to induce crime. However, many individuals committed crimes prior to the use of opioids, and they do not necessarily stop when opioid use begins. In addition, many individuals who did not engage in crime previously may begin to do so in order to obtain money to buy opioids, since the cost is generally beyond the amount they can obtain legitimately. In general, the number of crimes goes up while addicts are using illicit opioids. For a discussion of the complex relationship between the use of opioids and crime, see National Commission (1973) and McGlothlin (1979).

Tolerance, Physical Dependence, and Withdrawal Symptoms. A remarkable degree of tolerance develops to the respiratory depressant, analgesic, sedative, emetic, and euphorigenic effects of opioids; however, the rate at which this tolerance develops, in either the addict or the medical patient, depends on the pattern of use. With intermittent use, it is possible to obtain desired analgesic and sedative effects from doses in the therapeutic range for an indefinite period. It is only when there is a more or less continuous drug action that significant tolerance develops. Thus, if the drug is used frequently, the addict who is primarily seeking to get a "rush" or to maintain a state of dreamy indifference (a "high") must constantly increase the dose. In this way, some addicts can build up to phenomenally large doses. In one verified case a dose of 5 g of morphine was used each day. With the development of tolerance, the lethal dose is greatly altered. A case is recorded in which an addict was injected intravenously with 2 g of morphine over a period of 2.5 hours without significant change in blood pressure, pulse rate, or respiration; the usual dose for this individual was 0.25 g. However, tolerance is not absolute. With all opioid analgesics a dose always exists that is capable of producing death from respiratory depression, even in tolerant individuals.

Tolerance does not develop equally or at the same rate to all the effects of opioids, and even users highly tolerant to respiratory depressant effects continue to exhibit miosis and to complain of constipation. Addicts who self-administer heroin in an investigational laboratory setting develop tolerance to the euphorigenic effects within 1 to 2 weeks and thereafter seem dysphoric and depressed, except for a brief period following each intravenous dose (Meyer and Mirin, 1979). Subjects who are maintained on daily oral doses of 100 mg of methadone for more than 8 weeks still seem sedated and apathetic and have constricted pupils and decreased respiratory rates (Martin *et al.,* 1973). However, experience with thousands of patients maintained on methadone for periods of several years suggests that, while constipation is a continuing problem, substantial sedation and apathy are easily managed by reductions in dosage. Indeed, without laboratory technics, even skilled clinicians cannot distinguish between patients maintained on methadone and patients who are drug free. Some patients are eager to be withdrawn from methadone, which again underscores the distinction between physical dependence and addiction.

Meperidine addicts may use large daily doses (3 to 4 g per day), but significant tolerance does not develop to the drug's excitant and atropine-like actions. When very high doses of meperidine are used, even the tolerant addict may show dilated pupils, in-

creased muscular activity, twitching, tremors, mental confusion, and, occasionally, grand mal seizures (Isbell and White, 1953).

In general, there is a high degree of cross-tolerance between drugs with morphine-like actions. However, the development of opioid drugs such as nalbuphine, which appear to exert their primary agonistic actions at the κ rather than the μ receptor (*see* Chapter 22), makes it necessary to qualify generalizations about cross-tolerance and cross-dependence. Studies in animals suggest that κ-receptor agonists do not induce cross-tolerance to agents that act primarily on the μ receptor.

Tolerance to opioids largely disappears when withdrawal has been completed, and many addicts have taken fatal overdoses by returning to their previous dosage immediately after undergoing withdrawal.

The character and the severity of the withdrawal symptoms that appear when an opioid is discontinued depend upon many factors, including the particular drug, the total daily dose used, the interval between doses, the duration of use, and the health and personality of the addict.

It is helpful to view the total clinical picture of the abstinence syndrome as made up of *purposive behavior,* which is goal oriented, highly dependent on the observer and the environment, and directed at getting more drug, and *nonpurposive behavior,* which is not goal oriented and relatively independent of the observer and the environment. The purposive phenomena, including complaints, pleas, demands, manipulations, and simulations, are as varied as the imagination of the drug-using population. In the hospital setting, they are considerably less pronounced when the patient is certain that his behavior does not affect the decision to give him a drug.

In the case of morphine or heroin, nonpurposive symptoms, such as lacrimation, rhinorrhea, yawning, and sweating, appear about 8 to 12 hours after the last dose. About 12 to 14 hours after the last dose, the addict may fall into a tossing, restless sleep known as the "yen," which may last several hours but from which he awakens more restless and more miserable than before. As the syndrome progresses, additional signs and symptoms appear, consisting in dilated pupils, anorexia, gooseflesh, restlessness, irritability, and tremor. With morphine and heroin, nonpurposive symptoms reach their peak at 48 to 72 hours. As the syndrome approaches peak intensity, the patient exhibits increasing irritability, insomnia, marked anorexia, violent yawning, severe sneezing, lacrimation, and coryza. Weakness and depression are pronounced. Nausea and vomiting are common, as are intestinal spasm and diarrhea. Heart rate and blood pressure are elevated. Marked chilliness, alternating with flushing and excessive sweating, is characteristic. Pilomotor activity resulting in waves of gooseflesh is prominent, and the skin resembles that of a plucked turkey. This feature is the basis of the expression "cold turkey" to signify abrupt withdrawal without treatment. Abdominal cramps and pains in the bones and muscles of the back and extremities are also characteristic, as are the muscle spasms and kicking movements that may be the basis for the expression "kicking the habit." Other signs of CNS hyperexcitability include ejaculation in men and orgasm in women. The respiratory response to CO_2, which is decreased during opioid administration, is exaggerated during withdrawal. Rebound phenomena are also observed in the endocrine system. During addiction, urinary concentrations of 17-ketosteroids are decreased; during withdrawal, they increase markedly (Eisenman et al., 1958). Leukocytosis is common, and white-cell counts above 14,000/cu mm are often seen.

The failure to take food and fluids, combined with vomiting, sweating, and diarrhea, results in marked weight loss, dehydration, ketosis, and disturbance in acid-base balance. Occasionally there is cardiovascular collapse. At any point in the course of withdrawal, the administration of a suitable opioid will completely and dramatically suppress the symptoms of withdrawal. Obviously, administration of a drug cannot immediately restore body fluids or acid-base balance, and in this sense the syndrome is not completely reversible. Without treatment, the morphine withdrawal syndrome runs its course and most of the grossly observable symptoms disappear in 7 to 10 days, but it is not certain how long it takes to restore physiological equilibrium completely.

It is now clear that the recovery process is complex and protracted, and that the early opioid abstinence syndrome characterized by the signs and symptoms described above is followed by a *protracted abstinence syndrome*, during which a number of physiological variables attain subnormal values. For example, a period of hyposensitivity to the respiratory stimulant effects of CO_2 persists for many weeks after the exaggerated sensitivity of the early abstinence period subsides. In addition, there seem to be subtle behavioral manifestations of protracted abstinence that include an incapacity to tolerate stress, a poor self-image, and overconcern about discomfort. It is not unreasonable to postulate that these altered states contribute to the tendency of compulsive opioid users to relapse after withdrawal (see Dole, 1972; Martin et al., 1973).

The *abrupt withdrawal of methadone* produces a syndrome that is qualitatively similar to that of morphine, but it develops more slowly and is more prolonged, although usually less intense. The addict has few or no symptoms until 24 to 48 hours after the last dose, and then complains of weakness, anxiety, anorexia, insomnia, abdominal discomfort, headache, sweating, pain in muscles and bones, and hot and cold flashes. As with morphine withdrawal, there is

nausea, vomiting, and an increase in body temperature, blood pressure, pulse, respiratory rate, and pupillary size. In general, after abrupt withdrawal, the primary or early abstinence syndrome reaches its maximal intensity by about the third day and may not begin to decrease until the third week, and apparent recovery may not occur until the sixth or seventh week. The early abstinence syndrome is followed by a secondary or protracted abstinence syndrome in which a number of previously elevated physiological parameters attain and remain at subnormal values through the twenty-fourth postwithdrawal week, and there are concomitant psychological disturbances such as tiredness, weakness, hypochondriasis, and feelings of lessened efficiency (Martin et al., 1973). Even with very slow reduction in dosage, patients who have been maintained on high doses of methadone experience qualitatively similar withdrawal symptoms during and following the period of dosage reduction (Cushman and Dole, 1973; Senay et al., 1977).

The *meperidine abstinence syndrome* usually develops within 3 hours after the last dose, reaches its peak within 8 to 12 hours, and then declines, so that few symptoms are apparent after 4 to 5 days. Craving may be intense, but the nonpurposive autonomic signs, while present, are not as prominent; the pupils may not be widely dilated, and there is usually little nausea, vomiting, or diarrhea. However, at peak intensity the muscle twitching, restlessness, and nervousness may be worse than during morphine withdrawal (Isbell and White, 1953).

Although *codeine* can partially suppress morphine withdrawal, withdrawal symptoms after codeine (1200 to 1800 mg per day), while qualitatively similar to those of morphine, are considerably less intense.

Withdrawal symptoms after semisynthetic and synthetic opioids are qualitatively similar to those after morphine, and they seem to follow the general rule that drugs with shorter durations of action tend to produce shorter, more intense abstinence syndromes while those drugs that are slowly eliminated produce withdrawal syndromes that are prolonged but mild. Some differences between the opioid withdrawal syndrome and those seen with agonist-antagonists are described in Chapter 22.

Withdrawal in the Newborn. Babies born to mothers who have been taking opioids regularly prior to delivery will be physically dependent. The signs of withdrawal include irritability and excessive and high-pitched crying, tremors, frantic sucking of fists, hyperactive reflexes, increased respiratory rate, increased stools, sneezing, yawning, vomiting, and fever. With heroin, signs most commonly appear within the first day of life; they may not appear for several days with methadone. The intensity of the syndrome does not always correlate with the duration of maternal opioid use or dose. There is no consensus on the best method of managing such withdrawal. Although clinicians have used paregoric, phenobarbital, diazepam, and chlorpromazine, the use of paregoric (0.2 ml orally every 3 to 4 hours, increased as needed) seems to be the most rational and effective approach when there is no question of simultaneous dependence on alcohol or other sedatives. While withdrawal symptoms when untreated are generally more severe in babies born to mothers who have been maintained on methadone, compared to those who have been using heroin, the greater opportunity to provide prenatal care to the mother maintained on methadone results in a significant decrease in overall fetal distress and mortality (*see* Zelson *et al.,* 1973; Stimmel and Adamsons, 1976; Finnegan, 1979).

Opioid Antagonists. The abstinence syndromes described above are those seen when the drugs are abruptly withdrawn. If, however, the drug is not withdrawn but simply displaced from its site of action by an antagonist such as naloxone, a withdrawal syndrome develops within a few minutes after parenteral administration and reaches its peak intensity within 30 minutes. Until the antagonist is eliminated, even large doses of previously used opioid cannot suppress the syndrome; partial suppression is possible, but only by using extremely large doses of opioid, which may then produce respiratory depression as the action of the antagonist wanes. The intensity of naloxone-precipitated withdrawal is usually more severe than that seen after abrupt withdrawal of the drug. Withdrawal from methadone produced by an antagonist is especially severe.

GENERAL CNS DEPRESSANTS: BARBITURATES AND RELATED SEDATIVE-HYPNOTIC DRUGS

In general, the subjective effects of barbiturates and related sedatives and antianxiety agents are similar but not identical to those of alcohol, and the effects vary considerably with the dose, the situation, and the personality of the user.

Prevalence, Agents Employed, and Patterns of Use. The incidence and prevalence of nonmedical and compulsive use of barbiturates, benzodiazepines, and related drugs cannot be stated with accuracy, but it is believed to exceed greatly that of the opioids. In 1977, 18% of young adults reported nonmedical use of sedatives, with 2.5% reporting some use in the preceding month. About 13% indicated some experience with nonmedical use of tranquilizers. The incidence has been relatively stable over the past 5 years (Abelson *et al.,* 1977).

Opioid users frequently take barbiturates, benzodiazepines, or other sedatives to augment the effects of weak illicit heroin, and many heroin users are physically dependent on both heroin and sedatives. Some alcoholics use these agents to relieve the alcohol withdrawal syndrome or to produce a state of intoxication devoid of the odor of alcohol. The short-acting barbiturates such as pentobarbital ("yellow jackets") or secobarbital ("red devils") are preferred to long-acting agents such as phenobarbital. Since the user is more interested in the pharmacological effects than in chemical classifications, it is not surprising that nonbarbiturates such as meprobamate, glutethimide, methyprylon, methaqualone, and some of the benzodiazepines are also abused. Paraldehyde and chloral hydrate, subject to considerable abuse in the past, have now been largely replaced by the other agents mentioned. Meprobamate seems less acceptable as a barbiturate substitute; and chlordiazepoxide, with its minimal euphoriant actions and slow onset of effects, is quite uncommon as a drug of abuse. However, the shorter-acting diazepam is used widely for nonmedical purposes.

The patterns of nonmedical use are exceedingly varied. They range from infrequent sprees of gross intoxication, lasting a few days, to the prolonged, compulsive, daily use of huge quantities and a preoccupation with securing and maintaining adequate supplies. Some users may never exhibit gross intoxication but may, nevertheless, take drugs several times a day. The original contact with the drug may have been through a physician's prescription or through illicit drug trade. In the medical patient, the development of the problem may be a gradual one, beginning with prolonged use for insomnia or anxiety and progressing through increased dosage at night to a few capsules for sedation in the morning. Eventually, the drug is a major part of the user's life. In such situations, what at one point could be considered a habituation at another is clearly an addiction. Neither the patient taking benzodiazepines over a period of months nor his physician may recognize the existence of dependence. Both may assume that the anxiety, tremulousness, and insomnia that emerge when the drug is discontinued is a return of the original anxiety. There is no sharp line that can be drawn between appropriate use, abuse, habituation, and addiction. Most users take the drugs orally, but there are a few individuals who inject barbiturates intravenously or intramuscularly. Such users can be recognized by the large abscesses that cover the accessible areas of their bodies.

The combination of amphetamines and barbiturates produces more elevation of mood than either drug alone. The mechanisms of this supra-additive effect are not yet clear, but competition for the same microsomal enzyme system and hence production of higher blood concentrations of the drugs could be involved.

The amount of hypnotic that may be taken varies considerably, but an average daily dose of 1.5 g of short-acting barbiturate is not uncommon, and some individuals have consumed as much as 2.5 g daily over many months. Similar multiples of the usual daily therapeutic doses are taken by the compulsive users of meprobamate, glutethimide, methyprylon, methaqualone, and diazepam. The abuse of sedative agents has been reviewed by Essig (1968), Smith (1977), and Wesson and Smith (1977b).

Signs and Symptoms. Because tolerance develops to most of the actions of this group of drugs, there may be no apparent signs of chronic use. For the patient taking regular doses of sleeping pills the only manifestation may be a rebound insomnia when the drug is stopped. The patient taking benzodiazepines may experience insomnia and rebound increase in anxiety several days after stopping. Some users, however, attempt to maintain a state of intoxication. In these individuals, the acute and the chronic effects of mild intoxication with CNS depressants resemble those of intoxication with alcohol. The individual who is intoxicated with a barbiturate shows a general sluggishness, difficulty in thinking, slowness and slurring of speech, poor comprehension and memory, faulty judgment, narrowed range of attention, emotional lability, and exaggeration of basic personality traits. Irritability, quarrelsomeness, and moroseness are common. There may be laughing or crying without provocation, untidiness in personal habits, hostile and paranoid ideas, and suicidal tendencies (*see* Isbell *et al.,* 1950; Fraser *et al.,* 1954; Smith, 1977). Chronic intoxication with pharmacologically similar agents has not been studied in as controlled a manner, but the clinical descriptions of isolated cases of abuse of high doses of meprobamate, glutethimide, methaqualone, chlordiazepoxide, and diazepam are quite similar to the picture of chronic barbiturate intoxication. Neurological effects described here are those for barbiturates. These effects include thick, slurred speech, nystagmus, diplopia, strabismus, difficulty in visual accommo-

dation, vertigo, ataxic gait, positive Romberg's sign, hypotonia, dysmetria, and decreased superficial reflexes; deep reflexes, pupillary responses, and sensation are usually unaltered. Occasionally transient ankle clonus and Babinski's signs are elicitable. Nutrition is usually unimpaired. Skin rashes may develop; they may be erythematous, urticarial, purpuric, or scarlatiniform. The urine may contain albumin and casts.

Tolerance, Physical Dependence, and Withdrawal Symptoms. Chronic intoxication with short-acting barbiturates and related hypnotics results in both drug-disposition and pharmacodynamic tolerance. Pharmacodynamic tolerance also develops to most of the actions of benzodiazepines, but drug-disposition tolerance is less marked. Indeed, the slow accumulation of active metabolites of certain benzodiazepines tends to obscure the development of adaptive changes in the CNS. The overall tolerance that is attained has an upper limit that gives chronic intoxication with hypnotics a very characteristic picture. For example, an individual tolerant to 1.2 g of pentobarbital per day may show little evidence of intoxication on that dose; however, if the dose is raised by as little as 0.1 g per day, prolonged and perhaps cumulative intoxication may occur (Isbell and White, 1953). It is also characteristic of adaptation to this class of agents that, while there may be considerable tolerance to the sedative and intoxicating effects, the lethal dose is not much greater in addicts than in normal individuals. Consequently, acute barbiturate or meprobamate poisoning may be accidentally or willfully superimposed on chronic intoxication at any time.

Benzodiazepines appear to be considerably safer than barbiturates and related sedatives, since acute overdosage is much less likely to produce fatal respiratory depression. Cross-tolerance between various agents in this group is common, but not all combinations have been studied. Tolerance develops most readily to effects on behaviors that are impaired by drugs and for which there is the greatest motivation to perform. This suggests an element of learning as an important aspect of tolerance (*see* Smith, 1977; Kalant, 1978).

There are marked similarities between the withdrawal syndromes seen with barbiturates and those seen with meprobamate, glutethimide, methaqualone, benzodiazepines, and related drugs. It seems justified, therefore, to use the term *general depressant withdrawal syndrome* to refer to the manifestations of withdrawal from any of these agents. In its mildest form, the general depressant withdrawal syndrome may consist in only paroxysmal EEG abnormalities, rebound increases in rapid-eye-movement (REM) sleep, insomnia, or anxiety. Somewhat greater degrees of physical dependence result in tremulousness and weakness, in addition to anxiety and insomnia. When the syndrome is severe, there may be, in addition, grand mal seizures and delirium.

Former addicts can ingest 0.2 g of pentobarbital per day over many months without the development of any obvious manifestations of physical dependence on abrupt withdrawal. However, after a daily dose of 0.4 g for 3 months, abrupt withdrawal produces paroxysmal EEG changes without other significant symptoms in about 30% of subjects. After 0.6 g per day for 1 to 2 months, 50% of subjects show minor withdrawal symptoms such as insomnia, anorexia, tremor, and EEG changes, and 10% may have a single seizure. When subjects are continuously intoxicated (0.9 to 2.2 g per day) for several months, 75% may have seizures and 66% delirium, and all experience insomnia, tremor, and anorexia on abrupt withdrawal (Fraser *et al.*, 1958). Significant symptoms, similar to those described for barbiturates, are seen during withdrawal from meprobamate (3.2 to 6.4 g per day for 40 days).

If sleep patterns and electrical activity of the brain during sleep are used as measures of physical dependence, it becomes apparent that very little drug given over relatively short periods is sufficient to produce the effect. Subjects given hypnotic drugs in ordinary doses for several weeks show tolerance to the hypnotic effects. Rebound increases in percentage of REM sleep and insomnia are often seen when such drugs are discontinued. A similar rebound disturbance in sleep is seen upon withdrawal of shorter-acting benzodiazepines administered for as little as 1 to 2 weeks, although REM sleep does not rebound above baseline levels (Kales *et al.*, 1974, 1978).

The typical course of withdrawal from large amounts of short-acting barbiturates is as follows: over the first 12 to 16 hours, as the concentration of the drug in blood declines and the intoxication clears, the patient seems to improve but then becomes increasingly restless, anxious, tremulous, and weak. There may be complaints of abdominal cramps, nausea, and vomiting. Orthostatic hypotension is characteristic and may produce fainting if the patient stands up quickly. Within the first 24 hours, he may become too weak to get out of bed; coarse tremors of the hands are prominent, deep reflexes may be hyperactive, and the blink reflex is increased. During this period, *purposive behavior* is prominent

and the patient may plead for his drug. With the short-acting barbiturates and meprobamate, the symptoms usually reach their peak during the second and third days of abstinence; convulsions, when they occur, are usually seen within this period. The number of seizures varies from a single one to *status epilepticus*.

With the longer-acting barbiturates and the longer-acting benzodiazepines, symptoms reach their peak more slowly, and seizures may not occur at all or may occur as late as the seventh to eighth day (Wulff, 1959; Smith, 1977). In Wulff's (1959) series, when the rate of elimination of the barbiturate was slower than 20% per day, EEG changes and withdrawal symptoms were not seen. Thus, clinical studies are consistent with laboratory studies that show that the onset and intensity of withdrawal are related to the rate at which active drug leaves the CNS. Some patients who have seizures may begin to show improvement after the third day, but more than half go on to develop delirium. Anxiety mounts with time, and frightening dreams may be succeeded by a refractory insomnia. Visual hallucinations, usually of a persecutory nature, may occur, generally at the same time that sensorial clouding begins. Disorientation for time and place completes the picture of a full-blown delirium. Once the delirium develops, even the administration of large doses of barbiturate may not supress it immediately. This is also true of the delirium that develops during the withdrawal of alcohol. The reason for this relative irreversibility is not clear.

During the delirium, which usually occurs between the fourth and seventh day, agitation and hyperthermia can lead to exhaustion, cardiovascular collapse, and death. The withdrawal syndrome, even if untreated, usually clears by about the eighth day; this is generally preceded by a period of prolonged sleep. When hallucinations persist for several months, the situation would seem analogous to chronic alcoholic hallucinosis, which is felt by many investigators to be a manifestation of an underlying psychosis.

The spontaneous EEG during the second and third days of withdrawal from a short-acting barbiturate is characterized by dysrhythmias in the form of diffuse slowing, random slow waves, recurrent spikes, and high-voltage paroxysmal discharges of various sorts. Wulff (1959) has shown that photic stimulation will produce paroxysmal EEG changes in many patients who show no abnormalities in the resting EEG. Such changes were seen in over 90% of patients who exhibited abstinence phenomena.

Babies born to mothers physically dependent on general CNS depressants will manifest withdrawal syndromes of varying severity (Desmond *et al.*, 1972). The signs are similar to those seen in the opioid withdrawal syndrome of the newborn.

ALCOHOL

Prevalence and Patterns of Use. In Western society, alcohol has the unique distinction of being the only potent pharmacological agent with which obvious self-induced intoxication is socially acceptable.

In the United States, two thirds of all adults use alcohol occasionally, and at least 12% of the users can be considered "heavy" drinkers. If cigarette smoking is excluded, alcoholism is by far the most serious drug problem in the United States and most other countries. Measured in terms of accidents, lost productivity, crime, death, or damaged health, the combined social costs of problem drinking in the United States were estimated in 1979 to exceed 43 billion dollars annually. The cost in broken homes, wasted lives, loss to society, and human misery is beyond calculation.

There are different patterns of alcoholism in which there are varying degrees of psychological and nutritional complications, physical dependence (inability to abstain), "loss of control," and episodic use. In addition, problem drinkers may also abuse other drugs, such as sedatives, opioids, marihuana, and amphetamines. Sometimes these are used in combination with alcohol; at other times, such drugs are taken in preference to alcohol, and alcohol is used only when the drug of choice is not available (see Freed, 1973; Goodwin et al., 1975).

The wide spectrum of alcohol use associated with adverse consequences makes it difficult to formulate any simple definition of problem drinking or alcoholism. Different people use alcohol for different reasons. For some it produces euphoria and releases emotions; for others it temporarily relieves depression or anxiety. However, other modes of reinforcement must come into play with chronic use since, after the first few days of drinking, alcoholics in laboratory settings often become more anxious and more depressed as drinking continues (see Mello and Mendelson, 1977).

Tolerance, Physical Dependence, and Special Complications.

Chronic use of alcohol results in an increased capacity to metabolize alcohol, which declines after several weeks of abstinence, so that abstinent alcoholics and normal individuals metabolize alcohol at about the same rate. Chronic use of alcohol also produces pharmacodynamic tolerance, so that a higher blood concentration is necessary to produce intoxication in tolerant than in normal individuals. Some alcoholics can perform well on difficult tasks when their blood alcohol concentrations are above 200 mg/dl, twice the value that in most states is legally defined as significant intoxication. However, as is the case with barbiturates, there is no marked elevation of the lethal dose, and severe acute intoxication with respiratory depression may be superimposed on chronic alcoholic intoxication at any time (see Mello and Mendelson, 1977).

Cross-tolerance between alcohol and other drugs may be due to pharmacodynamic tolerance in the CNS or to more rapid metabolism, since the use of alcohol increases hepatic microsomal enzyme activity. Individuals tolerant to alcohol usually show cross-tolerance to general anesthetics; this cross-tolerance is probably a result of pharmacodynamic tolerance. There is also cross-tolerance to a variety of other sedative-hypnotics, including the benzodiazepines, which results from both pharmacodynamic (CNS) tolerance and from more rapid metabolism. However, cross-tolerance is seen only in the relatively sober alcoholic. When concentrations of alcohol in blood are high, the effects of other drugs are additive to those of alcohol. In addition, there is some mutual inhibition of metabolism as a result of competition for shared enzymatic systems (see Kalant et al., 1971; Hawkins and Kalant, 1972; Lieber, 1972; Sellers et al., 1972; Smith, 1977, 1978). There is no obvious cross-tolerance between alcohol and opioid drugs.

Chronic maintenance of high concentrations of alcohol in blood produces a state of physical dependence. The signs and symptoms of the alcohol withdrawal syndrome are quite similar to those described for barbiturate withdrawal (see above). The intensity of the alcohol withdrawal syndrome correlates only partially with the amount of alcohol consumed and the duration of use. The poor correlation is probably due to the way in which alcohol is metabolized. The body is able to metabolize the alcoholic content of about 30 ml (1 oz) of whisky in an hour (see Chapter 18). If the intake is sufficiently spread out over the day, each dose of alcohol may be metabolized without any substantial increase in blood concentration. On the other hand, the ingestion of only modestly larger amounts, but spaced so that the body's metabolic capacity is exceeded (e.g., 120 ml [4 oz] of whisky every 3 hours), can produce much higher blood concentrations, which can induce clinically significant physical dependence in a matter of a few days (see above). Withdrawal phenomena most commonly appear within 12 to 72 hours after total cessation of drinking. However, even a relative decline in blood concentration (e.g., from 300 to 100 mg/dl) may precipitate the syndrome, and such declines may occur with changes in the pattern of drinking, as well as with decreases in the total daily intake (*see* Mello and Mendelson, 1977).

With minimal levels of dependence, the entire syndrome may consist in disturbed sleep, nausea, weakness, anxiety, and mild tremors that last for less than a day. When dependence is severe, these symptoms are only prodromal.

The clinical picture of alcohol withdrawal in patients with severe physical dependence described by Victor and Adams (1953) is still the basis for the delineation of three somewhat distinct withdrawal states—the tremulous syndrome, alcohol-related seizure disorders, and delirium tremens. However, there is much *overlapping*, as the following description indicates.

Tremulousness, which appears within a few hours after the last drink, is often accompanied by nausea, weakness, anxiety, and sweating. Purposive behavior directed toward obtaining alcohol or a suitable substitute is prominent. There may be cramps and vomiting. Hyperreflexia is prominent. Tremors may be mild or so marked that the patient may be unable to lift a glass. The subject may begin to "see things," at first only when the eyes are closed but later even while the eyes are open. Insight is at first retained, and the subject remains oriented. The syndrome at this point is often referred to as *acute alcoholic hallucinosis*. However, some experts feel that hallucinosis is not necessarily an index of the severity of the withdrawal syndrome; it is sometimes seen while alcoholics are severely intoxicated (*see* Mello and Mendelson, 1977). Grand mal seizures can occur, but they are less common in alcohol withdrawal than in barbiturate withdrawal. The spontaneous EEG shows mild but definite dysrhythmias, in contrast to the major alterations seen during withdrawal of short-acting barbiturates (Wikler *et al.,* 1956). As in the case of barbiturates, however, photic stimulation often reveals paroxysmal abnormalities, even when the spontaneous record appears normal. The REM phase of sleep that is depressed by alcohol shows a rebound increase during alcohol withdrawal.

The tremulous state reaches peak intensity within 24 to 48 hours, and seizures are most likely to occur within the first 24 hours after cessation of drinking. If the syndrome progresses further, insight is lost; the subject becomes weaker, more confused, disoriented, and agitated. He may be terrified by his persecutory hallucinations. They are often so vivid that the subject, even after recovery, sometimes doubts their unreality. At this stage, which appears around the third day of withdrawal, the picture is that of the *tremulous delirium,* which was described by Thomas Sutton in 1813. Hyperthermia is common, and exhaustion and cardiovascular collapse may occur.

The alcohol abstinence syndrome is self-limited. If the patient does not die, recovery usually occurs within 5 to 7 days, without treatment. Those patients in whom the sensorium is clear but hallucinations persist well beyond the usual period of recovery are frequently found to be paranoid schizophrenics.

Babies born to mothers who drink heavily during pregnancy not only experience alcohol withdrawal after delivery but also, in some cases, are believed to suffer permanent mental retardation (Jones *et al.,* 1974; Chapter 18).

A number of special problems are seen in chronic alcoholism that are not apparent with other types of drug abuse. Most of these special problems are now thought to be related to multiple nutritional deficiencies, that are, in turn, the result of the capacity of alcohol to supply calories and depress appetite without supplying essential vitamins and amino acids. They include peripheral polyneuropathies, pellagra, nutritional amblyopia, Wernicke's encephalopathy, and Korsakoff's psychosis. However, other disorders, such as fatty liver, cirrhosis of the liver, and damage to cardiac and skeletal muscle, once thought to be related to nutritional aberrations, are due, at least in part, to direct toxic effects of alcohol itself (*see* Lieber, 1972; Chapter 18). Cerebral atrophy with accompanying mental impairment is far more common among alcoholics (even those who are apparently well nourished) than previously believed (Epstein *et al.,* 1977; Carlen *et al.,* 1978).

CNS SYMPATHOMIMETICS: AMPHETAMINE, COCAINE, AND RELATED DRUGS

The subjective effects of CNS sympathomimetics, like those of all centrally active drugs, are dependent on the user, the environment, the dose of the drug, and the route of administration. For example, moderate doses of amphetamine given orally to normal subjects commonly produce an elevation of mood, a sense of increased energy and alertness, and decreased appetite; task performance that has been impaired by fatigue or boredom is improved. Some individuals may become anxious, irritable, or loquacious. A few may experience transient drowsiness (Tecce and Cole, 1974), but insomnia is more common. As the dose is increased toward toxic levels, the effects of individual experiences and of environment become less significant. The general pharmacology of these agents is described in Chapter 8. When equated for differences in potency, a number of other CNS sympathomimetics and related agents can produce subjective effects that resemble those of amphetamine. These drugs include dextroamphetamine, methamphetamine, phenmetrazine, methylphenidate, and diethylpropion.

Some congeners with substitutions in the aromatic ring (*e.g.*, fenfluramine, chlorphentermine) do not produce amphetamine-like subjective effects and have little or no potential for reinforcement (*see* Martin *et al.*, 1971; Griffith, 1977; Griffiths *et al.*, 1978).

Cocaine addicts describe the euphoric effects of cocaine in terms that are almost indistinguishable from those used by amphetamine addicts. In the laboratory, subjects familiar with cocaine cannot distinguish between the subjective effects of 8 to 10 mg of cocaine and those of 10 mg of dextroamphetamine when both are given intravenously (Fischman *et al.*, 1976), and the toxic syndrome seen with cocaine seems clinically indistinguishable from that produced by amphetamines. In addition, animals exhibit similar patterns of self-administration of cocaine and amphetamine. In short, while it is commonly assumed that the subjective effects of cocaine are more intense and its abuse potential more significant than those of the amphetamines, the similarities in terms of subjective behavioral, pharmacological, and toxic effects are more striking than the differences. Amphetamine is thus taken as the prototype of this group of drugs.

Consideration of these drugs as a class does not imply that they have identical mechanisms of action or that drug abusers cannot distinguish among them. For example, after intravenous administration of cocaine the effects are brief, lasting only a matter of minutes, whereas those of methamphetamine may last for hours. With appropriate selected doses and tasks it is possible to demonstrate differences between the effects of amphetamine and cocaine on motor performance, aggression, and facilitation of self-stimulation with electrical current. It is often assumed that cocaine's local anesthetic actions are unrelated to its euphorigenic and reinforcing properties, but animals will administer procaine to themselves and subjects who have had experience with cocaine are unable to distinguish lidocaine from cocaine when both are used intranasally; they produce a similar degree of euphoria (Van Dyke *et al.*, 1978a). It is not clear whether all local anesthetics are euphorigenic.

Elevation of mood is the typical, rather than the atypical, response to CNS sympathomimetics. Perhaps it is the capacity of so many normal individuals to experience the drug-induced mood elevation without becoming compulsive users that made it difficult fully to appreciate the potential for abuse of the amphetamine-like drugs. However, this attitude has been revised as a result of both the waves of amphetamine abuse that have occurred throughout the United States and a number of Western European countries, and the belated appreciation of the significance of the epidemic of intravenous methamphetamine addiction that occurred in Japan immediately after World War II (*see* Kalant, 1966). Amphetamines and several related drugs are now covered by the same federal regulations applicable to the opioids and cocaine, and illicit transactions are subject to the same penalties.

Incidence and Patterns of Use. Nonmedical use of CNS sympathomimetics fluctuates widely over time in response to cycles of popularity. Presently, in the United States there seems to be a substantial increase in the use of cocaine, but the *intravenous* use of amphetamines has decreased sharply compared to the period of the late 1960s. In 1977, 21% of young adults, but only 5% of adults over 26 years of age, admitted nonmedical use of stimulants at some time in their lives; 2.5% reported use within the past month. In the same survey, 19% of those 18 to 25 years old reported some experience with cocaine, and 4% had used the drug within the preceding month (Abelson *et al.*, 1977).

There are a number of different patterns of amphetamine abuse. One involves those who first obtain the drug from a physician in the course of treatment for obesity or depression and then pass through a phase of habituation as described for barbiturates. Truck drivers and students who use the drug to stay awake may also follow this pattern. More often, the individual obtains the drug specifically for its euphoric effects. "Uppers," "dexies" (dextroamphetamine), and "ups" are terms commonly used to refer to oral preparations. Those who inject the drugs intravenously may dissolve oral tablets or use crystalline methamphetamine ("crystal") manufactured in illegal laboratories. Used intravenously, amphetamine and methamphetamine are known as "speed."

During the early phases of intravenous use, three or four doses of 20 to 40 mg of amphetamine are usually considered sufficient. In addition to the marked euphoria, the user experiences a sense of markedly enhanced physical strength and mental capacity, and feels little need for either sleep or food. Difficult to substantiate by objective means is the claim made by many users that orgasm in both male and female is delayed, permitting extended periods of sexual activity finally culminating in orgasms reported to be more intense and pleasurable (*see* Kramer *et al.*, 1967). The sensation of "flash" or "rush" that immediately follows intravenous administration, while qualitatively distinct from the opioid "rush," is nevertheless described as being intensely pleasurable and somewhat akin to sexual orgasm.

With time, tolerance develops to the euphorigenic effects; higher and more frequent doses are used, and toxic symptoms and signs then appear. These include bruxism, touching and picking of the face and extremities, suspiciousness, and a feeling of being watched. In addition, the user seems fascinated or preoccupied with his own thinking processes and with philosophical concerns about "meanings" and "essences." Stereotypical, repetitious behavior is common. Many patients who later show a full-blown toxic psychosis exhibit a compulsion to take apart mechanical objects. They also have a compulsion to put them together, but are usually too disorganized to do so. Both cocaine and amphetamine users commonly attempt to antagonize these effects with other drugs. The mixture of an opioid (the preferred antagonist) and either cocaine or an amphetamine is known as a "speedball." Many amphetamine users simultaneously consume large amounts of barbiturates or alcohol. Interestingly, subjects taking high doses of amphetamine in experimental settings generally exhibit depression and irritability rather than euphoria (Griffith *et al.*, 1972). Nevertheless, the amphetamine user continues his drug in spite of the toxic effects. The drug may be injected every 2 to 3 hours around the clock for periods of several days, during which time he may eat little and remain awake continuously. Such an episode or "run" commonly ends when the user is out of drug or too disorganized or paranoid to continue. Stopping is followed within a few hours by a deep sleep, which usually lasts 12 to 18 hours but which may last longer if the "run" has been an unusually long one. Upon awakening, users are extremely hungry and lethargic. Some are depressed. Much of the paranoid ideation is gone. The lethargy may persist for many days; reinitiation of drug use eliminates the lethargy and also starts a new cycle. During a "run" some addicts are reported to use as much as 1 g of methamphetamine intravenously every few hours.

Patterns of *cocaine* use show similar variability. The leaves of the coca bush (*Erythroxylon coca*), from which cocaine is obtained, have been chewed by the natives living high in the Andes for untold generations. Used in this way, cocaine appears to produce a sense of decreased hunger and fatigue and increased well-being. Cases of acute overdosage, chronic toxicity, psychosis, or patterns of dependence in which users neglect responsibilities and focus on the use of coca are exceedingly rare. Andean natives appear to have little difficulty in discontinuing use of

the drug when they move to lower altitudes. In contrast, the smoking of coca paste (60 to 80% cocaine sulfate) by younger people living in urban areas of Peru is associated with a variety of psychopathological states (euphoria, hypertalkativeness, irritability, stereotypical behaviors, insomnia, weight loss, and toxic psychosis); neglect of work, and a preoccupation with obtaining money to purchase coca paste. The paste is inexpensive, but it is reported that some users may smoke more than 40 g each day (Jeri *et al.*, 1978) and engage in criminal activity to get money. The use of cocaine has increased in developed countries, where it is commonly taken intranasally ("snorted"), but is sometimes used intravenously. Cocaine (also called coke, snow, gold dust, and lady) is sold as a powder, often diluted with procaine, and varies greatly in purity. The powder is usually arranged on a glass in thin lines 3 to 5 cm long, each containing about 25 mg. The line is then inhaled into the nose through a straw or rolled paper. While the high price of the material makes it a special treat for most users, some with special access engage in "runs" or sprees of use like those described for amphetamine (Wesson and Smith, 1977a).

The euphoric effects of cocaine decay more rapidly after intravenous or intranasal administration than do concentrations of the drug in plasma, suggesting some form of acute tolerance (Javaid *et al.*, 1978; Van Dyke *et al.*, 1978a). Cocaine users who try to maintain the euphoric state will take the drug repeatedly every 30 to 40 minutes if it is available.

Stereotypical behavior is also seen in animals given large doses of amphetamines or cocaine. It is thought to involve dopaminergic structures in the corpus striatum and is blocked by selective lesions or dopaminergic antagonists (*see* Lewander, 1977; Ellinwood, 1979). Animals self-administering cocaine or amphetamines often show a cyclic pattern of use, with periods of spontaneous abstinence interposed between periods of use. A small priming dose during abstinence will reinitiate self-administration. With round-the-clock access to the drugs there is weight loss, self-mutilation, and death within about 2 weeks. Given a choice between cocaine and food over a period of 8 days, monkeys consistently select cocaine (Aigner and Balster, 1978).

The reinforcing and euphorigenic effects of amphetamine, methylphenidate, and cocaine appear to involve potentiation of the actions of catecholamines in the CNS, especially those of dopamine. They can be blocked, at least partially, by pimozide and other dopaminergic antagonists but are relatively unaffected by phenoxybenzamine. Furthermore, both amphetamine and apomorphine (a dopaminergic agonist) facilitate electrical self-stimulation of "reward" areas of the brain. However, the mechanisms of reinforcement are still uncertain. Amphetamine, methylphenidate, and cocaine all block the reuptake of catecholamines, but so do the tricyclic antidepressants, which do not produce euphoria or stereotypy and are not abused. Amphetamine and phenmetrazine appear to release newly synthesized neurotransmitter selectively, and their effects can be blocked by inhibition of tyrosine hydroxylase, a procedure that does not block the central effects of methylphenidate or cocaine. Prior treatment with reserpine blocks the effects of the last-named drugs but not those of amphetamine (*see* Gunne, 1977; Lewander, 1977; Ellinwood, 1979). Clinicians report that lithium produces a variable attenuation of euphoria caused by both amphetamine and cocaine; euphoria induced by methylphenidate is not prevented by lithium (Wald *et al.*, 1978).

Unlike the user of morphine, whose drives are usually decreased, the user of CNS sympathomimetics is hyperactive and during a toxic episode may act in response to persecutory delusions. Some individuals seem able to use the drug for months or years without developing a toxic paranoid syndrome, yet such symptoms can develop in the course of a single "run."

Many of those who use amphetamine and cocaine are best described as recreational or occasional users, but some become dependent. A small percentage of the latter (*e.g.*, those taking the drugs for control of obesity) seem able to restrict drug intake and function productively (stabilized addicts). Others show progressive social and occupational deterioration, punctuated by periods of hospitalization for toxic psychosis. In terms of the compulsion to continue use, the degree to which a drug pervades the life of the user, and the tendency to relapse following withdrawal, some compulsive users of amphetamine or cocaine are addicts. It is not clear whether the amphetamine syndrome is as persistent as that produced by opioids. In the United States the waves of amphetamine use did not leave large numbers of chronic users in their wake. However, many intravenous users eventually become heroin users. Most observers have noted considerable psychopathology in compulsive amphetamine users and their families, which appeared to have antedated the drug use (*see* Connell, 1958; Kramer *et al.*, 1967; Angrist and Gershon, 1969; Ellinwood, 1969; Ellinwood and Kilbey, 1977; Petersen and Stillman, 1977).

Tolerance, Toxicity, Physical Dependence, and Withdrawal Symptoms. Tolerance develops to some of the central effects of amphetamines (*e.g.*, its euphorigenic, anorectic, hyperthermic, and lethal actions), and the chronic user often increases the dose to continue to obtain the desired effect. Some users are able to take several hundred milligrams per day over prolonged periods. By suppressing appetite, high doses of amphetamine may foster ketosis; and, since amphetamine is excreted much more rapidly in acidic urine, some of the apparent tolerance may be due to more rapid elimination of the drug. At the same time there is increased sensitivity to other effects on the CNS (*see* below). Although tolerance to the convulsant and cardiorespiratory effects of cocaine has been reported (Matsuzaki, 1978), the preponder-

ant view is that there may be an increased sensitivity of the CNS to the effects of cocaine when the drug is administered repeatedly (Castellani *et al.*, 1978; Ellinwood, 1979). The possibility of acute tolerance to the effects of cocaine was mentioned above. Cross-tolerance between the amphetamine-like sympathomimetic agents has been observed clinically, and cross-tolerance between the anorectic effect of cocaine and amphetamine has been demonstrated in rats (Woolverton *et al.*, 1978).

Tolerance does not develop to certain of the toxic effects of amphetamine on the CNS, and a toxic psychosis may occur after periods of weeks to months of continued use. Those who develop such a psychosis may have a lowered threshold during subsequent episodes if they resume use of amphetamine (*see* Ellinwood, 1979).

The fully developed toxic syndrome from amphetamine is characterized by vivid visual, auditory, and sometimes tactile hallucinations; picking and excoriation of the skin and delusions of parasitosis are not uncommon. There is also paranoid ideation, loosening of associations, and changes in affect occurring in association with a *clear sensorium*. In chronic users, there may be a striking paucity of sympathomimetic effects, and the blood pressure is not unduly elevated. It is often extremely difficult to differentiate this syndrome from a schizophrenic reaction (Connell, 1958; Angrist and Gershon, 1969; Ellinwood, 1969). The syndrome may be seen as early as 36 to 48 hours after the ingestion of a single large dose of amphetamine; in apparently sensitive individuals, psychosis may be produced by 55 to 75 mg of dextroamphetamine. With high enough doses, psychosis can probably be induced in anyone (Griffith *et al.*, 1972). Unless the individual continues to use the drug, the psychosis usually clears within a week, the hallucinations being the first symptoms to disappear. Acidification of the urine facilitates excretion of amphetamine (*see* Chapter 8), and the psychosis clears more rapidly. The toxic syndrome observed with cocaine is almost identical to that caused by amphetamine.

Chronic use of high doses of amphetamines has been reported to produce microvascular damage, neuronal chromatolysis (primarily in brain areas rich in adrenergic neurons), and profound and long-lasting (or permanent) depletion of dopamine in the caudate nucleus (*see* Ellinwood, 1979). In rats, continuous administration of amphetamine for 10 days can cause a significant decrease in the activity of tyrosine hydroxylase in the nigrostriatum that lasts for more than 3 months (Ellison *et al.*, 1978). After chronic use, animals (including man) begin to exhibit behaviors not seen after initial doses; these include exaggerated "startle" reactions, dyskinesias, and postural abnormalities. Since chronic intoxication with amphetamine renders the neurons of the caudate more sensitive to dopaminergic agonists, a form of supersensitivity may be responsible. Chronic administration of cocaine also results in increased stereotypical behavior.

Craving for the drug, prolonged sleep, general fatigue, lassitude, hyperphagia, and depression commonly follow abrupt cessation of chronic administration of amphetamine-like drugs and cocaine. Suppression of REM sleep and rebound after abrupt withdrawal have been reported. While these effects have not been consistently confirmed for amphetamine (*see* Gunne, 1977), they do appear to occur with cocaine (Post *et al.,* 1974). Such signs and symptoms appear to meet the criteria for a withdrawal syndrome. However, since abrupt discontinuation of the use of sympathomimetic amines does not cause major, grossly observable, physiological disruption that necessitates the gradual withdrawal of the drug, there is reluctance to accept the withdrawal syndrome as evidence of physical dependence on amphetamine. The role of withdrawal hyperphagia, lethargy, and depression in perpetuating the use of the drug is unclear. Ellinwood (1977) suggests the use of tricyclic antidepressants to treat this stage of lethargy and depression.

Acute Toxicity. Because tolerance develops to the hyperthermic and cardiovascular effects of amphetamine, acute intoxication is more likely to occur in the neophyte. The syndrome includes dizziness, tremor, irritability, confusion, hallucinations, chest pain, palpitations, hypertension, sweating, and cardiac arrhythmias. There may be hyperpyrexia and convulsions. Death is usually preceded by hyperpyrexia, convulsions, and shock. Chlorpromazine will antagonize many of the effects of amphetamine and will also prevent shivering and reduce blood pressure. Diazepam is administered to control convulsions, and acidification of the urine is also indicated (*see* Chapter 8). Since cocaine is also a local anesthetic, acute intoxication is more frequently characterized by convulsions and cardiac arrhythmias.

NICOTINE AND TOBACCO

The chemistry and the acute pharmacological effects of nicotine are considered in Chapter 10. In this section, the discussion centers on the use and effects of *tobacco products.*

History. Crewmen who accompanied Columbus to the New World were the first Europeans to observe the smoking of tobacco. In the following century the smoking of tobacco spread throughout the world, despite vigorous official opposition and, in some cases, draconian penalties. The tobacco plant was named *Nicotiana tabacum* in honor of Jean Nicot, who promoted its importation and cultivation in the belief that it had medicinal values. Nicotine was first isolated from the leaves by Posselt and Reiman in 1828. In the mid-nineteenth century, new varieties of tobacco, changes in the technology of curing the leaf, and machinery for mass production facilitated the spread of a new product—the cigarette—cheaper and neater than cigars and yielding a smoke so mild that it could be inhaled. In the United States, the consumption of cigarettes rose rapidly, and by the 1960s more than 600 billion cigarettes were consumed each year. The rate of increase in the consumption of cigarettes has been slowed but not reversed by official pronouncements of links between smoking and a number of serious diseases; however, despite educational campaigns and warning labels, 38% of the adult population in the United States were still smokers in 1978.

Chemical Composition of Tobacco. About 4000 compounds are generated by the burning of tobacco; the smoke can be separated into gaseous and particulate phases. The composition of the actual smoke delivered to the smoker depends not only on the composition of the tobacco but also on how densely it is packed, the length of the column of tobacco, the characteristics of the filter and the paper, and the temperature at which the tobacco is burned. Rapid drawing of the smoke raises the temperature of the burning tip and changes the size of the particles and the composition of both the gaseous and particulate phases. These changes may in turn alter what is trapped in the filter. It is possible to specify the amounts of nicotine, "tar," and carbon monoxide delivered by a given cigarette when it is smoked by a machine under constant conditions, as is now done by governmental agencies in many countries. However, smokers may not conform to the smoking style of the machine.

Among the components of the gaseous phase that produce undesirable effects are carbon monoxide, carbon dioxide, nitrogen oxides, ammonia, volatile nitrosamines, hydrogen cyanide, volatile sulfur-containing compounds, nitriles and other nitrogen-containing compounds, volatile hydrocarbons, alcohols, and aldehydes and ketones (*e.g.,* acetaldehyde, formaldehyde, and acrolein). Some of the last-named substances are potent inhibitors of ciliary movement (Surgeon General, 1979). The particulate phase contains nicotine, water, and "tar"; "tar" is what remains after the moisture and nicotine are subtracted and consists primarily of polycyclic aromatic hydrocarbons, some of which are documented carcinogens. Among these are nonvolatile nitrosamines and aromatic amines, which are believed to play an etiological role in bladder cancer, and polycyclic hydrocarbons such as benzo[a]pyrene, an exceedingly potent carcinogen. The "tar" also contains numerous other compounds, including metallic ions and several radioactive compounds (*e.g.,* polonium 210). According to experts, the components most likely to contribute to the health hazards of smoking are carbon monoxide, nicotine, and "tar"; probable contributors to the health hazards of smoking are acrolein, hydrocyanic acid, nitric oxide, nitrogen dioxide, cresols, and amphenols; suspected hazards include acetaldehyde, acetone, acetonitrile, acrylonitrile, ammonia, benzene, and other gases, and, in the particulate phase, butylamine, dimethylamine, DDT, endrin, furfural, and others. Additional components of smoke are potentially toxic, but their concentrations are quite low (*see* Surgeon General, 1979; Wynder and Hoffman, 1979).

When a cigarette is smoked on a standard machine, the delivery of "tar" varies from 0.5 to 35 mg (1976 average, 17 mg) and that of nicotine from 0.05 to 2.5 mg (1976 average, 1.1 mg). The actual content of nicotine in tobacco can vary from 0.2 to 5%, but is generally between 1 and 2% for smoking tobaccos. It is present in the protonated form in almost all cigarette tobaccos. Because of a more alkaline pH, it is present in the more readily absorbed, unprotonated form in cigars and in pipe tobaccos (*see* Surgeon General, 1979).

Effects on the CNS.   Although nicotine is self-administered by animals, it is far less powerful as a reinforcer than is amphetamine or cocaine (Yanagita, 1977). Nicotine appears to have very specific stimulant properties; its effects are not confused with those of other drugs. These properties appear to involve both specific receptors for nicotine and dopaminergic pathways. They can be blocked with mecamylamine, but not with muscarinic cholinergic or adrenergic blocking agents (*see* Rosecrans, 1979). Nicotine, as absorbed by the typical smoker, causes an alerting pattern in the EEG (low-voltage, fast activity); however, at the same time, there is decreased skeletal muscle tone, decreased amplitude in the electromyogram, and a decrease in deep-tendon reflexes. The latter effects may involve stimulation of the Renshaw cells in the spinal cord (*see* Domino, 1973). The smoking of one or two cigarettes produces a significant rise in the concentrations of growth hormone, cortisol, antidiuretic hormone, norepinephrine, epinephrine, and glycerol in plasma (Cryer *et al.*, 1976). Nicotine causes nausea and vomiting, in part, by stimulating the chemoreceptor trigger zone of the medulla oblongata and by activating the vagal reflexes involved in the act of vomiting.

Animal studies indicate that nicotine stimulates the release of norepinephrine and dopamine from brain tissue and, depending on the dose, increases or inhibits the release of acetylcholine. The alkaloid appears to facilitate memory and reduce aggression (*see* Larson and Silvette, 1975; Jaffe and Jarvik, 1978).

Many of nicotine's effects could, in theory, be reinforcing. These include the alerting and muscle relaxant effects, the facilitation of memory or attention, and the decrease in appetite and irritability.

Absorption from Smoke.   The nicotine in cigarette smoke, suspended on minute particles of "tar," is quickly absorbed from the lung, almost with the efficiency of intravenous administration. The compound reaches the brain within 8 seconds after inhalation. Nicotine in cigarette smoke, which is somewhat acidic, is not well absorbed from the mouth; pipe and cigar smoke, which is more alkaline (pH 8.5), is probably better absorbed, but the concentration of nicotine in the plasma of those who do not inhale cigars is still low compared to those who do inhale cigarettes (Turner *et al.*, 1977; Armitage *et al.*, 1978). Peak concentrations of nicotine in plasma after a cigarette is smoked are typically 25 to 50 ng/ml (*see* Russell and Feyerabend, 1978; Surgeon General, 1979). The half-time for elimination of nicotine is 30 to 60 minutes (*see* Chapter 10). Thus, the frequency of smoking is usually such that concentrations in plasma are somewhat higher at the end of the day for the average smoker (Russell and Feyerabend, 1978; Surgeon General, 1979). Enough nicotine is found in breast milk to affect nursing infants.

Chronic Toxicity of Tobacco.   Chronic use of tobacco is causally linked to a variety of serious diseases, ranging from coronary artery disease to lung cancer. The likelihood of developing any one of these disorders increases with the degree of exposure (measured in cigarettes per day, or "pack years"). For example, for all male smokers, the overall mortality ratio is about 1.7 compared to nonsmokers. The ratio is 2.0 for those who smoke two packs daily, and it is higher among inhalers than noninhalers. Cigar smoking increases mortality in proportion to the number smoked, but not as sharply as for cigarettes. Those who smoke pipes exclusively show a very slight increase in mortality. The differences between cigarette, pipe, and cigar smokers is probably related to the lesser inhalation among the latter two groups, which leads to lower exposure to all constituents of smoke. The smoking of tobacco has been described as the largest preventable cause of death in the United States, and it has been estimated that, each year, 80,000 deaths from lung cancer, 22,000 deaths from other cancers, 19,000 deaths from chronic pulmonary disease, and 225,000 deaths from cardiovascular disease are directly linked to smoking.

Evidence indicates that the different diseases that are related to the use of tobacco may be caused, at least in part, by different constituents of tobacco or tobacco smoke. This raises the possibility that changes in the composition of cigarettes or selective filtration might lower the probability of one disorder, while having little effect on another. The catalog of tobacco-related diseases is extensive, and only the more important in terms of prevalence and seriousness can be mentioned here. Cardiovascular diseases related to tobacco include coronary artery disease, cerebrovascular disease, peripheral vascular disease, and Buerger's disease. Carbon monoxide (and related hypoxia) and the effects of nicotine on cardiac rhythm, free fatty acids in plasma, lipoproteins, and the coagulability of blood may play a role in the acceleration of atherosclerosis and in sudden cardiac death (*see* Aronow, 1976; McGill, 1977; Surgeon General, 1979). Neoplastic diseases (cancer of the lung, larynx, oral cavity, esophagus, bladder, and pancreas) are probably due to one or more of the known carcinogens in the smoke, rather than to nicotine or carbon monoxide. Chronic obstructive lung disease is probably caused by effects on proteolytic enzymes, interference with immune mechanisms, and inhibition of clearance mechanisms. Impairment of respiratory function can be detected in young adults after only a few years of smoking (Surgeon General, 1979). The ciliotoxic actions of tobacco smoke and its ability to inhibit pulmonary clearance mechanisms probably account for the remarkable synergism between tobacco smoke and such environmental carcinogens as asbestos in increasing mortality for lung cancer (*see* Cohen *et al.,* 1979). The mechanisms by which smoking leads to an increased incidence of abortion, significantly reduces the birth weight of children born to women who smoke during pregnancy, and increases the likelihood of perinatal mortality and of sudden death of infants are unclear.

The likelihood of development of a disorder related to smoking is reduced by cessation. Over a period of 5 to 10 years, the risk falls to a level only slightly above that of the nonsmoker. Destruction of lung tissue is not reversible, but, with cessation, the rate of decline in pulmonary function begins to resemble that of the nonsmoker.

Smokers metabolize a wide variety of drugs more rapidly than do nonsmokers, probably as a result of induction of enzymes in the intestinal mucosa or the liver by components of tobacco smoke. Among the drugs affected are theophylline, warfarin, phenacetin, propranolol, imipramine, caffeine, and antipyrine (*see* Kuntzman *et al.,* 1977; Vestal *et al.,* 1979). Clinical reports suggest that smokers require more opioids to obtain relief from pain and are less sedated by benzodiazepines, but it is not clear that all differences arise from altered rates of metabolism (Miller, 1977).

Tolerance, Physical Dependence, and Relapse. Tolerance develops to some of the effects of nicotine. Following one or two cigarettes, even the chronic smoker still exhibits an increase in blood pressure and pulse rate, decreased skin temperature, and increases in the plasma concentrations of antidiuretic hormone, cortisol, norepinephrine, and growth hormone. However, the dizziness, nausea, and vomiting experienced by nontolerant individuals do not occur. Furthermore, while regular smokers report that injections of nicotine are pleasant, nonsmokers describe unpleasant reactions (*see* Jarvik, 1979). Although smokers appear to metabolize nicotine more rapidly than do nonsmokers, it is likely that tolerance is due primarily to pharmacodynamic changes rather than to alterations in drug disposition. In rats, marked tolerance develops to the depressant effects of nicotine after a few closely spaced doses. There are conflicting reports on the duration of tolerance. In some studies of animals it appeared to disappear within 24 to 48 hours of abstinence; in others it persisted for months (*see* Abood *et al.,* 1979; Jarvik, 1979; Surgeon General, 1979). In human smokers, some aspects of tolerance wax and wane rapidly. The first cigarette of the day produces a much greater cardiovascular and subjective response than do those that follow.

Cessation of the use of tobacco may be followed by a *withdrawal syndrome,* but it varies greatly from person to person in intensity and in specific signs and symptoms. There is uncertainty about what factors are responsible for its variability and virtually no information on what levels of exposure are required to induce physical dependence in man. The most consistent signs and symptoms (in addition to "craving" for tobacco, which subsides over a period of days to weeks) are nausea, headache, constipation, diarrhea, and increased appetite. Drowsiness, fatigue, sleep disturbances (insomnia), irritability (increased hostility), and inability to concentrate are also common. The syndrome is prompt in onset, usually within the first 24 hours, and some smokers complain that certain problems, such as increased appetite and inability to concentrate, persist for weeks or months. In some cases it is uncertain whether the specific problem represents an effect of withdrawal or a return to the *status quo* that existed before the individual started smoking. Among the objective findings that quickly follow cessation of smoking are changes in the EEG, with a decrease in high-frequency activity characteristic of arousal and an increase in low-frequency activity characteristic of drowsiness and hypoarousal. Decreases in performance on tests of vigilance and psychomotor performance and increases in hostility are detectable within hours. There is a decrease in heart rate and blood pressure, and peripheral blood flow increases. In time, weight gain is a common finding, cough and other respiratory difficulties show improvement, and, over a period of weeks to months, smoking-induced acceleration in degradation of other drugs approaches the norm for nonsmokers. There is some evidence that a higher intake of nicotine is associated with more severe withdrawal and more difficulty in giving up cigarettes, but other factors are probably just as important. Women smokers report more symptoms than do men. Craving for cigarettes seems to exhibit a diurnal variation and is low on arising and rises to a peak in the evening. Unlike those who are dependent on opioids, individuals who try to cut down gradually may simply extend the period of discomfort as compared to those who stop abruptly. The syndrome of withdrawal from tobacco can be suppressed to some degree by nicotine, but related drugs such as lobeline appear to be ineffective (*see* Jaffe and Jarvik, 1978; Schacter, 1978; Shiffman, 1979; Surgeon General, 1979). To what degree the craving (either caused directly by withdrawal or elicited by environmental stimuli that have become conditioned to the use of tobacco) contributes to relapse among smokers is uncertain. Of those who seek some sort of formal help with their problem, about two thirds actually stop for at least a few days; but of these, only 20 to 40% are still abstinent 12 months later.

Titration. Many heavy smokers behave as if they are attempting to adjust their concentration of nicotine within relatively narrow limits. When given cigarettes with a high content of nicotine, they reduce the number smoked and alter their puffing patterns and, thereby, achieve concentrations of nicotine in plasma close to those to which they are accustomed. When given cigarettes with exceedingly low nicotine content, they change patterns of puffing or increase the number of cigarettes smoked in order to avoid declines in plasma nicotine concentrations, but the regulation is less precise. The avoidance of decreases is thought to be linked to avoidance of early withdrawal phenomena (*see* Russell and Feyerabend, 1978; Schachter, 1978). Titration is of considerable clinical significance, since smokers who switch to "low tar and nicotine" cigarettes may alter their puffing patterns in a manner that minimizes the potential benefit. Although delivery of carbon monoxide is correlated with those of "tar" and nicotine, carbon monoxide is not selectively filtered and "switchers" may take in almost as much of the gas as they did previously.

CANNABINOIDS (MARIHUANA)

History and Source. *Cannabis,* obtained from the flowering tops of *hemp* plants, is a very ancient drug. Other names for cannabis or its products include *hashish, charas, bhang, ganja, dagga,* and *marihuana.* The common hemp is an herbaceous annual, of which *Cannabis sativa* is the sole species and *Cannabis sativa* var. *indica* and var. *americana* are two varieties. While all parts of both the male and the female plant contain psychoactive substances (cannabinoids), the highest cannabinoid concentrations are found in the flowering tops. In the Middle East and North Africa the dried resinous exudate of the tops is called *hashish;* in the Far East it is called *charas.* The dried leaves and flowering shoots of the plant, containing smaller amounts of the active substance, are called *bhang,* and the resinous mass from the small leaves and brackets of inflorescence is called *ganja.* In the United States, the term *marihuana* is used to refer to any part of the plant or extract therefrom that induces somatic and psychic changes in man. Most commonly, the plant is cut, dried, chopped, and incorporated into cigarettes.

Chemistry. Among the cannabinoids synthesized by the hemp plant are cannabinol, cannabidiol, cannabinolic acid, cannabigerol, cannabicyclol, and several isomers of tetrahydrocannabinol. The isomer believed responsible for most of the characteristic psychological effects of marihuana is l-Δ^9-tetrahydrocannabinol (Δ^9-THC), also referred to as l-Δ^1-THC. The effects of l-Δ^8-THC, which occurs in minute amounts in marihuana, are similar to those of l-Δ^9-THC. Both isomers are viscous, noncrystalline, water-insoluble compounds.

Δ^9-THC has the following structure:

Tetrahydrocannabinol (Δ^9-THC)

Many derivatives of tetrahydrocannabinol have been synthesized and studied; some of these are more potent than the natural plant products and may have potential therapeutic uses.

Pharmacological Effects in Animals. In rats and mice, Δ^9-THC or extracts of cannabis produce a decrease in spontaneous behavior associated with an altered responsivity to stimuli. There is a dose-dependent hypothermia. In monkeys, both Δ^9-THC and Δ^8-THC produce sedation, decrease in aggressive behavior, loss of ability or motivation to perform complex tasks, and apparent hallucinations. Chronic high dosage produces a dose-related depression of ovarian function, decreases in concentrations of luteinizing hormone (LH) and follicle-stimulating hormone (FSH), and anovulatory cycles. Decreased spermatogenesis has also been reported. Δ^9-THC and several of its synthetic congeners have a number of actions not unlike those of the barbiturates. They prolong hexobarbital sleeping time, exhibit anticonvulsant activity, raise the threshold for EEG and behavioral arousal, and depress polysynaptic reflexes. Yet they may also prolong the stimulant action of amphetamine (*see* Harris *et al.,* 1977).

Pharmacological Effects in Man. Δ^9-THC exerts its most prominent effects on the CNS and cardiovascular system. Because of differences due to dose, route of administration, setting, and the experience and expectations of subjects, condensed descriptions of the behavioral responses to Δ^9-THC are difficult and sometimes misleading.

In the United States, the Δ^9-THC content of marihuana ranges broadly from 0.5 to 6%. Furthermore, as with tobacco, the amount of active material that reaches the blood stream is highly dependent on the smoking technic and the amount destroyed by pyrolysis.

Oral doses of 20 mg of Δ^9-THC or the smoking of a cigarette containing 2% Δ^9-THC produces effects on mood, memory, motor coordination, cognitive ability, sensorium, time sense, and self-perception. Most commonly there is an increased sense of well-being or euphoria, accompanied by feelings of relaxation and sleepiness when subjects are alone; where users can interact, sleepiness is less pronounced and there is often spontaneous laughter (Hollister, 1971; Jones, 1971). The sleepiness contrasts with the effects of LSD and related hallucinogens, which induce a state of arousal. With oral doses of Δ^9-THC that are equivalent to several cigarettes, short-term memory is impaired and there is a deterioration in capacity to carry out tasks requiring multiple mental steps to reach a specific goal. This effect on memory-dependent, goal-directed behavior has been called "temporal disintegration," and is correlated with a tendency to confuse past, present, and future, and with depersonalization—a sense of strangeness and unreality about the self (Melges *et al.,* 1970).

Balance and stability of stance are affected even at low doses (Evans *et al.,* 1973), effects that are more apparent when the eyes are closed. Decreases in muscle strength and hand steadiness can be demonstrated. Performance of relatively simple motor tasks and simple reaction times are relatively unimpaired until higher doses are reached. More complex processes, including perception, attention, and information processing, which are involved in driving and flying, are impaired by doses equivalent to one or two cigarettes. While the results from simulated driving situations are inconsistent, they tend to show impaired performance (*see* Rafaelsen *et al.,* 1973; Klonoff, 1974; Janowsky *et al.,* 1976; McBay, 1977; Moskowitz, 1977). The rate of recovery of the eye from glare is slowed by low doses of marihuana. The

impairment produced by alcohol is additive to that induced by marihuana (Belgrave *et al.,* 1979).

Marihuana smokers frequently report increased hunger, dry mouth and throat, more vivid visual imagery, and a keener sense of hearing. Subtle visual and auditory stimuli previously ignored may take on a novel quality, and the nondominant senses of touch, taste, and smell seem to be enhanced. Yet, in usual social doses, marihuana decreases empathy and the perception of emotions in others (Clopton *et al.,* 1979). Altered perception of time is a consistent effect of cannabinoids. Time seems to pass more slowly—minutes may seem like hours (*see* Hollister, 1971; Jones, 1976). The effects on the surface EEG are not prominent, resembling those seen in the drowsy state. In a single case, electrodes in deep brain structures recorded high-voltage, slow-wave activity in septal leads, corresponding to the subjective elevation of mood (Heath, 1972). Similar changes in the EEG from the septal area, hippocampus, and amygdala of monkeys with implanted electrodes were observed after daily exposure to marihuana smoke or intravenous administration of Δ^9-THC; these were more pronounced after several months of daily administration and persisted for several months after cessation. The surface EEG was relatively normal (Heath, 1976).

Higher doses of Δ^9-THC can induce frank hallucinations, delusions, and paranoid feelings. Thinking becomes confused and disorganized; depersonalization and altered time sense are accentuated. Anxiety reaching panic proportions may replace euphoria, often as a result of the feeling that the drug-induced state will never end. With high enough doses, the clinical picture is that of a toxic psychosis with hallucinations, depersonalization, and loss of insight; this can occur acutely or only after months of use (*see* Nahas, 1973; Chopra and Smith, 1974; Thacore and Shukla, 1976). Because of the rapid onset of effects when marihuana is smoked and the low Δ^9-THC content of marihuana grown in the United States, most users are able to regulate their intake in order to avoid the excessive dosage that produces these unpleasant effects; psychiatric emergencies as a result of smoking marihuana are uncommon. Use of marihuana may, however, cause an acute exacerbation of symptomatology in stabilized schizophrenics.

The most consistent effects on the cardiovascular system are an increase in heart rate, an increase in systolic blood pressure, and a marked reddening of the conjunctivae. Propranolol, a β-adrenergic blocking agent, prevents the tachycardia produced by Δ^9-THC, but it does not interfere with the subjective and behavioral effects (*see* Drew *et al.,* 1972; Bachman *et al.,* 1979). The increase in heart rate is dose related, and its onset and duration correlate well with concentrations of Δ^9-THC in blood. Increases of 20 to 50 beats per minute are usual, but a tachycardia of 140 beats per minute is not uncommon. There are no consistent changes in respiratory rate or deep-tendon reflexes. There is a very slight tendency toward lowered oral temperature. Pupillary size is not significantly altered, but intraocular pressure is decreased and this effect may be useful in the treatment of glaucoma. With chronic use, there is an unexplained increase in plasma volume.

While there are similarities between the subjective effects of Δ^9-THC at high doses and those of LSD, there are also substantial differences, and cannabinoids should therefore be considered as a separate and distinct pharmacological class. The mechanism of action of Δ^9-THC is unknown. The psychological effects are not prevented by pretreatment with α-methyltyrosine (Hollister, 1974), which reduces brain concentrations of dopamine and norepinephrine, although such pretreatment does eliminate the euphoria produced by amphetamine and partially eliminates the euphoria produced by ethanol. Patients maintained on lithium or methadone continue to experience the effects of marihuana without apparent alteration.

Various cannabinoids suppress cellular and humoral immune responses in animals, although findings in human subjects smoking marihuana have been inconsistent. There is little correlation between the potency of these compounds in producing psychic effects and their capability to suppress immune response or inhibit protein synthesis (*see* Jakubovic and McGeer, 1976; Nahas *et al.*, 1976; Smith *et al.*, 1978). The possibility that cannabinoids may have antineoplastic activity is under study.

Conflicting data have been reported on the effects of chronic high doses of marihuana on human sexual function (*see* Secretary, 1977; Mendelson *et al.*, 1978). However, field studies of predominantly male, long-term users have not revealed any noticeable decreases in sexual potency or fertility (Rubin and Comitas, 1975; Stefanis *et al.*, 1977).

Chronic smoking of marihuana and hashish has long been associated with bronchitis and asthma; such smoking adversely affects pulmonary function and the bronchial epithelium even in young people (*see* Secretary, 1977). However, the acute response to Δ^9-THC (given orally, intravenously, or by aerosol) is a significant and relatively long-lasting bronchodilatation. This effect is seen in both normal subjects and asthmatics. The "tar" produced by pyrolysis of marihuana is more carcinogenic to animals than is that derived from tobacco. Smoking marihuana or the oral or topical administration of Δ^9-THC produces a significant decrease in intraocular pressure. This is due to effects on efferent and afferent blood vessels, and both α- and β-adrenergic receptors seem to be involved.

Some United States Army enlisted men using high doses of hashish on a chronic basis exhibited apathy, dullness, and impairment of judgment, concentration, and memory, associated with a loss of interest in personal appearance, hygiene, and diet. After discontinuation, memory, alertness, concentration, and calculating ability returned to normal within 2 to 4 weeks, but several men seemed to exhibit continued intermittent residual symptoms (memory loss, confusion, inability to calculate and concentrate) similar to those seen with organic brain disease (Tennant and Groesbeck, 1972). Such *chronic high-dosage* use is not common in the United States, but some clinicians have described subtle changes in personality and decreased interest in achievement and pursuit of conventional goals (the amotivational syndrome) in young marihuana users who regularly smoke a few cigarettes a day. At present, there is no evidence to suggest that any such personality changes are due to irreversible organic brain damage. The possibility of an adverse effect of frequent or chronic low levels of intoxication on developing personality cannot be dismissed.

Absorption, Fate, and Excretion. It is estimated that, even when smoked with maximal efficiency, no more than 50% of Δ^9-THC in a marihuana cigarette is actually absorbed. Thus, a 1-g cigarette containing 1% Δ^9-THC would deliver at most 5.0 mg of Δ^9-THC to the lungs. Pharmacological effects occur within minutes after smoking begins, and plasma concentrations reach their peak at 10 to 30 minutes. Unless more is smoked, the effects of a cigarette seldom last longer than 2 or 3 hours. After oral administration, the onset of effects usually occurs at about 0.5 to 1 hour; peak effects may not occur until the second or third hour and correlate well with plasma concentrations. Effects may persist for 3 to 5 hours. Although gastrointestinal absorption is largely complete, Δ^9-THC is approximately three times more potent when smoked than when taken by mouth (*see* Hollister, 1971; Secretary, 1977).

Δ^9-THC is rapidly converted into an active metabolite, 11-hydroxy-Δ^9-THC, which produces effects identical to those of the parent compound. 11-Hydroxy-Δ^9-THC is, in turn, converted into a more polar, inactive metabolite (8,11-dihydroxy-THC), which is then excreted in the urine and feces. Metabolites excreted in the bile may be reabsorbed. Very little unmetabolized Δ^9-THC is found in the urine. After reaching their peaks, plasma concentrations of Δ^9-THC and 11-hydroxy-Δ^9-THC fall rapidly at first (half-time of minutes), reflecting the redistribution of these lipophilic compounds to lipid-rich tissues, including the CNS. This first phase of rapid decline is followed by a much slower phase (half-time of days), reflecting the gradual metabolism and elimination of the drug from the body. Traces of Δ^9-THC and its metabolites persist in the plasma of man for several days and can be detected in the fat and brain of animals for days after a single administration. Metabolites can be found in the urine for days or weeks (*see* Hollister, 1971; Lemberger *et al.*, 1972; Perez-Reves *et al.*, 1972; Secretary, 1977). Δ^9-THC crosses the placental barrier. Consumption of repeated oral doses of Δ^9-THC by man for several days or its daily smoking for several weeks does not seem to produce clinically detectable evidence of accumulation. Chronic marihuana smokers metabolize Δ^9-THC more rapidly than do nonsmokers (Lemberger *et al.*, 1971). Marihuana also alters the metabolism of barbiturates, antipyrine, and ethanol.

Tolerance and Physical Dependence. In animals, tolerance develops to the lethal, hypothermic, and some of the behavioral effects of cannabinoids. While in certain species the degree of tolerance is remarkable, it may not develop to all the effects of the drug. Most of the tolerance is due to functional or pharmacodynamic adaptations of the CNS, rather than to a more rapid metabolic disposition (*see* Wikler, 1976; Harris *et al.,* 1977; Secretary, 1977).

Reports from many countries throughout the world indicate that a number of regular users of hashish consume amounts of Δ^9-THC that would produce toxic effects in most Western users. Some American soldiers in Europe smoked amounts of hashish that were equivalent to 5000 to 6000 marihuana cigarettes per month (Tennant and Groesbeck, 1972). When volunteers are given Δ^9-THC orally every 4 hours (maximal dose of 210 mg per day), tolerance develops to drug-induced changes of mood, tachycardia, decrease in skin temperature, increase in body temperature, decrease in intraocular pressure, changes in the EEG, and impairment of performance on psychomotor tests. Tolerance to the cardiac effects develops within a few days and decays relatively quickly (48 hours) (*see* Jones *et al.,* 1976; Wikler, 1976; Jones, 1977). If, however, the total dosage used is low, subjects continue to experience a "high" after the first cigarette of the day (Mendelson and Meyer, 1972). Daily use of low doses may not be sufficient to induce any remarkable degree of tolerance. Experienced users may actually report more subjective effects from smoking marihuana than naive subjects. However, they generally show less impairment of perceptual and motor functions, as well as smaller increases in heart rate.

Some degree of cross-tolerance between alcohol and Δ^9-THC has been observed in rats. However, there is no cross-tolerance between cannabinoids and the psychedelics (hallucinogens).

Abrupt discontinuation of cannabinoids after chronic use of high dosage is followed by irritability, restlessness, nervousness, decreased appetite, weight loss, and insomnia. There is a rebound increase in REM sleep, which is suppressed by marihuana. Tremor, increased body temperature, and chills may also occur. This syndrome, observed under laboratory conditions when high doses of the drug have been used every few hours for several weeks, is relatively mild, begins within a few hours after cessation of drug administration, and lasts about 4 to 5 days (*see* Jones *et al.,* 1976; Wikler, 1976).

Therapeutic Uses. Although not currently approved for any clinical use, marihuana, Δ^9-THC, and certain synthetic analogs have several potential therapeutic applications. These include antiemetic effects (especially against nausea and vomiting caused by cancer chemotherapeutic agents; Sallan *et al.,* 1980), bronchodilatation, and the capability to lower intraocular pressure. The natural cannabinoids have inconsistent effects as analgesics, but some synthetic agents are active (*see* Harris, 1979). Some cannabinoids may have useful anticonvulsant actions. Work with synthetic compounds shows that the psychological effects (both euphorigenic and psychotogenic) can be separated to some degree from the potential therapeutic actions. *Nabilone* is a synthetic analog that may be significantly better than prochlorperazine in reducing nausea and vomiting associated with cancer chemotherapy; its side effects include somnolence, dizziness, and dry mouth, but only minimal euphoria. At higher dosage nabilone does produce euphoria and tachycardia, but tolerance develops to these effects. Nabilone also lowers intraocular pressure, perhaps synergistically with agents currently used for the treatment of glaucoma, and appears to work when applied topically.

Patterns of Use. In the United States and in many other countries the smoking of marihuana (also known as grass, pot, tea, weed, and reefer) has been on the increase since the early 1960s. In 1977, 60% of young adults in the United States reported some experience with marihuana; during the month prior to the survey 28% had used marihuana at least once and 19% had used it on 5 or more days. Among younger people (ages 12 to 17), 16% reported use within the past month and an increasing number were reporting daily use. While still more common in large urban areas, marihuana is now used among all socioeconomic and ethnic groups and in rural as well as urban areas (Abelson *et al.,* 1977). There continues to be a consensus that criminal penalties and jail sentences for possession of small amounts of marihuana are unduly harsh deterrents, but there is also a growing recognition that the prevalent and heavy use of marihuana, particularly among adolescents, will have adverse effects on health and productivity.

PSYCHEDELICS (HALLUCINOGENS, PSYCHOTOMIMETICS, PSYCHOTOGENS)

There is no sharp line that divides the psychedelics from other classes of centrally active drugs. Under certain conditions, or at toxic dosage, several classes of drugs (anticholinergics, bromides, antimalarials, opioid antagonists, cocaine, amphetamines, and corticosteroids) can induce illusions, hallucinations, delusions, paranoid ideations, and other alterations of mood and thinking that are observed in spontaneously occurring psychotic states. However, despite the legal terminology that defines lysergic acid diethylamide (LSD) and related drugs as hallucinogens, the production of hallucinations is not the most useful way to describe the very interesting pharmacological effects of this group of drugs.

The psychedelic drugs to be discussed here can, indeed, produce such pathological effects as the terms *hallucinogenic, psychotomimetic,* and *psychotogenic* imply, but the feature that distinguishes the psychedelic agents from other classes of drugs is their capacity reliably to induce or compel states of altered perception, thought, and feeling that are not (or cannot be) experienced otherwise except in dreams or at times of religious exaltation.

Most descriptions of the "psychedelic state" include several major effects. There is heightened awareness of sensory input, often accompanied by an enhanced sense of clarity, but a diminished control over what is experienced. Frequently there is a feeling that one part of the self seems to be a passive observer (a "spectator ego") rather than an active organizing and directing force, while another part of the self participates and receives the vivid and unusual sensory experiences. The environment may be perceived as novel, often beautiful, and harmonious. The attention of the user is turned inward, preempted by the seeming clarity and portentous quality of his own thinking processes. In this state the slightest sensation may take on profound meaning. Indeed, "meaningfulness" seems more important than what is meant, and the "sense of truth" more significant than what is true. Commonly, there is a diminished capacity to differentiate the boundaries of one object from another and of the self from the environment. Associated with the loss of boundaries there may be a sense of union with "mankind" or the "cosmos." To the extent that these drugs reveal this innate capacity of the mind to see more than it can tell and to experience and believe more than it can explain, the term *mind expanding* is not entirely inappropriate (Freedman, 1968).

As with any scheme of classification, the choice of agents to include or exclude is somewhat arbitrary. Most of the drugs that are generally included among the psychedelics are related either to the indolealkylamines, such as LSD, psilocybin, psilocin, dimethyltryptamine (DMT), and diethyltryptamine (DET), or to the phenylethylamines (mescaline) or phenylisopropylamines, such as 2,5-dimethoxy-4-methylamphetamine (DOM, "STP"). However, even when a drug produces a profile of pharmacological effects that is quite similar to those of LSD at one dose level, it may produce other effects as the dose is raised. Thus, at low dosage, dimethoxyamphetamine (DMA) has primarily LSD-like effects, but it is more like amphetamine as the dose is raised. Martin and Sloan (1977b) have proposed three criteria for categorizing LSD-like drugs: (1) subjective effects and neurophysiological actions; (2) cross-tolerance between compounds; and (3) response to selective antagonists. By application of these criteria they

have classified a variety of compounds that produce changes in perception and mood into five categories: (I) LSD-like: LSD, mescaline, psilocybin, psilocin; (II) probably LSD-like: DMA, DOM, tryptamine, DMT, numerous congeners of lysergic acid; (III) probably LSD-like but with other properties: 3,4-methylenedioxyamphetamine (MDA), 5-methoxy-3,4-methylenedioxyamphetamine (MMDA); (IV) probably not LSD-like: D-2-bromlysergic acid diethylamide (BOL), 5-hydroxytryptophan; and (V) not LSD-like: amphetamine, β-phenethylamine (PEA), 2,5-dimethoxy-4-ethylamphetamine (DOET), bufotenine, L-LSD, scopolamine, Δ^9-THC.

A number of compounds produce alterations of mood and perception that are so obviously distinct as to merit separate discussion. Included among these are phencyclidine, certain opioid agonist-antagonists (considered in Chapter 22), and inhalants such as nitrous oxide and certain volatile solvents.

LSD and Related Compounds. *History.* Drugs that induce psychedelic effects have been used for centuries. The peyote cactus (containing mescaline) and mushrooms (containing psilocin) were being used by the natives of Mexico and the Southwestern United States at the time of the Spanish conquest. There was a brief period of scientific interest in mescaline at the beginning of this century and again in the 1930s. However, Hoffman's discovery in 1947 of the psychedelic effects of LSD and its remarkable potency stimulated interest among scientists who felt its study might help facilitate understanding of mental illness. In the 1950s hundreds of scientific papers were written on the effects of LSD on biological systems *in vitro*, animal behavior, patients with a wide range of physical and mental illnesses, and normal human volunteers. The effects of LSD then caught the attention of students, writers, and others more interested in its possibilities for self-exploration than for scientific investigation. Within a matter of a few years its use spread among young people, abetted by persuasive advocates who counseled young people to "turn on, tune in, and drop out." More conservative elements of society, made anxious as much by the unconventional life style associated with the use of LSD as by its known and suspected toxicities, passed laws and regulations designed to limit its availability. By 1970, LSD was included in the same regulatory category as heroin. Despite such laws the drug, which is relatively easy to manufacture, remains available and is still used. Chemists have also produced dozens of congeners of indoleamine and phenethylamine that cause subjective effects similar to those of LSD. The burdensome regulations and the recognition that LSD does not produce a "model psychosis" have markedly diminished its use in scientific investigations.

Chemistry. The structures of LSD, mescaline, psilocin, and several related compounds are shown in Table 23-1. The diversity of compounds included here precludes a consideration of structure-activity relationships (but *see* comments under Mechanism of Action).

Mechanism of Action. LSD and related psychedelic drugs have actions at multiple sites in the CNS, from the cortex to the spinal cord. Some of the best

Table 23–1. STRUCTURAL FORMULAS AND CLASSIFICATION OF SELECTED PSYCHEDELIC DRUGS *

LSD-LIKE

Indoleamines

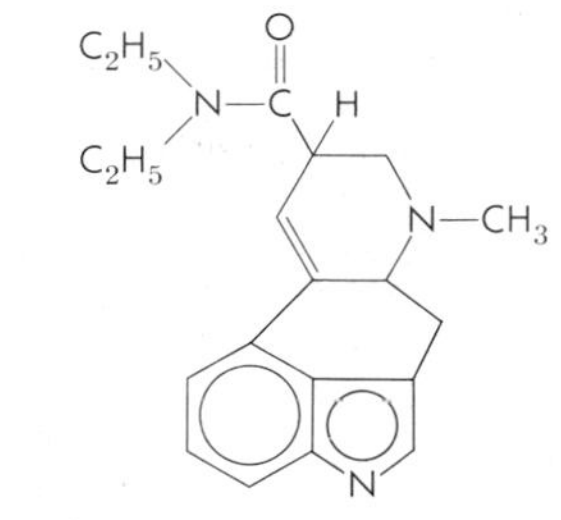

LSD

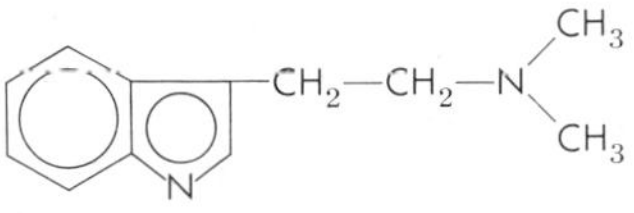

DMT

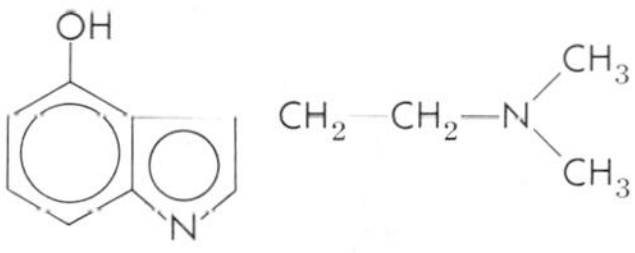

Psilocin

β-Phenethylamines

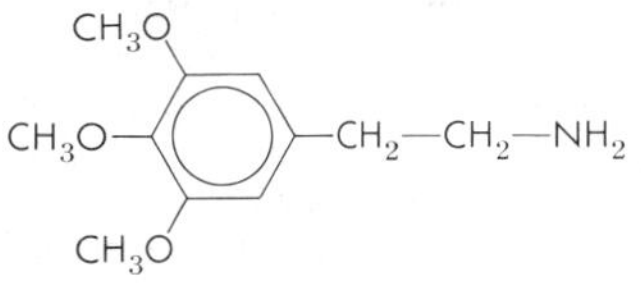

Mescaline

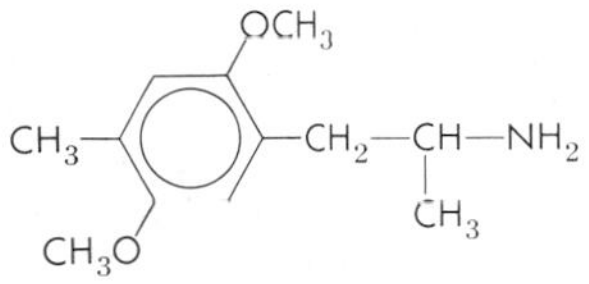

DOM

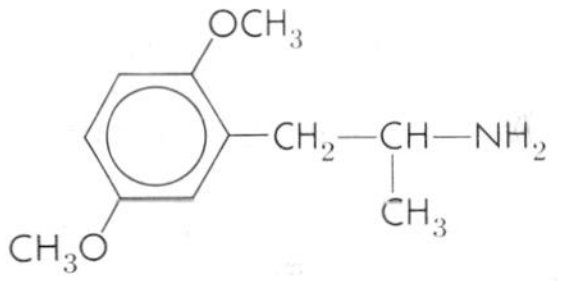

DMA

MIXED

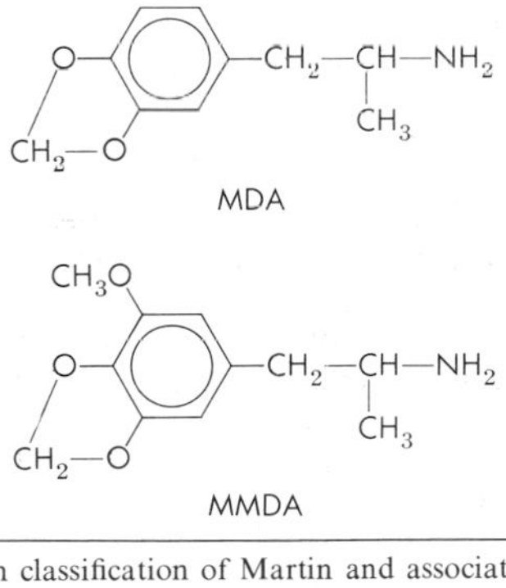

MDA

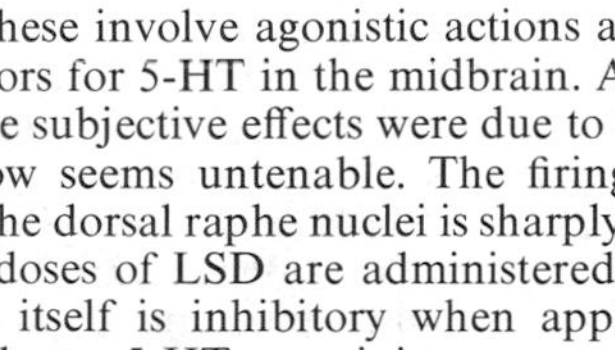

MMDA

AMPHETAMINE-LIKE

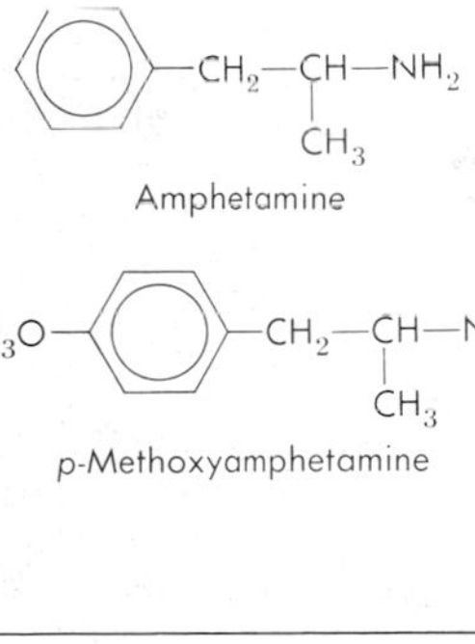

Amphetamine

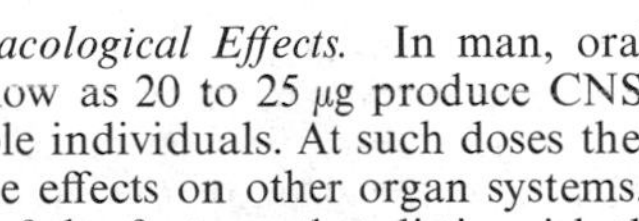

p-Methoxyamphetamine

* Based on classification of Martin and associates, 1978b.

studied of these involve agonistic actions at presynaptic receptors for 5-HT in the midbrain. An earlier view that the subjective effects were due to blockade of 5-HT now seems untenable. The firing rate of neurons in the dorsal raphe nuclei is sharply reduced after small doses of LSD are administered systemically. 5-HT itself is inhibitory when applied iontophoretically to 5-HT-containing neurons in the dorsal raphe nuclei or to those neurons of the forebrain to which the dorsal raphe neurons project. While tryptamine produces inhibition about equally at both sites, LSD, psilocin, and DMT are considerably more potent in producing inhibition at the presumed presynaptic sites on the dorsal raphe neurons (Haigler and Aghajanian, 1977).

Pharmacological Effects. In man, oral doses of LSD as low as 20 to 25 µg produce CNS effects in susceptible individuals. At such doses there are few detectable effects on other organ systems.

Some of the features that distinguish the psychedelic state from other effects produced by drugs have already been described. In addition, LSD produces somatic effects largely sympathomimetic in nature, such as pupillary dilatation, increase in blood pressure, tachycardia, hyperreflexia, tremor, nausea, piloerection, muscular weakness, and increased body temperature.

Following oral doses of 0.5 to 2 µg/kg the somatic symptoms are usually perceived within a few minutes. These include dizziness, weakness, drowsiness, nausea, and paresthesias. They may be followed by a feeling of inner tension relieved by laughing or crying. Several feelings may seem to coexist at the same time, although euphoric effects tend to predominate. In the second or third hour, visual illusions, wavelike recurrences of perceptual changes (*e.g.*, micropsia, macropsia), and affective symptoms may occur. There may be difficulty in locating the source of a sound; the user may be hypervigilant or withdrawn, or may alternate between these states. With many subjects there is a fear of fragmentation or disintegration of the self. Afterimages are prolonged, and the overlapping of present and preceding perceptions occurs. Some subjects recognize these confluences, whereas others elaborate them into hallucinations. In contrast to naturally occurring psychoses, auditory hallucinations are rare. Synesthesias, the overflow from one sensory modality to another, may occur. Colors are heard and sounds may be seen. Subjective time is also seriously altered, so that clock time seems to pass extremely slowly. The loss of boundaries and the fear of fragmentation create a need for a structuring or supporting environment; and, in the sense that they create a need for experienced companions and an explanatory system, these drugs are "cultogenic." During the "trip," thoughts and memories can vividly emerge under self-guidance or unexpectedly, to the user's distress. There may be a crossover of the affect of what is recalled with the content of what is presently perceived. Mood may be labile, shifting from depression to gaiety, from elation to fear. Tension and anxiety may mount and reach panic proportions. After about 4 to 5 hours, if a major panic episode does not occur, there may be a sense of detachment and the conviction that one is magically in control.

Between the dose ranges of 1 to 16 μg/kg, the intensity of the psychophysiological effects of LSD is proportional to the dose. The entire syndrome, including the pupillary dilatation, begins to clear after about 12 hours, although the half-life of the drug in man is approximately 3 hours. (For references and more detailed description, *see* Cohen, 1967; Freedman, 1969.)

While the user may be greatly impressed with the drug experience and feel a greater sensitivity for art, music, human feelings, and the harmony of the universe, there is little evidence for long-term changes in personality, beliefs, values, or behavior (McGlothlin and Arnold, 1971).

Although the patterns of psychological and biochemical effects seen with other agents are quite similar to those with LSD, there are significant differences in potency, absorption, metabolism, duration of action, and the slope of the dose-response curves. DMT, for example, is inactive by mouth and must be injected, sniffed, or smoked to produce effects. LSD is longer acting and more than 100 times as potent as psilocybin and psilocin, the active alkaloids in the Mexican "magic mushroom"; it is 4000 times as potent as mescaline in producing altered states of consciousness. There may also be some differences in the frequency of somatic effects, such as more vomiting with mescaline. The effects of an oral dose of mescaline (about 5 mg/kg) persist for about 12 hours. DOM and DOET are particularly

interesting in that at low doses they produce mild euphoria and enhanced self-awareness without perceptual distortion or hallucinogenic effects. At higher doses DOM has typical psychedelic activity, but with DOET there appears to be a rather wide dose range over which euphoria and self-awareness are produced without perceptual distortions (Snyder *et al.*, 1971). Infusions of tryptamine produce a profile of actions quite similar to those of LSD, including facilitation of spinal flexor reflexes, increases in respiratory rate, blood pressure, pulse, and pupillary diameter, wakefulness, desynchronization of the EEG, suppression of REM sleep, and perceptual distortions (*see* Martin and Sloan, 1977b; Kay and Martin, 1978). Most of the pharmacological actions of LSD, tryptamine, and, presumably, drugs with similar profiles are antagonized by chlorpromazine and cyproheptadine but not by α-adrenergic antagonists such as phenoxybenzamine.

Incidence and Patterns of Use. In the United States, the use of LSD ("acid") and related psychedelics reached a peak of popularity in the late 1960s and thereafter gradually declined. Psychedelic drugs are manufactured illegally and are still available through illicit channels. In 1977, approximately 20% of people in the United States aged 18 to 25 indicated use of hallucinogens at some time in their lives; only 1 or 2% had used such drugs during the preceding 30 days (Abelson *et al.*, 1977).

In general, these drugs do not give rise to patterns of repetitive use over prolonged periods. Used more by college students, the affluent, and the artistic than by the poor or the sociopathic, the most common psychedelic-use pattern is the occasional "trip," separated by intervals of weeks or months during which marihuana is used with variable frequency. The "acid head," or chronic user, is quite uncommon, and even among this group "trips" are rarely more frequent than biweekly. Chronic users may complain of memory difficulties and seem to exhibit extreme passivity. They tend to avoid competitive situations, equating these with anger and aggression. The relationship of such characteristics to the repeated drug experience is still not clear (*see* Blacker *et al.*, 1968). For most users the "psychedelic scene" tends to become less interesting with time. Even though the smoking of marihuana may continue, the use of the potent psychedelics is generally discontinued (*see* McGlothlin and Arnold, 1971).

Tolerance, Toxicity, and Physical Dependence. A high degree of tolerance to the behavioral effects of LSD develops after three or four daily doses; sensitivity returns after a comparable drug-free interval. Tolerance to the cardiovascular effects is less pronounced. There is considerable cross-tolerance between LSD, mescaline, and psilocybin, but none between LSD and the amphetamines or between LSD-like drugs and scopolamine or Δ^9-THC. Curiously, DMT induces little cross-tolerance to LSD, perhaps because of the short duration of action of DMT. Withdrawal phenomena are not seen after abrupt discontinuation of LSD-like drugs. In man, deaths attributable to *direct* effects of LSD are unknown, although fatal accidents and suicides during states of LSD intoxication have occurred. Death due to overdosage in animals results from respiratory failure, but in rabbits there is a marked hyperthermia as well. In spite of the concern about chromosomal aberrations and teratogenic effects induced by LSD, the evidence is contradictory and of uncertain significance (*see* Kato and Jarvik, 1969; Gilmour *et al.,* 1971). Among women who received pure LSD in medical settings months or years prior to conception, there was a slightly higher risk of spontaneous abortion, but no significant increase in birth defects. However, the effects of LSD during pregnancy are still uncertain (*see* Jacobson and Berlin, 1972). Among American Indian tribes that have used mescaline for several generations there appears to be no striking increase in genetic abnormalities or congenital malformations.

The evidence for significant psychological hazards in the use of psychedelic agents is unambiguous. The most common adverse effect is a temporary (24-hour) episode of panic—a "bad trip." This can be treated by reassurance in a supportive and familiar environment ("talking down"), antianxiety agents, or induction of sleep with barbiturates. Although phenothiazines antagonize the effects of LSD, they are usually not needed. Such "bad trips" cannot be reliably prevented and have been experienced even by users who had previous "good trips." Recurrences of drug effects without the drug, "flashbacks," are a puzzling but treatable phenomenon. In some individuals the use of psychedelics can precipitate serious depressions, paranoid behavior, or prolonged psychotic episodes. Whether such episodes would have occurred without the drug is not clear (*see* Cohen, 1967; Freedman, 1969). Prolonged psychotic episodes following repeated use of LSD tend to resemble the schizophreniform psychotic state and may require large doses of a phenothiazine for their control (Bowers, 1972). There is the possibility that repeated use of LSD can induce subtle deficits in the capacity for abstract thinking (McGlothlin *et al.,* 1969; Tucker *et al.,* 1972), although reviews examining the same clinical findings have tended to minimize this risk (*see* McWilliams and Tuttle, 1973).

Therapeutic Uses. Over the past 30 years, LSD has been proposed as an aid in psychotherapy, as an adjunct to the treatment of alcoholism and opioid addiction, and as a device to induce tranquility and reduce the need for opioid analgesics in cases of terminal cancer. In each situation, the use has been abandoned either because controlled studies have failed to demonstrate the value of LSD or because the elaborate precautions required to minimize adverse psychological reactions dampened enthusiasm and rendered its therapeutic use impractical.

ARYLCYCLOHEXYLAMINES

Phencyclidine and Related Compounds. *History and Source.* Phencyclidine, developed in the 1950s, was first used as an anesthetic for animals and, for a short time, as a general anesthetic in man. It fell into disuse quickly because patients experienced delirium when they emerged from anesthesia. Sporadic abuse of the compound by the oral route occurred in the 1960s, but the production of psychotic-like symptoms and other toxic effects gave the drug a "bad reputation." Phencyclidine became popular again in the early 1970s, when it was introduced as a drug to be smoked or "snorted." By the mid-1970s it was one of the most widely abused drugs in the United States. The compound is relatively easy to synthesize, and it is known among drug abusers by a number of street names, among which are angel dust, crystal, horse tranquilizer, PCP, and peace pill. Although it is still used as a veterinary anesthetic (SERNYLAN), almost all of the drug that is used illicitly is produced in clandestine laboratories and varies widely in purity. Phencyclidine is frequently misrepresented as LSD, mescaline, or Δ^9-THC.

Chemistry. Phencyclidine is one of a group of arylcyclohexylamines. A related compound, ketamine, is still used as an anesthetic in man. The structural formula of phencyclidine is as follows:

Phencyclidine

Pharmacological Actions. Phencyclidine and related arylcyclohexylamines have CNS stimulant, CNS depressant, hallucinogenic, and analgesic actions. The term *dissociative anesthetic* has been used to describe these drugs; they appear to represent a distinct category of agents in terms of their actions, as well as in terms of their properties in animal models.

In man, small doses produce a subjective sense of intoxication, with staggering gait, slurred speech, nystagmus, and numbness of the extremities. Users may exhibit sweating, catatonic muscular rigidity, and a blank stare; they may also experience changes in body image and disorganized thought, drowsiness, and apathy. There may be hostile and bizarre behavior. Amnesia for the episode may occur. With increasing dosage analgesia is more marked, and anesthesia, stupor, or coma may occur, although the eyes may remain open. Sensory impulses reach the cortex, but the individual experiences them in a distorted form. Heart rate and blood pressure are elevated; there is hypersalivation, sweating, fever, repetitive movements, and muscle rigidity on stimulation. At even higher doses prolonged coma, muscle rigidity, and convulsions may occur (*see* Domino, 1978; Petersen and Stillman, 1978).

Monkeys with implanted catheters do not administer LSD to themselves, but they do self-administer phencyclidine (Balster and Chait, 1978). Few drugs seem to induce so wide a range of subjective effects. Among those that users seem to like are increased sensitivity to external stimuli, stimulation, mood elevation, and a sense of intoxication. Other effects, some of which appear to occur with every use, are described as unwanted; these include perceptual disturbances, restlessness, disorientation, and anxiety. The typical "high" from a single dose lasts 4 to 6 hours and is followed by an extended "coming-down" period (Siegel, 1978).

At the cellular level, interactions of phencyclidine

have been described with several neurotransmitter systems. This is perhaps in keeping with its multiple effects on the CNS. Its fundamental actions remain obscure (*see* Domino, 1978; Johnson, 1978).

Absorption, Fate, and Excretion. Phencyclidine is well absorbed following all routes of administration. The parent compound may be hydroxylated, and these metabolites are conjugated with glucuronic acid. The pharmacological activity of the metabolites is unclear. Only a small fraction of the drug is excreted unchanged. Phencyclidine is a weak base, and lowering urinary pH (to below 5.0) with ammonium chloride markedly accelerates its excretion. Decreases in plasma pH produce decreases in the concentration of the drug in the cerebrospinal fluid; signs of intoxication referable to the CNS are thereby reduced. There is considerable gastroenteric recirculation, and continuous gastric suction is thus of value in the treatment of overdosage. In cases of overdose, the half-life of phencyclidine appears to be about 3 days, but this value can be shortened to about 1 day by continuous gastric suction and acidification of the urine (Aronow and Done, 1978; Domino, 1978; Done *et al.*, 1978).

Patterns of Use, Tolerance, and Physical Dependence. A 1977 survey indicated that 14% of 18- to 25-year-olds in the United States had used phencyclidine at least once. However, because the drug is often misrepresented, the true extent of use is uncertain and is probably underestimated. About half of current users claim to take phencyclidine about once a week. "Runs" also occur and consist in use for 2 to 3 days, during which the users do not sleep and eat very little. There is then a prolonged sleep, from which the user often awakens depressed and disoriented. A few take the drug several times per day. Most commonly, several users participate; the drug is often sprinkled on tobacco, marihuana, or parsley and smoked after making the material into a cigarette. The drug may also be snorted or taken orally or intravenously. The amount of phencyclidine in a cigarette varies from 1 to 100 mg, and chronic users may ingest up to 1 g in 24 hours.

In animals, tolerance develops to the behavioral and toxic effects of phencyclidine, but the extent varies with the species. In monkeys, there is no clear withdrawal syndrome even after several months of chronic administration. Clinical observations suggest that tolerance also develops in man. However, some chronic users make vague complaints about craving after stopping. Chronic users of large doses report persistent difficulties with recent memory, speech, and thinking that last from 6 months to 1 year after stopping. Personality changes ranging from social withdrawal and isolation to states of anxiety, nervousness, and severe depression have also been reported (*see* Balster and Chait, 1978; Lerner and Burns, 1978; Petersen and Stillman, 1978).

Toxicity and Treatment of Overdose. The frequency of adverse effects is uncertain, but deaths due to direct toxicity, violent behavior, and accidents have been reported. Phencyclidine can cause acute behavioral toxicity (intoxication, aggression, brief confusional states), coma or convulsions (from severe overdosage), and psychotic states. The last-named condition may be long lasting. In one study about 25% of those who exhibited a schizophrenic-like reaction were seen again with a similar syndrome in the absence of phencyclidine.

Treatment of overdosage is symptomatic and directed at protecting the patient and others from the effects of impaired behavior and judgment, supporting vital functions, and hastening the excretion of the drug by continuous gastric suction and acidification of urine. As mentioned, the half-life of the drug can be shortened to 1 day by such procedures. Hypersalivation may require suction, respiratory depression may require artificial ventilation, and fever may require external cooling. Convulsions have been treated with diazepam and hypertension with hydralazine. "Talking down" is not helpful, and clinicians advise isolation of patients from external stimuli to the degree compatible with support of vital functions and control of violent or self-destructive behavior. Where possible, four or five burly aides are superior to mechanical restraints, since excessive muscle contractions may lead to rhabdomyolysis and myoglobinuria (*see* Domino, 1978). Coma may be preceded or followed by delirium, paranoia, and assaultive behavior, and clinical arrangements must take this into consideration. A psychotic phase may last for several weeks after a single dose of phencyclidine. For the treatment of schizophrenic-like syndromes, clinicians prefer haloperidol to phenothiazines; the latter are believed to potentiate the anticholinergic actions of phencyclidine (*see* Burns and Lerner, 1976; Aronow and Done, 1978; Domino, 1978; Lerner and Burns, 1978).

MISCELLANEOUS SUBSTANCES USED FOR SUBJECTIVE EFFECTS

The catalog of agents that have been used to produce subjective changes is impressive, and each generation not only adds a few new substances but seems impelled to reevaluate the old.

Inhalants: Anesthetic Gases and Solvents. The intoxicating and euphorigenic effects of both nitrous oxide and ethyl ether were recognized before their potential as anesthetics was appreciated. In the nineteenth century, efforts to reduce alcoholism in Ireland by means of ether were markedly successful, but the use of ether became so widespread that it was necessary to take steps to reeducate the public to the use of alcohol. When access to alcohol or other intoxicants is restricted by finances, laws, or incarceration, substances with marked toxicity such as antifreeze, paint thinner, and other industrial solvents may be used. Since adolescents are usually prohibited from using alcoholic beverages, "glue sniffing" falls into this category. However, prohibition of alcohol cannot fully explain such behavior. Physicians, dentists, and nurses with access to a wide variety of drugs have been known to inhale anesthetic gases, sometimes with catastrophic outcomes for themselves and their patients. In 1977, about 11% of young adults (aged 18 to 25) indicated some experience with inhalants.

Animals will administer nitrous oxide, chloroform, and solvents (*e.g.,* toluene) to themselves; however, only a few of the many compounds have been systematically studied. There appears to be cross-tolerance and cross-dependence between barbiturates and chloroform (*see* Sharp and Brehm, 1977). While high doses of these substances produce depression of the CNS, low doses of most of these "anesthetics" and solvents produce increased activity that is usually thought to be due to disinhibition.

Because toxicity varies greatly with the specific substance, it can be discussed only in general terms. The causes of fatalities are not clear; most appear to involve cardiac arrhythmias. Inhalation of volatile material from a plastic bag (a common practice) may result in hypoxia as well as an extremely high concentration of vapor. Aerosol propellants containing fluorinated hydrocarbons produce cardiac arrhythmias, and ischemia increases sensitivity to fluorocarbon-induced arrhythmias. Chlorinated solvents (*e.g.,* trichloroethylene) depress myocardial contractility, and sympathetic activity is thereby increased reflexly. Ketones can produce pulmonary hypertension. Neurological impairment may occur with a variety of solvents. Peripheral neuropathies and progressive, fatal neurological deterioration have followed the "huffing" of lacquer thinner; however, because of the complexity of the mixture, the specific etiological agents are unknown. Studies of inhalers of aerosol paints have found indications of long-lasting brain damage (*see* Sharp and Brehm, 1977; Sharp and Carroll, 1978; Cohen, 1979).

Other Agents. In large amounts, the common household spice *nutmeg* produces marked subjective changes. It is commonly used for this purpose by the inmates of prisons. The oral ingestion of the equivalent of two grated nutmegs produces, after a latency of several hours, leaden feelings in the extremities and a mental state that may include feelings of depersonalization and unreality. Agitation and apprehension are also common. Dry mouth, thirst, rapid heart rate, and red, flushed face are common and may mimic atropine poisoning (*see* Weil, 1967).

Khat leaves (*Catha edulis*) are widely used for their stimulant effects in several countries of East Africa and in Yemen. The active principles in khat leaves are cathine (*d*-norisoephedrine) (a minor component in fresh leaves), cathinone ([−]-*s*-α-aminopropiophenone), and norephedrine. Animals will self-administer cathinone. The fresh khat leaves are chewed in a social setting, and amphetamine-like increased sense of well-being, talkativeness, and sociability occur. Effects on the heart, blood pressure, metabolism, appetite, and sleep are also like those of amphetamine (*see* Lugman and Danowski, 1976).

The medically inappropriate, excessive use of *nonopioid analgesic mixtures* (containing aspirin, phenacetin, caffeine, etc.) has been reported. Such use, however, is not characterized by extreme psychological dependence. Conceivably, excessive use of such drugs may be related to the mood-elevating effects of the *caffeine,* or to certain misconceptions about the capacity of such mixtures to relieve tension and increase the user's ability to concentrate on tedious tasks. Most investigators feel that tolerance and a limited degree of psychological dependence develop with caffeine and a withdrawal headache has been described repeatedly (*see* Greden *et al.,*

1978). Caffeine as a drug of abuse has been reviewed by Gilbert (1976).

For untold generations, *peyote, ololiuqui* (from the seeds of the morning glory, *Rivea corymbosa*), and *"magic mushrooms"* have been used to produce altered states of consciousness by the Indians of the North American continent. Throughout the world, many other substances are used for similar mind- and mood-changing effects. These include the use of *kava* in the South Pacific, *indole-containing snuff* among the Amazonian Indians in Brazil, and *fly agaric* among the Uralic-speaking tribes of Siberia. A discussion of the pharmacology and the use patterns of these substances is beyond the scope of this chapter. The interested reader should consult Efron and associates (1967).

TREATMENT

The indications for treatment vary with the drugs being used as well as with the social and cultural factors determining the particular pattern of drug use. Some patterns of drug use, such as the "recreational" use of marihuana, do not require treatment any more than does the occasional smoking of tobacco or the social use of alcohol. Such casual use is not without hazard, but this does not imply a treatable disorder. It is likely that changing views about drug use will continue to create gray areas where the indications for treatment are unclear. However, there is general agreement that treatment is appropriate for the adverse consequences of drug use and for the compulsive drug user who voluntarily seeks help.

WITHDRAWAL TECHNICS

Over the past decade, many views about withdrawal of drugs have been modified. No longer do all clinicians adhere to the view that drug withdrawal must be the first step in treatment or that it requires a carefully controlled, drug-free environment. Under appropriate circumstances successful withdrawal from opioids, alcohol, barbiturates, and amphetamines has been accomplished on an ambulatory basis. However, successful ambulatory withdrawal requires the establishment of a positive therapeutic relationship and considerable clinical experience. Withdrawal from tobacco is an exception and is typically an outpatient procedure. For the other drugs, withdrawal is usually more easily and more rapidly accomplished in an inpatient or residential setting where access to drugs can be controlled, the withdrawal syndrome observed, and appropriate treatment provided. When many addicted patients are being treated in the same treatment unit, drug smuggling can cause problems. However, when only an occasional patient is involved, it merely delays or prevents the completion of withdrawal; it should not unduly discourage attempts at treatment. Withdrawal in a controlled setting is obviously considerably more costly.

Certain general principles apply irrespective of the particular drug or drugs the patient has been using. (1) The *degree of physical dependence,* if any, that may have developed to each drug the patient has been using should be estimated. (2) A *medical history* should be taken and a physical examination carried out, to determine if there are any indications that the usual withdrawal technics should be modified. For example, a more gradual reduction of opioids would be appropriate in patients with angina pectoris, ulcerative colitis, pulmonary insufficiency, or other debilitating illness. Needless to say, patients who are experiencing severe pain from obvious causes are not appropriate candidates for withdrawal of opioid analgesics until some alternative method of managing the pain is available. (3) The patient should be given sufficient quantities of whichever *drugs* are necessary *to suppress severe withdrawal symptoms,* and the dose of these drugs is then gradually reduced.

Estimating the degree of physical dependence to opioids or to general CNS depressants from the history alone is difficult, since patients often distort their history of drug use. However, their motives vary widely, and so does the manner in which the history is distorted. For example, heroin users are usually unaware of the purity of the drugs they have been using. They tend to exaggerate their usage considerably and may also claim to be using large quantities of barbiturates or other sedatives in the hope that the doctor will then provide them with more generous amounts of opioids or hypnotics. Conversely, some individuals who use illicit drugs may completely deny the intake of barbiturates, even when they have been using a sufficient quantity to produce a dangerous degree of physical dependence. Others, who have used paregoric or cough medicines in an alcoholic vehicle, are often unaware of the large amounts of alcohol they consume. The possibility of physical dependence on general CNS depressants should always be considered when a patient who has had sufficient opioids to suppress withdrawal symptoms remains sleepless and jittery. In striking contrast are those addicts, such as physicians and nurses, who do not obtain their drugs through illicit traffic and who may attempt to mimimize the extent of their use. The difficulty in getting an accurate history means that the physician must place great reliance on observation of the patient and on his familiarity with the symptoms of withdrawal from both opioids and general depressants.

Withdrawal of Opioids. Even with very gradual reduction in dosage, most patients will perceive some withdrawal symptoms. It may be possible, of course, to continue to give the patient the drug he was using (heroin, morphine, meperidine, etc.) and simply reduce the dose over a period of several days. However, for reasons already discussed, methadone is quite suitable for suppressing withdrawal symptoms and can be substituted for any of the natural or synthetic opioid analgesics currently in use. With *methadone substitution,* in an inpatient or residential setting, now considered the standard technic, the opioid withdrawal symptoms are rarely worse than those of a moderate "influenza-like" syndrome. There are, however, newer methods that use other drugs, settings, and time frames that may have advantages (*see* below).

The dose of methadone will vary with the degree of physical dependence and the medical condition of the patient. The patient is observed and, if significant withdrawal symptoms appear, an initial dose of methadone that rarely needs to exceed 15 to 20 mg is given orally. Additional methadone can be given if the symptoms are not suppressed or each time withdrawal symptoms reappear. It is rarely necessary to give more than 80 mg of methadone over the first 24 hours. After the patient has been observed for 24 to 36 hours and given methadone as described, it becomes a relatively simple matter to calculate a stabilization dose. Usually 1 mg of methadone can substitute for 4 mg of morphine, 2 mg of heroin, or 20 mg of meperidine. Reduction can be started immediately. A reduction each day of 20% of the total daily dose is well tolerated and causes little discomfort. If the patient is not vomiting, methadone should be given by mouth and need not be given more frequently than twice a day. The majority of inpatients can be completely withdrawn from opioids in less than 10 days, although very mild abstinence symptoms may persist for a number of days after the last dose of methadone. The protracted abstinence syndrome has been described above.

A number of clinicians have found that after a period of social stabilization (usually 6 to 18 months) many former heroin addicts maintained on methadone can be gradually withdrawn from methadone entirely on an ambulatory basis. Even though the dosage is reduced very slowly (*e.g.,* by less than 10% of the stabilization dose per week or by as little as 3 mg per week), many of these patients experience opioid withdrawal symptoms when the daily dosage of methadone is reduced to about 10 to 30 mg. Some patients are able to tolerate the discomfort and the psychological difficulties, complete the withdrawal process, and do not relapse to opioid use. Others complete the withdrawal process but later relapse to heroin use, and still others elect to discontinue withdrawal and remain on maintenance doses of methadone. Exceedingly gradual reduction of dosage is more likely to be successful (Senay et al., 1977). Among the symptoms experienced over a period lasting up to several months after withdrawal are insomnia, irritability, restlessness, malaise, pain, fatigue, premature ejaculation, and gastrointestinal hyperactivity (Cushman and Dole, 1973).

Many nonopioids have been used for the opioid withdrawal syndrome; few have proven to have significant value. Certain drugs such as reserpine have a demonstrably aggravating effect on the course of withdrawal. The phenothiazines have not been demonstrated to be of significant help. Nighttime sedation with the barbiturates or related sedative-hypnotics is helpful, but complete suppression of opioid withdrawal symptoms with such agents alone cannot be achieved short of anesthetic doses. Clonidine, a centrally acting α-adrenergic agonist, can suppress the opioid withdrawal syndrome in patients who are withdrawn from low-to-moderate doses of methadone. Clonidine (5 μg/kg twice a day) can be given for 1 to 2 weeks to suppress symptoms. Naloxone does not precipitate withdrawal once subjects are free of opioids. The primary side effects appear to be dry mouth and sedation. No analgesia or euphoria has been observed during the clinical trials of this regimen (Gold et al., 1978). The theoretical basis for the treatment has been discussed above.

Some patients have difficulty in tolerating the persistent low level of discomfort that is associated with slow withdrawal of methadone and express a preference to "get it over with faster." Once patients require only low doses of methadone (5 to 10 mg per day), this can be accomplished by administration of repeated doses (1.2 mg) of naloxone every 30 minutes for several hours. While the withdrawal can be quite uncomfortable, the severity of the syndrome subsides after the first 3 to 6 hours and it is then possible to give the patients a longer-acting antagonist such as naltrexone (Resnick et al., 1977). The antagonist displaces methadone from receptor sites in the CNS and elsewhere; the displacement briefly intensifies the withdrawal syndrome but also permits the recovery process to begin.

Withdrawal of General CNS Depressants (Barbiturates and Related Drugs). Abrupt withdrawal of general CNS depressants that have been used in high doses over prolonged periods can be fatal. Nevertheless, some European clinicians with considerable experience feel that abrupt withdrawal has its advantages; they administer sedatives only if a delirium develops or if the patient has more than one seizure. In the United States, where there is considerably more abuse of short-acting barbiturates, abrupt withdrawal is not considered a safe technic, and the administration of a suitable general CNS depressant is usually started before major withdrawal symptoms develop. Pentobarbital (orally) can be substituted for any barbiturate the patient has been using. Clinical observations suggest that it is also a suitable substitute for glutethimide, paraldehyde, chloral hydrate, and meprobamate and for the suppression of the alcohol withdrawal syndrome. Sufficient pentobarbital should be given to produce mild intoxication, that is, slight ataxia, nystagmus, and slurred speech. Most patients require from 0.2 to 0.4 g every 6 hours, but some may need up to 2.5 g over a 24-hour period. The daily dose can be estimated from the response to a 200-mg pentobarbital test dose (Wikler, 1968). Once a level of mild intoxication has been achieved, the dosage of pentobarbital should be maintained for at least 24 to 36 hours. At this level, the patient should be free of tremulousness, irritability, and insomnia. The amount of barbiturate required for this initial period becomes the *stabilization level.*

Once the above-described stabilization level has been reliably established and the patient observed for 1 to 2 days, gradual withdrawal can be started. Clinical experience has shown that most patients can tolerate reductions of 0.1 g of pentobarbital per day without significant discomfort. However, the patient should be observed daily; if insomnia, tremulousness, or orthostatic hypotension occurs, further withdrawal should be suspended for 1 to 2 days. If such symptoms are severe, a single extra dose of 0.2 g will usually suppress them. However, once a withdrawal delirium develops, increasing the amount of pentobarbital will not immediately restore equilibrium; the delirium and disorientation may persist for several days. With the use of the pentobarbital-substitution technic, withdrawal may take from 10 days to 3 weeks. It cannot safely be hurried. Patients who are taking large amounts of lesser-known sedatives or longer-acting benzodiazepines should probably be gradually withdrawn from the original drug of abuse without substitution therapy (*see* Wikler, 1968).

Some clinicians feel that the longer duration of action of phenobarbital has advantages for managing withdrawal of general CNS depressants, and use 30 mg of phenobarbital for each hypnotic dose of the drug of dependence (*e.g.,* for each 100 mg of pentobarbital), divided and given four times each day. Phenobarbital is then reduced by 30 mg per day (Wesson and Smith, 1977b).

Withdrawal of Alcohol.   There are certain distinctions between the overall effects of chronic abuse of alcohol and those of other general CNS depressants, which necessitate differences in the therapeutic approach. Chronic ingestion of large amounts of alcohol is very frequently associated with various degrees of malnutrition and avitaminosis, especially vitamin B deficiencies. Whereas the well-nourished alcoholic may sometimes be overhydrated (Beard and Knott, 1968), others may be severely dehydrated because of vomiting caused by alcoholic gastritis or withdrawal and also, perhaps, because of the diuretic effects of alcohol. Pneumonitis is also a frequent complication. Thus, injections of vitamins, attention to fluid balance, and administration of antibiotics are often a necessary part of treatment, but *these are obviously not substitutes for measures that suppress the general-depressant withdrawal syndrome.*

As is the case with mild degrees of physical dependence of any type, in the milder forms of alcohol withdrawal a wide variety of drugs (phenothiazines, sedatives, antianxiety agents) will provide some symptomatic relief. Indeed, although screening is a problem and the procedure involves risk for patients with medical problems or significant physical dependence, many alcoholics are now routinely withdrawn on an outpatient or day hospital basis without the use of any pharmacological agent.

When there is a significant degree of physical dependence, drugs that show cross-dependence with alcohol are demonstrably superior in reducing mortality and morbidity to those that do not show such cross-dependence. Unfortunately, the tremulousness, which in some patients may be the most severe manifestation of physical dependence, may in others be the prodrome of the more severe epileptiform and delirious states. It is not possible to know in advance which patients are only mildly physically dependent and which patients will develop delirium tremens. Since delirium tremens always carries with it a certain risk of a fatal outcome, it seems appropriate to treat all but the mildest cases of alcoholic withdrawal with agents that show cross-dependence with alcohol.

Theoretically, alcohol itself should be quite effective in the suppression of the alcohol withdrawal syndrome. However, its short duration of action and narrow range of safety make it a poor therapeutic agent. In practice, alcohol is usually abruptly stopped and longer-acting agents are substituted. If given in adequate quantities, pentobarbital, pheno-barbital, chloral hydrate, paraldehyde, chlordiazepoxide, and diazepam have all been shown to be effective in preventing the development of withdrawal symptoms or suppressing the syndrome once it develops. The general technic is similar to that used in the management of physical dependence on barbiturates, in that the patient is brought to a level of stabilization in which he exhibits either no withdrawal symptoms or only mild intoxication and the drug is then gradually withdrawn. Chlordiazepoxide, diazepam, and flurazepam are now the most widely used drugs for withdrawal, even though in some well-controlled studies they were not superior to a combination of paraldehyde and chloral hydrate. The long duration of action and slow elimination of most benzodiazepines make their use in the treatment of physical dependence on alcohol analogous to the use of methadone in the treatment of physical dependence on opioids. The rate at which the dosage of the benzodiazepine should subsequently be reduced has not been carefully studied; the clinician's adjustment of doses should be guided by the degree of intoxication and the appearance of tremulousness and insomnia. If seizures occur, diazepam should probably be given, but chlordiazepoxide is less likely to lead to its abuse if treatment continues on an ambulatory basis. Sodium valproate and clormethiazole (used in Europe but not in the United States) are also effective. Magnesium sulfate, propranolol, the amino acid taurine, and lithium have also all been reported to reduce some of the symptoms and signs of withdrawal from alcohol (*see* Sellers and Kalant, 1976; Smith, 1978; Gessner, 1979). When physical dependence is at all severe, the use of phenothiazines does not prevent the development of delirium tremens and the mortality rate is significantly higher than in patients treated with paraldehyde or chlordiazepoxide (*see* Gessner, 1979).

Withdrawal Technics in Mixed Patterns of Abuse.   It is not uncommon to encounter individuals who are physically dependent on both opioids and general CNS depressants. The therapeutic regimen in such situations combines the procedures described above. General CNS depressants are given in sufficient quantity to produce mild intoxication, and a stabilization dose is determined. At the same time the patient is observed for the autonomic signs of opioid withdrawal, and sufficient methadone or another suitable opioid is given to suppress such symptoms. While the dose of the CNS depressant is held constant, the opioid is reduced as previously described. When withdrawal from opioids is complete, the dose of the CNS depressant is then reduced gradually. Simultaneous withdrawal of both classes of drugs at appropriate rates is not contraindicated, but this procedure requires considerable experience, since insomnia, weakness, and restlessness occur in both syndromes. Although the abrupt withdrawal of psychedelics, sympathomimetic drugs, and tobacco does not cause syndromes that require medical treatment, these syndromes do cause unpleasant physiological and psychological disturbances that may contribute to relapse. Administration of tricyclic antidepressants has been suggested for the treatment of the fatigue, irritability, and depression that may persist after withdrawal of amphetamines, and chewing gum containing nicotine may prove useful when the withdrawal syndrome from tobacco is severe or protracted.

APPROACHES TO BEHAVIORAL MODIFICATION

A number of very different approaches are currently in use for modification of patterns of compulsive drug abuse. They differ not only in the way the problem is conceptualized but also in the goals given priority, the methods used, and the patterns of change induced. No longer do all approaches use total abstinence as the sole criterion of successful treatment. Instead, there is a growing emphasis on achieving productive and socially acceptable behavior and on improving physical health and interpersonal relationships. Sometimes marked changes occur in these areas even when the pattern of drug use has only been modified rather than eliminated.

Some treatments place emphasis on emotional problems that are believed to increase vulnerability to compulsive drug use; others aim at providing alternative gratifications or modifying life styles; still others use various forms of external pressure and threats of adverse consequences to change drug-use patterns; some employ pharmacological agents to modify the response to the drugs themselves. In practice, several of these methods are combined in any one treatment program (*see* Glasscote *et al.*, 1972). Although similar themes appear in programs designed to modify compulsive use of different drugs, the great differences in pharmacological effects and social attitudes make it convenient to discuss treatment approaches to each drug separately. The nonpharmacological methods can be only briefly summarized here.

In assessing the value of any form of treatment it is essential to recognize that the recovery rate for all forms of drug dependence is sometimes surprisingly high even though there is little or no intervention

(*see* Armor *et al.*, 1976; Edwards *et al.*, 1977; Sells, 1979). For some young people, major changes in associates and environment lead to rapid abandonment of illicit use of opioids (Robins, 1974). Cessation of opioid use does not necessarily mean total abstinence from all substances. Former users may be dependent on a variety of other drugs (*see* O'Donnell, 1968).

Hospitalization and Psychotherapy. Measured by the percentage of patients who remain abstinent, the results of prolonged hospital or institutional rehabilitation are disappointing, not only for opioid users but also for patients addicted to alcohol, barbiturates, or amphetamines. The use of prolonged hospitalization (more than 3 weeks) is now on the decline, and questions have even been raised about the need for brief hospitalization in the absence of medical complications.

There is little evidence to show that traditional individual *psychotherapy* is of any value in the treatment of the compulsive drug user. Over the past decade specialized forms of group psychotherapy have been developed, but there is no way of predicting the type of drug user who will be helped by one or another of the many technics now in use. Furthermore, the repeated finding that some alcoholics can drink without immediately relapsing to compulsive, socially damaging use has raised questions about the view once generally held that compulsive drug users cannot regain the ability to employ the drug of abuse in moderation (*see* Armor *et al.*, 1976; Edwards *et al.*, 1977; Smith, 1978).

Voluntary Groups and Self-Regulatory Communities. Alcoholics Anonymous, Narcotics Anonymous, Synanon, Daytop Village, and similar groups have been helpful in the rehabilitation of certain types of compulsive drug users. Their efficacy may be due to a number of factors, including a reduction in the sense of isolation and a gratification of the need to belong. Equally important is the absence of a hard line between "patient" and "staff." The organizations are usually operated by former drug users, and the new member is immediately confronted by individuals who at once convey understanding and concern, and provide role models for responsible behavior. Also important is the participation itself, which keeps the individual away from the environment in which drug use occurred and in the company of people who share his concerns about drug use in a way that amounts to a ritualization of sobriety. Although a substantial proportion of treated alcoholics make contact with Alcoholics Anonymous at some point, it is not clear what proportion derive benefit. Only a small percentage of compulsive opioid users seem motivated to seek admission to self-regulating residential centers; fewer still actually enter after learning what is expected of members, and many leave within weeks after joining. Those who remain in residential programs do well while they are members, and many continue to do well after they leave. Indeed, the level of improvement seems directly related to the length of stay for up to 18 months, but controlled studies are lacking (*see* Sells, 1979).

Supervisory-Deterrent Approaches. Some approaches emphasize the maintenance of abstinence and involve a period in a hospital, prison, or special facility followed by careful supervision of the individual in the community. If the chemical analysis of urine specimens or other information indicates return to drug use, the supervisee, who has usually been paroled or civilly committed to the program, is reinstitutionalized. The critical element of the system is thought to be the deterrent effect of reinstitutionalization. In theory, this approach can be used with all types of compulsive drug abuse. While it is believed that this system was highly effective in Japan in controlling serious epidemics of amphetamine and heroin addiction, the experience in the United States has been far less impressive. Very few individuals under such supervision who were dependent on opioids were able to remain totally abstinent, and by the end of the first year after discharge more than two thirds had been reinstitutionalized. The economic and social cost of such an approach has led to a major decline in its use for compulsive drug users. However, there is now increasing use of external pressure (*e.g.,* threat of job loss) to motivate the working problem drinker to remain in treatment. The use of monitoring and external pressure with less draconian consequences for drug users who have been arrested or convicted of crimes appears to reduce the frequency of drug abuse (*see* McGlothlin, 1979).

Role of Pharmacological Agents.

With every form of drug dependence, other drugs have been tried as therapeutic agents on a variety of theoretical grounds. Sometimes the therapeutic agents are directed at some postulated underlying psychological difficulty (*e.g.,* anxiety or depression) that is felt to contribute to the motivation to use the drug of dependence. Sometimes the therapeutic agent is intended to be a less toxic substitute, in whole or in part, for the effects of the drug being used, or at least to suppress any subclinical withdrawal phenomena (*e.g.,* oral nicotine for inhaled tobacco, oral methadone or acetylmethadol for injected heroin). Still other agents are intended to interfere in a variety of ways with the reinforcing or satisfying properties of the dependence-producing drug (*e.g.,* opioid antagonists), or to create situations where their use becomes unpleasant (*e.g.,* disulfiram).

Opioid Maintenance. Methadone maintenance was originally based on the hypothesis that, as a result of repeated use of opioids, the addict has sustained a metabolic alteration such that opioids produce a euphoria not experienced by nonaddicts, and that for months or years after withdrawal the addict experiences a feeling of abnormality (opioid hunger) relieved only by opioids. Since the original pilot studies of Dole and Nyswander, the use of this approach has been greatly expanded and the procedures and dosages have been substantially modified. Most commonly the procedure consists in the daily administration of 40 to 100 mg of methadone, orally in a flavored vehicle, combined with efforts at social rehabilitation. At the stabilization level (achieved by gradually increasing the dose over a period of several weeks), there is a high degree of cross-tolerance to all opioids so that the euphoric effects of even high doses of intravenous opioid are generally not experienced. Dole and coworkers (1966) have referred to this state as "narcotic blockade." While many patients report little or no craving for illicit opioids, in most treatment programs and under experimental conditions there are usually some patients who continue to seek out and use intravenous opioids despite the attenuated effects. This treatment explicitly emphasizes law-abiding and productive behavior rather than abstinence *per se,* and its relative efficacy in reaching its goals is well documented (Wilmarth and Goldstein, 1974; Sells, 1979; Simpson *et al.,* 1979). The methadone-maintenance approach is no longer considered experimental, but it is subject to special regulations and is still criticized by some.

The use of methadone should not be confused with the British practice of prescribing heroin for self-administration. With methadone the route is exclusively oral, thus eliminating both the sharp ups and downs that characterize the effects of repeated doses of intravenous heroin and the complications that occur when addicts inject themselves without benefit of hygienic technic. Equally important, the duration of action of methadone is such that it need be given only once a day. Although the concentrations of methadone in plasma do change over the course of 24 hours (*see* Chapter 22), the decline is usually not great enough to produce perceptible withdrawal phenomena. Therefore, the ingestion of all medication can be supervised by scheduled visits to the clinic. Since nonmedical use of opioids seems to increase with greater availability of drugs, control of illicit redistribution from treatment programs is an important and controversial issue. In Great Britain, the prescribing of heroin for addicts is now restricted to clinics staffed by specialists. However, the existence of these clinics has not prevented the development of an illicit traffic in heroin that serves those who do not use the clinics and those who feel the clinics are not generous enough in their prescribing habits (*see* Stimson, 1973). In practice, most methadone treatment programs permit patients to take some drug home, and there has been some illicit diversion. Concern about this has led to efforts to develop longer-acting opioids for clinical use. One such drug is *acetylmethadol,* which suppresses opioid withdrawal for up to 72 hours after a single dose and, theoretically, all doses can be ingested under direct supervision when patients come to the clinics three times per week. In clinical trials it appears to be similar to methadone in its overall effects (*see* Ling *et al.,* 1978). It is still an investigational drug.

Opioid Antagonists. When the opioid receptors in the CNS are continuously occupied by antagonists, the effects of ordinary doses of opioids are attenuated or entirely blocked, and even the repeated administration of opioids for several weeks does not induce a significant degree of physical dependence.

Theoretically, the use of opioid antagonists might be helpful in several ways. If compulsive use of opioids is a result of the reinforcement of drug-seeking behavior due to drug effects, then the repeated use of opioids without effect (as would be the case if the patient were taking adequate amounts of an antagonist) would tend to produce extinction. Furthermore, if the development of physical dependence could be prevented, then conditioned abstinence phenomena should also be extinguished and the protracted abstinence syndrome should eventually subside. It is important to point out that, independent of the reinforcement model, prevention of the development of physical dependence in ambulatory patients may be of considerable value in that it may stop occasional illicit use from progressing quickly into regular and compulsive use. The patient who takes an antagonist behaves as if opioids are, for practical purposes, unavailable. This serves to decrease craving (Meyer and Mirin, 1979). A number of specific opioid antagonists (cyclazocine, naloxone, and naltrexone) have been subjected to clinical trial. Patients must first be withdrawn from opioids, since antagonists precipitate severe abstinence symptoms in individuals who are physically dependent.

Cyclazocine is relatively long acting, and significant blockade of intravenous opioids persists for approximately 24 hours after a 4- to 6-mg oral dose. Its use is associated with psychotomimetic side effects, to which tolerance develops. *Naloxone* is relatively free of the side effects that commonly occur with cyclazocine, but its short duration of action and low oral efficacy make it impractical for treatment. There is currently some optimism about *naltrexone*, since it is orally effective, seems relatively free of side effects, and, depending on the dose, can produce blockade for more than 24 hours. Depot preparations of naltrexone have also been developed but have not yet been tested adequately. Clinical trials of naltrexone have shown that it may have value for selected populations of patients (National Research Council, 1978). *Buprenorphine* (*see* Chapter 22) has also been suggested as a drug that may have advantages for maintenance purposes.

Other Pharmacological Procedures. Maintenance approaches for compulsive users of general CNS depressants and amphetamine-like drugs have not been well studied. With the exception of patients dependent on very small doses of such drugs, most practitioners strive for total withdrawal. Drugs that interfere with the synthesis or effects of catecholamines can attenuate or antagonize the effects of amphetamines, but the clinical significance of this observation is uncertain. Tricyclic antidepressants have been recommended for relief of postwithdrawal lethargy, but clinical studies are lacking. For the very heavy smoker, drugs such as nicotine in the form of chewing gum may prove to have some value in alleviating withdrawal and, in some cases, may serve as a less toxic substitute for nicotine inhaled in tobacco smoke.

Disulfiram and related agents have been used in the treatment of alcoholism for a number of years. When an individual who has been taking disulfiram ingests alcohol, a syndrome characterized by nausea, vomiting, flushing and hypotension, anxiety, and palpitations develops within minutes. The details of the administration and the potential hazards of disulfiram and related agents are discussed in Chapter 18. Disulfiram can be administered only with the patient's cooperation and, therefore, is useful only for selected patients. Other factors being equal, patients who take disulfiram relapse less rapidly than those who do not. Depot forms of disulfiram have also been employed. The pharmacology and use of disulfiram have been reviewed by Baekeland (1977) and Kwentus and Major (1979).

Conditioned aversion technics have been tried in alcoholism, smoking, and other forms of drug abuse. This usually involves the administration of an emetic agent (apomorphine or ipecac), followed shortly thereafter by a dose of the drug (*e.g.,* a small amount of whisky or other agent) so that nausea and vomiting occur soon after the drug is ingested. In this way, the taking of alcohol or the drug of abuse becomes a conditioned stimulus that produces a sensation of nausea. Enthusiasm for the aversion technics has declined as their limitations have become clearer. However, there is a renewed interest in the use of apomorphine in subemetic doses as a drug that reduces anxiety and craving, and there have been several optimistic clinical reports (*see* Smith, 1978).

Because of the risk of dependence, most practitioners avoid the use of benzodiazepines or other sedatives in the management of alcoholism after initial withdrawal. Although a substantial proportion of alcoholics are depressed and suicide among this group is not uncommon, there are relatively few studies that demonstrate efficacy of tricyclic antidepressants. Lithium has been reported to reduce the rate of relapse to problem drinking, but there is uncertainty about what kinds of alcoholics are most likely to respond (*e.g.,* perhaps it helps only those with symptoms of depression or those who have a history of affective disorder) (*see* Merry *et al.,* 1976; Smith, 1978).

ROLE OF THE MEDICAL PROFESSION IN PREVENTION

Since there is a relationship between availability of certain drugs and the prevalence of their self-administration, consideration must be given to regulation of the manufacture, prescription, and dispensing of those drugs considered to have a liability for abuse. Developing reasonable regulations requires efforts in several areas, including (1) methods for assessing the likelihood that a particular drug will be self-administered, (2) guidelines for classifying drugs in order to provide for different degrees of control at the levels of manufacturing, prescribing, and dispensing, and (3) general guidelines for medical practitioners who must prescribe these drugs for patients. The use of drugs with potential for abuse in the treatment of compulsive drug users creates special problems because of the belief that such individuals are particularly likely to sell or give some of their prescribed medication to others. While special concern about prescribing drugs for this group is often based on moral and political issues, there is a core of legitimate concern linked to the effort to control availability of drugs used illicitly.

Addicting and Nonaddicting Drugs: Assessing Liability for Abuse. In most cases it is not possible to predict from the chemical structure the likelihood that a given drug will produce effects that might lead to its abuse. At present such evaluations are accomplished by determining whether animals will administer the new drug to themselves and how many properties it shares with prototypical drugs known to be abused. Both of these approaches have limitations. For example, animals do not self-administer psychedelics, but they will do so with caffeine, procaine, and apomorphine.

The technics used with opioid-like agents are well established. Thus, a drug is considered to be non-opioid with respect to liability for abuse (1) if it does not suppress the opioid withdrawal syndrome when tested in subjects physically dependent on morphine, (2) if it does not produce morphine-like physical dependence when given chronically, and (3) if postaddicts neither consistently identify it as "dope" (morphine-like) nor repeatedly request it when offered the opportunity to do so. On the other hand, if a compound is found to share all of these key characteristics with morphine, it is considered to have a high liability for abuse and is recommended for appropriate controls. However, some drugs share a few characteristics but not others. For example, cyclazocine produces a variety of physical dependence in which the withdrawal symptoms are not associated with drug-seeking behavior. Other drugs, such as nalbuphine, may be somewhat morphine-like with respect to one or two characteristics; however, because of differences in solubility or toxicity or because they appear to exhibit a ceiling effect in inducing euphoria, they are considered to present a lower order of risk. Such agents may be recommended for less stringent controls than those applied to the opioids. The difficulties in assessing liability for abuse of agonist-antagonists are described in Chapter 22.

It is possible to estimate the cross-dependence of a drug with barbiturates in both man and animals. The assessment of the potential for abuse of other classes of drugs is less well established. Until recently, procedures for estimating potential for abuse were employed routinely prior to release only for the opioids. New drugs that have pharmacological actions similar to those of amphetamines or general CNS depressants are now required to be evaluated for potential for abuse prior to marketing for general use. (The procedures for assessing potential for abuse have been reviewed by Jasinski, 1977; *see also* Thompson and Unna, 1977.)

Treating the Compulsive Drug User. In the United States, the effort to control drug availability previously included severe restrictions on the use of opioids and certain other controlled drugs in the treatment of compulsive drug users. Musto (1973) has documented the history of the interactions between the medical profession and regulatory authorities. This situation has changed substantially since 1970, and opioids are now used both for easing withdrawal and for maintenance. However, it is likely that further changes will be made in laws and rules as practitioners and regulators strive for a balance between flexibility for treatment and control of illicit diversion. At present, continued administration of opioids to patients with chronic, incurable, and painful conditions is not considered "maintenance of an addiction" and, although the practice varies from state to state, such individuals are not generally reported to health authorities as opioid addicts.

The treatment of compulsive opioid users who do not have an obvious medical problem is more complicated. Methadone and similar drugs for both the ambulatory withdrawal and maintenance treatment of heroin addiction are now used in the treatment of more than 80,000 individuals at several hundred separate centers throughout the United States. While such a treatment system has many advantages, already discussed, it also creates certain problems and public health risks. Patients participating in programs can be sources of illicit diversion of the drug prescribed (especially if they are permitted to take home substantial quantities), thus creating the potential of primary addiction to methadone in others. In addition, some intermittent heroin users may become severely physically dependent if inappropriately admitted to maintenance programs. In an attempt to reduce such problems, the federal government promulgated regulations that legitimized the use of methadone, but at the same time attempted to minimize the amount of take-home medication permitted in such programs and to reduce the likelihood that patients would obtain methadone from more than one source. It is still medically appropriate to administer an opioid to relieve acute withdrawal symptoms. However, it is expected that, where there are nearby specialized detoxication or maintenance programs, the patient will be referred to these specialized facilities. The use of opioid maintenance is restricted to specially licensed centers and to clinicians affiliated with them. Since there are also state regulations, interested clinicians should contact the appropriate state agencies.

Thus far there are no specific regulations or constraints at the federal level that would prohibit the use of CNS stimulants or general CNS depressants in the treatment of compulsive users of nonopioid drugs. However, there is a prevalent view that with few exceptions chronic maintenance programs for these drugs are of little benefit to the patient, and a number of state medical boards have taken disciplinary actions against physicians who were too casual in prescribing CNS depressants and stimulants for purposes other than the traditional.

In practice, the physician must often administer potent analgesics or sedatives even to persons who seem predisposed to develop dependence on such drugs. There are a few general rules applicable to opioids that, if followed in all cases, will reduce, but obviously not eliminate, the probability of such a complication. The patient should not be given an opioid when another drug of lower potential for abuse will suffice. The patient should not be permitted to self-administer such drugs parenterally. Only a few days' supply should be dispensed at any given time, and a return to nonopioids should be undertaken as soon as the situation permits. If the drug has been administered repeatedly for more than a few weeks, a change to a long-acting drug a few days prior to discontinuation will minimize withdrawal symptomatology. On the other hand, the tendency to avoid the use of opioid analgesics should not be carried to unwarranted extremes; the patient who needs a potent analgesic should not be left in pain because of the physician's fear of causing addiction.

Most physicians now exercise great care in prescribing potent opioids. They are beginning to exercise similar prudence in the prescription of sedatives, antianxiety agents, and CNS sympathomimetics. New regulations limiting the number of times a prescription order for controlled drugs can be renewed should result in more careful periodic reassessment of the need for such drugs.

Drugs given for the relief of fluctuating levels of pain, anxiety, or feelings of depression can be taken in several ways. They can be requested or taken by the patient each time the distress becomes too intense to tolerate, that is, for *relief* of distress; or they can be taken in anticipation of the recurrence of distress, that is, to *avoid* distress. With respect to inducing drug dependence, both ways carry risks. When used for *relief,* minimal amounts of drug will be used, since the time of drug action will correspond to the time when its action is required. However, each time relief is promptly obtained, the act of self-administration of the drug will be reinforced. Drugs with slower onset and longer duration of action may minimize this reinforcement process. Self-administration to *avoid* distress may be less reinforcing of each drug-taking act, but the patient never waits long enough to find out whether the drug is needed at all. Even the idea of discontinuing may cause anticipation of the return of distress. From a pharmacological viewpoint, the avoidance schedule leads to the regular and frequent use of unnecessary amounts of drug, maximizing the development of physical dependence (where this phenomenon is relevant). Although there are no easy solutions to this therapeutic dilemma, the physician should be aware of the factors that may be operative and suggest to the patient the approach best suited to the individual situation. It would also be helpful if the physician took advantage of his own relationship with the patient to reinforce efforts other than the use of drugs to cope with psychic and physical distress and advised the patient's family to do likewise. Lastly, physicians cannot escape their responsibilities as role models. Doctors who smoke, drink too much, or use any drug to excess obviously do not present the proper model to their patients.

A final caveat is in order. Undoubtedly, whether drugs are used for producing pleasure or for the avoidance or relief of distress, it is the *self-administration* of drugs and the *self-induced* changes in mood that are the critical factors in the development of compulsive abuse. The physician would do well to remember this, not only in his treatment of patients but also when he considers treating himself.

IMPACT OF LEGISLATION AND SOCIAL ATTITUDES ON THE PATTERNS AND TREATMENT OF DRUG ABUSE

Every measure taken to regulate drug use has its social costs as well as its potential benefits. For example, harsh penalties for the possession of small amounts of certain drugs (*e.g.,* heroin, cocaine, marihuana) undoubtedly retard their acceptance as substances for social and "recreational" purposes, in the sense that alcohol and tobacco are so used. Whatever the advantages of such a retardation may be, costs must be measured in money, in the criminal stigmatization of many otherwise law-abiding citizens, and in the development of systems of illicit drug distribution. The eventual impact of restrictive laws and criminal sanctions is usually difficult to predict. To the extent that they may foster the development of socially stigmatized drug-using subcultures where there is social reinforcement of both drug use and deviant behavior, the problems of treating compulsive drug users are made more difficult. Experience seems to show that, within a culture that accepts the use of some psychoactive agents, total prohibition of selected classes of drugs tends to produce a shift toward the use of other agents, at least among individuals who have already developed patterns of compulsive drug use. Furthermore, prohibitions against specific classes of drugs and the social attitudes associated with such prohibitions create selective processes that determine the characteristics of users of prohibited drugs. For example, if the penalties and attitudes are such that a particular drug (*e.g.,* heroin) is available only by interacting with a deviant and antisocial subculture, then only those willing to engage in such interaction are likely to persist in the use of that particular drug. The effects of membership in a subculture, the drug-using experience, and the initial selective process interact to produce many of the characteristics sometimes thought to be due to the drug experience alone. Against these costs must be placed the finding that high price, inconvenience, and social disapproval produce major reductions in the overall amount of any drug that is consumed; the proportion of individuals who develop problems with the use of drugs and who become dependent on them decreases as overall consumption is reduced.

Abood, L. G.; Lowy, K.; and Booth, H. Acute and chronic effects of nicotine in rats and evidence for a noncholinergic site of action. In, *Cigarette Smoking as a Dependence Process.* (Krasnegor, N. A., ed.) National Institute on Drug Abuse. Department of Health, Education, and Welfare Publication No. (ADM) 79-800, U.S. Government Printing Office, Washington, D. C., **1979,** pp. 136-149.

Aghajanian, G. K. Tolerance of locus coeruleus neurones to morphine and suppression of withdrawal response by clonidine. *Nature,* **1978,** *276,* 186-188.

Aigner, T. G., and Balster, R. L. Choice behavior in rhesus monkeys: cocaine versus food. *Science,* **1978,** *201,* 534-535.

Alexander, E. J. Withdrawal effects of SODIUM AMYTAL. *Dis. Nerv. Syst.,* **1951,** *12,* 77-82.

Angrist, B. M., and Gershon, S. Amphetamine abuse in New York City—1966-1968. *Semin. Psychiatry,* **1969,** *1,* 195-207.

Armitage, A.; Dollery, C.; Houseman, T.; Kohner, E.; Lewis, P. J.; and Turner, D. Absorption of nicotine from small cigars. *Clin. Pharmacol. Ther.,* **1978,** *23,* 143-151.

Aronow, R., and Done, A. Phencyclidine overdose; an emergency concept of management. *J.A.C.E.P.,* **1978,** *7,* 56-59.

Bachman, J. A.; Benowitz, N. L.; Herning, R. I.; and Jones, R. T. Dissociation of autonomic and cognitive effects of THC in man. *Psychopharmacology,* **1979,** *61,* 171-175.

Beard, J. D., and Knott, D. H. Fluid and electrolyte balance during acute withdrawal in chronic alcoholic patients. *J.A.M.A.,* **1968,** *204,* 133-138.

Belgrave, B. E.; Bird, K. D.; Chesher, G. B.; Jackson, D. M.; Lubbe, K. E.; Starner, G. A.; and Teo, R. K. C. The effect of (−)trans-Δ⁹-tetrahydrocannabinol alone and in combination with ethanol on human performance. *Psychopharmacology,* **1979,** *62,* 53-60.

Blacker, K. H.; Reese, T. J.; Stone, G. C.; and Pfefferbaum, D. Chronic users of LSD: the "acidheads." *Am. J. Psychiatry,* **1968,** *125,* 341-351.

Boisse, N. R., and Okamoto, M. Physical dependence to barbital compared to pentobarbital. IV. Influence of elimination kinetics. *J. Pharmacol. Exp. Ther.,* **1978,** *204,* 526-540.

Bowers, M. B., Jr. Acute psychosis induced by psychotomimetic drug abuse. I. Clinical findings. II. Neurochemical findings. *Arch. Gen. Psychiatry,* **1972,** *27,* 437-442.

Burns, R. S., and Lerner, S. E. Perspectives: acute phencyclidine intoxication. *Clin. Toxicol.,* **1976,** *9,* 477-501.

Carlen, P. L.; Wortzman, G.; Holgate, R. C.; Wilkinson, D. A.; and Rankin, J. G. Reversible cerebral atrophy in recently abstinent chronic alcoholics measured by computed tomography scans. *Science,* **1978,** *200,* 1076-1078.

Castellani, S.; Ellinwood, E. H., Jr.; and Kilbey, M. M. Behavioral analysis of chronic cocaine intoxication in the cat. *Biol. Psychiatry,* **1978,** *13,* 203-215.

Chopra, G. S., and Smith, J. W. Psychotic reactions following cannabis use in East Indians. *Arch. Gen. Psychiatry,* **1974,** *30,* 24-27.

Clopton, P. L.; Janowsky, D. S.; Clopton, J. M.; Judd, L. L.; and Huey, L. Marihuana and the perception of affect. *Psychopharmacology,* **1979,** *61,* 203-206.

Cohen, D.; Arai, S. F.; and Brain, J. D. Smoking impairs long-term dust clearance from the lung. *Science,* **1979,** *204,* 514-517.

Collier, H. O. J. Tolerance, physical dependence and receptors: a theory of the genesis of tolerance and physical dependence through drug-induced changes in the number of receptors. *Adv. Drug Res.,* **1966,** *3,* 171-188.

Cryer, P. E.; Haymond, M. W.; Santiago, J. V.; and Shah, S. D. Norepinephrine and epinephrine release and adrenergic mediation of smoking-associated hemodynamic and metabolic events. *N. Engl. J. Med.,* **1976,** *295,* 573-577.

Cushman, P., and Dole, V. P. Detoxification of rehabilitated methadone-maintained patients. *J.A.M.A.,* **1973,** *226,* 747-752.

Desmond, M. M.; Schwaneke, R. P.; Wilson, G. S.; Yasunaga, S.; and Burgdorff, I. Maternal barbiturate utilization and neonatal withdrawal symptomatology. *J. Pediatr.,* **1972,** *80,* 190-197.

Dews, P. B. Behavioral tolerance. In, *Behavioral Tolerance: Research and Treatment Implications.* (Krasnegor, N. A., ed.) National Institute on Drug Abuse. Department of Health, Education, and Welfare Publication No. (ADM) 78-551, U.S. Government Printing Office, Washington, D. C., **1977,** pp. 18-26.

Dole, V. P. Narcotic addiction, physical dependence and relapse. *N. Engl. J. Med.,* **1972,** *286,* 988-992.

Dole, V. P.; Nyswander, M. E.; and Kreek, M. J. Narcotic blockade. *Arch. Intern. Med.,* **1966,** *118,* 304-309.

Done, A. K.; Aronow, R.; and Miceli, J. N. The pharmacokinetics of phencyclidine in overdosage and its treatment. In, *PCP Phencyclidine Abuse: An Appraisal.* (Petersen, R. C., and Stillman, R. C., eds.) National Institute on Drug Abuse. Department of Health, Education, and Welfare Publication No. (ADM) 78-728, U.S. Government Printing Office, Washington, D.C., **1978,** pp. 18-43.

Drew, W. G.; Kiplinger, G. F.; Miller, L. L.; and Marx, M. Effects of propranolol on marihuana-induced cognitive dysfunctioning. *Clin. Pharmacol. Ther.,* **1972,** *13,* 526-533.

Edwards, G.; Orford, J.; Egert, S.; Hawker, A.; Hensman, C.; Mitcheson, M.; Oppenheimer, E.; and Taylor, C. Alcoholism; a controlled trial of "treatment" and "advice." *J. Stud. Alcohol,* **1977,** *38,* 1004-1031.

Eisenman, A. J.; Fraser, H. F.; Sloan, J.; and Isbell, H. Urinary 17-ketosteroid excretion during a cycle of addiction to morphine. *J. Pharmacol. Exp. Ther.,* **1958,** *124,* 305-311.

Ellinwood, E. H., Jr. Amphetamine psychosis: a multidimensional process. *Semin. Psychiatry,* **1969,** *1,* 208-226.

Elliot, H. W.; Parker, K. D.; Crim, M.; Wright, J. A.; and Nomof, N. Actions and metabolism of heroin administered by continuous intravenous infusion to man. *Clin. Pharmacol. Ther.,* **1971,** *12,* 806-814.

Ellison, G.; Eison, M. S.; Huberman, H. S.; and Daniel, F. Long-term changes in dopaminergic innervation of caudate nucleus after continuous amphetamine administration. *Science,* **1978,** *201,* 276-278.

Epstein, P. S.; Pisani, V. D.; and Fawcett, J. A. Alcoholism and cerebral atrophy. *Alcoholism,* **1977,** *1,* 61-65.

Evans, M. A.; Martz, R.; Brown, D. J.; Rodda, B. E.; Kiplinger, G. F.; Lemberger, L.; and Forney, R. B. Impairment of performance with low doses of marihuana. *Clin. Pharmacol. Ther.,* **1973,** *14,* 936-940.

Fischman, M. W.; Schuster, C. R.; Rosnekov, L.; Shick, J. F. E.; Krasnegor, N. A.; Fennell, W.; and Freedman, D. X. Cardio-vascular and subjective effects of intravenous cocaine administration in humans. *Arch. Gen. Psychiatry,* **1976,** *33,* 983-989.

Frankel, D.; Khanna, J. M.; Kalant, H.; and LeBlanc, A. E. Effect of *p*-chlorophenylalanine on the acquisition of tolerance to the hypothermic effects of ethanol. *Psychopharmacology,* **1978,** *57,* 239-242.

Fraser, H. F.; Isbell, H.; Eisenman, A. J.; Wikler, A.; and Pescor, F. T. Chronic barbiturate intoxication: further studies. *Arch. Intern. Med.,* **1954,** *94,* 34-41.

Fraser, H. F.; Wikler, A.; Essig, C. F.; and Isbell, H. Degree of physical dependence induced by secobarbital or phenobarbital. *J.A.M.A.,* **1958,** *166,* 126-129.

Fraser, H. F.; Wikler, A.; Isbell, H.; and Johnson, N. K. Partial equivalence of chronic alcohol and barbiturate intoxications. *Q. J. Stud. Alcohol,* **1957,** *18,* 541-551.

Freedman, D. X. The use and abuse of LSD. *Arch. Gen. Psychiatry,* **1968,** *18,* 300–347.

Gilmour, D. G.; Bloom, A. D.; Lele, K. P.; Robbins, E. S.; and Maximilian, C. Chromosomal aberrations in users of psychoactive drugs. *Arch. Gen. Psychiatry,* **1971,** *24,* 268–272.

Gold, M. E.; Redmond, D. C.; and Kleber, H. D. Clonidine blocks acute opiate-withdrawal symptoms. *Lancet,* **1978,** *2,* 599–602.

Goldstein, A., and Goldstein, D. B. Enzyme expansion theory of drug tolerance and physical dependence. *Proc. Assoc. Res. Nerv. Ment. Dis.,* **1968,** *46,* 265–267.

Goldstein, D. B. Alcohol withdrawal reaction in mice: effects of drugs that modify neurotransmission. *J. Pharmacol. Exp. Ther.,* **1973,** *186,* 1–9.

———. Sodium bromide and sodium valproate: effective suppressants of ethanol withdrawal reactions in mice. *Ibid.,* **1979,** *208,* 223–227.

Goodwin, D. W. Alcoholism and heredity. *Arch. Gen. Psychiatry,* **1979,** *36,* 57–61.

Goodwin, D. W.; Davis, D. H.; and Robins, L. N. Drinking amid abundant illicit drugs. *Arch. Gen. Psychiatry,* **1975,** *32,* 230–233.

Greden, J. F.; Fontaine, P.; Lubetsky, M.; and Chamberlain, K. Anxiety and depression associated with caffeinism among psychiatric inpatients. *Am. J. Psychiatry,* **1978,** *135,* 963–966.

Griffith, J. D.; Cavanaugh, J.; Held, J.; and Oates, J. A. Dextroamphetamine. *Arch. Gen. Psychiatry,* **1972,** *26,* 97–100.

Griffiths, R. R.; Brady, J. V.; and Snell, J. D. Progressive-ratio performance maintained by drug infusions: comparison of cocaine, diethylpropion, chlorphentermine, and fenfluramine. *Psychopharmacology,* **1978,** *56,* 5–13.

Haigler, H. J., and Aghajanian, G. K. Serotonin receptors in the brain. *Fed. Proc.,* **1977,** *36,* 2159–2164.

Harris, L. S. Cannabinoids as analgesics. In, *Mechanisms of Pain and Analgesic Compounds.* (Beers, R. F., Jr., and Bassett, E. G., eds.) Raven Press, New York, **1979,** pp. 467–473.

Heath, R. G. Marihuana. *Arch. Gen. Psychiatry,* **1972,** *26,* 577–584.

———. Cannabis sativa derivatives: effects on brain function of monkeys. In, *Marihuana: Chemistry, Biochemistry, and Cellular Effects.* (Nahas, G. G., ed.) Springer-Verlag, Berlin, **1976,** pp. 507–519.

Hepler, R. S., and Petrus, R. Experiences with administration of marihuana to glaucoma patients. In, *The Therapeutic Potential of Marihuana.* (Cohen, S., and Stillman, R. C., eds.) Plenum Medical Book Co., New York, **1976,** pp. 63–75.

Hollister, L. E. Interactions in man of delta-9-tetrahydrocannabinol. I. Alphamethylparatyrosine. *Clin. Pharmacol. Ther.,* **1974,** *15,* 18–21.

Holmstedt, B.; Lindgren, J. E.; Rivier, L.; and Plowman, T. Cocaine in blood of coca chewers. *J. Ethnopharmacol.,* **1979,** *1,* 69–78.

Hughes, P.; Barker, N.; Crawford, G.; and Jaffe, J. H. The natural history of a heroin epidemic. *Am. J. Public Health,* **1972,** *62,* 995–1001.

Isbell, H.; Altschul, S.; Kornetsky, C. H.; Eisenman, A. J.; Flanary, H. G.; and Fraser, H. F. Chronic barbiturate intoxication: an experimental study. *Arch. Neurol. Psychiatry,* **1950,** *64,* 1–28.

Isbell, H., and White, W. M. Clinical characteristics of addictions. *Am. J. Med.,* **1953,** *14,* 558–565.

Jacobson, C. B., and Berlin, C. M. Possible reproductive detriment in LSD users. *J.A.M.A.,* **1972,** *222,* 1367–1373.

Jaffe, J. H., and Sharpless, S. K. Pharmacological denervation supersensitivity in the central nervous system: a theory of physical dependence. *Proc. Assoc. Res. Nerv. Ment. Dis.,* **1968,** *46,* 226–246.

Jakubovic, A., and McGeer, P. L. *In vitro* inhibition of protein and nucleic acid synthesis in rat testicular tissue by cannabinoids. In, *Marihuana: Chemistry, Biochemistry, and Cellular Effects.* (Nahas, G. G., ed.) Springer-Verlag, Berlin, **1976,** pp. 223–241.

Janowsky, D. S.; Meacham, M. P.; Blaine, J. D.; Schoor, M.; and Bozzetti, L. P. Marihuana effects on simulated flying ability. *Am. J. Psychiatry,* **1976,** *133,* 384–388.

Jarvik, M. E. Tolerance to the effects of tobacco. In, *Cigarette Smoking as a Dependence Process.* (Krasnegor, N. A., ed.) National Institute on Drug Abuse. Department of Health, Education, and Welfare Publication No. (ADM) 79-800, U.S. Government Printing Office, Washington, D. C., **1979,** pp. 150–157.

Javaid, J. I.; Fischman, M. W.; Schuster, C. R.; Dekirmenjian, H.; and Davis, J. M. Cocaine plasma concentration: relation to physiological and subjective effects in humans. *Science,* **1978,** *202,* 227–228.

Jeri, F. R.; Sanchez, C. C.; del Pozo, T.; Fernandez, M.; and Carbajal, C. Further experience with the syndromes produced by coca paste smoking. *Bull. Narc.,* **1978,** *30,* 1–11.

Johnson, K. M. Neurochemical pharmacology of phencyclidine. In, *PCP Phencyclidine Abuse: An Appraisal.* (Petersen, R. C., and Stillman, R. C., eds.) National Institute on Drug Abuse. Department of Health, Education, and Welfare Publication No. (ADM) 78-728, U.S. Government Printing Office, Washington, D. C., **1978,** pp. 44–52.

Johnson, S. M.; Westfall, D. P.; Howard, S. A.; and Fleming, W. W. Sensitivities of the isolated ileal longitudinal smooth muscle–myenteric plexus and hypogastric nerve–vas deferens of the guinea pig after chronic morphine pellet implantation. *J. Pharmacol. Exp. Ther.,* **1978,** *204,* 54–66.

Jones, K. L.; Smith, D. W.; Streissguth, A.; and Myrianthopoulos, N. C. Outcome in offspring of chronic alcoholic women. *Lancet,* **1974,** *1,* 1076–1077.

Jones, R. T. Marihuana-induced "high": influence of expectation, setting and previous drug experience. *Pharmacol. Rev.,* **1971,** *23,* 359–369.

———. Behavioral tolerance: lessons learned from cannabis research. In, *Behavioral Tolerance: Research and Treatment Implications.* (Krasnegor, N. A., ed.) National Institute on Drug Abuse. Department of Health, Education, and Welfare Publication No. (ADM) 78-551, U.S. Government Printing Office, Washington, D. C., **1977,** pp. 118–126.

Jones, R. T.; Benowitz, N.; and Bachman, J. Clinical studies of cannabis tolerance and dependence. *Ann. N. Y. Acad. Sci.,* **1976,** *282,* 221–239.

Kalant, H.; Engel, J. A.; Goldberg, L.; Griffiths, R. R.; Jaffe, J. H.; Krasnegor, N. A.; Mello, N. K.; Mendelson, J. H.; Thompson, T.; and Van Ree, J. M. Behavioral aspects of addiction: group report. In, *The Bases of Addiction: Report of the Dahlem Workshop on the Bases of Addiction.* (Fishman, J., ed.) Abakon Verlagsgesellschaft, Berlin, **1978,** pp. 463–495.

Kales, A.; Bixler, E. O.; Tan, T. L.; Scharf, M. B.; and Kales, J. D. Chronic hypnotic use: ineffectiveness, drug withdrawal insomnia and hypnotic drug dependence. *J.A.M.A.,* **1974,** *227,* 513–517.

Kales, A.; Scharf, M. B.; and Kales, J. D. Rebound insomnia: a new clinical syndrome. *Science,* **1978,** *201,* 1039–1041.

Kato, T., and Jarvik, L. LSD-25 and genetic damage. *Dis. Nerv. Syst.,* **1969,** *30,* 42–46.

Kay, D. C., and Martin, W. R. LSD and tryptamine effects on sleep/wakefulness and electrocorticogram patterns in intact cats. *Psychopharmacology,* **1978,** *58,* 223–228.

Klonoff, H. Marijuana and driving in real-life situations. *Science,* **1974,** *186,* 317–324.

Korf, J.; Bunney, B. S.; and Aghajanian, G. K. Noradrenalin neurons: morphine inhibition of spontaneous activity. *Eur. J. Pharmacol.,* **1974,** *25,* 165–169.

Kornetsky, C.; Esposito, R. U.; McLean, S.; and Jacobson, J. O. Intracranial self-stimulation thresholds. *Arch. Gen. Psychiatry,* **1979,** *36,* 289–292.

Kramer, J. C.; Fischman, V. S.; and Littlefield, D. C. Amphetamine abuse. *J.A.M.A.,* **1967,** *201,* 305–309.

Kreek, M. J. Medical safety and side effects of methadone in tolerant individuals. *J.A.M.A.,* **1973,** *223,* 665–668.

Kuntzman, R.; Pantuck, E. J.; Kaplan, S. A.; and Conney, A. H. Phenacetin metabolism: effect of hydrocarbons and cigarette smoking. *Clin. Pharmacol. Ther.,* **1977,** *22,* 757–764.

Lemberger, L.; Crabtree, R. E.; and Rowe, H. M. 11-Hydroxy-Δ⁹-tetrahydrocannabinol: pharmacology, disposition, and metabolism of a major metabolite of marihuana in man. *Science,* **1972,** *177,* 62–64.

Lemberger, L.; Tamarkin, N. R.; Axelrod, J.; and Kopin, I. J. Delta-9-tetrahydrocannabinol: metabolism and disposition in long-term marihuana smokers. *Science,* **1971,** *173,* 72–73.

Lerner, S. E., and Burns, R. S. Phencyclidine use among youth: history, epidemiology, and acute and chronic intoxication. In, *PCP Phencyclidine Abuse: An Appraisal.* (Petersen, R. C., and Stillman, R. C., eds.) National Institute on Drug Abuse. Department of Health, Education, and Welfare Publication No. (ADM) 78-728, U.S. Government Printing Office, Washington, D. C., **1978,** pp. 66–119.

Ling, W.; Klett, C. J.; and Gillis, R. D. A cooperative clinical study of methadyl acetate. *Arch. Gen. Psychiatry,* **1978,** *35,* 345–353.

Ludwig, A. M.; Wikler, A.; and Stark, L. H. The first drink: psychological aspects of craving. *Arch. Gen. Psychiatry,* **1974,** *30,* 539–547.

Lugman, W., and Danowski, T. S. The use of khat (*Catha edulis*) in Yemen. Social and medical observations. *Ann. Intern. Med.,* **1976,** *85,* 246–249.

McGlothlin, W. H. Drugs and crime. In, *Handbook on Drug Abuse.* (DuPont, R. I.; Goldstein, A.; and O'Donnell, J.; eds.) National Institute on Drug Abuse, U.S. Government Printing Office, Washington, D. C., **1979,** pp. 357–364.

McGlothlin, W. H., and Arnold, D. O. LSD revisited. *Arch. Gen. Psychiatry,* **1971,** *24,* 35–49.

McGlothlin, W. H.; Arnold, D. O.; and Freedman, D. X. Organicity measures following repeated LSD ingestion. *Arch. Gen. Psychiatry,* **1969,** *21,* 704–709.

McQuarrie, D. G., and Fingl, E. Effects of single doses and chronic administration of ethanol on experimental seizures in mice. *J. Pharmacol. Exp. Ther.,* **1958,** *124,* 264–271.

Martin, W. R. A homeostatic and redundancy theory of tolerance to and dependence on narcotic analgesics. *Proc. Assoc. Res. Nerv. Ment. Dis.,* **1968,** *46,* 206–225.

Martin, W. R., and Fraser, H. F. A comparative study of physiological and subjective effects of heroin and morphine administered intravenously in postaddicts. *J. Pharmacol. Exp. Ther.,* **1961,** *133,* 388–399.

Martin, W. R.; Haertzen, C. A.; and Hewitt, B. B. Psychopathology and pathophysiology of narcotic addicts, alcoholics and drug abusers. In, *Psychopharmacology: A Generation of Progress.* (Lipton, M. A.; DiMascio, A.; and Killam, K. F.; eds.) Raven Press, New York, **1978a,** pp. 1591–1602.

Martin, W. R.; Jasinski, D. R.; Haertzen, C. A.; Kay, D. C.; Jones, B. E.; Mansky, P. A.; and Carpenter, R. W. Methadone—a reevaluation. *Arch. Gen. Psychiatry,* **1973,** *28,* 286–295.

Martin, W. R.; Sloan, J. W.; Sapira, J. D.; and Jasinski, D. R. Physiologic, subjective, and behavioral effects of amphetamine, methamphetamine, ephedrine, phenmetrazine, and methylphenidate in man. *Clin. Pharmacol. Ther.,* **1971,** *12,* 245–258.

Martin, W. P.; Vaupel, D. B.; Nozaki, M.; and Bright, L. D. The identification of LSD-like hallucinogens using the chronic spinal dog. *Drug Alcohol Depend.,* **1978b,** *3,* 113–123.

Matsuzaki, M. Alteration in pattern of EEG activities and convulsant effect of cocaine following chronic administration in the rhesus monkey. *Electroencephalogr. Clin. Neurophysiol.,* **1978,** *45,* 1–15.

Melges, F. T.; Tinklenberg, J. R.; Hollister, L. E.; and Gillespie, H. K. Temporal disintegration and depersonalization during marihuana intoxication. *Arch. Gen. Psychiatry,* **1970,** *23,* 204–210.

Mello, N. K. Stimulus self-administration: some implications for the prediction of drug abuse liability. In, *Predicting Dependence Liability of Stimulant and Depressant Drugs.* (Thompson, T., and Unna, K. R., eds.) University Park Press, Baltimore, **1977,** pp. 243–260.

Mendelson, J. H.; Ellingboe, J.; Kuehnle, J. C.; and Mello, N. K. Effects of chronic marihuana use on integrated plasma testosterone and luteinizing hormone levels. *J. Pharmacol. Exp. Ther.,* **1978,** *207,* 611–617.

Mendelson, J. H., and Meyer, R. E. Behavioral and biological concomitants of chronic marihuana smoking by heavy and casual users. In, *Technical Papers of the First Report of the National Commission on Marihuana and Drug Abuse.* Appendix, Vol. I. U.S. Government Printing Office, Washington, D. C., **1972,** pp. 68–98.

Merry, J.; Reynolds, C. M.; Bailey, J.; and Coppen, A. Prophylactic treatment of alcoholism by lithium carbonate: a controlled study. *Lancet,* **1976,** *2,* 481–482.

National Research Council Committee on Clinical Evaluation of Narcotic Antagonists. Clinical evaluation of naltrexone treatment of opiate-dependent individuals. *Arch. Gen. Psychiatry,* **1978,** *35,* 335–340.

O'Brien, C. P.; Testa, T.; O'Brien, T. J.; Brady, J. P.; and Wells, B. Conditioned narcotic withdrawal in humans. *Science,* **1977,** *195,* 1000–1002.

O'Donnell, J. A. Social factors and follow-up studies in opioid addiction. *Proc. Assoc. Res. Nerv. Ment. Dis.,* **1968,** *46,* 333–346.

Okamoto, M.; Boisse, N. R.; Rosenberg, H. C.; and Rosen, R. Characteristics of functional tolerance during barbiturate physical dependency production. *J. Pharmacol. Exp. Ther.,* **1978,** *207,* 906–915.

Oldendorf, W. H. Factors affecting passage of opiates through the blood-brain barrier. In, *Factors Affecting the Action of Narcotics.* (Adler, M. W.; Manara, L.; and Samanin, R.; eds.) Raven Press, New York, **1978,** pp. 221–231.

Paalzow, G. Development of tolerance to the analgesic effect of clonidine in rats. Cross tolerance to morphine. *Naunyn Schmiedebergs Arch. Pharmacol.,* **1978,** *304,* 1–4.

Perez-Reyes, M.; Timmons, M. C.; Lipton, M. A.; Davis, K. H.; and Wall, M. E. Intravenous injection in man of Δ⁹-tetrahydrocannabinol and 11-OH-Δ⁹-tetrahydrocannabinol. *Science,* **1972,** *177,* 633–634.

Post, R. M.; Kotin, J.; and Goodwin, F. K. The effects of cocaine on depressed patients. *Am. J. Psychiatry,* **1974,** *131,* 511–517.

Rafaelsen, O. J.; Bech, P.; Christiansen, J.; Christrup, H.; Nyboe, J.; and Rafaelsen, L. Cannabis and alcohol: effects on simulated car driving. *Science,* **1973,** *179,* 920–923.

Resnick, R. B.; Kestenbaum, R. S.; Washton, A.; and Poole, D. Naloxone-precipitated withdrawal: a method for rapid induction onto naltrexone. *Clin. Pharmacol. Ther.,* **1977,** *21,* 409–413.

Rosecrans, J. A. Nicotine as a discriminative stimulus to behavior: its characterization and relevance to smoking behavior. In, *Cigarette Smoking as a Dependence Process.* (Krasnegor, N. A., ed.) National Institute on Drug Abuse. Department of Health, Education, and Welfare Publication No. (ADM) 79-800, U.S. Government Printing Office, Washington, D. C., **1979,** pp. 58–69.

Rosenberg, H. C., and Okamoto, M. Loss of inhibition in the spinal cord during barbiturate withdrawal. *J. Pharmacol. Exp. Ther.*, **1978**, *205*, 563–568.

Sallan, S. E.; Cronin, C.; Zelen, M.; and Zinberg, N. E. Antiemetics in patients receiving chemotherapy for cancer. *N. Engl. J. Med.*, **1980**, *302*, 135–138.

Schachter, S. Pharmacological and psychological determinants of smoking. *Ann. Intern. Med.*, **1978**, *88*, 104–114.

Sellers, E. M.; Lang, M.; Koch-Weser, J.; LeBlanc, E.; and Kalant, H. Interaction of chloral hydrate and ethanol in man. I. Metabolism. *Clin. Pharmacol. Ther.*, **1972**, *13*, 37–49.

Senay, E. C.; Dorus, W.; Goldberg, F.; and Thornton, W. Withdrawal from methadone maintenance: rate of withdrawal and expectation. *Arch. Gen. Psychiatry*, **1977**, *34*, 361–367.

Sharma, S. K.; Klee, W.`A.; and Nirenberg, M. Dual regulation of adenylate cyclase account for narcotic dependence and tolerance. *Proc. Natl. Acad. Sci. U.S.A.*, **1975**, *72*, 3092–3096.

Shiffman, S. M. The tobacco withdrawal syndrome. In, *Cigarette Smoking as a Dependence Process.* (Krasnegor, N. A., ed.) National Institute on Drug Abuse. Department of Health, Education, and Welfare Publication No. (ADM) 79-800, U.S. Government Printing Office, Washington, D. C., **1979**, pp. 158–184.

Siegel, R. K. Phencyclidine and ketamine intoxication: a study of four populations of recreational users. In, *PCP Phencyclidine Abuse: An Appraisal.* (Petersen, R. C., and Stillman, R. C., eds.) National Institute on Drug Abuse. Department of Health, Education, and Welfare Publication No. (ADM) 78-728, U.S. Government Printing Office, Washington, D. C., **1978**, pp. 119–147.

Siegel, S. A Pavlovian conditioning analysis of morphine tolerance. In, *Behavioral Tolerance: Research and Treatment Implications.* (Krasnegor, N. A., ed.) National Institute on Drug Abuse. Department of Health, Education, and Welfare Publication No. (ADM) 78-551, U.S. Government Printing Office, Washington, D. C., **1977**, pp. 27–53.

Simpson, D. D.; Savage, L. J.; and Lloyd, M. R. Follow-up evaluation of treatment of drug abuse during 1969 to 1972. *Arch. Gen. Psychiatry*, **1979**, *36*, 772–780.

Smith, S. H.; Harris, L. S.; Uwaydah, I. M.; and Munson, A. E. Structure activity relationships of natural and synthetic cannabinoids in suppression of humoral and cell-mediated immunity. *J. Pharmacol. Exp. Ther.*, **1978**, *207*, 165–170.

Snyder, S. H.; Weingartner, H.; and Faillace, L. A. DOET (2,5-dimethoxy-4-ethylamphetamine), a new psychotropic drug. Effects of varying doses in man. *Arch. Gen. Psychiatry*, **1971**, *24*, 50–55.

Stimmel, B., and Adamsons, K. Narcotic dependency in pregnancy. Methadone maintenance compared to use of street drugs. *J.A.M.A.*, **1976**, *235*, 1121–1124.

Stimson, G. V.; Oppenheimer, E.; and Thorley, A. Seven-year follow-up of heroin addicts: drug use and outcome. *Br. Med. J.*, **1978**, *1*, 1190–1192.

Tabakoff, B.; Yanai, J.; and Ritzmann, R. F. Brain noradrenergic systems as a prerequisite for developing tolerance to barbiturates. *Science*, **1978**, *200*, 449–451.

Tecce, J. J., and Cole, J. O. Amphetamine effects in man: paradoxical drowsiness and lowered electrical brain activity (CNV). *Science*, **1974**, *185*, 451–453.

Tennant, F. S., Jr., and Groesbeck, C. J. Psychiatric effects of hashish. *Arch. Gen. Psychiatry*, **1972**, *27*, 133–136.

Thacore, V. R., and Shukla, S. R. P. Cannabis psychosis and paranoid schizophrenia. *Arch. Gen. Psychiatry*, **1976**, *33*, 383–386.

Thompson, T., and Pickens, R. Stimulant self-administration by animals: some comparisons with opiate self-administration. *Fed. Proc.*, **1970**, *29*, 6–12.

Tseng, L. F.; Loh, H. H.; and Wei, E. T. Effects of clonidine on morphine withdrawal signs in the rat. *Eur. J. Pharmacol.*, **1975**, *30*, 93–99.

Tucker, G. J.; Quinlan, D.; and Harrow, M. Chronic hallucinogenic drug use and thought disturbance. *Arch. Gen. Psychiatry*, **1972**, *27*, 443–447.

Turner, J. A. M.; Sillett, R. W.; and McNicol, M. W. Effect of cigar smoking on carboxyhaemoglobin and plasma nicotine concentrations in primary pipe and cigar smokers and ex-cigarette smokers. *Br. Med. J.*, **1977**, *2*, 1387–1389.

Van Dyke, C.; Jatlow, P.; Ungerer, J.; Barash, P.; and Byck, R. Comparative psychological effects after intranasal application of local anesthetics: lidocaine and cocaine. In, *Problems of Drug Dependence 1978.* Proceedings of the Fortieth Annual Scientific Meeting. Committee on Problems of Drug Dependence, Inc., **1978a**, pp. 322–332.

———. Oral cocaine: plasma concentrations and central effects. *Science*, **1978b**, *200*, 211–213.

Vestal, R. E.; Wood, A. J. J.; Branch, R. A.; Shand, D. G.; and Wilkinson, G. R. Effects of age and cigarette smoking on propranolol disposition. *Clin. Pharmacol. Ther.*, **1979**, *26*, 8–20.

Victor, M., and Adams, R. D. The effect of alcohol on the nervous system. *Res. Publ. Assoc. Res. Nerv. Ment. Dis.*, **1953**, *32*, 526–573.

Wald, D.; Ebstein, R. P.; and Belmaker, R. H. Haloperidol and lithium blocking of the mood response to intravenous methylphenidate. *Psychopharmacology*, **1978**, *57*, 83–87.

Weil, A. T. Nutmeg as a psychoactive drug. In, *Ethnopharmacologic Search for Psychoactive Drugs.* (Efron, D. H.; Holmstedt, B.; and Kline, N. S.; eds.) Public Health Service Publication No. 1645, U.S. Government Printing Office, Washington, D. C., **1967**, pp. 188–201.

Weissman, M. M.; Slobetz, F.; Prusoff, B.; Mezritz, M.; and Howard, P. Clinical depression among narcotic addicts maintained on methadone in the community. *Am. J. Psychiatry*, **1976**, *133*, 1434–1438.

Wesson, D. R., and Smith, D. E. Cocaine: its use for central nervous system stimulation including recreational and medical uses. In, *Cocaine: 1977.* (Petersen, R. C., and Stillman, R. C., eds.) NIDA Research Monograph No. 13, U.S. Government Printing Office, Washington, D. C., **1977a**, pp. 137–150.

Wikler, A. Diagnosis and treatment of drug dependence of the barbiturate type. *Am. J. Psychiatry*, **1968**, *125*, 758–765.

———. Dynamics of drug dependence. Implications of a conditioning theory for research and treatment. *Arch. Gen. Psychiatry*, **1973**, *28*, 611–616.

———. Opioid antagonists and deconditioning in addiction treatment. In, *Drug Dependence—Treatment and Treatment Evaluation.* Skandia International Symposia. Almqvist & Wiksell International, Stockholm, **1975**, pp. 157–182.

Wikler, A.; Pescor, F. T.; Fraser, H. F.; and Isbell, H. Electroencephalographic changes associated with chronic alcoholic intoxication and the alcohol abstinence syndrome. *Am. J. Psychiatry*, **1956**, *113*, 106–114.

Woods, J. H., and Carney, J. Narcotic tolerance and operant behavior. In, *Behavioral Tolerance: Research and Treatment Implications.* (Krasnegor, N. A., ed.) National Institute on Drug Abuse. Department of Health, Education, and Welfare Publication No. (ADM) 78-551, U.S. Government Printing Office, Washington, D. C., **1977**, pp. 54–66.

Woolverton, W. L.; Kandel, D.; and Schuster, C. R. Tolerance and cross-tolerance to cocaine and *d*-amphetamine. *J. Pharmacol. Exp. Ther.*, **1978**, *205*, 525–535.

Wynder, E. L., and Hoffman, D. Tobacco and health. A societal challenge. *N. Engl. J. Med.*, **1979**, *300*, 894–903.

Yaksh, T. L.; Kohl, R. L.; and Rudy, T. A. Induction of

tolerance and withdrawal in rats receiving morphine in the spinal subarachnoid space. *Eur. J. Pharmacol.,* **1977,** *41,* 275–284.

Yanagita, T. Brief review on the use of self-administration techniques for predicting drug dependence potential. In, *Predicting Dependence Liability of Stimulant and Depressant Drugs.* (Thompson, T., and Unna, K. R., eds.) University Park Press, Baltimore, **1977,** pp. 231–260.

Zelson, C.; Lee, S. J.; and Casalino, M. Neonatal narcotic addiction: comparative effects of maternal intake of heroin and methadone. *N. Engl. J. Med.,* **1973,** *289,* 1216–1220.

Monographs and Reviews

Abelson, H. I.; Fishburne, P. M.; and Cisin, I. H. *National Survey on Drug Abuse: 1977. A Nationwide Study—Youth, Young Adults and Older Adults.* Vol. I, *Main Findings.* National Institute on Drug Abuse. Department of Health, Education, and Welfare Publication No. (ADM) 78-618, U.S. Government Printing Office, Washington, D. C., **1977.**

Armor, D. J.; Polich, J. M.; and Stambul, H. B. *Alcohol and Treatment.* The Rand Corporation, Santa Monica, Calif., **1976.**

Aronow, W. S. Effect of cigarette smoking and of carbon monoxide on coronary heart disease. *Chest,* **1976,** *70,* 514–518.

Baekeland, F. Evaluation of treatment methods in chronic alcoholism. In, *The Biology of Alcoholism.* Vol. 5, *Treatment and Rehabilitation of the Chronic Alcoholic.* (Kissin, B., and Begleiter, H., eds.) Plenum Press, New York, **1977,** pp. 385–440.

Balster, R. L., and Chait, L. D. The behavioral effects of phencyclidine in animals. In, *PCP Phencyclidine Abuse: An Appraisal.* (Petersen, R. C., and Stillman, R. C., eds.) National Institute on Drug Abuse. Department of Health, Education, and Welfare Publication No. (ADM) 78-728, U.S. Government Printing Office, Washington, D. C., **1978,** pp. 53–65.

Braude, M., and Szara, S. (eds.). *Pharmacology of Cannabis.* Raven Press, New York, **1976.**

Brecher, E. M. *Licit and Illicit Drugs.* Consumers Union of United States, Inc., Mt. Vernon, N.Y., **1972.**

Clouet, D. H. The role of brain proteins and peptides in opiate actions. In, *Factors Affecting the Actions of Narcotics.* (Adler, M. L.; Manara, L.; and Samanin, R.; eds.) Raven Press, New York, **1978,** pp. 379–386.

Cohen, S. Psychotomimetic agents. *Annu. Rev. Pharmacol.,* **1967,** *7,* 301–316.

———. Inhalants. In, *Handbook on Drug Abuse.* (DuPont, R. I.; Goldstein, A.; and O'Donnell, J.; eds.) National Institute on Drug Abuse, U.S. Government Printing Office, Washington, D. C., **1979,** pp. 213–220.

Collier, H. O. J., and Francis, D. L. A pharmacological analysis of opiate tolerance/dependence. In, *The Bases of Addiction: Report of the Dahlem Workshop on the Bases of Addiction.* (Fishman, J., ed.) Abakon Verlagsgesellschaft, Berlin, **1978,** pp. 281–297.

Connell, P. H. *Amphetamine Psychosis: Maudsley Monographs, No. 5, Institute of Psychiatry.* Chapman & Hall, Ltd., London, **1958.**

Domino, E. F. Neuropsychopharmacology of nicotine and tobacco smoking. In, *Smoking Behavior: Motives and Incentives.* (Dunn, W. L., Jr., ed.) V. H. Winston & Sons, Inc., Washington, D. C., **1973,** pp. 5–31.

———. Neurobiology of phencyclidine—an update. In, *PCP Phencyclidine Abuse: An Appraisal.* (Petersen, R. C., and Stillman, R. C., eds.) National Institute on Drug Abuse. Department of Health, Education, and Welfare Publication No. (ADM) 78-728, U.S. Government Printing Office, Washington, D. C., **1978,** pp. 18–43.

DuPont, R. I.; Goldstein, A.; and O'Donnell, J. (eds.). *Handbook on Drug Abuse.* National Institute on Drug

Abuse, U.S. Government Printing Office, Washington, D. C., **1979.**

Efron, D. H.; Holmstedt, B.; and Kline, N. S. (eds.). *Ethnopharmacologic Search for Psychoactive Drugs.* Public Health Service Publication No. 1645, U.S. Government Printing Office, Washington, D. C., **1967.**

Ellinwood, E. H., Jr. Amphetamine and cocaine. In, *Psychopharmacology in the Practice of Medicine.* (Jarvik, M. E., ed.) Appleton-Century-Crofts, New York, **1977,** pp. 467–479.

———. Amphetamines/anorectics. In, *Handbook on Drug Abuse.* (DuPont, R. I.; Goldstein, A.; and O'Donnell, J.; eds.) National Institute on Drug Abuse, U.S. Government Printing Office, Washington, D. C., **1979,** pp. 221–231.

Ellinwood, E. H., Jr., and Kilbey, M. M. (eds.). *Cocaine and Other Stimulants.* Plenum Press, New York, **1977.**

Essig, C. F. Addiction to barbiturate and nonbarbiturate sedative drugs. *Proc. Assoc. Res. Nerv. Ment. Dis.,* **1968,** *46,* 188–198.

Finnegan, L. P. (ed.). *Drug Dependence in Pregnancy: Clinical Management of Mother and Child.* Department of Health, Education, and Welfare Publication No. (ADM) 79-678, U.S. Government Printing Office, Washington, D. C., **1979.**

Fishman, J. (ed.). *The Bases of Addiction: Report of the Dahlem Workshop on the Bases of Addiction.* Abakon Verlagsgesellschaft, Berlin, **1978.**

Freed, E. X. Drug abuse by alcoholics: a review. *Int. J. Addict.,* **1973,** *8,* 451–473. (150 references.)

Freedman, D. X. The psychopharmacology of hallucinogenic agents. *Annu. Rev. Med.,* **1969,** *20,* 409–418.

Gessner, P. K. Drug therapy of the alcohol withdrawal syndrome. In, *The Biochemistry and Pharmacology of Ethanol.* (Majchrowicz, E., and Noble, E., eds.) Plenum Press, New York, **1979,** pp. 375–435.

Gilbert, R. M. Caffeine as a drug of abuse. In, *Research Advances in Alcohol and Drug Problems,* Vol. III. (Gibbins, R. J.; Israel, Y.; Kalant, H.; Popham, R. E.; Schmidt, W.; and Smart, K. G.; eds.) John Wiley & Sons, Inc., New York, **1976,** pp. 49–176.

Glasscote, R.; Sussex, J. N.; Jaffe, J. H.; Ball, J.; and Brill, L. *The Treatment of Drug Abuse: Programs, Problems, Prospects.* Joint Information Service, Washington, D. C., **1972.**

Griffith, J. D. Amphetamine dependence; clinical factors. In, *Drug Addiction II: Amphetamine, Psychotogen, and Marihuana Dependence.* (Martin, W. R., ed.) *Handbuch der Experimentellen Pharmakologie,* Vol. 45, Pt. 2. Springer-Verlag, Berlin, **1977,** pp. 277–304.

Gunne, L.-M. Effects of amphetamines in humans. In, *Drug Addiction II: Amphetamine, Psychotogen, and Marihuana Dependence.* (Martin, W. R., ed.) *Handbuch der Experimentellen Pharmakologie,* Vol. 45, Pt. 2. Springer-Verlag, Berlin, **1977,** pp. 247–275.

Harris, L. S.; Dewey, W. L.; and Razdan, R. K. Cannabis: its chemistry, pharmacology, and toxicology. In, *Drug Addiction II: Amphetamine, Psychotogen, and Marihuana Dependence.* (Martin, W. R., ed.) *Handbuch der Experimentellen Pharmakologie,* Vol. 45, Pt. 2. Springer-Verlag, Berlin, **1977,** pp. 371–429.

Hawkins, R. D., and Kalant, H. The metabolism of ethanol and its metabolic effects. *Pharmacol. Rev.,* **1972,** *24,* 67–157. (641 references.)

Herz, A., and Schulz, R. Changes in neuronal sensitivity during addictive processes. In, *The Bases of Addiction: Report of the Dahlem Workshop on the Bases of Addiction.* (Fishman, J., ed.) Abakon Verlagsgesellschaft, Berlin, **1978,** pp. 375–393.

Hollister, L. E. Marihuana in man: three years later. *Science,* **1971,** *172,* 21–29.

Jaffe, J. H. Factors in the etiology of drug use and dependence. In, *Rehabilitation Aspects of Drug Dependence.*

(Schecter, A., ed.) CRC Press, Cleveland, **1977**, pp. 23–68.

Jaffe, J. H., and Jarvik, M. E. Tobacco use and tobacco use disorder. In, *Psychopharmacology: A Generation of Progress.* (Lipton, M. A.; DiMascio, A.; and Killam, K. F.; eds.) Raven Press, New York, **1978**, pp. 1665–1676.

Jasinski, D. R. Assessment of the abuse potentiality of morphine-like drugs (methods in man). In, *Drug Addiction I: Morphine, Sedative/Hypnotic and Alcohol Dependence.* (Martin, W. R., ed.) *Handbuch der Experimentellen Pharmakologie,* Vol. 45, Pt. 1. Springer-Verlag, Berlin, **1977**, pp. 179–258.

Jessor, R. Psychosocial factors in the patterning of drinking behavior. In, *The Bases of Addiction: Report of the Dahlem Workshop on the Bases of Addiction.* (Fishman, J., ed.) Abakon Verlagsgesellschaft, Berlin, **1978**, pp. 67–79.

Jones, R. T. Human effects. In, *Marihuana Research Findings: 1976.* (Petersen, R. C., ed.) National Institute on Drug Abuse. Department of Health, Education, and Welfare Publication No. (ADM) 78-501, U.S. Government Printing Office, Washington, D. C., **1976**, pp. 128–178.

Kalant, H. Behavioral criteria for tolerance and physical dependence. In, *The Bases of Addiction: Report of the Dahlem Workshop on the Bases of Addiction.* (Fishman, J., ed.) Abakon Verlagsgesellschaft, Berlin, **1978**, pp. 199–220.

Kalant, H.; LeBlanc, A. E.; and Gibbins, R. J. Tolerance to and dependence on some non-opiate psychotropic drugs. *Pharmacol. Rev.,* **1971**, *23,* 135–191. (402 references.)

Kalant, O. J. *The Amphetamines: Toxicity and Addiction.* Charles C Thomas, Pub., Springfield, Ill., **1966**.

Kreek, M. J. Methadone in treatment: physiological and pharmacological issues. In, *Handbook on Drug Abuse.* (DuPont, R. I.; Goldstein, A.; and O'Donnell, J.; eds.) National Institute on Drug Abuse, U.S. Government Printing Office, Washington, D. C., **1979**, pp. 57–86.

Kwentus, M. D., and Major, L. F. Disulfiram in the treatment of alcoholism. *J. Stud. Alcohol,* **1979**, *40,* 428–446.

Larson, P. S., and Silvette, H. *Tobacco: Experimental and Clinical Studies,* Suppl. 3. The Williams & Wilkins Co., Baltimore, **1975**.

Lewander, T. Effects of amphetamine in animals. In, *Drug Addiction II: Amphetamine, Psychotogen, and Marihuana Dependence.* (Martin, W. R., ed.) *Handbuch der Experimentellen Pharmakologie,* Vol. 45, Pt. 2. Springer-Verlag, Berlin, **1977**, pp. 33–246.

Lieber, C. S. Chemical characteristics of drugs inducing physical and/or psychic dependence to alcohol. In, *Chemical and Biological Aspects of Drug Dependence.* (Mulé, S. J., and Brill, H., eds.) CRC Press, Cleveland, **1972**, pp. 135–161. (206 references.)

McBay, A. Marihuana; other drugs. In, *Drugs and Driving.* (Willette, R. E., ed.) National Institute on Drug Abuse. Department of Health, Education, and Welfare Publication No. (ADM) 77-432, U.S. Government Printing Office, Washington, D. C., **1977**, pp. 91–99.

McGill, H. C., Jr. Atherosclerosis: problems in pathogenesis. *Atherosclerosis Rev.,* **1977**, *2,* 27–65.

McWilliams, S. A., and Tuttle, R. J. Long-term psychological effects of LSD. *Psychol. Bull.,* **1973**, *79,* 341–351.

Martin, W. R., and Sloan, J. W. Neuropharmacology and neurochemistry of subjective effects, analgesia, tolerance, and dependence produced by narcotic analgesics. In, *Drug Addiction I: Morphine, Sedative/Hypnotic and Alcohol Dependence.* (Martin, W. R., ed.) *Handbuch der Experimentellen Pharmakologie,* Vol. 45, Pt. 1. Springer-Verlag, Berlin, **1977a**, pp. 43–158.

———. Pharmacology and classification of LSD-like hallucinogens. In, *Drug Addiction II: Amphetamine, Psychotogen, and Marihuana Dependence.* (Martin, W. R., ed.)

Handbuch der Experimentellen Pharmakologie, Vol. 45, Pt. 2. Springer-Verlag, Berlin, **1977b**, pp. 305–368.

Mello, N. K., and Mendelson, J. H. Clinical aspects of alcohol dependence. In, *Drug Addiction I: Morphine, Sedative/Hypnotic and Alcohol Dependence.* (Martin, W. R., ed.) *Handbuch der Experimentellen Pharmakologie,* Vol. 45, Pt. 1. Springer-Verlag, Berlin, **1977**, pp. 613–666.

Meyer, R. E., and Mirin, S. M. *The Heroin Stimulus: Implication for a Theory of Addiction.* Plenum Press, New York, **1979**.

Miller, R. R. Effects of smoking on drug action. *Clin. Pharmacol. Ther.,* **1977**, *22,* 743–756.

Moskowitz, H. Marihuana; general hallucinogens. In, *Drugs and Driving.* (Willette, R. E., ed.) National Institute on Drug Abuse. Department of Health, Education, and Welfare Publication No. (ADM) 77-432, U.S. Government Printing Office, Washington, D. C., **1977**, pp. 77–90.

Musto, D. F. *The American Disease.* Yale University Press, New Haven, **1973**.

Nahas, G. G. *Marihuana: Deceptive Weed.* Raven Press, New York, **1973**.

Nahas, G. G.; Paton, W. D. M.; and Idänpään-Heikkilä, J. E. (eds.). *Marihuana. Chemistry, Biochemistry, and Cellular Effects.* Springer-Verlag, Berlin, **1976**.

National Commission on Marihuana and Drug Abuse. Second Report. *Drug Use in America: Problem in Perspective.* U.S. Government Printing Office, Washington, D. C., **1973**.

Petersen, R. C., and Stillman, R. C. (eds.). *Cocaine: 1977.* National Institute on Drug Abuse. Department of Health, Education, and Welfare Publication No. (ADM) 77-471, U.S. Government Printing Office, Washington, D. C., **1977**.

———. (eds.). Phencyclidine: an overview. In, *PCP Phencyclidine Abuse: An Appraisal.* National Institute on Drug Abuse. Department of Health, Education, and Welfare Publication No. (ADM) 78-728, U.S. Government Printing Office, Washington, D. C., **1978**, pp. 1–17.

Platt, J. J., and Labate, C. *Heroin Addiction. Theory, Research, and Treatment.* John Wiley & Sons, Inc., New York, **1976**.

Robins, L. *The Vietnam Drug User Returns: Final Report, Sept. 1973.* Special Action Office Monograph, Ser. A, No. 2, U.S. Government Printing Office, Washington, D. C., **1974**.

Rubin, V., and Comitas, L. *Ganja in Jamaica.* Mouton, The Hague, **1975**.

Russell, M. A. H., and Feyerabend, C. Cigarette smoking: a dependence on high-nicotine boli. *Drug Metab. Rev.,* **1978**, *8,* 29–57.

Sapira, J. D. The narcotic addict as a medical patient. *Am. J. Med.,* **1968**, *45,* 555–588.

Schuster, C. R., and Thompson, T. Self administration of and behavioral dependence on drugs. *Annu. Rev. Pharmacol.,* **1969**, *9,* 483–502.

Secretary of Health, Education, and Welfare. *Marihuana and Health.* Seventh Annual Report to the U.S. Congress. National Institute on Drug Abuse, U.S. Government Printing Office, Washington, D. C., **1977**.

Sellers, E. M., and Kalant, H. Alcohol intoxication and withdrawal. *N. Engl. J. Med.,* **1976**, *294,* 757–762.

Sells, S. B. Treatment effectiveness. In, *Handbook on Drug Abuse.* (DuPont, R. L.; Goldstein, A.; and O'Donnell, J.; eds.) National Institute on Drug Abuse, U.S. Government Printing Office, Washington, D. C., **1979**, pp. 105–118.

Sharp, C. W., and Brehm, M. L. (eds.). *Review of Inhalants: Euphoria to Dysfunction.* National Institute on Drug Abuse. Department of Health, Education, and Welfare Publication No. (ADM) 77-553, U.S. Government Printing Office, Washington, D. C., **1977**.

Sharp, C. W., and Carroll, L. T. (eds.). *Voluntary Inhalation of Industrial Solvents.* National Institute on Drug

Abuse. Department of Health, Education, and Welfare Publication No. (ADM) 79-779, U.S. Government Printing Office, Washington, D. C., **1978.**

Shuster, L. Tolerance and physical dependence. In, *Narcotic Drugs: Biochemical Pharmacology.* (Clouet, D. H., ed.) Plenum Press, New York, **1971,** pp. 408–423.

Simon, E. J., and Hiller, J. M. The opiate receptors. *Annu. Rev. Pharmacol. Toxicol.,* **1978,** 18, 371–394.

Smith, C. M. The pharmacology of sedative/hypnotics, alcohol, and anesthetics: sites and mechanisms of action. In, *Drug Addiction I: Morphine, Sedative/Hypnotic and Alcohol Dependence.* (Martin, W. R., ed.) *Handbuch der Experimentellen Pharmakologie,* Vol. 45, Pt. 1. Springer-Verlag, Berlin, **1977,** pp. 413–587.

————. *Alcoholism: Treatment,* Vol. 2. Eden Press, Montreal, **1978.**

Stefanis, C.; Dornbush, R.; and Fink, M. (eds.). *Hashish: Studies of Long-Term Use.* Raven Press, New York, **1977.**

Stimson, G. V. *Heroin and Behavior: Diversity among Addicts Attending London Clinics.* John Wiley & Sons, Inc., New York, **1973.**

Surgeon General. *Smoking and Health.* (Office of Smoking and Health, eds.) Department of Health, Education, and Welfare Publication No. (PHS) 79-50066, U.S. Government Printing Office, Washington, D. C., **1979.**

Thompson, T., and Unna, K. R. (eds.). *Predicting Dependence Liability of Stimulant and Depressant Drugs.* University Park Press, Baltimore, **1977.**

Thornton, W. E., and Thornton, B. P. Narcotic poisoning: a review of the literature. *Am. J. Psychiatry,* **1974,** *131,* 867–869.

Way, E. L. Common and selective mechanisms in drug dependence. In, *The Bases of Addiction: Report of the Dahlem Workshop on the Bases of Addiction.* (Fishman, J., ed.) Abakon Verlagsgesellschaft, Berlin, **1978,** pp. 333–352.

Wesson, D. R., and Smith, D. E. *Barbiturates: Their Use, Misuse, and Abuse.* Human Sciences Press, New York, **1977b.**

Wikler, A. Aspects of tolerance to and dependence on cannabis. *Ann. N.Y. Acad. Sci.,* **1976,** *282,* 126–147.

Wilmarth, S. S., and Goldstein, A. *Therapeutic Effectiveness of Methadone Maintenance Programs in the U.S.A.* Offset Publication No. 3, World Health Organization, Geneva, **1974.**

Woods, J. H. Behavioral pharmacology of drug administration. In, *Psychopharmacology: A Generation of Progress.* (Lipton, M. A.; Di Mascio, A.; and Killam, K. F.; eds.) Raven Press, New York, **1978,** pp. 595–607.

World Health Organization. *Youth and Drugs.* Technical Report No. 516, WHO, Geneva, **1973.**

————. *Expert Committee on Drug Dependence: Twentieth Report.* Technical Report No. 551, WHO, Geneva, **1974.**

Wulff, M. H. The barbiturate withdrawal syndrome: a clinical and electroencephalographic study. *Electroencephalogr. Clin. Neurophysiol.,* **1959,** Suppl. 14, 1–173.

24 CENTRAL NERVOUS SYSTEM STIMULANTS

Strychnine, Picrotoxin, Pentylenetetrazol, and Miscellaneous Agents (Doxapram, Ethamivan, Nikethamide, Methylphenidate)

Donald N. Franz

Stimulation of the central nervous system (CNS) can be produced in man and animals by a large number of natural and synthetic substances. Only a few have been used therapeutically. Some drugs exhibit prominent central stimulation at toxic levels, and others produce mild stimulation as a side effect. This chapter includes discussion of those drugs that produce central stimulation as their most prominent action and are generally classified as *analeptics* or *convulsants*.

Although some analeptics were formerly used in attempts to counteract severe intoxication by general depressants, *this practice has been overwhelmingly discredited* by the far greater success achieved with more conservative measures that stress intensive supportive care. All of the analeptics are capable of producing generalized convulsions in sufficient doses. Unfortunately, the margin of safety of doses for stimulation of central respiratory centers is generally very narrow and unpredictable. No safe, selective respiratory stimulant is currently available. Thus, only a few very specialized applications remain for these agents.

The excitability of the CNS reflects a balance between excitatory and inhibitory influences that is normally maintained within relatively narrow limits. Drugs can increase excitability either by blocking inhibition or by enhancing excitation. Strychnine and picrotoxin selectively block inhibition in the CNS; these drugs are important research tools employed to study inhibitory transmitters and receptor types (*see* Chapter 12). The other analeptics described in this chapter do not affect inhibitory processes and, therefore, presumably act by enhancing excitation. The pharmacology of analeptics has been re-viewed by Hahn (1960), Esplin and Zablocka-Esplin (1969), and Wang and Ward (1977). The structure-activity relationship of convulsants that block inhibition has been reviewed by Smythies (1974).

STRYCHNINE

Strychnine has no demonstrated therapeutic value, despite a long history of unwarranted popularity. However, strychnine holds a singular position as the only centrally acting drug for which the detailed mechanism of action is thoroughly understood in terms of central synaptic transmission.

Source and Chemistry. Strychnine is the principal alkaloid present in *nux vomica,* the seeds of a tree native to India, *Strychnos nux-vomica.* The term *nux vomica* has been erroneously translated as "emetic nut." Actually, strychnine is not an emetic, and the word *vomica* means depression or cavity, a feature of the strychnos seed attributed by legend to the digital imprint of the Creator.

Nux vomica was introduced into Germany in the sixteenth century as a poison for rats and other animal pests. Its use as a pesticide persists to this day and is a source of accidental strychnine poisoning of children. Strychnine was first employed in medicine in 1540, but it did not gain wide usage until 200 years later.

In addition to strychnine, the closely related alkaloid *brucine* is found in nux vomica. Brucine is much less potent than strychnine. The structural formula of strychnine is as follows:

Strychnine

Pharmacological Actions. *Central Nervous System.* Strychnine produces excitation of all portions of the CNS. This effect, however, does not result from direct synaptic excitation. Strychnine increases the level of neuronal excitability by selectively blocking inhibition. Nerve impulses are normally confined to appropriate pathways by inhibitory influences. When inhibition is blocked by strychnine, ongoing neuronal activity is enhanced and sensory stimuli produce exaggerated reflex effects.

Strychnine is a powerful convulsant, and the convulsion has a characteristic motor pattern. Inasmuch as strychnine reduces inhibition, including the reciprocal inhibition existing between antagonistic muscles, the pattern of convulsion is determined by the most powerful muscles acting at a given joint. In most laboratory animals, this convulsion is characterized by tonic extension of the body and of all limbs. Tonic extension is preceded and followed during the phase of postictal depression by phasic *symmetrical* extensor thrusts that may be initiated by any modality of sensory stimulus. The sloth presents an interesting exception. In this animal, the powerful antigravity muscles are flexors, and the strychnine convulsion is characterized by tonic flexion of all limbs (Esplin and Woodbury, 1961). The pattern of the strychnine convulsion therefore contrasts sharply with that produced by drugs that directly excite central neurons.

Typical strychnine convulsions also occur in spinal animals. For this reason the effects of strychnine are often ascribed to a spinal locus of action, and the convulsion is frequently termed a *spinal convulsion*. In fact, other portions of the CNS are fully excited by doses that produce the characteristic motor manifestations in a spinal animal. The tonic extensor convulsion reflects the action of strychnine to reduce inhibition, rather than the characteristic response of the spinal cord to a convulsant drug. Convulsions in spinal animals produced by drugs that directly excite neurons are asymmetrical and incoordinated, in contrast to the pattern observed with strychnine. The medulla, likewise, is affected by strychnine at dosages that produce hyperexcitability throughout the CNS. However, strychnine does not selectively stimulate the medulla, and the drug is not therapeutically useful as a respiratory analeptic.

Cardiovascular System. The complex changes in blood pressure that occur during strychnine convulsions are related to the effects of the drug on vasomotor centers, including those in the spinal cord.

Gastrointestinal Tract. Strychnine was at one time employed for atonic constipation on the basis of a presumed stimulatory effect of the drug on the gastrointestinal tract. Experiments in both animals and man have failed to demonstrate such stimulation with concentrations of the agent that can be obtained clinically. The bitter taste of strychnine, which is detectable in very dilute solutions, led to its use as a stomachic and bitter. Bitters supposedly stimulate the taste buds, increase the appetite, and reflexly stimulate gastric secretion. Strychnine has no place in this type of therapy, which is of very dubious value.

Skeletal Muscle. Convulsive doses of strychnine have no detectable effect on skeletal muscle. Increased muscle tone is the result purely of the central actions of the drug. In supraconvulsive doses, a curariform action on the neuromuscular junction is observed.

Mechanism of Action. Strychnine has been the object of many experimental investigations. The convulsant action of the drug has often been attributed to interference with central inhibitory processes. Blockade of spinal inhibition by subconvulsive doses of strychnine was first demonstrated by Eccles and coworkers (Bradley *et al.*, 1953). Strychnine interferes only with *postsynaptic* inhibition. Postsynaptic inhibition is mediated by many known pathways in the brain and spinal cord, and, when allowances are made for differences in functional organization, the pathways appear to be about equally sensitive to blockade by strychnine. Well-known examples of postsynaptic inhibition are the inhibitory influences existing between the motoneurons of antagonistic muscle groups and recurrent spinal inhibition mediated by the Renshaw cell. Renshaw cells are excited by intraspinal collaterals of motoneuron axons that liberate acetylcholine. Strychnine blocks recurrent inhibition at the Renshaw cell–motoneuron synapse.

Glycine is the predominant postsynaptic inhibitory transmitter to motoneurons and interneurons in the spinal cord. An important part of the evidence for this fact is the ability of strychnine to block selectively both synaptically evoked postsynaptic inhibition and the identical inhibitory effects of glycine on spinal neurons. Strychnine acts as a competitive antagonist of the inhibitory transmitter at postsynaptic inhibitory sites in the same manner as curare blocks acetylcholine at the neuromuscular junction (Kuno and Weakly, 1972). Receptor-binding studies indicate that both strychnine and glycine interact with the same receptor complex, although possibly at different sites (*see* Johnston, 1978). Tetanus toxin also blocks postsynaptic inhibition, but it acts by preventing release of glycine from inhibitory interneurons. Strychnine-sensitive postsynaptic inhibition in higher centers of the CNS is also mediated by glycine. The pharmacology of postsynaptic inhibition has been reviewed by Curtis (1969).

Absorption, Fate, and Excretion. Strychnine is rapidly absorbed from the gastrointestinal tract and parenteral sites of injection. The CNS does not contain a higher concentration of the drug than do other organs. Strychnine is readily metabolized, mainly by the enzymes of hepatic microsomes (Adamson and Fouts, 1959). Approximately 20% of the alkaloid escapes into the urine. The rate of destruction of strychnine is such that approximately two lethal doses can be given over a period of 24 hours without noticeable toxic symptoms or cumulative effects.

Toxicology. Despite the fact that strychnine preparations are less available than formerly, poisoning by strychnine still occurs from rodenticides and sugar-coated proprietary cathartic and tonic tablets. An increasing source of unwitting poisoning stems from the adulteration of "street drugs" with strychnine. There is no pharmacological rationale for this dangerous practice.

Many cases of accidental poisoning are in children, who may succumb to as little as 15 mg. The fatal adult oral dose is about 50 to 100 mg, but 30 mg has been lethal (Polson and Tattersall, 1969; Gosselin *et al.*, 1976).

Symptoms of Strychnine Poisoning. The effects of strychnine in man closely resemble those described above for laboratory animals. The first effect that is noticed is stiffness of the face and neck muscles. Heightened reflex excitability soon becomes evident. Any sensory stimulus may produce a violent motor response. In the early stages this is a coordinated extensor thrust, and in the later stages it may be a full tetanic convulsion. In this convulsion, the body is arched in hyperextension (opisthotonos) so that only the crown of the head and the heels of the patient may be touching the ground. All voluntary muscles, including those of the face, are in full contraction. Respiration ceases due to the contraction of the diaphragm and the thoracic and abdominal muscles. Convulsive episodes may recur repeatedly with intermittent periods of depression; the frequency and severity of the convulsions are increased by sensory stimulation. Death results from medullary paralysis, which is due primarily to the hypoxia resulting from the periods of impaired respiration. In the early stages the patient not only is conscious but also is acutely perceptive to all stimuli. The muscle contractions are quite painful, and the patient is extremely apprehensive and fearful of impending death as he awaits the next tetanic spasm. If untreated, death from strychnine often occurs after the second to fifth full convulsion, but the first may be fatal if sustained.

Treatment of Strychnine Poisoning. The most urgent objectives in the treatment of strychnine poisoning are the prevention of convulsions and the support of respiration. *Diazepam* is the most useful agent for this purpose. It antagonizes the convulsions without potentiating postictal depression, as may be the case with barbiturates or other nonselective depressants of the CNS (Hardin and Griggs, 1971; Jackson *et al.,* 1971; Maron *et al.,* 1971; Herishanu and Landau, 1972). In adults, convulsions may be terminated by 10 mg of diazepam, intravenously, which should be repeated as subsequent prodromal symptoms appear. Children may require smaller doses. All forms of sensory stimulation should be minimized. If adequate respiratory ventilation is not restored by the termination of convulsions, intubation and mechanical assistance are essential. After convulsions are controlled, activated charcoal is an effective method of reducing absorption when used as a slurry in gastric lavage. Iodine tincture diluted with water (1:250), tannic acid solution (2.0%, or in the form of strong tea), or potassium permanganate (1:5000) may also be employed.

Therapeutic Uses. Strychnine has an undeserved reputation as a useful therapeutic agent. To the drug have been ascribed properties that it does not possess or that it exhibits only when administered in toxic doses. There is no current justification for its presence in any medication. However, preliminary experimental reports suggest that judicious treatment with strychnine may modify the neurological deterioration in some infants with *nonketotic hyperglycinemia,* a rare metabolic disorder characterized by abnormally high concentrations of glycine in the brain and cerebrospinal fluid (Gitzelmann *et al.,* 1978a, 1978b; Arneson *et al.,* 1979).

PICROTOXIN

Picrotoxin is obtained from *Anamirta cocculus,* a climbing shrub indigenous to Malabar and the East Indies. The drug is present in the seeds of the plant, commonly known as fishberries, a name derived from the practice of throwing the bruised berries upon the water as a means of catching fish. The fish, after devouring the berries, are incapacitated and rise to the surface.

Chemistry. Picrotoxin is a nonnitrogenous neutral compound that can be broken down into two dilactones, *picrotoxinin* and *picrotin;* the latter is inactive. Picrotoxinin, the active component, has the following structural formula:

Picrotoxinin

Pharmacological Actions. Picrotoxin is a powerful stimulant and affects all portions of the CNS. Larger doses of picrotoxin are required to produce convulsions in a spinal animal than in an intact animal; in this respect picrotoxin differs strikingly from strychnine.

No appreciable effect of picrotoxin is seen until convulsive doses are given. The resultant convulsion is clonic and incoordinated, and the pattern resembles that produced by pentylenetetrazol (*see* below). With large doses of picrotoxin a tonic clonic seizure may occur in which tonic flexion precedes tonic extension. Accompanying the convulsive movements are salivation, elevation of blood pressure due to vasomotor stimulation, and frequently emesis. Respiratory stimulation with picrotoxin is quite evident, but only in doses approaching convulsant levels.

Mechanism of Action. In mammals it has been shown that picrotoxin blocks *presynaptic* inhibition and strychnine-resistant *postsynaptic* inhibition in the CNS. Picrotoxin has been known for some time to antagonize the inhibitory transmitter gamma-aminobutyric acid (GABA) in invertebrates. Subsequently such antagonism has been convincingly demonstrated at many sites in the mammalian CNS. The nearly identical effects of GABA and natural inhibition and the selective antagonism of both by picrotoxin have made GABA a leading candidate as a central inhibitory transmitter, both in the spinal cord and in higher centers. Another convulsant and more selective GABA antagonist, *bicuculline,* has also contributed to this evidence. The two drugs appear to interact somewhat differently with presumed receptors for the transmitter (*see* Johnston, 1978). The relative importance of blockade of presynaptic or postsynaptic inhibition for the convulsant activity of picrotoxin is unknown (*see* Davidson, 1976).

Toxicology. Although picrotoxin is absorbed by all routes, the full effect on the CNS is not seen for several minutes, even when the drug is administered intravenously. Its duration of action is relatively brief. Picrotoxin is a highly toxic substance, and a dose of 20 mg may produce symptoms of severe poisoning. The fatal dose for man is unknown. *Diazepam* is an effective antidote for poisoning by picrotoxin and should be given as described above in the discussion of strychnine.

Therapeutic Uses. Formerly employed in the treatment of poisoning by CNS depressants, picrotoxin is not a selective respiratory stimulant (Hirsh and Wang, 1975) and is not regarded as a useful therapeutic agent.

PENTYLENETETRAZOL

Pentylenetetrazol (pentamethylenetetrazol) is a synthetic compound with the following structural formula:

Pentylenetetrazol

Pharmacological Actions. Pentylenetetrazol has been widely studied in man and experimental animals. The actions of the drug are exerted primarily on the CNS. All levels of the cerebrospinal axis are stimulated by the drug; however, the dose required to produce convulsive movements in an animal with the spinal cord transected is several times that needed in the intact animal.

Pentylenetetrazol is a useful laboratory tool for screening anticonvulsant drugs. In experimental animals, threshold convulsive doses of the drug produce motor activity characterized by forelimb and jaw clonus. This convulsion resembles that produced by electrical stimulation of the brain with current of just threshold intensity. With slightly larger doses of pentylenetetrazol, generalized, asynchronized clonic movements are observed. This phase is usually superseded by a tonic convulsion; such a convulsion resembles that produced by supramaximal brain stimulation in that the movements of the limbs consist in flexion followed by extension. Thus, the pentylenetetrazol convulsion contrasts markedly with that produced by strychnine (*see* above), which is characterized by extension only.

Mechanism of Action. Pentylenetetrazol does not block either presynaptic or postsynaptic inhibition. Studies of the drug on single spinal motoneurons and interneurons have thus far failed to reveal the mechanism of its stimulant action. There is evidence that the excitatory effect of pentylenetetrazol may be due to a decrease in neuronal recovery time. Lewin and Esplin (1961) demonstrated that pentylenetetrazol decreased the time for recovery in the monosynaptic pathway of the spinal cord. Pentylenetetrazol and trimethadione exhibit markedly antagonistic actions, both in the whole animal and in simple neuronal systems; the prominent action of trimethadione on spinal synaptic systems is prolongation of the time required for synaptic recovery (Esplin and Curto, 1957).

In a novel approach toward elucidating its mechanism of action, Gross and Woodbury (1972) found that pentylenetetrazol increased the permeability of toad bladder to potassium ions; this effect was antagonized by trimethadione in the same dose ratio that protects against pentylenetetrazol-induced convulsions in animals. The relative potencies of a series of related structural analogs on toad bladder bore a strong correlation to their convulsant potencies. Similar permeability changes in the CNS could raise extraneuronal potassium, which would partially depolarize neuronal membranes and thereby increase their excitability. Such a mechanism may account for the convulsive activity of pentylenetetrazol.

Absorption, Fate, and Excretion. Pentylenetetrazol is readily absorbed from all sites of administration and is rapidly and equally distributed throughout the tissues. It is rapidly metabolized by the liver to inactive products, 75% of which are excreted in the urine (Esplin and Woodbury, 1956; Rowles *et al.*, 1971).

Preparations. *Pentylenetetrazol* (METRAZOL, NIORIC, others) is available as oral tablets (0.1 g), a sterile 10% solution in 1-ml ampuls, and an elixir (100 mg/5 ml).

Therapeutic Uses. Pentylenetetrazol, administered intravenously, has a valid use to activate the EEG as a diagnostic aid in *epilepsy*. Subconvulsive doses of the drug, alone or together with stroboscopic light, will often activate latent epileptogenic foci. In addition, the pentylenetetrazol-induced convulsions are of value in characterizing the underlying cerebral disorders in patients with proven epilepsy.

Pentylenetetrazol has received extensive trial in the management of regressed geriatric patients. However, there is no convincing evidence that either pentylenetetrazol or any other CNS stimulant is of value in treating mental symptoms associated with senility (Medical Letter, 1978).

Pentylenetetrazol has no selective action on respiratory centers (Hirsh and Wang, 1974) and is no longer used as a respiratory stimulant.

DOXAPRAM, ETHAMIVAN, AND NIKETHAMIDE

Several pharmacological agents remain in use because of their supposedly selective ability to stimulate central respiratory centers. The purpose is to treat poisoning in which respiratory depression is prominent. Without questioning the value of this goal, it is apparent that direct, supportive measures, such as mechanical ventilation and maintenance of cardiovascular functions, are more useful.

The chemical structures of doxapram, ethamivan, and nikethamide are as follows:

Doxapram

Ethamivan

Nikethamide

Pharmacological Actions. Doxapram, ethamivan, and nikethamide stimulate all levels of the cerebrospinal axis. Tonic-clonic convulsions, similar to those that follow the administration of pentylenetetrazol, can be produced readily. These drugs appear to act by enhancing excitation rather than by blocking central inhibition.

Respiration can be stimulated by each of the three agents in doses that produce little generalized excitation. Doxapram administered intravenously in low doses selectively stimulates respiration and increases tidal volume by activating carotid chemoreceptors, but higher doses stimulate both respiratory and nonrespiratory neurons in the medulla oblongata of the cat about equally (Hirsh and Wang, 1974). In contrast, ethamivan causes no activation of carotid chemoreceptors, no selective stimulation of respiration, and no increase in tidal volume (Hirsh and Wang, 1975); nikethamide is probably similar to ethamivan. These distinctions have also been observed in man (*see* Winnie, 1973). The duration of respiratory stimulation by these drugs is transient after a single intravenous dose and seldom lasts for more than 5 or 10 minutes. The brief duration of action may reflect a "bolus effect," in which a large fraction of the drug is initially delivered to the CNS followed by redistribution to other organs and tissues. This may in part account for the greater likelihood of seizures after repeated doses, since the convulsant dose is generally not much larger than that required to stimulate respiration. Limited clinical experience indicates that the margin of safety is greater and the incidence of side effects is less for doxapram than for ethamivan and nikethamide (Wolfson *et al.,* 1965; Edwards and Leszczynski, 1967; Winnie, 1973). However, side effects indicative of subconvulsive CNS stimulation are common with all three: hypertension, tachycardia, arrhythmias, coughing, sneezing, vomiting, itching, tremors, muscle rigidity, sweating, flushing, and hyperpyrexia. Excessive CNS stimulation or convulsions may be controlled by intravenous administration of diazepam. Where needed most, in deeply comatose patients, analeptics are virtually ineffective in doses below those producing convulsions; postictal depression following convulsions further intensifies the coma (*see* Mark, 1967).

Preparations and Dosage. *Doxapram Hydrochloride,* U.S.P. (DOPRAM), is supplied for injection in 20-ml vials containing 20 mg/ml. Single or divided intravenous doses in the range of 0.5 to 1.5 mg/kg are employed to attempt to produce the desired effect. The drug may also be given by intravenous infusion at an initial rate of 5 mg per minute, later reduced 50% or more.

Ethamivan, U.S.P., is no longer available commercially in the United States.

Nikethamide (CORAMINE, NIKORIN) is available in 25% aqueous solution, marketed in bulk for oral use and in 1.5-ml sterile ampuls for parenteral administration. Intravenous or intramuscular doses range from 1 to 15 ml of the 25% parenteral solution.

Therapeutic Uses and Status. Successful treatment of *acute sedative-hypnotic intoxication* emphasizes an orderly regimen of supportive therapy *without* the use of respiratory stimulants (Clemmesen and Nilsson, 1961; *see* Chapter 17). Systematic improvements in physiological support during 3 decades have reduced mortality rates from 25% during the height of analeptic therapy to a present rate of less than 1%. Mechanical assistance to depressed respiration is established as being far safer, more reliable, and more effective than erratic stimulation by drugs. Present opinion is unanimous in the condemnation of analeptics for the management of poisoning from any sedative-hypnotic drug (Mark, 1967; Lawson and Proudfoot, 1971; Picchioni, 1971; Frank, 1974).

Doxapram, ethamivan, and nikethamide have been used as temporary measures to correct acute respiratory insufficiency in patients with *chronic obstructive pulmonary disease.* Intermittent or continuous infusion is necessary for sustained respiratory stimulation and reduction in carbon dioxide tension; however, potential improvement in oxygen tension is offset by a disproportionate increase in oxygen consumption. Typical side effects are common. Consequently, the value of analeptics in the therapy of pulmonary disease is very limited (Bader and Bader, 1965; Bickerman and Chusid, 1970). They may be of some short-term value to alleviate respiratory depression induced by oxygen therapy in these patients (Woolf, 1970; Moser *et al.,* 1973). Recommended oral doses of analeptics are ineffective.

METHYLPHENIDATE

Methylphenidate is a piperidine derivative that is structurally related to amphetamine and has the following formula:

Methylphenidate

Pharmacological Actions. In contrast to the other drugs discussed in this chapter, methylphenidate is a mild CNS stimulant with more prominent effects on mental than on motor activities. However, large doses produce signs of generalized CNS stimulation that may lead to convulsions in man and animals. Its pharmacological properties are essentially the same as those of the amphetamines. Methylphenidate also shares the abuse potential of the amphetamines.

Absorption, Fate, and Excretion. Methylphenidate is readily absorbed after oral administration and reaches peak concentrations in plasma in about 2 hours. Its half-life in plasma is 1 to 2 hours, but concentrations in the brain exceed those in plasma. The main urinary metabolite is a deesterified product, ritalinic acid, which accounts for 80% of the dose; microsomal oxidation in man is minimal (Faraj *et al.,* 1974).

Preparations and Dosage. *Methylphenidate Hydrochloride,* U.S.P. (RITALIN), is available as official tablets that contain 5, 10, or 20 mg of drug. The usual adult dose is 10 mg, given two or three times daily. The dosage recommended for hyperkinetic children initially is 0.25 mg/kg daily (Millichap, 1968). This dose is doubled each week, if untoward effects are not observed, until the optimal daily dosage of 2 mg/kg is reached. The drug is given in equal portions before breakfast and lunch.

Therapeutic Uses and Status. Methylphenidate has received extensive trial in various types of mental depression, in the treatment of overdosage from depressant drugs, and in relieving lassitude from various causes. Its effectiveness for these uses is doubtful.

Methylphenidate is an important adjunct in the therapy of *hyperkinetic syndromes* in children characterized as having *minimal brain dysfunction* (MBD). Millichap (1968, 1973) has concluded that methylphenidate is superior to amphetamine and is the drug of choice in such children. Double-blind studies with placebo control (*see* Knights and Hinton, 1969) have clearly demonstrated that methylphenidate can improve both behavior and learning ability in 50 to 75% of these children. However, indiscriminate use of stimulant drugs for "problem" children and sole dependence on drug therapy for MBD should be discouraged (*see* Erenberg, 1972; Sroufe and Stewart, 1973). Reports of growth suppression (Safer *et al.,* 1972) and increases in heart rate (Knights and Hinton, 1969) by methylphenidate, especially after the administration of high doses, further emphasize the advisability of judicious therapy. Acute episodes of hallucinosis early in therapy with methylphenidate may represent idiosyncratic reactions (Lucas and Weiss, 1971). It has been generally assumed that the effects of methylphenidate and amphetamine on the behavior of patients with MBD are selective for this condition. However, the behavioral responses of normal boys to short-term administration of amphetamine appear to be similar to those observed in patients with MBD (Rapoport *et al.,* 1978; *see also* Weiss and Hechtman, 1979).

Methylphenidate may be effective in the treatment of *narcolepsy,* either alone or in combination with a tricyclic antidepressant (Zarcone, 1973).

Pemoline. *Pemoline* (CYLERT) is structurally dissimilar to methylphenidate but elicits similar changes in CNS function with minimal effects on the cardiovascular system. It is employed in treating MBD and can be given once daily because of its long half-life. However, clinical improvement is delayed by 3 to 4 weeks.

Adamson, R. H., and Fouts, J. R. Enzymatic metabolism of strychnine. *J. Pharmacol. Exp. Ther.,* **1959,** *127,* 87–91.

Arneson, D.; Ch'ien, L. T.; Chance, P.; and Wilroy, R. S. Strychnine therapy in nonketotic hyperglycinemia. *Pediatrics,* **1979,** *63,* 369–373.

Bader, M. E., and Bader, R. A. Respiratory stimulants in obstructive lung disease. *Am. J. Med.,* **1965,** *38,* 165–171.

Bickerman, H. A., and Chusid, E. L. The case against the use of respiratory stimulants. *Chest,* **1970,** *58,* 53–56.

Bradley, K.; Easton, D. M.; and Eccles, J. C. An investigation of primary or direct inhibition. *J. Physiol. (Lond.),* **1953,** *122,* 474–488.

Clemmesen, C., and Nilsson, E. Therapeutic trends in the treatment of barbiturate poisoning—the Scandinavian method. *Clin. Pharmacol. Ther.,* **1961,** *2,* 220–229.

Edwards, G., and Leszczynski, S. O. A double-blind trial of five respiratory stimulants in patients in acute ventilatory failure. *Lancet,* **1967,** *2,* 226–229.

Erenberg, G. Drug therapy in minimal brain dysfunction: a commentary. *J. Pediatr.,* **1972,** *81,* 359–365.

Esplin, D. W., and Curto, E. M. Effects of trimethadione on synaptic transmission in the spinal cord; antagonism of trimethadione and pentylenetetrazol. *J. Pharmacol. Exp. Ther.,* **1957,** *121,* 457–467.

Esplin, D. W., and Woodbury, D. M. The fate and excretion of C14-labeled pentylenetetrazol in the rat, with comments on analytical methods for pentylenetetrazol. *J. Pharmacol. Exp. Ther.,* **1956,** *118,* 129–138.

———. Spinal reflexes and seizure patterns in the two-toed sloth. *Science,* **1961,** *133,* 1426–1427.

Faraj, B. A.; Israili, Z. H.; Perel, J. M.; Jenkins, M. L.; Holtzman, S. G.; Cucinell, S. A.; and Dayton, P. G. Metabolism and disposition of methylphenidate-14C: studies in man and animals. *J. Pharmacol. Exp. Ther.,* **1974,** *191,* 535–547.

Frank, J. T. Barbiturate intoxication. In, *Principles of Clinical Pharmacy Illustrated by Clinical Case Studies.* (McCarron, M. M., ed.) Drug Intelligence Publications, Inc., Hamilton, Ill., **1974,** pp. 104–111.

Gitzelmann, R.; Steinmann, B.; and Cu'enod, M. Strychnine for the treatment of nonketotic hyperglycinemia. *N. Engl. J. Med.,* **1978a,** *298,* 1424.

Gitzelmann, R.; Steinmann, B.; Otten, A.; Dumermuth, G.; Herdan, M.; Reubi, J. C.; and Cu'enod, M. Nonketotic hyperglycinemia treated with strychnine, a glycine receptor antagonist. *Helv. Paediat. Acta,* **1978b,** *32,* 517–525.

Gosselin, R. E.; Hodge, H. C.; Smith, R. P.; and Gleason, M. N. *Clinical Toxicology of Commercial Products,* 4th ed., Sect. III. The Williams & Wilkins Co., Baltimore, **1976,** pp. 303–307.

Gross, G. J., and Woodbury, D. M. Effects of pentylenetetrazol on ion transport in the isolated toad bladder. *J. Pharmacol. Exp. Ther.,* **1972,** *181,* 257–272.

Hardin, J. A., and Griggs, R. C. Diazepam treatment in a case of strychnine poisoning. *Lancet,* **1971,** *2,* 372–373.

Herishanu, Y., and Landau, H. Diazepam in the treatment of strychnine poisoning. *Br. J. Anaesth.,* **1972,** *44,* 747–748.

Hirsh, K., and Wang, S. C. Selective respiratory stimulating action of doxapram compared to pentylenetetrazol. *J. Pharmacol. Exp. Ther.,* **1974,** *189,* 1–11.

———. Respiratory stimulant effects of ethamivan and picrotoxin. *Ibid.,* **1975,** *193,* 657–663.

Jackson, G.; Ng, S. H.; Diggle, G. E.; and Bourke, I. G. Strychnine poisoning treated successfully with diazepam. *Br. Med. J.,* **1971,** *3,* 519–520.

Knights, R. M., and Hinton, G. S. The effects of methylphenidate (RITALIN) on the motor skills and behaviour of children with learning problems. *J. Nerv. Ment. Dis.,* **1969,** *148,* 643–653.

Kuno, M., and Weakly, J. N. Quantal components of the inhibitory synaptic potential in spinal motoneurones of the cat. *J. Physiol. (Lond.),* **1972,** *224,* 287–303.

Lawson, A. A. H., and Proudfoot, A. T. Medical management of acute barbiturate poisoning. In, *Acute Barbiturate Poisoning.* (Matthew, H., ed.) Excerpta Medica, Amsterdam, **1971,** pp. 175–193.

Lewin, J., and Esplin, D. W. Analysis of the spinal excitatory action of pentylenetetrazol. *J. Pharmacol. Exp. Ther.,* **1961,** *132,* 245–250.

Lucas, A. R., and Weiss, M. Methylphenidate hallucinosis. *J.A.M.A.,* **1971,** *217,* 1079–1081.

Mark, L. C. Analeptics: changing concepts, declining status. *Am. J. Med. Sci.,* **1967,** *254,* 296–302.

Maron, B. J.; Krupp, J. R.; and Tune, B. Strychnine poisoning successfully treated with diazepam. *J. Pediatr.,* **1971,** *78,* 697–699.

Medical Letter. Stimulants and other drugs for treatment of mental symptoms in the elderly. **1978,** *20,* 75.

Millichap, J. G. Drugs in management of hyperkinetic and perceptually handicapped children. *J.A.M.A.,* **1968,** *206,* 1527–1530.

———. Drugs in management of minimal brain dysfunction. *Ann. N.Y. Acad. Sci.,* **1973,** *205,* 321–334.

Moser, K. M.; Luchsinger, P. C.; Adamson, J. S.; McMahon, S. L.; Schlueter, D. P.; Spivack, M.; and Weg, J. G. Respiratory stimulation with intravenous doxapram in respiratory failure. *N. Engl. J. Med.,* **1973,** *288,* 427–431.

Picchioni, A. L. Clinical status and toxicology of analeptic drugs. *Am. J. Hosp. Pharm.,* **1971,** *28,* 201–203.

Polson, C. J., and Tattersall, R. N. *Clinical Toxicology,* 2nd ed. J. B. Lippincott Co., Philadelphia, **1969,** pp. 558–568.

Rapoport, J. L.; Buchsbaum, M. S.; Zahn, T. P.; Weingartner, H.; Ludlow, C.; and Mikkelsen, E. J. Dextroamphetamine: cognitive and behavioral effects in normal prepubertal boys. *Science,* **1978,** *199,* 560–563.

Rowles, S. G.; Born, G. S.; Russell, H. T.; Kessler, W. V.; and Christian, J. E. Biological disposition of pentylenetetrazol-10-^{14}C in rats and humans. *J. Pharm. Sci.,* **1971,** *60,* 725–727.

Safer, D.; Allen, R.; and Barr, E. Depression of growth in hyperactive children on stimulant drugs. *N. Engl. J. Med.,* **1972,** *287,* 217–220.

Sroufe, L. A., and Stewart, M. A. Treating problem children with stimulant drugs. *N. Engl. J. Med.,* **1973,** *289,* 407–413.

Winnie, A. P. Chemical respirogenesis: a comparative study. *Acta Anaesthesiol. Scand.,* **1973,** Suppl. 51, 1–32.

Wolfson, B.; Siker, E. S.; and Ciccarelli, H. E. A double blind comparison of doxapram, ethamivan and methylphenidate. *Am. J. Med. Sci.,* **1965,** *249,* 391–398.

Woolf, C. R. The use of "respiratory stimulant" drugs. *Chest,* **1970,** *58,* 49–53.

Zarcone, V. Narcolepsy. *N. Engl. J. Med.,* **1973,** *288,* 1156–1166.

Monographs and Reviews

Curtis, D. R. The pharmacology of postsynaptic inhibition. *Prog. Brain Res.,* **1969,** *31,* 171–189.

Davidson, N. *Neurotransmitter Amino Acids.* Academic Press, Inc., New York, **1976.** (477 references.)

Esplin, D. W., and Zablocka-Esplin, B. Mechanisms of action of convulsants. In, *Basic Mechanisms of the Epilepsies.* (Jasper, H. H.; Ward, A. A., Jr.; and Pope, A.; eds.) Little, Brown & Co., Boston, **1969,** pp. 167–183.

Hahn, F. Analeptics. *Pharmacol. Rev.,* **1960,** *12,* 447–530. (724 references.)

Johnston, G. A. R. Neuropharmacology of amino acid inhibitory transmitters. *Annu. Rev. Pharmacol. Toxicol.,* **1978,** *18,* 269–289. (173 references.)

Smythies, J. R. Relations between the chemical structure and biological activity of convulsants. *Annu. Rev. Pharmacol.,* **1974,** *14,* 9–21.

Wang, S. C., and Ward, J. W. Analeptics. *Pharmacol. Ther. [B],* **1977,** *3,* 123–165. (229 references.)

Weiss, G., and Hechtman, L. The hyperactive child syndrome. *Science,* **1979,** *205,* 1348–1354.

25 CENTRAL NERVOUS SYSTEM STIMULANTS

[*Continued*]

The Xanthines

Theodore W. Rall

THEOPHYLLINE, CAFFEINE, AND THEOBROMINE

Source and History. Theophylline, caffeine, and theobromine are three closely related alkaloids that occur in plants widely distributed geographically. It is believed that paleolithic man discovered the principal caffeine-containing plants throughout the world and made beverages from them. In South America, caffeine-containing beverages of great antiquity include *guaraná* (from the seeds of either *Paullinia cupana* or *Paullinia sorbilis*), *yoco* (from the bark of *Paullinia yoco*), and *maté* (from *Ilex paraguariensis,* a species of holly). At least half the population of the world consumes *tea* (containing caffeine and small amounts of theophylline and theobromine), prepared from the leaves of *Thea sinensis,* a bush native to southern China and now extensively cultivated in other countries. Cocoa and chocolate, from the seeds of *Theobroma cacao,* contain theobromine and some caffeine. *Coffee,* the most important source of caffeine in the American diet, is extracted from the fruit of *Coffea arabica* and related species. Cola-flavored drinks popular in the United States contain considerable amounts of caffeine, in part because of their content of extracts of the nuts of *Cola acuminata* (the guru nuts chewed by the natives of the Sudan) and in part because of the addition of caffeine as such in their production (*see* Graham, 1978).

The basis for the popularity of all the caffeine-containing beverages has been the ancient belief that these beverages had stimulant and antisoporific actions that elevated mood, decreased fatigue, and increased capacity for work. For example, legend credits the discovery of coffee to a prior of an Arabian convent. Shepherds reported that goats that had eaten the berries of the coffee plant gamboled and frisked about all through the night instead of sleeping. The prior, mindful of the long nights of prayer that he had to endure, instructed the shepherds to pick the berries so that he might make a beverage from them.

Classical pharmacological studies, principally of caffeine, during the first half of this century have confirmed these beliefs and have revealed that methylxanthines possess other important pharmacological properties as well. These properties were exploited for a number of years in a variety of therapeutic applications; many of these have now been replaced by more effective agents. However, in recent years there has been a resurgence of interest in the therapeutic use of the natural methylxanthines and synthetic derivatives thereof, principally as a result of increased knowledge of their cellular basis of action and their pharmacokinetic properties.

Chemistry. Caffeine, theophylline, and theobromine are methylated xanthines. They are often spoken of as *xanthine derivatives, methylxanthines,* or merely *xanthines.* Xanthine itself is dioxypurine and is structurally related to uric acid. Caffeine is 1,3,7-trimethylxanthine; theophylline, 1,3-dimethylxanthine; and theobromine, 3,7-dimethylxanthine. The structural formulas of xanthine and the three naturally occurring xanthine derivatives are as follows:

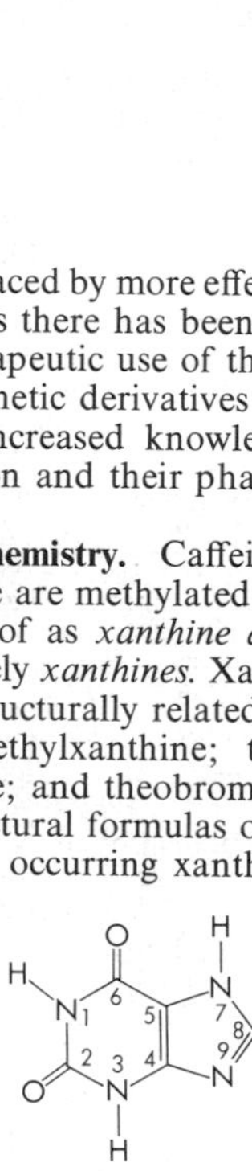

Xanthine

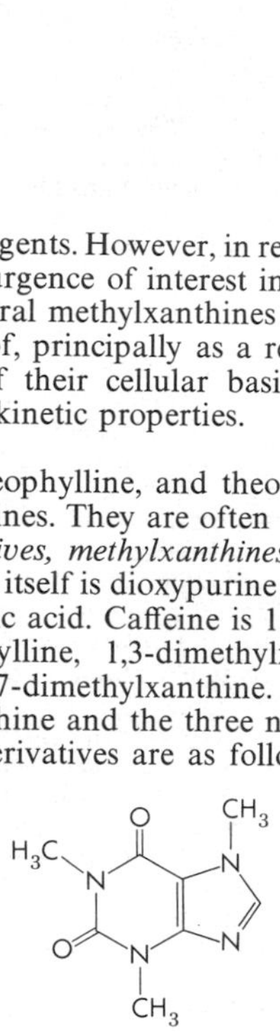

Caffeine

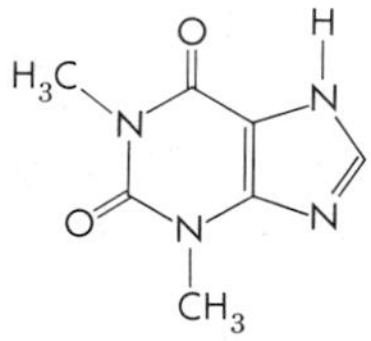

Theophylline

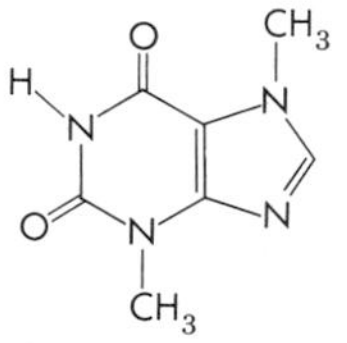

Theobromine

The solubility of the methylxanthines is low and is much enhanced by the formation of complexes (usually 1:1) with a wide variety of compounds. The most notable of such complexes is that between theophylline and ethylenediamine (to form *aminophylline*). The formation of complex double salts (*e.g.,* caffeine and sodium benzoate) or true salts (*e.g., choline theophyllinate, oxtriphylline*) also enhances aqueous solubility. These salts or complexes dissociate to yield the parent methylxanthines when dissolved in biological fluids and should not be confused with covalently modified derivatives such as *dyphylline* (1,3-dimethyl-7-(2,3-dihydroxypropyl)-xanthine).

Studies of the actions of congeners of the methylxanthines in whole animals or other relatively complex biological systems have revealed a structure-activity relationship that is difficult to interpret (*e.g.*, Goodsell *et al.*, 1971). On the other hand, studies of the inhibition of the cyclic nucleotide phosphodiesterases, a well-known cellular action of the methylxanthines, have shown that activity is associated with small nonpolar substitutions at positions 1 and 3. 1-Methyl-3-isobutylxanthine is particularly potent (Beavo *et al.*, 1970), and the addition of a benzyl group at position 7 or the substitution of sulfur for oxygen at position 6 of this compound further enhances potency (Garst *et al.*, 1976). The addition of aliphatic groups at position 8 of theophylline also enhances enzyme inhibitory potency (Goodsell *et al.*, 1971). Theophylline is considerably more potent than caffeine both as an inhibitor of cyclic nucleotide phosphodiesterases (Butcher and Sutherland, 1962) and of receptor-mediated actions of adenosine (*see* below). Although the methylxanthines and their congeners have been useful as experimental tools, no synthetic compound has yet emerged to challenge theophylline and caffeine as therapeutic agents.

PHARMACOLOGICAL PROPERTIES

Theophylline, caffeine, and theobromine share in common several pharmacological actions of therapeutic interest. They stimulate the central nervous system (CNS), act on the kidney to produce diuresis, stimulate cardiac muscle, and relax smooth muscle, notably bronchial muscle. Because the various xanthines differ markedly in the intensity of their actions on various structures, one particular xanthine has been used more than another for a particular therapeutic effect. Since theobromine displays a low potency in these pharmacological actions, it has all but disappeared from the therapeutic scene.

Central Nervous System. Theophylline and caffeine are potent stimulants of the CNS; theobromine is virtually inactive in this respect. Traditionally, caffeine has been considered the most potent of the methylxanthines; however, theophylline produces more profound and potentially more dangerous CNS stimulation than does caffeine.

Persons ingesting caffeine or caffeine-containing beverages usually experience less drowsiness, less fatigue, and a more rapid and clearer flow of thought. Under experimental conditions, caffeine produces an increased capacity for sustained intellectual effort, decreased reaction time, and a more perfect association of ideas. Typists, for example, work faster and with fewer errors. However, recently acquired motor skill in a task involving delicate muscular coordination and accurate timing may not be improved or may even be adversely affected (Goldstein *et al.*, 1965). The above-mentioned effects may be produced by the administration of 85 to 250 mg of caffeine, the amount contained in 1 to 3 cups of coffee. Comparable effects of theophylline have not been carefully investigated, owing in part to the fact that CNS stimulatory actions of this agent have been observed principally as side effects in the therapy of bronchial asthma, in which the minimal adult dose is above 250 mg. As the dose is increased, methylxanthines produce nervousness, restlessness, insomnia, tremors, hyperesthesia, and other signs of CNS stimulation. At still higher doses, focal and generalized convulsions are produced; theophylline is clearly more potent than caffeine in this regard. Such seizures, occasionally refractory to anticonvulsant agents, have sometimes occurred in patients when the blood concentration of theophylline was only about 50% above the top of the accepted therapeutic range (*see* Kordash *et al.*, 1977).

Methylxanthines also stimulate the *medullary respiratory centers*. This action is particularly prominent in certain pathophysiological states, such as in Cheyne-Stokes respiration and in apnea of preterm infants, and when respiration is depressed by certain drugs, such as barbiturates and opioids. The methylxanthines appear to increase the sensitivity of medullary centers to the stimulatory actions of CO_2, and respiratory minute volume is increased at any given value of alveolar P_{CO_2} (Stroud *et al.*, 1955). The potencies of caffeine and theophylline have not been adequately compared; however, approximately 2 mg/kg of caffeine does not appear to produce respiratory stimulation in normal human subjects (Bellville *et al.*, 1962), whereas significant effects are observed with slightly higher doses of theophylline (Stroud *et al.*, 1955). In the presence of therapeutic doses of opioids, both methylxanthines are capable of stimulating respiration at even lower doses; for example, caffeine at about 0.5 mg/kg produces significant stimulatory effects in the presence of 10 mg of morphine (Bellville *et al.*, 1962). Both methylxanthines may produce nausea and vomiting; this probably involves CNS actions, at least in part, since emesis occurs even after parenteral administration. Theophylline-induced emesis is common when concentrations in plasma exceed 15 µg/ml, which includes the upper part of the recommended range of therapeutic concentrations (Jacobs et al., 1976; Kordash et al., 1977).

It is difficult to find acceptable experimental data to substantiate the traditional view that caffeine is a more powerful CNS stimulant than theophylline. Moreover, a number of studies indicate that theophylline is at least as potent as caffeine and may produce more intense signs of CNS stimulation. For example, theophylline is more potent and effective than caffeine in lowering thresholds for production of motor and vocalization responses to electrical stimuli in rats (hyperalgesia) (Paalzow and Paalzow, 1973); significant effects are noted at theophylline concentrations in blood of 15 µg/ml (Paalzow, 1975). Some workers have suggested that the behavioral effects of methylxanthines are related to their capability to increase the turnover of monoamines in the CNS; such changes have been noted following administration of 3 to 10 mg/kg of theophylline (Karasawa et al., 1976). Related electrophysiological observations include marked increases in firing rates of neurons in the brain stem reticular formation of rats after oral administration of 1 to 2 mg/kg of caffeine (Foote et al., 1978).

Cardiovascular System. Caffeine and theophylline, especially the latter, have prominent actions on the circulatory system. The capacity of theophylline to produce modest decreases in peripheral vascular resistance, sometimes powerful cardiac stimulation, and increased perfusion of most organs was exploited until recently for the emergency treatment of congestive heart failure. However, the unpredictable absorption and distribution of theophylline in patients with compromised circulatory function led all too often to serious CNS toxicity (Piafsky et al., 1977). More effective vasodilators and specific inotropic agents are now preferred (see Cohn and Franciosa, 1977).

The actions of the methylxanthines on the circulatory system are complex and sometimes antagonistic, and the resultant effects largely depend upon the conditions prevailing at the time of their administration and the dose used. In addition to the traditional but poorly documented view that methylxanthines have appreciable capability to stimulate vagal and vasomotor centers in the brain stem, there is an array of more or less direct actions on vascular and cardiac tissues in combination with indirect peripheral actions that are mediated by catecholamines and possibly by the renin-angiotensin system. Therefore, the observation of a single function, for example, the blood pressure, is deceiving because the drugs may act on a variety of circulatory factors in such a way that the blood pressure may remain essentially unchanged.

Heart. At therapeutic plasma concentrations (10 to 20 µg/ml), theophylline produces a modest increase in heart rate in normal individuals (Ogilvie et al., 1977). Low concentrations of caffeine may produce small decreases in heart rate (Starr et al., 1937), presumably a consequence of stimulation of the medullary vagal nuclei. At higher concentrations, both methylxanthines produce definite tachycardia; sensitive individuals may experience other arrhythmias, such as premature ventricular contractions. Arrhythmias may also be encountered in persons who use caffeine-containing beverages to excess. Theophylline at 10 to 20 µg/ml in plasma also reduces the left ventricular ejection time index and isovolumetric contraction time, consistent with an increase in contractile force and a decrease in cardiac preload (Ogilvie et al., 1977). The decrease in the venous filling pressure may be caused in part by the more complete emptying of the heart. In normal individuals, any rise in cardiac output may be brief and may be followed by a fall below the initial level. In patients with heart failure, however, the venous pressure is initially rather high; consequently the cardiac stimulation, together with the lowering of venous pressure produced by theophylline, leads to a marked increase in cardiac output that occurs almost immediately and persists for 30 minutes or more after intravenous administration.

The effects of theophylline at therapeutic plasma concentrations may be mediated in part by the augmented release of catecholamines from the sympathoadrenal system. For example, the infusion of 485 mg of theophylline into normal subjects provokes an increased urinary excretion of epinephrine and, to a lesser extent, norepinephrine, which presumably reflects augmented concentrations of these amines in plasma (Atuk et al., 1967). The ingestion of 250 mg of caffeine, leading to plasma concentrations averaging about 10 µg/ml, has been observed to increase concentrations of epinephrine and norepinephrine in plasma by about 100% and 50%, respectively (Robertson *et al.*, 1978). Furthermore, the intravenous administration of as little as 200 mg of theophylline in human subjects can enhance the exocytosis of storage granules for catecholamines, as evidenced by an increase in dopamine β-hydroxylase activity in plasma (Aunis *et al.*, 1975). Plasma renin activity and both systolic and diastolic blood pressure are also increased, while the heart rate is significantly reduced during the initial rise in blood pressure.

Theophylline can cause an increase in isometric tension developed by cat papillary muscle *in vitro* at concentrations as low as 2.5 μM (about 0.5 μg/ml) (Marcus *et al.*, 1972). However, β-adrenergic antagonists shift the dose-response curve for this effect to the right, suggesting that endogenous catecholamines participate in the response. At concentrations above 0.1 mM (18 μg/ml), theophylline potentiates the inotropic response to norepinephrine in isolated left atria of rabbits (Rall and West, 1963). Since tissue from reserpinized animals yields similar results and because caffeine is much less effective, this interaction may be a consequence of the ability of methylxanthines to inhibit the degradation of cyclic adenosine 3′, 5′-monophosphate (cyclic AMP) (*see* below). At still higher concentrations of methylxanthines (1 to 10 mM), a variety of effects have been noted on myocardial tissue *in vitro;* alterations in the cellular metabolism of calcium may be involved (*see* below).

Blood Vessels. After therapeutic doses of caffeine or theophylline in man, the peripheral vascular resistance declines, regardless of the change, if any, of arterial blood pressure (Starr *et al.*, 1937; Ogilvie *et al.*, 1977). Oncometric studies in animals show that there is a definite increase in organ volume following the administration of xanthines. Vasodilatation, coupled with an augmented cardiac output, results in an increased blood flow. However, in man the increase in peripheral blood flow is short lived.

In contrast to their dilating effect upon the systemic blood vessels, the xanthines cause a marked increase in *cerebrovascular resistance* with an accompanying decrease in cerebral blood flow and in the oxygen tension of the brain (Wechsler *et al.*, 1950; Moyer *et al.*, 1952a, 1952b). It is this vasoconstriction, rather than the decrease in cerebrospinal fluid pressure that may also occur, that is believed to be responsible for the relief of hypertensive headache by the xanthines.

Experimentally, it can be demonstrated that the xanthines dilate coronary arteries and increase coronary blood flow. This led to their use in the treatment of coronary artery disease. However, opinion as to their value is divided and the evidence in this field is controversial. There seems to be general agreement in the studies on man that under certain conditions the xanthines increase coronary blood flow. There is also abundant evidence that the drugs increase the work of the heart. The outstanding question is whether the blood supply to the myocardium increases to a greater extent than does the oxygen demand. Regardless of controversial claims and disappointing clinical results, the xanthines continue to be employed by some physicians in the treatment of coronary insufficiency.

In vitro, it has generally been found that methylxanthines (about 0.5 mM or above) cause relaxation of vascular smooth muscle in the presence of various stimulators of contraction (*e.g.*, norepinephrine, angiotensin, K^+). While relaxation probably results from a reduction of the cytosolic concentration of Ca^{2+}, it is not clear to what extent the methylxanthines alter calcium binding and transport directly or influence these functions indirectly by means of changes in cyclic nucleotide metabolism. However, at concentrations close to those in the therapeutic range, the effects of methylxanthines are variable and depend upon the locale of the vascular bed and the experimental conditions employed. For example, theophylline (18 μg/ml) inhibits the vasoconstriction produced by nerve stimulation or by infusion of norepinephrine in the isolated, perfused rabbit kidney (Hedqvist *et al.*, 1978). This occurs despite the fact that theophylline promotes release of norepinephrine during nerve stimulation. These effects appear to involve specific antagonism of the actions of adenosine, rather than inhibition of cyclic nucleotide phosphodiesterase (*see* below). On the other hand, caffeine and theophylline (1 to 10 μg/ml) *augment* contractions of aortic strips in the presence of epinephrine (Kalsner, 1971). A similar potentiation of the effects of catecholamine is observed with bovine coronary artery (Kalsner *et al.*, 1975); however, in this case it is β-adrenergic receptor-mediated *relaxation* that is enhanced by methylxanthines. Lammerant and Becsei (1975) infused theophylline into the coronary artery of dogs and noted no changes in coronary blood flow until the heart rate was elevated to approximately 150 beats per minute by right atrial pacing. The *reduction* of coronary blood flow that was then caused by the methylxanthines may be due to antagonism of the coronary-dilating action of endogenously released adenosine (*see* Berne, 1964; Berne and Rubio, 1974).

Smooth Muscle. The xanthines relax various smooth muscles other than those of blood vessels. The most important action in this respect is their ability to relax the smooth muscles of the *bronchi*, especially if the bronchi have been constricted either experimentally by histamine or clinically in asthma.

Theophylline is the most effective and produces a definite increase in vital capacity. It is, therefore, of value in the treatment of bronchial asthma.

It is not clear to what extent therapeutic responses that occur when concentrations of theophylline in plasma are 5 to 20 μg/ml involve the release of or synergistic interactions with β-adrenergic agonists. Theophylline (4 mg/kg) reduces the bronchoconstriction induced by acetylcholine in anesthetized guinea pigs within 30 seconds of intravenous administration (James, 1967). This response is markedly reduced after adrenalectomy or in the presence of a β-adrenergic blocking agent. However, the capacity of theophylline to decrease spontaneous tension in guinea pig tracheal chains is apparently not affected by propranolol (Foster, 1966). While synergistic interactions between theophylline and β_2-adrenergic agonists have been noted when relaxation of certain airway muscle preparations has been studied *in vitro* (Bertelli *et al.,* 1973), examination of other model systems *in vitro* and studies in man have failed to indicate that such combinations produce synergistic therapeutic responses (Wolfe *et al.,* 1978; Ziment and Steen, 1978).

Theophylline (4 to 8 mg/kg) also inhibits the canine ureter *in situ* (Boatman *et al.,* 1967; Wein *et al.,* 1972), relaxes the bladder, and, in relatively high concentrations, abolishes spontaneous contractions of the rat uterus and guinea pig taenia coli (Mitznegg *et al.,* 1974; Pfaffman and McFarland, 1978). This last-named effect may account for the observation that intravenous injection of theophylline in man causes a transient suppression of motility in the large and small bowel. In guinea pig vas deferens muscle, as little as 0.1 mM theophylline reduces the contractile response to α-adrenergic agonists without altering that to acetylcholine (Iso, 1973); this is correlated with the ability of adenosine to augment the effects of adrenergic agonists (but not those of acetylcholine) and with the action of theophylline to abolish the actions of adenosine.

Methylxanthines appear to be able to antagonize rather specifically a number of the actions of opioids in both the CNS and the gastrointestinal tract. For example, the injection of about 3 mg/kg of theophylline in man inhibits transiently the spasm of the biliary tract produced by opioids (Butsch *et al.,* 1936). Theophylline also reduces the contractile response to morphine but not that to acetylcholine in isolated segments of dog intestine (Grubb and Burks, 1975). On the other hand, theophylline can antagonize morphine-induced *inhibition* of contractions produced by electrical stimulation of guinea pig myenteric plexus–longitudinal muscle preparations at concentrations that do not affect catecholamine-induced inhibition of contractions (Sawynok and Jhamandas, 1976).

Skeletal Muscle. Caffeine has been shown by objective measurements to increase the capacity for muscular work in man (Foltz *et al.,* 1942); significant effects are seen in some subjects with doses of 3.5 mg/kg. At approximately the same dose, caffeine increases twitch tension of the indirectly stimulated quadriceps muscle of cats (Huidobro and Amenbar, 1945). While there is no effect on tetanic tension, caffeine causes marked increases in tension at frequencies slightly below those producing tetanus. This is accompanied by fusion of individual contractions, perhaps owing to a prolonged contraction time (Goffart and Ritchie, 1952). Theophylline is considerably less potent in these actions (Huidobro, 1945). Such observations may be explained in part by the ability of caffeine to increase the release of acetylcholine, as judged by augmentation of the amplitude and rate of rise of end-plate potentials in curarized rat diaphragm (Goldberg and Singer, 1969). Caffeine can also increase the resting tension of *denervated* muscle (Huidobro, 1945). The possible role of the translocation of Ca^{2+} in the effects of caffeine on striated muscle is discussed below.

Diuretic Actions. Methylxanthines, especially theophylline, increase the production of urine, and the patterns of enhanced excretion of water and electrolytes are very similar to those produced by the thiazides (Maren, 1961). In normal man, theophylline may cause a transient increase in renal blood flow and glomerular filtration rate. However, in patients with congestive heart failure, theophylline produces small and inconsistent changes in glomerular filtration rate, suggesting that inhibition of renal tubular reabsorption of sodium is a major factor in the diuretic action of methylxanthines in this setting (Davies and Schock, 1949). During chronic treatment with high-ceiling diuretic agents, the administration of either theophylline or a thiazide diuretic produces additional excretion of sodium, chloride, and potassium ions (Sigurd and Olesen, 1978). More details on diuretic actions are given in Chapter 36.

Secretion. Methylxanthines augment release of the secretory products of a number of endocrine and exocrine tissues. One exception to this general statement is the ability of methylxanthines to inhibit secretion by mast cells and possibly other sources of mediators of inflammation. A number of the therapeutic and toxic properties of methylxanthines probably involve actions on secretory processes. However, the quantitative contribution of such actions has not often been delineated.

Gastric Secretion. The pattern of effects of methylxanthines on gastric secretion is dependent upon the species and conditions employed. Man is relatively sensitive, and moderate oral or parenteral doses of caffeine cause secretion of both acid and pepsin (*see* Debas *et al.,* 1971). Although never directly compared, theophylline would appear to be at least as potent as caffeine in this regard

(Krasnow and Grossman, 1949). While atropine may partially inhibit caffeine-induced secretion of acid, the prior administration of cimetidine, an H_2-receptor antagonist, completely prevents the response to even relatively high doses of caffeine (Cano et al., 1976).

It has been long known (and perhaps forgotten) that beverages made from roasted grain containing no caffeine stimulate acid secretion in man as much as does coffee (Öhnell and Berg, 1931); similarly, decaffeinated coffee is only slightly less potent than the natural product, and both are about twice as effective as is an equivalent amount of caffeine (Cohen and Booth, 1975). The effects of a combination of caffeine and pentagastrin upon acid and pepsin secretion in man are about equal to the sum of the effects of the individual agents (Cohen et al., 1971), and histamine and caffeine also produce only additive effects on pepsin secretion (Grossman et al., 1945). The evidence purporting to show that caffeine potentiates secretion of acid induced by histamine or alcohol in man is not convincing. However, in view of the responsiveness of the human gastric mucosa to caffeine and other substances in various beverages, cognizance must be taken of the ubiquitous use of coffee and colas in the pathogenesis of peptic ulcer and in the management of the patient with an ulcer.

Both in the cat (a species less sensitive than man to caffeine) and in the dog (in which methylxanthines alone cannot induce secretion), there is no doubt that methylxanthines *can potentiate* the actions of various gastric secretagogues, including histamine, cholinergic agonists, pentagastrin, and food (Roth and Ivy, 1944; Bieck et al., 1973; Gabrys et al., 1973). Despite intensive investigation, such issues as the mechanism of action of methylxanthines, the function of histamine, and the role of cyclic AMP in the regulation of gastric secretion are only poorly understood (*see* Jacobson and Thompson, 1976).

Secretion of Other Substances. As noted above, therapeutic concentrations of methylxanthines can increase the concentration of circulating catecholamines. Such concentrations of both caffeine (Robertson et al., 1978) and theophylline (Lowder et al., 1975, 1976) also elevate plasma renin activity in man. Since the administration of β-adrenergic blocking agents does not prevent this response (Zehner et al., 1975), mediation by epinephrine is not an essential part of this action of methylxanthines. Administration of theophylline also results in increases in the plasma concentrations of gastrin (Feurle et al., 1976) and parathyroid hormone

(Bowser et al., 1975). Since epinephrine can produce similar effects, it is not clear whether this represents a direct action of the methylxanthine.

Perfusion of the isolated rat pancreas with theophylline (25 μg/ml) augments glucose-induced release of insulin more than twofold (Somers et al., 1976). This concentration of theophylline is above the therapeutic range. While very low doses of theophylline (3 to 3.5 mg/kg) infused into human subjects cause little or no increase in concentration of insulin in plasma (Serrano-Ríos et al., 1974; Arnman et al., 1975), they do appear to potentiate the insulinemic responses to infusions of secretin and cholecystokinin-pancreozymin.

Theophylline inhibits the release of histamine from rat peritoneal mast cells *in vitro* under several different circumstances. In one case, theophylline (36 μg/ml) inhibited dextran-induced histamine release by 50% (Baxter, 1972); in another, theophylline (18 μg/ml) abolished the twofold augmentation by a calcium ionophore of the release of histamine produced by low concentrations of adenosine (Marquardt et al., 1978). These observations may relate to the therapeutic actions of theophylline in bronchial asthma, as well as to the observations that caffeine displays anti-inflammatory activity in various model systems (Vinegar et al., 1976). Small doses of caffeine (5 to 10 mg/kg) also appear to reduce the ED50 for aspirin, indomethacin, and phenylbutazone by more than threefold.

Metabolism. Caffeine, ingested orally at doses of 3 to 9 mg/kg, can produce a slight increase (10%) in the basal metabolic rate in man (Means et al., 1917; Haldi et al., 1941). Comparable observations with theophylline have not been reported. Infusion of theophylline at low doses (3 to 3.5 mg/kg) can elevate the concentration of free fatty acids and glycerol in the plasma of man within 10 minutes (Arnman et al., 1975). While such effects of caffeine in man have not been reported, similar observations have been made in dogs (Bellet et al., 1968). It is not clear if the release and action of catecholamines is essential for the production of these metabolic responses.

Cellular Basis for the Action of Methylxanthines. Three basic cellular actions of the methylxanthines have received major attention in studies to explain their diverse effects. Listed in order of their increasing sensitivity to methylxanthines, they are: (1) those associated with translocations of intracellular calcium; (2) those mediated by increasing accumulation of cyclic nucleotides, particularly cyclic AMP; and (3) those mediated by blockade of receptors for adenosine. Of particular importance is the question of what types of actions contribute appreciably to the effects of methylxanthines in the therapeutic dose range. The concentration of free theophylline in plasma rarely exceeds 50 μM during therapy (*see* below). At the present state of knowledge, this fact alone appears to limit severely the possible contribution of the first two categories of actions to the therapeutic effects of theophylline and leaves the anti-adenosine action as the leading candidate. There are also several other types of actions that have received relatively little attention to date but that might prove to be very important in certain effects of the methylxanthines. These include their potentiation of inhibitors of prostaglandin synthesis (*see* Vinegar *et al.,* 1976), and the possibility that methylxanthines reduce the uptake and/or metabolism of catecholamines in nonneural tissues (*see* Kalsner, 1971; Kalsner *et al.,* 1975). Further investigation will be required to establish the contribution of these actions to both the immediate effect of the methylxanthines and those involving the release of catecholamines.

Studies of the actions of methylxanthines on translocation of intracellular Ca^{2+} have involved principally those of caffeine on skeletal muscle. Caffeine (0.5 to 1 mM) augments the twitch response of the isolated frog sartorius muscle to stimulation of the motor nerve. The twitch is increased in height and is more rapid in onset and duration, probably because of sensitization of the mechanism for the release of Ca^{2+} from the terminal cisternae of the sarcoplasmic reticulum. Higher concentrations of caffeine produce contracture without nerve stimulation, owing probably to an increase in Ca^{2+} permeability of the sarcoplasmic reticulum, which normally participates in the termination of the contractile process by active uptake and sequestration of Ca^{2+} (*see* reviews by Bianchi, 1968, 1975). Caffeine-induced contractures characteristically do not require the presence of extracellular Ca^{2+} and are antagonized by certain local anesthetic agents. Under certain circumstances, effects of caffeine on Ca^{2+} release by purified preparations of skeletal muscle sarcoplasmic reticulum can be observed at concentrations as low as 0.25 mM (Katz *et al.,* 1977). Data on the relative potency of theophylline and caffeine are rarely presented, but theophylline has been stated to be less potent in producing contractures (Axelsson and Thesleff, 1958). At concentrations above 2 mM, the effects of methylxanthines on contraction and Ca^{2+} distribution in cardiac muscle resemble in general those observed with skeletal muscle (Blinks *et al.,* 1972); in cardiac muscle, little or no distinction can be made between caffeine and theophylline. Similar mechanisms may be important in the actions of methylxanthines upon certain secretory processes, notably the release of catecholamines from the adrenal medulla. In this case, theophylline (1 mM) can induce some secretion in the absence of extracellular Ca^{2+} (Peach, 1972). Since the *threshold* for phenomena related to alterations in the permeability to or binding of Ca^{2+} in intracellular organelles appears to be considerably greater than *maximal* therapeutic concentrations for methylxanthines, it is doubtful that these mechanisms play an important role in their desirable pharmacological actions.

Soon after the initial demonstration of the involvement of a heat-stable factor (later identified as cyclic AMP) in the regulation of glycogen phosphorylase activity and hormone-induced glycogenolysis (Rall *et al.,* 1957), caffeine was found to potentiate the actions of epinephrine and glucagon in homogenates of liver (Berthet *et al.,* 1957). This effect was later found to be due to the inhibition of cyclic nucleotide phosphodiesterase, the enzyme that catalyzes the hydrolysis of cyclic AMP to 5′-AMP (Sutherland and Rall, 1958); theophylline is considerably more potent than caffeine as an inhibitor of this enzyme system (Butcher and Sutherland, 1962). Over the years, a large number of hormones, neurotransmitters, and autacoids have been found to accelerate the synthesis of cyclic AMP in their target tissues, and the methylxanthines, especially theophylline, have been useful tools in investigations aimed at evaluating the role of cyclic AMP in the actions of a particular hormone on its target tissue. Accordingly, one important indication that cyclic AMP functions as an intracellular mediator is *evidence* that methylxanthines potentiate both the effects of the hormone in question and the accumulation of cyclic AMP (Sutherland *et al.,* 1968; Robison *et al.,* 1971). As a corollary, it has frequently been proposed that a variety of actions of methylxanthines, particularly those in which theophylline is more potent than caffeine, are also mediated by the cyclic AMP that accumulates as a consequence of inhibition of phosphodiesterase. However, theophylline at 50 μM and caffeine at 100 μM (the maximal therapeutic concentrations of free drug in plasma) inhibit phosphodiesterase activity in many tissues by only about 10% and 5%, respectively, when 1 μM cyclic AMP (the average tissue concentration) is used as substrate (*see* Beavo *et al.,* 1970). Furthermore methylxanthines in this concentration range have only rarely been observed to potentiate hormone-induced effects, even in those instances where other evidence exists for the involvement of cyclic AMP. Thus, until more convincing data become available, it would seem prudent to be skeptical about the frequently expressed view that a given therapeutic action of a methylxanthine is achieved by inhibition of cyclic nucleotide phosphodiesterase.

It was later observed that theophylline, added for the purpose of enhancing cyclic AMP accumulation in brain slices subjected to electrical stimulation, produced marked inhibition of the accumulation of the nucleotide (Kakiuchi *et al.,* 1969). Subsequently, this inhibition was found to be due to competitive antagonism by theophylline of the actions of adenosine that is released from brain cells under such conditions (Sattin and Rall, 1970); caffeine is a considerably less potent inhibitor. Numerous investigations over the past decade have provided evidence that adenosine functions as an autacoid, acting through receptors in the plasma membranes of a wide variety of cells (*see* Symposium, 1978).

Adenosine dilates blood vessels, particularly in the coronary and cerebral circulation, and slows the rate of discharge of cardiac pacemaker cells and of a variety of neurons in the CNS. In addition, it strongly inhibits hormone-induced lipolysis, reduces the release of norepinephrine from autonomic nerve endings, and in some cases probably inhibits the release of excitatory neurotransmitters in the CNS. Adenosine can also potentiate certain of the actions of norepinephrine, leading to increased contraction of some smooth muscles or to augmented accumulation of cyclic AMP in brain tissue.

Depending upon the type of cell involved, activation of receptors for adenosine can lead to either stimulation or inhibition of cyclic AMP synthesis. Furthermore, in a number of instances, adenosine receptors probably function without directly influencing the accumulation of the cyclic nucleotide. Although examination of the relative effectiveness of adenosine analogs has revealed differences in the characteristics of adenosine receptors in various tissues, theophylline thus far has proven to be a universal antagonist. However, *adenosine* receptors should not be confused with the putative *purinergic* receptors of the gastrointestinal tract and other tissues that are characterized by much greater sensitivity to ATP than to adenosine and by insensitivity to methylxanthines (*see* Burnstock, 1972). Complete antagonism of adenosine-induced effects has been achieved with about a 20-fold molar excess of theophylline in every system examined to date. Thus, depending upon the sensitivity of the particular system to adenosine and upon the amount of endogenous adenosine present in the experimental preparation, marked effects of theophylline have been observed at concentrations ranging from 20 to 100 μM. Hence, the anti-adenosine effects of methylxanthines must be considered seriously even in those instances in which a regulatory function for adenosine has yet to be established.

Toxicology. Fatal poisoning in man by the ingestion of caffeine is extremely rare (*see* Dimaio and Garriott, 1974). While emesis and convulsions are usually prominent consequences of caffeine overdosage, neither symptom was observed in at least one case of fatal poisoning. The concentration of caffeine in post-mortem blood has ranged from 80 μg/ml to over 1 mg/ml. Untoward reactions, however, may be observed following the ingestion of 1 g (15 mg/kg) or more of caffeine, leading to plasma concentrations above 30 μg/ml. These are mainly referable to the central nervous and circulatory systems. Insomnia, restlessness, and excitement are the early symptoms, which may progress to mild delirium. Sensory disturbances such as ringing in the ears and flashes of light are common. The muscles become tense and tremulous. Tachycardia and extrasystoles are frequent, and respiration is quickened.

Fatal intoxications with theophylline have been much more frequent than with caffeine. Rapid intravenous administration of therapeutic doses of *aminophylline* (500 mg) sometimes results in sudden death that is probably cardiac in nature. It is believed that this may be a consequence of precipitation of free theophylline at the pH of the blood, with the resultant production of high local concentrations. Most toxicity is the result of repeated administration of the drug by both oral and parenteral routes. Aminophylline should be injected slowly over 20 to 40 minutes to avoid severe toxic symptoms, which include headache, palpitation, dizziness, nausea, hypotension, and precordial pain. Additional symptoms of toxicity are tachycardia, severe restlessness, agitation, and emesis; these effects are associated with plasma concentrations of more than 20 μg/ml (Jacobs *et al.,* 1976). Focal and generalized seizures can also happen, sometimes without prior signs of toxicity. Seizures usually occur when concentrations in plasma exceed 40 μg/ml (Yarnell and Chu, 1975; Zwillich *et al.,* 1975; Kordash *et al.,* 1977), although convulsions and death have resulted at plasma concentrations as low as 25 μg/ml. Seizures caused by intoxication with methylxanthines can usually be treated with diazepam. However, in some cases of theophylline toxicity, the seizures have been refractory to intravenous diazepam, phenytoin, and phenobarbital. In a unique case a patient with a plasma concentration of theophylline of 190 μg/ml was reported to have survived, albeit with permanent neurological deficits; in this case, hemoperfusion through charcoal cartridges was probably lifesaving (Ehlers *et al.,* 1978). Premature infants may be relatively resistant to poisoning by theophylline; concentrations in plasma of up to 80 μg/ml have resulted in sustained tachycardia as the only sign of toxicity (Cole and Davies, 1980).

Mutagenic Effects. Caffeine induces chromosomal abnormalities both in plant cells and in mammalian cells in culture and has potent mutagenic effects on microorganisms either alone or in combination with other mutagens (*see* Timson, 1977). These effects seem to be associated with inhibition of DNA-repair processes. They are observed only with concentrations of caffeine that are much in excess of those that follow the ingestion of beverages and medications. Furthermore, available evidence suggests that caffeine is neither mutagenic by itself nor in combination with known mutagens in mammals. At very high doses, caffeine appears to have some teratogenic activity in mammals. One retrospective study indicated that pregnant women who ingest more than 600 mg of caffeine per day in beverages may have an increased incidence of spontaneous abortion, stillbirth, or premature delivery (Weathersbee *et al.*, 1977). Thus, while mutagenic effects would seem to pose little hazard in man, potential developmental toxicity for the human fetus and neonate warrants further investigation.

Relation to Myocardial Infarction. Much interest has developed concerning a possible deleterious effect of caffeine in the etiology of acute myocardial infarction. Jick and coworkers (1973) reported that individuals drinking more than 5 to 6 cups of coffee per day are about twice as liable to suffer myocardial infarction. However, in an equally careful study Klatsky and associates (1973) found no independent association between coffee drinking and a subsequent first myocardial infarction; they suggest that the discrepancy in the findings of the two groups may be related to factors such as cigarette smoking or the selection of control subjects. Further studies have confirmed that coffee drinking is associated with little, if any, increased incidence of coronary heart disease (Dawber *et al.*, 1974; Hennekens *et al.*, 1976).

Absorption, Fate, and Excretion. The methylxanthines are readily absorbed after oral, rectal, or parenteral administration. The oral absorption of theophylline is of particular importance because of its use in the treatment of chronic asthma. It had been believed that the absorption of the simple alkaloid was sometimes erratic because of its poor solubility in water and that its oral administration was especially apt to produce gastric irritation, nausea, and vomiting. This led to the marketing of more soluble salt forms of theophylline (*e.g.*, theophylline sodium glycinate, choline theophyllinate) with claims that they were better absorbed and less irritating to the gastric mucosa. Rectal administration of aminophylline was also employed to avoid gastric irritation. It is now clear that uncoated tablets of anhydrous theophylline are completely absorbed, as are some, but not all, sustained-released formulations (Weinberger *et al.*, 1978). Furthermore, parenteral administration does *not* obviate production of gastrointestinal distress, nausea, and vomiting. These symptoms are clearly a function of the concentration of theophylline in plasma. It is also possible that lack of appreciation of the proportion of the active principle in various preparations has resulted in lower actual doses of theophylline and thus a lower apparent incidence of gastric irritation. Any additional propensity of oral preparations to produce symptoms caused by local irritation of the gastrointestinal tract can probably be avoided by their administration with food, which slows but does not reduce absorption. In the absence of food, solutions or uncoated tablets of theophylline produce maximal concentrations in plasma within 2 hours; caffeine is more rapidly absorbed, and maximal plasma concentrations are achieved within 1 hour. Theophylline is rapidly but incompletely absorbed when administered by retention enema; concentrations in plasma are maximal within 1 hour, but never reach values found after oral administration of the same dose to a given individual (Lillehei, 1968). Use of rectal suppositories results in slow and erratic absorption (Truitt *et al.*, 1950). Intramuscular injection of soluble preparations of theophylline (*e.g.*, aminophylline) produces long-lasting local pain; this route of administration should not be used.

Methylxanthines are distributed into all body compartments, and they cross the placenta. The apparent volume of distribution is similar for both caffeine and theophylline and usually is between 400 and 550 ml/kg. Theophylline is about 50% bound to plasma proteins, more so than is caffeine. The difference in protein binding may account in part for the greater concentration of caffeine than theophylline in cerebrospinal fluid and brain tissue relative to that in blood. The substantially greater lipid solubility of caffeine may also be a factor.

Methylxanthines are eliminated primarily by metabolism in the liver. About 10% and 1% of administered theophylline and caffeine, respectively, are recovered in the urine unchanged. Limited data indicate that caffeine has a half-life in plasma of about 3.5 hours in man. The disposition of theophylline in both children and adults has been investigated more intensively (*see* Hendeles *et al.*, 1978). While there is considerable variability, the half-life of theophylline in young children averages about 3.5 hours, while values of 8 or 9 hours are more typical of adults. In patients with hepatic cirrhosis or acute pulmonary edema, the rate of elimination is variable and much slower; values of more than 60 hours have been observed. Similar prolongation of the half-life for theophylline is seen in premature babies treated for apnea

(Aranda *et al.,* 1976), while the value for caffeine ranges from 36 to 144 hours in such infants. Presumably, this reflects the relative renal clearance of these two substances in the absence of appreciable hepatic metabolism.

In addition to developmental and genetic factors, disposition of theophylline appears to be accelerated by smoking and by other agents that increase the capacity of drug-metabolizing systems in the liver, and to be slowed by certain macrolide antibiotics (Weinberger *et al.,* 1977). Furthermore, the elimination kinetics for theophylline displays dose dependency. Thus, increases in dosage sometimes produce concentrations in plasma that are higher than those predicted from the rate of elimination determined previously for a given patient (Weinberger and Ginchansky, 1977). Adjustments in dosage should therefore be made in small increments. In cases of theophylline overdosage or poisoning, the decline in plasma concentration to nontoxic levels may require a protracted period of time (*see* Ehlers *et al.,* 1978).

The principal metabolites of caffeine in the urine are 1-methyluric acid and 1-methylxanthine. Much smaller amounts of 1,3-dimethyluric acid, 7-methylxanthine, and 1,7-dimethylxanthine are detected (Cornish and Christman, 1957). While the chief urinary metabolite of theophylline is 1,3-dimethyluric acid (Brodie *et al.,* 1952), considerable amounts of 1-methyluric acid and 3-methylxanthine are also excreted. The latter compound accumulates to concentrations that approximate 25% of that of theophylline (Thompson *et al.,* 1974). Since 3-methylxanthine is about 50% as potent as theophylline in relaxing airway smooth muscle *in vitro* (Persson and Andersson, 1977; Williams *et al.,* 1978), it may contribute to some extent to the therapeutic effects of theophylline.

Because uric acid excretion does not increase appreciably after ingestion of methylxanthines, it has been long believed that these substances could not be converted to uric acid. However, the known products excreted can account for only between 65 and 80% of the administered agent. It thus remains possible that both xanthine and uric acid are produced but that the conversion of endogenous hypoxanthine to urate is reduced by competition with a metabolite of a methylxanthine. In any case, there is no evidence that the ingestion of methylxanthines exacerbates gout.

Preparations and Routes of Administration. The xanthines are weakly basic alkaloids. For oral administration either the free base or one of the double salts may be used; for parenteral administration, however, it is necessary to employ one of the salts.

Caffeine, U.S.P., is a white crystalline substance soluble in water to the extent of 1:50. *Caffeine and Sodium Benzoate Injection,* U.S.P., is a mixture of approximately equal parts of caffeine and sodium benzoate. It is available for intramuscular injection in ampuls containing 500 mg/2 ml, equivalent to 250 mg of caffeine.

Theophylline, U.S.P., is a white, bitter powder that is only slightly soluble in water (1%). Theophylline (anhydrous) is available in tablets (100, 125, 200, 225, and 250 mg), in capsules containing uncoated drug in suspension (100, 200, and 250 mg), and in capsules containing coated pellets for timed release (60, 65, 125, 130, 250, and 260 mg). The bioavailability of some timed-release preparations has not been documented. Elixirs (80 or 112.5 mg/15 ml), liquids (80, 150, or 160 mg/15 ml), syrups (80 mg/15 ml), and suspensions (100 mg/5 ml) are also available, as are rectal suppositories (120 and 500 mg).

Aminophylline, U.S.P. (*theophylline ethylenediamine*), is the most widely used of the soluble theophylline salts. It occurs as a whitish powder with a slightly ammoniacal odor and a bitter taste; 1 g dissolves in about 5 ml of water. The following preparations are available: solutions for injection, in ampuls that contain 250 mg/10 ml, 500 mg/2 ml, and 500 mg/20 ml for intravenous administration; tablets (enteric coated and uncoated), 100 and 200 mg; elixirs, 100 and 250 mg/15 ml; solutions for both oral (315 mg/15 ml) and rectal (60 and 100 mg/ml) administration; rectal suppositories in 125-, 250-, 350-, and 500-mg sizes; and extended-release tablets (300 mg).

Theophylline Olamine, U.S.P. (*theophylline monoethanolamine*), contains 75% anhydrous theophylline. It is available only in solutions for rectal administration (312 or 625 mg/37 ml).

Oxtriphylline, U.S.P., also called *choline theophyllinate,* contains 64% anhydrous theophylline. It is freely soluble in water to yield a solution of pH 9.7. Tablets (partially enteric coated) in 100- and 200-mg sizes and an elixir (100 mg/5 ml with 20% alcohol) are available.

Theophylline Sodium Glycinate, U.S.P., contains 51% anhydrous theophylline and is freely soluble in water. It is available in tablets (330 mg) and an elixir (330 mg/15 ml) for oral administration.

Dyphylline is 7-(2,3-dihydroxypropyl) theophylline. This substance is a chemical entity distinct from theophylline, and *no* evidence exists for its transformation to theophylline to *any* degree after administration. Unfortunately, this substance is often considered as "a theophylline" and is sometimes mistakenly assigned a theophylline "equivalence" of 70% (*see* Webb-Johnson and Andrews, 1977). Since its introduction in 1946, dyphylline has been extensively used in the treatment of asthma; however, investigation of its efficacy and pharmacokinetic properties has begun only recently (*see* Simons *et al.,* 1975). Oral doses of 15 mg/kg, leading to peak concentrations in plasma of 12 μg/ml after 40 minutes, were required to produce a barely detectable therapeutic response. Both the doses recommended and the claims made for this compound seem unjustified. Nevertheless, dyphylline is marketed under no fewer than seven trademarked names.

THERAPEUTIC USES

The diverse pharmacological actions of the methylxanthines have found many therapeutic applications. Caffeine has been incorporated into a number of "over-the-counter" preparations that are widely used for analgesia, presumably for its effect on mood. Its use as a stimulant of the CNS in the treatment of overdosage with barbiturates or opioids has markedly diminished. Theophylline preparations are primarily employed to relax bronchial smooth muscle in the treatment of asthma and chronic obstructive pulmonary disease, and they are of particular importance in the treatment of *status asthmaticus* refractory to the administration of adrenergic agonists. In recent years, theophylline has been found helpful in the treatment of the prolonged apnea sometimes observed in preterm infants; caffeine may also be of value in this regard. The use of theophylline to stimulate the myocardium in the treatment of acute episodes of congestive heart failure has become virtually extinct. The use of the diuretic actions of the methylxanthines is principally confined to the inclusion of caffeine in subtherapeutic amounts in "over-the-counter" preparations.

Bronchial Asthma.   Theophylline compounds, particularly aminophylline, play an important role in the management of the asthmatic patient. They are useful as prophylactic drugs and are valuable adjuncts in the treatment of prolonged attacks and in the management of status asthmaticus. Although adrenocorticosteroids may be necessary for the treatment of prolonged attacks of asthma, bronchodilator drugs occupy a dominant place in therapy. The successful treatment of status asthmaticus calls for a variety of measures, including the use of oxygen, sympathomimetic drugs, expectorants, sedatives, and bronchial aspiration (*see* Webb-Johnson and Andrews, 1977). One of the most effective bronchodilating agents is theophylline.

Studies on asthmatic subjects reveal that therapeutic effects of theophylline require a plasma concentration of at least 5 to 8 μg/ml. Toxic effects become apparent at about 15 μg/ml and are frequent above 20 μg/ml. Accordingly, most therapeutic strategies are aimed at achieving and maintaining average concentrations in plasma of about 10 μg/ml. In view of the wide range of rates of elimination of theophylline, this is an impossible task without careful titration of dosage against therapeutic and toxic effects and the aid of periodic determination of concentrations of drug in plasma. For treatment of episodes of severe bronchospasm and status asthmaticus, aminophylline is administered intravenously. A loading dose of 6 mg/kg (equivalent to about 5 mg/kg of theophylline) is infused over 20 to 40 minutes. In the absence of the desired therapeutic response and signs or symptoms of toxicity, an additional 3 mg/kg of aminophylline can be slowly infused. Continued therapy for acute symptoms can be maintained initially by the infusion of 0.5 to 0.6 mg/kg per hour of aminophylline to otherwise-healthy adults who are nonsmokers. Children below the age of 12 and adults who are smokers will probably require higher infusion rates of about 0.9 mg/kg per hour to maintain therapeutic concentrations. Patients with reduced hepatic function or perfusion should receive lower maintenance doses. In any event, infusions should not be continued beyond 10 to 12 hours without knowledge of the concentration of the drug. Chronic bronchodilator therapy, accomplished by the oral administration of *theophylline*, must also be individualized. Based on the values for clearance of theophylline from plasma (*see* Leung *et al.*, 1977; Hendeles *et al.*, 1978), mean plasma concentrations of 10 μg/ml would be achieved with daily doses of 9.4 mg/kg for nonsmoking adults and 23 mg/kg for children below the age of 12. However, in view of marked interindividual variations in clearance rates, initial daily doses should not exceed 6 mg/kg and 13 mg/kg, respectively. Initial daily doses for adults who smoke should be about 10 mg/kg, even though an average dose is about 16 mg/kg. Any increase in dosage should be made in small increments after about 3 days on a given regimen. These adjustments are guided by both clinical response and determination of the concentration of theophylline in plasma. The interval between doses also presents a problem in individuals who have high rates of elimination of theophylline. For example, when an 8-hour interval is used for compatibility with a reasonably normal sleep schedule in young children, doses determined to produce mean concentrations in plasma that are within the therapeutic range could also produce cyclical overdosage and underdosage in a significant fraction of patients. Sustained-release formulations that are completely absorbed would provide considerable therapeutic advantage for such patients (Weinberger *et al.*, 1978). While rectal instillation of theophylline solutions represents an alternative to oral administration, the limited amount of data available indicates that a given dose produces a lower concentration in plasma when given by this route.

The administration of the β_2-adrenergic agonists metaproterenol or terbutaline concurrently with doses of theophylline that result in *peak* concentrations in plasma of no greater than 10 μg/ml can provide therapeutic responses that are at least as great as those achieved with higher doses of theophylline. Such regimens apparently do not increase the incidence of adverse effects above that observed with theophylline alone (Galant *et al.*, 1978; Wolfe *et al.*, 1978). Although evidence for *greater-than-additive* therapeutic responses to combinations of β_2-adrenergic agonists and theophylline is not convincing (Wolfe *et al.*, 1978; Ziment and Steen, 1978), individualized regimens of combinations of these two classes of agents may well achieve effective bronchodilatation with less risk of toxicity than is currently experienced. Although there is some controversy, the combined use of ephedrine and theophylline appears to offer no therapeutic advantage over theophylline alone (*see* Weinberger, 1978). The use of preparations with fixed-dose combinations of components is irrational unless they happen by chance to correspond to an optimized regimen previously established with the individual agents. The addition of barbiturates in order to counteract the CNS effects of theophylline entails the risk of increasing the rate of elimination of theophylline, as well as possible interference with the determination of concentrations of the xanthine in plasma by certain analytical procedures. Although the literature is silent on the issue, common sense interdicts the use of caffeine-containing beverages and proprietary medications during therapy with theophylline. The following interactions would thereby be avoided: the additive CNS, cardiovascular, and gastrointestinal effects of caffeine; the effects of caffeine on the elimination of theophylline by competition for common metabolic enzymes; and the interference by caffeine with the determination of theophylline by certain analytical procedures.

Chronic Obstructive Pulmonary Disease. Theophylline is also used in the treatment of this disorder. The therapeutic approach is similar to that for asthma. However, the treatment of cardiovascular sequelae of chronic obstructive pulmonary disease (pulmonary hypertension, cor pulmonale, and right-heart failure) is more complex, and theophylline does not appear to play a prominent role in current approaches (see Fishman, 1976). It is probable that theophylline does not have appreciable direct dilating effects on pulmonary arteries, but perhaps can assist in reducing the hypoxemia that apparently is the primary cause of pulmonary hypertension. With appreciation of the reduced rates of theophylline elimination that occur in patients with compromised cardiac function, the inclusion of theophylline in future therapeutic approaches might prove beneficial without the relatively high risk of serious toxicity that was experienced in the past.

Apnea of Preterm Infants. Episodes of prolonged apnea, lasting more than 20 seconds, are not infrequent occurrences in premature infants and pose the threat of recurrent hypoxemia and neurological damage. While they are often associated with serious systemic illness, no specific cause is found in many instances. Beginning with the work of Kuzemko and Paala (1973), methylxanthines have undergone clinical trials for the treatment of apnea of undetermined origin. A number of studies have shown that oral or intravenous administration of aminophylline eliminates episodes of apnea that last more than 20 seconds and markedly reduces those of shorter duration (see Shannon et al., 1975). Therapeutic responses occur with concentrations of theophylline in plasma of 2 to 10 μg/ml (Dietrich et al., 1978); there is no indication that higher concentrations improve the response. Therapeutic concentrations are achieved with loading doses of 5 to 6 mg/kg of aminophylline (4 to 5 mg/kg of theophylline). Because of the highly variable and slow rates of elimination that are observed in these infants, maintenance doses of more than 2.4 mg/kg per 24 hours should not be used without determination of concentrations of the drug in plasma (Aranda et al., 1976). Since the effects of methylxanthines on development are not known,

drug-free periods are used intermittently. Therapy usually is required for only a few weeks and rarely for more than a few months. The relationship of apnea of preterm infants to "sleep apnea" or sudden infant death that occurs in apparently healthy term infants during the first year of life is not known. However, there has been one reported case in which a 3-month-old infant had a nearly fatal apneic episode and was later observed to have periodic breathing and severe bradycardia during rapid-eye-movement (REM) sleep. These episodes were eliminated by theophylline when concentrations in plasma were maintained between 9 and 10 μg/ml (Boutroy et al., 1978).

Miscellaneous Uses. Caffeine is rarely used in treating cases of poisoning by central depressants. The drug is given by intramuscular injection, usually as caffeine and sodium benzoate (0.5 to 1.0 g). Other approaches are preferred (see Chapters 17 and 68).

Caffeine in combination with an analgesic, such as aspirin, is widely employed in the treatment of ordinary types of headache. There are few data to substantiate this use. Caffeine is also used in combination with an ergot alkaloid in the treatment of migraine. The ability of methylxanthines to produce constriction of cerebral blood vessels may improve the therapeutic response.

After the claim that coffee could substitute for amphetamine or methylphenidate in the treatment of hyperkinetic behavior in children (Schnackenberg, 1973), there have been a number of reports both confirming and denying the original observations (see Reichard and Elder, 1977; Firestone et al., 1978). However, these studies involved the use of single doses of caffeine unadjusted for body weight. In addition, while there is no information on the rate of elimination of caffeine in young children, it is probable that its metabolism would be both rapid and variable in this population. It will require careful clinical trials to determine whether caffeine is a useful alternative for some patients who display rather intense side effects when the more powerful CNS stimulants are administered.

XANTHINE BEVERAGES

Various means of estimation lead to the conclusion that the per-capita intake of caffeine in the United States averages above 200 mg daily (see Graham, 1978). About 90% of this amount results from drinking coffee. Depending upon the alkaloid content of the coffee bean and the method of brewing, 1 cup of coffee contains about 85 mg of caffeine, while 1 cup of tea contains about 50 mg of caffeine and 1 mg of theophylline; cocoa contains about 250 mg of theobromine and 5 mg of caffeine per cup. A 12-oz (360-ml) bottle of a cola drink contains about 50 mg of caffeine, half of which is added by the manufacturer as the alkaloid.

The xanthine beverages present a medical problem in that a large fraction of the population consumes enough caffeine to produce substantial effects on a number of organ systems. Accordingly, the physician should be aware of the caffeine intake of patients and should secure a dietary history. Due consideration should be given to the possible contribution of caffeine to the presenting signs and symptoms, as well as to its potential interaction with any contemplated therapeutic regimen. Patients with active peptic ulcer should restrict their intake of both caffeine-containing and roasted-grain beverages. It is puzzling that a substance that can produce seizures in sufficient dosage is sometimes urged upon patients to counteract the sedative effects of anticonvulsant agents such as phenytoin (*see* Stephenson, 1977). In the absence of convincing evidence that caffeine does *not* reduce the effectiveness of phenytoin, it makes more sense to be suspicious of a possible interaction and to remove caffeine from the diet of patients who fail to respond adequately to therapeutic concentrations of phenytoin before proceeding to change the drug regimen.

There is little doubt that the popularity of the xanthine beverages depends on their stimulant action, although most people are unaware of any stimulation. The degree to which an individual is stimulated by a given amount of caffeine varies. For example, some persons boast of their ability to drink several cups of coffee in the evening and yet "sleep like a log." On the other hand, there are rare persons who are so sensitive to caffeine that even a single cup of coffee will cause a response bordering on the toxic.

Overindulgence in xanthine beverages may lead to a condition that might be considered one of chronic poisoning. Central nervous stimulation results in restlessness and disturbed sleep; myocardial stimulation is reflected in premature systoles and tachycardia. The essential oils of coffee may cause some gastrointestinal irritation, and diarrhea is a common symptom. The high tannin content of tea, on the other hand, is apt to cause constipation.

There is no doubt that a certain degree of tolerance (Colton *et al.,* 1968) and of psychic dependence (*i.e.,* habituation) develops to the xanthine beverages. This is probably true even in those individuals who do not partake to excess. However, the morning cup of coffee is so much a part of American and European dietary habit that one seldom looks upon its consumption as a drug habit. The feeling of well-being and the increased performance it affords, although possibly obtained at the expense of decreased efficiency later in the day, are experiences that few individuals would care to give up.

Aranda, J. V.; Sitar, D. S.; Parsons, W. D.; Loughman, P. M.; and Neims, A. H. Pharmacokinetic aspects of theophylline in premature newborns. *N. Engl. J. Med.,* **1976,** *295,* 413–416.

Arnman, K.; Carlström, S.; and Thorell, J. I. The effect of norepinephrine and theophylline on blood glucose, plasma FFA, plasma glycerol, and plasma insulin in normal subjects. *Acta Med. Scand.,* **1975,** *197,* 271–274.

Atuk, N. O.; Blaydes, M. C.; Westervelt, F. B.; and Wood, J. E. Effect of aminophylline on urinary excretion of epinephrine and norepinephrine in man. *Circulation,* **1967,** *35,* 745–753.

Aunis, D.; Mandel, P.; Miras-Portugal, M. T.; Coquillat, G.; Rohmer, F.; and Warter, J M. Changes of human plasma dopamine-beta-hydroxylase activity after intravenous administration of theophylline. *Br. J. Pharmacol.,* **1975,** *53,* 425–427.

Axelsson, J., and Thesleff, S. Activation of the contractile mechanism in striated muscle. *Acta Physiol. Scand.,* **1958,** *44,* 55–66.

Baxter, J. H. Histamine release from rat mast cells by dextran: effects of adrenergic agents, theophylline, and other drugs. *Proc. Soc. Exp. Biol. Med.,* **1972,** *141,* 576–581.

Beavo, J. A.; Rogers, N. L.; Crofford, O. B.; Hardman, J. G.; Sutherland, E. W.; and Newman, E. V. Effects of xanthine derivatives on lipolysis and on adenosine 3′,5′-monophosphate phosphodiesterase activity. *Mol. Pharmacol.,* **1970,** *6,* 597–603.

Bellet, S.; Feinberg, L. J.; Sandberg, H.; and Hirabayashi, M. The effects of caffeine on free fatty acids and blood coagulation parameters of dogs. *J. Pharmacol. Exp. Ther.,* **1968,** *159,* 250–254.

Bellville, J. W.; Escarraga, L. A.; Wallenstein, S. L.; Wang, K. C.; Howland, W. S.; and Houde, R. W. Antagonism by caffeine of the respiratory effects of codeine and morphine. *J. Pharmacol. Exp. Ther.,* **1962,** *136,* 38–42.

Berne, R. M., and Rubio, R. Regulation of coronary blood flow. *Adv. Cardiol.,* **1974,** *12,* 303–317.

Bertelli, A.; Bianchi, C.; and Beani, L. Interaction between β-adrenergic stimulant and phosphodiesterase inhibiting drugs on the bronchial muscle. *Experientia,* **1973,** *29,* 300–302.

Berthet, J.; Sutherland, E. W.; and Rall, T. W. The assay of glucagon and epinephrine with use of liver homogenates. *J. Biol. Chem.,* **1957,** *229,* 351–361.

Bieck, P. R.; Oates, J. A.; Robison, G. A.; and Adkins, R. B. Cyclic AMP in the regulation of gastric secretion in dogs and humans. *Am. J. Physiol.,* **1973,** *224,* 158–164.

Blinks, J. R.; Olson, C. B.; Jewell, B. R.; and Braveny, P. Influence of caffeine and other methylxanthines on mechanical properties of isolated mammalian heart muscle. Evidence for a dual mechanism of action. *Circ. Res.,* **1972,** *30,* 367–392.

Boatman, D. L.; Lewin, M. L.; Culp, D. A.; and Flocks, R. H. Pharmacologic evaluation of ureteral smooth muscle: a technique for monitoring ureteral peristalsis. *Invest. Urol.,* **1967,** *4,* 509–520.

Boutroy, M. J.; Monin, P.; Andre, M.; and Vert, P. Treatment with theophylline in near-miss sudden infant death. (Letter.) *Lancet,* **1978,** *1,* 1257.

Bowser, E. W.; Hargis, G. K.; Henderson, W. J.; and Williams, G. A. Parathyroid hormone secretion in the rat: effect of aminophylline. *Proc. Soc. Exp. Biol. Med.,* **1975,** *148,* 344–346.

Brodie, B. B.; Axelrod, J.; and Reichenthal, J. Metabolism of theophylline (1,3 dimethylxanthine) in man. *J. Biol. Chem.,* **1952,** *194,* 215–222.

Butcher, R. W., and Sutherland, E. W. Adenosine 3′,5′-phosphate in biological materials. *J. Biol. Chem.,* **1962,** *237,* 1244–1250.

Butsch, W. L.; McGowan, J. M.; and Walters, W. Clinical studies on influence of certain drugs in relation to biliary pain and to variations in intrabiliary pressure. *Surg. Gynecol. Obstet.,* **1936,** *63,* 451–456.

Cano, R.; Isenberg, J. I.; and Grossman, M. I. Cimetidine inhibits caffeine-stimulated gastric acid secretion in man. *Gastroenterology,* **1976,** *70,* 1055–1057.

Cohen, M. M.; Debas, H. T.; Holubitsky, I. B.; and Harrison, R. C. Caffeine and pentagastrin stimulation of human gastric secretion. *Gastroenterology,* **1971,** *61,* 440–444.

Cohen, S., and Booth, G. H. Gastric acid secretion and lower-esophageal-sphincter pressure in response to coffee and caffeine. *N. Engl. J. Med.,* **1975,** *293,* 897–899.

Cole, G. F., and Davies, D. P. Theophylline poisoning. *Br. Med. J.,* **1980,** *280,* 52.

Colton, T.; Gosselin, R. E.; and Smith, R. P. The tolerance of coffee drinkers to caffeine. *Clin. Pharmacol. Ther.,* **1968,** *9,* 31–39.

Cornish, H. H., and Christman, A. A. A study of the

metabolism of theobromine, theophylline, and caffeine in man. *J. Biol. Chem.,* **1957,** *228,* 315–323.

Davies, J. O., and Schock, N. W. The effect of theophylline ethylenediamine on renal function in controlled subjects and in patients with congestive heart failure. *J. Clin. Invest.,* **1949,** *28,* 1459–1468.

Dawber, T. R.; Kannell, W. B.; and Gordon, T. Coffee and cardiovascular disease. Observations from the Framingham Study. *N. Engl. J. Med.,* **1974,** *291,* 871–874.

Debas, H. T.; Cohen, M. M.; Holubitsky, I. B.; and Harrison, R. C. Caffeine-stimulated gastric acid and pepsin secretion: dose-response studies. *Scand. J. Gastroenterol.,* **1971,** *6,* 453–457.

Dietrich, J.; Krauss, A. N.; Reidenberg, M.; Drayer, D. E.; and Auld, P. A. M. Alterations in state in apneic preterm infants receiving theophylline. *Clin. Pharmacol. Ther.,* **1978,** *24,* 474–478.

Dimaio, V. J. M., and Garriott, J. C. Lethal caffeine poisoning in a child. *Forensic Sci.,* **1974,** *3,* 275–278.

Ehlers, S. M.; Zaske, D. E.; and Sawchuk, R. J. Massive theophylline overdose; rapid elimination by charcoal hemoperfusion. *J.A.M.A.,* **1978,** *240,* 474–475.

Feurle, G.; Arnold, R.; Helmstädter, V.; and Creutzfeldt, W. The effect of intravenous theophylline ethylenediamine on serum gastrin concentration in control subjects and patients with duodenal ulcers and Zollinger-Ellison syndrome. *Digestion,* **1976,** *14,* 227–231.

Firestone, P.; Poitras-Wright, H.; and Douglas, V. The effects of caffeine on hyperactive children. *J. Learn. Disabil.,* **1978,** *11,* 133–141.

Foltz, E.; Ivy, A. C.; and Barborka, C. J. The use of double work periods in the study of fatigue and the influence of caffeine on recovery. *Am. J. Physiol.,* **1942,** *136,* 79–86.

Foote, W. E.; Holmes, P.; Pritchard, A.; Hatcher, C.; and Mordes, J. Neurophysiological and pharmacodynamic studies on caffeine and on interactions between caffeine and nicotinic acid in the rat. *Neuropharmacology,* **1978,** *17,* 7–12.

Foster, R. W. The nature of the adrenergic receptors of the trachea of the guinea pig. *J. Pharm. Pharmacol.,* **1966,** *18,* 1–12.

Gabrys, B. F.; Nyhus, L. M.; Van Meter, S. W.; and Bombeck, C. T. The effect of aminophylline on pentagastrin-induced gastric secretion in the dog. *Am. J. Dig. Dis.,* **1973,** *18,* 563–566.

Galant, S. P.; Groncy, C. F.; Duriseti, S.; and Strick, L. The effect of metaproterenol in chronic asthmatic children receiving therapeutic doses of theophylline. *J. Allergy Clin. Immunol.,* **1978,** *61,* 73–79.

Garst, J. E.; Kramer, G. L.; Wu, Y. J.; and Wells, J. N. Inhibition of separated forms of phosphodiesterases from pig coronary arteries by uracils and by 7-substituted derivatives of 1-methyl-3-isobutylxanthine. *J. Med. Chem.,* **1976,** *19,* 499–503.

Goffart, M., and Ritchie, J. M. The effect of adrenaline on the contraction of mammalian skeletal muscle. *J. Physiol. (Lond.),* **1952,** *116,* 357–371.

Goldberg, A. L., and Singer, J. J. Evidence for a role of cyclic AMP in neuromuscular transmission. *Proc. Natl. Acad. Sci. U.S.A.,* **1969,** *64,* 134–140.

Goldstein, A.; Kaizer, S.; and Warren, R. Psychotropic effects of caffeine in man. II. Alertness, psychomotor coordination, and mood. *J. Pharmacol. Exp. Ther.,* **1965,** *150,* 146–151.

Goodsell, E. B.; Stein, H. H.; and Wenzke, K. J. 8-Substituted theophyllines. *In vitro* inhibition of 3',5'-cyclic adenosine monophosphate phosphodiesterase and pharmacological spectrum in mice. *J. Med. Chem.,* **1971,** *14,* 1202–1205.

Grossman, M. I.; Roth, J. A.; and Ivy, A. C. Pepsin secretion in response to caffeine. *Gastroenterology,* **1945,** *4,* 251–256.

Grubb, M. N., and Burks, T. F. Selective antagonism of the intestinal stimulatory effects of morphine by isopro-

terenol, prostaglandin E$_1$, and theophylline. *J. Pharmacol. Exp. Ther.,* **1975,** *193,* 883–891.

Haldi, J.; Bachman, G.; Ensor, C.; and Wynn, W. The effect of various amounts of caffeine on the gaseous exchange and the respiratory quotient in man. *J. Nutr.,* **1941,** *21,* 307–320.

Hedqvist, P.; Fredholm, B. B.; and Ölundh, S. Antagonistic effects of theophylline and adenosine on adrenergic neuroeffector transmission in the rabbit kidney. *Circ. Res.,* **1978,** *43,* 592–598.

Hendeles, L.; Weinberger, M.; and Bighley, L. Disposition of theophylline after a single intravenous infusion of aminophylline. *Am. Rev. Respir. Dis.,* **1978,** *118,* 97–103.

Hennekens, C. H.; Drolette, M. E.; Jesse, M. J.; Davies, J. E.; and Hutchison, G. B. Coffee drinking and death due to coronary heart disease. *N. Engl. J. Med.,* **1976,** *294,* 633–636.

Huidobro, F. A comparative study of the effectiveness of 1,3,7 trimethylxanthine and certain dimethylxanthines (1,3 dimethylxanthine and 3,7 dimethylxanthine) against fatigue. *J. Pharmacol. Exp. Ther.,* **1945,** *84,* 380–386.

Huidobro, F., and Amenbar, E. Effectiveness of caffeine (1,3,7 trimethylxanthine) against fatigue. *J. Pharmacol. Exp. Ther.,* **1945,** *84,* 82–92.

Iso, T. Effects of cyclic 3',5'-AMP and related compounds on catecholamine-induced contractions of isolated guinea-pig vas deferens. *Jpn. J. Pharmacol.,* **1973,** *23,* 717–721.

Jacobs, M. H.; Senior, R. M.; and Kessler, G. Clinical experience with theophylline: relationships between dosage, serum concentration, and toxicity. *J.A.M.A.,* **1976,** *235,* 1983–1986.

James, G. W. L. The role of the adrenal glands and of α- and β-adrenergic receptors in bronchodilatation of guinea-pig lungs *in vivo. J. Pharm. Pharmacol.,* **1967,** *19,* 797–802.

Jick, J.; Miettinen, O. S.; Neff, R. K.; Shapiro, S.; Heinonen, O. P.; and Slone, D. Coffee and myocardial infarction. *N. Engl. J. Med.,* **1973,** *289,* 63–67.

Kakiuchi, S.; Rall, T. W.; and McIlwain, H. The effect of electrical stimulation upon the accumulation of adenosine 3',5'-phosphate in isolated cerebral tissue. *J. Neurochem.,* **1969,** *16,* 485–491.

Kalsner, S. Mechanism of potentiation of contractor responses to catecholamines by methylxanthines in aortic strips. *Br. J. Pharmacol.,* **1971,** *43,* 379–388.

Kalsner, S.; Frew, R. D.; and Smith, G. M. Mechanism of methylxanthine sensitization of norepinephrine responses in a coronary artery. *Am. J. Physiol.,* **1975,** *228,* 1702–1707.

Karasawa, T.; Furukawa, K.; Yoshida, K.; and Shimizu, M. Effect of theophylline on monoamine metabolism in the rat brain. *Eur. J. Pharmacol.,* **1976,** *37,* 97–104.

Katz, A. M.; Repke, D. I.; and Hasselbach, W. Dependence of ionophore- and caffeine-induced calcium release from sarcoplasmic reticulum vesicles on external and internal calcium ion concentrations. *J. Biol. Chem.,* **1977,** *252,* 1938–1949.

Klatsky, A. L.; Friedman, G. D.; and Siegelaub, A. B. Coffee drinking prior to acute myocardial infarction. Results from the Kaiser-Permanente epidemiologic study of myocardial infarction. *J.A.M.A.,* **1973,** *226,* 540–543.

Kordash, T. R.; Van Dellen, R. G.; and McCall, J. T. Theophylline concentrations in asthmatic patients after administration of aminophylline. *J.A.M.A.,* **1977,** *238,* 139–141.

Krasnow, S., and Grossman, M. I. Stimulation of gastric secretion in man by theophylline ethylenediamine. *Proc. Soc. Exp. Biol. Med.,* **1949,** *71,* 335–336.

Kuzemko, J. A., and Paala, J. Apnoeic attacks in the newborn treated with aminophylline. *Arch. Dis. Child.,* **1973,** *48,* 404–406.

Lammerant, J., and Becsei, I. Inhibition of pacing-induced

coronary dilation by aminophylline. *Cardiovasc. Res.,* **1975,** *9,* 532–537.

Leung, P.; Kalisker, A.; and Bell, T. D. Variation in theophylline clearance rate with time in chronic childhood asthma. *J. Allergy Clin. Immunol.,* **1977,** *59,* 440–444.

Lillehei, J. P. Aminophylline. Oral vs. rectal administration. *J.A.M.A.,* **1968,** *205,* 530–533.

Lowder, S. C.; Frazer, M. G.; and Liddle, G. W. Effect of insulin-induced hypoglycemia upon plasma renin activity in man. *J. Clin. Endocrinol. Metab.,* **1975,** *41,* 97–105.

Lowder, S. C.; Hamet, P.; and Liddle, G. W. Contrasting effects of hypoglycemia on plasma renin activity and cyclic adenosine 3′,5′-monophosphate (cyclic AMP) in low renin and normal renin essential hypertension. *Circ. Res.,* **1976,** *38,* 105–108.

Marcus, M. L.; Skelton, C. L.; Grauer, L. E.; and Epstein, S. E. Effects of theophylline on myocardial mechanics. *Am. J. Physiol.,* **1972,** *222,* 1361–1365.

Maren, T. H. The additive renal effect of oral aminophylline and trichlormethiazide in man. *Clin. Res.,* **1961,** *9,* 57.

Marquardt, D. L.; Parker, C. W.; and Sullivan, T. J. Potentiation of mast cell mediator release by adenosine. *J. Immunol.,* **1978,** *120,* 871–878.

Means, J. H.; Aub, J. C.; and DuBois, E. F. The effect of caffeine on heat production. *Arch. Intern. Med.,* **1917,** *19,* 832–839.

Mitznegg, P.; Schubert, E.; and Heim, F. The influence of low and high doses of theophylline on spontaneous motility and cyclic 3′,5′ AMP content in isolated rat uterus. *Life Sci.,* **1974,** *14,* 711–717.

Moyer, J. H.; Miller, S. I.; Tashnek, A. B.; and Bowman, R. The effect of theophylline with ethylenediamine (aminophylline) on cerebral hemodynamics in the presence of cardiac failure with and without Cheyne-Stokes respiration. *J. Clin. Invest.,* **1952a,** *31,* 267–272.

Moyer, J. H.; Tashnek, A. B.; Miller, S. I.; Snyder, H.; and Bowman, R. O. The effect of theophylline with ethylenediamine (aminophylline) and caffeine on cerebral hemodynamics and cerebrospinal fluid pressure in patients with hypertension headaches. *Am. J. Med. Sci.,* **1952b,** *224,* 377–385.

Ogilvie, R. I.; Fernandez, P. G.; and Winsberg, F. Cardiovascular response to increasing theophylline concentrations. *Eur. J. Clin. Pharmacol.,* **1977,** *12,* 409–414.

Öhnell, H., and Berg, H. Zur Frage über die Ventrikelfunktion nach verabreichung verschiedener Arten von Kaffee. *Acta Med. Scand.,* **1931,** *76,* 491–520.

Paalzow, G., and Paalzow, L. K. The effects of caffeine and theophylline on nociceptive stimulation in the rat. *Acta Pharmacol. Toxicol.* (Kbh.), **1973,** *32,* 22–32.

Paalzow, L. K. Pharmacokinetics of theophylline in relation to increased pain sensitivity in the rat. *J. Pharmacokinet. Biopharm.,* **1975,** *3,* 25–38.

Peach, M. J. Stimulation of release of adrenal catecholamine by adenosine 3′,5′-cyclic monophosphate and theophylline in the absence of extracellular Ca^{2+}. *Proc. Natl. Acad. Sci. U.S.A.,* **1972,** *69,* 834–836.

Persson, C. G. A., and Andersson, K.-E. Respiratory and cardiovascular effects of 3-methylxanthine, a metabolite of theophylline. *Acta Pharmacol. Toxicol.* (Kbh.), **1977,** *40,* 529–536.

Pfaffman, M. A., and McFarland, S. A. Relationship between theophylline-induced relaxation and excitation-contraction coupling in intestinal smooth muscle. *Arch. Int. Pharmacodyn. Ther.,* **1978,** *232,* 180–191.

Piafsky, K. M.; Sitar, D. S.; Rango, R. E.; and Ogilvie, R. I. Theophylline kinetics in acute pulmonary edema. *Clin. Pharmacol. Ther.,* **1977,** *21,* 310–316.

Rall, T. W.; Sutherland, E. W.; and Berthet, J. The relation of epinephrine and glucagon to liver phosphorylase. IV. Effect of epinephrine and glucagon on the reactivation of phosphorylase in liver homogenates. *J. Biol. Chem.,* **1957,** *224,* 463–475.

Rall, T. W., and West, T. C. The potentiation of cardiac inotropic responses to norepinephrine by theophylline. *J. Pharmacol. Exp. Ther.,* **1963,** *139,* 269–274.

Reichard, C. C., and Elder, S. T. The effects of caffeine on reaction time in hyperkinetic and normal children. *Am. J. Psychiatry,* **1977,** *134,* 144–148.

Robertson, D.; Jürgen, C.; Frölich, M. D.; Carr, R. K.; Watson, J. T.; Hollifield, J. W.; Shand, D. G.; and Oates, J. A. Effects of caffeine on plasma renin activity, catecholamines and blood pressure. *N. Engl. J. Med.,* **1978,** *298,* 181–186.

Roth, J. A., and Ivy, A. C. The synergistic effect of caffeine upon histamine in relation to gastric secretion. *Am. J. Physiol.,* **1944,** *142,* 107–113.

Sattin, A., and Rall, T. W. The effect of adenosine and adenine nucleotides on the adenosine 3′,5′-phosphate content of guinea pig cerebral cortex slices. *Mol. Pharmacol.,* **1970,** *6,* 13–23.

Sawynok, J., and Jhamandas, K. H. Inhibition of acetylcholine release from cholinergic nerves by adenosine, adenine nucleotides and morphine: antagonism by theophylline. *J. Pharmacol. Exp. Ther.,* **1976,** *197,* 379–390.

Schnackenberg, R. Caffeine as a substitute for schedule II stimulants in hyperkinetic children. *Am. J. Psychiatry,* **1973,** *130,* 796–798.

Serrano-Ríos, M.; Hawkins, F. G.; Esobar-Jiménez, F.; and Rodriguez-Miñón, J. L. The effect of aminophylline on insulin release induced by secretin and cholecystokinin-pancreozymin in normal humans. *J. Clin. Endocrinol. Metab.,* **1974,** *38,* 194–199.

Shannon, D. C.; Gotay, F.; Stein, I. M.; Rogers, M. C.; Todres, I. D.; and Moylan, F. M. B. Prevention of apnea and bradycardia in low-birthweight infants. *Pediatrics,* **1975,** *55,* 589–594.

Sigurd, B., and Olesen, K. H. Comparative naturetic and diuretic efficacy of theophylline ethylenediamine and of bendroflumethiazide during long-term treatment with the potent diuretic bumetanide. *Acta Med. Scand.,* **1978,** *203,* 113–119.

Simons, F. E. R.; Simons, K. J.; and Bierman, C. W. The pharmacokinetics of dihydroxypropyltheophylline: a basis for rational therapy. *J. Allergy Clin. Immunol.,* **1975,** *56,* 347–355.

Somers, G.; Devis, G.; Van Obberghen, E.; and Malaisse, W. J. Calcium antagonists and islet function. II. Interaction of theophylline and verapamil. *Endocrinology,* **1976,** *99,* 114–124.

Starr, I.; Gamble, C. F.; Margolies, A.; Donal, J. S.; Joseph, N.; and Eagle, E. A clinical study of the action of 10 commonly used drugs on cardiac output, work and size; on respiration, on metabolic rate and on the electrocardiogram. *J. Clin. Invest.,* **1937,** *16,* 799–823.

Stephenson, P. E. Physiologic and psychotropic effects of caffeine on man. *J. Am. Diet. Assoc.,* **1977,** *71,* 240–247.

Stroud, M. W.; Lambertsen, C. J.; Ewing, J. H.; Kough, R. H.; Gould, R. A.; and Schmidt, C. F. The effects of aminophylline and meperidine alone and in combination on the respiratory response to carbon dioxide inhalation. *J. Pharmacol. Exp. Ther.,* **1955,** *114,* 461–469.

Sutherland, E. W., and Rall, T. W. Fractionation and characterization of a cyclic adenine ribonucleotide formed by tissue particles. *J. Biol. Chem.,* **1958,** *232,* 1077–1091.

Thompson, R. D.; Nagasawa, H. T.; and Jenne, J. W. Determination of theophylline and its metabolites in human urine and serum by high-pressure liquid chromatography. *J. Lab. Clin. Med.,* **1974,** *84,* 584–593.

Truitt, E. B., Jr.; McKusick, V. A.; and Krantz, J. C. Theophylline blood levels after oral, rectal, and intravenous administration, and correlation with diuretic action. *J. Pharmacol. Exp. Ther.,* **1950,** *100,* 309–315.

Vinegar, R.; Truax, J. F.; Selph, J. L.; Welch, R. M.; and White, H. L. Potentiation of the anti-inflammatory and analgesic activity of aspirin by caffeine in the rat. *Proc. Soc. Exp. Biol. Med.,* **1976,** *151,* 556–560.

Weathersbee, P. S.; Olsen, L. K.; and Lodge, J. R. Caffeine and pregnancy: a retrospective study. *Postgrad. Med.*, **1977**, *62,* 64–69.

Wechsler, R. L.; Kleiss, L. M.; and Kety, S. S. The effects of intravenously administered aminophylline on cerebral circulation and metabolism in man. *J. Clin. Invest.*, **1950**, *29,* 28–30.

Wein, A. J.; Gregory, J. G.; Sansone, T. C.; and Schoenberg, H. W. The effects of aminophylline on ureteral and bladder contractility. *Invest. Urol.*, **1972**, *9,* 290–293.

Weinberger, M., and Ginchansky, E. Dose-dependent kinetics of theophylline disposition in asthmatic children. *J. Pediatr.*, **1977**, *91,* 820–824.

Weinberger, M.; Hendeles, L.; and Bighley, L. The relation of product formulation to absorption of oral theophylline. *N. Engl. J. Med.*, **1978**, *299,* 852–857.

Weinberger, M.; Hudgel, D.; Spector, S.; and Chidsey, C. Inhibition of theophylline clearance by troleandomycin. *J. Allergy Clin. Immunol.*, **1977**, *59,* 228–231.

Williams, J. F.; Lowitt, S.; Polson, J. B.; and Szentivanyi, A. Pharmacological and biochemical activities of some monomethylxanthines and methyluric acid derivatives of theophylline and caffeine. *Biochem. Pharmacol.*, **1978**, *27,* 1545–1550.

Wolfe, J. D.; Tashkin, D. P.; Calvarese, B.; and Simmons, M. Bronchodilator effects of terbutaline and aminophylline alone and in combination in asthmatic patients. *N. Engl. J. Med.*, **1978**, *298,* 363–367.

Yarnell, P. R., and Chu, N-S. Focal seizures and aminophylline. *Neurology (Minneap.)*, **1975**, *25,* 819–822.

Zehner, J.; Klaus, D.; Klumpp, F.; and Lemke, R. The influence of propranolol, practolol, and theophylline on the plasma renin activity. *Res. Exp. Med. (Berl.)*, **1975**, *166,* 275–282.

Ziment, I., and Steen, S. N. Synergism of metaproterenol and theophylline. *Chest*, **1978**, *73,* Suppl. 6, 1016–1017.

Zwillich, C. W.; Sutton, F. D.; Neff, T. A.; Cohn, W. M.; Matthay, R. A.; and Weinberger, M. M. Theophylline-induced seizures in adults: correlation with serum concentrations. *Ann. Intern. Med.*, **1975**, *82,* 784–787.

Monographs and Reviews

Berne, R. M. Regulation of coronary blood flow. *Physiol. Rev.*, **1964**, *44,* 1–27.

Bianchi, C. P. Pharmacological actions on excitation-contraction coupling in striated muscle. *Fed. Proc.*, **1968**, *27,* 126–131.

————. Cellular pharmacology of contraction of skeletal muscle. In, *Cellular Pharmacology of Excitable Tissues.* (Narahashi, T., ed.) Charles C Thomas, Pub., Springfield, Ill., **1975**.

Burnstock, G. Purinergic nerves. *Pharmacol. Rev.*, **1972**, *24,* 509–581.

Cohn, J. N., and Franciosa, J. A. Vasodilator therapy of cardiac failure. (Second of two parts.) *N. Engl. J. Med.*, **1977**, *297,* 254–258.

Fishman, A. P. State of the art—chronic cor pulmonale. *Am. Rev. Respir. Dis.*, **1976**, *114,* 775–794.

Graham, D. M. Caffeine—its identity, dietary sources, intake and biological effects. *Nutr. Rev.*, **1978**, *36,* 97–102.

Jacobson, E. D., and Thompson, W. J. Cyclic AMP and gastric secretion: the illusive second messenger. In, *Advances in Cyclic Nucleotide Research*, Vol. 7. (Greengard, P., and Robison, G. A., eds.) Raven Press, New York, **1976**, pp. 199–224. (125 references.)

Robison, G. A.; Butcher, R. W.; and Sutherland, E. W. *Cyclic AMP.* Academic Press, Inc., New York, **1971**.

Sutherland, E. W.; Robison, G. A.; and Butcher, R. W. Some aspects of the biological role of adenosine 3′,5′-monophosphate (cyclic AMP). *Circulation*, **1968**, *37,* 279–306.

Symposium. (Various authors.) *Physiological and Regulatory Functions of Adenosine and Adenine Nucleotides.* (Baer, H. P., and Drummond, G. I., eds.) Raven Press, New York, **1978**.

Timson, J. Caffeine. *Mutat. Res.*, **1977**, *47,* 1–52.

Webb-Johnson, D. C., and Andrews, J. L., Jr. Bronchodilator therapy. *N. Engl. J. Med.*, **1977**, *297,* 476–482, 758–764.

Weinberger, M. Theophylline for treatment of asthma. *J. Pediatr.*, **1978**, *92,* 1–17.

Autacoids

INTRODUCTION

William W. Douglas

Assembled for consideration in this section are a number of substances with widely differing structures and pharmacological activities; although disparate in these respects, they are grouped together here because they have in common a natural occurrence in the body. At the same time, the opportunity is taken to discuss drugs antagonizing their actions, wherever such drugs are available. The oldest and most familiar substances in the group, *histamine* and the histamine antagonists, are dealt with in Chapter 26. The same chapter is concerned with another endogenous amine, *5-hydroxytryptamine (5-HT, serotonin, enteramine)*, and its antagonists. Chapter 27 is devoted to the polypeptides—*angiotensin, bradykinin, kallidin,* and others. Chapter 28 is concerned with *prostaglandins* and other derivatives of arachidonic acid. The section thus includes a motley of substances of intense pharmacological activity that are normally present in the body or may be formed there, and that cannot conveniently be classed with other members of this broad group, such as the neurohumors and hormones. These different substances have been variously described as *local hormones, autopharmacological agents,* and the like; but a generic term that is at once shorter, more accurate, and euphonious is *autacoid,* a word derived from the Greek *autos* ("self") and *akos* ("medicinal agent" or "remedy"). This term was devised by Sir Edward Schäfer (1916), later Sharpey-Schafer, as a substitute for Starling's word *hormone,* which, being derived from the Greek *hormaein* (meaning "to stir up"), is a misnomer for the inhibitory substances that also came to be embraced by this designation. However, Starling's term *hormone,* albeit unsatisfactory from the etymological standpoint, has won the day, and Schäfer's has passed into limbo. Such a good word deserves a better fate, and hence its revival here. Most of the substances described in this section can probably lay claim to the title without distortion of its sense.

What of the significance of this group of autacoids? What is their role in the body? What is their value as drugs and what is their place in therapeutics? Unfortunately, only rather imprecise answers can be given to these questions. The very fact that the substances have been classified under the noncommittal title of *autacoids* is, in a sense, a confession that the evidence does not at present permit a more precise functional classification such as, for example, hormone or neurohumor. This is not to say that such functions are foreign to the autacoids. On the contrary, as the evidence concerning their possible roles in the body is unfolded, it will be apparent to the reader that both such functions may be displayed by the substances under consideration. But the core of the matter is that, while the autacoids possess an astonishingly wide range of pharmacological activities and in vanishingly small amounts, there are comparatively few instances where a physiological role can be stated with assurance. After the example of Pirandello, who named one of his plays *Six Characters in Search of an Author,* the present section might well have been entitled "Various Autacoids in Search of a Function." The problem, as will become clear from what follows, is not so much with a dearth of hypotheses as with a surfeit of them. But while scientists dispute the rival claims of the different hypotheses, there is general agreement that each of the autacoids to be discussed is of importance in the body's economy. All are agents that the body employs in the execution of various functions in health and disease; they are clearly part and parcel of the physiological and pathological phenomena that provide the rationale for drug therapy; and their existence provides numerous possibilities for therapeutic intervention by the use of drugs that mimic or antagonize their action or interfere in one way or another with their metabolism. Together these facts thrust the autacoids squarely to the center of interest for those who are concerned with the pharmacological basis of therapeutics.

CHAPTER

26 HISTAMINE AND 5-HYDROXYTRYPTAMINE (SEROTONIN) AND THEIR ANTAGONISTS

William W. Douglas

HISTAMINE

History. The history of β-aminoethylimidazole, or histamine, shows several close parallels with that of acetylcholine (ACh). Both compounds were synthesized as chemical curiosities before their biological significance was recognized; both were first detected as uterine stimulants in extracts of ergot, from which they were subsequently isolated; and both proved to be casual contaminants of ergot, resulting from bacterial action.

When Dale and Laidlaw (1910, 1911) subjected histamine to intensive pharmacological study, they discovered, *inter alia*, that it stimulated a host of smooth muscles and had an intense vasodepressor action. With rare acumen they drew attention to the observation that the pharmacological activity of histamine resembled that of many tissue extracts and, further, that the immediate symptoms with which an animal responds to an injection of a normally inert protein, to which it has been sensitized, are to a large extent those of poisoning by β-aminoethylimidazole (histamine). Their prescient comments anticipated by many years the events that were to thrust histamine to the center of physiological interest, namely, the discovery of its occurrence in the body and its release during hypersensitivity (allergic) reactions and upon cellular injury. Although histamine had been identified chemically in tissue extracts previously, it was suspected that it might have arisen from putrefaction. It was not until 1927 that Best, Dale, Dudley, and Thorpe isolated histamine from impeccably fresh samples of liver and lung, thereby establishing beyond doubt that this amine is a natural constituent of the body. Demonstrations of its presence in a variety of other tissues soon followed—hence the name *histamine* after the Greek word for tissue, *histos*.

Meanwhile, Lewis and his colleagues, in a series of brilliant experiments, had amassed evidence that a substance with the properties of histamine ("H-substance") was liberated from the cells of the skin by injurious stimuli, including the union of antigen and antibody (Lewis, 1927). Given the chemical evidence of histamine's presence in the body, there remained little impediment to supposing that Lewis' "H substance" was histamine itself. This conception was advanced with telling force by Dale in his Croonian lectures of 1929 and stimulated the growth of interest in histamine to a rare luxuriance. Now, half a century later, it is evident that endogenous histamine is involved in diverse physiological processes quite apart from allergic reactions and injury. Thus, histamine clearly participates in the physiological regulation of gastric secretion, and there are strong indications that it serves as a chemical transmitter or modulator within the brain. Early suspicions that histamine acts through more than one receptor (Folkow *et al.,* 1948; Furchgott, 1955) have now been borne out, and it is clear that two distinct subclasses of histamine receptor exist, H_1 (Ash and Schild, 1966) and H_2 (Black *et al.,* 1972). The former type of receptor is blocked selectively by the classical "antihistamines" (such as pyrilamine) developed around 1940 and the latter by the H_2-blocking drugs introduced in the early 1970s. The discovery of H_2 antagonists has contributed enormously to the current resurgent interest in histamine in biology and clinical medicine.

Chemistry. Histamine is 2-(4-imidazolyl)ethylamine (or β-aminoethylimidazole). It may be formed by decarboxylation of the amino acid histidine, a reaction effected by the enzyme L-histidine decarboxylase (Figure 26–1, page 618).

There are many drugs with histamine-like properties, and most contain the following fragment:

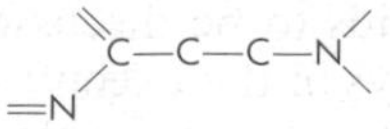

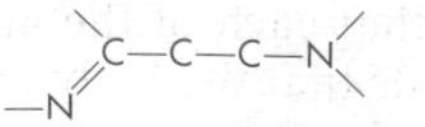

However, there are a number of exceptions, and one can say only that compounds with appreciable histamine-like activity generally consist of small, nitrogen-containing heterocyclic rings to which are attached 2-aminoethyl side chains. Among the histamine analogs there is a striking lack of correlation between their action on gastric secretion and their other histamine-like actions. This reflects the existence of two subclasses of receptor for the amine, termed H_1 and H_2, that show different structural requirements for both binding and activation. Structure-activity relationships are discussed by Durant and coworkers (1975, 1977).

PHARMACOLOGICAL EFFECTS:
H_1 AND H_2 RECEPTORS

Histamine contracts many smooth muscles, such as those of the bronchi and gut, but powerfully relaxes others, including those of fine blood vessels. It is also a very potent stimulus to gastric acid production and elicits various other exocrine secretions. Effects attributable to these actions dominate the overall response to the drug; however, there are several others, of which edema formation and stimulation of sensory nerve endings are perhaps the most familiar. Some of these effects, such as bronchoconstriction and contraction of the gut, are mediated by one type of histamine receptor, the H_1 receptors (Ash and Schild, 1966), which are readily blocked by pyrilamine and other such classical antihistamines, now more properly described as histamine H_1-receptor blocking drugs or simply H_1 blockers. Other effects, most notably gastric secretion, are completely refractory to such antagonists, involve activation of H_2 receptors, and are susceptible to inhibition by newly developed histamine H_2-receptor blocking drugs (Black *et al.*, 1972). Still others, such as the hypotension resulting from vascular dilatation, are mediated by receptors of both H_1 and H_2 types, and are annulled only by a combination of H_1 and H_2 blockers.

The two classes of histamine receptors also reveal themselves by differential responses to various histamine-like agonists. Thus, 2-methylhistamine preferentially elicits responses mediated by H_1 receptors, whereas 4-methylhistamine has a correspondingly preferential effect mediated through H_2 re-

ceptors (Black *et al.*, 1972). These compounds are representatives of two newly recognized classes of histamine-like drugs, the H_1- and H_2-receptor agonists. The structures of some are indicated in Table 26–1. The availability of these H_1 and H_2 agonists and of the corresponding antagonists has greatly enriched understanding of the pharmacology and physiology of histamine and has allowed new therapeutic approaches. This is reflected in a recent handbook edited by Rocha e Silva (1978a) (*see also* Rocha e Silva, 1966; Chand and Eyre, 1975; Symposium, 1977a, 1978a; Beaven, 1978; Hirschowitz, 1979).

Table 26–1. STRUCTURE OF HISTAMINE AND PROTOTYPICAL AGONISTS THAT ACT AT H_1 AND H_2 RECEPTORS

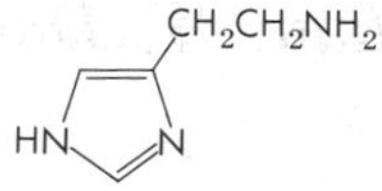

Histamine

Histamine H_1-Receptor Agonists

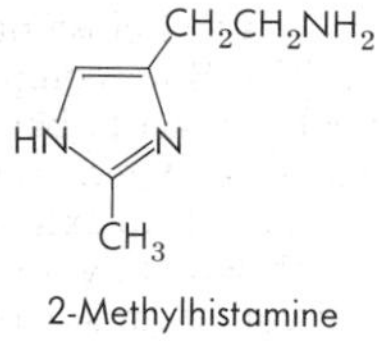

2-Methylhistamine

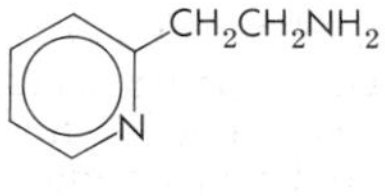

2-(2-Pyridyl)ethylamine

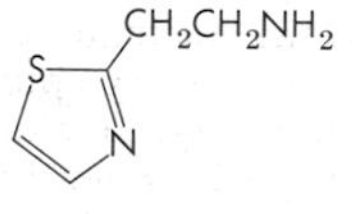

2-(2-Thiazolyl)ethylamine

Histamine H_2-Receptor Agonists

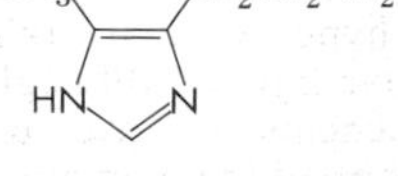

4-Methylhistamine

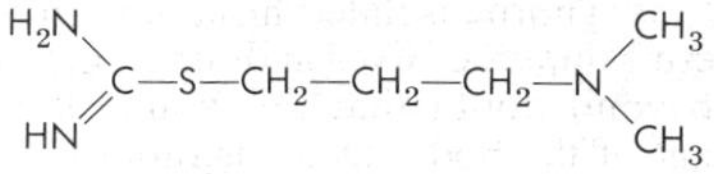

Dimaprit

Cardiovascular System. Histamine in man and most other animals characteristically exerts a predominantly dilator effect on the vasculature that involves the finer blood vessels; this results in flushing, lowered total peripheral resistance, and a fall in systemic blood pressure. In addition, histamine tends to increase capillary permeability. Its effects on the heart are generally less important.

Significant species differences in the cardiovascular responses became evident in the earliest studies performed by Dale and Laidlaw, who observed that histamine rapidly lowered blood pressure in dogs and cats (as it does in man) but that it had a biphasic effect on blood pressure in rabbits, causing a prominent rise before the fall. From their analysis Dale and Laidlaw (1919) concluded that histamine has two opposite actions on the blood vessels, dilatation, involving the finer vessels and tending to lower blood pressure, and vasoconstriction, involving somewhat larger vessels and tending to have the opposite effect. The tendency for the latter to predominate in rabbits and other rodents under certain conditions explained the pressor responses. Later, Dale (1929) pointed out that the response of arterioles changes as one ascends the zoological scale. The predominant effect in rodents is strong arterial constriction; in cats, slight constriction; and in the dog, monkey, and man, arteriolar dilatation. Even in this last group, however, where dilatation of the finer vessels dominates the overall response, some constrictor effects can be discerned in certain vessels and particular vascular beds. The overall response, nevertheless, is vasodilatation and fall in blood pressure mediated by both H_1 and H_2 receptors. Extensive reviews on the cardiovascular actions of histamine and the involvement of the different receptors are available (*see* Rocha e Silva, 1966, 1978a; Owen, 1977).

"Capillary" Dilatation. This is the most characteristic action of histamine on the vascular tree and by far the most important in man. It results from a direct action of histamine on the blood vessels mediated by both H_1 and H_2 receptors and is thus independent of innervation. Most regions in the body are involved, but the response following parenteral injection in man is most obvious in the skin of the face and upper part of the body, the so-called blushing area, which becomes hot and flushed.

Increased "Capillary" Permeability. This is the second of the classical effects of histamine on the fine vessels and results in outward passage of plasma protein and fluid into the extracellular spaces, an increase in the flow of lymph and its protein content, and formation of edema. H_1 receptors are clearly important for this response; participation of H_2 receptors is uncertain.

While it is traditional to ascribe these effects to an action of histamine on "capillaries," it should be understood that, when so used, the word is a generic term for the vessels of the microcirculation. Neither the fall in resistance nor the increase in permeability following histamine is attributable to the very finest vessels that are capillaries in the most rigorous morphological sense and devoid of smooth muscle. *Dilator responses* are mainly attributable to inhibitory effects of histamine on the smooth muscle of somewhat larger vessels of the microcirculation—the metarterioles, arterioles, and precapillary sphincters upstream, and the muscular venules downstream. Such dilatation as occurs in the smallest postcapillary venules, devoid of smooth muscle, seems to be mainly passive, due both to the fall in resistance upstream (and increased blood flow) and to a rise in pressure in larger veins, which histamine tends to constrict. Within the microcirculation, vessels larger than about 80 μm, both arterioles and venules, tend to constrict in response to histamine, and these effects are mainly mediated by H_1 receptors.

Increased permeability results mainly from actions of histamine on postcapillary venules, mostly those of about 20 to 30 μm in diameter, where histamine causes the endothelial cells to separate at their boundaries and thus to expose the basement membrane, which is freely permeable to plasma protein and fluid. The gaps between endothelial cells may also permit passage of particles such as platelets or injected colloidal drugs and dyes that become trapped between the cells and the basement membrane. Although the separation of the endothelial cells is doubtless favored by the dilatation of the small venules, it is not the primary cause. Rather, the endothelial cells seem to contract actively and shrink in response to histamine. An additional factor favoring increased transcapillary movement of fluid and macromolecules may be increased transcapillary vesicular transport (*see* Majno *et al.,* 1969; Altura and Halevy, 1978).

Triple Response. When histamine is injected intradermally, the above actions combine with a third to produce a characteristic triad of phenomena known as the "triple response" (Lewis, 1927). This is comprised of the following: (1) a localized red spot, extending for a few millimeters around the site of injection, appearing within a few seconds, reaching a maximum in about a minute, and soon acquiring a bluish tint; this results from the direct, vasodilatory effect of histamine on the minute blood vessels; (2) a brighter red flush or "flare," of irregular outline, extending about 1 cm or so beyond the original red spot and developing more slowly; this is due to histamine-induced axon reflexes that cause vasodilatation indirectly; and (3) a wheal that is discernible in 1 to 2 minutes and occupies the same area as the original small red spot at the injection site; this reflects histamine's effect to increase "capillary" permeability, thereby causing edema.

Heart. Histamine increases both the rate and force of myocardial contraction as well as cardiac output. It also tends to slow A-V conduction and, especially in high concentrations, may cause various arrhythmias. H_2 receptors seem largely responsible for positive chronotropic effects, participate (along with H_1 receptors) in the positive inotropic effects, and contribute importantly to the arrhythmias. Slowed A-V conduction mainly involves H_1 receptors. In addition to direct actions on cardiac tissue, histamine also appears to stimulate sympathetic nerve endings to release norepinephrine and thus elicits indirect effects.

In the intact animal given conventional doses of histamine, direct cardiac effects of histamine are not prominent and tend to be overshadowed by baroreceptor reflexes elicited by the reduced blood pressure, which stimulate heart rate and force through enhanced sympathetic outflow. Such effects, coupled with some constriction of the large veins and augmented venous return, may cause a prompt but transient rise in cardiac output; thereafter, cardiac output is generally little altered or may even fall as blood pools in the periphery.

Blood Pressure. Only small depressor responses to histamine are effectively inhibited by H_1 antagonists, which have only modest effects on responses to larger doses of the autacoid. The residual effects can, however, be blocked by adding an H_2 blocker. Thus, both H_1 and H_2 receptors are involved (*see* Owen, 1977).

An interestingly different pattern is observed in the rabbit, where the response of the systemic blood pressure to large doses of histamine is biphasic in time, first pressor then depressor. The rise is mediated by H_1 receptors and the fall by H_2 receptors (Carroll *et al.,* 1974).

Histamine Shock. Histamine in large doses causes a profound and progressive fall in blood pressure. Dale and Laidlaw (1919), who called the phenomenon "histamine shock," showed that as the minute blood vessels dilate, they trap large amounts of blood and, as their permeability increases, plasma escapes from the circulation. These effects diminish the effective blood volume, reduce venous return, and greatly lower cardiac output. The condition resembles surgical or traumatic shock.

Regional Vascular Responses. In addition to the interspecies differences already noted, responses to histamine vary in different vascular beds within a single species. For the most part, the differences are quantitative and reflect varying degrees of dilatation in the skeletal, mesenteric, coronary, cerebral, and renal beds. But sometimes, even where the overall response is clearly vasodilatation (*e.g.,* in cats), vasoconstriction is evident in liver, spleen, and skin. Within the pulmonary circulation, both constrictor and dilator effects (involving H_1 and H_2 receptors, respectively) have been demonstrated. The effect varies with species and dose and sometimes even with the duration of exposure to the drug. Variable effects have also been noted on pulmonary arterial pressure; some of the variability (like the corresponding effects on pulmonary venous pressure) may reflect changes in venous return and cardiac output rather than local vascular actions. In man, a fall in pulmonary arterial pressure has been demonstrated after subcutaneous injection of histamine (*see* Storstein *et al.,* 1959; *see also* Owen, 1977).

Vascular Tissue in Vitro. Isolated blood vessels from various species and regions (cranial, mesenteric, aortic, and umbilical arteries as well as umbilical vein and other large veins, including vena cava) commonly show constrictor responses to histamine *in vitro.* Under such conditions the vessels usually have little of the tone that is evident *in vivo,* a tone that facilitates demonstration of dilator effects. These constrictor responses, which are mediated by H_1 receptors, are thus of doubtful relevance to conditions *in vivo* (*see* Owen, 1977).

Extravascular Smooth Muscle. Histamine stimulates, or more rarely relaxes, various smooth muscles. Contraction is due to activation of H_1 receptors and relaxation (for the most part) to activation of H_2 receptors. Responses of different tissues, species, and even individuals vary widely. *Bronchial muscle* of guinea pigs is exquisitely sensitive, and bronchoconstriction leads to death. Minute doses of histamine will also evoke intense bronchoconstriction in patients with bronchial asthma and certain other pulmonary diseases. In normal man and many animals, the effect is much less pronounced and exceptionally, as in the sheep bronchus or cat trachea, histamine causes relaxation (*see*

Eyre, 1973). Likewise, the *uterus* of some species contracts to histamine while that of the rat relaxes; in the human uterus, gravid or not, the response is negligible. Responses of *intestinal muscle* also vary with species and region, but the classical effect is contraction; the contractile response of the terminal ileum of the guinea pig forms the basis for a common bioassay of histamine. *Bladder, gallbladder, iris,* and many other smooth muscle preparations are affected little or inconsistently by histamine.

Exocrine Glands. *Gastric Glands.* Histamine is a remarkably powerful gastric secretagogue and evokes a copious secretion of gastric juice of high acidity in doses below those that influence the blood pressure. Its effect on the composition of gastric juice varies somewhat with species and dose (Ivy and Bachrach, 1966), but in man the output of pepsin and instrinsic factor of Castle is increased along with that of acid. The effect is well maintained during prolonged intravenous infusions of histamine. While these actions are believed to be exerted directly on the gland cells (both parietal and chief), the presence of an intact vagus permits a higher rate of secretion. After vagotomy in man the maximal secretory response to histamine may fall to about one third of the value found before the operation (Payne and Kay, 1962). After cholinergic blockade by atropine the response to histamine is likewise reduced. It appears that a "background" of cholinergic effect on the secretory cells enhances their responsiveness to histamine. A similar potentiating effect can be shown with gastrin. From all this it has been concluded that the three gastric secretagogues are mutually interdependent (*see* Soll and Walsh, 1979, and below).

Other Exocrine Glands. The effects of histamine on glands outside the stomach are relatively unimportant. The drug has some stimulant actions on salivary, pancreatic, intestinal, bronchial, and lacrimal secretions, but these are generally inconstant, fleeting, and feeble. In salivary glands, where the action of histamine has been most closely studied, it is possible to show some stimulation after chronic denervation, which is thus direct; however, in normally innervated glands, much of the effect seems to be mediated through the nerves (*see* below and Emmelin, 1966). Histamine stimulates secretion of

bile even after removal of the stomach (*see* Jones and Meyers, 1979).

Nerve Endings: Pain and Itch. The "flare" component of the triple response is but one example of histamine's capacity to stimulate nerve endings. Histamine also causes itching when introduced into the most superficial layers of the skin by a variety of technics, including pricking, injection, and iontophoresis; when administered more deeply in the skin, especially in higher doses, it evokes pain, sometimes accompanied by itching. Afferent discharges evoked by histamine have been recorded in cutaneous nerves (*see* Keele and Armstrong, 1964).

Stimulant effects on nerve endings, motor as well as sensory, contribute to the indirect effects of histamine on smooth muscle preparations and glands that are blocked, for example, by atropine or hexamethonium; a stimulatory action on sympathetic nerve endings would explain the release of norepinephrine from the isolated heart provoked by histamine in high doses (*see* Paton and Vane, 1963; Rocha e Silva, 1966). An opposite effect has also been observed, in which histamine inhibits the release of norepinephrine from sympathetic nerve endings (McGrath and Shepherd, 1978).

Adrenal Medulla and Ganglia. Many substances that excite nerve endings also stimulate ganglion cells and chromaffin cells in the adrenal medulla and elsewhere. This is true of histamine (Euler, 1966; Brezenoff and Gertner, 1972). However, these cells respond vigorously only when histamine is administered in large amounts or by close arterial injection, and not when conventional doses are given intravenously. Nevertheless, a secondary rise in blood pressure attributable to adrenal medullary stimulation is seen in experimental animals given large doses of histamine intravenously and in patients with pheochromocytoma given modest doses. In addition to its direct action on the chromaffin cells, demonstrable by intracellular recording (Douglas *et al.,* 1967), histamine can also evoke medullary secretion indirectly by reflex effects mediated through the splanchnic nerves (Staszewska-Barczak and Vane, 1965).

Central Nervous System. Histamine does not penetrate the blood-brain barrier to any significant degree, and effects on the central nervous system (CNS) are not usually evident in response to parenteral injections of the autacoid. However, when injected directly into the cerebral ventricles or given by iontophoretic application into certain regions of the brain, histamine may elicit behavioral responses, elevate blood pressure, increase heart rate, lower body temperature, increase secretion of antidiuretic hormone, cause arousal or emesis, and increase or decrease firing of neurons. These central effects seem to involve both H_1 and H_2 receptors, and some, at least, may reflect the existence of endogenous central histaminergic mechanisms (see Chapter 12; Schwartz, 1977; Green et al., 1978).

White Blood Cells. H_2 receptors have been found to be distributed nonrandomly on leukocytes of mice, rats, and humans, and, in most instances, histamine acts to inhibit the secretion by these cells of substances that ordinarily contribute to the immune or inflammatory response. In the case of neutrophils, histamine prevents the release of lysosomal enzymes that normally occurs during phagocytosis. Histamine also inhibits the release of antibody from B lymphocytes and lymphokines from T cells, and the autacoid prevents cytolysis by T effector cells of allogeneic target cells. Of general interest has been the hypothesis that histamine and other mediators of inflammation may, by virtue of inhibition of such functions, also play an anti-inflammatory role. An important clinical implication is that antagonists of histamine might actually enhance some inflammatory process or modify immune responses (see Bourne et al., 1974; Melmon et al., 1977; Jorizzo et al., 1980).

Mechanism of Action. Receptors for histamine are presumed to be a component of the cell surface. They have not yet been identified by physical or chemical means, and the knowledge of their structural properties is restricted to such inferences as can be drawn from pharmacological studies of structure-activity relationships of histaminergic agonists and antagonists (see Durant, et al., 1975; Ganellin, 1978a, 1978b; Rocha e Silva, 1978b; van den Brink and Lien, 1978). How interaction of histamine with its receptors elicits the appropriate cellular responses is also uncertain.

Broadly speaking, there are two principal lines of evidence that bear on the problem of stimulus-response coupling for histamine, as well as for most other autacoids and many drugs. The first concerns actions leading to altered permeability of the plasma membrane to common inorganic ions, particularly increased permeability to sodium and calcium, which allows them to enter the cell along electrochemical gradients; actions also tend to promote elevation of the concentration of free intracellular calcium by its release from intracellular stores. The intracellular concentration of free calcium ions is a critical factor in determining muscle tension (see Weber and Murray, 1973) and secretion (see Douglas, 1968, 1978). Changes in permeability to ions in response to histamine are reflected in the smooth muscle depolarizing responses that accompany contraction, in the depolarization of chromaffin cells, in the generation of nerve impulses, and in an increased calcium component of the cardiac action potential during the positive inotropic effect. It should be noted, however, that both contraction and relaxation can be induced with histamine (as with other substances) in smooth muscles that are fully depolarized by potassium. Here, contraction reflects an effect of histamine that is clearly not dependent on voltage but that presumably involves the "opening" of calcium channels in the membrane to allow influx of the cation or the mobilization of calcium from cellular sources. Contractile responses to histamine in the absence of extracellular calcium clearly must be explained by such utilization of intracellular calcium.

The second line of evidence concerning stimulus-response coupling relates to effects of extracellular regulators on adenylate cyclase and, perhaps, on guanylate cyclase. Several effects of histamine, including gastric secretion, stimulation of cardiac contraction, and inhibition of secretion from basophils, have all been associated with elevated concentrations of cyclic adenosine 3',5'-monophosphate (cyclic AMP). These responses are all mediated through H_2 receptors. It is also of interest that histamine stimulates the accumulation of cyclic AMP in brain tissue through an action on H_2 receptors (see Greengard, 1976). Whether smooth muscle relaxation, which again involves H_2 receptors, also involves a rise in the concentration of cyclic AMP is uncertain. While elevated concentrations of cyclic guanosine 3',5'-monophosphate (cyclic GMP) have been demonstrated in smooth muscle contracted through H_1 receptors, the physiological actions of this nucleotide are unknown. Of course, these two lines of evidence may converge, since cyclic AMP may modulate ionic permeability, and calcium may regulate the activity of enzymes responsible for cyclic nucleotide synthesis and degradation (see Beaven, 1978; Rocha e Silva, 1978a). It should be clear that there are many uncertainties concerning the involvement of cyclic AMP and cyclic GMP in the mediation of various cellular responses to histamine and other autacoids (*e.g., see* Jacobson and Thompson, 1976; Busis *et al.,* 1978; Conference, 1978; Diamant *et al.,* 1978; Diamond, 1978).

ENDOGENOUS HISTAMINE:
DISTRIBUTION AND BIOSYNTHESIS

Distribution. Histamine is widely, if unevenly, distributed throughout the animal kingdom and is present in many venoms, noxious secretions, bacteria, and plants (Reite, 1972). Almost all mammalian tissues contain preformed histamine. The concentration is particularly high in the skin, intestinal mucosa, and lungs. Of no less importance than concentration, and often unrelated to it, is histamine-synthesizing capacity. Some tissues synthesize and turn over histamine at a remarkably high rate.

Origin, Synthesis, and Storage. Histamine that is ingested or formed by bacteria in the gastrointestinal tract does not contribute significantly to the endogenous pool. Most histamine that is absorbed is catabolized in the gut wall and liver and eliminated in the urine (*see* below). Every mammalian tissue that contains histamine is capable of synthesizing it from histidine by virtue of its content of a decarboxylase specific for the L-amino acid. In most tissues the chief site of histamine *storage* is the mast cell or, in the blood, its circulating counterpart, the basophil. These cells synthesize histamine and store it in secretory granules. The turnover rate of histamine here is slow, and, when tissues rich in mast cells are depleted of their stores of histamine, it may take weeks before concentrations of the autacoid return to normal. Nonmast-cell sites of histamine formation or storage include cells of the human epidermis, enterochromaffin-like cells in the rat gastric mucosa, cells within the CNS (probably neurons), and cells in regenerating or rapidly growing tissues. At these sites turnover is rapid, since the histamine is continuously released rather than stored. This contributes significantly to the daily excretion of histamine and its metabolites in the urine. Since L-histidine decarboxylase is an inducible enzyme, the histamine-forming capacity at such nonmast-cell sites is subject to regulation by various physiological and other factors. Conjecture on the functions of nonmast-cell histamine is therefore abundant.

ENDOGENOUS HISTAMINE:
FUNCTIONS

In the following discussion the now-classical involvement of histamine release from mast cells and basophils in various pathological processes will be considered before the later work implicating nonmast-cell histamine in various physiological processes. There is no significance to this order

other than convenience and approximation to the historical sequence of development of the field.

Histamine Release in Anaphylaxis and Allergy. Although Dale and Laidlaw had drawn attention to the close correspondence between the effects of poisoning with histamine and anaphylactic shock as early as 1910, many years elapsed before the meaning of this correspondence became apparent. Three major clues were provided by (1) the work of Dale (1913), which showed convincingly that the hypersensitivity phenomenon involved a reaction of antigen with cell-fixed antibody; (2) the work of Lewis (1927), demonstrating that a histamine-like agent ("H-substance") was liberated in the skin during the local anaphylactic reaction; and (3) the work of Best and associates (1927), establishing beyond doubt that histamine is a natural constituent of the tissues of the body. The first two clues prompted Lewis (1927) to enunciate the hypothesis that the antigen-antibody reaction caused the cells to liberate a substance with the properties of histamine that was responsible for the characteristic physiological accompaniments of the phenomenon, that is, vasodilatation, itching, and edema formation. The third clue allowed Dale (1929) to argue forcibly that this "H-substance" was histamine itself. Within a few years, the release of histamine during the antigen-antibody reaction had been successfully demonstrated by Bartosch and coworkers (1932) and by Dragstedt and Gebauer-Fuelnegg (1932), and the histamine hypothesis of the mediation of hypersensitivity phenomena won wide acceptance. When, following World War II, the newly discovered histamine antagonists were found to reduce the intensity of various hypersensitivity reactions, the involvement of histamine was established beyond all reasonable doubt. During this same period, however, it became increasingly evident from the failure of these antagonists to suppress the reactions completely that histamine was not the only factor involved.

Mechanism. The principal target cells of the hypersensitivity reactions of the immediate type are the mast cells and basophils. Within the secretory granules of these cells, the histamine is stored along with a heparin-protein complex to which it is loosely bound by ionic forces, probably involving carboxyl groups. The secretion (or "release") of histamine from sensitized mast cells or basophils in response to specific antigen is believed to be initiated when the antigen combines with and bridges adjacent molecules of reaginic antibodies (IgE) that have become attached to the cell surface (*see* Bach, 1978; Ishizaka and Ishizaka, 1978). The ensuing perturbation seemingly sets in motion a series of reactions that show a critical requirement for calcium and metabolic energy and terminate in the extrusion of the contents of secretory granules by the process of exocytosis. In these several respects the secretory behavior of mast cells and basophils is identical with that of various gland cells, endocrine and exocrine. The specific secretory response to antigen is an active process that must be distinguished from the passive loss of histamine that may occur in response to nonspecific cell damage (cytolysis). When studies on endocrine, exocrine, and other secretory cells led to the concept of stimulus-secretion coupling in which secretagogues of different sorts are thought to act by promoting an influx of calcium into their target cells and thereby inducing exocytosis, the suggestion was made that specific antigen acting on its sensitized target cells might release histamine in the same way (see Douglas and Rubin, 1961; Douglas, 1968). In this view the agonist or secretagogue (in this case, specific antigen) combines with its receptors (here cell-bound IgE molecules) to promote an increase in membrane permeability and the influx of calcium ions. There is now much evidence to sustain this hypothesis: the secretory response to antigen fails if extracellular calcium is removed; calcium chelators arrest ongoing secretion if added during the response to antigen; in the absence of calcium the interaction of antigen and cell-bound IgE still proceeds and causes an activation such that calcium will elicit histamine secretion when subsequently added; exposure to antigen causes increased uptake of calcium; and various other procedures that promote calcium influx or otherwise raise intracellular concentrations of calcium (e.g., microinjection of calcium or exposure to calcium ionophores) suffice to initiate histamine secretion by exocytosis (see Foreman et al., 1976; Douglas, 1978; Lichtenstein and Austen, 1978; Morrison and Henson, 1978).

As in other secretory systems, further details on the cellular events involved in stimulus-secretion coupling and the critical function of calcium are obscure. There have been suggestions that changes in cyclic nucleotide concentrations may participate, since a reduction in cyclic AMP or an increase in cyclic GMP both favor secretion, but this is controversial (Diamant et al., 1978). There are indications that crucial protein phosphorylation reactions are activated by calcium (Sieghart et al., 1978; see also Chapter 4, page 80) and that arachidonic acid and its metabolites may be involved (Sullivan and Parker, 1979). Despite these uncertainties it is evident that considerable *modulation* of the secretion of histamine from mast cells and basophils can be achieved with drugs that regulate concentrations of cyclic nucleotides. Thus, some inhibition can be achieved with epinephrine (acting through β-adrenergic receptors) and with theophylline, both of which have long been used in therapy of allergic states such as asthma (although their main benefit probably reflects their dilator actions on smooth muscle). Moreover, histamine itself also tends to reduce its own release, acting through H_2 receptors, thereby suggesting the operation of a negative feedback mechanism; the potentiating effects of H_2 blockers on the release of histamine are consistent with this observation. All these inhibitory responses may involve an elevation of concentrations of cyclic AMP. In addition, cromolyn, by some ill-defined actions, clearly reduces the allergic secretion from mast cells in the lungs. In contrast, cholinergic drugs, acting at muscarinic receptors, appear to potentiate allergic secretion, possibly by elevating concentrations of cyclic GMP.

Limitations of the Histamine Hypothesis of Hypersensitivity Reactions. *Involvement of Other*

Autacoids. It is now evident that the classical histamine hypothesis provides only a partial explanation for the effects that accompany hypersensitivity (antigen-antibody) reactions. During such reactions numerous other autacoids are liberated or produced. They include slow-reacting substance of anaphylaxis (SRS-A), prostaglandins, and other products of arachidonic acid metabolism; kallikrein and kinins; eosinophil leukocytic chemotactic factor; and (in some animals) 5-hydroxytryptamine and dopamine. The nature and relative importance of these substances vary with species and tissue, and this accounts largely for the widely variable efficacies of histamine blockers in combating allergic responses (Assem, 1976; Bach, 1978; see below).

Direct Effects of Antigen. An additional explanation for the anaphylactic and allergic responses that are apparently independent of histamine or other known autacoids may lie in the observation that antigens can act directly on the membranes of sensitized muscle cells to cause depolarization and contraction (Alonso–De Florida et al., 1968).

Histamine Release by Drugs, Peptides, Venoms, and Other Agents.

Many compounds, including numerous therapeutic agents, release histamine directly and quite independently of the presence of hypersensitization. Among them are many basic drugs, including amides, amidines, diamidines, quaternary ammonium compounds, piperidine derivatives, pyridinium compounds, various alkaloids, and antibiotic bases. Not uncommonly, therapeutic administration of such substances, especially by the intravenous route, has rather dramatic consequences that are attributable to the release of histamine. Drugs that can elicit this effect are discussed throughout the text. (For reviews, see Paton, 1957; Rocha e Silva, 1966; 1978a; Lorenz and Doenicke, 1978.)

Histamine Liberators. There are certain basic compounds with histamine-releasing activity that so far transcends their other pharmacological actions that they are commonly referred to as histamine liberators. The prototype and most thoroughly studied is compound 48/80, a low-molecular-weight polymer of *p*-methoxy-N-methylphenethylamine. Drugs of this class elicit the syndrome of histamine release in its purest form. Within seconds of their intravenous injection, human subjects experience a burning, itching sensation, as if a bundle of nettles had been placed on the skin. This effect, most marked in the palms of the hand and in the face, scalp, and ears, is soon followed by a feeling of intense warmth. The skin reddens, and the color rapidly spreads over the trunk. Blood pressure falls, the heart rate accelerates, and the subject complains of headache, often intense. After a few minutes, blood pressure recovers, and edema and crops of giant hives appear in the skin, particularly over the thorax and abdomen. There is colic, nausea, hypersecretion of acid with acid vomitus, and moderate bronchospasm. Such an "anaphylactoid" reaction may occasionally be seen following the administration of therapeutic agents with potent histamine-releasing effects. The effect becomes less intense with successive injections as the mast-cell stores of histamine are depleted. Histamine liberators do not deplete tissues of nonmast-cell histamine.

Mechanism. Studies on rat peritoneal mast cells show that the prototypical histamine liberator, compound 48/80, is preferentially bound to receptors on these cells and thereby sets in motion an active secretory process (exocytosis) that resembles that induced by the immediate hypersensitivity reaction in its dependence on energy and calcium; there is, however, less dependence on extracellular calcium, since the drug can readily mobilize calcium from intracellular stores (Douglas, 1974; Uvnäs, 1978). Some other basic compounds with surfactant properties, such as decylamine, seem to have a nonspecific membrane-disrupting, detergent-like effect or may even displace histamine from intracellular granules without frank rupture. These nonspecific effects require neither calcium ions nor energy.

Many *basic polypeptides* and *proteins* release histamine mainly by setting in motion the noncytolytic secretory response (exocytosis). Some of these substances are themselves released by tissue damage and could be regarded as pathophysiological stimuli that participate in the release of histamine that follows injury. The list includes cationic peptides from polymorphonuclear leukocyte granules, kinins, substance P, and components of the complement system (C_3a, C_5a), as well as substances such as polylysine, protamine, histones, and others (*see* Bach, 1978; Goth, 1978). Curiously, somatostatin, known for its inhibitory effects in various secretory systems, is among the most potent peptides known to release histamine (Theoharides and Douglas, 1978).

Other agents causing exocytotic release of histamine include dextrans and certain other plasma substitutes (*see* Lorenz and Doenicke, 1978). *Venoms* and *toxins* of many sorts also release histamine because of their content of basic polypeptides or enzymes such as phospholipase A, which may initiate exocytosis or lyse cells (*see* Beraldo and Dias da Silva, 1966; Goth, 1973, 1978).

Histamine Release by Physical or Chemical Insult. Mechanical, thermal, or radiant energies sufficiently intense to damage mast cells will liberate histamine. The redness and urtication seen when the skin is scratched is a familiar example, as is "cold urticaria." Histamine release also occurs on overexposure to sunlight or intense ionizing radiation. Chemicals causing gross cell damage, such as detergents, bile salts, and lysolecithin, will also release histamine, as will osmotic shock.

Injury, Stress, "Induced Histamine," and Microcirculation. Schayer (1963) suggested that "induced histamine," which is not stored but immediately freed, has a role in *regulating the microcirculation* to satisfy locally increased requirements for blood re-

sulting from injurious stimuli. Such histamine was also proposed to account for the delayed phase of vasodilatation occurring in *inflammation*. However, kinins, prostaglandins, and other factors participate. Thus, the humoral regulation of the microcirculation remains a complex puzzle (*see* Zweifach, 1973; Altura and Halevy, 1978).

Tissue Growth and Repair. Kahlson and colleagues have marshaled evidence that a conspicuously high histamine-forming capacity is present in many tissues undergoing rapid growth or repair, such as embryonic tissue, regenerating liver, bone marrow, wound and granulation tissue, and malignant growths in various species, principally the rat. The histamine formed, which they refer to as "nascent histamine," is not stored but free to diffuse (compare with Schayer's "induced histamine," above). They have shown that inhibition of L-histidine decarboxylase arrests fetal development in the rat and, conversely, that drugs elevating histamine-forming capacity accelerate wound healing. Their evidence has led them to suggest that "nascent histamine" has a role in anabolic processes (*see* Kahlson and Rosengren, 1971). More recently the focus of attention has been on the polyamines, putrescine, spermidine, and spermine.

Gastric Secretion. In 1920, Keeton and associates and also Popielski reported that histamine stimulates gastric secretion, and the former investigators proposed that endogenous histamine might mediate some of the stimulatory effects of the vagus. MacIntosh, in 1938, showed that histamine was released from the stomach during vagal stimulation and thus provided essential experimental support for the idea. Nearly 50 years were to pass, however, before sufficient evidence accumulated to allow Code (1965), Kahlson and Rosengren (1968), and others to mount persuasive arguments that histamine is involved in the regulation of normal gastrosecretory function. The difficulty then, and until recently, was that no drug existed that would block the effect of histamine on gastric secretion and thereby allow a critical test of the possibility. For this reason the idea was vigorously challenged (Johnson, 1971). With the development of the H_2 antagonists, the importance of histamine could no longer be doubted, since these drugs inhibit not only gastric secretion elicited by injected histamine but also basal secretion and that elicited by various physiological stimuli. The major problems that remain are to identify the cells that synthesize, store, and release histamine in the stomach; to learn how these cells are activated; and to characterize the function of histamine and its regulation by other physiological secretagogues such as gastrin and ACh. At issue is whether histamine is the final common mediator of secretory responses to all physiological influences, nervous or hormonal, or whether, as seems more likely at present, it is but one of three physiological stimuli to the parietal cell. These may interact at the level of their respective receptors in a complex, mutually interdependent manner, such that the efficacies of vagally released ACh and of gastrin are greatly heightened by concomitant activation of histamine receptors and correspondingly weakened when these receptors are blocked by H_2 antagonists (*see* reviews by Code, 1977; Sachs *et al.,* 1977; Johnson, 1978; Soll and Walsh, 1979).

Nerves and Brain. *Afferent Nerves.* Histamine, liberated by one means or another, is frequently involved in initiation of sensory impulses evoking *pain and itch* (Keele and Armstrong, 1964).

Efferent Nerves. The possibility that reflex vasodilatation involves an active component in addition to inhibition of sympathetic vasoconstrictor activity and that this *"active reflex vasodilatation"* may be mediated by histamine liberated by efferent nervous function continues to be debated. There is, as yet, no convincing evidence of peripheral histaminergic nerves. Although histamine has been shown in peripheral nerve trunks, much seems to be present there in mast cells (*see* Brody, 1978; Green *et al.,* 1978).

Brain. Evidence supports the idea that histamine serves as a chemical transmitter of certain "histaminergic" nerves in the brain (*see* reviews by Schwartz, 1977; Green *et al.,* 1978; Chapter 12).

Headache. Endogenous histamine has been implicated in the genesis of headaches, particularly the syndrome named *histaminic cephalalgia* by Horton (1941). The headache encountered in this syndrome is, however, quite different from that which occurs in response to histamine injections in the normal individual and cannot be mimicked in the patient. Involvement of histamine in "Horton's headache" is therefore unlikely (Lecomte, 1957).

Growths of Mast Cells and Basophils. In *urticaria pigmentosa,* mast cells aggregate in the upper corium and give rise to pigmented cutaneous lesions in the form of macules, papules, or nodules that urticate when stroked. In *systemic mastocytosis,* similar aggregates are found in other organs. Patients with these syndromes excrete abnormally high amounts of histamine and its metabolites in the urine. They also suffer a constellation of signs and symptoms attributable to excessive histamine release, including, in addition to urticaria and dermographism, pruritus, headache, weakness, hypotension, flushing of the face, and a variety of gastrointestinal effects such as peptic ulceration. The signs and symptoms are precipitated or exacerbated by a variety of stimuli—the friction of toweling the skin or exposure to drugs that release histamine directly or to which patients are allergic. Excessive numbers of basophils are present in the blood in *myelogenous leukemia* and raise its histamine content to high levels. *Gastric carcinoid* tumors secrete histamine, and this apparently contributes to the patchy "geographical" flush.

Additional Considerations

Absorption, Fate, and Excretion. Histamine is readily absorbed after parenteral injection and acts rapidly when given by the subcutaneous or intramuscular route. Its action is evanescent, since it diffuses into tissues and is rapidly metabolized. Very large amounts of histamine can be given orally, however, without causing effects, since much is converted by intestinal bacteria to inactive N-acetylhistamine, and the free histamine absorbed is mostly inactivated as it traverses the intestinal wall or circulates through the liver.

In man, there are two major paths of histamine metabolism (*see* Figure 26-1). The more important one involves ring methylation and is catalyzed by the enzyme histamine-N-methyltransferase (imidazole-N-methyltransferase, INMT). Most of the product, N-methylhistamine, is converted by monoamine oxidase (MAO) to N-methyl imidazole acetic acid. In the other path, histamine undergoes oxidative deamination catalyzed mainly by diamine oxidase (DAO), also called "histaminase," which actually comprises nonspecific enzymes found in most tissues that deaminate various aromatic or aliphatic diamines. The products are imidazole acetic acid and, eventually, its riboside. The various metabolites, which have little or

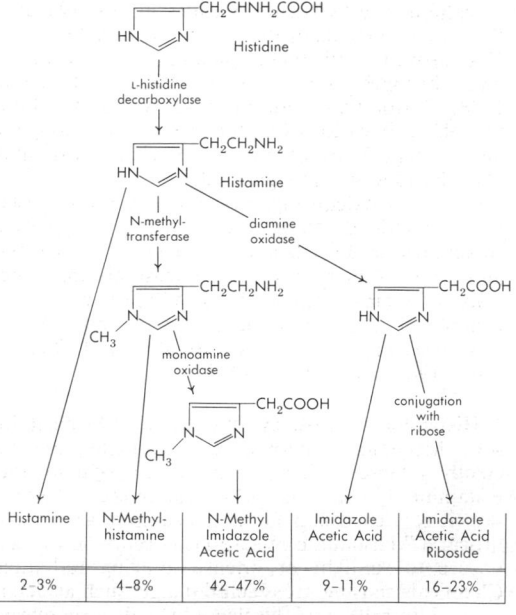

Histamine	N-Methyl-histamine	N-Methyl Imidazole Acetic Acid	Imidazole Acetic Acid	Imidazole Acetic Acid Riboside
2–3%	4–8%	42–47%	9–11%	16–23%

Figure 26-1. *Synthesis and catabolism of histamine.*

Percent recovery of histamine and metabolites in the urine in 12 hours following intradermal ^{14}C-histamine in human males. (Modified from Schayer and Cooper, 1956.)

no pharmacological activity, are excreted in the urine. The relative roles of these enzymes in the metabolism of endogenous histamine have not yet been established. Some inhibitors of INMT and DAO are known, but their significance is mainly experimental and their contribution to clinical responses uncertain. Amodiaquine and some other antimalarials inhibit INMT. DAO activity can be inhibited by aminoguanidine, by many MAO inhibitors, and by isoniazid and hydralazine.

The DAO activity of plasma rises sharply during the first trimester of pregnancy and remains high until term. Its origin is the maternal placenta, but its function is uncertain (Torok *et al.*, 1970). High activities of DAO are also found in the plasma of patients with medullary carcinoma of the thyroid, a tumor that synthesizes large amounts of the enzyme (Baylin *et al.*, 1972). (For reviews, *see* Maśliński, 1975a, 1975b; Schayer, 1978; Wetterquist, 1978.)

Toxicity. Overdosage with histamine is rare, and symptoms are generally not dangerous. However, massive doses cause intense headache, flushing, profound fall of blood pressure, bronchospasm, dyspnea, a metallic taste, vomiting, and diarrhea. The prompt injection of histamine antagonists will suppress these reactions, especially if absorption of the histamine can be delayed by application of a tourniquet. An H_1-receptor blocker alone may be adequate, but the addition of an H_2-receptor blocker may be worthwhile.

Preparations. *Histamine Phosphate,* U.S.P., and *histamine dihydrochloride* are water-soluble, colorless crystals. *Histamine Phosphate Injection,* U.S.P., is available in preparations containing 0.275, 1, or 2.75 mg in 1 ml (equivalent to 0.1, 0.36, or 1 mg of histamine base).

CLINICAL USES

The practical applications of histamine fall into two categories: first, its uses as a diagnostic agent, which for the most part are on a sound physiological basis; and, second, its more controversial uses in therapy, especially of diseases of allergy.

Diagnostic Uses. Histamine has been much used to assess the ability of the stomach to secrete acid and to determine parietal cell mass. Thus, anacidity or hyposecretion in response to histamine may reflect *pernicious anemia, atrophic gastritis,* or *gastric carcinoma,* whereas a hypersecretory response may be found in patients with *duodenal ulcer* or with the *Zollinger-Ellison syndrome.* Administered by itself, histamine causes distressing side effects; but these can be greatly reduced by giving beforehand an H_1 antagonist, which does not oppose histamine's actions as a gastric secretagogue. However, there are other, more suitable stimulants of gastric secretion (*see* below).

The fact that intradermal histamine causes a "flare" that is mediated by axon reflexes allows a test for the *integrity of sensory nerves,* of value in certain neurological conditions.

The stimulant effect of histamine on chromaffin cells has been applied in a provocative test for *pheochromocytoma.* Positive results may also be due to direct and indirect effects of histamine on adrenergic nerve terminals, which contain excessive quantities of catecholamines because of uptake from the circulation. The test may thus remain positive for a week or more after the tumor is removed. If measurement of the excretion of catecholamines and their metabolites in the urine yields equivocal results, release provoked by histamine can be quantified after administration of an α-adrenergic blocking agent.

Therapeutic Uses. In various diseases in which histamine is suspected of being involved in the etiology, such as in allergies, Ménière's disease, and various vascular headaches, attempts have been made to desensitize the patient with courses of histamine injections. There is no experimental evidence that such regimens induce significant tolerance, however, and the procedure is not recommended.

BETAZOLE

Betazole is an isomer of histamine with preferential effects on gastric secretion (Rosière and Grossman, 1951). It has the following structure:

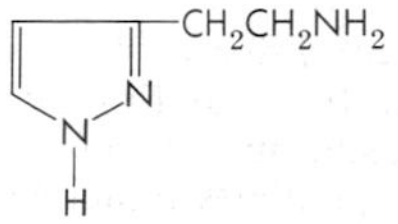

CH_2CH_2NH_2 — [structure]

Betazole

Pharmacological Properties. Betazole possesses, in attenuated form, the characteristic actions of histamine on gastric acid secretion, smooth muscle, and blood pressure. However, its effect on gastric secretion is about ten times more potent than is its effect as a vasodilator.

Clinical Use. Betazole is a convenient alternative to histamine in tests of gastric function; its use obviates the need for concomitant administration of an H_1 antagonist (*see* above and Figure 26–2, page 630). However, betazole is not devoid of side effects attributable to its other histamine-like actions, and it may cause flushing, weakness, syncope, headache, and urticaria. It should be avoided in individuals who have atopic allergy.

Preparation. *Betazole Hydrochloride,* U.S.P. (HISTALOG), is a water-soluble powder, available in ampuls containing 50 mg in 1 ml. The usual adult dose is 50 mg, given intramuscularly or subcutaneously.

Other H$_2$-Receptor Agonists. Drugs in this category, such as dimaprit (*see* above), are much more selective in their action on gastric secretion and may supplant betazole in tests of gastric secretory function. However, no such agent has yet been approved for clinical use in the United States.

PENTAGASTRIN

Largely due to the work of Gregory and Tracy (1966), the potent physiological gastric secretagogue, *gastrin,* released from the pyloric antrum by vagal and local gastric responses to feeding, was shown to be a heptadecapeptide. Their work and also that of Morley (1968) demonstrated that the full spectrum of gastrin-like activity is present in smaller fragments of the peptide, the smallest effective compound being the C-terminal tetrapeptide amide: Trp-Met-Asp-Phe-NH$_2$. This has about 10% of the potency of gastrin. A synthetic pentapeptide derivative, *pentagastrin,* proved still more active and has been adopted for gastric function tests as an alternative to histamine or betazole; pentagastrin causes fewer and less severe reactions.

Chemistry. Pentagastrin is N-*t*-butyloxycarbonyl-β- alanyl - L - tryptophyl - L - methionyl - L - aspartyl - L - phenylalanine amide. It has the structural formula:

Pentagastrin

Pharmacological Effects. The most prominent action of pentagastrin is to stimulate the secretion of gastric acid, pepsin, and intrinsic factor of Castle; additionally, it stimulates pancreatic secretion, inhibits absorption of water and electrolytes from the ileum, contracts the smooth muscle of the lower esophageal sphincter and stomach (but delays gastric emptying time), relaxes the sphincter of Oddi, increases blood flow in the gastric mucosa, stimulates L-histidine decarboxylase activity in rat gastric mucosa, and, *in high doses,* stimulates a variety of smooth muscles in different species. It also mimics or blocks the effects of the polypeptides pancreozymin-cholecystokinin, secretin, and caerulin, a naturally occurring decapeptide that, together with pancreozymin-cholecystokinin, shares a common C-terminal heptapeptide sequence with gastrin. The half-life of pentagastrin in the circulation appears to be about 10 minutes.

Clinical Use. Pentagastrin elicits reproducible gastric secretory responses comparable to those in-duced by histamine or betazole and offers several advantages. The pentagastrin test requires only a single subcutaneous or intramuscular injection; it is relatively short in duration of action, and side effects are usually minor and transient. These may include various gastrointestinal phenomena, such as nausea, borborygmi, and the urge to defecate, and circulatory effects, including flushing, tachycardia, faintness, and dizziness. Allergic reactions are rare. Gastric secretion begins within 10 minutes, and peak responses occur within 30 minutes (*see* Baron, 1972).

Preparation. *Pentagastrin* (PEPTAVLON) is marketed in vials containing 0.25 mg/ml in 2 ml of physiological saline solution. The diagnostic dose is 6 μg/kg, administered by subcutaneous injection.

INHIBITION OF ALLERGIC RELEASE OF HISTAMINE AND OTHER AUTACOIDS

Therapy aimed at controlling the symptoms of immediate hypersensitivity reactions with antagonists of histamine is useful but only partially effective. This is because histamine is but one of a battery of autacoids released or formed during the reaction, which together elicit the symptoms (*see* above). To suppress the effects of all these agents would require a corresponding battery of blocking agents; even if these were all available, such an approach would be cumbersome. It is for this reason that treatment of allergic reactions often necessitates the use of nonspecific "physiological antagonists" such as epinephrine or ephedrine, which essentially counter responses to the antigen-induced flood of autacoids by eliciting responses of an opposite nature. But this approach, like the use of blocking drugs, does not address the underlying cause. An attractive and advantageous procedure, uniquely applicable to *prophylaxis,* is to prevent production or release of the autacoids by inhibiting responses of sensitized mast cells and basophils to specific antigens. It has been mentioned above that adrenergic drugs and theophylline, beside their many other actions, tend to inhibit such allergic responses; this may contribute to their clinical utility. A much more specific inhibition is possible, however, with the type of antiallergic drug exemplified by *cromolyn.* This agent inhibits antigen-induced secretion of histamine from human pulmonary mast cells and from mast cells at certain other sites. Although the usefulness of cromolyn is circumscribed (human basophils, curiously, are not protected), the drug is a valuable adjunct in the prophylactic management of certain cases of asthma and certain other atopic states. Scarcely less important than the clinical value of cromolyn is the evidence thereby provided of the feasibility of inhibiting hypersensitivity reactions.

CROMOLYN SODIUM

History. Cromolyn was synthesized after a long search, the initial purpose of which was to enhance the smooth muscle relaxant, particularly bronchodilator, properties of the drug khellin, a chromone (benzopyrone) of plant origin. Successive modifications in structure yielded *bis*-chromones, the most important being cromolyn, which was not a bronchodilator but, surprisingly, effectively prevented allergic bronchospasm. Analysis revealed a novel mechanism of action, namely, inhibition of release of histamine and other autacoids (Altounyan, 1967; Cox *et al.*, 1970).

Chemistry. Cromolyn sodium, the disodium salt of 1,3-*bis*(2-carboxychromone-5-yloxy)-2-hydroxy-propane, has the following structure:

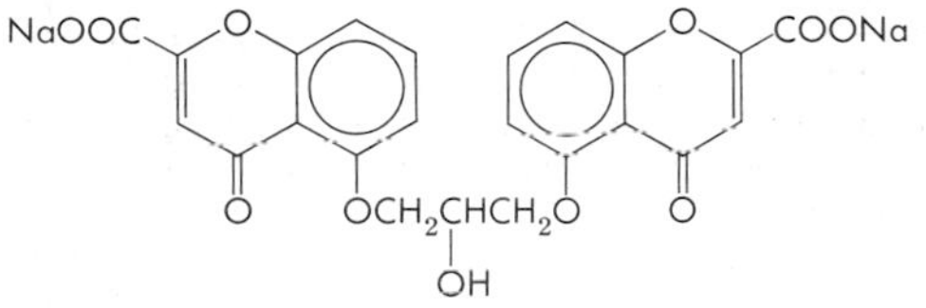

Cromolyn Sodium

Pharmacological Effects. Cromolyn does not relax bronchial or other smooth muscle. Nor does it inhibit significantly responses of these muscles to any of a variety of pharmacological spasmogens. It does, however, inhibit the secretion of histamine and other autacoids (including the potent spasmogen SRS-A) from human lung during allergic responses mediated by IgE and thereby reduces the stimulus for bronchospasm. It is believed to act on the pulmonary mast cells, the primary target cells for the immediate hypersensitivity reaction. Inhibition of antigen-induced release of histamine and production of SRS-A can readily be demonstrated in mast cells isolated from the rat peritoneal cavity. Cromolyn does not inhibit the binding of IgE to peritoneal mast cells nor the interaction between cell-bound IgE and specific antigen; rather, it suppresses the secretory response to this reaction. How it does so is uncertain. The effect is not restricted to the antigen-antibody reaction, although this may be preferentially affected, and it can also be observed when other secretagogues are tested (such as 48/80, dextran, phospholipase A, and the calcium ionophore A23187).

Attempts to explain the action of cromolyn in terms of changes in concentrations of cyclic nucleotides have been unrewarding and have prompted vague statements that cromolyn has a "membrane-stabilizing" action. More precisely, it may block calcium channels in the membrane (*see* reviews by Church, 1978; Johnson, 1978). Cromolyn has been shown to promote the phosphorylation of a single mast-cell protein, and this action has been advanced as a further possible explanation for its effect (Theoharides *et al.,* 1980). There are remarkable species and tissue differences in responsiveness to cromolyn, and it appears to have little influence on the allergic responses of human basophils or mast cells in human skin.

Absorption, Fate, and Excretion. Cromolyn is very poorly absorbed after oral administration and is therefore given, for asthma, by inhalation. A special turbo inhaler is used to disperse the finely powdered drug (mixed with lactose). By this route, some 10% penetrates deep into the lungs and is absorbed into the blood, where its half-life is about 80 minutes. The drug is not metabolized and is excreted unchanged, about half in the urine and half in the bile. Aqueous solutions are available for nasal and ophthalmic uses.

Toxicity. The acute toxicity of cromolyn given intravenously to animals is low. No hematological, biochemical, or renal abnormalities have been reported. Generally the drug is well tolerated by patients, and adverse reactions are minor. The most frequent reactions, probably related to the direct irritant effect of the powder, include bronchospasm, wheezing, cough, nasal congestion, and pharyngeal irritation. Sometimes dizziness, dysuria, joint swelling and pain, nausea, headache, and rash are encountered. More serious and rare effects, probably attributable to hypersensitivity to the drug, include laryngeal edema, angioedema, urticaria, and anaphylaxis. The drug is clearly contraindicated in patients who show hypersensitivity to it. Another indication for withdrawal of the drug is eosinophilic pneumonitis. The safety of cromolyn for use during pregnancy has not been established. Interactions with other drugs have not been noted.

Preparation and Dosage. *Cromolyn Sodium for Inhalation,* U.S.P. (INTAL), is available in capsules that contain 20 mg of the finely powdered drug mixed with lactose. The contents of the capsule are inhaled by means of a special turbo inhaler, usually four times daily.

Clinical Use. The main use of cromolyn is in the *prophylactic treatment* of bronchial asthma. This is based on the experimental observation that, when given before an antigenic challenge, it will inhibit bronchoconstriction and prevent the objective signs and the symptoms of the acute asthmatic attack. This protective effect can last for hours (*see* Altounyan, 1970). By contrast, if cromolyn is administered even as soon as 1 minute after the antigenic challenge, it has little effect on the course of the response. For this reason, *cromolyn has no place in the treatment of the acute asthmatic attack, nor in status asthmaticus.*

Clinical trials leave no doubt that, when given prophylactically, cromolyn benefits many asthmatic patients by improving pulmonary function and reducing the frequency and intensity of asthmatic episodes; the need for administration of corticosteroids or bronchodilators is thus reduced (Bernstein *et al.,* 1972; Collaborative Trial, 1972, 1976; Toogood *et al.,* 1978). Patients of different ages and with various types of asthma may be benefited. The effectiveness of the drug is not restricted to patients with extrinsic, atopic, IgE-mediated asthma; intrinsic asthma and dust- and exercise-induced asthmas may also be benefited. However, the drug is ineffective in many patients, and it is difficult to predict who will respond. Moreover, benefit may only become evident after 4 or more weeks of medication. Some indications of probable usefulness include onset of asthma before adulthood, family history of atopy, positive skin test to suspected allergens, forced expiratory volume (FEV_1) less than 80% of predicted normal value and improvement by 20% or more after inhalation of a clinical dose of a bronchodilator, eosinophilia of sputum, raised concentrations of specific IgE, and good responses to oral corticosteroids (*see* Kingsley and Cox, 1978).

Other clinical conditions in which beneficial effects of cromolyn may occur include *allergic rhinitis,* both *perennial* and *seasonal.* The drug may also be of benefit in some patients with vernal keratoconjunctivitis. Its value in various other conditions such as food allergies, ulcerative colitis, and systemic mastocytosis is presently being assessed. Numerous reviews covering basic and clinical aspects of cromolyn are available (Cox *et al.,* 1970; Brogden *et al.,* 1974; Cox, 1977; Kingsley and Cox, 1978; Toogood *et al.,* 1978; also *see* Symposium, 1979).

HISTAMINE ANTAGONISTS: H_1- AND H_2-BLOCKING AGENTS

History It was long obvious that drugs able to antagonize the actions of histamine would be of great interest both as investigative tools and as therapeutic agents. Histamine-blocking activity was first detected by Bovet and Staub (1937) in one of a series of amines with a phenolic ether function synthesized by Fourneau. This substance, 2-isopropyl-5-methylphenoxyethyldiethylamine, protected guinea pigs against several lethal doses of histamine, antagonized histamine-induced spasms of various smooth muscles, and, most significantly, lessened the symptoms of anaphylactic shock (Staub and Bovet, 1937). Although the drug was too weak and too toxic for clinical use, this was a most exciting beginning. A more effective drug was uncovered in diethylaminoethyl-N-ethylaniline. This, too, was rather toxic, but a dimethylamine derivative prepared by Mosnier and investigated by Halpern (1942) proved acceptable for clinical use. This substance, ANTERGAN, was the first histamine blocking drug to be employed in therapy. NEO-ANTERGAN, introduced shortly thereafter (Bovet *et al.,* 1944), the official name of which is *pyrilamine maleate,* is still one of the most specific and effective histamine blockers of this category. While these developments were taking place in wartime France, the leads offered by the original Fourneau compounds were also being followed in the United States and resulted in the discovery of the highly effective histamine antagonists *diphenhydramine* (Loew *et al.,* 1946) and *tripelennamine* (Yonkman *et al.,* 1946).

By the late 1940s, it was obvious that numerous compounds possessed significant histamine blocking properties. This circumstance, coupled with the unrestrained enthusiasm of some early clinical reports, encouraged a frenzy of syntheses. Most of the efforts were successful, and the physician was shortly confronted with scores of such drugs to choose from, mostly offering little or no advantage over the original compounds.

All these drugs, while effectively reducing many important responses to histamine, uniformly failed to inhibit others, most conspicuously gastric acid secretion. The introduction by Black and colleagues in 1972 of drugs that selectively inhibit gastric secretion and the several other responses to histamine that are refractory to the older antagonists of the autacoid signaled a breakthrough in the field. The discovery at once offered important new tools for probing the significance of histamine in physiological and pathophysiological processes and held out promise of a new and potentially important class of therapeutic agents.

Terminology. Depending on what responses to histamine are prevented, antagonists that act at receptors for histamine are classified as H_1- or H_2-receptor blocking agents, or simply as H_1 or H_2 blockers. The precedent for such a terminology has been long established in the adrenergic field, where the terms α-adrenergic and β-adrenergic blockers have now become common medical parlance (*see* Chapter 9).

Mechanism of Action. Drugs that block histamine receptors fall into that large group of pharmacological antagonists that appear to act by occupying receptors on the effector cell, to the exclusion of agonist molecules, without themselves initiating a response. In the case of the antagonists of histamine, the action is competitive and reversible (*see* Ganellin, 1978b; Rocha e Silva, 1978b; van den Brink and Lien, 1978).

H₁-BLOCKING AGENTS

Structure-Activity Relationship. Like histamine, most H₁ antagonists contain a substituted ethylamine moiety, $-\overset{|}{C}-\overset{|}{C}-N\overset{\diagup}{\diagdown}$; unlike histamine, which has a primary amino group and a single aromatic ring, most H₁ blockers have a tertiary amino group linked by a two- or three-atom chain to two aromatic substituents and conform to the general formula:

$$\begin{matrix} Ar_1 \\ \diagdown \\ \quad X-C-C-N \diagup \\ \diagup \\ Ar_2 \end{matrix}$$

where Ar is aryl and X is a nitrogen or carbon atom or a —C—O— ether linkage to the β-aminoethyl side chain. Sometimes the two aromatic rings are bridged, as in the tricyclic derivatives, or the ethylamine may be part of a ring structure. Other variations are also possible (*see* Table 26–2 and the structure of cyproheptadine, below). Extensive reviews of this complex field are available (*see* Casy, 1978; Nauta and Rekker, 1978).

Pharmacological Properties. Most H₁ blockers have similar pharmacological actions and therapeutic applications and can be conveniently discussed together. Individual compounds will be mentioned only in those few instances where they depart significantly from the pattern of the group. The characteristic pharmacological activity of this class of drugs is largely predictable from the foregoing presentation of the responses to histamine that involve interaction with H₁ receptors.

Smooth Muscle. H₁-blocking drugs inhibit

Table 26–2. REPRESENTATIVE H₁-RECEPTOR BLOCKING DRUGS

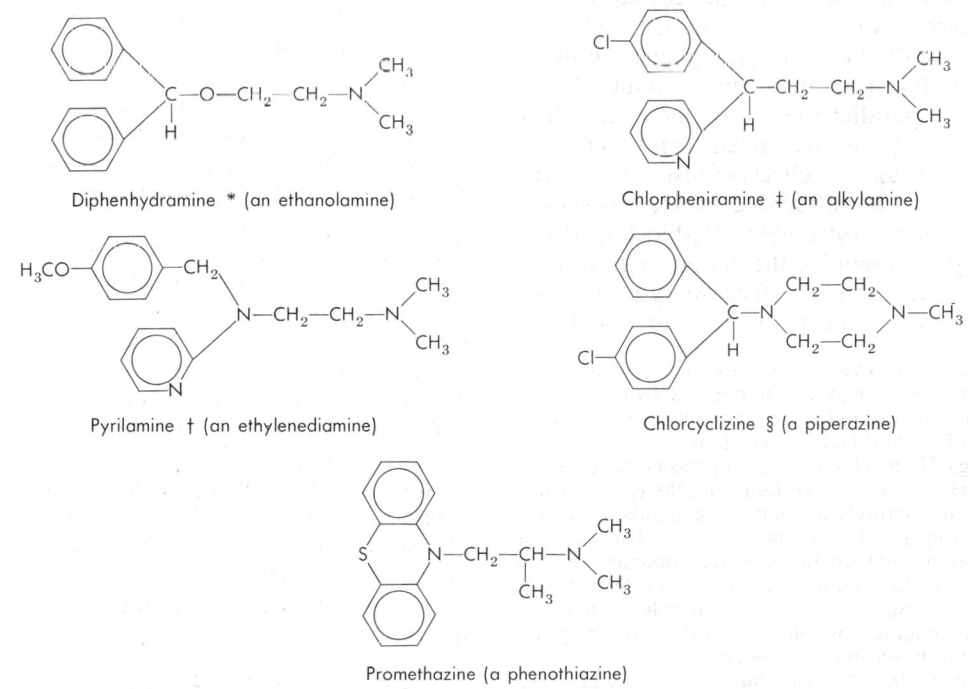

Diphenhydramine * (an ethanolamine)

Chlorpheniramine ‡ (an alkylamine)

Pyrilamine † (an ethylenediamine)

Chlorcyclizine § (a piperazine)

Promethazine (a phenothiazine)

---

* Dimenhydrinate is a combination of diphenhydramine and 8-chlorotheophylline in equal molecular proportions.
† Tripelennamine is the same less H₃CO.   ‡ Pheniramine is the same less Cl.   § Cyclizine is the same less Cl.

most responses of smooth muscle to histamine. Within the *gastrointestinal tract,* the guinea pig ileum has been extensively studied *in vitro.* This preparation illustrates the competitive and surmountable nature of the block as well as its specificity. Similar antagonism is also readily demonstrable *in vivo* and in other regions of the gastrointestinal tract.

Antagonism of the constrictor action of histamine on *respiratory smooth muscle* is easily shown *in vivo,* in isolated lungs, or in strips of tracheal, bronchial, or bronchiolar muscle of various species including man. In guinea pigs, death by asphyxia follows quite small doses of histamine, yet the animal may survive a hundred lethal doses of histamine if given an H_1-blocking drug. In the same species, striking protection is also afforded against anaphylactic bronchospasm, but this is not so in man, in whom allergic bronchoconstriction is mediated less by histamine than by other autacoids, such as SRS-A.

Within the *vascular tree,* the H_1-blocking drugs inhibit both the vasoconstrictor effects of histamine and, to a degree, the more important vasodilator effects. Residual vasodilatation reflects the involvement of H_2 receptors and can only be suppressed by the concurrent administration of an H_2 blocker. Effects of the histamine antagonists on histamine-induced changes in systemic blood pressure parallel these vascular effects. The variable, species-dependent, and generally minor stimulatory effects of histamine on the heart are little influenced by H_1 blockers.

Capillary Permeability. H_1-blocking drugs strongly antagonize the action of histamine that results in increased capillary permeability and formation of edema and wheal.

"Flare" and Itch. The "flare" component of the triple response and the itching caused by intradermal injection of histamine are two different manifestations of a stimulant action of histamine on nerve endings. H_1-blocking drugs suppress both. Although most H_1 blockers have local anesthetic properties, this cannot entirely account for their effectiveness in countering these effects of histamine. There is little correlation between the anesthetic potency of these drugs and their ability to inhibit neural responses to histamine. Such drugs act apparently in a rather specific manner by blocking histamine receptors, presumably on the nerve endings.

Adrenal Medulla and Autonomic Ganglia. H_1-blocking drugs selectively suppress the stimulant effects of histamine on adrenal chromaffin cells and autonomic ganglia.

Failure to Inhibit Gastric Secretion. Histamine stimulates gastric secretion via H_2 receptors. This effect is *not* inhibited at all by H_1 blocking agents; indeed, H_1 blockers are used in conjunction with histamine in diagnostic tests of gastric secretory function to lessen circulatory and other side effects (*see* above).

Other Exocrine Glands. H_1-blocking drugs inconstantly suppress histamine-evoked salivary, lacrimal, and other exocrine secretions. The atropine-like properties of many of these agents may, however, contribute to lessened secretion in cholinergically innervated glands and reduce ongoing secretion in, for example, the respiratory tree.

Failure to Inhibit Release of Endogenous Histamine. It is essential to note that neither the H_1 nor the H_2 blockers inhibit histamine release. Indeed, the effects of histamine antagonists tend to be in the opposite direction, namely, to facilitate release (*see* below). Any beneficial effects of histamine blockers are thus confined to antagonism of responses to the histamine that is released.

Immediate Hypersensitivity Reactions: Anaphylaxis and Allergy. During hypersensitivity reactions, histamine is but one of several potent autacoids that are released, and its relative importance for the ensuing symptoms varies widely with species and tissue. It follows that the protection afforded by histamine antagonists, which do not prevent responses to these other autacoids, is also variable with species and tissue. In man, some phenomena, including edema formation and itch, are fairly well controlled; others, such as hypotension, are less so; and bronchoconstriction is blocked little if at all (SRS-A is the principal autacoid responsible for allergic bronchoconstriction in man). Thus, the clinical usefulness of H_1-blocking drugs in allergic conditions revolves mainly around their effects on mucous membranes and skin. Moreover, even when histamine is clearly involved, some conditions may be so severe that they call for the more potent physiological antagonism offered by epinephrine; this is true, for example, of anaphylactic edema of the larynx (*see* below).

Responses to Histamine-Releasing Drugs. These are somewhat better controlled by H_1-blocking drugs in man than are the allergic responses. Fewer autacoids are presumably involved, and histamine is relatively more important.

Central Nervous System. The H_1 blockers can both stimulate and depress the CNS. Stimulation is occasionally encountered in patients given conventional doses, who become restless, nervous, and unable to sleep. Moreover, quite small doses may evoke EEG activation and epileptiform seizures in patients with focal lesions of the CNS. Central excitation is also a striking feature of poisoning, which not uncommonly results in convulsions, particularly in infants. Central depression, on the other hand, is the usual accompaniment of therapeutic doses of the H$_1$ antagonists, although patients vary in their susceptibility and responses to individual drugs. The ethanolamines (Table 26–2) are particularly prone to depress. Diphenhydramine, for example, causes somnolence in about half of those taking the drug (see Carruthers et al., 1978). An antitussive effect reflects another and, perhaps, unrelated central action (Lilienfield et al., 1976).

An interesting and useful property of certain H$_1$ blockers is the ability to counter motion sickness. This effect was first observed with dimenhydrinate and subsequently with diphenhydramine (the active moiety of dimenhydrinate), promethazine, and various piperazine derivatives.

Mechanism of Central Action. How the various H$_1$-blocking drugs produce their depressant and stimulant effects is not known. Although histaminergic nerves may be present in the brain, there is no obvious correlation between the peripheral histamine-blocking ability of these drugs and their central effects (see Schwartz, 1977; Faingold, 1978; Green et al., 1978). Only the antimotion sickness actions have been studied intensively, and even here there is no precise answer. Physiologists debate the causes of motion sickness. All that seems clear is that stimulation of the vestibular apparatus is necessary and sufficient (although the respective roles of semicircular canals and otoliths are uncertain), and that the vestibular cerebellar midbrain "integrative vomiting center" and medullary chemoreceptive trigger zone are somehow involved. Probably the effective drugs exert their action somewhere in these centers (Money, 1970). Electrophysiological recordings in dogs have shown that diphenhydramine diminishes excitability of the vestibular nuclear complex to vestibular afferent activity induced by motion or electrical stimulation of the vestibular nerve. Similar effects have been obtained with lower doses of scopolamine, a more potent antimotion sickness drug (see Jaju and Wang, 1971). Possibly, as suggested by Chinn and Smith (1955), the H$_1$ blockers effective in motion sickness act by central antagonism of ACh, as does scopolamine. Promethazine, which is perhaps the H$_1$-blocking drug with the strongest ACh-blocking action, is one of the most effective in combating motion sickness (see below).

Anticholinergic Effects. Many of the H$_1$ antagonists also prevent responses to ACh that are mediated by muscarinic receptors. These atropine-like actions are sufficiently prominent in some of the drugs to be manifest during clinical usage (see below). Among the H$_1$ blockers, pyrilamine is one of the *least* liable to produce this effect. Its relatively high degree of specificity has rendered it a favorite pharmacological tool (see Rocha e Silva and Antonio, 1978).

Local Anesthetic Effect. The H$_1$-blocking drugs possess local anesthetic activity. Some are more potent than procaine. Promethazine and pyrilamine are especially active. However, the concentrations required for this effect are several orders higher than those that antagonize histamine.

Cardiovascular System. Rapid intravenous injection of an H$_1$-blocking agent causes a transient fall in blood pressure, probably related to local anesthetic activity. Blood pressure is well maintained or may even be elevated when the drug is given slowly. With the usual oral dose the drugs have no significant cardiovascular effect; higher doses have quinidine-like effects on myocardial conduction, consistent with their other local anesthetic properties.

Absorption, Fate, and Excretion. The H$_1$ blockers are well absorbed from the gastrointestinal tract. Following oral administration, the effects develop within 15 to 30 minutes, are maximal within 1 to 2 hours, and last about 3 to 6 hours, although some of the drugs are much longer acting (Table 26–3, page 628).

Extensive studies of the metabolic fate of H$_1$-blocking drugs have been limited to a few compounds. *Diphenhydramine,* given orally, reaches a maximal concentration in the blood in about 2 hours, remains at about this level for another 2 hours, and then falls exponentially with a plasma elimination half-time of about 3.5 hours. Concentrations of the drug in plasma correlate with both its histamine-antagonizing effect (suppression of wheal) and its sedative effect (see Carruthers et al., 1978). The drug is widely distributed throughout the body, including the CNS. Little, if any, is excreted unchanged in the urine; most appears there as degradation products that are almost completely excreted within 24 hours. The main site of metabolic transformation is the liver. *Tripelennamine* and the other H$_1$ blockers appear to be eliminated in much the same way (see review by Witiak and Lewis, 1978).

Side Effects. In therapeutic doses, all H$_1$ blockers elicit side effects. Although these are rarely serious and often disappear with continued therapy, they are sometimes so troublesome that the drug must be withdrawn.

Some difference in the incidence and severity of the side effects with different preparations is discernible, but there is such marked variation in the responses of individual subjects that acccurate figures of relative incidence of side effects in the population as a whole, even if they were available, would be of doubtful value in assisting the physician to choose among these drugs. One notable exception is in the tendency to cause somnolence, which is clearly more marked in some of the drugs than in others. About one person in four will experience some bothersome reaction during treatment with a given H_1 blocker.

The side effect with the highest incidence, and the one common to all drugs in this group, is *sedation* (*e.g., see* Carruthers *et al.,* 1978). Although this may be a desirable adjunct in the treatment of some patients in the hospital or about to retire for the night, it interferes with the patient's daytime activities and can so dull the mind and slow reflex activity that accidents may occur. Alcohol heightens this danger. Decrease in dosage, the use of a different H_1 blocker, and combined therapy with stimulants such as caffeine may circumvent this undesirable effect. Other untoward reactions referable to *central actions* include dizziness, tinnitus, lassitude, incoordination, fatigue, blurred vision, diplopia, euphoria, nervousness, insomnia, and tremors.

The next most frequent side effects involve the *digestive tract* and include loss of appetite, nausea, vomiting, epigastric distress, and constipation or diarrhea. Their incidence may be reduced by giving the drug with meals. Other side effects include dryness of the mouth, throat, and respiratory passages, sometimes inducing cough; urinary frequency and dysuria; palpitation; hypotension; headache; tightness of the chest; and tingling, heaviness, and weakness of the hands. The atropine-like actions of many of the H_1 blockers clearly account for some of these side effects.

Allergy may develop when H_1 blockers are given orally, but more commonly it results from topical application. Allergic dermatitis is not uncommon. In addition, histamine-liberating properties have been demonstrated for several of the drugs (Rothschild, 1966) and may contribute to some adverse reactions encountered during therapy. For-

tunately, grave complications such as *leukopenia* and *agranulocytosis* are very rare.

The piperazine compounds—cyclizine, chlorcyclizine, and meclizine—have been demonstrated to have *teratogenic effects in laboratory animals,* and their use is contraindicated in pregnant women (*see* Sadusk and Palmisano, 1965).

Acute Poisoning. Although the H_1-blocking drugs have a relatively high margin of safety, acute poisoning with them is common. These drugs are frequently found in medicine cabinets, and all too often they are the cause of accidental poisoning in young children or the instrument of suicide in adults. In children, 20 to 30 tablets or capsules provide a lethal or near-lethal dose.

The central effects of the H_1 blockers constitute their greatest danger and, in a severely poisoned individual, give rise to a constellation of signs and symptoms in which both the depressant and stimulant properties of the drug are in evidence. In the small child, the dominant effect is excitation, and the syndrome of poisoning includes *hallucinations, excitement, ataxia, incoordination, athetosis,* and *convulsions.* The convulsions, sometimes heralded by muscular tremors and athetoid movements, are of the intermittent tonic-clonic type and difficult to control. *Fixed, dilated pupils* with a *flushed face* and *fever* are common and lend the syndrome a remarkable similarity to that of atropine poisoning. Terminally, there is deepening coma with cardiorespiratory collapse and death, usually within 2 to 18 hours. In the adult, fever and flushing are not usually in evidence, and the phase of excitement leading to convulsions and postictal depression is not uncommonly preceded by drowsiness and coma, so that there is a cycle of depression followed by stimulation and postictal depression. Inasmuch as the treatments of the two types of depression are different, they must be distinguished.

Treatment. There is no specific therapy for poisoning with H_1 blockers, and treatment is along general symptomatic and supportive lines. The central depressant effect of the drugs is not as profound as that of the barbiturates. Respiration is usually not seriously embarrassed, and blood pressure is fairly well maintained. Mechanical support of ventilation is obviously essential if respiration should fail. If convulsions develop, they are best countered by a short-acting depressant such as thiopental, to provide a rapid, transient, and controllable effect; diazepam is also worthy of a trial.

Preparations. There is a needlessly large number of H_1 blockers, and little distinction can be made between them on the basis of efficacy as histamine antagonists. They do vary somewhat, however, with respect to potency, dosage, relative incidence of side effects, and the types of preparations available. Naturally, the physician is desirous of choosing a preparation that will assure the greatest opportunity for therapeutic success with the minimal chance of side effects. Unfortunately, none of the H_1 antagonists can be said to be outstanding. The difficulty lies not only in the quantitative assessment of both therapeutic efficacy and incidence and severity of side effects, but also in the fact that individual variations in response are prominent. Such factors tend to undermine the value of generalizations, with the result that the physician must often approach the problem in a tentative manner, trying first a thoroughly tested drug known to have the desired pattern of effect in most patients, and using other drugs only in the event that the first proves unsatisfactory. Since there are many advantages to using the older and well-tried drugs, it would seem wise for the physician to become familiar with a few representative compounds from the different classes, and to base his therapy upon these. Few, if any, of the "newer" drugs have any conspicuous therapeutic advantage, and most are more costly (*see* Medical Letter, 1977). The brief discussion that follows is intended to provide only an indication of the different classes of H_1-blocking drugs and their properties. The statements should be interpreted in the light of the foregoing comments. Preparations are listed in Table 26–3.

Ethanolamines (Prototype: Diphenhydramine). The drugs in this group are potent and effective H_1 blockers that possess significant antimuscarinic activity and have a pronounced tendency to induce sedation. With conventional doses, about half of those who are treated with these drugs experience somnolence, although with carbinoxamine the proportion is rather less. The incidence of gastrointestinal side effects, however, is low in this group.

Ethylenediamines (Prototype: Pyrilamine). These include some of the most specific and active H_1 antagonists. Although their central effects are relatively feeble and of no therapeutic value, somnolence occurs, nevertheless, in a fair proportion of patients. Gastrointestinal side effects are quite common. This group contains some of the oldest and best-known H_1-blocking drugs.

Alkylamines (Prototype: Chlorpheniramine). These are among the most potent H_1-blocking agents and are generally effective in relatively low doses. The drugs are not so prone to produce drowsiness and are among the more suitable agents for daytime use; but again, a significant proportion of patients do experience this effect. Side effects involving CNS stimulation are more common in this than in other groups.

Piperazines (Prototype: Chlorcyclizine). The oldest member of this group, chlorcyclizine, is an H_1 blocker with prolonged action and a comparatively low incidence of drowsiness. The others have been used primarily to counter motion sickness, although it appears from extensive trials that other H_1 blockers, promethazine and diphenhydramine (dimenhydrinate), are more effective (as is scopolamine; *see* below). CNS depressant and anticholinergic effects compare favorably with those of other H_1-blocking drugs, but side effects attributable to these phenomena may nevertheless be disturbing.

Phenothiazines (Prototype: Promethazine). Most drugs of this class are H_1 blockers and also possess considerable anticholinergic activity. The prototype, promethazine, was introduced in 1946 for the management of allergic conditions. The prominent sedative effects of this compound and its value in motion sickness were early recognized. Promethazine and its many congeners are now used primarily for their antiemetic effects (*see* Chapter 19).

Therapeutic Uses. H_1-blocking drugs have an established and valued place in the symptomatic treatment of various allergic diseases, in which their usefulness is attributable to their antagonism of endogenously released histamine, one of several autacoids that together elicit the allergic response. In addition, the central properties of *some* of the series are of considerable therapeutic value, particularly in suppressing motion sickness.

Diseases of Allergy. H_1 antagonists are most useful in acute exudative types of allergy such as *pollinosis* and *urticaria*. Their effect, however, is purely palliative and confined to the suppression in varying degree of symptoms attributable to the pharmacological activity of histamine released by the antigen-antibody reaction. The drugs do not diminish the intensity of this reaction, which is the root cause of the various hypersensitivity diseases. This can be achieved only by other means, such as the removal or avoidance of allergen, specific desensitization, suppression of the reaction by corticosteroids, or, in restricted instances, use of cromolyn. This limitation must be clearly recognized because no histamine-blocking drug, or combination of such drugs, is effective against the various autacoids other than histamine. In *bronchial asthma,* histamine blockers are singularly ineffectual. They have no role in the therapy of the severe attack, in which chief reliance must be placed on "physiological antagonists" such as epinephrine, isoproterenol, and theophylline. Equally, in the treatment of *systemic anaphylaxis,* in which autacoids other than histamine are again important, the mainstay of therapy is once more epinephrine, with histamine antagonists having only a subordinate and adjuvant role. The same is true for severe *angioedema,* in which laryngeal swelling constitutes a threat to life. However, the subordination of histamine blockers to physiological antagonists in these allergic crises is not based solely on the grounds that autacoids other than histamine are involved. The superiority of physiological antagonists lies in the immediacy of the relief they afford and in the fact that they do not merely reduce the undesirable effects but tend to reverse them.

Other allergies of the respiratory tract are more amenable to therapy with H_1 blockers. The best results are obtained in *seasonal rhinitis* and *conjunctivitis* (hay fever, pollinosis), in which these drugs relieve the sneezing, rhinorrhea, and itching of eyes, nose, and throat. A gratifying response is obtained in most patients, especially at the beginning of the

Table 26–3.   PREPARATIONS AND DOSAGE OF REPRESENTATIVE OFFICIAL H$_1$-BLOCKING AGENTS *

CLASS AND NONPROPRIETARY NAME	TRADE NAME	DURATION OF ACTION (HOURS)	USUAL PREPARATION	OTHER PREPARATIONS AVAILABLE	SINGLE DOSE (ADULT)
Ethanolamines					
Diphenhydramine Hydrochloride	BENADRYL and others	4–6	Capsules, 25 and 50 mg	Injection (syringes, vials, and ampuls); elixir	50 mg
Dimenhydrinate	DRAMAMINE	4–6	Tablets, 50 mg	Injection; suppositories; liquid	50 mg
Carbinoxamine Maleate	CLISTIN	3–4	Tablets, 4 mg; repeat-action tablets, 8 and 12 mg	Elixir	4 mg
Ethylenediamines					
Tripelennamine Hydrochloride	PBZ	4–6	Tablets, 25 and 50 mg; long-action tablets, 50 mg	Cream (topical), 2%; ointment (topical), 2%	50 mg
Tripelennamine Citrate	PBZ		Elixir, 37.5 mg/5 ml		75 mg
Pyrilamine Maleate	ALLERTOC, NEO-ANTERGAN	4–6	Tablets, 25 and 50 mg	Various (in combinations)	25–50 mg
Antazoline Phosphate	VASOCON-A	3–4	Ophthalmic solution, 0.5% (with 0.05% naphazoline)		
Alkylamines					
Chlorpheniramine Maleate	CHLOR-TRIMETON and others	4–6	Tablets, 4 mg; repeat-action tablets, 8 and 12 mg	Injection; syrup	2–4 mg
Brompheniramine Maleate	DIMETANE, DISOMER	4–6	Tablets, 4 mg	Elixir	4–8 mg
Piperazines					
Cyclizine Hydrochloride	MAREZINE	4–6	Tablets, 50 mg		50 mg
Cyclizine Lactate	MAREZINE	4–6	Injection, 50 mg/ml in 1-ml ampul		50 mg
Meclizine Hydrochloride	ANTIVERT, BONINE	12–24	Tablets (chewing), 12.5 and 25 mg		25–50 mg
Phenothiazines					
Promethazine Hydrochloride	PHENERGAN and others	4–6	Tablets, 12.5, 25, and 50 mg	Injection; suppositories; syrup	25–50 mg

* For a discussion of phenothiazines, *see* Chapter 19.

season when pollen counts are low; however, the drugs are rather less effective when the allergens are in abundance, when exposure to them is prolonged, and when nasal congestion has become prominent. Such chronic congestion and the accompanying headache from edema of the paranasal sinus mucosa are rather refractory to treatment with H$_1$ blockers. In *perennial vasomotor rhinitis,* H$_1$ blockers are of limited value. Although H$_1$-blocking drugs have long been used in elixirs and syrups for controlling *cough,* especially in asthmatic children, any benefit from their specific antiallergic action or sedation may be offset by the anticholinergic properties of these drugs, which, by excessive drying of the respiratory tree, can render bronchial secretion viscid and make expectoration difficult.

Certain of the *allergic dermatoses* respond favorably to H$_1$ blockers. Benefit is most striking in *acute urticaria,* although the itching in this condition is perhaps better controlled than are the edema and the erythema. *Chronic urticaria* is less responsive, but some measure of benefit may be had in a fair proportion of patients. *Angioedema* is also responsive to treatment with antihistamines, but the paramount importance of epinephrine in the severe attack must be reemphasized, especially in the life-threatening involvement of the larynx. Here, however, it may be appropriate to administer *additionally* an H$_1$ antagonist by the intravenous route. H$_1$ blockers also have a place in the treatment of *itching pruritides.* Some relief may be obtained in many patients suffering from *atopic dermatitis* and *contact dermatitis,* although topical corticosteroids seem to be more valuable, and in such diverse conditions as *insect bites* and *ivy poisoning.* Various other pruritides without allergic basis sometimes respond to antihistamine therapy, usually when the drugs are applied topically but sometimes when they are given orally. However, the considerable danger of producing allergic dermatitis with local application of H$_1$ blockers must be recognized. Since these drugs inhibit allergic dermatoses, *they should be withdrawn before skin testing for allergies.*

The value of H$_1$-blocking drugs in *systemic allergies* is variable. As described above, they have only an adjuvant role in severe systemic anaphylaxis. The urticarial and edematous lesions of *serum sickness,* however, respond to H$_1$ blockers, but fever and arthralgia often do not. *Gastrointestinal allergies* are seldom benefited significantly by these drugs.

Many *drug reactions* attributable to allergic phenomena respond to therapy with H$_1$ blockers, particularly those characterized by itch, urticaria, and angioedema; reactions of the serum-sickness type also respond to intensive treatment. However, explosive release of histamine generally calls for treatment with epinephrine, with H$_1$-blocking drugs being accorded a subsidiary role. Nevertheless, prophylactic treatment with an H$_1$ blocker may suffice to reduce symptoms to a tolerable level when a drug known to be a powerful histamine liberator is to be given. Extensive discussion of the effects of H$_1$ antagonists in allergic and related conditions are supplied by Assem (1976), Pearlman (1976), Beaven (1978), and Hahn (1978). (*See also* Medical Letter, 1978a.)

Common Cold. Despite early claims and persistent popular belief, H$_1$-blocking drugs are without value in combating the common cold. Their weak anticholinergic effects may tend to lessen rhinorrhea, but this drying effect may do more harm than good, as may also their tendency to induce somnolence (*see* West *et al.,* 1975).

Motion Sickness and Other Conditions. By far the most common application of the central effects of certain H$_1$ antagonists is in the prophylaxis and treatment of *motion sickness.* In recent years there has been a tendency to restrict drug therapy to two types of agent, H$_1$ blockers and scopolamine. Early

claims that the former are superior have been rebutted by careful studies showing that, of all the *single* agents, scopolamine is the most effective in preventing motion sickness (Brand and Perry, 1966). More recent studies, while confirming this, have again demonstrated the usefulness of H$_1$ blockers, particularly diphenhydramine (dimenhydrinate) and promethazine. They have also shown that the effectiveness of these H$_1$ blockers (and of scopolamine) is increased by concurrent use with ephedrine or amphetamine (Wood and Graybiel, 1970; Graybiel *et al.,* 1975). Since individuals vary in their responsiveness to the different drugs and combinations, failure to control motion sickness with one does not preclude success with another.

The H$_1$-blocking drugs effective in motion sickness may have some beneficial effect in vestibular disturbances such as *Ménière's disease* and other types of *vertigo* (*see* Cohen and deJong, 1972). They are usually of no value in *benign positional vertigo.*

The tendency of certain of the H$_1$ blockers, particularly the ethanolamines, to produce somnolence has led to their use as *hypnotics.* They are by no means as powerful or effective as the barbiturates, for example, but they may have some value in selected patients. H$_1$ blockers, particularly pyrilamine, are often present in various proprietary remedies for insomnia that are sold "over the counter." While these remedies are generally ineffective in the recommended doses, some singularly sensitive individuals may derive benefit (*see* Faingold, 1978).

The *local anesthetic activity* of H$_1$-blocking drugs has often been used to counter itching or painful conditions of skin and mucous membranes. However, as already emphasized, there is danger of drug sensitization following topical application.

H$_2$-BLOCKING AGENTS

The search for drugs to oppose the several actions of histamine that are resistant to block by the original group of antagonists of the autacoid (the H$_1$ blockers) was lent special impetus by the many indications of involvement of endogenous histamine in gastric secretion and the clinical evidence that hypersecretion of gastric acid and peptic ulceration account for much illness (as many as 4,000,000 hospital days per year in the United States alone). The discovery and introduction of such drugs, the histamine H$_2$-receptor blocking drugs, soon provided incontrovertible evidence of the importance of endogenous histamine in the physiological control of gastric secretion. They have also provided a new and effective therapeutic approach to the treatment of gastric hypersecretory states.

Chemistry. The synthesis of H$_2$ antagonists was achieved by stepwise modifications of the histamine molecule, which resulted, some 200 compounds later, in the first highly effective drug with potent H_2-blocking activity, *burimamide* (Black *et al.,* 1972). This, like later compounds, retained the imidazole ring of histamine but possessed a much bulkier side chain. Burimamide was poorly absorbed orally, and better absorption and higher activity were achieved by introducing a methyl group in the ring to yield *metiamide*. This compound, while effective clinically, was withdrawn when it was found to cause granulocytopenia. Replacement of the thione ($=S$) sulfur atom of metiamide by a cyanimino group yielded *cimetidine,* a potent H_2 antagonist that is not known to cause this toxic effect. The structure of cimetidine is as follows:

$$CH_3 \quad CH_2SCH_2CH_2N\!\!=\!\!CNHCH_3$$
$$HN\!\!-\!\!C\!\!\equiv\!\!N$$

Cimetidine

Unlike the H_1 blockers, which are typically lipophilic amines, H_2 blockers such as cimetidine are very polar, hydrophilic molecules. The imidazole ring is believed to be important for receptor recognition, while both the cyanoguanidine and imidazole portions of the molecule contribute to affinity. (For detailed discussion of the development of H_2 blockers and the structure-activity relationship and physicochemical properties of cimetidine, *see* Ganellin *et al.,* 1976; Brimblecombe *et al.,* 1978; Ganellin, 1978a, 1978b.)

Pharmacological Properties. Cimetidine is a reversible, competitive antagonist of the actions of histamine that are exerted on H_2 receptors. It is selective in its action and is virtually without influence on those effects of histamine that are mediated through H_1 receptors. Moreover, it is not known to influence responses to drugs or autacoids acting through other receptors. The spectrum of pharmacological activity of cimetidine is thus to a large extent predictable from the preceding account of the actions of histamine mediated through H_2 receptors. The most prominent of these is the stimulation of gastric secretion, and it is the ability of cimetidine to inhibit this response that lends it particular interest and clinical importance. Detailed discussion of the pharmacological properties of the drug is presented in recent reviews and symposia (*see* Symposium, 1977a, 1978a; Brogden *et al.,* 1978).

Gastric Secretion. Cimetidine, administered intravenously or orally, inhibits histamine-evoked gastric acid secretion in a dose-dependent manner wherein the degree

of inhibition parallels closely the concentrations of the drug in blood (Brimblecombe and Duncan, 1977; Binder and Donaldson, 1978; Richardson, 1978; Figure 26–2). It also potently inhibits secretion induced by gastrin or pentagastrin and partially inhibits that stimulated by ACh or muscarinic drugs such as bethanechol. This breadth of effect is not due to any nonspecific actions at the receptors for these other secretagogues. Rather, it seems to reflect one of two possibilities. Histamine may be the common mediator of responses to these agents or, more probably, there may be mutual interdependence, such that these other secretagogues lose their efficacy when the ongoing stimulus provided by histamine is removed (*see* above). Whatever the explanation, this breadth of effect makes cimetidine a highly efficient inhibitor of

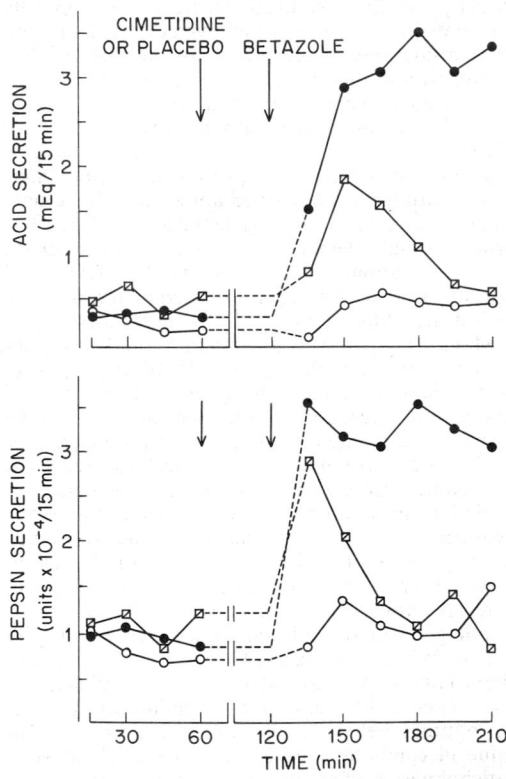

Figure 26–2. *Effect of cimetidine on betazole stimulation of secretion of acid* (upper panel) *and of pepsin* (lower panel) *in man.*

A placebo (●) or cimetidine (200 mg, ▨; 300 mg, ○) was given orally 1 hour prior to the subcutaneous administration of betazole (1.5 mg/kg). (Modified from Binder and Donaldson, 1978.)

physiological secretion of gastric juice stimulated by any of the three endogenous secretagogues. Cimetidine is thus a potent inhibitor of all *phases* of physiological secretion of gastric acid. In man, a single dose (300 mg) will inhibit basal (fasting) secretion and also secretion induced by solid, liquid, or peptone meals, sham feeding, fundic distention, pentagastrin, bethanechol, insulin, and caffeine, as well as the physiological stimulus provided by eating. It is noteworthy that this spectrum includes the cephalic or vagal phase.

Cimetidine reduces both the volume of gastric juice secreted and its hydrogen ion concentration. Output of pepsin generally falls in parallel with the diminished volume of gastric secretion. Output of intrinsic factor of Castle in response to betazole is inhibited by cimetidine, but basal secretion of the protein is only slightly affected and no evidence of deficient absorption of vitamin B_{12} has been noted, even during long-term treatment. Cimetidine does not alter basal concentrations of gastrin but tends to potentiate postprandial increases in the concentration of gastrin, possibly by reducing the negative feedback that is normally provided by decreased pH in the gastrointestinal tract; elevated concentrations of gastrin in plasma have sometimes been noted during prolonged treatment. Whether parietal-cell hyperplasia occurs is unknown. The reduction of gastric secretion caused by cimetidine protects experimental animals from gastric ulceration induced by stress, pyloric ligation, treatment with aspirin and related inhibitors of cyclooxygenase (*see* Chapter 29), or histaminergic and cholinergic drugs. Effects on peptic ulceration in man are described below. Cimetidine has no consistent effect on the rate of gastric emptying, lower esophageal sphincter pressure, or pancreatic secretion.

Other Effects. In doses that are more than adequate to depress gastric secretion profoundly, cimetidine has few obvious effects on the circulation. Histamine released during the hypersensitivity reaction is suspected of exerting some negative feedback on the mast cells or basophils from which it is discharged (*see* above), but cimetidine does not augment immediate hypersensitivity reactions except in doses 50 to 100 times higher than those needed to block the secretion of gastric acid (Brimblecombe and Duncan, 1977).

Absorption, Fate, and Excretion. Cimetidine is well absorbed (about 60%) by the oral route. Concentrations in blood are maximal in 1 to 1.5 hours, and a single oral dose yields an effective concentration for about 4 hours. Food delays absorption of cimetidine, so that the effect of the drug is prolonged when it is given with meals (and, of course, food will tend to buffer acidity during the latent period of absorption). Most of an oral dose of cimetidine is excreted unchanged in the urine within 24 hours. Some is excreted in the bile and, with the unabsorbed drug, escapes in the feces. Cimetidine crosses the placental barrier and is excreted in milk. It is distibuted widely in almost all tissues except the brain.

Toxicity. Cimetidine is generally well tolerated, and side effects are infrequent and usually minor. They include headache, dizziness, fatigue, muscle pains, constipation or diarrhea, and skin rashes. Sometimes an elevation in plasma creatinine concentration or aminotransferase activities may occur. Despite poor penetration to the CNS, neural dysfunction has been encountered, particularly with high doses in elderly patients and in association with impaired renal excretion. The effects include confusion, slurred speech, delirium, hallucinations, and coma. Fever has also been reported. The effects of cimetidine given for periods longer than 8 weeks, the currently approved duration of treatment, remain to be fully elucidated, but few important adverse reactions have been noted in patients treated with the drug for a year or more. A weak antiandrogenic effect has been noted in rats and dogs given high doses of cimetidine, and gynecomastia in men and galactorrhea in women have sometimes occurred in patients given high doses of the drug for long periods to treat, for example, the Zollinger-Ellison syndrome. A reduction in sperm count (by 40%) has also been noted in human males who received cimetidine for 9 weeks. This was associated with a reduced response of luteinizing hormone to the administration of gonadotropin-releasing hormone and elevated concentrations of testosterone in plasma (Van Thiel *et al.*, 1979). In some instances, withdrawal of cimetidine after a period of treatment has been followed by relapses in the symptoms of ulcer and even by perforation of duodenal, esophageal, or gastric ulcers. Whether such relapses or complications are more frequent after withdrawal of cimetidine than other forms of treatment is not clear. Accidental ingestion of up to 10 g of cimetidine in man has had no untoward effect. (*See* Bodemar and Walan, 1978; Kruss and Littman, 1978; Medical Letter, 1978b.)

Preparations, Routes of Administration, and Dosage. *Cimetidine* (TAGAMET) is available for *oral* use as tablets containing 300 mg. Recommended dosage for adults with duodenal ulcer is 300 mg four times a day with meals and at bedtime; the bedtime dose inhibits acid secretion throughout the night. Where oral administration is impractical, cimetidine may be given parenterally (intramuscularly or intravenously). For this purpose the drug is prepared in 2-ml vials containing cimetidine hydrochloride equivalent to 300 mg of cimetidine. These preparations are diluted with physiological saline solution before injection. Gastric acid secretion is reduced by approximately 50% when blood concentrations of the drug are 1 to 2 μM (0.25 to 0.5 μg/ml). Rectal administration is also efficacious; when given by this route, the concentrations of the drug in blood are lower but the effect is more sustained.

Therapeutic Uses. Clinical use of cimetidine obviously centers on its capacity to inhibit the secretion of gastric acid in hypersecretory states, particularly those involving peptic ulceration.

Duodenal Ulcer. Cimetidine has proven value in the treatment of duodenal ulcer disease in which most, but not all, patients show hypersecretion of gastric acid. It profoundly lowers basal and noctural secretion and that stimulated by meals and other factors, reduces both daytime and nighttime pain and the consumption of antacids, and hastens healing. The incidence of healing in 4- to 6-week periods is, in some trials, more than twice that of patients taking a placebo. Most duodenal ulcers are healed after 8 weeks of therapy with cimetidine. Healing rates of this order can be achieved by the use of highly efficacious antacids given at short intervals (Ippoliti *et al.*, 1978; Chapter 42), but cimetidine has the advantage of convenience in administration and lack of effect on the motility of the bowel. Possible advantages of concomitant therapy with antacids, anticholinergic agents, and other drugs that promote healing of peptic ulcers are being explored (*see* Wormsley, 1977). There are indications that cimetidine reduces the rate of recurrence of ulcer if given in maintenance doses after the acute episode. This is potentially important, since it is generally recognized

that it is easier to heal duodenal ulcers than to keep them healed. The merits and safety of such long-term maintenance therapy are being assessed, and it seems probable that the use of the drug for this purpose will be approved.

Zollinger-Ellison Syndrome (Gastrinoma) and Other Gastric Hypersecretory States. Hypersecretion of acid accounts for much of the morbidity and discomfort in the Zollinger-Ellison syndrome. Cimetidine is a useful adjunct to surgery or an alternative if surgery is impractical or contraindicated.

Other gastric hypersecretory states arising from *systemic mastocytosis, basophilic leukemia with hyperhistaminemia,* and *short-bowel syndrome* may also benefit. Conditions in which the drug has been used without clear evidence of benefit include *reflux esophagitis* (where cimetidine may offer some relief of heartburn and promote healing) and the prevention and treatment of *stress-related erosive gastritis, ulceration,* and *hemorrhage,* notably in patients with fulminant hepatic failure. Whether cimetidine is of any value in *benign gastric ulcer* is uncertain. The clinical uses of cimetidine are discussed at length in several reviews (Symposium, 1977a, 1978a; Brogden *et al.,* 1978; Feldman and Richardson, 1978; Koch-Weser *et al.,* 1978; Malagelada and Cortot, 1978; Hirschowitz, 1979).

5-HYDROXYTRYPTAMINE (SEROTONIN)

History. Mammalian physiologists have known for about a century that a vasoconstrictor material appears in serum when blood is allowed to clot. This unidentified vasoconstrictor material, which went by a variety of names, such as *vasotonin,* was a frequent nuisance in perfusion experiments in which defibrinated blood was used, although physiologists discovered empirically that it could be eliminated by passing the blood through the lungs, a phenomenon now understood to be due to uptake and enzymatic destruction. In the late 1940s, the substance appeared in another context during a search for humoral pressor agents such as angiotensin that might explain arterial hypertension. In this work the serum vasoconstrictor was a "pest," to be eliminated before the other enquiry could proceed. In 1948, investigators at the Cleveland Clinic isolated this vasoconstrictor substance as a crystalline complex and named it *serotonin* (Rapport *et al.,* 1948); shortly thereafter, Rapport (1949) deduced that the active moiety of this complex (for which he retained the name *serotonin*) was 5-hydroxytryptamine (5-HT). This compound, when prepared synthetically by Hamlin and Fischer (1951) and others, proved to have all the properties of natural serotonin.

Quite independently, studies had been proceeding in Italy that would soon reveal 5-HT as an autacoid whose occurrence and activities range far beyond the cardiovascular system. This work was begun in the 1930s by Erspamer and colleagues (*see* Erspamer, 1954), whose original purpose was to extract and characterize the substance that imparts peculiar histochemical properties to enterochromaffin cells of the gastrointestinal mucosa. Their experiments led them to discover, first in the mucosa and later in other tissues, a gut-stimulating factor of basic nature, which they termed *enteramine*. By the late 1940s, Erspamer had accumulated a great deal of information on the pharmacological activity of enteramine, had shown that it was present in many tissues of vertebrates and invertebrates, and had suggested that it was an indole alkylamine (Erspamer, 1946). In 1952, Erspamer and Asero identified enteramine as 5-hydroxytryptamine.

Thus, by the time 5-HT had been recognized as such, there already existed a mass of evidence indicating that it was widely distributed in nature and possessed a variety of pharmacological actions. It is therefore not surprising that the introduction of synthetic 5-HT in 1951 touched off an explosion of research. This was further fueled when 5-HT was discovered in the brain (Twarog and Page, 1953; Amin *et al.*, 1954), when lysergic acid diethylamide (LSD) and other potent hallucinogens were recognized to be structurally similar to 5-HT and were found to block smooth muscle responses to 5-HT (Gaddum, 1953; Woolley and Shaw, 1954), and when the potent tranquilizing drug reserpine was observed to lower concentrations of 5-HT in brain (*see* Brodie and Shore, 1957). All this suggested that 5-HT serves as a neurotransmitter, a function now established, and focused attention on a possible role of 5-HT in mental illnesses (*see* Woolley, 1962). These events, as much as any other, contributed greatly to the development of the still-burgeoning subdiscipline of psychopharmacology (*see* Chapter 19).

Source and Chemistry. 5-HT (serotonin) is 3-(β-aminoethyl)-5-hydroxyindole. Like histamine, it is widely distributed in the animal and plant kingdoms. It occurs, for example, in vertebrates; in tunicates, mollusks, arthropods, and coelenterates; in fruits such as pineapples, bananas, and plums; and in various nuts. It is also present in numerous stings and venoms, including those of the common stinging nettle, cowhage (the prankster's "itching powder"), wasps, and scorpions (*see* Erspamer, 1966a). It is formed enzymatically from the amino acid tryptophan by hydroxylation, followed by decarboxylation (*see* below and Figure 26–3, page 637).

Numerous synthetic or naturally occurring congeners of 5-HT have varying degrees of peripheral and central pharmacological activity. Particularly noteworthy are the "tryptamines" of plant origin with potent effects on brain function. For example, N,N-dimethyltryptamine (DMT) and its 5-hydroxy derivative (bufotenine) are active principles of the cahobe bean found along the shores of the Caribbean and used in aboriginal rites to induce mental changes. Both of these compounds can be formed in the mammal by N-methylation of tryptamine and 5-HT, respectively. Also, the active ingredients of various Mexican hallucinogenic mushrooms (*e.g., Psilocybe mexicana*) used for related purposes are 4-substituted tryptamine derivatives (*psilocine* is 4-hydroxy-N,N-dimethyltryptamine, and *psilocybin* is 4-phosphoryloxy-N,N-dimethyltryptamine). Furthermore, a 4-substituted tryptamine moiety can be recognized in the most potent known psychotomimetic drug, LSD. (*See* Woolley, 1962; Mantegazzini, 1966; Cerletti *et al.*, 1968; Symposium, 1968a, 1968b, 1973, 1974a, 1974b; Bosin, 1978; Weil-Malherbe, 1978; *see also* Chapters 12, 19, and 23.)

PHARMACOLOGICAL ACTIONS

5-HT stimulates or inhibits a variety of smooth muscles and nerves. These and other actions result in a wide spectrum of responses involving, in particular, the cardiovascular, respiratory, and gastrointestinal systems. Characteristically, responses to 5-HT are variable; they differ not only between species but also between animals of the same species and even in successive tests in the individual. This variability, which is responsible for many discrepant reports and much controversy, is attributable in large part to two factors: (1) many of the effects of 5-HT are reflexly mediated and hence subject to influences such as pattern of innervation, route and speed of injection, anesthetic state, and spontaneous tone; and (2) tachyphylaxis is common when tests are made at frequent intervals. What follows is a description of some of the more prominent effects of 5-HT. Detailed accounts will be found in the handbook edited by Erspamer (1966b), in the series of monographs edited by Essman (1977, 1978a, 1978b, 1978c), and in the other reviews cited.

Respiratory System. *Stimulation of Afferent Nerves.* Intravenous injection of 5-HT in the dog and man commonly causes a short-lived increase in respiratory minute volume accompanied by variable changes in respiratory rate. With lower doses, the effect is due to stimulation of carotid and aortic chemoreceptors. With higher doses, other ill-defined effects contribute to the responses observed. Sometimes, particularly in the cat, respiratory movements are inhibited through stimulation of vagal afferent fibers.

Bronchoconstriction. 5-HT causes bronchoconstriction in many animals, but rarely in man, except in asthmatic patients. The effect is partly reflex but mainly due to direct stimulation of bronchial smooth muscle (*see* Rodbard and Kira, 1972).

Cardiovascular System. The effects of 5-HT on this system are uniquely complex. By acting directly on vascular smooth muscle, the drug may evoke vasoconstriction or vasodilatation, depending on the vascular bed, its resting tone, and the dose given. By its actions on a variety of sensory nerve endings, it activates pressor and depressor reflexes; by direct and reflex mechanisms, it either stimulates or depresses cardiac output; and in high doses it influences ganglionic transmission, adrenal medullary secretion, and transmitter release from nerve endings.

Blood Vessels. Direct vasoconstriction is the classical effect of 5-HT that is responsible for the synonyms *vasotonin* and *serotonin*. In animals, such vasoconstriction is revealed in its purest form after pithing the spinal cord or performing other maneuvers to obviate indirect effects. The effect of 5-HT is then to cause a prompt, uncomplicated rise in blood pressure lasting several minutes. The splanchnic and renal beds are particularly affected, and in some laboratory animals necrosis of the renal cortex results. Placental, uterine, and umbilical vessels also constrict, thereby interrupting pregnancy in some rodents. Cerebral blood vessels are constricted powerfully in several species (*see* Edvinsson and MacKenzie, 1977). Pulmonary vasoconstriction is prominent in dogs and cats but less so in man.

Vasodilatation occurs in skeletal muscle, especially with lower doses of 5-HT. The drug acts directly on the smooth muscle, but it can also reduce the output of norepinephrine from sympathetic nerve terminals (*see* below). In the forearm, where muscle is preponderant, vasodilatation tends to increase blood flow. Superficial vessels of the human skin also dilate following intradermal or intra-arterial injection of 5-HT. The resulting flush, at first bright red, assumes a dusky hue indicating stagnation, probably as a result of venoconstriction. However, the overall response to 5-HT given intra-arterially is a rise in cutaneous vascular resistance. In the hand, where skin is preponderant, this effect reduces blood flow. *Capillary permeability* is not much affected by 5-HT, except in rats, where it increases.

Heart. 5-HT has positive inotropic and chronotropic effects of varying intensity. These are evident in isolated preparations and reflect in part direct actions on cardiac tissue and indirect actions mediated by the release of norepinephrine from sympathetic nerve terminals. *In vivo,* such effects are commonly blunted or overshadowed by autonomic reflexes arising from changes in blood pressure or direct actions of 5-HT on baroreceptors, chemoreceptors, and vagal endings in the coronary bed. The last-mentioned action is particularly noteworthy. It initiates the coronary chemoreflex (Bezold-Jarisch reflex), characterized by inhibition of sympathetic outflow and increased activity of the cardiac (efferent) vagus, leading to profound bradycardia and hypotension. Occasionally cardiovascular collapse and fainting occur from such causes when 5-HT is given to man. No significant changes in the electrical properties of the heart have been attributed to 5-HT.

Blood Pressure. In contrast to the pithed animal (*see* above), the intact animal responds to an intravenous injection of 5-HT with changes in blood pressure that are notoriously variable, since they represent the outcome of several opposed and capricious influences, direct and reflex. In most species, including man, it is nevertheless possible to discern three successive phases: a brief depressor phase immediately following the injection; a succeeding pressor phase; and finally, within 1 or 2 minutes of the injection, a prolonged depressor phase. The *early depressor phase* results from the coronary chemoreflex; it is abolished by cutting the vagi (which contain both the afferent and efferent limbs of the reflex) or by the administration of a combination of parasympathetic and sympathetic blocking agents. The *pressor phase* is due mainly to the direct effects of 5-HT to increase total peripheral resistance and cardiac output. The *late depressor phase* is attributable mainly to the direct vasodilator effects of 5-HT, principally in skeletal muscle; it persists after block of sympathetic outflow.

Veins are strongly constricted by 5-HT, and intense venospasm commonly accompanies intravenous infusions.

Platelets. 5-HT promotes platelet aggregation without inducing the "release reaction." The effect, which is small and reversible, seems to be due to activation of specific receptors on the platelet surface (*see* Born and Michal, 1975).

Smooth Muscle. *Alimentary Tract.* Intravenous injections of 5-HT stimulate motility of the small intestine. Man is particularly sensitive and often responds to doses insufficient to affect the cardiovascular or respiratory system; typically, the response consists in an initial intense spasm followed first by heightened tone with rhythmic propulsive contractions and then by a period of inhibition of spontaneous activity. Motility of the stomach and large intestine may also be increased by 5-HT; but in most animals, and in man, the usual response is inhibition. Isolated segments of gastrointestinal tract *in vitro* generally exhibit responses qualitatively similar to those obtained *in vivo,* namely, contraction, inhibition, or mixtures of these. The complexity of the pattern is in large measure due to the variety of elements, neural and muscular, responding to 5-HT.

The most thorough analysis of the stimulant effect of 5-HT has been carried out on the isolated guinea pig ileum, where 5-HT contracts the longitudinal muscle partly by acting directly upon it and partly by exciting intramural ganglion cells (Gaddum and Picarelli, 1957). The direct action is blocked by 5-HT antagonists such as LSD, methysergide, and cyproheptadine (*see* below). The indirect effect mediated through ganglion cells is countered by tetrodotoxin or cocaine, both of which block the nerves; by atropine, which blocks the action of ACh that the neurons liberate; and by morphine, which has the dual property of opposing the excitatory effect of 5-HT on the ganglion cells and of diminishing the output of ACh from their terminals. In addition, 5-HT can also increase peristaltic activity by stimulating or sensitizing intramural nerve endings.

The inhibitory actions of 5-HT in guinea pig stomach are due mainly to excitation of ganglion cells that have an inhibitory function (Bülbring and Gershon, 1968). Inhibition in isolated human colon is more complex; ganglion cells in both muscle layers participate, and, in addition, both muscle layers, circular and longitudinal, are directly relaxed (Burleigh, 1977).

Other Smooth Muscle. In addition to the actions on bronchi, blood vessels, and gut, 5-HT stimulates numerous other smooth muscles. The isolated uterus of the estrus rat is exquisitely sensitive, but isolated strips of human uterus in various functional states are not, and large doses of 5-HT given intravenously have minor and equivocal actions on the contractile activity of the human pregnant uterus. As in the intestine, the responses of the other viscera are complicated by diverse actions on nervous elements as well as muscle.

Exocrine Glands. Intravenous infusion of 5-HT in the dog reduces the volume, acidity, and pepsin content of *gastric juice* secreted spontaneously or in response to vagal activation, cholinergic drugs, or histamine, but at the same time it increases the production of mucus. Somewhat similar effects have been described in man and various other species and apparently involve reflex as well as direct actions (*see* Thompson, 1971). Variable effects on salivary, pancreatic, and other exocrine secretions have been reported in mammals.

Nerve Endings. Stimulatory effects of 5-HT on sensory nerve endings of several sorts have been mentioned above in connection with respiratory and circulatory reflexes. These are but illustrations of a general property of 5-HT, shown also by its tendency, upon intravenous administration, to produce pain at the site of injection, gasping, hyperventilation, substernal "pressure," coughing, and "tingling and pricking all over" (Hollander *et al.*, 1957). Stimulant effects of 5-HT on *autonomic efferent nerves,* with release of norepinephrine or ACh, seem to participate in the responses of some tissues, for example, the heart and gut (Ádám-Vizi and Vizi, 1978); but inhibition of transmitter output of nerve endings has also been noted (McGrath, 1977).

Autonomic Ganglia. In high dose, 5-HT elicits firing of ganglion cells; lower doses facilitate or inhibit ganglionic transmission, depending on experimental conditions (*see* Saum and de Groat, 1973).

Adrenal Medulla and Other Endocrine Glands. High doses of 5-HT cause secretion of catecholamines from the adrenal gland by depolarizing chromaffin cells (*see* Douglas *et al.*, 1967). The drug has capricious stimulatory or inhibitory effects on many other endocrine systems, including the adrenal cortex, pancreatic β cells, and adenohypophyseal cells; in the last mentioned the action may be to modulate action-potential activity (Taraskevich and Douglas, 1979).

Central Nervous System. Although 5-HT serves as a neurotransmitter within the brain, and sites responsive to 5-HT are abundant and easily demonstrated by microiontophoretic application of the drug (*see* below), central effects are not usually encountered when 5-HT is given parenterally, for it poorly penetrates the blood-brain barrier. When injected directly into the lateral cerebral ventricles of cats, 5-HT causes muscular weakness, a swaying gait, a tendency to adopt a sleeping posture, and a catatonic-like state (Feldberg and Sherwood, 1954). Intracisternal administration also results in tremor and changes in body temperature—fever in some animals, hypothermia in others (*see* Feldberg, 1968). Applied by microiontophoresis to randomly encountered neurons throughout the CNS from neocortex to spinal cord, 5-HT inhibits some cells and stimulates others (*see* Symposium, 1973, 1974a). However, when the transmitter is similarly applied to neurons known to receive tryptaminergic input, 5-HT has so far been observed only to inhibit. Moreover, it is inhibitory to the same neurons that release it by acting through autoreceptors (*see* Aghajanian and Wang, 1978).

Mode of Action. Receptors for 5-HT, located on the cell surface, are less well characterized than are those for histamine (*see* Berridge, 1972; Christian and Smythies, 1978). That distinct types of receptors for 5-HT exist is evident from their wide range of susceptibilities to different blocking drugs, some of which have been mentioned. Again, as with histamine, transduction of receptor occupancy into a functional response seems often to involve changes in membrane permeability to inorganic ions, which thereby influence ion fluxes; membrane potential, excitability, and spiking activity; or change in the intracellular concentration of free calcium ions, which is critical to excitation-contraction coupling (*see* Weber and Murray, 1973) or stimulus-secretion coupling (*see* Douglas, 1968, 1978). In neurons of mollusks, where the most detailed studies of the effects of 5-HT on membrane properties have been performed, excitation results from two independent actions of 5-HT, the first increasing conductance to Na^+, the second reducing conductance to K^+; likewise, 5-HT–induced inhibition may arise from an increase in K^+ conductance or from an increase in Cl^- conductance (*see* Gerschenfeld and Paupardin-Tritsch, 1974; Cottrell, 1977). In vertebrates, events may be simpler, with excitation and inhibition perhaps involving only increased conductance to Na^+ and K^+, respectively. A depolarizing action leading to influx of Ca^{2+} seems to account for the stimulant effect of 5-HT on chromaffin cells (Douglas *et al.*, 1967) and on certain cells in the adenohypophysis (pars intermedia), where 5-HT elicits action potentials (Taraskevich and Douglas, 1979). Smooth muscle contraction elicited by 5-HT may involve an influx of Ca^{2+} or mobilization of Ca^{2+} from cellular sources, whereas 5-HT–induced relaxation may involve actions that reduce the free intracellular concentration of Ca^{2+} or decrease the sensitivity of the contractile proteins to Ca^{2+} (*see* Symposium, 1977b). With regard to smooth muscle, evidence points to an association between elevated concentrations of cyclic AMP and relaxation on the one hand and elevated concentrations of cyclic GMP and contraction on the other. Nevertheless, there are many discrepancies to suggest that these nucleotides are not mandatory intermediates in such responses of smooth muscle (*see* Diamond, 1978). The possible involvement of cyclic nucleotides in other 5-HT–sensitive systems has been reviewed for neurons (Bloom, 1975; Kebabian, 1977; Nathanson, 1977) and for secretory and other cells (Berridge, 1975).

ENDOGENOUS 5-HYDROXYTRYPTAMINE: DISTRIBUTION AND BIOSYNTHESIS

Distribution. In mammals, about 90% of the 5-HT present in the body, which in an adult human probably amounts to 10 mg, is lodged in the gastrointestinal tract, mainly in enterochromaffin cells and enterochromaffin-like cells. A few such 5-HT–containing cells are also present in other tissues. Of the remaining 5-HT, most is present in platelets and the CNS. Mast cells of rodents and cattle contain 5-HT, but mast cells of other species, including man, do not normally contain 5-HT; however, some has been found in human mast-cell tumors (Morishima, 1970). For detailed accounts of the distribution of 5-HT in various tissues and body fluids, *see* Erspamer (1966a, 1966b) and Essman (1978d).

Origin, Synthesis, Uptake, and Storage. Although considerable amounts of 5-HT are present in the diet (*see* above), much is metabolized as it crosses the intestinal wall and the rest is destroyed by the liver and lungs (*see* Gillis and Roth, 1976). The 5-HT found in enterochromaffin cells, neurons, and most other 5-HT–containing cells is synthesized *in situ* from tryptophan. Platelets, an important exception, acquire 5-HT from their environment (*see* below). In cells that synthesize 5-HT, tryptophan is first hydroxylated to 5-hydroxytryptophan (5-HTP) by the enzyme tryptophan-5-hydroxylase (the activity of which is rate limiting), and is then decarboxylated to 5-HT by the nonspecific aromatic L-amino acid decarboxylase that is also involved in the synthesis of catecholamines (*see* Figure 26–3, page 637; Erspamer, 1966b). In the cytoplasm, 5-HT, whether synthesized or acquired (as by platelets), is taken up into secretory granules (or vesicles) and stored therein as a nondiffusible complex with adenosine triphosphate (ATP) and other substances to await the signal for secretion. The molecular events involved in pumping the amine into its granular storage sites and sequestering it there are presumably very similar to those involved in the storage of the catecholamines. Drugs that disrupt the storage of catecholamines, such as reserpine, impair that of 5-HT similarly (*see* Garattini and Samanin, 1978). Platelets take up 5-HT during their passage through the intestinal blood vessels, where they encounter relatively high concentrations of 5-HT that result from its secretion by enterochromaffin cells and possibly other sources. The important mechanism is a high-affinity uptake that allows accumulation of 5-HT against an enormous concentration gradient. A high-affinity uptake mechanism like that of platelets is also present in tryptaminergic nerve endings, thereby permitting them to recapture released transmitter. These uptake mechanisms are also similar to those for re-uptake of catecholamines by adrenergic and dopaminergic neurons; for example, both are influenced by the tricyclic antidepressant drugs. Because platelets are relatively easy to isolate and study, they are frequently used as models for study of the transport and storage of monoamine neurotransmitters (*see* Sneddon, 1973; Symposium 1975). (For recent reviews on the metabolism of 5-HT and drugs affecting it, *see* Bosin, 1978; Garattini and Samanin, 1978.)

Turnover. An amount of 5-HT roughly equal to that present in the body is synthesized each day (Erspamer, 1966b). Turnover times of 5-HT in brain and gastrointestinal tract have been estimated at about 1 and 17 hours, respectively. However, 5-HT in rodent mast cells turns over very slowly and that bound in platelets appears to be released only on their destruction or during the "release reaction" induced by thrombin or other agents (Holmsen *et al.*, 1973).

ENDOGENOUS 5-HYDROXYTRYPTAMINE: FUNCTIONS

A major function of 5-HT is to serve as the chemical transmitter of neurons within the brain that are referred to as "tryptaminergic" (or "serotonergic"). In addition, 5-HT serves as a precursor for the pineal hormone, *melatonin.* Less evident is its function in platelets, enterochromaffin cells, and other cells with established or suspected endocrine function.

Nervous System. Within the CNS the cell bodies of the 5-HT–containing neurons are located almost exclusively in the raphe nuclei of the brain stem, from which axons project to other portions of the brain stem, to the spinal cord, and to the forebrain (*see* Aghajanian and Wang, 1978). At all the synapses where 5-HT has been implicated as the transmitter, its effect on the postsynaptic cell appears to be inhibitory. It also inhibits the tryptaminergic neurons from which it is released through "autoreceptors." At both these sites, presynaptic and postsynaptic, LSD *mimics* 5-HT in producing inhibition. The role of 5-HT as a central neurotransmitter is discussed further in Chapter 12. There is also growing evidence that tryptaminergic fibers may be present in the *peripheral nervous system* of mammals, particularly in the gut (*see* Gershon *et al.,* 1977; Furness and Costa, 1978).

Hypothalamic–Anterior Pituitary Function. The hypothalamic neuroendocrine cells that release hypophysiotropic hormones to regulate adenohypophyseal secretion seem to be controlled themselves, in part, by tryptaminergic neurons. Thus, 5-HT has been implicated as a possible physiological factor in the stimulation of release of ACTH, growth hormone, and prolactin and in the inhibition of the secretion of luteinizing hormone (LH), follicle-stimulating hormone (FSH), and thyroid-stimulating hormone (TSH) (*see* Baumgarten *et al.,* 1978; Krieger, 1978; Symposium, 1978b). At the level of the adenohypophysis itself, the only prominent effects are on the pars intermedia, where 5-HT can diminish or increase the secretion of melanocyte-stimulating hormone (MSH), depending on species, and can inhibit or stimulate action potentials (Taraskevich and Douglas, 1979).

Endocrine Cells Secreting Polypeptide Hormones. In various species, 5-HT (or another arylethylamine such as dopamine or histamine) occurs in a host of cells known or believed to secrete polypeptide hormones, for example, the parafollicular cells (C cells) of the thyroid, α and β cells of the endocrine pancreas, and various cells secreting gastrointestinal hormones. In other species, where the endogenous amine is not readily apparent, it can be demonstrated after administering the corresponding amine precursor, 5-HTP, dopa, or histidine. Whereas the amine is stored and released along with the polypeptide hormone in the secretory granules, its function is unknown (*see* Pearce, 1977; Gylfe, 1978).

Enterochromaffin System. The physiological function of enterochromaffin cells is still uncertain.

Beside 5-HT, they contain the peptides substance P and motilin, which are potent autacoids in their own right. It is interesting that *some* 5-HT–containing neurons in the brain also contain substance P (Chan-Palay *et al.,* 1978). Intestinal enterochromaffin cells show a basal release of 5-HT that is augmented by mechanical stimulation (Bülbring, 1961); by hypertonicity and acidity; by norepinephrine (Burks and Long, 1966); and also by vagal influences, apparently mediated by adrenergic fibers contributed to the vagal trunk by sympathetic ganglia in the neck (*see* Ahlman *et al.,* 1978).

Tumors of 5-HT–Forming Cells: Malignant Carcinoid. Tumors of enterochromaffin or related cells (*carcinoid tumors*), in the gastrointestinal or respiratory tract or elsewhere, may synthesize and release large amounts of 5-HT along with varying amounts of other autacoids. With massive tumors, so much tryptophan may be diverted to 5-HT synthesis that niacin synthesis suffers and *pellagra* results. The symptoms of recurrent and severe diarrhea and abdominal cramps and the signs of malabsorption seen in many patients with the carcinoid syndrome are reversed by the use of competitive antagonists of 5-HT; the cardiovascular instability (flushes) is not affected by these drugs.

Pineal Gland and Melatonin Formation. The pineal gland is rich in 5-HT synthesized by the pinealocytes to serve as a precursor for the synthesis of the hormone *melatonin* (5-methoxy-N-acetyltryptamine). Synthesis of melatonin shows a remarkable diurnal rhythm accompanied by fluctuating concentrations of 5-HT (*see* Axelrod and Wurtman, 1968).

Platelet 5-HT. The function of 5-HT in platelets is obscure. As noted earlier, its potentiating effect on platelet aggregation is small and platelets depleted of 5-HT by reserpine function normally; bleeding time is unchanged (Mustard and Packham, 1970). One view is that platelets serve simply to sequester the 5-HT escaping from cells, such as those in the enterochromaffin system. Discharge of 5-HT from platelets may contribute to the pathophysiology of pulmonary embolism (*see* Spodick, 1972; Symposium, 1975).

ADDITIONAL CONSIDERATIONS

Absorption, Fate, and Excretion. For experimental purposes, 5-HT is usually given intravenously, but it is also well absorbed after intramuscular injection. Given orally, it is rapidly degraded and is ineffective. In man, most 5-HT, endogenous or ingested, undergoes oxidative deamination by MAO to form 5-hydroxyindoleacetaldehyde. This is promptly degraded, mainly by further oxidation to 5-hydroxyindoleacetic acid (5-HIAA) by aldehyde dehydrogenase, but also in small part by reduction, by alcohol dehydrogenase, to 5-hydroxytryptophol (5-HTOL) (*see* Figure 26–3). The three enzymes are present in liver and in various tissues that contain 5-HT, including the brain. Following intravenous injection of 5-HT, its uptake and degradation by the lung are important; depending on the rate of infu-

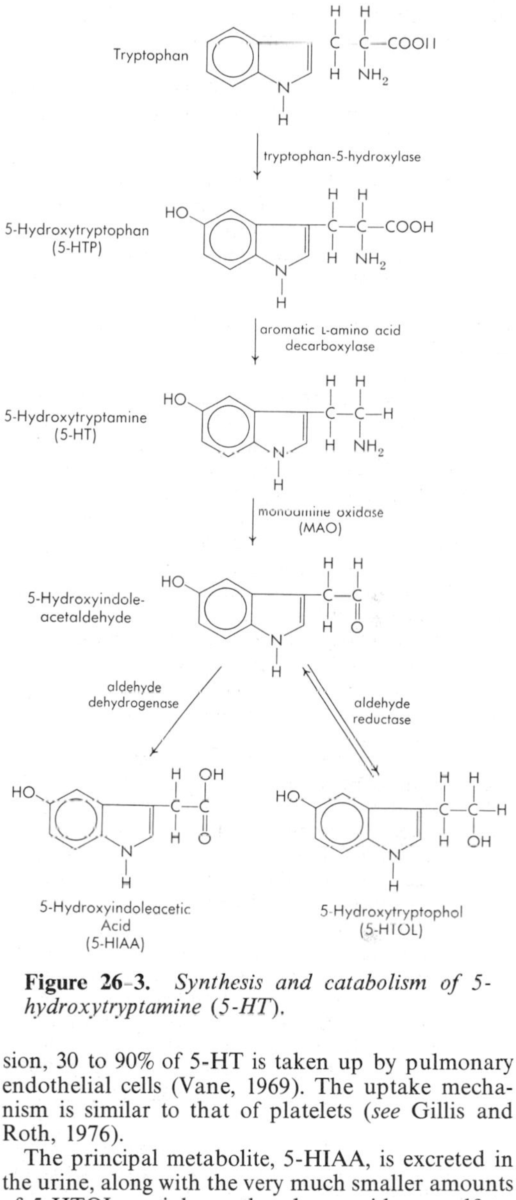

Figure 26–3. *Synthesis and catabolism of 5-hydroxytryptamine (5-HT).*

sion, 30 to 90% of 5-HT is taken up by pulmonary endothelial cells (Vane, 1969). The uptake mechanism is similar to that of platelets (*see* Gillis and Roth, 1976).

The principal metabolite, 5-HIAA, is excreted in the urine, along with the very much smaller amounts of 5-HTOL, mainly as the glucuronide or sulfate, and traces of other metabolites. About 2 to 10 mg of 5-HIAA is excreted daily by the normal adult as a result of metabolism of endogenous 5-HT. Larger amounts are excreted by patients with malignant carcinoid, a fact of diagnostic value. It must be remembered, however, that ingestion of 5-HT–containing foods also leads to increased excretion of 5-HT metabolites (*see* Erspamer, 1966a; Levine, 1974; Brown, 1977; Bosin, 1978).

The pattern of metabolism of 5-HT is strikingly affected by ingestion of ethyl alcohol, which diverts 5-hydroxyindoleacetaldehyde from the normally predominant oxidative route to the reductive pathway because of the elevated concentration of NADH. This greatly increases excretion of 5-HTOL and correspondingly reduces that of 5-HIAA (*see* Symposium 1968a; Bosin, 1978).

Preparations. There is no official preparation, but 5-HT is available as the creatinine sulfate complex for investigational use.

Clinical Use. From a clinical standpoint, the principal interest in 5-HT lies in its role in physiological and pathological processes (*see* above). To date, the drug has not found an accepted therapeutic application. Oral administration of 5-HT followed by measurement of 5-HIAA in the urine provides a simple means of testing the degree of inhibition of MAO (Sjoerdsma *et al.,* 1958).

Drugs Affecting Endogenous 5-HT. Many of these compounds are described fully in other chapters. The following is but an outline. The drugs fall into several categories. (1) Administration of the *precursor of 5-HT,* tryptophan, can increase endogenous concentrations of the amine (*see* Wurtman and Fernstrom, 1976) and may be of value in phenylketonuria. (2) *Inhibitors of synthesis* include p-chlorophenylalanine (PCPA), which blocks the rate-limiting enzyme tryptophan hydroxylase. The compound is a valuable experimental tool but is too toxic for clinical use. Another inhibitor of this enzyme is p-chloroamphetamine (PCA); this agent is less specific and more complex in its actions. The amino acid analog 6-fluorotryptophan is a more specific inhibitor. (3) *Inhibitors of membrane uptake* include the tricyclic antidepressant drugs, which also inhibit catecholamine uptake. The tertiary amines chloroimipramine, imipramine, and amitriptyline preferentially block 5-HT uptake over narrow concentration ranges. All of these are more effective in blocking the uptake of 5-HT than are the secondary amines of this class; however, like the latter, they also inhibit the uptake of catecholamines. A more potent and selective inhibition of 5-HT uptake is obtained with fluoxetine (*see* Lemberger *et al.,* 1978). (4) *Inhibitors of granule uptake and storage* include reserpine, tetrabenazine, and other benzoquinolizines, all of which deplete stores of 5-HT. A long-lasting depletion of 5-HT can also be achieved with the anorectic drug fenfluramine; the mechanism of its action is uncertain (*see* Symposium, 1978b). (5) *Inhibitors of degradation* include principally the MAO inhibitors. (6) *Neurotoxins* that preferentially destroy 5-HT–containing neurons include 5,6-dihydroxytryptamine (5,6-DHT) and 5,7-DHT. Their action is complex (*see* Symposium, 1978b). (7) *Antagonists of 5-HT* at the level of the receptor are discussed below.

5-HT ANTAGONISTS

Ergot alkaloids and related compounds were early recognized as antagonists at receptors for 5-HT, particularly on smooth muscle (*see* Chapter 39); in this group the *lysergic acid derivatives* such as the diethylamide (LSD), 2-bromo-LSD, and 1-methyl-*d*-lysergic acid butanolamide (methysergide, *see* below) are especially potent. Also, many *indole compounds* are 5-HT antagonists, including derivatives of gram-

ine, harmine, tryptamine (and tryptamine itself), quaternary ammonium salts of N,N-dialkyltryptamines, and indoleacetamidines. These last two indole groups, along with some *arylguanidines and biguanides,* are principally effective against a variety of 5-HT actions on ganglion cells and peripheral nerve endings, including those in the carotid body. In addition, 5-HT blocking activity, mainly demonstrated on smooth muscle and often of a high order, is present in a host of other drugs, including histamine H$_1$ blockers of the ethylenediamine type and also, most notably, cyproheptadine (*see* below), *phenothiazines* (particularly chlorpromazine), and *β-haloalkylamines* such as phenoxybenzamine and various other *adrenergic blocking drugs* (*see* Gyermek, 1966; Garattini and Samanin, 1978).

Several different mechanisms are involved in suppression of responses to 5-HT. Many drugs, such as LSD, methysergide, and cyproheptadine, are classical antagonists of the surmountable competitive type, and their blocking effect on 5-HT receptors is achieved without evidence of stimulation. With some others, such as tryptamine (or 5-HT itself in high dose), blockade follows activation and involves specific receptor desensitization. Much the same holds for the indoleacetamidines and guanidines. For example, phenylbiguanide, which blocks the actions of 5-HT on nerve endings, including those actions initiating the Bezold-Jarisch reflex, has long been remarkable as a drug precisely because it stimulates the same endings and induces this same reflex. While the effects of most of the 5-HT antagonists are rapidly reversible, those of the β-haloalkylamines are not (*see* Chapter 9).

5-HT antagonists that are active on peripheral structures fall, by and large, into two categories: those that are mainly effective in opposing effects on smooth muscle and those that preferentially block peripheral neural responses. For this reason, Gyermek (1966) has classified them as "musculotropic" and "neurotropic." This indicates at least two types of 5-HT receptors, but in fact there seem to be many types. A substance known to act as a 5-HT antagonist at one site cannot be assumed to act similarly at another, a consideration often ignored in experiments in which these drugs are used as tools without appropriate controls. Particularly, it is fitting to emphasize that none of the many drugs, such as methysergide or cyproheptadine, that antagonizes effects of 5-HT on peripheral tissues acts as a 5-HT antagonist at sites in the brain where 5-HT has been identified as a transmitter and where the effect of 5-HT is inhibitory (*see* Symposium 1974a, 1974b; Aghajanian and Wang, 1978). This is not to say that such "peripheral" 5-HT antagonists cannot act centrally. On the contrary, methysergide and cyproheptadine (and other such drugs, including methergoline and cinanserine) block responses to 5-HT at a wide range of central sites where, however, there is no evidence of *physiological* involvement of 5-HT, and the meaning of the antagonism is therefore unclear.

Methysergide. This drug (1-methyl-*d*-lysergic acid butanolamide) is a congener of methylergonovine and of LSD. Its structure is depicted in Table 39–1. It inhibits the vasoconstrictor and pressor effects of 5-HT as well as the action of the amine on a variety of extravascular smooth muscles and other cells. Unlike LSD, however, it has comparatively little action on the nervous system in usual doses. Although methysergide is an ergot derivative, it has only feeble vasoconstrictor and oxytocic activity. Nevertheless, such effects may contraindicate its use during pregnancy.

Methysergide is useful for the prophylactic treatment of migraine and other vascular headaches, including Horton's syndrome (Sicuteri, 1959; Friedman and Elkind, 1963). The protective effect of methysergide takes 1 to 2 days to develop and as long to pass off when treatment is terminated. Rebound headaches not uncommonly occur when the drug is withdrawn. Methysergide is without benefit when given during the acute attack and, indeed, may be contraindicated. For comparative evaluation of the prophylactic effects of methysergide and other agents, including cyproheptadine, *see* Speight and Avery (1972).

It is not clear why methysergide or any of the other effective agents should be of value in migraine or other vascular headaches. The mechanism of such headaches is unknown. Numerous attempts to correlate headaches of this type with some derangement in 5-HT metabolism have yielded equivocal results, and a variety of other autacoids have been incriminated (Symposium, 1968a, 1968b; Speight and Avery, 1972; Fozard, 1975, 1977; Sjaastad, 1975; Sicuteri, 1976).

Methysergide is useful in combating diarrhea and malabsorption in patients with *carcinoid* and may be beneficial in the *postgastrectomy dumping syndrome*. Both these conditions have a 5-HT-mediated component (*see* Levine, 1974).

Some ergot derivatives, notably bromocriptine, have dopamine-like properties and will, for example, inhibit the secretion of prolactin in man (*see* Chapter 59). Methysergide has some depressant effect on human prolactin secretion that may perhaps be explained in the same way (Oppizzi *et al.*, 1977).

Untoward Effects. These are usually mild and transient, but may be severe enough to require withdrawal of the drug. The most common are gastrointestinal and include heartburn, diarrhea, cramps, nausea, and vomiting. Effects attributable to central actions include unsteadiness, drowsiness, weakness, light-headedness, nervousness, insomnia, confusion, excitement, euphoria, hallucinations, and even frank psychotic episodes. Attention has been drawn to the drug's abuse potential and "street use" (Persyko, 1972). There may be either loss of appetite or weight gain. Reactions suggestive of vascular insufficiency have been observed in a few patients with peripheral vascular disease, and exacerbation of angina pectoris has been noted. One infrequent, but potentially serious, complication of prolonged treatment is *inflammatory fibrosis*. This gives rise to various syndromes, depending on the site, including retroperitoneal fibrosis, pleuropulmonary fibrosis, and coronary and endocardial fibrosis. Usually the fibrosis retrogresses after withdrawal of the drug, but this is not always so and persistent cardiac valvular damage has been reported (Graham, 1967). These pathological effects are interesting because of the structural similarities

of methysergide and 5-HT and the suggested causal relationship between endogenous 5-HT and fibrosis in the carcinoid syndrome.

Preparation and Dosage. Methysergide Maleate, U.S.P. (SANSERT), is available in 2-mg tablets. The adult dose is about 2 mg, two to four times per day.

Cyproheptadine. This compound has the following structural formula:

Cyproheptadine

Its structure resembles that of the phenothiazine H_1 antagonists.

Although several substances block receptors for both histamine and 5-HT, cyproheptadine stands out in both regards. The compound does not have exceptional interest as an H_1 blocker, for it is but one of a plethora of such drugs (*see* above); rather, it is noteworthy for blocking responses to 5-HT in vascular, intestinal, and other smooth muscles. In addition, it has weak anticholinergic activity and possesses mild central depressant properties (Stone *et al.*, 1961).

Preparations, Uses, and Side Effects. Cyproheptadine Hydrochloride, U.S.P. (PERIACTIN), is available as tablets (4 mg) and as a syrup (2 mg/5 ml). The dose for adults is 4 mg, three or four times per day.

Cyproheptadine shares the properties and uses of other H_1 blockers (*see* above). In allergic conditions its actions as a 5-HT antagonist are irrelevant, since 5-HT is not involved in human allergic responses. Mast cells contain 5-HT only in rodents and some other species. The 5-HT–antagonizing properties of cyproheptadine are, however, of benefit in the *postgastrectomy dumping syndrome, intestinal hypermotility of carcinoid,* and some other conditions involving the release of 5-HT (*see* Levine, 1974).

Side effects of cyproheptadine include drowsiness, dry mouth, and many other effects common to H_1 blockers (*see* above). Weight gain and increased growth in children have been observed. The mechanism is not understood. However, methysergide occasionally produces similar effects, and both drugs can distort secretion of insulin and growth hormone (*see* Baldridge *et al.*, 1974; Hintze *et al.*, 1977).

Ádám-Vizi, V., and Vizi, E. S. Direct evidence of acetylcholine releasing effect of serotonin in the Auerbach plexus. *J. Neural Transm.*, **1978**, *42*, 127–138.

Aghajanian, G. K., and Wang, R. Y. Physiology and pharmacology of central serotonergic neurons. In, *Psychopharmacology: A Generation of Progress.* (Lipton, M. A.; DiMascio, A.; and Killam, K. F.; eds.) Raven Press, New York, **1978**, pp. 171–183.

Ahlman, B. H.; Lundberg, J. M.; Dahlström, A.;

Larsson, I.; Pettersson, G.; Kewenter, J.; and Nyhus, L. M. Evidence for innervation of the small intestine from the cervical sympathetic ganglia. *J. Surg. Res.*, **1978**, *24*, 142–149.

Alonso-De Florida, F.; Del Castillo, J.; García, X.; and Gijón, E. Mechanism of the Schultz-Dale reaction in the denervated diaphragmatic muscle of the guinea pig. *J. Gen. Physiol.*, **1968**, *51*, 677–693.

Altounyan, R. E. C. Inhibition of experimental asthma by a new compound, disodium cromoglycate, "INTAL." *Acta Allergol. (Kbh.)*, **1967**, *22*, 487–489.

————. Changes in histamine and atropine responsiveness as a guide to diagnosis and evaluation of therapy in obstructive airways disease. In, *Proceedings of the Symposium on Disodium Cromoglycate in Allergic Airways Disease.* Bullveoulte, London, **1970**, pp. 47–53.

Amin, A. H.; Crawford, T. B. B.; and Gaddum, J. H. The distribution of substance P and 5-hydroxytryptamine in the central nervous system of the dog. *J. Physiol. (Lond.)*, **1954**, *126*, 596–618.

Ash, A. S. F., and Schild, H. O. Receptors mediating some actions of histamine. *Br. J. Pharmacol.*, **1966**, *27*, 427–439.

Axelrod, J., and Wurtman, R. J. Photic and neural control of indoleamine metabolism in the rat pineal gland. *Adv. Pharmacol.*, **1968**, *6A*, 157–166.

Baldridge, J. A.; Quickel, K. E.; Feldman, J. M.; and Lebovitz, H. E. Potentiation of tolbutamide-mediated insulin release in adult onset diabetes by methysergide maleate. *Diabetes*, **1974**, *23*, 21–24.

Baron, J. H. Gastric functions tests. In, *Chronic Duodenal Ulcer.* (Wastell, C., ed.) Appleton-Century-Crofts, New York, **1972**, pp. 82–114.

Bartosch, R.; Feldberg, W.; and Nagel, E. Das Freiwerden eines histaminähnlichen Stoffes bei der Anaphylaxie des Meerschweinchens. *Pfluegers Arch.*, **1932**, *230*, 120–153.

Baumgarten, H. G.; Bjorklund, A.; and Wuttke, W. Neural control of pituitary LH, FSH and prolactin secretion. In, *Brain-Endocrine Interaction III: Neural Hormones and Reproduction.* (Scott, D. E.; Kozlowski, G. P.; and Weindl, A.; eds.) S. Karger, Basel, **1978**, pp. 327–343.

Baylin, S. B.; Beavan, M. A.; Buja, L. M.; and Kreiser, H. R. Histaminase activity: a biochemical marker for medullary carcinoma of the thyroid. *Am. J. Med.*, **1972**, *53*, 723–732.

Bernstein, I. L.; Siegel, S. C.; Brandon, M. L.; Brown, E. B.; Evans, R. R.; Feinberg, A. R.; Friedlaender, S.; Krumholz, R. A.; Hadley, R. A.; Handelman, N. I.; Thurston, D.; and Yamate, M. A controlled study of cromolyn sodium sponsored by the Drug Committee of the American Academy of Allergy. *J. Allergy Clin. Immunol.*, **1972**, *50*, 235–245.

Best, C. H.; Dale, H. H.; Dudley, H. W.; and Thorpe, W. V. The nature of the vasodilator constituents of certain tissue extracts. *J. Physiol. (Lond.)*, **1927**, *62*, 397–417.

Binder, H. J., and Donaldson, R. M., Jr. Effect of cimetidine on intrinsic factor and pepsin secretion in man. *Gastroenterology*, **1978**, *74*, 371–375.

Black, J. W.; Duncan, W. A. M.; Durant, C. J.; Ganellin, C. R.; and Parsons, E. M. Definition and antagonism of histamine H₂-receptors. *Nature*, **1972**, *236*, 385–390.

Bodemar, G., and Walan, A. Maintenance treatment of recurrent peptic ulcer by cimetidine. *Lancet*, **1978**, *1*, 403–407.

Born, G. V. R., and Michal, F. 5-Hydroxytryptamine receptors of platelets. In, *Biochemistry and Pharmacology of Platelets.* Ciba Foundation Symposium, Vol. 35. Elsevier/Excerpta Medica/North Holland, Amsterdam, **1975**, pp. 287–307.

Bourne, H. R.; Lichtenstein, L. M.; Melmon, K. L.; Hennery, C. S.; Weinstein, Y.; and Shearer, G. M. Modulation of inflammation and immunity by cyclic AMP. *Science*, **1974**, *184*, 19–28.

Bovet, D.; Horclois, R.; and Walthert, F. Propriétés antihistaminiques de la N-*p*-méthoxybenzyl-N-diméthylaminoéthyl α amino-pyridine. *C. R. Soc. Biol. (Paris)*, **1944**, *138*, 99–100.

Bovet, D., and Staub, A. Action protectrice des éthers phénoliques au cours de l'intoxication histaminique. *C. R. Soc. Biol. (Paris)*, **1937**, *124*, 547–549.

Brand, J. J., and Perry, W. L. M. Drugs used in motion sickness. *Pharmacol. Rev.*, **1966**, *18*, 895–924.

Brezenoff, H. E., and Gertner, S. B. The actions of polymyxin and histamine on ganglionic transmission. *Can. J. Physiol. Pharmacol.*, **1972**, *50*, 824–831.

Brimblecombe, R. W., and Duncan, W. A. M. The relevance to man of pre-clinical data for cimetidine. In, *Cimetidine: Proceedings of the Second International Symposium on Histamine H₂-Receptor Antagonists.* (Burland, W. L., and Simkins, M. A., eds.) Excerpta Medica, Amsterdam, **1977**, pp. 54–65.

Brimblecombe, R. W.; Duncan, W. A. M.; Durant, G. J.; Emmett, J. C.; Ganellin, C. R.; Leslie, G. B.; and Parsons, M. E. Characterization and development of cimetidine as a histamine H₂-receptor antagonist. *Gastroenterology*, **1978**, *74*, 339–347.

Brodie, B. B., and Shore, P. A. A concept for a role of serotonin and norepinephrine as chemical mediators in the brain. *Ann. N.Y. Acad. Sci.*, **1957**, *66*, 631–642.

Bülbring, E. The intrinsic nervous system of the intestine and local effects of 5-hydroxytryptamine. In, *Regional Neurochemistry.* (Kety, S. S., and Elkes, J., eds.) Pergamon Press, Ltd., Oxford, **1961**, pp. 437–441.

Bülbring, E., and Gershon, M. D. Serotonin participation in the vagal inhibitory pathway to the stomach. *Adv. Pharmacol.*, **1968**, *6A*, 323–333.

Burks, T. F., and Long, J. P. 5-Hydroxytryptamine release into dog intestinal vasculature. *Am. J. Physiol.*, **1966**, *211*, 619–625.

Burleigh, D. E. Evidence for more than one type of 5-hydroxytryptamine receptor in the human colon. *J. Pharm. Pharmacol.*, **1977**, *29*, 538–541.

Busis, N. A.; Weight, F. F.; and Smith, P. A. Synaptic potentials in sympathetic ganglia: are they mediated by cyclic nucleotides? *Science*, **1978**, *200*, 1079–1081.

Carroll, P. R.; Glover, W. E.; and Latt, N. Cardiovascular histamine receptors in the rabbit. *Aust. J. Exp. Biol. Med. Sci.*, **1974**, *52*, 577–582.

Carruthers, S. G.; Shoeman, D. W.; Hignite, C. E.; and Azarnoff, D. L. Correlation between plasma diphenhydramine level and sedative and antihistamine effects. *Clin. Pharmacol. Ther.*, **1978**, *23*, 375–382.

Cerletti, A.; Taeschler, M.; and Weidmann, H. Pharmacologic studies on the structure-activity relationship of hydroxyindole alkylamines. *Adv. Pharmacol.*, **1968**, *6B*, 233–246.

Chand, N., and Eyre, P. Classification and biological distribution of histamine receptor sub-types. *Agents Actions*, **1975**, *5*, 277–295.

Chan-Palay, V.; Jonsson, G.; and Palay, S. L. Serotonin and substance P coexist in neurons of the rat's central nervous system. *Proc. Natl. Acad. Sci. U.S.A.*, **1978**, *75*, 1582–1586.

Cohen, B., and deJong, J. M. B. V. Meclizine and placebo in treating vertigo of vestibular origin. Relative efficacy in a double-blind study. *Arch. Neurol.*, **1972**, *27*, 129–135.

Collaborative Trial. Long-term study of disodium cromoglycate in treatment of severe extrinsic or intrinsic bronchial asthma in adults. *Br. Med. J.*, **1972**, *4*, 383–388.

Collaborative Trial. Sodium cromoglycate in chronic asthma. *Br. J. Med.*, **1976**, *1*, 361–364.

Cottrell, G. A. Identified amine-containing neurons and their synaptic connexions. *Neuroscience*, **1977**, *2*, 1–18.

Dale, H. H. The anaphylactic reaction of plain muscle in the guinea-pig. *J. Pharmacol. Exp. Ther.*, **1913**, *4*, 167–223.

————. Some chemical factors in the control of the circulation. *Lancet*, **1929,** *1,* 1179–1183, 1233–1237, 1285–1290.

Dale, H. H., and Laidlaw, P. P. The physiological action of β-imidazolylethylamine. *J. Physiol. (Lond.),* **1910,** *41,* 318–344.

————. Further observations on the action of β-imidazolylethylamine. *Ibid.,* **1911,** *43,* 182–195.

————. Histamine shock. *Ibid.,* **1919,** *52,* 355–390.

Diamant, B.; Kazimerczak, W.; and Patkar, S. A. Does cyclic AMP play any role in histamine release from mast cells? *Allergy,* **1978,** *33,* 50–51.

Diamond, J. Role of cyclic nucleotides in control of smooth muscle contraction. *Adv. Cyclic Nucleotide Res.,* **1978,** *9,* 327–340.

Douglas, W. W. Stimulus-secretion coupling: the concept and clues from chromaffin and other cells. The First Gaddum Memorial Lecture. *Br. J. Pharmacol.,* **1968,** *34,* 451–474.

————. Involvement of calcium in exocytosis and the exocytosis-vesiculation sequence. *Biochem. Soc. Symp.,* **1974,** *39,* 1–28.

————. Stimulus-secretion coupling: variations on the theme of calcium activated exocytosis involving cellular and extracellular sources of calcium. In, *Respiratory Tract Mucus.* Ciba Foundation Symposium, Vol. 54. Elsevier/Excerpta Medica/North Holland, Amsterdam, **1978,** pp. 61–90.

Douglas, W. W.; Kanno, T.; and Sampson, S. R. Effects of acetylcholine and other medullary secretagogues and antagonists on the membrane potential of adrenal chromaffin cells: an analysis employing techniques of tissue culture. *J. Physiol. (Lond.),* **1967,** *188,* 107–120.

Douglas, W. W., and Rubin, R. P. The role of calcium in adrenal medullary secretion evoked by acetylcholine or potassium. *J. Physiol. (Lond.),* **1961,** *159,* 24P–25P.

Dragstedt, C. A., and Gebauer-Fuelnegg, E. Studies in anaphylaxis. I. The appearance of a physiologically active substance during anaphylactic shock. *Am. J. Physiol.,* **1932,** *102,* 512–519.

Durant, G. J.; Ganellin, C. R.; and Parsons, M. E. Chemical differentiation of histamine H₁- and H₂-receptor antagonists. *J. Med. Chem.,* **1975,** *18,* 905–909.

————. Dimaprit [S-[3-(N,N-dimethylamino)propyl]isothiourea], a highly specific histamine H₂-receptor agonist. Part 2. Structure-activity considerations. *Agents Actions,* **1977,** *7,* 39–43.

Edvinsson, L., and MacKenzie, E. T. Amine mechanisms in the cerebral circulation. *Pharmacol. Rev.,* **1977,** *28,* 275–348.

Erspamer, V. Richerche farmacoligiche sull' enteramina. VII. Enteramina e indolalchilamine del veleno di rospo. *Arch. Sci. Biol. (Bologna),* **1946,** *31,* 86–95.

————. Occurrence of indolealkylamines in nature. In, *5-Hydroxytryptamine and Related Indolealkylamines.* (Erspamer, V., ed.) *Handbuch der Experimentellen Pharmakologie,* Vol. 19. Springer-Verlag, Berlin, **1966a,** pp. 132–181.

Erspamer, V., and Asero, B. Identification of enteramine, the specific hormone of the enterochromaffin cell system, as 5-hydroxytryptamine. *Nature,* **1952,** *169,* 800–801.

Eyre, P. Histamine H₂-receptors in the sheep bronchus and cat trachea: the action of burimamide. *Br. J. Pharmacol.,* **1973,** *48,* 321–323.

Feldberg, W. The monoamines of the hypothalamus as mediators of temperature responses. In, *Recent Advances in Pharmacology,* 4th ed. (Robson, J. M., and Stacey, R. S., eds.) J. & A. Churchill, Ltd., London, **1968,** pp. 349–397.

Feldberg, W., and Sherwood, S. L. Injections of drugs into the lateral ventricle of the cat. *J. Physiol. (Lond.),* **1954,** *123,* 148–167.

Folkow, B.; Haeger, K.; and Kahlson, G. Observations on reactive hyperaemia as related to histamine, on drugs antagonising vasodilatation induced by histamine and on vasodilator properties of adenosine triphosphate. *Acta Physiol. Scand.,* **1948,** *15,* 264–278.

Foreman, J. C.; Garland, L. G.; and Mongar, J. L. The role of calcium in secretory processes: model studies in mast cells. *Symp. Soc. Exp. Biol.,* **1976,** *30,* 193–218.

Fozard, J. R. The mechanism by which migraine prophylactic drugs modify vascular reactivity *in vitro.* In, *Headache: New Vistas.* Biomedical Press, Florence, **1977,** pp. 259–278.

Friedman, A. P., and Elkind, A. H. Appraisal of methysergide in treatment of vascular headaches of migraine type. *J.A.M.A.,* **1963,** *184,* 125–128.

Fuller, R. W., and Wong, D. T. Inhibition of serotonin reuptake. *Fed. Proc.,* **1977,** *36,* 2154–2158.

Furness, J. B., and Costa, M. Distribution of intrinsic nerve cell bodies and axons which take up aromatic amines and their precursors in the small intestine of the guinea pig. *Cell Tissue Res.,* **1978,** *188,* 527–543.

Gaddum, J. H. Antagonism between LSD and 5-hydroxytryptamine. *J. Physiol. (Lond.),* **1953,** *121,* 15P.

Gaddum, J. H., and Picarelli, Z. P. Two kinds of tryptamine receptor. *Br. J. Pharmacol.,* **1957,** *12,* 323–328.

Ganellin, C. R.; Durant, G. J.; and Emmett, J. C. Some chemical aspects of histamine H₂-receptor antagonists. *Fed. Proc.,* **1976,** *35,* 1924–1930.

Gerschenfeld, H. M., and Paupardin-Tritsch, D. Ionic mechanisms and receptor properties underlying the responses of molluscan neurones to 5-hydroxytryptamine. *J. Physiol. (Lond.),* **1974,** *243,* 427–456.

Gershon, M. D.; Dreyfus, C. F.; Pickel, V. M.; Joh, T. H.; and Reis, D. J. Serotonergic neurons in the peripheral nervous system: identification in gut by immunohistochemical localization of tryptophan hydroxylase. *Proc. Natl. Acad. Sci. U.S.A.,* **1977,** *74,* 3086–3089.

Graham, J. R. Cardiac and pulmonary fibrosis during methysergide therapy for headache. *Am. J. Med. Sci.,* **1967,** *254,* 1–12.

Graybiel, A.; Wood, C. D.; Knepton, J.; Hoche, J. P.; and Perkins, G. F. Human assay of antimotion sickness drugs. *Aviat. Space Environ. Med.,* **1975,** *46,* 1107–1118.

Gylfe, E. Association between 5-hydroxytryptamine release and insulin secretion. *J. Endocrinol.,* **1978,** *78,* 239–248.

Hamlin, K. E., and Fischer, F. E. The synthesis of 5-hydroxytryptamine. *J. Am. Chem. Soc.,* **1951,** *73,* 5007–5008.

Hintze, K. L.; Grow, A. B.; and Fischer, L. J. Cyproheptadine-induced alterations in rat insulin synthesis. *Biochem. Pharmacol.,* **1977,** *26,* 2021–2027.

Hollander, W.; Michelson, A. L.; and Wilkins, R. W. Serotonin and antiserotonins. I. Their circulatory, respiratory and renal effects in man. *Circulation,* **1957,** *16,* 246–255.

Holmsen, H.; Østvold, A.-C.; and Day, J. H. Behaviour of endogenous and newly absorbed serotonin in the platelet release reaction. *Biochem. Pharmacol.,* **1973,** *22,* 2599–2608.

Horton, B. T. The use of histamine in the treatment of specific types of headaches. *J.A.M.A.,* **1941,** *116,* 377–383.

Ippoliti, A. F., and others. Cimetidine versus intensive antacid therapy for duodenal ulcer. *Gastroenterology,* **1978,** *74,* 393–395.

Ishizaka, T., and Ishizaka, K. Triggering of histamine release from rat mast cells by divalent antibodies against IgE-receptors. *J. Immunol.,* **1978,** *120,* 800–805.

Jacobson, E. D., and Thompson, W. J. Cyclic AMP and gastric secretion: the illusive second messenger. *Adv. Cyclic Nucleotide Res.,* **1976,** *7,* 199–224.

Jaju, B. P., and Wang, S. C. Effects of diphenhydramine and dimenhydrinate on vestibular neuronal activity of cat: a search for the locus of their antimotion sickness action. *J. Pharmacol. Exp. Ther.,* **1971,** *176,* 718–724.

Jorizzo, J. L.; Sams, W. M.; Jegasothy, B. V.; and Olansky,

A. J. Cimetidine as an immunomodulator: chronic mucocutaneous candidiasis as a model. *Ann. Intern. Med.*, **1980**, *92*, 192–195.

Koch-Weser, J.; Finkelstein, W.; and Isselbacher, K. J. Drug therapy: cimetidine. *N. Engl. J. Med.*, **1978**, *299*, 992–996.

Kruss, D. M., and Littman, A. Safety of cimetidine. *Gastroenterology*, **1978**, *74*, 478–483.

Lecomte, J. Liberation of endogenous histamine in man. *J. Allergy*, **1957**, *28*, 102–112.

Lemberger, L.; Rowe, H.; Carmichael, R.; Crabtree, R.; Horng, J. S.; Bymaster, F.; and Wong, D. Fluoxetine, a selective serotonin uptake inhibitor. *Clin. Pharmacol. Ther.*, **1978**, *23*, 421–429.

Levine, R. J. Serotonin and the carcinoid syndrome; histamine and mastocytosis. In, *Duncan's Diseases of Metabolism: The Genetic and Biochemical Basis of Disease,* 7th ed., Vol. II. (Bondy, P. K., and Rosenberg, L. E., eds.) W. B. Saunders Co., Philadelphia, **1974**, pp. 1651–1684.

Lilienfield, L. S.; Rose, J. C.; and Princiotto, J. V. Antitussive activity of diphenhydramine in chronic cough. *Clin. Pharmacol. Ther.*, **1976**, *19*, 421–425.

Linnoila, M. Effect of antihistamines, chlormezanone and alcohol on psychomotor skills related to driving. *Eur. J. Clin. Pharmacol.*, **1973**, *5*, 247–254.

Loew, E. R.; MacMillan, R.; and Katser, M. E. The antihistamine properties of BENADRYL, β-dimethylaminoethyl benzhydryl ether hydrochloride. *J. Pharmacol. Exp. Ther.*, **1946**, *86*, 229–238.

Lorenz, W., and Doenicke, A. Histamine release in clinical conditions. *Mt. Sinai J. Med. N.Y.*, **1978**, *45*, 357–386.

McGrath, M. A. 5-Hydroxytryptamine and neurotransmitter release in canine blood vessels. Inhibition by low and augmentation by high concentrations. *Circ. Res.*, **1977**, *41*, 428–435.

McGrath, M. A., and Shepherd, J. T. Histamine and 5-hydroxytryptamine—inhibition of transmitter release mediated by H_2- and 5-hydroxytryptamine receptors. *Fed. Proc.*, **1978**, *37*, 195–198.

Majno, G.; Shea, S. M.; and Leventhal, M. Endothelial contraction induced by histamine-type mediators. An electron microscopic study. *J. Cell Biol.*, **1969**, *42*, 647–672.

Malagelada, J. R., and Cortot, A. H_2-receptor antagonists in perspective. *Mayo Clin. Proc.*, **1978**, *53*, 184–190.

Medical Letter. Azatadine (OPTIMINE)—a new antihistamine. **1977**, *19*, 77–79.

Medical Letter. Drugs for asthma. **1978a**, *20*, 69–72.

Medical Letter. Cimetidine (TAGAMET): update on adverse effects. **1978b**, *20*, 77–78.

Melmon, K. L.; Weinstein, Y.; Poon, T.; Bourne, H. R.; Shearer, G. M.; Coffino, P.; and Insel, P. A. Receptors for low molecular weight hormones on lymphocytes. In, *Immunopharmacology.* (Hadden, J. W.; Spreafico, F.; and Garattini, S.; eds.) Plenum Press, New York, **1977**, pp. 331–356.

Morishima, T. 5-Hydroxytryptamine (serotonin) and 5-hydroxytryptophan in mast cells of human mastocytosis. *Tohoku J. Exp. Med.*, **1970**, *102*, 121–126.

Morley, J. S. Structure-function relationships in gastrin-like peptides. *Proc. R. Soc. Lond. [Biol.]*, **1968**, *170*, 97–111.

Oppizzi, G.; Verde, G.; De Stefano, L.; Cozzi, R.; Botalla, L.; Liuzzi, A.; and Chiodini, P. G. Evidence for a dopaminergic activity of methysergide in humans. *Clin. Endocrinol. (Oxf.)*, **1977**, *7*, 267–272.

Paton, W. D. M., and Vane, J. R. An analysis of the responses of the isolated stomach to electrical stimulation and to drugs. *J. Physiol. (Lond.)*, **1963**, *165*, 10–46.

Payne, R. A., and Kay, A. W. The effect of vagotomy on the maximal acid secretory response to histamine. *Clin. Sci.*, **1962**, *22*, 373–382.

Pearse, A. G. E. The diffuse neuro-endocrine system and the APUD concept; related "endocrine" peptides in brain, intestine, pituitary, placenta and anuran cutaneous glands. *Med. Biol.*, **1977**, *55*, 115–125.

Persyko, I. Psychiatric adverse reactions to methysergide. *J. Nerv. Ment. Dis.*, **1972**, *4*, 299–301.

Popielski, L. β-Imidazolyläthylamin und die Organextrakte. Erster Teil: β-Imidazolyläthylamin als mächtiger Erreger der Magendrüsen. *Pflügers Arch. Ges. Physiol.*, **1920**, *178*, 214–236.

Rapport, M. M. Serum vasoconstrictor (serotonin). V. The presence of creatinine in the complex: a proposed study of the vasoconstrictor principle. *J. Biol. Chem.*, **1949**, *180*, 961–969.

Rapport, M. M.; Green, A. A.; and Page, I. H. Serum vasoconstrictor (serotonin). IV. Isolation and characterization. *J. Biol. Chem.*, **1948**, *176*, 1243–1251.

Richardson, C. T. Effect of H_2-receptor antagonists on gastric acid secretion and serum gastrin concentration. *Gastroenterology*, **1978**, *74*, 366–370.

Rodbard, S., and Kira, S. Lobar, airway, and pulmonary vascular effects of serotonin. *Angiology*, **1972**, *23*, 188–197.

Rosière, C. E., and Grossman, M. I. An analog of histamine that stimulates gastric acid secretion without other actions of histamine. *Science*, **1951**, *113*, 651.

Sadusk, J. F., and Palmisano, P. A. Teratogenic effect of meclizine, cyclizine, and chlorcyclizine. *J.A.M.A.*, **1965**, *194*, 987–989.

Saum, W. R., and de Groat, W. C. The actions of 5-hydroxytryptamine on the urinary bladder and on vesical autonomic ganglia in the cat. *J. Pharmacol. Exp. Ther.*, **1973**, *185*, 70–83.

Schayer, R. W., and Cooper, J. A. D. Metabolism of C^{14} histamine in man. *J. Appl. Physiol.*, **1956**, *9*, 481–483.

Schöön, I. M., and Olbe, L. Inhibitory effect of cimetidine on gastric acid secretion vagally activated by physiological means in duodenal ulcer patients. *Gut*, **1978**, *19*, 27–31.

Sicuteri, F. Prophylactic and therapeutic properties of 1-methyl-lysergic acid butanolamide in migraine (preliminary report). *Int. Arch. Allergy Appl. Immunol.*, **1959**, *15*, 300–307.

———. Headache: disruption of pain modulation. In, *Advances in Pain Research and Therapy*, Vol. 1. (Bonica, J. J., and Albe-Fessard, D., eds.) Raven Press, New York, **1976**, pp. 871–880.

Sieghart, W.; Theoharides, T. C.; Alper, S.; Douglas, W. W.; and Greengard, P. Calcium-dependent protein phosphorylation during secretion by exocytosis in the mast cell. *Nature*, **1978**, *275*, 329–331.

Sjaastad, O. The significance of blood serotonin levels in migraine. *Acta Neurol. Scand.*, **1975**, *51*, 200–210.

Sjoerdsma, A.; Gillespie, L.; and Udenfriend, S. A simple method for the measurement of monoamine-oxidase inhibition in man. *Lancet*, **1958**, *2*, 159–160.

Spodick, D. H. Electrocardiographic responses to pulmonary embolism. Mechanisms and sources of variability. *Am. J. Cardiol.*, **1972**, *30*, 695–699.

Staszewska-Barczak, J., and Vane, J. R. The release of catecholamines from the adrenal medulla by histamine. *Br. J. Pharmacol.*, **1965**, *25*, 728–742.

Staub, A.-M., and Bovet, D. Action de la thymoxyéthyldiéthylamine (929F) et des éthers phénoliques sur le choc anaphylactique du cobaye. *C. R. Soc. Biol. (Paris)*, **1937**, *125*, 818–823.

Stone, C. A.; Wenger, H. C.; Ludden, C. T.; Stavorski, I. M.; and Ross, C. A. Antiserotonin-antihistaminic properties of cyproheptadine. *J. Pharmacol. Exp. Ther.*, **1961**, *131*, 73–84.

Storstein, O.; Calabresi, M.; Nims, R. G.; and Gray, F. D., Jr. The effect of histamine on the pulmonary circulation in man. *Yale J. Biol. Med.*, **1959**, *32*, 197–208.

Sullivan, T. J., and Parker, C. W. Possible role of arachidonic acid and its metabolites in mediator release from rat mast cells. *J. Immunol.,* **1979,** *122,* 431–436.

Taraskevich, P. S., and Douglas, W. W. Stimulant effect of 5-hydroxytryptamine on action potential activity in pars intermedia cells of the lizard *Anolis carolinensis:* contrasting effects in pars intermedia of rat and rostral pars distalis of fish *(Alosa pseudoharengus). Brain Res.,* **1979,** *178,* 584–588.

Theoharides, T. C., and Douglas, W. W. Somatostatin induces histamine secretion from rat peritoneal mast cells. *Endocrinology,* **1978,** *102,* 1637–1640.

Theoharides, T. C.; Sieghart, W.; Greengard, P.; and Douglas, W. W. Antiallergic drug cromolyn may inhibit histamine secretion by regulating phosphorylation of a mast cell protein. *Science,* **1980,** *207,* 80–82.

Torok, E. E.; Brewer, J. I.; and Dolkart, R. E. Serum diamine oxidase in pregnancy and in trophoblastic diseases. *J. Clin. Endocrinol. Metab.,* **1970,** *30,* 59–65.

Twarog, B. M., and Page, I. H. Serotonin content of some mammalian tissues and urine and a method for its determination. *Am. J. Physiol.,* **1953,** *175,* 157–161.

Van Thiel, D. H.; Gavaler, B. S.; Smith, W. I., Jr.; and Paul, G. Hypothalamic-pituitary-gonadal dysfunction in men using cimetidine. *N. Engl. J. Med.,* **1979,** *300,* 1012–1015.

West, S.; Brandon, B.; Stolley, P.; and Rumrill, R. A review of antihistamines and the common cold. *Pediatrics,* **1975,** *56,* 100–107.

Wood, C. D., and Graybiel, A. A theory of motion sickness based on pharmacological reactions. *Clin. Pharmacol. Ther.,* **1970,** *11,* 621–629.

Woolley, D. W., and Shaw, E. A biochemical and pharmacological suggestion about certain mental disorders. *Science,* **1954,** *119,* 587–588.

Wormsley, K. G. Testing anti-ulcer drugs. *Lancet,* **1977,** *2,* 719.

Wurtman, R. J., and Fernstrom, J. D. Control of brain neurotransmitter synthesis by precursor availability and nutritional state. *Biochem. Pharmacol.,* **1976,** *25,* 1691–1696.

Yonkman, F. F.; Chess, D.; Mathieson, D.; and Hansen, N. Pharmacodynamic studies of a new antihistamine agent, N′-pyridyl-N′-benzyl-N-dimethylethylene diamine HCl, pyribenzamine HCl. Effects on salivation, nictitating membrane, lachrymation, pupil and blood pressure. *J. Pharmacol. Exp. Ther.,* **1946,** *87,* 256–264.

Monographs and Reviews

Adler, S. Serotonin and the kidney. In, *Clinical Correlates.* Vol. 4, *Serotonin in Health and Disease.* (Essman, W. B., ed.) Spectrum Publications, Inc., New York, **1978,** pp. 99–137.

Altura, B. M., and Halevy, S. Cardiovascular actions of histamine. In, *Histamine II and Anti-Histaminics: Chemistry, Metabolism and Physiological and Pharmacological Actions.* (Rocha e Silva, M., ed.) *Handbuch der Experimentellen Pharmakologie,* Vol. 18, Pt. 2. Springer-Verlag, Berlin, **1978,** pp. 1–39.

———. Circulatory shock, histamine, and antihistamines: therapeutic aspects. In, *Histamine II and Anti-Histaminics: Chemistry, Metabolism and Physiological and Pharmacological Actions.* (Rocha e Silva, M., ed.) *Handbuch der Experimentellen Pharmakologie,* Vol. 18, Pt. 2. Springer-Verlag, Berlin, **1978,** pp. 575–602.

Assem, E. S. K. Current aspects in the immunopharmacology of asthma. *Med. Biol.,* **1976,** *54,* 369–382.

Bach, M. K. *Immediate Hypersensitivity: Modern Concepts and Developments.* Marcel Dekker, Inc., New York, **1978.**

Beaven, M. A. *Histamine: Its Role in Physiological and Pathological Processes.* S. Karger, Basel, **1978.**

Beraldo, W. T., and Dias da Silva, W. Release of histamine by animal venoms and bacterial toxins. In, *Histamine: Its Chemistry, Metabolism and Physiological and Pharmaco-*

logical Actions. (Rocha e Silva, M., ed.) *Handbuch der Experimentellen Pharmakologie,* Vol. 18, pt. 1. Springer Verlag, Berlin, **1966,** pp. 334–366.

Berridge, M. J. The mode of action of 5-hydroxytryptamine. *J. Exp. Biol.,* **1972,** *56,* 311–321.

———. The interaction of cyclic nucleotides and calcium in the control of cellular activity. *Adv. Cyclic Nucleotide Res.,* **1975,** *6,* 1–98.

Bloom, F. E. The role of cyclic nucleotides in central synaptic function. *Rev. Physiol. Biochem. Pharmacol.,* **1975,** *74,* 1–103.

Bosin, T. R. Serotonin metabolism. In, *Availability, Localization and Disposition.* Vol. 1, *Serotonin in Health and Disease.* (Essman, W. B., ed.) Spectrum Publications, Inc., New York, **1978,** pp. 181–300.

Brand, J. J., and Perry, W. L. M. Drugs used in motion sickness. *Pharmacol. Rev.,* **1955,** *7,* 33–82.

Brody, M. J. *Histaminergic and Cholinergic Mechanisms of Vasodilatation.* (Vanhoutte, P. M., and Leusen, I., eds.) S. Karger, Basel, **1978,** pp. 266–277.

Brogden, R. N.; Heel, R. C.; Speight, T. M.; and Avery, G. S. Cimetidine: a review of its pharmacological properties and therapeutic efficacy in peptic ulcer disease. *Drugs,* **1978,** *15,* 93–131.

Brogden, R. N.; Speight, T. M.; and Avery, G. S. Sodium cromoglycate (cromolyn sodium): a review of its mode of action, pharmacology, therapeutic efficacy and use. *Drugs,* **1974,** *7,* 164–282.

Brown, H. Serotonin-producing tumors. In, *Clinical Correlates.* Vol. 4, *Serotonin in Health and Disease.* (Essman, W. B., ed.) Spectrum Publications, Inc., New York, **1977,** pp. 393–423.

Casy, A. F. Chemistry of anti-H_1 histamine antagonists. In, *Histamine II and Anti-Histaminics: Chemistry, Metabolism and Physiological and Pharmacological Actions.* (Rocha e Silva, M., ed.) *Handbuch der Experimentellen Pharmakologie,* Vol. 18, Pt. 2. Springer-Verlag, Berlin, **1978,** pp. 175–214.

Chakravarty, N. Metabolic changes in mast cells associated with histamine release. In, *Histamine II and Anti-Histaminics: Chemistry, Metabolism and Physiological and Pharmacological Actions.* (Rocha e Silva, M., ed.) *Handbuch der Experimentellen Pharmakologie,* Vol. 18, Pt. 2. Springer-Verlag, Berlin, **1978,** pp. 93–108.

Chinn, H. I., and Smith, P. K. Motion sickness. *Pharmacol. Rev.,* **1955,** *7,* 33–82.

Christian, S. T., and Smythies, J. R. Molecular interactions with serotonin. In, *Availability, Localization and Disposition.* Vol. 1, *Serotonin in Health and Disease.* (Essman, W. B., ed.) Spectrum Publications, Inc., New York, **1978,** pp. 363–374.

Church, M. K. Cromoglycate-like anti-allergic drugs: a review. *Medicamentos Actualidad/Drugs of Today,* **1978,** *14,* 281–341.

Code, C. F. Histamine and gastric secretion: a later look, 1955–1965. *Fed. Proc.,* **1965,** *24,* 1311–1325.

———. Reflections on histamine, gastric secretion and the H_2 receptor. *N. Engl. J. Med.,* **1977,** *296,* 1459–1462.

Conference. (Various authors.) *Proceedings of the Third International Conference on Cyclic Nucleotides.* (Greengard, P., and Robison, G. A., eds.) *Adv. Cyclic Nucleotide Res.,* **1978,** *9,* 1–799.

Cox, J. S. G. Cromolyn sodium. *Pharmacol. Biochem. Prop. Drug Subst.,* **1977,** *1,* 277–310.

Cox, J. S. C.; Beach, J. E.; Blair, A. M.; Clarke, A. J.; King, J.; Lee, T. B.; Loveday, D. E. E.; Moss, G. F.; Orr, T. S. C.; Ritchie, J. R.; and Sheard, P. Disodium cromoglycate (INTAL). *Adv. Drug Res.,* **1970,** *5,* 115–196.

Emmelin, N. Action of histamine upon salivary glands. In, *Histamine: Its Chemistry, Metabolism and Physiological and Pharmacological Actions.* (Rocha e Silva, M., ed.) *Handbuch der Experimentellen Pharmakologie,* Vol. 18, Pt. 1. Springer-Verlag, Berlin, **1966,** pp. 294–301.

Erspamer, V. Pharmacology of indolealkylamines. *Pharmacol. Rev.*, **1954**, *6*, 425–487.

——— (ed.). *5-Hydroxytryptamine and Related Indolealkylamines. Handbuch der Experimentellen Pharmakologie,* Vol. 19. Springer-Verlag, Berlin, **1966b.**

Essman, W. B. *Serotonin in Health and Disease,* Vol. 4. *Clinical Correlates.* Spectrum Publications, Inc., New York, **1977.**

———. *Serotonin in Health and Disease,* Vol. 1. *Availability, Localization and Disposition.* Spectrum Publications, Inc., New York, **1978a.**

———. *Serotonin in Health and Disease,* Vol. 2. *Physiological Regulation and Pharmacological Action.* Spectrum Publications, Inc., New York, **1978b.**

———. *Serotonin in Health and Disease,* Vol. 3. *The Central Nervous System.* Spectrum Publications, Inc., New York, **1978c.**

———. Serotonin distribution in tissues and fluids. In, *Availability, Localization and Disposition.* Vol. 1, *Serotonin in Health and Disease.* (Essman, W. B., ed.) Spectrum Publications, Inc., New York, **1978d,** pp. 15–179.

Euler, U. S. von. Relationship between histamine and the autonomic nervous system. In, *Histamine: Its Chemistry, Metabolism and Physiological and Pharmacological Actions.* (Rocha e Silva, M., ed.) *Handbuch der Experimentellen Pharmakologie,* Vol. 18, Pt. 1. Springer-Verlag, Berlin, **1966,** pp. 318–333.

Faingold, C. L. Antihistamines as central nervous system depressants. In, *Histamine II and Anti-Histaminics: Chemistry, Metabolism and Physiological and Pharmacological Actions.* (Rocha e Silva, M., ed.) *Handbuch der Experimentellen Pharmakologie,* Vol. 18, Pt. 2. Springer-Verlag, Berlin, **1978,** pp. 561–573.

Feldman, M., and Richardson, C. T. Histamine H_2-receptor antagonists. *Adv. Intern. Med.,* **1978,** *23,* 1–24.

Fozard, J. R. The animal pharmacology of drugs used in the treatment of migraine. *J. Pharm. Pharmacol.,* **1975,** *27,* 297–321.

Furchgott, R. F. The pharmacology of vascular smooth muscle. *Pharmacol. Rev.,* **1955,** *7,* 183–265.

Ganellin, C. R. Selectivity and the design of histamine H_2-receptor antagonists. *J. Appl. Chem. Biotechnol.,* **1978a,** *28,* 183–200.

———. Chemistry and structure-activity relationships of H_2-receptor antagonists. In, *Histamine II and Anti-Histaminics: Chemistry, Metabolism and Physiological and Pharmacological Actions.* (Rocha e Silva, M., ed.) *Handbuch der Experimentellen Pharmakologie,* Vol. 18, Pt. 2. Springer-Verlag, Berlin, **1978b,** pp. 251–294.

Garattini, S., and Samanin, R. Drugs affecting serotonin: a survey. In, *Physiological Regulation and Pharmacological Action.* Vol. 2, *Serotonin in Health and Disease.* (Essman, W. B., ed.) Spectrum Publications, Inc., New York, **1978,** pp. 247–293.

Gillis, C. N., and Roth, J. A. Pulmonary disposition of circulating vasoactive hormones. *Biochem. Pharmacol.,* **1976,** *25,* 2547–2553.

Goth, A. Histamine release by drugs and chemicals. In, *Histamine and Antihistamines,* Vol. 1. *International Encyclopedia of Pharmacology and Therapeutics,* Sect. 74. (Schachter, M., ed.) Pergamon Press, Ltd., Oxford, **1973,** pp. 25–43.

———. On the general problems of the release of histamine. In, *Histamine II and Anti-Histaminics: Chemistry, Metabolism and Physiological and Pharmacological Actions.* (Rocha e Silva, M., ed.) *Handbuch der Experimentellen Pharmakologie,* Vol. 18, Pt. 2. Springer-Verlag, Berlin, **1978,** pp. 57–74.

Green, J. P.; Johnson, C. L.; and Weinstein, H. Histamine as a neurotransmitter. In, *Psychopharmacology: A Generation of Progress.* (Lipton, M. A.; DiMascio, A.; and Killam, K. F.; eds.) Raven Press, New York, **1978,** pp. 319–332.

Greengard, P. Possible role for cyclic nucleotides and phosphorylated membrane proteins in postsynaptic actions of neurotransmitters. *Nature,* **1976,** *260,* 101–108.

———. *Cyclic Nucleotides, Phosphorylated Proteins, and Neuronal Function.* Vol. 1, *Distinguished Lecture Series of the Society of General Physiologists.* Raven Press, New York, **1978.**

Gregory, R. A., and Tracy, H. J. A review of recent progress in the chemistry of gastrin. *Am. J. Dig. Dis.,* **1966,** *11,* 97–102.

Gyermek, L. Drugs which antagonize 5-hydroxytryptamine and related indolealkylamines. In, *5-Hydroxytryptamine and Related Indolealkylamines.* (Erspamer, V., ed.) *Handbuch der Experimentellen Pharmakologie,* Vol. 19. Springer-Verlag, Berlin, **1966,** pp. 471–528.

Hahn, F. Antianaphylactic and antiallergic effects. In, *Histamine II and Anti-Histaminics: Chemistry, Metabolism and Physiological and Pharmacological Actions.* (Rocha e Silva, M., ed.) *Handbuch der Experimentellen Pharmakologie,* Vol. 18, Pt. 2. Springer-Verlag, Berlin, **1978,** pp. 439–504.

Halpern, B. N. Les antihistaminiques de synthèse: essais de chimiothérapie des états allergiques. *Arch. Int. Pharmacodyn. Ther.,* **1942,** *68,* 339–408.

Hirschowitz, B. I. H-2 histamine receptors. *Annu. Rev. Pharmacol. Toxicol.,* **1979,** *19,* 203–244.

Ivy, A. C., and Bachrach, W. H. Physiological significance of the effect of histamine on gastric secretion. In, *Histamine: Its Chemistry, Metabolism and Physiological and Pharmacological Actions.* (Rocha e Silva, M., ed.) *Handbuch der Experimentellen Pharmakologie,* Vol. 18, Pt. 1. Springer-Verlag, Berlin, **1966,** pp. 810–891.

Johnson, H. G. Specific inhibitors of mediator release and their modes of action. In, *Immediate Hypersensitivity: Modern Concepts and Developments.* (Bach, M. K., ed.) Marcel Dekker, Inc., New York, **1978,** 533–560.

Johnson, L. R. Control of gastric secretion: no room for histamine? *Gastroenterology,* **1971,** *61,* 106–118.

———. Histamine and gastric secretion. In, *Histamine II and Anti-Histaminics: Chemistry, Metabolism and Physiological and Pharmacological Actions.* (Rocha e Silva, M., ed.) *Handbuch der Experimentellen Pharmakologie,* Vol. 18, Pt. 2. Springer-Verlag, Berlin, **1978,** pp. 41–56.

Jones, R. S., and Meyers, W. C. Regulation of hepatic biliary secretion. *Annu. Rev. Physiol.,* **1979,** *41,* 67–82.

Kahlson, G., and Rosengren, E. New approaches to the physiology of histamine. *Physiol. Rev.,* **1968,** *48,* 155–196.

———. *Biogenesis and Physiology of Histamine.* Edward Arnold, Ltd., London, **1971.**

Kaliner, M., and Austen, K. F. Immunological release of chemical mediators from human tissues. *Annu. Rev. Pharmacol.,* **1975,** *15,* 177–189.

Kebabian, J. W. Biochemical regulation and physiological significance of cyclic nucleotides in the nervous system. *Adv. Cyclic Nucleotide Res.,* **1977,** *8,* 421–508.

Keele, C. A., and Armstrong, D. *Substances Producing Pain and Itch.* The Williams & Wilkins Co., Baltimore, **1964.**

Keeton, R. W.; Luckhardt, A. B.; and Koch, F. C. Gastrin studies. IV. The response of the stomach mucosa to food and gastrin bodies as influenced by atropine. *Am. J. Physiol.,* **1920,** *51,* 469–481.

Kingsley, P. J., and Cox, J. S. G. Cromolyn sodium (sodium cromoglycate) and drugs with similar activities. In, *Allergy: Principles and Practice,* Vol. 1. (Middleton, E.; Reed, C.; and Ellis, E. F.; eds.) C. V. Mosby Co., St. Louis, **1978,** pp. 481–498.

Krieger, D. T. Endocrine processes and serotonin. In, *The Central Nervous System.* Vol. 3, *Serotonin in Health and Disease.* (Essman, W. B., ed.) Spectrum Publications, Inc., New York, **1978,** pp. 51–67.

Lewis, T. *The Blood Vessels of the Human Skin and Their Responses.* Shaw & Sons, Ltd., London, **1927.**

Lichtenstein, L. M., and Austen, K. F. *Asthma, Physiology, Immunopharmacology and Treatment.* Academic Press, Inc., New York, **1978**.

MacIntosh, F. C. Histamine as a normal stimulant of gastric secretion. *Q. J. Exp. Physiol.,* **1938,** *28,* 87–98.

Mantegazzini, P. Pharmacological actions of indolealkylamines and precursor amino acids on the central nervous system. In, *5-Hydroxytryptamine and Related Indolealkylamines.* (Erspamer, V., ed.) *Handbuch der Experimentellen Pharmakologie,* Vol. 19. Springer-Verlag, Berlin, **1966,** pp. 424–470.

Maśliński, C. Histamine and its metabolism in mammals. Part I: Chemistry and formation of histamine. *Agents Actions,* **1975a,** *5,* 89–107.

———. Histamine and its metabolism in mammals. Part II: Catabolism of histamine and histamine liberation. *Ibid.,* **1975b,** *5,* 183–225.

Metzger, H. Early molecular events in antigen-antibody cell activation. *Annu. Rev. Pharmacol. Toxicol.,* **1979,** *19,* 427–445.

Metzger, H., and Bach, M. K. The receptor for IgE on mast cells and basophils: studies on IgE binding and on the structure of the receptor. In, *Immediate Hypersensitivity: Modern Concepts and Developments.* (Bach, M. K., ed.) Marcel Dekker, Inc., New York, **1978,** pp. 561–588.

Money, K. E. Motion sickness. *Physiol. Rev.,* **1970,** *50,* 1–39.

Morrison, D. C., and Henson, P. M. Release of mediators from mast cells and basophils induced by different stimuli. In, *Immediate Hypersensitivity: Modern Concepts and Developments.* (Bach, M. K., ed.) Marcel Dekker, Inc., New York, **1978,** pp. 431–502.

Mustard, J. F., and Packham, M. A. Factors influencing platelet function: adhesion, release and aggregation. *Pharmacol. Rev.,* **1970,** *22,* 97–187.

Nathanson, J. A. Cyclic nucleotides and nervous system function. *Physiol. Rev.,* **1977,** *57,* 157–256.

Nauta, W. T., and Rekker, R. F. Structure-activity relationships of H_1-receptor antagonists. In, *Histamine II and Anti Histaminics: Chemistry, Metabolism and Physiological and Pharmacological Actions.* (Rocha e Silva, M., ed.) *Handbuch der Experimentellen Pharmakologie,* Vol. 18, Pt. 2. Springer-Verlag, Berlin, **1978,** pp. 215–249.

Owen, D. A. A. Histamine receptors in the cardiovascular system. *Gen. Pharmacol.,* **1977,** *8,* 141–156.

Paton, W. D. M. Histamine release by compounds of simple chemical structure. *Pharmacol. Rev.,* **1957,** *9,* 269–328.

Pearlman, D. S. Antihistamine: pharmacology and clinical use. *Drugs,* **1976,** *12,* 258–273.

Plaut, M., and Lichtenstein, L. M. Pharmacologic control of mediator release. In, *Immediate Hypersensitivity: Modern Concepts and Developments.* (Bach, M. K., ed.) Marcel Dekker, Inc., New York, **1978,** pp. 503–532.

Reite, O. B. Comparative physiology of histamine. *Physiol. Rev.,* **1972,** *52,* 778–819.

Rocha e Silva, M. (ed.). *Histamine: Its Chemistry, Metabolism and Physiological and Pharmacological Actions. Handbuch der Experimentellen Pharmakologie,* Vol. 18, Pt. 1. Springer-Verlag, Berlin, **1966.**

——— (ed.). *Histamine II and Anti-Histaminics: Chemistry Metabolism and Physiological and Pharmacological Actions. Handbuch der Experimentellen Pharmakologie,* Vol. 18, Pt. 2. Springer-Verlag, Berlin, **1978a.**

———. Kinetics of antagonist action. In, *Histamine II and Anti-Histaminics: Chemistry, Metabolism and Physiological and Pharmacological Actions.* (Rocha e Silva, M., ed.) *Handbuch der Experimentellen Pharmakologie,* Vol. 18, Pt. 2. Springer-Verlag, Berlin, **1978b,** pp. 295–332.

Rocha e Silva, M., and Antonio, A. Bioassay of antihistaminic action. In, *Histamine II and Anti-Histaminics: Chemistry, Metabolism and Physiological and Pharmacological Actions.* (Rocha e Silva, M., ed.) *Handbuch der*

Experimentellen Pharmakologie,* Vol. 18, Pt. 2. Springer-Verlag, Berlin, **1978,** pp. 381–438.

Rothschild, A. M. Histamine release by basic compounds. In, *Histamine: Its Chemistry, Metabolism and Physiological and Pharmacological Actions.* (Rocha e Silva, M., ed.) *Handbuch der Experimentellen Pharmakologie,* Vol. 18, Pt. 1. Springer-Verlag, Berlin, **1966,** pp. 386–430.

Sachs, G.; Spenney, J. G.; and Rehm, W. S. Gastric secretion. In, *Gastrointestinal Physiology II,* Vol. 12. (Crane, R. K., ed.) University Park Press, Baltimore, **1977,** pp. 128–171.

Schachter, M. (ed.). *Histamine and Antihistamines,* Vol. 1. *International Encyclopedia of Pharmacology and Therapeutics,* Sect. 74. Pergamon Press, Ltd., Oxford, **1973.**

Schäfer, E. A. *The Endocrine Organs: An Introduction to the Study of Internal Secretion.* Longmans, Green & Co., New York, **1916.**

Schayer, R. W. Induced synthesis of histamine, microcirculatory regulation and the mechanism of action of the glucocorticoid hormones. *Prog. Allergy,* **1963,** *7,* 187–212.

———. Histamine and microcirculation. *Life Sci.,* **1974,** *15,* 391–401.

———. Biogenesis of histamine. In, *Histamine II and Anti-Histaminics: Chemistry, Metabolism and Physiological and Pharmacological Actions.* (Rocha e Silva, M., ed.) *Handbuch der Experimentellen Pharmakologie,* Vol. 18, Pt. 2. Springer-Verlag, Berlin, **1978,** 109–129.

Schwartz, J.-C. Histaminergic mechanisms in brain. *Annu. Rev. Pharmacol. Toxicol.,* **1977,** *17,* 325–339.

Sneddon, J. Blood platelets as a model for monoamine-containing neurones. *Prog. Neurobiol.,* **1973,** *1,* 153–198.

Soll, A., and Walsh, J. H. Regulation of gastric acid secretion. *Annu. Rev. Physiol.,* **1979,** *41,* 35–53.

Speight, T. M., and Avery, G. S. Pizotifen (B.C.–105): a review of pharmacological properties and its therapeutic efficacy in vascular headaches. *Drugs,* **1972,** *3,* 159–203.

Symposium. (Various authors.) Biological role of indolealkylamine derivatives. (Garattini, S., and Shore, P., eds.) *Adv. Pharmacol.,* **1968a,** *6A,* 1–440, *6B,* 1–323.

Symposium. (Various authors.) 5-Hydroxytryptamine. (Paasonen, M. K., and Klinge, E., eds.) *Ann. Med. Exp. Biol. Fenn.,* **1968b,** *46,* 361–519.

Symposium. (Various authors.) *Serotonin and Behavior.* (Barchas, J. D., and Usdin, E., eds.) Academic Press, Inc., New York, **1973,** pp. 1–642.

Symposium. (Various authors.) Serotonin—new vistas: histochemistry and pharmacology. (Costa, E.; Gessa, G. L.; and Sandler, M.; eds.) *Adv. Biochem. Psychopharmacol.,* **1974a,** *10,* 1–329.

Symposium. (Various authors.) Serotonin—new vistas: biochemistry and behavioural and clinical studies. (Costa, E.; Gessa, G. L.; and Sandler, M.; eds.) *Adv. Biochem. Psychopharmacol.,* **1974b,** *11,* 1–428.

Symposium. (Various authors.) *Biochemistry and Pharmacology of Platelets.* Ciba Foundation Symposium, Vol. 35. Elsevier/Excerpta Medica/North Holland, Amsterdam, **1975,** pp. 1–352.

Symposium. (Various authors.) *Proceedings of the Second International Symposium on Histamine H_2-Receptor Antagonists: Cimetidine.* (Burland, W. L., and Simkins, M. A., eds.) Excerpta Medica, Amsterdam, **1977a,** pp. 1–392.

Symposium. (Various authors.) Excitation-contraction coupling in smooth muscle. (Casteels, R.; Godfraind, T.; and Ruegg, J. C.; eds.) *Proceedings of the International Symposium on Excitation Contraction Coupling in Smooth Muscle and the Erwin-Riesch Symposium.* Elsevier/North Holland Biomedical Press, Amsterdam, **1977b.**

Symposium. (Various authors.) Third symposium on histamine H_2-receptor antagonists: clinical results with cimetidine. (Fordtran, J. S., and Grossman, M. I., eds.) *Gastroenterology,* **1978a,** *74,* 1–488.

Symposium. (Various authors.) Serotonin neurotoxins.

(Jacoby, J. H., and Lytle, L. D., eds.) *Ann. N.Y. Acad. Sci.,* **1978b,** *305,* 1–702.

Symposium. (Various authors.) *The Mast Cell: Its Role in Health and Disease.* (Petys, J., and Edwards, A. M., eds.) Pitman Medical, Kent, England, **1979.**

Thompson, J. H. Serotonin and the alimentary tract. *Res. Commun. Chem. Pathol. Pharmacol.,* **1971,** *2,* 687–781.

Toogood, J. H.; Lefcoe, N. M.; Wonnacott, T. M.; McCourtie, D. R.; and Mullin, J. K. Cromolyn sodium therapy: predictors of response. *Adv. Asthma Allergy,* **1978,** *5,* 2–15.

Uvnäs, B. The mechanism of histamine release from mast cells. In, *Histamine II and Anti-Histaminics: Chemistry, Metabolism and Physiological and Pharmacological Actions.* (Rocha e Silva, M., ed.) *Handbuch der Experimentellen Pharmakologie,* Vol. 18, Pt. 2. Springer-Verlag, Berlin, **1978,** pp. 75–92.

van den Brink, F. G., and Lien, E. J. Competitive and noncompetitive antagonism. In, *Histamine II and Anti-Histaminics: Chemistry, Metabolism and Physiological and Pharmacological Actions.* (Rocha e Silva, M., ed.) *Handbuch der Experimentellen Pharmakologie,* Vol. 18, Pt. 2. Springer-Verlag, Berlin, **1978,** pp. 333–367.

Vane, J. R. The release and fate of vaso-active hormones in the circulation. *Br. J. Pharmacol.,* **1969,** *35,* 209–242.

Weber, A. M., and Murray, J. M. Molecular control mechanism in muscular contraction. *Physiol. Rev.,* **1973,** *53,* 612–673.

Weil-Malherbe, H. Serotonin and schizophrenia. In, *The Central Nervous System.* Vol. 3, *Serotonin in Health and Disease.* (Essman, W. B., ed.) Spectrum Publications, Inc., New York, **1978,** pp. 231–291.

Wetterquist, H. Histamine metabolism and excretion. In, *Histamine II and Anti-Histaminics: Chemistry, Metabolism and Physiological and Pharmacological Actions.* (Rocha e Silva, M., ed.) *Handbuch der Experimentellen Pharmakologie,* Vol. 18, Pt. 2. Springer-Verlag, Berlin, **1978,** pp. 131–150.

Witiak, D. T., and Lewis, N. J. Absorption, distribution, metabolism, and elimination of antihistamines. In, *Histamine II and Anti-Histaminics: Chemistry, Metabolism and Physiological and Pharmacological Actions.* (Rocha e Silva, M., ed.) *Handbuch der Experimentellen Pharmakologie,* Vol. 18, Pt. 2. Springer-Verlag, Berlin, **1978,** 513–560.

Woolley, D. W. *The Biochemical Basis of Psychoses; or, the Serotonin Hypothesis about Mental Illness.* John Wiley & Sons, Inc., New York, **1962.**

Zweifach, B. W. Microcirculation. *Annu. Rev. Physiol.,* **1973,** *35,* 117–150.

POLYPEPTIDES—ANGIOTENSIN, PLASMA KININS, AND OTHERS

William W. Douglas

ANGIOTENSIN

History. In 1898, Tiegerstedt and Bergman found that crude saline extracts of the kidney contained a pressor principle, which they named *renin.* Their discovery had an obvious bearing on the problem of arterial hypertension and its relation to kidney disease that had been posed by Richard Bright's work some 60 years earlier; however, relatively little interest was generated until 1934, when Goldblatt and his colleagues showed convincingly that it was possible to produce persistent hypertension in dogs by constricting the renal arteries. Within a few years, several investigators had detected pressor activity in renal venous blood following renal artery constriction and had attributed the effect to renin. Renin thus came to occupy a central position in the field of experimental hypertension. It was subsequently determined that renin was not itself a pressor substance but was an enzyme that initiated the formation of the pharmacologically active material, a peptide, from a protein substrate present in the plasma (Braun-Menéndez *et al.,* 1940; Page and Helmer, 1940). Two names for the peptide, *angiotonin* and *hypertensin,* persisted until 1958, when it was agreed to rename the pressor substance *angiotensin* and to call the plasma substrate *angiotensinogen* (Braun-Menéndez and Page, 1958). Meanwhile in the mid-1950s, Skeggs, Peart, and their respective colleagues determined the amino acid composition and sequence of the active material. Two forms of angiotensin were recognized, the first a decapeptide (angiotensin I) and the second an octapeptide (angiotensin II) formed from angiotensin I by enzymatic cleavage by another enzyme termed *converting enzyme.* The octapeptide was shown to be the pharmacologically active form, and its synthesis in 1957 by Schwyzer and by Bumpus made the material available for intensive study (*see* Page and Bumpus, 1974).

A further impetus to research came in 1958, when Gross suggested that the renin-angiotensin system was involved in electrolyte balance and the regulation of aldosterone secretion by the adrenal cortex (*see* Gross, 1968). It was soon shown that the kidneys are important for the increase in aldosterone secretion in response to hemorrhage; that saline extracts of kidney stimulate aldosterone release (Davis *et al.,* 1961; Ganong and Mulrow, 1961); and that synthetic angiotensin, in minute amounts, stimulates the output of aldosterone in man (Genest *et al.,* 1960; Laragh *et al.,* 1960). Moreover, elevated rates of renin secretion were noted after experimental reduction of sodium concentration in plasma. Thus, the renin-angiotensin system was recognized as a mechanism to stimulate aldosterone secretion and thereby to conserve sodium and maintain blood volume. Such an action, clearly complementary to the usual vasoconstrictor actions, led to a broadening of the concept of the renin-angiotensin system as an important physiological mechanism in the interrelated homeostatic functions concerned with the volume, pressure, and electrolyte composition of body fluids. More recent findings, to be discussed below, have reinforced this interpretation by implicating the system in a variety of additional functions, central and peripheral, that influence electrolyte balance, vascular tone, and other processes.

Progress in the field has accelerated rapidly in the last few years. The pharmacological activities of the angiotensins are better understood, and the heptapeptide designated as angiotensin III is known to rival angiotensin II in its potency to produce certain effects (Blair-West *et al.,* 1971). Drugs have been developed that act effectively *in vivo* to inhibit the formation or actions of the angiotensins. Such inhibitors have provided powerful tools for assessing the physiological and pathophysiological roles of the renin angiotensin system. They have also made possible promising therapeutic approaches to the diagnosis and therapy of disease, notably certain hypertensive states.

Chemistry. The synthesis and degradation of the angiotensins *in vivo* are complex processes that are outlined in Figure 27–1 and treated in greater detail below (*see* page 652). Nomenclature follows recent recommendations (Nomenclature Committee, 1978). Briefly, the process is initiated when the enzyme renin acts on angiotensinogen (renin substrate), an α-globulin, to yield the decapeptide angiotensin I (angiotensin-[1-10]decapeptide). This decapeptide has limited pharmacological activity, but it is cleaved by converting enzyme, alternatively referred to as peptidyl dipeptidase (PDP; peptidyldipeptide carboxyhydrolase), to yield the highly active octapeptide angiotensin II (angiotensin-[1-8]octapeptide). This, in turn, undergoes hydrolysis by aminopeptidase to yield the heptapeptide angiotensin III (angiotensin-[2-8]heptapeptide), known alternatively as [des-Asp[1]]angiotensin II, which is also pharmacologically active. Further cleavage yields peptides with little activity. An alternative route of metabolism has been discovered wherein converting enzyme and aminopeptidase act in the opposite sequence such that the decapeptide, angiotensin I, is hydrolyzed first to [des-Asp[1]] angiotensin I, which like the

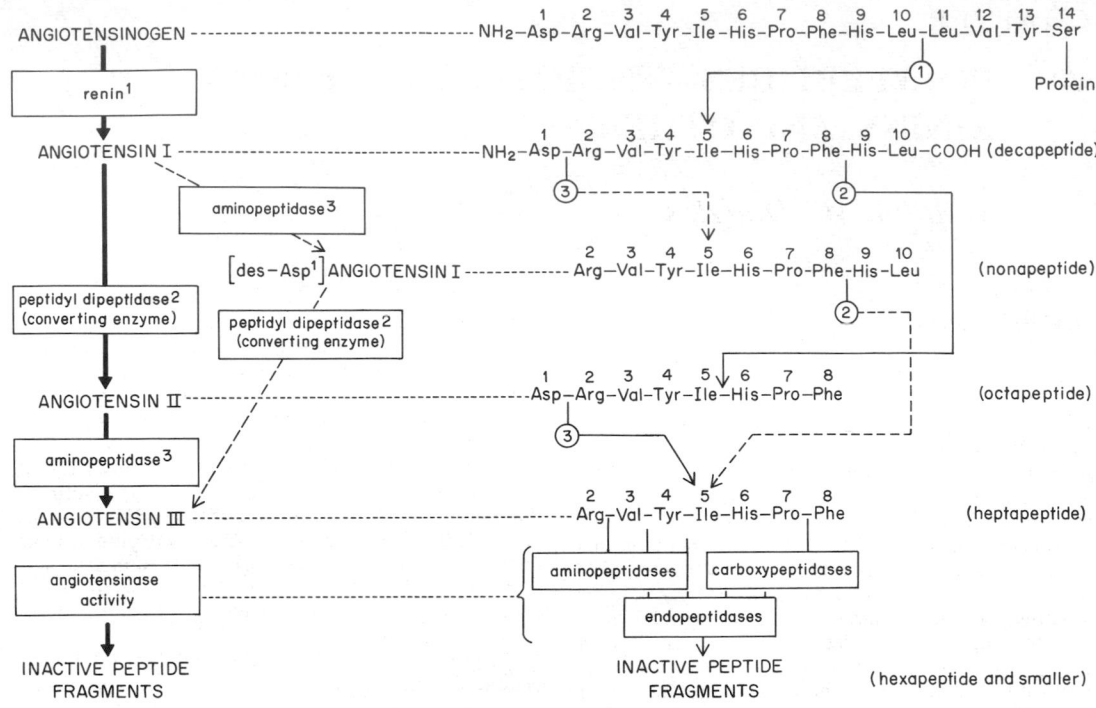

Figure 27–1. *Formation and destruction of angiotensins.*

The left-hand scheme is complemented by the diagram on the right of structures and sites of enzymatic cleavage (the numbers within circles correspond to those assigned to the enzymes within the boxes). The solid arrows show the classical paths, while the dashed arrows indicate the more recently described reactions. The structures of the angiotensins shown are those found in man, horse, rat, and pig; the bovine forms have valine in the 5 position.

parent compound has limited pharmacological activity. It is then cleaved by converting enzyme to form the active angiotensin III.

Many analogs of angiotensin II have been synthesized, and considerable information on the structure-activity relationship is available. As is evident from the activity of angiotensin III, most of the essential information resides in the C-terminal heptapeptide. Phenylalanine in position 8 is critical. Its removal from any of the angiotensins abolishes *agonist* (but not necessarily antagonist) activity, which, however, can be restored to some extent by substituting other aromatic amino acids. The other aromatic residues in positions 4 and 6, the guanido group in position 2, and the C-terminal carboxyl are involved mainly in binding to the receptor site. Position 1 is not critical (thus the efficacy of angiotensin III), but replacement of aspartic acid in position 1 with sarcosine (N-methylglycine) enhances binding and slows hydrolysis by rendering the peptide refractory to an important subgroup of aminopeptidases that are specific for aspartic or glutamic acid ("Asp-aminopeptidase"; "angiotensinase A") (Hall *et al.,* 1974). Such a substitution, combined with that of alanine in place of phenylalanine in position 8, was shown by Pals and associates (1971) to yield a potent angiotensin II blocking agent, *saralasin*, whose properties will be described below. Further

information on the chemistry of the angiotensins is available in the reviews by Page and Bumpus (1974), Regoli and coworkers (1974), and Bumpus (1977).

PHARMACOLOGICAL PROPERTIES

The most familiar and best-studied effects of angiotensin II are vasoconstriction and stimulation of the synthesis and secretion of aldosterone by the adrenal cortex. However, the peptide has numerous other effects. Some involve stimulation of the heart and the sympathetic nervous system; these complement the direct vasomotor effects and contribute to the increase in blood pressure caused by angiotensin. Others, such as stimulation of drinking and increased secretion of antidiuretic hormone, complement the effects of aldosterone and contribute to retention of sodium and water. In the following discussion the description refers to the octapeptide angiotensin II. As will become apparent from a brief description of the effects of the other angiotensins, only the heptapeptide angiotensin III shares most of the effects of angiotensin II; with the exception of the effects on the adrenal cortex, angiotensin III is generally weaker. The decapeptide angiotensin I and its nonapeptide derivative, [des-Asp[1]]-angiotensin, are much more restricted in their actions (*see* reviews by Severs and Daniels-Severs, 1973; Page and Bumpus, 1974; Regoli *et al.*, 1974; Peach, 1977).

Cardiovascular System. The strong pressor activity that led to the discovery of the renin-angiotensin system involves a constellation of effects, among which are direct stimulation of vascular and cardiac muscle, facilitation of sympathetic transmission in the periphery, and stimulation of central sympathetic outflow. Moreover, reflex responses, especially those involving baroreceptors, may obtund or mask the primary effects of angiotensin, such that the overall responses of the intact individual may be quite complex.

Blood Vessels. Vasoconstriction in response to angiotensin involves precapillary arterioles and, to a lesser but significant extent, postcapillary venules. The peptide has a direct action on the vascular smooth muscle and indirectly stimulates contraction by means of the sympathetic nervous system. The relative importance of the effects depends on species, vascular bed, route of injection, and dose of the compound. With intravenous infusions in man, the direct action seems to account for most of the increase in total peripheral resistance; however, in certain vascular beds, such as those of the hand and the foot, vasoconstriction has a large sympathetic component, since it is much reduced by α-adrenergic antagonists.

The vasoconstrictor effect of angiotensin given intravenously is strongest in the vessels of the skin, splanchnic region, and kidney; blood flow in these regions falls sharply. The effect is less in the vessels of the brain and still weaker in skeletal muscle. In both these regions blood flow may actually increase, especially following low doses, since the relatively weak vasoconstrictor response is opposed by the elevated systemic blood pressure. Nevertheless, with high doses cerebral blood flow tends to fall. Vasoconstriction prejudicial to flow may also occur in coronary vessels (*see* Gavras *et al.*, 1977).

Heart. Experiments with various isolated cardiac preparations have shown that angiotensin acts directly on the membrane of atrial and ventricular muscle to prolong the plateau phase of the action potential and hence increase the inward calcium current that drives the contractile elements. This effect is opposed by substances such as manganese or verapamil that block calcium channels. Angiotensin has no direct effect on the heart rate. *In vivo*, however, angiotensin tends to increase heart rate and force of contraction by its central and peripheral stimulant and facilitatory actions on sympathetic outflow (*see* below). However, by increasing systemic blood pressure and baroreceptor discharge, angiotensin may initiate reflex vagal activity sufficient to slow the heart and raise end-diastolic pressure. The rise in central venous pressure is generally modest, since angiotensin has a comparatively feeble constrictor effect on the larger veins and hence reduces venous capacity much less than does, for example, norepinephrine. As a result of these various factors cardiac output generally falls. Despite this, the work of the heart often increases as a result of the elevated systemic blood pressure and increased mechanical load, and there may be coronary insufficiency.

Blood Pressure. Angiotensin is by far the most potent pressor agent known; on a molar basis, it is about 40 times more so than norepinephrine. When a single moderate dose is injected intravenously, systemic blood pressure begins to rise within about 10 seconds, rapidly reaches maximum, and returns to normal in a few minutes. When the drug is infused continuously, blood pressure is maintained at an elevated level for hours or days, provided the concentration is not so high as to produce tachyphylaxis. Furthermore, with such continuous infusion the effectiveness of angiotensin may increase with time, so that pressor responses are observed with amounts that initially had no effect.

In the lesser circulation, angiotensin commonly causes a moderate rise in pulmonary arterial pressure that is due less, perhaps, to its feeble pulmonary vasoconstrictor action than to an increase of pressure in the pulmonary vein as end-diastolic pressure rises.

Blood Volume, Capillary Permeability, and Lymph Flow. Angiotensin appears to constrict postcapillary venules and thus increases filtration pressure in the capillaries. In addition, it increases vascular permeability in the larger arterioles by causing separation of the endothelial cells, possibly by some contractile response. There is a significant diminution in blood volume and increases in extravascular fluid and the flow of lymph.

Extravascular Smooth Muscle. Effects of angiotensin on smooth muscle other than that in blood vessels are generally feeble, but contractions are readily elicited in preparations such as guinea pig ileum and rat uterus *in vitro.* Beside direct stimulation of the smooth muscle cells, angiotensin can elicit indirect effects, contraction or relaxation, by exciting cholinergic or adrenergic ganglion cells or nerve endings. An unusual, seemingly direct, relaxant effect of angiotensin has been noted on tracheal muscle contracted by 5-hydroxytryptamine in dogs and cats.

Central Nervous System. Because the blood-brain barrier is considered generally to be impermeable to peptides, the possibility that angiotensin might have central actions was overlooked for many years. In 1961, however, Bickerton and Buckley demonstrated a centrally mediated hypertensive response in dogs. Since then, many other examples of actions of angiotensin on the central nervous system (CNS) have appeared, and it is evident that often quite small and probably physiological amounts suffice.

Central Sympathetic Stimulation. Small amounts of angiotensin infused into the vertebral arteries, including those of man, cause a rise in systemic blood pressure that has been maintained for up to a week. This is mediated by sympathetic vasoconstriction and cardiac stimulation, and is demonstrably due to effects of the drug on the medulla in the area postrema. Ablation of this region in experimental animals blunts the response and, interestingly, reduces somewhat the pressor response to *intravenous* injections of angiotensin.

Drinking and Hydration. Angiotensin has a centrally mediated dipsogenic effect that can be observed following intravenous injection as well as after injection of the peptide into the third ventricle or surrounding areas. The preoptic region and subfornical organ seem particularly sensitive. Hunger for food is suppressed in favor of drinking (*see* Sym-

posium, 1978a; *see also* Fitzsimons and Kucharczyk, 1978).

Release of Antidiuretic Hormone. Angiotensin increases activity in supraoptic neurons when injected into the brain or third ventricle and can thus stimulate secretion of antidiuretic hormone (ADH). This response, in contrast to the central effects previously mentioned, is not seen after intravenous injections because the supraoptic region, unlike the area postrema, is protected by the blood-brain barrier. However, angiotensin stimulates the release of ADH from the isolated neurohypophysis, and such an effect could conceivably occur *in vivo.* Angiotensin can also enhance the release of ACTH, apparently by a central action.

Peripheral Autonomic Nervous System. In addition to central enhancement of sympathetic outflow, angiotensin can stimulate sympathetic ganglion cells and facilitate ganglionic transmission. The effects are variable, and their contribution to the overall response to circulating angiotensin is capricious. A more consistent response to angiotensin is facilitation of sympathetic neuroeffector transmission. Increased responsiveness of the innervated organ to norepinephrine has been demonstrated; more important is an increased output of norepinephrine from the sympathetic nerve terminals. Several mechanisms may contribute, among them increased biosynthesis of norepinephrine, decreased re-uptake of the transmitter, and increased output of norepinephrine per impulse (*see* Zimmerman, 1978). As is the case with cardiac muscle, the last-named response may involve an increased duration of the nerve action potential and influx of Ca^{2+}.

Adrenal Medulla. Angiotensin stimulates the release of catecholamines from the adrenal medulla by directly depolarizing the chromaffin cells. Moderate doses of angiotensin given intravenously to normal subjects produce a small effect that does not contribute substantially to the overall cardiovascular response. But intense and dangerous responses to analogs of angiotensin have been noted in individuals with pheochromocytoma (*see* below).

The Adrenal Cortex and Secretion of Aldosterone. Angiotensin directly stimulates the synthesis and secretion of aldosterone; its effects on the output of other corticosteroids are dependent on species, variable, and usually minor. Increased output of aldosterone is elicited by very low concentrations of angiotensin that have little or no effect on blood pressure. The effect begins within a few minutes of injection and may be maintained indefinitely by infusion; indeed, the response tends to increase somewhat with time, at least in part as the zona glomerulosa hypertrophies. Increased output of aldosterone, in turn, acts on the kidney to cause retention of sodium and excretion of potassium and hydrogen ions. The stimulant effect of angiotensin on the output of aldosterone is enhanced when the concentration of sodium in plasma is low or when that of potassium is high. The peptide's effects are reduced when concentrations of these cations in plasma are altered in the opposite direction. Such changes in sensitivity to the drug are believed to be due to alterations of the number of receptors for angiotensin on the zona glomerulosa cells as well as to adrenocortical hyperplasia in the sodium-depleted state (see Davis and Freeman, 1976).

The Kidney and Formation of Urine. In addition to its indirect effect on tubular function mediated by aldosterone, angiotensin can influence urine formation through its hemodynamic actions. However, the effects are complex and variable. The outcome depends on the interplay between the effects of angiotensin on systemic blood pressure (renal perfusion pressure) and the renal vasculature. A preponderant constriction of the afferent or efferent glomerular arterioles may cause either a decrease or increase in glomerular filtration rate. Moreover, the indirect effects of the peptide mediated through aldosterone depend on the state of sodium balance. For all these reasons diverse patterns of response are observed (Gross and Mohring, 1973). In man, however, the usual response is prompt antidiuresis and antinatriuresis accompanied by reduction in effective renal plasma flow and glomerular filtration rate. However, certain hypertensive individuals and patients with hepatic cirrhosis and ascites respond in contrary fashion with diuresis and natriuresis. Angiotensin, unlike ADH, has weak and inconsistent effects on the transport of water and electrolytes in model epithelial systems, such as toad skin and bladder. The peptide may reduce the reabsorptive capacity of the proximal renal tubule (Leyssac, 1976).

Actions of the Other Angiotensins. The pharmacological properties so far described are those of angiotensin II. Much less is known of the other angiotensins, for it is only comparatively recently that angiotensin I and the nonapeptide [des-Asp[1]]angiotensin I have been studied. The heptapeptide metabolite of angiotensin II, [des-Asp[1]]-angiotensin II, is now known to be a potent agent in

its own right, deserving the appellation angiotensin III. *In vivo*, the decapeptide angiotensin I and the nonapeptide [des-Asp[1]]angiotensin I can, of course, exert the full panoply of angiotensin effects as they are cleaved to angiotensin II and angiotensin III (see Figure 27–1). Whether each peptide has direct actions has become of practical importance as potent inhibitors of peptidyl dipeptidase (converting enzyme) have been developed and introduced into clinical medicine.

Angiotensin I has little or no effect (less than 1% of that of angiotensin II) on smooth muscle, heart, or adrenal cortex but acts like angiotensin II on the adrenal medulla and sympathetic and central nervous systems. Little is known of the direct actions of [des-Asp[1]]angiotensin I, save that its potency on vascular smooth muscle is very low. On the other hand, angiotensin III retains most of the activity of angiotensin II. In most instances it is somewhat weaker; its pressor activity, for example, is about 25 to 50% of that of angiotensin II, and its stimulant action on the adrenal medulla is perhaps only about 10% of that of angiotensin II; however, it is as potent or more potent than angiotensin II in stimulating the output of aldosterone (Blair-West *et al.*, 1971; Davis and Freeman, 1977; Peach, 1977).

Mechanism of Action. High-affinity binding sites for angiotensin have been identified in a variety of tissues, and all of the effects of angiotensin are believed to be exerted through specific receptors on cell surfaces (see Devynck and Meyer, 1978). These receptors can be distinguished readily from those for other hormones and autacoids, and they are specifically blocked by selected analogs of angiotensin (see below). How the action at the receptor level is translated into the appropriate cellular response is, for the most part, obscure. The peptide depolarizes the membranes of chromaffin, ganglion, and smooth muscle cells. However, smooth muscle continues to respond to angiotensin (as it does to several other agonists) when it has been depolarized by excess potassium, presumably due to both facilitation of the entry of calcium into cells and mobilization of stores of intracellular calcium (see Deth and van Breeman, 1977). Possible mechanisms of action of angiotensin on the heart and on adrenergic nerve endings have already been mentioned. The stimulant action on the output of aldosterone is due to increased synthesis of the steroid. Again, angiotensin increases this synthesis through a calcium-dependent mechanism that facilitates the initial reaction in the biosynthetic path, conversion of cholesterol to pregnenolone.

Both prostaglandins and cyclic nucleotides, particularly cyclic adenosine 3′,5′-monophosphate (cyclic AMP), have been implicated in the mediation of responses to angiotensin. However, even for the best-studied effects, namely, increased secretion of aldosterone and cardiac stimulation, it is still quite uncertain that cyclic nucleotides are involved. The role of prostaglandins is also obscure, although there is abundant evidence that they can be formed in response to angiotensin, and sometimes (*e.g.*, with renal vasoconstriction) it is possible to reduce responses to angiotensin with indomethacin and other drugs that block the synthesis of prostaglandins.

There is, as yet, no satisfactory explanation why certain tissues, particularly vascular smooth muscle, may develop tachyphylaxis to angiotensin (*see* Moore *et al.*, 1977; Paiva *et al.*, 1977).

ENDOGENOUS RENIN-ANGIOTENSIN SYSTEM

The renin-angiotensin system exists in each of the vertebrate classes studied. The richest source of renin is the kidney, from which it is secreted by the granular juxtaglomerular cells (JG cells) that lie in the walls of the afferent arterioles as they enter the glomeruli. These are endocrine cells in the sense that they secrete renin directly into the renal arterial blood stream. Their "peculiarity" lies in the fact that the substance liberated, renin, is not itself a hormone but is an enzyme that initiates the formation of the active hormones, the angiotensins. Moreover, renin and the other components of the renin-angiotensin system are found at extrarenal sites. Of particular interest is their presence in the brain.

Synthesis and Catabolism of Elements of the Renin-Angiotensin System in Vivo. *Renin.* Renin, an acid protease, specifically cleaves a leucine-leucine peptide bond between residues 10 and 11 of its angiotensinogen substrate (Figure 27–1). It has no further hydrolytic acivity on angiotensin I. The enzyme is a glycoprotein with a molecular weight of about 40,000; after its release into the blood, renin is metabolized relatively slowly, mainly by the liver and kidney, and has a half-life in the circulation of about 15 to 30 minutes. Inactive forms of renin have been isolated from the kidney and found in plasma. These are sometimes of larger size ("big renins") and can be activated by trypsin or following acidification or storage of plasma in the cold. The significance of these inactive forms of renin is not yet known. There is continuing uncertainty, too, about the precise identity and function of the renin-like activity that is present at many extrarenal sites. Whether these renin-like enzymes ("tissue renins") are isoenzymes to renal renin or distinct entities is uncertain, but the term *isorenin* has some currency (Ganten *et al.*, 1976; Skeggs *et al.*, 1977; Millar *et al.*, 1978; Reid *et al.*, 1978).

Angiotensinogen(s). These are glycoproteins present in abundance in the plasma globulin fraction and synthesized by the liver. The molecular weight has been variously estimated at from 50,000 to 110,000. The relevant portion of this large molecule is the amino terminus, from which angiotensin I is cleaved (Figure 27–1). Human angiotensinogen serves as a substrate only for the renin of man or primates, whereas the angiotensinogens of other animals are substrates for the renins of all species examined, including man. Since the normal concentra-

tion of angiotensinogen in plasma is close to or less than the concentration required for maximal reaction velocity, variations in the concentration of angiotensinogen in plasma may conceivably alter the rate of angiotensin formation. It is thus noteworthy that the production of angiotensinogen by the liver is increased by glucocorticoids and by estrogens and that concentrations of angiotensin in plasma tend to rise during pregnancy and during use of oral contraceptive agents (*see* Reid *et al.*, 1978).

Angiotensin I and Peptidyl Dipeptidase (*Converting Enzyme; Kininase II*). Although slow conversion of angiotensin I to angiotensin II occurs in plasma, the very rapid mctabolism that occurs *in vivo* is due largely to the activity of tissue-bound enzyme present on the luminal aspect of vascular endothelial cells. For example, in man the lung converts some 20 to 40% of angiotensin I to angiotensin II in a single circulation. Extrapulmonary conversion is also brisk; thus, intra-arterial injection of angiotensin I into the forearm causes immediate distal vasocenstriction, attributable to local formation of angiotensin II. Peptidyl dipeptidase is also present in soluble form in most body fluids and in bound form in the brush border of epithelial cells of renal tubules and intestinal mucosa.

The enzyme is a Zn-containing exopeptidase that catalyzes the cleavage of dipeptide residues from the carboxyl terminus of various oligopeptide substrates. It has many important functions; in addition to its action on angiotensin I, it participates in the degradation and inactivation of kinins such as bradykinin (which it cleaves much more readily than angiotensin I). Peptidyl dipeptidase is indeed identical with kininase II (*see* below). Moreover, it degrades other potent peptide autacoids such as the enkephalins. The enzyme does not cleave a peptide bond with the imino group of a prolyl residue. Hence, after removal of the first dipeptide from angiotensin I, it does not act further, although it sequentially degrades other substrates, for example, bradykinin. Information on the enzyme is accumulating rapidly as possible clinical applications of its inhibition emerge (*see* Skeggs *et al.*, 1976; Soffer, 1976; Cushman *et al.*, 1977; Erdös, 1979).

Angiotensin II and Metabolites (*Including Angiotensin III*). Angiotensin II is quite rapidly catabolized, mainly by widely distributed aminopeptidases, which by sequential actions form the heptapeptide angiotensin III, the hexapeptide Val^3-Phe^8, and the pentapeptide Tyr^4-Phe^8 (*see* Figure 27–1). Only the heptapeptide has significant pharmacological activity. In man the half-life of angiotensin II is about 4 minutes, while those of the shorter peptides are about 2 minutes.

Angiotensin II can be formed directly from angiotensinogen by an enzyme termed *tonin*, which cleaves the Phe-His bond at position 8–9. Tonin also cleaves this bond in angiotensin I and [des-Asp^1] angiotensin I. It is widely distributed in the body and found in high concentration in certain salivary glands, from which it may be released to saliva or to venous blood. Its activity is normally masked by inhibitors present in the plasma; its physiological significance is obscure (*see* Boucher *et al.*, 1977).

The term *angiotensinase* is applied to various peptidases involved in the degradation and inactivation of angiotensin II; none is specific. Among them are aminopeptidases, the activity of which may also contribute to the formation of active angiotensins. One aminopeptidase, "Asp-aminopeptidase" or "angiotensinase A," is specific for aspartic (or glutamic) acid, and its action terminates with the formation of the [des-Asp[1]] compounds. In some tissues a considerable portion of angiotensin I is converted to [des-Asp[1]]angiotensin I; in the adrenal gland the fraction is as large as one half. Other reactions are shown in Figure 27-1.

Functions of the Renin-Angiotensin System. The main events that led to the prevalent view that the renin-angiotensin system is a part of the interrelated homeostatic mechanisms regulating hemodynamics and water and electrolyte balance are described in the historical introduction to this section. Most simply stated, factors that lower blood volume, renal perfusion pressure, or the sodium concentration in plasma tend to stimulate the secretion of renin, while factors that increase these parameters tend to inhibit its secretion (*see* Figure 27-2). Moreover, the hypothesis that derangement of the renin-angiotensin system contributes to hypertension has received additional support by observation of the effects of specific blocking agents (*see* below).

Control of Renin Secretion. The secretory cells in the kidney that synthesize and discharge renin are modified myoepithelial cells, and, as mentioned, these JG cells are found in clusters in the wall of each afferent glomerular arteriole. Their secretion is controlled by three influences—two acting locally within the kidney and the third acting through the CNS and mediated by sympathetic secretomotor nerves.

The first intrarenal influence is mechanical; factors that tend to lower renal perfusion pressure elicit the secretion of renin. These include a fall in systemic blood pressure from any cause, such as diminished cardiac output, lowered total peripheral resistance, or reduction in blood volume through sodium deficiency or hemorrhage. The mechanical stimulus to secretion may also arise from local vascular effects

such as renal arterial or aortic stenosis. The factor common to each of these events and the immediate stimulus to secretion is believed to be reduction in the *tension* within the wall of the glomerular afferent arterial vessel. The manner by which such reduced tension causes the JG cells to secrete is uncertain (Peart, 1978).

The second intrarenal influence is ionic; reduction in sodium load to the kidney stimulates the secretion of renin. This effect is *not* exerted directly on the JG cells but is apparently mediated by events in the renal tubule of the same glomerulus, particularly the macula densa region located at the end of the loop of Henle and at the beginning of the distal tubule. It is generally believed that the macula densa somehow monitors the ionic environment in the tubular fluid and relays to the JG cells the stimulus for secretion. The macula densa cells abut the JG cells and constitute with the latter (and some other specialized cells) the "juxtaglomerular apparatus." Just what it is in the tubule that is sensed by the macula densa cells is uncertain, but present evidence points to a decreased concentration of sodium chloride as the signal (*see* Davis and Freeman, 1976; but contrast with Thurau, 1974, and Leyssac, 1976).

The third influence—the sympathetic nervous control of renin output—is also complex and not fully understood, but the main influence is clearly secretomotor, as witness the increased output of renin when renal nerves are stimulated. The nerves innervate the JG cells directly and act through β_2-adrenergic receptors. The sympathetic secretomotor innervation mediates various central nervous influences on renin secretion that are determined by reflex and other factors. A fall in systemic blood pressure will, for example, activate sympathetic secretomotor activity through baroreceptors and volume receptors. The sympathetic outflow also stimulates release of renin in response to painful stimuli (including the cold pressor test) or certain stressful emotional states.

Other factors of uncertain physiological significance that can influence the release of renin include angiotensin II, which has an inhibitory effect that may reflect the existence of a negative-feedback

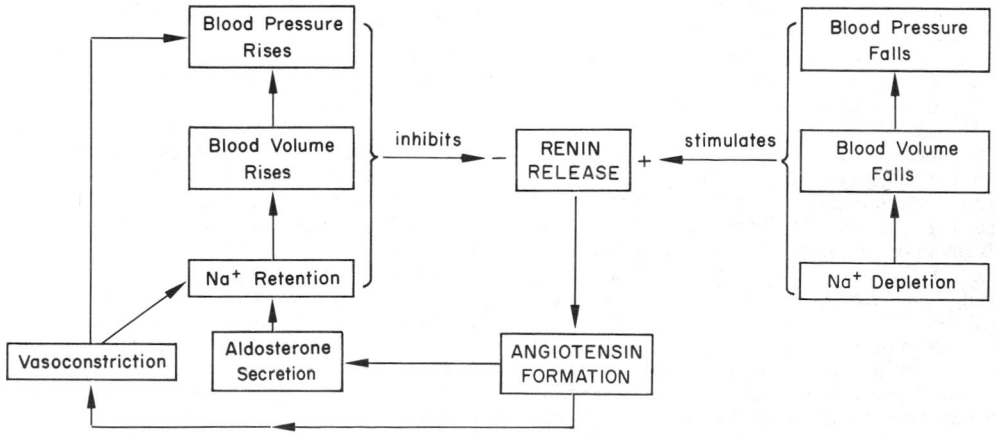

Figure 27-2. *A schematic portrayal of the possible homeostatic role of the renin-angiotensin system.*

mechanism. ADH and circulating adrenal catecholamines stimulate secretion (*see* Davis and Freeman, 1976; Peart, 1978; Wright and Briggs, 1979).

Role in Secretion of Aldosterone. Angiotensin is clearly an important factor in promoting the secretion of aldosterone in response to sodium depletion; it must be emphasized, however, that the zona glomerulosa can also be stimulated directly by low concentrations of sodium or elevated potassium, by ACTH, and possibly by other factors. Moreover, control of the secretion of aldosterone is not lost in animals and patients from whom both kidneys have been removed. However, control is then blunted, and direct responses of the adrenal cortex to sodium, potassium, and ACTH (as well as to angiotensin) are reduced and sluggish. Thus, angiotensin appears to exert some permissive and trophic effects on the adrenal cortex (Sealey *et al.,* 1978). The appreciation of the very potent stimulatory effect of angiotensin III on aldosterone synthesis and secretion suggests that this heptapeptide may also be an important physiological factor controlling the secretion of aldosterone (Blair-West *et al.,* 1971; Davis and Freeman, 1976; Peach, 1977). Receptors for angiotensin II and angiotensin III on the glomerulosa cells appear to be distinct and differ in their sensitivity to antagonists such as saralasin (*see* below).

It should be noted that activation of secretion of renin and aldosterone occurs with quite small negative sodium balances (about 200 mEq in man), which involve no change in the concentrations of sodium in plasma (*see* Peart, 1978). The increased secretion of renin that is seen when a patient is ingesting a low-sodium diet can be reduced by β-adrenergic antagonists. The renin-aldosterone axis may therefore be activated centrally or reflexly by changes too subtle to be sensed within the kidney or by the adrenal cortex. Stimulation of the renin-angiotensin system seems to be a major factor in the excess secretion of aldosterone by patients with decompensated hepatic cirrhosis (*see* Epstein *et al.,* 1977).

Possible Intrarenal Functions. It has long been suspected that the renin-angiotensin system is involved locally and directly in the regulation of urine formation. Angiotensin can clearly be formed locally within the kidney itself, and, through its vasoconstrictor actions on afferent or efferent glomerular arterioles, could influence the rate of glomerular filtration. In addition, evidence has been advanced that angiotensin can directly affect tubular reabsorption (Thurau, 1974; Leyssac, 1976). All the ingredients for local control of urine formation by the renin-angiotensin system would seem to be present. Despite this, the details of the operation of the suspected single-nephron feedback mechanism and the involvement of angiotensin are quite uncertain. (For detailed discussion of this complex situation, *see* Thurau, 1974; Leyssac, 1976; Wright and Briggs, 1979.)

Involvement in Circulatory Responses and Homeostasis. As indicated in Figure 27-2, factors that *lower* blood pressure or volume tend to *stimulate* renin secretion, while factors that *raise* blood pressure or volume have the opposite effect. Vigorous stimuli, such as severe hemorrhage, stimulate the release of renin directly by the intrarenal tension-receptive mechanism and indirectly by means of the sympathetic secretomotor system. Milder physiological stimuli, such as the assumption of the upright position, appear to operate mainly through the sympathetic reflex mechanism. Additional factors that activate renin secretion through the sympathetic system include exercise, hypoglycemia, the cold pressor test, and emotional stress.

Involvement in Hypertensive States. The renin-angiotensin system contributes to hypertension in some individuals. It is also a factor in experimental renal hypertension induced by partially occluding the renal arteries (Goldblatt hypertension). The main questions at issue are how many, or few, hypertensive conditions, clinical or experimental, involve increased renin-angiotensin activity and what is the magnitude and duration of this involvement. At the outset it must be recognized that hypertension is a spectrum of diseases that can arise by many mechanisms; the renin-angiotensin system is but one possible contributor to pathogenesis. There is no simple relationship between renin secretion, as reflected by plasma renin activity (PRA), and blood pressure. Although elevated PRA is found in most individuals with *malignant hypertension* and is commonly found in patients with *hypertension resulting from stenosis of the renal artery,* most patients with hypertension do *not* have high PRA. Thus, in the great majority of hypertensive patients, those with *essential hypertension,* PRA and plasma concentrations of angiotensin II are generally normal, not uncommonly subnormal, and elevated in only about one patient in six. Such evidence, by itself, might suggest that the role of the renin-angiotensin system in human hypertensive disease is rather limited. Nevertheless, there is other evidence that suggests a much wider involvement. It has long seemed that the "normal" values of PRA encountered in most individuals with essential hypertension are indeed inappropriately high, given the fact that they occur in the presence of conditions (high blood pressure and perhaps sodium retention and expansion of blood volume) that normally suppress the secretion of renin. Moreover, it has long been recognized that a more effective index than PRA might be provided by drugs that block the renin-angiotensin system. Now that such agents have been developed and tested (*see* below), they have been found to lower blood pressure in a broad range of hypertensive conditions, often where there is no evidence of elevated PRA (Case *et al.,* 1977; Gavras *et al.,* 1978). Various aspects of this problem have been discussed in many reviews and monographs (*see* Page and Bumpus, 1974; Gavras *et al.,* 1976; Hypertension Meeting, 1976, 1978; Stokes and Edwards, 1976; Symposium, 1976b; Brown *et al.,* 1978).

Possible Functions in the Central Nervous System. Conjecture concerning possible functions of angiotensin within the CNS has naturally stemmed from the various pharmacological effects of the peptide. These include *increased thirst, appetite for sodium, release of ADH (and possibly ACTH),* and stimulation of *central sympathetic outflow* resulting in pressor responses (*see* Symposium, 1978a). Angiotensin is dipsogenic when given in minute amounts directly into the third ventricle and surrounding areas or when administered intravenously in concentrations that fall well within the physiological range observed during mild sodium depletion (Fitzsimons and Kucharczyk, 1978). Moreover, drinking responses have been attenuated by administration of antagonists of angiotensin II. Compulsive thirst in some patients with renal disease, even when they are edematous, may reflect high concentrations of angiotensin II in the blood. Increase in appetite for sodium also seems to be a consistent response when angiotensin is given directly into the cerebral ventricles. Whether release of ADH occurs with physiological concentrations of angiotensin given intravenously is controversial, but this is a consistent phenomenon when angiotensin is placed in the cerebral ventricles (see Phillips et al., 1977). Each of these three responses—increased drinking, increased appetite for sodium, and increased secretion of ADH—tends to expand or conserve blood volume. This has led to the view that angiotensin is "a hormone with a consistent physiology concerned in the maintenance and restoration of the blood volume" (Fitzsimons, 1978). The central actions of angiotensin are only now being elucidated. New perspective on the roles of the system has been provided by evidence that the brain contains all of the components of a renin-angiotensin system wholly independent of the classical renal system: renin-like activity (isorenin), angiotensinogen and angiotensin I, angiotensin I converting enzyme, angiotensin II, angiotensin II receptors, and angiotensinases. Moreover, histochemical methods have allowed visualization of angiotensin-like immunoreactivity at many sites within the CNS, including nerve terminals, thus raising the possibility that angiotensin II serves as a neurotransmitter or modulator (Ganten et al., 1978). Clearly these central effects may reflect physiological functions of an angiotensin system endogenous to the brain. Moreover, the central renin-angiotensin system must now be considered a locus of potential pathological function. A particularly provocative finding is that an antagonist of angiotensin II (see below) can lower blood pressure in some spontaneously hypertensive rats when it is infused into the cerebral ventricles; the antagonist has no such effect when given intravenously (Sweet et al., 1976).

Extrarenal Sources of Renin. Other tissues, beside the brain, that show renin-like (isorenin) activity include blood vessels, uterus, placenta, amniotic fluid, salivary glands, and adrenal cortex. The physiological meaning is as yet obscure (see Page and Bumpus, 1974; Ganten et al., 1976). Such sources, however, account for the renin-like activity that sometimes persists in the blood of nephrectomized animals and patients. Isorenin has also been demonstrated in some lung tumors and seemingly can be responsible for the concomitant high levels of circulating "renin" and the production of malignant hypertension (see Genest et al., 1975).

Physiological Significance of the "Other" Angiotensins. The functions of angiotensins other than angiotensin II have yet to be defined. In the rat, concentrations of angiotensin III in plasma may approach those of angiotensin II; they are much lower in man and dog (Semple and Morton, 1976).

Moreover, angiotensin III is in the venous effluent from tissues such as the adrenal and heart, upon which it has demonstrably potent effects. Its potency on the adrenal cortex, which equals or exceeds that of angiotensin II, certainly permits conjecture on its physiological function at that site (see Davis and Freeman, 1977; Peach, 1977). Moreover, it should be recalled that this active heptapeptide can be formed directly from the nonapeptide without the need for prior formation of angiotensin II.

CLINICAL CONSIDERATIONS

Preparation. *Angiotensin amide,* the amide of angiotensin II (1-L-asparaginyl-5-L-valyl angiotensin octapeptide), is the preparation that has been used clinically. It is not available commercially in the United States. The drug may be given slowly intravenously at a rate each minute of about 0.01 to 0.2 μg/kg. Blood pressure must be monitored at short intervals until a safe rate of infusion is determined.

Precautions and Untoward Effects. Although considerable elevation of blood pressure may occur without symptoms, angiotensin sometimes causes dizziness and headache. Evidence of coronary insufficiency is occasionally encountered with S-T depression in the ECG and pain in the chest, and it has been held responsible for occasional negative inotropic effects. Profound bradycardia and, occasionally, ventricular irregularities may be encountered from overdosage. These are attributable to excessively high blood pressures and intense vagal reflex activity. Angiotensin has no direct arrhythmogenic effects. Mild urticarial reactions have been reported. The greatest danger lies in the powerful pressor activity of the drug; too rapid infusion may easily raise blood pressure to dangerous levels.

Clinical Uses. Since angiotensin has become available, interest has centered on its unique pressor properties. It differs from norepinephrine not only in its greater potency but also in a number of qualitative respects that seem to be advantageous in a pressor agent. Thus, its pressor effect is better sustained during prolonged infusion and is less liable to be followed by hypotension. It has little or no tendency to evoke disturbing arrhythmias and, indeed, has been used successfully during anesthesia with cyclopropane and halogenated hydrocarbon agents. Furthermore, it does not cause spasm of the infused vein, nor has it caused tissue necrosis and sloughing when extravasation has occurred at the site of injection. However, angiotensin shares with norepinephrine the disadvantage that it diminishes blood volume by promoting the loss of fluid from the circulation to tissue spaces. It is inferior to norepinephrine as a constrictor of capacitance vessels, and does not reduce the venous reservoir as effectively. Its lack of prominent stimulant effect on cardiac muscle may also be disadvantageous in certain circumstances.

Angiotensin has been used to restore blood pressure in a variety of hypotensive conditions. It must be emphasized, however, that its value in the treatment of shock is highly controversial, as is that of pressor agents of the sympathomimetic type (*see* Chapter 8). Where hypotension is the consequence of blood loss, treatment, of course, should be aimed at restoring blood volume, and angiotensin must be regarded as only an interim expedient until this can be done.

ANTAGONISTS OF THE RENIN-ANGIOTENSIN SYSTEM

Drugs that specifically antagonize actions of biologically active endogenous substances or prevent their formation have traditionally provided some of the most powerful tools for the analysis of the physiological and pathophysiological functions of these substances. Of course, such drugs may also have valuable therapeutic applications. For many years, therefore, inhibitors of the renin-angiotensin system have been sought, with a particular impetus provided by the possibility of discovering effective antihypertensive drugs. Blocking agents of current interest fall into two main classes: those that block receptors for angiotensin (angiotensin II antagonists) and those that slow the rate of formation of angiotensin II by inhibiting peptidyl dipeptidase (converting enzyme). In addition, stimulation of the secretion of renin mediated by the sympathetic secretomotor innervation is inhibited by β-adrenergic antagonists, and there are indications that the antihypertensive drug clonidine may decrease secretomotor impulses to the JG cells by an action within the CNS.

ANTAGONISTS OF ANGIOTENSIN II

For more than a decade after the synthesis of angiotensin II, many analogs of the peptide were prepared without discovery of a specific antagonist. The structural requirements for agonist activity were defined, and the importance of the aromatic amino acid phenylalanine at position 8 was appreciated (*see* above). In 1970, one analog in which this essential amino acid had been replaced by alanine ([Ala[8]]angiotensin II) was reported to antagonize the stimulatory effects of angiotensin II on the guinea pig ileum *in vitro* (Khairallah *et al.*, 1970). Shortly thereafter several investigators described analogs that effectively antagonized the classical pressor effect of angiotensin II *in vivo*. The archetypical and best studied of these antagonists of angiotensin II combines alanine in position 8 with sarcosine (N-methylglycine) in position 1; the "blocked" amino acid sarcosine not only slows degradation of the peptide but also increases its affinity for the receptor. This substance, [Sar[1], Val[5], Ala[8]]angiotensin-(1-8)octapeptide or *saralasin,* was introduced by Pals

and associates in 1971, who showed that it effectively antagonized the pressor effects of angiotensin II in rats, demonstrated that it lowered blood pressure in the hypertensive rat with a single kidney in the acute, renin-dependent phase of its hypertension, and suggested that the drug could be used to examine the role of endogenous angiotensin II in the regulation of blood pressure. The possible utility of saralasin in man soon became apparent when it was shown not only to block responses to injected angiotensin but also to lower blood pressure in certain renin-dependent hypertensive patients. In normal subjects who are depleted of sodium, saralasin lowers blood pressure somewhat (especially if the individual is sitting or standing rather than lying); this effect reflects the contribution of endogenous angiotensin to the maintenance of blood pressure in such conditions (*see* Anderson *et al.*, 1977; Laragh *et al.*, 1977).

Pharmacological Properties. Antagonists of angiotensin II, exemplified by saralasin, block responses to angiotensin II in a competitive manner and with high specificity; thus, they leave uninfluenced responses to biogenic amines and unrelated vasoactive peptides. However, their antagonism extends with varying efficacy to the other angiotensins, particularly angiotensin III (*see* Peach 1977). Angiotensin II antagonists block all the familiar effects of angiotensin II described above. They are, however, not themselves devoid of intrinsic activity, and thus they are classified as partial agonists (Chapter 2). *In vitro,* for example, where angiotensin II may be excluded, saralasin, like angiotensin II, will elicit contraction of aortic smooth muscle, although it has less than 1% of the activity of angiotensin II. In normal individuals in whom endogenous renin and angiotensin have been suppressed by administration of sodium, saralasin will elicit pressor responses. And pressor responses due to this agonist activity are particularly prominent in a subclass of hypertensive individuals with subnormal PRA (Anderson *et al.*, 1977; Laragh *et al.*, 1977). Analysis of this pressor activity reveals a pattern precisely like that to be expected of an angiotensin II–like drug (MacGregor and Dawes, 1976). Moreover, as with angiotensin II, the pressor effects seemingly reflect both direct actions on the vasculature and potentiation of the release of norepinephrine from sympathetic nerves. Another important agonist action of the antagonists of angiotensin II is stimulation of the secretion of aldosterone, which is readily observed in normal man ingesting a high-sodium diet (Williams *et al.*, 1978).

The characteristic blocking actions of the angiotensin II antagonists such as saralasin are seen whenever significant amounts of angiotensin II are present *in vitro* or *in vivo*. Although there are exceptions, there is a broad correspondence between high concentrations of renin in plasma and hypotensive responses to these antagonists. Indeed, when renin levels are particularly high, as they may be in patients with malignant hypertension or renal arterial stenosis, the hypotensive action of saralasin may be profound and even dangerous. The hypotensive response involves diminution of both total peripheral resistance and cardiac output (De Carvalho *et al.*, 1977). The other prominent antagonistic effect of saralasin is reduction of the secretion of aldosterone in sodium-depleted subjects. Although saralasin is by far the most extensively studied compound of its class, other antagonists of angiotensin II, for example [Sar[1], Thr[8]]angiotensin II, may be more potent as blocking agents and have less inherent, undesirable agonist activity (*see* Bumpus, 1977).

Since saralasin and related compounds are peptides, they must be given intravenously. Their half-lives are short (for saralasin, about 4 minutes), and infusion is thus necessary for sustained action.

Inhibitors of Peptidyl Dipeptidase

The discovery of potent inhibitors of peptidyl dipeptidase arose from observations by Ferreira and colleagues in the 1960s that the venoms of pit vipers are not only capable of forming bradykinin (*see* below) but also contain factors that intensify responses to bradykinin. These bradykinin potentiating factors (BPFs) proved to be a family of peptides of 5 to 13 amino acid residues, which were identified and subsequently synthesized. They were shown to inhibit an enzyme that catalyzes the degradation and inactivation of bradykinin (now known as kininase II). In 1968, Bakhle observed that these same peptides also inhibit the converting enzyme responsible for forming angiotensin II. Soon thereafter Erdös and associates established the identity of these two enzymatic activities; thus, its designation as peptidyl dipeptidase (PDP) is appropriate. It is important to recognize that PDP catalyzes both the *synthesis* of angiotensin II, the most potent pressor substance known, and the *destruction* of bradykinin, the most potent vasodilator. To lose sight of this fact is to risk misinterpretation of the effects and uses of inhibitors of this enzyme.

Chemistry. The most thoroughly studied of the peptide inhibitors of PDP is the nonapeptide (BPF$_{9a}$) known as *teprotide;* it has the following structure: pyroGlu-Trp-Pro-Arg-Pro-Gln-Ile-Pro-Pro (*see* Cushman *et al.,* 1977). Teprotide (like other BPFs) acts as a competitive inhibitor of PDP, with an affinity for the enzyme much higher than that of angiotensin II. It is not itself a substrate for the enzyme. Although PDP will cleave many different C-terminal dipeptide residues, it will not cleave peptides with proline in the penultimate position, as with teprotide and other BPFs. As noted, the penultimate proline in angiotensin II is, indeed, responsible for its refractoriness to further cleavage by PDP. Moreover, the presence of pyroGlu at the N-terminus renders teprotide refractory to aminopeptidases; this confers further stability and effectiveness *in vivo.*

Teprotide has been studied extensively, and its effects have generated intense clinical interest. However, it is a peptide and therefore is ineffective when given orally. The search for orally active compounds culminated in the development of the highly active and orally effective PDP inhibitor *captopril* (Cushman *et al.,* 1977). Based on analogy with carboxypeptidase A, which was known to be inhibited by

D-benzylsuccinic acid, Ondetti, Cushman, and their colleagues argued that inhibitors of PDP might be produced by succinyl amino acids that corresponded in length to the dipeptide cleaved by PDP. This proved to be true and led ultimately to the synthesis of a series of carboxy alkanoyl or mercapto alkanoyl derivatives that acted as potent competitive inhibitors of the enzyme. Most active (with a K_i of 1.7 nM) was D-3-mercapto-methylpropanoyl-L-proline or captopril, which has the following structure:

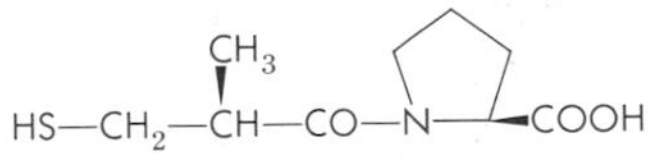

Captopril

Pharmacological Properties. The essential effect of these agents on the renin-angiotensin system is to block conversion of the relatively inactive angiotensin I to the active angiotensin II (or the conversion of [des-Asp[1]]angiotensin I to angiotensin III). In this way they blunt or annul responses to angiotensin I, whether administered or formed endogenously. In this respect they resemble the antagonists of angiotensin II. Unlike the latter, however, they do not block responses to angiotensin II and they are devoid of agonist activity. As would be expected, PDP inhibitors *in vivo* have their most profound hypotensive effects in those hypertensive states where the renin-angiotensin system is most active (*e.g.,* in some types of malignant and renal hypertension). However, the PDP inhibitors have hypotensive activity in a much broader spectrum of situations than might have been expected from the long-held view that secretion of renin accounts for a relatively small fraction of hypertension or, indeed, than might have been expected from the more limited effectiveness of angiotensin II antagonists. This unexpected efficacy in, for example, many patients with so-called normal-renin essential hypertension intensifies interest in the possible mechanisms of action of PDP inhibitors and their utility in the treatment of a broad spectrum of hypertensive conditions.

To date, the pharmacological activity of these drugs seems attributable entirely to their inhibitory effect on PDP. Thus, when tested on smooth muscle preparations *in vitro,* they selectively reduce responsiveness to angiotensin I without influencing that to angiotensin II or indeed to any of many other pharmacological agents, with the notable exception of bradykinin, which, of course, is potentiated. Similar responses are obtained *in vivo,* although PDP inhibitors tend to enhance responses to *exogenous* angiotensin II (Murthy *et al.,* 1977; Rubin *et al.,* 1978). Systemic blood pressure in *normal* individuals in sodium balance is not generally affected by inhibition of PDP. However, when endogenous angiotensin contributes to the maintenance of blood pressure, as, for example, in sodium depletion, PDP inhibitors reduce blood pressure as do antagonists of angiotensin II (Anderson *et al.,* 1977).

The broader efficacy of the PDP inhibitors, compared to antagonists of angiotensin II, requires explanation. It is probable that much of the difference is attributable to the lack of agonist activity of teprotide and captopril (Laragh *et al.,* 1977; Gavras *et al.,* 1978; Symposium, 1978b). There are, however, additional possible explanations for the greater hypotensive activity of PDP inhibitors, including potentiation of endogenous bradykinin (Ferguson *et al.,* 1977). While the role of bradykinin in hypertension is not yet clear, inhibitors of PDP increase concentrations of endogenous bradykinin severalfold in some hypertensive patients (Williams and Hollenberg, 1977; *see also* Thurston and Swales, 1978). Since PDP cleaves many substrates, conjecture need not be limited to the renin-angiotensin or bradykinin systems. All this notwithstanding, it is clear that PDP inhibitors exert much of their hypotensive effect by blocking the formation of angiotensin II initiated by circulating renin.

Another major effect of the PDP inhibitors is depression of the secretion of aldosterone. This is evident in both hypertensive individuals and normal subjects in negative sodium balance. This provides further testimony of the importance of the renin-angiotensin system in mediating the stimulus to aldosterone secretion provided by the deprivation of sodium (*see* Case *et al.,* 1978; Gavras *et al.,* 1978).

CLINICAL APPLICATIONS

Early demonstrations of the pharmacological properties of PDP inhibitors and competitive antagonists of angiotensin II led to the hypothesis that the drugs would be useful in *assessing the participation of the renin-angiotensin system in hypertensive disease,* in *screening for overactivity of this system,* and in *treating patients with hypertension.* In fact, the hypoten-

sive effects of these drugs in hypertensive patients have helped to identify renin-dependent "angiotensinogenic" hypertensive patients. Such agents assist, for example, in the *diagnosis of surgically remediable renovascular hypertension* (Re *et al.,* 1978).

The frequency with which PDP inhibitors lower blood pressure in the absence of renovascular diseases is surprising. In one study with a mixed population of hypertensive patients, teprotide yielded so many positive responses that the authors concluded that "an absolute or relative excess of angiotensin is actively involved in maintenance of the elevated blood pressure in about 70% of all patients with so called essential hypertension including those in which renin levels are within normal limits" (Laragh *et al.,* 1977). The more recent results with captopril (Case *et al.,* 1978; Gavras *et al.,* 1978) continue to provide evidence of PDP inhibitor–induced hypotensive effects in individuals whose plasma renin levels fall within the normal range. There is, however, an awareness that such a high incidence of depressor responses may overestimate the involvement of the renin-angiotensin system in hypertension, not only because other systems, such as the kallikrein-kinin system, may participate (*see* below) but also because there are factors that complicate the conduct of such tests whether carried out with PDP inhibitors or angiotensin II antagonists. Sodium depletion, for example, which has sometimes been used to facilitate demonstration of the angiotensinogenic component of hypertension, sets into operation the normal physiological mechanism of increased secretion of renin and may therefore lead to false-positive responses, especially when measurements of blood pressure are made when the patients are sitting or standing. It must be recognized, however, that a depressor response observed in the presence of "normal" plasma renin levels cannot be dismissed as the consequence of some action of the drug beyond the renin-angiotensin system. It has long been suspected that the persistence of "normal" renin and angiotensin levels in the presence of hypertension (or sodium retention or both) may in fact be inappropriate, and recent evidence has tended to support this idea (Brunner *et al.,* 1978; Gavras *et al.,* 1978). Moreover, there is evidence that an increased responsiveness to angiotensin II can occur. It is precisely because of such possibilities that blockers of the renin-angiotensin system, provided they are specific, should better assess the participation of this system in hypertension than can measurements of renin activity in plasma.

Because the peptide inhibitors of PDP, such as teprotide, must be given intravenously, they are likely to be practically useful only for the treatment of acute hypertensive episodes involving excess angiotensin, such as may occur in *malignant hypertension* or *renovascular emergencies.* By contrast, the orally effective PDP inhibitor captopril seems, from the clinical trials to date, well suited to long-term therapy of hypertension of various types. When given orally to normal individuals it inhibits PDP within 15 minutes. Profound inhibition is observed shortly thereafter and lasts for hours (Ferguson *et al.,* 1977). In normal individuals, the drug does not have obvious effects. In patients with high blood pressure for a variety of causes associated with elevated, normal, or even low activities of renin in plasma, captopril given orally two to four times per day for periods up to 26 weeks causes considerable lowering in blood pressure. This effect is evident in most instances without adjuvant treatment with diuretic drugs.

Additional uses of drugs that block the renin-angiotensin system include assessment of the contribution of the system to hypertension in patients with chronic renal disease whose blood pressure does not decrease after hemodialysis. Vasodilators are increasingly used in congestive heart failure to diminish the work of the heart by lowering total peripheral resistance (see Chapter 33). However, administration of vasodilators tends to increase renin output; PDP inhibitors therefore may be useful to prevent this response and, indeed, have been shown to be helpful by themselves in the treatment of selected cases of congestive heart failure secondary to angiotensinogenic hypertensive states (see Gavras et al., 1977). In a more recent study of ten patients with stable congestive heart failure poorly controlled by digitalis and diuretics, a single dose of captopril (25 to 150 mg) increased cardiac index and lowered both mean arterial and pulmonary wedge pressures over a period of 4 hours. Three patients were maintained on therapy for 4 to 8 weeks (25 to 100 mg every 8 hours). The drug was well tolerated and improvement in cardiac function was maintained, as measured by performance in exercise stress tests. Although hemodynamic measurements indicated that the increase in cardiac index was due to a decrease in both preload and afterload, the basic mechanism of action remains to be defined, since there was no correlation between the degree of improvement in cardiac function and control measurements of plasma renin activity (Davis et al., 1979). The blockers may also be beneficial for *prophylaxis or therapy of shock due to acute renal failure* arising from renovascular surgery, trauma, or surgery that requires extracorporeal circulation (see Stokes and Edwards, 1976; Symposium, 1976b). Dramatic reversal of vascular and renal crises of scleroderma has also been reported to follow the oral administration of captopril (Lopez-Ovejero et al., 1979).

Untoward Effects. In addition to side effects already mentioned, saralasin may evoke dangerous hypertensive episodes through its agonist activity, especially if given as a bolus to individuals with "low-renin" hypertension. Saralasin may also cause massive release of catecholamines in patients with pheochromocytoma. Dangerous "rebound hypertension" can occur when the effects of any of the blocking drugs wane. By contrast, blood pressure may fall to dangerously low levels in patients with marked angiotensinogenic hypertension who are given these drugs. The incidence and seriousness of the untoward effects of captopril have yet to be evaluated in a large population of patients. Those directly related to the actions of the drug include a slight elevation in plasma potassium and plasma renin activity and an increase in pulse rate. Fever, rash, and proteinuria have also been observed (Case et al., 1978; Gavras et al., 1978).

CENTRAL AND PERIPHERAL SYMPATHETIC BLOCKADE OF RENIN RELEASE

Several drugs have inhibitory effects on the central or peripheral sympathetic secretomotor control of the secretion of renin. Among these are the antihypertensive agent clonidine and β-adrenergic antagonists such as propranolol (see Gross, 1977; Peart, 1978; Reid et al., 1978; Weber et al., 1978). These are discussed elsewhere (see Index).

PLASMA KININS (KALLIDIN, BRADYKININ)

History. The discovery of the plasma kinins had its origins in the old observation that urine, injected intravenously, lowers blood pressure. In the 1920s and 1930s, Frey and associates characterized the hypotensive substance and showed that similar material could be obtained from saliva, plasma, and a variety of tissues. Since the pancreas was a rich source, they named this material *kallikrein* after an old Greek synonym for that organ, *kallikréas* (see Galen, c. 168). By 1937, Werle, Götze, and Keppler had established that kallikreins have an indirect effect and, behaving as enzymes, split off a pharmacologically active substance from some inactive precursor present in plasma. Their discovery preceded by 2 years the analogous finding that renin acts similarly. In 1948, Werle and Berek named the active substance *kallidin* and showed it to be a polypeptide cleaved from a plasma globulin that they termed *kallidinogen* (see Frey et al., 1968; Werle, 1970).

Interest in the field intensified when Rocha e Silva and associates (1949) reported that the venoms of certain snakes, as well as the enzyme trypsin, acted on plasma globulin to produce a substance, probably a polypeptide, that also lowered blood pressure and caused a slowly developing contraction of the gut. Because of the slow response of the gut, they named this substance *bradykinin*, a term derived from the Greek words *bradys*, meaning "slow," and *kinein*, meaning "to move." Since bradykinin and kallidin were formed under similar conditions and had similar pharmacological actions, it was early suspected that they were closely related. Identification of the pure materials some 10 years later confirmed this suspicion. In 1960, bradykinin, formed by reacting trypsin with globulin, was isolated by Elliott and coworkers and synthesized by Boissonnas and associates (see Elliott, 1970). It proved to be a nonapeptide of the structure shown below. Shortly thereafter, this same nonapeptide was found to be a constituent of kallidin, which, however, also contained a pharmacologically similar decapeptide with the same sequence of amino acids but with an additional N-terminal lysine residue (Webster and Pierce, 1963). These substances are now recognized to be but two of a large number of polypeptides that have related chemical structures and pharmacological properties and that are widely distributed in nature. For the whole group the generic term *kinins* has been adopted, and kallidin and bradykinin are referred to as *plasma kinins* (see Bertaccini, 1976; Rocha e Silva, 1977; Werle, 1977; Schachter and Barton, 1979).

Synthesis and Catabolism of Kinins and Other Chemical Considerations. Because two separate experimental paths led to the identification of the plasma kinins, nomenclature has been confused. The terms adopted here are those recommended by an international committee (*see* Webster, 1970). The term *kallidin* (which formerly embraced both the nonapeptides and decapeptides) is now restricted to the decapeptide, while the term *bradykinin* has been retained for the nonapeptide. Bradykinin has the following amino acid sequence: Arg-Pro-Pro-Gly-Phe-Ser-Pro-Phe-Arg. Kallidin has an additional lysine molecule in the N-terminal position and is sometimes referred to as lysyl-bradykinin. The two peptides are cleaved from precursors, referred to as *kininogens,* in the plasma α_2-globulin fraction (Figure 27–3). This cleavage may be effected by enzymes collectively referred to as *kininogenases.* Among these the greatest interest attaches to the *kallikreins,* a group of proteolytic enzymes of high substrate specificity present in plasma, lymph, various other body fluids (including urine and salivary, pancreatic, and other exocrine secretions), and diverse tissues. Other kininogenases include trypsin, plasmin, and various proteolytic enzymes in certain snake and insect venoms and bacteria. Plasma kallikrein (like trypsin and snake venoms) forms the nonapeptide kinin *bradykinin* directly from a kininogen of high ($\sim$100,000) molecular weight (HMW kininogen). Glandular and other tissue kallikreins form the decapeptide kinin *kallidin* from a kininogen of lower ($\sim$50,000) molecular weight (LMW kininogen).

The half-life of kinins in plasma is less than 15 seconds. Indeed, in a single passage through the pulmonary bed, some 60 to 90% is inactivated. Other tissues also metabolize kinins rapidly. There are two principal kininases: kininase I (carboxypeptidase N or arginine carboxypeptidase), which removes the C-terminal arginine, and kininase II, which removes the C-terminal dipeptide, Phe-Arg. Either cleavage

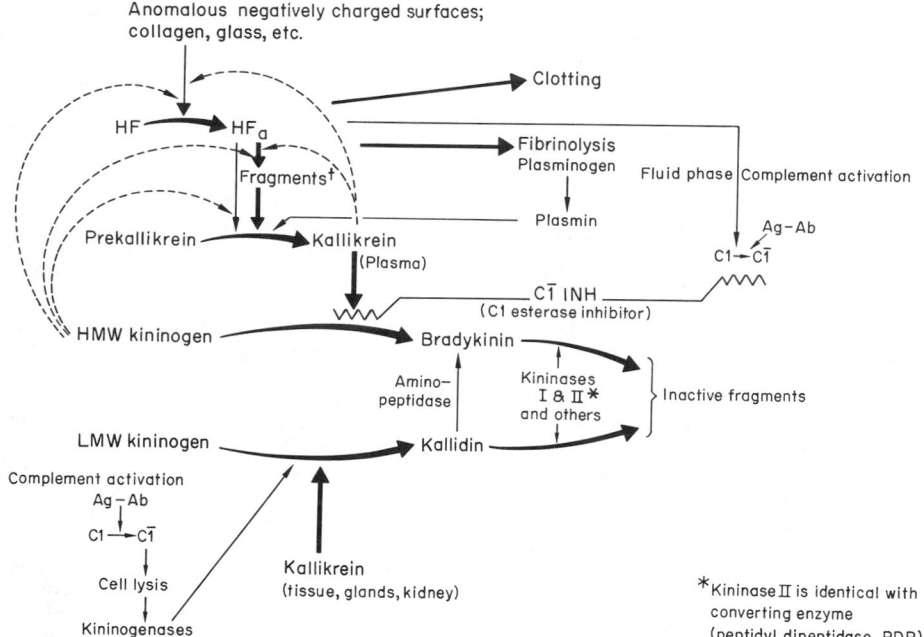

Figure 27-3. *Formation and destruction of the kinins.*

Bradykinin and kallidin are formed, respectively, by plasma and tissue kallikreins. Note the relationship of the plasma kinin–forming system to other Hageman factor (HF)–dependent processes, notably blood clotting and fibrinolysis. Observe that two components of the kinin cascade, prekallikrein and high-molecular-weight (HMW) kininogen, are essential for HF activation and function and hence are also clotting factors. Their points of interaction are indicated by the dashed arrows; note especially the strong positive feedback provided by kallikrein, which is a major HF activator in the fluid phase and mainly responsible for the formation of the HF fragments (†) that are potent "kallikrein activators." The kallikrein-inhibiting effect of complement C1 esterase inhibitor (C1 INH) is indicated; other plasma protease inhibitors, α_2-macroglobulin and α_1-antitrypsin, act at the same site. The activation of complement by antigen-antibody complexes (Ag-Ab), leading to cell lysis liberating kininogenases, is indicated, along with fluid-phase activation of complement by HF_a. Negative-feedback, "restraining" mechanisms and many other complexities are omitted. Note that kininase II is the same enzyme (peptidyl dipeptidase) elsewhere referred to as converting enzyme (*see* text and Figure 27–1).

yields virtually inactive peptides. Kininase II is the same as peptidyl dipeptidase (PDP; *see* above). Indeed, kinins are the preferred substrate for this enzyme (K_m of 0.1 μM for bradykinin versus 10 μM for angiotensin I). Kininase I is not inhibited by inhibitors of PDP but is inhibited by some substituted succinic acid derivatives that inhibit pancreatic carboxypeptidase B. The synthesis and destruction of kinins have been extensively reviewed (Erdös, 1970, 1976, 1979; Pisano, 1975; Pisano and Austen, 1977; Schachter and Barton, 1979).

Normal blood contains all essential ingredients for the formation of massive amounts of bradykinin. Usually, very little bradykinin is formed, mainly because plasma kallikrein is present in an inactive form, prekallikrein. Conversion of prekallikrein to kallikrein, with resultant formation of bradykinin, is, however, readily brought about by various factors. These include substantial changes in pH or temperature and contact with negatively charged surfaces, such as occur on glass and kaolin or on biological material such as collagen, which is readily exposed by tissue damage. Many of the factors that activate kallikrein are involved in Hageman factor (HF)–initiated coagulation and fibrinolysis (*see* Figure 27–3; Chapter 58). Thus, formation of bradykinin involves a cascade of enzymatic reactions triggered by activation of HF. Indeed, the three systems not only share this common triggering factor but also show further broad overlap and integration. Additional discussion of these interesting interrelationships is beyond the scope of this text. (For details, *see* Cochrane, 1976; Colman and Wong, 1977; Donaldson *et al.*, 1977; Chan *et al.*, 1978; Erdös, 1979.)

Hundreds of congeners of the kinins have been synthesized, and a considerable amount of information on the structure-activity relationship has emerged. The minimal effective compound is the nonapeptide. Arginine is essential at both positions 1 and 9. However, in contrast to the comparable studies on angiotensin II, this work has so far not led to the discovery or development of any congener with kinin-blocking activity (*see* Barabé *et al.*, 1977; Pisano and Austen, 1977).

PHARMACOLOGICAL PROPERTIES

The plasma kinins possess an extraordinarily high degree of pharmacological activity. They are the most potent vasodilator autacoids of mammals, and in very low concentration they increase capillary permeability, produce edema, evoke pain and reflexes by acting on nerve endings, contract or relax various smooth muscles (directly or through short or longer nervous paths), and elicit sundry other responses. In all these respects bradykinin and kallidin behave very similarly (*see* Erdös, 1970, 1976, 1979; Rocha e Silva and Garcia Leme, 1972; Pisano and Austen, 1977; Schachter and Barton, 1979).

Cardiovascular System. *Blood Vessels.* On a molar basis, kinins are about ten times as active as histamine in causing vasodilatation. Intravenously in man they cause flushing in the blush area and conjunctival injection. Blood vessels in muscle, kidney, viscera, and various glands are also dilated, as are coronary and cerebral vessels; throbbing headache may occur. Certain of these direct effects may be complemented by the ability of kinins to stimulate the release of histamine from mast cells. Effects on pulmonary vessels vary with dose, species, and state of development. These dilator effects, resulting from a direct action of the peptides on arteriolar smooth muscle, cause a sharp fall in systolic and diastolic blood pressures. In contrast to the fine-resistance vessels, large arteries and most veins, large and small, tend to be contracted by the kinins. Kinins promote dilatation of the fetal pulmonary artery, closure of the ductus arteriosus, and constriction of the umbilical vessels, all of which occur in the adjustment from fetal to neonatal circulation. Since identical responses can be elicited by prostaglandins, this autacoid may be the final mediator (*see* below).

Heart. Cardiac muscle is not directly affected by bradykinin, but the fall in total peripheral resistance and systemic blood pressure due to vasodilatation, combined with contraction of the large veins and increased venous return, causes a reflex increase in heart rate and increased cardiac output. Additional stimulant actions of bradykinin on coronary chemoreflex afferent nerve endings and on autonomic efferent nerve endings and ganglia may complicate the cardiac responses (*see* Staszewska-Barczak and Dusting, 1977).

Vascular Permeability and Edema Formation. The plasma kinins increase permeability in the microcirculation. The effect, like that of histamine and 5-hydroxytryptamine (5-HT), is exerted on the small venules rather than on the true capillaries and involves separation of the junctions between endothelial cells. Additionally, there may be increased vesicular transport by the endothelium. These effects, together with an increased hydrostatic pressure gradient, cause edema to form (*see* Kline *et al.*, 1973). Such edema, coupled with stimulation of nerve endings (*see* below), results in a "wheal-and-flare" response to intradermal injections in man.

Extravascular Smooth Muscle. Various isolated smooth muscle preparations contract in response to the kinins. The rat uterus is especially sensitive and responds to as little as 0.1 ng/ml. It was the characteristically slow response of the isolated guinea pig ileum that prompted the name *bradykinin*. Certain smooth muscles, such as the rabbit aorta or mammary smooth muscle, are little affected; still others, such as the rat duodenum, are relaxed. Tracheobronchial constriction is prominent in guinea pigs, but dilatation as well as constriction may occur in other species. In man, respiratory distress is encountered in asthmatics, especially when the kinins are inhaled (Newball *et al.*, 1975; Chand and Eyre, 1977).

Stimulation of Nerve Endings and Production of Pain. The plasma kinins are powerful algesic agents. They cause an intense, burning pain when applied to the exposed base of a blister, and a throbbing, burning pain in the hand when injected into the brachial artery. Nociceptive responses or pain occurs when the kinins are injected into animals or man either intraperitoneally or into arteries supplying skin, muscle, or various viscera. Such a nociceptive response can be elicited from the coronary vasculature and is accompanied by sympathetically mediated tachycardia and pressor effects (*see* Staszewska-Barczak and Dusting, 1977).

Stimulation of Autonomic Ganglia and Chromaffin Cells. The kinins, usually in relatively high concentration, stimulate ganglion cells and elicit discharge of catecholamines from the adrenal medulla (*see* Lewis and Reit, 1966); they depolarize chromaffin cells (Douglas *et al.*, 1967). Such actions occasionally contribute significantly to the excitatory and inhibitory responses of the intestine and other organs. Kinins, unlike angiotensin, do not stimulate the release of norepinephrine from sympathetic nerve terminals; rather, they tend to reduce it (Starke *et al.*, 1977).

Central Nervous System. The injection of bradykinin into the cerebral ventricles causes a wide spectrum of behavioral, autonomic, and EEG effects (*see* Walaszek, 1970; Ribeiro *et al.*, 1971).

Mechanism of Action. Little is known of the receptors for bradykinin or other kinins, save that they may be distinguished pharmacologically from receptors for various other peptides (*see* Barabé *et al.*, 1977). Some responses appear to be mediated by generation of prostaglandins, seemingly as a result of stimulation of phospholipase A_2. Release of prostaglandins in response to bradykinin was first demonstrated in guinea pig lung (Piper and Vane, 1969), where they contribute to bronchoconstriction. A similar mechanism may underlie the later phases of vasodilatation, the slowly developing nociceptive responses, and other effects of kinins that are reduced by inhibitors of prostaglandin synthesis, including the prominent renal vasodilator effects. Both cyclic AMP and cyclic GMP have also been suggested as mediators of some kinin-induced responses (*see* Erdös, 1976; 1979; Symposium, 1976a; Nustad *et al.*, 1978).

ENDOGENOUS KININ-GENERATING SYSTEMS

In considering physiological functions and pathological involvements of endogenous kininogen-kallikrein-kinin systems, it must be recognized that, despite common descriptors, two distinct entities are involved: the plasma system and the tissue ("glandular" or "exocrine") system. Although in each there is a similarly named plasma substrate, a kininogen, these substrates are clearly different, not only in molecular weight but also in the position of the kinin sequences within the molecules and thus in the different cleavages needed for the appearance of free kinins. The kallikreins too, although similarly named, have different features: the plasma enzyme preferentially cleaves HMW kininogen to produce bradykinin, and the tissue enzyme acts on LMW kininogen to produce kallidin. Other distinctive features of the tissue and plasma kinin-generating systems are described in the reviews cited above. The following brief discussion touches on only a few of the possible functions of these interesting systems.

Numerous suggestions have been made with regard to roles of the plasma kinin system. Proteins such as HMW kininogen and prekallikrein are critical for the functioning of HF-dependent blood coagulation and fibrinolysis. Familial deficiency of HMW kininogen (Fletcher trait) or prekallikrein (Fitzgerald, Flaujeac, Williams traits) thus results in defects in intrinsic clotting and fibrinolytic mechanisms as well as in kinin formation. *Hereditary angioedema* is characterized by a deficiency of the C1-esterase inhibitor of the complement system. This plasma protease inhibitor is also an inhibitor of kallikrein, and the episodes of edema that occur in this condition may be due in part to excess formation of bradykinin (*see* Donaldson *et al.*, 1977). Episodic flushing syndromes and carcinoid may be associated with hyperbradykininemia, and some such conditions may be caused by deficiency of kininase I (Streeten *et al.*, 1972). Other pathological circumstances that may be accompanied by excess formation of kinins are septic and anaphylactic shock, inflammatory reactions including various arthritides, and some immune reactions. A deficiency of kinins, resulting from reduced hepatic synthesis of precursors, has been implicated in the acute hepatorenal syndrome in patients with cirrhosis of the liver.

The long enigmatic function of the glandular and renal kallikreins has been lent particular interest by observation of correlations between renal kallikrein secretion, electrolyte balance, and systemic blood pressure. Renal kallikrein output rises during salt deprivation or potassium loading, and the evidence suggests that this response is mediated by enhanced secretion of aldosterone, itself the result of elevated concentrations of angiotensin. Furthermore, secretion of urinary kallikrein is influenced by postural changes. Together, these observations point to a link between the renin-angiotensin-aldosterone axis and kallikrein secretion. Moreover, this link may extend also to regulation of blood pressure. As early as 1936 it was noted that urinary kallikrein concentrations were subnormal in hypertensive individuals. This has recently been confirmed and extended to various animal models of the disease. Epidemiological surveys have demonstrated that secretion of kallikrein in the urine may be familially aggregated and that there is an inverse relation between urinary kallikrein and blood pressure in normotensive children. There are also provocative indications, discussed above, that some of the hypotensive effects of the inhibitors of peptidyl dipeptidase may be due to accumulation of kinins. No firm conclusions can be drawn at present, but current interest and puzzlement on the relationship between urinary kallikrein, blood pressure, regulation of electrolytes, and the renin-angiotensin-aldosterone axis are neatly illustrated by the title of a recent editorial, "Kallikrein, Kinins, and the Kidney: What's Going on in There?" (Margolius, 1978; *see also* Symposium, 1976a; Carretero *et al.*, 1978; Editorial, 1978).

Therapeutic Considerations. As with most other autacoids, therapeutic interest in the kinins focuses particularly on attempts to modulate their metabolism *in vivo*. The kinins themselves have an extremely short life, and no therapeutic use has been found for them. On the other hand, potentiation of endogenous kinins by slowing their destruction may prove to be useful. As described, PDP inhibitors have this effect; the full significance and utility of this action have yet to be defined, but the recent development of effective inhibitors of kininase I lends the approach increasing interest.

The opposite approach, that of blocking the endogenous kinin system, has potential applications because of the involvement of excess kinins in numerous clinical conditions. The lack of specific antagonists is a current frustration. Nevertheless, in certain conditions where kinins have been implicated, such as inflammatory states, some of the beneficial effects of aspirin and other nonsteroidal anti-inflammatory agents may reflect suppression of prostaglandin synthesis initiated by the kinins. In the light of increasing evidence that several of the effects of kinins may be mediated by prostaglandins or facilitated by concurrent kinin-induced prostaglandin formation, such inhibitors of prostaglandin synthesis may have broader, albeit nonspecific, antikinin activity than has been suspected (*see* Chapter 28). Blockade of kinin formation with inhibitors of kallikrein is another potential approach. A polypeptide inhibitor of kallikrein, *aprotinin* (TRASYLOL), has been used with some success to treat acute pancreatitis, (Trapnell, 1977), carcinoid syndrome, and some other conditions involving excess kinin formation (*see* Haberland, 1978).

OTHER ACTIVE POLYPEPTIDES

Erspamer, his colleagues, and others have described many small polypeptides in a broad range of nonmammalian species; they have remarkable pharmacological activity. Some resemble the mammalian kinins discussed above. A second group, also active vasodilator and hypotensive agents, somewhat resembles substance P (*see* below). A third group is similar to mammalian gastrointestinal hormones such as cholecystokinin-pancreozymin. A fourth group has unique stimulant actions in releasing mammalian gastrointestinal hormones and has recently been found in the mammalian gastrointestinal tract. These and other pharmacologically active peptides cannot be described here but are discussed in recent reviews (*see* Bertaccini, 1976; Pisano and Austen, 1977; Grossman *et al.*, 1978; Schachter and Barton, 1979).

A remarkable feature of these comparative studies is that they have not only revealed substances of pharmacological activity and great interest in their own right but have also emphasized the commonality of distribution of active peptides in the animal kingdom. The importance of such discoveries is heightened by the developing awareness that many—perhaps most—peptides that have been isolated from the gastrointestinal tract and associated with endocrine function there are also found in the brain, where they are suspected of subserving neurotransmitter as well as neuroendocrine functions (*see* Chapter 12). Some examples include cholecystokinin-pancreozymin, somatostatin, enkephalin, and gastrin (*see* Index), as well as vasoactive intestinal

polypeptide (VIP) and substance P (*see* Neuropeptide Symposium, 1977; Pearse, 1977; Grossman *et al.*, 1978).

Substance P. This is an undecapeptide with the following structure: Arg-Pro-Lys-Pro-Gln-Gln-Phe-Phe-Gly-Leu-Met-NH$_2$. Substance P was originally detected by Euler and Gaddum in 1931 in extracts of gut and brain; it was purified, characterized, and synthesized 40 years later (*see* Tregear *et al.*, 1971). It can now be recognized as the prototype of many other peptides more recently discovered that are also distributed between gut and brain. The pharmacological effects of substance P include vasodilatation, stimulation of intestinal and other smooth muscles, stimulation of salivary secretion, diuresis and natriuresis, and a variety of effects on the peripheral and central nervous systems apparently attributable to depolarization of neurons. Substance P has been localized within nerves in the peripheral and central nervous systems and is suspected of being a neurotransmitter (*see* Barker, 1977; Bury and Mashford, 1977; Euler and Pernow, 1977; Neuropeptide Symposium, 1977).

Substance P is also present, along with 5-HT and other autacoids, in enterochromaffin cells of the gastrointestinal and biliary tracts. It is therefore one of the autacoids secreted by tumors of these cells and contributes to the signs and symptoms of the carcinoid syndrome (*see* Skrabanek *et al.*, 1978).

Vasoactive Intestinal Polypeptide (VIP). This compound was isolated from small intestine by Said and Mutt (1972). It is a potent vasodilator and pancreatic secretagogue. Originally thought of as a gastrointestinal hormone, it is known to be widely distributed in central and peripheral nerves, including those to the pancreas. Its production by the nonbeta cells of the endocrine pancreas and by ganglioneuromata is believed to be responsible for the watery diarrhea syndrome (Verner-Morrison syndrome) (*see* Fahrenkrug and Schaffalitzky de Muckadell, 1978; Grossman *et al.*, 1978; Modlin *et al.*, 1978).

Anderson, G. H., Jr.; Streeten, D. H. P.; and Dalakos, T. G. Pressor response to 1-Sar-8-Ala-angiotensin II (saralasin) in hypertensive subjects. *Circ. Res.,* **1977**, *40,* 243–250.

Barabé, J.; Drouin, J.-N.; Regoli, D.; and Park, W. K. Receptors for bradykinin in intestinal and uterine smooth muscle. *Can. J. Physiol. Pharmacol.,* **1977**, *55,* 2170–2185.

Blair-West, J. R.; Coghlan, J. P.; Denton, D. A.; Funder, J. W.; Scoggins, B. A.; and Wright, R. D. The effect of the heptapeptide (2–8) and hexapeptide (3–8) fragments of angiotensin II on aldosterone secretion. *J. Clin. Endocrinol. Metab.,* **1971**, *32,* 575–578.

Boucher, R.; Demassieux, S.; Garcia, R.; and Genest, J. Tonin, angiotensin II system. *Circ. Res.,* **1977**, *41,* Suppl. II, 26–29.

Braun-Menéndez, E.; Fasciolo, J. C.; Leloir, L. F.; and Munoz, J. M. The substance causing renal hypertension. *J. Physiol. (Lond.),* **1940**, *98,* 283–298.

Braun-Menéndez, E., and Page, I. H. Suggested revision of nomenclature—angiotensin. *Science,* **1958**, *127,* 242.

Brunner, H. R.; Wauters, J. P.; McKinstry, D.; Waeber, B.; Turini, G.; and Gavras, H. Inappropriate renin secretion unmasked by captopril (SQ 14,225) in hypertension of chronic renal failure. *Lancet,* **1978**, *2,* 704–707.

Carretero, O. A.; Amin, V. M.; Ocholik, T.; Scicli, A. G.; and Koch, J. Urinary kallikrein in rats bred for their susceptibility and resistance to the hypertensive effect of salt. *Circ. Res.*, **1978**, *42*, 727–731.

Case, D. B.; Atlas, S. A.; Laragh, J. H.; Sealey, J. E.; Sullivan, P. A.; and McKinstry, D. N. Clinical experience with blockade of the renin-angiotensin-aldosterone system by an oral converting enzyme inhibitor (SQ 14,225, captopril) in hypertensive patients. *Prog. Cardiovasc. Dis.*, **1978**, *21*, 195–206.

Case, D. B.; Wallace, J. M.; Keim, H. J.; Weber, M. A.; Sealey, J. E.; and Laragh, J. H. Possible role of renin in hypertension as suggested by renin-sodium profiling and inhibition of converting enzyme. *N. Engl. J. Med.*, **1977**, *296*, 641–646.

Chan, J. Y. C.; Burrowes, C. E.; and Movat, H. Z. Surface activation of factor XII (Hageman factor)—critical role of high molecular weight kininogen and another potentiator. *Agents Actions*, **1978**, *8*, 65–72.

Chand, N., and Eyre, P. Bradykinin relaxes contracted airways through prostaglandin production. *J. Pharm. Pharmacol.*, **1977**, *29*, 387–388.

Cushman, D. W.; Cheung, H. S.; Sabo, E. F.; and Ondetti, M. A. Design of potent competitive inhibitors of angiotensin-converting enzyme. Carboxyalkanoyl and mercaptoalkanoyl amino acids. *Biochemistry*, **1977**, *16*, 5484–5491.

Davis, J. O.; Carpenter, C. C. J.; Ayers, C. R.; Holman, J. E.; and Bahn, R. C. Evidence for secretion of an aldosterone-stimulating hormone by the kidney. *J. Clin. Invest.*, **1961**, *40*, 684–696.

Davis, R.; Ribner, H. S.; Keung, E.; Sonnenblick, E. H.; and LeJemtel, T. H. Treatment of chronic congestive heart failure with captopril, an oral inhibitor of angiotensin-converting enzyme. *N. Engl. J. Med.*, **1979**, *301*, 117–121.

De Carvalho, J. G. R.; Dunn, F. G.; Kem, D. C.; Chrysant, S. G.; and Frohlich, E. D. Hemodynamic correlates of saralasin-induced arterial pressure changes. *Circulation*, **1977**, *57*, 373–378.

Deth, R., and van Breeman, C. Agonist induced release of intracellular Ca^{2+} in the rabbit aorta. *J. Membr. Biol.*, **1977**, *30*, 363–380.

Devynck, M. A., and Meyer, P. Angiotensin receptors. *Biochem. Pharmacol.*, **1978**, *27*, 1–5.

Donaldson, V. H.; Rosen, F. S.; and Bing, D. H. Role of the second component of complement (C2) and plasmin in kinin release in hereditary angioneurotic edema (H.A.N.E.) plasma. *Trans. Assoc. Am. Physicians*, **1977**, *90*, 174–183.

Douglas, W. W.; Kanno, T.; and Sampson, S. R. Effects of acetylcholine and other medullary secretagogues and antagonists on the membrane potential of adrenal chromaffin cells: an analysis employing techniques of tissue culture. *J. Physiol. (Lond.)*, **1967**, *188*, 107–120.

Editorial. Kinins and blood-pressure. *Lancet*, **1978**, *2*, 663–665.

Epstein, M.; Levinson, R.; Sancho, J.; Haber, E.; and Re, R. Characterization of the renin-aldosterone system in decompensated cirrhosis. *Circ. Res.*, **1977**, *41*, 818–829.

Fahrenkrug, J., and Schaffalitzky de Muckadell, O. B. Distribution of vasoactive intestinal polypeptide (VIP) in the porcine central nervous system. *J. Neurochem.*, **1978**, *31*, 1445–1451.

Ferguson, R. K.; Brunner, H. R.; Turini, G. A.; Gavras, H.; and McKinstry, D. N. A specific orally active inhibitor of angiotensin-converting enzyme in man. *Lancet*, **1977**, *1*, 775–778.

Fitzsimons, J. T., and Kucharczyk, J. Drinking and haemodynamic changes induced in the dog by intracranial injection of components of the renin-angiotensin system. *J. Physiol. (Lond.)*, **1978**, *276*, 419–434.

Ganong, W. F., and Mulrow, P. J. Evidence of secretion of an aldosterone-stimulating substance by the kidney. *Nature*, **1961**, *190*, 1115–1116.

Gavras, H.; Brunner, H. R.; Turini, G. A.; Kershaw, G. R.; Tifft, C. P.; Cuttlelod, S.; Gavras, I.; Vukovich, R. A.; and McKinstry, D. N. Antihypertensive effect of the oral angiotensin converting–enzyme inhibitor SQ 14,225 in man. *N. Engl. J. Med.*, **1978**, *298*, 991–995.

Gavras, H.; Flessas, A.; Ryan, T. J.; Brunner, H. R.; Faxon, D. P.; and Gavras, I. Angiotensin II inhibition. Treatment of congestive cardiac failure in a high-renin hypertension. *J.A.M.A.*, **1977**, *237*, 880–882.

Genest, J.; Rojo-Ortega, J. M.; Kuchel, O.; Boucher, R.; Nowaczynski, W.; Lefebvre, R.; Chretien, M.; and Cantin, M. Malignant hypertension with hypokalemia in a patient with renin-producing pulmonary carcinoma. *Clin. Res.*, **1975**, *18*, 448A.

Hall, M. M.; Khosla, M. C.; Khairallah, P. A.; and Bumpus, F. M. Angiotensin analogs: the influence of sarcosine substituted in position 1. *J. Pharmacol. Exp. Ther.*, **1974**, *188*, 222–228.

Khairallah, P. A.; Toth, A.; and Bumpus, F. M. Analogs of angiotensin II. II. Mechanism of receptor interaction. *J. Med. Chem.*, **1970**, *13*, 181–184.

Kline, R. L.; Scott, J. B.; Haddy, F. J.; and Grega, G. J. Mechanism of edema formation in canine forelimbs by locally administered bradykinin. *Am. J. Physiol.*, **1973**, *225*, 1051–1056.

Laragh, J. H.; Angers, M.; Kelly, W. G.; and Lieberman, S. Hypotensive agents and pressor substances; the effect of epinephrine, norepinephrine, angiotensin II and others on the secretory rate of aldosterone in man. *J.A.M.A.*, **1960**, *174*, 234–240.

Laragh, J. H.; Case, D. B.; Wallace, J. M.; and Keim, H. Blockade of renin or angiotensin for understanding human hypertension: a comparison of propranolol, saralasin and converting enzyme blockade. *Fed. Proc.*, **1977**, *36*, 1781–1787.

Lewis, G. P., and Reit, E. Further studies on the actions of peptides on the superior cervical ganglia and suprarenal medulla. *Br. J. Pharmacol.*, **1966**, *26*, 444–460.

Lopez-Ovejero, J. A.; Saal, S. D.; D'Angelo, W. A.; Cheigh, J. S.; Stenzel, K. H.; and Laragh, J. H. Reversal of vascular and renal crises of scleroderma by oral angiotensin-converting-enzyme blockade. *N. Engl. J. Med.*, **1979**, *300*, 1417–1419.

MacGregor, G. A., and Dawes, P. M. Agonist and antagonist effects of Sar^1–Ala^8–angiotensin II in salt-loaded and salt-depleted normal man. *Br. J. Clin. Pharmacol.*, **1976**, *3*, 483–487.

Millar, J. A.; Leckie, B. J.; Semple, P. F.; Morton, J. J.; Sonkodi, S.; and Robertson, J. I. S. Active and inactive renin in human plasma. Renal arteriovenous differences and relationships with angiotensin and renin-substrate. *Circ. Res.*, **1978**, *43*, Suppl. I, 120–127.

Modlin, I. M.; Bloom, S. R.; and Mitchell, S. VIP: the cause of the watery diarrhea syndrome. *Adv. Exp. Med. Biol.*, **1978**, *106*, 195–201.

Moore, A. F.; Bumpus, F. M.; and Khairallah, P. A. New approaches to the study of angiotensin tachyphylaxis. *Mayo Clin. Proc.*, **1977**, *52*, 446–448.

Murthy, V. S.; Waldron, T. L.; Goldberg, M. E.; and Vollmer, R. R. Inhibition of angiotensin converting enzyme by SQ 14,225 in conscious rabbits. *Eur. J. Pharmacol.*, **1977**, *46*, 207–212.

Newball, H. H.; Keiser, H. R.; and Pisano, J. J. Bradykinin and human airways. *Respir. Physiol.*, **1975**, *24*, 139–146.

Nomenclature Committee. Nomenclature of the renin-angiotensin system. *Clin. Sci. Mol. Med.*, **1978**, *55*, Suppl. 4, 113s–116s.

Page, I. H., and Helmer, O. M. Angiotonin-activator, renin- and angiotonin-inhibitor and the mechanism of angiotonin tachyphylaxis in normal, hypertensive and nephrectomized animals. *J. Exp. Med.*, **1940**, *71*, 485–519.

Paiva, T. B.; Miyamoto, M. E.; Juliano, L.; and Paiva, A. C. M. Requirements for angiotensin tachyphylaxis in smooth muscles. *J. Pharmacol. Exp. Ther.*, **1977**, *202*, 294–300.

Pals, D. T.; Masucci, F. D.; Denning, G. S., Jr.; Sipos, F.; and Fessler, D. C. Role of the pressor action of angiotensin II in experimental hypertension. *Circ. Res.*, **1971**, *29*, 673–681.

Phillips, M. I.; Mann, J. F. E.; Haebara, H.; Hoffman, W. E.; Dietz, R.; Schelling, P.; and Ganten, D. Lowering of hypertension by central saralasin in the absence of plasma renin. *Nature*, **1977**, *270*, 445–447.

Piper, P. J., and Vane, J. R. Release of additional factors in anaphylaxis and its antagonism by anti-inflammatory drugs. *Nature*, **1969**, *223*, 29–35.

Re, R.; Novelline, R.; Escourrou, M. T.; Athanasoulis, C.; Burton, J.; and Haber, E. Inhibition of angiotensin-converting enzyme for diagnosis of renal-artery stenosis. *N. Engl. J. Med.*, **1978**, *298*, 582–586.

Ribeiro, S. A.; Carrado, A. P.; and Graeff, F. G. Antinociceptive action of intraventricular bradykinin. *Neuropharmacology*, **1971**, *10*, 725–731.

Rocha e Silva, M.; Beraldo, W. T.; and Rosenfeld, G. Bradykinin, a hypotensive and smooth muscle stimulating factor released from plasma globulin by snake venoms and by trypsin. *Am. J. Physiol.*, **1949**, *156*, 261 273.

Rubin, B.; Laffan, R. J.; Kotler, D. G.; O'Keefe, E. H.; DeMaio, D. A.; and Goldberg, M. E. SQ 14,225 (D-3-mercapto-2-methylpropanoyl-L-proline), a novel orally active inhibitor of angiotensin I–converting enzyme. *J. Pharmacol. Exp. Ther.*, **1978**, *204*, 271–280.

Said, S. I., and Mutt, V. Isolation from porcine intestinal wall of a vasoactive octacosapeptide related to secretin and glucagon. *Eur. J. Pharmacol.*, **1972**, *28*, 199–204.

Sealey, J. E.; White, W. R.; Laragh, J. H.; Case, D. B.; and Rubin, A. L. Studies of plasma aldosterone in anephric people: evidence for the fundamental role of the renin system in maintaining aldosterone secretion. *J. Clin. Endocrinol. Metab.*, **1978**, *47*, 52–60.

Semple, P. F., and Morton, J. J. Angiotensin II and angiotensin III in rat blood. *Circ. Res.*, **1976**, *38*, 122–126.

Skeggs, L. T.; Dorer, F. E.; Kahn, J. R.; Lentz, K. E.; and Levine, M. The biochemistry of the renin-angiotensin system and its role in hypertension. *Am. J. Med.*, **1976**, *60*, 737–748.

Skeggs, L. T.; Levine, M.; Lentz, K. E.; Kahn, J. R.; and Dorer, F. E. New developments in our knowledge of the chemistry of renin. *Fed. Proc.*, **1977**, *36*, 1755–1759.

Skrabanek, P.; Cannon, D.; Kirrane, J.; and Powell, D. Substance P secretion by carcinoid tumours. *Ir. J. Med. Sci.*, **1978**, *147*, 47–49.

Starke, K.; Peskar, B. A.; Schumacher, K. A.; and Taube, H. D. Bradykinin and postganglionic sympathetic transmission. *Naunyn Schmiedebergs Arch. Pharmacol.*, **1977**, *299*, 23–32.

Staszewska-Barczak, J., and Dusting, G. J. Sympathetic cardiovascular reflex initiated by bradykinin-induced stimulation of cardiac pain receptors in the dog. *Clin. Exp. Pharmacol. Physiol.*, **1977**, *4*, 443–452.

Streeten, D. H. P.; Kerr, L. P.; Kerr, C. B.; Prior, J. C.; and Kalakos, T. G. Hyperbradykininism: a new orthostatic syndrome. *Lancet*, **1972**, *2*, 1048–1053.

Sweet, C. S.; Columbo, J. M.; and Gaul, S. L. Central antihypertensive effects of inhibitors of the renin-angiotensin system in rats. *Am. J. Physiol.*, **1976**, *231*, 1794–1799.

Thurston, H., and Swales, J. D. Converting enzyme inhibitor and saralasin infusion in rats. Evidence for an additional vasodepressor property of converting enzyme inhibitor. *Circ. Res.*, **1978**, *42*, 588–592.

Trapnell, J. E. Clinical trials with kallikrein inhibition. In, *Chemistry and Biology of the Kallikrein-Kinin System in Health and Disease.* (Pisano, J. J., and Austen, K. F., eds.) Department of Health, Education, and Welfare Publication No. (NIH) 76-791, U.S. Government Printing Office, Washington, D. C., **1977**, pp. 573–577.

Tregear, G. W.; Niall, H. D.; Potts, J. T., Jr.; Leeman, S. E.; and Chang, M. M. Synthesis of substance P. *Nature* [*New Biol.*], **1971**, *232*, 87–89.

Weber, M. A.; Drayer, J. I. M.; and Laragh, J. H. The effects of clonidine and propranolol, separately and in combination, on blood pressure and plasma renin activity in essential hypertension. *J. Clin. Pharmacol.*, **1978**, *18*, 233–240.

Williams, G. H., and Hollenberg, N. K. Accentuated vascular and endocrine response to SQ 20,881 in hypertension. *N. Engl. J. Med.*, **1977**, *297*, 184–188.

Williams, G. H.; Hollenberg, N. K.; Brown, C.; and Mersey, J. H. Adrenal responses to pharmacological interruption of the renin-angiotensin system in sodium-restricted normal man. *J. Clin. Endocrinol. Metab.*, **1978**, *47*, 725–731.

Zimmerman, B. G. Actions of angiotensin on adrenergic nerve endings. *Fed. Proc.*, **1978**, *37*, 199–202.

Monographs and Reviews

Barker, J. L. Physiological roles of peptides in the nervous system. In, *Peptides in Neurobiology.* (Gainer, H., ed.) Plenum Press, New York, **1977**, pp. 295–343.

Bertaccini, G. Active polypeptides of nonmammalian origin. *Pharmacol. Rev.*, **1976**, *28*, 127–177.

Brown, J. J.; Fraser, R.; Leckie, B.; Lever, A. F.; Morton, J. J.; Padfield, P. L.; Semple, P. F.; and Robertson, J. I. S. Significance of renin and angiotensin. In, *Hypertension: Mechanisms, Diagnosis, and Treatment*, Vol. 9. (Onesti, G., and Brest, A. N., eds.) F. A. Davis Co., Philadelphia, **1978**, pp. 55–89.

Bumpus, F. M. Mechanisms and sites of action of newer angiotensin agonists and antagonists in terms of activity and receptor. *Fed. Proc.*, **1977**, *36*, 2128–2132.

Bury, R. W., and Mashford, M. L. Substance P: its pharmacology and physiological roles. *Aust. J. Exp. Biol. Med. Sci.*, **1977**, *55*, 671–735.

Cochrane, C. G. The Hageman factor pathways of kinin formation, clotting and fibrinolysis. In, *The Role of Immunological Factors in Infectious, Allergic, and Autoimmune Processes.* (Beers, R. F., and Bassett, E. G., eds.) Raven Press, New York, **1976**, pp. 237–245.

Colman, R. W., and Wong, P. Y. Participation of Hageman factor dependent pathways in human disease states. *Thromb. Haemostas.*, **1977**, *38*, 751–775.

Davis, J. O. The pathogenesis of chronic renovascular hypertension. *Circ. Res.*, **1977**, *40*, 439–444.

Davis, J. O., and Freeman, R. H. Mechanisms regulating renin release. *Physiol. Rev.*, **1976**, *56*, 1–56.

———. The other angiotensins. *Biochem. Pharmacol.*, **1977**, *26*, 93–97.

Elliott, D. F. The discovery and characterization of bradykinin. In, *Bradykinin, Kallidin and Kallikrein.* (Erdös, E. G., ed.) *Handbuch der Experimentellen Pharmakologie*, Vol. 25. Springer-Verlag, Berlin, **1970**, pp. 7–13.

Erdös, E. G. (ed.). *Bradykinin, Kallidin and Kallikrein. Handbuch der Experimentellen Pharmakologie*, Vol. 25. Springer-Verlag, Berlin, **1970**.

———. The kinins. *Biochem. Pharmacol.*, **1976**, *25*, 1563–1569.

——— (ed.). *Bradykinin, Kallidin and Kallikrein. Handbuch der Experimentellen Pharmakologie*, Vol. 25, Suppl. Springer-Verlag, Berlin, **1979**.

Euler, U. S. von, and Pernow, B. (eds.). *Substance P.* Raven Press, New York, **1977**.

Fitzsimons, J. T. The role of the renin-angiotensin system in the regulation of extracellular fluid volume. In, *Osmotic and Volume Regulation.* Alfred Benzon Symposium XI. (Jørgensen, C. B., and Skadhauge, E., eds.) Munksgaard, Copenhagen, **1978**, pp. 100–122.

Frey, E. K.; Kraut, H.; and Werle, E. *Das Kallikrein-Kinen System.* Ferdinand Enke Verlag, Stuttgart, **1968**.

Galen, C. On the anatomy of veins and arteries (*c.* 168). In, *Opera Medicorum Graecorum*, Vol. 2. (Kuhn, D. C. G., ed.) Offisina Libraria Cnoblochii, Lipsiae, **1821**, p. 781.

Ganten, D.; Fuxe, K.; Phillips, M. I.; Mann, J. F. E.; and Ganten, U. The brain isorenin-angiotensin system: biochemistry, localization, and possible role in drinking and blood pressure regulation. In, *Frontiers in Neuroendocrinology,* Vol. 5. (Ganong, W. F., and Martini, L., eds.) Raven Press, New York, **1978,** pp. 61–99.

Ganten, D.; Hutchinson, J. S.; Schelling, P.; Ganten, U.; and Fischer, H. The iso-renin angiotensin systems in extrarenal tissue. *Clin. Exp. Pharmacol. Physiol.,* **1976,** *3,* 103–126.

Gavras, H.; Oliver, J. A.; and Cannon, P. J. Interrelations of renin, angiotensin II, and sodium in hypertension and renal failure. *Annu. Rev. Med.,* **1976,** *27,* 485–521.

Genest, J.; Nowaczynski, W.; Koiw, E.; Sandor, T.; and Biron, P. Adrenocortical function in essential hypertension. In, *Essential Hypertension: An International Symposium.* (Buchborn, C., and Bock, K. D., eds.) Springer-Verlag, Berlin, **1960,** pp. 126–146.

Gross, F. The regulation of aldosterone secretion by the renin-angiotensin system under various conditions. *Acta Endocrinol. (Kbh.),* **1968,** Suppl. 124, 41–64.

———. Beta-adrenergic blockade, blood pressure, and the renin-angiotensin system. *Eur. J. Clin. Invest.,* **1977,** *7,* 321–322.

Gross, F., and Mohring, J. Renal pharmacology, with special emphasis on aldosterone and angiotensin. *Annu. Rev. Pharmacol.,* **1973,** *13,* 57–90.

Grossman, M. I.; Speranza, V.; Basso, N.; and Lezoche, E. (eds.). Gastrointestinal hormones and pathology of the digestive system. *Adv. Exp. Med. Biol.,* **1978,** *106,* 1–326.

Guyton, A. C.; Coleman, T. G.; and Granger, H. J. Circulation: overall regulation. *Annu. Rev. Physiol.,* **1972,** *34,* 13–46.

Haberland, G. L. The role of kininogenases, kinin formation and kininogenase inhibition in post traumatic shock and related conditions. *Klin. Wochenschr.,* **1978,** *56,* 325–331.

Hypertension Meeting. Proceedings of the fourth meeting of the International Society of Hypertension. (Flenley, D. C., ed.) *Clin. Sci. Mol. Med.,* **1976,** *51,* Suppl. 3, 1s–708s.

———. Proceedings of the fifth meeting of the International Society of Hypertension. (Flenley, D. C., ed.) *Ibid.,* **1978,** *55,* Suppl. 4, 1s–414s.

Khosla, M. C.; Smeby, R. R.; and Bumpus, F. M. Structure-activity relationship in angiotensin II analogs. In, *Angiotensin.* (Page, I. H., and Bumpus, F. M., eds.) *Handbuch der Experimentellen Pharmakologie,* Vol. 37. Springer-Verlag, Berlin, **1974,** pp. 126–161.

Leyssac, P. P. The renin angiotensin system and kidney function. A review of contributions to a new theory. *Acta Physiol. Scand.,* **1976,** Suppl. 442, 1–52.

Margolius, H. S. Kallikrein, kinins, and the kidney: what's going on in there? *J. Lab. Clin. Med.,* **1978,** *91,* 717–720.

Neuropeptide Symposium. (Various authors.) The role of peptides in neuronal function. In, *Approaches to the Cell Biology of Neurons,* Vol. II. (Cowan, W. H., and Ferrendelli, J. A., eds.) Society for Neuroscience, Bethesda, **1977,** pp. 241–373.

Nustad, K.; Ørstavik, T. B.; Gautvik, K. M.; and Pierce, J. V. Glandular kallikreins. *Gen. Pharmacol.,* **1978,** *9,* 1–9.

Page, I. H., and Bumpus, F. M. (eds.). *Angiotensin. Handbuch der Experimentellen Pharmakologie,* Vol. 37. Springer-Verlag, Berlin, **1974.**

Page, I. H., and McCubbin, J. W. *Renal Hypertension.* Year Book Medical Publishers, Inc., Chicago, **1968.**

Peach, M. J. Renin-angiotensin system: biochemistry and mechanisms of action. *Physiol. Rev.,* **1977,** *57,* 313–370.

Peach, M. J., and Ackerly, J. A. Angiotensin antagonists and the adrenal cortex and medulla. *Fed. Proc.,* **1976,** *35,* 2502–2507.

Pearse, A. G. E. The diffuse neuro-endocrine system and the APUD concept; related "endocrine" peptides in brain, intestine, pituitary, placenta and anuran cutaneous glands. *Med. Biol.,* **1977,** *55,* 115–125.

Peart, W. S. The kidney as an endocrine organ. *Lancet,* **1977,** *2,* 543–547.

———. Renin release. *Gen. Pharmacol.,* **1978,** *9,* 65–72.

Pisano, J. J. Chemistry and biology of the kallikrein-kinin system. In, *Proteases and Biological Control.* (Reich, E.; Rifkin, D. B.; and Shaw, E.; eds.) Cold Spring Harbor Laboratory, Cold Spring Harbor, N.Y., **1975,** pp. 199–222.

Pisano, J. J., and Austen, K. F. (eds.). *Chemistry and Biology of the Kallikrein-Kinin System in Health and Disease.* Department of Health, Education, and Welfare Publication No. (NIH) 76-791, U.S. Government Printing Office, Washington, D. C., **1977.**

Regoli, D.; Park, W. K.; and Rioux, F. Pharmacology of angiotensin. *Pharmacol. Rev.,* **1974,** *26,* 69–123.

Reid, I. A.; Morris, B. J.; and Ganong, W. F. The renin-angiotensin system. *Annu. Rev. Physiol.,* **1978,** *40,* 377–410.

Rocha e Silva, M. Bradykinin and bradykininogen—introductory remarks. In, *Chemistry and Biology of the Kallikrein-Kinin System in Health and Disease.* (Pisano, J. J., and Austen, K. F., eds.) Department of Health, Education, and Welfare Publication No. (NIH) 76-791, U.S. Government Printing Office, Washington, D. C., **1977,** pp. 7–15.

Rocha e Silva, M., and Garcia Leme, J. *Chemical Mediators of the Acute Inflammatory Reaction.* Pergamon Press, Ltd., Oxford, **1972.**

Schachter, M. Kinins: a group of active peptides. *Annu. Rev. Pharmacol.,* **1964,** *4,* 281–292.

Schachter, M., and Barton, S. Kallikreins (kininogenases) and kinins. In, *Endocrinology: Metabolic Basis of Clinical Practice.* (Cahill, G., Jr., and de Groot, L. J., eds.) Grune & Stratton, Inc., New York, **1979.**

Severs, W. B., and Daniels-Severs, A. E. Effects of angiotensin on the central nervous system. *Pharmacol. Rev.,* **1973,** *25,* 415–449.

Sicuteri, F.; Back, N.; and Haberland, G. L. (eds.). Kinins: pharmacodynamics and biological roles. Symposium on kinins. *Adv. Exp. Med. Biol.,* **1976,** *70,* 1–398.

Soffer, R. L. Angiotensin-converting enzyme and the regulation of vasoactive peptides. *Annu. Rev. Biochem.,* **1976,** *45,* 73–94.

Stokes, G. S., and Edwards, K. D. G. Drugs affecting the renin-angiotensin-aldosterone system. *Prog. Biochem. Pharmacol.,* **1976,** *12,* 1–258.

Symposium. (Various authors.) Kinins, renal function and blood pressure regulation. *Fed. Proc.,* **1976a,** *35,* 172–206.

Symposium. (Various authors.) *Proceedings of the Council for High Blood Pressure Research. Hypertension: Neural, Vascular and Hormonal Factors.* (Cohn, J. N., ed.) *Circ. Res.,* **1976b,** *38,* Suppl. II, 1–128.

Symposium. (Various authors.) The pharmacology of angiotensin antagonists. *Fed. Proc.,* **1976c,** *35,* 2486–2525.

Symposium. (Various authors.) Advances in our knowledge of the renin-angiotensin system. *Ibid.,* **1977,** *36,* 1753–1787.

Symposium. (Various authors.) Angiotensin-induced thirst: peripheral and central mechanisms. *Ibid.,* **1978a,** *37,* 2667–2771.

Symposium. (Various authors.) Captopril. (Sonnenblick, E. H., and Lesch, M., eds.) *Prog. Cardiovasc. Dis.,* **1978b,** *21,* 159–206.

Thurau, K. Intrarenal action of angiotensin. In, *Angiotensin.* (Page, I. H., and Bumpus, F. M., eds.) *Handbuch der Experimentellen Pharmakologie,* Vol. 37. Springer-Verlag, Berlin, **1974,** pp. 475–499.

Walaszek, E. J. The effect of bradykinin and kallidin on smooth muscle. In, *Bradykinin, Kallidin and Kallikrein.* (Erdös, E. G., ed.) *Handbuch der Experimentellen Pharmakologie,* Vol. 25. Springer-Verlag, Berlin, **1970,** pp. 430–433.

Webster, M. E. Recommendations for nomenclature and units. In, *Bradykinin, Kallidin and Kallikrein.* (Erdös, E. G., ed.) *Handbuch der Experimentellen Pharmakologie,* Vol. 25. Springer-Verlag, Berlin, **1970,** pp. 659–665.

Webster, M. E., and Pierce, J. V. The nature of the

kallidins released from human plasma by kallikreins and other enzymes. *Ann. N.Y. Acad. Sci.,* **1963,** *104,* 91–107.

Werle, E. Discovery of the most important kallikreins and kallikrein inhibitors. In, *Bradykinin, Kallidin and Kallikrein.* (Erdös, E. G., ed.) *Handbuch der Experimentellen Pharmakologie,* Vol. 25. Springer-Verlag, Berlin, **1970,** pp. 1–6.

————. A short history of the kallikrein-kinin system. In, *Chemistry and Biology of the Kallikrein-Kinin System in Health and Disease.* (Pisano, J. J., and Austen, K. F., eds.) Department of Health, Education, and Welfare Publication No. (NIH) 76-791, U.S. Government Printing Office, Washington, D. C., **1977,** pp. 1–6.

Wright, F. S., and Briggs, J. P. Feedback control of glomerular blood flow, pressure and filtration rate. *Physiol. Rev.,* **1979,** *59,* 958–1006.

CHAPTER

28 PROSTAGLANDINS, PROSTACYCLIN, AND THROMBOXANE A$_2$

Salvador Moncada, Roderick J. Flower, and John R. Vane

History. There are few substances that currently command more widespread interest in biological circles than do the prostaglandins. Although their history extends back to the early 1930s, it was the isolation, characterization, and synthesis of the representative compounds in the early 1960s that generated such intense interest. The reasons are not hard to find. The prostaglandins are among the most prevalent of autacoids and have been detected in almost every tissue and body fluid; their production increases in response to astonishingly diverse stimuli; they produce, in minute amounts, a remarkably broad spectrum of effects that embraces practically every biological function; and inhibition of their biosynthesis is now recognized as a mechanism of some of the most widely used therapeutic agents, the nonsteroidal anti-inflammatory drugs such as aspirin (*see* Chapter 29).

A harbinger of this remarkable development was the observation made by two American gynecologists, Kurzrok and Lieb (1930), that strips of human uterus relax or contract when exposed to human semen. A few years later, Goldblatt in England and Euler in Sweden independently reported smooth-muscle-contracting and vasodepressor activity in seminal fluid and accessory reproductive glands, and Euler identified the active material as a lipid-soluble acid, which he named "prostaglandin" (*see* Goldblatt, 1935; Euler, 1936, 1973). More than 20 years were to pass before technical advances allowed the demonstration that prostaglandin was in fact a family of compounds of unique structure, permitted the isolation in crystalline form of two prostaglandins, prostaglandin E$_1$ (PGE$_1$) and PGF$_{1\alpha}$, and led to the elucidation of their structures in 1962 (*see* Bergström and Samuelsson, 1968). Soon, more prostaglandins were characterized and, like the others, proved to be 20-carbon unsaturated carboxylic acids with a cyclopentane ring.

When the general structure of the prostaglandins became apparent, their kinship with essential fatty acids was recognized, and in 1964 Bergström and coworkers and van Dorp and associates independently achieved the biosynthesis of PGE$_2$ from arachidonic acid using homogenates of sheep seminal vesicle (*see* Samuelsson, 1972).

Until recently it was believed that PGE$_2$ and PGF$_{2\alpha}$ were the most important prostaglandins. Indeed, thousands of analogs of these compounds were made in the largely frustrated hope that compounds of therapeutic value with a greater selectivity of action would emerge. However, since 1973, several

discoveries have caused a radical shift in emphasis away from PGEs and PGFs. The first was the isolation and identification of two unstable cyclic endoperoxides, prostaglandin G$_2$ (PGG$_2$ or 15-OOH PGH$_2$) and prostaglandin H$_2$ (PGH$_2$) (Hamberg and Samuelsson, 1973; Nugteren and Hazelhof, 1973). Later came the elucidation of the structure of thromboxane A$_2$ (TXA$_2$) and that of its degradation product, thromboxane B$_2$ (TXB$_2$) (Hamberg *et al.*, 1975), and then the discovery of prostacyclin (PGI$_2$) (Moncada *et al.*, 1976). These findings, coupled with the elucidation of ·a different enzymatic pathway (a lipoxygenase), which converts arachidonic acid to compounds such as 12-hydroperoxyarachidonic acid (HPETE) and 12-hydroxyarachidonic acid (HETE), have led to the realization that the "classically known" prostaglandins constitute only a fraction of the physiologically active products of arachidonic acid metabolism. Furthermore, interest in the newer compounds is particularly heightened by observations of their very high potency (*see* Moncada and Vane, 1977; Marcus, 1978; Samuelsson *et al.*, 1978a).

Chemistry. The prostaglandins and related compounds are derived from 20-carbon essential fatty acids that contain three, four, or five double bonds: 8,11,14-eicosatrienoic acid (dihomo-γ-linolenic acid), 5,8,11,14-eicosatetraenoic acid (arachidonic acid) (*see* Figure 28–2), and 5,8,11,14,17-eicosapentaenoic acid. The prostaglandins can be considered as analogs of an unnatural compound with the trivial name *prostanoic acid,* the structure of which is as follows:

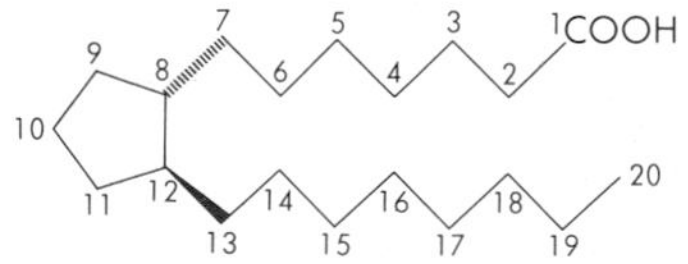

They fall into several main classes, designated by letters and distinguished by substitutions on the cyclopentane ring. These structures are shown in Figure 28–1. The main classes are further subdivided in accord with the number of double bonds in the side chains. This is indicated by subscript 1, 2, or 3, and reflects the fatty acid precursor. Thus, prostaglandins derived from 8,11,14-eicosatrienoic acid carry the subscript 1; those derived from arachidonic acid carry the subscript 2; and those derived from 5,8,11,14,17-eicosapentaenoic acid carry the sub-

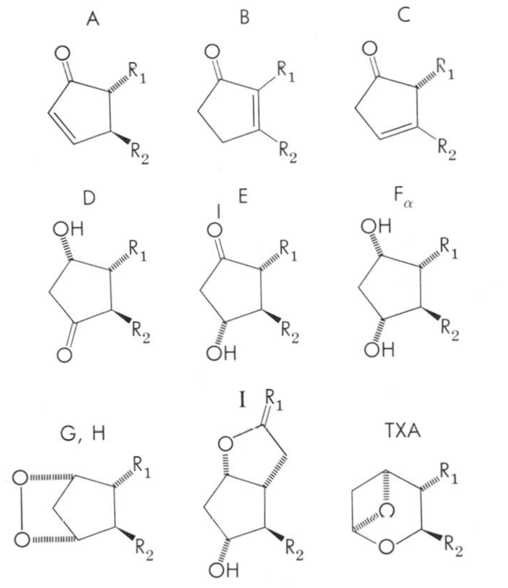

Figure 28-1. *Ring structures of the six "primary" prostaglandins (A-F), the cyclic endoperoxides (G, H), prostacyclin (I), and thromboxane A (TXA).*

In the stereochemical convention followed, the groups indicated by ⚊⚊⚊ lie behind the plane of the cyclopentane ring, while those indicated by ◀ lie in front of it.

script 3. In man, arachidonic acid is the most abundant precursor, and there is little evidence that prostaglandins of the 1 or 3 series are important. However, prostaglandins of the 3 series may have greater significance in fish and marine animals, where 5,8,11,14,17-eicosapentaenoic acid is the predominant precursor.

Prostaglandins of the E and F_α series are sometimes referred to as the "primary prostaglandins." They were believed to be the most abundant (especially E_2 and $F_{2\alpha}$) and have been the most intensively studied. The As, Bs, and Cs are all derivatives of the corresponding Es. Representative formulas are presented in Figure 28-2. (*See* Andersen and Ramwell, 1974.)

Biosynthesis. In man, arachidonic acid is either derived from dietary linoleic acid (octadecadienoic acid) or is ingested as a constituent of meat. It is then esterified as a component of the phospholipids of cell membranes or is found in ester linkage in other complex lipids.

Arachidonic acid is released from membrane phospholipids by the action of the enzyme phospholipase A_2. The concentration of free arachidonic acid is low, and it is therefore generally believed that endogenous biosynthesis of prostaglandins and related compounds depends on this phospholipase-catalyzed release of precursor acid from cellular phospholipid stores. Indeed, activation of phospholipase A_2 has been hypothesized to be the common rate-limiting step in the enhanced biosynthesis that occurs in response to widely divergent physical,

chemical, hormonal, and neurohumoral influences (Flower, 1978a; Marcus, 1978).

Once released, arachidonic acid is rapidly metabolized to oxygenated products by two distinct enzymatic mechanisms, a cyclooxygenase and a lipoxygenase (Figure 28-2).

Cyclooxygenase. Synthesis of the primary prostaglandins is accomplished in stepwise manner by a ubiquitous complex of microsomal enzymes, the first of which is referred to as *fatty acid cyclooxygenase.* The unesterified precursor acids are oxygenated and cyclized to form the cyclic endoperoxide derivatives, prostaglandin G (PGG) and prostaglandin H (PGH). There is an absolute requirement for heme as a cofactor for the formation of PGG, whereas the enzyme that converts PGG to PGH requires tryptophan or a similar substance. These endoperoxides, which are chemically unstable (*e.g.,* PGG_2 and PGH_2 have half-lives of 5 minutes at 37° C and pH 7.5), are then isomerized enzymatically or nonenzymatically into different products, PGE, PGF, or PGD (*see* Figure 28-2; Flower, 1978b). PGA, PGB, and PGC, which arise from the corresponding PGE by dehydration and isomerization, are formed chemically during extraction; probably none of them occurs biologically.

The endoperoxide PGH_2 is also metabolized into two unstable and highly biologically active compounds with structures that differ from those of the primary prostaglandins. One of these is thromboxane A_2 (TXA_2), formed by an enzyme, *thromboxane synthetase,* first isolated from human and equine platelets. TXA_2 has a very short half-life ($t_{1/2} = 30$ seconds at 37° C and pH 7.5), and it contains an oxane ring instead of the cyclopentane of the prostaglandins; it breaks down nonenzymatically into the stable thromboxane B_2 (TXB_2) (Figure 28-2).

The other route of metabolism of PGH_2 is to prostacyclin (PGI_2), yet another unstable compound ($t_{1/2} = 3$ minutes at 37° C and pH 7.5) formed by an enzyme, *prostacyclin synthetase,* first discovered in vascular tissue. PGI_2 has a double-ring structure, closed by an oxygen bridge between carbons 6 and 9. It is hydrolyzed nonenzymatically to a stable compound, 6-keto-PGF_1 (Figure 28-2).

The endoperoxides are also transformed into a 17-carbon hydroxy acid (HHT) with the concomitant formation of malondialdehyde, and, although HHT can be formed nonenzymatically, it is also generated by a purified preparation of thromboxane synthetase.

While tissues seem to be able to synthesize the intermediate prostaglandin endoperoxides from free arachidonic acid, the fate of these endoperoxides in each tissue depends on several factors that have not been clearly defined. Certainly, the presence of the different isomerases varies from tissue to tissue. For example, lung and spleen are able to synthesize the whole range of products, but other tissues cannot; platelets synthesize mainly TXA_2, whereas the blood vessel wall primarily produces PGI_2.

Even though PGE_2, PGD_2, and $PGF_{2\alpha}$ can be formed nonenzymatically, isomerases for the synthesis of PGE_2 and PGD_2 have been identified. However, the existence of a reductase for the synthesis of $PGF_{2\alpha}$ is in doubt. Moreover, the biochemical con-

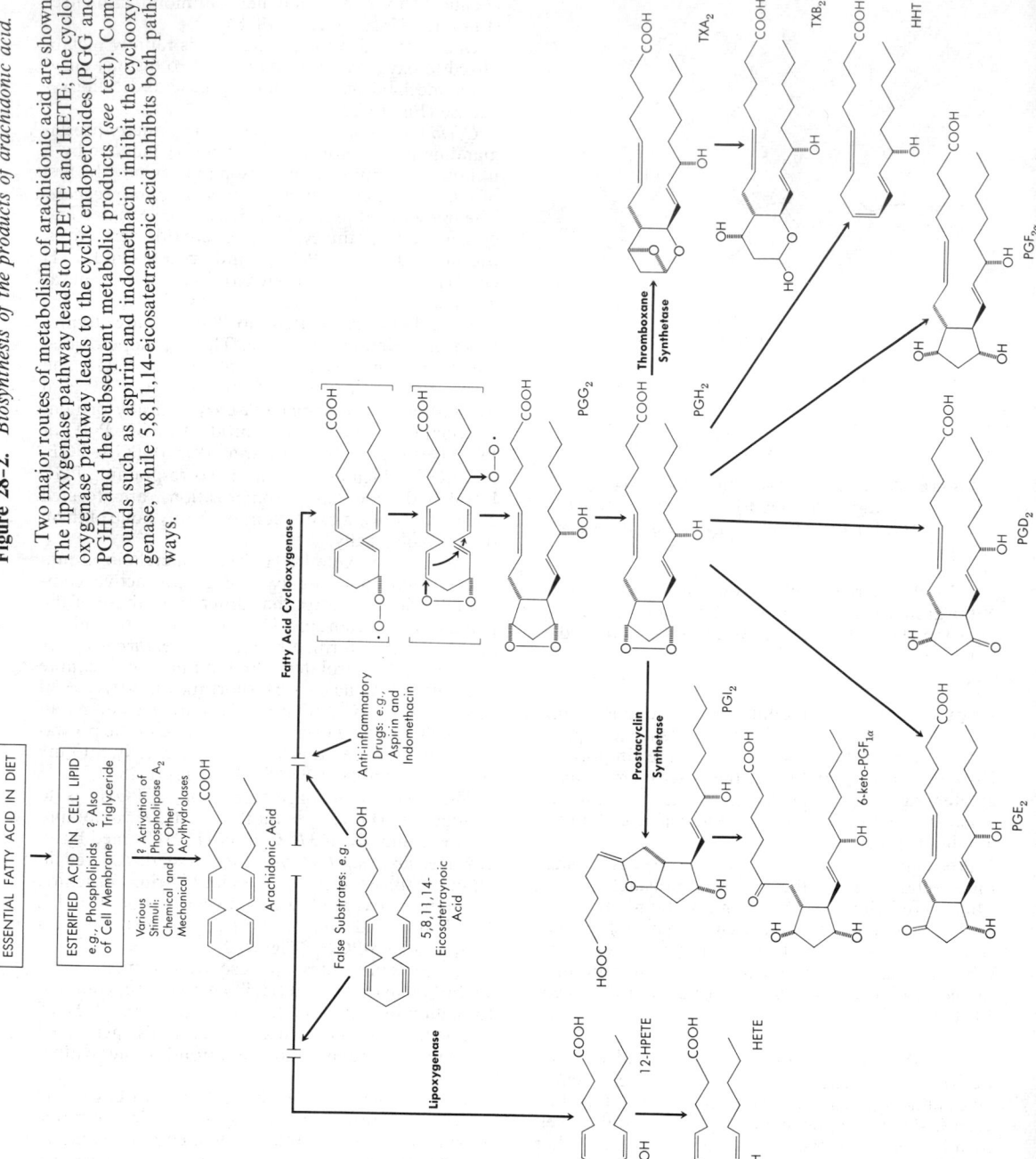

Figure 28–2. *Biosynthesis of the products of arachidonic acid.*

Two major routes of metabolism of arachidonic acid are shown. The lipoxygenase pathway leads to HPETE and HETE; the cyclooxygenase pathway leads to the cyclic endoperoxides (PGG and PGH) and the subsequent metabolic products (*see* text). Compounds such as aspirin and indomethacin inhibit the cyclooxygenase, while 5,8,11,14-eicosatetraenoic acid inhibits both pathways.

ditions under which the enzymes are studied influence the range of products obtained. For example, the production of $PGF_{2\alpha}$ is enhanced in the presence of reducing agents, while certain proteins increase the rate of isomerization of the endoperoxide to PGD_2. Interestingly, glutathione favors the generation of PGE_2.

Lipoxygenase. Despite extensive knowledge of lipid peroxidation and the identification of lipoxygenases in plants, the discovery of mammalian enzymes that catalyze the oxidation of polyunsaturated fatty acids to the corresponding hydroperoxides is relatively novel (Hamberg and Samuelsson, 1974a, 1974b; Nugteren, 1975, 1977). In contrast to fatty acid cyclooxygenase, which is widely distributed, lipoxygenases have so far been found only in lung, platelets, and white cells.

The compounds formed by these enzymes include 12-hydroperoxyarachidonic acid (HPETE) and its degradation product, 12-hydroxyarachidonic acid (HETE) (Figure 28–2). Little is known about the pharmacological activity or the further metabolism of these compounds, although HETE has been shown to be chemotactic for polymorphonuclear leukocytes and alveolar macrophages. This, coupled with the fact that these compounds have been identified in inflammatory exudates, suggests that they might be involved in the process of cellular invasion during inflammation.

There have been several indications in the last few years that slow-reacting substance of anaphylaxis (SRS-A) might be a product of the metabolism of arachidonic acid. Recently, a slow-reacting substance (SRS) produced by mouse mastocytoma cells has been reported to be a novel product of a lipoxygenase pathway. It is formed by the addition of glutathione to an unstable epoxide intermediate (leukotriene A) during the formation of dihydroxylated metabolites of arachidonic acid. The name *leukotriene* has been introduced as a generic name for compounds like SRS that are noncyclized, 20-carbon carboxylic acids with one or two oxygen substituents and three conjugated double bonds (*see* Figure 28–3; Borgeat and Samuelsson, 1979; Murphy *et al.,* 1979; Corey *et al.,* 1980). It is not known if leukotriene C is identical to SRS-A, which is released from lungs, but these findings highlight the importance of the products of the different lipoxygenases in various inflammatory states.

Inhibitors of Prostaglandin Biosynthesis. The association between aspirin-like drugs and prostaglandins became clear in 1971 (Vane, 1971). In retrospect, several observations can be recognized as providing critical clues. Piper and Vane (1969) discovered that an unknown autacoid, which they named rabbit aorta contracting substance (later identified as thromboxane A_2), was released along with other compounds from guinea pig lungs during anaphylaxis; aspirin prevented its escape. Aspirin had also been shown to counter responses to arachidonic acid in some preparations, and arachidonic acid was also found to release rabbit aorta contracting substance (RCS). In 1971, a series of critical observations was made indicating that aspirin and related anti-inflammatory drugs interfere with the liberation of prostaglandins and, in fact, prevent their biosynthesis. The anti-inflammatory agents prevent release of prostaglandins from spleen (Ferreira *et al.,* 1971) and platelets (Smith and Willis, 1971) and prevent the synthesis of prostaglandins from arachidonic acid in tissue homogenates (Vane, 1971). Aspirin and related anti-inflammatory drugs prevent production of the prostaglandin endoperoxides by the cyclooxygenase enzyme and, as a result, all the products below them in the metabolic pathway (*see* Chapter 29; Flower, 1974). Vane (1971) proposed that inhibition of prostaglandin synthesis provides an explanation for both the therapeutic effects and several side effects of aspirin and other anti-inflammatory substances of the nonsteroid type. All these anti-inflammatory compounds inhibit prostaglandin synthesis, and their therapeutic efficacy parallels their ability to inhibit fatty acid cyclooxygenase to a remarkable extent. A clear-cut inhibition of prostaglandin synthesis, as measured by the prostaglandin content of synovial fluid, urine, or semen, is evident in man treated with conventional doses of these anti-inflammatory agents.

It should be noted that analogs of the natural fatty acid precursors serve as competitive inhibitors of prostaglandin production. Among them is the acetylenic analog of arachidonic acid, 5,8,11,14-eicosatetraynoic acid (Figure 28–2) (*see* Lands *et al.,* 1973). The therapeutic potential of agents of this

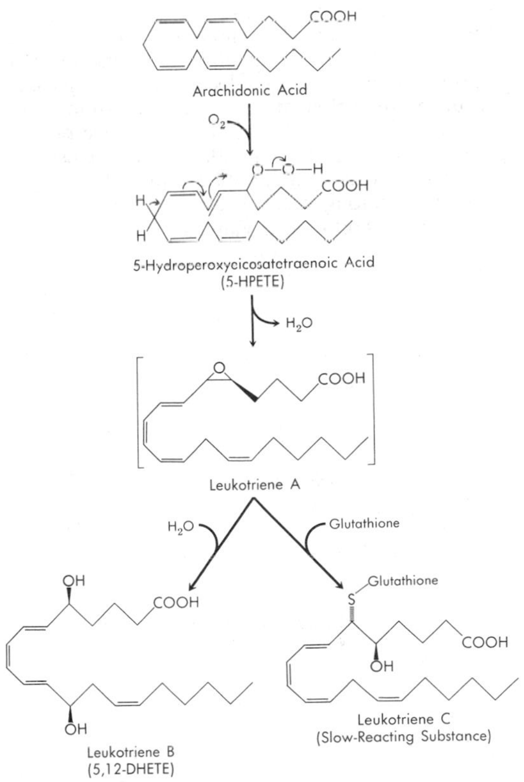

Figure 28–3. *Synthesis and structure of leukotrienes A, B, and C. (See* text for explanation.*)*

type remains to be assessed. Another exciting possibility lies in the development of drugs with preferential inhibitory actions on the enzymes that isomerize the endoperoxides. Compounds such as imidazole and some of its analogs preferentially inhibit thromboxane synthetase. Some chemical analogs of the prostaglandin endoperoxides are also powerful inhibitors of this enzyme. On the other hand, lipid peroxides, such as 15-hydroperoxyarachidonic acid, and their methyl esters preferentially inhibit the formation of PGI$_2$ in vitro. Selective inhibitors of PGE$_2$ or PGD$_2$ isomerases have not yet been described. The potential advantage of such compounds over the aspirin-like drugs lies in the possibility of interfering with formation of, for example, TXA$_2$ while leaving intact or enhanced the formation of other products, such as PGI$_2$ (Moncada and Vane, 1977, 1978a, 1978b).

Catabolism. Efficient mechanisms exist for the catabolism and inactivation of most prostaglandins. Such activity in certain vascular beds, for example, that of the lung, is well illustrated by the observation that 95% of infused PGE$_2$ is inactivated during one passage through the pulmonary circulation (Ferreira and Vane, 1967). Hamberg and Samuelsson (1971) showed that only 3% of an intravenous dose of PGE$_2$ remained in the plasma after 90 seconds. Selective cellular uptake of certain prostaglandins precedes their metabolism during passage through the pulmonary circulation. Because of the unique position of the lungs between the venous and arterial circulation, the pulmonary vascular bed constitutes an important filter for many substances (including some prostaglandins) that might be released from tissues into the venous circulation. The clearance of these potent, smooth-muscle-stimulating substances protects the cardiovascular system and other organs from their prolonged effects due to recirculation (*see* Vane, 1969; Bakhle and Vane, 1977).

Broadly speaking, the enzymatic catabolic reactions are of two types: an initial (relatively rapid) step, catalyzed by prostaglandin-specific enzymes, wherein prostaglandins lose most of their biological activity, and a second (relatively slow) step in which these metabolites are oxidized by enzymes probably identical to those responsible for the β and ω oxidation of most fatty acids. This sequence of reactions, which leads to the appearance of the metabolites in the urine, has been investigated in man (Hamberg and Samuelsson, 1971); the degradation of PGE$_2$ is summarized in Figure 28-4.

The initial step is the oxidation of the 15-OH group to the corresponding ketone by prostaglandin 15-OH dehydrogenase (PGDH) (Anggard and Samuelsson, 1964; Hamberg and Samuelsson, 1971). The 15-keto compound is then reduced to the 13,14-dihydro derivative, a reaction catalyzed by prostaglandin Δ^{13}-reductase (Anggard et al., 1971). While these first two reactions occur very rapidly, subsequent steps are slower. These consist of β and ω oxidation of the side chains of the prostaglandins, giving rise to a polar dicarboxylic acid, which is excreted in the urine as the major metabolite of both PGE$_1$ and PGE$_2$.

Enzymes that catalyze the degradation of prostaglandins are widely distributed in the body and are present in the spleen, kidney, adipose tissue, intestine, liver, and testicle, as well as in the lung. The enzymes responsible for β or ω oxidation are found in the liver, lung, kidney, and intestine. The liver is probably the major site for side chain oxidation (*see* Samuelsson et al., 1975; Flower, 1978b).

Studies on the metabolism of TXB$_2$ in monkeys have shown that a minor fraction of the compound is excreted unchanged after intravenous infusion and approximatly 30% is excreted as the product of single β oxidation, dinor TXB$_2$ (Kindahl, 1977; Roberts et al., 1977a). In man, the major urinary metabolite following an infusion of TXB$_2$ is also dinor TXB$_2$;

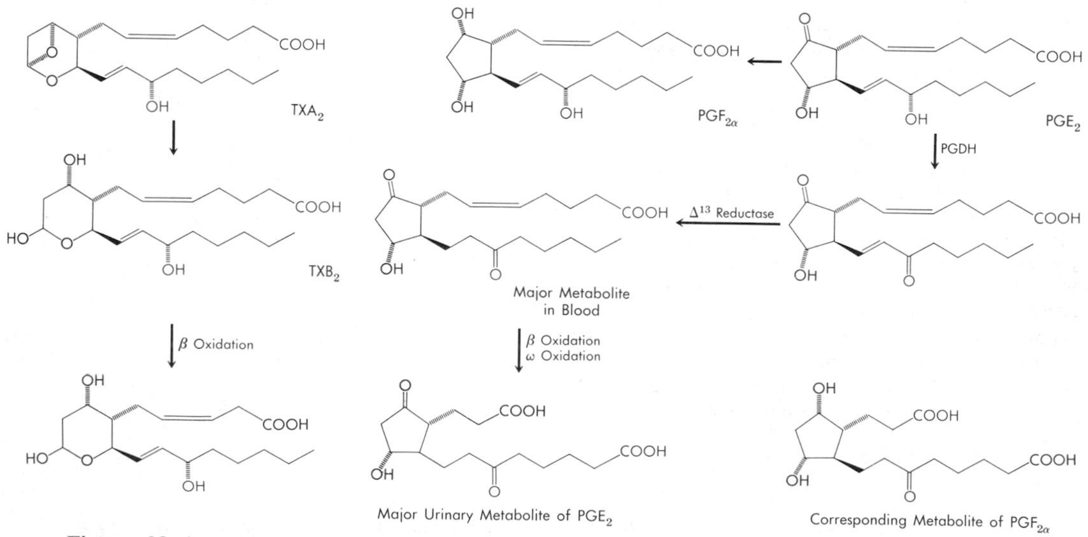

Figure 28-4. *Metabolism of PGE$_2$, PGF$_{2\alpha}$, and thromboxane A$_2$ (TXA$_2$). (See text for* explanation.)

other metabolic transformations also occur (Roberts *et al.*, 1977b).

The metabolism of PGI_2 has, to date, been studied only in rats. The compound is extensively metabolized; the fact that the majority of the metabolites have a keto group at carbon 15 suggests that a substantial fraction of the compound is metabolized by 15-OH prostaglandin dehydrogenase (Sun and Taylor, 1978).

PHARMACOLOGICAL PROPERTIES

No other autacoids show more numerous and diverse effects than do prostaglandins and related products. Those who have reviewed the field have remarked on this "awesome" and "bewildering" diversity. Not only is the spectrum of actions broad, but also different prostaglandins show different activities, both qualitatively and quantitatively. It would be confusing to present the myriad of pharmacological effects that have been ascribed to the natural prostaglandins and even more so to delve into the activities of their synthetic analogs. This discussion is limited to those activities that are thought to be the most important.

Cardiovascular System. In most species and in most vascular beds PGEs and PGAs are potent vasodilators; when injected into the femoral arterial bed in dogs, their potency exceeds that of acetylcholine or histamine, although it is less than that of bradykinin. Responses to $PGF_{2\alpha}$ show species variation, but vasodilatation has been observed following injection into the human brachial artery of $PGF_{2\alpha}$ and PGs A_1, A_2, B_1, E_1, and E_2 (Robinson *et al.*, 1973). PGA_1 has vasodilatory effects on coronary and other human vascular beds (Barner *et al.*, 1973). Dilatation in response to prostaglandins seemingly involves arterioles, precapillaries, sphincters, and postcapillary venules. PGEs are not universally vasodilatory; constrictor effects have been noted at selected sites. Superficial veins of the hand are contracted by $PGF_{2\alpha}$, but not by PGEs. The behavior of other large-capacitance veins in various animals is similar (*see* Nakano, 1973).

Cardiac output is generally increased by PGs E, F, and A. Weak, direct inotropic effects have been noted in various isolated preparations. In the intact animal, however, increased force of contraction as well as increased heart rate is in large measure a reflex consequence of fall in total peripheral resistance. Systemic blood pressure generally falls in response to PGs E and A, and blood flow to most organs, including the heart and kidney, is increased. These effects are particularly striking in some patients with hypertensive disease (*see* Lee, 1974).

Prostaglandin endoperoxides (both being roughly equipotent) have variable effects in vascular beds ranging from vasodilatation to vasoconstriction, and sometimes they induce constriction followed by dilatation (*see* Dusting *et al.*, 1979). Since the endoperoxides are substrates for conversion to other potent prostaglandins, their effects are a result of intrinsic vasoconstrictor activity coupled with some vasodilatation due to rapid conversion to a prostaglandin that is a vasodilator (most probably prostacyclin

[PGI_2]). They are rapidly converted into PGI_2 during passage through the lungs; PGH_2 is thus less active as a hypotensive agent when injected intra-arterially than when given intravenously (Armstrong *et al.*, 1976).

While very few studies have been performed with thromboxane A_2 (TXA_2) because of its intrinsic instability, it contracts all vascular smooth muscle strips tested; indeed, TXA_2 was first detected as the rabbit aorta contracting substance (RCS) (Piper and Vane, 1969). It appears to be a powerful vasoconstrictor in the whole animal and in isolated vascular beds (Dusting *et al.*, 1978; Samuelsson *et al.*, 1978b). TXB_2 is inactive when effects on the cardiovascular system are tested.

The administration of PGI_2 causes prominent hypotension in animals, including man. It is about five times more potent than PGE_2 in producing this effect. The compound causes dilatation in various vascular beds, including the coronary, renal, mesenteric, and skeletal muscle, and it relaxes essentially all isolated preparations of vascular smooth muscle that have been tested. Its degradation product, 6-keto-$PGF_{1\alpha}$, is at least 1000 times less active than PGI_2. Because it is not inactivated by the pulmonary circulation, PGI_2 is equipotent as a vasodilator when given either intra-arterially or intravenously (Moncada and Vane, 1978a; Szczeklik *et al.*, 1978).

Blood. The prostaglandins and related products exert powerful actions on platelets. Some of them, like PGE_1 and PGD_2, are inhibitors of the aggregation of human platelets *in vitro* at concentrations around 0.1 μM. PGI_2 is some 30 to 50 times more potent, inhibiting aggregation at concentrations between 1 and 10 nM. This fact and the observation that PGI_2 is generated by the vascular wall (particularly by the vascular endothelium) have led to the suggestion that the substance controls the aggregation of platelets *in vivo*. PGE_2 exerts variable effects on platelets; it is a potentiator of some forms of aggregation at low concentrations (below 1 μM) and an inhibitor at higher concentrations.

One of the products of arachidonic acid metabolism in platelets, TXA_2, is a very powerful inducer of platelet aggregation and the platelet release reaction. The endoperoxides, although active, are much less so than TXA_2. This physiological pathway of platelet aggregation, dependent on the generation of TXA_2, is sensitive to the inhibitory action of aspirin (*see* Chapter 29; Smith and Macfarlane, 1974; Smith *et al.*, 1977; Moncada and Vane, 1978b).

FGA_2, PGE_1, and PGE_2 induce erythropoiesis by stimulating the release of erythropoietin from the renal cortex (*see* Fisher and Gross, 1977). Moreover, PGE_1 and PGE_2 produce variable effects on the fragility of red cells; at very low concentrations (10 to 100 pM) they decrease fragility, while at higher concentrations (1 nM) they increase it (Rasmussen and Lake, 1977).

Smooth Muscle. Prostaglandins contract or relax many smooth muscles beside those of the vasculature. Again, responses may vary with species, type of prostaglandin, endocrine status of the tissue, and experimental conditions. However, few smooth muscles are uninfluenced, and many display intense and consistent responses.

Bronchial and Tracheal Muscle. In general, PGFs contract and PGEs relax bronchial and tracheal muscle from various species, including man. Asthmatic individuals are particularly sensitive, and PGF$_{2\alpha}$ has caused intense bronchospasm. In contrast, both PGE$_1$ and PGE$_2$ are potent bronchodilators when given to such patients by aerosol; the potency of PGE$_1$ may exceed that of isoproterenol (*see* Cuthbert, 1973; Parker and Snider, 1973; Zurier, 1974). Prostaglandin endoperoxides and TXA$_2$ are constrictors of guinea pig tracheal strips *in vitro.* TXA$_2$ is the more potent and induces bronchoconstriction in guinea pigs when given by aerosol (Hamberg *et al.,* 1976). PGI$_2$, on the other hand, is without effect or induces slight bronchodilatation; it antagonizes bronchoconstriction produced by other agents in man (Bianco *et al.,* 1978).

Uterus. PGEs and PGFs produce strong contraction of isolated guinea pig uteri in estrus or diestrus. Strips of nonpregnant human uterus are contracted by PGFs but relaxed by PGs E, A, and B. The contractile response is most prominent before menstruation, whereas relaxation is greatest at mid-cycle. Uterine strips from pregnant women are uniformly contracted by PGEs and PGFs. In contrast to the *in-vitro* behavior, the human uterus *in vivo,* whether pregnant or not, is always contracted by PGE$_1$, PGE$_2$, and PGF$_{2\alpha}$ administered intravenously. The response is prompt and dose dependent, and takes the form of a sharp rise in tonus with superimposed rhythmic contractions, which long outlast the tonic phase. Intravenous infusion results in sustained labor-like contractions with tone falling between each. In contrast to oxytocin (*see* Chapter 39), this effect is observed at all stages of pregnancy, although as with oxytocin sensitivity does increase at term (*see* Karim, 1972; Karim and Hillier, 1973; Behrman and Anderson, 1974). PGI$_2$, 6-keto-PGF$_{1\alpha}$, the prostaglandin endoperoxides, and TXA$_2$ are much less active in causing contractions of uterine muscle *in vitro* (Omini *et al.,* 1978). Indeed, PGI$_2$ antagonizes contractions of strips from pregnant human uterus induced by other prostaglandins.

Gastrointestinal Muscle. *In-vitro* responses vary widely with species, segment, type of muscle, and the particular prostaglandin. In the main, longitudinal muscle from stomach to colon is contracted by both PGEs and PGFs, while circular muscle generally relaxes to PGEs and contracts to PGFs. Prostaglandins of the A and D series generally have little activity. The *in-vivo* effects are also variable in man. Shortened transit times have been observed in the small intestine and colon. Diarrhea, cramps, and reflux of bile have been noted in response to oral PGE; these are common side effects (along with nausea and vomiting) in patients given prostaglandins for abortion (*see* Wilson, 1974; Bennett, 1977). Prostaglandin endoperoxides and TXA$_2$ contract longitudinal smooth muscle but are less active than the PGEs or PGFs. PGI$_2$ weakly contracts longitudinal smooth muscle strips of the rat stomach but has little effect on or decreases spontaneous rhythmic movements of the rat colon.

Gastric, Pancreatic, and Intestinal Secretions. PGEs, PGAs, and PGI$_2$ inhibit gastric acid secretion stimulated by feeding, histamine, or gastrin (Robert, 1977; Whittle *et al.,* 1978). Certain methylated analogs of prostaglandins likewise inhibit gastric secretion in man following oral or intravenous administration (Karim and Fung, 1976), raising the possibility of their therapeutic utility for peptic ulcer. Volume of secretion, acidity, and content of pepsin are all reduced, probably by an action exerted directly on the secretory cells. In addition, these prostaglandins are vasodilators in the gastric mucosa and may be involved in the local regulation of blood flow. In the pancreas, PGE$_1$ inhibits the secretion of fluid and electrolytes in both the resting gland and that stimulated by secretin or pancreozymin; the secretion of pancreatic enzymes may be stimulated (Rudick *et al.,* 1971). Mucus secretion in the stomach and small intestine is increased by prostaglandins, and there is substantial movement of water and electrolytes into the intestinal lumen. Such effects may underlie the watery diarrhea noted in animals and man following the oral or parenteral administration of prostaglandins. Effects of prostaglandins on water and electrolyte transport in other epithelial systems are mentioned below (*see* Bennett, 1972; Wilson, 1974). In contrast to PGE$_2$ and PGF$_{2\alpha}$, PGI$_2$ does not induce diarrhea in animals or man; indeed, it prevents that provoked by other prostaglandins and inhibits the toxin-induced accumulation of intestinal fluid in experimental models.

Kidney and Urine Formation. PGEs, PGAs, and PGI$_2$, but not 6-keto-PGF$_{1\alpha}$, infused directly into the renal arteries of dogs increase renal blood flow and provoke diuresis, natriuresis, and kaliuresis; there is little change in the rate of glomerular filtration (Zins, 1975; Dunn and Hood, 1977; Bolger *et al.,* 1978; Hill and Moncada, 1979). These effects of prostaglandins seem to result from a direct action on tubular transport processes (Grenier and Smith, 1978) or through changes in the distribution of renal blood flow. In addition, there is evidence that PGI$_2$ may mediate the release of renin from the renal cortex (Gerber *et al.,* 1978). In certain human subjects with hypertension, the intravenous injection of PGA$_1$ in amounts below those affecting systemic blood pressure causes a substantial increase in renal plasma flow, glomerular filtration rate, urine flow, and output of sodium and potassium. When PGA$_1$ is infused at higher rates in these individuals, parameters of renal function return toward normal as peripheral resistance falls. (*See* Arendshorst *et al.,* 1974; McGiff *et al.,* 1974.) PGEs inhibit water reabsorption induced by antidiuretic hormone (ADH) in toad bladder and in rabbit collecting tubules (*see* Nakano and Koss, 1973).

Central Nervous System. Many stimulant and depressant effects of prostaglandins on the central nervous system (CNS) have been reported (*see* Horton, 1969, 1972; Coceani, 1974). Among them is sedation; stupor, catatonia, and other behavioral changes follow injection of PGEs (but not PGFs) into the cerebral ventricles in cats. Many of these effects require rather high concentrations of prostaglandins. The firing rates of individual brain cells may be increased or decreased after application of PGE or PGF by microiontophoresis. Especially noteworthy is fever caused in various species in response to intracerebroventricular injection of PGE but not PGF or PGA. Release of PGE_2 into the CNS may explain the genesis of pyrogen-induced fever and symptoms related to it, such as malaise (*see* below; Feldberg, 1974).

Afferent Nerves and Pain. In man, PGEs cause pain when injected intradermally, and they irritate the mucous membranes of the eyes and respiratory passages. These effects are generally not as immediate or intense as those caused by bradykinin or histamine, but they outlast those caused by the other autacoids and are accompanied by tenderness and hyperalgesia. PGEs and PGI_2 sensitize the afferent nerve endings to the effects of chemical or mechanical stimuli; the release of these prostaglandins during the inflammatory process thus serves as an amplification system for the pain mechanism (*see* Ferreira *et al.*, 1974). The role of PGE_2 and PGI_2 in inflammation is discussed in Chapter 29.

Endocrine System. A variety of endocrine tissues respond to prostaglandins. In the rat, PGE_1 and PGFs stimulate the release of ACTH *in vivo,* and PGFs enhance the release of growth hormone *in vitro.* $PGF_{2\alpha}$ also has a stimulatory effect on the secretion of prolactin and gonadotropins. PGE_2 facilitates the release of luteinizing hormone (LH) and thyrotropin (*see* Hodge and Walters, 1975). Other effects include stimulation of steroid production by the adrenals, stimulation of insulin release (Johnson *et al.*, 1973), thyrotropin-like effects on the thyroid (Mashiter and Field, 1974), and LH-like effects on isolated ovarian tissue, causing increased progesterone secretion from the corpus luteum. This last effect, observed *in vitro,* contrasts with what is perhaps the most remarkable of all the effects of prostaglandins in the endocrine system, namely, luteolysis. This property is possessed especially but not uniquely by $PGF_{2\alpha}$.

Luteolysis. Prompt subsidence of progesterone output and regression of the corpus luteum follows parenteral injection of $PGF_{2\alpha}$ in a wide variety of mammals. This effect interrupts early pregnancy, which is dependent on luteal rather than placental progesterone (*see* Pharriss and Behrman, 1973). The mechanism of luteolysis is uncertain, but it may involve block of the normal ovarian response to circulating gonadotropin. The abortifacient action of prostaglandins in early human pregnancy does not seem to be accompanied by any demonstrable fall in plasma progesterone concentrations, and luteolysis is not a significant factor (*see* Goldberg and Ramwell, 1975; Horton and Poyser, 1976).

Metabolic Effects. PGEs, notably PGE_1, inhibit the basal rate of lipolysis from adipose tissue *in vitro* and also lipolysis stimulated by exposure to catecholamines or other lipolytic hormones. Such effects have also been noted *in vivo* in various species, including man, but are more capricious. Indeed, low doses of PGE_1 in man tend to stimulate lipolysis,

seemingly by an indirect effect mediated by sympathetic stimulation. PGEs also have some insulin-like effects on carbohydrate metabolism (Nakano, 1973) and exert parathyroid hormone-like effects that result in mobilization of calcium from bone in tissue culture (Klein and Raisz, 1970).

Autonomic Nervous System. Effects of prostaglandins on autonomic ganglia and the adrenal medulla have generally been negligible. On the other hand, prostaglandins often modify sympathetic neuroeffector junctions, sometimes in exceedingly low concentration. PGEs inhibit norepinephrine output from adrenergic nerve endings and depress the response of the innervated structures. However, such effects are not uniformly observed and vary with species, tissue, and experimental conditions. Moreover, contrary effects leading to increased output of norepinephrine or heightened responsiveness of the effector organ have been noted, particularly with PGFs. Such facilitatory effects could contribute to the arteriolar-constricting and venoconstricting actions of $PGF_{2\alpha}$. Prostaglandin endoperoxides inhibit the release of transmitter in some preparations *in vitro*, such as the vas deferens, probably due to conversion to PGE_2. PGI_2 does not inhibit transmitter release but depresses the responses to agonists in preparations such as isolated spiral strips of veins (*see* Hedqvist, 1973, 1976; Brody and Kadowitz, 1974; Herman *et al.*, 1978).

Mechanism of Action. The acidic lipid nature of prostaglandins places them in a unique chemical class of autacoids and raises the question whether their diverse actions can be accommodated within the familiar concept of specific membrane-bound receptors of the sort invoked to explain the actions of autacoids of the classical amine or peptide type. Nevertheless, receptors for PGE_1, PGE_2, and $PGF_{2\alpha}$ have been identified by ligand binding studies.

In many tissues prostaglandins stimulate the synthesis of cyclic adenosine $3',5'$-monophosphate (cyclic AMP) by activating adenylate cyclase. It has been proposed that prostaglandins are released by hormonal stimulation and in turn stimulate the enzyme. On the other hand, stimulation of prostaglandin biosynthesis by cyclic AMP has also been demonstrated in different types of tissues. A positive feedback between prostaglandins and the cyclic AMP system has thus been suggested. There are, however, effects of prostaglandins that are independent of cyclic AMP. Relationships between prostaglandins and cyclic guanosine $3',5'$-monophosphate (cyclic GMP) have also been described, but their significance is far less clear (Ramwell and Shaw, 1970; Katz and Katz, 1974; Samuelsson *et al.*, 1978a; Vapaatalo and Parantainen, 1978).

The mechanism of action of prostaglandins and related substances has been studied intensively in platelets. PGI_2, PGE_1, and PGD_2 appear to inhibit platelet aggregation by increasing the concentrations of cyclic AMP (although PGD_2 acts on a different receptor than do PGE_1 and PGI_2). PGE_2, which has a weak biphasic effect on platelet aggregation, increases cyclic AMP concentrations at inhibitory concentrations of the prostaglandin and lowers these values at concentrations that facilitate aggregation. The prostaglandin endoperoxides and TXA_2, which cause platelet clumping, also reduce the activity of adenylate cyclase, demonstrable as an inhibition of the increase in cyclic AMP induced by PGE_1 or PGI_2. There is some suggestion that PGH_2 or TXA_2 lowers basal concentrations of cyclic AMP in platelets. Whether these effects are exerted directly or through an effect on intracellular calcium is still debated. However, there is some evidence that TXA_2 acts as a calcium ionophore (Gerrard *et al.*, 1976; Smith *et al.*, 1977; Gorman *et al.*, 1978). Stimulation of smooth muscle by prostaglandins appears to be associated with the depolarization of cellular membranes and the release of bound calcium.

Inhibitors of Responses to Prostaglandins. There are presently no universally effective, potent antagonists of responses to the prostaglandins. However, some compounds are effective in selected *in-vitro* tests, and a few of these may be of practical value *in vivo*. Contractions in response to $PGF_{2\alpha}$ in isolated human bronchial muscle are inhibited by *fenamates, phenylbutazone,* and, less potently, *aspirin* (*see* Collier, 1971a, 1971b). The most important prostaglandin antagonists are of three types: the 7-oxa analogs of the prostaglandin molecule (*e.g.,* 7-oxa-13-prostanoic acid); the dibenzoxazepine hydrazide derivatives, of which SC-19220 is the most representative; and polyphloretin phosphate, a polyanionic polyester of phloretin and phosphoric acid, and related compounds. While these compounds block the effects of prostaglandins on certain cells, they fail to do so uniformly. This presumably reflects heterogeneity of receptors for this complex class of autacoids. Attempts are also being made to develop antagonists of the actions of prostaglandin endoperoxides and TXA_2 by alteration of the structure of the parent compounds (Bennett, 1974; Sanner and Eakins, 1976; Gorman *et al.*, 1978).

ENDOGENOUS PROSTAGLANDINS: POSSIBLE FUNCTIONS IN PHYSIOLOGICAL AND PATHOLOGICAL PROCESSES

With some autacoids, the scope of permissible conjecture on their possible involvement in normal and abnormal functions is limited by their restricted distribution. This is not so with the prostaglandins. Because these substances can probably be formed by virtually every tissue and cell type, it is not unreasonable to suspect that each pharmacological effect observed may reflect a physiological or pathophysiological function. And such suspicions have been nurtured and presented in countless hypotheses bearing on just about every bodily function (*see* appended list of monographs and reviews).

Platelets. An area in which there has been considerable interest is the elucidation of the role played by prostaglandin endoperoxides and TXA_2 in platelet aggregation and by PGI_2 in the prevention of such aggregation. It is generally accepted that stimulation of platelets to aggregate leads to activation of a membrane phospholipase with the consequent release of arachidonic acid and its transformation into

prostaglandin endoperoxides and TXA_2. These substances induce platelet aggregation. However, this pathway is not the only mechanism for the induction of platelet aggregation, since, for example, thrombin aggregates platelets without the release of arachidonic acid. The importance of the thromboxane pathway is, however, implied by the fact that aspirin inhibits the second phase of platelet aggregation and induces a mild hemostatic defect (Jobim, 1978).

PGI_2 generated in the vessel wall may be the physiological antagonist of this system in platelets. It has been suggested that PGI_2 is present in low concentrations in the circulation and is responsible for lack of aggregation of normal platelets. According to this concept, PGI_2 and TXA_2 represent biologically opposite poles of a mechanism for regulating platelet–vessel wall interaction and the formation of hemostatic plugs and intra-arterial thrombi (Moncada and Vane, 1978b). In this respect, there is evidence that the cyclooxygenase in the platelets is more sensitive to inhibition by aspirin than is the enzyme that synthesizes PGI_2 in the vessel wall. Aspirin in small doses has an antithrombotic effect and increases bleeding time in man; these effects disappear when high doses of aspirin are administered (*see* Moncada and Vane, 1978b).

Endocrine and Reproductive Systems. Much interest is attached to the possible involvement of prostaglandins in *reproductive physiology* (*see* Karim and Hillier, 1973; Behrman and Anderson, 1974). Their very high concentrations in human semen, coupled with the substantial absorption of prostaglandins by the vagina, have encouraged speculation that prostaglandins deposited during coitus may facilitate conception by actions on the cervix, uterine body, Fallopian tubes, and transport of semen. However, it should be pointed out that prostaglandins are sparse or absent in the semen of some species. Moreover, antifertility properties can be recognized in some effects of prostaglandins on ovum transport and implantation. Although there does seem to be correlation between the amounts of prostaglandins in the semen and some cases of male infertility, the role of the autacoids in semen remains obscure.

Prostaglandins cause contractions of the uterus of several species, including the human pregnant uterus, and they are luteolytic in many subprimate species. Concentrations of prostaglandins in blood and amniotic fluid are elevated in many species, including man, during labor. This has led to the suggestion that an increased intrauterine synthesis of a prostaglandin ($F_{2\alpha}$) initiates and maintains uterine contractions during labor. Moreover, since prostaglandins that contract the uterus have been found in the human endometrium, it has been suggested that increased synthesis of prostaglandins explains the pathophysiology of dysmenorrhea. This suggestion is strengthened by the finding that inhibitors of cyclooxygenase reduce pain in this condition.

$PGF_{2\alpha}$ produced in the uterus is the long-sought luteolytic hormone in some subprimate species. This knowledge has led to the development of prostaglandin analogs for veterinary use in synchronizing estrus in farm animals such as sheep, cattle, pigs, and horses. This method has simplified breeding procedures and is used to provide safe, early abortions before the animals are sent to market. However, a luteolytic prostaglandin analog for human use has not been developed.

Plasma concentrations of prostaglandins are elevated during labor in sheep, goats, and human subjects. Treatment with inhibitors of cyclooxygenase delays parturition in pregnant rats. A similar effect has been observed in women; Waltman and associates (1973) observed that the time between intra-amniotic instillation of hypertonic saline solution and the ensuing abortion was almost doubled in women treated with indomethacin. In a retrospective survey of 103 patients taking high doses of aspirin during the last two trimesters of pregnancy, Lewis and Shulman (1973) found a very significant increase in the average length of gestation and in the mean duration of spontaneous labor.

There is also considerable evidence implicating prostaglandins in premature labor. Inhibitors of prostaglandin biosynthesis such as indomethacin, sodium salicylate, or aspirin reduce contractions of the uterus in premature labor and may allow delivery to be postponed until adequate fetal maturity is achieved. However, it has not been established whether these drugs are superior to other therapeutic measures. Moreover, potential side effects, such as increases in ante- and post-partum blood loss, stillbirths, and neonatal hemorrhage, have not been evaluated. Inhibitors of cyclooxygenase can also interfere with the cardiovascular system of the fetus (*see* below). The possible roles of prostaglandins in reproductive processes have been reviewed by Goldberg and Ramwell (1975), Horton and Poyser (1976), and Karim (1978).

Increased biosynthesis of prostaglandins has been associated with Bartter's syndrome. This is a rare disease characterized by low to normal blood pressure, decreased sensitivity to angiotensin, high activity of renin in plasma, hyperaldosteronism, and excessive loss of potassium. There is also an increased granulation of renal medullary interstitial cells and an increased excretion of prostaglandins in the urine. After chronic administration of inhibitors of cyclooxygenase, sensitivity to angiotensin, plasma renin values, and the concentration of aldosterone in plasma return to normal. Although plasma potassium rises, it remains low, and urinary potassium wasting persists. Whether an increase in prostaglandin biosynthesis is the cause of Bartter's syndrome or a reflection of a more basic physiological defect is not known (Gill *et al.,* 1976; Ferris, 1978). However, PGI_2 has been implicated as an obligatory mediator in at least one pathway leading to the secretion of renin by the kidney (*see* below).

Vascular and Pulmonary Smooth Muscle. Local generation of PGE_2 and PGI_2 has been implicated in the maintenance of patency of the ductus arteriosus. This hypothesis has been strengthened by the fact that aspirin-like drugs induce closure of a patent ductus in animals and neonates (*see* Chapter 29). Prostaglandins might also play a role in the maintenance of placental blood flow (Friedman *et al.,* 1978; Heymann and Rudolph, 1978; Rankin, 1978).

The interesting notion has been advanced that an abnormal preponderance or imbalance of $PGF_{2\alpha}$ (constrictor) over PGE_2 (dilator) could contribute to high bronchial tone in asthma (*see* Cuthbert, 1973). TXA_2 and PGI_2 are also now recognized as products of metabolism in the lung. They are generated in different sites—TXA_2 mainly in the parenchyma and PGI_2 mainly in the vascular tissue; an imbalance between these products could also contribute to asthma (Mathe *et al.,* 1977; Boot *et al.,* 1978). Moreover, it has been suggested that the lung releases PGI_2 into the circulation. Such a release could control platelet aggregability *in vivo* and could be a physiological mechanism for dispersing clumps of platelets trapped in the fine vessels of the pulmonary circulation (Gryglewski *et al.,* 1978; Moncada *et al.,* 1978).

Kidney. Several signs point to functions within the kidney, including mediation of reactive (ischemic) hyperemia, modulation of renal blood flow (Herbaczynska-Cedro and Vane, 1973, 1974) and of the intrarenal effects of the renin-angiotensin system (Aiken and Vane, 1973), and renovascular and tubular effects regulating urine formation. There is, moreover, the possibility that the well-known antihypertensive property of the normally functioning kidney may be related to its capacity to synthesize and release, locally or into the systemic circulation, natriuretic and blood pressure–lowering PGE_2 or PGI_2. PGI_2, but not 6-keto-$PGF_{1\alpha}$, is a potent, direct stimulus for the secretion of renin from the kidney *in vitro* (Whorton *et al.,* 1977) and *in vivo* (Gerber *et al.,* 1978); this effect is not convincingly elicited by other prostaglandins. It is thus possible that endogenous PGI_2 regulates this important function *in vivo* (*see* Dusting *et al.,* 1978).

Inflammatory and Immune Responses. Prostaglandins are released by a host of mechanical, thermal, chemical, bacterial, and other insults and contribute importantly to the genesis of the signs and symptoms of the inflammatory process (Ferreira *et al.,* 1974; *see* Vane, 1978). PGEs and PGI_2 enhance the pain-producing activity and the edema-inducing effect of bradykinin and other autacoids (*see* Chapter 27). However, PGEs suppress the secretion of mediators of inflammation by mast cells in anaphylactic reactions and inhibit the participation of lymphocytes in delayed hypersensitivity reactions. Moreover, they inhibit the release of hydrolases and lysosomal enzymes from human neutrophils as well as from mouse peritoneal macrophages.

Prostaglandins have also been implicated in the control of the immunological response. PGE_1 has been claimed to regulate the functions of B lymphocytes selectively and to act synergistically with procarbazine to depress immune responsiveness. In addition, the humoral antibody response is decreased by PGE_1. Prostaglandins also affect T lymphocytes. The T ("killer") lymphocyte, active in slowing tumor growth and killing malignant cells, is inhibited by PGEs in its ability to reject allogenic thymus cells *in vitro*. Exogenously administered prostaglandins have been reported to cause an enhanced graft-versus-host reaction and to prolong skin allograft survival. Concentrations of PGE in plasma increase in proportion to the hypersensitized state and return to normal with acceptance of the graft. It has thus been suggested that prostaglandins, by inhibiting T- and B-cell functions, might facilitate graft acceptance. Finally, PGE is also active in inhibiting production and release of lymphokines by sensitized T lymphocytes.

Some experimental tumors in animals and certain spontaneous human tumors (medullary carcinoma of the thyroid, renal-cell adenocarcinoma, carcinoma of the breast) are accompanied by increased concentrations of local or circulating prostaglandins, bone metastasis, and hypercalcemia. The immunosuppressive activity of certain of these tumors may be related to their ability to produce prostaglandins. Furthermore, since prostaglandins of the E series have potent osteolytic activity, it has been suggested that they are implicated in the process of hypercalcemia. Consequently, aspirin or indomethacin has been used to treat this syndrome, with success in some patients. A current hypothesis is that patients with tumors, metastasis, and hypercalcemia can be divided into two subgroups: those with increased concentrations of prostaglandins, who will respond to treatment with aspirin-like drugs; and those with low concentrations of prostaglandins, who will not respond. It is probable that prostaglandins are only one of the mechanisms by which a tumor can induce hypercalcemia (Tashjian *et al.,* 1974; Jaffe and Santoro, 1977; Oates *et al.,* 1977). The capacity of prostaglandins to cause bone resorption has also been invoked as a cause of alveolar bone loss in peridontal disease. (For possible roles of prostaglandins in immunological mechanisms, *see* reviews by Bourne, 1974; Goldyne, 1977; Pelus and Strausser, 1977.)

Therapeutic Uses

As described above, there has been intense interest in the effects of the prostaglandins on the female reproductive system. The clinical value of the agents, particularly PGF$_{2\alpha}$ and PGE$_2$, is being assessed in numerous clinics throughout the world. Their actions as *abortifacients* is already clearly established. Given early in pregnancy they are abortifacient, but initial hopes that they might provide a simple, convenient means of postimplantation "contraception," perhaps given as a vaginal suppository, have not yet been fulfilled. Moreover, the abortifacient action of prostaglandins in the early weeks of pregnancy is inconstant and often incomplete, and may be accompanied by distressing side effects. Nevertheless, prostaglandins appear to be of value in missed abortion and molar gestation, and they have been considered as the agents of choice for inducing midtrimester abortion. They also offer alternatives to oxytocin for induction of labor at term. These actions of prostaglandins are considered more fully in Chapter 39.

The use of prostaglandins for other purposes is currently experimental. PGE$_2$ has been tried as an alternative to isoproterenol in bronchial asthma. However, its value when given by inhalation is limited by its irritant effect on the respiratory mucosa (*see* Cuthbert, 1973).

The capacity of several prostaglandins to suppress gastric ulceration in experimental animals is a property of potential therapeutic importance. Some markedly inhibit gastric secretion when given orally to man and have antiulcer activity. However, all the PGE analogs have caused undesirable side effects, especially diarrhea. Analogs of PGI$_2$, which appear to cause fewer side effects, are being developed for this use.

PGE$_1$ has been administered by intra-arterial or intravenous infusion to patients with severe peripheral vascular disease, and dramatic and long-lasting improvement has been observed after short-term infusion (Olsson and Carlsson, 1976). Similar results have been obtained with PGI$_2$ (Szczeklik *et al.,* 1979). The mechanism of this effect is at present unclear.

Infusions of PGI$_2$ to dogs have been shown to protect against the loss of platelets and formation of microthrombi that occur during extracorporeal circulation of blood in such procedures as dialysis, cardiopulmonary bypass, and hemoperfusion through charcoal. Clinical trials are at present underway. The use of PGI$_2$ or its analogs might well become important in the control of platelet aggregation, not only in extracorporeal circulation systems but also in thromboembolic disorders, especially arterial thrombosis (Moncada and Vane, 1978b). PGE$_1$ was proven valuable for improving the harvest and storage of blood platelets for therapeutic transfusion (*see* Allen and Valeri, 1974). The use of PGI$_2$ and its analogs for this purpose is developing rapidly.

The available preparations of the prostaglandins are described in Chapter 39.

Aiken, J. W., and Vane, J. R. Intrarenal prostaglandin release attenuates the renal vasoconstrictor activity of angiotensin. *J. Pharmacol. Exp. Ther.,* **1973,** *184,* 678–687.

Anggard, E.; Larsson, C.; and Samuelsson, B. The distribution of 15-hydroprostaglandin dehydrogenase and prostaglandin-Δ^{13}-reductase in tissues of the swine. *Acta Physiol. Scand.,* **1971,** *81,* 396–404.

Anggard, E., and Samuelsson, B. Prostaglandins and related factors. 28. Metabolism of prostaglandin E$_1$ in guinea pig lung: the structures of two metabolites. *J. Biol. Chem.,* **1964,** *239,* 4087–4102.

Arendshorst, W. J.; Johnson, P. A.; and Selkurt, E. E. Effect of prostaglandin E on renal hemodynamics in nondiuretic and volume-expanded dogs. *Am. J. Physiol.,* **1974,** *226,* 218–225.

Armstrong, J. M.; Boura, A. L. A.; Hamberg, M.; and Samuelsson, B. A comparison of the vasodepressor effects of the cyclic endoperoxides PGG$_2$ and PGH$_2$ with those of PGD$_2$ and PGE$_2$ in hypertensive and normotensive rats. *Eur. J. Pharmacol.,* **1976,** *39,* 251–258.

Barner, H. B.; Kaiser, G. C.; Jellinek, M.; and Lee, J. B. Effect of prostaglandin A on several vascular beds in man. *Am. Heart J.,* **1973,** *85,* 584–592.

Bianco, S.; Robuschi, M.; Ceserani, R.; and Gandolfi, C. Prevention of aspecifically induced bronchoconstriction by prostacyclin (PGI$_2$) in asthmatic subjects. *Int. Res. Commun. Syst. Med. Sci.,* **1978,** *6,* 256.

Bolger, P. M.; Eisner, G. M.; Ramwell, P. W.; and Slotkoff, L. M. Renal actions of prostacyclin. *Nature,* **1978,** *271,* 457–469.

Boot, J. R.; Cockerill, A. F.; Dawson, W.; Mallen, D. N. B.; and Osborne, D. J. Modification of prostaglandin and thromboxane release by immunological sensitization and successive immunological challenge for guinea pig lung. *Int. Arch. Allergy Appl. Immunol.*, **1978**, *57*, 159–164.

Borgeat, P., and Samuelsson, B. Metabolism of arachidonic acid in polymorphonuclear leukocytes. Structural analysis of novel hydroxylated compounds. *J. Biol. Chem.*, **1979**, *254*, 7865–7869.

Corey, E. J.; Clark, D. A.; Goto, G.; Marfat, A.; Mioskowski, C.; Samuelsson, B.; and Hammarström, S. Stereospecific total synthesis of a slow reacting substance of anaphylaxis, leukotriene C-1. *J. Am. Chem. Soc.*, **1980**, *102*, 1436–1439.

Dusting, G. J.; Moncada, S.; and Vane, J. R. Vascular actions of arachidonic acid and its metabolites in the perfused mesenteric and femoral beds of the dog. *Eur. J. Pharmacol.*, **1978**, *49*, 65–72.

Euler, U. S. von. On the specific vasodilating and plain muscle stimulating substance from accessory genital glands in man and certain animals (prostaglandin and vesiglandin). *J. Physiol. (Lond.)*, **1936**, *88*, 213–234.

Ferreira, S. H.; Moncada, S.; and Vane, J. R. Indomethacin and aspirin abolish prostaglandin release from the spleen. *Nature [New Biol.]*, **1971**, *231*, 237–239.

Gerber, J. G.; Branch, R. A.; Nies, A. S.; Gerkens, J. F.; Shand, D. G.; Hollifield, J.; and Oates, J. A. Prostaglandins and renin release. II. Assessment of renin secretion following infusion of PGI$_2$, E$_2$ and D$_2$ into the renal artery of anaesthetised dogs. *Prostaglandins*, **1978**, *15*, 81–88.

Gerrard, J. M.; Peterson, D.; Townsend, D.; and White, J. G. Prostaglandins and platelet contraction. *Circulation*, **1976**, *54*, Suppl. II, 196.

Goldblatt, M. W. Properties of human seminal fluid. *J. Physiol. (Lond.)*, **1935**, *84*, 208–218.

Grenier, F. C., and Smith, W. L. Formation of 6-keto-PGF$_1$ by collecting tubule cells isolated from rabbit renal papillae. *Prostaglandins*, **1978**, *16*, 759–772.

Gryglewski, R. J.; Korbut, R.; and Ocetkiewicz, A. Generation of prostacyclin by lungs *in vivo* and its release into the arterial circulation. *Nature*, **1978**, *273*, 765–767.

Hamberg, M., and Samuelsson, B. On the metabolism of prostaglandins E$_1$ and E$_2$ in man. *J. Biol. Chem.*, **1971**, *246*, 6713–6721.

———. Detection and isolation of an endoperoxide intermediate in prostaglandin biosynthesis. *Proc. Natl. Acad. Sci. U.S.A.*, **1973**, *70*, 899–903.

———. Prostaglandin endoperoxides. Novel transformations of arachidonic acid in human platelets. *Ibid.*, **1974a**, *71*, 3400–3404.

———. Prostaglandin endoperoxides. VII. Novel transformations of arachidonic acid in guinea pig lung. *Biochem. Biophys. Res. Commun.*, **1974b**, *61*, 942–949.

Hamberg, M.; Svensson, J.; and Samuelsson, B. Thromboxane: a new group of biologically active compounds derived from prostaglandin endoperoxides. *Proc. Natl. Acad. Sci. U.S.A.*, **1975**, *72*, 2994–2998.

Harms, P. G.; Ojeda, S. R.; and McCann, S. M. Prostaglandin-induced release of pituitary gonadotrophins: central nervous system and pituitary sites of action. *Endocrinology*, **1974**, *94*, 1459–1464.

Herbaczynska-Cedro, K., and Vane, J. R. Contribution of intrarenal generation of prostaglandin to autoregulation of renal blood flow in the dog. *Circ. Res.*, **1973**, *33*, 428–436.

———. Prostaglandins as mediators of reactive hyperaemia in kidney. *Nature*, **1974**, *247*, 492.

Herman, A. G.; Verbeuren, T. J.; Moncada, S.; and Vanhoutte, P. M. Effect of prostacyclin on myogenic activity and adrenergic neuroeffector interaction in canine isolated veins. *Prostaglandins*, **1978**, *16*, 911–921.

Hill, T. W. K., and Moncada, S. The renal haemodynamic and excretory actions of prostacyclin and 6-oxo-PGF$_1$ in anaesthetized dogs. *Prostaglandins*, **1979**, *17*, 87–98.

Johnson, D. G.; Fujimoto, W. Y.; and Williams, R. W. Enhanced release of insulin by prostaglandins in isolated pancreatic islets. *Diabetes*, **1973**, *22*, 658–663.

Kindahl, H. Metabolism of thromboxane B$_2$ in the cynomolgus monkey. *Prostaglandins*, **1977**, *13*, 619–629.

Klein, D. C., and Raisz, L. G. Prostaglandins: stimulation of bone resorption in tissue culture. *Endocrinology*, **1970**, *86*, 1436–1440.

Kurzrok, R., and Lieb, C. C. Biochemical studies of human semen. II. The action of semen on the human uterus. *Proc. Soc. Exp. Biol. Med.*, **1930**, *28*, 268–272.

Leslie, C. A., and Levine, L. Evidence for the presence of prostaglandin E$_2$-9-keto reductase in rat organs. *Biochem. Biophys. Res. Commun.*, **1973**, *52*, 717–724.

Lewis, R. B., and Shulman, J. D. Influence of acetylsalicylic acid, an inhibitor of prostaglandin synthesis on the duration of human gestation and labor. *Lancet*, **1973**, *2*, 1159–1160.

Mashiter, K., and Field, J. B. Prostaglandins and the thyroid gland. *Fed. Proc.*, **1974**, *33*, 78–80.

Moncada, S.; Gryglewski, R.; Bunting, S.; and Vane, J. R. An enzyme isolated from arteries transforms prostaglandin endoperoxides to an unstable substance that inhibits platelet aggregation. *Nature*, **1976**, *263*, 663–665.

Moncada, S.; Korbut, R.; Bunting, S.; and Vane, J. R. Prostacyclin is a circulating hormone. *Nature*, **1978**, *273*, 767–768.

Murphy, R. C.; Hammarström, S.; and Samuelsson, B. Leukotriene C: a slow-reacting substance from murine mastocytoma cells. *Proc. Natl. Acad. Sci. U.S.A.*, **1979**, *76*, 4275–4279.

Nugteren, D. H. Arachidonate lipoxygenase in blood platelets. *Biochim. Biophys. Acta*, **1975**, *380*, 299–307.

Nugteren, D. H., and Hazelhof, E. Isolation and properties of intermediates in prostaglandin biosynthesis. *Biochim. Biophys. Acta*, **1973**, *326*, 448–461.

Olsson, A. G., and Carlsson, A. L. Clinical, hemodynamic and metabolic effects of intraarterial infusions of prostaglandin E$_1$ in patients with peripheral vascular disease. *Adv. Prostaglandin Thromboxane Res.*, **1976**, *1*, 429–432.

Omini, C.; Pasargiklian, R.; Folco, G. C.; Fano, M.; and Berti, F. Pharmacological activity of PGI$_2$ and its metabolite 6-oxo-PGF$_1$ on human uterus and Fallopian tube. *Prostaglandins*, **1978**, *15*, 1045–1054.

Piper, P. J., and Vane, J. R. Release of additional factors in anaphylaxis and its antagonism by anti-inflammatory drugs. *Nature*, **1969**, *223*, 29–35.

Roberts, L. J.; Sweetman, B. J.; Morgan, J. L.; Payne, N. A.; and Oates, J. A. Identification of the major urinary metabolite of thromboxane B$_2$ in the monkey. *Prostaglandins*, **1977a**, *13*, 631–647.

Roberts, L. J.; Sweetman, B. J.; Payne, N. A.; and Oates, J. A. Metabolism of thromboxane B$_2$ in man. *J. Biol. Chem.*, **1977b**, *252*, 7415–7417.

Robinson, B. F.; Collier, J. G.; Karim, S. M. M.; and Somers, K. Effect of prostaglandins A$_1$, A$_2$, B$_1$, E$_2$ and F$_2$ on forearm arterial bed and superficial hand veins in man. *Clin. Sci.*, **1973**, *44*, 367–376.

Rudick, J.; Gonda, M.; Dreiling, D. A.; and Janowitz, H. D. Effects of prostaglandin E$_1$ on pancreatic endocrine function. *Gastroenterology*, **1971**, *60*, 272–278.

Smith, J. B., and Willis, A. L. Aspirin selectively inhibits prostaglandin production in human platelets. *Nature [New Biol.]*, **1971**, *321*, 235–237.

Sun, F. F., and Taylor, B. Metabolism of prostacyclin in rats. *Biochemistry*, **1978**, *17*, 4096–5101.

Szczeklik, A.; Gryglewski, R. J.; Nizankowski, R.; Musial, J.; Pieton, R.; and Mruk, J. Circulatory and anti-platelet effects of intravenous prostacyclin in healthy men. *Pharmacol. Res. Commun.*, **1978**, *10*, 545–556.

Szczeklik, A.; Nizankowski, R.; Splawinski, J.; Szczeklik, J.; Gluszko, P.; and Gryglewski, R. Successful therapy of advanced arteriosclerosis obliterans with prostacyclin. *Lancet*, **1979**, *1*, 1111–1114.

Vane, J. R. Inhibition of prostaglandin synthesis as a

mechanism of action for aspirin-like drugs. *Nature* [*New Biol.*], **1971,** *231,* 232–235.

Waltman, R.; Tricomi, V.; Shabanah, E. H.; and Arenas, R. The effect of anti-inflammatory drugs on parturition parameters in the rat. *Prostaglandins,* **1973,** *4,* 93–106.

Weber, P. C.; Larsson, C.; Anggard, E.; Hamberg, M.; Corey, E. J.; Nicolaou, K. C.; and Samuelsson, B. Stimulation of renin release from rabbit renal cortex by arachidonic acid and prostaglandin endoperoxides. *Circ. Res.,* **1976,** *39,* 868–874.

Whittle, B. J. R.; Boughton-Smith, N. K.; Moncada, S.; and Vane, J. R. Actions of prostacyclin (PGI$_2$) and its product 6-oxo-PGF$_1$ on the rat gastric mucosa *in vivo* and *in vitro. Prostaglandins,* **1978,** *15,* 955–967.

Whorton, A. R.; Misono, K.; Hollifield, J.; Frolich, J. C.; Inagami, T.; and Oates, J. A. Prostaglandins and renin release. I. Stimulation of renin release from rabbit renal cortical slices by PGI$_2$. *Prostaglandins,* **1977,** *14,* 1095–1104.

Monographs and Reviews

Allen, J. E., and Valeri, C. R. Prostaglandins in hematology. *Arch. Intern. Med.,* **1974,** *133,* 86–96.

Andersen, N. H., and Ramwell, P. W. Biological aspects of prostaglandins. *Arch. Intern. Med.,* **1974,** *133,* 30–50.

Bakhle, Y. S., and Vane, J. R. (eds.). *Metabolic Functions of the Lung.* Marcel Dekker, Inc., New York, **1977.**

Behrman, H. R., and Anderson, G. G. Prostaglandins in reproduction. *Arch. Intern. Med.,* **1974,** *133,* 77–84.

Bennett, A. Effects of prostaglandins on the gastrointestinal tract. In, *The Prostaglandins: Progress in Research.* (Karim, S. M. M., ed.) John Wiley & Sons, Inc., New York, **1972,** pp. 205–222.

———. Prostaglandin antagonists. *Adv. Drug Res.,* **1974,** *8,* 83–118.

———. The role of prostaglandins in gastrointestinal tone and motility. In, *Prostaglandins and Thromboxanes.* (Berti, F.; Samuelsson, B.; and Velo, G. P.; eds.) Plenum Press, New York, **1977,** pp. 275–285.

Bergström, S., and Samuelsson, B. The prostaglandins. *Endeavour,* **1968,** *27,* 109–113.

Bourne, H. R. Immunology, In, *The Prostaglandins.* (Ramwell, P. W., ed.) Plenum Press, New York, **1974,** pp. 277–292.

Brody, M. J., and Kadowitz, P. J. Prostaglandins as modulators of the autonomic nervous system. *Fed. Proc.,* **1974,** *33,* 48–60.

Coceani, F. Prostaglandins and the central nervous system. *Arch. Intern. Med.,* **1974,** *133,* 119–129.

Collier, H. O. J. Kinins and prostaglandins. *Proc. R. Soc. Med.,* **1971a,** *64,* 1–16.

———. Prostaglandins and aspirin. *Nature,* **1971b,** *232,* 17–19.

Cuthbert, M. F. Prostaglandins and respiratory smooth muscle. In, *The Prostaglandins: Pharmacological and Therapeutic Advances.* (Cuthbert, M. F., ed.) J. B. Lippincott Co., Philadelphia, **1973,** pp. 253–286.

Dunn, M. J., and Hood, V. L. Prostaglandins in the kidney. *Am. J. Physiol.,* **1977,** *233,* F169–F184.

Dusting, G. J.; Moncada, S.; and Vane, J. R. Prostaglandins, their intermediates and precursors, their cardiovascular actions and regulatory roles in normal and abnormal circulatory systems. *Prog. Cardiovasc. Dis.,* **1979,** *21,* 405–430.

Euler, U. S. von. Some aspects of the actions of prostaglandins. The First Heymans Memorial Lecture. *Arch. Int. Pharmacodyn. Ther.,* **1973,** *202,* Suppl., 295–307.

Feldberg, W. Fever, prostaglandins and antipyretics. In, *Prostaglandin Synthetase Inhibitors.* (Robinson, H. J., and Vane, J. R., eds.) Raven Press, New York, **1974,** pp. 197–203.

Ferreira, S. H.; Moncada, S.; and Vane, J. R. Prostaglandins and signs and symptoms of inflammation. In,

Prostaglandin Synthetase Inhibitors. (Robinson, H. J., and Vane, J. R., eds.) Raven Press, New York, **1974,** pp. 175–187.

Ferreira, S. H., and Vane, J. R. Prostaglandins: their disappearance from and release into the circulation. *Nature,* **1967,** *216,* 868–873.

Ferris, T. F. Prostaglandins, potassium and Bartter's syndrome. *J. Lab. Clin. Med.,* **1978,** *92,* 663–668.

Fisher, J. W., and Gross, D. M. Effects of prostaglandins on erythropoiesis. In, *Prostaglandins in Haematology.* (Silver, M.; Smith, B. J.; and Kocsis, J. J.; eds.) Spectrum Publications, Inc., New York, **1977,** pp. 159–185.

Flower, R. J. Drugs which inhibit prostaglandin biosynthesis. *Pharmacol. Rev.,* **1974,** *26,* 33–67.

———. Steroidal anti-inflammatory drugs as inhibitors of phospholipase A$_2$. *Adv. Prostaglandin Thromboxane Res.,* **1978a,** *3,* 105–112.

———. Prostaglandins and related compounds. In, *Handbook of Experimental Pharmacology,* Vol. 50. (Vane, J. R., and Ferreira, S. H., eds.) Springer-Verlag, Berlin, **1978b,** pp. 374–422.

Friedman, W. F.; Printz, M. P.; and Kirkpatric, S. E. Blocker of prostaglandin synthesis. A novel therapy in the management of the premature human infant with patent ductus arteriosus. *Adv. Prostaglandin Thromboxane Res.,* **1978,** *4,* 373–381.

Gill, J. R.; Frolich, J. C.; Bowden, R. E.; Raylor, A. A.; Keiser, H. R.; Seyberth, H. W.; Oates, J. A.; and Bartter, F. C. Bartter's syndrome, a disorder characterized by high urinary prostaglandins and a dependence of hyperreninemia on prostaglandin synthesis. *Am. J. Med.,* **1976,** *61,* 43–51.

Goldberg, V. J., and Ramwell, P. W. Role of prostaglandins in reproduction. *Physiol. Rev.,* **1975,** *55,* 325–351.

Goldyne, M. E. Prostaglandins and the modulation of immunological responses. *Int. J. Dermatol.,* **1977,** *16,* 701–712.

Gorman, R. R.; Fitzpatrick, F. A.; and Miller, O. V. Reciprocal regulation of human platelet cAMP levels by thromboxane A$_2$ and prostacyclin. *Adv. Cyclic Nucleotide Res.,* **1978,** *9,* 597–609.

Hamberg, M.; Svensson, J.; Hedqvist, P.; Strandberg, K.; and Samuelsson, B. Involvement of endoperoxides and thromboxanes in anaphylactic reactions. *Adv. Prostaglandin Thromboxane Res.,* **1976,** *1,* 495–501.

Hedqvist, P. Autonomic neurotransmission. In, *The Prostaglandins,* Vol. 1. (Ramwell, P. W., ed.) Plenum Press, New York, **1973,** pp. 101–132.

———. Prostaglandin action on transmitter release at adrenergic neuroeffector junctions. *Adv. Prostaglandin Thromboxane Res.,* **1976,** *1,* 357–363.

Heymann, M. A., and Rudolph, A. M. Effects of prostaglandins and blockers of prostaglandin synthesis on the ductus arteriosus: animal and human studies. *Adv. Prostaglandin Thromboxane Res.,* **1978,** *4,* 363–371.

Hodge, R. L., and Walters, S. The physiology and pharmacology of prostaglandins. *Aust. J. Pharm. Sci.,* **1975,** *NS5,* 42–48.

Horton, E. W. Hypotheses on physiological roles of prostaglandins. *Physiol. Rev.,* **1969,** *49,* 122–161.

———. *Prostaglandins. Monographs on Endocrinology,* Vol. 7. Springer-Verlag, Berlin, **1972.**

Horton, E. W., and Poyser, N. L. Uterine luteolytic hormone. A physiological role for prostaglandin F$_{2\alpha}$. *Physiol. Rev.,* **1976,** *56,* 595–651.

Jaffe, B. M., and Santoro, M. G. Prostaglandins and cancer. In, *The Prostaglandins,* Vol. 3. (Ramwell, P. W., ed.) Plenum Press, New York, **1977,** pp. 329–351.

Jobim, F. Acetylsalicylic acid, hemostasis and human thromboembolism. *Semin. Thromb. Hemostas.,* **1978,** *4,* 199–240.

Karim, S. M. M. Prostaglandins and human reproduction: physiological roles and clinical uses of prostaglandins in relation to human reproduction. In, *The Prostaglandins: Progress in Research.* (Karim, S. M. M., ed.) John Wiley & Sons, Inc., New York, **1972**, pp. 71–164.

———. On the use of blockers of prostaglandin synthesis in the control of labor. *Adv. Prostaglandin Thromboxane Res.,* **1978**, *4,* 301–306.

Karim, S. M. M., and Fung, W.-P. Effects of some naturally occurring prostaglandins and synthetic analogues on gastric secretion and ulcer healing in man. *Adv. Prostaglandin Thromboxane Res.,* **1976**, *2,* 529–539.

Karim, S. M. M., and Hillier, K. Pharmacology and therapeutic applications of prostaglandins in the human reproductive system. In, *The Prostaglandins: Pharmacological and Therapeutic Advances.* (Cuthbert, M. F., ed.) J. B. Lippincott Co., Philadelphia, **1973**, pp. 167–200.

Katz, R. L., and Katz, G. J. Prostaglandins—basic and clinical considerations. *Anesthesiology,* **1974**, *40,* 471–493.

Lands, W. E. M.; Le Tellier, P. R.; Rome, L. H.; and Vanderhoek, J. Y. Inhibition of prostaglandin biosynthesis. In, *International Conference on Prostaglandins. Advances in the Biosciences,* Vol. 9. Pergamon Press, Ltd., Oxford, **1973**, pp. 15–28.

Lee, J. B. Cardiovascular renal effects of prostaglandins. *Arch. Intern. Med.,* **1974**, *133,* 56–76.

McGiff, J. C.; Crowshaw, K.; and Itskovitz, H. D. Prostaglandins and renal function. *Fed. Proc.,* **1974**, *33,* 39–47.

Marcus, A. J. The role of lipids in platelet function with particular reference to the arachidonic acid pathway. *J. Lipid Res.,* **1978**, *19,* 793–826.

Mathe, A. A.; Hedqvist, P.; Strandberg, K.; and Leslie, C. A. Aspects of prostaglandin function in the lung. *N. Engl. J. Med.,* **1977**, *296,* 850–855, 910–914.

Moncada, S., and Vane, J. R. The discovery of prostacyclin—a fresh insight into arachidonic acid metabolism. In, *Biochemical Aspects of Prostaglandins and Thromboxanes.* (Kharasch, N., and Fried, J., eds.) Academic Press, Inc., New York, **1977**, pp. 155–177.

———. Prostacyclin (PGI$_2$) the vascular wall and vasodilatation. In, *Mechanisms of Vasodilatation.* (Vanhoutte, P. M., and Leusen, I., eds.) S. Karger, Basel, **1978a**, pp. 107–121.

———. Unstable metabolites of arachidonic acid and their role in haemostasis and thrombosis. *Br. Med. Bull.,* **1978b**, *34,* 129–136.

Nakano, J. General pharmacology of prostaglandins. In, *The Prostaglandins: Pharmacological and Therapeutic Advances.* (Cuthbert, M. F., ed.) J. B. Lippincott Co., Philadelphia, **1973**, pp. 23–124.

Nakano, J., and Koss, M. C. Pathophysiologic roles of prostaglandins and the action of aspirin-like drugs. *South. Med. J.,* **1973**, *66,* 709–721.

Nugteren, D. H. Arachidonate lipoxygenase. In, *Prostaglandins in Hematology.* (Silver, M.; Smith, B. J.; and Kocsis, J. J.; eds.) Spectrum Publications, Inc., New York, **1977**, pp. 11–25.

Oates, J. A.; Hannsjorg, W. S.; and Sweetman, B. Prostaglandins as mediators of the hypercalcaemia associated with certain human cancers. In, *Biochemical Aspects of Prostaglandins and Thromboxanes.* (Kharasch, N., and Fried, J., eds.) Academic Press, Inc., New York, **1977**, pp. 95–102.

Parker, C. W., and Snider, D. E. Prostaglandins and asthma. *Ann. Intern. Med.,* **1973**, *78,* 963–965.

Pelus, L. M., and Strausser, H. R. Prostaglandins and the immune response. *Life Sci.,* **1977**, *20,* 903–914.

Pharriss, B. B., and Behrman, H. R. Gonadal function. In, *The Prostaglandins,* Vol. 1. (Ramwell, P. W., ed.) Plenum Press, New York, **1973**, pp. 347–364.

Ramwell, P. W., and Shaw, J. E. Biological significance of the prostaglandins. *Recent Prog. Horm. Res.,* **1970**, *26,* 139–197.

Rankin, J. H. G. Role of prostaglandins in the maintenance of the placental circulation. *Adv. Prostaglandin Thromboxane Res.,* **1978**, *4,* 261–269.

Rasmussen, H., and Lake, W. Prostaglandins and the mammalian erythrocyte. In, *Prostaglandins in Hematology.* (Silver, M.; Smith, B. J.; and Kocsis, J. J.; eds.) Spectrum Publications, Inc., New York, **1977**, pp. 187–202.

Robert, A. Effect of prostaglandins and the mammalian erythrocyte. In, *Prostaglandins in Hematology.* (Silver, M.; Smith, B. J.; and Kocsis, J. J.; eds.) Spectrum Publications, Inc., New York, **1977**, pp. 187–202.

Samuelsson, B. Biosynthesis of prostaglandins. *Fed. Proc.,* **1972**, *31,* 1442–1460.

Samuelsson, B.; Folco, G.; Granstrom, E.; Kindahl, H.; and Malmsten, C. Prostaglandins and thromboxanes: biochemical and physiological consideration. *Adv. Prostaglandin Thromboxane Res.,* **1978a**, *4,* pp. 1–25.

Samuelsson, B.; Goldync, M.; Granstrom, E.; Hamberg, M.; Hammarstrom, S.; and Malmsten, C. Prostaglandins and thromboxanes. *Annu. Rev. Biochem.,* **1978b**, *47,* 997–1029.

Samuelsson, B.; Granstrom, E.; Green, K.; and Hamberg, M. Metabolism of prostaglandins. *Ann. N.Y. Acad. Sci.,* **1971**, *180,* 138–163.

Samuelsson, B.; Granstrom, E.; Green, K.; Hamberg, M.; and Hammarstrom, S. Prostaglandins. *Annu. Rev. Biochem.,* **1975**, *44,* 669–694.

Sanner, J. H., and Eakins, K. E. Prostaglandin antagonists. In, *Prostaglandins: Chemical and Biochemical Aspects.* (Karim, S. M. M., ed.) M. T. P. Press, Lancaster, England, **1976**, pp. 139–189.

Smith, J. B., and Macfarlane, D. C. Platelets. In, *The Prostaglandins.* (Ramwell, P. W., ed.) Plenum Press, New York, **1974**, pp. 293–343.

Smith, M.; Ingerman, C. M.; and Silver, M. J. Effects of arachidonic acid and some of its metabolites on platelets. In, *Prostaglandins in Hematology.* (Silver, M.; Smith, B. J.; and Kocsis, J. J.; eds.) Spectrum Publications, Inc., New York, **1977**, pp. 277–292.

Tashjian, A. H.; Voelkel, E. F.; Goldhaber, P.; and Levine, L. Prostaglandins, calcium metabolism and cancer. *Fed. Proc.,* **1974**, *33,* 81–86.

Vane, J. R. The release and fate of vasoactive hormones in the circulation. *Br. J. Pharmacol.,* **1969**, *35,* 209–242.

———. The mode of action of aspirin-like drugs. *Agents Actions,* **1978**, *8,* 430–431.

Vapaatalo, H., and Parantainen, J. Prostaglandins, their biological and pharmacological role. *Med. Biol.,* **1978**, *56,* 163–183.

Wilson, D. C. Prostaglandins. Their actions on the gastrointestinal tract. *Arch. Intern. Med.,* **1974**, *133,* 112–118.

Wolfe, L. S.; Poppius, H. M.; and Marion, J. The biosynthesis of prostaglandins by brain tissue *in vitro. Adv. Prostaglandin Thromboxane Res.,* **1976**, *1,* 345–355.

Zins, G. R. Renal prostaglandins. *Am. J. Med.,* **1975**, *58,* 14–24.

Zurier, R. B. Prostaglandins, inflammation and asthma. *Arch. Intern. Med.,* **1974**, *133,* 101–110.

V Drug Therapy of Inflammation

In this section drugs that are anti-inflammatory, analgesic, and antipyretic will be considered; their mechanisms of action differ from those of the anti-inflammatory steroids and the opioid analgesics. Also included are miscellaneous anti-inflammatory agents and drugs used in the treatment of gout, such as colchicine and allopurinol. Several other agents are employed to suppress the manifestations of inflammation but are considered more conveniently in other sections of the textbook. These especially include the adrenocorticosteroids; also in this category are immunosuppressive agents, chloroquine, and penicillamine.

CHAPTER

29 ANALGESIC-ANTIPYRETICS AND ANTI-INFLAMMATORY AGENTS; DRUGS EMPLOYED IN THE TREATMENT OF GOUT

Roderick J. Flower, Salvador Moncada, and John R. Vane

The anti-inflammatory, analgesic, and antipyretic drugs are a heterogeneous group of compounds, often chemically unrelated (although most of them are organic acids), which nevertheless share certain therapeutic actions and side effects. The prototype is aspirin; hence these compounds are often referred to as *aspirin-like drugs*.

There has been considerable recent progress in elucidating the mechanism of action of aspirin-like drugs, and it is now possible to hypothesize why such heterogeneous agents have the same basic therapeutic activities and often the same side effects. Indeed, their therapeutic activity appears to depend to a large extent upon the inhibition of a defined biochemical pathway responsible for the biosynthesis of the prostaglandins and related autacoids. The mechanism of action of aspirin-like drugs and some of their shared properties will first be considered; then the more important drugs will be discussed in some detail.

History. The medicinal effect of the bark of willow and certain other plants has been known to several cultures for centuries. In England in the mid-eighteenth century, Reverend Edmund Stone described in a letter to the president of the Royal Society "an account of the success of the bark of the willow in the cure of agues" (fever). Edmund Stone had accidentally tasted the bark of the common white willow (*Salix alba vulgaris*), and the bitterness was, to him, strongly reminiscent of *Cinchona* bark (the source of quinine). He rationalized his finding on the grounds that since the willow grew in damp or wet areas "whereas agues chiefly abound," it would probably possess curative properties appropriate to that condition.

The active ingredient in the willow bark was a bitter glycoside called *salicin,* first discovered by Leroux in 1827. On hydrolysis, salicin liberates glucose and *salicylic alcohol* (saligenin). Piria, in 1838, made *salicylic acid* from salicin. Six years later, salicylic acid was prepared from *oil of gaultheria* (oil of wintergreen) by Cahours. The synthetic manufacture of this acid from phenol was accomplished in 1860 by Kolbe and Lautemann. *Sodium salicylate* was first used as an antipyretic and for rheumatic fever by Buss in 1875, and in the following year its value in *rheumatic fever* was discovered independently by Stricker and MacLagan. In 1879, Sée observed that salicylates increased the urinary excretion of uric acid, and this property was utilized in the treatment of gout by Campbell in 1879. *Phenyl salicylate* was introduced into medicine in 1886 by Nencki, and *aspirin* (acetylsalicylic acid) in 1899 by Dreser. The synthetic salicylates soon completely displaced the more expensive compounds obtained from natural sources.

No doubt early researchers were partially motivated by the search for effective substitutes for quinine, which became scarce (and consequently extremely expensive) near the end of the nineteenth century.

MECHANISM OF ACTION OF ASPIRIN-LIKE DRUGS

An explanation of the therapeutic action of aspirin and its congeners has long been sought in terms of enzyme inhibition (of a specific enzyme or group of enzymes). Although this class of drugs was known to inhibit a wide variety of reactions *in vitro,* no convincing relationship could be established with their known anti-inflammatory, antipyretic, and analgesic effects. In 1971, Vane and associates and Smith and Willis demonstrated that low concentrations of aspirin and indomethacin inhibited the enzymatic production of prostaglandins (*see* Chapter 28; Ferreira *et al.,* 1971; Smith and Willis, 1971; Vane, 1971). There was, at that time, some evidence that prostaglandins participated in the pathogenesis of inflammation and fever, and this reinforced the suggestion that inhibition of the biosynthesis of these autacoids could explain a considerable number of the clinical actions of the drugs (*see* Moncada and Vane, 1979). In the subsequent years the following major points have been established: (1) All mammalian cell types studied (with the possible exception of the erythrocyte) have microsomal enzymes for the synthesis of prostaglandins. (2) Prostaglandins are always released when cells are damaged and have been detected in increased concentrations in inflammatory exudates. All available evidence indicates that cells do not store prostaglandins, and their release thus depends on biosynthesis *de novo.* (3) All aspirin-like drugs inhibit the biosynthesis and release of prostaglandins in all cells tested. (4) Other classes of drugs do not, generally speaking, affect the biosynthesis of prostaglandins.

Inflammation. While it is difficult to give an adequate description of the inflammatory phenomenon in terms of underlying cellular events in the injured tissue, there are certain features of the process that are generally agreed to be characteristic. These include fenestration of the microvasculature, leakage of the elements of blood into the interstitial spaces, and migration of leukocytes into the inflamed tissue. On a macroscopic level, this is usually accompanied by the familiar clinical signs of erythema, edema, tenderness (hyperalgesia), and pain. During this complex response, chemical mediators such as histamine, 5-hydroxytryptamine (5-HT), slow-reacting substance of anaphylaxis (SRS-A), various chemotactic factors, bradykinin, and prostaglandins are liberated locally. Phagocytic cells migrate into the area, and cellular lysosomal membranes may be ruptured, releasing lytic enzymes. All these events may contribute to the inflammatory response. However, aspirin-like drugs have little or no effect upon the release or activity of histamine, 5-HT, SRS-A, or lysosomal enzymes, and, similarly, potent antagonists of 5-HT or histamine have little or no therapeutic effect in inflammation. Consequently, one must question the importance of these mediators in the initiation or maintenance of the inflammatory response.

Inflammation in patients with rheumatoid arthritis probably involves the combination of an antigen (gamma globulin) with an antibody (rheumatoid factor) and complement, causing the local release of chemotactic factors that attract leukocytes. The leukocytes phagocytize the complexes of antigen, antibody, and complement and also release the many enzymes contained in their lysosomes. These lysosomal enzymes then cause injury to cartilage and other tissues, and this furthers the degree of inflammation. Cell-mediated immune reactions may also be involved. Prostaglandins are also released during this process.

The effects produced by intradermal, intravenous, or intra-arterial injections of prostaglandins are strongly reminiscent of inflammation. In nanogram amounts, prostaglandin E_2 (PGE$_2$) and prostacyclin (PGI$_2$), which are likely to be generated in inflammation, cause erythema and increase local blood flow. Two important vascular effects of prostaglandins of the E series are not generally shared by other mediators of inflammation—a long-lasting vasodilator action and the capacity to counteract the vasoconstrictor effects of substances such as norepinephrine and angiotensin. The erythema induced by intradermal injection of prostaglandins clearly illustrates their long-lasting action (up to 10 hours). In contrast to their long-lasting effects upon cutaneous vessels and superficial veins, vasodilatation produced by prostaglandins in other vascular beds vanishes within a few minutes.

Prostaglandins, like other putative mediators of inflammation, increase vascular permeability (leakage) in the postcapillary and collecting venules. Unlike erythema, which is caused by local pooling of blood due to relaxation of smooth muscle in arterioles and venules, increased vascular permeability may result from the *contraction* of the venular endothelial cells. In fact, prostaglandins produce vasodilatation more effectively than they do edema. However, PGE_1, PGE_2, and PGA_2 (but not $PGF_{2\alpha}$) cause edema when injected into the hind paw of the rat. In addition, there is a clear synergism between PGE_1 and bradykinin when these two mediators are given together. Interestingly, some of the vascular effects of bradykinin appear to be due to stimulation of the synthesis of prostaglandins.

Migration of leukocytes into an inflamed area is an important aspect of the inflammatory process. It is not clear to what extent prostaglandins contribute to this event. There have been reports that various prostaglandins are *chemotactic*, but the major chemotactic product of the metabolism of arachidonic acid is probably 12-hydroxyarachidonic acid (HETE). (*See* Chapter 28; Kaley and Weiner, 1971; Ferreira *et al.*, 1973.)

Pain. Aspirin-like drugs are mild analgesics and are effective against pain of low-to-moderate intensity. Consideration of the *type* of pain is also important. In some situations, for example, chronic postoperative pain, aspirin may be superior to the opioid analgesics. According to Beecher (1957), there are clear differences in the effectiveness of analgesic drugs against pathological and experimental pain, and aspirin-like drugs are more effective against the former. Karim (1971) observed that milligram doses of PGE_2 or $PGF_{2\alpha}$, given to women by intramuscular or subcutaneous injection to induce abortion, caused intense local pain. Prostaglandins can also cause headache and vascular pain when infused intravenously in man. Intraperitoneal injection of PGE_1, PGE_2, or $PGF_{2\alpha}$ in mice causes abdominal constrictions characteristic of nociception. This effect is antagonized by morphine, but not by aspirin-like drugs, which do, however, block the pain induced by several other agents (Collier and Schneider, 1972). While the doses of prostaglandins required to elicit pain are high in comparison with the concentrations expected *in vivo*, induction of hyperalgesia (*i.e.,* a state in which pain can be elicited by normally painless mechanical or chemical stimulation) seems to be a typical response to low concentrations of prostaglandins. A long-lasting hyperalgesia occurs when minute amounts of PGE_1 are given intradermally to man. Furthermore, in experiments in man where separate subdermal infusions of PGE_1, bradykinin, or histamine (or a mixture of bradykinin and histamine) caused no overt pain, marked pain was experienced when PGE_1 was added to bradykinin or histamine. When PGE_1 was infused with histamine, itching was also noted.

The analgesic action of morphine occurs centrally, whereas the work of Lim and colleagues (1964) clearly shows that aspirin acts mainly peripherally. Thus, by preventing the synthesis and release of prostaglandins in inflammation, aspirin may avert the sensitization of pain receptors to mechanical stimulation or to other mediators. This hypothesis explains why aspirin is ineffective as an analgesic in noninflamed tissues, as shown by the Randall-Selitto test (1957). Most data are consistent with the presumption that aspirin is only effective as an analgesic in pathological conditions or experimental models in which prostaglandins are synthesized locally. This concept also explains why aspirin-like drugs are ineffective against sharp, "stabbing" pain, which is caused by direct stimulation of sensory nerves, but are effective in the dull, "throbbing" pain of inflammation, where prostaglandins apparently sensitize the nerve endings.

As mentioned previously, aspirin-like drugs do not affect the hyperalgesia or the pain caused by direct action of prostaglandins, consistent with the notion that it is their synthesis that is inhibited. A possible exception to this is the fenamates, which may have some antagonistic action against prostaglandins, as well as potent capability to inhibit their synthesis (*see* Ferreira, 1972; Ferreira *et al.*, 1973; Moncada *et al.*, 1975).

Fever. Fever may be a result of infection or one of the sequelae of tissue damage, inflammation, graft rejection, malignancy, or other disease states. A multitude of microorganisms can cause fever. There is evidence that bacterial endotoxins (lipopolysaccharides from the cell wall) act by stimulating the biosynthesis and release by neutrophils and other cells of an *endogenous pyrogen,* a protein with a molecular weight in the range of 10,000 to 20,000 daltons.

Once released into the general circulation, the endogenous pyrogen apparently passes into the central nervous system (CNS) and stimulates the release of prostaglandins from discrete sites within the brain, probably including the preoptic hypothalamic area. It is this latter step that is sensitive to aspirin-like drugs. Regulation of body temperature requires a delicate balance between the production and loss of heat, and the hypothalamus regulates the set point at which body temperature is maintained. In fever, this set point is obviously elevated, and aspirin-like drugs promote its return to normal. Heat production is not inhibited, but dissipation of heat is augmented by increased blood flow through the skin and by sweating. Fever is often associated with an inflammatory process, and most prostaglandins (with the possible exception of PGI_2) are themselves pyrogenic. Fever is a frequent side effect of intravenous infusions of $PGF_{2\alpha}$ or PGE_2 given to women as an abortifacient (Hendricks *et al.*, 1971). Several prostaglandins are pyrogenic when injected into the third ventricle of conscious cats and rabbits; PGE_2 is among the most potent. Thus, the generation of a prostaglandin in some areas of the CNS or its presence in the general circulation may induce fever (*see* Feldberg and Saxena, 1971; Milton and Wendlandt, 1971; Feldberg and Gupta, 1973; Milton, 1973).

Inhibition of Prostaglandin Biosynthesis by Aspirin-like Drugs. The inhibition of prostaglandin biosynthesis by aspirin and indomethacin was demonstrated simultaneously in three different systems: cell-free homogenates of guinea pig lung, perfused dog spleen, and human platelets (Ferreira *et al.*, 1971; Smith and Willis, 1971; Vane, 1971). There are now numerous systems *in vitro* and *in vivo* in which inhibition of prostaglandin biosynthesis by aspirin, indomethacin, or similar compounds has been demonstrated, and it is evident that this effect is not restricted to any one species or tissue. It is dependent only on the drug reaching the enzyme, prostaglandin synthetase (cyclooxygenase); the distribution and pharmacokinetics of each agent thus have an important bearing on the drug's activity (*see* Graf *et al.*, 1975).

Aspirin-like drugs inhibit or interfere with a variety of other enzymes and cellular systems; indeed, some of their clinical effects may be explained by these actions. A telling objection to many of the proposals, however, is the unrealistically high concentrations of drug that are required. Few of the other enzymes known to be susceptible to aspirin-like drugs are affected at concentrations that inhibit prostaglandin synthetase, although inhibition of other enzymes may contribute to the toxic effects of these drugs, particularly with overdosage.

Any hypothesis that purports to explain the action of a drug in terms of inhibition of an enzyme must satisfy at least two basic criteria. First, the free concentrations achieved in plasma during therapy must be sufficient to inhibit the enzyme in question. Second, there must be a reasonable correlation between antienzyme activity and therapeutic potency.

Certainly, there is good evidence that therapeutic doses of aspirin-like compounds reduce prostaglandin biosynthesis in man. Such doses of aspirin or indomethacin inhibit the production of prostaglandins by human platelets and reduce the prostaglandin content of human semen. The most persuasive evidence, however, arises from the work of Hamberg (1972), who monitored the concentrations of the major metabolite of PGE_1 and PGE_2 in urine before and after treatment with therapeutic doses of indomethacin, aspirin, and salicylate. In females, almost maximal inhibition (63 to 92%) of prostaglandin turnover was obtained after 1 day; however, in males (who generally excrete more metabolite than do females), the initial reduction was less but the output continued to decline throughout the 3-day period of treatment. Two days after treatment was discontinued, excretion of the metabolite had returned nearly to control levels.

There is a reasonably good rank-order correlation between the antienzyme activity of these drugs and their anti-inflammatory activity (estimated by a popular laboratory model of inflammation, the carrageenin edema test in rat hind paw). The only outstanding exception is indomethacin, which is apparently more potent against paw edema than in the enzyme inhibition assay. Ham and associates (1972) found a similar correlation for individual members of structurally related groups of aspirin-like drugs (except for the fenamates). More interesting is that the high degree of stereospecificity for anti-inflammatory activity among several pairs of enantiomers of α-methyl arylacetic acids is also evident in their inhibitory effect on prostaglandin synthetase. In each instance the *d* isomer was more potent. Tomlinson and colleagues (1972) obtained similar results with enantiomers of naproxen. Another example of this type of selectivity is provided by the drug *sulindac*. It is a prodrug that is only weakly active; it is metabolized *in vivo* to a highly active anti-inflammatory metabolite. Likewise, the drug itself has little ability to inhibit prostaglandin

biosynthesis, but the sulfide metabolite is a potent inhibitor.

The degree to which microsomal preparations of prostaglandin synthetase from different tissues are inhibited by aspirin-like drugs also varies considerably, and it is possible that the synthetase system (or at least one component protein) exists in multiple forms within the organism. Investigation of this possibility may permit design of drugs with greater specificity.

As mentioned before, the migration of leukocytes into inflamed areas is an important component of inflammation. Although the classical aspirin-like drugs (salicylates, pyrazolone derivatives, indomethacin, etc.) block prostaglandin biosynthesis, they do not inhibit the formation of the major chemotactic metabolite of arachidonic acid, HETE, and may even increase concentrations of this compound in tissues. It is not clear whether treatment with these drugs enhances the migration of leukocytes in clinical situations. Clearly, a drug that blocks the formation of HETE by the lipoxygenase, as well as prostaglandin formation by the cyclooxygenase, may have advantages, since leukocytic infiltration is perhaps responsible for much of the damage in chronic joint disease.

Mode of Inhibitory Action. The generalization has been used that aspirin-like drugs block "prostaglandin synthetase." However, as described in Chapter 28, there are multiple steps between the fatty acid precursor, arachidonic acid, and, for example, PGE_2. The first enzyme cyclizes and oxygenates arachidonic acid to form the unstable endoperoxide intermediate PGG_2. It is this first step, catalyzed by the cyclooxygenase, that is inhibited by aspirin-like drugs. Individual agents have differing modes of inhibitory activity on the cyclooxygenase. Aspirin itself acetylates a serine at the active site of the enzyme (Roth and Siok, 1978). Platelets are especially susceptible to this action because (unlike most other cells) they are incapable of regenerating the cyclooxygenase enzyme, presumably because they have little or no capacity for protein biosynthesis. In practical terms this means that a single dose of aspirin will inhibit the platelet cyclooxygenase for the life of the platelet (8 to 11 days). In contrast to aspirin, salicylic acid has no acetylating capacity and, although closely related to aspirin, must produce its anti-inflammatory activity in a different manner. Salicylic acid is almost inactive against cyclooxygenase *in vitro* but is as active as aspirin *in vivo* in reducing the synthesis of prostaglandins (Hamberg, 1972).

Aspirin is rapidly hydrolyzed to salicylic acid *in vivo* (half-life in human plasma, approximately 15 minutes); evidently the acetylated and the nonacetylated species act as pharmacologically distinct entities, and aspirin probably has a dual mechanism of action.

Most of the other common aspirin-like drugs are "irreversible" inhibitors of the cyclooxygenase, although there are some exceptions (*see* Flower, 1974). For indomethacin, the mode of inhibition is particularly complex and probably involves a site on the enzyme different from that which is acetylated by aspirin.

SHARED THERAPEUTIC ACTIVITIES
AND SIDE EFFECTS OF
ASPIRIN-LIKE DRUGS

All aspirin-like drugs are antipyretic, analgesic, and anti-inflammatory, but there are important differences in their activities. For example, acetaminophen is antipyretic and analgesic but is only weakly anti-inflammatory. The reasons for such differences are not clear; variations in the sensitivity of enzymes in the target tissues may be important.

When employed as *analgesics,* these drugs are only effective against pain of low-to-moderate intensity, particularly that associated with inflammation. They have much lower maximal effects than do the opioids. However, they do not lead to addiction and are mainly free of the unwanted effects of the opioids on the CNS. Aspirin-like drugs do not change the perception of sensory modalities other than pain. As mentioned, the type of pain is important; chronic postoperative pain or pain arising from inflammation is particularly well controlled by aspirin-like drugs, whereas pain arising from the hollow viscera is usually not relieved.

As *antipyretics,* aspirin-like drugs reduce the body temperature in febrile states. Although all such drugs are antipyretics and analgesics, some are not suitable for either routine or prolonged use because of toxicity; phenylbutazone is an example.

This class of drugs finds its chief clinical application as *anti-inflammatory agents* in the treatment of musculoskeletal disorders, such as rheumatoid arthritis, osteoarthritis, and ankylosing spondylitis. In general, aspirin-like drugs provide only symptomatic relief from the pain and inflammation associated with the disease and do not arrest the progression of pathological injury to tissue. It has even been said that the use of these drugs may aggravate the disease by allowing movement of arthritic joints that is not otherwise possible, thereby further injuring the synovium.

In addition to sharing many therapeutic activities, aspirin-like drugs share several unwanted effects. The most common is a propensity to induce *gastric* or *intestinal ulceration* that can sometimes be accompanied by a secondary anemia from the resultant blood loss. Aspirin-like drugs vary considerably in their tendency to cause such erosions (*see* individual sections). It is not clear whether this side effect is closely related to the capacity of aspirin-like drugs to interfere with the biosynthesis of prostaglandins. The gastric mucosa synthesizes PGI_2, which may well be involved in functional hyperemia. The gastric erosions induced by indomethacin (and many other ulcerogenic agents) in experimental animals are most effectively prevented by oral or parenteral administration of prostaglandins or their analogs. Certainly, the fact that this side effect is shared, to a greater or lesser degree, by the common inhibitors of prostaglandin synthetase suggests that it is related to the withdrawal of a protective prostaglandin.

There are other side effects of these drugs that probably depend upon their capacity to block endogenous prostaglandin biosynthesis; these include disturbances in platelet function and the prolongation of gestation or spontaneous labor. *Platelet function* appears to be disturbed because aspirin-like drugs prevent the formation by the platelets of thromboxane A_2 (TXA_2), a potent aggregating agent. This accounts for the tendency of these drugs to increase the bleeding time. *Prolongation of gestation* may occur, because biosynthesis of prostaglandins by the uterus leads to uterine contractions and, hypothetically, this is one mechanism by which the fetus is expelled at birth. Prostaglandins of the E and F series are potent uterotropic agents, and their biosynthesis by the uterus increases dramatically in the hours before parturition. That administration of inhibitors of prostaglandin synthesis can prolong gestation was first demonstrated in rats, but a retrospective survey in 1973 by Lewis and Schulman has established that such an effect is also seen in the human female.

In addition to their toxic effect on the gastrointestinal tract, many aspirin-like drugs may affect renal function, perhaps in part because prostaglandins play a role in the control of the renal circulation. People who take large daily doses of these analgesics for a period of years, especially those who use "over-the-counter" analgesic mixtures, may develop *analgesic abuse nephropathy.* The primary lesion appears to be *papillary necrosis,* with secondary *chronic interstitial nephritis.* The injury is often insidious in onset, is usually manifest initially as reduced tubular function and concentrating ability, and may progress to irreversible renal insufficiency if misuse of analgesics continues. The lesion is often seen in conjunction with other symptoms of chronic toxicity of aspirin-like drugs. Females are involved more frequently than are males, and there is often a history of recurring urinary tract infection. Emotional disturbances are common, and other drugs may be abused concurrently. Despite numerous clinical observations and experimental studies in animals and man, crucial details of the problem remain uncertain. Critical analyses of analgesic nephropathy have been provided by Schreiner (1962), Gilman (1964), Shelley (1967), Gault and coworkers (1968), Abel (1971), and Arger and associates (1976). Phenacetin has been suggested by some to be the nephrotoxic component and, therefore, has been replaced in many analgesic mixtures by other agents; the use of phenacetin by itself has been restricted in some countries. In the United States, warning labels are required on all analgesic drug mixtures containing phenacetin. However, it is premature to single out any particular ingredient as the causative factor. Indeed, there is evidence that the substitution of acetaminophen for phenacetin in such mixtures does not reduce the incidence of renal damage. It is possible that chronic abuse of any of the analgesic-antipyretics or analgesic mixtures may cause renal injury in the susceptible individual.

Two other features of aspirin-like drugs that depend upon their capacity to block prostaglandin biosynthesis also deserve mention. Prostaglandins have been implicated in the maintenance of patency of the *ductus arteriosus,* and indomethacin and related agents have been used with mixed success in neonates to close the ductus when it has remained patent. *Bartter's syndrome* is an unusual and complex disorder of children, characterized by hypokalemia, hyperreninemia, hyperaldosteronism, juxtaglomerular hyperplasia, normotension, and resistance to the pressor effect of angiotensin II. Excessive production of renal prostaglandins may play an important role in the pathogenesis of this syndrome, and it has been successfully treated with aspirin-like drugs.

Aspirin-like drugs may have undesirable effects on *male fertility.* Human seminal fluid is probably the richest natural source of prostaglandins, and there is a group of subfertile males in whom the concentration of prostaglandin in seminal fluid correlates positively with fertility. Thus, it could be unwise to treat males of marginal fertility with aspirin-like drugs for any protracted length of time.

Choice of Drug to Be Prescribed. The choice of an agent as a simple antipyretic or analgesic is seldom a problem. It is in the field of *rheumatology* that the decision becomes complex. The choice between aspirin-like agents for the treatment of arthritides is largely empirical. A drug may be chosen and given for a week; if the therapeutic effect is adequate, treatment should be continued unless toxicity supervenes. There is a large variation in the response of individuals to different aspirin-like drugs, even when they are closely allied members of the same chemical family. Thus, a patient may do well on one propionic acid derivative (such as ibuprofen) but not on another. This may indicate that these drugs share (unequally) different types of therapeutic actions. Sound discussion of principles of the use of aspirin-

like drugs is provided by Hart (1976), Kaye and Pemberton (1976), Huskisson (1977, 1978), and Miller and associates (1978).

All the drugs in this chapter, with the exception of the *p*-aminophenol derivatives, have a tendency to cause gastrointestinal side effects, which may range from mild dyspepsia and heartburn to ulceration of the stomach or duodenum (or reactivation of latent ulcers), sometimes with fatal results. Generally speaking, the newer drugs such as the propionic acid derivatives are probably the best tolerated. *Hypersensitivity to aspirin* is a contraindication to therapy with any of the drugs discussed in this chapter. Patients who are sensitive to aspirin react to all inhibitors of prostaglandin biosynthesis; administration of any one of these could provoke a life-threatening hypersensitivity reaction reminiscent of anaphylactic shock. The problem is discussed more fully below.

When dealing with a child or a pregnant woman, the choice of drugs is considerably restricted. Only drugs that have been extensively tested in children should be used; this commonly means that only aspirin, indomethacin, or ibuprofen should be prescribed. If drugs must be given to a pregnant woman, low doses of aspirin are probably the safest. There is not much evidence to suggest that salicylates in moderate doses have teratogenic effects in humans, although the birth weights of children born to chronic users of salicylates are lower than normal. In any case, aspirin should be discontinued prior to the anticipated time of parturition in order to avoid prolonging labor, increasing postpartum hemorrhage, and other complications (*see* above).

Most aspirin-like drugs bind firmly to plasma proteins and thus may displace other drugs from the binding sites. This can cause serious problems if the patient is receiving, for example, warfarin, a sulfonylurea hypoglycemic agent, or methotrexate; the dosage of such agents may require adjustment, or concurrent administration should be avoided. The problem with warfarin is accentuated because almost all of the aspirin-like drugs disturb normal platelet function (*see* Chapter 58).

Having determined that the likelihood of side effects is acceptably low, one can choose a drug regimen. Initially, fairly low doses of the agent chosen should be prescribed to determine the patient's reaction. Some investigators suggest that the patient should be allowed use of mild analgesics (*e.g.*, acetaminophen) to control sporadic pain. When the patient has problems with sleeping because of pain or morning stiffness, a larger single dose of the drug may be given at night; as an alternative, single doses of another drug (*e.g.*, 50 to 100 mg of indomethacin) may be given to supplement existing medication without much danger of serious side effects. A week is generally long enough to determine the effect of a given drug. If the drug is effective, treatment should be continued, reducing the dose if possible and stopping it altogether if it is no longer necessary. Side effects usually appear in the first weeks of therapy. If the patient does not respond, another compound should be tried, since there is a marked variation in the response of individuals to different but closely related drugs.

For mild arthropathies, the scheme outlined above, together with rest and physiotherapy, will probably be effective. However, patients with a more debilitating disease may not respond adequately. In such cases, more aggressive therapy should be initiated with aspirin, indomethacin, or phenylbutazone. In general, indomethacin and phenylbutazone are effective for acute attacks of gout and ankylosing spondylitis, whereas aspirin, indomethacin, and phenylbutazone are probably equally effective in rheumatoid arthritis and osteoarthritis.

For the seriously debilitated patient who cannot tolerate these drugs or in whom they are not adequately effective, other forms of therapy should be considered. Gold is discussed in a separate section of this chapter. The pharmacology of chloroquine and hydroxychloroquine is described in Chapter 45, while that of penicillamine is presented in Chapter 69; glucocorticoids are discussed in Chapter 63.

A final important consideration is the cost of therapy, particularly since these agents are frequently used chronically. Generally speaking, aspirin is very inexpensive; phenylbutazone and indomethacin are more expensive; the cost of the newer drugs is very high.

THE SALICYLATES

Aspirin (acetylsalicylic acid) is probably still the most extensively employed analgesic-antipyretic and anti-inflammatory agent, and it is the standard for comparison and evaluation of the others.

As a therapeutic agent, aspirin presents something of a paradox. Prodigious amounts of the drug are consumed in the United States; some estimates place the quantity as high as 10 to 20 thousand tons annually. The layman relies upon it as the common household analgesic; yet, because the drug is so generally available, he often underrates its usefulness. Likewise, the pharmacologist and clinician praise the efficacy and safety of aspirin as an analgesic and antirheumatic agent; yet they find it necessary to warn constantly of its role as a common cause of lethal drug poisoning in young children and its potential for serious toxicity if it is used improperly.

The older literature on salicylates has been summarized by Hanzlik (1927); subsequent developments have been reviewed extensively (*see* Gross and Greenberg, 1948; Randall, 1963; Symposium, 1963, 1966b; Smith and Smith, 1966). Cohen (1976) and Miller and coworkers (1978) have provided more recent reviews of some of the clinical pharmacology.

Chemistry. Salicylic acid (orthohydroxybenzoic acid) is so irritating that it can only be used externally, and, therefore, various derivatives of this acid have been synthesized for systemic use. These comprise two large classes, namely, *esters of salicylic acid* obtained by substitution in the carboxyl group, and *salicylate esters of organic acids* in which the carboxyl group of salicylic acid is retained and substitution is made in the OH group. For example, aspirin is an ester of acetic acid. In addition, there are salts of salicylic acid. The chemical relationships can be seen clearly from the structural formulas shown in Table 29–1.

Structure-Activity Relationship. Salicylates generally act by virtue of their salicylic acid content, although some of the effects of aspirin are due to its capacity to acetylate proteins (*see* below). Substitutions on the carboxyl or hydroxyl groups change the potency or toxicity of the compound. The *ortho* position of the OH group is an important feature for the action of salicylate. Benzoic acid, C_6H_5COOH, shares many of the actions of salicylic acid but is much weaker. The effects of simple substitutions on the benzene ring have been extensively studied, and

Table 29–1. STRUCTURAL FORMULAS OF THE SALICYLATES

Salicylic Acid — Sodium Salicylate — Aspirin — Methyl Salicylate

new salicylate derivatives are still being synthesized. Recently, a difluorophenyl derivative, *diflunisal,* has been introduced for clinical use in some parts of the world; its efficacy has not yet been appraised.

PHARMACOLOGICAL PROPERTIES

Analgesia. The types of pain amenable to relief by salicylates are those of low intensity, whether circumscribed or widespread in origin; particularly amenable are headache, myalgia, arthralgia, and other pains arising from integumental structures rather than from viscera. The salicylates have lower maximal effects than do the opioid analgesics and hence are used only for pain of slight-to-moderate intensity. The salicylates are more widely used for pain relief than is any other class of drugs. Chronic use does not lead to tolerance or addiction, and toxicity is lower than that of more potent analgesics. The salicylates alleviate pain by virtue of both a peripheral and a CNS effect. The peripheral action of aspirin-like drugs has been discussed above.

Direct effects of salicylates on the CNS have been described and suggest a hypothalamic site of action for some of the analgesic as well as for the antipyretic effect. This is supported by the fact that analgesic doses do not cause mental disturbances, hypnosis, or changes in modalities of sensation other than pain. Neither do salicylates appear to affect the reticular pathways involved in arousal and in domination of attention caused by pain. Both peripheral and CNS factors appear to contribute significantly to the pain relief afforded by this class of drugs (*see* Winder, 1959; Paalzow, 1969; Dubas and Parker, 1971).

Antipyresis. Salicylates lower an elevated body temperature, as discussed above. The antipyretic effect is usually rapid and effective. Whereas moderate doses of salicylates lower an elevated body temperature, they also increase oxygen consumption and metabolic rate. In toxic doses, these compounds have a pyretic effect that results in sweating; this enhances the dehydration that occurs in salicylate intoxication (*see* below).

Miscellaneous Neurological Effects. In high doses, salicylates have toxic effects on the CNS, consisting in stimulation (including convulsions) followed by depression. Confusion, dizziness, tinnitus, high-tone deafness, delirium, psychosis, stupor, and coma may occur. The *tinnitus* and *hearing loss* caused by salicylate poisoning are similar to those seen in Ménière's disease and are due to increased labyrinthine pressure or an effect on the hair cells of the cochlea. There is a close relation between the hearing loss in decibels and the concentration of salicylate in plasma. The loss is completely reversible within 2 or 3 days after withdrawal of the drug.

Nausea and *vomiting* are induced by salicylates and result from stimulation of sites that are accessible from the cerebrospinal fluid (CSF), probably in the medullary chemoreceptor trigger zone (CTZ). In man, centrally induced nausea and vomiting generally appear at plasma salicylate concentrations of about 270 μg/ml, but these same effects may occur at much lower plasma values as a result of local gastric irritation.

Respiration. The effects of salicylate on respiration are of paramount importance because they contribute to the serious acid-base balance disturbances that characterize poisoning by this class of compounds. Salicylates stimulate respiration directly and indirectly. Full therapeutic doses of salicylates increase oxygen consumption and CO_2 production in experimental animals and man. This effect of salicylate occurs primarily in skeletal muscle and is a result of salicylate-induced uncoupling of oxidative phosphorylation (*see* below). The increased production of CO_2 stimulates respiration. The increased alveolar ventilation balances the increased CO_2 production, and thus plasma CO_2 tension (P_{CO_2}) does not change. The *initial* increase in alveolar ventilation is characterized mainly by an increase in depth of respiration and only a slight increase in rate, a pattern similar to that produced by inhalation of CO_2 and by exercise. If a barbiturate or morphine is administered to depress the respiratory response to CO_2, plasma P_{CO_2} increases markedly and a respiratory acidosis develops.

As salicylate gains access to the medulla, it directly stimulates the respiratory center. This results in marked hyperventilation, characterized by an increase in depth and a pronounced increase in rate. During the initial phase of salicylate toxicity in dogs, alveolar ventilation and respiratory rate may double; during the later phase of direct central stimulation, respiratory minute volume is increased as much as tenfold, alveolar and plasma P_{CO_2} fall, the latter to as low as 16 mm Hg, and *respiratory alkalosis* ensues. Similarly, dramatic changes occur in patients with salicylate poisoning. Plasma salicylate concentrations of 350 μg/ml are nearly always associated with hyperventilation in man, and marked hyperpnea occurs when the level approaches 500 μg/ml.

A *depressant* effect of salicylate on the medulla appears after high doses or after prolonged exposure. Toxic doses of salicylates cause central respiratory paralysis as well as circulatory collapse secondary to vasomotor depression. Since enhanced CO_2 production continues, respiratory acidosis ensues (*see* below).

Acid-Base Balance and Electrolyte Pattern. Therapeutic doses of salicylate produce definite changes in the acid-base balance and electrolyte pattern. The initial event, as discussed above, is an extracellular and intracellular *respiratory alkalosis. Compensation* for the respiratory alkalosis promptly ensues. Renal excretion of bicarbonate accompanied by sodium and potassium is increased, plasma bicarbonate is thus lowered, and blood pH returns toward normal. This is the stage of *compensated respiratory alkalosis.*

This phase of the acid-base sequence is most often seen in adults given intensive salicylate therapy and seldom proceeds further. The severity of the respiratory alkalosis is proportional to the dose of salicylate and the duration of medication. In ten healthy adults given 12 g of aspirin over a period of 9 hours, Farber and coworkers (1949) observed the following changes: an average increase of 4 liters per minute in respiratory volume, and a respiratory alkalosis with an increase in plasma pH of 0.06 unit, a decrease in plasma P_{CO_2} of 10.5 mm Hg, and a decrease in plasma bicarbonate of 3.0 mEq per liter. The maximal acid-base change occurred 2 to 4 hours after the

peak plasma salicylate concentration (390 μg/ml) was reached; significant alterations were still discernible 20 hours after the last dose of drug. Salicylism occurred in eight of the ten subjects.

Subsequent changes in acid-base status generally occur only when toxic doses of salicylates are ingested by infants and children and occasionally after large doses in adults. In infants and children, the phase of respiratory alkalosis may not be observed by the physician, since the child with salicylate intoxication is rarely seen early enough. The stage generally present is characterized by a decrease in blood pH, a low plasma bicarbonate concentration, and a normal or nearly normal plasma P_{CO_2}, changes consistent, except for P_{CO_2}, with the picture of metabolic acidosis. However, in reality there is a *combination of respiratory acidosis and metabolic acidosis* produced as follows. The respiratory depression from toxic doses of salicylate permits the enhanced production of CO_2 to outstrip its alveolar excretion; consequently, plasma P_{CO_2} increases and blood pH decreases. Since the concentration of bicarbonate in plasma is already low due to increased renal bicarbonate excretion, the acid-base status at this stage is essentially an uncompensated respiratory acidosis. Superimposed, however, is a true metabolic acidosis caused by accumulation of acids as a result of three processes. First, salicylic acid derivatives dissociate at plasma pH, and in toxic doses displace about 2 to 3 mEq per liter of plasma bicarbonate. Second, vasomotor depression caused by toxic doses of salicylate impairs renal function with consequent accumulation of strong acids of metabolic origin, namely, sulfuric and phosphoric acids. Third, organic acids accumulate secondary to salicylate-induced derangement of carbohydrate metabolism, especially pyruvic, lactic, and acetoacetic acids. Hence, metabolic acidosis is further enhanced.

The series of events that produce acid-base disturbances in salicylate intoxication also cause alterations of *water and electrolyte balance.* The low plasma P_{CO_2} leads to decreased renal tubular reabsorption of bicarbonate and increased renal excretion of sodium, potassium, and water (*see* introduction to Section VIII). In addition, water is lost by salicylate-induced sweating and by insensible water loss through the lungs during hyperventilation, and dehydration rapidly occurs. Since more water than electrolyte is lost by way of the sweat and lungs, the dehydration is associated with hypernatremia.

Prolonged exposure to high doses of salicylate also causes *potassium depletion* due to both renal and extrarenal factors.

Cardiovascular Effects. Ordinary therapeutic doses of salicylates have no important direct cardiovascular actions. The peripheral vessels tend to dilate after large doses, due to a direct effect on their smooth muscle. Toxic amounts depress the circulation directly and by central vasomotor paralysis.

In patients given large doses of sodium salicylate or aspirin, such as are used in acute rheumatic fever, the circulating plasma volume increases (about 20%), the hematocrit falls, and cardiac output and work are increased. Consequently, in patients with clear evidence of carditis, such alterations can cause congestive failure and pulmonary edema, and high doses are best avoided in such individuals (Alexander and Smith, 1962).

Gastrointestinal Effects. The ingestion of salicylate may result in epigastric distress, nausea, and vomiting. The mechanism of the emetic effect is discussed above. Salicylate may also cause gastric ulceration and even hemorrhage in experimental animals and in man. Exacerbation of peptic ulcer symptoms (heartburn, dyspepsia), gastrointestinal hemorrhage, and erosive gastritis have all been reported in patients on high-dose therapy, but may rarely occur with low doses as a hypersensitivity response. The salicylate-induced gastric bleeding is painless and frequently leads to blood loss in the stool and occasionally to an iron-deficiency anemia. In most cases, however, blood loss is not significant.

The occurrence of these effects in *man* has been demonstrated by many investigators (for reviews, *see* Symposium, 1963; Smith and Smith, 1966; Paulus and Whitehouse, 1973). For example, ingestion of 4 or 5 g of aspirin per day for 26 days, a dose that produces plasma salicylate concentrations in the usual range for anti-inflammatory therapy (120 to 350 μg/ml), results in an average fecal blood loss of about 3 to 8 ml per day as compared with approximately 0.6 ml per day in untreated subjects (Leonards and Levy, 1973). Gastroscopic or direct examination in salicylate-treated subjects reveals discrete ulcerative and hemorrhagic lesions of the gastric mucosa; in many cases, multiple hemorrhagic lesions with sharply demarcated areas of focal necrosis are observed.

The mechanism by which salicylates injure gastric mucosal cells is complex. Gastric acidity plays an important role, and other factors are also involved. Salicylates break down the normal gastric mucosal barrier against back diffusion of hydrogen ions and leakage of other ions, resulting in injury to the submucosal capillaries with subsequent necrosis and bleeding. Other salicylate-induced responses include reduction in the formation of PGI_2, which inhibits gastric acid secretion and regulates blood flow. There may be an increased bleeding tendency, secondary to impaired platelet aggregation, and a reduction in the biosynthesis and secretion of protective mucus. The incidence of bleeding is highest with salicylates that dissolve slowly and deposit as particles in the gastric mucosal folds. Occult blood loss might be reduced or prevented by administering aspirin in a solution that is made just before it is ingested or in a dosage form that provides reliable disintegration and dissolution. Ethanol ingestion may increase the occult blood loss induced by aspirin.

Hepatic and Renal Effects. There are increasingly frequent reports in the literature that salicylates have a deleterious effect on hepatic function (*e.g., see* Halla, 1976), but it is not absolutely clear whether this dysfunction is caused by salicylates *per se* or whether an underlying disease is intensified by salicylate therapy. The usual clinical findings (seen when the concentration of salicylate in plasma exceeds 250 μg/ml) are elevated enzyme activities in plasma, indicative of hepatic damage (SGOT, SGPT, alkaline phosphatase), occasional hepatomegaly, low-level periportal mononuclear infiltration, and decreased synthesis of cholic acid. The amount of damage appears to be minimal, is readily reversible, and should not preclude further salicylate therapy. Patients with a preexisting history of liver disease are more likely to develop changes in hepatic function in response to aspirin.

The salicylates cause an increase in the volume of bile, but they decrease the total excretion of cholate; the choleretic effect is apparently due to a direct action on hepatic cells. In severe salicylate intoxication, fatty infiltration of the liver and kidney may occur. Urinary changes are infrequent, and, even after high therapeutic doses and prolonged use of salicylate, normal renal function is usually unaltered.

Uricosuric Effects. Appropriate doses of salicylate increase the urinary excretion of urates, and the drug was once used in acute and chronic gout. The uricosuric action is markedly dependent on the dose. Low doses (1 or 2 g per day) may actually decrease urate excretion and elevate plasma urate concentrations; intermediate doses (2 or 3 g per day) usually do not alter urate excretion; large doses (over 5 g per day) induce uricosuria and lower plasma urate levels. Such large doses are poorly tolerated. Even small doses of salicylate should not be given concomitantly with probenecid and other uricosuric agents that decrease tubular reabsorption of uric acid, because it annuls their effect.

Effects on the Blood. Ingestion of aspirin by normal individuals causes a definite prolongation of the bleeding time; this is not due to hypoprothrombinemia and can occur with a dose as small as 0.3 g. For example, a single dose of 0.65 g of aspirin approximately doubles the mean bleeding time of normal persons for a period of 4 to 7 days. This effect is probably due to acetylation of platelet cyclooxygenase, as described above.

Aspirin should be avoided in patients with severe hepatic damage, hypoprothrombinemia, vitamin K deficiency, or hemophilia, because the inhibition of platelet hemostasis can result in hemorrhage. Also, aspirin therapy should be stopped at least 1 week prior to surgery. Additionally, care should be exercised in the use of aspirin during long-term treatment with oral anticoagulant agents, because of the possible danger of blood loss from the gastric mucosa. However, the intentional use of aspirin and other drugs inhibiting platelet aggregation, in conjunction with oral anticoagulants, is being actively explored for the prophylaxis of coronary and cerebral arterial thrombosis (*e.g., see* Aspirin Myocardial Infarction Study, 1980).

Salicylate medication does not ordinarily alter the *leukocyte* or *erythrocyte* count, the hematocrit, or the hemoglobin content, nor does it produce methemoglobinemia. The mechanism of the salicylate reduction in leukocytosis and in the elevated *erythrocyte sedimentation rate* in acute rheumatic fever is not understood. The *plasma iron concentration* is markedly decreased and *erythrocyte survival time* shortened by doses of 3 to 4 g per day. Aspirin is included among the drugs that can cause a mild degree of hemolysis in individuals with a glucose-6-phosphate dehydrogenase deficiency.

Effects on Rheumatic, Inflammatory, and Immunological Processes, and on Connective Tissue Metabolism.
For almost 100 years the salicylates have retained their preeminent position in the treatment of the rheumatic diseases. Although they suppress the clinical signs and even improve the histological picture in acute rheumatic fever, subsequent tissue damage such as cardiac lesions and other visceral involvement is unaffected. In addition to their action on prostaglandin biosynthesis, the mechanism of action of the salicylates in rheumatic disease may also involve effects on other cellular and immunological processes in mesenchymal and connective tissues.

Because of the known relationship between rheumatic fever and immunological processes, attention has been directed to the effects of salicylates on *antigen-antibody* reactions. These agents suppress a variety of such reactions. Several different mechanisms are involved, including suppression of antibody production, interference with antigen-antibody aggregation, inhibition *in vitro* of antigen-induced release of histamine, and nonspecific stabilization of changes in capillary permeability in the presence of immunological insults. The concentrations of salicylates needed to produce these effects are high, and the relationship of the suppressive effects of salicylates on immunological processes to their antirheumatic efficacy in man is yet to be determined.

Drugs useful as antirheumatic and anti-inflammatory agents influence the metabolism of *connective tissue,* and these effects may be involved in their anti-inflammatory action. For example, salicylates can affect the composition, biosynthesis, or metabolism of connective tissue mucopolysaccharides concerned with the ground substance that provides barriers to spread of infection and inflammation. (*See* Whitehouse, 1965; Smith and Smith, 1966; Paulus and Whitehouse, 1973.)

Metabolic Effects. The salicylates have a multiplicity of effects on metabolic processes, some of which have already been discussed. Only a few pertinent aspects will be presented here. (*See* Symposium, 1963; Whitehouse, 1965; Smith and Smith, 1966; Smith and Dawkins, 1971; Paulus and Whitehouse, 1973.)

Oxidative Phosphorylation. The uncoupling of oxidative phosphorylation by salicylate is similar to that induced by 2,4-dinitrophenol. The effect occurs in man with doses of salicylate used in the treatment of rheumatoid arthritis.

As a result of the uncoupling action of salicylates, a number of adenosine triphosphate (ATP)–dependent reactions are inhibited. The salicylate-induced increase in oxygen uptake and carbon dioxide production, described above, is due to the uncoupling action of the drug and the enhanced oxidation compensatory to the relative inefficiency of the phosphorylating mechanisms. The salicylate-induced depletion of hepatic glycogen can also be explained by this mechanism. The pyretic effect of toxic doses of salicylate can be similarly explained since the oxidatively derived energy normally used for the conversion of inorganic phosphate to ATP is dissipated principally as heat. Salicylate in toxic doses may decrease aerobic metabolism as a result of inhibition of various dehydrogenases, by competing with the pyridine nucleotide coenzymes, and inhibition of some oxidases that require nucleotides as coenzymes, such as xanthine oxidase.

Carbohydrate Metabolism. The effects of salicylate on carbohydrate metabolism are complex. Multiple factors appear to be involved, some tending to lower and others to raise the blood glucose concentration. In both animals and man, large doses of salicylates may cause hyperglycemia and glycosuria and deplete liver and muscle glycogen; these effects are partly explained by the release of epinephrine, through activation of central sympathetic centers. Such large doses also reduce aerobic metabolism of glucose, increase glucose-6-phosphatase activity, and promote the secretion of glucocorticoids.

Nitrogen Metabolism. Salicylate in toxic doses causes a significant negative nitrogen balance, characterized by an aminoaciduria. Adrenocortical activation may contribute to the negative nitrogen balance by enhancing protein catabolism. The mechanism of the aminoaciduria produced by salicylates is not known.

Fat Metabolism. Salicylates reduce lipogenesis by partially blocking incorporation of acetate into fatty acids; they also inhibit epinephrine-stimulated lipolysis in fat cells and displace long-chain fatty acids from binding sites on human plasma proteins. The combination of these effects leads to increased entry and enhanced oxidation of fatty acids in muscle, liver, and other tissues, and to the lowering of concentrations of plasma free fatty acids, phospholipid, and cholesterol; the oxidation of ketone bodies is also increased.

Endocrine Effects. Salicylate directly or indirectly influences the function of a number of endocrine systems; such effects are in part responsible for some of the metabolic and pharmacological responses to the drug.

Adrenal Cortex. Very large doses of salicylate stimulate steroid secretion by the adrenal cortex through an effect on the hypothalamus and increase transiently the plasma concentrations of free adrenocorticosteroids by displacement from plasma proteins. However, there is abundant evidence that the anti-inflammatory effects of salicylate are independent of these effects on adrenocorticosteroids (*see* Domenjoz, 1966; Smith and Smith, 1966; Paulus and Whitehouse, 1973).

Thyroid Gland. Chronic administration of salicylate decreases the plasma protein-bound iodine and thyroidal uptake and clearance of iodine, but increases oxygen consumption and rate of disappearance of thyroxine and triiodothyronine from the circulation. These effects are probably due to the competitive displacement by salicylate of thyroxine and triiodothyronine from prealbumin and the thyroxine-binding globulin in plasma.

Salicylates and Pregnancy. There is no evidence that therapeutic doses of salicylates cause fetal damage in human beings, although babies born to women who ingest salicylates chronically may have significantly reduced weights at birth. In addition, there is a definite increase in perinatal mortality, anemia, ante-partum and post-partum hemorrhage, prolonged gestation, and complicated deliveries (Lewis and Schulman, 1973; Collins and Turner, 1975; Turner and Collins, 1975).

Local Irritant Effects. Salicylic acid is quite irritating to skin and mucosa and destroys epithelial cells. The keratolytic action of the free acid is employed for the local treatment of warts, corns, fungal infections, and certain types of eczematous dermatitis. The tissue cells swell, soften, and desquamate. The salts of salicylic acid are innocuous to the unbroken skin; however, if the free acid is released in the stomach, the gastric mucosa may be irritated. Methyl salicylate (oil of wintergreen) is irritating to both skin and gastric mucosa and is only used externally, in liniments as a counterirritant.

Pharmacokinetics and Metabolism. These important aspects of the salicylates have been reviewed by Davison (1971).

Absorption. Orally ingested salicylates are absorbed rapidly, partly from the stomach but mostly from the upper small intestine. Appreciable concentrations are found in plasma in less than 30 minutes; after a single dose, a peak value is reached in about 2 hours and then gradually declines. Rate of absorption is determined by many factors, particularly the disintegration and dissolution rates if tablets are given, the pH at the mucosal surfaces, and gastric emptying time.

Salicylate absorption occurs by passive diffusion primarily of the nondissociated lipid-soluble molecules (salicylic acid and acetylsalicylic acid) across gastrointestinal membranes and hence is influenced by gastric pH. If the pH is increased, salicylate is more ionized and this tends to decrease rate of absorption; however, a rise in pH also increases solubility of salicylate, enhancing its absorption. Actually, there is little meaningful difference between the rates of absorption of sodium salicylate, aspirin, and the numerous buffered preparations of salicylates. For example, in man the absorption half-time for unbuffered aspirin is about 30 minutes, for buffered aspirin about 20 minutes, and for an aspirin solution only slightly less. What differences do exist probably have no therapeutic significance, since the rate-limiting factor in the onset of effects is accumulation of these drugs at their sites of action. The presence of food delays absorption of salicylates.

Rectal absorption of salicylate is usually slower, incomplete, and unreliable; rectal administration is therefore not advisable when high plasma concentrations of the drug are required. Salicylic acid is rapidly absorbed from the intact *skin,* especially when applied in oily liniments or ointments, and systemic poisoning has occurred from its application to large areas of skin. Methyl salicylate is likewise speedily absorbed when applied cutaneously; its gastrointestinal absorption may be delayed many hours, and, therefore, gastric lavage should be performed even in cases of poisoning that are seen late.

When the nonionized salicylate molecules in the gastric lumen enter the mucosal cells, they dissociate predominantly to the ionized form at the intracellular pH of 7.0 and accumulate there in large amounts; for example, the concentration of salicylate anion in mucosal cells may be 15 to 20 times that in the gastric lumen. As a result, gastric mucosal damage may occur.

Distribution. After absorption, salicylate is distributed throughout most body tissues and most transcellular fluids, primarily by pH-dependent passive processes. For example, it can be detected in synovial, spinal, and peritoneal fluid, and in saliva and milk. Salicylate is actively transported by a low-capacity, saturable system out of the CSF across the choroid plexus. Salicylate crosses the blood-brain barrier only slowly because of the large fraction of drug in the ionized form. The drug readily crosses the placental barrier. It is not secreted in gastric juice. Only traces of salicylate are present in sweat, bile, and feces.

The volumes of distribution of aspirin and sodium salicylate in normal subjects average about 150 ml/kg of body weight, a value equivalent to that of the extracellular space; since salicylate is present within cells in various tissues, this suggests a markedly uneven distribution of salicylate in the body.

Ingested aspirin is mainly absorbed as such, but some enters the systemic circulation as salicylic acid, consequent to hydrolysis by esterases in the gastrointestinal mucosa and the liver. Aspirin can be detected in the plasma only for a short time; for example, 30 minutes after a dose of 0.65 g, only 27% of the total plasma salicylate is in the acetylated form. The absorbed ester is rapidly hydrolyzed to salicylic acid in plasma, liver, and erythrocytes, and more slowly in synovial fluid. As a result of the rapid hydrolysis, plasma concentrations of aspirin are always low and rarely exceed 20 μg/ml at ordinary therapeutic doses. Aspirin *per se* is pharmacologically active and does not require hydrolysis to salicylic acid for its effects. Methyl salicylate is also rapidly hydrolyzed to salicylic acid, mainly in the liver.

At concentrations encountered clinically, from 80 to 90% of the salicylate is bound to plasma proteins, especially albumin. Hypoalbuminemia, as may occur in rheumatoid arthritis, is associated with a proportionately higher level of free salicylate in the plasma. Salicylate competes with thyroxine, triiodothyronine, penicillin, thiopental, phenytoin, sulfinpyrazone, bilirubin, trytophan, certain peptides, possibly steroids, uric acid, and naproxen for plasma protein binding sites. Aspirin as such is bound to a more limited extent; however, it acetylates human plasma albumin *in vivo* by reaction with the ϵ-amino group of lysine. Hormones, DNA, platelets, and hemoglobin and other proteins are also acetylated. The binding of phenylbutazone and flufenamic acid to albumin is modified as a result of acetylation of this protein by aspirin. The acetylation of human plasma albumin by aspirin is inhibited by salicylate anion.

Biotransformation and Excretion. The biotransformation of salicylate takes place in many tissues, but particularly in hepatic endoplasmic reticulum and mitochondria. The three chief metabolic products are salicyluric acid (the glycine conjugate), the ether or phenolic glucuronide, and the ester or acyl glucuronide. In addition, a small fraction is oxidized to gentisic acid (2,5-dihydroxybenzoic acid) and to 2,3-dihydroxybenzoic and 2,3,5-trihydroxybenzoic acids. Wilson and associates (1978) have found a new metabolite of salicylic acid in man—gentisuric acid, the glycine conjugate of gentisic acid. The metabolism of salicylate normally follows first-order kinetics. However, after very large doses, enzymes that metabolize the drug become saturated.

Salicylates are *excreted* mainly by the kidney. Studies in man indicate that salicylate is excreted in the urine as free salicylic acid (10%), salicyluric acid (75%), salicylic phenolic (10%) and acyl (5%) glucuronides, and gentisic acid ($<$1%). However, excretion of free salicylate is extremely variable. In alkaline urine up to 85% of the ingested drug is eliminated as free salicylate, whereas in acidic urine this may be as low as 5%.

The plasma half-life for aspirin is approximately 15 minutes; that for salicylate is 2 to 3 hours in low doses and 15 to 30 hours at high doses. This dose-dependent elimination is the result of the limited ability of the liver to form salicyluric acid and the phenolic glucuronide (Levy *et al.*, 1972).

The plasma concentration of salicylate is increased by conditions that decrease glomerular filtration rate or reduce the secretory Tm of the proximal tubules, such as renal disease or the presence of inhibitors that compete for the transport system (*e.g.*, probenecid). Changes in urinary pH in the acid range have negligible effects on salicylate clearance; however, the mean clearance is about four times as great at pH 8.0 as at pH 6.0. The clearance is well above the glomerular filtration rate at pH 8.0 but considerably below it when the urine is acidic. This is due to the fact that salicylate and salicylurate are highly ionized at pH 8.0, and little diffuses back from the renal tubular lumen. At a urinary pH of 6.0, a large fraction of salicylate is nonionized and readily back-diffuses. High rates of urine flow decrease tubular back diffusion, whereas the opposite is true in oliguria. The conjugates of salicylic acid with glycine and glucuronic acid are water-soluble organic acids that do not readily back-diffuse across the renal tubular cells. Their excretion, therefore, is both by glomerular filtration and proximal tubular secretion and is not pH dependent.

Although not metabolized to salicylate in the body, *salicylamide* has antipyretic, analgesic, and anti-inflammatory effects similar to those of salicylate. It also has sedative and hypotensive effects. However, the drug is very rapidly inactivated during absorption and the initial circulation through the liver. Concentrations of active drug in the systemic

THE SALICYLATES **695**

circulation are markedly influenced by the dosage form, and they are disproportionately low after low doses. Salicylamide may inhibit the metabolism of other drugs by the liver.

Preparations, Routes of Administration, and Dosage. The two most commonly used preparations of salicylate for systemic effects are *sodium salicylate* and *aspirin (acetylsalicylic acid)*.

Sodium Salicylate, U.S.P., is a white, water-soluble powder with a sweet, saline taste. It is available as official tablets that contain 300 or 600 mg of drug.

Aspirin, U.S.P., is a white powder, poorly soluble in water (1:300). It is available as official tablets ranging from 65 to 650 mg, capsules (300 mg), and suppositories ranging from 65 to 1300 mg.

Methyl salicylate (sweet birch oil, wintergreen oil, gaultheria oil, betula oil) is a colorless, yellowish, or reddish liquid having the characteristic odor and taste of wintergreen. It is employed only for cutaneous counterirritation in the form of salves and liniments.

Salicylic Acid, U.S.P., is a white powder poorly soluble in water (1:460) but quite soluble in alcohol (1:3). Its use is reserved for local application as a keratolytic agent, in official plasters and collodion, and as a component of *Benzoic and Salicylic Acids Ointment,* U.S.P., and *Zinc Oxide and Salicylic Acid Paste,* U.S.P.

Salicylamide, the amide of salicylic acid, is no longer an official drug. Its effects in man are not reliable, and its use is not recommended. The small doses included in "over-the-counter" analgesic and sedative mixtures are probably ineffective.

The *dose* of salicylate depends on the condition being treated. The usual single dose of sodium salicylate or aspirin in adults is 300 mg to 1.0 g. This may be repeated every 4 hours. In acute rheumatic fever and rheumatoid arthritis more intensive medication is employed (*see* below).

The *route of administration* is practically always oral. There is rarely any necessity for parenteral administration. The *rectal* administration of aspirin suppositories or sodium salicylate (2%) in thin starch or acacia solution may be necessary in infants or when oral medication is not retained. Salicylates are conveniently taken in tablets or capsules with a full glass of water to minimize gastric irritation. Aspirin is poorly soluble, has many chemical incompatibilities, and should be dispensed only in solid dry form.

Timed-release preparations are of limited value, since the half-time for elimination of salicylate is so long. Absorption from *enteric-coated* tablets is sometimes incomplete.

Preparations of aspirin containing alkali or buffer are sometimes better tolerated, but alkalinization of the urine, which may occur, can shorten the plasma half-life of salicylates considerably (*see* above).

Toxic Effects

Salicylates are widely used in medicine and are indiscriminately employed by the laity for every conceivable ailment. Over 10,000 cases of serious salicylate intoxication are seen in the United States every year. Some of them are fatal, and many occur in children. Considering their abuse and their availability, the high incidence of toxic reactions to salicylate is not surprising, and the drug should not be viewed as a harmless household remedy.

Hypersensitivity is also a cause of untoward responses to salicylate. Furthermore, renal or hepatic insufficiency or hypoprothrombinemia or other bleeding disorders enhance the possibility of salicylate toxicity. Children with fever and dehydration are particularly prone to intoxication from relatively small doses of salicylate.

Salicylate Intoxication. The *fatal dose* varies with the preparation of salicylate. From 10 to 30 g of sodium salicylate or aspirin has caused death in adults, but much larger amounts (130 g of aspirin, in one case) have been ingested without fatal outcome. The lethal dose of methyl salicylate is considerably less than that of sodium salicylate. As little as 4 ml (4.7 g) of methyl salicylate may be fatal in children.

Symptoms and Signs. Mild chronic salicylate intoxication is termed *salicylism.* The condition usually occurs only after repeated administration of large doses. When fully developed, the syndrome consists chiefly in headache, dizziness, ringing in the ears, difficulty in hearing, dimness of vision, mental confusion, lassitude, drowsiness, sweating, thirst, hyperventilation, nausea, vomiting, and occasionally diarrhea. Care should be exercised in prescribing salicylate to patients with aural disease. A more severe degree of salicylate intoxication is characterized by CNS disturbances (including EEG abnormalities), skin eruptions, and marked alterations in acid-base balance. The above-mentioned CNS effects are more pronounced; in addition, restlessness, garrulity, incoherent speech, apprehension, vertigo, tremor, diplopia, maniacal delirium, hallucinations, generalized convulsions, and coma may occur. The mental disturbances, sometimes referred to as "salicylate jag," simulate alcoholic inebriation; euphoria and elation are absent, however, and the experience is rather a melancholy affair.

A pustular acneform *skin eruption* simulating that of bromism may develop, but it is usually not observed unless salicylate medication has been continued for longer than 1 week. Other salicylate-induced cutaneous lesions are erythematous, scarlatiniform, pruritic, eczematoid, or desquamative in character. Rarely, the eruptions may be bullous or purpuric, and hemorrhages may occur from mucous membranes. Fever is usually prominent, especially in children. Dehydration often occurs as a result of hyperpyrexia, sweating, vomiting, and the loss of water vapor during hyperventilation.

Gastrointestinal symptoms are often conspicuous and include epigastric distress, nausea, vomiting, anorexia, and occasionally abdominal pain. Approximately 50% of all individuals with plasma salicylate concentrations of more than 300 µg/ml experience nausea.

A most prominent feature of salicylate intoxication is the *disturbance in acid-base balance and electrolyte composition of the plasma,* the characteristics of which have already been presented. The most severe metabolic disturbances occur in infants and very young children who become intoxicated as the result of therapeutic overdosage for some febrile illness, usually a minor respiratory infection; most of the acidotic patients seen with salicylate intoxication are in this group. Higher doses of the drug and a longer duration of intoxication intensify the metabolic effects and the acidosis. In older patients the intoxication is generally due to accidental or suicidal ingestion of a large single dose.

Hemorrhagic phenomena are occasionally seen during salicylate poisoning, the mechanism and significance of which have been discussed. Petechial hemorrhages are a prominent post-mortem feature. Thrombocytopenic purpura is a rare complication. While hyperglycemia may occur during salicylate intoxication, *hypoglycemia* may be a serious consequence of toxicity in young children. It should be seriously considered in any young child with coma, convulsions, or cardiovascular collapse.

Severe toxic *encephalopathy* may be a prominent feature of salicylate poisoning and may be difficult to differentiate from chorea or rheumatic encephalopathy. As poisoning progresses, central stimulation is replaced by increasing depression, stupor, and coma. Cardiovascular collapse and respiratory insufficiency ensue, and terminal asphyxial convulsions and pulmonary edema sometimes appear. Death usually results from respiratory failure after a period of unconsciousness.

Symptoms of poisoning by *methyl salicylate* differ little from those just described. Poisoning occurs most frequently in children who mistake this aromatic oil for candy. Central excitation, intense hyperpnea, and hyperpyrexia are prominent features. The odor of the drug can easily be detected on the breath and in the urine and vomitus. *Methyl salicylate should always be kept where children cannot gain access to it.* Poisoning by *salicylic acid* differs only in the increased prominence of gastrointestinal symptoms due to the marked local irritation. *Phenyl salicylate* intoxication is unique in that the most conspicuous symptoms are due to the phenol that is liberated by hydrolysis, probably in the tissues.

Treatment. Salicylate poisoning represents an acute medical emergency. The treatment is largely symptomatic. Death may result despite all recommended procedures. Salicylate medication is withdrawn as soon as intoxication is suspected. The patient should be hospitalized. *Hospitalization is particularly advisable in the case of methyl salicylate poisoning because children have been known to succumb within a few hours after the parents had been informed that recovery seemed assured or that the intoxication was inconsequential.* Blood should be obtained for plasma salicylate determinations and acid-base and electrolyte studies. The salicylate concentration is reasonably well correlated with clinical severity, when corrected for the duration of the in-

toxication, and is of value in assessing the type of therapy to be instituted. Absorption of salicylate from the gastrointestinal tract can be reduced by emesis, gastric lavage, administration of activated charcoal, or a combination of these.

Hyperthermia and dehydration are the immediate threats to life, and the initial therapy must be directed to their correction and to the maintenance of adequate renal function. External sponging with tepid water or alcohol should be provided quickly to any child with very high fever. Adequate amounts of intravenous fluids must be given promptly. The type and amount of repair solutions to be employed depend upon the interpretation of the laboratory data on acid-base balance. If the patient presents with an acidosis, correction of the low blood pH is essential, especially since acidosis results in a shift of salicylate from plasma into brain and other tissues; alkalosis reverses this process and also increases salicylate excretion (Hill, 1973). Bicarbonate solution should be infused intravenously, if possible, in sufficient quantity to maintain alkaline diuresis. Excessively rapid infusion of bicarbonate can cause pulmonary edema or other unwanted effects. Frequent monitoring of blood pH, plasma P_{CO_2}, and plasma glucose concentration are necessary. Correction of ketosis and hypoglycemia by administration of glucose is also essential for complete control of the metabolic acidosis; however, the ketosis clears only slowly. If potassium deficiency occurs during salicylate intoxication, it should be treated by adding the cation to the intravenous fluids once it has been determined that urine formation is adequate. Plasma transfusion may be beneficial, especially if the shock syndrome intervenes. Any attempt to obtund the salicylate-induced hyperventilation by giving a barbiturate or an opioid is dangerous and may rapidly lead to respiratory acidosis and coma. Hemorrhagic phenomena may necessitate whole-blood transfusion and vitamin K (phytonadione).

Measures to rid the body rapidly of salicylate should be immediately undertaken. Sodium bicarbonate administration is effective and rapid, if an alkaline urine can be produced. Forced diuresis with alkalinizing solution appears to be better than alkali alone; acetazolamide can be added to this combination if a more rapid effect is necessary and only if systemic acidosis is avoided (Hill, 1973). Potassium should be administered with the bicarbonate to prevent further depletion of intracellular potassium.

In severe intoxication, extrarenal measures such as exchange transfusion, peritoneal dialysis, hemodialysis, and hemoperfusion are the most effective measures available for the removal of salicylate. Hemodialysis in adults and older children and exchange transfusion or peritoneal dialysis in infants should be considered seriously in all salicylate-intoxicated patients whose clinical condition is deteriorating despite otherwise appropriate therapy and in those who have associated serious disease. (*See* Smith and Smith, 1966; Symposium, 1968; Done and Temple, 1971; Hill, 1973.)

Aspirin Hypersensitivity. Aspirin hypersensitivity or intolerance is a rather uncommon syndrome, but one that it is important to recognize, since the administration of aspirin and many other aspirin-like drugs may result in severe and possibly fatal toxic reactions.

It is difficult to estimate what proportion of the population exhibits this hypersensitivity reaction, but a total figure of a quarter of a million persons in the United States has been quoted (Abrishami and Thomas, 1977). The syndrome usually occurs in middle-aged patients, and there is a preponderance of females; intolerance is rare in children. A previous history of hypersensitivity reaction to other chemicals, endogenous asthma, and (especially) the occurrence of nasal polyps are warning signs.

The clinical manifestations of the syndrome may appear within minutes of ingestion of the drug. They range from vasomotor rhinitis with profuse watery secretions, angioneurotic edema, urticaria, and bronchial asthma to laryngeal edema and broncho-constriction, hypotension, shock, loss of consciousness, and complete vasomotor collapse. This reaction may occur in response to tiny amounts of aspirin. Other features, such as an abnormal prolongation of bleeding time, may also be seen.

Aspirin is the dominant *salicylate* that commonly provokes this response (reports of sodium salicylate having this effect are rather uncommon), but many other aspirin-like drugs can produce similar reactions. The underlying mechanism is unknown; despite the resemblance to anaphylaxis, it does *not* appear to be immunological in nature. The only common factor among the drugs that provoke the reaction appears to be that they are all potent inhibitors of prostaglandin biosynthesis (Szceklik *et al.,* 1975). Treatment of such responses to salicylates does not differ from that ordinarily employed in acute anaphylactic reactions. Epinephrine is the drug of choice and usually controls angioedema and urticaria without difficulty; asthma induced by aspirin may at times prove refractory to therapy (*see* Abrishami and Thomas, 1977).

THERAPEUTIC USES

There are many *systemic* and a few *local* uses of the salicylates. Several are based on tradition and empirical results rather than on a clear understanding of the mechanism of therapeutic benefit. The laity often attributes properties to the salicylates that have no existence in fact.

Systemic Uses. *Antipyresis.* Antipyretic therapy is reserved for patients in whom fever in itself may be deleterious, and for those who experience considerable relief when a fever is lowered. Little is known concerning the relationship between fever and the acceleration of immune processes; it may at times be a protective physiological mechanism. The course of the patient's illness may be obscured by the relief of symptoms and the reduction of fever from the use of antipyretic drugs; otherwise the effect of salicylate is nonspecific and does not influence the course of the underlying disease. The antipyretic dose of salicylate for adults is 325 mg to 1 g, orally every 3 to 4 hours;

for children, 10 to 20 mg/kg every 6 hours, not to exceed a total daily dose of 3.6 g.

Analgesia. Salicylate is valuable for the nonspecific relief of certain types of pain, for example, *headache, arthritis, dysmenorrhea, neuralgia,* and *myalgia.* For this purpose, it is prescribed in the same doses and manner as for antipyresis. The use of salicylate in combination with other analgesics, sedatives, and so forth is discussed later in the chapter.

Acute Rheumatic Fever. In this disease, the salicylates suppress the acute exudative inflammatory process of the disease but do not affect the progression of the disease or the later phases of granulomatous inflammation or scar formation. Within 24 to 48 hours after adequate doses of salicylate, there is usually considerable or complete relief of pain, swelling, immobility, local heat, and redness of the involved joints; fever and pulse rate are lowered and the patient feels much improved. Further joint involvement usually does not occur while appropriate salicylate medication is being given. Other aspects of the management of acute rheumatic fever are not altered as a result of medication with salicylates. Thus, cardiac complications, chorea, encephalopathy, subcutaneous nodules, and other features are not prevented or benefited, and the duration of the disease is not shortened. However, if a patient has severe carditis and heart failure, the nonspecific anti-inflammatory effect of salicylates and particularly of adrenocorticosteroids may be invaluable in reducing the burden upon the heart.

Dosage. For maximal suppression of rheumatic inflammation, doses that provide a plasma salicylate concentration of 250 to 350 µg/ml should be maintained, but polyarthritis and fever usually respond to smaller amounts. For adults, a total daily dosage of 5 to 8 g, given at intervals in 1-g amounts, usually suffices. Children are given 100 to 125 mg/kg per day, in divided portions every 4 to 6 hours, for up to 1 week; the dose is then reduced in stepwise fashion at weekly intervals to 60 mg/kg per day (10 mg/kg every 4 hours, or 15 mg/kg every 6 hours) and maintained as long as necessary. Anorexia, tinnitus, nausea, and vomiting are common during the first 3 or 4 days of therapy, but tend to subside despite continuation of medication. There is no fixed dose or schedule that will give optimal results in all patients. Large doses should be employed only if smaller amounts fail to give relief; indeed, relatively small doses (5 g per day) may occasionally cause very high plasma salicylate levels. Ordinarily, full doses are continued until at least 2 weeks after the patient is asymptomatic and all evidence of active inflammation has disappeared. The drug is then gradually discontinued over a period of 7 to 10 days. If symptoms and signs of the disease reappear, salicylate therapy is reinstituted. Aspirin is recommended and sodium salicylate should be avoided, because restricted sodium intake may be advisable if there is evidence of active cardiac involvement. Therapy with adrenocorticosteroids does not yield overall results superior to those obtained with the salicylates. Salicylate and adrenocorticosteroid are additive in their effects; an advantage of their concurrent use is the reduction of dosage of the steroid and thereby its side effects. If carditis is not evident, salicylates and not steroids should be used. However, if acute severe carditis is present, most investigators believe adreno-corticosteroids should be given instead of salicylates, at least initially. (*See* McEwen, 1959; Combined Rheumatic Fever Study Group, 1960, 1965; United Kingdom and United States Joint Report, 1960.)

Rheumatoid Arthritis. Despite the development of the newer anti-inflammatory agents, salicylates are still regarded as the standard with which other drugs should be compared for the treatment of rheumatoid arthritis. In addition to the analgesia that allows more effective therapeutic exercises, there is improvement in appetite and a feeling of well-being. Salicylates also reduce the inflammation in joint tissues and surrounding structures. Damage to joints is the most difficult aspect of rheumatoid arthritis to manage, and any agent that reduces the inflammation is important in lessening or delaying the development of crippling. Salicylates can be shown to produce objectively measurable anti-inflammatory changes when given in large doses for long periods to patients with active rheumatoid disease (*see* Boardman and Hart, 1967a; Deodhar *et al.,* 1973). If necessary, other drugs that favorably affect the course of the arthritis can be used concurrently to good advantage. Fairly large doses of salicylate slightly below those that produce tinnitus (5 to 6 g daily) are advised, but some patients respond well to 3.6 g daily (Multz *et al.,* 1974).

The majority of patients with rheumatoid arthritis can be controlled with salicylates alone or with other aspirin-like anti-inflammatory agents. Some require more aggressive therapy with more toxic drugs, such as gold salts, hydroxychloroquine, penicillamine, adrenocorticosteroids, or immunosuppressive agents.

Other Uses. Aspirin has been used successfully to treat children with *Bartter's syndrome* (*see* above), a disease of complex etiology apparently due to excessive production of renal prostaglandins. Norby and coworkers (1976) found that treatment of a 22-month-old girl with aspirin (100 mg/kg per day) reversed most of the subjective and objective manifestations of the disease.

Closure of a *patent ductus arteriosus* in neonates may sometimes be achieved with inhibitors of prostaglandin biosynthesis (*see* above). Heymann and associates (1976) treated three premature infants with cardiac failure due to a patent ductus with four doses of buffered aspirin (20 mg/kg) administered by orogastric tube every 6 hours. Two of the three infants responded to this treatment, one with a permanent closure and the other with a partial constriction and an improvement in clinical symptoms. There has been more extensive experience with indomethacin (*see* below).

Because of the potent and long-lasting effect of low doses of aspirin on platelet function, it has been suggested that this drug could be of use in the treatment or prophylaxis of diseases associated with platelet hyperaggregability, such as coronary artery disease, myocardial infarction, and postoperative deep-vein thrombosis (*see* Chapter 58).

Relationship of Plasma Salicylate Concentration to Therapeutic Effect and Toxicity. For optimal anti-inflammatory effect for patients with rheumatic diseases, plasma salicylate concentrations of 150 to 300 μg/ml are required. Elimination of salicylate that is free in plasma is dose dependent in this range because saturation of metabolic enzymes is approached. The clearance of the unbound drug thus decreases over the therapeutic range of concentrations. However, *total* clearance of the drug remains unchanged because the fraction of drug that is free and thus available for metabolism also increases as binding sites on plasma proteins are saturated. The total concentration of salicylate in plasma is thus a relatively linear function of dose (Furst *et al.,* 1979). Optimal intensive salicylate therapy can be achieved only by individualizing the total dose of aspirin. This is especially important since the range of plasma salicylate concentrations needed for optimal anti-inflammatory effects may overlap that at which tinnitus is noted. In a study of patients with rheumatoid arthritis by Mongan and coworkers (1973), the range of plasma salicylate concentrations at which tinnitus occurred varied from 196 to 458 μg/ml. Daily dosage varied from 3.6 to 10.8 g. Tinnitus was a reliable index of therapeutic plasma concentration in those patients with normal hearing, but not in those with a preexisting hearing loss. In the latter patients, plasma salicylate concentrations may be a useful guideline. Hyperventilation generally occurs at concentrations greater than 350 μg/ml and other signs of intoxication, such as acidosis, at concentrations greater than 460 μg/ml. Single analgesic-antipyretic doses of salicylate usually yield plasma concentrations below 60 μg/ml.

The plasma concentration of salicylate is generally little affected by other drugs, but concurrent administration of aspirin lowers the concentrations of indomethacin, naproxen, and fenoprofen, at least in part by displacement from plasma proteins. Important adverse interactions of aspirin with warfarin and methotrexate are mentioned above (page 687). Other interactions of aspirin include the antagonism of spironolactone-induced natriuresis and the blockade of the active transport of aminosalicylic acid and penicillin from CSF to blood.

Local Uses. *Salicylic acid* is applied topically as a *keratolytic agent.* In combination with benzoic acid, it is often prescribed for *epidermophytosis.* Salicylic acid is also employed as a *wart* and *corn* remover (10 to 20% in collodion). It is sometimes prescribed in talc (2 to 4%) for *hyperhidrosis.*

Methyl salicylate is reserved for external use as a *counterirritant.* It is employed for painful muscles or joints, in an ointment or liniment. Absorption of methyl salicylate can occur through the skin, and death has resulted from systemic poisoning from the local misapplication of the drug. It is a common *pediatric poison,* and its use should be strongly discouraged. It is also used as a *flavoring agent.*

PYRAZOLON DERIVATIVES

This group of drugs includes phenylbutazone, oxyphenbutazone, antipyrine, aminopyrine, dipyrone, and a recent addition, apazone (azapropazone). With the exception of apazone, these drugs have been in clinical use for many years; phenylbutazone is the most important from the therapeutic viewpoint, while antipyrine and aminopyrine are seldom used today. Apazone is not yet available in the United States.

PHENYLBUTAZONE

Phenylbutazone, employed originally as a solubilizing agent for aminopyrine, was introduced in 1949 for the treatment of rheumatoid arthritis and allied disorders. It is an effective anti-inflammatory agent, but serious toxicity limits its use in long-term therapy. Its structural formula is as follows:

Phenylbutazone

Pharmacological Properties. The anti-inflammatory effects of phenylbutazone are similar to those of the salicylates, but its toxicity differs significantly. Like aminopyrine, phenylbutazone can cause agranulocytosis. The pharmacology and toxicology of phenylbutazone and its metabolites and congeners have been reviewed by Randall (1963) and, more recently, in a symposium (1977b).

Anti-inflammatory Effects. Phenylbutazone has prominent anti-inflammatory effects and is used frequently in, for example, race horses to enhance their performance; somewhat comparable effects are demonstrable in patients with rheumatoid arthritis and related disorders.

Antipyretic and Analgesic Effects. The antipyretic effect of phenylbutazone has been little studied in man. For pain of nonrheumatic origin, its analgesic efficacy is inferior to that of salicylates. Because of its toxicity, phenylbutazone should not be used routinely as an analgesic or antipyretic.

Uricosuric Effect. In doses of about 600 mg per day, phenylbutazone has a mild uricosuric effect in man, probably attributable to one of its metabolites. This results from diminished tubular reabsorption of uric acid. Low concentrations of the drug inhibit tubular secretion of uric acid and cause retention of urate. A congener, *sulfinpyrazone*, is much more effective than phenylbutazone as a uricosuric agent and is useful for the treatment of chronic gout (*see* below and Chapter 38).

Effects on Water and Electrolytes. Phenylbutazone causes significant retention of sodium and chloride, accompanied by a reduction in urine volume; edema may result. The excretion of potassium is not changed. Plasma volume frequently increases as much as 50%, and, as a result, cardiac decompensation and acute pulmonary edema have occurred in patients given the drug. The expansion of plasma volume accounts, in part, for the anemia observed during medication. The retention of sodium and chloride represents a reversible, direct effect of the drug on the renal tubules. The mechanism has not been elucidated.

Other Effects. Phenylbutazone reduces the uptake of iodine by the thyroid gland, apparently secondary to inhibition of biosynthesis of organic iodine compounds. Goiter and myxedema may occasionally result from this effect.

Pharmacokinetics and Metabolism. Phenylbutazone is rapidly and completely absorbed from the gastrointestinal tract or the rectum, and the peak concentration in plasma is reached in 2 hours. After therapeutic doses, phenylbutazone is 98% bound to plasma proteins. The half-time of phenylbutazone in plasma is very long—50 to 100 hours. The drug penetrates into the synovial spaces and reaches a concentration about one half of that in the plasma; significant concentrations may persist in the joints for up to 3 weeks after treatment is discontinued.

Phenylbutazone undergoes extensive metabolic transformation in man. Contrary to early reports, the most significant primary reactions involve glucuronidation and hydroxylation of the phenyl rings or the butyl side chain (Faigle and Dieterle, 1977). The conjugates are excreted in the urine and represent the bulk of the excreted drug. Oxidative pathways are more important in various experimental animals, the half-life of drug in plasma is substantially shorter, and the autoinduction of enzymes that accelerate the degradation of the drug is of greater significance. *Oxyphenbutazone*, a metabolite of phenylbutazone, has antirheumatic and sodium-retaining activities similar to those of the parent drug. Oxyphenbutazone is also extensively bound to plasma proteins and has a half-life in plasma of several days. It accumulates significantly during chronic administration of phenylbutazone and contributes to the pharmacological and toxic effects of the parent drug.

Phenylbutazone and oxyphenbutazone are slowly excreted in the urine, since binding to plasma proteins limits their glomerular filtration and both have a relatively high pK_a, which favors passive reabsorption in the distal tubule. Only a trace of unchanged phenylbutazone is excreted in the urine. Oxyphenbutazone is excreted mainly as the O-glucuronide.

Drug Interactions. Other *anti-inflammatory* agents, *oral anticoagulant* agents, *oral hypoglycemics, sulfonamides,* and other drugs may be displaced from binding to plasma proteins by phenylbutazone. The net result may be increased pharmacological or toxic effects of the displaced drug, depending upon the drug and its disposition after being displaced. The well-documented increased risk of bleeding associated with concurrent phenylbutazone-warfarin medication involves such displacement, but phenylbutazone also modifies the action of the oral anticoagulant agent and influences platelet function. The gastrointestinal effects of phenylbutazone also contribute to the hazard. Displacement of plasma protein–bound thyroid hormone complicates the interpretation of *thyroid function tests.*

Phenylbutazone may cause induction of hepatic microsomal enzymes, and it may also inhibit inactivation of other drugs that are hydroxylated by the microsomal system. It has been said to increase the effect of *insulin.* Oral absorption of phenylbutazone is reduced by concurrently administered *cholestyramine.* The anabolic steroid *methandrostenolone* increases plasma concentrations of administered oxyphenbutazone, but features of the interaction have been inconsistent.

Toxic Effects. Phenylbutazone is poorly tolerated by many patients. Some type of side effect is noted in 10 to 45% of patients, and medication may have to be discontinued in 10 to 15%. Nausea, vomiting, epigastric discomfort, and skin rashes are the most frequently reported untoward effects. Diarrhea, vertigo, insomnia, euphoria, nervousness, hematuria (enhanced by concomitant administration of an anticoagulant), and blurred vision have also been observed. In addition, water and electrolyte retention and edema formation occur.

More serious forms of adverse effects include peptic ulcer (or its reactivation) with hemorrhage or perforation, hypersensitivity reactions of the serum-sickness type, ulcerative stomatitis, hepatitis, nephritis, aplastic anemia, leukopenia, agranulocytosis, and thrombocytopenia. *A number of deaths have occurred, especially from aplastic anemia and agranuloctytosis.*

When phenylbutazone is given, the patient should be closely supervised and his blood should be examined frequently; weight should also be checked to warn of undue retention of sodium. The drug should only be given for short periods (not more than 1 week). Even then, the incidence of disturbing side effects is about 10%. The patient must be told to discontinue the drug and promptly report to the physician if he develops fever, sore throat or other oral lesions, skin rash, pruritus, jaundice, weight increase, or tarry stools. The drug is contraindicated in patients with hypertension; cardiac, renal, or hepatic dysfunction; or a history of peptic ulcer or hypersensitivity to the drug. The toxic effects of the drug are more severe in elderly persons, and its use in this group is inadvisable. (*See* Mauer, 1955; Clinicopathologic Conference, 1961; and many others.)

Preparations, Route of Administration, and Dosage. *Phenylbutazone,* U.S.P. (BUTAZOLIDIN), is available in 100-mg coated tablets for oral adminis-

tration. Daily doses of 300 to 600 mg for brief periods provide maximal therapeutic effects (higher doses only increase toxicity), but the disease may subsequently be adequately controlled by doses of 100 to 400 mg per day. The drug should be taken with meals to lessen gastric irritation.

Therapeutic Uses. Phenylbutazone is used for the therapy of *acute gout* and for the treatment of *rheumatoid arthritis and allied disorders.* Acute exacerbations of these conditions respond particularly well to the drug, and its use should be reserved for such episodes.

Phenylbutazone should be employed only after other drugs have failed and then only after careful consideration of the risks involved as compared with the advantage to the patient. Indiscriminate use of phenylbutazone in the therapy of trivial acute or chronic *musculoskeletal disorders* can only be condemned. It should not be employed as a general analgesic or antipyretic.

Phenylbutazone is an effective alternative to colchicine in *acute gout.* Excellent relief can be attained with a brief course of medication, and about 85 to 95% of acute attacks are controlled within 24 to 36 hours. Phenylbutazone causes fewer gastrointestinal side effects than does colchicine and is more reliable when initiation of medication has been delayed. Dosage recommendations have varied: 800 mg daily for 2 days; 800 mg the first day, followed by 300 mg daily for 3 days; or an initial dose of 400 mg, followed by 100 mg every 4 hours until articular inflammation subsides. The relative merits and dangers of phenylbutazone, compared with colchicine, have been discussed by Goldfinger (1971) and Yü (1974). The drug should not be used prophylactically nor as a uricosuric agent.

Phenylbutazone has a *limited* role in the therapy of *rheumatoid arthritis,* primarily for relief of acute exacerbations of the disorder that are not relieved by other measures (Gifford, 1973). Synovitis is often reduced by a brief regimen (600 mg on the first day, followed by 400 mg daily for 3 days). Because of the high incidence of adverse effects, long-term therapy is not recommended. Brief courses of therapy, *if justified,* may be of similar benefit for acute exacerbations of *ankylosing spondylitis* and *osteoarthritis.*

OXYPHENBUTAZONE

Oxyphenbutazone is a *p*-hydroxy analog of phenylbutazone (on the N-1 phenyl group) and one of the active metabolites of the parent drug. Various aspects of its pharmacology and metabolism are discussed above, in comparison with phenylbutazone. Oxyphenbutazone has the same spectrum of activity, therapeutic uses, interactions, and toxicity as the parent compound, and it shares the same indications, dangers, and contraindications for clinical use. Oxyphenbutazone is said to cause somewhat less gastric irritation.

Oxyphenbutazone, U.S.P. (OXALID, TANDEARIL), is marketed in 100-mg tablets. It should be taken in three or four divided portions after meals to lessen gastric irritation. Dosage of oxyphenbutazone is the same as that of phenylbutazone.

ANTIPYRINE AND AMINOPYRINE

Antipyrine (*phenazone*) and *aminopyrine* (*amido-pyrine*) were introduced into medicine in the late nineteenth century as antipyretics and subsequently were also widely used as analgesics and anti-inflammatory agents. However, clinical use of aminopyrine was sharply curtailed after its potentially fatal bone-marrow toxicity, *agranulocytosis,* was recognized, and antipyrine has also lost favor. Both drugs have virtually disappeared from the therapeutic scene in the United States, but antipyrine is still employed in some countries, usually in analgesic mixtures. A variety of related pyrazolon derivatives have also enjoyed sporadic popularity, for example, *dipyrone.* It, too, can cause agranulocytosis. A full description of the pharmacological properties of these drugs may be found in *earlier editions* of this textbook.

APAZONE (AZAPROPAZONE)

Apazone is a new pyrazolon, aspirin-like agent with a spectrum of activity very similar to that of phenylbutazone. Thus, it is anti-inflammatory, analgesic, and antipyretic. In addition, apazone is a potent uricosuric agent and thus may be particularly useful for the treatment of acute gout. The drug is not currently available in the United States. The structural formula of apazone is as follows:

Apazone

Apazone is rapidly and probably almost completely absorbed from the gastrointestinal tract following oral administration to man; peak concentrations in plasma are achieved 4 hours later. The compound is extensively bound to plasma proteins (about 95%), and the half-life is thus long (20 to 24 hours). Most of the drug (about 65%) is excreted in the urine unchanged, while approximately 20% is present as the 6-hydroxy derivative.

Clinical experience to date suggests that apazone is generally well tolerated. Gastrointestinal side effects occur in about 3% of patients, with nausea, epigastric pain, dyspepsia, and heart burn being the most frequent complaints. These are seldom sufficiently serious to compel withdrawal of the drug. Skin rashes are also observed in 3% of patients, while CNS effects (headache, vertigo) are reported less frequently. The overall incidence of untoward reactions is probably 6 to 10%.

Because apazone is an inhibitor of prostaglandin synthetase, all precautions discussed above for the group are applicable; it can be assumed that the drug is ulcerogenic. It should not be given to patients who have experienced aspirin-induced bronchospasm. Since the drug binds extensively to albumin, its adverse interactions with other agents may resemble those of phenylbutazone. There is no evidence that apazone causes agranulocytosis, but assurance will come only from further experience.

Apazone has been advocated for the treatment of rheumatoid arthritis and osteoarthritis. It is available in other countries as *azapropazone* (RHEUMOX) in 300-mg capsules. The usual dose is 1200 mg per day (in two portions), but this may be reduced to 900 mg for maintenance therapy or increased to 1800 mg if required. A useful collection of reports on apazone may be found in a symposium (1976b).

PARA-AMINOPHENOL DERIVATIVES

The so-called coal tar analgesics, *phenacetin* and its active metabolite, *acetaminophen,* are effective alternatives to aspirin as analgesic-antipyretics; however, unlike aspirin, their anti-inflammatory activity is weak and seldom clinically useful. Acetaminophen probably has less overall toxicity and is thus usually preferred to phenacetin.

Because acetaminophen is well tolerated, lacks many of the side effects of aspirin, and is available without prescription, it has earned a place as a "common household analgesic." However, acute overdosage causes fatal hepatic damage, and the number of self-poisonings and suicides with acetaminophen has grown alarmingly in recent years.

History. *Acetanilid* is the parent member of this group of drugs. It was introduced into medicine in 1886 under the name of *antifebrin* by Cahn and Hepp, who had accidentally discovered its antipyretic action. However, acetanilid proved to be excessively toxic, and the early reports of poisoning from acetanilid prompted the search for less toxic compounds. *Para-aminophenol* was tried in the belief that the body oxidized acetanilid to this compound. Toxicity was not lessened, however, and a number of chemical derivatives of para-aminophenol were then tested. One of the more satisfactory of these was *phenacetin* (*acetophenetidin*). It was introduced into therapy in 1887 and is still extensively employed, although largely in analgesic mixtures.

Acetaminophen (*paracetamol;* N-acetyl-*p*-aminophenol) was first used in medicine by von Mering in 1893. However, it has gained popularity only since 1949, after it was recognized as the major active metabolite of both acetanilid and phenacetin. It has been available in the United States without a prescription since 1955.

Chemistry. The relationship between the drugs of this group and their metabolites is shown in Table 29–2. The antipyretic activity of the compounds resides in the aminobenzene structure. Introduction of other radicals into the hydroxyl group of para-aminophenol and into the free amino group of ani-

Table 29–2. STRUCTURAL FORMULAS OF MAJOR PARA-AMINOPHENOL DERIVATIVES, AND THEIR INTERRELATIONS

NHCOCH$_3$ NHCOCH$_3$ NHCOCH$_3$

OH   OC$_2$H$_5$

Acetanilid   Acetaminophen   Phenacetin

NH$_2$ NHCOCH$_3$ NH$_2$

O—R   OC$_2$H$_5$

Aniline   Conjugated Acetaminophen   Para-Phenetidin
R = glucuronate (major)
sulfate (minor)

Methemoglobin-Forming and Other Toxic Metabolites

partly account for its well-documented ability to reduce fever (a central action) and to induce analgesia.

Subjective Effects and Liability for Abuse. Phenacetin has been said to cause relaxation, drowsiness, euphoria, stimulation, and increased efficiency; such effects have been thought to contribute to its liability for abuse. In patients, minor subjective effects may well occur secondary to relief of pain or fever. In healthy subjects the subjective effects of a single 2-g dose of acetaminophen or aspirin could not be distinguished from those of placebo (Eade and Lasagna, 1967). In the same dose, phenacetin produced a sedative effect characterized as less prominent but more unpleasant than that of pentobarbital (150 mg). Similar subjective effects of phenacetin, often with light-headedness, dizziness, and a sense of unreality and detachment, have also been noted during pharmacokinetic studies. Restlessness and excitement may occur for 3 or 4 days after discontinuation of chronic administration of phenacetin.

Other Effects. Single or repeated therapeutic doses of phenacetin or acetaminophen have no effect on the cardiovascular and respiratory systems. Acid-base changes do not occur. Neither drug produces the gastric irritation, erosion, or bleeding that may occur after salicylates. They have only a weak effect upon platelets and no effect on bleeding time or the excretion of uric acid.

line reduces toxicity without loss of antipyretic action. Best results are obtained with phenolic alkyl ethers (ethyl in phenacetin) and with the amides (acetyl in phenacetin and acetaminophen).

Pharmacological Effects. Acetaminophen and phenacetin have analgesic and antipyretic effects that do not differ significantly from those of aspirin. However, as mentioned, they have only weak anti-inflammatory effects. The pharmacological effects of phenacetin are a combination of its inherent activity (Conney *et al.*, 1966) and those of acetaminophen, its major metabolite. Minor metabolites contribute significantly to the toxic effects of both drugs. The pharmacological properties of acetaminophen and phenacetin have been reviewed by Beaver (1965, 1966) and by Ameer and Greenblatt (1977).

Exactly why acetaminophen is an effective analgesic-antipyretic but only a weak anti-inflammatory agent has not been satisfactorily explained. An anti-inflammatory effect can be demonstrated in animal models, but only at doses considerably in excess of those required for analgesia. Acetaminophen is only a weak inhibitor of prostaglandin biosynthesis, although there is some evidence to suggest that it may be more effective against enzymes in the CNS than those in the periphery. This fact may

Pharmacokinetics and Metabolism. Acetaminophen and phenacetin are metabolized primarily by the hepatic microsomal enzymes (*see* Brodie and Axelrod, 1949; Prescott, 1969; Abel, 1971; Mrochek *et al.*, 1974; Margetts, 1976). The metabolic pathways for the two drugs are rather different, except, of course, that a considerable proportion of phenacetin is dealkylated to acetaminophen.

Acetaminophen is rapidly and almost completely absorbed from the gastrointestinal tract. The concentration in plasma reaches a peak in 30 to 60 minutes, and the half-life in plasma is 1 to 4 hours after therapeutic doses. Acetaminophen is relatively uniformly distributed throughout most body fluids. Binding of the drug to plasma proteins is variable; 20 to 50% may be bound at the concentrations encountered during acute intoxication. Following therapeutic doses, 90 to 100% of the drug may be recovered in the urine within the first day. However, practically no acetaminophen is excreted unchanged, and the bulk is excreted after hepatic conjugation with glucuronic acid (about 60%), sulfuric acid (about 35%), or cysteine (about 3%); small amounts of hydroxylated and deacetylated metabolites have also been detected. Children have less capacity for glucuronidation of the drug than do adults. When high doses are ingested, acetaminophen undergoes N-hydroxylation followed by spontaneous dehydration to form N-acetyl-*p*-benzoquinone, the metabolite generally believed to be responsible for the hepatotoxicity.

In the normal individual, 75 to 80% of *phenacetin* is rapidly metabolized to acetaminophen (Table 29–2). The peak concentration of phenacetin in plasma usually occurs in about 1 hour and that of acetaminophen derived therefrom in 1 to 2 hours. However, oral absorption of phenacetin is markedly influenced by the size of the particles in the preparation, and the concentrations of phenacetin and acetaminophen in plasma are correspondingly variable. Extensive first-pass metabolism of the drug occurs after oral ingestion of the usual doses.

Phenacetin is converted to at least a dozen other metabolites, by N-deacetylation to para-phenetidin and by hydroxylation and further metabolism of phenacetin and para-phenetidin. An unknown metabolite, but an oxidizing agent, is responsible for formation of methemoglobin and hemolysis of red blood cells. Metabolites of phenacetin in urine may darken upon standing to a red-brown or brown-black pigment. Less than 1% of phenacetin is excreted unchanged in the urine.

Individuals with a genetically determined limitation in their ability to metabolize phenacetin to acetaminophen convert a greater fraction of phenacetin to toxic metabolites, possibly with propensity for serious methemoglobin formation and hemolysis. Administration of acetaminophen or phenacetin to patients with impaired renal function results in increased accumulation of conjugated acetaminophen in plasma but only minor changes in the plasma concentrations of phenacetin and free acetaminophen.

Drug Interactions. Acetaminophen and phenacetin may induce synthesis of the hepatic microsomal enzymes, but the effect is not seen with usual doses. As a result, the prothrombinopenic effect of the oral anticoagulant agents may be slightly increased by chronic administration of full doses of acetaminophen, but intermittent doses of the drug have only little such effect.

Toxic Effects. In recommended therapeutic dosage, acetaminophen and phenacetin are usually well tolerated. *Skin rash* and other allergic reactions occur occasionally. The rash is usually erythematous or urticarial, but sometimes it is more serious and may be accompanied by *drug fever* and *mucosal lesions.* Patients who are sensitive to the salicylates may also exhibit sensitivity to these drugs. In a few isolated cases, the use of acetaminophen has been associated with *neutropenia, pancytopenia,* and *leukopenia.*

Despite the fact that acetaminophen is a metabolite of phenacetin, the signs and symptoms of acute intoxication with the two compounds are markedly different. The most serious adverse effect of acute overdosage of acetaminophen is a dose-dependent, potentially fatal *hepatic necrosis. Renal tubular ne-*crosis (also seen with phenacetin) and *hypoglycemic coma* may also occur. Phenacetin may cause *methemoglobinemia* and *hemolytic anemia* as a form of acute toxicity, but more commonly as a consequence of chronic overdosage. Lethal doses of phenacetin are not associated with hepatic damage, but with *cyanosis, respiratory depression,* and *cardiac arrest.* Acetaminophen is much less likely to cause the formation of methemoglobin and has not been incriminated in the hemolytic reactions, but it may cause thrombocytopenia. The nephrotoxicity associated with chronic abuse of acetaminophen, phenacetin, and other analgesics has been discussed above.

Hepatotoxicity. In adults, hepatotoxicity may occur after ingestion of a single dose of 10 to 15 g (200 to 250 mg/kg) of acetaminophen; a dose of 25 g or more is potentially fatal. Symptoms during the first 2 days of acute poisoning by acetaminophen do not reflect the potential seriousness of the intoxication. Nausea, vomiting, anorexia, and abdominal pain occur during the initial 24 hours and may persist for a week or more. Concurrent ingestion of alcohol or other drugs with acetaminophen may enhance its toxicity by reducing the metabolic capacity of the liver. Clinical indications of hepatic damage manifest themselves within 2 to 6 days of ingestion of toxic doses. Initially, plasma transaminases and lactic dehydrogenase activity may be elevated, but alkaline phosphatase activity and the albumin concentration may be normal. The concentration of bilirubin in plasma may be increased, and prothrombin time is prolonged. The hepatotoxicity may precipitate jaundice and coagulation disorders and progress to encephalopathy, coma, and death. Transient azotemia is apparent in most patients, and acute renal failure occurs in some. Hypoglycemia may occur, but glycosuria and impaired glucose tolerance have also been reported. Both metabolic acidosis and metabolic alkalosis have been noted; cerebral edema and nonspecific myocardial depression have also occurred. Biopsy of the liver reveals centrilobular necrosis with sparing of the periportal area. In nonfatal cases, the hepatic lesions are reversible over a period of weeks or months.

Measurement of the half-life of acetaminophen in plasma during the first day of acute poisoning provides an early indication of the severity of the hepatic injury. Hepatic necrosis should be anticipated if the half-time exceeds 4 hours, and hepatic coma is likely if the half-time is greater than 12 hours. A single determination of the concentration of acetaminophen in plasma is a less reliable predictor of hepatic injury. However, only minimal hepatic damage develops when the value is below 120 μg/ml at 4 hours or less than 50 μg/ml at 12 hours after ingestion of the drug, whereas concentrations greater than 300 μg/ml at 4 hours are generally associated with serious hepatic damage. Enzyme activities in plasma are perhaps a more reliable measure of hepatic injury; hepatic damage is indicated by aspartate aminotransferase levels in excess of 80 I.U. per liter (Prescott and Wright, 1973). Encephalopathy should also be anticipated if the concentration of bilirubin in plasma exceeds 4 mg/dl during the first 5 days.

Toxic doses of acetaminophen in animals produce hepatic injury with histological features similar to those in man. The hepatotoxicity has been attributed to a metabolite, possibly N-acetyl-p-benzoquinone, that binds covalently to cellular constituents. Since the severity of the injury can be varied by pretreatments that modify the rate of biotransformation of acetaminophen or that alter the hepatic stores of glutathione, it has been suggested that hepatotoxicity occurs when production of the toxic metabolite exceeds the quantity of glutathione available for its inactivation (*see* Chapter 1).

The enzyme system that is responsible for the formation of the hepatotoxic metabolite of acetaminophen is similar, if not identical, to the system that converts phenacetin to acetaminophen. This probably explains why phenacetin is not hepatotoxic, since the quantity of acetaminophen formed never exceeds the ability of the conjugation systems to remove it.

Treatment. Early diagnosis is vital in the treatment of overdosage with acetaminophen, and methods are now available for the rapid determination of concentrations of the drug in plasma (Kendall *et al.,* 1976). Vigorous supportive therapy is essential when intoxication is severe. Procedures to limit continuing absorption of the drug must be initiated promptly; induction of vomiting or gastric lavage should be performed in all cases and should be followed by oral administration of activated charcoal. Hemodialysis, if it can be initiated within the first 12 hours, has been advocated for all patients with a plasma concentration of acetaminophen greater than 120 μg/ml 4 hours after drug ingestion. Forced diuresis has also been advocated but has not been shown to increase drug elimination significantly and could be hazardous if renal function is impaired.

A promising method of treatment is the administration of sulfhydryl compounds, which probably act, in part, by replenishing hepatic stores of glutathione. L-Methionine, L-cysteine, and N-acetylcysteine have a protective action in animals. Methionine and another sulfhydryl compound, cysteamine (possibly a source of sulfate for conjugation), have been given to man with some success (*see* Crome *et al.,* 1976; Prescott *et al.,* 1976). N-acetylcysteine is apparently particularly effective and well tolerated when given orally. The drug is recommended if less than 24 hours has elapsed since ingestion of acetaminophen. A loading dose of 140 mg/kg is given, followed by the administration of 70 mg/kg every 4 hours for 17 doses. Dosage is terminated if assays of acetaminophen in plasma indicate that the risk of hepatotoxicity is low. *Acetylcysteine,* U.S.P. (MUCO-MYST), is available as a sterile 10 or 20% solution in vials containing 4, 10, and 30 ml. The solution is diluted with cola, fruit juice, or water to achieve a 5% solution and should be consumed within 1 hour of preparation. This use of N-acetylcysteine is considered experimental in the United States. Consultation

may be obtained from the Rocky Mountain Poison Center, Denver, Colorado (Tel.: 800-525-6115). (*See* Symposium, 1976a, for a comprehensive discussion of the management of overdosage with acetaminophen.)

Hemolytic Anemia. Phenacetin-induced hemolytic anemia is most frequently associated with chronic ingestion of the drug. Hemolysis is apparently caused by metabolites that oxidize glutathione and components of the red-blood-cell membrane and shorten erythrocyte survival. The anemia is usually mild, with slight reticulocytosis, but it may be progressive and severe in the presence of uremia or other exacerbating factors. Splenomegaly has been reported. Methemoglobinemia, sulfhemoglobin formation, and Heinz bodies are not consistently present; the blood film may contain characteristic irregularly contracted and fragmented erythrocytes.

Hemolytic anemia may also occur following acute administration of phenacetin. Although such a reaction is not common, the anemia is usually severe and may be accompanied by intravascular hemolysis, hemoglobinuria, and acute anuria. These reactions may occur in patients with glucose-6-phosphate dehydrogenase deficiency in erythrocytes or as an immunological reaction. Although the antibodies are directed to the drug or metabolite, adsorption of the antigen-antibody complexes on the surface of the red blood cell leads to activation of complement and damage to the membrane.

Methemoglobinemia. Marked methemoglobinemia, sulfhemoglobin formation, cyanosis, and functional anemia are prominent characteristics of poisoning by acetanilid. Phenacetin causes much less methemoglobinemia and sulfhemoglobin formation, and acetaminophen even less. The formation of methemoglobin is dependent upon the oxidation of aromatic amines, such as para-phenetidin, to quinones or aromatic nitrosoamines. Since a single 2-g dose of phenacetin in adults converts only 1 to 3% of the total hemoglobin to methemoglobin, the methemoglobinemia produced by therapeutic doses of acetaminophen or phenacetin is not usually of clinical significance. However, in acute overdosage or during chronic abuse, methemoglobinemia may contribute to the total toxicity. Methemoglobinemia may be prominent in individuals who are genetically variant so that they convert a greater fraction of phenacetin to the hydroxylated metabolites or in those with variations in the primary structure of hemoglobin that make the molecule more susceptible to oxidation.

Preparations, Routes of Administration, and Dosage. *Acetaminophen,* U.S.P. (*paracetamol;* N-acetyl-p-aminophenol), is marketed under many trade names (*e.g.,* TEMPRA, TYLENOL). Preparations include tablets (120, 325, and 500 mg), chewable tablets (80 mg), and an elixir and syrup (120 mg/5 ml); a solution (60 mg/0.6 ml) is also available.

The conventional oral dosage is 325 to 650 mg every 4 hours for adults and older children. For young children, the single dose is 60 to 120 mg, depending upon age and weight; total daily dosage should not exceed 1.2 g. Acetaminophen should not be administered for more than 10 days or to young children except upon advice of a physician.

Phenacetin, U.S.P., is too insoluble to be prescribed in aqueous solution and is usually administered orally in powder, capsule, or tablet form. In recent years it has been employed primarily in analgesic mixtures. The average single dose for adults is 300 mg; the total daily dose should not exceed 2.4 g.

Therapeutic Uses. Acetaminophen or phenacetin is a suitable substitute for aspirin for its analgesic or antipyretic uses in patients in whom aspirin is contraindicated (*e.g.,* those with peptic ulcer) or when the prolongation of bleeding time caused by aspirin would be a disadvantage. Acetaminophen has somewhat less overall toxicity and is preferred over phenacetin. An additional minor convenience of acetaminophen is its availability in a liquid dosage form for oral ingestion.

INDOMETHACIN AND SULINDAC

Indomethacin was the product of a laboratory search for drugs with anti-inflammatory properties. It was introduced in 1963 for the treatment of rheumatoid arthritis and related disorders. Although indomethacin is widely used and is effective, toxicity often limits its use. Sulindac was developed in an attempt to find a less toxic but effective congener of indomethacin. It remains uncertain to what extent this goal has been accomplished. The development, chemistry, and pharmacology of both drugs have been reviewed by Shen and Winter (1977).

INDOMETHACIN

Chemistry. The structural formula of indomethacin, a methylated indole derivative, is as follows:

Indomethacin

Pharmacological Properties. Indomethacin has prominent anti-inflammatory and analgesic-antipyretic properties in experimental animals similar to those of the sa-

licylates, and comparable effects have been demonstrated in man.

The anti-inflammatory effects of indomethacin are evident in patients with rheumatoid and other types of arthritis, including acute gout. Although indomethacin is more potent than aspirin, doses that are tolerated by patients with rheumatoid arthritis usually do not produce effects that are superior to those of salicylate. Contrary to early belief, indomethacin has *analgesic* properties distinct from its anti-inflammatory effects, and there is evidence for both a central and a peripheral effect. The *antipyretic* effect of indomethacin is also demonstrable in patients with fever.

Indomethacin is one of the most potent inhibitors of the prostaglandin-forming cyclooxygenase. Like colchicine, it inhibits motility of polymorphonuclear leukocytes. Like many other of the aspirin-like drugs, indomethacin uncouples oxidative phosphorylation in supratherapeutic concentrations and depresses the biosynthesis of mucopolysaccharides.

Pharmacokinetics and Metabolism. Indomethacin is rapidly and almost completely absorbed from the gastrointestinal tract following oral ingestion. The peak concentration in plasma is attained within 3 hours in the fasting subject but may be somewhat delayed when the drug is taken after meals. The concentrations in plasma required for an anti-inflammatory effect have not been accurately determined but are probably less than 1 μg/ml. Steady-state concentrations in plasma after chronic administration are approximately 0.5 μg/ml (Alvan *et al.,* 1975). Indomethacin is 90% bound to plasma proteins and also extensively bound to tissues. The concentration of the drug in the CSF is low.

Indomethacin is largely converted to inactive metabolites (Duggan *et al.,* 1972). About half of a single oral dose is O-demethylated and about 10% is conjugated with glucuronic acid by the hepatic microsomal enzymes. A portion is also N-deacylated by a nonmicrosomal system. Some of these metabolites are detectable in plasma, and free and conjugated metabolites are eliminated in the urine, bile, and feces. Enterohepatic cycling of the conjugates occurs. Ten to 20% of the drug is excreted unchanged in the urine, in part by tubular secretion. The plasma half-life of the unchanged drug is 2 to 3 hours.

Drug Interactions. The reported antagonism between indomethacin and *aspirin* in some laboratory tests for anti-inflammatory activity seems to have little clinical relevance, but the question remains whether the effects that result when the two drugs are administered concurrently for the therapy of rheumatoid arthritis are beneficial.

The total plasma concentration of indomethacin plus its inactive metabolites is increased by concurrent administration of *probenecid,* possibly because of reduced tubular secretion of the former. However, it has not been determined whether the concentration of free indomethacin in plasma is altered or whether the dosage of indomethacin must be adjusted when the two drugs are employed together. Indomethacin does not interfere with the uricosuric effect of probenecid. Indomethacin is said not to modify the effect of the *oral anticoagulant agents.* However, concurrent administration could be hazardous because of the increased risk of gastrointestinal bleeding. Indomethacin antagonizes the natriuretic effect of *furosemide.*

Toxic Effects. A very high percentage (35 to 50%) of patients receiving usual therapeutic doses of indomethacin experience untoward symptoms, and about 20% must discontinue its use. Most adverse effects are dose related (Boardman and Hart, 1967b).

Gastrointestinal complaints and complications consist in anorexia, nausea, and abdominal pain. Single ulcers or multiple ulceration of the entire upper gastrointestinal tract, sometimes with perforations and hemorrhage, has been reported. Occult blood loss may lead to anemia in the absence of ulceration. Acute pancreatitis has also been reported. Diarrhea may occur and is sometimes associated with ulcerative lesions of the bowel. Hepatic involvement has been rare, although some fatal cases of hepatitis and jaundice have been reported. The most frequent CNS effect (indeed, the most common side effect) is severe frontal headache, occurring in 25 to 50% of patients who take the drug chronically. Dizziness, vertigo, light-headedness, and mental confusion are also frequent. Severe depression, psychosis, hallucinations, and suicide have occurred. Early reports of corneal opacities and pallor of the optic disc seem to have been largely erroneous, but the signs should be sought in anyone taking the drug.

Hematopoietic reactions include neutropenia, thrombocytopenia, and, rarely, aplastic anemia. Deaths in children have occurred from what was probably overwhelming sepsis due to activation of latent infections. *Hypersensitivity* reactions are manifested as rashes, itching, urticaria, and, more seriously, acute attacks of asthma. Patients sensitive to *aspirin* may exhibit cross-reactivity to indomethacin. Indomethacin should not be used in pregnant women, persons operating machinery, or patients with psychiatric disorders, epilepsy, or parkinsonism. It is also contraindicated in individuals with renal disease or ulcerative lesions of the stomach or intestines.

Preparations, Route of Administration, and Dosage. *Indomethacin,* U.S.P. (INDOCIN), is available for oral use in capsules containing 25 or 50 mg of the drug.

The initial dose is 25 mg, twice daily, and this can be increased by 25-mg increments at weekly intervals until the total daily dose is 100 to 200 mg. Few patients tolerate more than 100 mg per day without severe side effects. Most patients respond within 4 to 6 days, but some require substantially longer treatment. The drug should be taken in divided portions with food or immediately after meals, to lessen gastric distress. A dose of indomethacin taken with milk at bedtime is said to reduce the incidence of morning headache.

Therapeutic Uses. Because of the high incidence and severity of side effects associated with chronic administration, indomethacin must not be routinely used as an analgesic or antipyretic. However, it has proven useful as an antipyretic in Hodgkin's disease when the fever has been refractory to other agents. Indomethacin has become an accepted part of the rheumatologist's armamentarium and a standard (together with aspirin and phenylbutazone) against which to measure the activity of other, newer drugs.

Clinical trials of indomethacin as an anti-inflammatory agent have been reviewed by O'Brien (1968), Gifford (1973), and Shen and Winter (1977). The majority of these trials have demonstrated that indomethacin relieves pain, reduces swelling and tenderness of the joints, increases grip strength, and decreases the duration of morning stiffness. In these actions the drug is superior to placebo and equivalent to phenylbutazone; estimates of its potency relative to salicylates vary between 10 and 40 times (Pitkeathly *et al.,* 1966; Pinals and Frank, 1967). Overall, about two thirds of patients benefit from treatment with indomethacin; however, if 75 to 100 mg of the drug fails to provide benefit within 2 to 4 weeks, alternative therapy must be considered. The incidence and severity of side effects with indomethacin are particularly annoying, but a useful way of employing the undoubted potency of the drug, perhaps in combination with other and better-tolerated daytime therapy, is to give a large single dose (100 mg) at bedtime (Huskisson, 1976). This enables the patient to obtain a better-quality sleep, reduces the severity and length of morning stiffness, and provides good analgesia until mid-morning. The side effects of indomethacin are apparently better tolerated when it is given at night.

Indomethacin is as effective as phenylbutazone and more effective than aspirin in the treatment of *ankylosing spondylitis* (Godfrey *et al.,* 1972), *osteoarthrosis,* and *acute gout,* although it does not promote uricosuria (Smyth and Percy, 1973).

Uveitis and the pain and inflammation following *ophthalmic surgery* are reported to respond favorably to oral indomethacin (Perkins and MacFaul, 1965). Indomethacin is also useful in the treatment of soft-tissue lesions (Burry, 1976). Various authors have reported indomethacin to be effective in reducing the pain, fever, and inflammation of *pleurisy, pericarditis,* and *pericardial effusion.*

Patients with *Bartter's syndrome* have been successfully treated with indomethacin, as well as with other inhibitors of prostaglandin synthetase (*see* Verberckmoes *et al.,* 1976; Zancan *et al.,* 1976; Halushka *et al.,* 1977). The results are frequently dramatic; however, the condition of the patients may deteriorate rapidly when therapy is discontinued, and the long-term therapy necessary to control the disease requires administration of a drug that is better tolerated.

Cardiac failure in neonates caused by a *patent ductus arteriosus* may sometimes be controlled with single doses of indomethacin as low as 0.1 to 0.3 mg/kg; larger doses (2 to 3.75 mg/kg, given for 2 days) appear to be more effective (Heymann *et al.,* 1976; Harinck *et al.,* 1977). In some cases renal insufficiency has been observed, and in one report moderate-to-severe gastrointestinal side effects were noted.

Indomethacin has been used to prevent spontaneous labor (Zuckerman *et al.,* 1974), as discussed above. The drug also appears to be more effective than aspirin in relieving the pain of dysmenorrhea.

SULINDAC

Chemistry. Sulindac is closely related to indomethacin; its structural formula is as follows:

Sulindac

It is unlikely, however, that sulindac itself has much therapeutic efficacy; most of its pharmacological activity apparently resides in its sulfide metabolite.

Pharmacological Properties.

In laboratory studies, sulindac exhibits the classical activities of aspirin-like drugs (Van Arman *et al.,* 1976). In all tests, sulindac is less than half as potent as indomethacin.

Because sulindac is a prodrug, it appears to be either inactive or relatively weak in many tests, whereas its sulfide metabolite may be very active. This especially applies to tests where little or no metabolism can occur. The sulfide metabolite is more than 500 times more potent than sulindac as an inhibitor of cyclooxygenase (Van Arman *et al.,* 1976). These observations may help to explain the somewhat lower incidence of gastrointestinal toxicity of sulindac, since the gastric or intestinal mucosa is not exposed to high concentrations of an active drug during oral administration.

The development, pharmacology, and therapeutic activities of sulindac have been reviewed by Shen and Winter (1977), Brogden and associates (1978a), and others (Symposium, 1978).

Pharmacokinetics and Metabolism.

The metabolism and pharmacokinetics of sulindac are complex and vary enormously between species. After oral administration to man, about 90% of the drug is absorbed. When taken with meals, the absorption of the drug is retarded and peak concentrations in plasma are attained more slowly and are lower.

Sulindac undergoes two major biotransformations in addition to conjugation reactions. It is oxidized to the sulfone and then reversibly reduced to the sulfide. It is this latter metabolite that is the active moiety, although all three compounds are found in comparable concentrations in human plasma. The half-life of sulindac itself is about 7 hours, but the active sulfide has a half-life as long as 18 hours. There seems to be little or no placental transfer of the drug, but it is present in breast milk. Sulindac and the sulfone and sulfide metabolites are all more than 93% bound to plasma protein; the sulfone is the most highly bound, and sulindac is the least.

Little of the sulfide or its conjugates is found in urine. The principal components that are so excreted are the sulfone and its conjugate, which account for nearly 30% of an administered dose; sulindac and its conjugates account for about 20%. Up to 25% of an oral dose may appear as metabolites in the feces.

The pharmacokinetics and metabolism of sulindac are discussed by Hucker and coworkers (1973), Van Arman and associates (1976), and Duggan and colleagues (1977).

Preparations, Route of Administration, and Dosage. *Sulindac* (ARTHROCINE, ARTRIBID, CLINORIL) is available as 150- and 200-mg tablets. The most common dosage for adults is 150 to 200 mg twice a day, although dosage should be optimized for each individual. The maximal daily dose is 400 mg. The drug may be given with food if gastric discomfort is experienced, although this could delay absorption and reduce the concentration in plasma.

Toxic Effects.

While the incidence of toxicity is lower than with indomethacin, untoward reactions to sulindac are common. Some estimate the incidence to be 25% (Rooney *et al.,* 1978).

Gastrointestinal side effects are seen in nearly 20% of patients, although these are generally mild. Abdominal pain and nausea are the most frequent complaints, followed by constipation. Gastric bleeding appears to be relatively uncommon. CNS side effects are seen in up to 10% of patients, with drowsiness, dizziness, headache, and nervousness being those most frequently reported. Skin rash and pruritus occur in 5% of patients. Transient elevations of hepatic enzymes in plasma are less common. As with other aspirin-like drugs, there is a danger that sulindac could precipitate a severe reaction in patients who are sensitive to aspirin; platelet function may also be impaired and bleeding time prolonged.

Drug Interactions. All drugs that bind tightly to plasma proteins have the capacity to displace drugs such as warfarin and oral hypoglycemic agents. To date, this problem has not been noted with sulindac.

Therapeutic Uses. Sulindac has been utilized mainly for the treatment of rheumatoid arthritis, osteoarthrosis, and ankylosing spondylitis. A few studies have also been carried out in patients with acute gout. In patients with *rheumatoid arthritis,* most investigators have compared sulindac (200 to 400 mg per day) with aspirin (3 to 4.8 g per day) in either short-term studies (2 months or less) (*e.g.*, Borrachero del Campo, 1978; Caruso *et al.*, 1978; Huskisson and Scott, 1978) or long-term trials (18 months) (Fasching and Eberl, 1976). Sulindac exerted analgesic and anti-inflammatory effects comparable to aspirin or sometimes superior. Sulindac and aspirin have been compared with similar results in patients with osteoarthritis (*see* Symposium, 1978). While tolerance of the drug by patients was good, most studies have been relatively brief. More experience with this agent is required before its place in therapy can be assessed.

THE FENAMATES

The fenamates are a family of aspirin-like drugs that are derivatives of N-phenylanthranilic acid. The group includes mefenamic, meclofenamic, flufenamic, tolfenamic, and etofenamic acids.

Although the biological activity of this group of drugs was discovered in the 1950s, the fenamates have not gained widespread clinical acceptance. They cause side effects frequently; diarrhea, in particular, may be very severe. Therapeutically, they also have no clear advantages over several other aspirin-like drugs.

Mefenamic acid is the only member of the series available in the United States, and its use is indicated only for analgesia. Flufenamic acid is used in many other countries, as is mefenamic acid, for its anti-inflammatory effects. Other members of the series will not be discussed further.

Chemistry. Mefenamic acid and flufenamic acid are both N-substituted phenylanthranilic acids. The structure of mefenamic acid is as follows:

Mefenamic Acid

Pharmacological Properties. In the tests of anti-inflammatory activity, mefenamic acid is about half as potent and flufenamic acid about 1.5 times as potent as phenylbutazone. Both drugs also have antipyretic and analgesic properties. In tests of analgesia, mefenamic acid was the only fenamate to display a central as well as a peripheral action.

The fenamates appear to owe these properties to their capacity to inhibit cyclooxygenase. Unlike the other aspirin-like drugs, certain of the fenamates (especially meclofenamic acid) appear to antagonize certain effects of prostaglandins, such as $PGF_{2\alpha}$-induced contraction of isolated bronchial smooth muscle (Collier and Sweatman, 1968).

Much of the basic pharmacology, pharmacokinetics, and early clinical experience with the fenamates has been summarized in a symposium (1966a).

Pharmacokinetics and Metabolism. *Mefenamic acid* is fairly rapidly absorbed following a single oral dose, and peak concentrations in plasma are reached in about 2 hours; the half-life in plasma is 3 to 4 hours. In man, approximately 50% of a dose of mefenamic acid is excreted in the urine. Of this, approximately half is the conjugated 3-hydroxymethyl metabolite, a little less than half is the 3-carboxyl metabolite and its conjugates, and the remaining few percent is mostly conjugated mefenamic acid. Twenty percent of the drug is recovered in the feces, mainly as the unconjugated 3-carboxyl metabolite.

Flufenamic acid is absorbed slowly following oral administration. Peak concentrations in plasma are reached in about 6 hours, and the half-life of the drug is about 9 hours. Little of the drug is eliminated unchanged. Hydroxylated metabolites and their conjugates are eliminated in the urine and feces. Only trace amounts of these drugs are present in the milk of lactating women; metabolites readily cross the placental barrier. Both drugs are tightly bound to plasma proteins.

Preparations, Routes of Administration, and Dosage. *Mefenamic acid* (PONSTEL) is available in 250-mg capsules for oral administration and also, in some countries, as a pediatric suspension containing 10 mg/ml. For adults, the recommended dose is 250 mg four times daily; the drug should be given with food. The drug is not recommended for use in children or pregnant women in the United States, nor should it be given for longer than 7 days. Flufenamic acid is not available in the United States.

Toxic Effects and Precautions. The most common side effects (occurring in approximately 25% of all patients) involve the gastrointestinal system. Usually these take the form of dyspepsia or upper gastrointestinal discomfort, although diarrhea, which may be severe and associated with inflammation of the bowel, or constipation is also relatively common. There have also been reports of bleeding ulcers following treatment with mefenamic acid (*see* Wolfe *et al.*, 1976). Steatorrhea may also be associated with diarrhea.

Other reactions that have been noted less frequently include transient abnormalities of hepatic and renal function, CNS effects, and skin rashes. A potentially serious side effect seen in isolated cases is a hemolytic anemia, which may be of an autoimmune type (Jackson *et al.*, 1970; Kennedy and Robertson, 1971).

The fenamates are contraindicated in patients with a history of gastrointestinal disease. If diarrhea or skin rash appears, the drug should be stopped at once. The physician and patient should watch for signs of hemolytic anemia. The fenamates can cause bronchoconstriction in patients who are sensitive to aspirin. Like all inhibitors of prostaglandin synthetase, these drugs affect platelet function.

Drug Interactions. The fenamates bind strongly to plasma proteins, and there is thus the possibility of displacement of other drugs from nonspecific binding sites on plasma albumin. This possibility has been confirmed for oral anticoagulants when mefenamic acid is administered (Sellers and Koch-Weser, 1970).

Therapeutic Uses. As an *analgesic agent,* mefenamic acid has been used to relieve pain arising from rheumatic conditions, soft-tissue injuries, other painful musculoskeletal conditions, and dysmenorrhea. While mefenamic acid clearly possesses analgesic activity, toxicity limits its utility. It appears to offer no advantage over other analgesic agents. As an *anti-inflammatory agent,* mefenamic acid has been mainly tested in short-term trials in the treatment of osteoarthritis and rheumatoid arthritis. Again, advantages of this agent or of flufenamic acid are not apparent.

TOLMETIN

Tolmetin is a relatively new anti-inflammatory, analgesic, and antipyretic agent that was introduced into clinical practice in the United States in 1976. Tolmetin, in recommended doses, appears to be approximately equivalent in efficacy to moderate doses of aspirin; it is usually better tolerated. The structural formula of tolmetin is as follows:

Tolmetin

Pharmacological Properties. Tolmetin is an effective anti-inflammatory agent; it is more potent than aspirin and less potent than indomethacin or phenylbutazone (Wong, 1975). Tolmetin also exerts antipyretic and analgesic effects in experimental animals and man. Like most of the other drugs considered in this chapter, tolmetin causes gastric erosions and prolongs bleeding time.

Pharmacokinetics and Metabolism. Tolmetin is rapidly and completely absorbed following its oral administration to man, and the concentrations achieved in plasma are not reduced by the concomitant administration of gastric antacids. Peak concentrations are achieved 20 to 60 minutes after oral administration, and the half-life in plasma is between 1 and 3 hours.

After absorption, tolmetin is extensively (99%) bound to plasma proteins. Virtually all of the drug can be recovered in the urine after 24 hours; some is unchanged (17%), but most is conjugated (10%) or otherwise metabolized. The major metabolic transformation is decarboxylation. The pharmacokinetics and metabolism of tolmetin are discussed by Brogden and associates (1978b).

Preparations, Route of Administration, and Dosage. *Tolmetin sodium* (TOLECTIN) is supplied as 200-mg tablets for oral use. The recommended initial dose is 400 mg three times daily, and it is suggested that one of these doses be taken on retiring and another on awakening. The response to the drug is usually seen within a week, and the dose can then be adjusted to suit individual requirements; the usual range is 600 to 800 mg per day in divided doses, and the maximal recommended dose is 2 g per day. The drug may be given with meals, milk, or antacids to lessen abdominal discomfort. The recommended initial daily dose for children is 20 mg/kg.

Toxic Effects. Some 25 to 40% of patients who take tolmetin experience side effects, and 5 to 10% discontinue use of the drug. Gastrointestinal side effects are the most common, with epigastric pain (15% incidence), dyspepsia, nausea, and vomiting being the chief manifestations. Gastric and duodenal ulceration has also been observed. CNS side effects, including nervousness, anxiety, insomnia, drowsiness, and visual disturbance, are less common and are said to be neither as frequent nor severe as those caused by indomethacin. Similarly, the incidence of tinnitus, deafness, and vertigo is less than with aspirin. There is an occasional skin rash or urticaria. Because of its potential for gastrointestinal toxicity, tolmetin should be used cautiously in patients with gastrointestinal problems. Likewise, the effect of the drug on platelets should be considered. It should be assumed that tolmetin will probably precipitate bronchoconstriction in those patients who are hypersensitive to aspirin.

Drug Interactions. Despite its extensive binding to albumin, Whitsett and associates (1975) found no change in prothrombin time when warfarin and tolmetin were given together. Tolmetin differs in this regard from many other drugs of this type.

Therapeutic Uses. Tolmetin is approved in the United States only for use in the treatment of rheumatoid arthritis and the juvenile form of the disease; elsewhere it has been used in the treatment of osteoarthritis and ankylosing spondylitis.

In rheumatoid arthritis many investigators have compared tolmetin (1.2 to 1.5 g per day) with aspirin (4 to 4.5 g per day) or indomethacin. In general, there has been little difference in therapeutic efficacy. Tolmetin may be tolerated somewhat better than is aspirin in equieffective doses (see Aylward et al., 1976; Klemp and Meyers, 1977). Similarly, Huskisson and coworkers (1974a) compared tolmetin (1.6 g per day) with phenylbutazone (400 mg per day) and found little difference in therapeutic efficacy and patient preference. Tolmetin is also probably as effective as ibuprofen in the usual therapeutic doses (Clark et al, 1977; McMillen, 1977). Levinson and associates (1977) found little difference between tolmetin (22.7 mg/kg daily) and aspirin (90.7 mg/kg daily) in terms of therapeutic efficacy in the treatment of juvenile rheumatoid arthritis. Side effects were slightly more severe with aspirin.

ALCLOFENAC

Alclofenac is another new aspirin-like drug with all of the features that are characteristic of the class (see Brogden et al., 1977a). It is not available in the United States, although it is utilized elsewhere. In general, it may be equivalent in therapeutic potency to moderate doses of aspirin. While the incidence and severity of gastrointestinal side effects are perhaps less, the drug causes a severe rash with systemic manifestations in a high percentage of cases.

PROPIONIC ACID DERIVATIVES

These drugs represent a new group of effective, useful aspirin-like agents. They may offer significant advantages over aspirin, indomethacin, and the pyrazolon derivatives for many patients, since they are usually better tolerated. Nevertheless, propionic acid derivatives share all of the detrimental features of the entire class of drugs. Furthermore, their rapid proliferation in number and heavy promotion have made difficult the physician's task of making a rational choice between members of the group and between propionic acid derivatives and the more established agents. The similarities between drugs in this class (and certain of the others discussed above) are far more striking than are the differences.

Ibuprofen, naproxen, fenoprofen, flurbiprofen, and ketoprofen are described individually below. Of these, the first three are currently available in the United States. Ibuprofen was the first of these agents to come into general use, and experience with this drug is correspondingly greater. The most distinctive feature among the others may probably be claimed by naproxen; its longer half-life makes twice-daily administration feasible. The structural formulas of these drugs are shown in Table 29–3.

Pharmacological Properties. The pharmacodynamic properties of propionic acid derivatives do not differ significantly. While they do vary in potency, this is not of obvious clinical significance. All are effective anti-inflammatory agents in various experimental models of inflammation in animals; all have useful anti-inflammatory, analgesic, and antipyretic activity in man.

All of these compounds can cause gastrointestinal erosions (gastric, duodenal, and intestinal) in experimental animals. All produce gastrointestinal side effects in man, although these are usually less severe than with aspirin. However, it is not yet known if the incidence of peptic ulceration during chronic administration of these drugs will be less than with aspirin or indomethacin.

The propionic acid derivatives are all effective inhibitors of the cyclooxygenase responsible for the biosynthesis of prostaglandins, although there is considerable variation in their potency. For example, flurbiprofen is approximately 600 times more potent than aspirin, while ibuprofen, fenoprofen, and aspirin are roughly equipotent in this action. It is thus not surprising that all of these agents alter platelet function and prolong bleeding time, as described above. It should also be assumed that any patient who is hypersensitive to aspirin may also suffer a

Table 29-3. STRUCTURAL FORMULAS OF ANTI-INFLAMMATORY PROPIONIC ACID DERIVATIVES

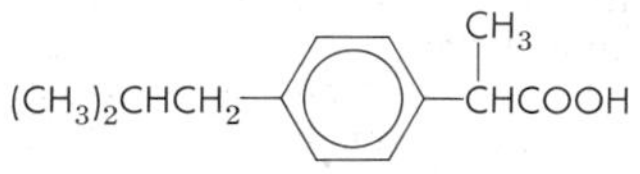

Ibuprofen

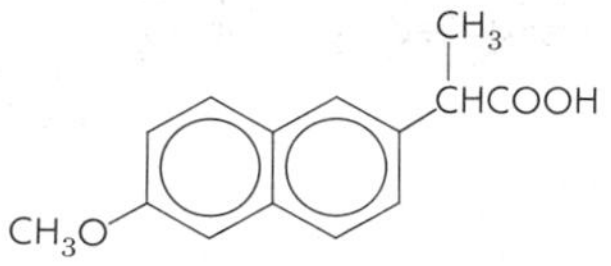

Naproxen

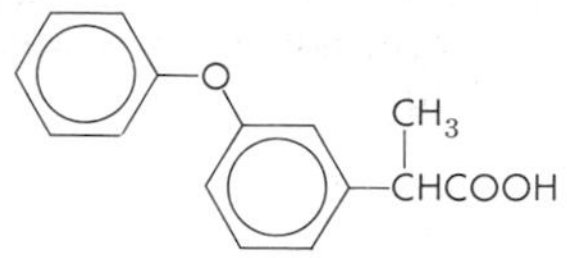

Fenoprofen

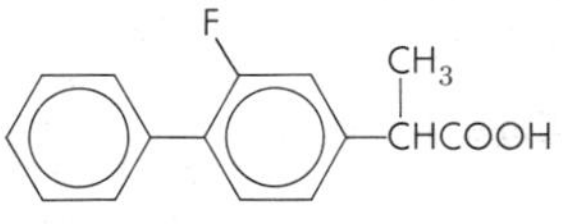

Flurbiprofen

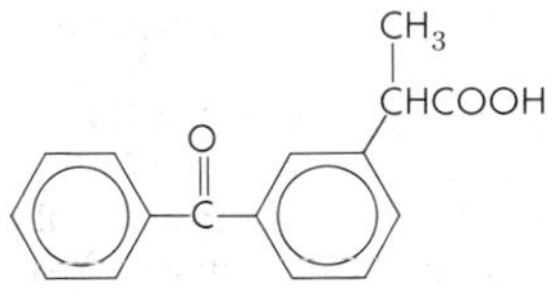

Ketoprofen

severe reaction following administration of one of these drugs.

Drug Interactions. The adverse drug interactions of particular concern with this group derive from their high degree of binding to albumin in plasma. The physician should adjust the dosage of warfarin accordingly, especially since platelet function is also impaired with these drugs and they may cause gastrointestinal lesions. This interaction has been found *not* to occur with ibuprofen, possibly because this drug occupies only a small number of the binding sites on albumin (Goncalves, 1973; Boekhout-Mussert and Loeliger, 1974; Thilo *et al.*, 1974). There are insufficient data on interactions with other drugs that are protein bound to a great extent, such as the oral hypoglycemic agents. Of the propionic acid derivatives, ketoprofen is itself bound to albumin to the least extent (less than 90%).

Simultaneous administration of aspirin and naproxen results in displacement of the latter from albumin and an increased rate of its clearance. However, this effect is of little clinical relevance (Willkens and Segre, 1976).

IBUPROFEN

Ibuprofen has been discussed in detail in a symposium (1975a) and by Adams and Buckler (1979).

Pharmacokinetics and Metabolism. Ibuprofen is rapidly absorbed following oral administration to man, and peak concentrations in plasma are observed after 1 to 2 hours. The half-life in plasma is about 2 hours. Absorption is also efficient, although slower, from suppositories.

Ibuprofen is extensively (99%) and firmly bound to plasma proteins, but probably occupies only a fraction of the total drug binding sites at usual concentrations. Ibuprofen passes slowly into the synovial spaces and may remain there in higher concentration for long after the concentrations in plasma have declined. In experimental animals, ibuprofen and its metabolites pass easily across the placenta.

The excretion of ibuprofen is rapid and complete. About 60 to 90% of an ingested dose is excreted in the urine as metabolites or their conjugates, and no ibuprofen *per se* is found in the urine. The major metabolites are a hydroxylated and a carboxylated compound.

Preparations, Route of Administration, and Dosage. *Ibuprofen* (BRUFEN, MOTRIN) is supplied as 200-, 300-, and 400-mg tablets and also as a suspension containing 20 mg/ml. Only tablets are available in the United States.

Daily doses of up to 2400 mg in divided portions may be given, although the usual total dose is 1200 to 1600 mg. It may also be possible to reduce the dose for maintenance purposes. The drug may be given with food to minimize gastrointestinal side effects. The pediatric dose is 20 mg/kg but should not exceed 500 mg per day in children weighing less than 30 kg.

Toxic Effects. Ibuprofen has been used in patients with known peptic ulceration, or a history of gastric intolerance to other aspirin-like agents. Nevertheless, therapy must usually be discontinued in 10 to 15% of patients because of intolerance to the drug (*see* Cardoe, in Symposium, 1975a).

Gastrointestinal side effects are experienced by 5 to 15% of patients taking ibuprofen; epigastric pain, nausea, heartburn, abdominal discomfort, and sensations of "fullness" in the gastrointestinal tract are the usual difficulties. However, the incidence of these side effects is less with ibuprofen than with aspirin or indomethacin. Occult blood loss is uncommon.

Other side effects of ibuprofen have been reported less frequently. They include thrombocytopenia, skin rashes, headache, dizziness and blurred vision, and, in a few cases, toxic amblyopia, fluid retention, and edema. Patients who develop ocular disturbances should discontinue the use of ibuprofen.

Ibuprofen is not recommended for use by pregnant women, nor by those who are breast-feeding their infants.

NAPROXEN

The pharmacological properties and therapeutic uses of naproxen have been reviewed by Brogden and associates (1975) and in a symposium (1975b).

Pharmacokinetics and Metabolism. Naproxen is fully absorbed when administered orally. The rapidity, but not the extent, of absorption is influenced by the presence of food in the stomach. Absorption may be accelerated by the concurrent administration of sodium bicarbonate or reduced by magnesium oxide or aluminum hydroxide. Naproxen is also absorbed rectally, but peak concentrations in plasma are achieved more slowly. The half-life of naproxen in plasma is 12 to 15 hours and is unrelated to the dose in the therapeutic range. In children, the half-life is probably slightly shorter.

Naproxen and its metabolites are almost entirely excreted in the urine. About 30% of the drug undergoes 6-demethylation, and most of this metabolite is excreted as the glucuronide or other conjugates.

Naproxen is almost completely (98 to 99%) bound to plasma protein following normal therapeutic doses. Naproxen crosses the placenta and appears in the milk of lactating women at approximately 1% of the maternal plasma concentration.

Preparations, Routes of Administration, and Dosage. *Naproxen* (NAPROSYN, others) is available in 250-mg tablets for oral administration and also, in some countries, as a suspension containing 25 mg/ml and in 500-mg suppositories. Because of the long half-life of naproxen, the most usual initial and maintenance dosage is 250 mg, given twice a day. The drug may be given with meals if gastric discomfort is experienced.

Toxic Effects. The incidence of gastrointestinal and CNS side effects is about equal, although naproxen is better tolerated than indomethacin in both regards. Gastrointestinal complications have ranged from relatively mild dyspepsia, gastric discomfort, and heartburn to nausea, vomiting, and gastric bleeding. CNS side effects range from drowsiness, headache, dizziness, and sweating to fatigue, depression, and ototoxicity. Less common reactions include pruritus and a variety of dermatological problems. A few instances of jaundice have also occurred.

FENOPROFEN

The pharmacological properties and therapeutic uses of fenoprofen have been reviewed by Brogden and associates (1977b).

Pharmacokinetics and Metabolism. Oral doses of fenoprofen are readily, if incompletely (85%), ab-

sorbed. The presence of food in the stomach retards absorption and lowers peak concentrations in plasma. The sodium salt may be absorbed somewhat better than the calcium salt. The concomitant administration of antacids does not seem to alter concentrations that are achieved.

After absorption, fenoprofen is extensively (>90%) metabolized and excreted almost entirely in the urine. Fenoprofen undergoes metabolic transformation to the 4-hydroxy analog. The glucuronic acid conjugate of fenoprofen itself and 4-hydroxy fenoprofen are formed in almost equal amounts and together account for 90% of the excreted drug.

Preparations, Route of Administration, and Dosage. *Fenoprofen Calcium,* U.S.P. (NALFON, others), is available in capsules containing 300 and 600 mg of the active drug for oral administration. The recommended dosage to treat rheumatoid arthritis is 600 mg, given four times a day, but this may be increased to a maximum of 3 g per day. Fenoprofen should be administered before meals. The drug is not recommended for children.

Toxic Effects. Gastrointestinal side effects have been the most frequently reported; abdominal discomfort and dyspepsia occur in about 15% of patients. Constipation and nausea have also been reported. These side effects are almost always less intense than with equipotent doses of aspirin and force discontinuation of therapy in a few percent of patients. Nevertheless, care should be exercised when giving the drug to patients having a history of gastrointestinal ulceration or other pathology. Other side effects include skin rash and, less frequently, CNS effects, such as tinnitus, dizziness, lassitude, confusion, and anorexia.

FLURBIPROFEN

This agent is not currently available in the United States. Further information on flurbiprofen is discussed in a symposium (1977a) and by Adams and Buckler (1979).

Pharmacokinetics and Metabolism. Flurbiprofen is rapidly and completely absorbed following oral administration in man, and peak concentrations in plasma are achieved about 90 minutes after a single dose. Flurbiprofen is extensively (99%) bound to plasma proteins; the half-life in plasma is about 4 hours.

Flurbiprofen is recovered quantitatively in the urine as the unchanged drug and a number of metabolites. Included in the latter are 4-hydroxy, 3,4-dihydroxy, and 3-hydroxy,4-methoxy compounds. The 4-hydroxy metabolite and its conjugate account for nearly half of the excreted dose.

Preparations, Route of Administration, and Dosage. *Flurbiprofen* (FROBEN) is available in 50- or 100-mg tablets. The usual daily dose is 150 to 200 mg, taken in divided doses of 50 mg. The maximal daily dose is 300 mg.

Toxic Effects. The total incidence of patients who

experience side effects while receiving flurbiprofen is very high—25 to 50%—but only about 5% are forced to stop therapy. Gastrointestinal side effects (dyspepsia, nausea, vomiting) are again the most common and occur in nearly 40% of patients (*see* Sheldrake *et al.,* 1977). CNS side effects (usually headache) are also common (16% of cases). Other untoward reactions include skin rash (6%) and various signs and symptoms referable to the renal, hematological, cardiovascular, and respiratory systems (4% or less).

KETOPROFEN

Further information on the pharmacological properties and therapeutic uses of ketoprofen may be found in the publications of Julou and associates (1971), Rahbek (1976), and Mason and Bolton (1977).

Pharmacokinetics and Metabolism. Rapid and virtually complete absorption occurs after oral administration of therapeutic doses of ketoprofen, and peak concentrations in plasma are reached within 1 to 2 hours. The half-life of ketoprofen in plasma varies enormously (1 to 35 hours) and appears to depend upon whether or not the drug has been administered previously.

In man, hepatic conjugation of the drug with glucuronic acid occurs, but ketoprofen itself may also be excreted by the kidneys. Most of the drug and its metabolites is ultimately excreted in the urine.

Preparations, Route of Administration, and Dosage. *Ketoprofen* (ALRHEUMAT, ORUDIS) is available as capsules containing 50 mg for oral administration. The recommended dose is 100 to 150 mg per day in divided doses. This can be increased to 200 mg per day if therapeutic control is inadequate. The drug should be taken with food to avoid gastrointestinal effects. Ketoprofen is not yet available in the United States.

Toxic Effects. The total incidence of side effects is approximately 15%. In about one third of these cases, their severity may require withdrawal of the drug. The untoward reactions are mainly gastrointestinal effects of the type described above. CNS side effects are much less common and generally take the form of light-headedness or vertigo. Very occasionally skin rashes, pruritus, or renal dysfunction may occur.

THERAPEUTIC USES

The propionic acid derivatives are useful for the symptomatic treatment of *rheumatoid arthritis, juvenile rheumatoid arthritis, osteoarthritis, ankylosing spondylitis,* and related conditions. Comparative clinical studies indicate that they are comparable to aspirin for the control of the signs and symptoms of these diseases. In patients with rheumatoid arthritis there is a reduction in joint swelling,

pain, and duration of morning stiffness. By objective measurements, strength, mobility, and stamina are improved. In general, the intensity of untoward effects is less than that associated with the ingestion of indomethacin or high doses of aspirin. However, aspirin is considerably less expensive for those who can tolerate it.

These agents are also effective for symptomatic relief from pain associated with injuries to soft tissues, and they have been used to relieve pain post partum and following oral, ophthalmic, and other types of surgery. The use of ibuprofen as an analgesic for such conditions has been approved in the United States. This drug also appears to be more effective than aspirin for relief of pain from dysmenorrhea (*see* Medical Letter, 1979).

It is difficult to find data on which to base a rational choice between the members of this group of drugs, if in fact one can be made. However, Reynolds and Whorwell (1974) and Huskisson and associates (1976) compared the activity of several members of this group. Although different doses of the drugs were used, patients in both studies preferred *naproxen* (with *fenoprofen* next) in terms of analgesia and relief of morning stiffness. With regard to side effects, naproxen was the best tolerated, followed by ibuprofen, ketoprofen, and fenoprofen. Huskisson and co-workers (1976) also observed that there was considerable interpatient variation in the preference for a single drug and also between the designation of the best drug and the worst agent. Unfortunately, it is probably impossible to predict *a priori* which drug will be most suitable for any given individual.

GOLD

Gold, in elemental form, has been employed for centuries as an antipruritic to relieve the itching palm. In more modern times, the observation by Robert Koch in 1890 that gold inhibited *Mycobacterium tuberculosis in vitro* led to trials in arthritis and lupus erythematosus, thought by some to be tuberculous manifestations. The favorable observations of Forestier (1929) were largely responsible for stimulating interest in gold therapy (chrysotherapy). At present, gold is employed to a moderate extent in the treatment of rheumatoid arthritis.

Chemistry. The significant preparations of gold are all aurous salts in which the gold is attached to sulfur. The water-soluble compounds employed in therapy all contain hydrophilic groups in addition to the aurothio group. The structural formulas of *aurothioglucose* and *gold sodium thiomalate* are as follows:

Aurothioglucose

CH₂COONa
|
AuSCHCOONa

Gold Sodium Thiomalate

Monovalent gold has a relatively strong affinity for sulfur, weak affinities for carbon and nitrogen, and almost no affinity for oxygen, except in chelates. The strong affinity for sulfur and the inhibitory effect of gold salts on various enzymes suggest that the therapeutic effects of gold salts derive from inhibition of sulfhydryl systems. However, other sulfhydryl inhibitors do not appear to have therapeutic actions in common with gold.

Pharmacological Actions.

Gold compounds can suppress or prevent, but not cure, experimental arthritis and synovitis due to a number of infections and chemical agents. While many effects of gold compounds have been observed, which, if any, is related to the therapeutic effects of gold in rheumatoid arthritis is unknown. Perhaps the best hypotheses relate to the uptake of gold by macrophages with resultant inhibition of phagocytosis and the activities of lysosomal enzymes (Persellin and Ziff, 1966; Jessop *et al.*, 1973) and also to its ability to influence immunological responses (Strong *et al.*, 1973; Gottlieb *et al.*, 1975). Gold can decrease concentrations of rheumatoid factor and immunoglobulins and impair mitogen-induced proliferation of lymphocytes. By several indices, gold suppresses cellular immunity (Strong *et al.*, 1973).

Gold salts administered *in vivo* alter the properties of collagen in rats, presumably by increasing cross-linkages (*see* Adam and Kühn, 1968). Gold is entrained in lysosomes and phagosomes in the synovial membrane, kidney, mesentery, skin, and other tissues. It does not affect the release of lysosomal hydrolases, but it inhibits these enzymes. Gold suppresses the anaphylactic release of histamine more effectively than do glucocorticoids (Norn, 1971). It

also prevents prostaglandin synthesis *in vitro* (Deby *et al.*, 1973; Stone *et al.*, 1975).

Aurothioglucose, but not other compounds of gold, in toxic doses induces obesity in dogs and certain strains of mice. Gold-induced necrosis of the oligodendroglia in the ventromedial hypothalamus occurs in both rats and mice. Gold is deposited in the scar. The gold of gold thiomalate, which does not induce obesity, is not found in hypothalamic loci. These effects of gold are not observed in human subjects.

Absorption, Distribution, and Excretion. The water-soluble gold salts are rapidly absorbed after intramuscular injection, peak concentrations in blood being reached in 2 to 6 hours (*see* Freyberg, 1966; Mascarenhas *et al.*, 1972), unless the salt is suspended in oil. Currently marketed gold preparations are erratically absorbed by the oral route. Some chloro (trialkylphosphine) gold compounds appear to be better absorbed orally, and preparations for oral use may be available in the near future. Less is known about the distribution of gold in man than in animals (*see* Grahame *et al.*, 1974; Vernon-Roberts *et al.*, 1976). Tissue distribution depends not only on the type of compound administered but also on the time after administration and probably on the duration of treatment. Early in the course of therapy, several percent of the total body content of gold is in the blood. However, the fraction in blood of the normal trace body burden is only about 2×10^{-8} (*see* Schroeder and Nason, 1971). In the blood, soluble gold is first bound (about 95%) to albumin; during the course of the first week, a substantial fraction may be transferred to the erythrocytes in about one third of patients (Smith *et al.*, 1973). During treatment, the concentration in the synovial fluid is about half that in plasma (Gerber *et al.*, 1972); equilibrium occurs in less than 4 hours.

With continued therapy, the concentration of gold in the synovium of affected joints is about ten times that of skeletal muscle, bone, or fat. Gold deposits are also found in macrophages of many tissues, as well as in renotubular epithelium, seminiferous tubules, hepatocytes, and adrenocortical cells. After therapy with gold is stopped, the metal remains in tissues for many years.

The pharmacokinetics of gold is complex and varies with the dose and the duration of treatment. The plasma half-life is about 7 days for a 50-mg dose (Gottlieb *et al.*, 1974; Sharp *et al.*, 1977). With successive doses the half-life lengthens, and values of weeks or months may be observed after prolonged therapy.

The excretion of gold is 60 to 90% renal and 10 to 40% fecal, the latter probably mostly by biliary secretion. The gold concentration in urine varies among patients. In the first day after injection it ranges from about equal to twice that in plasma; after 7 days it may be slightly above to slightly below the plasma concentration. The half-time for the fall in urine concentration after the first two or three weekly injections appears to be shorter than that of plasma concentration, but it eventually approaches that of the plasma half-life. Fecal excretion is erratic but tends to be low in the first day after injection and to increase during the next several days.

By a double-labeling technic, Gottlieb and co-workers (1972) discovered that during maintenance the total amount excreted during a week is about 40% from the most recent dose and 60% from previous doses. They reported that, with a biweekly to monthly maintenance dosage schedule, the average weekly excretion is approximately 40%. Although they did not state the mean interval, it is evident that during the 2 weeks or more of excretion most of a dose would have been eliminated; this disagrees sharply with the earlier data of Smith and associates (1958), which indicated that approximately 85% of a dose accumulates. Gottlieb and associates also reported that, after a cumulative dose of 1 g of gold, urinary excretion of gold can be detected for as long as a year. However, blood concentrations fall to the normal trace amounts in about 40 to 80 days (*see* the data of Mascarenhas *et al.,* 1972). Thus, the true cumulative potential of gold is not yet clearly ascertained. Sulfhydryl agents, such as dimercaprol, penicillamine, and N-acetylcysteine, increase the excretion of gold (*see* Lorber *et al.,* 1973b). It is of interest that penicillamine also tends to correct the abnormalities in copper and iron metabolism in rheumatoid arthritis as well as the pathological indices (*see* Jaffe, 1970; Zuckner *et al.,* 1970; Multicentre Trial Group, 1973). Details of the pharmacokinetics of gold can be found in reports by Lorber and associates (1968, 1973a), Gerber and coworkers (1972), Mascarenhas and colleagues (1972), Rubinstein and Dietz (1973), Gottlieb and colleagues (1974), and others.

Preparations, Routes of Administration, and Dosage. *Aurothioglucose,* U.S.P. (SOLGANAL), contains approximately 50% gold. Although it is water soluble, it is employed mainly as *Sterile Aurothioglucose Suspension,* U.S.P., a sterile suspension in a suitable fixed oil. Commercial preparations contain 50 mg/ml in 10-ml vials. *Gold Sodium Thiomalate,* U.S.P. (MYOCHRYSINE), also contains approximately 50% gold and is very soluble in water. *Gold Sodium Thiomalate Injection,* U.S.P., is a sterile aqueous solution of the drug that is marketed in 1-ml ampuls containing 10, 25, 50, or 100 mg of the salt and in 10-ml multiple-dose vials containing 50 mg/ml.

The optimal intramuscular dosage schedule for the treatment of rheumatoid arthritis is still not agreed upon. The usual dose is 10 mg of gold in the first week as a test dose, 25 mg in the second and third weeks, and 50 mg a week thereafter, up to a total of 750 mg. While doses of 100 to 150 mg weekly have been used for rheumatoid arthritis, this higher dose is no more effective than 50 mg weekly and leads to more side effects (*see* Furst *et al.,* 1977). If a remission occurs, treatment is continued but reduced to 50 mg biweekly for four doses, then every 3 weeks for four doses, and finally every 4 weeks for a year. If a relapse occurs during this time, the dosage interval should be shortened; if not, therapy may be discontinued. Many rheumatologists prefer to base dosage on concentrations of gold in urine and plasma. Lorber and associates (1973a) adjust each dose to maintain the plasma concentration at 3 mg per liter. However, the general concensus is that such values do not correlate well with the response to therapy, course of the disease, or development of toxicity. For a variety of other dosage regimens, *see* Research Sub-committee of the Empire Rheumatism Council (1960, 1961a, 1961b), Lockie (1961), Smyth (1972), Cooperating Clinics Committee of the American Rheumatism Association (1973), Bluhm (1975), Cats (1976), Gottlieb (1976–1977), Furst and associates (1977), and Sharp and coworkers (1977).

Aurothioglucose in oil is absorbed more slowly than gold sodium thiomalate and also appears to yield somewhat lower concentrations of gold in plasma (*see* Rubinstein and Dietz, 1973), but the posological and therapeutic implications of these findings are unknown. Preparations of aurothioglucose and gold sodium thiomalate appear to be equally effective and are used in similar dosages. An oral preparation of gold (*auranofin*) has been used in Europe and appears to be approximately equivalent to the parenteral preparations in efficacy and toxicity.

Clinical Toxicity. The incidence of toxicity in the therapeutic use of gold presently ranges from about 25 to 50% of patients, serious toxicity occurring in about 10%. The estimated mortality due to chrysotherapy is about 0.4%. It is commonly believed that clinical remission and toxicity are positively related and that some degree of toxicity is inevitable in any effective treatment with gold (*see* Freyberg, 1966, 1972). However, Gottlieb and coworkers (1972) found the toxicity to be lower among patients undergoing remission than among those refractory to treatment. Smith and associates (1958) marshal strong evidence that toxicity need not be a serious hazard if the maintenance dosage schedule is based upon considerations of the rate of elimination of gold from the body. The incidence of toxic reactions is generally felt to be unrelated to the concentration of gold in plasma; however, Jessop and Johns (1973) state that the incidence and seriousness of dermatological reactions are correlated with these values when they exceed 3.4 mg per liter. Toxicity may be better correlated with the total body content of gold (Smith *et al.,* 1958).

The most common toxic effects are those involving the skin and the mucous membranes, usually of the mouth. Early transient pruritus is an indication that the tolerance level has been exceeded. A rapid improvement in joint swelling and pain also indicates that the tolerance level is being closely approached. Cutaneous reactions may vary in severity from simple *erythema* to severe *exfoliative dermatitis*. The skin lesions have a characteristic histopathology, and biopsy is important for a differential diagnosis (*see* Gottlieb *et al.,* 1972). Cutaneous reactions have been characterized as manifestations of a type-1 hypersensitivity, in which IgE becomes elevated in reactors (Davis *et al.,* 1973). Lesions of the mucous membranes include *stomatitis, pharyngitis, tracheitis, gastritis, colitis,* and *vaginitis; glossitis* is fairly common. As with silver, a gray-to-blue pigmentation (*chrysiasis*) may occur in the skin and mucous membranes, especially in areas exposed to light (Cox and Marich, 1973).

Severe *blood dyscrasias* may result from aurotherapy. *Thrombocytopenia* occasionally occurs and accounts for many of the fatalities. Thrombocytopenia may develop many months after the gold is administered and is due to accelerated degradation of platelets; present evidence suggests that this is due to an immunological mechanism (Levin *et al.,* 1975). *Leukopenia, agranulocytosis,* and *aplastic anemia* may also occur. When panmyelopathy results from aurotherapy, the concentrations of coproporphyrin and δ-aminolevulinic acid (δ-ALA) in urine may increase, as in lead poisoning. Eosinophilia is common, and many rheumatologists temporarily discontinue gold therapy when it occurs.

Transient and mild proteinuria is frequent during therapy. Heavy albuminuria and microscopic hematuria occur in 1 to 3% of cases. The site of damage is usually the proximal tubules. Although there are only a few reports in the world literature of gold-induced *nephrosis,* the number reported in some series suggests an incidence of several percent. The nephrosis is usually reversible, and the predominant lesion is membranous glomerulonephritis.

Gold may cause a variety of other severe toxic reactions, including *encephalitis, peripheral neuritis, hepatitis, pulmonary infiltrates,* and *nitritoid crisis* (*see* Gordon *et al.,* 1975; Gottlieb, 1976–1977). Fortunately, the incidence of serious reactions is low, and they generally are the result of failure to discontinue therapy when earlier, less serious symptoms occur.

Avoidance and Treatment. Regular examination of the skin, buccal mucosa, urine, and blood, including cell and platelet counts, should be made. It is the practice in many arthritis clinics to initiate therapy with small doses of gold and to increase the dose

gradually. Although untoward effects are not eliminated by this procedure, the severity of those reactions that occur early is somewhat reduced. If an untoward response occurs, therapy should be withheld until it subsides completely. If the reaction is a rash or stomatitis, antihistamines and adrenocorticosteroids may be administered, the latter systemically and/or topically. Glucocorticoids are also indicated in gold-induced nephrosis. Although it has been claimed that glucocorticoids administered during the course of gold therapy increase toxicity (Ramos *et al.,* 1963) and interfere with the therapeutic efficacy of gold (Hill, 1968), not all authorities recognize these claims (*e.g., see* Freyberg, 1972). If gold therapy is initiated in a patient receiving adrenocorticosteroids, the latter should be withdrawn when the accumulated dose of gold is 400 to 600 mg.

If the reaction to gold therapy is not of a serious type, injections may be cautiously resumed 2 or 3 weeks after the toxic reaction has subsided and the steroid has been withdrawn. Maintenance dosage should be two thirds to three fourths that previously planned. However, many experts decline to use the drug again, once toxicity has occurred.

If a severe reaction to gold occurs or if the above-mentioned steps fail to control the toxic effects, treatment with dimercaprol or penicillamine (Bluhm *et al.,* 1962) should be instituted. The administration of dimercaprol may shorten a therapeutic remission induced by gold.

Chrysiasis is treated with strong iodine solution (Lugol's solution) (Silverberg *et al.,* 1970).

Therapeutic Uses. Gold compounds find their chief therapeutic application in *rheumatoid arthritis.* Their exact status continues to be unsettled, in part because of concern over their toxicity and in part because the status of immunosuppressive and other agents is still uncertain.

At present, gold is used in early, active arthritis that progresses despite an adequate regimen of salicylates, rest, and physical therapy. Both subjective and objective manifestations of rheumatoid arthritis are improved. Gold salts often arrest the progression of the disease in involved joints, at least temporarily; prevent involvement of unaffected joints; improve grip strength and morning stiffness; and decrease the erythrocyte sedimentation rate and abnormal plasma glycoprotein and fibrinogen levels. Gold should not be used if the disease is mild and is usually of little benefit when the disease is advanced. It is estimated that chrysotherapy will induce a protracted or permanent remission in about 15% of patients, improve symptoms in 60 to 70% of patients, and must be discontinued in 15 to 20% of patients because of toxicity (*see* Lorber *et al.,* 1975; Cats, 1976); about 10 to 15% of patients do not respond.

Therapy with gold is sometimes beneficial in juvenile rheumatoid arthritis, palindromic rheumatism, psoriatic arthritis, Sjörgren's syndrome, nondisseminated lupus erythematosus, and pemphigus (*see*

Pennys *et al.*, 1973; Gordon *et al.*, 1975; Gottlieb, 1976–1977). Gold should not be used to treat patients with disseminated lupus.

The duration of the remissions after discontinuation of treatment with gold is extremely variable (from 1 to 18 months). The recurrence is said to be usually not as severe as the original disease, and a high percentage of patients responds favorably to a second course of gold therapy, especially if marked benefits resulted from the first course. In patients who receive gold continuously over many years and who respond favorably, there is little doubt that remissions can be maintained over long periods (*see* Hill, 1968; Cats, 1976).

There is no unanimity of opinion as to the best therapeutic regimen to follow after the completion of a course. Some rheumatologists give no further gold until a relapse occurs; some give a second or even a third course to patients in remission, with rest periods of 6 weeks between courses, and others continue uninterrupted treatment indefinitely, so long as the remission continues (*see* Smyth, 1972). Because of the long period of treatment, requirement for office visits, intramuscular administration, and laboratory tests, patient compliance is poor and there is a high rate of dropout.

Contraindications. Gold therapy is contraindicated in patients with *renal disease, hepatic dysfunction* or a *history of infectious hepatitis,* or *hematological disorders.* Gold should not be readministered to patients who have developed severe hematological or renal toxicity during a course of chrysotherapy. It is contraindicated during pregnancy or breast feeding. Patients who have recently had *radiation* should not receive gold because of its depressant action on hematopoietic tissue. Concomitant use of *antimalarials, immunosuppressants, phenylbutazone,* or *oxyphenbutazone* is contraindicated because of the potential of these drugs to cause blood dyscrasias. *Urticaria, eczema,* and *colitis* are also considered to be contraindications to the use of the metal. Finally, gold is poorly tolerated by aged individuals.

Other Therapy for Rheumatoid Arthritis. In addition to aspirin-like drugs and gold, which have been discussed in this chapter, other agents are also used in the therapy of rheumatoid arthritis. These include glucocorticoids (Chapter 63), immunosuppressive agents (azathioprine and cyclophosphamide; Chapter 55), penicillamine (Chapter 69), and antimalarials (chloroquine and hydroxychloroquine; Chapter 45). These drugs are generally reserved for patients who are re-fractory to therapeutic regimens that include rest, physiotherapy, and aspirin-like drugs. Glucocorticoids (administered intra-articularly) and gold are usually considered to be the next therapeutic choices, followed by steroids given systemically.

Despite the dramatic symptomatic improvement in rheumatoid arthritis caused by glucocorticoids, they too do *not* arrest the progress of the disease and are at least as toxic as gold. Consequently, gold is usually used in preference to glucocorticoids. Gold is about as effective as penicillamine (Huskisson *et al.*, 1974b) but appears to be somewhat less effective than cyclophosphamide (Currey *et al.*, 1974). However, the use of immunosuppressants can be associated with serious toxicity, and such treatment is considered to be investigational and should be considered only for patients with rheumatoid arthritis and other collagen diseases who are refractory to other forms of therapy. It may be possible to optimize dosage schedules for immunosuppressive agents by monitoring counts of B lymphocytes in peripheral blood (Horwitz, 1974).

DRUGS EMPLOYED IN THE TREATMENT OF GOUT

An acute attack of gout occurs as a result of an inflammatory reaction to crystals of sodium urate (the end product of purine metabolism in man) that are deposited in the joint tissue. The inflammatory response involves local infiltration of granulocytes, which phagocytize the urate crystals. Lactate production is high in synovial tissues and in the leukocytes associated with the inflammatory process, and this favors a local decrease in pH that fosters further deposition of uric acid.

Several therapeutic strategies can be used to counter attacks of gout. *Uricosuric drugs* increase the excretion of uric acid, thus reducing concentrations in plasma. *Colchicine* has a specific efficacious action in gout, probably secondary to an effect on the mobility of granulocytes. *Allopurinol* is a selective inhibitor of the terminal steps of the biosynthesis of uric acid. Although prostaglandins may be implicated in the pain and inflammation, there is no evidence that they contribute to the pathogenesis of gout; nevertheless, *aspirin-like drugs* may afford symptomatic relief, and some of them are uricosuric as well.

The pharmacology of aspirin-like drugs is described in the previous section. Discussion in this section is limited to colchicine, allopurinol, and the clinical use of the uricosuric agents. The basic pharmacology of uricosuric drugs is presented in Chapter 38. Progress in the treatment of gout during the past 25 years has been authoritatively reviewed by Yü (1974). More recently, a most useful volume on uric acid has appeared that contains major sections on the pathogenesis and therapy of gout (*see* Kelley and Weiner, 1978).

COLCHICINE

Colchicine is a unique anti-inflammatory agent in that it is effective essentially only against gouty arthritis. It provides dramatic relief of acute attacks of gout and is an effective prophylactic agent against such attacks.

History. Colchicine is an alkaloid of *Colchicum autumnale* (autumn crocus, meadow saffron), a plant so named because it grew in Colchis in Asia Minor. Although the poisonous action of colchicum was known to Dioscorides, preparations of the plant were not recommended for pain of articular origin until the sixth century A.D. Colchicum was introduced for the therapy of acute gout by von Störck in 1763, and its specificity for this syndrome soon resulted in its incorporation in a number of "gout mixtures" popularized by charlatans. Benjamin Franklin, himself a sufferer from gout, is reputed to have introduced colchicum therapy in the United States. The alkaloid *colchicine* was isolated from colchicum in 1820 by Pelletier and Caventou.

Chemistry. The structural formula of colchicine is as follows:

Colchicine

The structure-activity relationship of colchicine and related agents has been discussed by Wallace (1961).

Pharmacological Properties. The anti-inflammatory effect of colchicine in acute gouty arthritis is selective for this disorder. Colchicine is only occasionally effective in other types of arthritis; it is not an analgesic and does not provide relief of other types of pain.

Colchicine is also an antimitotic agent and has been widely employed as an experimental tool in the study of normal and abnormal cell division and cell function.

Effect in Gout. Colchicine does not influence the renal excretion of uric acid, its concentration in blood, or the miscible pool of uric acid. By virtue of its ability to bind to microtubular protein, colchicine interferes with the function of the mitotic spindles and causes depolymerization and disappearance of the fibrillar microtubules in granulocytes and other motile cells. This action is apparently the basis of the long-accepted view of the beneficial effect of colchicine (*see* Malawista, 1975), namely, the inhibition of the migration of granulocytes into the inflamed area. This reduces the release of lactic acid and pro-inflammatory enzymes that occurs during phagocytosis and breaks the cycle that leads to the inflammatory response. However, there are a number of apparently contradictory observations that cannot be accommodated by this simple hypothesis (*see* Wallace and Ertel, 1978).

Neutrophils exposed to urate crystals ingest them and produce a glycoprotein, which may be the causative agent of acute gouty arthritis. Injected into joints, this substance produces a profound arthritis that is histologically indistinguishable from that caused by direct injection of urate crystals. Spilberg and associates (1979) found that colchicine does not prevent phagocytosis of urate crystals but appears to prevent either the production by or release from leukocytes of the glycoprotein that causes the joint pain and inflammation.

Effect on Cell Division. Colchicine can arrest plant and animal cell division *in vitro* and *in vivo*. Pernice in 1889 was the first to note that colchicum influenced mitosis, but the details were first elucidated by Lits (1934) and Amoroso (1935). Mitosis is arrested in the metaphase, due to failure of spindle formation. Bizarre and abnormal nuclear configurations ensue, and the cells often die. Cells with the highest rates of division are affected earliest. High concentrations may completely prevent cells from entering mitosis. Both normal and cancer cells are similarly affected. The effect is not specific for colchicine and is exhibited by the vinca alkaloids (vincristine and vinblastine), podophyllotoxin, griseofulvin, and other agents. The extensive studies of the effects of colchicine on cell division and its use as a pharmacological tool have been summarized by Dustin (1963).

Other Effects. Colchicine inhibits the release of histamine-containing granules from mast cells, the secretion of insulin from beta cells of pancreatic islets, and the movement of melanin granules in melanophores; all of these processes may involve the translocation of granules by the microtubular system.

Colchicine also exhibits a variety of other pharmacological effects. It lowers body temperature, increases the sensitivity to central depressants, depresses the respiratory center, enhances the response to sympathomimetic agents, constricts blood vessels, and induces hypertension by central vasomotor stimulation. It enhances gastrointestinal activity by neurogenic stimulation but depresses it by a direct effect, and alters neuromuscular function.

Absorption, Distribution, Biotransformation, and Excretion. Colchicine is rapidly absorbed after oral administration, and peak concentrations occur in plasma by 0.5 to 2 hours. Large amounts of the drug and metabolites enter the intestinal tract in the bile and intestinal secretions, and this fact, plus the rapid turnover of intestinal epithelium, probably explains the prominence of intestinal manifestations in colchicine poisoning. Administered intravenously, colchicine rapidly leaves the blood and distributes in an apparent space larger than that of the body water. The kidney, liver, spleen, and intestinal tract contain high concentrations of colchicine, but it is apparently largely excluded from heart, skeletal muscle, and brain. The drug can be detected in leukocytes and in the urine for at least 9 days after a single intravenous dose.

Colchicine is metabolized to a mixture of compounds *in vitro,* but such metabolites have not been detected in urine, cells, or plasma. Most of the drug is excreted in the feces; however, in normal individuals, 10 to 20% of the drug is excreted in the urine. In patients with liver disease, hepatic uptake and elimination are reduced and a greater fraction of the drug is excreted in the urine (*see* Wallace *et al.,* 1970).

Toxicity. *Nausea, vomiting, diarrhea,* and *abdominal pain* are the most common and earliest untoward effects of colchicine overdosage. To avoid more serious toxicity, administration of the drug is discontinued as soon as these symptoms occur. A latent period of several hours or more occurs between the administration of the drug and the onset of symptoms. This interval is not altered by dosage or route of administration. For this reason, and because of individual variation, adverse effects may be unavoidable during an initial course of colchicine medication. However, the patient often remains relatively consistent in his response to the drug, and therefore toxicity can be minimized or avoided during subsequent courses of therapy. The drug is as effective when given intravenously as orally; the onset of the therapeutic effect may be faster, and the gastrointestinal side effects may be almost completely avoided when the drug is given intravenously.

In *acute poisoning,* the diarrhea soon becomes profuse, watery, and bloody due to a *hemorrhagic gastroenteritis.* Considerable fluid, electrolyte, and plasma are lost through the bowel. Altered function of the ileal mucosa results in reversible malabsorption of cyanocobalamin and the actively transported sugars. Even when given by injection, colchicine causes gastrointestinal irritation. Burning of the throat and skin are also prominent symptoms. Because of the extensive vascular damage, shock occurs. The *kidney* is also injured, and hematuria and oliguria ensue. *Muscular depression* is pronounced, an ascending *paralysis* of the CNS develops, and death results from respiratory arrest usually within 1 to 2 days.

The *fatal dose* varies considerably. As little as 7 mg of colchicine has proved fatal. *Treatment* of acute colchicine poisoning should be directed very early against shock. The remaining measures are purely symptomatic and supportive. Atropine and morphine aid in relieving abdominal pain.

Colchicine produces a temporary leukopenia that is soon replaced by a leukocytosis, sometimes due to a striking increase in the number of basophilic granulocytes. The site of action is apparently directly on the bone marrow. *Chronic administration* of colchicine entails some risk of *agranulocytosis, aplastic anemia, myopathy,* and *alopecia.*

Preparations. *Colchicine,* U.S.P., is available as official tablets (0.5 or 0.6 mg); they should be stored in tight, light-resistant containers. Sterile solution (0.5 mg/ml) is also available for injection.

Therapeutic Uses. Colchicine provides dramatic relief of *acute attacks* of gout. The effect is sufficiently selective that the drug has been used for diagnostic purposes, but the test is not infallible. Colchicine also has an established role to *prevent* and to *abort* acute attacks of gout. (*See* Seegmiller and Grayzel, 1960; Yü and Gutman, 1961; Gutman, 1973; Yü, 1974.)

Acute Attacks. When colchicine is given promptly within the first few hours of an attack, less than 5% of patients fail to obtain relief. A patient who is in helpless agony with a tumefied, red, hot joint is sufficiently relieved so that he can walk about in a few hours. Pain, swelling, and redness abate within 12 hours and are completely gone in 48 to 72 hours.

The former practice of administering colchicine at hourly intervals is no longer recommended (Yü, 1974). An initial dose of 1 mg is followed by 0.5 mg every 2 to 3 hours; drug administration is stopped as soon as the pain disappears or gastrointestinal symptoms develop. The total dose usually required to alleviate an attack is 4 to 10 mg, and the latter amount should not be exceeded. Opioids or other drugs may be required for the diarrhea. In subsequent attacks, the patient may be able to stop medication short of the amount causing toxic reactions. To avoid cumulative toxicity, the course of colchicine should not be repeated within 3 days. Colchicine may be administered intravenously, and there may be distinct advantages to this route of administration. A single dose of 2 mg, diluted in 10 to 20 ml of 0.9% sodium chloride solution, is usually adequate. The solution is very irritating if extravasation occurs.

Great care should be exercised in prescribing colchicine for aged or feeble patients, and for those with cardiac, renal, or gastrointestinal disease. In these patients and in those who do not tolerate or respond to colchicine, a short course of phenylbutazone (*see* above), followed by prophylactic doses of colchicine, may be employed.

Prophylactic Uses. For patients with chronic gout, colchicine has established value as a prophylactic agent during the asymptomatic intercritical period. It has a preeminent place in the prevention of acute gout when there is frequent recurrence of attacks. The regular ingestion of colchicine effectively minimizes the frequency and the intensity of acute episodes; by reducing stiffness and aching, it often permits relatively normal activity in a person who otherwise would be incapacitated. Prophylactic medication is also indicated upon initiation of chronic medication with allopurinol or the uricosuric agents, since acute attacks often increase in frequency during the early months of such therapy.

The usual *prophylactic dose* of colchicine is 0.5 to 2.0 mg or more every night or every other night, as required by the individual patient. Tolerance does not develop to the alkaloid.

Colchicine should be taken in larger abortive doses immediately upon the first twinge of articular pain or the appearance of any prodrome of an acute attack. Thus, the patient should always have the drug with him. The judicious ingestion of colchicine during the premonitory, incipient, and inflorescent stages of acute gouty arthritis will abort paroxysms and prevent chronic gouty arthritis.

Prior to and following surgery in patients with gout, colchicine should be given for a few days (0.5 mg, three times a day); this greatly reduces the very high incidence of acute attacks of gouty arthritis precipitated by operative procedures.

Daily administration of colchicine is useful for the prevention of attacks of *familial Mediterranean fever* (familial paroxysmal polyserositis).

ALLOPURINOL

Allopurinol is an effective drug for the therapy of both the primary hyperuricemia of gout and that secondary to hematological disorders or antineoplastic therapy. In contrast with the uricosuric agents that increase the renal excretion of urate, allopurinol inhibits the terminal steps in uric acid biosynthesis. Since overproduction of uric acid is a contributing factor in most patients with gout and a characteristic of most types of secondary hyperuricemia, allopurinol represents a rational approach to therapy.

History. The introduction of allopurinol by Hitchings, Elion, and associates provides an elegant example of the development of a drug on a rational biochemical basis. Originally synthesized as a candidate antineoplastic agent, allopurinol was found to lack antimetabolite activity but, by *in-vitro* test, it proved to be a substrate for and an inhibitor of xanthine oxidase. Inhibition of xanthine oxidase *in vivo* was initially established in leukemic patients receiving therapy with the antimetabolite 6-mercaptopurine. Allopurinol delayed inactivation of 6-mercaptopurine by xanthine oxidase and also reduced the plasma concentration and renal excretion of uric acid. Subsequent clinical trial for treatment of gout by Rundles and coworkers was successful and quickly confirmed. (*See* Elion *et al.*, 1963; Rundles *et al.*, 1963; Elion, 1978.)

Chemistry and Pharmacological Effects. Allopurinol, an analog of hypoxanthine, has the following structural formula:

Allopurinol

Both allopurinol and its primary metabolite, alloxanthine (oxypurinol), are inhibitors of xanthine oxidase. Inhibition of this enzyme accounts for the major pharmacological effects of allopurinol (*see* Elion, 1978).

In man, uric acid is formed primarily by the xanthine oxidase–catalyzed oxidation of hypoxanthine and xanthine. At low concentrations, allopurinol is a substrate for and competitive inhibitor of the enzyme; at high concentrations, it is a noncompetitive inhibitor. Alloxanthine, the metabolite of allopurinol formed by the action of xanthine oxidase, is a potent noncompetitive inhibitor of the enzyme; the formation of this compound, together with its long persistence in tissues, is undoubtedly responsible for much of the pharmacological activity of allopurinol. Inhibition of the penultimate and ultimate steps in uric acid biosynthesis reduces the plasma concentration and urinary excretion of uric acid and increases the plasma concentrations and renal excretion of the more soluble oxypurine precursors.

Before allopurinol treatment of hyperuricemia, the urinary content of purines is almost solely uric acid. During such treatment, the urinary purines are divided among hypoxanthine, xanthine, and uric acid. Since each has its independent solubility, the concentration of uric acid in plasma is reduced without exposing the urinary tract to an excessive load of uric acid and the likelihood of calculus formation.

The alterations in purine metabolism produced by allopurinol explain its salutary effects in gout. By lowering the uric acid concentration in plasma below its limit of solubility, the dissolution of tophi is facilitated and the development or progression of chronic gouty arthritis is prevented. The formation of uric acid stones virtually disappears with therapy, and this prevents the development of nephropathy. The incidence of acute attacks of arthritis may increase during the early months of therapy but is subsequently reduced.

Tissue deposition of xanthine and hypoxanthine usually does not occur during allopurinol therapy because the renal clearance of the oxypurines is rapid; their plasma concentrations are only slightly increased and do not exceed their solubility. Although xanthine constitutes about 50% of total oxypurine excreted in the urine and is relatively insoluble, xanthine stone formation during allopurinol therapy has occurred only in an occasional patient with very high uric acid production prior to treatment. The risk can be minimized by alkalinization of the urine and by increasing the daily fluid intake during the administration of allopurinol. In some patients, the allopurinol-induced increase in excretion of oxypurines is less than the reduction in uric acid excretion; this disparity is primarily a result of reutilization of oxypurines and feedback inhibition of de-novo purine biosynthesis. Increased oxypurine excretion matches the reduction in uric acid excretion in patients with phosphoribosyltransferase deficiency; such individuals are unable to reutilize oxypurines.

Absorption, Distribution, Biotransformation, and Excretion. Allopurinol is relatively rapidly absorbed after oral ingestion, and peak plasma concentration is reached within 30 to 60 minutes. About 20% is excreted in the feces in 48 to 72 hours, presumably as unabsorbed drug. Allopurinol is rapidly cleared from plasma with a half-time of 2 to 3 hours, primarily by conversion to alloxanthine. Less than 10% of a single dose or about 30% of the drug ingested during chronic medication is excreted unchanged in the urine. Self-inhibition of the metabolism of allopurinol to alloxanthine explains this dose-dependent elimination. Alloxanthine is slowly excreted in the urine by the net balance of glomerular filtration and probenecid-sensitive tubular reabsorption. The plasma half-time of alloxanthine is 18 to 30 hours in patients with normal renal function and increases in proportion to the reduction of glomerular filtration in patients with renal impairment. Although alloxanthine is a less potent inhibitor of xanthine oxidase than is the parent drug, the metabolite accumulates in the body during chronic administration of allopurinol and contributes significantly to the therapeutic effects of the medication. Patients with a genetic deficiency of xanthine oxidase (xanthinuria) do not convert allopurinol to alloxanthine.

Allopurinol and its metabolite alloxanthine are distributed in total tissue water, with the exception of brain, in which their concentration is about one third that in other tissues. Neither compound is bound to plasma proteins.

Drug Interactions. Interactions between allopurinol and *probenecid* and other *uricosuric* agents and those between allopurinol and *6-mercaptopurine* (and its derivative *azathioprine*) have been alluded to above. Allopurinol may also interfere with the hepatic inactivation of other drugs, including the *oral anticoagulant* agents. Although the effect is variable and of clinical significance only in some patients, increased monitoring of prothrombin activity is recommended in patients receiving both medications.

Whether the increased incidence of skin rash in patients receiving concurrent allopurinol-ampicillin medication, compared with that of these agents administered individually, should be ascribed to allopurinol or to hyperuricemia remains to be established.

The reported interference by allopurinol with mobilization of hepatic iron has not been confirmed, and the proposed role of xanthine oxidase in iron metabolism remains unestablished. Nevertheless, concurrent administration of iron during allopurinol medication is not recommended.

Toxicity. Allopurinol is well tolerated by most patients. The most common adverse effects are hypersensitivity reactions. They may occur even after months or years of chronic medication. These usually subside within a few days after medication is discontinued. Serious reactions preclude further use of the drug.

Attacks of acute gout may occur more frequently during the initial months of allopurinol medication and may require concurrent prophylactic therapy with colchicine (*see* above).

The cutaneous reaction is predominantly a pruritic, erythematous, or maculopapular eruption, but occasionally the lesion is exfoliative, urticarial, or purpuric. Fever, malaise, and muscle aching may also occur. Such effects are noted in about 3% of patients with normal renal function but more frequently in those with renal impairment.

Transient leukopenia or leukocytosis and eosinophilia are rare reactions but may require cessation of therapy. A few cases of hepatomegaly and elevated levels of serum glutamic oxalacetic acid transaminase have been recorded, and there have been isolated reports of peripheral neuritis, bone-marrow depression, and cataract. Eosinophilia with epidermal necrolysis has resulted in renal failure.

Undesirable side effects such as headache, drowsiness, nausea, vomiting, vertigo, diarrhea, and gastric irritation occur occasionally but usually do not require that therapy be stopped.

Preparations, Route of Administration, and Dosage. *Allopurinol*, U.S.P. (ZYLOPRIM), is available as 100- and 300-mg scored tablets for oral use.

For control of hyperuricemia in gout, the aim of therapy is to reduce plasma uric acid concentration below 6 mg/dl. Medication must not be initiated during an acute attack of gouty arthritis, and it is started at low doses to minimize the risk of precipitating such attacks. Concurrent prophylactic colchicine therapy is also recommended during and sometimes beyond the initial months of therapy. Fluid intake should be sufficient to maintain daily urinary volume above 2 liters; slightly alkaline urine is preferred. An initial daily dose of 100 mg is increased by 100-mg increments at weekly intervals. The usual daily maintenance dose for adults is 300 mg; a single daily dose is satisfactory. Dosage must be reduced in patients with renal impairment in proportion to the reduction in glomerular filtration; 100 mg daily or 300 mg twice weekly is often satisfactory.

In the treatment of secondary hyperuricemias, as for the prevention of uric acid nephropathy during vigorous therapy of certain neoplastic diseases, a dose of 200 to 800 mg daily for 2 to 3 days or longer is advisable, together with a high fluid intake. In children with secondary hyperuricemias associated with malignancies, the usual daily dose is 150 to 300 mg, depending upon age.

Therapeutic Uses. Allopurinol provides effective therapy for both the primary *hyperuricemia* of gout and that secondary to polycythemia vera, myeloid metaplasia, or other blood dyscrasias. (*See* Rundles *et al.,* 1963, 1966; Yü and Gutman, 1964; Klinenberg *et al.,* 1965; Krakoff, 1967; Muggia *et al.,* 1967; Gutman, 1973; Yü, 1974.)

Allopurinol is contraindicated in patients who have exhibited serious adverse effects from the medication, nursing mothers, and children, except those with malignancy.

In *gout,* allopurinol is generally used in the severe chronic forms characterized by one or more of the following conditions: gouty nephropathy, tophaceous deposits, renal urate stones, impaired renal function, or hyperuricemia not readily controlled by the uricosuric drugs. In the absence of these indications, the uricosuric agents should be favored.

When given in effective doses and over prolonged periods, allopurinol fosters resorption of tophi and improvement of joint function in patients with tophaceous gout; this occurs *pari passu* with the reduction in plasma uric acid concentration. By decreasing the amount of uric acid excreted and thereby preventing the development of nephrolithiasis, allopurinol eliminates the major cause of renal injury in patients with gout. It also appears likely that gouty nephropathy can be reversed by the drug if therapy is begun at a reasonably early stage, before renal function is severely compromised; however, there is little evidence of improvement in advanced renal disease.

Since attacks of acute gout occur in patients taking allopurinol, particularly during the initial stage of treatment, colchicine is used prophylactically when therapy is begun and continued if necessary to prevent such attacks. Concurrent allopurinol and uricosuric therapy is also employed occasionally, especially in patients with large tophaceous deposits in whom it is desirable both to reduce production and to increase elimination of uric acid. Such combined medication is valid, but interaction between these drugs is sometimes complex. The uricosuric agents increase the renal excretion of alloxanthine and thus cause a reduction in allopurinol effect. Conversely, allopurinol may delay elimination of probenecid and increase its concentration in plasma.

Allopurinol is also administered prophylactically to reduce the hyperuricemia and to prevent urate deposition or renal calculi in patients with leukemias, lymphomas, or other malignancies, particularly when *antineoplastic* or *radiation* therapy is initiated. Allopurinol inhibits the enzymatic inactivation of 6-mercaptopurine by xanthine oxidase. Thus, when allopurinol is used concomitantly with 6-mercaptopu-

rine or azathioprine, dosage of the antineoplastic agent must be reduced to one fourth to one third of the usual dose. The risk of bone-marrow suppression is also increased when allopurinol is administered with cytotoxic agents that are not metabolized by xanthine oxidase, particularly cyclophosphamide.

The *iatrogenic hyperuricemia* sometimes induced by the thiazides and other drugs can be prevented or reversed by concurrent allopurinol medication, although this is rarely necessary. Allopurinol is also useful in lowering the high plasma concentrations of uric acid in patients with the *Lesch-Nyhan syndrome* and thereby prevents the complications resulting from hyperuricemia; there is no evidence that it alters the progressive neurological and behavioral abnormalities characteristic of the disease.

CLINICAL USE OF URICOSURIC AGENTS

As described in Chapter 38, the uricosuric agents act directly on the renal tubule to increase the rate of excretion of uric acid. While many agents share this property, only a few—probenicid, sulfinpyrazone, and benzbromarone—are used clinically as uricosuric agents. The last-named compound is not yet available for general use in the United States. In the clinical use of the available uricosuric drugs, it must be kept in mind that they can alter the plasma binding, distribution, and renal excretion of other organic acids, whether these be naturally occurring substances or drugs and drug metabolites.

Gout. The use of probenecid and sulfinpyrazone for the mobilization of uric acid in *chronic gout* is well established. In about two thirds of patients, these agents cause uric acid to be excreted at a rate sufficient to exceed that of formation and thereby promptly lower the plasma uric acid concentration. Although the intravenous administration of large doses of these drugs can cause a fivefold to sevenfold increase in the renal clearance of urate, continuous oral administration to patients with tophaceous gout approximately doubles the daily excretion of urates. In such patients, continued administration prevents the formation of new tophi and causes gradual shrinkage, or even disappearance, of old tophi. In gouty arthritis, there is a reduction in the swelling of chronically enlarged joints and a dramatic degree of rehabilitation may be achieved in patients who suffer severe pain and limitation of joint movement. In those patients who do not respond well to uricosuric agents because of impaired renal function, allopurinol is especially useful, as described above. In patients with gouty nephropathy, allopurinol offers the additional advantage over the uricosuric agents in that the daily excretion of uric acid is reduced rather than increased. Its administration is compatible with the simultaneous use of the uricosuric agents if necessary.

Neither the uricosuric agents nor allopurinol alters the course of acute attacks of gout or supplants the use of colchicine and anti-inflammatory agents in their management. Indeed, the acute attacks may increase in frequency or severity during the early months of therapy when urate is being mobilized from affected joints. Therefore, therapy with uricosuric agents should *not be initiated* during an acute attack but may be continued if already begun. Colchicine in small doses (0.5 to 2 mg per day) may be administered at this period (or at any time) to reduce the frequency of attacks. When an acute attack occurs, it is treated with full doses of colchicine or whatever agent has proven most satisfactory in the management of previous attacks (phenylbutazone, indomethacin, etc.). The use of salicylates is contraindicated because they antagonize the action of probenecid and sulfinpyrazone. However, for analgesia, acetaminophen may be used. Later in the course of therapy, acute attacks become less frequent or may cease altogether.

In the treatment of gout, the uricosuric drugs are given continually in the lowest dose that will maintain satisfactory plasma uric acid concentrations. Since the pK_a of uric acid is 5.6 and the solubility of the undissociated form is very low, maintaining the output of a large volume of alkaline urine minimizes its intrarenal deposition. This precaution is essential during the early weeks of therapy when uric acid excretion is large, especially in patients with a history of renal disease associated with the passage of urate stones or gravel. It is believed that renal disease of any etiology is a predisposing factor in the development of gouty nephropathy. Eventual improvement in renal function in patients with gouty nephropathy has been reported, but it is uncommon. The use of allopurinol permits a more favorable prognosis in such patients. (For detailed evaluations of uricosuric agents, see Gutman, 1966; Yü and Gutman, 1967; Yü, 1974; Boss and Seegmiller, 1979.)

Other Hyperuricemic States. Uricosuric agents are useful for the control of the hyperuricemia resulting from the use of the cytotoxic antineoplastic agents or from diseases that involve accelerated formation and destruction of blood cells. The use of other drugs, such as diuretics, levodopa, and ethambutol, as well as certain disease states, including toxemia of pregnancy, diabetic ketosis, and uremia, may be accompanied by moderate-to-marked elevation of plasma uric acid. The hyperuricemia may remain asymptomatic, but attacks of gout or renal precipitation of urate may occur. The management of such hyperuricemic states has been outlined by Yü (1974).

Selection of Agents for the Treatment of Gout and Hyperuricemia. Acute attacks of gout are effectively treated with colchicine, phenylbutazone, or indomethacin, as discussed above. While there is little advantage to the selection of one agent over another, colchicine is more commonly used (see Boss and Seegmiller, 1979).

After the acute arthritis has responded to therapy, the patient should be evaluated in order to select a rational regimen for long-term management. Elevated concentrations of uric acid in plasma and the observation of crystals of urate in the aspirated fluid from an affected joint establish the diagnosis of hyperuricemia and symptomatic gout. When evaluated on a diet that is low in purines, patients with

hyperuricemia can be categorized with regard to quantities of uric acid excreted in the urine. About 80 to 90% of such individuals excrete less than 600 mg of uric acid daily; the remainder excrete more than this amount due to excessive synthesis of urate. The former group can be managed effectively with uricosuric agents; the latter, however, is logically treated with allopurinol. If deposits of urate are evident as tophi, renal stones, or renal insufficiency, allopurinol is generally the preferred drug. During the first several months of treatment with allopurinol, colchicine may be given simultaneously to prevent acute attacks of gout. Patients with mild-to-moderate hyperuricemia (7 to 9 mg/dl) who do not have arthritis should be advised to take liberal amounts of fluids and a diet low in purines. Drug-induced hyperuricemia is most commonly caused by diuretics (see Chapter 36); acute attacks of gout are only rarely caused by such agents. However, hyperuricemia that accompanies chemotherapy or radiotherapy for various neoplasms may be considerably more severe and is usually treated prophylactically with allopurinol and hydration.

Abel, J. A. Analgesic nephropathy—a review of the literature, 1967–1970. *Clin. Pharmacol. Ther.,* **1971,** *12,* 583–598.

Abrishami, M. A., and Thomas, J. Aspirin intolerance—a review. *Ann. Allergy,* **1977,** *39,* 28–37.

Adam, M., and Kühn, K. Investigations on the reactions of metals with collagen *in vivo.* I. Comparison of the reaction of gold thiosulfate with collagen *in vivo* and *in vitro. Eur. J. Biochem.,* **1968,** *3,* 407–410.

Alexander, W. D., and Smith, G. Disadvantageous circulatory effects of salicylate in rheumatic fever. *Lancet,* **1962,** *1,* 768–771.

Alvan, G.; Orme, M.; Bertilsson, L.; Ekstrand, R.; and Palmer, L. Pharmacokinetics of indomethacin. *Clin. Pharmacol. Ther.,* **1975,** *18,* 364–373.

Amoroso, E. C. Colchicine and tumour growth. *Nature,* **1935,** *135,* 266–267.

Arger, P. H.; Bluth, E. I.; Murray, T.; and Goldberg, M. Analgesic abuse nephropathy. *Urology,* **1976,** *7,* 123–128.

Aspirin Myocardial Infarction Study Research Group. A randomized controlled trial of aspirin in persons recovered from myocardial infarction. *J.A.M.A.,* **1980,** *243,* 661–669.

Aylward, M.; Maddock, J.; Parker, R. J.; Thomas, S. R.; and Holly, F. Evaluation of tolmetin in the treatment of active chronic rheumatoid arthritis: open and controlled double-blind studies. *Curr. Med. Res. Opin.,* **1976,** *4,* 158–169.

Bluhm, G. B.; Sigler, J. W.; and Ensign, D. C. D-Penicillamine therapy of thrombocytopenia secondary to chrysotherapy: a case report. *Arthritis Rheum.,* **1962,** *5,* 638.

Boardman, P. L., and Hart, E. D. Clinical measurement of the anti-inflammatory effects of salicylates in rheumatoid arthritis. *Br. Med. J.,* **1967a,** *4,* 264–268.

―――. Side-effects of indomethacin. *Ann. Rheum. Dis.,* **1967b,** *26,* 127–132.

Boekhout-Mussert, J. J., and Loeliger, E. A. Influence of ibuprofen on oral anti-coagulation with phenprocoumon. *J. Int. Med. Res.,* **1974,** *2,* 279–283.

Borrachero del Campo, J. Comparative double-blind and open trials of sulindac and acetylsalicylic acid in the treatment of rheumatoid arthritis. *Eur. J. Rheumatol. Inflam.,* **1978,** *1,* 16–17.

Brodie, B. B., and Axelrod, J. The fate of acetophenetidin (phenacetin) in man and methods for the estimation of acetophenetidin and its metabolites in biological material. *J. Pharmacol. Exp. Ther.*, **1949**, *97*, 58–67.

Brogden, R. N.; Heel, R. C.; Speight, T. M.; and Avery, G. S. Alclofenac: a review of its pharmacological properties and therapeutic efficacy in rheumatic arthritis and allied rheumatic disorders. *Drugs*, **1977a**, *14*, 241–259.

Burry, H. C. Indomethacin in the management of soft tissue lesions. In, *Inflammatory Arthropathies.* (Huskisson, E. C., and Velo, G. P., eds.) Excerpta Medica, Amsterdam, **1976**, pp. 225–229.

Caruso, I.; Fumagalli, M.; Tirrito, M.; Montrone, F.; Vernazza, M.; Carratelli, L.; and Serio, A. A double-blind study with a new anti-rheumatic drug, sulindac, in the treatment of rheumatoid arthritis. Comparison with acetylsalicylic acid. *Eur. J. Rheumatol. Inflam.*, **1978**, *1*, 58–65.

Cats, A. A multicentre controlled trial of the effects of different dosages of gold therapy followed by a maintenance dosage. *Agents Actions*, **1976**, *6*, 355–363.

Clark, G. M.; Ricca, L. R.; Albert, M.; and Termulo, C. Evaluation of tolmetin sodium in the treatment of rheumatoid arthritis not responding to ibuprofen. *Curr. Ther. Res.*, **1977**, *21*, 697–703.

Clinicopathologic Conference. Agranulocytosis and anuria during phenylbutazone therapy of rheumatoid arthritis. *Am. J. Med.*, **1961**, *30*, 268–280.

Collier, H. O. J., and Schneider, C. Nociceptive response to prostaglandins and analgesic actions of aspirin and morphine. *Nature [New Biol.]*, **1972**, *236*, 141–143.

Collier, H. O. J., and Sweatman, W. J. F. Antagonism by fenamates of prostaglandin $F_{2\alpha}$ and of slow reacting substance on human bronchial muscle. *Nature*, **1968**, *219*, 864–865.

Collins, E., and Turner, G. Maternal effects of regular salicylate ingestion in pregnancy. *Lancet*, **1975**, *2*, 335–338.

Combined Rheumatic Fever Study Group. A comparison of the effect of prednisone and acetylsalicylic acid on the incidence of residual rheumatic heart disease. *N. Engl. J. Med.*, **1960**, *262*, 895–902.

———. A comparison of short-term, intensive prednisone and acetylsalicylic acid therapy in the treatment of acute rheumatic fever. *Ibid.*, **1965**, *272*, 63–70.

Conney, A. H.; Sansur, M.; Soroko, F.; Koster, R.; and Burns, J. J. Enzyme induction and inhibition in studies on the pharmacological actions of acetophenetidin. *J. Pharmacol. Exp. Ther.*, **1966**, *151*, 133–138.

Cooperating Clinics Committee of the American Rheumatism Association. A controlled trial of gold salt therapy in rheumatoid arthritis. *Arthritis Rheum.*, **1973**, *16*, 353–358.

Cox, A. J., and Marich, K. W. Gold in the dermis following gold therapy for rheumatoid arthritis. *Arch. Dermatol.*, **1973**, *108*, 655–657.

Crome, P.; Volans, G. N.; Vale, J. A.; Widdop, B.; Goulding, R.; and Williams, R. S. The use of methionine for acute paracetamol poisoning. *J. Int. Med. Res.*, **1976**, *4*, Suppl. 4, 105.

Currey, H. L. F.; Harris, J.; Mason, R. M.; Woodland, J.; Beveridge, T.; Roberts, C. J.; Vere, D. W.; Dixon, A. S.; Davies, J.; and Owen-Smith, B. Comparison of azathioprine, cyclophosphamide, and gold in treatment of rheumatoid arthritis. *Br. Med. J.*, **1974**, *3*, 763–766.

Davis, P.; Ezeoke, A.; Munro, J.; Hobbs, J. R.; and Hughes, G. R. V. Immunological studies on the mechanism of gold hypersensitivity reactions. *Br. Med. J.*, **1973**, *3*, 676–678.

Deby, C.; Bacq, Z.-M.; and Simon, D. *In vitro* inhibition of the biosynthesis of a prostaglandin by gold and silver. *Biochem. Pharmacol.*, **1973**, *22*, 3141–3143.

Deodhar, S. D.; Dick, W. C.; Hodgkinson, R.; and Buchanan, W. W. Measurement of clinical response to

anti-inflammatory drug therapy in rheumatoid arthritis. *Q. J. Med.*, **1973**, *42*, 387–401.

Done, A. K., and Temple, A. R. Treatment of salicylate poisoning. *Mod. Treat.*, **1971**, *8*, 528–551.

Dubas, T. S., and Parker, J. M. A central component in the analgesic action of sodium salicylate. *Arch. Int. Pharmacodyn. Ther.*, **1971**, *194*, 117–122.

Duggan, D. E.; Hogans, A. F.; Kwan, K. C.; and McMahon, F. G. The metabolism of indomethacin in man. *J. Pharmacol. Exp. Ther.*, **1972**, *181*, 563–575.

Duggan, D. E.; Hooke, K. F.; Risley, E. A.; Shen, T. Y.; and Van Arman, C. G. Identification of the biologically active form of sulindac. *J. Pharmacol. Exp. Ther.*, **1977**, *201*, 8–13.

Eade, N. R., and Lasagna, L. A comparison of acetophenetidin and acetaminophen. II. Subjective effects in healthy volunteers. *J. Pharmacol. Exp. Ther.*, **1967**, *155*, 301–308.

Elion, G. B.; Callahan, S.; Rundles, R. W.; and Hitchings, G. H. Relationship between metabolic fates and antitumor activities of thiopurines. *Cancer Res.*, **1963**, *23*, 1207–1217.

Faigle, J. W., and Dieterle, W. The biotransformation of phenylbutazone (butazolidin). *J. Int. Med. Res.*, **1977**, *5*, Suppl. 2, 2–14.

Farber, H. R.; Yiengst, M. J.; and Shock, N. W. The effect of therapeutic doses of aspirin on the acid-base balance of the blood in normal adults. *Am. J. Med. Sci.*, **1949**, *217*, 256–262.

Fasching, U., and Eberl, R. Sulindac: clinical test of a new anti-inflammatory agent in rheumatoid arthritis. *Wien. Klin. Wochenschr.*, **1976**, *59*, Suppl. 88, 1–10.

Feldberg, W., and Gupta, K. P. Pyrogen fever and prostaglandin-like activity in cerebrospinal fluid. *J. Physiol. (Lond.)*, **1973**, *228*, 41–53.

Feldberg, W., and Saxena, P. N. Fever produced by prostaglandin E_1. *J. Physiol. (Lond.)*, **1971**, *217*, 547–556.

Ferreira, S. H. Prostaglandins, aspirin-like drugs and analgesia. *Nature [New Biol.]*, **1972**, *240*, 200–203.

Ferreira, S. H.; Moncada, S.; and Vane, J. R. Indomethacin and aspirin abolish prostaglandin release from the spleen. *Nature [New Biol.]*, **1971**, *231*, 237–239.

———. Prostaglandins and the mechanism of analgesia produced by aspirin-like drugs. *Br. J. Pharmacol.*, **1973**, *49*, 86–97.

Forestier, J. L'aurothérapie dans les rhumatismes chronique. *Bull. Mém. Soc. Méd. Hôp. Paris*, **1929**, *53*, 323–327.

Furst, D. E.; Levine, S.; Srinwason, R.; Metzger, A. L.; Bangert, R.; and Paulus, H. E. A double-blind trial of high versus conventional dosages of gold salts for rheumatoid arthritis. *Arthritis Rheum.*, **1977**, *20*, 1473–1480.

Furst, D. E.; Tozer, T. N.; and Melmon, K. L. Salicylate clearance, the resultant of protein binding and metabolism. *Clin. Pharmacol. Ther.*, **1979**, *26*, 380–389.

Gault, M. H.; Rudwal, T. C.; Engles, W. D.; and Dossetor, J. B. Syndrome associated with abuse of analgesics. *Ann. Intern. Med.*, **1968**, *68*, 906–925.

Gengos, D. Long-term experience with sulindac in the treatment of osteoarthritis. *Eur. J. Rheumatol. Inflam.*, **1978**, *1*, 51.

Gerber, R. C.; Paulus, H. E.; Bluestone, R.; and Lederer, M. Kinetics of aurothiomalate in serum and synovial fluid. *Arthritis Rheum.*, **1972**, *15*, 625–629.

Gifford, R. H. Chemotherapy for rheumatoid arthritis. *Ration. Drug Ther.*, **1973**, *7*, No. 12, 1–7.

Gilman, A. Analgesic nephrotoxicity: a pharmacological analysis. *Am. J. Med.*, **1964**, *36*, 167–173.

Godfrey, R. G.; Calabro, J. J.; Mills, D.; and Maltz, B. A. A double-blind crossover trial of aspirin, indomethacin and phenylbutazone in ankylosing spondylitis. *Arthritis Rheum.*, **1972**, *15*, 110.

Goldfinger, S. E. Treatment of gout. *N. Engl. J. Med.*, **1971**, *285*, 1303–1306.

Goncalves, L. Influence of ibuprofen on haemostasis in patients on anticoagulant therapy. *J. Int. Med. Res.,* **1973,** *1,* 180–183.

Gordon, M. H.; Tiger, L. H.; and Ehrlich, G. E. Gold reactions are not more common in Sjögrens syndrome. *Ann. Intern. Med.,* **1975,** *82,* 47–49.

Gottlieb, N. L.; Kiem, I. M.; Penneys, N. S.; and Schultz, D. R. The influence of chrysotherapy on serum protein and immunoglobulin levels, rheumatoid factor, and anti-epithelial antibody titers. *J. Lab. Clin. Med.,* **1975,** *86,* 962–972.

Gottlieb, N. L.; Smith, P. M.; and Smith, E. M. Gold excretion correlated with clinical course during chrysotherapy in rheumatoid arthritis. *Arthritis Rheum.,* **1972,** *15,* 582–592.

——. Pharmacodynamics of ^{197}Au and ^{195}Au labeled aurothiomalate in blood. Correlation with course of rheumatoid arthritis, gold toxicity and gold excretion. *Ibid.,* **1974,** *17,* 171–183.

Graf, P.; Glatt, M.; and Brune, K. Acidic nonsteroid anti-inflammatory tissue. *Experientia,* **1975,** *31,* 951–953.

Grahame, R.; Billings, R.; Lawrence, M.; Marks, V.; and Wood, P. J. Tissue gold levels after chrysotherapy. *Ann. Rheum. Dis.,* **1974,** *33,* 536–539.

Gutman, A. B. The past four decades of progress in the knowledge of gout, with an assessment of the present status. *Arthritis Rheum.,* **1973,** *16,* 431–445.

Halla, J. T. Aspirin, liver, and rheumatic diseases. *J. Med. Assoc. State Ala.,* **1976,** *46,* 23–25.

Halushka, P. V.; Wohltmann, H.; Privitera, P. J.; Hurwitz, G.; and Margolius, H. S. Bartter's syndrome: urinary prostaglandin E-like material and kallikrein; indomethacin effects. *Ann. Intern. Med.,* **1977,** *87,* 281–286.

Ham, E. A.; Cirrillo, V. J.; Zanetti, M.; Shen, T. Y.; and Kuehl, F. A., Jr. Studies on the mode of action of non-steroidal anti-inflammatory agents. In, *Prostaglandins in Cellular Biology.* (Ramwell, P. W., and Pharris, B. B., eds.) Plenum Press, New York, **1972,** pp. 345–352.

Hamberg, M. Inhibition of prostaglandin synthesis in man. *Biochem. Biophys. Res. Comm.,* **1972,** *49,* 720–726.

Harinck, E.; van Ertbruggen, I.; Senders, R. C.; and Moulaert, A. J. Problems with indomethacin for ductus closure. (Letter.) *Lancet,* **1977,** *2,* 245.

Hart, F. D. Which anti-rheumatic drug? *Drugs,* **1976,** *11,* 451–460.

Hendricks, C. H.; Brenner, W. E.; Ekbladh, L.; Brotanek, V.; and Fishburne, J. I., Jr. Efficacy and tolerance of intravenous prostaglandins $F_{2\alpha}$ and E_2. *Am. J. Obstet. Gynecol.,* **1971,** *111,* 564–579.

Heymann, M. A.; Rudolph, A. M.; and Silverman, N. H. Closure of the ductus arteriosus in premature infants by inhibition of prostaglandin synthesis. *N. Engl. J. Med.,* **1976,** *295,* 530–533.

Hill, J. B. Salicylate intoxication. *N. Engl. J. Med.,* **1973,** *288,* 1110–1113.

Horwitz, D. A. Selective depletion of B lymphocytes by cyclophosphamide in patients with rheumatoid arthritis and systemic lupus erythematosus: guidelines for dosage. *Arthritis Rheum.,* **1974,** *17,* 363–374.

Hucker, H. B.; Stauffer, S. C.; White, S. D.; Rhodes, R. E.; Arison, B. H.; Umbenhauer, E. R.; Bower, R. J.; and McMahon, F. G. Physiologic disposition and metabolic fate of a new anti-inflammatory agent, *cis-*5-fluoro-2-methyl-1-[*p*-(methylsulfinyl)-benzylidenyl]-idene-3-acetic acid, in the rat, dog, rhesus-monkey, and man. *Drug Metab. Dispos.,* **1973,** *1,* 721–736.

Huskisson, E. C. Chronopharmacology of anti-rheumatic drugs with special reference to indomethacin. In, *Inflammatory Arthropathies.* (Huskisson, E. C., and Velo, G. P., eds.) Excerpta Medica, Amsterdam, **1976,** pp. 99–105.

——. Anti-inflammatory drugs. *Semin. Arthritis Rheum.,* **1977,** *7,* 1–20.

——. Non-steroidal anti-inflammatory analgesics: basic clinical pharmacology and therapeutic use. *Drugs,* **1978,** *15,* 387–392.

Huskisson, E. C.; Berry, H.; Scott, J.; and Halme, H. W. Tolectin for rheumatoid arthritis. *Rheumatol. Rehabil.,* **1974a,** *13,* 132–134.

Huskisson, E. C.; Gibson, T. J.; Balme, H. W.; Berry, H.; Burry, H. C.; Grahame, R.; Dudleyhart, F.; Henderson, D. R. F.; and Wojtulewski, M. A. Trial comparing D-penicillamine and gold in rheumatoid arthritis. *Ann. Rheum. Dis.,* **1974b,** *33,* 532–535.

Huskisson, E. C., and Scott, J. Sulindac: trials of a new anti-inflammatory drug. *Ann. Rheum. Dis.,* **1978,** *37,* 89–92.

Huskisson, E. C.; Wojtulewski, J. A.; Berry, H.; Scott, J.; Hart, F. D.; and Balme, H. W. Treatment of rheumatoid arthritis with fenoprofen: comparison with aspirin. *Br. Med. J.,* **1974,** *1,* 176–180.

Huskisson, E. C.; Woolf, D. L.; Balme, H. W.; Scott, J.; and Franklyn, S. Four new anti-inflammatory drugs: responses and variations. *Br. Med. J.,* **1976,** *1,* 1048–1049.

Jackson, J. M.; Quinlan, J.; and Goatcher, P. Mefenamic acid-induced haemolytic anaemia. *Br. Med. J.,* **1970,** *2,* 297–298.

Jaffe, I. A. The treatment of rheumatoid arthritis and necrotizing vasculitis with penicillamine. *Arthritis Rheum.,* **1970,** *13,* 436–443.

Jessop, J. D., and Johns, R. G. S. Serum gold determinations in patients with rheumatoid arthritis receiving sodium aurothiomalate. *Ann. Rheum. Dis.,* **1973,** *32,* 228–232.

Jessop, J. D.; Vernon-Roberts, B.; and Harris, J. Effects of gold salts and prednisolone on inflammatory cells. Phagocytic activity of macrophages and polymorphs in inflammatory exudates studied by a skin-window technique in rheumatoid and control patients. *Ann. Rheum. Dis.,* **1973,** *32,* 294–300.

Julou, L.; Guyonnet, J. C.; Dugrot, R.; Carret, C.; Bardone, M. C.; Maignan, G.; and Pasquet, J. Étude des propriétés pharmacologiques d'un nouvel anti-inflammatoire, l'acide (benzoyl-3 phenyl)-2-propiónique (19583 RP). *J. Pharmacol.,* **1971,** *2,* 259–286.

Kaley, G., and Weiner, R. Prostaglandin E_1—as potential mediator of the inflammatory response. *Ann. N. Y. Acad. Sci.,* **1971,** *180,* 338–350.

Karim, S. M. M. Action of prostaglandin in the pregnant woman. *Ann. N. Y. Acad. Sci.,* **1971,** *180,* 483–498.

Kaye, R. L., and Pemberton, R. G. Treatment of rheumatoid arthritis. *Arch. Intern. Med.,* **1976,** *136,* 1023–1028.

Kendall, S.; Lloyd-Jones, G.; and Smith, C. F. The development of a blood paracetamol estimation kit. *J. Int. Med. Res.,* **1976,** *4,* Suppl. 4, 83–88.

Kennedy, C. C., and Robertson, J. H. Haemolytic reaction to mefenamic acid. *Lancet,* **1971,** *2,* 607–608.

Klemp, P., and Meyers, O. L. Clinical trial of tolmetin and aspirin in the treatment of rheumatoid arthritis. *S. Afr. Med. J.,* **1977,** *52,* 167–169.

Klinenberg, J. R.; Goldfinger, S. E.; and Seegmiller, J. E. The effectiveness of the xanthine oxidase inhibitor allopurinol in the treatment of gout. *Ann. Intern. Med.,* **1965,** *62,* 639–647.

Krakoff, I. H. Clinical pharmacology of drugs which influence uric acid production and excretion. *Clin. Pharmacol. Ther.,* **1967,** *8,* 124–138.

Leonards, J. R., and Levy, G. Gastrointestinal blood loss during prolonged aspirin administration. *N. Engl. J. Med.,* **1973,** *289,* 1020–1022.

Levin, H. A.; McMillan, R.; Tavassoli, M.; Longmire, R. L.; Yelenosky, R.; and Sacks, P. V. Thrombocytopenia associated with gold therapy: observations on the mechanism of platelet destruction. *Am. J. Med.,* **1975,** *59,* 274–280.

Levinson, J. E.; Baum, J.; Brewer, E.; Fink, C. W.; Hanson, V.; and Schaller, J. Comparison of tolmetin and aspirin in the treatment of juvenile rheumatoid arthritis. *J. Pediatr.,* **1977,** *91,* 799–804.

Levy, G.; Tsuchiya, T.; and Amsel, L. P. Limited capacity

for salicyl phenolic glucuronide formation and its effect on the kinetics of salicylate elimination in man. *Clin. Pharmacol. Ther.,* **1972,** *13,* 258–268.

Lewis, R. B., and Schulman, J. D. Influence of acetylsalicylic acid, an inhibitor of prostaglandin synthesis on the duration of human gestation and labour. *Lancet,* **1973,** *2,* 1159–1161.

Lim, R. K. S.; Guzman, F.; Rodgers, D. W.; Goto, K.; Braun, G. D.; Dickerson, G. D.; and Engle, R. J. Site of action of narcotic and nonnarcotic analgesics determined by blocking bradykinin-evoked visceral pain. *Arch. Int. Pharmacodyn. Ther.,* **1964,** *152,* 25–58.

Lits, F. J. Contribution à l'étude des réactions cellulaires provoquées par la colchicine. *C. R. Soc. Biol. (Paris),* **1934,** *115,* 1421–1423.

Lorber, A.; Atkins, C. J.; Chang, C. C.; Lee, Y. B.; Starrs, J.; and Bovy, R. A. Monitoring serum gold values to improve chrysotherapy in rheumatoid arthritis. *Ann. Rheum. Dis.,* **1973a,** *32,* 133–139.

Lorber, A.; Baumgartner, W. A.; Bovy, R. A.; Chang, C. C.; and Hollcraft, R. Clinical application for heavy metal-complexing potential of N-acetylcysteine. *J. Clin. Pharmacol.,* **1973b,** *13,* 332–336.

Lorber, A.; Cohen, R. L.; Chang, C. C.; and Anderson, H. E. Gold determination in biological fluids by atomic absorption spectrometry; application to chrysotherapy in rheumatoid arthritis patients. *Arthritis Rheum.,* **1968,** *11,* 170–177.

Lorber, A.; Simon, T. M.; Leeb, J.; and Carroll, P. E., Jr. Chrysotherapy: pharmacological and clinical correlates. *J. Rheumatol.,* **1975,** *2,* 401–410.

McEwen, C. Current status of therapy in rheumatic fever. *J.A.M.A.,* **1959,** *170,* 1056–1062.

McMillen, J. I. Tolmetin sodium vs ibuprofen in rheumatoid arthritic patients previously treated with either drug: a double-blind crossover study. *Curr. Ther. Res.,* **1977,** *22,* 266–275.

Malawista, S. E. The action of colchicine in acute gouty arthritis. *Arthritis Rheum.,* **1975,** *18,* Suppl. 6, 835–846.

Margetts, G. Phenacetin and paracetamol. *J. Int. Med. Res.,* **1976,** *4,* Suppl. 4, 55–70.

Mascarenhas, B. R.; Granda, J. L.; and Freyberg, R. H. Gold metabolism in patients with rheumatoid arthritis treated with gold compounds—reinvestigated. *Arthritis Rheum.,* **1972,** *15,* 391–402.

Mason, J., and Bolton, M. S. A general practice assessment of ALRHEUMAT (ketoprofen) in the treatment of rheumatic conditions. *Br. J. Clin. Pract.,* **1977,** *31,* 127–134.

Mauer, E. F. The toxic effects of phenylbutazone (BUTAZOLIDIN): review of literature and report of the twenty-third death following its use. *N. Engl. J. Med.,* **1955,** *253,* 404–410.

Milton, A. S. Prostaglandin E_1 and endotoxin fever, and the effects of aspirin, indomethacin and 4-acetamidophenol. In, *Advances in the Biosciences.* Vol. 9, *International Conference on Prostaglandins.* (Bergstrom, S., and Bernhard, S., eds.) Pergamon Press, Ltd., Oxford, **1973,** pp. 495–500.

Milton, A. S., and Wendlandt, S. Effect on body temperature of prostaglandins of the A, E and F series on injection into the third ventricle of unanaesthetized cats and rabbits. *J. Physiol. (Lond.),* **1971,** *218,* 325–336.

Moncada, S.; Ferreira, S. H.; and Vane, J. R. Inhibition of prostaglandin biosynthesis as the mechanism of analgesia of aspirin-like drugs in the dog knee joint. *Eur. J. Pharmacol.,* **1975,** *31,* 250–260.

Moncada, S., and Vane, J. R. Mode of action of aspirin-like drugs. *Adv. Intern. Med.,* **1979,** *24,* 1–22.

Mongan, E.; Kelly, P.; Nies, K.; Porter, W. W.; and Paulus, H. E. Tinnitus as an indication of therapeutic serum salicylate levels. *J.A.M.A.,* **1973,** *226,* 142–145.

Mrochek, J. E.; Katz, S.; Christie, W. H.; and Dinsmore, S. R. Acetaminophen metabolism in man as determined by high resolution liquid chromatography. *Clin. Chem.,* **1974,** *20,* 1086–1096.

Muggia, F.; Ball, T. J., Jr.; and Ultmann, J. E. Allopurinol in the treatment of neoplastic disease complicated by hyperuricemia. *Arch. Intern. Med.,* **1967,** *120,* 12–18.

Multicentre Trial Group. Controlled trial of D(−) penicillamine in severe rheumatoid arthritis. *Lancet,* **1973,** *1,* 275–280.

Multz, C. V.; Bernhard, G. C.; Blechman, W. C.; Zane, S.; Restifo, R. A.; and Varady, J. C. A comparison of intermediate-dose aspirin and placebo in rheumatoid arthritis. *Clin. Pharmacol. Ther.,* **1974,** *15,* 310–315.

Norby, L.; Flamenbaum, W.; Lentz, R.; and Ramwell, P. Prostaglandins and aspirin therapy in Bartter's syndrome. *Lancet,* **1976,** *2,* 604–606.

Norn, S. Anaphylactic histamine release and influence of antirheumatics. *Acta Pharmacol. Toxicol. (Kbh.),* **1971,** *30,* Suppl. 1, 1–59.

O'Brien, W. M. Indomethacin: a survey of clinical trials. *Clin. Pharmacol. Ther.,* **1968,** *9,* 94–107.

Paalzow, L. An electrical method for estimation of analgesic activity in mice. *Acta Pharm. Suec.,* **1969,** *6,* 207–226.

Pennys, N. S.; Eaglestein, W. H.; Indgin, S.; and Frost, P. Gold sodium thiomalate treatment of pemphigus. *Arch. Dermatol.,* **1973,** *108,* 56–60.

Perkins, E. S., and MacFaul, P. A. Indomethacin in the treatment of uveitis. A double-blind trial. *Trans. Ophthalmol. Soc. U.K.,* **1965,** *85,* 53–58.

Persellin, R. H., and Ziff, M. The effect of gold salt on lysosomal enzymes of the peritoneal macrophage. *Arthritis Rheum.,* **1966,** *9,* 57–65.

Pinals, R. S., and Frank, S. Relative efficacy of indomethacin and acetylsalicylic acid in rheumatoid arthritis. *N. Engl. J. Med.,* **1967,** *276,* 512–514.

Pitkeathly, D. A.; Banerjee, N. R.; Harris, R.; and Sharp, J. Indomethacin in in-patient treatment of rheumatoid arthritis. *Ann. Rheum. Dis.,* **1966,** *25,* 334–339.

Prescott, L. F. The metabolism of phenacetin in patients with renal disease. *Clin. Pharmacol. Ther.,* **1969,** *10,* 383–394.

Prescott, L. F.; Park, J.; Sutherland, G. R.; Smith, I. J.; and Proudfoot, A. T. Cysteamine, methionine, and penicillamine in the treatment of paracetamol poisoning. *Lancet,* **1976,** *2,* 109–113.

Prescott, L. F., and Wright, N. The effects of hepatic and renal damage on paracetamol metabolism and excretion following overdosage. A pharmacokinetic study. *Br. J. Pharmacol.,* **1973,** *49,* 602–613.

Rahbek, I. Gastroscopic evaluation of the effect of a new antirheumatic compound, ketoprofen (19.583 R.P.), on the human gastric mucosa. A double-blind cross-over trial against acetylsalicylic acid. *Scand. J. Rheumatol. [Suppl.],* **1976,** *14,* 63–72.

Ramos, F. H.; Barrós, B.; Larrosa, R. A.; Dighiero, M.; and Batista, V. Present status of gold in the treatment of rheumatoid arthritis. *A.I.R.,* **1963,** *6,* 105–112.

Randall, L. O., and Selitto, J. J. A method for measurement of analgesic activity on inflamed tissue. *Arch. Int. Pharmacodyn. Ther.,* **1957,** *111,* 409–419.

Research Sub-committee of the Empire Rheumatism Council. Gold therapy in rheumatoid arthritis: report of a multicentre controlled trial. *Ann. Rheum. Dis.,* **1960,** *19,* 95–117.

———. Gold therapy in rheumatoid arthritis: final report of a multicentre controlled trial. *Ibid.,* **1961a,** *20,* 315–334.

———. Relation of toxic reactions in gold therapy to improvement in rheumatoid arthritis. *Ibid.,* **1961b,** *20,* 335–340.

Reynolds, P. M. G., and Whorwell, P. J. A single-blind comparison of fenoprofen, ibuprofen and naproxen in rheumatoid arthritis. *Curr. Med. Res. Opin.,* **1974,** *2,* 461–464.

Rooney, P.; Buchanan, W.; Haigh, B. S.; Roylance, P. J.; and Rhymer, A. R. A clinical assessment in general practice of sulindac. *Eur. J. Rheumatol. Inflam.,* **1978,** *1,* 66–68.

Roth, G. R., and Siok, C. J. Acetylation of the NH_2-

terminal serine of prostaglandin synthetase by aspirin. *J. Biol. Chem.*, **1978**, *253*, 3782–3784.

Rubinstein, H. M., and Dietz, A. A. Serum gold. II. Levels in rheumatoid arthritis. *Ann. Rheum. Dis.*, **1973**, *32*, 128–132.

Rundles, R. W.; Metz, E. N.; and Silberman, H. R. Allopurinol in the treatment of gout. *Ann. Intern. Med.*, **1966**, *64*, 229–258.

Rundles, R. W.: Wyngaarden, J. B.; Hitchings, G. H.; Elion, G. B.; and Silberman, H. R. Effects of a xanthine oxidase inhibitor on thiopurine metabolism, hyperuricemia and gout. *Trans. Assoc. Am. Physicians*, **1963**, *76*, 126–140.

Schreiner, G. E. The nephrotoxicity of analgesic abuse. *Ann. Intern. Med.*, **1962**, *57*, 1047–1052.

Schroeder, H. A., and Nason, A. P. Trace-element analysis in clinical chemistry. *Clin. Chem.*, **1971**, *17*, 461–473.

Seegmiller, J. E., and Grayzel, A. I. Use of the newer uricosuric agents in the management of gout. *J.A.M.A.*, **1960**, *173*, 1076–1080.

Sellers, E. M., and Koch-Weser, J. Displacement of warfarin from human albumin by diazoxide and ethacrynic, mefenamic and nalidixic acids. *Clin. Pharmacol. Ther.*, **1970**, *11*, 524–529.

Sharp, J. T.; Lindsky, M. D.; Duffy, J.; Thompson, H. K.; Person, B. D.; Masri, S. F.; and Andrianakos, A. A. Comparison of two dosage schedules of gold salts in the treatment of rheumatoid arthritis. *Arthritis Rheum.*, **1977**, *20*, 1179–1187.

Sheldrake, F. E.; Webber, J. M.; and Marsh, B. D. A long-term assessment of flurbiprofen. *Curr. Med. Res. Opin.*, **1977**, *5*, 106–116.

Shelley, J. H. Phenacetin, through the looking glass. *Clin. Pharmacol. Ther.*, **1967**, *8*, 427–471.

Silverberg, D. S.; Kidd, E. G.; Shnitka, T. S.; and Ulan, R. A. Gold nephropathy. A clinical and pathologic study. *Arthritis Rheum.*, **1970**, *13*, 812–825.

Smith, J. B., and Willis, A. L. Aspirin selectively inhibits prostaglandin production in human platelets. *Nature [New Biol.]*, **1971**, *231*, 235–237.

Smith, P. M.; Smith, E. M.; and Gottlieb, N. Gold distribution in whole blood during chrysotherapy. *J. Lab. Clin. Med.*, **1973**, *82*, 930–937.

Smith, R. T.; Peak, W. P.; Kron, K. M.; Hermann, I. F.; and Del Toro, R. A. Increasing the effectiveness of gold therapy in rheumatoid arthritis. *J.A.M.A.*, **1958**, *167*, 1197–1204.

Smyth, C. J. Therapy of rheumatoid arthritis. *Postgrad. Med.*, **1972**, *51*, Suppl., 23–31.

Smyth, C. J., and Percy, J. S. Comparison of indomethacin and phenylbutazone in acute gout. *Ann. Rheum. Dis.*, **1973**, *32*, 351–353.

Spilberg, I.; Mandell, B.; Mehta, J.; Simchowitz, L.; and Rosenberg, D. Mechanism of colchicine action in acute urate crystal-induced arthritis. *J. Clin. Invest.*, **1979**, *64*, 775–780.

Stone, K. J.; Mather, S. J.; and Gibson, P. O. Selective inhibition of prostaglandin biosynthesis by gold salts and phenylbutazone. *Prostaglandins*, **1975**, *10*, 241–251.

Strong, J. S.; Bartholomew, B. A.; and Smyth, C. J. Immunoresponsiveness of patients with rheumatoid arthritis receiving cyclophosphamide or gold salts. *Ann. Rheum. Dis.*, **1973**, *32*, 233–237.

Szczeklik, A.; Gryglewski, R. J.; and Czerniawska-Mysik, G. Relationship of inhibition of prostaglandin biosynthesis by analgesics to asthma attacks in aspirin-sensitive patients. *Br. Med. J.*, **1975**, *1*, 67–69.

Thilo, D.; Nyman, D.; and Duckert, F. A study of the effects of the antirheumatic drug ibuprofen (BRUFEN) on patients being treated with the oral anticoagulant phenprocoumon. *J. Int. Med. Res.*, **1974**, *2*, 276–278.

Tomlinson, R. V.; Ringold, H. J.; Qureshi, M. C.; and Forchielli, E. Relationship between inhibition of prostaglandin synthesis and drug efficacy: support for the current theory on mode of action of aspirin-like drugs. *Biochem. Biophys. Res. Commun.*, **1972**, *46*, 552–559.

Turner, G., and Collins, E. Fetal effects of regular salicylate ingestion in pregnancy. *Lancet*, **1975**, *2*, 338–339.

United Kingdom and United States Joint Report. The evaluation of rheumatic heart disease in children: five-year report of a cooperative clinical trial of ACTH, cortisone and aspirin. *Circulation*, **1960**, *22*, 503–515.

Van Arman, C. G.; Risley, E. A.; Nuss, G. W.; Hucker, H. B.; and Duggan, D. E. Pharmacology of sulindac. In, *Clinoril in the Treatment of Rheumatic Disorders: A New Nonsteroidal Anti-inflammatory/Analgesic Agent*. Proceedings of a Symposium, VIII European Rheumatology Congress. (Huskisson, E. C., and Franchimont, P., eds.) Raven Press, New York, **1976**, pp. 9–15.

Vane, J. R. Inhibition of prostaglandin synthesis as a mechanism of action for aspirin-like drugs. *Nature [New Biol.]*, **1971**, *231*, 232–235.

Verberckmoes, R.; Van Damme, B.; Clement, J.; Amery, A.; and Michielsen, P. Bartter's syndrome with hyperplasia of renomedullary cells: successful treatment with indomethacin. *Kidney Int.*, **1976**, *9*, 302–307.

Vernon-Roberts, B.; Dore, J. L.; Jessop, J. D.; and Henderson, W. J. Selective concentration and localization of gold in macrophages of synovial and other tissues during and after chrysotherapy in rheumatoid patients. *Ann. Rheum. Dis.*, **1976**, *35*, 477–486.

Wallace, S. L. Colchicine: clinical pharmacology in acute gouty arthritis. *Am. J. Med.*, **1961**, *30*, 439–448.

Wallace, S. L.; Omokoku, B.; and Ertel, N. H. Colchicine plasma levels: implications as to pharmacology and mechanism of action. *Am. J. Med.*, **1970**, *48*, 443–448.

Whitsett, T. L.; Barry, J. P.; Czerwinski, A. W.; Hall, W. M.; and Hampton, J. W. Interaction of tolmetin and warfarin: a clinical investigation to determine if interaction exists. In, *Tolmetin-A New Non-Steroidal Anti-Inflammatory Agent*. (Ward, J. R., ed.) Excerpta Medica, Amsterdam, **1975**, pp. 160–167.

Willkens, R. F., and Segre, E. J. Combination therapy with naproxen and aspirin in rheumatoid arthritis. *Arthritis Rheum.*, **1976**, *19*, 677–682.

Wilson, J. T.; Howell, R. L.; Holladay, M. W.; Brilis, G. M.; Chrastil, J.; Watson, J. T.; and Taber, D. V. Gentisuric acid; metabolic formation in animals and identification as a metabolite of aspirin in man. *Clin. Pharmacol. Ther.*, **1978**, *23*, 635–643.

Winder, C. V. Aspirin and algesimetry. *Nature*, **1959**, *184*, 494–497.

Wolfe, J. A.; Plotzker, R.; Safina, F. J.; Ross, M.; Popky, G.; and Rubin, W. Gastritis, duodenitis, and bleeding duodenal ulcer following mefenamic acid therapy. *Arch. Intern. Med.*, **1976**, *136*, 923–925.

Wong, W. Chemistry and pharmacology of tolmetin, 1-methyl-5-*p*-toluoylpyrrole-2-acetic acid. In, *Tolmetin—A New Non-Steroidal Anti-Inflammatory Agent*. (Ward, J. R., ed.) Excerpta Medica, Amsterdam, **1975**, pp. 1–22.

Yü, T.-F., and Gutman, A. B. Efficacy of colchicine prophylaxis in gout: prevention of recurrent gouty arthritis over a mean period of five years in 208 gouty subjects. *Ann. Intern. Med.*, **1961**, *55*, 179–192.

———. Effect of allopurinol (4-hydroxypyrazolo-[3,4-*d*] pyrimidine) on serum and urinary uric acid in primary and secondary gout. *Am. J. Med.*, **1964**, *37*, 885–898.

Zancan, L.; Zacchello, F.; and Mantero, F. Indomethacin for Bartter's syndrome. (Letter.) *Lancet*, **1976**, *2*, 1354.

Zuckerman, R.; Reiss, U.; and Rubenstein, I. Inhibition of human premature labor by indomethacin. *Obstet. Gynecol.*, **1974**, *44*, 787–792.

Zuckner, J.; Ramsey, R. H.; Dorner, R. W.; and Gantner, G. E., Jr. D-Penicillamine in rheumatoid arthritis. *Arthritis Rheum.*, **1970**, *13*, 131–138.

Monographs and Reviews

Adams, S. S., and Buckler, J. W. Ibuprofen and flurbiprofen. *Clin. Rheum. Dis.*, **1979**, *5*, 359–379.

Ameer, B., and Greenblatt, D. J. Acetaminophen. *Ann. Intern. Med.*, **1977**, *87*, 202–209.

Beaver, W. T. Mild analgesics: a review of their clinical pharmacology. *Am. J. Med. Sci.,* **1965,** *250,* 577–604; **1966,** *251,* 576–599. (392 references.)

Beecher, H. K. The measurement of pain. Prototype for the quantitative study of subjective responses. *Pharmacol. Rev.,* **1957,** *9,* 59–209. (687 references.)

Bluhm, J. B. The treatment of rheumatoid arthritis with gold. *Semin. Arthritis Rheum.,* **1975,** *5,* 147–166.

Boss, G. R., and Seegmiller, J. E. Hyperuricemia and gout; classification, complications, and management. *N. Engl. J. Med.,* **1979,** *300,* 1459–1468.

Brogden, R. N.; Heel, R. C.; Speight, T. M.; and Avery, G. S. Sulindac: a review of its pharmacological properties and therapeutic efficacy in rheumatic diseases. *Drugs,* **1978a,** *16,* 97–114.

———. Tolmetin: a review of its pharmacological properties and therapeutic efficacy in rheumatic diseases. *Ibid.,* **1978b,** *15,* 429–450.

Brogden, R. N.; Pinder, R. M.; Sawyer, P. R.; Speight, T. M.; and Avery, G. S. Naproxen: a review of its pharmacological properties and therapeutic efficacy and use. *Drugs,* **1975,** *9,* 326–363.

Brogden, R. N.; Pinder, R. M.; Speight, T. M.; and Avery, G. S. Fenoprofen: a review of its pharmacological properties and therapeutic efficacy in rheumatic diseases. *Drugs,* **1977b,** *13,* 241–265.

Cohen, L. S. Clinical pharmacology of acetylsalicylic acid. *Semin. Thromb. Hemostas.,* **1976,** *2,* 146–175.

Davison, C. Salicylate metabolism in man. *Ann. N.Y. Acad. Sci.,* **1971,** *179,* 249–268.

Domenjoz, R. Synthetic anti-inflammatory drugs: concepts of their mode of action. *Adv. Pharmacol.,* **1966,** *4,* 143–217. (520 references.)

Dustin, P., Jr. New aspects of the pharmacology of antimitotic agents. *Pharmacol. Rev.,* **1963,** *15,* 449–480.

Elion, G. B. Allopurinol and other inhibitors of urate synthesis. In, *Uric Acid. Handbuch der Experimentellen Pharmakologie,* Vol. 51. (Kelley, W. N., and Weiner, I.M., eds.) Springer-Verlag, Berlin, **1978,** pp. 485–514.

Flower, R. J. Drugs which inhibit prostaglandin biosynthesis. *Pharmacol. Rev.,* **1974,** *26,* 33–67.

Freyberg, R. H. Gold therapy for rheumatoid arthritis. In, *Arthritis and Allied Conditions,* 7th ed. (Hollander, J. L., ed.) Lea & Febiger, Philadelphia, **1966,** pp. 302–332.

———. Gold therapy for rheumatoid arthritis. In, *Arthritis and Allied Conditions,* 8th ed. (Hollander, J. L., and McCarty, D. J., Jr., eds.) Lea & Febiger, Philadelphia, **1972,** pp. 455–482.

Gottlieb, N. L. Chrysotherapy. *Bull. Rheum. Dis.,* **1976–1977,** *27,* 912–917.

Greenberg, L. A. *Antipyrine: A Critical Bibliographic Review.* Hillhouse Press, New Haven, Conn., **1950.** (1735 references.)

Gross, M., and Greenberg, L. A. *The Salicylates: A Critical Bibliographic Review.* Hillhouse Press, New Haven, Conn., **1948.** (4093 references.)

Gutman, A. B. Uricosuric drugs, with special reference to probenecid and sulfinpyrazone. *Adv. Pharmacol.,* **1966,** *4,* 91–142.

Hanzlik, P. J. *Actions and Uses of the Salicylates and Cinchophen in Medicine.* The Williams & Wilkins Co., Baltimore, **1927.**

Hill, D. F. Gold therapy for rheumatoid arthritis. *Med. Clin. North Am.,* **1968,** *52,* 733–738.

Kelley, W. N., and Weiner, I. M. (eds.). *Uric Acid. Handbuch der Experimentellen Pharmakologie,* Vol. 51. Springer-Verlag, Berlin, **1978.**

Lockie, L. M. Current methods of treatment. Adult peripheral rheumatoid arthritis: stages I and II. *Arthritis Rheum.,* **1961,** *4,* 404–407.

Medical Letter. Drugs for dysmenorrhea. **1979,** *21,* 81–84.

Miller, R. L.; Insel, P. A.; and Melmon, K. L. Inflammatory disorders. In, *Clinical Pharmacology: Basic Principles in Therapeutics,* 2nd ed. (Melmon, K. L., and Morrelli, H. F., eds.) Macmillan Publishing Co., Inc., New York, **1978,** pp. 657–708.

Paulus, H. E., and Whitehouse, M. W. Nonsteroid anti-inflammatory agents. *Annu. Rev. Pharmacol.,* **1973,** *13,* 107–125.

Randall, L. O. 2. Non-narcotic analgesics. In, *Physiological Pharmacology.* Vol. 1, *The Nervous System—Part A: Central Nervous System Drugs.* (Root, W. S., and Hofmann, F. G., eds.) Academic Press, Inc., New York, **1963,** pp. 313–416. (231 references.)

Rieselbach, R. E., and Steele, T. H. Influence of the kidney upon urate homeostasis in health and disease. *Am. J. Med.,* **1974,** *56,* 665–675.

Shen, T. Y., and Winter, C. A. Chemical and biological studies on indomethacin, sulindac and their analogues. *Adv. Drug Res.,* **1977,** *12,* 90–245.

Smith, M. J. H., and Dawkins, P. O. Salicylate and enzymes. *J. Pharm. Pharmacol.,* **1971,** *23,* 729–744.

Smith, M. J. H., and Smith, P. K. (eds.). *The Salicylates: A Critical Bibliographic Review.* John Wiley & Sons, Inc., New York, **1966.**

Smith, P. K. *Acetophenetidin: A Critical Bibliographic Review.* Interscience Publishers, Inc., New York, **1958.** (529 references.)

Symposium. (Various authors.) *Salicylates: An International Symposium.* (Dixon, A. St. J.; Martin, B. K.; Smith, M. J. H.; and Wood, P. H. N.; eds.) J. & A. Churchill, Ltd., London, **1963.**

Symposium. (Various authors.) *Fenamates in Medicine.* (Kendall, P. H., ed.) Baillière, Tindall & Cassell, London, **1966a.**

Symposium. (Various authors.) *Proceedings of the Conference on Effects of Chronic Salicylate Administration.* (Lamont-Honers, R. W., and Wagner, B. M., eds.) National Institutes of Health, NIAMD, Bethesda, **1966b.**

Symposium. (Various authors.) Aspirin and salicylates. *Clin. Toxicol.,* **1968,** *1,* 379–473.

Symposium. (Various authors.) Symposium on ibuprofen (BRUFEN). *Curr. Med. Res. Opin.,* **1975a,** *3,* 475–606.

Symposium. (Various authors.) Proceedings of an international medical symposium on naproxen. *J. Clin. Pharmacol.,* **1975b,** *14,* 305–378.

Symposium. (Various authors.) Symposium on paracetamol and the liver (overdosage and its management). *J. Int. Med. Res.,* **1976a,** *4,* Suppl. 4, 1–157.

Symposium. (Various authors.) Recent advances in clinical rheumatology: a review and clinical assessment of azapropazone. *Curr. Med. Res. Opin.,* **1976b,** *4,* 3–100.

Symposium. (Various authors.) Symposium on flurbiprofen (FROBEN). *Curr. Med. Res. Opin.,* **1977a,** *5,* 3–140.

Symposium. (Various authors.) Rheumatology workshop. A modern review of Geigy pyrazoles. *J. Int. Med. Res.,* **1977b,** *5,* Suppl. 2, 2–120.

Symposium. (Various authors.) Symposium on sulindac. *Eur. J. Rheumatol. Inflam.,* **1978,** *1,* 1–66.

Vane, J. R., and Ferreira, S. H. (eds.) *Anti-inflammatory Drugs. Handbuch der Experimentellen Pharmakologie,* Vol. 50. Springer-Verlag, Berlin, **1979.**

Wallace, S. L., and Ertel, N. H. Pharmacology of drugs used in the treatment of acute gout. In, *Uric Acid. Handbuch der Experimentellen Pharmakologie,* Vol. 51. (Kelley, W. N., and Weiner, I. M., eds.) Springer-Verlag, Berlin, **1978,** pp. 525–555.

Whitehouse, M. W. Some biochemical and pharmacological properties of anti-inflammatory drugs. *Prog. Drug Res.,* **1965,** *8,* 301–429. (404 references.)

Yü, T.-F. Milestones in the treatment of gout. *Am. J. Med.,* **1974,** *56,* 676–683.

Yü, T.-F., and Gutman, A. B. Principles of current management of primary gout. *Am. J. Med. Sci.,* **1967,** *254,* 893–907.

SECTION VI

Cardiovascular Drugs

A major pharmacological action of a number of drugs is their ability to alter cardiovascular function; these agents will be considered in this section. Many additional drugs, however, also markedly influence the heart and blood vessels; they are described elsewhere in connection with their other important pharmacodynamic properties.

CHAPTER 30 DIGITALIS AND ALLIED CARDIAC GLYCOSIDES

Brian F. Hoffman and J. Thomas Bigger, Jr.

Digitalis and certain other cardiac glycosides have in common a powerful action on the myocardium that is unrivaled in value for the treatment of heart failure. These drugs are found in a number of plants, and a few also are present in the venom of certain toads. The preparations commonly employed are obtained from digitalis and strophanthus; older preparations also came from squill. In the following discussion, the term *digitalis* is used to designate the entire group of *cardiac glycosides* rather than only those obtained from digitalis. The general descriptions of the pharmacology and the uses of digitalis apply to all related cardiac glycosides unless otherwise stated.

History. A large number of plant extracts containing cardiac glycosides have been used by natives in various parts of the world as arrow and ordeal poisons. *Squill* was known as a medicine to the ancient Egyptians. The Romans employed it as a diuretic, heart tonic, emetic, and rat poison. *Strophanthus* was introduced into medicine in 1890 by Sir Thomas Fraser, who discovered its digitalis-like action while studying African arrow poisons. The dried skin of the common toad has been used for centuries as a drug by the Chinese. Digitalis, or foxglove, was mentioned in 1250 in the writings of Welsh physicians. It was described botanically 300 years later by Fuchsius, who gave it the name *Digitalis purpurea*.

In 1785, William Withering published his famous book, entitled *An Account of the Foxglove and Some of Its Medical Uses: with Practical Remarks on Dropsy and Other Diseases.* Withering was aware that digitalis was effective only in certain forms of dropsy (edema) but apparently did not associate this with the cardiac actions of the drug. He recognized that the heart was affected, however, for he wrote, "It has a power over the motion of the heart to a degree yet unobserved in any other medicine, and this power may be converted to salutary ends." Apparently, John Ferriar in 1799 was the first to ascribe to digitalis a primary action on the heart and to relegate the diuretic effect to a position of secondary importance. Whereas Withering recorded the benefits to be derived from the proper use of foxglove, his advice was not always heeded. Even during the nineteenth century, digitalis was used indiscriminately for many disorders, often in toxic doses. During the early twentieth century, as a result of the work of Cushny, Mackenzie, Lewis, and others, the drug gradually came to be looked upon as a specific in the treatment of atrial fibrillation. Only within the last 60 years has it become firmly established that the main value of digitalis is in the therapy of congestive heart failure.

Sources and Composition of the Digitalis Principles. Official digitalis is the dried leaf of the foxglove plant, *Digitalis purpurea*. Seeds and leaves of a number of other digitalis species also contain active cardiac principles. *Digitalis lanata* leaves are used in

Europe and are the source of certain purified preparations employed in the United States. The formerly official strophanthus is obtained from the seeds of the *Strophanthus Kombé* or *hispidus.* Official ouabain is derived from *Strophanthus gratus.* Squill, the dried, fleshy bulb of the "sea onion," comes from *Urginea (Scilla) maritima.* Another member of this same family, *Convallaria majalis* (lily of the valley), yields a cardiac glycoside, convallatoxin, which is not employed clinically but which possesses potent characteristic digitalis-like activity. Belonging to the same family as the *Strophanthus* plant is a tropical tree, *Thevetia neriifolia* (yellow oleander), the fruit of which contains thevetin, a glycoside that has had desultory clinical trial. Many other plants, including certain members of the Helleborus family, contain cardiac glycosides, but none has clinical value.

Chemical Nature and Properties of the Cardiac Glycosides. Each glycoside represents the combination of an *aglycone,* or *genin,* with from one to four molecules of sugar. Pharmacological activity resides in the aglycone, but the particular sugars attached to the aglycone modify water and lipid solubility and potency of the resulting glycoside. The major contributions to this field have been reviewed by Chen and Henderson (1954), Fieser and Fieser (1959), Marshall (1970), and Fullerton and associates (1979).

The aglycones can be released from the cardiac glycosides by hydrolysis. They are chemically related to bile acids, sterols, and sex and adrenocortical hormones. The basic structure is a cyclopentanoperhydrophenanthrene nucleus to which is attached an unsaturated lactone ring at C 17. In addition, methyl, hydroxyl, and aldehyde groups are attached in specific positions that vary with the particular aglycone. All the naturally occurring aglycones carry OH groups at position 14, and many have additional OH groups, particularly at position 3, where the sugar moieties usually are attached. The hydroxyl group at C 3 is highly reactive, and semisynthetic derivatives have been made by reaction of aglycones with organic acids, sugars, xanthine, and other agents. *Acetylstrophanthidin,* one such semisynthetic derivative, is usually not employed clinically but is widely used for experimental purposes because of its rapid onset and relatively short duration of action. The number and the position of other OH groups are important for determining aqueous versus lipid solubility, protein binding, metabolic disposition, and duration of action. Most cardiac aglycones have an angular CH_3 group at C 10, but an aldehyde or alcohol grouping is present in a few. Favorable spatial arrangement in the steroid ring system is also required (Tamm, 1963). In general, the aglycones have more transient and less potent myocardial actions than the glycosides but cause similar toxic effects.

The unsaturated lactone ring attached to C 17 possesses the $\Delta^{\alpha,\beta}$ structure, and may be five or six membered. Saturation of the lactone ring reduces activity by tenfold or more, and increases the speed of development of the cardiac actions (Vick *et al.,* 1957); opening of the ring completely abolishes activity.

The structural formulas of *digoxigenin* and *digitoxigenin* are as follows:

Digoxigenin

Digitoxigenin

Digoxin and digitoxin, the cardiac glycosides in predominant clinical use, consist of the corresponding aglycone with three molecules of digitoxose, a 2,6-dideoxyhexose, joined in glycosidic linkage and attached at position 3. The chemical constituents of various other glycosides are described in *earlier editions* of this textbook.

PHARMACODYNAMICS

Digitalis is used most frequently to increase the adequacy of the circulation in patients with congestive heart failure and to slow the ventricular rate in the presence of atrial fibrillation and flutter. *The main pharmacodynamic property of digitalis is its ability to increase the force of myocardial contraction.* The beneficial effects of the drug in patients with heart failure—increased cardiac output; decreased heart size, venous pressure, and blood volume; diuresis and relief of edema—are all explained on the basis of increased contractile force, *a positive inotropic action.* The second important action of digitalis is to slow the ventricular rate in atrial fibrillation or flutter.

Because digitalis often dramatically slows the ventricular rate in atrial fibrillation, it was believed for many years that the main effect of the drug was to slow the heart rate. Starting perhaps with Wenckebach (1910) and as a result of numerous subsequent clinical studies, the conviction grew and finally became firmly established that digitalis is effective in congestive heart failure regardless of the cardiac rhythm, and that the beneficial effect is brought about *not* by virtue of cardiac slowing but by its direct action to increase the force of myocardial contraction. The mechanisms responsible for these beneficial effects of digitalis are complex. Digitalis exerts direct effects on the heart that modify both its mechanical and electrical activity. It also acts directly on the smooth muscle of the vascular system. In addition, digitalis exerts a number of effects on neural tissue and thus indirectly influences the mechanical and electrical activity of the heart and modifies vascular resistance and capacitance. Finally, changes in the circulation brought about by digitalis often result in reflex alterations in autonomic activity and hormonal balance that indirectly influence cardiovascular function. In describing the effects of digitalis on the heart and circulation, it is convenient to discuss the *direct and indirect actions* on the heart before considering the integrated effects of digitalis on the entire cardiovascular system.

DIRECT EFFECTS

Myocardial Contractility. Digitalis increases the contractility of cardiac muscle in a dose-dependent manner—a *positive inotropic effect.* The effects are similar for both atrial and ventricular muscle and are *qualitatively* the same for muscle obtained from either normal or failing hearts. The effects of digitalis on mechanical activity can be demonstrated for both isometric and isotonic contractions. If an isolated preparation of cardiac muscle is studied under *isometric conditions* and the resting length is set at the peak of the length-tension relationship, an appropriate concentration of digitalis increases the peak force developed. In addition, it increases the rate of development of force, decreases the time to peak tension, and speeds relaxation. The total duration of the contraction is thus decreased. These changes occur without any alteration in resting tension. The effects are similar qualitatively at all points on the length-tension relationship; for any given end-diastolic fiber length, digitalis increases the tension that can be generated.

The extent to which digitalis increases isometric tension depends strongly on the initial condition of the muscle. If the capacity to develop force is severely depressed, the effect is much larger than would occur in normal muscle (*see* Figure 30-1).

If the preparation of cardiac muscle is studied under *isotonic conditions,* digitalis shifts the force-velocity curve upward. The maximal load and rate of shortening both increase. As in the case of isometric contractions, the magnitude of the change produced by digitalis is greater if, under control conditions, the muscle is abnormally weak. Digitalis thus increases the rate at which work can be done and also the maximal work that the muscle can perform.

Concentrations of digitalis considerably higher than those needed to demonstrate the positive inotropic effect cause an increase in resting tension and partial *contracture.* Usually this is associated with a decrease in shortening velocity and peak isometric tension. It is almost certain that this effect is a toxic one and is unrelated to therapeutic actions.

The direct positive inotropic effect of digitalis also can be demonstrated in studies on the isolated supported mammalian heart or on the mammalian heart-lung preparation. These preparations present an advantage in that the effects of digitalis on the systemic vasculature and autonomic nervous system do not complicate the interpretation of its direct cardiac actions. With the isolated heart it is possible to keep heart rate and end-diastolic intraventricular pressures constant so that inotropic effects caused by changes in rate or end-diastolic fiber length need not be considered. Under these conditions, appropriate

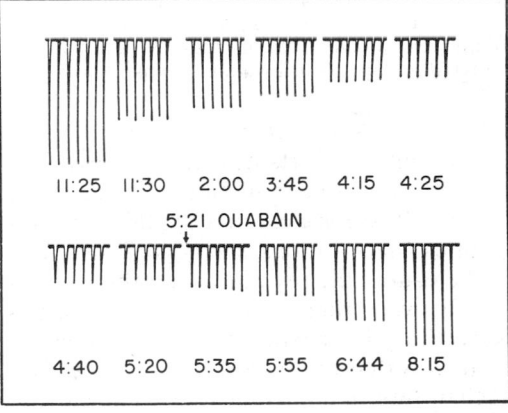

Figure 30-1. *The effect of ouabain on force of contraction of an isolated papillary muscle from the right ventricle of a cat heart.*

The muscle was prepared for isometric recording of contractions induced by rhythmic electrical stimulation. Systolic tension of the muscle, recorded as a downward deflection, decreased spontaneously during 6 hours of perfusion. The addition of ouabain in a concentration of 13 μg per liter (22 nM) restored the force of contraction. (After Gold and Cattell, 1940. Courtesy of the *Archives of Internal Medicine.*)

concentrations of digitalis increase the maximal rate of development of intraventricular pressure, decrease the duration of isovolumic contraction, increase ejection velocity, increase peak systolic pressure, and decrease the duration of contraction. Usually, stroke volume and aortic flow increase and, because the ventricle empties more completely during systole, end-systolic volume is reduced. In the canine heart-lung preparation, it is possible to demonstrate the major effects of digitalis on a failed heart. In this preparation failure can be induced by a variety of means; and among these, perhaps the simplest to study is failure induced by increasing resistance to aortic flow. A sufficient increase in aortic resistance reduces stroke volume; as a consequence, end-systolic volume is increased. With reasonably constant ventricular filling during diastole, end-diastolic pressure and volume increase. Because of the length-tension relationship, the increase in end-diastolic fiber length initially compensates for the elevated resistance to ejection. However, with time the contraction of the ventricle weakens; there is a progressive decrease in stroke volume and progressive increases in both end-diastolic pressure and volume. Because heart rate is constant and stroke volume decreased, aortic flow necessarily decreases. Under these conditions, administration of digitalis brings about most dramatic changes. Because digitalis increases the capacity of the fibers to develop tension and to shorten, the ventricle is able to develop sufficient pressure during systole to eject an increased stroke volume in spite of the increased aortic resistance. The increased stroke volume results in a decrease in end-systolic volume and a progressive decrease in end-diastolic volume and end-diastolic pressure. These changes in pressure and ventricular volume are demonstrated in Figure 30–2 in terms of intraventricular pressure-volume loops.

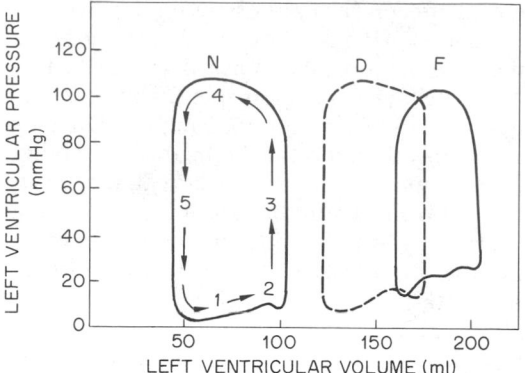

Figure 30–2. *Schematic representation of pressure-volume loops for the normal and failing left ventricle and the effects of digitalis.*

For the control loop (*N*), the arrows show the changes in ventricular pressure and volume with time during a single cardiac cycle. The numbers on the control loop indicate the phases of the cardiac cycle: *1* = diastasis, *2* = atrial systole, *3* = isovolumic contraction, *4* = ejection, *5* = isovolumic relaxation. End-diastolic pressure is relatively low, for the control curve pressure develops rapidly, and ejection is well maintained during systole. The loop labeled *F* shows the types of change that result from failure. End-systolic and end-diastolic volumes are greatly increased, as is end-diastolic pressure. During isovolumic contraction, pressure develops less rapidly and stroke volume is reduced. When digitalis has exerted its positive inotropic effect (*D*), the loop shifts to lower diastolic pressures and volumes and stroke volume increases.

Mechanism of Action. The manner in which digitalis exerts its direct positive inotropic effect has been studied by a variety of technics. It seems clear that digitalis, in therapeutic concentrations, exerts no *direct* effect on the contractile proteins or on the interactions between them. Also, it seems most unlikely that the positive inotropic effect of digitalis is due to any action on the cellular mechanisms that provide the chemical energy for contraction. The most probable explanation for the direct positive inotropic effect is the ability of digitalis to inhibit the *membrane-bound Na^+,K^+-activated adenosine triphosphatase (Na^+,K^+-ATPase)*. The hydrolysis of adenosine triphosphate (ATP) by this enzyme provides the energy for the so-called sodium pump—the system in the sarcolemma of cardiac fibers that actively extrudes sodium and transports potassium into the fibers. Digitalis glycosides bind specifically to the Na^+,K^+-ATPase, inhibit its enzymatic activity, and impair the active transport of these two monovalent cations. As a result, there is a gradual increase in intracellular sodium ($[Na^+]_i$) and a gradual small decrease in $[K^+]_i$. These changes are small at therapeutic concentrations of the drug. It is the former change, the increase in $[Na^+]_i$, that at present is judged to be crucially related to the positive inotropic effect of digitalis. This is so because cardiac fibers possess a mechanism for exchange of intracellular Na^+ for extracellular Ca^{2+}. When inhibition of the pump by digitalis causes $[Na^+]_i$ to increase, there is an augmented exchange of intracellular sodium for extracellular calcium. This causes an increase in net influx of Ca^{2+} and, presumably, an increase in the concentration of calcium ($[Ca^{2+}]_i$) in the sarcoplasm (*see* Figure 30–3).

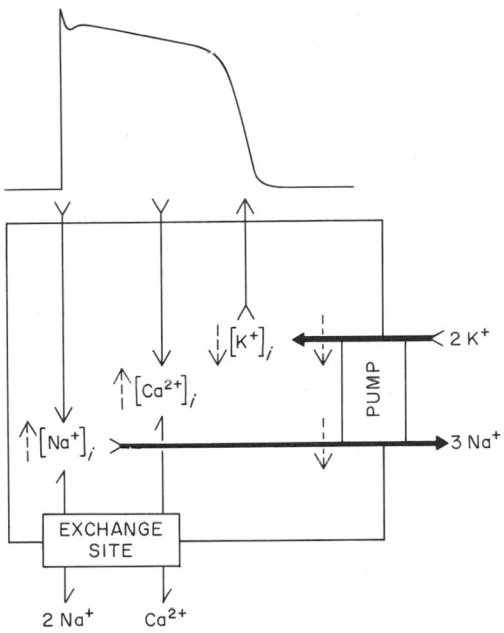

Figure 30-3. *Schematic representation of fluxes of Na^+, K^+, and Ca^{2+} across the cardiac cell membrane and the effects of digitalis thereon.*

During the transmembrane action potential, shown at the top, there is a net entry of Na^+ and Ca^{2+} and a net loss of K^+. The intracellular concentrations of Na^+ ($[Na^+]_i$) and K^+ ($[K^+]_i$) are maintained by the activity of the Na^+,K^+ pump, shown at the right. The intracellular concentration of calcium ($[Ca^{2+}]_i$) is in part regulated by exchange for sodium (exchange site). The effects of digitalis are shown by the dashed arrows. Active extrusion of Na^+ is decreased; this probably leads to an increase in $[Na^+]_i$, which in turn causes an increase in $[Ca^{2+}]_i$.

One difficulty in obtaining an unequivocal demonstration of the mechanism for the positive inotropic effect of digitalis is that the exact mechanism for excitation-contraction coupling in cardiac muscle is not completely understood. This results in part from the fact that there are quantitative and perhaps qualitative differences between hearts of different species and clear quantitative differences between atrial and ventricular muscle and, probably, Purkinje fibers within any one species. In spite of uncertainties, it is reasonable to assume that contraction of most mammalian hearts is initiated by the influx of Ca^{2+} that occurs during the transmembrane action potential (AP). This, in turn, causes the release of additional Ca^{2+} from the sarcoplasmic reticulum (SR) (Fabiato and Fabiato, 1977). Evidence from chemically "skinned" cardiac fibers strongly supports the concept that an increase in $[Ca^{2+}]$ does in fact cause release of Ca^{2+} from SR; in contrast, evidence that supports other mechanisms, such as depolarization-induced release of Ca^{2+} from SR, is

less convincing. Furthermore, voltage-clamp experiments on intact preparations have demonstrated that the development of tension is proportional to the influx of Ca^{2+} during the AP (Beeler and Reuter, 1970).

In addition, there are uncertainties about the metabolism of Ca^{2+} by cardiac fibers. Voltage-clamp experiments have established beyond doubt that the AP in both cardiac muscle and Purkinje fibers is associated with an inward current (i_{si}) carried in large part by Ca^{2+} (*see* Chapter 31). The extent to which this net influx of Ca^{2+} increases $[Ca^{2+}]_i$ is not sufficient, except perhaps in frog heart (Anderson *et al.*, 1977), to activate the contractile elements (*see* below). In the steady state, therefore, mechanisms must be available to extrude from the cell an amount of Ca^{2+} equal to the net gain during each AP. Most evidence indicates that such extrusion is accomplished by exchange between extracellular Na^+ and intracellular Ca^{2+} (*see* Figure 30-3). This exchange mechanism may result from the operation of a carrier in the membrane (*see* Katz, 1977). In terms of this mechanism, either an increase in $[Ca^{2+}]_o$ or an increase in $[Na^+]_i$ would cause an increase in $[Ca^{2+}]_i$. The same mechanism would explain the well-known observation that force of cardiac contraction is roughly proportional to the extracellular ratio of $[Ca^{2+}]/[Na^+]^2$.

The mechanism described thus assumes that the Na^+,K^+-ATPase is the pharmacological receptor for digitalis and that when digitalis binds to this enzyme it induces a conformational change that decreases the active transport of sodium. Schatzman (1953) first described this enzymatic system in red-cell membranes and its specific inhibition by digitalis. In 1957, Skou prepared a Na^+,K^+-ATPase from crab nerve membrane. The enzyme was specifically inhibited by ouabain and appeared to be an integral part of the Na^+,K^+ pump (*see* Skou, 1965). Wilbrandt (1955) proposed that the digitalis-induced positive inotropic effect on the myocardium was due to an increase in $[Ca^{2+}]_i$ and that this resulted from inhibition of Na^+ and K^+ transport. Many studies have provided evidence that digitalis binds to the ATPase in a specific and saturable manner, that the binding results in a conformational change of the enzyme, that the rate of binding is increased by $[Na^+]$ and decreased by $[K^+]$, and that the binding site for digitalis is probably on the external surface of the membrane (*see* Schwartz, 1976). Furthermore, the magnitude of the inotropic effect of digitalis is proportional to the degree of inhibition of the enzyme (Akera *et al.*, 1970). Digitalis has little direct effect on the uptake or release of Ca^{2+} by SR or mitochondria (Besch *et al.*, 1970).

Although a number of studies have provided data that are not readily explained by the following model (*see* Okita *et al.*, 1973; Besch and Watanabe, 1978), it seems most reasonable at present to assume that the following sequence of events occurs. Digitalis binds to a specific site on the membrane ATPase and decreases the active extrusion of Na^+. The consequent increase in $[Na^+]_i$ increases the exchange of intracellular Na^+ for extracellular Ca^{2+}. (Concomitant changes in $[K^+]_i$ are described below, in relation to effects of digitalis on electrical activity.) The elevated value of $[Ca^{2+}]_i$ might increase contractility by several mechanisms. For instance, Ca^{2+} binds to troponin in rat ventricle at concentrations that are too low to cause release of Ca^{2+} from SR. An elevated myoplasmic $[Ca^{2+}]$ thus might partially saturate binding sites on troponin and augment the change elicited by release of a fixed amount of Ca^{2+} from the SR. It has also been shown that the rate of release of Ca^{2+} from the SR may be increased in a graded fashion by elevation of $[Ca^{2+}]$ outside the SR (see Katz, 1977). An increase in $[Ca^{2+}]_i$ thus might increase the rate and amount of Ca^{2+} released from the SR in response to the AP and bring about a more rapid and more forceful contraction. Finally, an elevated $[Ca^{2+}]_i$ might increase the stores of Ca^{2+} in the SR that are available for release. Whatever the details of the mechanisms may be, it is certain that digitalis increases the uptake of Ca^{2+} by cardiac fibers and also that a positive inotropic effect is not prominent until there has been some inhibition of the active transport of Na^+ and K^+ (Hougen and Smith, 1978).

Electrical Activity. Because some of the therapeutic and most of the serious toxic effects of digitalis can be related to actions upon the electrophysiological properties of the heart, these actions of the drug have been studied extensively. Understanding of the cellular mechanisms involved has been greatly enhanced in recent years through the application of microelectrode technics to the study of isolated, superfused preparations of cardiac tissue. The results obtained have been supplemented by intracardiac records of the electrical activity of the heart *in situ*, both in experimental animals and in man, and by study of the response of the heart to electrical stimulation.

Purkinje Fibers. The direct effects of digitalis on the electrical activity of cardiac fibers will be described first in terms of the changes caused by digitalis in the transmembrane potentials of mammalian cardiac Purkinje fibers. These cells have been studied most intensively. In addition, most attempts to explain the toxic effects of digitalis on the electrical activity of the heart have been based on data for Purkinje fibers.

The effects of digitalis on the transmembrane AP and resting potential (RP) of the canine cardiac Purkinje fiber are dependent on both the time of exposure to digitalis and its concentration. The following sequence of changes can be observed (Vassalle *et al.*, 1962; Kassebaum, 1963; Müller, 1965; Rosen *et al.*, 1973a). Initially, if the preparation is stimulated at a low rate, there is a small increase in action potential duration (APD). This is not seen if the rate of stimulation is high. Subsequently, there is a decrease in APD that results largely from a shortening of the duration of the plateau (phase 2). Usually, this is associated with an increase in the slope of phase-4 depolarization. Later, there is a decrease in RP or maximal diastolic potential (MDP) and a further decrease in APD (see Figure 30-4). Largely because of the less negative RP, or because phase-4 depolarization causes the upstroke of the AP (phase 0) to start at a less negative potential, the maximal rate of rise of phase 0 ($\dot{V}_{max}$) decreases as does the amplitude of the AP (see Chapter 31). Finally, when toxic effects are fully developed, the RP is markedly reduced, there is a directly induced decrease in $\dot{V}_{max}$ (Kassebaum, 1963), conduction velocity is reduced, and ultimately the fibers become inexcitable.

The effects of digitalis on phase 4 vary as a function of $[K^+]_o$ and probably other factors. At low values of $[K^+]_o$, the most consistent effect is an increase in the slope of phase 4. This results in *increased automaticity* that can be demonstrated if the driving stimulus is terminated. At somewhat higher levels of $[K^+]_o$ (>4 mM), a different change in the time course of membrane potential can be observed during phase 4. This is the appearance of *delayed afterdepolarizations* (Davis, 1973; Ferrier *et al.*, 1973; Rosen *et al.*, 1973b). This change in membrane potential also is called a transient depolarization (Ferrier *et al.*, 1973; Lederer and Tsien, 1976). The delayed afterdepolarization initially appears as a subthreshold depolarization early during phase 4 or as a damped train of afterdepolarizations (see Chapter 31). As toxicity progresses, the afterdepolarization increases in amplitude until it attains the threshold for initiation of an AP. When this occurs, the delayed afterdepolarization caused by the *extra* response is also quite likely to reach the threshold because, within limits, the amplitude of the delayed afterdepolarization increases as the interval between APs decreases. Clearly, then, digitalis can initiate ectopic impulses by two quite different means: enhancement of normal phase-4 depolarization or the development of delayed afterdepolarization. At

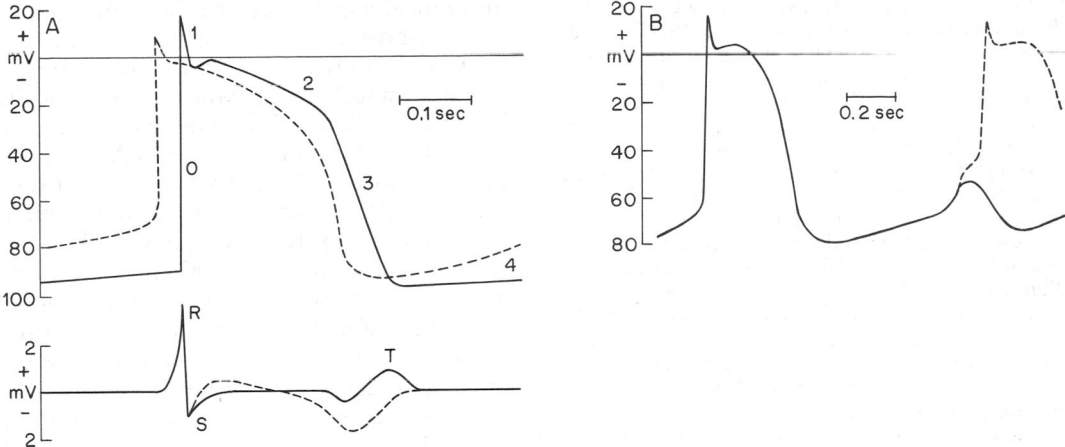

Figure 30-4. *Effects of digitalis on transmembrane potentials and electrograms.*

A. Schematic representation of a transmembrane action potential recorded from a cardiac Purkinje fiber (top trace) and a unipolar electrogram recorded from the same preparation (bottom trace) under control conditions (solid lines) and in the presence of digitalis (dashed lines). Phases 0, 1, 2, 3, and 4 have their usual meaning. After the effects of digitalis have developed, there is a decrease in maximal diastolic potential, an increase in the slope of phase-4 depolarization, and a decrease in action potential duration. Because of the increase in phase-4 depolarization, the fiber becomes automatic. Voltage at which activation occurs shifts to a more positive value, and the amplitude of the action potential decreases. Because of the change in the slope and duration of phases 2 and 3, there is a change in the S-T segment and T wave of the electrogram and a decrease in the R-T interval.

B. Schematic representation of the appearance of delayed afterdepolarizations caused by digitalis in the record of transmembrane potential from a Purkinje fiber. The delayed afterde-polarizations are shown as being subthreshold (solid line) and suprathreshold (dashed line); the latter initiates an extra action potential. *See* text for further explanation.

present, the clinical differentiation between these two mechanisms often is not possible.

As is the case for the mechanism by which digitalis increases cardiac contractility, there still is some uncertainty about the exact mechanisms by which direct effects of digitalis alter the transmembrane potentials of cardiac fibers (Rosen *et al.,* 1975b). It may be helpful to consider changes in electrical activity in relation to the concentration of glycoside or the intensity of its effect. At low concentrations, digitalis does not significantly influence the fast inward channel for Na^+. The increase in APD seen at very low concentrations of drug might be due to changes in the passive properties of the membrane (Kassebaum, 1963). The typical effects, a decrease in APD and an increase in the slope of phase-4 depolarization, can be attributed to the following. As digitalis decreases active extrusion of Na^+, there is a decrease in net outward background current (Isenberg and Trautwein, 1974; *see* Chapter 31), because, under many conditions, the pump is electrogenic; this is true because of the stoichiometry of transport of Na^+ and K^+. This decrease in outward current causes an increase in the slope of phase-4 depolarization. It might also cause the increase in APD, mentioned above, as well as some decrease in RP (Gadsby and Cranefield, 1979). As $[Na]_i$ increases

because of depressed active transport, there is an increase in $[Ca^{2+}]_i$. This can cause an increase in K^+ permeability (Bassingthwaighte *et al.,* 1976), an increased outward current during the plateau, and result in the typical decrease in APD. Higher concentrations of glycoside seem to decrease directly the magnitude of the current responsible for normal phase-4 depolarization in Purkinje fibers (i_{K_2}; *see* Chapter 31) (Aronson and Gelles, 1977). This effect would further increase the slope of phase 4. Also, in sufficiently high concentrations, digitalis can shift the inactivation curve for the fast inward channel to more negative transmembrane potentials (Kassebaum, 1963) and thus decrease the maximal rate of rise of the transmembrane AP (*See* Chapter 31).

With toxic concentrations of digitalis, inhibition of the pump has other effects on electrical activity. There is a small increase in $[Na^+]_i$ and a decrease in $[K^+]_i$ (Deitmer and Ellis, 1978; Miura and Rosen, 1978). The altered concentration gradients, by altering the sodium and potassium equilibrium potentials, will decrease slightly the rate of rise and amplitude of the AP and decrease the RP or maximal diastolic potential.

The mechanism responsible for the delayed afterdepolarizations is less certain but definitely occurs at concentrations of digitalis that clearly cause toxicity. Agents that block the inward current carried primarily by Ca^{2+} (i_{si}) are effective in abolishing delayed afterdepolarizations; this led to the suggestion that the delayed afterdepolarizations are due to an abnormal inward movement of Ca^{2+}. More recent studies with the use of voltage-clamp methods strongly support a different mechanism (Aronson and Gelles, 1977; Kass et al., 1978a, 1978b). It seems that the augmented $[Ca^{2+}]_i$ may cause transient oscillatory changes in $[Ca^{2+}]_i$; these result in transient increases in membrane permeability to Na^+ and other ions. The resultant transient inward currents are responsible for the delayed afterdepolarizations. One other effect of highly toxic concentrations of digitalis is also due to the increase in $[Ca^{2+}]_i$; this is an increase in the intercellular resistance. An elevated $[Ca^{2+}]_i$ causes "uncoupling" at gap junctions (DeMello, 1975; Weingart, 1977). This decreases the spread of excitatory current from one cell to another and impairs conduction.

One other observation should be mentioned. Over the years, several studies have demonstrated what appears to be *stimulation* of the active transport of Na^+ and K^+ when very low concentrations of digitalis are used. Data supporting this concept have been obtained from studies with voltage-clamp methods (Cohen et al., 1976) and also by measurement of intracellular Na^+ activity with a sodium-sensitive microelectrode (Deitmer and Ellis, 1978). This hypothesis does not seem to be supported by direct measurement of inhibition of active uptake of Rb^+ in the canine heart *in situ* caused by quite low (1 nM) concentrations of ouabain (Hougen and Smith, 1978).

The results of studies of effects of digitalis on isolated preparations of cardiac muscle (particularly Purkinje fibers) must be interpreted with care because some effects may be dependent on the nature of the preparation and can be modified by the experimental conditions. Nevertheless, Purkinje fibers are more sensitive to the toxic actions of digitalis than are ventricular muscle fibers (Vassalle et al., 1962). For both, toxicity develops more rapidly if the fibers are stimulated at a more rapid rate. The development of toxicity is inhibited by an increase in $[K^+]_o$ and facilitated by an increase in $[Ca^{2+}]_o$. When toxicity has developed, it can to a certain extent be reversed by elevating $[K^+]_o$. The effect of rate is not surprising, since the active transport required of the Na^+,K^+-ATPase is a function of the number of APs per unit of time. The influence of increasing $[K^+]_o$ may result from the stimulatory effect of extracellular potassium on the pump, as well as from decreased binding of digitalis to the ATPase. The interaction between Ca^{2+} and digitalis may reflect the effect of a higher concentration of this ion on the sodium-calcium exchange process, mentioned above, direct inhibition of the Na^+,K^+ pump by Ca^{2+} (Brown et al., 1978), or some effect of digitalis on the binding of Ca^{2+} to the ATPase.

Other Specialized Fibers. Digitalis exerts direct effects on the fibers of the sinoatrial (S-A) node and the atrioventricular (A-V) node, and on the specialized atrial fiber system. At concentrations that may obtain during clinical use, digitalis has little direct effect on the transmembrane potentials of the rabbit S-A node (Toda and West, 1966; Ten Eick and Hoffman, 1969a). Most of the clinically important effects of digitalis on the rate of formation of impulses by the S-A node are due to indirect effects that the drug exerts through the parasympathetic and sympathetic nervous system (*see* below). Nevertheless, concentrations of digitalis that cause toxicity can partially depolarize S-A nodal fibers and stop the generation of impulses. High concentrations of digitalis directly depress conduction of impulses through the A-V node. However, as for the S-A node, the clinically important actions of cardiac glycosides on the A-V node are mediated by the autonomic nervous system. The direct actions decrease conduction velocity, increase the effective refractory period (ERP), and ultimately cause complete A-V block. These changes in conduction are associated with a decrease in maximal diastolic potential and in the rate of rise and amplitude of the A-V nodal AP. The *specialized atrial fibers* respond to digitalis in much the same manner as do Purkinje fibers. Most importantly, digitalis causes not only an increase in automaticity due to enhanced phase-4 depolarization but also generation of ectopic impulses due to production of delayed afterdepolarizations (Hashimoto and Moe, 1973).

Atrial and Ventricular Muscle Fibers. The direct effects of digitalis on the transmembrane potentials of ventricular muscle have been studied fairly extensively. The changes in the duration of the AP resemble those described for Purkinje fibers. The decrease in this value is not marked but probably accounts for the decrease in the Q-T interval of the ECG (*see* Figure 30–4 and below). The ventricular transmembrane APs also show an increase in slope of the plateau and a decrease in the slope of phase 3. These alterations in the transmembrane potential cause changes in the S-T segment and the T wave in the ECG (*see* Figure 30–4 and below). In sufficiently high concentration, digitalis decreases both the RP and the amplitude of the AP of atrial and ventricular fibers and decreases the maximal rate of depolarization during phase 0. High concentrations thus can decrease conduction velocity and ultimately cause inexcitability. These drastic effects are not seen in clinical settings. Digitalis does not cause phase-4 depolarization in atrial or ventricular muscle fibers, but delayed after-depolarizations may occur (Ferrier, 1976).

INDIRECT EFFECTS

Electrical Activity. There is no doubt that many of the effects of digitalis on the electrical and mechanical activity of the mammalian heart result from glycoside-induced modification of both autonomic neural activity and the sensitivity of the heart to the vagal and sympathetic neurotransmitters. The decrease in sinus rate in the presence of heart failure is caused in large part by a glycoside-induced increase in efferent vagal impulses and a reflexly induced decrease in sympathetic tone; these changes are associated with improvement of the circulation. Other alterations of autonomic activity are more complex and less well understood (*see* Rosen *et al.*, 1975b; Mudge *et al.*, 1978).

Most experimental and clinical evidence supports the concept that efferent vagal activity is enhanced by digitalis; in both experimental animals and man, sinus slowing caused by therapeutic concentrations of a cardiac glycoside can be largely abolished by atropine. The increase in vagal activity appears to result from effects at several sites in the nervous system. The arterial baroceptors are sensitized (Gaffney *et al.*, 1958), possibly because of an effect of digitalis on active transport of cations in the afferent nerve terminals (Saum *et al.*, 1976). Pace and Gillis (1976) have shown an increase in afferent impulse traffic in carotid sinus nerves in cats given digoxin. Digitalis also affects the central vagal nuclei and the nodose ganglion (Chai *et al.*, 1967) and may modify the excitability of efferent vagal fibers (Ten Eick and Hoffman, 1969b). Effects that modify transmission in autonomic ganglia also have been described (Perry and Reinhert, 1954; Ten Eick and Hoffman, 1969a). Studies on isolated preparations suggest that the sensitivity of the sinus node to the negative chronotropic effect of acetylcholine is increased by digitalis (Toda and West, 1966). Most data indicate that administration of digitalis will intensify the effects of the vagus on the heart through several or all of the mechanisms mentioned above as well as by effects on the

heart and circulation that modify input to the autonomic nervous system (*see* below).

Changes in sympathetic activity caused by digitalis also have been described and are complex. Studies on both the S-A node (Nadeau and James, 1963) and the A-V node (Mendez *et al.*, 1961) indicate that sufficiently high concentrations of glycoside can decrease the sensitivity of these tissues to catecholamines and efferent sympathetic impulses. Other studies have shown enhancement of efferent sympathetic activity induced by toxic concentrations of digitalis (McLain, 1969; Gillis *et al.*, 1972; Pace and Gillis, 1976). Whether the increased sympathetic activity is caused by a peripheral or central effect of digitalis is still uncertain, as is also the importance of increased efferent sympathetic impulse traffic as a cause of cardiac arrhythmias (*see* Levitt *et al.*, 1970; Mudge *et al.*, 1978). Although it is certain that digitalis exerts direct effects on some parts of the central nervous system (CNS) (Chai *et al.*, 1973; Holloway *et al.*, 1976), other studies have demonstrated neither preferential uptake of glycosides in the CNS (Dutta *et al.*, 1977) nor significant inhibition of brain Na^+, K^+-ATPase activity (Weaver *et al.*, 1977). It has also been shown that if a highly polar semisynthetic glycoside is used to induce arrhythmias in dogs, there is no appreciable accumulation of the glycoside in the cerebrospinal fluid (Mudge *et al.*, 1978). The importance of norepinephrine in promoting arrhythmias caused by digitalis is suggested by studies on isolated cardiac Purkinje fibers (Tse and Han, 1978) and also by the capacity of β-adrenergic blocking drugs to attenuate or prevent some digitalis-induced disturbances of ventricular rhythm.

The combined effects of these indirect actions of digitalis on the *normal* heart and circulation are reasonably clear. However, when the circulation is abnormal, as when a patient has congestive heart failure, the net effects may be quite different. When the heart is normal, the augmented vagal activity typically decreases the rate of generation of impulses in the S-A node; other effects of digitalis on this node probably are not significant with usual therapeutic concentrations of the drug. In normal man at rest, a decrease in sinus rate may not occur when digitalis is given. However, the vagal effect of digitalis is still present, since the maximal heart rate achieved during exercise is significantly diminished (Horwitz *et al.,* 1977). If the sinus rate is increased, as in heart failure, the negative chronotropic effect of digitalis is usually quite prominent. Here withdrawal of compensatory sympathetic activity contributes to the net effect.

Atrial fibers, both specialized and nonspecialized, are quite sensitive to the actions of acetylcholine. The indirect action of digitalis thus causes prominent changes in the electrical activity of the atrium in experimental animals. At what may be assumed to be therapeutic concentrations, the indirect effects predominate over the direct effects. The liberated acetylcholine causes an increase in RP, a decrease in latent automaticity of specialized atrial fibers, and a marked decrease in the duration of the atrial AP and ERP. The indirect effect of digitalis on conduction in normal atrial fibers cannot be predicted with certainty because conduction velocity is dependent on so many variables. Nevertheless, if hyperpolarization is significant, conduction is slowed. What should be remembered is that the indirect effects tend to oppose the direct effects of digitalis (decrease in RP, increase in APD) on the atrium. Also, the most significant effects at therapeutic concentrations of digitalis are the decrease in atrial APD and ERP. These changes permit the atria to respond to stimulation at much higher rates. Thus, if digitalis is given during atrial flutter or atrial fibrillation, the net rate of atrial impulses may increase (*see* below).

If the RP of human atrial muscle is significantly decreased due to disease, digitalis can cause hyperpolarization and improvement in APs and conduction (Hordof *et al.,* 1978). This is due to liberation of acetylcholine, and the effect is abolished by atropine. If there is phase-4 depolarization, automaticity is decreased. Such findings demonstrate the importance of the initial condition of the tissue in relation to the net effect of digitalis. Toxic concentrations of ouabain cause delayed afterdepolarization in human atrial muscle fibers.

The *A-V node* is strongly influenced by the indirect actions of digitalis. The enhanced vagal activity and the decrease in sensitivity to catecholamines have pronounced effects on both the generation of the A-V nodal AP and the transmission of impulses through the node. Acetylcholine causes some hyperpolarization of certain fibers in the A-V node (Cranefield *et al.,* 1959) but, more importantly, decreases the rate of rise and amplitude of APs at these sites. Also, the recovery of excitability is delayed. Because of these changes, conduction is slowed and the ERP is greatly prolonged. The impairment of conduction may progress to complete heart block. A decreased sensitivity to norepinephrine would intensify these effects. In the A-V node, therefore, the direct and indirect effects of digitalis bring about similar changes. The most important result is to diminish the rate at which atrial impulses can be transmitted to the ventricles. Thus, in atrial tachycardias, atrial flutter, and atrial fibrillation, administration of digitalis will decrease the ventricular rate because of block of an increased fraction of atrial impulses in the A-V junction.

The effectiveness of the A-V block due to the direct and indirect effects on the A-V node is enhanced in atrial flutter and fibrillation because digitalis, through its indirect effect on the atria, usually *increases* the rate at which impulses enter the atrial margin of the node. Those impulses that enter the node but fail to propagate through it spread slowly and leave the tissue refractory in their wake (concealed conduction); this *repetitive concealed conduction* increases the fraction of time during which the node is effectively refractory (*see* below).

The *His-Purkinje system* is certainly strongly influenced by the sympathetic nervous system but ordinarily is thought not to be particularly sensitive to changes in vagal activity. Thus, in contrast to the S-A node, atria, and A-V node, the indirect effects of digitalis mediated through the sympathetic nervous system most likely influence electrical activity of the specialized ventricular conducting system.

Acetylcholine clearly can have effects on the electrical activity of the His bundle (Bailey *et al.,* 1972) and cardiac Purkinje fibers; it causes an increase in RP, a decrease in automatic rate, and some effect on the duration of the AP (Danilo *et al.,* 1978; Gadsby *et al.,* 1978; Tse and Han, 1978). Also, when impulses arise from partially depolarized Purkinje fibers, acetylcholine may either slow the rate of impulse generation or increase the transmembrane potential toward the normal value. Finally, acetylcholine antagonizes the effects of isoproterenol on Purkinje fibers. However, it does not modify the effects of digitalis on the transmembrane AP (Bailey *et al.,* 1979). In spite of these findings, until there is more convincing evidence for important functional vagal innervation of the ventricular conducting system, it is reasonable to emphasize only the indirect effects of digitalis that are mediated through the sympathetic efferent fibers.

Exactly how digitalis interacts with endogenous norepinephrine probably depends on the concentration of the glycoside. There is no strong evidence that the antiadrenergic effect of digitalis is prominent when its concentration is in the therapeutic range. On the other hand, enhanced efferent sympathetic activity may be important in relation to the drug-initiated arrhythmias that occur when the concentration of digitalis is high. If the heart is deprived of sympathetic innervation, toxic doses of digitalis usually cause cardiac arrest rather than ventricular arrhythmias and fibrillation (Erlij and Mendez, 1964; Ten Eick and Hoffman, 1969b). It seems reasonable to conclude, therefore, that the indirect and direct effects may at times act synergistically to cause disturbances of rhythm. Conversely, there is evidence that catecholamines stimulate the active transport of cations across the cardiac sarcolemma (Carpentier and Vassalle, 1971). In this sense, enhanced sympathetic activity might be expected to antagonize the depression of active transport caused by digitalis.

The indirect effects of digitalis probably result in only minor changes in the electrical activity of *ventricular fibers;* only extremely high concentrations of acetylcholine affect canine ventricular transmembrane RPs and APs. Similarly, catecholamines cause only small changes in the duration of the ventricular AP.

In *summary,* the indirect effects of digitalis, mediated primarily through the vagus, result in prominent changes in the activity of the sinus node, the atria, and the A-V node. Neurally mediated indirect effects on the functions of the specialized ventricular conducting system and the ventricles are much less important.

Mechanical Activity. The *direct* action of digitalis is primarily responsible for its positive inotropic effect on the heart. Nevertheless, certain of the drug's indirect effects do contribute to alterations of mechanical activity. For example, the decrease in heart rate due to sinus slowing influences contractility because of a change in end-diastolic fiber length; there is also a direct inotropic effect due to the change in rate. A decrease in ventricular rate caused by partial A-V block has similar effects. Enhanced vagal activity decreases the force of atrial contraction, but this negative inotropic effect, which might slightly reduce atrial transfer of blood, probably does not significantly attenuate the direct positive inotropic effect of digitalis on ventricular function.

Similarly, although vagal stimulation can decrease the force of ventricular contraction in experimental animals, particularly when contractility has been enhanced by sympathetic activation (Levy, 1971), it is not likely that acetylcholine liberated by enhanced vagal activity significantly attenuates the direct positive inotropic effect of cardiac glycosides. Interactions between digitalis and the sympathetic nervous system also are not crucially important in relation to the positive inotropic effect of digitalis. The glycoside can exert a strong positive inotropic effect after complete blockade of cardiac β-adrenergic receptors.

EFFECTS ON ELECTRICAL ACTIVITY OF THE HEART IN SITU

The effects of digitalis on the electrical activity of the heart *in situ* have been studied extensively. There is a reasonable correspondence between the toxic effects of digitalis on the canine and the human heart, and observations made on experimental animals have thus contributed importantly to our understanding of the therapeutic and toxic effects of digitalis in man.

The Canine Heart in Situ. Digitalis has a biphasic effect on the *electrical excitability* of both the atria and the ventricles. Low doses cause a slight increase in excitability, while higher doses decrease it (Mendez and Mendez, 1957). Unfortunately, there is no description of the effects of a therapeutic concentration of digitalis in plasma on the excitability of the canine heart during chronic left ventricular failure. The increased excitability may be accounted for by two mechanisms. Inhibition of active extrusion of sodium by digitalis decreases the net outward current across the membrane. This in itself would decrease the requirement for an effective stimulus. In addition, if inhibition of the sodium pump resulted in a small reduction in resting transmembrane potential, the stimulus requirement would also be diminished. The decreased excitability caused by higher concentrations of digitalis presumably results from the direct effect of digitalis on voltage-dependent inactivation of the fast inward channel (Kassebaum, 1963) and possibly also from a further reduction in RP sufficient to cause partial inactivation of the fast inward channel. Sufficiently high concentrations of digitalis can cause inexcitability of all cardiac tissues. The atria are more sensitive than ventricular muscle, and Purkinje fibers are much more sensitive than ventricular muscle to these toxic actions of digitalis (*see* Trautwein, 1963; Hoffman and Singer, 1964).

The effects of digitalis on *conduction velocity* in the different cardiac tissues is variable. Digitalis directly decreases the RP and slows conduction in atrial fibers. These effects are antagonized by the indirect vagal effects as long as the concentrations of glycoside are low. The increased liberation of acetylcholine tends to increase the RP. Also, conduction velocity depends, among other factors, not only on the level of the RP but also on the degree of inactivation of the fast inward channel, the membrane resistance, and the resistance between cardiac cells at gap junctions. Since high concentrations of digitalis can decrease RP, shift the curve describing inactivation of the fast inward channel in a depolarizing direction, decrease membrane resistance, and increase the resistance of the gap junctions, it becomes clear that sufficiently toxic concentrations of the drug can decrease conduction velocity in atrial and ventricular muscle fibers and cardiac Purkinje fibers. For the heart *in situ,* as for isolated ventricular and Purkinje tissue, conduction in the Purkinje system is seriously impaired at a lower concentration of drug than is required to affect ventricular muscle (Moe and Mendez, 1951; Swain and Weidner, 1957). Since digitalis typically does *not* prolong the QRS complex in the human ECG, the meaning of slowing of impulse propagation in the specialized conducting system of the canine heart is difficult to evaluate. The depression of conduction through the A-V node has been described in the previous section. Records of His bundle electrograms show that the prolongation of the P-R interval and the production of heart block are due primarily to actions on the A-V node and not to direct effects on the His bundle or bundle branches.

The effects of digitalis on the *refractoriness* of atrial muscle depend upon the relative predominance of the indirect (vagal) effects and the direct effects. Ordinarily, because of the enhanced vagal effects, the atrial refractory period is shortened. This is paralleled by a decrease in the duration of the atrial transmembrane action potential. However, if the

heart has been denervated or if atropine has been given, digitalis increases the duration of refractory periods in the atria, most likely because of its direct action. The effects of digitalis on the *ERP of the A-V node* have been described in detail. The vagal effect, the antiadrenergic effect, and the direct effect all increase the effective and functional refractory periods of the A-V junction. In the *ventricle,* digitalis shortens the duration of refractoriness, in parallel with the decrease in duration of the transmembrane AP. The change is modest in magnitude and proportional to the change in the Q-T interval in the ECG. Digitalis also alters the response of ventricular muscle to a single stimulus applied after the end of the T wave, such that a single stimulus can elicit repetitive ventricular responses (Lown *et al.,* 1967).

The effects of digitalis on impulse generation and conduction in the canine heart *in situ* provide a reasonably good picture of the usual changes brought about by therapeutic and toxic concentrations of cardiac glycosides in man. If sequential doses of digitalis are given gradually to an anesthetized dog to increase the body store and concentration in cardiac tissues, first to therapeutic and then to toxic levels, the sequence of changes in electrical activity is reasonably reproducible. Small doses of drug decrease the sinus rate and minimally increase the P-R interval. If premature stimuli are delivered to the atrium or if the atria are paced at progressively higher rates, it can be noted that the ERP of the A-V node is increased. Also, if the vagus is stimulated to cause A-V block, it can be seen that digitalis increases the automaticity of the specialized ventricular conducting system. This is evidenced by a decrease in the interval between the block and the first ventricular escape beat and by an increase in the rate of the escape rhythm as the dose of digitalis increases. The escape rhythms that occur after administration of digitalis are particularly interesting. They do not show the phenomenon of overdrive suppression. If a normal pacemaker in the His-Purkinje system is paced at a rate considerably in excess of the spontaneous rate, suppression of automatic activity results. When the pacing is discontinued, there is a pause, which is then followed by a spontaneous rhythm that increases slowly in rate. This overdrive suppression is not observed in the presence of digitalis; after overdrive, the rate of the ectopic pacemaker is usually increased (Wittenberg *et al.*, 1972).

The Human Heart in Situ. Perhaps surprisingly, most studies of the human atrium have shown only minimal effects of digitalis on the duration of refractoriness. This is true of normal atria (Dhingra *et al.*, 1975; Wu *et al.*, 1975) and those that have been denervated by cardiac transplantation (Goodman *et al.*, 1975). Refractoriness of the A-V node is increased, and A-V nodal conduction is slowed. The mechanism for this is similar to that described for the dog (Kosowsky *et al.*, 1968; Przybyla *et al.*, 1974). Refractoriness of the His-Purkinje system in man can be studied only by retrograde activation, because A-V nodal refractoriness usually prevents premature supraventricular impulses from propagating to the His bundle. When this method is used, intravenous ouabain in nontoxic doses does not cause any change in refractoriness or conduction in the His-Purkinje system (Gomes *et al.*, 1978). In contrast, the functional and effective refractory periods of ventricular muscle are decreased slightly but significantly. This may increase the interval during which ventricular premature depolarizations can induce reentrant excitation through the specialized conducting system.

Mechanism of Cardiac Slowing in Atrial Fibrillation. In typical atrial fibrillation the impulse spreads through the atrial synctium in a manner that may best be described as random reentry. Most atrial fibers are reexcited as soon as they recover sufficiently from refractoriness. The impulses arriving at the A-V node as a result of this activity are rapid (as many as 500 per minute) and random in time. Most of these impulses either fail to enter the A-V node because it is refractory or propagate only partway through it and give rise to the phenomenon of concealed conduction. The concealed conduction of these impulses increases the time during which nodal tissues are partially or totally refractory. The minimal interval between ventricular responses is determined by the ERP of the A-V node. Longer ventricular cycles occur when one or more successive atrial impulses enter the node but fail to propagate to the His bundle. The average frequency of the ventricular contractions during atrial fibrillation thus is determined by the refractoriness of the A-V junction. When atrial fibrillation is accompanied by congestive heart failure, the resulting reduction in vagal tone and increase in sympathetic tone increase the

ventricular rate. In rapid atrial fibrillation, the ventricular rate is grossly irregular and frequently, after short R-R intervals, stroke volume may be very small. The major effect of digitalis on ventricular rate during atrial fibrillation results from its actions on the A-V node. The ERP of the A-V node is prolonged by the increase in vagal effects, the direct effect of the glycoside, and perhaps by the antiadrenergic effect of digitalis described above. The net result of these actions is to decrease ventricular rate and, very often, to improve ventricular function.

In addition to its effects on A-V transmission, digitalis reduces ventricular rate during atrial fibrillation by another mechanism that operates simultaneously. Through its indirect action on the atria, mediated by acetylcholine, digitalis decreases the duration of the atrial transmembrane AP and decreases the ERP of atrial fibers. The result is that there is an increase in the mean frequency at which atrial fibers are excited. Because of the increase in the rate at which impulses enter the atrial margin of the A-V node, a greater proportion of them are extinguished as a result of concealed conduction and a smaller proportion propagate to excite the ventricles.

Action in Atrial Flutter. A circus-movement flutter about an obstacle of crushed atrial tissue in the dog heart will sustain itself at a stable frequency for hours, provided the path length (perimeter of the obstacle) is long enough to permit expiration of the refractory period between circuits. When such a flutter is established in an animal in which the vagi have been blocked with atropine, the administration of digitalis slows the flutter frequency and eventually restores normal sinus rhythm. In similar preparations in which the vagus nerves are intact, digitalis often converts the atrial flutter to atrial fibrillation. Administration of atropine may now restore normal rhythm. The explanation of these results may be found in the direct and indirect effects of digitalis upon the atrial refractory period. When the vagi are blocked, digitalis prolongs the refractory period; however, when the nerves are not blocked, the ERP is abbreviated (Farah and Loomis, 1950). The vagal effects are not uniformly distributed; the atrial refractory period is greatly reduced at some points and not at all at others. As a result, the flutter wave front becomes fractionated and fibrillation occurs.

Effect in Patients with the Wolff-Parkinson-White Syndrome. Effects of digitalis on conduction in and refractoriness of anomalous A-V bypass tracts are variable. Wellens and Durrer (1973) found that ouabain *decreased* refractoriness of the accessory pathways but did not change refractoriness of atrial muscle. In contrast, Sellers and coworkers (1977) found variable effects among different subjects. The important point to remember is that digitalis can decrease the ERP of the bypass tract sufficiently so that rapid atrial impulses can cause *ventricular fibrillation.* This decrease in refractoriness is seen in about 30% of patients with Wolff-Parkinson-White syndrome given the drug. This effect constitutes a clear *contraindication* to the use of digitalis.

Electrocardiographic Effects. Digitalis has characteristic effects on the ECG that may assist in determining whether a patient is taking digitalis. However, these changes cannot be used to estimate digitalis dosage or the degree of digitalization. Furthermore, the effects of digitalis are often superimposed on changes resulting from the basic cardiac disease. The ECG must be evaluated with these facts in mind. As mentioned previously, even toxic doses of digitalis do not cause an increase in the duration of the QRS complex.

Within 2 to 4 hours after a large oral dose of digitalis, definite alterations may appear in the ECG. Changes are first noted in the S-T segment or in the T wave itself. The normally upright T wave becomes diminished in amplitude, isoelectric, or inverted in one or more leads. The S-T segment may also show depression when the main QRS complex is upward; occasionally the S-T segment is elevated by digitalis when the main QRS deflection is downward. The changes in the S-T segment and the T wave may occur alone or may coincide. In precordial leads, these changes can simulate those resulting from coronary artery disease or recent coronary occlusion. After exercise in digitalized patients the J point may show depression similar to that caused by myocardial ischemia.

The P-R interval may be prolonged by digitalis. This effect occurs somewhat later than changes described above. The interval rarely becomes greater than 0.25 second, unless there is disease of the conduction system. Atropine can abolish lower degrees of A-V block produced by digitalis, but the direct (or antiadrenergic) actions of the drug are not overcome by atropine.

The Q-T interval is shortened by digitalis because ventricular repolarization is accelerated. Large doses occasionally cause changes in the size and the shape of the P wave. Digitalis can widen the abnormal QRS complex in the Wolff-Parkinson-White syndrome, probably by slowing A-V nodal propagation without affecting conduction time in the anomalous A-V pathway. This effect may be reversed by atropine. Almost every type of ECG tracing associated with cardiac disorders can be simulated by the effects of digitalis on the heart. However, if QRS widening occurs during normal sinus rhythm, it almost certainly is the result of concurrent disease, since digitalis does not cause this change.

Effects on the Cardiovascular System

The overall effects of digitalis on the cardiovascular system not only are a composite of changes in the force of ventricular contraction and heart rate but also result from effects on the autonomic nervous system and on vascular smooth muscle; furthermore, reflex adjustments to the initial hemodynamic changes caused by the drug are also important. The effects of digitalis on cardiovascular function differ depending on whether the heart and circulation are normal or whether there is congestive heart failure.

The extent to which digitalis changes systemic arterial pressure, cardiac output, heart size, and end-diastolic and venous pressure depends on whether the measurements are made while the subject is at rest or during exercise, as well as on other variables such as the use of anesthetics, the presence or absence of stress, and the work required of the heart at the time of measurement. For these reasons, there has been disagreement and argument for many years about many of the effects of digitalis on both the normal circulation and the circulation during congestive heart failure. It probably is helpful to consider first the changes brought about by the administration of digitalis to a conscious experimental animal or to a normal human subject and then deal with the effects of the drug in the presence of heart failure.

The Normal Heart and Circulation. When a rapidly acting drug like ouabain is injected intravenously into a *normal* conscious dog, the effects are reasonably clear and consistent (McRitchie and Vatner, 1976; Horwitz *et al.,* 1977). Usually there are increases in both systolic and mean arterial pressures that reach their maxima in 5 minutes and decline slowly over 30 minutes. All indices of ventricular contractility increase, but not markedly; these include the maximal rate of development of left intraventricular systolic pressure and the maximal rate of fiber shortening during systole. The increase in contractility can be demonstrated after doses of propranolol that block cardiac β-adrenergic receptors. It occurs in the absence of an increase in end-diastolic ventricular pressure or diameter and thus does not result from increased fiber length. The increase in contractility thus clearly results from the direct positive inotropic effect of digitalis. Heart rate usually decreases moderately, stroke volume increases, end-systolic ventricular volume decreases somewhat, and cardiac output is diminished slightly. If ouabain is injected after denervation of the arterial baroreceptors, usually there is little decrease in sinus rate even though the vagus nerves are intact; this indicates that a major cause of the sinus slowing is a reflex response to both the rate and the extent of increase in arterial pressure. If heart rate is maintained at the pretreatment value by atrial pacing, ouabain does not cause a decrease in cardiac output; however, there often is a decrease in heart size from the control value. The demonstration that the left ventricle can maintain or increase stroke volume and maintain cardiac output without an increase in end-diastolic fiber length and in spite of an increase in aortic pressure provides additional evidence that ouabain exerts a direct positive inotropic effect.

Since mean systemic arterial pressure is elevated without an increase in cardiac output, there must be an *increase in systemic vascular resistance.* This results from a direct effect of digitalis to cause contraction of the smooth muscle in the arterial resistance vessels. Digitalis also augments sympathetic outflow from the CNS, but this probably causes only minimal change in arterial resistance. After baroreceptor denervation, the glycoside-induced increase in systemic arterial pressure is enhanced; reflexes are thus important in modulating but not in causing the vasopressor effect of digitalis.

Digitalis also acts directly on *smooth muscle in veins* to cause constriction; in the dog, this effect is quite prominent in the hepatic veins and may result in venous pooling in the portal vessels. This action has been thought to be responsible for the decrease in cardiac output that often is observed after intravenous injection of digitalis into normal subjects.

If the effects of ouabain are evaluated in dogs during exercise, it can be shown that digitalis decreases maximal running speed, maximal cardiac index, and heart rate but causes no significant modification of the changes in left ventricular contractility, stroke volume, or end-diastolic diameter that result from the exercise. If the decrease in maximal heart rate is prevented with atropine, ouabain causes no significant change in any of these variables during exercise. If the effects of norepinephrine on the heart are blocked by propranolol, ouabain increases the maximal rate of development of pressure during exercise and improves exercise capacity. These findings indicate that the bradycardia caused by digitalis limits the capacity of the normal heart to do work. Furthermore, in the presence of very high levels of sympathetic activity, the positive inotropic effect of digitalis is negligible (Horwitz *et al.,* 1977).

Studies of the effects of digitalis on the heart and circulation of *normal human subjects* show that, in general, the changes are similar to those described above for the dog (Mason *et al.,* 1969; Smith and Haber, 1973). Digitalis exerts a direct positive inotropic effect on the normal human heart (Braunwald *et al.,* 1961). It causes a modest increase in systemic arterial pressure, an increase in systemic vascular resistance, and some venous constriction (Mason and Braunwald, 1964). Usually there is either no increase in cardiac output or a modest decrease; cardiac slowing is not prominent (Dresdale *et al.,* 1959; Selzer *et al.,* 1959). Overall, the increase in ventricular contractility is countered by the combined effect of increased systemic vascular resistance and decreased heart rate. Thus, cardiac output remains constant. The effects of the drug on patients with heart failure are quite different.

Heart Failure. To understand the effects of digitalis in patients with congestive heart failure, it is important to consider the factors that regulate cardiac contractility and their alteration in this disease. Furthermore, it is essential to appreciate other changes that are secondary to heart failure, such as retention of salt and water and reflex adjustments to impaired cardiac function.

The force developed by the ventricles during systole is regulated both by extrinsic factors, such as the level of sympathetic tone, and intrinsic factors, which include the frequency of contraction and the length of the fibers just before the onset of systole. In addition, the external work done by the ventricles is determined by their volume and the interaction between the afterload (the impedance met by the ventricle during ejection) and the contracting ventricle.

To describe the effects of digitalis on the failed ventricle it is essential first to consider the *pressure-volume relationship* described by Patterson and Starling in 1914 and extended by others in the form of the cardiac function curve (*see* Figure 30–5). For any given state of the ventricles, when end-diastolic fiber length and end-diastolic volume increase because of an increase in filling pressure, the force of ventricular contraction increases, up to a limit. Usually this results in an increase in the force developed during systole and in the stroke volume and stroke work. The absolute value of stroke volume or work for a given end-diastolic volume depends on the inotropic state of the ventricles. In the failing heart, the capacity to develop force during systole is reduced and thus a greater end-diastolic volume is needed to perform any given level of external work. In cardiac failure, therefore, one can imagine the following sequence of events. Reduced systolic ejection, caused by a mismatch of work capacity and load, results in decreased systolic ejection and an increased end-systolic volume. With constant filling, end-diastolic pressure and volume increase. If this sequence progresses, the ventricular volume will increase progressively. At the same time, because of the Laplace relationship, the effectiveness of increased wall tension in developing intraventricular pressure and the extent to which fiber shortening results in systolic ejection will both diminish. Further dilatation thus may be needed to maintain aortic flow. (At an excessive end-diastolic fiber length the force of contraction decreases; whether this occurs in the failed human heart *in situ* is doubtful.)

If, by means of the pressure-volume relation, the heart is unable to compensate for the load imposed, other mechanisms must be recruited; these usually include increased sympathetic and decreased vagal activity. These changes increase heart rate, myocardial contractility, systemic vascular resistance, and venous tone. Retention of salt and water may increase circulating blood volume. The retention of salt and water is due to decreased renal blood flow, in part because of increased activity in efferent sympathetic nerves. The increase in venous pressure is due in part to the venoconstriction, in part to the increased intravascular volume, and in part to the increase in end-diastolic right ventricular pressure.

If severe congestive heart failure involves both right and left ventricles, the following changes from normal usually will be found. Heart rate is elevated, end-diastolic ventricular pressures and volumes are increased, stroke volume is diminished, and end-systolic volume is increased. Cardiac output is decreased at rest and increases minimally with exertion. Systemic arterial resistance is elevated, primarily because of increased efferent sympathetic activity; tone in venous beds may be elevated. Because of the elevated diastolic left ventricular pressure, pulmonary capillary pressure is increased; if this capillary pressure exceeds a critical value, pulmonary edema develops. Because of edema and venous congestion, the lungs become stiffened and the work of breathing is increased; this results in dyspnea, orthopnea, and tachypnea. Because of the elevated right ventricular diastolic pressure, systemic venous pressure is increased and there is peripheral congestion, hepatomegaly, and edema. The increased sympathetic effect on renal vessels decreases renal perfusion, and this directly and indirectly results in retention of salt and water, increases blood volume, and contributes to the formation of edema. Systemic arterial pressure usually is not changed markedly as a result of failure and may be normal or elevated. Because of the decrease in cardiac output, perfusion of tissue is inadequate; hepatic blood flow may be decreased enough to slow elimination of some drugs, and cerebral perfusion may be impaired and result in confusion and other abnormalities of function of the CNS.

When digitalis is administered to patients with heart failure, its beneficial effects are primarily due to its direct positive inotropic action. A second important effect is the indirect action to decrease sinus rate. Because of the direct positive inotropic effect, the ventricles shift from one ventricular function curve to another (*see* Figure 30–5). They are thus able to develop more tension, empty more adequately, and eject more blood against the existing afterload. The increased stroke volume causes a decrease in end-systolic volume; since the ventricles contain less blood at the onset of diastole, end-diastolic pressure and volume both decrease if filling is constant. In spite of the decrease in fiber length, the ventricles can still do enough work to increase stroke volume because of the improved inotropic state. The decrease in heart size and the increase in output occur in spite of the decrease in heart rate. The direct positive inotropic effect thus increases cardiac output, decreases cardiac filling pressures, and decreases heart size and venous and capillary pressures. The decrease in ventricular volume increases the efficiency of contraction. Because of the improvement in the circulation, sympathetic activity is reduced; this, in turn, results in a decrease in systemic arterial resistance and venous tone. The former change decreases the afterload on the left ventricle and permits a further improvement in cardiac function.

Many factors are likely involved in the retention of salt and water in heart failure, but their consideration is not essential to the present discussion. However, the mechanism by which digitalization relieves edema is of interest. In addition to the fact that cardiac output is increased, the improved hemodynamic state that follows the administration of

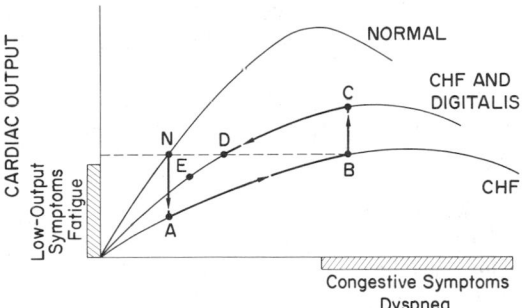

Figure 30-5. *Diagrammatic representation of the use of the Frank-Starling mechanism as a compensation for congestive heart failure.*

The three curves depict ventricular function in normal subjects and in those with congestive heart failure (*CHF*) and heart failure after treatment with digitalis. The points *N* through *D* represent in sequence: initial reduction of contractility due to congestive heart failure (*N* to *A*); use of Frank-Starling compensation to maintain cardiac output (*A* to *B*); increase in contractility when digitalis is administered (*B* to *C*); and reduction in the use of Frank-Starling compensation, which digitalis allows (*C* to *D*). Any factor that reduces ventricular filling pressure (decreased venous return) will lower cardiac output in spite of an inotropic effect (*D* to *E*). Of note is the fact that points *N, B,* and *D* all lie on the same line in the vertical axis and thus all represent the same cardiac output, but each is on a different end-diastolic pressure on the horizontal axis. The levels at which symptoms of congestion, such as dyspnea, and symptoms of low cardiac output, such as fatigue, occur are represented by the cross-hatched areas. (After Mason, 1973. Courtesy of *The American Journal of Cardiology.*)

digitalis causes a reduction in efferent sympathetic nerve impulse traffic and thus improves renal perfusion. However, in large part, the decrease in sympathetic impulses to the kidney may result primarily from a direct effect of digitalis on afferent nerve fiber endings in the heart. Acetylstrophanthidin applied to the ventricular epicardium or injected into the coronary circulation of dogs causes an almost immediate decrease in sympathetic nerve activity in the kidneys (Thames, 1979). This action appears to be mediated through neural receptors in the heart with vagal afferent connections. This mechanism might account for a number of other responses to digitalis that are manifest before the positive inotropic action is fully developed.

Effects on the Veins. In spite of repeated demonstrations of the action of digitalis on the contractile force of the heart muscle in many varied experimental preparations, it took many years to overcome arguments that the salutary action of the drug in congestive heart failure in man is due to some other action of the drug. After all, Withering himself believed its primary effect was on the kidneys. Mention has already been made of the emphasis long placed upon cardiac slowing as the primary therapeutic action. Harrison and Leonard (1926) showed that digitalis *decreased* the output of the nonfailing heart in normal dogs. Repeated confirmation of this observation resulted in the conclusion that digitalis reduces venous return, presumably by an action upon the venous capacitance vessels of the circulation (Cohn and Stewart, 1928; Dock and Tainter, 1930; Katz *et al.,* 1938; Cotten and Stopp, 1958). Similar results were obtained in normal human subjects (Stewart and Cohn, 1932; Bing *et al.,* 1950; Williams *et al.,* 1958). In the meantime, many observations showed beyond question that digitalis increases the cardiac output in patients with ventricular failure. As a result of these observations, the conviction grew that digitalis, although useful in heart failure, had an action on the peripheral veins that obscured or opposed its myocardial effects in the normal subject.

The concept of an extracardiac action upon the peripheral veins received its greatest impetus when it was reported that intravenous administration of digoxin to patients with congestive heart failure caused a reduction of central venous pressure before a measurable increase of cardiac output occurred (McMichael and Sharpey-Schafer, 1944). When the same laboratory reported that venesection also reduced the right atrial pressure and increased cardiac output in patients in advanced heart failure, it was again suggested that the primary action of digitalis was to diminish venomotor tone, resulting in a "physiological venesection." Explanation of these results was sought in the observations of Patterson and Starling: the output of the isolated heart increases to a maximum and then declines as the venous filling pressure is increased. The failing human heart was assumed to be "over the hump" of the Starling curve, that is, in a state in which reduction of venous pressure could result in an increased cardiac output (*see* Figure 30-5).

If digitalis acted primarily to increase the capacity of the veins, then it could increase cardiac output *only* if the heart were "over the hump," that is, in a state in which cardiac reserve is exhausted. At any level of filling pressure less than that at which maximal output is achieved, a primary reduction of venous pressure would reduce the output. This concept ignores the fact that the direct positive inotropic effect of digitalis shifts the heart from one function curve to another.

The effects of digitalis on venous tone and capacitance are important because they modify the pressure available to fill the ventricles. An understanding of this relationship is essential because treatment of congestive heart failure often includes, in addition to digitalis, the use of diuretics (which decrease blood volume and ventricular filling pressure) and vasodilators (which reduce afterload, preload, or both). This problem is considered in a subsequent section. However, it is clear from Figure 30–5 that a reduction in filling pressure (sufficient to shift ventricular function from *D* to *E*) would reduce cardiac output in spite of an improvement in contractility due to a direct positive inotropic effect.

Effects on the Coronary Circulation. The effects of digitalis on the coronary circulation depend on a number of actions, which can be described as direct and indirect. Digitalis glycosides constrict coronary arteries, presumably by a direct action on their smooth muscle. This effect may not be prominent when concentrations of drug in the plasma and tissues are kept at levels required to exert an optimal positive inotropic effect in heart failure.

Studies in man (Bing *et al.*, 1950) showed no significant change in coronary blood flow or cardiac oxygen consumption in normal subjects or those with heart failure given strophanthus glycosides intravenously. More recent studies in conscious dogs (Vatner *et al.*, 1978) have shown that ouabain can increase the perfusion of segments of the ventricle rendered ischemic by coronary occlusion and, in addition, can increase contractility of the ischemic parts of the myocardium.

Once again one faces the problem of discriminating between what digitalis can do and what it does do. This is quite important, because it may often be desirable to give digitalis to patients who have heart failure and reasonably severe coronary atherosclerosis. If the heart is dilated because of failure, it is likely that digitalis will improve the relationship between coronary flow and the needs of the myocardium for perfusion. The larger the heart during diastole, the greater the wall tension required to produce a given intraventricular pressure during systole. If digitalis decreases heart size during diastole, it is likely that this effect will more than compensate for any increase in oxygen consumption and requirement for perfusion that may result from the direct inotropic effect. If digitalis causes a decrease in heart rate and a decrease in the duration of systole, both of these changes will augment coronary perfusion. In *summary*, if the heart is dilated in failure, it seems most likely that the therapeutic effect of digitalis will improve the relationship between coronary flow and myocardial demand for perfusion.

In the case of regional ischemia, it probably is reasonable to assume that digitalis may exert its usual effect on the coronary vessels that provide blood to the nonischemic parts of the heart and cause constriction. At the same time the vessels that deliver blood to the ischemic regions may not respond to the same concentration of digitalis by constriction (Vatner *et al.*, 1978).

PHARMACOKINETICS

A detailed consideration of pharmacokinetics will be restricted to digoxin and digitoxin; these are the two most widely used preparations and have been studied most thoroughly in relation to clinical use. Some information on other preparations will be found below under Choice of Preparations. The significant data for digoxin and digitoxin are summarized in Table 30–1 (*see also* Appendix II).

Absorption. Absorption of *digoxin* after oral administration is somewhat variable; the fraction of the administered dose that is absorbed depends strongly on the type of preparation used and varies from 40 to 90%. Absorption is best with the preparation in a hydroalcoholic vehicle. Variation in bioavailability with tablets has been recognized as a significant clinical problem. Absorption of some preparations may be as low as 40%; with others the fraction reaches 75%. This variability is most prominent with tablets from different manufacturers; this does not result from differences in the content of active glycoside but from differences in the rate and extent of dissolution (Lindenbaum *et al.*, 1971, 1973; Wagner *et al.*, 1973). The problems of bioavailability of digoxin have been reviewed thoroughly (Harter *et al.*, 1974; New York Heart Association Task Force on Digitalis Preparations, 1974). It is advisable for physicians to use a preparation with which they are familiar and to indicate the commercial source if the drug is prescribed by a nonproprietary name. Absorption of digoxin also can be retarded by the presence of food in the gastrointestinal tract, by delayed gastric emptying, and by malabsorption syndromes. Antibiotics such as neomycin decrease absorption, as can steroid-binding resins (*see* below).

After oral administration, the concentration of digoxin in plasma typically reaches a peak in 2 to 3 hours; the maximal effect is apparent in 4 to 6 hours (Table 30–1). If a loading dose of digoxin is not given, up to 1 week can elapse before steady-state plasma concentrations are attained, since the half-life of the drug in the body is 1 to 2 days.

Absorption of *digitoxin* is much more complete (90 to 100%) than is that of digoxin because digitoxin is more lipid soluble. No significant problems with bioavailability have been noted for digitoxin, but its rate of absorption is also influenced by the factors mentioned above for digoxin. Because of its long half-life, steady-state concentrations in plasma are attained slowly and recovery from toxicity is protracted.

Distribution. The glycosides are distributed slowly in the body, in part due to their large volume of distribution. As for other drugs, the presence of congestive heart failure can influence the rate at which steady-state distribution is attained. About 25% of digoxin in the plasma is bound to proteins; in contrast, most (90% or more) digitoxin is so bound. These differences in binding account in part for the differences in apparent volume of distribution of the glycosides and in the concentrations in plasma that are associated with therapeutic effects. Digitalis glycosides are distributed to most body tissues, including red blood cells, skeletal muscle, and heart. At equilibrium, the concentrations in cardiac tissue are 15 to 30 times those in the plasma; the concentration in skeletal muscle is about half that in the heart. Binding to tissue is decreased by an increase in extracellular concentration of potassium, and the volume of distribution may be altered in some disease states. The time required to attain peak concentrations of digitalis glycosides in the heart and plasma is usually *less* than the time required for maximal effect; peak effect may not occur until 1 hour or more after levels in the heart reach their maximal value.

Elimination. *Digoxin* is eliminated primarily by the kidney. The drug is both filtered at the glomerulus and secreted by the tubules. There is some reabsorption from the tubular lumen, and this may become significant when the rate of flow of tubular fluid is markedly reduced. A very few patients form an inactive metabolite of digoxin, dihydrodigoxin; it is almost impossible to obtain a therapeutic effect with digoxin in such individuals. Also, a rare patient seems to form antibodies to the glycoside, and this prevents its therapeutic effect. *Digitoxin* is actively metabolized by hepatic microsomal enzymes; one of the products is digoxin. Metabolism of digitoxin may be accelerated by drugs that induce microsomal enzymes, including phenylbutazone, phenobarbital, phenytoin, and rifampin; the magnitude of this effect is variable among patients.

The half-time for elimination of *digoxin,* which averages 1.7 days, is strongly dependent on renal function; in most instances, there is a close correlation between the decrease in creatinine clearance and the concentration of digoxin in plasma that is attained with any given maintenance dose. The half-time for elimination of *digitoxin* is nearly 7 days and is *not* appreciably changed by hepatic disease; this probably reflects the huge reserve capacity of the liver for metabolic degradation of this drug. There is an enterohepatic circulation of digitoxin, but only a minor fraction of unchanged drug is eliminated through the intestine.

Dosage and Administration. Digitalis is used almost exclusively for two purposes—either to restore an adequate circulation in patients with congestive heart failure or to slow ventricular rate in patients with atrial fibrillation or flutter. Other uses are much less frequent. Since both conditions require chronic therapy, it is necessary to establish and to maintain an adequate concentration of digitalis in the heart. If there is no urgent need for an immediate effect, a maintenance dose can be given daily by mouth and its effect evaluated after appropriate intervals. A maximal effect will be achieved in approximately four elimination half-lives. On the other hand, if it is desired to achieve a full therapeutic effect fairly rapidly, it is necessary to give a large initial dose because of the relatively long half-time for elimination (*see* Table 30–1).

By tradition, the initial loading dose is called the *digitalizing dose.* The size of this dose may be difficult to estimate. In theory, it is the steady-state total body store sufficient to cause the desired therapeutic effect. However, the estimate of the loading dose must be adjusted for the condition of the individual patient. Depending on the state of the heart and the cause of the cardiac abnormality, the "digitalizing" dose may be much less than the dose that is likely to cause toxicity or it may be almost equal to it.

In practice, the digitalizing dose is selected from prior estimates (Table 30–1), with consideration of factors that increase or decrease the requirement for the individual patient (*see* below). If the need for a partial effect of digitalis is urgent, the initial dose is often given intravenously. If it is certain that the patient has *not* been taking digitalis, 1.0 mg of dig-

Table 30-1. DOSAGES, TIME OF EFFECT, AND FATE OF DIGOXIN AND DIGITOXIN IN MAN *

	DIGOXIN	DIGITOXIN
Average digitalizing dose		
Oral	1.0–2.5 mg	0.8–1.2 mg
IV	0.5–2.0 mg	0.8–1.2 mg
Average daily maintenance dose		
Oral	0.125–0.75 mg	0.05–0.2 mg
IV	0.25 mg	0.10 mg
Onset of action		
Oral	1.5–6 hr †	3–6 hr
IV	5–30 min	30–120 min
Maximal effect		
Oral	4–6 hr	6–12 hr
IV	1.5–3 hr	4–8 hr
Intestinal absorption	<40–90% ‡ (75%)	90–100%
Plasma protein binding	25%	90%
Disposition half-time	1.7 days	7 days
Route of elimination	Renal excretion of unchanged drug; limited hepatic metabolism	Hepatic degradation of molecule; renal excretion of metabolites
Enterohepatic circulation	Small	Large
"Therapeutic" plasma concentration	0.5–2.0 ng/ml	10–35 ng/ml

* *See also* Appendix II.

† Dependent on relationship of dose to meals, gastric emptying time, and type of preparation.

‡ About 90% of digoxin in an alcoholic elixir is absorbed from a normal enteric tract; about 75% of a tablet with high bioavailability is absorbed by a normal enteric tract. Absorption may be poor with certain tablets or when there is gastrointestinal malabsorption.

oxin can be given intravenously over a period of 10 to 20 minutes. Very often the loading dose is divided into two doses of 0.5 mg, given 3 to 4 hours apart. After the initial dose, a maintenance dose is administered daily and, after an appropriate interval, this may be increased or decreased as indicated by the therapeutic response and the concentration of drug in plasma. Because digitalis causes serious toxic effects so frequently and because digitalis toxicity is often lethal, it always is essential to observe the patient carefully, and it is frequently necessary to adjust the maintenance dose to achieve an optimal effect.

The maintenance dose must be equal to the daily loss. For *digoxin,* this is approximately 35% of the total body store; for *digitoxin,* approximately 10%. Regardless of the size of the initial dose, after a sufficient time (four to five times the $t_{1/2}$) the concentration in plasma and the total body store will be determined solely by the maintenance dose. Whether or not the desired effect has been obtained can be evaluated by careful and frequent observation of the patient. In patients with atrial fibrillation, the dose can be adjusted to produce the desired decrease in ventricular rate. Evaluation of effects in pa-

tients with heart failure is more difficult and should include quantification of changes in the signs and symptoms of failure, measurement of changes in body weight, venous pressure, and systolic time intervals, and evaluation of changes in exercise tolerance. The ECG and measurement of the concentration of cardiac glycoside in plasma may be helpful in adjusting the dosage.

Choice of Preparations and Routes of Administration. These decisions are made with consideration of the desired speed of onset of the therapeutic effect, the suitability of various routes of administration for the individual patient, the need for a stable concentration in plasma, and the likelihood of toxicity. Two preparations have a fairly rapid onset of action when they are administered intravenously—*ouabain* and *lanatoside C;* their rapid action is matched by a relatively short duration of action. Use of these preparations is infrequent and is probably more hazardous than use of digoxin. *Digoxin* can be given intravenously or orally; after intravenous administration there will be an appreciable effect in 5 to 30 minutes and a maximal effect in 1.5 to 2 hours. Digoxin should not be given intramuscularly because it causes severe pain and muscle necrosis. After oral administration, an effect usually will be evident in 1 to 2 hours and the peak effect will occur in 4 to

6 hours. Because of its relatively short $t_{1/2}$, the steady-state concentration of digoxin in plasma can be changed reasonably rapidly. The disadvantage of the use of this drug is that the therapeutic effect may be greatly diminished or lost if the patient fails to take several doses. Its advantage is that toxic effects disappear relatively rapidly after the drug is discontinued. *Digitoxin* is not associated with problems of bioavailability. Absorption is virtually complete after oral administration, and, compared with digoxin, concentrations in plasma are better maintained, particularly if a patient's compliance is sporadic. Elimination of the parent drug is ordinarily independent of renal function, and at times this may be an important consideration. On the other hand, because of the long $t_{1/2}$ of digitoxin, it may take days after discontinuation of therapy for a sufficient fraction of the total body store to be eliminated if there is toxicity. The major active glycoside in *digitalis leaf* is digitoxin. The preparation is standardized by bioassay. Variability in the potency of the preparation is likely, and, in most cases, there is no compelling reason to use it.

Assay and Unitage of Digitalis Preparations. The U.S.P. requires spectrophotometric assay of digitoxin, digoxin, and ouabain against appropriate reference standards. *Powdered Digitalis,* U.S.P., requires bioassay, by determination of the lethal dose in pigeons in comparison with that of a reference standard. Tablets or capsules of digitalis powder are prescribed by weight or in units. The official U.S.P. unit represents the potency of 100 mg of the U.S.P. *Digitalis Reference Standard Powder* and is roughly equivalent to 0.1 mg of digitoxin.

Preparations Available for Clinical Use. *Digitoxin,* U.S.P. (CRYSTODIGIN, PURODIGIN). As officially described, the drug is either pure digitoxin or a mixture of cardioactive glycosides obtained from *Digitalis purpurea, D. lanata,* or other species and consisting chiefly of digitoxin. *Digitoxin Tablets,* U.S.P., are available for oral use, each tablet containing 0.05, 0.1, 0.15, or 0.2 mg of drug. *Digitoxin Injection,* U.S.P., is available for *intravenous* administration and consists of a sterile solution of digitoxin in 40 to 50% alcohol; glycerin may also be present. Each milliliter contains 0.2 mg of the drug. There is evidence that market preparations of crystalline digitoxin may differ somewhat in potency.

Digoxin, U.S.P. (LANOXIN). This drug is a glycoside obtained from the leaves of *Digitalis lanata.* It is available for both oral and intravenous administration. *Digoxin Tablets,* U.S.P., contain 0.125, 0.25, 0.375, or 0.5 mg each. *Digoxin Elixir,* U.S.P., contains 0.05 mg/ml. *Digoxin Injection,* U.S.P., is a sterile solution of digoxin in 10% alcohol, each milliliter of solution containing 0.25 mg of drug. Because both the digoxin and the alcohol are tissue irritants, the appropriate dose should be diluted with 10 ml of sterile 0.9% sodium chloride solution before injection. The solution should be administered slowly (5 to 10 minutes), and care taken to avoid extravenous injection.

Lanatoside C (CEDILANID). This drug is no longer official. It is a precursor glycoside obtained from the leaves of *Digitalis lanata.* It is marketed only for oral administration in tablets that contain 0.5 mg of the glycoside. Lanatoside C is assayed in pigeons by the U.S.P. method for digitalis.

Deslanoside, U.S.P. (*desacetyl-lanatoside C;* CEDILANID-D). This precursor glycoside is derived from lanatoside C by alkaline hydrolysis, and is more soluble than the parent substance. Deslanoside exhibits the same pharmacological properties as lanatoside C, and for practical purposes merely constitutes the available injectable form of the latter. Deslanoside is assayed spectrophotometrically against a standard preparation. It is marketed as *Deslanoside Injection,* U.S.P., for intramuscular or intravenous use, in a sterile solution containing 10% ethanol. It is available in 2- and 4-ml ampuls containing 0.2 mg/ml of drug.

Acetyldigitoxin (ACYLAND). This is a crystalline glycoside derived from *Digitalis lanata.* It is supplied in tablets of 0.1 mg for oral use only.

Powdered Digitalis, U.S.P. This powder can be administered in pill, tablet, or capsule form. *Digitalis Tablets,* U.S.P., contain 32.5, 48.75, 65, or 100 mg of powder. *Digitalis Capsules,* U.S.P., contain 100 mg of powder.

Digitalis Tincture. This galenical preparation, formerly in wide use, is no longer official.

Ouabain, U.S.P. (*G-strophanthin*). This glycoside is available as *Ouabain Injection,* U.S.P., a sterile aqueous solution for intravenous injection; it is marketed as 2-ml ampuls containing 0.25 mg/ml. Various galenical preparations of *strophanthus* and of *squill* are no longer official.

THERAPEUTIC USES

Heart Failure. By far the most important use of digitalis is to treat heart failure. Digitalis is useful regardless of whether the failure is predominantly of the left or right ventricle or involves both. With very few exceptions, the type of rhythm exhibited by the decompensated heart neither indicates nor contraindicates the use of digitalis. Nevertheless, arrhythmias may modify the response to the drug.

Effectiveness. The effectiveness of digitalis in treating heart failure depends in part on the cause of the failure and in part on the severity of the cardiac damage. Failure can result from an increase in the requirement for blood flow, as in patients with anemia or left-to-right shunts; from an increase in the impedance to flow, as in patients with hypertension or valvular stenosis; or from a decrease in the capacity of the heart to do work, as in patients with coronary artery disease. In the first two cases, digitalis might exert a strong positive inotropic effect but still not restore the circulation to normal. In the third case, even with a maximal inotropic effect, the performance of the heart may be limited. Since it seems that toxic effects of digitalis on the heart are more likely if the heart is severely damaged, it is important to estimate the degree of improvement in the circulation that can be expected from an optimal concentration of drug in plasma and to recognize the need to correct abnormalities that increase the work required of the heart. Also, during maintenance therapy there may be changes in the condition of the patient that increase the concentration of digitalis in plasma or increase the sensitivity of the heart to its therapeutic or toxic effects (see below); usually it is desirable to use the lowest maintenance dose that provides the desired results.

Digitalis is particularly useful in patients with heart failure that results from an absolute or relative chronic overload (such as that caused by hypertension, valvular lesions, or atherosclerotic heart disease). Digitalis may not be of value in thyrotoxicosis, hypoxia, and severe thiamine deficiency. Experimental failure caused by poisons that reduce high-energy phosphate stores (cyanide, azide, dinitrophenol, etc.) is not relieved by digitalis (Gruhzit and Farah, 1955).

Once digitalis has restored compensation, its continued use often will do much to prevent the recurrence of heart failure. Usually it is unwise to omit the drug in patients with diminished cardiac reserve who previously have experienced an episode of failure, even though they are subsequently free of symptoms. Exceptions, of course, exist. Cardiac failure may be temporary following myocardial infarction; surgical correction of valvular lesions or successful therapy of hypertension may eliminate the need for continuing administration of digitalis.

The best results with digitalis are obtained in patients with *hypertensive* or *atherosclerotic* heart disease. In rheumatic, luetic, and congenital heart disease there is no specific defect that either indicates or contraindicates the use of digitalis. In forms of reversible heart disease, such as that associated with infections, anemia, thyrotoxicosis, thiamine deficiency, and arteriovenous fistula, correction of the underlying disease is of greater import than the administration of digitalis. Poor response to digitalis is to be expected in cases of active rheumatic and other forms of infectious or toxic myocarditis, and in advanced cardiomyopathy. Digitalis is not indicated in shock or in cardiac tamponade. When shock and congestive failure exist together, as they may after myocardial infarction, digitalis may be indicated for therapy of the failure. In the final analysis, improvement of cardiac function by digitalis depends on the cardiac reserve. In badly damaged hearts digitalis cannot provide much benefit.

The treatment of heart failure may require more than the administration of digitalis. For many patients, it is advisable to decrease sodium intake. If failure does not respond satisfactorily to digitalization and salt restriction, diuretics may be needed (see Chapter 36). There is little justification for using diuretics before digitalis in patients with heart failure. There is even less justification for using extremely potent diuretics when less potent ones are as effective and safer. There are two major clinical problems associated with the use of diuretics to treat congestive heart failure. Many decrease total body

stores of potassium, and this increases the likelihood of digitalis toxicity (see below). Furthermore, potent diuretics can cause such a large decrease in circulating blood volume that end-diastolic ventricular pressure may decrease markedly. If the heart requires an elevated filling pressure to perform its external work, this may increase the severity of failure (see Figure 30–5).

There has been renewed interest in the use of *vasodilators* to treat congestive heart failure. These agents may be particularly useful in emergency situations while waiting for digitalis to exert its effects. The drugs used for this purpose—nitroprusside, nitroglycerin, phentolamine, and others—are discussed in Chapter 33.

Use of Digitalis to Prevent Heart Failure. Numerous studies have shown improved cardiac function in subjects with heart disease without overt clinical evidence of failure (Selzer and Malborg, 1962). Also, it is possible and perhaps even likely that digitalization can decrease the rate of progression of cardiac damage in patients in whom the requirement for cardiac work, in relation to the work capacity of the heart, is such that a progressive increase in end-diastolic pressure and volume will occur. This may be particularly important in patients with inadequate coronary flow in whom the increase in ventricular volume and wall tension will decrease perfusion but increase the need for such perfusion. In all patients, if an increase in heart rate is needed to compensate for a diminished stroke volume, the energy requirement of the heart will be increased. Finally, it seems likely that marked overdistention of the ventricles causes structural changes that subsequently are not fully reversed by digitalization.

Atrial Fibrillation. Even in the absence of congestive heart failure, digitalis is indicated in most cases of atrial fibrillation. The inappropriately rapid ventricular rate in this disorder results in palpitation that may cause great discomfort, and a reduction in cardiac work capacity that may lead to heart failure. The aim of digitalis therapy in patients with atrial fibrillation is to reduce the ventricular rate. The mechanism of ventricular slowing by digitalis in this disorder has been discussed. The fibrillation is rarely halted by digitalis, and the drug should not be employed with this objective. The dosage should be adjusted to maintain the ventricular rate in the range of 60 to 80 per minute at rest, and not to exceed 100 with moderate exercise. If digitalis fails to cause a sufficient decrease in ventricular rate, a β-adrenergic blocking drug such as propranolol may also be used (see Chapter 31). Digitalis occasionally may be indicated as a prophylactic agent in patients in whom atrial fibrillation is likely.

Atrial Flutter. Digitalis can be used to manage atrial flutter. The primary effect of the drug is to increase the ERP of the A-V node. This almost always decreases the ventricular rate by increasing the degree of A-V block. Furthermore, digitalis prevents sudden increases in ventricular rate when exercise, excitement, or other factors decrease vagal and enhance sympathetic effects on A-V transmission. Digitalis can terminate atrial flutter. However, quite large doses are usually required, and cardioversion is preferable. Digitalis also may convert atrial flutter to fibrillation, and this, too, facilitates control of ventricular rate. Finally, if such conversion to fibrillation occurs, withdrawal of digitalis may result in the return of sinus rhythm. The change from flutter to fibrillation and the conversion to normal sinus rhythm probably result from digitalis-induced changes in vagal effects. If digitalis is used prior to attempts to convert atrial flutter to sinus rhythm with quinidine, there is an increased risk of digitalis toxicity (*see* below and Chapter 31).

Paroxysmal Tachycardia. Atrial and A-V nodal paroxysmal tachycardia are the most common tachyarrhythmias next to atrial fibrillation. Attacks are often abruptly terminated by measures that enhance vagal activity. Digitalis is often successful, probably by virtue of reflex vagal stimulation; intravenous administration of a rapidly acting preparation may be required. It should be remembered that *paroxysmal supraventricular tachycardia with partial A-V block may be a result of serious intoxication with digitalis.* It is extremely important to be certain of the diagnosis and etiology before digitalis is used.

Effects in Patients with the Sick Sinus Syndrome (Sinoatrial Dysfunction). In dogs, digoxin and ouabain slow conduction into and out of the sinus node, increase the sinus escape interval after overdrive, and increase the likelihood of sinus node reentry (Paulay and Damato, 1975). In man, however, digoxin decreases corrected sinus node recovery times and does not decrease sinus rate (Zakauddin *et al.,* 1978; Reiffel *et al.,* 1979). These findings suggest that digoxin does not have an adverse effect on the function of the sinus node in patients with the sick sinus syndrome. On the other hand, there has been one report (Margolis *et al.,* 1975) of severe toxicity in this condition. It would seem appropriate, if digitalization of such patients is required, to evaluate the effects of digitalis either by electrophysiological testing or by careful clinical monitoring.

DIGITALIS INTOXICATION

Withering recognized many of the signs of digitalis toxicity: "The foxglove when given in very large and quickly repeated doses, occasions sickness, vomiting, purging, giddiness, confused vision, objects appearing green or yellow; increased secretion of urine, with frequent motions to part with it; slow pulse, even as low as 35 in a minute, cold sweats, convulsions, syncope, death."

Toxic effects of digitalis are frequent and can be severe or lethal. The overall incidence of digitalis toxicity is not certain, but estimates have been made for some populations (Beller *et al.,* 1971; Smith, 1975); approximately 25% of hospitalized patients taking digitalis show some signs of toxicity. The single most frequent cause of intoxication with digitalis is the concurrent administration of diuretics that cause potassium depletion. As might be expected from the mode of action of digitalis, the manifestations of toxicity are varied and can involve most organ systems in the body. The most important toxic effects, in terms of risk to the patient, are those that involve the heart. If unrecognized or improperly treated, such reactions frequently cause fatality.

Digitalis is one of the most frequently prescribed drugs, and the number of patients for whom it is prescribed will increase as the proportion of older individuals in the population increases. Furthermore, all digitalis preparations have comparably low margins of safety and all can cause similarly severe toxic reactions. This is to be expected in view of their mechanism of action. The only difference among preparations is the duration of toxicity; for preparations that are more rapidly eliminated, the duration of toxicity will be comparatively short. *Because digitalis intoxication can be fatal and because it occurs frequently, physicians must exercise every precaution in prescribing digitalis; patients should be monitored carefully. Physicians must be familiar with the early signs of toxicity, the conditions or drugs likely to bring it about, and the means to treat intoxication. Patients should be educated about these matters as much as is deemed possible.*

Toxic Effects on the Heart. There is little evidence that excessive amounts of digitalis in patients have direct, deleterious effects on the mechanical activity of the heart. Concentrations in blood that are associated with toxicity typically cause abnormalities of cardiac rhythm and disturbances of A-V conduction, including complete A-V block. Ordinarily, abnormalities of conduction in the ventricular specialized conducting system and in the ventricles are not seen and, thus, digitalis does not directly prolong the QRS complex. Very high concentrations of the drug may impair conduction in the atria and prolong the P wave.

It is important to realize that all disturbances of rhythm associated with high concentrations of digitalis in plasma or tissues are *not* necessarily manifestations of digitalis toxicity and that low concentrations of the drug in plasma do not preclude the possibility of drug-induced arrhythmias or other toxicity. The concentrations measured in plasma serve only as crude, although useful, guides to the likelihood of efficacy and toxicity. Digitalis is used to treat patients with diseased hearts, and such hearts are likely to develop arrhythmias and conduction abnormalities. For example, an increase in the severity of heart failure often itself is a cause of atrial or ventricular arrhythmias. The demonstration that digitalis is the cause of such an arrhythmia or conduction abnormality depends on noting the response when administration of the drug is stopped, evaluation of the ECG, and measurement of the concentration of digitalis in plasma (Smith, 1975). In some instances, measurement of salivary Ca^{2+} and K^+ concentration may be of help (Wotman et al., 1971).

Although digitalis toxicity can mimic almost any arrhythmia or disturbance of conduction, certain abnormalities are of special importance (Bigger, 1972). Digitalis can cause marked *sinus bradycardia* and can also bring about *complete S-A block*. Both abnormalities probably result from a combination of enhanced vagal effects, a decreased sympathetic influence, and the direct effects of the drug. The likelihood is greater in patients with disease involving the sinus node. Toxicity can also be expressed as *disturbances of atrial rhythm*, including premature depolarizations and paroxysmal and nonparoxysmal tachycardias. The premature depolarizations and ectopic rhythms can result from enhanced automaticity brought about by the effects of digitalis on phase-4 depolarization, from the generation of delayed afterdepolarizations, or from reentrant excitation. Sufficiently precise tests are not yet available to identify each mechanism in patients.

The effects of digitalis on the *A-V junction* are important in relation to both its therapeutic and toxic effects. Toxicity is manifested by *high levels of A-V block* and by the appearance of *accelerated A-V junctional rhythms;* the most typical disturbances appear as either escape beats or as a nonparoxysmal *A-V junctional tachycardia.* This arrhythmia is almost always due to digitalis but occasionally can be caused by acute inferior myocardial infarction or acute carditis. The development of A-V block is due in part

to the vagal effects of digitalis and sometimes can be overcome by atropine; at other times the depression of A-V conduction almost certainly results from the direct effect of digitalis on the A-V node, perhaps intensified by its antiadrenergic action.

The accelerated rhythms originating in the A-V junction usually have been assumed to result from enhanced phase-4 depolarization, but more recent studies support delayed afterdepolarization as a cause of some types of escape beats. An A-V junctional tachycardia caused by toxic levels of digitalis may be quite difficult to recognize in patients with atrial fibrillation (Kastor and Yurchak, 1967).

The *disturbances of ventricular rhythm* most frequently caused by digitalis are *premature depolarizations* that appear as coupled beats (bigeminy, trigeminy); these arrhythmias are not specific for digitalis. Digitalis toxicity also can cause *ventricular tachycardia* and *ventricular fibrillation.* The premature depolarizations usually are not caused by increased automaticity; some very likely are due to reentry and some to delayed afterdepolarizations. Ventricular tachycardia probably results from increased automaticity of Purkinje fibers.

As mentioned above, digitalis decreases the ERP of human ventricular muscle but not that of the His-Purkinje system; it thus increases the interval during which reentrant excitation can be elicited (Gomes et al., 1978). In addition, it has been shown in experiments on dogs that certain disturbances of rhythm caused by digitalis respond to alterations in the dominant heart rate and rhythm in a manner that suggests they are due to delayed afterdepolarizations (Wittenberg et al., 1972). This makes it difficult to identify the mechanisms responsible for ventricular arrhythmias caused by digitalis. Sometimes, when digitalis causes a ventricular tachycardia, the polarity of the major QRS deflection in the ECG reverses for alternate complexes. This so-called *bidirectional tachycardia* once was thought to be a certain indication of excessive digitalis; however, the same ECG abnormality can be caused by other factors. The alternation in QRS polarity probably results from alternate excitation of the ventricles over one and then the other bundle branch.

Two further points about cardiac toxicity are of particular importance. First, the *likelihood* and probably also the *severity* of the arrhythmia are directly related to the severity of the underlying heart disease. If subjects with normal hearts ingest large but not lethal quantities of digitalis, either in an attempt at suicide or by accident, premature impulses and rapid arrhythmias are infrequent. The only typical findings are sinus bradycardia and A-V block. These disturbances probably result in large part from the marked increase in the concentration of potassium in plasma that is caused by severe, acute intoxication with digitalis. Second, infants and children seem to tolerate higher concentrations of digitalis in their plasma and myocardium than do adults. Studies on preparations isolated from canine hearts indicate that this results, at least in part, from real differences in sensitivity of the young specialized fibers to toxic effects of digitalis (Rosen *et al.*, 1975a). Also, the volume of distribution and the half-time for elimination of digitalis may be age dependent (Glantz *et al.*, 1976; Berman *et al.*, 1977).

Other Untoward Effects. *Gastrointestinal Effects. Anorexia, nausea,* and *vomiting* are among the earliest evidences of digitalis overdosage if digitalis leaf is used. Anorexia is most common with digoxin. Vomiting may occasionally develop without preliminary anorexia or nausea. This is especially likely if a large dose is given rapidly. The episodes of nausea and emesis may start and stop abruptly, only to recur with greater severity. Vomiting requires much physical effort, which the patient with congestive heart failure can ill afford. Nausea and vomiting may be transitory or entirely absent in some patients. *Diarrhea* may also be noted, and in rare cases it is the only gastrointestinal manifestation of digitalis toxicity. *Abdominal discomfort* or *pain* often accompanies the gastrointestinal symptoms. Once the drug is stopped, gastrointestinal symptoms disappear in a few days.

The *mechanism* of nausea and vomiting caused by cardiac glycosides has been investigated extensively (*see* review by Borison and Wang, 1953). Formerly, it was widely believed that gastrointestinal irritation from galenical preparations was the main cause of these symptoms. Subsequently, it was shown that emesis can be elicited by parenteral administration of digitalis and can be observed (retching movements) after complete removal of the gastrointestinal tract in animals. Local irritation thus is not the major factor in its production. The definitive studies of Borison, Wang, and their associates have demonstrated that vomiting induced shortly after intravenous administration of cardiac glycosides results from excitation of a chemoreceptor trigger zone

(CTZ), located in the area postrema of the medulla. However, gastric irritation may play a contributory role, since the incidence of nausea and vomiting is higher if digitalis leaf rather than a pure glycoside is prescribed.

Neurological Effects. Headache, fatigue, malaise, and *drowsiness* are common symptoms and can occur early in the course of digitalis intoxication; generalized muscle weakness and easy fatigability may be particularly prominent. *Neuralgic pain,* usually involving the lower third of the face and simulating trigeminal neuralgia, may be the earliest, most severe, and even the sole manifestation of digitalis intoxication; the extremities and lumbar area may also be involved, and paresthesias often accompany the pain. *Mental symptoms* include disorientation, confusion, aphasia, and even delirium and hallucinations ("digitalis delirium"); rarely, *convulsions* have occurred. Neuropsychiatric effects are especially likely to develop in elderly patients with atherosclerotic disease. The exact role played by digitalis is uncertain.

Vision. Vision is often blurred. White borders or halos may appear on dark objects ("white vision"), and objects may appear frosted. Color vision can be disturbed; chromatopsia is most common for yellow and green, but less frequently red, brown, and blue vision can occur. Transitory amblyopia, diplopia, and scotomata may also ensue. It has also been reported that digitalis can affect the papillomacular fibers of the optic nerve and cause retrobulbar neuritis. In an epidemic of accidental digitoxin intoxication, 95% of 179 patients complained of visual disturbances; 95% complained of extreme fatigue and weakness. ECG signs considered characteristic of digitalis poisoning were observed in 70% of the subjects (Lely and Enter, 1970).

Skin Rashes, Eosinophilia, and *Gynecomastia.* These are rare reactions to digitalis. The *skin lesions* may be urticarial or scarlatiniform in character, and are usually not aided by antihistamines. The increase in the number of *eosinophils* is often quite pronounced. *Gynecomastia* may be induced in men by digitalis therapy; it has been suggested that the drug, on the basis of its chemical similarity to the sex hormones, may exert estrogenic activity in certain cases.

Blood Coagulation. Experimental observations in animals suggest that digitalis preparations increase blood coagulability. Nevertheless, most carefully controlled clinical investigations indicate that digitalis has no adverse effect on coagulation time or heparin tolerance. Very rarely, digitalis can cause thrombocytopenia.

Factors Influencing the Likelihood of Toxicity. The most *obvious* cause of digitalis toxicity is the ingestion of too large a maintenance dose. The most *frequent* cause is concurrent administration of a diuretic that decreases body stores of potassium. Overdosage may result from the physician's decision, from the fact that the patient has independently increased the dose, or from improved absorption of the drug. The last-named cause might result from a change to a formulation with greater bioavailability. A decreased rate of elimination also could increase the concentration of drug in plasma to the toxic range. For digoxin, this can result from a decrease in renal function. Even quite marked abnormalities of hepatic function do not significantly decrease the metabolism of digitoxin. However, since one metabolite of digitoxin is digoxin, changes in renal elimination of the latter might contribute to toxicity when a patient is taking digitoxin.

Many factors are important in modifying the sensitivity of the heart to digitalis. A decrease in the plasma concentration of potassium is perhaps the most important cause of toxicity because many patients with congestive heart failure receive diuretics. Dialysis also can result in depletion of potassium. An abnormally high concentration of calcium in plasma can also contribute to toxicity. This could result from prolonged bed rest, myeloma, or parathyroid disease. A low concentration of magnesium in plasma has effects similar to those of high calcium. This change might result from diuretic therapy or dialysis. Hypothyroidism increases the likelihood of toxicity because elimination of digitalis is depressed and because in this condition the heart is more sensitive to cardiac glycosides. Conversely, hyperthyroid patients may require larger doses of digitalis to achieve a therapeutic effect. If hyperkalemia occurs in a patient taking maintenance doses of digitalis, complete A-V block may result.

It is important to remember that almost any worsening of the condition of the heart or circulation may increase the sensitivity of the heart to toxic actions of digitalis. Cardiac ischemia has this effect, as does an increase in the severity of congestive heart failure. With ischemia, there will very likely be a decrease in availability of chemical energy, and this can further depress the Na^+,K^+ pump. With severe impairment of ventilation or circulation there will be hypoxia and acidosis. The latter certainly contributes to toxicity, since a decrease in pH, like an increase in $[Ca^{2+}]_o$, depresses the Na^+,K^+-pump in cardiac tissues (Brown and Noble, 1978). With severe circulatory impairment, renal perfusion may be depressed. In addition, there likely will be an increase in heart rate in spite of the action of digitalis. The increase in rate can intensify the effects of digitalis by increasing the requirement of the pump for the transport of

cations. Finally, with severe heart failure there may be either an increase in sympathetic activity or additional depletion of cardiac stores of norepinephrine. Both changes might contribute to toxicity.

Advanced age almost always decreases the required maintenance dose of digitalis, and, as suggested above, infants and children often require larger doses than would be estimated from body size. In contrast, premature infants may be unusually sensitive to digitalis. During the first 24 to 48 hours after the onset of myocardial infarction there is an increased likelihood of toxic effects on rhythm and conduction from any dose of digitalis.

Diagnosis of Digitalis Intoxication. Digitalis is often used in situations in which the toxic effects of the drug are difficult to distinguish from the effects of cardiac disease. The diagnostic problem arises most frequently with the hospital admission of a patient with serious arrhythmia and congestive failure from whom a history of recent digitalis therapy cannot be elicited. Administration of a loading dose of a cardiac glycoside to such a patient obviously could be lethal if the arrhythmia were caused by digitalis. The use of the extremely short-acting glycoside *acetylstrophanthidin* as a provocative test to detect previous digitalization is hazardous and no longer should be employed (Lown *et al.,* 1972).

Other means to diagnose latent or overt toxicity have been suggested but not widely adopted. Lown showed that introduction of a single electrical stimulus to the ventricles after the end of the T wave caused repetitive ventricular responses in patients who were marginally toxic (Lown *et al.,* 1967). The intravenous administration of edrophonium will cause A-V block and the appearance of ventricular premature depolarizations in patients on the verge of overt toxicity. However, these tests are not without risk.

Sensitive specific methods for the estimation of the concentration of digitalis glycosides in plasma have now been developed to the stage where they are routinely used. The laboratory result can indicate whether or not the patient has recently received digitalis, and whether the concentration in plasma is within an unquestionably toxic range. However, the therapeutic and toxic ranges, not surprisingly, overlap. *Careful and judicious clinical appraisal is still the most important diagnostic tool* (Smith, 1975).

Treatment of Digitalis Intoxication. The treatment of digitalis toxicity is almost always successful if appropriate means are used (Fisch and Surawicz, 1969; Bigger and Strauss, 1972; Butler *et al.,* 1973; Smith and Haber, 1973; Smith, 1975). Thus, it is vitally important to make the correct diagnosis. The patient should be admitted to an intensive care unit and the ECG monitored. No additional digitalis should be given. Diuretics that cause potassium depletion should be withheld. If severe arrhythmias are present, additional treatment is needed. Phenytoin, lidocaine, and potassium salts are the most effective agents. Administration of K^+, either orally or intravenously, decreases the binding of digitalis to the heart and directly antagonizes certain cardiotoxic effects of the glycoside. If intravenous infusions are utilized, the ECG must be monitored frequently. It is essential, in addition, to measure the concentration of K^+ in plasma before and during the administration of potassium. If this value is low or normal, an increase will usually suppress many ectopic beats and abnormal rhythms caused by digitalis and improve depressed A-V conduction. In contrast, if the initial concentration of potassium in plasma is high, a further increase will *intensify* A-V block and depress the automaticity of ventricular pacemakers. *The result may be complete A-V block and cardiac arrest.* Potassium is contraindicated if A-V block is severe.

Among the antiarrhythmic drugs, *phenytoin* and *lidocaine* are quite effective in suppressing *ventricular arrhythmias* caused by digitalis (*see* Chapter 31). Phenytoin is also effective for the treatment of *atrial arrhythmias* caused by digitalis. The other antiarrhythmic drugs (quinidine, procainamide, propranolol) are effective at times but are associated with a higher probability of producing new arrhythmias. *Atropine* can be used to control sinus bradycardia, sinoatrial arrest, and second- or third-degree A-V block.

When toxicity is extreme, as when a very large amount has been taken in an attempt at suicide, it is possible to treat the toxicity experimentally with antibodies to the glycoside (Ochs and Smith, 1977). Very high doses of digitalis cause a progressive increase in the plasma concentration of potassium that is uniformly lethal. This can be reversed by administration of Fab fragments of digitalis-specific antibody. These fragments are not too likely to cause allergic reactions, and they bind digitalis effectively. Thus, they decrease the concentration of free drug available to interact with the heart cell membrane.

Several types of experiments have demonstrated the ability of antibodies to digitalis to reverse toxicity in isolated systems and in intact animals (*see* Ochs and Smith, 1977), and Fab fragments of digoxin-specific antibodies have been used clinically with success. In experimental animals, *digitoxin*-specific antibodies have similar desirable effects. This is important because 15 to 20% of patients in the United States who require digitalis are given digitoxin and because the elimination of this glycoside is quite slow. The Fab fragments of specific antibody have a very high affinity for the glycoside. After they are given, the total concentration of glycoside in plasma rises markedly because of binding to the antibody, but the fraction of drug in the plasma that is free is reduced to extremely low levels. The Fab-digitalis complex is eliminated readily in the urine. This is particularly important in settings where toxicity is caused by digitoxin.

A few other means for the treatment of cardiotoxicity due to digitalis should be mentioned. Certain binding resins (cholestyramine, colestipol; *see* Chapter 34) can decrease the reabsorption of digitoxin from the intestine. Dialysis is generally ineffective in lowering total body stores rapidly. For reasons that are not completely clear, electrical countershock is quite likely to result in conduction abnormalities and other serious arrhythmias in patients who are digitalized. It thus should not be employed indiscriminately to treat arrhythmias caused by digitalis toxicity, and, if used, the energy of the shock must be as low as possible.

Drug Interactions. Recent investigations have revealed a potentially important interaction between digoxin and *quinidine*. The administration of quinidine results in an increase in the plasma concentration of the glycoside in over 90% of digitalized patients (Ejvinsson, 1978; Leahey *et al.,* 1978). The degree of change is proportional to the dose of quinidine; however, there is marked individual variation in the magnitude (Doering, 1979). While the rise in the concentration of digoxin in plasma may be as great as fourfold, the average change is twofold. The concentration of digoxin in plasma apparently starts to rise within 24 hours after initiation of the administration of quinidine and reaches a new steady state in about 4 days. Thereafter it remains elevated for as long as quinidine is administered, unless the dose of digoxin is reduced appropriately (Doering, 1979; Leahey *et al.,* 1979). The effect of quinidine may be due to the displacement of digoxin from binding sites in tissues. Thus, there is a large decrease in the volume of distribution of digoxin. Since there is no change in the half-time for elimination, clearance of the drug apparently falls (Hager *et al.*, 1979).

It is not known if the concentration of digoxin in plasma correlates with its effects on the heart under these conditions (*e.g.*, drug may also be displaced from cardiac sites of action). However, data do suggest that effects of the cardiac glycoside are intensified (Leahey *et al.*, 1979). The digitalized patient who receives quinidine should be followed closely with respect to changes in the ECG and, if possible, the concentration of digoxin in plasma in order to make an appropriate adjustment of dosage; it may be advisable to reduce the dose of digoxin in anticipation of such changes (*see* Bigger, 1979). The use of antiarrhythmic drugs in conjunction with digitalis is further discussed in Chapter 31.

Interactions between cardiac glycosides and *diuretics* have been discussed above. *Amphotericin B,* which can also cause hypokalemia, may similarly provoke manifestations of digitalis intoxication. Administration of β-*adrenergic agonists* or *succinylcholine* may increase the likelihood of arrhythmias in digitalized patients. Agents that impair the absorption or alter the elimination of digitalis glycosides are mentioned elsewhere (*see* Appendix III).

AMRINONE

A recently discovered bipyridine derivative, *amrinone,* has been shown to exert a strong inotropic effect in a variety of preparations *in vitro* and *in vivo* (Alousi *et al.*, 1978; Farah and Alousi, 1978). Amrinone has the following structural formula:

Amrinone

This drug has had a very limited therapeutic trial in patients with congestive heart failure (Benotti *et al.*, 1978). When administered to patients maintained on digoxin who still showed evidence of congestive failure, the intravenous injection of amrinone increased cardiac output at rest, decreased left ventricle end-diastolic and pulmonary capillary wedge pressures, decreased right atrial pressure, and de-

creased systemic vascular resistance. In addition, the maximal rate of development of left ventricular pressure was augmented, as was left ventricular stroke work. More studies are needed to evaluate the role of amrinone in the treatment of heart failure and its safety for chronic administration.

Akera, T.; Larsen, F. S.; and Brody, T. M. Correlation of cardiac sodium- and potassium-activated adenosine triphosphatase activity with ouabain-induced inotropic stimulation. *J. Pharmacol. Exp. Ther.,* **1970,** *173,* 145–151.

Alousi, A. A.; Farah, A. E.; Lesher, G. Y.; and Opalka, C. J., Jr. Cardiotonic activity of amrinone (Win 40680): 5-amino-3,4′-bipyridin-6(IH)-one. *Fed. Proc.,* **1978,** *37,* 914.

Anderson, T. W.; Hirsch, C.; and Kavaler, F. Mechanism of activation of contraction in frog ventricle. *Circ. Res.,* **1977,** *41,* 472–480.

Aronson, R. S., and Gelles, J. H. The effect of ouabain, dinitrophenol and lithium on the pacemaker current in sheep cardiac Purkinje fibers. *Circ. Res.,* **1977,** *40,* 517–524.

Bailey, J. C.; Greenspan, K.; Elizari, M. V.; Anderson, G. J.; and Fisch, C. Effects of acetylcholine on automaticity and conduction in the proximal portion of the His-Purkinje specialized conduction system of the dog. *Circ. Res.,* **1972,** *30,* 210–216.

Bailey, J. C.; Watanabe, A. M.; Besch, H. R.; and Lathrop, D. A. Acetylcholine antagonism of the electrophysiological effects of isoproterenol on canine cardiac Purkinje fibers. *Circ. Res.,* **1979,** *44,* 378–383.

Bassingthwaighte, J. B.; Fry, C. H.; and McGuigan, J. A. S. Relationship between internal calcium and outward current in mammalian ventricular muscle: a mechanism for the control of the action potential duration? *J. Physiol. (Lond.),* **1976,** *262,* 15–37.

Beeler, G. W., and Reuter, H. The relationship between membrane potential, membrane currents and activation of contraction in ventricular myocardial fibers. *J. Physiol. (Lond.),* **1970,** *207,* 211–229.

Beller, G. A.; Smith, T. W.; Abelman, W. H.; Haber, E.; and Hood, W. B., Jr. Digitalis intoxication. A prospective clinical study with serum level correlations. *N. Engl. J. Med.,* **1971,** *284,* 989–997.

Benotti, J. R.; Grossman, W.; Braunwald, E.; Davalos, D. D.; and Alousi, A. A. Hemodynamic assessment of amrinone. A new inotropic agent. *N. Engl. J. Med.,* **1978,** *299,* 1373–1377.

Berman, W., Jr.; Ravenscroft, P. J.; Sheiner, L. B.; Hayman, M. A.; Melmon, K. L.; and Rudolph, A. M. Differential effects of digoxin at comparable concentrations in tissues of fetal and adult sheep. *Circ. Res.,* **1977,** *41,* 635–642.

Besch, H. R., Jr.; Allen, J. C.; Glick, G.; and Schwartz, A. Correlation between the inotropic action of ouabain and its effects on subcellular enzyme systems from canine myocardium. *J. Pharmacol. Exp. Ther.,* **1970,** *171,* 1–12.

Besch, H. R., Jr., and Watanabe, A. M. The positive inotropic effect of digitoxin: independence from sodium accumulation. *J. Pharmacol. Exp. Ther.,* **1978,** *207,* 958–965.

Bigger, J. T., Jr. The quinidine-digoxin interaction. What do we know about it? *N. Engl. J. Med.,* **1979,** *301,* 779–781.

Bigger, J. T., Jr., and Strauss, H. C. Digitalis toxicity: drug interactions promoting toxicity and the management of toxicity. *Semin. Drug Treat.,* **1972,** *2,* 147–177.

Bing, R. J.; Maraist, F. M.; Dammann, J. F.; Draper, A.; Heimbecker, R.; Daley, R.; Gerard, R.; and Calazel, P. Effect of strophanthus on coronary blood flow and cardiac oxygen consumption of normal and failing human hearts. *Circulation,* **1950,** *2,* 513–516.

Braunwald, E.; Bloodwell, R. D.; Goldberg, L. I.; and

Morrow, A. G.   Studies on digitalis. IV. Observations in man on the effects of digitalis preparations on the contractility of the nonfailing heart and on total vascular resistance. *J. Clin. Invest.,* **1961,** *40,* 52–59.

Brown, R. H.; Cohen, I.; and Noble, D.   The interactions of protons, calcium and potassium ions on cardiac Purkinje fibers. *J. Physiol. (Lond.),* **1978,** *282,* 345–352.

Brown, R. H., and Noble, D.   Displacement of activation thresholds in cardiac muscle by protons and calcium ions. *J. Physiol. (Lond.),* **1978,** *282,* 333–343.

Chai, C. Y.; Hsu, P. L.; and Wang, S. C.   Central locus of emetic action of digitalis substances in cats. *Neuropharmacology,* **1973,** *12,* 1187–1193.

Chai, C. Y.; Wang, H. H.; Hoffman, B. F.; and Wang, S. C.   Mechanisms of bradycardia induced by digitalis substances. *Am. J. Physiol.,* **1967,** *212,* 26–34.

Cohen, I.; Daut, J.; and Noble, D.   An analysis of the action of low concentrations of ouabain on membrane currents in Purkinje fibers. *J. Physiol. (Lond.),* **1976,** *260,* 75–104.

Cohn, A. E., and Stewart, H. J.   Relation between cardiac size and cardiac output per minute following administration of digitalis in normal dogs. *J. Clin. Invest.,* **1928,** *6,* 53–77.

Cotten, M. de V., and Stopp, P. E.   Action of digitalis on the non-failing dog heart. *Am. J. Physiol.,* **1958,** *192,* 114–120.

Cranefield, P. F.; Hoffman, B. F.; and Paes de Carvalho, A.   Effects of acetylcholine on single fibers of the atrioventricular node. *Circ. Res.,* **1959,** *7,* 19–23.

Danilo, P.; Rosen, M. R.; and Hordof, A. J.   Effects of acetylcholine on the ventricular specialized conducting system of neonatal and adult dogs. *Circ. Res.,* **1978,** *43,* 777–784.

Davis, L. D.   Effect of changes in cycle length on diastolic depolarization produced by ouabain in canine Purkinje fibers. *Circ. Res.,* **1973,** *32,* 206–214.

Deitmer, J. W., and Ellis, D.   The intracellular sodium activity of cardiac Purkinje fibers during inhibition and reactivation of the Na-K pump. *J. Physiol. (Lond.),* **1978,** *284,* 241–259.

DeMello, W. C.   Effect of intracellular injection of calcium and strontium on cell communication in heart. *J. Physiol. (Lond.),* **1975,** *250,* 231–245.

Dhingra, R. C.; Amat-y-Leon, F.; Wyndham, C.; Wu, D.; Denes, P.; and Rosen, K.   The electrophysiological effects of ouabain on sinus node and atrium in man. *J. Clin. Invest.,* **1975,** *56,* 555–562.

Dock, W., and Tainter, M. L.   The circulatory changes after full therapeutic doses of digitalis with a critical discussion of views on cardiac output. *J. Clin. Invest.,* **1930,** *8,* 467–484.

Doering, W.   Quinidine-digoxin interaction: pharmacokinetics, underlying mechanism and clinical implications. *N. Engl. J. Med.,* **1979,** *301,* 400–404.

Dresdale, P. T.; Yuceoglu, Y. Z.; Michton, R. J.; Schultz, M.; and Lunger, M.   Effects of lanatoside C on cardiovascular hemodynamics—acute digitalizing doses in subjects with normal hearts and with heart disease without failure. *Am. J. Cardiol.,* **1959,** *4,* 88–99.

Dutta, S.; Marks, B. H.; and Schoener, E. P.   Accumulation of radioactive cardiac glycosides by various brain regions in relation to the dysrhythmogenic effect. *Br. J. Pharmacol.,* **1977,** *59,* 101–106.

Ejvinsson, G.   Effect of quinidine on plasma concentrations of digoxin. *Br. Med. J.,* **1978,** *1,* 279–280.

Erlij, D., and Mendez, R.   The modification of digitalis intoxication by excluding adrenergic influences on the heart. *J. Pharmacol. Exp. Ther.,* **1964,** *144,* 97–103.

Fabiato, A., and Fabiato, F.   Calcium release from the sarcoplasmic reticulum. *Circ. Res.,* **1977,** *40,* 119–129.

Farah, A. E., and Alousi, A. A.   New cardiotonic agents: a search for a digitalis substitute. *Life Sci.,* **1978,** *22,* 1139–1148.

Farah, A. E., and Loomis, T. A.   The action of cardiac glycosides on experimental auricular flutter. *Circulation,* **1950,** *2,* 742–748.

Ferrier, G. R.   Effects of tension on acetylstrophanthidin-induced transient depolarizations and after-contractions in canine myocardial and Purkinje tissues. *Circ. Res.,* **1976,** *38,* 156–161.

Ferrier, G. R.; Saunders, J. H.; and Mendez, C.   A cellular mechanism for the generation of ventricular arrhythmias by acetylstrophanthidin. *Circ. Res.,* **1973,** *32,* 600–609.

Fullerton, D. S.; Yoshioka, K.; Rohrer, D. C.; From, A. H. L.; and Ahmed, K.   Digitalis genin activity: side-group carbonyl oxygen is a major determinant. *Science,* **1979,** *205,* 917–919.

Gadsby, D. C., and Cranefield, P. F.   Direct measurement of changes in sodium pump current in canine cardiac Purkinje fibers. *Proc. Natl. Acad. Sci. U.S.A.,* **1979,** *76,* 1783–1787.

Gadsby, D. C.; Wit, A. L.; and Cranefield, P. F.   The effects of acetylcholine on the electrical activity of canine cardiac Purkinje fibers. *Circ. Res.,* **1978,** *43,* 29–35.

Gaffney, T. E.; Kahn, J. B., Jr.; Van Maanen, E. F.; and Acheson, G. H.   A mechanism of the vagal effect of cardiac glycosides. *J. Pharmacol. Exp. Ther.,* **1958,** *122,* 423–429.

Gillis, R. A.; Raines, A.; Sohn, Y. J.; Levitt, B.; and Standaert, F. G.   Neuroexcitatory effects of digitalis and their role in the development of cardiac arrhythmias. *J. Pharmacol. Exp. Ther.,* **1972,** *185,* 154–168.

Glantz, J. A.; Kernoff, R.; and Goldman, R. H.   Age-related changes in ouabain pharmacology: ouabain exhibits a different volume of distribution in adult and young dogs. *Circ. Res.,* **1976,** *39,* 407–414.

Gold, H., and Cattell, M.   Mechanism of digitalis action in abolishing heart failure. *Arch. Intern. Med.,* **1940,** *65,* 263–278.

Gomes, J. A. C.; Dhatt, M. S.; Akhtar, M.; Carambas, C. R.; Rubenson, D. S.; and Damato, A.   Effects of digitalis on ventricular myocardial and His-Purkinje refractoriness and reentry in man. *Am. J. Cardiol.,* **1978,** *42,* 931–939.

Goodman, D. J.; Rossen, R. M.; Cannom, D. S.; Rider, A. K.; and Harrison, D. C.   Effects of digoxin on atrioventricular conduction. Studies in patients with and without cardiac autonomic innervation. *Circulation,* **1975,** *51,* 251–256.

Gruhzit, C. C., and Farah, A. E.   A comparison of the positive inotropic effects of ouabain and epinephrine in heart failure induced in the dog heart-lung preparation by sodium-pentobarbital, dinitrophenol, sodium cyanide, and sodium azide. *J. Pharmacol. Exp. Ther.,* **1955,** *114,* 334–342.

Hager, W. D.; Fenster, P.; Mayersohn, M.; Perrier, D.; Graves, P.; Marcus, F. I.; and Goldman, S.   Digoxin-quinidine interaction: pharmacokinetic evaluation. *N. Engl. J. Med.,* **1979,** *300,* 1238–1241.

Harrison, T. R., and Leonard, B. W.   The effects of digitalis on the cardiac output of dogs and its bearing on the action of the drug in heart disease. *J. Clin. Invest.,* **1926,** *3,* 1–36.

Harter, J. G.; Skelly, J. P.; and Steers, A. W.   Digoxin—the regulatory viewpoint. *Circulation,* **1974,** *49,* 395–398.

Hashimoto, K., and Moe, G. K.   Transient depolarizations induced by acetylstrophanthidin in specialized tissues of dog atrium and ventricle. *Circ. Res.,* **1973,** *32,* 618–624.

Holloway, L. S.; Bradley, I. B.; Janssen, H.; and O'Brien, L. J.   Cardiovascular effects of cerebroventricular ouabain perfusion in the adult dog. *Am. J. Physiol.,* **1976,** *230,* 1168–1172.

Hordof, A. J.; Spotnitz, A.; Mary-Rabine, L.; Edie, R. N.; and Rosen, M. R.   The cellular electrophysiologic effects of digitalis on human atrial fibers. *Circulation,* **1978,** *57,* 223–229.

Horwitz, L. D.; Atkins, J. M.; and Saito, M.   Effects of

digitalis on left ventricular function in exercising dogs. *Circ. Res.,* **1977,** *41,* 744–749.

Hougen, T. J., and Smith, T. W. Inhibition of myocardial cation active transport by subtoxic doses of ouabain in the dog. *Circ. Res.,* **1978,** *42,* 856–863.

Isenberg, G., and Trautwein, W. The effect of dihydro-ouabain and lithium ions on the outward current in cardiac Purkinje fibers. Evidence for electrogenicity of active transport. *Pfluegers Arch.,* **1974,** *350,* 41–54.

Kass, R. S.; Lederer, W. J.; Tsien, R. W.; and Weingart, R. Role of calcium ions in transient inward currents and aftercontractions induced by strophanthidin in cardiac Purkinje fibers. *J. Physiol. (Lond.),* **1978a,** *281,* 187–208.

Kass, R. S.; Tsien, R. W.; and Weingart, R. Ionic basis of transient inward current induced by strophanthidin in cardiac Purkinje fibers. *J. Physiol. (Lond.),* **1978b,** *281,* 209–226.

Kassebaum, D. G. Electrophysiological effects of strophanthin in the heart. *J. Pharmacol. Exp. Ther.,* **1963,** *140,* 329–338.

Kastor, J. A., and Yurchak, P. M. Recognition of digitalis intoxication in the presence of atrial fibrillation. *Ann. Intern. Med.,* **1967,** *67,* 1045–1054.

Katz, L. N.; Rodbard, S.; Friend, M.; and Rottersman, W. The effect of digitalis in the anesthetized dog. 1. Action on the splanchnic bed. *J. Pharmacol. Exp. Ther.,* **1938,** *62,* 1–15.

Kosowsky, B. D.; Haft, J. I.; Stein, E.; and Damato, A. N. The effects of digitalis on atrioventricular conduction in man. *Am. Heart J.,* **1968,** *75,* 736–742.

Leahey, E. B., Jr.; Reiffel, J. A.; Drusin, R. E.; Heissenbuttel, R. H.; Lovejoy, W. P.; and Bigger, J. T., Jr. Interaction between quinidine and digoxin. *J.A.M.A.,* **1978,** *240,* 533–534.

Leahey, E. B., Jr.; Reiffel, J. A.; Heissenbuttel, R. H.; Drusin, R. E.; Lovejoy, W. P.; and Bigger, J. T., Jr. Enhanced cardiac effect of digoxin during quinidine treatment. *Arch. Intern. Med.,* **1979,** *139,* 519–521.

Lederer, W. J., and Tsien, R. W. Transient inward current underlying arrhythmogenic effects of cardiotonic steroids in Purkinje fibers. *J. Physiol. (Lond.),* **1976,** *263,* 73–100.

Lely, A. H., and Enter, C. H. J. van. Large scale digitoxin intoxication. *Br. Med. J.,* **1970,** *3,* 737–740.

Levitt, B.; Raines, A.; Sohn, Y. J.; Standaert, F. G.; and Hirshfield, J. W. The nervous system as a site of action for digitalis and antiarrhythmic drugs. *Mt. Sinai J. Med. N.Y.,* **1970,** *37,* 227–240.

Levy, M. N. Sympathetic-parasympathetic interactions in the heart. *Circ. Res.,* **1971,** *29,* 437–445.

Lindenbaum, J.; Butler, V. P.; Murphy, J. E.; and Cresswell, R. M. Correlation of digoxin-tablet dissolution rate with biological availability. *Lancet,* **1973,** *1,* 1215–1217.

Lindenbaum, J.; Mellow, M. H.; Blackstone, M. O.; and Butler, V. P., Jr. Variability in biological availability of digoxin from four preparations. *N. Engl. J. Med.,* **1971,** *285,* 1344–1347.

Lown, B.; Cannon, R. L.; and Rossi, M. A. Electrical stimulation and digitalis drugs: repetitive response in diastole. *Proc. Soc. Exp. Biol. Med.,* **1967,** *126,* 698–701.

McLain, P. L. Effects of cardiac glycosides on spontaneous efferent activity in vagus and sympathetic nerves of cats. *Int. J. Neuropharmacol.,* **1969,** *8,* 379–387.

McMichael, J., and Sharpey-Schafer, E. P. The action of intravenous digoxin in man. *Q. J. Med.,* **1944,** *13,* 123–135.

McRitchie, R. J., and Vatner, S. F. The role of the arterial baroceptors in mediating cardiovascular responses to cardiac glycosides in conscious dogs. *Circ. Res.,* **1976,** *38,* 321–326.

Margolis, J. R.; Strauss, H. C.; Miller, H. C.; Gilbert, M.; and Wallace, A. G. Digitalis and the sick sinus syndrome: clinical and electrophysiologic documentation of a severe toxic effect on sinus node function. *Circulation,* **1975,** *52,* 162–169.

Mason, D. T. Regulation of cardiac performance in clinical heart disease: interactions between contractile state mechanical abnormalities and ventricular compensatory mechanisms. *Am. J. Cardiol.,* **1973,** *32,* 437–448.

Mason, D. T., and Braunwald, E. Studies on digitalis. X. Effects of ouabain on forearm vascular resistance and venous tone in normal subjects and in patients in heart failure. *J. Clin. Invest.,* **1964,** *43,* 532–543.

Mason, D. T.; Spann, J. F., Jr.; and Zelis, R. New developments in the understanding of the actions of the digitalis glycosides. *Prog. Cardiovasc. Dis.,* **1969,** *11,* 443–478.

Mendez, C.; Aceves, J.; and Mendez, R. Inhibition of adrenergic cardiac acceleration by cardiac glycosides. *J. Pharmacol. Exp. Ther.,* **1961,** *131,* 191–198.

Mendez, C., and Mendez, R. The action of cardiac glycosides on the excitability and conduction velocity of the mammalian atrium. *J. Pharmacol. Exp. Ther.,* **1957,** *121,* 402–413.

Miura, D. S., and Rosen, M. R. The effects of ouabain on the transmembrane potentials and intracellular potassium activity of canine cardiac Purkinje fibers. *Circ. Res.,* **1978,** *42,* 333–338.

Moe, G. K., and Mendez, R. The action of several cardiac glycosides on conduction velocity and ventricular excitability in the dog heart. *Circulation,* **1951,** *4,* 729–734.

Mudge, G. H.; Lloyd, B. L.; Greenblatt, D. J.; and Smith, T. W. Inotropic and toxic effects of a polar cardiac glycoside derivative in the dog. *Circ. Res.,* **1978,** *43,* 847–854.

Müller, P. Ouabain effects on cardiac contraction, action potential and cellular potassium. *Circ. Res.,* **1965,** *17,* 46–56.

Nadeau, R. A., and James, T. N. Antagonistic effects on the sinus node of acetyl strophanthidin and adrenergic stimulation. *Circ. Res.,* **1963,** *13,* 338–391.

New York Heart Association Task Force on Digitalis Preparations. What should the practicing physician know about digoxin bioavailability and how will FDA action affect him? *Circulation,* **1974,** *49,* 399–400.

Ochs, H. R., and Smith, T. W. Reversal of advanced digoxin toxicity and modification of pharmacokinetics by specific antibodies and Fab fragments. *J. Clin. Invest.,* **1977,** *60,* 1303–1313.

Okita, G. T.; Richardson, F.; and Roth-Schechter, B. F. Dissociation of the positive inotropic actions of digitalis from inhibition of sodium- and potassium-activated adenosine triphosphatase. *J. Pharmacol. Exp. Ther.,* **1973,** *185,* 1–11.

Pace, D. B., and Gillis, R. A. Neuroexcitatory effects of digoxin in the cat. *J. Pharmacol. Exp. Ther.,* **1976,** *199,* 583–600.

Paulay, K. L., and Damato, A. N. Effect of digoxin on sinus nodal reentry in the dog. *Am. J. Cardiol.,* **1975,** *35,* 370–375.

Perry, W. L. M., and Reinhert, H. The action of cardiac glycosides on autonomic ganglia. *Br. J. Pharmacol.,* **1954,** *9,* 324–328.

Przybyla, A. C.; Paulay, K. L.; Stein, E.; and Damato, A. N. Effects of digoxin on atrioventricular conduction patterns in man. *Am. J. Cardiol.,* **1974,** *33,* 344–350.

Reiffel, J. A.; Bigger, J. T., Jr.; and Cramer, M. The effects of digoxin on sinus nodal function before and after vagal blockade in patients with sinus nodal dysfunction: a clue to the mechanisms of the action of digitalis on the sinus node. *Am. J. Cardiol.,* **1979,** *43,* 983–989.

Rosen, M. R.; Gelband, H.; and Hoffman, B. F. Correlation between effects of ouabain on the canine electrocardiogram and transmembrane potentials of isolated Purkinje fibers. *Circ. Res.,* **1973a,** *47,* 65–72.

Rosen, M. R.; Gelband, H.; Merker, C.; and Hoffman, B. F. Mechanisms of digitalis toxicity: effects of ouabain on phase 4 of canine Purkinje fiber transmembrane potentials. *Circ. Res.,* **1973b,** *47,* 681–689.

Rosen, M. R.; Hordof, A. J.; Hodess, A. B.; Verosky, M.; and Vulliemoz, Y. Ouabain-induced changes in electrophysiologic properties of neonatal, young and adult canine cardiac Purkinje fibers. *J. Pharmacol. Exp. Ther.,* **1975a,** *194,* 255–263.

Rosen, M. R.; Wit, A. L.; and Hoffman, B. F. Electrophysiology and pharmacology of cardiac arrhythmias. IV. Cardiac antiarrhythmic and toxic effects of digitalis. *Am. Heart J.,* **1975b,** *89,* 391–399.

Saum, R. W.; Brown, A. M.; and Tuley, F. H. An electrogenic sodium pump and baroceptor function in normotensive and spontaneously hypertensive rats. *Circ. Res.,* **1976,** *39,* 497–505.

Schatzmann, H. J. Herzglycoside als Hemmstoffe für den aktiven Kalium- und Natriumtransport durch die Erythrocytenmembran. *Helv. Physiol. Pharmacol. Acta,* **1953,** *11,* 346–354.

Schwartz, A. Is the cell membrane Na$^+$,K$^+$-ATPase enzyme system the pharmacological receptor for digitalis? *Circ. Res.,* **1976,** *39,* 2–7.

Sellers, T. D., Jr.; Bashore, T. M.; and Gallagher, J. J. Digitalis in the preexcitation syndrome: analysis during atrial fibrillation. *Circulation,* **1977,** *56,* 260–270.

Selzer, A.; Hultgren, H. N.; Ebnother, C. L.; Bradley, H. W.; and Stone, A. O. Effects of digoxin on the circulation in normal man. *Br. Heart J.,* **1959,** *21,* 335–342.

Selzer, A., and Malmborg, R. O. Hemodynamic effects of digoxin in latent cardiac failure. *Circulation,* **1962,** *25,* 695–702.

Smith, T. W. Digitalis toxicity: epidemiology and clinical use of serum concentration measurements. *Am. J. Med.,* **1975,** *58,* 470–476.

Smith, T. W., and Haber, E. Medical progress: digitalis. *N. Engl. J. Med.,* **1973,** *289,* 945–952, 1010–1015, 1063–1072, 1125–1129.

Stewart, H. J., and Cohn, A. E. Studies on effect of action of digitalis on output of blood from heart; effect on output in normal human hearts; effect on output of hearts in heart failure with congestion in human beings. *J. Clin. Invest.,* **1932,** *11,* 917–955.

Swain, H. H., and Weidner, C. L. A study of substances which alter intraventricular conduction in isolated dog heart. *J. Pharmacol. Exp. Ther.,* **1957,** *120,* 137–146.

Ten Eick, R. E., and Hoffman, B. F. Chronotropic effect of cardiac glycosides in cats, dogs and rabbits. *Circ. Res.,* **1969a,** *25,* 365–378.

———. The effect of digitalis on the excitability of autonomic nerves. *J. Pharmacol. Exp. Ther.,* **1969b,** *169,* 95–108.

Thames, M. D. Acetylstrophanthidin-induced reflex inhibition of canine renal sympathetic nerve activity mediated by cardiac receptors with vagal afferents. *Circ. Res.,* **1979,** *44,* 8–15.

Toda, N., and West, T. C. Influence of ouabain on cholinergic responses in the sinoatrial node. *J. Pharmacol. Exp. Ther.,* **1966,** *153,* 104–113.

Tse, W., and Han, J. Interaction of epinephrine and ouabain on automaticity of canine Purkinje fibers. *Circ. Res.,* **1978,** *34,* 777–782.

Vassalle, M.; Karis, J.; and Hoffman, B. F. Toxic effects of ouabain on Purkinje fibers and ventricular muscle fibers. *Am. J. Physiol.,* **1962,** *203,* 433–439.

Vatner, J. F.; Haig, B. W.; Manders, T.; and Murray, P. A. Effect of a cardiac glycoside on regional function, blood flow and electrograms in conscious dogs with myocardial ischemia. *Circ. Res.,* **1978,** *43,* 413–423.

Vick, R. L.; Kahn, J. B., Jr.; and Acheson, G. H. Effects of dihydrodigoxin and dihydrodigitoxin on the heart-lung preparation of the dog. *J. Pharmacol. Exp. Ther.,* **1957,** *121,* 330–339.

Wagner, J. G.; Christensen, M.; Sakmar, E.; Blair, D.; Yates, J. D.; Willis, P. W., III; Sedman, A. J.; and Stall, R. G. Equivalence lack in digoxin plasma levels. *J.A.M.A.,* **1973,** *224,* 199–204.

Weaver, L. C.; Akera, T.; and Brody, T. M. Digitalis toxicity: lack of marked effect on brain Na$^+$-K$^+$ adenosine triphosphatase in the cat. *J. Pharmacol. Exp. Ther.,* **1977,** *200,* 638–646.

Weingart, R. The actions of ouabain on intercellular coupling and conduction velocity in mammalian ventricular muscle. *J. Physiol. (Lond.),* **1977,** *264,* 341–365.

Wellens, H. J., and Durrer, D. Effect of digitalis on atrioventricular conduction and circus movement tachycardias in patients with Wolff-Parkinson-White syndrome. *Circulation,* **1973,** *47,* 1229–1233.

Wenckebach, K. F. Discussion on the effects of digitalis on the human heart. *Br. Med. J.,* **1910,** *2,* 1600–1605.

Wilbrandt, W. Zum Wirkungmechanismus des Herzglykoside. *Schweiz. Med. Wochenschr.,* **1955,** *85,* 315–320.

Williams, M. H.; Zohman, L. R.; and Ratner, A. C. Hemodynamic effects of cardiac glycosides on normal human subjects during rest and exercise. *J. Appl. Physiol.,* **1958,** *13,* 417–421.

Wittenberg, S. M.; Gandel, P.; Hogan, P. M.; Kreuger, W.; and Klocke, F. J. Relationship of heart rate to ventricular automaticity in dogs during ouabain administration. *Circ. Res.,* **1972,** *30,* 167–176.

Wotman, S.; Bigger, J. T.; Mandel, I. D.; and Bartelstone, H. J. Salivary electrolytes in the detection of digitalis toxicity. *N. Engl. J. Med.,* **1971,** *285,* 871–876.

Wu, D.; Wyndham, C.; Amat-y-Leon, F.; Denes, P.; Dhingra, R.; and Rosen, K. The effects of ouabain on induction of atrioventricular nodal re-entrant paroxysmal supraventricular tachycardia. *Circulation,* **1975,** *52,* 201–207.

Zakauddin, V.; Miller, R. R.; McMillin, D.; and Mason, D. T. Effects of digitalis on sinus nodal function in patients with sick sinus syndrome. *Am. J. Cardiol.,* **1978,** *41,* 318–375.

Monographs and Reviews

Bigger, J. T., Jr. Mechanisms of digitalis toxic arrhythmias and the clinical recognition of toxicity. In, *Controversies in Clinical Pharmacology and Drug Development.* (Palmer, W., ed.) Futura Publishing Co., Inc., Mount Kisco, N.Y., **1972.**

Borison, H. L., and Wang, S. C. Physiology and pharmacology of vomiting. *Pharmacol. Rev.,* **1953,** *5,* 193–230.

Butler, V. P., Jr.; Watson, J. F.; Schmidt, D. H.; Gardner, J. D.; Mandel, W. J.; and Skelton, C. L. Reversal of pharmacological and toxic effects of cardiac glycosides by specific antibodies. *Pharmacol. Rev.,* **1973,** *25,* 239–248.

Carpentier, R., and Vassalle, M. Enhancement and inhibition of a frequency-activated electrogenic sodium pump in cardiac Purkinje fibers. In, *Research in Physiology.* (Kao, F. F.; Koizumi, K.; and Vassalle, M., eds.) Aulo Gaggi, Bologna, **1971.**

Chen, K. K., and Henderson, F. G. Pharmacology of sixty-four cardiac glycosides and aglycones. *J. Pharmacol. Exp. Ther.,* **1954,** *111,* 365–383.

Fieser, L. F., and Fieser, M. *Steroids.* Reinhold Publishing Corp., New York, **1959.**

Fisch, C., and Surawicz, B. *Digitalis.* Grune & Stratton, Inc., New York, **1969.**

Hoffman, B. F., and Singer, D. H. Effects of digitalis on electrical activity of cardiac fibers. *Prog. Cardiovasc. Dis.,* **1964,** *7,* 226–260.

Katz, A. M. *Physiology of the Heart.* Raven Press, New York, **1977.**

Lown, B.; Hagemeijer, F.; Barr, I.; and Klein, M. Digitalis intoxication: clinical and experimental assessment of the degree of digitalization. In, *Basic and Clinical Pharma-*

cology of Digitalis. (Marks, B. H., and Weissler, A. M., eds.) Charles C Thomas, Pub., Springfield, Ill., **1972,** pp. 299–318.

Marshall, P. G. Steroids: cardiotonic glycosides and aglycones: toad poisons. In, *Rodd's Chemistry of Carbon Compounds,* 2nd ed., Vol. 2 D. (Coffey, S., ed.) Elsevier Publishing Co., Amsterdam, **1970,** pp. 360–421.

Skou, J. C. Enzymatic basis for active transport of sodium and potassium across cell membranes. *Physiol. Rev.,* **1965,** *45,* 596–617.

Tamm, C. The stereochemistry of the glycosides in relation to biological activity. In, *Proceedings of the First International Pharmacological Meeting.* Vol. 3, *New Aspects of Cardiac Glycosides.* (Wilbrandt, W., and Lindgren, P., eds.) Pergamon Press, Ltd., Oxford, **1963,** pp. 11–26.

Trautwein, W. Generation and conduction of impulses in the heart as affected by drugs. *Pharmacol. Rev.,* **1963,** *15,* 277–332.

Withering, W. *An Account of the Foxglove and Some of Its Medicinal Uses: with Practical Remarks on Dropsy and Other Diseases.* C. G. J. & J. Robinson, London, 1785. Reprinted in *Med. Class.,* **1937,** *2,* 305–443.

31 ANTIARRHYTHMIC DRUGS

J. Thomas Bigger, Jr., and Brian F. Hoffman

Drug therapy of cardiac arrhythmias is based on a complex group of considerations. First, knowledge of the mechanism, consequences, and natural history of the arrhythmia to be treated is enormously helpful. The response of an arrhythmia to drugs is as much a function of pathophysiological condition as it is to drug action. Second, a clear understanding of the pharmacology of the drugs to be used is needed. This includes detailed knowledge of drug action on the electrophysiological properties of normal and abnormal cardiac tissues, of their effects on the mechanical properties of the heart and vasculature, and of their interactions with the autonomic nervous system and their effects on other organ systems. Optimal therapy of disturbances of cardiac rhythm requires considerable knowledge of the pharmacokinetics of antiarrhythmic drugs and how these parameters are affected by disease. Finally, a broad knowledge of adverse effects of the agents and their potential interactions with other drugs is necessary to monitor the course of therapy.

CARDIAC ELECTROPHYSIOLOGY

Resting Potential. There is a voltage difference across the surface membrane of all cardiac cells, the *resting transmembrane voltage* or potential (*Vm*). For most cardiac cells, the resting transmembrane potential difference is about -80 to -90 mV relative to the extracellular fluid. The resting transmembrane concentration gradients for ions such as Na^+ and K^+ are established by active transport. Typical values for concentrations of ions in the myocardium (in millimoles per liter of cell water) are: $[K]_o = 4.0$, $[K]_i = 150$, $[Na]_o = 140$, and $[Na]_i = 30$. If there were no voltage gradient across the membrane and the membrane were semipermeable to an ion, such as K^+, K^+ would have diffused out of the cell until the concentrations inside and outside were equal. However, fixed negative charges in the cell attract K^+ and counteract the concentration gradient that promotes diffusion (Noble, 1975). When these forces are equal, no net flux will occur. The Nernst equation can be solved for the voltage that will maintain the existing transmembrane concentration gradient at a constant value—the equilibrium voltage, V_X, for an ion, X:

$$V_X = \frac{RT}{F} \ln \frac{[X]_o}{[X]_i}$$

where $[X]_o$ is the concentration of the ion in extracellular fluid and $[X]_i$ is the intracellular concentration. (R is the gas constant, T is the absolute temperature, and F is Faraday's constant.) Given the ion concentrations listed above, $V_K = -97$ mV and $V_{Na} = +40$ mV. Since the resting membrane is permeable primarily to K^+, the resting transmembrane voltage is close to V_K. However, other ions, such as Na^+, do make a small contribution to resting transmembrane voltage.

Action Potentials. When cardiac cells are excited, a complex sequence of voltage changes occurs as a function of time, due to changes in ionic conductances across the membrane. A typical transmembrane *action potential* of a Purkinje fiber is diagrammed in Figure 31–1, *A*. The action potential is divided into *phases* for purposes of description and discussion. Phase 0 = rapid depolarization and reversal of transmembrane voltage; phase 1 = rapid repolarization to the plateau level of voltage; phase 2 = long-sustained depolarization or the plateau of the action potential; phase 3 = rapid repolarization to resting (diastolic) levels of transmembrane voltage; and phase 4 = the diastolic voltage time course. Many cells in the normal heart have action potentials that differ substantially from those of the Purkinje fiber. For example, sinus and A-V nodal cells have a very slowly rising phase 0, and phases 1, 2, and 3 cannot be distinguished clearly from one another. Also, many cells have a steady transmembrane voltage during phase 4, while others show spontaneous depolarization during this period. Automatic fibers in the sinus node and His-Purkinje system reach a maximal negative value of *Vm* at the end of the repolarization of phase 3. Then, these fibers may begin progressive spontaneous depolarization. If *Vm* achieves the critical *threshold voltage*, excitation occurs. The firing rate of an automatic cell is determined by: (1) the value of maximal diastolic voltage, (2) the slope of phase-4 depolarization, and (3) the value of the threshold voltage. When a cell or group of cells undergoes self-excitation by this process and initiates an impulse that propagates to the rest of the heart, it is known as a *pacemaker*. Although many fibers may undergo phase-4 depolarization, propa-

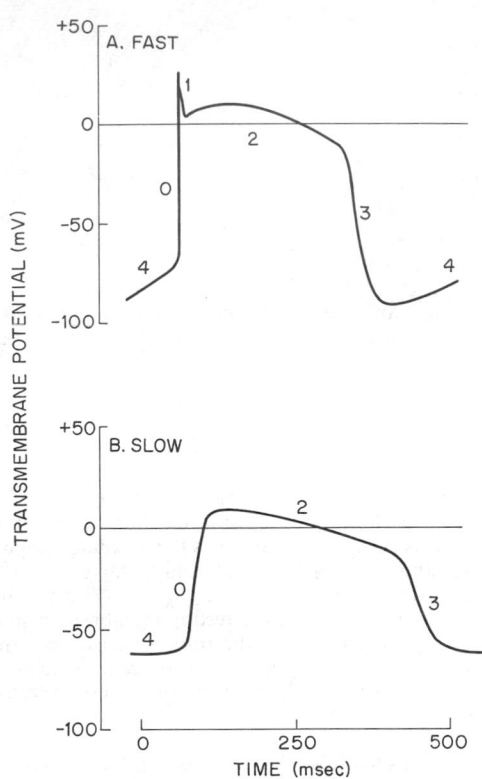

Figure 31-1. *Diagrammatic representation of fast and slow responses from mammalian cardiac Purkinje fibers.*

A. Fast Response. The phases of the normal fast response are shown: depolarization (*0*), repolarization (*1, 2, 3*), and the diastolic phase (*4*). Note the spontaneous phase-4 depolarization in this example. The rate of rise of phase 0 is rapid, and propagation will be rapid.

B. Slow Response. The slow response is initiated from a reduced (less negative) level of diastolic transmembrane voltage, shows slow depolarization, and has a long duration. Such an action potential propagates exceedingly slowly and leaves a long refractory wake.

gation of the excitation of the sinus impulse will interrupt this process in most cells before they attain threshold; such cells are called *latent pacemakers*.

The ionic basis for the cardiac action potential is still a subject of debate and active study. Although the voltage clamp technic has revealed clearly the ionic basis of the action potential of nerve, there are serious technical problems in the application of this technic to cardiac muscle (Fozzard and Beeler, 1975). It has been most successfully used in cardiac Purkinje fibers. Current concepts on the genesis of the cardiac action potential have been reviewed by Trautwein (1973), McAllister and associates (1975), and Noble (1975). The ionic currents that are thought to contribute to the action potential of the

Purkinje fiber are summarized in Table 31-1 and are discussed in the following sections.

Phase 0. In most cardiac cells, phase 0 is generated by the movement of Na^+ through channels that selectively allow permeation of this ion; they are activated in a voltage-dependent manner when the propagating cardiac impulse or spontaneous phase-4 depolarization causes the so-called *m* gate in the channel to open. The inward Na^+ current, i_{Na}, is very intense but very brief; it is terminated by a process called *inactivation*—the closing of an hypothetical gate (the *h* gate) in the Na^+ channel because of depolarization. After inactivation, the Na^+ channel cannot be opened again until it is *reactivated* during and after phase-3 repolarization.

Phase 1. Quick repolarization to the plateau of the action potential is brought about by several factors: the passive electrical properties of Purkinje fibers, inactivation of i_{Na}, and activation of a chloride current.

Phase 2. The plateau of the action potential is one of the most unusual characteristic features of the *cardiac* action potential. Membrane conductance is reduced during the plateau, due to inwardly directed rectification of the K^+ background current, i_{K_1}. Also, the Ca^{2+} or slow channel is activated in the range of voltage found during the plateau; this secondary inward current, i_{si}, is inactivated in a manner analogous to that for i_{Na}, but the time constant for inactivation of i_{si} is much greater (50 milliseconds compared to 0.5 millisecond). Therefore, i_{si} turns off slowly during the plateau.

Phase 3. A time-dependent outward current, i_{X_1}, plays an important role in terminating the plateau and causing the fiber to repolarize to normal diastolic values of transmembrane voltage. This current is carried primarily by K^+, but also by another unspecified ion or ions. The i_{X_1} activates (*i.e.*, the X_1 channel opens) at about -40 mV, with a time constant of about 0.5 second. By the end of the plateau, i_{X_1} has waxed to a considerable value, while i_{si} has waned. Phase 3 is primarily the product of activated i_{X_1} in the presence of inactivating i_{si} and some contribution from increasing i_{K_1} as the transmembrane voltage moves to more negative voltages. In the steady state, i_{X_1} is completely deactivated (*i.e.*, the X_1 channel is closed) at values of Vm more negative than -50 mV. This means that i_{X_1} deactivates quickly at the end of repolarization. The X_1 channel behaves as if it contains only one ion gating site, which activates or deactivates to control i_{X_1}; that is, it does not inactivate.

Phase 4. In many cells (*e.g.*, ordinary atrial or ventricular muscle), Vm is constant during diastole; these cells will rest indefinitely until activated by a propagating impulse or an external stimulus. However, as mentioned above, other cells exhibit spontaneous phase-4 depolarization and self-excitation (*see* Figure 31–1, *A*). This type of behavior is often seen in the His-Purkinje system and has been studied extensively. Several ionic currents modulate normal automaticity in the His-Purkinje system: two currents that do not change in time—an outward background current (i_{K_1}) and an inward background current (i_{bi})—and a time-dependent outward current (i_{K_2}); i_{K_2} has been called the pacemaker cur-

Table 31-1. IONIC CURRENTS AND THE PURKINJE FIBER ACTION POTENTIAL

CURRENT	MAJOR ION RESPONSIBLE FOR THE CURRENT	PHASE OF ACTION POTENTIAL *	REVERSAL VOLTAGE	DIRECTION OF CURRENT FLOW	PHYSIOLOGICAL ROLE
i_{Na}	Na^+	0	+40	Inward	Depolarizes fiber during phase 0
i_{qr}	Cl^-	1	−25	Outward	Rapid repolarization in phase 1; not present in ventricular muscle
i_{si}	Ca^{2+}	1, 2	+100	Inward	Contributes to plateau of action potential; triggers the release of internal Ca^{2+}
i_{X_1}	K^+, ?	3	−70	Outward	Repolarizes fiber during phase 3
i_{K_2}	K^+	4	−100	Outward	Deactivates during phase 4, permitting spontaneous depolarization
i_{bi}	Na^+, Ca^{2+}	0, 1, 2, 3, 4	+40 †	Inward	Depolarizes fiber during phase 4
i_{K_1}	K^+	0, 1, 2, 3, 4	−100	Outward	Outward background current

* The phases of the action potential during which the current makes its most important physiological contribution.
† Presumed.

rent. At the beginning of phase 4, i_{K_2}, which is rapidly activated during the plateau of the previous action potential, is almost fully activated. At diastolic values of Vm, i_{K_2} deactivates to its steady-state value of about 0, with a time constant of about 1 second. The progressive decrease in the outward current, i_{K_2}, as diastole proceeds will cause Purkinje fibers to depolarize if i_{bi} is greater than i_{K_2} plus i_{K_1}. Electrogenic extrusion of Na^+ may be an important part of background outward current.

Interestingly, pacemaker activity in the sinus node has a completely different ionic mechanism (Brown and Noble, 1974; Noma and Irisawa, 1976). The outward current i_{K_2} seems to be absent from the sinus node pacemaker cells. Spontaneous phase-4 depolarization relics on deactivation of an outward current, i_p, which is similar to i_{X_1} in Purkinje fibers (but more selective for K^+) and an i_{si} that is carried by Na^+ and Ca^{2+}. Background currents and electrogenic Na^+ pumping also play a role in the automaticity of the sinus node (Noma and Irisawa, 1974). The faster spontaneous activity of sinus nodal cells than Purkinje fibers is a function of the relative rates of deactivation of i_p and i_{K_2} (Noma and Irisawa, 1976).

Fast and Slow Responses. Cranefield and colleagues (1972) divided cardiac action potentials into *fast* and *slow* responses. Depolarization in the *fast response* (see Figure 31-1, *A*) is generated by an intense inward current, i_{Na}; has a large, fast-rising phase 0; propagates very rapidly; and has a large safety factor for conduction. Normal atrial, ventricular, and Purkinje fiber action potentials are examples of the fast response. Depolarization in the *slow response* is generated by a weak inward current, i_{si}; has a slowly rising phase 0; propagates very slowly; and has a low safety factor for conduction (Figure 31-1, *B*). Action potentials in sinus and A-V nodal cells and cells in the A-V rings are examples of slow responses seen under normal conditions. For a discussion of abnormal conditions that may generate

slow responses, *see* the section on reentrant arrhythmias below.

Excitability and Refractoriness. *Excitability* is traditionally measured in terms of the strength of an electrical pulse required to excite the heart when applied at selected times in the cardiac cycle. The functional significance of changes in excitability is usually difficult to determine. Therefore, little emphasis is placed here on the effects of antiarrhythmic drugs on excitability. *Refractoriness* has been defined in many different ways; in this discussion, refractoriness is usually used to refer to the duration of the *effective refractory period* (ERP), which is the minimal interval between two propagating responses. In most cardiac cells the ERP is closely linked to action potential duration (APD), because recovery from inactivation of the Na^+ channel closely parallels repolarization. However, sinus and A-V nodal cells (slow responses) have strikingly different characteristics. In nodal cells, refractoriness outlasts full repolarization, so that the ERP is much longer than the APD (Hoffman and Cranefield, 1960; Strauss and Bigger, 1972). Antiarrhythmic drugs can prolong the ERP relative to APD in many types of cardiac cells.

A period often can be found during the latter part of repolarization when the threshold for electrical stimulation is less than the value found in diastole after full recovery; this period of *supernormal excitability* has been regarded as a paradoxical response. An explanation for this phenomenon has been found for cardiac Purkinje fibers and may hold for some other types of cells as well. In Purkinje fibers, toward the end of repolarization, Vm is closer to threshold than it is after full repolarization. Therefore, a smaller electrical pulse may carry the membrane to threshold during the late portion of phase-3 repolarization than would be required in diastole.

Responsiveness and Conduction. The term *membrane responsiveness* is used to describe the response of a cardiac fiber to a stimulus (*e.g.*, a propagating action potential or applied electrical pulse). Cardiac fibers do not regain their full ability to develop a normal response until repolarization is complete (Lewis and Drury, 1926). Weidmann (1955) showed that changes in the maximal rate of depolarization during phase 0 ($\dot{V}_{max}$) provided an index of changes in availability of the Na^+ conductance system or the degree of recovery from inactivation of the Na^+ channel. Although there is controversy about the degree to which $\dot{V}_{max}$ reflects i_{Na} in cardiac muscle (Hondeghem, 1978), there is little doubt about the importance of phase-0 $\dot{V}_{max}$ in relation to conduction velocity and block of premature impulses. In cardiac Purkinje fibers, the $\dot{V}_{max}$ of a response is very strongly dependent on Vm at the instant of excitation (*see* Figure 31-2). In normal fibers, the time constant for recovery from inactivation of the Na^+ channel is quite short, so that $\dot{V}_{max}$ is similar when a cardiac fiber is stimulated at a given level of Vm, regardless of whether this level of Vm is achieved during the course of phase-3 repolarization or during phase-4 depolarization. The time constant for such recovery of Na^+ channels is likely to be significantly longer: (1) at low (more positive) values of Vm; (2) during treatment with antiarrhythmic drugs; and (3) in membranes altered by disease. Under these circumstances, a more complex scheme must be used to account for $\dot{V}_{max}$ as a function of Vm and the time-voltage history of Vm. The relationship between $\dot{V}_{max}$ and Vm is of considerable importance since $\dot{V}_{max}$ is one determinant of the efficacy of an action potential as an excitatory stimulus to adjacent resting membrane, propagation velocity, and the likelihood that the propagating cardiac impulse will undergo decrement or block. The S-shaped relationship between $\dot{V}_{max}$ and Vm (Figure 31-2) is typical not only of cardiac Purkinje fibers but also of atrial and ventricular muscle. Cells of the sinus node and the A-V node do not show this typical relationship; like excitability, responsiveness does not return in nodal cells (slow responses) until well after repolarization is complete (Hoffman, 1961; Strauss *et al.*, 1968). There is a considerable safety factor in cardiac muscle, since $\dot{V}_{max}$ must be reduced to half or less of normal before conduction velocity decreases (Peon *et al.*, 1978).

MECHANISMS RESPONSIBLE FOR CARDIAC ARRHYTHMIAS

An arrhythmia is an abnormality of rate, regularity, or site of origin of the cardiac impulse or a disturbance in conduction that causes an alteration in the normal sequence of activation of the atria and ventricles. Arrhythmias may arise because of alterations in automaticity, conduction, or both. The number of possible mechanisms for arrhythmias in each category is now large. The more important possible mechanisms will be discussed briefly.

ARRHYTHMIAS DUE TO ABNORMALITIES OF AUTOMATICITY

There are many examples of arrhythmias that arise because of either enhancement or failure of

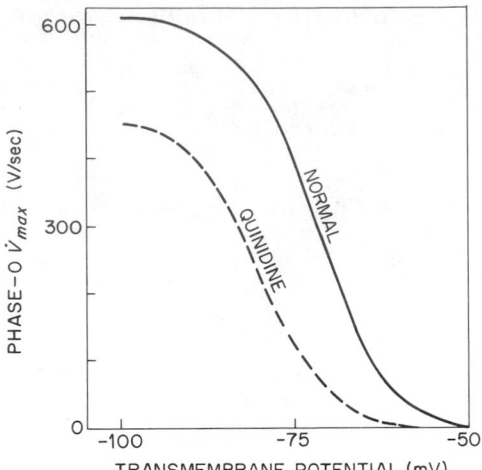

Figure 31-2. *Membrane responsiveness.*

Membrane responsiveness in a cardiac Purkinje fiber is depicted. The maximal rate of rise of depolarization during phase 0 is plotted as a function of transmembrane voltage at the time of activation. The solid line shows the relationship under normal conditions, and the dashed line depicts the effect of a moderate to high concentration of quinidine. Quinidine shifts the relationship on its voltage axis so that a reduced response is obtained at any given level of transmembrane voltage. Also, the maximal rate of depolarization is reduced.

normal automaticity. Mechanisms of abnormal impulse generation are also subjects of ongoing experimental interest.

Altered Normal Automaticity. When considering this topic, it is important to recall that only a few types of cardiac cells have the capacity to perform automatically under normal conditions: sinus node, distal A-V node, and the His-Purkinje system (Hoffman and Cranefield, 1960). There is some evidence that other cell types may develop automaticity, for example, specialized atrial fibers in the internodal tracts and fibers near the ostium of the coronary sinus (Wit and Cranefield, 1977).

Sinus Node. In the sinus node, rate can be altered by autonomic activity or intrinsic disease. Increased vagal activity can slow or stop sinus nodal pacemakers by increasing potassium conductance (g_K), which increases outward K^+ currents, hyperpolarizes the pacemaker cells, and prevents them from depolarizing (Harris and Hutter, 1956; Giles and Noble, 1976). Increased sympathetic traffic to the sinus node may cause sinus tachycardia either by increasing the magnitude of i_{si} or by causing an increase in the magnitude of i_{x_1}, thereby increasing maximal diastolic Vm and shortening the duration of the action potential (Brown and Noble, 1974). Intrinsic disease of sinus nodal pacemaker cells seems to be responsible for faulty pacemaker activity in the sick sinus syndrome in man. The precise mechanism and pathogenesis are still unknown.

Purkinje Fibers. Augmented automaticity in the His-Purkinje system is a common cause of arrhythmias in human subjects. Increased sympathetic nerve activity to the His-Purkinje system can cause a substantial increase in the rate of spontaneous firing. This increase is brought about by an ionic mechanism that is totally different from the changes causing sinus tachycardia. In cardiac Purkinje fibers, catecholamines enhance automaticity by substantially shifting the steady-state pacemaker current (i_{K_2}) activation curve toward depolarization on its voltage axis and decreasing the time constant for deactivation of i_{K_2} (Tsien, 1974). The inward background current (i_{bi}), which flows in the diastolic voltage range, does not appear to be altered by catecholamines. Although norepinephrine and other catecholamines cause substantial changes in the outward current (i_{x_1}) and in the secondary inward current (i_{si}) in cardiac Purkinje fibers, these changes are not essential for alterations in automaticity. It is possible for A-V junctional pacemakers to usurp control of the ventricles in the presence of a normal sinus node and normal A-V conduction. This could occur because of selectivity of traffic in sympathetic nerves (Randall, 1977), increase of release of catecholamines locally, or enhanced responsiveness of β-adrenergic receptors. Also, higher neural activity and neural activity associated with cardiovascular reflexes alter cardiac rate and produce disturbances of rhythm primarily by changing the pattern of firing of various subunits of the cardiac autonomic nerves (Levitt *et al.*, 1976). The effect of the vagus on the His-Purkinje system in man is not well understood. The response of Purkinje fibers to acetylcholine varies with species; acetylcholine slows normal pacemaker activity in the dog but accelerates it in sheep. In addition, many questions about functional vagal innervation of the His-Purkinje system are unsettled; it appears that vagal innervation of the proximal system may be significant, whereas that of the peripheral system is more sparse (Levy, 1977).

In disease, automaticity in the His-Purkinje system may become reduced. In the sick sinus syndrome it is typical for the ventricular pacemakers to be depressed as well as the sinus node (*see* Bigger and Reiffel, 1979). Thus, very long pauses in cardiac rhythm may occur when the sinus node fails as a pacemaker. In A-V block due to widespread bundle-branch disease, the rate of ventricular pacemakers may also be abnormally slow. In neither of these examples has a mechanism been identified.

Abnormal Generation of Impulses. In addition to the arrhythmias caused by alterations of normal automaticity, numerous abnormal mechanisms for the generation of impulses have been observed in experimental preparations (Hoffman and Cranefield, 1960; Bigger, 1973; Cranefield, 1977). Many of these mechanisms appear to fit into one of two categories—early afterdepolarization or delayed afterdepolarization. Both of these mechanisms can be distinguished from those responsible for normal automaticity. Moreover, abnormal automaticity can occur in fibers that ordinarily are incapable of automatic function, for example, atrial or ventricular muscle cells. Abnormal automaticity is currently receiving much attention as a potential explanation of coupled extrasystoles.

Early Afterdepolarizations. Early afterdepolarizations are secondary depolarizations that occur before repolarization is complete. Characteristically, the secondary depolarization starts from the level of the plateau (*see* Figure 31-3, *A*). Often, a burst of depolarizations occurs followed by a few damped oscillations, until, finally, *Vm* either rests at the range of the plateau voltage (about −20 to −40 mV) or returns to the resting value. Experimentally, early afterdepolarizations have been produced in cardiac Purkinje fibers by stretching or crushing, hypoxia, cooling, low $[K]_o$, high $[Ca]_o$, high concentrations of catecholamines, and certain chemicals (such as veratrine or aconitine) (*see* Trautwein, 1963; Bigger, 1973; Cranefield, 1975). Early afterdepolarizations are promoted by: (1) decreased background outward current, (2) increased background inward current, (3) increased residual i_{Na} during the plateau, (4) increased magnitude and/or duration of i_{si}, and (5) changes in i_{x_1}. Cardiac Purkinje fibers tend to have two stable resting potentials, one at about −80 to −90 mV and another at −30 to −50 mV (Carmeliet, 1961; Noble, 1975; Cranefield, 1977). Also, cardiac muscle shows inwardly directed rectifi-

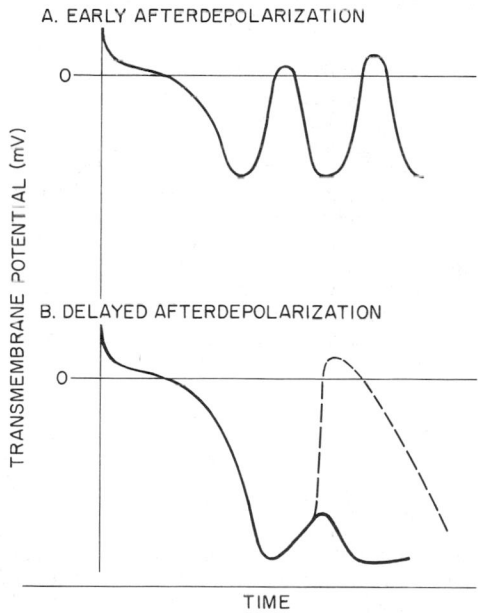

A. EARLY AFTERDEPOLARIZATION

B. DELAYED AFTERDEPOLARIZATION

TRANSMEMBRANE POTENTIAL (mV)

TIME

Figure 31-3. *Two forms of abnormal automaticity in a cardiac Purkinje fiber.*

A. Early Afterdepolarization. Repolarization is interrupted by secondary depolarizations. Such responses may excite neighboring fibers and be propagated.

B. Delayed Afterdepolarization. After full repolarization is achieved, *Vm* again transiently depolarizes. If the delayed afterdepolarization reaches threshold, a propagating response can occur (dashed line).

cation; when Vm is in the range of the plateau voltage, tiny inward currents cause substantial depolarization. Conditions such as stretch, cooling, and low $[K]_o$ probably act by decreasing membrane conductance to K^+ (*i.e.*, decreasing background outward currents). Aconitine increases the residual i_{Na} (Peper and Trautwein, 1967); high $[Ca]_o$ and catecholamines probably act by increasing i_{si}. The early afterdepolarizations associated with stretch or crush injury in cardiac Purkinje fibers have been studied with voltage clamp technics (Hauswirth *et al.*, 1969). This form of early afterdepolarization is due to increased background inward current and decreased background outward current coupled with phasic variations in i_{x_1}.

Delayed Afterdepolarizations. A delayed afterdepolarization is a secondary depolarization occurring in diastole, that is, after full repolarization has been achieved (*see* Figure 31–3, *B*). The delayed afterdepolarization is dependent on a prior action potential. The typical sequence leading to a delayed afterdepolarization is as follows. An action potential occurs, and repolarization leads to a more or less prominent *afterhyperpolarization;* that is, at the end of repolarization, Vm transiently swings negative to the resting diastolic level. However, rather than merely returning to the resting level of Vm, a secondary depolarization may occur in diastole—the delayed afterdepolarization. Delayed afterdepolarizations may be seen when certain cell types are exposed to catecholamines (Wit *et al.*, 1970; Wit and Cranefield, 1977), or digitalis (Ferrier, 1977), or perfusates containing low $[Na]_o$ and high $[Ca]_o$ (Cranefield, 1977). Delayed afterdepolarizations can reach threshold and give rise to a single extrasystole. However, if the extrasystole is also followed by a delayed afterdepolarization, a second extrasystole may result. In this way, delayed afterdepolarizations can cause either coupled extrasystoles or runs of tachyarrhythmias. A number of factors have been identified that tend to increase the amplitude of delayed afterdepolarizations, thus increasing the likelihood that they will reach threshold. They include increases in the basic driven or spontaneous rate, premature systoles, increased $[Ca]_o$, catecholamines, and certain other drugs, particularly digitalis. The delayed afterdepolarizations that arise in digitalis toxicity have been studied most and are discussed at greater length in Chapter 30. Delayed afterdepolarizations can readily be induced by digitalis in the His-Purkinje system and, with more difficulty, in specialized atrial fibers or in ordinary ventricular cells (Ferrier, 1977). The delayed afterdepolarizations induced by digitalis in Purkinje fibers are caused by an abnormal transient inward current that is carried mainly by Na^+ (Lederer and Tsien, 1976). It is reasonable to speculate that some clinical arrhythmias caused by digitalis, for example, coupled ventricular premature depolarizations and atrial or ventricular tachycardias, result from delayed afterdepolarizations. Also, some supraventricular tachycardias may be triggered rhythms that arise from delayed afterdepolarizations.

Triggered Arrhythmias. A single premature stimulus can cause a delayed afterdepolarization to reach threshold and may trigger sustained repetitive firing of the cell. Activation by this mechanism must be initiated by an action potential; thus, it cannot arise *de novo,* as can a normal automatic rhythm. Triggered rhythms in cells that have delayed afterdepolarizations have many characteristics that are often associated with reentrant tachyarrhythmias. A tachycardia may be triggered by a single premature stimulus and may also be terminated by a single premature stimulus. These characteristics make it difficult to assign a mechanism for a clinical tachyarrhythmia. The attempt to define mechanisms becomes even more difficult when one considers that an action potential caused by normal automaticity may initiate a tachyarrhythmia due to delayed afterdepolarization or that a single extrasystole arising from a delayed afterdepolarization may initiate a genuine reentrant rhythm.

REENTRANT ARRHYTHMIAS

Reentrant arrhythmias are caused by *recirculating activation* that is incited by an initiating depolarization. Thus, reentrant arrhythmias, like triggered rhythms, are self-sustained but are not self-initiated. For reentry to be initiated, one-way block of conduction must occur—an anatomical or functional "barrier" to conduction that forms a circuit (Cranefield *et al.*, 1972; Bigger, 1973). Another critical condition for reentry is that the pathlength of the circuit must be greater than the wavelength of the cardiac impulse, where wavelength is the product of conduction velocity and the refractory period (*see* Figure 31–4). The principal difficulty in attributing cardiac arrhythmias to reentry is that, usually, the cardiac refractory period is very long, cardiac conduction is rapid, and the pathways available are reasonably short. For reentry to occur, normal conduction must be greatly slowed, refractoriness markedly shortened, or both. Nevertheless, reentry does serve as an explanation for cardiac arrhythmias. The sinus and A-V nodes are regions in which conduction is normally very slow; further slowing by premature activation or by disease easily creates conditions that permit reentry. Disease processes may also create conditions that permit reentry even in those types of fibers that usually conduct the cardiac impulse at very rapid rates, such as cardiac Purkinje fibers. Usually, marked slowing of conduction is the alteration that permits reentry. However, marked abbreviation of action potentials and of refractoriness can play a role as well (Sasyniuk and Méndez, 1971). Conduction may be slowed due either to alterations in the *fast response* or development of *slow responses.*

Altered Fast Response. As mentioned in the discussion of responsiveness, phase-0 $\dot{V}_{max}$ and conduction velocity of impulses are critically dependent on the Vm at the time of activation (*see* Figure 31–2). When resting Vm is reduced to values more positive than -75 mV (as with stretch or high $[K]_o$), V_{max} and conduction velocity decrease substantially because of voltage-dependent inactivation in the fast Na^+ channel. When resting Vm is between -50 and -65 mV, i_{Na} is greatly reduced and the altered fast

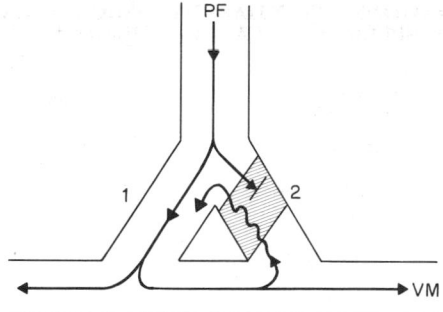

Figure 31-4. *Reentry.*

The diagram shows one of the forms of reentrant reexcitation in the ventricle (Schmitt and Erlanger, 1928–29). A branched Purkinje fiber (*PF*) terminates on a strip of ventricular muscle (*VM*). The shaded area in branch 2 represents a depolarized area that is the site of a *one-way block;* thus, orthograde sinus impulses are blocked in this area, but retrograde responses are propagated successfully. Retrograde conduction in branch 2 is slow enough for cells in branch 1 to recover and respond to the reentering impulse. A single reactivation of branch 1 will produce a single ventricular premature depolarization; continuous conduction around the circuit will cause ventricular tachycardia.

Antiarrhythmic drugs can abolish such reentrant activity by producing *two-way block* in branch 2 or by improving conduction in branch 2, that is, by removing the one-way block.

response can propagate slowly enough to permit reentry. If *Vm* is more positive than approximately −50 mV, i_{Na} is almost totally inactivated and fast responses cannot be elicited. At low values of *Vm,* fast responses may conduct decrementally; that is, the adequacy of the propagating response as a stimulus to resting tissue in its path lessens progressively as it propagates in depolarized tissues. Also, as conduction slows, the capacitance that must be filled by local circuit current will increase, causing further slowing of conduction. Under such conditions, a delicate balance exists that determines whether conduction succeeds or fails.

Slow Responses and Very Slow Conduction. Slow action potentials were discovered in cardiac Purkinje fibers exposed to increased $[K]_o$ and catecholamines by Carmeliet and Vereeke (1969). In the voltage range at which slow potentials emerge, i_{Na} is inactivated and the pacemaker current, i_{K_2}, is fully activated; these currents are thus unlikely to play a role in the genesis of the slow response. The inward current that causes the slow potential is i_{si}. Since i_{si} is relatively small in magnitude, slow responses are more likely to develop when background outward currents are decreased. Typically, slow responses are 40 to 80 mV in amplitude, depolarize at 1 to 2 V per second (*i.e.,* about 0.002 the rate of the fast response), and last for 0.4 to 1 second (*see* Figure 31-1, *B*). The

small-amplitude and very low phase-0 $\dot{V}_{max}$ of slow responses lead to very slow conduction, which increases the likelihood of reentry. Also, slow responses are less critically dependent on spatial distribution of a decreased resting potential for successful propagation than are fast responses. Slow responses can arise and propagate successfully in tissues too depolarized to generate a fast response. The slow response can easily overcome the chief difficulty for the production of reentry in heart muscle; it propagates so slowly that reentry can occur in very short pathways (Cranefield *et al.,* 1972; Wit *et al.,* 1972a, 1972b). Reentry in relatively small circuits of Purkinje fibers has been demonstrated directly (Wit *et al.,* 1972a, 1972b). As noted above, the duration of the action potential and refractoriness may shorten dramatically at the site of block due to local-circuit current flow (Sasyniuk and Méndez, 1971). Thus, premature stimulation can produce sufficient heterogeneity in the duration of the action potential and in refractoriness to permit reentry of subsequent impulses.

Significance of Reentry. Reentry may occur in many sites in the heart. The slow conduction in reentrant circuits may be due either to depressed fast responses or to slow responses. Reentry is relatively easy to elicit in the vicinity of the sinus or A-V nodes by the use of premature stimulation to slow conduction and to produce a functional one-way block, even in normal hearts (Moe and Méndez, 1966; Han *et al.,* 1968; Bigger and Goldreyer, 1970; Weisfogel *et al.,* 1975). It should be mentioned again that reentrant arrhythmias are very difficult to distinguish from triggered arrhythmias. Also, reentry in the His-Purkinje system is thought to be one cause of coupled ventricular premature depolarizations and ventricular tachycardia in man. This idea was well articulated by Schmitt and Erlanger (1928–29) and is supported by extensive experimentation (Wit *et al.,* 1972a, 1972b; Wellens *et al.,* 1976). For example, Durrer and coworkers (1971) and El-Sherif and associates (1977) have shown, in experimental acute myocardial infarction in the dog, that the cardiac impulse can meander through the infarcted region and emerge much later to produce ventricular premature depolarizations, ventricular tachycardia, or ventricular fibrillation.

INDIVIDUAL ANTIARRHYTHMIC AGENTS

Discussion of the individual drugs that are most useful for the treatment or prophylaxis of cardiac arrhythmias follows. The effects of these agents on the electrophysiological properties of specialized cardiac fibers are summarized in Table 31-2, while drug-induced alterations in the ECG are listed in Table 31-3. The clinical utility of each agent is described in the text, and an overall estimate of their value in the management of

Table 31–2. EFFECTS OF THERAPEUTIC CONCENTRATIONS OF ANTIARRHYTHMIC DRUGS ON ELECTROPHYSIOLOGICAL PROPERTIES OF SPECIALIZED CARDIAC FIBERS *

	QUINIDINE, PROCAINAMIDE, DISOPYRAMIDE	LIDOCAINE, PHENYTOIN	PROPRANOLOL	BRETYLIUM
Sinus Node				
Automaticity	→	→	↓	↑[†], ↓
A-V Node				
Effective refractory period (ERP) ‡	↑, →, ↓	↑, →, ↓	↑	↑, →, ↓
Purkinje Fibers				
Action potential duration (APD)	↑	↓	↓	↑
Effective refractory period (ERP)	↑	↓	↓	↑
ERP/APD	↑	↑	↑	→
Membrane responsiveness	**↓**	↓	↓	→
Automaticity	↓	↓	↓	↑[†], →

* Changes are indicated as follows: ↓, decreased; →, no change; ↑, increased; where multiple arrows are shown, there is variability in the direction of change. Bold-faced arrows indicate effects of greater magnitude.

† Due to release of catecholamines on initial exposure to the drug.

‡ Due to a complex balance of direct and indirect autonomic effects.

specific arrhythmias is presented in Table 31–4. Pharmacokinetic parameters for the major agents are summarized in Appendix II.

QUINIDINE

Quinidine is the dextrostereoisomer of quinine; it shares all of the pharmacological actions of quinine, including its antimalarial, antipyretic, and oxytocic effects. However, the actions of quinidine on cardiac muscle are more intense than are those of quinine.

History. Quinidine, an optical isomer of quinine, was first described in 1848 by van Heyningen, and was prepared and given its present name by Pasteur in 1853. In the use of quinine and quinidine for

malaria, it was noted many years ago that patients with malaria who also had atrial fibrillation would occasionally be cured of arrhythmia by these drugs.

Perhaps the earliest recorded reference to the use of cinchona in atrial fibrillation is that of the French physician Jean-Baptiste de Sénac of Paris, in 1749 (*see* Willius and Keys, 1942). Years later Wenckebach (1914) reported on the effect of quinine alkaloids in certain cardiac arrhythmias. Frey (1918), impressed by the report of Wenckebach, studied quinine, cinchonine, and quinidine in patients with atrial fibrillation and found quinidine to be the most effective. His observations were quickly confirmed by others, and the use of quinidine was extended to additional disorders of cardiac rhythm.

Chemistry. The chemistry of the cinchona alkaloids is presented in the discussion of quinine (Chapter 45). Quinidine differs from quinine only in the steric configuration of the secondary alcohol group.

Table 31–3. EFFECTS OF THERAPEUTIC CONCENTRATIONS OF ANTIARRHYTHMIC DRUGS ON THE ECG *

	P-R	QRS	Q-T$_c$ †	VENTRICULAR RATE IN ATRIAL FIBRILLATION
Quinidine	→, ↑	↑	↑	↑
Procainamide	→, ↑	↑	↑	↑
Disopyramide	→	→, ↑	→, ↑	↑
Lidocaine	→	→	→, ↓	↑, →, ↓
Phenytoin	→, ↓	→	→, ↓	↑, →, ↓
Propranolol	→, ↑	→	→, ↓	↓
Bretylium	→, ↑	→	→, ↑	↑, ↓

* Changes are indicated as follows: ↓, decreased; →, no change; ↑, increased; where multiple arrows are shown, there is variability in the direction of change.

† The Q-T$_c$ interval is the Q-T interval corrected for heart rate.

Table 31–4. UTILITY OF ANTIARRHYTHMIC AGENTS IN THE TREATMENT OF SPECIFIC CARDIAC ARRHYTHMIAS *

ARRHYTHMIA	QUINI-DINE	PROCAIN-AMIDE	DISOPY-RAMIDE	LIDO-CAINE	PHENY-TOIN	PROPRAN-OLOL	BRETY-LIUM
Supraventricular							
Conversion of atrial fibrillation	2	2	1	0	0	1	0
Prophylaxis	4	4	4	0	0	2	0
Conversion of atrial flutter	1	1	—	0	0	1	0
Paroxysmal supraventricular tachycardia	3	3	3	0	1	3	0
Atrial premature depolarizations	3	3	3	0	1	3	0
Ventricular							
Ventricular premature depolarizations	3	3	3	4	2	1	1
Ventricular tachycardia	2	4	3	4	2	1	3
Digitalis-Induced Arrhythmias							
Atrial tachycardia with block	1	1	1	3	3	2	0
Nonparoxysmal A-V junctional tachycardia	1	1	1	3	3	2	0
Ventricular arrhythmias	1	1	1	3	3	2	0

* Utility is based on an estimate of efficacy, convenience, and toxicity. The scale of relative utility is as follows: 0, none; 1, poor; 2, fair; 3, good; 4, excellent.

PHARMACOLOGICAL PROPERTIES

Cardiac Electrophysiological Effects. Quinidine has powerful direct effects on most types of cells in the heart. In addition, drug-induced alterations of autonomic regulation of the heart also influence the electrical properties of cardiac cells.

Automaticity. Therapeutic concentrations of quinidine have little effect on the action potential or the firing rate of the isolated rabbit *sinus node;* very high concentrations decrease the automaticity of the sinus node. In the human denervated heart, quinidine slows sinus rate very slightly (Mason *et al.,* 1977). Indirect effects of quinidine can increase sinus rate by cholinergic blockade or by reflexly increasing sympathetic activity (*see* Mason *et al.,* 1977). Quinidine can also cause severe depression of the sinus node in patients with the *sick sinus syndrome* (*see* Bigger and Reiffel, 1979). Therapeutic concentrations of quinidine substantially decrease the firing rate of *cardiac Purkinje fibers* by a direct action; quinidine decreases the slope of phase-4 depolarization and shifts the threshold voltage toward zero. The ionic mechanism of this action of quinidine is not completely understood. The shift in threshold is due to a shift in the i_{Na} reactivation curve. The decrease in the slope of phase 4 is not yet explained. These effects on automaticity are responsible for the ability of quinidine to suppress arrhythmias caused by enhanced normal automaticity. The potent effect of quinidine on the normal automaticity in the His-Purkinje system presents a hazard in the treatment of arrhythmias in the presence of A-V block. Therapeutic concentrations of quinidine have little effect on *abnormal automaticity* in markedly depolarized Purkinje fibers or on delayed after-depolarizations. However, quinidine may prevent triggered tachyarrhythmias by preventing the inciting of premature depolarization.

Excitability and Threshold. Quinidine increases the diastolic electrical current threshold in atrial and ventricular muscle and in Purkinje fibers; it also increases the fibrillation threshold in atria and ventricles (Wallace *et al.,* 1966a). As mentioned above, the threshold voltage is shifted by quinidine.

Responsiveness and Conduction. Quinidine decreases the amplitude, overshoot, and $\dot{V}_{max}$ of phase 0 in atrial, ventricular, and Purkinje cells. These effects become progressively more intense as the concentration of the drug is increased, and they are not accompanied by significant change in the resting Vm. The upstroke of premature responses is particularly depressed by quinidine because the drug causes changes in the voltage and time dependence of reactivation; for any steady-state value of Vm, $\dot{V}_{max}$ is reduced and, during dynamic changes in Vm, $\dot{V}_{max}$ takes longer to reach its steady-state value. The time-dependent changes are most marked at low (less negative) values of Vm.

Duration of the Action Potential and Re-

fractoriness. Quinidine causes minimal increases in the duration of the action potential of ordinary atrial, ventricular, or Purkinje fibers. The effective refractory period (ERP) of all of these cell types increases much more than would be expected from the changes in the duration of the action potential. This finding is explained by the changes in responsiveness discussed above.

Effect on Reentrant Arrhythmias. Quinidine can abolish reentrant arrhythmias because of its effect on ERP, responsiveness, and conduction. For example, when ventricular premature depolarizations are caused by reentry in loops of Purkinje fibers, quinidine can convert one-way block to two-way block, thus making reentry impossible.

The mechanism of its antiarrhythmic action in atrial flutter or fibrillation is more complex.

Atrial Flutter. Prolongation of the ERP of the atrium is commonly cited as the one desirable attribute of an "antiflutter" drug. The situation is by no means simple, for the effects of antiarrhythmic drugs upon ERP and upon conduction velocity are inextricably linked. When quinidine is administered to a dog in which a circus-movement flutter has been established, or to a patient with atrial flutter, the frequency invariably declines before reversion abruptly ensues. Quinidine slows conduction velocity in atrial muscle, which could account for the reduction of rate; but it also increases the atrial refractory period which could reduce the rate by forcing the circulating impulse to travel in relatively refractory tissue. The two actions are opposed. If the predominant effect of quinidine were a primary reduction of conduction velocity, reversion to sinus rhythm should not be expected to occur until the flutter frequency diminished to less than the prevailing rate of the sinus node. But if the action is primarily upon the ERP, then the conduction velocity will be secondarily depressed until some minimal value is reached below which successful impulse propagation is no longer possible. This may well be the mechanism of action of quinidine in the experimental situation, but the details of the process are still not clearly defined. Méndez and associates (1969) have emphasized the importance of the "wavelength" (*i.e.,* the product of ERP and conduction velocity) in termination of circus-movement flutter. Agents that prolong the ERP without specifically depressing conduction velocity are more effective than those with both actions.

Atrial Fibrillation. If atrial fibrillation were due to a single circus movement about an obstacle so limited in size that activation of the surrounding tissue is irregular and fractionated, then the circuit pathway itself would be unstable. This mechanism seems unlikely, for fibrillation can be, and often is, a very stable arrhythmia. If, however, fibrillation is due to

the random wandering of numerous fractionated wavelets, changing in breadth, direction, and number from moment to moment, as suggested by Burn (1961) and by Moe and Abildskov (1959), then the persistence of the arrhythmia is critically related to the degree of inhomogeneity of the tissue and to the mean ERP. Vagal stimulation or cholinomimetic drugs should tend to perpetuate the arrhythmia by reducing the mean ERP and by increasing the range of variation of the ERPs. The action of quinidine here is twofold. By virtue of its direct and antivagal actions, quinidine may increase the mean ERP and also reduce the inhomogeneity. The mathematical basis of these actions has been treated in detail by Moe and associates (1964). The action of quinidine, in terms of these concepts, is based not on its ability to snuff out a dominant circus movement but on its ability to reduce the number of wavelets possible in a given mass of tissue.

Electrocardiographic Effects. At therapeutic concentrations in man, quinidine causes a small increase in heart rate and in the P-R, QRS, and Q-T intervals. Clinical electrophysiological studies reveal that quinidine prolongs the ERP of the atrium, shortens the A-H interval (A-V nodal conduction), and usually prolongs the H-V interval slightly (His-Purkinje system conduction) (Josephson *et al.,* 1974). Careful studies reveal that widening of the QRS begins at low concentrations of quinidine in plasma and increases progressively as the concentration is increased (Heissenbuttel and Bigger, 1970). This effect is useful for monitoring the progress of therapy.

Autonomic Nervous System. In experimental animals, quinidine has a very significant atropine-like action, blocking the effects of vagal stimulation or of acetylcholine (Mason *et al.,* 1977). Quinidine also has α-adrenergic blocking properties. This action can cause vasodilatation and, via baroreceptors, activate sympathetic efferent activity (Roberts *et al.,* 1962; Schmid *et al.,* 1974b). Together, the cholinergic blockade and increased β-adrenergic activity caused by quinidine can increase sinus rate and enhance A-V nodal conduction in some human subjects (Josephson *et al.,* 1974; Mason *et al.,* 1977).

Absorption, Distribution, and Elimination. When administered orally, quinidine sulfate is absorbed rapidly and peak concentrations in plasma are attained in 60 to 90 minutes.

The absorption of quinidine gluconate is somewhat slower, and maximal concentrations are not observed until 3 or 4 hours after an oral dose. Quinidine can be given intramuscularly, but it causes pain at the injection site and a substantial increase in creatine kinase activity in plasma.

About 70 to 80% of quinidine in plasma is bound to plasma albumin. The drug enters erythrocytes and apparently binds to hemoglobin; at steady state, concentrations of quinidine in plasma and erythrocytes are approximately equal (Conn and Luchi, 1961). Quinidine accumulates rapidly in most tissues except brain, and the apparent volume of distribution is 2 to 3 liters per kilogram. In the heart, autoradiographic studies suggest that tritiated quinidine is localized in the sarcolemma and in mitochondria.

Quinidine is metabolized by the liver and excreted in the urine; the elimination halftime is about 6 hours. The greater portion of quinidine is eliminated by hepatic metabolism, but renal excretion is significant and about 20% of the parent drug is eliminated by this route.

Although quinidine is extensively metabolized in man, knowledge about its metabolic fate is still incomplete. Most urinary metabolites are hydroxylated at only one site, either on the quinoline ring or on the quinuclidine ring; small amounts of dihydroxy compounds are also found (Palmer et al., 1969; Drayer et al., 1977). The fraction of a dose of quinidine that is metabolized and the metabolic pathway appear to vary considerably from patient to patient. Unfortunately, preparations of quinidine are not pure and may contain other cinchona alkaloids; these can be mistaken for metabolic products when recovered from the urine. There is some controversy about whether the concentration of quinidine in plasma rises in patients with renal failure or congestive heart failure (see Kessler et al., 1974; Conrad et al., 1977; Drayer et al., 1977). The situation is complicated by the observation that at least some of quinidine's major metabolites are probably cardioactive (Conn, 1964; Drayer et al., 1977).

The free fraction of quinidine in plasma is filtered at the glomerulus, and quinidine is probably also actively secreted by the proximal renal tubule; passive back diffusion of the unchanged molecule occurs in the distal nephron. Since quinidine is a weak base, excretion is enhanced if the urine is acidic. When the urinary pH is increased from the 6–7 range to the 7–8 range, renal clearance of quinidine decreases by as much as 50% and concentration in the plasma increases (Gerhardt et al., 1969). This usually is not a problem clinically unless the patient takes sodium bicarbonate or acetazolamide concurrently or has renal tubular acidosis.

Routes of Administration, Dosage, and Preparations. For practical purposes, quinidine is only given orally, although it can be administered either intramuscularly or intravenously under special circumstances. The usual oral dose of quinidine sulfate is 300 to 500 mg four times a day. In most patients, quinidine will reach a steady state on such a schedule in about 24 hours and its concentration in plasma will fluctuate less than 50% between doses. Because of the large interindividual variation, drug interactions, and other causes of variability, it is wise to examine the ECG carefully after the initial dose of quinidine and to measure the plasma concentration of the drug at steady state (see Appendix II). Adjustment of dosage is often necessary. If an effective concentration must be achieved rapidly, a loading dose of 600 to 1000 mg can be given.

Quinidine Sulfate, U.S.P., *Quinidine Gluconate,* U.S.P., and *quinidine polygalacturonate* are available in a variety of preparations. Tablets and capsules of the sulfate contain 100, 200, or 300 mg of the drug (CIN-QUIN, QUINORA); tablets of quinidine polygalacturonate (CARDIOQUIN) contain 275 mg, equivalent to 200 mg of quinidine sulfate. Preparations for slow absorption are also available; these include a 300-mg extended-release tablet of quinidine sulfate (QUINIDEX) and a 324-mg tablet of the gluconate (QUINAGLUTE). For intravenous use, quinidine gluconate is provided in 10-ml vials containing 80 mg/ml. Quinidine sulfate is also available as an injection in 1-ml ampuls containing 200 mg/ml. The necessary dose is diluted to 800 mg/50 ml in 5% glucose solution and is injected at the rate of 16 mg per minute, with continuous observation of the patient and of the ECG. It is important to record the arterial pressure at frequent intervals.

THERAPEUTIC USES

Quinidine is a broad-spectrum drug; it is effective for acute and chronic treatment of supraventricular and ventricular arrhythmias. Quinidine is primarily used chronically to prevent recurrences of supraventricular tachyarrhythmias or to suppress ventricular premature depolarizations. Almost invariably some adjustment of the dose is required at the outset of therapy because the same dosage regimen will produce very different plasma concentrations in different individuals and because the same arrhythmia will be more or less responsive to a given concentration of the drug in different patients. Because the response to drug therapy is so variable, several 24-hour Holter ECG recordings are usually required to ensure adequate control of arrhythmias. Vigilance must be maintained to detect toxic reactions.

Supraventricular Arrhythmias. Quinidine is useful as chronic oral therapy for supraventricular arrhythmias. The objective of therapy usually is to prevent or to reduce the frequency of arrhythmic episodes.

Paroxysmal Supraventricular Tachycardia (PSVT). Quinidine can be effective against recurrent, aggravating PSVT, either the usual A-V nodal reciprocating tachycardia or the PSVT seen in the Wolff-Parkinson-White syndrome. In the A-V nodal form of PSVT, digitalis and other methods usually are utilized before quinidine because of the very significant toxicity of the latter drug. The mode of action of quinidine in PSVT is not certain. It may suppress the atrial premature depolarizations that trigger the arrhythmia or alter conduction and refractoriness of the atrium and A-V node so that PSVT no longer occurs. In the Wolff-Parkinson-White syndrome, quinidine often slows conduction and increases refractoriness in the accessory A-V connection and, therefore, prevents attacks of PSVT.

Atrial Flutter or Fibrillation. Quinidine was used for many years as the drug of choice for conversion of atrial flutter or atrial fibrillation to sinus rhythm. Since the advent of DC cardioversion, quinidine has been relegated to a supporting role in the management of these two arrhythmias. Patients scheduled for cardioversion are given oral maintenance doses of quinidine (*e.g.,* 400 mg every 6 hours) 1 or 2 days before the anticipated cardioversion. About one third of patients with atrial fibrillation will convert to sinus rhythm because of the effect of quinidine; others require DC shock. Maintenance of quinidine therapy helps to prevent recurrence of atrial fibrillation (*see* Sodermark *et al.,* 1975). If atrial premature depolarizations occur soon after cardioversion, the dose of quinidine should be increased until the arrhythmia is abolished or quinidine toxicity is encountered. If uninterrupted sinus rhythm resumes after cardioversion, the concentration of quinidine in plasma should be adjusted to plateau between 2 and 4 μg/ml.

Ventricular Arrhythmias. Quinidine is one of the most useful drugs for chronic treatment of ventricular arrhythmias (ventricular premature depolarization, ventricular tachycardia) or for the prevention of ventricular fibrillation.

Ventricular Premature Depolarizations. The ventricular premature depolarization (VPD) is the most common of these disturbances of rhythm. VPDs are treated when they cause discomfort (palpitations), impair hemodynamic performance, or increase the likelihood of death. When treating VPDs or brief recurrent bursts of ventricular tachycardia, the dose of quinidine is adjusted while 24-hour Holter ECG recordings are analyzed to establish the intensity of drug effect. Usually, the dose of quinidine is increased until complex forms (pairs or runs of VPDs) are abolished and the frequency of VPDs is reduced by 75 to 80%; this dose is then maintained. When the arrhythmia is caused by an acute process, such as open-heart surgery, acute myocardial infarction, or acute myocarditis, quinidine can be discontinued when the acute process is resolved. If the arrhythmia is life threatening, quinidine should be discontinued while the patient is in the hospital and can be monitored carefully for recurrence.

Ventricular Tachycardia. The treatment of sustained ventricular tachycardia is quite different. Prior to the advent of DC cardioversion, heroic and skilled dosage with quinidine was used to convert ventricular tachycardia to sinus rhythm. There were many problems associated with this approach, and the incidence of toxicity was high; it has been abandoned. The arrhythmia usually responds readily to DC conversion. After conversion, drug therapy can be used to prevent recurrences.

Digitalis-Induced Arrhythmias. The complex rhythm disturbances that can attend the use of digitalis are discussed in Chapter 30. Although quinidine can be effective for the treatment of a variety of digitalis-induced arrhythmias, it is not the preferred drug, since adverse effects on cardiac rhythm are more likely to occur with quinidine than with other effective treatments (*e.g.,* phenytoin).

UNTOWARD EFFECTS

About one third of the patients who receive quinidine will have immediate adverse effects that necessitate discontinuation of therapy. If this initial hurdle is passed, few extracardiac adverse effects are encountered during chronic therapy. However, excessive concentration of the drug in plasma will cause adverse effects in any patient because quinidine has a low therapeutic ratio. Constant vigilance is thus required in every patient taking this drug.

Cardiotoxicity. As the concentration of quinidine in plasma rises above 2 μg/ml, the QRS complex and the Q-T$_c$ interval will widen progressively (Heissenbuttel and Bigger, 1970). These changes are useful in monitoring quinidine therapy. A 25% increase in the duration of the QRS complex is cause for concern; a 50% increase should prompt a reduction in dosage. At high plasma concentrations of the drug, cardiac toxicity may become severe; S-A block or arrest, high-grade A-V block, ventricular arrhythmias, or asystole may result. Conduction is slowed tremendously in all parts of the heart. In addition, Purkinje fibers can become depolarized and develop abnormal automaticity. These changes are responsible for the bizarre arrhythmias seen in severe poisoning with quinidine. Ventricular tachycardia in quinidine toxicity is a life-threatening event and must be treated with the utmost speed and caution. The challenge for the therapist is to realize that the toxicity of the drug can mimic the disease it is used to treat. Appropriate criteria that can separate drug effects from spontaneous worsening of the disease must be used. The ECG is one such aid and must be closely monitored while the patient is in an intensive care unit. Sodium lactate, catecholamines, and glucagon may be useful in counteracting some of the arrhythmias caused by quinidine (Bellet *et al.*, 1959; Wasserman *et al.*, 1959). Quinidine and its hydroxy metabolites can be removed by dialysis (Conrad *et al.*, 1977).

Quinidine Syncope. Occasionally patients taking quinidine experience syncope or sudden death. In some instances, this reaction may be the result of high concentrations of quinidine in plasma or the result of coexisting digitalis toxicity. However, ventricular tachyarrhythmias may occur in susceptible individuals while the concentrations of quinidine in plasma are low (Selzer and Wray, 1964). Individuals with the long Q-T syndrome or those who respond to quinidine with marked lengthening of the Q-T interval appear to be particularly at risk and should not be treated with this drug (Koster and Wellens, 1976).

"Paradoxical" Ventricular Response to Atrial Fibrillation. A frequently mentioned complication of quinidine when the drug is used to treat atrial fibrillation is the so-called paradoxical increase in ventricular rate. In many instances of atrial fibrillation, quinidine causes a substantial decrease in the atrial rate. If the atrial rate decreases sufficiently, the ventricular rate may abruptly rise because of the decrease in concealed conduction of atrial impulses in the A-V node. Paradoxical increase in ventricular rate is not common in patients treated only with quinidine. However, the effect is so dramatic in some patients that it is traditional and prob-ably wise to digitalize patients prior to administration of quinidine in order to avoid this event.

Blood Pressure. Quinidine can cause significant hypotension, particularly when given intravenously. This response is probably due to the α-adrenergic blocking effect of the drug. Hemodynamic studies have revealed that hypotension due to quinidine is caused by vasodilatation without significant decrease in cardiac output (Ferrer *et al.*, 1948); therapeutic concentrations of quinidine have no significant adverse effects on myocardial performance (Markiewicz *et al.*, 1976; White *et al.*, 1977). Very high concentrations may adversely affect myocardial contractility.

Arterial Embolism. The risk of embolism following conversion of atrial fibrillation to sinus rhythm is a source of concern, particularly in patients with rheumatic heart disease. The fibrillating atria do not contract, and thrombi often develop in the left atrium, particularly in the atrial appendage. After the resumption of sinus rhythm, atrial contraction may dislodge thrombi; stroke is the most dreaded sequela of the resultant arterial embolization. However, the risk of systemic embolization is greater if atrial fibrillation persists than if conversion to sinus rhythm occurs. If cardioversion is performed as an elective procedure, patients are usually given anticoagulants for 1 to 2 weeks prior to conversion. Because the risk of embolization is reasonably small even without anticoagulation, it has not been possible to demonstrate unequivocally that anticoagulation significantly reduces the risk of embolism.

Cinchonism. Like other cinchona alkaloids and the salicylates, quinidine can cause cinchonism. Symptoms of mild cinchonism include tinnitus, loss of hearing, slight blurring of vision, and gastrointestinal upset. If toxicity is severe, headache, diplopia, photophobia, and altered color perception may occur, as can confusion, delirium, and psychosis. The skin may be hot and flushed; nausea, vomiting, diarrhea, and abdominal pain are likely.

Gastrointestinal Symptoms. The most common adverse reactions to quinidine are referable to the gastrointestinal tract—nausea, vomiting, and diarrhea. Gastrointestinal symptoms often occur, even when drug concentrations in plasma are low. This type of adverse reaction is apparent immediately after quinidine is first administered and forces discontinuation of the drug in almost one third of patients so treated.

Hypersensitivity Reactions. Hypersensitivity to quinidine can cause *fever;* this reaction is rare and disappears when the drug is discontinued. Rarely, quinidine causes *anaphylactic reactions,* which require the usual emergency measures. *Thrombocytopenia* is an uncommon but potentially lethal outcome of treatment with quinidine. Thrombocytopenia usually occurs after several weeks or months of therapy and is due to formation of drug-platelet complexes that evoke a circulating antibody. When quinidine, platelets, and antibody are all present in the circulation, platelets agglutinate and lyse (Larson, 1953; Schulman, 1958). Thrombocytopenia can be profound, and severe bleeding may ensue. If quinidine is stopped, the platelet count will return to near normal in 2 to 7 days. Until the bleeding time is normal, patients should be kept in the hospital and, if necessary, treated with adrenocorticosteroids and transfusions of platelets. Asthma-like *respiratory difficulty* or *vascular collapse* can occur as a result of hypersensitivity. Artificial ventilation and supportive measures usually will control the drug-induced respiratory difficulties; norepinephrine may be required to restore blood pressure.

DRUG INTERACTIONS

Drugs such as phenobarbital or phenytoin that induce drug-metabolizing enzymes in the liver may significantly shorten the duration of action of quinidine by increasing its rate of elimination (Data *et al.,* 1976). Since patients vary tremendously in their susceptibility to enzyme induction, it is difficult to predict which individuals will be affected. When quinidine is given to patients who have stable concentrations of digoxin in plasma, the digoxin concentration often increases substantially (Leahey *et al.,* 1978). The precise mechanism of this interaction is unknown, but it undoubtedly involves a

pharmacokinetic alteration (*see* Chapter 30). Occasionally, patients who are receiving warfarin or other oral anticoagulants show an increase in prothrombin time after quinidine is administered (Koch-Weser, 1968); the mechanism of this reaction is not clear. Since quinidine is an α-adrenergic blocking agent, it can interact additively with drugs that cause vasodilatation or decrease blood volume. For example, nitroglycerin can cause severe postural hypotension in patients who are taking quinidine. The effect of any given concentration of quinidine on the heart is greater when the concentration of K^+ in plasma is increased.

PROCAINAMIDE

Procainamide is useful for the treatment of a variety of arrhythmias, and it can be administered by several routes. Unfortunately its potency and versatility are marred by its short duration of action and a high incidence of adverse reactions when it is used chronically.

History. In 1936, Mautz demonstrated that direct application of procaine to the myocardium elevated the threshold of ventricular muscle to electrical stimulation. Extension of this observation by numerous workers established that the cardiac actions of procaine resemble those of quinidine. However, the therapeutic value of procaine as an antifibrillatory and antiarrhythmic agent is limited by rapid enzymatic hydrolysis and prominent adverse effects on the central nervous system. A systematic study of congeners and metabolites of procaine was undertaken to find a compound with clinically useful quinidine-like actions; procainamide was discovered as a result (Mark *et al.,* 1951).

Chemistry and Preparations. Procainamide has the following structural formula:

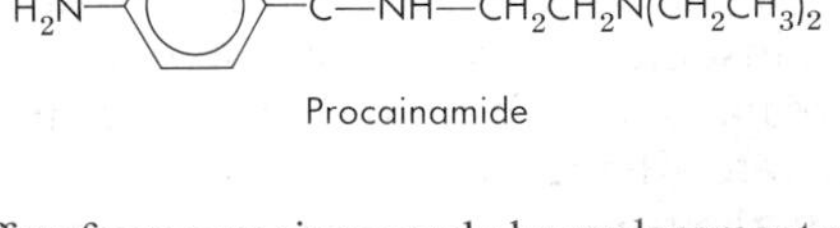

Procainamide

It differs from procaine merely by replacement of the ester linkage by the amide. *Procainamide Hydrochloride,* U.S.P., is a white to tan, odorless, crystalline salt that is readily soluble in water. For oral administration the drug is available as capsules and tablets containing 250, 375, or 500 mg (PROCAMIDE, PROCAPAN, PRONESTYL). *Procainamide Hydrochloride Injection,* U.S.P., is supplied in 10-ml vials containing 100 mg/ml and 2-ml vials containing 500 mg/ml and is suitable for intramuscular and intravenous injection.

PHARMACOLOGICAL PROPERTIES

Cardiac Electrophysiological Effects. The direct effects of procainamide on the electrical activity of the heart are very similar to those produced by quinidine. However, the indirect effects, that is, those resulting from interaction with the autonomic nervous system, are significantly different. The effects of procainamide on automaticity, excitability, responsiveness, and conduction are virtually the same as those of quinidine (Table 31-2). As a result, the effects of procainamide on the ECG are also quite similar.

Autonomic Nervous System. The anticholinergic action of procainamide is somewhat weaker than that of quinidine. Procainamide does not produce α-adrenergic blockade, but, in the dog, it can block autonomic ganglia weakly and cause a measurable impairment of cardiovascular reflexes (Schmid *et al.*, 1974a).

Absorption, Distribution, and Elimination. Procainamide is quickly and nearly completely absorbed following oral administration (Appendix II). The peak concentration in plasma is reached 45 to 75 minutes after ingestion of the capsule, but significantly later if tablets are administered. In the first week after acute myocardial infarction, oral absorption may be poor, the peak plasma concentration may be quite delayed, and concentrations of the drug may be inadequate to control arrhythmias (Koch-Weser *et al.*, 1969). Several sustained-release formulations of procainamide have been studied in man (Karlsson, 1973; Graffner *et al.*, 1975). In general, their bioavailability is somewhat lower than that of standard capsules. However, absorption is delayed sufficiently that the duration of action usually can be extended to at least 8 hours.

About 20% of the procainamide in plasma is bound to proteins. Procainamide is rapidly distributed into most body tissues except the brain, and the apparent volume of distribution is about 2 liters per kilogram. However, this value can decrease to 1.3 to 1.8 liters per kilogram in patients with cardiac failure or shock. Compensation for this change should be made in calculating dosage.

Procainamide is eliminated by renal excretion and hepatic metabolism. The biotransformation of procainamide has been intensively studied since the discovery that its major metabolic pathway is N-acetylation (Dreyfuss *et al.*, 1972). It is thought that there is bimodal genetic variation in the activity of the N-acetyltransferase for procainamide, similar to the situation for isoniazid, dapsone, and other drugs (Karlsson *et al.*, 1974; Gibson *et al.*, 1975; Reidenberg *et al.*, 1975). However, there is another acetylase system that does not show such variation and that also may contribute to the metabolism of procainamide (Giardina *et al.*, 1977). In fast acetylators or in renal insufficiency, as much as 40% of a dose of procainamide may be excreted as N-acetylprocainamide (NAPA), and concentrations of NAPA in plasma may equal or exceed those of the parent drug. Two other metabolites of procainamide, the structures of which are not yet known, account for 8 to 15% of a dose of procainamide (Giardina *et al.*, 1976). NAPA is cardioactive and, in fact, may be a useful antiarrhythmic drug. Clinical trials are in progress to explore this question. In patients with renal failure, concentrations of NAPA in plasma can become dangerously high. Furthermore, the rate of acetylation may be related to the probability that a lupus erythematosus–like syndrome will develop (*see* below). For optimal patient management, information should be available about the concentrations of both procainamide and NAPA in plasma.

A large fraction (up to two thirds) of a dose of procainamide is eliminated unchanged in the urine. Procainamide is a weak base that is filtered, secreted by the proximal tubule, and partially reabsorbed. Moderate changes in the pH of the urine cause little change in the renal excretion of procainamide (Galeazzi *et al.*, 1976). When intrinsic renal function or renal perfusion decreases, the concentration of procainamide in plasma rises significantly (Koch-Weser and Klein, 1971). However, as the blood urea nitrogen rises, the fraction of a dose of procainamide that is excreted unchanged decreases. The elimination of NAPA is nearly entirely by renal excretion, and its rate of renal clearance is lower than that for procainamide. NAPA thus tends to accumulate when renal failure or congestive heart failure is present.

Dosage and Routes of Administration. Procainamide is one of the most versatile of all antiarrhythmic drugs with respect to the variety of routes of administration that can be used and the flexibility of dosing schedules. Procainamide can be administered by intravenous injection or infusion, intramuscularly, and orally. The concentration in plasma needed for antiarrhythmic effects is usually 3 to 10 μg/ml, occasionally higher. The probability of toxicity becomes greater as the concentration rises above 8 μg/ml. As with quinidine, the cardiac effects of procainamide are enhanced if the concentration of K^+ in plasma is elevated.

Intravenous Administration. In acute or unstable situations, intravenous administration is desirable for speed (injection or rapid infusion), precision (constant infusion), and reliability of effect. The total loading dose is *never* given as a single intravenous injection because it can cause hypotension. One rapid and safe method to establish effective concentrations in plasma is *intermittent intravenous administration:* 100 mg is injected over 1 minute, and this dose is repeated every 5 minutes until the arrhythmia is controlled or adverse effects are seen or until the size of the total dose (about 1000 mg) suggests that the arrhythmia under treatment is resistant (Bigger and Heissenbuttel, 1969; Giardina *et al.,* 1973). The 5-minute dosing interval permits examination of the blood pressure and ECG after each dose. Serious hypotension or excessive widening of the QRS interval can thus be avoided. Alternatively, the same dose can be given over a similar period by *rapid intravenous infusion.* For example, 600 mg can be infused at a rate of 20 mg per minute (Bigger, 1975). The same precautions should be taken. When the arrhythmia is controlled, a *constant-rate intravenous infusion* is often used to maintain effective concentrations in plasma. The infusion rate can be estimated as the product of the desired concentration (3 to 10 μg/ml) and the estimated total clearance of procainamide (about 9 ml/kg per minute) (*see* Appendix II). The effective concentration can be roughly estimated from the response to the initial dosing.

Oral Administration. For chronic therapy, oral administration is the only practical route. Total daily doses of 3 to 6 g usually are required for therapeutic efficacy. Because its elimination half-life is short (about 3 hours in normal subjects), the drug must be given fairly frequently. Fortunately, most patients can take procainamide orally at intervals of 6 or more hours because the elimination half-time is often in the range of 5 to 8 hours in patients with cardiac disease and the accumulation of NAPA during administration of procainamide contributes to antiarrhythmic action. The best way to evaluate the efficacy of an oral regimen is to perform 24-hour Holter ECG recordings. If difficulty is encountered in controlling an arrhythmia, determination of the concentrations of procainamide and NAPA may help to distinguish inadequate concentrations of drug from drug-resistant arrhythmias.

When oral therapy is begun, a loading dose is occasionally desirable; a dose of twice the anticipated maintenance dose should be given. Oral loading doses usually are not required because of the short half-life of the drug.

One special circumstance is worthy of comment—the change from intravenous infusion to oral dosage. This transition often is required in the management of patients with acute myocardial infarction (Bigger, 1975). The infusion should be stopped and about one elimination half-time permitted to elapse before administration of the first oral dose. In this situation, the oral dose can be chosen very precisely based on the previous requirements for the drug.

Intramuscular Administration. Procainamide is well absorbed after intramuscular injection. Absorption is somewhat more rapid than that after oral administration.

THERAPEUTIC USES

Procainamide has been employed to treat a wide variety of cardiac arrhythmias. In general, the effectiveness of the drug parallels that of quinidine, and some investigators consider the two agents to be interchangeable. However, procainamide may be effective in patients who have failed to respond to maximally tolerated doses of quinidine and *vice versa.*

Ventricular Arrhythmias. The most favorable results have been reported in ventricular arrhythmias (except those resulting from digitalis intoxication). Ventricular premature depolarizations and paroxysmal ventricular tachycardia are abolished in a large percentage of cases within a few minutes after intravenous injection or within an hour after oral or intramuscular administration (Kayden *et al.,* 1957).

Digitalis-Induced Arrhythmias. Although ventricular premature depolarizations and tachycardia caused by digitalis intoxication can be suppressed by procainamide, its efficacy and toxicity are unpredictable; fatalities have occurred. If ventricular tachycardia induced by digitalis is accompanied by marked disturbances of A-V conduction, procainamide readily precipitates ventricular asystole or fibrillation. The complexities and dangers of the combined effects of digitalis and procainamide have been discussed by Zapata-Diáz and coworkers (1952).

Supraventricular Arrhythmias. Early reports suggested that procainamide was relatively ineffective for the treatment of atrial arrhythmias. Careful subsequent studies have documented that the efficacy of procainamide against atrial arrhythmias is comparable to that of quinidine (Miller *et al.,* 1952; Schack *et al.,* 1952). Often, however, high doses (4 to 8 g per day) are required to control atrial arrhythmias. Like quinidine, procainamide is only moderately effective in converting atrial flutter or chronic atrial fibrillation to sinus rhythm. Procainamide can be used to prevent recurrences of atrial flutter or atrial fibrillation after cardioversion.

UNTOWARD EFFECTS

Cardiotoxicity. The incidence of adverse effects is high when procainamide is used as an antiarrhythmic drug. Excessive concentrations in plasma produce ECG changes very similar to those seen during quinidine therapy. The same rules and precautions for using and discontinuing quinidine (*see* above) pertain to procainamide. High concentrations of procainamide in plasma can also produce ventricular premature depolarizations, ventricular tachycardia, or ventricular fibrillation. Interestingly, the syndrome of marked prolongation of the Q-T interval and severe ventricular arrhythmias produced by quinidine has not been observed with procainamide. Procainamide, like quinidine, will slow the rate of atrial fibrillation and can thereby cause a "paradoxical" increase in the rate of the ventricular response.

Blood Pressure. If procainamide is administered intravenously, it can cause hypotension. Intermittent or rapid intravenous infusion can be adjusted so that significant hypotension is unusual, provided that doses are less than 600 mg. Toxic concentrations of procainamide depress myocardial performance and promote hypotension.

Extracardiac Adverse Effects. During oral administration of procainamide, gastrointestinal symptoms (anorexia, nausea, vomiting, and, rarely, diarrhea) may occur; these symptoms are much more common with quinidine. Although procainamide has fewer adverse effects on the central nervous system than does procaine or lidocaine, a variety of symptoms, including giddiness, psychosis, hallucinations, and mental depression, can result from the drug.

Hypersensitivity Reactions. This class of adverse effects is the most common and troublesome. Occasionally, *fever* occurs during the first few days of therapy and forces discontinuance of procainamide. *Agranulocytosis* may occur in the early weeks of therapy; fatal infections may follow. Leukocyte

and differential blood counts should be performed regularly during the course of therapy, and complaints of sore throat should receive prompt evaluation. Myalgias, angioedema, skin rashes, digital vasculitis, and Raynaud's phenomenon have all been attributed to procainamide (*see* Bigger and Heissenbuttel, 1969).

Systemic Lupus Erythematosus–like Syndrome. Ladd (1962) first described a syndrome caused by procainamide that superficially resembled authentic systemic lupus erythematosus (SLE). Arthralgia is the most common symptom; pericarditis, pleuropneumonic involvement, fever, and hepatomegaly are common signs. The most serious complication is hemorrhagic pericardial effusion with tamponade. Drug-induced SLE is different from the naturally occurring disease. In the drug-induced syndrome, there is no predilection for females; the brain and kidney are spared; leukopenia, anemia, thrombocytopenia, and hyperglobulinemia are rare; and false-positive serologic tests for syphilis do not occur. The drug-induced syndrome is reversible when procainamide is discontinued. About 60 to 70% of patients who receive procainamide will develop antinuclear antibodies after 1 to 12 months of therapy. Only 20 to 30% of these individuals will develop the clinical symptoms and signs of the SLE syndrome if treatment is continued. When symptoms occur, LE-cell preparations are often positive. The development of antinuclear antibodies alone is insufficient reason to discontinue therapy with procainamide. However, procainamide usually should be stopped if patients become symptomatic. An exception should be made if the patient has a life-threatening arrhythmia for which alternative therapy is not available. In this circumstance, symptoms of SLE may be controlled with aspirin or adrenocorticosteroids. It is not yet clear if individuals who acetylate procainamide slowly have an increased risk of developing the SLE-like syndrome (Karlsson *et al.*, 1974; Davies *et al.*, 1975), but slow acetylators of hydralazine are more susceptible to hydralazine-induced lupus.

DISOPYRAMIDE

Disopyramide has been available in the United States since 1978 for oral treatment of some ventricular arrhythmias in adults.

Chemistry and Preparations. Disopyramide has the following structural formula:

$$(CH_3)_2CH-NCH_2CH_2-\overset{|}{C}-CONH_2$$
$$(CH_3)_2CH$$

Disopyramide

Disopyramide Phosphate, U.S.P. (NORPACE), is available as capsules containing 100 or 150 mg of the base. A preparation for intravenous administration is not available in the United States.

PHARMACOLOGICAL PROPERTIES

Cardiac Electrophysiological Effects. Disopyramide has not yet been studied extensively. The direct effect of the drug on the sinus node is to slow its rate of discharge (Sekiya and Vaughan Williams, 1963). In patients with the sick sinus syndrome, disopyramide can depress the automaticity of the sinus node (Seipel and Breithardt, 1976; LaBarre *et al.,* 1979). Therapeutic concentrations will decrease the slope of phase-4 depolarization in Purkinje fibers and decrease their spontaneous rate of firing (Kus and Sasyniuk, 1975); the mechanism of the change in pacemaker activity is unknown. The effects of disopyramide on the duration of the action potential, refractoriness, and membrane responsiveness are entirely comparable to the effects of quinidine or procainamide (Kus and Sasyniuk, 1975; Danilo and Rosen, 1976). Disopyramide reduces the differences in the duration of the action potential between normal and infarcted tissues by lengthening the action potential of normal cells (Sasyniuk and Kus, 1976). Disopyramide seems somewhat more potent than quinidine in increasing atrial or ventricular refractoriness and less potent in the His-Purkinje system.

Electrocardiographic Effects. Disopyramide usually causes little change in the sinus rate. The P-R interval does not change as much as with quinidine or procainamide; the QRS rarely increases by more than 20% when concentrations of the drug are in the therapeutic range; and the Q-T_c consistently lengthens by a small amount. Electrophysiological studies in man show that disopyramide shortens the recovery time of the sinus node. It consistently increases atrial refractoriness, but conduction and refractoriness in the A-V node do not change. Similarly, conduction in the His-Purkinje system is usually unaltered. The effective refractory period (ERP) of the ventricle is increased (Josephson *et al.,* 1973; Spurrell *et al.,* 1975; Marrott *et al.,* 1976). Birkhead and Vaughan Williams (1977) studied the effects of disopyramide on human atrial and A-V nodal conduction and refractoriness after cholinergic blockade. Under these circumstances, disopyramide (2 mg/kg) substantially decreased the sinus rate and increased recovery time of the sinus node; the drug

also increased the ERP of the atrium and the functional refractory period of the A-V node. Apparently, the atropine-like action of disopyramide nullifies some of its direct effects. Patients with bundle-branch disease seem more likely to develop an increase in the H-V interval after disopyramide than do patients with normal intraventricular conduction (Desai *et al.,* 1979).

Autonomic Nervous System. Disopyramide has antimuscarinic activity (about 10% as potent as atropine). The drug is neither an α- nor a β-adrenergic antagonist (Mathur, 1972).

Absorption, Distribution, and Elimination. About 90% of an oral dose of disopyramide is absorbed, of which a small fraction is subject to first-pass metabolism by the liver (Karim, 1975; Hinderling and Garrett, 1976). Concentrations in plasma peak at 1 to 2 hours after a dose.

At normal therapeutic concentrations (3 µg/ml) about 30% of disopyramide is bound to plasma proteins (Chien *et al.,* 1974); the bound fraction varies with the total concentration of drug in plasma (Hinderling *et al.,* 1974). The apparent volume of distribution of disopyramide is nearly 1 liter per kilogram.

About 50% of a dose of disopyramide is excreted by the kidney unchanged, 20% as the mono-N-dealkylated metabolite, and another 10% as unidentified metabolites (Karin, 1975). The monodealkylated metabolite has less antiarrhythmic and atropine-like activity than does the parent compound. The half-time for elimination is 7 to 8 hours, and this value is markedly prolonged in patients with renal insufficiency (up to 20 hours or more).

Dosage and Route of Administration. In the United States, disopyramide is approved only for oral administration. The usual total daily dose is 400 to 800 mg; this amount is divided into four doses. Loading doses of 200 to 400 mg will rapidly produce effective concentrations. For adult patients who weigh less than 50 kg, a loading dose of 200 mg, followed by 100-mg maintenance doses, is recommended. The maintenance dose must be carefully adjusted for patients with renal failure according to the creatinine clearance; efficacy, toxic manifestations, and plasma concentration should be carefully monitored in such individuals.

THERAPEUTIC USES

In the United States, disopyramide is approved only for the treatment of ventricular arrhythmias in adults. Its efficacy against atrial and ventricular arrhythmias caused by digitalis has not been established by controlled trials. Experience in Europe indicates that disopyramide is about as efficacious as quinidine or procainamide in converting atrial arrhythmias to sinus rhythm and that it is useful for the maintenance of sinus rhythm after cardioversion (Hartel *et al.,* 1974; Luoma *et al.,* 1978). The efficacy of intravenous and oral disopyramide in acute myocardial infarction is under investigation. Preliminary studies show a reduction in frequency of ventricular premature depolarizations, but protection from ventricular tachycardia or primary ventricular fibrillation has not been demonstrated.

TOXICITY

The anticholinergic action of disopyramide produces a significant incidence of dry mouth, constipation, blurred vision, urinary hesitancy, and, occasionally, urinary retention. Disopyramide can cause nausea, abdominal pain, vomiting, or diarrhea, but gastrointestinal symptoms are significantly less common than when quinidine is used. Disopyramide reduces cardiac output and left ventricular performance in patients who have well-compensated ventricular function. The adverse effects on ventricular function are significantly more pronounced in patients who have preexisting ventricular failure (Jensen *et al.*, 1975). Great caution should be exercised when such patients are treated with disopyramide. The *adverse hemodynamic effects* seem to be more marked than those characteristic of quinidine, procainamide, lidocaine, or phenytoin. The *blood pressure* usually increases transiently after intravenous administration of disopyramide, even though the cardiac output falls; total peripheral vascular resistance thus increases markedly. The cause of this unusual reaction is not known.

LIDOCAINE

Lidocaine is widely used as a local anesthetic (*see* Chapter 15). It has also achieved prominence as an antiarrhythmic agent and is now commonly used, particularly as emergency treatment, for ventricular arrhythmias that are encountered during cardiac surgery or acute myocardial infarction. Its mechanism of action differs in some respects from that of quinidine and procainamide, and it possesses certain advantages over the older drugs. Chief among these, especially for use in the coronary care unit, is that its antiarrhythmic action can be established very rapidly and safely by intravenous administration, and its effects decline quickly when the infusion is terminated. This permits moment-to-moment titration of ventricular ectopic activity.

Chemistry and Preparations. The structural formula of lidocaine is shown in Chapter 15. *Lidocaine Hydrochloride Injection,* U.S.P. (XYLOCAINE), is available for intravenous administration as a 5-ml prefilled syringe or a 5-ml ampul, each containing 20 mg/ml; the injection contains no preservative, sympathomimetic, or other vasoconstrictor, and *it is the only preparation of lidocaine that should be given intravenously.*

PHARMACOLOGICAL PROPERTIES

Cardiac Electrophysiological Effects. Unlike quinidine and procainamide, lidocaine exerts most of its electrophysiological effects on the heart by a direct action; no important interactions between lidocaine and the autonomic nervous system have been described.

Automaticity. Therapeutic concentrations of lidocaine have no effect on the action potentials or firing rate of the isolated sinus node of the rabbit (Mandel and Bigger, 1971). Depression of the human sinus node by lidocaine is distinctly unusual but can occur in subjects with preexisting disease of the sinus node (Cheng and Wadhwa, 1973; Bigger and Reiffel, 1979). Therapeutic concentrations of lidocaine decrease the slope of normal phase-4 depolarization in Purkinje fibers (Davis and Temte, 1969; Bigger and Mandel, 1970). This action is caused by a substantial increase in the background outward current (i_{K_1}), sometimes accompanied by a decrease in background inward current (i_{bi}) (Weld and Bigger, 1976). Preliminary studies indicate that lidocaine also can counteract automaticity in depolarized, stretched Purkinje fibers and delayed afterdepolarizations caused by digitalis. This is probably a result of the increase in i_{K_1}, which overcomes small inward currents that cause depolarization.

Excitability and Threshold. Lidocaine causes an increase in the diastolic electrical current threshold in cardiac Purkinje fibers by increasing K^+ conductance (g_{K_1}) without changing resting *Vm* or the voltage threshold (Arnsdorf and Bigger, 1975). Lidocaine also increases the threshold for ventricular fibrillation (Gerstenblith *et al.*, 1972).

Responsiveness and Conduction. Lidocaine has complex effects on membrane responsiveness, and studies of this relationship have yielded conflicting results.

The steady-state relationship between $\dot{V}_{max}$ and *Vm* is little altered in normal Purkinje fibers by therapeutic concentrations of lidocaine. However, therapeutic concentrations of lidocaine prevent fast responses at low (less negative) values of *Vm* (Davis and Temte, 1969; Bigger and Mandel, 1970). This effect can be explained by the large increase in i_{K_1} caused by lidocaine, which counteracts small inward-going excitatory currents. Also, the effect of lidocaine on responsiveness depends on $[K]_o$; at $[K]_o$ up to 4.5 mM, therapeutic concentrations have little effect on responsiveness (Obayashi *et al.*, 1975). At $[K]_o$ of 5.6 or 6.0, therapeutic concentrations of lidocaine reduce V_{max} at any level of Vm (Singh and Vaughan Williams, 1971; Obayashi *et al.*, 1975). Toxic concentrations clearly shift responsiveness in much the same way as quinidine (Bigger and Mandel, 1970). Abnormal ventricular muscle fibers that survive experimental infarction show reduced responsiveness when exposed to therapeutic concentrations of lidocaine (Kupersmith *et al.*, 1975). Even therapeutic concentrations of lidocaine delay reactivation of i_{Na}, so that responsiveness may decrease at fast heart rates (Weld and Bigger, 1975).

Because of the large safety factor for conduction, lidocaine usually has no effect on conduction velocity in normal tissues of the His-Purkinje system or ventricular muscle. Under abnormal circumstances, lidocaine may either decrease or increase conduction velocity in the His-Purkinje system or in ventricular muscle; in ischemic tissues, conduction usually decreases substantially (Kupersmith *et al.*, 1975); in tissues depolarized by stretch or low $[K]_o$ (both of which depress g_K), lidocaine causes hyperpolarization and significant increases in conduction velocity (Arnsdorf and Bigger, 1972).

Duration of the Action Potential and Refractoriness. Lidocaine causes almost no change in the duration of the action potential of ordinary or specialized atrial fibers. It very substantially decreases the duration of the action potential in Purkinje fibers and ventricular muscle. The greatest change is seen in portions of the His-Purkinje system, where the duration of the action potential is normally longest (Wittig *et al.*, 1973). Thus, lidocaine tends to reduce the temporal and spatial dispersion of refractoriness. The effective refractory period (ERP) also shortens after lidocaine, but this effect is less pronounced than that on the duration of the action potential. This difference may be due to decreased responsiveness (because of delayed reactivation) and/or the tendency for increased outward current to quell small responses.

Effect on Reentrant Arrhythmias. Lidocaine can abolish ventricular reentry, either by improving conduction or by causing two-way block. Conduction can be improved by lidocaine if depolarization and slow conduction are due to decreased g_{K_1} (*e.g.*, stretch or low $[K]_o$) or if slow conduction depends on the long and unequal action potential dura-

tions in portions of the reentrant circuit. Lidocaine can increase resting Vm in the former case or selectively shorten the duration of the action potential in the latter case. Alternatively, if one-way block occurs in ischemic, depolarized elements of a reentry circuit, lidocaine would be likely to abolish reentry by producing two-way block.

Lidocaine is much less effective than quinidine or procainamide in slowing the atrial rate in patients with atrial flutter or atrial fibrillation or in converting these arrhythmias to sinus rhythm. This lack of effect is expected, since lidocaine has so little effect on either refractoriness or responsiveness in the atria.

Electrocardiographic Effects.   In striking contrast to quinidine and procainamide, lidocaine causes negligible change in the ECG; the Q-T interval may shorten, but the QRS does not widen. Lidocaine has quite variable effects on the refractory period of the A-V node; there is usually no change, but some individuals show substantial shortening (Josephson *et al.*, 1972). The latter action is probably responsible for the marked increase in ventricular response that can occur in patients with atrial flutter and A-V block who are treated with lidocaine (Adamson and Spracklen, 1968). Usually the effective refractory period in the His-Purkinje system shortens substantially during treatment with lidocaine (Josephson *et al.*, 1972). However, lidocaine can cause complete A-V block within the His-Purkinje system in patients with preexisting bundle-branch disease (Gupta *et al.*, 1974).

Autonomic Nervous System.   In contrast to quinidine, procainamide, disopyramide, propranolol, and bretylium, lidocaine does not interact significantly with the autonomic nervous system.

Absorption, Distribution, and Elimination. Although lidocaine is well absorbed after oral administration, it is subject to extensive first-pass hepatic metabolism, and only about one third of the drug reaches the general circulation. The concentrations of drug in plasma are thus low and unpredictable (Boyes *et al.*, 1971). In addition, many patients experience nausea, vomiting, and abdominal discomfort after oral administration of lidocaine, and this route is thus not used. The drug is almost completely absorbed after intramuscular administration.

About 50% of lidocaine in plasma is bound to albumin at therapeutic concentrations of the drug. Distribution is rapid, and the apparent volume of distribution for lidocaine is normally about 1 liter per kilogram; this volume is substantially reduced in patients with heart failure (Thomson *et al.*, 1973).

Essentially no lidocaine is excreted unchanged in the urine. Deethylation in the liver results in the appearance of monoethylglycylxylidine and then glycine xylidide (Strong *et al.*, 1973). The former metabolite has antiarrhythmic activity, while the latter has almost none (Burney *et al.*, 1974). Severe hepatic disease or reduced perfusion of the liver in heart failure decreases the rate of metabolism (Thomson *et al.*, 1973). The clearance of lidocaine approaches the rate of hepatic blood flow and is thus very sensitive to changes in this parameter (Nies *et al.*, 1976). The clearance of lidocaine also may decrease as a result of prolonged infusion (LeLorier *et al.*, 1977). The half-time for elimination of lidocaine is normally about 100 minutes.

Dosage and Routes of Administration. Lidocaine is only administered intravenously or intramuscularly. To achieve effective concentrations rapidly in plasma, intravenous administration of about 1 to 2 mg/kg of body weight is used. A second injection may be required in 20 to 40 minutes; this should be half the size of the first. Smaller doses should be used for patients who are in heart failure. Rapid infusion also may be employed to administer the loading dose. A constant rate of intravenous infusion is used to maintain an effective concentration. Infusions in the range of 1 to 5 mg per minute produce therapeutic concentrations in plasma of 1 to 5 μg/ml; in patients with heart failure or shock, the same rate of infusion will produce plasma concentrations two or more times higher (Appendix II). As the circulatory status changes, hepatic blood flow can change dramatically and shifts in the concentration of lidocaine in plasma will reflect these alterations (Stenson *et al.*, 1971; Nies *et al.*, 1976). Lidocaine can be given intramuscularly in emergencies to obtain effective concentrations in plasma quickly. A dose of 4 to 5 mg/kg will produce an effective concentration within 15 minutes, and this therapeutic level is maintained for about 90 minutes (Fehmers and Dunning, 1972; Lie *et al.*, 1978).

THERAPEUTIC USES

Lidocaine has a narrow antiarrhythmic spectrum. It is used almost exclusively to treat ventricular arrhythmias, primarily in intensive care units. Lidocaine is effective against ventricular arrhythmias caused by acute myocardial infarction, open-heart surgery, and digitalis. After many negative studies (*see* Bigger *et al.*, 1977), Lie and coworkers (1974) demonstrated that infusions at a rate of 3 mg per minute provided effective prophylaxis for primary ventricular fibrillation in the acute phase of myocardial infarction. The utility of the intramuscular administration of lidocaine to prevent primary ventricular fibrillation while patients with acute myocardial infarction are being transported to a hospital is in dispute (Valentine *et al.*, 1974; Lie *et al.*, 1978).

TOXICITY

Although it can adversely affect hemodynamics in patients who have severely compromised cardiac function, lidocaine has few undesirable cardiovascular effects. The main adverse effects are on the central nervous system. At concentrations in plasma near 5 μg/ml, symptoms are often subtle. They may include feelings of dissociation, paresthesias (often perioral), mild drowsiness, or mild agitation. Higher concentrations may cause decreased hearing, disorientation, muscle twitching, convulsions, or respiratory arrest (*see* Bigger and Heissenbuttel, 1969). The minor central nervous system effects are not dangerous but do severely disturb some patients. Such symptoms should prompt an adjustment of the infusion rate. The more severe toxic manifestations are life threatening.

Few drug interactions have been reported with lidocaine. Propranolol can decrease hepatic blood flow in patients with heart disease. This will cause a decrease in the rate of hepatic metabolism of lidocaine and an increase in its plasma concentration after any given dosage (Branch *et al.*, 1973; Nies *et al.*, 1976).

PHENYTOIN

Phenytoin has been used since 1938 in the treatment of epileptic seizures (*see* Chapter 20). Harris and Kokernot (1950) reported that phenytoin was an effective therapeutic agent for ventricular tachycardia in experimental acute myocardial infarction in the dog. Clinical studies have demonstrated its utility for ventricular arrhythmias in man; it is particularly noted for its efficacy against arrhythmias in patients with digitalis toxicity (see Damato. 1969; Atkinson and Davison, 1974). The history, chemistry, and preparations of phenytoin are discussed in Chapter 20.

PHARMACOLOGICAL PROPERTIES

Cardiac Electrophysiological Effects. The electrophysiological effects of phenytoin are very similar, but not identical, to those of lidocaine.

Automaticity. Therapeutic concentrations of phenytoin have no effect on the normal sinus node of the rabbit *in vitro;* toxic concentrations cause a modest slowing (Strauss *et al.,* 1968). Phenytoin can reverse experimental S-A block produced by digitalis in the isolated atrium. Rarely, phenytoin causes depression of the sinus node in patients with sinus node disease (see Bigger and Reiffel, 1979). Phenytoin has the same effect on normal automaticity in Purkinje fibers as does lidocaine, probably by the same mechanism—a marked increase in i_{K_1}. Phenytoin has been shown to be effective in abolishing abnormal automaticity due to digitalis-induced delayed afterdepolarizations in cardiac Purkinje fibers (Rosen *et al.,* 1976; Peon *et al.,* 1978). This action may underlie phenytoin's efficacy against certain arrhythmias caused by cardiac glycosides.

Excitability, Responsiveness, and Conduction. Phenytoin has effects on excitability that are virtually identical to those of lidocaine (Bigger *et al.,* 1970). Its effects on responsiveness and conduction are also very similar to those of lidocaine (Bigger *et al.,* 1968a). Phenytoin can repolarize cells that are depolarized because of decreased potassium conductance, g_{K_1}, and thus make it difficult to obtain responses at very low levels of *Vm.* The effects of phenytoin on responsiveness have the same interaction with $[K]_o$ as described for lidocaine (Singh and Vaughan Williams, 1971; Rosen *et al.,* 1976).

The discussion of the effects of lidocaine on the duration of the action potential and on *reentrant ventricular arrhythmias* applies to phenytoin as well (see Wit *et al.,* 1975).

Electrocardiographic Effects. Like lidocaine, phenytoin has little effect on the ECG; the Q-T interval often shortens slightly (Bigger *et al.,* 1968b). Clinical electrophysiological studies show that phenytoin has quite variable effects on the A-H interval and the A-V nodal refractory period of patients with normal A-V conduction (Caracta *et al.,* 1973). The A-V nodal refractory period usually shortens significantly when phenytoin is given to digitalized patients. The effective refractory period (ERP) of the His-Purkinje system shortens very significantly in man, presumably due to shortening of the duration of the action potential in Purkinje fibers (Damato, 1969; Bissett *et al.,* 1974).

Autonomic Nervous System. Phenytoin has complex interactions with the autonomic nervous system; most of the effects are central. Phenytoin decreases the traffic in cardiac sympathetic nerves caused by ouabain toxicity (Gillis *et al.,* 1971). The drug also may modulate vagal efferent activity via a central action. Phenytoin has no peripheral cholinergic or β-adrenergic blocking activity (Strauss *et al.,* 1968).

Absorption, Distribution, and Elimination. Only a few points that are crucial to the use of phenytoin as an antiarrhythmic drug will be discussed here. A more detailed discussion is presented in Chapter 20.

Absorption of phenytoin from the gastrointestinal tract is slow, somewhat erratic, and incomplete; there is also much interindividual variance. Absorption after intramuscular injection is also slow and may be incomplete. About 90% of the phenytoin in plasma is bound to albumin; the fraction is less in patients with uremia (Reidenberg *et al.,* 1971). After intravenous administration, phenytoin is distributed to tissues reasonably rapidly. The drug is eliminated by hepatic hydroxylation. Since the major metabolites of phenytoin lack anticonvulsant properties, it is presumed that they have no antiarrhythmic activity. Metabolism is relatively slow (half-time of elimination is about 24 hours) and not substantially altered by changes in hepatic blood flow. In some patients, the enzyme system that metabolizes phenytoin becomes saturated by concentrations of the drug in the therapeutic range; hence, dose-dependent kinetics of elimination can result and can cause unexpected toxicity (Atkinson and Shaw, 1973).

Dosage and Routes of Administration. Phenytoin should be given by intermittent intravenous injection or orally. The vehicle used for the injectable preparation has a pH of about 11, and causes severe phlebitis if infused. Critical arrhythmias should not be treated by the intramuscular route because absorption is too unreliable. The schedule for *intermittent intravenous injection* of phenytoin is almost identical to that described above for procainamide: 100 mg of phenytoin is given every 5 minutes until the arrhythmia is controlled or until adverse effects are encountered (Bigger *et al.*, 1968b). The rate of intravenous injection should not exceed 50 mg per minute. Usually about 700 mg is required; doses above 1000 mg are rarely needed. *Oral treatment* of arrhythmias usually is initiated with loading doses because of phenytoin's long elimination half-time. A dose of 15 mg/kg (about 1000 mg) is given the first day, 7.5 mg/kg on the second and third days, and 4 to 6 mg/kg per day for chronic maintenance (most often 400 mg per day). The oral maintenance dose can be given once a day or divided into two portions.

THERAPEUTIC USES

Phenytoin is clinically useful in relatively few arrhythmias. They include ventricular arrhythmias, paroxysmal atrial flutter or fibrillation, and supraventricular arrhythmias caused by digitalis. Phenytoin is usually effective against ventricular arrhythmias seen after open-heart surgery and acute myocardial infarction, but lidocaine is equally effective and is easier to use. Phenytoin seems relatively ineffective against recurrent, drug-resistant ventricular tachycardia in patients with chronic ischemic heart disease (Stone *et al.*, 1971). Phenytoin has been tested as a prophylactic agent against sudden death in the year following acute myocardial infarction. Overall, phenytoin was not beneficial; however, in a subgroup who had concentrations of the drug in plasma greater than $10 \mu g/ml$, phenytoin was beneficial (Vajda *et al.*, 1973; *see also* Bigger *et al.*, 1977); such concentrations are readily attained in epileptic patients given conventional doses of the drug. Phenytoin is highly effective against multiform and complex ventricular premature depolarizations, ventricular tachycardia, and atrial tachycardia with A-V block induced by digitalis; small doses of phenytoin will often cause striking effects. It is somewhat less effective against nonparoxysmal A-V junctional tachycardia; higher doses are needed, and a larger fraction of cases fail to respond. The effects of phenytoin on sinus arrest or S-A block caused by digitalis in human subjects are unknown. Phenytoin is relatively ineffective against the common atrial arrhythmias, such as atrial flutter, atrial fibrillation, and supraventricular tachycardia (*see* Bigger *et al.*, 1968b; Damato, 1969; Atkinson and Davison, 1974; Wit *et al.*, 1975).

TOXICITY

The most prominent adverse effects of phenytoin during acute treatment of an arrhythmia are referable to the central nervous system and include drowsiness, nystagmus, vertigo, ataxia, and nausea. The progression of such symptoms shows an orderly relationship to increasing concentrations in plasma (Kutt, 1971). In acute treatment of arrhythmias, neurological signs usually are indicative of concentrations in plasma in excess of $20 \mu g/ml$. This information is useful; if an arrhythmia has not responded to phenytoin at concentrations of $20 \mu g/ml$ or more, it is unlikely to respond at higher concentrations (Bigger *et al.*, 1968b). A myriad of adverse reactions and interactions with other drugs has been described during chronic therapy with phenytoin; these are presented in Chapter 20.

PROPRANOLOL

The pharmacology of the β-adrenergic blocking agents is discussed in Chapter 9. Only those properties of propranolol related to its use in the treatment of cardiac arrhythmias are considered here.

PHARMACOLOGICAL PROPERTIES

Cardiac Electrophysiological Effects. Most of the antiarrhythmic effects of propranolol can be explained by its selective β-adrenergic blocking action. Propranolol has two other direct actions that must be considered in connection with its antiarrhythmic activity: it increases background outward current (i_{K_1}) and, in high concentrations, it significantly depresses i_{Na}.

Automaticity. β-Adrenergic stimulation causes a marked increase in the slope of phase-4 depolarization and in the spontaneous firing rate in the *sinus node*. This effect is competitively blocked by propranolol (Lucchesi and Whitsitt, 1969). Propranolol has little effect on sinus rate when catecholamines are absent. In the dog or man, the resting heart rate is only slightly affected by propranolol, but the acceleration of sinus rate during exercise or as a result of emotion is blunted (Wallace *et al.*, 1966b; Bodem *et al.*, 1973; Seides *et al.*, 1974). Propranolol can severely slow the sinus rate in patients with preexisting sinus node disease (Strauss *et al.*, 1976). Also, propranolol has significant effects on automaticity in *Purkinje fibers*. The ventricular rate slows somewhat when dogs with complete A-V block are given propranolol, due to blockade of background sympathetic activity (Wallace *et al.*, 1967). As noted above, catecholamines increase the firing rate of Purkinje fibers by shifting the steady-state curve for activation of i_{K_2} in a depolarizing direction on its voltage axis; propranolol completely reverses this action and slows spontaneous firing (Tsien, 1974). Under some conditions, cardiac Purkinje fibers require the action of catecholamines to sustain their spontaneous activity. In this case, propranolol can totally abolish normal automaticity in the His-Purkinje system. At low concentrations, propranolol also increases outward background current, i_{K_1}, in Purkinje fibers, as do lidocaine and phenytoin; this action decreases automaticity as well (Stagg and Wallace, 1974).

Excitability and Threshold. The electrical threshold of the atria and ventricles is not much affected by propranolol, and the electrical threshold for ventricular fibrillation is not consistently increased by the drug (Rosati *et al.*, 1966; Wallace *et al.*, 1966b). Propranolol reverses the action of catecholamines to lower the threshold for fibrillation. Concentrations of propranolol that cause shortening of the action potential in Purkinje fibers will increase slightly the electrical current threshold of the fibers. Very high concentrations increase threshold in Purkinje fibers by an effect on i_{Na}.

Responsiveness and Conduction. Only very high concentrations of propranolol (*e.g.*, 1000 to 3000 ng/ml) affect responsiveness in Purkinje fibers (Davis and Temte, 1968). These concentrations are much greater than those needed for substantial β-adrenergic blockade (100 to 300 ng/ml). However, concentrations over 1000 ng/ml are often required for control of ventricular arrhythmias (Woosley *et al.*, 1977). After propranolol, premature responses can no longer be elicited at low values of *Vm;* in addition, low-amplitude premature responses are abolished by the drug (Davis and Temte, 1968). These effects are similar to those seen with lidocaine or phenytoin and are probably due to an increase in g_{K_1}. Different effects may occur in abnormal fibers. In the dog heart *in situ*, propranolol causes slowing of intramyocardial conduction in muscle that is made acutely ischemic. It has no such effect on normal portions of the ventricle (Kupersmith *et al.*, 1976). Slow responses can be dependent on catecholamines, as can afterdepolarizations (Carmeliet and Vereeke, 1969); when this is the case, propranolol should ameliorate arrhythmias caused by these mechanisms.

Duration of the Action Potential and Refractoriness. Propranolol has little effect on the duration of action potentials in the sinus node, atrium, or A-V node (Vaughan Williams, 1966; Pitt and Cox, 1968). In ventricular muscle, action potentials shorten slightly; in Purkinje fibers, action potentials often shorten substantially (Davis and Temte, 1968). Propranolol has little effect on refractoriness of normal atrial or ventricular muscle. It causes a substantial increase in the *effective refractory period* (ERP) of the A-V node due to its β-adrenergic blocking action (Wallace *et al.*, 1966b); *this action is the basis of the major uses of propranolol as an antiarrhythmic drug.* The ERP of Purkinje fibers is shortened substantially (Davis and Temte, 1968).

Effect on Reentrant Arrhythmias. Propranolol could interrupt reentrant activity in many ways. In paroxysmal supraventricular tachycardia due to A-V nodal reentry, the substantial increase in A-V nodal refractoriness may abolish reentry. In the ventricles, propranolol may abolish slow responses that are dependent on catecholamines, repolarize tissues depolarized by virtue of decreased g_{K_1}

(such as stretch or low $[K]_o$), or abolish depressed fast responses in ischemic ventricular muscle. In higher concentration, propranolol has "quinidine-like" effects on phase-0 depolarization and responsiveness of Purkinje fibers. In addition, propranolol may favorably influence arrhythmias by its effect on the relationship between myocardial oxygen supply and demand and by decreasing the extent of ischemia.

Electrocardiographic Effects. Propranolol often causes an increase in the P-R interval and slight shortening of the $Q-T_c$ without any effect on the duration of the QRS segment (Stern and Eisenberg, 1969; Seides *et al.*, 1974). Clinical electrophysiological studies reveal little effect of propranolol, except for the dramatic increase in the ERP of the A-V node; there is no increase in the H-V interval after conventional doses of the drug (Seides *et al.*, 1974).

Autonomic Nervous System. Propranolol causes β-adrenergic blockade and leaves vagal and α-adrenergic mechanisms intact. A detailed discussion of β-adrenergic antagonists is presented in Chapter 9.

Absorption, Distribution, and Elimination. Intestinal absorption of propranolol is excellent, but extensive first-pass metabolism reduces bioavailability considerably (*see* Chapter 9; Appendix II). Propranolol is nearly entirely metabolized, but many of its metabolites have not been identified with certainty. One, 4-hydroxypropranolol, is about equipotent to propranolol as a β-adrenergic antagonist (Fitzgerald and O'Donnell, 1971). The half-time for elimination of propranolol is about 4 hours. As with lidocaine, the hepatic extraction of propranolol is very high and elimination is significantly reduced when hepatic blood flow decreases. Propranolol may decrease its own elimination rate by decreasing cardiac output and hepatic blood flow, particularly in patients with heart disease (Nies and Shand, 1975).

Dosage and Routes of Administration. Propranolol is given orally for long-term treatment of cardiac arrhythmias. Concentrations in plasma that are associated with therapeutic effects vary widely (20 to 1000 ng/ml) and are particularly dependent on the arrhythmia being treated. The dose ranges from 40 to 80 mg per day for treatment of arrhythmias that are sensitive to effects of the drug. More than 1000 mg a day may be needed to treat resistant arrhythmias. Propranolol is usually effective when given four times a day. The duration of action can be prolonged by the administration of large doses, since propranolol has a greater margin of safety than do the other antiarrhythmic drugs. For emergency use, propranolol can be given intravenously; one strategy is analogous to those discussed above for procainamide and phenytoin: 1 mg is administered intravenously every 3 to 5 minutes during careful monitoring of the ECG, arterial blood pressure, and left atrial pressure (by means of a Swan-Ganz catheter). Much lower doses are needed to achieve a given plasma concentration by this method than with oral administration because first-pass hepatic extraction is avoided.

THERAPEUTIC USES

Supraventricular Arrhythmias. Propranolol is used primarily to treat supraventricular tachyarrhythmias such as atrial fibrillation, atrial flutter, or paroxysmal supraventricular tachycardia (Gibson and Sowton, 1969). For these arrhythmias, the objective of therapy usually is to slow the ventricular rate rather than to abolish the arrhythmia. Propranolol accomplishes this objective by blocking β-adrenergic influences on the A-V node, thereby increasing refractoriness of the A-V node. Occasionally, as a bonus, the supraventricular arrhythmia will convert to sinus rhythm. Not infrequently, propranolol and digitalis successfully control the ventricular rate in patients with atrial fibrillation or flutter when maximal doses of digitalis alone do not (Stock and Dale, 1963); this additive effect may result from the fact that digitalis increases vagal tone, while propranolol blocks β-adrenergic influences on the A-V node.

Combination therapy with quinidine and propranolol has been advocated for the conversion of atrial fibrillation to sinus rhythm (Stern, 1967; Hillestad and Storstein, 1969); however, the efficacy and safety of this combination for such a purpose are still unproven. Propranolol is used to prevent paroxysmal supraventricular tachycardia due to A-V nodal reciprocation and the paroxysmal supraventricular tachycardia of the Wolff-Parkinson-White syndrome (Gettes and Yoshonis, 1970; Wu *et al.*, 1974). In the latter condition, quinidine increases the refractoriness of the accessory A-V connection and both drugs increase the refractoriness of the A-V node.

Ventricular Arrhythmias. Propranolol can be effective against ventricular arrhythmias. When ventricular arrhythmias are triggered by exercise or emotion, small doses of propranolol (*e.g.,* 80 to 160 mg per day) are very likely to prevent them (Gibson and Sowton, 1969). Even when the relationship between β-adrenergic influences and ventricular arrhythmias is not apparent, ventricular arrhythmias may respond to modest doses of propranolol. In patients with ischemic heart disease, propranolol may ameliorate ventricular arrhythmias by preventing or reducing ischemia. However, many ventricular arrhythmias do not respond to conventional doses of propranolol. Large doses of propranolol (500 to 1000 mg a day) may be required to control ventricular arrhythmias (Woosley *et al.,* 1977). Propranolol is the drug of choice for severe ventricular arrhythmias in the prolonged Q-T syndrome. When propranolol fails, removal of the left stellate ganglion may be effective (Vincent *et al.,* 1974). In 1975, a large controlled trial with another β-adrenergic blocking agent, *practolol,* showed promise for effective prophylaxis during the year after an acute myocardial infarction (Green *et al.,* 1975). A similar trial is currently underway in the United States with propranolol.

Digitalis-Induced Arrhythmias. Propranolol abolishes ventricular arrhythmias induced by digitalis by effects both directly on the heart and, probably, on the central nervous system (Gillis, 1969). However, the incidence of adverse effects during treatment of digitalis-induced arrhythmias with propranolol is higher than with phenytoin or lidocaine.

TOXICITY

Propranolol usually is well tolerated; most of its undesirable effects are related to β-adrenergic blockade. In patients with ventricular failure, the level of sympathetic activity is high and provides significant support to the ventricle. Therefore, when propranolol is used as an antiarrhythmic drug, particularly when it is given intravenously, significant hypotension, left ventricular failure, or even cardiovascular collapse can occur. Occasionally, propranolol will precipitate left ventricular failure in a patient who has not previously had heart failure (Stephen, 1966). Many patients who have ventricular failure can tolerate chronic oral therapy with propranolol if digitalis and diuretic agents are also used carefully. The potent effect of propranolol on conduction in the A-V node can also lead to serious adverse effects, such as A-V block or asystole (Stephen, 1966; Gibson and Sowton, 1969). Sudden withdrawal of propranolol in patients with angina pectoris can precipitate worsening of angina, cardiac arrhythmias, and acute myocardial infarction. Other untoward effects of propranolol are described in Chapter 9.

BRETYLIUM

Bretylium was introduced into medicine as an antihypertensive agent in the 1950s; however, for a number of reasons, it was supplanted by guanethidine (*see* Chapter 9). Bretylium also has antiarrhythmic properties and, in 1978, was approved in the United States for intramuscular and intravenous administration in emergency situations when other antiarrhythmic drugs prove to be ineffective.

Chemistry and Preparations. Bretylium has the following structural formula:

Bretylium

Bretylium tosylate (BRETYLOL) is available for intravenous or intramuscular administration in a 10-ml ampul containing 500 mg of bretylium tosylate in water.

PHARMACOLOGICAL PROPERTIES

Cardiac Electrophysiological Effects. Bretylium directly affects the electrical properties of heart muscle. In addition, it has important interactions with the autonomic nervous system (*see* Chapter 9).

Automaticity. The effects of bretylium on cardiac automaticity are complex and not fully understood. Bretylium has little direct effect on automaticity of the isolated perfused *sinus node* (Papp and Vaughan Williams, 1969). It somewhat decreases the sinus rate in dogs with surgically denervated hearts (Waxman and Wallace, 1972). Of the drugs discussed in this chapter, bretylium is the only one that *lacks* potent effects on normal automaticity in the *His-Purkinje system.* Immediately after administration, the firing rate of Purkinje fibers *in vitro* increases and quiescent fibers may become automatic (Wit *et al.,* 1970; Bigger and Jaffe, 1971). These effects are thought to be caused by release of catecholamines from adrenergic nerve terminals because they are abolished by pretreatment with either reserpine or propranolol.

Excitability and Threshold. Bretylium has little effect on the diastolic electrical current threshold (Waxman and Wallace, 1972). However, the drug significantly increases the threshold for ventricular fibrillation (Bacaner, 1968; Allen *et al.,* 1972; Kniffen *et al.,* 1975). This action probably does not depend on its adrenergic neuron blocking action. Other blockers of adrenergic neurons (such as guanethidine) do not elevate this threshold (Bacaner, 1968); conversely, quaternary ammonium analogs that are not blockers of adrenergic neurons do elevate the threshold for ventricular fibrillation (Kniffen *et al.,* 1975).

Responsiveness and Conduction. Therapeutic concentrations of bretylium have no significant effect on membrane responsiveness or conduction in either Purkinje fibers or ventricular muscle. Toxic concentrations cause mild depression of these parameters.

Duration of the Action Potential and Refractori-

ness. Bretylium causes no change in either the duration of action potentials or the effective refractory period (ERP) of isolated rabbit atria (Papp and Vaughan Williams, 1969). However, atrial ERP increases after the administration of bretylium to both intact and sympathectomized dogs. Bretylium causes marked prolongation of action potentials in canine Purkinje and ventricular muscle fibers (Wit *et al.,* 1970; Bigger and Jaffe, 1971; Waxman and Wallace, 1972). The distribution of this change within the conducting system is such that the normal disparity in the duration of the action potential is reduced. Also, bretylium minimizes the disparity in the duration of the action potential and ERP between normal and infarcted regions in experimental models of acute myocardial infarction in dogs (Cardinal and Sasyniuk, 1978).

Effect on Reentrant Arrhythmias. Bretylium could terminate reentrant arrhythmias either by its marked capacity to prolong refractoriness without affecting propagation of the cardiac impulse or by releasing catecholamines. The latter effect may cause repolarization and increased conductivity in abnormal depolarized tissues.

Electrocardiographic Effects. In human subjects, bretylium decreases the sinus rate and increases the P-R and Q-T intervals; the duration of the QRS complex does not change. There have been no clinical electrophysiological studies with bretylium in man, but Waxman and Wallace (1972) did such studies in the dog. The direct effects were to slow the sinus rate and conduction in the A-V node. Conduction in the His-Purkinje system was not altered.

Autonomic Nervous System. Bretylium has no effect on vagal reflexes and does not alter the responsiveness of cardiac cholinergic receptors. However, the drug profoundly affects the sympathetic nervous system. It is taken up and concentrated in adrenergic nerve terminals. Initially, as it is taken up, bretylium releases norepinephrine from nerve terminals; later, it prevents release of norepinephrine when the nerve terminal is depolarized by a nerve action potential (*see* Chapter 9). It does *not* depress preganglionic or postganglionic sympathetic nerve conduction, impair transmission across sympathetic ganglia, deplete the adrenergic neuron of norepinephrine, or decrease the responsiveness of adrenergic receptors (*see* Bigger and Jaffe, 1971). During chronic treatment with bretylium, the adrenergic receptors show increased responsiveness to circulating catecholamines.

Hemodynamic Effects. Even very high concentrations of bretylium do not decrease the contractility of the mammalian myocardium; contractility increases as catecholamines are released from adrenergic nerve terminals (Papp and Vaughan Williams, 1969; Markis and Koch-Weser, 1971; Heissenbuttel and Bigger, 1979). Although bretylium can increase myocardial contractility, it also may cause hypotension, even while the patient is supine (Chatterjee *et al.,* 1973). The hypotension seen after treatment with bretylium is aggravated by standing and is maximal during upright exercise, because bretylium blocks vital reflexes and prevents both vasoconstriction during standing and tachycardia during exercise.

Absorption, Distribution, and Elimination. There is a paucity of critically needed information on the pharmacokinetics of bretylium. Oral absorption of bretylium is notoriously poor, as would be expected of a quaternary amine. Bretylium is eliminated almost entirely by renal excretion without significant metabolism (Kuntzman *et al.,* 1970). The half-time for elimination is 6 to 10 hours; longer half-lives are to be expected in patients with renal insufficiency (*see* Heissenbuttel and Bigger, 1979).

Dosage and Routes of Administration. In the United States, bretylium is approved only for intravenous or intramuscular use. The contents of the 10-ml ampul should be diluted to a volume of 50 ml or more, and a dose of 5 to 10 mg/kg should be infused over 10 to 20 minutes. In extreme emergencies, such as during cardiac resuscitation, a dose of 5 mg/kg of the undiluted solution can be injected intravenously; this dose can be repeated at intervals of 15 to 30 minutes, but not to exceed a total of 30 mg/kg. For intramuscular administration, undiluted bretylium tosylate should be used, and doses are usually repeated every 6 to 8 hours. The patient should be kept supine during treatment and carefully observed for postural hypotension.

THERAPEUTIC USES

Currently, bretylium tosylate is recommended only for treatment of life-threatening ventricular arrhythmias that fail to respond to the more commonly used antiarrhythmic drugs, such as lidocaine or procainamide. Use of bretylium should be limited to intensive care facilities. Although experience with bretylium is limited and the published studies do not contain adequate controls, the response of severe, refractory ventricular arrhythmias has been impressive. Even ventricular fibrillation that has failed to respond to repeated DC countershock may respond to bretylium tosylate and countershock (*see* Heissenbuttel and Bigger, 1979).

TOXICITY

Hypotension is the principal undesirable effect of bretylium tosylate when it is used intravenously to treat acute arrhythmias. Orthostatic hypotension of significant magnitude usually occurs, and hypotension in the supine position is not rare. Hypotension is occasionally so severe that bretylium must be discontinued. Rapid intravenous administration may cause *nausea* and *vomiting.* During prolonged oral therapy, many patients develop tachyphylaxis to the hypotensive but not to the antiarrhythmic effects of bretylium. *Parotid pain* is an additional relatively common untoward effect during chronic oral therapy.

Adamson, A. R., and Spracklen, F. H. H. Atrial flutter with block: contraindication to use of lignocaine. *Br. Med. J.,* **1968,** *2,* 223–224.

Allen, J. D.; Zaidi, S. A.; Shanks, R. G.; and Pantridge, J. F. The effects of bretylium on experimental cardiac dysrhythmias. *Am. J. Cardiol.,* **1972,** *29,* 641–649.

Arnsdorf, M. F., and Bigger, J. T., Jr. Effect of lidocaine hydrochloride on membrane conductance in mammalian cardiac Purkinje fibers. *J. Clin. Invest.,* **1972,** *51,* 2252–2263.

———. The effect of lidocaine on components of excitability in long mammalian cardiac Purkinje fibers. *J. Pharmacol. Exp. Ther.,* **1975,** *195,* 206–215.

Atkinson, A. J., and Davison, R. Diphenylhydantoin as an antiarrhythmic drug. *Annu. Rev. Med.,* **1974,** *25,* 99–113.

Atkinson, A. J., and Shaw, J. M. Pharmacokinetic study of a patient with diphenylhydantoin toxicity. *Clin. Pharmacol. Ther.,* **1973,** *14,* 521–528.

Bacaner, M. B. Quantitative comparison of bretylium with other antifibrillatory drugs. *Am. J. Cardiol.,* **1968,** *21,* 504–512.

Bellet, S.; Hamdan, G.; Somlyo, A.; and Lara, R. The reversal of cardiotoxic effects of quinidine by molar sodium lactate: an experimental study. *Am. J. Med. Sci.,* **1959,** *237,* 165–176.

Bigger, J. T., Jr. Pharmacologic and clinical control of antiarrhythmic drugs. *Am. J. Med.,* **1975,** *58,* 479–488.

Bigger, J. T., Jr.; Bassett, A. L.; and Hoffman, B. F. The electrophysiological effects of diphenylhydantoin on canine Purkinje fibers. *Circ. Res.,* **1968a,** *22,* 221–236.

Bigger, J. T., Jr., and Goldreyer, B. N. The mechanism of supraventricular tachycardia. *Circulation,* **1970,** *42,* 673–688.

Bigger, J. T., Jr., and Heissenbuttel, R. H. The use of procaine amide and lidocaine in the treatment of cardiac arrhythmias. *Prog. Cardiovasc. Dis.,* **1969,** *11,* 515–534.

Bigger, J. T., Jr., and Jaffe, C. C. The effect of bretylium tosylate on the electrophysiologic properties of ventricular muscle and Purkinje fibers. *Am. J. Cardiol.,* **1971,** *27,* 82–92.

Bigger, J. T., Jr., and Mandel, W. J. Effects of lidocaine on the electrophysiological properties of ventricular muscle and Purkinje fibers. *J. Clin. Invest.,* **1970,** *49,* 63–77.

Bigger, J. T., Jr.; Schmidt, D. H.; and Kutt, H. Relationship between the plasma level of diphenylhydantoin sodium and its cardiac antiarrhythmic effects. *Circulation,* **1968b,** *38,* 363–374.

Bigger, J. T., Jr.; Weinberg, D. I.; Kovalik, A. T. W.; Harris, P. D.; Cranefield, P. F.; and Hoffman, B. F. Effects of diphenylhydantoin on excitability and automaticity in the canine heart. *Circ. Res.,* **1970,** *26,* 1–15.

Birkhead, J. S., and Vaughan Williams, E. M. Dual effect of disopyramide on atrial and atrioventricular conduction and refractory periods. *Br. Heart J.,* **1977,** *39,* 657–660.

Bissett, J. K.; de Soyza, N. D. B.; Kane, J. J.; and Murphy, M. L. Improved intraventricular conduction of premature beats after diphenylhydantoin. *Am. J. Cardiol.,* **1974,** *33,* 493–497.

Bodem, G.; Brammell, H. L.; Weil, J. V.; and Chidsey, C. A. Pharmacodynamic studies of beta adrenergic antagonism induced in man by propranolol and practolol. *J. Clin. Invest.,* **1973,** *52,* 747–754.

Boyes, R. N.; Scott, D. B.; Jebson, P. J.; Godman, M. J.; and Julian, D. G. Pharmacokinetics of lidocaine in man. *Clin. Pharmacol. Ther.,* **1971,** *12,* 105–116.

Branch, R. A.; Shand, D. G.; Wilkinson, G. R.; and Nies, A. S. The reduction of lidocaine clearance by *dl*-propranolol: an example of hemodynamic drug interaction. *J. Pharmacol. Exp. Ther.,* **1973,** *184,* 515–519.

Brown, H. F., and Noble, S. J. Effects of adrenaline on membrane currents underlying pacemaker activity in frog atrial muscle. *J. Physiol. (Lond.),* **1974,** *238,* 51–53.

Burn, J. H. The cause of fibrillation. *Can. Med. Assoc. J.,* **1961,** *84,* 625–627.

Burney, R. G.; DiFazio, C. A.; Peach, M. J.; Petrie, K. A.; and Silvester, M. J. Antiarrhythmic effects of lidocaine metabolites. *Am. Heart J.,* **1974,** *88,* 765–769.

Caracta, A. R.; Damato, A. N.; Josephson, M. E.;

Ricciutti, M. A.; Gallagher, J. J.; and Lau, S. H. Electrophysiologic properties of diphenylhydantoin. *Circulation,* **1973,** *47,* 1234–1241.

Cardinal, R., and Sasyniuk, B. I. Electrophysiologic effects of bretylium tosylate on subendocardial Purkinje fibers from infarcted canine hearts. *J. Pharmacol. Exp. Ther.,* **1978,** *204,* 159–174.

Carmeliet, E. E. Chloride ions and the membrane potential of Purkinje fibers. *J. Physiol. (Lond.),* **1961,** *156,* 375–388.

Carmeliet, E. E., and Vereeke, J. Adrenaline and the plateau phase of the cardiac action potential. *Pfluegers Arch.,* **1969,** *313,* 300–315.

Chatterjee, K.; Mandel, W. J.; Vyden, J. K.; Parmley, W. W.; and Forrester, J. S. Cardiovascular effects of bretylium tosylate in acute myocardial infarction. *J.A.M.A.,* **1973,** *223,* 757–760.

Cheng, T. O., and Wadhwa, K. Sinus standstill following intravenous lidocaine administration. *J.A.M.A.,* **1973,** *223,* 790–792.

Chien, Y. W.; Lambert, H. J.; and Karim, A. Comparative binding of disopyramide phosphate and quinidine sulfate to human plasma proteins. *J. Pharm. Sci.,* **1974,** *63,* 1877–1879.

Conn, H. L., Jr. Quinidine as an antiarrhythmic agent: basic and clinical considerations. In, *Advances in Cardiopulmonary Diseases,* Vol. 2. (Bengai, A. I., and Gordon, B. L., eds.) Year Book Medical Publishers, Inc., Chicago, **1964,** pp. 286–304.

Conn, H. L., Jr., and Luchi, R. J. Some quantitative aspects of the binding of quinidine and related quinoline compounds by human serum albumin. *J. Clin. Invest.,* **1961,** *40,* 509–516.

Conrad, K. A.; Molk, B. L.; and Chidsey, C. A. Pharmacokinetic studies of quinidine in patients with arrhythmias. *Circulation,* **1977,** *55,* 1–7.

Cranefield, P. F. Action potentials, afterpotentials, and arrhythmias. *Circ. Res.,* **1977,** *41,* 415–423.

Cranefield, P. F.; Wit, A. L.; and Hoffman, B. F. Conduction of the cardiac impulse. III. Characteristics of very slow conduction. *J. Gen. Physiol.,* **1972,** *59,* 227–246.

Damato, A. N. Diphenylhydantoin: pharmacological and clinical use. *Prog. Cardiovasc. Dis.,* **1969,** *12,* 1–15.

Danilo, P., Jr., and Rosen, M. R. Cardiac effects of disopyramide. *Am. Heart J.,* **1976,** *92,* 532–536.

Data, J. L.; Wilkinson, G. R.; and Nies, A. S. Interaction of quinidine with anticonvulsant drugs. *N. Engl. J. Med.,* **1976,** *294,* 699–702.

Davies, D. M.; Beedie, M. A.; and Rawlins, M. D. Antinuclear antibodies during procainamide treatment and drug acetylation. *Br. Med. J.,* **1975,** *3,* 682–683.

Davis, L. D., and Temte, J. V. Effects of propranolol on the transmembrane potentials of ventricular muscle and Purkinje fibers of the dog. *Circ. Res.,* **1968,** *22,* 661–667.

———. Electrophysiological actions of lidocaine on canine ventricular muscle and Purkinje fibers. *Ibid.,* **1969,** *24,* 639–655.

Dawes, G. S. Synthetic substitutes for quinidine. *Br. J. Pharmacol.,* **1946,** *1,* 90–112.

Desai, J. M.; Scheinman, M.; Peters, R. W.; and O'Young, J. Electrophysiological effects of disopyramide in patients with bundle branch block. *Circulation,* **1979,** *59,* 215–225.

Drayer, D. E.; Lowenthal, D. T.; Restivo, K. M.; Schwartz, A.; Cook, C. E.; and Reidenberg, M. M. Steady-state serum levels of quinidine and active metabolites in cardiac patients with varying degrees of renal function. *Clin. Pharmacol. Ther.,* **1978,** *24,* 31–39.

Drayer, D. E.; Restivo, K.; and Reidenberg, M. M. Specific determination of quinidine and (3S)-3-hydroxy-quinidine in human serum by high pressure liquid chromatography. *J. Lab. Clin. Med.,* **1977,** *90,* 816–822.

Dreyfuss, J.; Bigger, J. T., Jr.; Cohen, A. I.; and Schreiber, E. C. Metabolism of procainamide in rhesus monkey and man. *Clin. Pharmacol. Ther.,* **1972,** *13,* 366–371.

Durrer, D.; Van Dam, R. T.; Freud, G. E.; and Janse, M. J. Reentry and ventricular arrhythmias in local ischemia and infarction in the intact dog heart. *Proc. K. Ned. Akad. Wet.* [*Biol. Med.*], 1971, 74, 321–334.

El-Sherif, N.; Scherlag, B. J.; Lazzara, R.; and Hope, R. R. Reentrant ventricular arrhythmias in the late myocardial infarction period. 1. Conduction characteristics in the infarction zone. *Circulation*, 1977, 55, 686–702.

Fehmers, M. C. O., and Dunning, A. J. Intramuscularly and orally administered lidocaine in the treatment of ventricular arrhythmias in acute myocardial infarction. *Am. J. Cardiol.*, 1972, 29, 514–519.

Ferrer, M. I.; Harvey, R. M.; Werko, L.; Dresdale, D. T.; Cournand, A.; and Richards, D. W., Jr. Some effects of quinidine sulfate on the heart and circulation in man. *Am. Heart J.*, 1948, 36, 816–837.

Fitzgerald, J. D., and O'Donnell, S. R. Pharmacology of 4-hydroxypropranolol, a metabolite of propranolol. *Br. J. Pharmacol.*, 1971, 43, 222–235.

Fozzard, H. A., and Beeler, G. W., Jr. The voltage clamp and cardiac electrophysiology. *Circ. Res.*, 1975, 37, 403–413.

Frey, W. Weitere Erfährungen mit Chinidin bei absoluter Herzunregelmässigkeit. *Wien Klin. Wochenschr.*, 1918, 55, 849–853.

Galeazzi, R. L.; Sheiner, L. B.; Lockwood, T.; and Benet, L. Z. The renal elimination of procainamide. *Clin. Pharmacol. Ther.*, 1976, 19, 55–62.

Gerhardt, R. E.; Knouss, R. F.; Thyrum, P. T.; Luchi, R. J.; and Morris, J. J., Jr. Quinidine excretion in aciduria and alkaluria. *Ann. Intern. Med.*, 1969, 71, 927–933.

Gerstenblith, G.; Spear, J. F.; and Moore, E. N. Quantitative study of the effect of lidocaine on the threshold for ventricular fibrillation in the dog. *Am. J. Cardiol.*, 1972, 30, 242–247.

Gettes, L. S., and Yoshonis, K. F. Rapidly recurring supraventricular tachycardia; a manifestation of reciprocity tachycardia and an indication for propranolol therapy. *Circulation*, 1970, 41, 689–700.

Giardina, E. G. V.; Dreyfuss, J.; Bigger, J. T., Jr.; Shaw, J. M.; and Schreiber, E. C. Metabolism of procainamide in normal and cardiac subjects. *Clin. Pharmacol. Ther.*, 1976, 19, 339–351.

Giardina, E. G. V.; Heissenbuttel, R. H.; and Bigger, J. T., Jr. Intermittent intravenous procainamide to treat ventricular arrhythmias; correlation of plasma concentration with effect on arrhythmia, electrocardiogram, and blood pressure. *Ann. Intern. Med.*, 1973, 78, 183–193.

Giardina, E. G. V.; Stein, R. M.; and Bigger, J. T., Jr. The relationship between the metabolism of procainamide and sulfamethazine. *Circulation*, 1977, 55, 388–394.

Gibson, D., and Sowton, E. The use of beta-adrenergic receptor blocking drugs in dysrhythmias. *Prog. Cardiovasc. Dis.*, 1969, 12, 16–39.

Gibson, T. P.; Matusik, J.; Matusik, E.; Nelson, H. A.; Wilkinson, J.; and Briggs, W. A. Acetylation of procainamide in man and its relationship to isonicotinic acid hydrazide acetylation phenotype. *Clin. Pharmacol. Ther.*, 1975, 17, 395–399.

Giles, W., and Noble, S. J. Changes in membrane currents in bullfrog atrium produced by acetylcholine. *J. Physiol.* (*Lond.*), 1976, 261, 103–123.

Gillis, R. A. Cardiac sympathetic nerve activity; changes induced by ouabain and propranolol. *Science*, 1969, 166, 508–510.

Gillis, R. A.; McClellan, J. R.; Sauer, T. S.; and Standaert, F. G. Depression of cardiac sympathetic nerve activity by diphenylhydantoin. *J. Pharmacol. Exp. Ther.*, 1971, 179, 599–610.

Graffner, C.; Johnsson, G.; and Sjogren, J. Pharmacokinetics of procainamide intravenously and orally as conventional and slow-release tablets. *Clin. Pharmacol. Ther.*, 1975, 17, 414–423.

Green, K.; Chamberlin, D. A.; Fulton, R. M.; and others. Improvement in prognosis of myocardial infarction by long term beta-adrenergic blockade using practolol. A multicenter, international study. *Br. Med. J.*, 1975, 3, 735–740.

Gupta, P. K.; Lichstein, E.; and Chadda, K. D. Lidocaine-induced heart block in patients with bundle branch block. *Am. J. Cardiol.*, 1974, 33, 487–492.

Han, J.; Malozzi, A. M.; and Moe, G. K. Sino-atrial reciprocation in the isolated rabbit heart. *Circ. Res.*, 1968, 22, 355–362.

Harris, A. S., and Kokernot, R. H. Effects of diphenylhydantoin sodium (DILANTIN SODIUM) and phenobarbital sodium upon ectopic ventricular tachycardia in acute myocardial infarction. *Am. J. Physiol.*, 1950, 163, 505–516.

Harris, E. J., and Hutter, O. F. The action of acetylcholine on the movements of potassium ions in the sinus venosus of the heart. *J. Physiol.* (*Lond.*), 1956, 133, 58P.

Hartel, G.; Louhija, A.; and Konttinen, A. Disopyramide in the prevention of recurrence of atrial fibrillation after electroconversion. *Clin. Pharmacol. Ther.*, 1974, 15, 551–555.

Hauswirth, O.; Noble, D.; and Tsien, R. W. The mechanism of oscillatory activity at low membrane potentials in cardiac Purkinje fibers. *J. Physiol.* (*Lond.*), 1969, 200, 255–265.

Heissenbuttel, R. H., and Bigger, J. T., Jr. The effect of oral quinidine on intraventricular conduction in man. Correlation of plasma quinidine with changes in intraventricular conduction time. *Am. Heart J.*, 1970, 80, 453–462.

———. Bretylium tosylate: a newly available antiarrhythmic drug for ventricular arrhythmias. *Ann. Intern. Med.*, 1979, 90, 229–238.

Hillestad, L., and Storstein, O. Conversion of chronic atrial fibrillation to sinus rhythm with combined propranolol and quinidine treatment. *Am. Heart J.*, 1969, 77, 137–139.

Hinderling, P. H.; Bres, J.; and Garrett, E. R. Protein binding and erythrocyte partitioning of disopyramide and its monodealkylated metabolite. *J. Pharm. Sci.*, 1974, 63, 1684–1690.

Hinderling, P. H., and Garrett, E. R. Pharmacokinetics of the antiarrhythmic disopyramide in healthy humans. *J. Pharmacokinet. Biopharm.*, 1976, 4, 199–230.

Hoffman, B. F. Electrical activity of the A-V node. In, *The Specialized Tissues of the Heart.* (Paes de Carvalho, A., and Hoffman, B. F., eds.) Elsevier Publishing Co., Amsterdam, 1961, pp. 143–155.

Hondeghem, L. M. Validity of $\dot{V}_{max}$ as a measure of the sodium current in cardiac and nervous tissues. *Biophys. J.*, 1978, 18, 147–152.

Jensen, G.; Sigurd, B.; and Uhrenholt, A. Hemodynamic effects of intravenous disopyramide in heart failure. *Eur. J. Clin. Pharmacol.*, 1975, 8, 167–173.

Josephson, M. E.; Caracta, A. R.; Lau, S. H.; Gallagher, J. J.; and Damato, A. N. Effects of lidocaine on refractory periods in man. *Am. Heart J.*, 1972, 84, 778–786.

———. Electrophysiological evaluation of disopyramide in man. *Ibid.*, 1973, 86, 771–780.

Josephson, M. E.; Seides, S. F.; Batsford, W. P.; Weisfogel, G. M.; Akhtar, M.; Caracta, A. R.; Lau, S. H.; and Damato, A. N. The electrophysiological effects of intramuscular quinidine on the atrioventricular conducting system in man. *Am. Heart J.*, 1974, 87, 55–64.

Karim, A. The pharmacokinetics of NORPACE. *Angiology*, 1975, 26, 85–98.

Karlsson, E. Plasma levels of procaine amide after administration of conventional and sustained-release tablets. *Eur. J. Clin. Pharmacol.*, 1973, 6, 245–250.

Karlsson, E.; Molin, L.; Norlander, B.; and Sjoqvist, F. Acetylation of procainamide in man studied with a new gas chromatographic method. *Br. J. Clin. Pharmacol.*, 1974, 1, 467–475.

Kayden, H. J.; Brodie, B. B.; and Steele, J. M. Procaine amide. A review. *Circulation*, 1957, 15, 118–126.

Kessler, K. M.; Lowenthal, D. T.; Warner, H.; Gibson, T.; Briggs, W.; and Reidenberg, M. M. Quinidine elimination in patients with congestive heart failure or poor renal function. *N. Engl. J. Med.*, **1974**, *290*, 706–709.

Kniffen, F. J.; Lomas, T. E.; Counsell, R. E.; and Lucchesi, B. R. The antiarrhythmic and antifibrillatory actions of bretylium and its *o*-iodobenzyl trimethylammonium analog, UM-360. *J. Pharmacol. Exp. Ther.*, **1975**, *192*, 120–128.

Koch-Weser, J. Quinidine-induced hypoprothrombinemic hemorrhage in patients on chronic warfarin therapy. *Ann. Intern. Med.*, **1968**, *68*, 511–517.

Koch-Weser, J., and Klein, S. W. Procainamide dosage schedules, plasma concentrations, and clinical effects. *J.A.M.A.*, **1971**, *215*, 1454–1460.

Koch-Weser, J.; Klein, S. W.; Foo-Canto, L. L.; Kastor, J. A.; and DeSanctis, R. W. Antiarrhythmic prophylaxis with procainamide in acute myocardial infarction. *N. Engl. J. Med.*, **1969**, *281*, 1253–1260.

Koster, R. W., and Wellens, H. J. J. Quinidine-induced ventricular flutter and fibrillation without digitalis therapy. *Am. J. Cardiol.*, **1976**, *38*, 519–523.

Kuntzman, R.; Tsai, I.; Chang, R.; and Conney, A. H. Disposition of bretylium in man and rat. *Clin. Pharmacol. Ther.*, **1970**, *11*, 829–837.

Kupersmith, J.; Antman, E. M.; and Hoffman, B. F. *In vivo* electrophysiological effects of lidocaine in canine acute myocardial infarction. *Circ. Res.*, **1975**, *36*, 84–91.

Kupersmith, J.; Shiang, H.; Litwak, R. S.; and Herman, M. V. Electrophysiological and antiarrhythmic effects of propranolol in canine acute myocardial ischemia. *Circ. Res.*, **1976**, *38*, 302–307.

Kus, T., and Sasyniuk, B. I. Electrophysiological actions of disopyramide phosphate on canine ventricular muscle and Purkinje fiber. *Circ. Res.*, **1975**, *37*, 844–854.

Kutt, H. Biochemical and genetic factors regulating DILANTIN metabolism in man. *Ann. N.Y. Acad. Sci.*, **1971**, *179*, 704–722.

LaBarre, A.; Strauss, H. C.; Scheinman, M. M.; Evans, G. T.; Bashore, T.; Tiedeman, J. S.; and Wallace, A. G. Electrophysiologic effects of disopyramide phosphate on sinus node function in patients with sinus node dysfunction. *Circulation*, **1979**, *59*, 226–235.

Ladd, A. T. Procainamide-induced lupus erythematosus. *N. Engl. J. Med.*, **1962**, *267*, 1357–1358.

Larson, R. K. The mechanism of quinidine purpura. *Blood*, **1953**, *8*, 16–25.

Leahey, E. B., Jr.; Reiffel, J. A.; Drusin, R. E.; Heissenbuttel, R. H.; Lovejoy, W. P.; and Bigger, J. T., Jr. Interaction between quinidine and digoxin. *J.A.M.A.*, **1978**, *240*, 533–534.

Lederer, W. J., and Tsien, R. W. Transient inward current underlying arrhythmogenic effects of cardiotonic steroids in Purkinje fibers. *J. Physiol. (Lond.)*, **1976**, *263*, 73–100.

LeLorier, J.; Moisan, R.; Gagne, J.; and Caille, G. Effect of the duration of infusion on the disposition of lidocaine in dogs. *J. Pharmacol. Exp. Ther.*, **1977**, *203*, 507–511.

Levitt, B.; Cagin, N.; Kleid, J.; Somberg, J.; and Gillis, R. A. Role of the nervous system in the genesis of cardiac rhythm disorders. *Am. J. Cardiol.*, **1976**, *37*, 1111–1113.

Levy, M. N. Parasympathomimetic control of the heart. In, *Neural Regulation of the Heart.* (Randall, W. C., ed.) Oxford University Press, New York, **1977**, pp. 95–130.

Lewis, T., and Drury, A. N. Revised views of the refractory period, in relation to drugs reputed to prolong it, and in relation to circus movement. *Heart*, **1926**, *13*, 95–100.

Lie, K. I.; Liem, K. L.; Louridtz, W. J.; Janse, M. J.; Willebrands, A. F.; and Durrer, D. Efficacy of lidocaine in preventing primary ventricular fibrillation within one hour after a 300 mg intramuscular injection. *Am. J. Cardiol.*, **1978**, *42*, 486–488.

Lie, K. I.; Wellens, H. J. J.; van Capelle, F. J.; and Durrer, D. Lidocaine in the prevention of primary ventricular fibrillation. A double-blind, randomized study of 212 consecutive patients. *N. Engl. J. Med.*, **1974**, *291*, 1324–1326.

Lucchesi, B. R., and Whitsitt, L. S. The pharmacology of beta-adrenergic blocking agents. *Prog. Cardiovasc. Dis.*, **1969**, *11*, 410–430.

Luoma, P. V.; Kujala, P. A.; Juustila, H. J.; and Takkunen, J. T. Efficacy of intravenous disopyramide in the termination of supraventricular arrhythmias. *J. Clin. Pharmacol.*, **1978**, *18*, 293–301.

McAllister, R. E.; Noble, D.; and Tsien, R. W. Reconstruction of the electrical activity of cardiac Purkinje fibers. *J. Physiol. (Lond.)*, **1975**, *251*, 1–59.

Mandel, W. J., and Bigger, J. T., Jr. Electrophysiologic effects of lidocaine on isolated canine and rabbit atrial tissue. *J. Pharmacol. Exp. Ther.*, **1971**, *178*, 81–93.

Mark, L. C.; Kayden, H. J.; Steele, J. M.; Cooper, J. R.; Berlin, I.; Rovenstine, E. A.; and Brodie, B. B. The physiological disposition and cardiac effects of procaine amide. *J. Pharmacol. Exp. Ther.*, **1951**, *102*, 5–15.

Markiewicz, W.; Winkle, R.; Binetti, G.; Kernoff, R.; and Harrison, D. C. Normal myocardial contractile state in the presence of quinidine. *Circulation*, **1976**, *53*, 101–106.

Markis, J. E., and Koch-Weser, J. Characteristics and mechanism of inotropic and chronotropic actions of bretylium tosylate. *J. Pharmacol. Exp. Ther.*, **1971**, *178*, 94–102.

Marrott, P. K.; Ruttley, M. S. T.; Winterbottam, J. T.; and Muir, J. R. A study of the acute electrophysiological and cardiovascular action of disopyramide in man. *Eur. J. Cardiol.*, **1976**, *4*, 303–312.

Mason, J. W.; Winkle, R. A.; Rider, A. K.; Stinson, E. B.; and Harrison, D. C. The electrophysiologic effects of quinidine in the transplanted human heart. *J. Clin. Invest.*, **1977**, *59*, 481–489.

Mathur, P. P. Cardiovascular effects of a newer antiarrhythmic agent, disopyramide phosphate. *Am. Heart J.*, **1972**, *84*, 764–770.

Mautz, F. R. The reduction of cardiac irritability by the epicardial and systemic administration of drugs as a protection in cardiac surgery. *J. Thorac. Surg.*, **1936**, *5*, 612–628.

Méndez, C.; Mueller, W. J.; Merideth, J.; and Moe, G. K. Interaction of transmembrane potentials in canine Purkinje fibers and at Purkinje fiber-muscle junctions. *Circ. Res.*, **1969**, *24*, 361–372.

Miller, G.; Weinberg, S. L.; and Pick, A. The effect of procaine amide (PRONESTYL) in clinical auricular fibrillation and flutter. *Circulation*, **1952**, *6*, 41–50.

Moe, G. K., and Abildskov, J. A. Atrial fibrillation as a self-sustaining arrhythmia independent of focal discharge. *Am. Heart J.*, **1959**, *58*, 59–70.

Moe, G. K., and Méndez, C. The physiologic basis of reciprocal rhythm. *Prog. Cardiovasc. Dis.*, **1966**, *8*, 461–482.

Moe, G. K.; Rheinboldt, W. C.; and Abildskov, J. A. A computer model of atrial fibrillation. *Am. Heart J.*, **1964**, *67*, 200–220.

Nies, A. S., and Shand, D. G. Clinical pharmacology of propranolol. *Circulation*, **1975**, *52*, 6–15.

Nies, A. S.; Shand, D. G.; and Wilkinson, G. R. Altered hepatic blood flow and drug disposition. *Clin. Pharmacokinet.*, **1976**, *1*, 135–155.

Noma, A., and Irisawa, H. Electrogenic sodium pump in rabbit sinoatrial node cell. *Pfluegers Arch.*, **1974**, *351*, 177–182.

———. Membrane currents in the rabbit sinoatrial node cell as studied by the double microelectrode method. *Ibid.*, **1976**, *364*, 45–52.

Obayashi, K.; Hayakawa, H.; and Mandel, W. J. Interrelationships between external potassium concentration and lidocaine: effects on canine Purkinje fiber. *Am. Heart J.*, **1975**, *89*, 221–226.

Palmer, K. H.; Martin, B.; Baggett, B.; and Wall, M. E. The metabolic fate of orally administered quinidine gluconate in humans. *Biochem. Pharmacol.*, **1969**, *18*, 1845–1860.

Papp, J. G., and Vaughan Williams, E. M. The effect of bretylium on intracellular cardiac action potentials in relation to its antiarrhythmic and local anesthetic activity. *Br. J. Pharmacol.*, **1969**, *37*, 380–390.

Peon, J.; Ferrier, G. R.; and Moe, G. K. The relationship of excitability to conduction velocity in canine Purkinje tissue. *Circ. Res.*, **1978**, *43*, 125–135.

Peper, K., and Trautwein, W. The effect of aconitine on the membrane current in cardiac muscle. *Pfluegers Arch.*, **1967**, *296*, 328–336.

Pitt, W. A., and Cox, A. R. The effect of the beta-adrenergic antagonist propranolol on rabbit atrial cells with the use of the ultramicroelectrode technique. *Am. Heart J.*, **1968**, *76*, 168–172.

Randall, W. C. Sympathetic control of the heart. In, *Neural Regulation of the Heart.* (Randall, W. C., ed.) Oxford University Press, New York, **1977**, pp. 43–94. (164 references.)

Reidenberg, M. M.; Drayer, D. E.; Levy, M.; and Warner, H. Polymorphic acetylation of procainamide in man. *Clin. Pharmacol. Ther.*, **1975**, *17*, 722–730.

Reidenberg, M. M.; Odar-Cederlof, I.; von Bahr, C.; Borga, O.; and Sjoqvist, F. Protein binding of diphenylhydantoin and desmethylimipramine in plasma from patients with poor renal function. *N. Engl. J. Med.*, **1971**, *285*, 264–267.

Roberts, J.; Stadter, R. P.; Cairoli, V.; and Modell, W. Relationship between adrenergic activity and cardiac actions of quinidine. *Circ. Res.*, **1962**, *11*, 758–764.

Rosati, R. A.; Alexander, J. A.; Wallace, A. G.; Sealy, W. C.; and Young, W. G., Jr. Failure of beta-adrenergic blockade to alter ventricular fibrillation threshold in the dog. *Circ. Res.*, **1966**, *19*, 721–725.

Rosen, M. R.; Danilo, P., Jr.; Alonso, M. B.; and Pippenger, C. E. Effects of therapeutic concentrations of diphenylhydantoin on transmembrane potentials of normal and depressed Purkinje fibers. *J. Pharmacol. Exp. Ther.*, **1976**, *197*, 594–604.

Sasyniuk, B. I., and Kus, T. Cellular electrophysiologic changes induced by disopyramide phosphate in normal and infarcted hearts. *J. Int. Med. Res.*, **1976**, *4*, 20–25.

Sasyniuk, B. I., and Méndez, C. A mechanism for reentry in canine ventricular tissue. *Circ. Res.*, **1971**, *28*, 3–15.

Schack, J. A.; Hoffman, I.; and Vesell, H. The response of arrhythmias and tachycardias of supraventricular origin to oral procaine amide. *Br. Heart J.*, **1952**, *14*, 465–469.

Schmid, P. G.; Nelson, L. D.; Heistad, D. D.; Mark, A. L.; and Abboud, F. M. Vascular effects of procaine amide in the dog. Predominance of the inhibitory effect on ganglionic transmission. *Circ. Res.*, **1974a**, *35*, 948–960.

Schmid, P. G.; Nelson, L. D.; Mark, A. L.; Heistad, D. D.; and Abboud, F. M. Inhibition of adrenergic vasoconstriction by quinidine. *J. Pharmacol. Exp. Ther.*, **1974b**, *188*, 124–134.

Schmitt, F. O., and Erlanger, J. Directional differences in the conduction of the impulse through heart muscle and their possible relation to extrasystolic and fibrillary contractions. *Am. J. Physiol.*, **1928–29**, *87*, 326–347.

Schulman, N. R. Immunoreactions involving platelets. *J. Exp. Med.*, **1958**, *107*, 665–690.

Seides, S. F.; Josephson, M. E.; Batsford, W. P.; Weisfogel, G. M.; Lau, S. H.; and Damato, A. N. The electrophysiology of propranolol in man. *Am. Heart J.*, **1974**, *88*, 733–741.

Seipel, L., and Breithardt, G. Sinus recovery time after disopyramide phosphate. *Am. J. Cardiol.*, **1976**, *37*, 1118.

Sekiya, A., and Vaughan Williams, E. M. A comparison of the antifibrillatory actions and effects on intracellular cardiac potentials of pronethalol, disopyramide and quinidine. *Br. J. Pharmacol.*, **1963**, *21*, 473–481.

Selden, R., and Sasahara, A. A. Central nervous toxicity induced by lidocaine. *J.A.M.A.*, **1967**, *202*, 908–909.

Selzer, A., and Wray, H. W. Quinidine syncope. Paroxysmal ventricular fibrillation occurring during treatment of chronic atrial arrhythmias. *Circulation*, **1964**, *30*, 17–26.

Singh, B. N., and Vaughan Williams, E. M. Effect of altering potassium concentration on the action of lidocaine and diphenylhydantoin on rabbit atrial and ventricular muscle. *Circ. Res.*, **1971**, *29*, 286–295.

Sodermark, T.; Jonsson, B.; Olsson, A.; Oro, L.; Wallin, H.; Edhag, O.; Sjogren, A.; Danielsson, M.; and Rosenhamer, G. Effect of quinidine on maintaining sinus rhythm after conversion of atrial fibrillation or flutter. A multicenter study from Stockholm. *Br. Heart J.*, **1975**, *37*, 486–492.

Spurrell, R. A. J.; Thorburn, C. W.; Camm, J.; Sowton, E.; and Deuchar, D. C. Effects of disopyramide on electrophysiological properties of specialized conduction system in man and on accessory atrioventricular pathway in Wolff-Parkinson-White syndrome. *Br. Heart J.*, **1975**, *37*, 861–867.

Stagg, A. L., and Wallace, A. G. The effect of propranolol on membrane conductance in canine cardiac Purkinje fibers. *Circulation*, **1974**, *50*, Suppl. III, 145.

Stenson, R. E.; Constantino, R. T.; and Harrison, D. C. Interrelationships of hepatic blood flow, cardiac output, and blood levels of lidocaine in man. *Circulation*, **1971**, *43*, 205–211.

Stephen, S. A. Unwanted effects of propranolol. *Am. J. Cardiol.*, **1966**, *18*, 463–468.

Stern, S. Conversion of chronic atrial fibrillation to sinus rhythm with combined propranolol and quinidine treatment. *Am. Heart J.*, **1967**, *74*, 170–178.

Stern, S., and Eisenberg, S. The effect of propranolol (INDERAL) on the electrocardiogram of normal subjects. *Am. Heart J.*, **1969**, *77*, 192–195.

Stock, J. P. P., and Dalc, N. Beta-adrenergic receptor blockade in cardiac arrhythmias. *Br. Med. J.*, **1963**, *2*, 1230–1233.

Stone, N.; Klein, M. D.; and Lown, B. Diphenylhydantoin in the prevention of recurring ventricular tachycardia. *Circulation*, **1971**, *43*, 420–427.

Strauss, H. C., and Bigger, J. T., Jr. Electrophysiologic properties of the rabbit sino-atrial perinodal fibers. *Circ. Res.*, **1972**, *31*, 490–509.

Strauss, H. C.; Bigger, J. T.; Bassett, A. L.; and Hoffman, B. F. Actions of diphenylhydantoin on the electrical properties of isolated rabbit and canine atria. *Circ. Res.*, **1968**, *23*, 463–477.

Strauss, H. C.; Gilbert, M.; Svenson, R. H.; Miller, H. C.; and Wallace, A. G. Electrophysiological effects of propranolol on sinus node function in patients with sinus node dysfunction. *Circulation*, **1976**, *54*, 452–459.

Strong, J. M.; Parker, M.; and Atkinson, A. J. Identification of glycine xylidide in patients treated with intravenous lidocaine. *Clin. Pharmacol. Ther.*, **1973**, *14*, 67–72.

Thomson, P. D.; Melmon, K. L.; Richardson, J. A.; Cohn, K.; Steinbrunn, W.; Cudihee, R.; and Rowland, M. Lidocaine pharmacokinetics in advanced heart failure, liver disease, and renal failure in humans. *Ann. Intern. Med.*, **1973**, *78*, 499–508.

Tsien, R. W. Effects of epinephrine on the pacemaker potassium current of cardiac Purkinje fibers. *J. Gen. Physiol.*, **1974**, *64*, 293–319.

Vajda, F. J. E.; Prineas, R. J.; Lovell, R. R. H.; and Sloman, J. G. The possible effect on long-term high plasma levels of phenytoin on mortality after acute myocardial infarction. *Eur. J. Clin. Pharmacol.*, **1973**, *5*, 138–144.

Valentine, P. A.; Frew, J. L.; Mashford, M. L.; and Sloman, J. G. Lidocaine in the prevention of sudden death in the pre-hospital phase of acute infarction. A double-blind study. *N. Engl. J. Med.*, **1974**, *291*, 1327–1331.

Vaughan Williams, E. M. Mode of action of beta receptor antagonists on cardiac muscle. *Am. J. Cardiol.*, **1966**, *18*, 399–405.

Vincent, G. M.; Abildskov, J. A.; and Burgess, M. J. Q-T interval syndromes. *Prog. Cardiovasc. Dis.*, **1974**, *16*, 523–530.

Wallace, A. G.; Cline, R. E.; Sealy, W. C.; Young, W. G., Jr.; and Troyer, W. G., Jr. Electrophysiologic effects of quinidine. Studies using chronically implanted electrodes in awake dogs with and without cardiac denervation. *Circ. Res.*, **1966a**, *19*, 960–969.

Wallace, A. G.; Schaal, S. F.; Sugimoto, T.; Rozear, M.; and Alexander, J. A. The electrophysiologic effects of beta-adrenergic blockade and cardiac denervation. *Bull. N.Y. Acad. Med.*, **1967**, *43*, 1119–1137.

Wallace, A. G.; Troyer, W. G.; Lesage, M. A.; and Zotti, E. F. Electrophysiologic effects of isoproterenol and beta blocking agents in awake dogs. *Circ. Res.*, **1966b**, *18*, 140–148.

Wasserman, F.; Brodsky, L.; Kathe, J. H.; Rodensky, P. L.; Dick, M. M.; and Denton, P. S. The effect of molar sodium lactate in quinidine intoxication. *Am. J. Cardiol.*, **1959**, *3*, 294–299.

Waxman, M. B., and Wallace, A. G. Electrophysiologic effects of bretylium tosylate on the heart. *J. Pharmacol. Exp. Ther.*, **1972**, *183*, 264–274.

Weidmann, S. The effect of the cardiac membrane potential on the rapid availability of the sodium-carrying system. *J. Physiol. (Lond.)*, **1955**, *127*, 213–224.

Weisfogel, G. M.; Batsford, W. P.; Paulay, K. L.; Josephson, M. E.; Ogunkelu, J. B.; Akhtar, M.; Seides, S. F.; and Damato, A. N. Sinus node re-entrant tachycardia in man. *Am. Heart J.*, **1975**, *90*, 295–304.

Weld, F. M., and Bigger, J. T., Jr. Effect of lidocaine on the early inward transient current in sheep cardiac Purkinje fibers. *Circ. Res.*, **1975**, *37*, 630–639.

———. The effect of lidocaine on diastolic transmembrane currents determining pacemaker depolarization in cardiac Purkinje fibers. *Ibid.*, **1976**, *38*, 203–208.

Wellens, H. J. J.; Duren, D. R.; and Lie, K. I. Observations on mechanisms of ventricular tachycardia in man. *Circulation*, **1976**, *54*, 237–244.

Wenckebach, K. F. *Die unregelmässige Herztätigkeit und ihre klinische Bedeutung.* W. Engelmann, Leipzig, **1914**.

White, D.; Crawford, M.; O'Rourke, R.; Karliner, J.; and Gorwit, J. Effects of quinidine on left ventricular performance in normals and patients with congestive cardiomyopathy. *Circulation*, **1977**, *56*, Suppl. III, 180.

Willius, F. A., and Keys, T. E. Cardiac clinics. XCIV. A remarkably early reference to the use of cinchona in cardiac arrhythmia. *Proc. Staff Meet. Mayo Clin.*, **1942**, *17*, 294–296.

Wit, A. L., and Cranefield, P. F. Triggered activity in cardiac muscle fibers of the simian mitral valve. *Circ. Res.*, **1976**, *38*, 85–98.

———. Triggered and automatic activity in the canine coronary sinus. *Ibid.*, **1977**, *41*, 435–445.

Wit, A. L.; Cranefield, P. F.; and Hoffman, B. F. Slow conduction and reentry in the ventricular conducting system. II. Single and sustained circus movement in networks of canine and bovine Purkinje fibers. *Circ. Res.*, **1972a**, *30*, 11–22.

Wit, A. L.; Hoffman, B. F.; and Cranefield, P. F. Slow conduction and reentry in the ventricular conducting system. I. Return extrasystole in canine Purkinje fibers. *Circ. Res.*, **1972b**, *30*, 1–10.

Wit, A. L.; Rosen, M. R.; and Hoffman, B. F. Electrophysiology and pharmacology of cardiac arrhythmias. VIII. Cardiac effects of diphenylhydantoin. *Am. Heart J.*, **1975**, *90*, 265–272, 397–404.

Wit, A. L.; Steiner, C.; and Damato, A. N. Electrophysiologic effects of bretylium tosylate on single fibers of the canine specialized conducting system and ventricle. *J. Pharmacol. Exp. Ther.*, **1970**, *173*, 344–356.

Wittig, J.; Harrison, L. A.; and Wallace, A. G. Electrophysiological effects of lidocaine on distal Purkinje fibers of canine heart. *Am. Heart J.*, **1973**, *86*, 69–78.

Woosley, R. L.; Shand, D.; Kornhauser, D.; Nies, A. S.; and Oates, J. A. Relation of plasma concentration and dose of propranolol to its effect on resistant ventricular arrhythmias. *Clin. Res.*, **1977**, *25*, 262A.

Woske, H.; Belford, J.; Fastier, F. N.; and Brooks, C. McC. The effect of procaine amide on excitability, refractoriness and conduction in the mammalian heart. *J. Pharmacol. Exp. Ther.*, **1953**, *107*, 134–139.

Wu, D.; Denes, P.; Dhingra, R.; Kahn, A.; and Rosen, K. M. The effects of propranolol on induction of A-V nodal reentrant paroxysmal tachycardia. *Circulation*, **1974**, *50*, 665–677.

Zapata-Diáz, J.; Cabrera, C. E.; and Méndez, R. An experimental and clinical study on the effects of procaine amide (pronestyl) on the heart. *Am. Heart J.*, **1952**, *43*, 854–870.

Monographs and Reviews

Bigger, J. T., Jr. Electrical properties of cardiac muscle and possible causes of cardiac arrhythmias. In, *Cardiovascular Arrhythmias.* (Dreifus, L. S., and Likoff, W., eds.) Grune & Stratton, Inc., New York, **1973**, pp. 13–34.

Bigger, J. T., Jr.; Dresdale, R. J.; Heissenbuttel, R. H.; Weld, F. M.; and Wit, A. L. Ventricular arrhythmias in ischemic heart disease: mechanism, prevalence, significance and management. *Prog. Cardiovasc. Dis.*, **1977**, *19*, 255–300. (258 references.)

Bigger, J. T., Jr., and Reiffel, J. A. Sick sinus syndrome. *Annu. Rev. Med.*, **1979**, *30*, 91–118. (150 references.)

Boura, A. L. A., and Green, A. F. Adrenergic neurone blocking agents. *Annu. Rev. Pharmacol.*, **1965**, *5*, 183–212.

Cranefield, P. F. *The Conduction of the Cardiac Impulse.* Futura Publishing Co., Inc., Mount Kisco, N.Y., **1975**.

DiPalma, J. R., and Schults, J. E. Antifibrillatory drugs. *Medicine (Baltimore)*, **1950**, *29*, 123–168. (236 references.)

Ferrier, G. R. Digitalis arrhythmias: role of oscillatory afterpotentials. *Prog. Cardiovasc. Dis.*, **1977**, *19*, 459–474.

Hoffman, B. F., and Cranefield, P. F. *Electrophysiology of the Heart.* McGraw-Hill Book Co., New York, **1960**.

Noble, D. *The Initiation of the Heartbeat.* Clarendon Press, Oxford, **1975**.

Trautwein, W. Generation and conduction of impulses in the heart as affected by drugs. *Pharmacol. Rev.*, **1963**, *15*, 277–332. (352 references.)

———. Membrane currents in cardiac muscle fibers. *Physiol. Rev.*, **1973**, *53*, 793–835. (120 references.)

CHAPTER

32 ANTIHYPERTENSIVE AGENTS AND THE DRUG THERAPY OF HYPERTENSION

Terrence F. Blaschke and Kenneth L. Melmon

Despite advances in the understanding of central and peripheral mechanisms involved in the control of arterial blood pressure, drugs for the treatment of hypertension have largely evolved empirically. Yet there is enough information on which to base a rational approach to therapy (Hypertension Detection and Follow-Up Program Cooperative Group, 1979a, 1979b; Relman, 1980). The appropriate use of antihypertensive drugs requires a knowledge of the sites of action of these compounds and the physiological reflexes that occur in response to a

Table 32–1. CLASSIFICATION OF ANTI-HYPERTENSIVE DRUGS ACCORDING TO THEIR PRIMARY SITE OR MECHANISM OF ACTION

Drugs That Alter Central Sympathetic Nervous System Activity
    Methyldopa
    Clonidine
    Propranolol (?)
    Reserpine (?)

Vasodilators
  Arteriolar
    Hydralazine
    Diazoxide
    Minoxidil
    Thiazides and phthalimidines
  Arteriolar and venular
    Nitroprusside
    Prazosin

Adrenergic Receptor Blocking Drugs
  β-Adrenergic blocking drugs
    Propranolol
    Nadolol
    Metoprolol
  α-Adrenergic blocking drugs
    Prazosin
    Phentolamine
    Phenoxybenzamine

Drugs That Act at Postganglionic Sympathetic Nerve Endings
    Guanethidine
    Reserpine
    Monoamine oxidase inhibitors

Drugs That Interfere with the Renin-Angiotensin System
    Saralasin
    Captopril

change in blood pressure. All currently available hypotensive compounds act by interfering with normal homeostatic mechanisms, and this provides a useful basis for the classification of the drugs. Efficacy, toxicity, and suitable combinations of drugs can often be predicted by consideration of both the sites and the mechanisms of action of the agents. Table 32–1 shows such a classification for a number of commonly used antihypertensive agents that are available in the United States. Because there is a great diversity of proven and postulated mechanisms of action of antihypertensive drugs, the effectiveness of a given drug cannot necessarily be taken as evidence that its mechanism of action relates to the pathogenesis of the elevated blood pressure.

Several antihypertensive agents that act predominantly on the peripheral sympathetic nervous system, at adrenergic receptor sites, on autonomic ganglia, and on the renin-angiotensin system are described in Chapters 4, 9, 10, and 27. The present chapter focuses on additional important agents not covered in those chapters, on the pathophysiology of hypertension, and on the approach to therapy for the hypertensive patient.

I. Antihypertensive Agents

METHYLDOPA

Methyldopa (L-α-methyl-3,4-dihydroxyphenylalanine) was found to be an effective inhibitor of L-aromatic amino acid (dopa) decarboxylase in the mid-1950s, but it attracted major attention only after its hypotensive properties were noted during studies of aromatic amino acid metabolism in man (Oates *et al.*, 1960). It has since gained widespread popularity in the treatment of essential hypertension. However, the search for its mechanism of action has progressed much less smoothly than has its clinical application. Several blind alleys have held the spotlight, apparently because known biochemical mechanisms that could have been responsible for the antihypertensive effect were accepted without sufficient pharmacological evidence that they were causally involved. Data now available indicate that the major antihypertensive effect of methyldopa is not due to decarboxylase inhibition or to any other effect on peripheral sympathetic nerves; consequently, it should no longer be classified as a peripheral adrenergic neuron blocking agent (Chavdarian *et al.,* 1978; Freed *et al.,* 1978).

Locus and Mechanism of Action. Theories of the mechanism of action of methyldopa as an antihypertensive drug have undergone considerable revision. The earlier views deserve brief mention because they illustrate the potential danger of extrapolation of data derived *in vitro* to the more complex events that occur *in vivo.*

Methyldopa effectively inhibits the decarboxylation of both dopa and 5-hydroxytryptophan *in vitro* and *in vivo,* and decreases the concentrations of 5-hydroxytryptamine (5-HT), dopamine, and norepinephrine in the central nervous system (CNS) and in most peripheral tissues. It was first postulated that methyldopa reduced the blood pressure by inhibiting dopa decarboxylation in sympathetic nerves, which would in turn decrease stores of norepinephrine and, thus, decrease vasomotor tone.

Reductions of the concentrations of dopamine and 5-HT in tissues correlated with inhibition of decarboxylase, but depletion of norepinephrine was accomplished without complete inhibition of the enzyme. Furthermore, partial inhibition of decarboxylation *per se* (by other drugs) did not decrease the rate of synthesis of catecholamines. Finally, the depletion of catecholamines far outlasted the inhibition of the enzyme and did not correlate with the hypotensive response. α-Methyldopamine causes a greater reduction in the norepinephrine content of peripheral tissues than does methyldopa, but does not lower blood pressure. Because methyldopa is itself metabolized to α-methylnorepinephrine, which can be stored in sympathetic nerve endings, it was next hypothesized that the latter displaced norepinephrine and acted as an inadequate "false transmitter" (*see* Kopin, 1968). α-Methylnorepinephrine fully meets the definition of a false transmitter, but its pharmacological significance is questionable. The hypotensive effect of methyldopa is not well correlated with the production or tissue content of α-methylnorepinephrine in a variety of circumstances, and the α-methylnorepinephrine formed is readily

released by sympathetic nerve activity and effectively constricts peripheral blood vessels in most circumstances. (*See* Sjoerdsma *et al.,* 1963; Altura, 1975.) While investigators were preoccupied with the norepinephrine-depletion and false-transmitter theories of the action of methyldopa, little attention was paid to the early observation that cardiovascular reflexes and responses to sympathetic nerve stimulation are only slightly inhibited at the time of the maximal hypotensive response (Goldberg *et al.,* 1960). This has been repeatedly confirmed.

The current, generally accepted interpretation is that the major antihypertensive action of methyldopa is on the CNS. Early important evidence for this was that decarboxylase inhibitors that penetrate the CNS abolish the hypotensive response to methyldopa, but those that act only peripherally are ineffective (Henning, 1969; Kersting *et al.,* 1977). This observation also indicates that the effect is due to a metabolic product of methyldopa. Methyldopa enters the CNS, where it is decarboxylated and β-hydroxylated to α-methylnorepinephrine in central adrenergic neurons. When released, α-methylnorepinephrine potently stimulates central α-adrenergic receptors, and this inhibits sympathetic outflow (*see* Chapter 9). That the centrally active substance is α-methylnorepinephrine has been demonstrated by blockade of the hypotensive effects of methyldopa with inhibitors of CNS decarboxylation or β-hydroxylation. Furthermore, the hypotensive effect of intravenously or centrally administered methyldopa is blocked by the central administration of α-adrenergic blocking agents in animals. This theory is an expansion of the false-transmitter hypothesis and accounts for many of the heretofore-unexplained observations about methyldopa (Henning and Rubenson, 1971; Day *et al.,* 1973; Heise and Kroneberg, 1973; Ames *et al.,* 1977; Kersting *et al.,* 1977; Chavdarian *et al.,* 1978; Freed *et al.,* 1978).

Although it appears that the major antihypertensive effect of methyldopa is due to its action on the CNS, some contribution of peripheral mechanisms cannot be ruled out. The reduction in renal vascular resistance may be related to the fact that, at least in rats, α-methylnorepinephrine is a much weaker vasoconstrictor in this vascular bed than is norepinephrine (Finch and Haeusler, 1973). In addition, the observation that methyldopa lowers the blood pressure effectively in immunosympathectomized rats suggests some more direct peripheral action (Ayitey-Smith and Varma, 1970). It thus appears that several mechanisms of action account for the clinically useful effects of methyldopa (Gaffney *et al.*, 1969).

Pharmacological Properties. The hemodynamic effects of methyldopa consist in significant reductions in blood pressure and total peripheral resistance, while cardiac output and renal blood flow are maintained (Morin *et al.*, 1964; Mohammed *et al.*, 1968; Safar *et al.*, 1979). The change in blood pressure is maximal within 4 to 6 hours after an oral dose and persists for as long as 24 hours. However, one detailed study of mildly hypertensive patients given methyldopa for a year showed a predominant decrease in cardiac output, and the decrease in mean blood pressure was well correlated with the change in cardiac index (Lund-Johansen, 1972). Bradycardia, which is noted early in the response to methyldopa, persisted, and there was little change in stroke volume. The antihypertensive effect was decreased rather than increased during exercise. However, at present it is not possible to explain these divergent observations, which may be related to differences between acute and chronic effects of sympathetic blocking agents (*see* Sannerstedt and Conway, 1970).

The secretion of renin is slightly decreased by methyldopa but not sufficiently to result in misclassification of a patient's level of renin secretion if measurements are made while the patient is taking the drug. The decrease in renin may contribute to the antihypertensive action of methyldopa under some circumstances, but this action certainly is not the dominant one, nor is it necessary for the efficacy of the drug (Halushka and Keiser, 1974; Lowder and Liddle, 1975).

Functional competence of sympathetic nerves during acute hypotensive effects of methyldopa is indicated by normal responses to nerve stimulation and to most cardiovascular reflexes in both laboratory animals and man. Responses to the Valsalva maneuver and cold pressor test have been reported to be inhibited after more prolonged administration of methyldopa.

Because methyldopa does not work solely by its effects on the sympathetic nervous system, a moderate decrease in supine blood pressure is usually not accompanied by orthostatic hypotension. When the patient stands, his sympathetic reflexes are well maintained. When orthostatic hypotension appears, it is usually less severe than that caused by drugs that act predominantly on peripheral adrenergic nerves (Oates *et al.*, 1965). Hypotension does not usually occur after exercise. Consequently, it must be assumed that reflex venoconstriction is relatively intact. Other differences from responses to adrenergic neuron blocking drugs such as guanethidine are the absence of most of the signs of sympathetic inadequacy such as miosis, ptosis, and relaxation of the nictitating membrane.

Methyldopa regularly produces *sedation* in laboratory animals and man, and has a number of other effects on the CNS. In contrast to the sedative effect, the drug can lighten sleep and increase rapid-eye-movement (REM) sleep in man (Baekeland and Lundwall, 1971). It can prevent the rise in body temperature usually induced by bacterial and leukocytic pyrogens, and in large doses it can cause hypothermia (*see* Miert and Duin, 1972). Methyldopa also augments amphetamine-induced hyperactivity in mice, and it increases secretion of prolactin and induces lactation in human subjects. These various effects have been consistently attributed to or interpreted as evidence for the involvement of central adrenergic mechanisms of one type or another. However, most of the evidence is indirect.

Absorption, Fate, and Excretion. The extent of absorption of unchanged methyldopa is only approximately 25%, and there is considerable variability (Kwan *et al.*, 1976). Differences in metabolites that are found after oral and intravenous administration suggest the possibility of first-pass intestinal metabolism (Saavedra *et al.*, 1975). Disappearance of the drug from plasma after intravenous administration is biphasic, and the terminal half-time of elimination from the plasma is about 2 hours (Kwan *et al.*, 1976; Barnett *et al.*, 1977). Renal excretion accounts for about two thirds of the clearance of drug from plasma. Some accumulation of methyldopa may occur in patients with impaired renal function (Myhre *et al.*, 1972), but there is no evidence that the dosage regimen should be substantially adjusted when the drug is given to patients with hepatic or renal disease.

Methyldopa for intravenous use (methyl-dopate) is the hydrochloride of the ethyl ester of methyldopa. This preparation may not have effects equivalent to those of methyldopa given as the amino acid. In man and the monkey, some of the ester is excreted unchanged. From the animal experiments, it is apparent that less than half of the ester is hydrolyzed to methyldopa. The clinical importance of these observations is undetermined (Walson *et al.*, 1975). However, paradoxical hypertensive responses to the intravenous administration of methyldopate may be related to the direct effects of this ester.

Methyldopa and its metabolites may interfere with some of the standard chemical tests for catecholamines. Their presence in blood and urine can cause false-positive tests for pheochromocytoma.

Preparations, Routes of Administration, and Dosage. *Methyldopa*, U.S.P. (ALDOMET), is available for oral administration in tablets containing 125, 250, or 500 mg. The more soluble preparation, *Methyldopate Hydrochloride*, U.S.P. (ALDOMET ESTER HYDROCHLORIDE), is available in 5-ml vials (50 mg/ml) for parenteral use. The average daily oral dose of methyldopa is 1 g. There appears to be little additional effect with doses over 2 g. Methyldopa is given in divided doses, usually three times per day. In many patients, however, one daily dose may be adequate (Wright *et al.*, 1976). Single parenteral doses are 500 mg to 1 g, usually given by intravenous infusion and adjusted to the needs of the individual patient.

Toxicity and Precautions. Methyldopa, given either orally or parenterally, regularly causes *sedation*. After a single dose this is of shorter duration than the hypotensive effect and it tends to decrease with continued medication. However, a persistent lassitude and drowsiness, particularly disturbing to individuals doing mental work, represent the overall most important side effects. Other unwanted effects referable to the CNS include vertigo, extrapyramidal signs, nightmares, and psychic depression; the last three of these effects are less common with methyldopa than with reserpine. Dry mouth and nasal stuffiness may also be central in origin. Various gastrointestinal upsets occur, but they are only occasionally severe. *Postural hypotension* can develop, but it is considerably less frequent and less severe than during treatment with guanethidine. Exercise-induced hypotension is relatively infrequent.

Retention of salt and water with weight gain and *edema* may occur with methyldopa, as with most other antihypertensive drugs. Methyldopa does not cause bradycardia or decreased salivary flow to the same extent as does clonidine. Sexual dysfunction, primarily *impotence*, occurs in some males, but this problem also occurs frequently in hypertensive patients who are not receiving drugs. An adequate history can often prevent the unjustified discontinuation of a drug because of false attribution of an unwanted effect.

Methyldopa has several unique side effects that are unrelated to its other actions. *Drug fever* can be severe and mimic sepsis, with shaking chills and high, spiking temperatures (Glontz and Saslaw, 1968). Fever sometimes is associated with changes in metabolism of methyldopa (Valnes *et al.*, 1978) or *hepatic dysfunction*, reflected by elevation of hepatic enzymes in plasma and, occasionally, by the appearance of jaundice (Elkington *et al.*, 1969). Although usually reversible, the hepatic injury caused by the drug can progress to hepatic necrosis (Rehman *et al.*, 1973; Toghill *et al.*, 1974; Rodman *et al.*, 1976). In up to 25% of patients taking 1000 mg of methyldopa daily for 6 months or more, a *positive direct Coombs' test* develops (Carstairs *et al.*, 1966; Hunter *et al.*, 1971). Other than causing difficulties in the cross-matching of blood, this side effect does not usually cause clinical problems. *Hemolytic anemia* occurs in less than 5% of those with a positive Coombs' test. The drug should be stopped if hemolysis is detected. The antibody responsible for the positive Coombs' test is an IgG directed at the red-cell membrane. It does not react with methyldopa. The hemolytic anemia and Coombs' test positivity are reversible, but several weeks may be required after discontinuation of the drug before the test becomes normal (LoBuglio and Jandl, 1967). If hemolysis is severe, corticosteroids may be useful. As mentioned, methyldopa-induced *lactation* can appear in either sex. It is associated with high concentrations of prolactin in plasma. This uncommon side effect is usually reversible (Horwitz *et al.*, 1967). Sudden withdrawal of methyldopa therapy can cause *rebound hypertension*. However, the incidence of this complication is apparently much less than that observed after withdrawal of clonidine.

Therapeutic Uses. The major clinical use of methyldopa is for the treatment of essential hypertension, as discussed below. It has also been employed in a few patients with *carcinoid disease.*

CLONIDINE

Clonidine hydrochloride is a potent antihypertensive drug closely related chemically to tolazoline (peripheral vasodilator and α-adrenergic blocking agent), naphazoline and tetrahydrozoline (sympathomimetics), and antazoline (an antihistamine). Clonidine has the following structural formula:

Clonidine Hydrochloride

It was originally studied as an α-adrenergic agonist and was tested for its efficacy as a nasal decongestant. Small amounts of the drug given intranasally produced hypotension. Subsequent studies in animals and man confirmed its therapeutic efficacy as a centrally acting antihypertensive agent (*see* Lowenstein, 1980). These studies have substantially increased our knowledge of the central control of the sympathetic nervous system.

Pharmacological Properties. As expected from the pharmacology of the many 2-imidazoline derivatives previously studied, clonidine has many diverse actions. Although clinical use of the drug is almost entirely on a chronic basis, almost all of the available data on effects in both laboratory animals and man are from acute experiments. After intravenous injection of a few micrograms per kilogram, clonidine produces a brief rise and a subsequent more persistent fall in blood pressure, both of which are prolonged by anesthesia. The initial pressor response to clonidine is due to direct stimulation of peripheral α-adrenergic receptors; this action has also been demonstrated on the nictitating membrane and other structures. Clonidine also produces significant peripheral α-adrenergic blockade. Thus, it is a *partial agonist.*

The pressor response is accentuated and prolonged by drugs and procedures that interfere with reflex adjustments of blood pressure (*e.g.,* ganglionic blockade).

The hypotensive action of clonidine is a result of the direct action of the unchanged drug. The current hypothesis about central regulation of blood pressure stems from the observations that stimulation of α-adrenergic receptors in the vasomotor centers results in inhibition of peripheral sympathetic activity; when these receptors are blocked, there is increased peripheral sympathetic outflow (Van Zweiten, 1973; Haeusler, 1975). Clonidine presumably stimulates α-adrenergic receptors in the CNS. Indeed, the central effect of clonidine in animals is antagonized by α-adrenergic blocking drugs administered either intravenously or directly into the cerebral ventricles (Schmitt and Schmitt, 1970). In man, the α-adrenergic antagonist tolazoline can reverse the hypotensive effect of clonidine (Merguet *et al.,* 1968). There is a limited amount of evidence that clonidine is a more potent agonist at presynaptic α_2-adrenergic receptors than at postsynaptic α_1 receptors (Titeler *et al.,* 1978), but the relevance of this difference to the therapeutic effect of the drug is uncertain (*see* Chapter 9). Study of animals with lesions at various levels of the CNS indicates that a major site of action for clonidine is the medulla oblongata. The hypotension produced after acute administration of clonidine is associated with a clear reduction of the discharge rate of preganglionic adrenergic nerves, as well as by bradycardia. The latter is due to both a decrease in sympathetic and an increase in vagal tone, as would be expected from the known central interactions of these two mechanisms. The increase in vagal discharge involves an increased sensitivity of baroreceptor reflexes (Nayler and Stone, 1970). Whether adrenergic neurons in the CNS are necessary for the baroreceptor reflex arc and for the action of clonidine are unknown (Dollery and Reid, 1973; Reid *et al.,* 1973; Haeusler, 1974, 1975). Clonidine may also depress sympathetic transmission by peripheral actions, but this effect seems unimportant relative to its effects on the CNS.

Clonidine has many effects on the CNS, a number of which are similar to those of chlorpromazine.

They include marked sedation, decreased spontaneous motor activity and conditioned avoidance behavior, increased chloral hydrate sleeping time, lowered body temperature, and antipsychotic properties (Laverty and Taylor, 1969). Centrally but not peripherally induced salivation is inhibited, which probably explains the very frequent occurrence of dry mouth in hypertensive patients receiving clonidine (Putzeys and Hoobler, 1972). The antihypertensive effect in man is largely abolished by concomitant administration of desipramine (Briant et al., 1973).

Acute intravenous injection of clonidine induces a biphasic hemodynamic response. The systolic and diastolic blood pressures transiently increase and later fall (see above). The maximal decrease occurs in about 20 minutes and persists for several hours. This fall in blood pressure is due to a fall in cardiac output, with little change in peripheral resistance. After oral administration, the pressor phase is usually not seen. Pulmonary arterial pressure and cardiopulmonary blood volume are decreased, which indicates a relaxation of capacitance vessels. Glomerular filtration rate is usually decreased, but even when filtration is unaltered sodium excretion is considerably reduced. Clonidine causes an acute increase in cerebral vascular resistance and a decrease in cerebral blood flow in man (James et al., 1970). This was previously noted in laboratory animals (Sherman et al., 1968), and has received surprisingly little attention; changes in cerebral blood flow can have important effects on blood pressure. The acute effects of clonidine on cardiovascular reflexes are variable. It can block the carotid occlusion reflex but not the response to tilting in laboratory animals, and appears not to alter responses to exercise or to the Valsalva maneuver in man. Reflex control of capacitance vessels is not abolished, and postural hypotension is considerably less than with an adrenergic neuron blocking agent such as guanethidine.

There are few data concerning the hemodynamic effects that result from the chronic administration of clonidine. After 1 week of therapy, the effects are similar to those seen just after the drug is started (Safar et al., 1974). Even after treatment for a year, the effects of clonidine given alone seem constant (Lund-Johansen, 1974). The cardiac index, heart rate, and blood pressure increase during exercise. Postural hypotension occurs, but

it is not marked and responses to exercise indicate that reflex control of capacitance vessels is not abolished (see Muir et al., 1969; McRaven et al., 1971; Onesti et al., 1971).

Clonidine's central action results in suppression of the level of renin activity in plasma, although a direct action of clonidine on the kidney may also be important (Hokfelt et al., 1970; Reid et al., 1975; Karlberg and Tolagen, 1976; Pettinger et al., 1976). Renal vascular resistance decreases and renal blood flow is maintained when arterial blood pressure is lowered by clonidine (Brod et al., 1972).

Absorption and Elimination. Almost all of the available pharmacokinetic data for clonidine have been obtained from normal volunteers given single doses of the drug. In five normal individuals the bioavailability of clonidine averaged approximately 75%. The clearance from plasma is 3 ml/kg per minute, and 60% of the clearance is due to renal elimination of the unchanged drug. The elimination half-life averages 8.5 hours (Davies et al., 1977). The duration of the hypotensive effect after a single oral dose is 8 hours in normal volunteers (Dollery et al., 1976) and from 4 to more than 24 hours in patients with hypertension (Pettinger, 1975).

Preparations, Route of Administration, and Dosage. *Clonidine hydrochloride* (CATAPRES) is marketed in 100- and 200-µg tablets. The total daily dose is from 200 µg to 2 mg. In most patients, a single daily dose of clonidine is inadequate to control blood pressure; furthermore, unwanted effects, especially drowsiness, can be minimized by administering the drug twice daily in unequal doses. The larger dose should be given at bedtime and the smaller dose at noon (Jain et al., 1977).

Toxicity and Precautions. The most frequent side effects of clonidine in man are dry mouth and sedation. They are very common and frequently severe. Except for decreased salivation, the side effects improve somewhat when therapy is continued. Impotence occurs occasionally and orthostatic hypotension rarely (Hoobler and Sagastume, 1971; Onesti et al., 1971). As with other antihypertensive drugs, retention of sodium and fluid often occur when clonidine is given; diuretic therapy in combination with clonidine is usually necessary for optimal care. When compared with equihypotensive doses of methyldopa, clonidine produces an equal or greater incidence of side effects (Conolly *et al.,* 1972).

When clonidine is the sole drug used to control hypertension, its sudden withdrawal can result in a *hypertensive crisis* that can be life threatening (Conolly *et al.,* 1972; Webster *et al.,* 1974). Patients with the syndrome often first develop symptoms of nervousness, headache, abdominal pain, tachycardia, and sweating. Their blood pressure increases within 8 to 12 hours after the last dose of chronic therapy. In some instances, the increased blood pressure overshoots the pretreatment level. The incidence of the syndrome is unknown, but it may be relatively high; 7 of 14 patients developed subjective symptoms after sudden withdrawal from clonidine (Geyskes *et al.,* 1979). The pathogenesis of the syndrome is not known. Concentrations of catecholamines in the plasma and urine are elevated in symptomatic patients (Hokfelt *et al.,* 1970; Conolly *et al.,* 1972; Hansson *et al.,* 1973). Treatment involves either reinstitution of clonidine or administration of a combination of α- and β-adrenergic antagonists (*e.g.,* phentolamine and propranolol). As in the treatment of patients with pheochromocytoma, one should not use a β-adrenergic blocking agent alone, since blockade of β receptors allows exaggeration of the hypertensive effect of excess catecholamines in the circulation (Bailey and Neale, 1976). All patients who receive clonidine must be warned of the possibility of a severe withdrawal syndrome and of the possible dire effects of poor compliance. If elective surgery is required, other antihypertensive drugs should be substituted for clonidine well in advance of the procedure.

The tricyclic antidepressants, imipramine and desipramine, can nullify the effects of clonidine and therefore should not be prescribed when clonidine is being used (Briant *et al.,* 1973; Van Zweiten, 1976). Clonidine should not be employed in patients with depression, and an alternative antihypertensive drug should be used in patients who become depressed while taking clonidine.

Therapeutic Uses. The ability of clonidine to lower pressure without paralysis of the peripheral autonomic homeostatic control mechanisms is highly desirable in the treatment of hypertension; however, the incidence of unpleasant side effects and the potential for the withdrawal syndrome limit its use as a first-line drug. The use of clonidine in essential hypertension is discussed later in this chapter.

Although oral dosage with clonidine has been advocated for patients with hypertensive emergencies who require reduction in blood pressure over a period of several hours, its use for this purpose cannot be recommended because of the acute hemodynamic effects (including a fall in cardiac index without a decrease in peripheral vascular resistance) and the peripheral α-adrenergic agonistic activity of the drug (Mroczek *et al.,* 1973). Clonidine can be effective in some patients with *migraine headache* (Shafar *et al.,* 1972).

HYDRALAZINE

The effectiveness of *hydralazine* for the treatment of hypertension was documented in 1950. Although a considerable number of phthalazine derivatives produce significant hypotension, hydralazine is the only one used clinically in North America. It has the following structural formula:

Hydralazine

Locus and Mechanism of Action. Early studies on hydralazine attributed its antihypertensive effect successively to specific renal vasodilatation and to an action on the CNS. However, present evidence indicates that the major action of hydralazine is direct relaxation of vascular smooth muscle; the effect on arterioles is greater than on veins. In man, intraarterial is more effective than intravenous administration in raising skin temperature and blood flow of the extremities. Intravenous injection causes a greater vasodilatation in limbs to which vasomotor control has been chronically impaired by sympathectomy or by spinal cord section than in normally innervated limbs. Patients with chronic spinal cord transections as high as T_1 to T_5 and normal blood pressures respond to small doses of hydralazine with a drop in diastolic pressure comparable to that induced in normal subjects. (*See* Åblad, 1963.)

Cardiac stimulation by hydralazine probably involves a reflex response to the fall in blood pressure, but it is somewhat more marked than would be expected on this basis alone and is not well correlated with changes in blood pressure. Tachycardia can be induced by very small doses injected into the cerebral ventricles (Gupta and Bhargava, 1965), and hydralazine tachycardia can be prevented by ganglionic or β-adrenergic blocking agents.

Pharmacological Properties. All major effects of hydralazine are on the *cardiovascular system*. In both laboratory animals and man, adequate doses decrease arterial blood pressure, diastolic often more than systolic, and peripheral vascular resistance. The drug increases heart rate, stroke volume, and cardiac output. The preferential dilatation of arterioles, as compared to veins, minimizes postural hypotension and promotes the increase in cardiac output. When hydralazine is given alone, the latter may limit the reduction in mean blood pressure produced by the drug. The effect of hydralazine develops gradually over 15 to 20 minutes even after intravenous administration. The peripheral vasodilatation is widespread but not uniform. Splanchnic, coronary, cerebral, and renal blood flows increase unless the fall in blood pressure is very marked. Glomerular filtration, renal tubular function, and urine volume are not consistently affected; however, in common with many other antihypertensive agents, hydralazine can cause retention of sodium and water and decreased urine volume. Hydralazine usually increases renin activity in plasma, presumably as a result of increased secretion of renin by the renal juxtaglomerular cells in response to reflex sympathetic discharge. Vascular resistance in the cutaneous and muscle beds may decrease, but this is usually in parallel with the fall in blood pressure and blood flow does not increase. (*See* Freis *et al.,* 1953; Åblad, 1963.)

Absorption and Elimination. Because of extensive first-pass metabolism in the liver, the bioavailability of hydralazine is relatively low after oral administration. However, precise definition of the disposition of hydralazine has been hampered by its instability in biological fluids. It can be metabolized by multiple pathways, but acetylation seems to be a major route (Reidenberg *et al.,* 1973). The acetylation phenotype of a patient appears to be an important determinant of the bioavailability of the drug. Rapid acetylators have lower bioavailability (about 30%) than

do slow acetylators (about 50%) after oral administration of hydralazine; there is limited evidence that first-pass acetylation may be saturable in the slow acetylators (Talseth, 1977). The simultaneous ingestion of food and hydralazine can increase the bioavailability of the drug (Melander *et al.,* 1977). The elimination half-time of hydralazine from plasma ranges from 2 to 8 hours (averaging about 3 hours). Less than 15% of an intravenous dose is excreted unchanged in the urine.

During multiple oral dosing, slow acetylators attain higher concentrations of hydralazine in plasma than do those who acetylate the drug rapidly. Patients with renal failure may retain hydralazine, but the precise kinetics of elimination of the drug in healthy and diseased patients is unknown. The large first-pass metabolism of hydralazine suggests that there might be alterations in the bioavailability and decreased clearance of the drug in patients with hepatic cirrhosis. At present there are no data to support or refute this suggestion.

Preparations, Routes of Administration, and Dosage. *Hydralazine Hydrochloride,* U.S.P. (APRESOLINE, others), is available in 10-, 25-, 50-, and 100-mg tablets for oral administration, and in 1-ml ampuls containing 20 mg of the drug for intravenous or intramuscular injection. Parenteral administration is usually started with 20 or 40 mg, but the amount and the frequency of administration required to produce a satisfactory lowering of blood pressure are highly variable. The usual oral dose is 100 to 200 mg per day, starting with 10 or 20 mg two to four times daily; this is increased gradually until the desired effect is obtained or unacceptable side effects develop. The dose should not exceed 400 mg per day for any extended period, since the chance of development of a lupus erythematosus–like syndrome is unacceptably high. The validity of the suggestion that the drug need be given only twice rather than four times a day has been established (O'Malley *et al.,* 1975). Since compliance by the patient is greater as the regimen becomes simpler, such a dosage scheme might be beneficial.

Toxicity and Precautions. The incidence of untoward effects of hydralazine therapy is high. Headache, palpitation, anorexia, nausea, dizziness, and sweating are common. Nasal congestion, flushing, lacrimation, conjunctivitis, paresthesias, edema, tremors, and muscle cramps occur less frequently. Side effects are less frequent and less severe when the dose is increased slowly, and tolerance to them may develop with continued administration. Drug fever, urticaria, skin rash, polyneuritis, gastrointestinal hemorrhage, anemia, and pancytopenia are rare, but require termination of hydralazine therapy. Peripheral neuropathies have been corrected by giving pyridoxine (Raskin and Fishman, 1965). The myocardial stimulation associated with administration of hydralazine can produce anginal attacks and changes in the ECG characteristic of myocardial ischemia. The drug must be used carefully in patients with coronary artery disease. Not surprisingly, many of the unwanted effects are obtunded or prevented by the concurrent administration of a β-adrenergic antagonist; two mechanisms are operative. Propranolol, for example, is a hypotensive agent that is additive to hydralazine. Thus, less hydralazine is required to produce adequate reduction of blood pressure. In addition, β-adrenergic blockade *per se* limits the reflex cardiovascular response to hydralazine.

A drug-induced *lupus-like syndrome* occurs in 10 to 20% of patients who receive prolonged therapy with hydralazine at doses exceeding 400 mg daily. This syndrome can also occur at doses of 200 mg per day or less; while the mechanisms are obscure, it apparently is the result of a complex interplay of genetic, pathophysiological, and possibly other factors (Alarcon-Segovia, 1976). The syndrome occurs almost exclusively in Caucasians who are slow acetylators. Since the lupus syndrome is reversible (Perry, 1973), it seems reasonable to use doses of hydralazine larger than 200 mg per day if required, particularly in blacks and in Caucasians who are fast acetylators. Even in slow acetylators, the larger doses may be used if the patients are carefully followed for symptoms of hydralazine-induced lupus.

Therapeutic Use. Despite the availability of hydralazine since the early 1950s, the drug has become popular for the long-term management of hypertension only in the past few years. It is now clear that previous problems with the apparent lack of efficacy of hydralazine were caused by drug-induced reflex activation of the sympathetic nervous system. When the drug is used alone, the increased sympathetic activity not only opposes its hypotensive effects but also accounts for many of the untoward effects of the drug.

The use of hydralazine has now been optimized by concurrent administration of an inhibitor of the β-adrenergic nervous system; thereby both tachycardia and increased secretion of renin are prevented. When used concurrently with a thiazide and a β-adrenergic blocking drug, hydralazine is effective in small doses for long periods, and it does not often cause the symptoms that previously limited its use. Additional information on the use of hydralazine in essential hypertension is presented later in this chapter.

In a recent limited study of four patients, hydralazine was very effective in the treatment of primary pulmonary hypertension (Rubin and Peter, 1980). In response to a dose of 50 mg, four times daily, the following responses were observed: a fall in pulmonary arteriolar resistance, both at rest and after exercise; an increase in cardiac output, both at rest and after exercise; a decrease in arteriovenous oxygen difference; and a striking decrease in dyspnea. Benefit was maintained during the 6-month observation period of the study, the drug was well tolerated, and no change in dosage was necessary. Although heart rate increased, patients did not experience palpitations. The authors attributed the salutary responses to decreased pulmonary arteriolar resistance, since no change in preload was observed and all patients had unimpaired left ventricular function.

DIAZOXIDE

Diazoxide is closely related chemically to the thiazide diuretics, as can be seen from their structural formulas.

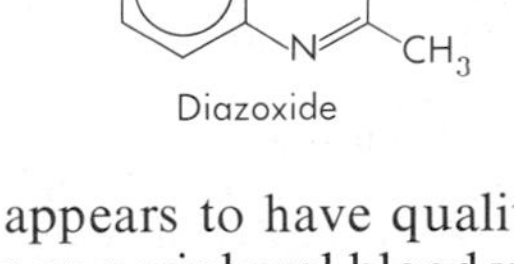

Chlorothiazide

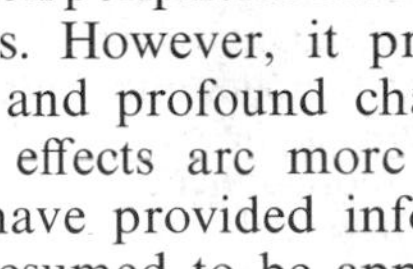

Diazoxide

Diazoxide appears to have qualitatively the same effects on peripheral blood vessels as do the thiazides. However, it produces much more rapid and profound changes. Consequently, its effects are more amenable to study and have provided information that has been presumed to be applicable to the related diuretics. Intravenous administration of diazoxide to a hypertensive subject causes a prompt fall in both systolic and diastolic pressures associated with a considerable increase in cardiac output and some tachycardia. When the drug is used appropriately (*see* below), the pressure rarely falls below the normal range and postural hypotension does not develop. These characteristics indicate that the function of the sympathetic nervous system is not impaired and that the major action is on resistance rather than capacitance vessels. The differential effect on blood vessels has been confirmed by a variety of detailed studies that show that diazoxide directly dilates arterioles but has very little effect on large veins (Gaskell and Diosy, 1959; Thirwell and Zsotér, 1972), although it can affect small postcapillary resistance vessels (Ogilvie and Mikulic, 1972).

The major effects of diazoxide on water and electrolyte balance are opposite to those of the diuretic thiazides. It causes marked *retention of sodium and water* in both normotensive and hypertensive individuals, expands plasma volume, and can produce frank edema in patients with myocardial inadequacy (Thomson *et al.*, 1962). These effects can be readily antagonized by a diuretic thiazide. When diazoxide causes a considerable reduction in blood pressure, glomerular filtration rate and renal plasma flow are also decreased, but retention of sodium can occur without any change in blood pressure or renal hemodynamics (Johnson, 1971). In common with its diuretic congeners, diazoxide inhibits tubular excretion of uric acid and can decrease free-water clearance.

Diazoxide is a relatively weak inhibitor of responses of vascular smooth muscle to a variety of stimulants, including norepinephrine and angiotensin. It appears to be a competitive antagonist of barium, and somewhat indirect evidence indicates that it may similarly antagonize the action of calcium (Wohl *et al.*, 1968). The antagonism of calcium may be complex. In a preparation of mesenteric vein that contracts spontaneously with the generation of calcium-dependent action potentials, diazoxide blocks the generation of potentials and inhibits responses to agonists that act through these potentials; when the muscle is depolarized, it blocks contractions produced by calcium (Rhodes and Sutter, 1971). As in hemodynamic studies, the weaker effects of diuretic thiazides make it more difficult to study their mechanism of action on vascular smooth muscle, but the evidence available to date is not incompatible with the assumption that it is similar to that of diazoxide.

Diazoxide inhibits the spontaneous activity and responses of many smooth muscles in addition to those in blood vessels. It is a powerful relaxant of both the gravid and nongravid human uterus, and this has led to the suggestion that it might be used to treat dysmenorrhea and to arrest premature labor (Landesman *et al.*, 1968).

Disposition and Elimination. In adults, the apparent volume of distribution of diazoxide averages 20% of body weight, and the clearance from plasma is approximately 7 ml per minute. Of this, about one third is renal. In plasma, 90% of the drug is bound to albumin, although the extent of binding decreases as the concentration in plasma rises or as renal failure progresses. Uremic patients are likely to have a greater-than-ordinary fall in blood pressure after diazoxide is given intravenously, and the dosage should thus be reduced (Pearson and Breckenridge, 1976).

Side Effects and Precautions. The major unwanted effects of diazoxide are those on the cardiovascular system. Excessive hypotension and reflex sympathetic stimulation can occur. These may be the effects of the drug that are largely responsible for the reported episodes of myocardial ischemia and infarction (Kanada *et al.*, 1976). When given for short periods, diazoxide has a relatively wide margin of safety. It inhibits release of insulin from the pancreas and raises the concentration of glucose in plasma. As mentioned, it causes retention of sodium. These actions rarely cause clinical problems when the drug is used for a brief time. Rare cases of severe hyperglycemia with or without ketoacidosis have been reported when use of the drug has been prolonged in patients with renal failure. Since the drug is dissolved in an alkaline vehicle, local extravasation can lead to severe pain at the injection site, but tissue necrosis apparently does not occur.

Preparations, Routes of Administration, and Dosage. *Diazoxide*, U.S.P. (HYPERSTAT I.V.), is available for intravenous use in 20-ml ampuls containing 300 mg of the drug. Preparations for oral use (50- and 100-mg capsules and a suspension of 50 mg/ml) are available for the management of hypoglycemia (*see* Chapter 64).

Recent evidence suggests that the drug may not have to be given as rapidly as was previously recommended (300 mg by intravenous bolus), and it may thus be possible to reduce the incidence of adverse effects associated with rapid administration (Gifford, 1977). The dose of diazoxide should be titrated by monitoring the effect on blood pressure. This method is effective in lowering the blood pressure quickly and safely (Ram and Kaplan, 1979).

Therapeutic Use. Diazoxide is occasionally used to treat hypoglycemia due to hyperinsulinemia, but its major use is for *hypertensive emergencies*. Its therapeutic use is discussed below.

MINOXIDIL

Minoxidil is a potent, orally administered vasodilator, recently released in the United States for use in severe hypertension. Its chemical structure is as follows:

Minoxidil

Pharmacological studies in animals and man demonstrate that its hypotensive action results from direct relaxation of arteriolar smooth muscle. The decrease in renal vascular resistance is not associated with reduction in glomerular filtration rate.

After oral administration of radiolabeled minoxidil, 97% can be recovered in the urine, but less than 10% is unchanged drug. The half-life of the drug in plasma is just over 4 hours (Gottlieb *et al.*, 1972a); since the duration of action of the drug is longer than this, the possibility is raised that one or more of its metabolites may be pharmacologically active (Shen *et al.*, 1975). However, the metabolites of minoxidil have not been identified. Dosage requirements seem to be similar in patients with and without renal failure.

Many of the untoward effects of minoxidil are similar to those of hydralazine and diazoxide and relate to reflex activation of the sympathetic nervous system. Fluid retention can be pronounced, particularly in patients with some degree of renal failure (Dormois *et al.*, 1975). A potentially serious adverse reaction to minoxidil is the development of *pericardial effusion*. Although there is a substantial incidence of spontaneous pericardial effusion in the population likely to receive minoxidil (many have renal failure), the high rate of occurrence in patients without uremia who take the drug suggests that the cause may be minoxidil. Patients taking minoxidil should probably be examined by echocardiography until the incidence and severity of this adverse effect are clarified (Marquez-Julio and Uldall, 1977). Hypertrichosis, most noticeable around the face, arms, and back, is a side effect that is particularly unpleasant for females. Since the drug has been marketed only recently and since it has not been widely used, additional unanticipated effects are likely to appear.

Treatment with minoxidil should be limited to patients with moderate-to-severe hypertension who are refractory to conventional therapy (Devine *et al.*, 1977; Hall *et al.*, 1978). It has greater efficacy as an antihypertensive than does hydralazine (Gottlieb *et al.*, 1972b) and may be particularly useful in patients with advanced renal disease that is complicated by hypertension (Pettinger and Mitchell, 1973). The drug should be used in combination with a β-adrenergic blocking agent and a diuretic in order to minimize the dosage requirement (Dargie *et al.*, 1977).

Minoxidil (LONITEN) is supplied in tablets containing either 2.5 or 10 mg. For patients over 12 years of age, the initial daily dose is 5 mg. Dosage is then increased, if necessary, to 10, 20, and then 40 mg in single or divided doses. The effective range is usually 10 to 40 mg per day. Maximal recommended daily dosage is 100 mg.

DIURETIC AGENTS

Chlorothiazide was the first of a now-extensive series of benzothiadiazide (thiazide) drugs that are used as diuretics and for the treatment of hypertension. Although the two actions may have a similar time course and may be dependent on a similar molecular effect in different tissues, they can be separated clinically. The drugs are highly effective after oral administration, and their use has greatly simplified long-term management of various conditions requiring treatment of hypertension and/or the elimination of salt and water. The antihypertensive effects augment responses to other antihypertensive drugs. The thiazides and closely related phthalimidine derivatives (*e.g.*, chlorthalidone) have become a mainstay of antihypertensive therapy. Details of the pharmacology of these agents are presented in Chapter 36. Only their antihypertensive effects and other properties specifically related to their use for the treatment of hypertension will be considered here.

BENZOTHIADIAZIDES

The precise mechanism of action of thiazide diuretics as antihypertensive agents is unknown, although the beneficial effects appear to result from an altered sodium balance. Upon initiation of treatment with a thiazide or phthalimidine alone, cardiac output is decreased and blood volume is diminished. During chronic therapy, the cardiac output returns to normal, peripheral vascular resistance falls, and there is a persistent, small reduction in extracellular water and plasma volume (Leth, 1970; Dustan *et al.,* 1973).

The importance of the drug-induced sodium excretion as a determinant of reduction of blood pressure is suggested by the demonstration that an infusion of dextran will not reverse the antihypertensive effects of a thiazide even after the blood volume is returned to normal, but a large intake of salt or an infusion of saline solution will return the blood pressure to pretreatment levels (Winer, 1961; Tobian, 1967).

Because hemodynamic measurements indicate that peripheral vascular resistance is decreased by thiazides, a direct action of these drugs on arteriolar smooth muscle has been suggested (Peters, 1966; Tobian, 1967). However, studies of anephric animals and man indicate that depletion of sodium by means other than diuretics initially causes a decrease in cardiac output that returns to normal in a few days and that is accompanied by a decrease in peripheral resistance. In contrast, diuretics do not produce any hemodynamic effects in anephric animals (Coleman *et al.,* 1970; Freis, 1976). Therefore, the decreased peripheral vascular resistance induced by a thiazide seems to be the result of sodium depletion, and such depletion may have secondary effects on the vasculature. The mechanism of action of thiazides may thus be different from that of diazoxide, which produces salt and water retention while substantially reducing peripheral resistance (*see* above). Nevertheless, diazoxide might differ from the thiazides only in its ability to modify the sodium content of arterioles directly. Clinically, one can produce about the same degree of antihypertensive effect using agents that differ in their diuretic potency. With the less potent agents, the change in plasma volume and salt may be minimal. A minimum of change would be clinically advantageous, since some of the side effects of the thiazides are related to the degree of depletion of sodium and potassium. Such depletion also compounds the difficulty of administration of cardioactive agents that are often required in the management of hypertensive patients.

Side effects of the diuretic thiazides are discussed in detail in Chapter 36. Those that most frequently complicate their use in the treatment of hypertension are *hypokalemia, hyperglycemia,* and *hyperuricemia.* The last-named effect may cause particular concern because many hypertensive patients have somewhat elevated concentrations of uric acid in blood. Some hypokalemia occurs in almost all patients on chronic treatment with a thiazide diuretic, but it is rarely of clinical significance in patients on an adequate diet. Routine potassium supplements are not indicated and may represent a greater hazard than the hypokalemia. In fact, if a patient develops hypokalemia while taking a thiazide for hypertension, the clinician should consider decreasing the dosage of thiazide rather than adding a potassium supplement. Special care is necessary to ensure adequate dietary intake of potassium by patients receiving a thiazide and digitalis concurrently.

OTHER DIURETICS

Many drugs that are used clinically to promote diuresis, including spironolactone, furosemide, and ethacrynic acid, have antihypertensive properties. However, sufficient reduction of plasma and extracellular volumes by any mechanism will reduce the blood pressure, and in most cases the available data do not allow differentiation between effects of the drugs on fluid volume *per se* and their action on arteriolar vascular resistance.

Spironolactone has been extensively studied. The antihypertensive effects of spironolactone are qualitatively and quantitatively very similar to those of a thiazide. Both drugs increase the activity of renin in plasma and are most effective in patients with low plasma renin activity. When administered chronically in appropriate doses, spironolactone and a thiazide produce similar small reductions in plasma volume and sodium concentration (Acchiardo *et al.,* 1972). It has been reported that the antihypertensive effect of spironolactone, but not that of hydrochlorothiazide, is correlated with weight loss (Adlin *et al.,* 1972). Unfortunately, there appear to be no hemodynamic measurements to indicate whether there is an early or late reduction in peripheral resistance during the administration of spironolactone. Some reports suggested that the antihypertensive effects of spironolactone and a thiazide are additive, but with adequate doses of each this does not appear to be the case (Ogilvie and Ruedy, 1969). At the present time the choice between a thiazide and spironolactone in the treatment of hypertension appears to be predominantly on the basis of anticipated side effects in the individual patient. Both drugs produce some gastrointestinal irritation and hypersensitivity reactions, and both can increase the blood urea nitrogen in patients with renal insufficiency. Spironolactone does not cause hypokalemia, hyperglycemia, or hyperuricemia, but amenorrhea, gynecomastia, and hyperkalemia can occur; the last-named effect is particularly hazardous in patients with impaired renal function.

The common occurrence of urate retention, hyperuricemia, and, in the rare patient, attacks of gout while receiving benzothiadiazides for hypertension has stimulated a search for diuretics that are simultaneously uricosuric. One such agent, *ticrynafen*, was for a brief time marketed in the United States. While it is effective as both an antihypertensive and a uricosuric agent, an unacceptable incidence of hepatotoxicity led to its withdrawal from the market.

Furosemide is a powerful diuretic that is used extensively and often inappropriately in the treatment of hypertension. The antihypertensive effect of furosemide is apparently solely related to its effect on blood volume and is less than that of the thiazides (Healy *et al.*, 1970; Anderson *et al.*, 1971). It thus reduces blood pressure substantially but does not lower peripheral resistance. In fact, if sufficient furosemide is given to lower blood pressure rapidly, a resultant reflex increase in peripheral vascular resistance may result. Since furosemide can cause *hypokalemia, hyperglycemia,* and *hyperuricemia* and has a considerably greater potential for producing *serious electrolyte disturbances,* there appears to be no rational role for furosemide in the treatment of the great majority of cases of essential hypertension. It may be useful in special cases, such as those in which renal function is so inadequate that a thiazide or spironolactone cannot prevent accumulation of sodium.

Therapeutic Uses. The current role of diuretics in the therapy of essential hypertension and their interactions with other drugs used to lower blood pressure are discussed at the end of this chapter. Other uses of diuretics are covered in Chapter 36.

NITROPRUSSIDE

Sodium nitroprusside (sodium nitroferricyanide) is a powerful, directly acting vasodilator that has been used sporadically as a hypotensive agent in man for over 5 decades but has not been marketed as a drug until recently (*see* Johnson, 1929). An important difference between this vasodilator and those discussed above is that nitroprusside relaxes both arteriolar and venous smooth muscle; furthermore, it has little effect on the gastrointestinal tract or uterus. Venodilatation results in a decreased cardiac preload. In the supine patient, the cardiac response depends on the state of myocardial function. In the absence of heart failure, the cardiac output either falls or does not change (Schlant *et al.*, 1962; Bhatia and Frohlich, 1973). However, if cardiac output is decreased because of myocardial disease, nitroprusside usually increases output (*see* Chapter 33). The drug lowers blood pressure in patients who are either in the supine or upright positions. However, because nitroprusside causes venous dilatation, more venous pooling occurs when the patient is upright. The heart rate of such patients often increases unless heart failure or tachycardia are already present; under these circumstances the heart rate may fall as the drug is given (Guiha *et al.*, 1974; Miller *et al.*, 1975). Renal blood flow and the glomerular filtration rate are maintained, and secretion of renin is increased during the use of nitroprusside. Angina often improves when this agent is given. This effect is in marked contrast to that of arteriolar vasodilators that do not affect veins; as noted earlier, diazoxide, hydralazine, and minoxidil may cause myocardial ischemia, since preload is maintained and there is reflex activation of the sympathetic nervous system.

The onset of action of nitroprusside is seen shortly after an infusion is started; when the infusion is stopped, the effects are rapidly dissipated as the drug is inactivated. The half-life of the drug is only a few minutes. The patient's arterial pressure can easily be titrated to almost any level by altering the rate of infusion. Tolerance or unresponsiveness to the drug is rare (Tuzel, 1974).

Toxicity, Precautions, and Contraindications. The acute toxicity of nitroprusside is entirely secondary to excessive vasodilatation and hypotension. Symptoms include nausea, vomiting, sweating, restlessness, headache, palpitation, and substernal distress; they disappear promptly when the infusion is stopped or the rate reduced. Patients receiving antihypertensive drug therapy are more sensitive to the anion. Elderly persons should be given lower-than-usual doses. Nitroprusside treatment is a hospital procedure and requires meticulous attention to details of administration (*see* below). The safety of the drug in children and pregnant women has not yet been established. A case of methemoglobinemia developing during prolonged infusion has been reported (Bower and Peterson, 1975).

Cyanide is an intermediate in the metabolism of nitroprusside, and the final metabolic product is thiocyanate. Although significantly elevated concentrations of cyanide in blood can be observed during prolonged therapy, cyanide toxicity is extremely uncommon (Vesey *et al.*, 1976). Thiocyanate is cleared slowly by the kidney; its half-life is normally 4 days and is prolonged in patients with renal failure. Thus, thiocyanate accumulates during prolonged therapy. If the concentration of thiocyanate exceeds 10 mg/dl, weakness, hypoxia, nausea, tinnitus, muscle spasms, disorientation, and psychosis are likely to occur. These problems should signal the need for alternative therapy. If the drug is continued for long periods, hypothyroidism can result, since thiocyanate interferes with transport of iodine by the thyroid gland (Nourok *et al.*, 1964).

Preparations, Route of Administration, and Dosage. *Sodium Nitroprusside*, U.S.P. (NIPRIDE), is a reddish-brown, water-soluble powder, marketed in 5-ml amber-colored, rubber-stoppered vials, each containing 50 mg of the drug. Only fresh solutions should be used, and those more than 4 hours old should be discarded. The solution is made by first adding 2 or 3 ml of 5% dextrose solution in water to the vial and then transferring the contents to an infusion bottle containing 500 ml of the same diluent. Because the compound decomposes in light, the bottle should be covered with an opaque wrapping. Nitroprusside solution must be administered only by intravenous infusion; an infusion pump or a microdrip regulator should be used to ensure a precise flow rate. Other drugs should not be added to the solution. Care should be taken to prevent extravasation. The average adult dose is 3 µg/kg per minute (about 200 µg per minute) for patients not receiving other antihypertensive drugs, but the range of dosage is broad. The maximal dose should not exceed 800 µg per minute. *Continuous monitoring of the patient's blood pressure and the flow rate are absolutely essential.* With careful supervision, the diastolic blood pressure can be maintained at almost any desired level. Some tolerance to the hypotensive

effect of nitroprusside is occasionally observed, but absolute resistance does not occur.

Therapeutic Uses. Nitroprusside is used when short-term, rapid reduction in blood pressure is required. There is no report of any condition in which the blood pressure cannot be lowered by this drug. Its use in *hypertensive emergencies* is mentioned at the end of this chapter, and the drug is also used where hypotension is required to minimize bleeding during surgery (*see* Mani, 1971). In addition, nitroprusside can improve left ventricular function following *acute myocardial infarction,* and vasodilators including nitroprusside are emerging as important adjuncts in the treatment of *acute congestive heart failure* (*see* Chapter 33).

PRAZOSIN

Prazosin is classified as both an arterial dilator and a venodilator. It has the following structural formula:

Prazosin

Although its mechanism of action is incompletely understood, it appears to act predominantly as an α-adrenergic blocking agent on vascular smooth muscle.

Several mechanisms have been proposed to explain the hypotensive actions of prazosin. The major current hypothesis is that the drug is a selective blocking agent at postsynaptic α_1-adrenergic receptors; it is thought to have relatively low affinity for presynaptic α_2 receptors. Prazosin thus inhibits the vasoconstriction produced by norepinephrine that is released from the sympathetic nerve endings, while its relative lack of effect on α_2 receptors allows norepinephrine to exert negative feedback control of its own release, thus reducing the cardiac stimulation that follows nonselective α-adrenergic blockade (*see* Chapter 9). However, this hypothesis is not entirely consistent with all of the cardiovascular effects of prazosin, and further investigations may reveal additional mechanisms and effects. Prazosin reduces peripheral vascular resistance without secondary reflex tachycardia or increase in renin activity in the plasma, as occur when hydralazine, diazoxide, or minoxidil is used. Although their mechanisms of action may be different, the hemodynamic effects of prazosin are similar to those of nitroprusside: each decreases arterial pressure and reduces arterial resistance and venous tone. During chronic administration of prazosin to hypertensive patients, the cardiac index is increased, peripheral vascular resistance is reduced, and the heart rate is modestly increased (Lund-Johansen, 1975). As would be predicted from its action on venous capacitance, prazosin has a greater effect when the patient is upright rather than in the supine position (Bolli et al., 1976). Fluid retention occurs during chronic therapy (Koshy et al., 1977). This could in part explain the finding that the initial hypotensive effect often dissipates by the fourth day of treatment when prazosin is given alone (Graham et al., 1976).

Information about the *disposition* of prazosin is limited. More than 99% of the drug is metabolized, and there may be substantial first-pass metabolism. Bioavailability averages 57%. In normal man, the half-life of the drug is about 3 hours (Bateman et al., 1979); this value is probably not altered in renal failure. However, when prazosin is given orally to patients with congestive heart failure, concentrations in the blood are higher and the half-life is prolonged. Smaller-than-usual doses are required for such patients.

The *side effects* of prazosin are usually well tolerated. They include drowsiness, dizziness, palpitations, headache, and easy fatigability. Sexual dysfunction is uncommon. A recent report suggests that one third of patients taking prazosin may develop a positive test for antinuclear factor (Marshall et al., 1979). Potentially the most troublesome effect is postural hypotension and syncope that often occur with the first dose. The likelihood of syncope is related to the size of the dose, and it occurs more readily in patients who are already salt depleted. This so-called first-dose phenomenon is probably due to inadequate venous return to the right side of the heart and is preceded by a precipitous fall in heart rate. Release of catecholamines is normal at the time of syncope. To minimize the possibility of the first-dose phenomenon, treatment with the drug should be instituted slowly, at a dose of 1 mg three times daily. The first dose should be no larger than 1 mg and preferably should be given at bedtime.

Preparations. *Prazosin hydrochloride* (MINIPRESS) is available in capsules containing 1, 2, or 5 mg.

Therapeutic Use. The efficacy of prazosin for the treatment of mild-to-moderate hypertension is well documented. Whether it is more efficacious or better tolerated than other useful vasodilators is not known. There is a dearth of controlled comparative trials with this agent. As is true with any recently marketed drug, the full spectrum of its activity and toxicity is not yet known.

Some data indicate that prazosin is often more effective when combined with a diuretic and/or a β-adrenergic blocking agent than when used alone. Up to 20 mg per day may eventually be required for maximal efficacy, although drug combinations should be tried before approaching the maximal recommended dosage. Prazosin is also currently under investigation to reduce afterload in patients with *severe chronic congestive heart failure*. Its efficacy in this condition has not been established.

OTHER AGENTS USED TO TREAT HYPERTENSION

Drugs that interfere with the renin-angiotensin-aldosterone system are currently under investigation for utility in the treatment of hypertension, especially in patients whose renin activity in plasma is high. Agents in this category have already proven useful in enhancing our understanding of the role of the renin-angiotensin system in the regulation of blood pressure (*see* Chapter 27). *Saralasin,* a structural analog of angiotensin II, has been extensively used as an investigative tool. Although it may be an effective antihypertensive drug in some patients, its partial agonistic activity and the necessity to give it intravenously limit its clinical utility. A second group of agents acts by inhibition of peptidyl dipeptidase, the enzyme that converts angiotensin I to angiotensin II (so-called converting enzyme inhibitors). One such compound that can be taken orally is *captopril* (Chapter 27). The drug is currently undergoing extensive trials in man (Haber, 1978; Brunner et al., 1979). The role of inhibitors of peptidyl dipeptidase or other antagonists of the renin-angiotensin system in the treatment of hypertension is not yet clear (Haber, 1978).

Although monoamine oxidase (MAO) inhibitors have been used to treat hypertension, there is currently no reason to employ them for this purpose, since safer and more effective drugs are available (*see* Chapter 9). MAO inhibitors do have a place in the management of depression (*see* Chapter 19). Since the two diseases are prevalent and often occur in the same patient, MAO inhibitors may be given to a patient for depression and greatly complicate the adjustment of the antihypertensive regimen. MAO inhibitors interact with foods that contain tyramine and with many drugs, particularly those that release catecholamines; the resultant hypertension can sometimes be severe. When an otherwise consistently effective antihypertensive regimen suddenly loses its efficacy, the physician should rule out the possibility that the patient is receiving an MAO inhibitor. A more complete discussion of MAO inhibitors can be found in Chapters 9 and 19 and in the *fifth edition* of this textbook. The reader is similarly referred to *earlier editions* of this textbook for discussion of the *veratrum alkaloids*, an interesting class of hypotensive drugs that are no longer used clinically (*see also* Benforado, 1967).

II. Drug Therapy of Hypertension

A relatively small proportion of patients develop hypertension as a manifestation of an identifiable and specifically treatable underlying cause. Pheochromocytoma, renal arterial stenosis, and endocrine diseases that cause hypertension are rare. Although these forms of hypertension are potentially curable by surgical measures, the vast majority of patients will respond to medical therapy that is not necessarily directed at reversal of the (still-unknown) mechanisms responsible for the increase in blood pressure (Nies, 1977). At least 80% of patients with sustained high blood pressure have no discernible underlying causative factor. These patients are said to have "essential" hypertension, a term introduced by Ludwig Traube in 1856, who believed that the elevation in blood pressure in these individuals was essential to maintain adequate perfusion of their vital organs.

The etiology of essential hypertension is almost certainly multifactorial. Although the sympathetic nervous system may contribute to the high blood pressure caused by dysfunction of other systems, there is no definitive evidence that it plays a primary etiological role in the pathogenesis of essential hypertension. The quantitation of sympathetic nervous activity has been attempted by a variety of methods. Measurement of the concentrations of catecholamines in the plasma of patients with essential hypertension has shown that their mean value is probably higher than that of normotensives (Louis *et al.*, 1973). Nevertheless, the ranges of concentrations in the normotensive and hypertensive groups overlap extensively. The pathophysiological meaning and mechanisms of these elevations are uncertain, but it is interesting that sympathetic blockade produces a greater fall in the arterial pressure of hypertensive patients than it does in normal individuals.

Baroreceptor function is abnormal in individuals with sustained hypertension, but the abnormality probably is a result rather than a cause of the sustained increase in blood pressure (Bristow *et al.*,

1969; Gribbin *et al.*, 1971). Denervation of the baroreceptors in animals or man results in lability of the blood pressure and evidence of imbalance in the autonomic nervous system with excessive sympathetic activity.

Patients with recent onset of labile hypertension also may have decreased parasympathetic activity and relative overactivity of the sympathetic nervous system. These patients, in addition, have detectable abnormalities in baroreceptor function that are not readily explained by sustained hypertension (Julius *et al.*, 1971; Takeshita *et al.*, 1975; Ripley *et al.*, 1977).

Intriguing as these data are, they do not provide sufficient evidence to establish or refute a definite etiological role for the sympathetic or parasympathetic nervous system in essential hypertension. It follows that any proposed relationship of abnormalities of the autonomic nervous system to the abnormalities in renin secretion or hemodynamic function found in patients with essential hypertension is unproven.

The renin-angiotensin-aldosterone system is one of the major physiological regulators of blood pressure and fluid balance. This system is described in Chapter 27. In the past several years the relationship of this system to various types of hypertension has been defined, and an important new group of agents that antagonize some aspect of the renin-angiotensin system has been developed (Chapter 27). While it is too soon to appraise fully the therapeutic worth of these new agents, it is already certain that they are of enormous investigative value and constitute an important advance in our potential to treat high blood pressure with pharmacological agents.

Approach to the Patient with Hypertension. Who should be treated? Hypertension is a sign of one of many underlying processes that can be expressed as abnormal blood pressure. The levels of systolic and diastolic blood pressure, both within and above the "normal" range, correlate with the incidence of death from cardiovascular disease. Furthermore, the effect of elevated blood pressure adds to the negative prognosis of other "cardiovascular risk factors," such as hypercholesterolemia, diabetes, cigarette smoking, and obesity (Kannel, 1977). As a result of well-controlled clinical trials, there is firm evidence that reducing diastolic blood pressure that is greater than 90 mm Hg in middle-age patients is associated with a decrease in cardiovascular morbidity and mortality, including intracerebral hemorrhage, thrombotic cerebrovascular disease, malignant hypertension, dissecting aneurysm, and congestive heart failure (*see* Veterans Administration Cooperative Study Group on Antihypertensive Agents, 1967, 1970, 1972). Even partial return of the blood pressure toward normal is associated with decreased morbidity (Taguchi and Freis, 1974; Hypertension Detection and Follow-Up Program Cooperative Group, 1979a, 1979b). To date, there is no evidence that treatment of hypertension reduces the risk of coronary artery disease. The evidence to prove or disprove this will have to be obtained by studying younger patients than those who have been utilized to date. The value of treating patients with "borderline" hypertension has been established recently (Hypertension Detection and

Follow-Up Program Cooperative Group, 1979a, 1979b; Relman, 1980).

Both the diagnosis itself (Haynes *et al.*, 1978) and the drug therapy of hypertension are associated with adverse effects. A very large scale investigation (18,000 subjects) of the efficacy of treatment of mild hypertension has been initiated by the Medical Research Council in Great Britain. The results probably will not be available until the mid-1980s but may provide new information on how to select patients for treatment (*see* Medical Research Council Working Party on Mild to Moderate Hypertension, 1977). In the meantime, the physician can rationally suggest treatment for most patients whose diastolic blood pressures are consistently above 90 mm Hg. *When treatment is suggested, a long-term agreement for care should be made between the patient and his physician.* If the treatment is successful, it will last over many years, a span that may reveal as-yet-unanticipated efficacy and toxicity of the drugs in current use.

The initial step in approaching a patient with potential hypertensive disease is to establish the presence and severity of the abnormality of blood pressure. In patients with severe hypertension, this task is not difficult. Not only is the blood pressure markedly elevated, but there are often signs of damage of target organs (*e.g.*, kidney, retina, or heart). However, when patients are encountered whose blood pressures are above the arbitrary level of 140/90 mm Hg but who have no vascular complications, some attempt must be made to establish how consistently the blood pressure is elevated. This often cannot be accomplished with accuracy by making multiple casual determinations of blood pressure while the patient is in the clinic or office or, for that matter, even during hospitalization. Blood pressures taken by the patient or his family for several days are usually accurate and reliable. They serve as a good index of the severity of hypertension and correlate better with the occurrences of complications of hypertension than do values obtained casually (Kain *et al.*, 1964; Sokolow and Perloff, 1966). However, blood pressures measured in the outpatient clinic were used to determine the efficacy of antihypertensive therapy in the Veterans Administration cooperative studies. Blood pressures measured during hospitalization are often significantly lower than the average ambulatory blood pressure. Such low blood pressures in an otherwise consistently hypertensive patient cannot be used to exclude the diagnosis of hypertension or to excuse the physician from offering therapy to his patient (Moutsos *et al.*, 1967). Patients who after repeated visits to the doctor have only intermittent elevation of blood pressure are not usually considered candidates for therapy. However, this does not relieve the physician of the responsibility of following such patients with labile hypertension, since, in time, a sizable proportion of them will develop fixed and treatable hypertension. There are no studies to indicate whether therapy of labile hypertensives will prevent fixed hypertension and its complications.

Many clinical studies have demonstrated that in almost all cases of hypertensive cardiovascular disease the blood pressure can be successfully controlled by skillful use of the drugs currently available. However, it has also been estimated that only a small percentage of all hypertensive patients under treatment are even close to optimal control. This disparity emphasizes the fact that *effective use of antihypertensive drugs is not "routine."* Therapy must be tailored to the needs of the individual patient and adjusted as necessary to maintain an optimal balance between therapeutic and side effects; the importance of this principle increases directly with the severity of the disease.

In all but the mildly hypertensive patient who might respond to a diuretic or to a β-adrenergic blocking agent, combinations of drugs are used. The goal of combination drug therapy is to lower the blood pressure toward normal by using less of any given agent in a combination than would be necessary to lower the blood pressure to the same extent with a single drug. A successful combination is one whose components give additive or synergistic therapeutic effects, while causing minimal toxicity because relatively small doses of any single drug are used. Ideally, antihypertensive therapy should lower blood pressure effectively without producing side effects that become so unacceptable to the patient that compliance to the regimen is threatened or that compromise the vital functions of the brain, heart, or kidneys. The physician who knows both the pharmacology of antihypertensive drugs and the physiological determinants of blood pressure can often predict the regimen likely to have optimal benefit and minimal toxicity in a given patient.

A very difficult and important problem in the treatment of hypertension is to determine what constitutes "acceptable" side effects, particularly in the long-term management of relatively mild, asymptomatic cases. All the effective antihypertensive drugs can produce quite significant adverse effects, and the reports of several studies have included a comment that, although side effects did not interfere with the management of most cases, the patients very frequently "felt better" while taking a placebo. *The physician treating patients with asymptomatic hypertension should remember the difference between prolonging life and making life seem longer.*

The drug treatment of hypertension can be obviated in some patients and aided in all by weight control and avoidance of excessive salt (*see* Coleman *et al.*, 1972). In addition, mild elevations of blood pressure can be controlled at least for short periods by physical training (Boyer and Kasch, 1970; Choquette and Ferguson, 1973). Oral contraceptive drugs can increase blood pressure, and the use of other contraceptive measures may be desirable in susceptible patients. Since the aim of treatment is primarily to prevent the cardiovascular complications of hypertension, other contributing factors, including obesity, hyperlipidemia, and smoking, should not be neglected.

THERAPEUTIC REGIMENS

Mild Hypertension. Initial drug therapy for most patients with mild hypertension should be with either a thiazide or a β-adrenergic blocking agent. Although there is evidence that the renin status of the patient correlates with the probability of satisfactory response (Dunn and Tannen, 1974), renin profiling is generally unnecessary. The choice between a thiazide and a β-adrenergic blocking agent usually rests on the clinical characteristics of the individual patient. Thus, the insulin-dependent diabetic probably should receive a thiazide first, since a drug of this type will not prolong the duration or attenuate the patient's awareness of hypoglycemia (Lager *et al.*, 1979). Similarly, the patient with asthma, chronic obstructive pulmonary disease, or congestive heart failure initially should receive a thiazide rather than propranolol. The latter could intensify the underlying disease regardless of its efficacy for hypertension. Metoprolol, a cardioselective β-adrenergic blocking agent, may eventually be found to be useful for such patients. Although preliminary evidence indicates that thiazide-induced increases in the concentrations of glucose and uric acid in plasma may not aggravate the condition of the patient with maturity-onset diabetes or with symptomatic gout, therapy with a β-adrenergic blocking agent may be more rationally and readily managed than a thiazide. The young hypertensive patient will often respond dramatically to small doses of propranolol (Buhler *et al.*, 1975). However, for many patients, either a thiazide or propranolol is appropriate and adequate when given alone.

Thiazides and Phthalimidines. Therapy may begin with oral administration of a thiazide or phthalimidine and avoidance of excessive sodium intake. Since all of the thiazides and related phthalimidines have very similar pharmacological actions (*see* Chapter 36), the choice of agent should be based on factors such as cost and convenience. The maximal antihypertensive action of a thiazide does not necessarily require doses that produce diuresis. Small doses of thiazide (*e.g.*, 25 mg of hydrochlorothiazide) will produce little change in plasma electrolytes but have about as much antihypertensive action as do much larger doses (Berglund and Andersson, 1976). Similarly, chlorthalidone in a single daily dose of 25 mg is at least as effective for the treatment of mild hypertension as are doses three times as large (Materson *et al.*, 1978). The higher doses of diuretic almost always result in noticeable diuresis, major loss of potassium in the urine, and symptoms that could eventually lead to poor compliance. Small doses are often sufficient to manage the patient with mild hypertension either when given alone or in combination with other drugs.

There is no reason to use the high-ceiling diuretics (ethacrynic acid and furosemide) to manage mild hypertension in a patient who has normal renal function. These drugs produce a high incidence of electrolyte disturbances that can complicate the use of cardioactive drugs often required by such patients. They should be reserved for patients who have reduced glomerular filtration rates or those in whom sodium retention is not reversed by less potent diuretics.

Spironolactone may occasionally be effective as the sole therapy for patients with low-renin hypertension. In patients with normal-renin hypertension in whom dose-response relationships were studied, 100 mg of spironolactone produced a significant fall in blood pressure and did not cause adverse effects. Larger doses of spironolactone (400 mg per day) were associated with frequent adverse effects and somewhat better control of blood pressure (Ogilvie *et al.*, 1978). These latter observations suggest that it might be preferable to combine spironolactone with other antihypertensive agents.

β-Adrenergic Blocking Agents. A β-adrenergic blocking agent can be tried as an alternative to a thiazide in the management of mild hypertension with a single agent. Although the proportion of patients who respond to propranolol is directly correlated with their plasma renin activity, the activity *per se* does not reliably predict the usefulness of the β-adrenergic blocker (Dunn and Tannen, 1974). Since propranolol appears to have multiple mechanisms of antihypertensive action (Dean *et al.*, 1980), its efficacy when given alone may not be predictable by its action on any single determinant of blood pressure.

Both cardioselective (β_1) and noncardioselective β-adrenergic blocking agents have antihypertensive activity (*see* Chapter 9). The selection of one agent in preference to another is thus based on other considerations. For example, use of a β_1-adrenergic blocking agent such as metoprolol should be advantageous when patients are susceptible to bronchospasm.

The doses of β-adrenergic blocking agents required for hypertensive patients are similar to those used to treat angina pectoris (*e.g.*, 80 to 240 mg per day for propranolol and 50 to 400 mg per day for metoprolol). The lowest effective dose should be sought. Because the acute hemodynamic effects of these drugs differ from those seen during chronic administration, adjustments of dosage should be made only after the patient has been given the same dose for several days. It may be possible to administer propranolol or metoprolol once a day and still maintain adequate reduction of blood pressure; the half-life of nadolol is considerably longer. Relative or absolute contraindications to the use of β-adrenergic antagonists for hypertension include the presence of cardiac failure, asthma, obstructive airway disease, heart block, and diabetes.

Combination Therapy. If the sole use of a thiazide or a β-adrenergic blocker is insufficiently effective at doses that begin to produce side effects, a combination of drugs should be employed. Most patients with mild hypertension can be managed by a combination of two drugs. Unless they are contraindicated for specific reasons, a thiazide or related drug should be part of every antihypertensive drug combination, since most of the other hypotensive agents cause retention of salt and water, which limits their effectiveness. The choice of the second drug is somewhat arbitrary. All hypotensive agents have side effects that are more or less tolerated by different patients. A logical first combination is that of a β-adrenergic blocking agent and a thiazide (Drayer *et al.*, 1975; Geyskes *et al.*, 1975). A major advantage of this combination is that orthostatic hypotension is uncommon. Another useful combination is that of a thiazide plus an adrenergic neuron blocking agent such as *methyldopa, clonidine, guanethidine,* or, possibly, *reserpine.*

If methyldopa is chosen, it is usually used at a dose of 250 mg twice daily. The dose can be increased as necessary at intervals of not less than 2 days. Maximal antihypertensive effects are usually seen when the dose reaches 2 g per day. When such a high dose is contemplated, another agent should ordinarily be tried instead. Whenever any drug that modulates sympathetic activity is given, such effects should be assessed independently of its hypotensive action. Only after such assessment can it be decided whether to increase the dose or to switch to another class of drugs. If high doses of an agent that interferes with sympathetic effects neither reduce blood pressure nor interfere with sympathetic reflexes, more of the same drug or a different member of the same group should be tried. If the drug interferes with baroreceptor reflexes but does not lower blood pressure, even a much larger dose is not likely to be helpful. Another drug that works by a different mechanism must be considered (*see* section below on "Refractory" Hypertension). The side effects of methyldopa, discussed above, are numerous. Some patients develop tolerance to the hypotensive effects of the drug even after they have had an initial satisfactory response.

Although the site of action of clonidine appears to be similar to that of methyldopa, each has a characteristic spectrum of side effects. Thus, while clonidine is less likely than methyldopa to produce orthostatic hypotension and impotence, it is more likely to produce sedation and dry mouth. Other limitations to the use of clonidine are discussed above. Clonidine therapy should be initiated at a dose of 0.1 mg, taken twice daily. The usual dose that eventually will be required is between 0.2 and 0.8 mg daily. Doses above this range are generally associated with an increasing incidence of side effects for a given decrement in blood pressure.

The combination of a thiazide and reserpine (0.1 mg twice daily) was proven highly effective in the Veterans Administration cooperative studies (1967, 1970). The relatively high incidence of side effects caused by reserpine include severe depression,

and there is current concern about its possible association with an increased incidence of carcinoma of the breast. These factors have reduced its use as an antihypertensive agent. However, in the most recent Veterans Administration multiclinic cooperative study, the combination of a thiazide and a *low dose* of reserpine was *not* associated with a higher incidence of adverse reactions than was observed when propranolol was used alone or in combination with a thiazide or a more effective arteriolar vasodilator (*see* Veterans Administration Cooperative Study on Antihypertensive Agents, 1977). Reserpine usually costs less than propranolol and should be considered for patients who do not have contraindications to its use (*e.g.,* mental depression or peptic ulcer) (McMahon, 1978).

Moderate-to-Severe Hypertension. Treatment for the patient with moderate-to-severe hypertension (*e.g.,* diastolic pressures consistently greater than 105 mm Hg) is often identical to that for the patient with mild hypertension. However, administration of a single agent often cannot be attempted because the disease may be rapidly progressive. It is also important to remember that even partial reduction of blood pressure toward normal is still associated with decreased morbidity. Since retention of sodium and water is a prominent feature in most patients with moderate-to-severe hypertension, thiazides should be part of a therapeutic regimen unless there is evidence of depletion of intravascular volume.

Most arterial vasodilators are reserved for the treatment of moderate-to-severe hypertension. Administration of a vasodilator (*e.g.,* hydralazine or minoxidil) is uniformly and predictably associated with reflex tachycardia and somewhat less predictably with a rise in the secretion of renin. Both effects are mediated primarily by the sympathetic nervous system and may partially or completely abolish the hypotensive effect of the vasodilator. Despite a significant reduction of peripheral resistance produced by a vasodilator such as hydralazine, there is virtually no fall in blood pressure until the reflex increase in heart rate (and cardiac output) and enhanced secretion of renin are blocked by propranolol. Arterial vasodilators should thus be combined with drugs that inhibit the sympathetic nervous system. In addition, a diuretic may be required to avoid fluid retention.

Prazosin has different (additional) mechanisms of action than do hydralazine and minoxidil. It may produce less reflex tachycardia and less of an increase in the activity of renin in plasma (Graham and Pettinger, 1979). Nevertheless, there is ample clinical evidence that prazosin is most useful when combined with a diuretic and an inhibitor of sympathetic activity. As with other vasodilators, this combination allows the use of smaller doses of each drug and thereby minimizes their side effects (Brogden *et al.,* 1977).

Agents able to produce profound inhibition of the sympathetic nervous system are often required to achieve adequate control of blood pressure. Because many of these patients have both high activity of renin in their plasma and high peripheral vascular resistance, combinations of vasodilators and agents that inhibit release of renin (propranolol, methyl-dopa, or clonidine) may be useful. Patients who have renal insufficiency may need a high-ceiling diuretic to promote excretion of sodium salts. Administration of such a diuretic may not be simple. If intravascular volume is depleted too rapidly, renal function may worsen and venous return to the heart may be impaired. If the drug is given without adequate inhibition of the sympathetic nervous system, rapid depletion of intravascular volume and arteriolar dilatation may result in profound reflex vasoconstriction, even to the point of *raising* the blood pressure.

Patients with moderate-to-severe hypertension should have their blood pressure reduced over a period of a few days, and this usually can be accomplished with oral therapy. Except in true hypertensive emergencies (*see* below), the rapid reduction of blood pressure (over minutes to a few hours) is unnecessary. Patients who have renal insufficiency before treatment may have a transient further decrease in their renal function as therapy is initiated. However, the long-term effect of a reduction in blood pressure is unequivocally to preserve renal function (Mroczek *et al.*, 1969; Woods *et al.*, 1974).

Hypertensive Emergencies. A hypertensive emergency may be defined as a clinical syndrome that results from or is complicated by very high, sustained levels of blood pressure. It necessitates aggressive treatment. These syndromes may be categorized and, fortunately, are infrequent (*see* Table 32–2). The starting level of systolic or diastolic pressure *per se* should *not* be used to determine how fast the blood pressure should be lowered. Rather, evidence of a recent and rapid increase in blood pressure or deterioration of the vasculature of the eye or function of the kidneys or brain are the signals for rapid inter-

Table 32–2. HYPERTENSIVE EMERGENCIES

SYNDROME	DRUGS OFTEN USED FOR MANAGEMENT *
Malignant hypertension (no previous therapy)	N, D
Hypertensive encephalopathy	N, D
Hypertension associated with:	
acute left ventricular failure	N
intracranial hemorrhage	N
aortic dissection or leaking aneurysm	N + P
coronary insufficiency	N + P
Eclampsia	D, N
Severe hypertension associated with excess catecholamines (pheochromocytoma or MAO inhibitor interactions)	PH, N
Withdrawal of clonidine, propranolol, and sometimes other antihypertensive agents	P + PH, N †

* N = nitroprusside;   D = diazoxide;   P = propranolol; PH = phentolamine.

† Alternatively, the drug that has been withdrawn can be readministered.

vention. Parenteral therapy usually is indicated, and several useful agents are available. Certain drugs may have advantages in specific situations. They are indicated in Table 32–2. Sodium nitroprusside and diazoxide have become the mainstays of therapy for most hypertensive emergencies. The actions of both begin soon after administration. Neither interferes with the clinical evaluation of CNS function nor precludes the administration of antihypertensive agents that take some time to act. Diazoxide may be more easily administered than nitroprusside, because, when properly titrated, blood pressure rarely falls to dangerously low levels. The use of smaller-bolus doses (100 to 150 mg) than has been traditionally suggested (300-mg bolus) and separation of successive doses by intervals of 10 to 15 minutes usually produce a controlled fall in blood pressure. When the drug is given as a 300-mg bolus, overshoot of the return of blood pressure to higher than pretreatment levels and other complications are observed in a number of patients (Gifford, 1977; Ram and Kaplan, 1979). There are several clinical contraindications to the use of diazoxide. Because it increases cardiac work, coronary insufficiency can be worsened; myocardial infarction or increased ischemia can result (Kanada *et al.*, 1976). Not surprisingly, pulmonary edema can also worsen. Dissecting aortic aneurysm may be another condition in which diazoxide is contraindicated. The tear in the aorta may be worsened not only by the absolute levels of blood pressure but also by the rate of rise of blood pressure in the aorta during the cardiac cycle (shear force) (Wheat *et al.*, 1969). Since diazoxide increases the cardiac output and the stroke volume as a result of reflex sympathetic stimulation, it can increase the shear force produced by ejected blood and may extend the tear in the aorta. Treatment with diazoxide may need to be combined with the administration of a diuretic, since diazoxide causes retention of salt and water. Nevertheless, most patients with accelerated or malignant hypertension are not hypervolemic at the time they are first seen. Therefore, the need for a diuretic should be assessed in the individual patient. The patient's concentrations of glucose in plasma should be monitored as diazoxide is used. Diabetic ketoacidosis and hyperosmolar coma can appear subtly as diazoxide is administered.

The use of sodium nitroprusside is preferable to that of diazoxide if patients with accelerated or malignant hypertension also have coronary insufficiency or pulmonary edema. Because nitroprusside increases venous capacitance, the drug decreases preload and, therefore, cardiac oxygen demand is lessened for any given output. Cardiac failure and angina can thus be rapidly improved as the blood pressure falls (Cohn and Franciosa, 1977). Nitroprusside has other inherent advantages in the treatment of unstable situations. For instance, if a hypertensive patient is having a myocardial infarction, his hypertension should also be treated, but long-acting drugs should be avoided in order to accommodate to any sudden hemodynamic change caused by the infarction. Otherwise, protracted hypotension could result. Nitroprusside has been recommended for patients with dissecting aneurysm. In such cases it is used in combination with propranolol, which blocks the reflex increase in sympathetic cardiac stimulation that occurs if the vasodilator is used alone (Palmer and Lasseter, 1975). Since experience with nitroprusside to treat aortic dissection is limited, trimethaphan is still the drug with the most predictable and documented effects (Palmer and Lasseter, 1976). The major disadvantage in the use of nitroprusside is the absolute necessity to monitor the patient's blood pressure and the rate of infusion constantly. Intensive care units are the ideal setting for the use of nitroprusside.

Although nitroprusside is effective while the patient is supine or prone, the blood pressure will fall more if the patient sits or stands or if his body is tilted toward the head-upward position. Thus, the blood pressure must be monitored very carefully when the patient moves or is transported for diagnostic procedures. Tilt is an inexpensive and effective way to amplify the hypotensive effects of most antihypertensive drugs.

The nearly automatic parenteral administration of diuretics to patients with hypertensive emergencies can lead to undesirable results. As stated above, hypervolemia is usually absent at the time of presentation unless cardiac failure has occurred. Although most of the agents used to treat hypertensive emergencies can cause sodium retention, this can be modulated if intake of sodium is restricted. Restriction of sodium from the diet is preferable to the use of diuretics in the acute management of very high blood pressure. When the patient is ready for oral feeding and medication, the details of long-range care can be devised so that compliance and the effects of the drugs are optimized.

When malignant hypertension is not associated with complications such as encephalopathy, left ventricular cardiac failure, or renal failure, it may be treated as a moderate, but real, emergency. Oral therapy designed to reduce the pressure below 160 mm Hg systolic and 110 mm Hg diastolic within 24 hours may be preferable to parenteral therapy. Possible regimens include a diuretic, a potent vasodilator, and propranolol or a diuretic plus methyldopa. Methyldopa should be given in an initial dose of 500 mg to 1 g and, if a satisfactory response does not occur within 6 hours, another drug should be used. It is important to note that both diazoxide and nitroprusside may be effective in very small doses if the patient has also received other drugs (Berdoff et al., 1977). If parenteral therapy is used, oral antihypertensive drugs should be started as soon as possible so that the duration of parenteral therapy will not be unnecessarily prolonged.

"Refractory" Hypertension. As a wide variety of potent hypotensive agents with many different sites and mechanisms of action have become available, the occurrence of true resistance to the effects of these drugs has fallen to the point where it should now be rare. Yet the incidence of uncontrolled hypertension is still common (Stamler, 1974). The fault must lie with the health profession. Many patients who are qualified for therapy are not being convinced to take drugs, and the drugs are frequently given inappropriately once a patient is convinced (Gifford and Tarazi, 1978; Relman, 1980). The correction of these problems requires a critical evaluation of the patient, the drug regimen, and the physicians who care for the patient, as well as a long-term commitment for responsibility to the patient and an understanding of factors that are known to be associated with "refractory" hypertension.

A major reason why a patient's blood pressure does not fall is that he is not complying with the prescribed drug regimen. The importance of this problem can hardly be overemphasized. In part, this may be because patients with hypertension are often asymptomatic until there is damage to vital organs. Also, those who take their prescribed drugs often experience side effects; such patients have little inherent motivation to remain on drug therapy. In addition to the general measures to improve compliance discussed in Appendix I, the following points should be remembered: if thiazides are given only once a day, administer them in the morning so that any diuretic effect will not require the patient to get up at night. Discuss the potential side effects of the drugs with the patient; if the effects become annoying or intolerable, the drug regimen should be altered. The patient or a member of his family should monitor his blood pressure; the positive feedback this procedure can give might counter the disadvantages of side effects of drug therapy (Haynes et al., 1978). If a patient is not responding well to his therapeutic regimen, consider noncompliance and attempt to document or refute it; pill counts, inquiries as to the number of times the patient has had the prescription filled, and measurement of the concentration of the drugs in blood or urine are helpful.

Other causes that make hypertension seem to be refractory to treatment are the use of inappropriate drugs or combinations of drugs or inadequate doses. A combination of drugs that act at the same site is inappropriate. Failure to take into account the reflex homeostatic mechanisms that result from drug-induced decreases in blood pressure can greatly reduce the efficacy of a therapeutic regimen. For example, the combination of two drugs that reduce sympathetic activity (such as clonidine and methyldopa) or two vasodilators (such as hydralazine and prazosin) is usually inappropriate. Conversely, omission of a thiazide when a drug such as methyldopa or clonidine is given can lead either to a requirement for an unnecessarily high dose of the latter drug or to excessive retention of salt and water. Therapeutic failure may be the result.

Adverse drug interactions may be another cause of therapeutic failure (see Appendix III). Antagonism of the antihypertensive effects of guanethidine or clonidine by tricyclic antidepressants or even phenothiazines is well established; the adverse drug interactions that are provoked by MAO inhibitors have resulted in their virtual abandonment for antihypertensive therapy. Other drug combinations may lead to an excessive fall in blood pressure or loss of control of the high blood pressure when one member of the combination is discontinued.

In some patients the failure to achieve adequate control of blood pressure is the result of administration of insufficient doses of hypotensive agents. If a carefully planned, appropriate combination of drugs, used in normally effective doses, does not produce the desired fall in blood pressure, one should seek to determine whether some pharmacological effects are evident, even though the blood pressure is not controlled. As discussed above, assessment of sympathetic function can be performed at the bedside by measuring the response to the Valsalva maneuver or the orthostatic changes in blood pressure and heart rate.

Given the extent of the data demonstrating the progressive increase in morbidity and mortality associated with hypertension, the evidence documenting the benefits of treatment, and the availability of a wide variety of potent hypotensive agents, inadequate control of blood pressure should be thought of as a serious but surmountable challenge for the physician.

Åblad, B. A study of the mechanism of the hemodynamic effects of hydralazine in man. *Acta Pharmacol. Toxicol. (Kbh.)*, **1963**, *20*, Suppl. 1, 1–53.

Acchiardo, S.; Dustan, H. P.; and Tarazi, R. C. Similar effects of hydrochlorothiazide and spironolactone on plasma renin activity in essential hypertension. *Cleve. Clin. Q.*, **1972**, *39*, 153–162.

Adler, S. Methyldopa-induced decrease in mental activity. *J.A.M.A.*, **1974**, *230*, 1428–1429.

Adlin, V.; Marks, A. D.; and Channick, B. J. Spironolactone and hydrochlorothiazide in essential hypertension. Blood pressure response and plasma renin activity. *Arch. Intern. Med.*, **1972**, *130*, 855–865.

Alarcon-Segovia, D. Drug-induced antinuclear antibodies and lupus syndromes. *Drugs*, **1976**, *12*, 69–77.

Altura, B. M. Pharmacological effect of alpha-methyldopa, alpha-methylnorepinephrine, and octopamine on rat arteriolar, arterial and terminal vascular smooth muscle. *Circ. Res.*, **1975**, *36*, Suppl. 1, 223–246.

Ames, M. D.; Melmon, K. L.; and Castagnoli, N., Jr. Stereochemical course *in vivo* of alpha methyldopa decarboxylation in rat brains. *Biochem. Pharmacol.*, **1977**, *26*, 1757–1762.

Anderson, J.; Godfrey, B. E.; Hill, D. M.; Munro-Faure, A. D.; and Sheldon, J. A comparison of the effects of hydrochlorothiazide and of furosemide in the treatment of hypertensive patients. *Q. J. Med.*, **1971**, *40*, 541–560.

Ayitey-Smith, E., and Varma, D. R. Mechanism of the hypotensive action of methyldopa in normal and immunosympathectomized rats. *Br. J. Pharmacol.*, **1970**, *40*, 186–193.

Baekeland, F., and Lundwall, L. Effects of methyldopa on sleep patterns in man. *Electroencephalogr. Clin. Neurophysiol.*, **1971**, *31*, 269–273.

Bailey, R. R., and Neale, T. J. Rapid clonidine withdrawal with blood pressure overshoot exaggerated by beta-blockade. *Br. Med. J.*, **1976**, *1*, 942–943.

Barnett, A. J.; Bobok, A.; Carson, V.; Korman, J. S.; and McLean, A. J. Pharmacokinetics of methyldopa. *Clin. Exp. Pharmacol. Physiol.*, **1977**, *4*, 331–339.

Bateman, D. N.; Hobbs, D. C.; Twomey, T. M.; Stevens, E. A.; and Rawlins, M. D. Prazosin, pharmacokinetics and concentration effect. *Eur. J. Clin. Pharmacol.*, **1979**, *16*, 177–181.

Berdoff, R. L.; Chalal, R. L.; and Madden, M. Hazards in antihypertension therapy. (Letter.) *Ann. Intern. Med.*, **1977**, *86*, 111.

Berglund, G., and Andersson, O. Low doses of hydrochlorothiazide in hypertension. Antihypertensive and metabolic effects. *Eur. J. Clin. Pharmacol.*, **1976**, *10*, 177–182.

Bhatia, S. K., and Frohlich, E. D. Hemodynamic comparison of agents useful in hypertensive emergencies. *Am. Heart J.*, **1973**, *55*, 365–373.

Bolli, P.; Wood, A. J.; and Simpson, F. O. Effects of prazosin in patients with hypertension. *Clin. Pharmacol. Ther.*, **1976**, *20*, 138–218.

Bower, P. J., and Peterson, J. N. Methemoglobinemia after sodium nitroprusside therapy. *N. Engl. J. Med.*, **1975**, *293*, 865.

Boyer, J. L., and Kasch, F. W. Exercise therapy in hypertensive men. *J.A.M.A.*, **1970**, *211*, 1668–1671.

Briant, R. H.; Reid, J. L.; and Dollery, C. T. Interaction between clonidine and desipramine in man. *Br. Med. J.*, **1973**, *1*, 522–523.

Bristow, J. D.; Honour, A. J.; Pickering, G. W.; Sleight, P.; and Smyth, H. S. Diminished baroreflex sensitivity in high blood pressure. *Circulation*, **1969**, *39*, 48–54.

Brod, J.; Horbach, L.; Just, H.; Rosenthal, J.; and Nicolescu, R. Acute effects of clonidine on central and peripheral haemodynamics and plasma renin activity. *Eur. J. Clin. Pharmacol.*, **1972**, *4*, 107–114.

Brogden, R. N.; Heel, R. C.; Speight, T. M.; and Avery, G. S. Prazosin: a review of its pharmacologic properties and therapeutic efficacy in hypertension. *Drugs*, **1977**, *14*, 163–197.

Brunner, H. R.; Gavras, H.; Waeber, B.; Kershaw, G.; Turini, G. A.; Vukovich, R. A.; McKinstry, D. N.; and Gavras, I. Oral angiotensin-converting enzyme inhibitor in long-term treatment of hypertensive patients. *Ann. Intern. Med.*, **1979**, *90*, 19–23.

Buhler, F. R.; Burkart, F.; Lutold, B. E.; Kung, M.; Marbet, G.; and Pfisterer, M. Antihypertensive beta blocking action as related to renin and age: a pharmacologic tool to identify pathogenetic mechanisms in essential hypertension. *Am. J. Cardiol.*, **1975**, *36*, 653–659.

Carstairs, K. C.; Breckenridge, A.; Dollery, C. T.; and Worlledge, S. M. Incidence of positive direct Coombs' test in patients on alpha methyldopa. *Lancet*, **1966**, *2*, 133–135.

Chavdarian, C. G.; Karashima, D.; and Castagnoli, N. Oxidative and cardiovascular studies on natural and synthetic catecholamines. *J. Med. Chem.*, **1978**, *21*, 548–554.

Choquette, G., and Ferguson, R. J. Blood pressure reduction in "borderline" hypertensives following physical training. *Can. Med. Assoc. J.*, **1973**, *108*, 699–703.

Coleman, T. G.; Bower, J. D.; Langford, H. G.; and Guyton, A. C. Regulation of arterial pressure in the anephric state. *Circulation*, **1970**, *42*, 509–514.

Coleman, T. G.; Manning, R. D., Jr.; Norman, R. A., Jr.; Granger, H. J.; and Guyton, A. C. The role of salt in experimental and human hypertension. *Am. J. Med. Sci.*, **1972**, *264*, 103–110.

Conolly, M. E.; Briant, R. H.; George, C. F.; and Dollery, C. T. A crossover comparison of clonidine and methyldopa in hypertension. *Eur. J. Clin. Pharmacol.*, **1972**, *4*, 222–227.

Dargie, H. J.; Dollery, C. T.; and Daniel, J. Minoxidil in resistant hypertension. *Lancet*, **1977**, *2*, 515–518.

Davies, D. S.; Wing, L. M. H.; Reid, J. L.; Neil, E.; Tippett, P.; and Dollery, C. T. Pharmacokinetics and concentration-effect relationships of intravenous and oral clonidine. *Clin. Pharmacol. Ther.*, **1977**, *21*, 593–601.

Day, M. D.; Roach, A. G.; and Whiting, R. L. The mechanism of the antihypertensive action of α-methyldopa in hypertensive rats. *Eur. J. Pharmacol.*, **1973**, *21*, 271–280.

Dean, C. R.; Maling, T.; Dargie, H. J.; Reid, J. L.; and Dollery, C. T. Effect of propranolol on plasma norepinephrine during sodium nitroprusside–induced hypotension. *Clin. Pharmacol. Ther.*, **1980**, *27*, 156–163.

Devine, B. L.; Fife, R.; and Trust, P. M. Minoxidil for severe hypertension after failure of other hypotensive drugs. *Br. Med. J.*, **1977**, *2*, 667–669.

Dollery, C. T.; Davies, D. S.; Draffan, G. H.; Dargie, H. J.; Dean, C. R.; Reid, J. L.; Clare, R. A.; and Murray, S.

Clinical pharmacology and pharmacokinetics of cloni-dine. *Clin. Pharmacol. Ther.,* **1976,** *19,* 11–17.

Dollery, C. T., and Reid, J. L. Central noradrenergic neurones and the cardiovascular actions of clonidine in the rabbit. *Br. J. Pharmacol.,* **1973,** *47,* 206–216.

Dormois, J. C.; Young, J. L.; and Nies, A. S. Minoxidil in severe hypertension: value when conventional drugs have failed. *Am. Heart J.,* **1975,** *90,* 360–368.

Drayer, J. I. M.; Kloppenberg, P. W. C.; Festen, J.; Van't Laar, A.; and Benraad, T. J. Inpatient comparison of treatment with chlorthalidone, spironolactone and pro-pranolol in normoreninemic essential hypertension. *Am. J. Cardiol.,* **1975,** *36,* 716–721.

Dunn, M. J., and Tannen, R. L. Low-renin hypertension. *Kidney Int.,* **1974,** *5,* 317–325.

Dustan, H. P.; Bravo, E. L.; and Tarazi, R. C. Volume-dependent essential and steroid hypertension. *Am. J. Cardiol.,* **1973,** *31,* 606.

Elkington, S. G.; Schreiber, W. M.; and Conn, H. O. Hepatic injury caused by L-alpha-methyldopa. *Circulation,* **1969,** *40,* 589–594.

Finch, L., and Haeusler, G. Further evidence for a central hypotensive action of α-methyldopa in both the rat and cat. *Br. J. Pharmacol.,* **1973,** *47,* 217–228.

Freed, C. R.; Quintero, E.; and Murphy, C. Hypotension and hypothalamic amine metabolism after long term α-methyldopa infusions. *Life Sci.,* **1978,** *23,* 313–322.

Freis, E. D. Salt, volume and the prevention of hyperten-sion. *Circulation,* **1976,** *53,* 589–595.

Freis, E. D.; Rose, J. C.; Riggins, T. F.; Finnerty, F. A., Jr.; Kelley, R. T.; and Partenop, E. A. The hemodynamic effects of hypotensive drugs in man. IV. I-Hydrazino-phthalazine. *Circulation,* **1953,** *8,* 188–204.

Gaskell, P., and Diosy, A. Persistence of abnormally high vascular tone in vessels of the finger after digital nerve block in patients with chronic high blood pressure. *Circ. Res.,* **1959,** *7,* 1006–1010.

Geyskes, G. G.; Boer, P.; and Dorhout Mees, E. J. Clonidine withdrawal. Mechanism and frequency of rebound hypertension. *Br. J. Clin. Pharmacol.,* **1979,** *7,* 55–62.

Geyskes, G. G.; Boer, P.; Vos, J.; Leenan, F. H. H.; and Dorhout Mees, E. J. Effect of salt depletion and pro-pranolol on blood pressure and plasma renin activity in various forms of hypertension. *Circ. Res.,* **1975,** *36,* Suppl. 1, 248–256.

Glontz, G. E., and Saslaw, S. Methyldopa fever. *Arch. Intern. Med.,* **1968,** *122,* 445–447.

Goldberg, L. I.; DaCosta, F. M.; and Ozaki, M. Actions of the decarboxylase inhibitor α-methyldopa-3,4-dihydroxy-phenylalanine, in the dog. *Nature,* **1960,** *188,* 502–504.

Gottlieb, T. B.; Katz, F. H.; and Chidsey, C. A. Combined therapy with vasodilator drugs and beta-adrenergic blockade. A comparative study of minoxidil and hydral-azine. *Circulation,* **1972b,** *45,* 571–582.

Gottlieb, T. B.; Thomas, R. C.; and Chidsey, C. A. Phar-macokinetic studies of minoxidil. *Clin. Pharmacol. Ther.,* **1972a,** *13,* 436–441.

Graham, R. M.; Thornell, I. R.; Gain, J. M.; Bagnoli, C.; Oates, H. F.; and Stokes, G. S. Prazosin: the first-dose phenomenon. *Br. Med. J.,* **1976,** *2,* 1293.

Gribbin, B.; Pickering, T. G.; Sleight, P.; and Peto, R. Effect of age and high blood pressure on baroreflex sensitivity in man. *Circ. Res.,* **1971,** *49,* 424–431.

Guiha, N. H.; Cohn, J. N.; Mikulic, E.; Franciosa, J. A.; and Limas, C. J. Treatment of refractory heart failure with infusion of nitroprusside. *N. Engl. J. Med.,* **1974,** *291,* 587.

Gupta, K. P., and Bhargava, K. P. Mechanism of tachy-cardia induced by intracerebroventricular injection of hydralazine (1-hydrazinophthalazine). *Arch. Int. Pharma-codyn. Ther.,* **1965,** *155,* 84–89.

Haber, E. Renin inhibitors. *N. Engl. J. Med.,* **1978,** *298,* 1023–1025.

Haeusler, G. Clonidine-induced inhibition of sympathetic nerve activity: no indication for a central presynaptic or an indirect sympathomimetic mode of action. *Naunyn Schmiedebergs Arch. Pharmacol.,* **1974,** *286,* 97–111.

————. Cardiovascular regulation by central adrenergic mechanisms and its alteration by hypotensive drugs. *Circ. Res.,* **1975,** *37,* Suppl. 1, 223–232.

Hall, D.; Charcopos, F.; Froer, K. L.; and Rudolph, W. Use of minoxidil in resistant hypertension. *Herz,* **1978,** *3,* 313–324.

Halushka, P. V., and Keiser, H. R. Acute effects of alpha-methyldopa on mean blood pressure and plasma renin activity. *Circ. Res.,* **1974,** *35,* 458–463.

Hansson, L.; Hunyor, S. N.; Julius, S.; and Hoobler, S. W. Blood pressure crisis following withdrawal of clonidine (CATAPRES, CATAPRESAN), with special reference to arte-rial and urinary catecholamine levels, and suggestion for acute management. *Am. Heart J.,* **1973,** *85,* 605–610.

Haynes, R. B.; Sackett, D. L.; Taylor, D. W.; Givson, E. S.; and Johnson, A. L. Increased absenteeism from work after detection and labelling of hypertensive patients. *N. Engl. J. Med.,* **1978,** *299,* 741–744.

Healy, I. J.; McKenna, T. J.; Canning, B. St. J.; Brien, T. G.; Duffy, G. J.; and Muldowney, F. P. Body compo-sition changes in hypertensive subjects on long term oral diuretic therapy. *Br. Med. J.,* **1970,** *1,* 716.

Heise, A., and Kroneberg, G. Central nervous α-adrenergic receptors and the mode of action of α-methyl-dopa. *Naunyn Schmiedebergs Arch. Pharmacol.,* **1973,** *279,* 285–300.

Henning, M. Studies on the mode of action of α-meth-yldopa. *Acta Physiol. Scand.,* **1969,** *76,* Suppl. 322, 1–37.

Henning, M., and Rubenson, A. Evidence that the hypo-tensive action of methyldopa is mediated by central actions of methylnoradrenaline. *J. Pharm. Pharmacol.,* **1971,** *23,* 407–411.

Hokfelt, B.; Hedeland, H.; and Dymling, J. F. Studies on catecholamines, renin and aldosterone following CAT-APRESN^R [(2,6-dichlor-phenylamine)-2-imidazolene hy-drochloride] in hypertensive patients. *Eur. J. Pharmacol.,* **1970,** *10,* 389–397.

Hoobler, S. W., and Sagastume, E. Clonidine hydrochlo-ride in the treatment of hypertension. *Am. J. Cardiol.,* **1971,** *23,* 67–73.

Horwitz, D.; Pettinger, W. A.; Orvis, H.; and Sjoerdsma, A. Effects of methyldopa in fifty hypertensive patients. *Clin. Pharmacol. Ther.,* **1967,** *8,* 224–234.

Hunter, E.; Raik, E.; Gordon, S.; and Taylor, K. B. Inci-dence of positive Coombs' test, LE cells and antinuclear factor in patients on alpha-methyldopa therapy. *Med. J. Aust.,* **1971,** *2,* 810–812.

Hypertension Detection and Follow-Up Program Coopera-tive Group. Five-year findings of the hypertension de-tection and follow-up program. I. Reduction in mortality of persons with high blood pressure, including mild hypertension. *J.A.M.A.,* **1979a,** *242,* 2562–2571.

————. Five-year findings of the hypertension detection and follow-up program. II. Mortality by race-sex and age. *Ibid.,* **1979b,** *242,* 2572–2577.

Jain, A. K.; Ryan, J. R.; Vargas, R.; and McMahon, F. G. Efficacy and acceptability of different dosage schedules of clonidine. *Clin. Pharmacol. Ther.,* **1977,** *21,* 382–387.

James, I. M.; Larbi, E.; and Zaimis, E. The effect of the acute intravenous administration of clonidine (ST 155) on cerebral blood flow in man. *Br. J. Pharmacol.,* **1970,** *39,* 198P–199P.

Johnson, B. F. Diazoxide and renal function in man. *Clin. Pharmacol. Ther.,* **1971,** *12,* 815–824.

Julius, S.; Paxcual, A. V.; and London, R. Role of para-sympathetic inhibition in the hyperkinetic type of bor-derline hypertension. *Circulation,* **1971,** *44,* 413–418.

Kain, H. K.; Hinman, A. T.; and Sokolow, M. Arterial blood pressure measurements with a portable recorder in hypertensive patients. I. Variability and correlation with "casual" pressures. *Circulation,* **1964,** *30,* 882–892.

Kanada, S. A.; Kanada, D. J.; Hutchinson, R. A.; and Wu, D. Angina-like syndrome with diazoxide therapy for hypertensive crisis. *Ann. Intern. Med.,* **1976,** *84,* 696–699.

Karlberg, B. E., and Tolagen, K. Different antihypertensive effect of beta-blocking drugs in low and normal-high renin hypertension. *Am. J. Med.,* **1976,** *60,* 891–896.

Kersting, F.; Reid, J. L.; and Dollery, C. T. Clinical and cardiovascular effects on alpha methyldopa in combination with decarboxylase inhibitors. *Clin. Pharmacol. Ther.,* **1977,** *21,* 547–555.

Koshy, M. C.; Mickey, D.; Bourgoignie, J.; and Blauforx, M. D. Physiologic evaluation of a new antihypertensive agent: prazosin HCl. *Circulation,* **1977,** *55,* 533–536.

Kwan, K. C.; Foltz, E. L.; Breault, G. O.; Baer, J. E.; and Totaro, J. A. Pharmacokinetics of methyldopa in man. *J. Pharmacol. Exp. Ther.,* **1976,** *198,* 264–277.

Lager, I.; Blohme, G.; and Smith, U. Effect of cardioselective and non-selective β-blockade on the hypoglycaemic response in insulin-dependent diabetics. *Lancet,* **1979,** *1,* 458–462.

Landesman, R.; Coutinho, E. M.; Wilson, K. H.; and Vieira Lopes, A. C. The relaxant effect of diazoxide on nongravid human myometrium *in vivo. Am. J. Obstet. Gynecol.,* **1968,** *102,* 1080–1084.

Laverty, R., and Taylor, K. M. Behavioural and biochemical effects of 2-(2,6-dichlorophenylamino)-2-imidazoline hydrochloride (ST 155) on the central nervous system. *Br. J. Pharmacol.,* **1969,** *35,* 253–264.

Leth, A. Changes in plasma and extracellular fluid volumes in patients with essential hypertension during long term treatment with hydrochlorthiazide. *Circulation,* **1970,** *42,* 479–485.

LoBuglio, A. F., and Jandl, J. H. Nature of alpha-methyldopa red cell antibody. *N. Engl. J. Med.,* **1967,** *276,* 658–665.

Louis, W. J.; Doyle, A. E.; and Anavekar, S. Plasma norepinephrine levels in essential hypertension. *N. Engl. J. Med.,* **1973,** *288,* 599–601.

Lowder, S. C., and Liddle, G. W. Effects of guanethidine and methyldopa on a standardized test for renin responsiveness. *Ann. Intern. Med.,* **1975,** *82,* 757–760.

Lund-Johansen, P. Hemodynamic changes in long term α-methyldopa therapy of essential hypertension. *Acta Med. Scand.,* **1972,** *192,* 221–226.

———. Hemodynamic changes at rest and during exercise in long term clonidine therapy of essential hypertension. *Ibid.,* **1974,** *195,* 111–115.

———. Hemodynamic changes at rest and during exercise in long term prazosin therapy for essential hypertension. *Postgrad. Med.,* **1975,** *58,* Suppl., 45–52.

McMahon, F. G. *Management of Essential Hypertension.* Futura Publishing Co., Inc., Mount Kisco, N.Y., **1978.**

McRaven, D. R.; Kroetz, F. W.; Kioschos, J. M.; and Kirkendall, W. M. The effect of clonidine on hemodynamics in hypertensive patients. *Am. Heart J.,* **1971,** *81,* 482–489.

Mani, M. K. Nitroprusside, revisited. *Br. Med. J.,* **1971,** *3,* 407–408.

Marquez-Julio, A., and Uldall, P. R. Pericardial effusions associated with minoxidil. *Lancet,* **1977,** *1,* 816.

Marshall, A. J.; McGraw, M. E.; and Barritt, D. W. Positive antinuclear factor tests with prazosin. *Br. Med. J.,* **1979,** *1,* 165–166.

Materson, B. J.; Oster, J. R.; Michael, U. F.; Bolton, S. M.; Burton, Z. C.; Stambaugh, J. E.; and Morledge, J. Dose response to chlorthalidone in patients with mild hypertension. Efficacy of a lower dose. *Clin. Pharmacol. Ther.,* **1978,** *24,* 192–198.

Medical Research Council Working Party on Mild to Moderate Hypertension. Randomised control trial of treatment for mild hypertension: design and pilot trial. *Br. Med. J.,* **1977,** *1,* 1437–1440.

Melander, A.; Danielson, K.; Hanson, A.; Rudell, B.; Schersten, B.; Thulin, T.; and Wahlin, E. Enhancement of hydralazine bioavailability by food. *Clin. Pharmacol. Ther.,* **1977,** *22,* 104.

Merguet, P.; Heimsoth, V.; Murata, T.; and Bock, K. D. Experimental study on the circulatory effects of [2-(2,6-dichlorophenylamino)-2-imidazoline-hydrochloride] in man. *Pharmacol. Clin.,* **1968,** *1,* 30.

Miert, A. S. J. P. A. M. van, and Duin, C. T. M. van. The antipyretic effect of methyldopa in experimental fever. *J. Pharm. Pharmacol.,* **1972,** *24,* 988.

Miller, R. R.; Vismara, L. A.; Zelis, R.; Amsterdam, E. A.; and Mason, D. T. Clinical use of sodium nitroprusside in chronic ischemic heart disease. Effects on peripheral vascular resistance and venous tone and on ventricular volume, pump and mechanical performance. *Circulation,* **1975,** *51,* 328.

Mohammed, S.; Gaffney, T. E.; Yard, C. A.; and Gomez, H. Effect of methyldopa, reserpine and guanethidine on hindleg vascular resistance. *J. Pharmacol. Exp. Ther.,* **1968,** *160,* 300–307.

Morin, Y.; Turmel, L.; and Fortier, J. Methyldopa: clinical studies in arterial hypertension. *Am. J. Med. Sci.,* **1964,** *248,* 633.

Moutsos, S. E.; Sapira, J. D.; Scheib, E. T.; and Shapiro, A. P. An analysis of the placebo effect on hospitalized hypertensive patients. *Clin. Pharmacol. Ther.,* **1967,** *8,* 676–683.

Mroczek, W. J.; Davidov, M.; and Finnerty, F. A., Jr. Intravenous clonidine in hypertensive patients. *Clin. Pharmacol. Ther.,* **1973,** *14,* 847–851.

Mroczek, W. J.; Davidov, M.; Gavrilovich, L.; and Finnerty, F. A., Jr. The value of aggressive therapy in hypertensive patients with azotemia. *Circulation,* **1969,** *40,* 893–904.

Muir, A. L.; Burton, J. L.; and Lawrie, D. M. Circulatory effects at rest and exercise of clonidine, an imidazoline derivative with hypotensive properties. *Lancet,* **1969,** *2,* 181–185.

Myhre, E.; Brodwall, E. K.; Stenbaek, O.; and Hansen, T. Plasma turnover of methyldopa in advanced renal failure. *Acta Med. Scand.,* **1972,** *191,* 343–347.

Nayler, W. G., and Stone, J. An effect of ST 155 (clonidine), 2-(2,6-dichlorophenylamino)2-imidazole hydrochloride, CATAPRES on relationship between blood pressure and heart rate in dogs. *Eur. J. Pharmacol.,* **1970,** *10,* 161–167.

Nourok, D. G.; Glassock, K. J.; Solomon, D. H.; and Maxwell, M. H. Hypothyroidism following prolonged sodium nitroprusside therapy. *Am. J. Med. Sci.,* **1964,** *248,* 129–138.

Oates, J. A.; Gillespie, L.; Udenfriend, S.; and Sjoerdsma, A. Decarboxylase inhibition and blood pressure reduction by α-methyl-3,4-dihydroxy-DL-phenylalanine. *Science,* **1960,** *131,* 1890–1891.

Oates, J. A.; Seligman, A. W.; Clark, M. A.; Rousseau, P.; and Lee, R. E. The relative efficacy of guanethidine, methyldopa and pargyline as antihypertensive agents. *N. Engl. J. Med.,* **1965,** *273,* 729–734.

Ogilvie, R. I., and Mikulic, E. Effects of diazoxide and ethacrynic acid on sequential vascular segments in the canine gracilis muscle. *J. Pharmacol. Exp. Ther.,* **1972,** *180,* 368–376.

Ogilvie, R. I.; Piafsky, K. M.; and Ruedy, J. Antihypertensive response to spironolactone in normal renin hypertension. *Clin. Pharmacol. Ther.,* **1978,** *24,* 525–530.

Ogilvie, R. I., and Ruedy, J. Treatment of hypertension with hydrochlorothiazide and spironolactone. *Can. Med. Assoc. J.,* **1969,** *101,* 591–594.

O'Malley, K.; Segal, J. L.; Israili, Z. H.; Boles, M.; McNay, J. L.; and Dayton, P. G. Duration of hydralazine action in hypertension. *Clin. Pharmacol. Ther.,* **1975,** *18,* 581–588.

Onesti, G.; Schwartz, A. B.; Kim, K. W.; Paz-Martinez, V.; and Swartz, C. Antihypertensive effect of clonidine. *Circ. Res.,* **1971,** *28,* Suppl. 2, 53–69.

Palmer, R. F., and Lasseter, K. C. Nitroprusside and aortic dissecting aneurysm. (Letter.) *N. Engl. J. Med.,* **1976,** *294,* 1403–1404.

Pearson, R. M., and Breckenridge, A. M. Renal function, protein binding and pharmacogical response to diazoxide. *Br. J. Clin. Pharmacol.,* **1976,** *3,* 169–175.

Perry, H. M. Late toxicity to hydralazine resembling systemic lupus erythematosus or rheumatoid arthritis. *Am. J. Med.,* **1973,** *54,* 58–72.

Pettinger, W. A.; Keeton, T. K.; Campbell, W. B.; and Harper, D. C. Evidence for a renal α-adrenergic receptor inhibiting renin release. *Circ. Res.,* **1976,** *38,* 338–346.

Pettinger, W. A., and Mitchell, H. C. Minoxidil—an alternative to nephrectomy for refractory hypertension. *N. Engl. J. Med.,* **1980,** *302,* 293–294.

Putzeys, M. R., and Hoobler, S. W. Comparison of clonidine and methyldopa on blood pressure and side effects in hypertensive patients. *Am. Heart J.,* **1972,** *83,* 464–468.

Ram, C. V. S., and Kaplan, N. M. Individual titration of diazoxide dosage in the treatment of severe hypertension. *Am. J. Cardiol.,* **1979,** *43,* 627–630.

Raskin, N. H., and Fishman, R. A. Pyridoxine-deficiency neuropathy due to hydralazine. *N. Engl. J. Med.,* **1965,** *273,* 1182–1185.

Rehman, O. U.; Keith, T. A.; and Gall, E. A. Methyldopa-induced submassive hepatic necrosis. *J.A.M.A.,* **1973,** *224,* 1390–1392.

Reid, I. A.; MacDonald, D. M.; Pachnis, B.; and Ganong, W. F. Studies concerning the mechanism of suppression of renin secretion by clonidine. *J. Pharmacol. Exp. Ther.,* **1975,** *192,* 1713–1721.

Reid, J. L.; Briant, R. H.; and Dollery, C. T. Desmethylimipramine and the hypotensive action of clonidine in the rabbit. *Life Sci.,* **1973,** *12,* Pt. 1, 459–467.

Reidenberg, M. M.; Drayer, D.; DeMarco, A.; and Bello, C. T. Hydralazine elimination in man. *Clin. Pharmacol. Ther.,* **1973,** *14,* 970–977.

Relman, A. S. Mild hypertension: no more benign neglect. *N. Engl. J. Med.,* **1980,** *302,* 293–294.

Rhodes, H. J., and Sutter, M. C. The action of diazoxide on isolated vascular smooth muscle. Electrophysiology and contraction. *Can. J. Physiol. Pharmacol.,* **1971,** *49,* 276–287.

Ripley, R. C.; Hollifield, J. W.; and Nies, A. S. Sustained hypertension after section of the glossopharyngeal nerve. *Am. J. Med.,* **1977,** *62,* 297–302.

Rodman, J. S.; Deutsch, D. J.; and Gutman, S. L. Methyldopa hepatitis. A report of six cases and review of the literature. *Am. J. Med.,* **1976,** *60,* 941–948.

Rubin, L. J., and Peter, R. H. Oral hydralazine therapy for primary pulmonary hypertension. *N. Engl. J. Med.,* **1980,** *302,* 69–73.

Saavedra, J. A.; Reid, J. L.; Jordan, W.; Rawlins, M. D.; and Dollery, C. T. Plasma concentration of alpha methyldopa and sulphate conjugate after oral administration of methyldopa hydrochloride ethyl ester. *Eur. J. Clin. Pharmacol.,* **1975,** *8,* 381–386.

Safar, M.; Corvol, P.; Weiss, Y.; Folliot, A.; and Ménard, J. Action antihypertensive de trois drogues inhibant le système nerveux sympathique. *Nouv. Presse Med.,* **1974,** *3,* 871–874.

Safar, M. E.; London, G. M.; Levenson, J. A.; Kheder, M. A.; Aboras, N. E.; and Simon, A. C. Effect of alpha-methyldopa on cardiac output in hypertension. *Clin. Pharmacol. Ther.,* **1979,** *25,* 266–272.

Schlant, R. C.; Tsagaris, T. S.; and Robertson, R. J. Studies on the acute cardiovascular effects of intravenous sodium nitroprusside. *Am. J. Cardiol.,* **1962,** *9,* 51–59.

Schmitt, H., and Schmitt, H. Interactions between 2-(2,6-dichlorophenylamine)2-imidazoline hydrochloride (ST 155, CATAPRESAN) and alpha-adrenergic blocking drugs. *Eur. J. Pharmacol.,* **1970,** *9,* 7–13.

Shafar, J.; Tallett, E. R.; and Knowlson, P. A. Evaluation

of clonidine in prophylaxis of migraine. Double-blind trial and follow-up. *Lancet,* **1972,** *1,* 403–407.

Sheiner, L., and Melmon, K. L. The utility function of antihypertensive therapy. *Ann. N.Y. Acad. Sci.,* **1978,** *304,* 112–122.

Shen, D.; Gibaldi, M.; Throne, M.; Bellward, G.; Cunningham, R.; Israili, Z.; and McNay, J. Pharmacokinetics of bethanidine in hypertensive patients. *Clin. Pharmacol. Ther.,* **1975,** *17,* 363–373.

Sherman, G. P.; Grega, G. J.; Woods, R. J.; and Buckley, J. P. Evidence for a central hypotensive mechanism of 2-(2,6-dichlorophenylamino)-2-imidazoline(CATAPRESAN, ST-155). *Eur. J. Pharmacol.,* **1968,** *2,* 326–328.

Sjoerdsma, A.; Vendsalu, A.; and Engelman, K. Studies on the metabolism and mechanism of action of methyldopa. *Circulation,* **1963,** *28,* 492–502.

Sokolow, M., and Perloff, D. Five-year survival of consecutive patients with malignant hypertension treated with antihypertensive agents. *Am. J. Cardiol.,* **1966,** *6,* 858–863.

Sourkes, T. L. Inhibition of dihydroxyphenylalanine decarboxylase by derivatives of phenylalanine. *Arch. Biochem. Biophys.,* **1954,** *51,* 444–456.

Stamler, J. High blood pressure in the United States—an overview of the problem and the challenge. In, *National Conference on High Blood Pressure Education: Report of Proceedings, 1973.* Department of Health, Education, and Welfare Publication No. (NIH) 73-486, U.S. Government Printing Office, Washington, D. C., **1974,** pp. 11-66.

Taguchi, J., and Freis, E. D. Partial reduction of blood pressure and prevention of complications in hypertension. *N. Engl. J. Med.,* **1974,** *291,* 329–331.

Takeshita, A.; Tanaka, S.; Kuroiwa, A.; and Nakamura, M. Reduced baroreceptor sensitivity in borderline hypertension. *Circulation,* **1975,** *51,* 738–742.

Talseth, T. Clinical pharmacokinetics of hydrallazine. *Clin. Pharmacokinet.,* **1977,** *2,* 317–329.

Thirwell, M. P., and Zsotér, T. T. The effect of diazoxide on the veins. *Am. Heart J.,* **1972,** *83,* 512–517.

Thomson, A. E.; Nickerson, M.; Gaskell, P. I.; and Grahame, G. R. Clinical observations on an antihypertensive chlorothiazide analogue devoid of diuretic activity. *Can. Med. Assoc. J.,* **1962,** *87,* 1306–1310.

Thomson, P. D., and Melmon, K. L. Clinical assessment of autonomic function. *Anesthesiology,* **1968,** *29,* 724–731.

Titeler, M.; Tedesco, J. L.; and Seeman, P. Selective labeling of pre-synaptic receptors by ³H-dopamine, ³H-apomorphine and ³H-clonidine; labeling of post-synaptic sites by ³H-neuroleptics. *Life Sci.,* **1978,** *23,* 587–592.

Toghill, P. J.; Smith, P. G.; Benton, P.; Brown, R. C.; and Matthews, H. L. Methyldopa liver damage. *Br. Med. J.,* **1974,** *3,* 545–548.

Tuzel, I. H. Sodium nitroprusside. A review of its clinical effectiveness as a hypotensive agent. *J. Clin. Pharmacol.,* **1974,** *14,* 494–503.

Valnes, K.; Hillestad, L.; Hansen, T.; and Arnold, E. Alpha-methyldopa and drug fever: study of the metabolism of alpha-methyldopa in patients and normal subjects. *Acta Med. Scand.,* **1978,** *204,* 21–25.

Van Zweiten, P. A. The central action of antihypertensive drugs mediated via central alpha-receptors. *J. Pharm. Pharmacol.,* **1973,** *25,* 89–95.

———. Reduction of the hypotensive effect of clonidine and alpha-methyldopa by various psychotropic drugs. *Clin. Sci. Mol. Med.,* **1976,** *51,* 4115–4155.

Vesey, C. J.; Cole, P. V.; and Simpson, P. J. Cyanide and thiocyanate concentrations following sodium nitroprusside infusion in man. *Br. J. Anaesth.,* **1976,** *48,* 651–660.

Veterans Administration Cooperative Study Group on Antihypertensive Agents. Effects of treatment on morbidity in hypertension: results in patients with diastolic blood pressures averaging 115 through 129 mm Hg. *J.A.M.A.,* **1967,** *202,* 1028–1034.

———. Effects of treatment on morbidity in hypertension. II. Results in patients with diastolic blood pressures averaging 90 through 114 mm Hg. *J.A.M.A.,* **1970,** *213,* 1143–1152.

——. Effects of treatment on morbidity in hypertension. III. Influence of age, diastolic pressure, and prior cardiovascular disease; further analysis of side effects. *Circulation,* **1972,** *45,* 991–1004.

——. Propranolol in the treatment of essential hypertension. *J.A.M.A.,* **1977,** *237,* 2303–2310.

Walson, P. D.; Marshall, K. S.; Forsyth, R. P.; Rapoport, R.; Melmon, K. L.; and Castagnoli, N., Jr. Metabolic disposition and cardiovascular effects of methyldopa in unanesthetized rhesus monkeys. *J. Pharmacol. Exp. Ther.,* **1975,** *195,* 151–158.

Webster, J. S.; Moberg, C.; and Rincon, G. Natural history of severe proximal coronary artery disease as documented by coronary cineangiography. *Am. J. Cardiol.,* **1974,** *33,* 195–200.

Wheat, M. W.; Prockop, E. K.; and Palmer, R. F. Management of acute dissecting aneurysms of the aorta. *Hosp. Pract.,* **1969,** *4,* 29–35.

Wohl, A. J.; Hausler, L. M.; and Roth, F. E. Mechanism of the antihypertensive effect of diazoxide: *in vitro* vascular studies in the hypertensive rat. *J. Pharmacol. Exp. Ther.,* **1968,** *162,* 109–114.

Woods, J. W.; Blythe, W. B.; and Huffines, W. D. Managements of malignant hypertension complicated by renal insufficiency. *N. Engl. J. Med.,* **1974,** *291,* 10–14.

Wright, J. M.; McLeod, P. J.; and McCullough, W. Antihypertensive efficacy of a single bedtime dose of methyldopa. *Clin. Pharmacol. Ther.,* **1976,** *20,* 733–737.

Monographs and Reviews

Benforado, J. M. The veratrum alkaloids. In, *Physiological Pharmacology.* Vol. 4, *The Nervous System—Part D: Autonomic Nervous System Drugs.* (Root, W. S., and Hofmann, F. G., eds.) Academic Press, Inc., New York, **1967,** pp. 331–398.

Cohn, J. N., and Franciosa, J. A. Vasodilator therapy of cardiac failure. *N. Engl. J. Med.,* **1977,** *297,* 27–31.

Gaffney, T. E.; Sigell, L. T.; Mohammed, S.; and Atkinson, A. J., Jr. The clinical pharmacology of antihypertensive drugs. *Prog. Cardiovasc. Dis.,* **1969,** *12,* 52–71.

Gifford, R. W. Management and treatment of malignant hypertension and hypertensive emergencies. In, *Hypertension: Pathophysiology and Treatment.* (Genest, J.; Koiw, E.; and Kuchel, O.; eds.) McGraw-Hill Book Co., New York, **1977,** pp. 1024–1038.

Gifford, R. W., and Tarazi, R. C. Resistant hypertension: diagnosis and management. *Ann. Intern. Med.,* **1978,** *88,* 661–665.

Graham, R. M., and Pettinger, W. A. Prazosin. *N. Engl. J. Med.,* **1979,** *300,* 232–236.

Hansten, P. D. *Drug Interactions,* 4th ed. Lea & Febiger, Philadelphia, **1979.**

Johnson, C. C. The actions and toxicity of sodium nitroprusside. *Arch. Int. Pharmacodyn. Ther.,* **1929,** *35,* 480–496.

Julius, S. Borderline hypertension—overview. *Med. Clin. North Am.,* **1977,** *61,* 495–511.

Kannel, W. B. Importance of hypertension as a major risk factor in cardiovascular disease. In, *Hypertension: Physiopathology and Treatment.* (Genest, J.; Koiw, E.; and Kuchel, O.; eds.) McGraw-Hill Book Co., New York, **1977,** pp. 888–910.

Kopin, I. J. False adrenergic transmitters. *Annu. Rev. Pharmacol.,* **1968,** *8,* 337–394.

Lowenstein, J. Clonidine. *Ann. Intern. Med.,* **1980,** *92,* 74–77.

Nies, A. S. Adverse reactions and interactions limiting the use of antihypertensive drugs. *Am. J. Med.,* **1975,** *58,* 495–503.

——. Clinical pharmacology of antihypertensive drugs. *Med. Clin. North Am.,* **1977,** *61,* 675–698.

Palmer, R. F., and Lasseter, K. C. Sodium nitroprusside. *N. Engl. J. Med.,* **1975,** *292,* 294–297.

Peters, W. G. Pharmacology of diuretics. In, *Antihypertensive Therapy, Principles and Practices: An International Symposium.* (Gross, F., ed.) Springer-Verlag, Berlin, **1966,** pp. 31–57.

Pettinger, W. A. Clonidine, a new antihypertensive drug. *N. Engl. J. Med.,* **1975,** *293,* 1179–1180.

Sackett, D. L. Hypertension in the real world: public reaction, physician response, and patient compliance. In, *Hypertension: Physiopathology and Treatment.* (Genest, J.; Koiw, E.; and Kuchel, O.; eds.) McGraw-Hill Book Co., New York, **1977,** pp. 1142–1149.

Sannerstedt, R., and Conway, J. Hemodynamic and vascular response to antihypertensive treatment with adrenergic blocking agents: a review. *Am. Heart J.,* **1970,** *79,* 122–127.

Tobian, L. Why do thiazide diuretics lower blood pressure in essential hypertension? *Annu. Rev. Pharmacol.,* **1967,** *7,* 399–408.

Winer, B. M. The antihypertensive actions of benzothiadiazines. *Circulation,* **1961,** *23,* 211–218.

CHAPTER

33 VASODILATORS AND THE TREATMENT OF ANGINA

Philip Needleman and Eugene M. Johnson, Jr.

Angina pectoris is the principal symptom of ischemic heart disease. Both the typical and the variant forms of angina are manifested by sudden, severe, pressing substernal pain, which often radiates to the left shoulder and along the flexor surface of the left arm. In typical angina, the pain is often brought on by exercise or emotion. The attacks may recur for years. Anginal attacks probably are the result of temporary ischemia of the myocardium; that is, the flow of blood is inadequate to maintain oxygenation, nutrition, and removal of metabolites.

Considerable new information has emerged regarding the cause of a variant angina (Prinzmetal's angina) (*see* Hillis and Braunwald, 1978). Vasospasm of the coronary arteries appears to be a primary feature, and it may be (but is not necessarily) superimposed on atherosclerotic coronary artery disease. The patient with variant angina develops chest pain while at rest rather than during exertion or stress, and electrocardiographic S-T segment elevation is more common than is S-T segment depression, which is characteristic of "typical angina." The chest pain of both types of angina is usually quickly relieved by *nitroglycerin* (glyceryl trinitrate).

Discussion in this chapter is particularly directed at the treatment of typical angina pectoris—initiated by exertion and associated with atherosclerotic lesions. The use of pharmacological agents to diagnose and treat variant angina is discussed separately.

The strategy for pharmacological relief of typical angina is based upon improving the balance between the delivery to and the utilization of oxygen by the myocardium. Numerous drugs have been used to treat angina; nevertheless, when agents have been evaluated rigorously, few have been found to be more effective than placebo. In fact, placebos have been reported to relieve symp-

toms in as many as 50% of patients with angina pectoris (Cole *et al.*, 1957). For over a century, however, nitroglycerin has been known to be useful to prevent or relieve acute anginal attacks. More recently, the efficacy of β-adrenergic antagonists, particularly *propranolol*, has been established for the long-term prophylaxis of typical angina. Antianginal agents provide only symptomatic treatment for ischemic heart disease; they have no beneficial effect on the underlying pathology.

ORGANIC NITRATES

History. Nitroglycerin was first synthesized by Sobrero in 1846, and he observed that a small quantity of the oily substance placed on the tongue elicited a severe headache. Constantin Hering, in 1847, developed the sublingual dosage form for nitroglycerin, which he advocated for a number of diseases. The eminent English physician, T. Lauder Brunton, was unable to relieve severe recurrent anginal pain except when he bled his patient, and he believed that phlebotomy provided relief by lowering arterial blood pressure. In 1857, Brunton administered amyl nitrite, a known vasodepressor, by inhalation, and he noted that anginal pain was relieved within 30 to 60 seconds. The action of amyl nitrite was transitory, however, and the dosage was difficult to adjust. In 1879, William Murrell decided that the action of nitroglycerin mimicked that of amyl nitrite, and he established the use of sublingual nitroglycerin for relief of the acute anginal attack and as a prophylactic agent to be taken prior to exertion. The empirical observation that organic nitrates could be used safely for the rapid and dramatic alleviation of the symptoms of angina pectoris led to their widespread acceptance by the medical profession (*see* Krantz, 1975).

Chemistry. Organic nitrates are polyol esters of nitric acid, whereas organic nitrites are esters of nitrous acid (Table 33–1, page 826). Nitrate esters ($-C-O-NO_2$) and nitrite esters ($-C-O-NO$) are characterized by a sequence of carbon-oxygen-nitrogen, whereas nitro compounds (which are not vasodilators) possess carbon-nitrogen bonds ($C-NO_2$). Thus, glyceryl trinitrate is not a nitro compound, and it is erroneously called nitroglycerin;

819

however, this nomenclature is both widespread and official. Amyl nitrite is a highly volatile liquid that is administered by inhalation. Organic nitrates of low molecular weight (such as nitroglycerin) are moderately volatile, oily liquids, whereas the high-molecular-weight nitrate esters (*e.g.*, mannitol hexanitrate, erythrityl tetranitrate, pentaerythritol tetranitrate, isosorbide dinitrate) are solids. The fully nitrated polyols are lipid soluble, whereas incompletely nitrated compounds (which are metabolites) are more soluble in water.

PHARMACOLOGICAL PROPERTIES

Cardiovascular Effects. *Hemodynamic Effects in Normal Individuals.* The organic nitrates and nitrites are dilators of arterial and venous smooth muscle. The mechanism by which they produce relaxation of smooth muscle is unknown. Low concentrations of nitroglycerin produce dilatation of the veins that predominates over that of arterioles. The venodilatation results in decreased left and right ventricular end-diastolic pressures, which are greater on a percentage basis than is the decrease in systemic arterial pressure. Net systemic vascular resistance is usually relatively unaffected; heart rate is unchanged or slightly increased; and pulmonary vascular resistance is consistently reduced (Ferrer *et al.*, 1966). In normal individuals or those with coronary artery disease (in the absence of heart failure), sublingual administration of nitroglycerin decreases cardiac output. Doses of nitroglycerin that do not alter systemic arterial pressure often produce arteriolar dilatation in the face and neck, resulting in a flush. The same doses may also cause headache, presumably due to dilatation of meningeal arterial vessels.

Rapid administration of high doses of organic nitrates decreases systolic and diastolic blood pressure and cardiac output, resulting in pallor, weakness, dizziness, and activation of compensatory sympathetic reflexes. The resultant tachycardia and peripheral arteriolar vasoconstriction tend to maintain peripheral resistance; this is superimposed on sustained venous pooling. Coronary blood flow increases transiently due to coronary vasodilatation but subsequently falls as arterial blood pressure decreases and cardiac output falls. A marked hypotensive effect may occasionally follow sublingual administration of nitroglycerin. This is especially likely when the individual is in the upright position,

which augments venous pooling and further decreases cardiac output.

Mechanism of Relief of Symptoms of Angina Pectoris. Typical attacks of angina are usually precipitated by exercise or stress, which increases cardiac work and myocardial demand for oxygen. Effective drugs could correct the inadequacy of myocardial oxygenation by (1) increasing the supply of oxygen to ischemic myocardium by direct dilatation of the coronary vasculature, or (2) decreasing the oxygen demand secondary to a reduction of cardiac work. Brunton ascribed the relief of anginal pain afforded by nitrates to a decrease in cardiac work secondary to the fall in systemic blood pressure. After demonstration of direct coronary vasodilatation in experimental animals, it became generally accepted that nitrates relieved anginal pain by dilating coronary arteries and thereby increasing coronary blood flow. This hypothesis was questioned by Gorlin and associates (1959), who were unable to demonstrate increases in coronary blood flow in patients with coronary insufficiency following the administration of nitroglycerin. Although the mode of action of organic nitrates to relieve typical angina is not fully understood, the preponderance of evidence favors a reduction in the myocardial requirement for oxygen as the major action. In contrast, the ability of nitrates to dilate large coronary vessels selectively may be the primary mechanism by which they benefit patients with angina caused by coronary spasm (*see* below).

Effects on Total and Regional Coronary Blood Flow. Increases in the myocardial requirement for oxygen are normally met by increasing blood flow, rather than by more complete extraction of oxygen from the blood. Ischemia is a powerful stimulus to coronary vasodilatation, and regional blood flow is adjusted by autoregulatory mechanisms that alter the tone of small resistance vessels. When there is atherosclerotic coronary occlusion, ischemia distal to the lesion is a stimulus for marked vasodilatation, and, if the degree of occlusion is severe, much of the *capacity* to dilate is utilized to maintain resting blood flow to the compromised area. When situations arise that increase demand, further dilatation may not be possible.

As mentioned, organic nitrates do not increase *total* coronary blood flow in patients with typical angina due to atherosclerosis (Gorlin *et al.*, 1959). This does not, however, preclude the possibility that a drug could produce a redistribution of blood flow in favor of more hypoxic regions of the myocardium. During systolic contraction the tension within the left ventricle increases progressively from the subepicardium to the subendocardium; during systole, coronary blood flow is thus highest in the epicardium and lowest in the endocardium. The endocardium is more vulnerable to ischemia and more susceptible to necrosis subsequent to infarction or coronary insufficiency (*see* Moir, 1972). Organic nitrates do appear to cause redistribution of coronary blood flow to the ischemic subendocardium by selective dilatation of large epicardial vessels. These normally contribute little to the overall coronary vascular resistance and are not involved in autoregulation (Cohen and Kirk, 1973). When flow through large epicardial and collateral vessels is increased and tone of coronary resistance vessels is unchanged (autoregulation is unimpaired by organic nitrates), blood is shunted to areas of myocardium where arteriolar resistance is low (ischemic subendocardium). Experimental evidence *in vitro* (Schnaar and Sparks, 1972), in animals (Fam and McGregor, 1964; Winbury *et al.*, 1969, 1971; Cohen and Kirk, 1973), and in man (Goldstein *et al.*, 1974) supports the hypothesis that nitrates do have a selective effect on large coronary vessels. Nitroglycerin administered sublingually increases the rate of washout of radioactive xenon injected directly into diseased regions of the ventricular wall of angina patients (Horwitz *et al.*, 1971), indicating that blood flow to regions of poorly perfused myocardium has been improved. Nitrates increase endocardial blood flow (Becker *et al.*, 1971) and the oxygenation of tissue (Winbury *et al.*, 1971) relative to epicardial regions in ischemic canine ventricle. Such redistribution of blood flow to subendocardial tissue is *not* typical of all vasodilators. Dipyridamole, for example, dilates resistance vessels nonselectively and inhibits autoregulation; it is ineffective in patients with typical angina.

Effects on Myocardial Oxygen Requirements. The organic nitrates reduce the requirement of the myocardium for oxygen by their effects on the systemic circulation. The major determinants of myocardial oxygen consumption include the stress on the ventricular wall during systole, the heart rate, and the state of contractility of the myocardium. The stress on the ventricular wall is affected by a number of factors that are generally considered under the categories of "preload" and "afterload." *Preload* is determined by the diastolic pressure that distends the relaxed ventricular wall (left ventricular end-diastolic pressure). Increasing end-diastolic pressure and volume augment the ventricular tension required to eject blood (by the law of Laplace, tension = pressure × radius). Decreasing venous resistance (which increases venous capacitance) decreases venous return to the heart, ventricular end-diastolic pressure and volume, and thereby oxygen consumption. *Afterload*, or ventricular systolic wall tension, is the force distributed in the ventricular wall during ejection of blood. It is related to the radius of the ventricle and to the aortic pressure (and therefore to peripheral resistance). Decreasing peripheral arteriolar resistance reduces afterload and thus myocardial consumption of oxygen.

Organic nitrates do not directly alter the inotropic or chronotropic state of the heart. The drugs do decrease both preload and afterload as a result of respective dilatation of venous capacitance and arteriolar resistance vessels (Williams *et al.*, 1965). Since the primary determinants of oxygen demand are reduced by the nitrates, their net effect usually is to decrease myocardial consumption of oxygen.

Paradoxically, however, high doses of organic nitrates may reduce diastolic blood pressure to such an extent that reflex tachycardia and adrenergic enhancement of contractility may override the salutary action of the drugs. The resultant negative effect on oxygen balance can aggravate ischemia and, potentially, initiate an anginal attack.

Relative Importance of the Actions of Organic Nitrates. Of the two general mechanisms by which nitrates can reduce myocardial ischemia, their ability to reduce the demand for oxygen (by reducing preload and afterload) appears to be the most important for patients with typical angina. When nitroglycerin is injected or infused directly into the coronary circulation of patients with coronary artery disease, anginal attacks (induced by electrical pacing) are not aborted, even when coronary blood flow is increased. Sublingual administration of nitroglycerin does relieve anginal pain in the same patients (Ganz and Marcus, 1972). Furthermore, venous phlebotomy that is sufficient to reduce left ventricular end-diastolic pressure can mimic the beneficial effect of nitroglycerin (Parker *et al.*, 1970; Strauer and Scherpe, 1978).

Patients are able to exercise for considerably longer periods after the administration of nitroglycerin. Nevertheless, angina occurs, with or without nitroglycerin, at the same value of the "triple product" (aortic pressure × heart rate × ejection time). The triple product can be determined experimentally and is proportional to the myocardial consumption of oxygen. The observation that angina occurs at the same level of myocardial oxygen consumption suggests that the beneficial effects of nitroglycerin are the result of a reduced cardiac oxygen demand, rather than the result of an increase in the delivery of oxygen to ischemic regions of myocardium (Goldstein and Epstein, 1972).

Other Effects. The organic nitrates and nitrites act on almost all smooth muscle structures. *Bronchial* smooth muscle is relaxed irrespective of the cause of the preexisting tone. The muscles of the *biliary tract,* including those of the gallbladder, biliary ducts, and sphincter of Oddi, are effectively relaxed. In patients with T-tube drainage, a nitrate can rapidly reduce biliary pressure, whether elevated spontaneously or in response to morphine, and can induce rapid emptying of biliary contents into the duodenum. Pain and other symptoms incident to increased pressure are transiently relieved. Smooth muscle of the *gastrointestinal tract,* including that of the esophagus, can be relaxed and its spontaneous motility decreased by nitrate both *in vivo* and *in vitro.* The effect may be transient and incomplete *in vivo,* but abnormal "spasm" is frequently reduced. Similarly, nitrate can relax *ureteral* and *uterine* smooth muscle, but these effects are somewhat unpredictable. Organic nitrates are singularly devoid of actions on tissues other than smooth muscle.

Nitrites, nitrates, and a variety of other nitrogen-containing compounds (including nitroprusside and hydralazine, Chapter 32) are capable of activating guanylate cyclase and causing marked increases in concentrations of cyclic guanosine 3',5'-monophosphate (cyclic GMP) in most tissues. This effect is apparently due to the action of nitric oxide (NO), which can be formed from such agents; nitric oxide probably activates the enzyme directly. It is not known if this action is causally related to the effects of these drugs on smooth muscle. Nitric oxide itself, however, is also a relaxant of smooth muscle (*see* review by Murad *et al.*, 1979).

Absorption, Fate, and Excretion. The biotransformation of organic nitrates is the result of reductive hydrolysis catalyzed by the hepatic enzyme glutathione–organic nitrate reductase. The enzyme converts the lipid-soluble organic nitrate esters into more water-soluble denitrated metabolites and inorganic nitrite. The partially and fully denitrated metabolites are considerably less potent vasodilators than are the parent compounds. However, under certain conditions their activity may become important. Since the liver has an enormous capacity to catalyze this reaction, the biotransformation of organic nitrates is a major factor in determining their duration of action *in vivo* and the relative efficacy of the drugs when given by various routes of administration. The pharmacokinetic properties of nitroglycerin and isosorbide dinitrate have been studied in the greatest detail.

Nitroglycerin. Investigation of biotransformation of organic nitrates began with the observation that inorganic nitrite was formed when organic nitrate esters were incubated with homogenates of rabbit liver (Oberst and Snyder, 1948). Studies in a variety of systems indicate that the reductive hydrolysis requires glutathione (Heppel and Hilmoe, 1950) and is rapidly catalyzed by glutathione–organic nitrate reductase (Needleman, 1975). One molecule of nitroglycerin reacts with two of reduced glutathione to release one inorganic nitrite ion from either the 2 or 3 position; the products are 1,3- or 1,2-glyceryl dinitrate and oxidized glutathione (Needleman and Harkey, 1971). A comparison of the maximal velocities of metabolism of the clinically used nitrates by hepatic glutathione–organic nitrate reductase indicates that mannitol hexanitrate and erythrityl tetranitrate are degraded seven and three times faster, respectively, than is nitroglycerin. Isosorbide dinitrate and pentaerythritol nitrate are denitrated at one sixth and one tenth of the rate of nitroglycerin (Needleman and Hunter, 1965).

In man, peak concentrations of nitroglycerin are found in plasma within 4 minutes of sublingual administration; the compound has a half-life of 1 to 3 minutes (Bogaert and Rosseel, 1972). Dinitrate metabolites, which are about ten times less potent as vasodilators, appear to have a half-life of approximately 2 hours (*see* Appendix II).

Isosorbide Dinitrate. Following intravenous administration of isosorbide dinitrate to dogs, rats, and rabbits, the concentration of unchanged drug in plasma decreases rapidly ($t_{1/2} \cong 5$ minutes) (Sisenwine and Ruelius, 1971). After intravenous or oral administration the primary metabolite in the plasma is 5-isosorbide mononitrate, which has only 1/30 to 1/100 the coronary vasodilating or vasodepressor activity of the parent compound. The mononitrate has a half-life of about 2.5 hours (Johnson *et al.*, 1972; Wendt, 1972). A quantitatively different clearance pattern is observed following *oral* administration of isosorbide dinitrate to dogs. Trace amounts of the intact molecule appear only transiently in the circulation, and the major metabolite, 5-isosorbide mononitrate, reaches its peak concentration at a later time (30 minutes) (Sisenwine and Ruelius, 1971).

The major route of metabolism of isosorbide dinitrate in man is also by enzymatic denitration followed by formation of glucuronides. Sublingual administration produces maximal concentrations of the drug in plasma by 6 minutes, and the fall in concentration is rapid (Rosseel and Bogaert, 1973). Only trace concentrations of the compound are found when it is given orally in relatively low doses (Chasseaud *et al.*, 1975; *see* below). Essentially all the drug is eliminated in the urine of human subjects, principally as isosorbide glucuronide.

Correlation of Plasma Concentrations of Drug and Biological Activity. Intravenous administration of nitroglycerin or the so-called long-acting nitrates (isosorbide dinitrate, pentaerythritol tetranitrate and trinitrate, erythrityl tetranitrate, and mannitol hexanitrate) in anesthetized animals produces the same transient decrease (1 to 4 minutes) in blood pressure (Needleman *et al.*, 1972). Relative to nitroglycerin, the potency of pentaerythritol trinitrate as a vasodepressor in dogs is about 20%, erythrityl tetranitrate 12%, and isosorbide dinitrate 3.5% (Parker *et al.*, 1975). Since denitration markedly reduces the activity of the organic nitrates, their rapid clearance from blood indicates that the transient duration of action under these conditions correlates with the concentrations of the parent compounds (Needleman *et al.*, 1972; Yap and Fung, 1978). The kinetics of hepatic denitration is characteristic of each nitrate. In addition, it appears to be influenced by hepatic blood flow or the presence of hepatic disease. In experimental animals, injection of moderate amounts of organic nitrates into the portal vein results in little or no vasodepressor activity (Needleman *et al.*, 1972; Commarato *et al.*, 1973). A substantial amount of drug can be metabolized during its first circulation through the liver.

Routes of Administration. *Sublingual Administration.* The sublingual route of administration of organic nitrates is rational and effective for the treatment of acute attacks of angina pectoris. Most of the drug bypasses the hepatic circulation initially, since only about 15% of the cardiac output is delivered to the liver. A transient but effective concentration of drug appears in the circulation. One expects and finds little difference in the *duration* of action of the various nitrates when relatively small doses are taken sublingually, since the metabolic capacity is high. Under this condition, their half-lives depend only on the rate at which they are delivered to the liver. Indeed, when equieffective doses of nitroglycerin and isosorbide dinitrate are given sublingually, there is no significant difference in their duration of action; effects on exercise tolerance wane with a half-time of about 20 minutes (Goldstein *et al.*, 1971). Pentaerythritol trinitrate and erythrityl tetranitrate are also able to prolong exercise tolerance and prevent depression of the S-T segment in the ECG when administered sublingually to patients with typical angina (Klaus *et al.*, 1973). However, the duration of action of these agents is also short when they are given in this way (10 to 45 minutes). *Thus, the sublingual administration of organic nitrates is most appropriate to alleviate acute attacks of angina and for the immediate prophylaxis of such attacks.*

Oral Administration. Organic nitrates have been administered orally in an attempt to provide convenient and prolonged prophylaxis against attacks of angina. The effectiveness of such administration was controversial until dosages were adjusted so that active drug would reach the systemic circulation.

The efficacy of *low doses* of organic nitrates (*e.g.*, 5 mg of isosorbide dinitrate) given orally for prophylaxis of angina is questionable (*see* Freis, 1970; Aronow, 1975). A review of 59 studies wherein low doses of oral nitrates were administered demonstrated that the majority of the investigations failed to include adequate controls, crossover protocols, double-blind design, and valid statistical analysis (Stipe and Fink, 1973). When only properly designed investigations were evaluated, oral nitrates were usually no more effective than placebos.

High doses of nitrates given orally can cause a small decrease in arterial blood pressure, a substantial decrease in left ventricular filling pressure, and an increase in the exercise tolerance of patients with angina (Franciosa *et al.,* 1974; Kasparian *et al.,* 1975; Willis *et al.,* 1976). High doses of isosorbide dinitrate (30 mg orally, given four times daily) produce sustained hemodynamic and antianginal effects (Danahy and Aronow, 1977; Danahy *et al.,* 1977). The hemodynamic effects that are observed after large doses of nitrates are swallowed likely result because of saturation of the capacity of the liver to denitrate the intact molecule. The active agent can thus reach the systemic circulation. Under these circumstances the activities of less potent metabolites may also contribute to the therapeutic effect. Chronic oral administration of isosorbide dinitrate (120 to 720 mg daily) has resulted in persistence of the parent compound and higher concentrations of metabolites in plasma (Shane *et al.,* 1978). However, such high doses are more likely to cause troublesome side effects and tolerance (*see* below; Danahy and Aronow, 1977).

Older work suggested prolonged pharmacological actions resulting from the oral administration of nitroglycerin, and a recent clinical trial has demonstrated significant, prolonged (up to 4 hours) improvement of exercise tolerance in patients with angina pectoris who are given a sustained-release oral form of nitroglycerin (Winsor and Berger, 1975). High doses (6.5 mg) of nitroglycerin are required to elicit prolonged hemodynamic responses (Blumenthal *et al.,* 1977).

Nitroglycerin Ointment. The topical administration of nitroglycerin in an ointment has been used to provide gradual absorption of the drug for prolonged prophylactic purposes. Patients with angina who used 2% nitroglycerin ointment (average dose of 5 mg) experienced improved and prolonged exercise capacity and showed decreased ischemic S-T segment changes in the ECG (Reichek *et al.,* 1974). Higher doses of ointment (equivalent to 15 mg) reduce arterial pressure and decrease left ventricular end-diastolic pressure (Parker *et al.,* 1976).

Tolerance. Sublingual organic nitrates are usually taken by the patient at the time of an anginal attack or in anticipation of exercise or stress. Such intermittent treatment results in reproducible cardiovascular effects. However, frequently repeated exposure to high doses of organic nitrates leads to a decrease in the magnitude of most of the pharmacological effects of these agents (*see* Needleman and Johnson, 1975). The therapeutic significance of this phenomenon is likely to increase as the oral administration of higher doses of organic nitrates becomes more prevalent. For example, the chronic oral use of isosorbide dinitrate (120 mg per day) led to the development of partial tolerance to the hemodynamic effects of the drug (Danahy and Aronow, 1977) and to cross-tolerance to the venodilatation produced by sublingual nitroglycerin (Zelis and Mason, 1975).

A special aspect of tolerance has been observed among individuals exposed to nitroglycerin in the manufacture of explosives. If protection is inadequate, workers may experience severe headaches, dizziness, and postural weakness during the first several days of employment. Tolerance then develops, but headache and other symptoms may reappear after a few days away from the job, the "Monday disease." The most serious effect of chronic exposure is a form of *organic nitrate dependence.* Individuals without demonstrable organic vascular disease have died suddenly or developed myocardial infarctions after a few days' break in chronic exposure, and there are now well-documented cases with typical subjective and objective findings of severe myocardial ischemia, relieved by nitroglycerin, during withdrawal from chronic exposure to an organic nitrate. Coronary and digital arteriospasm during withdrawal and its relaxation by nitroglycerin have also been demonstrated radiographically (*see* Lange *et al.,* 1972).

The mechanism of initiation and maintenance of tolerance to these drugs is due neither to an alteration of the biotransformation of organic nitrates nor to changes in sympathetic function. When blood vessels are removed from animals that have been made tolerant to organic nitrates, they too are hyposensitive to the effects of the agents, suggesting alteration in a specific vascular receptor. Of interest, exposure of vessels made tolerant either *in vivo* or *in vitro* to the disulfide reducing agent dithiothreitol restores sensitivity to the relaxant effect of nitroglycerin (Needleman and Johnson, 1975).

Toxicity and Untoward Responses. Untoward responses to the therapeutic use of organic nitrates are almost all secondary to actions on the cardiovascular system. *Headache* is common and can be severe. It usually decreases over a few days if treatment is continued, and often can be controlled by decreasing the dose. Transient episodes of *dizziness, weakness,* and other manifestations of the cerebral ischemia associated with *postural hypotension* may develop occasionally in many patients, particularly if standing immobile, and may occasionally progress to loss of consciousness. This reaction appears to be accentuated by alcohol. Even in the most severe nitrate syncope, positioning and other procedures to facilitate venous return are the only therapeutic measures required. It was widely believed that nitrates can increase intraocular pressure and precipitate glaucoma, but this fear appears to be completely unfounded (Whitworth and Grant, 1964). Drug *rash* is occasionally produced by all the organic nitrates, but it appears to occur most commonly with pentaerythritol tetranitrate.

Preparations and Dosage. Data for the nitrites and organic nitrates available for clinical use are given in Table 33–1. Sodium nitrite is obsolete except as an intravenous solution for use in the treatment of cyanide poisoning (*see* Chapter 70). Amyl nitrite acts very rapidly after inhalation and is occasionally used for very brief effects. Nitroglycerin is sufficiently unstable and volatile for the tablets to lose activity rapidly unless kept in a tightly sealed, dark-tinted glass container (without a cotton plug); plastic is unsatisfactory. Active tablets should produce a distinct burning sensation when placed under the tongue. Only nitroglycerin, erythrityl tetranitrate, and isosorbide dinitrate are available in sublingual tablets. Trolnitrate, which is irritant, and pentaerythritol tetranitrate, which has a very low aqueous solubility, cannot be administered sublingually.

THERAPEUTIC USES

Angina. Diseases that predispose to angina should be treated as part of a comprehensive therapeutic program. Such conditions as hypertension, anemia, thyrotoxicosis, obesity, heart failure, and chronic and acute anxiety can precipitate anginal symptoms in many patients. The patient should be asked to stop smoking, overeating, or exercising shortly after meals, and he should avoid exposure to certain sympathomimetic agents (*e.g.*, those used in nasal decongestants) that increase myocardial oxygen demand. The use of drugs that modify the perception of pain is a poor approach to the treatment of angina, since the underlying myocardial ischemia is not relieved.

Sublingual Administration. Because of its rapid action, long-established efficacy, and low cost, nitroglycerin is the most useful drug among the organic nitrates that can be given sublingually. An initial dose of 0.3 mg of nitroglycerin will often relieve pain within 3 minutes. Pain may be prevented when the drug is used prophylactically immediately prior to exercise or stress. The smallest effective dose should be prescribed. Patients should be taught to contact their physicians when more than three tablets taken over a 15-minute period do not relieve a sustained attack, since this situation may be indicative of myocardial infarction. The patient should be advised that there is no virtue in trying to avoid taking the sublingual nitroglycerin tablets for anginal pain; tolerance to the therapeutic effectiveness does not arise from proper intermittent usage (Cohn and Gorlin, 1974; Aronow, 1976).

Other nitrates that can be taken sublingually do not appear to be longer acting or more effective than nitroglycerin. They are often more expensive (Goldstein *et al.,* 1971; Aronow, 1976).

Oral Administration. Oral nitrates employed at usual dose (*e.g.,* 5 to 10 mg of isosorbide dinitrate) are no more effective than placebo in decreasing the frequency of angina or increasing the patient's exercise tolerance. Clinical studies that have used higher doses either of isosorbide dinitrate (*e.g.,* 20 mg or more orally every 4 hours) or sustained-release preparations of nitroglycerin (Winsor and Berger, 1975) indicate that such regimens decrease the frequency of attacks of angina, improve exercise tolerance, and favorably alter the determinants of myocardial oxygen demand. However, these high doses increase the risk of hypotension, tachycardia, and tolerance.

Topical Administration. Application of nitroglycerin ointment can relieve angina for up to 4 hours. Usually 2% nitroglycerin ointment is applied to the skin (2.5 to 5 cm [1 to 2 in.] as it is squeezed from the tube; it is then spread in a uniform layer); the dosage must be adjusted for each patient. The drug is well absorbed through the skin and produces hemodynamic effects within 15 minutes. The ointment is particularly useful for controlling nocturnal angina, which commonly develops within 3 hours after the patient goes to sleep.

Congestive Heart Failure. The goal of treatment of congestive heart failure is to increase cardiac output and reduce pulmonary and peripheral edema. Conventional therapy of heart failure involves the use of positive inotropic agents and diuretics (*see* Chapters 30 and 36). Vasodilators can improve cardiovascular function in congestive heart failure, even in some patients who are unresponsive to conventional therapy (*see* Symposium, 1978b). The acceptance of these drugs for the treatment of acute, refractory congestive failure has been aided by the development of bedside technics that allow fre-

Table 33–1. ORGANIC NITRATES AVAILABLE FOR CLINICAL USE

NONPROPRIETARY NAME AND TRADE NAMES	CHEMICAL STRUCTURE	PREPARATIONS *	DOSES AND ROUTES OF ADMINISTRATION
Amyl Nitrite, U.S.P. (isoamyl nitrite; VAPOROLE)	H_3C $\quad$CHCH$_2$CH$_2$ONO H_3C	P: 0.18, 0.3 ml	0.18 or 0.3 ml, inhalation
Nitroglycerin, U.S.P. (glyceryl trinitrate; NITRO-BID, NITROL, NITROSTAT, others)	H_2C—O—NO_2 HC—O—NO_2 H_2C—O—NO_2	T: 0.15, 0.3, 0.4, 0.6 mg C: 1.3, 2.5, 6.5, 9 mg O: 2%	0.15 to 0.6 mg 2.5 to 6.5 mg every 12 hr 1.25 to 5 cm (1/2 to 2 in.), topical to skin, every 4 hr
Isosorbide Dinitrate, U.S.P. (ISORDIL, LASERDIL, SORBITRATE, others)		T: 2.5, 5 mg T(C): 5, 10 mg T(O): 5, 10, 20 mg C: 40 mg	2.5 to 10 mg 5 to 10 mg every 2 to 3 hr 5 to 30 mg every 6 hr 40 mg every 6 to 12 hr
Erythrityl Tetranitrate, U.S.P. (CARDILATE)	H_2C—O—NO_2 HC—O—NO_2 HC—O—NO_2 H_2C—O—NO_2	T: 5, 10, 15 mg T(C): 10 mg	5 to 15 mg 30 to 90 mg every 8 hr
Pentaerythritol Tetranitrate, U.S.P. (DUOTRATE, PENTRITOL, PERITRATE, others)	O_2N—O—$H_2C\quad CH_2$—O—NO_2 C O_2N—O—$H_2C\quad CH_2$—O—NO_2	T(O): 10, 20, 40 mg C: 30, 45, 60, 80 mg	10 to 40 mg every 6 hr 30 to 80 mg every 12 hr
Mannitol hexanitrate (NITRANITOL)	H_2C—O—NO_2 O_2N—O—CH O_2N—O—CH HC—O—NO_2 HC—O—NO_2 H_2C—O—NO_2	Available only in fixed-dose combination.	

* P = pearl; T = tablet for sublingual use; C = sustained-release capsule; O = ointment; T(C) = chewable tablet; T(O) = oral tablet.

quent measurement of ventricular filling pressure and cardiac output. Thus, the effects of the drug have been objectively evaluated, and their doses and intervals of administration have been optimized (at least in some individuals) for the ability to improve left ventricular performance. Initial use of vasodilators (Burch, 1956; Johnson *et al.*, 1957) was aimed at reduction of preload by producing venodilatation, which reduced end-diastolic pressure and relieved pulmonary congestion. The utility of reduction of afterload (by dilatation of arterioles and reduction of peripheral resistance) to increase cardiac output has been described more recently (Majid *et al.*, 1971; Franciosa *et al.*, 1972).

The response of the cardiovascular system to vas-

odilators is different in patients with congestive failure than in normal individuals. In a normal subject the administration of a vasodilator produces venodilatation, which decreases preload and results in decreased cardiac output. The drugs also reduce afterload, which causes only a small increase in stroke volume. The net effect of vasodilators in a normal individual is a marked decrease in blood pressure and tachycardia.

Patients with congestive heart failure have elevated peripheral vascular resistance due to compensatory increases in adrenergic tone. This acts to maintain blood pressure and redistribute blood flow to vital organs, despite low cardiac output. Arteriolar resistance may be elevated to a degree that is greater than optimal to maintain maximal cardiac output (Ross, 1976). Drugs that reduce peripheral resistance in patients with congestive heart failure significantly increase the ejection fraction, stroke volume, cardiac output, and tissue perfusion. The increases in cardiac output may counterbalance the fall in peripheral resistance, and little or no change in the patient's blood pressure and heart rate may occur. If the reduction of preload is excessive (to below-normal levels), the cardiac output will fall. The hemodynamic effects of the drugs must, therefore, be monitored carefully. When this is done, the treatment can be individualized so that preload and afterload are appropriately reduced and cardiac output is increased in the face of a net reduction of myocardial oxygen demand. The use of conventional positive inotropic agents may allow a similar increase in cardiac output, but at the cost of increased consumption of oxygen.

The vasodilators most widely studied in the treatment of congestive heart failure are the organic nitrates (primarily nitroglycerin), nitroprusside (Chapter 32), and, to a lesser degree, the α-adrenergic antagonist phentolamine. Each drug produces a distinct pattern of vasodilatation (Miller et al., 1976). The organic nitrates primarily reduce preload and may relieve pulmonary congestion with only modest effects on cardiac output. Nitroprusside, administered intravenously, produces comparable dilation of both the arterial and venous beds. It thus can increase cardiac output significantly while relieving pulmonary congestion. Infusion of phentolamine has a greater effect on arteriolar than on venous tone; its ability to increase cardiac output is greater than its effect to lower diastolic filling pressure. Phentolamine also tends to cause tachycardia (Chatterjee and Parmley, 1977). Of the three types of agents, nitroprusside is the most widely used in patients with reduced cardiac output associated with elevated end-diastolic pressure (Miller et al., 1976).

The abrupt withdrawal of an infusion of nitroprusside from patients with severe chronic heart failure may be associated with a rebound in hemodynamic effects that produce a transient deterioration in cardiac performance. Presumably, this is due to the activation of baroreceptor reflexes, and its magnitude is related to the degree of preservation of compensatory vasoconstrictive mechanisms in individual patients (Packer et al., 1979).

The utility of the *chronic administration* of vasodilators for the treatment of congestive heart failure is not yet defined (Chatterjee and Parmley, 1977). Organic nitrates can be used orally, but this form of therapy suffers from their short duration and unreliable degree of effect. While such use may alleviate dyspnea, the drugs are relatively ineffective in increasing cardiac output substantially. *Hydralazine*, which is primarily an arteriolar dilator, can increase cardiac output when administered orally; it causes only slight changes in blood pressure or heart rate in patients with chronic congestive failure (Chatterjee et al., 1978). Orally administered *prazosin*, which appears to function primarily as an α-adrenergic antagonist, acts on both arterial and venous beds and more closely mimics the effects of parenteral nitroprusside. Moderately long-term treatment with

prazosin has resulted in sustained improvement in symptoms and exercise tolerance in patients with chronic congestive heart failure (Aronow et al., 1977, Awan et al., 1978). A similar response has been obtained with *captopril*, which blocks the conversion of angiotensin I to angiotensin II (*see* Chapter 27). Although these findings are encouraging, large-scale, controlled clinical trials will have to be performed to determine the duration of beneficial effects, the incidence of side effects, and the impact of such a mode of therapy on morbidity and mortality from this common disorder.

Myocardial Infarction. Some therapeutic maneuvers are directed at reducing the size of a myocardial infarction and preserving or retrieving viable tissue by reducing the oxygen demand of the myocardium. A drug that favorably alters the oxygen balance could decrease the area of myocardial damage if it were given soon after infarction.

In the past, nitroglycerin was considered to be contraindicated for use in patients with acute myocardial infarction. Its ability to induce hypotension and trigger a reflex tachycardia was feared. However, when the effects of nitroglycerin were carefully monitored, they were found to decrease left ventricular filling pressure, thus relieving pulmonary congestion in patients with heart failure following acute myocardial infarction (Gold et al., 1972). Since the effects of sublingual nitroglycerin are transient, investigators have tested the usefulness of intravenous infusions of the drug. This route allows precise control of dosage for long periods, and sudden and profound falls in arterial pressure can be avoided. When the dose is adjusted such that tachycardia does not occur, intravenous nitroglycerin can reduce the elevation of the S-T segment that follows acute coronary occlusion in both normal dogs and in those with preexisting multivessel coronary occlusive disease (Epstein et al., 1975). Furthermore, simultaneous administration of α-adrenergic agonists (methoxamine or phenylephrine) apparently can selectively eliminate the *arterial* vasodilatation and tachycardia produced by nitroglycerin. The combination of α-adrenergic agonist and nitroglycerin also appears to increase the threshold for ventricular fibrillation. Other vasodilators, such as nitroprusside or phentolamine, have been tested for their capacity to diminish ischemic injury but appear to have no advantage over nitroglycerin. The frequency of elevation of the S-T segment during acute coronary occlusion in dogs was reduced by nitroglycerin but increased by nitroprusside, and regional coronary blood flow was increased by nitroglycerin but reduced by nitroprusside (Chiariello et al., 1976). Furthermore, nitroglycerin is more effective than nitroprusside in reducing coronary collateral resistance, whereas phentolamine may have a deleterious effect (Capurro et al., 1977).

Intravenous infusion of nitroglycerin in patients with acute myocardial infarction at doses that maintain or improve stroke work can relieve pulmonary congestion by decreasing left ventricular filling pressure; there is also a reduction of myocardial oxygen demand (Flaherty et al., 1975). Additional clinical evidence demonstrates that nitroglycerin can decrease the electrophysiological signs of ischemic injury in patients with acute myocardial infarction. Nevertheless, considerable additional experience with larger experimental groups and with careful monitoring of hemodynamic parameters is required to define the utility of organic nitrates in myocardial infarction. At the moment, there is no convincing evidence that would favor the combined use of vasodilators plus α-adrenergic agonists for this purpose.

Variant (Prinzmetal's) Angina. Numerous studies of experimental animals have demonstrated that coronary blood flow can be modulated by stimulation of the adrenergic receptors of the large coronary arteries. These vessels normally contribute little to coronary resistance. However, neurogenic stimulation of the large vessels may cause marked coronary constriction, resulting in reduced blood flow and ischemic pain. Variant angina is now believed to be the result of coronary vasospasm, possibly resulting from neurogenic α-adrenergic stimulation; this may occur in the presence or absence of atherosclerotic coronary artery disease (Hillis and Braunwald, 1978). Ergonovine maleate, a vasoconstrictor (*see* Chapter 39), has been utilized intravenously during coronary arteriography as a provocative diagnostic test to induce coronary artery vasospasm and identify patients with variant angina (Heupler *et al.,* 1978). Ergonovine-induced coronary artery spasm is reversed by nitroglycerin.

Variant angina that occurs as a result of coronary artery spasm is quickly relieved by nitroglycerin. However, β-adrenergic blockade, which is beneficial in patients with typical angina, may be detrimental for patients with variant angina. This may result from the unopposed action of norepinephrine at α-adrenergic receptors, with resultant coronary vasoconstriction. α-Adrenergic blocking agents (*e.g.,* phenoxybenzamine or phentolamine) have been reported to be beneficial in patients with variant angina, as have perhexilene and the calcium antagonists verapamil and nifedipine (Hillis and Braunwald, 1978).

OTHER ANTIANGINAL AGENTS

PROPRANOLOL

The β-adrenergic antagonist *propranolol* (*see* Chapter 9) is effective in reducing the severity and frequency of attacks of typical angina pectoris. Conversely, it may worsen variant angina caused by coronary vasospasm. When propranolol alleviates the symptoms of angina, it reduces the requirement for nitroglycerin by decreasing myocardial oxygen consumption at rest and during exercise or stress (Hamer and Sowton, 1966; Elliott and Stone, 1969). The cardioprotective actions of propranolol include a negative chronotropic effect (especially during exercise), a decreased inotropic state, and

a minor depression of arterial pressure. All these effects can lessen cardiac demand for oxygen (Epstein and Braunwald, 1968). However, not all the actions of propranolol are beneficial. The decrease in cardiac contractility caused by propranolol tends to increase left ventricular end-diastolic pressure and thereby increase ventricular dilatation; this, in turn, can increase myocardial consumption of oxygen (Parker *et al.,* 1968). Fortunately, the concomitant reductions in heart rate and arterial pressure apparently negate this potentially deleterious effect.

Propranolol is readily absorbed from the gastrointestinal tract and is largely metabolized in the liver. Its availability to the systemic circulation can thus be restricted in the same way as is that of an orally administered organic nitrate (*see* Chapter 9). Clearance of propranolol is a direct function of hepatic blood flow, and the half-life of the drug is prolonged in patients with hepatic disease or congestive heart failure.

The dosage of propranolol required to reduce the number and severity of anginal attacks is highly variable and must be adjusted to the requirements of the individual. The initial dose is usually 10 mg, given three or four times daily. The dosage may be increased gradually at 3- to 7-day intervals, as needed, to control symptoms. For maintenance, most patients require 160 to 240 mg (or more) daily in four divided doses. Nitrates, administered sublingually, should be continued as needed. Long-term studies indicate that tolerance does not develop to the therapeutic effects of propranolol. However, abrupt discontinuation of chronic therapy with propranolol can cause a rebound increase in the frequency of angina and may even precipitate myocardial infarction. This untoward reaction, which could be due to the development of supersensitivity during the course of therapy, can be avoided by gradual withdrawal of the drug. Since the half-life of propranolol varies from 3 to 6 hours, intervals between doses should be maintained while individual doses are reduced over a period of 1 to 2 weeks.

The combined use of propranolol and organic nitrates can be very effective in the treatment of typical angina. Some of the negative aspects of the effects of each drug are reduced. For example, the reflex tachycardia and increased contractility induced by nitrates are blocked by propranolol, whereas the increased ventricular size, filling pressure, and end-diastolic pressure caused by β-adrenergic antagonists are opposed by the action of the nitrates (Russek, 1968).

Untoward effects of β-adrenergic blockade include cardiac complications, such as severe bradycardia and precipitation of congestive heart failure. β-Adrenergic blockade of pulmonary smooth muscle may cause bronchial constriction and precipitate asthma in susceptible individuals (Aronow, 1976). This and certain other side effects of propranolol may be avoided by the use of β_1-specific agents such as *metoprolol*. For a detailed consideration of the actions, side effects, and other uses of β-adrenergic antagonists, *see* Chapter 9.

PERHEXILENE

Perhexilene maleate (2-[2,2-dicyclohexylethyl]piperidine maleate; PEXID) is used in Europe and elsewhere as an antianginal agent and is under investigation in the United States. Many studies indicate that perhexilene (200 to 400 mg per day) reduces the number and severity of anginal attacks in patients with coronary artery disease (*see* Symposium, 1973, 1978a). Some patients who do not respond to other modes of therapy may respond favorably to perhexilene. However, the role of perhexilene in the treatment of angina is not yet clearly defined. Since the drug has neither bronchoconstrictor nor β-adrenergic blocking activity, it represents an alternative to propranolol in patients with left ventricular insufficiency or asthma.

Although the molecular mechanism of action of perhexilene is not fully understood, it behaves like a "calcium antagonist," similar to *verapamil* or *nifedipine* (*see* review by Fleckenstein, 1977). Calcium antagonists inhibit excitation-contraction coupling in myocardial and smooth muscle by blocking the transmembrane carrier of calcium. This results in decreased myocardial contractility and in vasodilatation. The relative effects of perhexilene on the coronary vasculature and on contractility are such that, in isolated hearts, coronary blood flow can increase greatly at doses that have little effect on contractility (Klaus and Güttler, 1978). In preparations *in vitro,* automaticity of ventricular pacemakers is reduced, but effects on atrial pacemakers are minimal. These effects are consistent with clinical studies, which show that perhexilene reduces ectopic ventricular electrical activity (Drake *et al.,* 1973; Sukerman, 1973).

The absorption, distribution, and excretion of perhexilene have not been studied thoroughly. Perhexilene is reported to be well absorbed, and it is metabolized to hydroxylated derivatives. The half-life of perhexilene and its metabolites in plasma is 2 to 6 days, but in some individuals this value may exceed 30 days. Hence, a considerable period of time is required for maximal concentrations and effects of a given dosage regimen of perhexilene (and metabolites) to be reached.

Mechanism of Antianginal Action. The antianginal effect of perhexilene appears to involve several aspects of the mechanisms previously discussed for nitrates and propranolol. The drug causes a decrease in exercise-induced tachycardia, a redistribution of coronary blood flow toward ischemic areas of the myocardium, decreased ventricular filling pressures, and, possibly, metabolic effects that are conducive to better utilization of oxygen by the myocardium. Perhexilene does not alter the resting heart rate, blood pressure, or total coronary blood flow. However, tachycardia and increases in ventricular filling pressures in response to exercise are reduced in patients with angina without affecting myocardial function. Patients treated with perhexilene tolerate higher heart rates (induced by pacing) before onset of pain or prior to depression of the S-T segment of the ECG (Pepine *et al.,* 1974). Increases in exercise tolerance are associated with increased oxygen utilization, suggesting improved delivery of oxygen to ischemic myocardium. In ischemic canine myocardium, perhexilene (infused at low concentrations into the pulmonary artery) causes a redistribution of blood flow to the subendocardium relative to the subepicardium and an enhanced utilization of lactate (Klassen *et al.,* 1976).

Adverse Effects. Both minor and serious untoward effects are associated with the use of perhexilene. Dizziness, insomnia, anorexia, and gastrointestinal upsets are frequent. These side effects often subside as the use of the drug is continued. Many patients complain of generalized weakness, which is dose related. Hypoglycemic episodes, occasionally serious, have been reported and may be associated with abnormalities of insulin secretion (Luccioni *et al.,* 1978). Polyuria is occasionally observed. Significant weight loss is often reported by patients taking perhexilene; the mechanism of this effect is not understood. Hepatotoxicity and neuropathy are more serious toxicities associated with perhexilene. About 20% of patients develop elevations of serum transaminase and lactate dehydrogenase activities, which reverse when the drug is discontinued. Serious neuropathies also have been reported (Bourrat *et al.,* 1975; Said, 1978). The signs and symptoms of neuropathy usually appear after more than a year of treatment with low doses of perhexilene (200 mg per day), but they may be seen earlier when higher doses are used (400 mg per day). Patients first complain of paresthesias and pain in the lower limbs. The protein content of the spinal fluid is often increased. Papilledema may be present. If treatment is continued, severe sensorimotor neuropathy may occur. The symptoms and morphological alterations associated with the neuropathy reverse when the drug is discontinued. The incidence of clinically significant neuropathies is not established, but it is relatively rare. It appears more commonly in those patients with slower rates of metabolism of perhexilene (Singlas *et al.,* 1978). (For detailed discussion of the basic and clinical pharmacology of perhexilene, *see* Symposium, 1973 and 1978a.)

DIPYRIDAMOLE

Dipyridamole (2,6-*bis*-[diethanolamino]-4,8-dipiperidinopyrimido-[5,4-*d*]-pyrimidine) is similar to papaverine in many of its pharmacological properties (*see* below). In therapeutic doses, dipyridamole usually produces only slight alteration of systemic blood pressure or peripheral blood flow. The drug does decrease coronary vascular resistance and increases coronary blood flow and oxygen tension in coronary sinus blood. However, dipyridamole appears to act predominantly on small resistance vessels of the coronary bed, and it alters transcapillary exchange in the same way as does severe hypoxemia. Thus, it appears to have little effect on vascular resistance in ischemic areas where small vessels are already maximally dilated.

The actions of dipyridamole seem to be linked, at least in part, to the metabolism and transport of adenosine and adenine nucleotides; in particular, dipyridamole inhibits the uptake of adenosine by erythrocytes and other cells. Adenosine, which is released from the hypoxic myocardium, is a coronary vasodilator and appears to be an important signal for the autoregulation of coronary blood flow.

In the doses usually employed clinically, dipyridamole is quite nontoxic. Gastrointestinal intolerance with nausea, vomiting, and diarrhea occurs occasionally, as do headache and vertigo. Excessive doses can cause peripheral vasodilatation and hypotension.

Dipyridamole has been used predominantly for the prophylaxis of *angina pectoris*. Although many conflicting observations have been reported, there is no convincing evidence that either acute or chronic administration decreases the frequency or severity of anginal attacks. There is no improvement of performance during standardized exercise tolerance tests. The effects of dipyridamole on platelets are described in Chapter 58.

Dipyridamole (PERSANTINE) is available in 25-mg tablets. The recommended dosage is 50 mg three times daily, taken at least 1 hour before meals.

VASODILATORS IN THE TREATMENT OF VASCULAR INSUFFICIENCY

Vasodilator drugs have been used in an attempt to increase peripheral blood flow to areas where perfusion is compromised by acute or chronic arterial obstruction or vasospasm. The drugs that have been used can be divided into agents that interfere with adrenergically mediated vasoconstriction (Chapter 9) and drugs that directly dilate vascular smooth muscle, such as *papaverine, isoxsuprine, nylidrin, cyclandelate,* and *niacin derivatives.* The pharmacological properties of this latter group are described briefly below and in more detail in *earlier editions* of this textbook.

Despite the fact that these drugs continue to be promoted and widely prescribed for the treatment of chronic occlusive vascular diseases of skeletal muscle (arteriosclerosis obliterans, thromboangiitis obliterans), there is no acceptable evidence that they are efficacious (*see* review by Coffman, 1975; Medical Letter, 1978; Coffman, 1979). Likewise, the utility of vasodilators in reversing or delaying the deleterious effects of acute or chronic cerebrovascular insufficiency is controversial, and the case for clinical efficacy is unimpressive. Direct-acting vasodilators can increase blood flow in normal resting skeletal muscle and in brain. However, it is unlikely that any vasodilator drug can significantly increase blood flow distal to a physical occlusion. Autoregulatory mechanisms in skeletal muscle and cerebral vascular beds produce dilatation in response to ischemia; hence vasodilators will increase blood flow primarily to nonischemic areas.

Vasospastic conditions affecting cutaneous circulation (*e.g.,* Raynaud's syndrome) may be responsive to α-adrenergic antagonists, but drug therapy is usually reserved for the most severe cases.

Papaverine. Papaverine (6,7-dimethoxy-1-veratrylisoquinoline) is an alkaloid present to the extent of about 1% in crude opium. It is, however, unrelated chemically or pharmacologically to the opioid alkaloids. Papaverine is a nonspecific smooth muscle relaxant. It can relax all smooth muscle structures *in vitro,* irrespective of the agent used to induce tone in the preparation. As with all musculotropic smooth muscle relaxants, the molecular mechanism of action is not known. It has been suggested that vasodilatation is related to its ability to inhibit cyclic nucleotide phosphodiesterase, an action for which it has been widely used as an experimental tool. Papaverine is capable of producing arteriolar dilatation in the systemic, coronary, and cerebral circulations. Large doses can depress A-V nodal and intraventricular conduction and produce arrhythmias. These direct effects on the myocardium are seen only after parenteral administration of high doses.

As described above, papaverine has not been demonstrated to be of therapeutic value in any condition. Furthermore, at least some of the widely promoted sustained-release preparations produce very low and erratic concentrations in blood when compared to conventional preparations (Arnold et al., 1977). Side effects associated with the use of papaverine include facial flushing, tachycardia, drowsiness, and gastrointestinal symptoms. Papaverine also frequently causes elevation of the activities of alkaline phosphatase and transaminases in plasma, indicative of hepatic toxicity (Ronnov-Jensen and Tjerlund, 1969; Driemen, 1973).

Papaverine Hydrochloride, U.S.P., is marketed in tablets (30 to 200 mg), sustained-release capsules (150, 200, and 300 mg), and an elixir (100 mg/15 ml), and as a 3% solution for injection. Despite lack of proof of efficacy, the compound is sold under more than 40 trade names, indicative of the extent of promotion of such products. The recommended dose is 100 to 300 mg, taken three to five times daily. *Dioxyline phosphate* is a synthetic derivative of papaverine; *ethaverine* is also closely related to papaverine and has similar actions.

Cyclandelate. *Cyclandelate* (3,3,5-trimethylcyclo-hexyl mandelate, CYCLOSPASMOL, others) is a musculotropic vasodilator; although quite different chemically, it appears to exert actions similar to those of papaverine (Bijlsma *et al.*, 1956). However, its pharmacological properties are scantily characterized. Cyclandelate appears to be a more potent vasodilator *in vitro* than is papaverine. As with the other vasodilators, reports in the literature are contradictory, and the therapeutic value of cyclandelate has never been convincingly demonstrated for any condition.

Cyclandelate is available in tablets (100 mg) and capsules (200 and 400 mg). Side effects include flushing, tachycardia, headache, a feeling of weakness, and gastrointestinal symptoms. The usual dose of cyclandelate is 100 to 200 mg, taken four times daily.

Isoxsuprine. Isoxsuprine is similar chemically to the sympathomimetic amines and has often been described as a β-adrenergic agonist. However, the drug appears to act as a musculotropic vasodilator, and its effects are not blocked by propranolol (Manley and Lawson, 1968). Objective studies do not support the use of this drug in obstructive arterial disease or in any other condition.

Isoxsuprine Hydrochloride, U.S.P. (VASODILAN, others), is available in 10- and 20-mg tablets and as an injection (5 mg/ml). The usual oral dose is 10 to 20 mg, taken three or four times daily. Side effects include hypotension, tachycardia, nausea, vomiting, dizziness, abdominal distress, and severe rash.

Nylidrin. The vasodilator activity of this compound appears to be a combination of direct musculotropic and β-adrenergic agonistic activity. It has been and is used in a variety of vascular disorders without proof of efficacy. Side effects include dizziness, weakness, palpitations, trembling, nervousness, and vomiting. *Nylidrin Hydrochloride*, U.S.P. (ARLIDIN, others), is available in 6- and 12-mg tablets. The usual dose is 3 to 12 mg, taken three or four times daily.

Nicotinic Acid and Nicotinyl Alcohol. These drugs (*see* Chapters 34 and 66) produce more dilatation of the vessels of the blush areas than of the extremities. There is no consistent increase in skin or muscle blood flow in patients with obstructive vascular disease. There is no basis for the use of these agents in such conditions, despite their promotion for this purpose.

Arnold, J. D.; Baldridge, J.; Riley, B.; and Brody, G. Papaverine hydrochloride: the evaluation of two new dosage forms. *Int. J. Clin. Pharmacol. Biopharm.*, **1977**, *15*, 230–233.

Aronow, W. S. Treatment of angina pectoris: pharmacologic approaches. *Postgrad. Med.*, **1976**, *60*, 100–106.

Aronow, W. S.; Greenfield, R. S.; Alimadadian, H.; and Danahy, D. T. Effect of the vasodilator trimazosin versus placebo on exercise performance in chronic left ventricular failure. *Am. J. Cardiol.*, **1977**, *40*, 789–793.

Awan, N. A.; Miller, R. R.; Miller, M. P.; Specht, K.; Vera, Z.; and Mason, D. T. Clinical pharmacology and therapeutic application of prazosin in acute and chronic refractory congestive heart failure: balanced systemic venous and arterial dilation improving pulmonary congestion and cardiac output. *Am. J. Med.*, **1978**, *65*, 146–154.

Becker, L. C.; Fortuin, N. J.; and Pitt, B. Effect of ischemia and antianginal drugs on the distribution of radioactive microspheres in the canine left ventricle. *Circ. Res.*, **1971**, *28*, 263–269.

Bijlsma, U. G.; Funcke, A. B. H.; Tersteege, H. M.; Rekker, R. F.; Ernsting, M. J. E.; and Nauta, W. T. The pharmacology of CYCLOSPASMOL. *Arch. Int. Pharmacodyn. Ther.*, **1956**, *105*, 145–174.

Blumenthal, H. P.; Fung, H. L.; McNiff, E. F.; and Yap, S. K. Plasma nitroglycerin levels after sublingual, oral and topical administration. *Br. J. Clin. Pharmacol.*, **1977**, *4*, 241–242.

Bogaert, M. G., and Rosseel, M. T. Plasma levels in man of nitroglycerin after buccal administration. *J. Pharm. Pharmacol.*, **1972**, *24*, 737–738.

Bourrat, C.; Viala, J. J.; and Guastala, J. P. Neuropathie périphérique après absorption prolongée de maléate de perhexiline. *Nouv. Presse Med.*, **1975**, *4*, 2528.

Burch, G. E. Evidence for increased venous tone in chronic congestive heart failure. *Arch. Intern. Med.*, **1956**, *98*, 750–766.

Capurro, N. L.; Kent, K. M.; and Epstein, S. E. Comparison of nitroglycerin-, nitroprusside-, and phentolamine-induced changes in coronary collateral function in dogs. *J. Clin. Invest.*, **1977**, *60*, 295–301.

Chasseaud, L. F.; Down, W. H.; and Grundy, R. K. Concentrations of the vasodilator isosorbide dinitrate and its metabolites in the blood of human subjects. *Eur. J. Clin. Pharmacol.*, **1975**, *8*, 157–160.

Chatterjee, K.; Massie, B.; Rubin, S.; Gelberg, H.; Brundage, B. H.; and Ports, T. A. Long-term vasodilator therapy of congestive heart failure: consideration of agents at rest and during exercise. *Am. J. Med.*, **1978**, *65*, 134–145.

Chiariello, M.; Gold, H. K.; Leinbach, R. C.; Davis, M. A.; and Maroko, P. R. Comparison between the effects of nitroprusside and nitroglycerin on ischemic injury during acute myocardial ischemia. *Circulation*, **1976**, *54*, 766–773.

Cohen, M. V., and Kirk, E. S. Differential response of large and small coronary arteries to nitroglycerin and angiotensin: autoregulation and tachyphylaxis. *Circ. Res.*, **1973**, *33*, 445–453.

Cohn, P. F., and Gorlin, R. Physiologic and clinical actions of nitroglycerin. *Med. Clin. North Am.*, **1974**, *58*, 407–415.

Cole, S. L.; Kay, H.; and Griffith, G. C. Assay of antianginal agents. I. A curve analysis with multiple control periods. *Circulation*, **1957**, *15*, 405–413.

Commarato, M. A.; Winbury, M. M.; and Kaplan, H. R. Glyceryl trinitrate and pentrinitrol (pentaerythritol trinitrate); comparative cardiovascular effects in dog, cat and rat by different routes of administration. *J. Pharmacol. Exp. Ther.*, **1973**, *187*, 300–307.

Danahy, D. T., and Aronow, W. S. Hemodynamics and antianginal effects of high dose oral isosorbide dinitrate after chronic use. *Circulation*, **1977**, *56*, 205–212.

Danahy, D. T.; Burwell, D. T.; Aronow, W. S.; and Prakash, R. Sustained hemodynamic and antianginal effect of high dose oral isosorbide dinitrate. *Circulation*, **1977**, *55*, 382–387.

Drake, F. T.; Haring, O.; Singer, D. H.; and Dirnberger, G. Evaluation of anti-arrhythmic efficacy of perhexiline maleate in ambulatory patients by Holter monitoring. *Postgrad. Med. J.*, **1973**, *49*, Suppl. 3, 52–63.

Driemen, P. M. Papaverine—hepatotoxic or not? *J. Am. Geriatr. Soc.*, **1973**, *21*, 202–205.

Elliott, W. C., and Stone, J. M. Beta-adrenergic blocking agents for the treatment of angina pectoris. *Prog. Cardiovasc. Dis.*, **1969**, *12*, 83–92.

Epstein, S. E., and Braunwald, E.   Inhibition of the adrenergic nervous system in the treatment of angina pectoris. *Med. Clin. North Am.,* **1968,** *52,* 1031–1039.

Epstein, S. E.; Kent, K. M.; Goldstein, R. E.; Borer, J. S.; and Redwood, D. R.   Reduction of ischemic injury by nitroglycerin during acute myocardial infarction. *N. Engl. J. Med.,* **1975,** *292,* 29–35.

Fam, W. A., and McGregor, M.   Effect of coronary vasodilator drugs on retrograde flow in areas of chronic myocardial ischemia. *Circ. Res.,* **1964,** *15,* 355–365.

Ferrer, M. I.; Bradley, S. E.; Wheeler, H. O.; Enson, Y.; Preiseg, R.; Brickner, P. W.; Conroy, R. J.; and Harvey, R. M.   Some effects of nitroglycerin upon the splanchnic, pulmonary, and systemic circulations. *Circulation,* **1966,** *33,* 357–373.

Flaherty, J. T.; Reid, P. R.; Kelly, D. T.; Taylor, D. R.; Weisfeldt, M. L.; and Pitt, B.   Intravenous nitroglycerin in acute myocardial infarction. *Circulation,* **1975,** *51,* 132–139.

Franciosa, J. A.; Limas, C. J.; Guiha, N. H.; Rodriguera, E.; and Cohn, J. N.   Improved left ventricular function during nitroprusside infusion in acute myocardial infarction. *Lancet,* **1972,** *1,* 650–654.

Franciosa, J. A.; Mikulic, E.; Cohn, J. N.; Jose, E.; and Fabie, A.   Hemodynamic effects of orally administered isosorbide dinitrate in patients with congestive heart failure. *Circulation,* **1974,** *50,* 1020–1024.

Freis, E. D.   Report of the panels on cardiovascular drugs from the drug efficacy study. *Circulation,* **1970,** *41,* 149–151.

Ganz, W., and Marcus, H. S.   Failure of intracoronary nitroglycerin to alleviate pacing-induced angina. *Circulation,* **1972,** *46,* 880–889.

Gold, H. K.; Leinbach, R. C.; and Sanders, C. A.   Use of sublingual nitroglycerin in congestive failure following acute myocardial infarction. *Circulation,* **1972,** *46,* 839–845.

Goldstein, R. E.; Douglas, M. D.; Rosing, M. D.; Redwood, D. R.; Beiser, G. D.; and Epstein, S. E.   Clinical and circulatory effects of isosorbide dinitrate. Comparison with nitroglycerin. *Circulation,* **1971,** *43,* 629–640.

Goldstein, R. E.; Stinson, E. B.; Scherber, J. L.; Seningen, R. P.; Grehl, T. M.; and Epstein, S. E.   Intraoperative coronary collateral function in patients with coronary occlusive disease: nitroglycerin responsiveness and angiographic correlations. *Circulation,* **1974,** *49,* 298–308.

Gorlin, R.; Brachfield, N.; MacLeod, C.; and Bopp, P.   Effect of nitroglycerin on the coronary circulation in patients with coronary artery disease or increased left ventricular work. *Circulation,* **1959,** *19,* 705–718.

Hamer, J., and Sowton, E.   Effects of propranolol on exercise tolerance in angina pectoris. *Am. J. Cardiol.,* **1966,** *18,* 354–363.

Heppel, L. A., and Hilmoe, R. J.   Metabolism of inorganic nitrate and nitrate esters. II. The enzymatic reduction of nitroglycerin and erythritol tetranitrate by glutathione. *J. Biol. Chem.,* **1950,** *183,* 129–138.

Heupler, F. A., Jr.; Proudfit, W. L.; Razavi, M.; Shirey, E. K.; Greenstreet, R.; and Sheldon, W. C.   Ergonovine maleate provocative test for coronary arterial spasm. *Am. J. Cardiol.,* **1978,** *41,* 631–640.

Horwitz, L. D.; Gorlin, R.; Taylor, W. J.; and Kemp, H. G.   Effects of nitroglycerin on regional myocardial blood flow in coronary artery disease. *J. Clin. Invest.,* **1971,** *50,* 1578–1584.

Johnson, E. M., Jr.; Harkey, A. B.; Blehm, D. J.; and Needleman, P.   Clearance and metabolism of organic nitrates. *J. Pharmacol. Exp. Ther.,* **1972,** *182,* 56–62.

Johnson, J. B.; Gross, J. F.; and Hole, E.   Effects of sublingual nitroglycerin on pulmonary artery pressure in patients with failure of the left ventricle. *N. Engl. J. Med.,* **1957,** *257,* 1114–1117.

Kasparian, H.; Wiener, L.; Duca, P. R.; Gottlieb, R. S.; and Brest, A. N.   Comparative hemodynamic effects of placebo and oral isosorbide dinitrate in patients with significant coronary artery disease. *Am. Heart J.,* **1975,** *90,* 68–75.

Klassen, G. A.; Sestier, F.; L'Abbate, A.; Mildenberger, R. R.; and Zborowska-Sluis, D. T.   Effects of perhexilene maleate on coronary flow distribution in the ischemic canine myocardium. *Circulation,* **1976,** *54,* 14–20.

Klaus, A. P.; Zaret, B. L.; Pitt, B. L.; and Ross, R. S.   Comparative evaluation of sublingual long acting nitrates. *Circulation,* **1973,** *48,* 519–525.

Klaus, W., and Güttler, K.   Functional and metabolic effects of perhexilene maleate on the isolated myocardium. In, *Perhexilene Maleate.* Excerpta Medica, Amsterdam, **1978,** pp. 23–32.

Lange, R. L.; Reid, M. S.; Tresch, D. D.; Keelan, M. H.; Bernhard, V. M.; and Coolidge, G.   Nonatheromatous ischemic heart disease following withdrawal from chronic industrial nitroglycerin exposure. *Circulation,* **1972,** *46,* 666–678.

Luccioni, R.; Vague, P.; Luccioni, F.; Balansard, P.; Simonia, R.; and Gerard, R.   Abnormalities of insulin secretion in coronary patients: effects of perhexilene maleate. In, *Perhexilene Maleate.* Excerpta Medica, Amsterdam, **1978,** pp. 71–88.

Majid, P. A.; Sharma, B.; and Taylor, S. H.   Phentolamine for vasodilator treatment of severe heart failure. *Lancet,* **1971,** *2,* 719–722.

Manley, E. S., and Lawson, J. W.   Effect of beta adrenergic receptor blockade on skeletal muscle vasodilation produced by isoxsuprine and nylidrin. *Arch. Int. Pharmacodyn. Ther.,* **1968,** *175,* 239–250.

Medical Letter.   Drugs for ischemic peripheral arterial disease. **1978,** *20,* 11.

Miller, R. R.; Vismara, L. A.; Williams, D. O.; Amsterdam, E. A.; and Mason, D. T.   Pharmacological mechanisms for left ventricular unloading in clinical congestive heart failure: differential effects of nitroprusside, phentolamine, and nitroglycerin on cardiac function and peripheral circulation. *Circ. Res.,* **1976,** *39,* 127–133.

Needleman, P., and Harkey, A. B.   Role of endogenous glutathione in the metabolism of glyceryl trinitrate by isolated perfused rat liver. *Biochem. Pharmacol.,* **1971,** *20,* 1867–1876.

Needleman, P., and Hunter, F. E., Jr.   The transformation of glyceryl trinitrate and other nitrates by glutathione-organic nitrate reductase. *Mol. Pharmacol.,* **1965,** *1,* 77–86.

Needleman, P., and Johnson, E. M., Jr.   Mechanism of tolerance development to organic nitrates. *J. Pharmacol. Exp. Ther.,* **1973,** *184,* 709–715.

Needleman, P.; Lang, S.; and Johnson, E. M., Jr.   Organic nitrates: relationship between biotransformation and rational angina pectoris therapy. *J. Pharmacol. Exp. Ther.,* **1972,** *181,* 489–497.

Nies, A. S., and Shand, D. G.   Clinical pharmacology of propranolol. *Circulation,* **1975,** *52,* 6–15.

Oberst, F. W., and Snyder, F. H.   Studies on nitrate esters. 1. Nitrite-producing systems in rabbit tissues. *J. Pharmacol. Exp. Ther.,* **1948,** *93,* 444–450.

Packer, M.; Meller, J.; Medina, N.; Gorlin, R.; and Herman, M. V.   Rebound hemodynamic events after the abrupt withdrawal of nitroprusside in patients with severe chronic heart failure. *N. Engl. J. Med.,* **1979,** *301,* 1193–1197.

Parker, J. C.; Di Carlo, F. J.; and Davidson, I. W. F.   Comparative vasodilator effects of nitroglycerin, pentaerythritol trinitrate and other organic nitrates. *Eur. J. Pharmacol.,* **1975,** *31,* 29–37.

Parker, J. O.; Augustine, R. J.; Burton, J. R.; West, R. O.; and Armstrong, P. W.   Effect of nitroglycerin ointment on the clinical and hemodynamic response to exercise. *Am. J. Cardiol.,* **1976,** *38,* 162–166.

Parker, J. O.; Case, R. B.; Khaja, F.; Ledwich, J. R.; and Armstrong, P. W.   The influence of changes in blood volume on angina pectoris: a study of the effect of phlebotomy. *Circulation*, **1970**, *16*, 593–604.

Parker, J. O.; West, R. O.; and Digiorgi, S. Hemodynamic effects of propranolol in coronary heart disease. *Am. J. Cardiol.*, **1968**, *21*, 11–19.

Pepine, C. J.; Schang, S. J.; and Bemiller, C. R. Effects of perhexilene on coronary hemodynamic and myocardial metabolic responses to tachycardia. *Circulation*, **1974**, *49*, 887–893.

Reichek, N.; Goldstein, R. E.; and Redwood, D. R. Sustained effects of nitroglycerin ointment in patients with angina pectoris. *Circulation*, **1974**, *50*, 348–352.

Ronnov-Jensen, V., and Tjernlund, A. Hepatotoxicity due to treatment with papaverine. *N. Engl. J. Med.*, **1969**, *281*, 1333–1335.

Rosseel, M. T., and Bogaert, M. G. GLC determination of nitroglycerin and isosorbide dinitrate in human plasma. *J. Pharm. Sci.*, **1973**, *62*, 754–758.

Russek, H. I. Propranolol and isosorbide dinitrate synergism in angina pectoris. *Am. J. Cardiol.*, **1968**, *21*, 44–54.

Said, G. Perhexilene neuropathy: a clinicopathological study. *Ann. Neurol.*, **1978**, *3*, 259–266.

Schnaar, R. L., and Sparks, H. V. Response of large and small coronary arteries to nitroglycerin, $NaNO_2$, and adenosine. *Am. J. Physiol.*, **1972**, *223*, 223–228.

Shane, S. J.; Iazzetta, J. J.; Chisholm, A. W.; Berka, J. F.; and Leung, D. Plasma concentrations of isosorbide dinitrate and its metabolites after chronic oral dosage in man. *Br. J. Clin. Pharmacol.*, **1978**, *6*, 37–41.

Singlas, E.; Goujet, M. A.; and Simon, P. Pharmacokinetics of perhexilene maleate in anginal patients with and without peripheral neuropathy. *Eur. J. Clin. Pharmacol.*, **1978**, *14*, 195–201.

Sisenwine, S. F., and Ruelius, H. W. Plasma concentrations and urinary excretion of isosorbide dinitrate and its metabolites in the dog. *J. Pharmacol. Exp. Ther.*, **1971**, *176*, 296–301.

Stipe, A. A., and Fink, G. B. Prophylactic therapy of angina pectoris with organic nitrates. relationship of drug efficacy and clinical experimental design. *J. Clin. Pharmacol.*, **1973**, *13*, 244–250.

Strauer, B. E., and Scherpe, A. Ventricular function and coronary hemodynamics after intravenous nitroglycerin in coronary artery disease. *Am. Heart J.*, **1978**, *95*, 210–219.

Sukerman, M. Clinical evaluation of perhexilene maleate in the treatment of chronic cardiac arrhythmias of patients with coronary heart disease. *Postgrad. Med. J.*, **1973**, *49*, Suppl. 3, 46–52.

Wendt, R. L. Systemic and coronary vascular effects of the 2- and the 5-mononitrate esters of isosorbide. *J. Pharmacol. Exp. Ther.*, **1972**, *180*, 732–742.

Whitworth, C. G., and Grant, W. M. Use of nitrite and nitrate vasodilators by glaucomatous patients. *Arch. Ophthalmol.*, **1964**, *71*, 492–496.

Williams, J. K.; Glick, G.; and Braunwald, E. Studies on cardiac dimensions in intact unanesthetized man. Effects of nitroglycerin. *Circulation*, **1965**, *32*, 767–771.

Willis, W. H., Jr.; Russell, R. O., Jr.; Mantle, J. A.; Ratshin, R. A.; and Rackley, C. E. Hemodynamic effects of isosorbide dinitrate vs. nitroglycerin in patients with unstable angina. *Chest*, **1976**, *69*, 15–22.

Winbury, M. M.; Howe, B. B.; and Hefner, M. A. Effect of nitrates and other coronary dilators on large and small coronary vessels: an hypothesis for the mechanism of action of nitrates. *J. Pharmacol. Exp. Ther.*, **1969**, *168*, 70–95.

Winbury, M. M.; Howe, B. B.; and Weiss, H. R. Effect of nitroglycerin and dipyridamole on epicardial and endocardial oxygen tension—further evidence for redistribution of myocardial blood flow. *J. Pharmacol. Exp. Ther.*, **1971**, *176*, 184–199.

Winsor, T., and Berger, H. J. Oral nitroglycerin as a prophylactic antianginal drug: clinical, physiologic, and statistical evidence of efficacy based on a three-phase experimental design. *Am. Heart J.*, **1975**, *90*, 611–626.

Yap, P. S. K., and Fung, H. L. Pharmacokinetics of nitroglycerin in rats. *J. Pharm. Sci.*, **1978**, *67*, 584–586.

Zelis, R., and Mason, D. T. Isosorbide dinitrate. Effect on the vasodilator response to nitroglycerin. *J.A.M.A.*, **1975**, *234*, 166–170.

Monographs and Reviews

Aronow, W. S. Use of nitrates as antianginal agents. In, *Organic Nitrates*. (Needleman, P., ed.) *Handbuch der Experimentellen Pharmakologie*, Vol. 40. Springer-Verlag, Berlin, **1975**, pp. 163–174.

Chatterjee, K., and Parmley, W. W. The role of vasodilator therapy in heart failure. *Prog. Cardiovasc. Dis.*, **1977**, *19*, 301–325.

Coffman, J. D. Vasodilator drugs in peripheral vascular disease. *Am. J. Hosp. Pharm.*, **1975**, *32*, 1276–1281.

———. Vasodilator drugs in peripheral vascular disease. *N. Engl. J. Med.*, **1979**, *300*, 713–717.

Di Carlo, F. J. Nitroglycerin revisited: chemistry, biochemistry, interactions. *Drug Metab. Rev.*, **1975**, *4*, 1–38.

Fleckenstein, A. Specific pharmacology of calcium in myocardium, cardiac pacemakers, and vascular smooth muscle. *Annu. Rev. Pharmacol. Toxicol.*, **1977**, *17*, 149–166.

Goldstein, R. E., and Epstein, S. E. Medical management of patients with angina pectoris. *Prog. Cardiovasc. Dis.*, **1972**, *14*, 360–398.

Hillis, L. D., and Braunwald, E. Coronary artery spasm. *N. Engl. J. Med.*, **1978**, *13*, 695–702.

Johnson, E. M., Jr. Chemistry of organic nitrates. In, *Organic Nitrates*. (Needleman, P., ed.) *Handbuch der Experimentellen Pharmakologie*, Vol. 40. Springer-Verlag, Berlin, **1975**, pp. 16–23.

Krantz, J. C., Jr. Historical background. In, *Organic Nitrates*. (Needleman, P., ed.) *Handbuch der Experimentellen Pharmakologie*, Vol. 40. Springer-Verlag, Berlin, **1975**, pp. 1–12.

Moir, T. W. Subendocardial distribution of coronary blood flow and the effect of anti-anginal drugs. *Circ. Res.*, **1972**, *30*, 621–627.

Murad, F.; Arnold, W. P.; Mittal, C. K.; and Braughler, J. M. Properties and regulation of guanylate cyclase and some proposed functions for cyclic GMP. *Adv. Cyclic Nucleotide Res.*, **1979**, *11*, 175–204.

Needleman, P. Biotransformation of organic nitrates. In, *Organic Nitrates*. (Needleman, P., ed.) *Handbuch der Experimentellen Pharmakologie*, Vol. 40. Springer-Verlag, Berlin, **1975**, pp. 57–96.

Needleman, P., and Johnson, E. M., Jr. The pharmacological and biochemical interaction of organic nitrates with sulfhydryls. In, *Organic Nitrates*. (Needleman, P., ed.) *Handbuch der Experimentellen Pharmakologie*, Vol. 40. Springer-Verlag, Berlin, **1975**, pp. 97–114.

Ross, J. Afterload mismatch and preload reserve: a conceptual framework for the analysis of ventricular function. *Prog. Cardiovasc. Dis.*, **1976**, *18*, 255–264.

Symposium. (Various authors.) Perhexilene. *Postgrad. Med. J.*, **1973**, *40*, Suppl. 3, 1–132.

Symposium. (Various authors.) *Perhexilene Maleate.* Excerpta Medica, Amsterdam, **1978a.**

Symposium. (Various authors.) Vasodilator and inotropic therapy of heart failure. (Mason, D. T., ed.) *Am. J. Med.*, **1978b**, *62*, 101–216.

Warren, S. E., and Francis, G. S. Nitroglycerin and nitrate esters. *Am. J. Med.*, **1978**, *65*, 53–62.

34 DRUGS USED IN THE TREATMENT OF HYPERLIPOPROTEINEMIAS

Robert I. Levy

Treatment of the patient with hyperlipidemia has become more precise as knowledge of lipid metabolism and of the mechanism of action of hypolipidemic drugs has increased. The routine clinical measurement of the concentrations of cholesterol and triglycerides in plasma, which has become widespread, permits identification of patients with asymptomatic hyperlipidemia and has allowed recognition of the association of hyperlipidemia with such conditions as abdominal pain, pancreatitis, xanthomatosis, and premature vascular disease. These factors have emphasized the need for means to manage hyperlipidemia in the safest and simplest manner.

Hyperlipidemia is a sign of a heterogeneous group of diseases that differ in etiology, clinical manifestations, prognosis, and response to therapy. Understanding of the various hyperlipidemias requires knowledge of the different types of *lipoproteins* that circulate in plasma, since it is in association with these proteins that nearly all lipids in plasma (except free fatty acids) are found. Thus, the measurement of total cholesterol and triglyceride concentrations in plasma is inadequate for diagnosis and as a guide to therapy, since reciprocal changes in the concentration of different classes of lipoproteins may mask the presence of an abnormality of an individual type of lipoprotein. The various disorders are classified in terms of the specific types of lipoproteins whose concentrations are altered, rather than simply in terms of the concentrations of the associated lipids. Particularly because none of the hypolipidemic agents currently available is useful for the management of all types of hyperlipidemia (hyperlipoproteinemia), such classification is essential for a rational approach to the formulation of effective therapy.

In the past, studies of drug efficacy focused primarily on how hypolipidemic agents affected the biosynthesis and catabolism of cholesterol and the formation of bile acids. Moreover, no distinction was made between the various forms of hypercholesterolemia and hypertriglyceridemia. Thus, successful treatment for one patient failed for another who might have a similar concentration of cholesterol or triglyceride in plasma. The principal drawbacks to these oversimplifications included the failure to appreciate the heterogeneity of disorders of plasma lipids as well as the inability to understand the mechanism of action and seemingly variable effectiveness of hypolipidemic drugs. For instance, nicotinic acid was recognized as a highly effective hypolipidemic agent, but one that had no clearly demonstrable influence on either the synthesis or catabolism of cholesterol; why cholesterol concentrations fell was totally unclear. The efficacy of cholestyramine was originally attributed to its capacity to bind bile acids in the gastrointestinal tract and to prevent their reabsorption, thereby increasing their turnover and the breakdown of cholesterol. This concept was challenged by demonstrations that *de novo* biosynthesis of cholesterol in the liver was increased concomitantly with the increased catabolism, so that the total cholesterol balance in the liver remained unchanged. Why then should cholesterol concentrations in plasma fall so dramatically? In seeking an answer to this question, the focus of pharmacological studies shifted away from lipid and fatty acid metabolism and toward the effects of drugs on the metabolism of lipoproteins. At the root of this change was knowledge that the plasma lipid concentrations are dependent upon concentrations of lipoproteins in the circulation, which in turn are determined by their rate of entry into and clearance from the plasma. Therefore, the utility of a hypolipidemic drug should be determined by its effects, whether primary or secondary, on the pattern and concentrations of lipoproteins rather than on the concentration of lipid *per se*.

RELATIONSHIP BETWEEN BLOOD LIPIDS AND VASCULAR DISEASE

Among the numerous recognized risk factors for the development of atherosclerosis, one of the best documented is the association between the concentrations of lipids in blood and the development of coronary heart disease. The evidence for the association between cholesterol concentrations in plasma and coronary heart disease is extensive and unequivocal (Task Force on Arteriosclerosis, 1977; Stamler, 1978). The strength of this evidence is based on numerous sources, including (1) the experimental production of atherosclerotic lesions in animals fed diets that induce hypercholesterolemia, (2) knowledge of the nature and dynamics of the human atherosclerotic plaque, (3) the occurrence of hyperlipidemia in groups of subjects with clinically manifested atherosclerotic disease, (4) the study of genetic hyperlipidemias associated with premature coronary heart disease, and (5) epidemiological studies of populations with differing concentrations of cholesterol in plasma (Levy *et al.,* 1979). Although elevated concentrations of triglycerides have been associated with an increased incidence of coronary heart disease in several cross-sectional studies, the evidence from prospective studies of a cause-and-effect relationship as yet remains inconclusive. In sharp contrast, a number of prospective studies have shown that, in an otherwise-healthy population, the risk of coronary heart disease is directly related to the concentration of cholesterol in plasma. Predictions of the risk of coronary heart disease from knowledge of cholesterol concentrations are more accurate, however, in individuals below age 65 than in the more elderly.

One of the most important results to emerge from these studies is the demonstration that there are multiple risk factors for the development of coronary heart disease, and no value of the concentration of cholesterol in plasma confers immunity on an individual (Stamler, 1978). However, the continuous relationship between concentrations of cholesterol and the incidence of coronary heart disease is of the utmost significance. When considering the risk for the development of coronary heart disease, there is little justification to use the Gaussian distribution to define "normal" levels. The higher the plasma cholesterol, the greater is the need for concern. Furthermore, the clinician should be aware of current systems that use arbitrary limits (usually the ninetieth or ninety-fifth percentile) for their definition of abnormalities of cholesterol, low-density lipoprotein cholesterol, or triglyceride. A clear distinction must be made between these arbitrary limits, which are used to define "types" of hyperlipoproteinemia, and the concept of cholesterol as a risk factor.

TRANSLATING HYPERCHOLESTEROLEMIA INTO HYPERLIPOPROTEINEMIA

The major plasma lipids, including cholesterol and triglycerides, do not circulate freely in solution but, rather, are transported in blood in the form of complexes with lipoproteins (Fredrickson *et al.,* 1967; Levy and Rifkind, 1977). The major families of lipoproteins are the chylomicrons, very-low-density lipoproteins (VLDL), intermediate-density lipoproteins (IDL), low-density lipoproteins (LDL), and high-density lipoproteins (HDL); they are usually classified in terms of physicochemical properties, such as density or electrophoretic mobility. Sufficient elevation in the concentration of any of the families of lipoproteins can result in hypercholesterolemia. Similarly, hypertriglyceridemia can result from increased concentrations of chylomicrons, VLDL, or IDL, either alone or in various combinations.

Concentrations of LDL in plasma correlate closely with the concentrations of cholesterol, since 60 to 75% of the total cholesterol in plasma is normally transported in association with this lipoprotein. Thus, concentrations of LDL or cholesterol carry more or less the same predictive power for assessment of risk of coronary heart disease.

There is a *negative correlation* between the plasma concentration of HDL, which normally accounts for 20 to 25% of the total plasma cholesterol, and the risk of coronary heart disease. In spite of numerous studies that have demonstrated this inverse relationship between HDL and atherosclerosis, quantification of HDL is only now becoming part of a standard "coronary profile" (*see* Gordon *et al.,* 1977; Kannel *et al.,* 1979).

LIPOPROTEIN METABOLISM

Concentrations of the lipoproteins in plasma are subject to dynamic change. The origins and fates of VLDL, IDL, and LDL are thus of particular interest in the study of hyperlipoproteinemia and the effects of hypolipidemic drugs (*see* Table 34–1). VLDL is the main carrier of endogenous triglyceride. It originates in the liver and small intestine and is catabolized rapidly into an intermediate with a short half-life (IDL), which is further degraded to LDL (Eisenberg and Levy, 1975). Thus, LDL (which is 50% cholesterol by weight) is in part, if not entirely, a remnant of the metabolism of VLDL.

It is now recognized that the lipid disorders are in fact related to abnormalities in the metabolism of lipoproteins (Fredrickson and Levy, 1972). Specifically, excess concentrations of lipids can occur because of either overproduction or faulty removal from the circulation of one or more lipoproteins.

There are many pathogenic mechanisms that may be responsible for the resulting hyperlipoproteinemia. These include primary defects that lead to increased influx of exogenous cholesterol or of triglyceride from the intestine as chylomicrons, increased release of VLDL containing cholesterol or triglyceride from the liver and small intestine, defects in enzymes that catabolize lipoproteins, and abnormalities of the solubility of lipoproteins or in their structures. Other modifying factors include the general state of carbohydrate or protein metabolism and the activity of hormones that promote lipogenesis or lipolysis in muscle, liver, and adipose tissue.

The hyperlipoproteinemias are a heterogeneous group of diseases, not only in etiology

Table 34–1. BIOCHEMICAL AND CLINICAL FEATURES OF LIPOPROTEINS AND LIPOPROTEINEMIAS

FAMILY	ORIGIN	FUNCTION	CATABOLISM	CHARACTERISTICS OF HYPERLIPOPROTEINEMIA	
				Appearance of Plasma *	*Clinical Features*
Chylomicrons	Intestine (from dietary fat)	Transport of dietary fat	Tissue lipoprotein lipase; chylomicron remnant cleared by liver	Creamy supernatant; clear infranatant	Eruptive xanthomata; organomegaly; pancreatitis
Very-Low-Density Lipoproteins (VLDL)	Liver and small intestine (from carbohydrates, free fatty acids, medium-chain triglycerides)	Transport of endogenous triglycerides	Complex; probably requires lipoprotein lipase for degradation	Turbid	Glucose intolerance; hyperuricemia; premature atherosclerosis
Intermediate-Density Lipoproteins (IDL)	VLDL	Unknown	Unclear; degradation to LDL	Turbid	Glucose intolerance; hyperuricemia; premature atherosclerosis; tuboeruptive, tendinous, and palmar planar xanthomata
Low-Density Lipoproteins (LDL)	VLDL, IDL (? other sources)	Unknown	Unclear; relative importance of liver and peripheral receptors (uptake sites) for LDL to be defined	Clear	Premature atherosclerosis; corneal arcus; tendinous and tuberous xanthomata, xanthelasma
High-Density Lipoproteins (HDL)	Liver and intestine	Unclear; facilitates intravascular triglyceride and cholesterol metabolism and clearance	Unclear; primary site of removal appears to be the liver	Clear	Decreased risk of cardiovascular disease

* The appearance of the plasma is evaluated after a sample has been held overnight at 4° C.

but also in clinical signs, prognosis, and responsiveness to therapy. The detection of hypercholesterolemia or hypertriglyceridemia does not identify either the site or the nature of the disorder. Quantitation of individual lipoproteins, however, has helped to eliminate much of the guesswork involved in the selection of appropriate therapy (Levy et al., 1974; Levy and Rifkind, 1977).

Chylomicrons. Chylomicrons are primarily triglyceride; they originate in the intestine from exogenous dietary fat. Seventy to one hundred grams of dietary fat are transported daily from the intestine to sites of utilization and storage. Chylomicrons are usually absent from the plasma after 12 to 14 hours of fasting. Their presence in plasma after such a fast should always be considered to be abnormal. These large particles produce turbidity and rise as a creamy layer to the top of a sample of blood that is held overnight at 4° C. When chylomicronemia is present, the ratio of triglyceride to cholesterol in the plasma can be as high as 20 to 1. Even marked chylomicronemia, which may be associated with abdominal pain, pancreatitis, and hepatosplenomegaly, does not appear to be associated with premature coronary artery disease.

Very-Low-Density Lipoprotein. VLDL is composed primarily of triglyceride that is derived endogenously from the liver and small intestine. Less than 10% of the mass of this species is actually protein, and its ratio of cholesterol to triglyceride is normally about 1 to 5. Between 15 and 25 g of VLDL glyceride is released into the blood stream daily. Diets high in carbohydrate will invariably increase the concentration of triglyceride in plasma, at least transiently. Other factors that contribute to variation of the concentrations of VLDL triglyceride include changes in weight, use of alcohol, the presence of stress, and patterns of exercise. As mentioned, the relationship between the concentration of triglycerides in plasma and the incidence of coronary heart disease is unclear, particularly because hypertriglyceridemia is often accompanied by hypertension, obesity, and glucose intolerance.

Intermediate-Density Lipoprotein. IDL is essentially an intermediate in the catabolism of VLDL to LDL. The average cholesterol content is 30%, while that of triglyceride is 40%. Some IDL may be identical to the abnormal form of lipoprotein that characterizes type-III hyperlipoproteinemia, but confirmation of this hypothesis is needed. In patients who have type-III hyperlipoproteinemia, excess concentrations of IDL-like particles are associated with an increased incidence of premature coronary and peripheral vascular disease.

Low-Density Lipoprotein. LDL is the product of the intravascular metabolism of the glyceride-rich lipoprotein, VLDL. Subjects with increased concentrations of LDL in plasma thus have accumulated the lipoprotein either because of overproduction of precursors (which is uncommon) or because of inadequate clearance of LDL.

Approximately 50% of the mass of LDL is cholesterol, and patients with elevated LDL will thus usually have an increased concentration of cholesterol in their plasma. The other lipoproteins also contain cholesterol, but in lesser amounts. It is important to quantitate concentrations of LDL, since elevated levels of this lipoprotein are directly correlated with the incidence of coronary heart disease. In a population with a normal range of concentrations of LDL, comparison of those with values below 119 mg/dl with those whose concentrations exceed 150 mg/dl (equivalent to a plasma cholesterol concentration of approximately 230 mg/dl) reveals a clear difference in the incidence of cardiovascular disease—measured either as overt myocardial infarctions or by other cardiac events, such as angina.

High-Density Lipoprotein. The role of HDL in lipid transport is unclear. It may serve to remove cholesterol from tissues or, alternatively, to accept it as a consequence of the metabolism of VLDL. Exciting recent findings have focused attention on this lipoprotein. Unlike the atherogenesis associated with LDL, the concentration of HDL is *inversely* correlated with the risk of development of coronary heart disease (Kannel et al., 1979). Moreover, this correlation is independent of other risk factors. While the mechanisms responsible for such a correlation are unclear, epidemiological findings do suggest that an increased concentration of HDL may be a protective factor in the development of vascular disease. HDL concentrations have been positively correlated with exercise and moderate ingestion of alcohol; they are inversely related to the degree of obesity, smoking, poor control of diabetes, and the use of oral contraceptives that contain progestins (Bradley et al., 1978). The prevalence of coronary heart disease in people whose concentration of HDL was 30 mg/dl was double that of individuals whose concentration was 60 mg/dl (Gordon et al., 1977). Mean values of cholesterol in HDL were *lower* in subjects with coronary heart disease. Familial excess of HDL or deficiency of LDL have been associated with decreased risk of coronary heart disease. These findings provide a cogent reason to determine whether elevated concentrations of cholesterol are due to increases in LDL or HDL. They also provide an incentive for the study of factors that might increase circulating concentrations of HDL (see Tall and Small, 1978).

Lipoprotein Apoproteins. Understanding of the functions and the regulation of the protein constituents of the plasma lipoproteins, the apoproteins, is of obvious importance (Morrisett et al., 1977; Schaefer et al., 1978). Immunological quantification of the apoproteins is becoming a practical technic that promises to improve the diagnosis of hyperlipoproteinemias and, potentially, the assessment of risk of coronary heart disease. At least seven different apoproteins have been isolated to date. Some of these appear to play a structural or stabilizing role, while others clearly have functional properties as well.

Apoproteins with primarily structural roles are A-II in HDL and apo B in chylomicrons, VLDL, and LDL. Apoprotein A-I is apparently bound very loosely to HDL by interaction with A-II and activates lecithin-cholesterol acyltransferase, the enzyme responsible for esterification of plasma cholesterol. The C apoproteins also have specific physiological functions. Apolipoprotein C-II (and possibly C-I) activates lipoprotein lipase, the enzyme primarily responsible for the hydrolysis of triglycerides. Apolipoprotein C-III appears to inhibit this enzyme.

Greater understanding of the activity of the apoproteins has helped clarify the function and metabolic fate of the plasma lipoproteins. This, in turn, has shed light on the underlying metabolic defects in hyperlipoproteinemia, as well as the mode of action of hypolipidemic drugs.

EVALUATION OF HYPERLIPO-PROTEINEMIA

Five patterns (types) of hyperlipoproteinemia have been described (Fredrickson et al., 1967; Fredrickson and Levy, 1972). Each constitutes an entity in which specific classes of lipoproteins are present in excess; they are listed in Table 34-2.

Since all the lipoprotein families have relatively fixed composition, and since two of them refract light and produce turbidity, the definition of hyperlipoproteinemia usually only requires inspection of the plasma (after storage overnight at 4° C) and precise measurement of the concentration of cholesterol and triglycerides. Hyperchylomicronemia can be differentiated from increased VLDL (both of which produce hypertriglyceridemia) by the appearance of the plasma. A creamy layer over a clear infranatant is generally diagnostic of a type-I abnormality. Hyperbetalipoproteinemia (type IIa) is characterized by a clear plasma with an elevated concentration of cholesterol. Turbid plasma may be observed in types IIb, III, IV, and V, and there may be a separate creamy layer of chylomicrons in types III and V.

Occasionally, additional procedures such as ultracentrifugation or the determination of HDL concentrations (or both) may be required to establish the type of lipoprotein responsible for hyperlipidemia; electrophoresis is usually not necessary. Frequently, the type of lipoprotein responsible can be related to the patient's history and to clinical features of the

Table 34-2. TYPES OF HYPERLIPOPROTEINEMIA

TYPE	LIPOPROTEIN CLASS INCREASED
I	Chylomicrons
IIa	LDL
IIb	LDL and VLDL
III	Abnormal IDL
IV	VLDL
V	Chylomicrons and VLDL

abnormality. There are simple quantitative technics to determine whether an elevated concentration of cholesterol is due to increased LDL or to other lipoproteins (see Lipid Research Clinics Program, 1974).

Several limitations must be kept in mind if measurements of lipids or lipoproteins are to be useful. (1) One should know which technic is used for the measurement, and allowance should be made for any systematic difference between various procedures. (2) Concentrations of lipids and lipoproteins increase with age. A value for cholesterol that is acceptable in a person 40 to 50 years old might be alarmingly high in a child. (3) Chylomicrons normally appear in the blood 2 to 10 hours after a meal; blood should be obtained after a fast of 12 to 16 hours. (4) Concentrations of lipoproteins are easily affected by diet, illness, drugs, and the gain or loss of weight. Dramatic changes occur immediately and for about 6 weeks after a myocardial infarction; the plasma concentrations of cholesterol and LDL may fall by as much as 60% in the first few days. Blood samples should be obtained from patients who are ingesting a regular diet; consumption of large quantities of eggs, butter, milk, cheese, and organ meat will increase concentrations of LDL. Other factors that can raise concentrations of lipids include hypothyroidism, nephrosis, myeloma, porphyria, hepatic disease, and alcoholism. If these disorders are ruled out and the diagnosis of *primary hyperlipoproteinemia* is made, family members should be examined to reveal possible genetic transmission of the disorder as well as to detect others at risk for coronary artery disease. Since the plasma lipid concentrations in patients with hyperlipidemia can often be reduced by proper dietary management, all such individuals should have an adequate trial on an appropriately designed diet before institution of treatment with drugs (see Handbook, 1974).

DRUGS AFFECTING THE CONCENTRATIONS OF PLASMA LIPOPROTEINS

With increased interest in the prevention of coronary heart disease and the recognition of the role of hyperlipoproteinemia as a risk factor, a number of drugs have become available for the treatment of hyperlipidemia (see Hunninghake and Probstfield, 1977). These agents vary markedly in both their clinical effects and their mechanisms of action. The hypolipidemic drugs currently available can be placed into three basic categories: (1) those that affect the production of lipoproteins (e.g., nicotinic acid); (2) those that affect the intravascular metabolism of lipoproteins (e.g., clofibrate); and (3) those that affect removal of lipoprotein from the circulation (e.g., cholestyramine).

Nicotinic Acid

In 1955, Altschul and coworkers showed that large doses of nicotinic acid lower the concentration of cholesterol in plasma. This property is not shared by nicotinamide and appears to have nothing to do with the role of these compounds as vitamins. The chemistry of nicotinic acid and its function as a vitamin are discussed in Chapter 66.

Effects on Plasma Lipids and Lipoproteins. Nicotinic acid rapidly reduces the concentrations of triglycerides in plasma by lowering concentrations of VLDL; effects are noted in 1 to 4 days. Concentrations of cholesterol (LDL) fall a bit more slowly, but the drop is clearly apparent within 5 to 7 days of the initiation of therapy. Plasma concentrations of triglycerides may be reduced by 20% to over 80%, and the degree of reduction is directly related to the initial concentration of VLDL. The magnitude of the fall in LDL is related to the dose, and the maximal effect is usually achieved 3 to 5 weeks after an appropriate dosage regimen has been established. Administration of nicotinic acid usually results in a mild-to-moderate *increase* in the concentration of HDL (especially HDL cholesterol). The drug clearly is effective in subjects with excesses of VLDL, IDL, and LDL (types II, III, IV, and V), although higher dosages are frequently required for the effective treatment of excess LDL (type II). In the Coronary Drug Project (1975), the administration of nicotinic acid (3 g per day) to men with coronary artery disease resulted in the reduction of cholesterol and triglyceride concentrations by 10% and 26%, respectively, regardless of the initial lipid concentration. Regression of eruptive, tuboeruptive, and tuberous xanthomata has been reported with prolonged therapy.

Mechanism of Action. The effects of nicotinic acid are diverse (Gey and Carlson, 1971). They include inhibition of lipolysis in adipose tissue, decreased esterification of triglycerides in the liver, and increased activity of lipoprotein lipase. The effects of nicotinic acid on the synthesis and catabolism of cholesterol in the liver are unclear. How all these changes relate to the alterations of plasma lipoproteins that follow the administration of nicotinic acid remains conjectural. Langer and Levy (1971) demonstrated that nicotinic acid reduces the rate of synthesis of LDL in normal subjects and in patients with type-II hyperlipoproteinemia. Subsequent evaluation has shown that the decreased synthesis is directly related to the decreased hepatic synthesis and release of the precursor of LDL—that is, VLDL (and apoprotein B).

Untoward Effects. There are several untoward effects of nicotinic acid that limit its usefulness. Notably, the drug produces intense cutaneous flush and pruritus. While these reactions decrease in intensity in most individuals after they have been on therapy for several weeks, they are unpleasant and result in poor patient compliance. Slow upward adjustment of dosage appears to ameliorate this problem. Gastrointestinal disturbances such as vomiting, diarrhea, and dyspepsia are also common, and peptic ulceration has been reported. Hyperpigmentation, acanthosis nigricans, and dry skin may occur after prolonged therapy.

Abnormalities of hepatic function occur in patients taking large doses of nicotinic acid. These include jaundice, a decrease in the excretion of BSP, and increases of plasma transaminase activities. Hyperglycemia and abnormal glucose tolerance occur in many nondiabetic patients taking nicotinic acid. Plasma concentrations of uric acid may also be elevated, and the incidence of acute gouty arthritis is increased. The drug should therefore be used with extreme caution, if at all, in patients who have hepatic disease, diabetes mellitus, or gout. The abnormalities of plasma glucose and uric acid and hepatic function are reversible when the drug is discontinued. Nicotinic acid may also increase the vasodilatation and postural hypotension caused by antihypertensive agents. Toxic amblyopia has also been reported.

Preparations, Dosage, and Therapeutic Uses. Preparations of *nicotinic acid* (*Niacin*, U.S.P.) are described in Chapter 66. *Aluminum nicotinate* (NICALEX) is also marketed; it is a complex of aluminum hydroxynicotinate and nicotinic acid. It is hydrolyzed to aluminum hydroxide and nicotinic acid in the gastrointestinal tract. There are no advantages to this preparation, and the aluminum hydroxide may interfere with the absorption of other drugs. The usual dosage of nicotinic acid is 2 to 9 g daily; the equivalent for aluminum nicotinate is 2 to 7.5 g per day. The daily dose is divided into three or four portions, taken orally with or just after meals. There are other preparations of nicotinic acid that produce sustained concentrations of the drug in blood, but they appear to cause gastrointestinal irritation and hepatotoxicity. To reduce gastric irritation and to enhance absorption of nicotinic acid, the drug is best given at mealtimes, initially in small doses (three 100-mg tablets per day). Over a 1- to 3-week period, additional tablets are added to the regimen until the maintenance dose is reached. This is usually considerably lower in children (55 to 87 mg/kg per day) than in adults.

Nicotinic acid fell into relative disrepute because of the variety of troublesome untoward effects associated with its use, but it has regained popularity as a result of its ability to reduce elevated concentrations of both VLDL and LDL. Because of these effects, nicotinic acid is useful in the management of all types of hyperlipoproteinemia except type I. If dietary management of the disease fails, the drug may be used cautiously while monitoring its untoward effects in type-II, -III, -IV, and -V abnormalities. The combination of nicotinic acid with a bile acid–sequestering resin may allow effective lowering of the concentration of LDL with more conservative doses of each drug than would be required if either was given alone. In primary type-V hyperlipoproteinemia (in subjects without gout or diabetes), a maintenance dosage of 3 g of nicotinic acid per day can prevent the recurrent bouts of pancreatitis and eruptive xanthomata that occur in this disorder.

In two different trials of secondary prevention, the long-term use of nicotinic acid significantly decreased the incidence of recurrent myocardial infarction. In both trials, however, there was no definitive effect on cardiovascular or overall mortality (Coronary Drug Project, 1975; Carlson *et al.,* 1977). Moreover, in the Coronary Drug Project, an increased incidence of atrial fibrillation and other cardiac arrhythmias was observed, in addition to the aforementioned gastrointestinal and dermatological effects. Thus, until the efficacy of lowering cholesterol is established in man, nicotinic acid should be used with caution and primarily in high-risk patients with hyperlipoproteinemia who have not responded dramatically to dietary measures.

CLOFIBRATE

In the course of screening tests in rats, Thorp and Waring (1962, 1963) found that a series of aryloxyisobutyric acids was effective in reducing plasma concentrations of total lipid and cholesterol. The compound that combined maximal effectiveness with minimal toxicity was clofibrate. Since then, it has been widely used in man and there is now evidence that, in specific cases, it is a very effective drug. However, its use has become increasingly circumscribed because its effectiveness for the primary or secondary prevention of atherosclerosis and its clinical sequelae have come into question (Coronary Drug Project, 1975; Report from the Committee, 1978); furthermore, awareness of latent untoward effects of clofibrate has grown (*see* below and Oliver, 1978).

Chemistry. Clofibrate, the ethyl ester of *p*-chlorophenoxyisobutyric acid, has the following structural formula:

Clofibrate

While a number of congeners of clofibrate have been developed, none appears to offer significant advantages.

Effects on Plasma Lipids and Lipoproteins.

Clofibrate characteristically reduces the plasma triglyceride concentration by lowering the levels of VLDL within 2 to 5 days after initiation of therapy. In most patients, plasma cholesterol and LDL concentrations also fall. However, a large fall in VLDL may be accompanied by a *rise* in LDL, such that the net effect on cholesterol may be slight. The mean value of plasma cholesterol was reduced only 6% in men treated chronically with clofibrate (1.8 g per day) during the Coronary Drug Project (1975); the reduction in plasma triglyceride was 22%.

In a similar trial of primary prevention involving asymptomatic men with hypercholesterolemia, clofibrate lowered the plasma cholesterol concentration by only 6 to 11% (Report from the Committee, 1978). This very modest effect can be contrasted with that in type-III hyperlipoproteinemia (dysbetalipoproteinemia), where concentrations of cholesterol and triglycerides may be lowered by approximately 50% and by as much as 80%, respectively (Levy *et al.,* 1972). In type-III disease, concentrations of IDL and VLDL are markedly lowered, while there is little effect on LDL. In such patients, administration of clofibrate results in the mobilization of deposits of cholesterol in tissues, accompanied by regression and disappearance of xanthomata. In subjects with isolated elevations of LDL (type IIa) or elevations in VLDL (types IIb, IV, and V), clofibrate has only a modest ability to lower concentrations of lipids and its utility is limited. The drug has no effect on chylomicronemia (type I), nor does it affect concentrations of HDL (except in some hypertriglyceridemic subjects in whom marked reduction of VLDL may be accompanied by modest increases in HDL). Thus, clofibrate appears to have specific efficacy only in patients with type-III hyperlipoproteinemia. Even in these patients, however, the lipid-lowering effects of clofibrate can be countered by weight gain.

Mechanism of Action. The sites of action of clofibrate are only partially established, and the details of its mechanism of action are largely lacking (*see* Kudchodkar *et al.,* 1977). It is known to cause inhibition of the hepatic synthesis of cholesterol in the rat. In man, clofibrate also causes inhibition of cholesterol synthesis and increased biliary execretion of neutral sterols (Grundy *et al.,* 1969). It appears to enhance the rate of intravascular catabolism of VLDL and IDL to LDL. In some cases, it may also hasten the rate of removal of these lipoproteins from the circulation (Segal *et al.,* 1972; Wolfe *et al.,* 1973; D'Costa *et al.,* 1977; Berman *et al.,* 1978). Hepatic synthesis and release of VLDL are not altered consistently.

Absorption, Fate, and Excretion. In man, clofibrate is completely absorbed from the intestine and appears in the plasma as the deesterified *p*-chlorophenoxyisobutyric acid (CPIB); peak concentrations of the acid occur in the plasma within 4 hours after the oral administration of clofibrate. The major fraction of CPIB is bound to plasma albumin. The elimination of CPIB proceeds in two kinetic phases, with the slower exponential phase having a mean half-time of nearly 15 hours. Essentially all the acid is excreted in the urine, about 60% as the glucuronide.

Untoward Effects and Drug Interactions. Clofibrate is usually well tolerated, but occasionally patients experience nausea, diarrhea, or weight gain (apparently related to increased appetite). Skin rash, alopecia, weakness, impotence, breast tenderness, and decreased libido also have been reported to occur occasionally. A more disturbing effect is a now well-characterized flulike syndrome, associated with severe muscle cramps and tenderness, stiffness, and weakness (Langer and Levy, 1968). The syndrome recurs whenever the drug is taken and is associated with elevated activities of creatine phosphokinase and glutamic-oxaloacetic transaminase in the plasma. These same enzymatic

activities are sometimes elevated even in asymptomatic patients who are receiving clofibrate. Administration of clofibrate also increases the lithogenicity of bile and has thus been associated with a high incidence of cholelithiasis and cholecystitis (Coronary Drug Project Research Group, 1977). Patients with existing or suspected coronary artery disease may be at risk from drug-induced cardiac arrhythmias (LaRosa *et al.,* 1969), cardiomegaly, increased angina, claudication, and thromboembolic phenomena (Coronary Drug Project, 1975). The drug enhances the effect (and toxicity) of other acidic drugs such as phenytoin and tolbutamide, presumably by displacing them from their binding sites on albumin. This same effect may in part explain the enhancement of the effects of coumarin anticoagulants by clofibrate (Bjornsson *et al.,* 1977). A reduction in the dosage of oral anticoagulants and frequent determinations of prothrombin time are usually required to control patients who are receiving both medications. Use of clofibrate may be associated with an increased incidence of various tumors, but this remains to be confirmed (Oliver, 1978). The drug is contraindicated in patients with impaired renal or hepatic function and in pregnant or nursing women.

Preparation, Dosage, and Therapeutic Uses. *Clofibrate,* U.S.P. (ATROMID-S), is available as official capsules containing 500 mg. The drug is administered orally in a dose of 2 g daily, in two or four portions. Increase in dosage above 2 g per day does not appear to increase its effects on lipids but does greatly increase the incidence of side effects. In all cases, its effects on lipids are enhanced by proper diet (Handbook, 1974). Clofibrate is indicated only in subjects with increased concentrations of VLDL and IDL who have failed to respond adequately to dietary therapy alone. Thus, the drug has clear utility in subjects with type-III hyperlipoproteinemia, as well as in some patients with type-IV or type-V abnormalities. Because clofibrate has only a modest effect on LDL and since there exist other more effective agents for lowering the concentration of LDL, the drug is of limited utility for patients with type-II hyperlipoproteinemia. Furthermore, since clofibrate may *increase* the concentration of LDL in some patients with elevations of VLDL, the effects of the drug should be monitored by sequential measurements of plasma lipoproteins. A shift from an excess of VLDL to one of LDL suggests the necessity to discontinue the drug.

The clinical evidence for the efficacy of clofibrate in preventing deaths from coronary artery disease is most discouraging. A number of clinical trials have now been completed. Early studies, especially in Great Britain, suggested that clofibrate might reduce the mortality rate in patients with a history of coronary artery disease (Dewar and Oliver, 1971). Reevaluation of those trials—as well as the completion of two other studies, one in secondary prevention (Coronary Drug Project, 1975) and the other in primary prevention (Report from the Committee, 1978)—has not shown any beneficial effect on mortality. However, the more recent study did show a significant decline in the rate of suspected and proven myocardial infarctions.

The association of clofibrate with hepatobiliary and other side effects further decreases its promise for the prevention or control of atherosclerosis and its sequelae. In fact, the long-term utility of clofibrate has been demonstrated only in subjects with type-III hyperlipoproteinemia, who experienced regression of xanthomata and an apparent increase in peripheral blood flow (Zelis et al., 1970).

BILE ACID–SEQUESTERING RESINS

The first of these agents, *cholestyramine*, was originally used to control pruritus in patients with elevated concentrations of plasma bile acid due to cholestasis. While this remains a valid use of the drug, greater interest now centers on the ability of this and similar agents to lower concentrations of plasma cholesterol.

Chemistry. Cholestyramine is the chloride salt of a basic anion-exchange resin. The ion-exchange sites are provided by trimethylbenzylammonium groups in a large copolymer of styrene and divinylbenzene. The average polymeric molecular weight is greater than 10^6. Cholestyramine has the following structural formula:

Cholestyramine

A second resin, colestipol hydrochloride, is a copolymer of diethyl pentamine and epichlorohydrin. The tentative structural formula of colestipol is as follows:

Colestipol

These agents are hydrophilic but insoluble in water. They are unaffected by digestive enzymes, remain unchanged in the gastrointestinal tract, and are not absorbed.

Effects on Plasma Lipids and Lipoproteins. Sequestrants of bile acids characteristically reduce the concentration of cholesterol in plasma by lowering the level of LDL. The fall in the concentration of LDL is usually apparent in 4 to 7 days and approaches 90% of the maximal effect within 2 weeks. The magnitude of the effect on LDL is related to the dose and may be as great as 25 to 35%. In most patients, concentrations of triglyceride in plasma (VLDL) increase by 5 to 20% during the first weeks of therapy with a sequestrant; this increase usually then disappears gradually, and, within 4 weeks, concentrations of VLDL and triglyceride return to pretreatment values (Levy et al., 1973). In patients with elevated concentrations of VLDL and IDL, the increase of triglycerides that follows the initiation of therapy with these agents may be greater and the increase in VLDL and IDL may be more sustained. Hence, sequestrants are most effective when only LDL is in excess (type IIa); they may, in fact, worsen the hyperlipidemia of disease of types III, IV, and V. Sequestrants have no predictable effect on the concentration of HDL. When therapy with the resin is discontinued, plasma concentrations of lipids rise rapidly and then slowly approach the pretreatment values over a period of 3 to 4 weeks.

Mechanism of Action. These resins, administered orally, are not absorbed. They act to bind bile acids in the intestine, and there is thus a large increase in the fecal excretion of the acids. Since bile acids inhibit the microsomal hydroxylase that catalyzes the rate-limiting step in the conversion of cholesterol to bile acids, their removal increases the rate of hepatic metabolism of cholesterol (*see* Mosbach, 1969). Furthermore, since bile acids are required for the intestinal absorption (and enterohepatic reabsorption) of cholesterol, there is some additional fecal loss of neutral sterol. Unfortunately, a compensatory increase occurs in the rate of hepatic biosynthesis of cholesterol, and *balance is maintained* (Myant, 1972). In man, the lowering of the concentration of LDL in plasma has been shown to result from an increase in the rate of catabolism of the lipoprotein (increased catabolism of apoprotein B) or the clearance of LDL from the blood stream. In both normal individuals and subjects with familial elevations of LDL (type-II familial hypercholesterolemia), administration of a sequestrant results in a decrease in the size of the pool of LDL and an increase in the rate of catabolism (without any noticeable change in the synthesis of LDL) (Levy and Langer, 1972). The precise mechanism by which the unabsorbed sequestrants increase the rate of removal of LDL is presently unclear. It may involve an increase in the number or activity of peripheral receptors for the lipoprotein. Such receptors are responsible for the uptake and removal of LDL from the circulation.

Untoward Effects and Drug Interactions. These preparations often have an unpleasant sandy or gritty quality, and patients may complain of this. Nausea, abdominal discomfort, indigestion, and constipation are frequent difficulties. Impaction may occur, and hemorrhoids are frequently aggravated. A large intake of fluid and a diet high in bulk minimize constipation. Beside increasing concentrations of triglycerides in plasma, the sequestrants often transiently increase activities of alkaline phosphatase and transaminases as well. Since cholestyramine is a chloride form of an anion-exchange resin, hyperchloremic acidosis can occur, especially in younger and smaller patients in whom the relative dosage is higher.

With high doses of resins steatorrhea may occur, and preexisting steatorrhea is aggravated by conventional doses. In such cases, the absorption of fat-soluble vitamins is also impaired and vitamin supplementation is recommended. Hypoprothrombinemia has been observed.

The resins obviously may also bind other compounds in the intestine, including drugs administered concurrently. This has been noted particularly with chlorothiazide, phenylbutazone, phenobarbital, anticoagulants, thyroxine, and various digitalis preparations. As a general rule, it is recommended that other drugs taken orally should be ingested at least 1 hour before or 4 hours after the resin.

Preparations, Dosage, and Therapeutic Uses. *Cholestyramine Resin,* U.S.P. (QUESTRAN), is available in packets that contain 9 g of powder (equivalent to 4 g of resin) or in cans that contain 378 g. *Colestipol hydrochloride* (COLESTID) is available in packets containing 5 g of resin and in bottles containing 500 g of drug. Both resins must be mixed with water or other fluids or pulpy fruits before ingestion. They should never be swallowed in the dry form. They are usually administered in daily dosages of 16 to 32 g (cholestyramine) or 15 to 30 g (colestipol), divided into two to four portions to be taken either before or during meals and at bedtime.

Cholestyramine and colestipol are most effective in patients with primary excesses of LDL (familial hypercholesterolemia, type II) and should be combined with a diet that lowers cholesterol in the treatment of this disorder. When dietary and drug therapy are combined, LDL concentrations in plasma may be reduced to normal in heterozygotes (Kuo *et al.,* 1979). Sequestrants may increase plasma concentrations of triglyceride-VLDL in patients with type-IIb disease (LDL and VLDL excess) and, although they are still very effective in reducing concentrations of LDL in these subjects, sequestrants should be combined with weight-reducing diets or other hypolipidemic agents. The sequestrants are of no known benefit to patients with excessive concentrations of chylomicrons, IDL, or VLDL, and they may indeed exacerbate the excess of triglycerides. They thus should not be used to treat hyperlipoproteinemias of types I, III, IV, or V.

Long-term prospective studies are only now being conducted in man to evaluate the efficacy of cholestyramine in reducing the incidence and consequences of coronary vascular disease. In the interim, these agents may be used with caution in subjects who are at high risk because of elevated concentrations of LDL. While the sequestrants are probably among the safest drugs currently available to treat hyperlipoproteinemia (because they are not absorbed from the gastrointestinal tract), their widespread use must await demonstration of their efficacy in preventing or controlling atherosclerosis and its sequelae in man.

PROBUCOL

This drug, which lowers concentrations of cholesterol in plasma, is the newest of such agents available for clinical use in the United States. Experience with the drug has thus far been limited (Heel *et al.,* 1978).

Chemistry. Probucol has no apparent structural similarity to other agents that lower cholesterol concentrations. It is a *bis*-phenol with the following structural formula:

Probucol

Effects on Plasma Lipids and Lipoproteins. Probucol lowers concentrations of cholesterol (LDL) in plasma by 10 to 15% when it is used in conjunction with an appropriate diet. In most studies, the maximal effect on plasma cholesterol occurred after 1 to 3 months of treatment. The effects on plasma concentrations of triglyceride

(VLDL) are variable. Because it has no apparent effect on HDL, probucol appears to be indicated solely for patients with elevated concentrations of LDL (type II). Details of its mechanism of action are currently lacking, although a possible effect on an early step in the synthesis of cholesterol has been noted. No late-stage products of cholesterol biosynthesis have been shown to accumulate. Its primary effect on LDL suggests that it probably acts to enhance removal of this lipoprotein from the circulation, but this remains to be demonstrated.

Absorption, Fate, and Excretion. Less than 10% of an oral dose of probucol is absorbed. Peak concentrations in blood are said to be higher and less variable when the drug is taken with food. Despite its limited absorption, probucol is lipid soluble and accumulates slowly in adipose tissue. It may persist in fat and blood for 6 months or longer after the last dose is taken. The major pathway of elimination is via the bile and feces; renal clearance is negligible.

Untoward Effects. Probucol has been well tolerated by man. Diarrhea, flatulence, abdominal pain, and nausea have occasionally been reported. However, experience with the drug is limited and its long-term effects are not known. The safety of probucol has not been established for children or during pregnancy. Because of its persistence in the body, it has been recommended that patients discontinue probucol and practice contraception for at least 6 months before attempting to become pregnant.

Preparation, Dosage, and Therapeutic Uses. *Probucol* (LORELCO) is available as 250-mg tablets. The recommended dosage (*for adults only*) is 500 mg twice daily, taken with morning and evening meals. Probucol can be considered to be an adjunct for lowering the concentration of cholesterol in patients with excessive LDL (type II) who cannot be controlled by dietary management. It is not presently recommended for other types of hyperlipoproteinemia or as a substitute for an appropriate diet. There is as yet no evaluation of the efficacy of probucol for prevention or control of atherosclerosis or its clinical sequelae.

THYROID HORMONES

Patients with hypothyroidism have elevated concentrations of plasma lipids; when such patients are treated with thyroid hormone, the plasma lipid concentrations decrease, often before there is a significant return of other measurements, such as pulse rate or basal metabolic rate, to normal. Patients with hyperthyroidism often have low concentrations of plasma cholesterol. These findings have led to the attempt to reduce plasma lipid and lipoprotein concentrations in euthyroid individuals by the administration of thyroid hormones. The amounts of hormone required are such as to increase tissue O_2 consumption appreciably, and in patients with coronary heart disease this often produces anginal attacks and can cause myocardial infarction.

The thyroid hormones exert a marked effect on cholesterol metabolism; they cause increased synthesis of cholesterol in the liver, but they also promote increased excretion of sterol in the feces and increased conversion of cholesterol to bile acids. Thus, increased hepatic synthesis of cholesterol is balanced by its increased catabolism. The concentration of cholesterol in plasma falls, however, because the clearance of LDL from the plasma is increased, whereas the synthesis of LDL is unchanged (Walton *et al.*, 1965). As with the bile acid sequestrants, an overall increase in cholesterol turnover is associated with enhanced clearance of LDL, possibly due to an increased number or activity of receptors for LDL on cells that are responsible for its uptake and removal from the circulation.

The report that thyroacetic acid analogs of thyroxine can produce a lowering of plasma cholesterol concentration without an increase in basal metabolic rate (Lerman and Pitt-Rivers, 1955) led to the study of a number of analogs of thyroid hormones in an attempt to find agents that affect plasma lipid concentrations without increasing metabolism. D-Thyroxine, the optical isomer of the naturally occurring hormone, was found to lower the plasma cholesterol concentration in rats by 50% at a dose between ¹⁄₁₀ and ¹⁄₄₀ of that which produces a 50% increase in O_2 consumption and heart rate. The doses of L-thyroxine required to produce these same effects on cholesterol and O_2 consumption are approximately equal (Boyd and Oliver, 1960).

When D-thyroxine is administered to man in doses of 4 to 8 mg per day, the concentration of LDL is reduced on the average by about 20%. Neither the concentration of VLDL nor the concentration of HDL is changed significantly (Strisower *et al.*, 1968). The most serious adverse effect of this drug is an increase in frequency or severity of anginal attacks in patients with coronary heart disease. The incidence increases with the dose, so that at doses of 10 mg per day the occurrence of angina is frequent whereas at 4 mg per day it is uncommon. Other adverse effects are cardiac arrhythmias and the hypermetabolic effects associated with administration of thyroid hormones, such as nervousness, sweating, tremor, and insomnia. The drug potentiates the effect of concurrently administered oral anticoagulants.

In the Coronary Drug Project (1972) a large number of patients (survivors of a first myocardial infarction) were treated with D-thyroxine in doses of 6 mg per day. Although the drug did result in reduction in plasma lipid concentrations, there was *increased* mortality from coronary disease in these patients, and hence this portion of the drug study was discontinued. In addition, individuals treated with D-thyroxine developed decreased glucose tolerance, increased plasma bilirubin concentrations, and increased serum glutamic oxaloacetic transaminase and alkaline phosphatase activities.

Preparations, Dosage, and Therapeutic Uses. *Dextrothyroxine Sodium,* U.S.P. (CHOLOXIN), is available as scored tablets containing 1, 2, 4, or 6 mg. The initial oral dose for adults is 1 mg daily for 1 month. This dose is increased by 1 mg at intervals of 1 month until a satisfactory effect is achieved or until a maximal daily dose of 8 mg is reached. For children, the initial daily dose is 0.05 mg/kg and the maximal dose is 4 mg.

Since dextrothyroxine has no consistent effect on VLDL, it is useful only for type-II hyperlipoproteinemia. In view of the results of the Coronary Drug Project described above, it is probably undesirable to use this drug in any but young individuals known to be free of coronary artery disease. Its use in hypothyroidism is reserved for patients in whom hypercholesterolemia persists despite adequate therapy with thyroid hormone.

OTHER DRUGS

Estrogens were used to treat hyperlipidemia after it was demonstrated that women have lower concentrations of LDL and higher values of HDL than do men, as well as decreased susceptibility to atherosclerosis and ischemic heart disease until after the menopause. However, *estrogens are no longer considered to be hypolipidemic agents.* Not only is their administration associated with an increased frequency of thromboembolic events, but also they have been shown to increase concentrations of VLDL and induce pancreatitis in susceptible patients (those with type-IV or -V hyperlipoproteinemia). In the Coronary Drug Project (1973), both high- and low-dose estrogen regimens (5 and 2.5 mg per day) were discontinued because of a host of side effects in men, including gynecomastia, impotence, loss of libido, depression, and problems involving several organ systems, including the cardiovascular. The progestin *norethindrone acetate* appears to cause a marked decrease in chylomicrons and VLDL in susceptible females with type-V hyperlipoproteinemia (Glueck *et al.,* 1969). However, progestins cannot be recommended for routine use, not only because they have systemic effects but also because they reduce concentrations of HDL (Bradley *et al.,* 1978).

β-Sitosterol is a plant sterol with a structure similar to that of cholesterol, except for the substitution of an ethyl group at C 24 of its side chain. Like most plant sterols, it is not absorbed by man. β-Sitosterol lowers plasma concentrations of LDL but has no effect of VLDL; its mechanism of action is not known. It is indicated only for treatment of excess of LDL. The long-term effects of β-sitosterol are unknown. Untoward reactions include a mild laxative effect and occasional nausea and vomiting. It is available as *sitosterols* (CYTELLIN) in suspension form; each 30 ml contains 6 g of the drug. The recommended dose is 30 ml (usually mixed with coffee, tea, fruit juice, or milk to increase palatability), taken 30 minutes before meals and at bedtime.

The antibiotic *neomycin* (*see* Chapter 51) has a hypolipidemic effect only when administered orally. The effect is not dependent on its antimicrobial activity but appears to be secondary to the formation of insoluble complexes with bile acids in the intestine (Faloon *et al.,* 1966). Its mechanism of action might thus be similar to that of the sequestrants of bile acids. Small doses of neomycin reduce the plasma concentration of LDL; effects on VLDL are variable. Neomycin is administered in divided doses of 0.5 to 2 g per day. While the drug is absorbed only to a minor extent, ototoxicity and nephrotoxicity may occur in patients with impaired renal function. Diarrhea and malabsorption are other complications. Neomycin should be considered only for patients with type-IIa lipoproteinemia who are unable or unwilling to follow other regimens.

Para-aminosalicylic acid recrystallized in vitamin C (aminosalicylic acid; PAS-C) is a highly purified preparation of this tuberculostatic agent. Para-aminosalicylic acid was first found to have a hypocholesterolemic effect in patients treated for tuberculosis. The newer preparation (Barter *et al.,* 1974) has been reported to lower plasma concentrations of cholesterol and triglycerides in patients with type-IIa and -IIb hyperlipoproteinemia. Although its effects on the metabolism of lipoproteins have yet to be studied, it reduces the concentration of both VLDL and LDL; it may therefore act on the synthesis of lipoproteins rather than on their clearance (Vessby *et al.,* 1978). Maintenance dosage is generally 8 to 9 g per day for adults and 5 to 6 g per day for children. Gastrointestinal problems have been reported (*see also* Chapter 53). Para-aminosalicylic acid requires further investigation.

BENEFITS OF REDUCTION OF THE CONCENTRATIONS OF PLASMA LIPIDS

Concentrations of lipids in plasma can be lowered considerably, frequently to normal values, in most subjects with primary hyperlipoproteinemia; several benefits of such therapy are apparent. Recurrent attacks of abdominal pain, with or without overt and sometimes fatal pancreatitis, may be controlled or averted in patients with type-V disease. Superficial xanthomata, which may accompany hyperlipoproteinemias, may disappear; the benefit is largely cosmetic or psychological. The major reason for the treatment of hyperlipoproteinemia is to reduce the risk of cardiovascular disease. Ample data exist on the risks associated with high plasma concentrations of LDL and, in nonhuman primates, atherosclerosis regresses when the plasma concentrations of this lipoprotein are lowered.

However, such benefits for man are still a presumption and not a fact (Ahrens, 1976; Stone, 1978). In view of this, the following guidelines are offered. Dietary manipulation should always be attempted before a drug is used for its effects on plasma lipids. Drugs should be administered only after dietary therapy of 3 to 6 months' duration and only to patients with hyperlipoproteinemia who are in the following categories: (1) those with premature coronary heart disease that is manifest clinically; (2) patients with a strong family history of coronary heart disease, hyperlipoproteinemia, or both; (3) individuals with one or more of the other established risk factors for coronary vascular disease beside hyperlipidemia, such as hypertension, cigarette smoking, and diabetes. Even in these patients, the drug should be discontinued after 1 to 2 months if the concentration of cholesterol in plasma is not lowered by at least an additional 10% over that achieved by dietary manipulation alone.

Ahrens, E. H.   The management of hyperlipidemia: whether rather than how. *Ann. Intern. Med.,* 1976, *85,* 87–93.

Altschul, R.; Hoffer, A.; and Stephen, J. D.   Influence of nicotinic acid on serum cholesterol in man. *Arch. Biochem. Biophys.,* 1955, *54,* 558–559.

Barter, P. J.; Connor, W. E.; Spector, A. A.; Armstrong, M. D.; Connor, S. L.; and Newman, M. A.   Lowering of serum cholesterol and triglyceride by para-aminosalicylic acid in hyperlipoproteinemia. *Ann. Intern. Med.,* 1974, *81,* 619–624.

Berman, M.; Hall, M.; Levy, R. I.; Eisenberg, S.; Bilheimer, D. W.; Phair, D.; and Goebel, R. H.   Metabolism of apo B and apo C lipoproteins in man: kinetic studies in normal and hyperlipoproteinemic subjects. *J. Lipid Res.,* 1978, *19,* 38–56.

Bjornsson, T. D.; Mellin, P. J.; and Blaschke, T. F.   Interaction of clofibrate with warfarin. I. Effect of clofibrate on the disposition of the optical enantiomorphs of warfarin. *J. Pharmacokinet. Biopharm.,* 1977, *5,* 495–505.

Bradley, R. D.; Wingred, J.; Petitti, D. B.; Krauss, R. M.; and Ramcharan, S.   Serum high-density-lipoprotein cholesterol in women using oral contraceptives, estrogens and progestins. *N. Engl. J. Med.,* 1978, *299,* 17–20.

Carlson, L. A.; Danielson, M.; Ekberg, I.; Klintemar, B.; and Rosenhamer, G.   Reduction of myocardial reinfarction by the combined treatment with clofibrate and nicotinic acid. *Atherosclerosis,* 1977, *28,* 81–86.

Coronary Drug Project.   Findings leading to further modification of its protocol with respect to dextrothyroxine. *J.A.M.A.,* 1972, *220,* 966–1008.

————.   Findings leading to discontinuation of the 2.5 mg/day estrogen group. *Ibid.,* 1973, *226,* 652–657.

————.   Clofibrate and niacin in coronary heart disease. *Ibid.,* 1975, *231,* 360–381.

Coronary Drug Project Research Group.   Gallbladder disease as a side effect of drugs influencing lipid metabolism. *N. Engl. J. Med.,* 1977, *296,* 1185–1190.

D'Costa, M. A.; Smigura, F. C.; Kulhay, K.; and Angel, A.   Effects of clofibrate on lipid synthesis, storage and plasma intralipid clearance. *J. Lab. Clin. Med.,* 1977, *90,* 823–836.

Dewar, H. A., and Oliver, M. F.   Secondary prevention trials using clofibrate. A joint commentary on the Newcastle and Scottish trials. *Br. Med. J.,* 1971, *4,* 784–786.

Faloon, W. W.; Paes, I. C.; Woodfolk, D.; Nankin, H.; Wallace, K.; and Haro, E. N.   Effect of neomycin and kanamycin upon intestinal absorption. *Ann. N.Y. Acad. Sci.,* 1966, *132,* 879–884.

Glueck, C. J.; Brown, W. V.; Levy, R.; Greten, H.; and Fredrickson, D. S.   Amelioration of hypertriglyceridemia by progestational drugs in familial type V hyperlipoproteinemia. *Lancet,* 1969, *1,* 1290–1291.

Gordon, T.; Castelli, W. P.; Hjortland, M.; Kannel, W. B.; and Dawber, T.   High density lipoprotein as a protective factor against coronary artery disease: the Framingham Study. *Am. J. Med.,* 1977, *62,* 704–714.

Grundy, S. M.; Ahrens, E. H., Jr.; Salen, G.; and Quintao, E.   Mode of action of ATROMID-S on cholesterol metabolism in man. *J. Clin. Invest.,* 1969, *48,* 33a.

Kannel, W. B.; Castelli, W. P.; and Gordon, T.   Cholesterol in the prediction of atherosclerotic disease. New perspectives based on the Framingham Study. *Ann. Intern. Med.,* 1979, *90,* 85–91.

Kudchodkar, B. J.; Sodhi, H. S.; Horlick, L.; and Mason, D. T.   Effects of clofibrate on cholesterol metabolism. *Clin. Pharmacol. Ther.,* 1977, *22,* 154–163.

Kuo, P. T.; Hayase, K.; Kostis, J. B.; and Moreyra, A. E.   Use of combined diet and colestipol in long-term (7–7½ years) treatment of patients with type II hyperlipoproteinemia. *Circulation,* 1979, *59,* 199–211.

Langer, T., and Levy, R. I.   Acute muscular syndrome associated with administration of clofibrate. *N. Engl. J. Med.,* 1968, *279,* 856–858.

————.   The effect of nicotinic acid on the turnover of low density lipoproteins in type II hyperlipoproteinemia. In, *Metabolic Effects of Nicotinic Acid and Its Derivatives.* (Gey, K. F., and Carlson, L. A., eds.) Hans Huber Pub., Bern, 1971, pp. 641–647.

LaRosa, J. C.; Brown, W. V.; Frommer, P. L.; and Levy, R. I.   Clofibrate-induced ventricular arrhythmia. *Am. J. Cardiol.,* 1969, *23,* 266–269.

Lerman, J., and Pitt-Rivers, R.   Physiological activity of triiodothyroacetic acid. *J. Clin. Endocrinol. Metab.,* 1955, *15,* 653–655.

Levy, R. I.; Fredrickson, D. S.; Shulman, R.; Bilheimer, D. W.; Breslow, J. L.; Stone, N. J.; Lux, S. E.; Sloan, H. R.; Krauss, R. M.; and Herbert, P. N.   Dietary and drug treatment of primary hyperlipoproteinemia. *Ann. Intern. Med.,* 1972, *77,* 267–294.

Levy, R. I., and others.   Cholestyramine in type II hyperlipoproteinemia. *Ann. Intern. Med.,* 1973, *79,* 51–58.

Levy, R. I., and Langer, T.   Hypolipidemic drugs and lipoprotein metabolism. In, *Drugs Affecting Lipid Metabolism: Pharmacological Control of Lipid Metabolism,* Vol. 26. (Holmes, W. L. S.; Paoletti, R.; and Kritchevsky, D.; eds.) Plenum Publishers, New York, 1972, pp. 155–163.

Oliver, M. F.   Cholesterol, coronaries, clofibrate and death. (Editorial.) *N. Engl. J. Med.,* 1978, *299,* 1360–1362.

Report from the Committee of Principal Investigators.   A co-operative trial in the primary prevention of ischaemic heart disease using clofibrate. *Br. Heart J.,* 1978, *40,* 1069–1118.

Segal, P.; Roheim, P. S.; and Eder, H. A.   Effect of clofibrate on lipoprotein metabolism in hyperlipidemic rats. *J. Clin. Invest.,* 1972, *51,* 1632–1638.

Stamler, J.   Lifestyles, major risk factors, proof and public policy. *Circulation,* 1978, *58,* 3–19.

Stone, N. J.   Cholesterol, colestipol and coronary heart disease. (Editorial.) *J. Chronic Dis.,* 1978, *31,* 1–3.

Strisower, E. H.; Adamson, G.; and Strisower, B.   Treatment of hyperlipidemia. *Am. J. Med.,* 1968, *45,* 488–501.

Thorp, J. M., and Waring, W. S.   Modification and distribution of lipids by ethyl chlorophenoxyisobutyrate. *Nature,* **1962,** *194,* 948–949.

———. An experimental approach to the problem of disordered lipid metabolism. *J. Atheroscler. Res.,* **1963,** *3,* 351.

Vessby, B.; Lithel, H.; Boberg, J.; and Hellsing, K. Para-aminosalicylic acid as a lipid-lowering agent. *Clin. Pharmacol. Ther.,* **1978,** *23,* 651–657.

Walton, K. W.; Scott, P. J.; Dykes, P. W.; and Davies, J. W. L. The significance of alterations in serum lipids in thyroid dysfunction. II. Alterations of the metabolism and turnover of ^{131}I low-density lipoproteins in hypothyroidism and thyrotoxicosis. *Clin. Sci.,* **1965,** *29,* 217–238.

Wolfe, B. M.; Kane, J. P.; Havel, R. J.; and Brewster, H. P. Mechanism of the hypolipidemic effect of clofibrate in postabsorptive man. *J. Clin. Invest.,* **1973,** *52,* 2146–2159.

Zelis, R.; Mason, D. T.; Braunwald, E.; and Levy, R. I. Effects of hyperlipoproteinemias and their treatment on the peripheral circulation. *J. Clin. Invest.,* **1970,** *49,* 1007–1015.

Monographs and Reviews

Boyd, G. S., and Oliver, M. F. Thyroid hormones and plasma lipids. *Br. Med. Bull.,* **1960,** *16,* 138–142.

Eisenberg, S., and Levy, R. I. Lipoprotein metabolism. *Adv. Lipid Res.,* **1975,** *13,* 1–89.

Fredrickson, D. S., and Levy, R. I. Familial hyperlipoproteinemia. In, *The Metabolic Basis of Inherited Disease,* 3rd ed. (Stanbury, J. B.; Wyngaarden, J. B.; and Fredrickson, D. S.; eds.) McGraw-Hill Book Co., New York, **1972,** pp. 545–614.

Fredrickson, D. S.; Levy, R. I.; and Lees, R. S. Fat transport in lipoproteins—an integrated approach to mechanisms and disorders. *N. Engl. J. Med.,* **1967,** *276,* 32–44, 94–103, 148–156, 215–226, 273–281.

Gey, K. F., and Carlson, L. A. (eds.). *Metabolic Effects of Nicotinic Acid and Its Derivatives.* Hans Huber Pub., Bern, **1971.**

Handbook. *The Dietary Management of Hyperlipoproteinemia: A Handbook for Physicians.* National Institutes of Health, NIILI, Bethesda, **1974.**

Heel, R. C.; Brogden, R. N.; Speight, T. M.; and Avery, G. S. Probucol: a review of its pharmacological properties and therapeutic use in patients with hypercholesterolemia. *Drugs,* **1978,** *15,* 409–428.

Hunninghake, D. B., and Probstfield, J. L. Drug treatment of hyperlipoproteinemia. In, *Hyperlipidemia: Diagnosis and Therapy.* (Rifkind, B. M., and Levy, R. I., eds.) Grune & Stratton, Inc., New York, **1977,** pp. 327–362. (366 references.)

Levy, R. I.; Morganroth, J.; and Rifkind, B. M. Treatment of hyperlipidemia. *N. Engl. J. Med.,* **1974,** *290,* 1295–1301.

Levy, R. I., and Rifkind, B. M. Lipid lowering drugs in hyperlipidemia. In, *Cardiovascular Drugs.* Vol. 1, *Antiarrhythmic, Antihypertensive and Lipid Lowering Drugs.* (Avery, G. S., ed.) ADIS Press, Sydney, Australia, **1977,** pp. 1–34.

Levy, R. I.; Rifkind, B. M.; Dennis, B. H.; and Ernst, N. (eds.). *Nutrition, Lipids, and Coronary Heart Disease—A Global View.* Raven Press, New York, **1979.**

Lipid Research Clinics Program. *Manual of Laboratory Operations.* Vol. 1, *Lipid and Lipoprotein Analysis.* Department of Health, Education, and Welfare Publication No. (NIH) 75-628, U.S. Government Printing Office, Washington, D. C., **1974.**

Morrisett, J. D.; Jackson, R. L.; and Gotto, A. M., Jr. Lipid-protein interactions in the plasma lipoproteins. *Biochim. Biophys. Acta,* **1977,** *472,* 93–133.

Mosbach, E. H. Effect of drugs on bile acid metabolism. *Adv. Exp. Med. Biol.,* **1969,** *4,* 421–441.

Myant, N. B. Effect of drugs on the metabolism of bile acids. *Adv. Exp. Med. Biol.,* **1972,** *26,* 137–154.

Schaefer, E. J.; Eisenberg, S.; and Levy, R. I. Lipoprotein apoprotein metabolism. *J. Lipid Res.,* **1978,** *19,* 667–687.

Tall, A. R., and Small, D. M. Plasma high-density lipoproteins. *N. Engl. J. Med.,* **1978,** *299,* 1232–1236.

Task Force on Arteriosclerosis. *Atherosclerosis.* Report of the 1977 Working Group to Review the 1971 Report by the National Heart, Lung, and Blood Institute Task Force on Arteriosclerosis. Department of Health, Education, and Welfare Publication No. (NIH) 78-1526, U.S. Government Printing Office, Washington, D. C., **1977.**

VII

Water, Salts, and Ions

Normal inorganic constituents of the body may be considered as pharmacological agents when they are administered to repair either acute or chronic states of depletion or deficiency. These compounds fall into several groups. Those that contribute to the osmolality, the pH, or the volume of the body fluids are considered in this section (Chapter 35), while those that have a more unique relationship to the function of specific organs are discussed in the appropriate organ-related sections of the text. Thus, calcium and phosphate are considered together with the agents that are primarily responsible for their regulation—vitamin D, parathyroid hormone, and calcitonin (Chapter 65); iodide is presented with other agents that are relevant to the function of the thyroid gland (Chapter 60), and the salts of iron are discussed in the context of hematopoiesis (Chapter 56). Drugs that are inorganic ions, such as lithium (Chapter 19), are described in chapters most appropriate to their therapeutic utility, while metallic ions that are primarily of toxicological importance are grouped in Chapter 69. It is not within the scope of this textbook to consider the role of trace elements in nutrition.

CHAPTER

35 AGENTS AFFECTING VOLUME AND COMPOSITION OF BODY FLUIDS

Gilbert H. Mudge

The volume and composition of the body fluids vary tremendously from one compartment to another and from one cell type to another, and are maintained remarkably constant despite the vicissitudes of daily life and the greater stresses imposed by disease. The organization of this remarkable system has developed over millions of years and permits the efficient regulation of homeostasis. The responsible mechanisms reside in a variety of organs and tissues, which include the central nervous system (CNS), the heart and the lungs, the gastrointestinal tract, the kidneys, and, to a remarkable extent, the cell membranes themselves. The failure of the kidney to repair a disordered state to a more nearly normal level is more commonly related to the unavailability of adequate raw material rather than to some primary renal

disturbance *per se*. To the extent that this is true, it follows that the wisdom with which the raw materials are supplied may be crucial.

Disturbances in fluid and electrolyte metabolism involve four major properties of the body fluids—volume, osmolality, hydrogen ion concentration (pH), and the concentrations of specific ions. In some disease states an abnormality in one property may dominate the picture. However, severely ill patients often manifest multiple disturbances that coexist and interact.

Throughout this chapter, guidelines for therapy are suggested, and, although exceedingly useful, the reader should be aware that they represent an approach that is an approximation toward an average patient. The physician must examine the details of management as carefully as in any other therapeutic regimen in clinical medicine.

DISTURBANCES OF VOLUME AND OSMOLALITY

THE DISTRIBUTION AND THE COMPOSITION OF BODY FLUIDS

Distribution of Body Fluids. Total body water in man varies between the approximate limits of 50% of the body weight in the obese to 70% in the lean. This total volume is divided into two major compartments, the intracellular and the extracellular, and into a much smaller compartment, referred to as the transcellular. This last-named includes fluids within the tracheobronchial tree, the gastrointestinal tract, the excretory system of the kidneys and glands, the cerebrospinal fluid, and the aqueous humor of the eye.

The volumes of these compartments may be estimated with the use of agents that distribute themselves uniformly throughout a particular compartment. In this fashion one can estimate the total volume of body water, the extracellular volume, and the plasma volume. The volume of the intracellular compartment can be calculated as the difference between total body water and the volume of the extracellular compartment (*see* Table 35–1).

Composition of Body Fluids. There are vast differences in the composition of the two major compartments. An average composition for *plasma* is as follows:

CATIONS		ANIONS	
	(mEq/liter)		
Sodium	135–145	Chloride	98–106
Potassium	3.5–5.0	Bicarbonate	24–28
Calcium	4.5–5.3	Phosphate and sulfate	2–5
Magnesium	1.5–2.0	Organic anions	3–6
		Protein	15–20

The concentration of the filterable ions in the *interstitial fluid* can be calculated from the values in serum with a correction for serum water (SW) and the Donnan ratio. Both of these corrections are necessary because of the contribution of protein. The Donnan ratio is 0.95 for cations and 1.05 for anions, and the calculation is made in the following fashion:

$$Na_{IF} = \frac{Na_S}{SW} \times 0.95$$

$$Cl_{IF} = \frac{Cl_S}{SW} \times 1.05$$

where the subscripts IF and s refer to interstitial fluid and serum, respectively. For precise measurements it should be emphasized that the significant datum is the concentration in serum water, whereas a clinical laboratory usually reports the concentration per liter of serum. Under most circumstances, this matters very little since the water content of serum (92%) is reasonably constant. Since the composition of the interstitial fluid is only slightly but predictably different from that of the plasma, the plasma and interstitial fluids may be considered together as *extracellular fluid.*

The composition of *intracellular fluid* is quite different. The major cations are potassium and magnesium with very little sodium, and the major anions are phosphate and protein with less bicarbonate and very little chloride. The composition of intracellular fluid is, of course, estimated with considerable indirection, since the only cells that can be simply obtained as such are erythrocytes and, to a lesser extent, leukocytes and platelets. Because muscle tissue represents the largest segment of intracellular fluid, its composition has been studied extensively. Even if one grants the validity of the figures thereby obtained by derived data, simple statements of concentrations per liter of in-

Table 35–1. THE MEASUREMENT AND DISTRIBUTION OF BODY WATER

COMPARTMENT	% TOTAL BODY WATER	AGENT USED FOR ESTIMATE *
Total Body Water (TBW)	100	DHO, THO, antipyrine
Intracellular Water (ICW)	55	By difference between TBW and ECW
Extracellular Water (ECW)	35	Inulin, SO_4^{2-}, Cl^-, Br^-
Plasma Volume (PV)	7.5	T1824, ^{131}I-albumin
Interstitial Fluid	27.5	By difference between ECW and PV
Inaccessible Bone Water	7.5	Special technics
Transcellular Water	2.5	Special technics

* DHO = deuterated water; THO = tritiated water; T1824 = plasma protein–bound dye.

tracellular water tell us little of the physico-chemical activity of these ions, the characteristics of the phosphate and protein anions, their valence, or other properties. The intracellular fluids of different tissues differ from each other, and, furthermore, intracellular fluid is not likely to be homogeneous but probably varies in the several cellular organelles. The data for *muscle-cell fluid* are as follows:

CATIONS		ANIONS	
		(mEq/liter)	
Sodium	10	Bicarbonate	10
Potassium	150	Phosphate and	
Magnesium	40	sulfate	150
		Protein	40

The composition of the body can also be studied by the use of radioactive isotopes and by calculation of the *total exchangeable quantity* of a given ion. The method involves the administration of a known quantity of radioactive material, the equilibration of the isotope with all the stable element with which it will readily equilibrate (usually 24 hours), the determination of the specific activity in serum, and the calculation of the total quantity of the ion that is exchangeable. The values determined by Moore and associates (1963) are as follows:

	MALE	FEMALE
	(mEq/kg of Body Weight)	
Sodium	39.5	38.3
Potassium	48	39.4
Chloride	29.3	28.6

It is known from other analyses that about 75% of total body sodium and 85% of total body potassium are exchangeable.

Another isotopic technic takes advantage of the presence in the body of the naturally occurring isotope of potassium, ^{40}K, from which one can compute the total quantity of potassium in the body. The values average 55 mEq/kg and 49 mEq/kg for male and female, respectively.

Cellular Mechanisms of Electrolyte Control. The manner by which the major compositional differences of the intracellular and extracellular fluids are maintained has been and continues to be under investigation. These ions are not at equilibrium but exist in a steady state away from equilibrium; this demands an energy-requiring series of operations, referred to in general as "active transport." In the steady-state condition, the concentration of sodium and potassium within the cell is dependent on the rate of pumping of sodium out and potassium in (by the Na^+,K^+-activated adenosine triphosphatase system) and the rates at which these ions move by passive diffusion along the established electrochemical gradients. These ionic transport mechanisms are partially responsible for the regulation of cell volume. In addition, they serve to establish and maintain the electrical potential gradients across the cell membrane that are essential for the generation and propagation of action potentials in excitable cells.

Osmotic Pressure. The chief determinant of the passage of fluid from one compartment to another is a change in osmotic pressure (activity of water molecules). Those solutes that can freely permeate a cell membrane influence the total osmotic pressure but do not promote a redistribution of water. Those solutes that cannot freely permeate membranes by diffusion contribute an *effective osmotic pressure* and one that is responsible for net movement of water.

INTERNAL EXCHANGES OF WATER AND SOLUTE

Intracellular and Extracellular Fluid Volumes. Almost all cell membranes are freely permeable to water. Exceptions include the sweat glands and the distal nephron. However, as a consequence of free diffusion of water in the major tissues of the body, it follows that the extracellular and intracellular fluids are of equal osmolality, and that any transient alteration in the effective osmolality of one fluid must influence a net redistribution of water between the two components until the two fluids are once again of equal osmolality. Primary changes in osmolality occur most often in the extracellular fluid; under some circumstances intracellular osmolality may be directly altered by marked changes in cell metabolism.

The principal determinant of the effective osmolality of the extracellular fluid is the concentration of sodium salts. These ions represent more than 90% of all extracellular solutes that contribute an *effective osmolality*.

Addition of Water. If a subject drinks water faster than he can excrete it, he develops a positive water balance. This water gains access initially to the extracellular phase, where it expands the volume and dilutes the solutes. The decrease in effective osmolality (increase in the activity of water) is accompanied by a net movement of water molecules from the extracellular space to the intracellular fluid. Obviously, this will cease when the two fluids are once again of equal osmolality, albeit lower than initially. The result is the distribution of the increment of water through the volume of total body water.

Addition of Salt. If a subject is administered a sodium salt in a concentration in excess of that in extracellular fluid, the concentration of sodium in the extracellular space will increase. Although more sodium tends to diffuse into cells, the rate of extrusion will match the enhanced entry. Thus, one can consider that the increment of salt is confined to the extracellular compartment. The addition of solute diminishes the activity of the molecules of extracellular water, and fewer water molecules enter intracellular fluid than leave it. Water thus redistributes from cells to extracellular space until the two fluids are once again of equal osmolality, albeit higher than initially.

These same net effects on intracellular volume are observed if *hypo*natremia results from a loss of salt in excess of water, or if *hyper*natremia results as a consequence of the loss of water in excess of salt. However, in the last two circumstances, in addition to a redistribution of water between the two major compartments, total body fluid will have been diminished.

The corollary is, of course, that a gain or loss of a saline fluid that is isosmotic with body fluids will cause no shift of water between the cells and the extracellular compartments, but it will expand or contract extracellular volume.

Interstitial and Plasma Fluid Volumes. The same basic principles apply to the steady-state distribution of volume between these two components of the extracellular phase. The determinants are those factors that influence the activity of the molecules of water in the two fluids. The vascular endothelium is permeable to water and to *most* of the solutes. However, it is relatively *im*permeable to the larger molecular species such as proteins. The segregation of these molecules within the vascular component tends to diminish the activity of the water molecules, and if there were no counteracting force all the extracellular fluid would move into the plasma volume. In the regulation of fluid distribution between the vascular and interstitial fluids, the counteracting force is the hydrostatic pressure within the vascular system. The hydrostatic pressure increases the activity of the molecules of water to such an extent as virtually to nullify the opposite effect on the activity of water exerted by the plasma proteins. In addition, there is a small colloidal osmotic force operating in the interstitial fluid and a minor pressure force referred to as "tissue tension." The *balance* of these forces—the Starling forces—is the determinant of the steady-state distribution of volume between the two compartments.

There is an additional influence that operates owing to the fact that the plasma proteins are charged molecules. Since they are unable to penetrate the endothelial membrane, an equilibrium is set up (the Gibbs-Donnan equilibrium) such that there is a slightly greater concentration of diffusible ions in the fluid associated with the charged impermeant anion. The total influence of the protein on the activity of plasma water is referred to as the "colloidal *oncotic* pressure."

All the above-described Starling forces are usually so adjusted that about one fourth of the extracellular fluid is within the confines of the vascular system and the remainder is in the interstitial space. Furthermore, these forces operate in such a fashion that there is a tendency for water and diffusible solutes to leave the vascular bed at the arteriolar end of the capillaries and return at the same rate at the venous end. In this fashion, there is a large turnover of water and diffusible solutes between the two compartments without a net change in volume. The importance of this turnover is obvious, because this is how the circulation can efficiently bring oxygen and nutrients to the cell and remove carbon dioxide and other end products of metabolism without relying solely on diffusion.

Net shifts can and do occur, however, when there is a dislocation of these Starling forces. An increase in the hydrostatic pressure transmitted to the capillaries may permit a greater rate of transudation than reabsorption. The same effect may be noted when there is hypoproteinemia and the influence of the colloidal oncotic pressure is thereby diminished. In both circumstances, there is a net movement of volume to the interstitial fluid compartment. The overall effect may be mitigated partially by another system of vessels, namely, the lymphatic system.

One of the important therapeutic implications is that the plasma volume cannot specifically be increased unless the administered fluid contains a colloidal agent. The administration of saline solution to a subject who has lost blood will reexpand the extracellular fluid volume, but virtually all the expansion will be confined to the interstitial compartment.

External Exchanges of Water and Solute

The Balance Principle. In the early decades of this century a great deal of research involved measuring the intake and output of various nutrients and their metabolites. While this method has properly become archaic for the study of intermediary metabolism, it nevertheless provides the conceptual basis for our understanding of the pathogenesis and proper therapy of many disturbances of fluid and electrolyte metabolism. With the exceptions that are noted below, one may consider that water and the major solutes do not undergo metabolic alteration. Hence, concentrations within the body fluids represent the balance between intake and output, both for water and the solute in question. By general usage, if a patient gains

or loses something, he is in *positive* or *negative* balance, respectively; if there are no significant changes, the balance is *neutral.* The latter is often referred to as "being in balance," and this is the condition of the normal subject who is neither gaining nor losing weight (Table 35–2).

In general, the greater the change in external balance and the more acutely it occurs, the more accurate is the estimate of the change itself. With large changes, insensible, unmeasured, or unestimated losses assume relatively less importance. Also, with large external changes, analytical errors become less important. This applies both to the quantitative analysis of either food or excreta and to clinical estimates based on history and physical examination. It is possible to get independent estimates that serve as checks—for example, the change in weight that accompanies a large change in fluid balance. The proper management of many patients includes an accurate record of *intake and output* and daily weights. This is particularly true of severely ill patients with complex disturbances. Intake includes oral intake, infusions, transfusions, and so forth. Output includes urine, vomitus, and fecal and other intestinal losses (*e.g.*, drainage from a common-bile-duct T tube). Except for research purposes, insensible losses through the lungs and skin are not measured, but they should be estimated. Solid food is rarely included in the estimate of intake even though it provides some water of oxidation. In acute renal failure, this assumes importance.

The *initial state* may have two connota-

Table 35-2. REPRESENTATIVE "NORMAL" VALUES OF FLUID AND ELECTROLYTE INTAKE AND OUTPUT *

	INTAKE		OUTPUT		
	Oral	*Metabolism*	*Urine*	*Feces*	*Insensible*
Water as fluid, ml	1200	0	1500	100	900
Water in food, ml	1000	300			
Nitrogen, g	13	0	12	1.0	0
Sodium, mEq	75	0	74	0.5	0.5
Potassium, mEq	50	0	45	5.0	0
Chloride, mEq	75	0	74	0.5	0.5
Nonvolatile acid, mEq	0	70	70	0	0
Volatile acid, mEq	0	14,000	0	0	14,000

* A single value is selected for each entry to facilitate comparison of intake and output, and all are adjusted to depict a zero net external balance. Nonvolatile acids are largely phosphoric and sulfuric acid residues of metabolism. Volatile acid is exclusively carbon dioxide. All values refer to the amount per 24 hours.

tions. It may refer to the value presumed to have been present in the state of health (*e.g.,* body water estimated from a patient's normal weight), or it may refer to any state during an illness prior to the initiation of a specific treatment. Balance is the difference between intake and output; for example, balance = infusions + dietary intake − urine − vomitus. The sign of the result obviously indicates if the patient is in positive or negative balance.

From an accurate knowledge of the external balance, or even from a thoughtful guess as to its probable value, it is possible to deduce many pathophysiological mechanisms. Changes in the balance of water and solute may occur simultaneously, but their independent contributions should be evaluated separately.

It should be emphasized that the effect of a change in external balance on the composition of the body fluids is independent of the discrete physiological mechanisms that may be involved. For example, the loss of 10 liters of water has essentially the same effect on the residual body fluids, whether due to excessive losses through the skin or to the passage of very dilute urine in uncontrolled diabetes insipidus. Because of this, the "black box" mechanisms of fluid and electrolyte balance warrant reemphasis.

Fixed and Labile Ions and Solutes. Provided the definitions are not extended too far or applied too rigidly, it is useful to bear in mind the distinction between fixed and labile solutes. This is based on physiological considerations. In the case of charged particles, a *fixed ion* is one that exists in the ionic form under all physiological circumstances. This holds true for strong electrolytes such as sodium, potassium, and chloride. Through metabolic alterations, *labile ions* may either be generated from nonionic precursors or converted to nonionic end products. Thus, labile ions may be added to or removed from the body fluids in a form other than that of the charged ion. For example, the ammonium cation (NH_4^+) can be converted to urea in the liver, and also synthesized from amino acids in the kidney. Bicarbonate ion (HCO_3^-) is labile since at the proper concentration of hydrogen ion (H^+) it can be converted to H_2CO_3, and thence to its volatile

form, CO_2. Another example would be the formation of lactate from glucose. In addition, the ion of an appropriate weak acid or base may be buffered so as to change its ionic equivalence (*e.g.,* monobasic and dibasic phosphate). Of course, this is not metabolic alteration in the usual sense, but it does denote a degree of partial lability.

The same considerations apply to nonelectrolytes. Mannitol does not undergo metabolic change and may be considered fixed. However, glucose, which has the same osmotic characteristics as mannitol, is highly labile.

It is a truism that in electrolyte metabolism the most important attribute of any solute relates to its actual concentration in solution in the body fluids. For many solutes, this is directly related to their external balance. However, this does not apply to those that may be either formed or catabolized within the body. It should be apparent that metabolism may change either ionic or osmotic characteristics.

Consideration of Basal Requirements. A summary of average values for the intake and output of water and the major electrolytes is given in Table 35–2. These values presuppose average diet and physical activity, a normal state of metabolism, and no abnormal losses. There is considerable variation from one individual to another and moderate variation from day to day. The composition of important fluids that may be lost from the body is given in Table 35–3.

Insensible Perspiration. Water is continuously lost from the surface of the skin and from the air that is exhaled by the lungs. This is pure water with no solute.

Sweat. This is a hypotonic solution. The rate of sweating is responsive to internal heat, and, therefore, it is difficult to assign a "daily average." Furthermore, it is exceedingly difficult to estimate, and in some circumstances represents a large and unidentifiable loss.

Gastrointestinal. Although there is a large turnover of ions and water between the gut lumen and the body fluid, the *net* loss from the gastrointestinal tract in the feces is usually trivial.

Urine. A liter of urine per day is adequate to contain the solutes destined for excretion.

Endogenous Water. A certain amount of water is produced by the body each day from the metabolism of nutrients.

Sodium Chloride. The average diet contains 4 to 10 g of NaCl a day. This value varies widely due to personal tastes. If salt is removed from the diet, the normal kidney excretes urine that is virtually free of sodium chloride within 3 to 5 days.

Potassium. In the face of reduced intake this cation is not quite so well conserved by the kidney as is sodium, and with chronic reduction of dietary intake it is important to guard against a deficit.

Magnesium. Renal and gastrointestinal conservation of magnesium is excellent.

Summary. These approximate daily basal requirements may be summarized as follows:

Water	1500–2000 ml
Potassium chloride	30–60 millimoles
Sodium chloride	75 millimoles
Magnesium salts	8 millimoles

These amounts relate specifically to the adult. Since the requirements for water and electrolytes are related more closely to the rate of metabolism than to age or body size, the following values may be helpful:

	PER 100 KCAL
Water	100 ml
Sodium	2–3 mEq
Potassium	2–3 mEq
Chloride	4–6 mEq

The probable average caloric expenditure per 24 hours may be estimated from the following:

KG	KCAL
0–10 kg	100/kg
11–20 kg	1000 + 50/kg, for each kg in excess of 10
>20 kg	1500 + 20/kg, for each kg in excess of 20

CLINICAL DISTURBANCES OF VOLUME AND OSMOLALITY

For purposes of classification, several points warrant emphasis. By common clinical usage, the terms *dehydration* and *overhydration* are often inadequate. For an appropriate description, as well as for correct therapy, each condition should be described with two terms—*volume* and *osmolality* (Table 35–4). However, for many purposes the changes in volume and osmolality may be considered independently. (1) The reference point for the classification system is the extracellular fluid. This is justified for two reasons. First, it is the plasma that is available for chemical analysis. Second, it is the extracellular com-

partment, or its close relative the transcellular compartment, from which abnormal fluid losses occur. (2) The classification is valid for acute changes occurring over hours or days. With more chronic disturbances, compensatory physiological adjustments make the classification less accurate. (3) These conditions may or may not be associated with disturbances in acid-base balance. (4) The primary classification refers to changes in *extracellular* volume. If, in response to changes in osmolality, there are secondary changes in *intracellular* volume, these may be in the same or opposite direction to the volume change in the extracellular compartment. (5) The classification is based on external changes in water or solute balance, but without any change in red-blood-cell mass or total circulating protein.

It is rare in clinical situations to find pure examples of the categories listed in Table 35–4. This is not surprising since each depends on two factors, which may be influenced by partially independent mechanisms.

Sodium Concentration as an Index of Plasma Osmolality. Since sodium is the major extracellular solute, its concentration may be used as an index of osmolality, directly for the extracellular fluid and indirectly for the intracellular. As a first approximation, osmolality is twice the sodium concentration. This estimate is not valid in two instances.

Pseudohyponatremia. This is a condition in which the concentration of sodium in the plasma is abnormally low when analyzed by conventional methods (which depend on aliquots measured volumetrically and thus determine molarity and not molality), but in which the concentration would be normal if referred to plasma water. The discrepancy occurs when there is an abnormally high concentration of large molecules and hence an abnormally low percentage of plasma water, most commonly with hyperlipemia or marked hyperproteinemia. A clue to the former is afforded by the lactescence of the serum; the latter occurs particularly in multiple myeloma but also in severe instances of volume depletion.

Sodium as a False Index. This occurs, even with corrections for plasma water, when there is an abnormally high concentration of another solute that is an effective extracellular osmotic particle. It may be seen with severe *hyperglycemia,* either occurring spontaneously in patients with diabetes mellitus or following the infusion of large amounts of glucose. It is also seen after the administration of a nonmetabolizable extracellular solute such as *mannitol.* Glucose slowly gains access to the intracellular space by carrier-mediated transport. Thus, if the concentration in plasma rises abruptly, glucose acts at least transiently as if it were confined to the extracellular space. This may lead to hyperosmolality without

Table 35-3. PRODUCTION RATES AND COMPOSITION OF VARIOUS BODY FLUIDS *

	VOLUME	COMPOSITION			
		Na^+	K^+	Cl^-	HCO_3^-
	ml/24 hr	mEq/liter			
Cutaneous sweat	100–200	50–80	5	40–85	—
Gastrointestinal					
Saliva	1500	10	30	10	10–20
Gastric fluid	2500	10–115	1–35	90–150	0–15
Bile	500	130–160	3–12	90–120	40–50
Pancreatic fluid	700	115–150	3–8	55–95	60–120
Intestinal fluids	3000				
Jejunum	—	85–150	2–10	45–125	—
Ileum	—	85–120	3–10	60–130	—
Ileostomy (old)	—	40–50	3–5	20–30	—
Cecostomy	—	45–135	5–45	20–90	—
Feces					
Normal	100	5	50	5	—
Diarrhea (cholera)	—	130	20	100	50

* Data are summarized from the literature for both average values and their ranges, and refer to an adult in a temperate climate engaging in mild physical activity.

hypernatremia and, indeed, due to shifts of water from the intracellular to the extracellular space, may be associated with hyponatremia. The simplest method of evaluation is to determine the concentrations of sodium and glucose separately, convert these to osmolar terms, and add them together. If hyperglycemia is rapidly corrected under the influence of insulin, a significant amount of extracellular solute may in effect disappear. This is accompanied by a redistribution of water between the extracellular and intracellular compartments. (*See* Katz, 1973.)

Isotonic Contraction. This occurs when *sodium and water are lost in isotonic propor-* tions. The most common example is the loss of fluid from the gastrointestinal tract, and cholera is the classical example. Indeed, it was W. B. O'Shaughnessy, in the cholera epidemic of 1831, who pioneered the modern study of fluid and electrolyte disorders by doing chemical analyses that, although crude and difficult, were essentially accurate. This type of disturbance may be complicated by acid base changes. Loss of strongly acidic fluid from the stomach leads to metabolic alkalosis; loss of alkaline bile and pancreatic

Table 35-4. TYPES OF ACUTE CHANGES IN VOLUME AND OSMOLALITY *

ACUTE EXTRACELLULAR CHANGE	CLINICAL EXAMPLE	Δ VOLUME		Δ CONC. PLASMA SODIUM	Δ HEMATOCRIT	Δ CONC. PLASMA PROTEIN
		Δ ECW	Δ ICW			
Isotonic contraction	Cholera	↓	0	0	↑	↑
Hypertonic contraction	Excessive sweating	↓	↓	↑	0	↑
Hypotonic contraction	Adrenal insufficiency	↓	↑	↓	↑	↑
Isotonic expansion	Isotonic saline solution	↑	0	0	↓	↓
Hypertonic expansion	Hypertonic saline solution	↑	↓	↑	↓	↓
Hypotonic expansion	Water intoxication	↑	↑	↓	0	↓

* For discussion of hematocrit, *see* text. Direction of change is shown by arrows. 0 = no change; ECW = extracellular water; ICW = intracellular water. Under clinical examples, isotonic and hypertonic saline solutions refer to infusions.

fluid, or the less alkaline fluid of severe diarrhea, leads to metabolic acidosis. The characteristic of this type of dehydration is a normal value for the concentration of sodium in serum. Therefore, regardless of the volume deficit of the extracellular phase, so long as the *concentration* of plasma sodium is normal, there will be no redistribution of water from or into the cellular compartment. The repair of the dehydration requires an expansion of the extracellular fluid volume with a solution that approximates the composition of that fluid. Although in many instances simple restoration of the volume of the extracellular space as a whole will serve to replace the plasma volume proportionately, there are occasions when more prompt and specific attention must be directed to plasma volume in particular, by providing a colloidal solution that will specifically ensure its expansion.

Hypertonic Contraction. This type of dehydration is observed in any circumstance in which there is a *loss of water in excess of sodium.* The classical example involves survival on a life raft under the unremitting impact of the tropical sun (Gamble, 1947). In more common clinical conditions it occurs when the patient is unable to drink water owing to a clouded sensorium and too little water has been provided parenterally. Other circumstances include diabetes insipidus, excessive sweating (of a hypotonic fluid), and osmotic diuresis. When this occurs in uncontrolled diabetes mellitus, the effect of glucose (a labile solute) in high concentrations is additive to the negative external balance of water in causing extracellular hypertonicity. Less commonly the disturbance may be produced by a high dietary intake of protein if unaccompanied by sufficient water intake to balance the increased urinary losses accompanying the excretion of large amounts of urea.

The effect of hypernatremia on the internal redistribution of water has already been described. In this fashion, the extracellular fluid volume, although diminished, is not as deprived as it would be if the total deficit were derived from this volume alone. On theoretical grounds there should be no change in hematocrit if there were a pure loss of water, since this would occur proportionately from the plasma and the erythrocytes. In most clinical examples, there is also a negative balance of sodium and the hematocrit would therefore rise.

Hypotonic Contraction. This occurs when there is a *loss of sodium in excess of water.* Chief among these conditions are chronic renal insufficiency and adrenocortical insufficiency. It also occurs commonly when isotonic fluid losses are treated with water (isotonic glucose solution) and too little or no salt. Essentially the same mechanism is involved when physical exercise in a hot, dry climate is associated with the drinking of water but without the ingestion of salt tablets to replace the loss of salt that occurred through perspiration. The distinguishing feature of this type of dehydration is, of course, a reduction in the concentration of sodium in serum. The consequence of this primary reduction in effective osmolality of the extracellular fluid is a passage of water from extracellular fluid into the cells. This type of dehydration greatly reduces the volume of the extracellular phase, for not only has this compartment suffered a loss of volume to the external environment but to the cells as well. In most instances of dehydration accompanied by hyponatremia, the intensity of the dehydration is of significant magnitude and warrants prompt and aggressive attention.

Isotonic Expansion. This is the *proportional retention of sodium and water* and is the basis of edema, most commonly due to cardiac, hepatic, or renal disease. The extracellular compartment may also be expanded by the injudicious use of isotonic saline solution in the overtreatment of dehydration. Even major fluctuations of dietary salt intake rarely give rise to isotonic expansion, at least in the adult. Normal renal function quite rapidly compensates for dietary changes. The changes described in Table 35–4 are most applicable to the rapid and excessive infusion of isotonic saline solution, since with spontaneous disease the slower development of edema is accompanied by changes in red-blood-cell mass and plasma protein. Indeed, the hypoproteinemia of hepatic and renal disease may be an important cause of edema. By definition, in all these examples the concentration of sodium in the plasma is normal.

There are no osmotically induced shifts of water between the extracellular and intracellular compartments.

If volume expansion is rapidly induced by infusions of saline solution, this may be accompanied by *dilutional acidosis*—the dilution of extracellular bicarbonate into an abnormally large volume (*see* section on Acid-Base Disturbances).

Hypertonic Expansion. This occurs when *sodium is retained in excess of water.* In its simplest form, it results from the rapid and excessive infusion of hypertonic saline solution. The most common clinical example probably occurs in infants improperly treated for diarrhea and involves the balance between input and output. When treatment consists in oral administration of salt and water, the concentration of salt may be erroneously excessive, or the total quantity administered may be too great to be excreted by the kidneys. Accidental salt poisoning has been reported in infants following the addition of sodium chloride instead of sugar to the formula. In these instances, hypertonicity is extreme, but volume expansion is more variable and dependent upon fluid intake and excretion (Finberg *et al.,* 1963). Fatality from severe hypernatremia is due primarily to damage to the CNS. Osmotically induced water shifts decrease intracellular volume. This contributes to the fall in hematocrit; expansion of plasma volume is obviously also involved.

Hypotonic Expansion. This occurs with *retention of water in excess of sodium.* The simplest example is water intoxication due to the excessive ingestion of water. The concentrations of sodium and protein in the plasma fall by dilution. Since water distributes itself throughout the body fluids in proportion to the compartment size, there is an increase in both the extracellular and the intracellular volumes. It is for this reason that on theoretical grounds the hematocrit does not change since the erythrocytes gain water and enlarge. In a sense, the hematocrit measures imbalances or nonproportional distribution of water between the two compartments. Careful studies provide data that are in close agreement with the theory (Wynn, 1955). Excessive ingestion of water is sometimes encountered in emotionally disturbed patients. The dominant symptoms are weakness and confusion or other signs of CNS dysfunction. This may progress from confusion and apathy to stupor and coma. In addition, generalized seizures may occur.

Another more complicated example of hypotonic expansion is seen in some patients with edema. In rare instances, during its spontaneous development, edema is associated with a greater retention of water than of salt, often referred to as dilutional hyponatremia. Far more frequently this results from the excessive use of diuretics, which may produce an imbalance between the losses of salt and water. The syndrome of the inappropriate secretion of antidiuretic hormone (ADH) also produces hypotonic expansion.

Regulation of Cell Volume. The preceding classification relies heavily on the traditional view that the net movement of water across cell membranes depends solely on osmotic gradients and that the cellular content of osmotically active solutes remains constant. While these assumptions provide a sound basis for therapeutics, it should be recognized that additional mechanisms may be involved that vary from one organ to another. These include the role of metabolism, the intracellular osmotic pressure, several transport mechanisms for solutes, and differential sensitivities to the cardiac glycosides and other drugs that alter the distribution of ions (Macknight and Leaf, 1977).

Evaluation of Intensity of Dehydration. It would be inappropriate in this textbook to dwell on the details of the clinical evaluation of the patient. However, it is exceedingly important to emphasize that a shrewd clinical appraisal of the patient's problem can permit the physician accurately to estimate the state of hydration in both qualitative and quantitative terms. One utilizes the same tools employed throughout clinical medicine, namely, a carefully obtained history, a physical examination, and the intelligent, discriminating choice and interpretation of laboratory data. Perhaps the most seriously neglected step is the correlation of the quantitative aspects of external fluid imbalance, as obtained by history, with the probable composition of those fluids (Table 35–3).

Treatment of Fluid and Electrolyte Deficits. The basic objective of therapy is to restore the volume and composition of the body fluids to normal. However, this requires extensive qualification insofar as priorities are concerned. The present discussion is limited to water and salt balance. The more complex derangements involving blood loss and protein depletion will be considered separately.

Volume Contraction. This is life threatening because it impairs the circulation. With a decreased circulating blood volume, cardiac output falls and the integrity of the micro-circulation is compromised. This occurs whether volume contraction is isotonic, hypertonic, or hypotonic, even though, as outlined above, there are important differences between them. It is urgent, therefore, that in a critical situation, attention be primarily directed to the deficit of volume. Given volume depletion of sufficient magnitude to threaten life, the prompt infusion of *isotonic sodium chloride solution is indicated;* indeed, it is difficult to contrive a contraindication.

The volume of fluid that needs to be replaced varies enormously. As a general rule, the greater and more acute the depletion, the more urgent the need for replacement. As an extreme example, intravenous therapy at the rate of 100 ml per minute for the first 1000 ml is considered necessary for the successful treatment of cholera (Carpenter, 1966). Most conditions require far less dramatic treatment. In addition to the factors outlined, attention should also be directed to the speed with which the volume depletion developed. For example, a 4-kg weight loss due to the loss of gastrointestinal fluids, from either vomiting or diarrhea, is far more debilitating if it occurs over 2 to 3 hours than over a period of days or weeks.

Disorders of Osmolality. Even with moderately severe hyponatremia or hypernatremia, frequently the disorder may be satisfactorily corrected with isotonic saline solution, provided there is normal renal function. The correction occurs as a result of the physiological adjustments made by the kidney, leading to the excretion of urine at a concentration appropriate to the underlying situation. As emphasized previously, given an adequate supply of raw materials (here best considered in terms of extracellular volume and renal blood flow) the kidney is a remarkably effective regulator of the osmolality of the body.

However, if the disturbance in osmolality is severe, producing symptoms in its own right, or threatening life, it is proper to treat this directly. Clinical judgment should be based on the actual physiological consequences of the disorder, and not on blood chemistry values considered in isolation. As is the case with disturbances of volume, a change in osmolality varies in importance depending on the speed of its development. There are examples of virtually asymptomatic extreme hyponatremia that have developed over periods of months, whereas the same degree of hyponatremia, if it appeared over hours, would invariably be accompanied by severe CNS dysfunction. If the plasma sodium concentration is lowered rapidly in infants with hypernatremia, seizures due to water intoxication may develop even though the plasma is still hypernatremic.

Intracellular osmolality within the CNS appears to be regulated by mechanisms in addition to the simple diffusion of water. In hyperosmotic states there is evidence for the appearance of osmotically active particles, sometimes referred to as "idiogenic osmoles." While these have not been identified chemically, this type of mechanism appears to explain why rapid changes in extracellular osmolality are poorly tolerated by the CNS (Kreisberg, 1978).

In the treatment of a disturbance in osmolality, a conservative goal is to return the plasma osmolality halfway to normal within 1 day. Except in extreme instances, this leads to major symptomatic and physiological improvement. In some cases of dilutional hyponatremia it is often debatable whether specific therapy is justified, either because of the absence of any detectable harm or because specific treatment may be of little use (*see* Chapter 36).

Salt or Water Requirements to Correct Disturbances in Osmolality. As an example, given a plasma sodium concentration of 120 mEq per liter, how much salt would be required to elevate this to 130 mEq per liter? For a 70-kg subject without gross volume deficits or excesses, one may assume a total body water of 50 liters. Although the administered sodium will distribute itself in an actual volume equivalent to that of the extracellular compartment, it will exert an osmotic effect to move fluid into that compartment from the intracellular space. This will diminish the induced increment in extracellular osmolality and will also increase intracellular osmolality. The concentration of sodium in the plasma will not rise by the desired increment of 10 mEq per liter until the osmolality of both the intracellular and extracellular compartments has been raised to a similar extent. Thus, 50 liters $\times$ 10 mEq per liter equals 500 mEq of sodium. In this example the volume that is added with the hypertonic saline solution is ignored. A calculation based exclusively on the extracellular volume would be in error. Using TBW for total body water, [Na] for sodium concentration in plasma, and subscripts 1 and 2 for the initial and final states, if TBW is kept constant and one solves for electrolyte balance, then:

$$(TBW_1 \times [Na]_1) + Na \text{ Balance} = TBW_2 \times [Na]_2$$
$$50 \times 120 \quad + 500 \quad\quad = 50 \quad \times 130$$

The same principle applies to the calculation of water requirements for the treatment of hypernatremia. Thus, for the same subject, if the initial concentration of sodium in the plasma were 175 mEq per liter and one desired to dilute this to 160 mEq per liter, this would require a positive water balance of 4.7 liters; with the same equation, now keeping electrolyte content constant, and solving for the change in fluid balance, then:

$$TBW_1 \times [Na]_1 = TBW_2 \times [Na]_2$$
$$50 \times 175 \quad = 54.7 \quad \times 160$$

This equation, or simple modifications for other situations, may be used to estimate requirements involving complex changes in both volume and osmolality.

Dialysis Disequilibrium Syndrome. This disorder is a complication of the use of hemodialysis for renal insufficiency and is characterized by neurological manifestations associated with the cerebral edema that results from the formation of idiogenic osmoles. The therapeutic effect of osmotically active solutes added to the dialysis fluid has been studied. While the picture is complicated by simultaneous changes in osmolality, pH, and cerebral metabolism, a number of osmotic agents do appear to be beneficial. Of these, glycerol may have particular utility because it is metabolized and therefore disappears from the plasma even in the total absence of renal function (Arieff *et al.,* 1978).

Technics of Administration of Fluid. Fluids can be administered by mouth, by intermittent gavage, by vein, and by hypodermoclysis. *Oral* intake or administration of fluids by *gavage* is proscribed whenever there is nausea or vomiting or when the therapy must be given relatively rapidly; the *parenteral* route is important when the patient is unconscious, since it is wise to eschew gavage feedings in the unconscious patient lest he vomit and aspirate. However, when it is possible, the oral route is desirable since this is truly the only way that adequate calories and other essential nutrients can be made available with ease.

Due consideration must be given to the status of the cardiovascular system in terms of the speed with which fluids are administered. If congestive heart failure is suspected or is likely to occur but relatively large volumes of fluid are needed as soon as possible, the central venous pressure, or, preferably, the pulmonary venous pressure, should be monitored. As fluid replacement progresses, boluses of the fluid should be injected rapidly to determine the effect on the venous pressure. If the effect is minimal and transient, the infusion can proceed unabated. If the venous pressure rises substantially and takes some time to return to normal, the rate of infusion must be decreased.

Fluids Available for the Repair of Dehydration. There are a variety of *commercially* available solutions that have been designed to repair the average deficits that one might anticipate in most clinical situations. It is suggested that they not be relied upon because their use tends to detract from a careful consideration of the individual problem at hand.

Appropriate fluid regimens can be designed from a small list of simple solutions. For the purposes discussed thus far, they include: (1) 5%, 10%, and 50% dextrose in water; (2) solutions of fructose in water; (3) 0.45% NaCl in water (77 mM); (4) 0.45% NaCl and 5% glucose in water; (5) 0.9% NaCl in water (154 mM); (6) 5.0% NaCl in water (855 mM); (7) 5% $NaHCO_3$ in water (595 mM); and (8) 7.5% $NaHCO_3$ in water (900 mM).

With these solutions one can administer water in excess of salt (solutions of dextrose or fructose in water), or 0.45% sodium chloride with or without dextrose; isotonic solutions of sodium chloride adequate, in most instances, for replacement of extracellular fluid *per se;* and solutions of hypertonic saline to correct hyponatremia, in which case about 25% of the sodium may be given as sodium bicarbonate to avoid dilutional acidosis.

Correction of Plasma Volume. When the plasma volume is contracted as the result of simple loss of fluid and electrolyte, as in cholera, diabetic ketoacidosis, or addisonian crisis, the defect may be corrected in many patients by simple replacement of fluid and electrolyte. These same solutions also have the capacity transiently to return cardiovascular function toward normal when the initial losses are of a more complex nature, as in hemorrhagic shock. In such a setting, the volume of saline (or equivalent) that is required is far greater than the initial loss of whole blood (Cervera and Moss, 1975). Furthermore, even when the volume is adequately replaced, the oxygen-carrying capacity will not be. Nevertheless, saline should be employed as an initial emergency measure until blood products are obtained.

The best substitute for the loss of whole blood is obviously suitable and adequately cross-matched whole blood. However, when plasma volume is critically jeopardized, the use of colloid-containing solutions is another interim measure that is much more efficacious than saline. These include individual units of plasma, which should have no more serious threat of homologous serum hepatitis (hepatitis virus B) than does a single transfusion of whole blood; a plasma protein solution (5%) prepared from pooled plasma (heated to 60° C for 10 hours by most manufacturers); 25% solutions of salt-poor human albumin, which may be used as such or diluted with saline; and solutions of dextran. The albumin and the plasma protein solutions are safe with respect to hepatitis virus B, but they are expensive. In addition, commercially prepared fractions of plasma proteins may contain low concentrations of prekallikrein activators (Hageman-factor fragments). Since these have a hypotensive action, they may worsen the clinical situation for which the plasma protein fractions are prescribed (Colman, 1978). For these reasons, there has been a widespread effort to find alternative substances that possess the properties desirable for a plasma expander.

Desirable Properties of a Plasma Expander. The major requirement to be sought in an ideal plasma expander is that it should have an oncotic pressure comparable to that of plasma. The substance should remain in the circulation for a period of time adequate to perform its function of immediate expansion of the plasma volume, and yet eventually be disposed of by excretion or metabolic degradation. This period of time is difficult to define and, in fact, would differ with circumstances. The ideal plasma expander should not affect adversely any visceral function, nor should it have an antigenic, allergenic, or pyretic effect. Indeed, except for its physical properties, it should be pharmacologically inert. It should not interfere with typing or cross-agglutination of blood, and it should be able to withstand long periods of storage and wide variations in environmental temperature and still be effective. It should be easily sterilized and have a viscosity suitable for infusion over a reasonable temperature range.

Many substances have been investigated as potential plasma expanders, including fluorocarbon-polyols (Geyer, 1973) and stroma-free crystalline hemoglobin (Nees *et al.*, 1978; Savitsky *et al.*, 1978). Dextran meets most of the above requirements, as does hetastarch, although there is less clinical experience with the latter agent (*see* Fox and Nahas, 1970).

Dextran. Dextran was originally described by the German carbohydrate-chemist Schleibler. The compound was first isolated from solutions of beet sugar, where it is formed by the action of a contaminating bacterium, *Leuconostoc mesenteroides.*

Chemistry. In its original form, dextran is a branched polysaccharide of about 200,000 glucose units, with a molecular weight of approximately 40 million. The glucose units in the main chain are bound together through 1:6 glucosidic linkages; those in the shorter branches, through 1:4 linkages. By means of partial hydrolysis and subsequent fractionation, native dextran can be converted to polysaccharides of any desired range of molecular weights.

There are two forms of dextran solution currently available. One has an average molecular weight of either 70,000 or 75,000 (depending on the pharmaceutical preparation), and the other has an average molecular weight of 40,000. Both agents expand plasma volume specifically. There is evidence to suggest that the lower-molecular-weight dextran may well have advantages (*see* Moore, 1963). Its administration not only corrects hypovolemia but also appears to improve the microcirculation independently of simple volume expansion. It seems to minimize the tendency for sludging of blood that may accompany many forms of shock.

Hemodynamic Action. The hemodynamic action of dextran is that expected of an effective plasma expander. When given to normal individuals, there is a temporary increase in cardiac output, stroke volume, right atrial pressure, and venous pressure. As a result of the hypervolemia, urine flow is increased. There is no reliable evidence that the dextrans influence renal function unfavorably. However, in the presence of hypotension and a reduction in filtration rate, the excessive tubular reabsorption of water may increase the concentration of dextran in the tubular fluid so that viscosity impedes the flow of fluid through the tubule (*see* Fox and Nahas, 1970). In an individual who has sustained a loss of whole blood or plasma, a single infusion of dextran increases the circulating blood volume and improves the hemodynamic status for 24 hours or longer. It has been successfully employed in the treatment of loss of blood and plasma in a variety of conditions.

Effects on Blood. Dextran has little effect on the blood. It may interfere with typing, cross-matching, or Rh determinations, but this is unpredictable. It may produce a hemostatic defect described as an acquired form of von Willebrand's disease (*see* Fox and Nahas, 1970). The uses of dextran for its antiplatelet and antithrombotic effects are described in Chapter 58.

Antigenic Action. Dextran is a potent antigen. This is true of the native polysaccharide and the hydrolysis products used clinically. Furthermore, dextran occurs in commercial sugar, and dextran-producing organisms can be found in the human gastrointestinal tract. Therefore, a small percentage of individuals who have never received dextran have precipitins to the polysaccharide in the circulation.

The antigenic activity of dextran would seem to preclude its repeated use. However, when given in the massive doses that are employed for infusion, antibody production does not occur, due presumably to the phenomenon of "immunological paralysis." Indeed, the incidence of anaphylactoid reactions to colloidal volume expanders such as plasma protein solutions, dextran, and hetastarch is remarkably low and is significantly less than that for transfusions or for many drugs (Ring and Messmer, 1977).

Distribution, Metabolic Fate, and Excretion. Following the infusion of dextran, the molecules of smaller molecular weight are excreted by the kidney. As much as 50% appears in the urine within 24 hours. However, the remainder traverses the capillary wall very slowly, as judged by its appearance in lymph. The portion that is not excreted is slowly oxidized over a period of a few weeks. The persistence of dextran and its ultimate metabolic disposal are desirable features of a plasma expander.

Untoward Reactions. Dextran appears to have no significant deleterious effects on renal, hepatic, or other vital functions. However, sensitivity reactions occur for reasons already mentioned. The incidence of such reactions is extremely variable, depending upon the preparation employed. As the technic of manufacture has improved, the number of untoward responses has diminished. These consist in itching, urticaria, joint pains, and other side effects, and are relatively mild in character. Their incidence in normal individuals is less than 10%.

Clinical Status. Dextran possesses most of the attributes of an ideal plasma expander, its chief defect being antigenicity. It has been successfully employed in the treatment of the circulatory inadequacies associated with the hypovolemia attending the loss of both whole blood and plasma. It must be realized that the use of a plasma expander is a temporary measure in the treatment of blood loss.

Hetastarch. This synthetic polymer, also known as hydroxyethyl starch, is prepared from amylopectin by the introduction of hydroxyethyl ether groups into its glucose residues. The purpose of the modification is to retard the rate of degradation of the polymer. This preparation bears many similarities to dextran. Hetastarch has an average molecular weight of 450,000, with a range from 10,000 to 1,000,000. Molecules with the lower molecular weights are readily excreted in the urine, and, with the usual preparation, about 40% of the dose is excreted within 24 hours. The molecules of higher molecular weight are metabolized slowly; only about 1% of a dose persists after 2 weeks. Hetastarch may have the same action as dextran on the blood coagulation mechanisms. Although hetastarch is said to have fewer antigenic properties than dextran, this assertion is not supported by clinical experience (Ring and Messmer, 1977).

Preparations of Fluids Available. Most of the following solutions are now generally available in glass vials, plastic bags, and prefilled syringes with various-sized needles. The pH ranges are important with respect to both stability and possible incompatibilities with drugs that may be added. The U.S.P. requires that the concentrations of solutions of dextrose and of dextrose and sodium chloride be labeled in terms of *milliosmoles* of the total solution, that is, the sum of each compound or ion in milligrams per liter divided by its molecular or atomic weight.

Glucose. Dextrose, U.S.P., is commonly referred to as *glucose. Dextrose Injection*, U.S.P., is a sterile solution, pH 3.5 to 6.5, for parenteral administration. It is marketed in concentrations varying from 2.5 to 70%. *Dextrose and Sodium Chloride Injection*, U.S.P., pH 3.5 to 6.0, is a sterile solution of glucose and sodium chloride. Available solutions consist of varying concentrations of glucose, 2.5 to 25%, in sodium chloride solution, 0.11 to 0.9%, a complete list of which is given in the U.S.P. Rapid intravenous administration of solutions of glucose may lead to glycosuria. When given at an hourly rate of 800 mg/kg, approximately 95% of the glucose is retained; at half this rate, 100% retention is achieved.

Fructose. Fructose Injection, U.S.P., is a sterile solution of fructose in water, available as a 10% solution, pH 3.0 to 6.0. One of the advantages of fructose is its rapid removal from the extracellular space, and, therefore, urinary excretion is minimized. *Fructose and Sodium Chloride Injection*, U.S.P., is a sterile solution of fructose and sodium chloride in water.

Sodium Salts. Sodium Chloride, U.S.P., is the

most important single salt for the maintenance or replacement of deficits of extracellular fluid. It is available in a variety of concentrations. Isotonic sodium chloride solution (0.9%) may be administered by different routes. For oral use, tablets or solutions may be used. For subcutaneous injection, an isotonic solution must be employed. *Sodium Chloride Injection,* U.S.P., is available in various volumes; its pH range is 4.5 to 7.0. Hypertonic solutions (3 and 5%) must be administered intravenously. Hypotonic sodium chloride solution (0.45%) is also available. Sodium chloride may also be incorporated into solutions of glucose and fructose, as described above. *Sodium Bicarbonate,* U.S.P., is available in the form of *Sodium Bicarbonate Tablets,* U.S.P. A solution of 1.4% is approximately isotonic with body fluids. A sterile solution, *Sodium Bicarbonate Injection,* U.S.P., is available in solutions of 4% (5-ml vials), 4.2% (10-ml disposable syringe), 5% (500 ml), 7.5% (50-ml ampuls; 50-ml disposable syringe), and 8.4% (10- and 50-ml vials; 50-ml disposable syringe); its pH range is up to 8.5.

Plasma Protein Fraction, U.S.P. (PLASMANATE, PLASMA-PLEX, PLASMATEIN, PROTENATE), is a sterile aqueous solution containing 5% human plasma proteins in sodium chloride solution (0.9%), of which not less than 83% is albumin and the remainder is α- and β-globulins; it is osmotically equivalent to plasma. The risk of transmitting hepatitis B virus is minimized by manufacturers by heating at 60° C for 10 hours. This preparation is available in 250- and 500-ml quantities.

Albumin Human, U.S.P. (ALBUTEIN, ALBUMINAR, ALBUMISOL, ALBUSPAN, BUMINATE, PROSERUM), is a sterile preparation of 5 or 25% serum albumin obtained by fractionating blood from healthy human donors. The 5% solution, which is osmotically equivalent to plasma, is available in 250- and 500-ml quantities; the 25% solution is supplied in units of 20, 50, and 100 ml. Risk of hepatitis B virus is minimized by heating in the same manner as described above. These preparations were formerly made with two concentrations of sodium chloride, one of which was erroneously referred to as "salt poor." All preparations now have 130 to 160 mEq per liter of sodium chloride.

Dextran. Two forms of dextran, which differ in molecular size, are available for use as plasma expanders. *Dextran 70 injection* (MACRODEX) contains 6% *dextran* (average molecular weight 70,000) in 0.9% sodium chloride solution or 5% dextrose in water, pH 4.0 to 6.5. *Dextran 75 injection* (GENTRAN) is virtually identical but with an average molecular weight of 75,000. *Dextran 40 injection* (GENTRAN 40, LMD 10%, RHEOMACRODEX) contains 10% *dextran 40* (average molecular weight 40,000) in 0.9% sodium chloride solution or 5% dextrose in water. The molecular weight of the former preparation approximates that of human plasma albumin; the smaller molecular size of the latter preparation is said to have the advantage of retarding rouleau formation and sludging of red blood cells. Both preparations are available in units of 500 ml.

Hetastarch injection (VOLEX) is prepared as a 6% solution in 0.9% sodium chloride in units of 500 ml.

PROBLEMS OF CARBOHYDRATES FATS, AND PROTEINS

In the absence of the normal dietary intake of calories and foodstuffs by mouth, intravenous dextrose solution serves to protect against the development of ketosis and to minimize the wasting of protein. For this purpose, on a short-term basis, isotonic or slightly hypertonic dextrose solution is a useful adjuvant, and one should administer approximately 100 g of carbohydrate per day to an adult. For more prolonged treatment, carbohydrate and protein hydrolysates may be given by gavage.

Intravenous Hyperalimentation. This technic has been developed within the last few decades and now represents an important contribution to the management of certain patients, particularly those with intestinal abnormalities or severe dysfunction, trauma, or various surgical complications, both in the pediatric and adult age groups. The success of these procedures justifies their use, but the complications are serious and can be avoided only by meticulous attention to detail involving the pharmacist, nurse, and physician. Such therapy accomplishes a positive nitrogen balance and can be continued for as long as 30 to 60 days. The basic nutrient solution consists of hypertonic dextrose (20 to 25%) and protein hydrolysates or crystalline amino acids in water, plus electrolytes and vitamins. The need for hypertonic solutions is dictated by the limits of water intake. This therapeutic approach should be undertaken only with the realization that long-term tactical planning is required for the management of a number of details; these include intravenous technics, frequency and nature of blood chemical determinations, and day-to-day estimates of requirements for water, electrolytes, and the nutritional components of the solutions.

The infusion is given through a percutaneous catheter inserted into a large branch of the superior vena cava. Delivery into a large vein permits prompt adjustment of osmolality by dilution. Rigid sterile surgical technic is essential. A peristaltic pump should be used to drive the infusion through the tubing, which contains a microfilter. Both tubing and filter should be changed frequently. Ancillary medications should be given by another route. Pharmaceutical incompatibilities must be avoided. These include incompatibilities of electrolytes that may involve bicarbonate, calcium, phosphate, and sulfate (for other details, *see* Fischer, 1977).

Infrequent mechanical complications are related to the insertion of the catheter. Undoubtedly the most serious complication is that of *infection*. To the extent that this results from the infusion, its incidence is greatly reduced by in-line filters. *Metabolic complications* are common, often mild, and are a direct consequence of the infusions themselves. Since these are acceptable if mild, the regimen should be initiated gradually, then kept constant from day to day and carefully monitored. Mild *glycosuria* is common but may subside after stimulation of endogenous insulin production as a result of the hyperglycemia. However, severe glycosuria may lead to excessive water loss and the undesirable development of hypertonic contraction of body fluids. With the addition of adequate amounts of sodium, potassium, magnesium, chloride, and bicarbonate, electrolyte imbalance may be avoided. Prolonged *hypophosphatemia* may lead to serious neurological and hematological complications, and phosphate is a requirement for prolonged therapy. *Hyperammonemia* may occur, particularly in infants, and can be prevented by reducing the nitrogenous components of the infusion. The rationale for the parenteral administration of fat does not involve total caloric requirements as much as it does the possibility that certain lipids may be essential nutritional requirements, particularly for the synthesis of various components of cellular membranes.

Preparations. In addition to the solutions of electrolytes and simple sugars, which have been previously mentioned, the following solutions are used in parenteral alimentation.

Protein Hydrolysates. Protein Hydrolysate Injection, U.S.P. (AMIGEN, AMINOSOL, CPH, HYPROTIGEN, PARENAMINE, TRAVAMIN), is a sterile solution of amino acids and short-chain peptides that represent the approximate nutritive equivalent of the casein, lactalbumin, plasma, fibrin, or other suitable protein from which it is derived by an acidic, enzymatic, or other method of hydrolysis. It may be modified by partial removal and restoration or addition of one or more amino acids. It may contain dextrose or other carbohydrate suitable for intravenous infusion. It is usually available in 5% solution in combination with dextrose, fructose, or alcohol in 500- and 1000-ml volumes. Preparations differ slightly in electrolyte content.

Amino Acids. Amino acid injection (AMINOSYN, FREAMINE, TRAVASOL, VEINAMINE) consists of approximately 15 amino acids (both essential and nonessential), with total amino acid content from 3.5 to 10%. Formulations vary as to total osmolality and are available with or without electrolytes. The proportion of amino acids also varies slightly between preparations. A solution of 3.5% amino acids is only slightly hypertonic and may be administered by peripheral vein; more concentrated solutions are intended for infusion by central vein and are usually mixed with hypertonic glucose solution to provide

additional caloric intake. *Essential amino acid injection* (NEPHRAMINE) is composed of eight essential amino acids in an almost electrolyte-free solution, prepared to be diluted with hypertonic glucose solution and administered by central vein. It is particularly intended for patients with potentially reversible acute renal failure.

Fat Emulsion. Emulsions of 10% fat (INTRALIPID 10%) are prepared from refined soy bean oil, egg-yolk phospholipids, and glycerin. The major fatty acids are linoleic, oleic, palmitic, and linolenic. The preparation is isotonic and may be administered into a peripheral vein. It should not be mixed with other solutions employed in parenteral alimentation.

ACID-BASE DISTURBANCES

Abnormalities of the pH of body fluids are just as important as pathological alterations of their volume or osmolality.

There are several definitions of the terms *acid* and *base;* for our purposes an acid is a substance that can provide a hydrogen ion (proton donor) and a base is a substance that can accept a hydrogen ion (proton acceptor), as follows:

$$\text{Acid} \rightleftharpoons \text{Base} + \text{H}^+$$

The negative logarithm of the equilibrium constant for this reversible reaction is termed the pK_a. Acids with lower values of pK_a have a greater tendency to dissociate or to donate a proton and are referred to as strong acids. The Henderson-Hasselbalch equation expresses the pH of a solution of an acid-base pair as a function of their concentrations and the value of pK_a (a measure of the intrinsic tendency of the acid to dissociate to form the conjugate base):

$$\text{pH} = pK_a + \log \frac{[\text{Base}]}{[\text{Acid}]}$$

This equation is derived in any fundamental textbook of chemistry. It makes clear the fact that the pH is determined by the pK_a and the *ratio* of the concentrations of the acid-base pair. Since many different substances may coexist in solution, and since a solution may have only a single hydrogen ion concentration or pH, it follows that the ratios of different buffer pairs must vary in order to satisfy the general equation:

$$\text{pH} = pK_{a_\text{I}} + \log \frac{[\text{Base}]_\text{I}}{[\text{Acid}]_\text{I}} = pK_{a_\text{II}} + \log \frac{[\text{Base}]_\text{II}}{[\text{Acid}]_\text{II}}$$

in which I and II refer to different chemical entities.

Carbonic acid and the ammonium ion are acids of physiological importance that dissociate as follows:

$$H_2CO_3 \rightleftharpoons HCO_3^- + H^+$$
$$NH_4^+ \rightleftharpoons NH_3 + H^+$$

For carbonic acid the conjugate base (bicarbonate) is charged (negatively), and for ammonia (a base) the conjugate acid is charged (positively). Since the charge of an ion is of major importance for many biological processes, it is often convenient to refer to *cations* (positively charged ions) and to *anions* (negatively charged ions). Thus, one may say that carbonic acid dissociates to an anion and a cation, or, since the specificity of the hydrogen ion is so important, it dissociates to an anion and a hydrogen ion.

Mechanisms of Compensation. The responses that tend to minimize any deviation in pH include buffer reactions, ion-exchange mechanisms, alterations in respiratory activity, and renal mechanisms. The physiological mechanisms that respond to a disturbance in acid-base equilibrium tend to restore pH toward normal.

Buffers. A buffered solution is one that is able to minimize a deviation in pH caused by the addition of H^+ or OH^-. For significant buffering to occur in biological fluids, the pK_a of the weak acid must be within the pH range of those fluids. According to the Henderson-Hasselbalch equation, buffering is maximally efficient when the ratio of base to acid is unity, that is, when one half of the weak acid is present as its conjugate base. By definition, this occurs when $pH = pK_a$.

Total buffering capacity also depends on the concentration of the buffer itself. The role of true buffer

reactions is often inadequately appreciated, particularly in the extent to which the intracellular buffers (principally proteins) are involved in the regulation of bicarbonate concentration in the presence of changing concentrations of carbon dioxide. In the following example, the diffusion reactions between the extracellular and intracellular spaces have been omitted.

$$H^+ + HCO_3^- + B^+Pr^- \rightleftharpoons HPr + B^+ + HCO_3^-$$
$$\Updownarrow$$
$$H_2CO_3$$

B^+Pr^- is the potassium salt of an intracellular protein. It may be seen that the generation of HCO_3^- is reversibly determined by the H_2CO_3 concentration, or the P_{CO_2}. This occurs without any change in the external balance of bicarbonate. This buffer reaction contributes to the changes in bicarbonate concentration that occur in primary respiratory disorders (Table 35-5).

The Bicarbonate–Carbonic Acid System. There are, of course, many buffers in the body fluids, including hemoglobin, phosphates, proteins, and the bicarbonate-carbonic acid pair, which can be expressed as follows:

$$pH = 6.1 + \log \frac{[HCO_3^-]}{[H_2CO_3] + [\text{dissolved } CO_2]}$$

This buffer system has many unique features. Of practical importance is the ease of measurement in serum of the components of the system, the concentrations of which deviate in acid-base disturbances. Such measurements are of great diagnostic value. Of major physiological importance is the manner by which the concentrations of carbonic acid and bicarbonate can be regulated. Since H_2CO_3 is readily converted from or to a gas, CO_2, its concentration is responsive to alveolar P_{CO_2} and can be altered by variations in pulmonary ventilation. Furthermore, the

Table 35-5. **TYPICAL PLASMA VALUES IN THE VARIOUS ACID-BASE DISORDERS** *

	pH	HCO_3^-	P_{CO_2}	Cl^-	ANION GAP
Respiratory acidosis	↓	↑	↑	↓	±
Respiratory alkalosis	↑	↓	↓	↑	±
Metabolic acidosis	↓	↓	↓	± or ↑	± or ↑
Metabolic alkalosis	↑	↑	↑	↓	± or ↑

* For calculation of anion gap, *see* text.

concentration of bicarbonate ion in extracellular fluid can be altered by changes in renal function. Indeed, the *bicarbonate–carbonic acid system is the major buffer system in the body that is subject to compensatory physiological regulation.* Following any alteration in this system, every other buffer pair in body fluids must alter, since the ratio of a buffer pair defines and in turn is defined by the pH. The ratio of the bicarbonate–carbonic acid system at a pH of 7.4 is 20:1. Although a buffer pair is more efficient when the ratio of the pair at body pH is close to 1, the unique qualities of this particular system make it highly effective even at a ratio of 20:1.

Ion Exchange. Cations such as sodium and potassium, and perhaps magnesium and calcium, from muscle, bone, and other tissues can exchange for hydrogen ions in the extracellular fluid, and this plays a significant role in the moderation of alterations in acid-base equilibrium. The exchange of anions probably plays a much less important role, except for the shift of chloride and bicarbonate that occurs across the red-cell membrane.

Respiratory Regulation. In terms of quantity alone, the lungs play the major role in the daily excretion of acid. Approximately 10 millimoles of CO_2 are generated and expired each minute. The mechanisms in the CNS that are responsible for the rate and the depth of respiratory activity are responsive to the partial pressure of CO_2 and to pH. A depression in pH or an increase of P_{CO_2} increases ventilatory exchange. This, in turn, serves to eliminate more acid as CO_2 and to minimize the acid-base disturbance.

Renal Regulation. The renal mechanisms contribute to acid-base regulation by varying the net rate of excretion of hydrogen ions and by selectively reabsorbing and rejecting cations and anions. In terms of combating an acidosis, one can view the major role of the kidney as reabsorbing all the filtered bicarbonate and, in addition, generating new bicarbonate that is formed by the excretion of hydrogen ion as either ammonium or titratable acid. Since the normal diet gives rise to nonvolatile acids that must be eliminated by the kidney, this mechanism is normally in operation. In the renal compensation for alkalosis, particularly metabolic alkalosis produced by the excessive intake of sodium bicarbonate, the amount of filtered bicarbonate

is increased and is only partially reabsorbed. Thus, bicarbonate is excreted in the urine, mainly as the sodium salt. The details of the manner by which the kidney can regulate the bicarbonate buffer system are presented in the Introduction to Section VIII.

Laboratory Diagnosis of Acid-Base Disturbances. There are *four primary acid-base disturbances* of clinical significance: respiratory acidosis and alkalosis, and metabolic acidosis and alkalosis. This classification is based on the original directional change of a single component of the bicarbonate–carbonic acid system. By reference to the Henderson-Hasselbalch equation, the initial change may be either a rise or fall in bicarbonate, or a rise or fall in carbonic acid (or P_{CO_2}). These changes, in turn, may be induced by multiple factors, depending upon the disease entity. There are several technics for the evaluation of these disturbances. The history and physical examination should be revealing as to the general nature of the underlying disorder. The simplest and most common laboratory measurements are the pH and P_{CO_2} of the blood, and the total CO_2 content of the serum. These data will usually indicate what sort of disturbance or disturbances are present.

The simple calculation of the *anion gap* is also exceedingly helpful and may provide important insight into etiology. On the basis of the normal cation-anion pattern of the plasma and assuming single normal values in mEq per liter, the difference between the concentration of sodium (140) and the sum of the concentrations of bicarbonate (25) and chloride (105) is 10. A normal range is 8 to 12. Since the anion gap represents the difference between two relatively large numbers, it is subject to accumulative analytical error. If the concentration of a normal anion, other than chloride or bicarbonate, is abnormally high, or if an abnormal anion has accumulated, the disorder may be detected by calculation of the anion gap. Major examples of anions that contribute to the anion gap include β-hydroxybutyrate, acetoacetate, lactate, phosphate, and sulfate. Much less commonly, and unrelated to acid-base disturbances, the anion gap may be decreased (Oh and Carroll, 1977).

The *potassium* ion plays a complex and

important role in many acid-base disturbances. This will be discussed in a separate section, below.

Respiratory Acidosis. In this situation the primary disorder is retention of carbon dioxide because of improper ventilation. The effect is to increase the denominator of the buffer ratio in the Henderson-Hasselbalch equation, and hence to lower the pH. The accession of acid (in this case, CO_2) is buffered, and the kidney responds by increasing the reabsorption of bicarbonate at the expense of chloride. The lungs play no compensatory role, since it is their disability that has induced the disturbance. The chemical characteristics of this disorder are listed in Table 35-5.

Retention of carbon dioxide results from two main causes: depression of the respiratory center in the medulla due to an overdose of central depressant drugs, such as morphine or barbiturates, and pathological changes in the alveoli or airways. In the first instance, respiratory minute volume declines progressively due to diminishing responsiveness of the medulla to changes in P_{CO_2} and pH. Respiratory drive is inadequate and totally dependent on impulses arising from the hypoxic carotid body. The administration of oxygen may result in apnea (*see* Chapter 16). A similar situation occurs with pathological changes in the lung. After a period of hyperpnea, the medulla becomes increasingly insensitive to hypercapnia and hypoxia becomes the major stimulus to respiration. Again, the administration of oxygen can result in apnea. This does not mean that patients with respiratory acidosis should not receive oxygen, but that artificial respiration is essential in the presence of inadequate respiratory drive. If ventilatory assistance is not possible and oxygen is required, it should be administered very cautiously and with the doctor *at the bedside.*

Obviously, the most important aspects of therapy relate to an improvement in the basic cause underlying the hypoventilation. However, in severe respiratory acidosis, particularly in asthmatic patients, it may be essential to correct the derangement of pH directly. This can be accomplished by the infusion of sodium bicarbonate solution. At a more normal pH the bronchodilator drugs become more effective and the basic pulmonary disorder may be alleviated (Mithoefer *et al.,* 1965).

Respiratory Alkalosis. In this situation the disturbance is caused by an increased excretion of CO_2 by way of the lungs, owing to hyperventilation. It is usually a consequence of an emotional disorder and much less frequently of a lesion of the CNS that stimulates the mechanisms that drive respiration. It can also be caused by drugs that stimulate respiration, such as the salicylates. The hyperventilation diminishes the P_{CO_2}, which increases the value of the buffer ratio and, therefore, increases the pH. At the same time the plasma concentration of bicarbonate falls as a direct result of the buffer reactions and compensatory mechanisms that come into play. The chemical characteristics are described in Table 35-5.

The therapeutic measures are several. In the patient with hysterical hyperventilation, rebreathing into a paper bag will tend to augment P_{CO_2} and combat the respiratory alkalosis. In the more severe form, in which there is sufficient alkalosis to induce carpopedal spasm, the use of sedation along with breathing a gas mixture with CO_2 (usually about a 5% concentration) may be very helpful. In instances of primary respiratory alkalosis due to a CNS lesion, the therapy must obviously be directed at the specific cause as well. Salicylate poisoning as a cause of respiratory alkalosis is discussed in Chapter 29.

Metabolic Acidosis. The disturbance results either from a loss of proton acceptors (such as bicarbonate during severe diarrhea) or from the accession of an acid load that may result from a metabolic disturbance such as diabetic ketoacidosis, renal insufficiency, lactic acidosis, or that caused by administration of an acidifying salt such as ammonium chloride. Insight into etiology may be obtained from the magnitude of the anion gap. The ketoacids and lactic acid play an obvious role. In renal insufficiency the abnormally large anion gap is attributable to phosphate and sulfate. If acidosis is the result of the ingestion of ammonium chloride, the anion gap is normal since the chloride anion is accounted for in the basic measurement. Whether due to the accession of an acidic load or to the primary loss of bicarbonate, the impact on the Henderson-Hasselbalch equation is to reduce the value of the numerator and, therefore, to decrease the pH. The buffers, ion-exchange mechanisms, and respiratory and renal responses tend to compensate for the acidosis and are more or less efficient, depending on the intensity of the disturbance on the one hand and the health of the lungs and kidneys on the other.

No effort is made herein to detail the specific therapy for the many types of acidosis. However, the role of adequate renal function should be emphasized. Since metabolic acidosis is often accompanied by volume depletion, renal blood flow may be compromised and the kidneys may be unable to excrete appropriate amounts of titratable acid and ammonium. This may be corrected by the administration of isotonic sodium chloride solution. When it is considered advisable to employ an alkalinizing salt, the use of a solution of sodium bicarbonate instead of sodium lactate is recommended. When sodium lactate is employed, it is converted to bicarbonate by cellular oxidative activity. If this is deficient, the therapeutic goal will not have been achieved. This is particularly important in view of the greater recognition of lactic acidosis itself as a disease entity.

The dose of bicarbonate necessary to correct an acute acidosis is exceedingly difficult to define antecedently. One suggestion has been to estimate the difference between the normal and the current total HCO_3^- content, expressed in mEq, and multiply this by 50% of the body weight in kilograms. Because of the persistent high rate of lactic acid production, undertreatment is more likely in lactic acidosis than in the other forms of metabolic acidosis. Overtreatment is to be avoided since the rapid conversion from acidosis to alkalosis may be harmful, perhaps because of the disequilibrium that arises between the pH of the cerebrospinal fluid and that of the plasma when abrupt changes occur (Kreisberg, 1978).

In more chronic diseases, such as chronic renal insufficiency, the metabolic acidosis is correctable with the use of sodium bicarbonate or preparations of sodium citrate. The latter is more palatable in the form of Shohl's solution (see below). In any event, the dose must be found empirically and small doses should be used initially so as not to overtreat.

Metabolic Alkalosis. This is characterized by an increase in the concentration of bicarbonate in the extracellular fluid, unassociated with a proportionate increase in the P_{CO_2} (see Table 35–5), so that the buffer ratio is in excess of 20 and the pH is accordingly increased. A metabolic alkalosis can be induced by the loss of hydrogen ions, as in vomiting hydrochloric acid, or by the administration of alkalinizing salts, such as sodium bicarbonate or sodium citrate.

The compensatory mechanisms that tend to minimize the deviation in pH may be anticipated from the Henderson-Hasselbalch equation, but in every instance there are serious limits imposed on their efficiency. For example, respiratory compensation may have serious limits imposed upon it, since the increase in pH would tend to suppress ventilation, thus permitting some accumulation of CO_2. However, this might very well be limited owing to hypoxia and hypercapnia, both of which independently tend to increase ventilatory activity. In addition, although CO_2 penetrates the brain rapidly, equilibration with bicarbonate is slow. Hence, if the cerebrospinal fluid bicarbonate is still relatively normal and the P_{CO_2} is increased, the pH of this fluid is reduced and the central receptors are thereby stimulated to increase ventilatory exchange. The renal response might be expected to promote the excretion of sodium bicarbonate. In fact, this will occur to the point at which a negative balance of sodium develops, in which case all the mechanisms available to promote the retention of sodium are implemented. Stated in different terms, the compensatory renal excretion of bicarbonate requires the obligatory excretion of a fixed cation, principally sodium. When a significant deficit of sodium develops, this ion is no longer excreted in the urine. Hence, bicarbonate excretion also declines despite the persistent alkalosis of the extracellular fluids. *It should be emphasized that sodium depletion is primarily responsible for the paradoxical aciduria of a metabolic alkalosis.* Little bicarbonate will be excreted without accompanying sodium ions. However, a deficit of potassium augments this phenomenon.

In severe metabolic alkalosis there is another mechanism that may be considered compensatory in nature since it tends to minimize the change in extracellular pH. This involves the accumulation of organic acids in the plasma, and it may be measured indirectly by the anion gap. If these endogenous organic acids did not accumulate, the bicarbonate concentration would be still higher.

The treatment of the metabolic alkalosis is dependent, in part, on removing the initiating circumstance that induced the sequence of events leading to the disturbance. When caused by the excessive use of alkalinizing salts, the intensity of the disorder may vary, but even if mild the intake of such salts should be halted. On the basis of early studies of Gamble and Ross (1925) that have been amply supported by subsequent experience, acute metabolic alkalosis may be corrected by the administration of adequate amounts of sodium chloride solution. The ability of a neutral salt to correct an acid-base disturbance is based on physiological rather than simple chemical mechanisms. In the case of alkalosis due to vomiting, the body is depleted of water, hydrogen ion, chloride, and, to a lesser extent, sodium. Once an adequate extracellular volume is reestablished, normal renal mechanisms become effective and sodium, along with bicarbonate, is excreted in the urine. This corrects the compositional abnormality in the plasma.

Severe metabolic alkalosis may be life threatening. In rare instances, the severity of symptoms requires direct correction of the abnormal pH itself. This can be accomplished with an acidifying salt such as ammonium chloride since, in the presence of normal hepatic function, the alkalosis can be corrected without waiting for renal mechanisms to come into play (see below). Hepatic failure is a contraindication to the administration of ammonium chloride. The administration of 0.1 N hydrochloric acid by catheter into a large central vein may be employed in instances of severe metabolic alkalosis in which it is desired to lower the systemic pH promptly and directly without reliance on either renal or hepatic mechanisms. The infused acid is immediately buffered by the circulating blood, although mild hemolysis may occur; if administered into a peripheral vein, severe thrombophlebitis can result. This procedure should be considered as a heroic measure that is to be used only when more conventional therapy has failed (Abouna et al., 1974).

Dilution Acidosis and Subtraction Alkalosis. These acid-base disturbances, which result from therapeutic maneuvers, occur when a large volume of isotonic sodium chloride, devoid of bicarbonate, is added to or removed from the extracellular space. In actual practice, dilution commonly results from large infusions of isotonic saline. In contrast, diuretics can remove a large volume of essentially isotonic sodium chloride from the edematous patient (see Chapter 36). In neither case is there a significant gain or loss of bicarbonate. The change in acid-base balance

occurs because the amount of bicarbonate initially present in the extracellular fluid remains constant—in one case (subtraction alkalosis) it is concentrated by the reduction in extracellular fluid volume, and in the other case (dilution acidosis) it is diluted by the expansion of that volume. A number of balance studies are consistent with this concept, particularly those of the pathogenesis of the alkalosis induced by the saluretic diuretics. However, the situation is complicated by a number of factors, such as the rate of production of carbon dioxide, changes in the intracellular distribution of bicarbonate, and the effect of the volume and osmolality of the extracellular fluid on renal bicarbonate reabsorption (Garella et al., 1975). Nevertheless, the basic concepts are valid and provide the basis for the evaluation of these frequently encountered disturbances.

Alkalinization or Acidification of the Urine. There are situations in which the primary purpose of therapy is to change the pH of the urine rather than to correct a systemic abnormality in acid-base balance. This is readily accomplished, when renal function is normal, by the administration of either alkalinizing or acidifying salts that are rapidly excreted in the urine. Such a maneuver produces only a modest distortion in systemic acid-base balance. However, in edema-forming states, when the renal reabsorption of sodium is inappropriately high, alkalinizing salts are poorly excreted. Furthermore, in the presence of renal insufficiency, there is a diminished capacity of the kidney to compensate for acidosis, and acidifying salts may have harmful systemic effects.

One goal of alkalinization of the urine (to a pH greater than 7.4) is to increase the solubility of certain of its constituents. This particularly involves weak acids that are more soluble as the salt and is generally utilized for conditions in which the acid is excreted in the urine in an excessively high concentration. Examples include cystine, in cystinuria; uric acid, in spontaneous hyperuricemia or following the administration of oncolytic or uricosuric agents; methotrexate, in high-dosage therapy; and the administration of certain sulfonamides. A second goal is to increase the excretory rate of lipid-soluble organic acids whose reabsorption is accomplished by diffusion of the nonionized species. Examples include the treatment of overdosage of salicylate or phenobarbital.

An alternate approach to the administration of an alkalinizing salt such as sodium bicarbonate is to utilize an inhibitor of carbonic anhydrase such as acetazolamide (see Chapter 36). When sodium bicarbonate is administered, large doses (10 to 15 g per day) are required to keep the urine persistently alkaline throughout the 24-hour period. When acetazolamide increases bicarbonate excretion, it depletes the body stores of the anion, which tends to reduce the efficacy of the drug. It thus may be logical to prescribe both acetazolamide and sodium bicarbonate. Their actions on the pH of the urine are complementary. However, it should be kept in mind that acetazolamide may competitively inhibit the tubular secretion of other organic acids.

The urine is purposely rendered more *acidic* than normal either to increase the renal excretion of lipid-soluble organic bases or to provide conditions appropriate for a specific pharmacological effect. There are no examples in which acidification is required to increase the solubility of a basic drug. A low urinary pH is required for the activation of methenamine, a urinary tract antiseptic; some other antimicrobials (*e.g.*, nitrofurantoin) are more potent in an acidic urine (Milne, 1978).

Preparations for the Treatment of Acid-Base Disturbances. *Sodium Bicarbonate.* This salt has already been discussed in a previous section. It should be emphasized that it is the preferred alkalinizing salt since it achieves the therapeutic goal promptly.
Sodium Lactate. *Sodium Lactate Injection,* U.S.P., is a sterile solution of sodium lactate in water. It is usually marketed as an isotonic ($\frac{1}{6}$ M; 1.9%) solution or as a molar solution that can be appropriately diluted. The reasons for preferring sodium bicarbonate in lieu of sodium lactate have been stated.
Shohl's Solution. This is a palatable form in which to prescribe an oral alkalinizing agent. It contains 140 g of citric acid and 90 g of hydrated crystalline salt of sodium citrate per liter of water (1 mEq/ml of sodium).
Tromethamine. Tromethamine, U.S.P. (THAM), is a synthetic buffer (*tris*-[hydroxymethyl]aminomethane); it is available as a 0.3 M solution adjusted to pH 8.6 with acetic acid. It is also supplied as a powder (THAM-E) to be dissolved in 1 liter of sterile water. Each liter contains 300 millimoles (36 g) of tromethamine, 30 millimoles of sodium chloride, and 5 millimoles of potassium chloride.
The use of tromethamine is contraindicated in pregnant women or patients with uremia or chronic respiratory acidosis. It should not be given for longer than 1 day. Preparations of acidifying salts are discussed in the section on Ammonium.

AMMONIUM AND ACID-FORMING SALTS

The ammonium ion is of particular interest because it is toxic in high concentrations and because it serves a major role in the maintenance of the acid-base balance of the body.

The ammonium ion is an acid that dissociates to H^+ and NH_3, and the dissociation constant (pK_a 9.3) is such that, in the pH range of body fluids, NH_4^+ constitutes about 99% of the total ammonia ($NH_3 + NH_4^+$) concentration.

Endogenous Metabolism. Ammonia in the body represents that which is liberated from the deamination of amino acids and the deamidation of amides, and there are several major sources. Portal venous blood contains a high concentration of ammonia. Normally about 20% of the urea produced in the body diffuses into the gut, where it is converted by bacteria to ammonia and carbon dioxide. Intestinal bacteria also produce ammonia from dietary proteins. The ammonia is absorbed and converted back to urea in the liver by way of the ornithine (urea) cycle. Another significant role of ammonia is in the synthesis of glutamine.

Renal Excretion. Normal renal venous blood contains a high concentration of ammonia that results from the liberation of ammonia from glutamine and certain other amino acids in the kidney. The ammonia that is formed by the kidney is eliminated from the body when the urine is acidic, but is largely returned to the systemic circulation if the urine is alkaline. In an acidic urine, NH_3 accepts a proton and exists almost entirely as NH_4^+. Under normal states of metabolism, about 70 mEq of nonvolatile acid is generated per day (Table 35–2); about one half of this is excreted in the urine in conjunction with NH_4^+, and the remainder is excreted as titratable acid. Renal production of ammonia is stimulated by acidosis; this represents a physiological compensation, since ammonia buffers urinary acid and allows further secretion of protons into the tubular fluid. Potassium depletion also results in a primary increase in the renal synthesis of ammonia, sometimes accompanied by slight alkalinization of the urine (Tannen, 1977). This may increase the amount of ammonia that is returned to the circulation via the renal vein and have a deleterious effect when potassium depletion coexists with hepatic failure.

It should be noted that normal physiological mechanisms are designed to keep the concentration of ammonia in blood as low as possible. Thus, ammonia added to the venous circulation by the kidney or gastrointestinal tract is converted to urea by the liver. The highest concentrations of ammonia are normally achieved in the urine. This is not derived from arterial ammonia but is synthesized by the kidney.

Toxicity. Patients with severe hepatic disease or with portacaval shunts often develop derangements of the CNS, which are manifested by disturbance of consciousness, tremor, hyperreflexia, and EEG abnormalities. Since the syndrome is most often associated with elevated concentrations of ammonia in blood, and since it can be provoked by feeding of protein as well as by ingestion of ammonium salts, it is thought to represent ammonia toxicity to the brain.

The occurrence of hyperammonemia in children and infants has been associated with defects of enzymes of the urea cycle. Hyperammonemia due to defects of ornithine transcarbamylase or carbamylphosphate synthetase may be related to cyclic vomiting and to at least one form of migraine. The mechanisms by which ammonia induces changes in the CNS are currently unknown. (*See* Russell, 1973.)

Pharmacological Actions. *Diuresis from Ammonium Salts.* Following the absorption of inorganic salts of ammonium, such as ammonium chloride, the conversion of the ammonium ion to urea frees hydrogen ion and bicarbonate is dissipated. This may result in severe acidosis. Acid-forming salts were formerly employed as primary diuretics, but they have become obsolete for this purpose.

Correction of Metabolic Alkalosis. Ammonium chloride is useful for this purpose, particularly when sodium chloride is contraindicated in the edematous patient. The acidifying action depends on the conversion of the ammonium ion to urea by the liver, and ammonium salts are thus contraindicated in hepatic insufficiency. It should be noted that ammonium chloride, which has a *fixed* anion, is an acidifying salt; ammonium carbonate and ammonium bicarbonate, which have a *labile* anion, are not acidifying.

Expectorant Action. The ammonium ion supposedly exerts an expectorant action, and its salts are extensively used for this purpose.

Local Actions. Solutions of ammonium hydroxide are local irritants. When applied to the skin in low concentration, they have a rubefacient action, and in high concentrations they are vesicant. Ammonia gas is very irritating, but when inhaled in dilute form it can stimulate reflexly the medullary respiratory and vasomotor centers through irritation of the sensory endings of the trigeminal nerve. High concentrations of ammonia vapor are injurious to the lungs, and death may result from pulmonary edema. Long exposure to low concentrations of ammonia may lead to chronic pulmonary irritation. The maximal concentration of ammonia vapor that can be tolerated without harmful effect is probably less than 250 ppm. High concentrations of neutral ammonium salts are irritating to the gastric mucosa and may produce nausea and vomiting.

Preparations. *Ammonium Chloride*, U.S.P., is available as an official injection, syrup, or tablet. *Ammonium Carbonate*, N.F., consists of a mixture of ammonium bicarbonate and ammonium carbamate. *Aromatic Ammonia Spirit*, U.S.P., is a solution of ammonia, ammonium carbonate, and various essential oils in 70% alcohol, and is often employed as a reflex stimulant. It is given by mouth in a dose of 2 ml, well diluted in water.

Reversal of Intoxication with Ammonia. Several measures have been advocated for the management of portal-systemic encephalopathy associated with hepatic failure. Dietary intake of protein should be curtailed. *Neomycin* may be used to reduce the number of ammonia-producing microorganisms in the intestine. *Lactulose* is a disaccharide that is metabo-lized by intestinal bacteria to organic acids in the lower intestinal tract. The acidification of the intestinal contents retards the nonionic diffusion of ammonia from the colon to the blood. Although lactulose is theoretically incompatible with neomycin because of the latter's action on the intestinal flora, clinical results suggest that the two agents may be administered concomitantly (Fischer and Baldessarini, 1976). Therapy with *arginine* has been advocated because it acts as a precursor of ornithine in the urea cycle in the liver; *glutamate* has been advocated because it reacts with ammonia in the enzymatic synthesis of glutamine. While these two amino acids have been used singly and in combination to attempt to lower plasma concentrations of ammonia, there is no proof of efficacy.

In a somewhat different context, the α-keto analogs of essential amino acids react with ammonia by transamination to give rise to the amino acids themselves. Several such analogs have been used to treat patients with chronic renal failure. Their action on nitrogen metabolism, acidosis, and potassium imbalance has apparently been favorable (Walser, 1978).

POTASSIUM

As the predominant intracellular cation, potassium is of obvious importance. Disorders of potassium homeostasis are particularly evident because of the vital role that the ion assumes in the maintenance of electrical excitability of nerve and muscle. Potassium also plays an important role in the genesis and correction of imbalances of acid-base metabolism. Potassium salts are thus important therapeutic agents, but they are extremely dangerous if used improperly.

PHYSIOLOGICAL REGULATION

Absorption and Distribution. Active ion transport systems maintain a high gradient of potassium across the plasma membrane; while the plasma concentration is 4 to 5 mEq per liter, the intracellular concentration of the ion is approximately 150 mEq per liter, although there is modest variation from one cell type to another. Potassium is a normal and essential dietary constituent and is derived from foods of both vegetable and animal origin. Almost all the dietary potassium is absorbed from the gastrointestinal tract, and in the steady state the amount of potassium excreted in the urine is thus essentially equal to that in the diet. In the fluids within the intestinal tract the potassium concentration is two to three times greater than that in the plasma (Table 35–3). In the adult, the daily intake varies with dietary habits and is usually in the range of 50 to 100 mEq per day.

Potassium is accumulated by cells by an energy-dependent mechanism that extrudes sodium. Potassium uptake is either coupled to this directly or is driven by the potential difference resulting from the extrusion of sodium. With relatively minor modifications, the same mechanism is operative in many different types of cells. Of particular significance for excitable tissues are the facts that there is a high concentration gradient for potassium from cell to extracellular fluid, a high gradient for sodium in the opposite direction, and elaborately regulated mechanisms for rapid and selective alterations in the permeability of these monovalent cations.

Excretion. Renal mechanisms are of paramount importance in maintaining both the total body potassium and its concentration in the plasma within narrow limits. Potassium is freely filtered at the glomerulus and is almost completely reabsorbed in the proximal tubule. The amount excreted in the urine, which is normally equivalent to 10% of the amount filtered, gains access to the tubular fluid by the process of tubular secretion. This occurs in the distal convoluted tubule and, under some circumstances, in the collecting duct. The secretory process is a passive one to the extent that potassium moves into tubular fluid down an electrochemical gradient.

Tubular reabsorption of sodium has a dual impact on the secretion of potassium. First, sodium reabsorption is active and thereby the tubular fluid becomes relatively negative with respect to the cell. This increases the electrical gradient for potassium secretion. Second, increased amounts of fluid may be delivered to the secretory segment as the result of inhibition of sodium reabsorption in the proximal segment. This can occur with increased filtered loads of sodium or as the result of the action of diuretics. The increased volume of distal fluid tends to lower the concentration of potassium present in the tubular fluid as the result of secretion. This enables the total *amount* of potassium that is secreted to increase, other factors remaining constant, albeit at a relatively low concentration in the voided urine. These two factors,

which are related to sodium reabsorption, play an important role in the regulation of potassium homeostasis. For example, any condition in which there is an acute increase in sodium excretion is associated with an increase in potassium excretion as well. In contrast, when little or no sodium is reabsorbed distally, potassium secretion is minimal.

Aldosterone markedly stimulates distal sodium reabsorption and hence potassium secretion. Clinical conditions that enhance the secretion of aldosterone are characterized by potassium loss. For example, in patients with heart failure, reduced renal blood flow leads to secretion of renin, elevated concentrations of angiotensin in plasma, increased secretion of aldosterone, and an enhanced but inappropriate reabsorption of sodium in the distal tubules. When diuretics are given, the increased delivery of sodium to the distal tubule further contributes to a negative potassium balance. To prevent such loss, potassium-sparing diuretics can be added to the therapeutic regimen (*see* Chapter 36).

The normal renal response to changes in intake is different for sodium and potassium. For illustration, assume that the intake of each ion is 100 mEq per day and that the kidneys and adrenals are normal. What then are the kinetics of renal adjustment when intake is increased or decreased by 100 mEq, that is, either doubled or reduced to zero? In this example, the intake of the other cation is assumed to remain constant. The increased amount of dietary sodium will be excreted rather slowly over several days. When sodium intake is reduced to zero, the urine will become sodium free within 3 to 4 days. In the case of potassium, the increased intake will be excreted more rapidly—in a matter of hours. When potassium intake is reduced, the amount of potassium excreted in the urine will fall, but this is a gradual process and even after weeks of reduced intake the urine will not become potassium free.

Adaptation to Potassium Loads. When the intake of potassium is increased, either by a high-potassium diet or by the administration of potassium salts, the resultant degree of hyperkalemia depends on the prior intake of potassium. If this had been low, the degree of hyperkalemia would be far greater than if potassium intake had been high. Since ingested potassium is virtually *completely* absorbed in the upper intestinal tract, it is apparent that adaptation involves mechanisms of excretion and redistribution.

The increased rate of urinary excretion is achieved by increased tubular secretion of potassium, either in the distal convoluted tubule or in the collecting duct, depending on the conditions. Hyperkalemia directly enhances Na^+,K^+-ATPase activity in the kidney and indirectly increases enzyme activity by stimulation of the production of aldosterone. The function of ATPase is critically involved in the adaptive response, since enhanced potassium excretion can be abolished in the isolated kidney by the administration of ouabain, a known inhibitor of the enzyme (Silva *et al.*, 1977).

The major extrarenal adaptation involves the uptake of potassium by tissues, principally muscle and liver. The amount of potassium that is involved is relatively small compared to endogenous intracellular stores and hence cannot readily be detected by analyses of tissue. However, the operation of these processes is readily discerned by their effect on extracellular concentrations of potassium. A number of endocrine systems are involved. Hyperkalemia stimulates the release of insulin, which in turn facilitates the cellular uptake of potassium. Insulin increases the uptake of potassium by muscle cells by hyperpolarizing the muscle membrane independently of any action of the hormone on carbohydrate metabolism; stimulation of Na$^+$,K$^+$-ATPase and a consequent effect on sodium efflux may be involved. Insulin also stimulates glycogen deposition in liver and muscle, which is accompanied by the intracellular sequestration of potassium, particularly in the liver. Hyperkalemia also stimulates the secretion of glucagon. Although this hormone increases plasma potassium in association with its action on hepatic glycogenolysis, it also has a hypokalemic effect that results from its stimulation of the renal excretion of potassium. Thus, both the adrenals and the pancreas have an endocrine function in the adaptation to potassium loads. When the function of both glands is compromised, subjects may be predisposed to hyperkalemia. This may occur when potassium loads are given to patients with diabetes mellitus who, at the same time, are subject to either spontaneous hypoaldosteronism or its iatrogenic equivalent in the form of potassium-sparing diuretics (Goldfarb *et al.*, 1975). Conversely, when a high-potassium intake is suddenly terminated, adrenocortical hyperfunction may persist, leading to hypokalemia that can cause paralysis (Duggin and Price, 1974).

During excessive intake of potassium the amount of the ion secreted into the colon increases; this is excreted in the feces. As in the distal tubule of the kidney, Na$^+$,K$^+$-ATPase is involved. However, in the colon an increase in enzyme activity appears to require aldosterone. As a mechanism of physiological compensation, the intestinal excretion of potassium is far less important in the normal subject than in the patient with chronic renal insufficiency, in whom a major fraction of dietary potassium may be eliminated by this route.

Potassium Metabolism and Acid-Base Balance. This subject is complicated by the fact that it involves both ion-exchange mechanisms across the membranes of many types of cells and the excretory function of the kidney. In addition, the physiological disposition of the hydrogen and potassium ions may be influenced, at least in part independently of each other, by the balance of other cations and anions. The following underlying principles have been reasonably well established, and their understanding is of particular importance for the therapeutic use of potassium.

Cellular Equilibria. The intracellular concentrations of both potassium *and hydrogen* ions are higher than those of the extracellular fluid. Attempts have been made to describe this distribution of ions across the cell membrane by application of the Donnan equilibrium. However, a simple and accurate formulation has not been possible, in part because of the technical difficulties of measurement of the exact intracellular concentrations of the ions involved. However, the following generalizations are valid in a qualitative sense. When the extracellular hydrogen ion concentration is raised, as in acidosis, there is a shift of potassium from cells to extracellular fluid. When the extracellular concentration of hydrogen ion is decreased, as in alkalosis, potassium moves into cells. Thus, extracellular acidosis produces hyperkalemia, and extracellular alkalosis produces hypokalemia. A change of 0.1 unit in plasma pH can be accompanied by a change of opposite sign of 0.6 mEq per liter in the plasma concentration of potassium.

When a change in the concentration of potassium is the initiating event, the distribution of hydrogen ion may also be affected. In severe potassium depletion, when K$^+$ leaves the cell it exchanges with extracellular Na$^+$ and H$^+$ to preserve electroneutrality. This redistribution of hydrogen ion results in extracellular alkalosis and intracellular acidosis. The opposite tends to occur in hyperkalemia (Adler and Fraley, 1977).

Renal Mechanisms. Deprivation of dietary potassium initially increases urinary pH slightly and also stimulates the renal synthesis of ammonia (Tannen, 1977). Since urinary pH controls the excretion of both titratable acid and ammonia, the immediate overall effect is to diminish net acid excretion. If the concomitant loss of potassium is mild, the decreased elimination of acid results in metabolic acidosis (Burnell *et al.*, 1974). However, if potassium depletion becomes more extensive, systemic metabolic alkalosis and intracellular acidosis develop. These results appear contradictory. The phenomenon has been observed in several species, including man, and species differences are not involved (Cooke *et al.*, 1952; Mudge and Hardin, 1956). Because of its strong kaluretic action, aldosterone, combined with a low-potassium diet, has been used to produce this condition experimentally; the production of aldosterone is increased in its clinical counterparts. However, there is no requirement for aldosterone for the occurrence of this phenomenon—only significant depletion of potassium.

Considered together, the data suggest that near the normal range of potassium balance, the potassium ion has a regulatory role in the determination of urinary pH and ammonia synthesis, but that with severe potassium depletion, additional mechanisms supervene. The initiating event that leads to extracellular alkalosis and intracellular acidosis is the entry of H^+ and Na^+ into cells in exchange for the lost K^+. However, the kidney fails to compensate for the alkalosis by excreting an alkaline urine; rather, the concentration of extracellular HCO_3^- continues to rise and that of Cl^- to fall because of the inappropriate renal secretion of H^+. The failure of renal compensation can be explained by two simplistic concepts. The first and most obvious is that the renal distal tubular cells are responding to their intracellular rather than their extracellular environment. The second proposes that competition exists between K^+ and H^+ for the electrochemical gradient produced by distal tubular Na^+ reabsorptive transport. Thus, when one ion is being secreted excessively, that of the other is reduced; or, conversely, when one ion is being conserved, the other may be secreted excessively and inappropriately.

The concept of competition is supported by many simple observations. For example, in response to an acute potassium load, renal secretion of K^+ increases rapidly, that of H^+ falls, and the urine becomes alkaline; conversely, when the kidney is compensating for acute alkalosis (diminished H^+ secretion), renal secretion of K^+ increases. In the case of hypokalemic alkalosis due to extrarenal loss of K^+, both the diminished tubular secretion of K^+ (conservation) and an increase in the concentration of intracellular H^+ presumably contribute to the failure of renal compensation. In the case of renal loss of K^+ as a result of the administration of chloruretic diuretics,

both subtraction alkalosis and intracellular acidosis are the initiating events that lead to extracellular alkalosis (*see* below). Failure of renal compensation is presumably due to intracellular acidosis. With large losses of potassium, the above-described abnormalities can only be corrected by restoration of the potassium deficit by the administration of KCl. K^+ then reenters the cell in exchange for H^+ and Na^+, intracellular acidosis and extracellular alkalosis are corrected, K^+ again competes for distal cationic exchange, and renal compensatory mechanisms become operative.

PATHOLOGICAL CONDITIONS

The metabolism of the potassium ion may be considered pathological when its concentration in either the extracellular or intracellular fluid is above or below normal. Since the concentrations in these two compartments may vary partially independently of each other, the concentration in both must be appraised for a complete understanding of potassium imbalance.

Measurement of Extracellular Potassium. The concentration of potassium in the plasma is readily measured directly. Factitiously low values may be encountered in the same conditions that produce pseudohyponatremia, that is, when the plasma water content is abnormal (*see* above). *Pseudohyperkalemia* is observed when concentrations are measured in the serum of patients with marked thrombocytosis or leukocytosis. Potassium leaks from the cells during the clotting process; true values are obtained with plasma from blood that is harvested with anticoagulants. Falsely high values are also obtained with samples that contain abnormal erythrocytes, as in sickle cell anemia, in the absence of hemolysis. Since the human erythrocyte has a high concentration of potassium, hemolysis in shed blood produces falsely high estimates of the plasma concentration of the ion. However, an elevated potassium concentration in serum or plasma from patients with intravascular hemolysis is a true representation of the extracellular concentration.

Since both hypokalemia and hyperkalemia directly influence the electrical activity of the heart, the ECG may be employed as a guide to the concentration in plasma. This is particularly useful when there is a diagnostic emergency and when the concentration must be monitored sequentially during therapy to replace potassium.

As a first approximation, the concentration of potassium in the fluids of the gastrointestinal tract is about three times that of plasma (Table 35–3). Direct measurement of fecal potassium is useful only in the exceptional case. Measurement of the urinary concentration of potassium is often uninterpretable unless many factors are taken into account, such as the concentration in plasma, previous or simultaneous drug treatment, dietary intake, and the rate of urine flow. Under normal circumstances the amount of potassium excreted in the urine shows less diurnal variation than does sodium.

Measurement of Intracellular Potassium. Because of the distribution of the ion, measurement of the intracellular concentration of potassium is virtually synonymous with measurement of total body potassium. Skeletal muscle obviously accounts for the bulk of the total intracellular store. However, the skeletal muscle cell is not necessarily representative of all types of cells. For example, in potassium depletion skeletal muscle shows a major loss of the ion while myocardial potassium remains virtually normal.

Attempts to obtain accurate measurements of intracellular stores have been frustrating. The concentration of potassium in the plasma is an index of only limited value. In those conditions in which extracellular and intracellular concentrations change in the same direction, that is, in otherwise-uncomplicated potassium depletion, there may be only a slight fall in the plasma concentration while the intracellular concentration may vary from almost normal to clearly low values. There are other conditions in which the extracellular and intracellular concentrations diverge because of the movement of potassium from one compartment to the other. Examples include acute alkalosis or acidosis without significant change in external potassium balance, untreated diabetic ketoacidosis, and hypokalemic periodic paralysis. Since the erythrocyte and leukocyte may be readily sampled, their potassium content may be measured directly. However, these data correlate poorly with total body stores. The total amount of potassium in the body may also be directly measured by quantitation of the naturally occurring isotope, ^{40}K. However, this is a research procedure and the errors are sufficiently great that small but physiologically important changes may not be detected. Although usually considered to be investigational procedures, careful determination of metabolic balance and biopsy of skeletal muscle may provide the most accurate means to assess intracellular stores (Patrick, 1977).

In the usual clinical situation, an evaluation of total body potassium must depend on other sources of information. A careful analysis of the patient's history is probably the single most important step. Particular attention must be given to the quantitative aspects of dietary intake and abnormal fluid losses, especially from the gastrointestinal tract, with the realization that significant changes in external balance rarely occur acutely but require days or weeks.

Hyperkalemia. *Causes.* Hyperkalemia results from a variety of causes: a sudden increase in potassium intake, either by mouth or by vein; severe tissue trauma; acute rhabdomyolysis; acute acidosis, but sometimes also chronic acidosis; untreated Addison's disease; the rare metabolic disorder hyperkalemic periodic paralysis; an acute increase in osmolality, as after the infusion of hypertonic mannitol or, in a more special case, with the induction of hyperglycemia in diabetic patients who are also deficient in aldosterone; the action of glucagon; the acute stimulation of α-adrenergic receptors; and the improper use of potassium-sparing diuretics (Goldfarb *et al.*, 1975; Knochel, 1977). Hyperkalemia is *not* observed during chronic renal failure, except as an almost terminal event (due to the effectiveness of both the renal and intestinal adaptive mechanisms). However, in each of the above-listed conditions the degree of hyperkalemia will be accentuated by renal insufficiency.

Consequences. Deleterious effects on the electrical activity of the heart are by far the most important consequences of hyperkalemia. At modest levels of elevation (plasma potassium 5 to 7 mEq per liter), a minor acceleration of conduction may be demonstrable; the T waves become increased in height or "tented"; the P-R interval lengthens and the P wave ultimately disappears. At higher concentrations of potassium (8 to 9 mEq per liter) there is a profound depression in impulse generation and conduction in all cardiac tissues, widening of the QRS complex, and eventual asystole, sometimes preceded by ventricular tachycardia or fibrillation (*see* Ettinger *et al.*, 1974). There is a moderate variation in the absolute concentration of potassium in plasma at which these changes occur.

Increase in Total Body Potassium. As indicated above in the discussion of adaptation to high-potassium intake, it is not possible to increase total body potassium significantly above normal.

Hypokalemia. *Causes.* The most common cause of hypokalemia is depletion of total body potassium, which is considered below. However, the plasma concentration may also fall without any change in external balance, and hence without depletion, as a result of acute alkalosis, treatment with insulin, hypokalemic periodic paralysis, and stimulation of β-adrenergic receptors.

Consequences. Since hypokalemia and

depletion of potassium often coexist, it is difficult to attribute the sequelae specifically to one condition or the other. It is probable that the abnormalities associated with neuromuscular dysfunction are primarily correlated with the degree of hypokalemia. These include impaired neuromuscular function, which may vary from minimal weakness to frank paralysis; intestinal dilatation and ileus; and abnormalities of myocardial function with disturbed ECG patterns such as prolongation of the Q-T interval, a broad and flat T wave, depression of the S-T segment, and defects in conduction.

Decrease in Total Body Potassium. *Types of Potassium Depletion.* Classification of potassium depletion into three subgroups has important implications for guidelines to therapy. First, *simple depletion* occurs when extracellular and intracellular concentrations are reduced to approximately the same extent. Transmembrane potentials are unchanged, and conduction abnormalities are not observed. Second, the intracellular stores may be excessively lowered relative to extracellular concentrations when there is a *disturbance in membrane function*. And third, a diminished capacity for potassium, or *pseudodepletion,* may occur when the total cellular mass is reduced with little or no change in the composition of the residual cells (Patrick, 1977).

This classification is admittedly an oversimplification but provides a useful framework for the consideration of many diverse situations. For example, mild starvation may lead to pseudodepletion, but severe starvation causes all three types. Examples of defects in the ability of the cell to maintain normal concentration gradients include uremia, thyrotoxicosis, severe and prolonged hypoxia, and simultaneous deficiencies in pancreatic and adrenocortical function. Cardiac glycosides also produce this type of defect. As a more complex example, depletion of potassium may produce rhabdomyolysis. If the depletion is sufficiently severe (approximately 25 to 30% of normal body stores), the integrity of the membrane of the muscle cell becomes secondarily impaired. This leads to a further loss of intracellular potassium, which may possibly alleviate the preexisting hypokalemia (Knochel, 1978).

Causes of Potassium Depletion. The common causes of potassium depletion are associated with an increased rate of excretion by either the kidneys or the gastrointestinal tract, or, more rarely, the skin. Increased renal excretion occurs in the following conditions: therapy with diuretics; the administration of large doses of anionic drugs that achieve high concentrations in the urine (*e.g.,* aminosalicylic acid and penicillin G and related antibiotics); primary disorders of renal function, such as renal tubular acidosis; secondary disorders of tubular function induced by amphotericin B or by deficiency of magnesium; primary hyperaldosteronism; and excessive ingestion of licorice or other compounds with mineralocorticoid activity. In each instance, particularly with the use of diuretics for conditions associated with edema, secondary hyperaldosteronism markedly enhances the potassium loss (*see* above). The administration of sodium bicarbonate acutely increases potassium excretion, but the effect may be short lived since both hypokalemia and expansion of extracellular volume suppress production of aldosterone (Sanderson, 1954).

Increased elimination of potassium via the gastrointestinal tract occurs with the loss of any gastrointestinal fluid (vomitus, diarrhea, or surgical drainage), chronic abuse of laxatives, the malabsorption syndromes, and mucus-secreting villous adenomas of the small intestine. Aldosterone accentuates some of these losses, but this is less well documented than are those from the kidney. Malabsorption syndromes are frequently accompanied by hypocalcemia, which tends to counterbalance the effect of hypokalemia on neuromuscular function.

Although the concentration of potassium in perspiration is only about 10 mEq per liter, cutaneous losses from excessive exercise in a hot environment can result in significant depletion (Knochel, 1978).

Relationship to Metabolic Alkalosis. The popular term *hypokalemic hypochloremic metabolic alkalosis* is an unfortunate collection of redundancies that does not denote what was intended. First, except in the most contrived experimental situation, all instances of metabolic alkalosis are hypochloremic. And second, due to shifts of potassium from the extracellular to the intracellular space, all instances of alkalosis are hypokalemic. The phrase was originally employed to describe cases of metabolic alkalosis in which the acid-base imbalance could be restored to normal *only* following the correction of the simultaneous depletion of potassium and chloride. In view of our present knowledge, this condition should be termed either *potassium-depletion alkalosis* or *saline-resistant alkalosis* (Garella *et al.*, 1970).

Consider, as an example, alkalosis in which there is a loss of chloride and hydrogen ions in vomitus. It has long been apparent that this could be corrected by the administration of sodium chloride, with the kidney making the appropriate adjustments in excretion. Subsequent measurements have shown a substantial loss of potassium in the urine and gastric juice. A potassium deficit of as much as 500 mEq may develop and be accompanied by hypokalemia (as in all types of alkalosis). However, the underlying acid-base imbalance may be corrected with sodium chloride without direct repair of the potassium deficit (Kassirer and Schwartz, 1966).

When potassium depletion is more severe, potassium salts are required to correct the alkalosis (Cooke *et al.*, 1952). In quantitative terms of potassium loss, the exact borderline between responsiveness and resistance to saline therapy is not known. With the greater degree of depletion, there is an intracellular acidosis of the muscle and probably also of the kidney (Anderson and Mudge, 1955), and the kidney fails to compensate for the acid-base imbalance. The sequence and basic mechanisms of these events are discussed above (page 872). The abnormalities may be corrected by the administration of potassium chloride. The amount of potassium that is required is less than the probable deficit, which has been estimated to be as high as 1000 mEq in the adult.

Potassium-depletion alkalosis may be suspected if the external losses of potassium and chloride have occurred over a long period and the degree of hypokalemia is extreme. However, the simple combination of hypochloremia and hypokalemia is not diagnostically conclusive. The most direct evidence, which is also quite simply obtained, is the continued excretion of chloride in the urine at a concentration greater than 10 mEq per liter, despite the presence of hypochloremia and an adequate intake of saline and in the absence of any diuretic drugs. The diagnosis is confirmed and the problem is solved when adequate replacement of potassium renders the urine alkaline and corrects the alkalosis.

Paradoxical aciduria is defined as the excretion of an acidic urine in the presence of metabolic alkalosis. When the plasma bicarbonate concentration is raised by the infusion of sodium bicarbonate and the renal threshold for bicarbonate is exceeded, bicarbonate is excreted in the urine along with sodium, thereby rendering the urine alkaline and correcting the systemic alkalosis. Under these conditions extracellular volume is expanded as the result of the administration of sodium bicarbonate. However, in the more common clinical situation, when alkalosis results from the loss of hydrogen and chloride ions and water, as in gastric alkalosis, extracellular volume is contracted and, in response to this, sodium is completely reabsorbed by the renal tubule and the urine is not alkalinized. This is the most common example of paradoxical aciduria. This also occurs in edema formation where there is avidity for sodium and in posthypercapneic alkalosis with inadequate replenishment of sodium chloride. With alkalosis induced by the high-ceiling diuretics, the urine is acidic during the diuretic phase, when sodium and chloride are excreted, as well as in the postdiuretic phase, when sodium is conserved. Thus, paradoxical aciduria occurs in many conditions. Misconceptions to the contrary, this finding is not diagnostic of potassium-depletion alkalosis.

Effect of Diuretics. As described in Chapter 36, several classes of diuretics increase the excretion of potassium. This is regularly observed acutely, but the consequences of chronic therapy with diuretics are more controversial. In patients with uncomplicated hypertension, the daily administration of diuretics produces a slight reduction in plasma potassium concentration and either little or no change in total body potassium, the latter result depending on the technic of measurement (Oh and Carroll, 1978). In edematous patients, the results are more variable. Some have failed to find any evidence for depletion of total body potassium (Wilkinson, 1978). Others suggest moderate depletion but emphasize the difficulty of interpretation, since this may also occur in patients with the same underlying diseases who are not maintained on diuretics (Kassirer and Harrington, 1977). On *a-priori* grounds one might anticipate that to the extent that edematous patients have secondary hyperaldosteronism, they would also be more prone to diuretic-induced losses of potassium. The validity of this concept is amply supported by the high incidence of severe potassium deficiency in a series of patients treated simultaneously with diuretics and carbenoxolone, an agent with mineralocorticoid activity (Knochel, 1978). In this group, chlorthalidone appeared particularly prone to produce potassium depletion.

The problem is further complicated by the effects of diuretics on acid-base balance. When edema fluid is rapidly mobilized by high-ceiling diuretics, the resulting alkalosis is largely of the subtraction type (*see* above). When the same diuretics are used chronically to maintain the patient free of edema, the genesis of the persistent alkalosis must involve the negative chloride balance itself, as well as the associated response of the renal acidification mechanisms (Strihou and Morales-Barria, 1969). With chronic diuretic therapy, despite the association of alkalosis and hypokalemia, there is no evidence in the vast majority of patients that potassium depletion itself is a cause of the alkalosis. However, exceptions have been noted (Kassirer and Harrington, 1977; Knochel, 1978).

Consequences of Potassium Depletion. The effects of hypokalemia, listed above, are also seen when there is depletion of intracellular potassium. The changes in acid-base balance are also discussed above. In addition, there is reduced tolerance to carbohydrate and a deficiency in glycogen deposition. Vasopressin-resistant polyuria is a prominent symptom. A deficit of potassium appears to increase the renal synthesis of prostaglandins, which in turn can decrease the permeability to water of the distal nephron and produce a diabetes insipidus–like syndrome. In experimental animals, the disorder is responsive to indomethacin, an inhibitor of prostaglandin synthesis (Galvez et al., 1977).

Morphological Changes. In skeletal muscle, so-called waxy degeneration is observed, which may progress to severe rhabdomyolysis. In the heart, patchy necrosis occurs, especially in the subendocardial region. In the kidney, there is a characteristic vacuolization of the epithelium of the proximal convolution, along with hyperplasia of certain cell types in the medulla.

PHARMACOLOGICAL CONSIDERATIONS

As a constituent of the normal diet, potassium is slowly absorbed from the intestinal tract. Following distribution and uptake by cells the kidney excretes an appropriate amount to maintain balance. As a consequence of the large volume of distribution and the rapid response of the kidney, the extracellular and intracellular concentrations of the ion are normally maintained within relatively narrow limits.

Transient Volume of Distribution. When potassium is administered as a drug, the factors that govern the rate and extent of its distribution are of major importance. It is not possible to increase the total body content of potassium significantly above normal. However, it is very easy to raise the extracellular concentration excessively. For example, if mild hypokalemia is treated injudiciously, one may suddenly find that the plasma concentration of potassium has risen alarmingly (*e.g.*, from 3 to 9 mEq per liter). This does not represent a significant increment in total body potassium, of which only about 2% is located extracellularly. However, *it is the concentration in the extracellular fluid that determines life-threatening toxicity*. Therefore, even though the administered potassium is eventually destined either to be excreted or taken up by cells, knowledge of the transient concentration achieved in the plasma must govern the use of potassium as a therapeutic agent.

Indications and Rationale for Treatment with Potassium. As a practical matter one should distinguish between prophylaxis and replacement and, in states of potassium depletion, between acute and chronic conditions. In addition, it is essential to consider as a separate group those patients who are receiving cardiac glycosides and some antiarrhythmic drugs and β-adrenergic agonists.

Indications. The unequivocal indication for the therapeutic administration of potassium is profound muscular weakness associated with hypokalemia, with or without corresponding abnormalities in cardiac conduction. One should include hypokalemia of all origins, including the specific disease entity of hypokalemic periodic paralysis. Also to be considered are those conditions, particularly diabetic ketoacidosis, in which standard treatment may be *antici-*

pated to produce acute and severe hypokalemia, either with or without symptoms. In these conditions, the rationale for treatment is to correct a life-threatening disturbance of neuromuscular function.

Replacement of potassium is also indicated in those cases of metabolic alkalosis that persist because of an inappropriate excretion of an acidic urine. The rationale is to correct the deficit of potassium and thereby the acid-base abnormality.

In either acute or chronic disorders of acid-base or fluid balance, potassium may be indicated either to correct or prevent the disturbances attributable to hypokalemia. The goal of therapy is to elevate the plasma concentration of the ion to the low normal range. Potassium supplementation should be considered if: (1) the concentration of potassium in plasma is less than 2.5 mEq per liter on repeated occasions, even if the patient is asymptomatic; (2) the concentration of potassium is between 2.5 and 3.0 mEq per liter with symptoms or ECG findings suggestive of hypokalemia; or (3) the plasma potassium concentration is consistently between 3.0 and 3.5 mEq per liter and there are clear-cut symptoms or ECG signs of hypokalemia.

Since digitalis and potassium have competitive affinities for myocardial Na^+,K^+-ATPase, the actions of digitalis are accentuated by hypokalemia (Schwartz *et al.,* 1975). Therefore, the criteria for supplementation with potassium are altered for patients who are receiving a digitalis glycoside. In such individuals it is advisable to maintain the plasma potassium concentration at 3.2 mEq per liter or higher. Although digitalis-related arrhythmias are accentuated by hypokalemia, there is no evidence that they are influenced by the absolute concentration of potassium within the normal range for plasma (*i.e.,* from 3.5 to 5.0 mEq per liter). The role of potassium in the treatment of digitalis intoxication is considered in Chapter 30.

The prophylactic administration of potassium cannot be justified when the plasma concentration is normal, except for patients with hypokalemic periodic paralysis. In this disorder the concentration of potassium is often normal during asymptomatic periods, but the frequency of attacks may be diminished by high-potassium intake.

Contraindications. Supplementation with potassium is either contraindicated or should be undertaken with great caution when potassium-sparing diuretics have been prescribed. In the presence of renal insufficiency it has often been asserted that it is essential to have adequate urinary excretion of potassium before parenteral administration in order to avoid the risk of hyperkalemia. This is true when renal insufficiency is due to severe dehydration (*e.g.,* diabetic acidosis) and correction of the fluid deficit can restore adequate excretory function. Such a maneuver will help prevent excessive fluctuations in extracellular concentration of potassium. However, potassium supplementation may be interdicted in patients with chronic renal insufficiency because a defective cellular uptake of potassium may be an accompanying abnormality. The result of giving standard doses could be life-threatening hyperkalemia. In acute tubular necrosis that is potentially

reversible, potassium intake should be reduced to the lowest possible level (*see* below).

Potassium salts have a somewhat unpleasant taste, and they can be irritating to the gastrointestinal tract; many patients do not take the prescribed dose. This assumes particular importance when an ambulatory noncompliant patient requires hospitalization and the same dose that was prescribed is continued under supervision that assures compliance. In addition, salt substitutes that contain potassium may be prescribed at the same time. Instances of severe hyperkalemia have resulted from such a sequence.

Misleading Indications. In the common situation in which diuretics are chronically prescribed for the prevention of edema formation, patients may also receive digitalis for underlying heart failure. As indicated above, alkalosis and hypokalemia may result. Potassium supplementation is warranted to control the plasma concentration of potassium; however, in the vast majority of patients, it may not be necessary to correct the alkalosis. If this distinction were more clearly kept in mind, the incidence of iatrogenic hyperkalemia might be reduced. In addition, small doses of ammonium chloride should be considered as a means to replenish chloride without sodium.

Dose, Route, and Rate of Administration of Potassium. Potassium chloride is the preferred salt for most situations because of the frequency with which deficits of chloride and potassium coexist. This salt has a moderately unpleasant taste, and preparations of other salts are available for oral use.

Oral Administration. For the prophylaxis of hypokalemia during chronic diuretic therapy, a total oral dose of potassium of 50 mEq per day in divided portions is effective for most patients. This is given in addition to dietary intake, which may be quite variable.

Intravenous Administration. In acute illness when the oral administration of potassium is not possible, it may be administered intravenously. The daily dose, the dose per hour, the concentration of potassium administered, and the total amount of drug in the infusion bottle must all be considered.

Daily Dose. Since the normal potassium intake is 50 to 100 mEq per day, it is rare that a larger amount is warranted. In patients with potassium depletion this amount slowly but adequately corrects the deficit. With extreme depletion or with high rates of ongoing loss, larger doses may be required. Some studies have suggested that these be given with glucose and insulin in order to enhance cellular uptake, but this has not been studied systematically (Clementsen, 1962).

Dose per Hour. The recommended maximal rate of administration varies from 10 to 30 mEq per hour. If an infusion rate of greater than 30 mEq per hour is considered to be essential, the ECG should be monitored continuously so that the earliest indication of hyperkalemia may be detected.

Concentration. When infused into a peripheral vein, concentrations of potassium chloride up to 40 mEq per liter are usually tolerated and do not produce localized pain. If higher concentrations are required because of the concomitant need to minimize fluid intake, a central vein should be employed. When high concentrations are used, even brief errors in the rate of administration can cause cardiotoxicity. It is therefore recommended that, when the potassium concentration in the infusion is 80 mEq per liter or higher, the *total amount* of ion in the infusion system should not exceed 10 mEq. In this case a fluid volume up to 100 ml can be conveniently administered by SOLUSET or similar device with a very low rate of infusion of fluid. The available dose of potassium may be renewed as indicated by the clinical situation.

Toxicity of Potassium Salts. The cardiac toxicity of hyperkalemia, which has been discussed above, is one of the leading causes of iatrogenic morbidity and mortality. Enteric-coated tablets of potassium chloride can be irritating to the small bowel and cause ulceration. The rather bad-tasting solutions of KCl may limit the patient's compliance.

Treatment of Hyperkalemia. The acute management of this problem includes, first and foremost, the termination of the administration of potassium, if this is the cause. Additional treatment includes the intravenous administration of a calcium salt, glucose, insulin, and sodium bicarbonate. Ion-exchange resins such as sodium polystyrene sulfonate, administered by mouth or by rectum, are also useful (*see* below). If the above measures fail, either peritoneal or extracorporeal dialysis may be lifesaving.

Preparations to Repair Potassium Depletion and to Control Hyperkalemia. *Potassium Chloride Oral Solution,* U.S.P., contains 20 mEq of potassium per 15 ml (1 tablespoonful). Preparations of potassium chloride for oral administration are supplied in a vast array of formulations (liquids, powders, and effervescent tablets) and flavors, a reflection of their lack of palatability. Enteric-coated tablets (4, 8.7, and 13.4 mEq) and tablets that contain a wax matrix (6.67 and 8 mEq) are also available. *Potassium Chloride Injection,* U.S.P., is a sterile solution of potassium chloride in water. It is usually marketed as a 7.5% (1 mEq/ml), 15% (2 mEq/ml), or 22.5% (3 mEq/ml) solution in 10-, 20-, or 30-ml ampuls. This solution should never be administered as such but must be suitably diluted. Various other potassium salts are also available.

Cation-Exchange Resins. Exchange resins are useful to lower concentrations of potassium in plasma and other body fluids. One of the most efficient is *Sodium Polystyrene Sulfonate,* U.S.P. (KAYEXALATE), which exchanges sodium for potassium. It may be given by mouth, instilled as an enema, or inserted in the rectum in a dialysis bag to facilitate recovery. The resin should be retained in the rectum for 30 to 45 minutes. When administered orally, a laxative should be given concurrently to avoid fecal impaction. The use of resins by mouth is frequently proscribed because there is nausea and vomiting. The usual oral dose is 15 g of the resin one to four times daily. It should be suspended in a palatable vehicle, or it may be incorporated into a candy. When used as an enema, 25 g of the resin in 100 ml of a suitable vehicle is inserted through a large Foley catheter with the 30-ml Foley bag inflated. The rectal tube is clamped and the material left in the rectum for the period indicated above. The clamp is then released and the material expelled by the patient. Such enemas are given at 1- to 2-hour intervals until the potassium concentration is within a safe range.

Calcium Gluconate, U.S.P. Calcium gluconate may be a very useful agent in combating the deleterious effects of hyperkalemia on the heart. It may be administered directly intravenously as a 10% solution while the ECG is monitored. As much as 50 ml of a 10% solution can be administered safely if given slowly. Following this, another 50 ml of the calcium gluconate (10%) can be placed in a larger volume of fluid (glucose in water, etc.) and administered more slowly. Available preparations are described in Chapter 65.

MAGNESIUM

Magnesium is the second most plentiful cation of the intracellular fluids. It is essential for the activity of many enzyme systems and plays an important role with regard to neurochemical transmission and muscular excitability. Deficits are accompanied by a variety of structural and functional disturbances.

The average 70-kg adult has about 2000 mEq of magnesium in his body. About 50% of this magnesium is found in bone, 45% exists as an intracellular cation, and 5% is in the extracellular fluid. Intracellular concentrations of magnesium range from 5 to 30 mEq/kg, depending on the tissue. The concentration in plasma is 1.5 to 2.2 mEq of magnesium per liter, with about two thirds as free cation and one third bound to plasma proteins. Intracellular and extracellular concentrations of magnesium can vary independently, and a deficit in one compartment may not be accompanied by a significant change in the other (Walser, 1967; Wallach and Dimich, 1969). Some form of exchange of magnesium occurs between plasma, the intracellular compartment, and bone; however, very little is known about the mechanisms involved. About 30% of the magnesium in the skeleton represents an exchangeable pool. Mobilization of the cation from this pool in bone is fairly rapid in children but not in adults. The larger fraction of magnesium in bone is apparently an integral part of bone crystal (Alfrey and Miller, 1973).

Absorption and Excretion. The average adult in the United States ingests about 20 to 40 mEq of magnesium a day, and of this approximately one third is absorbed from the gastrointestinal tract. Absorption occurs in the upper small bowel by means of an active process closely related to the transport system for calcium. Ingestion of low amounts of magnesium results in increased absorption of calcium and *vice versa.*

Magnesium is excreted principally by the kidney, and, under normal conditions, 3 to 5% of the filtered ion is excreted in the urine. Most of the reabsorption of magnesium occurs in the proximal tubule (Massry, 1977). Renal excretion of magnesium is increased during diuresis induced by glucose, ammonium chloride, furosemide, ethacrynic acid, and organic mercurials. Hypomagnesemia can occur as a complication of diuretic therapy. Small amounts of magnesium are excreted in milk and in saliva.

PHYSIOLOGICAL AND PHARMACOLOGICAL ACTIONS

Enzyme Systems. Magnesium is a cofactor of all enzymes involved in phosphate transfer reactions that utilize adenosine triphosphate (ATP) and other nucleotide triphosphates as substrates. Various phosphatases and pyrophosphatases also represent enzymes from an enormous list that are influenced by this ion.

Magnesium plays a vital role in the reversible association of intracellular particles and in the binding of macromolecules to subcellular organelles. For example, the binding of messenger RNA (mRNA) to ribosomes is magnesium dependent, as is the functional integrity of ribosomal subunits.

Central Nervous System. Certain of the effects of magnesium on the nervous system are similar to those of calcium. Hypomagnesemia causes increased CNS irritability, disorientation, convulsions, and psychotic behavior (Shils, 1969). Significantly elevated concentrations of magnesium in the plasma of manic-depressive and schizophrenic patients or low plasma magnesium values in patients with endogenous and neurotic depressions have been reported in some studies but not in others (Naylor *et al.,* 1972; Carney *et al.,* 1973).

The flaccid, anesthesia-like state that is produced by the acute intravenous administration of high doses of magnesium sulfate is probably due to peripheral neuromuscular blockade. In a carefully monitored study of two subjects in whom the plasma concentration of magnesium was raised to 15 mEq per liter, the ensuing profound muscular paralysis was unaccompanied by any significant loss of sensation or consciousness (Somjen *et al.,* 1966).

Neuromuscular System. Magnesium has a direct depressant effect on skeletal muscle. In addition, excess magnesium causes a decrease in acetylcholine release by motor-nerve impulses, reduces the sensitivity of the motor end-plate to applied acetylcholine, and decreases the amplitude of the motor end-plate potential. The most critical of these effects is inhibition of acetylcholine release (Hubbard, 1973). The actions of increased magnesium on neuromuscular function are antagonized by calcium. The administration of magnesium sulfate in preeclampsia and eclampsia potentiates neuromuscular blockade produced by *d*-tubocurarine, decamethonium, and succinylcholine (Ghoneim and Long, 1970). Abnormally low concentrations of magnesium in the extracellular fluid result in increased acetylcholine release and increased muscle excitability that can produce tetany.

Cardiovascular System. Certain of the cardiac effects of excess magnesium are similar to those of the potassium ion. High concentrations of magnesium (10 to 15 mEq per liter) cause increased conduction time with lengthened P-R and QRS intervals of the ECG (Randall *et al.,* 1964; Seelig, 1969). Magnesium slows the rate of S-A nodal impulse formation. Higher concentrations of magnesium (greater than 15 mEq per liter) produce cardiac arrest in diastole. Magnesium may abolish digitalis-induced premature ventricular contractions (Sodeman, 1965), but the ion is rarely used for this purpose unless hypomagnesemia is also present. States of magnesium deficiency may or may not be associated with decreased potassium in cardiac cells and enhanced toxicity to cardiac glycosides (Seller *et al.,* 1970). The ECG changes seen with magnesium depletion are similar to those seen with hypercalcemia (Seelig, 1969).

Excess magnesium causes vasodilatation by both a direct action on blood vessels and ganglionic blockade.

ABNORMALITIES OF MAGNESIUM METABOLISM

Hypomagnesemia. The *pathology* of magnesium depletion includes changes in skeletal and cardiac muscle and striking nephrocalcinosis. The latter is unique in that it consists in the formation of tiny microliths within the lumen of the nephron, almost entirely confined to the broad ascending limb of Henle's loop. There appears to be no direct initial damage to renal tubular cells, but damage does occur when the microliths grow sufficiently large to cause obstruction. In the course of several months on a magnesium-deficient regimen, volunteer subjects have developed hypomagnesemia, with inconsistent occurrence of hypokalemia and hypocalcemia. They may exhibit neuromuscular disorders akin to those seen in hypocalcemia.

Magnesium deficiency can occur in diarrhea and steatorrhea; in chronic alcoholism; with prolonged intravenous feeding with magnesium-free solutions; during hemodialysis; and in diabetes mellitus, pancreatitis, postdiuretic electrolyte imbalance, renal tubular damage, and primary aldosteronism. Magnesium deficiency is therefore often associated with hypokalemia and hypocalcemia (Martin, 1969).

Hypomagnesemia, as well as a decrease in total body stores of magnesium, frequently occurs in chronic alcoholic patients (*see* Flink, 1971). The factors responsible probably include increased renal excretion of magnesium, decreased dietary intake of magnesium, vomiting and diarrhea, and hyperaldosteronism in the presence of hepatic cirrhosis. This observation and the similarity between the signs and symptoms of experimental magnesium deficiency in experimental animals and those of delirium tremens have led to the hypothesis that hypomagnesemia is a causative factor in the latter condition. However, convincing evidence of this is lacking (*see* Wacker and Parisi, 1968). As part of the total treatment program for chronic alcoholism, the plasma concentrations of magnesium and of calcium, which is also frequently decreased, should be determined and corrected if found to be low.

During rapid growth periods in newborns and children, hypomagnesemia has been associated with poor intake or excessive losses. A low concentration of magnesium in plasma in newborns who are fed cow's milk or artificial formulas is apparently related to a high phosphate:magnesium ratio in these diets (Cockburn et al., 1973). In infancy the symptoms reliably associated with hypomagnesemia are seizures, hyperirritability, exaggerated tendon reflexes, and increased muscle tone. There is frequently a concomitant hypocalcemia that is resistant to therapy with calcium and vitamin D. Symptoms may be corrected by the replacement of magnesium (Coussons, 1969; Cockburn et al., 1973). Magnesium therapy also appears to be important in correcting hypocalcemia in infants. Oral administration of calcium for treatment of hypocalcemia without regard to decreased magnesium may only exacerbate a magnesium deficiency by reducing intestinal absorption of the cation. This is consistent with the proposed common transport mechanism for magnesium and calcium in the gastrointestinal tract.

Hypomagnesemia in protein-calorie malnutrition is well documented. Conflicting reports exist on the significance of magnesium therapy in reducing the mortality rate in such patients (Caddell, 1967; Rosen et al., 1970).

Magnesium deficiency, particularly if severe, can lead to a form of hypocalcemia that persists despite increased calcium intake until the deficit of magnesium is repaired. Several factors may be involved, including parathyroid dysfunction and an altered equilibrium between calcium in bone and extracellular fluid (Massry, 1977). If tetany is present, it is reversed by the administration of magnesium but not of calcium. Other interrelationships between magnesium, calcium, and the parathyroid glands are discussed in Chapter 65.

A high proportion of patients who form oxalate and phosphate renal stones have low excretion rates of magnesium. When compared to normal subjects, patients with primary hyperparathyroidism and renal stones have a low urinary magnesium concentration relative to calcium excretion. Hyperparathyroid patients with osteitis fibrosa excrete relatively high concentrations of magnesium, and it has been suggested that magnesium excretion may be a factor in the rarity of urinary calculi in these patients (Sutton and Watson, 1969). These and related observations indicate that magnesium therapy may be of value in preventing the formation of certain types of renal stones (Elliot and Ribeiro, 1973).

Conflicting reports exist regarding changes in magnesium metabolism in women taking oral contraceptive hormones (Goldsmith and Goldsmith, 1966; Simpson and Dale, 1972).

Hypomagnesemia is treated with parenteral fluids containing magnesium sulfate or chloride.

Hypermagnesemia. An elevated magnesium concentration in plasma is usually due to renal insufficiency. The use of magnesium sulfate as a cathartic in patients with impaired renal function can lead to severe toxicity, as can chronic ingestion of magnesium-containing antacids by such individuals. Hypermagnesemia is manifested by muscle weakness, hypotension, ECG changes, sedation, and confusion. As plasma concentrations of magnesium begin to exceed 4 mEq per liter, the deep-tendon reflexes are decreased and may be absent at levels approaching 10 mEq per liter. At 12 to 15 mEq per liter respiratory paralysis is a potential hazard; the respiratory effects can be antagonized to some extent by the intravenous administration of calcium salts. The concentration of magnesium in the plasma at which complete heart block occurs may be quite variable.

Plasma concentrations of magnesium increase in the fetus and approach the maternal blood values after magnesium sulfate administration in eclampsia and preeclampsia. The neonate may be drowsy and exhibit respiratory difficulties and diminished muscle tone (Lipsitz and English, 1967). However, Stone and Pritchard (1970) found no relationship between the plasma magnesium concentration of blood collected from the umbilical cord and the Apgar score. In infants who suffer hypoxia during delivery, hypermagnesemia can result, and the plasma magnesium concentration is inversely correlated with the Apgar score (Engel and Elin, 1970).

Preparations. Magnesium citrate and sulfate are the salts usually employed for their action on the gastrointestinal tract. There are many magnesium preparations used as antacids. For parenteral medication, magnesium sulfate is usually employed. The dosage is expressed in terms of the official U.S.P. hydrated salt, $MgSO_4 \cdot 7H_2O$. One gram of this salt is equivalent to 4.06 millimoles (8.12 mEq) of magnesium. *Magnesium Sulfate Injection,* U.S.P., is available in concentrations of 10, 12.5, 25, and 50%.

Therapeutic Uses. *Gastrointestinal Uses.* The uses of magnesium salts as cathartics (Chapter 43) and as antacids (Chapter 42) are discussed elsewhere.
Central Depression. Magnesium sulfate is used in the treatment of seizures associated with acute nephritis and with eclampsia of pregnancy. The dose for children is 0.1 to 0.2 ml/kg of body weight (0.16 to 0.32 mEq/kg) of a 20% solution administered intramuscularly. In the treatment of patients with toxemia of pregnancy, Rogers and associates (1969) have developed a system of initial and sustaining dosage, based on body weight. It is possible to attain unduly high plasma concentrations, and the patient must be carefully monitored both clinically and chemically. If magnesium therapy of this sort is to be used, a preparation of a calcium salt should be readily available for intravenous injection to counteract the potential serious hazard of magnesium intoxication. A clinical sign of significance is the presence of deep-tendon reflexes. As long as these are active, it is probable that the patient will not develop respiratory paralysis.
Hypomagnesemia. Intravenous administration of magnesium sulfate is the treatment for severe mag-

nesium deficiency; it should be injected extremely slowly with observance of the same precautions as described above. Two to 4 g (17 to 34 mEq) may be given daily in divided doses.

ACUTE RENAL INSUFFICIENCY

An acute deterioration in renal function may be transient and solely due to dehydration. This may be corrected as described above for the treatment of dehydration and hypovolemia.

However, acute tubular necrosis may be provoked by a variety of poisons and drugs, heavy metals, the products of hemolysis, shock, and perhaps other insults. The damage is often ultimately reversible, and the physician is faced with the problem of attempting to maintain the internal environment as nearly normal as possible in the absence of the excretory function of the kidney.

For the control of *fluid volume,* adults need about 500 ml of water per day to replace the difference between insensible loss and the amount of water produced from the metabolism of body tissues. Under such a program a patient *should* lose 0.2 to 0.4 kg per day, since without adequate caloric intake this amount of body substance will be consumed. *Calories* should be provided in the form of carbohydrate, and the usual procedure is to administer the daily allotment of fluid as hypertonic glucose. Additional fluid may be added, when necessary, to replace vomitus and the extra losses of water that may accompany fever and sweating. These additional fluids should contain electrolytes in the approximate concentration in which they are lost, with the exception of potassium and hydrogen ion.

Hyponatremia is most commonly a consequence of dilution, and the restoration toward normal should be accomplished by the restriction of water intake. The development of *metabolic acidosis* is inevitable, and, as long as the patient is not volume depleted, the administration of sodium bicarbonate would appear not to be indicated, since one of the complications to be avoided is hypervolemia. *Hyperkalemia* is usually controllable by ensuring that no potassium is administered, and by the use of exchange resins as outlined above. However, if high concentrations of potassium persist in plasma, more aggressive treatment may be indicated in the form of dialysis.

Peritoneal dialysis is a simple and useful technic. In general, the composition of the dialysis solutions should mimic extracellular fluid, with a somewhat higher level of potential bicarbonate and without potassium. The commercial preparations of dialytic fluid contain 1.5 or 4.25% glucose. The lower concentration is utilized when the extracellular fluid volume appears to be normal and it is not desirable to reduce it. The higher concentration of glucose is used to help remove fluid, osmotically, in excess of that which is instilled. Although glucose exchanges rapidly across the peritoneal membrane, it does so slowly relative to sodium salts and water, and, therefore, it can act as an effective osmotic agent.

In instances in which one wishes to reduce the plasma concentration of potassium and the degree of uremia more quickly, *extracorporeal hemodialysis* (the "artificial kidney") is a more efficient way to accomplish these ends.

Abouna, G. M.; Veazey, P. R.; and Terry, D. B., Jr. Intravenous infusion of hydrochloric acid for treatment of severe metabolic alkalosis. *Surgery,* **1974,** *75,* 194–202.

Adler, S., and Fraley, D. S. Potassium and intracellular pH. *Kidney Int.,* **1977,** *11,* 433–442.

Alfrey, A. C., and Miller, N. L. Bone magnesium pools in uremia. *J. Clin. Invest.,* **1973,** *52,* 3019–3027.

Anderson, H. M., and Mudge, G. H. The effect of potassium on intracellular bicarbonate in slices of kidney cortex. *J. Clin. Invest.,* **1955,** *35,* 1691–1697.

Arieff, A. I.; Lazarowitz, V. C.; and Guisado, R. Experimental dialysis disequilibrium syndrome: prevention with glycerol. *Kidney Int.,* **1978,** *14,* 270–278.

Burnell, J. M.; Teubner, E. J.; and Simpson, D. P. Metabolic acidosis accompanying potassium deprivation. *Am. J. Physiol.,* **1974,** *227,* 329–333.

Caddell, J. L. Studies in protein-calorie malnutrition. II. A double-blind clinical trial to assess magnesium therapy. *N. Engl. J. Med.,* **1967,** *276,* 533–535.

Carney, M. W. P.; Sheffield, B. F.; and Sebastian, J. Serum magnesium, diagnosis, ECT and season. *Br. J. Psychiatry,* **1973,** *122,* 424–429.

Carpenter, C. C. J. Clinical studies in Asiatic cholera. VI. Overall clinical observations. *Bull. Johns Hopkins Hosp.,* **1966,** *118,* 243–245.

Cervera, A. L., and Moss, G. Progressive hypovolemia leading to shock after continuous hemorrhage and 3:1 crystalloid replacement. *Am. J. Surg.,* **1975,** *129,* 670–674.

Clementsen, H. J. Potassium therapy, a break with tradition. *Lancet,* **1962,** *2,* 175–177.

Cockburn, F.; Brown, J. K.; Belton, N. R.; and Forfar, J. O. Neonatal convulsions associated with primary disturbances of calcium, potassium, and magnesium metabolism. *Arch. Dis. Child.,* **1973,** *48,* 99–108.

Colman, R. W. Paradoxical hypotension after volume expansion with plasma protein fraction. *N. Engl. J. Med.,* **1978,** *299,* 97–98.

Cooke, R. E.; Segar, W. E.; Cheek, D. B.; Coville, F. E.; and Darrow, D. C. Extrarenal correction of alkalosis associated with potassium deficiency. *J. Clin. Invest.,* **1952,** *31,* 798–805.

Coussons, H. Magnesium metabolism in infants and children. *Postgrad. Med.,* **1969,** *46,* 135–139.

Duggin, G. G., and Price, M. A. Hypokalemic muscular paresis in migratory Papua/New Guineans. *Lancet,* **1974,** *1,* 649–651.

Elliot, J. S., and Ribeiro, M. E. The effect of varying concentrations of calcium and magnesium upon calcium oxalate solubility. *Invest. Urol.,* **1973,** *10,* 295–297.

Engel, R. R., and Elin, R. J. Hypermagnesemia from birth asphyxia. *J. Pediatr.,* **1970,** *77,* 631–637.

Ettinger, P. O.; Regan, T. J.; and Oldewurtel, H. A. Hyperkalemia, cardiac conduction, and the electrocardiogram: a review. *Am. Heart J.,* **1974,** *88,* 360–371.

Finberg, L.; Kiley, J.; and Luttrell, C. N. Mass accidental salt poisoning in infancy. A study of a hospital disaster. *J.A.M.A.,* **1963,** *184,* 187–190.

Fischer, J. E. Hyperalimentation. *Adv. Surg.,* **1977,** *11,* 1–69.

Fischer, J. E., and Baldessarini, R. J. Pathogenesis and therapy of hepatic coma. *Prog. Liver Dis.,* **1976,** *5,* 363–397.

Flink, E. B. Mineral metabolism in alcoholism. In, *The Biology of Alcoholism,* Vol. 1. (Kissin, B., and Begleiter, H., eds.) Plenum Press, New York, 1971, pp. 377–395.

Galvez, O. G.; Bay, W. H.; Roberts, B. W.; and Ferris, T. F. The hemodynamic effects of potassium deficiency in the dog. *Circ. Res.,* **1977,** *40,* Suppl. I, 11–16.

Gamble, J. L. Physiological information gained from studies on the life raft ration. *Harvey Lect.,* **1947,** *62,* 247–273.

Gamble, J. L., and Ross, S. G. The factors in the dehydration following pyloric obstruction. *J. Clin. Invest.,* **1925,** *1,* 403–423.

Garella, S.; Chang, B. S.; and Kahn, S. I. Dilution acidosis and contraction alkalosis: review of a concept. *Kidney Int.,* **1975,** *8,* 279–283.

Garella, S.; Chazan, J. A.; and Cohen, J. J. Saline-resistant metabolic alkalosis or "chloride-wasting nephropathy." *Ann. Intern. Med.,* **1970,** *73,* 31–38.

Geyer, R. P. Fluorocarbon-polyol artificial blood substitutes. *N. Engl. J. Med.,* **1973,** *289,* 1077–1082.

Ghoneim, M. M., and Long, J. P. The interaction between magnesium and other neuromuscular blocking agents. *Anesthesiology,* **1970,** *32,* 23–27.

Goldfarb, S.; Strunk, B.; Singer, I.; and Goldberg, M. Paradoxical glucose-induced hyperkalemia. Combined aldosterone-insulin deficiency. *Am. J. Med.,* **1975,** *59,* 744–750.

Goldsmith, N. F., and Goldsmith, J. R. Epidemiological aspects of magnesium and calcium metabolism. Implication of altered magnesium metabolism in women taking drugs for the suppression of ovulation. *Arch. Environ. Health,* **1966,** *12,* 607–619.

Kassirer, J. P., and Harrington, J. T. Diuretics and potassium metabolism: a reassessment of the need, effectiveness and safety of potassium therapy. *Kidney Int.,* **1977,** *11,* 505–515.

Kassirer, J. P., and Schwartz, W. B. Correction of metabolic alkalosis in man without repair of potassium deficiency. *Am. J. Med.,* **1966,** *40,* 19–26.

Katz, M. A. Hyperglycemia-induced hyponatremia—calculation of sodium depression. *N. Engl. J. Med.,* **1973,** *289,* 843–844.

Knochel, J. P. Role of glucoregulatory hormones in potassium homeostasis. *Kidney Int.,* **1977,** *11,* 443–452.

——— Rhabdomyolysis and effects of potassium deficiency on muscle structure and function. *Cardiovasc. Med.,* **1978,** *3,* 247–261.

Kreisberg, R. A. Diabetic ketoacidosis: new concepts and trends in pathogenesis and treatment. *Ann. Intern. Med.,* **1978,** *88,* 681–695.

Lipsitz, P. J., and English, I. C. Hypermagnesemia in the newborn infant. *Pediatrics,* **1967,** *40,* 856–862.

Macknight, A. D. C., and Leaf, A. Regulation of cellular volume. *Physiol. Rev.,* **1977,** *57,* 510–573.

Milne, M. D. Influence of acid base balance on efficacy and toxicity of drugs. In, *Nephrotoxicity.* (Fillastre, J.-P., ed.) Masson Publishing USA, Inc., New York, **1978,** pp. 53–61.

Mithoefer, J. C.; Runser, R. H.; and Karetsky, M. S. The use of sodium bicarbonate in the treatment of acute bronchial asthma. *N. Engl. J. Med.,* **1965,** *272,* 1200–1203.

Moore, F. D. Tris buffer, mannitol, and low viscous dextran. *Surg. Clin. North Am.,* **1963,** *43,* 577–596.

Mudge, G. H., and Hardin, B. Response to mercurial diuretics during alkalosis: a comparison of acute metabolic and chronic hypokalemic alkalosis in the dog. *J. Clin. Invest.,* **1956,** *35,* 155–163.

Nahata, M. C.; Shrimp, L.; Lampman, T.; and McLeod, D. C. Effect of ascorbic acid on urine pH in man. *Am. J. Hosp. Pharm.,* **1977,** *34,* 1234–1237.

Naylor, G. J.; Fleming, L. W.; Stewart, W. K.; McNamee, H. B.; and Le Poidevin, D. Plasma magnesium and calcium levels in depressive psychosis. *Br. J. Psychiatry,* **1972,** *120,* 683–684.

Nees, J. E.; Hauser, C. J.; Skippy, C.; State, D.; and Shoemaker, W. E. Comparison of cardiorespiratory effects of crystalline hemoglobin, whole blood, albumin, and Ringer's lactate in the resuscitation of hemorrhagic shock in dogs. *Surgery,* **1978,** *83,* 639–647.

Oh, M. S., and Carroll, H. J. The anion gap. *N. Engl. J. Med.*, **1977**, *297*, 814–817.

———. The renin-aldosterone system and thiazide-induced depletion of total body potassium in essential hypertension. *Nephron*, **1978**, *21*, 269–276.

Patrick, J. Assessment of body potassium stores. *Kidney Int.*, **1977**, *11*, 476–490.

Randall, R. E., Jr.; Cohen, M. D.; Spray, C. C., Jr.; and Rossmeid, E. C. Hypermagnesemia in renal failure: etiology and toxic manifestations. *Ann. Intern. Med.*, **1964**, *61*, 73–88.

Ring, J., and Messmer, K. Incidence and severity of anaphylactoid reactions to colloid volume substitutes. *Lancet*, **1977**, *1*, 466–469.

Rogers, S. F.; Flowers, C. E., Jr.; and Alexander, J. A. Aggressive toxemia management. *Obstet. Gynecol.*, **1969**, *33*, 724–728.

Rosen, E. U.; Campbell, P. G.; and Moosa, G. M. Hypomagnesemia and magnesium therapy in protein-calorie malnutrition. *J. Pediatr.*, **1970**, *77*, 709–714.

Savitsky, J. P.; Doczi, J.; Black, J.; and Arnold, J. D. A clinical safety trial of stroma-free hemoglobin. *Clin. Pharmacol. Ther.*, **1978**, *23*, 73–80.

Schwartz, A.; Lindenmayer, G. E.; and Allen, J. C. The sodium-potassium adenosine triphosphatase: pharmacological, physiological and biochemical aspects. *Pharmacol. Rev.*, **1975**, *27*, 3–134.

Seelig, M. S. Electrographic patterns of magnesium depletion appearing in alcoholic heart disease. *Ann. N.Y. Acad. Sci.*, **1969**, *162*, 906–917.

Seller, R. H.; Cangiano, J.; Kim, K. E.; Mendelssohn, S.; Brest, A. N.; and Swartz, C. Digitalis toxicity and hypomagnesemia. *Am. Heart J.*, **1970**, *79*, 57–68.

Shils, M. E. Experimental human magnesium depletion. *Medicine (Baltimore)*, **1969**, *48*, 61–85.

Silva, P.; Brown, R. S.; and Epstein, F. H. Adaptation to potassium. *Kidney Int.*, **1977**, *11*, 466–475.

Simpson, G. R., and Dale, E. Serum levels of phosphorus, magnesium, and calcium in women utilizing combination oral or long-acting injectable progestational contraceptives. *Fertil. Steril.*, **1972**, *23*, 326–330.

Sodeman, W. A. Diagnosis and treatment of digitalis toxicity. *N. Engl. J. Med.*, **1965**, *273*, 35–37, 93–95.

Somjen, G.; Hilmy, M.; and Stephen, C. R. Failure to anesthetize human subjects by intravenous administration of magnesium sulfate. *J. Pharmacol. Exp. Ther.*, **1966**, *154*, 652–659.

Stone, S. R., and Pritchard, J. A. Effects of maternally administered magnesium sulfate on the neonate. *Obstet. Gynecol.*, **1970**, *35*, 574–577.

Strihou, C. V. Y. de, and Morales-Barria, J. The influence of dietary sodium and potassium intake on the genesis of induced alkalosis. *Clin. Sci.*, **1969**, *37*, 859–871.

Sutton, R. A., and Watson, L. Urinary excretion of calcium and magnesium in primary hyperparathyroidism. *Lancet*, **1969**, *1*, 1000–1003.

Tannen, R. L. Relationship of renal ammonia production and potassium homeostasis. *Kidney Int.*, **1977**, *11*, 453–465.

Wallach, S., and Dimich, A. Radiomagnesium turnover studies in hypomagnesemic states. *Ann. N.Y. Acad. Sci.*, **1969**, *162*, 963–972.

Walser, M. Keto acid therapy in chronic renal failure. *Nephron*, **1978**, *21*, 56–74.

Wilkinson, P. R. Potassium changes during diuretic therapy. *Cardiovasc. Med.*, **1978**, *3*, 181–183.

Wynn, V. A metabolic study of acute water intoxication in man and dogs. *Clin. Sci.*, **1955**, *14*, 669–680.

Monographs and Reviews

Black, D. A. K., and Milne, M. D. Experimental potassium depletion in man. *Clin. Sci.*, **1952**, *11*, 397–415.

Fox, C. L., Jr., and Nahas, G. G. *Body Fluid Replacement in the Surgical Patient.* Grune & Stratton, Inc., New York, **1970**.

Hubbard, J. I. Microphysiology of vertebrate neuromuscular transmission. *Physiol. Rev.*, **1973**, *53*, 674–723.

Martin, H. E. Clinical magnesium deficiency. *Ann. N.Y. Acad. Sci.*, **1969**, *162*, 891–900.

Massry, S. G. Pharmacology of magnesium. *Annu. Rev. Pharmacol. Toxicol.*, **1977**, *17*, 67–82.

Maxwell, M. H., and Kleeman, C. R. *Clinical Disorders of Fluid and Electrolyte Metabolism.* McGraw-Hill Book Co., New York, **1972**.

Moore, F. D.; Oleson, K. H.; McMurrey, J. D.; Parker, H. V.; Ball, M. R.; and Boyden, C. M. *The Body Cell Mass and Its Supporting Environment.* W. B. Saunders Co., Philadelphia, **1963**.

Russell, A. The implications of hyperammonemia in rare and common disorders, including migraine. *Mt. Sinai J. Med. N.Y.*, **1973**, *40*, 609–630, 723–735.

Sanderson, P. H. Renal response to massive alkali loading in the human subject. In, *Ciba Foundation Symposium on the Kidney.* (Lewis, A. A. G., and Wolstenholme, G. E. W., eds.) Little, Brown & Co., Boston, **1954**, pp. 165–174.

Wacker, W. E. C., and Parisi, A. F. Magnesium metabolism. *N. Engl. J. Med.*, **1968**, *278*, 658–663, 712–717, 772–776.

Walser, M. Magnesium metabolism. *Ergeb. Physiol.*, **1967**, *59*, 185–296.

Winters, R. W. *The Body Fluids in Pediatrics.* Little, Brown & Co., Boston, **1973**.

VIII

Drugs Affecting Renal Function and Electrolyte Metabolism

INTRODUCTION

Gilbert H. Mudge

The important homeostatic role of the kidney in maintaining the volume and the composition of the body fluids has already been stressed in the preceding chapter. It is not surprising, therefore, to find that drugs that alter renal function comprise a major and indispensable group of therapeutic agents. As knowledge of the fundamental physiological mechanisms of renal function has expanded, the number of drugs that affect specific renal tubular processes has grown. Indeed, in many instances the drug has provided the tool to elucidate the finer details of cellular mechanisms. Drugs that alter renal function fall into a variety of classes, depending on both the chemical nature of the drug and the specific renal function upon which it acts. As anticipated, these drugs have wider therapeutic applications than would be included under the designation of diuretics. Therefore, in the following section, drugs with widely different clinical uses will be discussed together because their basic action is on the kidney. It should also be noted that the kidney is the major excretory organ for many therapeutic agents and their metabolites. A knowledge of renal mechanisms is important, therefore, in evaluating the pattern of drug excretion, particularly since alteration of renal function may markedly affect the rate of excretion and hence the duration of drug action or the extent of drug toxicity.

PHYSIOLOGICAL CONSIDERATIONS

The majority of excretory products appear in the glomerular filtrate and are incompletely reabsorbed by the renal tubules. Other substances can also be secreted by the renal tubular cells into the tubular urine and in this manner be eliminated from the body. Certain substances, moreover, undergo both reabsorption and secretion. It should be emphasized that the terms *reabsorption* and *secretion* refer to the direction of net transport without any implication as to underlying cellular mechanisms. Therefore, the factors that are important in the determination of volume and composition of urine are: (1) glomerular filtration, (2) tubular reabsorption, and (3) tubular secretion.

Glomerular Filtration. The glomerulus of the kidney is similar to other capillary beds, and filtration is subject to the same physical laws that govern the transport of fluid and permeable solutes across any capillary membrane. The filtering force is the hydrostatic pressure of the blood derived from the work of the heart. The plasma proteins do not penetrate the normal glomerular membrane to an appreciable extent. All the plasma constituents gain access to the glomerular capsule with the exception of the proteins, lipids, and substances bound to proteins.

The hydrostatic pressure within the glomerular capillaries is approximately 60% of the arterial pressure. Thus, systemic blood pressure must be considerably reduced before the rate of glomerular filtration is significantly changed. For example, mean blood pressure must usually fall to a level of 40 mm Hg before filtration ceases. Theoretically, the rate of glomerular filtration may be altered by (1) the hydrostatic pressure within the glomerular capillaries, (2) the osmotic pressure of the nondiffusible constituents of the blood, (3) the number of functioning glomeruli, and (4) back pressure from those structures that drain the glomerular filtrate to the outside.

Urine formation begins in a prodigal way. Included in the glomerular filtrate are not only the waste products but also the essential constituents of the extracellular fluid such as water, electrolytes, and nutrients. Apparently the excretory function of the kidney demands the filtration of a large volume of extracellular fluid. In turn, the homeostatic function of the organ demands the reabsorption of most of the ingredients of the filtrate.

Although the rate of glomerular filtration is a very important aspect of renal function, drugs that affect the rate of filtration will not be discussed in this section. The most common cause of reduction in the filtration rate is organic change in the renal vascular bed. There is no drug available to correct this abnormality. Another common cause of reduction in filtration rate is the reduced renal blood flow secondary to heart failure. For its correction, attention is directed to the heart rather than to the kidney. Many drugs used in the treatment of hypertension reduce renal blood flow and filtration rate, but these represent undesirable side effects. Drugs with marked hemodynamic action, such as epinephrine, alter filtration rate and urine flow by affecting arterial pressure and afferent and efferent renal arteriolar resistance, but no therapeutic application is made of these actions. Finally, there are a few agents, such as dopamine, that significantly increase renal blood flow and filtration rate, but these have relatively limited therapeutic use. Experience has demonstrated that one can alter the rate of excretion of many substances much more effectively by drugs that alter tubular function than by those that change filtration rate.

Measurement of Glomerular Filtration. The rate of glomerular filtration can be determined very accurately in animals and man by measuring the renal clearance of substances that are freely filtered at the glomerulus and are neither secreted nor reabsorbed by the renal tubule. Thus, the amount of the substance excreted in the urine is a measure of the amount filtered by the glomeruli. It is only necessary to divide this by the concentration of the substance in the filtrate to determine the volume of filtrate from which the urine was derived. The polysaccharide inulin is accepted as the most valid substance for measuring the filtration rate under almost all circumstances, although there are other agents that behave in a similar manner.

Renal Plasma Flow. Certain substances at low concentrations in plasma are secreted by the renal tubules so efficiently, and undergo so little tubular reabsorption, that essentially all of the substance is removed from the blood in a single passage through the kidney. It therefore follows that the total amount of such a substance appearing in the urine over a given time divided by its concentration in plasma is an expression of renal plasma flow. The outstanding example of this type is para-aminohippuric acid.

Tubular Transport of Inorganic Compounds. The importance of the reabsorptive function of the renal tubules to the body economy cannot be overemphasized and can best be illustrated by a few numerical considerations. The rate of glomerular filtration in the average adult is approximately 125 ml per minute. In such an individual, the total extracellular fluid volume is approximately 12.5 liters. Thus, a volume equivalent to that of the extracellular fluid is filtered across the glomerular capillary bed within a period of 100 minutes. During this time approximately 100 ml of urine reaches the bladder. Therefore, the tubules normally reabsorb over 99% of the glomerular filtrate. Obviously the composition of the tubular reabsorbate must closely approximate that of the extracellular fluid; otherwise, extreme distortions in the composition of the extracellular fluid would soon result. Reabsorption is largely achieved by active transport of electrolyte and other solutes from tubular fluid to tubular cell and thence to the extracellular fluid. This involves the expenditure of energy derived from metabolic activity. Physical forces involving the oncotic pressure of the peritubular plasma may also contribute to the reabsorption of water. The magnitude of this component is relatively small and uncertain.

Although many of the intimate mechanisms of electrolyte transport are incompletely understood, for operational purposes it is possible to describe them in terms of the scheme summarized in Figure VIII-1. Considered primarily from the point of view of the action of pharmacological agents, the most important tubular mechanisms of electrolyte transport are (1) reabsorption of sodium and chloride, (2) secretion of hydrogen ion, and (3) secretion of potassium. In addition, there are related but separate mechanisms for the reabsorption of calcium, magnesium, phosphate, and sulfate. Previously it was thought that sodium was the primary ion actively reabsorbed against an electrochemical gradient throughout the nephron, accompanied by the back diffusion of an equivalent amount of fixed anion, mostly chloride. It has now been shown that in the ascending limb of the loop of Henle it is the chloride anion that is transported actively.

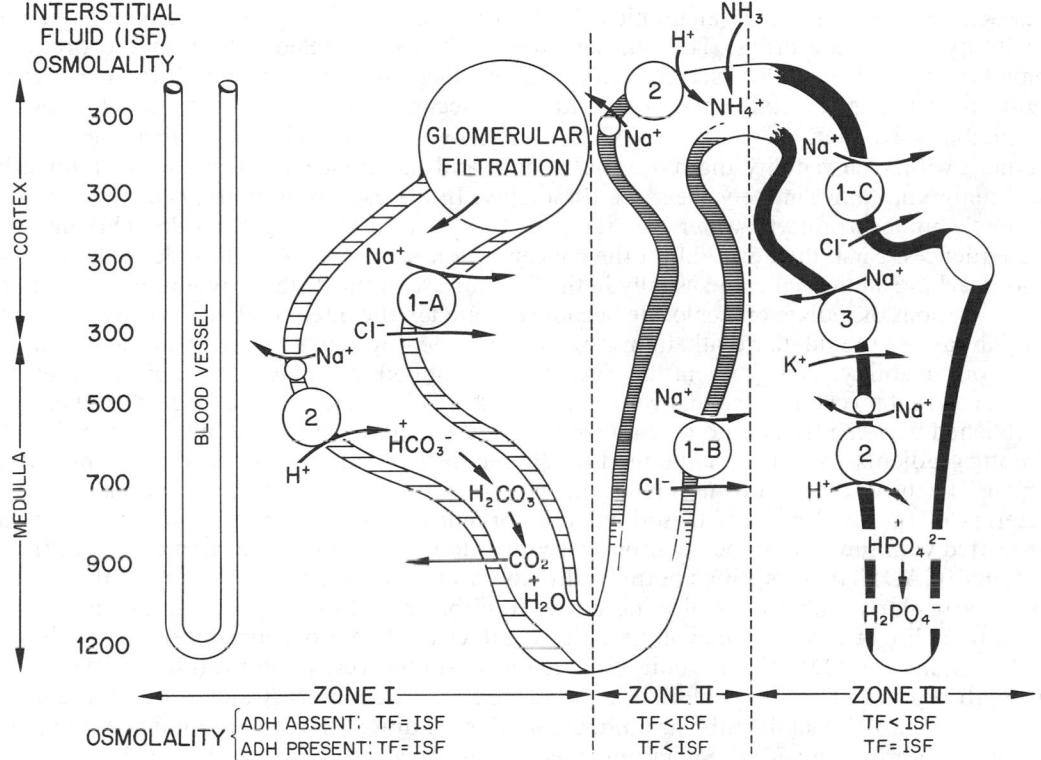

Figure VIII-1. *Schematic representation of the major electrolyte transport systems in the kidney that are susceptible to drug action.* Numbers coincide with the description in the text.

The functional organization of the nephron in relation to the countercurrent system is depicted on the vertical axis to show interstitial osmolality (isosmotic cortex; hypertonic medulla), and also on the horizontal axis to show the water permeability characteristics of the nephron segments. Interstitial osmolality is given in milliosmoles per kilogram of water. In zone I, osmolality of tubular fluid (TF) is approximately equal to that of interstitial fluid (ISF), both being isosmotic to plasma in the cortex but increasingly hypertonic to it in the medulla. The blood vessels are also isosmotic to the adjacent ISF. In zone II, chloride and sodium reabsorptive transport is relatively greater than outward diffusion of water. Hence, osmolality of TF is less than that of adjacent ISF. In zone III, water permeability is under the control of the antidiuretic hormone (ADH). Three types of tubular epithelium are schematically shown to indicate differences in water permeability; the associated mechanisms of sodium reabsorption are indicated by *1–A* and *1–C*, and of chloride reabsorption by *1–B*. The beginning and the end of epithelium in zone II (mostly the ascending limb of the loop of Henle) are left indeterminate because of uncertainty concerning exact functional boundaries.

Mechanisms are also shown for acidification of the urine (*2*) and secretion of potassium (*3*). For a full explanation of these tubular functions, *see* text.

The secretion of hydrogen and potassium ions has often been described in terms of an exchange mechanism by which the reabsorption of sodium is visualized as being coupled with the transport of either hydrogen or potassium in the opposite direction. Newer studies, however, cast doubt on the validity of an exchange reaction as an actual cellular mechanism and emphasize that reabsorption occurs by one process and secretion by another.

All but a very small fraction of the filtered sodium and water is normally reabsorbed, sodium by active transport and water by diffusion. On the basis of the quantitative relationship between these two processes, it is possible to identify three segments of the nephron on both an anatomical and functional basis. These are intimately related to the processes of concentration and dilution of the urine. As indicated in Figure VIII-1, the reabsorption of sodium and chloride, the major solutes of the glomerular filtrate, can be considered in terms of three different mechanisms: *1-A, 1-B,* and *1-C.* There are at least three criteria by which each of these can be distinguished: anatomical localization, concomitant water permeability, and sensitivity to diuretic drugs. The reabsorptive mechanism labeled *1-A* is in the proximal convolution; *1-B* is in the ascending limb of the loop of Henle; and *1-C* is in the distal nephron, in both the distal convolution and the collecting duct. At *1-A,* there is a high water permeability so that, as solute (Na^+Cl^-) is reabsorbed, water diffuses along the osmotic gradient with such rapidity that the tubular fluid and the adjacent peritubular or interstitial fluid maintain approximately the same osmolality. In the ascending limb (*1-B*) the tubule is relatively impermeable to water despite the active reabsorption of chloride. This has two consequences. First, there is a fall in the concentration of sodium and chloride in the tubular fluid, reaching a minimal value usually in the first portion of the distal convolution; second, the concentrations of sodium and chloride become elevated in the interstitial fluid. A concentration gradient across the tubular epithelium is thus established by active transport at the site of low water permeability. This gradient then becomes multiplied in a longitudinal direction by the countercurrent mechanism, so that within the interstitial fluid a large osmotic gradient becomes established between the isosmotic renal cortex and the hyperosmotic medulla and papilla. The osmotic gradients are partly maintained by the relatively meager blood flow to the medullary region. The third sodium transport mechanism (*1-C*) is probably less significant than the others in terms of the total amount of sodium reabsorbed, but is of unique importance in being associated with the area of the nephron susceptible to the antidiuretic hormone (ADH). In the presence of ADH, there is a high permeability to water in this segment. As a result, the tubular fluid, particularly within the collecting ducts, equilibrates with the hyperosmotic interstitium and is then discharged at the end of the collecting duct as a hypertonic or concentrated solution. In the absence of ADH, this portion of the nephron is relatively impermeable to water. Thus, the reabsorption of sodium chloride, as indicated by reactions *1-B* and *1-C,* progressively lowers the osmolality of the tubular fluid. Under this condition, the tubular fluid does not reach osmotic equilibration with the adjacent interstitium. As a result, in the absence of ADH, the voided urine is characteristically hypoosmotic, or dilute.

There are two other features that characterize distal sodium reabsorption. First, the absolute amount reabsorbed in this area is determined not only by the amount filtered but also by the proportion of the filtrate that has already undergone reabsorption at more proximal sites. This fraction may vary over a wide range, particularly in pathological conditions associated with edema formation or oliguria. Second, the distal mechanisms may have discrete sensitivities to the action of some drugs, including the adrenocortical hormones.

Free-Water Production. By definition, this term refers to the amount of distilled water (*i.e.,* water free of solute) that would have to be added to, or subtracted from, the urine voided over a period of time (usually calculated on a minute basis) in order to render that urine specimen isosmotic with a simultaneous sample of plasma. In arithmetical terms, free-water production equals urine volume (V) minus the osmolal clearance (C_{OSM}). The latter term has the usual dimensions of clearance (UV/P) and refers to the sum of the concentrations of all osmotically active solutes in plasma and urine. When the urine is more dilute than plasma, free-water production is positive; when the urine is more concentrated, free-water production is negative. In the first instance, solute-free water is actually excreted as part of the voided urine; in the latter instance, solute-free water can be considered as being returned to the body from the kidney. When the urine has the same osmolality as plasma, free-water production is zero regardless of the rate of urine flow.

Free-water production is an operational concept. At no time, and in no place, does distilled, or solute-free, water exist as such within the kidney. The concept is important in that it takes into account more than just the concentration of osmotically active solute in the urine. By introducing the dimensions of volume per unit time, the net rate at which either the concentrating or diluting mechanism is operating may be accurately described.

It should be emphasized that free-water production is *not* synonymous with diuresis. Some of the most potent diuretics may produce a massive diuresis of almost isosmotic urine, and hence with a minimal rate of free-water production. While it is true that free-water production must ultimately influence the solute concentration of the residual body fluids, nevertheless, in the clinical use of diuretics the free-water production has relatively minor therapeutic implications. This is partly due to the fact that urinary excretion is promptly balanced by a variable dietary intake of both solute and water.

The concept of free-water production has played an interesting role in localizing the site of diuretic action within the nephron. It must be strongly emphasized that, in order to infer intrarenal sites of action on the basis of the excretion of solute and water, observations must be made under one or the other of two physiological extremes—either in the absence of ADH or under its maximal influence. The former condition is obtained during unequivocal water diuresis or in patients with diabetes insipidus of posterior pituitary origin; the latter condition may be achieved by restriction of water, infusion of hypertonic solute, or administration of exogenous ADH. There is no evidence that the available diuretic drugs directly alter the action of ADH itself.

Figure VIII–2 shows the pattern obtained with three different diuretics. These can be evaluated in terms of the mechanisms and with the nomenclature previously described in Figure VIII–1. The interpretations that have been advanced are essentially as follows. If sodium reabsorption is inhibited in the proximal tubule (*i.e., 1–A*), an increased amount of solute will be delivered to the more distal segments, including the ascending limb (*1–B*). With the greater load to this latter site, an increased amount of sodium would be reabsorbed along with chloride, leading to an increase in either the positive or the negative free-water production. This is the result obtained with *mannitol*. In addition, in the case of positive free-water production, some of the increase might also be attributed to augmented reabsorption of sodium in the most distal nephron (*1–C*). A second pattern is illustrated by *ethacrynic acid*. If chloride and sodium reabsorption were to be inhibited predominantly in the ascending limb (*1–B*), the urine would tend to remain isosmotic. Despite the resultant diuresis, the production of both positive and negative free water would be impaired. A third possibility is illustrated with *chlorothiazide*. The findings have been interpreted in terms of the inhibition of sodium reabsorption at a distal site, that is, *1–C*. Since the rate of negative free-water production is normal, it is inferred that there is no inhibition of transport in the ascending limb (*1–B*). However, since positive free-water production is partially inhibited, it has been proposed that the drug acts at the most distal site of sodium reabsorption.

Although there is uncertainty about some of the interpretations that have been proposed, there can be no doubt that different diuretics act by distinct and separate mechanisms as judged by free-water production. Of course, the demonstration of an action at one site does not invariably exclude an action elsewhere. By these criteria, osmotic diuretics and acetazolamide act proximally, ethacrynic acid and furosemide act on the ascending limb, and chlorothiazide acts on the distal segment.

In this discussion, the term *free-water production* has been used instead of *free-water clearance*. In the literature, the term *clearance* has been employed, with positive free water being designated as C_{H_2O} and negative free water as $T^c_{H_2O}$. Despite auspicious precedent, the term C_{H_2O} is incorrect if literally translated as "the renal clearance of water," and the term $T^c_{H_2O}$ was initially based on premises that have become obsolete. Despite these semantic difficulties, the concept of free water remains valid, but the term *production* is preferable to that of *clearance*.

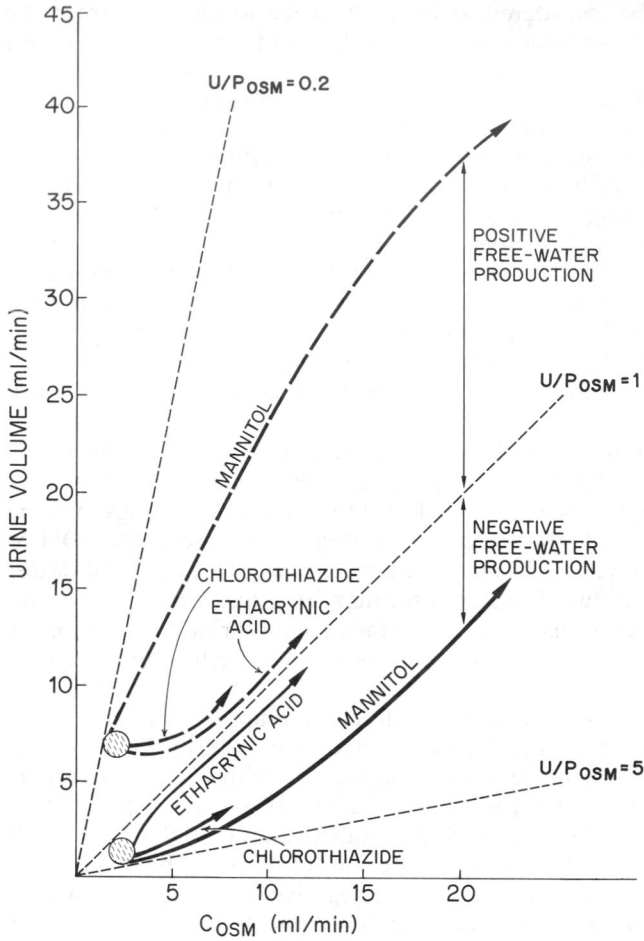

Figure VIII–2. *Relation of urine volume to osmolar clearance* (C_{OSM}).

The diuretic agents were given during a maximal water diuresis, that is, in the absence of ADH (dash lines), or to dehydrated subjects under maximal influence of ADH (solid lines). The magnitude of free-water production is given graphically as the vertical distance between any observed point and the isosmotic line ($U/P_{OSM} = 1$). The shaded circles indicate normal rates of solute excretion (*i.e.,* without diuretics) at extremes of ADH activity. Note that the maximal and minimal urinary osmolalities (as indicated by U/P_{OSM}) are achieved only at normal rates of solute excretion. These data from the literature were obtained in normal man.

Fine distinctions between actual generation and net production of free water are beyond the scope of the present discussion.

Hydrogen Ion Secretion. The concept of hydrogen ion secretion has played an important role in the development of modern theories of renal function and of the action of therapeutic agents. Under certain circumstances the amount of titratable acid in the voided urine cannot be accounted for by the selective reabsorption of constituents of the filtrate. This provides proof that hydrogen ion is added to or secreted into the tubular fluid by the tubular cells. The source of the secreted hydrogen ions is carbonic acid derived from the hydration of carbon dioxide. Present evidence strongly suggests that the primary event is the secretion of H^+ itself, rather than the reabsorption of anion (HCO_3^-).

It has long been known that the kidney plays an important role in maintaining acid-base balance. This applies to normal conditions but increases in importance as a homeostatic compensation to metabolic acidosis. The renal response can be described in four separate parameters, as follows: (1) the complete reabsorption of filtered sodium bicarbonate, (2) the acidification of the urinary buffers (*i.e.,* the production of titratable acid), (3) the excretion of fixed anions in combination with NH_4^+ rather than Na^+, and (4) the adjustment of urinary pH or H^+ ion concentration. Each process can be considered in terms of the same underlying mechanism.

In the process of bicarbonate reabsorption, H^+ is secreted into the tubular fluid while Na^+ is reabsorbed by a simultaneous but separate mechanism. The Na^+ combines with the HCO_3^- in the tubular cell and is returned to the extracellular fluid as $Na^+HCO_3^-$. The H^+ in the tubular urine combines with HCO_3^- to form H_2CO_3, which is rapidly broken down to CO_2 and H_2O. This CO_2 then readily back-diffuses across the tubular epithelium to become admixed with the carbonic acid–bicarbonate pool of the body. The overall reaction is the reabsorption of Na^+ and HCO_3^-.

When all the bicarbonate in the tubular urine has been removed, H^+ will be added to the buffer systems in the urine, primarily phosphate, with the conversion of HPO_4^{2-} to $H_2PO_4^-$. The reabsorbed Na^+ will be returned to the extracellular fluid as $Na^+HCO_3^-$ and thus contribute to the available fixed cation of the extracellular fluid. If secretion of H^+ proceeds at a rate insufficient to reabsorb the filtered bicarbonate, an alkaline urine containing large amounts of bicarbonate will be excreted. On the other hand, at maximal rates of H^+ transport, not only will all the bicarbonate disappear from the urine but also the titratable acidity of the urine will rise as a result of protonation of the buffer systems and more $Na^+HCO_3^-$ will be returned to extracellular fluid than was filtered at the glomerulus.

If bicarbonate and phosphate buffers were not present in the tubular urine, secretion of H^+ would increase the hydrogen ion concentration of the urine to such an extent that further transport of H^+ would be blocked because of the concentration gradient of H^+ thereby established between tubular cell and tubular urine. (The minimal pH that can be achieved in the urine of man is 4.4 to 4.5.) However, in response to the need for conservation of fixed cation, the kidney synthesizes ammonia. When ammonia is formed in the renal tubular cells, it diffuses readily into the tubular urine. If the urine is acidic, the ammonia that diffuses immediately reacts with H^+ to form NH_4^+. The renal tubule is impermeable to the charged particle (NH_4^+), and hence it does not diffuse back out of the tubular fluid. There are two important consequences of this reaction: first, H^+ is removed, and this permits further secretion of H^+ to occur; second, NH_3 is removed, and this permits more NH_3 to diffuse from tubular cell to tubular urine. In short, the two processes occur concurrently and can continue only by aiding and abetting each other. By this sequence of events, large amounts of Na^+ can be retrieved from neutral salts and returned to the extracellular fluid as sodium bicarbonate (2 in Figure VIII–1).

The above discussion is of pharmacological significance because the rate of H^+ secretion in the renal tubule can be greatly decreased by drugs that inhibit carbonic anhydrase. This enzyme catalyzes both the hydration of CO_2 and dehydration of H_2CO_3 and thus determines the relative concentrations of these molecular species. This, in turn, is an important determinant of both the availability of hydrogen ion for secretion and the disposition of the hydrogen ion within the tubular fluid.

Potassium Reabsorption and Secretion. Potassium is an unusual fixed cation in that it undergoes both tubular reabsorption and secretion. Reabsorption occurs largely in the proximal tubule, secretion in the distal tubule (3 in Figure VIII–1). Since the major fraction of the filtered potassium is reabsorbed, and since this process is relatively inflexible, it follows, therefore, that variations in the amount of potassium actually excreted may be attributed to the distal secretory mechanism. As judged by the action of many diuretic agents, the volume of unreabsorbed glomerular filtrate that flows through the distal tubule is one of the determinants of the rate of secretion of potassium. Thus, some drugs have the dual effect of increasing the urinary excretion of both sodium and potassium, the former by inhibition of reabsorption and the latter by augmentation of secretion (3 in Figure VIII–1).

Tubular Transport of Organic Compounds. In the preceding discussion the number of different chemical compounds (*i.e.,* inorganic electrolytes) that were considered is small compared to the total number of organic compounds that are present in the plasma and therefore are candidates for renal tubular transport.

In general, endogenous substances such as glucose, amino acids, and other essentials are filtered and then reabsorbed. They do not appear in the voided urine unless presented to the tubules in unusually large amounts so that transport capacity is exceeded. While reabsorption of such compounds occurs by highly specific mechanisms that can be affected experimentally by a variety of agents, these compounds have no application in therapeutics. Indeed, drug-induced glucosuria or aminoaciduria is a manifestation of nephrotoxicity.

Two major mechanisms for secretion of organic compounds have been identified—one for organic acids, the other for organic bases; both are localized in the proximal tubule. In general, substances that affect one system do not affect the other. Whereas the processes of filtration and secretion increase the amount of a substance presented to the tubular fluid, the amount ultimately excreted depends on the degree of reabsorption. This may occur both in the proximal tubule and in more distal segments.

In order to encompass all the foreign organic compounds that have been studied, it is essential to consider two separate mechanisms for their reabsorption. The first, diffusion, proceeds at a rate that is primarily dependent on the lipid solubility of the compound in question. If the molecule is an acid or a base, the pK_a of the compound and the pH of the tubular fluid are also important, since the nonionized form may be far better able to permeate the tubular epithelium. The rate of formation of urine (time available for reabsorption) is another important variable. These factors are fully discussed in Chapter 1. A carrier-mediated mechanism of *reabsorption* has been clearly shown for a few foreign compounds; this is usually difficult to demonstrate because of the quantitatively more important role of diffusion. In fact, little distinction need be made between endogenous and exogenous organic solutes with respect to carrier-mediated reabsorption and secretion. For example, uric acid, an endogenous product of metabolism, is both secreted and reabsorbed by the same carrier-mediated mechanisms as are many organic acids. The complications that arise from the effects of a drug on one or both components of a bidirectional transport system are discussed in Chapter 38.

CHAPTER

36 DIURETICS AND OTHER AGENTS EMPLOYED IN THE MOBILIZATION OF EDEMA FLUID

Gilbert H. Mudge

Diuretics are agents that increase the rate of urine formation. By common usage the term *diuresis* has two separate connotations: one refers to the increase in urine volume *per se,* the other to the net loss of solute and water. Under some conditions, the maintenance of an adequate urine volume in itself justifies the use of diuretic agents. However, by far the most important indication is the mobilization of edema fluid, that is, the production of a negative extracellular fluid balance. In general, the different types of diuretics are classified according to the manner by which they alter the excretion of solute.

Localization of Site of Drug Action. Most diuretics act directly on the kidney and, with few exceptions, on tubular rather than glomerular function. Extensive studies have been carried out to localize further the site of action to discrete segments of the nephron. A variety of methods has been employed.

These include the clearance technic, stop-flow analysis, micropuncture, histochemistry, enzyme assay, the direct determination of the composition of renal tissue, *in-vitro* studies with kidney slices and isolated tubules, and, by inference, examination of related systems, particularly preparations of frog skin and toad bladder.

Despite this intense activity, it is not possible to correlate all observations in a definitive manner. Brief comment on some of the complexities is warranted. First, a drug does not necessarily act at the site at which its concentration is maximal. Second, a drug may act on separate transport mechanisms at different sites—for example, the action of mercurials on the tubular secretion of organic acids proximally and on that of potassium distally. Third, there may be important species differences, most marked in the case of uricosuric agents but also observed with some diuretics. Fourth, although popularly simplified in terms of a single schematic nephron, the operation of the kidney is actually accomplished by millions of individual units that may respond differently both to physiological stress and to the action of diuretics. Fifth, modern concepts of renal function emphasize the architectural integrity of the nephron as an entire unit. This applies to many discrete functions, including solute reabsorption, the operation of the countercurrent system, and the determinants of bidirectional transport, that is, secretion in one segment and reabsorption in another. In the case of the countercurrent mechanism, for example, the magnitude of water reabsorption from the collecting duct is determined primarily by solute reabsorption in the ascending limb. And, sixth, particularly in the case of the quantitative interpretation of sodium and water reabsorption, a drug action at one site may be accompanied by secondary and compensatory changes in transport at another segment. These secondary effects may be mediated by normal mechanisms, rather than by drug action at both sites. Depending on the experimental technic, the compensatory changes may obscure the primary action. It has long been recognized that changes in solute reabsorption in one segment may influence tubular function at more distal sites that are "downstream." However, there is increasing evidence that the reverse may also be true. Distal events may influence more proximal transport. The mechanisms are both intrarenal and extrarenal in nature. Since sodium, the major solute of the tubular fluid, is reabsorbed throughout most portions of the nephron, it is quite possible that many drugs that inhibit its reabsorption act at more than a single site. The apparent localization of drug action to a particular locus may in large part be determined by experimental conditions, as well as by quantitative differences between the actions of the diuretic agent at different sites (see Jacobson and Kokko, 1976).

Extrarenal Sites of Drug Action. Many of the newer diuretics have proven to be useful in the investigation of electrolyte transport in organs other than the kidney, particularly under in-vitro conditions. Not surprisingly, these studies have revealed fundamental mechanisms common to many tissues. However, these are not reviewed systematically in this chapter unless the action at the extrarenal site occurs with reasonable dosages and is of sufficient magnitude to be clinically important.

WATER AND OSMOTIC DIURETICS

Normally the volume of urine is largely determined by the concentrations and types of solutes delivered to the renal tubule. Therefore, water and various electrolytes and nonelectrolytes can act as diuretic agents when given in excess.

WATER

Mechanism of Water Diuresis. Water is a true physiological diuretic. The mechanism of water diuresis is fully discussed in connection with the antidiuretic hormone (ADH) of the posterior pituitary (see Chapter 37).

Therapeutic Uses. It is often essential to limit or to force fluid intake. The problems of administration of water associated with parenteral alimentation are discussed in Chapter 35. There are many other circumstances when one must regulate the volume of fluid intake. For example, it may be necessary to restrict the intake of water when there is dilutional hyponatremia due to the inappropriate secretion of ADH (see Chapter 37). On the other hand, when drugs irritating to the urinary tract or of limited solubility are being employed, a higher water intake permits their excretion in sufficiently low concentrations to avoid renal damage. In addition, with many substances, either endogenous such as urea, or exogenous such as drugs or their metabolites, the rate of excretion is partially dependent on the rate of urine flow.

For a long time it was advocated that water should be restricted when edema fluid was present, in the belief that the ingestion of water contributed to the formation of edema. It is now known that the intake of extracellular electrolyte rather than of water is of primary importance in this regard and that, if sodium salts are restricted, under most circumstances little is gained by the simultaneous restriction of water.

SODIUM SALTS

Sodium salts occupy a unique position among diuretic salts. Under certain circumstances, the *administration* of sodium salts plays an important and irreplaceable role in assuring and promoting an adequate flow of urine. However, in other situations, the *restriction* of sodium intake is of paramount importance.

Renal Excretion of Sodium Salts. The source of the glomerular filtrate is extracellular fluid. The predominant cation of extracellular fluid is sodium; the predominant anions are chloride and bicarbonate. The average intake of sodium chloride is approximately 10 g daily, and this amount must be excreted in the urine to maintain electrolyte balance and the constancy of the extracellular environment. If the kidneys were to excrete sodium salts excessively with a concomitant loss of water, a rapid reduction in extracellular fluid volume would result. Conversely, an excessive reabsorption of sodium salts and water would soon result in overwhelming edema.

The several processes by which sodium is reabsorbed have been outlined in the Introduction to Section VIII. The anionic composition of the tubular fluid may also be of importance. If there is a high concentration of anion to which the tubule is impermeable, the amount of cation reabsorbed necessarily decreases; a large fraction of this cationic component is usually sodium. The active transport of Na^+ is the primary event in most of the tubule except the ascending limb of the loop of Henle, where Cl^- is actively reabsorbed.

The exact relationship of the filtered load of sodium to the amount reabsorbed is complex and incompletely understood. The absolute amount reabsorbed in the proximal tubule varies with the amount filtered, the concentration in plasma, and the extracellular fluid volume. In the reabsorption of sodium from the more distal portions of the nephron, acid-base balance and adrenocorticosteroids also play a very important role. In the development of edema, the renal adjustments fail and excretion of sodium decreases. This is true regardless of the nature of the primary disease—most commonly, cardiac, renal, or hepatic.

Therapeutic Uses. *Sodium chloride* is never employed as a diuretic agent in the treatment of edema. Rather, the restriction of sodium intake is of paramount importance. Sodium chloride is used primarily to treat deficits in extracellular fluid volume or concentration. When these are corrected, urinary excretion usually increases to normal rates.

Sodium bicarbonate may be useful in nonedematous states for the purposeful alkalinization of the urine (*see* Chapter 35).

OSMOTIC DIURETICS

The term *osmotic diuretic* is used for certain nonelectrolytes that have the following attributes in common: (1) they are freely filterable at the glomerulus; (2) they undergo limited reabsorption by the renal tubule; and (3) they are pharmacologically inert by conventional criteria. Taken together, these three characteristics permit the administration of such agents in sufficiently large quantities to contribute significantly to the osmolality of the plasma, the glomerular filtrate, and the tubular fluid. Their action within the kidney depends primarily upon the concentration of osmotically active particles in solution. In addition, most osmotic diuretics are resistant to metabolic alteration.

Mechanism of Diuretic Action. When there is a significant increase in the amount of any osmotically active solute in the voided urine, this is accompanied by an increase in urine volume. This generalization is subject to quantitative modification by several factors, including the compensatory effects of the rate of release of ADH, the magnitude of positive or negative free-water production, and the exact mechanisms by which solute excretion is increased (*see* Figure VIII-2, page 890).

It is important to appreciate the circumstances under which the osmotic diuretics may play a unique role in either maintaining or increasing urine volume. When the rate of glomerular filtration is acutely reduced, either experimentally in the laboratory or clinically as a result of hypovolemic shock, dehydration, or trauma, the solutes of the glomerular filtrate undergo more complete reabsorption so that there is a disproportionately large fall in the rate of urine flow and solute excretion. The administration of a normal solute, such as sodium chloride, may restore renal excretory function, but only if there is improvement in renal hemodynamics. If the rate of glomerular filtration remains severely reduced, administration of sodium chloride fails to augment urine flow because of the virtually complete tubular reabsorption of this normal electrolyte. Under these conditions, diuretics that normally act by inhibiting tubular transport may also be ineffective because they do not reduce tubular reabsorptive capacity sufficiently to compensate for the diminished filtered load.

However, under the same conditions, the osmotic diuretics retain their efficacy. To take mannitol as an example—even though the filtration rate is reduced, mannitol is still filtered at the glomerulus. The tubular impermeability to mannitol is not altered by acute renal ischemia of short duration. Hence, the mannitol that is filtered is also excreted in the voided urine. Unreabsorbed solute limits the back diffusion of water. As a consequence, urine volume can be maintained even in the presence of decreased glomerular function. As a first approximation, urine volume is proportional to the rate of solute excretion, which under these circumstances may be composed largely of the administered osmotic diuretic. Nephrotoxic agents and prolonged, severe renal ischemia may damage the tubular epithelium and produce acute tubular necrosis with oliguria. The tubule is then no longer selectively impermeable, and osmotic diuretics become ineffective.

An additional action of the osmotic diuretics is to increase the rate of excretion of electrolytes, particularly sodium, chloride, and potassium. However, this occurs only when large doses are given and is of little practical importance. Under normal conditions, sodium chloride is the major solute in the proximal tubular fluid and, as it is reabsorbed, water diffuses passively so that the tubular fluid remains isosmotic. Thus, the concentration of sodium in the tubular fluid is virtually unaltered, despite the fact that sodium itself is undergoing active reabsorption. However, in the presence of nonreabsorbable solute, the diffusion of water is reduced relative to the movement of sodium in order to maintain an isotonic fluid in the lumen of the tubule. As a consequence, the concentration of sodium in the fluid decreases. This increases the concentration gradient of sodium between the tubular fluid and the extracellular fluid. Net reabsorption of sodium diminishes because of decreased transport in the reabsorptive direction and increased flux back into the lumen (Gennari and Kassirer, 1974). With slight modification, a similar mechanism is applicable to reabsorption in the loop of Henle.

The same general considerations apply to all osmotic diuretics, even though they may be handled slightly differently by the renal tubule. Mannitol undergoes very little reabsorption. Sucrose is excreted in a similar manner. In the case of urea, about 50% of the amount filtered at the glomerulus is not reabsorbed. With elevated loads of urea, this fraction tends to increase. Glucose reabsorption is by an active transport mechanism in the proximal tubule and, at normal concentrations in plasma, is complete. However, as the glucose concentration is increased, the threshold and total reabsorptive capacity of the transport mechanism are exceeded and glucose appears in the voided urine. Hence, with severe hyperglycemia, glucose acts as an osmotic diuretic, even though a portion of the amount filtered continues to be reabsorbed.

The intestinal and renal tubular epithelia have many permeability characteristics in common. Most osmotic diuretics, which, by definition, are poorly reabsorbed by the renal tubules, are also not absorbed from the gastrointestinal tract. Thus, these agents must be administered parenterally in order to achieve effective concentrations in plasma. While urea is absorbed from the intestine, it is not given by this route. Glycerin and isosorbide are effective when administered orally. However, the onset of their action is slower and the extent of diuresis is less. These agents are particularly used to elevate the osmolality of plasma and thereby to decrease intraocular pressure, since they penetrate the eye poorly.

Therapeutic Uses. Osmotic diuretics may be used for several purposes that are distinct and separate, but all of which depend on the same fundamental characteristics.

Mannitol is the agent most extensively employed. Perhaps one of the clearest and most important indications is the *prophylaxis of acute renal failure.* It is used for this purpose in conditions as diverse as cardiovascular operations, severe traumatic injury, operations in the presence of severe jaundice, and management of hemolytic transfusion reactions. In each of these conditions, a precipitous fall in the flow of urine may be anticipated either as the result of an acutely reduced filtration rate or from acute changes in tubular permeability. The latter may be the consequence of the presence of a noxious agent within the tubular fluid in excessively high concentrations, in some instances sufficient to result in actual precipitation. In these situations, mannitol exerts an osmotic effect within the tubular fluid, inhibits water reabsorption, and maintains the rate of urine flow. As a consequence, the concentration of the toxic agent within the tubular fluid does not reach the excessively high levels that otherwise would have been achieved by the more complete reabsorption of water. Many of the mechanisms responsible for nephrotoxicity are incompletely understood. However, it is clear that under these conditions the use of osmotic diuretics protects the kidney against damage. The maintenance of an adequate flow of relatively dilute urine is probably the single most important factor. In the presence of hypotension mannitol is more effective than saline solution in maintaining glomerular filtration. If given in sufficiently large amounts, mannitol increases extracellular osmolality, which in turn may decrease cellular swelling and improve renal blood flow (Flores *et al.,* 1972).

A closely related but separate use of mannitol is in the *evaluation of acute oliguria.* With a partial reduction in glomerular function, as might occur from excessive loss of body fluids, urine flow may be increased toward normal by the administration of an osmotic diuretic, and this response may serve as a guide for the additional administration of parenteral fluids. However, if either glomerular or tubular function is too severely compromised, mannitol will not increase urine flow.

Mannitol is also used for the *reduction of the pressure and volume of the cerebrospinal fluid.* By elevating the osmolality of the plasma, one is able to enhance the diffusion of water from this fluid back into the plasma. However, the degree of success is quite variable (*see* Prockop, 1976). Mannitol, glycerin, and isosorbide are also used for the short-term reduction of intraocular pressure, particularly preoperatively and postoperatively in patients who require ocular surgery. They are also useful in certain other ophthalmological procedures.

Toxicity. Mannitol is distributed in the extracellular fluid, and consequently, the acute administration of hypertonic solutions in amounts sufficient to make a significant contribution to extracellular osmolarity will inevitably be accompanied by an acute expansion of extracellular fluid volume. In the patient with cardiac decompensation, this represents an undesirable hazard. A variety of signs and symptoms suggestive of hypersensitivity reactions has occurred in occasional patients. Urea is more irritating to tissues and may cause thrombosis or pain if extravasation occurs. Glycerin is metabolized and can cause hyperglycemia and glycosuria. Headache, nausea, and vomiting are relatively common sequelae of the administration of any osmotic diuretic.

Preparations and Dosage. *Mannitol,* U.S.P. (OSMITROL), is available for intravenous administration as *Mannitol Injection,* U.S.P., and *Mannitol and Sodium Chloride Injection,* U.S.P., in concentrations of 5, 10, 15, 20, or 25% mannitol in volumes ranging from 50 to 1000 ml of water or 0.3 to 0.45% sodium chloride solution. The adult dose for promotion of diuresis ranges from 50 to 200 g over a 24-hour period of infusion; the rate is generally adjusted to maintain a urinary output of at least 30 to 50 ml per hour. It should be preceded by a test dose in patients with marked oliguria or questionable adequacy of renal function. The recommended test dose is 200 mg/kg (approximately 75 ml of a 20% solution for an adult patient), infused over 3 to 5 minutes; if the first or a second test dose fails to promote a urinary flow greater than 30 ml per hour for 2 to 3 hours, the patient's status should be reevaluated prior to continuation of therapy. When used for the prevention of acute renal failure during various types of surgery or for the treatment of oliguria, the total dose is 50 to 100 g of mannitol for an adult patient. The dose for the reduction of intracranial pressure and brain mass prior to neurosurgery, or for the reduction of intraocular tension during an acute attack of congestive glaucoma or for ophthalmic surgery, is 1.5 to 2 g/kg, given as a 15 or 20% solution over a period of 30 to 60 minutes. Contraindications to the administration of mannitol include renal disease of sufficient severity to produce anuria, marked pulmonary congestion or edema, marked dehydration, and intracranial hemorrhage unless craniotomy is to be performed. The infusion of mannitol should be terminated if the patient develops signs of progressive renal dysfunction, heart failure, or pulmonary congestion.

Urea, U.S.P., is a white crystalline powder, with a slightly bitter taste, freely soluble in water. Sterile preparations (UREAPHIL, UREVERT) are available that may be reconstituted for intravenous use. When administered in this manner, the solution may contain up to 30% urea (w/w) and an isosmotic concentration of dextrose or invert sugar (equal parts of dextrose and levulose), the latter substances being necessary to prevent the hemolysis produced by pure solutions of urea. Intravenous doses of 1 to 1.5 g of urea per kilogram of body weight are optimal in preparation for neurosurgical procedures.

Glycerin, U.S.P. (GLYROL, OSMOGLYN), is given orally, particularly for use prior to ophthalmological procedures. Since the agent is rapidly metabolized, it produces relatively little diuresis. The dose is 1 to 1.5 g/kg, and it is usually given as a 50 or 75% solution. Maximal reduction of intraocular pressure occurs 1 hour after its administration, and the effect disappears after 5 hours.

Isosorbide (HYDRONOL, ISONOL) is also used orally for ophthalmological purposes. The effects observed are generally similar to those of glycerin, although diuresis is greater and hyperglycemia does not occur. A dose of 1.5 g/kg is given as an oral solution.

MERCURIAL DIURETICS

For a period of over 30 years the organic mercurials were the preeminent diuretics in clinical use. The drugs that have been introduced within the past 3 decades are effective by mouth, and some are also effective when renal blood flow and filtration rate are greatly reduced—attributes not possessed by the mercurials. As a consequence, the mercurials have virtually disappeared from clinical practice. A detailed description of their pharmacology is presented in the *fourth* and *fifth editions* of this textbook.

INHIBITORS OF CARBONIC ANHYDRASE

Acetazolamide is the prototype of a class of agents that have had limited usefulness as diuretics but have played a major role in the development of fundamental renal physiology and pharmacology.

History. In the early 1930s, Roughton demonstrated the presence in red blood cells of an enzyme, carbonic anhydrase, that catalyzes reaction I:

$$CO_2 + H_2O \overset{I}{\rightleftharpoons} H_2CO_3 \overset{II}{\rightleftharpoons} H^+ + HCO_3^-$$

Both the hydration and the dehydration reactions are under enzymatic control. Reaction II is an ionic dissociation that is virtually instantaneous and not subject to enzymatic acceleration. Carbonic anhydrase has subsequently been found in many sites—including the renal cortex, gastric mucosa, pancreas, eye, and central nervous system (CNS). When sulfanilamide was introduced as a chemotherapeutic agent, metabolic acidosis was recognized as a side effect. The drug was found to inhibit carbonic anhydrase *in vitro* and to inhibit the normal acidification of the urine *in vivo*. Subsequent studies established the role of carbonic anhydrase in renal transport.

Chemistry and Structure-Activity Relationship. An enormous number of sulfonamides have been synthesized and tested for their activity as carbonic anhydrase inhibitors and for their usefulness as diuretics. Acetazolamide has been studied the most extensively. The other three official drugs of this group are dichlorphenamide, ethoxzolamide, and methazolamide. Their structural formulas are as follows:

Acetazolamide

Dichlorphenamide

Ethoxzolamide

Methazolamide

The most important structure-activity relationship is that carbonic anhydrase inhibitory activity is abolished by N-sulfamyl substitutions (Maren, 1976).

Mechanism of Action. The major pharmacological action of acetazolamide is the inhibition of the enzyme carbonic anhydrase; the inhibition is noncompetitive. The noncatalyzed hydration or dehydration reaction can take place, of course, in the absence of the enzyme. However, the quantitative relationship between the two reaction rates depends on many complex factors. In general, the enzyme is normally present in tissues in huge excess. More than 99% of enzyme activity in the kidney must be inhibited before physiological effects become apparent. The enzyme itself is the dominant tissue component to which the inhibitors become bound.

Action on the Kidney. Following the administration of acetazolamide, the urine volume promptly

increases. The normally acidic pH becomes alkaline. The urinary concentration of the bicarbonate anion increases and is matched by sodium and substantial amounts of potassium. (*See* Table 36–1.) The urinary concentration of chloride falls. The increased alkalinity of the urine is necessarily accompanied by a decrease in the excretion of titratable acid and of ammonia.

The above sequence of events may be attributed to the inhibition of H^+ secretion by the renal tubule. This action was originally attributed exclusively to the distal segment. Current evidence indicates a greater effect on the proximal than on the distal tubule, with little or no effect on the ascending limb. This is supported by measurements of free-water production as well as by micropuncture studies (Goldberg, 1973). Carbonic anhydrase is probably located at the luminal border of the cells of the proximal but not of the distal tubule. Hence, inhibition of the enzyme at the former site may lead to transient changes in pH gradients that limit tubular secretion of H^+ (Rector, 1973).

Within recent years *phosphaturia* has been used as an index of localizing diuretic action since the phosphate anion is thought to be reabsorbed almost exclusively in the proximal tubule. For a given degree of natriuresis, the phosphaturia is greatest for acetazolamide, followed by the thiazides, mercurials, and high-ceiling diuretics in diminishing order. This is consistent with a largely proximal action for acetazolamide (Goldberg, 1973). The phosphaturia may be related to the stimulation by acetazolamide of cyclic adenosine 3',5'-monophosphate (cyclic AMP) production by the kidney. In this sense, the drug acts similarly to parathyroid hormone in enhancing the urinary excretion of phosphate and cyclic AMP, in contrast to its antagonism of the action of the hormone on bone (Rodriguez *et al.*, 1974).

Effect on Plasma Composition. Acetazolamide increases the urinary excretion of bicarbonate and fixed cation, mostly sodium. As a result, the concentration of bicarbonate in the extracellular fluid decreases and metabolic acidosis results. In metabolic acidosis, the renal response to acetazolamide is greatly reduced. However, with metabolic alkalosis the diuretic response is enhanced. Factors other than the amount of filtered bicarbonate must be determinants of drug action since the extracellular alkalosis of potassium depletion (with presumed intracellular acidosis) decreases the diuretic response.

Acetazolamide produces a marked increase in potassium excretion, attributable to enhanced secretion in the distal nephron. The effects on potassium are most prominent in acute experiments. With chronic administration, acetazolamide has less effect on potassium balance than do certain other agents.

Eye. The presence of carbonic anhydrase in a number of intraocular structures, including the ciliary processes, and the high concentration of bicarbonate in the aqueous humor have focused attention on the role that the enzyme might play in the secretion of aqueous humor. Acetazolamide reduces the rate of aqueous humor formation; intraocular pres-

Table 36-1.　URINARY ELECTROLYTE COMPOSITION DURING DIURESIS *

| | VOLUME (ml/min) | pH | Na$^+$ | K$^+$ | Cl$^-$ | HCO$_3^-$ |
				(mEq/l)		
Control	1	6	50	15	60	1
Mannitol	10	6.5	90	15	110	4
Mercurial	7	6	150	8	160	1
Acetazolamide	3	8.2	70	60	15	120
Benzothiadiazides (thiazides)	3	7.4	150	25	150	25
Ethacrynic acid	8	6	140	10	155	1
Furosemide	8	6	140	10	155	1
Triamterene	3	7.2	130	5	120	15
Amiloride	2	7.2	130	5	110	15
Aminophylline	3	6	150	15	160	1

* Data are representative of results that would be observed in man or dog during normal hydration and acid-base balance. Such findings are readily reproducible during the peak of diuresis and following a single maximally effective dose. However, a significant range of urinary values may be anticipated; *a single value is given here solely to facilitate comparison of one drug with another.* Excretion rates are obtainable as the product of urinary volume and composition.

sure in patients with glaucoma is correspondingly reduced. This action of the drug appears to be independent of systemic acid-base balance (*see* review by Maren, 1967).

Gastrointestinal Tract. Under appropriate experimental conditions, it is possible to implicate carbonic anhydrase in the formation of gastric and pancreatic juice and to block secretion by enzyme inhibition. These processes are relatively insensitive to ordinary doses of carbonic anhydrase inhibitors, and their pharmacological effect has no therapeutic applications. It is of interest that acetazolamide inhibits the absorption of sodium and chloride in the jejunum without affecting that of bicarbonate. It is possible that the drug is acting by a mechanism other than the inhibition of carbonic anhydrase (Gerson *et al.*, 1975).

Central Nervous System. An action of acetazolamide on the CNS was first suggested by the frequency of paresthesias and somnolence as side effects. Subsequently, the drug was found to inhibit epileptic seizures and to decrease the rate of formation of spinal fluid. Metabolic acidosis from ketogenic diets diminishes epileptic seizures, and acetazolamide, by virtue of its action on the kidney, leads to the production of a systemic acidosis. However, there is undoubtedly a more direct action on CNS function. An increase in local CO_2 tension may result from inhibition of the enzyme in the brain, the choroid plexus, or the erythrocytes of the cerebral blood. The exact role of carbonic anhydrase in brain function remains unknown. The concentration of the enzyme varies from one site to another within the brain. Acetazolamide may reduce the rate of cerebrospinal fluid formation by the choroid plexus, but it may also transiently elevate cerebrospinal fluid pressure as a result of an increase in intracranial blood flow (Maren, 1967; Laux and Raichle, 1978).

Respiration. The dynamic state of CO_2 in the blood and its transport between the blood and both the alveoli and the peripheral tissues are related to the carbonic anhydrase activity of the circulating

erythrocytes. Acetazolamide may create a disequilibrium in the CO_2 transport system, giving rise to increased CO_2 tensions in the tissues and a decreased tension in the expired gas. A decrease in the rate of elimination of CO_2 may therefore result from acetazolamide administration, but this appears to be transient due to compensatory mechanisms.

Absorption, Fate, and Excretion. Acetazolamide is readily absorbed from the gastrointestinal tract. Peak concentrations in plasma occur within 2 hours. The drug is excreted by the kidney, and both active tubular secretion and passive reabsorption are involved. Excretion is complete within 24 hours. Acetazolamide is tightly bound to carbonic anhydrase and, consequently, is present in greater amounts in those tissues in which the enzyme is present in high concentration, particularly the erythrocytes and the renal cortex. Some carbonic anhydrase inhibitors do not penetrate the erythrocyte. Thus, renal and systemic drug actions may be dissociated on the basis of drug distribution (*see* Maren, 1967). Acetazolamide is not metabolized. Other analogs have been found to be inactive *in vitro* but active *in vivo*, as the result of N-dealkylation to form an active metabolite.

Preparations and Dosage. *Acetazolamide,* U.S.P. (DIAMOX), is available as *Acetazolamide Tablets,* U.S.P., each containing 125 or 250 mg, and as sustained-release capsules containing 500 mg. An effective single oral dose is 250 to 500 mg. Vials of *acetazolamide sodium* are available for parenteral administration. When used as a diuretic, it should be given once daily or every other day. To achieve a sustained metabolic acidosis, the drug should be given at intervals of 8 hours. *Dichlorphenamide,* U.S.P. (DARANIDE), is available as official 50-mg tablets. Optimal effects have been achieved with doses of 200 mg per day. *Methazolamide,* U.S.P. (NEPTAZANE), is available as official 50-mg tablets; the usual dose is 100 to 300 mg per day. *Ethoxzolamide,* U.S.P. (CARDRASE, ETHAMIDE), is available as official 125-mg tablets. An effective dose appears to vary from 125 to 1000 mg per day, given orally in divided doses.

Clinical Toxicity. Serious toxic reactions are infrequent. With large doses, many patients exhibit drowsiness and paresthesias. In hepatic cirrhosis, episodes of disorientation may be induced; it has been postulated that urinary alkalinization diverts ammonia of renal origin from the urine into the systemic circulation. Hypersensitivity reactions are relatively rare. They consist in fever, skin reactions, bone-marrow depression, and sulfonamide-like renal lesions. Calculus formation and ureteral colic have been attributed to the marked reduction in urinary citrate produced by acetazolamide associated with either no change or even a rise in urinary calcium (Gordon and Sheps, 1957). Acetazolamide depresses the uptake of iodine by the thyroid gland. However, drugs of this class are not therapeutically useful as antithyroid agents. Teratogenic effects have been demonstrated in animals, and it is recommended that these drugs not be administered during pregnancy. Since carbonic anhydrase inhibitors alkalinize the urine, they interfere with the action of methenamine as a urinary tract antiseptic. Drug-induced osteomalacia has been reported in conjunction with the use of phenytoin.

Therapeutic Uses. Inhibitors of carbonic anhydrase are not used frequently as therapeutic agents. Their most common applications are to reduce intraocular pressure (in the treatment of glaucoma) and as an adjuvant for the management of petit mal and grand mal epilepsy. Acetazolamide is rarely administered as a diuretic but may be useful for alkalinization of the urine. The clinical situations in which such alkalinization is appropriate are discussed in Chapter 35. Acetazolamide appears to have a beneficial effect in the management of *periodic paralysis* even when associated with hypokalemia (Griggs *et al.,* 1970). It has been postulated that the induced acidosis raises the extracellular potassium concentration locally in the microcirculation of muscle. Acetazolamide is also effective in ameliorating the symptoms of *acute mountain sickness* (Gray *et al.,* 1971).

BENZOTHIADIAZIDES

History. This class of diuretics has an interesting history and provides an instructive example of the manner in which newly synthesized agents may be endowed with unanticipated efficacious properties. They were synthesized as an outgrowth of studies on inhibitors of carbonic anhydrase. In the examination of certain benzenedisulfonamides, ring closure was found to occur between an acylamino group and the sulfamyl group *ortho* to it. This changed fundamental characteristics of the diuresis. The voided urine contained increased amounts of chloride, a response significantly different from that evoked by the parent compounds (*see* Beyer, 1958). Subsequent studies indicated that the benzothiadiazides have a direct effect on the renal tubular transport of sodium and chloride that is independent of any effect on carbonic anhydrase.

Chlorothiazide was the first member of this class to be extensively studied. Although many analogs have been subsequently prepared, the basic pharmacological action is the same as for chlorothiazide.

Chemistry and Structure-Activity Relationship. Most compounds of this group are analogs of 1,2,4-benzothiadiazine-1,1-dioxide (*see* Table 36–2 for the parent structural formula and the substituents of the analogs that have received the most intensive study). As a group they can be designated as the "benzothiadiazide," or "thiazide," diuretics. The relationship between structure and activity is complex and is influenced by physiological and pharmacokinetic factors. The problem has been reviewed by Beyer and Baer (1961). Some compounds have hyperglycemic activity, for which the structural requirements differ from those for diuresis (Wales *et al.,* 1968).

It should be emphasized that all thiazides thus far carefully examined have parallel dose-response curves and comparable maximal chloruretic effects. This implies that they have a similar mechanism of action. The various analogs differ primarily in the dose required to produce a given effect and not necesarily in their optimal therapeutic response.

There are some other sulfonamide diuretics that differ chemically from the thiazides by the nature of the heterocyclic ring. However, their pharmacological action is indistinguishable from that of the thiazides. They have the following structures:

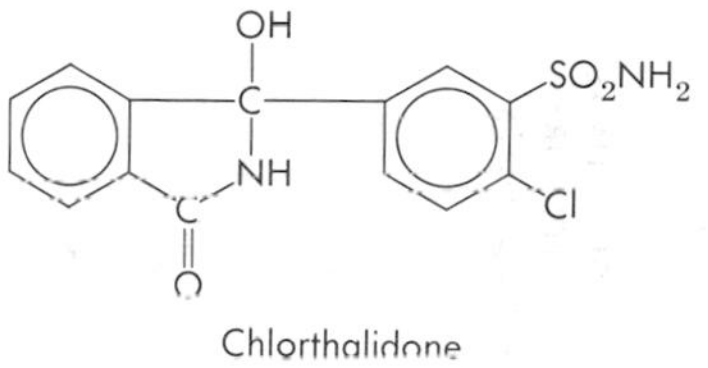

Chlorthalidone

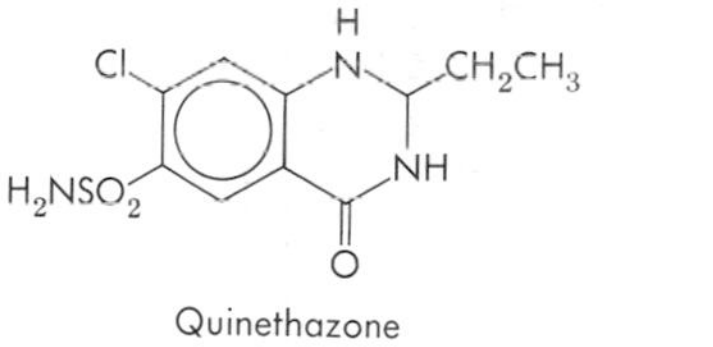

Quinethazone

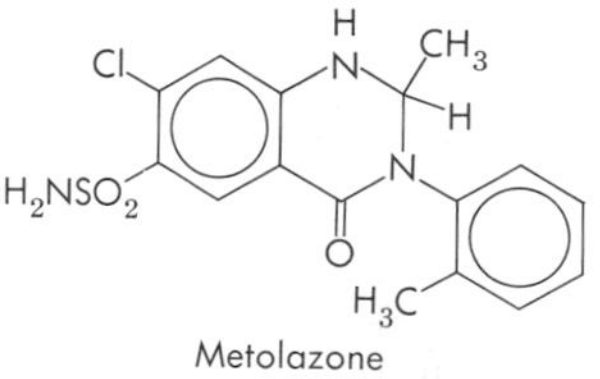

Metolazone

Because of the nature of their historical development, the thiazides and high-ceiling diuretics are often considered as clearly separate classes by both chemical and physiological criteria. As newly synthesized compounds have been studied, some of these distinctions have become blurred; drugs with intermediate characteristics may be anticipated (*see* Smith *et al.,* 1976).

Mechanism of Diuretic Action. The dominant action of the thiazides is to increase the

Table 36–2. SUMMARY OF CHEMICAL STRUCTURES AND DIURETIC PROPERTIES OF BENZOTHIADIAZIDES *

Agent †	R_2	R_3	R_6	RANGE OF OPTIMALLY EFFECTIVE ORAL DIURETIC DOSE IN MAN mg/day	RELATIVE ORAL NATRIURETIC MAXIMAL RESPONSE IN MAN	EQUIEFFECTIVE CHLORURETIC I.V. DOSE IN THE DOG mg/kg	CARBONIC ANHYDRASE 50% INHIBITION IN VITRO M	MARKET PREPARATION (TABLETS) mg
Chlorothiazide ‡	H	H	Cl	500–2000	1	1.25	2×10^{-6}	250,500
Hydrochlorothiazide	H	H	Cl	25–100	1.8	0.05	2×10^{-5}	25,50
Hydroflumethiazide	H	H	CF_3	25–50	1.6	0.25	2×10^{-4}	50
Bendroflumethiazide	H	CH_2—(phenyl)	CF_3	2.5–15	2.3	0.01	3×10^{-4}	2.5,5
Benzthiazide ‡	H	CH_2—S—CH_2—(phenyl)	Cl	50–200	1.6	0.01–0.05	ca. 10^{-7}	50
Trichlormethiazide	H	$CHCl_2$	Cl	2–8	2.1	0.01	6×10^{-5}	2,4
Methyclothiazide	CH_3	CH_2Cl	Cl	2.5–10	2.3			2.5,5
Polythiazide	CH_3	$CH_2SCH_2CF_3$	Cl	1–4	2.5	0.01–0.03	5×10^{-7}	1,2,4
Cyclothiazide	H	(norbornenyl CH_2)	Cl	1–6	—	—	—	2
Chlorthalidone	—	—	—	25–200	2.3	0.25	3×10^{-7}	25,50,100
Quinethazone	—	—	—	50–200	1			50
Metolazone	—	—	—	2.5–20	1	0.1	5×10^{-5}	2.5,5,10
Acetazolamide	—	—	—	250–500	0.3	—	7×10^{-8}	125,250,500

* Note the general agreement between the optimal oral dosage for man relative to the equieffective dosage by intravenous administration in the dog. The relative oral natriuretic response in man is based on the method of Ford (1961), who used careful metabolic regimens and doses in the general range indicated. The numerical values refer to potency ratios, with the natriuretic response to a standard dose of chlorothiazide being given the value of 1. Despite the extremely wide range of effective oral dosage, the usual natriuretic response by this assay varies less than threefold.

† The above-listed agents are available under the following nonproprietary and trade names: Chlorothiazide (U.S.P.): DIURIL. Hydrochlorothiazide (U.S.P.): ESIDREX, HYDRODIURIL, ORETIC. Hydroflumethiazide (U.S.P.): SALURON. Bendroflumethiazide (U.S.P.): NATURETIN. Benzthiazide (U.S.P.): EXNA. Trichlormethiazide (U.S.P.): METAHYDRIN, NAQUA. Methyclothiazide (U.S.P.): ENDURON. Polythiazide (U.S.P.): RENESE. Cyclothiazide (U.S.P.): ANHYDRON. Chlorthalidone (U.S.P.): HYGROTON. Quinethazone (U.S.P.): HYDROMOX. Metolazone: DIULO, ZAROXOLYN. Acetazolamide (U.S.P.): DIAMOX.

‡ Unsaturated between C 3 and N 4.

renal excretion of sodium and chloride and an accompanying volume of water. This effect is virtually independent of acid-base balance. The thiazides also evoke a significant augmentation of potassium excretion. They vary widely in their potency as inhibitors of carbonic anhydrase. Those that are active in this respect have the same action on bicarbonate transport by the kidney as does acetazolamide. The pharmacology and the therapeutic use of thiazides as hypotensive agents are considered in Chapter 32. In patients with diabetes insipidus, the thiazides *decrease* urinary volume. These actions are discussed in Chapter 37.

Effect on Renal Function. The unilateral renal intra-arterial injection of thiazides produces a unilateral diuretic response, indicating a direct renal action. Like many other organic acids, the thiazides are themselves actively secreted in the proximal tubule. This may be inhibited by probenecid. Depending on the thiazide, its dosage, and the solutes measured, its action on electrolyte transport may or may not be blocked (Beyer and Baer, 1961). The nature of the chemical interaction between the thiazides and specific renal receptors responsible for the chloruretic effect is not known; no critical enzymatic reactions have been identified. It is of interest that nondiuretic thiazide analogs can block the chloruretic action of chlorothiazide without inhibiting urinary alkalinization, a finding interpreted as a competitive reaction for critical renal receptor sites (Ross and Cafruny, 1963).

The thiazides inhibit the reabsorption of sodium and its attendant anion, chloride, in the distal segment. Bioelectrical studies suggest a direct action on the movement of sodium itself (Pendleton *et al.*, 1968).

As a class, the thiazides have an important action on the excretion of potassium that results from the increased secretion of the cation by the distal tubule (Giebisch, 1976). The kaliuresis is most readily seen in acute studies and may be negligible during chronic administration (*see* Table 36–1). Under some experimental conditions, and with selected thiazides, it has been possible partially to separate the effects on sodium and potassium. This can only be observed with doses that have minimal saluretic effects. At higher doses, all thiazides appear to share the same action on potassium.

The *glomerular filtration* rate may be reduced by the thiazides, particularly with intravenous administration for experimental purposes. This is presumably the result of a direct action on the renal vasculature. It has little significance in the interpretation of primary drug action but may be of clinical importance, particularly in patients with diminished renal reserve.

The thiazides may decrease the excretion of *uric acid* in man, thus increasing its concentration in plasma. The hyperuricemic effect results primarily from inhibition of the tubular secretion of urate. This increase of uric acid concentration may have little prognostic significance, since the incidence of acute attacks of gout is related more to the concentrations of uric acid in plasma before treatment with a thiazide.

Unlike most other natriuretic agents, the thiazides decrease the renal excretion of calcium relative to that of sodium, since its reabsorption is unaffected in the distal nephron whereas that of sodium is blocked. On the other hand, furosemide reduces the reabsorption of both cations proportionately (Edwards *et al.*, 1973). The excretion of *magnesium* is enhanced by the thiazides, leading to hypomagnesemia.

Iodide and *bromide* are excreted by renal mechanisms qualitatively similar to those for chloride. Diuretic agents that produce chloruresis fail to modify the discriminatory function of the tubule for the different halides. Thus, all chloruretic agents may be useful in the management of bromide intoxication. In addition, increased excretion of iodide, particularly with prolonged diuretic therapy, may produce slight iodine depletion.

Effect on Composition of Extracellular Fluid. The thiazides tend to produce less distortion in the extracellular fluid composition than do other diuretic agents. This results from their multiple action on renal tubular transport, affecting not only the reabsorption of sodium and chloride but also H^+ secretion. For example, in the dog preloaded with sodium bicarbonate, the urine excreted after the administration of a thiazide contains relatively more bicarbonate than chloride. On the other hand, after pretreatment with ammonium chloride, bicarbonate excretion is decreased and chloruresis is enhanced in response to the drug.

Absorption, Fate, and Distribution. The thiazides are rapidly absorbed from the gastrointestinal tract, and most agents show a demonstrable diuretic effect within an hour after oral administration. In general, thiazides with relatively long durations of action show a proportionately high degree of binding to plasma proteins and are reabsorbed to a greater extent by the renal tubules. Chlorothiazide is distributed throughout the extracellular space and does not accumulate in tissues other than the kidney. The drug passes readily through the placental barrier to the fetus. All thiazides probably undergo active secretion in the proximal tubule. The renal clearances of the drugs are high and may be either above or below the rate of filtration. Most compounds are rapidly excreted within 3 to 6 hours. Bendroflumethiazide and polythiazide have a longer duration of action that is correlated with their slower excretion. The same is true of chlorthalidone and metolazone. In the nephrectomized animal, chlorothiazide may be excreted in the bile.

Clinical Toxicity. In animal experiments, the demonstrable toxic dose of all the thiazides is manyfold that required for their pharmacological action. For example, large acute doses can depress CNS function. Clinical toxicity is relatively rare and usually results from unexpected hypersensitivity. Cases of purpura, dermatitis with photosensitivity, depression of the formed elements of the blood, and necrotizing vasculitis have been reported.

Thiazide-induced *hypokalemia* is discussed in Chapter 35 along with the indications for potassium supplementation. Alternatively, the thiazides have been prescribed in combination with a potassium-sparing diuretic (*see* below) in order to obtain an additive diuretic effect with maintenance of potassium balance. The plasma *uric acid* is frequently elevated. For reasons that are unexplained, isolated cases have been reported in which prolonged therapy with thiazides gave rise to hypercalcemia and hypophosphatemia simulating hyperparathyroidism (Christensson *et al.,* 1977).

Borderline *renal* and/or *hepatic insufficiency* may be unpredictably aggravated by the thiazides. In patients, particularly those with hypertensive disease and decreased renal reserve, the manifestations of renal insufficiency may be aggravated after intensive or prolonged courses of thiazides that lead to excessive depletion of fluid and electrolyte. In patients with cirrhosis of the liver, deterioration of mental function, including the onset of coma, has been attributed to thiazide therapy. Many observers have noted a correlation with hypokalemia and alkalosis. Increased concentrations of ammonia in the blood have been reported. Cholestatic hepatitis has also been observed.

The thiazides may induce *hyperglycemia* and aggravate preexisting diabetes mellitus (Dollery, 1973). Several mechanisms have been proposed, including inhibition of pancreatic release of insulin and blockade of peripheral utilization of glucose. However, the exact mechanism is in doubt and may involve several factors. The disturbance in carbohydrate metabolism is relatively common and is probably unrelated to the much rarer toxic reaction of acute pancreatitis.

Preparations and Dosage. The thiazides are available as tablets for oral administration. The wide range of dosage is indicated in Table 36–2. In a few instances, preparations of the sodium salt are available for intravenous administration. However, this route offers no advantage for most therapeutic purposes.

Most of the thiazides are given in divided daily doses for the treatment of hypertension and for diuresis. A single daily dose is often preferable for the mobilization of edema fluid and to improve patient compliance to a regimen of antihypertensive therapy. Trichlormethiazide, chlorthalidone, and polythiazide could be given less frequently, since they have a duration of action longer than 24 hours. The action of quinethazone and metolazone may also persist up to 24 hours. Combinations of thiazides in a fixed-dose ratio with other diuretics or with other antihypertensive agents or potassium supplements are usually not recommended. However, fixed-dose combinations of aldosterone antagonists (*see* below) and hydrochlorothiazide are available and can be employed to advantage where the maintenance of potassium balance presents a problem.

Therapeutic Uses. The thiazides are the diuretics of choice in the management of *edema* due to mild-to-moderate congestive heart failure. Edema due to chronic hepatic or renal disease may also respond favorably. The use of the thiazides to treat *hypertensive disease* is discussed in Chapter 32. Less common usage includes the treatment of *diabetes insipidus* (*see* Chapter 37) and the management of *hypercalci-*

uria in patients who have recurrent urinary calculi composed of calcium (Yendt and Cohanim, 1978).

HIGH-CEILING DIURETICS

The term *high-ceiling* has been used to denote a group of diuretics that have a distinctive action on renal tubular function. These drugs effect a peak diuresis far greater than that observed with other agents. Other features that such drugs share in common are: (1) prompt onset of action, (2) inhibition of sodium and chloride transport in the ascending limb of the loop of Henle, and (3) independence of their action from acid-base balance changes. Ethacrynic acid and furosemide have been studied the most extensively, both clinically and experimentally. Bumetanide and muzolimine have been used in Europe but are not yet available for clinical use in the United States.

Chemistry and Structure-Activity Relationship. These agents have the following chemical structures:

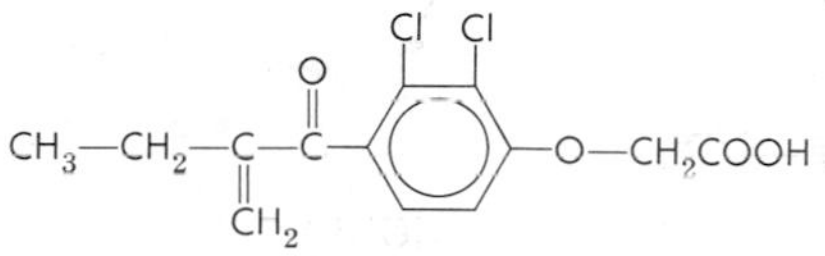

Ethacrynic Acid

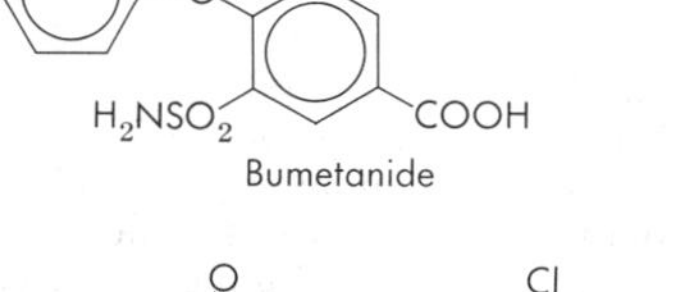

Furosemide

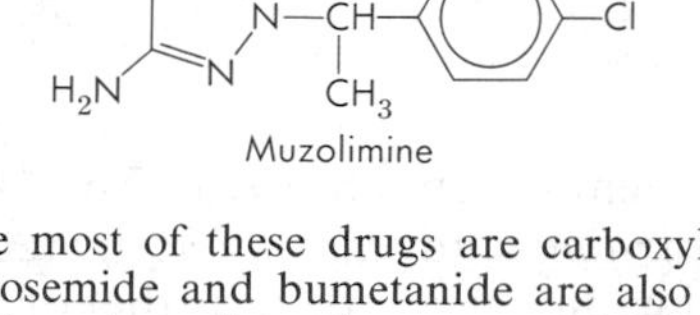

Bumetanide

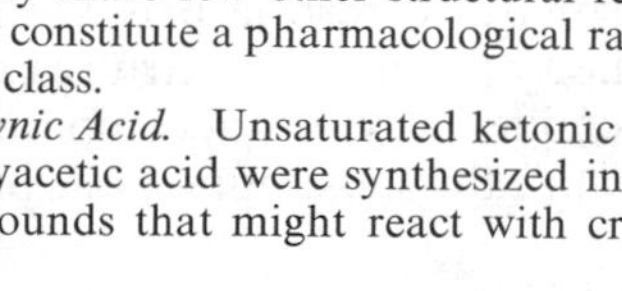

Muzolimine

While most of these drugs are carboxylic acids, and furosemide and bumetanide are also sulfonamides, they share few other structural features and appear to constitute a pharmacological rather than a chemical class.

Ethacrynic Acid. Unsaturated ketonic derivatives of aryloxyacetic acid were synthesized in the search for compounds that might react with critical renal sulfhydryl groups in a manner similar to that of the organic mercurials (Schultz *et al.*, 1962). Optimal diuretic activity depends on at least two structural requirements: (1) the methylene and adjacent ketone groups capable of reacting with sulfhydryl radicals of the presumed receptor, and (2) the substituents on the aromatic nucleus.

Furosemide. This drug is one of a series of anthranilic acid derivatives. Congeners differ in milligram potency but exhibit the same pharmacological spectrum.

Bumetanide. This compound is a 3-aminobenzoic acid derivative. Several analogs, which have various substituents, are about equally active in test animals (Feit, 1971). Bumetanide has a higher milligram potency than furosemide, but in other respects the compounds are similar.

Muzolimine. This amphoteric compound, the only one of the type of diuretic shown that is not a carboxylic acid, appears to be of a substantially new and different chemical class (Möller *et al.*, 1977).

Absorption, Distribution, and Excretion. The high-ceiling diuretics are readily absorbed from the gastrointestinal tract, and considerable proportions are bound to plasma proteins. They are rapidly excreted in the urine, by both glomerular filtration and tubular secretion. The rates of excretion are of such a magnitude that cumulation does not occur despite repeated administration. With oral ingestion, a diuretic response may be anticipated within an hour; with intravenous injection, within 2 to 10 minutes. (*See* Beyer *et al.*, 1965; Gayer, 1965; Østergaard *et al.*, 1972.)

Ethacrynic acid is bound to plasma protein. After intravenous injection, about one third of the dose is excreted by the liver and about two thirds by the kidney. The drug recovered from the urine is about equally divided into three fractions: the parent compound, a cysteine adduct, and an unstable metabolite of undetermined nature (Beyer *et al.*, 1965). Ethacrynic acid is secreted by the organic-acid secretory mechanism of the proximal tubule. The net rate of urinary secretion is also dependent on urinary pH. Thus, ethacrynic acid probably normally undergoes substantial back diffusion.

Furosemide is strongly bound to plasma proteins, and its urinary excretion is thus predominantly accomplished by proximal tubular secretion. However, nearly one third of the drug may be excreted in the feces, and a small fraction is metabolized by cleavage of the side chain (Beyer *et al.*, 1965; Gayer, 1965). An additional product, possibly a glucuronide conjugate, has also been found.

Bumetanide is strongly bound to plasma proteins. While the drug is largely excreted in the urine, in the nephrectomized animal the plasma concentration declines at an appreciable rate, presumably due to fecal excretion.

Mechanism of Diuretic Action. In general, the time of onset and duration of diuresis with the agents in this class are shorter than with other classes of diuretics, such as thiazides, but this depends to a considerable extent on concomitant changes in fluid balance. The duration of action varies with the particular renal function being measured (Figure 36–1).

The high-ceiling diuretics act primarily to inhibit chloride and sodium reabsorption in the ascending limb of the loop of Henle. This site has been localized as a result of the virtually complete inhibition of both positive and negative free-water production, and by micropuncture technics (*see* Edwards *et al.,* 1973; Goldberg, 1973; Suki *et al.,* 1973). The primary action appears to be inhibition of the active transport of chloride at the luminal border of the tubule of the ascending limb (Burg, 1976). The magnitude of peak electrolyte excretion is given in Table 36–1. Inhibition of electrolyte reabsorption has also been observed in the proximal tubule (Morgan *et al.,* 1970). Indeed, the magnitude of the inhibition of tubular reabsorption can be explained only by multiple sites of action. The effect at the proximal site of action has been studied by micropuncture experiments, but it is uncertain to what extent this contributes to the diuresis observed *in vivo.* Actions on the distal tubule and collecting duct are controversial and of a minor degree. The diuretic response is largely independent of acid-base balance.

Ethacrynic acid does not inhibit carbonic anhydrase *in vitro* and does not augment excretion of bicarbonate (Beyer *et al.,* 1965). Since furosemide and bumetanide have unsubstituted sulfonamide side chains, they might be expected to inhibit carbonic anhydrase; however, as judged by their effect on bicarbonate excretion, such an action, if any, must be extremely weak (Østergaard *et al.,* 1972).

The increase in *potassium* excretion results from its distal secretion and is approximately proportional to the increased rate of flow in

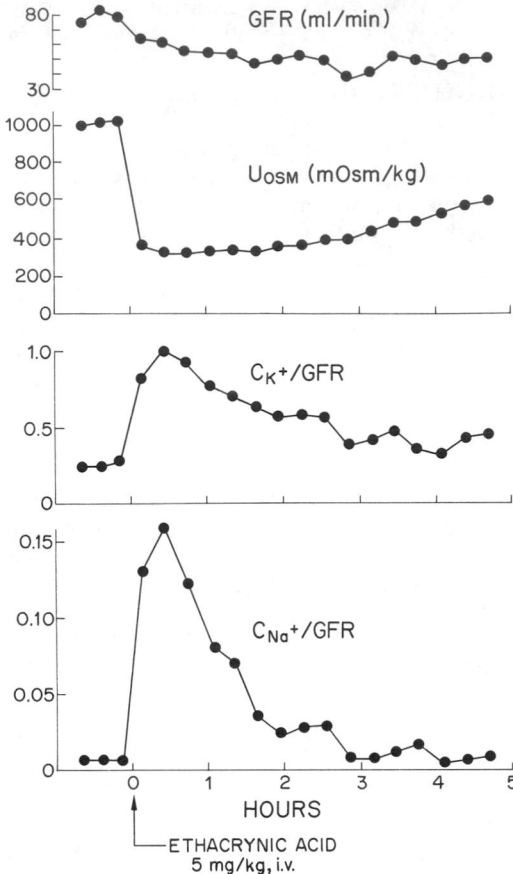

Figure 36–1. *Time course of ethacrynic acid diuresis.*

Observations were made in an anesthetized dog, infused with vasopressin and without volume replacement. Note the gradual reduction in glomerular filtration rate (GFR), which is probably the result of volume depletion. The immediate effect of the drug is a prompt fall in U_{OSM} to a U/P ratio of essentially unity, and an increase in the ratios C_{K^+}/GFR and C_{Na^+}/GFR. Note that the latter ratio returns toward control levels before the urinary concentrating ability is restored, as indicated by U_{OSM}. This discrepancy could be due either to the fact that, with a decrease in GFR, less sodium chloride is available for reabsorption by the ascending limb, or that there is a time lag involving the replenishment of solute to the medullary interstitium.

this segment (Giebisch, 1976). The excretion of *magnesium* and *calcium* is increased by about the same percentage as that of sodium. The phosphaturic response is variable; for unexplained reasons, the natriuresis induced by furosemide may be accompanied by a decrease in the excretion of phosphate

(Goldberg, 1973). The high-ceiling diuretics may cause *hyperuricemia* in man. Since these drugs are organic acids that are secreted in the proximal tubule, it is presumed that they act competitively to inhibit urate secretion at this site.

Effect on Renal Blood Flow. Depending on the experimental conditions, including the dose and speed of administration of the diuretic, either an increase or decrease in renal blood flow may occur. These hemodynamic changes are of interest, since they indicate that the renal actions of these drugs are more complicated than simply to increase the excretion of solute. When furosemide increases renal blood flow, there is a redistribution of flow from medulla to cortex and within the cortex. Acute diuresis increases intraluminal pressure and transiently reduces the filtration rate (Mudge *et al.,* 1975). This raises the possibility that diuretic-induced redistribution of blood flow might be directly mediated through changes in pressure. However, many studies have indicated a more complicated mechanism that involves both prostaglandins and renin. The renal secretion of these substances is increased by the high-ceiling diuretics. Stimulation of renin release results from both the effect of vascular dilatation on the juxtaglomerular apparatus and that of elevated sodium concentration in the region of the macula densa. Indomethacin, in doses adequate to inhibit the synthesis of prostaglandins, blocks the increase in renal blood flow and the increased secretion of prostaglandins and renin produced by furosemide. Although the natriuretic effect of furosemide is blunted by indomethacin, the overall contribution of the hemodynamic changes to natriuresis is minimal (*see* Hook and Bailie, 1977).

Extrarenal Sites of Action. In isolated systems and with high doses, these agents act upon electrolyte transport in a variety of tissues. However, with usual doses the high-ceiling diuretics have no significant pharmacological effects other than on renal function. For example, there may be a slight decrease in bile flow (Erlinger *et al.,* 1970) or changes in the ionic fluxes of isolated erythrocytes (Dunn, 1973). These actions have no known clinical implications. An exception is the action on the inner ear, consisting in a depression of the cochlear microphonic and neural potentials, and a transient increase in the sodium and potassium concentrations in the endolymph (Brusilow and Gordes, 1973). This may result from a direct toxic action on the hair cells (Prazma *et al.,* 1972).

Biochemical Mechanism of Action. Ethacrynic acid was developed as an agent that would combine with thiol groups. There is ample evidence for this type of reaction. For example, the drug irreversibly combines with two thiol groups of glyceraldehyde 3-phosphate dehydrogenase, thus inactivating the enzyme (Birkett, 1973). However, it is not possible to attribute diuretic action to this type of biochemical reaction, for at least three reasons. First, the other high-ceiling diuretics do not share the same reactivity with thiols. Second, the adduct of ethacrynic acid with cysteine is a more potent inhibitor of electrolyte transport than ethacrynic acid itself. And third, if one considers the thiol-dependent reactions of either aerobic or anaerobic metabolism, it is still unknown to what extent the overall rates of metabolism can be correlated with either electrolyte transport or drug action (Baer and Beyer, 1972; Bowman *et al.,* 1973; Klahr *et al.,* 1973). Some of the high-ceiling diuretics inactivate the Na^+,K^+-dependent adenosine triphosphatase (ATPase) of the kidney, but attempts to implicate this as the mechanism of drug action have encountered quantitative difficulties (Nechay, 1977). Since ATPase is presumably directly related to cation transport, the problem is further compounded by the demonstration that ethacrynic acid acts on the primary transport of the chloride anion, as well as on that of the sodium cation. On an experimental basis, the metabolic actions of furosemide have been used to enhance the preservation of transplanted kidneys (Panijayanond *et al.,* 1973).

Comparative Diuretic Action. From the available data the drugs of this class have remarkably similar actions upon the kidney in most species. Ethacrynic acid and bumetanide are almost inactive in the rat, except at extremely high doses. In the dog and man, bumetanide is effective in a dose about 2% that of furosemide, but its maximal effect is the same. The diuretic action of this group of drugs may be additive to that of less effective agents, but the high-ceiling diuretics themselves are not additive to each other. One of the major differences between furosemide and ethacrynic acid is that the former has a broader dose-response curve. Accordingly, the therapeutic regimen may be initiated with rather small doses and adjusted upward to meet the needs of the individual patient.

Effect on Composition of Extracellular Fluid. Metabolic alkalosis may result from the use of the high-ceiling diuretics. When the mobilization of edema fluid is rapid, the alkalosis largely results from a contraction of extracellular fluid volume. With chronic therapy, the dietary intake of salt and the urinary excretion of hydrogen ions and potassium become important factors. This is discussed in Chapter 35. Alkalosis is frequently accompanied by hyponatremia, but each is produced by separate mechanisms.

Clinical Toxicity. Two generalizations may be made from extensive experience with ethacrynic acid and furosemide: (1) abnormalities of fluid and electrolyte imbalance are the most common forms of clinical toxicity (*see* discussion at end of this chapter), and (2) side effects unrelated to the primary action of these drugs are quite rare. Hyperuricemia is relatively common, but in most patients it represents little more than a chemical abnormality. Other reactions include gastrointestinal disturbances (with or without bleeding), depression of formed elements in the blood, skin rashes, paresthesias, and hepatic dysfunction. Cross-sensitivity may occur between furosemide and other sulfonamides. Gastrointestinal side effects are much more frequent with ethacrynic acid than furosemide. Furosemide and the thiazides have been implicated as causes of allergic interstitial nephritis, leading to reversible renal failure (Lyons *et al.*, 1973). A decrease in tolerance to carbohydrate may occur, but to a lesser extent than when the thiazides are given (Dollery, 1973). Acute hypoglycemia of unexplained origin has been reported as a manifestation of overdosage. Because of their effect on offspring in experimental animals, the high-ceiling diuretics should not be prescribed during pregnancy unless absolutely necessary.

The development of deafness, either transient or permanent, is a serious and rare complication of treatment with ethacrynic acid. Transient deafness has also been reported with furosemide. Drug-induced changes in the electrolyte composition of the endolymph represent a possible mechanism. Due to the rarity of this complication it is difficult to evaluate the contention that it is more common in the presence of renal insufficiency and that it occurs with one drug more often than with the other. From available data, it appears that ototoxicity from diuretics is unique to this class of drugs. If another potentially ototoxic drug, such as an aminoglycoside antibiotic, is being administered and concurrent diuretic therapy is indicated, it is advisable to use a diuretic agent from another class, for example, a thiazide.

The high-ceiling diuretics may interact adversely with other drugs. Ethacrynic acid and furosemide are significantly bound to plasma albumin and may compete for sites on the protein with drugs such as warfarin and clofibrate (Sellers and Koch-Weser, 1970; Prandota and Pruitt, 1975). The renal clearance of lithium is decreased during chronic therapy with diuretics (when there is depletion of sodium), and their concurrent use should be avoided unless concentrations of lithium in plasma can be monitored very carefully. The nephrotoxicity produced by cephaloridine is increased by furosemide, and one should be judicious in the use of any cephalosporin in conjunction with furosemide or ethacrynic acid (Dodds and Foord, 1970).

Preparations. *Ethacrynic Acid*, U.S.P. (EDECRIN), is available for oral use as 25- and 50-mg tablets. The usual dose for adults is from 50 to 200 mg per day. The optimal dose should be determined for each patient, starting with minimal amounts. The sodium salt of ethacrynic acid is available for intravenous use as *Ethacrynate Sodium for Injection*, U.S.P. (EDECRIN SODIUM); the usual dose is 50 mg. *Furosemide*, U.S.P. (LASIX), is available as 20- and 40-mg tablets. In adults, the range of optimal dosage varies from 40 to 200 mg per day. A preparation is also available for parenteral administration, either intravenously or intramuscularly, in ampuls containing 20 mg/2 ml or 100 mg/10 ml of saline solution. The recommended adult dose by this route is 20 or 40 mg, repeated if necessary after not less than 2 hours.

Therapeutic Uses. Due to the lower incidence of gastrointestinal reactions and a less precipitous dose-response curve, furosemide is prescribed much more frequently than is ethacrynic acid. The high-ceiling diuretics are effective for the treatment of *edema* of cardiac, hepatic, or renal origin. The oral route should be used unless impractical or the clinical situation demands a very prompt diuresis, in which case intravenous or intramuscular administration may be employed. This applies particularly to the management of *acute pulmonary edema*. In this condition the rapid reduction of the volume of extracellular fluid is of sufficient magnitude to reduce venous return and right ventricular output. In the management of refractory edema, the high-ceiling agents may be used in conjunction with other types of diuretics, particularly the potassium-sparing drugs, but there is no rationale for administering two high-ceiling agents concomitantly.

In the presence of *nephrosis* or *chronic renal failure*, doses of furosemide far higher than usual may be required (Muth, 1973). The reason for this is not clear. Although a reduction in filtration rate clearly decreases the rate of drug excretion in the urine, there is no *a-priori* reason why the concentration in the residual tubular fluid should be decreased unless there is either a decrease in tubular secretion, an increased diuresis per residual nephron, or binding of the drug to protein within the tubular fluid. Patients with uremia do have a decreased rate of tubular secretion (Rose *et al.*, 1976). Furosemide is metabolized to a reactive intermediate that produces hepatic necrosis in experimental animals. At the usual clinical dose hepatic toxicity is not observed, but the possible occurrence of this undesirable effect should be kept in mind when the massive doses sometimes employed in renal failure must be given (Mitchell *et al.,* 1974). By conventional measurements, renal function is not compromised by high doses. However, the incidence of undesirable side effects may be increased (Allison and Kennedy, 1971). The high-ceiling diuretics have also been used in patients with early *acute renal failure,* but results are inconclusive (Kleinknecht *et al.,* 1976). The drugs are contraindicated once anuric renal failure is unequivocally established. In symptomatic *hypercalcemia,* the high-ceiling diuretics may lower the concentration of calcium in plasma by increasing its urinary excretion. When employed for this purpose, the replacement of urinary losses of sodium and chloride is required (Suki *et al.,* 1970).

ALDOSTERONE ANTAGONISTS

The role of adrenocorticosteroids in the regulation of electrolyte and water balance is discussed in Chapter 63. With greater insight into the chemistry of the steroids and with more complete knowledge of their physiological function, it has been possible to synthesize competitive antagonists that are useful as diuretics.

SPIRONOLACTONE

Chemistry. A number of 17-spirolactone steroids have been employed, of which *spironolactone* appears to have the greatest selectivity and efficacy. Its structural formula is as follows:

Spironolactone

Mechanism of Diuretic Action. Compounds of this type are considered as competitive antagonists of aldosterone, the most potent endogenous mineralocorticoid. Presumably they compete for receptor sites because they are homologs of the natural hormone, but they fail to evoke an active response. This concept is based on two general types of indirect evidence obtained from experiments *in vivo:* first, that the antagonist drug is effective only in the presence of either endogenous or exogenous aldosterone; second, that the action of the antagonist may be overcome by increasing the concentration of aldosterone (Kagawa *et al.,* 1959; Liddle, 1961).

The secretion of aldosterone is increased primarily by alterations in electrolyte balance, most importantly by a reduction in effective blood volume, hyponatremia, or hyperkalemia. In addition, angiotensin resulting from the release of renin by the kidney stimulates production of aldosterone (*see* Chapter 27). Assay of aldosterone antagonists is usually undertaken experimentally following sodium chloride restriction. In clinical disorders, augmented aldosterone production is commonly associated with cirrhosis and less consistently with cardiac or nephrotic edema. Advanced renal hypertensive disease is accompanied by very high rates of aldosterone secretion.

The mineralocorticoids normally act to augment the renal tubular reabsorption of sodium and chloride, and to increase the excretion of potassium. The latter effect is the result of the stimulation by the steroid of the uptake of potassium from the peritubular fluid by the cells of the distal nephron. This leads to a higher intracellular concentration of potassium and a steeper electrochemical gradient for the diffusion of potassium from the cell to the tubular fluid (Giebisch, 1976). Excessive mineralocorticoid activity leads to metabolic alkalosis, in which potassium depletion plays a major role.

In the absence of adrenal function, there is an increased excretion of sodium and chloride; or, stated more exactly, sodium and chloride excretion persists even in the presence of depleted body stores, whereas in the normal subject such a condition is associated with extremely low excretory rates due to a compensatory increase in the secretion of aldosterone. In heart failure, concentrations of aldosterone are also increased due to secretion of renin in response to diminished renal blood flow.

Under controlled conditions the urinary $Na^+:K^+$ ratio serves as an indirect index of aldosterone activity. The ratio can be greatly increased in response to the administration of spironolactone. Spironolactone also increases calcium excretion through a direct effect on tubular transport (Wills *et al.,* 1969).

Agents that inhibit the synthesis of aldosterone by the adrenal cortex theoretically have potential diuretic activity, but these are not clinically useful.

Clinical Toxicity. The most serious toxic effects of spironolactone result from hyperkalemia. Although hyperkalemia is almost certain to occur when the drug is injudiciously administered in conjunction with a high intake of potassium, it may also happen even when ordinary doses are given simultaneously with a thiazide to patients with severe renal insufficiency. A number of minor reactions have also been reported that are usually reversible when the drug is discontinued. Of these, the most common are gynecomastia, androgen-like side effects, and minor gastrointestinal symptoms.

Preparations. *Spironolactone,* U.S.P. (ALDACTONE), a microcrystalline preparation, is available in official 25-mg oral tablets. It is effective in an average daily dose of 100 mg, given in divided doses. A fixed-dose combination of spironolactone (25 mg) and hydrochlorothiazide (25 mg) is also available (ALDACTAZIDE); the usual dose is one tablet, given one to four times daily.

Therapeutic Uses. The aldosterone antagonists have been used mostly in the management of *refractory edema.* Frequently, they have been employed in conjunction with other diuretic agents rather than as the sole drug. On theoretical grounds, the potassium loss that occurs secondary to the use of other diuretics may be decreased by the coadministration of aldosterone antagonists. In general, this has been substantiated by clinical experience in the treatment of congestive heart failure, cirrhosis of the liver, and the nephrotic syndrome. However, the quantitative effects are not exactly predictable, due to the complex interactions of the primary disease, the degree of secondary hyperaldosteronism, and the actions of the diuretics given concomitantly.

Competitive aldosterone antagonists, as well as potassium-retaining agents, are also useful in both the diagnosis and the management of those rare metabolic and renal diseases associated with hypokalemia and potassium depletion (*see* Liddle, 1966).

POTASSIUM-SPARING DIURETICS

During the last several decades, the introduction of new natriuretic agents has been accompanied by parallel studies on the secretion of potassium. These have established (1) that potassium excretion is achieved by distal tubular secretion, (2) that excessive potassium losses may constitute an unfavorable consequence of diuretic action, (3) that

the excretion of potassium can be influenced by steroids with mineralocorticoid activity, and (4) that the loss of potassium may also be influenced by drugs that act directly on the distal nephron independently of adrenal steroids. While it is true that triamterene and amiloride possess moderate natriuretic activity, nevertheless their major importance lies in their effect on potassium excretion (Baer and Beyer, 1972).

TRIAMTERENE

Chemistry. Triamterene has the following structural formula:

Triamterene

It is a pteridine compound with a structural resemblance to the antimalarial diaminopyrimidines and folic acid. The diuretic activity of closely related homologs of triamterene has been examined, but no specific structural requirements have been established (Maass and Wiebelhaus, 1967). In another series of pteridine compounds, it is possible to demonstrate natriuretic activity with agents that have no potassium-retaining action (Rosenthale and Osdene, 1966). Triamterene is a weak competitive inhibitor of dihydrofolate reductase *in vitro,* but it has no significant antifolic activity *in vivo* (Maass *et al.,* 1967).

Absorption, Distribution, and Excretion. Triamterene is relatively insoluble in water and is administered only by the oral route. It is rapidly absorbed from the gastrointestinal tract and is then excreted in the urine, with a peak in renal excretion within 1 to 2 hours after oral ingestion. Most of the drug in the urine is in the form of metabolites, but certain of these compounds may be active (*see* Appendix II). In the plasma, about one half of triamterene is bound to protein. Renal excretion is accomplished by both filtration and tubular secretion.

Mechanism of Diuretic Action. Triamterene has no significant pharmacological actions other than those on the kidney. As indicated in Table 36–1, diuresis is characterized by an increase in the excretion of sodium, mostly accompanied by chloride as the anion, and under some circumstances by slight alkalinization of the urine. Compared to acetazolamide, this latter effect is quantitatively of little importance as far as extracellular electrolyte balance is concerned. Triamterene is not an inhibitor of carbonic anhydrase. The exact mechanisms by which it slightly alkalinizes the urine remain unexplained. Under normal circumstances, diuresis is accompanied either by no increase in potassium excretion or by only a slight increase. However, the effect of triamterene on potassium excretion may be greatly modified by pharmacological means, and a sharp reduction in potassium output is then observed. This is particularly noted when other natriuretic agents are given simultaneously, and when there is an excessive amount of mineralocorticoids (see Wiebelhaus et al., 1967). The action of triamterene is not significantly altered by alkalosis or acidosis.

Originally considered a nonsteroidal competitive antagonist of aldosterone, triamterene has subsequently been shown to have a natriuretic effect in the adrenalectomized animal that is not significantly different from that in the normal. It is presumed, therefore, that the action of triamterene is directly on tubular transport and is independent of aldosterone. The reduced rate of potassium excretion results from inhibition of the secretion of potassium in the distal nephron. This effect is achieved by a primary reduction in sodium reabsorption, which in turn leads to a drop in the transtubular electrical-potential difference. It is the latter that is normally the driving force for potassium secretion (Gatzy, 1971). The slight effect on urinary acidification is also probably distal. Under some circumstances, triamterene may be slightly uricosuric, but the mechanism of this action has not been examined. Unlike other diuretics, triamterene does not appear to cause retention of urate.

Clinical Toxicity. The most serious toxic effect is hyperkalemia, which is a direct consequence of the major action of the drug. Triamterene produces relatively few other side effects. The most common are nausea, vomiting, leg cramps, and dizziness. Slight-to-moderate azotemia is relatively common. This does not appear to be directly related to electrolyte and water imbalance and is reversible. Megaloblastic anemia has been reported in patients with alcoholic cirrhosis, presumably by inhibition of dihydrofolate reductase in patients with reduced stores and intake of folic acid.

Preparations. *Triamterene*, U.S.P. (DYRENIUM), is administered only by the oral route. It is marketed in capsules containing 100 mg. The usual initial dose is 100 mg, given twice daily. The maximal dose is 300 mg. The maintenance dose should be determined for the individual patient and may be as low as 100 mg every other day. The fixed-dose combination of triamterene (50 mg) and hydrochlorothiazide (25 mg) (DYAZIDE) is available in capsules, one of which is usually given one to four times daily.

Therapeutic Uses. Some patients with *edema* have a satisfactory diuretic response to triamterene alone. However, the available clinical data suggest that the greatest usefulness of this drug may be in conjunction with other diuretic agents. In general, the administration of triamterene with another natriuretic compound augments natriuresis and reduces potassium loss. With concurrent drug therapy, it is this latter effect that is more consistently observed. Therefore, the rationale of concomitant drug therapy is primarily in relation to potassium metabolism. Hansen and Bender (1967) summarized the experience obtained from several hundred patients maintained on long-term regimens with triamterene alone, chlorothiazide alone, and both drugs together, and showed that both drugs together provided the highest incidence of normal values of potassium in plasma. Because of the real possibility of inducing serious hyperkalemia, patients treated with triamterene should *not* receive supplements of potassium. Triamterene and spironolactone should *not* be prescribed together; an unexpectedly high degree of hyperkalemia has occurred when this was done.

AMILORIDE

Amiloride is an organic base with the following structural formula:

Amiloride

Absorption, Distribution, and Metabolism. After oral administration, from 15 to 26% of the drug is absorbed from the gastrointestinal tract. When given parenterally, amiloride is almost completely excreted in the urine. The urinary product appears to be identical to the parent compound. However, closely related congeners may become pharmacologically active by conversion to amiloride. After oral administration, the action of amiloride on the kidney reaches a peak within about 6 hours and usually ceases within 24 hours.

Pharmacological Actions. In the usual dosage, amiloride has no important pharmacological actions except those related to the renal tubular transport of electrolytes. Under normal conditions, amiloride slightly increases the renal excretion of sodium and chloride without a significant change in the glomerular filtration rate. At the same time, there may be a moderate increase in urinary pH, indicative of a lesser degree of hydrogen ion secretion. The finding of greatest interest is that, under all conditions tested, natriuresis is associated with either only a slight increase or sometimes an absolute decrease in potassium excretion. This effect of amiloride is undoubtedly most striking when it is given together with more potent saluretic agents. Under these conditions, the effect of amiloride is approximately additive as far as sodium and chloride excretion is concerned, but it is antagonistic with respect to potassium.

By analogy with the more direct studies of the mechanisms of electrolyte transport in the toad bladder, it is postulated that amiloride inhibits the secretion of potassium in essentially the same manner as does triamterene (Gatzy, 1971). The slight action of amiloride on hydrogen ion transport remains unexplained; the drug is not an inhibitor of carbonic anhydrase.

Although amiloride has an overall effect on electrolyte excretion qualitatively similar to that of antagonists of aldosterone, it does not act as a competitive antagonist. Since amiloride retains its activity in the absence of adrenal steroids, it is clear that its action at the cellular level of transport is independent of the presence of the steroid hormones (see Baer et al., 1967; Bull and Laragh, 1968).

Preparations and Clinical Use. While *amiloride hydrochloride* (MIDAMOR) is employed extensively in Europe, particularly in combination with hydrochlorothiazide, it is not yet available in the United States.

XANTHINES

The xanthines have long been known for their diuretic action. Their additional pharmacological properties are discussed in Chapter 25. Of the xanthines, theophylline has the greatest action on the kidney.

Mechanism of Diuretic Action. The stimulatory effect of the xanthines on cardiac function has raised the possibility that diuresis may result, in part, from the increased renal blood flow and glomerular filtration rate. However, all drugs of this class appear to have a direct action on the renal tubule. The urinary response involves an increase in the rate of excretion of sodium and chloride, with no significant effect on urinary acidification. Diuretic action is only slightly affected by changes in acid-base balance but is potentiated by the coadminstration of carbonic anhydrase inhibitors. It has been postulated that intracellular pH directly affects the intrarenal action of these agents. Augmentation of potassium excretion is not remarkable. Theophylline has been a useful agent in the study of water and electrolyte metabolism and the role of cyclic AMP to regulate these processes (Strewler and Orloff, 1977).

Clinical Application. The xanthines are rarely employed as primary diuretics. However, when used for other purposes, particularly as bronchodilators, the coexistence of their diuretic action should be kept in mind.

URICOSURIC DIURETICS

Interest in the development of diuretics that are simultaneously uricosuric stems from several considerations. Many of the currently available diuretics commonly lead to urate retention, hyperuricemia, and, in the rare subject, attacks of gout. Furthermore, hyperuricemia may itself be a risk factor for the development of cardiovascular disease, carbohydrate intolerance, and urate-induced nephropathy. Two uricosuric diuretics, *ticrynafen* and *indacrynic acid,* warrant mention. In the United States, ticrynafen was approved for use as an antihypertensive agent in 1979 and was widely prescribed. However, postmarketing surveillance revealed an incidence of hepatotoxicity sufficiently high (0.1 to 0.01%) to result in its withdrawal. Indacrynic acid is not yet available for therapeutic use. Nevertheless, both drugs will be discussed briefly for their heuristic value.

Like other uricosuric agents (see Chapter 38), these drugs are organic acids and have the potential to compete for sites for the transport of uric acid in the proximal tubule. Unlike the diuretics in current use, these compounds *increase* urate excretion rather than decrease it. The chemical basis for such disparate actions is not known. The new agents maintain the tradition that sensitivity to uricosuric agents in different species is unpredictable. The diuretic and uricosuric effects result from separate actions on different parts of the tubule.

TICRYNAFEN

Ticrynafen was developed in Europe, where it is referred to as tienilic acid. It has the following structural formula:

Ticrynafen

Ticrynafen is effective orally and produces a prompt diuresis with an increased excretion of sodium and chloride and a modest kaliuresis. There is no effect on urine pH or bicarbonate excretion. Continued use of the drug may cause alkalosis and hypokalemia. In these respects it is similar to the high-ceiling diuretics. However, as judged by free-water production, the diuretic action of ticrynafen is on the cortical diluting segment. In an extensive study in different species in which there is either net reabsorption or net secretion of uric acid, ticrynafen has essentially the same action as does probenecid (with the exception of the dog, where ticrynafen produces a marked increase in urate excretion). In man, when the effect of the drug is maximal, uric acid clearance increases about five-fold. This is blunted by pyrazinoate, but the latter has no effect on diuresis. The drug does not inhibit xanthine oxidase. (*See* Lemieux *et al.,* 1977; Prasad *et al.,* 1977; Lemieux *et al.,* 1978.) Ticrynafen is apparently equivalent in efficacy to the thiazides as an antihypertensive agent.

INDACRYNIC ACID

Indacrynic acid has the following structural formula:

Indacrynic Acid

It is effective orally in small doses. The agent undergoes tubular secretion, which is inhibited by probenecid, and is reabsorbed by nonionic diffusion. The diuretic action of indacrynic acid is prompt and, depending on the species, may be more prolonged than that of furosemide or ethacrynic acid. Micropuncture studies in the rat indicate that indacrynic acid inhibits urate reabsorption in the proximal tubule and sodium chloride reabsorption in the ascending limb of the loop of Henle. It has been studied most extensively in the chimpanzee, in which species it has remarkable diuretic and uricosuric actions, apparently more so than in man. Uricosuria is blunted but not abolished by pyrazinoate; this has no effect on diuresis (*see* Weimman *et al.,* 1976; Fanelli *et al.,* 1977a, 1977b).

THE CLINICAL USE OF DIURETICS

Pathological Physiology of Edema Formation. In a healthy subject, changes in dietary intake or variations in the extrarenal loss of fluid and electrolytes are accompanied by fine adjustments in the rate of renal excretion. Edema can obviously result either from an abnormally high intake of water and electrolyte or from abnormally low rates of their excretion. When fluids are administered parenterally with excessive vigor, edema can certainly be produced. However, when cardiac and renal function are normal, the condition is short lived. In the usual edematous states encountered in clinical medicine, the underlying abnormality involves a decreased rate of renal excretion, and the regulation of sodium excretion is the mechanism that is primarily disturbed. The retention of this cation is accompanied by retention of extracellular anion and a proportional amount of water and, as a result, the increased volume of extracellular fluid is usually of normal composition and osmolality. However, particularly in instances of severe cardiac or hepatic decompensation, retention of water may be relatively greater than that of electrolyte, and hypoosmolality results.

The exact mechanisms by which the kidney retains excessive amounts of sodium have been intensively examined. In many edematous states, increased rates of aldosterone secretion have been correlated with increased tubular reabsorption of sodium. In addition, particularly in cardiac decompensation, the glomerular filtration rate may be reduced. However, quantitative studies, both in disease and under experimental conditions, have failed to provide a predictable relationship between the rate of sodium excretion and either the amount of sodium filtered or the activity of aldosterone. For this reason, a "third factor" has been postulated that might regulate sodium reabsorption and excretion. However, at the moment, the nature of this factor is obscure and, indeed, several factors may be involved.

The normal relationship between the volumes of interstitial fluid and the circulating plasma depends on dynamic equilibria across the capillary membrane (*see* Chapter 35). In diseases of hepatic origin, particularly cirrhosis, the pressure relationships are disturbed primarily within the portal circulation, and the formation of edema becomes manifest as ascites. In congestive heart failure, pressure-flow relationships may be disturbed relatively more in either the systemic or the pulmonary circulation, and edema may be localized accordingly. In the nephrotic syndrome or other hypoproteinemic states, the equilibrium across all capillary membranes tends to be altered and edema fluid accumulates in a variety of tissues. However, in each instance the formation of significantly increased amounts of extracellular fluid is either preceded or accompanied by decreased rates of renal excretion.

Indications for the Use of Diuretics. When edema accumulates, three therapeutic approaches are available to mobilize the fluid and thereafter maintain the constancy of the extracellular fluid volume. The first is to correct the primary disease. This is, of course, the most desirable goal. The second is to suppress renal tubular reabsorptive capacity by the use of drugs. The third is to reduce the amount of sodium salts absorbed from the gastrointestinal tract. This is achieved primarily by a low-salt diet.

In all patients with *cardiac decompensation,* digitalis should be administered in full, adequate dosage and should be considered the primary therapeutic agent. Diuretic drugs acting directly on the kidney, irrespective of their potency or effectiveness, must be considered to have a secondary, albeit important, role.

The diuretics are extensively employed in the management of ascites, especially when associated with *cirrhosis* of the liver. Periodic administration either eliminates the necessity for or reduces the interval between paracenteses. Not only does a diuretic regimen contribute to the comfort of the patient, but also his meager protein reserves are spared inasmuch as significant amounts of protein are lost when ascitic fluid is mechanically withdrawn. With mild, asymptomatic, or residual ascites, no useful purpose is served in attempting to make the patient completely free of edema if this involves the persistent administration of diuretics and the production of hypovolemia or electrolyte imbalances.

As a general rule, *chronic renal disease* that causes edema may be treated in the same manner as other edematous states, with the recognition that these patients are more subject to electrolyte imbalance. In the presence of primary renal disease there is often a lesser effect of the diuretic on tubular function. In the case of the high-ceiling diuretics, particularly furosemide, an increased dose is required (Muth, 1973). The thiazides are relatively less effective and in high doses may decrease the glomerular filtration rate.

In the *nephrotic syndrome,* the response to diuretic agents is often disappointing. Although hypoproteinemia is a major etiological factor, the administration of albumin produces a minimal and unpredictable diuretic response. The important role of the corticosteroids in the management of the nephrotic syndrome is discussed in Chapter 63.

In incipient *acute renal failure,* diuretics have been used in the hope of diminishing further renal damage. Protection has been obtained in experimental models, and several intrarenal mechanisms may be involved (Thiel *et al.,* 1976). Unfortunately such administration of diuretics has been of limited clinical utility (Kleinknecht *et al.,* 1976).

Complications of Diuretic Therapy.

With the availability of powerful diuretics, there has been an increased incidence of complications in the management of the edematous state that may be directly attributed to the diuresis itself. It should be remembered that the goal of diuretic therapy is the mobilization of edema fluid in such a manner that the extracellular fluid is restored toward normal, in terms of both volume and composition. The *excessively rapid mobilization* of edema may lead to malaise and asthenia. Rapid changes in the pressure-flow relationships in the cardiovascular system may, even in the presence of an expanded extracellular fluid volume, give rise to symptoms usually associated with hypovolemia. In *intensive long-term therapy,* the diuretic-induced renal loss of sodium chloride may lead to *extracellular fluid depletion,* with or without hyponatremia. The condition usually responds to discontinuation of the diuretic agent and the liberalization of sodium chloride intake in the diet. Both these conditions are relatively rare.

A far more common condition, particularly in congestive heart failure and hepatic cirrhosis, is *chronic dilutional hyponatremia.* This is associated with persistent edema and expanded extracellular volume. It may occur solely as a result of the underlying disease, but is most often seen as a consequence of diuretic therapy. The physiological defect results from the inability of the patient to excrete an adequately dilute urine. The distal generation of positive free water is defective. This is attributed to an inadequate sodium load to this segment of the nephron. Water restriction is the most direct therapeutic approach, but may be complicated by uncontrollable thirst.

The problems of diuretic-induced *alkalosis* and *potassium depletion* are discussed in Chapter 35. In addition, *hyperkalemia* may result if potassium-sparing diuretics are used injudiciously or if potassium supplements are administered simultaneously.

Both extracellular and intracellular *magnesium depletion* may result from the use of diuretics. Since magnesium and potassium deficits may interact, the problem is complex and warrants more extensive evaluation (*see* Lim and Jacob, 1972).

Refractory Edema. The increasing attention being given to so-called refractory edema is, in fact, partly attributable to the high degree of success in the management of the less severely ill patient. This has enabled many patients with cardiac decompensation to survive longer in an edema-free state. With the progression of the underlying disease, these patients consequently tend to become edematous at a time when their cardiac reserve is significantly more impaired than in the earlier years of their illness.

With many drugs, diuretic efficacy is decreased by hyponatremia. An additional factor in drug refractoriness is the reduction in glomerular filtration rate. It should also be emphasized that diuresis is limited in an overall sense by the extracellular fluid volume. As edema subsides, the response to an individual dose of most drugs diminishes until, as the edema-free state is approached, the magnitude of diuresis is necessarily smaller than at the height of the edema.

When a patient becomes refractory to a diuretic, the entire regimen should be reevaluated. In some instances, minor adjustments of dosage may suffice. Bed rest itself may restore drug responsiveness, due to improvement in the renal circulation. Abnormalities of extracellular fluid composition should be sought for and corrected. The administration of additional diuretics may be appropriate. As a general rule, patients who are refractory to a diuretic of moderate efficacy, such as the thiazides, will show a more satisfactory response to high-ceiling diuretics.

Use of Multiple Diuretics and Adjuvant Agents. The availability of many different types of diuretics and many different compounds of the same type has provided the temptation to alter the diuretic regimen at frequent intervals. In the *initial management* of the edematous subject, when *mobilization* of edema fluid is the primary goal of therapy, the changing status of the patient warrants appropriate adjustments in dosage schedules and also in the agents selected for use. However, in the *chronic management* of edema, the best therapeutic results are often correlated with a purposefully constant therapeutic regimen.

Despite the widespread use of high-ceiling diuretics for the treatment of chronic edema, especially of cardiac origin, one may properly raise the question of their overuse in situations in which other diuretics, although less effective by conventional standards, might equally well achieve the desired therapeutic goal with less risk of overtreatment.

In the severely edematous patient, it is becoming apparent that, if a single diuretic agent proves ineffective, it is proper to use more than one type of diuretic agent. Of course, nothing is to be gained by the administration of two drugs of the same type, such as two different thiazides. Specific examples of rational concurrent therapy with diuretics have been cited in the discussion of individual drugs.

Allison, M. E. M., and Kennedy, A. C. Diuretics in chronic renal disease: a study of high dosage furosemide. *Clin. Sci.,* **1971,** *41,* 171–187.

Baer, J. E.; Jones, C. B.; Spitzer, S. A.; and Russo, H. F. The potassium-sparing and natriuretic activity of N-amidino-3,5-diamino-6-chloropyrazinecarboxamide hydrochloride dihydrate (amiloride hydrochloride). *J. Pharmacol. Exp. Ther.,* **1967,** *157,* 472–485.

Beyer, K. H. The mechanism of action of chlorothiazide. *Ann. N.Y. Acad. Sci.,* **1958,** *71,* 363–379.

Beyer, K. H.; Baer, J. E.; Michaelson, J. K.; and Russo, H. F. Renotropic characteristics of ethacrynic acid: a phenoxyacetic saluretic diuretic agent. *J. Pharmacol. Exp. Ther.,* **1965,** *147,* 1–22.

Birkett, D. J. Mechanism of inactivation of rabbit muscle glyceraldehyde 3-phosphate dehydrogenase by ethacrynic acid. *Mol. Pharmacol.,* **1973,** *9,* 209–218.

Bowman, R. H.; Dolgin, J.; and Coulson, R. Furosemide, ethacrynic acid, and iodoacetate on function and metabolism in perfused rat kidney. *Am. J. Physiol.,* **1973,** *224,* 416–424.

Brusilow, S. W., and Gordes, E. The mutual independence of the endolymphatic potential and the concentrations of sodium and potassium in endolymph. *J. Clin. Invest.,* **1973,** *52,* 2517–2521.

Bull, M. B., and Laragh, J. H. Amiloride, a potassium-sparing natriuretic agent. *Circulation,* **1968,** *37,* 45–53.

Burg, M. B. Tubular chloride transport and the mode of action of some diuretics. *Kidney Int.,* **1976,** *9,* 189–197.

Christensson, T.; Hellström, K.; and Wengle, B. Hypercalcemia and primary hyperparathyroidism. Prevalence in patients receiving thiazides as detected in a health screen. *Arch. Intern. Med.,* **1977,** *137,* 1138–1142.

Dodds, M. G., and Foord, R. D. Enhancement by potent diuretics of renal tubular necrosis induced by cephaloridine. *Br. J. Pharmacol.,* **1970,** *40,* 227–236.

Dollery, C. T. Diabetogenic effect of long-term diuretic therapy. In, *Modern Diuretic Therapy in the Treatment of Cardiovascular and Renal Disease.* (Lant, A. F., and Wilson, G. M., eds.) Excerpta Medica, Amsterdam, **1973,** pp. 320–330.

Dunn, M. J. Diuretics and red blood cell transport of cations. In, *Modern Diuretic Therapy in the Treatment of Cardiovascular and Renal Disease.* (Lant, A. F., and Wilson, G. M., eds.) Excerpta Medica, Amsterdam, **1973,** pp. 196–208.

Edwards, B. R.; Baer, P. G.; Sutton, R. A. L.; and Dirks, J. H. Micropuncture study of diuretic effects on sodium and calcium reabsorption in the dog nephron. *J. Clin. Invest.,* **1973,** *52,* 2418–2427.

Erlinger, S.; Dhumeaux, D.; Berthelot, P.; and Dumont, M. Effect of inhibitors of sodium transport on bile formation in the rabbit. *Am. J. Physiol.,* **1970,** *219,* 416–422.

Fanelli, G. M., Jr.; Bohn, D. L.; Scriabine, A.; and Beyer, K. H., Jr. Saluretic and uricosuric effects of (6,7-dichloro-2-methyl-1-oxo-2-phenyl-5-indanyloxy) acetic acid (MK-196) in the chimpanzee. *J. Pharmacol. Exp. Ther.,* **1977a,** *200,* 402–412.

Fanelli, G. M., Jr.; Bohn, D. L.; and Zacchei, A. G. Renal excretion of a saluretic-uricosuric agent (MK-196) and interaction with a urate-retaining drug, pyrazinoate, in the chimpanzee. *J. Pharmacol. Exp. Ther.,* **1977b,** *200,* 413–419.

Feit, P. W. Aminobenzoic acid diuretics. 2. 4-Substituted-3-amino-5-sulfamylbenzoic acid derivatives. *J. Med. Chem.,* **1971,** *14,* 432–439.

Flores, J.; DiBona, D. R.; Beck, C. H.; and Leaf, A. The role of cell swelling in ischemic renal damage and the protective effect of hypertonic solute. *J. Clin. Invest.,* **1972,** *51,* 118–126.

Ford, R. V. The new diuretics. *Med. Clin. North Am.,* **1961,** *45,* 961–972.

Gatzy, J. T. The effect of K⁺-sparing diuretics on ion transport across the excised toad bladder. *J. Pharmacol. Exp. Ther.,* **1971,** *176,* 580–594.

Gayer, J. Die renale Exkretion des neuen Diureticum Furosemide. *Klin. Wochenschr.,* **1965,** *43,* 898–902.

Gennari, F. J., and Kassirer, J. P. Osmotic diuresis. *N. Engl. J. Med.,* **1974,** *291,* 714–720.

Gerson, C. D.; Cohen, N.; Pinkel, M.; and Janowitz, H. D. Effect of parenteral acetazolamide on intestinal absorption of salt and water in man. *Proc. Soc. Exp. Biol. Med.,* **1975,** *149,* 950–952.

Giebisch, G. Effects of diuretics on renal transport of potassium. In, *Methods in Pharmacology,* Vol. 4A. (Martinez-Maldonado, M., ed.) Plenum Press, New York, **1976,** pp. 121–164.

Gordon, E. E., and Sheps, S. G. Effect of acetazolamide on citrate excretion and formation of renal calculi. *N. Engl. J. Med.,* **1957,** *256,* 1215–1219.

Gray, G. W.; Bryan, A. C.; Frayser, R.; Houston, C. S.; and Rennie, I. D. B. Control of acute mountain sickness. *Aerosp. Med.,* **1971,** *41,* 81–84.

Griggs, R. C.; Engel, W. K.; and Resnick, J. S. Acetazolamide treatment of hypokalemic periodic paralysis. Prevention of attacks and improvement of persistent weakness. *Ann. Intern. Med.,* **1970,** *73,* 39–48.

Hansen, K. B., and Bender, A. D. Changes in serum potassium levels occurring in patients treated with triamterene and triamterene-hydrochlorothiazide combination. *Clin. Pharmacol. Ther.,* **1967,** *8,* 392–399.

Hook, J. B., and Bailie, M. D. Release of vasoactive materials from the kidney by diuretics. *J. Clin. Pharmacol.,* **1977,** *17,* 673–680.

Kagawa, C. M.; Sturtevant, F. M.; and Van Arman, C. G. Pharmacology of a new steroid that blocks salt activity of aldosterone and desoxycorticosterone. *J. Pharmacol. Exp. Ther.,* **1959,** *126,* 123–130.

Klahr, S.; Bourgoignie, J.; and Yates, J. Effects of ethacrynic acid and furosemide on renal metabolism. In, *Modern Diuretic Therapy in the Treatment of Cardiovascular and Renal Disease.* (Lant, A. F., and Wilson, G. M., eds.) Excerpta Medica, Amsterdam, **1973,** pp. 241–252.

Kleinknecht, D.; Ganeval, D.; Gonzales-Duque, L. A.; and Fermanian, J. Furosemide in acute oliguric renal failure. A controlled trial. *Nephron,* **1976,** *17,* 51–58.

Laux, B. E., and Raichle, M. E. The effect of acetazolamide on cerebral blood flow and oxygen utilization in the rhesus monkey. *J. Clin. Invest.,* **1978,** *62,* 585–592.

Lemieux, G.; Gougoux, A.; Vinay, P.; Kiss, A.; and Baverel, G. Metabolic effects in man of tienilic acid, a new diuretic with uricosuric properties. *Nephron,* **1978,** *20,* 54–64.

Lemieux, G.; Kiss, A.; Vinay, P.; and Gougoux, A. Nature of the uricosuric effect of tienilic acid, a new diuretic. *Kidney Int.,* **1977,** *12,* 104–114.

Liddle, G. W. Specific and non-specific inhibition of mineralocorticoid activity. *Metabolism,* **1961,** *10,* 1021–1030.

Lim, P., and Jacob, E. Magnesium deficiency in patients on long-term diuretic therapy for heart failure. *Br. Med. J.,* **1972,** *3,* 620–622.

Lyons, H.; Pinn, V. W.; Cartell, S.; Cohen, J. J.; and Harrington, J. T. Allergic interstitial nephritis causing reversible renal failure in four patients with idiopathic nephrotic syndrome. *N. Engl. J. Med.,* **1973,** *288,* 124–128.

Maass, A. R., and Wiebelhaus, V. D. Die biologischen und diuretischen Eigenschaften von Triamterene. In, *Therapie mit Triamterene.* (Fellinger, K., ed.) George Thieme Verlag, Stuttgart, **1967,** pp. 2–21.

Maass, A. R.; Wiebelhaus, V. D.; Sosnowski, G.; Jenkins, B.; and Gessner, G. Effect of triamterene on folic reductase activity and reproduction in the rat. *Toxicol. Appl. Pharmacol.,* **1967,** *10,* 413–423.

Maren, T. H. Relations between structure and biological activity of sulfonamides. *Annu. Rev. Pharmacol. Toxicol.,* **1976,** *16,* 309–327.

Mitchell, J. R.; Potter, W. Z.; Hinson, J. A.; and Jollow, D. J. Hepatic necrosis caused by furosemide. *Nature,* **1974,** *251,* 508–511.

Möller, E.; Horstmann, H.; Meng, K.; and Loew, D. 3-Amino-1-(3,4-dichloro-α-methyl-benzyl)-2-pyrazolin-5-one (Bay g^{2821}), a potent diuretic from a new substance class. *Experientia,* **1977,** *33,* 382–383.

Morgan, T.; Tadokoro, M.; Martin, D.; and Berliner, R. W. Effect of furosemide on Na$^+$ and K$^+$ transport studied by microperfusion of the rat nephron. *Am. J. Physiol.,* **1970,** *218,* 292–297.

Mudge, G. H.; Cooke, W. J.; and Berndt, W. P. Electrolyte excretion and free-water production during onset of acute diuresis. *Am. J. Physiol.,* **1975,** *228,* 1304–1312.

Muth, R. G. Diuretics in chronic renal insufficiency. In, *Modern Diuretic Therapy in the Treatment of Cardiovascular and Renal Disease.* (Lant, A. F., and Wilson, G. M., eds.) Excerpta Medica, Amsterdam, **1973,** pp. 294–305.

Nechay, B. R. Biochemical basis of diuretic action. *J. Clin. Pharmacol.,* **1977,** *17,* 626–641.

Østergaard, E. H.; Magnussen, M. P.; Nielsen, C. K.; Eilertsen, E.; and Frey, H.-H. Pharmacological properties of 3-n-butylamino-4-phenoxy-5-sulfamylbenzoic acid (bumetanide), a new potent diuretic. *Arzneim. Forsch.,* **1972,** *22,* 66–72.

Panijayanond, P.; Cho, I.; Ulrich, F.; and Nabseth, D. C. Enhancement of renal preservation by furosemide. *Surgery,* **1973,** *73,* 368–373.

Pendleton, R. G.; Sullivan, L. P.; Tucker, J. M.; and Stephenson, R. E., III. The effect of benzothiadiazide on the isolated toad bladder. *J. Pharmacol. Exp. Ther.,* **1968,** *164,* 348–361.

Prandota, J., and Pruitt, A. W. Furosemide binding to human albumin and plasma of nephrotic children. *Clin. Pharmacol. Ther.,* **1975,** *17,* 159–166.

Prasad, D. R.; Weiner, I. M.; and Steele, T. H. Diuretic-induced uricosuria: interaction with pyrazinoate transport in man. *J. Pharmacol. Exp. Ther.,* **1977,** *200,* 58–64.

Prazma, J.; Thomas, W. G.; Fischer, N. D.; and Preslar, M. J. Ototoxicity of ethacrynic acid. *Arch. Otolaryngol.,* **1972,** *95,* 448–456.

Prockop, L. D. The pharmacology of increased intracranial pressure. In, *Clinical Neuropharmacology.* (Klawans, H. L., ed.) Raven Press, New York, **1976,** pp. 147–171.

Rodriguez, H. J.; Walls, J.; Yates, J.; and Klahr, S. Effects of acetazolamide on the urinary excretion of cyclic AMP

and on the activity of renal adenyl cyclase. *J. Clin. Invest.,* **1974,** *53,* 122–130.

Rose, H. J.; Pruitt, A. W.; Dayton, P. G.; and McNay, J. L. Relationship of urinary furosemide excretion rate to natriuretic effect in experimental azotemia. *J. Pharmacol. Exp. Ther.,* **1976,** *199,* 490–497.

Rosenthale, M. E., and Osdene, T. S. Renal pharmacology of the pteridine diuretic Wy-5356. *Arch. Int. Pharmacodyn. Ther.,* **1966,** *164,* 11–29.

Ross, C. R., and Cafruny, E. J. Blockade of the diuretic action of benzothiadiazines. *J. Pharmacol. Exp. Ther.,* **1963,** *140,* 125–132.

Schultz, E. M.; Cragoe, E. J., Jr.; Bicking, J. B.; Bolhofer, W. A.; and Sprague, J. A. Alpha, beta-unsaturated ketone derivatives of aryloxyacetic acids, a new class of diuretics. *J. Med. Pharm. Chem.,* **1962,** *5,* 660–662.

Sellers, E. M., and Koch-Weser, J. Displacement of warfarin from human albumin by diazoxide and ethacrynic, mefenamic, and nalidixic acids. *Clin. Pharmacol. Ther.,* **1970,** *11,* 524–529.

Smith, R. L.; Woltersdorf, O. W., Jr.; and Cragoe, E. J., Jr. Diuretics. In, *Annual Reports in Medicinal Chemistry,* Vol. 11. (Clarke, F. H., ed.) Academic Press, Inc., New York, **1976,** pp. 71–79.

Suki, W. N.; Yium, J. J.; Von Minden, M.; Saller-Hebert, C.; Eknoyan, G.; and Martinez-Maldonado, M. Acute treatment of hypercalcemia with furosemide. *N. Engl. J. Med.,* **1970,** *283,* 836–840.

Thiel, G.; Brunner, F.; Wunderlich, P.; Huguenin, M.; Bienko, B.; Torhorst, J.; Peters-Haefeli, L.; Kirchertz, E. J.; and Peters, G. Protection of rat kidneys against HgCl$_2$-induced acute renal failure by induction of high urine flow without renin suppression. *Kidney Int.,* **1976,** *10,* S 191–S 200.

Wales, J. K.; Krees, S. V.; Grant, A. M.; Viktora, J. K.; and Wolff, F. W. Structure-activity relationships of benzothiadiazine compounds as hyperglycemic agents. *J. Pharmacol. Exp. Ther.,* **1968,** *164,* 421–432.

Weinman, E. J.; Knight, T. F.; McKenzie, R.; and Eknoyan, G. Dissociation of urate from sodium transport in the rat proximal tubule. *Kidney Int.,* **1976,** *10,* 295–300.

Wiebelhaus, V. D.; Brennan, F. T.; Sosnowski, G.; Maass, A. R.; Weinstock, J.; and Bender, A. D. The natriuretic and diuretic characteristics of triamterene in the dog. *Arch. Int. Pharmacodyn. Ther.,* **1967,** *169,* 429–451.

Wills, M. R.; Gill, J. R., Jr.; and Bartter, F. C. The interrelationships of calcium and sodium excretions. *Clin. Sci.,* **1969,** *37,* 621–630.

Yendt, E. R., and Cohanim, M. Prevention of calcium stones with thiazides. *Kidney Int.,* **1978,** *13,* 397–409.

Monographs and Reviews

Baer, J. E., and Beyer, K. H. Subcellular pharmacology of natriuretic and potassium-sparing drugs. *Prog. Biochem. Pharmacol.,* **1972,** *7,* 59–93.

Beyer, K. H., and Baer, J. E. Physiological basis for the action of newer diuretic agents. *Pharmacol. Rev.,* **1961,** *13,* 517–562.

Colindres, R. E., and Gottschalk, C. W. Neural control of renal tubular sodium reabsorption in the rat: single nephron analysis. *Fed. Proc.,* **1978,** *37,* 1218–1221.

Goldberg, M. The renal physiology of diuretics. In, Sect. 8., *Renal Physiology. Handbook of Physiology.* (Orloff, J., and Berliner, R. W., eds.) American Physiological Society, Washington, D. C., **1973,** pp. 1003–1031.

Jacobson, H. R., and Kokko, J. P. Diuretics: sites and mechanisms of action. *Annu. Rev. Pharmacol. Toxicol.,* **1976,** *16,* 201–214.

Lassiter, W. E. Kidney. *Annu. Rev. Physiol.,* **1975,** *37,* 371–393.

Liddle, G. W. Aldosterone antagonists and triamterene. *Ann. N.Y. Acad. Sci.,* **1966,** *139,* 466–470.

Maren, T. H. Carbonic anhydrase: chemistry, physiology,

and inhibition. *Physiol. Rev.,* **1967,** *47,* 595–781.

Rector, F. C., Jr. Acidification of the urine. In, Sect. 8, *Renal Physiology. Handbook of Physiology.* (Orloff, J., and Berliner, R. W., eds.) American Physiological Society, Washington, D. C., **1973,** pp. 431–454.

Strewler, G. J., and Orloff, J. The role of cyclic nucleotides in the transport of water and electrolytes. *Adv. Cyclic Nucleotide Res.,* **1977,** *8,* 311–361.

Suki, W. N.; Ekonyan, G.; and Martinez-Maldonado, M. Tubular sites and mechanisms of diuretic action. *Annu. Rev. Pharmacol.,* **1973,** *13,* 91–106.

Valtin, H. *Renal Function: Mechanisms Preserving Fluid and Solute Balance in Health.* Little, Brown & Co., Boston, **1973.**

37 AGENTS AFFECTING THE RENAL CONSERVATION OF WATER

Richard M. Hays

ANTIDIURETIC HORMONE

Evolutionary Considerations. The earliest forms of life in the Cambrian sea had little concern with water balance. They were probably close to equilibrium with their environment with respect to both its osmolality and its ionic composition. With time, however, the environment changed; the salinity of the oceans increased manyfold, and, at the same time, fresh-water lakes and rivers formed. Primitive marine forms, such as the hagfish, simply maintained equilibrium with sea water. More imaginative species, notably the fish, employed their gills as well as their kidneys to retain their extracellular fluid near its original Cambrian composition. Salt-water species developed efficient pumps for sodium chloride in the gill, as well as renal pumps for magnesium and sulfate to excrete these ions. Fresh-water forms, threatened by salt loss, made the opposite adaptation and developed the capacity to reabsorb sodium chloride across their gills. Those species that alternate between fresh and salt water as part of their life cycle acquired the ability to switch their gill transport systems from salt reabsorption to salt secretion (*see* Schmidt-Nielsen, 1972).

Although gill-mediated salt transport was the primary mechanism for the regulation of volume, *vasotocin,* the evolutionary precursor of the antidiuretic peptides, was already present in the central nervous system (CNS) of the early aquatic species. Its role in fish is not completely understood, but includes such actions as modification of blood flow through the gill and control of glomerular filtration rate. The intriguing problem of the structural and functional evolution of the neurohypophyseal peptides has been reviewed recently (Sawyer and Pang, 1977).

With the emergence of life on land, antidiuretic hormone (ADH) became the mediator of a remarkable regulatory system for the conservation of water. ADH is released by the posterior pituitary under conditions of water deprivation (when plasma osmolality is elevated) or when extracellular volume is depleted (irrespective of the level of plasma osmolality). In amphibia, the target organs for ADH are skin and the urinary bladder; in other vertebrates, including man, the site of action is the renal collecting duct. In each of these target tissues, ADH acts by increasing the permeability of the cell membrane to water, thus permitting water to move passively down an osmotic gradient across skin, bladder, or collecting duct into the extracellular compartment.

In view of the long evolutionary history of the hormone, it is not surprising that ADH also has a number of nonrenal actions. It is a potent vasopressor; indeed, the name *vasopressin* was originally chosen on the basis of its vasoconstrictor action. More recently, it has been found to have effects within the CNS and on blood coagulation; these will be described briefly below.

Chemistry. duVigneaud and coworkers (1953, 1954) determined the structures of ADH and oxytocin and accomplished the complete synthesis of each. This was an unprecedented achievement at a time when the synthesis of even small peptides required years of effort, and duVigneaud was awarded the Nobel Prize in 1955. Studies in his laboratory established principles of the structure-activity relationship that underlie much of the current effort to design peptides for therapeutic purposes. The structures of 8-arginine vasopressin (the neurohypophyseal peptide found in all mammals except swine), 8-lysine vasopressin (*lypressin,* the swine peptide), and oxytocin (the oxytocic and milk-ejecting peptide, *see* Chapter 39) are shown in Table 37–1. All are nonapeptides with two cysteine residues forming a bridge between positions 1 and 6. Integrity of the ring is essential for biological activity, and amino acid substitutions dictate specific physiological actions. Thus, a basic amino acid residue in position 8 confers antidiuretic activity, while isoleucine in position 3 promotes oxytocic activity. Commercial preparations of ADH of pituitary origin are usually derived from both bovine and porcine pituitaries and, therefore, are mixtures of 8-arginine and 8-lysine vasopressin.

The natural hormones are subjected to rapid enzymatic degradation *in vivo.* Four sites of cleavage have been identified, the most important of which appear to be at positions 7–8 and 8–9 in the linear portion of the peptide; the disulfide bond and position 1–2 are also sites of modification by a variety of enzymes in kidney, brain, liver, and uterus (*see* Walter and Simmons, 1977). The kidney is probably the major site of enzymatic degradation.

Two synthetic antidiuretic peptides are also shown in Table 37–1. In accordance with the principles established by duVigneaud, oxytocic or antidiuretic activity is enhanced by deamination of the cysteine residue in position 1, and also by substitution of a more aliphatic amino acid in position 4 (Gilleson and duVigneaud, 1970). The development of technics for solid-phase peptide synthesis made it possible to synthesize and screen great numbers of analogs of ADH, and, in 1967, Zaoral and coworkers announced the synthesis of 1-deamino-8-D-arginine

Table 37-1. CHEMICAL STRUCTURES AND ACTIVITIES OF NATIVE AND SYNTHETIC ANTIDIURETIC PEPTIDES

	ACTIVITY * (Relative to Arginine Vasopressin)	
	Antidiuretic	Pressor

Native Peptides

Cys—Tyr—Phe—Glu—Asp—Cys—Pro—Arg—Gly(NH$_2$)
  1   2   3   4   5   6   7   8   9

8-Arginine Vasopressin
(ADH, AVP; mammals) — **100** / **100**

———————— Lys
8-Lysine Vasopressin
(lypressin, LVP; swine) — **80** / **60**

———Ile————Leu———
Oxytocin — **1** / **1**

Synthetic Antidiuretic Peptides

1-Deamino-8-D-Arginine Vasopressin
(desmopressin, dDAVP) — **1200** / **0.39**

1-Deamino-4-Valine-8-D-Arginine Vasopressin
(dVDAVP) — **1230** / **0**

* Assayed in the rat.

vasopressin (dDAVP, *desmopressin*), now the preferred drug for the treatment of ADH-sensitive diabetes insipidus (Zaoral *et al.*, 1967). Deamination at position 1 renders the molecule less subject to the action of peptidases; it is this resistance to degradation that is the most important factor in the superior antidiuretic activity of desmopressin. The substitution of D- for L-arginine in position 8 sharply decreases pressor activity and thus greatly increases the ratio of antidiuretic to pressor effects. An even more selective antidiuretic peptide is 1-deamino-4-valine-8-D-arginine vasopressin (dVDAVP). This compound, which has no detectable pressor activity, is effective in the treatment of human diabetes insipidus (Cort *et al.*, 1975) but is not yet commercially available. Synthetic peptides that have selective pressor activity have also been designed; one example, 2-phenylalanine-8-lysine vasopressin (*felypressin*), is in use in Europe as a vasoconstrictor. Finally, a series of peptides has been synthesized in which a

penicillamine group has been substituted at the β carbon of position 1. Such substitution converts 1-deamino oxytocin to a potent antagonist of oxytocin (1-deaminopenicillamine oxytocin). Attempts to design an equally potent antagonist of the antidiuretic action of ADH have to date had limited success (*see*, however, Lowbridge *et al.*, 1978). Progress in the design of peptides with selective activity has been reviewed by Manning and associates (1977).

PHYSIOLOGICAL AND PATHOPHYSIOLOGICAL CONSIDERATIONS

Antidiuresis in the mammal involves a hypothalamiconeurohypophyseal system for the synthesis, storage, and release of ADH and a renal system for hormonally regulated concentration of the urine. At almost every point, pharmacological agents, as well as disease, can modify the normal chain of events. The CNS components of the system will be considered first.

Anatomy. The hypothalamiconeurohypophyseal tract is an extended neurosecretory system; the perikarya are located in specific hypothalamic nuclei, and their long axons traverse the supraoptico-hypophyseal tract to terminate in the median eminence and pars nervosa of the posterior pituitary. Interruption of the tract at any level produces retrograde degeneration of the axons and nerve bodies. However, interruption below the level of the median eminence does not result in clinical diabetes insipidus, since axons terminating in the median eminence are spared and secrete adequate amounts of ADH. Lesions above this level generally result in diabetes insipidus.

Synthesis. In man, ADH and oxytocin are synthesized primarily at two hypothalamic sites: the supraoptic and paraventricular nuclei. However, recent studies with antisera to vasopressin have identified additional hypothalamic sites of synthesis (George, 1978). There is good evidence that ADH and oxytocin are synthesized predominantly in separate neurons, and painstaking studies with immunocytochemical technics have shown that the more ventral portion of the supraoptic nucleus and the more central portion of the paraventricular nucleus contain the neurons that synthesize ADH, while those that produce oxytocin are more dorsal and peripheral (Zimmerman, 1976; Zimmerman and Defendini, 1977). Relatively more ADH than oxytocin is synthesized in the supraoptic nucleus, while the reverse is true in the paraventricular nucleus.

Synthesis itself occurs in the perikaryon of the neuron and appears to follow the pattern established for many hormones. Thus, a relatively large and biologically inactive precursor is first synthesized on ribosomes. This prohormone may be a precursor of both the active hormone and its associated binding protein (*neurophysin*), or it may simply be the neurophysin with the hormone as its terminal element (*see* Sachs, 1969; Gainer *et al.,* 1977). Following synthesis, the prohormone is "packaged" into large (0.1- to 0.3-μm), membrane-enclosed granules in the Golgi apparatus. Much of the process of enzymatic cleavage of the prohormone takes place within the granules, and this proceeds as the granules move down the axon. The end products of maturation of the granules are the peptide hormones, the neurophysins to which they are bound, and a number of small peptide cleavage products. The neurophysins themselves are proteins with a molecular weight of approximately 30,000 that bind ADH and oxytocin electrostatically; their function, aside from this binding, is not known.

Transport and Storage. The process of axonal transport of the granules is relatively rapid; newly synthesized neurohypophyseal hormones arrive at the posterior lobe within 30 minutes of a stimulus such as hemorrhage (in rats) (Norstrom and Sjostrand, 1971). The axons involved in transport of granules may be of two types, carrying vasopressin and neurophysins not only to the classical terminations in the neurohypophysis but also to the external zone of the median eminence, where they may enter the adenohypophyseal portal circulation and play a role as corticotropin-releasing factors (*see* Zimmerman *et al.,* 1977; *see also* below).

Once the granules have arrived at the bulbous axonal terminations, they are stored until the need for secretion. The capacity to store hormone is important, since acute depletion of extracellular volume requires the immediate availability of ADH. Synthesis is too slow to meet instant needs, although it is accelerated under conditions of prolonged dehydration.

Secretion. Much of our current understanding of the secretion of ADH comes from the morphological studies of Douglas and associates (Douglas, 1973) and from technics for the study of the hypothalamiconeurohypophyseal system in organ culture (*see* Sladek and Knigge, 1977). Briefly, the neurosecretory system functions as a conventional neuron. Incoming impulses from osmoreceptors, higher cerebral centers, vascular baroreceptors, and other sites converge on the nerve bodies in the supraventricular or paraventricular nuclei. Stimulation leads to depolarization of the nerve membrane, which is propagated to the terminal bulb. The resultant influx of Ca^{2+} promotes fusion of granules with the membrane of the bulb and exocytosis of the granular contents. Neurophysins, as well as ADH or oxytocin, are released.

Physiological Stimuli for the Secretion of ADH.
The two principal physiological stimuli for the secretion of ADH are an increase in plasma osmolality and a decrease in extracellular volume. Other stimuli include pain, emotional stress, and an increase in the temperature of the blood perfusing the hypothalamus. A number of pharmacological agents stimulate or inhibit the secretion of ADH; they will be discussed separately.

Hyperosmolality. The classical experiments of Verney (1947) showed that an increase of less than 2% in the osmolality of blood perfusing the hypothalamus produced a sharp antidiuresis in dogs. Antidiuresis was stimulated by hypertonic saline or sucrose solution, but not by hypertonic urea, suggesting that actual osmotic shrinkage of some receptor cell was necessary. This concept of an "osmoreceptor" that communicates with the nerve bodies is still retained by physiologists, although some workers have proposed that even more remote receptors in the forebrain respond not only to hyperosmolality but also to hypoxia and sensory stimuli (*see* Hayward, 1972).

The pattern of secretion of ADH in response to hyperosmolality is shown in Figure 37-1, *A*. The threshold for secretion is approximately

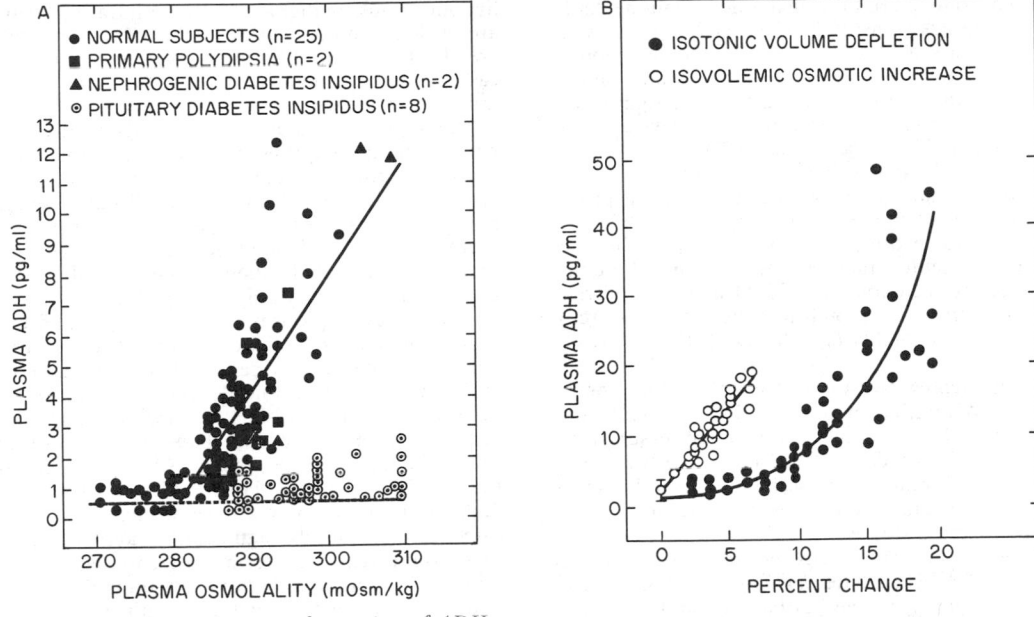

Figure 37-1. *Patterns of secretion of ADH.*

A. Effect of osmolality on the concentration of ADH in plasma. (After Robertson, Mahr, Athar, and Sinha, 1973. Courtesy of *Journal of Clinical Investigation.*)

B. Comparison of the effects of an increase in osmolality and a decrease in extracellular volume (both expressed as percent change) on the concentration of ADH in plasma. (After Dunn, Brennan, Nelson, and Robertson, 1973. Courtesy of *Journal of Clinical Investigation.*)

280 mOsm/kg; below this level, ADH is barely detectable in plasma. Above threshold, the concentration of ADH in plasma rises rapidly as osmolality increases. Patients with fully developed ADH-sensitive diabetes insipidus are unable to increase the rate of secretion of ADH, while patients with partial disease show a range of concentrations in plasma. Subjects with nephrogenic diabetes insipidus (failure of the kidney to respond to ADH) or psychogenic polydipsia secrete ADH normally in response to hyperosmolality.

Volume Depletion. The second major stimulus for the secretion of ADH is depletion of extracellular fluid volume. Hemorrhage, sodium depletion, or other acute causes of reduction of extracellular volume, irrespective of plasma osmolality, produce a discharge of ADH into the circulation. Secretion occurs from what appears to be a readily releasable "pool" of hormone, representing about 10 to 20% of the total ADH in the gland. Subsequent release takes place at a considerably slower rate. In addition to these acute stimuli, more chronic conditions in which effective circulating volume is reduced (*e.g.*, cardiac failure, hepatic cirrhosis with ascites, and excessive use of diuretics) may also be associated with abnormally high concentrations of ADH in plasma.

The receptors that mediate this type of release differ completely from those involved in the response to hyperosmolarity. They include the baroreceptors of the left atrium and pulmonary veins, as well as those in the carotid sinus and aorta. Impulses from these receptors are relayed to the hypothalamus via afferent pathways in the vagus and the glossopharyngeal nerves. Secretion of ADH is believed to be under tonic inhibitory control by the baroreceptors, so that hormone is released when blood pressure falls and release is inhibited when blood pressure rises. In addition to baroreceptors, the carotid body may contain chemoreceptors, sensitive to hypoxemia, which stimulate the secretion of ADH (*see* Schrier *et al.,* 1979).

The pattern of release of ADH during volume depletion in the rat is shown in Figure 37-1, *B*. Isotonic contraction of volume causes little change in plasma ADH until the loss approaches 10%, after which concentrations of ADH increase exponentially. This response eventually exceeds that of hypertonicity. The resultant concentrations of ADH are high enough to exert a direct pressor effect on arterioles and may help to maintain blood pressure under such conditions (Szczepanska-Sadowska, 1973). Indeed, on the basis of studies of the pressor effects of physiological concentrations of ADH in baroreceptor-denervated dogs, Cowley and colleagues (1974) have suggested that the hormone may contribute to the normal regulation of arterial blood pressure.

Renin-Angiotensin System. A question of current interest is the role of the renin-angiotensin system in stimulating the secretion of ADH under conditions of volume depletion. Angiotensin is a potent dipsogen, and there is evidence that it plays a role in the development of thirst that follows volume depletion (*see* Fitzsimons, 1976; Chapter 27). While angiotensin does appear to stimulate the secretion of ADH *in vitro*, a number of studies in intact animals and in man have failed to establish the significance of this observation (*see* Hays and Levine, 1976; Forsling, 1977; Schrier *et al.*, 1979).

Other Regulators. Pain, temperature, and emotional stress have already been mentioned as probable stimuli for the secretion of ADH. There is also evidence for a direct functional interplay between the neural centers that regulate thirst and those that control the secretion of ADH. Drinking appears to suppress ADH secretion before there is any decrease in plasma osmolality (*see* Hayward, 1975).

Pharmacological Agents and the Secretion of ADH. A number of pharmacological agents alter the osmolality of urine, and, in many cases, it has been hypothesized that their action involves stimulation or inhibition of the secretion of ADH. Experimental difficulties complicate the interpretation of many of these studies.

Stimulators. The agents believed to stimulate the release of ADH include *cholinergic agonists* (acetylcholine, methacholine, carbachol, and nicotine), *prostaglandin E$_1$* (note, however, that the dominant effect of the prostaglandin is to inhibit the action of ADH in the kidney), and large doses of barbiturates and meperidine. Morphine, which causes oliguria, was originally regarded as a stimulator of the release of ADH; however, it may inhibit secretion of the hormone by raising the osmotic threshold for release (Kamoi *et al.*, 1979). The oliguria caused by morphine (and possibly other opioids) may represent a direct renal or general hemodynamic effect.

Catecholamines alter the excretion of water; β-adrenergic agonists cause antidiuresis, while α-adrenergic agents promote diuresis. The catecholamines appear to act primarily by modulating baroreceptor-mediated alterations of secretion, but they may also play a role as neurotransmitters in the pathways that mediate osmotic and nonosmotic secretion of ADH (Miller *et al.*, 1978).

There is suggestive evidence that *vincristine, cyclophosphamide, clofibrate, chlorpropamide, tricyclic antidepressants,* and certain *anticonvulsants* may stimulate ADH release; some of the therapeutic implications will be discussed below.

Inhibitors. Ethanol and *phenytoin* inhibit the secretion of ADH, and there is evidence from both clinical and animal studies that *glucocorticoids* may play an inhibitory role in ADH release (Agus and Goldberg, 1971). *Chlorpromazine* and *reserpine* may also cause this effect.

Pathophysiology. *ADH-Sensitive Diabetes Insipidus.* ADH-sensitive diabetes insipidus, also referred to as central or neurogenic diabetes insipidus, results from the failure to secrete adequate quantities of ADH. The result is polyuria and the excretion of a dilute urine (specific gravity, 1.001 to 1.005). Any lesion that interrupts the supraopticoneurohypophyseal system and reduces the secretion of ADH to levels that are less than approximately 7% of normal will produce clinically apparent diabetes insipidus. Trauma or surgery in the region of the pituitary and

hypothalamus, malignancy, and infiltrative lesions are well-recognized causes of this condition; there are also familial and idiopathic varieties of the disease. Acute, postoperative diabetes insipidus may be transient in nature.

The appropriate diagnosis of ADH-sensitive diabetes insipidus requires differentiation from other causes of polyuria (diabetes mellitus; natriuretic syndromes, such as salt-losing nephritis and the diuretic phase of acute tubular necrosis; other types of osmotically induced polyuric states, such as those that occur in tube-fed patients receiving high-protein feedings; and primary polydipsia). Once the diagnosis of diabetes insipidus is established, it is confirmed by showing that the patient is unable to reduce urine volume and increase urine osmolality after a period of carefully observed fluid deprivation. Finally, it is necessary to distinguish the vasopressin-sensitive condition from nephrogenic diabetes insipidus (failure of the kidney to respond to ADH) by administration of the hormone. Patients with ADH-sensitive diabetes insipidus show a prompt increase in urine osmolality (to levels significantly above that of plasma) if given vasopressin intravenously (1 ml per minute of a solution containing 5 units per liter of aqueous vasopressin). Patients with nephrogenic diabetes insipidus show little or no response. For a more complete discussion of diagnostic procedures, *see* Hays and Levine (1976) and Moses (1977).

Inappropriate Secretion of ADH. Excessive production of ADH, with resultant retention of water and dilutional hyponatremia, may occur in patients with a variety of tumors or head injuries, meningitis or encephalitis, pulmonary infections, and other diseases. ADH is produced ectopically in the case of tumors and pulmonary disease, or by abnormal stimulation of the hypothalamiconeurohypophyseal system (head injury, meningitis, etc.). Concentrations of the hormone may be exceedingly high, as determined by radioimmunoassay, and unresponsive to normal control mechanisms. Drugs that stimulate the secretion of ADH (*e.g.*, vincristine, cyclophosphamide) or that sensitize the kidney to ADH (*e.g.*, chlorpropamide) may also produce abnormal water retention and dilutional hyponatremia (*see* Miller and Moses, 1976).

Nephrogenic Diabetes Insipidus. Nephrogenic diabetes insipidus, a failure of the renal tubule to respond to ADH, has many etiologies. As discussed above, drugs can interfere with the ability to produce a concentrated urine. Renal disease may cause hyposthenuria and polyuria especially when the structure or function of the distal tubule and collecting duct are disproportionately affected. Calcium nephropathy, hypokalemia, amyloidosis, sarcoidosis, polycystic and medullary cystic disease, pyelonephritis, myeloma, and ureteral obstruction are among the entities that can cause nephrogenic diabetes insipidus. Congenital forms of the disease are also well known, although rare (*see* Hays and Levine, 1976). *Diuretics* are the mainstay of treatment, since exogenous ADH is ineffective (*see* below).

Action of ADH on the Kidney. Upon release from the pituitary, ADH circulates in the vascular space with a half-time of disappearance of 5 to 10 minutes in the human adult. Several factors are responsible for removal of the hormone from the circulation. Enzymatic cleavage by peptidases has been mentioned above; in addition, there is some binding to receptors on smooth muscle. However, the affinity of such receptors for ADH is far less than that of the receptors of the renal distal tubule, and it is on this segment of the nephron that ADH exerts its principal action. ADH is bound by receptors on the basolateral (nutrient) surface of the cortical and medullary portions of the collecting duct. The critical role of the collecting duct in the conservation of water is described in the Introduction to Section VIII (*see* page 888). By the time tubular fluid arrives at the cortical segment of the collecting duct, it has been rendered hypotonic by the action of the chloride pump of the loop of Henle. In the well-hydrated subject, where concentrations of ADH are low, the entire collecting duct remains relatively impermeable to water; the urine thus remains dilute. A minimal osmolality of 50 mOsm/kg can be achieved, and as much as 15% of the filtered water can escape into the urine, virtually free of electrolytes. The osmotically unobligated water lost during the excretion of hypotonic urine is termed the *positive free-water production.* Under conditions of dehydration or volume depletion, on the other hand, concentrations of ADH are significantly elevated, and the cortical and medullary segments of the collecting duct become permeable to water. There is an osmotic gradient between the dilute tubular urine and the peritubular interstitial fluid, which becomes more pronounced in the medullary and papillary segments. Water moves passively down this concentration gradient and is reabsorbed from the tubule; the final osmolality of the urine may be as high as 1200 mOsm/kg in man and 4000 mOsm/kg in certain rodents. Free-water production is negative under these circumstances, and a significant saving of water is possible. Clearly, antidiuresis depends on the maintenance of medullary hypertonicity. This is largely achieved by the renal countercurrent system (*see* page 887; Jamison, 1976). The further requirement to achieve concentration of the urine, in addition to medullary hypertonicity, is a tubular epithelial cell that is capable of altering its permeability to water in response to ADH.

Cellular Action of ADH. The binding of ADH to cellular receptors initiates a sequence of steps that eventually increases the permeability of the opposite (luminal) cell surface to water. Permeability to urea may also increase in the medullary segment of the collecting duct. The sequence of steps is one of many examples in which cyclic adenosine 3′,5′-monophosphate (cyclic AMP) appears to serve as the intracellular mediator of the actions of a hormone on its target cell. ADH activates adenylate cyclase at the basolateral membrane, with resultant accumulation of cyclic AMP intracellularly. Cyclic AMP, in turn, initiates a series of events that ultimately increases the permeability of the luminal membrane. The exact nature of these events and their relationship to one another are not completely understood. However, the following is hypothesized: (1) a cyclic AMP–dependent protein kinase is activated; (2) a phosphoprotein phosphatase may also be activated; (3) microtubules and microfilaments appear to be important in the initiation and maintenance of the action of ADH (Taylor, 1977); and (4) aggregates of membrane-associated proteins appear on the luminal membrane surface. These aggregates were first described in freeze-fracture electron micrographic studies by Chevalier and associates (1974), and a series of observations has established their role in the movement of water across the membrane. Water may move through narrow protein-associated channels that are close to the size of the water molecule and can exclude solutes even as small as urea (Rosenberg and Finkelstein, 1978; Carvounis *et al.*, 1979). In segments of the collecting duct in which the movement of urea is also increased by ADH, transport appears to take place through channels that may differ from the water-conducting sites. The aggregates may be components of cytoplasmic vesicles that become inserted into the luminal membrane in response to ADH by a process that resembles exocytosis (Wade, 1978). The cellular actions of ADH have been reviewed by Strewler and Orloff (1977).

Prostaglandins appear to be important inhibitory modulators of the action of ADH (Grantham and Orloff, 1968). Zusman and associates (1977a) have shown that ADH stimulates the synthesis of prostaglandins by the toad bladder, and this has been demonstrated in the mammalian kidney as well (Dunn *et al.*, 1978). In effect, vasopressin initiates the production of its own inhibitor, and the system may thus be controlled by a negative-feedback loop. This observation may be relevant to the mechanism of action of chlorpropamide, a hypoglycemic sulfonylurea that has been employed as an antidiuretic agent in patients with vasopressin-sensitive diabetes insipidus (Arduino *et al.*, 1966). Chlorpropamide acts by sensitizing the kidney to low concentrations of ADH (Ingelfinger and Hays, 1969), and the drug has proven to be a potent inhibitor of ADH-stimulated production of prostaglandins by the toad bladder (Zusman *et al.*, 1977b). Other agents that enhance the effect of ADH (acetaminophen, indomethacin) probably have the same mechanism of action.

Pharmacological Agents That Modify the Renal Response to ADH. The ability of *chlorpropamide, acetaminophen,* and *indo-*

methacin to enhance the action of ADH has already been described. A number of pharmacological agents inhibit the antidiuretic action of the hormone to the point of producing ADH-resistant polyuria (nephrogenic diabetes insipidus). *Lithium carbonate,* used in the treatment of manic-depressive disorders, can cause a reversible polyuria (Lee *et al.,* 1971). *Methoxyflurane,* an anesthetic now in limited use, causes severe renal failure and associated polyuria, both of which may be irreversible (*see* Chapter 14). This is due to metabolites of the anesthetic, particularly including the fluoride ion. The antibiotic *demeclocycline* causes defects in the ability of the kidney to produce a concentrated urine in a high percentage of patients and can produce symptomatic polyuria and polydipsia (Singer and Rotenberg, 1973). The ability of demeclocycline to antagonize the action of ADH has been used successfully to promote diuresis in patients with water intoxication due to inappropriate secretion of ADH (Forrest *et al.,* 1978). *Colchicine* and the *vinca alkaloids,* which disrupt intracellular microtubules, also interfere with the action of ADH (Dousa and Barnes, 1974). These and other inhibitory effects have been reviewed by Forrest and Singer (1977).

Nonrenal Actions of ADH. ADH and related peptides are old hormones in evolutionary terms, and they are found in species that have no mechanisms for the concentration of urine. It is thus not surprising that there are actions of ADH in mammals in addition to that on the kidney.

Cardiovascular System. Reference has already been made to the pressor effect of ADH and to evidence that the concentrations of hormone that can be generated in response to volume depletion are high enough to exert a vasoconstrictor effect in man. This occurs only at concentrations that are significantly higher than those required for maximal antidiuresis. The pressor effect of ADH is a general one, and smooth muscle of all parts of the vasculature can be affected. The effect is a direct one on contractile elements. It is neither antagonized by adrenergic blocking agents nor prevented by vascular denervation. Circulation in the skin and the gastrointestinal tract is markedly reduced. The coronary vessels are not exempt from the vasoconstrictor effects of vasopressin, and pulmonary arterial pressure also rises.

The effects on *blood pressure* are conditioned by the reactivity of baroreceptor reflexes. Therefore, in normal conscious subjects, very large amounts of vasopressin must be administered to produce a marked and sustained rise in blood pressure. When the efficiency of baroreceptor reflexes is depressed by anesthesia, smaller amounts of the hormone elicit pressor responses. The blockade of autonomic vasomotor and cardioregulatory outflow by ganglionic blocking agents causes a marked increase in sensitivity to the pressor effects.

The effects of vasopressin on the *heart* are indirect and are the result of decreased coronary blood flow and of reflexly induced alterations in vagal and sympathetic tone. Aside from the reflex responses occasioned by the elevation of blood pressure, the effects observed are characteristic of myocardial ischemia.

The effects of ADH on the coronary blood flow can readily be demonstrated in man, provided large doses are employed. In patients with coronary insufficiency, ECG changes similar to those observed after exercise can be observed. The cardiac actions of the hormone are of more than academic interest. Some patients with coronary insufficiency experience anginal pain even in response to the relatively small amounts of ADH required to control diabetes insipidus. ADH-induced myocardial ischemia has led to severe reactions and even death (*see* Slotnick and Teigland, 1951). This is an important consideration in relation to the use of ADH in the control of gastrointestinal hemorrhage (*see* below).

Other Smooth Muscle. The effects of ADH on smooth muscle also occur in the *enteric tract.* The response is elicited only by large doses (5 to 20 units). Motility of the bowel is markedly increased. Peristaltic activity rather than tone is increased, and, therefore, the propulsive movements are greatly enhanced. The effect is greater on the large than on the small bowel. The smooth muscle of the *uterus* is stimulated by large doses of ADH at all stages of the menstrual cycle and during gestation.

Blood Coagulation. An unexpected action of ADH and its analogs was described by Mannucci and colleagues (1977), who noted that ADH or desmopressin was effective in the management of moderately severe hemophilia and von Willebrand's disease. Both peptides increase the level of factor VIII and can be administered prophylactically during surgical procedures to prevent bleeding. Their mechanism of action is unknown.

Secretion of ACTH. There has been a long debate about a role for ADH in the release of ACTH by the anterior pituitary. Zimmerman and associates (1977) have described a neural pathway from the paraventricular nucleus to the zona externa of the median eminence; its stimulation enhances the secretion of ADH and its associated neurophysin into the hypophyseal portal blood. Concentrations of ADH in the hypophyseal portal system are many times higher than in the systemic circulation (Zimmerman *et al.,* 1977). It appears possible that ADH plays some role in regulating the secretion of ACTH, although it does not seem to be potent enough to be the principal corticotropin-releasing factor.

Learning and Behavior. The supraopticoneurohypophyseal system may be involved in learning and memory. A number of experiments in animals have implicated ADH in the maintenance of learned avoidance behavior and in various aspects of memory consolidation (*see* deWied, 1976).

Water Permeability of Brain. ADH introduced into the lateral ventricle of the monkey increases the permeability of the brain to water (Raichle and Grubb, 1978). The finding suggests that the hormone, if released centrally, may modify the permeability of the vasculature of the brain to water.

Absorption, Fate, and Excretion. When ADH, lypressin, and their congeners are given orally, they are quickly inactivated by trypsin, which cleaves the 8-9 peptide link. ADH in aqueous solution may be given by the intravenous, intramuscular, or subcutaneous route and by the nasal insufflation of powders or sprays. Due to rapid inactivation by a number of enzymes that cleave the peptide at several sites (*see* above), the effects are brief after intravenous administration unless the hormone is given by continuous infusion. An exception is desmopressin, which has a prolonged half-life in the circulation when absorbed from the nasal mucous membranes. After intramuscular or subcutaneous injection, the effects last only a few hours. Repository forms, such as *vasopressin tannate in oil,* are effective for 24 to 48 hours after subcutaneous or intramuscular injection. An inefficient means of administration has been to apply rather large amounts of the hormone, in the form of posterior pituitary powder, to the nasal mucous membranes. The amounts of ADH absorbed are sufficient for the control of diabetes insipidus for a period of 6 to 12 hours. This procedure is, however, no longer recommended. Lypressin, in the form of a nasal spray, is administered for this purpose.

The half-life of ADH in the circulation is approximately 10 minutes, due particularly to inactivation by peptidases in various tissues. The kidney is of major importance in the removal of ADH from the circulation, accounting for one third to one half of the clearance (Lauson, 1974). In the rat, approximately 50% of the clearance of ADH is apparently by glomerular filtration, and the remainder is removed at peritubular sites beyond the glomerulus (Rabkin *et al.,* 1979). Thus, both the luminal and contraluminal surfaces are exposed to the hormone. Less than 20% of the total ADH removed from the circulation is excreted in the urine, indicating that most of the hormone is degraded within the kidney.

During pregnancy a peptidase appears in plasma that is capable of inactivating both ADH and oxytocin by cleavage at position 1-2.

Preparations, Bioassay, and Unitage. ADH is available in two types of preparations. One is an extract in which no separation of the antidiuretic and oxytocic principles has been made. It is assayed for its oxytocic activity, which parallels antidiuretic activity. Activity is compared to that of a U.S.P. bovine pituitary standard and is expressed in terms of U.S.P. *posterior pituitary units. Posterior pituitary* consists of desiccated posterior pituitary powder that contains the equivalent of 1 U.S.P. posterior pituitary unit in each milligram; it is marketed as capsules containing approximately 45 mg, and as an inhalator. *Posterior pituitary injection* (PITUITRIN) is a sterile aqueous extract of the gland that contains the equivalent of 10 U.S.P. posterior pituitary units per milliliter. *Posterior pituitary injection (S)* (PITUITRIN-S), for use as a local hemostatic agent in surgery, contains 20 U.S.P. units per milliliter.

Vasopressin Injection, U.S.P. (PITRESSIN), is prepared from the posterior pituitary glands of domestic animals by separation of ADH from the oxytocic hormone, or by synthesis. It is assayed for pressor activity rather than antidiuretic activity, but these are identical, unit for unit. The test method is the blood pressure of the rat. Activity is designated as *pressor units* and is determined by comparison with a U.S.P. standard. Theoretically, there should be no difference in antidiuretic activity between a U.S.P. posterior pituitary unit and a U.S.P. pressor unit. Vasopressin injection contains 20 pressor units and not more than 1 oxytocic unit per milliliter.

Desmopressin acetate (DDAVP) is marketed as a clear liquid solution containing 0.1 mg/ml of the synthetic peptide, with hydrochloric acid and chlorobutanol as preservatives. The preparation is available in a screw-top vial containing 2.5 ml; it includes a plastic catheter (rhynyle) for intranasal administration.

Lypressin, U.S.P. (DIAPID), is available as a nasal spray containing 50 U.S.P. posterior pituitary units (pressor) per milliliter. One spray into a nostril provides approximately 2 pressor units.

Vasopressin tannate (PITRESSIN TANNATE) is a water-insoluble tannate of the antidiuretic principle. It is marketed suspended in peanut oil (*vasopressin tannate oil suspension*). Each milliliter contains 5 pressor units.

THERAPEUTIC USES

The actions of ADH on the kidney and the circulation provide the basis for therapeutic applications of the hormone. Recent experience suggests a new use for ADH in the control of certain bleeding disorders.

Antidiuretic Action. Once the diagnosis of vasopressin-sensitive diabetes insipidus has been made, the administration of ADH provides effective and immediate therapy, with reduction of urine volume to normal. With the exception of patients who experience transient diabetes insipidus as a result of head injury or surgery in the area of the pituitary, therapy is lifelong. Until recently, the principal mode of therapy was intramuscular administration of *vasopressin tannate*. Desmopressin, administered intranasally, has now become the drug of choice.

Numerous clinical trials (*see* Cobb *et al.*, 1978) have confirmed the initial reports that *desmopressin* is an effective agent in both adults and children and has few side effects. The duration of effect from a single intranasal dose is from 6 to 20 hours, and twice-daily administration has proven to be effective in the majority of patients. There is considerable variability in the dose of desmopressin required to maintain normal urine volume (2.5 to 20 μg twice daily), and the dosage must be tailored to the needs of the individual patient. In view of the high cost of the drug and the importance of avoiding water intoxication, it has been suggested that the schedule of administration be adjusted to determine the minimal amount required (Cobb *et al.*, 1978). An initial dose of 2.5 μg can be used, and therapy should first be directed toward the control of nocturia. An equivalent or higher morning dose controls daytime polyuria in most patients, although a third dose may occasionally be needed in the afternoon. Resistance to desmopressin may develop (Cort *et al.*, 1975; Cobb *et al.*, 1978). Administration of more than 40 to 50 μg may cause headache. Rado and Marosi (1975) have reported prolongation of the duration of action of desmopressin by clofibrate, an observation that might be of importance in allowing reduction of dose of the drug required for control.

Vasopressin tannate oil suspension was the standard therapy for vasopressin-sensitive diabetes insipidus, and this preparation is still useful for the treatment of patients who are refractory to desmopressin or who experience significant side effects. Given as

an intramuscular injection (2 to 5 units every 2 or 3 days), it produces a satisfactory antidiuresis in virtually all patients. Care must be used in preparing the ampul for use; it should be warmed in the hand and mixed until the hormone is distributed in the solution. In view of the inconvenience of intramuscular injection and its side effects (*see* below), vasopressin tannate is less desirable than desmopressin, especially in children.

Vasopressin injection, the aqueous form of ADH, has no place in the chronic therapy of diabetes insipidus. Given intramuscularly, its rate of absorption and its duration of action are unpredictable. Given intravenously, it has two uses: in the initial diagnostic evaluation of patients with suspected diabetes insipidus and to control polyuria in the patient with diabetes insipidus who has experienced recent surgery (*e.g.,* hypophysectomy) or head trauma. Under these circumstances polyuria may be transient, and long-acting agents may produce water intoxication.

Lypressin, synthetic lysine vasopressin administered as a nasal spray, produces antidiuresis if administered approximately every 4 hours. Its short duration of action limits its effectiveness, especially in cases of severe diabetes insipidus.

Pressor Action. Despite its unfortunately chosen name, *vasopressin should not be employed as a pressor agent.* If it is desired to produce systemic peripheral vasoconstriction, preference should be given to appropriate sympathomimetic amines that can increase peripheral resistance without reducing coronary blood flow. However, justifiable exception may be made for the use of vasopressin as an adjunct in the control of bleeding *esophageal varices* and during abdominal surgery in patients with portal hypertension. When large doses (20 units in 5 minutes) are infused in normal subjects or in patients with cirrhosis and portal hypertension, there is a marked decrease in portal blood flow and pressure lasting approximately 30 minutes (Edmunds and West, 1962). Only a moderate rise in arterial pressure occurs. This effect on portal circulation is attributable to marked splanchnic vasoconstriction. As an alternative to systemic administration, infusion of vasopressin directly into the superior mesenteric artery has been advocated (Nusbaum *et al.*, 1968). The use of vasopressin to control gastrointestinal bleeding is not without hazard; cardiac and vascular complications have been reported, and it is not yet established whether superior mesenteric arterial administration is safer than systemic administration (*see* Freedman *et al.*, 1978; Getzen *et al.*, 1978).

Bleeding Disorders. Reference has been made above to the unexpected action of ADH and desmopressin in von Willebrand's disease and moderately severe hemophilia (Mannucci *et al.*, 1977). The beneficial effect of the peptides appears to be related to an increase in factor-VIII activity (*see also* Sutor *et al.*, 1978).

Untoward Reactions and Contraindications. Following the injection of large doses of vasopressin, marked facial pallor as a result of cutaneous vasoconstriction is commonly observed. Increased intestinal activity is likely to cause nausea, belching, cramps, and an urge to defecate. Women are apt to experience uterine cramps of a menstrual character. Most serious, however, is the effect on the coronary circulation. Individuals suffering from vascular disease, especially disease of the coronary arteries, should never receive vasopressin, except in the small doses needed for the treatment of diabetes insipidus. Sometimes even these small doses may cause difficulty in a patient who is subject to anginal attacks. Other cardiac complications include arrhythmias and decreased cardiac output. Peripheral vasoconstriction and gangrene have been encountered in patients receiving large doses of vasopressin.

When posterior pituitary powder is applied to the nasal mucosa, local irritation is common and hypersensitivity reactions may occur.

Allergic reactions, ranging from urticaria to anaphylaxis, may also occur in patients receiving vasopressin (*see* Schleyer, 1944; Lawrence *et al.*, 1972). Pulmonary fibrosis has been reported in a patient taking pituitary snuff (Mahon *et al.*, 1967).

Complications of the administration of vasopressin tannate include sterile abscesses and abdominal pain. Many of the untoward effects described above are not encountered with desmopressin, although headache and elevations of blood pressure may occur in patients taking large (40-μg) doses of the drug (Cobb *et al.*, 1978). As mentioned, there is a possibility of water intoxication with the use of any of these antidiuretic agents.

BENZOTHIADIAZIDES

Chlorothiazide and other benzothiadiazide (thiazide) diuretics paradoxically cause a reduction in the polyuria of patients with diabetes insipidus (Crawford and Kennedy, 1959). Their clinical use for this purpose is now well established. Other potent natriuretic agents, such as ethacrynic acid, have also been successfully employed.

Since effective agents are available for the treatment of vasopressin-sensitive diabetes insipidus, the principal use of the thiazide diuretics is in the treatment of the ADH-resistant (nephrogenic) disease.

Here, the change from a copius polyuria to the excretion of a smaller volume of urine can reduce or eliminate the handicap of the patient in the pursuit of daily activities. In infants with diabetes insipidus resistant to ADH, the antidiuretic effect may be of more crucial importance since the uncontrolled polyuria may exceed the child's capacity to imbibe and absorb fluids.

The mechanism of the antidiuretic effect is not yet completely understood. Most investigators agree that the natriuretic action of the thiazides plays an important role. When these agents are given continuously to nonedematous subjects, an initial loss of sodium, chloride, and water during the first 2 days is followed by a sustained, moderate state of electrolyte depletion and reduction of extracellular volume. A small reduction in filtration rate may occur, but this is not always observed. It has been proposed that, under these conditions, a significant increase in the fraction of glomerular filtrate reabsorbed in the proximal tubule leads to delivery of reduced amounts of sodium chloride and, most importantly, potential free water to the distal tubule. Thus, a fluid smaller in volume and less dilute leaves the distal tubule. This explanation is supported by the fact that reduction of filtration rate by dehydration or by drug-induced hypotension has a similar antidiuretic effect in diabetes insipidus. Also, it has been observed that restricted salt intake enhances, and high salt intake antagonizes, the antidiuretic effect of the thiazides. The common denominator among these effects is felt to be the reduction of the amount of filtered water reaching the distal segment (*see* Earley and Orloff, 1962).

Therapeutic Use. Chlorothiazide and its congeners are less effective than vasopressin in the treatment of pituitary diabetes insipidus but are useful for patients who experience undesirable side effects or allergic reactions after vasopressin and invaluable for those who have nephrogenic diabetes insipidus. Since their antidiuretic effects appear to parallel their ability to cause natriuresis, they are given in doses similar to those used for the mobilization of edema fluid. Chlorothiazide, 1.0 to 1.5 g, or hydrochlorothiazide, 50 to 150 mg, in daily divided doses, have been most frequently employed. Reduction of urine volume to 50% or less of pretreatment volumes is considered to be a good response. Moderate restriction of sodium chloride intake has been shown to enhance the antidiuretic effect. Representative clinical studies in adults are described by Havard and Wood (1961) as well as by Earley and Orloff (1962); in infants, by Schotland and associates (1963).

Among the most common of the side effects encountered is potassium depletion. Other untoward effects of the thiazides are described in Chapter 36, as are the chemistry, pharmacology, and preparations of these agents.

OTHER DRUGS

A number of agents have antidiuretic properties and have been administered as the sole therapy for vasopressin-sensitive diabetes insipidus. In general, they are only effective in patients with some residual circulating ADH; they are ineffective in nephrogenic diabetes insipidus. Recent studies (Zusman *et al.,* 1977b) suggest that some of these agents (notably chlorpropamide) act by suppressing the ADH-activated endogenous synthesis of prostaglandins by the kidney (*see* above).

Chlorpropamide impairs free-water excretion, and a number of cases of hyponatremia and water intoxication have resulted from its use. Webster and Bain (1970) reported an average reduction in urine volume of 70% in patients with diabetes insipidus, with urine becoming hypertonic during periods of low fluid intake. The major problem with chlorpropamide therapy is the incidence of hypoglycemic reactions, especially among children; its use is thus not advised (*see* Webster and Bain, 1970; Cobb *et al.,* 1978). Other agents (*e.g.,* clofibrate) may directly stimulate the secretion of ADH by the pituitary. Such stimulation has also been proposed as a second action of chlorpropamide (*see* Moses, 1977). The untoward effects that accompany the chronic administration of clofibrate should also be considered in those situations in which an oral agent must be employed (*see* Chapter 34). However, given the availability of desmopressin and the incidence of untoward side effects of agents such as chlorpropamide and clofibrate, the importance of these oral agents has declined (*see* Hays and Levine, 1976).

ADH ANTAGONISTS

Attempts to design a synthetic peptide antagonist to ADH have had limited success thus far. *Demeclocycline* is effective in producing a water diuresis in patients with water intoxication due to inappropriate secretion of ADH. At a dosage of 600 to 1200 mg per day, demeclocycline restores the concentration of Na^+ in plasma to normal within 5 to 14 days and affords symptomatic relief, according to the report of Forrest and coworkers (1978). A diminution in glomerular filtration rate was not reported in this study. Patients with cirrhosis may show a deterioration of renal function when demeclocycline is administered (Oster *et al.,* 1976). Demeclocycline appears to be superior to lithium carbonate in the treatment of inappropriate secretion of ADH.

Agus, Z. S., and Goldberg, M. Role of antidiuretic hormones in the abnormal water diuresis of anterior hypopituitarism in man. *J. Clin. Invest.,* **1971,** *50,* 1478–1489.

Arduino, F.; Ferraz, F. P. J.; and Rodrigues, J. Antidiuretic action of chlorpropamide in idiopathic diabetes insipidus. *J. Clin. Endocrinol. Metab.,* **1966,** *26,* 1325–1328.

Carvounis, C. P.; Levine, S. D.; Franki, N.; and Hays, R. M. Membrane pathways for water and solutes in the toad bladder. II. Reflection coefficients of the water and solute channels. *J. Membr. Biol.,* **1979,** *49,* 269–281.

Chevalier, J.; Bourguet, J.; and Hugon, J. S. Membrane associated particles: distribution in frog urinary bladder epithelium at rest and after oxytocin treatment. *Cell Tissue Res.,* **1974,** *152,* 129–140.

Cobb, W. E.; Spare, S.; and Reichlin, S. Neurogenic diabetes insipidus: management with dDAVP (1-desamino-8-D-arginine vasopressin). *Ann. Intern. Med.,* **1978,** *88,* 183–188.

Cort, J. H.; Shuck, O.; Stribrna, J.; Skopkova, J.; Jost, K.; and Mulder, J. L. Role of the disulfide bridge and the C-terminal tripeptide in the antidiuretic action of vasopressin in man and rat. *Kidney Int.,* **1975,** *8,* 292–302.

Cowley, A. W., Jr.; Monos, E.; and Guyton, A. C. Interaction of vasopressin and the baroreceptor reflex system in the regulation of arterial blood pressure in the dog. *Circ. Res.,* **1974,** *34,* 505–514.

Crawford, J. D., and Kennedy, G. C. Chlorothiazide in diabetes insipidus. *Nature,* **1959,** *183,* 891–892.

Dousa, T. P., and Barnes, L. D. Effect of colchicine and vinblastine on the cellular action of vasopressin in mammalian kidney. *J. Clin. Invest.,* **1974,** *54,* 252–262.

Dunn, F. L.; Brennan, T. J.; Nelson, A. E.; and Robertson, G. L. The role of blood osmolality and volume in regulating vasopressin secretion in the rat. *J. Clin. Invest.,* **1973,** *52,* 3212–3219.

Dunn, M. J.; Greely, H. P.; Valtin, H.; Kinter, L. B.; and Beewnokes, R., III. Renal excretion of prostaglandins E_1 and $F_{2\alpha}$ in diabetes insipidus in rats. *Am. J. Physiol.,* **1978,** *235,* E624–E627.

duVigneaud, V.; Gish, D. T.; and Katsoyannis, P. G. A synthetic preparation possessing biological properties associated with arginine vasopressin. *J. Am. Chem. Soc.,* **1954,** *76,* 4751–4752.

duVigneaud, V.; Ressler, C.; Swan, J. M.; Roberts, C. W.; Katsoyannis, P. G.; and Gordon, S. The synthesis of an octapeptide amide with the hormonal activity of oxytocin. *J. Am. Chem. Soc.,* **1953,** *75,* 4879–4880.

Earley, L. E., and Orloff, J. The mechanism of antidiuresis associated with the administration of hydrochlorothiazide to patients with vasopressin-resistant diabetes insipidus. *J. Clin. Invest.,* **1962,** *41,* 1988–1997.

Edmunds, R., and West, S. P. A study of the effect of vasopressin on portal and systemic blood pressure. *Surg. Gynecol. Obstet.,* **1962,** *114,* 458–462.

Forrest, J. M., Jr.; Cox, M.; Hong, C.; Morrison, G.; Bia, M.; and Singer, I. Superiority of demeclocycline over lithium in the treatment of chronic syndrome of inappropriate antidiuretic hormone. *N. Engl. J. Med.,* **1978,** *298,* 173–177.

Freedman, A. R.; Kerr, J. C.; Swan, K. G.; and Hobson, R. W. Primate mesenteric blood flow. Effect of vasopressin and its route of delivery. *Gastroenterology,* **1978,** *74,* 875–878.

Gainer, H.; Jarne, Y.; and Brownstein, M. J. Biosynthesis and axonal transport of rat neurohypophysial proteins and peptides. *J. Cell Biol.,* **1977,** *73,* 366–381.

George, J. M. Immunoreactive vasopressin and oxytocin: concentration in individual human hypothalamic nuclei. *Science,* **1978,** *200,* 342–343.

Getzen, L. C.; Brink, R. R.; and Wolfman, E. F. Survival following infusion of PITRESSIN into the superior mesenteric artery to control bleeding esophogeal varices in cirrhotic patients. *Ann. Surg.,* **1978,** *187,* 337–342.

Gilleson, D., and duVigneaud, V. Synthesis and pharmacological properties of 4-decarboxyamido-8-arginine-vasopressin and its 1-deamino analog. *J. Med. Chem.,* **1970,** *13,* 346–349.

Goldstein, A. Opioid peptides (endorphins) in pituitary and brain. *Science,* **1976,** *193,* 1081–1086.

Grantham, J. J., and Orloff, J. Effect of prostaglandin E_1 on the permeability response of the isolated collecting tubule to vasopressin, adenosine 3',5' monophosphate and theophylline. *J. Clin. Invest.,* **1968,** *47,* 1154–1161.

Havard, C. W. H., and Wood, P. H. N. The effect of diuretics on renal water excretion in diabetes insipidus. *Clin. Sci.,* **1961,** *21,* 321–332.

Hayward, J. N. Hypothalamic input to supraoptic neurons. *Prog. Brain Res.,* **1972,** *38,* 145–162.

Ingelfinger, J. R., and Hays, R. M. Evidence that chlorpropamide and vasopressin share a common site of action. *J. Clin. Endocrinol. Metab.,* **1969,** *29,* 738–740.

Kamoi, K.; White, K.; and Robertson, G. L. Opiates

elevate the osmotic method for vasopressin (VP) release in rats. *Clin. Res.,* **1979,** *27,* 254A.

Lawrence, G. D.; Hsu, T.-II., and Lichtenstein, L. M. Diabetes insipidus with hypersensitivity to PITRESSIN; an immunological study. *Johns Hopkins Med. J.,* **1972,** *131,* 172–177.

Lee, R. V.; Jampol, L. M.; and Braun, W. V. Nephrogenic diabetes insipidus and lithium intoxication—complications of lithium carbonate therapy. *N. Engl. J. Med.,* **1971,** *284,* 93–94.

Lowbridge, J.; Manning, M.; Haldar, J.; and Sawyer, W. H. [1-(β-Mercapto-β,β-cyclopentamethylenepropionic acid), 4-valine,-8-D-arginine] vasopressin, a potent and selective inhibitor of the vasopressor response to arginine-vasopressin. *J. Med. Chem.,* **1978,** *21,* 313–315.

Mahon, W. E.; Scott, D. J.; Ansell, G.; Manson, G. L.; and Fraser, N. Hypersensitivity to pituitary snuff with miliary shadowing in the lungs. *Thorax,* **1967,** *22,* 13–20.

Mannucci, P. M.; Pareti, F. I.; Ruggeri, Z. M.; and Capitano, A. 1-Deamino-8-D-arginine vasopressin: a new pharmacological approach to the management of haemophilia and von Willebrand's disease. *Lancet,* **1977,** *1,* 869–872.

Miller, T.; Schrier, R. W.; Molinoff, P.; and McDonald, K. Effect of central (CNS) catecholamine depletion of the hypovolemic and osmotic stimulation of vasopressin in the rat. *Clin. Res.,* **1978,** *26,* 140A.

Norstrom, A., and Sjostrand, J. Effect of haemorrhage on the rapid axonal transport of neurohypophysial proteins of the rat. *J. Neurochem.,* **1971,** *18,* 2017–2026.

Nusbaum, M.; Baum, S.; Kuroda, K.; and Blakemore, W. S. Control of portal hypertension by selective mesenteric arterial drug infusion. *Arch. Surg.,* **1968,** *97,* 1005–1013.

Oster, J. R.; Epstein, M.; and Ulano, H. B. Deterioration of renal function with demeclocycline administration. *Curr. Ther. Res.,* **1976,** *20,* 794–801.

Rabkin, R.; Share, L.; Payne, P. A.; Young, J.; and Crofton, J. The handling of immunoreactive vasopressin by the isolated perfused rat kidney. *J. Clin. Invest.,* **1979,** *63,* 6–13.

Rado, J. P., and Marosi, J. Prolongation of duration of action of 1-deamino-8-D-arginine vasopressin (DDAVP) by ineffective doses of clofibrate in diabetes insipidus. *Horm. Metab. Res.,* **1975,** *7,* 527–528.

Raichle, M. E., and Grubb, R. L. Regulation of brain water permeability by centrally-released vasopressin. *Brain Res.,* **1978,** *143,* 191–194.

Robertson, G. L.; Mahr, E. A.; Athar, S.; and Sinha, T. Development and clinical application of a new method for the radioimmunoassay of arginine vasopressin in human plasma. *J. Clin. Invest.,* **1973,** *52,* 2340–2352.

Rosenberg, P. A., and Finkelstein, A. Water permeability of gramicidin A–treated lipid bilayer membranes. *J. Gen. Physiol.,* **1978,** *72,* 341–350.

Schleyer, E. Anaphylactic shock after posterior pituitary extract injection. *Br. Med. J.,* **1944,** *1,* 255.

Schotland, M. G.; Grunbach, M. M.; and Strauss, J. The effects of chlorothiazides in nephrogenic diabetes insipidus. *Pediatrics,* **1963,** *31,* 741–753.

Singer, I., and Rotenberg, D. Demeclocycline-induced nephrogenic diabetes insipidus. *In vivo* and *in vitro* studies. *Ann. Intern. Med.,* **1973,** *79,* 679–683.

Sladek, L., and Knigge, M. Osmotic control of vasopressin release by rat hypothalamus—neurohypophysial explants in organ culture. *Endocrinology,* **1977,** *101,* 1834–1838.

Slotnick, I. L., and Teigland, J. D. Cardiac accidents following vasopressin injection (PITRESSIN). *J.A.M.A.,* **1951,** *146,* 1126–1129.

Sutor, A. H.; Uollman, H.; and Arends, P. Intranasal application of DDAVP in severe haemophilia. (Letter.) *Lancet,* **1978,** *1,* 446.

Szczepanska-Sadowska, E. Neurodynamic effects of a

moderate increase of the plasma vasopressin level in conscious dogs. *Pfluegers Arch.,* **1973,** *338,* 313–322.

Wade, J. B. Membrane structural specialization of the toad urinary bladder revealed by the freeze-fracture technique. III. Location, structure and vasopressin dependence of intramembranous particle arrays. *J. Membr. Biol.,* **1978,** *40,* 281–296.

Webster, B., and Bain, J. Antidiuretic effect and complications of chlorpropamide therapy in diabetes insipidus. *J. Clin. Endocrinol. Metab.,* **1970,** *30,* 215–227.

Zaoral, M.; Kole, J.; and Sorm, F. Amino acids and peptides. LXXI. Synthesis of 1-deamino-8-D-aminobutyrine-vasopressin, 1-deamino-8-D-lysine vasopressin, and 1-deamino-8-D-arginine vasopressin. *Coll. Czech. Chem. Commun.,* **1967,** *32,* 1250–1257.

Zimmerman, E. A., and Defendini, R. Hypothalamic pathways containing oxytocin, vasopressin and associated neurophysins. In, *Neurohypophysis: International Conference on the Neurohypophysis.* (Moses, A. M., and Share, L., eds.) S. Karger, Basel, **1977,** pp. 22–29.

Zimmerman, E. A.; Stillman, M. A.; Recht, L. D.; Antures, J. L.; and Carmill, P. W. Vasopressin and corticotropin releasing factor. An axonal pathway to portal capillaries in the zona externa of the median eminence containing vasopressin and its interaction with adrenal corticoids. *Ann. N.Y. Acad. Sci.,* **1977,** *297,* 405–419.

Zusman, R. M.; Keiser, H. R.; and Handler, J. S. Vasopressin-stimulated prostaglandin E biosynthesis in the toad urinary bladder. *J. Clin. Invest.,* **1977a,** *60,* 1339–1347.

———. Inhibition of vasopressin-stimulated prostaglandin E biosynthesis by chlorpropamide in the toad bladder. *Ibid.,* **1977b,** *60,* 1348–1353.

Monographs and Reviews

deWied, D. Hormonal influences on motivation, learning and memory processes. *Hosp. Pract.,* **1976,** *11,* 123–131.

Douglas, W. W. How do neurons secrete peptides? Exocytosis and its consequences, including "synaptic vesicle" formation in the hypothalamoneurohypophyseal system. *Prog. Brain Res.,* **1973,** *39,* 21–39.

Fitzsimons, J. T. The physiological basis of thirst. *Kidney Int.,* **1976,** *10,* 3–11.

Forrest, J. N., Jr., and Singer, I. Drug-induced interference with action of antidiuretic hormone. In, *Disturbances in Body Fluid Osmolality.* (Andreoli, T. E.; Grantham, J. J.; and Rector, F. C., Jr.; eds.) American Physiological Society, Bethesda, **1977,** pp. 309–340. (107 references.)

Forsling, M. L. *Anti-Diuretic Hormone.* Eden Press, Inc., Montreal, **1977.**

Hays, R. M., and Levine, S. D. Pathophysiology of water metabolism. In, *The Kidney,* 1st ed. (Brenner, B. M., and Rector, F. C., Jr., eds.) W. B. Saunders Co., Philadelphia, **1976,** pp. 533–614.

Hayward, J. N. Neural control of the posterior pituitary. *Annu. Rev. Physiol.,* **1975,** *37,* 191–210.

Jamison, R. L. Urine concentration and dilution. In, *The Kidney,* 1st ed. (Brenner, B. M., and Rector, F. C., Jr., eds.) W. B. Saunders Co., Philadelphia, **1976,** pp. 391–441.

Lauson, H. D. Metabolism of the neurohypophysial hormones. In, Sect. 7, *Endocrinology,* Vol. 4, Pt. 1. *Handbook of Physiology.* (Greep, R. O., and Astwood, E. B., eds.) American Physiological Society, Washington, D. C., **1974,** pp. 287–393. (251 references.)

Manning, M.; Lowbridge, J.; Holdon, J.; and Sawyer, W. H. Design of neurohypophyseal peptides that exhibit selective agonistic and antagonistic properties. *Fed. Proc.,* **1977,** *36,* 1848–1852.

Miller, M., and Moses, A. M. Drug-induced states of impaired water excretion in the mammalian kidney. *Kidney Int.,* **1976,** *10,* 96–103.

Moses, A. M. Diabetes insipidus and ADH regulation. *Hosp. Pract.,* **1977,** *12,* 37–44.

Sachs, H. Neurosecretion. *Adv. Enzymol.,* **1969,** *32,* 327–372.

Sawyer, W. H., and Pang, P. K. T. Evolution of neurohypophyseal hormones and their function. In, *Neurohypophysis: International Conference on the Neurohypophysis.* (Moses, A. M., and Share, L., eds.) S. Karger, Basel, **1977,** pp. 1–8. (27 references.)

Schmidt-Nielsen, B. Comparative physiology of electrolyte and water regulation with emphasis on sodium, potassium, chloride, urea and osmotic pressure. In, *Clinical Disorders of Fluid and Electrolyte Metabolism,* 2nd ed. (Maxwell, M. H., and Kleeman, C. R., eds.) McGraw-Hill Book Co., New York, **1972,** pp. 45–93. (188 references.)

Schrier, R. W.; Berl, T.; and Anderson, R. J. Osmotic and nonosmotic control of vasopressin release. *Am. J. Physiol.,* **1979,** *236,* F321–F332.

Strewler, G. J., and Orloff, J. Role of cyclic nucleotides in the transport of water and electrolytes. *Adv. Cyclic Nucleotide Res.,* **1977,** *8,* 311–361.

Symposium. (Various authors.) *Neurohypophysis: International Conference on the Neurohypophysis.* (Moses, A. M., and Share, L., eds.) S. Karger, Basel, **1977.**

Taylor, A. Role of microtubules and microfilaments in the action of vasopressin. In, *Disturbances in Body Fluid Osmolality.* (Andreoli, T. E.; Grantham, J. J.; and Rector, F. C., Jr.; eds.) American Physiological Society, Bethesda, **1977,** pp. 97–124. (116 references.)

Verney, E. B. Croonian lecture: The antidiuretic hormone and the factors which determine its release. *Proc. R. Soc. Lond. [Biol.],* **1947,** *135,* 25–106.

Walter, R., and Simmons, W. H. Metabolism of neurohypophyseal hormones: considerations from a molecular viewpoint. In, *Neurohypophysis: International Conference on the Neurohypophysis.* (Moses, A. M., and Share, L., eds.) S. Karger, Basel, **1977,** pp. 167–188. (94 references.)

Zimmerman, E. A. Localization of hypothalamic hormones by immunocytochemical techniques. In, *Frontiers in Neuroendocrinology,* Vol. 4. Raven Press, New York, **1976,** pp. 25–62.

CHAPTER

38 INHIBITORS OF TUBULAR TRANSPORT OF ORGANIC COMPOUNDS

Gilbert H. Mudge

The physiological factors that influence the renal excretion of organic compounds have been considered in Chapter 1 and in the Introduction to Section VIII. Pharmacological agents can influence the rates of these processes by several mechanisms. Drugs that alter the quantity of an organic compound that is filtered at the glomerulus may change its rate of excretion; thus, agents that impair or enhance glomerular filtration or that compete with the molecule in question for binding sites on plasma proteins can have this effect. Diuretics that enhance urine flow by inhibition of tubular reabsorption of ions and water can also increase the rate of excretion of compounds that are at least partially reabsorbed during their transit through the renal tubule, and agents that alter the pH of the urine may influence the rate of excretion of lipid-soluble organic acids and bases. In this chapter, however, there is described a class of drugs that act directly to influence tubular transport systems for organic molecules and thus alter the rate of elimination of compounds that are excreted or reabsorbed by such mechanisms.

In theory, a drug may act on tubular transport systems to either increase or decrease the rate at which a compound is excreted. Furthermore, since transport can be bidirectional, it is possible that an observed effect could be achieved either by stimulation of transport in one direction or inhibition of transport in the opposite direction. While many critical observations cannot be made for technical reasons, it is generally held that drugs inhibit carrier-mediated transport and do not stimulate it. Thus, decreased excretion of an organic compound can be attributed to inhibition of its secretion rather than to enhancement of its reabsorption.

The mechanisms by which drugs inhibit carrier-mediated transport have been studied extensively. A drug may act relatively non-specifically on the steps by which the cell generates energy or more specifically and directly at the site of transport itself. General metabolic inhibitors have played an important role in experimental studies but have no therapeutic application. The useful therapeutic agents interfere directly with the transport mechanism—in some instances competitively, in others probably noncompetitively, and in still others in a manner not fully understood.

To illustrate the complexity of the problem, consider the action of probenecid, the prototypical drug in this group, on the renal excretion of three different organic acids—penicillin, uric acid, and salicylate. Probenecid itself is a highly lipid-soluble carboxylic acid. In an acidic urine it is completely reabsorbed, while in an alkaline urine net tubular secretion of the drug is apparent. Penicillin is also secreted by the tubule, but it is a much more polar compound and is not reabsorbed. The effect of probenecid is to *decrease* the excretion of penicillin by inhibition of its secretion. Uric acid, on the other hand, is largely reabsorbed in man by active transport, although there is also a simultaneous secretory component; it is not soluble in lipid. Probenecid *increases* the urinary excretion of uric acid by inhibition of reabsorption. Since such an action must be on a carrier-mediated process rather than on diffusion, it follows that probenecid and uric acid must share the same reabsorptive transport system. While such a mechanism is not demonstrable in studies limited to probenecid alone, it becomes apparent through the action of probenecid on other compounds. And finally, when the urine is acidic, the excretion of salicylate and probenecid are both minimal and there is *no effect* of one on the other. In an alkaline urine, however, both are excreted at a high rate and probenecid *inhibits* the excretion of salicylate by competition for the carrier-mediated transport system that is apparently shared by both compounds.

Action of Uricosuric Agents. A uricosuric agent is a drug that increases the rate of excretion of uric acid. There is probably no class of therapeutic agents in which the observations in their entirety appear so inconsistent and at times contradictory. This results from the complexity of the transport mechanisms and from the fact that for each individual mechanism there is a marked variation in the action of a drug from one animal species to another. Uricosuric agents have the following peculiarities: first, depending on the species of animal, a given uricosuric agent may increase, decrease, or have no effect on the excretion of uric acid; second, for a given drug and a given species, the dose of the drug may determine if the excretion of uric acid is increased or decreased; and third, depending on the exact conditions, the combined effect of two drugs may be either additive or antagonistic.

To understand these phenomena, a brief review of the renal physiology of uric acid is warranted. In man, uric acid is largely reabsorbed, and the amount that is excreted is thus but a small fraction of that which is filtered. The renal tubule of birds and reptiles secretes uric acid, and at one time it was believed that this capacity had been lost during mammalian evolution. For many years the Dalmatian coachhound was considered a unique exception in having retained the secretory capacity. Recently, considerable evidence has accumulated that most mammals have a similar secretory mechanism. It should be emphasized that, in the presence of bidirectional transport, secretion may occur even though the data on clearance indicate net overall reabsorption. Reasonable generalizations are: (1) secretion and reabsorption of uric acid occur in all mammals; (2) secretion always dominates in some and reabsorption in others; (3) in many species, including man, the relative importance of the two transport mechanisms is influenced by a variety of factors and can be affected by uricosuric drugs; (4) in all species, uric acid is transported by carrier-mediated mechanisms and not by diffusion; and (5) in those mammalian species in which the site of transport

has been satisfactorily studied, it is located in the proximal tubule, including both the convoluted and straight portions.

The *paradoxical effect of uricosuric agents* refers to the fact that, depending on dosage, a drug may either decrease or increase the excretion of uric acid. The former usually occurs at a low dose, the latter at a higher concentration. Not all agents show this phenomenon. With some drugs, such as aspirin, the biphasic effect may be seen within the normal dose range; with pyrazinamide, reduction of excretion of uric acid is the dominant action except at extremely high (experimental) doses (Weiner and Fanelli, 1975). The paradoxical effect results from differences in the sensitivity of the reabsorptive and secretory mechanisms for urate to the drug.

Although the tubular secretion of uric acid has been ascribed to the same system that secretes other organic acids, it is possible that more than a single transport mechanism is involved. However, this would mean that the two separate systems have overlapping affinities for many compounds. In addition, drugs may vary widely both in their affinity for a transport mechanism and in the capacity of that mechanism to transport the drug in question. In view of the complex transport patterns exhibited by these compounds, it is not surprising that there should be multiple regulatory factors. Several may be mentioned. First, there is considerable evidence that the critical concentration of a uricosuric agent is not that in the plasma but the concentration that develops within the tubular fluid (Mudge *et al.*, 1973; Weiner and Fanelli, 1975). This concentration is obviously subject to all the factors that influence both the reabsorption of the tubular fluid and the excretion of the drug in question. Second, if one considers the effects of multiple compounds, either endogenous or exogenous, on urate transport, it is apparent that any compound (or drug) could either act directly on the transport of uric acid or act indirectly by influencing the transport of another compound. The latter possibility is probably responsible for the often unpredictable results obtained when two uricosuric agents are administered together. And third, although a certain structure-activity relationship is apparent within a given series of drugs, it is remarkable that there is almost no sound basis on which to predict what type of effect, if any, a drug will have on the excretion of uric acid. Only a few drugs are prescribed as uricosuric agents; a far greater number have the same action but are prescribed primarily for other reasons. These include such diverse classes as anticoagulants, analgesics, and cholecystographic agents. In almost all instances the drugs in question are organic acids or give rise to acidic metabolites. In the few instances in which organic bases have been held suspect, the possibility of acidic metabolites has not been rigorously excluded. Indeed, any acidic drug, regardless of its primary pharmacological action, should be considered to have the potential to affect the excretion of uric acid until proven otherwise.

PROBENECID

History. Probenecid was developed as a result of a planned approach to achieve a specific objective. When penicillin was first introduced, it was in critically short supply and the rapid renal excretion of the antibiotic was thus of practical significance. For this reason, Beyer and associates began a study to find an organic acid that would depress the tubular secretion of penicillin in the manner described above. The first compound to be evaluated clinically was CARINAMIDE. It proved to be effective, but the drug was secreted by the renal tubules fairly rapidly so that it was necessary to give frequent doses. This problem was overcome with the discovery of probenecid (Beyer et al., 1951).

Chemistry. Probenecid is a highly lipid-soluble benzoic acid derivative (pK_a 3.4) with the following structural formula:

Probenecid

Various congeners of probenecid have been studied. Increasing the size of the N-alkyl substitution results in more efficient compounds. Optimal activity appears in probenecid, the N-dipropyl derivative. Gutman (1966) has reviewed the structure-activity relationship of probenecid congeners and that of other uricosuric drugs.

Pharmacological Actions. The actions of probenecid are largely confined to inhibition of the transport of organic acids across epithelial barriers. This is most important for the *renal tubule*, in which tubular secretion of many drugs and drug metabolites is inhibited

(Weiner et al., 1964; Diamond, 1978). The renal action of probenecid reduces the concentrations of certain compounds in the urine and raises them in the plasma. This is a desirable therapeutic effect in the case of penicillin and related antibiotics that have a beneficial systemic action, but it may be undesirable with an agent such as nitrofurantoin when it is employed as a urinary antiseptic. When tubular secretion of a substance is inhibited, its final concentration in the urine is determined by the degree of filtration, which in turn is a function of binding to plasma protein, and by the degree of reabsorption. The significance of each of these factors varies widely with different compounds.

Uric Acid. Uric acid is the only important endogenous compound whose excretion is known to be increased by probenecid. This results from inhibition of its reabsorption (*see* above). The uricosuric action of probenecid is blunted by the administration of aspirin.

Miscellaneous Substances. Probenecid inhibits the tubular secretion of a number of drugs such as indomethacin and methotrexate, but there is no clinical indication for the coadministration of probenecid. In the case of a number of endogenous or exogenous organic acids whose rate of excretion is determined for diagnostic purposes, misleading values may be obtained if the patient is receiving probenecid. Substances of interest include para-aminohippurate (PAH), phenolsulfonphthalein (PSP), and 5-hydroxyindoleacetic acid (5-HIAA). In contrast to the older agent iodopyracet (DIODRAST), the excretion of modern urographic contrast agents, such as diatrizoate, is not inhibited by probenecid since tubular secretion is not involved.

Cerebrospinal Fluid. Probenecid inhibits the transport of 5-HIAA and other acidic metabolites of cerebral monoamines from the subarachnoid space to the plasma. This has been the subject of recent interest in psychopharmacology (*see* Van der Poel et al., 1977). The transport of drugs such as penicillin G may also be affected (Spector and Lorenzo, 1974; *see* Chapter 50).

Biliary Excretion. Since probenecid and some of its metabolites may be secreted into the bile, it is not surprising that probenecid depresses the biliary secretion of other compounds, including the diagnostic agents indocyanine green and sulfobromophthalein (BSP). The inhibition of biliary secretion also has implications in the use of rifampin for the treatment of tuberculosis. Higher concentrations of the antibiotic are achieved in plasma if probenecid is administered concurrently; this may be of economic significance (Guarino and Schanker, 1968; Kenwright and Levi, 1973).

Absorption, Fate, and Excretion. Probenecid is completely absorbed after oral administration. Peak concentrations in plasma are reached in 2 to 4 hours. While their rate of decline is rather variable, the half-life of the drug in the plasma is about 9 hours. Between 85 and 95% of the drug is bound to plasma albumin. The small unbound portion gains access to the glomerular filtrate; a much larger portion is actively secreted by the proximal tubule. The high lipid solubility of the undissociated form results in virtually complete absorption by back diffusion unless the urine is markedly alkaline. A small amount of probenecid glucuronide appears in the urine. It is also hydroxylated to metabolites that retain their carboxyl function and have uricosuric activity (Israeli *et al.*, 1972).

Preparations and Dosage. *Probenecid*, U.S.P. (BENEMID), is a white crystalline, odorless powder. The free acid is insoluble in water, but the sodium salt is freely soluble. The compound is marketed as oral tablets (500 mg). The dosage schedule depends upon the objectives of therapy. To block effectively the renal excretion of penicillin, a total daily dose of 2 g is employed in adults. This is administered in four divided doses. The total daily dose for children is from 10 to 25 mg/kg of body weight. In the treatment of chronic gout, a single daily dose of 250 mg is given for 1 week, following which 500 mg is administered twice daily. In some patients it may be necessary to increase the daily dose gradually to a maximum of 2 g, given in four divided portions.

Adjunct in Penicillin Therapy. The oral administration of probenecid in conjunction with penicillin G results in higher and more prolonged concentrations of the antibiotic in plasma than when penicillin is given alone. The elevation in the plasma level is at least twofold and sometimes much greater. Although the reduction of a daily dose of penicillin G from 1 million to 500,000 units has very little significance, a reduction by 50% or more may be of importance for convenience in the treatment of resistant infections that may require the administration of penicillin G in very large doses.

Probenecid is also included in regimens that can be completed during one visit to the physician for the treatment and prophylaxis of gonococcal infections (*see* Chapter 50).

Untoward Reactions and Precautions. Probenecid is well tolerated by most patients. Some degree of gastrointestinal irritation is experienced by at least 2% of patients; the incidence is considerably higher after large doses. Cautious administration is advised in patients with a history of peptic ulcer. Most reports place the incidence of hypersensitivity reactions, usually mild skin rashes, between 2 and 4%. More serious hypersensitivity reactions occur, but they are rare. The nephrotic syndrome has been reported as a toxic reaction. The appearance of a rash during the concurrent administration of probenecid and penicillin G or a congener presents the physician with an awkward diagnostic dilemma. The compound also increases to some degree the concentration of sulfonamide in the blood. Huge overdosage of probenecid results in stimulation of the central nervous system, convulsions, and death from respiratory failure (McKinney *et al.*, 1951).

SULFINPYRAZONE

History. Despite its therapeutic efficacy as an anti-inflammatory and uricosuric agent, phenylbutazone (*see* Chapter 29) has undesirable side effects severe enough to preclude its continuous use. For this reason, a number of congeners were evaluated for uricosuric and anti-inflammatory activity. One of these, in which a phenyl-thioethyl configuration replaces the butyl side chain of the parent compound, displayed promising activity. When the metabolites of the new compound were studied, it was found that side chain oxidation *in vivo* led to the formation of the sulfoxide, *sulfinpyrazone*, which was a potent uricosuric agent (Gutman *et al.*, 1960).

Chemistry. The chemical structure of sulfinpyrazone is as follows:

Sulfinpyrazone

It is a strong organic acid (pK_a 2.8) that readily forms soluble salts. Burns and coworkers (1958) studied a number of congeners; they found that a low pK_a and polar side chain substitutions favor uricosuric activity (*see also* Gutman, 1966).

Pharmacological Actions. Sulfinpyrazone in sufficient dosage is a potent inhibitor of the renal tubular reabsorption of uric acid. As with other uricosuric agents, small doses may reduce the excretion of uric acid. Like probenecid, sulfinpyrazone reduces the renal tubular secretion of many other organic anions. The drug may induce hypoglycemia by decreasing the excretion of the sulfonylurea oral hypoglycemic agents. The uricosuric action of sulfinpyrazone is additive to that of probenecid and phenylbutazone but is mutually antagonistic to that of the salicylates (Yü et al., 1963). Sulfinpyrazone is strongly bound to site I of human plasma albumin and therefore displaces other anionic drugs that have their highest binding affinity for the same site (Sudlow et al., 1975).

Sulfinpyrazone lacks the anti-inflammatory and analgesic properties of its congener, phenylbutazone.

Platelet Aggregation. The effect of sulfinpyrazone on platelet function is discussed in Chapter 58.

Absorption, Fate, and Excretion. Sulfinpyrazone is well absorbed after oral administration. It is bound to plasma proteins to the extent of 98 to 99%. The half-life of the drug in plasma after its intravenous injection is about 3 hours. After oral administration, however, its uricosuric effect may persist for as long as 10 hours. Although little sulfinpyrazone is available for filtration at the glomerulus, it is secreted by the proximal tubule and undergoes little passive back diffusion. Approximately half of the orally administered dose appears in the urine within 24 hours. Most of the drug (90%) in the urine is unchanged; the remainder is eliminated as the N^1-*p*-hydroxyphenyl metabolite, which also is a potent uricosuric substance. (For details, *see* Burns et al., 1957; Gutman et al., 1960; Dayton et al., 1961.)

Preparations and Dosage. *Sulfinpyrazone,* U.S.P. (ANTURANE), is available as official 100-mg tablets and 200-mg capsules. For the treatment of *chronic gout,* the initial dosage is 100 to 200 mg per day. After the first week, the dose may be gradually increased until a satisfactory lowering of plasma uric acid is achieved and maintained. This may require from 100 to 400 mg per day, divided in two to four doses and preferably given with meals. Occasional resistant patients have been treated successfully with doses as high as 800 mg per day. Larger doses are poorly tolerated and unlikely to produce a further uricosuric effect in the resistant patient.

Untoward Reactions and Precautions. *Gastrointestinal irritation* occurs in 10 to 15% of all patients receiving sulfinpyrazone, and an occasional patient may require discontinuance of its use. Gastric distress is lessened when the drug is taken in divided doses with meals. Sulfinpyrazone should be given to patients with a history of peptic ulcer only with the greatest caution. *Hypersensitivity* reactions, usually a rash with fever, do occur, but less frequently than with probenecid. The severe blood dyscrasias and salt and water retention, hazards of phenylbutazone therapy (*see* Chapter 29), have not been observed during sulfinpyrazone therapy. However, depression of hematopoiesis has been demonstrated experimentally, and periodic blood-cell counts are therefore advised during prolonged therapy.

BENZBROMARONE

This is a potent uricosuric agent that has been used in Europe and is currently undergoing clinical trials in the United States. It has the following structural formula:

Benzbromarone

The drug is readily absorbed after oral ingestion, and peak concentrations in blood are achieved in about 4 hours. It is metabolized to the monobromine and dehalogenated derivatives, both of which have uricosuric activity, and is principally excreted in the bile. The uricosuric action is blunted by aspirin or sulfinpyrazone and is abolished by pyrazinamide. No paradoxical retention of urate has been observed. At clinically effective doses there is no effect on the synthesis of urate. Therefore, benzbromarone probably reduces the concentration of urate in plasma solely by inhibiting its tubular reabsorption. Its action on the tubular transport of other organic acids has not been systematically examined.

Benzbromarone (EXURATE) is of interest as a member of a new chemical class of uricosuric agents. As the micronized powder it is effective in a single daily dose of 40 to 80 mg, which makes it significantly more potent than other uricosuric drugs. It may be useful clinically in patients who are either allergic or refractory to other drugs used for the treatment of gout (Delbarre et al., 1967; Sinclair and Fox, 1975; Yü, 1976).

THE CLINICAL USE OF URICOSURIC AGENTS

This subject is described in Chapter 29 in conjunction with the discussion of other types of drugs that are also used for the treatment of gout and other syndromes characterized by hyperuricemia.

Beyer, K. H.; Russo, H. F.; Tillson, E. K.; Miller, A. K.; Verwey, W. F.; and Gass, S. R. BENEMID, *p*-(di-*n*-propylsulfamyl)-benzoic acid: its renal affinity and its elimination. *Am. J. Physiol.,* **1951**, *166*, 625–640.

Burns, J. J.; Yü, T.-F.; Dayton, P. G.; Berger, L.; Gutman, A. B.; and Brodie, B. B. Relationship between pK_a and uricosuric activity in phenylbutazone analogues. *Nature,* **1958**, *182*, 1162–1163.

Burns, J. J.; Yü, T.-F.; Ritterbrand, A.; Perel, J. M.; Gutman, A. B.; and Brodie, B. B. A potent new uricosuric agent, the sulfoxide metabolite of the phenylbutazone analogue G25671. *J. Pharmacol. Exp. Ther.,* **1957**, *119*, 418–426.

Dayton, P. G.; Secam, L. E.; Landrau, M.; and Burns, J. J. Metabolism of sulfinpyrazone and other thio analogues of phenylbutazone in man. *J. Pharmacol. Exp. Ther.,* **1961**, *132*, 287–390.

Delbarre, F.; Auscher, C.; Oliver, J.; and Rose, A. Traitement des hyperuricémics et de la goutte par des dérivés du benzofuranne. *Sem. Hop. Paris,* **1967**, *43*, 1127–1133.

Diamond, H. S. Uricosuric drugs. In, *Uric Acid.* (Kelley, W. N., and Weiner, I. M., eds.) Springer-Verlag, Berlin, **1978**, pp. 459–484.

Guarino, A. M., and Schanker, L. S. Biliary excretion of probenecid and its glucuronide. *J. Pharmacol. Exp. Ther.,* **1968**, *164*, 387–395.

Gutman, A. B.; Dayton, P. G.; Yü, T.-F.; Berger, L.; Chen, W.; Sicam, L. E.; and Burns, J. J. A study of the inverse relationship between pK_a and rate of renal excretion of phenylbutazone analogues in man and dogs. *Am. J. Med.,* **1960**, *29*, 1017–1033.

Israeli, Z. H.; Perel, J. M.; Cunningham, R. F.; Dayton, P. G.; Yü, T.-F.; Gutman, A. B.; Long, K. R.; Long, R. C., Jr.; and Goldstein, J. H. Metabolites of probenecid. Chemical, physical, and pharmacological studies. *J. Med. Chem.,* **1972**, *15*, 709–716.

Kenwright, S., and Levi, A. J. Impairment of hepatic uptake of rifamycin antibiotics by probenecid and its therapeutic implications. *Lancet,* **1973**, *2*, 1401–1405.

McKinney, S. E.; Peck, H. M.; Bochey, J. M.; Byham, B. B.; Schuchardt, G. S.; and Beyer, K. H. BENEMID, *p*-(di-*n*-propylsulfamyl)-benzoic acid: toxicological properties. *J. Pharmacol. Exp. Ther.,* **1951**, *102*, 208–214.

Sinclair, D. S., and Fox, I. H. The pharmacology of hypouricemic effect of benzbromarone. *J. Rheumatol.,* **1975**, *2*, 437–445.

Spector, R., and Lorenzo, A. V. The effects of salicylate and probenecid on the cerebrospinal fluid transport of penicillin, aminosalicylic acid and iodide. *J. Pharmacol. Exp. Ther.,* **1974**, *188*, 55–65.

Sudlow, G.; Birkett, D. J.; and Wade, D. N. The characterization of two specific drug binding sites on human serum albumin. *Mol. Pharmacol.,* **1975**, *11*, 824–832.

Van der Poel, F. W.; Van Praag, H. M.; and Korf, J. Evidence for a probenecid-sensitive transport system of acid monamine metabolites from the spinal subarachnoid space. *Psychopharmacology,* **1977**, *52*, 35–40.

Weiner, I. M.; Blanchard, K. C.; and Mudge, G. H. Factors influencing renal excretion of foreign organic acids. *Am. J. Physiol.,* **1964**, *207*, 953–963.

Weiner, I. M., and Fanelli, G. M., Jr. Renal urate excretion in animal models. *Nephron,* **1975**, *14*, 33–47.

Yü, T.-F. Pharmacokinetic and clinical studies of a new uricosuric agent—benzbromarone. *J. Rheumatol.,* **1976**, *3*, 305–312.

Yü, T.-F.; Dayton, P. G.; and Gutman, A. B. Mutual suppression of the uricosuric effects of sulfinpyrazone and salicylate: a study in interactions between drugs. *J. Clin. Invest.,* **1963**, *42*, 1330–1339.

Monographs and Reviews

Fanelli, G. M., Jr. Drugs affecting the renal handling of uric acid. In, *Methods in Pharmacology,* Vol. 4A. (Martinez-Maldonado, M., ed.) Plenum Press, New York, **1976**, pp. 269–292.

Gutman, A. B. Uricosuric drugs, with special reference to probenecid and sulfinpyrazone. *Adv. Pharmacol.,* **1966**, *4*, 91–142.

Kelley, W. N., and Weiner, I. M. (eds.). *Uric Acid.* Springer-Verlag, Berlin, **1978**.

Mudge, G. H.; Berndt, W. O.; and Valtin, H. Tubular transport of urea, glucose, phosphate, uric acid, sulfate, and thiosulfate. In, Sect. 8, *Renal Physiology. Handbook of Physiology.* (Orloff, J., and Berliner, R. W., eds.) American Physiological Society, Washington, D. C., **1973**, pp. 587–652.

Rennick, B. R. Proximal tubular transport and renal metabolism of organic cations and catechol. In, *Methods in Pharmacology,* Vol. 4A. (Martinez-Maldonado, M., ed.) Plenum Press, New York, **1976**, pp. 335–356.

Torretti, J., and Weiner, I. M. The renal excretion of drugs. In, *Methods in Pharmacology,* Vol. 4A. (Martinez-Maldonado, M., ed.) Plenum Press, New York, **1976**, pp. 357–379.

Weiner, I. M. Transport of weak acids and bases. In, Sect. 8, *Renal Physiology. Handbook of Physiology.* (Orloff, J., and Berliner, R. W., eds.) American Physiological Society, Washington, D. C., **1973**, pp. 521–554.

Drugs Affecting Uterine Motility

In this section, only the uterine-stimulating and uterine-relaxing agents are discussed. The effects of estrogens, androgens, and anterior pituitary hormones on the reproductive system are presented elsewhere.

39 OXYTOCIN, PROSTAGLANDINS, ERGOT ALKALOIDS, AND OTHER AGENTS

Theodore W. Rall and Leonard S. Schleifer

Many drugs have the capacity to stimulate the smooth muscle of the uterus. However, only a few have effects that are sufficiently selective and predictable to justify their use as uterine-stimulating (or oxytocic) agents in obstetrical practice. These are *oxytocin,* certain of the *prostaglandins,* and the ergot alkaloids *ergonovine* and *methylergonovine.* Each, in appropriate doses during pregnancy, is capable of eliciting graded increases in uterine motility from a moderate increase in the rate and force of spontaneous motor activity to sustained "tetanic" contraction, while causing minimal side effects in healthy subjects. Although these agents have other physiological and pharmacological effects that will be described, the dangers as well as the value of their use in obstetrics reside largely in this single common action.

The prostaglandins are the latest group of uterine-stimulating agents to be studied. Discussion in this chapter will be limited to the effects of prostaglandins of the E and F types on the uterus and their potential for use as abortifacients and as uterine-stimulating agents at term. The general discussion of the prostaglandins appears in Chapter 28.

Several drugs, including β-adrenergic agonists, alcohol, and inhibitors of prostaglandin synthesis, have been used to inhibit uterine contractility. The general discussion of the pharmacology of these compounds appears in Chapters 8, 18, and 29, respectively. Only their therapeutic use in obstetrics is discussed below.

Physiological and Anatomical Considerations. Uterine smooth muscle is characterized by a high degree of spontaneous electrical and contractile activity. Waves of decreased membrane potential with superimposed spike activity are associated with contraction. Cell-to-cell spread of excitation occurs. Increased frequency and duration of spike activity in "pacemaker" areas and more extensive spread of excitation are associated with increases in force of contraction. Widespread depolarization of the myometrium, for example, by high concentrations of potassium ion *in vitro,* results in sustained contracture. As in most excitable tissues, movement of sodium ions appears to play the primary role in depolarization, whereas calcium ions are required for excitation-contraction coupling. The availability of calcium ion strongly influences the response of uterine smooth muscle to physiological and pharmacological stimulation and inhibition.

The uterus has parasympathetic and sympathetic innervation, the former by way of the pelvic nerve and the latter by way of postganglionic fibers from the inferior mesenteric and hypogastric ganglia. Both can elicit increased activity in the mature human uterus, but denervation causes little change in uterine motor activity. Both α-(excitatory)- and β-(inhibitory, hyperpolarizing)-adrenergic receptors are clearly demonstrable in the myometrium of mammals. Stimulation of sympathetic nerves supplying the uterus also causes vasoconstriction. Uterine contractile activity is inhibited by local anesthetics and by direct-acting smooth muscle relaxants such as papaverine, nitroglycerin, and caffeine. However, these drugs lack selectivity.

Uterine smooth muscle is unusually susceptible to endocrine influence, especially that of the estrogens. Thus, spontaneous activity, as well as responsiveness to neurogenic, hormonal, and pharmacological stimulation, increases greatly at puberty and varies thereafter with the ovulatory cycle. In some species, progesterone markedly inhibits uterine activity. Whether progesterone has an important physiological role in regulating the motor activity of the human uterus has yet to be clearly demonstrated.

Experimental Evaluation of Drugs Affecting Uterine Motility. The study of the uterus is complicated by many factors, such as the alterations in its behavior occasioned by physiological variables (maturity, endocrine milieu, period of gestation, etc.). Confusion is compounded by the marked species variations among the experimental animals that have been studied and between these and the human female. *In vitro*, the responses of uterine smooth muscle are strongly influenced by the concentrations not only of calcium but also of magnesium, potassium, and other ions in the bathing medium. The smooth muscle of the cervical region often responds differently than that of the body of the uterus. It is not surprising that there are many conflicting reports of the effects of drugs on this organ. Unless otherwise stated, the effects of the drugs to be discussed are those that have been confirmed in human beings.

OXYTOCIN AND POSTERIOR PITUITARY EXTRACTS

The structure, formation, storage, and release of the neurohypophyseal hormones, oxytocin and antidiuretic hormone (ADH), and a comparison of their biological activities have been presented in Chapter 37. The following discussion will deal in more detail with the physiological and pharmacological properties of oxytocin. This hormone has slight, but not insignificant, antidiuretic and vascular activity that may become manifest when large doses are used (*see* below).

Physiological Role of Oxytocin. Oxytocin has stimulant effects on the smooth muscle of the uterus and mammary gland so potent and selective as to suggest that the polypeptide serves a true hormonal function at these sites. Oxytocin elicits contractions of the fundus that are indistinguishable in amplitude, duration, and frequency from those seen in late pregnancy and during spontaneous labor. However, a direct link between endogenous oxytocin and the onset of labor has been difficult to establish. While it is clear that the appropriate sensory stimuli, arising in the cervix and vagina or in the mammillae, reflexly cause oxytocin to be released from the posterior pituitary, the concentration of oxytocin in plasma is not elevated at the onset of labor. The sensitivity of the uterus to oxytocin does, however, increase as pregnancy progresses (*see* below), and this may be important in the regulation of human parturition. Consistent with this hypothesis is the observation that the number of receptors for oxytocin increases dramatically in the rat myometrium at this time (Soloff *et al.*, 1979). It has not been shown that parturition or lactation fails to occur in the complete absence of oxytocin. However, prolonged labor has been observed and the milk-ejection reflex is absent. It is known that in domestic animals the uterine stimulation, resulting from the release of oxytocin (and ADH), facilitates the ascent of spermatozoa. A corresponding effect in the human reproductive tract has not been established. Oxytocin can thus be considered to play a facilitatory role, at least, in parturition and an essential role in the milk-ejection reflex. Its function, if any, in males is not known. (For detailed discussions, *see* Symposium, 1961; Harris and Donovan, 1966; Vasicka *et al.*, 1978.)

PHARMACOLOGICAL PROPERTIES

Uterus. Oxytocin stimulates both frequency and force of contractile activity in uterine smooth muscle. With higher concentrations, sustained decreases in resting membrane potential occur. At threshold concentrations, where there is no change in membrane potential, oxytocin initiates spike discharges, increases the frequency and number of spikes in a burst discharge, and increases the amplitude of spike discharges (*see* Kao, 1977). These effects are highly dependent on the presence of estrogen. When concentrations of estrogen are low, the effect of oxytocin is much reduced. The immature uterus is quite resistant (*see* Csapo, 1959). Although progesterone antagonizes the stimulant effect of oxytocin *in vitro*, the corresponding effect in the pregnant human uterus has been difficult to demonstrate. However, progestins have been widely used clinically to attempt to reduce uterine activity in cases of threatened or habitual abortion (*see* Chapter 61).

A very low level of motor activity prevails in the human uterus during the first and second trimesters of pregnancy. During the third trimester, spontaneous motor activity increases progressively until the sharp rise that constitutes the initiation of labor and delivery. The responsiveness of the uterus to oxytocin roughly parallels the increase in spontaneous activity. Oxytocin can initiate or enhance rhythmic contractions at any time, but in early pregnancy only very high doses elicit a response. In a study in which the effect of oxytocin infusions was carefully quantitated in terms of force, duration, and frequency of contractions, Caldeyro-Barcia and Posiero (1959) found an eightfold increase in responsiveness between the twentieth and thirty-ninth week. Most of this increase occurred during the last 9 weeks. Thus, slow intravenous infusion of a few units of oxytocin usually is effective in initiating labor at term. However, there is considerable variability among individuals and labor has been observed to occur after infusion of as little as 25 milliunits (0.05 μg) of oxytocin (*see* below).

Mechanism of Action. Binding sites for oxytocin have been demonstrated in the myometrium of a variety of mammals, including the human female (Soloff *et al.,* 1977). These sites are located on the plasma membrane of the smooth muscle cells and show the appropriate specificity of the physiological receptor for oxytocin. The mechanism for translation of receptor binding into increased frequency and force of contraction is unknown. While oxytocin causes the release of prostaglandins in several species, it is unclear if this effect is primary or if it is a result of uterine contraction. Inhibitors of prostaglandin synthesis can abolish the contractile effect of oxytocin in human myometrium *in vitro* without affecting the contractile response to prostaglandin $F_{2\alpha}$ ($PGF_{2\alpha}$) (Garrioch, 1978). The effects of prostaglandins on uterine muscle are discussed below.

Mammary Gland. The alveolar ramifications of the mammary gland are surrounded by a network of modified smooth muscle, the myoepithelium. Contraction of these cells forces milk from the alveolar channels into the large sinuses, where it is easily available to the suckling infant. This function is known as milk ejection (milk letdown, in domestic animals). The myoepithelium is highly responsive to oxytocin. Although the catecholamines inhibit milk ejection, the contraction of the myoepithelium is not believed to be dependent on autonomic innervation, but is considered to be under the control of oxytocin and the reflex pathways that initiate the release of the hormone. Oxytocin is occasionally employed to promote milk ejection when this component of lactation appears to be inefficient in nursing mothers.

Cardiovascular System. Oxytocin has a marked but transient, direct relaxing effect on vascular smooth muscle when large amounts are administered to man. A decrease in systolic and especially diastolic blood pressure, flushing, and an increase in limb blood flow are observed (Kitchin *et al.,* 1959). A reflexly induced tachycardia and increase in cardiac output accompany the depressor phase. When high doses are infused continuously, the brief fall in blood pressure is followed by a small but much more sustained rise. With decreased activity of buffer reflexes, for example, during the concomitant use of ganglionic or sympathetic blocking agents, the fall in blood pressure may be more pronounced. The amounts of oxytocin administered for most obstetrical purposes are insufficient to produce marked alterations of blood pressure. However, when very large doses are administered for therapeutic abortion or during uterine surgery, a marked fall in arterial pressure may occur, particularly in deeply anesthetized patients.

The vasodilator effect of oxytocin is independent of autonomic receptors. Infusions of oxytocin within a "physiological" dose range have sometimes been found to cause a marked increase in renal blood flow in dogs (especially in hypophysectomized dogs). (For further details of the cardiovascular effects of oxytocin, *see* Pickford, 1961; Andersen *et al.,* 1965; Nakano, 1973.)

Other Actions. No predictable changes in electrolyte excretion by the kidney occur in man during the administration of oxytocin, although an increase in sodium excretion is regularly seen when the hormone is given intravenously in experimental animals. When large doses are required for therapeutic purposes, an antidiuretic effect can occur due to the slight intrinsic ADH-like activity of the hormone. Signs of water intoxication have been observed when excessive volumes of intravenous fluids have been administered during such procedures (Saunders and Munsick, 1966). The smooth muscle of tissues other than the uterus, blood vessels, and mammary myoepithelium is not sensitive to oxytocin. In experimental studies, oxytocin, like vasopressin, in high concentrations has effects in numerous tissues that are apparently irrelevant to its primary hormonal actions (for references, *see* Farrell *et al.,* 1968).

Absorption, Fate, and Excretion. Oxytocin is effective after administration by any parenteral route. A less efficient but convenient route is the intranasal application of drops or a spray. The ready absorption of oxytocin from buccal lozenges also permits the use of the oral mucosa as a route of administration. The nasal or buccal routes of administration are reserved for uses post partum.

The distribution and fate of oxytocin in the body are much like those of ADH (*see* Chapter 37). Its half-life in plasma is short. Various investigators have estimated it to be from 1 to several minutes, and even briefer in late pregnancy and during lactation. Its rapid removal from plasma is accomplished largely by the kidney and the liver. The lactating mammary gland also inactivates a significant portion of the circulating hormone. During pregnancy, a glycoprotein aminopeptidase referred to as both "oxytocinase" and "vasopressinase" appears in plasma and is capable of inactivating either hormone by cleavage of the 1-cysteine to 2-tyrosine peptide bond. Enzyme activity in plasma increases gradually until, as term approaches, it rises steeply to high levels; these then decline after delivery. High "oxytocinase" activity is also found in the placenta and in uterine tissue during this period. These tissues are thought by most investigators to be the source of the circulating enzyme. (For details, *see* Sawyer, 1954; Berde, 1959; Lauson, 1970.)

Bioassay and Unitage. The uterine-stimulating potency of posterior pituitary extracts is determined by bioassay of their avian vasodepressor activity, which parallels uterine-stimulating activity. Activity is expressed in terms of *U.S.P. units*. The strength of the preparations of synthetic oxytocin now in use is still expressed in these units, each unit being the equivalent of approximately 2 μg of the pure hormone.

Preparations and Routes of Administration. *Oxytocin Injection,* U.S.P. (PITOCIN, SYNTOCINON), contains 10 U.S.P. units per milliliter and may be administered intravenously or intramuscularly. All commercial preparations of oxytocin are now synthetic. Oxytocin is also available in the form of *Oxytocin Nasal Solution,* U.S.P., containing 40 U.S.P. units per milliliter. For sublingual administration of the hormone, *oxytocin citrate buccal tablets* (PITOCIN CITRATE), each containing 200 U.S.P. units, are available.

THERAPEUTIC USES

The uses of oxytocin in *obstetrics* are discussed below.

Use during Lactation. Theoretically oxytocin should be of value for the relief of engorgement of the breasts during lactation and in cases of inadequacy of breast feeding in which insufficient milk ejection is felt to be a contributing factor. The hormone is administered most conveniently by the intranasal route. In cases of inadequacy of breast feeding, it is given by a single burst of the nasal spray in each nostril 2 to 3 minutes before a feeding is to begin. The procedure is often not successful. However, it is simple and without risk to the patient, and when effective it resolves a frustrating and sometimes painful problem for the patient. Oxytocin does not possess galactopoietic properties and is not useful when inadequate production of milk is the underlying problem.

PROSTAGLANDINS

The sources, chemistry, and physiological actions of this ubiquitous group of autacoids are presented in Chapter 28. They have numerous types and sites of direct action and can influence (or be influenced by) the effects of other autacoids, neurotransmitters, hormones, and drugs at these sites. In the female reproductive system, prostaglandins are found in the ovary, myometrium, and menstrual fluid in concentrations that vary with the ovulatory cycle. Following coitus, accessible portions of the female reproductive tract are also exposed to prostaglandins, which occur in high concentrations in human seminal fluid. Seminal prostaglandins can also be absorbed from the vagina in amounts sufficient to produce physiologically active concentrations in plasma. At term and during labor, prostaglandin concentrations rise in amniotic fluid and umbilical cord blood, and prostaglandin may also appear in maternal blood.

In spite of the clearly demonstrable effectiveness of the prostaglandins in stimulating (or, in a few instances, relaxing) smooth muscle in reproductive organs, their physiological role in menstruation and conception remains debatable. The semen of a number of mammalian species is devoid of prostaglandins. Although the widely used drugs aspirin and indomethacin profoundly depress prostaglandin synthesis, their use has not yet been clearly shown to influence menstruation or reproduction in patients receiving therapeutic doses.

The prostaglandins have been shown in experimental animals to participate in ovulation and luteolysis and to influence the hormonal events associated with these processes, including the pituitary release of luteinizing hormone. The possible usefulness of prostaglandins or their inhibitors for the control of fertility is under active investigation. (For reviews, *see* Horton, 1969; Higgins and Braunwald, 1972; Behrman and Anderson, 1974.)

Physiological Role of Prostaglandins in Human Parturition.

There is considerable evidence to suggest that prostaglandins play an important role in human parturition. In contrast to oxytocin, prostaglandins can induce labor if given at any time during pregnancy. Concentrations of prostaglandins in peripheral blood and amniotic fluid increase during the course of spontaneous labor, and inhibitors of prostaglandin synthesis can delay the onset of or prolong spontaneous labor (*see* Chapters 28 and 29; Thiery and Amy, 1977).

PHARMACOLOGICAL PROPERTIES

The prostaglandins can be considered to be local hormones since, with few exceptions, they exert their effects and are inactivated principally in the tissues or organs in which they are synthesized. Those found in the uterus, and in the menstrual and amniotic fluid, are of the E and F types. Clinical investigation for obstetrical use has been limited almost entirely to PGE_2 and $PGF_{2\alpha}$.

The members of the PGF series consistently stimulate contractions of both the pregnant or nonpregnant uterus. Although PGE_2 causes relaxation of nonpregnant uterine tissue *in vitro*, it has a considerably more potent uterine-stimulating action than $PGF_{2\alpha}$ during the last two trimesters of pregnancy. For the induction of labor at term, PGE_2 has been shown to be as effective as the more widely used $PGF_{2\alpha}$ or oxytocin (Karim *et al.*, 1970). The physiological response of the uterus in late pregnancy to these prostaglandins is probably indistinguishable from that to oxytocin (*see* Anderson, 1973). Some investigators have indicated that prostaglandins may show a narrower dose-response range for production of physiological contractions and the occurrence of uterine hypertonus, a potential hazard that may be avoided by very cautious stepwise increments in the rate of infusion.

Although the response of the uterus to prostaglandins also increases as gestation progresses, these agents are much more effective than oxytocin in the earlier months. For abortion in the second trimester, intra-uterine instillation by way of a cervical catheter or intra-amniotic injection of PGE_2 or $PGF_{2\alpha}$ results in a high success rate, with frequent but tolerable side effects. However, for very early abortion (menses delayed up to several weeks), the rate of success is low and serious side effects have resulted from the doses required.

The *side effects* attending the use of prostaglandins in the second and third trimester and at term are caused by their stimulatory action on the smooth muscle of the alimentary tract, that is, nausea, vomiting, and diarrhea.

Preparations and Routes of Administration. *Dinoprost tromethamine* (PROSTIN F2 ALPHA) is a solution containing the equivalent of 5 mg of prostaglandin $F_{2\alpha}$ per milliliter; it is available in 4- and 8-ml ampuls for intra-amniotic administration to induce abortion. Dosage is discussed in the final section of this chapter. *Dinoprostone* (PROSTIN E2) is available in official vaginal suppositories containing 20 mg of prostaglandin E_2. It is used to induce abortion, to evacuate the uterus in the management of missed abortion, and for treatment of benign hydatidiform mole. Dosage of these preparations is discussed in the final section of this chapter.

ERGOT AND THE ERGOT ALKALOIDS

The dramatic effect of ergot ingested during pregnancy has been recognized for over 2000 years, and it was first used by physicians as a uterine-stimulating agent almost 400 years ago. In the early years of this century, the isolation and chemical identification of the active principles of ergot were accomplished and detailed study of their biological activity was begun. The elucidation of the constituents of ergot and their complex actions comprises a most important chapter in the evolution of modern pharmacology. The ergot alkaloids are therefore discussed in detail in this and other chapters, even though the very complexity of their actions limits their therapeutic uses.

Source. *Ergot* is the product of a fungus (*Claviceps purpurea*) that grows upon rye and other grains. Rye is the most susceptible. The parasite can be found in the grainfields of North America and Europe. Rye destined for commercial sale is subject to government inspection and is rejected if it contains more than 0.3% infected grain. In dry years the rejection rate is usually less than 1%, but in other years it has been as high as 36%. Infection of other edible grain by *Claviceps purpurea* or other fungi that produce pharmacologically active alkaloids occurs, but it is less common.

The spores are carried by insects or the wind to the ovaries of young rye, where they germinate into hyphal filaments. As the hyphal filaments penetrate deep into the ovary of the rye, a dense tissue forms. This tissue gradually consumes the entire substance of the grain and hardens into a purple, curved body called the *sclerotium*. This sclerotium is still a major commercial source of ergot alkaloids.

Constituents of Ergot. Ergot has been termed a "veritable treasure house of pharmacological constituents." The substances isolated from ergot have been divided by Barger (1931) into two main groups. In the first group are those products peculiar to ergot and not obtainable from any other source. Among these are the ergot alkaloids. The second group consists of a heterogeneous collection of compounds, including several amines of pharmacological importance (*e.g.*, histamine, tyramine, isoamylamine, choline, and acetylcholine). *Claviceps purpurea* and related fungi have also been successfully grown *in vitro* by means of fermentation technics that resemble those used for the antibiotic-producing fungi. Biosynthetic pathways have been established and biosynthetic structural modifications induced.

History. The contamination of an edible grain by a poisonous, parasitic fungus spread death and destruction for centuries. As early as 600 B.C., an Assyrian tablet alluded to a "noxious pustule in the ear of grain"; and in one of the sacred books of the Parsees (400 to 300 B.C.) the following pertinent passage occurs, "Among the evil things created by Angro Maynes are noxious grasses that cause pregnant women to drop the womb and die in childbed." It was fortunate for the ancient Greeks that they objected to the "black malodorous product of Thrace and Macedonia," and therefore did not eat rye. Rye was also comparatively unknown to the early Romans, for it was not introduced into Southwest Europe until after the beginning of the Christian era. Consequently, there is no undisputed reference to ergot poisoning in the early Greek and Roman literature. It was not until the Middle Ages that written descriptions of ergot poisoning first appeared, although it is probable that the disease was prevalent long before this time. Strange epidemics were described in which the characteristic symptom was gangrene of the feet, legs, hands, and arms. In severe cases, the tissue became dry and black and the mummified limbs separated off without loss of blood. Limbs were said to be consumed by the Holy Fire and blackened like charcoal. Mention was also made of agonizing burning sensations in the extremities. The disease was called Holy Fire or St. Anthony's fire, the latter name being in honor of the saint at whose shrine relief was said to be obtained. The relief that followed migration to the shrine of St. Anthony was probably real, for the sufferers received a diet free of contaminated grain during their sojourn at the shrine. The symptoms of ergot poisoning were not restricted to the limbs. Indeed, a frequent complication of ergot poisoning was abor-

tion. A convulsive type of ergotism was also known. There still is no proven explanation as to why, in certain instances, ergotism was associated with symptoms referable to the central nervous system (CNS). The effects of ergot poisoning were described most effectively in paintings and woodcuts during the late Middle Ages (*e.g.*, Grünewald's altar paintings, now located in the museum at Colmar, France).

Ergot was known as an obstetrical herb before it was identified as the cause of St. Anthony's fire. It was mentioned as early as 1582 by Lonicer as a proven means of producing pains in the womb. It was used by midwives long before it was recognized by the medical profession. The first physician to employ ergot was Desgranges, but he did not publish his observations until 1818. Ten years before, a letter published by John Stearns in the *Medical Repository* of New York, entitled "Account of the Pulvis Parturiens, a Remedy for Quickening Childbirth," marked the official introduction of ergot into medicine (Thoms, 1931). This communication is of sufficient historical interest to quote certain pertinent portions of it:

It [pulvis parturiens] expedites lingering parturition and saves to the accoucheur a considerable portion of time, without producing any bad effects on the patient. . . . Previous to its exhibition it is of the utmost consequence to ascertain the presentation . . . as the violent and almost incessant action which it induces in the uterus precludes the possibility of turning. . . . If the dose is large it will produce nausea and vomiting. In most cases you will be surprised with the suddenness of its operation; it is, therefore, necessary to be completely ready before you give the medicine. . . . Since I have adopted the use of this powder I have seldom found a case that detained me more than three hours. . . .

The use of ergot spread rapidly in the United States, but its adoption in Europe was delayed, perhaps, as Barger (1931) has suggested, because the Old World had suffered too much from the poisonous properties of ergot. The dangers attending the use of the drug, however, were soon recognized. In 1824, Hosack wrote that the number of stillborn children had increased so greatly since the introduction of ergot that the Medical Society of New York instituted an inquiry. Said Hosack, "The ergot has been called . . . *pulvis ad partum;* as it regards the child, it may, with almost equal truth be denominated the *pulvis ad mortem.*" This astute observer recommended that the drug be used only to control post-partum hemorrhage. Thus, more than a century and a half ago, the indications and contraindications of ergot were accurately defined.

Chemistry. The ergot alkaloids can all be considered to be derivatives of the tetracyclic compound 6-methylergoline. The naturally occurring alkaloids contain a substituent in the β configuration at position 8 and a double bond in ring D (Table 39-1). The natural alkaloids of therapeutic interest are amide derivatives of *d-lysergic acid;* these compounds contain a double bond between C 9 and C 10 and thus belong to the family of 9-ergolene compounds. Many alkaloids, containing either a methyl or a hydroxymethyl group at position 8, are present in ergot in small quantities. These have been called

Table 39-1. NATURAL AND SEMISYNTHETIC ERGOT ALKALOIDS

A. AMINE ALKALOIDS AND CONGENERS

ALKALOID	X	Y
d-Lysergic acid	—COOH	—H
d-Isolysergic acid	—H	—COOH
d-Lysergic acid diethylamide (LSD)	—C(=O)—N(CH₂CH₃)₂	—H
Ergonovine (ergometrine)	—C(=O)—NH—CH(CH₃)—CH₂OH	—H
Methylergonovine	—C(=O)—NH—CH(CH₂CH₃)—CH₂OH	—H
Methysergide [1]	—C(=O)—NH—CH(CH₂CH₃)—CH₂OH	—H
Lisuride	—H	—NH—C(=O)—N(CH₂CH₃)₂
Lysergol [2,3]	—CH₂OH	—H
Lergotrile [2,3]	—CH₂CN	—H
Methergoline [1,2]	—CH₂—NH—C(=O)—O—CH₂—phenyl	—H

B. AMINO ACID ALKALOIDS

ALKALOID [4]	R(2')	R''(5')
Ergotamine	—CH₃	—CH₂—phenyl
Ergosine	—CH₃	—CH₂CH(CH₃)₂
Ergostine	—CH₂CH₃	—CH₂—phenyl
Ergotoxine group:		
Ergocornine	—CH(CH₃)₂	—CH(CH₃)₂
Ergocristine	—CH(CH₃)₂	—CH₂—phenyl
α-Ergokryptine	—CH(CH₃)₂	—CH₂CH(CH₃)₂
β-Ergokryptine	—CH(CH₃)₂	—CH₂CH₂CH₃
Bromocriptine [5]	—CH(CH₃)₂	—CH₂CH(CH₃)₂

[1] Contains methyl substitution at N 1.
[2] Contains hydrogen atoms at C 9 and C 10.
[3] Contains chlorine atom at C 2.
[4] Dihydro derivatives contain hydrogen atoms at C 9 and C 10.
[5] Contains bromine atom at C 2.

clavine alkaloids and consist principally of both 9-ergolenes (*e.g., lysergol*) and 8-ergolenes (*e.g., elymoclavine,* the 8-ergolene isomer of lysergol). A crystalline, pharmacologically active preparation was first isolated from ergot in 1906 by Barger, Carr, and Dale as well as by Kraft. This material was called *ergotoxine*. It is now known to be a mixture of four alkaloids, *ergocornine, ergocristine, α-ergokryptine,* and *β-ergokryptine*. The first pure ergot alkaloid, *ergotamine,* was obtained by Stoll in 1920. Moir reported the discovery of the "water soluble uterotonic principle of ergot" in 1932. This was subsequently determined to be *ergonovine* (also designated *ergometrine*).

The chemical structures of the alkaloids of ergot have been elucidated primarily by Stoll and associates and by Jacobs and Craig and their coworkers (*see* Rutschmann and Stadler, 1978). Optical isomerism is due to the presence of two asymmetrical carbon atoms (positions 5 and 8) in the lysergic acid portion of the molecule. Derivatives of *l*-lysergic acid (the epimer at position 5) and of *d*-isolysergic acid (the epimer at position 8) display relatively little biological activity. Upon hydrolysis, ergonovine and its derivatives yield lysergic acid and an amine; consequently they are designated as *amine alkaloids*. The alkaloids of higher molecular weight yield lysergic acid, ammonia, pyruvic acid (or a derivative thereof), proline, and one other amino acid (either phenylalanine, leucine, isoleucine, or valine) and are thus known as *amino acid alkaloids* or *ergopeptines*.

Numerous semisynthetic derivatives of the ergot alkaloids have been prepared, and several are of therapeutic interest (*see* Rutschmann and Stadler, 1978). The earliest derivatives were prepared by the catalytic hydrogenation of the natural alkaloids, yielding a series of compounds that are saturated in ring D of lysergic acid. These have been designated *dihydroergotamine, dihydroergocristine,* and so forth, and possess somewhat different pharmacological properties than do the parent alkaloids. Another ergopeptine derivative is *bromocriptine* (2-bromo-α-ergokryptine). In addition, it is possible to prepare different amides of lysergic acid. Two products of this series, lysergic acid diethylamide (LSD; Chapter 23) and lysergic acid hydroxybutylamide (*methylergonovine*), are of pharmacological interest. Methylation of the indole nitrogen of the latter compound yields 1-methylmethylergonovine (*methysergide;* Chapter 26). A large number of related compounds that are not derivatives of lysergic acid have also been prepared. These include *lisuride* (N-[6-methyl-8α-(9-ergolenyl)]-N′,N′-diethylurea), *lergotrile* (2-chloro-6-methyl-8β-cyanomethyl-ergoline), and *methergoline* (1,6-dimethyl-8β-carbobenzoxyamino-methyl-ergoline) (*see* Chapter 21).

Pharmacological Properties

The pharmacological actions of the ergot alkaloids are varied and complex; some actions are completely unrelated, and some are even mutually antagonistic. The marked effects of ergotamine on the cardiovascular system, for example, are due to simultaneous peripheral vasoconstriction, depression of vasomotor centers, and peripheral adrenergic blockade. The following presentation will be concerned primarily with the responses of the smooth muscle of the uterus and blood vessels. The actions on adrenergic receptors and vasomotor reflexes are discussed in Chapter 9; CNS effects are discussed in Chapters 21 and 23. The use of bromocryptine to control the secretion of prolactin is described in Chapter 59. A summary of the actions of representative ergot alkaloids is presented in Table 39–2.

The stimulation of vascular and uterine smooth muscle by ergot alkaloids was once thought to reflect an action that was exerted independently of receptors for other substances that cause such contractile responses. However, there is now convincing evidence that mediation by α-adrenergic receptors, tryptaminergic receptors, or both, is involved (*see* Berde and Stürmer, 1978; Müller-Schweinitzer and Weidmann, 1978). In general, the effects of all the ergot alkaloids appear to result from their actions as partial agonists or antagonists at adrenergic, dopaminergic, and tryptaminergic receptors (Table 39–2). The spectrum of effects depends on the agent, dosage, species, tissue, and experimental or physiological conditions. However, there are some aspects of the actions of ergot alkaloids that are not entirely compatible with this view: (1) while agonistic effects are generally apparent only at concentrations that are lower than those required to observe antagonism, this is not always the case (*e.g.,* the action of methysergide on cerebral blood vessels); (2) the effects of full agonists (*e.g.,* norepinephrine) are usually augmented by low concentrations of ergot alkaloids, even those with weak efficacy as partial agonists (*e.g.,* the action of ergonovine on arterioles); and (3) the contractile responses to other agents, such as acetylcholine or angiotensin, are sometimes also augmented by low concentrations of ergot alkaloids, and such synergistic effects are not always prevented by adrenergic or tryptaminergic blocking agents. These and other observations emphasize the importance of the physiological or pathophysiological state in determining the spectrum and intensity of effects produced in animals or patients.

Aside from the stereochemical considerations mentioned above, few rules governing structure-activity relationships have emerged. In general, small amide derivatives of lysergic acid are potent and relatively selective antagonists of 5-hydroxytryptamine (5-HT), while the amino acid alkaloids are usually less selective and show similar affinities as blocking agents at α-adrenergic and tryptaminergic receptors. Dihydrogenated derivatives usually have fewer and less intense agonistic actions than do the parent alkaloids. Finally, insertion of a methyl group at position 1 usually results in compounds with less affinity for receptors for catecholamines and with more selective ability to block tryptaminergic receptors.

Table 39-2. PHARMACOLOGICAL ACTIONS OF SELECTED ERGOT ALKALOIDS

	PHARMACOLOGICAL ACTIONS			
COMPOUND	Interactions with Tryptaminergic Receptors	Interactions with Dopaminergic Receptors	Interactions with α-Adrenergic Receptors	Uterine Stimulation
Ergotamine	Partial agonist in certain blood vessels; nonselective antagonist in various smooth muscles; poor agonist/antagonist in CNS	No notable actions on central or peripheral structures, but high emetic potency after intravenous administration	Partial agonist and antagonist in blood vessels and various smooth muscles; mainly antagonist in peripheral and central nervous systems	Highly active
Dihydroergotamine	Partial agonist and antagonist in a few smooth muscles; may be agonist in lateral geniculate nucleus	Nonselective antagonist in sympathetic ganglia; low emetic potency	Partial agonist in veins; antagonist in blood vessels, various smooth muscles, and peripheral and central nervous systems	Active on pregnant human uterus
Bromocriptine	Only a few weak antagonistic actions reported	Partial agonist and antagonist in various areas of CNS; presumed agonist in inhibiting secretion of prolactin; less emetic potency than ergotamine	No agonistic effects; somewhat less potent antagonist than dihydroergotamine in various tissues	Inactive
Ergonovine and methylergonovine	Partial agonists in human umbilical and placental blood vessels; selective and fairly potent antagonists in various smooth muscles; partial agonists and antagonists in some areas of CNS	Weak antagonists in certain blood vessels; partial agonists and antagonists in various areas of CNS; less potent than bromocriptine in producing emesis or inhibiting secretion of prolactin	Partial agonists in blood vessels (less than ergotamine); little antagonistic action	Very highly active
Methysergide	Partial agonist in certain blood vessels and areas of CNS; selective and very potent antagonist in many tissues and areas of CNS	Little evidence for agonistic or antagonistic activity; no emetic activity	Little or no agonistic or antagonistic action	Very little activity

943

Uterus. All the natural alkaloids of ergot markedly increase the motor activity of the uterus. The character of the changes elicited is related to the dose administered. After small doses, contractions are increased in force or frequency, or both, but are followed by a normal degree of relaxation. After larger doses, contractions become forceful and prolonged and resting tonus is markedly increased. Although this characteristic precludes their use for induction or facilitation of labor, it is quite compatible with their use post partum or post abortion to control bleeding and maintain uterine contraction. Very high doses can cause sustained contracture. The sensitivity of the uterus to ergot alkaloids varies, especially with the degree of maturity and the stage of gestation, but even an immature uterus is stimulated. The gravid uterus, however, is very sensitive, and small doses of ergot alkaloids can be given immediately post partum to obtain a marked uterine response, usually without significant side effects.

All natural ergot alkaloids have qualitatively the same effect on the uterus, but they exhibit important differences in potency. Ergonovine is the most active. It is superior to ergotamine, the most potent of the amino acid alkaloids, with respect to rapidity of onset of the uterine response following intravenous administration and activity following oral administration, and it is less toxic. For these reasons ergonovine and its semisynthetic derivative, methylergonovine, have replaced other ergot preparations as clinical oxytocics.

Methylergonovine differs little from ergonovine in its uterine actions. The dihydrogenated alkaloids do not have the uterine-stimulating properties of the parent alkaloids when tested in experimental animals. However, they are capable of exerting a marked uterine-stimulating action on the pregnant human uterus at term.

The uterine-stimulating effect of ergot alkaloids apparently involves interactions with receptors for biogenic amines, in that cyproheptadine blocks the effects of both 5-HT and ergonovine in the rat uterus (Hashimoto *et al.*, 1977), while phentolamine blocks the effects of both norepinephrine and ergotamine, but not of oxytocin, in the rabbit uterus (*see* Berde and Stürmer, 1978).

Cardiovascular System. Ergotamine, the other natural amino acid alkaloids, and the dihydrogenated derivatives exert complex actions on the cardiovascular system. These are discussed further in Chapter 9.

The natural amino acid alkaloids, particularly ergotamine, produce constriction of both arteries and veins. While dihydroergotamine retains appreciable vasoconstrictor activity, it is far more effective on capacitance than on resistance vessels. This property is the basis for investigation of its usefulness in the treatment of postural hypotension. The dihydrogenated derivatives of the ergotoxine group are considerably less active and usually produce hypotension because of effects in the CNS. In doses used in the treatment of migraine, ergotamine usually produces only small increments in blood pressure but does increase peripheral vascular resistance and decrease blood flow in various organs. These effects result in part from reduced flow through nonnutritive arteriovenous anastomoses (*see* Saxena, 1978). While less potent than ergotamine, the amine alkaloids can also raise blood pressure slightly and decrease blood flow in the extremities when administered in therapeutic doses. The intensity of pressor effects is greater when the blood pressure is elevated.

Ergot alkaloids that produce peripheral vasoconstriction can also damage the capillary endothelium. The mechanism of this toxic action is not clearly understood. Vascular stasis, thrombosis, and gangrene result and are prominent features of ergot poisoning. The propensity of these alkaloids to cause gangrene appears to parallel their vasoconstrictor activity.

Vascular Responses Related to the Therapy of Migraine. Ergotamine is effective in relieving migraine headaches, even though it is neither sedative nor analgesic. The etiology of migraine is complex and poorly understood, but it now seems clear that an attack begins with a period of unexplained diminished blood flow in some region of the cerebrum (Sakai and Meyer, 1978), during which some patients experience a subjective "aura" or display objective neurological signs and symptoms. This is followed by increased blood flow in both intracerebral and extracranial vessels and results in greatly increased amplitude of pulsations of the cranial arteries, chiefly the meningeal branches of the external carotid. These pulsations are believed to be the chief source of the pain. Factors that decrease the amplitude of pulsation, for example, digital pressure on the carotid artery, reduce the intensity of the headache, and there is a parallel decline in arterial pulsation when ergotamine provides relief from pain (*see* Wolff, 1972; Saper, 1978a). In addition to reducing extracranial blood flow, ergotamine markedly decreases hyperperfusion of regions served by the basilar artery but does not decrease cerebral hemispheric flow, which may remain elevated for several days following an attack (Sakai and Meyer, 1978). There is also some evidence that opening of arteriovenous anastomoses during an attack contributes both to regional cerebral hypoxemia and the marked decrease in resistance to flow in areas served by the carotid artery (*see* Saxena, 1978). Therapeutic doses of ergotamine, acting perhaps as a tryptaminergic agonist, cause decreased shunting of blood from the carotid artery to the jugular vein in experimental animals.

Absorption, Fate, and Excretion. The amino acid alkaloids, such as ergotamine, are slowly and incompletely absorbed from the gastrointestinal tract. Peak concentrations in plasma are achieved in 2 hours. For unexplained reasons, the concurrent administration of caffeine (100 mg per 1 mg of ergotamine) increases both the rate of absorption and the peak plasma concentration about twofold; oral and rectal preparations used in the treatment of migraine often contain such a combination. The effective intramuscular dose of ergotamine is about 10% of the oral dose, but absorption from the site of injection is slow, as judged by a latent period of about 20 minutes before the onset of the uterine response. The effective intravenous dose is about 50% of the intramuscular dose, and a uterine-stimulating effect is observed within 5 minutes.

Ergotamine is metabolized in the liver by largely undefined pathways, and 90% of the metabolites are excreted in the bile (*see* Eckert *et al.*, 1978). Only traces of unmetabolized drug can be found in urine and feces. There is evidence that ergotamine is sequestered in various tissues. This probably accounts for its long-lasting therapeutic and toxic actions, despite a half-time of about 2 hours for disappearance from plasma.

Bromocriptine is absorbed more completely after oral administration and is eliminated more slowly than ergotamine. Dihydroergotamine and dihydroergotoxine are much less completely absorbed and are eliminated more rapidly than is ergotamine. The amine alkaloids are rapidly and virtually completely absorbed after oral administration and reach peak concentrations in plasma within 60 to 90 minutes that are more than tenfold those achieved with an equivalent dose of ergotamine. A uterotonic effect can be observed within 10 minutes after oral administration of 0.2 mg of ergonovine to women post partum. Judging from the relative durations of action, ergonovine and methylergonovine are metabolized and/or eliminated more rapidly than is ergotamine. Studies on animals indicate that the principal metabolites of the amine alkaloids are hydroxylated in the A ring, while the metabolism of the amino acid alkaloids primarily involves alterations in the tricyclopeptide moiety. Nearly all of the metabolites recovered after the administration of methysergide to human subjects are devoid of the methyl group at position 1.

Ergot Poisoning. The ergot alkaloids are highly toxic and may cause acute or chronic poisoning. The former is rare and usually results from large amounts of ergot ingested in attempts at abortion. The symptoms consist in vomiting, diarrhea, unquenchable thirst, tingling, itching, and coldness of the skin, a rapid and weak pulse, confusion, and unconsciousness. The natural amino acid alkaloids are many times more toxic than their dihydrogenated derivatives. Fatal poisoning has occurred after the oral administration of 26 mg of ergotamine over a period of several days, and also following single injections of only 0.5 to 1.5 mg.

At present the epidemic form of chronic ergot poisoning arising from the ingestion of contaminated grain is seldom seen. However, the alkaloids of ergot are extensively employed in therapeutics, and poisoning from their injudicious administration is not rare. Poisoning is usually due to overdosage. There are indications, however, that increased sensitivity to ergot alkaloids may accompany febrile and septic states and disease of the liver. Several fatalities from gangrene have occurred in patients with hepatic damage who received ergotamine for relief of the accompanying pruritus. Patients with occlusive peripheral vascular disease are extremely susceptible to the vascular complications of ergotamine therapy.

In chronic ergotism, whether due to overdosage or to unusual susceptibility, striking circulatory changes develop. The feet and legs, and somewhat less frequently the hands, become cold, pale, and numb. Muscle pain occurs while walking and later at rest. Arterial pulses in the affected limbs become faint or even disappear. Eventually gangrene develops, beginning usually in the toes but sometimes in the fingers. Two factors are involved in the impairment of the circulation, vasoconstriction and intimal lesions; the latter may result in thrombi that completely occlude the smaller arteries. Additional circulatory disturbances may include anginal pain, tachycardia or bradycardia, and elevation or lowering of the blood pressure.

The most common other symptoms are *headache, nausea, vomiting, diarrhea,* and *dizziness.* Also, there may be noticeable weakness, formication, itching, and coldness of the skin. Symptoms particularly referable to the CNS are confusion, depression, drowsiness, and, rarely, convulsions, hemiplegia, tabetic manifestations, and a fixed miosis.

Methysergide has been implicated in the initiation and exacerbation of fibrotic disease of several types (*see* Chapter 26).

Complications of Ergotamine Therapy. When ergotamine is prescribed in correct dosage in the absence of contraindications, it is a safe and useful drug; few serious complications have been reported from its use in the migraine syndrome.

Nausea and vomiting occur in approximately 10% of patients after oral administration and in about twice that number after parenteral administration; there is a direct effect of the drug on CNS emetic centers. However, severe nausea is common during attacks of migraine regardless of treatment. Weakness in the legs is common, and muscle pains, which occasionally are quite severe, may occur in the extremities. Numbness and tingling of the fingers and toes are other reminders of the ergotism that this alkaloid may cause. Precordial distress and pain suggestive of angina pectoris, as well as transient tachycardia or bradycardia, have also been noted. Localized edema and itching may occur in an occasional hypersensitive patient. Most of these effects are not alarming and ordinarily do not necessitate interruption of ergotamine therapy.

Treatment. The treatment of ergotism consists in complete withdrawal of the offending drug and symptomatic measures. The latter include attempts to maintain an adequate circulation to the affected parts. Pharmacological agents that have been employed include anticoagulants, low-molecular-weight dextran, and potent vasodilator drugs. Carliner and associates (1974) have reported the successful treatment of a severe case of ergotism by the intravenous infusion of sodium nitroprusside. The initial rate of infusion was 50 μg per minute. Increase in dosage and the duration of infusion were determined by the response of the ischemic limbs and the systemic blood pressure. (*See* Chapter 32 for a further discussion of nitroprusside.)

Nausea and vomiting may be relieved by atropine or by antiemetic compounds of the phenothiazine type.

Preparations and Routes of Administration. Only a few of the purified ergot alkaloids are available for therapeutic application. *Ergotamine Tartrate,* U.S.P. (ERGOMAR, ERGOSTAT, GYNERGEN, others), is usually dispensed in the form of *Ergotamine Tartrate Tablets,* U.S.P., which contain either 1 mg (oral) or 2 mg (sublingual) of the salt, or as an aqueous solution containing 0.5 mg/ml (*Ergotamine Tartrate Injection,* U.S.P.). The drug is also available as a solution for inhalation (MEDIHALER-ERGOTAMINE); each dose delivers 0.36 mg of salt. *Ergotamine Tartrate and Caffeine Tablets,* U.S.P., and *Ergotamine Tartrate and Caffeine Suppositories,* U.S.P. (CAFERGOT, others), are also available; the official tablets contain 1 mg of ergotamine tartrate and 100 mg of caffeine, and the corresponding suppositories contain 2 mg and 100 mg, respectively. *Dihydroergotamine Mesylate,* U.S.P. (D.H.E. 45), is supplied as a solution (1 mg/ml) for injection. *Methysergide Maleate,* U.S.P. (SANSERT), is available as oral tablets containing 2 mg.

Ergonovine Maleate, U.S.P. (ERGOTRATE), is available in the form of *Ergonovine Maleate Injection,* U.S.P., which contains 0.2 mg of the salt per milliliter, and in the form of *Ergonovine Maleate Tablets,* U.S.P., which contain 0.2 mg of the alkaloidal salt. Ergonovine preparations should be kept at temperatures of 0° to 12° C and protected from light. *Methylergonovine Maleate,* U.S.P. (METHERGINE), is marketed in solution in 1-ml ampuls and in oral tablets, each containing 0.2 mg.

Ergot alkaloids, dihydrogenated (CIRCANOL, DEAPRIL-ST, HYDERGINE), are available in 0.5- or 1.0-mg tablets. Each 0.5-mg tablet contains 0.167 mg each of dihydroergocornine, dihydroergocristine, and dihydroergokryptine (dihydro-α-ergokryptine and dihydro-β-ergokryptine in the proportion of 2:1) as the mesylates.

Bromocriptine mesylate (PARLODEL) is supplied in tablets that contain 2.5 mg of the drug.

THERAPEUTIC USES

The major therapeutic uses of the ergot alkaloids fall into two categories: (1) applications in obstetrics (discussed later in this chapter), and (2) treatment of migraine. The use of bromocriptine in the treatment of Parkinson's disease is discussed in Chapter 21, while the uses related to the suppression of the secretion of prolactin are presented in Chapter 59.

Migraine. Ergotamine remains an important agent for symptomatic relief of the pain of migraine. However, before reliance is placed on ergotamine or other medications, it is important that the physician attempt to assess and correct any underlying emotional or physical stresses, dietary or hormonal factors, or ingestion of drugs that may influence the incidence and severity of attacks (*see* Saper, 1978b).

Dosage and Route of Administration. Subcutaneous or intramuscular injection is the usual method of administering ergotamine tartrate. The dose is 0.25 to 0.5 mg, and this may be repeated if the migraine is not relieved or if it recurs. No more than 1 mg should be given in 1 week. Occasionally, ergotamine may be given *intravenously,* but this route should be employed only by those who are thoroughly familiar with the use of the drug. The intravenous dose is usually 0.25 mg and must not be more than 0.5 mg. The latter amount is the maximum allowable in any 1-week period.

Tablets of ergotamine may be administered *orally* or *sublingually;* the dose is 2 mg, given as soon as the headache starts. Doses of 2 mg may be given at intervals of 30 minutes thereafter, if necessary, until a total of 6 mg has been taken. No more than 10 mg should be ingested per week.

Ergotamine may also be administered by inhalation. A single inhalation (about 0.36 mg) is used at the onset of an attack, and this may be repeated at intervals of 5 minutes to a total of six doses in 24 hours. The maximal dosage in 1 week is 12 mg (about 36 inhalations).

If a patient cannot tolerate ergotamine orally, rectal administration of a mixture of caffeine and ergotamine tartrate may be attempted. At the onset of an attack, one-half to one suppository (1 to 2 mg) may be used, and another suppository may be used in 1 hour, if necessary. No more than two suppositories per attack or five suppositories per week should be administered.

Since overdosage is the chief cause of untoward effects from ergotamine, the smallest amount effective for relief of the headache should be employed. The speed and thoroughness of the relief from pain are directly proportional to the promptness with which medication is started after the onset of an attack. If the drug is given early, the dose may be decreased considerably. If the headache has reached its peak, larger amounts of ergotamine are needed. Not only is a longer time then required for effective action but also unpleasant side effects from medication are more pronounced. It is believed by some that the use of ergotamine during the period of vasoconstriction associated with neurological symptoms is potentially dangerous, since it may promote or exacerbate cerebral ischemia. However, the available evidence indicates that ergotamine does not reduce blood flow in the cerebral hemispheres, although it may do so in the brain stem and cerebellar region (Sakai and Meyer, 1978). Nevertheless, it is advisable to use ergotamine with caution while the patient is experiencing neurological disturbances.

Efficacy. Ergotamine is effective in the vast majority of cases. The specificity of the drug for migraine is indicated by the fact that only occasionally are other types of headaches influenced. Relief is often dramatic. After parenteral injection of ergotamine, the headache may disappear in 15 minutes, but sometimes only after 2 hours or more. Oral medication is much slower in bringing relief, an average of 5 hours being required, and it may fail in severe attacks. The drug is not useful in preventing attacks. In fact, it has been claimed that, if the drug is given before the onset of the prodromal stage, an attack may be precipitated, possibly because the migraine attack is preceded by marked constriction of the involved arteries; ergotamine might tend to exaggerate such vasoconstriction. Observance of the specified maximal weekly doses is important, not only to minimize the untoward effects of the drug but also to avoid possible dependence. Patients who take ergotamine daily for prolonged periods may require increased dosage to achieve relief and may experience rebound attacks of migraine.

Dihydroergotamine in Migraine. Dihydroergotamine has also been used for the treatment of migraine, but fewer patients respond to it than to ergotamine. It is given intramuscularly in a dose twice that of ergotamine, and it is not effective orally.

Ergonovine in Migraine. Lennox reported in 1938 that ergonovine administered intravenously completely relieved the headache of patients about one half as often as did ergotamine. Since 0.2- to 0.4-mg doses of ergonovine were compared with 0.5-mg doses of ergotamine and in view of the relatively rapid oral absorption of ergonovine, it is surprising that the intervening years have seen little investigation of the possible usefulness of this agent, particularly in patients who do not require parenteral administration of ergotamine for relief. In any event, neither ergonovine nor methylergonovine is approved for the treatment of migraine in the United States, and neither agent has been mentioned in dissertations on the subject in recent years.

Methysergide and Propranolol in Migraine. While methysergide is not useful for the treatment of acute attacks of migraine, it has been found to be effective prophylactic medication. A beneficial response (reduction of the number and/or severity of attacks) has been observed in 50 to 65% of patients (*see* Saper, 1978b). There are a number of unsubstantiated hypotheses as to its mode of action. Because methysergide has prominent actions as an antagonist of 5-HT, other such blocking agents have been investigated; they are only marginally effective. Attention has also been focused on the partial agonistic actions of methysergide.

Propranolol, a β-adrenergic antagonist, has also been demonstrated to be effective for the prophylaxis of migraine and has been approved for this use in the United States (*see* Chapter 9).

Combination with Caffeine. Caffeine enhances the action of the ergot alkaloids in the treatment of migraine, a discovery that must be credited to the sufferers from the disease who observed that strong coffee gave symptomatic relief, especially when combined with the ergot alkaloids. As mentioned, caffeine increases the oral and rectal absorption of ergotamine, and it is widely believed that this accounts for the enhancement of therapeutic effects. Caffeine may also contribute to vasoconstriction in both extracranial and intracranial vessels by its capacity to increase the release of catecholamines and to antagonize adenosine-induced vasodilatation,

respectively (*see* Chapter 25). Whatever the contributing factors, some physicians prefer to obtain the augmented therapeutic response by administration of caffeine and ergotamine separately, rather than by use of fixed-dose combinations.

Contraindications. Because gangrene due to ergotamine has occurred in a number of patients with infection, sepsis is a definite contraindication. It should not be used in patients with vascular disease, such as syphilitic arteritis, marked atherosclerosis, coronary artery disease, thrombophlebitis, and Raynaud's or Buerger's syndrome. Diseases of the liver or kidney are also contraindications. Serious toxicity has been reported from the use of ergotamine in patients with pruritus (Kenney, 1946), especially when the symptom is secondary to hepatic disease. Although very large amounts of ergotamine are required to produce abortion, pregnancy constitutes an objection to use.

Other Uses. The mixture of dihydrogenated ergot alkaloids (dihydroergotoxine) has been widely employed in the treatment of senile dementias. In a few apparently well-controlled studies, patients treated with dihydroergotoxine have displayed slight improvement in some behavioral or other psychological measure (*see* Yesavage *et al.,* 1979). The mechanisms that could possibly underlie any beneficial responses are not understood, and the subject remains controversial.

Ergonovine has been used as a provocative agent during coronary arteriography to aid in the diagnosis of angina pectoris secondary to coronary artery spasm (*Prinzmetal's variant angina*) (*see* Chapter 33).

THE CLINICAL USE OF DRUGS THAT INFLUENCE UTERINE MOTILITY

There are many indications for, and contraindications to, the clinical use of agents that stimulate uterine contractions. In brief, the clearest indications are: (1) to induce or augment labor in *selected* individuals, (2) to control post-partum hemorrhage, (3) to correct post-partum uterine atony, (4) to cause uterine contraction after cesarean section or during other uterine surgery, and (5) to induce therapeutic abortion after the first trimester.

Induction of Labor. The indications for the use of uterine-stimulating agents for the induction of labor have been the subject of intense debate. As the result of hearings on the subject, the United States Food and Drug Administration issued a ruling that oxytocin is no longer indicated for the *elective* termination of pregnancy and should be reserved for those cases where continuation of the pregnancy is considered to be a greater risk to the mother or fetus than the concomitant risks of pharmacological induction. At present, evidence indicates that the benefits of elective induction are usually outweighed by the known hazards, including delivery of a premature infant, rupture of the uterus, and fetal hypoxia secondary to hypertonic uterine contractions (*see* Flaksman *et al.,* 1978).

When it is determined that a medical indication exists for the termination of pregnancy (*e.g.,* maternal diabetes, isoimmunization, hypertensive states, anemia, prolonged pregnancy with placental insufficiency), a careful assessment of the clinical variables must be made. Objective determination of fetal maturity must also be made, and the possibility of fetopelvic disproportion should be considered. Other potential contraindications to induction of labor include abnormal fetal position, evidence of fetal distress, placental abnormalities, and previous uterine surgery.

The drug of choice for the induction of labor in most cases is oxytocin. For all ante-partum indications except abortion, oxytocin should be given by intravenous infusion of a dilute solution, preferably by means of a variable-speed infusion pump. A suitable concentration for use in induction of labor at term is 10 milliunits per milliliter (10 units added to 1 liter of 5% dextrose). The infusion is started at the slow rate of 0.2 ml (2 milliunits) per minute. If no response is obtained within 15 minutes, the rate of administration can be slowly increased in increments of 0.1 to 0.2 ml (1 to 2 milliunits) per minute to a maximum of 2.0 ml (20 milliunits) per minute. The total dose required to initiate labor ranges from 600 to 12,000 milliunits, with an average of 4000.

During the entire procedure trained personnel must be present and uterine activity should be carefully monitored. If contractions become too forceful or frequent or resting tone is elevated, the infusion should be immediately discontinued. The short half-life of oxytocin (1 minute to several minutes) accounts for the rapid disappearance of the uterine-stimulating effect. Changes in fetal heart rate are useful indicators of fetal distress. Occasionally, even the cautious use of oxytocin will stimulate the uterus to a sustained tetanic contraction, which may so interfere with the placental circulation that it may be necessary to administer a general anesthetic to effect uterine relaxation. As labor progresses, it may be necessary to decrease the dosage of oxytocin or to terminate the infusion. The infusion should be maintained at the lowest possible rate that will allow adequate progression of labor (*see* Baxi *et al.,* 1980).

When employed at term, oxytocin induces labor in the majority of cases. If amniotomy is also used, as it is by many obstetricians, successful induction occurs in 80 to 90% of cases.

The prostaglandins ($PGF_{2\alpha}$ and PGE_2) are potential alternatives to oxytocin for the induction of labor. Although they have not yet been approved for this use in the United States, numerous clinical studies have demonstrated their efficacy. Because individual responses to prostaglandins, such as $PGF_{2\alpha}$ and PGE_2, are highly variable and involve a long lag period, induction of labor with these agents should be carried out by stepwise increments of the intravenous infusion of dilute solutions. As an example, Behrman and Anderson (1974) reported a schedule in which $PGF_{2\alpha}$ or PGE_2 was infused in appropriate

dosage over a period of 10 hours. In comparison with results obtained in patients who received infusions of oxytocin by a similar schedule, the prostaglandins showed no firm advantages. Efficacy was approximately equal, and an occasional patient who received $PGF_{2\alpha}$ developed uterine hypertonus. The precautions with regard to close monitoring of uterine response and fetal heart rate are the same for the prostaglandins as for oxytocin. The prostaglandins have the potential advantage of stimulating uterine contractions at any stage of pregnancy; thus, they are useful for the treatment of most cases of missed abortion, late intrauterine death, molar gestation, and premature rupture of the membranes (*see* Thiery and Amy, 1977).

Augmentation of Labor. Oxytocin should not be used for the augmentation of labor if labor is progressing, albeit slowly. The type of contraction produced often is too forceful and sustained to be compatible with the safety of mother and fetus. In normal labor, events move in an orderly and purposeful manner. Each period of uterine contraction is followed by one of relaxation that not only allows a rest period for the uterine musculature but also assures adequate placental circulation. During the first stage of labor, the cervix gradually dilates. When the uterus, under the stimulus of a drug, contracts too forcibly against an incompletely dilated and rigid cervix, the following accidents may occur: (1) the force of the contraction may drive the presenting part through the incompletely dilated cervical tissues and cause severe laceration of the mother and trauma to the infant; (2) if the soft tissues are unyielding, the uterus may rupture; and (3) the forceful tetanic contraction of the uterus may asphyxiate the fetus.

There are occasions, however, when oxytocin can be used advantageously by the experienced obstetrician to manage *dysfunctional labor.* Cases must be selected carefully and dosage regulated continuously. Oxytocin is usually effective in those patients where there is a very prolonged latent phase of cervical dilatation as well as in those cases where there is a significant arrest of dilatation or descent. When there is protracted dilatation or descent without actual arrest, a response to uterine-stimulating agents will generally not be obtained (*see* Friedman, 1978).

Third Stage of Labor and Puerperium. After delivery of the fetus, it is desirable to have the uterus firm and active. This reduces greatly the incidence and extent of post-partum hemorrhage. The use of uterine-stimulating agents for this purpose has declined in recent years, in part because of the decreased utilization of general anesthetics during delivery. When used, the usual procedure is to await delivery of the placenta before the administration of a uterine-stimulating agent. However, a recent study that compared the administration of either oxytocin or ergonovine prior to delivery of the placenta with the administration of ergonovine after placental delivery suggests that early administration of the uterine-stimulating agent may be more effective in reducing the incidence of post-partum hemorrhage

(Sorbe, 1978). In any case, it is necessary to exclude the possibility of a multiple pregnancy before the drug is given. Before the introduction of ergonovine, oxytocin was usually given intramuscularly to control post-partum bleeding. It was the drug of choice because of the rapid onset of its action. Ergonovine (or methylergonovine) is now preferred for this use because of its sustained duration of action. The intramuscular injection of 0.2 to 0.3 mg produces a rapid and lasting response. Either alkaloid may also be given intravenously in a dose of 0.2 mg if immediate action is desirable.

In the normal individual, the period of uterine involution is 8 to 10 weeks, but the process is most rapid during the first 10 days. Although it has not been definitely established whether uterine-stimulating drugs are of material benefit if involution proceeds normally, some obstetricians use small doses of either ergonovine or methylergonovine orally (0.2 mg, three times daily for 7 days) in order to lessen the possibility of bleeding and infection. However, both alkaloids at these doses have been shown to produce small but significant decreases in the concentration of prolactin in the circulation (see Flückiger et al., 1978). The possibility of interference with lactation must be considered. If involution is delayed, stimulation of the uterus is definitely helpful because delayed involution is usually associated with uterine atony. Under such conditions, ergonovine may be given orally or sublingually in doses of 0.2 to 0.4 mg, three times daily, for as long a period as is necessary to accomplish the desired results. If infection develops in the post-partum uterus, there is evidence that the use of ergonovine may limit its spread. Caution must be observed in the use of ergonovine for an extended period of time.

Therapeutic Abortion. Abortion during the *first trimester* is most commonly accomplished by means of suction curettage. No satisfactory form of drug-induced abortion during this period is yet available. Beyond the first few weeks of the *second trimester,* several alternative procedures for abortion are available. Intra-amniotic injection of a hypertonic (20%) solution of sodium chloride has been widely employed, but numerous failures occur and the procedure entails serious potential hazards for the patient. Oxytocin is not generally effective, even with infusion of relatively large doses (20 to 30 units). The *prostaglandins* have been used effectively for second-trimester abortion. For example, of the various modifications tested by Behrman and Anderson (1974), the most satisfactory results were obtained with the intra-amniotic instillation of 40 mg of dinoprost ($PGF_{2\alpha}$), followed by an additional 20 mg 6 hours later. Under these conditions, complete abortion was obtained in over 80% of 70 patients treated, and partial abortion occurred in all the remainder; most patients aborted within 24 and all within 48 hours. Dinoprostone (PGE_2) has also been used effectively in the form of a vaginal suppository. Nausea, vomiting, or diarrhea is a frequent side effect of both the intra-amniotic and intravaginal use of prostaglandins. Dilatation and evacuation may also be used to achieve abortion during the second trimester (Grimes et al., 1977). Comparison of large controlled studies of technics for second-trimester abortion has led to the conclusion that dilatation and evacuation is a safer and more effective procedure than intra-amniotic injection of either hypertonic saline or dinoprost (see Cates et al., 1978).

After spontaneous or therapeutic abortion or premature delivery, the post-partum indications for ergonovine and oxytocin to control bleeding and maintain uterine tone are similar to those after delivery at term.

Oxytocin-Challenge Test. Oxytocin has recently been used for an ante-partum test of uteroplacental insufficiency in high-risk pregnancies. Oxytocin is infused initially at the rate of 0.5 milliunit per minute; this rate is increased slowly until uterine contractions occur every 3 to 4 minutes. Concurrent monitoring of the pattern of the fetal heart rate indicates whether the contractions result in signs of fetal distress. The outcome of the oxytocin-challenge test is helpful in determining whether there exists adequate placental reserve for continuation of a high-risk pregnancy (see Freeman, 1975).

Premature Labor. A variety of pharmacological agents, including progesterone, β-sympathomimetic drugs, ethanol, and inhibitors of prostaglandin synthesis, has been used in the attempt to prevent premature labor. The ability of these drugs to improve the outcome for the infant has yet to be established clearly. In view of the obvious and potential side effects of these agents on the mother and infant, there is a need for further studies to determine the usefulness of such drugs in the treatment or prevention of premature labor (Hemminki and Starfield, 1978).

Andersen, I. W.; De Padua, C. B.; Stenger, V.; and Prystowsky, H. Cardiovascular effects of rapid intravenous injection of synthetic oxytocin during elective cesarean section. *Clin. Pharmacol. Ther.,* **1965,** *6,* 345–349.

Anderson, G. G. Induction of term labor with intravenous PGF_2: a review. *Prostaglandins,* **1973,** *4,* 765–774.

Barger, G.; Carr, F. H.; and Dale, H. H. An active alkaloid from ergot. *Br. Med. J.,* **1906,** *2,* 1792.

Baxi, L. V.; Petrie, R. H.; and Caritis, S. N. Induction of labor with low-dose prostaglandin $F_{2\alpha}$ and oxytocin. *Am. J. Obstet. Gynecol.,* **1980,** *136,* 28–31.

Behrman, H. R., and Anderson, G. G. Prostaglandins in reproduction. *Arch. Intern. Med.,* **1974,** *133,* 77–84.

Caldeyro-Barcia, R., and Posiero, J. J. Oxytocin and the contractility of the human uterus. *Ann. N.Y. Acad. Sci.,* **1959,** *75,* 813–830.

Carliner, N. H.; Denune, D. P.; Finch, C. S., Jr.; and Goldberg, L. I. Sodium nitroprusside treatment of ergotamine-induced peripheral ischemia. *J.A.M.A.,* **1974,** *227,* 308–309.

Csapo, A. Function and regulation of the myometrium. *Ann. N.Y. Acad. Sci.,* **1959,** *75,* 790–808.

Flaksman, R. J.; Vollman, J. H.; and Benfield, D. G. Iatrogenic prematurity due to elective termination of the uncomplicated pregnancy: a major perinatal health care problem. *Am. J. Obstet. Gynecol.,* **1978,** *132,* 885–888.

Freeman, R. K. The use of the oxytocin challenge test for antepartum clinical evaluation of uteroplacental respiratory function. *Am. J. Obstet. Gynecol.,* **1975,** *121,* 481–489.

Garrioch, D. B. The effect of indomethacin on spontaneous activity in the isolated human myometrium and on the response to oxytocin and prostaglandin. *Br. J. Obstet. Gynaecol.,* **1978,** *85,* 47–52.

Grimes, D. A.; Schulz, K. F.; Cates, W., Jr.; and Tyler, C. W., Jr. Mid-trimester abortion by dilatation and evacuation: a safe and practical alternative. *N. Engl. J. Med.,* **1977,** *296,* 1141–1145.

Hashimoto, H.; Hayashi, M.; Nakahara, Y.; Niwaguchi, T.; and Ishii, H. Actions of D-lysergic acid diethylamide (LSD) and its derivatives on 5-hydroxytryptamine receptors in the isolated uterine smooth muscle of the rat. *Eur. J. Pharmacol.,* **1977,** *45,* 341–348.

Hemminki, E., and Starfield, B. Prevention and treatment of premature labor by drugs: review of controlled clinical trials. *Br. J. Obstet. Gynaecol.,* **1978,** *85,* 411–417.

Karim, S. M. M.; Hillier, K.; Trussell, R. R.; Patel, R. C.; and Tamusange, S. Induction of labour with prostaglandin E$_2$. *J. Obstet. Gynaecol. Br. Commonw.,* **1970,** *77,* 200–210.

Kenney, F. R. Gangrene of the hand following treatment for pruritus of hepatotoxic origin. *N. Engl. J. Med.,* **1946,** *235,* 35–39.

Kitchin, A. H.; Lloyd, S. M.; and Pickford, M. Some actions of oxytocin on the cardiovascular system in man. *Clin. Sci.,* **1959,** *18,* 399–406.

Kraft, F. Über das Mutterkorn. *Arch. Pharm.,* **1906,** *244,* 336–359.

Lennox, W. G. Ergonovine versus ergotamine as a terminator of migraine headaches. *Am. J. Med. Sci.,* **1938,** *195,* 458–468.

Moir, C. The action of ergot preparations on the puerperal uterus. *Br. Med. J.,* **1932,** *1,* 1119–1122.

Pickford, M. Some extra-uterine actions of oxytocin. In, *Oxytocin.* (Caldeyro-Barcia, R., and Heller, H., eds.) Pergamon Press, Ltd., Oxford, **1961,** pp. 68–83.

Sakai, F., and Meyer, J. S. Regional cerebral hemodynamics during migraine and cluster headaches measured by the ^{133}Xe inhalation method. *Headache,* **1978,** *18,* 122–132.

Sanner, J. H. Substances that inhibit the actions of prostaglandins. *Arch. Intern. Med.,* **1974,** *133,* 133–146.

Saunders, W. G., and Munsick, R. A. Antidiuretic potency of oxytocin in women post partum. *Am. J. Obstet. Gynecol.,* **1966,** *95,* 5–11.

Sawyer, W. H. Inactivation of oxytocin by homogenates of uteri and other tissues from normal and pregnant rats. *Proc. Soc. Exp. Biol. Med.,* **1954,** *87,* 463–465.

Soloff, M. S.; Alexandrova, M.; and Fernstrom, M. J. Oxytocin receptors: triggers for parturition and lactation? *Science,* **1979,** *204,* 1313–1315.

Soloff, M. S.; Schroeder, B. T.; Chakraborty, J.; and Pearlmutter, A. F. Characterization of oxytocin receptors in the uterus and mammary gland. *Fed. Proc.,* **1977,** *36,* 1861–1866.

Sorbe, B. Active pharmacologic management of the third stage of labor: a comparison of oxytocin and ergometrine. *Obstet. Gynecol.,* **1978,** *52,* 694–697.

Stoll, A. Zur Kenntnis der Mutterkornalkaloide. *Verh. Naturf. Ges. (Basel),* **1920,** *101,* 190–191.

Thoms, H. John Stearns and pulvis parturiens. *Am. J. Obstet. Gynecol.,* **1931,** *22,* 418–423.

Vasicka, A.; Kumaresan, P.; Han, G. S.; and Kumaresan, M. Plasma oxytocin in initiation of labor. *Am. J. Obstet. Gynecol.,* **1978,** *130,* 263–273.

Monographs and Reviews

Barger, G. *Ergot and Ergotism.* Gurney & Jackson, Edinburgh, **1931.**

Berde, B. *Recent Progress in Oxytocin Research.* Charles C Thomas, Pub., Springfield, Ill., **1959.**

Berde, B., and Stürmer, E. Introduction to the pharmacology of ergot alkaloids and related compounds as a basis of their therapeutic application. In, *Ergot Alkaloids and Related Compounds.* (Berde, B., and Schild, H. O., eds.) *Handbuch der Experimentellen Pharmakologie,* Vol. 49. Springer-Verlag, Berlin, **1978,** pp. 1–28.

Cates, W., Jr.; Grimes, D. A.; Schulz, K. F.; Ory, H. W.; and Tyler, C. W., Jr. World Health Organization studies of prostaglandins versus saline as abortifacients: a reappraisal. *Obstet. Gynecol.,* **1978,** *52,* 493–498.

Eckert, H.; Kiechel, J. R.; Rosenthaler, J.; Schmidt, R.; and Schreier, E. Biopharmaceutical aspects: analytical methods, pharmacokinetics, metabolism and bioavailability. In, *Ergot Alkaloids and Related Compounds.* (Berde, B., and Schild, H. O., eds.) *Handbuch der Experimentellen Pharmakologie,* Vol. 49. Springer-Verlag, Berlin, **1978,** pp. 719–803.

Farrell, G.; Fabre, L. F.; and Rauschkolb, E. The neurohypophysis. *Annu. Rev. Physiol.,* **1968,** *30,* 557–588.

Flückiger, E.; del Pozo, E.; and Richardson, B. P. Influence on the endocrine system. In, *Ergot Alkaloids and Related Compounds.* (Berde, B., and Schild, H. O., eds.) *Handbuch der Experimentellen Pharmakologie,* Vol. 49. Springer-Verlag, Berlin, **1978,** pp. 615–690.

Friedman, E. A. *Labor: Clinical Evaluation and Management,* 2nd ed. Appleton-Century-Crofts, New York, **1978.**

Harris, G. W., and Donovan, B. T. (eds.). *The Pituitary Gland,* Vol. 3. University of California Press, Berkeley, **1966.**

Higgins, C. B., and Braunwald, E. The prostaglandins. *Am. J. Med.,* **1972,** *53,* 92–112.

Horton, E. W. Hypotheses on physiological roles of prostaglandins. *Physiol. Rev.,* **1969,** *49,* 122–161.

Kao, C. Y. Electrophysiological properties of the uterine smooth muscle. In, *Biology of the Uterus.* (Wynn, R. M., ed.) Plenum Press, New York, **1977,** pp. 423–496.

Lauson, H. D. Fate of the neurohypophysial hormones. In, *Pharmacology of the Endocrine System and Related Drugs,* Vol. 1. *International Encyclopedia of Pharmacology and Therapeutics,* Sect. 41. (Heller, H., and Pickering, B. T., eds.) Pergamon Press, Ltd., Oxford, **1970,** pp. 377–397.

Müller-Schweinitzer, E., and Weidmann, H. Basic pharmacological properties. In, *Ergot Alkaloids and Related Compounds.* (Berde, B., and Schild, H. O., eds.) *Handbuch der Experimentellen Pharmakologie,* Vol. 49. Springer-Verlag, Berlin, **1978,** pp. 87–232.

Nakano, J. Cardiovascular actions of oxytocin. *Obstet. Gynecol. Surv.,* **1973,** *28,* 75–92.

Rutschmann, J., and Stadler, P. A. Chemical background. In, *Ergot Alkaloids and Related Compounds.* (Berde, B., and Schild, H. O., eds.) *Handbuch der Experimentellen Pharmakologie,* Vol. 49. Springer-Verlag, Berlin, **1978,** pp. 29–85.

Saper, J. R. Migraine. I. Classification and pathogenesis. *J.A.M.A.,* **1978a,** *239,* 2380–2383.

———. Migraine. II. Treatment. *Ibid.,* **1978b,** *239,* 2480–2484.

Saxena, P. R. Arteriovenous shunting and migraine. *Res. Clin. Stud. Headache,* **1978,** *6,* 89–102.

Symposium. (Various authors.) *Oxytocin.* (Caldeyro-Barcia, R., and Heller, H., eds.) Pergamon Press, Ltd., Oxford, **1961.**

Thiery, M., and Amy, J. Spontaneous and induced labor: two roles for the prostaglandins. *Obstet. Gynecol. Annu.,* **1977,** *6,* 127–171.

Wolff, H. G. *Wolff's Headache and Other Pain,* 3rd ed. (Dalessio, D. J., rev.) Oxford University Press, New York, **1972.**

Yesavage, J. A.; Tinklenberg, J. R.; Hollister, L. E.; and Berger, P. A. Vasodilators in senile dementias. *Arch. Gen. Psychiatry,* **1979,** *36,* 220–223.

SECTION
X

Locally Acting Drugs

CHAPTER

40 SURFACE-ACTING DRUGS

Ewart A. Swinyard and Madhu A. Pathak

A large number of drugs act locally in a purely mechanical or physical manner. Although they possess both therapeutic and pharmaceutical usefulness, their pharmacological properties warrant only brief discussion. Their effects are confined to the site of application when the compounds are employed in reasonable dosage. These effects are described adequately by the names that are applied to the groups into which the drugs can be classified, namely, *demulcents, emollients, protectives, adsorbents,* and *absorbable hemostatics.* Other drugs act primarily at the site of application but have a chemical rather than a physical basis of action; they are *astringents, irritants, sclerosing agents, caustics, keratolytics, antiseborrheics, melanizing and demelanizing agents, sunscreening agents, mucolytics,* and certain *enzymes.*

DEMULCENTS

The demulcents comprise a group of compounds of high molecular weight that form aqueous solutions having the ability to alleviate irritation, particularly of mucous membranes or abraded surfaces. When applied locally to irritated or abraded tissues, the demulcents tend to coat the surface and, by mechanical means, protect the underlying cells from stimuli that result from contact with air or irritants in the environment. The demulcents are applied to the skin in the form of lotions, ointments, or wet dressings; to the gastrointestinal tract in the form of demulcent drinks or enemas; and to the throat in the form of lozenges or gargles. The demulcents also have valuable pharmaceutical properties. They mask the obnoxious taste of certain drugs, and solutions of demulcents are often used as vehicles for this purpose. They are also employed to provide stable emulsions or suspensions of drugs immiscible with or insoluble in aqueous vehicles. Chemically, the more important demulcents are either gums, synthetic cellulose derivatives, or polyhydroxy compounds; their principal uses will be briefly described.

The two most commonly employed demulcent gums are *acacia* and *tragacanth. Acacia*, N.F. (gum arabic), either in the form of the powder or as *Acacia Syrup,* N.F. (a vanilla-flavored syrup that contains 10% acacia), is employed chiefly to suspend or emulsify drugs. It is also incorporated in lozenges. *Tragacanth,* N.F. (gum tragacanth), a gum that in the presence of sufficient water swells to 50 times its original volume, is used as a demulcent base for cutaneous medication, a suspending agent for insoluble powders, and an emulsifying agent for oils administered orally. Other natural plant hydrocolloids used to a lesser extent than acacia and tragacanth include *Agar,* N.F., *Glycyrrhiza,* N.F., and *Sodium Alginate,* N.F.

The synthetic cellulose derivatives, *Methylcellulose,* U.S.P., and *Carboxymethylcellulose Sodium,* U.S.P., are widely used in contact-lens solutions and other ophthalmic preparations, and as suspending agents for nosedrops and other drugs that act locally. In addition, they are used as hydrophilic colloid laxatives (*see* Chapter 43).

The demulcent polyhydroxy compounds include *Glycerin,* U.S.P. (glycerol), *Propylene Glycol,* U.S.P., and the *polyethylene glycols.* Glycerin is a trihydric alcohol, $CH_2OHCHOHCH_2OH$, and consists of a clear, colorless, syrupy liquid that has a sweet taste. Glycerin is miscible with water and alcohol. It is extensively employed as a vehicle for many drugs applied to the skin. Diluted with rose water it is an effective lotion for chapped and roughened hands. In combination with starch it forms a jelly base known as *Starch Glycerite,* N.F., a preparation sometimes employed as an emollient and a vehicle.

Glycerin absorbs water, and, therefore, in high concentration it is somewhat dehydrating and irri-

951

tating to exposed tissue. The irritant action of glycerin accounts for its efficacy in promoting evacuation
of the bowel when used rectally in the form of a
suppository (*Glycerin Suppositories,* U.S.P.). It is also
available as *Glycerin Oral Solution,* U.S.P. (50 and
75%). When given orally, glycerin is readily absorbed
and serves as a source of calories (4.32 kcal/g).
Glycerin by oral administration is used for the management of cerebral edema, to lower ocular tension
in glaucoma, and to decrease cerebrospinal fluid
pressure (Tourtellotte *et al.,* 1972; *see* Chapter 36). It
may be employed as a sweetening agent or vehicle in
place of syrups.

Glycerin can exert systemic toxic effects when
given orally or parenterally in very large doses. The
major toxic effects (hemolysis, hemoglobinuria, and
renal failure) are a function of concentration and
route of administration. For example, glycerin does
not hemolyze red blood cells when it is prepared in
concentrations up to 40% in isotonic sodium chloride
solution (Tourtellotte *et al.,* 1972). Systemic effects do
not follow copious application to the skin.

Various congeners of glycerin are much more toxic
than the parent compound. They exert a nephrotoxic
effect and also may damage the liver. Indeed, deaths
have resulted from the ingestion of drugs dissolved
in *diethylene glycol* for oral administration (Bowie
and McKenzie, 1972), and poisonings from *ethylene
glycol* continue to occur (Parry and Wallach, 1974);
propylene glycol is said to be less toxic (however, *see*
Genel, 1978).

Propylene Glycol, U.S.P., is a clear, colorless, viscous liquid with a slightly acrid taste. It is completely
miscible with water and dissolves in many essential
oils. It is used as a solvent for oral and injectable
drugs, and is also employed in cosmetics, lotions, and
ointments, as in the water-washable *Hydrophilic
Ointment,* U.S.P. The topical application of a 40 to
60% aqueous solution of propylene glycol with occlusion has been reported to clear the skin in X-
linked ichthyosis and ichthyosis vulgaris (Goldsmith
and Baden, 1972).

Polyethylene glycols are high-molecular-weight
polymers produced by reacting ethylene oxide with
ethylene glycol or water. They have the general
formula $H(OCH_2CH_2)_nOH$. The *n* may range from 1
to a large number; hence, the molecular weights of
these substances range from 150 to about 20,000.
Substances with molecular weights up to 600 are
liquids at room temperature and resemble highly
refined petroleum oils in appearance and consistency. Those with molecular weights of 1000 to 9000
are solids at room temperature and resemble petroleum waxes such as paraffin. *Polyethylene Glycol,*
N.F. is a hard, tough solid. The polyethylene glycols
are of growing importance to the drug industry,
because of their blandness, water solubility, wide
compatibility, and low order of toxicity. They are
employed as water-soluble ointment bases similar to
Polyethylene Glycol Ointment, N.F., as ingredients of
lotions and suppositories, and as tablet coatings.
Various preparations of polyethylene glycol range in
molecular weight from 300 to 20,000.

Several proprietary water-miscible (oil-in-water)
ointment bases, such as CETAPHIL, DERMABASE, MULTI-
BASE, NEOBASE, and VANIBASE, are also available.

These bases can be readily removed from the skin by
washing and are valuable when large quantities of
liquid are to be incorporated into an ointment.

EMOLLIENTS

Emollients are fats or oils used for their local
action on the skin and, occasionally, the mucous
membranes. They are employed as protectives and as
agents for softening the skin and rendering it more
pliable, but chiefly as vehicles for more active drugs.
These oleaginous substances soften the skin by
forming an occlusive oil film on the stratum corneum, thus preventing drying from evaporation of
the water that diffuses to the surface from the underlying layers of skin. Only the commonly employed
emollients are described below.

Vegetable Oils. Official vegetable oils include
Olive Oil, N.F., *Cottonseed Oil,* N.F., *Corn Oil,* N.F.,
Almond Oil, N.F., *Peanut Oil,* N.F. *Persic Oil,* N.F.,
and *Cocoa Butter,* N.F. (*cacao butter, theobroma oil*).
With the exception of the last-named preparation, all
are fluids. When taken internally, they act as mild
cathartics and as protectives for the gastrointestinal
tract in cases of corrosive poisoning. When applied
externally, they are emollient to the skin and mucous
membranes. They also provide the vehicles for many
drugs that are injected in oily solution or suspension.
Cocoa butter is a solid that melts at body temperatures. It is widely used as a suppository and an
ointment base.

Animal Fats. The animal fat of particular pharmacological interest is *Anhydrous Lanolin,* U.S.P.
(*wool fat*). This is a yellow, unctuous mass obtained
from the wool of sheep. Wool fat is usually employed
mixed with 25 to 30% water, in which form it is
known as *Lanolin,* U.S.P. (*hydrous wool fat*). These
two semisolids are used principally as bases for ointments. Because certain individuals are allergic to
wool fat, it has been deleted from many official
formulations.

Hydrocarbons. The important emollient hydrocarbons are *Paraffin,* N.F., *Petrolatum,* U.S.P., *White
Petrolatum,* U.S.P., *Mineral Oil,* U.S.P., and *Light
Mineral Oil,* U.S.P. *Hydrophilic Petrolatum,* U.S.P., is
an ointment (water-in-oil) base characterized by the
capacity to take up large amounts of water; it contains cholesterol, stearyl alcohol, white wax, and
white petrolatum. Many official ointments have a
base composed of either white wax (5%) and white
petrolatum (95%) or yellow wax (5%) and petrolatum
(95%). The former combination is official under the
name *White Ointment,* U.S.P.; the latter, *Yellow
Ointment,* U.S.P. *Paraffin* is used mainly in ointments
to raise their melting points. *White petrolatum* is a
common ointment base and also is employed as an
emollient and a lubricant. *Light mineral oil* has been
used as a vehicle for drugs to be applied to the nasal
mucous membranes; however, aqueous vehicles are
preferred for this purpose. The more viscous *mineral
oil* is an ingredient in various pharmaceutical preparations and is used also as a laxative.

Waxes. *White Wax,* N.F. (*bleached beeswax*), and *Yellow Wax,* N.F. (*beeswax*), are employed to harden ointment bases. A base composed of lard hardened with wax is known as a *cerate. Spermaceti,* a waxy substance obtained from the head of the sperm whale, is used to raise the melting point of ointments. A mixture of oil and wax is sometimes used as a vehicle for drugs when slow absorption and sustained effect are desired; the drugs are suspended in the oil-wax vehicle, and the resulting suspension is injected intramuscularly.

A widely employed, pleasant-smelling, soft emollient preparation is *Rose Water Ointment,* U.S.P. It consists essentially of spermaceti, white wax, almond oil, rose water, and rose oil. Most of the commercial *cold creams* are modifications of this basic preparation. For example, *Cold Cream,* U.S.P., contains mineral oil in place of the almond oil.

Other proprietary water-miscible (water-in-oil) emulsion bases, such as AQUAPHOR, HYDROSORB, PLASTIBASE, POLYSORB, and QUALATUM, are also available. Although large amounts of liquids can be incorporated in these bases, they cannot be readily removed from the skin by washing.

PROTECTIVES AND ADSORBENTS

Protectives are designed to cover the skin or mucous membranes in order to prevent contact with possible irritants. Although demulcents and emollients are also protective, common usage restricts the term to certain insoluble and chemically inert substances in a very fine state of subdivision, for example, *dusting powders,* and to the several materials that form an adherent, continuous, flexible or semirigid coat when applied to the skin. Some chemically inert powders also adsorb dissolved or suspended substances, such as gases, toxins, and bacteria; these are known as *adsorbents.* Substances used internally for this purpose are described below, under *gastrointestinal protectives and adsorbents.* Unfortunately, there are no all-purpose effective protective agents; it is essential, therefore, to choose a particular substance for protection against a specific hazard.

Dusting Powders. These relatively innocuous (inert and insoluble) substances are used to cover and to protect epithelial surfaces, ulcers, and wounds. Those with a smooth surface act mainly by preventing friction; those with a porous structure, by absorbing moisture. The absorption of skin moisture also decreases friction and discourages growth of certain bacteria. The more important dusting powders include *Talc,* U.S.P., *Zinc Oxide,* U.S.P., *Zinc Stearate,* U.S.P., *Magnesium Stearate,* N.F., *Starch,* N.F., *Boric Acid,* N.F., and *insoluble salts of bismuth.* Water-absorbent powders should not be used on raw surfaces with profuse exudate, as they tend to cake and form adherent crusts. Starch becomes doughy when it absorbs moisture and requires the addition of an antiseptic (2 to 4% boric acid or 1% salicylic acid) to prevent fermentation. Zinc stearate and magnesium stearate are not wetted by moisture, and thus they permit seepage and evaporation and do not crust.

Medicated or perfumed *talc* (mainly magnesium silicate) is widely used as a dusting powder under the name *talcum powder.* Although *talc* is a benign substance when applied to the intact skin, it can induce severe granulomatous reactions when introduced into wounds or an operative field. For this reason, *talc* should never be used as a dusting powder for surgical gloves. *Absorbable Dusting Powder,* U.S.P. (BIO-SORB, EZON), is an absorbable powder prepared from cornstarch. The resulting product is mixed with 2% magnesium oxide and contains residual amounts of sodium sulfate and sodium chloride. It is used as a dusting powder for surgical gloves. It has no deleterious effect on rubber gloves, appears to produce no appreciable reaction in tissues, and is absorbed completely in a short time. This product is used only in surgery and does not replace the other uses of talc.

Dextranomer (DEBRISAN) is a new product promoted for the debridement of secreting wounds, such as *venous stasis ulcers, decubitus ulcers, infected traumatic* and *surgical wounds,* and *infected burns.* It consists of spherical hydrophilic beads of dextranomer, 0.1 to 0.3 mm in diameter. The beads, composed of a three-dimensional network of macromolecular chains of cross-linked dextran, allow substances with a molecular weight of less than 1000 to enter freely; those with a molecular weight of 1000 to 5000 enter less freely, and higher-molecular-weight substances are excluded from the beads. Each gram of dextranomer absorbs approximately 4 ml of water; this action is continuous as long as unsaturated beads are in proximity to the wound. The rapid and continuous removal of exudate from the surface of the wound results in a marked reduction in *inflammation, edema,* and *pain* and appears to enhance the formation of granulation tissue and reduce the time for wound healing.

Mechanical Protectives. Agents in this category are used to provide occlusive protection from the external environment, to give mechanical support, and as vehicles for various medicaments. *Collodion,* U.S.P., pyroxylon (5%) in an ether-alcohol vehicle, and *Flexible Collodion,* U.S.P., composed of collodion with camphor (2%) and castor oil (3%), are occasionally used to seal small wounds and as vehicles for medicated collodions. *Zinc Gelatin,* U.S.P., a smooth jelly composed of zinc oxide (10%) and gelatin (15%) in a glycerin-water vehicle, is spread between layers of bandage and used as a protective dressing and support for varicosities and similar lesions. The dressing may be removed by soaking with warm water.

Dimethicone (SILICOTE), a relatively inert silicone oil with skin-adherent and water-repellent properties, is used to protect the skin against exposure to ordinary soap, water, and dermal irritants such as cleansers, decomposition products of urine, and other substances. It is available as an ointment (30%), cream (30%), or spray (33⅓%).

Gastrointestinal Protectives and Adsorbents. The principal gastrointestinal protectives and adsorbents include *magnesium trisilicate, aluminum hydroxide, activated charcoal, kaolin,* and *pectin.*

Magnesium Trisilicate, U.S.P., a relatively weak

antacid, is an effective gastrointestinal adsorbent. The gelatinous silicon dioxide, formed by the reaction of magnesium trisilicate with the gastric contents, is said to protect ulcerated mucosal surfaces and favor healing. The salt also interferes with the absorption of tetracyclines, anticholinergics, and other drugs. It is usually given orally suspended in water, in a dose of 1 g four times a day. Chronic use may rarely result in silica kidney stones.

A number of aluminum compounds, such as *Aluminum Hydroxide Gel*, U.S.P., *Dried Aluminum Hydroxide Gel*, U.S.P., and *Aluminum Phosphate Gel*, U.S.P., are used as adsorbents. These substances also decrease the absorption of tetracyclines, anticholinergics, and other drugs. Since they neutralize hydrochloric acid so efficiently, they are discussed under the gastric antacids (Chapter 42).

Activated Charcoal, U.S.P., an odorless, tasteless, fine black powder, is the residue from the destructive distillation of various organic materials, treated to increase its adsorptive power. The adsorptive capacity of various brands of activated charcoal differs enormously; a finely powdered activated charcoal with a high adsorptive capacity, such as ACTIVATED CHARCOAL–MERCK, NORIT A, and NUCHAR C, has been reported to be satisfactory (Picchioni *et al.*, 1974); however, AMOCO GRADE PX-21 has been reported to adsorb nearly three times as much sodium salicylate from simulated gastric juice as does the first-named brand (Cooney, 1977). Activated charcoal, because of its broad spectrum of adsorptive activity and its rapidity of action, is considered to be the most valuable single agent for the emergency treatment of oral drug poisoning (*see* Chapter 68).

Kaolin, U.S.P., is a native, hydrated aluminum silicate, powdered and freed from gritty particles by elutriation. It is used internally and externally for its adsorbent properties.

Pectin, U.S.P., is a purified carbohydrate product obtained from the acid extraction of the rind of citrus fruits or from apple pomace. Chemically, it consists chiefly of polygalacturonic acid, some of the hydroxyl groups of which are methylated. It dissolves in 20 parts of water; the resulting colloidal solution is viscous, opalescent, and acidic. Pectin may be administered simply and conveniently in the form of ground raw apple. Kaolin mixture with pectin usually contains 3 g of kaolin and 0.67 g of pectin in each 15 ml. It is claimed to act as an adsorbent and demulcent in the treatment of diarrhea. However, adequately controlled clinical studies that demonstrate the efficacy of these popular but minimally effective antidiarrheal mixtures are lacking.

Simethicone, U.S.P. (MYLICON), a light-gray, translucent liquid of greasy consistency, is a mixture of liquid dimethylpolysiloxanes with antifoaming and water-repellent properties. It is promoted as an adjunct in the treatment of conditions in which gas is a problem, such as flatulence, functional gastric bloating, and postoperative gaseous distention. It has also been used to reduce gas shadows in radiography of the bowel and to improve visualization in gastroscopy. Clinical studies in support of these recommendations are not convincing. Simethicone is available as an official oral suspension (40 mg in 0.6 ml) and in official tablets (40 and 80 mg). The usual adult oral dose is 160 to 400 mg daily in divided doses, given after each meal and at bedtime. Simethicone is also used in combination with antacids, antispasmodics, sedatives, and digestants.

ANTIPERSPIRANTS AND DEODORANTS

Antiperspirants and *deodorants*, applied as aerosol sprays, pads, sticks, and roll-on creams, liquids, or semisolids, are vigorously promoted to the public for the control of excessive perspiration and body odor. The average adult produces from 0.5 to 1.5 liters of perspiration a day. Under normal conditions this secretion is odorless. The unpleasant odor sometimes associated with skin secretions results from chemical and bacterial degradation of the components of perspiration. Consequently, proper skin hygiene is essential to the control of body odors. Many individuals find skin hygiene inadequate and resort to preparations that decrease the flow and/or inhibit the degradation of perspiration (*see* Robinson, 1973).

Antiperspirants.   The agents most commonly used topically as *antiperspirants* include *Aluminum Chloride*, U.S.P., *aluminum hydroxychloride, aluminum phenolsulfonate, Aluminum Sulfate*, U.S.P., *zinc phenolsulfonate*, and *zirconyl hydroxychloride*. Aluminum hydroxychloride (aluminum chlorohydrate) is the most frequently employed agent. The use of aluminum chloride has declined markedly; it hydrolyzes in aqueous solution to produce aluminum hydroxide and hydrochloric acid. The acidity of such preparations has a deleterious effect on fabrics that come in contact with treated skin. Similar hydrolysis occurs with other aluminum salts of strong inorganic acids such as aluminum sulfate. Aluminum hydroxychloride has a lower acidity than aluminum chloride or sulfate but is still active as an antiperspirant; it is also an effective deodorant, possibly because of an antibacterial effect against gram-positive microorganisms. Aluminum and zinc phenolsulfonate not only are useful astringents with moderate acidity but also are soluble in alcohol, an advantage in liquid aerosol preparations. Aluminum salts are known to cause allergic reactions in susceptible individuals. Zirconium salts, except for the hydroxychloride, have been discarded because of the marked incidence of associated granulomas of the skin.

The effectiveness of metallic salt antiperspirants results from their ability to diffuse into the sweat duct and to form an obstructive hydroxide gel *in situ*. Secondarily, the more acidic $AlCl_3$ has a necrotic effect on the sweat duct.

Deodorants.   *Deodorants* reduce the number of resident bacteria on the skin and thus inhibit bacterial decomposition of perspiration. The agents most commonly employed include *Benzalkonium Chloride*, N.F., *Methylbenzethonium Chloride*, U.S.P., and *Neomycin Sulfate*, U.S.P. These agents are not devoid of untoward side effects. Quaternary ammonium compounds such as benzalkonium are inactivated by soaps and irritate the skin if used in concentrations exceeding 1%, and the use of antibiotics may sensitize the individual and/or result in the production of resistant strains of bacteria.

Available proprietary preparations are either antiperspirant or deodorant or both, depending on the ingredients in the formulation. Consequently, allergic reactions may be induced by any of the above-mentioned agents as well as by the perfume used to scent the preparations. Diagnosis of allergic manifestations is usually not difficult, inasmuch as the allergic response is usually confined to the axilla.

ABSORBABLE HEMOSTATICS

The absorbable hemostatics arrest bleeding either by the formation of an artificial clot or by providing a mechanical matrix that facilitates clotting when applied directly to denuded or bleeding surfaces. Since they are absorbed from the site of application after varying periods of time, they are referred to as absorbable hemostatics. The agents to be described are used to *control oozing from minute vessels* and will not effectively combat bleeding from arteries or veins when there is appreciable intravascular pressure. The absorbable hemostatics include *absorbable gelatin sponge, oxidized cellulose, thrombin,* and *thromboplastin.*

Absorbable Gelatin Sponge, U.S.P. (GELFOAM), is a sterile, absorbable, water-insoluble, gelatin-base sponge. It is used for the control of capillary oozing and frank hemorrhage, particularly from highly vascular areas that are difficult to suture. For this purpose it is frequently moistened with sterile isotonic sodium chloride solution or with thrombin solution before use. Since it is completely absorbed in 4 to 6 weeks, it may be left in place after the closure of an operative wound. Contact with tissue does not produce excessive scar formation or untoward cellular reactions. It is usually available as cones, packs, and sponges.

Oxidized Cellulose, U.S.P. (OXYCEL SURGICEL), is a specially treated form of surgical gauze or cotton that promotes clotting by a reaction between hemoglobin and cellulosic acid. Hence, it does not interact with the normal physiological clotting mechanism. Absorption of oxidized cellulose usually occurs within 2 to 7 days after application of the dry material, but complete absorption of large amounts of blood-soaked material may take 6 weeks or longer. It should not be used in combination with thrombin because the low pH interferes with the activity of the thrombin. Oxidized cellulose should not be employed for permanent packing or implantation in fractures because it interferes with bone regeneration and may result in cyst formation. The preparation also inhibits epithelialization and hence should not be used as a surface dressing except for the immediate control of hemorrhage. It is marketed as sterile cotton pledgets, gauze pads, and gauze strips.

Thrombin, U.S.P., is obtained from bovine plasma and is standardized on the basis of National Institutes of Health (N.I.H.) units. One N.I.H. unit is that amount of thrombin required to clot 1 ml of standard fibrinogen solution in 15 seconds. Thrombin is used to control the oozing of blood from accessible small capillaries and small venules, such as occurs in parenchymatous tissues, cancellous bone, and dental

sockets, and as a consequence of laryngeal, nasal, and plastic surgery. *Thrombin should be used only topically.* It is marketed as a powder in vials containing 1000, 5000, or 10,000 N.I.H. units. Despite its bovine origin, official thrombin appears to be non-antigenic when employed topically.

Thromboplastin (thrombokinase) is a powder prepared from the acetone-extracted brain and/or lung tissue of freshly killed rabbits. It contains thrombokinase, a factor necessary for the conversion of prothrombin to thrombin. It is used for the determination of prothrombin time, an important guide in oral anticoagulant therapy. Thromboplastin is also employed in surgery as a local hemostatic.

ASTRINGENTS

Astringents are locally acting drugs that precipitate proteins but have so little penetrability that only the surface of cells is affected. Many germicidal protein precipitants exert an astringent effect in high dilutions. Certain metallic ions, such as those of zinc and aluminum, are primarily astringent. *Tannic acid* is also astringent. However, there are few if any legitimate medical uses for this substance. Sufficient tannic acid may be absorbed from the gastrointestinal tract, denuded surfaces, and mucous membranes to cause severe centralobular necrosis of the liver (*see* Eshchar and Friedman, 1974).

IRRITANTS

The irritants are drugs that act locally on cutaneous or mucosal tissue to produce "inflammation." The first response to local irritation is an increased circulation to the injured part. The localized vasodilatation, mediated by way of an axon reflex, is attended by the feeling of comfort, warmth, and sometimes itching. Localized hyperesthesia also occurs. Drugs that evoke only reactive hyperemia are known as *rubefacients.* If the irritant action progresses, the capillaries dilate widely and become more permeable. Plasma escapes into the extracellular spaces, fluid collects under the epidermis, and blisters are formed. Drugs capable of causing this degree of irritation are known as *vesicants.* Irritants of another type readily penetrate into the orifices of the sebaceous glands and cause small multiple abscesses that may become confluent if the irritant action proceeds. Such drugs are called *pustulants.* The pustulants have few if any valid therapeutic applications.

Drugs are the *least* useful means available for producing hyperemia and irritation. Heat is often the rubefacient of choice; the hot-water bottle or heating pad, the moist hot pack, and the heat lamp are simple means for applying heat. Short-wave diathermy also is an effective method for producing localized hyperemia.

Camphor is employed exclusively for its local actions. Natural camphor is obtained from the wood and bark of a tree, *Cinnamomum camphora,* growing especially in Japan and Taiwan. Camphor is also obtained synthetically. The compound is a rubefacient when rubbed on the skin. When not vigorously applied, however, it may produce a feeling of coolness. Camphor also has a mild local anesthetic action, and its application to the skin may be followed by numbness. Camphor has a hot, bitter taste and, when taken in small amounts, produces a feeling of warmth and comfort in the stomach. In large doses it is irritating and causes nausea and vomiting. Large doses of the drug, as can occur from ingestion of solid camphor by children, may cause convulsions. Treatment is the same as for poisoning by other central stimulants.

Camphor, U.S.P., a transparent, aromatic, crystalline substance, is an ingredient in *paregoric* and a number of proprietary preparations for external application. Official camphor preparations for local application are *Camphor Spirit,* U.S.P. (10% in alcohol), and *Camphorated Parachlorophenol,* U.S.P. (35% parachlorophenol and 65% camphor). Camphor spirit is used as a local irritant. Camphor, applied topically as a 1 to 3% lotion or ointment, is used as an antipruritic and an irritant. Camphorated parachlorophenol has *antibacterial* properties and is used in dentistry for the treatment of infected root canals.

Cantharidin, the active irritant in cantharides (*Spanish fly, Russian flies*), is used locally only for its irritant and vesicant action on the skin. This white crystalline substance has been shown by Einbinder and associates (1969) to poison mitochondria and to cause changes in cell membranes, epidermal cell dyshesion, and acantholysis. It is available as *cantharidin collodion* (CANTHARONE), cantharidin (0.7%) in a film-forming vehicle containing acetone, ethocel, flexible collodion, ether (35%), and alcohol (11%). It is used for the removal of benign epithelial growths: warts (ordinary, periungal, subungal, plantar, and palpebral) and molluscum contagiosum (Epstein and Kligman, 1958). Thick hyperkeratotic lesions should be pared down, painted with cantharidin collodion, allowed to dry, and covered with a nonporous occlusive tape. The blisters induced by this agent heal rapidly, without leaving a scar.

SCLEROSING AGENTS

Sclerosing agents are irritating substances that are used to obliterate varicose veins and fibrose uncomplicated hemorrhoids. For a review of treatment methods for the former, *see* Nabatoff (1976); for the latter, *see* Symposium (1973). Numerous irritants have been used as sclerosing agents. Only three, however, warrant even the brief description given below.

Morrhuate Sodium Injection, U.S.P., is a sterile solution of the sodium salts of the fatty acids of cod liver oil. It is marketed as a 5% aqueous solution; the intravenous dose is 1 to 5 ml injected into a localized segment of vein. Hypersensitivity reactions occasionally occur, and appropriate measures should be taken to avoid such effects. *Quinine and urea hydrochloride injection* is a sterile solution of the double salt. One to two milliliters of a 5% solution is injected for sclerosing hemorrhoids, especially those that cannot be treated surgically. *Sodium tetradecyl sulfate* (SOTRADECOL) is an anionic surface-active agent used to sclerose varicose veins. The preparation for

this purpose is a 1 or 3% aqueous solution with 2% benzyl alcohol and buffered to a pH of 7 to 8. Not more than 0.5 to 2.0 ml should be injected at any one site; total volume should not exceed 10 ml of a 3% solution (*see* Perchuk, 1974). The drug may cause pain at the site of the injection and sloughing of the tissue if the solution is allowed to extravasate. Since allergic reactions have been reported, the possibility of an anaphylactic reaction should be kept in mind, and the physician should be prepared to treat it appropriately.

CAUSTICS, ESCHAROTICS, KERATOLYTICS, AND ANTISEBORRHEICS

Caustics and Escharotics. A *caustic* (or *corrosive*) is a topical agent that causes destruction of tissues at the site of application. If the agent also precipitates cell proteins and the inflammatory exudate forms a scab (or eschar) that is later organized into a scar, it is also known as an *escharotic* (or *cauterizant*). Most, but not all, caustics are also escharotics. Certain caustics, especially the alkalis, redissolve precipitated proteins, partly by hydrolysis, so that no scab or only a soft scab forms; such agents penetrate deeply and are generally unsuitable for therapeutic use. Caustics are used to destroy *warts, condylomata, keratoses, certain moles,* and *hyperplastic tissue.* They have also been used in the management of *fungal infections* and *eczematoid dermatitis.* Agents commonly classified in this category include the following: *glacial acetic acid, exsiccated alum, podophyllum, podophyllum resin, phenol,* and *trichloroacetic acid.*

Keratolytics (Desquamating Agents). *Benzoic acid, salicylic acid, resorcinol,* various thiols, and certain other substances are frequently used as keratolytic agents. Salicylic acid produces desquamation by solubilizing the intercellular cement that binds scales in the stratum corneum. An effective keratolytic therapy involves the use of 40% propylene glycol under plastic occlusion. The addition of 6% salicylic acid to the former results in a very effective keratolytic preparation (KERALYT) that is effective in a variety of skin diseases associated with hyperkeratosis (*e.g., ichthyosis, seborrheic dermatitis, psoriasis, chronic eczematous dermatitis, hyperkeratosis* of the palms and soles, *keratosis pilaris, warts, actinic keratosis,* etc.).

Antiseborrheics. Seborrheic dermatitis is an inflammatory, erythematous, and scaling eruption that occurs primarily in those areas with a large number and high activity of sebaceous glands, such as the scalp, face, and trunk. A number of drugs, including *benzoic acid, salicylic acid, resorcinol, sulfur,* and some *mercurial compounds,* are sometimes used in the management of disorders of the scalp. Drugs prepared in pharmaceutical forms especially designed for the treatment of seborrheic dermatitis are considered here.

Selenium Sulfide, U.S.P., is a bright-orange, insoluble powder that is used externally for control of seborrheic dermatitis, dandruff, and nonspecific dermatoses. Its antidandruff effectiveness is thought to result from its antimitotic activity and substantivity (residual adherence after shampoo and rinse) to the skin (Kligman *et al.,* 1976). The toxicity of insoluble selenium sulfide contrasts sharply with the highly toxic soluble selenites, selenates, and organic selenium compounds (Henschler and Kirschner, 1969). Indeed, Cummins and Kimura (1971) have shown in rats that the oral LD50 for the insoluble selenium sulfide is quite comparable to that for other substances commonly employed in shampoos. Comparatively little absorption occurs after local application of selenium sulfide to normal skin, but the drug is absorbed more readily from inflamed or damaged epithelium. Prolonged contact with skin surfaces may result in burns and dermatitis venenata. Selenium sulfide is employed as *Selenium Sulfide Lotion,* U.S.P. (EXSEL, IOSEL 250, SELSUN), a therapeutic shampoo containing 2.5% of the active ingredient in a detergent vehicle. It is also available as a nonprescription drug in a 1% detergent suspension (SELSUN BLUE) in a scented, detergent vehicle. The preparation should not be used more frequently than required to maintain control. Adverse effects include chemical conjunctivitis if the preparation enters the eyes, increased oiliness or dryness of the hair, and orange tinting of gray hair. The latter effect may be minimized by thoroughly rinsing the hair immediately after each treatment.

Zinc pyrithione is widely used in nonprescription formulations (DANEX, ZINCON, others) that are temporarily effective for the management of dandruff. Like selenium sulfide, zinc pyrithione is thought to act by reducing the turnover of epidermal cells (Kligman *et al.,* 1976); the two agents are equally effective and more effective than a nonmedicated shampoo. Zinc pyrithione has little or no toxicity when applied as directed to normal skin and hair.

MELANIZING AND DEMELANIZING AGENTS

Many characteristics of normal and abnormal skin pigmentation and achromasia are of importance in pharmacology. Skin alterations resulting from untoward effects of drugs are discussed in connection with the agents responsible for such changes. The drugs discussed in this section have clinically useful melanizing (hyperpigmenting) or demelanizing (hypopigmenting and depigmenting) properties. Many details relating to the etiology and management of vitiliginous and lentiginous skin disorders are presented in the reviews by Fitzpatrick and coworkers (1961) and by Fitzpatrick and Mihm (1971), and in the monograph edited by Kawamura and associates (1971).

TRIOXSALEN

Trioxsalen (4,5′,8-trimethylpsoralen), a congener of methoxsalen, is used to facilitate repigmentation in vitiligo, increase tolerance to solar exposure, and enhance pigmentation. Recently, it has also been used as a photochemotherapeutic agent in the treatment of psoriasis, but it is less effective than me-

thoxsalen. The structural formula of this furocoumarin is shown below.

Trioxsalen

Pharmacological Actions. The mode of action of trioxsalen in inducing repigmentation of the vitiliginous skin is not yet known. It is believed, however, that its action depends upon the presence of functional melanocytes and their proliferation (mitotic activation) by the photoactivated trioxsalen. Well-controlled exposure of the skin either to sunlight or to ultraviolet radiation from artificial sources (320 to 400 nm) is essential for the stimulation of melanin pigmentation. Repigmentation may begin after a few weeks; however, significant results may take as long as 6 to 9 months to occur. The drug activates the few functional and dopa-positive melanocytes present in the vitiliginous skin area (Jarrett and Szabó, 1956) and evokes a mitotic response in these cells; the latter is indicated by the autoradiographic studies of Africk and Fulton (1971) and the light- and electron-microscopic studies of Pathak and associates (1974, 1976b). The increase in perifollicular and epidermal pigment is thought to occur by one or more of the following mechanisms: (1) an increase in the number of functional melanocytes and also, possibly, by activation of dormant or resting melanocytes; (2) the augmentation of melanosome (melanin granule) synthesis, (3) an increase in the activity of tyrosinase, the enzyme that catalyzes the conversion of tryosine to dihydroxyphenylalanine, a precursor of melanin; and (4) the hypertrophy of melanocytes and increased arborization of their dendrites. The metabolism of trioxsalen has been studied by Mandula and Pathak (1979).

Side Effects and Contraindications. Side effects are minimal; an occasional patient may experience gastric irritation and nausea. The drug is contraindicated in patients with photosensitizing diseases, such as erythropoietic protoporphyria or acute lupus erythematosus. No other photosensitizing drug should be administered with trioxsalen. The safety of this drug in children under 12 years of age has not been established.

Preparations. *Trioxsalen,* U.S.P. (TRISORALEN), is available as *Trioxsalen Tablets,* U.S.P. (5 mg). The usual oral dose is 10 mg, 2 hours before exposure to sunlight or ultraviolet light. Higher doses (0.6 mg/kg) have, however, been used in the treatment of vitiligo. If a patient is treated on alternate days and follicular repigmentation is not apparent after 3 to 4 months, the drug should be discontinued as a failure. Exposure times should be limited to the manufacturer's recommended schedule, except at low latitudes (0 to 20°), where exposure times should be reduced.

Therapeutic Uses. Trioxsalen is used in *idiopathic vitiligo,* to *increase tolerance to sunlight,* and to enhance *skin pigmentation* (tanning). The drug is a potent skin photosensitizing agent and should be used only under medical supervision. Its effectiveness in the photochemotherapy of psoriasis remains to be established.

METHOXSALEN

Methoxsalen (8-methoxypsoralen) is used in combination with exposure to ultraviolet radiation (320 to 400 nm) to increase skin tolerance to sunlight, to facilitate repigmentation in vitiligo, and to treat skin diseases such as psoriasis, eczema, and mycosis fungoides. The chemistry of the psoralens has been reviewed by Fowlks (1959) and by Pathak and associates (1974, 1976a). Methoxsalen has the following structural formula:

OCH$_3$
Methoxsalen

Pharmacological Actions. Methoxsalen is a potent photosensitizer of the skin, particularly to long-wavelength (320 to 400 nm) ultraviolet light (Pathak *et al.,* 1967). Patients with psoriasis or vitiligo are treated with methoxsalen orally (0.3 to 0.6 mg/kg) and approximately 2 hours later are exposed to a measured dose of UV-A radiation (320 to 400 nm). Exposure is carried out with a specially designed ultraviolet lamp system. After oral ingestion, increased sensitivity of the skin to such radiation appears in 1 hour, reaches a maximum in 2 hours, and disappears in about 8 hours. The therapeutic effect in psoriasis is believed to result from the photochemically induced covalent binding of methoxsalen to pyrimidine bases. This photoconjunction appears to involve first the formation of monofunctional C-4 cycloadducts of methoxsalen at the 5,6 double bond of pyrimidine bases in DNA. Subsequently, bifunctional adducts involving interstrand cross-links between two pyrimidine bases on opposite strands of DNA are formed (Cole, 1970; Dall'Aqua *et al.,* 1972; Pathak *et al.,* 1974). The light-dependent conjugation of epidermal DNA with psoralens is believed to inhibit DNA synthesis and cell division, thereby leading to clinical improvement in diseases such as psoriasis.

Exposure of methoxsalen-treated patients to ultraviolet light thickens the stratum corneum, induces an inflammatory reaction in the skin, and increases the amount of melanin in the exposed area (Becker, 1960). Repigmentation persists for 8 to 14 years without further treatment (Kenney, 1971). Topical therapy is recommended for the repigmentation of small macules of vitiligo. The topical application of methoxsalen (0.1 to 1%) renders the skin very sensitive to ultraviolet radiation; blistering occurs frequently, and photosensitivity may persist for several days. The mechanism of repigmentation or hyperpigmentation in patients with vitiligo appears to be similar to that of trioxsalen, as discussed above.

Side Effects and Contraindications. The most common side effects after oral therapy are excessive erythema (burns), nausea, and pruritus. Although abnormal hepatic function was originally reported in a few patients taking methoxsalen, this apparently is not a danger (*e.g., see* Melski *et al.,* 1977). It would seem prudent, however, to perform tests of hepatic function prior to the initiation of therapy and at intervals thereafter. While occular effects have not been reported in man, annual ophthalmic examinations are recommended in patients who are receiving long-term therapy with methoxsalen. The potential long-term side effects of methoxsalen plus UV-A treatment are the same as those known to occur from ultraviolet exposure; they include actinic alterations of the skin (aging), skin cancer, and cataracts.

Stern and associates (1979) have evaluated the risk of cutaneous carcinoma in a 2-year prospective study of nearly 1400 patients receiving photochemotherapy with 8-methoxypsoralens for psoriasis. Their data suggested that patients having skin types I and II (who sunburn easily and tan poorly) and a previous history of receiving ionizing radiation were at a high risk for the development of cutaneous carcinoma. A higher-than-expected proportion of squamous-cell carcinomas that arose in areas not habitually exposed to the sun were seen. In view of these findings, the benefits of such treatment for patients with psoriasis, especially those with skin types I and II, should be carefully weighed against the possible risks. This treatment must be considered to be experimental (Epstein, 1979).

Preparations. *Methoxsalen,* U.S.P. (OXSORALEN), is available in 10-mg capsules and as *Methoxsalen Topical Solution,* U.S.P. (1%). For vitiligo the capsules are given orally to adults in a dose of 20 mg once a day, followed in 2 hours with a 5-minute exposure to sunlight or ultraviolet light (1 to 2 joules/cm^2); exposure may be gradually increased to 30 minutes (15 to 20 joules/cm^2). For increased tolerance to sunlight and enhanced pigmentation, the same dosage is employed but should be limited to 14 days of treatment. If the 1% topical solution is used, it is applied at weekly intervals to well-defined vitiliginous lesions followed with a 1-minute exposure to ultraviolet light. Subsequent exposures should be increased with caution. *The topical solution should never be dispensed to the patient for home use.* The beneficial effects of orally administered methoxsalen photochemotherapy can be achieved in patients with either vitiligo or psoriasis by well-controlled exposure to ultraviolet light that is less than that which produces grossly observable phototoxic reactions in skin.

Therapeutic Uses. Methoxsalen should be employed only under strict medical supervision. It may be effective for the treatment of *idiopathic vitiligo* when employed in conjunction with exposure of affected areas of the skin to ultraviolet light. If the vitiligo is extensive and is associated with total destruction of melanocytes, the drug is ineffective. It may be effective when used to enhance skin tolerance to sunlight. Well-controlled clinical studies in several university medical centers suggest that oral methoxsalen, followed by exposure to high-intensity, long-wavelength ultraviolet light, is effective in the management of *psoriasis* (Parrish *et al.,* 1974; Melski *et al.,* 1977).

MONOBENZONE

Monobenzone, the monobenzyl ether of hydroquinone, is an amelanotic agent used topically for the induction of complete, often irreversible depigmentation of severely affected patients with pigmentary problems. The use of monobenzone should be restricted to situations in which it is desired to achieve *complete* amelanosis. Monobenzone (*p*-benzyloxyphenol) has the following structural formula:

Monobenzone

Pharmacological Actions. The mechanism of action of monobenzone is not fully understood. The histology of the skin after depigmentation is the same as that seen in vitiligo; the epidermis is normal except for the absence of identifiable melanocytes. Electron microscopy reveals the absence of melanocytes and melanosomes. The selective destruction of melanocytes is accompanied by increased degradation of melanosomes, destruction of membranous organelles, and inhibition of the enzyme tyrosinase, which catalyzes the oxidation of tyrosine to dihydroxyphenylalanine, a precursor of melanin. Response to therapy is usually not apparent for 1 to 4 months, and complete depigmentation may require 9 to 12 months of treatment. Untoward effects, including mild erythema, dermatitis, and eczematous reactions, have been reported. Unless carefully applied, unsightly depigmented patches may result from its use. Systemic toxicity has not been observed after its local application.

Preparations. *Monobenzone,* U.S.P. (BENOQUIN), is marketed as *monobenzone lotion,* a 5% solution in isopropyl alcohol and propylene glycol, and *Monobenzone Ointment,* U.S.P., which contains 20% of the active ingredient in a suitable base. It is applied to hyperpigmented areas two or three times daily for up to 4 months, or until depigmentation has occurred, and then twice weekly to maintain the effect. Treated areas should not be exposed to sunlight; the depigmenting site should be protected with a topical sunscreen. If a satisfactory response is not observed within 4 to 6 months, treatment should be discontinued.

Therapeutic Uses. Monobenzone is a potent depigmenting chemical, more effective than hydroquinone, and is a useful agent for permanent depigmentation in patients with generalized vitiligo who are unresponsive to methoxsalen or trioxsalen photochemotherapy and who wish to be one color (Mosher *et al.,* 1977). Monobenzone should *not* be used as a hypopigmenting agent in melasma or in hyperpigmentation caused by the excessive formation of melanin, such as occurs in generalized lentigo, severe freckling, or melasma of pregnancy, or in hyperpigmentation that follows inflammation of the skin. Monobenzone is of no value in the treatment of *café au lait* spots, pigmented nevi, malignant melanoma, or pigmentation resulting from substances other than melanin.

HYDROQUINONE

Hydroquinone (*p*-dihydroxybenzene) is a safe but weak depigmenting agent used topically in the treatment of hypermelanosis (*e.g.,* circumscribed brown hypermelanotic macules of melasma, in women taking progestational agents, in Berlock dermatitis caused by certain perfumes, in postinflammatory hyperpigmentation, severe freckling, and melasma of pregnancy). Although percutaneous application does not, in most instances, completely remove the hyperpigmentation, results are good enough to help the majority of patients become less self-conscious about their abnormality.

Pharmacological Actions. Histochemical and electron-microscopic studies reveal that hydroquinone affects the nonfollicular and follicular melanocyte system. It decreases the formation and increases the degradation of melanosomes, causes structural changes in the membranous organelles of the melanocytes, and inhibits tyrosinase (Jimbow *et al.,* 1974). Depigmentation is not immediate, since hydroquinone interferes only with the formation of new melanin. Cutaneous depigmentation is reversible, since the production of melanin is resumed when the drug is discontinued. It should be emphasized that hydroquinone does not produce the confetti-like depigmentation often seen after the application of monobenzone.

Side Effects and Contraindications. Side effects are usually mild; burning, stinging, rash, and irritation have been reported. Possible allergic reactions have been noted. Therefore, patients should be patch-tested for sensitivity before initiating therapy. The drug should not be used near the eyes, on open cuts, or on children under 12 years of age.

Preparations. *Hydroquinone,* U.S.P., is marketed as *hydroquinone ointment* (ELDOPAQUE), 2% and 4%, in an opaque base to protect treated areas from ultraviolet light; *Hydroquinone Cream,* U.S.P. (ELDOQUIN), 2%; and *hydroquinone lotion,* 2%, in a stabilized base. These preparations are applied to the area to be lightened once or twice daily and rubbed in well, for up to 4 to 6 months. Hydroquinone lotion (2% and 4%) in propylene glycol, in combination with retinoic acid (0.05%), appears to be more effective in the treatment of melasma than is hydroquinone cream.

Therapeutic Uses. Hydroquinone is used to bleach and lighten localized areas of darkened skin (melasma, postinflammatory hyperpigmentation, and severe freckling).

SUNSCREENING AGENTS

Sunscreens are formulated to protect the user against the sunburn reaction normally evoked by ultraviolet radiation (290 to 320 nm) and are also used to prevent skin cancer, premature aging of the skin (*actinic elastosis*), and various forms of photosensitivity diseases (*e.g.*, polymorphic light eruptions, drug-induced phototoxic and photoallergic reactions). Sunscreens protect the viable cells of the skin by absorbing and reflecting the solar radiation that impinges upon them. Topical sunscreens that absorb and filter the solar radiation exhibit a wide range of effectiveness, depending upon the ultraviolet absorption spectrum and the extinction coefficient of the agent itself, its concentration, the vehicle in which it is formulated, and its substantivity to remain on the skin after sweating or swimming. The sunscreens may be grouped into three broad categories. (1) Para-aminobenzoic acid and its derivatives are common constituents of many preparations. Lotions containing 5% para-aminobenzoic acid in 50 to 70% ethanol offer a particularly high degree of protection. Those containing lower concentrations of such compounds as amyl *p*-dimethylaminobenzoate and octyl *p*-dimethylaminobenzoate are somewhat less effective. (2) Sunscreens that rely on the absorptive capacity of other compounds include those that contain benzophenones and cinnamates. These agents are also highly effective when present in adequate concentration. Preparations that contain lower concentrations of these compounds or those mentioned previously are intended for use by those who want to become tan but not burned. (3) Physical sunscreens include heavy creams or pastes containing such compounds as titanium dioxide, zinc oxide, kaolin, or talc. While they are opaque to light of all wavelengths, they lack cosmetic appeal. Preparations of sunscreens have been listed in the Medical Letter (1979).

In prescribing sunscreen agents, the most important consideration should be the individual's reactivity to sunlight. People with fair skin and blue eyes, who burn easily and tan poorly or minimally (skin types I and II), should use sunscreens that are highly protective. Most formulations are not water resistant and should be reapplied after swimming or during prolonged sunbathing. Drug-induced photosensitization reactions can be prevented by prescribing topical sunscreens containing benzophenones. To avoid cross-sensitization reactions, individuals who have experienced phototoxic or allergic reactions to drugs such as sulfonamides, thiazide diuretics, or local anesthetics that are derivatives of para-aminobenzoic acid should not utilize sunscreens that contain para-aminobenzoic acid or its derivatives. Patients who are sensitive to ultraviolet radiation (290 to 400 nm) and also to visible radiation (400 to 760 nm) should use opaque sunscreens that contain zinc oxide and other light-scattering agents. Artificial tanning preparations containing dihydroxyacetone provide no protection against sunburn unless a sunscreen is also incorporated in the formulation.

MUCOLYTICS

Although iodides, ammonium chloride, and other drugs have been used orally for many years to loosen viscid sputum and to improve expectoration, the use of nebulized mucolytic agents for this purpose is a comparatively recent development. A number of substances have been reported to be effective mucolytic agents, but more definitive studies have shown them to be either ineffective or undesirable for a variety of clinical reasons (*see* Lieberman, 1970). Only acetylcysteine will be mentioned here.

Acetylcysteine, U.S.P. (MUCOMYST), liquefies mucus and DNA (the component of pus responsible for its viscosity) but has no effect on fibrin, blood clots, or living tissue. It exerts its mucolytic activity through its free sulfhydryl group, which acts directly on the mucoproteins to open the disulfide bonds and lower the viscosity of the mucus. The mucolytic activity is greatest at pH 7 to 9. Liquefaction after inhalation is apparent within 1 minute; maximal effect occurs in 5 to 10 minutes; after direct application, the effect is immediate. It is used by inhalation and direct application as adjunct therapy in patients with abnormal, viscid, or inspissated mucous secretions. The agent is marketed as *Acetylcysteine Solution*, U.S.P. (10 and 20% sterile solution). A nebulized solution, 1 to 10 ml of a 20% solution or 2 to 20 ml of a 10% solution, is inhaled three to four times daily. By direct instillation, 1 or 2 ml of a 10 or 20% solution is used every 1 to 4 hours. Untoward effects are not common but include bronchospasm, stomatitis, severe rhinorrhea and bronchorrhea, nausea, and vomiting. Consequently, asthmatic patients under treatment with acetylcysteine should be watched closely. Acetylcysteine is also used in the treatment of poisoning with acetaminophen (*see* Chapter 29).

ENZYMES

This discussion is limited to enzymes that act at local sites after either topical application or hypodermic injection.

HYALURONIDASE

Hyaluronidase is a soluble enzyme product prepared from mammalian testes.

Pharmacological Actions. Hyaluronidase hydrolyzes hyaluronic acid by splitting the glucosaminidic bond between C 1 of the glucosamine moiety and C 4 of glucuronic acid. This temporarily decreases the viscosity of the cellular cement, promotes diffusion of injected fluids or of localized transudates or exudates, and in this way facilitates their absorption. Sensitivity to hyaluronidase occurs, although infrequently; a test for sensitivity should be conducted prior to administration.

Preparations and Bioassay. *Hyaluronidase for Injection*, U.S.P. (ALIDASE, HYAZYME, WYDASE), is supplied as a sterile, white, amorphous solid in ampuls containing 150 or 1500 units and as *Hyaluronidase Injection*, U.S.P., containing 150 units per milliliter. Its solutions are colorless, odorless, and unstable. Hyaluronidase activity is assayed on the basis of the ability of the enzyme to decrease the turbidity of colloidal suspensions of hyaluronate and protein *in vitro*.

Therapeutic Uses. Hyaluronidase is effective for enhancing the dispersion and absorption of other injected drugs, for hypodermoclysis, as an adjunct in subcutaneous urography, for improving resorption of radiopaque agents, and to enhance absorption of drugs in tissue spaces and in transudates of fluids. Kloner and associates (1978) have shown that the myocardium of the dog subjected to experimental coronary occlusion can be protected by the infusion of the enzyme. Hyaluronidase has been selected for a national clinical study designed to determine if its administration can limit the size of myocardial infarction in man.

STREPTOKINASE AND STREPTODORNASE

Pharmacological Actions. Streptokinase and streptodornase are enzymes produced during the growth of certain strains of hemolytic streptococci. Streptokinase is a plasminogen activator and dissolves blood clots and the fibrinous portion of exudates. Streptodornase hydrolyzes deoxyribonucleoprotein and hence liquefies the viscous nucleoprotein of dead cells; it has no effect on living cells. These enzymes are used together to aid in the removal of clotted blood and fibrinous or purulent accumulations following trauma or inflammation.

Preparations. *Streptokinase-streptodornase* (VARIDASE) is marketed as a *jelly* (100,000 units of streptokinase and 25,000 units of streptodornase in 15 ml), as a *powder* for preparation of sterile solution for intramuscular injection (20,000 units of streptokinase and 5000 units of streptodornase in each vial), and as *oral tablets* (10,000 units of streptokinase and 2500 units of streptodornase per tablet). Solutions deteriorate at room temperature but remain active for 7 days at 10° C. *Streptokinase* (STREPTASE), a highly purified preparation for intravenous use, is sometimes employed in lieu of surgery in pulmonary embolism and deep-vein thrombosis (*see* Chapter 58).

Therapeutic Uses and Dosage. Streptokinase-streptodornase is employed to remove clotted blood and fibrinous or purulent exudate resulting from trauma or inflammation. It is also used as an adjunct in the treatment of *hemothorax, hematoma,* and *empyema,* and of chronic suppurations involving draining sinuses, osteomyelitis, and infected wounds or ulcers. Such therapy can be considered only as a supplement to appropriate antibiotic therapy and surgical debridement and drainage.

Adverse reactions include nausea, vomiting, diarrhea, skin rash, and urticaria following oral administration; a pyrogenic reaction after topical application; and pain at the site of the injection or a febrile reaction after intramuscular injection. The last-named reaction has been attributed to pyrogenic substances in the enzyme mixture.

Streptokinase-streptodornase is administered by injection into cavities and by topical application in the form of a jelly or wet dressings. It must not be administered intravenously. It is essential that the mixture be placed in intimate contact with the substrate. In enclosed areas, provision must be made for release of increased fluid resulting from the liquefying action of the enzymes. For a *hemothorax* or *thoracic empyema,* the initial dose is 200,000 units of streptokinase and 50,000 units of streptodornase in not less than 10 ml of isotonic sodium chloride solution. A suitable initial dose in *maxillary sinus empyema* is 10,000 to 15,000 units of streptokinase and 2500 to 3750 units of streptodornase in 2 to 3 ml of solution. Similar concentrations may be applied in wet dressings when enzymatic debridement is indicated. Orally, the suggested dose is one tablet (streptokinase 10,000 units and streptodornase 2500 units) four times a day. The value of oral administration of the enzyme mixture has not been established.

PROTEOLYTIC ENZYMES

Chymotrypsin, crystalized from an extract of bovine pancreas, is an endopeptidase that hydrolyzes ester and peptide bonds. The enzyme can be shown to have an anti-inflammatory action in experimental animals, but only when administered parenterally in very large doses and *prior* to the production of the inflammation. The systemic clinical usefulness of this enzyme is thus very questionable. Furthermore, since chymotrypsin is a foreign protein, severe anaphylactic reactions have followed its systemic use.

Chymotrypsin, U.S.P. (AVAZYME), is a white to yellowish-white, odorless, crystalline or amorphous powder. It is also official as *Chymotrypsin for Ophthalmic Solution,* U.S.P. (ALPHA CHYMAR, CATARASE, ZOLYSE). Each milligram of chymotrypsin contains not less than 1000 U.S.P. chymotrypsin units. It is marketed in vials containing 300 and 750 U.S.P. units (75 and 150 units per milliliter when reconstituted), and as tablets (50,000 U.S.P. units). It is also available in combination with trypsin in oral tablets (ORENZYME) containing 4000 units of chymotrypsin and 50,000 units of trypsin or 8000 units of chymotrypsin and 100,000 units of trypsin. The usual dosage is 1 to 2 tablets four times a day.

Chymotrypsin is used in cataract operations to loosen the lens after incision of the cornea. After the corneoscleral or corneoscleral-conjunctival incision, the posterior chamber is irrigated with 1 or 2 ml of enzyme solution (1:5000 dilution) to fragment the fibers of the zonule (enzymatic zonulolysis). Untoward effects include temporary glaucoma, moderate uveitis, corneal edema, and striation. Delayed healing has been reported. Chymotrypsin is not recommended for use in ophthalmic surgery in patients under 20 years of age because of possible loss of vitreous humor.

Collagenase is an enzymatic debriding agent derived from the fermentation of *Clostridium histolyticum.* It has the capacity to digest native collagen as well as the denatured protein. Since collagen accounts for approximately 75% of the dry weight of skin, the enzyme is utilized for debridement for severely burned areas and dermal lesions (Boxer *et al.,* 1969; Varma *et al.,* 1973). The usefulness of this agent in other necrotic skin lesions remains to be determined. The enzyme's optimal pH range is 7 to 8. Detergents, hexachlorophene, and ions of heavy metals (mercury and silver) inhibit enzymatic activity; cleansing materials such as hydrogen peroxide, Dakin's solution, and buffered (pH 7.0 to 7.5) normal saline solution do not. Collagenase, as an ointment containing 250 units per gram (SANYTL OINTMENT), is applied to the lesion every day or every other day and is covered with a sterile dressing. Should infection intervene, appropriate antimicrobial therapy should be used. The collagenase is discontinued when sufficient debridement of necrotic tissue has taken place.

Fibrinolysin-deoxyribonuclease (ELASE) is a topical debriding agent composed of two hydrolytic enzymes—fibrinolysin, derived from bovine plasma, and deoxyribonuclease, isolated from bovine pancreas. The former acts principally on fibrin of blood clots and fibrinous exudates, whereas the latter hydrolyzes deoxyribonucleic acid (DNA). This combination of enzymes is indicated for topical use as a debriding agent in general surgical wounds, ulcerative lesions, and second- and third-degree burns, and following circumcision and episiotomy; it is also used intravaginally in cervicitis (benign, post-partum, and postconization), and vaginitis and as an irrigating agent in infected wounds, otorhinolaryngological wounds, and superficial hematomas. Adverse reactions are usually minimal and include local irritation with hyperemia after higher concentrations. The agent should not be used in patients with a history of hypersensitivity reactions to either of the components. Fibrinolysin-deoxyribonuclease is available as a lyophilized sterile powder (25 units of fibrinolysin and 15,000 units of deoxyribonuclease per 30-ml vial) and as an ointment containing fibrinolysin (30 units) and deoxyribonuclease (20,000 units) in 10 and 30 g.

Sutilains, U.S.P., is a proteolytic enzyme elaborated by *Bacillus subtilis*. At body temperature it has optimal activity at a pH range of 6.0 to 6.8. It is available as *Sutilains Ointment*, U.S.P. (TRAVASE), 1 g of which contains approximately 82,000 casein units of proteolytic activity. The ointment is used for wound debridement as adjunct therapy to established methods of wound care (Garrett, 1969). It is indicated in second- and third-degree burns; decubitus ulcers; incisional, traumatic, and pyogenic wounds; and ulcers secondary to peripheral vascular disease. Patients should be warned to keep the enzyme away from the eyes. Untoward local effects include mild and transient pain, paresthesia, bleeding, and dermatitis; if bleeding or dermatitis occurs, therapy should be discontinued. Systemic toxicity has not been observed from the topical application of the ointment.

Africk, J., and Fulton, J. Treatment of vitiligo with topical trimethylpsoralen and sunlight. *Br. J. Dermatol.*, **1971**, *84*, 151–156.

Antopol, W. Lycopodium granuloma. *Arch. Pathol.*, **1933**, *16*, 326–331.

Barnes, J. M., and Rossiter, R. J. Toxicity of tannic acid. *Lancet*, **1943**, *2*, 218–222.

Becker, S. W., Jr. Use and abuse of psoralens. *J.A.M.A.*, **1960**, *173*, 1483–1485.

Bowie, M. D., and McKenzie, D. Diethylene glycol poisoning in children. *S. Afr. Med. J.*, **1972**, *46*, 931–934.

Boxer, A. M.; Gottesman, N.; Bernstein, H.; and Mandl, I.

Debridement of dermal ulcers and decubiti with collagenase. *Geriatrics*, **1969**, *24*, 75–86.

Chain, E., and Duthie, E. S. Identity of hyaluronidase and spreading factor. *Br. J. Exp. Pathol.*, **1940**, *21*, 324–338.

Cole, R. S. Light-induced cross-linking of DNA in the presence of a furocoumarin (psoralen). *Biochim. Biophys. Acta*, **1970**, *217*, 30–39.

Colman, R. W. Proteolytic enzymes in clinical medicine. *Clin. Pharmacol. Ther.*, **1965**, *6*, 598–630.

Cooney, D. O. A "superactive" charcoal for antidotal use in poisonings. *Clin. Toxicol.*, **1977**, *11*, 387–390.

Cummins, L. M., and Kimura, E. T. Safety evaluation of selenium sulfide antidandruff shampoos. *Toxicol. Appl. Pharmacol.*, **1971**, *20*, 89–96.

Dall'Aqua, F.; Marciani, S.; Vedaldi, D.; and Rodighiero, G. Formation of interstrand cross-linkings on DNA of guinea pig skin after application of psoralen and irradiation at 365 nm. *FEBS Lett.*, **1972**, *27*, 192–194.

Duran-Reynals, F. The effect of extracts of certain organs from normal and immunized animals on the infecting power of vaccine virus. *J. Exp. Med.*, **1929**, *50*, 327–340.

Einbinder, J. M.; Parshley, M. S.; Walzer, R. A.; and Sanders, S. L. The effect of cantharidin on epithelial cells in tissue culture. *J. Invest. Dermatol.*, **1969**, *52*, 291–303.

Elliott, J. A., Jr. Clinical experiences with methoxsalen in the treatment of vitiligo. *J. Invest. Dermatol.*, **1959**, *32*, 311–313.

Epstein, J. H. Risks and benefits of the treatment of psoriasis. *N. Engl. J. Med.*, **1979**, *300*, 852–853.

Epstein, W. L., and Kligman, A. M. Treatment of warts with cantharidin. *Arch. Dermatol.*, **1958**, *77*, 508–511.

Eshchar, J., and Friedman, G. Acute hepatotoxicity of tannic acid added to barium enemas. *Am. J. Dig. Dis.*, **1974**, *19*, 825–829.

Fitzpatrick, T. B.; Arndt, K. A.; ElMofty, A. M.; and Pathak, M. A. Hydroquinone and psoralens in the therapy of hypermelanosis and vitiligo. *Arch. Dermatol.*, **1966**, *93*, 589–600.

Fitzpatrick, T. B., and Mihm, M. C. Abnormalities of the melanin pigmentary system. In, *Dermatology in General Medicine*. (Fitzpatrick, T. B.; Arndt, K. A.; Clark, W. H., Jr.; Eisen, A. Z.; Van Scott, E. J.; and Vaughan, J. H.; eds.) McGraw-Hill Book Co., New York, **1971**, pp. 1591–1637.

Fitzpatrick, T. B.; Parrish, J. A.; Pathak, M. A.; and Tanenbaum, L. The risks and benefits of oral PUVA photochemotherapy and psoriasis. In, *Psoriasis: Proceedings of the Second International Symposium*. (Farber, E. M., and Cox, A. J., eds.) Yorke Medical Books, New York, **1976**, pp. 320–327.

Fitzpatrick, T. B.; Seiji, M.; and McGugan, A. D. Melanin pigmentation. *N. Engl. J. Med.*, **1961**, *265*, 328–332, 374–378, 430–434.

Fowlks, W. L. The chemistry of the psoralens. *J. Invest. Dermatol.*, **1959**, *32*, 249–254.

Garrett, T. A. *Bacillus subtilis* protease: a new topical agent for debridement. *Clin. Med.*, **1969**, *76*, No. 5, 11–15.

Genel, M. Central nervous system toxicity associated with ingestion of propylene glycol. *J. Pediatr.*, **1978**, *93*, 515–516.

Goldsmith, L. A., and Baden, H. P. Propylene glycol with occlusion for treatment of ichthyosis. *J.A.M.A.*, **1972**, *220*, 579–580.

Hayden, J. W., and Comstock, E. G. Use of activated charcoal in acute poisoning. *Clin. Toxicol.*, **1975**, *8*, 515–533.

Henschler, D., and Kirschner, U. Zur Resorption und Toxität von Selensulfid. *Arch. Toxicol. (Berl.)*, **1969**, *24*, 341–344.

Jarrett, A., and Szabó, G. The pathological varieties of vitiligo and their response to treatment with MELADININE. *Br. J. Dermatol.*, **1956**, *68*, 313–326.

Jimbow, K.; Pathak, M. A.; Obata, H.; and Fitzpatrick,

T. B. Mechanism of depigmentation by hydroquinone. *J. Invest. Dermatol.,* **1974,** *62,* 436–449.

Kabacoff, B. L.; Wohlman, A.; Zombley, M.; and Avakian, S. Absorption of chymotrypsin from the intestinal tract. *Nature,* **1963,** *199,* 815–817.

Kawamura, T.; Fitzpatrick, T. B.; and Seiji, M. (eds.). *Biology of Normal and Abnormal Melanocytes.* University of Tokyo Press, Tokyo, **1971.**

Kenney, J. A., Jr. Vitiligo treated by psoralens. *Arch. Dermatol.,* **1971,** *103,* 475–480.

Kligman, A. M., and Goldstein, F. P. Oral dosage in methoxsalen phototoxicity. *Arch. Dermatol.,* **1973,** *107,* 548–550.

Kligman, A. M.; McGinley, K. J.; and Leyden, J. J. The nature of dandruff. *J. Soc. Cosmet. Chem.,* **1976,** *27,* 111–139.

Kloner, R. A.; Braunwald, E.; and Maroko, P. R. Longterm preservation of ischemic myocardium in the dog with hyaluronidase. *Circulation,* **1978,** *58,* 220–226.

Krezanoski, J. Z. Tannic acid: chemistry, analysis, and toxicology. *Radiology,* **1966,** *87,* 655–657.

Labby, D. H.; Imbrie, J. D.; and Fitzpatrick, T. B. Studies of liver function in subjects receiving methoxsalen. *J. Invest. Dermatol.,* **1959,** *32,* 273–275.

Lieberman, J. The appropriate use of mucolytic agents. *Am. J. Med.,* **1970,** *49,* 1–4.

Mandula, B. B., and Pathak, M. A. Metabolic reactions *in vitro* of psoralens with liver and epidermis. *Biochem. Pharmacol.,* **1979,** *28,* 127–132.

Masters, E. J. Allergies to cosmetic products. *N.Y. State J. Med.,* **1960,** *60,* 1934–1940.

Medical Letter. Sunscreens. **1979,** *21,* 46–48.

Melski, J. W.; Tanenbaum, L.; Parrish, J. A.; Fitzpatrick, T. B.; Bleich, H. L.; and 28 Participating Investigators. Oral methoxsalen photochemotherapy for the treatment of psoriasis: a cooperative clinical trial. *J. Invest. Dermatol.,* **1977,** *68,* 328–335.

Mosher, D. B.; Parrish, J. A.; and Fitzpatrick, T. B. Monobenzyl ether of hydroquinone: a retrospective study of treatment of 18 vitiligo patients and a review of the literature. *Br. J. Dermatol.,* **1977,** *97,* 669–679.

Nabatoff, R. A. Surgical versus injection treatment for varicose veins. *Mt. Sinai J. Med. N.Y.,* **1976,** *43,* 447–453.

Orentreich, N.; Taylor, E. H.; Berger, R. A.; and Auerbach, R. Comparative study of two antidandruff preparations. *J. Pharm. Sci.,* **1969,** *58,* 1279–1280.

Parrish, J. A.; Fitzpatrick, T. B.; Tanenbaum, L.; and Pathak, M. A. Photochemotherapy of psoriasis with oral methoxsalen and long-wave ultraviolet light. *N. Engl. J. Med.,* **1974,** *291,* 1207–1211.

Parry, M. F., and Wallach, R. Ethylene glycol poisoning. *Am. J. Med.,* **1974,** *57,* 143–150.

Pathak, M. A.; Fitzpatrick, T. B.; and Parrish, J. A. Pharmacologic and molecular aspects of psoralen photochemotherapy. In, *Psoriasis: Proceedings of the Second International Symposium.* (Farber, E. M., and Cox, A. J., eds.) Yorke Medical Books, New York, **1976a,** pp. 262–271.

Pathak, M. A.; Jimbow, K.; Parrish, J. A.; Kaidbey, K. H.; Kligman, A. L.; and Fitzpatrick, T. B. In, *Pigment Cell—Unique Properties of Melanocytes: Proceedings of the Ninth International Pigment Cell Conference.* Pt. II, Vol. 3. (Riley, V., ed.) S. Karger, Basel, **1976b,** pp. 291–298.

Pathak, M. A.; Kramer, D. M.; and Fitzpatrick, T. B. Photobiology and photochemistry of furocoumarins (psoralens). In, *Sunlight and Man.* (Pathak, M. A.; Harber, L. C.; Seiji, M.; and Kukita, A.; eds.) University of Tokyo Press, Tokyo, **1974,** pp. 335–368.

Pathak, M. A.; Worden, L. R.; and Kaufman, K. D. Effect of structural alterations on the photosensitizing potency of furocoumarins (psoralens) and related compounds. *J. Invest. Dermatol.,* **1967,** *48,* 103–118.

Perchuk, E. Injection therapy of varicose veins. A method of obliterating huge varicosities with small doses of sclerosing agent. *Angiology,* **1974,** *25,* 393–405.

Picchioni, A. L.; Chin, L.; and Laird, H. E. Activated charcoal preparations relative antidotal efficacy. *Clin. Toxicol.,* **1974,** *7,* 97–108.

Robinson, J. R. Deodorants and antiperspirants. In, *Handbook of Nonprescription Drugs.* (Griffenhagen, G. B., and Hawkins, L. L., eds.) American Pharmaceutical Association, Washington, D. C., **1973,** pp. 209–214.

Stern, R. S.; Thibodeau, L. A.; Kleinerman, R. A.; Parrish, J. A.; Fitzpatrick, T. B.; and 22 Participating Investigators. Risk of cutaneous carcinoma in patients treated with oral methoxsalen photochemotherapy for psoriasis. *N. Engl. J. Med.,* **1979,** *300,* 809–813.

Symposium. (Various authors.) Diverse methods of managing hemorrhoids. *Dis. Colon Rectum,* **1973,** *16,* 171–192.

Tourtellotte, W. W.; Reinglass, J. L.; and Newkirk, T. A. Cerebral dehydration action of glycerol. *Clin. Pharmacol. Ther.,* **1972,** *13,* 159–171.

Tucker, H. A. Clinical and laboratory tolerance studies in volunteers given oral methoxsalen. *J. Invest. Dermatol.,* **1959,** *32,* 277–280.

Varma, A. D.; Bugatch, E.; and German, F. M. Debridement of dermal ulcers with collagenase. *Surg. Gynecol. Obstet.,* **1973,** *136,* 281–282.

Wells, D. B.; Humphrey, H. D.; and Coll, J. J. The relation of tannic acid to the liver necrosis occurring in burns. *N. Engl. J. Med.,* **1942,** *226,* 629–636.

Wohlman, A.; Kabacoff, R. L.; and Avakian, S. Comparative stability of trypsin and chymotrypsin in human intestinal juice. *Proc. Soc. Exp. Biol. Med.,* **1962,** *109,* 26–28.

41 ANTISEPTICS AND DISINFECTANTS; FUNGICIDES; ECTOPARASITICIDES

Stewart C. Harvey

I. Antiseptics and Disinfectants

Once the germ theory of disease was accepted by the medical profession and antisepsis by chemical agents was demonstrated scientifically, topical antimicrobial drugs were employed with naive enthusiasm by both physicians and laymen. Astute physicians early learned the limitations of antiseptics, but the vast majority of physicians and laymen alike employed such drugs uncritically and often inappropriately, encouraged by promotional propaganda almost from the very beginning. Although several effective and useful antiseptics, such as iodine, were known quite early, in the first half of this century there was a rush to accept a host of lesser and even useless drugs. The euphoria surrounding the discovery of the sulfonamides and antibiotics obscured the need for a thoroughgoing appraisal of the value of antiseptics, collectively and individually. Only a few of the antiseptics have been subjected to controlled clinical comparison with other agents, and clinical standards have yet to be accepted. Both laymen and many physicians still continue to employ the topical antimicrobial drugs in a ritual manner that is often irrational, usually ineffective, and occasionally harmful.

Nevertheless, there are indispensable uses of disinfectants in the household, in hospital sanitation, and in public health measures. Likewise, antiseptics find many legitimate therapeutic applications. Even though systemic antimicrobial drugs have quite properly caused a decline in the use of topical anti-infective agents, antiseptics are sometimes still of value in treating local infections caused by microorganisms refractory to systemic chemotherapy and in the supplementation of such therapy. Antiseptics are especially useful in the preoperative preparation of both patient and surgeon and in some cases for chemoprophylaxis. It is the problem

of the physician to choose wisely from the vast number of available drugs and to delineate the beneficial and the harmful uses of germicides.

History. Centuries before the basic researches of Pasteur, Koch, and others established the pathogenicity of bacteria, chemicals were used to control the suppuration of wounds and the spread of contagious diseases. By the time the true significance of microorganisms was appreciated, many drugs were already available as germicides. The earliest written records of man contain references to the use of germicidal agents. Egyptian embalmers found excellent preservatives among the spices, vegetable oils, and gums, as attested by the fine state of preservation of Egyptian mummies. Persian laws instructed the populace to store drinking water in bright copper vessels. The practice of salting, smoking, and spicing foods is older than recorded history. The use of wine and vinegar in the dressing of wounds dates back at least to Hippocrates.

During the nineteenth century, the agents used empirically for their germicidal action included several compounds still employed. For example, iodine was used in treating wounds several decades before the bacterial etiology of suppuration was suspected. Because it was then believed that there was an association between putrefaction and the spread of disease, chlorine occupied a prominent place due to the fact that it was a deodorant. Semmelweiss decreased the incidence of puerperal fever in the obstetrical ward of the Allgemeines Krankenhaus of Vienna from about 10 to 1% by ordering the medical students (who were prone to come directly from the autopsy room to the obstetrical ward) to wash their hands in chlorinated lime before examining patients. Following the introduction of the technic of aseptic surgery by Lister (1867a, 1867b), the importance of disinfection of the skin of the patient, the hands of the surgeon, the instruments, and the hospital environment was readily appreciated. Some of the early drugs employed for these purposes are still valuable today. During the early part of this century, the use of germicides in purification of water supplies and in the sanitization of utensils and containers in multiple use by the public became widespread. An interesting review of the ancient and modern uses of germicidal substances is given by Block (1968).

Terminology. The terminology used to describe the actions of drugs on microorganisms is unfortunately somewhat confusing due to the discrepancy between the strict definitions of the terms employed and their usage in loose medical parlance. The origins of these terms, together with their current precise and imprecise connotations, are fully described by Davis (1968) and Lawrence (1968a).

Antiseptics are substances that kill or prevent the growth of microorganisms. This term is used especially for preparations *applied to living tissue.* The definition derives from the original meaning of the term *antiseptic* as a substance that opposes sepsis, putrefaction, or decay. A *disinfectant* is an agent that prevents infection by the destruction of pathogenic microorganisms. It is commonly used in reference to substances *applied to inanimate objects.* A *sanitizer* represents a particular kind of disinfectant; it is an agent that reduces the number of bacterial contaminants to levels judged safe by public health requirements. *Sterilization,* in contrast to *sanitization,* refers to the complete destruction of all forms of life, especially microorganisms, by some chemical or physical process. Under appropriate conditions, a disinfectant may produce complete sterilization. A *germicide,* in the broad and most useful sense, is an agent that destroys microorganisms. Germicides may be further defined by the appropriate use of self-evident terms such as *bactericide, fungicide, virucide,* and *amebicide.*

Properties Desirable in Germicides.
The properties of germicides that determine the usefulness and applicability of these agents may appropriately be divided into those desirable for purposes of *disinfection* and those useful in *antiseptics.*

Properties Desirable in Disinfectants. Agents used for disinfection should obviously have high germicidal efficacy. A wide antimicrobial spectrum is also desired, and the most valuable agents are those that are lethal to bacteria, including bacterial spores, as well as fungi, viruses, and protozoa. Rapidly lethal action is a useful property. The ability of the disinfectant to penetrate into crevices and cavities and beneath films of organic matter is desirable. It is also essential that lethal concentrations of the agent can be obtained in the presence of organic matter such as blood, sputum, and fecal material. The agent should be compatible with soaps and with other chemical substances likely to be encountered in the material to be disinfected.

The disinfectant must possess certain physical and chemical properties. A high degree of chemical stability is desired. A universal disinfectant should be noncorrosive to surgical instruments and nondestructive to other materials. Esthetic factors, such as odor, color, or staining quality, are sometimes determinants in the choice of a disinfectant. Cost is often an important consideration.

Properties Desirable in Antiseptics. A high degree of germicidal potency is also an important factor in an antiseptic, and a drug that is lethal to microorganisms is obviously superior to one that merely inhibits growth. The clinical usefulness of an antiseptic is related to the breadth of the antimicrobial spectrum; however, agents with narrow spectra find usefulness against infections caused by sensitive microorganisms. Low surface tension is desired in antiseptic solutions for topical application. It is of importance that the drugs retain their activity in the presence of

the body fluids, including the exudate present in infection. Rapid germicidal action is desired, but sustained action is likewise of value.

A prime consideration determining the usefulness of an antiseptic is the *therapeutic index*—the relationship between the concentration that is effective against microorganisms and one that produces such harmful effects as local tissue irritation and interference with the processes of healing and tissue repair. Also to be considered are the incidence of hypersensitivity reactions and the degree to which absorption of the drug leads to systemic toxicity. Unfortunately, the chemical properties that give most antiseptics their broad spectrum of activity may make them not only toxic to human tissues but often allergenic as well.

Evaluation of Antimicrobial Activity. Many different procedures are presently employed to test germicides. However, there are many inadequacies in the existing methods, and the procedures are not fully standardized. Detailed aspects of this subject are discussed in the monograph edited by Lawrence and Block (1968).

Numerous *in-vitro* tests are employed at the present time to evaluate activity of the different chemical classes of germicides against various microorganisms. However, the information obtained from such tests is applicable primarily to the use of the agents in the *disinfection* of inanimate objects.

Methods of testing *antiseptics* are even more varied and less standardized than those employed in testing disinfectants. Two types of information are sought by such tests: evaluation of antimicrobial efficiency under conditions of use and indications of tissue toxicity. A commonly employed test, representative of those designed to estimate antimicrobial efficiency, is that designed by Price for estimating *degermation* of the skin. (*See* Price, 1968, for details and for comparative data on various antiseptics.) In this method, at various times after the skin is treated with an antiseptic agent, culture plates are attached to the skin in a manner such that the culture medium contacts the epidermis. In the handwash method, hand washings are sampled for inocula. In the gloved-hand method, the surgical glove becomes the collector of the bacteria (*e.g., see* Michaud *et al.,* 1972). In the finger-streak test, the index finger is drawn across the culture plate. Persistent effects are sometimes evaluated by introducing an inoculum of *Staphylococcus aureus* or *Escherichia coli* onto the skin at various times after application of the antiseptic (*e.g., see* Lowbury and Lilly, 1973). Antiseptics are also tested against bacteria on the abraded or incised skin of animals in "infection-prevention" tests. Many other methods have been devised for assessing antiseptics under conditions designed to simulate those of actual use (*see* Miller, 1971). The details of these methods and of the procedures for evaluating tissue toxicity are given by Leary and Stuart (1968) and Ortenzio and Stuart (1968).

Testing of *virucidal agents* requires technics different from those employed in assessing bactericides. Inactivation of bacteriophages and reduction in infectivity of specific viral inocula for chick embryos and for experimental animals are among the procedures employed. The details concerned with testing antiviral agents are given by Koski and Stuart (1968).

Estimates of *antifungal activity* again require methods different from those used for testing agents against bacteria or viruses. The methods of evaluation of antifungal agents are considered subsequently.

In spite of the many tests for evaluating activity and toxicity of antiseptics, laboratory methods fail to give enough information to determine efficacy of a drug in actual use. It is difficult to ascertain from such tests whether one agent is superior to another. A number of well-controlled clinical trials of surgical and urinary tract antiseptics have been made, but there have been few valid comparisons of antiseptics in the treatment of cutaneous infections. Many commonly used antiseptics are exceedingly weak germicides. Their continued use has the character of folk medicine.

Status of Antiseptics in Relation to Systemic Chemotherapeutic Agents. Most germicides have been employed at one time or another in the local treatment of *wounds* and *infections.* Because of tissue toxicity, inadequate penetration into foci of infection, and reduced activity in the presence of body fluids, dramatic benefit from this use of germicides is the exception rather than the rule. The importance of antiseptics in treating infections is now secondary to that of systemic antimicrobial agents. In experienced hands, selected germicides may be useful in cleansing wounds and in reducing bacterial contamination. However, the common belief that substantial benefit is obtained from the application of antiseptics to wounds, cuts, and abrasions is not supported by the considerable evidence in this field. The various applications of surgical antiseptics have been considered in detail by Price (1968).

In *dermatological infections,* systemic treatment will usually provide more dramatic results than topical therapy. Nevertheless, there are also barriers to the outward movement of systemic drugs, especially into the stratum corneum, so that both systemic and topical treatment may be of value. Also, where resistance or intolerance to systemic antimicrobial drugs exists, topical antiseptics may be indicated. However, topical therapy is not the only recourse; debridement and various cleansing, dressing, and surgical procedures are vital to good management. Germicidal drugs are sometimes useful in prophylaxis against specific infections.

Importance of Germicidal Kinetics. The rate of germicidal action approximates first-order kinetics and is dependent upon the concentration, temperature, pH, and vehicle in which the drug is applied. On the skin of the hands and arms, the time necessary for a 50% reduction in bacterial count is about 0.6 minute for 70% ethanol and 7 minutes for 1:1000 benzalkonium chloride. Obviously, where time is a critical factor, the kinetics are of the utmost importance. The medical and promotional literature frequently neglects this important aspect of the pharmacology of antiseptics.

The conditions in which antiseptics are used are usually much more complex than implied above, because of diffusion, penetration, binding, redistribution, and other factors. The rate of action is often not directly proportional to the concentration, and for many antiseptics there is an optimal concentration. Furthermore, many antiseptics fall far short of complete antisepsis; neither of the two agents used in the example above can reduce the bacterial count of the skin by much more than 90%. The pharmacokinetics of antifungal drugs in relation to efficacy has been reviewed by Drouhet (1978).

Mechanisms of Antimicrobial Action. The mechanisms by which drugs kill or inhibit the growth of microorganisms are so varied and complex that little can be gained by a general discussion. The monograph edited by Lawrence and Block (1968) and the reviews by Russell (1969) and Drouhet (1970) present general mechanisms of antimicrobial action as well as information on specific germicides. The mechanisms of action of the individual agents will be discussed in the sections that follow.

Antimicrobial Spectra of Germicides. Many germicides exhibit a broad antimicrobial spectrum. Iodine exemplifies a germicide of this type. However, some germicides show marked selectivity. For example, hexachlorophene is toxic primarily to gram-positive bacteria. In general, antiseptics are broad-spectrum agents, so that attention will be called only to those drugs that depart significantly from this generalization. For detailed information and references on the antimicrobial spectra of germicides, *see* the monograph edited by Lawrence and Block (1968).

It may be stated as a general rule that *bacterial spores* are less readily killed by germicides than are vegetative forms of bacteria. In order to destroy spores it is necessary greatly to increase the time of contact, the concentration of the germicide, or both, above that necessary to kill nonsporulating bacteria. The susceptibility of bacterial spores will be mentioned only in those instances in which the agent is unusually sporicidal or in which it is virtually ineffective against spore forms.

Viruses and vegetative forms of *fungi* seem to exhibit approximately the same degrees of sensitivity to chemical agents as do vegetative forms of bacteria (*see* Spaulding, 1968). Improvements in methods of testing for antiviral activity have contributed to the development of a number of agents effective locally or systemically against viral infections. Many germicides have sufficient antifungal activity to warrant their use in the treatment of mycotic diseases. Antifungal agents effective locally are considered subsequently.

Classification. In a discussion of such heterogeneous compounds as the antiseptics and disinfectants, some method of classification is desirable. So varied are the compounds with respect to chemical structure, mechanism of action, and therapeutic use, however, that too strict a classification may be more confusing than elucidating. Thus, by elimination, a chemical classification is the least objectionable.

PHENOLS, CRESOLS, AND RESORCINOLS

PHENOL

Phenol itself deserves exposition here only because of its historical importance. Certain derivatives are currently of considerably greater importance. The germicidal efficacy of phenol (carbolic acid) was dramatically demonstrated by Lister in 1867, although the compound had been occasionally employed in medicine prior to that time.

Pharmacological Action. Both the local and the systemic actions of phenol require consideration.

Local Actions. Phenol is bacteriostatic in a concentration of approximately 0.2%, bactericidal above 1%, and fungicidal above 1.3%. The efficacy is greatly reduced at low temperatures and in alkaline media. The drug is much more effective in aqueous solution than in glycerin or lipids. It is relatively inactive when incorporated in soaps.

Phenol presumably exerts its germicidal action by denaturing protein. The protein-phenol complex is a loose one. Therefore, phenol is diffusible and penetrates into tissues. The compound has a markedly toxic action, and because of its penetrability affects even the unabraded skin. When the drug is applied directly to the skin, a white pellicle of precipitated protein is formed. This soon turns red and eventually sloughs, leaving the cutaneous surface stained a light brown. If phenol remains in contact with the skin, it penetrates deeply and may cause extensive necrosis.

When applied locally, phenol exerts a local anesthetic action. A 5% solution, even on the unabraded epithelial surface, produces a feeling of warmth and tingling and, eventually, rather complete local anesthesia. Phenol in this concentration is very irritating to exposed tissue and may cause necrosis.

Systemic Actions. When taken orally, phenol causes extensive corrosion of the mucous membranes, severe pain, and vomiting. Once in the body, it stimulates and then depresses the *central nervous system (CNS)*. In man, brief stimulation is observed, and the prominent effects are those of CNS depression, which is usually the cause of death. The *circulation* is also markedly depressed by phenol. The blood pressure falls, partly as a result of central vasomotor depression but mainly due to a direct toxic action of phenol on the myocardium and the smaller blood vessels. Urine output is scanty, and the urine may contain casts and hemoglobin.

Absorption, Distribution, and Elimination. Phenol is absorbed by all routes of administration and can reach the circulation even when applied to the intact skin. A portion of the absorbed drug is oxidized to hydroquinone and pyrocatechol. Approximately 80%

is excreted by the kidney, either unchanged or conjugated with glucuronic and sulfuric acids.

Preparations. *Phenol,* U.S.P. (*carbolic acid*), consists of colorless crystals with a somewhat aromatic odor. It is soluble in water 1:15. *Liquefied Phenol,* U.S.P. (*liquefied carbolic acid*), is phenol maintained in a liquid state by the presence of 10% distilled water. *Phenolated Calamine Lotion,* U.S.P. (*compound calamine lotion*), contains 1% phenol.

Therapeutic Uses. Phenol has few legitimate uses as an antiseptic. Crude carbolic acid is sufficiently inexpensive to use for disinfection of excrement. Phenol is sometimes used as an antipruritic, either in the form of phenolated calamine lotion or as an ointment or simple aqueous solution. Aqueous solutions stronger than 2%, however, should not be applied to the surface of the body. Solutions containing 4% phenol in glycerin may be employed if necessary.

SUBSTITUTED PHENOLS

A number of phenol derivatives are more bactericidal than phenol itself. The most important of these are the *halogenated phenols* and bis-*phenols,* the *alkyl-substituted phenols,* and the *resorcinols.*

Relation of Chemical Structure to Pharmacological Action. Lipid solubility is a prerequisite of most antiseptics, especially those that interact with or pass through the bacterial membrane into the cell. Therefore, chemical modifications of phenol that increase lipid solubility, such as halogenation or alkylation, tend to increase activity, provided that aqueous solubility does not diminish below the level for effective transport. Additional polar groups, as in resorcinol, decrease potency but can be compensated for by alkyl or other nonpolar groups, as in hexylresorcinol. Phenols are less effective in alkaline solution because the phenolate ion is less lipid soluble. The structure-activity relationship of phenol derivatives has been reviewed by Gump and Walter (1968) and Prindle and Wright (1968).

Cresols. Cresol is usually marketed as a mixture of the three isomers of methylphenol. It is a fairly efficient bactericide against the common pathogenic organisms, including *Mycobacterium* species. The pharmacological properties of cresol are almost identical with those of phenol and do not warrant separate discussion. It is three to ten times more potent as a germicide than phenol and about equally toxic, so that it has a higher therapeutic index. However, advantage is not taken of this to lower the concentration employed; instead, it is used in high concentration to realize a superior effect. Consequently, cresol preparations should not be used with a false sense of security. Many cases of poisoning from cresol have been reported.

Cresol is soluble in water only to the extent of 1:60. Therefore, it is commonly used in the form of *saponated cresol solution (compound cresol solution),* which is 50% cresol in saponified linseed or other suitable oil. In this form it is miscible with water. Compound cresol solution is used widely for disinfecting inanimate objects. It is superior to and cheaper than phenol. It is probably the preparation of choice for the disinfection of excrement.

Resorcinol. Resorcinol, *m*-dihydroxybenzene, is both bactericidal and fungicidal but is only about one third as active as phenol. Locally, resorcinol is a protein precipitant. It also has keratolytic properties. The compound resembles phenol in its systemic actions. Central stimulation is more prominent than with phenol. *Resorcinol,* U.S.P., is a colorless crystalline substance, freely soluble in water and in alcohol and other organic solvents. It is employed in the treatment of *acne, ringworm, eczema, psoriasis, seborrheic dermatitis,* and other cutaneous lesions. Its mild irritant and keratolytic properties may be important to whatever erratic efficacy resorcinol has in these disorders. It is usually applied as a 10% ointment or lotion. It is also used as *Compound Resorcinol Ointment,* U.S.P., which contains 6% resorcinol. Its monoacetylated derivative, *Resorcinol Monoacetate,* U.S.P., gradually liberates resorcinol and, therefore, exerts a milder but more lasting action. It is used for the same purposes as resorcinol. Resorcinol monoacetate is compounded with sulfur in antifungal preparations.

Hexylresorcinol. *Hexylresorcinol,* U.S.P., is a useful antiseptic that is relatively odorless and does not stain. It is commonly employed in a 1:1000 solution or glycerite in mouthwashes or pharyngeal antiseptic preparations. It is quite irritating to tissue, and an occasional individual exhibits marked sensitivity to its local application.

Hexachlorophene. *Hexachlorophene,* U.S.P., is a polychlorinated *bis*-phenol with the following structure:

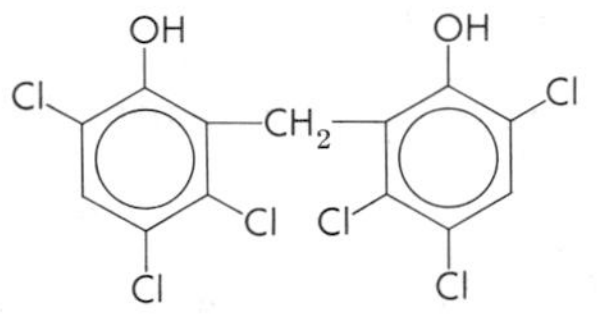

Hexachlorophene

Hexachlorophene is more effective against gram-positive than gram-negative bacteria. The drug exhibits high bacteriostatic activity, but considerable time is required to kill microorganisms and there is little effect on spores. A 3% solution may kill *Staphylococcus aureus* within 15 to 30 seconds, but as long as 24 hours or more may be required for some gram-negative bacteria. Indeed, epidemics have been caused by gram-negative bacteria actually growing in hexachlorophene solutions. For this reason and also to attempt to prevent suprainfections with gram-negative microorganisms, 4-chloro-3,5-xylenol (parachlorometaxylenol) or 4-chloro-3-cresol (parachlorometacresol) is included in some preparations. Nevertheless, such combinations may still require as long as 3 hours to kill gram-negative bacteria. The

additives enhance the efficacy against gram-positive bacteria.

Development of resistance of microorganisms to hexachlorophene has not been reported. The presence of organic matter such as pus or serum reduces the efficiency of hexachlorophene, but activity is retained in the presence of soaps, oils, and vehicles for topical application. The actions of low concentrations of hexachlorophene appear to include interruption of the bacterial electron-transport chain and inhibition of other membrane-bound enzymes. Higher concentrations actually rupture bacterial membranes.

Hexachlorophene accumulates in the skin. Immediately after a hand scrub with 3% hexachlorophene, the cutaneous bacterial population may be decreased by only 30 to 50%, compared to 99% following use of an iodophor (*see* Michaud *et al.,* 1976). However, 60 minutes later the population surviving hexachlorophene will have fallen further to about 4%, whereas with the iodophor the population will have recovered to about 16% of normal. Repeated daily applications over a period of 2 to 4 days create a steady-state reservoir of drug in the skin that maintains the bacterial population at about 1 to 5% of normal during the 24-hour interval between applications (Kundsin and Walter, 1973). Removal of the hexachlorophene film and regrowth of the normal flora begin promptly when a soap not containing hexachlorophene is substituted.

Since most of the potentially pathogenic bacterial residents of the skin are gram positive, hexachlorophene is commonly used by surgeons, physicians, dentists, food handlers, pediatric nurses, and others who routinely are in a position to spread contaminants from their own hands. The drug is also used to degerm the skin of patients scheduled for certain surgical procedures. Because iodophors (*see* below) are bactericidal and also initially decrease the skin bacterial population more than does hexachlorophene, the above-named uses of hexachlorophene have been criticized (*see* Price, 1968). However, as noted, the effect of hexachlorophene is more durable. White and Duncan (1972) have shown that the surgical infection rate is the same with either antiseptic in the surgical scrub.

Routine use of hexachlorophene preparations is effective in reducing the incidence and severity of pyogenic skin infections. However, when hexachlorophene is the only antibacterial drug in the preparation, an excess of gram-negative microorganisms appears in about a week, and the incidence of infections with such bacteria increases. Candidal infections also occur with greater frequency during chronic use of hexachlorophene.

In the early 1960s, the daily bathing of neonates with hexachlorophene was widely adopted in hospital nurseries as a prophylactic measure against fatal staphylococcal infections. This measure appeared to decrease the incidence of such infections but also to increase somewhat the incidence of gram-negative infections. Some observers argue in retrospect that the appearance of effective prophylaxis was an illusion caused by normal fluctuations in staphylococcal ecology, but most authoritative medical opinion holds that the prophylactic value of hexachlorophene is real. Within a decade, evidence mounted that daily bathing of infants with hexachlorophene could cause brain damage (*see* below). Consequently, the practice was discontinued in many hospitals, with the result that numerous staphylococcal epidemics in nurseries were reported. Increased emphasis was placed on disinfection of hospital personnel by means of hexachlorophene or iodophor handwashes, without demonstrable effect on the incidence of infection (*see* Steere and Mallison, 1975, for references). In some nurseries the concentration of hexachlorophene in the bathing solution was lowered to as little as 0.2%, but the apparent degree of protection was not that afforded by the 3% concentration. This is consistent with the findings of Michaud and coworkers (1976) that a concentration of 0.375% causes only a transient minor decrease in the cutaneous bacterial population. In some nurseries the use of the 3% hexachlorophene bath was continued, but the infant was immediately rinsed with ethanol to remove the hexachlorophene from the skin, which of course also prevented the salutary persistent antiseptic effect. Presently, it is common practice to delay the hexachlorophene bath until the third day (*see* Hyams *et al.,* 1975) or to bathe only the umbilical stump, which is the most common site for initial staphylococcal colonization. In the latter practice, isopropyl alcohol or iodophors are sometimes employed instead of hexachlorophene. Meanwhile, other antiseptics and hygienic practices are under investigation. It is probable that chlorhexidine will replace hexachlorophene in this controversial but important use. For various perspectives of this problem, *see* Gluck (1973), Bressler and associates (1977), Cooperman (1977), and Kimbrough (1977).

Hexachlorophene is sometimes used in the treatment of *acne vulgaris* to suppress the associated staphylococci. However, it does not affect the anaerobic, gram-negative *Propionibacterium* (*Corynebacterium*) *acnes,* and thus is not as effective as topical benzoyl peroxide or systemic tetracyclines or erythromycin.

Although hexachlorophene and the other *bis*-phenols are less toxic to tissue than is phenol, hexachlorophene causes moderate histological damage in experimental models (Faddis *et al.,* 1977); solutions containing detergents are the most toxic. Hexachlorophene is toxic by the oral route. Acute effects include anorexia, nausea, vomiting, abdominal cramps, asthenia, miosis, absence of light reflex, cerebrospinal tract signs, elevated intracranial pressure, and death. Systemic toxicity can also occur from topical use when the drug is applied daily to the skin of underweight, premature infants or infants with excoriated skin, or several times a day to the skin or vagina of adults. Confusion, diplopia, lethargy, twitching, convulsions, respiratory arrest, and death have occurred. Diffuse status spongiosus of the brain has been demonstrated, especially in the brain stem reticular formation. Endoneurial pressure is increased (Powell *et al.,* 1978). In experimental animals this condition appears to be slowly reversible, but damage in some children appears to be permanent. The routine use of hexachlorophene by pregnant nurses has been reported to be teratogenic (*see* Check, 1978). Details of the toxicity of hexachloro-

phene may be found in publications by Kimbrough (1971, 1973, 1977), Lockhart (1972, 1973), Plueckhahn (1973), and Powell and coworkers (1973), and in a conference (1973).

Hexachlorophene is available as a 0.25% liquid soap, 0.23% tincture foam, 3% sponge, and 3% cleansing (detergent) emulsion. Some detergent emulsions also contain parachlorometaxylenol.

Parabens. *Methylparaben,* N.F., *Ethylparaben,* N.F., *Propylparaben,* N.F., and *Butylparaben,* N.F., aliphatic esters of parahydroxybenzoic acid, are used as preservatives in a great variety of pharmaceutical preparations. Their actions are both those of phenols and an antimetabolite effect of parahydroxybenzoic acid. They have antifungal properties. All are effective in low concentrations (usually 0.1 to 0.3%) that are devoid of systemic toxic effects. However, as constituents of antibacterial ointments, dermatological preparations, and proprietary lotions and skin creams, they are recognized causes of severe and intractable contact dermatitis.

Parabens have been identified as the cause of chronic dermatitis in numerous instances. Patients sensitive to one paraben show cross-sensitivity to the others. The first step in treatment is to eliminate contact with parabens, a difficult task since they are so widely used in proprietary preparations, and their presence is often not indicated on the label.

Miscellaneous Phenols. *Thymol,* N.F., is both antibacterial and antifungal. It is presently used in a 1% concentration in vaginal deodorants. It is also present in some mouthwashes; in the concentrations used, it is not effective within any practical contact time. *Chlorothymol* is incorporated into some dental preparations for application to the gingiva and buccal mucosae and into anorectal preparations. *Parachlorometaxylenol* in concentrations of 0.25 to 2% is incorporated into preparations for the treatment of superficial burns, acne vulgaris, eczema, seborrheic dermatitis, and diaper rash. It is also used in combination with hexachlorophene to enhance its antimicrobial spectrum and to prevent contamination by gram-negative bacteria. *Orthophenylphenol* is contained in several dermatological preparations and in hospital disinfectants. Each of the above-named drugs is more potent than phenol; the true efficacy of none is known, because clinical testing has been desultory. *p-Tertiarybutylphenol, p-tertiaryamylphenol,* and *o-benzyl-p-chlorophenol* are employed as hospital disinfectants. The latter two plus orthochlorophenol are combined in the detergent disinfectant, VESTAL I.PH, which has been implicated in epidemics of neonatal hyperbilirubinemia (Wysowski *et al.,* 1978).

Parachlorophenol, U.S.P., is similar to phenol in its properties and uses. It is a more potent antiseptic than phenol, but the toxicity and caustic actions are also greater. *Camphorated Parachlorophenol,* U.S.P., a mixture of approximately 1 part parachlorophenol to 2 parts camphor, is used in root canal therapy; however, it is inferior to sodium hypochlorite and locally instilled antibiotics for this purpose. Blood and necrotic tissue markedly decrease its efficacy. *Triclosan* (2[2,4-dichlorophenoxy]-5-chlorophenol) is bacteriostatic mainly against gram-positive bacteria. It is incorporated into antiseptic soaps and solutions such as IRGASAN DP300. It has been reported to be effective in the treatment of acne. *Tetrabromo-methylphenol* in a concentration of 0.1% is as effective as 3% hexachlorophene in decreasing the number of cutaneous bacteria. *2,6-Dimethyl-4-chlorophenol* has an antibacterial efficacy equal to that of hexachlorophene (Borchardt *et al.,* 1978). It is the active agent in DERMA-CLEAN.

TARS

The medicinal tars are sometimes considered to be antiseptic because of various phenolic components. However, whatever efficacy they have in their uses mainly results from a mild irritant effect. The tars are used in the treatment of diseases of the skin, such as *psoriasis* and *eczema-dermatitis. Coal Tar,* U.S.P., is used in 1 to 5% strengths in creams, gels, lotions, ointments, pastes, and shampoos and in 5, 20, or 30% concentrations in topical solutions, emulsions, or suspensions, and as a 50% bath emulsion. Coal tar is also combined with salicylic acid and sulfur in antifungal preparations. *Juniper Tar,* U.S.P., is used as a 1 to 5% ointment, 4% shampoo, or 35% bath emulsion.

ALCOHOLS

The aliphatic alcohols are germicidal in varying degree, roughly in logarithmic proportion to their lipid solubility. Thus, potency increases with chain length until solubility limits availability, and branching and additional hydroxyl groups diminish potency.

ETHANOL

Ethanol is an antimicrobial drug of low potency but moderate efficacy in appropriate concentrations. It is bactericidal to all of the common pathogenic bacteria, but some rare species survive and can grow in otherwise-optimal concentrations of the chemical. It is erratic as a fungicide and virucide; it is virtually inactive against dried spores.

Against staphylococci, concentrations between 40 and 60% are the most effective, but they act more slowly than 70% ethanol (*Rubbing Alcohol,* U.S.P.). On the skin, 70% ethanol kills nearly 90% of the cutaneous bacteria within 2 minutes, provided the area is kept moist during that time. The user deludes himself if he expects more than a 75% reduction in cutaneous bacterial count when 70% ethanol is applied by a single wipe of ethanol-wetted cotton and left to evaporate. An ethanol foam not only prevents premature evaporation but also does not seem to cause the residual dry sensation that a soap wash does (Beck, 1978). Concentrations above 80% have a low efficacy.

The germicidal activities of chlorhexidine, quaternary ammonium antiseptics, and hexachlorophene are increased by ethanol. Alcohol is also combined with acetone to make an effective antiseptic and cleansing mixture.

Ethanol precipitates protein. Briefly applied to the skin it does no damage, but it is irritating if left on for long periods of time. Applied to wounds or raw surfaces it not only increases the injury but also forms a coagulum under which bacteria may subsequently thrive. It is thus not used to disinfect open lesions.

Other uses of ethanol are described in Chapter 18.

ISOPROPANOL

In concentrations above 70%, isopropanol is slightly more germicidal than ethanol, and it is effective in undiluted form. It causes vasodilatation beneath the surface of application, so that needle punctures and incisions at the site bleed more than with ethanol. It is used in any strength from 70% by weight (*Isopropyl Rubbing Alcohol,* U.S.P.) to 100% (*Isopropyl Alcohol,* U.S.P.). Isopropanol is used as a vehicle for other germicidal compounds, and it increases their efficacies.

ALDEHYDES

Several aldehydes possess bactericidal activity. The aldehyde group condenses with amino groups to form azomethines, and other types of linkages are also formed. In low concentrations, a toxic action is exerted on cells, including microorganisms; in higher concentrations, proteins are precipitated.

FORMALDEHYDE

Formaldehyde is effective against bacteria, fungi, and viruses, but the action is slow. In a concentration of 0.5%, 6 to 12 hours is required to kill bacteria and 2 to 4 days to kill spores; even in 8% concentration, 18 hours is required to kill spores. Organic matter is erroneously said not to interfere with the effectiveness of formaldehyde. The aldehyde is bound to organic matter, and a large excess of formaldehyde must be applied to compensate for depletion. In sufficient concentrations, proteins are precipitated.

As a germicide, formaldehyde is mainly used in 2 to 8% concentration to disinfect inanimate objects, such as surgical instruments and gloves. To sterilize tuberculous sputum, it is employed as an 8% solution in 65 to 70% isopropanol. Formaldehyde cannot be applied safely to the mucous membranes or most of the skin in concentrations high enough to kill microbes rapidly; hence it is seldom used as an antiseptic. However, intraperitoneal solutions of compounds that liberate formaldehyde have been reported to decrease the incidence of adhesions in experimental bowel surgery (Gilmore, 1977) and to control peritonitis in human patients (Browne *et al.,* 1978). The urinary antiseptic methenamine (Chapter 49) is effective because of the formaldehyde released. Some areas of the skin can tolerate fungicidal concentrations.

The astringent properties of 20 to 30% formaldehyde are employed in the treatment of hyperhidrosis; the soles of the feet and palms of the hands can usually tolerate these concentrations. The protein-precipitant action is used in the fixation of histological specimens and in the alteration of bacterial toxins to toxoids for vaccines. Preservation of cadavers with formaldehyde rests more on the antimicrobial effects than on hardening of the tissues. It is also used to desensitize teeth.

Alteration of tissue proteins by formaldehyde causes local toxicity and promotes allergic reactions. Repeated contact with solutions of formaldehyde may cause an eczematoid dermatitis. Dermatitis from clothing treated with formaldehyde for crease resistance has occurred.

Formaldehyde Solution, U.S.P., contains 37% of the aldehyde and 10 to 15% of methanol to retard polymerization.

GLUTARALDEHYDE

Glutaraldehyde is superior to formaldehyde as a sterilizing agent. It is effective against all microorganisms, including viruses and spores. It is less volatile than formaldehyde and hence causes less odor and irritant fumes, although it can cause contact dermatitis. It has been marketed as a 2% alkaline solution in 70% isopropanol, which is promoted as rapidly acting. However, a period of 10 hours is necessary to sterilize dried spores. Furthermore, in neutral or alkaline solution, glutaraldehyde polymerizes and thus has a useful shelf-life of less than 14 days. An acid-stabilized solution not only polymerizes more slowly but also kills dried spores in 20 minutes. Neutral emulsifying agents, such as polyethylene glycol and poloxamers, stabilize and increase the activity of both acidic and alkaline solutions of glutaraldehyde. Neither alkaline nor acidic solutions are damaging to most surgical instruments and endoscopes. As a sterilizing agent for endoscopes, it is superior to iodophors and hexachlorophene. In the gas-aerosol phase, glutaraldehyde is effective against airborne and surface resident microorganisms (Bovallius and Ånäs, 1977). *Succinic dialdehyde* is also effective as a disinfectant.

ACIDS

Acids have been used in the preservation of foods since antiquity. At present, several acids are employed as antiseptics or cauterizing agents. While the germicidal action of some acids is due to hydrogen ions, others have a more selective type of action.

Acetic Acid. This acid in 5% concentration is bactericidal to many types of microorganisms and bacteriostatic at lower concentrations. It is occasionally used in 1% solution on the skin for surgical dressings. *Pseudomonas aeruginosa* is particularly susceptible to acetic acid, and the acid may be employed in burn therapy. It is used in vaginal douches to suppress infections with *Trichomonas, Candida,* and *Haemophilus.* It is also a spermatocide. In con-

centrations of 0.25% applied to donor sites in skin grafting, it does not appear to retard healing (Gruber *et al.,* 1975).

Benzoic Acid. This compound has been widely used as a *food preservative.* In a concentration of 0.1% it prevents bacterial and fungal growth if the medium is slightly acidic. It is much less effective at an alkaline pH. Benzoic acid is relatively nontoxic and almost tasteless, and for these reasons it can be added to food. After ingestion, the benzoic acid is conjugated with glycine and excreted in the urine as hippuric acid. A daily intake of 4 to 6 g does not cause toxic symptoms aside from slight gastric irritation. Larger doses have systemic effects not unlike those of the salicylates.

Benzoic Acid, U.S.P., is a component of *Benzoic and Salicylic Acids Ointment,* U.S.P., which is discussed with the antifungal drugs (page 984). Benzoic acid can be safely applied to the skin in high concentrations.

Boric Acid. Boric acid has an unwarranted reputation as a germicide. It is primarily bacteriostatic, even in saturated aqueous solution. There is little to warrant its continued use in an era of potent antiseptics. Solutions are nonirritating and, therefore, have been applied to delicate structures such as the cornea; however, since they do not kill bacteria and secretions quickly wash the acid away, little antibacterial effect results. There is no clinical evidence of a significant effect on vaginal flora. Boric acid is also included in otic preparations. Its use as a buffer in various topical preparations is valid.

Toxicity. In the past, boric acid was considered to be a relatively benign and nontoxic substance, and the compound was once a common item in both hospital and home. However, the many cases of serious boric acid poisoning have focused attention on the toxic potentialities of the compound. With repeated applications of the powder to the abraded or inflamed skin, sufficient amounts can be absorbed to cause acute poisoning, especially in infants. Lethal amounts can also be absorbed from wound cavities irrigated with boric acid solutions. Approximately half of the persons accidentally intoxicated die. The slow excretion of boric acid contributes to cumulation of the compound and ultimate toxic effects consequent to repeated application. Thus, the chronic use of boric acid in rectal suppositories and in vaginal deodorants carries the risk of intoxication. A description of the toxicity of boric acid and appropriate references can be found in the *fifth edition* of this textbook.

Preparations and Therapeutic Uses. Boric Acid, N.F., occurs as colorless, odorless crystals or as a white powder. It is now usually colored to prevent error. Containers of boric acid should bear an autoclavable "poison" label. Boric acid is soluble to the extent of approximately 5% in water and 25% in glycerin. Most hospitals limit the use of boric acid to the *ophthalmic ointment.* The use of *boric acid solution* or *powder* on extensive inflamed surfaces or in body cavities is no longer practiced. The substance is included in rectal suppositories for hemorrhoids and in vaginal deodorants. Few dermatological preparations contain supposedly antiseptic concentrations of boric acid today. Boric acid and sodium borate are included as buffers in many products.

Lactic Acid. *Lactic Acid,* U.S.P., is less volatile than acetic acid; solutions applied topically thus persist longer on the skin or in the vagina. In the United States, lactic acid is used primarily in spermatocides in concentrations of 1 to 2%, but it is employed more widely elsewhere as a mild antiseptic. It can be used for the same purposes as acetic acid. A 10.5% solution has been reported to suppress pathogenic bacteria on the skin of neonates and to decrease the rate of infection (*e.g., see* Hnatko, 1977), but the conclusions are not statistically sound. The acid can be corrosive to tissues after prolonged contact; in a 16.7% concentration in flexible collodion it is combined with salicylic acid for the removal of warts and benign epithelial tumors.

Miscellaneous Acids. Propionic, salicylic, and undecylenic acids are discussed under Antifungal Drugs.

HALOGENS AND HALOGEN-CONTAINING COMPOUNDS

IODINE

Tincture of iodine was first used as an antiseptic by a French surgeon in 1839, and it was employed in treating battle wounds in the U.S. Civil War (*see* Gershenfeld, 1968). Despite the present wide choice of antiseptics, iodine is still among the most valuable agents. The drug has survived on the basis of efficacy, economy, and low toxicity to tissues.

Germicidal Action. Elemental iodine is lethal to both microflora and microzoa and to viruses. It is potent and rapidly acting. In the absence of organic matter, most bacteria are killed within 1 minute by exposure to a 1:20,000 solution of iodine; a period of approximately 15 minutes is required to kill wet bacterial spores with this concentration, but certain dry spores may require hours, even at much higher concentrations. A dilution as high as 1:200,000 will destroy all vegetative forms of bacteria in 15 minutes. On the skin, a 1% tincture will kill 90% of the bacteria in 90 seconds, a 5% solution in 60 seconds, and a 7% tincture in 15 seconds. The germicidal properties of iodine are reviewed by Gershenfeld (1968).

In the presence of organic matter, some iodine is bound covalently, but most of it forms loose complexes from which the iodine is slowly released. Thus, the immediate efficacy is somewhat diminished, but over a period of 15 minutes to 1 hour the efficacy is only moderately diminished. All commercial preparations contain iodine in great excess, so that organic matter does not adversely influence immediate efficacy. Even a solution as dilute as 0.1%

exerts adequate bactericidal actions in the presence of serum and tissue debris. Although penetration is limited by interaction with organic matter, dissociation of the complexes allows for slow diffusion below the surface.

Preparations. *Iodine Tincture,* U.S.P., contains 2% iodine and 2.4% sodium iodide diluted in 50% ethanol. The function of NaI is to increase solubility through formation of I_3^- ions. Aqueous solutions of iodine are *Strong Iodine Solution,* U.S.P. (*compound iodine solution, Lugol's solution*), and *Iodine Topical Solution,* U.S.P. The former contains 5% iodine and 10% potassium iodide; the latter, 2% iodine and 2.4% sodium iodide.

Toxicity. The local toxicity of iodine is quite low compared to its germicidal potency. Most of the iodine burns that gave iodine a bad reputation were caused by a 7% tincture. Iodine tinctures sting strongly when applied to raw surfaces, but iodine solution stings only slightly.

In rare instances, an individual may exhibit hypersensitivity to iodine and react markedly to moderate amounts of the element applied to the skin. Symptoms usually take the form of a severe constitutional reaction with fever and a generalized skin eruption of varying type. Iodine has a relatively low toxicity when therapeutic preparations are ingested. Few patients succumb to the effects of the drug. Fatalities have occurred only when large amounts (30 to 250 ml) of iodine tincture have been taken orally.

The toxic effects of iodine are largely due to the local actions of the element in the gastrointestinal tract. Iodine is corrosive, but it is also readily inactivated by combination with gastrointestinal contents. Little free iodine is absorbed from the intestinal tract; the element reaches the blood stream mainly in the form of iodide. It is probable that the pathological changes recorded in fatal cases of iodine poisoning and attributed to the systemic effects of iodine are largely the result of shock due to massive loss of fluid from the gastrointestinal tract, tissue hypoxia, and sometimes ethanol intoxication. Iodine can be inactivated in the stomach by gastric lavage with solutions of starch or 5% sodium thiosulfate.

Therapeutic Uses. The chief use of solutions of elemental iodine is in the *disinfection of the skin.* In this regard iodine is probably superior to any other agent. It is best employed in the form of the tincture, for the alcoholic vehicle facilitates spreading and penetration. Iodine may also be employed in the treatment of *wounds* and *abrasions.* Applied to abraded tissue, aqueous solutions are less irritating than the tincture. Aqueous solutions of 0.5 to 1.0% iodine with iodide are suitable for wounds and abrasions and a 0.1% solution may be used for irrigations. These concentrations can readily be made by proper dilution of the official solutions with water. For application to *mucous membranes,* a 2% solution of iodine in glycerin is the preparation of choice. In the treatment of *cutaneous infections* due to bacteria and fungi, the U.S.P. tincture or solution of iodine may be employed. Strong iodine solution has keratolytic properties, probably because of the iodide content, and it is sometimes used in the treatment of keratoscleritis.

Iodine may be used to render contaminated water safe for drinking. The addition of 3 drops of iodine tincture to each quart of water will kill not only amebae but also bacteria within 15 minutes without making the water unpalatable.

IODOPHORS

An iodophor is a loose complex of elemental iodine with a carrier that serves not only to increase the solubility of iodine but also to provide a sustained-release reservoir of the element. The iodine-carrying substances in medicinal iodophors are neutral polymers with amphipathic properties.

The most widely used iodophor is povidone-iodine, in which the carrier molecule is polyvinylpyrrolidone (povidone). A 10% solution contains 1% of available iodine, but the free iodine concentration is less than 1 ppm. This is low enough so that very little staining of the skin occurs, although starched linen will be stained. Because of the low concentration, the immediate bactericidal action is only moderate compared to that of iodine solutions. A standard surgical scrub with a 10% solution (1% available iodine) will decrease the usual cutaneous bacterial population by about 85%; it returns to normal in about 6 to 8 hours but effective control is lost in about 1 hour, which is a much shorter time than with hexachlorophene or chlorhexidine. However, when the hands are contaminated by gram-negative bacteria, povidone-iodine is a more effective scrubbing disinfectant than is aqueous chlorhexidine (Dineen, 1978). It is not as effective as 1% tincture of iodine. Blood on the hands moderately decreases its efficacy. For the disinfection of endoscopes and other instruments, even quite low concentrations of povidone-iodine are superior to 3% hexachlorophene (Dunkerley *et al.*, 1977).

Povidone-iodine *per se* has a low toxicity to tissues (*see* Gilmore, 1977), but the detergent in povidone-iodine cleansing solutions (surgical scrubs) has been reported to increase toxicity considerably (Faddis *et al.*, 1977). Povidone-iodine penetrates through the eschar of burned patients, which is therapeutically advantageous; however, it is also absorbed from the burned surface and thus causes elevated concentrations of iodine in plasma, which may be the cause of occasional intoxication (Lavelle *et al.*, 1975). Hypo-

thyroidism can result from topical application of povidone-iodine to neonates.

Various poloxamers also make effective carriers for iodine. When PLURONIC F68 is used as the poloxamer, a 10% solution provides a free-iodine concentration twice that of 10% povidone-iodine and has a higher *in-vitro* germicidal potency (Rodeheaver *et al.*, 1976). The germicidal activity of *poloxamer-iodine* has been reported to be equal to that of *povidone-iodine*.

Povidone-Iodine, U.S.P. (BETADINE, ISODINE), is available in a variety of forms, such as a 10% applicator solution, 2% cleansing solution (scrub), aerosol spray, aerosol foam, vaginal gel (for trichomonal and candidal infections), ointment, mouthwash, perineal wash, whirlpool concentrate, and so forth (all 2%). Concentrations are expressed as percent of the complex; to obtain the available content of iodine, this figure must be divided by ten. *Poloxamer-iodine* (PREPODYNE, SEPTODYNE) is available as a cleansing solution (scrub) containing 0.75% of available iodine, a solution containing 1% of available iodine, and other forms.

CHLORINE AND CHLOROPHORS

Chlorine became widely used in the sterilization of water supplies during the first decade of the twentieth century, and in World War I chlorine-containing compounds became extensively employed in medicine and surgery. Today, they are used mainly as sanitizing agents.

CHLORINE

Elemental chlorine is a potent germicidal agent. It exerts its antibacterial action in both the elemental form and as undissociated hypochlorous acid (HOCl), which is formed by the hydrolysis of chlorine. The concentration of undissociated HOCl and hence the bactericidal activity of chlorine are pH dependent. Thus, the bactericidal action of chlorine is ten times greater at pH 6.0 than at pH 9.0. At pH 7.0, the concentration of chlorine necessary to kill most microorganisms in 15 to 30 seconds varies between 0.10 and 0.25 ppm. However, mycobacteria are uniquely resistant to chlorine; 500 times the concentrations cited are necessary to destroy *Mycobacterium tuberculosis*. Chlorine is also virucidal and amebicidal.

Chlorine is a highly reactive element and thus can be bound by organic material, which decreases bactericidal efficacy. In the presence of excessive organic matter, chlorine is not the disinfectant of choice. In the disinfection of inanimate objects, for example, water, the uptake of chlorine by the organic matter present is known as the *chlorine demand*. It is generally considered that a residual chlorine content of 0.2 to 0.4 ppm of water affords a generous margin of safety. In order to attain this concentration of chlorine in relatively pure water, it is sufficient to add only 0.5 ppm; in grossly polluted waters, 20 ppm is scarcely sufficient.

Elemental chlorine has no medical uses. Its principal relevance to public health is its use in the treatment of community water supplies, although chlorinated lime is often used instead.

CHLOROPHORS

Chlorine itself has limited usefulness as an antiseptic because of difficulties in handling the element in its gaseous state and because chlorine water is very unstable. Many compounds, however, slowly yield hypochlorous acid, and these can be employed for the disinfection of inanimate objects and in surgery. Such compounds may be regarded as chlorophors, even though the ultimate product is hypochlorous acid. The germicidal efficiency of such compounds is related to the ease and extent of the liberation of HOCl.

Hypochlorite Solutions. There are a number of solutions in which chlorine is present in the form of hypochlorites. They are known under various names, such as Dakin's solution, Dakin-Carrel solution, and Labarraque's solution. *Sodium Hypochlorite Solution,* U.S.P., is a preparation of this type. It contains 5% NaOCl. This concentration is too high to be employed on tissues, except that it is a useful agent in root canal therapy. For surgical purposes *diluted sodium hypochlorite solution (modified Dakin's solution)* is employed. This preparation contains 0.45 to 0.5% of NaOCl. It may be diluted 1:3.

Solutions of sodium hypochlorite are relatively unstable and should be freshly prepared. They are not only germicidal but also dissolve necrotic tissues. A disadvantage of the hypochlorites is that they dissolve blood clots and delay clotting. Hypochlorite antiseptics are also somewhat irritating to the skin.

Oxychlorosene (CLORPACTIN) is a mixture of HOCl and alkylbenzene sulfonates; sodium oxychlorosene contains NaOCl, which is more stable. The surfactant properties of the alkylbenzene sulfonates promote penetration and the antibacterial actions.

Chlorinated Lime. Chlorinated lime consists of a mixture of calcium chloride and calcium hypochlorite and should contain a minimum of 30% available chlorine. It is too irritating to be used on tissues, but it is widely employed for the *disinfection* of inanimate objects and drinking water. Chlorinated lime is relatively unstable, even in solid form, and loses much of its activity over a period of a year.

Chloramines. The chloramines are amines, amides, or imides containing an N-chloro substituent. They are unstable in water and slowly release chlorine. Some chloramines also have a direct germicidal action. Chloramines are no longer employed for the irrigation of wounds or as antiseptics but are used in the emergency sterilization of drinking water and for sanitization. In the United States, *Halazone,* U.S.P., is the only chloramine of importance.

OXIDIZING AGENTS

A number of antiseptic drugs are toxic to microorganisms because they are oxidizing agents. Some compounds release oxygen as an active intermediate, and others probably directly oxidize vulnerable microbial constituents. Their individual properties differ considerably and are influenced by penetration, the rate at which oxygen is liberated, the actions of the cation linked with the oxygen-containing anion, and the effects of the substance remaining after oxygen has been released. For these reasons the drugs require separate discussion.

PEROXIDES

Hydrogen Peroxide. Hydrogen peroxide is very unstable and breaks down readily to form molecular oxygen and water. It is used as *Hydrogen Peroxide Topical Solution,* U.S.P., which contains 3% hydrogen peroxide in water. When hydrogen peroxide is applied to tissue, catalase causes rapid decomposition and effervescence, and the germicidal action is brief. Furthermore, solutions of hydrogen peroxide have poor penetrability and are relatively feeble germicides. Consequently, they have a very limited use. The continued use of hydrogen peroxide solution as a mouthwash, even in half strength, may cause the development of hypertrophied filiform papillae of the tongue ("hairy tongue"), but these disappear after the drug is discontinued.

Benzoyl Peroxide. *Hydrous Benzoyl Peroxide,* U.S.P., slowly releases oxygen and hence is bactericidal, especially to anaerobic and microaerophilic bacteria. It is also keratolytic, antiseborrheic, and irritant. As *Benzoyl Peroxide Lotion,* U.S.P., *gel,* or *cream,* all of which contain 5 or 10% hydrous benzoyl peroxide, it is used in the treatment of *acne vulgaris* and *acne rosacea.* The bactericidal action on *Propionibacterium (Corynebacterium) acnes* decreases the production of irritating fatty acids in sebum, and the keratolytic action helps peel the caps from the comedones. After application, there may be transient stinging or burning sensations, which disappear after continued use. Vasodilatation and perivascular lymphocytic infiltration occur. It is especially irritating to skin on the neck and circumoral areas. It must be kept away from the eyes. Excess dryness of the skin and desquamation may occur after 1 to 2 weeks of use. Benzoyl peroxide can cause contact dermatitis. It also bleaches clothing.

PERMANGANATES

Potassium Permanganate, U.S.P., has a limited topical efficacy against bacteria and fungi. Concentrations of 1:5000 or more are necessary for an effective bactericidal action, but they are irritating to tissues. Consequently, solutions of 1:10,000 are usually used. However, up to an hour may be required to kill many bacteria, and some strains survive exposure to this concentration. For this reason, permanganate has been made obsolete by much superior antiseptic and antifungal drugs. Because of the astringency of the manganous and manganic ions that result from reduction of the permanganate anion, the substance is occasionally used to suppress the vesicular stage of *eczema-dermatitis.* A wet dressing of permanganate may be employed in the treatment of *ivy poisoning.* Permanganate solution can oxidize many drugs, but it is seldom used as an antidote in poisoning.

CHLORHEXIDINE

Chlorhexidine is one of a number of biguanides with potent antiseptic activity. Its structure is as follows:

Chlorhexidine

It is used mainly as the gluconate, but the acetate is also employed for some purposes. In British Commonwealth countries, chlorhexidine has been in use for nearly 2 decades, but, strangely, it was approved for use in the United States only in 1976. It seems certain to become a most important compound in the antiseptic armamentarium.

Chlorhexidine is effective against both gram-positive and gram-negative bacteria, although it is somewhat less effective against the latter. The agent disrupts the plasma membrane of the bacterial cell. The activity is maintained even in the presence of blood.

As a handwash or surgical scrub, 4% chlorhexidine causes a greater initial decrease in the number of normal cutaneous bacteria than does either 7.5% povidone-iodine or 3% hexachlorophene, and it has a persistent effect equal to or greater than that of hexachlorophene (Smylie *et al.,* 1973; Lilly and Lowbury, 1974; Ojajärvi, 1976; Peterson *et al.,* 1978). A 0.5% solution in 95% ethanol exerts a greater effect than 4% chlorhexidine emulsion, 3% hexachlorophene solution, or IRGASAN DP300 (Lowbury *et al.,* 1974; Ayliffe *et al.,* 1975; Rosenberg *et al.,* 1976). A 1% aqueous solution is more erratic and has a less persistent action than do the other preparations. In experiments in which gloved hands were inoculated with large numbers (10^{14}) of *Providencia, Serratia, Pseudomonas,* and *Escherichia,* 4% chlorhexidine appeared to be somewhat less effective than 7.5% povidone-iodine (Dineen, 1978). Some gram-negative organisms are apparently completely resistant to the drug; epidemic infections caused by *Pseud. maltophilia* have been traced to contaminated aqueous preparations of chlorhexidine (Wishart and Riley, 1976).

Although chlorhexidine is mainly employed for the *preoperative preparation* of the surgeon and patient, it is also used to treat *superficial infections* caused especially by gram-positive bacteria and to *disinfect wounds.* The 4% solution has been successfully employed to decrease the rate of staph-ylococcal and streptococcal infections among neonates (Hnatko, 1977). Mouthwashes containing chlorhexidine gluconate appear to be effective in the treatment of *aphthous ulcers.* Both the gluconate and acetate decrease the amount of bacterial plaque on teeth and have been used successfully in the *prophylaxis of dental caries;* chlorhexidine appears to be adsorbed onto the enamel and dentine.

Chlorhexidine is poorly absorbed from the gastrointestinal tract and negligibly absorbed from the skin of adults. The extent of absorption from the skin of neonates is not known, but the physicochemical properties of the drug suggest that it should be slight. The oral toxicity is quite low; in rats, oral doses of 2 g/kg are hepatotoxic and nephrotoxic, but they are not lethal. In blood, very low concentrations can cause hemolysis.

Chlorhexidine gluconate is available in the United States only as the 4% aqueous emulsion (HIBICLENS) and 1% aqueous solution (HIBITANE).

HEAVY METALS AND THEIR SALTS

MERCURY COMPOUNDS

The inorganic mercury compounds were among the earliest antiseptics to be used and were highly regarded as potent germicides by Robert Koch. By the end of the last century, discerning bacteriologists had presented evidence that mercury compounds are primarily bacteriostatic, a finding that has been amply confirmed for the inorganic mercurials as well as for the organic mercury compounds introduced in this century. Nevertheless, the belief still persists that these agents are highly effective germicides.

Although mercuric ion can combine with a number of biologically significant chemical groups, the most probable mechanism of action is the inhibition of sulfhydryl enzymes. The inhibition is reversible, and bacteria inactivated on the skin, if subsequently carried into a wound or body fluid, may retain their virulence. Plasma and tissue thiols, such as glutathione and cysteine, compete for the mercury and thus assist in the reactivation. Bacterial spores exposed to mercurials for many months resume multiplication when the inhibitor is removed.

The mercury antiseptics inhibit the sulfhydryl enzymes of tissue cells as well as those of bacteria, and the therapeutic index of mercury compounds is therefore low.

It is obvious that mercury compounds fall far short of being ideal germicides. However, some are effective bacteriostatic agents and, as such, find medicinal applications. It should be noted that in many preparations of organic mercurials the vehicle contains ethyl or benzyl alcohol and/or acetone, which contribute to germicidal activity. With some mercurials it has been shown that the vehicle alone is more active than the mercurial plus the vehicle.

Inorganic Mercurial Antiseptics. The inorganic mercurials have all been rendered obsolete by more efficacious and less toxic agents. Only *Ammoniated Mercury,* U.S.P., persists. It is water insoluble and hence is applied as *Ammoniated Mercury Ointment,* U.S.P., which contains 5 or 10% $HgNH_2Cl$ in liquid petrolatum and white ointment. The mercurial is slowly transferred from the ointment base into the skin, where it exerts its actions over long periods of time. It is used chiefly as a skin antiseptic, especially in *impetigo contagiosa, dermatomycoses,* and certain other dermatoses. It is also employed for scaling in *psoriasis,* in *pruritus ani,* and in *pinworm* and *crab louse infestation.* Sensitization is a common occurrence. Furthermore, not only can mercury pass through the skin into the body but also inunction can force the ointment through the skin. Thus, chronic application can cause systemic mercury intoxication.

Organic Mercurial Antiseptics. As a group, the organic mercurials are more bacteriostatic, less irritating, and less toxic than the inorganic mercurial salts. Their mechanism of action and limitations have already been discussed.

Merbromin (MERCUROCHROME) was the first organic mercurial antiseptic to be introduced and for some time had official status. It is only feebly active, even as a bacteriostatic agent. It is the least effective of the commercial mercurial antiseptics. It also has the lowest therapeutic index. The continued inclusion of this drug in first-aid kits is regrettable.

Five organic mercurial antiseptics—*Nitromersol,* U.S.P. (METAPHEN), *phenylmercuric acetate, phenylmercuric nitrate, hydroxyphenyl mercuric chloride,* and *Thimerosal,* U.S.P. (MERTHIOLATE)—have many features in common and thus can be discussed together conveniently. They have the structural formulas shown below.

Nitromersol   Phenylmercuric {Nitrate / Acetate}

Hydroxyphenyl Mercuric Chloride   Thimerosal

Because organic mercurials are less irritating than soluble inorganic mercurial salts, they can be applied directly to tissue. However, they penetrate poorly, and the tissues fix the mercury so that it is unavailable to the microorganisms. Organic mercurials have been used to disinfect instruments and as antiseptics on cutaneous and mucosal surfaces in concentrations from 0.01 to 0.5%. It should be emphasized that these agents are primarily bacteriostatic and are relatively ineffective in killing spores. They are not as efficient in disinfecting instruments as is commonly believed. Sensitization to the organic mercurials occasionally occurs. The organic mercurial antiseptics are marketed in various types of proprietary solutions, tinctures, aerosols, creams, gels, glycerites, and ointments, and in powder form. They are also included as preservatives in many pharmaceutical products.

SILVER COMPOUNDS

Many silver compounds have antiseptic properties, but only a few have been used clinically. Soluble, highly ionizable silver salts have astringent and caustic actions as well. Only the local actions of silver are discussed here.

Actions. The silver ion combines with sulfhydryl, carboxyl, phosphate, amino, and other biologically important chemical groups. Such interactions involving a protein alter its physical properties and often cause it to precipitate. This is the basis of the astringent and caustic actions of silver ions. This may, in part, explain the antibacterial actions. Yet several poorly ionizable or poorly soluble silver compounds that do not provide enough ion for precipitation of proteins are good antiseptics nevertheless. Silver ions act on the bacterial cell surface to cause drastic alterations in the cell wall and plasma membrane. When solutions of inorganic silver salts are applied to tissue, they exert an immediate germicidal effect. Thereafter, small amounts of ionic silver are liberated from the silver proteinate formed, and this results in a sustained bacteriostatic action.

An interesting bacteriological phenomenon is that distilled water becomes markedly bactericidal after contact with metallic silver. Despite the fact that the concentration of silver ions reaches only 1 part in 20 million, even heavy suspensions of bacteria succumb within a few hours. This action of silver is shared by many heavy metals and is known as *oligodynamic action.* Although diverse theories have been proposed (*see* Romans, 1968), the mechanism of this action is obscure.

Inorganic silver salts are highly germicidal in solution. For example, silver nitrate destroys most microorganisms in a concentration of 0.1%. Lower concentrations are bacteriostatic. Silver nitrate is toxic to tissue cells in bactericidal concentrations.

Silver Nitrate. Silver nitrate is the most commonly employed of the inorganic silver salts and is used as a caustic, antiseptic, and astringent agent. The degree of action depends upon the concentration employed and the period of time during which the compound is allowed to act. The silver ion is precipitated by chloride; consequently, solutions of ionizable salts of silver do not readily penetrate into tissue. Silver salts stain tissue black due to the deposition of reduced silver. Most of the stain slowly disappears spontaneously, but some may persist indefinitely at some sites.

Silver Nitrate, U.S.P., is employed either in solid form or in solution. The solid form, *Toughened Silver Nitrate,* U.S.P. *(lunar caustic),* is used for the cauterization of wounds and for removing granulation tissue and warts. It is conveniently dispensed in pencils that should be moistened before use.

Solutions of silver nitrate, in strengths of 0.01 to 10%, are also employed for local application. When a strong germicidal action is desired, as for local treatment of infected aphthous ulcers, a 10% solution may be carefully applied. Silver salts are particularly germicidal for gonococci, and *Silver Nitrate Ophthalmic Solution,* U.S.P. (1%), is routinely employed for the *prophylaxis of ophthalmia neonatorum.* A few drops are instilled in the conjunctival sac in newborn infants. If a stronger solution is used, the eyes should be washed immediately with an isotonic sodium chloride solution. At one time, this treatment of the newborn was the established practice in the United States, but the laws were repealed in certain states because some authorities consider penicillin to be superior. However, not only can penicillin cause sensitization but also many gonococci have become resistant to the antibiotic. Hence silver nitrate continues to be used.

Silver nitrate as a 0.5% solution is used in the treatment of *extensive burns,* usually in conjunction with gentamicin, kanamycin, and/or mafenide. However, since the silver ion combines with chloride to yield insoluble silver chloride, serious hypochloremia can occur. Hyponatremia also results because the cations that accompany the serum chloride are lost into the exudate. Furthermore, absorbed nitrate can cause methemoglobinemia.

Other Silver Compounds. *Silver sulfadiazine* has been introduced to replace silver nitrate in the topical treatment of *extensive burns.* It readily penetrates the eschar. Its solubility is low enough that insufficient silver ion is released to precipitate significant amounts of chloride ion or proteins. Hypochloremia, hyponatremia, and eschars that adhere to dressings are thus avoided. Despite its low solubility, silver sulfadiazine exerts a prominent antibacterial action against *Pseudomonas.* The compound is painless upon application. Furthermore, unlike silver nitrate, it does not cause argyrial staining of wounds or bed linens. Insufficient sulfadiazine is absorbed to cause crystalluria. Bacterial resistance to sulfonamides can result from the use of silver sulfadiazine. *Silver allantoinate* and *silver uracil* have actions similar to silver sulfadiazine.

In the past, a number of colloidal suspensions of insoluble silver compounds or of elemental silver were marketed. Because of the low silver ion concentrations of such preparations, they did not precipitate chloride or protein, and they were usually nonastringent and nonirritating. *Mild silver protein* (19 to 23% silver) is still marketed. It is mostly bacteriostatic. It is nonirritating, even mildly demulcent. Claims that mild silver protein penetrates tissue at the site of application because chloride ion does not precipitate the silver are misleading. The large-carrier protein molecule penetrates poorly. Fortunately, the colloidal silver preparations are now in a deserved oblivion.

ZINC SALTS

The salts of zinc are employed as astringents, antiperspirants, styptics, corrosives, and mild antiseptics. They probably owe their action to the ability of the zinc ion to precipitate protein, but other mechanisms may be involved in the effect on bacteria. The highly ionizable, soluble salts, such as zinc chloride, are quite irritating and can be used as escharotics.

Zinc Sulfate, U.S.P., is used as *Zinc Sulfate Ophthalmic Solution,* U.S.P. (OP-THAL-ZIN) (0.25%), in angular (diplobacillary) *conjunctivitis.* For application to the skin, zinc sulfate is used in a concentration of 4%. It is often incorporated with sulfurated potash in equal concentration in a lotion known as *White Lotion,* U.S.P. Zinc sulfate has been used in such skin diseases and infections as *acne, ivy poisoning, lupus erythematosus,* and *impetigo.* The compound also forms the basis for some deodorant anhidrotics (*see* Chapter 40). Zinc sulfate is used in vaginal deodorants in concentrations of 0.25 to 4%. The compound accelerates the rate of healing of leg ulcers, other lesions, and acrodermatitis enteropathica, especially in patients with low plasma concentrations of zinc; the salt has been applied topically or given orally in a dose of 220 mg three times a day.

Zinc Chloride, U.S.P., is occasionally used as an astringent in solutions of 0.5 to 2%. A 10% solution applied to the teeth is sometimes used to make the teeth less sensitive. *Zinc Acetate,* U.S.P., is used as an astringent and styptic and occasionally as an emetic.

Zinc Oxide, U.S.P., is incorporated in powders, ointments, and pastes. It has a mild astringent and antiseptic action. It is used in skin diseases and infections such as *eczema, impetigo, ringworm, varicose ulcers, pruritus,* and *psoriasis.* Zinc oxide can alter skin pigmentation. Preparations containing zinc oxide include *Zinc Oxide Ointment,* U.S.P. (20% zinc oxide), *Zinc Oxide Paste,* U.S.P. (25% zinc oxide), and *Zinc Oxide and Salicylic Acid Paste,* U.S.P. (2% salicylic acid in paste of zinc oxide). *Calamine,* U.S.P., consists of a pink powder containing zinc oxide (not less than 98%) and a small amount of ferric oxide. It is incorporated into *Calamine Lotion,* U.S.P. (8% calamine and 8% zinc oxide), and *Phenolated Calamine Lotion,* U.S.P. (*compound calamine lotion*) (1% phenol in calamine lotion). *Zinc Stearate,* U.S.P., and *zinc oleate* have actions similar to those of zinc oxide.

Zinc pyrithione, in concentrations of 0.1 to 2%, is employed in the treatment of *seborrhea* and *dandruff.*

QUATERNARY AMMONIUM COMPOUNDS

Surface-active agents are widely used in industry and in the home as wetting agents, detergents, and emulsifiers. Some compounds possess the ability to precipitate or denature protein and to destroy microorganisms. In this category, only the quaternary ammonium compounds are much used as germicides.

Chemistry. Detergents are characterized by a structural balance between one or more hydrophilic and hydrophobic centers and may be ionic or nonionic. The structural formulas of the major cationic agents used in medicine are shown below.

Germicidal Properties. Quaternary ammonium agents in low concentrations are bactericidal *in vitro* to a wide variety of gram-positive and gram-negative bacteria; the gram-positive microorganisms are the more sensitive. Some gram-negative bacteria, especially *Pseud. cepacia,* are resistant, and epidemics have been caused by using instruments supposedly sterilized by quaternary ammonium agents or by contaminated commercial preparations (*see* Frank and Schaffner, 1976). *Mycobacterium tuberculosis* is also relatively resistant. Many fungi and viruses are susceptible. Ethanol enhances the germicidal activity, so that tinctures are more effective than aqueous solutions. The major site of action of these compounds appears to be the cell membrane, where the agents cause changes in permeability.

Anionic surface-active agents antagonize the effect of cationic agents. Thus, within certain time limits, bacteriostatic actions of cationic compounds can be reversed by soaps and other anionic agents. Germicidal activity of the cationic compounds is reduced by organic matter and by other reactive substances; Lawrence (1968b) lists the more important chemicals that are incompatible with cationic agents. Of special importance is the fact that these agents are adsorbed to a significant degree by cotton, rubber, and other porous materials. This adsorption reduces the effective concentration of the agent and thereby decreases its germicidal efficiency (*see* below).

Preparations. Only the cationic surface-active agents are employed in medicine. *Benzalkonium chloride* (ZEPHIRAN) is freely soluble in water, alcohol, or acetone. Aqueous solutions are slightly alkaline. It is available as a 0.133% solution, tincture, and tincture spray. Other commonly used agents are *Benzethonium Chloride,* U.S.P. (PHEMEROL CHLORIDE), available as 0.133 and 3% solutions, 0.2% tincture, and 0.2% vaginal foam; *Cetylpyridinium Chloride,* U.S.P. (CEEPRYN, CEPACOL), available as a 0.1% solution, 0.067% mouthwash-gargle, and 1.5-mg (0.067%) lozenges; *domiphen bromide* (BRADOSOL BROMIDE), available as a lozenge containing 1.5 mg (0.067%); and *Methylbenzethonium Chloride,* U.S.P. (DIAPARENE, others), available as 0.1% ointment or powder. These agents are also compounded with others in a variety of mouthwashes and gargles and dermatological and vaginal preparations.

Actions and Uses. Quaternary ammonium agents are detergents as well as sanitizers, and they were once widely used in sanitation. In medicine they have been overly employed as all-purpose antiseptics for application to skin, tissue, and mucous membranes and as disinfectants for medical and surgical materials.

Antiseptic Uses. Quaternary ammonium antiseptics are relatively nonirritating to tissue in effective concentrations. They have a rapid onset of action. They wet and penetrate tissue surfaces and possess detergent, keratolytic, and emulsifying actions. They have a relatively low systemic toxicity, but poisoning from oral ingestion has occurred. Nevertheless, certain serious shortcomings must be kept in mind. Their activity is antagonized by soaps, tissue constituents, and pus. Also, when applied to the skin, they tend to form a film under which bacteria may remain viable; the inner surface of the film has low bactericidal power whereas the outer surface is strongly bactericidal. They do not kill spores. Their action is rather slow when compared to that of iodine. A 0.1% solution of benzalkonium chloride applied to the human skin requires about 7 minutes to decrease the bacterial population by a mere 50%; the 0.1% tincture has a slower action than 70% ethanol. Even in

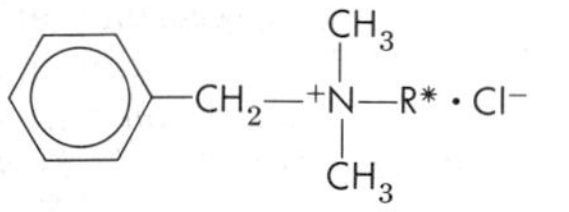

Benzalkonium Chloride

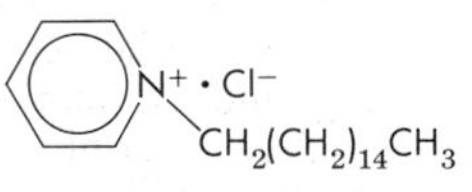

Cetylpyridinium Chloride

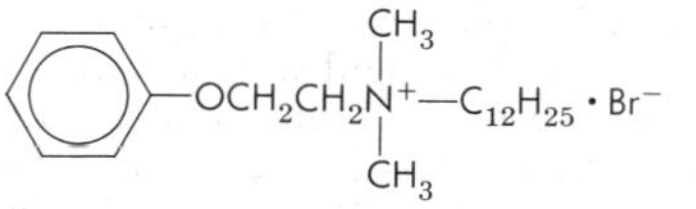

Domiphen Bromide

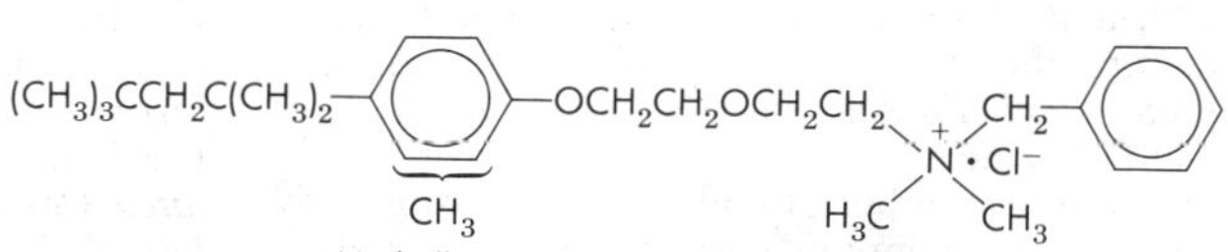

Methylbenzethonium Chloride †

---

* *R* represents any alkyl from C_8H_{17} to $C_{18}H_{37}$; the preparation is thus a mixture of molecules in which the alkyls differ.

† Benzethonium differs from methylbenzethonium in lacking the CH_3 in the position indicated by the brace.

the absence of antagonistic tissue constituents, a 0.002% solution requires 9 hours to kill 98% of *Escherichia coli;* this poorly effective concentration is close to that advocated for irrigation and lavage of the urinary tract. The cationic surfactants interact with keratin and cause epidermal damage, although this is minor except during continued use. Lastly, these drugs can cause occasional allergic responses with chronic use, as with certain deodorant preparations and diaper washes; cutaneous necrosis has been reported. In aggregate, the disadvantages would appear greatly to outweigh the advantages. Since superior agents are available, there seems little reason to use the cationic surfactants as antiseptics. Despite this fact, their use as antiseptics and as spermatocides and deodorants persists.

Disinfectant Uses. Surface-active agents have been widely used for the sterilization of instruments and other materials such as cotton pledgets and rubber gloves. However, skin, rubber gloves, surgical sponges of various materials, endoscopes, and objects made of polyethylene or polypropylene adsorb quaternary ammonium antiseptics to such a degree that the concentration of the solution may be materially reduced. Thus, repeated use of the same solution for disinfection of porous materials can reduce the concentration of the agent below the bactericidal limit. Hospital infections have been traced to materials stored in ineffective solutions of benzalkonium chloride. The actions, uses, and abuses of quaternary ammonium antiseptics have been reviewed by Dixon and coworkers (1976).

NITROFURAZONE

Derivatives of furan possess antimicrobial activity. The presence of a nitro group in the 5 position of the furan ring confers antibacterial activity on many 2-substituted furans. The structural formula of nitrofurazone is:

$$O_2N\!-\!\langle\!\langle\,O\,\rangle\!\rangle\!-\!CH\!=\!N\!-\!\underset{\underset{H}{|}}{N}\!-\!\underset{\underset{O}{\|}}{C}\!-\!NH_2$$

Nitrofurazone

Antibacterial Actions. Nitrofurazone affects a variety of gram-positive and gram-negative microorganisms. A bacteriostatic action is exerted upon most bacteria in the concentration range of $1:100,000$ to $1:200,000$. Bactericidal concentrations are approximately twice as great. Certain strains of bacteria, however, are insensitive to concentrations of the agents far in excess of those mentioned. The mechanism of the antibacterial action of the furan derivatives is unknown. Heavy inocula of microorganisms as well as plasma and blood reduce the activity of the drugs. Bacteria develop only a limited resistance to nitrofurazone, and cross-resistance between it and sulfonamides or antibiotics does not occur.

Preparations and Therapeutic Uses. *Nitrofurazone,* U.S.P. (FURACIN), is used as a broad-spectrum

topical antibacterial agent in the treatment of mixed infections of superficial wounds and diseases of the skin. The effects are generally favorable; the bacterial population is greatly reduced, and adverse effects on healing are not observed. Its efficacy in the treatment of burns is high (*see* Crenshaw *et al.,* 1976). It is available in the form of a 0.2% cream, ointment, powder, soluble dressing, or topical solution. The compound produces sensitization in approximately 0.5 to 2% of patients, and this sometimes occurs within a few days after the initial application. The systemic toxicity of nitrofurazone is relatively low, and, furthermore, the drug is not significantly absorbed from mucosal or burned surfaces.

DYES

There is little in common among the clinically used dyes with respect to chemical class or mechanism of action, and their inclusion together expresses a want of a better system of classification. Some of the dyes are not antimicrobial and, therefore, receive only brief mention here.

Gentian Violet. *Gentian Violet,* U.S.P. (*crystal violet, hexamethylrosaniline chloride*), is a triphenylmethane (rosaniline) dye with the following structure:

Gentian Violet

Marketed products often contain up to 4% of the tetramethyl and pentamethyl congeners. The pure compound is known as *crystal violet.*

Gentian violet is bacteriostatic and bactericidal to gram-positive bacteria and to many fungi. Gram-negative and acid-fast bacteria are very resistant to the drug.

Gentian Violet Topical Solution, U.S.P., contains 1% of the drug in 10% ethanol, and *Gentian Violet Cream,* U.S.P., contains 1.35% in an absorbable base. Gentian violet was once widely employed in the control of many types of infections. It has been used for superficial pyogenic infections, impetigo, Vincent's infection, and chronic and irritative lesions and dermatitides. It is still occasionally employed in treatment of fungal infections. For direct application to tissues, the dye is used in concentrations of 0.02% to 1%. Vaginal suppositories contain 17 mg, while vaginal tablets contain 2 mg. For instillations in closed cavities, the concentration is reduced to 0.01%. It may be used for infected wounds, mucous membranes, and serous surfaces. Permanent pigmentation of the skin can result from contact of gentian violet with granulation tissue, and the dye should not be applied to ulcerative lesions of the face. The staining properties are a distinct disadvantage.

Methylene Blue. Methylene blue is tetramethyl-thionine chloride. It has the following structural formula:

Methylene Blue

The compound can be reduced to a colorless (leuko) form; consequently, methylene blue and leuko-methylene blue comprise a reversible oxidation-reduction system.

Actions and Uses. Although methylene blue has weak bacteriostatic activity, it is no longer used as a topical or urinary antiseptic. *In vitro,* it has an effect to retard crystal formation; consequently, it has recently had brief but unproductive popularity in the treatment of nephrolithiasis. The dye continues to be of value in the treatment of *methemoglobinemia.*

Methylene blue has two interesting and opposite actions on hemoglobin. In high concentrations it oxidizes the ferrous iron of reduced hemoglobin to the ferric form, and, as a result, methemoglobin is produced. Conversely, *in vivo,* low concentrations of methylene blue or the chemically related thionine are capable of hastening the conversion of methemoglobin to hemoglobin. The reduction of methemoglobin within the intact erythrocyte is accomplished by methemoglobin reductases, which are pyridine-nucleotide dependent. Methylene blue can act as an electron acceptor in the transfer of electrons from reduced pyridine nucleotides to methemoglobin. In the reaction, methylene blue is reduced by pyridine nucleotides, and the leukomethylene blue, in turn, reduces methemoglobin to hemoglobin. The dye will not affect methemoglobinemia in persons with glucose-6-phosphate dehydrogenase deficiency. When the formation of reduced pyridine nucleotides is prevented, methylene blue acts purely as an oxidant.

Absorption, Fate, and Excretion. Methylene blue is poorly absorbed from the gastrointestinal tract. In the tissues, methylene blue is rapidly reduced to the leuko form, which is excreted slowly into the urine and the bile. A portion of the leukomethylene blue may be partially demethylated.

Untoward Reactions. The intravenous administration of very large doses of methylene blue (500 mg) causes nausea, abdominal and precordial pain, dizziness, headache, profuse sweating, mental confusion, and methemoglobinemia.

Preparations and Dosage. Methylene Blue, U.S.P. (*methylthionine chloride*), consists of dark-green crystals that are moderately soluble in water and alcohol and form deep-blue solutions. The compound is marketed as a 1% injection and in 65-mg tablets. For *idiopathic methemoglobinemia,* it is given orally in the daily dose of 300 mg in conjunction with large amounts of ascorbic acid. For acute, drug-induced methemoglobinemia, 1 to 2 mg/kg of *Methylene Blue Injection,* U.S.P., can be given intravenously.

Miscellaneous Dyes. *Aminacrine hydrochloride* exerts germicidal actions against both gram-positive and gram-negative bacteria and against fungi and trichomonads. It is not inactivated by pus, secretions, or body fluids. In the treatment of *vaginal candidiasis, trichomoniasis,* or *Haemophilus infections* it is employed as a 0.1% powder or 0.2% cream, jelly, or suppository. It is also used as a 2% cream for application to the skin.

Triple dye contains brilliant green, crystal violet, and proflavine hemisulfate in a 2:2:1 ratio. A 0.5% solution is bactericidal to both gram-positive and gram-negative bacteria. Although it was used as early as 1958 for antisepsis of the umbilical stump of the neonate, triple dye was not carefully studied until the toxicity of hexachlorophene occasioned the reappraisal of antisepsis of the skin in neonates. From a study with 531 neonates, Pildes and associates (1973) reported that triple dye was as effective as daily baths of 3% hexachlorophene in decreasing colonization by staphylococci.

MISCELLANEOUS GERMICIDES

Acetone. Acetone is bactericidal and virucidal; it is not sporicidal. Concentrations of acetone below 40% have little effect, and the optimal concentration is pure acetone. In concentrations above 85%, bacteria are killed in 5 to 30 seconds. On the skin, pure acetone is less effective than 70% ethanol, possibly because rapid evaporation limits the contact time. However, a brief sojourn on the skin is an advantage in allergy testing and immunization. Undiluted acetone has been reported to be an excellent and convenient sterilizing agent (Drews, 1977), provided that the object to be sterilized is free of clots, which resist penetration. Acetone is mixed with ethanol for antiseptic and presumed keratolytic purposes.

Sulfur and Thiosulfates. Sulfur must be converted to pentathionic acid ($H_2S_5O_6$) in order to exert germicidal action. Presumably the oxidation of sulfur to pentathionic acid is accomplished by certain microorganisms or by epidermal cells when the element is applied to the skin. Sulfur possesses a keratolytic property, which may be the basis for the therapeutic action of the element in certain cutaneous disorders unassociated with infection.

Sublimed Sulfur, U.S.P. (*flowers of sulfur*), is a fine, yellow crystalline, water-insoluble powder. *Precipitated Sulfur,* U.S.P., is a much finer powder and, therefore, has a greater reactive surface than sublimed sulfur. *Colloidal sulfur* is the most active form of sulfur and is available as elemental sulfur in stable aqueous colloidal solutions. Precipitated sulfur is the form that is most used in topical preparations. It is available in a 10% soap, 10% ointment, and 2% gel (which also contains 37% ethanol). Sublimed sulfur is used in the preparation of *sulfurated lime,* which is applied as a 25% topical solution.

Sulfur is used as a fungicide and parasiticide (*see* below). Sulfur alone, or in combination with other keratolytic agents (often 2% salicylic acid, resorcinol, or coal tar), is widely used in the treatment of cutaneous disorders such as *psoriasis, seborrhea,* and *eczema-dermatitis.* The percentage of sulfur employed may be that of the full-strength ointment, or less if the patient's skin exhibits intolerance. Prolonged local use of sulfur may result in a characteristic dermatitis venenata.

Thiosulfates readily generate free sulfur, especially in acidic solution. The pH of the skin is usually low enough to favor a slow release of elemental sulfur, and bacteria also favor the conversion. *White Lotion,* U.S.P., contains sulfurated potash, which is a complex polysulfide and thiosulfate. *Sodium Thiosulfate,* U.S.P., is marketed for parenteral use in the treatment of cyanide poisoning, but it may be applied to the skin in various forms.

Ichthammol. *Ichthammol,* U.S.P. (*ammonium ichthosulfonate*), is the product obtained from sulfonating and neutralizing with ammonia, the distillate of certain bituminous schists. The compound contains approximately 10% sulfur in the form of organic sulfonates. It is a brown, viscous fluid with a strong characteristic odor and is soluble in both aqueous and organic solvents. Ichthammol is mildly irritant and somewhat antiseptic. It is used alone, or in combination with other antiseptics, for the treatment of cutaneous disorders and to promote healing in chronic inflammations. The drug is commonly employed in the form of *Ichthammol Ointment,* U.S.P. (10% in a petrolatum base). At one time the drug was used widely, but it has deservedly lost much popularity.

Anthralin. *Anthralin,* U.S.P. (1,8,9-anthratriol), is a mild irritant with weak antimicrobial activity. The compound is employed in the treatment of *psoriasis and chronic dermatoses.* Anthralin is available as *Anthralin Ointment,* U.S.P., and in proprietary creams or ointments in concentrations of 0.1 to 1.0%. The weakest preparation is first employed, and the strength is then increased according to the tolerance of the patient. Weigand and Everett (1967) found that anthralin was quite effective in cases of psoriasis that had not responded to other treatment. It should be kept away from the eyes and other sensitive surfaces. Anthralin stains the skin yellow.

Salicylanilides and Carbanilides. *Dibromsalan* and *tribromsalan* are brominated derivatives of salicylanilide. Tribromsalan is a component of IRGASAN DP300 soap and washing cream; on the skin, the soap is slightly less effective than 3% hexachlorophene against staphylococci, but it suppresses the overgrowth of gram-negative organisms. *Cloflucarban* is a polychlorofluoro derivative and *triclocarban* a trichloro derivative of carbanilide. They are effective against both gram-positive and gram-negative bacteria and also against fungi. Their principal use is in deodorant soaps, for which they appear to be effective. Cloflucarban is also contained in the antiseptic emulsion IRGASAN CF3. Triclocarban in DIAL soap has been reported to be as effective as 3% hexachlorophene solution (Borchardt *et al.,* 1978). However, claims that such soaps reduce the incidence of cutaneous infections require substantiation. All these

drugs can cause occasional hypersensitivity; the salicylanilides, especially, may cause photosensitization (*see* Ison and Tucker, 1968). There is a spate of literature on the absorption and fate of triclocarban.

Ethylene and Propylene Oxides. *Ethylene oxide* is a gaseous alkylating germicide with a broad spectrum of activity. It is sporicidal and virucidal. It is used to disinfect and sterilize heat-labile surgical instruments. It alkylates tissue constituents and is thus toxic. Inhalation causes nausea, vomiting, neurological disorders, and even death. Traces of the gas in gloves or clothing may cause burns. Desorption for 8 hours at 50° C is much more effective than for 24 hours at room temperature. Residues in vascular catheters can cause thrombophlebitis; in endotracheal tubes, tracheitis. The gas is explosive in concentrations above 3% and must be mixed with CO_2 or fluorocarbons. The optimal humidity is 30 to 40%. An exposure of 3 hours is used to guarantee killing of desiccated spores. For further information, *see* Borick (1968) and Boucher (1972).

Propylene oxide, a liquid, is also an effective sterilizing agent (*see* Hart and Brown, 1974).

II. Antifungal Drugs

In temperate climates, fungal infections comprise a minor fraction of human diseases caused by microorganisms. Nevertheless, the incidence, particularly of superficial infections such as tinea pedis, is appreciable. The list of chemicals reputed to have some degree of antifungal activity is long, and a number of preparations of low efficacy are successfully foisted upon both the lay public and the medical profession, despite the existence at the present time of drugs that are demonstrably beneficial in dermatophytosis.

Many antibacterial agents possess fungistatic or fungicidal properties. Therefore, many of the drugs discussed under antiseptics and disinfectants have been employed in the local treatment of fungal infections, and their uses in such mycoses have already been noted in some instances. The present discussion will be restricted to *nonsystemic antifungal drugs;* systemic antifungal drugs are discussed in Chapter 54. The antifungal drugs have been reviewed by Drube (1972), Kobayashi and Medoff (1977), and Drouhet (1978).

Mechanisms of Antifungal Action. Drugs exert fungistatic and fungicidal actions by a variety of mechanisms (*see* references cited above). In addition, many agents used in the treatment of superficial mycoses are virtually devoid of either fungistatic or fungicidal actions in the concentrations employed, and their beneficial effects probably depend upon factors not related to any direct effect on fungi. The keratolytic agents exert their effect mainly by promoting desquamation of the stratum corneum, especially in hyperkeratotic locations. The fungus resides in the stratum corneum, where keratin is its substrate, not in the toxin-induced lesion. Thus, keratolysis removes the offending fungus as well as aids in the penetration of drugs. Drugs that prevent hyperhidrosis indirectly retard proliferation of the fungus by altering the conditions of growth. Astringent drugs exert a palliative effect by allaying the symptoms of acute inflammation and irritation.

FATTY ACIDS AND THEIR SALTS

It has long been known that fatty acids and their salts possess antifungal activity. The antifungal activity of sweat is due to the fatty acids contained therein.

Propionates. Sodium and calcium propionates have long been incorporated in bread dough as nontoxic inhibitors of mold growth. *Sodium propionate* is promoted for the treatment of dermatomycoses. It is relatively weak and possesses only fungistatic activity; both *in vitro* and in human infections, viable fungi can be recovered after exposure to it. Both its low efficacy and exaggerated price make it an irrational choice for treatment. Sodium propionate is used in proprietary preparations in concentrations of 5 to 10%. It is also compounded with the more active *undecylenic acid. Caprylic acid* and its salts are similar in actions to sodium propionate and are used for the same medical purposes.

Undecylenic Acid. Undecylenic acid is 10-undecenoic acid, an 11-carbon, unsaturated compound. It is a yellow liquid with a characteristic rancid odor. It is primarily fungistatic, although fungicidal activity may be observed with long exposure to high concentrations of the agent. The drug is active against a variety of fungi, including the common pathogens in superficial mycoses. It is usually compounded with its zinc salt, but it is also available alone as a 2% soap, which has dubious efficacy. *Zinc Undecylenate,* U.S.P., is a fine white powder that has antifungal properties similar to those of the acid. It is usually used as *Compound Undecylenic Acid Ointment,* U.S.P., which contains 5% undecylenic acid and 20% zinc undecylenate in a polyethylene glycol base, and as *compound undecylenic powder* and a *topical aerosol powder,* both of which contain 2% undecylenic acid and 20% zinc undecylenate. The zinc provides an astringent action that aids in the reduction of inflammation. *Calcium undecylenate* is also marketed.

Undecylenic acid preparations are employed in the treatment of various *dermatomycoses,* especially *tinea pedis.* Concentrations of the acid as high as 10%, as well as in the compound ointment, may be applied to the skin. For use on mucous membranes the concentration of the acid should not exceed 1%. The preparations are usually not irritating to tissue

in the stated concentrations, and sensitization to them is uncommon. It is of undoubted benefit in retarding fungus growth in *tinea pedis,* but the infection frequently persists despite intensive treatment with preparations of the acid and the zinc salt. At best, the clinical "cure" rate is about 50% (Smith *et al.,* 1977) and is thus much lower than that obtained with miconazole, haloprogin, or tolnaftate. The efficacy in the treatment of *tinea capitis* is marginal, and the drug is no longer used for that purpose.

IMIDAZOLES

Several related imidazoles have broad-spectrum antifungal activity and also some antibacterial activity. The group includes the most effective drugs for several of the superficial mycoses. Some are also effective systemically for treatment of certain deep mycoses.

Miconazole Nitrate. Miconazole is an imidazolinylmethyl derivative of *bis*-(2,4-dichlorobenzyl) ether. It has the following structure:

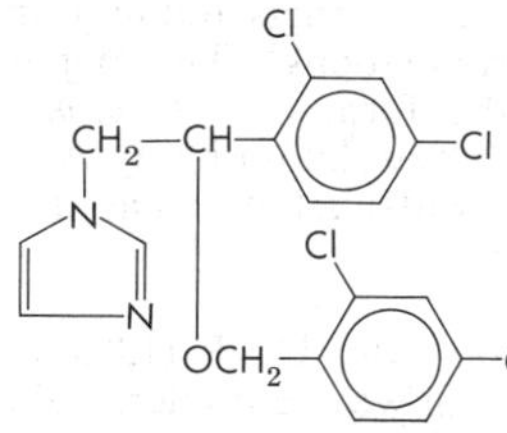

Miconazole

The compound has a broad antifungal spectrum; it is fungicidal to various species of *Trichophyton, Epidermophyton, Microsporum, Candida, Cryptococcus, Aspergillus, Coccidioides, Paracoccidioides, Cladosporium, Phialophora, Madurella, Blastomyces,* and *Histoplasma.* The drug permeates the chitin of the fungal cell wall and increases the membrane permeability to various intracellular substances. Miconazole is also effective against gram-positive bacteria. The drug readily penetrates the stratum corneum of the skin and persists there for more than 4 days after application.

In the treatment of *tinea pedis,* topical miconazole relieves itching within a few days; vesicles and fissures heal rapidly, but desquamation may continue for several weeks. In one double-blind study in which progress was verified by microscopic examination and cultures (Brugmans *et al.,* 1970), the cure rate was 96%. In the treatment of *tinea curis,* the drug is comparably effective. *Tinea versicolor, ringworm, onychomycosis,* and *cutaneous candidiasis* also respond to topical miconazole. In the treatment of *vulvovaginal candidiasis,* the mycological cure rate at the end of 1 month is about 80 to 95%, compared to about 65% with nystatin (Proost *et al.,* 1972; Culbertson, 1974; Hilton *et al.,* 1978). Pruritus sometimes is relieved after a single application. Some vaginal infections caused by *T. glabratus* also respond. The free base is used to treat ophthalmic mycoses (*see* Jones, 1978). The actions and uses of miconazole have been reviewed by Sawyer and associates (1975a) and Kobayashi and Medoff (1977).

Miconazole is colorless and odorless. Rarely, burning and maceration follow cutaneous application. Burning, itching, urticaria, rash, headache, and pelvic cramps may occur after intravaginal application, especially during the first week of treatment; the incidence of such side effects is about 7%. Although the drug penetrates rapidly, only trace amounts can be found in the blood or urine. Miconazole is considered safe for use during pregnancy.

Miconazole nitrate is available as a 2% cream or lotion (MICATIN) for use on the skin and nails or as a 2% vaginal cream (MONISTAT-7). It is applied once or twice daily to the skin for 4 weeks or once daily intravaginally for 7 days. The systemic and intrathecal uses, doses, and adverse effects of miconazole are discussed in Chapter 54.

Clotrimazole. Clotrimazole is a close chemical congener of miconazole. It has the following structure:

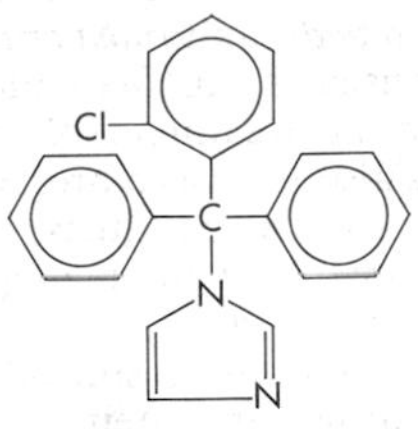

Clotrimazole

Its antifungal and antibacterial spectra and mechanism of action are essentially the same as those of miconazole, except that it has activity against cutaneous *Corynebacterium* and against the ameba *Naegleria fowleri*. In the United States, it has been approved for cutaneous application in the treatment of *tinea pedis, cruris,* and *corporis* due to *T. rubrum, T. mentagrophytes, E. floccosum,* and *M. canis* and *tinea versicolor* due to *Malassezia furfur,* and for cutaneous or vulvovaginal application in infections caused by *C. albicans.* Clotrimazole certainly appears to be as effective as miconazole in treating the epidermophytoses and candidosis and somewhat superior to nystatin in candidosis. It has been successfully utilized as a troche in the treatment of oral candidiasis and orally in the treatment of pulmonary and urinary candidiasis, although the concentrations achieved in blood are low. Despite scleroconjunctival irritant effects that discourage ophthalmological use, clotrimazole has been employed successfully in the treatment of difficult-to-manage ocular mycoses, such as *aspergillosis* (*see* Jones, 1975).

Clotrimazole is applied as a 1% topical cream or solution (LOTRIMIN) or 100-mg foaming vaginal tablet (GYNE-LOTRIMIN) once a day.

On the skin, in a small fraction of recipients, clotrimazole may cause stinging, erythema, edema, vesication, desquamation, pruritus, and urticaria. Applied to the vagina, about 1.5% of recipients complain of a mild burning sensation and, rarely, of

lower abdominal cramps, slight urinary frequency, or skin rash. Occasionally, the sexual partner may experience penile or urethral irritation. By the oral route, clotrimazole causes gastrointestinal irritation. The details of the pharmacology and clinical uses of clotrimazole may be found in Symposium (1974) and the review by Sawyer and associates (1975b).

TOLNAFTATE

Tolnaftate was the first chemical compound to be found effectively fungicidal when applied topically. It has the following structural formula:

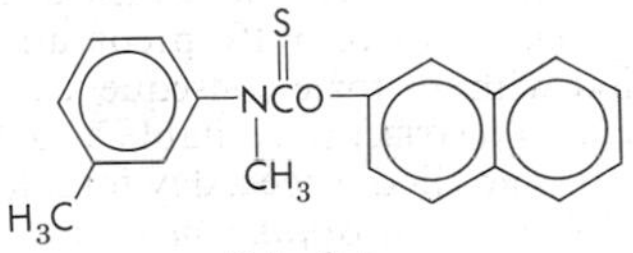

Tolnaftate

In vitro, it inhibits the growth of *T. mentagrophytes* in a concentration of 7.5 to 75 ng/ml; it is also active against *T. rubrum, T. tonsurans, M. canis, M. gypseum,* and *E. floccosum.* It is without effect on *Candida* species and bacteria. Tolnaftate is effective in the treatment of the majority of cutaneous mycoses caused by *T. rubrum, T. mentagrophytes, T. tonsurans, E. floccosum, M. canis, M. audouini, M. gypseum,* and *Malassezia furfur.* The drug is less effective in the presence of hyperkeratotic lesions, and these should be treated with 10% salicylic acid ointment alternating with tolnaftate. The clinical results produced by the topical application of this agent are thought to be better than those that follow the parenteral administration of griseofulvin in the infections listed above, but it is less effective than miconazole. For example, in tinea pedis the cure rate is around 80%, compared to about 95% for miconazole. Lesions on the scalp due to *T. tonsurans* and *M. audouini* do not respond. The drug does not alter the course of onychomycosis. Relapse may occur after cessation of therapy and approximates the rate observed when griseofulvin is employed; it is not due to development of drug resistance in the microorganisms. Retreatment is usually successful. Toxic or allergic reactions to tolnaftate have not been reported.

Tolnaftate, U.S.P. (TINACTIN), is available in 1% concentration as an official cream, gel, powder, aerosol powder, or topical solution, or as a topical aerosol solution. The preparations are applied locally twice a day. When pruritus is present, it is usually relieved in 24 to 72 hours. Involution of interdigital lesions due to susceptible fungi is very often complete in 7 to 21 days.

HALOPROGIN

Haloprogin is a halogenated phenolic ether with the following structure:

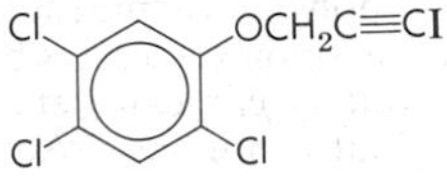

Haloprogin

It is fungicidal to various species of *Epidermophyton, Malassezia, Microsporum, Trichophyton,* and *Candida.* During treatment with this drug, irritation, pruritus, burning sensations, vesiculation, increased maceration, and "sensitization" (or exacerbation of the lesion) occasionally occur, especially on the foot if occlusive footgear is worn. It is possible that the sensitization indicates a rapid therapeutic response in which the release of toxins makes the lesion temporarily worse. Haloprogin is poorly absorbed through the skin; it is converted to trichlorophenol in the body. The systemic toxicity from topical application appears to be low. Hughes and coworkers (1974) have reported a case in which a 4-year-old child was given 12 kg of a 1% preparation over a 3-year period without toxic consequence.

Haloprogin (HALOTEX) is available as a 1% cream or solution. It is applied twice a day for 2 to 4 weeks. Its principal use is against *tinea pedis,* for which the cure rate is about 80%; it is thus approximately equal in efficacy to tolnaftate. It is also used against *tinea cruris, tinea corporis, tinea manuum,* and *tinea versicolor.* For the results of two double-blind comparative clinical studies, *see* the reports by Hermann (1972) and Katz and Cahn (1972). It is equal in efficacy to nystatin in the treatment of *cutaneous candidiasis.*

Benzoic Acid and Salicylic Acid

Benzoic and Salicylic Acids Ointment, U.S.P., is known as *Whitfield's ointment.* It combines the fungistatic action of benzoate with the keratolytic action of salicylate. It contains benzoic acid and salicylic acid in a ratio of 2:1 (usually 12%:6%). It is used mainly in the treatment of *tinea pedis.* Since benzoic acid is only fungistatic, eradication of the infection occurs only after the infected stratum corneum is shed, and continuous medication is required for several weeks to months. The salicylic acid accelerates the desquamation. The ointment is also sometimes used to treat *tinea capitis.* Mild irritation may occur at the site of application.

Miscellaneous Antifungal Agents

Acrisorcin, U.S.P. (AKRINOL), 9-aminoacridinium 4-hexylresorcinolate, is effective against *Malassezia furfur.* Therefore, it is used in the treatment of *tinea versicolor* (*pityriasis versicolor*). The drug is available as *Acrisorcin Cream,* U.S.P. (0.2%). It is applied twice daily to the affected areas; application is continued for 6 weeks after clearing of the lesions. Relapses sometimes occur. Although acrisorcin has mild antibacterial actions, it is not used as an antiseptic. The topical toxicity is low, but it includes production of hives, blisters, and erythematous vesicles. The drug may cause burning sensations when applied to eczematous lesions. Its use may result in photo-induced pruritus. It should be kept away from the eyes.

Candicidin is a polyene (heptaene) antibiotic obtained from a soil actinomycete. It is both fungistatic and fungicidal and is clinically effective only for treatment of vaginal candidiasis. Adverse reactions to candicidin have been rare. The antibiotic is used topically, twice a day for 2 weeks. *Candicidin,* U.S.P. (CANDEPTIN, VANOBID), is available as a vaginal ointment (0.06%) with an applicator for insertion; vaginal tablets and capsules containing 3 mg are also supplied.

Chlordantoin (SPOROSTACIN) is mainly antifungal against the yeasts, and its use is limited to treatment of *candidiasis* of the skin, nails, buccal mucosa, and vagina. Many such infections fail to respond to the drug. Local irritation and hypersensitivity can occur. It is applied to the vagina as a 1% cream, inserted twice daily for 2 weeks.

Natamycin (*pimaricin;* MYPROZINE, NATACYN) is a pentaenic macrolide. It has a broader antifungal spectrum than does amphotericin B, especially against ocular pathogens. It is also much less irritating to the eye and hence is used to treat fungal keratitis, especially when caused by myceliating fungi. It is the drug of choice in infections caused by *Fusarium solani.* However, it penetrates poorly and may not reach deep corneal mycoses. It is used as a 5% suspension or 1% ophthalmic ointment.

Carbol-Fuchsin Topical Solution, U.S.P., contains 0.3% basic fuchsin, 4.5% phenol, 10% resorcinol, 5% acetone, and 10% ethanol. It is still marketed for the treatment of *tinea pedis* and *tinea cruris. Orthochlormercuriphenol* is used as a 0.1% solution, generally in isopropanol, for the treatment of *tinea pedis* and *tinea capitis.* It is also used as a preservative in pharmaceutical and cosmetic products. *Salicylanilide* is used in a 5% ointment for the management of *tinea capitis.* Its efficacy is erratic.

Sulfur and the *thiosulfates* still offer useful alternatives to other drugs, and their value in the treatment of the superficial cutaneous mycoses is probably underrated. Sulfur is used in combination with salicylic acid or resorcinol. *Sodium Thiosulfate,* U.S.P. (2 to 8%), is incorporated into a number of dermatological preparations. Its use in the treatment of *tinea versicolor* is well established, but its value in the treatment of other cutaneous mycoses is largely unexplored. The uses of *selenium sulfide* are described in Chapter 40. It is effective in the treatment of *tinea versicolor.*

Many of the agents discussed in the section on antiseptics and disinfectants are antifungal, and the antimycotic uses of some are mentioned in that section. *Acetic acid* and *aminacrine* require no further discussion. *Gentian violet* (1.35%) is probably used more in the topical treatment of *vaginal candidiasis* than in any other fungal infection. The pure form, *crystal violet,* is used as the *bismuth crystal violet salt* in the treatment of *tinea pedis;* a 1% solution or ointment is applied. The excellent fungicidal properties of *iodine* are usually overlooked. The tincture can be used to treat various dry forms of cutaneous superficial mycoses, and the solution may be applied to wet forms.

Iodoquinol, U.S.P. (*diiodohydroxyquin*), and *Clioquinol,* U.S.P. (*iodochlorohydroxyquin*), are incorporated into vaginal preparations to suppress candidal and monilial infections and into dermatological preparations for the treatment of various dermatomycoses and other skin diseases; as amebicides, they are discussed more fully in Chapter 46.

III. Ectoparasiticides

The ectoparasiticides are both ectozoic and ectophytic. In common usage, however, the term *ectoparasiticides* connotes only those drugs that are used against the animal parasites. In the human, these are primarily pediculocides and miticides.

LINDANE (GAMMA BENZENE HEXACHLORIDE)

Lindane is the gamma isomer of hexachlorocyclohexane. It is lipid soluble, is absorbed through chitin, and is insecticidal by producing seizures. It can also cause convulsions in humans, even by the topical route (Lee and Groth, 1977; *see* Chapter 70); in children, especially, the seizures are of the grand mal type. Diazepam is an appropriate antagonist. Nervousness, irritability, insomnia, vertigo, amblyopia, stupor, and coma have also been observed following excessive cutaneous application. The drug can sensitize the heart to arrhythmias. It is irritant to the skin, eyes, and mucosae, and care must be taken to keep the drug away from the face and eyes. Fatal cases of aplastic anemia have resulted from prolonged exposure to vaporized lindane (Loge, 1965). The compound is readily absorbed through the skin, even of adults, and about 10% ultimately appears in the urine (Feldmann and Mailbach, 1974).

Lindane, U.S.P. (*gamma benzene hexachloride;* KWELL), is an excellent miticide in the treatment of *scabies*. It is employed in 1% concentration in a vanishing cream, lotion, or shampoo. The mixture is applied in a thin layer over the entire cutaneous surface (15 to 25 g for an adult) and is not removed for 24 hours. Pruritus is usually relieved within 24 hours, and the great majority of patients do not require a second treatment. If necessary, however, second and third applications can be made at weekly intervals.

The drug is also a very active pediculocide and is effective in the treatment of *pediculosis pubis, capitis,* and *corporis*. A single application of the 1% ointment or shampoo usually suffices to eradicate the ectoparasite. Lindane is also used to treat infestation by *Phthirus pubis* (crab lice).

MISCELLANEOUS ECTOPARASITICIDES

Benzyl benzoate is a relatively harmless substance that in high concentration is toxic to *Acarus scabiei*. The compound has been widely employed in the treatment of *scabies* and is also useful in the treatment of *pediculosis. Benzyl Benzoate*, U.S.P., is used as a 25% lotion (*Benzyl Benzoate Lotion*, U.S.P.). In the treatment of *scabies*, the lotion is applied to the entire body, except the face, after thorough cleansing. When the first application is dry, a second coat is applied. After 24 hours, the residue is then washed off.

Pyrethrins, which are discussed in Chapter 70, are moderately effective as pediculocides. Commercial preparations contain piperonylbutoxide, which enhances the effectiveness by inhibiting enzymatic destruction in the insect. Commercial preparations contain 0.165 to 0.333% pyrethrins, 1.65 to 4% piperonylbutoxide, and 0.8 to 5% petroleum distillate. They are available as a gel, shampoo, and various liquid suspensions. Preparations should be kept away from the eyes and mucous membranes.

Crotamiton, U.S.P. (N-ethyl-*o*-crotonyltoluide; EURAX), is an effective scabicide. It is available as a cream or lotion containing 10% crotamiton (and also oxyquinoline sulfate). It occasionally causes irritation, especially on inflamed skin or when applied over a prolonged period of time. It can cause sensitization. Paradoxically, the preparations also have antipruritic properties.

A combination of 31% *tetrahydronaphthalene* and 0.03% *cupric oleate* (CUPREX) is promoted, as a pediculocide and niticide, but its true efficacy remains to be determined.

Isobornyl thiocyanoacetate (BARC) can eradicate both adult forms and nits of crab, head, and body lice. It is applied as an emulsion containing 4.1% of isobornyl thiocyanoacetate, 0.9% related compounds, and 35% propylene glycol or as a cream. No more than two applications should be made. The drug is irritant to the eyes and mucous membranes and to the skin of some persons.

Sulfur Ointment, U.S.P., and other preparations containing sulfur are employed in the treatment of *scabies* and, less frequently, of *pediculosis. Sulfurated Lime Topical Solution*, U.S.P. (16.5% lime, 25% sublimed sulfur), is also used in both types of infestations.

Thiabendazole, U.S.P., can be applied to the skin as a 10% suspension in the treatment of cutaneous *larva migrans*. It has scabicidal activity, for which it is used outside of the United States. It is also reputed to be mildly antifungal.

Ayliffe, G. A. J.; Babb, J. R.; Bridges, K.; Lilly, H. A.; Lowbury, E. J. L.; Varney, J.; and Wilkins, M. D. Comparison of two methods for assessing the removal of total organisms and pathogens from the skin. *J. Hyg. (Camb.)*, **1975**, *75*, 259–274.

Beck, W. C. Handwashing substitute for degerming. *Am. J. Surg.*, **1978**, *135*, 728.

Borchardt, K. A.; Jenkins, W.; and Moffa, J. An evaluation of surgical scrubs in a dental clinic. *Milit. Med.*, **1978**, *43*, 347–348.

Bovallius, Å., and Ånäs, A. Surface-decontaminating action of glutaraldehyde in the gas-aerosol phase. *Appl. Environ. Microbiol.*, **1977**, *34*, 129–134.

Bressler, R.; Walsen, P. D.; and Fulginitti, V. A. Hexachlorophene in the newborn nursery. *Clin. Pediatr. (Phila.)*, **1977**, *16*, 342–351.

Browne, M. K.; MacKenzie, M.; and Doyle, P. J. A controlled trial of taurolin in established peritonitis. *Surg. Gynecol. Obstet.*, **1978**, *146*, 721–724.

Brugmans, J. P.; van Cutsem, J. M.; and Thienpont, D. C. Treatment of long-term tinea pedis with miconazole. Double-blind clinical evaluation. *Arch. Dermatol.*, **1970**, *102*, 428–432.

Check, W. New study shows hexachlorophene is teratogenic in humans. (Editorial.) *J.A.M.A.*, **1978**, *240*, 513–514.

Cooperman, E. M. Hexachlorophene in the nursery. *Can. Med. Assoc. J.*, **1977**, *117*, 205–206.

Crenshaw, C. A.; Glanges, E.; Stuart, B. H.; and Pierce, J. Nitrofurazone therapy in "middle burns": a review. *Curr. Ther. Res.,* **1976,** *19,* 487–492.

Crowder, V. H., Jr.; Welsh, J. S.; Bornside, G. H.; and Cohn, I. Bacteriological comparison of hexachlorophene and polyvinylpyrrolidone-iodine surgical scrub soaps. *Am. Surg.,* **1967,** *33,* 906–911.

Culbertson, C. Monistat: a new fungicide for treatment of vulvovaginal candidiasis. *Am. J. Obstet. Gynecol.,* **1974,** *120,* 973–976.

Dineen, P. Hand-washing degerming: a comparison of povidone-iodine and chlorhexidine. *Clin. Pharmacol. Ther.,* **1978,** *23,* 63–67.

Drews, R. C. Acetone sterilization in ophthalmic surgery. *Ann. Ophthalmol.,* **1977,** *9,* 781–784.

Dunkerley, R. C.; Cromer, M. D.; Edmiston, C. E., Jr.; and Dunn, G. D. Practical technique for adequate cleansing of endoscopes: a bacteriological study of PHISOHEX and BETADINE. *Gastrointest. Endosc.,* **1977,** *23,* 148–149.

Epstein, S. Paraben sensitivity: subtle trouble. *Ann. Allergy,* **1968,** *26,* 185–189.

Faddis, D.; Daniel, D.; and Boyer, J. Tissue toxicity of antiseptic solutions. A study of rabbit articular and periarticular tissues. *J. Trauma,* **1977,** *17,* 895–897.

Feldmann, R. J., and Maibach, H. I. Percutaneous penetration of some pesticides and herbicides in man. *Toxicol. Appl. Pharmacol.,* **1974,** *28,* 126–132.

Frank, M. J., and Schaffner, W. Contaminated aqueous benzalkonium chloride. An unnecessary hospital infection hazard. *J.A.M.A.,* **1976,** *236,* 2418–2419.

Gilmore, O. J. A. A reappraisal of the use of antiseptics in surgical practice. *Ann. R. Coll. Surg. Engl.,* **1977,** *59,* 93–103.

Gluck, L. A. Perspective on hexachlorophene. *Pediatrics,* **1973,** *51,* 400–406.

Gruber, R. P.; Vistnes, L. P.; and Pardoe, R. The effect of commonly used antiseptics on wound healing. *Plast. Reconstr. Surg.,* **1975,** *55,* 472–476.

Hart, A., and Brown, M. W. Propylene oxide as sterilizing agent. *Appl. Microbiol.,* **1974,** *28,* 1069–1070.

Hermann, H. W. Clinical efficacy studies of haloprogin, a new topical antimicrobial agent. *Arch. Dermatol.,* **1972,** *106,* 839–842.

Hilton, A. L.; Warnock, D. W.; Milne, J. D.; and Scott, A. J. Treatment of vaginal candidiasis with miconazole. *Curr. Med. Res. Opin.,* **1978,** *5,* 295–298.

Hnatko, S. I. Alternatives to hexachlorophene bathing of newborn infants. *Can. Med. Assoc. J.,* **1977,** *117,* 223–226.

Hughes, W. T.; Feldman, S.; and Hermann, H. W. Safety of megadosage haloprogin. *Arch. Dermatol.,* **1974,** *110,* 926–928.

Hyams, P. J.; Counts, G. W.; Monkus, E.; Feldman, R.; Kicklighter, J. L.; and Gonzales, C. Staphylococcal bacteremia and hexachlorophene bathing. Epidemic in a newborn nursery. *Am. J. Dis. Child.,* **1975,** *129,* 595–599.

Ison, A. E., and Tucker, J. B. Photosensitive dermatitis from soaps. *N. Engl. J. Med.,* **1968,** *278,* 81–84.

Katz, A., and Cahn, B. Haloprogin therapy for dermatophyte infections. *Arch. Dermatol.,* **1972,** *106,* 837–838.

King, T. C., and Zimmerman, J. M. Skin degerming practices: chaos and confusion. *Am. J. Surg.,* **1965,** *109,* 695–698.

Kundsin, R. B., and Walter, C. W. The surgical scrub—practical consideration. *Arch. Surg.,* **1973,** *107,* 75–77.

Lavelle, K. J.; Doedens, D. J.; Kleit, S. A.; and Forney, R. B. Iodine absorption in burn patients treated topically with povidone-iodine. *Clin. Pharmacol. Ther.,* **1975,** *17,* 355–362.

Lawrence, C. A. Definition of terms. In, *Disinfection, Sterilization, and Preservation.* (Lawrence, C. A., and Block, S. S., eds.) Lea & Febiger, Philadelphia, **1968a,** pp. 9–10.

Lee, B., and Groth, P. Scabies: transcutaneous poisoning during treatment. *Pediatrics,* **1977,** *59,* 643.

Lilly, H. A., and Lowbury, E. J. L. Disinfection of the skin with detergent preparations of IRGASAN DP 300 and other antiseptics. *Br. Med. J.,* **1974,** *4,* 372–374.

Lister, J. On a new method of treating compound fractures, abscesses, etc. *Lancet,* **1867a,** *1,* 326–329.

———. On the antiseptic principle in the practice of surgery. *Ibid.,* **1867b,** *2,* 353–356.

Loge, J. P. Aplastic anemia following exposure to benzene hexachloride (lindane). *J.A.M.A.,* **1965,** *193,* 110–114.

Lowbury, E. J. L., and Lilly, H. A. Use of 4% chlorhexidine solution (HIBISCRUB) and other methods of skin disinfection. *Br. Med. J.,* **1973,** *1,* 510–515.

Lowbury, E. J. L.; Lilly, H. A.; and Ayliffe, G. A. J. Preoperative disinfection of surgeons' hands: use of alcoholic solutions and effects of gloves on skin flora. *Br. Med. J.,* **1974,** *4,* 369–372.

Mathews, K. P. Immediate type hypersensitivity of phenylmercuric compounds. *Am. J. Med.,* **1968,** *44,* 310–318.

Michaud, R. N.; McGrath, M. B.; and Goss, W. A. Improved experimental model for measuring skin degerming activity on the human hand. *Antimicrob. Agents Chemother.,* **1972,** *2,* 8–15.

———. Application of a gloved-hand model for multiparameter measurements of skin-degerming activity. *J. Clin. Microbiol.,* **1976,** *3,* 406–413.

Ojajärvi, J. An evaluation of antiseptics used for hand disinfection in wards. *J. Hyg. (Camb.),* **1976,** *76,* 75–82.

Peterson, A. F.; Rosenberg, A.; and Alatery, S. D. Comparative evaluation of surgical scrub. *Surg. Gynecol. Obstet.,* **1978,** *146,* 63–65.

Pildes, R. S.; Ramamurthy, R. S.; and Vidyasagar, D. Effect of triple dye on staphylococcal colonization in the newborn infant. *Pediatrics,* **1973,** *82,* 987–990.

Powell, H. C.; Myers, R. R.; Zweifach, B. W.; and Lampert, P. W. Endoneurial pressure in hexachlorophene neuropathy. *Acta Neuropathol. (Berl.),* **1978,** *41,* 139–144.

Powell, M. B.; Swarner, O.; and Lampert, P. Hexachlorophene myelinopathy in premature infants. *J. Pediatr.,* **1973,** *82,* 976–981.

Proost, J. M.; Maes-Dockx, F. M.; Nelis, M. O.; and van Cutsem, J. M. Miconazole in the treatment of mycotic vulvovaginitis. *Am. J. Obstet. Gynecol.,* **1972,** *112,* 688–692.

Rodeheaver, G.; Turnbull, V.; Edgerton, M. T.; Kurtz, L.; and Edlich, R. F. Pharmacokinetics of a new skin wound cleanser. *Am. J. Surg.,* **1976,** *132,* 67–74.

Rosenberg, A.; Alatary, S. D.; and Peterson, A. F. Safety and efficacy of the antiseptic chlorhexidine gluconate. *Surg. Gynecol. Obstet.,* **1976,** *143,* 789–792.

Schorr, W. F. Paraben allergy: a cause of intractable dermatitis. *J.A.M.A.,* **1968,** *204,* 107–110.

Smith, E. B.; Powell, R. F.; Graham, J. L.; and Ulrich, J. A. Topical undecylenic acid in tenia pedis: a new look. *Int. J. Dermatol.,* **1977,** *16,* 52–56.

Smylie, H. G.; Logie, J. R. C.; and Smith, G. From PHISOHEX to HIBISCRUB. *Br. Med. J.,* **1973,** *4,* 586–589.

Steere, A. C., and Mallison, G. F. Handwashing practices for the prevention of nosocomial infections. *Ann. Intern. Med.,* **1975,** *83,* 683–690.

Weigand, D. A., and Everett, M. A. Clearing of resistant psoriasis with anthralin. *Arch. Dermatol.,* **1967,** *96,* 554–559.

White, J. J., and Duncan, A. The comparative effectiveness of iodophor and hexachlorophene surgical scrub solutions. *Surg. Gynecol. Obstet.,* **1972,** *135,* 890–892.

Wishart, M. M., and Riley, T. V. Infection with *Pseudomonas maltophilia:* hospital outbreak due to contaminated disinfectant. *Med. J. Aust.,* **1976,** *2,* 710–712.

Wysowski, D. K.; Flynt, J. W., Jr.; Goldfield, M.; Altman, R.; and Davis, A. T. Epidemic neonatal hyperbilirubinemia and use of a phenolic disinfectant detergent. *Pediatrics,* **1978**, *61,* 165–170.

Monographs and Reviews

Block, S. S.   Historical review. In, *Disinfection, Sterilization, and Preservation.* (Lawrence, C. A., and Block, S. S., eds.) Lea & Febiger, Philadelphia, **1968**, pp. 3–8.

Borick, P. M.   Chemical sterilizers (chemosterilizers). *Adv. Appl. Microbiol.,* **1968**, *10,* 291–312. (83 references.)

Boucher, R. M.   Advances in sterilization techniques: state of the art and recent breakthroughs. *Am. J. Hosp. Pharm.,* **1972**, *29,* 661–672.

Conference.   Hexachlorophene—its usage in the nursery. *Pediatrics,* **1973**, *51,* Pt. II, 329–434.

Davis, J. G.   Chemical sterilization. *Prog. Ind. Microbiol.,* **1968**, *8,* 141–208. (307 references.)

Dixon, R. E.; Kaslow, R. A.; Mackel, D. C.; Fulkerson, C. C.; and Mallison, G. F.   Aqueous quaternary ammonium antiseptics and disinfectants. Use and misuse. *J.A.M.A.,* **1976**, *236,* 2415–2417.

Drouhet, E.   Basic mechanisms of antifungal chemotherapy. *Mod. Treat.,* **1970**, *7,* 539–564.

———.   Antifungal agents. *Antibiot. Chemother.,* **1978**, *25,* 253–288. (87 references.)

Drube, C. G.   Antifungal agents. In, *Annual Reports in Medicinal Chemistry,* Vol. 8. (Heinzelman, R. V., ed.) Academic Press, New York, **1972**, pp. 116–127.

Gershenfeld, L.   Iodine. In, *Disinfection, Sterilization, and Preservation.* (Lawrence, C. A., and Block, S. S., eds.) Lea & Febiger, Philadelphia, **1968**, pp. 329–347.

Gump, W. S., and Walter, G. R.   The *bis*-phenols. In, *Disinfection, Sterilization, and Preservation.* (Lawrence, C. A., and Block, S. S., eds.) Lea & Febiger, Philadelphia, **1968**, pp. 257–277.

Jones, B. R.   Principles in the management of oculomycosis. XXXI Edward Jackson Memorial Lecture. *Am. J. Ophthalmol.,* **1975**, *79,* 719–751.

Jones, D. B.   Therapy of postsurgical fungal endophthalmitis. *Ophthalmology,* **1978**, *85,* 357–373.

Kimbrough, R. D.   Review of the toxicity of hexachlorophene. *Arch. Environ. Health,* **1971**, *23,* 119–122.

———.   Review of the toxicity of hexachlorophene, including its neurotoxicity. *J. Clin. Pharmacol.,* **1973**, *13,* 439–444.

———.   Hexachlorophene: toxicity and use as an antibacterial agent. In, *Essays in Toxicology,* Vol. 8. (Hayes, W. J., Jr., ed.) Academic Press, Inc., New York, **1977**, pp. 99–120.

Kobayashi, G. S., and Medoff, G.   Antifungal agents: recent developments. *Annu. Rev. Microbiol.,* **1977**, *31,* 291–308.

Koski, T. A., and Stuart, L. S.   Methods of testing virucides. In, *Disinfection, Sterilization, and Preservation.* (Lawrence, C. A., and Block, S. S., eds.) Lea & Febiger, Philadelphia, **1968**, pp. 194–206.

Lawrence, C. A.   Quaternary ammonium surface-active disinfectants. In, *Disinfection, Sterilization, and Preservation.* (Lawrence, C. A., and Block, S. S., eds.) Lea & Febiger, Philadelphia, **1968b**, pp. 430–452.

Lawrence, C. A., and Block, S. S. (eds.).   *Disinfection, Sterilization, and Preservation.* Lea & Febiger, Philadelphia, **1968**.

Leary, J. S., and Stuart, L. S.   Safety evaluations on antimicrobial chemicals. In, *Disinfection, Sterilization, and Preservation.* (Lawrence, C. A., and Block, S. S., eds.) Lea & Febiger, Philadelphia, **1968**, pp. 221–233.

Lockhart, J. D.   How toxic is hexachlorophene? *Pediatrics,* **1972**, *50,* 229–235.

———.   Hexachlorophene and the Food and Drug Administration. *J. Clin. Pharmacol.,* **1973**, *13,* 445–450.

Miller, A. K.   *In vivo* evaluation of antibacterial chemotherapeutic substances. *Adv. Appl. Microbiol.,* **1971**, *14,* 151–183. (149 references.)

Ortenzio, L. F., and Stuart, L. S.   Methods of testing antiseptics. In, *Disinfection, Sterilization, and Preservation.* (Lawrence, C. A., and Block, S. S., eds.) Lea & Febiger, Philadelphia, **1968**, pp. 179–198.

Plueckhahn, V. D.   Hexachlorophene and skin care of newborn infants. *Drugs,* **1973**, *5,* 97–107.

Price, P. B.   Surgical antiseptics. In, *Disinfection, Sterilization, and Preservation.* (Lawrence, C. A., and Block, S. S., eds.) Lea & Febiger, Philadelphia, **1968**, pp. 532–542.

Prindle, R. F., and Wright, E. S.   Phenolic compounds. In, *Disinfection, Sterilization, and Preservation.* (Lawrence, C. A., and Block, S. S., eds.) Lea & Febiger, Philadelphia, **1968**, pp. 401–429.

Reddish, G. F. (ed.).   *Antiseptics, Disinfectants, Fungicides, and Chemical and Physical Sterilization.* Lea & Febiger, Philadelphia, **1957**.

Romans, I. B.   Oligodynamic metals. In, *Disinfection, Sterilization, and Preservation.* (Lawrence, C. A., and Block, S. S., eds.) Lea & Febiger, Philadelphia, **1968**, pp. 372–400.

Russell, A. D.   The mechanism of action of some antibacterial agents. *Prog. Med. Chem.,* **1969**, *6,* 135–199. (426 references.)

Sawyer, P. R.; Brogden, R. N.; Pinder, R. M.; Speight, T. M.; and Avery, G. S.   Miconazole: a review of its antifungal activity and therapeutic efficacy. *Drugs,* **1975a**, *9,* 406–423. (44 references.)

———.   Clotrimazole: a review of its antifungal activity and therapeutic efficacy. *Ibid.,* **1975b**, *9,* 424–447. (78 references.)

Spaulding, E. H.   Chemical disinfection of medical and surgical materials. In, *Disinfection, Sterilization, and Preservation.* (Lawrence, C. A., and Block, S. S., eds.) Lea & Febiger, Philadelphia, **1968**, pp. 517–531.

Symposium. (Various authors.)   Biological effects of pesticides in mammalian systems. *Ann. N.Y. Acad. Sci.,* **1969**, *160,* 1–946.

Symposium. (Various authors.)   Clotrimazole. *Postgrad. Med. J.,* **1974**, *50,* Suppl. 1, 1–108.

CHAPTER
42 GASTRIC ANTACIDS AND DIGESTANTS

Stewart C. Harvey

GASTRIC ANTACIDS

Gastric antacids are agents that neutralize or remove acid from the gastric contents. They are employed by physicians chiefly in the treatment of reflux esophagitis and peptic ulcer, and by the laity in self-medication for a wide variety of symptoms.

The gastric antacids are a much-abused group of drugs. As a result of irresponsible advertising, the public has come to believe that man is constantly fighting a battle against acidity and that every little belch or upper gastrointestinal upset calls for an antacid. The substantial incidence of placebo responsiveness of individuals with minor gastrointestinal upsets, and even with peptic ulcer, further deludes the laity and often the physician into inappropriate use of antacids. Yet when indicated, they are often used too casually to be of optimal value.

Actions and Effects of Gastric Antacids. The common gastric antacids all contain a weakly basic moiety. The weaker bases, such as the several oxyaluminum compounds, hardly raise the pH of the gastric contents above 4, some not above 3, whereas the mildly strong bases, such as magnesium hydroxide, can raise the pH to about 9 but rarely do so in clinical settings.

The presence of an antacid in the gastric contents increases the volume of gastric juice secreted and the output of HCl. An elevated pH induces the pyloric antrum to release gastrin. In patients with duodenal ulcer the effect is remarkably pronounced. If sodium bicarbonate is continuously administered so that the intragastric pH remains above 4, the 24-hour output of HCl is 6 to 20 times the control continuous-fasting secretion in such patients (Price and Sanderson, 1956). If the pH is kept at 5.5, the gastrin and acid secretory outputs after a meal are approximately doubled (Fordtran and Walsh, 1973).

Acid rebound (i.e., continued hypersecretion of HCl after the intragastric pH has recovered to normal) consequent to antacid ingestion is usually thought to occur only with calcium carbonate, but evidence for a slight-to-moderate rebound after $Mg(OH)_2$ or $NaHCO_3$ can be found in the data published by Posey and coworkers (1965), Fordtran (1968), and Barreras (1970). Two mechanisms for the rebound are suggested: (1) a non-pH-related effect of the product salts ($MgCl_2$, $AlCl_3$, $CaCl_2$) to stimulate gastrin secretion and hence production of acid (*see* Feurle, 1975) and (2) an effect of alkalinization in the proximal jejunum to increase gastric secretion of acid (*see* Alday and Goldsmith, 1974). The latter mechanism would only obtain when an excess of an alkaline antacid was ingested in an amount sufficient to reach the jejunum in an unreacted state. Chronic ingestion of antacids does not induce hyperactivity of the antral gastrin-producing system (Caldwell *et al.,* 1976).

All antacids *indirectly* suppress peptic activity when given in sufficient quantity to elevate the pH of human gastric contents above 5 (Piper and Fenton, 1965). Between pH 7 and 8, pepsin is irreversibly inactivated. Although there have been a number of claims that aluminum-, calcium-, and bismuth-containing antacids have *direct* antipeptic activity, such claims have not been supported by studies in which the pH effect was used for control (*see* Kuruvilla, 1971).

Neutralization of the gastric contents increases gastric motility through the action of gastrin; aluminum hydroxide, however, greatly delays gastric emptying (Hurwitz *et al.,* 1976). Neutralization also increases lower-esophageal sphincter pressure, but by a mechanism that is independent of gastrin.

Individual gastric antacids may bring about effects that are unique to the particular compound or to one of its constituent groups.

Except for the systemic alkalotic effects of some gastric antacids, other properties and effects are discussed under the individual agents.

Systemic and Nonsystemic Antacids. Systemic antacids, such as sodium bicarbonate, have the disadvantage of producing metabolic alkalosis because of appreciable absorption of the cationic moiety. A compound of this type, even if administered in doses that only partially neutralize the gastric contents, may disturb the acid-base balance of the body fluids. A *nonsystemic* antacid is one in which the cationic moiety in the intestine forms insoluble basic compounds that are not subsequently absorbed.

Effects of Systemic Antacids. If a systemic antacid such as sodium bicarbonate is administered, the gastric acid is neutralized by exogenous bicarbonate in lieu of intestinal bicarbonate. The spared equivalent amount of intestinal bicarbonate is then absorbed. The net effect is the same as though the exogenous sodium bicarbonate had been directly transported into the extracellular fluid. The effect on extracellular bicarbonate is the same whether the antacid is an oxide, carbonate, or any alkaline-reacting compound of an absorbable cation. The kidney must then excrete the excess bicarbonate and cation in order to restore the acid-base balance of the body fluids. Consequently, the urine becomes alkaline. Failure of the renal mechanisms to function adequately would result in a more enduring metabolic alkalosis. Even when the excretory disposal of the bicarbonate is adequate, the repeated alkalinization of the urine during chronic administration of systemic antacids predisposes to phosphatic nephrolithiasis.

For the calcium and magnesium compounds that are partly systemic, the pharmacological and toxicological effects of the cations themselves are of more concern than the alkalosis. The nature of the adverse systemic effects will be discussed under the individual agents.

Effects of Nonsystemic Antacids. A nonsystemic antacid neutralizes the gastric contents but does not tend to cause systemic alkalosis, because not only is the cation very little absorbed but it regains a basic anion in the small intestine. For example, in gastric acid, $CaCO_3$ is converted to Ca^{2+}, CO_2, and H_2O, with the loss of $2H^+$; in the small intestine, Ca^{2+} combines with CO_3^{2-} to yield insoluble $CaCO_3$, and the equivalent of $2HCO_3^-$ is lost. Since the loss of H^+ is equal to the loss of HCO_3^-, the net effect on acid-base balance is zero. At the pH of the jejunum (about 8), there is sufficient CO_3^{2-} in equilibrium with HCO_3^- to precipitate more than 99% of calcium ion present. In the small intestine, calcium ion also combines with fatty acid anions to form insoluble calcium soaps. Were the fatty acid anions not so removed, they would be absorbed and ultimately metabolized to bicarbonate. Thus, it follows that the

formation of calcium soaps has the same overall effect to prevent systemic alkalosis as does the intra-intestinal precipitation of $CaCO_3$. At the pH of the lower colon (5 to 7.5), some of the $CaCO_3$ will redissolve, but little absorption takes place. Continued formation of insoluble calcium soaps will tend to offset the acid-base effects of the carbonate liberated. Insoluble calcium phosphate also forms in the intestine and contributes to the nonsystemic antacid properties.

Other substances are nonsystemic antacids by virtue of similar mechanisms. The basic aluminum compounds regenerated in the small intestine are probably a mixture of hydrated aluminum oxide, oxyaluminum hydroxide, basic aluminum carbonates of variable composition, and aluminum soaps. Magnesium carbonate is too soluble to precipitate in the intestines; however, since Mg^{2+} is poorly absorbed, its bases act as nonsystemic antacids because of the obligatory retention of anions in the intestine and their eventual excretion. The formation of soaps also accounts in part for the nonsystemic properties of magnesium-containing antacids.

pH-Related Adverse Effects. The only adverse effects in common among the antacids are those resulting from changes in gastric and urinary pH and alterations in acid-base status. Gastric alkalinization has been suggested as a cause of increased susceptibility to various acid-sensitive microbial pathogens, such as *Brucella abortus*. In the presence of renal failure, all antacids except aluminum compounds can cause metabolic alkalosis. The disturbance in acid-base balance *per se* is usually of minor consequence; nevertheless, when there is a high phosphate intake along with chronic alkalosis, the milk-alkali syndrome can occur (*see* under Calcium Carbonate, below), even when the antacid contains no calcium (*see* Ansari, 1970). Usually of greater consequence are the specific effects of the absorbed cation and the elevation of urinary pH. Even small therapeutic doses of $Mg(OH)_2$ and $CaCO_3$ can cause significant elevations in the pH of the urine that may persist for longer than 1 day after discontinuation of the antacid (*see* Gibaldi *et al.*, 1974, 1975). Elevation of the urinary pH can affect the renal elimination of drugs and may also predispose to certain urinary tract infections; chronic urinary alkalinization predisposes to urolithiasis.

Drug Interactions. Antacids interact with other drugs by pH-related and other mechanisms. Since gastric alkalinization hastens gastric emptying, antacids other than aluminum compounds will hasten the delivery of a drug into the small intestine. This may speed the absorption of drugs that are poorly absorbed from the stomach, or it may shorten the total time available for absorption. The dissolution rate of solid preparations of weak acids and of enteric coatings is increased, which accelerates absorption. The rate of absorption of salicylates, indomethacin, naproxen, pseudoephedrine, sulfadiazine, and enteric-coated phenylbutazone or aspirin is increased at elevated pH. The absorption of dicumarol, but not warfarin, is also facilitated by the formation of a rapidly absorbed complex. Aluminum hydroxide accelerates the absorption and increases the bioavailability of diazepam by an unknown mechanism.

Gastric alkalinization slows the dissolution rate of solid dosage forms of amine drugs and may cause the precipitation of poorly soluble agents such as quinine and quinidine, but the potential retarding effect on absorption is evidently compensated by the increased rate of gastric emptying. Gastric alkalinization interferes with the dissolution of tetracyclines. It also causes the conversion of dietary and administered ionic iron to poorly absorbable polymeric iron oxides.

Aluminum hydroxide delays gastric emptying and has been shown to slow the rate of absorption of indomethacin, dicumarol, isoniazid, barbiturates, and some benzodiazepines. In addition, the drug decreases the bioavailability of indomethacin and isoniazid.

The bioavailability of a number of drugs is decreased because of their capacity to form complexes with various antacids. Magnesium trisilicate and SiO_2 formed therefrom strongly bind and interfere with the bioavailability of iron, digoxin, certain benzodiazepines, and phenothiazines; this antacid also decreases the bioavailability of antimuscarinic drugs. Magnesium-containing antacids bind to and decrease the bioavailability of digoxin and tetracyclines. Aluminum hydroxide adsorbs and decreases the bioavailability of propranolol, antimuscarinic drugs, digoxin, tetracyclines, chlorpromazine, and sulfadiazine.

Antacids that increase urinary pH delay the elimination and elevate the blood concentrations of some amines, such as quinidine and amphetamines.

Drug interactions with antacids have been reviewed by Romankiewicz (1976) and Hurwitz (1977).

ALUMINUM HYDROXIDE

So-called aluminum hydroxide is actually a mixture of aluminum hydroxide and aluminum oxide hydrates, and it usually contains some fixed CO_2 (i.e., carbonate). Products differ with respect to antacid efficacy, according to the process of manufacture and to age. The differences are due in part to the formation of polymers and anhydrous alumina, which dissolve exceedingly slowly in acid. Liquid preparations react faster than do solids. Furthermore, proteins, peptides, amino acids, and certain dietary organic acids greatly impair the neutralizing capacity of aluminum hydroxide.

Although aluminum hydroxide is considered to be nonsystemic, some absorption from the gastrointestinal tract occurs. The fraction absorbed is quite small, and concentrations of the drug in blood remain relatively low in normal recipients; the amount of aluminum excreted in the urine is less than 0.33 mg per day (Kaehny et al., 1977). However, patients with renal failure who chronically ingest $Al(OH)_3$ accumulate the metal in a variety of tissues (Alfrey et al., 1976); the concentration of aluminum in plasma may be as high as 56 μg/ml (Berlyne et al., 1970).

Among the compounds formed in the intestine from aluminum hydroxide are insoluble aluminum phosphates, which pass through the intestinal tract unabsorbed. Hypophosphatemia, hypophosphaturia, and hypopyrophosphaturia result. All aluminum-containing antacids except aluminum phosphate have this property. This provides the basis of the occasional therapeutic use of aluminum hydroxide in the treatment of phosphatic nephrolithiasis (see below). Phosphate depletion is occasionally observed after the chronic ingestion of aluminum hydroxide, especially if phosphate intake is limited. Decreased phosphate absorption is accompanied by increased calcium absorption, which, along with resorption of bone salts, causes hypercalciuria and sometimes nephrolithiasis (Cooke et al., 1978). Hypomagnesemia and hypomagnesiuria also occur.

Aluminum ion forms coordinate complexes with a wide variety of substances. Reactions with proteins account for its astringent properties. Mucus secretion is supposedly stimulated by the irritant action of Al^{3+}. Aluminum compounds cause constipation, an effect often attributed to the astringent aluminum ion; inasmuch as the concentration of aluminum ion in the intestine is extremely low, it is difficult to attribute the effect to an astringent action. Aluminum hydroxide adsorbs pepsin, but the adsorbed enzyme remains active. The compound decreases uropepsin excretion. Aluminum hydroxide is an effective adsorbent and interacts with many drugs in the gastrointestinal tract (see above). It interferes with the defoaming action of simethicone. Particles of wet aluminum hydroxide are somewhat adhesive, and the compound is demulcent. The role that the demulcent action plays in the treatment of peptic ulcer is contestable. Dried aluminum hydroxide gel probably does not disperse sufficiently to cover the mucosa. A concentrated suspension has been claimed to provide appreciable coating, but this finding is controversial (*e.g., see* Morrissey *et al.,* 1967).

Preparations. Since aluminum hydroxide is a poorly effective antacid, it is marketed mostly in combination with other antacids. Of the suspensions listed in Table 42–1, the only preparation containing *aluminum hydroxide gel* alone is AMPHOJEL. The details of the neutralizing capacity of this product have not been published; however, the manufacturer's literature states that 10 ml, containing 640 mg of $Al(OH)_3$, neutralizes 13 mEq of acid in 60 minutes. The average single dose is 15 ml, which is usually insufficient. *Dried Aluminum Hydroxide Gel Tablets,* U.S.P., each contain 300 or 600 mg of Al_2O_3 equivalent. The 600-mg tablet will neutralize 9 mEq of acid in 60 minutes. The average single dose is 600 mg.

Therapeutic Uses. The use of aluminum hydroxide in the treatment of peptic ulcer is discussed on page 995. Mention has already been made of the application of the demulcent and adsorbent properties of aluminum hydroxide. The hypophosphatemic effect has been used in the treatment of *calcinosis universalis* (Nassim and Connolly, 1970) and in hyperparathyroidism secondary to prolonged hemodialysis (*see* Goldsmith *et al.,* 1971). Individuals who suffer from recurrent *phosphatic nephrolithiasis* often can be benefited if their urine is kept relatively free of phosphate. A low-phosphate diet and enough aluminum hydroxide (about 40 ml of gel four times a day) to reduce the 24-hour urinary phosphorus excretion to 200 mg or less are prescribed. Some experts are reluctant to continue treatment for long periods of time because of the possibility of mobilizing bone salts. Furthermore, objections to the unpalatable and constipating gel foster noncompliance.

Untoward Reactions. Aluminum hydroxide itself is relatively safe. However, prolonged use by persons ingesting a diet low in phosphate may cause osteomalacia and proximal myopathy (David and Robson, 1976). Alfrey and coworkers (1976) suggested that the encephalopathy seen in certain patients undergoing hemodialysis may be due to intoxication with aluminum. Some individuals are intolerant of the astringent action of the drug and experience nausea and vomiting. Constipation can be circumvented by concurrent therapy with a magnesium-containing antacid. Concretions of fatty acid salts of

Table 42–1.   COMPOSITION AND NEUTRALIZING CAPACITY OF REPRESENTATIVE PROPRIETARY "NONSYSTEMIC" ANTACID SUSPENSIONS *

PRODUCT	CONTENT (*mg/5 ml*)					CAPACITY [3] (*per 5 ml*)
	$Al(OH)_3$	$Mg(OH)_2$	$CaCO_3$	Si [1]	Na [2]	
DELCID	600	665	0	0	15	42
MYLANTA-II	400	400	0	30	1.4	25
GELUSIL-II	400	400	0	30	1.3	24
BASALJEL XS [4]		1000 $Al_2(CO_3)_3$ [5]		0	17	22
TITRALAC	0	0	1000	0	11	20
CAMALOX	225	200	250	0	2.5	18
MARBLEN		See footnote [6]		0	3.2	18
TRISOGEL	150	585 $Mg_2Si_3O_8$ [7]		0	9.3	17
SILAIN-GEL	282	285	0	25	4.4	15
ALUDROX	307	103	0	0	1.5	14
BASALJEL		400 $Al_2(CO_3)_3$ [5]		0	2.4	14
MAALOX	225	200	0	— [8]	2.5	13
CREAMALIN	320	75	0	0	2.3	13
MYLANTA	200	200	0	20	0.7	12
A-M-T		$Al(OH)_3 + Mg_2Si_3O_8$ [7]		0	7.5	11
GELUSIL	200	200	0	25	0.9	11
RIOPAN		400 magaldrate [5]		— [9]	<0.7	11
KOLANTYL GEL	150	150	0	0	5.0	10
WIN GEL	180	160	0	0	2.0	10
AMPHOJEL	320	0	0	0	6.9	6

* Solid dosage forms (mostly tablets) are also available for most preparations. Their composition per tablet is similar to that listed per 5 ml.

[1] Si = simethicone.

[2] Data mostly from Yokel, 1977.

[3] Milliequivalents of acid neutralized in 60 minutes. Obtained from manufacturer's physician-directed literature; up-to-date independent figures have not been published in the scientific literature.

[4] XS = extra strength.

[5] Indicated composition is in lieu of $Al(OH)_3$, $Mg(OH)_2$, and/or $CaCO_3$.

[6] Contains $CaCO_3$, $MgCO_3$, $Mg_3(PO_4)_2$, and $Mg_2Si_3O_8$.

[7] Contains $Mg_2Si_3O_8$ in lieu of $Mg(OH)_2$.

[8] MAALOX PLUS contains 25 mg of simethicone.

[9] RIOPAN PLUS contains 20 mg of simethicone.

aluminum may occur in the stools. Several cases of intestinal obstruction by a large mass composed of clotted blood and aluminum hydroxide have been reported.

BASIC ALUMINUM CARBONATE

Basic aluminum carbonate is an aluminum oxycarbonate of indefinite composition. It is marketed in the form of a suspension that contains the equivalent of 400 or 1000 mg of $Al(OH)_3$ per 5 ml and as tablets or capsules containing 500 mg of equivalent. Its pharmacological properties are similar to those of aluminum hydroxide gel, but its capacity for neutralization is greater (see BASALJEL, Table 42–1). It may bind one third more phosphate than does the hydroxide; the reason for the supposed greater phosphate-retaining power of the carbonate is obscure, but it may be the best of the aluminum-containing antacids for the management of phosphatic nephrolithiasis. For use as an antacid the dose is 10 ml of the suspension or two tablets. To decrease phosphate absorption, the dose is 40 ml 1 hour after each meal and at bedtime.

OTHER ALUMINUM COMPOUNDS

Dihydroxyaluminum sodium carbonate combines in a single chemical entity properties of both sodium bicarbonate and aluminum hydroxide. The drug is a partially systemic antacid. The sodium carbonate moiety reacts rapidly with hydrogen ion, with the evolution of carbon dioxide and aluminum hydroxide. The aluminum hydroxide supposedly exerts a sustained, moderate buffering action that is more reliable than the action of some aluminum hydroxide suspensions. However, present published data on the *in-vivo* properties of dihydroxyaluminum sodium carbonate are unreliable, so that a true comparison is not possible. The only product of this entity (ROLAIDS) is available in tablets, each of which contains 334 mg of the compound and 53 mg of sodium. The recommended dose of one or two tablets is inadequate for treatment of ulcer.

Dihydroxyaluminum aminoacetate is a basic salt of aluminum and glycine. In neutralization four hydrogen ions are used—one for each hydroxyl group, one for the carboxyl group, and one for the amino group. The aminoacetic acid may possibly delay gastric emptying, but it may also increase gastric secretion. Claims that the substance is less constipating than aluminum hydroxide are not objective, but there is less aluminum per chemical equivalent. The only product containing this entity (ROBALATE) is available in tablets, each of which contains 500 mg of the antacid. The capacity for neutralization is low.

Aluminum phosphate reacts slowly with the hydrochloric acid in gastric juice to yield aluminum chloride and phosphoric acid. In the small intestine aluminum phosphate is largely regenerated from the original constituents of the antacid, so that endogenous phosphate is spared. The compound is intended for use as an antacid in preference to aluminum hydroxide when interference with phosphate absorption should be avoided, but it is an ineffective antacid. Although the drug has negligible effects on concentrations of aluminum in the plasma and urine

(Kaehny *et al.*, 1977), it can cause hyperphosphatemia in patients with impaired renal function. It is marketed as PHOSPHALJEL, an aqueous suspension that contains 233 mg/5 ml; this amount neutralizes about 5 mEq of acid. The recommended dose is 15 to 45 ml, but no practical dose is sufficient to neutralize the gastric acid in a patient with peptic ulcer.

CALCIUM CARBONATE

As chalk, calcium carbonate ($CaCO_3$) was the first gastric antacid to be used. It has remained popular for a century and a half. Its antacid effects are rapid in onset and relatively prolonged in duration. $CaCO_3$ has a high capacity for neutralizing acid *in vivo*. Kirsner and Palmer (1940) found it to be the most effective gastric antacid of those they studied, and for nearly 30 years thereafter most authorities considered it to be the antacid of choice in the treatment of peptic ulcer. Today, $CaCO_3$ is used much less frequently, for reasons that are cited below and elsewhere in this chapter.

$CaCO_3$ has long been considered to be the epitome of a nonsystemic antacid. However, enough is absorbed to cause systemic and renal effects in certain circumstances. A slight-to-moderate metabolic alkalosis occurs during treatment with $CaCO_3$, but it is slow to develop.

The amount of calcium absorbed from $CaCO_3$ is usually stated to be 10%, but it probably depends upon the amount of gastric acid; in one study, 0 to 2% of a single 2-g dose was found to be absorbed in achlorhydric persons, 9 to 16% in normal subjects, and 11 to 37% in patients with peptic ulcer (Ivanovich *et al.*, 1967). The fraction absorbed seems to be nearly the same when $CaCO_3$ is given chronically in daily doses of 20 g. A dose-absorption relationship has not been established for $CaCO_3$; however, by analogy with other forms of calcium, the amount absorbed probably reaches a plateau at a dose of about 20 g. Dietary fat decreases absorption.

After a single 4-g dose in normal subjects, the concentration of calcium in plasma rises and may be maintained for nearly 3 hours; after an 8-g dose, the hypercalcemia is more persistent. A normal individual can ingest 20 g per day without developing chronic hypercalcemia, but clinically dangerous hypercalcemia may follow the administration of as little as 3.4 g per day to patients with uremia. Excretion of calcium varies directly with the creatinine clearance. The amount excreted falls far short of the amount absorbed, even after weeks of treatment. Normal persons excrete an average of 7% of a daily intake of 50 mg/kg (approximately equivalent to 8 g of $CaCO_3$). Some individuals appear to be hyperexcretors of calcium and are prone to nephrolithiasis. Although increased calcium excretion almost always follows the administration of antacid doses of $CaCO_3$, alkaluria does not invariably occur.

The administration of $CaCO_3$ promotes positive phosphate balance; plasma phosphate concentrations may or may not be increased, but hyperphosphatemia is the usual finding in patients with the milk-alkali syndrome. Increased intake of calcium decreases absorption of magnesium. Various details of the absorption, excretion, and systemic effects of

$CaCO_3$ can be found in the reports by Wenger and coworkers (1957), McMillan and Freeman (1965), Clarkson and colleagues (1966), Vincent and Radcliff (1966), Ivanovich and associates (1967), and Makoff and coworkers (1969).

Doses of $CaCO_3$ as low as 0.5 g may cause acid rebound (*see* above) (*e.g., see* Levant *et al.,* 1973). Various studies suggest that neither a local effect of alkalinization or calcium ions in the antrum nor hypercalcemia account for the rebound; the rebound primarily results from an action of Ca^{2+} in the small intestine to release gastrin (*see* Peterson and Fordtran, 1978).

$CaCO_3$ is considered to be constipating. However, Clemens and Feinstein (1977) argue cogently that $CaCO_3$ may actually be a laxative.

Untoward Effects. The chalky taste of $CaCO_3$ is clinically disadvantageous. Disturbances resulting from the liberation of carbon dioxide are not a serious problem, although belching occurs in some individuals. Nausea is also an occasional complaint. The possible constipating effect is discussed above. More serious are the infrequent instances of hypercalcemia with alkalosis, calcinosis (including nephrocalcinosis), and azotemia that occur during chronic usage of $CaCO_3$, especially in conjunction with milk and cream (milk-alkali syndrome; *see* McMillan and Freeman, 1965); renal dysfunction, gastrointestinal hemorrhage, and vomiting or aspiration of the gastric contents through a nasogastric tube seem to predispose to the disorder. When phosphate intake is low, hypophosphatemia may occur. Hypercalciuria and alkaluria predispose to nephrolithiasis. If no more than 160 mEq (8 g) a day is administered, nephrolithiasis and the milk-alkali syndrome can be avoided (Fordtran, 1966; *see also* Schmidt, 1974). The gastric hypersecretory action is counterproductive and may possibly account for various reports that $CaCO_3$ is less efficacious than other antacids. $CaCO_3$ has been known to cause fecal concretions.

Preparations. *Precipitated Calcium Carbonate,* U.S.P., is usually dispensed as *Calcium Carbonate Tablets,* U.S.P., which generally contain 650 mg of $CaCO_3$; chewable tablets contain 350, 420, or 500 mg. A magma, which also includes glycine (*see* TITRALAC, Table 42–1), contains 1 g of $CaCO_3$ per 5 ml; 1 g neutralizes 13 mEq of acid in 30 minutes. The usual dose of $CaCO_3$ for peptic ulcer is 1 to 2 g; however, 2-g doses in an effective schedule will exceed the recommended 8-g daily limit, and preparations containing lesser amounts of $CaCO_3$ in combination with other antacids are thus to be preferred.

MAGNESIUM CARBONATE

The rate of reaction of $MgCO_3$ with acid is considerably slower than that of $CaCO_3$; when the gastric emptying time is short, the requirement for $MgCO_3$ may be as much as ten times that of $CaCO_3$. Nevertheless, $MgCO_3$ appears to be an excellent antacid under clinical conditions. The absorption of magnesium and the systemic effects are largely those of $Mg(OH)_2$. The release of CO_2 in the stomach may cause belching.

Magnesium Carbonate, U.S.P., is available as a bulky hydrated powder. Although 1 g contains approximately 20 mEq, only a fraction may be available for neutralization *in vivo*. The usual antacid dose of 500 mg to 2 g may be inadequate.

MAGNESIUM HYDROXIDE AND OXIDE

Magnesium hydroxide, $Mg(OH)_2$, as milk of magnesia has long been popular among the laity as an antacid and a cathartic, and is also somewhat popular among physicians. The compound is practically insoluble, and solution is not effected until the hydroxide reacts with hydrochloric acid to form magnesium chloride. Nevertheless, its neutralizing action is nearly as prompt and complete as that of sodium bicarbonate. When the dose is in excess of that required to neutralize the acid, intragastric pH may reach 8 or 9. Acid rebound following $Mg(OH)_2$ is clinically insignificant.

In water, MgO hydrates to $Mg(OH)_2$; consequently, its pharmacology is that of the hydroxide. However, unneutralized MgO may not be completely converted to $Mg(OH)_2$ in the stomach.

In man, a mixture of magnesium and aluminum hydroxide possibly decreases antral motility (Khan *et al.,* 1970); in dogs, the magnesium content of the gastric mucosa and muscularis is increased, and it is possible that the effect to decrease antral motility and uropepsin secretion is from a direct local action. Presumably it is not due to a decrease in gastric secretion, since $Mg(OH)_2$ increases lower-esophageal sphincter pressure and acid secretion in Heidenhain pouches (Posey *et al.,* 1965).

A disadvantage of the use of $Mg(OH)_2$ as an antacid in some patients is its cathartic effect (*see* Chapter 43). Consequently, $Mg(OH)_2$ is usually coadministered or alternated with constipating antacids, such as $Al(OH)_3$ and $CaCO_3$, although the constipating action of $CaCO_3$ is now in doubt (*see* above). Although $Mg(OH)_2$ is classified as a nonsystemic antacid, 5 to 10% of the magnesium can be absorbed; retention of any absorbed magnesium can cause neurological, neuromuscular, and cardiovascular impairment and even death in persons with renal insufficiency (*see* Randall *et al.,* 1964). Ordinarily the absorbed magnesium ion is rapidly excreted by the kidney. In normal persons, absorption is attended by little or no danger of systemic alkalosis, but the urine may become alkaline. Prolonged use of $Mg(OH)_2$ may rarely cause fecal stones composed of $MgCO_3$ and $Mg(OH)_2$.

Preparations. *Milk of Magnesia,* U.S.P., is an aqueous suspension of magnesium hydroxide containing 7.0 to 8.5% of $Mg(OH)_2$. Each milliliter is capable of neutralizing approximately 2.7 mEq of acid. The antacid dose is 5 to 15 ml. Suspensions of other strengths are also marketed. Magnesium hydroxide is also available as *magnesia tablets;* such tablets generally contain 325 mg each, which can neutralize 11.2 mEq of acid. Magnesium hydroxide is usually marketed in combination with other antacids.

Magnesium Oxide, U.S.P., is usually incorporated into various mixtures. When it is used alone, the official dose is 250 mg to 1 g. Although 1 g contains approximately 50 mEq of base, only 8 to 20 mEq may react with the gastric acid in 30 minutes. MgO is available in suspensions of various strengths, as a powder, and in capsules and tablets that contain 140 to 500 mg of the drug.

MAGALDRATE

Magaldrate is a complex hydroxymagnesium aluminate with the approximate formula $[Mg(OH)^+]_4$ $[Al_2(OH)_{10}^{4-}] \cdot 2H_2O$. It reacts with acid in stages. The hydroxymagnesium is relatively rapidly converted to magnesium ion and the aluminate to hydrated aluminum hydroxide; the aluminum hydroxide then reacts more slowly to give a sustained antacid effect. Magaldrate does not simply simulate physical mixtures of magnesium and aluminum hydroxides, since the aluminum hydroxide freshly generated in the gastric acid does not have time to convert to less reactive forms. Consequently, magaldrate more consistently buffers the gastric contents than do the mixtures. The pH is usually maintained between 3.5 and 4.0. Its systemic effects are those of $Mg(OH)_2$.

Preparations. *Magaldrate,* U.S.P. (RIOPAN), is available as tablets (to be chewed or swallowed) containing 400 mg of antacid or as a suspension containing 400 mg/5 ml. The dose is 400 to 800 mg.

MAGNESIUM TRISILICATE

Magnesium Trisilicate, U.S.P., is the magnesium salt of mesotrisilicic acid ($Mg_2Si_3O_8 \cdot nH_2O$). It functions as a nonsystemic antacid. Magnesium trisilicate reacts with acid in the following manner:

$$Mg_2Si_3O_8 \cdot nH_2O + 4H^+ \longrightarrow 2Mg^{2+} + 3SiO_2 + (n+2)H_2O$$

Magnesium trisilicate has too slow a rate of reaction with acid to be useful for the management of peptic ulcer; even in normal persons, it rarely elevates the intragastric pH above 2.7. As a single entity, $Mg_2Si_3O_8$ cannot meet the pH requirement for nonprescription antacids that currently prevails in the United States.

Both hydrous SiO_2 and magnesium trisilicate are good adsorbents. Not only does magnesium trisilicate adsorb pepsin, but it also interferes with the absorption of dietary protein and a number of drugs (*see* page 990).

The principal side effect of magnesium trisilicate is the laxation caused by high doses. However, hypermagnesemia and systemic toxicity can occur in patients with renal insufficiency. Approximately 5% of the magnesium is absorbed. This results in a slight alkaluria. Approximately 7% of the silica may be

absorbed. Since 1960, there have been a number of reports of siliceous nephroliths caused by chronic ingestion of magnesium trisilicate (*see* Joekes *et al.,* 1973). The stones have a low radiopacity and hence may easily be overlooked. It is probable that the phenomenon occurs moderately often during chronic use. Silica deposits and glomerular and tubular interstitial nephropathy occur in individuals who ingest silicates chronically and in dogs treated chronically with magnesium trisilicate in doses comparable to doses that are *effective* in man. Intestinal impaction from concretions or sediments of magnesium trisilicate also occurs, especially if there is gastrointestinal bleeding.

Products that contain only magnesium trisilicate have been discontinued in the United States; the antacid is available only in combinations with other drugs.

SODIUM BICARBONATE

Because of the solubility of sodium bicarbonate ($NaHCO_3$), it exerts an immediate and rapid antacid action in the stomach. Any excess, however, rapidly enters the intestine, so that the substance has a shorter duration of action than do other antacids.

The formerly wide use of $NaHCO_3$ has greatly declined, owing not only to the "over-the-counter" promotion of other antacids but also to medical concern about its systemic effects. Chronic use of $NaHCO_3$ alone as an antacid (along with milk) can cause the milk-alkali syndrome (*e.g., see* Ansari, 1970). The systemic toxicity of $NaHCO_3$ in persons with normal renal function has perhaps been overly stressed. Van Goidsenhoven and coworkers (1954) administered daily doses up to 25 mEq/kg to patients for 3 weeks. Although there were changes in the plasma electrolyte concentrations, they were not remarkable; plasma total CO_2 increased by only 5 mEq per liter with the largest dose. Considerable weight gain was the most prominent effect. One of 33 patients developed albuminuria and hematuria with these massive doses. Dehydration with consequent renal ischemia, rather than alkalosis or fluid retention, was the primary cause of complications. Kirsner and Palmer (1942) reported that even with a combination of 380 mEq of $NaHCO_3$ and 640 mEq of $CaCO_3$ per day only 10% of 1350 patients developed alkalosis. However, volume expansion can increase the blood pressure and promote edema, so that the use of even moderate amounts of $NaHCO_3$ may be a hazard to persons with renal insufficiency or incipient or active hypertension or cardiac failure. Alkalinization of the urine may be detrimental. Consequently, a daily limit of 200 mEq in persons under 60 years of age and 100 mEq in those who are older has been established as guidelines (*see* Schmidt, 1974). Belching and an uncomfortable but rarely dangerous gastric distention occur after ingestion of $NaHCO_3$.

Preparations. *Sodium Bicarbonate,* U.S.P., is available as a powder and as tablets that contain 325, 488, 527, or 650 mg of the drug. One gram of sodium bicarbonate neutralizes 12 mEq of acid. The usual dose is 300 mg to 2 g, but up to 4 g may be needed in some patients. As a prophylactic against stress and traumatic ulceration, a 0.05-N solution may be used as a continuous irrigant (Morrissey and Barreras, 1974).

Other Therapeutic Uses. The use of sodium bicarbonate in combating systemic acidosis is discussed elsewhere (*see* Chapter 35). The drug is of great value when it is desired to render the urine alkaline. Sodium bicarbonate is used locally on the skin for various disorders, particularly as an antipruritic, in the form of a moist paste or a solution; there is doubt whether the antipruritic effect derives from anything more than its cooling wetness. Sodium bicarbonate is an ingredient of many solutions employed as douches, mouthwashes, and enemas.

ANTACID MIXTURES

Antacids are combined for a variety of reasons: laxative and constipating compounds can correct the disadvantages of each other; a fast-acting ingredient can be combined with a slow-acting ingredient to increase the total buffering time; the daily dose of a single entity can be decreased to reduce the risk of toxicity; patient compliance can be improved by combining agents, rather than by giving multiple separate preparations. Simethicone, supposed demulcents, and antipeptic substances are sometimes included in these products.

The patient and physician can search for one preparation or combination that is best suited to the needs of the case. A mixture that causes laxation in one patient may constipate another. However, mixtures should be selected not only on the basis of the effect on the bowel but also on a knowledge of the efficacy of the antacid and the potential toxic effects of the separate components in relation to the condition of the patient.

Preparations. The most common mixtures of antacids are those of $Al(OH)_3$ and $Mg(OH)_2$. The U.S.P. describes oral suspensions and tablets for two such mixtures, namely, *Alumina and Magnesia* and *Magnesia and Alumina*. In suspensions of the former, the gravimetric ratio of $Al(OH)_3$ to $Mg(OH)_2$ is approximately 2:1; of the latter, close to 1:1. Most of the $Al(OH)_3$-$Mg(OH)_2$ suspensions listed in Table 42–1 approximate the 1:1 ratio. Simethicone is a common ingredient; it is included to defoam the gastric juice, in order to decrease the tendency toward gastroesophageal reflux. Details of the composition, dosage forms, sodium content, and cost index for these preparations can be found in *Facts and Comparisons,* edited by Kastrup and Boyd (1979).

MISCELLANEOUS GASTRIC ANTACIDS

GAVISCON is a mixture containing small amounts of $NaHCO_3$, $Al(OH)_3$, $Mg_2Si_3O_8$, and alginic acid. CO_2 released from $NaHCO_3$ is entrained by the alginic acid to make a foam ("raft"), which floats the mixture on top of the gastric juice. It is intended that, in gastroesophageal reflux, the floating mixture is the first material to make contact with the esophagus. The mixture has a negligible effect on gastric acid below the raft.

The mineral *hydrotalcite* ($Mg_6Al_2(OH)_{16}CO_3 \cdot 4H_2O$; ALTACITE) has an acid-neutralizing capacity about 84% of that of $Mg(OH)_2$. It buffers the gastric contents at pH 4 for sustained periods, during which time it inactivates pepsin by adsorption. It also effectively adsorbs bile acids.

Although milk has often been extolled as a gastric acid buffer, the traditional 90 ml of milk has very little effect on the intragastric pH. After a brief buffer effect, the contained *proteins* induce hypersecretion. The use of milk for this purpose is thus no longer tenable.

GASTRIC ANTACIDS IN THE TREATMENT OF PEPTIC ULCER

The status of antacids is presently in a stage of evolution. The use of *cimetidine* (*see* Chapter 26) will undoubtedly decrease but not abolish the need for antacids. Cimetidine and appropriate intensive antacid treatment have comparable effects on the mean intragastric pH, the amount of acid that is delivered to the duodenum (Deering and Malagelada, 1977), and the healing of both duodenal and gastric ulcers (Englert *et al.,* 1978; Ippoliti *et al.,* 1978) Treatment with cimetidine is much more convenient, is advantageous in that bowel function is not altered, and is no more expensive. However, there may be a group of patients with duodenal ulcer who are relatively refractory to its therapeutic effects (Ippoliti *et al.,* 1978). Regimens have been designed that combine the use of cimetidine and antacids. This approach may be especially useful in the treatment of patients with the Zollinger-Ellison syndrome, in which gastric acid production can be enormous.

There has long been a controversy over whether antacid therapy is more ritualistic than beneficial and whether it does, in fact, aid in the healing of the lesion. Present evidence, while sparse, indicates that therapeutic regimens that incorporate large doses and appropriate schedules do in fact hasten healing.

In 1977, Peterson and coworkers reported that, in a double-blind study, a high-dose liquid antacid regimen considerably accelerated the healing of *duodenal ulcers.* Hollander and Harlan (1973) reported that $CaCO_3$ promoted healing of *gastric ulcers,* but their data were equivocal with respect to duodenal ulcer. However, Butler and Gersh (1975) did not find that moderately intensive antacid therapy benefited patients with gastric ulcer. Two double-blind studies have indicated that appropriate antacid treatment promotes healing of both duodenal (Ippoliti *et al.*, 1978) and gastric (Englert *et al.*, 1978) ulcers, although placebo controls were not used. Most expert gastroenterologists now hold that antacids are efficacious if used properly. For further discussions of this subject and references to the older literature, *see* Peterson and Fordtran (1978) and the *fifth edition* of this textbook.

There is an older literature that indicates that antacids relieve the pain of peptic ulcer when the pH is raised above 2, but subsequent reports (Butler and Gersh, 1975; Sturdevant *et al.*, 1977) state that antacids relieve pain no better than does a placebo (but *see* Hollander and Harlan, 1973).

Neutralization and pH. If the pathogenic role of gastric acid is a *direct* attack on the mucosa to generate a lesion, then any degree of neutralization should be of benefit. Fordtran and coworkers (1973) cite studies in experimental animals that suggest that control of acidity alone, and not peptic activity, is sufficient to confer a therapeutic benefit. The implication that the attack factor is acid and not acid-pepsin is critical to establishing the tenets of effective antacid treatment. For example, to neutralize 80% of gastric acid of pH 1.3, it is necessary only to raise the pH to 2, which most antacids can do. But to inhibit peptic activity of human gastric juice by 80% it is necessary to raise the pH to about 5.5 (*see* Piper and Fenton, 1965). Moreover, the peptic activity is maximal at pH 2, where it is nearly four times what it is at pH 1.3. Therefore, if acid-pepsin is the attack factor, it would be better to leave the gastric acid undisturbed than to neutralize it partially. Not until the pH is elevated to about 5 does the peptic activity drop below that at pH 1.3. Perhaps this explains in part why an effect of antacid treatment on healing has so long eluded conclusive demonstration. At present, it is common to accept an end point of pH 3 or 3.5 as a reasonable goal for antacid treatment. At this pH the acid concentration is only 0.6% that at pH 1.3, but the peptic activity is still three times that at pH 1.3. In this connection, it is of interest that gastric juice buffered to pH 3.5 has nevertheless caused an acidic pulmonary aspiration syndrome (Taylor, 1975).

Dose. Neutralization of the gastric contents stimulates acid secretion, so that a dose cannot be prescribed on the basis of the basal secretory rate. The maximal augmented rate has been estimated to be 30 to 80 mEq per hour in patients with duodenal ulcer (Price and Sanderson, 1956; Fordtran and Walsh, 1973). From the augmented rate and the kinetics of gastric emptying, Myhill and Piper (1964) calculated that 50 mEq per hour of *available* antacid would be required to neutralize continuously the gastric juice of 90% of patients with duodenal ulcer. This is consistent with the hourly 40- to 80-mEq dose of $CaCO_3$ that Kirsner and Palmer (1940) found necessary to maintain the intragastric pH above 4.0. Translated

into the volume of some of the antacid suspensions listed in Table 42–1, 50 mEq would require 6 ml of DELCID, 10 ml of MYLANTA-II, 19 ml of MAALOX, and 40 ml of AMPHOJEL. The 50-mEq requirement may not obtain in all cases, since there are hyposecretors among patients with duodenal ulcer who may require only one fifth as much antacid as the average patient (*e.g.*, *see* Fordtran *et al.*, 1973).

Dose Interval. If antacids are prescribed only with the intent to relieve pain, then they may be taken only as needed. However, if the intent is to promote healing, a continuous buffering would be ideal. Except with intragastric drip, continuous buffering is difficult to achieve, and practical considerations force a compromise in which buffering is achieved discontinuously. Gastric emptying limits the duration of action of even the most potent and persistent antacids. The buffering effects of the recommended single dose of a nonconcentrated antacid disappear in an empty stomach in 5 to 40 minutes and those of a concentrated antacid in 45 to 60 minutes (end point, pH 3.5). However, the sojourn in the stomach is prolonged if the antacid is administered while food is in the stomach; if a large dose (more than 80 mEq for duodenal ulcer and 40 mEq for gastric ulcer) is given 1 hour after a steak meal, its buffering action may persist for more than 2 hours (Fordtran and Collyns, 1966; Texter *et al.*, 1975; but *see* Smyth *et al.*, 1976); an additional dose given 3 hours after eating will extend the period of buffering for another hour (*see* Peterson and Fordtran, 1978). But steak is not eaten at every meal, and it remains to be shown how long buffering persists after various kinds and quantities of meals. Certain observations suggest the effect is not universal. Nevertheless, it is now common practice to administer large doses of antacids *1 and 3 hours after eating and at bedtime,* and as needed for pain; the minimal number of daily doses is thus seven. The apparent efficacy of this dose regimen in the treatment of duodenal ulcer (*see* Peterson *et al.*, 1977) seems to justify it. Hourly doses or intragastric drip are recommended for the effective prophylaxis of the erosive gastritis, stress ulcers, and acute gastrointestinal bleeding that occur in critically ill patients (Morrissey and Barreras, 1974; Hastings *et al.*, 1978). In a carefully matched group of critically ill patients, the continuous administration of an antacid (MYLANTA-II) proved to be superior to cimetidine for such prophylaxis (Priebe *et al.*, 1980).

Choice of Preparation. The following guidelines are offered to assist in the selection of an antacid product. (1) Choose only products with a proven high neutralization capacity. The data in Table 42–1 rank well-known proprietary products in decreasing order of the capacity of the suspensions to neutralize HCl. There is more than a sixfold range in these capacities. It would require only 10 ml of DELCID but 36 ml of A-M-T to provide one 80-mEq dose. The data do not show the rapidity of onset. It is high for $Mg(OH)_2$, MgO, hydrotalcite, and $CaCO_3$; intermediate for magaldrate and $MgCO_3$; and slow for $Mg_2Si_3O_8$ and aluminum compounds, except hexitol-stabilized $Al(OH)_3$ suspensions. (2) Although

NaHCO$_3$ and effervescent antacids react very rapidly, they are also easily emptied from the stomach and hence have short durations of action. (3) In adequate doses, MgO, Mg(OH)$_2$, and NaHCO$_3$ can raise the gastric pH above 8 and CaCO$_3$ can raise it above 5. A pH of approximately 4 can sometimes be achieved with magaldrate and dihydroxyaluminum sodium carbonate, but the action is brief and erratic. (4) The antacid capacity, rate of onset, and pH achieved depend upon the proportions of the various constituents in mixtures. When Al(OH)$_3$ is included, the acid reaction of Al^{3+} prevents a high pH from being reached, unless the proportion of Al(OH)$_3$ in the mixture is small. (5) The long-standing precept that suspensions have greater capacities for neutralization than tablets is not necessarily true, especially for chewable tablets; however, the rate of neutralization by suspensions is usually faster and their shelf-life is better. (6) High doses of CaCO$_3$ should be avoided. (7) Although simethicone may relieve some gastrointestinal discomfort and decrease gastroesophageal reflux, it does not lessen the requirement for antacids. (8) The renal and cardiovascular status should always be assessed before a daily dose of an antacid is established. Consideration may have to be given to the added intake of sodium and potassium, as well as to disturbances of acid-base balance. The sodium and potassium contents of antacid products have been tabulated by Yokel (1977). (9) In considering the cost to the patient, the physician should compare products on the basis of chemical equivalence and not on cost per volume or tablet.

For opinions on the appropriate use of antacids, *see* the reviews by Piper and Heap (1972), Piper (1973), Morrissey and Barreras (1974), Littman and Pine (1975), Grossman and coworkers (1976), and Peterson and Fordtran (1978).

Other Therapeutic Uses. Neutralization of gastric acid in patients who have gastroesophageal reflux both decreases the erosive activity of the secretion and increases lower-esophageal pressure. Antacid can be used intermittently to relieve mild symptoms, or hourly or occasionally continuously by intraesophageal drip to manage severe disease. Vigorous treatment can increase the patient's tolerance to intraesophageal acid for as long as 3 days after treatment has ceased (Serebro *et al.*, 1973). In double-blind trials, GAVISCON can effectively relieve the symptoms of reflux esophagitis (Beeley and Warner, 1972; Barnardo *et al.*, 1975). Benefit can persist for weeks after discontinuation of the regimen. This preparation can also decrease output of gastric acid and promote the healing of duodenal ulcers (Moshal, 1973; Chaput de Saintonge *et al.*, 1978). Other drugs used in the treatment of reflux esophagitis are bethanechol, cimetidine, and metoclopramide (*see* Fox and Behar, 1979).

Antacids are occasionally employed in patients undergoing anesthesia or during labor to lessen the danger from aspiration of gastric contents.

OTHER ANTIULCER DRUGS

The subject of antiulcer agents has been reviewed by Peterson and Fordtran (1978) and Ippoliti and

Peterson (1979), and drugs other than antacids will only be highlighted here.

Cimetidine promises to be the most important single agent in the treatment of peptic ulcer, and a valuable drug for the management of reflux esophagitis. The pharmacology and clinical uses of cimetidine are discussed in Chapter 26.

Carbenoxolone sodium, an oleandane derivative obtained from glycerrhiza, may be efficacious in ambulatory but not in hospitalized patients with gastric ulcer (*see* Lewis, 1974). In capsule form, it also appears to promote healing of duodenal ulcers (Davies and Reed, 1977). It protects the mucosal barrier from bile acids and also selectively inhibits the synthesis of prostaglandin F$_{2\alpha}$. It has mineralocorticoid activity, and it may be necessary to administer a diuretic and potassium concomitantly. Carbenoxolone is not available for general use in the United States.

Prostaglandin E$_2$ and several of its derivatives inhibit gastric secretion in man to the same extent as that observed with cimetidine. These compounds prevent ulcers and bile-induced erosive gastritis and mucosal hemorrhage in experimental animals. *15(R),15-Methylprostaglandin E$_2$ methyl ester* may promote healing of gastric ulcers in humans (Fung *et al.*, 1974). Diarrhea is the principal side effect of the prostaglandins but is minimal when proper doses are used.

A colloidal *bismuth* preparation, tripotassium dicitratobismuthate, can accelerate the healing of gastric and duodenal ulcers, but the number of patients who have as yet been given this drug is small (*see* Ippoliti and Peterson, 1979). Micronized bismuth subnitrate has a similar effect (Sezer *et al.*, 1975). The mechanism of its action is unknown.

Antimuscarinic drugs can delay gastric emptying and decrease gastric secretion (*see* Chapter 7). Atropine and other belladonna alkaloids are exceptionally poor in this respect, but certain quaternary antimuscarinic drugs (*e.g.*, anisotropine methylbromide, glycopyrrolate, clidinium bromide, and methscopolamine bromide) in doses that are tolerated can considerably suppress gastric secretion, and some patients have been successfully medicated for several years. In a recent small study it was found that small doses of antacids and nighttime medication with anisotropine methylbromide increased the number of healed duodenal ulcers by 40% within the first 2 weeks (Bowers *et al.*, 1978). Even quaternary ammonium antimuscarinic drugs with annoying side effects can often be used at night to retard gastric emptying and hence increase the retention of antacids in the stomach. However, gastric stasis may favor duodenal-gastric reflux of bile, and some gastroenterologists thus consider antimuscarinic drugs to be contraindicated in the treatment of benign gastric ulcer. The uses of antimuscarinic drugs to manage ulcers have been reviewed by Littman and Pine (1975), Peterson and Fordtran (1978), and Ippoliti and Peterson (1979).

Even though the reflux of bile acids may play a role in the pathophysiology of erosive gastritis and gastric ulcer, the usefulness of *cholestyramine* to treat these conditions has been slight. The effect of *metoclopramide* to stimulate orthograde peristalsis has been employed in attempts to suppress the reflux of bile; it appears to promote healing of gastric ulcers and to prevent relapse, but not to accelerate healing of duodenal ulcers.

DIGESTANTS

Digestants are drugs that supposedly promote the process of digestion in the gastrointestinal tract in conditions characterized by a lack of one or more of the specific substances that function in the digestion of food.

HYDROCHLORIC ACID

The only use of hydrochloric acid is in the treatment of gastric *achlorhydria*. Conventional doses after a meal do not increase the free hydrochloric acid in the stomach; the occasional relief of the symptoms of distress may thus be a placebo effect. Glutamic acid hydrochloride is even less effective; however, because it can be administered in capsules, damage to the teeth is avoided. The free acid is administered as *diluted hydrochloride acid* (10%) in a dose of 5 to 10 ml in 125 to 250 ml of water, often in several divided doses at 15-minute intervals. It must be sipped through a tube. The dose of *glutamic acid hydrochloride* (ACIDULIN) is 340 mg to 1 g.

PEPSIN

Pepsin may be administered when there is gastric achylia, as in patients with pernicious anemia or gastric carcinoma. However, hydrochloric acid is often used alone in the treatment of achylia, since the proteolytic enzymes of the intestinal tract function sufficiently to prevent serious digestive disturbances.

PANCREATIC ENZYMES

The enzymes of the pancreas are obtainable in a preparation known as *pancreatin,* which is obtained from fresh hog pancreas. It contains principally amylase, trypsin, and lipase. Pancreatin is employed in the treatment of conditions in which the secretion of pancreatic juice is deficient, for example, pancreatitis and mucoviscidosis. The administration of pancreatin provides some benefit; for example, the nitrogen and fat content of the stool can be decreased. Pancreatin should be given in enteric capsules to prevent its destruction by pepsin. The average dose is 0.5 to 1 g. Cimetidine increases the amount of pancreatin delivered into the duodenum.

BILE ACIDS AND SALTS

The salts of the bile acids and their conjugates are important constituents of bile. The important bile acids in human bile are cholic acid (3,7,12-trihydroxycholanic acid) and chenodeoxycholic acid ($3\alpha,7\alpha$-dihydroxycholanic acid); these are mainly present as the glycine and taurine conjugates (glycocholic, taurocholic, glycochenodeoxycholic, and taurochenodeoxycholic acids), the salts of which are often referred to as the *bile salts.* The structure of cholanic acid is as follows:

Cholanic Acid

Bile salts are strongly amphiphilic and, with the aid of biliary phospholipids, they readily form micelles with and emulsify lipids. They are important not only for the emulsification of cholesterol and other lipids in bile but also for the emulsification of dietary lipids preparatory to digestion and absorption.

Pharmacological and Toxic Effects. Bile acids increase the output of bile and hence are called *choleretic* drugs; the bile salts have little choleretic activity. Dehydrocholic acid, a semisynthetic cholate, is especially active and evokes the secretion of a bile of low specific gravity; it is therefore called a *hydrocholeretic drug.* The increase in bile flow is not the result of true cholepoiesis, since the augmented flow is only that necessary to secrete the increased load of bile acid imposed by that administered. The secretion of preformed bile pigment is not increased, and any increase in bile pigments in the intestine is the result of its flushing from dead spaces and/or the hemolytic actions of the drugs themselves. Dehydrocholate actually decreases the excretion of bilirubin. Therefore, bile acids are ineffective in attenuating jaundice.

Chenodeoxycholic and ursodeoxycholic acids, but not cholic acid, decrease the cholesterol content of bile. If the bile is supersaturated with cholesterol, it will become unsaturated when the content of chenodeoxycholate reaches approximately 70% of the total bile acids. The mechanism is twofold: (1) absorption of cholesterol by the small intestine is impaired, possibly as the result of a decrease in the output of bile salts, and (2) synthesis of cholesterol is diminished through inhibition of hydroxymethylglutaryl-CoA reductase. The agent also inhibits cholesterol 7α-hydroxylase and thus decreases the synthesis of the other bile acids and, *pari passu,* their conjugates. The decrease in cholesterol concentration in bile may not only halt the formation of cholesterolic gallstones but also promote their dissolution during sustained treatment.

Prolonged treatment with chenodeoxycholic acid causes patchy loss of microvilli in the biliary epithelium and an increase in sinusoidal lipocytes (Bateson *et al.,* 1977). Dehydrocholic and taurocholic acids cause similar effects. Some patients have increases in plasma SGOT and aspartate aminotransferase activities. Diarrhea may occur, probably as a result of inhibition of glucose uptake, loss of electrolytes into the lumen of the small intestine, and inhibition of colonic mucosal membrane ATPase. Bile salts can impair the resistance to acid of the mucosal barrier of the stomach and esophagus and probably also the upper duodenum. This fact has pathophysiological implications in gastritis, peptic ulcer, and reflux esophagitis, and it also brings into question the propriety of the oral administration of these agents. Choleretic bile acids may cause biliary colic if a dislodged stone obstructs the bile duct. Following intravenous injection, bile acids can cause hypotension, bradycardia, and skeletal muscle hyperactivity with twitching and spasms. Anaphylaxis occurs rarely.

Preparations and Dosage. *Dehydrocholic Acid,* U.S.P. (DECHOLIN), is available in tablets containing 250 mg. The usual dose is 250 to 750 mg, three times a day. *Dehydrocholate Sodium Injection,* U.S.P. (DECHOLIN SODIUM), is marketed as a 20% solution in ampuls containing 3, 5, or 10 ml. The intravenous dose is 3 to 5 ml. *Ox bile extract* resembles that from human bile and is available in tablets. The bile acid content is equivalent to about 45% cholic acid. The usual dose is 250 to 500 mg. *Chenodeoxycholic acid* is given initially in divided doses that total 8 to 10 mg/kg per day; this is then adjusted upward to 13 to 15 mg/kg (or 18 to 20 mg/kg in obese patients).

Therapeutic Uses. Because of their physiological role in the absorption of dietary lipids, the bile salts were once used widely for so-called replacement therapy in pathological conditions in which the concentration of bile acids in the upper intestine is low (such as biliary fistula, disease or resection of the ileum, hepatic or extrahepatic cholestasis). However, the usual preparations are generally ineffective and sometimes harmful. They are little used today. Hydrocholeretic drugs are sometimes used after gallbladder surgery to facilitate T-tube drainage. Hydrocholeresis may also be used to assist roentgenographic visualization of the gallbladder and bile ducts; the intravenous route is used.

Chenodeoxycholic and ursodeoxycholic acids are employed for the dissolution of radiolucent gallstones. Complete dissolution occurs within 12 months in 15 to 50% of patients treated with daily doses of 0.75 to 1.5 g of chenodeoxycholic acid. When partial dissolution is included, the overall response rate is about 60%. This treatment has been reviewed by Watts and coworkers (1975), Batey (1977), Dowling and Hofmann (1978), Thistle (1978), and Pearlman and associates (1979).

Alday, E. S., and Goldsmith, H. S. Gastric hypersecretion after antacid infusion into the small intestine. *Surg. Gynecol. Obstet.,* **1974,** *139,* 333–336.

Alfrey, A. C.; LeGendre, G. R.; and Kaehny, W. S. The dialysis encephalopathy syndrome. Possible aluminum intoxication. *N. Engl. J. Med.,* **1976,** *294,* 184–188.

Ansari, A. Antacid-induced phosphorus depletion and repletion. *Minn. Med.,* **1970,** *53,* 837–838.

Barnardo, D. E.; Lancaster-Smith, M.; Strickland, I. D.; and Wright, J. T. A double-blind controlled trial of GAVISCON in patients with symptomatic gastro-esophageal reflux. *Curr. Med. Res. Opin.,* **1975,** *3,* 388–391.

Barreras, R. F. Acid secretion after calcium carbonate in patients with duodenal ulcer. *N. Engl. J. Med.,* **1970,** *282,* 1402–1405.

Bateson, M. C.; Hopwood, D.; and Bouchier, I. A. D.

Effect of gallstone-dissolution therapy on human liver structure. *Am. J. Dig. Dis.,* **1977,** *22,* 293–299.

Beeley, M., and Warner, J. O. Medical treatment of symptomatic hiatus hernia with low-density compounds. *Curr. Med. Res. Opin.,* **1972,** *1,* 63–69.

Berlyne, G. M.; Ben-Ari, J.; Pest, D.; Weinberger, J.; Stern, M.; Gilmore, G. R.; and Levine, R. Hyperaluminaemia from aluminum resins in renal failure. *Lancet,* **1970,** *2,* 494–496.

Bowers, J. H.; Forbes, J. A.; and Freston, J. W. Effect of nighttime anisotropine methylbromide on duodenal ulcer healing and pain: a double-blind controlled trial. *J. Clin. Pharmacol.,* **1978,** *18,* 365–371.

Butler, M. L., and Gersh, H. Antacid vs. placebo in hospitalized gastric ulcer patients: a controlled therapeutic study. *Am. J. Dig. Dis.,* **1975,** *20,* 803–807.

Caldwell, J. H.; Cline, C. T.; Fox, A. W.; and Cataland, S. Effect of chronic antacid ingestion on serum gastrin and gastric secretion. *Am. J. Dig. Dis.,* **1976,** *21,* 863–866.

Castell, D. O., and Levine, S. M. Lower esophageal sphincter response to gastric neutralization. A new mechanism for treatment of heartburn with antacids. *Ann. Intern. Med.,* **1971,** *74,* 223–227.

Chaput de Saintonge, D. M.; Earlam, R. J.; Wright, T. J.; Evans, S. J. W.; Hillenbrand, P.; Lancaster-Smith, M. J.; Balme, R. H.; and Barnardo, D. E. An antacid preparation in the treatment of duodenal ulcer. *Practitioner,* **1978,** *220,* 321–324.

Clarkson, E. M.; McDonald, S. J.; and de Wardener, H. E. The effect of high intake of calcium carbonate in normal subjects with chronic renal failure. *Clin. Sci.,* **1966,** *30,* 425–438.

Clemens, J. D., and Feinstein, A. R. Calcium carbonate and constipation: a historical review of medical mythopoeia. *Gastroenterology,* **1977,** *72,* 957–961.

Cooke, N.; Teitelbaum, S.; and Avioli, L. V. Antacid-induced osteomalacia and nephrolithiasis. *Arch. Intern. Med.,* **1978,** *138,* 1007–1009.

David, M., and Robson, M. Proximal myopathy caused by iatrogenic phosphate depletion. *J.A.M.A.,* **1976,** *236,* 1380–1381.

Davies, W. A., and Reed, P. I. Controlled trial of DUOGASTRONE in duodenal ulcer. *Gut,* **1977,** *18,* 78–83.

Deering, T. B., and Malagelada, J. R. Comparison of an H2-receptor antagonist and a neutralizing antacid on postprandial acid delivery into the duodenum in patients with duodenal ulcer. *Gastroenterology,* **1977,** *73,* 11–14.

Englert, E., Jr.; Freston, J. W.; Graham, D. Y.; Finklestein, W.; Kruss, D. M.; Priest, R. J.; Raskin, J. B.; Rhodes, J. B.; Rogers, A. I.; Wenger, M. D.; Wilcox, L. L.; and Crossley, R. J. Cimetidine, antacid, and hospitalization in the treatment of benign gastric ulcer. A multicenter double blind study. *Gastroenterology,* **1978,** *74,* 416–425.

Feurle, G. Effect of rising intragastric pH induced by several antacids on serum gastrin concentrations in duodenal ulcer patients and in a control group. *Gastroenterology,* **1975,** *68,* 1–7.

Fordtran, J. S. Comparison of antacids for peptic ulcer. *N. Engl. J. Med.,* **1966,** *275,* 1316.

Fordtran, J. S., and Collyns, J. A. H. Antacid pharmacology in duodenal ulcer. Effect of antacids on postcibal gastric acidity and peptic activity. *N. Engl. J. Med.,* **1966,** *274,* 921–927.

Fordtran, J. S.; Morawski, S. G.; and Richardson, C. T. *In vivo* and *in vitro* evaluation of liquid antacids. *N. Engl. J. Med.,* **1973,** *288,* 923–928.

Fordtran, J. S., and Walsh, J. H. Gastric acid secretion rate and buffer content of the stomach after eating. Results in normal patients and in patients with duodenal ulcer. *J. Clin. Invest.,* **1973,** *52,* 645–657.

Fung, W. P.; Karim, S. M.; and Tye, C. Y. Effect of 15(R)15 methylprostaglandin E2 methylester on healing of gastric ulcers—controlled endoscopic study. *Lancet*, **1974**, *2*, 10–12.

Gibaldi, M.; Grundhofer, B.; and Levy, G. Effect of antacids on pH of urine. *Clin. Pharmacol. Ther.*, **1974**, *16*, 520–525.

———. Time course and dose dependence of antacid effect on urine pH. *J. Pharm. Sci.*, **1975**, *64*, 2003–2004.

Goidsenhoven, G. M. -T. van; Gray, O. V.; Price, A. V.; and Sanderson, P. H. The effect of prolonged administration of large doses of sodium bicarbonate in man. *Clin. Sci.*, **1954**, *13*, 383–401.

Goldsmith, R. S.; Furszyfer, J.; Johnson, W. J.; Fournier, A. E.; and Arnaud, C. D. Control of secondary hyperparathyroidism during long-term hemodialysis. *Am. J. Med.*, **1971**, *50*, 692–699.

Hastings, P. R.; Skillman, J. J.; Bushnell, L. S.; and Silen, W. Antacid titration in the prevention of acute gastrointestinal bleeding. A controlled, randomized trial in 100 critically ill patients. *N. Engl. J. Med.*, **1978**, *298*, 1041–1045.

Hollander, D., and Harlan, J. Antacids vs placebos in peptic ulcer therapy. A controlled double-blind investigation. *J.A.M.A.*, **1973**, *226*, 1181–1185.

Hurwitz, A.; Robinson, R. G.; Vats, T. S.; Whittier, F. C.; and Herrin, W. F. Effects of antacids on gastric emptying. *Gastroenterology*, **1976**, *71*, 268–273.

Ippoliti, A. F., and others. Cimetidine versus intensive antacid therapy for duodenal ulcer. A multicenter trial. *Gastroenterology*, **1978**, *74*, 393–395.

Ivanovich, P.; Fellows, H.; and Rich, C. The absorption of calcium carbonate. *Ann. Intern. Med.*, **1967**, *66*, 917–923.

Joekes, A. M.; Rose, G. A.; and Sutor, J. Multiple renal silica calculi. *Br. Med. J.*, **1973**, *1*, 146–147.

Kaehny, W. D.; Hegg, A. P.; and Alfrey, A. C. Gastrointestinal absorption of aluminum from aluminum-containing antacids. *N. Engl. J. Med.*, **1977**, *296*, 1389–1390.

Kastrup, E. K., and Boyd, J. R. (eds.). *Facts and Comparisons*. Facts and Comparisons, Inc., St. Louis, **1979**, pp. 291a–297a.

Khan, A. A.; Englert, E., Jr.; and Moore, J. G. Tissue magnesium and gastric motility after antacids. *Clin. Res.*, **1970**, *18*, 127.

Kirsner, J. B., and Palmer, W. L. The effect of various antacids upon hydrogen-ion concentration of the gastric contents. *Am. J. Dig. Dis.*, **1940**, *7*, 85–93.

———. Alkalosis complicating the Sippy treatment of peptic ulcer. *Arch. Intern. Med.*, **1942**, *69*, 789–807.

Knapp, E. L. Factors influencing the urinary excretion of calcium. I. In normal persons. *J. Clin. Invest.*, **1947**, *26*, 182–202.

Kuruvilla, J. T. Antipeptic activity of antacids. *Gut*, **1971**, *12*, 897–898.

Levant, J. A.; Walsh, J. H.; and Isenberg, J. I. Stimulation of gastric secretion and gastrin release by single oral doses of calcium carbonate in man. *N. Engl. J. Med.*, **1973**, *289*, 555–558.

McMillan, D. E., and Freeman, R. B. The milk-alkali syndrome: a study of the acute disorder with comments on the development of the chronic condition. *Medicine* (Baltimore), **1965**, *44*, 485–501.

Makoff, D. L.; Gordon, A.; Franklin, A. S.; and Gerstein, A. R. Chronic calcium carbonate therapy in uremia. *Arch. Intern. Med.*, **1969**, *123*, 15–21.

Morrissey, J. F.; Honda, T.; and Tanaka, Y. Gastric mucosal coating and gastric emptying time of antacids. *Arch. Intern. Med.*, **1967**, *119*, 510–517.

Moshal, M. G. Trials with GAVISCON*: its mode of action and its use in the treatment of duodenal ulcers (a double-blind trial). *S. Afr. J. Surg.*, **1973**, *11*, 139–144.

Myhill, J., and Piper, D. W. Antacid therapy of peptic ulcer. Part 1. A mathematical definition of an adequate dose. *Gut*, **1964**, *5*, 581–585.

Nassim, J. R., and Connolly, C. K. Treatment of calcinosis

universalis with aluminum hydroxide. *Arch. Dis. Child.*, **1970**, *45*, 118–121.

Peterson, W. L.; Sturdevant, R. A. L.; Frankl, H. D.; Richardson, C. T.; Isenberg, J. I.; Elashoff, J. D.; Sones, J. Q.; Gross, R. A.; McCallum, R. W.; and Fordtran, J. S. Healing of duodenal ulcer with an antacid regimen. *N. Engl. J. Med.*, **1977**, *297*, 341–345.

Piper, D. W., and Fenton, B. H. pH stability and activity curves of pepsin with special reference to their clinical importance. *Gut*, **1965**, *6*, 506–508.

Posey, E. L.; Smith, P.; Turner, C. I.; and Aldridge, J. Effects of anticholinergics, antacids, and antrectomy on gastrin production and relation of antral motility to gastrin release. *Am. J. Dig. Dis.*, **1965**, *10*, 399–410.

Price, A. V., and Sanderson, P. H. Alkali requirement for continuous neutralization of gastric contents in gastric and duodenal ulcer. *Clin. Sci.*, **1956**, *15*, 285–295.

Priebe, H. J.; Skillman, J. J.; Bushnell, L. S.; Long, P. C.; and Silen, W. Antacid versus cimetidine in preventing acute gastrointestinal bleeding. *N. Engl. J. Med.*, **1980**, *302*, 426–430.

Randall, R. E.; Cohen, M. D.; Spray, C. C.; and Rossmeissl, E. C. Hypermagnesemia in renal failure. Etiology and toxic manifestations. *Ann. Intern. Med.*, **1964**, *61*, 73–88.

Schmidt, A. M. Over-the-counter drugs: antacid and anti-flatulent products. *Federal Register*, **1974**, *39*, 19862–19877.

Serebro, H. A.; Friedman, M.; and Beck, I. T. Efficacy of continuous intraoesophageal antacid drip therapy in the treatment of reflux esophagitis. A quantitative assessment using the acid perfusion test. *S. Afr. Med. J.*, **1973**, *47*, 1656–1659.

Sezer, R.; Özman, M.; and Karaagac, M. Clinical, radiological and laboratory findings in patients with duodenal ulcer, treated with micronized bismuth subnitrate, singly and in combination with antacids. *Br. J. Clin. Pract.*, **1975**, *29*, 227–233.

Smyth, R. D.; Herczeg, T.; Wheatley, T. A.; Hause, W.; and Reavey-Cantwell, N. H. Correlation of in vitro and in vivo methodology for evaluation of antacids. *J. Pharm. Sci.*, **1976**, *65*, 1045–1047.

Sturdevant, R. A. L.; Isenberg, J. I.; Secrist, D.; and Ansfield, J. Antacid and placebo produced similar pain relief in duodenal ulcer patients. *Gastroenterology*, **1977**, *72*, 1–5.

Taylor, G. Acid pulmonary aspiration syndrome after antacids. *Br. J. Anaesth.*, **1975**, *47*, 615–617.

Vincent, P. C., and Radcliff, F. J. Effect of large doses of calcium carbonate on serum and urinary calcium. *Am. J. Dig. Dis.*, **1966**, *11*, 286–295.

Wenger, J.; Kirsner, J. B.; and Palmer, W. L. The milk alkali syndrome: hypercalcemia, alkalosis, and azotemia following calcium carbonate and milk therapy of peptic ulcer. *Gastroenterology*, **1957**, *33*, 745–769.

Wenger, J., and Sundy, M. Pepsin adsorption by commercial antacid mixtures. *In vitro* studies. *J. Clin. Pharmacol.*, **1972**, *12*, 136–141.

Yokel, R. A. Sodium and potassium levels in antacids. *Am. J. Hosp. Pharm.*, **1977**, *34*, 200–202.

Monographs and Reviews

Batey, R. G. Chenodeoxycholic acid in the management of gallstones. *Drugs*, **1977**, *14*, 116–119.

Dowling, R. H., and Hofmann, A. F. *The Medical Treatment of Gallstones*. University Park Press, Baltimore, **1978**.

Fordtran, J. S. Acid rebound. *N. Engl. J. Med.*, **1968**, *279*, 900–905.

Fox, S., and Behar, J. Control of lower oesophageal sphincter pressure and acid reflux. *Clin. Gastroenterol.*, **1979**, *8*, 37–52.

Grossman, M. I.; Guth, P. H.; Isenberg, J. I.; Passaro, E. P., Jr.; Roth, B. E.; Sturdevant, R. A. L.; and Walsh,

J. H.   A new look at peptic ulcer. *Ann. Intern. Med.,* **1976,** *84,* 57–67.

Hurwitz, A.   Antacid therapy and drug kinetics. *Clin. Pharmacokinet.,* **1977,** *2,* 269–280. (75 references.)

Ippoliti, A., and Peterson, W.   The pharmacology of peptic ulcer disease. *Clin. Gastroenterol.,* **1979,** *8,* 53–67.

Lewis, J. R.   Carbenoxolone sodium in the treatment of peptic ulcer. *J.A.M.A.,* **1974,** *229,* 460–462.

Littman, A., and Pine, B. H.   Antacids and anticholinergic drugs. *Ann. Intern. Med.,* **1975,** *82,* 544–551.

Morrissey, J. F., and Barreras, R. F.   Drug therapy: antacid therapy. *N. Engl. J. Med.,* **1974,** *290,* 550–554.

Pearlman, B. J.; Marks, J. W.; Bonorris, G. G.; and Schoenfield, L. J.   Gallstone dissolution—a progress report. *Clin. Gastroenterol.,* **1979,** *8,* 123–140. (69 references.)

Peterson, W. L., and Fordtran, J. S.   Reduction of gastric acidity. In, *Gastrointestinal Disease: Pathophysiology, Diagnosis, Management,* 2nd ed. (Sleisenger, M. H., and Fordtran, J. S., eds.) W. B. Saunders Co., Philadelphia, **1978,** pp. 891–917. (135 references.)

Piper, D. W.   Antacid and anticholinergic drug therapy. *Clin. Gastroenterol.,* **1973,** *2,* 361–377.

Piper, D. W., and Heap, T. R.   Medical management of peptic ulcer with reference to anti-ulcer agents in other gastro-intestinal diseases. *Drugs,* **1972,** *3,* 366–403. (172 references.)

Romankiewicz, J. A.   Effects of antacids on gastrointestinal absorption of drugs. *Primary Care,* **1976,** *3,* 537–550. (31 references.)

Texter, E. C.; Smart, D. F.; and Butler, R. C.   Antacids. *Am. Fam. Physician,* **1975,** *11,* No. 4, 111–118.

Thistle, J. L.   Therapy of gallstones. *Ration. Drug Ther.,* **1978,** *12,* No. 3, 1–5.

Watts, J. McK.; Jablonski, P.; and Toouli, J.   Medical treatment of gallstones. *Drugs,* **1975,** *10,* 342–350.

43 LAXATIVES AND CATHARTICS

Edward Fingl

Laxatives and cathartics are drugs that promote defecation. Valid indications for the use of these agents are limited. The contrasting extensive misuse of self-prescribed cathartic nostrums by the public is a result of the many misconceptions concerning bowel function and of the mistaken notions of the value of cathartic medication. Persistence of this misuse reflects the failure of the medical and ancillary health professions to counter the proprietary drug advertising designed to perpetuate these erroneous beliefs.

The terms *laxative* and *cathartic* correctly imply different intensities of drug effect. Laxative effect suggests the elimination of a soft, formed stool, whereas cathartic effect implies a more fluid evacuation. When applied to the *effect* of a drug, this distinction is convenient and should be preserved. Most drugs that promote defecation produce a laxative effect in low dosage but a cathartic effect in higher dosage. Consequently, when applied to the *drugs* themselves, the terms are often employed interchangeably.

The numerous laxative-cathartic preparations available for "over-the-counter" use have been reviewed by the United States Food and Drug Administration Advisory Review Panel (FDA, 1975).

GENERAL CONSIDERATIONS

Laxatives and cathartics constitute a varied group of drugs. The major common characteristics are oral efficacy and activity that is primarily due to their physical properties within the intestinal lumen or to contact with the intestinal mucosa. Interestingly, the effects of several of the laxative-cathartics are due to products of biotransformation of the drug by the intestinal microflora.

Mechanisms of Laxative-Cathartic Effects. Laxatives and cathartics increase the water content of the feces and speed transit of the intestinal contents by one or more of three general mechanisms: (1) Water and electrolytes may be retained in the intestinal lumen by the *hydrophilic* or *osmotic* properties of the drug or its metabolites, with intestinal transit being increased indirectly due to increased intestinal bulk. (2) The laxative-cathartic may act on the mucosa to decrease normal *net absorption of electrolytes and water,* with intestinal transit being increased indirectly by the fluid bulk. (3) The laxative-cathartic may increase transit by primary effects on *intestinal motility,* with net absorption of electrolytes and water being decreased indirectly because of the reduced time for absorption.

Views about the mechanism of action of the individual laxative-cathartics are changing (*see* FDA, 1975; Gaginella and Phillips, 1975; Binder, 1977; Fingl and Freston, 1979). Traditional explanations have been reexamined, and most have been modified, if not discarded. Unfortunately, the mechanism of action of all laxative-cathartics remains uncertain. For example, it is now recognized that a primary effect of many cathartics is inhibition of the net absorption of electrolytes and water by the intestine. Yet, at least some of these agents also influence intestinal motility directly, and the relative contributions of the two types of actions to the laxative-cathartic effect *in vivo* remain to be determined. Moreover, analysis of the biochemical mechanisms that underlie laxative-cathartic effects is still rudimentary. The possible role of the gastrointestinal hormones, prostaglandins, and cyclic nucleotides as mediators of laxative-cathartic effects is just beginning to be explored in a systematic manner. However, as this analysis proceeds, the laxative-cathartic agents can be expected to be useful tools for defining the role of these mediators in intestinal physiology and pathology and for clarifying the interrelationship between intestinal transport of electrolytes and water and intestinal motility. The mechanisms of laxative-cathartic effects are considered further in subsequent discussions of the individual agents.

The term *stimulant cathartic,* previously employed to refer to drugs that increase intestinal motility, should be abandoned. These drugs are now known also to have primary effects on the absorption of electrolytes and water, and the effects on motility are a combination of excitatory and inhibitory actions. A suitable substitute term is *contact cathartic.* It is appropriately noncommittal with regard to the relative contributions of the various actions to the laxative-cathartic effects *in vivo,* and it correctly implies that these drugs act on the intestine, as contrasted with those that act primarily by their hydrophilic or osmotic properties.

Classification and Choice of Laxatives and Cathartics. The laxatives and cathartics are classified and discussed in the text to emphasize mechanism of action. However, the more commonly used agents are listed in Table 43–1 without regard to mechanism of action in order to identify the major groups of drugs and to indicate the pattern of laxative-cathartic effects produced in *usual clinical dosage.* It must be emphasized, however, that the effect and latency of all laxatives and cathartics vary with dosage. The major groups of drugs (*e.g.,* bulk-forming agents, docusates) often have distinguishing pharmacological characteristics that influence their choice for a specific patient. Nevertheless, agents within a group usually have similar clinical usefulness and limitations.

DIETARY FIBER AND RELATED BULK-FORMING LAXATIVES

A fiber-rich diet, in conjunction with other nonpharmacological measures, is the most appropriate method for prevention and treatment of functional constipation. Dietary fiber is also of benefit for patients in whom it is desired that the feces be maintained soft, to avoid straining at the stool, and in the management of irritable bowel disease and diverticular disease of the colon. The related bulk-forming agents are natural and semisynthetic polysaccharides and cellulose derivatives similar to those characterized as dietary fiber. They are useful as a supplement to dietary adjustment or when a constipating, fiber-poor diet cannot be corrected.

The term *dietary fiber* has supplanted the older term *crude fiber.* Dietary fiber is defined physiologically as the portion of plant food that escapes digestion in the human small intestine. Chemically, it consists of cellulose and lignin, the components measured by the method for crude fiber, and also gums, pectins, hemicelluloses, and other polysaccharides. The polysaccharide components are now considered to be more important. The content of total dietary fiber of many foods is three to four times that of the crude fiber.

Because of differences in their component polysaccharides, dietary fiber from various sources and the related bulk-forming agents vary somewhat in their pharmacological characteristics. Unfortunately, these differences are as yet poorly defined, and choice among these preparations often depends upon preference of the individual patient. An excellent review of dietary fiber has been provided by Cummings (1973); the properties of the bulk-forming laxatives have been summarized by Tainter and Buchanan in a symposium (1954).

Table 43–1. CLASSIFICATION AND COMPARISON OF REPRESENTATIVE LAXATIVES AND CATHARTICS

LAXATIVE-CATHARTIC EFFECT AND LATENCY IN USUAL CLINICAL DOSAGE *

Softening of Feces, *1 to 3 Days*	*Soft or Semifluid Stool,* *6 to 8 Hours*	*Watery Evacuation,* *1 to 3 Hours*

Bulk-forming laxatives
  Bran
  Psyllium preparations
  Methylcellulose
	Diphenylmethane cathartics
	  Phenolphthalein
	  Bisacodyl
		Saline cathartics †
		  Sodium phosphates
		  Magnesium sulfate
		  Milk of magnesia

Docusates (dioctyl
  sulfosuccinates)
	Anthraquinone cathartics
	  Senna
	  Cascara sagrada
	  Danthron
		Castor oil

Lactulose		
Mineral oil		

* Effect and latency of all laxatives and cathartics vary with dosage.
† Also employed in lower dosage for laxative effect.

Effects on the Intestinal Tract. Dietary fiber and related agents increase the mass of stool, its water content, and the rate of colonic transit. These effects are usually apparent within 24 hours, but full effect during repeated use may be delayed for several days or longer. Alterations of the metabolism of bile acids and cholesterol, gas production, and other effects are variable. The laxative effect is commonly attributed to the hydrophilic bulk-forming properties of the component polysaccharides. However, a likely additional factor is metabolism of the polysaccharides by the intestinal microflora, with accumulation of metabolites that are osmotically active. Active metabolites may also alter intestinal transport of electrolytes and/or motility and cause subtle changes in fecal bile acids and fecal flora.

Bran and other bulk-forming agents reduce intraluminal rectosigmoid pressure and relieve symptoms in patients with irritable bowel disease and diverticular disease of the colon. Relief of pain and other symptoms occurs progressively over several months (see Parks, 1974; Brodribb, 1977). However, a causal role for lack of dietary fiber in disorders of the large bowel and other diseases remains to be established (see Goldstein, 1972; Cummings, 1973; Painter and Burkitt, 1975; Mendeloff, 1977).

Because of their ability to absorb water and to provide an emollient intestinal mass, the bulk-forming laxatives have some usefulness for the symptomatic relief of *acute diarrhea* and to modify the effluent in patients with an *ileostomy* or *colostomy*. However, loss of sodium, potassium, and water may be increased in such patients. The alleged effectiveness of the bulk-forming agents as appetite suppressants in the management of *obesity* has *not* been established.

Adverse Effects. The bulk-forming laxatives have minimal systemic effects. However, possible alterations of glucose tolerance and calcium metabolism are still incompletely defined. Allergic reactions have been reported for several of the natural products.

Flatulence may also occur, particularly if the dosage of dietary fiber or bulk-forming agent is increased abruptly; it can sometimes be relieved by adjusting the dosage, switching to a different preparation or different source of fiber, or increasing the fluid intake. The bulk-forming agents potentially adsorb other drugs administered concurrently, thereby interfering with their intestinal absorption, but solid evidence is lacking.

Intestinal obstruction has been reported after administration of the bulk-forming agents, and *impaction* may result when there is gross intestinal pathology. These agents should not be employed in individuals with intestinal ulceration, stenosis, or adhesions. Occasional cases of *esophageal obstruction* have also occurred when these agents have been swallowed dry or when the tablets were chewed. *Patients who have difficulty swallowing should be warned not to take these preparations dry, and generous amounts of water should be prescribed with all bulk-forming laxatives.*

Bran and Other Dietary Fiber. Bran, a by-product of the milling of wheat, contains more than 40%

dietary fiber and is the most convenient source of intestinal bulk. Crude bran is rather unpalatable, but the processed form makes a pleasant cereal or may be taken in the form of cookies and muffins. Bran-rich cereals contain 25% dietary fiber.

A helpful guide to the fiber content of foods has been provided by Burkitt and Meisner (1979). For prevention of constipation, they recommend substitution of wholemeal bread for white bread and sufficient bran or breakfast cereal to provide 6 to 10 g of dietary fiber daily.

Psyllium (Plantago) Preparations. *Plantago Seed*, U.S.P., is obtained from various species of plantain. The seeds contain a large amount of natural mucilage and form a gelatinous mass on contact with water. However, the whole seeds have now been largely replaced by powdered preparations of the mucilaginous component. Typical preparations are *plantago ovata coating* (KONSYL) and *psyllium hydrophilic mucilloid* (METAMUCIL, L.A. FORMULA). The latter preparation also contains dextrose as a dispersing agent and provides 14 kcal per 7-g dose. The usual dose of these preparations is 4 to 10 g, one to three times daily, stirred in a glassful of water or other liquid.

Chronic administration of the psyllium preparations may produce modest reduction of plasma cholesterol concentration, apparently by interference with reabsorption of bile acids. Sensitization, with asthmatic symptoms upon inhalation of psyllium powder, has been reported in atopic individuals chronically exposed to the powder during its manufacture.

Methylcellulose and Carboxymethylcellulose Sodium. *Methylcellulose*, U.S.P., and *Carboxymethylcellulose Sodium*, U.S.P., are hydrophilic semisynthetic cellulose derivatives. They are marketed under many trade names. Methylcellulose has the following structure:

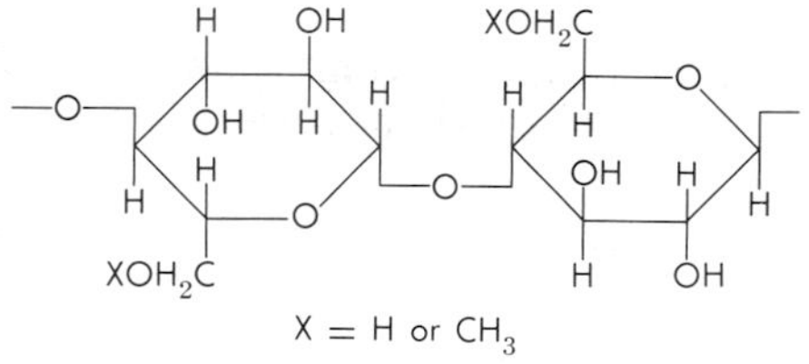

X = H or CH$_3$

Methylcellulose

Methylcellulose and carboxymethylcellulose sodium have similar laxative properties. Methylcellulose is available as official tablets (500 mg) and oral solution (450 mg/5 ml) and also as a syrup (985 mg/5 ml) and powder; carboxymethylcellulose sodium is available largely in combination with other laxatives and as a powder. The usual adult dose is 1 to 6 g daily, in divided dosage. During chronic medication, smaller doses may be satisfactory. The dosage for children is 500 mg, two or three times daily. Both preparations should be taken with ample water.

Other Bulk-Forming Agents. Other hydrophilic substances that differ little from those described include *Polycarbophil*, U.S.P., and *powdered karaya* (*sterculia*) *gum. Allergic reactions,* characterized by urticaria, rhinitis, dermatitis, and asthma, have been attributed to the latter preparation. Daily adult dosage for these preparations is 4 to 6 g and 5 to 10 g, respectively.

SALINE CATHARTICS

The saline cathartics include various magnesium salts and several sulfates and phosphates. These salts are often employed in full dosage when prompt, thorough evacuation of the bowel is desired, as prior to certain diagnostic procedures. They are also used in lower dosage for a laxative effect, but frequent administration should be avoided. Since they have many common characteristics, the saline cathartics are conveniently considered as a group. The distinctive features of the individual drugs are mainly palatability, cost, and risk of untoward systemic effects.

Laxative-Cathartic Effects. Full doses of the saline cathartics (15 g of magnesium sulfate or its equivalent) produce a semifluid or watery evacuation in 3 hours or less. Low doses produce a laxative effect with greater latency. The saline cathartics are incompletely absorbed from the digestive tract and retain water in the intestinal lumen by their osmotic properties. Intestinal transit is increased indirectly. However, since magnesium salts cause the secretion of cholecystokinin from the duodenal mucosa, Harvey and Read (1975) have suggested that cholecystokinin-mediated pancreatic secretion and increased secretion and motility of the small intestine and colon may contribute to the cathartic effect.

Systemic Effects. Some absorption of the component ions of the saline cathartics does occur, and in certain instances they may produce systemic toxicity. In an individual with impaired renal function, the accumulation of magnesium ions in the body fluids may be sufficient to cause intoxication (*see* Chapter 35). Magnesium cathartics should thus be administered only if renal function is adequate. Similarly, sodium salts may be contraindicated in patients with congestive heart failure, and phosphate salts may reduce the concentration of ionized calcium in plasma.

The luminal contents of the intestinal tract remain essentially isosmotic. Consequently, hypertonic solutions of the saline cathartics can produce significant dehydration. For this reason, the saline salts should be administered with sufficient water by mouth to ensure that no net loss of body water occurs.

Magnesium Salts. *Magnesium Sulfate*, U.S.P. (*Epsom salt*), is one of the traditional saline cathartics. The official dose is 15 g, but 5 g (about 40 mEq of magnesium ion) or less produces a significant laxative effect when the salt is administered in dilute solution to a fasting individual. The intensely bitter taste may be partially masked by taking the salt in lemon juice.

Milk of Magnesia, U.S.P., is a 7.0 to 8.5% aqueous suspension of magnesium hydroxide. The usual adult dose is 15 to 30 ml (about 40 to 80 mEq of magnesium ion); the dose for children is 0.5 ml/kg. *Magnesium Hydroxide*, U.S.P., is also available as tablets. The usual dose is 2 to 4 g (80 to 160 mEq). Other magnesium salts commonly employed as gastric antacids have similar laxative properties (*see also* Chapter 42).

Magnesium Citrate Oral Solution, U.S.P., is a pleasant-tasting, but expensive, saline cathartic. It is a flavored, effervescent solution that provides the equivalent of 3 to 4 g of magnesium hydroxide in the official 200-ml dose.

Sodium Phosphates. Phosphate salts are relatively pleasant-tasting saline cathartics. The most frequently employed preparation is *Sodium Phosphates Oral Solution*, U.S.P. Each 10 ml contains 1.8 g of sodium phosphate and 4.8 g of sodium biphosphate. The official dose is 10 to 20 ml, taken diluted and with ample additional water. *Sodium Phosphates Enema*, U.S.P., is employed for rectal administration. The official 120-ml dose contains 7.2 g and 19.2 g of the two salts, respectively. Sodium phosphate is also available as citrate-flavored sodium phosphate solution. The usual 10-ml dose provides 7.5 g of sodium phosphate.

Other Saline Cathartics. *Sodium Sulfate*, U.S.P. (*Glauber's salt*), is one of the cheapest saline cathartics, but it is the most objectionable as far as taste is concerned. The usual dose is 15 g. *Potassium Sodium Tartrate*, U.S.P. (*Rochelle salt*), *Effervescent Sodium Phosphate*, U.S.P., and other saline cathartics that contain tartrates are pleasant-tasting agents. However, there is insufficient evidence to establish safe and effective dosage for the tartrates (FDA, 1975).

A large number of proprietary saline cathartic preparations are available. They range from expensive natural mineral waters, for which extravagant claims are made, to salts that differ little from those described above.

CONTACT CATHARTICS

The contact cathartics are agents that act on the intestinal mucosa and have effects both on the net absorption of electrolytes and water and on motility. Included in this group are the *diphenylmethane* derivatives, the *anthraquinones, castor oil,* the *docusates* (dioctyl sulfosuccinates), and the *bile acids.* Despite similarity of their mechanism of action, the clinical uses and limitations of these agents are sufficiently varied to require separate description. These differences depend largely upon dosage and whether the drug acts primarily upon the small intestine or colon. The contact cathartics are the agents commonly involved in cathartic abuse. These agents have been reviewed by Travell in a symposium (1954).

Mechanism of Laxative-Cathartic Effects. The effects of the contact cathartics on intestinal fluxes of electrolytes and water are readily demonstrated *in vitro* and *in situ* under conditions in which effects secondary to motility are excluded. Concentrations of the contact cathartics that reduce net absorption of electrolytes and water also increase the permeability of the mucosa. The latter effect may result from increased permeability of the normally tight intercellular junctions and/or patchy damage to the mucosal surface (*see* Rummel *et al.,* 1975; Gaginella *et al.,* 1977; Gullikson *et al.,* 1977; Saunders *et al.,* 1977). Whatever the specific mechanism, the increased mucosal permeability is at least partially reversible and can explain the alterations of the absorption of electrolytes and water. Net movement of electrolytes and water across the mucosa is determined in part by passive back diffusion to the lumen down a hydrostatic gradient. If permeability is increased, back diffusion is increased, and net absorption is reduced or may even be converted to net accumulation of fluid in the lumen. However, since the contact cathartics also release prostaglandins and cause an increase in the mucosal concentration of cyclic adenosine 3'5'-monophosphate (cyclic AMP), increased secretion of electrolytes, as occurs in diarrhea induced by cholera toxin, may contribute to the total cathartic effect. The inhibition of Na^+,K^+-activated adenosine triphosphatase (ATPase) observed *in vitro* appears to be of doubtful significance (Wanitschke *et al.,* 1977).

The diphenylmethane and anthraquinone cathartics are contact agents that act primarily on the large bowel. They increase transit of the colonic contents by causing a coordinated increase in the frequency of periodic mass movements and a decrease in segmenting activity that impedes transit (*see* Hardcastle and Wilkins, 1970; Ritchie, 1972; Symposium, 1975; Waller, 1975). Since the motor effects that follow the direct application of these agents to the mucosa are inhibited by prior topical administration of a local anesthetic, they are thought to reflect stimulation of the submucosal or myenteric plexus, but additional

evidence is needed to support this view. More importantly, the relative contributions of primary effects on motility and those secondary to reduced absorption of electrolytes and water remain uncertain. Castor oil is a contact cathartic that acts on the small intestine. The effects of ricinoleic acid, its active metabolite, on motility of the small intestine are poorly defined, but they too appear to involve inhibitory as well as excitatory effects. The interesting suggestion by Stewart and Bass (1976) that they are mediated by cholecystokinin requires experimental verification.

Structure-activity relationship among the contact cathartics has been summarized by Loewe (1948), Hubacher and Doernberg (1964), and Fairbairn and Moss (1970).

DIPHENYLMETHANE CATHARTICS

The primary diphenylmethane cathartics are *phenolphthalein* and *bisacodyl.* These agents have similar pharmacological characteristics and clinical uses. Bisacodyl is available for rectal as well as oral administration.

Laxative-Cathartic Effects. Individual effective doses of the diphenylmethane derivatives vary as much as fourfold to eightfold. Consequently, recommended doses that promote a laxative effect in the majority of patients can be expected to be relatively ineffective in some patients and to produce griping and excessively fluid evacuation in others. Since the diphenylmethane derivatives act primarily on the colon, laxative effects are not usually produced in less than 6 hours. They are frequently taken at bedtime to produce their effect the next morning.

Absorption and Excretion. As much as 15% of a therapeutic dose of phenolphthalein is absorbed and eliminated by the kidney, most of it in conjugated form. The urine becomes pink or red if it is sufficiently alkaline. Some absorbed drug is also excreted in the bile, and the resulting enterohepatic cycle may contribute to prolongation of the cathartic effect.

Bisacodyl is rapidly converted by intestinal and bacterial enzymes to its active desacetyl metabolite. As much as 5% of an orally administered dose is absorbed and excreted in the urine as the glucuronide. This inactive metabolite is also excreted in the bile and may be hydrolyzed to active drug in the colon.

Adverse Effects. The major danger of overdosage of the diphenylmethane derivatives is fluid and electrolyte deficits resulting from excessive cathartic effect. However, allergic reactions, including fixed-drug eruption, Stevens-Johnson syndrome, and a syndrome that resembles lupus erythematosus, have been reported to follow the use of *phenolphthalein.*

Phenolphthalein. The cathartic effect of phenolphthalein was discovered in 1902 by Vamossy, during a study undertaken for the Hungarian government to determine its safety as an additive for identification of artificial wines. It has since been widely employed as a cathartic. The structural formula of phenolphthalein is as follows:

Phenolphthalein

Phenolphthalein, U.S.P., is available as tablets and in numerous proprietary preparations. The usual dose is 60 mg for adults and 15 to 30 mg for children. Phenolphthalein usually acts in 6 to 8 hours. The patient should be warned of possible pink coloring of the urine and feces.

Bisacodyl. Bisacodyl, 4,4′-(2-pyridylmethylene) diphenol diacetate, was introduced as a clinical cathartic in 1953 on the basis of structure-activity studies of compounds related to phenolphthalein. Bisacodyl has the following structural formula:

Bisacodyl

Bisacodyl, U.S.P. (DULCOLAX), is available as 5-mg enteric-coated tablets for oral administration and as 10-mg suppositories and in solution (10 mg/30 ml) for rectal administration. It is also supplied in kits, with other agents, for evacuation of the bowel prior to diagnostic procedures or surgery.

The usual *oral dosage* is 10 to 15 mg for adults and 5 to 10 mg for children (0.3 mg/kg). To avoid gastric irritation, tablets should be swallowed without chewing or crushing and should not be taken within 1 hour of antacid medication. One or two soft, formed stools are usually produced within 6 to 12 hours. Recommended *rectal dosage* is 10 mg for adults and for children over 2 years, and 5 mg for children under 2 years. After rectal administration, the drug usually acts in 15 to 60 minutes. Bisacodyl suppositories may produce a burning sensation in the rectum; mild proctitis has been reported after use of the suppositories for several weeks.

Isatin Derivatives. *Oxyphenisatin acetate* is a cathartic with pharmacological properties similar to those of bisacodyl. However, oxyphenisatin acetate, particularly when administered with the docusates, has been incriminated as a cause of hepatic injury (*see* Goldstein *et al.,* 1973) and has been withdrawn from the market in many countries.

The interesting claim that an isatin derivative is the active cathartic constituent of prunes has been challenged (*see* Hubacher and Doernberg, 1964).

ANTHRAQUINONE CATHARTICS

The anthraquinone cathartics are also known as the anthracene or emodin cathartics. The principal agents in this group are *senna, cascara sagrada,* and *danthron.* Their clinical uses and limitations are similar to those of the diphenylmethane derivatives.

Laxative-Cathartic Effects. The major active constituents of the anthraquinone cathartics are anthraquinone or anthrone derivatives related to 1,8-dihydroxyanthraquinone. The effects of the individual cathartics vary, depending upon their anthraquinone content and the ease of liberation of the active constituents from their inactive precursor glycosides by the intestinal microflora. In addition, the galenical preparations often employed may contain other active ingredients. The cathartic effect of the anthraquinone cathartics is limited mainly to the large intestine. Consequently, they are seldom effective before 6 hours after oral administration.

Adverse Effects. Untoward results of the administration of the anthraquinone cathartics are mainly excessive cathartic effects. Despite suggestions to the contrary, it is unlikely that the active anthraquinone derivatives appear in the milk during lactation in sufficient amount to affect the nursing infant. Certain constituents of the drugs are also excreted by the kidney and may color the urine; patients should be informed of this possibility. A melanotic pigmentation of the colonic mucosa (*melanosis coli*) has been observed in individuals who have taken anthraquinone cathartics over extended periods of time. The pigmentation is benign and is usually reversible within 4 to 12 months after medication is discontinued. Its presence may help confirm a suspicion of cathartic abuse.

Senna. Senna is obtained from the dried leaflets or pods of *Cassia acutifolia* or *Cassia angustifolia.* It was introduced into Arabian medicine as early as the ninth century A.D. The official (U.S.P.) preparations of senna leaf—*Senna, Senna Fluidextract,* and *Senna Syrup*—usually produce a single, thorough bowel evacuation within 6 hours, but with considerable griping. Other preparations are usually preferred. *Concentrates of senna pods,* standardized by chemical or biological assay, are more stable and more reliable than the preparations of senna leaf, and they are alleged to cause less cramping and griping than does crude senna. Preparations of senna pods are available as granules, syrup, oral solution, suppositories, and tablets. The dosage is as labeled. Purified senna glycosides, *Sennosides A and B,* U.S.P. (GLYSENNID), are available as 12-mg tablets; the adult dose is 12 to 24 mg.

Cascara Sagrada. *Cascara Sagrada,* U.S.P. (*sacred bark*), is obtained from the bark of the buckthorn tree, *Rhamnus purshiana.* It was used as a cathartic by the Indians of California. The most commonly employed official preparation is *Aromatic Cascara Fluidextract.* The conventional 5-ml dose usually causes a single soft or semifluid evacuation of the bowel in approximately 8 hours. Other official (U.S.P.) preparations are not recommended. *Cascara Sagrada Fluidextract* is very bitter; *Cascara Sagrada Extract* and *Cascara Tablets* are less reliable. Proprietary preparations of the cascara sagrada glycosides (*casanthranol*) are also available. The adult dose is 30 mg.

Danthron. *Danthron*, U.S.P. (DORBANE), is 1,8-dihydroxyanthraquinone. Its structural formula is as follows:

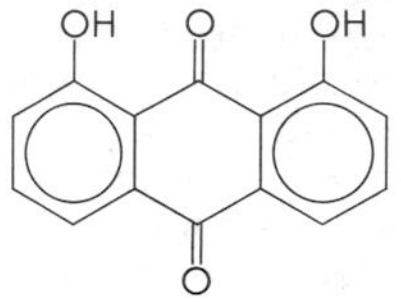

Danthron

Although danthron is a free anthraquinone rather than a glycoside, its pharmacological properties, uses, and limitations are similar to those of the anthraquinone glycosides. Danthron is available as 37.5- and 75-mg tablets and in solution (37.5 mg/5 ml). The usual adult dose of 75 to 150 mg produces a soft or semifluid stool in 6 to 8 hours.

Other Anthraquinone Cathartics. Proprietary preparations contain anthraquinone derivatives from a number of other plant sources. None is superior to the preparations described; most should be abandoned (*see* FDA, 1975).

CASTOR OIL

Castor oil, obtained from the seeds of *Ricinus communis,* is composed primarily of the triglyceride of ricinoleic acid. The cathartic effects of the seeds were known to the ancient Egyptians. Castor oil acts upon the small intestine. For this reason, it is usually prescribed only when prompt, thorough evacuation of the bowel is desired, as in preparation for certain radiological examinations. Chronic use is not recommended, since absorption of nutrients may be reduced.

Metabolism. Castor oil itself is a bland oil and is employed locally on the skin for its emollient properties. However, it is hydrolyzed in the intestine by pancreatic lipases to glycerol and ricinoleic acid. The latter substance is an unsaturated hydroxy fatty acid; like other anionic surfactants, it reduces net intestinal absorption of electrolytes and water and increases intestinal transit. A portion of the ricinoleic acid is absorbed and is metabolized much like other fatty acids.

Preparations and Dosage. Castor oil is usually administered on an empty stomach, and as little as 4 ml may produce a laxative effect in the fasting adult. However, the usual dose for a cathartic effect is 15 to 60 ml for adults, 5 to 15 ml for children over 2 years of age, and 1 to 5 ml for younger children. Full doses of castor oil cause the evacuation of one or two copious, semifluid stools within 2 to 6 hours.

Official preparations are *Castor Oil,* U.S.P., and *Aromatic Castor Oil,* U.S.P. Although the objectionable taste of the oil is partially masked in the latter preparation, flavored *castor oil emulsions* are somewhat more palatable. Castor oil is also available as official capsules in sizes (0.6 and 2.5 ml) suitable for pediatric dosage.

DOCUSATES (DIOCTYL SULFOSUCCINATES)

Docusate sodium, the prototype for this group of anionic surfactants, is widely employed in the pharmaceutical industry as an emulsifying agent and as a wetting and dispersing agent in formulations for external application. It has the following structural formula:

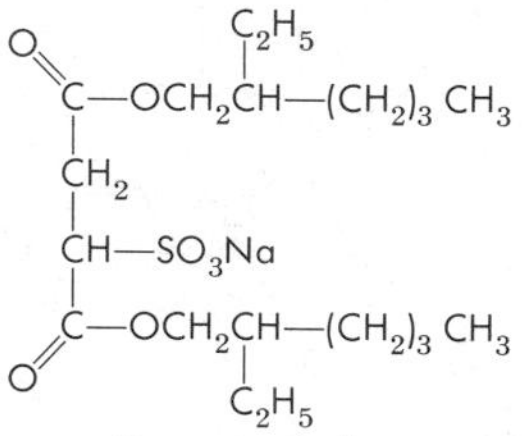

Docusate Sodium

In recommended dosage, the docusates have minimal laxative effects; their clinical usefulness is limited to situations in which it is desired that the feces be kept soft and that straining at the stool be avoided. Many details of their pharmacology remain uncertain.

Laxative Effects. In recommended oral dosage, the docusates produce minimal softening of the feces with a latency of 1 to 3 days. Hydration of the stool has been attributed to their surfactant effect on the *intestinal contents,* which was assumed to facilitate penetration of the fecal mass by water and fats. However, *in vitro* and *in situ,* docusate sodium alters net intestinal absorption of electrolytes and water and has other effects on the *intestinal mucosa* similar to those described for ricinoleic acid and other contact cathartics (*see* Binder, 1977; Gullikson *et al.,* 1977).

Adverse Effects. Recommended oral doses of the docusates are well tolerated. Cramping pains have been reported occasionally, and the liquid preparations sometimes cause nausea. Nevertheless, the safety of the docusates has been questioned because they increase the intestinal absorption and/or hepatic uptake of other drugs administered concurrently and may increase their toxicity. Of particular concern are the observations that docusate sodium is absorbed, appears in the bile in significant concentration, has cytotoxic effects on liver cells in tissue culture, and may contribute to the hepatotoxicity of oxyphenisatin and danthron (Dujovne and Shoeman, 1972; Goldstein *et al.,* 1973; Tolman *et al.,* 1976). Although the evidence is insufficient to warrant restriction of the use of the docusates, periodic reevaluation is indicated (FDA, 1975).

Preparations and Dosage. *Docusate Sodium,* U.S.P. (*dioctyl sodium sulfosuccinate;* COLACE, DOXINATE), *Docusate Calcium,* U.S.P. (*dioctyl calcium sulfosuccinate;* SURFAK), and *docusate potassium* (*dioctyl potassium sulfosuccinate;* KASOF) are available as capsules and tablets of various sizes. Docusate sodium is also available in solution (10 and 50 mg/ml) and as a syrup (20 mg/5 ml). The three salts have not been compared carefully but are presumed to have similar pharmacological properties, clinical uses, and limitations.

The usual *oral* dose for adults is 50 to 250 mg daily, as a single or divided dose; for children, 1.25 mg/kg, four times daily. The solutions should be administered in milk or fruit juice to mask the bitter taste. The usual *rectal* dose is 50 to 100 mg, as a 0.1% solution.

Mixtures of a docusate with mineral oil are contraindicated, since the surfactant may enhance absorption of the oil. Mixtures with other contact cathartics are also available but cannot be recommended until they have been demonstrated to provide clinical advantages over the other agent given alone.

BILE ACIDS

Bile acids reduce net absorption of electrolytes and water and have other effects on the intestine similar to those of the other anionic surfactants. They cause diarrhea if they escape absorption in the terminal ileum; in addition, diarrhea occurs in most patients when cholic acid or chenodiol (chenodeoxycholic acid; chenic acid) is employed for dissolution of gallstones in doses that exceed 1.5 g daily. Nevertheless, there is insufficient evidence of efficacy and safety to recommend use of the *natural bile* acids as laxatives (FDA, 1975). However, *Dehydrocholic Acid* U.S.P., is considered effective and safe for adults at a dosage of 750 mg to 1.5 g daily (*see also* Chapter 42).

OTHER LAXATIVES AND CATHARTICS

MINERAL OIL

Mineral oil is a mixture of liquid hydrocarbons obtained from petroleum. The oil is indigestible and absorbed only to a limited extent. It penetrates and softens the stool; it may also interfere with absorption of water.

Mineral oil can cause a variety of untoward effects, and its use as a laxative requires appreciation of its potential hazards (*see* Becker, 1952). Habitual use of mineral oil must be avoided.

Adverse Effects. Mineral oil acts as a lipid solvent; administered with meals, it may interfere with the *absorption of essential fat-soluble substances.* The regular ingestion of mineral oil during pregnancy may reduce absorption of vitamin K and produce hypoprothrombinemia.

Mineral oil is *absorbed* to a limited extent from the intestinal tract, and it elicits a typical foreign-body reaction in the intestinal mucosa, mesenteric lymph nodes, liver, and spleen. Although no physiological disturbances have been related to the presence of the oil at these sites, it must be questioned whether the substance can be used safely over long periods of time.

If it gains access to the lungs, mineral oil produces *lipid pneumonitis.* Although more frequently observed when the oil was used as a vehicle for application of drugs to the nasal mucous membranes, lipid pneumonitis can also occur following the *oral ingestion* of the oil, particularly if it is taken at bedtime. The indiscriminate use of mineral oil by elderly, debilitated, or dysphagic individuals should be discouraged.

Leakage of the oil past the anal sphincter is an annoying side effect and an occasional cause of pruritus ani. It is also claimed that the oil interferes with the healing of postoperative wounds in the anorectal region and that continuous presence of the oil in the rectum disturbs normal defecatory reflexes.

Preparations and Dosage. *Mineral Oil,* U.S.P. (*liquid petrolatum*), is available in numerous preparations, often under various trade names. The dose is 15 to 45 ml, usually taken at night before retiring.

Mineral oil is somewhat more palatable if it is taken with fruit juice or as *Mineral Oil Emulsion,* U.S.P. Stable emulsions of the oil penetrate and soften the stool more effectively than does the non-emulsified oil, and they cause less difficulty with leakage of the oil through the anal sphincter. However, emulsification enhances absorption of the oil. Mineral oil is also available for rectal administration as *mineral oil enema.*

LACTULOSE

Lactulose is a semisynthetic disaccharide (4-O-β-D-galactopyranosyl-D-fructofuranose) that is not hydrolyzed by intestinal enzymes. In the United States, it is available only by prescription and is approved for management of portal-systemic encephalopathy in patients with chronic liver disease; it is also employed for its laxative effects. Lactulose has the following structure:

Lactulose

The pharmacological properties of lactulose have been reviewed by Avery and co-workers (1972).

Laxative Effects. Since lactulose is not hydrolyzed in the small intestine, it is not absorbed, and water and electrolytes are retained in the lumen because of the osmotic activity of the disaccharide. The osmotic effect is augmented in the distal ileum and colon, where the unabsorbed disaccharide is metabolized by the intestinal microflora to lactate and other organic acids, which are only partially absorbed. Whether the concomitant reduction in luminal pH has additional effects on intestinal transport of electrolytes or motility has not been clarified.

Efficacy in Portal-Systemic Encephalopathy. In adequate dosage, lactulose provides symptomatic improvement and some normalization of the EEG in about three fourths of patients with portal-systemic encephalopathy associated with chronic liver disease. Concentrations of ammonia in blood are reduced by 25 to 50%; favorable effects are observed in 1 to 7 days after initiation of therapy. Chronic medication reduces recurrences and may permit liberalization of protein intake. Lactulose is more effective than sorbitol in equivalent laxative dosage, and equal or somewhat more effective than the concurrent administration of sorbitol and neomycin. Neomycin acts more promptly than does lactulose and may be favored in acute episodes. Despite theoretical antagonism, combined therapy with lactulose and neomycin has been effective in some patients who failed to respond to either drug alone. However, dosage schedules for such therapy have not yet been established (see Avery et al., 1972; Conn et al., 1977).

The beneficial effects of lactulose are related to bacterial metabolism of the disaccharide and reduction in fecal pH. The more important factors appear to be reduced production and increased utilization of ammonia by the intestinal microflora. Increased fecal excretion of ammonia, the laxative effect, and reduction in ammonia-producing bacteria in the stool, if it occurs, may contribute to the total effect of the drug (see Avery et al., 1972; Conn, 1978).

Adverse Effects. Lactulose may cause flatulence, cramps, and abdominal discomfort, especially when therapy is initiated; these symptoms occur in about 20% of patients receiving full doses of the drug. Nausea and vomiting have also been reported, particularly with higher dosage. Excessive dosage can cause diarrhea, loss of fluid and potassium, and exacerbation of encephalopathy.

Preparations and Dosage. *Lactulose* (CEPHULAC, DUPHALAC) is available as a syrup; each 15 ml contains 10 g of lactulose and not more than 2.2 g of galactose, 1.2 g of lactose, or 1.2 g of other sugars. The sweet taste is considered unpalatable by some patients but can be masked by mixing the syrup with fruit juice or other foods. The drug should be taken with ample water. Since the syrup also contains other sugars, it is contraindicated in patients who require a galactose-free diet, and it must be administered with care to diabetic patients.

For management of *chronic portal-systemic encephalopathy,* the usual maintenance dose is 20 to 30 g (30 to 45 ml), three or four times daily, adjusted to produce two or three soft stools daily and an acidic fecal pH. Acidification of the stool (pH 5 to 5.5) is essential, and excessive diarrhea must be avoided. Other laxatives should not be employed concurrently in order to avoid inadequate acidification of the stool. Additional aspects of the management of the underlying hepatic disease must, of course, not be neglected. Therapy may be initiated with 20 to 30 g of lactulose at hourly intervals until the desired effect upon the stools is attained.

The daily maintenance dose for a *laxative effect* for management of constipation has varied widely but may be as low as 7 to 10 g (10 to 15 ml), as a single dose or divided. Larger doses (up to 30 g) are sometimes required initially, and the full effect of lactulose may not be attained for several days or longer.

USES AND ABUSES OF LAXATIVES AND CATHARTICS

Laxatives and cathartics have no role in the management of constipation associated with intestinal pathology, and they are of only secondary importance to a fiber-rich diet and other nonpharmacological measures for the prevention and treatment of functional constipation. Other valid uses include maintenance of soft feces, to prevent straining at the stool or in patients with anorectal disorders, and evacuation of the bowel prior to diagnostic procedures or surgery. *All laxatives and cathartics are contraindicated in a patient with cramps, colic, nausea, vomiting,*

*or other symptoms of appendicitis or any un-
diagnosed abdominal pain.*

Constipation. Many of the causes of functional
constipation are simple to correct, once recognized,
and therapy is first attempted without the use of
drugs. A fiber-rich diet, the establishment of a proper
"habit time," the reminder that "haste does not make
waste," adequate fluid intake, appropriate physical
activity, reassurance to overcome emotional factors,
and similar measures are often successful. Correction
of underlying disease should not be neglected. In
cases of drug-induced constipation, such as that
produced by chronic therapy with antimuscarinic
agents or certain antihypertensive agents, correction
by readjustment of drug dosage or by use of alternative drugs should be attempted before resorting to
concurrent laxative medication.

If nonpharmacological measures alone are inadequate, they may be supplemented by use of the
bulk-forming agents. The docusates or mineral oil
may sometimes be helpful but are often ineffective.
Laxative doses of the contact cathartics may be necessary in the more refractory cases. When laxatives
are employed in the treatment of constipation, they
should be administered in the lowest effective dosage, as infrequently as possible, and medication
should be discontinued promptly and completely
upon termination of the need.

Principles of the management of constipation and
the use of laxatives and cathartics have been summarized in a symposium (1954), by Erle (1976), and
by Burkitt and Meisner (1979).

Other Valid Uses. The use of laxatives is justified
to prevent straining at the stool by patients with
hernia or *cardiovascular disease.* In addition, they are
frequently indicated, both before and after surgery,
to maintain soft feces in patients with *hemorrhoids
and other anorectal disorders.* Most laxatives have
been recommended for these purposes, but dietary
fiber or the bulk-forming agents are generally satisfactory and should be preferred. A fiber-rich diet
and related drugs also have an established role in the
management of *diverticular disease* of the colon and
irritable bowel disease.

Cathartics are frequently employed prior to *radiological examination* of the gastrointestinal tract or
other abdominal structures and prior to *elective
bowel surgery.* The contact cathartics or full doses of
the saline cathartics are usually employed. Contact
cathartics, either orally or rectally, may also be used
instead of enemas for emptying the large bowel prior
to *proctological examination.*

In cases of *drug and food poisoning,* full doses of
the saline cathartics are sometimes administered
after gavage to flush the offending substance from
the intestinal tract. Sodium sulfate is safer than
magnesium sulfate if the toxic substance causes central nervous system depression, and especially if
renal function is impaired. Cathartics are also sometimes employed with certain *anthelmintics* (*see*
Chapter 44).

The Cathartic Habit. The occasional taking of a
laxative, even for an ill-advised reason, can hardly

be considered harmful. However, the continued use
of these drugs is to be deplored. Many individuals
have unusual notions regarding the frequency,
quantity, and consistency of stools necessary for
health, and they readily resort to self-prescribed
cathartic medication to achieve these goals. More
importantly, even the casual use of these drugs can
develop into the cathartic habit. After a thorough
evacuation of the colon by a cathartic, several days
may elapse before a normal bowel movement can
again occur. Nevertheless, in the interim, the patient
becomes convinced that he is constipated, and he
again turns to his favorite remedy. After a time, his
bowel habits become so abnormal that he comes to
rely entirely on a daily dose of cathartic for a bowel
movement.

The patient suffering from the cathartic habit
presents a difficult therapeutic problem. Initially, all
cathartic medication should be discontinued, and the
patient should be informed not to expect a bowel
movement for several days. The underlying cause for
constipation, if one exists, must be found and eliminated, and the patient's misconceptions pertaining to
bowel function must be corrected. If necessary, a
contact cathartic in minimally effective dosage may
be employed during the period in which reestablishment of normal colonic function and defecatory
reflexes is being attempted. Unfortunately, many
individuals suffering from the cathartic habit often
promptly return to the use of cathartics, despite the
full remedial efforts of the physician.

Dangers of Cathartic Abuse. In addition to perpetuating dependence upon drugs, the cathartic
habit may provide the basis for serious *gastrointestinal disturbances.* Spastic colitis and other functional
ills have been traced to the habitual use of the contact cathartics; after prolonged abuse, the appearance of the digestive tract by x-ray examination may
resemble that of enterocolitis. Surreptitious ingestion
of cathartics can cause signs and symptoms that are
mistaken for gastrointestinal disease and lead to
unnecessary surgery.

Repeated misuse of the contact cathartics may also
result in excessive *fecal loss of water and electrolytes.*
Hypokalemia, sodium depletion, and dehydration
have been reported most frequently, and secondary
aldosteronism may occur if volume depletion is
prominent. Steatorrhea and protein-losing gastro-
enteropathy with hypoalbuminemia have been observed, as has excessive excretion of calcium in the
stools and osteomalacia of the vertebral column.

Much more dangerous than the cathartic habit is
the practice of taking a cathartic for the relief of
abdominal pain. An inflamed appendix can be ruptured by the resulting intestinal motor activity, and
patients who take purgatives subsequent to the onset
of symptoms of acute appendicitis have a mortality
rate manyfold higher than the rate for those who do
not receive cathartics.

The dangers of cathartic abuse have been reviewed by Cummings (1974) and Cooke (1977).

Avery, G. S.; Davies, E. F.; and Brogden, R. N. Lactulose:
a review of its therapeutic and pharmacological properties with particular reference to ammonia metabolism

and its mode of action in portal systemic encephalopathy. *Drugs,* **1972,** *4,* 7–48.

Becker, G. L. The case against mineral oil. *Am. J. Dig. Dis.,* **1952,** *19,* 344–348.

Brodribb, A. J. M. Treatment of symptomatic diverticular disease with a high-fibre diet. *Lancet,* **1977,** *1,* 664–666.

Burkitt, D. P., and Meisner, P. How to manage constipation with high-fiber diet. *Geriatrics,* **1979,** *34,* No. 2, 33–40.

Conn, H. O. Lactulose: a drug in search of a modus operandi. *Gastroenterology,* **1978,** *74,* 624–626.

Conn, H. O.; Leevy, C. M.; Vlahcevic, Z. R.; Rodgers, J. B.; Maddrey, W. C.; Seeff, L.; and Levy, L. L. Comparison of lactulose and neomycin in the treatment of chronic portal-systemic encephalopathy. *Gastroenterology,* **1977,** *72,* 573–583.

Dujovne, C. A., and Shoeman, L. W. Toxicity of a hepatic laxative preparation in tissue culture and excretion in bile in man. *Clin. Pharmacol. Ther.,* **1972,** *13,* 602–608.

Fairbairn, J. W., and Moss, M. J. R. The relative purgative activities of 1,8-dihydroxyanthracene derivatives. *J. Pharm. Pharmacol.,* **1970,** *22,* 584–593.

Gaginella, T. S.; Chadwick, V. S.; Debongnie, J. C.; Lewis, J. C.; and Phillips, S. F. Perfusion of rabbit colon with ricinoleic acid: dose-related mucosal injury, fluid secretion, and increased permeability. *Gastroenterology,* **1977,** *73,* 95–101.

Gaginella, T. S., and Phillips, S. F. Ricinoleic acid: current view of an ancient oil. *Am. J. Dig. Dis.,* **1975,** *20,* 1171–1177.

Goldstein, F. Diet and colonic disease. *J. Am. Diet. Assoc.,* **1972,** *60,* 499–503.

Goldstein, G. B.; Lam, K. C.; and Mistilis, S. P. Drug-induced active chronic hepatitis. *Am. J. Dig. Dis.,* **1973,** *18,* 177–184.

Gullikson, G. W.; Cline, W. S.; Lorenzsonn, V.; Benz, L.; Olsen, W. A.; and Bass, P. Effects of anionic surfactants on hamster small intestinal membrane structure and function: relationship to surface activity. *Gastroenterology,* **1977,** *73,* 501–511.

Hardcastle, J. D., and Wilkins, J. L. The action of sennosides and related compounds on human colon and rectum. *Gut,* **1970,** *11,* 1038–1042.

Harvey, R. F., and Read, A. E. Mode of action of the saline purgatives. *Am. Heart J.,* **1975,** *89,* 810–812.

Hubacher, M. H., and Doernberg, S. Laxatives. II. Relationship between structure and potency. *J. Pharm. Sci.,* **1964,** *53,* 1067–1072.

Loewe, S. Studies on the laxative activity of triphenylmethane derivatives. I. Relationship between structure and activity of phenolphthalein congeners. *J. Pharmacol. Exp. Ther.,* **1948,** *94,* 288–298.

Mendeloff, A. I. Dietary fiber and human health. *N. Engl. J. Med.,* **1977,** *297,* 811–814.

Painter, N. S., and Burkitt, D. P. Diverticular disease of the colon, a 20th century problem. *Clin. Gastroenterol.,* **1975,** *4,* 3–21.

Parks, T. G. Diverticular disease. *Proc. R. Soc. Med.,* **1974,** *67,* 29–32.

Ritchie, J. Mass peristalsis in the human colon after contact with oxyphenisatin. *Gut,* **1972,** *13,* 211–219.

Rummel, W.; Nell, G.; and Wanitschke, R. Action mechanisms of antiabsorptive and hydragogue drugs. In, *Intestinal Absorption and Malabsorption.* (Csáky, T. Z., ed.) Raven Press, New York, **1975,** pp. 209–227.

Saunders, D. R.; Sillery, J.; Rachmilewitz, D.; Rubin, C. E.; and Tytgut, G. N. Effect of bisacodyl on the structure and function of rodent and human intestine. *Gastroenterology,* **1977,** *72,* 849–856.

Stewart, J. J., and Bass, P. Effect of intravenous C-terminal octapeptide of cholecystokinin and intraduodenal ricinoleic acid on contractile activity of the dog intestine. *Proc. Soc. Exp. Biol. Med.,* **1976,** *152,* 213–217.

Tolman, K. G.; Hammar, S.; and Sannella, J. J. Possible hepatotoxicity of DOXIDAN. *Ann. Intern. Med.,* **1976,** *84,* 290–292.

Waller, S. L. Differential measurement of small and large bowel transit times in constipation and diarrhoea: a new approach. *Gut,* **1975,** *16,* 372–378.

Wanitschke, R.; Nell, G.; Rummel, W.; and Specht, W. Transfer of sodium and water through isolated rat colonic mucosa under the influence of deoxycholate and oxyphenisatin. *Naunyn Schmiedebergs Arch. Pharmacol.,* **1977,** *297,* 185–190.

Monographs and Reviews

Binder, H. J. Pharmacology of laxatives. *Annu. Rev. Pharmacol. Toxicol.,* **1977,** *17,* 355–367.

Cooke, W. T. Laxative abuse. *Clin. Gastroenterol.,* **1977,** *6,* 659–673.

Cummings, J. H. Dietary fibre. *Gut,* **1973,** *14,* 69–81.

———. Laxative abuse. *Ibid.,* **1974,** *15,* 758–766.

Erle, H. R. Constipation. *Primary Care,* **1976,** *3,* 301–310.

FDA. Over-the-counter drugs: proposed establishment of monographs for OTC laxative, antidiarrheal, emetic, and antiemetic products. *Federal Register,* **1975,** *40,* 12902–12944.

Fingl, E., and Freston, J. W. Antidiarrheal agents and laxatives: changing concepts. *Clin. Gastroenterol.,* **1979,** *8,* 161–185.

Symposium. (Various authors.) The colon: its normal and abnormal physiology and therapeutics. *Ann. N.Y. Acad. Sci.,* **1954,** *58,* 293–540.

Symposium. (Various authors.) Colonic function. *Gut,* **1975,** *16,* 298–329.

Chemotherapy of Parasitic Diseases

CHAPTER

44 DRUGS USED IN THE CHEMOTHERAPY OF HELMINTHIASIS

Ian M. Rollo

Anthelmintics are drugs used to rid the body of parasitic worms known as helminths. These drugs are of great importance because helminthiasis is the most common disease in the world. Several billion people are hosts to various types of worms, and this number is increasing rather then decreasing. For example, with increased agricultural use of land and artificial irrigation, multiplication of aquatic snails has occurred. In endemic areas, this has resulted in a marked increase in the number of people infected with schistosomes. Furthermore, as a result of migration and travel, worms may appear in countries where previously they had been unknown.

The term *anthelmintic* is not restricted to drugs that act locally to expel worms from the *gastrointestinal tract*. There are several types of worms that penetrate *tissues,* and drugs used to combat systemic infections are also included under the general term *anthelmintic.*

Worms parasitic for man belong to widely different zoological species and vary with respect to bodily structure, physiology, habitat in the human host, and sensitivity to drugs. There are available now to the physician effective drugs that will bring about a cure in most instances. Considerable advances have been made in the last several years in discovering drugs that surpass the older remedies both in selectivity of action and in relative lack of toxicity, thus relegating the older drugs to a deserved obsolescence. Increase in selectivity, however, puts greater responsibility on the physician to make an accurate diagnosis and to make proper use of the available agents. Physicians and technicians who have few opportunities to deal with specimens in which parasites are presumed to be present should have their findings corroborated by an expert.

In the following presentation, no attempt has been made to group drugs with respect to relative importance or therapeutic application. Rather, individual anthelmintics are presented in *alphabetical order.* A discussion of antimonials then follows. Finally, treatment of specific helminthic infections is discussed.

BEPHENIUM HYDROXYNAPHTHOATE

Bephenium was introduced for the treatment of hookworm infections on the basis of laboratory trials of a series of quaternary ammonium compounds showing activity against a broad range of parasitic nematodes (Copp *et al.,* 1958). The drug is now only occasionally used against infections due to *Necator americanus* and *Ancylostoma duodenale* (Goodwin *et al.,* 1958; Standen, 1963).

Chemistry. Bephenium is usually employed as the hydroxynaphthoate salt. It has the following structural formula:

Bephenium Hydroxynaphthoate

Standen (1963) has reported the structure-activity relationship of a large series of analogs of bephenium.

Anthelmintic Action. Bephenium hydroxynaphthoate is highly effective, even when given in a single dose, against both species of human hookworms and against human infections with *Ascaris lumbricoides* (roundworm) and *Trichostrongylus orientalis.* It is ineffective against *Strongyloides stercoralis* and has only moderate activity against *Trichuris trichiura.*

Bephenium is a cholinergic agonist, and *Ascaris* exposed to the compound first contract and then relax. Hookworms in the gastrointestinal tract lose their attachment in the presence of the drug and are expelled.

Absorption, Fate, and Excretion. Very little bephenium is absorbed from the gastrointestinal tract, and after oral administration of a therapeutic dose of the drug not more than 0.5% is excreted in the urine within 24 hours.

Preparations, Route of Administration, and Dosage. *Bephenium Hydroxynaphthoate,* U.S.P. (ALCO-PARA), is available in single-dose sachets of 5 g, containing the equivalent of 2.5 g of bephenium base. Bephenium hydroxynaphthoate is given orally on an empty stomach, and food is then withheld for at least 2 hours. The dosage for adults is 5 g twice daily for 1 day for *Ancylostoma duodenale* and for 3 days for *Necator americanus.* In cases of severe diarrhea associated with hookworm disease, daily treatment for 4 to 7 days may be necessary. Purging is not required either before or after the administration of bephenium and may even reduce the response obtained. Since residual eggs may be excreted for some days after the adult worms have been eliminated, assessment of the effects of the drug should be deferred until 2 or 3 weeks after treatment.

Toxicity and Side Effects. Bephenium hydroxynaphthoate seems to produce no serious side effects. Because of its bitter taste, the drug may provoke nausea and vomiting; however, most adults and children can take it without difficulty, particularly if the dose is given suspended in a strong sugar solution.

Therapeutic Uses. The primary indication for the use of bephenium is in *hookworm disease.* Against *Ancylostoma duodenale,* single-dose treatment results in cure rates of from 80 to 98%, with major reduction of worm burden in the remainder. While fairly high cure rates follow single-dose treatment of patients who are infected with *Necator americanus,* some investigators have found that larger doses and more extended treatment were necessary for a high order of radical cure. In infections with *Ascaris lumbricoides* or when this roundworm occurs, as it often does, in association with hookworm, bephenium has proven effective in removing or causing a major reduction in the worm burden. Single-dose treatments have resulted in about 80% cures in infections due to *Trichostrongylus orientalis.*

DICHLOROPHEN

Because *dichlorophen* is a useful drug against the large tapeworms of cats and dogs, successful trials were carried out to assess its usefulness in *Taenia saginata* and *T. solium* infections of man.

Chemistry. Dichlorophen has the following structural formula:

Dichlorophen

Anthelmintic Action. Dichlorophen is primarily effective against the large tapeworms of man and domestic animals. The mechanism of action of dichlorophen is not known. Shortly after the administration of an effective dose, the scolex detaches itself from the wall of the intestine, and the worm is killed and digested. For this reason, usually nothing recognizable or only partially disintegrated mature segments can be seen in the stool. This presents difficulty in diagnosing cure, and, therefore, careful follow-up of the patient is required.

Preparations, Route of Administration, and Dosage. *Dichlorophen* (ANTHIPHEN) is not marketed in the United States. It is supplied as scored tablets containing 500 mg of active material. Dichlorophen is given orally without preliminary fasting or other prior preparation of the patient. Satisfactory results have been obtained by giving 2 to 3 g every 8 hours for three doses (children, 1 to 2 g). Alternatively, a single dose of 6 g (children, 2 to 4 g) may be given on each of 2 successive days. If mass treatment of adults is undertaken, a single dose of 6 to 9 g may be given.

Toxicity and Side Effects. An appreciable proportion of treated patients experience colic, diarrhea, and nausea lasting from 4 to 6 hours. Vomiting may occur occasionally. Lassitude is another common symptom.

Therapeutic Uses. Dichlorophen is effective in clearing a large proportion of infections by *T. saginata. Taenia solium* is also susceptible; however, there may be a danger of cysticercosis from liberated ova. Available data suggest it may be useful against *Diphyllobothrium latum* and *Hymenolepis nana* infections. Its lack of serious side effects may recommend its use in patients who are undernourished, weak, or convalescent.

DIETHYLCARBAMAZINE

During World War II, over 15,000 cases of filariasis occurred in American military personnel quartered on the islands of the Western Pacific. This stimulated the search for effective filaricides. The most promising group of antifilarial compounds to emerge were piperazine derivatives.

Chemistry. *Diethylcarbamazine* has the following structural formula:

Diethylcarbamazine

The drug is marketed as the dicitrate salt, a colorless, crystalline solid, highly soluble in water.

Anthelmintic Action. Diethylcarbamazine causes rapid disappearance of microfilariae of *Wuchereria bancrofti, W. (Brugia) malayi,* and *Loa loa* from the blood of man. The drug is inactive *in vitro;* rather, it appears to sensitize the microfilariae so that they become susceptible to phagocytosis by the fixed macrophages of the reticuloendothelial system. There is no phagocytosis by the circulating phagocytes of the blood (Hawking *et al.,* 1950). The drug causes microfilariae of *Onchocerca volvulus* to disappear from the skin but does not kill microfilariae in the nodules. Nor does it affect the microfilariae of *W. bancrofti* when they are in a hydrocele. There is presumptive evidence that diethylcarbamazine kills adult worms of *W. bancrofti* and definite evidence that it kills adult *W. malayi* and *Loa loa.* However, it has little action against adult *O. volvulus* (*see* Hawking, 1963). The mechanism of the filaricidal action of diethylcarbamazine is unknown.

Absorption, Fate, and Excretion. Diethylcarbamazine is readily absorbed from the gastrointestinal tract. After a single oral dose, a peak blood concentration appears in 3 hours; this falls to zero within 48 hours. Excretion is almost entirely urinary, most of the drug appearing as metabolites. The compound is distributed almost equally throughout all body compartments with the exception of fat, and there is little tendency to accumulation when repeated doses are given.

Preparations, Route of Administration, and Dosage. *Diethylcarbamazine Citrate,* U.S.P. (BANOCIDE, HETRAZAN), is available as tablets, each containing 50 mg. The product is stable even under conditions of high temperature and humidity, such as occur in the tropics. The dosage of diethylcarbamazine used to treat filarial disease has varied considerably. The following are representative of the dosages used most frequently. They may be modified effectively according to individual experience.

Wuchereria bancrofti and *W. malayi.* For mass treatment with the objective of reducing microfilaremia to subinfective levels for mosquitoes, the dose is 2 mg/kg, three times daily after meals, for 7 days. For treatment directed toward possible cure, the dose is 2 mg/kg, three times daily after meals, for 10 to 30 days. Much experience has shown that, if people can be persuaded to take an adequate amount of diethylcarbamazine, the microfilariae and probably some of the adult worms will be destroyed. For practical purposes, an adequate amount seems to be a total dose of about 72 mg of the citrate salt per kilogram of body weight. The period over which this amount is administered has varied from area to area; spaced doses of 6 mg/kg once a week or once a month give as good an effect as daily doses, and are less likely to cause adverse reaction (World Health Organization, 1967).

Loa loa. Two to 4 mg/kg should be given three times daily after meals for 10 days. If repeated courses are required to produce cure, they should be separated by periods of 3 to 4 weeks.

Onchocerca volvulus. Treatment is effective in removing microfilariae from the skin; however, since the adult worms are not killed, they usually return after some weeks. It may be possible to hold both forms in check by periodic short courses of treatment. When lesions of the eye are present, the initial dose of diethylcarbamazine should not exceed 0.5 mg/kg. This is given once on the first day and twice on the second. The dose is then increased to 1 mg/kg, three times daily for the third day, and therapy is continued up to a total of 21 days with a dose of 2 mg/kg three times daily.

In patients infected with *O. volvulus* or *W. malayi,* and to a lesser extent in those infected with *W. bancrofti* and *Loa loa,* the initial systemic reactions provoked by the massive destruction of microfilariae, macrofilariae, or both during treatment may be severe. In such cases the dosage should be lowered or the drug stopped temporarily. Relief of these symptoms is afforded by the use of antihistamines, but, exceptionally, corticosteroids may be required. Once the initial reactions have subsided, continued treatment should not provoke a further series of reactions.

Toxicity and Side Effects. Untoward reactions to diethylcarbamazine, although fairly frequent, are not severe and usually disappear within a few days despite continuation of therapy. Reactions believed to result directly from the drug are headache, general malaise, weakness, joint pains, anorexia, nausea, and vomiting. Other untoward responses result from the filaricidal action. In patients with onchocerciasis, there is usually a violent reaction that is well marked within 16 hours after the first oral dose. This includes swelling and edema of the skin, intense itching, enlargement and tenderness of the inguinal lymph nodes, sometimes a fine papular rash, hyperpyrexia, tachycardia, and headache. These symptoms persist for 3 to 7 days and then subside, after which quite high doses can be tolerated without further reaction. Nodular swellings may occur along the course of the lymphatics, and there is often an accompanying lymphadenitis. The nodules may be the sites of dead worms. The reaction subsides within a few days. Almost all patients receiving therapy exhibit a leukocytosis, first evident on the second day, reaching its peak on the fourth or fifth day, and gradually subsiding over a period of a few weeks. The eosinophilia that frequently occurs in patients with filariasis is intensified for a brief period by diethylcarbamazine therapy.

Precautions and Contraindications. With the exception of the caution that must be exercised in initial treatment with diethylcarbamazine and management of allergic symptoms, particularly in the case of onchocerciasis, there are apparently no contraindications to the use of this drug in recommended doses. In onchocerciasis it is advisable, when treating patients with ocular complications, to have 5% hydrocortisone eyedrops available; when the eye complications are marked, 25 mg of cortisone (or equivalent) may be given with advantage four times a day, 2 days before starting treatment and continued for the first 4 days of treatment. As a precaution in preparing patients for treatment, it may be advisable to give an antimalarial agent if the patient has had a recent history of malaria. This is to prevent relapses that might be provoked by the systemic response to therapy with diethylcarbamazine.

Therapeutic Uses. Diethylcarbamazine can be used effectively to treat infections with *W. bancrofti,* *W. (Brugia) malayi, Loa loa,* and *O. volvulus.* In the first three, radical cure can be achieved by either single or multiple courses of treatment. In onchocerciasis, radical cure is unlikely, but control can be achieved by short periodic courses of treatment. The drug has also been used effectively in the treatment of cutaneous *larva migrans,* although the total number of reported cases is small. Diethylcarbamazine is also effective in clearing *Ascaris* infections, but it has been replaced by other agents for this purpose. In patients with *eosinophilic lung* (*tropical eosinophilia*), treatment with diethylcarbamazine causes a rapid disappearance of symptoms. This, and the finding of microfilariae in lung biopsies, suggest an association between filariasis and one of the eosinophilic pulmonary syndromes.

HYCANTHONE

The group of xanthones and thioxanthones known as the "MIRACILS" was first synthesized in Germany and studied during World War II as potential chemotherapeutic agents for the treatment of *schistosomiasis* (Kikuth *et al.,* 1946; Mauss, 1948). *Lucanthone* (MIRACIL D) was found to be the most active. This compound was studied extensively in the postwar years in England and the United States and used successfully in the treatment of infections with *Schistosoma haematobium* and *S. mansoni.* However, intolerance to the drug in a high proportion of patients, particularly in adults, proved to be a considerable disadvantage and led to further investigation of the chemical series. Of the several metabolites of lucanthone appearing in the urine of treated patients, the hydroxymethyl derivative, *hycanthone,* was shown to have very high schistosomicidal activity (Rosi *et al.,* 1965). Early clinical trials provided encouraging results (Katz *et al.,* 1968). Since then the agent has been used in several programs to control schistosomiasis in the Middle East, Africa, and South America.

Chemistry. Hycanthone has the following structural formula:

Hycanthone

A solution for injection is stable for at least 24 hours at temperatures of 37° C or lower.

Anthelmintic Action. Hycanthone acts primarily against the adult forms of *S. haematobium* and *S. mansoni.* The drug interferes with the laying of eggs, induces separation of paired worms, produces degenerative changes, and induces a shift of worms to the liver within a period of 3 to 7 days. Death of the adult worm follows. The mechanism of action is unknown but may be associated with stimulation of the worm's low-affinity 5-hydroxytryptamine (5-HT) uptake into nonneuronal tissue. At the same time, there is an impairment of the ability of neuronal structures to store this putative excitatory neurotransmitter (Chou *et al.,* 1973). Hycanthone also stimulates motor activity in worms by an anticholinergic mechanism (Hillman and Senft, 1975). Clinically, reduced egg excretion becomes most apparent during the second week after treatment.

Absorption, Fate, and Excretion. Hycanthone is well absorbed after oral administration if the tablet is enteric coated to protect it from degradation by gastric acidity. However, after it was shown that a single intramuscular injection provided the same results as several days of oral treatment, only the parenteral preparation was made available. The drug is well absorbed from the site of intramuscular injection. Peak concentration in the blood is reached in 30 minutes, and in tissues within 1 hour. Only traces remain at the site of injection after 24 hours. The drug appears unchanged in the blood and in all organs with the exception of the liver, where several metabolites of hycanthone have been identified. The main route of excretion is through the bile and feces in the form of conjugated metabolites.

Preparations, Route of Administration, and Dosage. *Hycanthone mesylate* (ETRENOL) is supplied in vials, each containing 200 mg of base to be dissolved in 2 ml of water for injection. The drug is not available in the United States. Hycanthone is given by deep intramuscular injection in a single dose of 2.5 to 3.0 mg of base per kilogram of body weight, up to a maximal adult dose of 200 mg of base. Since there is a high incidence of dose-related side effects, close attention should be paid to the dosage table supplied by the manufacturer. Re-treatment of patients reinfected or harboring a residual infection may be carried out after 1 to 3 months.

In highly endemic areas in the West Indies and East Africa, half the recommended dose has been used to produce very substantial reductions in egg output; side effects are markedly decreased with this regimen.

Toxicity and Side Effects. The administration of hycanthone is associated with a high incidence of side effects, varying from 22 to 60% in various trials. These are generally self-limiting and include nausea, vomiting, abdominal discomfort, headache, dizziness, weakness, myalgia, anorexia, diarrhea, and weight loss. Transient, minimal ECG changes have been reported in a few patients, but these appear to have little clinical significance. Vomiting is the most common reaction and usually begins 4 to 8 hours after treatment. In general, side effects rarely persist beyond 24 hours. The onset of severe, persistent vomiting within 2 to 3 hours after injection suggests possible hepatotoxicity, for which treatment should be started promptly. The most serious adverse effect is acute hepatic necrosis, and death may occur in 2 to

5 days. Estimates of the frequency of this complication vary, but in general they are low. The cause is unknown.

Hycanthone has been shown to be both mutagenic and carcinogenic in several experimental systems *in vitro* and *in vivo* (*see* Batzinger and Bueding, 1977). The significance of this in the treatment of human schistosomiasis has not yet been determined. It may be wise, since alternative drugs are available, to avoid the use of hycanthone at least in children and young adults. Several analogs of hycanthone have been shown to retain chemotherapeutic activity with much reduced *in-vitro* mutagenic activity (Hulbert *et al.,* 1974). The potential clinical value of these or other derivatives has yet to be determined.

Precautions and Contraindications. Hycanthone should not be administered to pregnant women or to those who have recently given birth until at least 1 month after parturition. As mentioned, it is prudent to use alternative agents in children and young adults. Patients should be under close medical supervision for at least 2 days after treatment.

Absolute contraindications to treatment with hycanthone are suspected or confirmed jaundice in the present or recent past, hepatic tenderness or nonschistosomal hepatic disease, or recent or concurrent use of drugs known to affect the liver. In particular, phenothiazines should not be administered for the relief of side effects such as nausea or vomiting. Hycanthone should not be given to patients with serious bacterial infection or any acute febrile state. It is also contraindicated when there is a history of previous allergic reaction to the drug, to lucanthone, or to other thioxanthone derivatives.

Therapeutic Uses. Because a single intramuscular injection represents the full course of treatment, hycanthone has had great value in mass treatment where schistosomiasis is endemic. Both *S. haematobium* and *S. mansoni* infections are susceptible; *S. japonicum* is not. The potential for serious, long-term side effects has led to very close examination of the properties of hycanthone by two international consultant groups of the World Health Organization. They found no reason sufficient to justify discontinuation of the use of hycanthone for the treatment of schistosomiasis. However, the decision to use the drug, especially in mass control programs, should be based on the conditions prevailing in each population to be treated and a realistic assessment of possible benefit against the risks involved.

MEBENDAZOLE

This drug was introduced for the treatment of roundworm infections as a result of research carried out in Belgium (Brugmans *et al.,* 1971).

Chemistry. *Mebendazole* has the following structural formula:

Mebendazole

It is a yellowish amorphous powder, very slightly soluble in water and most organic solvents, and not unpleasant to taste.

Anthelmintic Action. Mebendazole is an effective and versatile anthelmintic agent. It is highly effective against ascariasis, capillariasis, enterobiasis, trichuriasis, and hookworm infection in single or in mixed infection. Variable results have been obtained against *Strongyloides stercoralis*. It has shown promise in the treatment of hydatid disease and trichinosis and in infections with both beef and pork tapeworms (Keystone and Murdoch, 1979). The effect of the drug is due to its ability to inhibit glucose uptake irreversibly (*see* Fierlafijn, 1971), but it does not affect blood glucose concentrations in the host, even in high doses (Van den Bossche, 1972). Parasite immobilization and death occur slowly, and clearance from the gastrointestinal tract may not be complete up to 3 days after treatment. The drug inhibits the development of larval hookworms *in vitro* at 50 μg/ml. Much higher concentrations have no effect on fully formed larvae. Shortly after treatment is started, eggs of *Trichuris* and hookworm fail to develop to the larval stage (Wagner and Chavarria, 1974). (*See also* Miller *et al.*, 1974; Wolfe and Wershing, 1974.)

Absorption, Fate, and Excretion. Only a small proportion of an orally administered dose is absorbed, and up to 10% may be recovered in the urine within 24 to 48 hours. Most of the material excreted by the kidney is the decarboxylated metabolite.

Preparations, Route of Administration, and Dosage. *Mebendazole*, U.S.P. (VERMOX), is available as tablets, each containing 100 mg of the drug. Mebendazole is given orally, and the same dosage schedule applies to adults and children. For control of enterobiasis, a single 100-mg tablet is given; a second should be given after 2 weeks. For control of ascariasis, trichuriasis, and hookworm infection, 100 mg is administered morning and evening on 3 consecutive days. If the patient is not cured 3 weeks after treatment, a second course should be given. Fasting or purging is not required.

Infections with *Capillaria philippinensis* are more resistant to treatment; 400 mg of the drug should be given per day in divided doses for at least 20 days. The drug has caused complete regression of intrahepatic hydatid cysts when given in a course of 400 to 600 mg three times a day for 21 to 30 days.

Toxicity and Side Effects. Probably as a result of its poor absorption, mebendazole has not caused systemic toxicity in clinical use, even in the presence of anemia and malnutrition. Transient symptoms of abdominal pain and diarrhea have occurred in cases of massive infestation and expulsion of worms. Mebendazole has, however, caused embryotoxic and teratogenic effects in pregnant rats at single oral doses as low as 10 mg/kg. Its parafluoro analog, *flubendazole*, is an effective anthelmintic and has no teratogenic effects in rats or in rabbits (Thienpont *et al.*, 1978).

Precautions and Contraindications. Mebendazole should not be given to pregnant women, nor should it be used in patients who have experienced allergic reactions to the agent.

Therapeutic Uses. Mebendazole is the drug of choice in the treatment of *Trichuris trichiura*. It produces a large proportion of cures and, in those not cured with a first course of treatment, a marked reduction in egg production. It is also the drug of choice for infection with *Ancylostoma duodenale*. It is particularly valuable in the treatment of double or triple infections since it also has high activity, and is a highly recommended alternative to pyrantel pamoate, against *ascariasis, enterobiasis,* and *Necator americanus* infection (Chavarria *et al.*, 1973; Sargent *et al.*, 1974). In the Philippines, mebendazole has been used in high dosage successfully in the treatment of intestinal capillariasis (Singson *et al.*, 1975); in even higher dosage successful cure of hydatid disease has been achieved (Bekhti *et al.*, 1977; *see* Editorial, 1979).

METRIFONATE

Metrifonate (BILARCIL) is an organophosphorus inhibitor of cholinesterases, used first as an insecticide (DIPTEREX, DYLOX) and later as an anthelmintic. The original trials in man arose from the hope that the anticholinesterase activity of organophosphorus compounds in arthropods would extend to other invertebrates, including the helminths. Metrifonate was selected for trial on the basis of *in-vitro* tests carried out with *Ascaris lumbricoides*. In 1962 it was shown to have high anthelmintic activity in several different human infections. The substance has the following structural formula:

Metrifonate

The drug is, indeed, a potent inhibitor of nematode cholinesterase; 0.1 μM metrifonate inhibits the enzyme from *Schistosoma haematobium* by 50%, and lower concentrations inhibit that from *S. mansoni*. In clinical practice, however, the order is reversed, since infections with *S. haematobium* respond much better to metrifonate. Given in therapeutic doses, metrifonate produces rapid and almost complete inhibition of plasma cholinesterase activity of the host; this recovers to almost normal levels within a few weeks of stopping treatment. Erythrocyte acetylcholinesterase is inhibited to a lesser degree but recovers more slowly. Despite these changes the drug is well tolerated. Treated individuals should, of course, be free from recent exposure to insecticides that might add to the anticholinesterase effect and not receive depolarizing neuromuscular blocking agents for at least 48 hours after treatment.

Metrifonate is recommended only for the treatment of *S. haematobium* infection. Its low cost, effectiveness, and ready acceptance have placed it in an important role in the treatment of urinary schistosomiasis in North and East Africa. The dose employed is 5 to 15 mg/kg, given orally three times at intervals of 2 weeks. It is supplied in 100-mg scored tablets. Successful prophylaxis has been carried out in a highly endemic area with a dosage of 7.5 mg/kg, given once every 4 weeks (Jewsbury *et al.*, 1977). Protection was established at a cost less than that incurred with molluscicidal technics or single courses of treatment with established drugs. In the United States, metrifonate is available from the Parasitic Diseases Division, Center for Disease Control, Atlanta, Georgia 30333.

NICLOSAMIDE

Niclosamide was introduced as a taeniacide after laboratory trials in rats with *Hymenolepis diminuta* as a test organism (Gönnert and Schraufstätter, 1960). In the intervening years so much impressive evidence of its high activity and safety has accumulated that it is generally regarded as the most effective agent for the treatment of most infections with cestodes (Keeling, 1968).

Chemistry. Niclosamide has the following structural formula:

Niclosamide

It occurs as a yellowish-white powder that is tasteless and odorless. It is insoluble in water.

Anthelmintic Action. Niclosamide has prominent activity against most of the cestodes that infect man; *Enterobius* (*Oxyuris*) *vermicularis* is also susceptible. Very little of the drug is absorbed by *H. diminuta in vitro*, but if a homogenate of intestine is added, the amount of drug taken up by the worms is greatly increased. Niclosamide stimulates oxygen uptake by *H. diminuta* at low concentrations, but at higher concentrations respiration is inhibited and glucose uptake is blocked. A more prominent effect of the drug may be to inhibit anaerobic metabolism, on which many helminths are particularly dependent. Worms affected by the drug either in the gut or *in vitro* are more susceptible to proteolytic enzymes. After effective doses of the drug, the scolex and segments may be partially digested and unrecognizable.

Preparations, Route of Administration, and Dosage. *Niclosamide* (YOMESAN) is supplied in vanilla-flavored tablets, each containing 500 mg of the drug. In the United States, this drug is available from the Parasitic Diseases Division, Center for Disease Control, Atlanta, Georgia 30333. Niclosamide is given orally. The patient may be prepared by fasting overnight, but there is no conclusive evidence that this is necessary. Those with chronic constipation should be given a laxative before administering the drug. The recommended dose for an adult is 2 g, the tablets to be chewed thoroughly and washed down with water. The dosage for children who weigh between 11 and 34 kg is 1 g and for children under 2 years, 0.5 g. For small children it is advisable to grind the tablets as finely as possible and to mix the powder with a little water. A purge may be given 2 hours after the dose in the hope of obtaining less damaged lengths of the worm and an identifiable scolex.

In infections with *H. nana*, which are usually multiple, the recommended dose of 2 g should be taken once daily for 5 days after breakfast. Discharge of intestinal mucus can be promoted by the administration of sour fruit juices. Worms lodging under accumulations of mucus thus become more readily accessible to the drug.

Toxicity and Side Effects. Niclosamide seems to be singularly free from any undesirable effects, other than very occasional gastrointestinal upset. Very little is absorbed from the gastrointestinal tract, and it has no direct irritant effect. No side effects were observed when niclosamide was given to debilitated or pregnant patients (Gönnert and Schraufstätter, 1960). Follow-up studies showed no alteration in hepatic or renal function or in blood counts of treated patients (Abdallah and Saif, 1961).

Precautions and Contraindications. There are no contraindications to the use of niclosamide as a taeniacide. However, it is important to note that the lethal action of the drug against the adult worm does not extend to the ova contained within the tapeworm segments. This means that the use of niclosamide in *T. solium* infections may expose the patient to the risk of cysticercosis, since, following digestion of the dead segments, viable ova will be liberated into the lumen of the gut. It is mandatory to give an adequate purge within 1 to 2 hours after the drug has been given, to clear the bowel of all dead segments before they can be digested. In *T. saginata* infections in which there is no risk of cysticercosis, purging is unnecessary unless immediate proof of cure by finding the scolex is desired.

Therapeutic Uses. Niclosamide can be considered an agent of choice in the treatment of *D. latum, H. nana,* and *T. saginata* infections (Brown, 1968). It is also very effective in the treatment of *T. solium* infection, but the danger of cysticercosis following its administration must be recalled. The ready acceptance of niclosamide by patients, together with the fact that fasting is not necessary, is valuable, particularly in the treatment of children.

NIRIDAZOLE

Chemistry. *Niridazole* was developed from the synthesis of a large number of nitrothiazole derivatives. The nitrothiazole nucleus was chosen because heterocyclic compounds bearing a nitro group as a characteristic substituent occupy an important position in chemotherapy. Of the many preparations synthesized and tested, derivatives of 5-nitrothiazole substituted by a cyclic urea group in position 2 displayed optimal chemotherapeutic properties. From this category the ethylene-urea derivative, 1-(5-nitro-2-thiazolyl)-2-imidazolidinone (niridazole), was selected for clinical investigation. Niridazole has the following structural formula:

Niridazole

The substance is a yellow crystalline powder that is odorless and tasteless. It is sparingly soluble in water and most organic solvents.

Anthelmintic Action. Niridazole is both schistosomicidal and amebicidal. Anthelmintic activity is observed first on the vitellogenic gland. The vitelline cells become depleted of egg-shell substance, and there is complete arrest of shell formation in the ootype. Eventually no eggs can be seen in the uterus. Destruction of the vitellogenic gland coincides with a decrease in body length of both male and female worms, and the size of the ovary in the female. The gonads of male worms are less sensitive than those of females. In affected worms, spermatogenesis is stopped; this is followed by complete destruction of the testes. In the liver the female worm is destroyed by leukocytes and the male is immobilized by connective tissue and eventually undergoes autolysis. Niridazole has been shown to decrease the uptake of exogenous glucose by *S. mansoni,* and to promote the breakdown of glycogen by the organism.

In addition to its action on schistosomes, niridazole is an effective amebicide both *in vitro* and in the treatment of intestinal and extraintestinal amebiasis. It is effective in the treatment of guinea worm infection and has been reported to have some therapeutic effect against the adult worms of *O. volvulus.* It has proven useful in treating a few cases of cutaneous leishmaniasis.

Other Actions. Niridazole has been shown to possess marked anti-inflammatory properties. Although the drug is not cytotoxic, it is a potent and long-acting suppressant of cell-mediated immune responses; it has only a minor, transient effect on the humoral immune response (Mahmoud *et al.,* 1975). Consequently, it has been tested successfully in the rat for its ability to prolong the survival of cardiac allografts; profound immunosuppression was obtained when niridazole was combined with azathioprine and prednisolone (Salaman *et al.,* 1977). Some delayed hypersensitivity responses are also suppressed in schistosome-infected human subjects receiving therapeutic doses of niridazole (Webster *et al.,* 1975).

Tests *in vitro* with bacteria have shown that mutagenic activity appears in the urine of patients treated with niridazole. Carcinogenic effects have also been demonstrated in mice and hamsters, both uninfected and infected with *S. mansoni,* fed a diet containing high concentrations of the drug. The clinical implications remain to be established, and this is an important objective, considering the size of the population that receives this drug.

Further details on the pharmacological effects of niridazole may be found in the proceedings of a symposium (*see* Symposium, 1969a).

Absorption, Fate, and Excretion. Following oral administration, niridazole is absorbed almost entirely over a period of several hours. The drug is largely metabolized during its first passage through the liver. Owing to slow absorption and rapid metabolism, a low but uniform concentration of parent drug is maintained in the peripheral blood for several hours. The metabolites attain high concentration in the blood and persist there for a long time because they are firmly bound to plasma albumin. The parent compound and its metabolites are uniformly distributed throughout the tissues. The drug is eliminated largely, and almost equally, in the urine and feces, in the latter by way of the bile. The urine becomes dark in color, and there is an unpleasant body odor. The schistosomicidal activity of niridazole is attributable to the parent compound. At least part of its effectiveness must be due to the high concentration in the portal blood and the fact that the various species of *Schistosoma* live mainly or exclusively in the vascular bed supplied by portal blood.

Preparations, Route of Administration, and Dosage. *Niridazole* (AMBILHAR) is supplied in scored tablets of 100 and 500 mg. In the United States it is available from the Parasitic Diseases Division, Center for Disease Control, Atlanta, Georgia 30333. Niridazole is administered orally. The usual daily dose is 25 mg/kg (maximum of 1.5 g), which may or may not be divided into two portions, depending on the local experience of the physician and practical considerations for ambulatory patients. Treatment is usually continued for 5 days, but may be extended to 7 or even 10 days. These longer periods should probably be the rule in *S. mansoni* infection, which is rather less responsive to therapy than is *S. haematobium,* and also in *S. japonicum* infection, although the most that can be expected in the latter condition is a reduction in the egg count. The dosage schedule of niridazole in dracontiasis is 25 mg/kg daily for 7 days.

Toxicity and Side Effects. In patients, niridazole produces changes in the ECG after several days of treatment. Flattening or inversion of the T wave occurs. This reverts to normal within 1 to 2 weeks after completion of treatment and has never been associated with clinical evidence of cardiac impairment. The drug may produce EEG changes and may cause agitation, confusional states, visual and auditory hallucinations, and localized or generalized convulsions. These effects appear to occur largely in patients in whom some degree of impairment of hepatic function exists as a result of the hepatosplenic form of schistosomiasis, concurrent disease, malnutrition, or anemia. As a consequence, the drug is not well metabolized and the concentration of parent substance in the blood is high. Niridazole, in common with some nitrofurazone derivatives, inhibits spermatogenesis in experimental animals by a direct effect on the germinal epithelium of the testes. The effect is reversible on stopping treatment. Human subjects receiving standard doses of niridazole occasionally display a transitory reduction in the number of spermatozoa in ejaculate. Administration of the drug has not been known to impair the fertility of either male or female patients. Treatment with niridazole can provoke hemolysis in individuals with red cells deficient in glucose-6-phosphate dehydrogenase (Doyen *et al.,* 1967).

Niridazole also causes the following less specific effects: abdominal spasm and discomfort, nausea, vomiting, diarrhea, loss of appetite, and headache. Less frequently encountered are insomnia, skin rash, and paresthesias. The incidence and the severity of these side effects are considerably less in children, with the exception of those infected with *S. japonicum.* In this condition, hepatic impairment is seen more frequently than in *S. mansoni* or *haematobium* infection, with consequent increase in the amount of circulating niridazole.

Precautions and Contraindications. Since the toxicity of niridazole appears to depend on the amount of parent drug circulating in the blood, any impairment of hepatic function demands the greatest care in its use and contraindicates its employment at least in the ambulatory patient. Evidence of epilepsy or neurotic or psychotic behavior may also be regarded as a contraindication, unless it is deemed necessary to utilize niridazole and the means are at hand to control any symptoms of central nervous system (CNS) excitation. In general, those in poor general condition due to malnutrition, marked anemia, and severe concomitant infections or parasitoses, notably tuberculosis and ancylostomiasis, should not be treated with niridazole. To this group may be added those suffering from the hyperacute exudative form of schistosomiasis. In the presence of genetically determined glucose-6-phosphate dehydrogenase deficiency, additional care is required, and the physician must be aware of the possibility of hemolytic anemia.

Therapeutic Uses. Niridazole is particularly useful in the treatment of schistosomiasis. *Schistosoma haematobium* infections respond particularly well. *Mansoni* schistosomiasis is not as consistent in its response, but quite good results have followed a slightly more extended course of treatment. Infections due to *S. japonicum* have given quite varied responses, but reductions in egg count usually follow an adequate course of treatment. Niridazole is also effective in the treatment of infections with guinea worm (*D. medinensis*).

OXAMNIQUINE

Oxamniquine is a metabolic derivative of the most active of a novel series of 2-aminomethyltetrahydroquinoline compounds that showed promising schistosomicidal activity and low toxicity in laboratory animals (*see* Foster, 1973). It is prepared by microbial (*Aspergillus sclerotiorum*) hydroxylation of its synthetic precursor.

Chemistry. Oxamniquine has the following structural formula:

Oxamniquine

It is a light-orange crystalline solid.

Anthelmintic Action. *Schistosoma mansoni* is highly susceptible to oxamniquine; therapeutically useful activity has not been demonstrated against either *S. haematobium* or *japonicum*. Effective treatment with the drug causes a shift of worms from the mesentery to the liver within a few days. Later, surviving unpaired females return to the mesentery but do not lay eggs. Egg loads in primate hosts have been found to be due to only one or two surviving·

pairs of worms. Male worms are retained in the liver by tissue reactions, and the vast majority are dead.

Absorption, Fate, and Excretion. Oxamniquine is readily absorbed following oral administration, and a peak concentration in plasma occurs within about 3 hours. The presence of food significantly delays absorption and limits the concentration achieved in plasma during the first several hours after administration of the drug. Most of an administered dose is excreted in the urine. Only a small proportion is excreted unchanged; most appears as a single metabolite, a 6-carboxyl derivative, and there are traces of a second compound, a 2-carboxylic acid. The major metabolite is predominantly excreted in the first 12 hours; it is devoid of schistosomicidal activity (Kaye and Woolhouse, 1976).

Preparations, Route of Administration, and Dosage. *Oxamniquine* (MANSIL in Brazil, VANSIL in Africa) is available as capsules, each of which contains 250 mg of the drug, and as a syrup (50 mg/ml). Because of severe local pain following intramuscular injection, oxamniquine is administered orally; the dosage depends on the geographical location. For the treatment of all forms of *S. mansoni* infections in Brazil, the recommended dose is 12 to 15 mg/kg, given as a single dose. For children weighing less than 30 kg, the dose is 20 mg/kg (in two doses of 10 mg/kg with an interval of 2 to 8 hours between them). The drug is tolerated better after food. In Africa, the recommended total dose ranges from 15 to 60 mg/kg, given over 1 to 3 days. The most appropriate regimen within this range is determined by the geographical location and the particular strain of *S. mansoni*. In the treatment of mixed *mansoni* and *haematobium* infections, metrifonate, in divided doses, has been used satisfactorily in conjunction with oxamniquine.

Toxicity and Side Effects. Dizziness and drowsiness have been reported after the administration of oxamniquine. Convulsions have occurred in a small number of patients, particularly in individuals with a history of epilepsy. Minor and transient elevation of transaminase activities may also be observed. However, since oxamniquine has been used safely in patients with severe hepatosplenic disease, these changes are considered to be of doubtful clinical significance. Minor elevations of the number of circulating eosinophils are seen after treatment. These changes are likely due to the host's reaction to dead and dying worms. Orange-to-red discoloration of the urine may follow treatment.

Therapeutic Uses. Oxamniquine is currently used in the treatment of infections with *Schistosoma mansoni*. Its value as an orally administered, readily accepted schistosomicide has been proven, both for the treatment of individual patients and in mass-treatment and control programs (*see* Clarke *et al.*, 1976; Katz *et al.*, 1977; Pedro *et al.*, 1977; Bassily *et al.*, 1978; Omer, 1978). It is effective in all stages of infection, including the acute phase and the chronic phase with hepatosplenic involvement. Recommended dosages differ in various geographical areas as a consequence of differing sensitivity of various strains of *S. mansoni* and not to differences in the pharmacokinetics of the drug in different racial groups. It has been used successfully in combination with metrifonate in the treatment of mixed *mansoni* and *haematobium* infections.

PIPERAZINE

Piperazine was used early in this century for the treatment of gout because a solution of piperazine is an excellent solvent for uric acid. Although the drug proved to be ineffective as a uricosuric agent, extensive clinical experience indicated that it was nontoxic. The discovery of the anthelmintic properties of piperazine is usually credited to Fayard (1949), but these were first observed by Boismare, a Rouen pharmacist, whose recipe is quoted in Fayard's thesis. Clinical studies have shown that the drug is highly effective against both *Ascaris lumbricoides* and *Enterobius (Oxyuris) vermicularis*. A large number of substituted piperazine derivatives exhibit anthelmintic activity, but apart from diethylcarbamazine none has found a place in human therapeutics (*see* Standen, 1963).

Chemistry. Piperazine has the following structural formula:

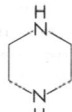

Piperazine

It is available as the hexahydrate, which contains about 44% of base, and, in addition, as various salts such as citrate, adipate, phosphate, calcium edetate, and tartrate. These salts occur as stable, nonhygroscopic, white crystals, freely soluble in water. Aqueous solutions are slightly acidic.

Anthelmintic Action. The predominant effect of piperazine on *Ascaris* is to cause flaccid paralysis of muscle that results in expulsion of the worm by peristalsis. Affected worms recover if incubated in drug-free medium. Piperazine blocks the response of *Ascaris* muscle to acetylcholine, apparently by altering the permeability of the cell membrane to ions that are responsible for the maintenance of the resting potential. The drug causes hyperpolarization and suppression of spontaneous spike potentials with accompanying paralysis (*see* Saz and Bueding, 1966). The basis for its selectivity of action is not entirely clear.

Absorption, Fate, and Excretion. Piperazine is readily absorbed from the gastrointestinal tract. A portion of the absorbed drug is degraded, and the remainder is excreted in the urine. Rogers (1958) observed no significant difference between the rates of urinary excretion of the citrate, phosphate, and adipate. However, there was a wide variation in the rates at which piperazine was excreted by different individuals.

Preparations, Route of Administration, and Dosage. Piperazine salts are available as tablets and wafers, each containing 500 mg, and as syrups and suspensions containing 100 mg/ml, calculated as the hexahydrate. Of the various preparations, one is probably as good as another. The liquid preparations are more acceptable for children. *Piperazine Citrate*, U.S.P., and *Piperazine Phosphate*, U.S.P., are the official preparations. Trade names include ANTEPAR (citrate and phosphate), MULTIFUGE, and PIPIZAN CITRATE.

Piperazine preparations are always given orally. It is unnecessary to supplement treatment with cathartics or enemas. Prior fasting is not necessary. Many different dosage schedules have been investigated, and all have resulted in a considerable measure of success. In *ascariasis,* accepted therapy is to give 75 mg/kg (maximum of 3.5 g) as a single daily dose for 2 consecutive days. Children should be treated in the same way. This dosage schedule will cure almost 100% of patients. A single dose of 4 g has been shown to cure about 50% of patients and to reduce markedly the worm burden in the remainder (Goodwin and Standen, 1958). In *oxyuriasis,* single daily doses of 65 mg/kg, with a maximum of 2.5 g, given for 8 days, will result in 95 to 100% cure. One study in hospital patients showed that a single dose of 4 g of piperazine, with or without senna, cured more than 90% of patients (White and Scopes, 1960). Because of the possibility of autoinfection, a second dose should be given to ambulatory patients 2 weeks after the first.

Toxicity and Side Effects. There is a wide range between effective therapeutic and overtly toxic doses of piperazine. Laboratory studies on patients receiving treatment for several days have showed no abnormality. Very occasionally gastrointestinal upset, transient neurological effects, and urticarial reactions have attended its use. Piperazine has been used without ill effect during pregnancy. Lethal doses cause convulsions and respiratory depression.

Precautions and Contraindications. Piperazine is contraindicated in patients with a history of epilepsy. Neurotoxic effects have occurred in individuals with renal dysfunction; because urinary excretion is the main route of elimination, care should be exercised in the treatment of such patients.

Therapeutic Uses. In the treatment of *ascariasis*, piperazine has the advantage of greatly reducing the motility of the worms, thereby reducing the hazard of migration. Since the worms are usually alive when passed, there is little chance of absorption of disintegration products. Where partial intestinal obstruction is a complication of infection, conservative management together with the administration of piperazine syrup through a drainage tube may obviate the need for surgical intervention.

Treatment of *oxyuriasis* is complicated by the readiness with which reinfection may occur. Many authorities advocate the simultaneous treatment of the entire household with piperazine in lieu of investigation of each member by anal swabs. The palatability of the various preparations, ease of administration to children, and low toxicity make piperazine an agent of choice in pinworm infections.

PRAZIQUANTEL

Praziquantel was developed from a series of novel pyrazinoisoquinolines that were studied in an attempt to find compounds with wide cestocidal activity. It was found to be highly effective not only against all juvenile and adult cestodes tested but also against larval cestodes and all species of schistosomes that are parasitic in man (Andrews, 1977; Thomas and Gönnert, 1977).

Chemistry. Praziquantel has the following structural formula.

Praziquantel

It is a colorless crystalline powder with a bitter taste.

Anthelmintic Action. At very low concentrations *in vitro* (1 to 10 ng/ml), praziquantel stimulates the motility of cestodes and impairs the function of their suckers. At concentrations of 10 to 100 ng/ml and above, it causes a strong contraction of the entire strobila. When concentrations exceed 1 μg/ml, this contraction occurs instantaneously; the effect is reversible. The effectiveness of the drug *in vivo* thus appears in part to be due to dislocation of the worm in the intestine. Irreparable damage is probably due to a drug-induced sensitivity of the tegument to proteolytic enzymes (Thomas and Andrews, 1977).

Absorption, Fate, and Excretion. In man, praziquantel is readily absorbed after oral administration. Maximal concentrations in plasma occur in 1 to 2 hours. Rapid metabolism after oral administration limits the half-life of praziquantel to 1 hour. Those of the metabolites are longer, although 70% is eliminated in the urine during the first day following administration of the drug (Leopold *et al.*, 1977).

Preparations, Route of Administration, and Dosage. *Praziquantel* (DRONCIT) is administered orally. Clinical trials are currently being conducted in the treatment of cestode infections and of infections due to all three species of schistosomes that inhabit man. A cure rate of 100% of infections with *Diphyllobothrium latum* has followed the administration of a single oral dose of 25 mg/kg; treatment of infections from *Taenia saginata* with doses of 10 mg/kg has been just as successful, while nearly 95% of patients infected with *Hymenolepis nana* have been cured by 25 mg/kg of the drug (Canzonieri *et al.*, 1977).

Toxicity and Side Effects. Although data are as yet sparse, investigators remark on the lack of side effects that follows the administration of praziquantel in doses up to 50 mg/kg. *In vitro*, the drug has been shown to have an inotropic effect on rat atria.

Therapeutic Uses. The cestocidal effect of praziquantel has been demonstrated against both cyclophyllidea and pseudophyllidea, and this property has been exploited in both medical and veterinary practice. Its schistosomicidal effect extends to all three species that infect man, and this property, which is unique among schistosomicides, should make the drug especially valuable as an agent for all endemic areas and for the treatment of mixed infections.

PYRANTEL PAMOATE

Pyrantel pamoate was introduced first into veterinary practice as a broad-spectrum anthelmintic effective against pinworm, roundworm, and hookworm (Austin *et al.*, 1966). Its effectiveness and lack of toxicity led to its trial against related helminths that infect the human digestive tract (Bumbalo *et al.*, 1969). Success in these and other trials has resulted in its recognition as an important agent for the treatment of infections with various nematodes. *Oxantel,* a *m*-oxyphenol analog of pyrantel, has been used successfully in the single-dose treatment of trichuriasis.

Chemistry. Pyrantel is employed as the pamoate salt. It has the following structural formula:

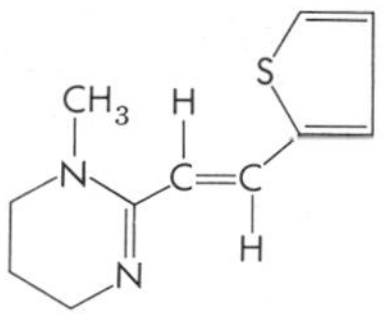

Pyrantel

The pamoate is a white crystalline salt practically insoluble in either alcohol or water. It is tasteless and stable.

Anthelmintic Action.

Pyrantel and its analogs are depolarizing neuromuscular blocking agents. They induce marked, persistent nicotinic activation, which results in spastic paralysis of the worm. Pyrantel also inhibits cholinesterases. It causes a slowly developing contracture of preparations of *Ascaris* at $\frac{1}{100}$ the concentration of acetylcholine required to produce the same effect. In single muscle cells of the helminth, pyrantel causes depolarization and increased spike-discharge frequency, accompanied by increase in tension. In contrast, piperazine causes hyperpolarization with reduction in spike-discharge frequency and relaxation in identical preparations. In the *Ascaris* preparations, pyrantel and piperazine are mutually antagonistic (Aubry *et al.*, 1970; Eyre, 1970). Pyrantel is effective against hookworm, pinworm, and roundworm; however, unlike its analog oxantel, it is ineffective against the whipworm.

Absorption, Fate, and Excretion.

Pyrantel pamoate is poorly absorbed from the gastrointestinal tract. Less than 15% is excreted in the urine as parent drug and metabolites. The major proportion of an administered dose may be recovered in the feces. Poor absorption contributes to the selectivity of the action of the drug on nematodes.

Preparations, Route of Administration, and Dosage. *Pyrantel Pamoate*, U.S.P. (ANTIMINTH, COMBANTRIN), is supplied as an oral suspension (50 mg of the base per milliliter) and as tablets (125 mg of the base). Pyrantel pamoate is given orally at any time without regard to ingestion of food or beverages. A single dose of 11 mg/kg, to a maximum of 1 g, should be given to treat infections with *Ascaris lumbricoides, Enterobius (Oxyuris) vermicularis, Ancylostoma duodenale, Necator americanus,* or *Trichostrongylus.* In the case of pinworm, it is often wise to repeat the treatment after an interval of 2 weeks.

Toxicity and Side Effects. When administered parenterally to rabbits, pyrantel can produce complete neuromuscular blockade; if given orally, toxic effects are produced only by very large dosage. Gastrointestinal upset is occasionally observed in man, as are headache and dizziness; however, these effects do not persist and are not severe enough to require treatment.

Precautions and Contraindications. Pyrantel pamoate has not been studied in pregnant women, and its use in such patients is thus normally contraindicated. It is also not recommended for children less than 1 year of age. Since pyrantel pamoate and piperazine appear to be mutually antagonistic, it would be unwise to use them together.

Therapeutic Uses. Pyrantel pamoate may be regarded as an agent of choice in the treatment of *ascariasis* and *enterobiasis.* High cure rates have been achieved after single-dose treatment. Similarly, high rates of cure have been achieved against *Ancylostoma, Necator americanus,* and *Trichostrongylus.*

PYRVINIUM PAMOATE

Early studies in experimental infection showed that a series of cyanine dyes possessed marked antifilarial activity (Welch *et al.*, 1947; Peters *et al.*, 1949). One of these, *pyrvinium chloride,* was reported to be active against canine ascarids, trichurids, and hookworm. Weston and associates (1953) first observed that the drug was highly effective against pinworm infections of mice and rats. Its activity against human pinworm infections was confirmed by Royer (1956) and Sawitz and Karpinski (1956). The chloride, however, produced nausea, abdominal pain, and vomiting, and was later replaced by the pamoate.

Chemistry. The structural formula of pyrvinium is as follows:

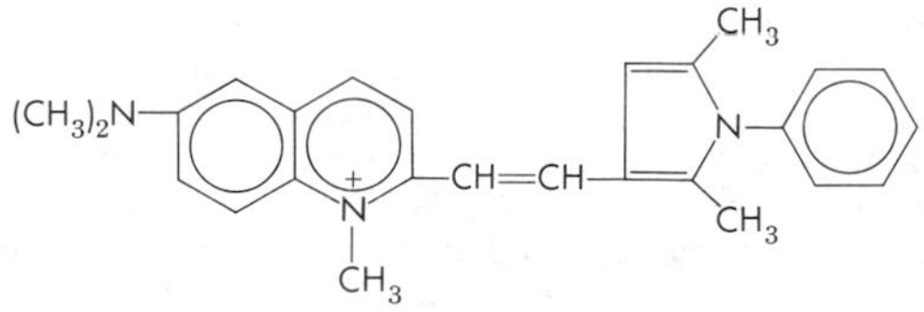

Pyrvinium

Pyrvinium pamoate is a deep-red crystalline solid, insoluble in water.

Anthelmintic Action. Inhibition of oxygen uptake of adult *Litomosoides* is effected by many compounds containing the amidinium ion system, in which a quaternary nitrogen is separated from a tertiary nitrogen by a resonating carbon chain of alternating double and single bonds. This respiratory inhibition is associated with a compensatory increase in aerobic glycolysis. Concentrations of cyanine dyes a thousand times greater than those exerting an inhibitory effect on the respiration of *Litomosoides* have no effect on the oxygen uptake of mammalian tissues or on the activities of cytochrome *c* or of cytochrome oxidase. In *Trichuris vulpis,* dog whipworms, cyanine dyes in low concentrations interfere with the anaerobic transport of exogenous glucose; this effect is not seen with *L. carinii.* The dependence of *T. vulpis* on anaerobic metabolism is suggested not only by the low oxygen tension of its habitat, the colon of the dog, but also by the fact that the motility of the parasite is not reduced during incubation for 24 hours in an atmosphere of nitrogen. Hence, the anthelmintic activity of these compounds is associated with inhibition of respiration in aerobes, and interference with the absorption of exogenous glucose in intestinal helminths. Such interference may account for the anthelmintic effects of the cyanines in trichuriasis and in other intestinal helminthiases.

Standen (1963) has reviewed the effects of pyrvinium pamoate on helminth infections in man and animals. It possesses a marked oxyuricidal action. In trials against *Trichuris* and *Necator* in man, however, repeated treatments gave unimpressive results.

Absorption. When given by the oral route, pyrvinium pamoate is not absorbed from the gastrointestinal tract to any appreciable extent.

Preparations, Route of Administration, and Dosages. *Pyrvinium Pamoate,* U.S.P. (POVAN, VANQUIN), is available as a suspension containing the equivalent of 10 mg of pyrvinium base per milliliter, and as tablets each containing the equivalent of 50 mg of pyrvinium base. For control of *pinworm infection* in children and adults, pyrvinium pamoate is given orally in a single dose equivalent to 5 mg of pyrvinium base per kilogram of body weight, up to a maximum of 350 mg. A second dose should be administered 2 weeks later, to eliminate worms that have developed from ova ingested after the first dose. As in the case of piperazine, occupants of an entire household may be treated rather than investigating each member by anal swabs. Investigations on the effect of this drug on *strongyloidiasis* have shown promising results. In one series, doses from 2 to 6.4 mg/kg, given daily for 7 days, resulted in a high proportion of cures. Doses of 5 mg/kg, administered for 5 days, cured a smaller proportion but reduced considerably the worm burden in the remainder. Because of the staining quality of the drug, the tablets should be swallowed immediately without chewing. Parents and patients should be informed that the drug will color the stools a bright red, and that the suspension, if spilled, will stain.

Toxicity and Side Effects. Pyrvinium pamoate is well tolerated; the side effects are minimal and should not interfere with therapy. Side effects reported in a small proportion of treated patients included nausea, vomiting, and cramping; the majority of these patients were older children or adults who had received a relatively large dose of either suspension or tablets. Emesis was the most frequent side effect associated with the suspension, but it did not occur in patients who were given tablets.

Therapeutic Uses. Pyrvinium pamoate is an effective alternative drug in treating oxyuriasis. A high cure rate has been achieved following single-dose therapy. However, because of the considerable risk of reinfection, chemotherapy should be combined with vigorous sanitation procedures and a follow-up examination for eggs at the anus at least 5 weeks after the end of treatment. Its usefulness against strongyloidiasis has been established, but at least 7 days of therapy appears necessary to effect a high proportion of cures. Results obtained in combating infections by *Trichuris* and *Necator* are unimpressive.

TETRACHLOROETHYLENE

Although *tetrachloroethylene* replaced carbon tetrachloride as an anthelmintic because of the toxicity of the latter, its physical properties are much like those of carbon tetrachloride. However, the drug is only one fifth as soluble in water and, in the absence of fat in the intestine, it is not absorbed to an appreciable extent. This probably accounts for its relatively low toxicity. Tetrachloroethylene is useful in the treatment of hookworm infections. However, since more effective and less toxic agents are now available, the drug is now seldom used in the United States. For a fuller description of its properties, *earlier editions* of this textbook should be consulted.

TETRAMISOLE AND LEVAMISOLE

Tetramisole (ANTHELVET, RIPERCOL) was introduced into veterinary practice in 1966 as a nematocidal agent, and it has subsequently been used for the treatment of infections in man. The *l* isomer is more active than the racemic mixture, and it is now marketed separately in some countries as *levamisole* (KETRAX). It has the following structural formula:

Levamisole

The substance is highly active against a wide range of nematodes. The primary anthelmintic action of levamisole is due to ganglionic stimulation, which produces a rapid, reversible muscular paralysis. It also inhibits fumarate reductase in higher concentrations, and this may contribute to its anthelmintic effect.

There is unanimity about the effectiveness of levamisole in *ascariasis.* A single oral dose of 120 to 150 mg is well tolerated and produces a very high incidence of cure. The drug is moderately effective for hookworm disease at higher dosage.

Levamisole has been shown, in both experimental animals and man, to be an immunostimulant (*see* Renoux, 1978), and it has been used as an adjunct for therapy of malignancies (*see* Chirigos, 1978). It appears to act by restoring cell-mediated immune mechanisms in peripheral leukocytes; precursor T lymphocytes are also stimulated to differentiate into mature T cells.

THIABENDAZOLE

Thiabendazole was the product of investigation of several hundred substituted benzimidazole compounds. Some of these are among the most potent chemotherapeutic agents known, complete larvicidal activity being manifested *in vitro* at 10 pg/ml. This potency, coupled with the absence of activity toward other microorganisms and negligible mammalian toxicity, suggests a unique interference with a metabolic pathway essential to a variety of helminths (Brown *et al.*, 1961). The drug has been reviewed at length in a symposium (*see* Symposium, 1969b).

Chemistry. Thiabendazole has the following structural formula:

Thiabendazole

The drug occurs as a stable, white crystalline compound. It is almost insoluble in water but readily soluble in dilute acid or alkali.

Anthelmintic Action. Thiabendazole is reported to possess a high degree of activity against a wide range of nematodes that infect the gastrointestinal tract of domestic animals and to be larvicidal *in vitro* at very high dilution (Brown *et al.*, 1961; Standen, 1963). A concentration of 1 ppm has been shown to prevent the embryonic development of *Ascaris* eggs *in vitro* (Egerton, 1961). Its mechanism of action is unknown, although the compound inhibits the helminth-specific enzyme fumarate reductase. Of particular interest are the reports that thiabendazole kills larvae in the muscle of pigs experimentally infected with *Trichinella spiralis*. Several cases of human trichinosis have been treated with thiabendazole and have shown marked clinical improvement. However, in some patients biopsy of deltoid muscle after comple-

tion of a course of treatment has revealed actively motile larvae. Generally the drug seems to allay symptoms and reduce eosinophilia, but its effect on larvae that have migrated to muscle is questionable. Anti-inflammatory, antipyretic, and analgesic effects, demonstrated in laboratory animals, may have contributed to the clinical responses. Thiabendazole has no effect on *filariasis*. It is active *in vitro* against a variety of *saprophytic and pathogenic fungi,* particularly against strains of *Trichophyton* and *Microsporum.* Clinically, however, response to treatment of superficial fungal infections has been equivocal.

Absorption, Fate, and Excretion. After oral administration of thiabendazole in man, absorption is rapid. Peak concentrations in plasma occur about 1 hour after treatment. Most of the drug is excreted in the urine within 24 hours as 5-hydroxythiabendazole, conjugated either as the glucuronide or as the sulfate.

Preparations, Route of Administration, and Dosage. *Thiabendazole*, U.S.P. (MINTEZOL), is available as an oral suspension containing 500 mg/5 ml, as a topical suspension, and in 500-mg chewable tablets. The drug is preferably given after meals. The maximal daily recommended dose is 3 g. The standard dose for treating all roundworm infections is 25 mg/kg. This is administered twice daily for 1 day for pinworms, and for 2 successive days for all other infections. Single-day courses have been utilized quite successfully for all but the treatment of cutaneous larva migrans and trichinosis. A 2-day course is required in treating the former; this may be repeated in 2 days if active lesions are still present. This condition has been treated successfully by the topical application of thiabendazole. In trichinosis, treatment may be continued for 2 or 3 additional days, according to the response of the patient. For pinworms, the initial course should be repeated 2 weeks later to decrease the likelihood of reinfection due to the presence of viable ova in the environment. In disseminated strongyloidosis, treatment with thiabendazole should be continued for at least 5 days. Thiabendazole may be tried in the treatment of visceral larva migrans at the usual dosage until either the symptoms subside or toxic effects intervene. Since this is usually a self-limiting disease, however, treatment should be restricted to severe cases.

Toxicity and Side Effects. Side effects frequently encountered are anorexia, nausea, vomiting, and dizziness. Less frequently, diarrhea, epigastric distress, pruritus, weariness, drowsiness, giddiness, and headache occur. Side effects that are experienced rarely include tinnitus, collapse, abnormal sensation in the eyes, numbness, hyperglycemia, xanthopsia, enuresis, decrease in pulse rate and systolic blood pressure, and transitory changes in liver function tests. Fever, facial flush, chills, conjunctival injection, angioneurotic edema, lymphadenopathy, perianal rash, and skin rash occur infrequently, but it is not certain whether these represent hypersensitivity to the drug, hypersensitivity to the parasite, or a manifestation of the disease. Appearance of live *Ascaris* in the mouth and nose has been reported on rare occasions. Some patients may excrete a metabolite that imparts an odor to urine. This is much like that occurring after ingestion of asparagus, and is noted during and for about 24 hours after completion of therapy. Crystalluria without hematuria has been reported on occasion; it promptly subsides with discontinuation of therapy. Transient leukopenia has been noted in a few patients on thiabendazole therapy.

It has been reported that up to one third of patients treated with the recommended dosage have been incapacitated for several hours by one or more symptoms; half were incapacitated for as long as 24 hours by doses of about 50 mg/kg.

Precautions and Contraindications. There are no absolute contraindications to the use of thiabendazole. Because CNS side effects occur quite frequently, activities requiring mental alertness should be prohibited during therapy. Since thiabendazole has hepatotoxic potentialities, it should be used with caution in patients with hepatic disease or decreased hepatic function. No special diet or purgation is needed.

Therapeutic Uses. Administration of thiabendazole is a major advance in the therapy of *S. stercoralis* infections and of *cutaneous larva migrans.* A 2-day course of treatment produces a better-than-90% cure rate in strongyloidiasis. Pseudohookworm infection (*trichostrongyliasis*) also responds well. In the United States its use for this purpose, for *strongyloidosis,* and for *dracontiasis* is considered investigational. The majority of patients experience marked relief of symptoms of creeping eruption. Progression of the disease should cease after 2 successive days of treatment. If active lesions persist after a 2-day interval, a second course of treatment is recommended. There is circumstantial evidence that the drug is also beneficial in the treatment of *visceral larva migrans.* Although thiabendazole is effective against *trichinosis* in ani-

mals, its value in the human disease is as yet unproven. It seems to allay symptoms and to reduce eosinophilia, but its effect on larvae that have migrated to muscle is open to doubt. Thiabendazole produces a cure rate of more than 90% in *enterobiasis* and a lesser, and more variable, rate in *ascariasis* and *hookworm disease.* The efficacy of the drug against *whipworm* varies greatly, depending on the size of the dose and the duration of treatment. A single 2-day course of treatment produces up to 35% cures. An advantage of thiabendazole is its effectiveness against *Ascaris, Enterobius, Strongyloides,* and *Trichuris* and, consequently, its usefulness in patients with multiple infections.

ANTIMONY COMPOUNDS

Trivalent antimonials are used in the treatment of *trematode* infections, while the pentavalent antimonial sodium stibogluconate is used to treat leishmaniases, which are protozoal infections (*see* Chapter 47). The following discussion relates only to the uses of antimony compounds in helminthiasis.

Anthelmintic Action. Trivalent antimonials inhibit phosphofructokinase in schistosomes. This enzyme catalyzes the rate-limiting step in the glycolytic pathway. The inhibition of phosphofructokinase activity can be reversed by increasing the concentration of fructose-6-phosphate and removing the antimony from the supporting medium. This reversibility manifests itself during treatment of the host with subcurative doses of antimonials. Initially the schistosomes migrate from mesenteric veins to the liver, and egg production ceases. After termination of treatment, however, the worms eventually recover and shift back to the mesenteric veins. Mammalian phosphofructokinase is much less sensitive (nearly 100-fold) to the action of antimonials, and, therefore, the chemotherapeutic usefulness of antimonials in schistosomiasis is due, in part at least, to differences in the nature of these two enzymes (*see* Saz and Bueding, 1966; Bueding and Schiller, 1968).

Absorption, Distribution, and Excretion. Antimony compounds are only slowly absorbed from the gastrointestinal tract. Moreover, they cause marked irritation of the intestinal mucosa. Consequently, they are given only parenterally.

Trivalent and pentavalent antimonials differ greatly in their distribution and excretion. The trivalent compounds have a high affinity for cells. Consequently, they rapidly leave the plasma but remain in the circulation bound in some manner to erythrocytes, where they interfere with the function of hemoglobin. Comparatively little is known of the distribution of trivalent antimony in the tissues of man. In animals, abnormally high concentrations are found in the liver and the thyroid.

The trivalent antimonials are excreted for the most part by the kidney. Renal excretion is slow, presumably because of the low plasma concentrations. Therefore, following a single therapeutic dose of a trivalent antimonial, only about 10% is recovered in the urine within 24 hours, and only about 30% within a week. As a result, when antimonials are given in courses, the patient is usually in positive antimony balance; plasma and erythrocyte concentrations and urinary excretion increase progressively so that as much as 50% of the preceding dose of antimony may be excreted within 48 hours. When injections are discontinued, plasma and erythrocyte concentrations fall slowly, and antimony can still be detected in the urine after 100 days.

The pentavalent antimonials are not bound by erythrocytes and attain much higher plasma concentrations than do the trivalent compounds. Consequently, they are excreted more rapidly by the kidney. As much as 50% of a pentavalent antimonial may appear in the urine in the 24 hours following a single injection. When the drug is given in courses, the plasma concentration and the urinary excretion both rise, but the patient remains in positive antimony balance. Small amounts of pentavalent antimony are reduced to trivalent antimony in the liver.

Toxicity. Certain untoward reactions to antimonials are elicited much more frequently by the trivalent than by the pentavalent compounds and appear most often during therapy with antimony potassium tartrate (tartar emetic). Severe coughing, sometimes associated with vomiting, is likely to develop immediately after intravenous injection. Pneumonia is not an unusual sequel to a therapeutic course of tartar emetic. It is definitely a reaction to the drug and not a complication of the disease being treated. It has not been encountered in the use of pentavalent compounds. Pains in the joints and muscles are common; they do not occur, however, until near the end of a therapeutic course. Acute arthritis is a less common reaction. It generally involves the wrist, knee, and ankle joints. Marked bradycardia occasionally occurs late in a course of antimony therapy. It necessitates the discontinuation of medication. ECG studies in patients receiving medication with trivalent antimonials reveal significant changes during therapy in a high percentage of individuals. These are unassociated with cardiovascular symptoms and disappear within 30 to 60 days after cessation of therapy. Miscellaneous untoward reactions are headache, fainting, dyspnea, apnea, facial edema, abdominal pain, vascular collapse, and mild rashes. Hepatic function may be somewhat depressed during treatment and for several months after its cessation. Hepatitis is a rare but serious reaction and necessitates immediate cessation of medication. An anaphylactoid response, characterized by urticarial rash, husky voice, and, in severe cases, collapse, may be encountered after the sixth or seventh injection in a therapeutic course. Hemolytic anemia, sometimes fatal, may occasionally occur during treatment with stibophen.

ANTIMONY POTASSIUM TARTRATE

Antimony potassium tartrate was introduced in 1918 as the first of the trivalent antimony compounds to be used in the treatment of schistosomiasis.

Chemistry. Antimony potassium tartrate has the following structural formula:

Antimony Potassium Tartrate

The compound occurs as colorless crystals or as a granular powder containing 36.5% trivalent antimony. It is soluble 1 : 12 in water. Such solutions are stable and may be sterilized by autoclaving or filtration.

Preparations, Routes of Administration, and Dosage. *Antimony Potassium Tartrate*, U.S.P. (*tartar emetic*), is available in crystalline form or in sterile solution in ampuls. The drug is normally administered intravenously, and such treatment is started with 8 ml of a 0.5% solution. If this is well tolerated, subsequent doses are given on alternate days, each dose being increased by 4 ml until the maximal single dose of 28 ml has been reached. A course normally consists of a maximum of 360 ml of the solution.

Precautions and Contraindications. Tartar emetic must be given very slowly by means of a fine needle, and care should be taken to avoid leakage into the perivascular tissue. Too rapid injection may produce a hacking cough, vomiting, and severe or even fatal reactions. The use of antimony potassium tartrate is contraindicated in the presence of severe hepatic, renal, or cardiac insufficiency.

Therapeutic Uses. Antimony potassium tartrate has been used effectively against all three species of *Schistosoma*. Its use against *S. haematobium* and *S. mansoni* has largely been replaced by more easily employed and less toxic schistosomicides. It remains, however, the drug of choice against *S. japonicum*, which is relatively less susceptible to other agents. For cure of this infection, a total of 500 ml of 0.5% solution has been used. The drug has also proven valuable in the treatment of *granuloma inguinale*. A small percentage of patients have shown marked improvement after treatment of *mycosis fungoides* with antimony potassium tartrate.

ANTIMONY SODIUM TARTRATE

This compound possesses the same schistosomicidal activity as the potassium salt, but it is claimed to be rather less toxic. Nevertheless, the same precautions must be taken in its use. Antimony sodium tartrate is employed much more widely than the potassium salt in some countries in various parts of the world.

ANTIMONY SODIUM-α,α'-DIMERCAPTO-SUCCINATE (STIBOCAPTATE)

Antimony sodium-α,α'-dimercaptosuccinate was reported by Friedheim and coworkers (1954) and Friedheim (1956) to be as effective as stibophen in the treatment of *S. mansoni* and *S. haematobium* infections and to be less toxic. Subsequent trials have shown high cure rates against both species. It is effective in a smaller proportion of cases of *S. japonicum*.

Chemistry. Antimony sodium-α,α'-dimercaptosuccinate has the following structural formula:

Antimony Sodium Dimercaptosuccinate

It is a white crystalline substance, readily soluble in water. The aqueous solution is unstable and should be used within 24 hours; if refrigerated, the solution may be used as long as it remains colorless and transparent.

Preparation, Route of Administration, and Dosage. The drug is supplied as a white crystalline powder in ampuls, each containing 0.5 g. The trade name is ASTIBAN. It is prepared for injection by adding 5 ml of water to the ampul, to give a 10% solution. In the United States the compound is available from the Parasitic Diseases Division, Center for Disease Control, Atlanta, Georgia 30333.

The drug should be given intramuscularly in a course of five injections, at the rate of one or two per week. Particularly fit hospitalized patients may be given injections on alternate or even on consecutive days with a pause of 1 or 2 days after any injection, if necessary, according to tolerance. The total dose in adults should be between 30 and 50 mg/kg, with a maximum of 2.5 g. In children under 20 kg, total doses of 40 to 60 mg/kg may be given. The higher doses are indicated in *S. mansoni* and *S. japonicum* infections. There is some evidence that better therapeutic results, greater activity, and less intolerance are obtained if the injection is given once or twice weekly, rather than on 5 consecutive days. Patients with heart disease of various etiologies have been treated successfully and without apparent harm with a total of 50 mg/kg, divided into five weekly intramuscular injections. In areas with highly endemic schistosomiasis, Friedheim and de Jongh (1959) and others have shown that "suppressive management" of *S. haematobium* infections may be achieved by the monthly injection of the drug. Such treatment, while not providing radical cure, may suppress the production of eggs by the female parasites and thereby interrupt transmission. Ata and Mousa (1961) have used antimony potassium tartrate and stibophen, given weekly, to the same end. Antimony sodium-α,α'-dimercaptosuccinate is ineffective in the "suppressive management" of *S. mansoni* infections.

Precautions and Contraindications. The appearance of rashes, excessive vomiting, pronounced fatigue, and pyrexia is an indication for temporary suspension of treatment. The drug is contraindicated in the presence of bacterial as well as *herpes simplex* and *zoster* infections; in patients with hepatic, renal, or cardiac insufficiency; and if treatment with antimonials has been carried out within the previous 2 months. It is also contraindicated if there is massive infection with intestinal helminths.

STIBOPHEN

Chemistry. Stibophen has the following structural formula:

Stibophen

The drug occurs as colorless crystals that are freely soluble in water. It is stable in solution after autoclaving but may dissociate and become toxic after prolonged storage. Stibophen oxidizes when the solution is exposed to air for any length of time; hence, unused portions of opened ampuls should be discarded.

Preparation, Route of Administration, and Dosage. Stibophen (FUADIN) is available in ampuls, each containing 300 mg in 5 ml of a 6.3% aqueous solution with 0.1% sodium bisulfite as preservative. Each milliliter contains the equivalent of 8.5 mg of trivalent antimony. Stibophen is administered intramuscularly. Various dosage schedules are recommended. The best is probably that which best suits local conditions, except in the treatment of *S. japonicum* infections, for which the most intensive course should be instituted.

Conservative Dosage, Slow Therapy. A total volume of 40 ml is given as follows: 1.5 to 2.0 ml as a sensitivity test dose on the first day, 3.5 ml on the second, and 5 ml on the third; thereafter, six further doses of 5 ml each are given at 2- to 3-day intervals. This course should be repeated after 1 or 2 weeks. Some investigators give adults a total dose of 70 ml in 27 days. In these cases, the final 5-ml doses are given every other day for 12 doses.

Conservative Dosage, Rapid Therapy. A total dosage of 34 ml is given in one course of treatment. On the first day, a 2-ml dose is injected in the morning, followed by 4 ml at midday and 4 ml in the afternoon. On the second and third days, a 4-ml dose is injected three times daily. The course should be repeated after 1 or 2 weeks.

Intensive Therapy. A total dose of 100 ml, given over 14 days, has been used in the treatment of infections with *S. japonicum*. On the first, second, and third days, 2, 4, and 6 ml, respectively, are injected, followed by 8 ml daily for 11 days. A cure rate of about 80% may be achieved, but nearly all the patients will suffer from some toxic reactions.

Precautions and Contraindications. To test the susceptibility of the patient, it is advisable that the first dose be small, only 1.5 to 2.0 ml. Inadvertent intravenous injection should be carefully avoided. Treatment should be stopped in the event of recurrent vomiting, progressive albuminuria, severe and persistent joint pain, or intercurrent febrile infection. Blood dyscrasias, particularly thrombocytopenia with or without purpura, should be watched for and treatment stopped if they occur. The use of stibophen is contraindicated in the presence of renal or cardiac insufficiency or hepatic disease, except that caused by schistosomiasis.

Therapeutic Uses. Stibophen is particularly useful in the treatment of *S. haematobium* and *S. mansoni* infections. It can be successfully employed against *S. japonicum,* but the dosage used is of necessity high and patient cooperation is required because of toxic reactions.

TREATMENT OF WORM INFECTIONS

ROUNDWORMS

Ascaris lumbricoides. *Ascaris lumbricoides,* known as the "roundworm," is cosmopolitan. Although cases of ascariasis are not infrequent in temperate climates, the parasite flourishes best in warm localities. In the southern United States, the incidence of ascariasis is high in the children of poorer families.

Treatment. The older, less efficient, and more toxic ascaricides have largely been discarded in favor of more active, less toxic compounds. Both *mebendazole* and *pyrantel pamoate* are, without doubt, agents of first choice. *Piperazine* may also be considered. Cure can be achieved in nearly 100% of cases. If ascariasis is a complication of hookworm infection, great care should be taken in the treatment of the latter to avoid promoting unusual activity of the ascarids. Under such circumstances, the roundworms may block the lumen of the appendix and produce symptoms of appendicitis. They often occlude the common bile duct and occasionally invade the hepatic parenchyma. Perforation of the intestinal wall with subsequent peritonitis may rarely occur. If the worms are stirred to unusual activity, they may form a tangled mass and cause intestinal obstruction. In the treatment of such mixed infections the advantage lies with mebendazole and pyrantel pamoate, since both are effective against *Ascaris* and both species of hookworms. Mebendazole offers a further advantage in that it is also effective against the whipworm. Preference should probably be given to pyrantel pamoate, however, because single-dose treatment is effective and it does not possess the teratogenic potential of mebendazole. Pyrantel pamoate is also effective against *Ancylostoma duodenale,* but such use is considered investigational in the United States. *Bephenium* has been shown to remove or cause a major reduction in the *Ascaris* burden, but its prime indication is in the treatment of hookworm infection.

Hookworm: Necator americanus, Ancylostoma duodenale. These related species are commonly known as the *New World,* or *American, hookworm* and the *Old World hookworm,* respectively. The former species was imported into America from Africa. The parasites flourish chiefly between about latitudes 30° south and 40° north. Distribution much further north, into areas where a similar environment prevails, has been brought about by carriers. Such conditions occur in mines and large mountain tunnels, hence the terms *miner's disease* and *tunnel disease.*

Treatment. Treatment of hookworm disease involves two objectives. The first is to restore the blood values to normal, and the second is to expel the intestinal parasites. Often it is necessary to improve the patient's general condition before it is safe to administer an anthelmintic. Proper diet and iron medication are usually quite effective in this regard, but blood transfusion may occasionally be required. *Mebendazole* and *pyrantel pamoate* are now agents of first choice against both *Ancylostoma duodenale* and *Necator americanus* and have the advantage of effectiveness against roundworms when there is multiple infection. The use of pyrantel against *Ancylostoma* is considered investigational in the United States. Bephenium may also be considered, particularly in concurrent infection with *Ascaris.* However, in patients suffering from water and electrolyte imbalance, bephenium should not be used until these are corrected because of the possibility of vomiting induced by its bitter taste. *Thiabendazole,* while not a drug of first choice in any of the aforementioned infections, has the advantage of being effective in the treatment of all three. In addition, it is effective in the treatment of trichuriasis, oxyuriasis, and strongyloidiasis, and hence is of special value in patients with multiple infections.

Larva migrans or "creeping eruption," penetration of the skin of man by larvae of the dog hookworm *Ancylostoma braziliense,* has been successfully treated with *thiabendazole.*

Whipworm: Trichuris trichiura. Whipworm infection is encountered throughout the world, especially in warm, humid climates. It is frequently found in areas where ascaris and hookworm are endemic. The worm does not usually cause appreciable trouble except in heavily infected young children. Rarely, the worms may lodge in the appendix or may penetrate the bowel wall and give rise to peritonitis. Infected children may exhibit mild toxic symptoms and some degree of anemia.

Treatment. Mebendazole in a dosage of 100 mg twice daily for 3 days is considered the safest and most effective treatment against whipworm. *Thiabendazole* is also effective in an appreciable proportion of cases.

Threadworm: Strongyloides stercoralis.

Strongyloides stercoralis, sometimes called the threadworm or dwarf threadworm, is frequently found in tropical regions, and infection with this worm is common in parts of the southern United States. Similar environmental conditions are often found underground in the mining industry; hence the worm is occasionally found in mines even in temperate zones.

Treatment. Thiabendazole has been shown to be highly effective and is considered by most to be the drug of choice. In disseminated strongyloidosis, administration of thiabendazole should be continued for at least 5 days. *Pyrvinium pamoate* given for 7 days also results in a high proportion of cures.

Pinworm: Enterobius (Oxyuris) vermicularis.

Oxyuris is cosmopolitan. It is the most common helminthic infection in the United States, especially in school children. The systemic symptoms caused by this parasite are mild and often unnoticed. Pruritus in the perianal and perineal regions, however, is especially severe and irritating, and scratching may cause infection. In female patients, the worms may wander into the genital tract and can then penetrate into the peritoneal cavity. Salpingitis or even peritonitis may occur. Because of the ease with which the infection is distributed throughout the members of a family, a school, or an institution, the physician must decide whether to treat all persons in close contact with an infected person. The possibility of reinfection demands a rigid standard of personal hygiene, such as keeping nails short, washing hands before meals, and changing cotton undergarments twice a day. Pruritus can be treated symptomatically. It is important also to wash bedroom and bathroom floors at the end of the course of treatment. It is necessary to remember that the time required for development from the egg that is swallowed to the emergence of the sexually mature worm from the anus or to the laying of eggs by the worm is at least 35 days. For this reason it is necessary, in order to prove cure, to show that no eggs can be found at the anus during a period of at least 5 weeks after the end of treatment.

Treatment. Mebendazole and *pyrantel pamoate* are equally effective. When their use is allied with rigid standards of personal hygiene, a very high proportion of cures can be obtained. Treatment is simple and almost devoid of side effects. Mebendazole should not be used during pregnancy because of its teratogenic potential. Some have employed a single dose of *piperazine* combined with a laxative. Satisfactory results have been claimed. However, daily doses of piperazine for 1 week is a more usual course of treatment. Pyrantel pamoate, mebendazole, and piperazine have the added advantage of successfully clearing concurrent *Ascaris* infection. Also, a single dose of *pyrvinium pamoate* has been shown to produce a high proportion of cures, but its use may be associated with mild-to-severe vomiting. It will also stain clothing or other absorbent material. *Thiabendazole* has also been used as successfully, but associated with its use has been an appreciable incidence of side effects.

Trichinella spiralis.

The trichina worm does not live at any time outside a host and is found all over the earth, regardless of climate. It is found frequently in Canada, Eastern Europe, and the United States. The only mode of infection is the eating of raw, or insufficiently cooked, flesh of trichinous animals. All pork, not forgetting pork sausages, should be thoroughly cooked before being eaten. The encysted larvae are killed by exposure to a temperature of 60° C for 5 minutes.

Treatment. Corticosteroids are of considerable value in controlling the acute and dangerous systemic manifestations of established infection. Persons with mild cases may be ill only for a few days. The indefinite symptoms of fever, headache, muscle pain, and weakness seldom lead to a diagnosis of trichinosis. *Thiabendazole,* in well-tolerated doses, has been shown to kill *Trichinella* larvae in the muscle of experimental animals. In human cases, results have been variable. It appears to allay symptoms and to reduce eosinophilia, but its effect on larvae that have migrated to muscle is questionable. *Mebendazole* has been shown to kill encysted larvae in experimental animals. Clinical experience with mebendazole for this purpose is very limited.

Filariae: Wuchereria bancrofti.

Infection with this species is especially a risk in Central Africa, South America, India, and southern China. It is found also in the Mediterranean region of southern Spain, Tangier, the Nile Delta, and Turkey; in the Transvaal; and in Brisbane in Australia. The subspecies, *W. bancrofti var. pacifica,* which does not appear periodically in the peripheral blood of man, is found only in New Guinea and the islands of the Central and South Pacific.

Wuchereria (*Brugia*) *malayi* is restricted to Indonesia, the Malay peninsula, Vietnam, southern China, central India, and Ceylon. The migrating filaria, *Loa loa,* is a purely African species. It is found chiefly in western Central Africa, from Sierra Leone to Angola, and chiefly in the region of the large rivers, the Congo, the Niger, the Wellé, and the Ogowé.

Treatment. Although organic antimonials and arsenicals have been shown to have more effect in filariasis, *diethylcarbamazine* is the only agent that should be considered for both suppression and cure. It is advisable to start with a small initial dose to diminish the tendency to allergic reactions resulting from destruction of the microfilariae, particularly those of *Loa loa.* Prophylactic administration of *antihistamines* may diminish the severity of these reactions but will not abolish them altogether. *Corticosteroids* may be required to control acute reactions. In rare instances, serious cerebral allergic reactions have been observed in the treatment of loiasis, probably due to destruction of microfilariae in the brain. If headache is severe or if there is other evidence of an adult *Loa loa* near the orbit, extra care is advisable in initial dosing. The most satisfactory results are achieved in *W. bancrofti* and *W. malayi* infections if treatment is started early, before obstructive lesions in the lymphatics have occurred. Even in late cases, however, improvement may result. In long-standing *elephantiasis,* surgical measures are required to improve lymph drainage and remove redundant tissue.

Onchocerca volvulus. This filarial worm is very common all over West and Central Africa. It was presumably imported from there into Mexico, northeastern Venezuela, and Guatemala.

Treatment. Migrating microfilariae in the skin in onchocerciasis can readily be eliminated by treatment with *diethylcarbamazine.* Allergic reactions, however, are likely to be even more severe than those occurring in the treatment of *Loa loa.* Great care should be exercised in initial dosing, particularly in cases where lesions of the eye are present (*see* above). The adult worms have low susceptibility to the action of the drug. Elimination of adult worms can be achieved by the administration of *suramin* following the schedule recommended by the World Health Organization's Expert Committee on Onchocerciasis (1954). The committee recommended an intravenous dose of 1 g, given weekly for 5 weeks. One fourth of this dose should be given initially to test for intolerance in the patient. Other workers have continued weekly treatment to a total of 10 weeks. Suramin acts principally on the adult female worms; these die or degenerate by the fourth or fifth week of treatment. The male adults are more resistant and remain alive and motile much longer than do the females. In the longer course of treatment, the ova and embryos are destroyed by the sixth to the tenth week. Later, the free microfilariae are also killed. The reaction to suramin is similar to that provoked by diethylcarbamazine, but it appears much later and is more prolonged and less severe. Suramin may therefore be used after a course of diethylcarbamazine or as the initial treatment to destroy the adult worms and to eradicate the infection. However, since the infection is not dangerous to life and dangerous side effects may follow the prolonged administration of suramin (*see* Chapter 47), treatment should not be lightly undertaken.

Guinea Worm. *Dracunculus medinensis,* also known as the *dragon* or *Medina* worm, occurs in East and West Africa, India, Pakistan, Bangladesh, Arabia, and Iraq.

Treatment. Traditional treatment is to draw the adult worm out alive. Natives do this by rolling it onto a small piece of wood, drawing out a little of it day by day. If it is ruptured by this procedure, severe secondary infections may appear. It is therefore recommended that the site at which the worm has broken through should be continuously washed with water to cause the worm to discharge all the larvae. After this it may be more easily extracted. Alternatively the worm may be removed by incisions along its course, under a local anesthetic. Satisfactory healing with either extrusion of the worm or, if no worm was extruded, complete symptomatic and functional relief has been obtained by the administration of *niridazole.* No local reactions occur if the worm is ruptured on extrusion (*see* Kothari *et al.,* 1968). *Thiabendazole* has also been used with considerable success; such use is considered investigational in the United States. Similar results have been obtained with *metronidazole.* However, more credit is given to the anti-inflammatory properties of the drug than to a direct effect on the adult female worm.

TAPEWORMS

Taenia saginata. *Taenia saginata,* or the beef tapeworm, is the most common form of tapeworm. It is cosmopolitan.

Treatment. Niclosamide is the drug of choice for treatment of infection by *Taenia saginata.* It is very effective, simple to administer, and comparatively free from side effects. Assessment of cure can be difficult because the worm, segments as well as scolex, is usually passed in a partially digested state. Cure can be assumed only if no further segments have been passed by the end of 3 months. The antibiotic *paromomycin* (*see* Chapter 46), given in four doses of 1 g every 15 minutes, is also highly effective. Its use for this purpose, however, is considered investigational in the United States. Dichlorophen is used in some locations other than the United States.

Taenia solium. *Taenia solium,* or pork tapeworm, is also cosmopolitan. An attendant danger of *T. solium* infection, and one that is unique to this type of tapeworm, is that of *cysticercosis,* the harboring of the cysticerci (larvae) in the tissues of the human host. This usually results either from the ingestion of eggs of the parasite, as a result of the contamination of the hands with feces, or from the fact that eggs liberated from a gravid segment may pass upward into the duodenum, where the outer layers are digested. In either case, the free larvae gain access to the circulation and the tissues exactly as in their cycle in the intermediate host, the pig. The seriousness of the symptoms that result depends upon the particular tissue invaded. The usual sites are the brain, orbit, muscles, liver, and lungs.

Treatment. The treatment of infection with *T. solium* is the same as that with *T. saginata.* It is most important, however, that therapy be successful, for there is a small but real danger that the patient may develop cysticercosis. Because of the action of *niclosamide* and *paromomycin,* resulting in partial digestion of the worm, it is obligatory to follow anthelmintic treatment with an adequate purge to clear the bowel before the segments can be digested. Otherwise, autoinfection by the liberated ova may occur. If the scolex is not identified, courses should be repeated at suitable intervals.

Diphyllobothrium latum. *Diphyllobothrium latum,* the fish tapeworm, is a common parasite in many European countries, the Near East, Siberia, northern Manchuria, Japan, and the lake regions of Canada and the United States. In North America the pike is the most common second intermediate host. The eating of inadequately cooked infested fish introduces the larvae into the human intestine. The tasting of foods containing fish during their preparation is another common cause of infection. In countries where infection with fish tapeworm is common, there is a high incidence of megaloblastic anemia, which resembles addisonian pernicious anemia in all respects. This syndrome, which has been termed "bothriocephalus anemia," is especially prevalent in Finland, where in the past, 90% of the population of certain provinces harbored worms. The incidence of megaloblastic anemia in infected individuals has been placed as high as 1 case in 136 carriers. Expulsion of the worm results in a hematological remission.

Treatment. Treatment is again the same as that for *T. saginata.* The presence of eggs in the stool 18 or more days after treatment is indicative of drug failure or reinfection. The use of paromomycin for the treatment of fish tapeworm is considered investigational in the United States.

Hymenolepis nana. *Hymenolepis nana,* the dwarf tapeworm, with its subspecies *H. nana fraterna,* is the smallest of the tapeworms found in the small intestine of man. Children are infected more often than adults. It is cosmopolitan, but infection is more common in warm climates. It is the most frequently occurring tapeworm disease in the southern United States. *Hymenolepis nana* can develop from ovum to mature adult in man without an intermediate host. The cysticerci develop in the villi of the intestine for 3 to 4 days and then regain access to the intestinal lumen. Treatment must therefore be adapted to this form of development.

Treatment. Niclosamide is the agent of choice in North America. Failure of treatment or reinfection is indicated by the appearance of eggs in the stool about 4 weeks after the last dose. High cure rates have also been obtained with *paromomycin,* an investigational drug in this case, given in a dose of 45 mg/kg daily for 5 to 7 days.

FLUKES

Schistosoma haematobium, S. mansoni. Infection with these parasites, commonly known as the *blood flukes,* is termed *schistosomiasis* or *bilharziasis.* The disease is widespread throughout Africa and Brazil. Smaller foci also exist in the Near East.

Treatment. The success of therapy depends upon early diagnosis and prompt treatment. If the disease has reached the chronic stage characterized by tissue change, appropriate treatment will be required in addition to chemotherapy if infection is still present. The drugs of choice differ in the two infections. *Niridazole* is considered to be the best drug by many experts in the treatment of *S. haematobium* infection; others prefer an antimonial. Against *S. haematobium* but not *S. mansoni,* metrifonate has been used with considerable success. The treatment is well tolerated and has become widely used in many parts of East Africa and Egypt. Against *S. mansoni,* the antimonials may be preferred to niridazole. The response to the latter is not as consistently good as it is in the case of *S. haematobium.* The *antimonial tartrates* have been largely replaced by other trivalent antimony compounds because of a high incidence of side effects. Nevertheless, the employment of any of the drugs is complicated by a high incidence of side effects.

More recently, *oxamniquine* has proven extremely valuable in the treatment of *S. mansoni* infection, particularly in South America, where the sensitivity of the strains permits single-dose therapy. The drug has also been used successfully in Africa, but in somewhat greater dosage. It is ineffective against *S. haematobium* but may be given with metrifonate in the treatment of mixed infections. *Praziquantel* has also shown promise against all three species of schistosomes in early clinical trials.

In mass campaigns against both *S. haematobium* and *S. mansoni* in several parts of the world, single-dose intramuscular treatment with *hycanthone* has resulted in a high incidence of cure and reduction in egg output. While the controversy over the possible mutagenic and carcinogenic effects of the drug on the treated population is far from settled, the World Health Organization has found no justification to recommend cessation of its use. The large-scale control of schistosomiasis has been reviewed by the World Health Organization (1973).

Schistosoma japonicum. This species is restricted to East Asia. Treatment of *S. japonicum* infection differs from that of infection by the other species.

Treatment. *Schistosoma japonicum* is apparently insusceptible to *hycanthone* and *metrifonate*. This worm is also less sensitive to the more complex trivalent antimonials; therefore, the tartrates, possessing higher activity albeit greater toxicity for the host, are the agents of choice. *Stibophen* has been used successfully, although a most intensive course of treatment is necessary. Experience with *antimony sodium dimercaptosuccinate* is more limited, but some success has followed its use. There appears to be little consistency in the proportion of patients cured by *niridazole* in various trials. Most investigators are agreed, however, that a course of treatment is followed by a marked reduction in the egg count. *Praziquantel* also has shown promise in early clinical trials.

Paragonimus westermani, P. kellicotti. These two species of *lung fluke* differ morphologically from each other only slightly. *Paragonimus westermani* is prevalent in the Far East, while *P. kellicotti* probably occurs only in the Americas. Infection with lung fluke, species undetermined, has also been reported in West Africa.

Treatment. *Bithionol* (ACTAMER, BITIN) has been used successfully in the treatment of this infection. Patients are given 40 to 50 mg/kg orally, in divided doses on alternate days, for a total of 10 to 15 doses. In all cases, stools and sputum become free of eggs after 2 to 5 days of treatment and remain free for at least 12 months. Patients receiving this drug have experienced photosensitivity reactions, urticaria, and gastrointestinal distress. Bithionol is available from the Parasitic Diseases Division, Center for Disease Control, Atlanta, Georgia 30333. *Chloroquine,* in large doses over an extended period, has also had some success. Treatment with 250 mg three times daily should be continued for 6 weeks.

Clonorchis sinensis. *Clonorchis sinensis,* the *Chinese liver fluke,* is widely distributed in East Asia.

Treatment. There is no drug that will reliably clear infection with *C. sinensis.* Prolonged therapy

with *chloroquine* offers the best chance of success. However, treatment may have to be discontinued because of the side effects of the large doses required. Treatment with 250 mg, three times daily, should be continued for 6 weeks. Follow-up of treated cases for over 1 year will probably show a disappointing proportion of relapses in those apparently cured. Early cases respond quite well to intravenous *antimony sodium tartrate.* The technic outlined for the treatment of schistosomiasis is followed. *Bithionol,* in the regimen outlined under *P. westermani,* may also be tried. In heavy infections, therapy can do no more than reduce the number of invading organisms and hence the severity of symptoms. The closely related *Opisthorchis felineus,* the *cat liver fluke,* may develop equally well in man, dogs, and some other fish-eating mammals. No really reliable drug is known for the treatment of this infection. The therapy outlined for treatment of *C. sinensis* infection could be tried.

Fasciola hepatica. *Fasciola hepatica,* the *large liver fluke,* is relatively rare in man but common in sheep, cattle, goats, and other herbivorous animals throughout the world.

Treatment. *Emetine hydrochloride* is the drug of choice. It is given by deep subcutaneous injection in a daily dose of 1 mg/kg (maximum of 60 mg), for up to 10 days. The precautions necessary in treatment with emetine are outlined in Chapter 46. *Bithionol* has been found to be effective when given in the same dosage as in the treatment of lung fluke.

Fasciolopsis buski. *Fasciolopsis buski,* the giant intestinal fluke, occurs chiefly in Southeast Asia.

Treatment. The older drugs used in the treatment of hookworm infection, *tetrachloroethylene* and *hexylresorcinol,* are very effective against this infection. The value of *bephenium* is not known.

Heterophyes heterophyes, Metagonimus yokogawai, Watsonius watsoni, Gastrodiscus hominis, Echinostoma ilocanum, Echinostoma lindoënsis. These smaller *intestinal flukes,* occurring in various parts of the world, may cause clinical symptoms only if present as massive infections.

Treatment. *Tetrachloroethylene,* given in the usual manner, is effective in the treatment of these infections. *Bephenium* and *niclosamide* are helpful in combating *H. heterophyes.*

Dicrocoelium dendriticum. The small *liver fluke, Dicrocoelium dendriticum,* is primarily a parasite of ruminants, but occasionally it also occurs in man.

Treatment. If massive infection makes treatment necessary, a course of therapy with *emetine* as outlined above should be tried.

Abdallah, A., and Saif, M. The efficacy of N-2'-chloro-4'-nitrophenyl-5-chlorosalicylamide in the treatment of taeniasis. *J. Egypt. Med. Assoc.,* **1961,** *44,* 379–381.

Andrews, P. Praziquantel—a novel schistosomicide. *Parasitology,* **1977,** *75,* XVII–XVIII.

Ata, A. H. A., and Mousa, A. H. The evaluation of treating haematobium schistosomiasis in a controlled population with tartar emetic by the slow method. *J. Egypt. Med. Assoc.,* **1961,** *44,* 695–703.

Aubry, M. L.; Cowell, P.; Davey, M. J.; and Shevde, S. Aspects of the pharmacology of a new anthelmintic: pyrantel. *Br. J. Pharmacol.*, **1970,** *38,* 332–344.

Austin, W. C.; Courtney, W.; Danilewicz, J. C.; Morgan, D. H.; Conover, L. H.; Howes, H. L., Jr.; Lynch, J. E.; McFarland, J. W.; Cornwall, R. L.; and Theodorides, V. J. Pyrantel tartrate, a new anthelmintic effective against infections of domestic animals. *Nature,* **1966,** *212,* 1273–1274.

Bassily, S.; Farid, Z.; Higashi, G. I.; and Watten, R. H. Treatment of complicated schistosomiasis mansoni with oxamniquine. *Am. J. Trop. Med. Hyg.,* **1978,** *27,* 1284–1286.

Batzinger, R. P., and Bueding, E. Mutagenic activities *in vitro* and *in vivo* of five antischistosomal compounds. *J. Pharmacol. Exp. Ther.,* **1977,** *200,* 1–9.

Bekhti, A.; Schaaps, J.-P.; Capron, M.; Dessaint, J.-P.; Santoro, F.; and Capron, A. Treatment of hepatic hydatid disease with mebendazole: preliminary results in four cases. *Br. Med. J.,* **1977,** *2,* 1047–1051.

Brown, H. D.; Matzuk, A. R.; Ilves, I. R.; Peterson, L. H.; Harris, S. A.; Sarett, L. H.; Egerton, J. R.; Yakstis, J. J.; Campbell, W. C.; and Cuckler, A. C. Antiparasitic drugs. IV. 2-(4′-thiazolyl)-benzimidazole, a new anthelmintic. *J. Am. Chem. Soc.,* **1961,** *83,* 1764–1765.

Brugmans, J. P.; Thienpont, D. C.; van Wijngaarden, I.; Vanparijs, O. F.; Schuermans, V. L.; and Lauwers, H. L. Mebendazole in enterobiasis. Radiochemical and pilot clinical study in 1278 subjects. *J.A.M.A.,* **1971,** *217,* 313–316.

Bumbalo, T. S.; Fugazzoto, D. J.; and Wyczalek, J. V. Treatment of enterobiasis with pyrantel pamoate. *Am. J. Trop. Med. Hyg.,* **1969,** *18,* 50–52.

Canzonieri, C. J.; Rodrigues, R. R.; Castillo, H. E.; Ibanez de Balella, C.; and Lucena, M. Ensayos terapéuticos con praziquantel en infecciones por *Taenia saginata* e *Hymenolepis nana. Bol. Chil. Parasitol.,* **1977,** *32,* 41–42.

Chavarria, A. P.; Swartzwelder, J. C.; Villarejos, V. M.; and Zeledon, R. Mebendazole, an effective broad-spectrum anthelmintic. *Am. J. Trop. Med. Hyg.,* **1973,** *22,* 592–595.

Chirigos, M. A. (ed.). *Immune Modulation and Control of Neoplasia by Adjuvant Therapy,* Vol. 7. *Progress in Cancer Research and Therapy.* Raven Press, New York, **1978.**

Chou, T. T.; Bennett, J. L.; Pert, C.; and Bueding, E. Effect of hycanthone and of two of its structural analogs on levels and uptake of 5-hydroxytryptamine in *Schistosoma mansoni. J. Pharmacol. Exp. Ther.,* **1973,** *186,* 408–415.

Clarke, V. de V.; Blair, D. M.; Weber, M. C.; and Garnett, P. A. Dose finding trials of oxamniquine in Rhodesia. *S. Afr. Med. J.,* **1976,** *50,* 1867–1871.

Copp, F. C.; Standen, O. D.; Scarnell, J.; Rawes, D. A.; and Burrows, R. B. A new series of anthelmintics. *Nature,* **1958,** *181,* 183.

Doyen, A.; Léonard, J.; Mbendi, S.; and Sonnet, J. Influence des doses thérapeutique du CIBA 32644-Ba sur l'hématopoïèse des patients atteints de bilharziose et d'amibiase. *Acta Trop. (Basel),* **1967,** *24,* 59–77.

Editorial. Medical treatment for hydatid disease. *Br. Med. J.,* **1979,** *2,* 563.

Egerton, J. R. The effect of thiabendazole upon *Ascaris* and *Stephanurus* infections. *J. Parasitol.,* **1961,** *47,* Sect. 2, 37.

Eyre, P. Some pharmacodynamic effects of the nematocides: methyridine, tetramisole and pyrantel. *J. Pharm. Pharmacol.,* **1970,** *22,* 26–36.

Fayard, C. Ascaridiose et piperazine. Thesis, Paris, **1949.** (Quoted from *Sem. Hop. Paris,* **1949,** *35,* 1778.)

Fierlafijn, E. Mebendazole in enterobiasis. *J.A.M.A.,* **1971,** *218,* 1051.

Foster, R. The preclinical development of oxamniquine. *Rev. Inst. Med. Trop. Sao Paulo,* **1973,** *15,* 1–9.

Friedheim, E. A. H. Le traitement de la bilharziose urinaire à *S. haematobium* par le dimercaptosuccinate d'antimoine (TWSb). *Bull. Soc. Pathol. Exot.,* **1956,** *49,* 1247–1252.

Friedheim, E. A. H., and de Jongh, R. T. The effect of a single dose of TWSb in urinary bilharziasis: suggestions for suppressive management of bilharziasis. *Ann. Trop. Med. Parasitol.,* **1959,** *53,* 316–324.

Friedheim, E. A. H.; Rodrigues da Silva, J.; and Martins, A. V. Treatment of schistosomiasis mansoni with antimony-α,α′-dimercapto-potassium succinate (TWSb). *Am. J. Trop. Med. Hyg.,* **1954,** *3,* 714–727.

Gönnert, R., and Schraufstätter, E. Experimentelle Untersuchungen mit N-(2′-chlor-4′-nitrophenyl)-5-Chlorsalicylamid, einen neuen Bandwurmmittel. I. Mitterlung: Chemotherapeutische Versuche. *Arzneim. Forsch.,* **1960,** *10,* 881–884.

Goodwin, L. G.; Jayewardene, L. G.; and Standen, O. D. Clinical trials with bephenium hydroxynaphthoate against hookworm in Ceylon. *Br. Med. J.,* **1958,** *21,* 1572–1576.

Goodwin, L. G., and Standen, O. D. Treatment of ascariasis with various salts of piperazine. *Br. Med. J.,* **1958,** *1,* 131–133.

Hawking, F.; Sewell, P.; and Thurston, J. P. The mode of action of HETRAZAN on filarial worms. *Br. J. Pharmacol. Chemother.,* **1950,** *5,* 217–238.

Hillman, G. R., and Senft, A. W. Anticholinergic properties of the antischistosomal drug hycanthone. *Am. J. Trop. Med. Hyg.,* **1975,** *24,* 827–834.

Hulbert, P. B.; Bueding, E.; and Hartman, P. R. Hycanthone analogs: dissociation of mutagenic effects from antischistosomal effects. *Science,* **1974,** *186,* 647–648.

Jewsbury, J. M.; Cooke, M. J.; and Weber, M. C. Field trial of metrifonate in the treatment and prevention of schistosomiasis infection in man. *Ann. Trop. Med. Parasitol.,* **1977,** *71,* 67–83.

Katz, N.; Pellegrino, J.; Ferreira, M. T.; Oliveira, C. A.; and Dias, C. B. Preliminary clinical trials with hycanthone, a new antischistosomal agent. *Am. J. Trop. Med. Hyg.,* **1968,** *17,* 743–746.

Katz, N.; Zicker, F.; and Pereira, J. P. Field trials with oxamniquine in a schistosomiasis mansoni–endemic area. *Am. J. Trop. Med. Hyg.,* **1977,** *26,* 234–237.

Kaye, B., and Woolhouse, N. M. The metabolism of oxamniquine, a new schistosomicide. *Ann. Trop. Med. Parasitol.,* **1976,** *70,* 323–328.

Keystone, J. S., and Murdoch, J. K. Mebendazole. *Ann. Intern. Med.,* **1979,** *91,* 582–586.

Kikuth, W.; Gönnert, R.; and Mauss, H. MIRACIL, ein neues Chemotherapeuticum gegen die Darmbilharziose. *Naturwissenschaften,* **1946,** *33,* 253.

Kothari, M. L.; Pardnani, D. S.; and Anand, M. P. Niridazole in dracunculiasis. *Am. J. Trop. Med. Hyg.,* **1968,** *17,* 864–866.

Leopold, G. H.; Diekmann, H.; Nowak, H.; and Patzschke, K. Pharmakokinetik von Praziquantel. *Tropenmed. Parasitol.,* **1977,** *28,* 276.

Mahmoud, A. A. F.; Mandel, M. A.; Warren, K. S.; and Webster, L. T. Niridazole: a potent long-acting suppressant of cellular hypersensitivity. *J. Immunol.,* **1975,** *114,* 279–283.

Mauss, H. Ueber basisch substituierte Xanthon-und Thioxanthon-Abkömmlinge: MIRACIL, ein neues Chemotherapeuticum. *Chemie,* **1948,** *81,* 19.

Miller, M. J.; Krupp, I. M.; Little, M. D.; and Santos, C. Mebendazole. An effective anthelmintic for trichuriasis and enterobiasis. *J.A.M.A.,* **1974,** *230,* 1412–1414.

Omer, A. H. S. Oxamniquine for treating *Schistosoma mansoni* infection in Sudan. *Br. Med. J.,* **1978,** *2,* 163–165.

Pedro, R. de J.; Amato Neto, V.; Rodrigues, M. S. de M.; Magalhaes, L. A.; and Lucca, R. S. Treatment of schistosomiasis mansoni with oxamniquine: present state of our observations. *Rev. Inst. Med. Trop. Sao Paulo,* **1977,** *19,* 130–137.

Peters, L.; Bueding, E.; Valk, A. D., Jr.; Higachi, A.; and Welch, A. D. The antifilarial action of cyanine dyes. I. The relative antifilarial activity of a series of cyanine dyes against *Litomosoides carinii, in vitro* and in the cotton rat. *J. Pharmacol. Exp. Ther.,* **1949,** *95,* 212–239.

Renoux, G. Modulation of immunity by levamisole. *Pharmacol. Ther. [A],* **1978,** *2,* 397–423.

Rogers, E. W. Excretion of piperazine salts in urine. *Br. Med. J.,* **1958,** *1,* 136–137.

Rosi, D.; Peruzzotti, G.; Dennis, E. W.; Berberian, D. A.; Freele, H.; and Archer, S. A new, active metabolite of 'MIRACIL D.' *Nature,* **1965,** *208,* 1005–1006.

Royer, A. Preliminary report on a new antioxyuritic, POQUIL. *Can. Med. Assoc. J.,* **1956,** *74,* 297.

Salaman, J. R.; Bird, M.; Godfrey, A. M.; Jones, B.; Millar, D.; and Miller, J. Prolonged allograft survival with niridazole, azathioprine, and prednisolone. *Transplantation,* **1977,** *23,* 29–32.

Sargent, R. G.; Savory, A. M.; Mina, A.; and Lee, P. R. A clinical evaluation of mebendazole in the treatment of trichuriasis. *Am. J. Trop. Med. Hyg.,* **1974,** *23,* 375–377.

Sawitz, W. G., and Karpinski, F. E. Treatment of oxyuriasis with pyrrovinylquinium chloride (POQUIL). *Am. J. Trop. Med. Hyg.,* **1956,** *5,* 538–543.

Singson, C. N.; Banzon, T. C.; and Cross, J. H. Mebendazole in the treatment of intestinal capillariasis. *Am. J. Trop. Med. Hyg.,* **1975,** *24,* 932–934.

Thienpont, D.; Vanparijs, O.; Niemegeers, C.; and Marsboom, R. Biological and pharmacological properties of flubendazole. *Arzneim. Forsch.,* **1978,** *28,* 605–612.

Thomas, H., and Andrews, P. Praziquantel—a new cestocide. *Pestic. Sci.,* **1977,** *8,* 556–560.

Thomas, H., and Gönnert, R. The efficacy of praziquantel against cestodes in animals. *Z. Parasitenkd.,* **1977,** *52,* 117–127.

Wagner, E. D., and Chavarria, A. P. *In vivo* effects of a new anthelmintic, mebendazole (R-17,635) on the eggs of *Trichuris trichiura* and hookworm. *Am. J. Trop. Med. Hyg.,* **1974,** *23,* 151–153.

Welch, A. D.; Peters, L.; Bueding, E.; Valk, A. D., Jr.; and Higachi, A. A new class of antifilarial compounds. *Science,* **1947,** *105,* 486–488.

Weston, J. K.; Thompson, P. E.; Reinertson, J. W.; Fiskin, R. A.; and Reutner, T. F. Antioxyurid activity, toxicology and pathology in laboratory animals of a cyanine dye, 6-dimethyl-amino-2 (2,5-dimethyl-1-phenyl-3-pyrrol)-vinyl-1-methyl-quinilium chloride. *J. Pharmacol. Exp. Ther.,* **1953,** *107,* 315–324.

White, R. H. R., and Scopes, J. W. A single-dose treatment of threadworms in children. *Lancet,* **1960,** *1,* 256–258.

Wolfe, M. S., and Wershing, J. M. Mebendazole. Treatment of trichuriasis and ascariasis in Bahamian children. *J.A.M.A.,* **1974,** *230,* 1408–1411.

Monographs and Reviews

Brown, H. W. Anthelmintics, new and old. *Clin. Pharmacol. Ther.,* **1968,** *10,* 5–21.

Bueding, E., and Schiller, E. Mechanism of action of antischistosomal drugs. In, *Mode of Action of Antiparasitic Drugs,* Vol. 1. (Rodrigues da Silva, J., and Ferreira, M. J., eds.) Pergamon Press, Ltd., Oxford, **1968,** pp. 81–86.

Hawking, F. Chemotherapy of filariasis. In, *Experimental Chemotherapy,* Vol. I. (Schnitzer, R. J., and Hawking, F., eds.) Academic Press, Inc., New York, **1963,** pp. 893–912.

Katz, M. Anthelmintics. *Drugs,* **1977,** *13,* 124–136.

Keeling, J. E. D. The chemotherapy of cestode infections. *Adv. Chemother.,* **1968,** *3,* 109–152.

Lämmler, G. Chemotherapy of trematode infections. *Adv. Chemother.,* **1968,** *3,* 153–251.

Marsden, P. D. (ed.). *Clinics in Gastroenterology,* Vol. 7, No. 1. W. B. Saunders Co., Ltd., London, **1978,** pp. 1–243.

Saz, H. J., and Bueding, E. Relationships between anthelmintic effects and biochemical and physiological mechanisms. *Pharmacol. Rev.,* **1966,** *18,* 871–894.

Standen, O. D. Chemotherapy of helminthic infections. In, *Experimental Chemotherapy,* Vol. I. (Schnitzer, R. J., and Hawking, F., eds.) Academic Press, Inc., New York, **1963,** pp. 701–892.

Symposium. (Various authors.) The pharmacological and chemotherapeutic properties of niridazole and other antischistosomal compounds. *Ann. N.Y. Acad. Sci.,* **1969a,** *160,* 423–946.

Symposium. (Various authors.) Thiabendazole. *Tex. Rep. Biol. Med.,* **1969b,** *27,* 533–708.

Symposium. (Various authors.) Symposium on common parasitic diseases. (Zaman, V., ed.) *Drugs,* **1978,** *15,* Suppl. 1, 1–110.

Van den Bossche, H. Biochemical effects of the anthelmintic drug mebendazole. In, *Comparative Biochemistry of Parasites.* (Van den Bossche, H., ed.) Academic Press, Inc., New York, **1972,** pp. 139–157.

Webster, L. T.; Butterworth, A. E.; Mahmoud, A. A. F.; Mngola, E. N.; and Warren, K. S. Suppression of delayed hypersensitivity in schistosome-infected patients by niridazole. *N. Engl. J. Med.,* **1975,** *292,* 1144–1147.

World Health Organization. *Report of the Expert Committee on Onchocerciasis.* Technical Report No. 87, WHO, Geneva, **1954.**

———. *Report of the Expert Committee on Filariasis.* Technical Report No. 359, WHO, Geneva, **1967.**

———. *Report of the Expert Committee on Schistosomiasis Control.* Technical Report No. 515, WHO, Geneva, **1973.**

CHAPTER

45 DRUGS USED IN THE CHEMOTHERAPY OF MALARIA

Ian M. Rollo

In order to understand the actions and uses of antimalarial drugs, it is necessary to appreciate the basic features of the biology of the malarial infection and the major principles and objectives of its treatment, including the problem of multidrug-resistant strains of plasmodia. Accordingly, these aspects will be presented before the pharmacology of the individual drugs is considered.

The chief agents employed in malaria therapy are *chloroquine* and its congeners, inhibitors of dihydrofolate reductase such as *pyrimethamine* and *chloroguanide, primaquine,* and *quinine.* Sulfonamides, sulfones, and tetracyclines are also used concurrently with certain of these drugs. *Quinacrine,* a prior mainstay of antimalarial suppression and treatment, is now obsolete for this purpose, but it does have some uses in other infections. It has been replaced by chloroquine, the most important antimalarial and the prototype of those agents that suppress the malarial infection and control the overt clinical attacks. Quinine, the mainstay of malaria therapy until the 1920s when the more potent synthetic agents became available, remains important because of the prevalence of plasmodial strains that are resistant to many of the newer drugs. The lack of development of such resistance to quinine is ironic in view of the thousands of compounds that have been synthesized in the attempt to free physician and patient from reliance on this relatively toxic natural product.

Of considerable importance has been the development of *in-vitro* technics for the assessment of antimalarial activity with, for example, laboratory malarial strains (Richards and Williams, 1973) and strains of falciparum malaria (Rieckmann *et al.,* 1968; Desjardins *et al.,* 1979a). The opportunity for experimental chemotherapy of human malarias in a nonhuman, laboratory host has been provided by the successful passage of both falciparum and vivax malarias in the owl monkey (*see* World Health Organization, 1973; Schmidt, 1978).

BIOLOGY OF THE MALARIAL INFECTION

Inasmuch as the efficacy of drugs in the prevention and the treatment of malaria is related to the species of infecting parasite and its stage of development, it is essential to review briefly the nature of the malarial infection.

Species of the Genus Plasmodium Infecting Man. (1) *Plasmodium falciparum,* the cause of *malignant tertian* malaria, often produces a fulminating infection in the nonimmune patient; if untreated, the infection may progress rapidly to a fatal termination. Delay in treatment after the demonstration of parasites in the blood may lead to an irreversible state of shock, and death may occur even after the peripheral blood has been cleared of parasites. If treated early, the infection usually responds readily to the administration of effective antimalarial drugs, and relapses will not occur. If treatment is inadequate, however, recrudescence may result from parasites persisting in the blood. (2) *Plasmodium vivax* is the cause of *benign tertian* malaria, which produces milder clinical attacks than those of *P. falciparum* and has a low mortality rate in untreated adults. The infection is characterized by relapses that occur for a period of at least 2 years after primary infection. (3) *Plasmodium malariae* is the cause of *quartan* malaria, an infection that is common in localized areas in the tropics. Relapses do occur but are much rarer than after infection with *P. vivax.* Latent infections of many years' standing may give rise to transfusion-induced malaria. (4) *Plasmodium ovale* is the cause of a rare malarial infection with a periodicity like that of *P. vivax,* but it is milder and more readily cured.

Man is infected by *sporozoites* injected by the bite of infected mosquitoes. The sporozoites disappear rapidly from the circulation and localize in the parenchymal cells of the liver, where they grow, segment, and sporulate. This constitutes the *preerythrocytic stage* of infection, during which the subject remains symptom free. On reaching maturity, *merozoites* are released from the cells of the liver and enter erythrocytes to start the *blood cycle.* In all but falciparum malaria, a proportion of these parasites infects more tissue cells, and this stage of infection, the *exoerythrocytic cycle,* may continue for several

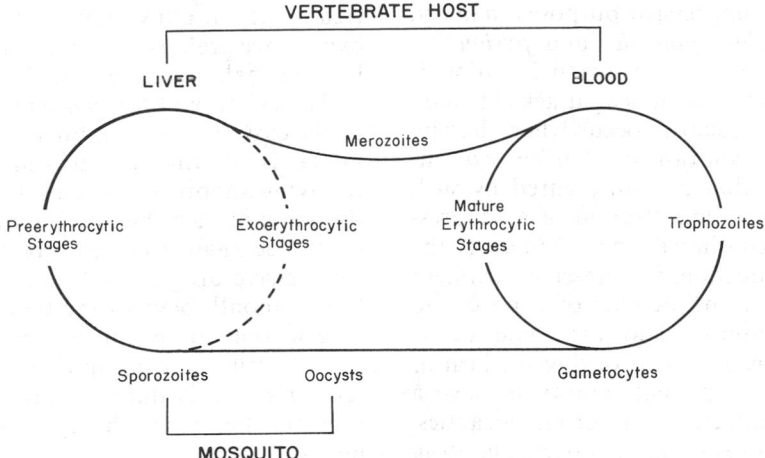

Figure 45-1. *Schematic representation of plasmodial life cycle.* For details, *see* text (———, all malarias; -----, relapsing malarias only). (After Rollo, 1964. Courtesy of Academic Press, Inc.)

years and result in clinical recrudescence or *relapse* in the infected patient. *Schizogony* occurs in the infected erythrocytes as a result of growth and segmentation of the merozoites. When the erythrocyte bursts, the liberated *merozoites* are capable of infecting more red blood cells and of starting the cycle anew. It is this periodic breaking of erythrocytes that causes the chill so characteristic of malaria. The fever following the chill is due to the liberated foreign protein and cell products. For reasons not yet understood, some of the merozoites invading erythrocytes fail to follow the asexual pattern of reproduction. They differentiate into male and female parasites known as *gametocytes*. No further development of these forms occurs until blood is ingested by a female mosquito. In the gut of the mosquito, exflagellation of the male gametocyte is followed by fertilization of the female gametocyte; the resulting *zygote,* developing in the gut wall as an *oocyst,* eventually gives rise to the infective *sporozoite*. The various stages are outlined in Figure 45-1.

CHEMOTHERAPY OF MALARIA IN RELATION TO THE BIOLOGY OF THE INFECTION

The chemotherapy of malaria may be conveniently considered under the following six categories: (1) causal prophylaxis, (2) suppressive treatment, (3) clinical cure or treatment of the acute attack, (4) radical cure, (5) suppressive cure, and (6) gametocytocidal therapy.

Causal Prophylaxis. A causal prophylactic is an agent that prevents demonstrable infection by exerting a lethal effect on the malarial parasites during their preerythro-

cytic stages. Inasmuch as man is his own reservoir of infection, causal prophylaxis also prevents the further transmission of malaria to mosquitoes. To be effective, such therapy must be continued as long as the individual remains in a region where malaria is endemic. The term *true causal prophylaxis* should be reserved for the killing of sporozoites before they can infect the cells of the reticuloendothelium. Unfortunately, no such agent is clinically practical.

Primaquine has causal prophylactic properties, most pronounced against falciparum malaria; unfortunately the possibility of serious side effects makes its use for this purpose unsafe and impracticable. *Chloroguanide* and *pyrimethamine* exert a marked prophylactic effect against falciparum parasites, but they are only partially active against vivax infections.

Suppressive Treatment. Because of the lack of an ideal causal prophylactic agent, attention must be centered on suppressive drug therapy. By suppression is meant the inhibition of the erythrocytic stage of development of the parasites so that the infected individual is kept free of clinical manifestations of the disease. Infection is not prevented by a suppressive drug. The exoerythrocytic stage persists and clinical attacks may supervene at varying intervals after suppressive medication is stopped, particularly in certain types of vivax malaria.

Three particularly effective drugs are

available for suppressive purposes, namely, *chloroquine, chloroguanide,* and *pyrimethamine.* Continued suppressive medication is necessary to prevent clinical attacks in *vivax* infections, and relapses occur when therapy is stopped. In contrast, most *falciparum* infections are rather promptly cured by such treatment; the administration of a suppressive drug is continued only if there is the hazard of reinfection. Suppressive treatment is employed during periods of exposure to infected mosquitoes and for some weeks thereafter. It is also used during medical or surgical crises in patients known to have a latent *vivax* infection. In certain localities, insensitivity or resistance to a particular drug may call for careful selection of the agent to be used.

Clinical Cure. Agents in this category interrupt erythrocytic schizogony of the malarial parasite and in this manner terminate the clinical attack. Such agents are called *schizontocides.* The 4-aminoquinoline derivatives, *chloroquine* and *amodiaquine,* are the drugs of choice. Both vivax and most falciparum malarias respond well. Chloroguanide and pyrimethamine are also highly active schizontocides, but their action is much slower than that of chloroquine. Other differences in therapeutic actions of these drugs are described subsequently. If satisfactory results are not obtained with one of these agents, therapy should be repeated with another. In certain parts of the world, strains of falciparum malaria may be resistant or insensitive to all synthetic antimalarial drugs (*see* above). Under these circumstances recourse must be had to *quinine* or to certain combination therapies to be described later.

Radical Cure. The term *radical cure* refers to eradicating not only the erythrocytic but also the exoerythrocytic parasites of an established infection. The only drugs that accomplish radical cure in *vivax malaria* are the 8-aminoquinoline derivatives, of which only *primaquine* is used now. Usually primaquine is employed concurrently with chloroquine, and a high proportion of cures can be expected (*see* below). Individuals living in endemic areas are not suitable candidates for radically curative therapy because of the considerable likelihood of reinfection. Such

treatment is usually reserved for persons who experience relapsing vivax malaria after leaving malarious regions.

Radical cure of *falciparum malaria* is relatively easy. Proper treatment of the clinical attack is all that is necessary. In persons receiving suppressive medication, mere continuation of such therapy is usually adequate insurance against clinical breakthrough; the suppressive drug should be continued for at least 1 month beyond the time of last exposure to potentially infected mosquitoes. Infection with falciparum sporozoites may recur repeatedly during suppressive medication, but the exoerythrocytic stage does not persist.

Suppressive Cure. The term *suppressive cure* refers to the complete elimination of malarial parasites from the body by continued suppressive treatment, the effect of which is longer than the life-span of the infection. The continued administration of pyrimethamine for 10 weeks after leaving a malarious area has been associated with suppressive cure of certain vivax infections.

Gametocytocidal Therapy. Drugs in this category destroy the sexual forms of malarial parasites in human blood and thereby eliminate the reservoir from which mosquitoes are reinfected. Causal prophylaxis, suppressive therapy, and prompt and adequate treatment of acute clinical attacks all prevent the development or persistence of vivax and falciparum gametocytes. Chloroguanide and pyrimethamine do not destroy gametocytes but prevent their development in mosquitoes. Small doses of primaquine eradicate both vivax and falciparum gametocytes within 3 days. The remaining antimalarial drugs are all effective against *vivax* gametocytes, but *falciparum* gametocytes are quite insensitive.

Mechanisms of Action. Antimalarial agents may be divided rather grossly into two quite distinct groups. The first of these includes the older agents, which may be recognized, even clinically, by the rapidity of their schizontocidal action and the relative difficulty with which resistance to them can be developed by many originally sensitive strains. Their fundamental mechanism of action appears to be, at least in part, not specific for the various species and remains somewhat obscure. Some evidence suggests that the ability of parasite DNA to serve as a template for replication is impaired by intercalation of drug molecules between appropriate base pairs. This occurs with *chloroquine, primaquine,* and *quinine,* but not with *mefloquine* (*see* Thompson and Werbel, 1972; Davidson *et al.,* 1977). Their selective toxicity seems to depend on accumulation of drug in the intracellular milieu of the parasite by means of a metabolically driven membrane-potential gradient or because of the presence of high-affinity binding sites in sensitive parasites (Fitch, 1970; Fitch *et al.,* 1974; Warhurst and Thomas, 1978).

Primaquine differs from the others in being much less active against the erythrocytic stage of the parasite. The fact that it produces much less change in certain properties of native DNA, when bound to it, than do other potent schizontocidal agents may account for this. Its high activity against the exoerythrocytic stages of the parasite is associated with cytological changes at concentrations that leave the host cells unaffected. Mefloquine and other quinoline-methanolamines do not intercalate with DNA and yet retain a high degree of antimalarial activity; multiple mechanisms of action may be important among this group of compounds.

Members of the second group of antimalarials are characterized by a schizontocidal effect that is slow in onset and dependent on the stage of multiplication of the parasite. Resistance to their action can be attained readily in experimental studies, and resistance in the field is not uncommon. Their mechanism of action is much more clearly defined. The biochemical pathway involved is the synthesis of folinic acid from para-aminobenzoic acid (PABA). Agents in this group either interfere with the incorporation of PABA into folic acid, a process that does not occur in mammals, or bind to and inhibit dihydrofolate reductases; such binding to plasmodial dihydrofolate reductase is very strong in comparison with that to the mammalian heteroenzyme (*see* Table 45 1, page 1049, and Chapter 49). This group includes *chloroguanide, pyrimethamine,* and their derivatives (inhibitors of dihydrofolate reductase), as well as *sulfonamides* and *sulfones* (inhibitors of folic acid synthesis). Mechanisms of action are discussed further under the individual drugs.

ACQUIRED RESISTANCE TO ANTIMALARIAL DRUGS

The foregoing section on mechanisms of action defined the two groups of antimalarial drugs partly in terms of the readiness with which resistance to those agents is achieved. As noted, a high degree of resistance to the *pyrimidines* and *biguanides* can be developed quite readily among malarial strains. Resistance to the *cinchona alkaloids* or to the 4- or 8-*aminoquinolines* develops less readily in many strains. Acquired drug resistance should not be confused, however, with insensitivity or natural refractoriness, which has nothing to do with previous exposure to a drug. The amount of quinine required to control primary attacks of Roman and Sardinian strains of *P. falciparum,* for example, is eight times more than is required to control infection with other strains. In these cases there is no evidence to suggest that the refractoriness is the result of selective pressure exerted by the drug.

The development of resistant strains is often due to the commonly accepted mechanism by which the drug acts simply as a selective agent, allowing the overgrowth of resistant mutants that are likely to occur in any large population. The situation may be complicated, however, by the occurrence, in a large population of parasites, of a small proportion of *less susceptible* plasmodia. Under the circumstances of either no treatment or intensive treatment, these would have little or no opportunity to predominate. During mass prophylaxis, however, a reversal of population pressure, due to the presence of only minimal concentrations of drug in the blood of some individuals of the community, would result in the predominance of the insensitive plasmodia and a change in the characteristic of the strain. Such conditions could occur either as a result of underdosage, malabsorption of the drug, or a combination of both.

Whatever the mechanism, and the foregoing presents the problem in the simplest of terms, the end result is the same. Infections appear, usually in distinct geographical areas, that will no longer respond to previously adequate doses of the antimalarial drug being used. Unfortunately, strains resistant to one drug may exhibit cross-resistance to other agents. For this reason, the utmost care should be exercised in the administration of antimalarial drugs in endemic areas. Schemes of mass prophylaxis either in small localities or over large areas should be designed with the possibility always in mind that improper dosage and methods of drug distribution are very likely to result in the emergence of resistant strains.

A high degree of acquired resistance to *chloroguanide* has been demonstrated conclusively in all species of plasmodia where it has been sought; the characteristic appears to be stable. Such strains retain their initial sensitivity to quinine and to 4- and 8-aminoquinoline antimalarials. Chloroguanide resistance of a high degree has occurred in *P. falciparum* found in Southeast Asia, West Africa, India, and elsewhere. Also, clinical evidence has accumulated that various strains of *P. vivax* and *P. malariae* may become resistant to the drug.

In several cases where chloroguanide resistance has developed, field observations have pointed to unduly low or too widely spaced doses as an important causal factor. In many areas of the world the development of resistant strains has seriously compromised the value of chloroguanide as a suppressive agent. West African strains of *P. falciparum* are relatively insensitive to the schizontocidal action of chloroguanide, but this is a *natural insensitivity.*

Resistance to *pyrimethamine* can be induced fairly readily in plasmodia of laboratory animals. Cross-resistance to chloroguanide and its derivatives, but not to any other antimalarial drug used clinically, is generally present. Lack of cross-resistance to sulfadiazine in chick malaria, although sulfadiazine-resistant strains are usually cross-resistant to both chloroguanide and pyrimethamine, led to Rollo's hypothesis (1955) on the mode of action of all three substances. Evidence from these experiments, together with data on synergism and antagonism, suggested that all three substances enter the parasite cell by some common mechanism other than passive diffusion. Cross-resistance, or the lack of it, may be explained by changes in the specificity of the uptake mechanism. Subsequently Ferone (1969) found altered dihydrofolate reductase with lesser affinity for the drug in a pyrimethamine-resistant strain of *P. berghei.*

Strains of *P. falciparum* have become resistant to pyrimethamine in several geographical areas, usually as a result of programs of mass suppression. The experimental production of resistance in *P. vivax* has also been demonstrated (*see* Rollo, 1964). Combinations of *pyrimethamine* with either dapsone or a long-acting sulfonamide have proven effective in suppression and treatment of pyrimethamine-resistant strains of *P. falciparum* and even of multiresistant strains (*see* below).

Resistance to *chloroquine* has become a grave problem in parts of South America and Southeast Asia. Formerly it was considered that chloroquine was one of the available antimalarial drugs to which resistance could not readily be attained. Chloroquine resistance has been associated with a decrease in drug-concentrating capacity of red cells infected with malarial parasites (Macomber *et al.,* 1966) and changes in high-affinity binding sites for the drug (Fitch, 1970).

Despite the widespread use of the drug, chloroquine resistance in the field was not reported until 1961, when Moore and Lanier described falciparum infections in Colombia, relapsing after normally adequate courses of treatment with chloroquine. The strain was normally sensitive to quinine. The strain was also insensitive to congeners of chloroquine, such as amodiaquine and hydroxychloroquine, but remained sensitive to quinine, quinacrine, and pyrimethamine. Since then, resistance to chloroquine has been reported from several parts of South America and Southeast Asia (*see* Powell and Tigertt, 1968) and, more recently, from Africa.

Many chloroquine-resistant falciparum strains are cross-resistant to other 4-aminoquinolines, quinacrine, chloroguanide, and pyrimethamine, and are termed *multiresistant strains.* Not infrequently, even quinine cannot be relied upon to effect a radical cure, although it can usually control the clinical attack. To date, mefloquine has been effective against all such strains. In response to a standard regimen of chloroquine, there is a spectrum of resistance or insensitivity. An initial response that appears to be adequate may be followed sooner or later by a recrudescence. With other strains, parasitemia may decrease but still remain patent, may show no change, or may even increase. The various categories have been characterized by the World Health Organization (1968). Schedules of treatment vary and obviously depend on the strains involved and local experience. Quinine has been the sheet anchor, given parenterally initially in severely ill patients who cannot tolerate oral medication. Against those strains known to respond inadequately to quinine alone, pyrimethamine in combination with either dapsone, sulfadiazine, or a long-acting sulfonamide such as sulfadoxine should be administered. The combination itself, without quinine, is also effective, although initial response to treatment is generally slower than

when quinine is included. A tetracycline given in a course of treatment with quinine has also been found effective. Details of the various regimens have been outlined by the World Health Organization (1973). If current trials confirm the effectiveness of mefloquine when administered alone, it likely will become the agent of choice for suppression and cure of falciparum malaria.

QUINACRINE

Quinacrine is obsolete as an antimalarial drug; nevertheless, it deserves brief mention because of its historical importance in antimalarial chemotherapy. Full descriptions of its properties can be found in *earlier editions* of this textbook. Its use for the treatment of *giardiasis* is described in Chapter 47.

Quinacrine is an acridine derivative introduced for malarial therapy in 1930 mainly as a result of the work of Kikuth. It was first prepared by Mauss and Mietzsch as part of an extensive research program on synthetic antimalarials in Germany, which started when normal supplies of quinine become unavailable during World War I. In World War II, quinine, up to that time the chief antimalarial, was no longer available to the Allies and large-scale production of quinacrine began.

Field experiences gained by the armed forces soon established the superiority of quinacrine over quinine, and quinacrine became the official drug for the treatment of malaria. However, its toxicity and inability to cure benign tertian malaria or to act as a true causal prophylactic provided the incentive for the search for more effective drugs (*see* Wiselogle, 1946).

CHLOROQUINE

History. Chloroquine is one of a large series of *4-aminoquinolines* investigated in connection with the extensive cooperative program of antimalarial research in the United States during World War II. The objective was to discover more effective and less toxic suppressive agents than quinacrine. Although the 4-aminoquinolines had previously been described as potential antimalarials by Russian investigators, serious attention was not paid to this chemical class until the French reported that 3-methyl-7-chloro-4-(4-diethylamino-1-methylbutylamino)quinoline (SN-6911; sontochin, sontoquin) was well tolerated and had high activity in human malarias. Beginning in 1943, thousands of these compounds were synthesized and tested for activity in avian malaria and for toxicity in mammals; ten of the series were then examined in human volunteers with experimentally induced malarias. Of these, chloroquine proved most promising and was released for field trial. When hostilities ceased, it was discovered that the chemical had been synthesized and studied under the name of resochin by the Germans as early as 1934.

Chemistry. Chloroquine has the following structural formula:

Chloroquine

The diphosphate is a white, bitter powder, soluble in water. Its solutions are stable.

Structure-Activity Relationship. Chloroquine contains the same alkyl side chain as quinacrine; it differs from the latter in having a quinoline instead of an acridine nucleus and in lacking the methoxy radical. Chloroquine also bears close resemblance to pamaquine and pentaquine (obsolete 8-aminoquinoline antimalarials); it differs from them in the position of the alkyl side chain and in having a chlorine instead of a methoxy nuclear substituent. The *d, l,* and *dl* forms of chloroquine are indistinguishable in potency tests in duck malaria, but the *d* isomer is somewhat less toxic than the *l* isomer in mammals. The 4-aminoquinolines showing the most marked antimalarial activity in both avian and human malarias have a chlorine atom in position 7 of the quinoline nucleus. Methyl substitution in position 3 of the nucleus reduces activity, and additional methyl substitution in position 8 completely eliminates activity. The details of the structure-activity relationship of chloroquine and its congeners are discussed by Berliner and coworkers (1948) and Coatney and colleagues (1953).

Pharmacological Effects. Although chloroquine was developed primarily as an antimalarial agent, it possesses several other pharmacological properties, some of which are useful. Its anti-inflammatory properties are well known, and the drug (or hydroxychloroquine) is used occasionally in the treatment of *rheumatoid arthritis* and frequently for *discoid lupus erythematosus.* Less well established is its efficacy in *systemic lupus erythematosus* (*see* Dubois, 1978). It has also been employed with success in the treatment of *porphyria cutanea tarda, solar urticaria,* and *polymorphous light eruption.* Treatment of these conditions requires the administration of much larger doses of the drug than are employed in prophylaxis and treatment of malaria, and involves proper consideration of the toxicity of such large amounts.

Antimalarial Actions. Chloroquine exerts no significant activity against the exoerythrocytic tissue stages of plasmodia, even when given in massive doses. The drug is thus not a causal prophylactic agent and does not prevent the establishment of infection. However, it is highly effective against the asexual erythrocytic forms of *P. vivax* and *P. falciparum,* and gametocytes of *P. vivax.* It is superior to quinine and quinacrine in suppressing vivax malarias. In the *acute malarial attack,* it rapidly controls parasitemia and clinical symptoms; most patients become completely afebrile within 24 to 48 hours after administration of therapeutic doses, and thick smears of peripheral blood are generally negative by 48 to 72 hours. With the exception of certain strains in Southeast Asia, Central and South America, Africa, and the Indian subcontinent (extending into adjacent land masses), it completely cures falciparum malaria. Chloroquine, like quinine and quinacrine, does not prevent relapses in vivax malaria, but it substantially lengthens the interval between relapses. Chloroquine is well tolerated and is thus easier to administer than quinine or quinacrine. It differs from quinine and quinacrine in that no therapeutic or toxic synergism is manifested when it is administered with primaquine.

Mechanism of Antimalarial Action. The mechanism of plasmodicidal action of chloroquine is not completely certain. While the drug can inhibit certain enzymes, its effect is believed to result, at least in part, from its interaction with DNA. Schellenberg and Coatney (1960) have shown that chloroquine inhibits the incorporation of ^{32}P-labeled phosphate into RNA and DNA by *P. gallinaceum in vitro* and *in vivo,* and by *P. berghei in vitro.* Subsequent study has demonstrated that chloroquine combines strongly with DNA, but only if it is double stranded. In addition, it inhibits DNA polymerase markedly and RNA polymerase less so, in both cases by combining with the DNA primer (Allison *et al.,* 1965; Cohen and Yielding, 1965). Changes in several physical parameters are consistent with an intercalation of chloroquine between base pairs of the double helix and, furthermore, with the necessary presence of guanine, more particularly its 2-amino group. Stabilization of the double helix is believed to occur by the formation of additional ionic bonds between the substituted amino side chain of chloroquine and the phosphate anions of complementary strands of DNA across the minor groove (Allison *et al.,* 1966). This appears to be a nonspecific reaction affecting vulnerable DNA regardless of its source.

Other studies indicate that chloroquine and related antimalarial drugs cause clumping of the malarial pigment that forms as the parasite digests the hemoglobin of the host erythrocyte. This clumping may in some way disrupt the amino acid metabolism of the parasite and lead to its death (*see* Warhurst *et al.*, 1972; Peters, 1973). Quinine and mefloquine, both effective against chloroquine-resistant strains of malaria, competitively antagonize the clumping produced by chloroquine.

The drug affects both microbial and mammalian cell growth at concentrations of about $10\,\mu M$. *In vitro*, erythrocyte-bound parasites are affected by concentrations of the order of $0.1\,\mu M$. The apparent anomaly can be explained in part by the accumulation of chloroquine within parasitized erythrocytes to the extent of at least two orders of magnitude greater than the concentration occurring outside (Macomber *et al.*, 1966; Polet and Barr, 1968). The usefulness of chloroquine as a selectively toxic agent is due, at least in part, to this preferential accumulation, since parasitized erythrocytes concentrate more of the drug than do most body organs. The mechanism of this accumulation is unclear; hypotheses envision the importance of ionic or potential gradients (Warhurst and Thomas, 1978), sequestration of drug in lysosomes (Homewood *et al.*, 1972), or the participation of high-affinity receptor sites (Fitch, 1970). However, it should be noted that certain tissues of the host can concentrate chloroquine to an even greater extent (*see* below), and other factors may be involved to cause the selective antiplasmodial action of the drug.

Absorption, Fate, and Excretion. Chloroquine is rapidly and almost completely absorbed from the gastrointestinal tract, and only a small proportion of the administered dose is found in the stools. Approximately 55% of the drug in the plasma is bound to nondiffusible plasma constituents. Excretion of chloroquine is quite slow, but is increased by acidification of the urine. Chloroquine is deposited in the tissues in considerable amounts. In animals, from 200 to 700 times the plasma concentration may be found in the liver, spleen, kidney, and lung; leukocytes also concentrate the drug. The brain and spinal cord, in contrast, contain only 10 to 30 times the amount present in plasma.

Chloroquine undergoes appreciable degradation in the body. The main metabolite is desethylchloroquine, which accounts for one fourth of the total material appearing in the urine; bisdesethylchloroquine, a carboxylic acid derivative, and other metabolic products as yet uncharacterized are found in small amounts. Seventy percent can be accounted for as unchanged chloroquine (McChesney *et al.*, 1967). Deethylation to the secondary amine results in a substance that is highly active against avian malaria. Metabolic products of chloroquine may thus be partially responsible for antimalarial activity.

Because of the avidity of tissues for the drug, a loading or priming dose is essential if effective plasma concentrations are to be reached and maintained. When the drug is discontinued, following daily dosage for 2 weeks, plasma concentrations and urinary excretion both decrease with a half-life of 6 to 7 days for the next 4 weeks; subsequently the half-life for urinary excretion increases to 17 days. Small amounts can be found in the urine for long periods of time, some claim for as long as 5 years. Daily oral dosage of 310 mg of chloroquine base results in a plasma plateau of about 125 μg per liter. With a weekly 0.5-g dose, the peak plasma concentration varies between 150 and 250 μg per liter; just prior to the succeeding dose, the range is between 20 and 40 μg per liter. After single or weekly doses, the half-life of the drug in plasma is about 3 days. Congeners of chloroquine such as amodiaquine or hydroxychloroquine interfere with its metabolism; with their concurrent use, plasma concentrations of chloroquine are elevated for prolonged periods.

Preparations. *Chloroquine Phosphate*, U.S.P. (ARALEN PHOSPHATE, AVLOCLOR, RESOCHIN), is available as tablets containing either 250 or 500 mg of the diphosphate. Approximately 60% of the diphosphate represents the base. Chloroquine is also available as *Chloroquine Hydrochloride Injection*, U.S.P. (ARALEN HYDROCHLORIDE) (50 mg/ml in 5-ml ampuls). It is also combined in tablets with pyrimethamine (DARACLOR) or with chloroproguanil (LAPAQUIN), a dihalogenated derivative of chloroguanide, for prophylactic and therapeutic use, and with primaquine for prophylactic use only.

Routes of Administration and Dosage. Chloroquine phosphate is administered in tablet form by the oral route, either before or after meals. The hydrochloride of chloroquine may be employed for parenteral (intramuscular) injection, if necessary.

For the purpose of *suppressive therapy* an oral dose of 500 mg of the phosphate is given on the same day of each week, continuing for at least 6 weeks after the last exposure in an endemic area. In some parts of the world where malaria transmission is intense, a weekly dose of 1 g is used for nonimmune persons. In certain areas, strains of *P. falciparum* exist that are less sensitive to 4-aminoquinolines than are most commonly encountered strains. In these circumstances, despite apparently adequate suppression, acute attacks may occur on stopping medication, even if maintained for several weeks after leaving the malarious area. With some strains patent infections and acute attacks of falciparum malaria may occur even during suppressive therapy. The management of infections arising from such strains is discussed above.

For the *treatment of the acute attack* of vivax or falciparum malaria, an initial priming or loading dose of 1 g is administered; this is followed by an additional 500 mg after 6 or 8 hours and a single dose of 500 mg on each of 2 consecutive days, so that a total of 2.5 g is given in 3 days. This dosage is usually sufficient to cure completely most *P. falciparum* infections and to terminate promptly fever and parasitemia in acute *P. vivax* infections. Freedom from clinical attacks in vivax malaria may then be maintained by suppressive doses of 500 mg weekly.

If parenteral therapy is required for the treatment of coma due to falciparum malaria, the equivalent of

200 mg of chloroquine *base* (250 mg of the hydrochloride) should be administered intramuscularly, half the dose in each buttock. This may be repeated at intervals of 6 hours, but the total dose for the first 24 hours should never exceed the equivalent of 800 mg of the base. Parenteral administration should be terminated as soon as the drug can be taken orally.

Dosages administered to infants or children, orally or intramuscularly, should not exceed 10 mg of chloroquine base per kilogram of body weight per day; the usual dose is 5 mg/kg of the base.

Toxicity and Side Effects. The amounts of chloroquine employed for therapy of the acute malarial attack may cause mild and transient headache, visual disturbances, gastrointestinal upset, and pruritus. Prolonged chronic medication for suppressive purposes causes few significant untoward effects, and only rarely must the drug be discontinued because of intolerance. None of the symptoms is serious, and all readily disappear when the drug is withheld. Chloroquine does not discolor the skin, as does quinacrine. It may, however, cause discoloration of nailbeds and mucous membranes. The chief untoward effects are pruritus and gastrointestinal discomfort.

Prolonged treatment with chloroquine causes a lichenoid skin eruption in a small percentage of patients; the condition is mild and subsides promptly when the drug is stopped. Readministration of chloroquine usually does not result in reappearance of the lesion. Large doses given for a year to a group of healthy volunteers occasionally caused some visual symptoms (blurring of vision due to difficulty in accommodation, diplopia), bleaching of the hair, diminution of T waves in some or all leads of the ECG (without evidence of cardiovascular impairment), mild skin eruptions, headache, and slight weight loss; the observed toxic effects caused no incapacity and were reversible upon withdrawal of the drug (Alving *et al.,* 1948). These findings emphasize the relative safety of chloroquine in the recommended dose range.

The administration of chloroquine in the long-term treatment of diseases other than malaria may involve the administration of 250 to 750 mg daily for many months or even years. Such long-term treatment has been shown to result, not infrequently, in a retinopathy. This is characterized by loss of central visual acuity, granular pigmentation of the macula, and retinal artery constriction. The visual loss is not necessarily progressive if the drug is discontinued, but it appears to be irreversible. Bernstein and colleagues (1963) have demonstrated that chloroquine is stored in the iris and choroid of laboratory animals in significantly higher concentrations than in other tissues. Rubin and coworkers (1963) have suggested acidifying the urine of affected patients with ammo-

nium chloride and administering dimercaprol intramuscularly to increase the urinary excretion of chloroquine. Ototoxicity has been reported in a few cases. Hart and Naunton (1964) have implicated chloroquine in the development of fetal abnormalities characterized by severe cochleovestibular paresis. Their single patient had received chloroquine in high dosage for the treatment of lupus erythematosus. There has been no report of an association between chloroquine administered during pregnancy as an antimalarial agent and fetal abnormalities.

Precautions and Contraindications. Because of the high concentration that occurs in the liver, chloroquine should be used with caution in the presence of hepatic disease. It should be used cautiously or not at all in the presence of severe gastrointestinal, neurological, or blood disorders. If such disorders occur during the course of therapy, the drug should be discontinued. Concomitant use of gold or phenylbutazone with chloroquine should be avoided because of the tendency of all three agents to produce dermatitis. For patients on long-term, large-dose therapy, ophthalmological examination is recommended before and periodically during treatment (Percival and Meanock, 1968).

Therapeutic Uses. *Malaria.* In human vivax malarias, choloquine has neither prophylactic nor radically curative value. However, in well tolerated doses it is highly effective in terminating acute attacks of vivax malaria, and when administered chronically it acts as an effective suppressive agent. When medication is discontinued, relapses may occur but the interval for their appearance is prolonged. In falciparum malaria, the drug is markedly effective in controlling acute attacks and as a rule it completely cures the disease. Chloroquine is superior to quinine in that it is more potent and less toxic and it need be given only once weekly as a suppressive agent. It is one of the most generally useful of the antimalarial drugs; however, in some parts of the world, certain strains of *P. falciparum* occur that are much less sensitive or even completely insensitive to the action of the drug.

Other Uses. Apart from the uses mentioned earlier, choloquine is valuable in the treatment of *extraintestinal amebiasis* (*see* Chapter 46). It has also been reported to be of value in *giardiasis* and to produce symptomatic improvement in *Babesia* infection.

CHLOROQUINE CONGENERS: AMODIAQUINE AND HYDROXYCHLOROQUINE

Of the more than 200 derivatives of 4-aminoquinoline found to be active against avian malarial parasites (Wiselogle, 1946), chloroquine has been the most adequately studied. Other congeners, however, are available for use. One of these is *Amodiaquine Hydrochloride,* U.S.P. (CAMOQUIN), the structure of which is as follows:

Amodiaquine

Amodiaquine is employed for the treatment of overt malarial attacks and for suppression, but it is not used as extensively as chloroquine. Amodiaquine is more active than chloroquine both *in vitro* and *in vivo* against certain strains of *P. falciparum* with decreased sensitivity to chloroquine. However, it cannot be recommended for routine use in the treatment of such infections.

The frequency and severity of adverse responses to amodiaquine are similar to those that follow the administration of chloroquine. Most commonly encountered are diarrhea, vomiting, and vertigo.

The dosage schedules for amodiaquine are analogous to those detailed above for chloroquine. For suppressive therapy, the unit dose is 520 mg of the dihydrochloride (400 mg of the base). For treatment of acute attacks, 600 mg of the base is given on the first day, followed by daily doses of 400 mg on the 2 subsequent days. Amodiaquine is supplied in tablets that contain the equivalent of 200 mg of the base.

Hydroxychloroquine Sulfate, U.S.P. (PLAQUENIL), in which one of the N-ethyl substituents of chloroquine is β-hydroxylated, is considered to be essentially equivalent to the parent molecule. It is supplied in tablets that contain 200 mg, equivalent to 155 mg of the base. For purposes of dosage, 400 mg of hydroxychloroquine sulfate is equivalent to 500 mg of chloroquine phosphate. The drug has been used successfully in place of chloroquine against normally sensitive strains.

CHLOROGUANIDE

History. Chloroguanide represents a distinctly British contribution to antimalarial research during World War II. The compound was synthesized by Curd and associates (1945), who have reviewed the chemical considerations that resulted in the synthesis of chloroguanide and its congeners. Suffice it to say that early members of the series were synthesized as *pyrimidine* derivatives because of the known importance of pyrimidine-containing compounds in cell metabolism. Later members of the series, of which chloroguanide is one, were simplified by opening the pyrimidine ring to give a biguanide. Metabolism in the body converts this biguanide to a triazine ring, the active form of the drug. Chloroguanide was first employed for the treatment of human vivax and falciparum malarias by Adams and coworkers (1945)

at the Liverpool School of Tropical Medicine. The compound was then given extensive clinical trial. Unfortunately, the value of the drug is now seriously compromised by the development of chloroguanide-resistant strains of plasmodia (*see* above).

Chemistry. Chloroguanide has the following structural formula:

Chloroguanide

It is a white powder with a bitter taste.

Pharmacological Effects. *Antimalarial Actions and Efficacy.* Chloroguanide exerts causal prophylactic and suppressive activity in sporozoite-induced falciparum malaria, adequately controls the acute clinical attack, and usually eradicates the infection. The drug exhibits suppressive activity against *P. vivax* infections, and controls the acute clinical attack. It is, however, not fully prophylactic against mosquito-induced vivax malaria because it does not affect the exoerythrocytic tissue stage of this infection. Also, in *P. vivax* infections, erythrocytic forms of the parasite often reappear in the blood shortly after suppressive doses of chloroguanide are withdrawn. Its action on erythrocytic forms of all malarias is slow compared to that of the 4-aminoquinoline antimalarials. Gametocytes are not destroyed, but the development of gametes encysted in the gut wall of the mosquito is prevented.

Resistance to chloroguanide, which greatly compromises its general usefulness, is discussed earlier in this chapter.

Mechanism of Antimalarial Action. The elucidation of the mechanism of action of chloroguanide was a rich reward from studies of its metabolic fate. The compound is converted in the body to a triazine derivative that is an active inhibitor of the enzyme dihydrofolate reductase. This observation led to a planned program for the synthesis and study of direct inhibitors of the enzyme and the introduction into chemotherapy of the diaminopyrimidines. The mechanism of the chemotherapeutic action of inhibitors of dihydrofolate reductase and the rationale for their concurrent use with sulfonamide compounds that interfere with folate metabolism by other means are discussed in detail under the diaminopyrimidines (*see* below; Rollo, 1970).

Absorption, Fate, and Excretion. Chloroguanide is slowly but adequately absorbed from the gastrointestinal tract. After single oral doses, peak plasma concentrations of the drug are attained at 2 to 4 hours; the concentration then declines rather rapidly and is practically zero at 24 hours. Approximately 75% of the chloroguanide in plasma is bound to protein, and the concentration of the drug in erythrocytes is six times that in the plasma.

During chronic administration of chloroguanide,

the drug accumulates only to a slight extent in the tissues. In man, from 40 to 60% of the chloroguanide absorbed is excreted in the urine, and approximately 10% is secreted directly into the intestinal tract and eliminated in the feces.

As stated above, the drug itself has little effect against plasmodia; activity is dependent upon the accumulation of a metabolite—2,4-diamino-1-*p*-chlorophenyl-1,6-dihydro-6,6-dimethyl-1,3,5-triazine (Carrington *et al.*, 1951; Crowther and Levi, 1953). Smith and colleagues (1961) found that, in man, 60% of the drug excreted in the urine is parent compound, and 30% is the triazine.

Preparations, Route of Administration, and Dosage. *Chloroguanide hydrochloride* (PALUDRINE) is available in tablets containing 25, 100, or 300 mg. Chloroguanide is always administered orally.

The *prophylactic* (and *suppressive*) dose for both vivax and falciparum malarias is 100 mg daily for nonimmune subjects, although twice this dose is necessary in some regions. Semi-immune individuals given 300 mg once weekly are moderately well protected; however, if possible, 200 mg should be given twice weekly. For the treatment of the *acute attack* of vivax malaria in semi-immune or nonimmune subjects, an initial dose of 300 to 600 mg should be followed by 300 mg daily for as long as is required. A single administration of 300 mg usually terminates the clinical attack in semi-immune persons, but many experts prefer to give a 5- or 10-day course. This course of treatment is rarely curative, and either suppressive doses must subsequently be employed or radical cure obtained as described below.

In considering the use of this agent, the sensitivity of local strains must be known. Resistance to chloroguanide is prevalent.

Toxicity and Side Effects. Chloroguanide is the most innocuous of the currently employed antimalarials; in therapeutic doses, it causes practically no untoward effects. Large doses (1 g daily) may cause vomiting, abdominal pain, and diarrhea. Excessive amounts may cause hematuria and the transient appearance of epithelial cells and casts in the urine; myelocytes to the extent of 10% may appear in the blood of patients with overt malaria.

Therapeutic Uses. Chloroguanide is employed only in *malaria*. In both falciparum and vivax malarias, the compound adequately controls the overt clinical attack, but it is slower in abolishing fever and parasitemia than are all other antimalarial drugs with the exception of pyrimethamine. For this reason, its use in the treatment of the acute attack of falciparum malaria is not recommended. In *falciparum* malaria, chloroguanide is a causal prophylactic, suppressive, and radically curative agent if the plasmodia have not developed resistance to the drug.

In *vivax* malaria, chloroguanide controls the acute clinical attack but has no advantage over more rapidly acting 4-aminoquinoline antimalarial agents. It is also an effective suppressive, but its use does not result in radical cure, particularly of infections caused by highly relapsing strains.

Chloroguanide represents an important chemotherapeutic advance because, in addition to being a potent schizontocide, the drug is lethal to actively developing preerythrocytic tissue forms of certain plasmodia and exerts a sterilizing action on gametocytes. Furthermore, it opened the field for the development of other antifolates.

CYCLOGUANIL PAMOATE

The fact that single doses of antimalarial drugs are effective for only brief periods stimulated Thompson and coworkers (1963) to synthesize compounds that might act for much longer periods of time. Their optimism stemmed from the remarkably high potency of the triazine metabolite of chloroguanide. Their objective was a single-dose, parenteral, repository preparation. Cycloguanil pamoate (embonate) (4,6-diamino-1-[*p*-chlorophenyl]-1,2-dihydro-2,2-dimethyl-*s*-triazine pamoate) was prepared and found to possess the desired properties. (It is also known as *chloroguanide triazine pamoate* and CAMOLAR.) The prolonged period of protection afforded by this preparation was found to be due to release of the active moiety from a depot formed at the site of injection and not to a systemic reservoir formed after administration of the drug (Waitz *et al.*, 1963).

Studies in man showed that a single intramuscular injection of 5 mg/kg protects against *P. falciparum* and *P. vivax* for several months. The results indicated that a single intramuscular injection of the drug provides the equivalent of a prolonged infusion of the soluble dihydrotriazine and appears to prevent the growth or even the survival of both the erythrocytic and the preerythrocytic parasites. Up to 80% of the drug remains at the injection site 2 weeks after administration, and small amounts can be found for as long as 56 weeks later (Thompson *et al.*, 1963).

While field trials with cycloguanil pamoate were at first encouraging, resistant strains were soon encountered. Furthermore, use of this compound may lead rapidly to the emergence and spread of drug-resistant strains. In the light of these shortcomings clinical trials have involved the use of two depot preparations in combination. The one is the triazine just described and the other is *acedapsone*, the diacetyl derivative of diaminodiphenylsulfone (N,N'-diacetyl-4,4'-diaminodiphenylsulfone, DADDS; HANSOLAR), which, on slow hydrolysis following intramuscular injection, yields the active antimalarial, diaminodiphenylsulfone (*see* Peters, 1968). There is some evidence that the use of the combination, a 1:1 mixture, may extend the period of protection, delay the emergence of resistant strains, and even provide some protection against strains already less sensitive to either drug alone. However, problems have been encountered with local reactions from its intramuscular administration. The combination is presently termed DAPOLAR. The rationale for the concurrent use of these drugs is discussed below. In the United States, cycloguanil is available only for investigational use and has been employed as an alternative drug in the treatment of American cutaneous *leishmaniasis*.

DIAMINOPYRIMIDINES

History. Of the many 2,4-diaminopyrimidines synthesized and tested for antimicrobial activity, two are outstanding. The first, *pyrimethamine,* was developed and used almost solely as an antimalarial agent; the second, *trimethoprim,* was created as an antibacterial agent and found later to have antimalarial properties. Several 2,4-diaminopyrimidines were found to antagonize competitively folic and folinic acids in the growth of *Lactobacillus casei.* The prediction was made that *L casei* would not be unique in its sensitivity to these substances and that eventually, from this group, useful chemotherapeutic agents would be developed. Experiments with the diaminopyrimidines in the treatment of malaria in experimental animals bore out prediction; a high degree of antimalarial activity was found in several members of the series. The most active, *pyrimethamine,* was later found to be highly effective against the plasmodia infecting man (*see* Falco *et al.,* 1951; Symposium, 1952), and has since been used widely for prophylaxis and suppression.

Chemistry. *Pyrimethamine* has the following structural formula:

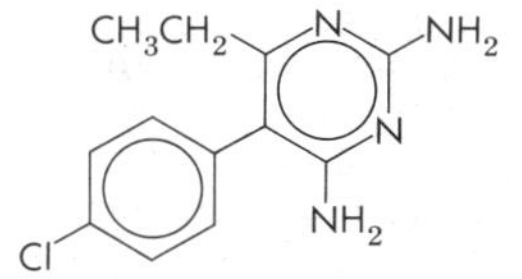

Pyrimethamine

It is a white powder, insoluble in water.

Trimethoprim has the following structural formula:

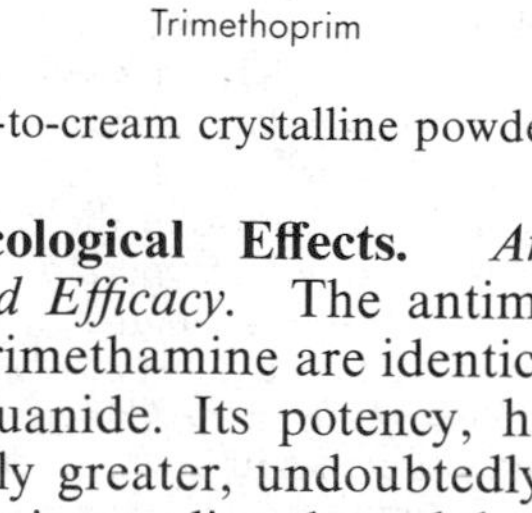

Trimethoprim

It is a white-to-cream crystalline powder.

Pharmacological Effects. *Antimalarial Actions and Efficacy.* The antimalarial effects of pyrimethamine are identical to those of chloroguanide. Its potency, however, is considerably greater, undoubtedly owing to the fact that it acts directly and the half-life is much longer than that of the active metabolite of chloroguanide. *Suppressive cure* of some vivax infections may be achieved by continuing prophylactic medication for 10 weeks after leaving a malarious area. There

is a possibility that some causal prophylactic activity may occur in vivax infections. The antimalarial effects of both chloroguanide and pyrimethamine have been reviewed by Davey (1963) and Hill (1963). The major use of pyrimethamine is in prophylaxis and suppression and in concurrent therapy.

Investigations into the antimicrobial activity of 2,4-diaminopyrimidines have resulted in novel and important concepts of the action of these chemotherapeutic agents. The enzyme dihydrofolate reductase, which catalyzes the reduction of dihydrofolate to tetrahydrofolate with NADPH, is of vital importance to cells in the biosynthesis of purines, pyrimidines, and certain amino acids (*see* Chapter 57). Methotrexate, a structural analog of dihydrofolate, is a potent inhibitor of the enzyme and an important chemotherapeutic agent in the treatment of neoplastic disease (*see* Chapter 55). Methotrexate, however, has little antimicrobial activity, although cell-free preparations of the enzyme from bacterial, protozoal, and mammalian sources are all inhibited by nanomolar concentrations of the drug (Ferone *et al.,* 1969). The apparent anomaly is explained by consideration of the permeability of the cell to folic acid. Mammalian cells, which utilize exogenous folate, must actively transport the vitamin; this uptake mechanism is shared by the folate analogs. Protozoa, like certain bacteria, do not have the ability to transport preformed folate, and they require a supply of PABA to synthesize the compound (Ferone and Hitchings, 1966). The dihydrofolate reductase in intact cells is thus not exposed to these inhibitors. The "small-molecule" antifolates, such as pyrimethamine and trimethoprim, seem to penetrate by nonionic diffusion, and their entrance is unrelated to the ability of the cell to assimilate folic acid (Hitchings and Burchall, 1965). Their selective effect must depend, therefore, on some mechanism other than selective permeability. The answer is found in the fact that dihydrofolate reductases from various sources exhibit differences in sensitivity to inhibition by the diaminopyrimidines. Table 45–1 summarizes the pertinent data of Ferone and coworkers. There is an obvious correlation between the inhibitory potency of the agents and their effect on the intact microorganism and the host. For ex-

Table 45-1. INHIBITION OF DIHYDROFOLATE REDUCTASES BY PYRIMETHAMINE AND TRIMETHOPRIM *

	CONCENTRATION (nM) FOR 50% INHIBITION OF DIHYDROFOLATE REDUCTASES FROM VARIOUS SOURCES		
INHIBITOR	Mammalian (rat liver)	Bacterial (E. coli)	Protozoal (P. berghei)
Pyrimethamine	700	2500	~0.5
Trimethoprim	260,000	5	70

* Modified from Ferone, Burchall, and Hitchings, 1969.

ample, pyrimethamine is ineffective as an antibacterial agent although extremely effective as an antimalarial. It has significant toxicity only at doses appreciably higher than the conventional. Trimethoprim, on the other hand, is effective both as an antibacterial and as an antimalarial agent. Its toxicity for the mammalian host seems to be minimal (Kahn et al., 1968).

Drug Combinations. The concept of inhibiting two steps in an essential metabolic pathway with separate drugs was developed by Hitchings and associates a decade before its practical application was to be realized (*see* Hitchings and Burchall, 1965; Rollo, 1970). Such "sequential blockade" should result in a supra-additive effect. The two steps investigated were the utilization of PABA in the synthesis of dihydropteroic acid, inhibited by sulfonamides, and the reduction of dihydrofolate to tetrahydrofolate, inhibited by pyrimethamine. About one eighth of the ED50 of pyrimethamine and sulfadiazine administered together was equivalent to the ED50 of either used alone in experimental malarial infections (Rollo, 1955). Hurly (1959) treated African children infected with *P. falciparum* and *P. malariae* with pyrimethamine and sulfadiazine, alone and in combination; clinical cure was obtained with the combination of less than one tenth of the curative dose of pyrimethamine plus less than one fourth of the curative dose of sulfadiazine. Subsequently, trials of several combinations of pyrimethamine and either sulfonamides or dapsone have attested to the value of the augmentative effect both in the suppression and in the treatment of acute falciparum infections (*see* Donno et al., 1969; Lucas et al., 1969).

The value of such combinations is not in reducing the dose of the pyrimidines, since therapeutic doses have a low order of toxicity, but in the possibility of preventing strains of plasmodia from developing resistance to these drugs. Such strains have arisen fairly readily when small doses of pyrimethamine alone were used for long periods of time. Suitable combinations have shown their value in the treatment of some multiresistant strains and in suppression where such strains have been encountered (World Health Organization, 1973). Combinations of trimethoprim with sulfamethoxazole are of particular value in the treatment of bacterial infections (*see* Chapter 49).

Absorption, Fate, and Excretion. Pyrimethamine is well absorbed after oral administration. The compound is eliminated slowly and has a half-life in plasma of about 4 days. Suppressive concentrations remain in the blood for 2 weeks (*see* Brooks et al., 1969; Stickney et al., 1973). Several metabolites of pyrimethamine appear in the urine, but few data are available on either their structure or their antimicrobial activity. Pyrimethamine is also excreted in the milk of nursing mothers.

Preparations, Route of Administration, and Dosage. *Pyrimethamine*, U.S.P. (DARAPRIM), is marketed in scored tablets, each containing 25 mg of the base. Pyrimethamine is recommended only for prophylaxis and suppression; hence a first dose of 50 mg should be taken just before entering an endemic area. An effective dose is 25 mg once weekly for adults. Dosage is continued weekly as long as residence in endemic areas continues and for 6 weeks after leaving the area, to afford a chance for suppressive cure of vivax infection. The drug is available in combination with *dapsone,* as MALOPRIM; this preparation is intended for *prophylactic use,* particularly in areas where multiresistant strains are known to occur. It is also available in certain countries in combination with *sulfadoxine,* as FANSIDAR, for use in the *treatment* of multiresistant infections. Sulfadoxine is a sulfanomide with a particularly long half-life (7 to 9 days).

Toxicity, Precautions, and Contraindications. With the recommended dosage of 25 mg once weekly, no significant toxic symptoms have been reported for *pyrimethamine*. Excessive doses may be expected to produce a megaloblastic anemia resembling that of folic acid deficiency and readily reversible on discontinuance of treatment or on administration of folinic acid. The dose of pyrimethamine should not be increased over that recommended for suppression, except when used in combination with other agents for the treatment of multiresistant strains. At the same time care should be taken to see that the dose is taken regularly to lessen the possibility of selective emergence of relatively insensitive or resistant strains. In general, the drug should not be used in areas where the plasmodia are predominantly insensitive to the recommended dosage or have become resistant through its misuse. Its use with either dapsone or a sulfonamide has proven beneficial, however, in areas where multiresistant strains are endemic. Used in this way, it is recommended that folinic acid in a daily dose of 10 mg/kg also be given to prevent possible hematological complications.

Therapeutic Uses. *Pyrimethamine* administered by itself has little value in the treatment of the acute primary attack of malaria. It is slow in clearing parasitemia, but it prevents development of the fertilized gamete and has some causal prophylactic activity. In combination with a short-acting sulfonamide (*e.g.,* sulfadiazine) or a sulfone, pyrimethamine is useful for the treatment of acute attacks of uncomplicated chloroquine-resistant *P. falciparum* malaria. Quinine should probably also be included in this regimen.

Pyrimethamine has had considerable use as a prophylactic and suppressive agent and has proven effective if given once weekly. It is not a radically curative agent in vivax malaria, although continuance of suppressive therapy for 10 weeks after leaving a malarious area will provide "suppressive cure" with certain strains of *P. vivax*. The combination of pyrimethamine and sulfadoxine is particularly appropriate for prophylaxis since, as mentioned, the half-life of sulfadoxine is long. This preparation is effective if given at intervals of 2 to 4 weeks.

Pyrimethamine given concurrently with triple sulfonamides has been found useful in the treatment of *toxoplasmosis* (*see* Feldman, 1968). Folinic acid should be given concurrently to obviate the hematological toxicity that may occur with continued daily use of pyrimethamine. Some success has followed the use of pyrimethamine in the treatment of *polycythemia vera* and in the prophylaxis of *meningeal leukemia*.

MEFLOQUINE

Mefloquine was developed in response to the proliferation of multidrug-resistant strains of *P. falciparum*, particularly in Southeast Asia. Such strains are variously resistant to available schizontocidal drugs and, in general, respond only to quinine or to certain drug combinations. As part of an extensive research program on malaria mounted by the U.S. Army, data collected during the course of World War II (Wiselogle, 1946) were examined to identify compounds with potential activity against these strains. Attention was focused on substances of proven antimalarial activity with some structural resemblance to quinine. These included quinolinemethanols and phenanthrene and pyridine carbinols. Unfortunately interest in these series, which contained many active compounds, had declined because of serious phototoxicity. Phototoxic potential, however, did not always parallel antimalarial activity. Of the many compounds that were then developed and tested for both phototoxicity and antimalarial activity, derivatives of 4-quinolinemethanol showed the most promise, and one of these, *mefloquine*, emerged from eventual clinical trial as a readily tolerated antimalarial drug that is highly active against both the usual and the multidrug-resistant strains of *P. falciparum* (*see* Schmidt *et al.,* 1978).

Chemistry. Mefloquine has the following structural formula:

Mefloquine

The hydrochloride is a white, odorless, bitter-tasting powder.

Pharmacological Effects. *Antimalarial Actions.* This new antimalarial drug was developed for the treatment and prevention of chloroquine-resistant strains of falciparum malaria. Such strains not only are resistant to chloroquine but also may show reduced sensitivity to antimalarials of different chemical types. While quinine alone will control an acute attack caused by these microorganisms, it not infrequently fails to prevent recurrence. Mefloquine in single, well-tolerated doses has been shown to eliminate fever and parasitemia rapidly in nonimmune volunteers infected with either chloroquine-sensitive or highly chloroquine-resistant strains of *P. falciparum* and to effect a radical cure. It has also been shown to effect suppressive cure against all strains of *P. falciparum* and suppression of *P. vivax*. In *P. vivax* infections, however, malarial attacks recur some time after the end of treatment (Rieckmann *et al.*, 1974; Trenholme *et al.*, 1975; Clyde *et al.*, 1976).

Mechanism of Antimalarial Action. The mechanism of action of mefloquine is unknown. It does not intercalate with DNA (Davidson *et al.*, 1977). It does interfere with the clumping of pigment in the parasite produced by chloroquine and related 4-amino-quinolines (Warhurst and Thomas, 1978), and it competes for accumulation of chloroquine by infected erythrocytes (Fitch *et al.*, 1979). The latter observation prompted Fitch and coworkers to hypothesize that accumulation of chloroquine and mefloquine is by a shared mechanism; while changes in chloroquine-resistant strains result in the exclusion of chloroquine, affinity for mefloquine appears to be retained.

Absorption, Fate, and Excretion. Studies in experimental animals have demonstrated that mefloquine is well absorbed after oral administration and is extensively bound to plasma proteins. Peak concentrations in plasma are attained in a few hours and decline slowly over a period of several days. Concentrations in tissues, particularly liver and lungs, are relatively high for extended periods of time. Excretion is mainly in the feces, and only very small amounts of drug appear in the urine. Several metabolites are formed. There is evidence of enterohepatic circulation (Mu *et al.*, 1975). Subsequent studies in man have confirmed the long sojourn of mefloquine in the body. After a single dose of 1 g, the half-life in blood averages 17 days (Desjardins *et al.*, 1979b).

Preparations, Route of Administration, and Dosage. Mefloquine is supplied in 250-mg tablets. It is a new drug, and in the United States its use is limited to investigational purposes. It is currently manufactured by the Walter Reed Army Institute of Research. Administered orally, single doses of 1 to 1.5 g have been effective in curing chloroquine-resistant *P. falciparum* infections in nonimmune patients (Trenholme *et al.*, 1975). Single oral doses of 250 mg weekly, 500 mg every 2 weeks, or 1000 mg every 4 weeks, given to nonimmune volunteers, are completely effective in producing suppressive cure of *P. falciparum* (Smith strain). The strain used for these tests is resistant to 4-aminoquinolines, pyrimethamine, and chloroguanide and has diminished susceptibility to quinine (Clyde *et al.*, 1976). In the same study doses of 250 mg of mefloquine, administered at weekly intervals, suppressed sporozoite-induced *P. vivax* infections. However, malaria developed some time after completing the course of treatment. Persistence of the drug is evident from the observation that exposure to infected mosquitoes 2 weeks after a single oral dose of 1 g did not result in parasitemia.

Toxicity and Side Effects. Mefloquine, given orally in single doses up to 1500 mg or in 500-mg doses each week for 1 year, is well tolerated in man. In dogs, repeated daily oral doses of 30 mg/kg and greater have produced occasional emesis and diarrhea, as well as lesions in the lymphoid tissue and liver (*see* Caldwell and Nash, 1977). Due to lack of

information, the use of mefloquine in women, infants, and children is not recommended. Its long-term use also is not recommended, since animal studies in one species with repeated high dosage have shown evidence of histological abnormalities of the retina and epididymal injury.

Therapeutic Use. Mefloquine is indicated only for the treatment and prevention of chloroquine-resistant falciparum malaria. Currently, it is the only agent that, when used alone, is capable of ensuring suppression and cure in infections due to multidrug-resistant strains. The drug should be used *only* for the treatment and prevention of infections with such strains, since its misuse could result in the development of mefloquine-resistant plasmodia.

PRIMAQUINE

History. In 1891, Ehrlich discovered that methylene blue exhibited weak plasmodicidal activity; the dye was tested because of his observation that it preferentially stained the parasite in the blood stream without staining other tissues. Later it was demonstrated that 8-aminoquinoline had weak schizontocidal activity in infected canaries and also that the slight antimalarial potency of methylene blue could be intensified by substitution of a dialkyl-aminoalkyl group for one of the N-methyl groups of the dye. Because the methoxy group on the quinoline ring, as in quinine, was believed important for antimalarial activity, a large series of quinoline derivatives was synthesized in which both the methoxy and substituted 8-amino groups were present. *Pamaquine* was the first of the 8-aminoquinoline antimalarials to be introduced into medicine (Muhlens, 1926). Its activity was outstanding, being 60 times that of quinine against canary malaria. During the course of the large-scale cooperative antimalarial research program conducted in the United States during World War II, several hundred derivatives of 8-aminoquinoline were explored in an attempt to discover compounds more potent and less toxic than pamaquine itself (*see* Elderfield *et al.*, 1946; Wiselogle, 1946). From this large number, three agents—*pentaquine, isopentaquine,* and *primaquine*—were selected for further study. Of these three, only primaquine, which received extensive field trials with United Nations forces in Korea, is widely used now. *Quinocide,* a substance very similar in structure to primaquine, is employed in some parts of the world.

Chemistry. Primaquine has the following structural formula:

$$H_2N(CH_2)_3CH \begin{matrix} CH_3 \\ | \\ \end{matrix}$$

Primaquine

The diphosphate is the commercially available salt; it is soluble in water, and its solutions are stable, although some decomposition may take place on exposure to light and air.

Structure-Activity Relationship. Since a low chemotherapeutic index was a main drawback to the use of pamaquine, the prime value of the newer 8-aminoquinoline derivatives was a reduction in toxicity without concomitant decrease in antimalarial activity. In a study on toxicity and curative activity against vivax infections, Edgcomb and coworkers (1950) showed that primaquine was the most active, followed by isopentaquine, and pamaquine the least active of the trio. Toxicity decreased as antimalarial activity increased. The degree of toxicity is related to the degree of substitution of the terminal amino group. Pamaquine has a tertiary terminal amine, while primaquine has a primary terminal amine. Intermediate between these two lies isopentaquine, isomeric with pamaquine but with a secondary terminal amine. (For a review, *see* Hill, 1963.)

Pharmacological Effects. Aside from its antimalarial actions, primaquine exerts few pharmacological effects at safe therapeutic doses. Its main actions are of a toxicological nature (*see* below), exerted particularly on the blood.

Antimalarial Actions and Efficacy. Primaquine is highly active against the primary exoerythrocytic forms of *P. vivax* and *P. falciparum,* especially the latter. Although its causal prophylactic effect is obtained with well-tolerated doses, this activity is of relatively little practical value. The drug is also active against the asexual blood forms of *P. vivax,* but its effect is too erratic to be useful for the treatment of frank clinical attacks of benign tertian malaria. The drug is almost completely ineffective against the asexual blood forms of *P. falciparum.* The 8-aminoquinolines do, however, exert a marked gametocytocidal activity against all four species of plasmodia that infect man, especially against the gametocytes of *P. falciparum.* The great clinical value of primaquine lies in the *radically curative treatment of vivax malaria* and, in certain exceptional circumstances where single-drug administration has proven less than fully effective, in its use as a supplement to chloroquine suppression.

Primaquine is the best-available drug for curative treatment of vivax malaria since it destroys the late tissue forms with greater effectiveness and less danger of toxicity than does any other drug.

Acquired Resistance of Plasmodia to Primaquine. Resistance to 8-aminoquinoline compounds has been developed in avian and monkey malarias (*see* Hill, 1963; Rollo, 1964). Arnold and colleagues (1961) produced primaquine resistance in *P. vivax* by treating partially immune volunteers with subcurative doses of the drug. The asexual erythrocytic forms became resistant to the maximal tolerated dose of the drug after 36 passages. Gametocytes could be transmitted to mosquitoes and developed to the stage of mature and apparently viable sporozoites. These, however, did not infect man. Thus, it appears that the development of primaquine-resistant strains may not become a problem. Nevertheless, it is of the utmost importance that misuse of the drug does not occur, because the 8-aminoquinolines are the only antimalarial agents that can eliminate the late tissue stages of relapsing malaria, and the development of resistant strains would be disastrous.

Mechanism of Antimalarial Action. Little is known of the mode of action of 8-aminoquinolines. Pentaquine, unlike quinine, chloroquine, and quinacrine, does not inhibit the incorporation of ^{32}P-labeled phosphate into DNA or RNA by *P. gallinaceum* or *P. berghei* (Schellenberg and Coatney, 1960). Nevertheless, binding of 8-aminoquinolines to DNA, similar to that observed with chloroquine, has been shown to occur (Whichard *et al.,* 1968). There is evidence that the parent 8-aminoquinoline compounds have only slight antimalarial activity and that metabolism *in vivo* results in more highly active substances (*see* Goodwin and Rollo, 1955).

Absorption, Fate, and Excretion. After oral administration, the 8-aminoquinoline antimalarial compounds, including primaquine, are readily absorbed. They are, however, rapidly metabolized, and only a small proportion of the administered dose is excreted as the parent drug. The plasma concentration reaches a maximum in about 6 hours, but it falls rapidly thereafter and is barely detectable after 24 hours. Considerable variation in peak plasma values is noted among individuals on the same dose schedule. However, neither the hemolytic effect on sensitive erythrocytes (*see* below) nor, probably, the antimalarial effect has much relation to the concentration of the parent drug in the plasma.

Tarlov and coworkers (1962) have outlined a degradation scheme for primaquine modeled after Smith's (1956) proposal for the degradation of pentaquine in monkeys. In this scheme the 6-methoxy group of primaquine is reduced to hydroxy, a second hydroxy group is added in the 5 position, and the resultant compound is converted to a quinonimine by way of the 5,6-quinone derivative of the parent compound. Such a derivative is, or may be, transformed into a resonating compound capable of acting as an oxidation-reduction mediator. Such an agent may accelerate the oxidation of essential substances in sensitive erythrocytes by acting as a hydrogen acceptor and thereby promote hemolysis.

Preparations, Route of Administration, and Dosage. *Primaquine Phosphate*, U.S.P., is supplied in tablets containing 26.3 mg of the salt, equivalent to 15 mg of base. The dosage is usually expressed in terms of the base.

Primaquine is always given orally. Extensive field trials carried out with the United Nations forces in Korea demonstrated the great value of the drug against vivax infections and permitted assessment of the optimal schedule of treatment. Primaquine base (15 mg daily for 14 days) combined with standard chloroquine therapy (1.5 g of base in 3 days) proved to be the regimen of choice for radical cure of Korean vivax malaria treated either during the acute clinical attack or during the late stage of clinical activity. With such a schedule, ambulatory treatment with only minimal medical supervision is possible, clinical toxicity is insignificant, and the relapse rate is less than 3%. Radical cure can be obtained by giving 15 mg of primaquine base alone, daily for 14 days, if administration is carried out during the long-term latent period of the infection.

The above schedule is currently recommended for the treatment and cure of the *temperate zone* variety of vivax malaria. Patients infected with the *Chesson* (*Southwest Pacific*) strain may be treated with two to three times this daily dose of primaquine, that is, 30 to 45 mg of base. Alving and coworkers (1960), however, introduced a schedule involving weekly rather than daily doses of primaquine because of the danger of hemolytic reactions arising from the increased dosage necessary to cure Chesson strain infections. They found that 60 mg of primaquine base together with 300 mg of chloroquine given weekly for 8 weeks resulted in 6% failure, compared with about 30% failure following 15 mg of primaquine base alone given daily for 14 days. The use of combinations containing 45 mg of primaquine base resulted in 10% failure; and 30 mg, 55% failure. The highest-dose regimen had negligible hemolytic effect upon the erythrocytes of primaquine-sensitive individuals. The recommended therapy for patients infected with this strain of malaria is, therefore, 600 mg of chloroquine base, followed 6 hours later by 300 mg of chloroquine base combined with 45 mg of primaquine base in one dose. Thereafter 300 mg of chloroquine combined with 45 mg of primaquine should be given as a single dose on the same day of each week for 7 additional weeks. Amodiaquine or hydroxychloroquine may be substituted for chloroquine.

Toxicity and Side Effects. In the usual therapeutic doses, primaquine has proven quite innocuous when given to Caucasians. Mild-to-moderate abdominal cramps and occasional epigastric distress have occurred in some individuals given the larger doses, and mild anemia, cyanosis (methemoglobi-

nemia), and leukocytosis have been observed. Higher doses (60 to 240 mg of primaquine base daily) accentuate the abdominal symptoms and cause methemoglobinemia and cyanosis in most subjects and leukopenia in some. Hepatic function is unaffected by primaquine, even in patients with infectious hepatitis. Abdominal distress can be alleviated by antacids and by taking the drug at mealtime. Granulocytopenia and even agranulocytosis are rare complications of therapy and are usually associated with overdosage. Also rare are hypertension, arrhythmias, and symptoms referable to the central nervous system (CNS).

The toxicity of primaquine in most blacks is as described above; however, there is a fraction of the black population (about 10% of black males in the United States) who develop anemia due to intravascular hemolysis at daily dose levels of 20 mg (base) and higher. Such primaquine sensitivity of erythrocytes is seen also in some darker-hued Caucasian ethnic groups, including Sardinians, Sephardic Jews, Greeks, and Iranians, in whom the sensitivity is greater than in blacks, so that the hemolytic reaction from a given dose of drug may well be more severe.

The incidence of hemolysis (and of the sickle trait) in general follows the same geographical pattern as the distribution of falciparum malaria; erythrocytes that reflect these genetic changes are less subject to malarial infection. A decrease in glucose-6-phosphate dehydrogenase activity has been shown to be characteristic of primaquine-sensitive erythrocytes and appears to represent their major enzymatic deficiency. In normal erythrocytes there are several mechanisms that protect the cells against injury by oxidative drugs such as metabolic derivatives of primaquine. These drugs are capable of accelerating the transfer of hydrogen from reduced nicotinamide adenine dinucleotide phosphate (NADPH), reduced glutathione, hemoglobin, the free sulfhydryl groups of proteins, and other donors. In normal erythrocytes under the stress of oxidant drugs, the rate of NADPH regeneration can be greatly accelerated by increasing the amount of glucose metabolized by means of the pentose phosphate pathway. Sufficient NADPH is therefore readily made available for reduction of oxidized glutathione and, directly and indirectly, for reduction of methemoglobin; reduced glutathione also protects the sulfhydryl groups of hemoglobin and the sulfhydryl-containing enzymes against oxidative destruction. Primaquine-sensitive erythrocytes, on the other hand, are incapable of sufficiently rapid regeneration of NADPH because of their deficiency of glucose-6-phosphate dehydrogenase; consequently, all the reductive processes within the cell that are dependent upon NADPH are impaired. Metabolic processes are diminished so that normal vital functions can no longer be carried out, and alterations in the lipoprotein membrane of the cell result in lysis (see Tarlov et al., 1962; Beutler, 1969). Brewer and colleagues (1960) have devised a simple test for detecting such primaquine sensitivity based on the observation that the rate of methemoglobin reduction by erythrocytes from these individuals is markedly slower than normal in the presence of methylene blue. Results from this test correlate very well with the severity of hemolysis. The World Health Organization (1967) and Beutler and Mitchell (1968) have described other simple tests. Since primaquine sensitivity is inherited by a gene carried on the X chromosome, the hemolysis is often of intermediate severity in heterozygous females; because of "variable penetrance," females may be affected less frequently than would be predicted.

At present more than 40 drugs and other substances are known to be capable of inducing hemolysis. These include antimalarials, sulfonamides, nitrofurans, antipyretics, analgesics, sulfones, vitamin K analogs, fava beans (favism), and certain other vegetables.

The severity of the hemolysis is dependent on the dose of drug used. If the initial dose is not too large, the hemolysis is self-limited even when the same dose of drug is continued. This is because older erythrocytes are most susceptible, and, after their destruction, the remaining younger cells and newly produced reticulocytes are relatively resistant to hemolysis. However, the severity of hemolysis can be enhanced or mitigated by many factors and is often unpredictable. For this reason the administration of primaquine or of any other potentially hemolytic drug should be discontinued immediately if marked darkening of the urine or a sudden decrease in hemoglobin concentration occurs (see Kellermeyer et al., 1962).

Precautions and Contraindications. Because of the possibility of hemolytic reactions (see above), one should watch for suggestive signs. If a daily dose of more than 30 mg of primaquine base (more than 15 mg daily in possibly sensitive patients such as blacks) is administered, repeated peripheral blood counts and at least gross examination of the urine should be performed during therapy. If the drug is used in schemes for mass administration, supervision is required.

Primaquine is contraindicated in acutely ill patients suffering from systemic disease characterized by a tendency to granulocytopenia, such as very active forms of rheumatoid arthritis and lupus erythematosus. It should not be given to subjects receiving, at the same time, other potentially hemolytic drugs or agents capable of depressing the myeloid elements of the bone marrow.

Therapeutic Uses. Primaquine is used mainly for the *radical cure* of vivax and other relapsing malarias. If it is administered during the long-term latent period of the infection, radical cure can be achieved. Its use during an acute clinical attack will prevent subsequent recrudescences. Primaquine should always be given in conjunction with full doses of a 4-aminoquinoline schizontocide, preferably chloroquine, in order to reduce the possibility of developing drug-resistant strains. In appropriate circumstances it may be used in combination with a 4-aminoquinoline for prophylaxis or for the interruption of transmission, especially of *P. falciparum*.

QUININE AND THE CINCHONA ALKALOIDS

History. Quinine is the chief alkaloid of cinchona, the bark of the cinchona tree indigenous to certain regions of South America. The bark is also called Peruvian, Jesuit's, or Cardinal's bark. It is not clear whether the natives were acquainted with the medicinal properties of cinchona. The first written record of the use of cinchona occurs in a religious book written in 1633 and published in Spain in 1639. The author, an Augustinian monk named Calancha, of Lima, Peru, wrote: "A tree grows which they call 'the fever tree' in the country of Loxa, whose bark, the color of cinnamon, is made into powder amounting to the weight of two small silver coins and given as a beverage, cures the fevers and tertians; it has produced miraculous results in Lima." A variety of colorful and fanciful versions of the discovery of the fever bark exist. A popular and persistent version is that the bark was employed in 1638 to treat Countess Anna del Chinchón, wife of the viceroy to Peru, and that her miraculous cure resulted in the introduction of cinchona into Spain in 1639 for the treatment of ague. There is no evidence that the countess ever used the bark; yet for many years the drug was called *los Polvos de la Condesa.* However, the viceroy did bring a large shipment of cinchona to Spain. By 1640, the drug was being employed for fevers in Europe. Its use was first mentioned in European medical literature in 1643 by a Belgian, Herman van der Heyden.

The term *cinchona* was chosen by Linné (who accidentally misspelled it) for the species of plants yielding the drug. Although this term is probably derived from the name of the countess whose alleged cure led to its wide use, some believe that it comes from a word of Incan origin, *kinia,* which means "bark." The Jesuit fathers were the main importers and distributors of cinchona in Europe, and the name *Jesuit bark* soon became attached to the drug. It was sponsored in Rome chiefly by the eminent philosoper Cardinal de Lugo; hence the drug came to be called *Cardinal's bark.* The conservative medical groups viewed the new antipyretic with disdain because its use did not conform to the teachings of Galen. Others looked upon it with suspicion because the Jesuits used it. For these reasons, the drug was dispensed for many years predominantly by charlatans and in the form of secret remedies. The most fabulous of these quacks was the incomparable

Robert Talbor. The first official recognition of cinchona came in 1677, when it was included in an edition of the *London Pharmacopoeia* as "Cortex Peruanus."

For almost 2 centuries the bark was employed for medicine as a powder, extract, or infusion. In 1820, Pelletier and Caventou isolated quinine and cinchonine from cinchona, and the use of the alkaloids as such gained favor rapidly.

Chemistry. While quinine has been synthesized, the procedure is too complex and expensive to provide a practical source of the drug. Quinine and the other alkaloids are, therefore, still obtained entirely from natural sources.

Cinchona contains a mixture of more than 20 alkaloids. The most important of these are two pairs of optical isomers, *quinine* and *quinidine*, and *cinchonidine* and *cinchonine*. Quinine and cinchonidine are levorotary.

Quinine has the following structural formula:

Quinine

Quinine contains a quinoline group attached through a secondary alcohol linkage to a quinuclidine ring. A methoxy side chain is attached to the quinoline ring and a vinyl to the quinuclidine. *Quinidine* has the same structure as quinine except for the steric configuration of the secondary alcohol grouping. The many natural alkaloids related to quinine and the semisynthetic chemicals derived from quinine differ mainly in the nature of the substitutions on the side chain. Each alteration in the chemical pattern of quinine causes corresponding quantitative but not qualitative changes in the pharmacological actions of the resulting compounds.

Structure-Activity Relationship. The effects of chemical alterations in the quinine molecule on various pharmacological actions have been studied, particularly with regard to antimalarial potency. Since none of the resulting compounds has an antimalarial action superior to that of quinine, the details will not be presented. To summarize, the data indicate that neither the methoxy nor the vinyl radical of the quinine molecule is required for antimalarial activity. In contrast, the secondary alcohol group is absolutely essential, and its reduction increases toxicity and abolishes antiplasmodial potency. Stereoisomerism is a relatively unimportant factor.

Further details of the structure-activity relationship in the cinchona alkaloids may be found elsewhere (*see* Oettingen, 1933; Wiselogle, 1946; and others). Historically, this important field has provided the necessary background for the search for more effective and less toxic antimalarials.

PHARMACOLOGICAL PROPERTIES

The typical actions of cinchona are largely attributable to its quinine content. The pharmacological properties of quinine are described in abbreviated form below. More complete descriptions and remarks on the properties of related cinchona alkaloids may be found in *earlier editions* of this textbook.

Local Actions. Quinine affects such a large variety of biological systems that it has been called a "general protoplasmic poison"; with some reservations this appraisal is probably correct. It is toxic to many bacteria and other unicellular organisms such as trypanosomes, infusoria, yeast, plasmodia, and spermatozoa. Despite this wide range of activity, quinine does exhibit considerable specificity in its action.

Local Anesthetic Action. Sensory nerves are briefly stimulated and then paralyzed by quinine. Concentrations only slightly higher than those necessary for anesthesia are likely to cause edema, pain, and reactive fibrosis. The anesthesia may last for many hours or days, and in this respect differs sharply from that produced by the conventional local anesthetics.

Irritant Action. Quinine is a marked local irritant. When taken orally, it may cause gastric pain, nausea, and vomiting. Subcutaneous or intramuscular injections of the drug are painful and may cause sterile abscesses. Intravenous administration may result in thrombosis of the injected vein from injury to the intima. Vascular damage is the basis for the occasional use of quinine solutions for sclerosing varicose veins.

Antimalarial Actions and Efficacy. Until the third decade of the present century, the cinchona alkaloids represented the sole chemotherapeutic agents for the specific treatment of malaria. While the advent of synthetic antimalarials brought the use of quinine to a low ebb, the emergence of resistant plasmodial strains has necessitated its continued availability.

Quinine is not a true causal prophylactic agent; it is incapable of preventing sporozoite-induced vivax or falciparum malaria in human volunteers. However, like chloroquine, it is effective both as a suppressive drug and in the control of overt clinical attacks. Its primary action is schizontocidal, and no lethal effect is exerted on sporozoites or preerythrocytic tissue forms. In addition, quinine is gametocytocidal for *P. vivax* and *P. malariae* but not for *P. falciparum*. As both a suppressive and a therapeutic agent, quinine is less well tolerated and less effective than chloroquine. However, a valuable current use of quinine is in the treatment of severe illness due to certain multiresistant strains of *P. falciparum*.

Central Nervous System. Therapeutic doses of quinine have few effects on the CNS other than to cause *analgesia* and *antipyresis*. The discovery that cinchona lowered the fever of malarial patients quickly led to its use in all forms of febrile illnesses. However, quinine is not a potent antipyretic.

Cardiovascular System. The actions of quinine on cardiac muscle are qualitatively similar to those of its isomer, quinidine. These are described in full in Chapter 31. Therapeutic doses of quinine have little, if any, effect on the normal heart or blood pressure in man. When given intravenously, quinine causes a definite and sometimes alarming hypotension, particularly when the injection is made rapidly.

Skeletal Muscle. Quinine and related cinchona alkaloids exert interesting effects on skeletal muscle that have some clinical applicability. Quinine increases the tension response to a single maximal stimulus delivered to the muscle directly or through the nerve, but it increases the refractory period of muscle so that the response to tetanic stimulation is diminished. Quinine also decreases the excitability of the motor end-plate region so that the responses to repetitive nerve stimulation and to acetylcholine are reduced. Thus, it has a curare-like effect on skeletal muscle, and can antagonize the actions of physostigmine on skeletal muscle as effectively as does curare.

The effects of quinine and related alkaloids on skeletal muscle remained purely a matter of academic interest until it was demonstrated that myotonia congenita could be symptomatically relieved by quinine (Wolf, 1936). This disease is the pharmacological antithesis of myasthenia gravis, and investigations soon revealed that drugs effective in one syndrome aggravate the other. Quinine may so aggravate the symptoms of myasthenia that alarming respiratory distress and dysphagia may ensue.

Gastrointestinal Tract. The soluble salts of quinine are extremely bitter, and very small amounts of cinchona preparations are occasionally used as *stomachics.* Larger doses may inhibit vagal-mediated gastric secretion. The irritant properties of the cinchona alkaloids cause considerable *gastric distress.* Nausea, vomiting, and diarrhea are prominent when large doses are taken orally. Toxic amounts also produce vomiting by a central action on the medulla. The *musculature* of the intestinal tract is not stimulated by concentrations of the drug reached clinically.

Absorption, Fate, and Excretion. Quinine and its congeners are readily absorbed when given orally. Absorption occurs mainly from the upper small intestine, and is almost complete even in patients with marked diarrhea. Subcutaneous or intramuscular injection of quinine is contraindicated because of local tissue damage.

Peak plasma concentrations of cinchona alkaloids occur within 1 to 3 hours after a single oral dose. After chronic administration of total daily doses of 1 g of drug, the average plasma quinine concentration is approximately 7 μg/ml. After termination of quinine therapy, the plasma level falls rapidly and only a negligible concentration is detectable after 24 hours. A large fraction (approximately 70%) of the plasma quinine is bound to proteins. This explains in part why the concentration of the alkaloid in cerebrospinal fluid is only 2 to 5% of that in the plasma. Quinine readily reaches the tissues of the fetus.

The cinchona alkaloids in large measure are metabolically degraded in the body, especially in the liver, so that less than 5% of an administered dose is excreted *unaltered* in the urine. There is no accumulation of the drugs in the body upon continued administration. The metabolic degradation products are excreted in the urine, where many of them have been identified as hydroxy derivatives (Brodie *et al.,* 1951). The cinchona alkaloids are excreted mainly in the urine, but small amounts also appear in the feces, gastric juice, bile, and saliva. Renal excretion of quinine is twice as rapid when the urine is acidic as when it is alkaline.

Toxicity. Poisoning by quinine is usually due to clinical overdosage or to hypersensitivity. The fatal oral dose of quinine for adults is approximately 8 g. When quinine is repeatedly given in full doses, a typical cluster of symptoms occurs to which the term *cinchonism* has been applied. Certain features of the syndrome are seen in salicylate poisoning. In its mildest form it consists in ringing in the ears, headache, nausea, and slightly disturbed vision; however, when medication is continued or after large single doses, symptoms also involve the gastrointestinal tract, the nervous and cardiovascular systems, and the skin.

Hearing and *vision* are particularly disturbed. Functional impairment of the eighth nerve results in tinnitus, decreased auditory acuity, and vertigo. The visual signs are those of blurred vision, disturbed color perception, photophobia, diplopia, night blindness, constricted visual fields, scotomata, and mydriasis. It is not known if the visual and auditory effects are directly neural or secondary to vascular changes. Attention has been directed repeatedly to the marked spastic constriction of the retinal vessels. The retina is ischemic, the discs are pale, and retinal edema may ensue. In severe cases, optic atrophy results. Degenerative changes in the spiral ganglion cells similar to those noted in the ganglion cells of the retina lend support to the belief that the cellular injury from quinine is direct. Perhaps both vascular and neural components of injury are involved.

Gastrointestinal symptoms are also prominent in cinchonism. Nausea, vomiting, abdominal pain, and diarrhea result from the local irritant action of quinine, but the nausea and emesis also have a central basis. The *skin* is often hot and flushed, and sweating is prominent. Rashes frequently appear. Angioedema, especially of the face, is occasionally observed.

CNS symptoms are noted in severer grades of poisoning, particularly headache, fever, vomiting, apprehension, excitement, confusion, delirium, and syncope. *Respiration* is first stimulated and then shallow and depressed. The skin becomes cold and cyanotic as poisoning progresses, the body temperature and the blood pressure fall, weakness is extreme, the pulse is feeble, coma ensues, and death occurs from respiratory arrest. *Death* may result in a few hours or be delayed 1 or 2 days. If the patient recovers, symptoms usually disappear completely except that there may be variable degrees of residual optic and auditory damage in some cases.

At times, *renal damage* may be caused by quinine, and anuria and uremia may ensue. *Acute hemolytic anemia* is a rare complication of quinine therapy; it apparently is caused by the drug only in pregnant women or in patients with malaria. Quinine, like salicylate, is capable of causing *hypoprothrombinemia;* the simultaneous administration of vitamin K counteracts the prolongation of the prothrombin time. Rarely, quinine may cause symptomatic *purpura* in hypersusceptible individuals, by a thrombocytolytic action. In a few instances, the drug appears to have caused *agranulocytosis. Abortion* may result from quinine overdosage, but this is not necessarily due to an oxytocic action of the drug. The alkaloid may cause *asthma* in hypersensitive individuals. Transient *ventricular tachycardia* may rarely be observed after massive acute overdosage.

When small doses of cinchona alkaloids cause toxic manifestations, the individual is usually hypersensitive to the drug. Cinchonism may appear after a single dose of quinine, but it is usually mild. Cutaneous flushing, pruritus, skin rashes, fever, gastric distress, dyspnea, ringing in the ears, and visual impairment are the usual expressions of hypersensitivity; extreme flushing of the skin accompanied by intense, generalized pruritus is the most common form. Hemoglobinuria and asthma from quinine are rare types of idiosyncrasy.

Contraindications. Quinine must be used with considerable caution, if at all, in patients who manifest idiosyncrasy to it, especially when this takes the form of cutaneous, angioedematous, visual, or auditory symptoms. Quinine should be stopped immediately if evidence of hemolysis appears. The drug should not be employed in patients with tinnitus or optic neuritis. In patients with atrial fibrillation, the administration of quinine requires the same precautions as outlined for quinidine (*see* Chapter 31).

Preparations, Routes of Administration, and Dosages. There are numerous preparations of cinchona alkaloids available to the practitioner, particularly in tropical communities where malaria is endemic and where inexpensive cinchona medication is essential. In the United States, the pure alkaloids are employed rather than the galenical preparations.

The most commonly used salts of quinine are *Quinine Sulfate,* U.S.P., and *quinine dihydrochloride.* Tablets and capsules of quinine sulfate contain 130, 200, or 325 mg.

The usual oral dose of quinine or its salts is 325 mg four times daily for 7 days. The drug is given after meals, preferably in capsules, to minimize gastric irritation. For young children, quinine may have to be given in solution. The syrup of licorice and the aromatic syrup of eriodictyon are vehicles helpful for this purpose.

Totaquine contains approximately 10% of anhydrous quinine and approximately 75% of the total anhydrous crystallizable cinchona alkaloids. The drug is cheaper than quinine and available in abundance in parts of the world where quinine is expensive or limited in supply. In proper doses, it is as effective as quinine in malaria inasmuch as it contains cinchona alkaloids with approximately the same order of antimalarial potency as quinine. The usual dosage of totaquine for malaria is 600 mg three times daily after meals, for 7 days.

The *oral route* should be employed for quinine administration whenever possible. Intravenous injection of quinine is to be reserved for certain emergencies such as pernicious or cerebral malaria. The dihydrochloride is employed and the injection should be made very slowly, preferably by the drip method; drugs should be available to counteract the untoward effects on the cardiovascular system.

THERAPEUTIC USES

While quinine has been employed in preparations as diverse as douches and hair tonics, it currently has two valid therapeutic applications—for the treatment of malaria and for the relief of nocturnal leg cramps.

Status as an Antimalarial. Quinine should not be employed alone as an antimalarial. It is more toxic and less effective than the synthetic antimalarial drugs. A valid antimalarial use of quinine is its administration in combination with primaquine for the radical cure of relapsing vivax malaria and for the treatment of malaria due to strains of *P. falciparum* resistant to chloroquine and cross-resistant to other antimalarial drugs. In patients very seriously ill from such resistant strains, the intravenous use of quinine is mandatory. However, it must be given slowly with constant monitoring of the pulse and blood pressure. Oral treatment should be substituted as soon as possible.

Nocturnal Leg Cramps. Recumbency leg muscle cramps (night cramps) are quickly and effectively relieved by quinine in most cases. The dose is 200 to 300 mg before retiring. In some patients, only a brief period of quinine therapy is required to provide long periods of freedom from muscle cramps; in a few individuals, even large doses of the drug may fail to give relief.

ANTIBACTERIAL AGENTS IN ANTIMALARIAL CHEMOTHERAPY

Shortly after their introduction into therapeutics, the sulfonamides were shown to possess antimalarial activity. The sulfones were also shown to be effective; the first trial of dapsone was against *P. falciparum* in 1943. Little attention was paid to the data because of the superiority of other drugs. Current interest stems from their use, usually in combination with pyrimethamine, against resistant strains of falciparum malaria. When antimalarial activity was found in several antibiotics, the tetracyclines and chloramphenicol were tried clinically. Although their action as schizontocides is slow, their activity against drug-resistant malarial parasites is proving useful.

Sulfonamides and Sulfones. Much of the important work on sulfonamides was carried out during the intensive antimalarial program during World War II. This and later work focused attention on sulfadiazine, because of its relatively high activity. It was found, however, to be active only against the asexual blood forms of the human malarial parasites, and to act slowly. Subsequently, two longer-acting sulfonamides, sulfadoxine (FANZIL) and sulfalene

(KELFIZINA), have been used for treatment and suppression, mainly in partially immune patients infected with fully sensitive strains of *P. falciparum*. Combinations of sulfadoxine with pyrimethamine are important for the prophylaxis of chloroquine-resistant strains of *P. falciparum*. A combination of sulfadiazine and pyrimethamine is preferable for the treatment of acute attacks that follow infection with such strains because of the shorter half-life of this sulfonamide.

Parallel studies have demonstrated the value of dapsone used in the same way as sulfonamides, either alone or given concurrently with dihydrofolate reductase inhibitors. Field trials have also shown the value of 4,4′-diacetyıdiaminodiphenylsulfone (*acedapsone*), a repository sulfone, given intramuscularly at intervals of several months, either alone or with cycloguanil, for suppression of falciparum infection. Another sulfone, 4,4′-diformamidodiphenylsulfone, is deformylated in the liver after oral administration to provide low sustained plasma concentrations of dapsone. Some success has followed its weekly use for suppression of malaria, in place of dapsone. The danger of producing resistant strains not only of malarial parasites but also of pathogenic bacteria by the use of such relatively low dosage has been expressed. Neither sulfonamides nor sulfones are as active against *P. vivax* as they are against *P. falciparum*.

Tetracyclines. The use of tetracyclines in the treatment of the acute attack of multiresistant strains of falciparum malaria reflects sadly the sparsity of primary antimalarial drugs effective in such conditions. Their relative slowness of action makes concurrent treatment with quinine mandatory for rapid control of parasitemia. While several tetracyclines appear equivalent, most data have accumulated for tetracycline itself, and this is recommended. Although tetracycline has shown marked activity against primary tissue schizonts of chloroquine-resistant *P. falciparum*, its long-term use as a prophylactic agent cannot be recommended because of the danger of producing antibiotic-resistant pathogenic bacteria (World Health Organization, 1973).

Adams, A. R. D.; Maegraith, B. G.; King, J. D.; Townshend, R. H.; Davey, T. H.; and Havard, R. E. Studies on synthetic antimalarial drugs. XIII. Results of a preliminary investigation of the therapeutic action of 4888 (PALUDRINE) on acute attacks of benign tertian malaria. *Ann. Trop. Med. Parisitol.*, **1945,** *39,* 225–231.

Allison, J. L.; O'Brien, R. L.; and Hahn, F. E. DNA: reaction with chloroquine. *Science,* **1965,** *149,* 1111–1113.

———. Nature of the deoxyribonucleic acid—chloroquine complex. In, *Antimicrobial Agents and Chemotherapy—1965.* (Sylvester, J. C., ed.) American Society for Microbiology, Ann Arbor, Mich., **1966,** pp. 310–314.

Alving, A. S.; Eichelberger, L.; Craige, B., Jr.; Jones, R., Jr.; Whorton, C. M.; and Pullman, T. N. Studies on the chronic toxicity of chloroquine (SN-7618). *J. Clin. Invest.,* **1948,** *27,* 60–65.

Alving, A. S.; Johnson, C. F.; Tarlov, A. R.; Brewer, G. J.; Kellermeyer, R. W.; and Carson, P. E. Mitigation of the hemolytic effect of primaquine and enhancement of its action against exo-erythrocytic forms of the Chesson strain of *Plasmodium vivax* by intermittent regimens of

drug administration. *Bull. WHO,* **1960,** *22,* 621–631.

Arnold, J.; Alving, A. S.; and Clayman, C. B. Induced primaquine resistance in vivax malaria. *Trans. R. Soc. Trop. Med. Hyg.,* **1961,** *55,* 345–350.

Bartonelli, P. J.; Sheehy, T. W.; and Tigertt, W. D. Combined therapy for chloroquine-resistant *Plasmodium falciparum* infection. *J.A.M.A.,* **1967,** *199,* 173–177.

Berliner, R. W.; Earle, D. P., Jr.; Taggart, J. V.; Zubrod, C. G.; Welch, W. J.; Conan, N. J.; Bauman, E.; Scudder, S. T.; and Shannon, J. A. Studies on the chemotherapy of the human malarias. VI. The physiological disposition, antimalarial activity, and toxicity of several derivatives of 4-aminoquinoline. *J. Clin. Invest.,* **1948,** *27,* 98–107.

Bernstein, H. N.; Svaifler, N. J.; Rubin, M.; and Mausour, A. M. The ocular deposition of chloroquine. *Invest. Ophthalmol. Visual Sci.,* **1963,** *2,* 384–392.

Beutler, E., and Mitchell, M. Special modifications of the fluorescent screening method for glucose-6-phosphate dehydrogenase deficiency. *Blood,* **1968,** *32,* 816–818.

Brewer, G. J.; Tarlov, A. R.; and Alving, A. S. Methemoglobin reduction test: a new simple, *in vitro* test for identifying primaquine-sensitivity. *Bull. WHO,* **1960,** *22,* 633–640.

Brodie, B. B.; Baer, J. E.; and Craig, L. C. Metabolic products of the cinchona alkaloids in human urine. *J. Biol. Chem.,* **1951,** *188,* 567–581.

Brooks, M. H.; Malloy, J. P.; Bartelloni, P. J.; Sheehy, T. W.; and Barry, K. G. Quinine, pyrimethamine, and sulphorthodimethoxine: clinical response, plasma levels, and urinary excretion during the initial attack of naturally acquired *falciparum* malaria. *Clin. Pharmacol. Ther.,* **1969,** *10,* 85–91.

Caldwell, R. W., and Nash, C. B. Pulmonary and cardiovascular effects of mefloquine methanesulfonate. *Toxicol. Appl. Pharmacol.,* **1977,** *40,* 437–448.

Carrington, H. C.; Crowther, A. F.; Davey, D. G.; Levi, A. A.; and Rose, F. L. A metabolite of PALUDRINE with high antimalarial activity. *Nature,* **1951,** *168,* 1080.

Clyde, D. F.; McCarthy, V. C.; Miller, R. M.; and Hornick, R. B. Suppressive activity of mefloquine in sporozoite-induced human malaria. *Antimicrob. Agents Chemother.,* **1976,** *9,* 384–386.

Cohen, R. J.; Sachs, J. R.; Wicker, D. J.; and Conrad, M. E. Methaemoglobinemia provoked by malarial chemoprophylaxis in Vietnam. *N. Engl. J. Med.,* **1968,** *279,* 1127–1131.

Cohen, S. N., and Yielding, K. L. Inhibition of DNA and RNA polymerase reactions by chloroquine. *Proc. Natl. Acad. Sci. U.S.A.,* **1965,** *54,* 521–527.

Crowther, A. F., and Levi, A. A. PROGUANIL: isolation of metabolite with high antimalarial activity. *Br. J. Pharmacol. Chemother.,* **1953,** *8,* 93–97.

Curd, F. H. S.; Davey, D. G.; and Rose, F. L. Studies on synthetic antimalarial drugs. II. General chemical considerations. *Ann. Trop. Med. Parasitol.,* **1945,** *39,* 157–164.

———. X. Some biguanide derivatives as new types of antimalarial substances with both therapeutic and causal prophylactic activity. *Ibid.,* **1945,** *39,* 208–216.

Davidson, M. W.; Griggs, B. G., Jr.; Boykin, D. W.; and Wilson, W. D. Mefloquine, a clinically useful quinolinemethanol antimalarial which does not significantly bind to DNA. *Nature,* **1975,** *254,* 632–634.

———. Molecular structural effects involved in the interaction of quinolinemethanolamines with DNA. Implications for antimalarial action. *J. Med. Chem.,* **1977,** *20,* 1117–1122.

Desjardins, R. E.; Canfield, C. J.; Haynes, J. D.; and Chulay, J. D. Quantitative assessment of antimalarial activity *in vitro* by a semiautomated microdilution technique. *Antimicrob. Agents Chemother.,* **1979a,** *16,* 710–718.

Desjardins, R. E.; Pamplin, C. L.; von Bredow, J.; Barry, K. G.; and Canfield, C. J. Kinetics of a new antimalarial, mefloquine. *Clin. Pharmacol. Ther.,* **1979b,** *26,* 372–379.

Donno, L.; Sanguineti, V.; Ricciardi, M. L.; and Soldati, M.

Antimalarial activity of kelfizina-trimethoprim and kelfizina-pyrimethamine versus chloroquine in field trials in Nigeria. *Am. J. Trop. Med. Hyg.*, **1969**, *18*, 182–187.

Edgcomb, J. H.; Arnold, J.; Yount, E. H., Jr.; Alving, A. S.; and Eichelberger, L. Primaquine, SN 13272, a new curative agent in *vivax* malaria: a preliminary report. *J. Natl. Malar. Soc.*, **1950**, *9*, 285–292.

Elderfield, R. C., and others. Alkylaminoalkyl derivatives of 8-aminoquinoline. *J. Am. Chem. Soc.*, **1946**, *68*, 1524–1529.

Fairley, N. H. Chemotherapeutic suppression and prophylaxis in malaria: an experimental investigation undertaken by medical research teams in Australia. *Trans. R. Soc. Trop. Med. Hyg.*, **1945**, *38*, 311–365.

————. Researches on PALUDRINE (M. 4888) in malaria: an experimental investigation undertaken by the L.H.Q. Medical Research Unit (A.I.F.), Cairns, Australia. *Ibid.*, **1946**, *40*, 105–153.

Falco, E. A.; Goodwin, L. G.; Hitchings, G. H.; Rollo, I. M.; and Russell, P. B. 2:4-Diaminopyrimidines—a new series of antimalarials. *Br. J. Pharmacol. Chemother.*, **1951**, *6*, 185–200.

Ferone, R. Altered dihydrofolate reductase in a strain of pyrimethamine-resistant *Plasmodium berghei. Fed. Proc.*, **1969**, *28*, 847.

Ferone, R.; Burchall, J. J.; and Hitchings, G. H. *Plasmodium berghei* dihydrofolate reductase: isolation, properties, and inhibition by antifolates. *Mol. Pharmacol.*, **1969**, *5*, 49–59.

Ferone, R., and Hitchings, G. H. Folate cofactor biosynthesis by *Plasmodium berghei:* comparison of folate and dihydrofolate as substrates. *J. Protozool.*, **1966**, *13*, 504–506.

Fitch, C. D. *Plasmodium falciparum* in owl monkeys: drug resistance and chloroquine binding capacity. *Science*, **1970**, *169*, 289–290.

Fitch, C. D.; Chan, R. L.; and Chevli, R. Chloroquine resistance in malaria: accessibility of drug receptors to mefloquine. *Antimicrob. Agents Chemother.*, **1979**, *15*, 258–262.

Fitch, C. D.; Yunis, N. G.; Chevli, R.; and Gonzalez, Y. High-affinity accumulation of chloroquine by mouse erythrocytes infected by *Plasmodium berghei. J. Clin. Invest.*, **1974**, *54*, 24–33.

Hart, C. W., and Naunton, R. F. The ototoxicity of chloroquine phosphate. *Arch. Otolaryngol.*, **1964**, *80*, 407–412.

Homewood, C. A.; Warhurst, D. C.; Peters, W.; and Baggaley, V. C. Lysosomes, *pH* and the anti-malarial action of chloroquine. *Nature*, **1972**, *235*, 50–52.

Hurly, M. G. D. Potentiation of pyrimethamine by sulphadiazine in human malaria. *Trans. R. Soc. Trop. Med. Hyg.*, **1959**, *53*, 412–413.

Kahn, S. B.; Fein, S. A.; and Brodsky, I. Effects of trimethoprim on folate metabolism in man. *Clin. Pharmacol. Ther.*, **1968**, *9*, 550–560.

Kellermeyer, R. W.; Tarlov, A. R.; Brewer, G. J.; Carson, P. E.; and Alving, A. S. Hemolytic effect of therapeutic drugs: clinical considerations of the primaquine-type hemolysis. *J.A.M.A.*, **1962**, *180*, 388–394.

Lucas, A. O.; Hendrickse, R. G.; Okubadejo, O. A.; Richards, W. H. G.; Neal, R. A.; and Kofie, B. A. K. The suppression of malarial parasitaemia by pyrimethamine in combination with dapsone or sulphormethoxine. *Trans. R. Soc. Trop. Med. Hyg.*, **1969**, *63*, 216–229.

McChesney, E. W.; Fasco, M. J.; and Banks, W. F., Jr. The metabolism of chloroquine in man during and after repeated oral dosage. *J. Pharmacol. Exp. Ther.*, **1967**, *158*, 323–331.

Macomber, P. B.; O'Brien, R. L.; and Hahn, F. E. Chloroquine: physiological basis of drug resistance in *Plasmodium berghei. Science*, **1966**, *152*, 1374–1375.

Moore, D. V., and Lanier, J. E. Observations on two *Plasmodium falciparum* infections with an abnormal response to chloroquine. *Am. J. Trop. Med. Hyg.*, **1961**, *10*, 5–9.

Mu, J. Y.; Israili, Z. H.; and Dayton, P. G. Studies of the disposition and metabolism of mefloquine HCl (WR 142490), a quinolinemethanol antimalarial, in the rat. *Drug Metab. Dispos.*, **1975**, *3*, 198–210.

Mühlens, P. Die Behandlung der naturlichen menschlichen Malaria-Infektion mit Plasmochin. *Naturwissenschaften*, **1926**, *14*, 1162–1166.

Percival, S. P. B., and Meanock, I. Chloroquine: ophthalmological safety and clinical assessment in rheumatoid arthritis. *Br. Med. J.*, **1968**, *3*, 579–584.

Peters, W. Antimalarial drugs and their actions. *Postgrad. Med. J.*, **1973**, *49*, 573–583.

Polet, H., and Barr, C. F. Chloroquine and dihydroquinine: *in vitro* studies of their antimalarial effect upon *Plasmodium knowlesi. J. Pharmacol. Ther.*, **1968**, *164*, 380–386.

Richards, W. H. G., and Williams, S. G. Malaria studies *in vitro*. II. The measurement of drug activities using leucocyte-free blood-dilution cultures of *Plasmodium berghei* and ³H-leucine. *Ann. Trop. Med. Parasitol.*, **1973**, *67*, 179–190.

Rieckmann, K. H.; McNamara, J. V.; Frischer, H.; Stockert, T. A.; Carson, P. E.; and Powell, R. D. Effects of chloroquine, quinine and cycloguanil upon the maturation of asexual erythrocytic forms of two strains of *Plasmodium falciparum in vitro. Am. J. Trop. Med. Hyg.*, **1968**, *17*, 661–671.

Rieckmann, K. H.; Trenholme, G. M.; Williams, R. L.; Carson, P. E.; Frischer, H.; and Desjardins, R. E. Prophylactic activity of mefloquine hydrochloride (WR 142490) in drug-resistant malaria. *Bull. WHO*, **1974**, *51*, 375–377.

Rollo, I. M. The mode of action of sulphonamides, PROGUANIL, and pyrimethamine on *Plasmodium gallinaceum. Br. J. Pharmacol. Chemother.*, **1955**, *10*, 208–214.

Rubin, M.; Bernstein, H. N.; and Zvaifler, N. J. Studies on the pharmacology of chloroquine. *Arch. Ophthalmol.*, **1963**, *70*, 474–481.

Schellenberg, K. A., and Coatney, G. R. The influence of antimalarial drugs on nucleic acid synthesis in *Plasmodium gallinaceum* and *Plasmodium berghei. Biochem. Pharmacol.*, **1960**, *6*, 143–152.

Schmidt, L. H. *Plasmodium falciparum* and *Plasmodium vivax* infections in the owl monkey (*Aotus trivirgatus*). *Am. J. Trop. Med. Hyg.*, **1978**, *27*, 671–737.

Schmidt, L. H.; Crosby, R.; Rasco, J.; and Vaughan, D. Antimalarial activities of various 4-quinolinemethanols with special attention to WR-142,490 (mefloquine). *Antimicrob. Agents Chemother.*, **1978**, *13*, 1011–1030.

Smith, C. C. Metabolism of pentaquine in the rhesus monkey. *J. Pharmacol. Exp. Ther.*, **1956**, *116*, 67–76.

Smith, C. C., and Ihrig, J. Persistent excretion of pyrimethamine following oral administration. *Am. J. Trop. Med. Hyg.*, **1959**, *8*, 60–62.

Smith, C. C.; Ihrig, J.; and Menne, R. Antimalarial activity and metabolism of biguanides. I. Metabolism of chloroguanide and chloroguanide triazine in rhesus monkeys and man. *Am. J. Trop. Med. Hyg.*, **1961**, *10*, 694–703.

Smith, C. C., and Schmidt, L. H. Observations on the absorption of pyrimethamine from the gastrointestinal tract. *Exp. Parasitol.*, **1963**, *13*, 178–185.

Stickney, D. R.; Simmons, W. S.; De Angelis, R. L.; Rundles, R. W.; and Nichol, C. A. Pharmacokinetics of pyrimethamine (PRM) and 2,4-diamino-5-(3′,4′-dichlorophenyl)-6-methyl pyrimidine (DMP) relevant to meningeal leukemia. *Proc. Am. Assoc. Cancer Res.*, **1973**, *14*, 52.

Thompson, P. E.; Olszewski, B. J.; Elslager, E. F.; and Worth, D. F. Laboratory studies on 4,6-diamino-1-(p-chlorophenyl)-1,2-dihydro-2,2-dimethyl-s-triazine pamoate (CI-501) as a repository antimalarial drug. *Am. J. Trop. Med. Hyg.*, **1963**, *12*, 481–493.

Trenholme, G. M.; Williams, R. L.; Desjardins, R. E.; Frischer, H.; Carson, P. E.; and Rieckmann, K. H.

Mefloquine (WR 142,490) in the treatment of human malaria. *Science,* **1975,** *190,* 792–794.

Waitz, J. A.; Olszewski, B. J.; and Thompson, P. E. Dialysis studies in rats on the long-acting antimalarial CI-501. *Science,* **1963,** *141,* 723–725.

Warhurst, D. C.; Homewood, C. A.; Peters, W.; and Baggaley, V. C. Pigment changes in *Plasmodium berghei* as indications of activity and mode of action of antimalarial drugs. *Proc. Helminthol. Soc. Wash.,* **1972,** *39,* 271–278.

Warhurst, D. C., and Thomas, S. C. The chemotherapy of rodent malaria. XXXI. The effect of some metabolic inhibitors upon chloroquine-induced pigment clumping (CIPC) in *Plasmodium berghei. Ann. Trop. Med. Parasitol.,* **1978,** *72,* 203–211.

Whichard, L. P.; Morris, C. R.; Smith, J. M.; and Holbrook, D. J., Jr. The binding of primaquine, pentaquine, pamaquine, and PLASMOCID to deoxyribonucleic acid. *Mol. Pharmacol.,* **1968,** *4,* 630–639.

Wolf, A. Quinine: an effective form of treatment for myotonia. *Arch. Neurol. Psychiatry,* **1936,** *36,* 382–383.

Young, M. D., and Moore, D. V. Chloroquine resistance in *Plasmodium falciparum. Am. J. Trop. Med. Hyg.,* **1961,** *10,* 317–320.

Monographs and Reviews

Albert, A. *Selective Toxicity: The Physico-Chemical Basis of Therapy,* 5th ed. Chapman & Hall, Ltd., London, **1973.**

Beutler, E. Drug-induced hemolytic anemia. *Pharmacol. Rev.,* **1969,** *21,* 73–103.

Coatney, G. R.; Cooper, W. C.; Eddy, N. B.; and Greenberg, J. *Survey of Antimalarial Agents: Chemotherapy of Plasmodium gallinaceum Infections; Toxicity; Correlation of Structure and Action.* Public Health Service Monograph No. 9, U.S. Government Printing Office, Washington, D. C., **1953.**

Davey, D. G. Chemotherapy of malaria. Part 1. Biological basis of testing methods. In, *Experimental Chemotherapy,* Vol. 1. (Schnitzer, R. J., and Hawking, F., eds.) Academic Press, Inc., New York, **1963,** pp. 487–511.

Dubois, E. L. Antimalarials in the management of discoid and systemic lupus erythematosus. *Semin. Arthritis Rheum.,* **1978,** *8,* 33–51.

Feldman, H. A. Toxoplasmosis. *N. Engl. J. Med.,* **1968,** *279,* 1370–1375, 1431–1437.

Goodwin, L. G., and Rollo, I. M. The chemotherapy of malaria, piroplasmosis, trypanosomiasis, and leishmaniasis. In, *Biochemistry and Physiology of Protozoa,* Vol. II.

(Hutner, S. H., and Lwoff, A., eds.) Academic Press, Inc., New York, **1955,** pp. 225–276.

Hill, J. Chemotherapy of malaria. Part 2. The antimalarial drugs. In, *Experimental Chemotherapy,* Vol. 1. (Schnitzer, R. J., and Hawking, F., eds.) Academic Press, Inc., New York, **1963,** pp. 513–601.

Hitchings, G. H., and Burchall, J. J. Inhibition of folate biosynthesis and function as a basis for chemotherapy. *Adv. Enzymol.,* **1965,** *27,* 417–468.

Modell, W. Malaria and victory in Vietnam. *Science,* **1968,** *162,* 1346–1352.

Oettingen, W. F. von. *The Therapeutic Agents of the Quinoline Group.* Chemical Catalog Co., New York, **1933.**

Peters, W. Chemotherapeutic agents in tropical diseases. In, *Recent Advances in Pharmacology.* (Robson, J. M., and Stacey, R. S., eds.) J. & A. Churchill, Ltd., London, **1968,** pp. 503–537.

Powell, R. D., and Tigertt, W. D. Drug resistance of parasites causing human malaria. *Annu. Rev. Med.,* **1968,** *19,* 81–102.

Rollo, I. M. The chemotherapy of malaria. In, *Biochemistry and Physiology of Protozoa,* Vol. III. (Hutner, S. H., ed.) Academic Press, Inc., New York, **1964,** pp. 525–561.

————. Dihydrofolate reductase inhibitors as antimicrobial agents and their potentiation by sulfonamides. *CRC Crit. Rev. Clin. Lab. Sci.,* **1970,** *1,* 565–583.

Symposium on DARAPRIM. (Various authors.) *Trans. R. Soc. Trop. Med. Hyg.,* **1952,** *46,* 467–508.

Symposium. (Various authors.) The synergy of trimethoprim and sulphonamides. *Postgrad. Med. J.,* **1969,** *45,* Suppl., 3–104.

Tarlov, A. R.; Brewer, G. J.; Carson, P. E.; and Alving, A. S. Primaquine sensitivity. *Arch. Intern. Med.,* **1962,** *109,* 209–234.

Thompson, P. E., and Werbel, L. M. *Antimalarial Agents: Chemistry and Pharmacology.* Academic Press, Inc., New York, **1972.**

Wiselogle, F. Y. (ed.). *A Survey of Antimalarial Drugs, 1941–1945.* J. W. Edwards, Pub., Inc., Ann Arbor, Mich., **1946.** (Two volumes.)

World Health Organization. *Standardization of Procedures for the Study of Glucose-6-Phosphate Dehydrogenase.* Technical Report No. 366, WHO, Geneva, **1967.**

————. *Fourteenth Report of the Expert Committee on Malaria.* Technical Report No. 382, WHO, Geneva, **1968.**

————. *Chemotherapy of Malaria and Resistance to Antimalarials.* Technical Report No. 529, WHO, Geneva, **1973.**

CHAPTER

46 DRUGS USED IN THE CHEMOTHERAPY OF AMEBIASIS

Ian M. Rollo

Amebiasis is worldwide in distribution. It can no longer be considered a tropical disease. Indeed, in some districts in the temperate climates where sanitary conditions are poor, the incidence may be almost as high as in warm countries. While endemic amebiasis is relatively rare among the general population of the United States, the disease may be very common where sanitation is poor—for example, in lower socioeconomic areas in the South, in mental institutions, and on certain Indian reservations.

Dysentery is only one of the protean clinical manifestations of amebiasis. The majority of patients with amebic infections do not have dysentery, but only mild symptoms recognized with difficulty as being caused by pathogenic amebae. Much of the difficulty arises partly from an inability to identify the parasite and partly from a failure to realize the fine interplay of host-parasite relations. The latter may take multiple forms: the parasite may remain as a commensal in the lumen of the bowel, producing cysts but with little or no disturbance to the well-being of the host; dysentery may occur, at which time motile trophozoites (which develop from the cysts) are found in the mucoid and bloody stools; or the protozoan may abuse the hospitality unwittingly offered and invade the extraintestinal tissues, producing, for example, hepatic abscesses (*see* Elsdon-Dew, 1968; Krogstad *et al.*, 1978). Disease is acquired by the ingestion of cysts. Before a definitive diagnosis of amebiasis is made, it is most important that other nonpathogenic amebae found in the human are not mistaken for *Entamoeba histolytica*. Differentiation from *Entamoeba hartmanni* is difficult. White blood cells are also often mistaken for trophozoites or cysts. The services of an experienced microscopist are required. Evidence of invasive amebiasis can be obtained serologi-

cally. *Entamoeba histolytica* antigen prepared from axenic cultures or a simple latex agglutination kit is available commercially. However, since antibody titers persist for months or years after a complete cure, positive serology is not proof of a current infection.

The physician has at his disposal a variety of amebicidal drugs. No one drug can as yet be said to be a cure-all, and treatment must be based on the state of the disease, the condition of the patient, local practice, experience of the practitioner, and, by no means least, the overall cost of a course, or possibly several courses, of treatment.

An important division of amebicides is into agents effective against *extraintestinal* infections and those effective against *intestinal* amebiasis. Of the drugs used to treat amebiasis, only emetine, the closely related dehydroemetine, chloroquine, and metronidazole are effective for the treatment of the more serious extraintestinal disease. While, in fact, the use of metronidazole has revolutionized the treatment of all forms of amebiasis (Powell, 1971), the eradication of microorganisms from asymptomatic patients who are passing cysts is difficult to achieve. Diloxanide furoate may be particularly useful for this purpose.

In recent years infection with free-living *Naegleria*, particularly *Naegleria fowleri*, and perhaps *Acanthamoeba* species has been recognized as presenting special problems in diagnosis and treatment. In man, the former amebae produce a generalized and rapidly progressing, fatal meningoencephalitis. Unfortunately, unless the microorganism is suspected, adequately early diagnosis cannot be made, since the amebae are not readily recognized in the customary gram-stained preparation of cerebrospinal fluid sediment. Evidence from both *in-vitro* and *in-vivo* experiments, and from sparse clinical data, suggests that treatment with amphotericin B may be successful (Duma *et al.*, 1971). Intravenous and intracisternal administration of the drug is probably essential.

PRINCIPLES OF CHEMOTHERAPY OF AMEBIASIS

The therapy of amebiasis includes the treatment of patients with all forms of the disease, including the asymptomatic passer of cysts. The latter individual is a source of infection for both himself and others and is an extremely serious public health problem, especially if he handles food. While unlikely, amebic abscesses of the liver, brain, and lung may develop in carriers who have had few or no previous symptoms of intestinal amebiasis. It is important also to remember that hepatic amebiasis has been known to occur during treatment with amebicides acting only at the intestinal site of infection.

The criterion of cure of intestinal amebiasis is based on laboratory, not clinical, examination. Disappearance of symptoms does not mean cure of amebiasis. Cure is considered accomplished if no amebae of the *histolytica* species are found in multiple stool specimens properly obtained and examined at intervals for 6 months. Repeated courses of medication are sometimes required to effect a cure. Treatment should be resumed whenever the stools again become positive for pathogenic amebae. It must be emphasized again, however, that many false diagnoses and much unnecessary therapy have resulted from incorrect laboratory reports.

Only the general principles of therapy of amebiasis with specific chemotherapeutic agents can be reviewed here. The details of treatment and of the adjuvant measures employed should be sought in the specialized literature, references to which are given at the end of this chapter.

Treatment of the Asymptomatic Carrier and Mild Case. Agents effective in these forms of the disease act by destroying trophozoites and thus eradicating amebic cysts. If one course of medication does not establish a cure, concurrent drug therapy or alternating courses of two different drugs should be prescribed. Both the asymptomatic cyst passer and the cyst passer who has mild intestinal symptoms may be treated in this manner. The preferred drugs are diloxanide furoate or an 8-hydroxyquinoline. Since the presence of cysts in the feces is presumptive evidence of trophozoite activity in the colon, a course of metronidazole or chloroquine may be given to eradicate any unsuspected concurrent hepatic infection, although few authorities actually follow this practice. Metronidazole has proven less effective in the asymptomatic cyst passer than might have been

expected from its success in the treatment of other forms of the disease. Although a relatively high rate of cure has resulted from its use, more reliable results can be achieved by the use of purely luminal amebicides. However, the drug has the advantage of dealing effectively with an unsuspected concurrent hepatic infection. Emetine and chloroquine are not useful in eradicating the passage of cysts by the asymptomatic carrier.

Patients with mild cases of diarrhea or enteritis may remain ambulatory and are best managed by treatment with metronidazole. If relapse occurs, the course of metronidazole may be repeated or drugs from different chemical classes may be alternated or used concurrently.

Treatment of Acute Amebic Dysentery. With the first successful use of metronidazole in 1966 for the treatment of invasive amebiasis, it became obvious that antiamebic therapy was greatly simplified. In place of, for example, emetine and an antibiotic followed by a course of an intestinal amebicide, a course of treatment with metronidazole, which is readily acceptable to the patient, provides a high percentage of cures. The drug eliminates not only the intestinal amebae but also any extraintestinal foci of infection.

While such therapy is undeniably effective, dehydroemetine should probably be used for the rapid relief of symptoms in severely ill patients. In this situation it is injected daily for not more than 10 days (5 days preferred), and the total daily dose should not exceed 60 mg. As a rule, symptoms subside within 4 to 6 days and the stools become formed. The drug is discontinued as soon as the acute symptoms are under control, and either metronidazole or a specific intestinal amebicide is substituted.

As an alternative to metronidazole or in cases of inadequate response to metronidazole, concurrent drug therapy may often be employed to advantage in patients with acute amebic dysentery, as well as in those with latent intestinal amebiasis with or without symptoms. For example, dehydroemetine plus tetracycline or paromomycin have been employed concurrently and then followed with a course of treatment with an intestinal amebicide, such as iodoquinol. Although dehydroemetine will most likely have destroyed any amebae reaching the liver, a course of treatment with chloroquine may be advisable to conclude therapy.

Symptoms and signs suggestive of acute appendicitis may be simulated by acute cecal amebiasis; this complication calls for immediate treatment with dehydroemetine, which, as a rule, affords prompt relief. Surgical intervention may cause serious or fatal complications, especially in patients with acute amebic dysentery.

Treatment of Amebic Hepatitis and Abscess. Amebic hepatitis and amebic abscess of the liver and other organs are always secondary to intestinal infection with *E. histolytica*, even though symptoms of intestinal amebiasis may never have been experienced by the patient. Abscesses may occur in asymptomatic passers of cysts. Only motile forms of amebae are found in abscesses.

Treatment with metronidazole is preferred for this severe form of amebiasis. A very high incidence of cure is achieved with a course of treatment readily tolerated by the large majority of patients. Treatment with a combination of dehydroemetine (or emetine) and chloroquine remains the alternative to metronidazole; despite their limitation in the therapy of intestinal amebiasis, they are extremely effective for treating amebic hepatitis or amebic abscess. If myocardial damage is present, emetine and dehydroemetine should be avoided, although the use of chloroquine alone carries a greater chance of relapse. While emetine and dehydroemetine are very similar, many believe that the latter compound is somewhat less toxic.

Early recognition of amebic hepatitis and initiation of appropriate treatment may prevent abscess formation. Usually, symptoms and signs of amebic hepatitis are relieved within a week; if not, suppuration has probably occurred. Decisions about the advisability of drainage of an hepatic abscess are difficult; there have been no convincing demonstrations that the procedure facilitates healing. It is probably necessary only if there is concern that rupture may occur, as evidenced by severe tenderness, marked elevation of the diaphragm, or other signs. Aspiration by needle is usually sufficient; surgical drainage is rarely necessary. Amebic brain abscess is very rare, and an etiological diagnosis is seldom made *in vivo*.

If the patient has been treated with metronidazole and cured of amebic hepatitis or amebic abscess, he will have been cured simultaneously of his intestinal infection. If an alternative course of treatment has been used, attention must be then given to eradicating the infection of the colon with an intestinal amebicide.

METRONIDAZOLE

Probably the most significant advance in the treatment of protozoal infection has been the introduction and successful use of *metronidazole* as an amebicide. Metronidazole was first introduced as a systemic trichomonacidal agent, effective when given orally in both male and female patients. The background of its development, its chemistry and pharmacology, and its other clinical uses are described in Chapter 47. The drug is exceedingly active against *E. histolytica*. In culture, the morphology of the microorganisms is altered markedly within 6 to 20 hours by concentrations of 1 to 2 μg/ml of metronidazole. Within 24 hours all microorganisms are killed. At a concentration of 0.2 μg/ml, the same effect is seen within 72 hours (Gordeeva, 1965). The significance of the advance lies in the usefulness of the drug in the treatment of all forms of amebiasis. The other agents described in this chapter are useful primarily in only one form of the disease, whether it be in the asymptomatic luminal stage, the intestinal invasive stage, or the extraintestinal stage.

In all geographical areas, regardless of the virulence of the strains or the form of amebiasis being treated, it is recommended that patients receive 750 mg of metronidazole, three times daily for 5 to 10 days. The daily dose for children is 35 to 50 mg/kg, given in three divided doses for 10 days. Treatment with metronidazole is least effective when the drug is administered to the *asymptomatic* passer of cysts. While metronidazole has proven effective in a large number of cases, it is generally felt that there are more failures than result from the use of purely luminal amebicides; the latter are thus preferred. Despite considerable clinical use over the last several years, resistance of *E. histolytica* to metronidazole has not occurred. Indeed, attempts to produce resistance to the drug *in vitro* have been unsuccessful. *Mass treatment* with a large dose once monthly for a few months and then on alternate months has resulted in a marked decrease in the incidence of amebic dysentery in relatively isolated communities with a high degree of endemicity.

In the relatively large doses used in treating amebiasis, nausea, headache, dry mouth, and metallic taste are frequently encountered but rarely necessitate interruption of treatment. Other toxic effects and preparations of metronidazole are described in Chapter 47.

8-HYDROXYQUINOLINES

A number of halogenated 8-hydroxyquinolines have been synthesized and utilized clinically for their amebicidal action. Two such compounds, *iodoquinol* (*diiodohydroxyquin*) and *clioquinol* (*iodochlorhydroxyquin*), are described here. Other derivatives available in various parts of the world include *broxyquinoline* (5,7-dibromo-8-quinolinol), *chlorquinaldol* (5,7-dichloro-2-methyl-8-quinolinol), and *chiniofon* (8-hydroxy-7-iodo-5-quinolinesulfonic acid). It is difficult to rank the halogenated 8-hydroxyquinoline amebicides in any order of superiority; authorities differ in their preferences, and each agent has its advocates.

Chemistry. Iodoquinol and clioquinol are both dihalogenated derivatives of 8-hydroxyquinoline (8-quinolinol). Their structural formulas are as follows:

Iodoquinol (X = Y = I)
Clioquinol (X = I; Y = Cl)

Pharmacological Effects. The 8-hydroxyquino-lines are directly amebicidal. They are active against both motile and cystic forms, but their efficacy in eliminating cysts is probably based on their ability to destroy trophozoites. They act only on amebae in the intestinal tract and are ineffective in amebic abscess and hepatitis. While these drugs are effective in the cyst-passing patient, they are much less effective in the treatment of acute amebic dysentery. The mechanism of the amebicidal action of the 8-hydroxy-quinolines is unknown.

Absorption, Fate, and Excretion. After oral administration, a variable but significant portion of the ingested dose is absorbed. In man, up to one fourth of an administered dose of clioquinol can be recovered in the urine, largely in the form of the glucuronide. The ethereal sulfate is also formed. Iodoquinol is the least well absorbed of this group of drugs—only one third as much as clioquinol (Berggren and Hansson, 1968). It is not known if the compounds are effective in intestinal amebiasis solely by virtue of their presence in the lumen of the bowel or also in part by their presence in the circulation.

After a single oral dose of 250 mg, the maximal concentration of clioquinol in the plasma averages 5 μg/ml within 4 to 8 hours. The half-life of the drug is 11 to 14 hours, and, after repeated, thrice-daily administration in man, a steady-state plasma concentration is reached within a few days (Jack and Riess, 1973).

Preparations. *Iodoquinol,* U.S.P. (*diiodohydroxy-quin;* YODOXIN), is available as tablets containing 210 or 650 mg of the drug and in packets containing 25 g of powder.

Clioquinol, U.S.P. (*iodochlorhydroxyquin;* VIO-FORM), is available in several official preparations: as a cream (3% in water-washable base), an ointment (3% in petrolatum base), a powder, and enteric-coated tablets (not currently available in the United States). Topical preparations that contain hydrocortisone are also available. The drug is used topically for inflammatory conditions such as eczema, athlete's foot, and other fungal infections.

Route of Administration and Dosage. In intestinal amebiasis, the dose of iodoquinol for adults is 650 mg, three times daily for 20 days. Children should receive 30 to 40 mg/kg daily in three divided doses for 20 days (to a maximal daily dose of 2 g). The initial course should not be repeated without an intervening rest period of 2 to 3 weeks. A daily dose of 650 mg may be adequate in asymptomatic carriers. In the treatment of symptomatic intestinal amebiasis, it is common practice to administer iodoquinol either concurrently with another effective intestinal amebicide or to give the two drugs in alternating courses.

Clioquinol is given for amebiasis in the form of oral tablets; a course consists of 500 to 750 mg, three times a day for 10 days. This regimen is repeated after an 8-day rest period. Clioquinol may be given with another effective intestinal amebicide, or the two drugs may be used in alternating courses. Clioquinol retention enemas have been employed

with considerable success, and rectal irritation does not occur; 2 g of clioquinol powder in a 1% suspension in water (200 ml) may be instilled on alternate nights for five doses.

Toxicity and Side Effects. While these compounds were thought to have a low order of toxicity and have been widely sold and used for such nonspecific entities as "traveler's diarrhea," such use is apparently associated with significant risk. The most important toxic reaction, ascribed particularly to clioquinol, is a *subacute myelo-optic neuropathy* (SMON), the incidence of which has had a peculiar geographic distribution. The disease is a myelitis-like illness that was first described in Japan, to whose inhabitants it is largely confined; only sporadic cases have been diagnosed elsewhere. As the number of afflicted patients rose to the thousands, a special research council was formed in Japan to investigate the matter. In its findings clioquinol was implicated as an important etiological factor. This resulted in cessation of sale of the drug in Japan in 1970, and restrictions were imposed on its sale and use in some other countries, including the United States. While there was considerable controversy over the role of the drug in the etiology of the disease, its discontinuation in Japan led to an immediate and dramatic reduction in the appearance of cases of the syndrome; its causative role is thus indicated (*see* Cavanagh, 1973; Oakley, 1973; Zbinden, 1973).

SMON is usually preceded by abdominal pain and persistent diarrhea, and it proceeds to bilateral sensory disturbances—paresthesias and dysesthesias, preferentially in the distal parts of the lower limbs. Other frequent symptoms are deep sensory disturbances, muscle weakness in the legs, pyramidal signs, and slight involvement of the upper limbs. Less common are blurred vision and blindness, disturbances of the autonomic nervous system, psychological changes, and greenish discoloration of the tongue.

While SMON was epidemic only in Japan and was apparently caused by the administration of clioquinol, similar toxic effects also have been observed with other 8-hydroxyquinolines in other countries (*see* Oakley, 1973). While the precise relationship is uncertain, administration of iodoquinol to children for chronic diarrhea has been associated with optic atrophy and permanent loss of vision.

Other side effects observed with 8-hydroxyquinolines include severe generalized furunculosis (iodine toxicoderma), chills, fever, mild-to-severe dermatitis, anal irritation and itching, transitory abdominal discomfort, diarrhea, and headache. These drugs are contraindicated in patients with hepatic damage or iodine intolerance. Thyroid enlargement has occasionally been noted, and these agents interfere with certain thyroid function tests for months because of their content of iodine.

Therapeutic Uses. The 8-hydroxyquinolines are effective for *intestinal amebiasis* and are particularly useful for treatment of asymptomatic passers of cysts. The drugs are useful for ambulatory and mass treatment. They are inexpensive. However, because of the apparent ability of at least some of these compounds to cause SMON, the administration of diloxanide furoate is probably preferable.

The use of these agents to treat "traveler's diarrhea" and chronic nonspecific diarrhea in children cannot be condoned, since such conditions are self-limited and any possible therapeutic benefit does not justify the risk of serious neurotoxicity.

Iodoquinol has been reported of value in intestinal infections due to *Dientamoeba fragilis*. It is also useful in cases of *lambliasis* resistant to treatment with quinacrine and in *balantidial dysentery;* such use is regarded as investigational in the United States. Both iodoquinol and clioquinol have been used for the treatment of various dermatological disorders, and large doses have been employed orally in the treatment of *acrodermatitis enteropathica*, a rare, potentially fatal pediatric condition (Deffner and Perry, 1973). Oral treatment with zinc sulfate has also been found to be effective in this condition.

EMETINE

History. The rational use of emetine as an amebicide dates from 1912, when Vedder showed that the drug killed amebae *in vitro;* since then emetine has been one of the most widely used agents in the treatment of both *intestinal* and *extraintestinal* amebiasis. Much of the early work has been reviewed by Craig (1944).

Chemistry and Preparations. *Emetine Hydrochloride,* U.S.P., is a hydrated hydrochloride of an alkaloid obtained from ipecac or prepared synthetically by methylation of cephaëline, another alkaloid in ipecac. The source of ipecac ("Brazil root") is the dried root or rhizome of *Cephaëlis ipecacuanha* or *acuminata,* plants native to Brazil and Central America but also cultivated in India and Malaysia. Emetine has the following structural formula:

Emetine

Emetine hydrochloride is very irritating and should not be allowed to come in contact with the cornea or with mucous membranes, especially of the conjunctiva. It is available in solution in ampuls for parenteral use (65 mg/ml).

The *structure-activity relationship* in several chemical series allied to emetine has been explored (*see* Woolfe, 1963). However, none of the many congeneric compounds tested by both *in-vitro* and *in-vivo* methods approaches emetine in amebicidal activity, with the exception of its dehydrogenated derivative (*see* below).

Mechanism of Amebicidal Action. Emetine has a direct lethal action on *E. histolytica.* The drug is much more effective against motile forms than against cysts. *In vitro,* emetine readily kills trophozoites at concentrations that are found in the systemic circulation after therapeutic doses. These values may not be attained in the lumen of the intestine.

Grollman (1966) has studied the structural basis for the emetine-induced inhibition of protein synthesis in certain mammalian and other cells. He demonstrated the configurational and conformational similarities of (−)-emetine to (−)-cycloheximide and other glutarimide antibiotics, findings that provide the basis for new synthetic approaches to potentially superior chemotherapeutic agents. Later work showed that emetine prevented protein synthesis by inhibiting the translocation of peptidyl-tRNA from the acceptor site to the donor site on the ribosome (Huang and Grollman, 1970). Emetine, like cycloheximide, inhibits protein synthesis in eukaryotes but not in prokaryotes.

Absorption, Fate, and Excretion. Oral administration of emetine results in considerable irritation of the gastrointestinal tract, and the drug cannot be given by this route. Emetine is absorbed from parenteral sites of administration and is excreted or metabolized slowly. Although the drug appears in the urine 20 to 40 minutes after injection, emetine can still be found there 40 to 60 days after treatment has been discontinued. Therefore, cumulative toxic action is an ever-present danger. The highest concentration of the alkaloid is found in the liver, a fact that may account for the greater efficacy of emetine in hepatic than in intestinal amebiasis; appreciable amounts are also found in the lung, kidney, and spleen.

Toxicity. The long persistence of the alkaloid in the body is the basis for cumulative toxicity, and repeated courses of emetine without adequate rest periods frequently result in serious intoxication. The nature, incidence, and mechanisms of the untoward reactions to emetine have been critically reviewed by Klatskin and Friedman (1948).

Gastrointestinal Effects. These manifestations of emetine toxicity include diarrhea, nausea, and vomiting. Diarrhea may be induced or aggravated in approximately 50% of patients; it is often associated with cramping abdominal pain and, rarely, with blood, mucus, or pus. It may cause marked prostration. The diarrhea is due to increased peristalsis caused by the direct action of emetine on the intestinal musculature. Emetine-induced diarrhea may be mistaken for an exacerbation of the amebic dysentery, from which it can usually be differentiated by the fact that a period of improvement initiated by emetine often precedes the diarrhea. Nausea occurs in approximately one third of patients receiving emetine and may be associated with vomiting; both are probably central in origin when the drug is administered parenterally. Dizziness and faintness often occur, especially in association with the nausea and vomiting. Headache may also be experienced. Gastrointestinal symptoms may disappear despite continued emetine therapy, but occasionally they are so severe that the drug must be discontinued.

Neuromuscular Effects. Neuromuscular manifestations consist in weakness, aching, tenderness, and stiffness of skeletal muscles, especially those of the neck and the extremities. Edema may also occur, perhaps secondary to the muscle injury or inactivity. Mild sensory disturbances and tremor may be observed, but the usual signs of neuritis are absent. Ng (1966) has observed a blocking action of emetine on the neuromuscular junction, which may account for some of the clinical findings. A direct effect on skeletal muscle fibers of treated rats has also been described (Bradley *et al.*, 1976). Weakness and muscular pain tend to persist until the drug administration is stopped; they usually appear before more serious symptoms develop and thus serve as a guide for avoiding overdosage.

Cardiovascular System. The most important toxic effects of emetine relate to the cardiovascular system, and include hypotension, precordial pain, tachycardia, dyspnea, and ECG abnormalities; the last two disturbances tend to persist until medication is discontinued, but the others may disappear despite continued emetine therapy. The incidence of cardiovascular involvement varies in different series, and some degree of toxicity may occur in the great majority of patients. Frequently, multiple symptoms are experienced. *Hypotension* is rarely marked. Its cause is unknown. *Precordial pain* caused by emetine may resemble that of coronary thrombosis, from which it requires differentiation; its cause is also unknown. *Tachycardia* may occur, especially if the patient is permitted to be ambulatory, and frequently precedes the appearance of ECG abnormalities. Emetine should be discontinued as soon as tachycardia is evident. *Dyspnea* is experienced by some patients, but in most cases it is probably not cardiac in origin. It may be related to the generalized weakness and tends to persist until the drug is stopped.

ECG changes induced by emetine may occur in from 25 to 50% or more of patients. The direct toxic effect of emetine on cardiac muscle has been repeatedly demonstrated in animals and man, and cardiac dilatation, failure, and death have been reported; the ECG affords a sensitive and early index of such toxicity. The major changes from therapeutic doses are flattening and inversion of the T waves in all leads, and prolongation of the Q-T interval (*see* Kent and Kingsland, 1950). ECG alterations tend to persist even after emetine is discontinued, in some cases for 2 months or more. In other patients, ECG abnormalities may not appear until the usual course of emetine is completed. Obviously, emetine medication should be stopped as soon as significant ECG changes are evident. To reduce the incidence of cardiotoxicity, patients should be sedentary and the cardiovascular status should be monitored carefully. Emetine should obviously be avoided if at all possible for patients with organic heart disease.

Local Reactions. A *local reaction* to emetine is very common. It is characterized by aching, tenderness, stiffness, and weakness of the muscles in the area of the injection site, and occurs even after subcutaneous injection. Evidence of local inflammation is lacking, and the reaction is believed to represent a regional myositis. Local eczematous lesions may result from subcutaneous injection of the drug; generalized urticarial and purpuric skin lesions also have been observed.

Routes of Administration and Dosage. The preferred routes of emetine administration are by deep subcutaneous or intramuscular injection. The intravenous use of emetine is contraindicated because it is dangerous and offers no therapeutic advantages. The dose of emetine hydrochloride for adults should not exceed 60 mg per day; treatment with 1 mg/kg per day (to this limit) for up to 5 days is recommended. Children should receive not more than 1 mg/kg daily in two divided doses for the same length of time. A course of emetine should not be repeated until a rest period of at least 6 weeks has intervened.

Therapeutic Uses. Emetine alone does not result in the *cure* of amebic infection in more than 10 to 15% of patients. Although clinical symptoms are greatly improved and both motile amebae and cysts disappear from the stools during emetine medication in patients with acute amebic dysentery, cysts reappear in approximately 50% of cases at varying periods after therapy has been discontinued. This fact indicates that trophozoites still exist in the bowel. Such patients often become asymptomatic carriers, with all the attendant dangers to themselves and the general public. Treatment of asymptomatic carriers with emetine is notoriously unsuccessful.

The valid uses of emetine in *intestinal amebiasis* are for severe cases of amebic diarrhea and acute amebic dysentery, that is, when trophozoites are found in the stool. The drug should be given only long enough to control the diarrhea or dysenteric symptoms. Dosage is discussed above. Emetine has great value in the treatment of *amebic abscesses* and *amebic hepatitis*. In such conditions, the alkaloid may be lifesaving; it should be used in combination with chloroquine and is an alternative to metronidazole.

DEHYDROEMETINE

The synthesis of emetine in 1959 led to the ready availability of various analogs (*see* Whittaker, 1969). Of these, dehydroemetine has been studied extensively both in the laboratory and in clinical trial. These studies suggest that dehydroemetine retains the amebicidal property of the parent compound but is less toxic. The substance is identical to emetine except for the lack of hydrogen atoms at positions 2 and 3.

Dehydroemetine is not marketed in the United States, but it can be obtained from the Parasitic Diseases Division, Center for Disease Control, Atlanta, Georgia 30333. The drug is available in single-dose, 2-ml ampuls, each containing 60 mg of the dihydrochloride in aqueous solution.

The uses of dehydroemetine are identical to those of emetine, which are discussed above. The recommended dosage is a single intramuscular or subcutaneous injection of 1 to 1.5 mg/kg, given daily for up to 5 days (90 mg per day maximal). The course of treatment should not be repeated in less than 14 days. Children should receive the same dosage up to a limit of 90 mg per day.

Side effects following the use of dehydroemetine are similar to those following emetine; of these, cardiotoxicity has been studied in some detail. While there is no unanimity of opinion, it appears that myocardial changes associated with the administration of dehydroemetine have been less frequent and less severe and have persisted for a shorter period of time than those following the administration of emetine. Nevertheless, the drug should be used cautiously, if at all, in patients with existing cardiac disease, or with primary muscular or neurological disorders.

CHLOROQUINE

History. The unique therapeutic value of chloroquine in *extraintestinal amebiasis* in man was first reported by Conan (1948, 1949) and Murgatroyd and Kent (1948). *In-vitro* studies with trophozoites of *E. histolytica* had revealed that chloroquine possesses amebicidal activity greater than that of the halogenated 8-hydroxyquinolines but less than that of emetine. This discovery, combined with the knowledge that chloroquine localizes in the liver in a concentration several hundred times greater than that in the plasma, suggested its use in *hepatic amebiasis*. Clinical trial then revealed that the signs and the symptoms of amebic hepatitis disappeared within a few days after the start of chloroquine therapy and that the disease was adequately controlled and often cured.

Pharmacological Properties. The pharmacology and the toxicology of chloroquine are fully presented in Chapter 45. Only those features of the drug pertinent to its use in amebiasis are described here.

The *clinical response* to chloroquine in patients with *hepatic amebiasis* is often as prompt and complete as that to emetine, and the drug is effective in some individuals who fail to respond to emetine. Chloroquine, like emetine, is not always curative, and, therefore, additional amebicidal therapy may be necessary. There is no evidence that amebae develop resistance to chloroquine. The drug is much less effective in amebiasis of the colon, partly because it attains a much lower concentration in the intestinal wall than in the liver and partly because it is almost completely absorbed from the small bowel. Since colonic infection with *E. histolytica* is always the source of extraintestinal amebiasis, it is also necessary routinely to administer a drug effective in intestinal amebiasis to all patients receiving chloroquine for hepatic amebiasis; such therapy reduces the relapse rate. Conversely, because of the clinical impossibility of determining with certainty whether individuals with colonic amebiasis also have hepatic involvement, it is often wise to administer metronidazole or chloroquine when a solely intestinal amebicide is prescribed. Although few cases of *pulmonary amebic abscess* have been treated with chloroquine, the results indicate that this type of infection also responds well to the drug.

The conventional course of treatment with chloroquine phosphate for extraintestinal amebiasis in adults is 1 g daily for 2 days, followed by 500 mg daily for 2 to 3 weeks. Because of the low toxicity of the drug, this dose schedule can be revised upward if necessary. The course of chloroquine may be repeated. Extended courses of treatment with chloroquine (10 weeks) have also been recommended (Cohen and Reynolds, 1975). Some authorities consider that chloroquine therapy should immediately follow a course of emetine, while others prefer to give the two drugs concurrently.

DILOXANIDE FUROATE

History. *Diloxanide* (ENTAMIDE) was introduced by Bristow and associates (1956) as a result of the examination of a series of substituted acetanilides for amebicidal activity. Clinical trials showed diloxanide to be effective in cyst-passing patients, but to be relatively ineffective in the treatment of acute intestinal amebiasis. This was attributed to the presence of inadequate concentrations of the drug at the sites of infection. Of the many derivatives prepared in attempts to offset this disadvantage, the furoate ester proved to be appreciably more active than the parent compound in experimentally infected rats (Main *et al.*, 1960). The results of clinical trials showed it to be effective in cases of acute intestinal amebiasis (Shaldon, 1960; Woodruff and Bell, 1960).

Chemistry and Preparations. *Diloxanide furoate* (FURAMIDE) has the following structural formula:

COO—⟨ring⟩—N—COCHCl$_2$
                  |
                  CH$_3$

Diloxanide Furoate

The ester is hydrolyzed to diloxanide and furoic acid. In the United States it is available in oral tablets containing 500 mg of the drug from the Parasitic Diseases Division, Center for Disease Control, Atlanta, Georgia 30333.

Pharmacological Effects. Diloxanide is directly amebicidal when tested *in vitro*. The furoate ester is active at 0.01 to 0.1 μg/ml, and it is thus considerably more potent than emetine. Little is known of its mechanism of action.

Absorption, Fate, and Excretion. In experimental animals, 60 to 90% of an oral dose of diloxanide furoate is excreted in the urine within 48 hours. More than half of this appears within 6 hours. Excretion in the feces accounts for 4 to 9% of the dose. Peak concentrations appear in the blood within 1 hour but fall to a fraction of this within 6 hours. Hence, a major part of an oral dose is rapidly absorbed from the gastrointestinal tract and is rapidly excreted in the urine. The ester is largely, if not wholly, hydrolyzed in the lumen or mucosa of the intestine, so that only diloxanide appears in the systemic circulation (Wilmshurst and Cliffe, 1964). The drug appears in the urine largely as the glucuronide.

Route of Administration and Dosage. Diloxanide furoate is given only orally. The recommended dosage is 500 mg, three times daily for 10 days. If necessary, a second course may be given immediately following the first. Children should be given 20 mg/kg per day in three divided doses for 10 days.

Toxicity and Side Effects. Reports of trials to date remark on the lack of serious side effects following the administration of diloxanide furoate; mild gastrointestinal symptoms have been noted, and in some cases there is increased flatulence (*see* Wolfe, 1973).

Therapeutic Uses. Diloxanide furoate is regarded by some authorities as an agent of first choice in the treatment of asymptomatic passers of cysts (administered alone) (Krogstad *et al.,* 1978), or in the treatment of invasive and extraintestinal amebiasis (administered with other appropriate drugs). It is ineffective when administered alone in the treatment of extraintestinal amebiasis. There is no unanimity of opinion on its efficacy when used alone in the treatment of acute amebiasis with frank dysentery. While good results have been reported from some areas, other trials have been less successful (*see* Suchak *et al.,* 1962; Wilmot *et al.,* 1962). In trials carried out primarily on asymptomatic subjects passing trophozoites or cysts, or on patients with nondysenteric, symptomatic intestinal amebiasis, treatment with diloxanide furoate resulted in a high percentage of cures (Woodruff and Bell, 1960; Wolfe, 1973). In all cases the drug was well tolerated and suited the cooperative, ambulatory outpatient. Forsyth (1962) compared the value of several forms of treatment and pointed out that the low cost of the drug might be a major factor in underdeveloped countries.

ANTIBIOTIC AMEBICIDES

A number of antibiotics have been found to be of value in the treatment of intestinal amebiasis, especially *erythromycin, paromomycin,* and some of the *tetracyclines.* Inasmuch as paromomycin is the only one that is directly amebicidal, it is the only one discussed in any detail here. Other antibiotics are not amebicidal directly, but act by interfering with the enteric flora essential for the proliferation of pathogenic amebae. The older tetracyclines—tetracycline itself, chlortetracycline, and oxytetracycline—are the most frequently used, their efficacy probably depending on the relatively large proportion of the administered dose that escapes absorption in the bowel. The better-absorbed agents are much less effective (*see* Chapter 52). If a tetracycline is used, it is recommended that it be administered together with the appropriate drugs for either intestinal or extraintestinal amebic infections.

Paromomycin. This aminoglycoside antibiotic, isolated from cultures of *Streptomyces rimosus,* is amebicidal both *in vitro* and *in vivo*. Many of its properties are similar to those of other antibiotics in this class (*see* Chapter 51). Paromomycin acts directly on amebae but is also antibacterial to normal

and pathogenic microorganisms in the gastrointestinal tract. Its structural formula is as follows:

Paromomycin

Paromomycin Sulfate, U.S.P. (HUMATIN), is supplied in capsules, each containing 250 mg, and in a syrup (125 mg/5 ml). The recommended dosage is 25 to 35 mg/kg each day, orally in three divided doses at mealtimes, for 5 to 10 days. Higher doses, up to 66 mg/kg, have been used by some investigators. After oral administration, little of the drug is absorbed into the systemic circulation. Side effects are mainly limited to gastrointestinal upset and diarrhea occurring during the course of therapy. Marked renal damage occurs in animals treated parenterally with the drug. A number of clinical trials have been carried out since the introduction of the drug (*see* review by Woolfe, 1965). Experience has shown paromomycin to be effective, but by no means infallible, in the treatment of *intestinal amebiasis;* it is ineffective against extraintestinal forms of the disease. Paromomycin is also effective in the treatment of infections with various tapeworms.

Berggren, L., and Hansson, O. Absorption of intestinal antiseptics derived from 8-hydroxyquinolines. *Clin. Pharmacol. Ther.,* **1968,** *9,* 67–70.

Bradley, W. G.; Fewings, J. D.; Harris, J. B.; and Johnson, M. A. Emetine myopathy in the rat. *Br. J. Pharmacol.,* **1976,** *57,* 29–41.

Bristow, N. W.; Oxley, P.; Williams, G. A. H.; and Woolfe, G. ENTAMIDE, a new amoebicide; preliminary note. *Trans. R. Soc. Trop. Med. Hyg.,* **1956,** *50,* 182.

Cohen, H. G., and Reynolds, T. B. Comparison of metronidazole and chloroquine for the treatment of amebic liver abscess: a controlled trial. *Gastroenterology,* **1975,** *69,* 35–41.

Conan, N. J., Jr. Chloroquine in amebiasis. *Am. J. Trop. Med. Hyg.,* **1948,** *28,* 107–110.

——. The treatment of hepatic amebiasis with chloroquine. *Am. J. Med.,* **1949,** *6,* 309–320.

Deffner, N. F., and Perry, H. O. Acrodermatitis enteropathica and failure to thrive. *Arch. Dermatol.,* **1973,** *108,* 658–662.

Duma, R. J.; Rosenblum, W. I.; McGehee, R. F.; Jones, M. M.; and Nelson, E. C. Primary amoebic meningoencephalitis caused by *Naegleria. Ann. Intern. Med.,* **1971,** *74,* 923–931.

Elsdon-Dew, R. The epidemiology of amoebiasis. *Adv. Parasitol.,* **1968,** *6,* 1–62.

Forsyth, D. M. The treatment of amoebiasis: a field study of various methods. *Trans. R. Soc. Trop. Med. Hyg.,* **1962,** *56,* 400–403.

Gordeeva, L. M. [A study of the effect of FLAGYL upon *Entamoeba histolytica* in culture.] *Med. Parazitol. (Mosk.),* **1965,** *34,* 325–329. (In, *Trop. Dis. Bull.,* **1965,** *62,* 1115.)

Grollman, A. P. Structural basis for inhibition of protein synthesis by emetine and cycloheximide based on an analogy between ipecac alkaloids and glutarimide antibiotics. *Proc. Natl. Acad. Sci. U.S.A.,* **1966,** *56,* 1867–1874.

Huang, T., and Grollman, A. P. Novel inhibitors of protein synthesis in animal cells. *Fed. Proc.,* **1970,** *29,* 609.

Jack, D. B., and Riess, W. Pharmacokinetics of iodochlorhydroxyquin in man. *J. Pharm. Sci.,* **1973,** *62,* 1929–1932.

Kean, B. H. The treatment of amebiasis. A recurrent agony. *J.A.M.A.,* **1976,** *235,* 501.

Kent, L., and Kingsland, R. C. Effects of emetine hydrochloride on the electrocardiogram in man. *Am. Heart J.,* **1950,** *39,* 576–587.

Main, P. T.; Bristow, N. W.; Oxley, P.; Watkins, T. I.; Williams, G. A. H.; Wilmshurst, E. C.; and Woolfe, G. Entamide. *Ann. Biochem. Exp. Med.,* **1960,** *20,* 441–448.

Murgatroyd, F., and Kent, R. P. Refractory amoebic liver abscess treated by chloroquine. *Trans. R. Soc. Trop. Med. Hyg.,* **1948,** *42,* 15–16.

Ng, K. K. F. Blockade of adrenergic and cholinergic transmissions by emetine. *Br. J. Pharmacol. Chemother.,* **1966,** *28,* 228–237.

Oakley, G. P., Jr. The neurotoxicity of the halogenated hydroxyquinolines. *J.A.M.A.,* **1973,** *225,* 395–397.

Powell, S. J. The cardiotoxicity of systemic amebicides: a comparative electrocardiographic study. *Am. J. Trop. Med. Hyg.,* **1967,** *16,* 447–450.

Shaldon, S. Entamide furoate in the treatment of acute amoebic dysentery. *Trans. R. Soc. Trop. Med. Hyg.,* **1960,** *54,* 469–470.

Suchak, N. G.; Satoskar, R. S.; and Sheth, U. K. Entamide furoate in the treatment of intestinal amoebiasis. *Am. J. Trop. Med. Hyg.,* **1962,** *11,* 330–332.

Vedder, E. B. An experimental study of the action of ipecacuanha on amoebae. In, *Transactions of the Second Biennial Congress, Far-Eastern Association of Tropical Medicine,* **1912,** *87.* (Abstracted in, *J. Trop. Med. Hyg.,* **1912,** *15,* 313–314.)

Whittaker, N. The synthesis of emetine and related compounds. Pt. IX. The use of Wittig-type reagents in the synthesis of 2,3-dehydroemetine. *J. Chem. Soc.,* **1969,** *1,* Sect. C, 94–100.

Wilmot, A. J.; Powell, S. J.; McLeod, I.; and Elsdon-Dow, R. Some newer amoebicides in acute amoebic dysentery. *Trans. R. Soc. Trop. Med. Hyg.,* **1962,** *56,* 85–86.

Wilmshurst, E. C., and Cliffe, E. E. Absorption and distribution of amoebicides. In, *Absorption and Distribution of Drugs.* (Binns, T. B., ed.) E. & S. Livingstone, Ltd., Edinburgh, **1964,** pp. 191–198.

Wolfe, M. S. Nondysenteric intestinal amebiasis. Treatment with diloxanide furoate. *J.A.M.A.,* **1973,** *224,* 1601–1604.

Woodruff, A. W., and Bell, S. Clinical trials with entamide furoate and related compounds. I. In a non-tropical environment. *Trans. R. Soc. Trop. Med. Hyg.,* **1960,** *54,* 389–395.

Monographs and Reviews

Anderson, H. H. Newer drugs in amebiasis. *Clin. Pharmacol. Ther.,* **1960,** *1,* 78–86.

Cavanagh, J. B. Peripheral neuropathy caused by chemical agents. *CRC Crit. Rev. Toxicol.,* **1973,** *2,* 365–417.

Craig, C. F. *The Etiology, Diagnosis and Treatment of Amebiasis.* The Williams & Wilkins Co., Baltimore, **1944.**

Juniper, K. Amoebiasis. In, *Clinics in Gastroenterology,* Vol. 7, No. 1. (Marsden, P. D., ed.) W. B. Saunders Co., Ltd., London, **1978,** pp. 3–29.

Klatskin, G., and Friedman, H. Emetine toxicity in man: studies on the nature of early toxic manifestations, their relation to the dose level, and their significance in determining safe dosage. *Ann. Intern. Med.,* **1948,** *28,* 892–915.

Krogstad, D. J.; Spencer, H. C., Jr.; and Healy, G. R. Amebiasis. *N. Engl. J. Med.,* **1978,** *298,* 262–265.

Powell, S. J. Therapy of amebiasis. *Bull. N.Y. Acad. Med.,* **1971,** *47,* 469–477.

Schneider, J. Traitement médical de l'amibiase. *Bull. Soc. Pathol. Exot.,* **1961,** *54,* 616–675.

Woolfe, G. Chemotherapy of amebiasis. In, *Experimental Chemotherapy,* Vol. 1. (Schnitzer, R. J., and Hawking, F., eds.) Academic Press, Inc., New York, **1963,** pp. 355–433.

———. The chemotherapy of amoebiasis. In, *Progress in Drug Research,* Vol. 8. (Jucker, E., ed.) Birkhäuser Verlag, Basel, **1965,** pp. 11–52.

Zbinden, G. Geographical toxicology. In, *Progress in Toxicology,* Vol. 1. Springer-Verlag, Berlin, **1973,** pp. 66–71.

47 MISCELLANEOUS DRUGS USED IN THE TREATMENT OF PROTOZOAL INFECTIONS

Ian M. Rollo

SURAMIN

Suramin is one of the few nonmetallic compounds effective in the treatment of *trypanosomiasis*. It was introduced into therapy in 1920 after several years of research in Germany, based on the observed trypanocidal activity of the dyestuffs *trypan red, trypan blue,* and *afridol violet.*

Chemistry and Preparations. *Suramin sodium* (GERMANIN) has the structural formula shown below. It is a white microcrystalline powder, readily soluble in water to yield a neutral solution. Only freshly prepared solutions should be employed. It is marketed in ampuls containing 1.0 g of the drug. Suramin is available in the United States only from the Parasitic Diseases Division, Center for Disease Control, Atlanta, Georgia 30333.

Antiprotozoal Effects. *Trypanocidal Action.* The mechanism of the trypanocidal action of suramin is unknown. The drug inhibits numerous enzyme systems in low concentrations, but trypanocidal activity has not been related to the inhibition of any specific enzyme. Suramin, a polyanion, forms firm complexes with protein; this possibly may be related to its chemotherapeutic activity. If trypanosomes are exposed to suramin and then washed, they are no longer infective for animals, although they remain active *in vitro* for over 24 hours. Williamson and Macadam (1965) observed morphological damage in suramin-treated trypanosomes characterized by damage to, or disappearance of, all intracellular membranous structures with the exception of lysosomes. This is remarkable in view of the low concentration of suramin that has been shown to occur in these organelles (*see* Allison, 1968).

Filaricidal Action. Suramin is active against *Onchocerca volvulus.* Its action is primarily against the adult filariae, although the maintenance of high concentrations in the blood is said also to eliminate the microfilariae. It is usually employed following a course of diethylcarbamazine, which is safer and more reliable in its effect on microfilariae (*see* Chapter 44).

Absorption, Fate, and Excretion. Suramin must be administered parenterally. Following its intravenous administration, a high concentration is achieved in the plasma. This falls fairly rapidly for a few hours, then more slowly for a few days, after which a low concentration is maintained for as long as 3 months. The persistence of suramin in the circulation is due to its firm binding to plasma protein. The large, polar compound apparently does not enter cells readily since none is present in erythrocytes, and tissue concentrations are uniformly lower than those in the plasma. In experimental animals, however, the kidneys have been found to contain considerably more suramin than other organs. This retention in the kidney may account for the fairly frequent occurrence of albuminuria following injection of the drug in man. Suramin does not penetrate into the cerebrospinal fluid in appreciable amounts. Metabolic destruction of the drug appears to be negligible. The protein-bound suramin dissociates slowly to yield effective concentrations of the drug over long periods of time. Thus, suramin has proven valuable in the *prophylaxis* of trypanosomiasis.

Routes of Administration and Dosage. Suramin is usually given by slow intravenous injection in 10% aqueous solution. Treatment of active *African trypanosomiasis* should not be started until 24 hours after diagnostic lumbar puncture, and caution is required if the patient has onchocerciasis. The normal single dose for adults is 1 g. It is advisable to employ a small dose of 200 mg initially to test for sensitivity, after which the normal dose is given on days 1, 3, 7, 14, and 21; weekly doses may be given for an additional 5 weeks. Patients in poor condition should be treated cautiously during the first week. A

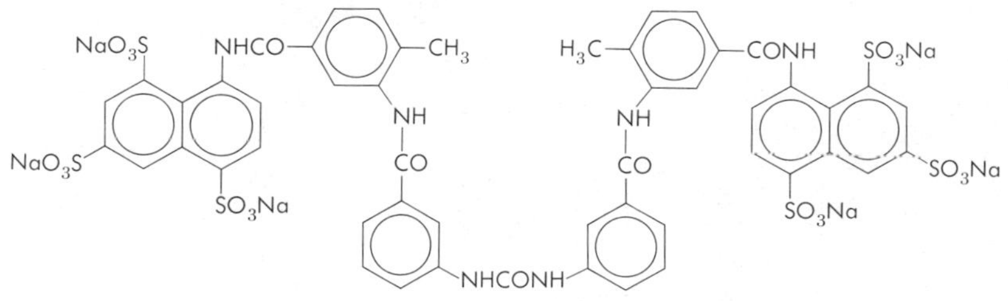

Suramin Sodium

second course of treatment should not be given earlier than 3 months after the first. Suramin may be used also as a chemoprophylactic agent. A single dose of 1 g gives protection for about 3 months.

In the treatment of *onchocerciasis,* after initial treatment with diethylcarbamazine, a trial dose of 200 mg should be followed 1 week later by a dose of 1 g; then 1 g is given weekly to a total dose of 4 to 6 g.

Toxicity and Side Effects. Suramin can cause a variety of untoward reactions. These vary in intensity and frequency with the nutritional status of the patient and reach rather serious proportions among the malnourished. The most serious immediate reaction consists in nausea, vomiting, shock, and loss of consciousness. Fortunately, the incidence is low (0.1 to 0.3%). Colic and acute urticaria are other immediate reactions. Later reactions, which occur up to 24 hours after drug administration, are papular eruptions, paresthesia, photophobia, lacrimation, palpebral edema, and hyperesthesia of the palms of the hands and the soles of the feet. Still later reactions consist in albuminuria, hematuria, and cylindruria. Rarely, agranulocytosis or hemolytic anemia may occur.

Precautions and Contraindications. Patients receiving suramin should be followed closely. Therapy should not be continued in patients who show intolerance to initial doses, and the drug should be employed with great caution in individuals with renal insufficiency. A moderate albuminuria is usual during the control of the acute phase, but persisting, heavy albuminuria calls for caution as well as modification of the schedule of treatment. If casts appear, treatment with suramin should be discontinued. The occurrence of palmar-plantar hyperesthesia necessitates caution since it may presage peripheral neuritis.

Therapeutic Uses. Suramin is employed in the treatment of *trypanosomiasis* caused by *T. gambiense* and *T. rhodesiense.* It is of no value in Chagas' disease (South American trypanosomiasis, caused by *T. cruzi*). When employed alone, the drug is effective only in the early stage of the disease. In the late stage of the disease with central nervous system (CNS) involvement, suramin is commonly used before, or in conjunction with, a course of arsenical therapy because only small amounts of suramin gain access to the cerebrospinal fluid. Suramin is effective in the *prophylaxis* of Rhodesian and Gambian trypanosomiasis. The dose schedule has been outlined. Pentamidine is also useful for this purpose and, indeed, may be a superior agent. Chemoprophylaxis is not recommended for travelers on occasional brief visits to endemic areas since the risk of serious drug toxicity outweighs the risk of acquiring the disease. Suramin is the most effective drug for clearing the adult filariae in *onchocerciasis.* The single dose of 1 g is repeated weekly for 5 or 6 weeks.

PENTAMIDINE

The discovery of chemotherapeutic activity in the diamidine group of drugs, of which pentamidine is a member, was quite fortuitous (*see* King *et al.,* 1938; Lourie and Yorke, 1939). Of the compounds of this type, three were found to possess outstanding activity: 4,4'-diamidinostilbene (*stilbamidine*), 4,4'-diamidinophenoxy pentane (*pentamidine*), and 4,4'-diamidinophenoxy propane (*propamidine*). Pentamidine is the most valuable because of its stability, low toxicity, and ease of administration. *Hydroxystilbamidine Isethionate,* U.S.P. (2-hydroxy-4,4'-diamidinostilbene diisethionate), is preferred by some and has proven useful in the treatment of North American blastomycosis (*see* Chapter 54) and visceral leishmaniasis.

Chemistry and Preparations. Pentamidine has the following structural formula:

Pentamidine

Pentamidine isethionate (LOMIDINE), the preparation available commercially, is a white powder, soluble in water to the extent of 10%. It is marketed as a dry powder, in ampuls containing 200 mg of the drug. It is available in the United States only from the Parasitic Diseases Division, Center for Disease Control, Atlanta, Georgia 30333.

Antiprotozoal Effects. The diamidines are toxic to a number of different protozoa, yet show rather marked selectivity of action. For example, the drugs are curative against *T. rhodesiense* and *T. congolense* infections in experimental animals. However, they are ineffective in curing mice infected with *T. cruzi.* They are also capable of curing *Babesia canis* infections in puppies and *Leishmania donovani* infections in hamsters. These results in animals provide the experimental background for the therapeutic application of diamidines in the treatment of human leishmaniasis and trypanosomiasis.

The diamidines are also fungicidal. This can be readily demonstrated *in vitro* against *Blastomyces dermatitidis,* and has led to the successful therapeutic trial of the drugs in systemic blastomycosis. The advent of amphotericin B has, however, reduced the value of the diamidines in the treatment of this disease. The antibiotic is to be preferred in initial therapy, but hydroxystilbamidine may prove useful if an inadequate response is obtained. Of particular significance are the excellent results obtained with pentamidine in the treatment of pneumonia caused by *Pneumocystis carinii* (*see* Ivady *et al.,* 1967).

Mechanism of Action. The susceptibility of different species of trypanosomes appears to be related to the relative importance of aerobic and anaerobic glycolysis in their metabolism. While the fundamental mechanism of action of pentamidine remains to be defined, related diamidines bind to DNA, particularly that of the trypanosomal kinetoplast. In trypanosomes this specialized rod-shaped, DNA-containing structure is a part of the mitochondrial system. Diamidines may inhibit the replication of kinetoplast DNA (Brack *et al.,* 1972).

Absorption, Fate, and Excretion. Pentamidine isethionate is fairly well absorbed from parenteral sites of administration. Following a single dose, the drug is detectable in the blood for only a very brief period. However, in experimental animals, the liver and the kidney are found to store the drug for months (*see* Waalkes *et al.*, 1970). Binding of pentamidine in tissues seems to be the most important factor in its use as a prophylactic agent in trypanosomiasis.

Routes of Administration and Dosage. Pentamidine is best given by intramuscular injection in individual doses of 4 mg/kg of body weight, daily or on alternate days. The intravenous route may also be used. In the *treatment of early African trypanosomiasis*, a course of ten injections should be given. The drug may be less effective in *T. rhodesiense* infections than in those caused by *T. gambiense*. Because of the rapidity with which *T. rhodesiense* may invade the CNS, treatment with pentamidine is contraindicated unless infection with this species is known with certainty to have occurred within the previous 3 or 4 weeks. Pentamidine has been widely used as a *prophylactic* agent in endemic areas. Single intramuscular injections should be given at intervals of not longer than 6 months; various dosages have been used, but all fall within the range of 3 to 5 mg/kg.

In the treatment of *visceral leishmaniasis* (*L. donovani* leishmaniasis, or *kala-azar*), pentamidine has been used successfully in courses of 12 to 15 doses. A second course, given after an interval of 1 to 2 weeks, may be necessary in areas where the infection is known to respond less well to treatment. The drug is particularly useful in cases that have failed to respond to antimonials—for example, in the Sudan, where the disease responds only to high doses of antimonials, and in China, where many patients with kala-azar are hypersensitive to antimony. Some success has followed the use of pentamidine in the treatment of *cutaneous* (*L. tropica*) *leishmaniasis*, or Oriental sore (*see* Beveridge, 1963). Hydroxystilbamidine is preferred by some practitioners; the choice probably depends upon the local availability of either compound.

Cases of *Pneumocystis carinii pneumonia* should be treated daily with 4 mg/kg intramuscularly, for 12 to 14 days. In severe cases the drug may be given by slow intravenous injection. If treatment is effective, clinical improvement will occur usually 4 to 6 days after the first injection. A high proportion of cures can be expected, depending on supportive therapy and, if possible, elimination of predisposing conditions. The prognosis is less favorable in debilitated patients with altered immunity or neoplastic disease.

Toxicity and Side Effects. The intravenous injection of pentamidine (and other diamidines) is often followed quickly by alarming reactions, which, fortunately, are not dangerous. They include breathlessness, tachycardia, dizziness or fainting, headache, and vomiting. These reactions are probably connected with the sharp fall in blood pressure that follows too rapid intravenous administration of the drug, and they may be due in part to the release of

histamine. Because pentamidine is better tolerated by intramuscular injection and causes little pain, this route is to be preferred. Pentamidine has not been observed to give rise to late neuropathies such as have been reported frequently after courses of stilbamidine. Both hypoglycemia and, paradoxically, hyperglycemia have been reported following administration of pentamidine. Reversible renal dysfunction has been associated with the use of the drug in a small proportion of treated patients (*see* DeVita *et al.*, 1969).

Therapeutic Uses. The diamidines, in particular pentamidine, have three important therapeutic applications. The first is in the treatment of *leishmaniasis*. Although antimonials are generally considered to be the drugs of choice, gratifying results can be obtained with diamidines in cases that fail to respond to antimonial therapy or in patients who cannot tolerate the metal. Pentamidine is given in courses as described above.

Pentamidine is also highly effective in the treatment of *early* cases of Gambian and Rhodesian *trypanosomiasis,* and it has been widely used as a prophylactic against *T. gambiense.* Because the drug does not gain access to the cerebrospinal fluid and cannot be given intrathecally, it should not be employed in the neurological stage of the disease.

Gratifying response may also be obtained in the treatment of *pneumonia* due to *Pneumocystis carinii.* This opportunistic protozoon is a cause of pneumonitis in the compromised host—usually a patient with a malignancy or one who is receiving therapy with immunosuppressive agents (Walzer *et al.*, 1974). The use of pentamidine has, for example, very markedly reduced mortality in the epidemic form of infection found in debilitated and premature infants. This treatment is considered investigational in the United States; an alternative is administration of the combination of trimethoprim and sulfamethoxazole.

The effectiveness of pentamidine in human *Babesia* infections is unknown but would seem likely in view of its activity against babesiosis in animals.

MELARSOPROL

In 1940, Friedheim described trypanocidal activity in an organic compound of arsenic containing the melamine nucleus. Two compounds made subsequently, the pentavalent melarsen and the trivalent melarsen oxide, were shown to be effective in advanced cases of trypanosomiasis but were considered to be more toxic than tryparsamide. In 1949, Friedheim demonstrated that a dimercaprol derivative of melarsen oxide also could be used effectively and with greater safety in the treatment of such cases; this compound was named *Mel B* and is now known as *melarsoprol.* Of considerable importance was the finding that trypanocidal arsenicals of the melamine type retained their activity against tryparsamide-resistant strains of trypanosomes (VanHoof, 1947).

Chemistry and Preparations. Melarsoprol has the following structural formula:

Melarsoprol

It is very slightly soluble in water but is readily soluble in propylene glycol. *Melarsoprol* (*Mel B;* ARSOBAL) is provided as a 3.6% (w/v) sterile solution in propylene glycol. It is available in the United States only from the Parasitic Diseases Division, Center for Disease Control, Atlanta, Georgia 30333. The dosage regimens below refer to the 3.6% solution.

Antiprotozoal Effects. Arsenicals react avidly with sulfhydryl groups, including those of proteins, and thereby inactivate a great number and variety of enzymes. As far as is known, the same mechanism by which melarsoprol is lethal to parasites is responsible for its toxicity to host tissues. However, Flynn and Bowman (1969) have demonstrated that arsenical drugs act differently upon the terminal glycolytic enzyme, pyruvate kinase, depending on whether the source of the enzyme is trypanosomal or mammalian. It is also possible that mammalian tissues oxidize the drug to nontoxic and readily excreted pentavalent compounds more rapidly than does the protozoan. Additionally, melarsoprol may be able to penetrate into the parasite more readily than into mammalian tissue cells. So-called arsenic-resistant parasites may resemble host cells in that they have become less permeable to organic arsenicals (*see* Eagle and Doak, 1951).

The pharmacological effects of melarsoprol in man are regarded as toxic effects, and are discussed below.

Absorption, Fate, and Excretion. Melarsoprol is usually administered intravenously. A small but therapeutically significant amount of the drug penetrates into the cerebrospinal fluid and has a lethal effect on trypanosomes infecting the CNS. The substance is excreted quite quickly, and its prophylactic action lasts no more than a few days (*see* Hawking, 1963).

Route of Administration and Dosage. Melarsoprol is administered by slow intravenous injection of the propylene glycol solution. It should be given through a fine needle, and care must be taken to avoid leakage into surrounding tissues, because it is intensely irritating. Patients with advanced meningoencephalitis, or those who are febrile or wasted, should receive preliminary treatment with suramin (two to four doses of 250 to 500 mg on alternate days). Adults in good condition weighing 50 kg or more and whose cerebrospinal fluid contains less than 40 mg of protein per 100 ml should be given up to 3.6 mg/kg daily for 3 or 4 days; this course should be repeated after an interval of 7 to 10 days. A third course may be given if required. Lesser doses should be given to children and more severely debilitated

patients. Following such regimens, about 80 to 90% of patients are cured. A proportion of those relapsing will be refractory to further treatment with melarsoprol.

Toxicity and Side Effects. Unfortunately, side effects are common during treatment with melarsoprol (*see* Robertson, 1962). Reactive encephalopathy is the most common. The clinical manifestation usually appears after the first 3- or 4-day course and then subsides; additional treatment does not produce further deterioration. The administration of dimercaprol produces little benefit, but it is not contraindicated and should perhaps be used if the encephalopathy is severe. The condition may be fatal. Deaths due to this cause, however, have become less frequent with increasing experience in the use of this drug. The reactive encephalopathy occurs more frequently and is more severe in those with pronounced cerebrospinal fluid changes. Hypersensitivity reactions are not common and generally occur during the second or subsequent course of treatment. After recovery, a small dose provokes a lesser reaction, so that desensitization may be carried out by starting with a small dose and increasing this slightly, allowing time for recovery, until it is possible to give a final 3- or 4-day course in full dosage. Corticosteroids may be used to control the symptoms during such a procedure. Hemorrhagic encephalopathy is uncommon during treatment, and agranulocytosis is very rare. Occasionally the appearance of numerous casts in the urine or evidence of hepatic disturbance may necessitate modification of treatment. Vomiting and abdominal colic may occur, but their incidence may be reduced by injecting the drug slowly in the supine, fasting patient. The patient should remain in bed and not eat for several hours after the injection is given.

Precautions and Contraindications. Melarsoprol should be given only to patients under hospital supervision so that the dosage regimen may be modified if necessary. It is most important that the initial dosage be based upon clinical assessment of the general condition of the patient, rather than on body weight. It should be recognized that the administration of melarsoprol to leprous patients may precipitate erythema nodosum. The use of the drug is contraindicated during epidemics of influenza. Severe hemolytic reactions have been reported in patients with glucose-6-phosphate dehydrogenase deficiency.

Therapeutic Uses. Because of its ability to penetrate into cerebrospinal fluid, melarsoprol is the drug of choice in the treatment of the meningoencephalitic stage of human trypanosomiasis. It is effective in both Gambian and Rhodesian varieties of the disease. Its value is in its quick action against both stages of trypanosomiasis, its effectiveness against tryparsamide-resistant strains of trypanosomes, and the absence of ocular toxicity. For these reasons, it has largely superseded tryparsamide. Melarsoprol is also effective in the treatment of the hemolymphatic stage of the disease; however, because of its toxicity, it is usually reserved for treatment of the late stage. For this reason also, it has no place in prophylaxis.

Cases of late-stage trypanosomiasis may be encountered that are refractory to treatment with melarsoprol and also to treatment with tryparsamide. *Nitrofurazone* may be tried in these difficult cases with some chance of success. A single course of treatment should not exceed 500 mg of the drug at 6-hour intervals for 1 week. Three courses may be given with a week's rest between each. This treatment is unsuitable for febrile or debilitated patients. The drug causes severe polyneuropathy and reversible degeneration of the seminiferous tubules. It produces hemolytic anemia in patients with glucose-6-phosphate dehydrogenase deficiency. *Furaltadone* and, presumably, *nifurtimox* may also be used.

OTHER ARSENICALS

The introduction of nonarsenical trypanocides and melarsoprol in the treatment of trypanosomiasis has left little place for the use of the older arsenicals. Of these compounds, tryparsamide is still employed in some parts of the world. The many others are described in *earlier editions* of this textbook (*see also* Chapter 69).

Tryparsamide. Tryparsamide is a pentavalent arsenical with the following structural formula:

$$O=As(OH)(ONa)-C_6H_4-N(H)-CH_2-C(=O)-NH_2$$

Tryparsamide

Tryparsamide is given *intravenously* in doses of 30 mg/kg in 10 ml of water, at 5- to 7-day intervals for 10 to 12 injections. Children do not tolerate the drug well. A course of treatment may be repeated after an interval of 1 month.

The overall incidence of toxic reactions to tryparsamide is 15% or higher. These include nausea, vomiting, optic atrophy, fever, dermatitides, and allergic reactions.

While tryparsamide was the mainstay of therapy for *Gambian trypanosomiasis* for several decades, it offers no advantage over melarsoprol. Furthermore, strains of *T. gambiense* resistant to tryparsamide are not infrequently encountered, and the drug can cause blindness. It is thus little used.

SODIUM STIBOGLUCONATE

The history of the development of leishmanicidal antimonial compounds can be divided into three distinct phases. At first, the use of *antimony potassium tartrate* (*tartar emetic*) in the treatment of trypanosomiasis was followed by its successful use against cutaneous leishmaniasis and, shortly afterward, in cases of kala-azar. Inconvenience in the use of this drug, however, led to the trial of several other trivalent antimonial compounds, notably *antimony sodium tartrate, stibophen,* and *anthiomaline.* These were found to be as effective as and less toxic than tartar emetic. During this period, the successful syntheses of pentavalent antimonial derivatives of phenylstibonic acid were followed by the introduction of a variety of drugs that were as effective as and much less toxic than tartar emetic, thus permitting the use of larger doses and reduction in the period of treatment. Subsequent syntheses reverted to the "tartar-emetic" type of compound in which trivalent antimony was replaced by pentavalent antimony. An early member of this type of compound was *sodium stibogluconate*. This drug is widely used today and, together with *meglumine antimonate* (GLUCANTIME), a compound of the same type that is preferred in countries formerly under French influence, is the mainstay of the treatment of leishmaniasis by antimony. Full details of the investigations of leishmanicides can be found in the reviews of Findlay (1950) and Beveridge (1963).

Chemistry. Sodium stibogluconate has the following structural formula:

$$\text{Sodium Stibogluconate} \quad 3Na^+$$

Sodium Stibogluconate

It is a colorless, amorphous powder, readily soluble in water, and contains 30 to 34% pentavalent antimony.

Antiprotozoal Effects. Pentavalent antimony compounds such as sodium stibogluconate have little effect on leptomonads growing in tissue culture. Such a marked contrast between *in-vitro* and *in-vivo* activity of these compounds suggests that reduction of antimony to the trivalent form is necessary for activity. However, the sensitivity of the free flagellated forms could be quite different from that of the morphologically different intracellular stage, which cannot be readily cultured. The mechanism of action of organic antimonials is discussed in chapter 44.

Preparations. *Sodium stibogluconate* (*sodium antimony gluconate;* PENTOSTAM) is available in sterile, aqueous solution for parenteral administration. Each milliliter contains 330 mg of the drug, equivalent to 100 mg of pentavalent antimony. It is available in the United States only from the Parasitic Diseases Division, Center for Disease Control, Atlanta, Georgia 30333.

Routes of Administration, Dosage, and Therapeutic Uses. Sodium stibogluconate may be given either intravenously or by the intramuscular route. In cases of *kala-azar,* in which the leishmania are normally sensitive to antimony, the large majority will be cured by a single course of treatment consisting of six daily injections of 6 ml. Against less sensitive strains, three courses, each consisting of ten daily doses of

6 ml intramuscularly and separated by intervals of 10 days, have proven satisfactory. In very debilitated individuals who appear to react unfavorably to the initial injections, it may be advisable to administer the drug on alternate days or at longer intervals. Reduced dosage is indicated in those who have recently received a course of antimony in another form, and in children. Infants and children, however, tolerate rather larger doses in proportion to body weight than do adults. In the treatment of *Oriental sore*, rapid disappearance of parasites has been reported following an infiltration of the solution around the edges of the lesions. The total volume used should not exceed more than 2 ml at any one time. Otherwise, a single course of treatment as outlined above should prove to be effective in nearly all cases. Less is known of the effectiveness of sodium stibogluconate in the treatment of *mucocutaneous leishmaniasis*. Cautious treatment with *amphotericin B* has proven successful in this condition (Sampaio *et al.*, 1960). Single injections of *cycloguanil pomoate* have cured a large proportion of patients in Costa Rica, Mexico, and Panama (*see* Johnson, 1968). Drug therapy of the leishmaniases has been reviewed by Steck (1974).

The toxicity of antimonial drugs as well as the precautions and contraindications to be observed in their use are described in Chapter 44. Untoward reactions to pentavalent antimonials are qualitatively similar to those that follow the administration of trivalent compounds, but they are less frequent and usually less severe. In general, sodium stibogluconate is tolerated relatively well.

METRONIDAZOLE

History. The discovery of *azomycin* (2-nitroimidazole) by Nakamura in 1955 and the demonstration of its trichomonacidal properties by Horie (1956) opened the way for the chemical synthesis and biological testing of many nitroimidazoles. In 1959, Cosar and Julou reported the trichomonacidal activity, both *in vitro* and *in vivo*, of 1-(β-hydroxyethyl)-2-methyl-5-nitroimidazole, now called *metronidazole*. Durel and associates (1960) found that oral doses of the drug imparted trichomonacidal activity to semen and urine, and showed that a high cure rate could be obtained in both male and female patients suffering from trichomoniasis. The success of this treatment spurred the synthesis and trial of many similar compounds. Two 5-nitroimidazoles closely related in structure and activity to metronidazole are currently available in some parts of the world. They are *tinidazole* (FASIGYN) and *nimorazole* (NAXOGIN, NULOGYL).

Up to the time of the introduction of metronidazole, topical therapy with many and varied agents effected cure in a large proportion of infected females, but left a hard core of chronic cases for which little could be done other than produce some measure of symptomatic relief. Furthermore, infection in the male forms a reservoir of parasites for reinfection of the female by sexual contact; males cannot be treated topically. By the employment of metronidazole, a high percentage of such patients can be cured.

The drug is also very useful in the treatment of *intestinal and extraintestinal amebiasis* (Chapter 46) and is effective in the treatment of *lambliasis*. Other uses of metronidazole are discussed below (*see* Roe; 1977; Symposium, 1977).

Chemistry. Metronidazole has the following structural formula:

Metronidazole

It occurs as pale-yellow crystals that are slightly soluble in water and alcohol.

Antimicrobial Effects. Metronidazole is directly trichomonacidal. It destroys 99% of the microorganisms in cultures of *Trichomonas vaginalis* within 24 hours at a concentration of 2.5 µg/ml. It is also directly amebicidal in very low concentrations (*see* Chapter 46) and is bactericidal *in vitro* for many anaerobic microorganisms, including *Bacteroides* species (Ralph and Kirby, 1975). Its mechanism of action is reflected in a selective toxicity to anaerobic or microaerophilic microorganisms and for other anoxic or hypoxic cells. In susceptible cells, the nitro group of metronidazole is reduced by electron-transport proteins with low redox potentials (such as ferredoxin in clostridia); these proteins play a much more important role in the metabolism of such cells than they do in aerobes. Metronidazole thus acts as an electron sink and deprives the cell of required reducing equivalents. It is currently thought, however, that it is the reduced form of the drug that actually produces the biochemical lesions that lead to death of the cell. While earlier work had established that the drug inhibits DNA synthesis in *T. vaginalis* and *Clostridium bifermentans* and causes degradation of existing DNA in the latter microorganism, further studies with calf thymus DNA indicate that reduced metronidazole causes a loss of the helical structure of DNA, strand breakage, and an accompanying impairment of its function as a template. Such findings are consistent with its antimicrobial effects and its ability to potentiate the effects of radiation on hypoxic tumor cells (*see* Edwards *et al.*, 1973; Tanowitz *et al.*, 1975; Knight *et al.*, 1978).

Absorption, Fate, and Excretion. Metronidazole is usually well absorbed after oral administration. Some patients fail to respond to treatment, however, and in such cases a low systemic concentration of the drug may be responsible. Whether this is due to relatively poor absorption from the gastrointestinal tract or to a rapid rate of metabolic transformation is open to question. The half-life of metronidazole in plasma approximates 8 hours. High concentrations are achieved in cerebrospinal fluid (Ralph *et al.,* 1974; Schwartz and Jeunet, 1976).

Both unchanged metronidazole and several metabolites are excreted in various proportions in the urine of experimental animals and man after oral administration of the parent compound (Stambaugh *et al.,* 1968). The principal metabolites result from oxidation of side chains and glucuronide formation. The urine of some patients may be reddish-brown in color due to the presence of water-soluble pigments derived from the drug. Low concentrations of metronidazole appear in the saliva and in breast milk during treatment.

Preparations. *Metronidazole,* U.S.P. (FLAGYL), is available as 250-mg tablets. The drug is also supplied for investigational purposes as a 0.5% solution for intravenous infusion. *Benzoyl metronidazole,* a tasteless form of metronidazole, is available in some countries as an oral suspension for children.

Routes of Administration and Dosage. Many different dosage schedules have been used in the treatment of trichomoniasis in the female. However, the currently accepted regimen is one 250-mg tablet, given orally three times daily for 7 to 10 days. When repeated courses of the drug are required for stubborn infections, it is recommended that intervals of 4 to 6 weeks elapse between courses. In such cases, leukocyte counts should be carried out before, during, and after each course of treatment. A single oral dose of 2 g of metronidazole has been reported to be equally effective. Vaginal inserts may be used concurrently with oral medication, although there is no evidence that their use yields a higher cure rate than oral medication alone. If their use seems justified because of persistence of infection after normally adequate oral administration, one insert should be used daily for 10 days. At the same time, oral dosage should be reduced to two 250-mg tablets daily. Lack of satisfactory response may indicate the necessity for surgical eradication of foci in the cervical glands or in Skene's and Bartholin's glands.

Reinfection by an infected male partner may also cause apparent lack of satisfactory response. If such is the case, the male may be treated by the oral administration of 250 mg twice daily for 7 to 10 days, both partners being treated over the same 10-day period. However, the male should be treated only when trichomonads are demonstrated in the urogenital tract.

While quinacrine is the drug of choice in the treatment of *lambliasis,* its administration is not without unpleasant side effects. Metronidazole is effective in the same dosage as that used in the treatment of trichomoniasis. Others have successfully used a daily dose of 2 g for 3 successive days. Metronidazole is also considered to be an alternative to niridazole for the elimination of the guinea worm in dracontiasis (Padonu, 1973). Recommended dosage is 250 to 500 mg of the drug three times daily for 5 to 7 days. Both of these uses are, however, still considered investigational in the United States. The various regimens of treatment for the several forms of amebiasis are discussed in Chapter 46.

Toxicity. Side effects are only rarely sufficiently severe to cause discontinuance of the drug. The most common are referable to the gastrointestinal tract. In particular, nausea, anorexia, diarrhea, epigastric distress, and abdominal cramping have occurred; headache and vomiting are occasionally experienced. A metallic, sharp, and unpleasant taste is not unusual. Furry tongue, glossitis, and stomatitis may occur during therapy and be associated with a sudden intensification of moniliasis. Neurotoxic effects of metronidazole have also been observed. Dizziness, vertigo, and very rarely, incoordination and ataxia may appear. Numbness or paresthesia of an extremity occurs occasionally. Reversal of serious sensory neuropathies may be slow or incomplete (Coxon and Pallis, 1976). Urticaria, flushing, pruritus, dysuria, cystitis, a sense of pelvic pressure, and dryness of the mouth, vagina, or vulva have been reported. Metronidazole has a well-documented disulfiram-like effect, and a few patients experience abdominal distress, vomiting, flushing, or headache if they drink alcoholic beverages during a course of treatment with metronidazole.

While related chemicals have caused blood dyscrasias, serious difficulties have not been recorded with metronidazole. However, in an appreciable proportion of treated patients, a significant neutropenia has been observed. In all cases the white-cell count returned to normal after the course of medication was completed (*see* Lefebvre and Hesseltine, 1965).

Treatment should be discontinued promptly if ataxia or any other symptom of CNS involvement occurs. Metronidazole is contraindicated in patients with active disease of the CNS or with evidence or a history of blood dyscrasia.

Metronidazole is carcinogenic in rodents and mutagenic in bacteria (Voogd *et al.,* 1974). Furthermore, mutagenic activity associated with metronidazole and several of its metabolites is found in the urine of patients treated with therapeutic doses of the drug (Speck *et al.*, 1976). While the clinical significance of these phenomena is difficult to evaluate, they should compel the prudent use of the drug. While metronidazole has been given with no apparent adverse effects during all stages of pregnancy (Peterson *et al.*, 1966), its use during the first trimester is now considered to be contraindicated.

Therapeutic Uses. Metronidazole cures genital infections with *T. vaginalis* in both males and females in a high percentage of cases. This efficacy and a probable low incidence of comparatively minor side effects have led to its adoption as the agent of choice. The development of resistance to metronidazole has not proven to be a therapeutic problem. There is also no doubt that persistent reinfection of the female can be prevented if the male partner harboring the parasite is treated concurrently. However, treatment of the male is recommended only if reinfection can be demonstrated to arise from this source.

Metronidazole also kills *Giardia lamblia* and has been shown to be effective in treating *lambliasis* in Europe and South America. Its use in the treatment of *dracontiasis* is discussed above. Metronidazole is an effective amebicide and has become the agent of choice in the treatment of the several forms of *amebiasis* (Chapter 46).

Several studies have indicated that metronidazole may be useful for the treatment of infections with various anaerobic bacteria, particularly *Bacteroides fragilis*. In this use the drug is an alternative to clindamycin and chloramphenicol. Metronidazole has been employed prophylactically, for postsurgical abdominal and pelvic infections, and for the treatment of endocarditis caused by *Bacteroides fragilis* (*see* Roe, 1977; Symposium, 1977; Galgiani *et al.*, 1978). While information is limited, the drug may also be effective for the treatment of brain abscesses that are not uncommonly caused by such microorganisms.

There is interest in the experimental use of metronidazole and other nitroimidazoles to sensitize more hypoxic tumor cells to the effects of ionizing radiation. Some success in this goal has been achieved *in vitro* and in mice *in vivo*.

NIFURTIMOX

In Latin America many millions of people are infected with *T. cruzi*, the infective agent of Chagas' disease. Approximately one tenth of those infected die, usually after a chronic and often asymptomatic course. Until recently, there was no drug that could be tolerated in doses sufficient to affect the intracellular, leishmanial stage. The nonmultiplying trypanosomes in the blood are more susceptible; primaquine has been found useful in eliminating this initial parasitemia.

Nitrofurans were known to be effective in experimental infections with *T. cruzi*, and numerous congeners have been investigated for their chemo-therapeutic usefulness; recent work has proven promising. One drug, 3-methyl-4(5'-nitrofurfurylidene-amino)-tetrahydro-4H-1,4-thiazine-1,1-dioxide, is effective clinically in acute and chronic Chagas' infection (Bock *et al.*, 1972).

Chemistry and Preparations. *Nifurtimox* (*Bayer 2502;* LAMPIT) has the following structural formula:

Nifurtimox

Nifurtimox is marketed in scored tablets that contain 100 mg of the drug; it is available in the United States only from the Parasitic Diseases Division, Center for Disease Control, Atlanta, Georgia 30333.

Antiprotozoal Effects. Nifurtimox is trypanocidal against both the trypamastigote and the amastigote forms of *T. cruzi*. Little is known of its mode of action. Concentrations of 1 μM have been shown to damage intracellular amastigotes *in vitro* and inhibit their development. Continuous exposure to this concentration of the drug lengthens considerably the intracellular cycle. Trypamastigotes are less sensitive; 10-μM concentrations of nifurtimox inhibit penetration of vertebrate cells by the parasites but do not eliminate this process (*see* Dvorak and Howe, 1977).

Absorption, Fate, and Excretion. Nifurtimox is well absorbed after oral administration. Despite this, only low concentrations of the drug are found in the blood and tissues, and little is present in the urine. High concentrations of several unidentified metabolites are found, however, and it is obvious that biotransformation occurs rapidly. The effect of biotransformation on trypanocidal activity is unknown.

Route of Administration and Dosage. The drug is given orally. *Children* (up to 15 years of age) with *acute* Chagas' disease should receive 25 mg/kg per day in four divided doses for 15 days, followed by 15 mg/kg per day in four divided doses for 75 days. Therapy should be extended to a total of 120 days for *chronic* disease. *Adults* with acute or chronic disease should receive 5 to 7 mg/kg daily for 2 weeks, and this dose is increased by 2 mg/kg at intervals of 2 weeks until 15 to 17 mg/kg is given daily by week 10. Treatment with this dose is continued until the patient has taken the drug for a total of 120 days. Gastric upset resulting from drug administration may be alleviated by simultaneous administration of aluminum hydroxide preparations. Weight loss is not uncommon during treatment. If it occurs, dosage should be reduced. The ingestion of alcohol should be avoided during treatment, since the incidence of side effects may increase.

Toxicity and Side Effects. The major toxic effects of nifurtimox in experimental animals given large doses for prolonged periods are referable to the CNS and to the male gonads. Treatment with large doses is associated with stiffness and weakness in the hindlimbs and transitory convulsive episodes. In man, the incidence of undesirable side effects has been high, and from 40 to 70% of patients have been affected. Children appear to tolerate the drug better than do adults. Symptoms are attributable to effects on the CNS and the gastrointestinal tract. All have been reversible on stopping treatment. Anticonvulsants afford symptomatic control of effects on the CNS. Because of the nature of the disease and the unique position of the drug, there are no absolute contraindications to its use.

Therapeutic Uses. Nifurtimox is employed in the treatment of *trypanosomiasis* caused by *T. cruzi* (Chagas' disease). It is effective in both the acute and the chronic stages of the infection, although treatment with nifurtimox has no effect on irreversible organ lesions brought about by the disease process. In the acute stage, drug therapy results in disappearance of parasitemia and amelioration of symptoms and cure in over 80% of those treated. In the chronic stage, a cure rate of over 90% has been achieved in trials in Argentina, southern Brazil, Chile, and Venezuela. Much poorer results have been obtained in the middle section of Brazil, where the character of the infection is somewhat different. However, there is no evidence that the intrinsic susceptibility of the parasite differs from that in the other regions.

QUINACRINE

Quinacrine is an acridine derivative widely used during World War II as an antimalarial agent. It has almost wholly been superseded for this purpose by other drugs with more desirable properties (*see* Chapter 45). Its use for the treatment of infections with tapeworms is also considered to be obsolete. Currently, the major indication for the administration of quinacrine is for the treatment of *giardiasis* (Wolfe, 1975). For a fuller description of its properties, *earlier editions* of this textbook should be consulted. Quinacrine has the following structural formula:

Quinacrine

Quinacrine is very readily absorbed from the intestinal tract. Even severe diarrhea does not interfere with absorption. It is widely distributed in the tissues and very slowly liberated. Therefore, the drug accumulates progressively in the tissues when it is administered chronically. Significant amounts of quinacrine can still be detected in the urine for at least 2 months after therapy is discontinued. The *metabolic fate* of quinacrine in the body is incompletely understood. Whether quinacrine exerts its antiparasitic actions *per se* or after metabolic transformation remains to be determined. However, its ready intercalation into DNA suggests that the parent drug is the active substance, and that its selective toxicity is a function of relative distribution rather than specificity of action (*see* Albert, 1973).

Quinacrine is available as the dihydrochloride, designated *Quinacrine Hydrochloride,* U.S.P. (*mepacrine hydrochloride;* ATABRINE). It contains approximately 80% quinacrine base and is supplied as tablets containing 100 mg of the dihydrochloride.

In the treatment of *giardiasis,* 100 mg should be given three times daily for 5 days. A second course of treatment may be given, if necessary, a week later. The dosage for children under 8 years of age should be proportionally reduced. The microorganisms disappear from the stools, and symptoms referable to the infection clear rapidly.

Because of its widespread use as an antimalarial drug, data on its toxicity are well documented. These have been reviewed extensively by Findlay (1951). The drug frequently causes headache, dizziness, and vomiting. Blood dyscrasias, urticaria, and exfoliative dermatitis may also follow its administration. The skin may acquire a yellow stain from deposition of the drug, and blue or black pigmentation of the nails can occur. Ocular toxicity, similar to that caused by chloroquine, occurs occasionally. The relatively large doses used in the treatment of cestode infection may cause the transitory *toxic psychosis* that is seen in a small proportion of patients receiving lower doses. The duration of the drug-induced psychosis is usually 2 to 4 weeks, and the course is relatively benign. Only symptomatic therapy is indicated.

Great caution should be exercised in administering quinacrine (and other antimalarial compounds) to patients with *psoriasis,* since pronounced exacerbation is frequently produced and exfoliative lesions have sometimes developed. Quinacrine is contraindicated in patients receiving antimalarial therapy with primaquine. Concurrent administration of the two drugs results in a markedly elevated concentration of primaquine (or other 8-aminoquinolines) in plasma and greatly enhances its toxicity. Quinacrine should not be given to pregnant women because the drug readily passes the placenta and reaches the fetus.

Bock, M.; Haberkorn, A.; Herlinger, H.; Mayer, K. H.; and Petersen, S. The structure-activity relationship of 4-(5′-nitrofurfurylidine-amino)-tetrahydro-4H-1,4-thiazine-1,1-dioxides active against *Trypanosoma cruzi. Arzneim. Forsch.,* **1972,** *22,* 1564–1569. (This issue, 9a of Vol. 22, is devoted to a full discussion of nifurtimox.)

Brack, C.; Delain, E.; and Riou, G. Replicating, covalently closed, circular DNA from kinetoplasts of *Trypanosoma cruzi. Proc. Natl. Acad. Sci. U.S.A.,* **1972,** *69,* 1642–1646.

Cosar, C., and Julou, L. Activité de 1′(hydroxy-2′ ethyl)-1 méthyl-2 nitro-5 imidazole (8,823 R.P.) vis-à-vis des infections expérimentales à *Trichomonas vaginalis. Ann. Inst. Pasteur* (*Paris*), **1959,** *96,* 238–241.

Coxon, A., and Pallis, C. A. Metronidazole neuropathy. *J. Neurol. Neurosurg. Psychiatry,* **1976,** *39,* 403–405.

DeVita, V. T.; Emmer, M.; Levine, A.; Jacobs, B.; and Berard, C. *Pneumocystis carinii* pneumonia. *N. Engl. J. Med.,* **1969,** *280,* 287–291.

Durel, P.; Roiron, V.; Siboulet, A.; and Borel, L. J. Systemic treatment of human trichomoniasis with a derivative of nitroimidazole, 8823 R.P. *Br. J. Vener. Dis.*, **1960**, *36*, 21–26.

Dvorak, J. A., and Howe, C. L. The effects of LAMPIT (Bayer 2502) on the interaction of *Trypanosoma cruzi* with vertebrate cells *in vitro*. *Am. J. Trop. Med. Hyg.*, **1977**, *26*, 58–63.

Edwards, D. I.; Dye, M.; and Carne, H. The selective toxicity of antimicrobial nitroheterocyclic drugs. *J. Gen. Microbiol.*, **1973**, *76*, 135–145.

Flynn, I. W., and Bowman, I. B. R. Further studies on the mode of action of arsenicals on trypanosome pyruvate kinase. *Trans. R. Soc. Trop. Med. Hyg.*, **1969**, *63*, 121.

Friedheim, E. A. H. L'acide triazine-arsinique dans le traitement de la maladie du sommeil. *Ann. Inst. Pasteur* (*Paris*), **1940**, *65*, 108–118.

————. Mel B in the treatment of human trypanosomiasis. *Am. J. Trop. Med.*, **1949**, *29*, 173–180.

Galgiani, J. N.; Busch, D. F.; Brass, C.; Rumans, L. W.; Mangels, J. I.; and Stevens, D. A. *Bacteroides fragilis* endocarditis, bacteremia and other infections treated with oral or intravenous metronidazole. *Am. J. Med.*, **1978**, *65*, 284–289.

Horie, H. Anti-*Trichomonas* effect of azomycin. *J. Antibiot.* (*Tokyo*) [*A*], **1956**, *9*, 168.

Ivady, G.; Paldy, L.; Koltay, M.; Toth, G.; and Kovaks, Z. *Pneumocystis carinii* pneumonia. *Lancet*, **1967**, *1*, 616–617.

Johnson, C. M. Cycloguanil pamoate in the treatment of cutaneous leishmaniasis: initial trials in Panama. *Am. J. Trop. Med. Hyg.*, **1968**, *17*, 819–822.

King, H.; Lourie, E. M.; and Yorke, W. Studies in chemotherapy. XIX. Further report on new trypanocidal substances. *Ann. Trop. Med. Parasitol.*, **1938**, *32*, 177–192.

Knight, R. C.; Skolimowski, I. M.; and Edwards, D. I. The interaction of reduced metronidazole with DNA. *Biochem. Pharmacol.*, **1978**, *27*, 2089–2093.

Launoy, L.; Guillot, M.; and Jonchère, H. [Storage and elimination of pentamidine in mice and white rats.] *Ann. Pharm. Fr.*, **1960**, *18*, 273–284, 424–439.

Lefebvre, I., and Hesseltine, H. C. The peripheral white blood cells and metronidazole. *J.A.M.A.*, **1965**, *194*, 15–18.

Lourie, E. M., and Yorke, W. Studies in chemotherapy. XXI. The trypanocidal action of certain aromatic diamidines. *Ann. Trop. Med. Parasitol.*, **1939**, *33*, 289–304.

Padonu, K. O. A controlled trial of metronidazole in the treatment of dracontiasis in Nigeria. *Am. J. Trop. Med. Hyg.*, **1973**, *22*, 42–44.

Peterson, W. F.; Stauch, J. E.; and Ryder, C. D. Metronidazole in pregnancy. *Am. J. Obstet. Gynecol.*, **1966**, *94*, 343–349.

Ralph, E. D.; Clarke, J. T.; Libke, R. D.; Luthy, R. P.; and Kirby, W. M. M. Pharmacokinetics of metronidazole as determined by bioassay. *Antimicrob. Agents Chemother.*, **1974**, *6*, 691–696.

Ralph, E. D., and Kirby, W. M. M. Unique bactericidal action of metronidazole against *Bacteroides fragilis* and *Clostridium perfringens*. *Antimicrob. Agents Chemother.*, **1975**, *8*, 409–420.

Richet, P. Le melarsonyl (TRIMELARSAN) en pathologie tropical. *Bull. Séanc. Acad. R. Sci. Colon.* (*Outre-Mer*), **1966**, No. 4, 759–785.

Robertson, D. H. H. A trial of Mel W in the treatment of *Trypanosoma rhodesiense* sleeping sickness. *Trans. R. Soc. Trop. Med. Hyg.*, **1963**, *57*, 274–289.

Sampaio, S. A.; Godoy, J. T.; Paiva, L.; Dillon, N. L.; and Lacas, C. da S. The treatment of American (mucocutaneous) leishmaniasis with amphotericin-B. *Arch. Dermatol.*, **1960**, *82*, 627–635.

Schwartz, D. E., and Jeunet, F. Comparative pharmacokinetic studies of ornidazole and metronidazole in man. *Chemotherapy*, **1976**, *22*, 19–29.

Speck, W. T.; Stein, A. B.; and Rosenkranz, H. S. Mutagenicity of metronidazole: presence of several active metabolites in human urine. *J. Natl. Cancer Inst.*, **1976**, *56*, 283–284.

Stambaugh, J. E.; Feo, L. G.; and Manthei, R. W. The isolation and identification of the urinary oxidative metabolites of metronidazole in man. *J. Pharmacol. Exp. Ther.*, **1968**, *161*, 373–381.

Steck, E. A. The leishmaniases. In, *Progress in Drug Research: Tropical Diseases*, Vol. 1. (Jucker, E., ed.) Birkhäuser Verlag, Basel, **1974**, pp. 289–351.

Tanowitz, H. B.; Wittner, M.; Rosenbaum, R. M.; and Kress, Y. *In vitro* studies on the differential toxicity of metronidazole in protozoa and mammalian cells. *Ann. Trop. Med. Parasitol.*, **1975**, *69*, 19–28.

VanHoof, L. M. J. J. Observations on trypanosomiasis in Belgium Congo. *Trans. R. Soc. Trop. Med. Hyg.*, **1947**, *40*, 728–761.

Voogd, C. E.; Van Der Stel, J. J.; and Jacobs, J. J. The mutagenic action of nitroimidazoles. I. Metronidazole, nimorazole, dimetridazole and ronidazole. *Mutat. Res.*, **1974**, *26*, 483–490.

Waalkes, T. P.; Denham, C.; and DeVita, V. T. Pentamidine: clinical pharmacological correlations in man and mice. *Clin. Pharmacol. Ther.*, **1970**, *11*, 505–512.

Walzer, P. D.; Perl, D. P.; Krogstad, D. J.; Rawson, P. G.; and Schultz, M. G. *Pneumocystis carinii* pneumonia in the United States. *Ann. Intern. Med.*, **1974**, *80*, 83–93.

Williamson, J., and Macadam, R. F. Effect of trypanocidal drugs on the fine structure of *Trypanosoma rhodesiense*. *Trans. R. Soc. Trop. Med. Hyg.*, **1965**, *59*, 367–368.

Monographs and Reviews

Albert, A. *Selective Toxicity: The Physico-Chemical Basis of Therapy*, 5th ed. Chapman & Hall, Ltd., London, **1973**.

Allison, A. C. Effects of drugs and toxic agents on lysosomes. In, *The Interaction of Drugs and Subcellular Components in Animal Cells*. (Campbell, P. N., ed.) J. & A. Churchill, Ltd., London, **1968**, pp. 218–235.

Beveridge, E. Chemotherapy of leishmaniasis. In, *Experimental Chemotherapy*, Vol. I. (Schnitzer, R. J., and Hawking, F., eds.) Academic Press, Inc., New York, **1963**, pp. 257–287.

Eagle, H., and Doak, G. O. The biological activity of arsenosobenzenes in relation to their structure. *Pharmacol. Rev.*, **1951**, *3*, 107–143.

Findlay, G. M. *Recent Advances in Chemotherapy*, Vol. I. J. & A. Churchill, Ltd., London, **1950**.

————. *Recent Advances in Chemotherapy*, Vol II. J. & A. Churchill, Ltd., London, **1951**.

Hawking, F. Chemotherapy of trypanosomiasis. In, *Experimental Chemotherapy*, Vol. I. (Schnitzer, R. J., and Hawking, F., eds.) Academic Press, Inc., New York, **1963**, pp. 129–256.

Robertson, D. H. H. Chemotherapy of African trypanosomiasis. *Practitioner*, **1962**, *188*, 80–83.

Roe, F. J. C. Metronidazole: review of uses and toxicity. *J. Antimicrob. Chemother.*, **1977**, *3*, 205–212.

Symposium. (Various authors.) *Proceedings of the International Metronidazole Conference*. International Congress Series No. 438. (Finegold, S. M., ed.) Excerpta Medica, Amsterdam, **1977**.

Williamson, J. Chemotherapy and chemoprophylaxis of African trypanosomiasis. *Exp. Parasitol.*, **1962**, *12*, 274–322.

Wolfe, M. S. Giardiasis. *J.A.M.A.*, **1975**, *233*, 1362–1365.

Chemotherapy of Microbial Diseases

48 ANTIMICROBIAL AGENTS
General Considerations

Merle A. Sande and Gerald L. Mandell

Historical Aspects and Introduction. The concept that substances derived from one living organism may kill another (antibiosis) is almost as old as the science of microbiology. Indeed, the application of antibiotic therapy, without recognition of it as such, is considerably older. The Chinese were aware, over 2500 years ago, of the therapeutic properties of moldy curd of soybean applied to carbuncles, boils, and similar infections and used this material as standard treatment in such disorders. The medical literature has for many centuries contained descriptions of beneficial effects from the application to infections of soil and various plants, most of which probably were sources of antibiotic-forming molds and bacteria.

The first investigators to recognize the clinical potentialities of microorganisms as therapeutic agents were Pasteur and Joubert, who recorded their observations and speculations in 1877. They noted that anthrax bacilli grew rapidly when inoculated into sterile urine but failed to multiply and soon died if one of the "common" bacteria of the air was introduced in the urine at the same time. The same type of experiment in animals produced similar results. They commented on the fact that life destroys life among the lower species even more than among higher animals and plants, and came to the astonishing conclusion that anthrax bacilli could be administered to an animal in large numbers, and it would not sicken, provided that "ordinary" bacteria were given at the same time. They stated that this

observation might hold great promise for therapeutics.

The clinical use of antibiotic agents represents the practical, controlled, and directed application of phenomena that occur naturally and continuously in soil, sewage, water, and other natural habitats of microorganisms. During the latter part of the nineteenth century and the early years of the twentieth century, several antimicrobial substances were demonstrated in bacterial cultures and some were even tested clinically but discarded because they proved to be highly toxic.

The modern era of the chemotherapy of infection started with the clinical use of sulfanilamide in 1936. The "golden age" of antimicrobial therapy began with the production of penicillin in 1941, when this compound was mass-produced and first made available for limited clinical trial. Although the earliest development of antibiotics involved considerable serendipity, from the discovery of streptomycin by Schatz, Bugie, and Waksman (1944) to the present, the search for such agents has been a highly planned, scientifically designed effort. These 40 years of antibiotic development and production have resulted in the introduction of dozens of antimicrobial agents with notable clinical utility. Approximately 30% of all hospitalized patients receive one or more courses of therapy with antibiotics, and millions of potentially fatal infections have been cured. However, at the same time, these pharmaceutical agents have become among the most misused of those available to the practicing physician. One result of widespread use of antimicrobial agents has been the emergence of antibiotic-resistant pathogens, which in turn has created an ever-increasing need for new drugs.

The history of antimicrobial agents has thus been dynamic, characterized by the constant emergence of new challenges followed by investigation, discovery, and the production of new drugs. The following pages present both a philosophical and a practical approach to the appropriate use of antimicrobial agents, as well as a discussion of the factors that influence the outcome of treatment with them.

Definition and Characteristics. Antibiotics are chemical substances produced by various species of microorganisms (bacteria, fungi, actinomycetes) that suppress the growth of other microorganisms and may eventually destroy them. The number of antibiotics that has been identified now extends into the hundreds, and more than 60 have been developed to the stage where they are of value in the therapy of infectious diseases. Antibiotics differ markedly in physical, chemical, and pharmacological properties, antibacterial spectra, and mechanisms of action. Most have been chemically identified, and some have been synthesized. A few are available only as crude or partially purified extracts.

The synthetic chemist has added greatly to our therapeutic armamentarium. Thus, drugs such as isoniazid and ethambutol represent important contributions and provide the mainstay for the treatment of tuberculosis. Indeed, little distinction should now be made between compounds of natural and synthetic origin. Chemotherapy of viral diseases is currently benefiting from a similar planned approach directed toward purely synthetic drugs as more is learned about mechanisms of viral replication.

Classification and Mechanism of Action. There are several methods used to classify and group antimicrobial agents, and all are hampered by exceptions and overlaps. Historically, the most common classification has

been based on chemical structure and proposed mechanism of action, as follows: (1) agents that inhibit synthesis of or activate enzymes that disrupt bacterial cell walls to cause loss of viability and, often, cell lysis; these include the penicillins and cephalosporins, which are structurally similar, and dissimilar agents such as cycloserine, vancomycin, ristocetin, and bacitracin; (2) agents that act directly on the cell membrane, affecting permeability and leading to leakage of intracellular compounds; these include the detergents, polymyxin and colistimethate, and the polyene antifungal agents, nystatin and amphotericin B, that bind to cell-wall sterols; (3) agents that affect the function of bacterial ribosomes to cause a reversible inhibition of protein synthesis; these bacteriostatic drugs include chloramphenicol, the tetracyclines, the macrolide antibiotics such as erythromycin, lincomycin, and its congener clindamycin; (4) agents that bind to the 30 S ribosomal subunit and cause the accumulation of protein synthetic initiation complexes, misreading of the mRNA code, and the production of abnormal polypeptides; these include the aminoglycoside group of antibiotics, which are bactericidal; (5) agents that affect nucleic acid metabolism, such as rifampin, which inhibits DNA-dependent RNA polymerase; (6) the antimetabolites, including trimethoprim and the sulfonamides, which block specific metabolic steps that are essential to the microorganism. Additional categories will likely emerge as more complex mechanisms are elucidated; at the present time, the precise mechanism of action of some antimicrobial agents is unknown.

Another classification with functional utility is based on the general antimicrobial activity of the various groups of drugs: (1) drugs primarily effective against the gram-positive cocci and bacilli, which tend to have a relatively narrow spectrum of activity, include penicillin G, the semisynthetic penicillinase-resistant penicillins, the macrolides, the lincomycins, vancomycin, and bacitracin; (2) drugs primarily effective against the aerobic gram-negative bacilli include the aminoglycosides and polymyxins; (3) relatively broad-spectrum drugs that affect both the gram-positive cocci and gram-negative bacilli include the broad-spectrum penicillins (ampicillin and carbenicillin), the cephalosporins, the tetracyclines, chloroamphenicol, trimethoprim, and the sulfonamides. While this classification has *many important exceptions,* it does help the physician to remember the antibiotic spectrum of each drug.

Factors That Determine the Susceptibility and Resistance of Microorganisms to Antimicrobial Agents. When antibiotics are used to treat an infection, a favorable therapeutic outcome is influenced by numerous factors. However, in simple terms, success is dependent on achieving a level of antibacterial activity at the site of infection that is sufficient to inhibit the bacteria in a manner that tips the balance in favor of the host. When host defenses are maximally effective, the alteration required may be minimal, for example, slowing protein synthesis or preventing microbial cell division. On the other hand, when host defenses are impaired, complete killing or lysis of the bacteria may be required to achieve a successful outcome. The dose of drug utilized must be sufficient to produce the necessary effect on the microorganisms; however, concentrations of the agent in plasma and tissues must remain below those that are toxic to human cells. If this can be achieved, the microorganism is said to be susceptible to the antibiotic. If the concentration of drug required to inhibit or kill the organism is greater than the concentration that can safely be achieved, the microorganism is considered to be resistant to the antibiotic. The precise information required to make accurate decisions about concentrations of drugs in various tissues or body fluids is frequently unavailable, and the concentrations vary from site to site. Thus, determination of antibiotic sensitivity of microorganisms is at best an inexact science. For example, group-A beta-hemolytic streptococci are inhibited and killed by exquisitely low concentrations of penicillin G (1 ng/ml), yet very high concentrations of penicillin (20 to 100 µg/ml) can be safely achieved in plasma. There is thus a very large margin of "overkill." On the other hand, many gram-negative aerobic bacilli, such as *Pseudomonas aeruginosa,* may require 2 to 4 µg/ml of gentamicin or tobramycin to be inhibited. Such bacilli are considered to be susceptible

to these antimicrobials, although peak concentrations in plasma above 6 to 10 µg/ml may result in ototoxicity or nephrotoxicity. Thus, the ratio of toxic to therapeutic concentrations is very low and such agents are difficult to use. Concentrations of these drugs at certain sites of infection (such as vitreous fluid or cerebrospinal fluid) may be much lower than those in plasma, and the drug may be only marginally effective or ineffective in such cases even though standardized *in-vitro* tests would likely report the microorganism as sensitive. Conversely, concentrations of drug in urine may be much higher than those in plasma. Microorganisms reported as "resistant" may thus respond to therapy when they are localized in the urinary tract. Most *in-vitro* sensitivity tests are standardized on the basis of the drug concentrations that can be safely achieved in plasma, and they do *not* reflect concentrations at sites of infection and local factors that affect the activity of the drug. The limitations of such *in-vitro* tests must be understood.

The factors that determine the relative antimicrobial activity of a drug against a specific microorganism are multiple. For an antibiotic to be effective, it must first gain access to the target sites of action on or in the bacterial cell. Microorganisms may resist this passage by several mechanisms. Some produce enzymes at or within the cell surface that inactivate the drug. Others possess impermeable cell membranes that prevent influx of the drug. Still others lack the transport systems that are required for entrance of the drug into the bacterial cell (Dickie *et al.,* 1978). Since many antibiotics are organic acids, their penetration may be pH dependent (Strausbaugh and Sande, 1978); in addition, permeation may be altered by osmolality or by various cations in the external milieu (Zimilis and Jackson, 1973). The transport mechanisms for certain drugs are energy dependent and are not operative in an anaerobic environment (Verklin and Mandell, 1977).

Once the drug has gained access to the target site, it must exert an effect that is deleterious to the microorganism. Multiple factors are involved. Each class of drug has its unique sites of action, and natural or acquired resistance to the drug may be explicable on the basis of differences in these targets.

Acquired Resistance to Antimicrobial Agents. When the antimicrobial activity of an agent is first tested, a pattern of sensitivity and resistance is usually defined. Unfortunately, this spectrum can subsequently vary remarkably, since microorganisms have evolved an array of ingenious alterations that allow them to survive in the presence of antibiotics. The phenomenon of drug resistance varies from microorganism to microorganism and from drug to drug. Strains of *Staphylococcus aureus* that were resistant to penicillin G appeared shortly after this antibiotic was introduced, and the frequency increased such that up to 80% of both hospital- and community-acquired strains of this bacterium are now insensitive. Emergence of resistance in other species has occurred much more slowly. The gonococcus acquired low-level resistance to penicillin G over a period of 20 years, especially in areas where this drug was used excessively. However, since 1974 many gonococcal strains have suddenly emerged that produce penicillinase (beta-lactamase), an enzyme that inactivates the drug. These strains are highly resistant to penicillin G, and infections produced by them are not cured even with high doses of the drug. Likewise, the pneumococcus (*Streptococcus pneumoniae*) has historically been exquisitely sensitive to penicillin G; however, in 1978, strains resistant to this drug emerged in South Africa, and several similar strains have subsequently been isolated in the United States.

The development of resistance to antibiotics involves a stable genetic change, heritable from generation to generation. Any of the mechanisms that result in alteration of bacterial genetic composition can operate. While *mutation* is frequently the cause, resistance to antimicrobial agents may be acquired through transfer of genetic material from one bacterium to another by *transduction, transformation,* or *conjugation.*

Mutation. Any large population of antibiotic-susceptible bacteria is likely to contain some mutants that are relatively resistant to the drug. Such variants can be isolated when the microorganisms are grown in medium containing the antibiotic, and analysis indicates that these strains have undergone a stable genetic change that may persist in the absence of the drug. There is, however, no evidence that these mutations are actually caused by exposure to the particular drug. Strains of some bacterial species isolated long before certain antibacterial agents were developed have been found to be naturally highly resistant to these drugs; such was the case with penicillinase-producing *Staph. aureus.* Such mutations are random events, and the resultant alteration is usually specific for a single drug or class of drugs.

Microorganisms that acquire resistance to a particular antimicrobial agent become important clinically because of *selection.* Thus, particularly when the use of an individual drug is widespread, sensitive strains are suppressed and resistant ones multiply unimpaired; in time, resistant microorganisms predominate.

The acquisition of resistance to antimicrobial agents can follow different temporal patterns. In some instances, a single-step mutation results in a high degree of resistance. For example, certain variants in a population of streptomycin-sensitive enteric bacilli contain an altered ribosomal protein that does not bind the drug; these bacilli are resistant to very high concentrations of streptomycin (Hahn, 1971). Likewise, when *Escherichia coli* or *Staph. aureus* are exposed to rifampin, highly resistant mutants emerge that contain an altered DNA-dependent RNA polymerase that does not bind the drug (Wehrli *et al.,* 1968; Sande and Johnson, 1975). In other cases the emergence of resistant mutants may be a slow stepwise process, with each step conferring only slight alterations in susceptibility. As mentioned, this has occurred with the gonococcus, where there has been a gradual reduction in accessibility of penicillin G to target sites in the cell envelope of the organism (Sparling *et al.,* 1976).

Mutational changes that confer resistance to a drug may simultaneously alter virulence factors and affect the pathogenicity of the microorganism. For example, strains of *Staph. aureus* that spontaneously develop resistance to rifampin also produce less catalase and are less virulent to animals

(Mandell, 1975). These resistant strains do not persist well in the environment (Sande and Mandell, 1975). Strains of *Neisseria gonorrhoeae* that have acquired stepwise, low-level resistance to penicillin G rarely disseminate from the genital sites of primary infection, but this is a frequent occurrence with their penicillin-sensitive counterparts (Handsfield *et al.*, 1976; Jaffe *et al.*, 1976). Unfortunately, all antibiotic-resistant mutants are *not* less virulent—for example, penicillinase-producing *Staph. aureus.*

Transduction. This process occurs by the intervention of a bacteriophage (a virus that infects bacteria) that can carry bacterial DNA incorporated into its protein coat. If this genetic material includes a gene for drug resistance, the newly infected bacterial cell may become resistant to the agent and capable of passing the trait on to its progeny. Transduction is particularly important in the transfer of antibiotic resistance among strains of *Staph. aureus,* where some phages can carry plasmids (extrachromosomal DNA) that code for penicillinase, while others transfer information for resistance to erythromycin, tetracycline, or chloramphenicol.

Transformation. This method of transfer involves incorporation into bacteria of DNA that is contained in its environment. Although some bacterial cells are capable of excreting transforming DNA during certain phases of growth, the importance of this method of transfer remains unknown.

Conjugation. The passage of resistant genes from cell to cell by direct contact through a sex pilus or bridge is termed conjugation. This is now recognized as an extremely important mechanism for spread of antibiotic resistance, since DNA that codes for resistance to *multiple* drugs may be so transferred. Conjugation was first recognized in Japan in 1959 after an outbreak of bacillary dysentery caused by *Shigella flexneri* that was resistant to four different classes of antibiotics (Watanabe, 1966). Resistance could be easily transferred to sensitive strains of both *Shigella* and other Enterobacteriaceae. The transferable material consisted of two different DNA sequences. The first sequence codes for resistance and is termed the resistance (R) factor, or the R determinant plasmid. For example, in the case of resistance to aminoglycosides or chloramphenicol,

the R factor codes for the synthesis of drug-inactivating enzymes (Davies *et al.*, 1971). The second sequence codes for a sex factor for the transfer apparatus and is termed resistance transfer factor (RTF), or transfer factor plasmid. This DNA specifies the synthesis of sexual apparatus or pili that are essential for the conjugal transfer of the genetic material (Wilson and Miles, 1977). Each of these two components can exist alone, but they must be joined in order to transfer antibiotic resistance successfully.

Transfer of such information by conjugation occurs predominantly among gram-negative bacilli, and resistance is conferred on a susceptible cell as a single event. Conjugation can take place in the intestinal tract between nonpathogenic and pathogenic microorganisms. While the efficiency of transfer is low *in vitro* and lower *in vivo,* antibiotics can exert a powerful selective pressure. The proportion of enteric bacteria that carry plasmids for multiple-drug resistance has thus risen slowly in the past 20 years. In some studies, greater than 50% of persons have been found to carry multiple-resistant coliform bacilli containing R factors, and such bacteria have been isolated in large numbers from rivers containing untreated sewage. Multiple-resistant Enterobacteriaceae have become a problem worldwide, taxing the physician and creating a constant need for new antibiotics. In several situations where antibiotic usage has been controlled, the rate of increase in these resistant strains was slowed; in some instances their incidence was actually reduced (Bulger and Sherris, 1968).

The worldwide emergence of *Haemophilus* and gonococci that produce beta-lactamase is a major therapeutic problem. The gene for production of this enzyme is carried on small plasmids. At least some of the gonococcal plasmids are similar in size to the *H. influenzae* gene, and a *Haemophilus* plasmid has been transferred to gonococci by conjugation *in vitro* (Sparling, 1978). Likewise, many gonococcal strains carry a conjugative plasmid that enables sexual transfer to other *Neisseria* and to *E. coli.* It is thus likely that beta-lactamase-producing gonococci initially obtained their plasmid from a *Haemophilus* species and may maintain the potential to transfer it to penicillin-sensitive species such as the meningococcus. Fortunately, some of these genes are unstable, which may explain the reduction in the incidence of these strains in England and their failure to become predominant in the United States.

SELECTION OF AN ANTIMICROBIAL AGENT

Optimal and judicious selection of antimicrobial agents for the therapy of infectious diseases is a complex procedure that requires clinical judgment and detailed knowledge of pharmacological and microbiological factors. Unfortunately, the decision to use antibiotics is frequently made lightly, without regard to the potential infecting microorganism or to the pharmacological features of the drug. *When an antimicrobial agent is indicated, the goal is to choose a drug that is selective for the infecting microorganism and that has the least potential to cause toxicity or allergic reactions in the individual being treated (see* Table 48–1).

The first decision a physician must make is whether administration of an antimicrobial agent is indicated. Many physicians reflexly associate fever with treatable infections and prescribe antimicrobial therapy without further evaluation. This practice is irrational and dangerous, since all antibiotics can cause serious toxicity and, as noted above, injudicious use of antimicrobial agents results in the selection of highly resistant microorganisms. On the other hand, one is not always blessed with the luxury of being able to identify a bacterial infection clearly before treatment must be initiated. In the absence of a clear indication, antibiotics may often be used if disease is severe and if it seems likely that withholding therapy will result in failure to manage a potentially life-threatening infection.

Optimal initiation of antibiotic therapy requires the identification of the infecting agent. Since therapy may be required before bacteriological confirmation of identity is available, the physician must make an educated guess, that is, identify the most likely microorganisms responsible for the infection. A number of technics are helpful in this process. Importantly, the clinical picture may suggest the agent: the therapist must know the microorganisms most likely to cause specific infections in a given host. In addition, simple and rapid laboratory technics are available for the examination of infected tissues. The most valuable and time-tested method for immediate identification of bacteria is the examination of the infected secre-

tion or body fluid with the gram stain. Such tests help to narrow the list of potential pathogens and permit rational selection of initial antibiotic therapy. However, in some situations, identification of the morphology of the infecting organism may not be adequate to arrive at a specific bacteriological diagnosis, and the selection of a single narrow-spectrum antibiotic may be inadequate. Broad antimicrobial coverage is then indicated, pending isolation and identification of the microorganism. *Whenever the clinician is faced with initiating therapy on a presumptive bacteriological diagnosis, cultures of blood and other body fluids should be taken prior to the institution of drug therapy.*

Testing for Microbial Sensitivity to Antimicrobial Agents. There may be wide variations in the susceptibility of different strains of the same bacterial species to antibiotics. Essential to the choice of drug is information about the pattern of sensitivity of the infecting agent. Several tests are now available for determination of bacterial sensitivity to antimicrobial agents.

The most commonly used test of sensitivity to antimicrobial agents is the Kirby Bauer or disc diffusion technic (Bauer *et al.,* 1966). Although it is simple to perform and relatively inexpensive, it provides only qualitative or semiquantitative information on the susceptibility of a given microorganism to a given antibiotic. The test is performed by applying commercially available filter-paper discs impregnated with specific quantities of the drug onto the surface of agar plates over which a culture of the microorganism has been streaked. After 18 hours of incubation, the size of a clear zone of inhibition around the disc is determined, and this correlates with the activity of the drug against the test strain. Standards for sensitivity vary for each microorganism and, as previously stated, are based on the concentration of drug that can safely be achieved in plasma without producing toxicity. Even though the concentration of the antibiotic in plasma is the standard used for these tests, it may not always reflect the drug concentration at the site of the infection.

Tests that are more reliable, quantitatively, involve serial dilutions of antibiotics in solid agar or broth media containing a culture of the test microorganism. The lowest concentration of the agent that prevents visible growth after 18 to 24 hours of incubation is known as the *minimal inhibitory concentration* (MIC), and the lowest concentration that sterilizes the medium or results in a 99.9% decline in bacterial numbers is known as the *minimal bactericidal concentration* (MBC). The latter test is used

Table 48-1. CURRENT USE OF ANTIMICROBIAL AGENTS IN THE THERAPY OF INFECTIONS

Presentation of choices of specific agents for the treatment of various infections is always provocative of discussion and disagreement because such choices often represent the distillate of personal experiences that are approximately equally effective makes an order of choice very difficult, if not impossible. To complicate matters, patterns of sensitivity of a number of microorganisms often vary with the hospital or clinic in which they are isolated; in some instances, this reflects a varying degree of exposure to specific agents. The material presented in this table represents not only the practice of the authors, based on their experience with the management of these infections, but also that of other experts in the United States. It is important to stress that, as more information accumulates, as recently introduced drugs are used for longer periods, and as entirely new agents are developed, some of the recommendations will require modification not only in the order of choice but even in the specific drugs that are suggested.

I. GRAM-POSITIVE COCCI	DISEASES		DRUG ORDER OF CHOICE		
			1st	2nd [1]	3rd [1]
Staphylococcus aureus *	Abscesses, Bacteremia, Endocarditis, Pneumonia, Meningitis, Osteomyelitis, Cellulitis, Other	Penicillin G [2] sensitive	Penicillin G	A cephalosporin [3], Vancomycin	Clindamycin [3]
		Penicillin G resistant	A penicillinase-resistant penicillin	A cephalosporin [3], Vancomycin	—
		Methicillin resistant	Vancomycin	Erythromycin [4] + rifampin	
Streptococcus pyogenes	Pharyngitis, Scarlet fever, Otitis media, sinusitis, Cellulitis, Erysipelas, Pneumonia, Bacteremia, Other systemic infections		Penicillin G, Penicillin V	A cephalosporin [5], Erythromycin	Vancomycin
Streptococcus * (viridans group)	Endocarditis, Bacteremia		Penicillin G ± streptomycin	A cephalosporin	Vancomycin
Streptococcus agalactiae (group B)	Septicemia, Meningitis		Ampicillin or penicillin G ± an aminoglycoside	A cephalosporin [3], Chloramphenicol	Erythromycin
Streptococcus faecalis * (enterococcus)	Endocarditis		Penicillin G + an aminoglycoside	Vancomycin + an aminoglycoside	—
	Urinary tract infection, Bacteremia		Ampicillin, Penicillin G + an aminoglycoside	Vancomycin	—

	Penicillin G	A cephalosporin	Vancomycin
Streptococcus bovis — Endocarditis, Urinary tract infection, Bacteremia	Penicillin G	A cephalosporin	Vancomycin
Streptococcus * (anaerobic species) — Bacteremia, Endocarditis, Brain and other abscesses, Sinusitis	Penicillin G [6]	A cephalosporin [3] / Clindamycin [3]	Chloramphenicol [7] / Erythromycin
Streptococcus pneumoniae (pneumococcus) — Pneumonia, Meningitis, Endocarditis, Arthritis, Sinusitis, Otitis	Penicillin G	A cephalosporin [3] / Erythromycin	Chloramphenicol [7] / Clindamycin [3]

DRUG ORDER OF CHOICE

DISEASES

		1st	*2nd* [1]	*3rd* [1]
II. GRAM-NEGATIVE COCCI				
Neisseria gonorrhoeae (gonococcus) — Genital infections	Penicillin sensitive	Ampicillin or amoxicillin / Penicillin G / A tetracycline	Erythromycin / Spectinomycin [8]	—
	Penicillinase producing	Spectinomycin [8]	Cefoxitin	Trimethoprim-sulfamethoxazole
	Arthritis-dermatitis syndrome	Ampicillin or amoxicillin / Penicillin G	A tetracycline	—
Neisseria meningitidis (meningococcus) — Meningitis, Bacteremia		Penicillin G	Chloramphenicol	—
Carrier state		Rifampin	Minocycline	—

* All strains must be examined *in vitro* for sensitivity to various antimicrobial agents.

[1] Drugs included for second and third choices are (a) indicated in patients hypersensitive to equally or more effective agents, (b) potentially more dangerous than equally active crugs, (c) less likely to produce the desired therapeutic response, or (d) in need, in some cases, of further study in order to allow a valid evaluation of their efficacy.

Lists of drugs within each box are given alphabetically since they are approximately equally effective.

[2] Minimal inhibitory concentration (MIC) is less than 0.2 µg/ml

[3] Therapeutic concentrations of this drug are not achieved in the cerebrospinal fluid, and alternative agents should be used to treat infections of the central nervous system (CNS).

[4] Rifampin is highly active against most strains of *Staph. aureus*, including some that are resistant to methicillin. Since resistance develops rapidly (one-step mutation) during therapy, a second active drug, such as erythromycin, should be used concurrently.

[5] Especially for bacteremia.

[6] Large doses of penicillin G may be required.

[7] Chloramphenicol is the drug of choice for infection of the CNS in patients who are allergic to penicillin.

[8] Spectinomycin is useful for genital infections only.

Table 48-1. CURRENT USE OF ANTIMICROBIAL AGENTS IN THE THERAPY OF INFECTIONS (Continued)

III. GRAM-POSITIVE BACILLI	DISEASES	DRUG ORDER OF CHOICE		
		1st	2nd [1]	3rd [1]
Bacillus anthracis *	"Malignant pustule" Pneumonia	Penicillin G	Erythromycin A tetracycline	A cephalosporin Chloramphenicol
Corynebacterium diphtheriae [9]	Pharyngitis Laryngotracheitis Pneumonia Other local lesions	Penicillin G	Erythromycin	A cephalosporin Rifampin
	Carrier state	Erythromycin	Penicillin G	—
Corynebacterium species, aerobic and anaerobic * (diphtheroids)	Endocarditis Infected foreign bodies	Penicillin G ± an aminoglycoside Vancomycin	Rifampin ± penicillin G	—
Listeria monocytogenes	Meningitis Bacteremia Endocarditis	Ampicillin ± an aminoglycoside	Chloramphenicol Erythromycin A tetracycline	—
Erysipelothrix rhusiopathiae	Erysipeloid	Penicillin G	Erythromycin A tetracycline	Chloramphenicol
Clostridium perfringens and other species	Gas gangrene [10]	Penicillin G	Chloramphenicol	A cephalosporin Clindamycin
Clostridium tetani	Tetanus [10]	Penicillin G [11]	A tetracycline	Erythromycin

IV. GRAM-NEGATIVE BACILLI	DISEASES	DRUG ORDER OF CHOICE		
		1st	2nd [1]	3rd [1]
Escherichia coli *	Urinary tract infection [12]	Ampicillin A sulfonamide Trimethoprim-sulfamethoxazole	A cephalosporin A tetracycline	Nitrofurantoin
	Other infections Bacteremia	Ampicillin Gentamicin	A cephalosporin Chloramphenicol	—

Organism	Disease	Drug of first choice	Alternative	
Enterobacter aerogenes *	Urinary tract [13] and other infections	Cefamandole / Gentamicin / Tobramycin	Carbenicillin / Ticarcillin	—
Proteus mirabilis *	Urinary tract [13] and other infections	Ampicillin / Gentamicin / Tobramycin	A cephalosporin	—
Proteus, other species *	Urinary tract [13] and other infections	Gentamicin / Tobramycin	Carbenicillin / Ticarcillin	Cefoxitin
Pseudomonas aeruginosa *	Urinary tract infection [13]	Carbenicillin / Ticarcillin	Gentamicin / Tobramycin	Colistimethate
	Pneumonia [14] / Bacteremia [14]	Carbenicillin or ticarcillin + gentamicin or tobramycin		—
Klebsiella pneumoniae *	Urinary tract infection [13]	A cephalosporin [15]	Gentamicin / Tobramycin	Chloramphenicol
	Pneumonia	A cephalosporin [15] + gentamicin or tobramycin		
Salmonella *	Typhoid fever / Paratyphoid fever / Bacteremia	Ampicillin [16] / Chloramphenicol [16]	Trimethoprim-sulfamethoxazole	—
	Acute gastroenteritis	No therapy		
Shigella *	Acute gastroenteritis [17]	Ampicillin / Trimethoprim-sulfamethoxazole	Chloramphenicol	—
Serratia *	Variety of nosocomial and opportunistic infections	Gentamicin	Amikacin	Cefoxitin

9 Antibiotics alone do not alter the clinical course of diphtheria, but drugs can eradicate the carrier state.

10 Adequate debridement is absolutely essential.

11 Ten to 20 million units of penicillin G daily, with debridement and adsorbed tetanus toxoid.

12 Sulfonamides, trimethoprim-sulfamethoxazole, and urinary tract antiseptics are useful for acute urinary tract infections, especially cystitis, in the patient without obstructive uropathy or in whom the disease has not become chronic. These agents also prove useful for chronic suppressive therapy in patients with recurrent urinary tract infection. Some clinicians prefer to reserve the antibiotics, such as ampicillin, for cases in which there are systemic manifestations—particularly in acute pyelonephritis.

13 Urinary tract infections caused by microorganisms other than *E. coli* are less usual and frequently occur in the setting of obstructive uropathy or an indwelling urinary catheter, or following recurrent infections and the use of antibiotics. Therapy must be individualized but is frequently unsuccessful unless the underlying condition is corrected.

14 While single-drug therapy with either carbenicillin or ticarcillin or an aminoglycoside (gentamicin or tobramycin) is adequate for most infections caused by *Pseud. aeruginosa*, the combination of the two classes of drug is recommended for therapy of bacteremia, especially in the neutropenic patient or in the individual with pneumonia.

15 An increasing number of strains are becoming resistant to the cephalosporins. Cefamandole appears to be the most active cephalosporin currently available. Many authorities would use a cephalosporin with an aminoglycoside for treatment of pneumonia.

16 Chloramphenicol is the drug of choice for the treatment of typhoid fever. Ampicillin may be used as initial treatment for other types of infections with *Salmonella*. However, many strains of this microorganism are presently resistant to a wide variety of drugs; sensitivity testing is mandatory.

17 Many strains of *Shigella* are now resistant to ampicillin, and some are also resistant to chloramphenicol.

Table 48-1. CURRENT USE OF ANTIMICROBIAL AGENTS IN THE THERAPY OF INFECTIONS (Continued)

DISEASES	DRUG ORDER OF CHOICE		
	1st	2nd [1]	3rd [1]
IV. GRAM-NEGATIVE BACILLI			
Acinetobacter * — Various nosocomial infections, Bacteremia	Gentamicin	Amikacin	Cefoxitin
Otitis media, Sinusitis, Bronchitis	Amoxicillin, Ampicillin	Trimethoprim-sulfamethoxazole	—
Haemophilus influenzae * — Epiglottitis, Pneumonia, Meningitis	Ampicillin [18], Chloramphenicol	Cefamandole [19]	—
Haemophilus ducreyi — Chancroid	A tetracycline	A sulfonamide	Streptomycin
Brucella — Brucellosis	A tetracycline ± streptomycin [20]	Chloramphenicol ± streptomycin [20]	Trimethoprim-sulfamethoxazole
Yersinia pestis — Plague	Streptomycin ± a tetracycline	A tetracycline	Chloramphenicol
Yersinia enterocolitica — Yersiniosis	Trimethoprim-sulfamethoxazole [21]	—	—
Francisella tularensis — Tularemia	Streptomycin	A tetracycline	Chloramphenicol
Pasteurella multocida — Wound infection, Abscesses, Bacteremia, Meningitis	Penicillin G	A tetracycline	—
Vibrio cholerae — Cholera	A tetracycline	Trimethoprim-sulfamethoxazole	Chloramphenicol
Flavobacterium meningosepticum — Meningitis	Erythromycin	Rifampin	—
Pseudomonas mallei — Glanders	Streptomycin + a tetracycline	Streptomycin + chloramphenicol	—
Pseudomonas pseudomallei — Melioidosis	A tetracycline ± chloramphenicol	Chloramphenicol	Trimethoprim-sulfamethoxazole
Campylobacter fetus * — Enteritis	No treatment or erythromycin	—	—
Campylobacter fetus * — Bacteremia	Chloramphenicol [22], Gentamicin	—	—
Bacteroides species (oral, pharyngeal) — Oral disease, Sinusitis, Brain abscess, Lung abscess	Penicillin G	Chloramphenicol, Clindamycin [3]	Erythromycin, A tetracycline

	DISEASES	DRUG ORDER OF CHOICE		
		1st	2nd [1]	3rd [1]
Bacteroides fragilis	Brain abscess Lung abscess Intra-abdominal abscess Empyema Bacteremia Endocarditis	Chloramphenicol [23] Clindamycin	Carbenicillin or ticarcillin Metronidazole [24] Penicillin G [25]	Cefoxitin
Fusobacterium nucleatum	Ulcerative pharyngitis Lung abscess, empyema Genital infections Gingivitis	Penicillin G	Chloramphenicol Clindamycin	A cephalosporin Erythromycin A tetracycline
Calymmatobacterium granulomatis	Granuloma inguinale	A tetracycline	Streptomycin	—
Streptobacillus moniliformis	Bacteremia Arthritis Endocarditis Abscesses	Penicillin G	Streptomycin A tetracycline	—
Legionella pneumophila	Legionnaires' disease	Erythromycin	Rifampin	—
V. ACID-FAST BACILLI				
Mycobacterium tuberculosis [26]	Pulmonary	Isoniazid – ethambutol Isoniazid – rifampin	—	—
	Miliary, renal, meningeal, and other tuberculous infections	Isoniazid + rifampin Isoniazid + rifampin + streptomycin [27] or ethambutol	—	—
Mycobacterium leprae	Leprosy	Dapsone = rifampin	Clofazimine Rifampin	—

18 Ampicillin-resistant strains are becoming increasingly common, and chloramphenicol should be given with ampicillin as initial therapy for life-threatening infections, especially meningitis, pending results of sensitivity testing.

19 Cefamandole cannot be recommended for the therapy of H. influenzae meningitis.

20 Such combined therapy is useful in severe infections.

21 Data on treatment are sparse, but therapy with trimethoprim-sulfamethoxazole has been successful in some cases.

22 Most strains are sensitive to aminoglycosides, but chloramphenicol is recommended in CNS infections.

23 Preferred antibiotic for CNS infections.

24 Metronidazole is the only drug with bactericidal activity against B. fragilis, and it is thus recommended in endocarditis; however, its use for this purpose is not yet approved in the United States.

25 Many strains of B. fragilis are resistant to conventional doses of penicillin G. Other species of Bacteroides (e.g., B. melaninogenicus) are sensitive to penicillin G.

26 Second- and third-choice drugs are available for the treatment of disease caused by M. tuberculosis; their use, which is complex, is discussed in Chapter 53. The choice of drugs for treatment of infections with atypical mycobacteria is also discussed in Chapter 53.

27 Recommended by many clinicians for more severe forms of tuberculosis, such as meningitis and the disseminated (miliary) disease. Other physicians use only two of these agents, combining isoniazid and rifampin.

Table 48-1. CURRENT USE OF ANTIMICROBIAL AGENTS IN THE THERAPY OF INFECTIONS (Continued)

VI. SPIROCHETES	DISEASES	DRUG ORDER OF CHOICE		
		1st	2nd[1]	3rd[1]
Treponema pallidum	Syphilis	Penicillin G	A tetracycline	Erythromycin
Treponema pertenue	Yaws	Penicillin G	A tetracycline	—
Borrelia recurrentis	Relapsing fever	A tetracycline	Penicillin G	—
Leptospira	Weil's disease / Meningitis	Penicillin G	A tetracycline[28]	—

VII. ACTINOMYCETES	DISEASES	DRUG ORDER OF CHOICE		
		1st	2nd[1]	3rd[1]
Actinomyces israelii	Cervicofacial, abdominal, thoracic, and other lesions	Penicillin G	A tetracycline	A cephalosporin / Chloramphenicol
Nocardia *	Pulmonary lesions / Brain abscess / Lesions of other organs	A sulfonamide ± ampicillin	A sulfonamide ± minocycline	A tetracycline + cycloserine / Trimethoprim-sulfamethoxazole

VIII. MISCELLANEOUS AGENTS	DISEASES	DRUG ORDER OF CHOICE		
		1st	2nd[1]	3rd[1]
Ureaplasma urealyticum	Nonspecific urethritis	A tetracycline	—	—
Mycoplasma pneumoniae (Eaton agent)	"Atypical pneumonia"	Erythromycin / A tetracycline	—	—
Rickettsia	Typhus fever / Murine typhus / Brill's disease / Rocky Mountain spotted fever / Q fever / Rickettsialpox	Chloramphenicol / A tetracycline	—	—
Chlamydia psittaci	Psittacosis (ornithosis)	A tetracycline	Chloramphenicol	—

		A tetracycline	Chloramphenicol	A sulfonamide
Chlamydia trachomatis	Lymphogranuloma venereum	A tetracycline	Chloramphenicol	A sulfonamide
	Trachoma	A sulfonamide + a tetracycline [29]	Erythromycin / A tetracycline	Chloramphenicol
	Inclusion conjunctivitis (blennorrhea)	A tetracycline [30]	Chloramphenicol [31]	—
	Nonspecific urethritis	A tetracycline	A sulfonamide	—
Pneumocystis carinii	Pneumonia in impaired host	Trimethoprim-sulfamethoxazole	Pentamidine	—

IX. FUNGI	DISEASES	DRUG ORDER OF CHOICE		
		1st	2nd [1]	3rd [1]
Candida albicans	Skin and superficial mucous membrane lesions	Amphotericin B / Nystatin	Flucytosine [32]	—
Cryptococcus neoformans	Meningitis	Amphotericin B + flucytosine [33]	Amphotericin B	—
Candida albicans Aspergillus Coccidioides immitis Histoplasma capsulatum Mucor	Pneumonia Meningitis Skin lesions Isolated lung lesions Bone lesions Disseminated disease	Amphotericin B	—	—
Blastomyces dermatitidis	Blastomycosis (North American)	Amphotericin B	Hydroxystilbamidine [34]	—
Sporothrix schenckii	Sporotrichosis	Iodides	Amphotericin B	—

X. VIRUSES	DISEASES	DRUG ORDER OF CHOICE		
		1st	2nd [1]	3rd [1]
Herpes simplex virus	Keratoconjunctivitis	Vidarabine [35]	Idoxuridine [35]	—
	Encephalitis	Vidarabine [36]	—	—
Influenza virus A	Influenza	Amantadine [37]	—	—

28 Some physicians favor a tetracycline over penicillin G as the drug of first choice.
29 A tetracycline may be given orally alone, or it may be applied locally in the conjunctiva sac while a sulfonamide is being administered orally.
30 Topical or oral administration.
31 Topical application.
32 A significant percentage of strains may be resistant.
33 The combination appears to give superior therapeutic results.
34 Should be used only in cutaneous blastomycosis.
35 Topical.
36 Parenteral.
37 Effective as prophylaxis for Asian A_2 influenza virus. Some authorities recommend amantadine for treatment of established disease, but the proven therapeutic efficacy is minimal.

only in special instances where very precise knowledge is required, as in the therapy of bacterial endocarditis.

In some instances, antibiotic sensitivity tests need not be carried out, since long experience has indicated that certain microorganisms have remained highly susceptible to specific antibiotics despite years of exposure. For example, group-A beta-hemolytic streptococci have fortunately remained remarkably sensitive to penicillin G; meningococci are always susceptible to penicillin G and to chloramphenicol.

Pharmacokinetic Factors. Although the knowledge that an antibiotic is active against the infecting microorganism is critical, it is not the only factor to be considered. Successful therapy depends upon achieving inhibitory or bactericidal activity at the site of the infection without significant toxicity to the host. To accomplish this, several pharmacokinetic and host factors must be evaluated.

The location of the infection may, to a large extent, dictate the choice of drug and the route of administration. The minimal drug concentration achieved at the infected site should be at least equal to the MIC for the infecting organism, although in most instances it is advisable to achieve multiples (four to eight times) of this concentration if possible. However, there is evidence to suggest that even subinhibitory concentrations of antibiotics may enhance phagocytosis and tip the balance in favor of the host. Scanning electron-microscopic studies of bacteria also demonstrate that effects of drugs on bacteria can be detected at much lower concentrations than those required to inhibit growth in broth (Lorian *et al.*, 1977). Although these observations may explain why some infections are cured even when inhibitory concentrations are not achieved, it should be the aim of antimicrobial therapy to produce a suprainhibitory or bactericidal concentration of drug at all times during treatment.

Access of antibiotics to sites of infection depends on multiple factors. If the infection is in the cerebrospinal fluid (CSF), the drug must pass the blood-brain barrier, and many antimicrobial agents that are polar at physiological pH do so poorly. For example, the concentrations of penicillins and cephalo-

sporins in the CSF are usually only 1 to 5% of steady-state values determined simultaneously in plasma (Sande *et al.*, 1978). However, the integrity of the blood-brain barrier is diminished during active bacterial infection, and penetration of polar drugs can increase markedly. As the infection is eradicated and the inflammatory reaction subsides, penetration reverts toward normal. Since this may occur while viable microorganisms persist in the CSF, drug dosage should not be reduced as the patient improves until the CSF is presumed or proven to be sterile.

Penetration of drugs into infected loci almost always depends on passive diffusion. The rate of penetration is thus proportional to the concentration of free drug in the plasma or extracellular fluid. Drugs that are extensively bound to protein thus do not penetrate to the same extent as do congeners that are bound to a lesser extent (Craig and Kunin, 1976).

Some feel that one should try to maintain inhibitory concentrations of antibiotics in the plasma at all times. This can only be achieved if the pharmacokinetic properties of the individual drugs and the pharmacokinetic principles presented in Chapter 1 are understood and employed. Knowledge of the status of the individual patient's mechanisms for elimination of drugs is also of course essential, especially when excessive plasma or tissue concentrations of the drugs cause serious toxicity.

Most antimicrobial agents are eliminated primarily by the kidneys. Specific nomograms are available to facilitate adjustment of dosage of many such agents in patients with renal insufficiency. These are discussed in the chapters dealing with the individual drugs and in Appendix II. One must be particularly careful when using the aminoglycosides, the polymyxins, vancomycin, and flucytosine in patients with impaired renal function, since these drugs are completely eliminated by renal mechanisms and their toxicity correlates directly with their concentrations in plasma and tissue. Furthermore, a vicious cycle may ensue if care is not exercised, since the toxicity of certain of these drugs is particularly manifested on the kidney. Administration of many tetracyclines is also complicated in patients with impaired renal function; elevated concentrations of these drugs in plasma may worsen uremia because of their catabolic effect.

The dosage of drugs excreted by the liver (erythromycin, chloramphenicol, lincomycin, clindamycin) must be reduced in patients with hepatic failure. Rifampin and isoniazid also have prolonged half-lives in patients with cirrhosis. If there is infection in the biliary tract, hepatic disease or biliary obstruction may reduce the access of drug to the site of the infection. This has been shown to occur with ampicillin, nafcillin, and other drugs that are normally excreted in high concentrations in the bile (Weinstein and Dalton, 1968).

Route of Administration. The discussion of choice of routes of administration that appears in Chapter 1 of course applies to antimicrobial agents. While oral administration is preferred whenever possible and efficacious, parenteral administration of antibiotics is usually recommended in seriously ill patients in whom predictable concentrations of drug must be achieved. Specific factors that govern the choice of route of administration for individual agents are discussed in the chapters that follow.

Host Factors. Innate host factors, which may be completely unrelated to the infectious disorder being treated, are often the prime determinants not only of the type of drug selected but also of its dose, route of administration, risk and nature of untoward effects, and therapeutic effectiveness.

Host Defense Mechanisms. An important determinant of the therapeutic effectiveness of antimicrobial agents is the functional state of the host's defense mechanisms. Both humoral and cellular immunity are involved. Inadequacy of type, quality, and quantity of the immunoglobulins, alteration of the cellular immune system, or either a qualitative or, most important, a quantitative defect in phagocytic cells may result in therapeutic failure despite the use of otherwise-appropriate and effective drugs. Frequently, the contribution of antimicrobial agents to the successful treatment of infection may be to halt multiplication of the microorganism and tip the balance in favor of the host. When the defenses of the host are impaired,

this action may be inadequate. Numerous examples of this phenomenon have been reported. In the normal host, bacteremia with *Pseud. aeruginosa* can be successfully treated with colistin, polymyxin, or gentamicin. These drugs are either bacteriostatic or slowly bactericidal against this microorganism *in vitro.* However, it is common to find persistent *Pseudomonas* septicemia in neutropenic, leukemic patients receiving therapeutic doses of these drugs. Concurrent administration of carbenicillin and gentamicin increases the bactericidal rate *in vitro* and is much more successful in eradicating the bacteremia (Schimpff *et al.,* 1971). Treatment is most successful when the host is again able to generate a polymorphonuclear response (Schimpff, 1977). White-blood-cell transfusions may be an effective adjunct to antibiotic therapy of severe bacterial infections in the neutropenic host. Antimicrobial therapy in these patients should consist in administration of the most rapidly bactericidal drug or combination of drugs possible (*see* below).

Local Factors. Cure of an infection with antibiotics depends on an understanding of how local factors at the site of infection affect the antimicrobial activity of the drug. Pus, which consists of phagocytes, cellular debris, fibrin, and protein, binds aminoglycosides, polymyxins, and vancomycin, resulting in a reduction in their antimicrobial activity. Large accumulations of hemoglobin in infected hematomas can bind penicillins and tetracyclines and may thus reduce their effectiveness (Craig and Kunin, 1976). The pH in abscess cavities, in other confined infected sites (pleural space, CSF), and in urine is usually low, resulting in a marked loss of antimicrobial activity of aminoglycosides, macrolides, and lincomycins (Strausbaugh and Sande, 1978). However, some drugs, such as chlortetracycline, nitrofurantoin, and methenamine, are more active in such an acidic environment. The anaerobic conditions found in abscess cavities may also impair activity of the aminoglycosides (Verklin and Mandell, 1977). Penetration of antimicrobial agents into infected areas such as abscess cavities is impaired, since the vascular supply is reduced. Successful therapy of abscesses usually requires drainage.

The presence of a foreign body in an infected site markedly reduces the likelihood of effective antimicrobial therapy. This factor has become increasingly important in the present era of prosthetic cardiac valves, prosthetic joints, pacemakers, vascular prostheses, and various vascular and central nervous system (CNS) shunts. The presence of the foreign body may produce a protected environment where host defenses are not able to eliminate the microorganisms completely, even if antimicrobial agents have inhibited their growth. Infections associated with foreign bodies are characterized by frequent relapses and failure, even with long-term, high-dose therapy with antibiotics. Successful therapy usually requires removal of the foreign material. Certain infectious agents that reside within phagocytic cells (intracellular parasites) may also be relatively resistant to the action of antimicrobial agents, since many of these drugs penetrate into cells only poorly. This may be a problem in infections with *Salmonella, Brucella, Toxoplasma,* and *Mycobacterium,* and, in some instances, even in infections caused by *Staph. aureus.* Rifampin is very soluble in lipid, penetrates cells well, and can kill many intraleukocytic microbes.

Age. The age of the patient is an important determinant of pharmacokinetic properties of antimicrobial agents (*see* Chapter 1). Mechanisms of elimination, especially renal excretion and hepatic biotransformation, are poorly developed in the newborn; this is particularly true of the premature infant. Failure to make adjustments for such differences can have disastrous consequences (*e.g., see* discussion of the "gray baby syndrome," caused by chloramphenicol, in Chapter 52). Elderly patients may also have significantly reduced rates of creatinine clearance, and slower rates of drug metabolism may be suspected.

Developmental factors may also determine the *type* of untoward response to a drug. Tetracyclines bind avidly to developing teeth and bones, and their use in young children can result in discoloration or hypoplasia of tooth enamel. Kernicterus may follow the use of sulfonamides in newborn infants because this class of drugs competes effectively with bilirubin for binding sites on plasma albumin.

Genetic Factors. Certain genetic or metabolic abnormalities must be considered when prescribing antibiotics. A number of drugs, including the sulfonamides, nitrofurantoin, and chloramphenicol, may produce acute hemolysis in patients with glucose-6-phosphate dehydrogenase deficiency; more common in black males, the defect is also occasionally found in Caucasians. Patients with hemoglobin

Zurich and hemoglobin H may also develop methemoglobinemia and hemolysis when given some of these agents.

Pregnancy. Pregnancy imposes an increased risk of reaction to some antimicrobial agents for both mother and fetus. For example, hearing loss in the child has been associated with administration of streptomycin to the mother during pregnancy. The tetracyclines cross the placenta readily and can cause injury to the developing teeth, particularly if given during the second and third trimester, when the crowns of the teeth are being formed. Tetracyclines can also be particularly toxic to the pregnant female. Pregnant women receiving these drugs may develop fatal acute fatty necrosis of the liver, pancreatitis, and associated renal damage (*see* review by Weinstein and Dalton, 1968).

Pregnancy also affects the pharmacokinetics of various antibiotics. Plasma concentrations of ampicillin and probably those of other penicillins are lower in pregnant than in nonpregnant females (Philipson, 1977). This phenomenon is likely related to a greater volume of distribution (increased plasma volume) and more rapid clearance of the drug during pregnancy.

The lactating female can transmit antimicrobial agents to her nursing child. Both nalidixic acid and sulfonamides in breast milk have been associated with hemolysis in children with glucose-6-phosphate dehydrogenase deficiency. In addition, sulfonamides, even in the small amounts received from breast milk, may predispose the nursing child to kernicterus (Vorherr, 1974).

Drug Allergy. Antibiotics, especially the penicillin derivatives, are notorious for provoking allergic reactions in man. Patients with a history of atopic allergy seem particularly susceptible to the development of these reactions. The sulfonamides, trimethoprim, nitrofurantoin, the macrolides, and aminoglycosides have particularly been associated with hypersensitivity reactions, especially rash (Arndt and Jick, 1976). When use of a penicillin is contemplated, a history of anaphylaxis (immediate reaction) or hives and laryngeal edema (accelerated reaction) precludes the use of the drug in all but extreme life-threatening situations. Skin testing, particularly of the penicillins and the cephalosporins, has become widespread and has some value in predicting the life-threatening reactions. However, the controversy over the utility of such tests is only partly resolved (*see* Chapter 50).

Disorders of the Nervous System. Patients with diseases of the nervous system that predispose to seizures are prone to develop localized or major motor seizures while taking high doses of penicillin G. Neurotoxicity of penicillin correlates with high concentrations of drug in the CSF and usually occurs in patients with renal insufficiency. Patients with myasthenia gravis or other neuromuscular problems appear to be particularly susceptible to the neuromuscular blocking effect of the aminoglycosides, polymyxins, and colistin. Patients undergoing general anesthesia who receive a neuromuscular blocking agent are also particularly liable to such antibiotic toxicity.

THERAPY WITH COMBINED ANTIMICROBIAL AGENTS

The simultaneous use of two or more antimicrobial agents has a certain rationale and is recommended in *specifically defined situations* (Table 48–1). However, selection of an appropriate combination requires an understanding of the potential for interaction between the antimicrobial agents. Such interactions may have consequences for *both* the microorganism and the host. Since the various classes of antimicrobial agents exert different actions on the microorganism, one drug has the potential to either *enhance or inhibit* the effect of the second. Similarly, combinations of drugs that might rationally be used to cure infections may have additive or supra-additive toxicities. For example, vancomycin when given alone has minimal nephrotoxicity, as does tobramycin; however, when the drugs are given in combination to experimental animals, they cause marked impairment of renal function.

Methods of Testing Antimicrobial Activity of Multiple Drugs. To predict the potential therapeutic efficacy of combinations of antibiotics, methods have been developed to quantitate their effects on bacterial growth *in vitro*. Two distinctly different methods are used. The first employs serial twofold dilutions of antibiotics in broth inoculated with a standard inoculum of the test microorganism in a checkerboard fashion, so that a large number of antibiotic concentrations in different proportions can be tested simultaneously (Figure 48–1). Inhibition of bacterial growth is quantified after 18 hours of incubation. This test determines whether the MIC of one drug is reduced, unchanged, or increased in the presence of another drug. Synergism between antibiotics is said to occur when inhibition results from a combination of one fourth or less of the MIC of each drug (FIC index less than 0.5). This implies that one drug is affecting the microorganism in such a way that it becomes more sensitive to the inhibitory effect of the other. If one half of the inhibitory concentration of each drug is required to produce inhibition, the result is called additive (FIC index = 1), suggesting that the two drugs are working independently of each other. If more than one half of the MIC of each drug is necessary to produce the inhibitory effect, the drugs are said to be antagonistic (FIC index > 1). When the drugs are tested in a variety of proportions, such as with the checkerboard technic, an isobologram may be constructed (Figure 48–1). Synergism is shown by a concave curve, the additive effect by a straight line, and antagonism by a convex curve.

The second method for evaluation of drug combinations involves quantitation of their *rate* of bactericidal action. Identical cultures are incubated simul-

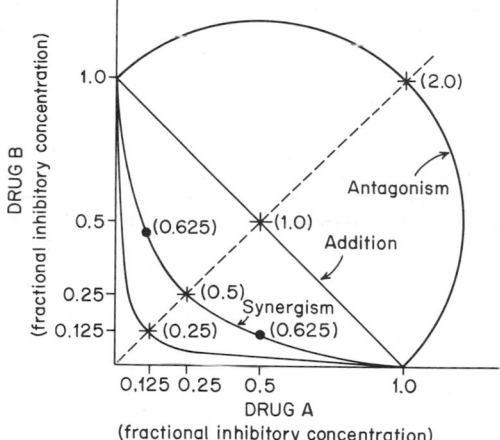

Figure 48–1. *Effect of combinations of two antimicrobial agents to inhibit bacterial growth.*

The effects are expressed as isobols and fractional inhibitory concentration (FIC) indices. The FIC index is equal to the sum of the values of FIC for the individual drugs. Points on concave isobols (FIC index < 1) are indicative of synergistic interaction between the two agents, and points on convex isobols (FIC index > 1) represent antagonism. The nature of the interaction is adequately revealed by testing combinations lying along the dotted line (marked +). *See text for further explanation.*

taneously with antibiotics added singly or in combination. If a combination of antibiotics is more rapidly bactericidal than either drug alone, the result is termed *synergism*. Moellering (1979) has recommended that the minimal criterion for synergism should be the observation of a 100-fold additional decrease in the number of microorganisms counted at any one time. If the bactericidal rate of the combination is less than that for either drug alone, *antagonism* is said to occur. If the bactericidal rate is as rapid as that for the more bactericidal drug, the result is called *indifference*. Comparative evaluation of these two distinctly different laboratory technics has, in general, demonstrated a good correlation between the results (Rahal, 1978).

There have been various attempts to predict synergism and antagonism from a knowledge of the action of the two drugs involved. A simple scheme, devised by Jawetz and Gunnison (1952), is still useful. They observed that bacteriostatic antibiotics frequently antagonize the action of a bactericidal drug and that two bactericidal drugs may exhibit synergism. In 1957, Dowling suggested that bactericidal drugs are neither synergistic nor antagonistic to each other, but that additive effects are sometimes observed. Although there are exceptions to this rule, the general principle remains sound. An up-to-date grouping of these bactericidal and bacteriostatic drugs was proposed by Rahal (1978), as follows. Group-1 drugs, which are primarily bactericidal, include the penicillins, cephalosporins, aminoglycosides, polymyxins, and the fixed-dose combination of trimethoprim and sulfamethoxazole. Group-2 agents, which are primarily bacteriostatic, include the tetracyclines, chloramphenicol, erythromycin, and the lincomycins. There is frequent antagonism between the drugs of group 1 and those in group 2 because most of the bactericidal agents require active cell division or protein synthesis for expression of their bactericidal activity, and many of the bacteriostatic drugs in group 2 inhibit these processes. However, drugs within group 1 may exhibit synergism by combination of their bactericidal actions. For example, Moellering and colleagues (1971) have demonstrated that the uptake of streptomycin into *Strep. faecalis* is increased markedly following exposure of the organism to penicillin G. It is suggested that the action of penicillin on the cell wall of the bacterium accelerates the uptake of the aminoglycoside, thereby allowing higher concentrations of the latter drug to reach the ribosome. The efficacy of the combination of trimethoprim and sulfamethoxazole is relatively unique, in that synergism results from sequential inhibition of two steps in the pathway of biosynthesis of tetrahydrofolate (*see* Chapter 49).

Indications for the Clinical Use of Combinations of Antimicrobial Agents. Numerous reasons have been given to justify the use of combinations of antimicrobial agents. These will be considered individually.

1. *Treatment of Mixed Bacterial Infections.* Some infections are caused by two or more microorganisms. These include intra-abdominal, pulmonary, hepatic, and brain abscesses and many of the genital tract infections. In such situations it may be necessary to administer different antibiotics with different antimicrobial spectra to obtain the necessary breadth of activity.

Following perforation of a viscus such as the colon, one can expect contamination and, frequently, infection with aerobic Enterobacteriaceae, anaerobic and aerobic gram-positive cocci (streptococci), anaerobic bacilli such as *Bacteroides fragilis,* and anaerobic gram-positive rods such as *Clostridium* species. A single drug would likely be ineffective against this mixed infection. A rational combination might include penicillin or ampicillin for the anaerobic and aerobic gram-positive microorganisms, an aminoglycoside such as gentamicin or tobramycin for the Enterobacteriaceae, and either clindamycin or chloramphenicol for the *B. fragilis.* In most intra-abdominal infections, therapy with antibiotics alone is rarely successful unless there is adequate drainage of pus. The importance of combined therapy has been demonstrated in an animal model of intraperitoneal infection produced by artificial contamination with stool (Weinstein *et al.,* 1975). Animals not treated with antimicrobial agents rapidly expired with sepsis due to *E. coli.* Those receiving gentamicin

alone were protected from the septic complications of the Enterobacteriaceae, but abscesses containing *B. fragilis* developed in the majority of cases. Treatment with clindamycin alone prevented abscess formation, but animals were again killed by the *E. coli.* When both drugs were used in combination, the majority of animals survived without formation of abscesses. While such studies lend support to the use of combination therapy in mixed microbial infections, not all such infections need to be treated with multiple drugs. For example, cellulitis due to the combination of *Staph. aureus* and group A streptococci can be treated with a penicillinase-resistant penicillin alone. A drug of this type has antimicrobial activity against both microorganisms. Once results of cultures of aspirated material are known, the minimal number of drugs that will be effective should be used.

2. *Therapy of Severe Infections in Which a Specific Etiology Is Unknown.* Combination chemotherapy is probably most frequently used in the treatment of infections in which the etiological agent has not been or cannot be identified. In these situations, the goal of treatment is to select antibiotic "coverage" for all microorganisms that are most likely involved. This selection of antimicrobials must be based on the physician's clinical judgment, which reflects a knowledge of the signs and symptoms of the various infectious diseases and of the microbiology of these diseases and an understanding of the antibiotic spectrum of available drugs. The breadth of the antibiotic blanket that is used is inversely related to one's ability to narrow the list of potential agents.

For example, when a patient has classical signs and symptoms of septic shock with associated upper urinary tract infection, the physician can be relatively certain that the systemic manifestations result from endotoxin released by the gram-negative bacilli disseminated from the kidney. If the patient has not received antibiotics in the immediate past or has not suffered from recurrent urinary tract infections, the agent is most likely *E. coli.* In some geographical locations, ampicillin would be expected to provide adequate initial coverage. In others, resistant strains are common and therapy with an aminoglycoside is indicated. If the patient had suffered from prior urinary tract infection or had structural abnormalities of the urinary tract, gentamicin or tobramycin plus ampicillin would constitute rational initial coverage. Broadened initial coverage is commonly employed in the severely ill where the penalty for "missing" the microorganism is high. In 24 to 48 hours, the initially obtained cultures of the urine and probably of the blood will likely contain the infecting microorganism, and, once sensitivity tests are available, the broad coverage can be narrowed and the infection treated specifically.

While the above approach to the severely ill patient can be justified, it may also lead, when abused, to a serious overuse of toxic antibiotics. This problem arises when the physician fails to obtain adequate cultures *prior* to the initiation of therapy or fails to discontinue the combination chemotherapy *after* identifying the microorganism and determining sensitivities. There is an understandable reluctance to change antimicrobial agents when a favorable clinical response has occurred. However, the goal of chemotherapy should always be to use the most selective drug that produces the least toxicity.

3. *Enhancement of Antibacterial Activity in the Treatment of Specific Infections.* As mentioned above, when two antimicrobial agents are administered together, they may produce a synergistic effect. This may permit a reduction in the dosage of one or both drugs with achievement of a similar therapeutic effect. Alternatively, the combination may produce a more rapid or complete bactericidal effect than could be achieved with either drug alone. There are specific clinical indications for the use of combinations of antimicrobial agents, and they are based on documented proof of efficacy.

Perhaps the best-documented need for a synergistic combination of antimicrobial agents is in the treatment of enterococcal endocarditis. *In vitro*, a combination of penicillin and streptomycin or gentamicin is bactericidal, while penicillin alone is bacteriostatic against most strains of *Strep. faecalis* (enterococci). Treatment of enterococcal endocarditis with penicillin alone frequently results in relapses, while combination therapy is curative at rates that are comparable to those achieved with endocarditis caused by streptococci that are more sensitive to penicillin (Mandell *et al.*, 1970; Moellering *et al.*, 1971). This is a clear-cut case where combination therapy produces superior clinical results. Antibiotic therapy of endocarditis caused by strains of penicillin-sensitive *Strep. viridans* may also be improved and the duration of treatment shortened when two drugs are used. Penicillin and streptomycin are synergistic *in vitro* against the vast majority of these strains. In animal models of endocarditis, this combination produces more rapid eradication of bacteria from infected vegetations on heart valves than does penicillin G alone. Wilson and associates (1978) reported a 100% cure rate of patients with this condition who received a short course (2 weeks) of combination chemotherapy; those who advocate treatment with penicillin G alone recommended treatment for 4 weeks.

Synergism *in vitro* by a combination of a penicillin and an aminoglycoside has also been demonstrated with *Staph. aureus*. Eradication of the microorganism from infected vegetations was found to be more rapid in an animal model of staphylococcal endocarditis treated with this combination; however, clinical studies have yet to support use of this combination in humans.

Synergistic antibiotic combinations are recommended in the therapy of infections with *Pseudomonas* in neutropenic patients. *In vitro*, carbenicillin or ticarcillin plus an aminoglycoside (usually either gentamicin or tobramycin) are synergistic against most strains of *Pseud. aeruginosa*. Studies in animals support the superiority of the combination over either drug alone, and clinical studies suggest improved survival with the combination. Despite the fact that the microorganism is sensitive to gentamicin *in vitro*, administration of gentamicin alone frequently does not cure the infection and may even allow sustained bacteremia. The addition of carbenicillin markedly increases the cure rate, a phenomenon that correlates with a more rapid bactericidal effect *in vitro*. This success may be a reflection of the importance of the use of antibiotics that produce bactericidal effects rapidly when infection occurs in the neutropenic patient.

Sulfonamides combined with trimethoprim are synergistic *in vitro* and are effective against infections caused by microorganisms that may be resistant to sulfonamides alone. A fixed combination of trimethoprim and sulfamethoxazole is available for clinical use and has been effective in the treatment of recurrent urinary tract infections, typhoid fever, shigellosis, and certain infections due to ampicillin-resistant *H. influenzae*. The therapy of brucellosis appears to be most effective when tetracycline and streptomycin are combined. Mecillinam, an experimental semisynthetic penicillin belonging to the 6-beta-amidinopenicillanic acid group, possesses a unique antibacterial action and is most effective when combined with another beta-lactam compound; the combination is effective against various strains of *E. coli, Klebsiella, Enterobacter, Salmonella, Proteus, Pseudomonas,* and *Serratia*. This new approach may result in successful therapy of severe gram-negative bacillary infections without utilization of the more toxic aminoglycoside antibiotics.

Advances have also been made by combination of synergistic agents in the antimicrobial therapy of fungal infections. Combinations of amphotericin B with other agents, including flucytosine, rifampin, or tetracycline, enhance antifungal activity (Kwan *et al.*, 1972). The mechanism of this synergism seems to involve damage to the fungal-cell envelope by amphotericin B, with resulting enhanced intracellular penetration of flucytosine or the other agents. The most significant clinical advance to date is in the therapy of cryptococcal meningitis. A combination of flucytosine and low-dose amphotericin B given for 6 weeks was as effective as therapy with a higher dose of amphotericin B for 10 weeks (Bennett *et al.*, 1979). In addition, the incidence of renal toxicity was reduced.

4. *Prevention of the Emergence of Resistant Microorganisms.* The use of combina-

tions of antimicrobial agents was first proposed as a method to prevent the emergence of resistant mutants during therapy. If spontaneous mutation were the predominant means by which microorganisms acquired resistance to antibiotics, combination chemotherapy would, in theory, be an effective means of prevention. For example, if the frequency of mutation for the acquisition of resistance to one drug is 10^{-7} and that for a second drug 10^{-6}, the probability of independent mutation to resistance to both drugs in a single cell is the product of the two frequencies, 10^{-13}. This makes the emergence of such mutant resistant strains statistically unlikely. In practice, however, this method has received extensive use only in the treatment of tuberculosis, where the concomitant use of two or more appropriate agents strikingly reduces the development of drug resistance by the tubercle bacillus.

Disadvantages of Combinations of Antimicrobial Agents. It is important that physicians understand the potential negative results of the use of combinations of antimicrobial agents. The most obvious are the risk of toxicity from two or more agents, the selection of microorganisms that are resistant to antibiotics that may not have been necessary, and increased cost to the patient. In addition, as noted above, antagonism of antibacterial effect may result when bacteriostatic and bactericidal agents are given concurrently. The clinical significance of antibiotic antagonism is not fully understood. Although antagonism of one antibiotic by another has been a frequent observation *in vitro,* well-documented clinical examples are relatively rare. The most notable of these involves the therapy of pneumococcal meningitis.

In 1951, Lepper and Dowling reported that the fatality rate among patients with pneumococcal meningitis who were treated with penicillin alone was 21%, while those patients who received the combination of penicillin and chloramphenicol had a fatality rate of 79%. This study was supported by Mathies and colleagues (1967), who treated children with bacterial meningitis of multiple etiologies with either ampicillin alone or with the combination of ampicillin, chloramphenicol, and streptomycin. The mortality rate among those treated with ampicillin was 4.3%, while those treated with the combination was significantly greater—10.5%. Several other clini-

cal reports suggest that such antagonism occurs and is detrimental in the therapy of urinary tract infections and streptococcal pharyngitis. The relative paucity of clinical studies that support the concept of a deleterious effect of antagonism between antibiotics has several possible explanations. First, few studies have been conducted to examine this question. Second, antagonism between antibiotics is probably relatively unimportant in *most* infections. This latter concept is particularly supported by studies in animals.

If an antagonistic interaction between two antibiotics is to occur, both agents must be active against the infecting microorganism. The addition of a bacteriostatic to a bactericidal drug frequently results in only a bacteriostatic effect. In many infections where host defenses are adequate, this may still be adequate to tip the balance in favor of the host. Where host defenses are impaired, as in patients with neutropenia, or with special infections, such as endocarditis and perhaps meningitis, the bactericidal effect may become more important. Certain studies in experimental animals and in the clinic support this contention. In animals with *Proteus mirabilis* peritonitis, gentamicin alone and a combination of gentamicin and chloramphenicol are equally effective in preventing death. However, if the animals are first irradiated and rendered neutropenic, the antagonistic combination of gentamicin and chloramphenicol is much less effective than gentamicin alone in preventing death (Sande and Overton, 1973). In clinical trials in man, the more rapidly bactericidal combinations of antibiotics have in general been more effective than less rapidly bactericidal or purely bacteriostatic drugs in the therapy of gram-negative infections in neutropenic patients (Klastersky, 1976; Lau *et al.,* 1977). In bacterial endocarditis, therapy limited to bacteriostatic drugs is frequently associated with relapse.

THE PROPHYLAXIS OF INFECTION
WITH ANTIBIOTICS

A large percentage (from 30 to 50%) of antibiotics administered in the United States are given to *prevent* infection rather than to treat established disease. This practice accounts for some of the most flagrant misuses of these drugs.

Clinical studies have demonstrated that there are some situations in which chemoprophylaxis is highly effective and others in which it is totally without value and may in fact be deleterious. There are still numerous situations where the attempt to use antimicrobial compounds to prevent bacterial infections is controversial. *In general, when a single effective drug is used to prevent infection by a specific microorganism or to eradicate it immediately or soon after it has become established, chemoprophylaxis is frequently successful. On the other hand, if the aim of prophylaxis is to prevent colonization or infection by any or all microorganisms represented in the environment of a patient, prophylaxis usually fails.*

Chemoprophylaxis has been employed primarily for three purposes. (1) Prophylaxis may be utilized to protect healthy persons, singly or in groups, from acquisition of or invasion by specific microorganisms to which they are exposed. Successful examples of this practice include the following: the use of penicillin G to prevent infection by group-A streptococci; prevention of gonorrhea or syphilis after contact; the use of ampicillin (in certain populations at risk) to prevent recurrent episodes of otitis media caused by *H. influenzae* or *Strep. pneumoniae;* the intermittent use of trimethoprim and sulfamethoxazole to prevent recurrent urinary tract infections usually caused by *E. coli* (Harding and Ronald, 1974); the use of rifampin, minocycline, or sulfadiazine to prevent meningococcal disease. (2) Attempts are often made to prevent secondary bacterial infection in patients who are ill with other diseases. Examples of this form of prophylaxis have been efforts to prevent bacterial infection in patients with measles or in those in coma. Likewise, antibiotics are given to prevent infection in patients on respirators. *This form of "total" chemoprophylaxis has been uniformly unsuccessful.* Resistant microorganisms, especially Enterobacteriaceae and fungi, emerge as pathogens and increase in frequency as prophylaxis is prolonged. The normal microbial flora of the host appears to represent an important defense in the prevention of colonization and infection with these pathogens. "Shotgun" chemoprophylaxis disrupts this barrier and in most cases is self-defeating; however, elaborate technics involving sterile food, life islands, and nonabsorbable antibiotics have shown modest success in decreasing infections in neutropenic patients with hematological malignancies. (3) Chemoprophylaxis *should* be attempted to prevent endocarditis in patients with valvular or other structural lesions of the heart who are undergoing surgical or other procedures that produce a high incidence of bacteremia. Endocarditis results from the bacterial colonization of the cardiac endothelium, particularly that of cardiac val-

ves. The area of colonization is probably a deposit of fibrin and platelets on a damaged valve or other area of turbulent blood flow. The prophylactic use of antibiotics is therefore recommended in patients who have cardiac lesions, such as those produced by rheumatic or congenital heart disease that produce turbulence in blood flow. Any procedure that injures a mucous membrane where there are large numbers of bacteria (such as in the oropharyngeal or gastrointestinal tract) will produce transient bacteremia. *Viridans* streptococci from the mouth, enterococci from the gastrointestinal or genitourinary tract, and staphylococci from the skin have a propensity to produce endocarditis, and chemoprophylaxis directed against these microorganisms is recommended (Kaplan *et al.*, 1977). Therapy should not begin until immediately before the procedure, since prolonged administration of antibiotics can lead to colonization by resistant strains. The American Heart Association has established criteria for the selection of specific drugs and patients who should receive chemoprophylaxis for various procedures (*see* Chapter 50).

Chemoprophylaxis to prevent wound infections after various surgical procedures has created considerable controversy. There are several well-controlled clinical studies that support the use of prophylactic antimicrobial agents in certain surgical procedures. The first such demonstration was by Bernard and Cole (1964), who showed the effectiveness of prophylactic antibiotics in patients undergoing operations involving the stomach, pancreas, and bowel. Wound infection results when a critical number of bacteria are present in the wound at the time of closure. Several factors determine the size of this critical inoculum, and these include the virulence of the bacteria, the presence of devitalized or poorly vascularized tissue, the presence of a foreign body, and the status of the host. Antimicrobial agents directed against the invading microorganisms may reduce the number of viable bacteria below the critical level and thus prevent infection.

Several factors are important to the effective and judicious use of antibiotics in this situation (Sandusky, 1979). First, antimicrobial activity must be present at the wound site at the time of its closure. This has led to the recommendation that the drug be given immediately preoperatively and, perhaps, intraoperatively. Second, the antibiotic must be active against *most* of the contaminating microorganisms. This has prompted the wide use of cephalosporins, broad-spectrum agents, in this form of chemoprophylaxis. Third, there is mounting evidence that the continued use of drugs after the surgical procedure is *unwarranted.* There are no data to suggest that the incidence of wound infections is lower if antimicrobial treatment is continued after the day of surgery. Prolonged use does, however, lead to the development of a more resistant flora and of wound infections caused by antibiotic-resistant strains. The risk of toxicity and unnecessary expense are, of course, additional disadvantages. In practice, however, this guideline is frequently broken. In a survey of the usage of antibiotics in Pennsylvania, where one third of all antimicrobial agents used were given for chemoprophylaxis, the median duration of such use was 7 days.

Chemoprophylaxis should be used in only a distinct minority of operative procedures. A number of studies indicate that it can be justified in dirty and contaminated surgical procedures (*e.g.,* resection of the colon), where the incidence of wound infections is high. These include less than 10% of all operations. In clean surgical procedures, which account for approximately 75% of the total, the expected incidence of wound infection is less than 5%, and antibiotics should not be used routinely. Exceptions are rational when the surgical procedure involves insertion of a permanent prosthetic implant. Although clear-cut data are not available to support the use of antibiotics during placement of prosthetic cardiac valves or artificial orthopedic devices, the complications of infection are so drastic that most authorities currently agree with this indication. Of course, the use of systemic antibiotics for chemoprophylaxis during surgical procedures does not reduce the need for clean and skilled surgical technic.

SUPRAINFECTIONS CAUSED BY ANTIMICROBIAL AGENTS

The reactions produced by anti-infective agents are of three general types. There is no difference in concept between *toxic effects* and *hypersensitivity reactions* caused by antimicrobial agents and other classes of drugs. These are discussed for individual agents in the chapters that follow. More distinctive, however, are *biological alterations in the host.*

All individuals who receive therapeutic doses of these agents undergo alterations in the normal microbial population of the intestinal, upper respiratory, and genitourinary tracts; some develop *suprainfection* as a result of such changes. This phenomenon may be defined as the appearance of bacteriological and clinical evidence of a new infection during the chemotherapy of a primary one. It is relatively common and potentially very dangerous because the microorganisms responsible for the new disease are, in many cases, *Proteus* strains, drug-resistant staphylococci, *Pseudomonas, Candida,* and true fungi; these may be very difficult to eradicate with the presently available anti-infective drugs. Suprainfection by these microorganisms is due to removal of the inhibitory influence of the flora that normally inhabits the oropharynx and other body orifices. Many members of the normal flora appear to produce antibacterial substance (bacteriocins), and they also presumably compete for essential nutrients. The more "broad" the effect of an antibiotic on microorganisms, the greater is the alteration in the normal microflora and the greater is the possibility that a single microorganism will become predominant, invade the host, and produce infection. Thus, the incidence of suprainfections is lowest with penicillin G and highest with the tetracyclines, cephalosporins, chloramphenicol, and mixtures of broad-spectrum antibiotics. The most specific antimicrobial agent to treat a given infection should be chosen whenever possible. The incidence of suprainfection also increases when administration of antibiotics is prolonged; and, except when clearly indicated (endocarditis, osteomyelitis, and other chronic infections), therapy should be as brief as possible. The uselessness of continued administration of antibiotics for certain prophylactic purposes for more than 1 to 2 days has been discussed above.

The fact that harmful effects may follow the therapeutic or the prophylactic use of anti-infective agents must never discourage the physician from their administration in any situation in which they are definitely indicated. It should, however, make him very careful in their use when they are required, and very hesitant to employ them in instances in which indications for their application are either entirely lacking or, at most, only suggestive. To do otherwise is to run the risk, at times, of converting a simple, benign, and self-limited disease into one that may be serious or even fatal.

MISUSES OF ANTIBIOTICS

The purpose of this introductory chapter has been to lay the groundwork for the maximally effective utilization of antimicrobial drugs. Unfortunately, in reality, these agents are frequently misused and overused (*see* Symposium, 1978).

Treatment of Untreatable Infections. A common misuse of these agents is in infections that have been proved by experimental and clinical observation to be untreatable. The vast majority of the diseases due to the true viruses will not respond to any of the presently available anti-infective compounds. Thus, the antimicrobial therapy of measles, chickenpox, mumps, and at least 90% of infections of the upper respiratory tract is totally ineffective and, therefore, worse than useless.

Therapy of Fever of Undetermined Origin. Fever of undetermined etiology may be of two types: one that is present for only a few days to a week and another that persists for an extended period. Both of these are frequently treated with antimicrobial agents when their etiology is unknown. Most instances of pyrexia of short duration, in the absence of localizing signs, are probably associated with undefined viral infections, often of the upper respiratory tract, and usually do not respond to such drugs; in the bulk of these cases, defervescence takes place spontaneously within a week or less. Studies of prolonged fever have shown that two common infectious causes are tuberculosis, often of the disseminated variety, and subacute bacterial endocarditis. Also, the so-called collagen disorders and various neoplasms, especially lymphoma (often undetectable because it is situated intra-abdominally), are frequently responsible for prolonged and significant degrees of fever. Various types of cancer, metabolic disorders, hepatitis, asymptomatic regional enteritis, atypical rheumatoid arthritis, and a number of other noninfectious disorders may present themselves as cases of fever of unknown etiology (Petersdorf and Beeson, 1961).

It has been suggested that fever of longer than 1-week duration merits the use of antimicrobial agents since, if a treatable condition has defied recognition, it will respond, and that failure to improve indicates the presence of nonbacterial disease. Experience has taught, however, that this approach is not only futile but dangerous for three reasons. (1) Untoward reactions to the drugs may occur. (2) The use of antimicrobial agents in an etiologically undefined situation that eventually proves to be noninfectious results in delay in application of more effective therapy, when this is available. Thus, the patient with a malignancy, who in the absence of a diagnosis is given antibacterial drugs, is denied the opportunity of cure or palliation. (3) Difficulty may arise from the nonspecific use of antimicrobial therapy even in instances of fever due to bacterial infection. This is well illustrated by experiences with subacute bacterial endocarditis when the only manifestation is an elevated temperature. Until the diagnosis is made, this situation is frequently treated empirically with one or another anti-infective agent, on and off, sometimes for weeks, before careful studies are finally carried out and blood cultures reveal the true nature of the disease. The dangers of prolonged delay in applying effective therapy in subacute bacterial endocarditis have been thoroughly documented.

It must be stressed that the anti-infective agents are not antipyretics. The most rational approach to the problem of fever of unknown etiology is not one that concentrates on the elevated temperature alone but one that involves a thorough search for its cause, before the patient is exposed to chemotherapy in the hope, often in vain, that, if one agent is not effective, another one or a combination of drugs will be helpful.

Improper Dosage. Erroneous dosage of antimicrobial agents is of two types: administration of excessive amounts and use of suboptimal quantities. There is little doubt that harm may be produced by overdoses of most antimicrobial agents. The difficulties that may arise from drug overdosage in patients with impairment of elimination have already been discussed.

A large area of misuse of antibacterial agents has been created by the administration of doses that are too small or that, although adequate in amount, are given for too short a period of time. As a general rule, the treatment of serious systemic infection requires that patients receive maximal quantities of drug rather than the relatively small amounts usually employed for the therapy of minor illnesses.

Reliance on Chemotherapy with Omission of Surgical Drainage. To rely on anti-infective agents alone to cure some types of infections is to place a demand on them that they cannot always satisfy. The conditions in which this is a problem are usually those with appreciable quantities of purulent exudate or necrotic or avascular infected tissues. Two of many possible examples will be cited. The patient with staphylococcal pneumonia with empyema often fails to be cured by the administration of large doses of an effective drug until constant catheter drainage of the involved area is established. The patient with renal lithiasis will frequently suffer recurrent episodes of acute pyelonephritis, regardless of the number of times he is treated with antimicrobial agents, until the stones are removed. As a generalization, it may be said that, when an appreciable quantity of pus, or necrotic tissue, or a foreign body is a problem, the most effective treatment is a combination of an antimicrobial agent given in adequate dose plus a properly performed surgical procedure.

Lack of Adequate Bacteriological Information. One half of the courses of antimicrobial therapy administered to hospitalized patients appear to be given in the absence of support from the microbiological laboratory. It is clear that the great bulk of the use of these drugs in hospitals is based on clinical judgment alone. A high proportion of the use is for chemoprophylaxis of questionable value. Bacterial cultures are obtained too infrequently, and the results, when available, are disregarded all too frequently in the selection and application of drug therapy. Frequent use of drug combinations is a cover for diagnostic imprecision. The agents selected are more likely to be those of habit rather than for specific indications, and the dosages employed are routine. Antimicrobial drug therapy must be individualized on the basis of the clinical situation, microbiological information, and the pharmacological considerations presented in this and the subsequent chapters of this section. (For discussions of patterns of antibiotic administration by physicians, *see* Symposium, 1978.)

Arndt, K. A., and Jick, H. Rates of cutaneous reactions to drugs. *J.A.M.A.,* **1976,** *235,* 918–922.

Bauer, A. W.; Kirby, W. M. M.; Sherris, J. C.; and Turck, M. Antibiotic susceptibility testing by a standardized single disc method. *Am. J. Clin. Pathol.,* **1966,** *45,* 493–496.

Bennett, J. E., and others. Amphotericin B–flucytosine in cryptococcal meningitis. *N. Engl. J. Med.,* **1979,** *301,* 126–131.

Bernard, H. R., and Cole, W. R. The prophylaxis of surgical infections: the effect of prophylactic antimicrobial drugs on the incidence of infection following potentially contaminated operations. *Surgery,* **1964,** *56,* 151–157.

Bulger, R. J., and Sherris, J. C. Decreased incidence of antibiotic resistance among *S. aureus. Ann. Intern. Med.,* **1968,** *69,* 1099–1108.

Davies, J.; Brzezinska, M.; and Benveniste, R. R factors: biochemical mechanisms of resistance to aminoglycoside antibiotics. *Ann. N.Y. Acad. Sci.,* **1971,** *182,* 226–233.

Dickie, P.; Bryan, L. E.; and Pichard, M. A. Effect of enzymatic adenylation on dehydrostreptomycin accumulation in *Escherichia coli* carrying an R-factor: model explaining aminoglycoside resistance by inactivating mechanisms. *Antimicrob. Agents Chemother.,* **1978,** *14,* 569–580.

Hahn, F. E. Streptomycin. In, *Antibiotics and Chemotherapy.* Vol. 17, *Mode of Action.* (Schonfeld, H., and DeWeck, A., eds.) S. Karger, Basel, **1971,** pp. 29–51.

Handsfield, H. H.; Wiesner, P. J.; and Holmes, K. K. Therapy of the gonococcal arthritis-dermatitis syndrome. *Ann. Intern. Med.,* **1976,** *84,* 661–667.

Harding, G. K. M., and Ronald, A. R. A controlled study of antimicrobial prophylaxis of recurrent urinary infection in women. *N. Engl. J. Med.,* **1974,** *291,* 597–601.

Jaffe, H. W.; Biddle, J. W.; Thornsberry, C.; Johnson, R. E.; Kaufman, R. E.; Reynolds, G. H.; and Wiesner, P. J. National gonorrhea therapy monitoring study: *in vitro* antibiotic susceptibility and its correlation with treatment results. *N. Engl. J. Med.,* **1976,** *294,* 5–9.

Jawetz, E., and Gunnison, J. B. Studies on antibiotic synergism and antagonism: the scheme of combined antimicrobial activity. *Antibiot. Chemother.,* **1952,** *2,* 243–248.

Kaplan, E. L.; Anthony, B. F.; Bisno, A.; Durack, D.; Houser, H.; Millard, H. D.; Sanford, J.; Shulman, S. T.; Stillerman, M.; Taranta, A.; and Wenger, N. Prevention of bacterial endocarditis. *Circulation,* **1977,** *56,* 139A–143A.

Klastersky, J. The use of synergistic combinations of antibiotics in patients with haematological diseases. *Clin. Haematol.,* **1976,** *5,* 361–377.

Kwan, C. N.; Medoff, G.; Kobayashi, G.; Schlessinger, D.; and Raskas, H. J. Potentiation of the antifungal effects of antibiotics by amphotericin B. *Antimicrob. Agents Chemother.,* **1972,** *2,* 61–65.

Lau, W. K.; Young, L. S.; Black, R. E.; Winston, D. J.; Linne, S. R.; Weinstein, R. J.; and Hewitt, W. L. Comparative efficacy and toxicity of amikacin/carbenicillin versus gentamicin/carbenicillin in leukopenic patients. *Am. J. Med.,* **1977,** *62,* 959–966.

Lepper, M. H., and Dowling, H. F. Treatment of pneumococcic meningitis with penicillin plus AUREOMYCIN: studies including observations on apparent antagonism between penicillin and AUREOMYCIN. *Arch. Intern. Med.,* **1951,** *88,* 489–494.

Lorian, V.; Koike, M.; Zak, O.; Zanon, U.; Sabath, L. D.; Grassi, G. G.; and Stille, W. Effects of subinhibitory concentrations of antibiotics on bacteria. In, *Current*

Chemotherapy: Proceedings of the Tenth International Congress of Chemotherapy, Vol. I. (Siegenthaler, W., and Lüthy, R., eds.) American Society for Microbiology, Washington, D. C., **1977**, pp. 72–78.

Mandell, G. L. Catalase, superoxide dismutase, and virulence of *Staphylococcus aureus. J. Clin. Invest.,* **1975**, *55,* 561–566.

Mandell, G. L.; Kaye, D.; Levison, M. L.; and Hook, E. W. Enterococcal endocarditis; a review of 38 cases. *Arch. Intern. Med.,* **1970**, *125,* 258–264.

Mathies, A. W., Jr.; Leedom, J. M.; Ivler, D.; Wehrle, P. F.; and Portnoy, B. Antibiotic antagonism in bacterial meningitis. *Antimicrob. Agents Chemother.,* **1967**, *7,* 218–224.

Moellering, R. C., Jr.; Wennersten, C.; and Weinberg, A. N. Studies on antibiotic synergism against enterococci. I. Bacteriologic studies. *J. Lab. Clin. Med.,* **1971**, *77,* 821–828.

Pasteur, L., and Joubert, J. Charbonne et septicemie. *C. R. Acad. Sci.* [*D*] (*Paris*), **1877**, *85,* 101–115.

Petersdorf, R. G., and Beeson, P. B. Fever of unexplained origin: report on 100 cases. *Medicine (Baltimore),* **1961**, *40,* 1–30.

Philipson, A. Pharmacokinetics of ampicillin during pregnancy. *J. Infect. Dis.,* **1977**, *136,* 370–376.

Rahal, J., Jr. Antibiotic combinations: the clinical relevance of synergy and antagonism. *Medicine (Baltimore),* **1978**, *57,* 179–195.

Sande, M. A., and Johnson, M. L. Antimicrobial therapy of experimental endocarditis caused by *Staphylococcus aureus. J. Infect. Dis.,* **1975**, *131,* 367–375.

Sande, M. A., and Mandell, G. L. Effect of rifampin on nasal carriage of *Staphylococcus aureus. Antimicrob. Agents Chemother.,* **1975**, *7,* 294–297.

Sande, M. A., and Overton, J. W. *In vivo* antagonism between gentamicin and chloramphenicol in neutropenic mice. *J. Infect. Dis.,* **1973**, *128,* 247–250.

Sande, M. A.; Sherertz, R. J.; Zak, O.; Dacey, R. G.; Bodine, J. A.; and Strausbaugh, L. J. Factors influencing the penetration of antimicrobial agents into the cerebrospinal fluid of experimental animals. *Scand. J. Infect. Dis.,* **1978**, Suppl. 14, 160–163.

Schatz, A.; Bugie, E.; and Waksman, S. A. Streptomycin, a substance exhibiting antibiotic activity against gram-positive and gram-negative bacteria. *Proc. Soc. Exp. Biol. Med.,* **1944**, *55,* 449–450.

Schimpff, S. C. Therapy of infection in patients with granulocytopenia. *Med. Clin. North Am.,* **1977**, *61,* 1101–1118.

Schimpff, S. C.; Satterlee, W.; Young, V. M.; and Serpick, A. Empiric therapy with carbenicillin and gentamicin for febrile patients with cancer and granulocytopenia. *N. Engl. J. Med.,* **1971**, *284,* 1061–1065.

Sparling, F. P. Current problems in sexually transmitted diseases. *Adv. Intern. Med.,* **1978**, *24,* 203–228.

Sparling, F. P.; Guymon, L.; and Biswas, G. Antibiotic resistance in the gonococcus. In, *Microbiology, 1976.*

(Schlessinger, D., ed.) American Society for Microbiology, Washington, D. C., **1976**, pp. 494–500.

Strausbaugh, L. J., and Sande, M. A. Factors influencing the therapy of experimental *Proteus mirabilis* meningitis in rabbits. *J. Infect. Dis.,* **1978**, *137,* 251–260.

Verklin, R. M., Jr., and Mandell, G. L. Alteration of effectiveness of antibiotics by anaerobiosis. *J. Lab. Clin. Med.,* **1977**, *89,* 65–71.

Vorherr, H. Drug excretion in breast milk. *Postgrad. Med.,* **1974**, *56,* 97–104.

Watanabe, T. Infectious drug resistance in enteric bacteria. *N. Engl. J. Med.,* **1966**, *275,* 888–894.

Wehrli, W.; Knüsel, F.; Schmid, K.; and Staehelin, M. Interaction of rifamycin with bacterial RNA polymerase. *Proc. Natl. Acad. Sci. U.S.A.,* **1968**, *61,* 667–673.

Weinstein, W. M.; Onderdonk, A. B.; Bartlett, J. G.; Louis, T. J.; and Gorbach, S. L. Antimicrobial therapy of experimental intra-abdominal sepsis. *J. Infect. Dis.,* **1975**, *132,* 282–286.

Wilson, G. S., and Miles, A. (eds.). Bacterial variation. In, *Topley and Wilson's Principles of Bacteriology, Virology, and Immunity,* 6th ed., Vol. 1. The Williams & Wilkins Co., Baltimore, **1977**, pp. 379–382.

Wilson, W. R.; Geraci, J. E.; Wilkowske, C. J.; and Washington, J. A., II. Short-term intramuscular therapy with procaine penicillin plus streptomycin for infective endocarditis due to *viridans* streptococci. *Circulation,* **1978**, *57,* 1158–1161.

Zimilis, V. M., and Jackson, G. G. Activity of aminoglycoside antibiotics against *Pseudomonas aeruginosa:* specificity and site of calcium and magnesium antagonism. *J. Infect. Dis.,* **1973**, *127,* 663–669.

Monographs and Reviews

Craig, W. A., and Kunin, D. M. Significance of serum protein and tissue binding of antimicrobial agents. *Annu. Rev. Med.,* **1976**, *27,* 287–300.

Handbook of Antimicrobial Therapy. Antimicrobial prophylaxis. The Medical Letter, Inc., New Rochelle, N.Y., **1978**, pp. 11–15.

Moellering, R. C., Jr. Principles of anti-infective therapy. In, *Principles and Practice of Infectious Diseases.* (Mandell, G. L.; Douglas, R. G., Jr.; and Bennett, J. E.; eds.) John Wiley & Sons, Inc., New York, **1979**, pp. 201–218.

Sandusky, W. R. Postoperative infections and antimicrobial prophylaxis for surgical infection. In, *Principles and Practice of Infectious Diseases.* (Mandell, G. L.; Douglas, R. G., Jr.; and Bennett, J. E.; eds.) John Wiley & Sons, Inc., New York, **1979**, pp. 2248–2256.

Symposium. (Various authors.) The impact of infections on medical care in the United States. (Kunin, C., and Edelman, R., eds.) *Ann. Intern. Med.,* **1978**, *89,* Suppl., Pt. 2, 737–866.

Weinstein, L., and Dalton, A. C. Host determinants of response to antimicrobial agents. *N. Engl. J. Med.,* **1968**, *279,* 467–473, 524–531, 580–588.

49 ANTIMICROBIAL AGENTS

[*Continued*]

Sulfonamides, Trimethoprim-Sulfamethoxazole, and Urinary Tract Antiseptics

Gerald L. Mandell and Merle A. Sande

SULFONAMIDES

The sulfonamide drugs were the first effective chemotherapeutic agents to be employed systemically for the prevention and cure of bacterial infections in man. The considerable medical and public health importance of their discovery and their subsequent widespread use were quickly reflected in the sharp decline in morbidity and mortality figures for the treatable infectious diseases. Before penicillin became generally available, the sulfonamides were the mainstay of antibacterial chemotherapy. While the advent of antibiotics has diminished the usefulness of the sulfonamides, they continue to occupy an important, although relatively small, place in the therapeutic armamentarium of the physician. However, the introduction in the mid-1970s of the combination of trimethoprim and sulfamethoxazole has resulted in increased use of sulfonamides for the treatment of specific microbial infections.

The term *sulfonamide* is herein employed as a generic name for derivatives of para-aminobenzenesulfonamide (sulfanilamide). More than 5400 congeneric substances were synthesized and studied in the decade that followed the discovery of sulfanilamide. Yet less than a score of them have attained any therapeutic importance.

History. Although sulfanilamide was first prepared in 1908 by Gelmo in the course of investigations of azo dyes, a quarter century was to pass before it was used in human bacterial infections. Investigations at the I. G. Farbenindustrie resulted, in 1932, in a German patent to Klarer and Mietzsch, covering PRONTOSIL and several other azo dyes containing a sulfonamide group. In the same year, Domagk, a research director of the I. G., work-

ing with Klarer and Mietzsch, observed that mice with streptococcal and other infections could be protected by PRONTOSIL (Domagk, 1935a, 1935b). To Domagk belongs the credit for the discovery of the chemotherapeutic value of PRONTOSIL, for which he was awarded the Nobel Prize in Medicine for 1938. In 1933, the first clinical case study was reported by Foerster, who gave PRONTOSIL to a 10-month-old infant with staphylococcal septicemia and obtained a dramatic cure.

In France, the Tréfouëls, Nitti, and Bovet (1935), working with Fourneau at the Pasteur Institute in Paris, soon communicated the important finding that in the tissues the azo linkage was split so that PRONTOSIL yielded para-aminobenzenesulfonamide, which they thought to be the chemotherapeutic moiety of the molecule. Fourneau then prepared this compound, and he and his associates (1936) demonstrated it to be as effective as PRONTOSIL in curing experimental infections. No great attention was paid elsewhere to these epoch-making advances in chemotherapy until the interest of English investigators was aroused. Colebrook and Kenny (1936) as well as Buttle and coworkers (1936) reported their favorable clinical results with PRONTOSIL and sulfanilamide in puerperal sepsis and meningococcal infections. These two reports awakened the medical profession to the new field of antibacterial chemotherapy, and experimental and clinical articles in great profusion soon appeared.

A vast number of derivatives of sulfanilamide were subsequently synthesized; many have been tested for their clinical value in various bacterial, protozoal, and viral diseases. Several achieved important, although temporary, clinical status; relatively few are valuable chemotherapeutic agents today. The major developments have been (1) the introduction of congeners that remain largely unabsorbed in the intestinal tract and hence produce local changes in bacterial flora, (2) the discovery of certain advantages of a combination of sulfonamides (*triple sulfonamides*), (3) the development of sulfonamides with high solubility in urine and hence low renal toxicity, and (4) the establishment of the value of a sulfonamide given in combination with trimethoprim in the therapy of specific infections. One interested in the history of sulfonamides is referred to *earlier editions* of this textbook and the references therein.

Chemistry. The structural formulas of selected sulfonamides are shown in Table 49–1. Most of them are relatively insoluble in water, but their sodium salts are readily soluble. Concentrations of sulfonamides in body fluids are determined by chemical technics (Rieder, 1972, 1973), rather than by bioassay; the latter technic is used for most antibiotics.

Structure-Activity Relationship. The number of sulfonamides is so vast and the structure-activity data are so complex that only the major features of this subject will be presented. The minimal structural prerequisites for antibacterial action are all embodied in sulfanilamide itself. The —SO_2NH_2 group is not essential as such, but the important feature is that the sulfur is directly linked to the benzene ring.

The para-NH_2 group (the N of which has been designated as N^4) is essential and can be replaced only by such radicals as can be converted in the tissues to a free amino group. Acylation of the para-NH_2 abolishes *in-vitro* activity; but deacylation may occur *in vivo* with a resulting return of potency, as in the case of the phthalyl derivative of sulfathiazole. Substitutions made in the amide NH_2 group (the N of which has been designated as N^1) have variable effects on antibacterial activity of the molecule. Substitution of heterocyclic aromatic nuclei at N^1 yields highly potent compounds. Bell and Roblin (1942) concluded that the more negative the SO_2 group of an N^1-substituted sulfonamide, the greater is the bacteriostatic activity. They hypothesized that optimal activity had thus been achieved in sulfadiazine. In the main, time has borne out the validity of this prediction. Acetylation at N^1 or its substitution by an amidine group does not interfere with chemotherapeutic activity and may result in compounds with novel properties; for example, the sodium salt of sulfacetamide is nearly neutral in solution, in contrast to the strong alkalinity of sodium salts of other sulfonamides. Substitution in the benzene ring of sulfonamides usually yields inactive compounds.

EFFECTS ON MICROBIAL AGENTS

Sulfonamides have a wide range of antimicrobial activity against both gram-positive and gram-negative microorganisms. With a few exceptions, there is a direct correlation between their efficacy *in vitro* and *in vivo*. In general, the sulfonamides exert only a bacteriostatic effect in the body, and cellular and humoral defense mechanisms of the host are essential for the final eradication of the infection.

Antibacterial Spectrum. Among the microorganisms highly susceptible *in vitro* to sulfonamides are *Streptococcus pyogenes, Strep. pneumoniae,* some strains of *Bacillus anthracis* and *Corynebacterium diphtheriae, Haemophilus influenzae, H. ducreyi, Brucella, Vibrio cholerae, Yersinia pestis, Nocardia, Actinomyces, Calymmatobacterium granulomatis,* and *Chlamydia trachomatis* (the agent responsible for trachoma, lymphogranuloma venereum, and inclusion conjunctivitis). Minimal inhibitory concentrations range from 0.1 µg/ml for *C. trachomatis* to 4 to 64 µg/ml for *Escherichia coli* (*see* below).

The widespread use of sulfonamides for the treatment of gonorrhea resulted in the appearance of a

Table 49–1. STRUCTURAL FORMULAS OF SELECTED SULFONAMIDES AND PARA-AMINOBENZOIC ACID *

* The N of the para-NH_2 group is designated as N^4; that of the amide NH_2, as N^1.

large number of cases of this disease in which the responsible microorganisms were resistant to these drugs. Therefore, therapy of this infection with the sulfonamides has been replaced completely with the penicillins and other antimicrobial agents. Consequently, there has been a gradual increase in the number of sulfonamide-sensitive *gonococci*, but this has not reached the point where the use of these compounds is warranted. Although sulfonamides were used successfully for the management of meningococcal infections for many years, a gradual increase in the prevalence of resistant strains became apparent after World War II. By 1963 it was evident that sulfonamide-insensitive strains of *Neisseria meningitidis* were becoming more numerous and producing both the carrier state and disease. The majority of isolates of *N. meningitidis* of serogroups B and C in the United States and group-A isolates from other countries are resistant to sulfadiazine (Eickhoff and Finland, 1965). A similar situation prevails with respect to *Shigella*. By 1965, nearly 60% of *Shigella flexneri* and 90% of *Shig. sonnei* were insensitive to this class of drugs (Haltalin and Nelson, 1965).

Most strains of *E. coli* isolated from patients with urinary tract infections that have not previously been treated are susceptible to sulfonamides. *Nocardia asteroides* is highly sensitive (Black and McNellis, 1971). *Enterobacter aerogenes, Pseudomonas aeruginosa,* and *Proteus* species, although occasionally sensitive *in vitro,* seldom respond favorably when they are producing disease. *Francisella tularensis, Bordetella pertussis, Leptospira, Borrelia, Treponema, Mycobacterium tuberculosis, M. leprae,* rickettsiae, amebae, plasmodia, fungi, and viruses are *not* inhibited by sulfonamides.

Mechanism of Action. Sulfonamides are structural analogs and competitive antagonists of para-aminobenzoic acid (PABA), and thus prevent normal bacterial utilization of PABA for the synthesis of folic acid (pteroylglutamic acid, PGA) (*see* Fildes, 1940; Woods, 1940). More specifically, sulfonamides are competitive inhibitors of the bacterial enzyme responsible for the incorporation of PABA into dihydropteroic acid, the immediate precursor of folic acid. Sensitive microorganisms are those that must synthesize their own PGA. Bacteria that do not require PGA or that can utilize preformed PGA are not affected. Bacteriostasis induced by sulfonamides is counteracted by PABA competitively. Sulfonamides do not affect mammalian cells by this mechanism, since they require *preformed* PGA and cannot synthesize it. They are, therefore, comparable to sulfonamide-insensitive bacteria that utilize preformed PGA.

The theory presented above does not explain all the known facts concerning the action of sulfonamides on bacteria. Brown (1962), using cell-free extracts of *E. coli,* found that sulfonamides can also be used as alternative substrates by the enzyme system to form products that are probably analogs of reduced forms of pteroic acid. These analogs could then exert inhibitory effects. The development of knowledge concerning the mode of action of the sulfonamides has been reviewed by Woods (1962).

Synergists and Antagonists of Sulfonamides. One of the most active agents that exerts a synergistic effect when used with a sulfonamide is *trimethoprim* (*see* Bushby and Hitchings, 1968). This compound is a potent and selective inhibitor of microbial dihydrofolate reductase, the enzyme that reduces dihydrofolate to tetrahydrofolate. It is this reduced form of folic acid that is required for one-carbon transfer reactions. The simultaneous administration of a sulfonamide and trimethoprim thus introduces *sequential blocks* in the pathway by which microorganisms synthesize tetrahydrofolate from precursor molecules. The expectation that such a combination would yield synergistic antimicrobial effects has been realized both *in vitro* and *in vivo* (*see* below; Reisberg *et al.,* 1967).

PABA is the most prominent among the sulfonamide antagonists. Certain local anesthetics, such as procaine, that are esters of PABA antagonize these drugs *in vitro* and *in vivo.* PABA may be added to cultures of blood or body fluids in order to block the inhibitory effect of sulfonamides on microbial growth; sensitivity to sulfonamides must be determined in media that are free of PABA. The antibacterial action of these drugs is also inhibited by blood, pus, and tissue breakdown products because the bacterial requirement for folic acid is reduced in media that contain purines and thymidine.

Effects of Sulfonamide Combined with Other Chemotherapeutic Agents. Investigations of the activity of combinations of sulfonamides and antibiotics *in vitro* and in experimental animals suggest an additive effect when sulfonamide is combined with bacteriostatic agents such as the tetracyclines and either an antagonistic or a synergistic effect when bacteria are exposed simultaneously to sulfonamides and a bactericidal antibiotic (*see* review by Jawetz and Gunnison, 1953). The combination of trimethoprim and sulfamethoxazole is discussed below.

Acquired Bacterial Resistance to Sulfonamides. Bacteria initially sensitive to sulfonamides can acquire resistance to the drug both *in vitro* and *in vivo.* The clinical importance of resistance to sulfonamides was first generally appreciated in the early 1940s, when the cure rate of gonorrhea treated with this class of drugs dropped sharply.

Bacteria resistant to sulfonamide are presumed to originate by random mutation and selection or by transfer of resistance by plasmids (Chapter 48). Such resistance, once it is maximally developed, is usually persistent and irreversible, particularly when produced *in vivo.* Acquired resistance to sulfonamide usually does not imply *cross-resistance* to chemotherapeutic agents of other classes. The *in-vivo* acquisition of resistance has little or no effect either on virulence or on antigenic characteristics of microorganisms.

Mechanism of Resistance. Resistance to sulfonamide is probably the consequence of an altered enzymatic constitution of the bacterial cell; the alteration may be characterized by (1) an alteration in the enzyme that utilizes PABA, (2) an increased capacity to destroy or inactivate the drug, (3) an alternative metabolic pathway for synthesis of an essential metabolite, or (4) an increased production of an essential metabolite or drug antagonist. The latter possibility has received most attention. Woods (1940) was the first to suggest that the resistance of some bacteria to sulfonamide may be based on their ability to synthesize enough PABA to antagonize the drug. Many data support this view. For example, some resistant staphylococci may synthesize 70 times as much PABA as do the susceptible parent strains. Further observations have confirmed this finding and have also substantiated the role of increased production of PGA by sulfonamide-resistant strains of *Staphylococcus aureus* (White and Woods, 1965). Nevertheless, an increased production of PABA is not a constant finding in sulfonamide-resistant bacteria, and resistant mutants may possess enzymes for folate biosynthesis that are less readily inhibited by sulfonamides.

Clinical Aspects and Significance of Resistance to Sulfonamide. Acquired bacterial resistance to sulfonamides plays a significant role in limiting the therapeutic efficacy of these drugs, particularly in infections caused by gonococci, staphylococci, meningococci, streptococci, and shigellae. Sulfonamide-resistant *Strep. pyogenes* emerged during the mass prophylactic use of sulfadiazine in military personnel during World War II. Outbreaks of streptococcal infections in U.S. military camps were caused by these sulfonamide-resistant strains and were a source of considerable concern. Although one would anticipate that the daily prophylactic use of a sulfonamide in patients who have had rheumatic fever (*see* below) might favor the development of drug-resistant hemolytic streptococci, resistance of clinical importance has not been documented from such medication.

ABSORPTION, FATE, AND EXCRETION

Absorption. Except for sulfonamides especially designed for their local effects in the bowel, this class of drugs is rapidly absorbed from the gastrointestinal tract. Approximately 70 to 100% of an oral dose is absorbed, and sulfonamide can be found in the urine within 30 minutes of ingestion. The small intestine is the major site of absorption, but some of the drug is absorbed from the stomach. Absorption from *other sites,* such as the vagina, respiratory tract, or abraded skin, is variable and unreliable, but a sufficient amount may enter the body to cause toxic reactions in susceptible persons or to produce sensitization.

Protein Binding. All sulfonamides are bound in varying degree to plasma proteins, particularly to albumin. The extent to which this occurs is determined by the hydrophobicity of a particular drug and its pK_a; at physiological pH, drugs with a high pK_a exhibit a low degree of protein binding, and *vice versa.* The extent of binding is decreased in patients with severe renal failure, a phenomenon not totally accounted for by low levels of plasma albumin (Andreasen, 1973). In general, a sulfonamide is bound to a somewhat greater extent in the acetylated than in the free form.

Distribution. Sulfonamides are distributed throughout all tissues of the body. The diffusible fraction of sulfadiazine is uniformly distributed throughout the total body water, while sulfisoxazole is largely confined to the extracellular space. The sulfonamides readily enter *pleural, peritoneal, synovial, ocular,* and similar body fluids, and may reach concentrations therein that are 50 to 80% of the simultaneously determined concentration in blood. Since the protein content of such fluids is usually low, the drug is present in the unbound active form.

Cerebrospinal Fluid. After systemic administration of adequate doses, sulfadiazine and sulfisoxazole attain concentrations in cerebrospinal fluid that may be effective in meningeal infections. At steady state, the concentration ranges between 10 and 80% of that in the blood. Rate and extent of diffusion vary with each drug and depend on many factors, such as the degree of binding by plasma albumin, extent of acetylation, and presence of meningeal inflammation. Inasmuch as the acetylated compounds are more extensively bound by plasma albumin and hence are less available for diffusion, the ratio of free to acetylated drug is higher in the cerebrospinal fluid than in the blood.

Fetus. Sulfonamides readily pass through the placenta and reach the fetal circulation. Equilibration between maternal and fetal blood is usually established within 3 hours after a single oral dose. The concentrations attained in the fetal tissues are sufficient to cause both antibacterial and toxic effects. The concentrations of sulfadiazine in the blood of the fetus are 50 to 90% of those in the maternal blood. The drug appears more slowly in amniotic fluid than in fetal blood.

Metabolism. The sulfonamides undergo metabolic alterations to a varying extent in the tissues, especially in the liver. The major metabolic derivative is the N^4-acetylated sulfonamide. Each sulfonamide is acetylated to a different extent. For example, the percentage of the total plasma sulfonamide that is acetylated ranges between 10 and 40 for sulfadiazine and its methylated derivatives. Acetylation is disadvantageous because the resulting product has no antibacterial activity and yet retains the toxic potentialities of the parent substance. Furthermore, the acetylated forms of some of the older sulfonamides are less soluble and hence contribute to crystalluria and renal complications. Since acetylation is a function of time and hepatic function, the conjugated fraction increases considerably when the sojourn of the drug in the body is prolonged, as in patients with impaired renal function, or decreases when hepatic failure is present. Because of varying degrees of acetylation and other factors, periodic determination of the plasma concentration of free drug is advisable when patients with severe bacterial infections are being treated with large doses of sulfonamide.

Excretion.   Sulfonamides are eliminated from the body partly as such and partly as metabolic products. The largest fraction is excreted in the urine, and the half-life of sulfonamides in the body is thus dependent on renal function. Small amounts are eliminated in the feces and in bile, milk, and other secretions.

Renal Elimination.   Each sulfonamide, free and acetylated, is handled by the kidney in a characteristic manner. In all cases, glomerular filtration is a major factor. Varying degrees of tubular reabsorption occur for most sulfonamides, although sulfacetamide is not appreciably reabsorbed. Tubular secretion also plays a role in some instances. Marked variations in the rate of renal excretion account for the differences in duration of action of the various sulfonamides, as discussed under the individual drugs. As a generalization, the rate of excretion of sulfonamides increases as their pK_a decreases.

Other Routes.   Except for sulfonamides that are poorly absorbed from the gastrointestinal tract, only small amounts of these drugs are found in the *feces* after oral medication. The concentration of sulfonamide in *human milk* is similar to that in plasma. These agents are also secreted in *sweat, tears, saliva, bile,* and *intestinal fluids.* The concentration in bile is similar to that in blood, but the *gastric juice* contains a much lower quantity.

PHARMACOLOGICAL PROPERTIES, PREPARATIONS, AND DOSAGE OF INDIVIDUAL SULFONAMIDES

The sulfonamides may be classified into four groups on the basis of the rapidity with which they are absorbed and excreted: (1) *agents absorbed rapidly and excreted rapidly,* such as sulfisoxazole and sulfadiazine; (2) *compounds absorbed rapidly but excreted slowly,* such as sulfamethoxypyridazine and sulfadimethoxine; (3) *agents absorbed very poorly when administered orally* and hence active in the bowel lumen, such as succinylsulfathiazole and phthalylsulfathiazole; and (4) *sulfonamides employed mainly for topical use,* such as sulfacetamide, mafenide, and silver sulfadiazine.

Rapidly Absorbed and Rapidly Eliminated Sulfonamides.   *Sulfisoxazole.*   Early studies of sulfisoxazole established that it was a rapidly absorbed and rapidly excreted sulfonamide with excellent antibacterial activity (equal to that of sulfadiazine). Since its high solubility eliminates much of the renal toxicity inherent in the use of the older sulfonamides, it has essentially replaced the less soluble agents. Sulfisoxazole should thus be regarded as the prototype of this group.

Sulfisoxazole is distributed only in extracellular body water, and this may explain the fact that the plasma concentration after a given dose is at least twice that for sulfadiazine. Following an oral dose of 2 to 4 g, peak concentrations in plasma of 110 to 250 μg/ml are found in 2 to 4 hours. Both the free and acetylated forms of the drug are much more soluble in urine at pH values encountered clinically than are the respective forms of sulfadiazine. From 28 to 35% of sulfisoxazole in the blood and about 30% in the urine is in the acetylated form. Approximately 95% of a single dose is excreted by the kidney in 24 hours. Concentrations of the drug in urine thus greatly exceed those in blood and may be bactericidal. The cerebrospinal fluid concentration averages about a third of that in the blood.

The recommended daily *oral dose* of sulfisoxazole for children is 150 mg/kg of body weight; one half of this is given initially, followed by one sixth of the daily dose every 4 hours (not to exceed 6 g in 24 hours). The oral dose for adults is 2 to 4 g initially, followed by 1 g every 4 to 6 hours. The *parenteral dose* for adults and children is 100 mg/kg per day, divided into three or four portions. The areas of *clinical usefulness* of sulfisoxazole are discussed below.

Less than 0.1% of patients receiving sulfisoxazole suffer serious *toxic reactions.* The untoward effects produced by this agent are similar to those that follow the administration of other sulfonamides, as discussed below. Because of its relatively high solubility in the urine as compared to sulfadiazine, sulfisoxazole only infrequently produces hematuria or crystalluria (0.2 to 0.3%) and the risk of anuria is very small. Despite this, it is advisable that patients taking this drug ingest an adequate quantity of water. Sulfisoxazole and all sulfonamides that are absorbed must be used with caution in patients with impaired renal function. Like all other sulfonamides, sulfisoxazole may produce hypersensitivity reactions, some of which are potentially lethal. Sulfisoxazole is presently preferred over other sulfonamides by most clinicians, when a rapidly absorbed and rapidly excreted sulfonamide is indicated.

Preparations. *Sulfisoxazole,* U.S.P. (GANTRISIN, SK-SOXAZOLE, others), is available in 500-mg tablets for *oral* use. It is also marketed as a vaginal cream (10%). *Sulfisoxazole Diolamine,* U.S.P., is available in 4% solution or ointment prepared for *topical* use in the eye; the same salt is marketed for *parenteral injection,* in 5- and 10-ml ampuls (400 mg/ml). Doses are given above. Intravenous administration requires the slow administration of dilute solutions of the drug. *Sulfisoxazole Acetyl,* U.S.P., is tasteless and hence preferred for *oral* use in children; it is available as a flavored syrup and pediatric suspension (100 mg/ml). The compound is deacetylated by the enzymes in the small intestine, and this results in a relatively slow absorption of the active form of the drug. A flavored emulsion of sulfisoxazole acetyl in vegetable oil (LIPO GANTRISIN) (1 g/5ml) is a longer-acting preparation. The dose for adults is 4 to 5 g every 12 hours. Sulfisoxazole is also marketed in a fixed-dose combination with phenazopyridine (sulfisoxazole, 500 mg; phenazopyridine, 50 mg; AZO GANTRISIN, others) as a urinary tract antiseptic and analgesic. The urine becomes orange-red soon after ingestion of this mixture because of the presence of phenazopyridine, an orange-red dye.

Sulfamethoxazole. Sulfamethoxazole, U.S.P. (GANTANOL), is a close congener of sulfisoxazole, but its rates of enteric absorption and urinary excretion are slower. It is employed for both systemic and urinary tract infections. Precautions must be observed to avoid sulfamethoxazole *crystalluria* because of the high percentage of the acetylated, relatively insoluble form of the drug in the urine. Sulfamethoxazole is available for oral use, as 500-mg and 1-g tablets and as a suspension (100 mg/ml). The *dosage schedule* of sulfamethoxazole for *children* is 50 to 60 mg/kg initially, followed by 25 to 30 mg/kg morning and evening thereafter. The dose for *adults* with mild infections is 2 g, followed by 1 g every 12 hours; for severe disease, the initial dose is 2 g and then 1 g every 8 hours. The half-life of sulfamethoxazole in babies during the first 10 days of life is considerably longer than in adults. It falls rapidly, being about 9 hours at 3 weeks of age and 4 to 5 hours at 1 year. It then increases toward the half-life characteristic for adults, namely, 6 to 12 hours. The clinical uses of sulfamethoxazole are the same as those for sulfisoxazole. It is presently marketed in fixed-dose combination with phenazopyridine (AZO GANTANOL) as a urinary antiseptic and analgesic, and with trimethoprim (*see* below).

Sulfadiazine. Sulfadiazine given orally is rapidly absorbed from the gastrointestinal tract, and peak blood concentrations are reached within 3 to 6 hours after a single dose. Following an oral dose of 3 g, peak concentrations in plasma are 50 μg/ml. About 55% of the drug is bound to plasma protein at a concentration of 100 μg/ml when plasma protein levels are normal. Therapeutic concentrations are attained in cerebrospinal fluid within 4 hours after a single oral dose of 60 mg/kg.

Sulfadiazine is *excreted* quite readily by the kidney in both the free and the acetylated form, rapidly at first and then more slowly over a period of 2 to 3 days. It can be detected in the urine within 30 minutes after oral ingestion. About 15 to 40% of the excreted sulfadiazine is in the *acetylated* form. This form of the drug is excreted more readily than the free fraction, and the administration of alkali accelerates the renal clearance of both forms by further diminishing their tubular reabsorption.

In *adults* who are being treated with sulfadiazine, the initial dose for oral administration is 2 to 4 g, followed by 1 g every 4 to 6 hours. *Children* over 2 months of age should receive one half of the calculated daily dose to initiate therapy and then 65 to 150 mg/kg (to a maximum of 6 g) daily in four to six divided doses. Every precaution must be taken to ensure fluid intake adequate to produce a urine output of at least 1200 ml in adults and a corresponding quantity in children. If this cannot be accomplished, sodium bicarbonate may be given to reduce the risk of crystalluria. Parenteral therapy with sodium sulfadiazine is not usually recommended.

Preparations. *Sulfadiazine,* U.S.P., is available as official tablets that usually contain 325 or 500 mg of the drug. *Sulfadiazine Sodium Injection,* U.S.P., is available for parenteral injection; it is a sterile aqueous solution and usually contains 250 mg/ml. It is rarely used anymore.

Sulfacytine. Sulfacytine (RENOQUID) is a rapidly excreted sulfonamide for the oral treatment of acute urinary tract infections (Moffat and Wenzel, 1971). The half-life in plasma is shorter than that of sulfisoxazole (4 hours versus 7 hours). Concentrations in blood are lower than those achieved with sulfisoxazole, and this agent should be used only for the treatment of urinary tract infections. A loading dose of 500 mg should be given, followed by 250 mg four times per day. Sulfacytine is supplied in 250-mg tablets.

Sulfamethizole. Sulfamethizole, U.S.P. (THIOSULFIL, others), is a rapidly eliminated sulfonamide; concentrations of the drug in blood are thus low after the administration of conventional doses. It is used for the treatment of urinary tract infections in a dosage of 500 to 1000 mg, given three or four times daily. Sulfamethizole is available in tablets containing 250, 500, or 1000 mg and in suspensions of 250 mg/5 ml or 500 mg/5 ml.

Sulfonamide Mixtures. A major and frequent toxic reaction to the older sulfonamides was urinary tract injury from precipitation of crystals, usually of acetylated drug, in the renal tubules and ureter. Alkalinization of the urine or intake of adequate fluid is effective in preventing such precipitation; however, these precautions are frequently neglected or undesirable. To offset and circumvent these disadvantages, sulfonamide mixtures were introduced into therapy. The principle that accounts for the value of sulfonamide mixtures is quite simple. Many substances can coexist in solution without interfering with each other's solubility. It is thus possible to saturate a solution with any one sulfonamide and still dissolve in it, almost to the limit of their individual solubilities, a second and a third sulfonamide. Because of the availability of newer agents such as sulfisoxazole that are appreciably more soluble than the older sulfonamides, mixtures of these drugs (*e.g., Trisulfapyrimidines,* U.S.P.) are now little used. However, numerous preparations containing sulfadiazine, sulfamerazine, and sulfamethazine remain available.

Rapidly Absorbed and Slowly Excreted Sulfonamides. *Sulfamethoxypyridazine* and *sulfameter* offer the potential advantage of maintenance of effective plasma concentrations when administered only once or twice a day because these agents are rapidly absorbed and slowly excreted. However, because of the high incidence of severe exudative erythema multiforme (Stevens-Johnson syndrome) resulting from their use, they are not recommended.

Poorly Absorbed Sulfonamides. *Phthalylsulfathiazole,* U.S.P. (SULFATHALIDINE), and *Sulfasalazine,* U.S.P. (AZULFIDINE, others), are very poorly absorbed from the gastrointestinal tract.

Phthalylsulfathiazole is conjugated at N^4 and thus is inactive until hydrolyzed by intestinal bacteria to sulfathiazole. For this reason, it has been employed to reduce the number of microorganisms in the bowel prior to surgery. However, there is no proof of efficacy for such prophylactic use of this drug (*see* Nichols and Condon, 1971). Despite very limited absorption of this drug or of the sulfathiazole derived in the colon, untoward systemic effects do occur. These include fever and allergic reactions. Interference with the normal flora of the intestine can jeopardize bacterial synthesis of vitamin K, and hypoprothrombinemia and hemorrhage may result. It is therefore advisable to administer vitamin K to patients receiving such agents.

Sulfasalazine is used in the therapy of *ulcerative colitis* and regional enteritis. Although improvement of ulcerative colitis follows the administration of 4 to 8 g of the drug per day, relapses tend to occur in about one third of patients who experience a satisfactory initial response. Sulfasalazine is preferred to corticosteroids by some gastroenterologists for treatment of patients mildly or moderately ill with ulcerative colitis (Zetzel, 1954; Riis *et al.,* 1973). The drug is also being employed as the first approach to treatment of relatively mild cases of *regional enteritis* and *granulomatous colitis* (Singleton, 1977; Summers *et al.,* 1979). Sulfasalazine is broken down in the gut to sulfapyridine, which is absorbed and eventually excreted in the urine, and 5-aminosalicylate, which reaches high levels in the feces (Peppercorn and Goldman, 1973). Toxic reactions include Heinz-body anemia, acute hemolysis in patients with glucose-6-phosphate dehydrogenase deficiency, and agranulocytosis. Nausea, fever, arthralgias, and rashes occur in up to 20% of patients treated with the drug. A daily dose of 2 g is also effective and is associated with fewer untoward effects (Dissanayake and Truelove, 1973). There is no evidence that the compound alters the intestinal microflora of persons with ulcerative colitis (Gorbach *et al.,* 1967). This suggests that any beneficial effect of the drug is probably due to some property other than its antibacterial activity.

Sulfonamides for Topical Use. *Sulfacetamide.* Sulfacetamide is the N^1-acetyl-substituted derivative of sulfanilamide. Its aqueous solubility (1:140) is approximately 90 times that of sulfadiazine. While this agent is no longer used in the therapy of urinary tract infections, solutions of the sodium salt of the drug are employed extensively in the management of *ophthalmic infections.* Although topical sulfonamide for most purposes is discouraged because of lack of efficacy and a high risk of sensitization, sulfacetamide has certain advantages. Very high aqueous concentrations are nonirritating to the delicate tissues of the eye and are effective against susceptible microorganisms. A 30% solution of the sodium salt has a pH of 7.4, whereas the solutions of sodium salts of other sulfonamides are highly alkaline. The drug penetrates into ocular fluids and tissues in high concentration. Sensitivity reactions to sulfacetamide are rare, but the drug should not be used in patients with known hypersensitivity to sulfonamides.

The *usual dose* of sodium sulfacetamide solution applied topically to the eye is 1 or 2 drops of a 10 to 30% solution every 2 hours for severe infections and the same amount three or four times a day for chronic conditions. An ophthalmic ointment may be used instead of the solution, provided there is no wound of the cornea; as a rule, the ointment is reserved for application at bedtime.

Preparations. *Sulfacetamide Sodium,* U.S.P. (BLEPH, ISOPTO CETAMIDE, SULAMYD SODIUM), is available only for topical application to the eye, as an *ophthalmic solution* (10, 15, and 30%) and an *ophthalmic ointment* (10%).

Silver Sulfadiazine (SILVADENE). This drug inhibits the growth *in vitro* of nearly all pathogenic bacteria and fungi, including some species resistant to sulfonamides (Rosenkranz and Rosenkranz, 1972). The compound is used topically to reduce microbial colonization and the incidence of infections of wounds from burns. It should not be used to treat an established infection. Silver is released slowly from the preparation in concentrations that are selectively toxic to the microorganisms (*see* Chapter 41). However, bacteria may develop resistance to silver sulfadiazine (Wenzel *et al.,* 1976). While little silver is absorbed, the plasma concentration of sulfadiazine may approach therapeutic levels if a large surface area is involved. Adverse reactions are infrequent and include burning, rash, and itching (*see* Ballin, 1974). Silver sulfadiazine is considered by most authorities to be the agent of choice for the prevention of infection of burns.

Mafenide. This sulfonamide (α-amino-*p*-toluenesulfonamide) is marketed as *Mafenide Acetate Cream,* U.S.P. (SULFAMYLON CREAM). It is effective, when applied topically, for the prevention of colonization of *burns* by a large variety of gram-negative and gram-positive bacteria. It should not be used in treatment of an established infection. Suprainfection with *Candida* may occasionally be a problem. The cream is applied once or twice daily to a thickness of 1 to 2 mm over the burned skin. Cleansing of the wound and removal of debris should be carried out before each application of the drug. Therapy is continued until skin grafting is possible. Mafenide is rapidly absorbed systemically and converted to para-carboxybenzenesulfonamide. Studies of absorption from the burn surface indicate that peak plasma concentrations are reached in 2 to 4 hours (*see* Harrison *et al.,* 1972). Adverse effects include intense pain at sites of application, allergic reactions, and loss of fluid by evaporation from the burn sur face, since occlusive dressings are not used. The drug and its primary metabolite inhibit carbonic anhydrase. The urine becomes alkaline, and a metabolic acidosis may ensue (White and Asch, 1971). Compensatory tachypnea and hyperventilation with respiratory alkalosis are also observed.

UNTOWARD REACTIONS TO SULFONAMIDES

The untoward effects that follow the administration of sulfonamides are numerous and varied. They may involve nearly every organ system. An untoward reaction increases the likelihood of a severe response to the subsequent administration of a member of this class of drugs. The overall incidence of reactions is about 5%. Certain of these interdict the subsequent use of any sulfonamide; included in this category are drug fever and reactions involving the blood, bone marrow, kidney, liver, skin, and peripheral nerves. (*See* Kutscher *et al.,* 1954; Weinstein *et al.,* 1960.)

Disorders of the Hematopoietic System. Blood dyscrasias are quite uncommon; however, when they do occur, they may be so serious that drug administration must be stopped promptly and appropriate therapy undertaken.

Acute Hemolytic Anemia. The mechanism of the acute hemolytic anemia produced by sulfonamides is not always readily apparent. In some cases, it has been thought to be a sensitization phenomenon. In other instances, the hemolysis is related to an erythrocytic deficiency of glucose-6-phosphate dehydrogenase activity, as discussed on page 1053.

The development of acute hemolytic anemia in the absence of a deficiency of glucose-6-phosphate dehydrogenase may not be dependent on dosage or the concentration of the drug in plasma. Readministration of sulfonamides to individuals who have had an episode of hemolysis provoked by these compounds is accompanied by a 65% incidence of recurrence. Blacks are more susceptible to this reaction than are white-skinned individuals, and children more so than adults. The hemolytic episode occurs abruptly, usually in the first week of therapy. Nausea, fever, vertigo, jaundice, pallor, hepatosplenomegaly, and shock may develop suddenly. There is a marked decrease in erythrocyte and hemoglobin levels, often by 50 to 70% within a few hours, and leukocytosis, reticulocytosis, bilirubinemia, urobilinuria, and hemoglobin casts are common laboratory findings. Acute renal tubular necrosis may follow the hemoglobinuria.

Hemolytic anemia is rare after sulfadiazine (0.05%); its exact incidence following therapy with sulfisoxazole is unknown.

Agranulocytosis. Agranulocytosis occurs in about 0.1% of patients who receive sulfadiazine; it also can follow the use of other sulfonamides. A myelotoxic effect is evident in the bone marrow by a maturation arrest at the myeloblast stage. The granulocytopenia is not related to the dose of drug. Most cases develop after 10 days of medication. The reaction may appear suddenly and without warning, or only after a period of progressive neutropenia. Although return of granulocytes to normal levels may be delayed for weeks or months after sulfonamide is withdrawn, most patients recover spontaneously with supportive care.

Aplastic Anemia. Complete suppression of bone-marrow activity with profound anemia, granulocytopenia, and thrombocytopenia is an extremely rare occurrence with sulfonamide therapy. It probably results from a direct myelotoxic effect, and may be fatal.

Thrombocytopenia. Severe thrombocytopenia rarely arises as a result of therapy with the sulfonamides. Transient, mild decreases in platelet counts are a more common occurrence. The mechanism is unknown.

Eosinophilia. Peripheral eosinophilia may occur as an isolated finding and usually disappears promptly after discontinuation of the sulfonamide. It may also accompany other manifestations of sulfonamide hypersensitivity.

Disturbances of the Urinary Tract. The primary factor responsible for the renal damage frequently produced by the older sulfonamides is the formation and deposition of *crystalline aggregates* in the kidneys, calyces, pelvis, ureters, or bladder; this leads to the development of irritation and obstruction. Anuria and death may occur in patients in whom no evidence of crystalluria or hematuria can be detected and in whom the lesion found at autopsy is tubular necrosis or necrotizing angiitis.

The risk of crystalluria is minimal with more soluble sulfonamides such as sulfisoxazole. Fluid intake should be such as to ensure a daily urine volume of at least 1200 ml (in adults). Alkalinization of the urine may be desirable if urine volume or pH is unusually low, since the solubility of sulfisoxazole increases greatly with slight elevations of pH.

Hypersensitivity Reactions. The incidence of hypersensitivity reactions to sulfonamides is quite variable. Reactions are seen with greater frequency when long-acting agents are used, and these drugs should thus be avoided.

Vascular lesions, involving various organs including the heart and resembling those present in periarteritis nodosa, may appear rarely in the course of sulfonamide administration. The use of sulfisoxazole has been associated with clinical activation of quiescent systemic lupus erythematosus. Eosinophilic migrating pneumonia may occur.

Among the *skin and mucous membrane manifestations* attributed to sensitization to sulfonamide are morbilliform, scarlatinal, urticarial, erysipeloid, pemphigoid, purpuric, and petechial rashes; and erythema nodosum, erythema multiforme of the Stevens-Johnson type, Behçet's syndrome, exfoliative dermatitis, and photosensitivity. Contact dermatitis is very uncommon today, as the result of discontinuation of topical application of most of these drugs. Although localized sensitization usually leads to a recurrence of the dermatitis when sulfonamide is again administered orally or parenterally, diffuse systemic hypersensitivity states may also develop. Drug eruptions occur most often after the first week of therapy, but may appear earlier in previously sensitized individuals. Fever, malaise, and pruritus are frequently present simultaneously. The incidence of untoward dermal effects is about 1.5% with sulfadiazine therapy and about 2% with sulfisoxazole.

A syndrome similar to *serum sickness* may appear after several days of sulfonamide therapy. Fever, joint pain, urticarial eruptions, conjunctivitis, bronchospasm, and leukopenia are the outstanding features. In persons previously sensitized to these drugs, immediate reactions of the *anaphylactoid type* are sometimes observed.

Drug fever is a common untoward manifestation of sulfonamide treatment. The incidence approximates 3% with sulfisoxazole. The fever is generally sudden in onset and develops between the seventh and tenth day of sulfonamide administration. It may occur earlier, however, especially if the patient has been previously sensitized to the drug. Headache, chills, malaise, pruritus, and skin rash may accompany the fever. It should be differentiated from the fever that heralds serious toxic reactions to the sulfonamides, such as agranulocytosis and acute hemolytic anemia.

Although *cross-sensitivity* between different sulfonamides does occur, this is not a universal phenomenon; the incidence of sensitivity manifestations following the subsequent administration of a compound other than the one that initially provoked the response is about 20%.

Hepatitis. Focal or diffuse necrosis of the liver due to direct drug toxicity or sensitization occurs in less than 0.1% of patients. Headache, nausea, vomiting, fever, hepatomegaly, jaundice, and laboratory evidence of hepatocellular dysfunction usually appear 3 to 5 days after sulfonamide administration is started, and the syndrome may progress to acute yellow atrophy and death (*see* Dujovne *et al.,* 1967). The development of hepatitis is not influenced by the dose of drug or by the presence of preexisting hepatic disease. Damage to the liver may increase even after drug withdrawal.

Miscellaneous Reactions to the Sulfonamides. Among other untoward effects that may follow the administration of various sulfonamides are *goiter* and *hypothyroidism, arthritis,* and various *neuropsychiatric disturbances.* Coordination and reaction time are not impaired. *Peripheral neuritis* is very rare. *Anorexia, nausea,* and *vomiting* occur in 1 to 2% of persons receiving sulfonamides, and these manifestations are probably central in origin.

The *age* of patients may be an important determinant of the risk of reactions associated with the use of various sulfonamides. The administration of sulfonamides to premature babies may lead to the development of kernicterus due to the displacement of bilirubin from plasma albumin. Sulfonamides should not be given to pregnant women near term.

Drug Interactions. Administration of a sulfonamide may increase the effect of oral anticoagulants and methotrexate, probably by displacement of these drugs from binding sites on plasma albumin. Potentiation of the action of sulfonylurea hypoglycemic agents, thiazide diuretics, and uricosuric agents may also be noted. This, too, may be due to displacement of the drugs from albumin, or a pharmacodynamic mechanism may play a role. Conversely, agents such as indomethacin, probenecid, and salicylates may displace sulfonamides from plasma albumin and increase the concentrations of free drug in plasma.

SULFONAMIDE THERAPY

The number of conditions for which the sulfonamides are therapeutically useful and constitute drugs of first choice has been sharply reduced by the development of more effective antimicrobial agents and by the gradual increase in the resistance of a number of bacterial species to this class of drugs. However, the use of sulfonamides has undergone a revival as a result of the introduction of the combination of trimethoprim and sulfamethoxazole (*see* below).

Urinary Tract Infections. The major utility of the sulfonamides in therapeutics is in the treatment of infections of the urinary tract. The vast majority of microorganisms responsible for acute urinary tract infections acquired in the community are *E. coli,* and these are usually sensitive to sulfonamides. Sulfisoxazole (2 g initially followed by 1 g, orally, four times a day for 5 to 10 days) is usually effective. When infections are recurrent, obstruction is present, or bacteremia is suspected, therapy with a sulfonamide alone may not be adequate. In these instances antibiotics may be preferred, and the choice of a specific agent is based on the results of tests of sensitivities of the causative microorganisms. It is important to attempt to distinguish between infections involving the kidney and those that are located in the lower urinary tract. *Acute pyelonephritis* with high fever and other severe constitutional manifestations and the risk of bacteremia and shock is best not treated with a sulfonamide. Most physicians prefer to administer an antibiotic parenterally, selected on the basis of the anticipated antimicrobial sensitivities and later modified, if necessary, by knowledge of the laboratory data. The sulfonamides should be reserved for the management of *acute and chronic cystitis, chronic infections of the upper urinary tract,* and *asymptomatic bacilluria.* Since acute cystitis is most often caused by *E. coli* or *Pr. mirabilis,* the sulfonamides are highly effective.

Recurrent infections of the urinary tract are much more difficult to manage successfully. An integral part of the study of patients with this kind of disease is first to establish whether the chronicity is due to *reinfection* with new microorganisms or whether the same microorganism(s) is persisting, causing *relapse* despite therapy (Turck *et al.,* 1966, 1968). Reinfection occurs most commonly in sexually active females and is related to repeated intraurethral inoculation of perineal bacteria during sexual intercourse. When recurrences are frequent (more than two or three per year), prophylaxis to reduce their number may be employed. Sulfonamides, nitrofurantoin, mandelamine, and trimethoprim-sulfamethoxazole have all been used successfully (Harding and Ronald, 1974; Vosti, 1975), but the last-named preparation is the most effective (*see* below).

Relapse with the same microorganism(s) is often more serious, suggesting a persistent focus of infection in the upper urinary tract that is difficult or impossible to eradicate. This type of infection is often associated with bacteriuria with antibody-coated microorganisms that can be detected by fluorescence microscopy (Thomas *et al.,* 1974). Reasons for this persistence include a functional or mechanical obstruction that interferes with the normal flow of urine or impairment of normal host defenses, as in patients with diabetes mellitus. These patients must be thoroughly evaluated to rule out remediable obstruction. The microorganisms involved include *Escherichia, Enterobacter, Klebsiella, Proteus,* grampositive cocci (including the enterococcus), and mixtures of microorganisms. Anaerobes are only rarely responsible for urinary tract infections. In some patients the focus of infection may be eradicated by prolonged (6 weeks or more) administration of an antimicrobial agent. However, the cure rate for this type of chronic infection of the urinary tract is relatively low, regardless of the type of antimicrobial therapy employed, and *chronic suppressive therapy or intermittent treatment of symptomatic relapses may eventually be the most reasonable goal.* Chronic suppressive therapy has been shown to decrease the number of symptomatic episodes but has no proven effect on preservation of renal function (Freeman *et al.,* 1975). Agents that have been used include sulfonamides, trimethoprim-sulfamethoxazole, antibiotics, and urinary tract antiseptics.

Bacillary Dysentery (Shigella Diarrhea). Because of the frequency of resistant strains, the sulfonamides are now only infrequently useful in the management of this disease. An antibiotic such as ampicillin or tetracycline should be administered, depending on the sensitivity of the microorganisms. For resistant bacteria, trimethoprim-sulfamethoxazole appears to be effective when given orally in daily doses of 8 to 12 mg/kg of trimethoprim plus 40 to 60 mg/kg of sulfamethoxazole (divided into two portions) for 5 days (Nelson *et al.,* 1976). In instances where the responsible microorganism is sensitive to a sulfonamide, sulfisoxazole or sulfadiazine may be given orally (4 g initially, followed by 1 g every 4 hours).

Meningococcal Infections. Resistance to sulfonamides is now common in the various serological groups of *N. meningitidis* (Feldman, 1967; Singer, 1967). All forms of disease produced by meningococci should now be treated with large doses of penicillin G or ampicillin; chloramphenicol has been recommended for patients who are allergic to the penicillins. If an epidemic is *proven* to be due to a sulfonamide-sensitive strain of meningococcus, sulfisoxazole or sulfadiazine may be given. In this case, initial sulfonamide therapy is by intravenous administration.

Chemoprophylaxis should be considered for close contacts of patients with meningococcal disease. If the strain of *N. meningitidis* is sensitive to sulfonamides, sulfadiazine (1 g every 12 hours for four doses) should be given. One half of this dose is administered to children 1 to 12 years of age. Penicillin G and several other antibiotics are *not* effective for prophylaxis. Rifampin is now considered the prophylactic agent of choice, since most strains are resistant to sulfonamides. Minocycline is also effective, but its use is not recommended because of a high incidence of vestibular toxicity.

Nocardiosis. Sulfonamides are of value in the treatment of infections due to *Nocardia* species. A number of instances of complete recovery from the disease after adequate treatment with a sulfonamide have been recorded. Sulfisoxazole or sulfadiazine may be given in doses of 6 to 8 g daily. Concentrations of sulfonamide in plasma should be 80 to 160 μg/ml. This schedule is continued for several months after all manifestations have been controlled. The administration of sulfonamide together with an antibiotic has been recommended, especially for advanced cases, and ampicillin, erythromycin, or streptomycin has been suggested for this purpose. The clinical response and the results of sensitivity testing may be helpful in choosing a companion drug. It should be emphasized, however, that there are no clinical data to show that combination therapy is better than therapy with a sulfonamide alone.

Streptococcal Infections. Sulfonamide therapy does not significantly alter the course of *pharyngitis* due to *Strep. pyogenes*. It neither eradicates the microorganisms from the throat nor prevents the development of the late nonsuppurative sequelae such as rheumatic fever and glomerulonephritis. Penicillin therapy, on the other hand, eradicates the microorganisms from practically all patients treated for 10 days and reduces the incidence of subsequent rheumatic fever.

There is presently no indication for the use of sulfonamides in therapy of streptococcal diseases such as erysipelas, cellulitis, bacteremia, and pneumonia. They are readily managed by administration of penicillin or erythromycin.

Trachoma and Inclusion Conjunctivitis. Systemic therapy with tetracycline (Hoshiwara *et al.,* 1973) or a sulfonamide for 3 weeks appears to be the most effective treatment for *trachoma*. While the topical use of such agents will often suppress signs of infection, it will not eradicate the microorganism. Therapeutic results are best when therapy is initiated early, but even chronic cicatricial cases may respond. The local symptoms may disappear in a few days. Pannus, keratitis, conjunctival granulations, entropion, trichiasis, iritis, and corneal ulcerations improve and may even disappear. Corneal lesions respond more rapidly than do those of the conjunctivae. Blindness may be prevented (*see* Siniscal, 1952). Dawson and associates (1968) reported that some of the alleged benefits of chemotherapy in trachoma might be attributable to control of bacterial suprainfection.

Many physicians prefer to treat *inclusion conjunctivitis* (inclusion blenorrhea) by the topical application of tetracycline or sulfacetamide ointment (10%), six times a day for 10 days. Administration of tetracycline or erythromycin systemically is also effective.

Lymphogranuloma Venereum and Chancroid. Oral administration of a sulfonamide (1 g of sulfisoxazole four times daily for 21 days) or tetracycline (500 mg four times daily for 21 days) has been successful for the treatment of lymphogranuloma venereum. A similar schedule is recommended for chancroid.

Dermatitis Herpetiformis (Duhring's Disease). Dapsone and sulfonamides have been used for the management of this skin disorder. The preferred sulfonamide appears to be sulfapyridine. Therapy is started with 0.5 g four times a day; this dose may be increased gradually until a total of 4 to 5 g per day is being given, unless intolerance develops. Dermatitis herpetiformis is the only indication for sulfapyridine, an older sulfonamide; it is available in 500-mg tablets for this purpose. Some physicians prefer to use dapsone; the initial dose is 25 to 50 mg per day. If this does not produce suppression of the disease and if there is no evidence of toxicity, the dose is increased by 50 mg per day over a period of several days. Usually a total daily dose of 200 mg is successful.

Toxoplasmosis. Although pyrimethamine is the agent of primary importance in the therapy of infections due to *Toxoplasma gondii,* most clinicians who have had experience with this disease prefer to give full doses of sulfadiazine simultaneously. In patients with severe chorioretinitis, it is advisable to add a corticosteroid to the therapeutic regimen (*see* Remington and Desmonts, 1976).

Use of Sulfonamides for Prophylaxis. The sulfonamides exhibit a degree of effectiveness equal to that of oral penicillin in *preventing streptococcal infections and recurrences of rheumatic fever* among susceptible subjects. Despite the efficacy of sulfonamides in the prevention of rheumatic fever recurrence, their toxicity and the possibility of infection by drug-resistant streptococci make them less desirable than penicillin for this purpose. They should be used, however, without hesitation in patients who are hypersensitive to penicillin. Chemoprophylaxis with sulfonamides for even long periods does not lead to important and potentially dangerous alterations in the microflora of the upper respiratory tract. The recommended dose of sulfisoxazole is 1 g twice daily; for children under 27 kg (60 lb), the dose is halved. If untoward responses occur, they usually do so during the first 8 weeks of therapy; serious reactions after this time are rare. White-cell counts should be carried out once weekly during the first 8 weeks.

TRIMETHOPRIM-SULFA-METHOXAZOLE

The introduction of trimethoprim in combination with sulfamethoxazole constitutes an important advance in the development of clinically effective antimicrobial agents and represents the practical application of a theoretical consideration; that is, if two drugs act on sequential steps in the pathway of an obligate enzymatic reaction in bacteria, the result of their combination will be synergistic (*see* Hitchings, 1961). Extensive biochemical studies of the mode of action of this combination of compounds clearly indicate that this is the case. The details of the mechanisms of action of this preparation were defined well before its range of clinical effectiveness was established.

Chemistry. Sulfamethoxazole has been discussed on page 1111, and its structural formula is shown in Table 49-1. The history and chemistry of trimethoprim, a diaminopyrimidine, are discussed in Chapter 45. In the United States, trimethoprim is available only in combination with sulfamethoxazole.

Antibacterial Spectrum. The antibacterial spectrum of trimethoprim is similar to that of sulfamethoxazole, although the former drug is usually 20 to 100 times more potent than the latter. The data presented here refer to the antimicrobial activity of the *combination* of the two agents.

All strains of *Strep. pneumoniae, C. diphtheriae,* and *N. meningitidis* are sensitive to trimethoprim-sulfamethoxazole. From 50 to 95% of strains of *Staph. aureus, Staph. epidermidis, Strep. pyogenes,* the *viridans* group of streptococci, *Strep. faecalis, E. coli, Pr. mirabilis, Pr. morganii, Pr. rettgeri, Enterobacter* species, *Salmonella, Shigella, Pseud. pseudomallei, Serratia,* and *Alcaligenes* species are inhibited. Also sensitive are *Klebsiella* species, *Brucella abortus, Pasteurella haemolytica, Yersinia pseudotuberculosis, Y. enterocolitica,* and *Nocardia asteroides.* Very few strains of *Pseud. aeruginosa* are sensitive. Methicillin-resistant strains of *Staph. aureus,* although also resistant to trimethoprim or sulfamethoxazole alone, are usually susceptible to the combination. A synergistic interaction between the components of the preparation is apparent *even* when microorganisms are resistant to sulfonamide or resistant to sulfonamide and moderately resistant to trimethoprim. However, a *maximal degree* of synergism occurs when microorganisms are sensitive to both components. The activity of trimethoprim-sulfamethoxazole *in vitro* depends on the medium in which it is determined; for example, low concentrations of thymidine almost completely abolish the antibacterial activity (*see* Symposium, 1969, 1973; Pelton *et al.,* 1977).

Mechanism of Action. The antimicrobial activity of the combination of trimethoprim and sulfamethoxazole results from its actions on two steps of the enzymatic pathway for the synthesis of tetrahydrofolic acid. Sulfonamide inhibits the incorporation of PABA into folic acid, and trimethoprim prevents the reduction of dihydrofolate to tetrahydrofolate. The latter is the form of folate essential for one-carbon transfer reactions, for example, the synthesis of thymidylate from deoxyuridylate. Selective toxicity for microorganisms is achieved in two ways. Mammalian cells utilize preformed folates from the diet and do not synthesize the compound. Furthermore, trimethoprim is a highly *selective* inhibitor of dihydrofolate reductase of lower organisms (*see* Chapter 45). This is vitally important, since this enzymatic function is a crucial one in all species.

The synergistic interaction between sulfonamide and trimethoprim is thus predictable from their respective mechanisms. There is an optimal ratio of the concentrations of the two agents for synergism, and this is equal to the ratio of the minimal inhibitory concentrations of the drugs acting independently. While this ratio varies for different bacteria, the most effective ratio for the greatest number of microorganisms is 20 parts of sulfamethoxazole to one part of trimethoprim. The combination is thus formulated to achieve a sulfamethoxazole concentration *in vivo* 20 times greater than that of trimethoprim. (*See* articles by Hitchings, Burchall, and Bushby in Symposium, 1973.) The pharmacokinetic properties of the sulfonamide chosen to be in combination with trimethoprim are thus important, since relative constancy of the concentrations of the two compounds in the body is desired.

Examination of the sensitivity pattern of a typical isolate of *E. coli* illustrates the extent of synergism. The minimal inhibitory concentration for sulfamethoxazole alone is $3\mu g/ml$, while that for trimethoprim is $0.3\mu g/ml$. When the combination is tested at a ratio of 20:1, inhibitory concentrations are $1.0\mu g/ml$ and $0.05\mu g/ml$, respectively.

Bacterial Resistance. The frequency of development of bacterial resistance to trimethoprim-sulfamethoxazole is lower than it is to either of the agents alone. This is logical, since a microorganism that has acquired resistance to one of the components may still be killed by the other. Trimethoprim-resistant microorganisms may arise by mutation. Resistance in gram-negative bacteria is often associated with the presence of R factors, which can be transferred to susceptible microorganisms by conjugation. Resistance to high concentrations of sulfonamides and to moderate concentrations of trimethoprim has been demonstrated to be transferred in this manner. Resistance to trimethoprim in *Staph. aureus* appears to be determined by a chromosomal gene rather than by a plasmid (Nakhla, 1973). The development of resistance to the combination also occurs *in vivo*. *Escherichia coli* resistant to trimethoprim and *H. influenzae* resistant to trimethoprim-sulfamethoxazole have been isolated from patients treated with the combination (Lacey *et al.,* 1972; May and Davies, 1972). While the incidence of resistance of *E. coli* to trimethoprim-sulfamethoxazole increased only from 0.2% to 1.5% over a 5-year period of use

(*see* McAllister, 1976), resistance of *Staph. aureus* increased from 0.4% to 12.6% during a similar time span (*see* Chattopadhyay, 1977).

Absorption, Distribution, and Excretion. The pharmacokinetic profiles of both sulfamethoxazole and trimethoprim are closely but not perfectly matched to achieve a constant ratio of 20:1 in their concentrations in blood and tissues. The ratio in blood is often greater than 20:1, and that in tissues is frequently less (Craig and Kunin, 1973). After a single oral dose of the combined preparation, trimethoprim is absorbed more rapidly than sulfamethoxazole. The concurrent administration of the drugs appears to slow the absorption of sulfamethoxazole. Peak blood concentrations of trimethoprim usually occur by 2 hours in most patients, while peak concentrations of sulfamethoxazole occur by 4 hours after a single oral dose. The half-lives of trimethoprim and sulfamethoxazole are approximately 10 and 9 hours, respectively.

When 800 mg of sulfamethoxazole is given with 160 mg of trimethoprim (the conventional 5:1 ratio), twice daily, the peak concentrations of the drugs in plasma are approximately 40 and $2\mu g/ml$, the optimal ratio that is sought.

Trimethoprim is rapidly distributed and concentrated in tissues, and about 70% is bound to plasma protein in the presence of sulfamethoxazole. The volume of distribution of trimethoprim is about six times that of sulfamethoxazole. The drug enters cerebrospinal fluid and sputum readily. High concentrations of each component of the mixture are also found in bile. About 65% of sulfamethoxazole is bound to plasma protein.

Up to 60% of administered trimethoprim and from 25 to 50% of sulfamethoxazole are excreted in the urine in 24 hours. Two thirds of the sulfonamide is unconjugated. Metabolites of trimethoprim are also excreted. The rates of excretion and the concentrations of both compounds in the urine are significantly reduced in patients with uremia.

(For details of the pharmacology of trimethoprim-sulfamethoxazole and its components, *see* Bushby and Hitchings, 1968; Sharpstone, 1969; Schwartz and Rieder, 1970; Bergan and Brodwall, 1972; Nolte and Büttner, 1973; Symposium, 1973.)

Preparations, Routes of Administration, and Dosage. *Sulfamethoxazole and Trimethoprim Tablets,* U.S.P. (BACTRIM, SEPTRA), are available in two sizes: 400 mg of sulfamethoxazole plus 80 mg of trimethoprim, and 800 mg of sulfamethoxazole plus 160 mg trimethoprim. An official oral suspension of 200 mg of sulfamethoxazole plus 40 mg of trimethoprim per 5 ml is also available. The usual *adult* dose is 800 mg of sulfamethoxazole plus 160 mg of trimethoprim every 12 hours for 10 to 14 days for management of most infections. Larger quantities have been given in special circumstances in patients with serious or life-threatening disease. Dosage must be reduced in patients with renal insufficiency (*see* Appendix II), and the preparation should not be administered if creatinine clearance is less than 15 ml per minute.

The recommended daily dose for children for treatment of urinary tract infections, otitis media, and shigellosis is 8 mg/kg of trimethoprim and 40 mg/kg of sulfamethoxazole, given in two divided doses every 12 hours for 10 days.

The combination should not be used in infants under 2 months of age, during pregnancy, and during the nursing period.

Untoward Effects. There is no evidence that trimethoprim-sulfamethoxazole, when given in the recommended doses, induces folate deficiency in normal persons. However, the margin between toxicity for bacteria and that for man may be relatively narrow when the cells of the patient are deficient in folate. In such cases, trimethoprim-sulfamethoxazole may cause or precipitate *megaloblastosis, leukopenia,* or *thrombocytopenia.* In routine use, the combination appears to exert little toxicity. About 75% of the untoward effects involve the *skin.* These are typical of those known to be produced by *sulfonamides,* as already described. However, trimethoprim-sulfamethoxazole has been reported to cause up to three times as many dermatological reactions as does sulfisoxazole when given alone (5.9% versus 1.7%; Arndt and Jick, 1976). *Exfoliative dermatitis, Stevens-Johnson Syndrome,* and *toxic epidermal necrolysis* (Lyell's syndrome) are rare, occurring primarily in older individuals. *Nausea* and *vomiting* constitute the bulk of gastrointestinal reactions; *diarrhea* is rare. *Glossitis* and *stomatitis* are relatively common. Mild and transient *jaundice* has been noted and appears to have the histological features of allergic cholestatic hepatitis. Central nervous system reactions consist in *headache, depression,* and *hallucinations,* manifestations known to be produced by sulfonamides. Hematological reactions, in addition to those mentioned above, are various types of *anemia* (including *aplastic, hemolytic,* and *macrocytic*), *coagulation disorders, granulocytopenia, agranulocytosis, purpura, Henoch-Schönlein purpura,* and *sulfhemoglobinemia.* Previous or simultaneous administration of diuretics with trimethoprim-sulfamethoxazole may carry an increased risk of thrombocytopenia, especially in elderly patients with heart failure; death may occur. Permanent impairment of renal function may follow the use of trimethoprim-sulfamethoxazole in patients with renal disease (Kalowski *et al.,* 1973), and a reversible decrease in creatinine clearance has been noted in patients with normal renal function (Symposium, 1973; Shouval *et al.,* 1978).

Therapeutic Uses. *Urinary Tract Infections.* Experience with the treatment of uncomplicated lower urinary tract infections with trimethoprim-sulfamethoxazole is now sufficiently extensive to indicate that it is often highly effective, even when the infecting agent is resistant to the sulfonamides alone. A dose of 800 mg of sulfamethoxazole plus 160 mg of trimethoprim every 12 hours for 10 days produces cure in the vast majority of cases. The preparation has been shown to produce a better therapeutic effect than does either of its components given separately when the infecting microorganisms are of the family Enterobacteriaceae.

The combination appears to have special efficacy in chronic and recurrent infections of the urinary tract (*see* Gleckman, 1975). In females, this may be related to the presence of therapeutic concentrations of trimethoprim in vaginal secretions (Stamey and Condy, 1975). Enterobacteriaceae surrounding the urethral orifice may be eliminated or reduced markedly in number, thus diminishing the chance of an ascending reinfection (*see* Stamey *et al.,* 1977). Trimethoprim is also found in therapeutic concentrations in prostatic secretions and is often effective for the treatment of bacterial prostatitis (Dabhiolwala *et al.,* 1976).

Small doses (200 mg of sulfamethoxazole plus 40 mg of trimethoprim per day, or two to four times these amounts once or twice per week) appear to be effective in reducing the number of recurrent urinary tract infections in females. This correlates with a reduction in the numbers of Enterobacteriaceae inhabiting the vaginal introitus.

It should be remembered that trimethoprim-sulfamethoxazole is a drug combination with toxic potential equal at least to that of the sulfonamide. Furthermore, the cost of a therapeutic course of this combination is considerably more than that of sulfisoxazole alone. Acute, nonrecurrent urinary tract infections need not be treated with the combination; a sulfonamide alone will suffice.

Bacterial Respiratory Tract Infections. Trimethoprim-sulfamethoxazole is effective for *acute exacerbations of chronic bronchitis.* Administration of

1200 mg of sulfamethoxazole plus 240 mg of trimethoprim twice a day appears to be very effective in decreasing fever, purulence and volume of sputum, and sputum bacterial count. The microorganisms involved have been *H. influenzae* and *Strep. pneumoniae* (*see* Carroll *et al.,* 1977; Tandon, 1977). Trimethoprim-sulfamethoxazole should *not* be used to treat streptococcal pharyngitis, since it does not eradicate the microorganism. It is effective for acute otitis media in children and acute maxillary sinusitis in adults caused by susceptible strains of *H. influenzae* and *Strep. pneumoniae* (*see* Cameron *et al.,* 1975; Willner *et al.,* 1978).

Gastrointestinal Infections. The combination has become useful for treatment of shigellosis, since many strains of the causative agent are now resistant to ampicillin (*see* Chang *et al.,* 1977). It is also effective for typhoid fever, but there is some difference of opinion concerning the precise role of trimethoprim-sulfamethoxazole for the management of this disease. The experience of Scragg and Rubidge (1971) suggests that, in children, this drug is not as effective as chloramphenicol. In adults, trimethoprim-sulfamethoxazole appears to be effective when the dose is 800 mg of sulfamethoxazole plus 160 mg of trimethoprim every 12 hours for 15 days. Chloramphenicol remains the drug of choice for typhoid fever (*see* Ramachandran *et al.,* 1978).

Trimethoprim-sulfamethoxazole appears to be effective in the management of carriers of *S. typhi* and other species of *Salmonella.* One proposed schedule is the administration of 800 mg of sulfamethoxazole plus 160 mg of trimethoprim twice a day for 3 months; however, failures have occurred. It has been suggested that the presence of chronic disease of the gallbladder is associated with a high incidence of failure to clear the carrier state (Brodie *et al.,* 1970). (*See* Symposium, 1969; 1973; Geddes, 1975.)

Infection by Pneumocystis carinii. High-dose therapy (trimethoprim, 20 mg/kg per day, plus sulfamethoxazole, 100 mg/kg per day, in two or three divided doses) is effective for this severe infection of impaired hosts. This combination has become the preferred treatment, since pentamidine is more toxic (Hughes *et al.,* 1975, 1978; Larter *et al.,* 1978).

Prophylaxis in Neutropenic Patients. Several studies have demonstrated the effectiveness of low-dose therapy (150 mg/m² of trimethoprim and 750 mg/m² of sulfamethoxazole) for the prophylaxis of infection by *Pneumocystis carinii* (*see* Hughes *et al.,* 1977). In addition, significant protection against sepsis caused by gram-negative bacteria was noted when 800 mg of sulfamethoxazole plus 160 mg of trimethoprim was given twice daily to severely neutropenic patients (Enno *et al.,* 1978; Gurwith, *et al.,* 1979).

Genital Infections. Trimethoprim-sulfamethoxazole is effective in the management of *acute gonococcal urethritis* in both men and women. Several regimens have been recommended. Among these are (1) two tablets (400 mg/80 mg) twice a day for 5 days; (2) four tablets twice a day for 2 days; (3) six tablets once a day for 3 days or three tablets twice a day for 3 days (Austin and Holmes, 1975). These regimens appear to be as effective as a single dose of 4.8 million units of procaine penicillin G plus 1 g of probenecid. The drug has no effect in preventing incubating *syphilis* or in curing the established disease (Svindland, 1973).

Miscellaneous Infections. Several reports have suggested that trimethoprim-sulfamethoxazole may be effective in the therapy of *brucellosis* even when localized lesions such as arthritis, endocarditis, or epididymo-orchitis are present. Doses have ranged from two tablets (400 mg/80 mg) three times a day for 1 week followed by two tablets a day for 2 weeks to four to eight tablets per day for 2 months. Most patients recover, particularly when the latter dosage schedule is employed; however, relapse has occurred in 4% of cases even with this regimen. Hassan and associates (1971) have suggested that therapy (two to four tablets per day) be continued for an additional 6 weeks to minimize the risk of relapse.

Although attempts have been made to treat *subacute bacterial endocarditis* with trimethoprim-sulfamethoxazole, this is not advisable in cases due to the *viridans* group of streptococci, other streptococci, or *Staph. aureus,* since experience is much too limited as yet and highly effective agents for the therapy of this disease are available. However, there is some evidence that valvular infection due to *Pseud. cepacia* may respond favorably, especially when polymyxin is given simultaneously (*see* Moody and Young, 1975).

URINARY TRACT ANTISEPTICS

The urinary tract antiseptics inhibit the growth of many species of bacteria. They cannot be used to treat systemic infections because effective concentrations are not achieved in plasma with safe doses. However, because they are concentrated in the renal tubules, they can be used to treat infections of the urinary tract. Furthermore, effective antibacterial concentrations reach the renal pelves and the bladder. Treatment with such drugs can be thought of as local therapy in that only in the kidney and bladder, with the rare exceptions mentioned below, are adequate therapeutic levels achieved. The drugs have therefore become known as urinary tract antiseptics (*see* Andriole, 1979).

Methenamine. Methenamine is a urinary tract antiseptic that owes its activity to formaldehyde.

Chemistry. Methenamine is hexamethylenetetramine (hexamethyleneamine). It has the following structure:

Methenamine

The compound decomposes in water to generate formaldehyde, according to the following reaction:

$$N_4(CH_2)_6 + 6H_2O + 4H^+ \rightleftharpoons 4NH_4^+ + 6HCHO$$

At pH 7.4 almost no decomposition occurs; however, 6% of the theoretical amount of formaldehyde is yielded at pH 6 and 20% at pH 5. Thus, acidification of the urine promotes the formaldehyde-dependent antibacterial action. The reaction is fairly slow, and 3 hours are required to reach 90% of equilibrium.

Antimicrobial Activity. Nearly all bacteria are sensitive to free formaldehyde at concentrations of about 20 μg/ml. Urea-splitting microorganisms (*e.g.*, *Proteus* species) tend to raise the pH of the urine and thus inhibit the release of formaldehyde. Microorganisms do not develop resistance to formaldehyde.

Pharmacology and Toxicology. Methenamine is absorbed orally, but 10 to 30% decomposes in the gastric juice unless the drug is protected by an enteric coating. Because of the ammonia produced, methenamine is contraindicated in hepatic insufficiency. Methenamine distributes widely into body fluids, but so little decomposes in the blood and tissues that there is no systemic toxicity from ammonia or formaldehyde. Excretion into the urine is nearly quantitative. When the urine pH is 6 and the daily urine volume is 1000 to 1500 ml, a daily dose of 2 g will yield a concentration of 18 to 60 μg/ml of formaldehyde; this is more than the minimal inhibitory concentration for most urinary tract pathogens. Some of the formaldehyde is bound to substances in the urine and in the surrounding tissues, so that daily doses below 0.5 g may not yield much free formaldehyde.

Various poorly metabolized acids can be used to acidify the urine. Low pH alone is bacteriostatic, so that acidification serves a double function. The acids commonly used are mandelic acid, hippuric acid, ascorbic acid, sodium biphosphate, and acid-producing foods such as cranberry juice. Doses of 3 to 6 g or more per day of the acids may be needed to keep the urinary pH at 5.5 or below. Both mandelic and hippuric acids are bacteriostatic *in vitro* in high concentrations, but these levels are not achieved in urine and there is little evidence that they contribute anything more than their effect on the pH (*see* Hamilton-Miller and Brumfitt, 1977).

Gastrointestinal distress frequently is caused by doses greater than 500 mg four times a day, even with enteric-coated tablets. Painful and frequent micturition, albuminuria, hematuria, and rashes may result from doses of 4 to 8 g a day given for longer than 3 to 4 weeks. Once the urine is sterile, a high dose should be reduced. Because systemic methenamine is nontoxic, renal insufficiency does not constitute a contraindication to the use of methenamine alone, but the acids may be detrimental. Methenamine mandelate is contraindicated in renal insufficiency. Crystalluria from the mandelate moiety can occur. Methenamine combines with sulfamethizole (Lipton, 1963) and perhaps other sulfonamides in the urine, which results in mutual antagonism.

Preparations and Dosage. Methenamine, U.S.P., is given as tablets in a dose of 0.5 to 2 (usually 1) g,

four times a day. *Methenamine Mandelate,* U.S.P. (MANDELAMINE, others), is given in an oral suspension or as tablets in the same dose as for methenamine, even though the methenamine equivalence is less. *Methenamine hippurate* (HIPREX, UREX) is usually given in a dose of 1 g, twice a day. The recommended dose of *Methenamine and Sodium Biphosphate Tablets,* U.S.P., 325 mg four times a day, cannot be considered to yield activity equivalent to the usual doses of the other preparations.

Therapeutic Uses and Status. Methenamine is not a primary drug for the treatment of acute urinary tract infections, but it is of value for chronic suppressive treatment (Freeman *et al.*, 1975). The agent is most useful when the causative organism is *E. coli*, but it can usually suppress the common gram-negative offenders and often *Staph. aureus* and *Staph. epidermidis* as well. *Enterobacter aerogenes* and *Proteus vulgaris* are usually resistant. Urea-splitting bacteria (mostly *Proteus*) make it difficult to control the urine pH. The physician should strive to keep the pH below 5.5. Patient compliance is poor because of the number of pills required with many products. Methenamine is sometimes employed prophylactically in instrumentation and catheterization of the urinary tract, but studies suggest that it is ineffective for this purpose (Gerstein *et al.*, 1968; Vainrub and Musher, 1977).

Nalidixic Acid. Nalidixic acid has the following chemical structure:

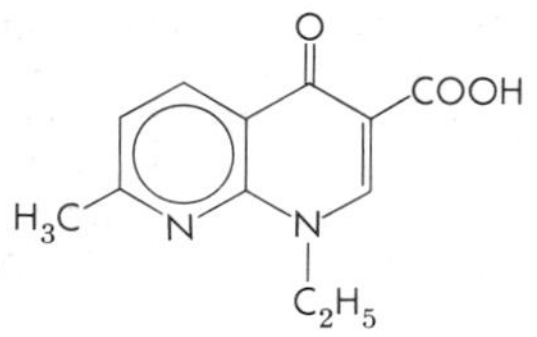

Nalidixic Acid

Antimicrobial Activity. Nalidixic acid is bactericidal to most of the common gram-negative bacteria that cause urinary tract infections. It appears to act by inhibiting DNA synthesis. Brumfitt and Pursell (1971) reported that 99% of strains of *E. coli*, 98% of *Pr. mirabilis* and 75 to 97% of other *Proteus* species, 92% of *Klebsiella-Enterobacter*, and 80% of other coliform bacteria are sensitive to concentrations of 16 μg/ml or less of the drug. *Pseudomonas* species are resistant. It is less active against gram-positive microorganisms. Acquired resistance to the drug occurs during therapy, but it does not seem to be transferable.

Pharmacology and Toxicology. Almost all of orally administered nalidixic acid is absorbed. Plasma concentrations of 20 to 50 μg/ml may be achieved, but the acid is 93 to 97% bound to plasma proteins. In the body some nalidixic acid is converted to an active hydroxynalidixic acid, and both are excreted into the urine. Very high concentrations of nalidixic acid plus its active metabolite are achieved in the urine—100 to 500 μg/ml. Antibacterial activity is not found in prostatic fluid (Stamey *et al.*, 1970). Some nalidixic acid is conjugated in the liver. The plasma half-life is normally about 8 hours, but it may be as long as 21 hours in the presence of renal failure.

Oral nalidixic acid is usually well tolerated, but nausea, vomiting, and abdominal pain may occur. Allergic reactions such as pruritus, urticaria, various rashes, photosensitivity, eosinophilia, and fever occasionally occur, and cholestasis, thrombocytopenia, leukopenia, and hemolytic anemia rarely occur. Liver function tests and blood-cell counts are advisable if treatment lasts longer than 2 weeks. Effects on the central nervous system (CNS), such as headache, drowsiness, malaise, vertigo, visual disturbances, asthenia, and myalgia, are experienced infrequently. In patients with cerebral vascular insufficiency, parkinsonism, or epilepsy, or in normal children given excessive doses, convulsions occur, perhaps as the result of intracranial hypertension (*see* Boréus and Sundström, 1967). Pseudotumor cerebri has been described (Rao, 1974). The presence of the drug results in false-positive responses in some tests for urinary glucose. Nitrofurantoin interferes with the therapeutic action of nalidixic acid.

Therapeutic Uses, Preparations, and Dosage. In the United States, nalidixic acid is approved only for the treatment of urinary tract infections caused by susceptible microorganisms (*see* above). The effectiveness against indole-positive *Proteus* is especially important. Failures in men may be, in part, the result of reinfection from the prostate gland. Whether nalidixic acid can effectively penetrate the renal medulla and be of direct value in the treatment of pyelonephritis is uncertain. Rapid development of bacterial resistance has been reported in a widely varying percentage of cases. Stamey and Bragonje (1976) noted the development of resistance in 7% of patients who were treated with 1 g of the drug four times daily. Others have reported that 25% of patients will harbor resistant microorganisms (Ronald *et al.*, 1966).

Nalidixic Acid, U.S.P. (NEGGRAM), is available in tablets containing 250, 500, or 1000 mg of the drug and in an oral suspension containing 250 mg/5 ml. The recommended dose for adults is 1 g four times a day for 1 to 2 weeks; thereafter a daily dose of 2 g is suggested. The recommended daily dose for children is 55 mg/kg of body weight. The drug should not be used in infants under 3 months of age.

Oxolinic Acid. This drug is very similar to nalidixic acid. Its structural formula is as follows:

Oxolinic Acid

The mechanism of action and spectrum of antimicrobial activity resemble those of nalidixic acid, and cross-resistance between the two agents can be demonstrated. Oxolinic acid is two to four times more potent than nalidixic acid *in vitro*. Adverse reactions are also similar, although oxolinic acid has been associated with a greater incidence of CNS toxicity. Side effects are most frequent in elderly patients, and these include restlessness, insomnia, dizziness, headache, and nausea (*see* Atlas *et al.*, 1969; Ghatikar, 1974).

Oxolinic acid (UTIBID) is available in 750-mg tablets. The usual dose is one tablet twice daily. Because of the increased incidence of CNS toxicity compared to nalidixic acid, the latter drug is usually preferred.

Nitrofurantoin. Nitrofurantoin is a synthetic nitrofuran that is used for the prevention and treatment of infections of the urinary tract. Its structural formula is as follows:

Nitrofurantoin

Antimicrobial Activity. Nitrofurantoin inhibits a number of bacterial enzymes, but the basis for its antimicrobial activity and specificity is not known. Bacteria that are susceptible to the drug rarely become resistant during therapy. Nitrofurantoin is active against many strains of *E. coli*. However, most species of *Proteus* and *Pseudomonas* and many of *Enterobacter* and *Klebsiella* are resistant. Nitrofurantoin is bacteriostatic for most susceptible microorganisms at concentrations of 32 μg/ml or less. The antibacterial activity is higher in an acidic urine.

Pharmacology and Toxicity. Nitrofurantoin is rapidly and completely absorbed from the gastrointestinal tract. The macrocrystalline form of the drug is absorbed and excreted more slowly. Antibacterial concentrations are not achieved in plasma following ingestion of recommended doses, because the drug is rapidly eliminated. The plasma half-life is 0.3 to 1 hour; about 40% is excreted unchanged into the urine. The average dose of nitrofurantoin yields a concentration in urine of approximately 200 μg/ml. This amount is soluble at pH values above 5, but the urine should not be alkalinized because this reduces antimicrobial activity. The rate of excretion is linearly related to the creatinine clearance (Sachs *et al.*, 1968), so that in patients with impaired glomerular function the efficacy of the drug may be decreased and the systemic toxicity increased. Nitrofurantoin colors the urine brown.

The most common untoward effects are *nausea, vomiting*, and *diarrhea*. The incidence is less if the drug is administered with milk or other food or is used in a smaller dosage. The macrocrystalline preparation is better tolerated. Various *hypersensitivity reactions* occasionally occur. They may involve the skin, blood, liver, or lungs. They include *chills, fever, leukopenia, granulocytopenia, hemolytic anemia* (when glucose-6-phosphate dehydrogenase deficiency exists in the erythrocyte), *cholestatic jaundice*, and *hepatocellular damage*. Chronic active hepatitis is a rare but serious side effect (Tolman, 1980). *Acute pneumonitis* with fever, chills, cough, dyspnea, chest pain, pulmonary infiltration, and eosinophilia may occur within hours to days of the initiation of therapy (*see* DeMasi, 1967; Strauss and Griffin, 1967); it usually resolves within hours after discontinuation of the drug. More insidious subacute reactions may also be noted, and *interstitial pulmonary fibrosis* can occur in patients on chronic medication. Elderly patients are especially susceptible to the pulmonary toxicity of nitrofurantoin. (*See* Dawson, 1966; Rosenow *et al.*, 1968; Hailey *et al.*, 1969.) Megaloblastic anemia is rare. Various *neurological disorders* are occasionally observed. Headache, vertigo, drowsiness, muscular aches, and nystagmus are readily reversible, but severe *polyneuropathies* with demyelination and degeneration of both sensory and motor nerves have been reported (*see* Roelsen, 1964); signs of denervation and muscle atrophy result. Neuropathies are most likely to occur in patients with impaired renal function and in persons on long-continued treatment. However, Lindholm (1967) has detected electromyographic signs of muscle denervation in 62% of nonuremic patients receiving nitrofurantoin chronically. Nitrofurantoin-induced polyneuropathy has been reviewed by Toole and Parrish (1973).

Nitrofurantoin, U.S.P. (FURADANTIN, others), is available in tablets containing 50 or 100 mg of the drug and in an oral suspension containing 25 mg/5 ml. Nitrofurantoin macrocrystals (MACRODANTIN) are available in 25-, 50-, and 100-mg capsules. The oral dose for adults is 50 mg four times a day, with meals and at bedtime, for infections caused by sensitive microorganisms and twice this dose if the microorganisms are relatively resistant. Alternatively, the daily dose is better expressed as 5 to 10 mg/kg in four divided doses. A single 50- to 100-mg dose at bedtime may be sufficient to prevent recurrences (Stamey *et al.*, 1977). The daily dose for children is 5 to 7 mg/kg, but it may be as low as 2 mg/kg for long-term therapy (Lohr *et al.*, 1977). A course of therapy should not exceed 14 days, and repeated courses should be separated by rest periods. Pregnant women at term, individuals with impaired renal function (creatinine clearance less than 40 ml per minute), and children below 1 month of age should not receive nitrofurantoin.

Nitrofurantoin is approved only for the treatment of urinary tract infections caused by microorganisms that are known to be sensitive to the drug, but it is not usually as effective as several antibiotics or sulfonamides in the eradication of infections. It has been used effectively to prevent recurrent infections and for the prevention of bacteriuria after prostatectomy (Matthew *et al.*, 1978).

Phenazopyridine. *Phenazopyridine Hydrochloride,* U.S.P. (PYRIDIUM), is *not* a urinary antiseptic. However, it does have an analgesic action on the urinary tract and alleviates symptoms of dysuria, frequency, burning, and urgency (Trickett, 1970). Phenazopyridine is supplied as *Phenazopyridine Hydrochloride Tablets,* U.S.P., containing 100 or 200 mg of the drug for oral administration. The usual dose is 200 mg three times daily. The compound is an azo dye, and the urine is colored orange or red; the patient should be so informed. Gastrointestinal upset is seen in up to 10% of patients; overdosage may result in methemoglobinemia (*see* Gould, 1975). Phenazopyridine is also marketed in combination with sulfisoxazole (AZO GANTRISIN) and sulfamethoxazole (AZO GANTANOL) (*see* above).

Andreasen, F. Protein binding in plasma from patients with acute renal failure. *Acta Pharmacol. Toxicol. (Kbh.),* **1973,** *32,* 417–429.

Andriole, V. T. Urinary tract agents: nalidixic acid, oxolinic acid, nitrofurantoin, methenamine. In, *Principles and Practice of Infectious Diseases.* (Mandell, G. L.; Douglas, R. G., Jr.; and Bennett, J. E.; eds.) John Wiley & Sons, Inc., New York, **1979,** pp. 317–328.

Arndt, K. A., and Jick, H. Rates of cutaneous reactions to drugs. *J.A.M.A.,* **1976,** *235,* 918–923.

Atlas, E.; Clark, H.; Silverblatt, F.; and Turck, M. Nalidixic acid and oxolinic acid in the treatment of chronic bacteriuria. *Ann. Intern. Med.,* **1969,** *70,* 713–722.

Austin, T. W., and Holmes, K. K. The use of trimethoprim-sulfamethoxazole in gonococcal infections. *Can. Med. Assoc. J.,* **1975,** *112,* Suppl., 375–395.

Bailey, R. R.; Gower, P. E.; Roberts, A. P.; and de Wardener, H. E. Prevention of urinary tract infections with low-dose nitrofurantoin. *Lancet,* **1971,** *3,* 1112–1114.

Ballin, J. C. Evaluation of a new topical agent for burn therapy. Silver sulfadiazine (SILVADENE). *J.A.M.A.,* **1974,** *230,* 1184–1185.

Bell, P. H., and Roblin, R. O., Jr. Studies in chemotherapy. VII. A theory of the relation of structure to activity of sulfanilamide type compounds. *J. Am. Chem. Soc.,* **1942,** *64,* 2905–2917.

Bergan, T., and Brodwall, E. K. Kidney transport in man of sulfamethoxazole and trimethoprim. *Chemotherapy,* **1972,** *17,* 320–333.

Black, W. A., and McNellis, D. A. Susceptibility of *Nocardia* species to modern antimicrobial agents. In, *Antimicrobial Agents and Chemotherapy—1970.* (Hobby, G. L., ed.) American Society for Microbiology, Bethesda, **1971,** pp. 346–349.

Boréus, L. O., and Sundström, B. Intracranial hypertension in a child during treatment with nalidixic acid. *Br. Med. J.,* **1967,** *2,* 744–745.

Brodie, J.; MacQueen, I. A.; and Livingstone, D. Effect of trimethoprim-sulfamethoxazole on typhoid and salmonella carriers. *Br. Med. J.,* **1970,** *3,* 318–319.

Brown, G. M. The biosynthesis of folic acid. II. Inhibition by sulfonamides. *J. Biol. Chem.,* **1962,** *237,* 536–540.

Brumfitt, W., and Pursell, R. Observations on bacterial sensitivities to nalidixic acid and critical comments on the 6-centre survey. *Postgrad. Med. J.,* **1971,** *47,* 16–18.

Bushby, S. R. M., and Hitchings, G. H. Trimethoprim, a sulphonamide potentiator. *Br. J. Pharmacol. Chemother.,* **1968,** *33,* 72–90.

Buttle, G. A. H.; Gray, W. H.; and Stephenson, D. Protection of mice against streptococcal and other infections by *p*-aminobenzenesulphonamide and related substances. *Lancet,* **1936,** *1,* 1286–1290.

Cameron, G. G.; Pomahac, A. C.; and Johnston, M. T. Comparative efficacy of ampicillin and trimethoprim-sulfamethoxazole in otitis media. *Can. Med. Assoc. J.,* **1975,** *112,* 87S–88S.

Carroll, P. G.; Krejci, S. P.; Mitchell, J.; Puranik, V.; Thomas, R.; and Wilson, B. A comparative study of co-trimoxazole and amoxycillin in the treatment of acute bronchitis in general practice. *Med. J. Aust.,* **1977,** *2,* 286–287.

Chang, M. J.; Dunkle, L. M.; Van Reken, D.; Anderson, D.; Wong, M. L.; and Feigin, R. D. Trimethoprim-sulfamethoxazole compared to ampicillin in the treatment of shigellosis. *Pediatrics,* **1977,** *51,* 726–729.

Chattopadhyay, B. Co-trimoxazole resistant *Staphylococcus aureus* in hospital practice. *J. Antimicrob. Chemother.,* **1977,** *3,* 371–374.

Colebrook, L., and Kenny, M. Treatment of human puerperal infections, and of experimental infections in mice, with PRONTOSIL. *Lancet,* **1936,** *1,* 1279–1286.

Craig, A., and Kunin, C. M. Distribution of trimethoprim-sulfamethoxazole in tissues of rhesus monkeys. *J. Infect. Dis.,* **1973,** *128,* Suppl., S575–S579.

Dabhiolwala, N. F.; Bye, A.; and Claridge, M. A study of concentrations of trimethoprim-sulfamethoxazole in the human prostate gland. *Br. J. Urol.,* **1976,** *48,* 77–81.

Dawson, C. R.; Hanna, L.; Wood, T. R.; and Jawetz, E. Double-blind treatment trials in chronic trachoma of American Indian children. In, *Antimicrobial Agents and Chemotherapy—1967.* American Society for Microbiology, Ann Arbor, Mich., **1968,** pp. 137–142.

Dawson, R. B. Pulmonary reactions to nitrofurantoin. *N. Engl. J. Med.,* **1966,** *274,* 522.

DeMasi, C. J. Allergic pulmonary infiltrates probably due to nitrofurantoin. *Arch. Intern. Med.,* **1967,** *120,* 631–634.

Dissanayake, A., and Truelove, S. A controlled therapeutic trial of long-term maintenance treatment of ulcerative colitis with sulphasalazine. *Gut,* **1973,** *14,* 818.

Domagk, G. Ein Beitrag zur Chemotherapie der bakteriellen Infektionen. *Dtsch. Med. Wochenschr.,* **1935a,** *61,* 250–253.

————. Eine neue Klasse von Desinfektionsmitteln. *Ibid.,* **1935b,** *61,* 829–832.

Dujovne, C. A.; Chan, C. H.; and Zimmerman, H. J. Sulfonamide liver injury: review of the literature and report of a case due to sulfamethoxazole. *N. Engl. J. Med.,* **1967,** *277,* 785–788.

Eickhoff, T. C., and Finland, M. Changing susceptibility of meningococci to antimicrobial agents. *N. Engl. J. Med.,* **1965,** *272,* 395–398.

Enno, A.; Catovsky, D.; Darrell, J.; Goldman, J. M.; Hows, J.; and Galton, D. A. G. Co-trimoxazole for prevention of infection in acute leukemia. *Lancet,* **1978,** *1,* 395–398.

Feldman, H. A. Sulfonamide-resistant meningococci. *Annu. Rev. Med.,* **1967,** *18,* 495–506.

Fildes, P. A rational approach to research in chemotherapy. *Lancet,* **1940,** *1,* 955–957.

Fourneau, E.; Tréfouël, J.; Tréfouël, J.; Nitti, F.; and Bovet, D. Chimiothérapie des infections streptococciques par les dérivés du *p*-aminophénylsulfamide. *C. R. Soc. Biol.* (Paris), **1936,** *122,* 652–654.

Freeman, R. B.; Smith, W. M.; and Richardson, J. A. Long-term therapy for chronic bacteriuria in men: U.S. Public Health Service Cooperative Study. *Ann. Intern. Med.,* **1975,** *83,* 133–147.

Geddes, A. M. Trimethoprim-sulfamethoxazole in the treatment of gastrointestinal infections, including enteric fever and typhoid carriers. *Can. Med. Assoc. J.,* **1975,** *112,* 35S–36S.

Gelmo, P. Sulphamides of *p*-aminobenzenesulphonic acid. *J. Prakt. Chem.,* **1908,** *77,* 369–382.

Gerstein, A. R.; Okun, R.; Gonick, H. C.; Howard, I. W.; Kleeman, C. R.; and Maxwell, M. H. The prolonged use of methenamine hippurate in the treatment of chronic urinary tract infections. *J. Urol.,* **1968,** *100,* 767–771.

Ghatikar, K. N. A multicenter trial of a new synthetic antibacterial in urinary infections. *Curr. Ther. Res.,* **1974,** *16,* 130–136.

Gleckman, R. A. Trimethoprim-sulfamethoxazole vs. ampicillin in chronic urinary tract infections. *J.A.M.A.,* **1975,** *233,* 427–431.

Gorbach, S. L.; Nahas, L.; Plaut, A.; Weinstein, L.; Patterson, J. F.; and Levitan, R. Studies of intestinal microflora. V. Fecal microbial ecology in ulcerative colitis and regional enteritis: relationship to severity of disease and chemotherapy. *Gastroenterology,* **1967,** *54,* 575–587.

Gould, S. Urinary tract disorders. Clinical comparison of flavonate and phenazopyridine. *Urology,* **1975,** *5,* 612–615.

Gurwith, M. J.; Brunton, J. L.; Lank, B. A.; Harding, G. K. M.; and Ronald, A. R. A prospective controlled investigation of prophylactic trimethoprim-sulfamethoxazole in hospitalized granulocytic patients. *Am. J. Med.,* **1979,** *66,* 248–256.

Hailey, F. J.; Glascock, H. W.; and Hewitt, W. F. Pleuropneumonic reactions to nitrofurantoin. *N. Engl. J. Med.,* **1969,** *281,* 1087–1090.

Haltalin, K. C., and Nelson, J. D. *In vitro* susceptibility of shigellae to sodium sulfadiazine and eight antibiotics. *J.A.M.A.,* **1965,** *193,* 705–710.

Hamilton-Miller, J. M., and Brumfitt, W. Methenamine and its salts as urinary tract antiseptics: variables affecting the antibacterial activity of formaldehyde, mandelic acid, and hippuric acid *in vitro. Invest. Urol.,* **1977,** *14,* 287–291.

Harding, G. K. M., and Ronald, A. R. Controlled study of antimicrobial prophylaxis of recurrent urinary infection in women. *N. Engl. J. Med.,* **1974,** *291,* 597–601.

Harrison, H. N.; Bales, H. W.; and Jacoby, F. J. The absorption into burned skin of SULFAMYLON ACETATE from 5 percent aqueous solution. *J. Trauma,* **1972,** *12,* 994–998.

Hassan, A.; Erian, M. M.; Farid, Z.; Hathout, S. D.; and Sorensen, K. Trimethoprim-sulfamethoxazole in acute brucellosis. *Br. Med. J.,* **1971,** *3,* 159–160.

Hitchings, G. H. A biochemical approach to chemotherapy. *Ann. N.Y. Acad. Sci.,* **1961,** *23,* 700–708.

Hoshiwara, I.; Oster, B.; Hana, V.; Cignett, F.; Colema, V. R.; and Jawetz, E. Doxycycline treatment of chronic trachoma. *J.A.M.A.,* **1973,** *224,* 220–223.

Hughes, W. T.; Feldman, S.; Chaudhary, S. C.; Ossi, M. J.; Cox, F.; and Sanyal, S. K. Comparison of pentamidine isethionate and trimethoprim-sulfamethoxazole in the treatment of *Pneumocystis carinii* pneumonia. *J. Pediatr.,* **1978,** *92,* 285–291.

Hughes, W. T.; Feldman, S.; and Sangal, S. K. Treatment of *Pneumocystis carinii* pneumonitis with trimethoprim-sulfamethoxazole. *Can. Med. Assoc. J.,* **1975,** *112,* 47–50.

Hughes, W. T.; Kuhn, S.; Chaudhary, S.; Feldman, S.; Verzosa, M.; Aur, J. A. R.; Pratt, C.; and George, S. L. Successful chemoprophylaxis for *Pneumocystis carinii* pneumonitis. *N. Engl. J. Med.,* **1977,** *297,* 1419–1426.

Kalowski, S.; Nanra, R. S.; Mathew, T. H.; and Kincaid-Smith, P. Deterioration in renal function in association with co-trimoxazole therapy. *Lancet,* **1973,** *2,* 394–397.

Kutscher, A. H.; Lane, S. L.; and Segall, R. The clinical toxicity of antibiotics and sulfonamides: a comparative review of the literature based on 104,672 cases treated systemically. *J. Allergy,* **1954,** *25,* 135–150.

Lacey, R. W.; Gillespie, W. A.; Bruten, D. M.; and Lewis, E. L. Trimethoprim-resistant coliforms. *Lancet,* **1972,** *1,* 409–410.

Larter, W. E.; John, T. J.; Sieber, O. F.; Johnson, H.; Corrigan, J. J.; and Fulginiti, V. A. Trimethoprim-sulfamethoxazole treatment of *Pneumocystis carinii* pneumonitis. *J. Pediatr.,* **1978,** *92,* 826–828.

Lindholm, T. Electromyographic changes after nitrofurantoin (FURADANTIN) therapy in nonuremic patients. *Neurology* (Minneap.), **1967,** *17,* 1017–1020.

Lipton, J. H. Incompatibility between sulfamethizole and methenamine mandelate. *N. Engl. J. Med.,* **1963,** *268,* 92–93.

Lohr, J. A.; Nunley, D. H.; Howards, S. S.; and Ford, R. F. Prevention of recurrent urinary tract infections in girls. *Pediatrics,* **1977,** *59,* 562–565.

McAllister, T. A. Resistance to co-trimoxazole. *Scand. J. Infect. Dis.,* **1976,** *29,* Suppl. 8, 29–35.

Matthew, A. D.; Gonzalez, R.; Jeffords, D.; and Pinto, M. H. Prevention of bacteriuria after transurethral prostatectomy with nitrofurantoin macrocrystals. *J. Urol.,* **1978,** *120,* 442–443.

May, J. R., and Davies, J. Resistance of *Haemophilus influenzae* to trimethoprim. *Br. Med. J.,* **1972,** *3,* 376–377.

Moffat, N. A., and Wenzel, F. J. The treatment of urinary tract infections with sulfacytine, a new soluble sulfonamide. *Curr. Ther. Res.,* **1971,** *13,* 286–291.

Moody, M. R., and Young, V. M. *In vitro* susceptibility of *Pseudomonas cepacia* and *Pseudomonas maltophilia* to trimethoprim and trimethoprim-sulfamethoxazole. *Antimicrob. Agents Chemother.,* **1975,** *7,* 836–839.

Nakhla, L. S. Genetic determinants of trimethoprim resistance in a strain of *Staphylococcus aureus. J. Clin. Pathol.,* **1973,** *26,* 712–715.

Nelson, J. D.; Kusmiesz, H.; and Jacobson, L. H. Comparison of trimethoprim-sulfamethoxazole and ampicillin therapy for shigellosis in ambulatory patients. *J. Pediatr.,* **1976,** *89,* 491–493.

Nichols, R. L., and Condon, R. E. Preoperative preparation of the colon. *Surg., Gynecol., Obstet.,* **1971,** *132,* 323–337.

Nolte, H., and Büttner, H. Pharmacokinetics of trimethoprim and its combination with sulfamethoxazole in man after single and chronic oral administration. *Chemotherapy,* **1973,** *18,* 274–284.

Pelton, S. I.; Shurin, P. A.; Klein, J. O.; and Finland, M. Quantitative inhibition of *Haemophilus influenzae* by trimethoprim-sulfamethoxazole. *Antimicrob. Agents Chemother.,* **1977,** *12,* 649–654.

Peppercorn, M. A., and Goldman, P. Distribution studies of salicylazosulfapyridine and its metabolites. *Gastroenterology,* **1973,** *64,* 240–245.

Ramachandran, S.; Godfrey, J. J.; and Lionel, N. D. W. A comparative trial of co-trimoxazole and chloramphenicol in typhoid and paratyphoid fever. *J. Trop. Med. Hyg.,* **1978,** *81,* 36–39.

Rao, K. G. Pseudotumor cerebri associated with nalidixic acid. *Urology,* **1974,** *4,* 204–207.

Reisberg, B.; Herzog, J.; and Weinstein, L. *In vitro* antibacterial activity of trimethoprim alone and in combination with sulfonamides. In, *Antimicrobial Agents and Chemotherapy—1966.* American Society for Microbiology, Ann Arbor, Mich., **1967,** pp. 424–427.

Remington, J. S., and Desmonts, G. Toxoplasmosis. In, *Infectious Diseases of the Fetus and Newborn Infant.* (Remington, J. S., and Klein, J. O., eds.) W. B. Saunders Co., Philadelphia, **1976,** pp. 191–332.

Rieder, J. Quantitative determination of the bacteriostatically active fraction of sulfonamides and the sum of their inactive metabolites in the body fluids. *Chemotherapy,* **1972,** *17,* 1–12.

———. Metabolism and techniques for assay of trimethoprim and sulfamethoxazole. *J. Infect. Dis.,* **1973,** *128,* S567–S573.

Riis, P.; Anthonisen, P.; Wulff, R.; Folkenborg, O.; Bonnevie, O.; and Binder, V. The prophylactic effect of salicylazosulphapyridine in ulcerative colitis during long-term treatment. *Scand. J. Gastroenterol.,* **1973,** *8,* 71–74.

Roelsen, R. Polyneuritis after nitrofurantoin (FURADANTIN) therapy: a survey and report of two new cases. *Acta Med. Scand.,* **1964,** *175,* 145–154.

Ronald, A. R.; Turck, M.; and Petersdorf, R. G. A critical evaluation of nalidixic acid in urinary-tract infections. *N. Engl. J. Med.,* **1966,** *275,* 1081–1089.

Rosenkranz, H. S., and Rosenkranz, S. Silver sulfadiazine: interaction with isolated deoxyribonucleic acid. *Antimicrob. Agents Chemother.,* **1972,** *2,* 373–383.

Rosenow, E. C.; DeRemee, R. A.; and Dines, D. E. Chronic nitrofurantoin pulmonary reaction: report of five cases. *N. Engl. J. Med.,* **1968,** *279,* 1258–1262.

Sachs, J.; Geer, T.; Noell, P.; and Kunin, C. M. Effect of renal function on urinary recovery of orally administered nitrofurantoin. *N. Engl. J. Med.,* **1968,** *278,* 1032–1035.

Schwartz, D. E., and Rieder, J. Pharmacokinetics of sulfa-

methoxazole plus trimethoprim in man and their distribution in the rat. *Chemotherapy,* **1970,** *15,* 337–355.

Scragg, J. N., and Rubidge, C. J. Trimethoprim and sulphamethoxazole in typhoid fever in children. *Br. Med. J.,* **1971,** *3,* 738–741.

Sharpstone, P. The renal handling of trimethoprim and sulphamethoxazole in man. *Postgrad. Med. J.,* **1969,** *45,* Suppl., 38–42.

Shouval, D.; Ligumsky, M.; and Ben-Ishay, D. Effect of co-trimoxazole on normal creatinine clearance. *Lancet,* **1978,** *2,* 244–245.

Singer, R. C. Sulfonamide-resistant meningococcal disease. *Med. Clin. North Am.,* **1967,** *51,* 719–727.

Singleton, J. W. National Cooperative Crohn's Disease Study (NCCDS). Results of drug treatment. *Gastroenterology,* **1977,** *72,* A110/1133.

Siniscal, A. A. The sulfonamides and antibiotics in trachoma. *J.A.M.A.,* **1952,** *148,* 637–639.

Stamey, T. A., and Bragonje, J. Resistance to nalidixic acid. A misconception due to underdosage. *J.A.M.A.,* **1976,** *236,* 1857–1860.

Stamey, T. A., and Condy, M. The diffusion and concentration of trimethoprim in human vaginal fluid. *J. Infect. Dis.,* **1975,** *131,* 261–266.

Stamey, T. A.; Condy, M.; and Mihara, G. Prophylactic efficacy of nitrofurantoin macrocrystals and trimethoprim-sulfamethoxazole in urinary infections. Biologic effects on the vaginal and rectal flora. *N. Engl. J. Med.,* **1977,** *296,* 780–783.

Stamey, T. A.; Meares, E. M.; and Winningham, D. G. Chronic bacterial prostatitis and the diffusion of drugs into prostatic fluid. *J. Urol.,* **1970,** *103,* 187–194.

Strauss, W. G., and Griffin, L. M. Nitrofurantoin pneumonia. *J.A.M.A.,* **1967,** *199,* 765–766.

Summers, R. W.; Switz, D. M.; Sessions, J. T., Jr.; Becktel, J. M.; Best, W. R.; Kern, F., Jr.; and Singleton, J. W. National cooperative Crohn's disease study: results of drug treatment. *Gastroenterology,* **1979,** *77,* 847–869.

Svindland, H. B. Treatment of gonorrhoea with sulphamethoxazole-trimethoprim. Lack of effect on concomitant syphilis. *Br. J. Vener. Dis.,* **1973,** *49,* 50–53.

Tandon, M. K. A comparative trial of co-trimoxazole and amoxycillin in the treatment of acute exacerbations of chronic bronchitis. *Med. J. Aust.,* **1977,** *2,* 281–284.

Thomas, V.; Shelokov, M.; and Furland, M. Antibody-coated bacteria in urine and site of urinary tract infections. *N. Engl. J. Med.,* **1974,** *290,* 588–590.

Tolman, K. G. Nitrofurantoin and chronic active hepatitis. *Ann. Intern. Med.,* **1980,** *92,* 119–120.

Toole, J. F., and Parrish, M. L. Nitrofurantoin polyneuropathy. *Neurology (Minneap.),* **1973,** *23,* 554–559.

Tréfouël, J.; Tréfouël, J.; Nitti, F.; and Bovet, D. Activité du *p*-aminophénylsulfamide sur les infections streptococciques expérimentales de la souris et du lapin. *C. R. Soc. Biol. (Paris),* **1935,** *120,* 756–758.

Trickett, P. C. Ancillary use of phenazopyridine (PYRIDIUM) in urinary tract infections. *Curr. Ther. Res.,* **1970,** *12,* 441–445.

Turck, M.; Anderson, K. N.; and Petersdorf, R. G. Relapse and reinfection in chronic bacteriuria. *N. Engl. J. Med.,* **1966,** *275,* 70–73.

Turck, M.; Ronald, A. R.; and Petersdorf, R. G. Relapse and reinfection in chronic bacteriuria. II. The correlation between site of infection and pattern of recurrence in chronic bacteriuria. *N. Engl. J. Med.,* **1968,** *278,* 422–427.

Vainrub, B., and Musher, D. M. Lack of effect of methenamine in suppression of, or prophylaxis against chronic urinary infection. *Antimicrob. Agents Chemother.,* **1977,** *12,* 625–629.

Vosti, K. L. Recurrent urinary tract infection. Prevention by prophylactic antibiotics after sexual intercourse. *J.A.M.A.,* **1975,** *231,* 934–940.

White, M. G., and Asch, M. J. Acid-base effects of topical

mafenide acetate in the burned patient. *N. Engl. J. Med.,* **1971**, *284,* 1281–1286.

White, P. J., and Woods, D. D. The synthesis of *p*-aminobenzoic acid and folic acid by staphylococci sensitive and resistant to sulphonamides. *J. Gen. Microbiol.,* **1965**, *40,* 243–253.

Willner, M. M.; Dull, T. A.; and McDonald, H. Comparison of trimethoprim-sulfamethoxazole and ampicillin in the treatment of acute bacterial otitis media in children. In, *Current Chemotherapy: Proceedings of the Tenth International Congress of Chemotherapy,* Vol. I. (Siegenthaler, W., and Lüthy, R., eds.) American Society for Microbiology, Washington, D. C., **1978**, pp. 125–127.

Woods, D. D. Relation of *p*-aminobenzoic acid to mechanism of action of sulphanilamide. *Br. J. Exp. Pathol.,* **1940**, *21,* 74–90.

————. The biochemical mode of action of the sulphonamide drugs. *J. Gen. Microbiol.,* **1962**, *29,* 687–702.

Zetzel, L. Ulcerative colitis. *N. Engl. J. Med.,* **1954**, *251,* 610–615, 653–658.

Monographs and Reviews

Jawetz, E., and Gunnison, J. B. Antibiotic synergism and antagonism: an assessment of the problem. *Pharmacol. Rev.,* **1953**, *5,* 175–192.

Symposium. (Various authors.) The synergy of trimethoprim and sulphonamides. *Postgrad. Med. J.,* **1969**, *45,* Suppl., 3–104.

Symposium. (Various authors.) Trimethoprim-sulfamethoxazole. *J. Infect. Dis.,* **1973**, *128,* Suppl., 425–816.

Weinstein, L.; Madoff, M. A.; and Samet, C. A. The sulfonamides. *N. Engl. J. Med.,* **1960**, *263,* 793–800, 842–849, 900–907.

Wenzel, R. P.; Hunting, K. J.; Ostermary, C. O.; and Sande, M. A. *Providencia stuartii,* a hospital pathogen: potential factors for its emergence and transmission. *Am. J. Epidemiol.,* **1976**, *104,* 170–180.

50 ANTIMICROBIAL AGENTS

[*Continued*]

Penicillins and Cephalosporins

Gerald L. Mandell and Merle A. Sande

THE PENICILLINS

Penicillin is one of the most important of the antibiotics. Its initial discovery was largely fortuitous, but its development and therapeutic application represent the result of a well-planned and executed program that brought about one of the major advances in medical therapeutics. Although numerous other antimicrobial agents have been produced since penicillin became available, it is still a widely used, major antibiotic, and new derivatives of the basic penicillin nucleus are being produced every year. Many of these have unique advantages, such that members of this group of antibiotics are presently the drugs of choice for a large number of infectious diseases.

History. The history of the discovery and the development of penicillin has become common knowledge. It has fortunately been recorded by the chief participants. (*See* Fleming, 1946; Florey, 1946, 1949; Abraham, 1949; Chain, 1954.) In 1896, Ernest Duchesne, a French medical student, demonstrated the antibacterial activity of *Penicillium glaucum* and published his findings in his thesis; the observation attracted no attention at the time. In 1928, while studying staphylococcus variants in the laboratory at St. Mary's Hospital in London, Alexander Fleming, a bacteriologist who had previously discovered lysozyme, observed that a mold contaminating one of his cultures caused the bacteria in its vicinity to undergo lysis. Broth in which the fungus was grown was markedly inhibitory and even bactericidal *in vitro* for many microorganisms. Because the mold belonged to the genus *Penicillium,* Fleming named the antibacterial substance *penicillin.*

A decade later penicillin was developed as a systemic therapeutic agent by the concerted and brilliant researches of a group of investigators at Oxford University headed by Florey, Chain, and Abraham. Starting in 1939, work on the biosynthesis and extraction of penicillin from broth cultures of *Penicillium notatum* was energetically pursued. Within a few months, many of the chemical, physical, and pharmacological properties of the antibiotic were established. By May, 1940, the crude material then available was found to produce dramatic therapeutic effects when administered parenterally to mice with experimentally produced streptococcal infections. Despite great obstacles to its laboratory production, enough penicillin was accumulated by 1941 to conduct therapeutic trials in several patients desperately ill with staphylococcal and streptococcal infections refractory to all other therapy. At this stage, the crude amorphous penicillin was only about 10% pure and it required nearly 100 liters of the broth in which the mold had been grown to obtain enough of the antibiotic to treat one patient for 24 hours. Herrell (1945) records that bedpans were actually used by the Oxford group for growing cultures of *P. notatum.* Case 1 in the 1941 report from Oxford was that of a policeman who was suffering from a severe mixed staphylococcal and streptococcal infection. He was treated with penicillin, some of which had been recovered from the urine of other patients who had been given the drug. It is said that an Oxford professor referred to penicillin as a remarkable substance, grown in bedpans and purified by passage through the Oxford Police Force.

Expansion of the clinical program required the production of larger amounts of penicillin than could be made in the laboratory, and a vast research program was soon initiated in the United States. During 1942, 122 million units of penicillin were made available, and the first clinical trials were conducted at Yale University and the Mayo Clinic with dramatic results (Figure 50–1). By the spring of 1943, 200 patients had been treated with the drug. The results were so impressive that the surgeon general of the United States Army authorized trial of the antibiotic in a military hospital. Soon thereafter, penicillin was adopted throughout the medical services of the United States Armed Forces. By the summer of 1943, the clinical results in 500 patients were reported (National Research Council, 1943).

The deep-fermentation procedure for the biosynthesis of penicillin developed at the Northern Regional Research Laboratories of the Department of Agriculture, Peoria, Illinois, marked a crucial advance in the large-scale production of the antibiotic. From a total production of a few-hundred million units a month in the early days, the quantity manufactured rose to over 200 trillion units (nearly 150 tons) by 1950. The first marketable penicillin cost several dollars per 100,000 units; today, the same dose costs only a few cents.

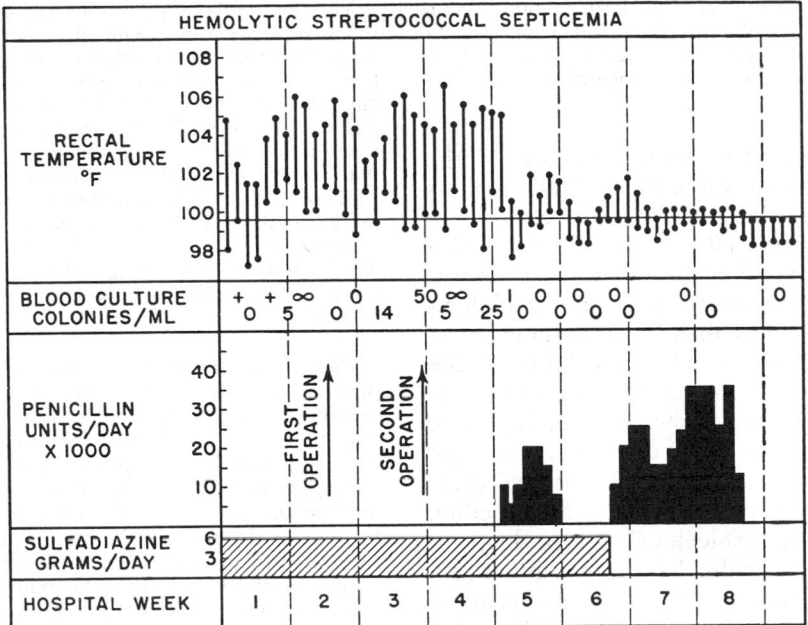

Figure 50-1. *First clinical trial of penicillin in the United States: penicillin therapy of beta-hemolytic streptococcal septicemia.*

The patient, a 33-year-old multiparous housewife, entered the New Haven Hospital (Yale University) on February 14, 1942, with the presumptive diagnosis of inevitable abortion of a 4-month-old fetus. Following emptying of the uterus, a chill developed and the temperature rose sharply. (The highest and lowest daily rectal temperature recordings are shown in the figure.) The patient was given sulfadiazine, 6 g daily. High spiking fever persisted despite adequate concentrations of sulfadiazine in plasma, repeated blood transfusions, and supportive therapy. Cultures of the blood and of the fluid aspirated from a septic ankle joint revealed *beta-hemolytic streptococcus* type 27. (An "infinite" number of colonies per milliliter of blood is indicated in the figure by the symbol ∞.) The diagnosis of infected abortion, streptococcal septicemia, and thrombophlebitis of the pelvic veins was made. On the eleventh hospital day, surgical exploration of the pelvis was performed (left arrow in figure); the right uterine veins were found to be thrombosed. The right common iliac and left internal iliac veins were ligated. Although blood cultures were negative for several days, the patient's course continued downhill. On the twenty-first hospital day (right arrow), a second operation was undertaken and supravaginal hysterectomy and bilateral salpingo-oophorectomy were performed. The patient's condition remained critical.

On the twenty-ninth hospital day, it was decided to give the patient the carefully husbanded, small supply of penicillin then available. It was injected intravenously every 4 hours day and night for 1 week, in the doses depicted in the figure, until the supply was exhausted. These doses are now known to have been quite small. (The urine was saved for extraction of penicillin for reuse.) The clinical response was dramatic. The temperature fell to normal within a few hours; the blood cultures became sterile and remained so. The persistence of moderate fever was attributable to a pyrogen present in the crude penicillin preparation. The skepticism prevalent at the time resulted in the continuation of sulfadiazine therapy. A new supply of more potent and purer penicillin became available and was given in the depicted doses for 2 weeks, starting on the forty-first hospital day. Convalescence was rapid and uneventful. In its first trial in the United States, penicillin had proved lifesaving. (After Blake, Craige, and Tierney, 1944. Courtesy of the *Transactions of the Association of American Physicians*.)

Source. In the early years of its production, all penicillin came from subcultures of Fleming's original strain of *P. notatum*. The urgent necessity of producing large amounts of the antibiotic during World War II prompted a vigorous worldwide search for other, more productive strains of *Penicillium*. One of the best was a strain of *P. chrysogenum* that was obtained from the stem of a moldy cantaloupe. Exposure of this organism to x-rays produced a mutant with a high penicillin yield (X-1612). The production of the antibiotic was enhanced manyfold by growing the mold in corn-steep liquor, a by-product of the manufacture of cornstarch. Several natural penicillins may be produced, depending on the chemical composition of the fermentation media. These include penicillins F, X, K, and G. Penicillin G (benzylpenicillin) has the greatest antimicrobial activity and is the only *natural* penicillin used clinically.

Chemistry. The basic structure of the penicillins, as shown in Figure 50–2, consists of a thiazolidine ring (*A*) connected to a beta-lactam ring (*B*), to which is attached a side chain (*R*). The penicillin nucleus itself is the chief structural requirement for biological activity; metabolic transformation or chemical alteration of this portion of the molecule causes loss of all significant antibacterial activity. The side chain (*see* Table 50–1, page 1134) determines many of the antibacterial and pharmacological characteristics of a particular type of penicillin. As mentioned, penicillin G is benzylpenicillin. While penicillin has been synthesized, the process has no commercial application.

Semisynthetic Penicillins. The discovery that 6-aminopenicillanic acid could be obtained from cultures of *P. chrysogenum* that were depleted of side chain precursors led to the development of the semisynthetic penicillins. Side chains can be added that alter the susceptibility of the resultant compounds to inactivating enzymes (beta-lactamases) and that change the antibacterial activity and the pharmacological properties of the drug.

The semisynthetic penicillins can be obtained by the incorporation of specific precursors in mold cultures, by chemical modification of wholly natural penicillins, and by synthesis from 6-aminopenicillanic acid; the last-named method is the most efficient. The steps leading to the commercial production of 6-aminopenicillanic acid have been summarized by Chain (1962) and reviewed by Klein and Finland (1963). The compound is now produced in large quantities with the aid of an amidase from *P. chrysogenum* (Figure 50–2). This enzyme splits the peptide linkage by which the side chain of penicillin is joined to 6-aminopenicillanic acid (*see* Hamilton-Miller, 1966).

Unitage of Penicillin. A standard system for expressing penicillin potency was adopted by the International Conference on the Standardization of Penicillin, held in London in 1944, which established the *international unit of penicillin* and the *international penicillin master standard.* The latter is a specimen of the crystalline sodium salt of penicillin G; the unit, by definition, is the specific penicillin activity contained in 0.6 μg of the master standard. One milligram of pure penicillin G sodium thus equals 1667 units. Because of the differences in molecular weight, 1.0 mg of pure penicillin G potassium represents 1595 units. The dosage and the antibacterial potency of the semisynthetic penicillins are usually expressed in terms of weight.

Assay. While various methods are available, microbiological assay is the method of choice for clinical purposes. This technic is widely employed for measurement of penicillin concentrations in blood, urine, and spinal and other body fluids, and for studies on the absorption, fate, and excretion of penicillin.

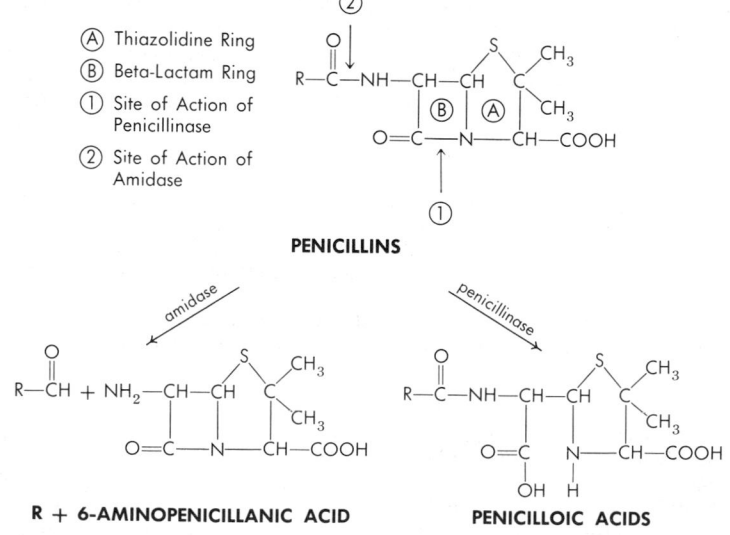

Figure 50–2. *Structure of penicillins and products of their enzymatic hydrolysis.*

Mechanism of Action of the Penicillins and Cephalosporins. The beta-lactam antibiotics (penicillins, cephalosporins, and cephamycins) can kill susceptible bacteria. Although knowledge of the mechanism of this action is incomplete, numerous researchers have supplied information that allows understanding of the basic phenomenon (*see* Perlman, 1977; Schlessinger, 1977).

The cell walls of bacteria are essential for their normal growth and development. Peptidoglycan is a heteropolymeric component of the cell wall that provides rigid mechanical stability by virtue of its highly cross-linked latticework structure. It is composed of glycan chains, which are linear strands of alternating pyranoside residues of two amino sugars (N-acetylglucosamine and N-acetylmuramic acid), that are cross-linked by peptide chains. The composition of the peptide cross-links is characteristic of individual microbial species. In *Staphylococcus aureus,* tetrapeptide units are bonded to the acetylmuramic acid residues, and pentaglycine chains bridge between the tetrapeptide moieties on adjacent strands (Figure 50–3).

The biosynthesis of the peptidoglycan involves about 30 bacterial enzymes and may be considered in three stages. The first stage, precursor formation, takes place in the cytoplasm. The product, uridine diphosphate (UDP)–acetylmuramyl-pentapeptide, called a "Park nucleotide" after its discoverer, accumulates in cells when subsequent synthetic stages are inhibited. The detection of this accumulation was a major step in the elucidation of the mechanism of action of penicillin (Park and Strominger, 1957). The last reaction in this stage is the addition of a dipeptide, D-alanyl-D-alanine. Synthesis of the dipeptide involves prior racemization of L-alanine and condensation catalyzed by D-alanyl-D-alanine synthetase. D-Cycloserine is a structural analog of D-alanine and acts as a competitive inhibitor of both the racemase and the synthetase (*see* Chapter 53).

During reactions of the second stage, UDP-acetyl-muramyl-pentapeptide and UDP-acetylglucosamine are linked (with the release of the uridine nucleotides) to form a long polymer. The sugar pentapeptide is first attached by a pyrophosphate bridge to a phospholipid in the cell membrane. The second sugar is then added, followed by the addition of five glycine residues as a branch of the heteropentapeptide. The first half of the pentaglycine cross-link is thus formed. The completed unit is then cleaved from the membrane-bound phospholipid, a reaction that is inhibited by vancomycin.

The third and final stage involves the completion of the cross-link. This is accomplished by a *transpeptidation reaction* that occurs outside the cell membrane. The transpeptidase itself is membrane bound. The terminal glycine residue of the pentaglycine bridge is linked to the fourth residue of the pentapeptide (D-alanine), releasing the fifth residue (also D-alanine) (Figure 50–3). It is this last step in peptidoglycan synthesis that is inhibited by the beta-lactam antibiotics. Stereomodels reveal that the conformation of penicillin is very similar to that of D-alanyl-D-alanine. The transpeptidase is probably acylated by penicillin; that is, penicilloyl enzyme is

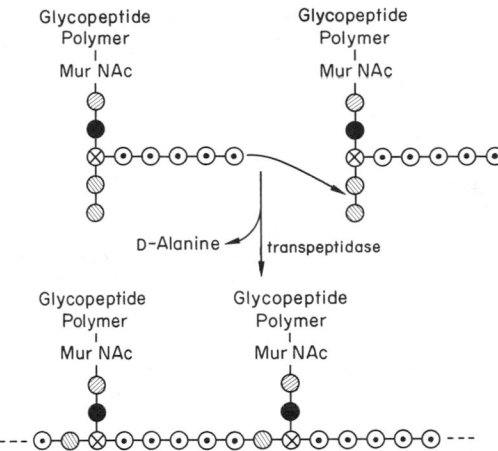

Figure 50-3. *The transpeptidase reaction in* Staphylococcus aureus *that is inhibited by penicillins and cephalosporins.*

See text for details. *Mur NAc* = N-acetyl-muramic acid; ⊘ = L-alanine; ● = D-glutamate; ⊗ = L-lysine; ◎ = D-alanine; ⊙ = glycine.

apparently formed, with cleavage of the —CO—N— bond of the beta-lactam ring (*see* Strominger, 1973).

Beta-lactam antibiotics produce certain characteristic morphological effects on bacteria. These changes are dependent on the antibiotic, its concentration, and the microbe. Bacteria may form long filamentous forms and fail to divide. Under certain conditions growth may take place at the midportion of a rod with formation of a bulge. Microorganisms may swell and then rupture, with extrusion of their contents. In medium that is isosmotic with bacterial cytoplasm, relatively stable cell-wall-deficient bacteria (protoplasts) may be formed. In general, at the lowest effective concentrations of a beta-lactam antibiotic, cell division is inhibited but elongation continues. As the concentration of the antibiotic is increased, growth is inhibited, bulges may form, and lysis is then observed.

Certain of these changes may result from effects of beta-lactam antibiotics on enzymes in addition to the transpeptidase that is involved in cell-wall synthesis (*see* Ghuysen, 1977; Spratt, 1977). It is probable that certain enzymes control increases in cell size and that others are involved in septum formation and normal fission into daughter cells. Thus, an antibiotic that interferes with an enzyme involved in septum formation may cause the appearance of filamentous nondividing bacteria (*see* Blumberg and Strominger, 1974).

Data suggest that *lysis* of bacteria is due to the activity of bacterial enzymes, autolysins, probably including murein hydrolases. These enzymes may function normally in processes related to cell division. Beta-lactam antibiotics appear to decrease the availability of an inhibitor of murein hydrolase. The uninhibited enzyme can then destroy the structural integrity of the cell. Certain bacterial strains (e.g., strains of *Staph. aureus* and *Streptococcus pneumoniae*) that lack these autolysins have been identified. Beta-lactam antibiotics inhibit the growth of the microorganisms, but lysis does not take place; these bacteria are thus "tolerant" to penicillin (*see* Tomasz and Holtje, 1977; Tomasz, 1979). Patients with staphylococcal endocarditis caused by such microorganisms have been described. Some of these patients may require therapy with agents that have a different mechanism of action, such as vancomycin, rifampin, or an aminoglycoside (*see* Greenwood, 1972; Sabath et al., 1977).

Mechanisms of Bacterial Resistance to Penicillins and Cephalosporins.

Beta-lactam antibiotics cannot kill or even inhibit all bacteria, and various mechanisms of bacterial resistance to these agents are operative. The microorganism may be intrinsically resistant because of structural differences in the enzymes that are the targets of these drugs. Furthermore, it is possible for a sensitive strain to acquire resistance of this type by mutation. However, in the case of the beta-lactam antibiotics this mechanism for the acquisition of resistance is probably relatively unimportant (*see* Benveniste and Davies, 1973).

Other instances of bacterial resistance to the beta-lactam antibiotics are caused by the inability of the agent to permeate to its site of action. In gram-positive bacteria the peptidoglycan polymer is very near the cell surface. Only surface macromolecules (capsule) are external to the peptidoglycan. The small beta-lactam antibiotic molecules can easily penetrate to the outer layer of the cytoplasmic membrane, where the final stages of the synthesis of the peptidoglycan take place. The situation is different with gram-negative bacteria. Their surface structure is more complex, and the inner membrane (which is analogous to the cytoplasmic membrane of gram-positive bacteria) is covered by the outer membrane, lipopolysaccharide, and capsule. The outer membrane functions as an impenetrable barrier for certain hydrophilic antibiotics (*see* Richmond, 1978).

Bacteria can destroy beta-lactam antibiotics enzymatically. While amidohydrolases may be present, these enzymes are relatively inactive and do not protect the bacteria. Beta-lactamases or penicillinases, however, are capable of inactivating certain of these antibiotics and may be present in large quantity (*see* Figure 50–2). The different penicillins and cephalosporins vary in their susceptibility to the beta-lactamases that are produced by different bacterial species.

In general, gram-positive bacteria produce a large amount of enzyme that is secreted extracellularly. The information for staphylococcal penicillinase is encoded in a plasmid, and this may be transferred by phage to other bacteria; the enzyme is inducible by substrates. In gram-negative bacteria, beta-lactamases are found in relatively small amounts but are located in the periplasmic space between the inner and outer cell membranes. Since the enzymes of cell-wall synthesis are on the outer surface of the inner membrane, these beta-lactamases are strategically located for maximal protection of the microbe. Beta-lactamases of gram-negative bacteria are encoded either in chromosomes or plasmids, and they may be constitutive or inducible. They may hydrolyze penicillins, cephalosporins, or both (*see* Sykes and Matthew, 1976). However, there is an inconsistent correlation between the susceptibility of an antibiotic to inactivation by beta-lactamase and the ability of that antibiotic to kill the microorganism. For example, certain antibiotics that are hydrolyzed by beta-lactamase (*e.g.,* ampicillin) are able to kill certain strains of beta-lactamase-producing microbes (*see* Richmond, 1978).

The beta-lactamase activity of microorganisms may be inhibited by drugs. If the enzyme binds a beta-lactam antibiotic that it cannot hydrolyze, such as cloxacillin or a cephalosporin, an inherently more potent but hydrolyzable antibiotic such as ampicillin may be able to exert an antibacterial effect. Thus, true synergism between two beta-lactam antibiotics may occasionally be demonstrable (Mandell and Hook, 1971). Clavulanic acid is a potent inhibitor of beta-lactamases that can protect susceptible penicillins and cephalosporins from destruction (Neu and Fu, 1978a). Thienamycin is a novel beta-lactam antibiotic that inhibits both bacterial cell-wall synthesis and beta-lactamase (Tally *et al.,* 1978).

The penicillinase from *Bacillus* species is produced commercially (NEUTRAPEN). It can be used to hydrolyze susceptible penicillins to augment growth of cultures from samples obtained from patients who are receiving the drug. Since it is a foreign protein, it must not be used to treat patients who are experiencing an allergic reaction to a penicillin.

Other Factors That Influence the Activity of Beta-Lactam Antibiotics. The density of the bacterial population and the age of an infection influence the activity of beta-lactam antibiotics. The drugs may be several thousand times more potent when tested against small bacterial inocula compared to their activity against a dense culture. Many factors are probably involved. Among these are the greater number of relatively resistant microorganisms in a large population, the amount of beta-lactamase produced, and the phase of growth of the culture. The clinical significance of this effect of inoculum size is uncertain. The intensity and the duration of penicillin therapy needed to abort or cure experimental infections in animals increase with the duration of the infection. The reason is primarily that the bacteria are no longer multiplying as rapidly as they are in a fresh infection. These antibiotics are most active against bacteria in the logarithmic phase of growth and have little effect on microorganisms in the lag phase, when there is no need to synthesize components of the cell wall (*see* Eagle, 1949, 1952; Durack and Beeson, 1972).

The presence of protein and pus does not appreciably decrease the ability of beta-lactam antibiotics to kill bacteria. However, bacteria that survive inside viable cells of the host are protected from the action of the beta-lactam antibiotics (*see* Mandell, 1973a). The antibiotics are active when pH or oxygen tension is low.

CLASSIFICATION OF THE PENICILLINS AND SUMMARY OF THEIR PHARMACOLOGICAL PROPERTIES

It is useful to classify the penicillins according to their spectrum of antimicrobial activity (*see* Table 50–1, page 1134; Neu, 1979a).

1. Penicillin G and its closely related congeners penicillin V and phenethicillin are highly active against gram-positive cocci, but they are readily hydrolyzed by penicillinase. Thus, they are ineffective against most strains of *Staph. aureus.*

2. The penicillinase-resistant penicillins (methicillin, nafcillin, oxacillin, cloxacillin, dicloxacillin, and floxacillin) have less potent antimicrobial activity against microorganisms that are sensitive to penicillin G, but they are the drugs of choice for infections caused by penicillinase-producing *Staph. aureus.*

3. Ampicillin, amoxicillin, and hetacillin comprise a group of penicillins whose antimicrobial activity is extended to include such gram-negative microorganisms as *Haemophilus influenzae, Escherichia coli,* and *Proteus mirabilis.* All of these drugs and the others listed below that are particularly effective against gram-negative bacteria are

readily hydrolyzed by staphylococcal penicillinase.

4. The antimicrobial activity of carbenicillin and its indanyl ester (carbenicillin indanyl), ticarcillin, and azlocillin is extended to include *Pseudomonas, Enterobacter,* and *Proteus* species.

5. A new group of penicillins whose members are as yet not available in the United States includes mezlocillin and piperacillin. These drugs have useful antimicrobial activity against *Klebsiella* species and certain other gram-negative microorganisms.

While the pharmacological properties of the individual drugs are discussed in detail below, certain generalizations are useful. Following absorption, penicillins are widely distributed throughout the body. Therapeutic concentrations of these agents are readily achieved in tissues and in such secretions as joint fluid, pleural fluid, pericardial fluid, and bile. However, only small amounts of these drugs are found in prostatic secretions, brain tissue, and intraocular fluid, and penicillins do not penetrate living phagocytic cells to a significant extent. Concentrations of penicillins in cerebrospinal fluid (CSF) are variable but are less than 1% of those in plasma when the meninges are normal. When there is inflammation, concentrations in CSF may rise to be as high as 5% of the plasma value. Penicillins are rapidly eliminated, particularly by glomerular filtration and renal tubular secretion, such that their half-lives in the body are short; values of 30 to 60 minutes are typical. Concentrations of these drugs in urine are thus high.

PENICILLIN G, PENICILLIN V, AND PHENETHICILLIN

Antimicrobial Activity. The antimicrobial spectrum of penicillin G (benzylpenicillin), penicillin V (the phenoxymethyl derivative), and phenethicillin (the phenoxyethyl analog) are very similar for aerobic gram-positive microorganisms. However, penicillin G is five to ten times more active against gram-negative microorganisms, especially *Neisseria* species, and certain anaerobes.

Penicillin G is highly effective *in vitro* against many, but not all, species of gram-positive and gram-negative cocci. Streptococci, with the exception of enterococci, are very susceptible to the drug, less than 0.01 μg/ml being effective. Whereas most strains of *Staph. aureus* were highly sensitive to similar concentrations of penicillin G when this agent was first employed therapeutically, an increasing number of strains that are resistant to the drug have been recovered over the years. At present, *most* staphylococci isolated from individuals outside of hospitals are resistant to penicillin G; in hospitalized patients, the incidence of such strains may be as high as 90 to 95%. Many strains of *Staph. epidermidis* are also resistant to penicillin. *Gonococci* are generally sensitive to penicillin G, although continued exposure of this microorganism to the antibiotic has led to a general decrease in sensitivity (Sparling, 1972). Rare strains are highly resistant to penicillin and produce penicillinase. *Meningococci* are quite sensitive to penicillin G. *Pneumococci* of all serological types are, in general, highly susceptible to penicillin G; however, some highly resistant strains have now been described, and hospitals should test their isolates of these bacteria as a means of surveillance.

Although the vast majority of strains of *Corynebacterium diphtheriae* are sensitive to penicillin G, some are highly resistant. This is also true for *Bacillus anthracis*. Most anaerobic microorganisms, including *Clostridium* species, are highly sensitive. *Bacteroides fragilis* is an exception; however, high doses of penicillin (20 million units per day) result in concentrations in blood that inhibit 50 to 80% of strains of this bacterium (*see* Tally *et al.*, 1975b). *Actinomyces israelii*, *Streptobacillus moniliformis*, *Pasteurella multocida*, and *Listeria monocytogenes* are inhibited by penicillin G. Most species of *Leptospira* are moderately susceptible to the drug. One of the most exquisitely sensitive microorganisms is *Treponema pallidum*. None of the penicillins is effective against *amebae, plasmodia, rickettsiae, fungi,* or *viruses*.

Although many species of *gram-negative bacilli* are resistant to penicillin G, some are affected by moderate-to-high concentrations. The majority of strains of *Pr. mirabilis* are inhibited by 10 μg/ml or less of the drug. Many strains of *E. coli* are also susceptible to high concentrations of penicillin G.

Absorption.   *Oral Administration of Penicillin G.*

About one third of an orally administered dose of penicillin G is absorbed from the intestinal tract under favorable conditions. Only a small portion is absorbed from the stomach. Gastric juice at pH 2 rapidly destroys the antibiotic. Because the gastric acidity of full-term newborn babies (after the first 24 to 48 hours) and of premature infants is relatively low, the oral administration of standard doses of penicillin yields higher concentrations of the drug in plasma than would be found in older children or adults. The decrease in gastric acid production with aging, as well as the development of achlorhydria in about 35% of persons over

60 years of age, accounts for better absorption of penicillin G from the gastrointestinal tract of older individuals. Absorption occurs mainly in the duodenum; it is rapid, and maximal concentrations in blood are attained in 30 to 60 minutes. The peak value is approximately 0.5 unit/ml after an oral dose of 400,000 units in an adult. Two thirds or more of an ingested dose is unabsorbed and passes into the colon, where it is largely inactivated by bacteria; only a small amount is excreted in the feces. The oral dose of penicillin G must be four to five times as large as the intramuscular in order to obtain concentrations in blood of comparable height and duration. The two important points to observe in prescribing penicillin G by mouth are to be certain that the dose is adequate, and that it is taken at least 0.5 hour before a meal and no earlier than 2 to 3 hours after a meal. Ingestion of food interferes with enteric absorption of penicillin, perhaps by adsorption of the antibiotic on food particles. Although oral preparations containing buffers are available, these offer no essential advantages over soluble salts of penicillin G taken orally in dry form or (preferably) in aqueous solution. Despite the convenience of oral administration of penicillin G, this route should be used only in those infections in which clinical experience has proven its efficacy; the dosage to be employed is also determined on this basis.

Oral Administration of Penicillin V.   The sole virtue of penicillin V in comparison with penicillin G is that it is more stable in an acidic medium and, therefore, is better absorbed from the gastrointestinal tract (*see* Klein and Finland, 1963). After oral ingestion, the drug escapes destruction in gastric juice, since it is both insoluble and stable at a low pH. It goes into solution in the more alkaline medium of the duodenum and is well but incompletely absorbed from the upper portion of the small intestine. On an equivalent oral-dose basis, the compound yields plasma concentrations two to five times greater than those provided by penicillin G. The peak concentration in the blood of an adult after an oral dose of 500 mg is nearly 3 μg/ml. There is some evidence that the drug is better absorbed when ingested after a meal than on an empty stomach.

Once absorbed, penicillin V is distributed in the body and excreted by the kidney in the same manner as penicillin G.

Oral Administration of Phenethicillin. This drug shares with penicillin V the property of stability in acidic media and better absorption from the gastro-intestinal tract (*see* Klein and Finland, 1963). It is available only for oral use as the potassium salt, which is freely soluble in water. Its antimicrobial spectrum is almost identical to that of penicillin V. Given orally, phenethicillin is well absorbed and escapes destruction in the acidic gastric contents; despite this fact, intestinal absorption is incomplete. In equal oral doses, it produces higher plasma concentrations than does penicillin G or penicillin V. But this seeming advantage can be overcome by appropriately larger doses of the other two agents. Food retards absorption and thereby prolongs the duration of action of the compound. Peak concentrations in plasma occur about 1 hour after oral administration of the drug and average 6 μg/ml after an oral dose of 500 mg. Once phenethicillin is absorbed, its protein binding, distribution, fate, and excretion are similar to those of penicillin G.

Parenteral Administration of Penicillin G. The speed of absorption of penicillin G after subcutaneous or intramuscular injection and hence the magnitude and persistence of the concentrations in plasma that are attained depend on many factors, including dose, vehicle, concentration, physical form, and solubility of the particular salt or ester of penicillin G. Other factors, especially renal excretion, are also important; for example, so rapid is elimination of penicillin G by the kidney that the concentration in plasma falls to half its peak value within 1 hour after injection of aqueous preparations (Figure 50–4). The speed of absorption of soluble penicillin salts is not significantly different after subcutaneous and intramuscular injection, and peak concentrations in plasma are reached within 15 to 30 minutes.

Many means for prolonging the sojourn of the antibiotic in the body and thereby reduc-

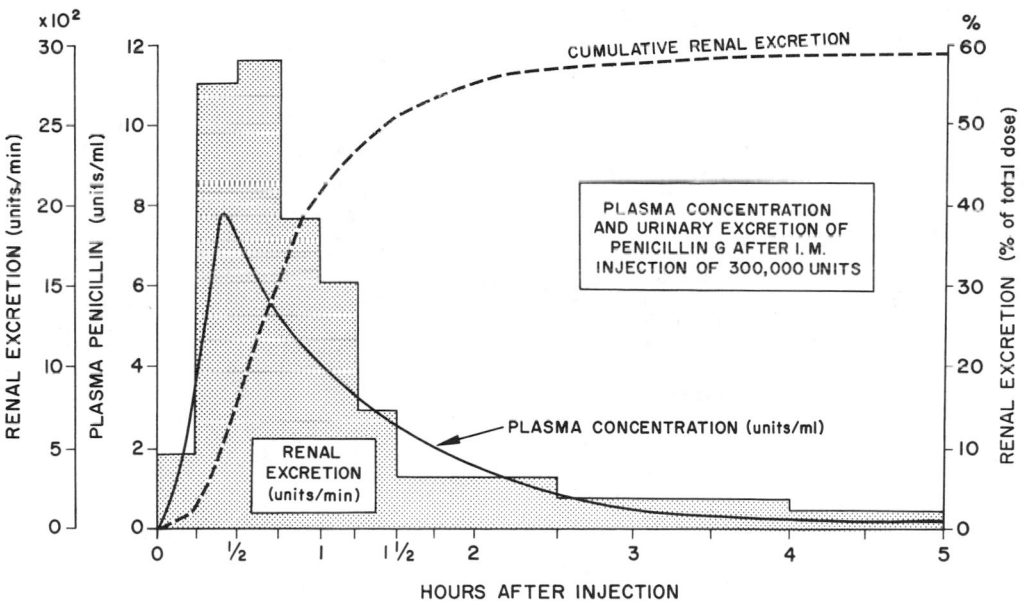

Figure 50–4. *Plasma concentration and renal excretion of penicillin G.*

This schematic chart is constructed from various reported data on the plasma concentration and the renal elimination of penicillin G in adults with normal renal function. Following an intramuscular injection of 300,000 units of an aqueous solution of sodium penicillin G, a peak plasma concentration of 8 units/ml is reached between 15 and 30 minutes after the injection; this value then falls quickly to 0.1 unit/ml by the end of 5 hours. The decline is the result of the rapid renal excretion of penicillin G, which is due primarily to tubular secretion. Within the 5-hour period depicted, nearly 60% (180,000 units) of the administered dose is eliminated in the urine. At the height of the excretory process, nearly 3000 units are excreted each minute and about 500 ml of plasma is cleared of penicillin during the same time span.

Table 50-1. CHEMICAL STRUCTURES AND MAJOR PROPERTIES OF VARIOUS PENICILLINS

SIDE CHAIN *	NONPROPRIETARY NAME	MAJOR PROPERTIES		
		Absorption after Oral Administration	*Resistance to Penicillinase*	*Useful Antimicrobial Spectrum*
[structure] —CH₂—	Penicillin G	Variable (poor)	No	*Streptococcus* species, *Neisseria* species, many anaerobes, spirochetes, others
[structure] —OCH₂—	Penicillin V	Good	No	
[structure] —OCH— CH₃	Phenethicillin	Good	No	
[structure] OCH₃ ... OCH₃	Methicillin	Poor (not given orally)	Yes	
[structure] R₁ ... R₂ O CH₃	Oxacillin (R₁ = R₂ = H) Cloxacillin (R₁ = Cl; R₂ = H) Dicloxacillin (R₁ = R₂ = Cl) Floxacillin (R₁ = Cl; R₂ = F)	Good	Yes	*Staphylococcus aureus*
[structure] OC₂H₅	Nafcillin	Variable	Yes	
[structure] R— —CH— NH₂	Ampicillin (R = H) Amoxicillin (R = OH)	Good / Excellent	No	*Haemophilus influenzae, Proteus mirabilis,* † *Escherichia coli, Neisseria* species
[structure] —CH— COOR	Carbenicillin (R = H) Carbenicillin indanyl (R = 5-indanol)	Poor (not given orally) / Good	No	Above plus *Pseudomonas* species, *Enterobacter* species, and *Proteus* (indole positive)
[structure] CH— COO— —CH₃ S	Ticarcillin	Poor (not given orally)	No	
[structure] CH— NHCO N O O N C₂H₅	Piperacillin	Poor (not given orally)	No	*Pseudomonas* species, *Enterobacter* species, many *Klebsiella*

* Equivalent to R in Figure 50–2 (page 1128).
† Up to 30% of strains may be resistant to ampicillin.

ing the frequency of injections have been explored. *Probenecid,* a drug that blocks renal tubular secretion of penicillin, is occasionally used for this purpose (*see* below and Chapter 38). More commonly, *repository preparations* of penicillin G are employed. The two such compounds currently favored are *penicillin G procaine* and *penicillin G benzathine* (*see* section on preparations). Such agents release penicillin G slowly from the area in which they are injected and produce relatively low but persistent concentrations of antibiotic in the blood.

The injection of 300,000 units of penicillin G procaine produces a peak concentration in plasma of about 1.5 units/ml within 1 to 3 hours; after 24 hours the concentration is reduced to 0.2 unit/ml, and by 48 hours it has fallen to 0.05 unit/ml. A larger dose (600,000 units) yields somewhat higher values that are maintained for as long as 4 to 5 days.

Penicillin G benzathine is very slowly absorbed from intramuscular depots and produces the longest duration of detectable antibiotic of all the available repository penicillins. For example, in adults, a dose of 1.2 million units given intramuscularly produces a concentration in plasma of 0.15 unit/ml on the first, 0.03 unit/ml on the fourteenth, and 0.003 unit/ml on the thirty-second day after injection. The average duration of demonstrable antimicrobial activity in the plasma is about 26 days. Similar pharmacokinetic data are available for newborn infants (Kaplan and McCracken, 1973; Klein *et al.,* 1973).

Absorption from Other Routes. Although suppositories of penicillin G yield detectable concentrations in plasma when inserted in the *rectum* or *vagina,* such therapy is undependable and not advised. The antibiotic is also absorbed from serous surfaces such as the *pleura, pericardium,* and *peritoneum,* and from *joint cavities,* the *subarachnoid space,* and the *respiratory tract.* Penicillin G is not absorbed through the unbroken *skin.*

Intrathecal administration of any of the penicillins is no longer recommended. Penicillin is a potent convulsant when given by this route. Bactericidal concentrations of the drug can be attained in the brain and meninges by the use of other parenteral routes.

Distribution. Penicillin G is widely distributed throughout the body, but the concentrations in various fluids and tissues differ widely. Its apparent volume of distribution is in about 50% of total body water. More than 90% of the penicillin G in blood is in the plasma and less than 10% is in the erythrocytes; approximately 65% is reversibly bound to plasma albumin. Significant amounts appear in liver, bile, kidney, semen, joint fluid, lymph, and intestine.

While probenecid markedly decreases the tubular secretion of the penicillins, this is not the only factor responsible for the elevated plasma concentrations of the antibiotic that follow its administration. Probenecid produces a significant decrease in the volume of distribution of the penicillins (Gibaldi *et al.,* 1970).

Cerebrospinal Fluid. Penicillin does not readily enter the cerebrospinal fluid (CSF) when the meninges are normal. A plasma concentration of less than 10 units/ml cannot be depended on to establish therapeutically effective concentrations in the CSF. When the meninges are acutely inflamed, penicillin penetrates into the CSF more easily. Although the concentrations attained vary and are unpredictable, they are usually in the range of 5% of the value in plasma and are often therapeutically effective. Fever appears to increase penetration of the blood-brain barrier by penicillin, probably as a result of vasodilatation and increased cerebral blood flow.

Penicillin and other organic acids are rapidly secreted from the CSF into the blood stream by an active transport process. Probenecid competitively inhibits this transport and thus elevates the concentration of penicillin in CSF (Spector and Lorenzo, 1974). In uremia, other organic acids accumulate in the CSF and compete with penicillin for secretion; the drug occasionally reaches toxic concentrations in brain and can produce convulsions (Spector and Snodgrass, 1976).

Excretion. Under normal conditions, penicillin G is rapidly eliminated from the body, mainly by the kidney but in small part in the bile and by other channels. The rapid renal excretion of the antibiotic is the reason for the use of measures to prolong its sojourn in the body, such as repository insoluble salts of the drug or the administration of probenecid.

Renal. Approximately 60 to 90% of an intramuscular dose of penicillin G in aqueous solution is eliminated in the urine, largely within the first hour after injection (Figure 50–4). The elimination half-time is about 30 minutes in normal adults. The antibiotic thus reaches high concentrations in the urine; for example, if a dose of 100,000 units of an aqueous solution is injected every 3 hours, the urine will contain from 300 to 1000 units/ml. Approximately 10% of the drug is eliminated by glomerular filtration and 90% by tubular secretion. Renal clearance approximates the total renal plasma flow. The maximal tubular secretory capacity (Tm) for penicillin in the normal male adult is about 3 million units (1.8 g) per hour. Obviously, this maximal transfer capacity is rarely, if ever, approached, even when massive doses of the antibiotic are injected intravenously. The rapid renal clearance accounts for the fact that the dose of penicillin G must be increased about fivefold in order to increase the persistence of a plasma concentration of 0.8 unit/ml by only 2 hours.

Clearance values are considerably lower in neonates and infants, because of incomplete development of renal function; as a result, after doses proportionate to surface area, the persistence of penicillin in the blood is several times as long in premature infants as in children and adults. The half-life of the antibiotic in children less than 1 week old is 3 hours; by 14 days of age it is 1.4 hours (McCracken et al., 1973). After renal function is fully established in young children, the rate of renal excretion of penicillin G is considerably more rapid than in adults. For example, following an intramuscular dose of 300,000 units of penicillin G in aqueous solution in a 3- to 4-year-old child, concentrations of the drug in plasma are no longer detectable after 2 to 3 hours. With increasing age and its accompanying decrease in renal tubular excretory function, the rate of elimination of the antibiotic by the kidney is decreased. The renal plasma clearance of penicillin is markedly diminished in the presence of other organic acids that are secreted by the renal tubules.

Approximately 20% of an *oral* dose of penicillin G is excreted in the urine, a reflection of the limited intestinal absorption of the drug; once penicillin has passed the intestinal mucosa, its fate and excretion are the same as for the injected antibiotic.

Anuria increases the half-life of penicillin G from a normal value of 0.5 hour to about 10 hours. When renal function is impaired, 7 to 10% of the antibiotic may be inactivated per hour by the liver. This probably accounts for its failure to accumulate in excessive concentrations in anuric persons given multiple doses. Patients with renal shutdown who require vigorous therapy with penicillin can be treated adequately with 3 million units of aqueous penicillin G followed by additional injections of 1.5 million units every 8 to 12 hours. The dose of the drug must be readjusted during the period of progressive recovery of renal function. If, in addition to renal failure, hepatic insufficiency is also present, the half-life will be prolonged further. It may be necessary to determine the half-life of the drug for the individual patient.

Once penicillin G is released from its repository forms (penicillin G procaine and penicillin G benzathine), it is excreted by the kidney as described above. However, because absorption into the blood from the injection site is continued over a long period, the excretion of active antibiotic in the urine is prolonged. For example, Wright and coworkers (1959) detected penicillin G in the urine of 100% of patients 84 days after an intramuscular injection of 1.2 million units of penicillin G benzathine.

6-Aminopenicillanic acid has been demonstrated in the urine of individuals given oral penicillin. It probably is produced by microbial hydrolytic conversion of penicillin in the intestinal tract, and subsequently it is absorbed and then excreted by the kidney.

Bile and Other Fluids. Penicillin G is present in human bile, from both the liver and gallbladder, where it is more concentrated and persists longer than in plasma. Indeed, a major site of extrarenal disposition of penicillin is the liver. Biliary excretion of the drug is directly proportional to the adequacy of hepatic function. Because the duodenum is the main site for the enteric absorption of the antibiotic, it is possible that some of the drug excreted in the bile is reabsorbed by the intestinal mucosa. Some inactivation of the antibiotic takes place in the bile.

A small amount of penicillin G is excreted in human milk and saliva, the concentrations being lower than in plasma. The drug does not appear in detectable quantities in the sweat or tears in man.

Preparations. Preparations of penicillin G that are available for parenteral use include aqueous solutions and repository forms that are slowly absorbed from intramuscular depots. In addition, there are many preparations of penicillin G, penicillin V, and phenethicillin for oral administration. Details of *dosage* of these preparations are presented subsequently, in the discussion of the treatment of specific infections. The use of penicillin G preparations for *inhalational therapy* and for *topical application* to skin and mucous membranes is not recommended because they are ineffective and because they produce a high incidence of hypersensitization. A possible exception is the instillation of penicillin G into the conjunctiva for prevention of gonococcal ophthalmitis in the neonate. This is used in some locales instead of silver nitrate.

Penicillin G in Aqueous Solution for Parenteral Use. This type of preparation, the first to be marketed, is still widely employed. It is designed for subcutaneous, intramuscular, or intravenous injection, although its use should be limited to the intravenous route. It can be given as a bolus or by constant drip. Because of the rapid rate of renal excretion of the drug, intravenous doses should be given at close intervals (usually every 2 to 4 hours) or by constant infusion. The potassium salts are most frequently used. The two official penicillin salts for injection are *Penicillin G Potassium for Injection,* U.S.P., and *Penicillin G Sodium for Injection,* U.S.P. The preparations listed are crystalline powders, marketed for parenteral use in sterile dry form in vials or ampuls containing 200,000 to 20 million units each. Solutions are prepared by adding the solvent (sterile distilled water, 0.9% sodium chloride solution, or 5% dextrose solution) directly to the container to yield the desired concentration, usually 100,000 or 200,000 units/ml. It should be remembered that each million units of penicillin G potassium contains about 1.7 mEq of potassium. Because the stability of penicillin G is affected by changes in pH (it is most stable at pH 6 to 7.2), it is physically incompatible with many drugs; other agents should not be mixed with the penicillin solution. Usual doses of intravenous penicillin G for adults are 6 to 20 million units per day.

Penicillin G Preparations for Parenteral Use in Repository Form for Prolonged Action. Repository penicillin preparations are designed for deep intramuscular injection, to provide a tissue depot from which the drug is slowly absorbed over a period of 12 hours to several days. The objective is to maintain therapeutic concentrations in plasma with as few injections as possible. *Repository penicillin should never be injected intravenously or subcutaneously or into body cavities.*

Sterile Penicillin G Procaine Suspension, U.S.P. (CRYSTICILLIN, DIURNAL-PENICILLIN, DURACILLIN A.S., WYCILLIN SUSPENSION, others), is an aqueous preparation of the crystalline salt that is soluble in water only to the extent of 0.4%. Penicillin G procaine preparations are marketed for intramuscular injection in 1-, 2-, and 4-ml cartridges and 10-ml vials, each milliliter usually containing 300,000, 500,000, or 600,000 units of the antibiotic.

Procaine combines with penicillin mole for mole; therefore, a dose of 300,000 units contains approximately 120 mg of procaine. When large doses of penicillin G procaine are given (*e.g.,* 4.8 million units), procaine may reach toxic concentrations in the plasma (*see* Green *et al.,* 1974). If the patient is believed to be hypersensitive to procaine, 0.1 ml of 1% solution of procaine should be injected intradermally; individuals exhibiting a positive local response should not be given penicillin G procaine. A slight anesthetic effect of the procaine accounts in part for the fact that injections of penicillin G procaine are virtually painless.

Sterile Penicillin G Benzathine Suspension, U.S.P. (BICILLIN, PERMAPEN), is the aqueous suspension of the salt obtained by the combination of 1 mole of an ammonium base and 2 moles of penicillin G to yield N,N'-dibenzylethylenediamine dipenicillin G. The salt itself is soluble in water only to the extent of 0.02%. It is provided for intramuscular injection in 10-ml vials containing 300,000 units/ml and in prefilled syringes (1, 1.5, 2, and 4 ml) containing 600,000 units/ml. The long persistence of penicillin in the blood after a suitable intramuscular dose reduces cost, need for repeated injections, and local trauma. The local anesthetic effect of penicillin G benzathine is comparable to that of penicillin G procaine. Penicillin G benzathine should be used only for treatment or prophylaxis of group-A beta-hemolytic streptococcal pharyngitis, treatment of group-A beta-hemolytic streptococcal pyoderma, or treatment of syphilis outside the central nervous system (CNS).

Certain nonofficial repository preparations for intramuscular use combine an insoluble penicillin G salt (procaine or benzathine) with a soluble salt of penicillin (sodium or potassium). They are designed to provide both the rapid establishment of high plasma concentrations and the prolonged effect of depot penicillin. Some question has been raised about the rationale underlying the use of these combinations. Bacteria eradicated by the repository penicillin are not more rapidly killed by the brief exposure to the higher concentration of drug afforded by the preparation; on the other hand, bacteria that can be eradicated only with a high concentration of penicillin G are not affected by the low persistent concentrations achieved with the repository preparation. These preparations are thus *not* recommended.

Preparations of Penicillin G, Penicillin V, and Phenethicillin for Oral Use. The official oral preparations of penicillin G are *Penicillin G Potassium Tablets,* U.S.P., *Penicillin G Potassium Tablets for Oral Solution,* U.S.P., and *Penicillin G Benzathine Tablets,* U.S.P. They are usually marketed as tablets containing from 100,000 to 800,000 units. Various buffer materials are sometimes added; these increase stability of the antibiotic but do not significantly protect against destruction of penicillin G in the acidic gastric contents. Dry salts of penicillin G mixed with flavoring material and various buffers are available for pediatric use. The requisite dose can be mixed with syrup, water, or milk, or added to the milk formula for infants.

Penicillin V Potassium, U.S.P. (COMPOCILLIN-V K, PEN-VEE K, V-CILLIN K, others), is supplied for oral use as official tablets (125, 250, or 500 mg each) and granules for solution (125 or 250 mg/5 ml). Suspensions (125 or 250 mg/5 ml) are also available. *Penicillin V,* U.S.P., is marketed under trade names and in official dosage forms and unitages similar to those for the potassium salt. *Penicillin V Benzathine,* U.S.P., and *Penicillin V Hydrabamine,* U.S.P., are additional official preparations.

The official preparations of phenethicillin are *Phenethicillin Potassium,* U.S.P. (MAXIPEN, SYNCILLIN), *Phenethicillin Potassium for Oral Solution,* U.S.P., and *Phenethicillin Potassium Tablets,* U.S.P. However, the drug is not available commercially in the United States at the present time.

Therapeutic Uses. Penicillin G is the antibiotic of choice for a wide variety of infectious diseases (*see* Table 48–1, page 1086). When therapy with an orally effective penicillin is indicated, advantage can be taken of the properties of its acid-stable congeners, particularly penicillin V.

Pneumococcal Infections. Penicillin G remains the agent of choice for the management of infections of all types caused by *Strep. pneumoniae.* However, rare strains of pneumococci resistant to usual doses of penicillin G have been encountered in several countries, including the United States (*see* Jacobs *et al.,* 1978).

Pneumococcal Pneumonia. A variety of dose schedules and types of penicillin have been employed successfully in the treatment of pneumococcal pneumonia. For parenteral therapy, penicillin G or penicillin G procaine are favored, and 300,000 to 600,000 units of procaine penicillin G, given intramuscularly every 12 hours, is adequate therapy for uncomplicated cases. Although oral treatment with 500 mg of penicillin V given every 6 hours has been used with success in this disease, it cannot be recommended for routine initial use. The doses of penicillin G currently used are, in all probability, excessive. Therapy should be continued for 7 to 10 days, including 3 to 5 days after the temperature has returned to normal.

Pneumococcal Empyema. The frequency of this complication of pneumococcal pneumonia has been sharply reduced by penicillin therapy of the primary lung disease. It is not necessary to instill the antibiotic intrapleurally when purulent exudate is present in the pleural sac; in such instances, however, the dose of penicillin should be increased to 10 to 20 million units per day, and adequate drainage must be ensured. Patients frequently develop nonpurulent pleural effusions that do not contain pneumococci; these can be treated by drainage, and it is not necessary to increase the dosage of penicillin G.

Pneumococcal Meningitis. Penicillin has reduced the death rate in this disease from nearly 100% to between 8 and 25%. The recommended therapy is 20 to 24 million units of penicillin G daily by constant intravenous drip or divided into boluses given every 2 to 3 hours. The usual duration of therapy is 14 days.

Other Pneumococcal Infections. Penicillin G provides optimal therapy for suppurative *arthritis, osteomyelitis, acute suppurative mastoiditis, endocarditis, peritonitis,* and *pericarditis* due to the pneumococcus. Because of poor penetration of the drug into purulent exudate, the plasma and tissue-fluid concentrations must be high; this is best accomplished by the intravenous administration of large doses of aqueous penicillin G. Doses of the order of 10 to 20 million units per day are probably required for cure. Oral and repository penicillins should not be used. The shortest period of treatment for any of these disorders should be 2 weeks. This should be prolonged to at least 4 weeks if there is infection of bone. Infections in the *middle ear* and *paranasal sinuses* caused by the pneumococcus may be treated

with 300,000 to 600,000 units of procaine penicillin G intramuscularly every 12 hours or with 250 to 500 mg of oral penicillin V every 6 hours.

Streptococcal Infections. Streptococcal Pharyngitis (Including Scarlet Fever). This is the most common disease produced by *Strep. pyogenes* (group-A beta-hemolytic streptococcus). The preferred oral therapy is with penicillin V, 500 mg every 6 hours for 10 days. Equally good results are produced by the administration of 600,000 units of penicillin G procaine intramuscularly, once daily for 10 days, or by a single injection of 1.2 million units of penicillin G benzathine. Penicillin therapy of streptococcal pharyngitis reduces the risk of subsequent acute rheumatic fever; however, present evidence suggests that the incidence of glomerulonephritis that follows streptococcal infections is not reduced to a significant degree by treatment with penicillin.

Streptococcal Pneumonia, Arthritis, Meningitis, and Endocarditis. While uncommon, when these conditions are caused by *Strep. pyogenes,* they should be treated with daily doses of 10 to 20 million units of penicillin G intravenously for 2 to 4 weeks. Such treatment of endocarditis should be continued for a full 4 weeks.

Streptococcal Otitis Media and Sinusitis. Treatment with an oral preparation, such as 250 to 500 mg of penicillin V every 6 hours for 2 weeks, is usually adequate. Streptococcal mastoiditis is now an uncommon complication of otitis media; it should be treated with high doses of parenteral penicillin G for at least 2 weeks.

Infections Due to Other Streptococci. Group-B (*Strep. agalactiae*) streptococcal infections, including meningitis and bacteremia, are frequent in neonates and should be treated with high doses of penicillin G given parenterally (150,000 to 250,000 units/kg per day).

The *viridans* streptococci are the most common cause of infectious endocarditis. These are nongroupable alpha-hemolytic microorganisms that are usually highly sensitive to penicillin G (minimal inhibitory concentration less than 0.1 μg/ml). Since enterococci may also be beta-hemolytic and certain other alpha-hemolytic strains may be relatively resistant to penicillin, it is important to determine quantitative microbial sensitivities to penicillin G in patients with endocarditis. Patients with penicillin-sensitive *viridans*-group streptococcal endocarditis have been successfully treated with 1.2 million units of procaine penicillin G, given four times daily for 4 weeks, or with daily doses of 6 to 10 million units of intravenous penicillin G for 4 weeks. Some physicians also administer streptomycin, 500 mg intramuscularly twice daily, for the first 2 weeks of a 4-week course of penicillin. Others have had good results with a 2-week course of treatment with both penicillin G and streptomycin.

Enterococcal endocarditis is one of the few diseases that is optimally treated with two antibiotics. The recommended therapy is 20 million units of penicillin G daily, administered intravenously in combination with an aminoglycoside. Some physicians prefer to initiate treatment with streptomycin, 1 g intramuscularly every 12 hours for 2 weeks followed by 500 mg intramuscularly every 12 hours for the next 4 weeks. In cases in which there is no demonstrable synergism (*in vitro*) between penicillin and streptomycin, gentamicin is substituted for streptomycin; the dose is 80 mg every 8 hours in patients with normal renal function. Synergism between penicillin and streptomycin may be determined with standard tests (*see* Chapter 48). Sometimes therapy is instituted with a combination of penicillin and gentamicin, since this combination is synergistic for more strains of enterococci than is that of penicillin and streptomycin.

Infections with Anaerobes. Many anaerobic infections are caused by mixtures of microorganisms. The majority are sensitive to penicillin G. An exception is *Bacteroides fragilis,* where 20 to 50% of strains may be resistant to high concentrations of this antibiotic. Pulmonary and periodontal infections respond well to penicillin G. Mild-to-moderate infections at these sites may be treated with oral medication (either penicillin G or penicillin V, 400,000 units four times daily). More severe infections should be treated with 10 to 20 million units of penicillin G intravenously. Anaerobic infections involving the gastrointestinal tract and certain pelvic infections may be due in part to *B. fragilis.* Either clindamycin or chloramphenicol should be given to treat infections that are caused by this microorganism. Because aerobic gram-negative bacteria may also be involved, an aminoglycoside should be included for the treatment of anaerobic infections originating from the gastrointestinal tract. Brain abscesses also frequently contain several species of anaerobes, and most authorities prefer to treat such disease with high doses of penicillin G (20 million units per day) plus chloramphenicol (2 to 4 g per day, intravenously).

Staphylococcal Infections. The majority of staphylococcal infections (60 to 80%) are caused by microorganisms that produce penicillinase and are thus resistant to therapy with most penicillins. A patient with a staphylococcal infection who requires treatment with an antibiotic should receive one of the penicillinase-resistant penicillins—for example, nafcillin, oxacillin, or methicillin. However, since penicillin G is more active than are the penicillinase-resistant penicillins against staphylococci that do not produce the enzyme, it should be utilized when staphylococcal sensitivity to penicillin G has been demonstrated. Severe infections should be treated with intravenous doses of 10 to 20 million units of penicillin G per day.

Several hospitals throughout the world have reported infections due to so-called methicillin-resistant staphylococci. These microorganisms are resistant to penicillin G, all of the penicillinase-resistant penicillins, and, usually, the cephalosporins. Vancomycin appears to be the therapy of choice for infections caused by these bacteria; rifampin is sometimes used concurrently.

Meningococcal Infections. Penicillin G remains the drug of choice for meningococcal disease. Patients should be treated with high doses of penicillin given intravenously, as described for pneumococcal meningitis. It should be remembered that penicillin G does not eliminate the meningococcal carrier state, and its administration is thus ineffective as a prophylactic measure.

Gonococcal Infections. Gonococci have gradually become more resistant to penicillin G, and thus higher doses of the antibiotic are now recommended for treatment of gonococcal infections. In addition, there are rare strains of penicillinase-producing gonococci that are totally resistant to the administration of penicillin G. In spite of this, a penicillin preparation remains the therapy of choice for most gonococcal infections. In view of the nature of the disease and the patient population in which it is most prevalent, it is desirable to complete treatment, if possible, in one visit. Uncomplicated gonococcal urethritis is most common, and, because of safety and acceptability to patients, the oral administration of amoxicillin (3 g) *plus* probenecid (1 g) or ampicillin (3.5 g) plus probenecid is recommended. A total of 4.8 million units of penicillin G procaine injected into two sites combined with oral probenecid (1 g) is equally efficacious. Oral penicillin V or penicillin G is *not* adequate therapy for gonococcal infections, and penicillin G benzathine does not provide adequate therapeutic concentrations. Treatment of contacts of known cases of gonorrhea is the same as is that for gonococcal urethritis. Patients with gonococcal pharyngitis respond better to intramuscular procaine penicillin G than to the oral regimens.

Pelvic inflammatory disease can be caused by the gonococcus. Mild cases respond well to treatment by a single administration of 4.8 million units of procaine penicillin G intramuscularly; equally effective is oral dosage with either amoxicillin (3 g) or ampicillin (3.5 g), followed by the same drug (0.5 g) taken orally four times a day for 10 days. Severely ill patients may require hospitalization; it may be necessary to drain abscesses and to administer parenteral doses of 10 to 20 million units of penicillin G per day.

Gonococcal arthritis has been treated with a variety of regimens, including those outlined for pelvic inflammatory disease. Some physicians prefer the intravenous administration of 10 million units of penicillin G daily for 3 days, followed by ampicillin or amoxicillin given orally for 5 to 7 additional days. Disseminated gonococcal infections with skin lesions and gonococcemia should be treated similarly. Gonococcal endocarditis is a very rare disease and requires treatment with 10 to 20 million units of penicillin G intravenously daily for at least 4 weeks. Ophthalmia neonatorum is readily cured by parenteral penicillin G. Some pediatricians prefer aqueous penicillin G for the neonate because of the possibility of adverse reactions to procaine penicillin.

Syphilis. Therapy of syphilis with penicillin G is highly effective. Primary, secondary, and latent syphilis of less than 1 year's duration should be treated with a single intramuscular dose of 2.4 million units of penicillin G benzathine. Patients with latent syphilis of more than 1 year's duration should also be treated with penicillin G benzathine, 2.4 million units weekly for 4 weeks. Penicillin G benzathine should not be used for the therapy of neurosyphilis, since concentrations of the drug in CSF may not be sufficient to eradicate the spirochetes. Patients with neurosyphilis or cardiovascular syphilis may be treated with a variety of regimens. Since these diseases are potentially lethal and their progression can be halted (but not reversed), intensive therapy with 20 million units of penicillin G daily for 14 days is recommended.

Infants with congenital syphilis discovered at birth or during the postnatal period should be treated for 10 days with 50,000 units/kg daily of aqueous penicillin G in two divided doses or 50,000 units/kg of procaine penicillin G in a single daily dose. If the CSF is normal and there is no evidence of neurological involvement, penicillin G benzathine can be given as a single dose (50,000 units/kg).

The vast majority (90% or more) of patients with secondary syphilis develop the Jarisch-Herxheimer reaction. This may also be seen in patients with other forms of syphilis. Several hours after the first injection of penicillin, the patient may develop chills, fever, headache, myalgias, and arthralgias. The syphilitic cutaneous lesions may become more prominent, edematous, and brilliant in color. Manifestations usually persist for a few hours, and the rash begins to fade within 48 hours. It does not recur with the second or subsequent injections of penicillin. This reaction is thought to be due to release of spirochetal antigens, with subsequent host reactions to the products. Therapy should be continued if the Jarisch-Herxheimer reaction occurs.

Actinomycosis. Penicillin G is the agent of choice for the treatment of all forms of actinomycosis. The dose should be 10 to 20 million units of penicillin G intravenously per day for 6 weeks. Some physicians continue therapy for 2 to 3 months with oral penicillin V (500 mg four times daily). Surgical drainage or excision of the lesion may be necessary before cure is accomplished.

Diphtheria. There is no evidence that penicillin or any other antibiotic alters the incidence of complications or the outcome of diphtheria; specific antitoxin is the only effective treatment. However, penicillin G eliminates the carrier state. The parenteral administration of 2 to 3 million units per day, in divided doses for 10 to 12 days, eliminates the diphtheria bacilli from the pharynx and other sites in practically 100% of cases. A single daily injection of penicillin G procaine for the same period produces about the same results. Erythromycin appears to be as effective, and some consider it to be preferable.

Anthrax. Penicillin G is the agent of choice in the treatment of all clinical forms of anthrax. However, strains of *B. anthracis* resistant to this antibiotic have been recovered from human infections. When penicillin G is used, the dose should be 10 to 20 million units per day.

Clostridial Infections. Penicillin G is the agent of choice for *gas gangrene;* the dose is in the range of 10 to 20 million units per day, given parenterally. Adequate debridement of the infected areas is essential. Antimicrobial drugs probably have no effect on the ultimate outcome of *tetanus.* Debridement and administration of human tetanus immune globulin may be indicated. Penicillin is administered, however, to eradicate the vegetative forms of the bacteria that may persist.

Fusospirochetal Infections. Gingivostomatitis, produced by the synergistic action of *Leptotrichia buccalis* and spirochetes that are present in the mouth, is readily treatable with penicillin. For simple "trench mouth," 500 mg of penicillin V given every 6 hours for several days is usually sufficient to clear the disease.

Rat-Bite Fever. The two microorganisms responsible for this infection, *Spirillum minor* in the Orient and *Streptobacillus moniliformis* in America and Europe, are sensitive to penicillin G, the therapeutic agent of choice. Since most cases due to the streptobacillus are complicated by bacteremia and, in many instances, by metastatic infections especially of the synovia and endocardium, the dose should be large; a daily dose of 12 to 15 million units given parenterally, for 3 to 4 weeks, has been recommended.

Listeria Infections. Penicillin G is regarded as the drug of choice in the management of infections due to *List. monocytogenes;* ampicillin is also effective. The recommended dose of penicillin G is 15 to 20 million units parenterally per day, for at least 2 weeks. When endocarditis is the problem, the dose is the same, but the duration of treatment should be no less than 4 weeks.

Pasteurella Infections. The only species of *Pasteurella* highly susceptible to penicillin is *Past. multocida.* Soft-tissue infection, bacteremia, and meningitis are the most common forms of the disease produced by this microorganism in man, and often follow animal bites. Penicillin G, 4 to 6 million units per day parenterally for at least 2 weeks, is effectively curative.

Erysipeloid. The causative agent of this disease, *Erysipelothrix rhusiopathiae,* is sensitive to penicillin. The uncomplicated infection responds well to a single injection of 1.2 million units of penicillin G benzathine. When endocarditis is present, penicillin G, 2 to 20 million units per day, has been found effective; therapy should be continued for 4 to 6 weeks.

Prophylactic Uses of the Penicillins. Demonstration of the effectiveness of penicillin in eradicating microorganisms was quickly, and quite naturally, followed by attempts to prove that it was also effective in preventing infection in susceptible hosts. As a result, the antibiotic has been administered in almost every situation in which a risk of bacterial invasion has been present. As prophylaxis has been investigated under controlled conditions, it has become clear that penicillin is highly effective in some situations, useless and potentially dangerous in others, and of questionable value in still others (*see* Chapter 48).

Streptococcal Infections. The administration of penicillin to individuals exposed to *Strep. pyogenes* affords a predictable and high order of protection. The oral ingestion of 200,000 units of penicillin G or penicillin V twice a day or a single injection of 1.2 million units of penicillin G benzathine has been found effective. Such therapy may promptly and markedly reduce the carrier rate. Some objections have been raised to the routine use of penicillin as prophylaxis in individuals who have had contact with *Strep. pyogenes* on the ground that the risks of reactions to the drug are as great as those associated with the disease. In addition, evidence indicating that the carrier state leads to the development of type-specific immunity has raised serious questions concerning prophylaxis with penicillin, since this tends to suppress or abolish immune responses to *Strep. pyogenes*. This type of prophylaxis finds a rational use in closed populations of young people who are experiencing a high incidence of streptococcal infection. Patients with extensive deep burns are at high risk of developing severe wound infections with *Strep. pyogenes;* several days of "low-dose" prophylaxis appears to be effective in reducing the incidence of this complication.

Recurrences of Rheumatic Fever. Although not all individuals who have had rheumatic fever have residual valvular damage, their susceptibility to recurrent episodes and the risk of cardiac injury in subsequent attacks make it imperative that everyone who has recovered from this disorder be protected against infection by the beta-hemolytic streptococcus. The oral administration of 200,000 units of penicillin G or penicillin V every 12 hours produces a striking decrease in the incidence of recurrences of rheumatic fever in susceptible individuals. Because of the difficulties associated with oral treatment, mainly the fact that patients neglect to take the drug, parenteral administration is preferable, especially in children. The intramuscular injection of 1.2 million units of penicillin G benzathine once a month yields excellent results. In cases of hypersensitivity to penicillin, sulfisoxazole or sulfadiazine, 1 g twice a day for adults, is also effective; for children weighing under 27 kg, the dose is halved. Prophylaxis must be continued throughout the year. The duration of such treatment is an unsettled question. It has been suggested that prophylaxis should be continued for life, because instances of acute rheumatic fever have been observed in the fifth and sixth decades. However, the necessity for such prolonged prophylaxis has not been established.

Gonorrhea. The conjunctival instillation of a penicillin G solution in neonates is highly effective in preventing *gonorrheal ophthalmia*. Sexual contacts of patients with gonorrhea should receive a course of antibiotics identical to that described for the treatment of gonococcal urethritis.

Syphilis. Prophylaxis for a contact with syphilis consists in the intramuscular administration of 4.8 million units of penicillin G procaine plus 1 g of oral probenicid (this is also effective for gonorrhea) or 2.4 million units of penicillin G benzathine within 24 hours after exposure. A serological test for syphilis should be performed at monthly intervals for at least 4 months thereafter.

Surgical Procedures in Patients with Valvular Heart Disease. About 25% of cases of subacute bacterial endocarditis follow dental extractions. This observation, together with the fact that up to 80% of persons who have teeth removed experience a transient bacteremia, emphasizes the potential importance of chemoprophylaxis for those who have congenital or acquired heart disease of any type and need to un-

dergo dental procedures. Even such mild manipulations as the scaling of teeth may result in transient bacteremia. This procedure should be "covered" by prophylaxis when it is performed in patients with known valvular lesions. Since transient bacterial invasion of the blood stream occurs occasionally after surgical procedures such as tonsillectomy and operations on the genitourinary and intestinal tracts and during childbirth, these too are indications for prophylaxis in patients with valvular heart disease. Bacteremia is not eliminated by the use of penicillin. Whether the incidence of bacterial endocarditis is actually altered to an appreciable degree by this type of chemoprophylaxis remains to be determined.

Detailed recommendations for both adults and children with valvular heart disease have been formulated by a committee of the American Heart Association (*see* Kaplan *et al.,* 1977). Briefly, for dental procedures that are likely to result in gingival bleeding or for surgery or instrumentation of the respiratory tract, two alternative regimens are recommended. Drugs are administered 30 minutes to 1 hour prior to the procedure and for 2 days thereafter. One regimen relies solely on penicillin (combinations of parenteral and oral preparations or oral administration alone), while the other utilizes both parenteral penicillin G and streptomycin, followed by penicillin V. The latter protocol is particularly recommended for patients with prosthetic heart valves. Alternative schemes for prophylaxis in patients who are allergic to penicillin are also offered. These rely on erythromycin or on a combination of vancomycin followed by erythromycin. For surgery or examination of the genitourinary or gastrointestinal tract, aqueous penicillin G or ampicillin plus gentamicin or streptomycin are recommended in courses that span approximately 1 day. For those who are allergic to penicillin, reliance is placed on a combination of vancomycin and streptomycin.

Penicillin Prophylaxis of No Value. A number of disorders in which penicillin has been used prophylactically have been shown by carefully controlled study to be unaffected by such treatment as far as secondary bacterial invasion is concerned. Among these are numerous viral infections, coma, shock, heart failure, elective and uncontaminated surgical procedures, "clean" wounds, normal obstetrical delivery, catheterization of the urinary tract, and prematurity.

THE PENICILLINASE-RESISTANT PENICILLINS

The penicillins described in this section are not hydrolyzed by staphylococcal penicillinase. Their appropriate use should be restricted to the treatment of infections that are known or suspected to be caused by staphylococci that elaborate the enzyme—the majority of strains of this bacterium that are encountered in the hospital *or* in the general community. These drugs are less active than is penicillin G against other penicillin-sensitive microorganisms, including non-penicillinase-producing staphylococci.

The penicillinase-resistant penicillins remain the agents of choice for most staphylococcal disease despite the increasing incidence of isolates of so-called methicillin-resistant microorganisms. As commonly used, this latter term denotes resistance of these bacteria to all of the penicillinase-resistant penicillins. Such strains are usually resistant as well to the cephalosporins, aminoglycosides, tetracyclines, erythromycin, and clindamycin. Vancomycin is considered to be the drug of choice for such infections, although some physicians use a combination of vancomycin and rifampin. The mechanism of resistance to methicillin is unknown, although it seems to be related to alterations in the cell wall of these strains. From 10 to 40% of strains of *Staph. epidermidis* are also insensitive to the penicillinase-resistant penicillins, but many of these are susceptible to the cephalosporins *in vitro*.

Methicillin. This semisynthetic penicillin is prepared from 6-aminopenicillanic acid. Its structural formula is shown in Table 50–1. The drug is highly resistant to cleavage by penicillinase.

Pharmacological Properties. Methicillin is bactericidal for nearly all strains of *Staph. aureus* at concentrations of 1 to 6 µg/ml. Microorganisms that are inhibited only by concentrations in excess of 12.5 µg/ml are considered to be resistant. Penicillinase-producing strains are from 15 to 80 times more susceptible to methicillin than to penicillin G, although it is not as effective as penicillin G against other gram-positive microorganisms. Methicillin is totally without effect on gram-negative bacteria, some of which may even inactivate it.

Methicillin is not employed by the oral route because it is poorly absorbed and readily destroyed by the acidic gastric contents. When the drug is given intramuscularly, peak concentrations in plasma are reached in about 30 minutes to 1 hour. After the conventional dose of 1 g in adults, plasma concentrations in excess of 10 µg/ml are demonstrable; a 2-g dose provides a peak concentration over 20 µg/ml, and approximately 8 µg/ml is still present after 4 hours. About 40% of the methicillin in plasma is bound to protein. The distribution and excretion of methicillin and penicillin G are essentially identical (*see* above).

Preparations and Routes of Administration. The official preparation is *Methicillin Sodium*, U.S.P. (AZAPEN, CELBENIN, STAPHCILLIN). The salt is stable in dry form and freely soluble in water. It is unstable in acidic media and loses potency when dissolved in 0.85% sodium chloride or in dextrose solution at room temperature. This instability, together with the fact that the drug is excreted rapidly, contraindicates continuous intravenous infusion unless the solutions are buffered to neutrality. The preparation employed for intramuscular or intravenous administration is *Methicillin Sodium for Injection*, U.S.P. The drug is marketed in ampuls containing 1, 4, or 6 g of the salt. The solution should be fresh, and other drugs should not be included, since many are incompatible with methicillin in solution. Intramuscular injection of methicillin is more painful than is the case for other penicillins; the need for frequent injections (every 2 to 3 hours) is a definite disadvantage when prolonged therapy by this route is required.

The Isoxazolyl Penicillins: Oxacillin, Cloxacillin, Dicloxacillin, Floxacillin. These four congeneric semisynthetic penicillins are similar pharmacologically and are thus conveniently considered together. Their structural formulas are shown in Table 50–1. All are relatively stable in an acidic medium and are adequately absorbed after oral administration. All are markedly resistant to cleavage by penicillinase. These drugs are not substitutes for penicillin G in the treatment of diseases amenable to it. Furthermore, because of variability in intestinal absorption, oral administration is not a substitute for the parenteral route in the treatment of serious staphylococcal infections that require a penicillin unaffected by penicillinase.

Pharmacological Properties. The isoxazolyl penicillins are potent inhibitors of the growth of most penicillinase-producing staphylococci. This is their valid clinical use. Dicloxacillin is the most active, and most strains of *Staph. aureus* are inhibited by concentrations of 0.05 to 0.8 µg/ml. Comparable values for cloxacillin and oxacillin are 0.1 to 3 µg/ml and 0.4 to 6 µg/ml, respectively. These differences may have little practical significance, however, since dosages are adjusted accordingly. These agents are, in general, less effective against microorganisms susceptible to penicillin G, and they are not useful against gram-negative bacteria. Microorganisms can become resistant to these drugs in a stepwise fashion, and cross-resistance to all of the penicillinase-resistant penicillins is usually complete.

These agents are rapidly but incompletely (30 to 80%) absorbed from the gastrointestinal tract. Absorption of the drugs is more efficient when they are taken on an empty stomach. Peak concentrations in plasma are attained by 1 hour and approximate 5 to 10 µg/ml after the ingestion of 1 g of oxacillin. Slightly higher concentrations are achieved after the administration of 1 g of cloxacillin, while the same oral dose of dicloxacillin or floxacillin yields peak plasma concentrations of 15 µg/ml. There is little evidence that these differences are of clinical significance. Since absorption is less than complete, higher plasma concentrations are achieved following intramuscular injection, and larger quantities of the drugs are recoverable in the urine. For example, a 500-mg dose of oxacillin given intramuscularly results in peak concentrations in plasma of approximately 15 μg/ml after 30 to 60 minutes. All these congeners are bound to plasma albumin to a great extent (approximately 90 to 95%); none is removed from the circulation to a significant degree by hemodialysis.

The isoxazolyl penicillins are rapidly excreted by the kidney, and the concurrent administration of probenecid results in higher and more persistent concentrations in plasma. Normally, 30 to 50% of any of these drugs is excreted in the urine in the first 6 hours after a conventional oral dose. There is also significant hepatic elimination of these agents in the bile. The half-lives for all are between 30 and 60 minutes. Intervals between doses of oxacillin, cloxacillin, and dicloxacillin do not have to be altered for patients with renal failure. The above-noted differences in plasma concentrations produced by the isoxazolyl penicillins are related mainly to differences in rate of urinary excretion and degree of resistance to degradation in the liver (Rosenblatt et al., 1968).

Preparations and Routes of Administration. *Oxacillin Sodium,* U.S.P. (BACTOCILL, PROSTAPHLIN), is available for oral use in official capsules containing 250 or 500 mg of drug, and as *Oxacillin Sodium for Oral Solution,* U.S.P. (250 mg/5 ml). It is readily soluble in water and stable in the dry state at room temperature. The drug is preferably administered 1 or 2 hours before meals, to ensure better absorption. The daily oral dose of oxacillin for adults is 2 to 4 g, divided into four portions; for children, 50 to 100 mg/kg per day is administered similarly. The injectable form of the drug, *Oxacillin Sodium for Injection,* U.S.P., is available in 250- and 500-mg and 1-, 2-, and 4-g vials. For adults a total of 2 to 12 g per day, and for children 100 to 300 mg/kg per day, may be given intravenously or intramuscularly, injections being given every 4 to 6 hours.

Cloxacillin Sodium, U.S.P. (CLOXAPEN, TEGOPEN), is available in capsules (250 and 500 mg) and as an oral solution (125 mg/5 ml). The dose for adults is 250 mg orally every 6 hours for mild-to-moderate infections; for severe infections, it is 500 mg or more every 6 hours. The dose for children is 50 mg/kg per day, divided into equal quantities and given every 6 hours; for those weighing more than 20 kg, adult doses have been recommended.

Dicloxacillin Sodium, U.S.P. (DYCILL, DYNAPEN, PATHOCIL, VERACILLIN), is quite stable at acidic pH, soluble in water, and stable at room temperature. The drug is available for oral use in capsules (125, 250, and 500 mg) and as a suspension (62.5 mg/5 ml). The dose for adults and for children weighing more than 40 kg is 250 mg or more every 6 hours; for children weighing less than 40 kg, the recommended daily dose is 25 mg/kg, given in four equal portions at intervals of 6 hours. Vials containing 250 mg of drug for intramuscular injection are also available; the adult dose is 200 to 500 mg every 6 hours. Because there is incomplete information at present, dicloxacillin should not be given to newborn infants.

Floxacillin is not currently available in the United States; it closely resembles cloxacillin.

Nafcillin. This semisynthetic penicillin, derived from 6-aminopenicillanic acid, is highly resistant to penicillinase and has proven effective against infections caused by penicillinase-producing strains of *Staph. aureus.* Its structural formula is shown in Table 50–1.

Pharmacological Properties. Nafcillin is slightly more active than oxacillin against penicillin G–resistant *Staph. aureus* (most strains are inhibited by 0.06 to 2 μg/ml). While it is the most active of the penicillinase-resistant penicillins against other microorganisms, it is not as potent as penicillin G.

Nafcillin is inactivated to a variable degree in the acidic medium of the gastric contents. Its absorption after oral administration is irregular, regardless of whether the drug is taken with meals or on an empty stomach. After parenteral administration, the concentration of nafcillin in plasma is lower than that produced by an equivalent dose of oxacillin. The peak plasma concentration is about 8 μg/ml 60 minutes after a 1-g intramuscular dose. This is due to a much larger apparent volume of distribution of nafcillin compared to oxacillin, resulting from a selective sequestration of the antibiotic in the liver and possibly in other tissues (Kind *et al.,* 1970). Nafcillin is bound to plasma protein to the extent of about 90%. Only approximately 10% of an oral dose of nafcillin is recoverable in the urine. Probenecid further reduces its excretion in the urine. Peak concentrations of nafcillin in bile are well above those found in plasma. Concentrations of the drug in CSF appear to be adequate for therapy of staphylococcal meningitis (*see* Ruiz and Warner, 1976).

Preparations and Routes of Administration. *Nafcillin Sodium,* U.S.P. (NAFCIL, UNIPEN), is available for oral and parenteral use. Capsules usually contain 250 mg of the drug, and a solution is also marketed for oral use. However, because of its variable absorption from the gastrointestinal tract, the oral route is not recommended. A sterile preparation for injection is supplied in vials containing 500 mg or 1, 2, or 4 g of the salt. The doses of nafcillin are the same as those described above for oxacillin. Serious staphylococcal infections should be treated with 8 to 12 g of the drug daily, given in divided doses every 4 hours. Nafcillin is not a substitute for penicillin G in the therapy of infections caused by microorganisms sensitive to the latter agent.

THE BROAD-SPECTRUM PENICILLINS: AMPICILLIN, AMOXICILLIN, AND THEIR CONGENERS

These agents have similar antibacterial activity and a spectrum that is broader than the antibiotics heretofore discussed. They are all destroyed by beta-lactamase (from both gram-positive and gram-negative bacteria) and thus are ineffective for most staphylococcal infections.

Antimicrobial Activity. Ampicillin and the related aminopenicillins are bactericidal for both gram-positive and gram-negative bacteria. They are somewhat less active than penicillin G against gram-positive cocci sensitive to the latter agent. The meningococcus, pneumococcus, gonococcus, and *List. monocytogenes* are sensitive to the drug. *Haemophilus influenzae* and the *viridans* group of streptococci are usually inhibited by very low concentrations of ampicillin. However, strains of type-b *H. influenzae* highly resistant to ampicillin have been recovered from children with meningitis. It is estimated that 5% of cases of *H. influenzae* meningitis are now caused by ampicillin-resistant strains, although some localities report that up to 30% of strains of type-b *H. influenzae* are resistant to the drug. Enterococci are about twice as sensitive to ampicillin, on a weight basis, as they are to penicillin G (minimal inhibitory concentration for ampicillin averages 1.5 $\mu g/ml$). Although most strains of *E. coli, Pr. mirabilis, Salmonella,* and *Shigella* were highly susceptible when ampicillin was first used in the early 1960s, an increasing percentage of these species is now resistant. From 30 to 50% of *E. coli,* a significant number of *Pr. mirabilis,* and practically all species of *Enterobacter* are presently insensitive. Resistant strains of *Salmonella* (episome mediated) have been recovered with increasing frequency in various parts of the world. Most strains of *Shigella* are now resistant. Most strains of *Pseudomonas, Klebsiella, Serratia, Acinetobacter,* and indole-positive *Proteus* are also resistant to this group of penicillins; these antibiotics are less active against *B. fragilis* than is penicillin G.

Ampicillin. This drug is the prototypical agent of the group. Its structural formula is shown in Table 50–1.

Pharmacological Properties. Ampicillin is stable in acid and is well absorbed after oral administration. An oral dose of 0.5 g produces peak concentrations in plasma of about 3 $\mu g/ml$ at 2 hours. The drug is detectable in the plasma for about 4 hours after a conventional oral dose. Intake of food prior to ingestion of ampicillin results in less complete absorption. Intramuscular injection of 0.5 or 1 g of sodium ampicillin yields peak plasma concentrations of about 7 or 10 $\mu g/ml$, respectively, at 1 hour; these decline exponentially with a half-time approximating 90 minutes (*see* Eickhoff *et al.,* 1965). Administration of equal doses of penicillin G and ampicillin results in higher plasma concentrations of the latter agent because of its slower rate of renal elimination.

The administration of probenecid leads to increased concentration and persistence of ampicillin in the plasma. About one half of an oral dose is cleared by the kidney in the first 6 hours following ingestion. Approximately 70% of an intramuscular or intravenous dose of 500 mg is eliminated in the urine in this time. Severe renal impairment markedly prolongs the persistence of ampicillin in the plasma. Peritoneal dialysis is ineffective in removing the drug from the blood, but hemodialysis removes about 40% of the body store in about 7 hours. Adjustment of the dose of ampicillin is required in the presence of renal dysfunction (*see* Appendix II).

Ampicillin appears in the bile, undergoes enterohepatic circulation, and is excreted in appreciable quantities in the feces. Biliary concentration of the drug is markedly dependent on the integrity of the gallbladder and its ducts (Mortimer *et al.,* 1969). When the common bile duct is obstructed, ampicillin is not detectable in the bile.

Preparations and Routes of Administration. Ampicillin, U.S.P. (AMCILL, OMNIPEN, PENBRITIN, POLYCILLIN, others), is available for oral use in capsules containing 250 or 500 mg or in 125-mg tablets; for parenteral use, as the sodium salt in vials containing from 125 mg to 10 g; as the sodium salt for oral suspension (125 or 250 mg/5 ml); and in pediatric drops (100 mg/ml). The dose varies with the type and the severity of the infection being treated, with renal function, and with age. For children, doses cannot be prescribed on the basis of body weight or surface area; because the drug is excreted mainly by the kidney, the state of renal function to a great extent determines the dose. Very young babies thus require small doses, while children 3 to 4 years old may receive quantities almost as large as those given to adults. For mild-to-moderately severe disease, the oral dose for adults is 2 to 4 g per day, divided into equal portions and given every 6 hours. For severe infections, it is best to administer the drug parenterally in doses ranging from 6 to 12 g per day. The treatment of meningitis requires the use of large doses, 300 to 400 mg/kg per day parenterally (in equally divided portions given every 4 hours) for children, and 12 g or more per day for adults. Solutions should be freshly prepared prior to injection.

Amoxicillin. This drug, a penicillinase-susceptible semisynthetic penicillin, is a close chemical and pharmacological relative of ampicillin (*see* Table 50–1). The drug is stable in acid and is designed for oral use. The antimicrobial spectrum of amoxicillin is essentially identical to that of ampicillin, with the important exception that amoxicillin appears to be less effective than ampicillin for shigellosis. (*See* International Symposium, 1974; Neu, 1979b.)

Amoxicillin is more rapidly and completely absorbed from the gastrointestinal tract than is ampicillin, which is the major difference between the two. Peak concentrations in plasma are two to two and one-half times greater for amoxicillin than for ampicillin after oral administration of the same dose; they are reached at 2 hours and average about 4 $\mu g/ml$ when 250 mg is administered. Food does not interfere with absorption. Perhaps because of more complete absorption of this congener, the incidence of diarrhea with amoxicillin is less than that following administration of ampicillin. The incidence of other adverse effects appears to be similar. While the half-life of amoxicillin is similar to that for ampicillin, effective concentrations of orally administered amoxicillin are detectable in the plasma for twice as long as with ampicillin, again because of the more complete absorption. About 20% of amoxicillin is protein bound in plasma, a value similar to that for ampicillin. Approximately 50% of a dose of the antibiotic is excreted in an active form in the urine, in contrast to only about 30% of ampicillin. This also correlates with the difference in absorption. Probenecid delays excretion of the drug. (See Gordon et al., 1972; Kerrebijn and Michel, 1973; Rolinson, 1973; see also Appendix II.)

Amoxicillin, U.S.P. (AMOXIL, LAROTID, others), is available for oral use in capsules (250 or 500 mg), as an oral suspension (125 or 250 mg/5 ml), and as pediatric drops (50 mg/ml). The recommended dose of amoxicillin is similar to that of ampicillin (250 to 500 mg in adults), except that it is given three instead of four times a day.

Hetacillin. This drug is also a chemical modification of ampicillin. Indeed, in the body, hetacillin is very rapidly hydrolyzed to ampicillin and acetone. It is acid resistant. The antibacterial spectrum is the same as that of ampicillin. Peak concentrations in plasma are reached 2 hours after an oral dose and are lower than those produced by an equal quantity of ampicillin. The ingestion of food prior to the drug slows absorption. After intramuscular or oral administration of 450 mg, maximal plasma concentrations are about 6 or 2.5 $\mu g/ml$, respectively. Antibacterial activity is still detectable in the blood 8 hours after an oral dose.

While hetacillin has been used successfully in the therapy of a variety of infections, it is doubtful that this congener has any advantages to recommend its use in place of ampicillin.

Hetacillin, U.S.P. (VERSAPEN), is available in capsules, suspension, and pediatric drops for oral use. When the drug is prepared for oral use as a suspension or as pediatric drops, it is stable for 7 days at room temperature and 14 days under refrigeration. The doses of hetacillin recommended are often too low; they should be at least as large as those of ampicillin.

Other Congeners. *Pivampicillin* is the pivaloyloxymethyl ester of ampicillin. It too is active only after conversion to ampicillin *in vivo*. Absorption after oral administration is similar to that for amoxicillin. There is no indication that the use of this drug will offer any advantage. *Bacampicillin* and *talampicillin* are two other similar esters of ampicillin. *Epicillin* and *cyclacillin* are newer aminopenicillins that are also similar to ampicillin and have no advantage over the parent compound. None of these drugs, with the exception of cyclacillin (CYCLAPEN), is currently available in the United States.

Therapeutic Indications for the Broad-Spectrum Penicillins. *Gonococcal Infections.* Ampicillin and amoxicillin are now considered to be agents of first choice for the treatment of gonococcal urethritis. The uses of these drugs for this and other forms of gonococcal disease are described in more detail above (page 1139).

Upper Respiratory Infections. Ampicillin and amoxicillin are active against *H. influenzae*, *Strep. pneumoniae*, and *Strep. pyogenes*, which are the major upper respiratory bacterial pathogens. The drugs constitute effective therapy for sinusitis, otitis media, acute exacerbations of chronic bronchitis, and epiglottitis. Bacterial pharyngitis should be treated with penicillin G or penicillin V, since *Strep. pyogenes* is the major pathogen.

Urinary Tract Infections. Most uncomplicated urinary tract infections are caused by Enterobacteriaceae, and *E. coli* is the most common species. A sulfonamide (see Chapter 49) or ampicillin is often considered to be the drug of choice. Enterococcal urinary tract infections are treated effectively with ampicillin alone.

Meningitis. Acute bacterial meningitis in children is most frequently due to *H. influenzae*, *Strep. pneumoniae*, or *Neisseria meningitidis*. Ampicillin is frequently used for therapy. Since 5 to 30% of strains of *H. influenzae* may be resistant to this antibiotic, it is recommended that chloramphenicol be given concurrently at first until the microorganism is identified and its sensitivities are determined. Alternatives include the use of chloramphenicol alone or a combination of penicillin G and chloramphenicol.

Salmonella Infections. Uncomplicated gastroenteritis caused by *Salmonella* probably should not be treated with antibiotics. Such therapy probably has little influence on the course of the disease and *prolongs* the period of postconvalescent excretion of the microorganisms. Disease associated with bacteremia, disease with metastatic foci, and the enteric fever syndrome (including typhoid fever) respond favorably to antibiotics. Chloramphenicol is still considered to be the drug of choice, but the administration of high doses of ampicillin (12 g per day for adults) is also effective. The typhoid carrier state has been successfully eliminated in patients without gallbladder disease who have been given 6 g of ampicillin daily for 1 to 3 months.

Other Infections. The dual administration of ampicillin and an aminoglycoside may be used to treat sepsis caused by gram-negative bacteria acquired in the general community. After sensitivities of infecting microorganisms are known, it is advisable to treat with a beta-lactam antibiotic and to discontinue the aminoglycoside, if possible. Thus, ampicillin may be used alone to treat a variety of serious gram-negative infections once the bacterial sensitivities have been determined.

CARBENICILLIN, TICARCILLIN,
AND RELATED PENICILLINS

These antibiotics are active against most isolates of *Pseudomonas aeruginosa* and certain indole-positive *Proteus* species that are resistant to ampicillin and its congeners. They are ineffective against most strains of *Staph. aureus. Bacteroides fragilis* is susceptible to high concentrations of these drugs, but penicillin G is actually more active on a weight basis (Maki *et al.,* 1978).

Carbenicillin and Carbenicillin Indanyl.
Carbenicillin. This drug is a penicillinase-susceptible derivative of 6-aminopenicillanic acid. Its structural formula is shown in Table 50–1. The major advantage of this agent is that it often cures serious infections caused by *Pseudomonas* species, *Proteus* strains resistant to ampicillin, and certain other gram-negative microorganisms.

Low concentrations of carbenicillin inhibit the growth of *Pr. mirabilis* and many microorganisms sensitive to penicillin G. *Escherichia coli, Enterobacter,* and *Salmonella* are less sensitive. The majority of strains of *Pr. vulgaris* and *Pseud. aeruginosa* are sensitive to 25 μg/ml or less of the drug; 70 to 80% of *Pseudomonas* are inhibited by 100 μg/ml. Penicillin G–resistant staphylococci, *Klebsiella,* and *Serratia* are usually resistant to carbenicillin. Enterococci are suppressed in the range of 50 to 100 μg/ml. Bacterial resistance may appear *in vivo* during treatment with suboptimal doses of carbenicillin.

Carbenicillin is not absorbed from the gastrointestinal tract and, therefore, must be given parenterally. Large doses are often necessary. Intramuscular injection of 1 g produces peak concentrations in plasma of 15 to 20 μg/ml in 0.5 to 2 hours; activity is practically gone at 6 hours. Maximal plasma concentrations are about four times higher after intravenous than after intramuscular administration of the antibiotic. Intravenous infusion at a rate of 1 g per hour results in average plasma concentrations of approximately 150 μg/ml. Intravenous infusion of 4 to 5 g over a 2-hour period every 4 hours will maintain blood concentrations above 100 μg/ml. About 50% of the antibiotic in plasma is protein bound. The distribution of carbenicillin is similar to that of other penicillins. The half-life of carbenicillin in individuals with normal renal function is about 1 hour; it is prolonged to about 2 hours in the presence of hepatic dysfunction. Hemodialysis reduces the concentration of the antibiotic in plasma.

Carbenicillin is excreted primarily by the renal tubules. About 75 to 85% of a dose is recoverable in active form in the urine in 9 hours. Probenecid, by delaying renal excretion of the drug, increases plasma concentrations by about 50%.

Preparations of carbenicillin may cause adverse effects in addition to those that follow use of the other penicillins. Congestive heart failure may result from the administration of excessive sodium. Hypokalemia may occur because of obligatory excretion of cation with the large amount of non-reabsorbable anion (carbenicillin) presented to the distal renal tubule. The drug interferes with platelet function, and bleeding may occur because of abnormal aggregation of platelets (*see* Shattil *et al.,* 1980).

Carbenicillin is available for parenteral injection as the disodium salt (GEOPEN, PYOPEN) in sterile vials containing 1, 2, 5, or 10 g. The daily dose for adults with serious infections is 25 to 30 g; some patients have been given as much as 35 to 40 g. When the drug is administered intravenously, the dosage may be as high as 2 to 2.5 g every 2 hours. Daily doses of 600 to 800 mg/kg have been used to treat very young infants with life-threatening infection. In patients with severe renal failure, the dose should not exceed 2 g every 8 to 12 hours; during hemodialysis, the interval between doses may be reduced to 4 to 6 hours. Available preparations of carbenicillin contain 4.7 mEq of sodium per gram.

Carbenicillin Indanyl. This congener is the indanyl ester of carbenicillin; it is acid stable and is suitable for oral administration. The ester is rapidly converted to carbenicillin *in vivo* by hydrolysis of the ester linkage. The antimicrobial spectrum of the drug is therefore that of carbenicillin, and bacterial resistance develops as to the parental compound. While relatively low plasma concentrations of carbenicillin are achieved, the active moiety is excreted rapidly in the urine. Thus, the main use of this drug clinically is for the management of urinary tract infections caused by *Proteus* species other than *Pr. mirabilis* and by *Pseud. aeruginosa* (Wallace *et al.,* 1971).

Carbenicillin indanyl is rapidly absorbed from the small intestine. The peak concentration in plasma, reached about 1 hour after ingestion of 500 mg of the drug, is approximately 5 μg/ml. About 30% of a dose of 500 mg is excreted in the urine in the first 12 hours; an additional 6% is eliminated in the urine over the next 12 hours. After the administration of 1 g, about 50% is excreted in the first 12 hours and an additional 10% in the next 12 hours. The urine thus contains antimicrobially effective concentrations of carbenicillin after recommended doses of carbenicillin indanyl. Some of the drug is excreted in the bile, and some is detoxified in the liver. (*See* Butler *et al.,* 1971; English *et al.,* 1972.)

Carbenicillin Indanyl Sodium, U.S.P. (GEOCILLIN), is available in tablets containing 500 mg of the drug (equivalent to 382 mg of carbenicillin). The recommended daily doses are 2 to 4 g, given in four divided portions. The higher end of this range is preferred for treatment of chronic infections or those caused by *Pseudomonas.*

Ticarcillin. This semisynthetic penicillin (Table 50–1) is very similar to carbenicillin, but it is two to four times more active against *Pseud. aeruginosa.* Doses are thus usually smaller, and, hopefully, the incidence of toxicity may be decreased. Ticarcillin may also be used in larger doses to inhibit strains of

Pseudomonas that are resistant to usual doses. *Ticarcillin disodium* (TICAR) is available for parenteral injection in sterile vials containing 1, 3, or 6 g. Daily doses of the drug are 200 to 300 mg/kg. Ticarcillin disodium contains about 5.1 mEq of sodium per gram (*see* Parry and Neu, 1976, 1978).

Other Related Agents. *Azlocillin* is an acylureido penicillin and is similar pharmacologically to carbenicillin. Of interest, it is about ten times more active against *Pseud. aeruginosa. Carbenicillin phenyl* is the phenyl ester of carbenicillin, intended for oral administration. It is thus similar to carbenicillin indanyl. Neither of these drugs is currently available in the United States.

Therapeutic Indications. Carbenicillin and the related penicillins are important agents for the treatment of patients with serious infections caused by gram-negative bacteria. These patients frequently have impaired immunological defenses, and their infections are often acquired in the hospital. Many authorities feel that a beta-lactam agent, often in combination with an aminoglycoside, should be employed for all such infections. Therefore, these penicillins find their greatest use in treating bacteremias, pneumonias, infections following burns, and urinary tract infections due to microorganisms resistant to penicillin G and ampicillin; the bacteria responsible especially include *Pseud. aeruginosa,* indole-positive strains of *Proteus,* and *Enterobacter* species. Since *Pseudomonas* infections are common in neutropenic patients, therapy for severe bacterial infections in such individuals should include carbenicillin or ticarcillin.

OTHER EXTENDED-SPECTRUM PENICILLINS

A new group of penicillin derivatives, none of which is yet available in the United States, are notable for activity against *Klebsiella* species in addition to those microorganisms also inhibited by carbenicillin. Some of these agents are more active than carbenicillin against *Pseud. aeruginosa.*

Mezlocillin is a acylureido penicillin that inhibits 75% of *Klebsiella* isolates at concentrations of 25 μg/ml and is ten times more active than carbenicillin against *Pseudomonas.* Its pharmacological properties are similar to those of carbenicillin.

Piperacillin (Table 50-1), a piperazine derivative, is the most active of the penicillins against *Pseudomonas;* it is also highly active against many genera of Enterobacteriaceae, including *Klebsiella.* Its antimicrobial activity is synergistic with that of the aminoglycosides (*see* Dickinson *et al.,* 1978; Tjandramaga *et al.,* 1978).

Mecillinam is a 6-β-acylaminopenicillanic acid. While it is relatively inactive against gram-positive cocci, it is highly active against *E. coli, Salmonella, Shigella, Klebsiella, Enterobacter,* and *Citrobacter.* However, it does *not* inhibit *Pseudomonas,* many strains of *Proteus,* or *B. fragilis.* Because of its novel mechanism of action (it appears to bind to different

proteins than do many other penicillins), it shows significant synergism with other beta-lactam antibiotics (*see* Neu, 1976).

UNTOWARD REACTIONS TO PENICILLINS

Hypersensitivity Reactions. Hypersensitivity reactions are by far the most common adverse effects noted with the penicillins, and these agents are probably the most common cause of drug allergy. There is no convincing evidence that any single penicillin differs from the group in its potential for causing true allergic reactions. In approximate order of decreasing frequency, manifestations of allergy to penicillins include maculopapular rash, urticarial rash, fever, bronchospasm, vasculitis, serum sickness, exfoliative dermatitis, Stevens-Johnson syndrome, and anaphylaxis (*see* Levine, 1972). The overall incidence of such reactions to the penicillins varies from 0.7 to 10% in different studies (Idsøe *et al.,* 1968).

Hypersensitivity reactions may occur with any dosage form of penicillin; the presence of allergy to one penicillin exposes the patient to a greater risk of reaction if another is given. On the other hand, the occurrence of an untoward effect does not necessarily imply repetition on subsequent exposures. For example, some patients who have had mild-to-moderate skin manifestations may later receive the same penicillin without experiencing a repetition of the allergic response. Hypersensitivity reactions may appear in the absence of previous known exposure to the drug. This may be caused by unrecognized prior exposure to penicillin in the environment (*e.g.,* in foods of animal origin or from the fungus producing penicillin). Although elimination of the antibiotic usually results in rapid clearing of the allergic manifestations, they may persist for 1 or 2 weeks or longer after therapy has been stopped. In some cases, the reaction is mild and disappears even while the use of penicillin is continued. In others, it is of serious import and necessitates immediate cessation of penicillin treatment. In a few instances, it is necessary to interdict the future use of penicillin because of the risk of death, and the patient should be so warned. It must be stressed that fatal episodes of anaphylaxis have followed the ingestion of very small doses of this antibiotic or skin testing with minute quantities of the drug.

Penicillins and breakdown products of penicillins act as haptens after their covalent reaction with proteins. The most important antigenic intermediate of penicillin appears to be the penicilloyl moiety, which is formed when the beta-lactam ring is opened. This is considered to be the *major* (predominant) determinant of penicillin allergy. In addition, *minor* determinants of allergy to penicillins are present. These include the intact molecule itself and penicilloate. These products are formed *in vivo* and can also be found in solutions of penicillin prepared for administration. The terms *major determinant* and *minor determinant* refer to the frequency with which antibodies to these haptens appear to be formed. They do *not* describe the severity of the reaction that may result.

Antipenicillin antibodies are detectable in virtually all patients who have received the drug and in many who have never knowingly been exposed to it. Studies on subjects of various ages indicate that 64% of persons have IgM antibodies that react with penicilloyl-polylysine, 13% have IgG antibodies for this compound, 5% have both types, and only 16% have neither (Klaus and Fellner, 1973). Recent treatment with the antibiotic induces an increase in major-determinant-specific antibodies that are skin sensitizing. The incidence of positive skin reactors is three to four times higher in atopic than in nonatopic individuals. Clinical and immunological studies suggest that immediate allergic reactions are mediated by skin-sensitizing or IgE antibodies, usually of minor-determinant specificities. Accelerated and late urticarial reactions are usually mediated by major-determinant-specific, skin-sensitizing antibodies. The recurrent-arthralgia syndrome appears to be related to the presence of skin-sensitizing antibodies of minor-determinant specificities. Some maculopapular and erythematous reactions may be due to toxic antigen-antibody complexes of major-determinant-specific IgM antibodies. Accelerated and late urticarial reactions to penicillin may terminate spontaneously because of the development of blocking antibodies (*see* Levine *et al.,* 1966).

Skin rashes of all types may be caused by allergy to penicillin. Scarlatiniform, morbilliform, urticarial, vesicular, and bullous eruptions may develop. Purpuric lesions are uncommon and are usually the result of a vasculitis; thrombopenic purpura may occur very rarely. Henoch-Schoenlein purpura with renal involvement has been a rare complication. *Contact dermatitis* is observed occasionally in pharmacists, nurses, and physicians who prepare penicillin solutions, even though they may have never received the drug either orally or parenterally; it also results from the ill-advised topical application of penicillin ointments. Fixed-drug reactions have also occurred. More severe reactions involving the skin are exfoliative dermatitis and exudative erythema multiforme of either the erythematopapular or vesiculobullous type; these lesions may be very severe and atypical in distribution and constitute the characteristic Stevens-Johnson syndrome. The incidence of skin rashes appears to be highest following the use of ampicillin, being about 9%; rashes follow the administration of ampicillin in nearly all patients with infectious mononucleosis. When allopurinol and ampicillin are administered concurrently, the incidence of rash also increases. Ampicillin-induced skin eruptions in such patients may represent a "toxic" rather than a truly allergic reaction. Positive skin reactions to the major and minor determinants of penicillin sensitization may be absent. The rash may clear even while administration of the drug is continued.

The most serious hypersensitivity reactions produced by the penicillins are *angioedema* and *anaphylaxis.* Angioedema with marked swelling of the lips, tongue, face, and periorbital tissues, frequently accompanied by asthmatic breathing and "giant hives," has been observed after topical, oral, or systemic administration of penicillins of various types.

Acute *anaphylactic* or *anaphylactoid* reactions induced by various preparations of penicillin constitute the most important immediate danger connected with their use. Among all drugs, the penicillins are the most often responsible for this type of untoward effect. Anaphylactoid reactions may occur at any age. Their incidence is thought to be 0.015 to 0.04% in persons treated with penicillins. About 0.002% of patients treated with these agents die from anaphylaxis. It has been estimated that there are at least 300 deaths per year due to this complication of therapy. About 15% of those who succumb have had other types of allergy; 70% have had penicillin previously, and one third of these reacted to it on a prior occasion (Idsøe *et al.,* 1968). Anaphylaxis has most often followed the *injection* of penicillin, although it has also been observed after *oral ingestion* of the drug, and has even resulted from the intradermal instillation of a very small quantity for the purpose of testing for the presence of hypersensitivity. The clinical pictures that develop vary in severity. The most dramatic is sudden, severe hypotension and rapid death. In other instances, bronchoconstriction with severe asthma, or abdominal pain, nausea, and vomiting, or extreme weakness and fall in blood pressure, or diarrhea and purpuric skin eruptions have characterized the anaphylactic episodes.

Serum sickness varies from mild fever, rash, and leukopenia to severe arthralgia or arthritis, purpura, lymphadenopathy, splenomegaly, mental changes, ECG abnormalities suggestive of myocarditis, generalized edema, albuminuria, and hematuria. It is mediated by IgG antibodies. This reaction usually appears after penicillin treatment has been continued for 1 week or more; it may be delayed, however, until 1 or 2 weeks after the drug has been stopped. Serum sickness caused by penicillin may persist for a week or longer.

Vasculitis of the skin or other organs may be related to hypersensitivity to penicillin. The Coombs' reaction frequently becomes positive during prolonged therapy with a penicillin or cephalosporin, but hemolytic anemia is rare. Reversible neutropenia may occur. It is not known if this is truly a hypersensitivity reaction; it has been noted with all of the penicillins and has been seen in up to 30% of patients treated with 8 to 12 g of nafcillin for longer than 21 days. The bone marrow shows an arrest of maturation.

Fever may be the only evidence of a hypersensitivity reaction to the penicillins. It may reach high levels and be maintained, remittent, or intermittent; chills occasionally occur. The febrile reaction usually disappears within 24 to 36 hours after administration of the drug is stopped, but may persist for days.

Eosinophilia is an occasional accompaniment of other allergic reactions to penicillin. At times, it may be the sole abnormality and eosinophils may reach levels of 10 to 20% or more of the total number of circulating white blood cells.

Interstitial nephritis may rarely be produced by the penicillins; methicillin has been implicated most frequently. Hematuria, albuminuria, pyuria, renal-cell and other casts in the urine, elevation of serum creatine, and even oliguria have been noted. Biopsy shows a mononuclear infiltrate with eosinophilia and tubular damage. IgG is present in the interstitium (*see* Ditlove *et al.,* 1977; Galpin *et al.,* 1978; Kancir *et al.,* 1978). This reaction is usually reversible.

Management of the Patient Potentially Allergic to Penicillin. Evaluation of the patient's history appears to be the most practical way to avoid the use of penicillin in patients who are at the greatest risk of developing an adverse reaction. The vast majority of patients who give a history of allergy to penicillin should be treated with a different type of antibiotic. In the unusual instance where treatment with a penicillin is essential, skin tests may be of some help. Lack of a response to *benzylpenicilloyl-polylysine* (PREPEN) makes it very unlikely that a patient will develop an immediate or accelerated reaction to penicillin; this preparation is not immunogenic, nor is it likely to provoke severe reactions. Furthermore, only 3% of such patients will develop a delayed reaction (usually rash). Patients with a positive response to benzylpenicilloyl-polylysine are at significant risk of developing a serious reaction, and two thirds of these patients will develop some form of allergic reaction. In order further to reduce the likelihood of an immediate severe reaction, sensitivity to the minor antigenic determinants probably should also be tested. Unfortunately, mixtures of the minor antigenic determinants are not commercially available. A scratch test with a solution of the penicillin to be administered (10,000 units/ml) can be performed; if this is negative, an intradermal test with 0.02 ml of a solution of 100 units/ml should also be done. If these are negative, penicillin may be administered cautiously. Administration of epinephrine is the therapy of choice for an immediate or accelerated reaction to penicillin.

"Desensitization" is occasionally recommended for patients who are allergic to penicillin and who it is felt must receive the drug. This procedure consists of administering gradually increasing doses of penicillin in the hope of avoiding a severe reaction. This may result in a subclinical anaphylactic discharge and the binding of all IgE before full doses are administered. Penicillin may be given in doses of 1, 5, 10, 100, and 1000 units intradermally in the lower arm with 60-minute intervals between doses. If this is well tolerated, then 10,000 units and 50,000 units may be given subcutaneously. When full doses are reached, penicillin should not be discontinued and then restarted, since immediate reactions may recur. *The patient should be observed constantly during the procedure, an intravenous line must be in place, and epinephrine and equipment and expertise for artificial ventilation must be on hand. It must be emphasized that this procedure may be dangerous and its efficacy is unproven.*

Patients with life-threatening infections (*e.g.*, endocarditis or meningitis) may be continued on penicillin despite the development of a maculopapular rash. The rash often clears as therapy is continued. This is thought to be due to the development of blocking antibodies of the IgG class. The rash may be treated with antihistamines or adrenocorticosteroids, although there is no evidence that this therapy is efficacious. Rarely, such patients develop exfoliative dermatitis with or without vasculitis if therapy with penicillin is continued. Therefore, alternative antimicrobial agents should be used where possible (*see* Green *et al.*, 1977).

Toxic Reactions.   The penicillins have minimal direct toxicity to man (*see* Parker, 1975). The actual limit of the dose of penicillin G that can be administered parenterally with safety still remains to be determined. A number of individuals have been treated intravenously with quantities ranging from 40 to 80 million units per day for as long as 4 weeks without untoward effects (Weinstein *et al.*, 1964).

Apparent toxic effects that have been reported include bone-marrow depression, granulocytopenia, and hepatitis. The latter is rare but is most commonly seen following the administration of oxacillin (*see* Onorato and Axelrod, 1978; Pollack *et al.*, 1978). The administration of carbenicillin or ticarcillin has been associated with a potentially significant defect of hemostatis that appears to be due to an impairment of platelet aggregation (Brown *et al.*, 1974).

Most common among the *irritative responses* to penicillin are *pain* and *sterile inflammatory reactions* at the sites of intramuscular injections, reactions that are related to concentration. Serum transaminases and lactic dehydrogenase may be elevated as a result of local damage to muscle. Whereas the administration of 1 million units of penicillin G dissolved in 1 ml of isotonic saline solution may produce severe discomfort for an appreciable period, the injection of the same quantity of drug dissolved in 5 ml is accompanied by only moderate pain that persists only for a short time. Some individuals who receive penicillin intravenously develop *phlebitis* or *thrombophlebitis*. Many persons who take various penicillin preparations by mouth experience nausea, with or without vomiting, and some have mild-to-severe diarrhea. These manifestations are often related to the dose of the drug.

When penicillin is injected accidentally into the sciatic nerve, severe pain occurs and dysfunction in the area of distribution of this nerve develops and persists for weeks. Intrathecal injection of penicillin G may produce *arachnoiditis* or severe and fatal *encephalopathy*. Because of this, intrathecal or intraventricular administration of penicillins should be avoided. The parenteral administration of large doses of penicillin G (greater than 20 million units per day, or less with renal insufficiency) may produce lethargy, confusion, twitching, multifocal myoclonus, or localized or generalized epileptiform seizures. These arc most apt to occur in the presence of renal insufficiency, localized CNS lesions, or hyponatremia. When the concentration of penicillin G in CSF exceeds 10 μg/ml, significant dysfunction of the CNS is frequent. The injection of 20 million units of penicillin G potassium, which contains 34 mEq of potassium, may lead to severe or even fatal hyperkalemia in persons with renal dysfunction.

Injection of penicillin G procaine may result in an immediate reaction, characterized by dizziness, tinnitus, headache, hallucinations, and sometimes seizures. This is due to the rapid liberation of toxic concentrations of procaine (Green *et al.*, 1974). It has been reported to occur in 1 of 200 patients receiving 4.8 million units of penicillin G procaine to treat their venereal disease.

Reactions Unrelated to Hypersensitivity or Toxicity.   The most important biological effect of penicillin, unrelated to hypersensitivity or to a toxic reaction, is alteration of the bacterial flora in areas of the body to which it gains access. Regardless of the route by which the drug is administered, but most strikingly when it is given by mouth, penicillin changes the composition of the microflora by eliminating sensitive microorganisms. Thus, profound alterations may be observed in the types and numbers of microorganisms present in the intestinal and upper respiratory tracts; the degree of alteration is related directly to the quantity of penicillin administered. Although this occurs in practically all individuals, it is usually of no clinical significance and the normal microflora is reestablished shortly after therapy is stopped. In some persons, however, *suprainfection* results from the changes in flora.

Fever and even vascular collapse and death may follow the use of penicillin in syphilis. This is one manifestation of the Jarisch-Herxheimer reaction. It is thought to be due to hypersensitivity to antigens released during rapid and massive lysis of spirochetes.

THE CEPHALOSPORINS

History and Source.   *Cephalosporium acremonium*, the first source of the cephalosporins, was isolated in 1948 by Brotzu from the sea near a sewer outlet off the Sardinian coast. Crude filtrates from cultures of this fungus were found to inhibit the *in-vitro* growth of *Staph. aureus* and to cure staphylococcal infections and typhoid fever in man. Culture fluids in which the Sardinian fungus was cultivated were found to contain three distinct antibiotics: (1) *cephalosporin P*, active only against gram-positive microorganisms; (2) *cephalosporin N*, a new type of penicillin with a side chain derived from D-α-aminoadipic acid, effective against both gram-positive and gram-negative bacteria; and (3) *cephalosporin C*, less potent than cephalosporin N but possessing the same range of antimicrobial effectiveness. (For a complete historical review and discussion of the biochemistry of the cephalosporins, *see* Abraham, 1962; Flynn, 1972.)

With the isolation of the active nucleus of cephalosporin C, 7-aminocephalosporanic acid, and with the addition of side chains, it became possible to produce semisynthetic compounds with antibacterial activity very much greater than that of the parent substance.

Chemistry. *Cephalosporin P* is a steroid compound related chemically to helvolic acid and to fusidic acid, an antibiotic elaborated by *Fusidium coccineum*. *Cephalosporin N* (penicillin N) is an N-acyl derivative of 6-aminopenicillanic acid and is inactivated by penicillinase. It has a polar side chain not previously demonstrated in an antibiotic and yields penicillamine when hydrolyzed. *Cephalosporin C* resembles cephalosporin N in containing a side chain derived from D-α-aminoadipic acid but differs from it because the side chain is condensed with a dihydrothiazine beta-lactam ring system (7-aminocephalosporanic acid) instead of a thiazolidine beta-lactam ring complex (Table 50–2). Compounds containing 7-aminocephalosporanic acid are relatively stable in dilute acid and highly resistant to penicillinase, regardless of the nature of their side chains and their affinity for the enzyme.

Cephalosporin C can be hydrolyzed by acid to 7-aminocephalosporanic acid. This compound has been subsequently modified by the addition of different side chains to create a whole family of cephalosporin antibiotics. It appears that modifications at position 7 of the beta-lactam ring are associated with alteration in antibacterial activity and that substitutions at position 3 of the dihydrothiazine ring are associated with changes in the metabolism and the pharmacokinetic properties of the drugs (*see* Huber *et al.,* 1972).

The *cephamycins* are similar to the cephalosporins, but they are derived from *Streptomyces* species. The cephamycins have a methoxyl group at position 7 of the beta-lactam ring of the 7-aminocephalosporanic acid nucleus. Cefoxitin is derived from cephamycin C, which is a product of *Streptomyces lactamdurans*. The structural formulas of representative cephalosporins, cefoxitin, and 7-aminocephalosporanic acid are shown in Table 50–2.

Mechanism of Action. Cephalosporins and cephamycins appear to inhibit bacterial cell-wall synthesis in a manner similar to that of penicillin. This is discussed in detail above (*see* page 1129).

Antibacterial Activity of the Cephalosporins. With the exception of cefamandole and cefoxitin, the cephalosporins currently available in the United States all have very similar antimicrobial activity *in vitro*, and a single antibiotic disc (a "cephalosporin disc") can be used to screen for bacterial sensitivity to these agents as a class. *Cephalothin* can be considered as the prototype; it is active against both gram-positive and gram-negative microorganisms. Group-A *Strep. pyogenes*, the *viridans* group and nonhemolytic streptococci, *Strep. pneumoniae*, penicillin-resistant and penicillin-sensitive *Staph. aureus*, *Staph. epidermidis*, *Cl. perfringens*, *List. monocytogenes*, *B. subtilis*, *C. diphtheriae*, *N. gonorrhoeae*, *N. meningitidis*, and *A. israelii* are highly sensitive to this agent, many being suppressed by concentrations of 0.004 to 1 µg/ml. Gram-negative bacteria are generally less susceptible, but the majority of strains of *Salmonella*, including *S. typhi*, most *Shigella*, and all *Pr. mirabilis* are inhibited by 1 to 6 µg/ml. About 75% of *E. coli*, 60% of paracolon strains, and only 50% of *H. influenzae* are inhibited by these concentrations. Almost all strains of *Klebsiella* are sensitive to 4 to 16 µg/ml. Cephalothin is not active against *Enterobacter*, other *Proteus* species (*vulgaris, rettgeri, morganii, inconstans*), *Pseud. aeruginosa*, *Past. multocida*, *Acinetobacter*, *Bacteroides*, *Serratia*, enterococci, viruses, yeasts, and fungi. While methicillin-resistant strains of *Staph. aureus* are usually resistant to the cephalosporins, many strains of methicillin-resistant *Staph. epidermidis* are sensitive to these drugs. However, the presence of antibiotic-resistant subpopulations of bacteria may diminish their effectiveness (*see* Archer, 1978). Cephalothin does not inhibit most strains of *B. fragilis*, although many other anaerobic microorganisms, especially anaerobic cocci, many strains of *Clostridium*, and *Bacteroides melaninogenicus*, are susceptible. (*See* Moellering *et al.,* 1974; Tally *et al.,* 1975a; Ernst *et al.,* 1976; Mandell, 1979.)

Cefamandole is more active than cephalothin against gram-negative microorganisms. Thus, more strains of *E. coli* and *Enterobacter* species are sensitive to cefamandole. However, *Pseudomonas* species are resistant to both drugs. The greatest advantage of cefamandole appears to be its increased activity against *Enterobacter* species, indole-positive *Proteus*, and *H. influenzae*. It is slightly less active than cephalothin against gram-positive bacteria, although most gram-positive microorganisms are still in the range of susceptibility (*see* Neu, 1974b).

Cefoxitin is less active than cefamandole against most gram-positive and many gram-negative microorganisms. However, it is more active for indole-positive species of *Proteus*, *Serratia marcescens*, and *B. fragilis* (*see* Eickhoff and Ehret, 1976).

Mechanisms of Bacterial Resistance to the Cephalosporins. Resistance to the cephalosporins (as to the penicillins) may be related to an incapacity of the antibiotic to penetrate to its site of action or to interact with its normal target. Bacteria also have the ability to produce enzymes—beta-lactamases (or cephalosporinases)—that can disrupt the beta-lactam ring and inactivate these antibiotics (*see* Farrar and Kruse, 1970).

The cephalosporins have differing susceptibilities to beta-lactamases. Cephaloridine is the most sensitive to these enzymes from both gram-positive and

Table 50–2. STRUCTURAL FORMULAS OF SELECTED CEPHALOSPORINS AND CEPHAMYCINS

COMPOUND	R_1	R_2
7-Aminocephalosporanic acid	H—	$-CH_2-O-C(=O)-CH_3$
Cephalothin	(thiophene)$-CH_2-C(=O)-$	$-CH_2-O-C(=O)-CH_3$
Cefazolin	(tetrazole)$N-CH_2-C(=O)-$	$-CH_2-S-$(thiadiazole)$-CH_3$
Cephapirin	(pyridine)$N-S-CH_2-C(=O)-$	$-CH_2-O-C(=O)-CH_3$
Cephalexin	(phenyl)$-CH(NH_2)-C(=O)-$	$-CH_3$
Cephradine	(cyclohexadienyl)$-CH(NH_2)-C(=O)-$	$-CH_3$
Cefoxitin *	(thiophene)$-CH_2-C(=O)-$	$-CH_2-O-C(=O)-NH_2$
Cefamandole	(phenyl)$-CH(OH)-C(=O)-$	$-CH_2-S-$(tetrazole)$-CH_3$

* Cefoxitin, a cephamycin, is further characterized by insertion of a methoxy residue ($-OCH_3$) at position 7 of the beta-lactam ring.

gram-negative bacteria; cefazolin is more susceptible to hydrolysis by beta-lactamases from *Staph. aureus* than is cephalothin (Farrar and O-Dell, 1978). Cefoxitin and, to a lesser extent, cefamandole seem to be the most resistant to hydrolysis by the beta-lactamases produced by gram-negative microorganisms. However, the correlation between antimicrobial activity and resistance to hydrolysis by beta-lactamases is not perfect. Some bacterial strains that fail to hydrolyze the cephalosporins are nevertheless resistant to them; conversely, some bacteria that can hydrolyze these antibiotics are still killed by them. The cephalosporins can protect the penicillins from hydrolysis by beta-lactamases by binding to these enzymes.

Absorption, Distribution, Fate, and Excretion of the Cephalosporins. The individual cephalosporins differ significantly in such factors as the extent of absorption following oral administration or the severity of pain produced by intramuscular injection. This is but one reason for the proliferation of individual agents and preparations that has occurred in the last decade. Of the agents currently available in the United States, the absorption of *cephalexin* and *cephradine* is adequate after oral administration, and these drugs can be given by this route. *Cefazolin, cefamandole, cefoxitin,* and *cephaloridine* are administered either intramuscularly or intravenously. *Cephalothin* and *cephapirin* cause pain after intramuscular injection, and their use is thus essentially restricted to the intravenous route.

Following absorption, the extent of binding of cephalosporins to plasma proteins is also quite dependent on the individual agent. Cefazolin (about 80% bound) and cephalothin and cefamandole (about 70% bound) interact with plasma proteins significantly, while cephalexin and cephradine are bound to the least extent (less than 15%). Cephalosporins cross the placenta readily, and they are also found in high concentrations in synovial (Nelson, 1971) and pericardial fluids. Penetration into the aqueous and vitreous humors of the eye is relatively poor, although it may be possible to achieve therapeutic concentrations of these drugs in the eye after their systemic administration. Concentration of cephalosporins in bile is high, particularly with cefazolin and cefamandole (*see* Mendelson *et al.,* 1974; Ratzan *et al.,* 1974). None of the cephalosporins currently available penetrates into CSF in sufficient amounts to be consistently useful for the treatment of meningitis.

All of the cephalosporins are excreted by the kidney by glomerular filtration and tubular secretion. Probenecid thus slows the elimination of these agents. The doses of these drugs must be altered in patients with renal insufficiency (*see* Appendix II).

Four cephalosporins (cephalothin, cephapirin, cephaloglycin, and cephacetrile) have acetylated methoxy residues at position 3 of the heterocyclic nucleus. These compounds are metabolized *in vivo* to deacetyl derivatives, which have less antimicrobial activity than the parent compounds; these metabolites are also excreted by the kidney. Some of the other cephalosporins also appear to be subject to metabolism to a significant extent.

Specific Agents: Unique Features, Preparations, Dosage, and Routes of Administration. *Cephalothin.* The antimicrobial activity of cephalothin has been described above. Since cephalothin is the cephalosporin most impervious to attack by staphylococcal beta-lactamase, many consider it to be the agent of choice when a cephalosporin is used to treat severe staphylococcal infection such as endocarditis.

This antibiotic is not well absorbed orally, and, because of pain following its intramuscular injection, cephalothin is usually administered only intravenously. Cephalothin has a half-life of about 40 minutes, slightly longer than that of the phenoxyalkyl penicillins. Approximately 70% of the drug is bound to plasma protein. While cephalothin is found in many tissues and fluids, it does not enter the CSF to a significant extent; this drug should not be used for the therapy of meningitis. Indeed, meningitis due to cephalothin-sensitive microorganisms has *developed* during the course of therapy with cephalothin. The administration of 0.5 g of cephalothin intramuscularly to adults produces plasma concentrations of about 10 μg/ml in 30 minutes; administration of 1 g, about 20 μg/ml. Approximately 50% of a dose of cephalothin is eliminated in unchanged form in the urine, by renal tubular secretion. Probenecid blocks tubular secretion of the antibiotic and thereby prolongs its sojourn in the body and elevates the plasma concentration attained by a given dose. Decreased tubular secretion of the drug also accounts for the higher plasma values observed in premature and newborn infants, because of the incomplete development of their renal function. Twenty to 30% is changed in the body to the weakly antibacterial O-deacetyl metabolite, which is excreted in the urine. The concentrations of cephalothin present in urine after administration of 1 g range from 0.7 to 5 mg/ml. Excretion is delayed in the presence of decreased renal function, and intervals between doses must be lengthened when renal failure is severe (*see* Appendix II). Peritoneal dialysis removes all of cephalothin from the blood in about 48 hours (*see* review by Weinstein and Kaplan, 1970). The drug is also removed from the circulation by hemodialysis; intravenous injections of 1 g at the start and at the conclusion of dialysis produce effective but not excessive concentrations in plasma for 48 to 72 hours (Venuto and Plaut, 1971).

Cephalothin Sodium, U.S.P. (KEFLIN), is available in vials containing either 1, 2, 4, or 20 g for intravenous or intramuscular injection. The dose varies with the severity of the infection being treated. For mild disease in *adults,* 1 g every 6 hours often suffices; for more serious infection, 1 g every 3 hours; for life-threatening infections, especially when bacteremia is present, 1 g every 2 hours, intravenously. Doses as large as 24 g per day have been administered to adults without apparent ill effects. When the drug is given intravenously, 1 g should be dissolved in 20 to 30 ml of isotonic sodium chloride solution and infused over a period of 20 to 30 minutes; for intramuscular injection, 1 g is dissolved in 4 ml of the saline solution. The daily dose of cephalothin for *infants* and *children* is 40 to 100 mg/kg. The intramuscular injection of this agent is quite painful.

Cefazolin. The antibacterial spectrum of cefazolin is similar to that of cephalothin. However, cefazolin is more active against *E. coli* and *Klebsiella* species (*see* Sabath *et al.,* 1973). Cefazolin is somewhat more sensitive to staphylococcal penicillinase than is cephalothin (*see* Regamey *et al.,* 1975; Fong *et al.,* 1976a). While the evidence of clinical importance is not firm, some authorities prefer not to use cefazolin for treatment of staphylococcal endocarditis.

Concentrations of cefazolin in plasma are higher after intramuscular (64 µg/ml after 1 g) and intravenous injections than they are following the administration of either cephaloridine or cephalothin. This is caused in part by a smaller volume of distribution for cefazolin. Cefazolin is highly (about 80%) bound to plasma proteins. The half-life of cefazolin is also appreciably longer—nearly 2 hours, compared to 30 to 40 minutes for cephalothin and 1 to 1.5 hours for cephaloridine (*see* Bergeron *et al.,* 1973). Cefazolin is primarily excreted by glomerular filtration and is not secreted to the same extent as is cephalothin. Cefazolin is not metabolized, and nearly all of an administered dose can be recovered in the urine within 24 hours (Kirby and Regamey, 1973). Cefazolin is relatively well tolerated after intramuscular or intravenous injection, and some prefer it, since it can be administered less frequently and in smaller doses because of its longer half-life (*see* Quintiliani and Nightingale, 1978).

Sterile Cefazolin Sodium, U.S.P. (ANCEF, KEFZOL), is available in vials containing 250, 500, or 1000 mg for intravenous or intramuscular injection. The dose of *cefazolin* for intramuscular or intravenous injection in *adults* with mild infections is 250 to 500 mg every 8 hours; for moderate-to-severe disease, it is 500 mg to 1 g every 6 to 8 hours; daily doses as high as 6 g have been administered. In *children,* the recommended daily dose of cefazolin is 25 to 50 mg/kg; this may be increased to 100 mg/kg if necessary.

Cephapirin. This cephalosporin is very similar to cephalothin. Like cephalothin it causes pain when it is injected intramuscularly. It is also similar in its metabolism, half-life, elimination, and propensity to cause phlebitis (*see* Renzini *et al.,* 1975).

Sterile Cephapirin Sodium, U.S.P. (CEFADYL), is available in vials containing 1, 2, or 4 g of the drug for intravenous or intramuscular use. The parenteral dose of *cephapirin* for *adults* is 500 mg to 1 g every 4 to 6 hours. For very serious and life-threatening infections, a daily dose of 12 g administered intravenously may be required. *Children* should be given 40 to 80 mg/kg each day, in four equally divided and spaced doses.

Cefamandole. As noted, this newer cephalosporin is more active than cephalothin and the other agents described above against certain species of gram-negative bacteria (*see* Moellering *et al.,* 1974; Meyers and Hirschman, 1978). This is particularly evident for *H. influenzae, Enterobacter* species, indole-positive strains of *Proteus, E. coli,* and *Klebsiella* species (*see* Ernst *et al.,* 1976). Although gram-positive cocci are less susceptible to cefamandole than to cephalothin, therapeutic concentrations of cefamandole can be achieved. The particular utility of cefamandole is for the treatment of gram-negative microorganisms that are resistant to other cephalosporins.

The half-life of cefamandole (40 to 50 minutes) is similar to that of cephalothin; the drug is excreted (and secreted) unchanged in the urine. Plasma concentrations are 20 to 35 µg/ml after a 1-g intramuscular dose (*see* Fong *et al.,* 1976b; Neu, 1978; Symposium, 1978).

Cefamandole nafate (MANDOL) is available in vials containing 0.5, 1, or 2 g of the drug for intravenous or intramuscular administration. For severe infections, adults can be given 1 to 2 g of cefamandole every 4 to 6 hours. Life-threatening infections should be treated with 12 g per day. Infants and children should receive 50 to 150 mg/kg per day, divided into four to six doses.

Cefoxitin. As noted above, cefoxitin is a cefamycin. It is highly resistant to beta-lactamases produced by gram-negative bacilli (*see* Neu, 1974a). This antibiotic is more active than cephalothin against certain gram-negative microorganisms, although it is less active than cefamandole against *Enterobacter* species and *H. influenzae* (*see* Moellering *et al.,* 1974). It is more active than cefamandole against species of *Serratia* and indole-positive *Proteus.* It is less active than cefamandole and the older cephalosporins against gram-positive bacteria. Cefoxitin's special role in clinical practice seems to be related to its increased activity against *B. fragilis* (*see* Sutter and Finegold, 1975; Tally *et al.,* 1975a;

Bach *et al.*, 1977; Chow and Bednorz, 1978). However, its place in the therapy of serious anaerobic infections remains to be determined. Cefoxitin is effective for the treatment of urethritis due to penicillinase-producing strains of *Neisseria gonorrhoeae* (Berg *et al.*, 1979).

After a 1-g intramuscular dose of cefoxitin, concentrations in plasma are about 20 μg/ml; the half-life of the compound is about 45 minutes. The drug is excreted unchanged in the urine by both glomerular filtration and tubular secretion. (For summaries of the properties and clinical utility of cefoxitin, *see* Williams *et al.*, 1978; Kass and Evans, 1979.)

Cefoxitin (MEFOXIN) is available in vials containing 1 or 2 g of the drug for intravenous or intramuscular administration. The dose of cefoxitin is the same as for cefamandole, although cefoxitin has not yet been approved for use in children. The intramuscular injection of cefoxitin is uncomfortable; the drug can be diluted with 0.5% lidocaine solution to reduce the pain.

Cephaloridine. This cephalosporin is poorly absorbed following oral ingestion. Its only significant advantage compared to cephalothin is less pain on intramuscular injection. It is not metabolized and is minimally bound to plasma proteins. The peak concentration in blood after the intramuscular administration of 1 g is about 35 μg/ml. Cephaloridine is the most *nephrotoxic* of the available cephalosporins, and, although toxicity can be avoided with care, the use of this compound is not recommended (*see* Mandell, 1973b).

Sterile Cephaloridine, U.S.P. (LORIDINE), is available in ampuls containing 250, 500, and 1000 mg for intravenous or intramuscular use. Because of nephrotoxicity, the maximal daily dose of cephaloridine must be limited to 4 g.

Cephalexin. This cephalosporin has essentially the same antibacterial spectrum as does cephalothin. However, it is somewhat less active against penicillinase-producing staphylococci.

Cephalexin is stable in acid and is well absorbed from the gastrointestinal tract. Peak concentrations in plasma, reached at about 1 hour after ingestion of the drug, are approximately 9 and 18 μg/ml after oral doses of 250 and 500 mg, respectively. The ingestion of food may delay absorption. Less than 10 to 15% of the antibiotic is bound to plasma protein, and drug concentrations in plasma fall rapidly, the half-life of cephalexin normally being about 50 minutes. More than 90% of the drug is excreted unaltered in the urine within 6 hours, primarily by renal tubular secretion. The peak concentration of cephalexin in the urine may exceed 1 mg/ml following a 250-mg dose, and therapeutically effective concentrations are still achieved in the urine of patients with decreased renal function. Probenecid is effective in slowing urinary clearance and enhancing the duration of systemic antimicrobial activity. Cephalexin is efficiently removed from the circulation by hemodialysis or peritoneal dialysis. Cephalexin is also excreted into the bile.

(For details of the clinical pharmacology of cephalexin, *see* Conference, 1970; Kunin and Finkelberg, 1970; Boothman *et al.*, 1973.)

Cephalexin, U.S.P. (KEFLEX), is marketed in several forms, including capsules of 250 and 500 mg, oral suspensions providing, after reconstitution, 125 mg/5 ml or 250 mg/5 ml, and pediatric drops, 100 mg/ml. Cephalexin is administered to *adults* in oral doses of 1 to 4 g daily, depending on the nature of the infection. The usual dose is 250 to 500 mg every 6 hours. The daily dose for *children* ranges from 25 to 50 mg/kg, divided into four portions. This may be doubled for more serious infections.

Cephradine. This compound is a close congener of cephalexin, and its activity *in vitro* is almost identical. Cephradine is not metabolized and, after rapid absorption from the gastrointestinal tract, is excreted unchanged in the urine. Cephradine can also be administered intramuscularly or intravenously. When administered orally, cephradine behaves very much like cephalexin, and some feel that these two drugs can be used interchangeably. Because cephradine is completely and rapidly absorbed, the concentrations in blood after an oral dose are nearly equivalent to those observed after intramuscular administration (about 10 to 18 μg/ml after 500 mg orally or intramuscularly) (*see* Neiss, 1973). Cephradine probably causes more pain following intramuscular injection than does cefazolin or cephaloridine.

Cephradine, U.S.P. (ANSPOR, VELOSEF), is available as an oral suspension (125 mg/5 ml and 250 mg/5 ml) and in 250- and 500-mg capsules. Cephradine (VELOSEF) for injection is available in vials of 250, 500, or 1000 mg for intravenous or intramuscular use and in 100 ml-containers holding 2 or 4 g of the drug for intravenous administration. The oral dosage of cephradine is the same as for cephalexin. The parenteral dose for adults is 500 to 1000 mg, given two to four times daily, depending on the severity of the infection. For severe disease, 8 g may be given daily. For infants and children, 50 to 100 mg/kg should be divided into equal portions and given every 6 hours. Daily doses up to 300 mg/kg have been used without apparent incident.

Cefaclor. Cefaclor, which differs from cephalexin by the substitution of Cl for CH_3 at position 3 (*see* Table 50–2), is administered orally. The concentrations that are achieved in blood are about 50% of those that follow an equivalent oral dose of cephalexin. However, cefaclor is more active against gram-negative bacilli. This may be especially important for *H. influenzae, E. coli,* and *Pr. mirabilis.* Because of its activity against strains of *H. influenzae* that produce beta lactamase, cefaclor is useful for the treatment of otitis media and upper respiratory infections caused by these microorganisms (*see* Silver *et al.,* 1977). *Cefaclor* (CECLOR) is available in 250- and 500-mg capsules and in oral suspensions containing 125 or 250 mg/5 ml.

Cefadroxil. This *p*-hydroxylated derivative of cephalexin resembles cephalexin closely, although its half-life is somewhat longer (*see* Hartstein *et al.,* 1977); it is intended for oral administration. There appears to be no advantage to the use of cefadroxil, and the drug is very expensive. *Cefadroxil,* U.S.P. (DURICEF), is available in 500-mg capsules.

Cephaloglycin. This antibiotic is administered only orally. However, absorption from the gastrointestinal tract is relatively poor and the concentrations that are achieved in plasma are low. Thus, despite the fact that the drug retains official status and is available commercially (KAFOCIN), there is no justification for its use.

Other Cephalosporins. A variety of other cephalosporins is under investigation. None of the following is yet available for clinical use in the United States.

Cefuroxime has a broad antimicrobial spectrum similar to that of cefamandole; like cefoxitin, it is resistant to beta-lactamases from gram-negative microorganisms. *Serratia marcescens,* indole-positive *Proteus, Pseud. aeruginosa,* and *B. fragilis* are often resistant (*see* Neu and Fu, 1978b). Cefuroxime is not metabolized and is excreted by the kidney (*see* Foord, 1976).

Ceforanide is administered parenterally and has a half-life of 3 hours. Peak concentrations in plasma of 60 μg/ml are achieved after a 1-g dose. Ceforanide is less active than cephalothin against staphylococci. Its antimicrobial activity is that of cefamandole against gram-negative bacilli, although it is less active against *H. influenzae* and *N. gonorrhoeae* (*see* Shadomy *et al.,* 1978).

Cefatrizine, a semisynthetic cephalosporin for oral administration, is slightly more active than cephalexin against gram-negative bacilli (*see* Actor *et al.,* 1975). However, concentrations in plasma are lower than those achieved after oral administration of cephalexin.

Cephacetrile is a cephalosporin for parenteral administration; it has a spectrum of antimicrobial activity similar to that of cephalothin.

Several new cephalosporins are being evaluated that appear to have useful activity against *Pseud. aeruginosa* (*see* Heymes *et al.,* 1978; Sosna *et al.,* 1978).These include *cefotaxime* (Chabbert and Lutz, 1978) and *moxalactam* (Trager *et al.,* 1979).

Modification of Dosage in Patients with Renal Insufficiency. The cephalosporins, although largely excreted by the kidney, require only moderate reduction of dosage in patients with impaired renal function (*see* Craig *et al.,* 1973; Levison *et al.,* 1973). An exception is *cephaloridine,* which should be avoided because of its greater potential to cause nephrotoxicity. Recommendations for adjustment of dosage in such patients are available in Appendix II

(and in the package insert for each drug). Dialysis removes some cephalosporin from the circulation, and a modest increase in dosage is required; this is not true for cefamandole.

Adverse Reactions. Hypersensitivity reactions to the cephalosporins are the most common systemic side effects (*see* Petz, 1978), and there is no evidence that any single cephalosporin is more or less likely to cause such sensitization. The reactions appear to be identical to those caused by the penicillins, and this may be related to the shared beta-lactam structure of both groups of antibiotics. Immediate reactions such as anaphylaxis, bronchospasm, and urticaria are observed. More commonly, patients develop maculopapular rash, usually after several days of therapy; this may or may not be accompanied by fever and eosinophilia. Fever and lymphadenopathy have been associated with the administration of cephalosporins in the absence of other manifestations of allergic phenomena (*see* Sanders *et al.,* 1974).

Because of the similarity in structure of the penicillins and cephalosporins, patients who are allergic to one class of agents may manifest cross-reactivity when a member of the other class is administered. Immunological studies have demonstrated cross-reactivity in as many as 20% of patients who are allergic to penicillin (*see* Levine, 1973), but clinical reports seem to indicate a lower frequency (5 to 10%) of such reactions. There are no skin tests that can reliably predict whether a patient will manifest an allergic reaction to the cephalosporins.

Patients with a history of a mild or a temporally distant reaction to penicillin appear to be at low risk of developing a rash or other allergic reaction following the administration of a cephalosporin. *However, patients who have had a recent severe, immediate reaction to a penicillin should be given a cephalosporin with great caution, if at all.* A positive Coombs' reaction appears frequently in patients who receive large doses of a cephalosporin. Hemolysis is not usually associated with this phenomenon, although it has been reported. Cephalothin has produced rare instances of bone-marrow depression, characterized by granulocytopenia. Thrombocytopenia has been described (Gralnick *et al.,*

1972), but this may be a toxic effect that resembles the defect in platelet aggregation caused by carbenicillin.

The cephalosporins have been implicated as potentially nephrotoxic agents, although they are not nearly as toxic to the kidney as are the aminoglycosides or the polymixins (*see* Barza, 1978). Renal tubular necrosis has followed the administration of cephaloridine in doses greater than 4 g per day. In recommended doses the other cephalosporins rarely produce significant renal toxicity when used by themselves. High doses of cephalothin have produced acute tubular necrosis in certain instances, and usual doses (8 to 12 g per day) of the drug have caused nephrotoxicity in patients with preexisting renal disease (*see* Pasternack and Stephens, 1975). There is evidence that the concurrent administration of cephalothin and gentamicin or tobramycin may cause nephrotoxicity (Wade *et al.*, 1978), particularly in patients over 60 years of age (Klastersky, 1976).

Intravenous administration of any of the cephalosporins can cause thrombophlebitis. All of the drugs appear to cause this problem with equal frequency (*see* Carrizosa *et al.*, 1973; Berger *et al.*, 1976).

Therapeutic Uses. The cephalosporins are widely used antibiotics. They are effective for the treatment of infections of the respiratory tract, skin and soft tissues, bones and joints, urinary tract, and blood stream. However, prior to the availability of cefamandole and cefoxitin in 1978, many infectious disease consultants felt that they were the drugs of choice only for infections caused by *Klebsiella pneumoniae*.

Cephalosporins have been useful alternatives to penicillins for patients who are allergic to the penicillins. Cephalosporins may be used for therapy of acute pneumonia acquired in the community. Cefamandole, with its increased activity against *H. influenzae* in addition to the usual activity of a cephalosporin against *Strep. pneumoniae*, *Staph. aureus*, and *K. pneumoniae*, is a suitable single-drug therapy for the majority of such cases of bacterial pneumonia. Initial treatment of a pneumonia acquired in the hospital might often involve the combination of a cephalosporin and an aminoglycoside, especially in situations where *Pseudomonas* is not thought to be the pathogenic agent. For patients with septicemia caused by a gram-negative microorganism, initial therapy with a broad-spectrum penicillin and an aminoglycoside or a cephalosporin and an

aminoglycoside is widely used. Many physicians prefer the cephalosporin-aminoglycoside combination in patients who are not at great risk to acquire an infection with *Pseudomonas*, since it offers better activity against both staphylococci and *Klebsiella* species. Cefoxitin appears to be an effective agent for mixed aerobic-anaerobic infections, such as occur in pelvic inflammatory disease.

Cephalosporins may also be useful when the sensitivities of infecting microorganisms have been ascertained. In some instances aminoglycosides may be avoided if, for example, a gram-negative bacterium is sensitive to a cephalosporin. This may be especially true of the newer, broader-spectrum agents such as cefamandole and cefoxitin.

Cephalosporins are widely used by surgeons for the prophylaxis of infection. *Staphylococcus aureus* and *Staph. epidermidis* are major pathogens in surgery that involves the implantation of a prosthesis. In these instances cephalosporins may be used rationally. Cephalosporins are effective prophylactic agents for a wide variety of abdominal, gynecological, urological, and orthopedic surgical procedures. Proper guidelines for such prophylactic use of antimicrobial agents are discussed in Chapter 48.

Actor, P.; Uri, J. V.; Phillips, L.; Sachs, C. S.; Guarini, J. R.; Zajac, I.; Berges, D. A.; Dunn, G. L.; Hoover, J. R. E.; and Weisbuck, J. E. Laboratory studies with cefatrizine (SK&F 6077): a new broad spectrum orally-active cephalosporin. *J. Antibiot. (Tokyo)*, **1975**, *28*, 594–601.
Applestein, J.; Crosby, E. B.; Johnson, W. D.; and Kaye, D. *In vitro* antimicrobial activity and human pharmacology of cephaloglycin. *Appl. Microbiol.*, **1968**, *16*, 1006–1010.
Archer, G. L. Antimicrobial susceptibility and selection of resistance among *Staphylococcus epidermidis* isolates recovered from patients with infections of indwelling foreign devices. *Antimicrob. Agents Chemother.*, **1978**, *14*, 353–359.
Bach, V. T.; Roy, I.; and Thadepalli, H. Susceptibility of anaerobic bacteria to cefoxitin and related compounds. *Antimicrob. Agents Chemother.*, **1977**, *11*, 912–913.
Barza, M. The nephrotoxicity of cephalosporins: an overview. *J. Infect. Dis.*, **1978**, *137*, 560–573.
Benveniste, R., and Davies, J. Mechanisms of antibiotic resistance in bacteria. *Annu. Rev. Biochem.*, **1973**, *42*, 471–506.
Berg, S. W.; Kilpatrick, M. E.; Harrison, W. O.; and McCutchan, J. A. Cefoxitin as a single-dose treatment for urethritis caused by penicillinase-producing *Neisseria gonorrhoeae*. *N. Engl. J. Med.*, **1979**, *301*, 509–511.
Berger, S.; Ernest, E.; and Barza, M. Comparative incidence of phlebitis due to buffered cephalothin, cephapirin, and cefamandole. *Antimicrob. Agents Chemother.*, **1976**, *9*, 575–579.
Bergeron, M. D.; Brusch, J. L.; Barza, M.; and Weinstein, L. Bactericidal activity and pharmacology of cefazolin. *Antimicrob. Agents Chemother.*, **1973**, *4*, 396–401.
Blake, F. G.; Craige, B., Jr.; and Tierney, N. A. Clinical experiences with penicillin. *Trans. Assoc. Am. Physicians*, **1944**, *58*, 67–74.
Boothman, R.; Kerr, M. M.; Marshall, M. J.; and Burland, W. L. Absorption and excretion of cephalexin in the newborn infant. *Arch. Dis. Child.*, **1973**, *48*, 147–150.
Brown, C. H., III; Natelson, E. A.; Bradshaw, M. W.; Williams, T. W., Jr.; and Alfrey, C. P., Jr. The hemostatic defect produced by carbenicillin. *N. Engl. J. Med.*, **1974**, *291*, 265–270.
Butler, K.; English, A. R.; Knirsch, A. K.; and Korst, J. J.

Metabolism and laboratory studies with indanyl carbenicillin. *Del. Med. J.,* **1971,** *43,* 366–375.

Carrizosa, J.; Levison, M. E.; and Kaye, D. Double-blind controlled comparison of phlebitis produced by cephapirin and cephalothin. *Antimicrob. Agents Chemother.,* **1973,** *3,* 306–307.

Chabbert, Y. A., and Lutz, A. J. HR 756, the syn isomer of a new methoxyimino cephalosporin with unusual antibacterial activity. *Antimicrob. Agents Chemother.,* **1978,** *14,* 749–754.

Chain, E. B. The development of bacterial chemotherapy. *Antibiot. Chemother.,* **1954,** *4,* 215–241.

Chow, A. W., and Bednorz, D. Comparative *in vitro* activity of newer cephalosporins against anaerobic bacteria. *Antimicrob. Agents Chemother.,* **1978,** *14,* 668–671.

Craig, W. A.; Welling, P. G.; Jackson, T. C.; and Kunin, C. M. Pharmacology of cefazolin and other cephalosporins in patients with renal insufficiency. *J. Infect. Dis.,* **1973,** *128,* S347–S353.

Dickinson, G. M.; Cleary, T. J.; and Hoffman, T. A. Comparative evaluation of piperacillin *in vitro. Antimicrob. Agents Chemother.,* **1978,** *14,* 919–921.

Ditlove, J.; Weidmann, P.; Bernstein, M.; and Massry, S. G. Methicillin nephritis. *Medicine (Baltimore),* **1977,** *56,* 483–491.

Durack, D. T., and Beeson, P. B. Experimental bacterial endocarditis. II. Survival of bacteria in endocardial vegetations. *Br. J. Exp. Pathol.,* **1972,** *53,* 50–53.

Eagle, H. The recovery of bacteria from the toxic effects of penicillin. *J. Clin. Invest.,* **1949,** *28,* 382–386.

———. Experimental approach to the problem of treatment failure with penicillin. I. Group A streptococcal infection in mice. *Am. J. Med.,* **1952,** *13,* 389–399.

Eickhoff, T. C., and Ehret, J. M. *In vitro* comparison of cefoxitin, cefamandole, cephalexin, and cephalothin. *Antimicrob. Agents Chemother.,* **1976,** *9,* 994–999.

Eickhoff, T. C.; Kislak, J. W.; and Finland, M. Sodium ampicillin—absorption and excretion of intramuscular and intravenous doses in normal young men. *Am. J. Med. Sci.,* **1965,** *249,* 163–171.

English, A. R.; Retsema, J. A.; Ray, V. A.; and Lynch, J. E. Carbenicillin indanyl sodium, an orally active derivative of carbenicillin. *Antimicrob. Agents Chemother.,* **1972,** *1,* 185–191.

Ernst, E. C.; Berger, S.; Barza, M.; Jacobus, N. V.; and Tally, F. P. Activity of cefamandole and other cephalosporins against aerobic and anaerobic bacteria. *Antimicrob. Agents Chemother.,* **1976,** *9,* 852–855.

Farrar, W. E., Jr., and Kruse, J. M. Relationship between β-lactamase activity and resistance of *Enterobacter* to cephalothin. *Infect. Immun.,* **1970,** *2,* 610–616.

Farrar, W. E., Jr., and O'Dell, N. M. Comparative beta-lactamase resistance and antistaphylococcal activities of parenterally and orally administered cephalosporins. *J. Infect. Dis.,* **1978,** *137,* 490–493.

Florey, H. W. The use of micro-organisms for therapeutic purposes. *Yale J. Biol. Med.,* **1946,** *19,* 101–118.

Fong, I. W.; Engelking, E. R.; and Kirby, W. M. M. Relative inactivation by *Staphylococcus aureus* of eight cephalosporin antibiotics. *Antimicrob. Agents Chemother.,* **1976a,** *9,* 939–944.

Fong, I. W.; Ralph, E. D.; Engelking, E. R.; and Kirby, W. M. M. Clinical pharmacology of cefamandole as compared with cephalothin. *Antimicrob. Agents Chemother.,* **1976b,** *9,* 65–69.

Foord, R. D. Cefuroxime: human pharmacokinetics. *Antimicrob. Agents Chemother.,* **1976,** *9,* 741–747.

Galpin, J. E.; Shinaberger, J. H.; Stanley, T. M.; Blumenkrantz, M. J.; Bayer, A. S.; Friedman, G. S.; Montgomerie, J. Z.; Guze, L. B.; Coburn, J. W.; and Glassock, R. J. Acute interstitial nephritis due to methicillin. *Am. J. Med.,* **1978,** *65,* 756–765.

Ghuysen, J. Penicillin-sensitive enzymes of peptidoglycan metabolism. In, *Microbiology—1977.* (Schlessinger, D.,

ed.) American Society for Microbiology, Washington, D. C., **1977,** pp. 195–202.

Gibaldi, M.; Davidson, D.; Plaut, M. E.; and Schwartz, M. A. Modification of penicillin distribution and elimination by probenecid. *Int. Z. Klin. Pharmakol. Ther. Toxikol.,* **1970,** *3,* 182–189.

Gordon, R. C.; Regamey, C.; and Kirby, W. M. M. Comparative clinical pharmacology of amoxicillin and ampicillin administered orally. *Antimicrob. Agents Chemother.,* **1972,** *1,* 504–507.

Goto, S.; Ogawa, M.; Kaneka, V.; Tsuchiya, K.; Kondo, M.; Nishi, T. J.; and Nagatomo, H. SCE-129, a new antipseudomonal cephalosporin; *in vitro* and *in vivo* antibacterial activity. In, *Current Chemotherapy: Proceedings of the Tenth International Congress of Chemotherapy,* Vol. II. (Siegenthaler, W., and Lüthy, R., eds.) American Society for Microbiology, Washington, D. C., **1978,** p. 835.

Gralnick, H. R.; McGinniss, M.; and Halterman, R. Thrombocytopenia with sodium cephalothin therapy. *Ann. Intern. Med.,* **1972,** *77,* 401–404.

Green, G. R.; Rosenblum, A. H.; and Sweet, L. C. Evaluation of penicillin hypersensitivity. *J. Allergy Clin. Immunol.,* **1977,** *60,* 339–345.

Green, R. L.; Lewis, J. E.; Kraus, S. J.; and Frederickson, E. L. Elevated plasma procaine concentrations after administration of procaine penicillin G. *N. Engl. J. Med.,* **1974,** *291,* 223–226.

Greenwood, D. Mucopeptide hydrolases and bacterial "persisters." *Lancet,* **1972,** *2,* 465–466.

Hamilton-Miller, J. M. T. Penicillinacylase. *Bacteriol. Rev.,* **1966,** *30,* 761–771.

Hartstein, A. I.; Patrick, K. E.; Jones, S. R.; Miller, M. J.; and Bryant, R. E. Comparison of pharmacological and antimicrobial properties of cefadroxil and cephalexin. *Antimicrob. Agents Chemother.,* **1977,** *12,* 93–97.

Heymes, R.; Lutz, A.; and Schrinner, E. Experimental cephalosporins. In, *Current Chemotherapy: Proceedings of the Tenth International Congress of Chemotherapy,* Vol. II. (Siegenthaler, W., and Lüthy, R., eds.) American Society for Microbiology, Washington, D. C., **1978,** p. 823.

Huber, F. M.; Chauvette, R. R.; and Jackson, B. G. Preparative methods for 7-aminocephalosporanic acid and 6-aminopenicillanic acid. In, *Cephalosporins and Penicillins.* (Flynn, E. H., ed.) Academic Press, Inc., New York, **1972,** p. 27.

Idsøe, O.; Guthe, T.; Willcox, R. R.; and DeWeck, A. L. Nature and extent of penicillin side-reactions, with particular reference to fatalities from anaphylactic shock. *Bull. WHO,* **1968,** *38,* 159–188.

Jacobs, M. R.; Koornhof, H. J.; Robins-Browne, R. M.; Stevenson, C. M.; Vermaak, Z. A.; Freiman, I.; Miller, G. B.; Witcomb, M. A.; Isaacson, M.; Ward, J. I.; and Austrian, R. Emergence of multiply resistant pneumococci. *N. Engl. J. Med.,* **1978,** *299,* 735–740.

Kancir, L. M.; Tuazon, C. U.; Cardella, T. A.; and Sheagren, J. H. Adverse reactions to methicillin and nafcillin during treatment of serious *Staphylococcus aureus* infections. *Arch. Intern. Med.,* **1978,** *138,* 909–911.

Kaplan, E. L.; Anthony, B. F.; Bisno, A.; Durack, D.; Houser, H.; Millard, H. D.; Sanford, J.; Shulman, S. T.; Stillerman, M.; Taranta, A.; and Wenger, N. Prevention of bacterial endocarditis. AHA committee report. *Circulation,* **1977,** *56,* 139A–143A.

Kaplan, J. M., and McCracken, G. H., Jr. Clinical pharmacology of benzathine penicillin G in neonates with regard to its recommended use in congenital syphilis. *J. Pediatr.,* **1973,** *82,* 1069–1072.

Kass, E. H., and Evans, D. A. (eds.). Future prospects and past problems in antimicrobial therapy: the role of cefoxitin. *Rev. Infect. Dis.,* **1979,** *1,* 1–244.

Kerrebijn, K. F., and Michel, M. F. Amoxycillin (BRL 2333) in children. *Chemotherapy,* **1973,** *18,* Suppl., 92–96.

Kind, A. C.; Tupasi, T. E.; Standiford, H. C.; and Kirby,

W. M. M. Mechanisms responsible for plasma levels of nafcillin lower than those of oxacillin. *Arch. Intern. Med.,* **1970,** *125,* 685–690.

Kirby, W. M. M., and Regamey, C. Pharmacokinetics of cefazolin compared with four other cephalosporins. *J. Infect. Dis.,* **1973,** *128,* S341–S346.

Klastersky, J. The use of synergistic combinations of antibiotics in patients with haematological diseases. In, *Clinics in Haematology,* Vol. 5, Sect. 2. (Bodey, G., ed.) W. B. Saunders, Ltd., London, **1976,** pp. 361–367.

Klaus, M. V., and Fellner, M. J. Penicilloyl-specific serum antibodies in man. Analysis in 592 individuals from the newborn to old age. *J. Gerontol.,* **1973,** *28,* 312–316.

Klein, J. O.; Schaberg, M. J.; Buntin, M.; and Gezon, H. M. Levels of penicillin in serum of newborn infants after single intramuscular doses of benzathine penicillin G. *J. Pediatr.,* **1973,** *82,* 1065–1068.

Kunin, C. M., and Finkelberg, Z. Oral cephalexin and ampicillin: antimicrobial activity, recovery in urine, and persistence of uremic patients. *Ann. Intern. Med.,* **1970,** *72,* 349–356.

Levine, B. B. Skin rashes with penicillin therapy: current management. *N. Engl. J. Med.,* **1972,** *286,* 42–43.

———. Antigenicity and cross reactivity of penicillins and cephalosporins. *J. Infect. Dis.,* **1973,** *128,* S364–S366.

Levine, B. B.; Redmond, A. P.; Fellner, M. J.; Voss, H. E.; and Levytska, V. Penicillin allergy and the heterogeneous immune responses of man. *J. Clin. Invest.,* **1966,** *45,* 1895–1906.

Levison, M. E.; Levison, S.; Ries, K.; and Kaye, D. Pharmacology of cefazolin in patients with normal and abnormal renal function. *J. Infect. Dis.,* **1973,** *128,* S354–S357.

McCracken, G. H., Jr.; Ginsberg, C.; Chrane, D. F.; Thomas, M. A.; and Horton, L. J. Clinical pharmacology of penicillin in newborn infants. *J. Pediatr.,* **1973,** *82,* 692–698.

Maki, D. G.; Karzynski, T. A.; and Agger, W. A. Carbenicillin for treatment of *Bacteroides fragilis* infections: why not penicillin? *J. Infect. Dis.,* **1978,** *138,* 859–864.

Mandell, G. L. Interaction of intraleukocytic bacteria and antibiotics. *J. Clin. Invest.,* **1973a,** *52,* 1673–1679.

———. The cephalosporins. In, *Principles and Practice of Infectious Diseases.* (Mandell, G. L.; Douglas, R. G., Jr.; and Bennett, J. E.; eds.) John Wiley & Sons, Inc., New York, **1979,** pp. 238–248.

Mandell, G. L., and Hook, E. W. Persistence of ampicillin-sensitive *Salmonella thompsoni* due to fecal penicillinase. *Arch. Intern. Med.,* **1971,** *127,* 137–138.

Mendelson, J.; Portnoy, J.; Sigman, H.; and Dick, V. Pharmacology of cephalothin in the biliary tract of humans. *Antimicrob. Agents Chemother.,* **1974,** *6,* 659–665.

Meyers, B. R., and Hirschman, S. Z. Antibacterial activity of cefamandole *in vitro. J. Infect. Dis.,* **1978,** *137,* 525–531.

Moellering, R. C.; Dray, M.; and Kunz, L. J. Susceptibility of clinical isolates of bacteria to cefoxitin and cephalothin. *Antimicrob. Agents Chemother.,* **1974,** *6,* 320–323.

Mortimer, P. R.; Mackie, D. B.; and Haynes, S. Ampicillin levels in human bile in the presence of biliary tract disease. *Br. Med. J.,* **1969,** *3,* 88–89.

National Research Council. Committee on Chemotherapeutic and Other Agents. Division of Medical Sciences. (Keefer, C. S., chrmn.) Penicillin in the treatment of infections; a report of 500 cases. *J.A.M.A.,* **1943,** *122,* 1217–1224.

Neiss, E. Cephradine—summary of preclinical studies and clinical pharmacology. *J. Ir. Med. Assoc.,* **1973,** *44,* S1–S12.

Nelson, J. D. Antibiotic concentration in septic joint effusion. *N. Engl. J. Med.,* **1971,** *284,* 349–353.

Neu, H. C. Cefoxitin, a semisynthetic cephamycin antibiotic: antibacterial spectrum and resistance to hydrolysis by gram-negative beta-lactamases. *Antimicrob. Agents Chemother.,* **1974a,** *6,* 170–176.

———. Cefamandole, a cephalosporin antibiotic with an unusually wide spectrum of activity. *Ibid.,* **1974b,** *6,* 177–182.

———. Mecillinam, a novel penicillanic acid and derivative with unusual activity against gram-negative bacteria. *Ibid.,* **1976,** *9,* 793–799.

———. Comparison of the pharmacokinetics of cefamandole and other cephalosporin compounds. *J. Infect. Dis.,* **1978,** *137,* S80–S87.

———. Penicillins. In, *Principles and Practice of Infectious Diseases.* (Mandell, G. L.; Douglas, R. G., Jr.; and Bennett, J. E.; eds.) John Wiley & Sons, Inc., New York, **1979a,** pp. 218–238.

Neu, H. C., and Fu, K. P. Clavulanic acid, a novel inhibitor of β-lactamases. *Antimicrob. Agents Chemother.,* **1978a,** *14,* 650–655.

———. Cefuroxime, a beta-lactamase resistant cephalosporin with a broad spectrum of gram-positive and negative activity. *Ibid.,* **1978b,** *13,* 657–664.

Onorato, I. M., and Axelrod, J. L. Hepatitis from intravenous high-dose oxacillin therapy. Findings in an adult inpatient population. *Ann. Intern. Med.,* **1978,** *89,* 497–500.

Park, J. T., and Strominger, J. L. Mode of action of penicillin. *Science,* **1957,** *125,* 99–101.

Parker, C. W. Drug allergy (third of three parts). *N. Engl. J. Med.,* **1975,** *292,* 957–960.

Parry, M. F., and Neu, H. C. Ticarcillin for treatment of serious infections with gram-negative bacteria. *J. Infect. Dis.,* **1976,** *134,* S476–S485.

———. A comparative study of ticarcillin plus tobramycin versus carbenicillin plus gentamicin for the treatment of serious infections due to gram-negative bacilli. *Am. J. Med.,* **1978,** *64,* 961–966.

Pasternack, D. P., and Stephens, B. G. Reversible nephrotoxicity associated with cephalothin therapy. *Arch. Intern. Med.,* **1975,** *135,* 599–602.

Pollack, A. A.; Berger, S. A.; Simberkoff, M. S.; and Rahal, J. J. Hepatitis associated with high-dose oxacillin therapy. *Arch. Intern. Med.,* **1978,** *138,* 915–917.

Quintiliani, R., and Nightingale, C. II. Cefazolin—diagnosis and treatment. *Ann. Intern. Med.,* **1978,** *89,* 650–656.

Ratzan, K.; Ruiz, C.; and Irvin, G., III. Biliary tract excretion of cefazolin, cephalothin and cephaloridine in the presence of biliary tract disease. *Antimicrob. Agents Chemother.,* **1974,** *6,* 426–431.

Regamey, C.; Libke, R. D.; Engelking, E. R.; Clarke, J. T.; and Kirby, W. M. M. Inactivation of cefazolin, cephaloridine, and cephalothin by methicillin-sensitive and methicillin-resistant strains of *Staphylococcus aureus. J. Infect. Dis.,* **1975,** *131,* 291–294.

Renzini, G.; Ravagnan, G.; and Oliva, B. *In vitro* and *in vivo* microbiological evaluation of cephapirin, a new antibiotic. *Chemotherapy,* **1975,** *21,* 289–296.

Richmond, M. H. Factors influencing the antibacterial action of β-lactam antibiotics. *J. Antimicrob. Chemother.,* **1978,** *4,* 1–14.

Rolinson, G. N. Laboratory evaluation of amoxycillin. *Chemotherapy,* **1973,** *18,* Suppl., 1–10.

Rosenblatt, J. E.; Kind, A. C.; Brodie, J. L.; and Kirby, W. M. M. Mechanisms responsible for the blood level differences of isoxazolylpenicillins. *Arch. Intern. Med.,* **1968,** *121,* 345–348.

Ruiz, D. E., and Warner, J. F. Nafcillin treatment of *Staphylococcus aureus. Antimicrob. Agents Chemother.,* **1976,** *9,* 554–555.

Sabath, L. D.; Wheeler, N.; Laverdiere, M.; Blazevic, D.; and Wilkinson, B. J. A new type of penicillin resistance. *Lancet,* **1977,** *1,* 443–447.

Sabath, L. D.; Wilcox, C.; Garner, C.; and Finland, M. *In vitro* activity of cefazolin against recent clinical bacterial isolates. *J. Infect. Dis.,* **1973,** *128,* S320–S326.

Sanders, W. E.; Johnson, J. E.; and Taggart, J. G. Adverse

reactions to cephalothin and cephapirin. *N. Engl. J. Med.,* **1974,** *290,* 424–429.

Schlessinger, D. (ed.). *Microbiology—1977.* American Society for Microbiology, Washington, D. C., **1977.**

Shadomy, S.; Wagner, G.; and Carver, M. *In vitro* and *in vivo* studies with BL-S786, cefoxitin and cefamandole. *Antimicrob. Agents Chemother.,* **1978,** *13,* 412–415.

Shattil, J. S.; Bennett, J. S.; McDonough, M.; and Turnbull, J. Carbenicillin and penicillin G inhibit platelet functions *in vitro* by impairing the interaction of agonists with the platelet surface. *J. Clin. Invest.,* **1980,** *65,* 329–337.

Silver, M. S.; Counts, G. W.; Zeleznik, D.; and Turck, M. Comparison of *in vitro* antibacterial activity of three oral cephalosporins: cefaclor, cephalexin, and cephradine. *Antimicrob. Agents Chemother.,* **1977,** *12,* 591–596.

Sosna, J. P.; Murray, P. R.; and Medoff, G. Comparison of the *in vitro* activities of HR756 with cephalothin, cefoxitin, and cefamandole. *Antimicrob. Agents Chemother.,* **1978,** *14,* 876–879.

Sparling, P. F. Antibiotic resistance in *Neisseria gonorrheae. Med. Clin. North Am.,* **1972,** *56,* 1133–1144.

Spector, R., and Lorenzo, A. V. Inhibition of penicillin transport from the cerebrospinal fluid after intracisternal inoculation of bacteria. *J. Clin. Invest.,* **1974,** *54,* 316–325.

Spector, R., and Snodgrass, S. R. The effect of uremia on penicillin flux between blood and cerebrospinal fluid. *J. Lab. Clin. Med.,* **1976,** *87,* 749–759.

Spratt, B. G. Penicillin-binding proteins of *Escherichia coli:* general properties and characterization of mutants. In, *Microbiology—1977.* (Schlessinger, D., ed.) American Society for Microbiology, Washington, D. C., **1977,** pp. 182–190.

Sutter, V. L., and Finegold, S. M. Susceptibility of anaerobic bacteria to carbenicillin, cefoxitin, and related drugs. *J. Infect. Dis.,* **1975,** *131,* 417–422.

Sykes, R. B., and Matthew, M. The β-lactamases of gram-negative bacteria and their role in resistance to β-lactam antibiotics. *J. Antimicrob. Chemother.,* **1976,** *2,* 115–157.

Tally, F. P.; Jacobus, N. V.; Bartlett, J. G.; and Gorbach, S. L. Susceptibility of anaerobes to cefoxitin and other cephalosporins. *Antimicrob. Agents Chemother.,* **1975a,** *7,* 128–132.

———. *In vitro* activity of penicillins against anaerobes. *Ibid.,* **1975b,** *7,* 413–414.

Tally, F. P.; Jacobus, N. V.; and Gorbach, S. L. *In vitro* activity of thienamycin. *Antimicrob. Agents Chemother.,* **1978,** *14,* 436–438.

Tjandramaga, T. B.; Muller, A.; Verbesselt, R.; DeSchepper, P. S.; and Verbist, L. Piperacillin: human pharmacokinetics after intravenous and intramuscular administration. *Antimicrob. Agents Chemother.,* **1978,** *14,* 829–837.

Tomasz, A., and Holtje, J. V. Murein hydrolases and lytic and killing action of penicillin. In, *Microbiology—1977.* (Schlessinger, D., ed.) American Society for Microbiology, Washington, D. C., **1977,** pp. 209–215.

Trager, G. M.; White, G. W.; Zimelis, V. M.; and Panwalker, A. P. LY-127935: a novel beta-lactam antibiotic with unusual antibacterial activity. *Antimicrob. Agents Chemother.,* **1979,** *16,* 297–300.

Venuto, R. C., and Plaut, M. E. Cephalothin handling in patients undergoing hemodialysis. In, *Antimicrobial Agents and Chemotherapy—1970.* (Hobby, G. L., ed.) American Society for Microbiology, Bethesda, **1971,** pp. 50–52.

Wade, J. C.; Petty, B. G.; and Conrad, G. Cephalothin plus an aminoglycoside is more nephrotoxic than methicillin plus an aminoglycoside. *Lancet,* **1978,** *2,* 604–606.

Wallace, J. F.; Atlas, E.; Bear, D. M.; Brown, N. K.; Clark, H.; and Turck, M. Evaluation of an indanyl ester of carbenicillin. In, *Antimicrobial Agents and Chemotherapy—1970.* (Hobby, G. L., ed.) American Society for Microbiology, Bethesda, **1971,** pp. 223–226.

Weinstein, L.; Lerner, P. I.; and Chew, W. H. Clinical and bacteriologic studies of the effect of "massive" doses of penicillin G on infections caused by gram-negative bacilli. *N. Engl. J. Med.,* **1964,** *271,* 525–533.

Williams, J. D.; Geddes, A. M.; and Neu, H. C. Cefoxitin: microbiology, pharmacology, and clinical use. *J. Antimicrob. Chemother.,* **1978,** *4,* Suppl. B, 1–256.

Wright, W. W.; Welch, H. W.; Wilner, J.; and Roberts, E. F. Body fluid concentrations of penicillin following intramuscular injection of single doses of benzathine penicillin G and/or procaine penicillin G. *Antibiotic Med. Clin. Ther.,* **1959,** *6,* 232–241.

Monographs and Reviews

Abraham, E. P. The action of antibiotics on bacteria. In, *Antibiotics,* Vol. II. (Florey, H. W., *et al.,* authors.) Oxford University Press, New York, **1949,** pp. 1438–1496.

———. The cephalosporins. *Pharmacol. Rev.,* **1962,** *14,* 473–500. (110 references.)

Barza, M. Penicillins. *J. Maine Med. Assoc.,* **1976,** *67,* 377–386.

Blumberg, P. M., and Strominger, J. L. Interaction of penicillin with the bacterial cell: penicillin-binding proteins and penicillin-sensitive enzymes. *Bacteriol. Rev.,* **1974,** *38,* 291–335.

Braude, A. I. *Antimicrobial Drug Therapy.* W. B. Saunders Co., Philadelphia, **1976.**

Chain, E. B. Penicillinase-resistant penicillins and the problem of the penicillin-resistant staphylococci. In, *Resistance of Bacteria to the Penicillins* (Ciba Foundation Study Group No. 13). (De Reuck, A. V. S., and Cameron, M. P., eds.) Little, Brown & Co., Boston, **1962,** pp. 3–19.

Conference. (Various authors.) Cephalosporins. *Postgrad. Med. J.,* **1970,** *46,* Suppl., 3–159.

Finland, M., and Weinstein, L. Complications induced by antimicrobial agents. *N. Engl. J. Med.,* **1953,** *248,* 220–226.

Fleming, A. History and development of penicillin. In, *Penicillin: Its Practical Application.* (Fleming, A., ed.) The Blakiston Co., Philadelphia, **1946,** pp. 1–33.

Florey, H. W. Historical introduction. In, *Antibiotics,* Vol. I. (Florey, H. W., *et al.,* authors.) Oxford University Press, New York, **1949,** pp. 1–73.

Flynn, E. H. (ed.). *Cephalosporins and Penicillins: Chemistry and Biology.* Academic Press, Inc., New York, **1972.**

Griffith, R. S., and Black, H. R. Cephalexin. *Med. Clin. North Am.,* **1970,** *54,* 1229–1244.

Herrell, W. E. *Penicillin and Other Antibiotic Agents.* W. B. Saunders Co., Philadelphia, **1945.**

International Symposium. (Various authors.) Amoxicillin: clinical perspectives. *J. Infect. Dis.,* **1974,** *129,* Suppl., S121–S274.

Klein, J., and Finland, M. The new penicillins. *N. Engl. J. Med.,* **1963,** *269,* 1019–1025. (214 references.)

Kucers, A., and Bennett, N. M. (eds.). *The Use of Antibiotics,* 2nd ed. William Heinemann Medical Books, Ltd., London, **1975.**

McHenry, M. C., and Gavan, T. L. Selection and use of antibacterial drugs. *Prog. Clin. Pathol.,* **1975,** *6,* 205–265.

Mandell, G. L. Cephaloridine. *Ann. Intern. Med.,* **1973b,** *79,* 561–565.

Moellering, R. C. Principles of anti-infective therapy. In, *Principles and Practice of Infectious Diseases.* (Mandell, G. L.; Douglas, R. G., Jr.; and Bennett, J. E.; eds.) John Wiley & Sons, Inc., New York, **1979,** pp. 201–218.

Neu, H. C. Amoxicillin. *Ann. Intern. Med.,* **1979b,** *90,* 356–360.

Perlman, D. (ed.). *Structure-Activity Relationship among the Semi-Synthetic Antibiotics.* Academic Press, Inc., New York, **1977.**

Petz, L. D. Immunologic cross-reactivity between penicillins and cephalosporins: a review. *J. Infect. Dis.,* **1978,** *137,* S74–S79.

Pratt, W. B. *Chemotherapy of Infection.* Oxford University Press, New York, **1977.**

Rahal, J., and Simberkoff, M. S. Adverse reactions to anti-infective agents. *D.M.,* **1978,** *25,* No. 1, 1–67.

Strominger, J. L. The action of penicillin and other antibiotics on bacterial wall synthesis. *Johns Hopkins Med. J.,* **1973,** *133,* 63–81.

Symposium. (Various authors.) Symposium on cefamandole. (Moellering, R. C., ed.) *J. Infect. Dis.,* **1978,** *137,* S1–S194.

Tomasz, A. From penicillin-binding proteins to the lysis and death of bacteria: a 1979 view. *Rev. Infect. Dis.,* **1979,** *1,* 434–467.

Weinstein, L., and Kaplan, K. The cephalosporins. Microbiological, chemical and pharmacological properties and use in chemotherapy of infection. *Ann. Intern. Med.,* **1970,** *72,* 729–739.

CHAPTER

51 ANTIMICROBIAL AGENTS

[*Continued*]

The Aminoglycosides

Merle A. Sande and Gerald L. Mandell

The aminoglycoside antibiotics—gentamicin, tobramycin, amikacin, kanamycin, streptomycin, and neomycin—are discussed in this chapter. As the group name adequately implies, all these drugs contain amino sugars in glycosidic linkage. They are polycations, and their polarity is in part responsible for pharmacokinetic properties shared by all members of the group. For example, none is adequately absorbed after oral administration, none penetrates into the cerebrospinal fluid (CSF) with ease, and all are relatively rapidly excreted by the normal kidney.

The aminoglycosides are used almost exclusively to treat infections caused by gram-negative bacteria. They act to interfere with protein synthesis in susceptible microorganisms; the mechanism of this action is best understood for streptomycin, but a similar action is probably shared by the others. Mutations affecting proteins in the bacterial ribosome, the target for these drugs, can confer marked and rapid resistance to their action. Resistance can also result from the acquisition of a plasmid, and this is associated with the elaboration of drug-metabolizing enzymes. Bacteria that acquire resistance to one aminoglycoside may exhibit resistance to the others.

Serious toxicity is a major limitation to the usefulness of the aminoglycosides, and the same spectrum of toxicity is shared by all members of the group. Most notable is ototoxicity, which can involve both the auditory and vestibular functions of the eighth cranial nerve. Nephrotoxicity is an additional important problem.

History and Source. The ineffectiveness of penicillin G in the treatment of infections due to gram-negative microorganisms was the primary stimulus for the search for antimicrobial agents effective against such bacteria. The development of streptomycin was the result of a well-planned, scientific search for antibacterial substances. Waksman and coworkers examined a number of soil actinomycetes between 1939 and 1943 and demonstrated the elaboration by such fungi of a number of potent antibiotics; however, none of these was clinically useful, being too toxic or not sufficiently active. In 1943, a strain of *Streptomyces griseus* was isolated that elaborated a potent antimicrobial substance. The first public announcement of the discovery of this new antibiotic—*streptomycin*—was made by Schatz, Bugie, and Waksman early in 1944, and it was soon shown to inhibit the growth of the tubercle bacillus and a number of gram-positive and gram-negative microorganisms *in vitro* and *in vivo*. In less than 2 years, extensive bacteriological, chemical, and pharmacological investigations of streptomycin had been carried out, and its clinical usefulness was established. Controlled studies of the therapeutic efficacy of the drug in man were supervised by the National Research Council and supported by large contributions from pharmaceutical and chemical companies; this constituted the first privately financed, nationally coordinated, clinical drug evaluation in history. (*See* Waksman, 1949, 1953.) However, streptomycin-resistant gram-negative bacilli emerged rapidly and limited its clinical usefulness. Today, it is usually administered in combination with other antimicrobial agents only for the treatment of relatively unusual diseases, such as certain types of bacterial endocarditis, tularemia, and plague; it is occasionally used for tuberculosis.

In 1949, Waksman and Lechevalier isolated a soil organism, *Streptomyces fradiae,* which produced a new antibiotic that in crude form contained an antifungal compound (*fradicin*) and a group of antibacterial substances that were labeled "neomycin." *Neomycin* was purified in the same year and found to be a complex of three compounds (neomycins A, B, and C) with different antimicrobial activities; commercial preparations consist almost entirely of neomycin B. Unfortunately, this drug proved to cause severe renal toxicity and ototoxicity when administered parenterally, and it is now used only topically and for its local effect in the bowel.

Kanamycin, an antibiotic produced by *Streptomyces kanamyceticus,* was first produced and isolated by Umezawa and coworkers at the Japanese National

Institutes of Health in 1957. It was shown to be active against a variety of microorganisms and, for several years, was an important antibiotic for the treatment of serious infections with gram-negative bacilli. Because of toxicity and the emergence of resistant microorganisms, kanamycin has largely been replaced by the three newer aminoglycosides, gentamicin, tobramycin, and amikacin.

Gentamicin is a broad-spectrum antibiotic derived from the actinomycete *Micromonospora purpurea.* This drug was first studied and described by Weinstein and coworkers in 1963, and isolated, purified, and characterized by Rosselot and colleagues (1964). It has a broader spectrum of activity than kanamycin and is currently the most widely used aminoglycoside for the treatment of severe infections due to gram-negative bacteria. Its heirs, tobramycin and amikacin, were introduced into clinical practice in the 1970s. *Tobramycin* is one of several components of a complex of aminoglycosides (nebramycin) elaborated by *Streptomyces tenebrarius* (Higgins and Kastners, 1967). It is most similar in antimicrobial activity and toxicity to gentamicin. In contrast to the

other aminoglycosides, *amikacin* is a semisynthetic product—a modification of kanamycin described by Kawaguchi and coworkers (1972). This agent was found to be resistant to inactivation by most of the bacterial enzymes known to metabolize aminoglycosides.

Chemistry. The aminoglycosides all consist of two or more amino sugars joined in glycosidic linkage to a hexose nucleus, which is usually in a central position (*see* Figure 51–1). This hexose, or *aminocyclitol,* is either streptidine (found in streptomycin) or 2-deoxystreptamine (characteristic of all other available aminoglycosides) (*see* formulas of neomycin B and streptomycin, below). These compounds are thus aminoglycosidic aminocyclitols, although the simpler term *aminoglycoside* is commonly used to describe them.

The aminoglycoside families are distinguished by the amino sugars attached to the aminocyclitol. In the neomycin family, which includes neomycin B, paromomycin (*see* Chapter 46), ribostamycin, and lividomycin (the last two compounds are not used

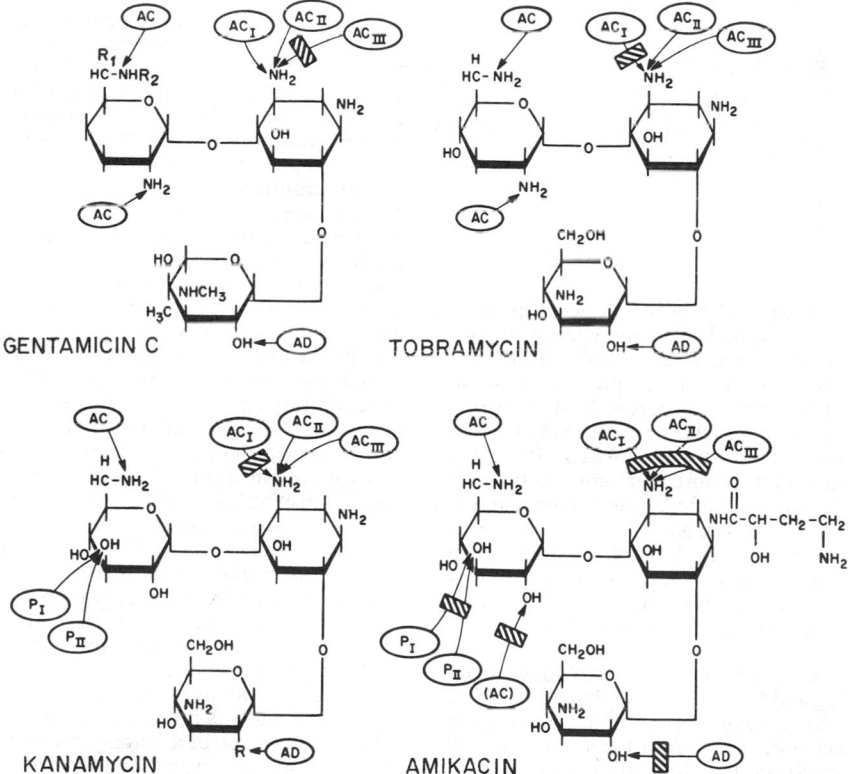

Figure 51–1. *Sites of activity of various plasmid-mediated enzymes capable of inactivating aminoglycosides.*

The symbol ▨ indicates regions of the molecule that are protected from the designated enzyme (*AC* = acetylase; *AD* = adenylylase; *P* = phosphorylase). In gentamicin C_1, $R_1 = R_2 = CH_3$; in gentamicin C_2, $R_1 = CH_3$, $R_2 = H$; in gentamicin C_{1a}, $R_1 = R_2 = H$. In kanamycin A, R = OH; in kanamycin B, R = NH_2. (Modified from Moellering, 1977. Courtesy of the *Medical Journal of Australia.*)

clinically in the United States), there are three amino sugars attached to the central 2-deoxystreptamine, which distinguishes it from the kanamycin and gentamicin families, which have only two such amino sugars. Neomycin B is a polybasic, water-soluble substance that readily forms salts with a variety of acids. Its structural formula is as follows:

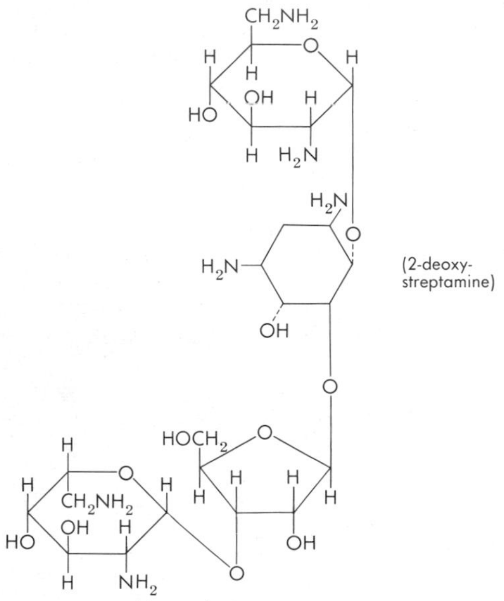

Neomycin B

In the kanamycin family, which includes kanamycins A and B, amikacin, and tobramycin, two amino sugars are linked to a centrally located 2-deoxystreptamine moiety; one of these (in position III) is a 3-aminohexose (*see* Figure 51–1 for structural formulas). Commercial preparations of kanamycin contain both kanamycins A and B; in the United States the latter must represent less than 5% of the total. Tobramycin differs from kanamycin B in the absence of a 3'-oxygen atom in the amino sugar in position I (Figure 51–1). As mentioned, amikacin is a semisynthetic derivative; it is prepared from kanamycin A by acylation of the 1-amino group of the 2-deoxystreptamine moiety with 2-hydroxy-4-aminobutyric acid.

The gentamicin family, which includes gentamicins C_1, C_{1a}, and C_2, sisomicin, and netilmicin, has a different 3-amino sugar (garosamine) in position III. Variations in methylation of the amino sugar in position I result in the different components of gentamicin. These modifications have little effect on biological activity.

Streptomycin and dihydrostreptomycin (the latter is no longer available because of excessive ototoxicity) differ from the other aminoglycoside antibiotics in that they contain streptidine rather than 2-deoxystreptamine and the aminocyclitol is not in a central position. The structural formula of streptomycin is as follows:

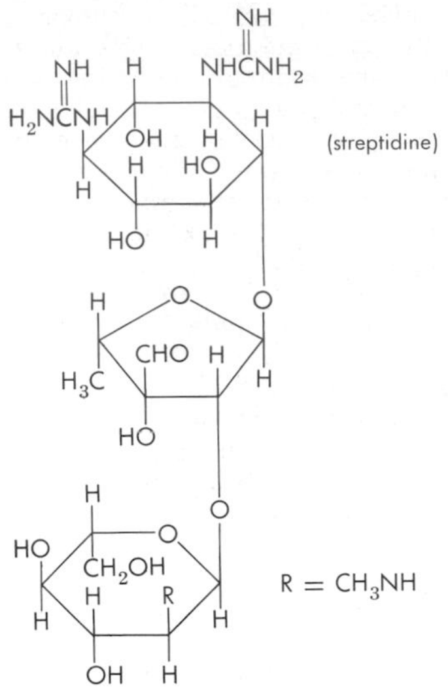

Streptomycin

Mechanism of Action. The aminoglycoside antibiotics are rapidly bactericidal; they act directly on the bacterial ribosome, where they inhibit protein synthesis and decrease the fidelity of translation of the genetic code. To reach the ribosome, the drugs must be transported across the cell membrane. Since these compounds are highly polar, there is little passive diffusion. Their transport appears to be an active process that is closely linked to electron transport, oxidative phosphorylation, and the respiratory quinones in the cell membrane.

Bryan and coworkers have proposed a model that includes two distinct phases of transport (*see* Bryan and Van Den Elzen, 1977). The first (energy-dependent phase I) is characterized by fortuitous, low-affinity binding of aminoglycosides to portions of respiratory energization complexes that are transported through the cell membrane. This phase is relatively inefficient and is inhibited by several divalent cations (including Ca^{2+} and Mg^{2+}); nevertheless, in sensitive bacteria it results in accumulation of adequate concentrations of the antibiotics to bind with high affinity to ribosomes that are associated with the membrane. This interaction triggers a second phase of transport (energy-dependent phase II) and corresponds to the onset of inhibition of protein synthesis. The second transport system is not well understood, but its operation appears to be associated with functional or architectural changes in the membrane; there is marked acceleration of intracellular accumulation of aminoglycoside. The efficiency of these transport systems and, thus, the rate of drug accumulation are the factors primarily responsible for variation in the sensitivity *in vitro* of different microbial strains to the aminoglycosides. In addition, the kinetics of transport can be significantly altered by pH, divalent cations, osmolality, and oxygen tension. Thus, antimicrobial activity of the aminoglycosides may be markedly reduced in the anaerobic environment of an abscess, in an acidic urine, and so forth.

The primary intracellular site of action of the aminoglycosides is the 30 S ribosomal subunit, which consists of 21 proteins and a single 16 S molecule of RNA (*see* Mitsuhashi, 1975). Alterations of at least three of these proteins markedly affects the action of streptomycin (Stöffler and Tischendorf, 1975). For example, a single amino acid substitution of asparagine for lysine at position 42 of one ribosomal protein (S_{12}) prevents binding of the drug; the resultant mutant is totally resistant to streptomycin. Another mutant, wherein glutamine is the amino acid at this position, is *dependent* on streptomycin. These microorganisms actually require the presence of the antibiotic for survival (*see* below). Most of the other aminoglycosides have also been shown to bind to the 30 S ribosomal subunit; these antibiotics also appear to bind to several sites on the 50 S ribosomal subunit (Davies and Courvalin, 1977; Le Goffic et al., 1979).

Aminoglycosides disrupt the normal cycle of ribosomal function by interfering, at least in part, with the first step of protein synthesis that occurs at the ribosome (initiation). Abnormal initiation complexes (or "streptomycin monosomes") accumulate in the cell (Luzzatto *et al.*, 1969). Other investigators have noted inhibitory effects at later points in the sequence (Tai *et al.*, 1973). Another effect of the aminoglycosides is their capacity to induce misreading of the genetic code of the mRNA template, and incorrect amino acids are incorporated into the growing polypeptide chains (*see* Tai *et al.*, 1978). The aminoglycosides vary in their capacity to cause misreading, and this property presumably depends on differences in their affinities for specific ribosomal proteins. The mutation to dependence on streptomycin probably results from misreading of the genetic code (*see* Stöffler and Tischendorf, 1975). If there is a mutation at some other site in the bacterial genome that would effectively prevent growth (*e.g.,* an amino acid substitution in a protein essential for normal metabolism), streptomycin-induced misreading of the mutation could result in an acceptable correction of the defect (phenotypic suppression). Bacteria could then resume growth only in the presence of the aminoglycoside. While this is a fascinating phenomenon, it is not of clinical significance.

None of the known actions of the aminoglycosides has been shown to account for the bactericidal effect of these drugs. It is thus not known why aminoglycosides are bactericidal, while other antibiotics that impair protein synthesis are usually only bacteriostatic. Differences may be related to the high affinity of these agents for the ribosome or, perhaps, to secondary effects on the cell envelope.

Microbial Resistance to the Aminoglycosides. Bacteria may be resistant to the antimicrobial activity of the aminoglycosides because of failure of permeation of the antibiotic, low affinity of the drug for the bacterial ribosome, or inactivation of the drug by microbial enzymes. The last-named mechanism is by far the most important explanation for the acquired microbial resistance to aminoglycosides that is encountered in clinical practice.

As mentioned above, the transport of aminoglycosides across the cell membrane is an oxygen-dependent, active process. Strictly anaerobic bacteria

are thus resistant to these drugs, since they lack the necessary transport system. Similarly, facultative bacteria are generally much more resistant when they are grown under anaerobic conditions (Bryan and Van Den Elzen, 1976). The significance of the so-called permeability barrier as an explanation for resistance to aminoglycosides among aerobic gram-negative bacilli is not known. This mechanism is responsible for low-level resistance to streptomycin in many strains of *Pseudomonas aeruginosa* (Tseng *et al.,* 1972). Natural resistance to amikacin by *Pseud. maltophilia* and certain other microorganisms appears to have a similar basis (Price *et al.,* 1976), as does the low-level resistance of gram-positive cocci, especially enterococci, to aminoglycosides. The addition of antibiotics such as penicillin that alter the structure of the cell wall can markedly increase the entrance of aminoglycosides into these cells; this is an excellent example of synergism between antibiotics (*see* Chapter 48; Moellering and Weinberg, 1971).

The second mechanism of resistance, which results from alterations in ribosomal structure, is less relevant clinically. Single-step mutations in *Escherichia coli* that result in the substitution of a single amino acid in a crucial ribosomal protein may prevent binding of the drug. While such strains are highly resistant to streptomycin (Stöffler and Tischendorf, 1975), they are not widespread in nature. Only 5% of strains of *Pseud. aeruginosa* exhibit such ribosomal resistance to streptomycin. However, from 18 to 40% of strains of enterococci isolated from patients with endocarditis are resistant to high concentrations of streptomycin, and ribosomes from these strains fail to bind streptomycin. For this reason there is no synergistic effect of penicillin and streptomycin against these strains. The vast majority of these enterococci are, however, sensitive to a combination of penicillin and gentamicin. Ribosomal resistance to gentamicin is rare among both gram-negative bacilli and gram-positive cocci (Zimmermann *et al.,* 1971).

Most acquired resistance to aminoglycosides results from their enzymatic inactivation. There are multiple enzymes involved, and they are localized in the bacterial membrane at or near the site of drug transport. They are capable of adenylylating, acetylating, or phosphorylating the aminoglycosides at numerous sites (Figure 51–1). Effort in the development of new aminoglycosides is being directed at the synthesis or isolation of agents that are poor substrates for these enzymes. Amikacin is the product of one such successful search and is remarkably resistant to inactivation. Only one of the common enzymes, an acetylase, is capable of inactivating this drug (*see* Price *et al.,* 1976; Moellering, 1977; Figure 51–1).

Antibacterial Activity of the Aminoglycosides. The antibacterial activity of gentamicin, tobramycin, kanamycin, and amikacin is primarily directed against aerobic, gram-negative bacilli. As noted above, these antibiotics have little activity against anaerobic microorganisms or facultative bacteria under anaerobic conditions. Their action against most gram-positive bacteria is limited. *Streptococcus pneumoniae* and *Strep. pyogenes* are highly resistant, and, in fact, gentamicin has been added to blood-

Table 51-1. ANTIBACTERIAL ACTIVITY OF THE AMINOGLYCOSIDES *

DRUG	PLASMA CONCENTRATION ACHIEVED ($\mu g/ml$)	BACTERIUM													
		Staphylococcus aureus		Escherichia coli		Proteus mirabilis		Pseudomonas aeruginosa		Klebsiella		Enterobacter		Serratia	
		MIC †	% ‡	MIC	%	MIC	%	MIC	%	MIC	%	MIC	%	MIC	%
Kanamycin	8–16	1	90%	4	90%	4	90%	>32	5%	4	60%	16	50%	>32	10%
Gentamicin	4–8	0.25	95%	1	95%	2	85%	4	90%	1	80%	2	90%	2	80%
Tobramycin	4–8	0.25	95%	2	95%	1	85%	1	95%	1	80%	2	90%	4	85%
Amikacin	8–16	1	95%	2	98%	2	95%	4	95%	2	96%	2	98%	4	90%

* Data from Korzeniowski and Hook (1979).
† Mean minimal inhibitory concentration (*see text*).
‡ Percentage of isolated strains considered sensitive to the drug. These values vary among hospitals; most resistant strains are found in hospitals, especially in intensive care units.

agar plates to aid in the isolation of these microorganisms from sputum and pharyngeal secretions (Dilworth et al., 1975). Streptomycin and gentamicin are active against enterococci and other streptococci at concentrations that can be achieved clinically only when combined with a penicillin. Such combinations result in a more rapid bactericidal effect than is produced by either drug alone. Both gentamicin and tobramycin are active in vitro against more than 95% of strains of Staphylococcus aureus and most strains of Staph. epidermidis. However, the clinical efficacy of these agents in the treatment of serious staphylococcal infections has not been documented, and they should not be used alone in such situations. Gentamicin-resistant mutant strains of staphylococci emerge rapidly during exposure to the drug in vitro or in experimental infections; these mutants exhibit a unique dwarf colonial morphology (Sande and Courtney, 1976).

The aerobic gram-negative bacilli vary in their susceptibility to the four major aminoglycosides. Sensitive microorganisms are defined as those inhibited by concentrations that can be achieved clinically in plasma but that are not associated with a high incidence of toxicity; this value is 4 to 8 μg/ml for gentamicin and tobramycin and 8 to 16 μg/ml for amikacin and kanamycin. The mean minimal inhibitory concentration (MIC) and the percentage of clinical isolates considered sensitive are listed in Table 51-1. In general, gentamicin, tobramycin, and amikacin are more active than kanamycin. The only exceptions may be some unusual strains of Proteus rettgeri, Providencia species, and Herellea vaginicola, which may be more susceptible to kanamycin. Tobramycin and gentamicin exhibit similar activity against most gram-negative bacilli, although tobramycin is usually more active against Pseud. aeruginosa and against some strains of Proteus species. Most gram-negative bacilli (except Pseud. aeruginosa) that are resistant to gentamicin because of plasmid-mediated inactivating enzymes will also inactivate tobramycin. However, approximately 50% of Pseud. aeruginosa that are resistant to gentamicin remain sensitive to tobramycin (Symposium, 1976b). In some hospitals, the nosocomial flora have undergone considerable alterations in susceptibility to antibiotics during the last 10 years, with a gradual increase in resistance to gentamicin and tobramycin. Fortunately, amikacin has retained its activity in this setting, a phenomenon attributed to this drug's resistance to the aminoglycoside-inactivating enzymes. While not as active against many gram-negative bacilli as are tobramycin and gentamicin, higher concentrations of amikacin can be achieved, and the drug has a broad spectrum of activity; it is thus particularly valuable in treating nosocomial infections.

ABSORPTION, DISTRIBUTION, AND ELIMINATION OF THE AMINOGLYCOSIDES

Absorption.　The aminoglycosides are highly polar cations; they are thus very poorly absorbed from the intestinal tract. Less than 1% of a dose is absorbed following either oral or rectal administration. The drugs are not inactivated in the intestine, and they are eliminated quantitatively in the feces. The effect of intestinal inflammation on absorption has not been clearly established. Absorption of gentamicin from the gastrointestinal tract may be increased considerably when there is bacillary dysentery (Cox, 1970), but that of neomycin is not altered in the presence of ulcers or inflammatory disease of the bowel (Breen et al., 1972). Repeated oral or rectal administration may, however, result in accumulation to toxic concentrations in patients with renal impairment. Instillation of these drugs into body cavities with serosal surfaces may result in rapid absorption and unexpected toxicity. Similarly, intoxication may occur when aminoglycosides are applied topically to large wounds, burns, or cutaneous ulcers, particularly if there is renal insufficiency (Kelley et al., 1969).

All of these antibiotics are absorbed rapidly from intramuscular and subcutaneous sites of injection. Intramuscular injection results in peak concentrations in plasma after 30 to 90 minutes. That peak is similar to the concentration observed 30 minutes after completion of an intravenous infusion of an equal dose over a 30-minute period. In critically ill patients, especially those in shock, absorption of drug may be reduced from intramuscular sites because of poor perfusion.

Distribution.　Because of their polar nature, the aminoglycosides are largely excluded from most cells, from the central nervous system (CNS), and from the eye. There is negligible binding of aminoglycosides to plasma albumin; while one third of streptomycin may be so bound, less than 10% of any of the newer aminoglycosides is associated with plasma proteins (Barza and Scheife, 1977). The volume of distribution of these drugs is therefore equal to the volume of extracellular fluid, which constitutes approximately 25% of lean body weight (Barza et al., 1975).

As would be expected, concentrations of aminoglycosides in secretions and tissues are low. High concentrations are found only in the renal cortex, a factor that presumably contributes to the nephrotoxicity caused by these drugs. Concentrations in bile approach 30% of those found in plasma as a result of active hepatic secretion, but this represents a very minor excretory route for the aminoglycosides. Concentrations may be lower if there is biliary obstruction (Mendelson et al., 1973). Penetration into respiratory secretions is likewise poor (Howley et al., 1974). Diffusion into pleural fluid is relatively slow, but concentrations that approximate those in the plasma may be achieved after repeated administration. Similarly, drug concentrations in synovial fluid are eventually more than 50% of those found in plasma (Dee and Kozin, 1977). Inflammation increases the penetration of aminoglycosides into peritoneal and pericardial cavities.

Penetration of aminoglycosides into CSF is very limited. In experimental animals and man, concentrations in CSF are less than 10% of those in plasma in the absence of inflammation; this value may approach 20% when there is meningitis (Strausbaugh et al., 1977). The concentrations achieved are usually *inadequate* for the treatment of gram-negative bacillary meningitis, especially in adults. Intrathecal or intraventricular administration of aminoglycosides is necessary in such cases (Rahal et al., 1974; Kaiser and McGee, 1975). Therapeutic results of systemic administration are better in the treatment of meningitis in neonates (perhaps because of immaturity of the blood-brain barrier), and controlled studies have not shown additional benefit of either intrathecal or intraventricular injection of these drugs (McCracken and Mize, 1976; McCracken et al., 1979). Similarly, penetration into ocular fluids is so poor that effective therapy of bacterial endophthalmitis requires periocular injections of aminoglycosides (Barza, 1978).

Administration of aminoglycosides to females late in pregnancy may result in accumulation of drug in fetal plasma and amniotic fluid.

Elimination. The aminoglycosides are excreted almost entirely by glomerular filtration, and concentrations in the urine of 50 to 200 μg/ml are achieved (Jackson, 1977). Approximately 50 to 60% of a parenterally administered dose is excreted unchanged during the first 24 hours, with most of this appearing in the first 12 hours. The half-lives of the aminoglycosides in plasma are similar and vary between 2 and 3 hours. Renal clearance is approximately two thirds of the simultaneous creatinine clearance (Barza and Scheife, 1977); this observation suggests some tubular reabsorption of these drugs, although probenecid has no detectable effect on their excretion (Chiu et al., 1976).

Following the initial doses of an aminoglycoside, disappearance from the plasma exceeds renal excretion by 10 to 20%; however, after 1 to 2 days of therapy, nearly 100% of subsequent doses is recovered in the urine. This lag period probably represents saturation of binding sites in tissues. The rate of disappearance of drug from these sites is considerably longer than from plasma; the half-life for tissue-bound aminoglycoside has been estimated to range from 30 to 700 hours (Schentag and Jusko, 1977). For this reason aminoglycosides can be detected in the urine for 10 to 20 days after dosage is discontinued. All of the administered dose is eventually recovered in the urine unaltered. Aminoglycoside bound to renal tissue appears to exhibit antibacterial activity and protects experimental animals against bacterial infections of the kidney after the drug can no longer be detected in plasma (Glauser et al., 1979).

The concentration of aminoglycoside in plasma produced by the initial or loading dose is not affected by renal function. However, elimination of aminoglycosides is almost entirely dependent on the kidney; a linear relationship exists between the concentration of creatinine in plasma and the half-life of all aminoglycosides in patients with moderately compromised renal function. In anephric patients, the half-life varies from 20 to 40 times that determined in normal individuals. *Since the incidence of nephrotoxicity and ototoxicity is directly related to the concentration to which an aminoglycoside accumulates, it is critical to reduce the maintenance dosage of these drugs in patients with impaired renal function.* This must be done with precision, since the concentration in plasma that is associated with toxicity is not much greater than that required for treatment of many bacterial infections. The size of the individual dose, the interval between doses, or both can be altered. There is no conclusive information on the best approach. A variety of specific recommendations and nomograms may be found in the literature (Chan et al., 1972; Hull and Sarubbi, 1976; Barza and Scheife, 1977; Korzeniowski and

Hook, 1979). The most consistent plasma concentrations are achieved when the recommended dosage is given in milligrams per kilogram of body weight, and, since aminoglycosides are minimally distributed in fatty tissue, the lean or expected body weight should be used (*see* Diem and Lentner, 1970, for calculation). Methods for calculation of dosage are also described in Appendix II.

However, there are obvious difficulties in utilizing any of these approaches for ill patients with rapidly changing renal function. In addition, even when known factors are taken into consideration, concentrations of aminoglycosides achieved in plasma after a given dose vary widely between patients (Barza *et al.,* 1975). If extracellular volume is expanded, concentrations will be reduced. For unknown reasons the half-lives of the aminoglycosides are reduced in patients with cystic fibrosis, and the volume of distribution is increased in patients with leukemia (Rosenthal, 1977; Spyker *et al.,* 1978). Patients with anemia (hematocrit <25%) have a concentration in plasma that is higher than expected, probably because of a reduction in the number of binding sites on red blood cells (Siber *et al.,* 1975).

Determination of the concentration of drug in plasma is an essential guide to the proper administration of aminoglycosides. Ideally, a plasma concentration at the trough of the fluctuating curve, collected just prior to a dose, and a peak concentration, collected 30 minutes after a dose, should be obtained to ensure adequacy of the antimicrobial activity (peak) and to protect against accumulation of drug (trough). Concentrations should be determined several times per week (more frequently if renal function is changing) and should always be determined within 24 hours after a change in dosage.

Aminoglycosides are removed from the body by either hemodialysis or peritoneal dialysis. Approximately 50% of the administered dose is removed in 12 hours by hemodialysis, and this technic has been used for the treatment of overdosage (*see* Danish *et al.,* 1974; Barza and Scheife, 1977). As a general rule, a dose equal to half of the loading dose administered after each hemodialysis should maintain the plasma concentration in the desired range; however, a number of variables make this a rough approximation at best. Frequent monitoring of drug concentrations in plasma is again crucial.

Peritoneal dialysis is less effective than hemodialysis in removing aminoglycosides. Clearance rates are approximately 5 to 10 ml per minute for the various drugs, but are highly variable (Atkins *et al.,* 1973; Appel and Neu, 1977). If there is bacterial peritonitis in a patient who requires dialysis, a therapeutic concentration of the aminoglycoside will probably not be achieved in the peritoneal fluid, since the ratio of the concentration in plasma to that in peritoneal fluid may be 10 to 1 (Smithivas *et al.,* 1971). It is thus recommended that antibiotic be added to the dialysate to achieve concentrations equal to those desired in plasma (*i.e.,* 4 µg/ml for gentamicin and tobramycin; 15 µg/ml for amikacin and kanamycin). This should be preceded by the parenteral administration of a loading dose.

Although excretion of aminoglycosides is similar in adults and children over 6 months of age, half-lives of the drugs may be significantly prolonged in the newborn (Nelson and McCracken, 1972). Newborn infants who weigh less than 2 kg have half-lives for aminoglycosides of 8 to 11 hours during the first week of life, while those who weigh over 2 kg eliminate these drugs with half-lives of about 5 hours (Yow, 1977). It is thus critically important to monitor concentrations of aminoglycosides during treatment of neonates.

UNTOWARD EFFECTS OF THE AMINOGLYCOSIDES

All aminoglycosides have the potential to produce *vestibular, cochlear,* and *renal* toxicity. These side effects reduce the usefulness of the compounds and make a difficult job of their proper administration. Toxicity varies between the drugs and, as previously emphasized, can be minimized by careful control of their concentrations in plasma (Appel and Neu, 1977).

Ototoxicity. Both vestibular and auditory dysfunction can follow the administration of any of the aminoglycosides. Studies of both animals and man have documented progressive accumulation of these drugs in the perilymph of the inner ear (Federspil, 1977). Penetration occurs predominantly when concentrations in plasma are high and diffusion back into the blood stream is slow; the half-lives of the aminoglycosides are five to six times longer in the otic fluids than in plasma. Back diffusion is obviously facilitated when the concentration of drug in plasma reaches a low trough. Thus, ototoxicity is more severe in patients with repeated trough concentrations of gentamicin in plasma that exceed 2 µg/ml (Barza and Scheife, 1977). However, even a single dose of tobramycin can produce slight cochlear dysfunction during periods when the concentration in plasma is at its peak (Wilson and Ramsden, 1977).

Ototoxicity is the result of progressive destruction of vestibular or cochlear sensory cells. Studies in guinea pigs exposed to large doses of gentamicin reveal degeneration of the sensory hair cells in the central part of the crista ampullaris (vestibular organ) and fusion of individual sensory hairs into giant hairs (Wersäll *et al.,* 1973). Similar studies with gentamicin and tobramycin also demonstrate loss of hair cells in the cochlea of the organ of Corti (Theopold, 1977). With increasing dosage and prolonged exposure, damage progresses from the base of the cochlea, where high-frequency sounds are processed, to the apex, necessary for the perception of low frequencies. These histologic changes correlate with the ability of the cochlea to generate an action potential in response to sound. While early changes induced by aminoglycosides may be reversible, cellular regeneration does not occur after sensory cells are lost. It has been suggested that aminoglycosides interfere with the active transport system essential for the maintenance of the ionic balance of the endolymph (Neu and Bendush, 1976); this leads to alteration in the normal concentrations of ions in the labyrinthine fluids, with impairment of electrical activity and nerve conduction. Eventually, the osmotic changes, or perhaps the drugs themselves, damage the hair cells irreversibly.

The degree of permanent dysfunction correlates with the number of destroyed or altered sensory hair cells, and this is directly related to sustained exposure to the drug. Repeated courses of aminoglycosides, each resulting in the loss of more cells, can lead to deafness. Since there appears to be a decrease in the number of cells with age, older patients are more susceptible to ototoxicity. Drugs such as ethacrynic acid (Mathog and Capps, 1977) furosemide, mannitol, and, probably, other diuretics potentiate the ototoxic effects of the aminoglycosides. Patients with preexisting auditory impairment are also more likely to develop hearing loss following exposure to these agents.

Although all of the aminoglycosides are capable of affecting both cochlear and vestibular function, some preferential toxicity is evident. Streptomycin and gentamicin predominantly produce vestibular effects, whereas amikacin, kanamycin, and neomycin primarily affect auditory function; tobramycin affects both equally. The exact incidence of ototoxicity is extremely difficult to determine. Data suggest that the incidence of overt ototoxicity is about 3% for amikacin, 2% for gentamicin, and 1% for tobramycin, streptomycin, and kanamycin in patients who are treated for less than 2 weeks (Barza and Scheife, 1977; Jackson, 1977; Korzeniowski and Hook, 1979). Prolonged use, high dosage, and preexisting renal disease markedly increase the incidence of toxicity. For example, up to 75% of patients who receive 2 g of streptomycin for more than 60 days show evidence of nystagmus or postural imbalance. Five to 30% of patients who receive kanamycin for long periods and 20% of very ill patients who receive amikacin exhibit ototoxicity. The incidence of subclinical toxicity, as revealed by sensitive tests for auditory and vestibular function, appears to be much higher.

Initial symptoms of cochlear damage induced by aminoglycosides include tinnitus and/or a sensation of pressure or fullness in the ears. Loss of perception of tones at high frequencies may be detected by audiometry before toxicity is overt; however, deafness may develop without warning. Vestibular dysfunction is manifested by nystagmus, vertigo, nausea, vomiting, or acute Ménière's syndrome. (The complete clinical picture is described in the section on Streptomycin; *see* page 1172.) However, functional impairment is frequently minimal because of rapid adaptation and compensation. A careful study of children born to women who received long-term treatment with streptomycin revealed a high incidence of subtle vestibular abnormalities, but none of the children had gross functional impairment (Conway and Boct, 1965).

It is recommended that patients receiving aminoglycosides be carefully monitored for ototoxicity, since the initial symptoms may be reversible; however, deafness may occur several weeks after therapy is discontinued.

Nephrotoxicity. Very high concentrations of aminoglycoside antibiotics accumulate in the renal cortex and urine, and this correlates with the potential of these drugs to cause nephrotoxicity. The true incidence of nephrotoxicity caused by the aminoglycosides is extremely difficult to determine. It appears to vary with the compound and, as with ototoxicity, depends on other factors. Neomycin is the most nephrotoxic aminoglycoside and is no longer administered systemically for this reason. When administered orally to patients with renal disease, neomycin may accumulate in plasma to concentrations that cause nephrotoxicity.

Gentamicin appears to be the most nephrotoxic of the commonly used drugs (Gary *et al.,* 1976). The incidence of renal toxicity in man varies in reported series from 2 to 10%, with most investigators reporting values of approximately 4%. Corresponding figures for the other aminoglycosides are amikacin and kanamycin, 3 to 8%; tobramycin, 1%; streptomycin, less than 1%. Prolonged therapy and excessively high trough concentrations of the drugs in plasma seem to correlate with the incidence and severity of renal damage, just as they do with ototoxicity. Nephrotoxicity does not correlate as well with the peak concentration of drug in plasma or with total daily dose. Periodic determination of the trough concentration of aminoglycoside is, in fact, a more sensitive indicator of renal function than is the concentration of creatinine. Gradual accumulation of drug occurs when there is a slight reduction in glomerular filtration, whereas the concentration of creatinine in plasma may not rise appreciably until creatinine clearance falls below 40 ml per minute.

Elderly patients are more susceptible to nephrotoxic effects of these drugs, as are patients with shock, dehydration, preexisting renal decrease, or oliguria. Other nephrotoxic drugs (*e.g.*, polymyxin B, amphotericin, and vancomycin) potentiate the toxicity of the aminoglycosides (Churchill and Seely, 1977). Concurrent therapy with cephalothin may also potentiate the nephrotoxic effect of gentamicin (Barza and Scheife, 1977), although this has not been a universal observation.

Nephrotoxicity from aminoglycosides is essentially a form of acute tubular necrosis and is initially manifested by the inability to concentrate the urine. This damage does not usually occur until after at least 5 to 7 days of therapy; it progresses as administration of the drug is continued. The urine then characteristically contains protein and tubular cell casts. A reduction in glomerular filtration rate follows and is associated with elevation in the concentrations of the aminoglycoside, creatinine, and urea in plasma. The histological features are those of acute tubular damage, with secondary interstitial damage (Bennet *et al.*, 1977; Luft *et al.*, 1977). These changes are usually reversible, and regeneration of renal cells occurs if the drug is discontinued. Treatment with an aminoglycoside should not be reinstituted soon, since these drugs can be detected in the renal medulla and urine for up to 25 days after their administration is stopped (Bergeron and Trottier, 1979).

Neuromuscular Blockade. The rather unique toxic reaction of acute muscular paralysis and apnea resulting from neuromuscular blockade has been attributed to the various aminoglycosides. A review of 83 reports of prolonged paralysis implicated neomycin as the most frequent cause (Pittinger *et al.*, 1970). In experimental systems the order of decreasing potency is neomycin, kanamycin, amikacin, gentamicin, and tobramycin.

In man, neuromuscular blockade has generally occurred after intrapleural or intraperitoneal instillation of large doses of an aminoglycoside; however, the reaction has followed the intravenous, intramuscular, and even the oral administration of these agents (Holtzman, 1976). Most episodes have occurred in association with anesthesia or the administration of other neuromuscular blocking agents. Patients with myasthenia gravis are particularly susceptible to this effect. However, others who depend on various degrees of hypoxemia to drive respiration (*e.g.*, patients with chronic obstructive pulmonary disease) should be observed carefully for signs of respiratory depression when an aminoglycoside is used.

Animal studies indicate that the aminoglycosides inhibit prejunctional release of acetylcholine while also reducing postsynaptic sensitivity to the transmitter (Pittinger and Adamson, 1972). Calcium overcomes the effect of the aminoglycoside at the neuromuscular junction, and the intravenous administration of a calcium salt is the preferred treatment of this toxicity. Inhibitors of cholinesterase (edrophonium, neostigmine) have also been used with varying degrees of success. Since physicians have become aware of this complication, it is now relatively uncommon.

Other Untoward Effects. In general, the aminoglycosides have little allergenic potential; both anaphylaxis and rash are unusual. Other reactions that have been attributed to these drugs are discussed below, particularly in the section on Streptomycin.

STREPTOMYCIN

Streptomycin is used today for the treatment of certain unusual infections, generally in combination with other antimicrobial agents. It is also occasionally administered for tuberculosis (*see* Chapter 53).

Preparations, Routes of Administration, and Dosage. *Streptomycin Sulfate*, U.S.P., is supplied for parenteral injection either as a sterile dry powder or in sterile solution. Each vial contains the equivalent of 1 or 5 g of the base; solutions, which are stable for months, contain 500 mg/ml.

Streptomycin can be administered by a variety of routes. *Intermittent, deep intramuscular injection* is the method most often used for parenteral administration. The total daily dose varies from 1 to 2 g (15 to 25 mg/kg); 500 mg to 1 g is injected every 12 hours. In adults, 1 g given intramuscularly produces a peak plasma concentration of 25 to 30 μg/ml. The intramuscular administration of 0.5 g of streptomycin every 8 hours produces *urinary concentrations* ranging from 200 to 1500 μg/ml, depending on renal function and urine volume. Children should receive 20 to 30 mg/kg daily, in two divided doses. Except in tuberculosis and subacute bacterial endocarditis, it is rarely necessary to give streptomycin for more than 7 to 10 days. Dosage schedules for tuberculosis are described in Chapter 53. Streptomycin has also been administered intravenously, intrathecally, and intraperitoneally. There is presently no indication for these methods of administration.

Untoward Effects. Since streptomycin has been available for over 35 years, the extent of its toxicity is more clearly defined than is that of the other aminoglycosides. It is believed that most toxicities are shared by all of the various congeners; detailed description is thus presented here.

Hypersensitivity Reactions. Skin rashes, eosinophilia, fever, blood dyscrasias, angioedema, exfoliative dermatitis, stomatitis, and *anaphylactic shock* are among the hypersensitivity reactions that may follow the administration of streptomycin. *Skin eruptions* have been reported in as many as 5% of persons so treated. Morbilliform, maculopapular, erythematous, and urticarial rashes have been observed. Mild cutaneous manifestations do not necessarily require cessation of treatment. *Pruritus, scaling, eosinophilia, lymphadenopathy,* and *fever* may accompany the eruptions, but classical serum sickness does not occur. *Eosinophilia* is common and may develop in 50% of patients receiving streptomycin for an extended period.

Exfoliative dermatitis occurs in less than 1% of individuals given the drug. Most of the allergic cutaneous phenomena subside promptly with cessation of therapy.

Drug fever as an isolated hypersensitivity phenomenon is relatively uncommon; elevations of temperature that occur during therapy more frequently result from sterile inflammatory reactions at the sites of injection of the antibiotic. Although rare, *acute anaphylaxis* may follow the administration of any quantity of streptomycin.

Several types of *blood dyscrasias* have been noted in patients receiving streptomycin. About 0.7% of individuals who receive streptomycin develop *neutropenia*. In a few, the process may progress to *agranulocytosis. Aplastic anemia, hemolytic anemia,* and *thrombopenia* with purpura have been described in a few instances.

Toxic and Irritative Reactions. The intramuscular administration of streptomycin commonly produces pain at the site of injection. Hot and tender masses may develop in the areas in which the antibiotic is injected. The inflammation is sterile and is frequently accompanied by fever.

Vestibular Toxicity. Nearly 75% of patients given 2 g of streptomycin daily for 60 to 120 days manifest some detectable vestibular disturbance; reduction of the dose to 1 g daily reportedly decreases the inci-

dence to approximately 25%. Moderately intense headache lasting 1 or 2 days may precede the onset of labyrinthine dysfunction. This is immediately followed by an *acute stage,* in which nausea, vomiting, and equilibratory difficulty develop and persist for 1 to 2 weeks. Vertigo in the upright position, inability to perceive termination of movement ("mental past pointing"), and difficulty in sitting or standing without visual cues are prominent symptoms. Drifting of the eyes at the end of a movement so that focusing and reading are difficult, positive Romberg test, and, rarely, pendular trunk movement and spontaneous nystagmus are outstanding signs. The acute stage ends suddenly and is followed by the appearance of manifestations consistent with *chronic labyrinthitis,* in which, although symptomless while in bed, the patient has difficulty when he attempts to walk or make sudden movements; ataxia is the most prominent feature. The chronic phase persists for approximately 2 months; it is gradually superseded by a *compensatory stage,* in which symptoms are latent and appear only when the eyes are closed. Adaptation to the impairment of labyrinthine function is accomplished by the use of visual cues and deep proprioceptive sensation for determining movement and position; it is more adequate in the young than in the old, but may not be sufficient to permit the high degree of coordination required in many special trades. Full recovery may require 12 to 18 months, and some patients have permanent residual damage. Although there is no specific treatment for the vestibular deficiency, early discontinuation of the drug may permit recovery prior to irreversible damage of the hair cells.

Deafness. Although the toxic effect of streptomycin is greater upon the vestibular than upon the auditory component of the eighth cranial nerve, disturbances in hearing occur, nevertheless, in an appreciable number of patients. Four to 15% of individuals receiving the drug for more than 1 week can be shown to have a measurable decrease in hearing, and complete deafness may ensue in rare cases. A high-pitched tinnitus is often the first symptom of impending difficulty. If the drug is not discontinued, auditory impairment may develop after a few days. The tinnitus may persist for several days to 2 weeks after therapy is stopped. Since perception of sound in the high-frequency range (outside the conversational range) is lost first, the affected individual is not aware of the difficulty, which is not detected unless careful audiometric examination is carried out. If the loss of hearing progresses, the lower sound ranges are affected, and conversation becomes difficult.

Other Effects on the Nervous System. The administration of streptomycin may produce dysfunction of the *optic nerve.* Scotomas, presenting as enlargement of the blind spot, have been induced by the drug.

Among the less common toxic reactions to streptomycin is *peripheral neuritis.* This may be due either to accidental injection of a nerve during the course of parenteral therapy or to toxicity involving nerves remote from the site of antibiotic administration. Paresthesia, most commonly perioral but also present in other areas of the face or in the hands, occasionally follows the use of the antibiotic and usually appears within 30 to 60 minutes after injection of the drug, it may persist for several hours.

Renal Effects. Streptomycin produces less nephrotoxicity than do the other aminoglycoside antibiotics, but albuminuria, cylindruria, and reduced urine output may develop as a result of streptomycin therapy. Renal dysfunction is infrequent after daily doses of 1 to 1.5 g of the drug, but it is common when doses of 3 to 4 g are administered daily.

Therapeutic Uses. *Bacterial Endocarditis.* Streptomycin and penicillin produce a synergistic bactericidal effect *in vitro* and in animal models of infection against enterococci, other group-D streptococci, and the various oral streptococci of the *viridans* group. Many authorities administer such antibiotics concurrently for treatment of endocarditis caused by these microorganisms. Penicillin G alone is ineffective in the therapy of enterococcal endocarditis, and either streptomycin (1 to 2 g per day) or gentamicin (1 mg/kg three times daily) must also be given to ensure cure. Gentamicin is preferred when the strain shows complete (ribosomal) resistance (MIC greater than 2 mg/ml) to streptomycin. Both penicillin G and the aminoglycoside are administered for 4 to 6 weeks. Endocarditis caused by penicillin-sensitive streptococci (MIC less than 0.1 µg/ml) has been successfully treated with penicillin G alone for 4 weeks (relapse rate 1 to 2%; Karchmer et al., 1979), penicillin G plus streptomycin (0.5 g twice a day) for 2 weeks (relapse rate 1 to 2%, Wilson et al., 1978), or penicillin G for 4 weeks combined with streptomycin for the first 2 weeks of therapy (relapse rate 0%; Wolfe and Johnson, 1974). The clinician thus has several options, one of which can be chosen based on the needs of the individual patient. For example, the elderly patient with streptococcal endocarditis due to a penicillin-sensitive strain should probably receive penicillin alone, because of the increased toxicity from streptomycin in this age group. Results with the short, 2-week course of therapy are exciting; however, since earlier studies suggested a higher rate of relapse, a controlled trial is needed before this regimen can be recommended (*see* Sande and Scheld, 1980).

Tularemia. All forms of tularemia benefit dramatically from the administration of streptomycin. The course of the disease is shortened, the fatality rate markedly lowered, the incidence of late relapses greatly reduced, and the incidence of complications such as suppuration of buboes and secondary bacterial infection minimized. The best results are obtained when therapy is instituted early; however, chronicity does not exclude the possibility of complete cure. The dose of streptomycin varies with the severity of the infection; most cases respond to the administration of 1 to 2 g per day for 7 to 10 days. The tetracyclines are also highly effective in tularemia and are preferred by some physicians for milder forms of the disease.

Plague. Streptomycin is highly specific and one of the most effective agents for the treatment of all forms of plague. The tetracyclines and chloramphenicol are also beneficial in this disease. When streptomycin is used, a dose of 4 g per day is given

for the first 2 days, followed by a 2-g amount each day for an additional 5 to 7 days.

Brucellosis. Mild cases of brucellosis respond well to the administration of a tetracycline. Severe cases, even when complicated, and especially those due to *Br. suis* or *Br. melitensis,* are best treated with a combination of a tetracycline and streptomycin (2 g per day), given for 14 to 21 days. Relapses are managed in the same fashion.

Miscellaneous Infections. Although the tetracyclines and chloramphenicol are the agents of choice at present in the treatment of *granuloma inguinale* and *chancroid,* streptomycin (2 g per day) is indicated in patients who have suffered reactions to the other drugs or in whom the response to these agents is unsatisfactory.

GENTAMICIN

Gentamicin is an important agent for the treatment of many serious gram-negative bacillary infections. However, emergence of resistant microorganisms in some hospitals has become a serious problem and may limit the future use of this agent.

Preparations, Routes of Administration, and Dosage. The official preparation is *Gentamicin Sulfate,* U.S.P. (GARAMYCIN). It is available in various official forms: vials and prefilled syringes containing 40 mg/ml (or 10 mg/ml for pediatric use), an *ointment* and *cream* (0.1%), an *ophthalmic ointment* (0.3%), and *ophthalmic solution* (0.3%). The preparation available for parenteral administration contains preservatives and is not suitable for intrathecal use. The recommended intramuscular dose for adults is 3 to 5 mg/kg per day, one third being given every 8 hours. Several dosage schedules have been suggested for *infants:* 2 to 2.5 mg/kg every 8 hours has been found to be safe for children up to 2 years of age; 6 mg/kg daily, divided into two equally spaced injections, has been recommended for neonates with severe infections.

While the peak concentration in plasma is approximately 4 µg/ml after the intramuscular administration of 1 mg/kg, careful studies by a number of investigators have emphasized that the recommended doses of gentamicin do not yield reproducible concentrations in plasma and that there is a considerable degree of individual variation. Gentamicin may be present in the plasma in only subinhibitory or undetectable concentrations for several hours after its injection in some patients given the "standard" dose every 8 hours. Periodic determinations of the plasma concentration of the antibiotic are strongly recommended. Although it has not yet been established exactly what plasma concentration is toxic, peak concentrations greater than 10 µg/ml and minimal (predose) values in excess of 2 µg/ml for longer than 10 days have been associated with nephrotoxicity.

The presence of any significant degree of renal insufficiency imposes additional difficulty in establishing a regimen of therapy that will yield maximal therapeutic benefit with minimal or no risk of toxic reactions. This problem has been discussed above.

Carbenicillin and gentamicin must never be mixed in the same bottle because the penicillin inactivates the aminoglycoside to a significant degree; similar incompatibilities exist *in vitro* between gentamicin and other penicillins, cephalosporins, amphotericin B, and heparin.

Gentamicin is very slowly absorbed when applied in an *ointment*, but absorption may be more rapid when a *cream* is used topically. When the antibiotic is applied to large areas of denuded body surface, as may be the case in burned patients, plasma concentrations can reach 1 µg/ml, and 2 to 5% of the drug used may appear in the urine.

Penetration of gentamicin into the CSF after intramuscular administration is not sufficient to produce therapeutic concentrations in the CNS, and intrathecal or intraventricular instillation is often used in the treatment of gram-negative bacillary meningitis in adults. Rahal and colleagues (1974) have reported that the simultaneous intramuscular injection of 3.5 mg/kg per day of gentamicin and the instillation of 4 mg into the lumbar sac produce antibiotic concentrations in the CSF of 20 to 45 µg/ml within 8 hours after the intrathecal injection.

Penetration into secretions of the respiratory tract is also poor. Klastersky and coworkers (1972) have instilled the drug directly into the trachea of patients with tracheostomy, to treat tracheobronchial infections. Therapeutic concentrations of gentamicin are achieved in the aqueous humor following subconjunctival administration; there is little drug in the vitreous or lens.

Untoward Effects. Untoward effects of gentamicin, which are similar to those of streptomycin, include *nausea, vomiting, headache, increase in serum transaminases and alkaline phosphatase,* and *transient macular skin eruptions. Overgrowth of Candida* may follow oral administration of the drug. The most important and serious side effect of the use of gentamicin is *ototoxicity.* This has been discussed in detail above (page 1169). Gentamicin may produce more *nephrotoxicity* than do the other aminoglycosides that are currently available (*see* page 1170).

Intrathecal or intraventricular administration may cause local inflammation and can result in radiculitis and other complications (Hollifield *et al.,* 1976). Persistent fever and pleocytosis of the CSF have also been attributed to the intrathecal administration of gentamicin (Buckley *et al.,* 1977).

Therapeutic Uses. A large variety of infections have been treated successfully with gentamicin. However, due to the high toxicity of this drug, its use *must* be restricted to the therapy of life-threatening infections and those for which a less toxic antimicrobial agent is ineffective. The antibiotic is frequently used (often in combination with a penicillin or a cephalosporin) for the therapy of proven or suspected serious gram-negative microbial infections, especially those due to *Pseud. aeruginosa, Enterobacter, Klebsiella, Serratia,* and other species resistant to less toxic antibiotics. Among these are urinary tract infections, bacteremia, meningitis, cerebral ventriculitis, infected burns, osteomyelitis, pneumonia, peritonitis, and otitis.

Urinary Tract Infections. Aminoglycosides are not indicated for the treatment of uncomplicated urinary tract infections. However, in the extremely ill patient with pyelonephritis, gentamicin alone or in combination with ampicillin offers broad and effective initial coverage. Once the microorganism is isolated and its sensitivities to antibiotics are determined, gentamicin should be discontinued if the infecting microorganism is sensitive to ampicillin or other less toxic antibiotics. The antibacterial activity of gentamicin, like other aminoglycosides, is markedly influenced by pH (Strausbaugh and Sande, 1978); all are most active in an alkaline environment. On the other hand, the very high concentrations achieved in urine in patients with normal renal function are usually sufficient to eradicate sensitive microorganisms.

Pneumonia. The frequency of pneumonia caused by various gram-negative bacilli is increasing, especially in hospitalized patients, patients on respirators, and those with impaired defenses (especially granulocytopenia). Selection of an antibiotic depends on the sensitivity of the microorganism. Gentamicin is used widely in this setting, but most authorities administer a penicillin or a cephalosporin concurrently, since therapy with an aminoglycoside alone is not very effective. Gentamicin or tobramycin, combined with carbenicillin or ticarcillin, constitutes optimal treatment of pneumonia caused by *Pseud. aeruginosa.* Gentamicin and a cephalosporin are used concurrently for sensitive strains of *Klebsiella,* and gentamicin plus ampicillin for pneumonia caused by *E. coli* or *Pr. mirabilis.* All selections should be based initially on the sensitivity patterns at the individual hospital. Use of gentamicin administered by aerosol to prevent pulmonary infections with gram-negative bacilli has been largely unsuccessful and is not recommended (Klastersky *et al.,* 1973; Levine *et al.,* 1978).

Gentamicin-resistant strains of *Klebsiella, Enterobacter, Serratia, Proteus,* and *Pseudomonas* have emerged in many hospitals. The major reservoirs for these microorganisms are burn units and intensive care units, where gentamicin is used extensively. Critically ill patients with tracheostomies and impaired host defenses and those with indwelling intravenous and urinary catheters all appear to acquire gentamicin-resistant bacteria with an increased frequency (Guerrant *et al.,* 1977; Symposium, 1977).

Gentamicin (or any other aminoglycoside) is totally ineffective for treatment of pneumonia due to *Strep. pneumoniae,* the most common cause of pneumonia acquired in the community. Gentamicin should not be considered to be active against any other gram-positive cocci (including *Staph. aureus* or streptococci) or anaerobic bacteria, the microorganisms commonly responsible for suppurative pneumonia or lung abscess. Thus, gentamicin (or other aminoglycosides) should never be used as the sole agent to treat pneumonia acquired in the community or as the initial treatment for pneumonia acquired in the hospital (Kunin, 1977).

Meningitis. Meningitis caused by gram-negative microorganisms presents a grave therapeutic problem. Therapy with gentamicin is frequently necessary; however, adequate concentrations can be obtained only by intrathecal administration. Rahal and associates (1974) have recommended intramuscular administration of gentamicin in combination with intrathecal injection of 4 to 12 mg every 18 hours for 5 to 10 days. However, even this regimen is associated with a significant number of treatment failures, probably because of coexistent ventriculitis. In such instances, direct administration of gentamicin (or other aminoglycosides) into the cerebral ventricles with an Ommaya reservoir has been suggested. However, a recent study in children with gram-negative bacillary meningitis failed to show a beneficial effect from such treatment. (For discussion, *see* Kaiser and McGee, 1975; Lee *et al.*, 1977; Pickering *et al.*, 1978; McCracken *et al.*, 1979.) Some authorities recommend the concurrent systemic administration of chloramphenicol because of superior penetration by this drug into the CNS. Unfortunately, chloramphenicol is only bacteriostatic against most gram-negative bacilli, and reports of therapeutic failures have been numerous when this drug is used alone. Chloramphenicol markedly *reduces* the bactericidal activity of the gentamicin *in vitro* and in experimental infections in animals (antibiotic antagonism) (Strausbaugh *et al.*, 1977). Its use in gram-negative bacillary meningitis in man could thus be deleterious; clinical studies of this combination are not available.

Other Infections. Patients who develop peritonitis as a result of peritoneal dialysis may require therapy with gentamicin. Since suboptimal intraperitoneal concentrations of the antibiotic may follow intramuscular administration in patients undergoing dialysis, the procedure should be continued with fluids containing 5 to 10 mg of gentamicin per liter of fluid (*see* Smithivas *et al.*, 1971; page 1169).

Gentamicin has been given parenterally and applied topically at the same time in the treatment of infected burns; some of the bacteria involved have become resistant to the drug during such therapy (Shulman *et al.*, 1971; Wyatt *et al.*, 1977). It has been suggested that this regimen be rigorously restricted to patients with thermal burns that are life endangering, and be used only when other topical agents have failed.

While there are very few indications for the use of gentamicin for gram-positive bacterial infections, it may at times be necessary and lifesaving. Methicillin-resistant staphylococci may be sensitive to gentamicin. In cases of enterococcal endocarditis, up to 30% of isolates of enterococci are not killed by penicillin plus streptomycin; these strains are nearly always sensitive to penicillin plus gentamicin (page 1139). However, this is not revealed by testing for sensitivity to a standard dose of gentamicin.

When a serious infection of unknown etiology is present, many physicians administer gentamicin with a penicillinase-resistant penicillin, until such time as bacteriological diagnosis is obtained and specific therapy can be planned. When a patient has granulocytopenia and infection (sepsis) with *Pseud. aeruginosa* is suspected, the administration of carbenicillin or ticarcillin in combination with gentamicin or tobramycin is recommended. Treatment of gram-negative bacillary sepsis, especially in neutropenic patients, has been improved by the use of such synergistic combinations (Bloomfield and Kennedy, 1974; Klastersky *et al.*, 1977; Schimpff, 1977).

TOBRAMYCIN

The antimicrobial activity and pharmacokinetic properties of tobramycin are very similar to those of gentamicin.

Preparations, Routes of Administration, and Dosage. *Tobramycin*, U.S.P. (NEBCIN), is available as the sulfate salt for parenteral administration in 2-ml vials and 1.5- or 2-ml disposable syringes, all of which contain 40 mg/ml. A pediatric injection (2-ml vials containing 10 mg/ml) is also supplied. Tobramycin may be given either intramuscularly or intravenously. Dosages are identical to those for gentamicin. When doses of 1 mg/kg are given intramuscularly every 8 hours, peak concentrations in plasma are typically 5 to 8 μg/ml and minimal concentrations are 1 to 2 μg/ml. Toxicity is most common at peak concentrations of 10 to 12 μg/ml or minimal concentrations that exceed 2 μg/ml for a prolonged period. The latter observation usually suggests impairment of renal function and requires reduction of dosage.

Untoward Effects. Tobramycin, like other aminoglycosides, causes both nephrotoxicity and ototoxicity, as discussed above. Numerous studies in rats, rabbits, guinea pigs, and dogs suggest that tobramycin is less toxic to hair cells in the cochlear and vestibular end organs and causes less renal tubular damage than does gentamicin (Symposium, 1976b, 1978). However, conclusive data with human subjects are not yet available.

Therapeutic Uses. Indications for the use of tobramycin are essentially identical to those for gentamicin. The superior activity of tobramycin against *Pseud. aeruginosa* makes it desirable in the treatment of bacteremia, osteomyelitis, and pneumonia caused by *Pseudomonas* species; it should usually be used in combination with carbenicillin or ticarcillin. In contrast to gentamicin, tobramycin shows poor activity in combination with penicillin against enterococci; essentially all strains of *Strep. faecium* are highly resistant (Moellering *et al.*, 1979). Tobramycin is ineffective against mycobacteria, although most other aminoglycosides are active against these microorganisms (Gangadharam *et al.*, 1977).

AMIKACIN

Amikacin is the newest of the aminoglycosides and is most similar to kanamycin in dosage and pharmacokinetic properties. The spectrum of antimicrobial activity of amikacin is the broadest of the group, and, because of its unique resistance to the aminoglycoside-inactivating enzymes, it has a special role in hospitals where gentamicin-resistant microorganisms are prevalent.

Preparations, Routes of Administration, and Dosage. *Amikacin,* U.S.P. (AMIKIN), is available as the sulfate in 2-ml vials containing either 100 or 500 mg of the drug and in 4-ml vials containing 1 g. The recommended dose is 15 mg/kg per day, divided into either two or three equal portions. The individual dose or the interval between doses must be altered in patients with renal failure. The drug is rapidly absorbed after intramuscular injection, and peak concentrations in plasma approximate 20 μg/ml after injection of 7.5 mg/kg. An intravenous infusion of the same dose over a 30-minute period produces a peak concentration in plasma of nearly 40 μg/ml at the end of the infusion; this falls to about 20 μg/ml 30 minutes later.

Untoward Effects. Like the other aminoglycosides, amikacin causes both ototoxicity and nephrotoxicity. Auditory deficits are most commonly produced, as discussed on page 1169.

Therapeutic Uses. Amikacin has become the preferred drug for initial treatment of serious nosocomial gram-negative bacillary infections in hospitals where resistance to gentamicin has become a significant problem. Some hospitals have restricted its use to avoid emergence of resistant strains.

Because of its unique resistance to aminoglycoside-inactivating enzymes, amikacin is active against the vast majority of aerobic gram-negative bacilli in both the community and the hospital (Symposium, 1976a, 1977). This includes most strains of *Serratia, Proteus,* and *Pseud. aeruginosa.* It is active against nearly all strains of *Klebsiella, Enterobacter,* and *E. coli* that are resistant to gentamicin and tobramycin. Most resistance to amikacin is found among strains of *Acinetobacter, Providencia,* and *Flavobacter* and strains of *Pseudomonas* other than *Psued. aeruginosa;* these are all unusual pathogens. While amikacin is not active against the majority of gram-positive anaerobic bacteria, it is effective against *Mycobacterium tuberculosis* (99% of strains inhibited by 4 μg/ml) and atypical mycobacteria (Gangadharam *et al.,* 1977).

KANAMYCIN

The use of kanamycin declined markedly throughout the 1970s because of its more limited spectrum of activity. It retains some popularity among pediatricians for the treatment of severe infections with gram-negative bacilli in children; it is also used orally as an adjunct in the treatment of hepatic coma.

Preparations, Routes of Administration, and Dosage. *Kanamycin Sulfate,* U.S.P. (KANTREX), is available as an official injection in vials containing 500 mg in a 2-ml or 1.0 g in a 3-ml volume, in pediatric vials (75 mg/2 ml), and for oral use in official capsules containing 500 mg. The daily oral dose of kanamycin for children is 50 mg/kg, divided equally and given at 6-hour intervals; adults may receive up to 8 g per day by this route. Great care must be exercised when such treatment is carried out in patients with renal insufficiency, and the oral dose must be reduced. The parenteral dose for adults is 15 mg/kg per day (two to three equally divided and spaced doses) with a maximum of 1.5 g per day. The total quantity administered over a period of treatment should not exceed 15 g. For neonates, the intramuscular dose, during the first 3 days of life, is 7.5 mg/kg per day, divided into two to four equal doses; for older infants, it is 5 to 15 mg/kg per day; children may be given up to 15 mg/kg per day. The intravenous dose is the same as the intramuscular; however, intravenous infusion is rarely employed because absorption of kanamycin from intramuscular sites is excellent. The parenteral dose of kanamycin must be lowered in patients with renal insufficiency.

Intramuscular injection of 1 g of kanamycin yields a peak plasma concentration of 20 to 35 μg/ml at about 1 hour; this falls to 1.2 μg/ml or less at 12 hours. The half-life of the drug in premature infants less than 2 days old is 18 hours; in babies 5 to 22 days of age, 6 hours.

Untoward Effects. The untoward effects of kanamycin administered parenterally are the same as those that follow the administration of the other aminoglycosides. Auditory function is affected more frequently than vestibular; nephrotoxicity is not uncommon (*see* Conference on Kanamycin, 1966). The untoward effects of the oral administration of aminoglycosides are considered under Neomycin, below.

Therapeutic Uses. Kanamycin is still occasionally used for the therapy of infections due to gram-negative microorganisms, especially *Klebsiella, Enterobacter, Proteus,* and *E. coli.* It is without effect on disease produced by *Pseudomonas* and most gram-positive bacteria. It has been used successfully for single-dose therapy of uncomplicated infections of the lower urinary tract (Ronald *et al.,* 1976). Kanamycin has also been employed to treat human tuberculosis in combination with other effective drugs. Since the therapy of this disease is long and involves the administration of large total doses of the drug, with the risk of ototoxicity and nephrotoxicity, it should be used only to treat patients who harbor microorganisms that are resistant to the more commonly used agents (*see* Chapter 53).

Prophylactic Uses. Kanamycin has been administered *orally* to *suppress the intestinal flora prior to* surgery and as adjunct therapy in cases of *hepatic coma.* The first of these uses is discussed in Chapter 48, and the rationale for such therapy in hepatic coma is described under Neomycin (*see* below). The dose usually employed for these purposes is 6 to 8 g per day; quantities as large as 12 g per day have been given. The effect on intestinal bacteria may not be sustained even when such large doses of kanamycin are administered.

NEOMYCIN

Antibacterial Activity. Neomycin is a broad-spectrum antibiotic. Susceptible microorganisms are usually inhibited by concentrations of 5 to 10 μg/ml or less. Gram-negative species that are highly sensitive are *E. coli, Enterobacter aerogenes, K. pneumoniae, Pasteurella, Pr. vulgaris, Salmonella, Shigella, Haemophilus influenzae, Neisseria meningitidis, Vibrio cholerae,* and *Bordetella pertussis.* Gram-positive microorganisms that are inhibited include *Bacillus anthracis, Corynebacterium diphtheriae, Staph. aureus, Strep. faecalis, Listeria monocytogenes,* and *M. tuberculosis. Borrelia* and *Leptospira interrogans* (*icterohaemorrhagiae*) are also suppressed. Strains of *Pseud. aeruginosa* are resistant to neomycin. *Streptococcus pyogenes,* the *viridans* group of streptococci, fungi, and viruses are also resistant. (*See* Waksman *et al.,* 1949, 1950.) Neomycin is active against *tubercle bacilli,* regardless of their susceptibility to streptomycin. Neomycin-resistant microorganisms are less susceptible to streptomycin; cross-resistance is induced to a greater degree by neomycin than by streptomycin. The enzyme involved in certain types of resistance is kanamycin phosphotransferase, which can inactivate kanamycin, neomycin, and paromomycin. Neomycin is also a substrate for kanamycin acetyltransferase, but inactivation of neomycin does not occur following this alteration.

Preparations, Routes of Administration, and Dosage. *Neomycin Sulfate,* U.S.P. (MYCIFRADIN, NEO-BIOTIC), is available for topical, oral, and parenteral administration. Another formulation (MYCIQUENT) is available only for topical use. Neomycin sulfate is marketed as 500-mg oral tablets, in a solution (125 mg/5 ml), in *dermatological* and *ophthalmic* ointments, and as a *sterile powder* in vials containing 500 mg or 5 or 10 g for dilution with isotonic saline solution for topical application or parenteral injection. Ointments or creams should contain 5 mg of neomycin sulfate per gram, and be applied two or three times a day. *Neomycin and Polymyxin B Sulfates Solution for Irrigation,* U.S.P. (NEOSPORIN), contains 40 mg of neomycin and 200,000 units of polymyxin B per milliliter. One milliliter of this preparation is added to 1000 ml of 0.9% sodium chloride solution and is used for continuous irrigation of the urinary bladder through appropriate catheter systems. The goal is to prevent bacteriuria and bacteremia associated with the use of indwelling catheters. The bladder is usually irrigated at the rate of 1000 ml every 24 hours. Neomycin is rarely used parenterally; the dose for intramuscular injection is 250 mg every 6 hours, and only in exceptional instances may this be increased to 500 mg every 6 hours. Oral therapy with neomycin sulfate either for

"preparation" of the bowel for surgery or for the management of hepatic coma requires the ingestion of 4 to 8 g daily, in divided doses.

Neomycin is presently available in at least 100 different brands of creams, ointments, and sprays, both alone and in combination with polymyxin, bacitracin, other antibiotics, and a variety of corticosteroids. One such preparation is *Neomycin and Polymyxin B Sulfates and Bacitracin Zinc Ointment,* U.S.P. The drug is also included in deodorants and in MYCOLOG, a preparation often used to treat "diaper rash." There is no evidence that these topical preparations shorten the time required for healing of wounds or that those containing a steroid are more effective.

Absorption and Excretion. Neomycin is poorly absorbed from the gastrointestinal tract and is excreted by the kidney, as are the other aminoglycosides. An *oral* dose of 3 g produces a peak plasma concentration of only 1 to 4 μg/ml; a total daily intake of 10 g for 3 days yields a blood concentration below that associated with systemic toxicity. About 97% of an oral dose of neomycin escapes absorption and is eliminated unchanged in the feces. Although neomycin can be given orally to very young children, in doses as high as 100 mg/kg per day, its use in such patients for longer than 3 weeks should be avoided because of partial absorption from the intestinal tract, especially if it is the site of disease.

Untoward Effects. *Hypersensitivity reactions,* primarily *skin rashes,* occur in 6 to 8% of patients when neomycin is applied topically. Individuals sensitive to this agent may develop cross-reactions when exposed to other aminoglycosides. The most important toxic effects of neomycin are *renal damage* and *nerve deafness.* These are most frequent when relatively large quantities of the antibiotic are used parenterally and are the reason the drug is almost never used in this way. Loss of hearing usually develops during the course of treatment. It has even occurred in patients with normal renal function following topical application or irrigation of wounds with 0.5% neomycin (Kelley *et al.,* 1969). Abnormal urine sediment and azotemia are quite common in patients treated with neomycin. Neuromuscular blockade with respiratory paralysis has also occurred after irrigation of wounds or serosal cavities.

The most important *biological effects* resulting from the oral administration of neomycin are *intestinal malabsorption* and *suprainfection.* Individuals treated with 4 to 6 g of the drug by mouth per day sometimes develop a *spruelike syndrome* with diarrhea, steatorrhea, and azotorrhea. The outstanding example of drug-induced *malabsorption* is that caused by neomycin. In man, the drug produces a moderate malabsorption syndrome for a variety of substances, including fat, protein, cholesterol, carotene, glucose, lactose, sodium, calcium, cyanocobalamin, and iron. This effect may be produced by as little as 3 g of the drug per day but is more marked with a dose of 12 g per day. Neomycin produces mild morphological changes of intestinal villi; precipitates bile salts within the lumen of the intestine; inhibits intraluminal hydrolysis of long-chain triglycerides, presumably by inhibition of pancreatic lipase activity; increases the fecal bile acid excretion, presumably by decreasing bile acid absorption; and reduces intestinal lactase activity. The antibiotic causes a marked decrease in plasma cholesterol concentrations. This is out of proportion to the moderate malabsorption produced, and small doses of the drug have been used for long periods of time for this purpose. The drug has been shown to produce intestinal crypt-cell necrosis, and, since cholesterol synthesis may occur at these sites, this may account for the effect. Parenterally administered neomycin in doses of 200 mg per day does not produce malabsorption nor does it lower plasma cholesterol (Dobbins, 1968). *Overgrowth of yeasts* in the intestine may also occur; this is not associated with diarrhea or other symptoms in most cases. The oral administration of even large doses of neomycin usually has no effect on blood levels of prothrombin.

Therapeutic Uses. Neomycin has been widely used for *topical application* in a variety of infections of the skin and mucous membranes caused by microorganisms susceptible to the drug. These include *burns, wounds, ulcers,* and *infected dermatoses.* However, such treatment does not eradicate bacteria from the lesions.

The *oral administration* of neomycin has been employed primarily for *"preparation" of the bowel for surgery* and as an adjunct to the therapy of *hepatic coma.* In a recent controlled study conducted by the Veterans Administration, concurrent administration of neomycin and erythromycin base to prepare the bowel for surgery was found to reduce the incidence of postoperative wound infections significantly (Clarke *et al.,* 1977).

While the importance of reducing the number of bacteria in the intestine in patients with hepatic coma has not been proved, general clinical experience suggests strongly that this may play an important role in producing a satisfactory outcome in this disease. Blood concentrations of ammonia are reduced during therapy. A daily dose of 4 to 8 g by mouth can be given without difficulty to such patients, provided renal function is normal. Because severe renal insufficiency may develop in the late stages of hepatic failure, treatment with neomycin must be followed with the greatest care and stopped if evidence of ototoxicity or further injury to the kidney appears.

There is presently little or no indication for the parenteral administration of neomycin. Other equally effective and safer antibiotics have almost completely replaced it.

Appel, G. B., and Neu, H. C. Nephrotoxicity of antimicrobial agents. *N. Engl. J. Med.,* **1977,** *296,* 722–728.

Atkins, R. C.; Mion, C.; Despaux, E.; Van-Hai, N.; Christian, J.; and Mion, H. Peritoneal transfer of kanamycin and its use in peritoneal dialysis. *Kidney Int.,* **1973,** *3,* 391–396.

Barza, M. Factors affecting the intraocular penetration of antibiotics, the influence of route, inflammation, animal species, and tissue pigmentation. *Scand. J. Infect. Dis.,* **1978,** *14,* 151–159.

Barza, M.; Brown, R. B.; Shen, D.; Gibaldi, M.; and Weinstein, L. Predictability of blood levels of gentamicin in man. *J. Infect. Dis.,* **1975,** *132,* 165–174.

Barza, M., and Scheife, R. T. Antimicrobial spectrum, pharmacology, and therapeutic use of antibiotics. *J. Maine Med. Assoc.,* **1977,** *68,* 194–210.

Bennet, W. M.; Gilbert, D. N.; Houghton, D.; and Porter, G. A. Gentamicin nephrotoxicity—morphologic and pharmacologic features. *West. J. Med.,* **1977,** *126,* 65–68.

Bergeron, M. G., and Trottier, S. Influence of single or multiple doses of gentamicin and netilmicin on their cortical, medullary, and papillary distribution. *Antimicrob. Agents Chemother.,* **1979,** *15,* 635–641.

Bloomfield, C. D., and Kennedy, B. J. Cephalothin, carbenicillin, and gentamicin combination therapy in febrile patients with acute non-lymphocytic leukemia. *Cancer,* **1974,** *34,* 431–437.

Breen, K. J.; Bryant, R. E.; Levinson, J. D.; and Schenker, S. Neomycin absorption in man. *Ann. Intern. Med.,* **1972,** *76,* 211–218.

Bryan, L. E., and Van Den Elzen, H. M. Streptomycin accumulation in susceptible and resistant strains of *E. coli* and *P. aeruginosa. Antimicrob. Agents Chemother.,* **1976,** *9,* 928–938.

———. Effects of membrane-energy mutations and cations on streptomycin and gentamicin accumulation by bacteria: a model for entry of streptomycin and gentamicin in susceptible and resistant bacteria. *Ibid.,* **1977,** *12,* 163–177.

Buckley, R. M.; Watters, W.; and MacGregor, R. R. Persistent meningeal inflammation associated with intrathecal gentamicin. *Am. J. Med. Sci.,* **1977,** *274,* 207–209.

Chan, R. A.; Benner, E. J.; and Hoeprich, P. D. Gentamicin therapy in renal failure: nomogram and dosage. *Ann. Intern. Med.,* **1972,** *76,* 773.

Chiu, P. J. S.; Brown, A.; Miller, G.; and Long, J. F. Renal excretion of gentamicin in anesthetized dogs. *Antimicrob. Agents Chemother.,* **1976,** *10,* 277–282.

Churchill, D. N., and Seely, J. Nephrotoxicity associated with combined gentamicin–amphotericin B therapy. *Nephron,* **1977,** *19,* 176–181.

Clarke, J. S.; Condon, R. E.; Bartlett, J. G.; Gorbach, S. L.; Nichols, R. L.; and Ochi, S. Preoperative oral antibiotics reduce septic complications of colon operations: results of prospective, randomized, double-blind clinical study. *Ann. Surg.,* **1977,** *186,* 251–259.

Conway, N., and Boct, B. D. Streptomycin in pregnancy: effect on foetal ear. *Br. Med. J.,* **1965,** *2,* 260–263.

Cox, C. E. Gentamicin. *Med. Clin. North Am.,* **1970,** *54,* 1305–1315.

Danish, M.; Schultz, R. E.; and Jusko, W. J. Pharmacokinetics of gentamicin and kanamycin during hemodialysis. *Antimicrob. Agents Chemother.,* **1974,** *6,* 841–847.

Davies, J., and Courvalin, P. Mechanisms of resistance to aminoglycosides. *Am. J. Med.,* **1977,** *62,* 868–872.

Dee, T. H., and Kozin, F. Gentamicin and tobramycin penetration into synovial fluid. *Antimicrob. Agents Chemother.,* **1977,** *12,* 548–549.

Dickie, P.; Bryan, L. E.; and Pichard, M. A. Effect of enzymatic adenylation on dihydrostreptomycin accumulation in *Escherichia coli* carrying an R-factor: model explaining aminoglycoside resistance by inactivating mechanisms. *Antimicrob. Agents Chemother.,* **1978,** *14,* 569–580.

Diem, K., and Lentner, C. Scientific tables. In, *Documenta Geigy,* 7th ed. J. R. Geigy, Basel, **1970,** p. 711.

Dilworth, J. A.; Hendley, J. O.; Gwaltney, J. M., Jr.; and Sande, M. A. Detection of pneumococci in clinical specimens. *J. Clin. Microbiol.,* **1975,** *2,* 453–455.

Dobbins, W. O., III. Drug-induced steatorrhea. *Gastroenterology,* **1968,** *54,* 1193–1195.

Federspil, P. Pharmacokinetics and ototoxicity of gentamicin, tobramycin, and amikacin. *Arch. Otolaryngol.,* **1977,** *217,* 147.

Gangadharam, P. R. J.; Candler, E. R.; and Ramakrishna, P. V. *In vitro* anti-mycobacterial activity of some new aminoglycoside antibiotics. *J. Antimicrob. Chemother.,* **1977,** *3,* 285–286.

Gary, N. E.; Buzzeo, L.; Solaki, J.; and Eisinger, R. P. Gentamicin-associated acute renal failure. *Arch. Intern. Med.,* **1976,** *126,* 1101–1104.

Glauser, M. P.; Lyons, J. M.; and Braude, A. I. Prevention of pyelonephritis due to *Escherichia coli* in rats with gentamicin stored in kidney tissue. *J. Infect. Dis.,* **1979,** *139,* 172–177.

Guerrant, R. L.; Strausbaugh, L. J.; Wenzel, R. P.; Hamory, B. H.; and Sande, M. A. Nosocomial bloodstream infections caused by gentamicin-resistant gram-negative bacilli. *Am. J. Med.,* **1977,** *62,* 894–901.

Hawley, H. B.; Lewis, R. M.; Swartz, D. R.; and Gump, D. W. Tobramycin therapy of pulmonary infections in patients with cystic fibrosis. *Curr. Ther. Res.,* **1974,** *16,* 414–423.

Higgins, C. E., and Kastners, R. E. Nebramycin, a new broad-spectrum antibiotic complex. II. Description of *Streptomyces tenebrarius. Antimicrob. Agents Chemother.,* **1967,** *7,* 324–331.

Hollifield, J. W.; Kaiser, A. B.; and McGee, Z. A. Gram-negative bacillary meningitis therapy. Polyradiculitis following intralumbar aminoglycoside administration. *J.A.M.A.,* **1976,** *236,* 1264–1266.

Holtzman, J. L. Gentamicin neuromuscular blockade. (Letter.) *Ann. Intern. Med.,* **1976,** *84,* 55.

Hull, J. H., and Sarubbi, F. A., Jr. Gentamicin serum concentrations: pharmacokinetic predictions. *Ann. Intern. Med.,* **1976,** *85,* 183–189.

Jackson, G. G. Present status of aminoglycoside antibiotics and their safe effective use. *Clin. Ther.,* **1977,** *1,* 200–215.

Kaiser, A. B., and McGee, Z. A. Aminoglycoside therapy of gram-negative bacillary meningitis. *N. Engl. J. Med.,* **1975,** *293,* 1215–1220.

Karchmer, A. W.; Moellering, R. C.; Maki, D. G.; and Swartz, M. N. Single-antibiotic therapy for streptococcal endocarditis. *J.A.M.A.,* **1979,** *241,* 1801–1806.

Kawaguchi, H.; Naito, T.; Nakagawa, S.; and Fugijawa, K. BBK8, a new semisynthetic aminoglycoside antibiotic. *J. Antibiot.* (*Tokyo*), **1972,** *25,* 695.

Kelley, D. R.; Nilo, E. R.; and Berggren, R. B. Deafness after topical neomycin wound irrigation. *N. Engl. J. Med.,* **1969,** *280,* 1338–1339.

Klastersky, J.; Cappel, R.; Noterman, J.; Snoeck, J.; Geuning, C.; and Mouawad, E. Endotracheal gentamicin for the prevention of bronchial infections in patients with tracheotomy. *Int. J. Clin. Pharmacol. Biopharm.,* **1973,** *74,* 279–286.

Klastersky, J.; Geuning, C.; Mouawad, E.; and Daneau, D. Endotracheal gentamicin in bronchial infections in patients with tracheostomy. *Chest,* **1972,** *61,* 117–120.

Klastersky, J.; Meunier-Carpentier, F.; and Prevost, J. M. Significance of antimicrobial synergism for the outcome of gram-negative sepsis. *Am. J. Med. Sci.,* **1977,** *273,* 157–167.

Korzeniowski, O. M., and Hook, E. W. Aminocyclitols: aminoglycosides and spectinomycin. In, *Principles and Practice of Infectious Diseases.* (Mandell, G. L.; Douglas, R. G., Jr.; and Bennett, J. E.; eds.) John Wiley & Sons, Inc., New York, **1979,** pp. 249–273.

Kunin, C. M. Blunder drug for pneumonia. (Letter.) *N. Engl. J. Med.,* **1977,** *297,* 113–114.

Le Goffic, F.; Capmau, M. L.; Tangy, F.; and Baillarge, M. Mechanism of action of aminoglycoside antibiotics. Binding studies of tobramycin and its 6'-N-acetyl derivative to the bacterial ribosome and its subunits. *Eur. J. Biochem.,* **1979,** *102,* 73–81.

Lee, E. L.; Robinson, M. J.; Thong, M. L.; Puthucheary, S. D.; Ong, T. H.; and Ng, K. K. Intraventricular chemotherapy in neonatal meningitis. *J. Pediatr.,* **1977,** *91,* 991–995.

Levine, B. A.; Petroff, P. A.; Slade, C. L.; and Pruitt, B. A., Jr. Prospective trials of dexamethasone and aerosolized gentamicin in the treatment of inhalation injury in the burned patient. *J. Trauma,* **1978,** *18,* 188–193.

Luft, F. C.; Yum, M. N.; Walker, P. D.; and Kleit, S. A. Gentamicin gradient patterns and morphological changes in human kidneys. *Nephron,* **1977,** *18,* 167–174.

Luzzatto, L.; Apirion, D.; and Schlessinger, D. Polyribosome depletion and blockage of the ribosome cycle by streptomycin in *Escherichia coli. J. Mol. Biol.,* **1969,** *42,* 315–335.

McCracken, G. H., and Mize, S. G. A controlled study of intrathecal antibiotic therapy in gram-negative enteric meningitis of infancy. *J. Pediatr.,* **1976,** *89,* 66–72.

McCracken, G. H.; Mize, S. G.; and the Neonatal Meningitis Cooperative Study Group. Intraventricular therapy of neonatal meningitis caused by gram-negative enteric bacilli. *Pediatr. Res.,* **1979,** *13,* 464.

Mathog, R. H., and Capps, M. J. Ototoxic interactions of ethacrynic acid and streptomycin. *Ann. Otol. Rhinol. Laryngol.,* **1977,** *86,* 158–163.

Mendelson, J.; Portnoy, J.; and Sigman, H. Pharmacology of gentamicin in the biliary tract of humans. *Antimicrob. Agents Chemother.,* **1973,** *4,* 538–541.

Mitsuhashi, S. (ed.). *Drug Action and Drug Resistance in Bacteria.* Vol. 2, *Aminoglycoside Antibiotics.* University Park Press, Baltimore, **1975.**

Moellering, R. C. Microbiological considerations in the use of tobramycin and related aminoglycosidic aminocyclitol antibiotics. *Med. J. Aust.,* **1977,** *2,* Suppl., 4–8.

Moellering, R. C.; Korzeniowski, O. M.; Sande, M. A.; and Wennersten, C. B. Species-specific resistance to antimicrobial synergism among enterococci. *J. Infect. Dis.,* **1979,** *140,* 203–208.

Moellering, R. C., and Weinberg, A. N. Studies on antibiotic synergism against enterococci. II. Effect of various antibiotics on the uptake of ^{14}C-labelled streptomycin by enterococci. *J. Clin. Invest.,* **1971,** *50,* 2580–2584.

Nelson, J. D., and McCracken, G. H., Jr. Current status of gentamicin for the neonate and young infant. (Editorial.) *Am. J. Dis. Child.,* **1972,** *124,* 13–14.

Neu, H. C., and Bendush, C. L. Ototoxicity of tobramycin: a clinical overview. *J. Infect. Dis.,* **1976,** *134,* S206–S218.

Pickering, L. K.; Ericsson, C. D.; Ruiz-Palacios, G.; Blevins, J.; and Miner, M. E. Intraventricular and parenteral gentamicin therapy for ventriculitis in children. *Am. J. Dis. Child.,* **1978,** *132,* 480–483.

Pittinger, C., and Adamson, R. Antibiotic blockade of neuromuscular function. *Annu. Rev. Pharmacol.,* **1972,** *12,* 169–184.

Pittinger, C. B.; Eryasa, Y.; and Adamson, R. Antibiotic-induced paralysis. *Anesth. Analg.* (*Cleve.*), **1970,** *49,* 487–501.

Price, K. E.; DeFuria, M. D.; and Pursiano, T. A. Amikacin, an aminoglycoside with marked activity against antibiotic-resistant clinical isolates. *J. Infect. Dis.,* **1976,** *134,* S249–S261.

Rahal, J. J., Jr.; Hyams, P. S.; Simberkoff, M. S.; and Rubenstein, E. Intrathecal and intramuscular gentamicin for gram-negative meningitis: pharmacologic study of 21 patients. *N. Engl. J. Med.,* **1974,** *290,* 1394–1398.

Ronald, A. R.; Boutros, P.; and Mourtada, H. Bacteruria localization and response to single-dose therapy in women. *J.A.M.A.,* **1976,** *235,* 1854–1856.

Rosenthal, A.; Button, L. N.; and Khaw, K. T. Blood volume changes in patients with cystic fibrosis. *Pediatrics,* **1977,** *59,* 588–594.

Rosselot, J. P.; Marquez, J.; Meseck, E.; Murawski, A.; Hamdan, A.; Joyner, C.; Schmidt, R.; Migliore, C.; and Herzog, H. L. Isolation, purification, and characterization of gentamicin. In, *Antimicrobial Agents and Chemotherapy—1963.* (Sylvester, J. C., ed.) American Society for Microbiology, Ann Arbor, Mich., **1964,** pp. 14–16.

Sande, M. A., and Courtney, K. B. Nafcillin-gentamicin synergism in experimental staphylococcal endocarditis. *J. Lab. Clin. Med.,* **1976,** *88,* 118–124.

Sande, M. A., and Scheld, M. Antibiotic combinations in infective endocarditis. *Ann. Intern. Med.,* **1980,** *92,* 390–395.

Schatz, A.; Bugie, S.; and Waksman, S. A. Streptomycin, a substance exhibiting antibiotic activity against gram-positive and gram-negative bacteria. *Proc. Soc. Exp. Biol. Med.,* **1944,** *57,* 244–248.

Scheld, W. M.; Fletcher, D. D.; Fink, F. N.; and Sande, M. A. Experimental *Listeria* meningitis: description of a model and response to therapy. *J. Infect. Dis.,* **1979,** *140,* 287–294.

Schentag, J. J., and Jusko, W. J. Renal clearance and tissue accumulation of gentamicin. *Clin. Pharmacol. Ther.,* **1977,** *22,* 364–370.

Schimpff, S. C. Therapy of infection in patients with granulocytopenia. *Med. Clin. North Am.,* **1977,** *61,* 1101–1118.

Shulman, J. A.; Terry, P. M.; and Hough, C. E. Colonization with gentamicin-resistant *Pseudomonas aeruginosa,* pyocine type 5, in a burn unit. *J. Infect. Dis.,* **1971,** *124,* Suppl., S18–S23.

Siber, G. R.; Echeverria, P.; Smith, A. L.; Paisley, J. W.; and Smith, D. H. Pharmacokinetics of gentamicin in children and adults. *J. Infect. Dis.,* **1975,** *132,* 637–651.

Smithivas, T.; Hyams, P. J.; Matalon, R.; Simberkoff, M. S.; and Rahal, J. J. The use of gentamicin in peritoneal dialysis. I. Pharmacologic results. *J. Infect. Dis.,* **1971,** *124,* Suppl., S77–S83.

Spyker, D. A., and Guerrant, R. L. Gentamicin dosage. *Ann. Intern. Med.,* **1977,** *86,* 357.

Spyker, D. A.; Sande, M. A.; and Mandell, G. L. Tobramycin pharmacokinetics in patients with cystic fibrosis and leukemia. In, *Eighteenth Interscience Conference on Antimicrobial Agents and Chemotherapy.* American Society for Microbiology, Washington, D. C., **1978,** p. 345.

Stöffler, G., and Tischendorf, G. W. Antibiotic receptor-sites in *E. coli* ribosomes. In, *Drug Receptor Interactions in Antimicrobial Chemotherapy.* Vol. I, *Topics in Infectious Diseases.* (Drews, J., and Hahn, F. E., eds.) Springer-Verlag, New York, **1975.**

Strausbaugh, L. J.; Mandaleris, C. D.; and Sande, M. A. Comparison of four aminoglycoside antibiotics in the therapy of experimental *E. coli* meningitis. *J. Lab. Clin. Med.,* **1977,** *89,* 692–701.

Strausbaugh, L. J., and Sande, M. A. Factors influencing the therapy of experimental *Proteus mirabilis* meningitis. *J. Infect. Dis.,* **1978,** *137,* 251–260.

Tai, P.-C.; Wallace, B. J.; and Davis, B. D. Streptomycin causes misreading of natural messenger by interacting with ribosomes after initiation. *Proc. Natl. Acad. Sci. U.S.A.,* **1978,** *75,* 275–279.

Tai, P.-C.; Wallace, B. J.; Herzog, E. L.; and Davis, B. D. Properties of initiation-free polysomes of *Escherichia coli. Biochemistry,* **1973,** *12,* 609–615.

Theopold, H. M. Comparative surface studies of ototoxic effects of various aminoglycoside antibiotics on the organ of Corti in the guinea pig. A scanning electron microscopic study. *Acta Otolaryngol. (Stockh.),* **1977,** *84,* 57–64.

Tseng, J. T.; Bryan, L. E.; and Van Den Elzen, H. M. Mechanisms and spectrum of streptomycin resistance in a natural population of *Pseudomonas aeruginosa. Antimicrob. Agents Chemother.,* **1972,** *2,* 136–141.

Waksman, S. A.; Hutchinson, D.; and Katz, E. Neomycin activity upon *Mycobacterium tuberculosis* and other mycobacteria. *Am. Rev. Tuberc. Pulm. Dis.,* **1949,** *60,* 78–89.

Waksman, S. A.; Katz, E.; and Lechavlier, H. Antimicrobial properties of neomycin. *J. Lab. Clin. Med.,* **1950,** *36,* 93–99.

Waksman, S. A., and Lechevalier, H. A. Neomycin, a new antibiotic active against streptomycin-resistant bacteria, including tuberculosis organisms. *Science,* **1949,** *109,* 305–307.

Weinstein, M. J.; Luedemann, G. M.; Oden, E. M.; Wagman, G. H.; Rosselot, J. P.; Marquez, J. A.; Coniglio, C. T.; Charney, W.; Herzog, H. L.; and Black, J.

Gentamicin, a new antibiotic complex from *Micromonospora. J. Med. Chem.,* **1963,** *6,* 463–464.

Wersäll, J.; Bjorkroth, B.; Flock, A.; and Lundquist, P.-G. Experiments on the ototoxic effects of antibiotics. *Adv. Otorhinolaryngol.,* **1973,** *20,* 14–41.

Wilson, P., and Ramsden, R. T. Immediate effects of tobramycin on human cochlea and correlation with serum tobramycin levels. *Br. Med. J.,* **1977,** *1,* 259–261.

Wilson, W. R.; Geraci, J. E.; Wilkowske, C. J.; and Washington, J. A., II. Short-term intramuscular therapy with procaine penicillin plus streptomycin for infective endocarditis due to *viridans* streptococci. *Circulation,* **1978,** *57,* 1158–1161.

Wolfe, J. C., and Johnson, W. D., Jr. Penicillin-sensitive streptococcal endocarditis. *Ann. Intern. Med.,* **1974,** *81,* 178–181.

Wyatt, T. D.; Ferguson, W. P.; Wilson, T. S.; and McCormick, E. Gentamicin-resistant *Staphylococcus aureus* associated with the use of topical gentamicin. *J. Antimicrob. Chemother.,* **1977,** *3,* 213–214.

Yow, M. O. An overview of pediatric experience with amikacin. *Am. J. Med.,* **1977,** *62,* 954–958.

Zimmermann, R. A.; Moellering, R. C., Jr.; and Weinberg, A. N. Mechanism of resistance to antibiotic synergism in enterococci. *J. Bacteriol.,* **1971,** *105,* 873–879.

Monographs and Reviews

Barza, M.; Brown, K. B.; Shen, D.; Gibaldi, M.; and Weinstein, L. Predictability of blood levels of gentamicin in man. In, *Clinical Pharmacy and Clinical Pharmacology.* (Gouveia, W. A.; Tognoni, G.; and van der Kleijn, E.; eds.) North-Holland Publications, Amsterdam, **1976,** pp. 207–222.

Conference on Kanamycin. (Various authors.) Appraisal after eight years of clinical application. *Ann. N.Y. Acad. Sci.,* **1966,** *132,* 773–1090.

Federspil, P., and Tiesler, E. Pharmacokinetics and ototoxicity of gentamicin, tobramycin, and amikacin. In, *Chemotherapy,* Vol. 2. (Williams, J. D., and Geddes, A. M., eds.) Plenum Press, New York, **1976,** pp. 427–429.

Hawkins, J. E., Jr. Conditions of the inner hair cells after aminoglycoside intoxication. In, *Inner Ear Biology.* (Portmann, M., and Aran, J. M., eds.) Inserm, Paris, **1977,** pp. 327–334.

Kucers, A., and Bennett, N. M. (eds.). *The Use of Antibiotics,* 2nd ed. William Heinemann Medical Books, Ltd., London, **1975.**

Murray, B. E., and Moellering, R. C., Jr. Patterns and mechanisms of antibiotic resistance. *Med. Clin. North Am.,* **1978,** *62,* 899–923.

Round-Table Discussion on Gentamicin and Tobramycin. Royal Society of Medicine International Congress and Symposium. (Richardson, R. G., ed.) Grune & Stratton, Inc., New York, **1979.**

Simberkoff, M. S., and Rahal, J. J. Parenteral aminoglycoside antibiotics—1977. Clinical use. *N.Y. State J. Med.,* **1977,** *77,* 81–85.

Symposium. (Various authors.) Advances in aminoglycoside therapy: amikacin. *J. Infect. Dis.,* **1976a,** *134,* S235–S460.

Symposium. (Various authors.) Tobramycin. *J. Infect. Dis.,* **1976b,** *134,* S1–S234.

Symposium. (Various authors.) Amikacin. *Am. J. Med.,* **1977,** *62,* 863–966.

Symposium. (Various authors.) Tobramycin—comparative toxicity of aminoglycoside antibiotics. *J. Antimicrob. Chemother.,* **1978,** *4,* Suppl. A, 1–101.

Waksman, S. A. (ed.). *Streptomycin, Nature and Practical Applications.* The Williams & Wilkins Co., Baltimore, **1949.**

———. Streptomycin: background, isolation, properties, and utilization. *Science,* **1953,** *118,* 259–266.

52 ANTIMICROBIAL AGENTS
[*Continued*]

Tetracyclines and Chloramphenicol

Merle A. Sande and Gerald L. Mandell

TETRACYCLINES

History. The development of the tetracycline antibiotics was the result of a systematic screening of soil specimens collected from many parts of the world for antibiotic-producing microorganisms. The first of these compounds, *chlortetracycline,* was introduced in 1948. Two years later, *oxytetracycline* became available. Elucidation of the chemical structure of these agents confirmed their similarity and furnished the basis for the production of a third member of this group, *tetracycline,* in 1952. In 1957, a new family of tetracyclines was developed, characterized chemically by the absence of the ring-attached CH_3 group present in the others. One of these, *demethylchlortetracycline,* subsequently given the official name *demeclocycline,* became available for general use in 1959. *Methacycline,* a derivative of oxytetracycline, was introduced in 1961; *doxycycline* became available in 1966; and *minocycline,* in 1972.

Soon after their initial development, the tetracyclines were found to be highly effective against rickettsiae, a number of gram-positive and gram-negative bacteria, and the agents responsible for lymphogranuloma venereum, inclusion conjunctivitis, and psittacosis, and hence became known as "broad-spectrum" antibiotics. With establishment of their *in-vitro* antimicrobial activity, effectiveness in experimental infections, and pharmacological properties, the tetracyclines rapidly became widely used in therapy. (*See* Dowling, 1955; Lepper, 1956; Musselman, 1956.)

Although there are specific and useful differences between the tetracyclines currently available in the United States, they are in the main very much alike. This permits discussion of these drugs as a group.

Source. *Chlortetracycline* and *oxytetracycline* are elaborated by *Streptomyces aureofaciens* and *Streptomyces rimosus,* respectively. The antibiotics are produced in broth by deep-tank fermentation. *Tetracycline* is produced semisynthetically from chlortetracycline; it has also been obtained from a species of *Streptomyces. Demeclocycline* is the product of a mutant of the strain of *Streptomyces aureofaciens* from which chlortetracycline was first obtained. *Methacycline, doxycycline,* and *minocycline* are all semisynthetic derivatives.

Chemistry, Stability, and Assay. The tetracyclines are closely congeneric derivatives of the polycyclic naphthacenecarboxamide. Their structural formulas are shown in Table 52-1.

The crystalline bases are faintly yellow, odorless, slightly bitter compounds. They are only slightly soluble in water at pH 7 (0.25 to 0.5 mg/ml), but they form soluble sodium salts and hydrochlorides. While the bases and the hydrochlorides are quite stable as dry powders, most of these agents lose activity relatively rapidly when in solution.

Determination of the concentration of tetracyclines in biological fluids and assay for their degree of antibacterial activity are accomplished by conventional microbiological methods. Because of the instability of solutions of most of these drugs, particularly chlortetracycline, the results of such determinations are only relative and are greatly modified by the assay conditions.

Effects on Microbial Agents. The tetracyclines possess a wide range of antimicrobial

Table 52-1. STRUCTURAL FORMULAS OF THE TETRACYCLINES

Tetracycline

CONGENER	SUBSTITUENT(S)	POSITION(S)
Chlortetracycline	—Cl	(7)
Oxytetracycline	—OH,—H	(5)
Demeclocycline	—OH,—H; —Cl	(6; 7)
Methacycline	—OH,—H; =CH_2	(5; 6)
Doxycycline	—OH,—H; —CH_3,—H	(5; 6)
Minocycline	—H,—H; —N(CH_3)$_2$	(6; 7)

activity against gram-positive and gram-negative bacteria, which overlaps that of many other antimicrobial drugs. They are also effective against some microorganisms innately insensitive to many chemotherapeutic agents, such as *rickettsiae, Mycoplasma, Chlamydia* (the agents of *urethritis, lymphogranuloma venereum, psittacosis, inclusion conjunctivitis,* and *trachoma*), some *atypical mycobacteria,* and *amebae.* Individually, they have little activity against true fungi; however, they may exert an antifungal action when combined with amphotericin (Lew *et al.,* 1977).

In vitro, these drugs are primarily bacteriostatic; in high concentrations, they are frequently bactericidal. In general, but not invariably, their efficacies *in vivo* and *in vitro* closely parallel each other. Only multiplying microorganisms are affected. The sensitivity or resistance of a particular microorganism to each of the congeners is similar. However, minocycline is usually the most active, followed by doxycycline. Tetracycline and oxytetracycline are the least active.

Bacteria. In general, gram-positive microorganisms are affected by lower concentrations of tetracycline than are gram-negative species. However, these agents are less useful for infections caused by gram-positive bacteria because of problems of resistance and the availability of superior antimicrobial agents (*see* Table 52-2). For example, in some geographical areas as many as 14% of strains of *Streptococcus pneumoniae* may be resistant to the tetracyclines (Gopalakrishna and Lerner, 1973); there is, however, an encouraging trend toward a decline in the number of resistant pneumococci (Neu, 1978). Forty percent of strains of *Strep. pyogenes* isolated in Israel are resistant (Bergner-Rabinowitz and Davies, 1970). The incidence of tetracycline-resistant staphylococci has also been declining, and minocycline appears to be active against strains of *Staphylococcus aureus* that are resistant to other tetracyclines (Finland, 1974). Several gram-positive bacilli are sensitive to these drugs (*see* Table 48-1, page 1088).

Neisseria gonorrhoeae and many strains of *N. meningitidis* are inhibited by tetracyclines.

Table 52-2. BACTERIAL SENSITIVITY TO TETRACYCLINES *

AEROBIC BACTERIA	PERCENTAGE OF SENSITIVE STRAINS (*Minimal Inhibitory Concentration* ≤ 3.1 $\mu g/ml$)	
	Tetracycline	*Doxycycline*
Staphylococcus aureus	65	65
Streptococcus pyogenes	87	95
Streptococcus pneumoniae †	100	—
Streptococcus (group B)	50	50
Streptococcus (group D)	0	0
Neisseria gonorrhoeae	88	92
Neisseria meningitidis ‡	100	—
Haemophilus influenzae	33	93
Escherichia coli §	5	5
Klebsiella pneumoniae	0	0
Enterobacter species §	50	0
Pseudomonas pseudomallei	100	—
Shigella species	50	—

ANAEROBIC BACTERIA	PERCENTAGE OF SENSITIVE STRAINS (*Minimal Inhibitory Concentration* ≤ 4 $\mu g/ml$)	
	Tetracycline	*Doxycycline*
Peptococcus	36	70
Peptostreptococcus	52	79
Streptococcus	90	90
Eubacterium	65	82
Propionibacterium	83	92
Clostridium perfringens	67	78
Other *Clostridium* species	52	68
Actinomyces	94	100
Bacteroides fragilis	42	75
Bacteroides melaninogenicus	87	96
Other *Bacteroides* species	50	68

* Modified from Standiford (1979).
† Tetracycline-resistant strains of *Strep. pneumoniae* are more common in some areas.
‡ All strains are inhibited by 1.6 µg/ml of minocycline.
§ The majority of strains are inhibited by 25 µg/ml of doxycycline, a concentration achieved in the urinary tract.

The order of efficacy of the tetracyclines *in vitro* against most gram-negative bacilli is similar to that of chloramphenicol, although a number of these microorganisms have become less susceptible to the tetracyclines as they have been widely used. Some gram-negative bacilli resistant to other congeners appear to be inhibited by clinically achievable concentrations of minocycline. Tetracylines are particularly useful for infections caused by *Haemophilus ducreyi, Brucella, Vibrio cholerae,* and *Pseudomonas mallei* and *pseudomallei.* These drugs also inhibit the growth of *Yersinia pestis, Yersinia enterocolitica, Francisella tularensis,* and *Pasteurella multocida.* Many strains of *Escherichia coli, Klebsiella, Enterobacter, H. influenzae,* and indole-producing strains of *Proteus* are resistant. Tetracycline is active against many strains of *Bacteroides* but is less active against *B. fragilis* than is chloramphenicol or clindamycin. Nearly all strains of *Pr. vulgaris* and *Pseud. aeruginosa* are resistant.

Rickettsiae. Like chloramphenicol, all the tetracyclines are highly effective against the rickettsiae responsible for *Rocky Mountain spotted fever, murine typhus, epidemic typhus, scrub typhus, rickettsialpox,* and *Q fever,* when they are tested *in vivo.*

Miscellaneous Microbial Agents. The tetracyclines are active against many spirochetes, including *Borrelia recurrentis, Treponema pallidum,* and *T. pertenue.* The activity of tetracyclines against *Chlamydia* and *Mycoplasma* has been mentioned. High concentrations of tetracyclines inhibit the growth of the protozoan *Entamoeba histolytica.*

Effects on Intestinal Flora. Since many of the tetracyclines are incompletely absorbed from the gastrointestinal tract, high concentrations are reached in the intestinal contents. Within 48 hours after daily administration of conventional doses of these agents, the enteric flora is markedly altered. Many aerobic and anaerobic coliform microorganisms and gram-positive spore-forming bacteria are sensitive and may be markedly suppressed during chronic medication, before resistant strains reappear. The stools become softer and odorless and acquire a yellow-green color. However, as the fecal coliform count declines, tetracycline-resistant microorganisms, particularly yeasts, enterococci, *Proteus,* and *Pseudomonas,* overgrow and the total fecal microbial count may actually increase. The overgrowth of antibiotic-resistant strains of coagulase-positive staphylococci may cause fatal enterocolitis, although the existence of this disease entity has been questioned (Gorbach and Bartlett, 1977). Tetracycline occasionally produces so-called antibiotic-associated colitis. Normal intestinal flora is restored several days after antibiotic medication is withdrawn. Doxycycline, in a daily dose of 100 mg, has been noted to exert a substantially smaller impact on the intestinal flora than does tetracycline (Hinton, 1970).

Effects of Combined Chemotherapeutic Agents. The results of concurrent therapy with tetracyclines and other antimicrobial agents are not predictable in most instances, and deleterious effects have occurred. Striking antagonism between penicillin and the tetracyclines has been observed clinically in pneumococcal meningitis, and the unfortunate therapeutic results emphasize the fact that such antibiotic therapy may be harmful (*see* Lepper and Dowling, 1951).

Mechanism of Action. The site of action of tetracyclines is the bacterial ribosome, but at least two processes appear to be required for these antibiotics to gain access to the ribosomes of gram-negative bacteria (Chopra and Howe, 1978). The first is passive diffusion through hydrophilic pores in the outer cell membrane. These structures have been specifically located within protein IA, one of three proteins in the envelope. Minocycline and perhaps doxycycline are more lipophilic than the other congeners and pass directly through the lipid bilayer. The second process involves an energy-dependent active transport system that pumps all tetracyclines through the inner cytoplasmic membrane. Such transport may require a periplasmic protein carrier. Although permeation of these drugs into gram-positive bacteria is less well understood, it too requires an energy-dependent system. Once the tetracyclines gain access to the bacterial cell, they inhibit protein synthesis and, like the aminoglycosides, bind specifically to 30 S ribosomes. They appear to prevent access of aminoacyl tRNA to the acceptor site on the mRNA-ribosome complex. This prevents the addition of amino acids to the growing peptide chain. Only a small portion of the drug is irreversibly bound, and the inhibitory effects of the tetracyclines can be reversed by washing. Therefore, it is probable that the reversibly bound antibiotic is responsible for the antibacterial action. These compounds also impair protein synthesis in mammalian cells at high concentrations; however, the host cells lack the active transport system found in bacteria. Tetracyclines, even in subinhibitory concentrations, have been shown to reduce the ability of *E. coli* to adhere to mammalian epithelial cells *in vitro.* The details of the extensive studies in this field have been reviewed by Pratt (1977).

Resistance to the Tetracyclines. Resistance to the tetracyclines produced *in vitro* appears slowly in a graded, stepwise fashion similar to that observed with penicillin. Microorganisms that have become insensitive to one tetracycline frequently exhibit resistance to the others. Gram-negative bacilli made resistant to tetracycline exhibit moderate-to-great insensitivity to chloramphenicol.

Resistance to the tetracyclines in *E. coli* and probably in other bacterial species is mediated by a plasmid and is an inducible trait; that is, the bacteria become resistant only after exposure to the drug. Plasmids that impart resistance contain genetic information for a number of proteins that appear to affect transport of the drug into the cell. In *E. coli,* at least one of these proteins has been located on the inner cytoplasmic membrane, where it may interfere with the energy-dependent accumulation of tetracycline (Chopra and Howe, 1978).

Absorption, Distribution, and Excretion.
Absorption. Most of the tetracyclines are adequately but incompletely absorbed from

the gastrointestinal tract. The percentage of an oral dose that is absorbed (when the stomach is empty) is lowest for chlortetracycline (30%); intermediate for oxytetracycline, demeclocycline, and tetracycline (60 to 80%); and high for doxycycline (95%) and minocycline (100%) (Barza and Scheife, 1977). The percentage that is not absorbed rises as the dose increases. Most absorption takes place from the stomach and upper small intestine and is greater in the fasting state; it is much less complete from the lower portions of the intestinal tract. Absorption of these agents is impaired, to a variable degree, by milk and milk products, and particularly by the concomitant administration of aluminum hydroxide gels, sodium bicarbonate, calcium and magnesium salts, and iron preparations (Neuvonen *et al.*, 1970). The mechanisms responsible for the decreased absorption appear to be chelation and an increase in gastric pH (Barr *et al.*, 1971).

The wide range of plasma concentrations present in different individuals following the oral administration of the various tetracyclines is related in large measure to the irregularity of their absorption from the gastrointestinal tract. These drugs can be divided into three groups based on the dosage and frequency of oral administration required to produce effective plasma concentrations.

Chlortetracycline, oxytetracycline, and *tetracycline* are, as mentioned, incompletely absorbed. After a single *oral* dose peak plasma concentrations are attained in 2 to 4 hours. These drugs have half-lives in the range of 6 to 9 hours, and they are frequently administered two to four times daily. The administration of 250 mg every 6 hours produces peak plasma concentrations of approximately 3 μg/ml.

Demeclocycline and *methacycline* are usually administered in lower daily dosage than are the above-mentioned congeners. Their absorption is also incomplete, but their half-lives are about 16 hours and effective plasma concentrations may thus persist for 24 to 48 hours. This is particularly true for demeclocycline. Poor absorption of methacycline may lead to lower plasma concentrations than with recommended doses of tetracycline, despite the difference in half-life. The peak concentration of methacycline is approximately 2 μg/ml after an oral dose of 500 mg.

Doxycycline and *minocycline* should be administered in even lower daily dosage by the oral route, since their half-lives are long (17 to 20 hours) and they are well absorbed. After an oral dose of 200 mg of doxycycline, plasma concentrations of the drug reach a maximum of 3 μg/ml at 2 hours and are maintained above 1 μg/ml for 8 to 12 hours. Plasma concentrations are equivalent when doxycycline is given by the oral or parenteral route (Leibowitz *et al.*, 1972). Food does not interfere with the absorption of doxycycline or minocycline.

Distribution. The volume of distribution of the tetracyclines is relatively larger than that of the body water. They are bound to plasma proteins in varying degree. The approximate values are as follows: *doxycycline,* 80 to 95%; *demeclocycline,* 65 to 90%; *methacycline,* about 80%; *minocycline,* 60 to 75%; *chlortetracycline,* 50 to 70%; *tetracycline,* 45 to 65%; and *oxytetracycline,* 20 to 40%. However, the values reported in the literature are highly variable (*see* Kunin, 1967; Appendix II).

All the tetracyclines are concentrated in the liver and excreted, by way of the bile, into the intestine, from which they are partially reabsorbed. Biliary concentrations of these agents average at least five to ten times higher than the simultaneous values in plasma (*see* Acocella *et al.*, 1968). Chlortetracycline is more dependent on biliary excretion for its elimination from the body than are the other tetracyclines. Decreased hepatic function or obstruction of the common bile duct results in reduction in the biliary excretion of these agents and their consequent persistence in the blood. Because of their enterohepatic circulation, the tetracyclines may be present in the blood for a long time after cessation of therapy.

Concentrations of *chlortetracycline* in spinal fluid average about one fourth those in the plasma; they vary considerably, however, regardless of dose. Inflammation of the meninges is not a prerequisite for the passage of tetracyclines into the cerebrospinal fluid; route and duration of treatment are major determinants. The intravenous injection of a tetracycline results in the gradual appearance of the drug in the spinal fluid over a period of 6 hours. Oral therapy yields very low spinal fluid concentrations.

Penetration of these drugs into most other fluids and tissues is excellent. Concentrations in synovial fluid and the mucosa of the maxillary sinus approach that of plasma (Parker and Schmid, 1971; Lundberg *et al.*, 1974). Minocycline reaches a sufficient concentration in tears and saliva to eradicate the meningococcal carrier state; this characteristic is unique to minocycline among the tetracyclines and has been attributed to its greater solubility in lipid (Hoeprich and Warshauer, 1974). The tetracyclines are stored in the reticuloendothelial cells of the liver, spleen, and bone marrow, and in bone and the dentine and enamel of unerupted teeth (*see* below). Tetracyclines cross the placenta and enter the fetal circulation and amniotic fluid. Concentrations of tetracycline in umbilical cord plasma reach 60% and in amniotic fluid 20% of those in the circulation of the mother. Relatively high concentrations of these drugs are also found in milk.

Excretion. All the tetracyclines are excreted in the urine and the feces, the primary route for most being the kidney. Since renal clearance of these drugs is by glomerular filtration, their excretion is significantly affected by the state of renal function (*see* below). Twenty to 60% of an intravenous dose of 0.5 g of *tetracycline* is excreted in the urine during the first 24 hours; from 20 to

55% of an oral dose, regardless of size, is excreted by this route. Ten to 35% of a dose of *oxytetracycline* is excreted in active form in the urine, in which it is detectable within 30 minutes and reaches a peak concentration in about 5 hours after it is administered. Only 10 to 15% of multiple or single oral doses of *chlortetracycline* is recoverable in the urine; intravenous injection leads to 60% urinary excretion during the first 12 hours. The clearance of chlortetracycline by the kidney is about 35% of the glomerular filtration rate and is less than that of oxytetracycline. The rate of renal clearance of *demeclocycline* is less than half that of tetracycline. About 50% of *methacycline* is excreted in unchanged form in the urine, while about 5% is excreted in the feces over a period of 72 hours.

Minocycline is recoverable both from urine and feces in significantly lower amounts than are the other tetracyclines, and it appears to be metabolized to a considerable extent. Renal clearance of minocycline is low. The drug persists in the body after its administration is stopped; this may be due to retention in fatty tissues. The half-life of minocycline is apparently not prolonged in patients with hepatic failure (Devine *et al.*, 1971).

An important distinction should be made in the case of *doxycycline*. It is clear that, with conventional doses, doxycycline is not eliminated via the same pathways as are other tetracyclines, and it does not accumulate significantly in the blood of patients with renal failure. It is thus one of the safest of the tetracyclines for the treatment of extrarenal infections in such individuals. The drug is excreted in the feces, largely as an inactive conjugate or perhaps as a chelate; for this reason it has relatively less impact on the intestinal microflora. The half-life of doxycycline may be shortened from approximately 20 to 7 hours in patients who are receiving chronic treatment with barbiturates or phenytoin (Neuvonen and Penttilä, 1974; Penttilä *et al.*, 1974).

As mentioned, the intestine is an important avenue of elimination of the tetracyclines. Because these agents are incompletely absorbed from the bowel when given orally or when excreted into the intestine in the bile, they are present, in varying concentrations, in the feces. Elimination from the intestinal tract occurs even when the drugs are given parenterally, as a result of excretion in the bile.

Preparations, Routes of Administration, and Dosage. *Chlortetracycline Hydrochloride*, U.S.P. (AUREOMYCIN), *Oxytetracycline Hydrochloride*, U.S.P. (TERRAMYCIN), *Tetracycline Hydrochloride*, U.S.P. (ACHROMYCIN, TETRACYN, others), *Demeclocycline Hydrochloride*, U.S.P. (DECLOMYCIN), *Methacycline Hydrochloride*, U.S.P. (RONDOMYCIN), *Doxycycline Hyclate*, U.S.P. (VIBRAMYCIN), and *Minocycline Hydrochloride*, U.S.P. (MINOCIN, VECTRIN), are available in a wide variety of forms for oral, topical, and parenteral administration.

The tetracyclines are usually prescribed for *oral* use, but they may be administered by intravenous injection. Topical administration is best avoided because of the high risk of sensitization, except for use in the eye. *The tetracyclines should never be injected intrathecally.*

Preparations for Oral Administration. All the tetracyclines listed above are available for oral administration, usually as capsules and occasionally in tablet form, in appropriate dosages ranging from 50 to 500 mg, depending on the preparation. Some of the tetracyclines are also marketed as flavored powders, ophthalmic solutions and ointments, solutions for injection, soluble salts for preparation of oral suspensions and drops, and syrups and elixirs for pediatric use.

The *oral dose* of the tetracyclines varies with the nature and the severity of the disease. For *tetracycline, oxytetracycline,* and *chlortetracycline,* it ranges from 1 to 2 g per day in adults. The recommended dose of *demeclocycline* is somewhat lower, being 150 mg every 6 hours in moderately severe infections and 300 mg every 6 hours when the disease is more serious. The doses for children and infants are calculated on a weight basis. The oral dose of *methacycline* for adults is 150 mg every 6 hours or 300 mg every 12 hours; for children it is 10 mg/kg per day, divided into equal-sized quantities given every 8 hours. The dose of *doxycycline* for adults is 100 mg every 12 hours during the first 24 hours, followed by 100 mg once a day, or twice daily when severe infection is present. Children should receive 4 to 5 mg/kg per day, divided into two equal doses given at a 12-hour interval during the first day, after which a single dose of half this amount is administered; in serious disease, the same quantity is given every 12 hours. The dose of *minocycline* for adults is 200 mg initially, followed by 100 mg every 12 hours; for children it is 4 mg/kg initially, followed by 2 mg/kg every 12 hours.

Because the incidence of gastrointestinal distress and particularly of tetracycline-resistant bacterial enteritis rises as the dose of the antibiotic is increased, the minimal dosage compatible with the desired therapeutic response is recommended. Gastrointestinal distress, nausea, and vomiting can be minimized by administration of the tetracyclines with meals. Milk, antacids containing aluminum or magnesium hydroxide or silicate, and iron interfere with the absorption of the drugs and should not be ingested at the same time as is a tetracycline.

Preparations for Parenteral Administration. Injectable preparations of chlortetracycline, oxytetracycline, tetracycline, doxycycline, and minocycline are designed for intravenous use, while preparations of tetracycline and oxytetracycline for intramuscular injection are also available. For intravenous use, vials usually contain 100, 250, or 500 mg of the dry, crystalline salt mixed with a suitable buffer. The contents of the vial are dissolved in a convenient volume of sterile distilled water, isotonic sodium chloride solution, or 5% dextrose solution and subsequently diluted to a final concentration of not more than 5 mg/ml of antibiotic. The solution should be injected slowly at a rate not exceeding 2 ml per minute. Oxytetracycline and tetracycline may be given by intermittent intravenous infusion, but chlortetracycline is not sufficiently stable to be administered in this manner. Infusion of doxycycline must be completed within 12 hours of reconstitution of the powder.

Intravenous administration of the tetracyclines can be used in severe illness in which the dose may be large and cause nausea and vomiting if given orally, in patients unable to ingest medication, and when the response to oral therapy is inadequate. However, it should be emphasized that there are currently very few indications for intravenous administration of these drugs, since better alternatives are usually available. The total daily intravenous dose of chlortetracycline, oxytetracycline, or tetracycline for most acute infections is 500 mg to 1 g, usually administered in two equal portions at 12-hour intervals. Up to 2 g per day may be given in severe infections, but this dose may cause difficulty in some patients (*see* below); quantities larger than 2 g per day must not be given parenterally. The recommended daily intravenous dose for children and infants is 10 to 20 mg/kg of body weight. Because of local irritation and poor absorption, *intramuscular administration* of these tetracyclines is generally unsatisfactory and is rarely indicated. Preparations containing a local anesthetic are better tolerated on intramuscular injection; the usual adult dose by this route is 100 mg at 8-hour intervals. The usual intravenous dose of doxycycline is 200 mg in one or two infusions on the first day and 100 to 200 mg on subsequent days. The dose for children who weigh less than 45 kg is 4.4 mg/kg on the first day, and this is then reduced correspondingly.

Preparations for Local Application. Except for local use in the eye, topical use of the tetracyclines is not recommended. Official ophthalmic preparations include *Chlortetracycline Hydrochloride Ophthalmic Ointment,* U.S.P., *Tetracycline Hydrochloride Ophthalmic Ointment,* U.S.P., and *Tetracycline Hydrochloride Ophthalmic Suspension,* U.S.P. Solutions should be freshly prepared every 7 days and kept refrigerated. One or 2 drops are instilled in the conjunctival sac every 2 hours. The usual concentration of a tetracycline for ophthalmic use is 0.5 to 1%.

Untoward Effects

Toxic Effects. *Gastrointestinal.* The tetracyclines all produce *gastrointestinal irritation* to a varying degree in some but not all individuals; such effects are more common after oral administration of the drugs. Epigastric burning and distress, abdominal discomfort, nausea, and vomiting may occur. The larger the dose, the greater is the likelihood of an irritative reaction. If troublesome, gastric distress can be controlled by administration of the tetracyclines with food (not milk or milk products), or antacids that do not contain aluminum, magnesium, or calcium. Nausea and vomiting often subside as medication continues and can frequently be controlled by temporary reduction in dose or by the use of smaller amounts at frequent intervals. Esophageal ulcers have, however, resulted (Schneider, 1977). *Diarrhea* may also result from the irritative effects of the tetracyclines given orally. In such cases, the stools, while frequent and fluid, do not contain blood or leukocytes. *It is imperative that this type of diarrhea be promptly distinguished from that which results from suprainfection of the bowel by staphylococci or pseudomembranous colitis caused by overgrowth of Clostridium difficile.* These are both potentially life-threatening complications (*see* below).

Phototoxicity. Demeclocycline may produce mild-to-severe reactions in the skin of treated individuals exposed to sunlight; this phenomenon is a *phototoxic reaction.* It appears to develop most frequently with a daily dose of 600 mg, but may also occur when smaller quantities are given. High fever, with or without eosinophilia, may be present in some patients. Onycholysis and pigmentation of the nails may develop simultaneously. The incidence of the "sunburn" reaction was found to be 40 in 2682 patients treated with demeclocycline (Carey, 1960), and doxycycline also is said to produce a high incidence. Phototoxicity is evident only when the skin is exposed to sunlight containing rays in the range of 270 to 320 nm; these are filtered out by ordinary window glass and are present in the sunlight of temperate zones only in the summer. Oxytetracycline and tetracycline also appear to cause photo-onycholysis and porphyria-like cutaneous changes, but the incidence is less than that with demeclocycline (Epstein and Seibert, 1976; Saunders et al., 1976; Hatch and Pascente, 1978).

Hepatic Toxicity. Hepatic toxicity due to tetracycline was first observed by Lepper (1951) in patients receiving large doses of tetracycline orally or intravenously. Microscopic study of the liver revealed fine vacuoles, cytoplasmic changes, and increase in fat. Oxytetracycline and tetracycline appear to be less hepatotoxic than are the other drugs of this group. Most reactions of this type develop in patients receiving 2 g or more of drug per day parenterally; however, this effect may also occur when large quantities are administered orally. *Pregnant women appear to be particularly susceptible to severe, tetracycline-induced hepatic damage* (Schultz *et al.,* 1963). Jaundice appears first, and azotemia, acidosis, and irreversible shock may follow. The livers are diffusely infiltrated with fat. Although hepatic fat is increased during pregnancy, the quantity appears to be even greater after exposure to a tetracycline. Disseminated intravascular coagulation has been reported in a pregnant woman who developed hepatorenal failure after being given only two doses of 100 mg each of tetracycline intramuscularly (Pride *et al.,* 1973).

Renal Toxicity. Use of tetracyclines for the treatment of renal infections may be particularly ill-advised, because it may lead to decreased renal function, reduced excretion of the drug, and accumulation of toxic concentrations.

Established renal insufficiency may be aggravated by the tetracyclines, and these drugs are not recommended in this setting. Doxycycline has been reported to be free of renal side effects; however, a possible association between this drug and the production of renal failure has been suggested (Orr *et al.,* 1978). The untoward effects are directly related to the particular tetracycline used, the dose, the duration of therapy, and the extent of renal disease. Among the toxic effects are azotemia, hyperphosphatemia, acidosis, weight loss, nausea, and vomiting. Kuzucu (1970) has called attention to the possibility of the development of severe renal failure in patients who receive tetracycline after being anesthetized with methoxyflurane; in those who died, the kidneys contained numerous calcium oxalate crystals. Transient diabetes insipidus has been observed in some patients receiving demeclocycline. Attempts to exploit this phenomenon for the treatment of chronic, inappropriate secretion of antidiuretic hormone have been reported (Forrest *et al.,* 1978; *see* Chapter 37).

A clinical picture characterized by nausea, vomiting, polyuria, polydipsia, proteinuria, acidosis, glycosuria, and gross aminoaciduria—a form of the *Fanconi syndrome*—has been observed in patients ingesting outdated and degraded tetracycline (Frimpter *et al.,* 1963; Fulop and Drapkin, 1965). All manifestations disappear in about a month after cessation of treatment. A facial lesion typical of systemic lupus erythematosus, as well as sensitivity to sunlight, has also been observed following ingestion of outdated and degraded tetracycline.

Effects on Calcified Tissues. Children receiving long- or short-term therapy with a tetracycline may develop *brown discolorations of the teeth.* The larger the dose of drug relative to body weight, the more severe the deformity, the deeper the color, and the more intense the hypoplasia of enamel. The duration of therapy appears to be less important than the total quantity of antibiotic administered. Repeated courses of tetracycline increase the discoloration; mild darkening of the permanent teeth occurred in 3 of 14 children who received five courses of the drug, whereas 4 of 6 who received eight courses had moderate darkening of the enamel (Grossman *et al.,* 1971). The risk of this untoward effect is highest when the tetracycline is given to neonates and babies prior to the first dentition. However, pigmentation of the permanent dentition may develop if the drug is given between the ages of 2 months and 5 years, when these teeth are being calcified. An early characteristic of this defect is a yellow fluorescence of the dental pigment, which has an ultraviolet spectrum with an absorption peak at 270 nm. The *deposition of the drug in the teeth and bones* is probably due to its chelating property and the formation of a tetracycline-calcium orthophosphate complex. As time progresses, the yellow fluorescence is replaced by a nonfluorescent brown color that may represent an oxidation product of the antibiotic, the formation of which is hastened by light. This discoloration is permanent.

Treatment of pregnant patients with tetracyclines may produce discoloration of the teeth in their offspring. The period of greatest danger to the teeth is from midpregnancy to about 4 to 6 months of the postnatal period for the deciduous anterior teeth, and from 6 months to 5 years of age for the permanent anterior teeth (Weyman, 1965), the periods when the crowns of the teeth are being formed. However, children up to 7 years old may be susceptible to this complication of tetracycline therapy.

Tetracyclines are deposited in the *skeleton* of the human fetus and young child. A 40% depression of bone growth, as determined by measurement of fibulas, has been demonstrated in premature infants treated with these agents (Cohlan *et al.*, 1963). This is readily reversible if the period of exposure to the drug is short.

Miscellaneous Effects. The tetracyclines exert a catabolic effect, perhaps due to a generalized inhibition of protein synthesis in mammalian cells. The severity of this effect is proportional to the concentration of drug and thus correlates with dosage, duration of therapy, and renal insufficiency (Shils, 1963). The administration of 2.5 to 3 g of chlortetracycline to undernourished adults results in weight loss, increased urinary but not fecal nitrogen excretion, negative nitrogen balance, and elevated serum nonprotein nitrogen concentrations (Gabuzda *et al.*, 1958).

The intravenous administration of the tetracyclines is frequently followed by *thrombophlebitis*, especially when a single vein is used for repeated infusion. The highly irritative effects of these agents are emphasized by the severe pain that they produce when injected intramuscularly without a local anesthetic.

Long-term therapy with tetracyclines may produce changes in the peripheral blood. *Leukocytosis, atypical lymphocytes, toxic granulation of granulocytes,* and *thrombopenic purpura* have been observed.

The tetracyclines may cause *increased intracranial pressure* and tense bulging of the fontanels (pseudotumor cerebri) in young infants, even when given in the usual therapeutic doses. Except for the elevated pressure, the spinal fluid is normal. Discontinuation of therapy results in prompt return of the pressure to normal. This complication may occur rarely in older individuals (Stuart and Litt, 1978).

Patients receiving *minocycline* may experience *vestibular toxicity*, manifested by dizziness, ataxia, nausea, and vomiting. The symptoms occur soon after the initial dose and generally disappear within 24 to 48 hours after drug administration is stopped (*see* Williams *et al.*, 1974). The frequency of this side effect is directly related to the dose

and has been noted more often in women than in men (Fanning *et al.*, 1977).

Hypersensitivity Reactions. Various skin reactions, including *morbilliform rashes, urticaria, fixed drug eruptions,* and generalized *exfoliative dermatitis,* may follow the use of any of the tetracyclines, but they are rare. Among the more severe allergic responses are *angioedema* and *anaphylaxis;* anaphylactoid reactions can occur even after the oral use of these agents. Other effects that have been attributed to hypersensitivity are *burning of the eyes, cheilosis, atrophic or hypertrophic glossitis, pruritus ani or vulvae, and vaginitis;* these effects often persist for weeks or months after cessation of tetracycline therapy. The exact cause of these reactions is unknown, but they could represent the results of subtle changes in the bacterial flora of the patient. *Fever* of varying degree and *eosinophilia* may occur when these agents are administered. Asthma has also been reported (Menon and Das, 1977).

It should be emphasized that *cross-sensitization among the various tetracyclines is extremely common* if not universal.

Biological Effects Other Than Allergic or Toxic.

Like all antimicrobial agents, the tetracyclines administered orally or parenterally may lead to the development of *suprainfections* that are usually due to strains of bacteria or yeasts resistant to these agents. Vaginal, oral, pharyngeal, and even systemic infections with yeasts and fungi, particularly *Candida,* are not uncommon; they tend to occur most often in individuals with disorders such as diabetes, leukemia, systemic lupus erythematosus, diffuse vasculitis, and lymphoma, especially if steroids are also being administered. The incidence of these infections appears to be much higher with the tetracyclines than with the penicillins.

Among the most important suprainfections associated with the administration of the tetracyclines are those that involve the intestinal tract; they may occur with either oral or parenteral therapy. The possibility that drug-induced diarrhea may be due to active infection of the bowel merits serious consideration in every instance.

Staphylococcal enterocolitis may appear at any time during or shortly after therapy with a tetracycline and is characterized by severe diarrhea with liquid stools that often contain blood and large numbers of polymorphonuclear leukocytes; staining reveals a very marked preponderance of gram-positive cocci, and culture yields almost a pure growth of large numbers of coagulase-positive staphylococci. Fever and leukocytosis are common features. Management must be prompt and consists in immediate cessation of tetracycline administration and oral treatment with vancomycin. In many instances, omission of the tetracycline and repair of water and electrolyte disturbances are sufficient to produce rapid cure. When there is any evidence of systemic involvement, *parenteral therapy* with full doses of an appropriate penicillin may be necessary. The incidence of this condition seems to be decreasing, and some investigators now feel that many cases previously diagnosed as *staphylococcal enterocolitis* may in fact have been *pseudomembranous colitis* (Fekety, 1979).

Pseudomembranous colitis is characterized by severe diarrhea, fever, and stools containing shreds of mucous membrane and a large number of neutrophils. It has been attributed to the overgrowth of toxin-producing bacteria (*Cl. difficile*). The toxin is cytotoxic to mucosal cells and causes shallow ulcerations that can be seen by sigmoidoscopy. Discontinuation of the drug, combined in some instances with the oral administration of vancomycin, is curative.

The oral administration of tetracyclines may result in an increase in the quantity of bilirubin and a decrease in the concentration of urobilinogen in the urine. This may cause diagnostic confusion in instances in which differentiation of obstructive from hepatocellular jaundice is important. Plasma prothrombin may be depressed to low levels by the oral administration of tetracyclines given for even moderate periods; this is probably related to the changes in intestinal flora induced by these drugs.

To decrease the incidence of toxic effects, the following precautions should be observed in the use of the tetracyclines. They should not be given to pregnant patients; they should not be employed for the therapy of the common infections in children under the age of 12 years, nor in patients with overt renal insufficiency; they should be given prophylactically with great care; unused supplies of these antibiotics should be discarded.

THERAPEUTIC USES

The tetracyclines have been used extensively both for the treatment of infectious diseases and as an additive to animal feeds to facilitate growth. Both uses have resulted in increasing bacterial resistance to these drugs. Because of this and the development of new antimicrobial agents that are more effective for specific infections and less toxic, the number of indications for the use of tetracyclines has declined (*see* Finland, 1974).

These agents are useful in rickettsial and bacterial diseases, in infections produced by some *Mycoplasma,* and in disorders caused by *Chlamydia.* Among the infectious diseases for which they are of proven value are *Rocky Mountain spotted fever, murine typhus, recru-*

descent epidemic typhus, scrub typhus, Q fever, lymphogranuloma venereum, psittacosis, tularemia, brucellosis, gonorrhea, certain urinary tract infections, ocular infections, granuloma inguinale, chancroid, syphilis, and *disease due to Bacteroides* and *Clostridium.*

The status of the tetracyclines for the therapy of various infections is given in Table 48–1 (page 1086).

Rickettsial Infections. The tetracyclines and chloramphenicol are effective and may be lifesaving in rickettsial infections, including Rocky Mountain spotted fever, recrudescent epidemic typhus (Brill's disease), murine typhus, scrub typhus, rickettsialpox, and Q fever. Fever usually subsides in 1 to 3 days, and the rash disappears in 3 to 5 days; striking clinical improvement is often evident within 24 hours after initiation of therapy.

Nonspecific Urethritis. Nonspecific urethritis is now known to be caused by *Chlamydia* or *Ureaplasma urealyticum.* These microorganisms are sensitive to tetracycline; the oral administration of 500 mg every 6 hours for 7 days is recommended.

Chlamydia. *Lymphogranuloma Venereum.* The tetracyclines are currently the treatment of choice in this infection. They exert markedly favorable effects in acute cases and are a valuable adjunct to surgery in management of chronic cases. Decided reduction in the size of buboes is observed within 4 days, and inclusion and elementary bodies entirely disappear from the lymph nodes within 1 week. Lymphogranulomatous proctitis is promptly improved. Rectal pain, discharge, and bleeding are markedly decreased. The most satisfactory results are obtained with prolonged medication; therapy is continued for 3 to 4 weeks in acute cases and for 1 to 2 months in chronic cases. When relapses occur, treatment is resumed with full doses and is continued for longer periods.

Psittacosis. The tetracyclines are also of value in proven cases of psittacosis. Fever and pneumonitis are controlled within 2 to 3 days, and convalescence is rapid and uneventful. Drug therapy for 12 to 14 days is usually adequate.

Inclusion Conjunctivitis. This disease responds clinically to topical administration of tetracycline, in ointment or liquid form, four times a day for 3 weeks. However, this treatment does not always eradicate the microorganisms. Systemic therapy with tetracycline or a sulfonamide for 3 weeks is preferred in adults. In infants, either a sulfonamide or erythromycin has been used systemically, but experience is limited (Bowie and Holmes, 1979).

Trachoma. Although the sulfonamides are preferred by some for the treatment of trachoma, the tetracyclines have proven very effective. While topical therapy has been used, oral administration of an antimicrobial agent is now recommended. The most effective regimen has been doxycycline given once daily for 40 days in a dose of 2.5 to 4 mg/kg (Hoshiwara et al., 1973).

Mycoplasma Infections. *Mycoplasma pneumoniae* is sensitive to the tetracyclines. Treatment of pneumonia with either tetracycline or erythromycin results in a shorter duration of fever, cough, malaise, fatigue, pulmonary rales, and roentgenographic changes in the lungs. Mycoplasma may persist in the sputum following cessation of therapy despite rapid resolution of the active infection (*see* Smith *et al.*, 1967).

Bacillary Infections. *Brucellosis.* Treatment with the tetracyclines produces excellent results in infections caused by *Brucella melitensis, suis,* and *abortus.* Both acute and chronic forms of the disease respond dramatically. The temperature becomes normal within 2 to 5 days, the blood is rapidly cleared of bacilli, palpable liver and spleen recede, and the clinical picture promptly improves. Good results are usually obtained in acute brucellosis with full doses of a tetracycline for 3 weeks. Clinical and bacteriological relapses are not the result of the development of resistant strains of *Brucella* and usually respond to a second course of therapy. The tetracyclines given with streptomycin (1 g daily, intramuscularly) also provide prompt results in patients severely ill with acute brucellosis. Whether such therapy results in a lower incidence of relapse than that observed with a tetracycline alone (for 6 weeks) is unsettled.

Tularemia. Although streptomycin is preferable, therapy with the tetracyclines also produces prompt results in tularemia. Both the ulceroglandular and typhoidal types of the disease respond well. Fever, toxemia, and clinical signs and symptoms are all improved; the bacteria rapidly disappear from blood, sputum, and pleural fluid; and complications are usually prevented.

Cholera. In a controlled trial of the effects of oral antibiotics in the management of cholera in children in Pakistan, Lindebaum and associates (1967) found that tetracycline was the most effective of the agents studied in reducing stool volume, intravenous fluid requirement, and the duration of diarrhea and positive stool culture. Only 1% of the children given tetracycline had diarrhea for more than 4 days. Treatment with tetracycline was significantly more effective than intravenous fluid therapy alone, regardless of the severity of the disease. When oral drug therapy was given for only 48 hours, bacteriological relapse developed in 20% of the cases despite a good clinical response. It must be emphasized that antimicrobial agents are not substitutes for fluid and electrolyte replacement in this disease. The effectiveness of tetracycline as a prophylactic agent in families of cholera patients was demonstrated by McCormack and coworkers (1968). They noted that the administration of the drug for 5 days was effective in preventing infection in contacts.

Other Bacillary Infections. Therapy with the tetracyclines is not uniformly effective in infections caused by *Shigella* and *Salmonella,* because of the increase in incidence of resistant strains; consequently, tetracyclines are not the drugs of choice. However, these drugs may prove beneficial in some cases (Pickering *et al.,* 1978). A similar situation holds for infections of various types caused by *E. coli* and *Enterobacter aerogenes.* Doxycycline has been used successfully to reduce the incidence of traveler's diarrhea, especially that caused by endotoxin-producing strains of *E. coli* (Sack *et al.,* 1978). Emergence of resistant strains and the potential for an increased incidence of salmonellosis will likely limit the usefulness of this approach (Guerrant and Hughes, 1978).

Coccal Infections. The tetracyclines are no longer indicated for infections caused by *staphylococci* or by *Strep. pyogenes* because of the high frequency of resistant strains. The recovery of tetracycline-resistant strains of *Strep. pneumoniae* has also decreased the utility of these drugs in the management of pneumococcal pneumonia. None of the tetracyclines should be used to treat meningococcal infections when other effective drugs are available. Although *minocycline* has been found, when given in a dose of 100 mg every 12 hours for 5 days, to *prevent the development of meningococcal disease* and markedly to *lower the carrier rate* (Guttler and Beatty, 1972), its use for this purpose is not recommended because of the vestibular disturbances that this drug can cause (*see* above).

Venereal Infections. Although penicillin G is the drug of choice in all clinical forms of *gonorrhea,* it cannot be used in some patients because of the presence of a dangerous degree of hypersensitivity. In such cases, the administration of 0.5 g of a tetracycline (0.3 g of demeclocycline) orally every 6 hours for 5 days is as effective as single-dose therapy with penicillin or ampicillin for *gonococcal urethritis.* For *gonococcal salpingitis* (pelvic inflammatory disease), tetracycline should be given for 10 days. *Epididymitis* in males less than 35 years of age is usually caused by the gonococcus or *Chlamydia trachomatis* and is effectively treated with tetracycline.

Tetracyclines are effective in the therapy of *syphilis* in patients unable to tolerate penicillin. A dose of 500 mg of tetracycline given every 6 hours for 15 days is recommended for early syphilis (less than 1-year duration), but therapy should be continued for 30 days if the disease has been present for longer than 1 year. Tetracyclines are also effective in *chancroid* and *granuloma inguinale,* but their use in these diseases entails the risk of masking a luetic infection that may have been contracted at the same time. If they are employed, the dose and duration of treatment should be the same as those used to treat syphilis.

Urinary Tract Infections. Although the tetracyclines were initially very valuable in the management of urinary tract infection due to gram-negative bacilli, their usefulness has been appreciably reduced by the increase in the number of drug-resistant microorganisms involved in this kind of infection. As a rule, these drugs are not active against *Proteus* and *Pseud. aeruginosa.* Therapy of urinary tract infections with a tetracycline *should* be undertaken only if the strain isolated from the urine is sensitive. Therapy is usually continued for 7 to 10 days. For severe acute pyelonephritis, tetracyclines should be used only if no other antimicrobial agent is effective. While doxycycline may be given to patients with high-grade renal dysfunction, the drug concentration in the urine will then not be sufficient for such therapy.

Amebiasis. A symptomatic intestinal infection may be treated with tetracycline (250 mg four times a day for 7 days) in combination with either iodoquinol or diloxanide furoate (*see* Chapter 46).

Other Infections. *Actinomycosis,* although most responsive to penicillin G, may be successfully treated with a tetracycline; in severe infections, intravenous therapy for 1 week, followed by oral administration of drug for a month or more, may be required. Minocycline has been suggested for the treatment of *nocardiosis* (Bach *et al.,* 1973), but a sulfonamide should be used concurrently. *Yaws* and *relapsing fever* respond favorably to the tetracyclines and penicillin (Salih and Mustafa, 1977). Although either tetracycline or penicillin is used to treat *leptospirosis,* evidence of efficacy is not convincing with these or any other antimicrobial agent.

The tetracyclines have recently been used to treat atypical mycobacterial diseases, including those caused by *Mycobacterium marinum* (Loria, 1976; Izumi *et al.,* 1977). Oxytetracycline has been given to patients with *lymphadenopathic toxoplasmosis* (Fertig *et al.,* 1977). Further studies are needed before tetracyclines can be recommended for treatment of these two types of infection.

Chronic Obstructive Pulmonary Disease. A large number of studies have suggested that the oral administration of 0.5 g per day of tetracycline or corresponding doses of the congeneric agents is effective in reducing the number of acute pulmonary infections in individuals with chronic lung disease, especially bronchitis or obstructive disorders such as emphysema (Francis *et al.,* 1964; Reynolds, 1979). In some instances, such prophylaxis has been used only during the winter months; in others, it has been more prolonged. Although many of the reports are enthusiastic about this procedure, universal agreement as to its effectiveness and safety is lacking. The danger of this kind of prophylaxis is suprainfection with drug-resistant bacteria and with fungi that may be very difficult or impossible to eradicate; death has occurred as a result of such a complication in a number of patients treated in this manner.

Intestinal Disease. Patients with *Whipple's disease* may respond to tetracycline with a prompt and dramatic cessation of fever, diarrhea, and arthralgia, and with a sustained gain of weight; relapses may disappear promptly on re-treatment. The administration of tetracycline to some patients with *tropical sprue* may be associated with repletion of folate, a favorable hematological response, decrease in diarrhea, improvement in the enzymatic activity and morphology of the superficial epithelium of the jejunal mucosa, gain in weight, and reversal of the abnormal pattern of lipid distribution. Tetracyclines may also be of value in the *blind-loop syndrome.*

Acne. Tetracyclines have been used for the therapy of acne, and good results have been reported by some workers. Benefit has been produced by very small doses. It has been suggested that these drugs may act by decreasing the fatty acid content of sebum. Although it is generally accepted that the tetracyclines or other antibiotics have a beneficial effect in acne, some placebo crossover studies raise doubt concerning the value of this kind of therapy (Crounse, 1965; Fry and Ramsay, 1966). Use of tetracycline seems to be associated with few side effects when given in doses of 250 mg orally twice a day (Sauer, 1976).

CHLORAMPHENICOL

History and Source. *Chloramphenicol* is an antibiotic produced by *Streptomyces venezuelae,* an organism first isolated by Burkholder in 1947 from a soil sample collected in Venezuela. Filtrates of liquid cultures of the organisms were found to possess marked effectiveness against several gram-negative bacteria and also to exhibit antirickettsial activity (*see* Ehrlich *et al.,* 1948); a crystalline antibiotic substance was then isolated (Bartz, 1948) and named CHLOROMYCETIN because it contained chlorine and was obtained from an actinomycete. When the structural formula of the crystalline material was determined, the antibiotic was prepared synthetically. Pharmacological studies in animals and man were soon undertaken by Smadel and Jackson (1947). Late in 1947, the small amount of available chloramphenicol was employed in an outbreak of epidemic typhus in Bolivia, with dramatic results. It was then tried with excellent success in cases of scrub typhus on the Malay peninsula. By 1948, chloramphenicol was produced in amounts sufficient for general clinical use, and was then found to be of value in the therapy of a variety of infections. By 1950, however, it became evident that the drug could cause *serious and fatal blood dyscrasias.* Nevertheless, two events of the 1970s have necessitated the increased use of chloramphenicol: the emergence of ampicillin-resistant strains of *H. influenzae* and a greater awareness of anaerobic bacteria, especially *B. fragilis,* as major pathogens.

Chemistry. Chloramphenicol has the following structural formula:

$$O_2N-\!\!\!\bigcirc\!\!\!-\overset{\overset{\displaystyle OH}{|}}{\underset{\displaystyle CHCH}{}}\!\!-\overset{\overset{\displaystyle CH_2OH}{|}}{}\!\!-NH-\overset{\overset{\displaystyle O}{\|}}{C}-CHCl_2$$

Chloramphenicol

The antibiotic is unique among natural compounds in that it contains a nitrobenzene moiety and is a derivative of dichloroacetic acid. The biologically active form is levorotatory. It is only slightly soluble in water (1:400). The antibiotic is extremely stable. Chloramphenicol is inactivated by enzymes present in filtrates of certain bacteria, which reduce the nitro group and hydrolyze the amide linkage; it is also acetylated (*see* below).

Mechanism of Action. Chloramphenicol inhibits protein synthesis in bacteria and, to a lesser extent, in eukaryotic cells. The drug readily penetrates into bacterial cells, probably by a process of facilitated diffusion. Chloramphenicol acts primarily by binding reversibly to the 50 S ribosomal subunit (near the site of action of the macrolide antibiotics and clindamycin). This prevents the binding of the amino acid–containing end of aminoacyl tRNA to one of its binding sites on the ribosome. It has been suggested that the drug specifically attaches either to the acceptor site (the initial site of binding of aminoacyl tRNA) (*see* Werner *et al.,* 1975) or to the peptidyl (or donor) site, which is the critical binding site for the elongating peptide chain during the translocation step (*see* Hahn and Gund, 1975). Chloramphenicol may act as an analog of a dipeptide and an antagonist of the peptidyl substrate for the enzyme. Peptide bond formation is prevented as long as the drug remains bound to the ribosome.

Chloramphenicol can also inhibit mitochondrial protein synthesis in mammalian cells (Wheeldon and Lehninger, 1966), perhaps because mitochondrial ribosomes resemble bacterial ribosomes (both are 70 S) more than they do the 80 S cytoplasmic ribosomes of mammalian cells. The peptidyl transferase of bovine mitochondrial ribosomes, but not cytoplasmic ribosomes, is susceptible to the inhibitory action of chloramphenicol (Denslow and O'Brien, 1978). Mammalian erythropoietic cells seem to be particularly sensitive to the drug (Skinnider and Ghadially, 1976; Hara *et al.,* 1978).

Effects on Microbial Agents. Chloramphenicol possesses a fairly wide spectrum of antimicrobial activity. It is primarily bacteriostatic, although it may be bactericidal to certain species, such as *H. influenzae* (Turk, 1977). Over 95% of strains of the following gram-negative bacteria are inhibited *in vitro* by 6.3 µg/ml of chloramphenicol: *H. influenzae, N. meningitidis, N. gonorrhoeae, Salmonella typhi, Brucella* species, and *Bordetella pertussis.* Likewise, all anaerobic bacteria, including gram-positive cocci and *Clostridium* species and gram-negative rods including *B. fragilis,* are inhibited by this concentration of the drug. Some aerobic gram-positive cocci, including *Strep. pyogenes, Strep. agalactiae* (group-B streptococci), and *Strep. pneumoniae,* are sensitive to 6.3 µg/ml, while fourfold higher concentrations are required to inhibit over 95% of strains of *Staph. aureus* (Standiford, 1979).

The Enterobacteriaceae have a variable sensitivity to chloramphenicol; while 95% of strains of *E. coli* are inhibited by 12.5 µg/ml, only 75% of *K. pneumoniae,* 50% of *Enterobacter,* and 33% of *Serratia marcescens* are inhibited. Ninety percent of strains of *Pr. mirabilis* are inhibited by 12.5 µg/ml. All strains of *Pseud. pseudomallei* are inhibited by this concentration, while *Pseud. aeruginosa* is resistant to even very high concentrations of chloramphenicol. Eighty-four percent of *V. cholerae* are inhibited by 6.3 µg/ml, as are 90% of *Shigella.* Chloramphenicol exerts marked prophylactic and therapeutic effects in experimental infections produced by all rickettsiae. The drug, as a rule, only suppresses rickettsial growth. Chloramphenicol is also effective against *Chlamydia* and *Mycoplasma.*

Resistance to Chloramphenicol. Some species of bacteria, but not rickettsiae, may be made resistant to chloramphenicol *in vitro* by serial culture in increasing concentrations of the drug. The resistance of gram-positive and gram-negative microorganisms to chloramphenicol *in vivo* is a problem of increasing *clinical* importance. Resistance of gram-negative bacteria to the drug is due to the presence of a specific resistance (R) factor acquired by conjugation. The resistance of such strains to chloramphenicol is due to the presence of a specific acetyltransferase, which inactivates the drug by using acetyl coenzyme A as the donor of the acetyl group (*see* Shaw, 1971). At least three types of enzyme have been characterized (Gaffney and Foster, 1978). Acetylated derivatives of chloramphenicol fail to bind to bacterial ribosomes (Piffaretti and Froment, 1978). Several strains of *H. influenzae* that are resistant to chloramphenicol contain resistance factors that can be transferred to *E. coli* and to other strains of *H. influenzae* (van Klingeren *et al.,* 1977). Plasmid-mediated resistance to chloramphenicol in *S. typhi* has become a worldwide problem. Resistance of staphylococci to this antibiotic has also increased in incidence; it varies from one hospital to another and is as high as 50% or more in some. Shaw and Brodsky (1968) demonstrated that resistant *Staph. aureus* contains an inducible form of chloramphenicol acetyltransferase.

Absorption, Distribution, Fate, and Excretion. Chloramphenicol is rapidly absorbed from the gastrointestinal tract, and peak concentrations are reached in plasma in 1 to 2 hours; this value is 10 to 13 µg/ml after a 1-g dose. The half-life of the drug in plasma varies from 1.5 to 3.5 hours (Kunin *et al.,* 1959), and therapeutic concentrations of 3 to 4 µg/ml are still present in plasma after 8 hours. The preparation of chloramphenicol for intravenous administration is the inactive succinate ester, which is rapidly hydrolyzed *in vivo* to the biologically active drug. Peak concentrations of chloramphenicol in plasma after intravenous injection are similar to those that follow oral administration. Absorption after intramuscular administration is unpredictable. Peak concentrations are about 5 to 7 µg/ml 2 hours after injection; this route is not recommended (DuPont *et al.,* 1970). When the concentration of chloramphenicol in blood is at its peak value, about 50% of the drug is bound to albumin.

Chloramphenicol is well distributed in body fluids and readily reaches therapeutic concentrations in cerebrospinal fluid; the drug is actually concentrated in brain tissue (Kramer *et al.*, 1969). Chloramphenicol is present in bile and milk and readily passes the placental barrier. It penetrates into the aqueous humor of the eye after subconjunctival injection. (*See* Brock, 1961.)

Chloramphenicol is inactivated primarily in the liver by glucuronyl transferase and is cleared from the plasma of patients with hepatic cirrhosis more slowly than normally. Its half-life can be correlated directly with the plasma concentration of bilirubin (Azzollini *et al.*, 1972). The dosage should be reduced for patients with hepatic insufficiency.

Chloramphenicol and its metabolites are rapidly excreted in the urine. Over a 24-hour period, 75 to 90% of an orally administered dose is so excreted; about 5 to 10% is in the biologically active form. The remainder consists of a hydrolysis product and a glucuronic acid conjugate. The unaltered antibiotic is eliminated mainly by glomerular filtration; the inactive degradation products are eliminated primarily by tubular secretion. The half-life of the active drug is only slightly prolonged by renal failure ($t_{1/2} = 3$ to 4 hours in anuric patients). The inactive conjugated metabolites accumulate and have a half-life in anuric patients of 75 to 150 hours (Sanford, 1979). It is not known whether the inactive metabolites contribute to toxicity, but the drug may be more toxic to the bone marrow of uremic patients (Kucers and Bennett, 1975). Full doses of chloramphenicol must still be given, however, to achieve therapeutic plasma concentrations of active drug in uremia (Kunin, 1967).

Preparations, Routes of Administration, and Dosage. *Chloramphenicol,* U.S.P. (CHLOROMYCETIN, MYCHEL), is marketed in capsules containing 50, 100, and 250 mg for oral use. *Chloramphenicol Ophthalmic Ointment,* U.S.P., contains 1% of the drug, and *Chloramphenicol Ophthalmic Solution,* U.S.P., is a sterile 0.5% aqueous solution. *Chloramphenicol Palmitate,* U.S.P., is a water-insoluble powder; 1.7 g of this preparation is equivalent to 1 g of chloramphenicol base. *Chloramphenicol Palmitate Oral Suspension,* U.S.P., contains an amount of chloramphenicol palmitate equivalent to 150 mg of chloramphenicol base, mixed with suitable dispersing and flavoring agents, in each 5 ml. This ester is hydrolyzed to free chloramphenicol in the gastrointestinal tract. Lower plasma concentrations may be achieved than those that follow administration of an equivalent dose of chloramphenicol itself. *Sterile*

Chloramphenicol Sodium Succinate, U.S.P., is marketed as the dry powder in 1-g quantities; it is intended for solution for *intravenous use,* and it may not be effective when given by the intramuscular route.

Chloramphenicol may be administered orally or intravenously. Dosage schedules for the therapy of specific infections are presented below. Adjustment in dose must be made when chloramphenicol palmitate is used, as indicated above.

Untoward Effects. *Hypersensitivity Reactions.* Although relatively uncommon, *macular* or *vesicular skin rashes* occur as a result of hypersensitization to chloramphenicol. *Fever* may appear simultaneously or be the sole manifestation. Angioedema is a rare complication. *Herxheimer reactions* have been observed shortly after institution of chloramphenicol therapy for syphilis, brucellosis, and typhoid fever.

Hematological Toxicity. The most important adverse effect of chloramphenicol is on the *bone marrow;* of all the drugs that may be responsible for *pancytopenia,* chloramphenicol is the most common cause (Erslev and Wintrobe, 1962; Wallerstein *et al.*, 1969). Changes in peripheral blood include *leukopenia, thrombocytopenia,* and *aplasia of the marrow* with *fatal pancytopenia.* These reactions may represent hypersensitization or an idiosyncratic reaction to the drug. The incidence is not related to dose; however, it seems to occur more commonly in individuals who undergo prolonged therapy and especially in those who are exposed to the drug on more than one occasion. Pancytopenia has occurred in identical twins, suggesting a genetic predisposition (Nagao and Mauer, 1969). Although the incidence of the reaction is low, one in approximately 30,000 or more courses of therapy, the fatality rate is high when bone-marrow aplasia is complete, and there is a high incidence of acute leukemia in those who recover.

A compilation of 576 cases of blood dyscrasia due to chloramphenicol indicates that aplastic anemia was the most common type reported, accounting for about 70% of the cases; hypoplastic anemia, agranulocytosis, thrombocytopenia, and bone-marrow inhibition made up the remainder. Among the patients with pancytopenia the outcome was apparently unrelated to the dose of chloramphenicol taken. However, the longer the interval between the last dose of chloramphenicol and the appearance of the first sign of the blood dyscrasia, the greater was the mortality rate; nearly all patients in whom this interval was longer than 2 months died. In most cases the condition for which chloramphenicol had been prescribed did not justify its use (Polak et al., 1972).

Holt (1967) noted the absence of reported instances of aplastic anemia following parenteral administration of chloramphenicol and suggested that absorption of a toxic breakdown product from the gastrointestinal tract might be responsible. Subsequently, four such cases have been described; however, in all instances, the association with parenterally administered chloramphenicol is not clear. In two patients other drugs known to affect the bone marrow were also given (phenylbutazone and glutethimide). The issue thus remains unsettled (Polin and Plaut, 1977), but it seems unlikely that the mode of administration influences the incidence of aplastic anemia (Kucers, 1980).

The risk of aplastic anemia does not contraindicate the use of chloramphenicol in situations in which it is necessary; however, it emphasizes that the drug should never be employed in diseases readily, safely, and effectively treatable with other antimicrobial agents or in undefined situations (see Erslev, 1953; Dameshek, 1960; Best, 1967).

A second hematological effect of chloramphenicol is probably due to its inhibitory action on mitochondrial protein synthesis. The result is a reduction of uptake of ^{59}Fe by normoblasts and, to a great extent, the incorporation of this isotope into heme (Ward, 1966). The clinical picture is featured by reticulocytopenia, decrease in hemoglobin, increase in plasma iron, cytoplasmic vacuolation of early erythroid forms and granulocyte precursors, and normoblastosis with a shift to early erythrocyte forms. Severe leukopenia and thrombocytopenia may also occur. The incidence and severity of this syndrome are related to dose. It occurs regularly when plasma concentrations are 25 μg/ml or higher and is observed during the use of large doses of chloramphenicol, prolonged treatment, or both (Yunis, 1973).

Toxic and Irritative Effects. Nausea, vomiting, unpleasant taste, diarrhea, and perineal irritation may follow the oral administration of chloramphenicol. Differentiation of the diarrhea from that due to suprainfection is critical (*see* below). Among the rare toxic effects produced by this antibiotic are *blurring of vision* and *digital paresthesias. Optic neuritis* occurs in 3 to 5% of children with mucoviscidosis who are given chloramphenicol; there is symmetrical loss of ganglion cells

from the retina and atrophy of the fibers in the optic nerve (Cogan et al., 1973).

Fatal chloramphenicol toxicity may develop in *neonates,* especially premature babies, when they are exposed to excessive doses of the drug. Iossifides and coworkers (1963) reported that the antibiotic accumulates in the blood of such children and reaches high concentrations at about the fourth day of treatment. In 1959, Sutherland described three newborn infants who died of "cardiovascular collapse" after receiving daily doses of chloramphenicol of about 200 mg/kg of body weight. Burns and associates (1959) have pointed out that the illness, the *"gray syndrome,"* usually begins 2 to 9 days (average, 4 days) after treatment is started. The manifestations in the first 24 hours are vomiting, refusal to suck, irregular and rapid respiration, abdominal distention, periods of cyanosis, and passage of loose green stools. All the children are severely ill by the end of the first day and, in the next 24 hours, develop flaccidity, an ashen-gray color, and a decrease in temperature. Death occurs in about 40% of the patients, most frequently on the fifth day of life. Those who recover exhibit no sequelae.

Two mechanisms are apparently responsible for this toxic effect in neonates (Weiss et al., 1960; Craft et al., 1974): (1) *failure of the drug to be conjugated with glucuronic acid,* due to inadequate activity of glucuronyl transferase in the liver, which is characteristic of the first 3 to 4 weeks of life; and (2) *inadequate renal excretion of unconjugated drug* in the newborn. Excessive plasma concentrations of the glucuronide conjugate are also present, despite low rate of formation, because tubular secretion, the pathway of excretion of this compound, is underdeveloped in the neonate. Children 1 month of age or younger should receive chloramphenicol in a daily dose no larger than 25 mg/kg of body weight; after this age, daily quantities up to 50 mg/kg may be given without difficulty. All babies treated with this antibiotic must be observed very carefully during the entire period of therapy and the drug discontinued at the first sign of toxicity. Toxic effects have not been observed in the newborn when as much as 1 g of the antibiotic has been given every 2 hours to women in labor.

Although the rate at which chloramphenicol is conjugated with glucuronic acid may be reduced in individuals with hepatic insufficiency, the overall metabolism of the drug is essentially normal. However, the administration of the drug in the *presence of hepatic disease* frequently results in *depression of erythropoiesis;* this is most intense when ascites and jaundice are present (Suhrland and Weisberger, 1963). About one third of patients with renal insufficiency exhibit the same reaction. Chloramphenicol is removed from the blood to only a very small extent by either peritoneal dialysis or hemodialysis.

Biological Effects Other Than Allergic or Toxic. The effects of chloramphenicol on the normal microflora and the consequences of such alterations are similar to those discussed above for the tetracyclines.

Drug Interactions. Chloramphenicol can inhibit hepatic microsomal enzymes (Adams *et al.,* 1977) and thus may prolong the half-life of drugs that are metabolized by this system. Such drugs include dicumarol, phenytoin, chlorpropamide, and tolbutamide. Severe toxicity and death have occurred because of failure to recognize such effects (Brunov *et al.,* 1977; Rose *et al.,* 1977). The inhibitory effect of chloramphenicol on hepatic enzymes may protect the liver from the toxic effects of carbon tetrachloride, since metabolism is apparently necessary to convert carbon tetrachloride to toxic products (Castro *et al.,* 1978; Dolci and Brabec, 1978).

Conversely, other drugs may alter the elimination of chloramphenicol. Chronic administration of phenobarbital shortens the half-life of the antibiotic, presumably because of enzyme induction (Bloxham *et al.,* 1979). Diuretics appear to increase the urinary excretion of chloramphenicol (Schuck *et al.,* 1978).

Therapeutic Uses. *Therapy with chloramphenicol must be limited to those infections for which the benefits of the drug outweigh the risks of the potential toxicities. When other antimicrobial drugs are available that are equally effective but potentially less toxic than chloramphenicol, they should be used (see Kucers, 1980).*

Typhoid Fever. Chloramphenicol is still the drug of choice for the treatment of typhoid fever and other types of systemic salmonella infections. However, epidemics in some parts of the world have been due to strains of *S. typhi* highly resistant to the drug. Although ampicillin is also effective in the management of these infections, studies indicate that, given orally, it is less effective than chloramphenicol in producing a clinical response. However, there appear to be fewer carriers and fewer relapses after ampicillin than after chloramphenicol (*see* Robertson *et al.,* 1968; Snyder *et al.,* 1976). The occurrence of resist-

ance to the drugs makes it necessary to determine the sensitivity of the microorganisms recovered from patients with these diseases.

Within a few hours after chloramphenicol is administered, *S. typhi* disappears from the blood. Stool cultures frequently become negative in a few days. Clinical improvement is often evident within 48 hours, and fever and other signs of the disease commonly abate within 3 to 5 days. The patient usually becomes afebrile before the intestinal lesions heal; as a result, intestinal hemorrhage and perforation may occur at a time when the clinical condition is rapidly improving. The incidence and the duration of the *carrier state* are not altered. The *dose* of chloramphenicol employed in adults with typhoid fever is 1 g every 6 hours for 4 weeks. Although both intravenous and oral routes have been used, the response is more rapid with oral administration (Kaye *et al.,* 1963). Relapses usually respond satisfactorily to retreatment; microorganisms isolated during recurrences are usually still sensitive to the antibiotic *in vitro*.

Bacterial Meningitis. Treatment with chloramphenicol produces excellent results in *H. influenzae meningitis* that are equal to or better than those achieved with ampicillin (Jones and Hanson, 1977; Koskinniemi, 1978). The total daily dose for children should be 50 to 75 mg/kg of body weight, divided into four equal doses given intravenously every 6 hours for 2 weeks. Such therapy is recommended for strains of *H. influenzae* that are resistant to ampicillin; furthermore, dual administration of ampicillin and chloramphenicol is now recommended for *initial* treatment of bacterial meningitis in *children* prior to evaluation of the results of cultures. Although chloramphenicol is bacteriostatic against most microorganisms, it kills *H. influenzae* rapidly. There is no evidence of antagonism when it is combined with ampicillin, and, in fact, an additive or synergistic effect may result (Feldman, 1978). Rare strains of *H. influenzae* resistant to chloramphenicol have produced meningitis (Kinmonth *et al.,* 1978), and sensitivity tests should be obtained on all isolates. Chloramphenicol remains the drug of choice for the therapy of meningitis caused by *N. meningitidis* and *Strep. pneumoniae* in patients who are allergic to penicillin. Since some strains of *Strep. pneumoniae* may be inhibited but not killed by chloramphenicol, lumbar puncture should be repeated 2 to 3 days after treatment has been initiated to ensure that an adequate response has occurred (Scheld *et al.,* 1979). Higher doses of chloramphenicol (100 mg/kg per day) may be required in some instances.

Anaerobes. Chloramphenicol is quite effective against most anaerobic bacteria; it may be used instead of clindamycin in patients with serious anaerobic infections originating from foci in the bowel or pelvis. Chloramphenicol, usually in combination with penicillin, is recommended for the treatment of brain abscesses. Most of these infections are caused by anaerobic or mixed aerobic-anaerobic bacteria, including *B. fragilis.* Since chloramphenicol is concentrated in brain tissue, it should be used; clindamycin is largely excluded from the brain and cerebrospinal fluid. Chloramphenicol may also be used in conjunction with a penicillin and an aminoglycoside for the treatment of intra-abdominal or pelvic abscesses, which are frequently caused by anaerobic bacteria (especially *B. fragilis*). Antimicrobial therapy should be accompanied by surgical drainage whenever possible.

Rickettsial Diseases. The tetracyclines are often the preferred agents for the treatment of rickettsial diseases. However, in patients sensitized to these drugs, in those with reduced renal function, in pregnant women, and in certain patients who require parenteral therapy because of severe illness, chloramphenicol is the drug of choice. The dramatic effect of chloramphenicol in rickettsial infections has been demonstrated by a number of investigators (*see* Woodward and Wisseman, 1958). *Epidemic, murine, scrub,* and *recrudescent typhus* as well as *Rocky Mountain spotted fever* and *Q fever* respond favorably to the antibiotic. The same dose schedule is applicable in all the rickettsial diseases. For adults, 1 g every 6 to 8 hours or 500 mg every 4 hours is recommended. Oral therapy is preferred, whenever possible. The succinate preparation of the drug is used in the same quantities when *intravenous* therapy is necessary. The daily dose of chloramphenicol for children with these diseases is 75 mg/kg of body weight, divided into equal portions and given every 6 to 8 hours; if chloramphenicol palmitate is used, the daily maintenance dose is 100 mg/kg, given at the same intervals. Therapy should be continued until the general condition has improved and fever has been absent for 24 to 48 hours. The duration of illness and the incidence of relapses and complications are greatly reduced.

Brucellosis. Chloramphenicol is not as effective as the tetracyclines in the treatment of brucellosis. In cases in which the use of a tetracycline is contraindicated, 750 mg to 1 g of chloramphenicol orally every 6 hours may produce a beneficial effect in both the acute and chronic forms of the disease. Relapses usually respond to re-treatment.

Urinary Tract Infections. Chloramphenicol, once commonly used for therapy in urinary tract infection, is now rarely indicated. It should be reserved for cases of acute pyelonephritis in which no other effective and safer agent is available.

Miscellaneous Uses. Rarely, chloramphenicol (1 g intravenously every 6 hours) may be useful therapy for infections caused by strains of *K. pneumoniae* resistant to cephalosporins and aminoglycosides. Although chloramphenicol therapy is quite effective in *lymphogranuloma venereum, psittacosis,* and infections caused by *Mycoplasma pneumoniae* and *Yersinia pestis,* other antimicrobial agents are preferred.

Acocella, G.; Mattiussi, R.; Nicolis, F. B.; Pallanza, R.; and Tenconi, L. T. Biliary excretion of antibiotics in man. *J. Br. Soc. Gastroenterol.,* **1968,** *9,* 536–545.

Adams, H. R.; Isaacson, E. L.; and Masters, B. S. Inhibition of hepatic microsomal enzymes by chloramphenicol. *J. Pharmacol. Exp. Ther.,* **1977,** *203,* 388–396.

Azzollini, F.; Gazzaniga, A.; Lodola, E.; and Natangelo, R. Elimination of chloramphenicol and thiamphenicol in subjects with cirrhosis of the liver. *Int. J. Clin. Pharmacol.,* **1972,** *6,* 130–134.

Bach, M. C.; Monaco, A. P.; and Finland, M. Pulmonary nocardiosis: therapy with minocycline and with erythromycin plus ampicillin. *J.A.M.A.,* **1973,** *224,* 1378–1381.

Barr, W. H.; Adir, J.; and Garnetson, L. Decrease of tetracycline absorption in man by sodium bicarbonate. *Clin. Pharmacol. Ther.,* **1971,** *12,* 779–784.

Bartz, Q. R. Isolation and characterization of CHLOROMYCETIN. *J. Biol. Chem.,* **1948,** *172,* 445–450.

Barza, M., and Scheife, R. T. Antimicrobial spectrum, pharmacology, and therapeutic use of antibiotics. *J. Maine Med. Assoc.,* **1977,** *68,* 194–210.

Bergner-Rabinowitz, S., and Davies, A. M. Sensitivity of *Streptococcus pyogenes* types to tetracycline and other antibiotics. *Isr. J. Med. Sci.,* **1970,** *6,* 393–398.

Best, W. R. Chloramphenicol-associated blood dyscrasias: a review of cases submitted to the American Medical Association Registry. *J.A.M.A.,* **1967,** *201,* 181–188.

Bloxham, R. A.; Durbin, G. M.; Johnson, T.; and Winterborn, M. H. Chloramphenicol and phenobarbitone—a drug interaction. *Arch. Dis. Child.,* **1979,** *54,* 76–77.

Brunov, A. E.; Slabochov, A. Z.; Platilov, A. H.; Pavlik, F.; Grafnetterov, A. J.; and Dvoracek, K. Interaction of tolbutamide and chloramphenicol in diabetic patients. *Int. J. Clin. Pharmacol. Biopharm.,* **1977,** *15,* 7–12.

Burns, L. E.; Hoggman, J. E.; and Cass, A. B. Fatal circulatory collapse in premature infants receiving chloramphenicol. *N. Engl. J. Med.,* **1959,** *261,* 1318–1321.

Carey, B. W. Photodynamic response of a new tetracycline. *J.A.M.A.,* **1960,** *172,* 1196.

Castro, J. A.; De Ferreyra, E. C.; De Castro, C. R.; De Fenos, O. M.; Gram, T. E.; Reagan, R. L.; and Guarino, A. M. Mechanism of chloramphenicol prevention of carbon tetrachloride–induced liver damage. *Exp. Mol. Pathol.,* **1978,** *28,* 395–405.

Cogan, D. C.; Truman, J. T.; and Smith, T. R. Optic neuropathy, chloramphenicol and infantile genetic agranulocytosis. *Invest. Ophthalmol.,* **1973,** *12,* 534–537.

Cohlan, S. Q.; Bevelander, G.; and Tiamsic, T. Growth inhibition of prematures receiving tetracycline: clinical and laboratory investigation. *Am. J. Dis. Child.,* **1963,** *105,* 453–461.

Craft, A. W.; Brocklebank, J. T.; Hey, E. N.; and Jackson, R. H. The "grey toddler": chloramphenicol toxicity. *Arch. Dis. Child.,* **1974,** *49,* 235–237.

Crounse, R. G. The response of acne to placebos and antibiotics. *J.A.M.A.,* **1965,** *193,* 906–910.

Dameshek, W. B. Editorial. Chloramphenicol—a new warning. *J.A.M.A.,* **1960,** *174,* 1853–1854.

Dawson, C. R.; Ostler, H. B.; Hanna, L.; Hoshiwara, I.; and Jawetz, E. Tetracyclines in the treatment of chronic trachoma in American Indians. *J. Infect. Dis.,* **1971,** *124,* 255–263.

Denslow, N. D., and O'Brien, T. W. Antibiotic susceptibility of the peptidyl transferase locus of bovine mitochondrial ribosomes. *Eur. J. Biochem.,* **1978,** *91,* 441–448.

Devine, L. F.; Johnson, D. P.; Hagerman, C. R.; Pierce, W. E.; Rhode, S. L.; and Peckinpaugh, R. O. The effect of minocycline on meningococcal nasopharyngeal carrier state in naval personnel. *Am. J. Epidemiol.,* **1971,** *93,* 337–345.

Dolci, E. D., and Brabec, M. J. Antagonism by chloramphenicol of carbon tetrachloride hepatotoxicity. Examination of microsomal cytochrome P-450 and lipid peroxidation. *Exp. Mol. Pathol.,* **1978,** *28,* 96–106.

DuPont, H. L.; Hornick, R. B.; Weiss, C. F.; Snyder, M. J.; and Woodward, T. E. Evaluation of chloramphenicol acid succinate therapy of induced typhoid fever and Rocky Mountain spotted fever. *N. Engl. J. Med.,* **1970,** *282,* 53.

Ehrlich, J.; Gottlieb, D.; Burkholder, P. R.; Anderson, L. E.; and Prindham, T. G. *Streptomyces venezuelae,* N. sp., the source of CHLOROMYCETIN. *J. Bacteriol.,* **1948,** *56,* 467–477.

Epstein, J. H., and Seibert, J. S. Porphyria-like cutaneous

changes induced by tetracycline hydrochloride photo-sensitization. *Arch. Dermatol.*, **1976**, *112*, 661–666.

Erslev, A.   Hematopoietic depression induced by CHLORO-MYCETIN. *Blood*, **1953**, *8*, 170–174.

Erslev, A. J., and Wintrobe, M. M.   Detection and prevention of drug-induced blood dyscrasias. *J.A.M.A.*, **1962**, *181*, 114–119.

Fabre, J.; Pitton, J. S.; and Kunz, J. P.   Distribution and excretion of doxycycline in man. *Chemotherapia*, **1966**, *11*, 73–85.

Fanning, W. L.; Gump, D. W.; and Safferman, R. A.   Side effects of minocycline: a double-blind study. *Antimicrob. Agents Chemother.*, **1977**, *11*, 712–717.

Fekety, R.   Vancomycin. In, *Principles and Practice of Infectious Diseases.* (Mandell, G. L.; Douglas, R. G., Jr.; and Bennett, J. E.; eds.) John Wiley & Sons, Inc., New York, **1979**, pp. 304–307.

Feldman, W. E.   Effect of ampicillin and chloramphenicol against *Haemophilus influenzae. Pediatrics*, **1978**, *61*, 406–409.

Fertig, A.; Selwyn, S.; and Tibble, M. J.   Tetracycline treatment in a food-borne outbreak of toxoplasmosis. *Br. Med. J.*, **1977**, *1*, 1064.

Finland, M.   Commentary. Twenty-fifth anniversary of the discovery of AUREOMYCIN: the place of the tetracyclines in antimicrobial therapy. *Clin. Pharmacol. Ther.*, **1974**, *15*, 3–8.

Forrest, J. N.; Cox, M.; Hong, C.; Morrison, G.; Bia, M.; and Singer, I.   Superiority of demeclocycline over lithium in the treatment of chronic syndrome of inappropriate secretion of antidiuretic hormone. *N. Engl. J. Med.*, **1978**, *298*, 173–177.

Francis, R. S.; May, J. R.; and Spicer, C. C.   Influence of daily penicillin, tetracycline, erythromycin, and sulphamethoxypyridazine on acute exacerbations of bronchitis: a report to the research committee of the British Tuberculosis Association. *Br. Med. J.*, **1964**, *1*, 728–732.

Frimpter, G. W.; Timpanelli, A. E.; Eisenmenger, W. J.; Stein, H. S.; and Ehrlich, L. I.   Reversible "Fanconi syndrome" caused by degraded tetracycline. *J.A.M.A.*, **1963**, *184*, 111–113.

Fry, L., and Ramsay, C. A.   Tetracycline in acne vulgaris: clinical evaluation and the effect on sebum production. *Br. J. Dermatol.*, **1966**, *78*, 653–660.

Fulop, M., and Drapkin, A.   Potassium depletion syndrome secondary to nephropathy apparently caused by "outdated tetracycline." *N. Engl. J. Med.*, **1965**, *272*, 986–989.

Gabuzda, G. J.; Gocke, T. M.; Jackson, G. G.; Grigsby, M. E.; Love, B. D., Jr.; and Finland, M.   Some effects of antibiotics on nutrition in man including studies of the bacterial flora of the feces. *Arch. Intern. Med.*, **1958**, *101*, 476–513.

Gaffney, D. F., and Foster, T. J.   Chloramphenicol acetyltransferase determined by R plasmids from gram-negative bacteria. *J. Gen. Microbiol.*, **1978**, *109*, 351–358.

Gopalakrishna, K. V., and Lerner, P. I.   Tetracycline-resistant pneumococci. Increasing incidence and cross resistance to newer tetracyclines. *Am. Rev. Respir. Dis.*, **1973**, *108*, 1007–1010.

Gorbach, S. L., and Bartlett, J. G.   Colitis associated with clindamycin therapy. *J. Infect. Dis.*, **1977**, *135*, S89–S94.

Grossman, E. R.; Walcheck, A.; and Freedman, H.   Tetracycline and permanent teeth: the relationship between doses and tooth color. *Pediatrics*, **1971**, *47*, 567–570.

Guerrant, R. L., and Hughes, J. M.   Doxycycline for traveler's diarrhea: risks and benefits. *N. Engl. J. Med.*, **1978**, *299*, 1412–1413.

Gussoff, B. D., and Lee, S. L.   Chloramphenicol-induced hematopoietic depression: a controlled comparison with tetracycline. *Am. J. Med. Sci.*, **1966**, *251*, 8–15.

Guttler, R. B., and Beatty, H. N.   Minocycline in the chemoprophylaxis of meningococcal disease. *Antimicrob. Agents Chemother.*, **1972**, *1*, 397–402.

Hahn, F. E., and Gund, P.   A structural model of the chloramphenicol receptor site. In, *Drug Receptor Interactions in Antimicrobial Chemotherapy*, Vol. I. (Drews, J., and Hahn, F. E., eds.) Springer-Verlag, New York, **1975**, pp. 245–266.

Hara, H.; Kohsaki, M.; Noguchi, K.; and Nagai, K.   Effect of chloramphenicol on colony formation from erythrocytic precursors. *Am. J. Hematol.*, **1978**, *5*, 123–130.

Hatch, D. J., and Pascente, R. W.   Photo-onycholysis associated with tetracycline. A case report and literature review. *J. Am. Podiatry Assoc.*, **1978**, *68*, 172–177.

Hinton, N. A.   The effect of oral tetracycline HCl and doxycycline on the intestinal flora. *Curr. Ther. Res.*, **1970**, *12*, 341–352.

Hoeprich, P. D., and Warshauer, D. M.   Entry of four tetracyclines into saliva and tears. *Antimicrob. Agents Chemother.*, **1974**, *5*, 330–336.

Holt, R.   The bacterial degradation of chloramphenicol. *Lancet*, **1967**, *1*, 1259–1260.

Hoshiwara, I.; Ostler, B.; Hanna, L.; Cignetti, F.; Coleman, V. R.; and Jawetz, E.   Doxycycline treatment of chronic trachoma. *J.A.M.A.*, **1973**, *224*, 220–223.

Iossifides, I. A.; Smith, I.; and Keitel, H. G.   Chloramphenicol-bilirubin interaction in premature babies. *J. Pediatr.*, **1963**, *62*, 735–741.

Izumi, A. K.; Hanke, C. W.; and Higaki, M.   *Mycobacterium marinum* infections treated with tetracycline. *Arch. Dermatol.*, **1977**, *113*, 1067–1068.

Jones, F. E., and Hanson, D. R.   *H. influenzae* meningitis treated with ampicillin or chloramphenicol, and subsequent hearing loss. *Dev. Med. Child Neurol.*, **1977**, *19*, 593–597.

Kaye, D.; Merselis, J. G.; and Hook, E. W.   Susceptibility of *Salmonella* species to four antibiotics. *N. Engl. J. Med.*, **1963**, *269*, 1084–1086.

Kinmonth, A. L.; Storrs, C. N.; and Mitchell, R. G.   Meningitis due to chloramphenicol-resistant *Haemophilus influenzae* type B. *Br. Med. J.*, **1978**, *1*, 694.

Koskinniemi, M.; Pettay, O.; Raivio, M.; and Sarna, S.   *Haemophilus influenzae* meningitis. A comparison between chloramphenicol and ampicillin therapy with special reference to impaired hearing. *Acta Paediatr. Scand.*, **1978**, *67*, 17–24.

Kramer, P. W.; Griffith, R. S.; and Campbell, R. L.   Antibiotic penetration of the brain: a comparative study. *J. Neurosurg.*, **1969**, *31*, 295–302.

Kucers, A.   Current position of chloramphenicol in chemotherapy. *J. Antimicrob. Chemother.*, **1980**, *6*, 1–9.

Kucers, A., and Bennett, N. M. (eds.).   *The Use of Antibiotics*, 2nd ed. William Heinemann Medical Books, Ltd., London, **1975**.

Kunin, C. M.   A guide to use of antibiotics in patients with renal disease. *Ann. Intern. Med.*, **1967**, *67*, 151–158.

Kunin, C. M., and Finland, M.   Restriction imposed on antibiotic therapy by renal failure. *Arch. Intern. Med.*, **1959**, *104*, 1030–1050.

Kunin, C. M.; Glazko, A. J.; and Finland, M.   Persistence of antibiotics in blood of patients with acute renal failure. II. Chloramphenicol and its metabolic products in the blood of patients with severe renal disease or hepatic cirrhosis. *J. Clin. Invest.*, **1959**, *38*, 1498–1508.

Kuzucu, E. Y.   Methoxyflurane, tetracycline and renal failure. *J.A.M.A.*, **1970**, *211*, 1162–1164.

Leibowitz, B. J.; Hakes, J. L.; Cohn, M. M.; and Levy, E. J.   Doxycycline blood levels in normal subjects after intravenous and oral administration. *Curr. Ther. Res.*, **1972**, *14*, 820–831.

Lepper, M. H.   Effect of large doses of AUREOMYCIN on human liver. *Arch. Intern. Med.*, **1951**, *88*, 271–283.

Lepper, M. H., and Dowling, H. F.   Treatment of pneumococcic meningitis with penicillin plus AUREOMYCIN: studies including observations on apparent antagonism between penicillin and AUREOMYCIN. *Arch. Intern. Med.*, **1951**, *88*, 489–494.

Lew, M. A.; Beckett, K. M.; and Levin, M. J.   Antifungal

activity of four tetracycline analogues against *Candida albicans in vitro:* potentiation by amphotericin B. *J. Infect. Dis.,* **1977,** *136,* 263–270.

Lindebaum, J.; Greenough, W. B.; and Islam, M. R. Antibiotic therapy of cholera in children. *Bull. WHO,* **1967,** *37,* 529–538.

Loria, P. R. Minocycline hydrochloride treatment for atypical acid-fast infection. *Arch. Dermatol.,* **1976,** *112,* 517–519.

Lundberg, C.; Malmburg, A.; and Ivemark, B. I. Antibiotic concentrations in relation to structural changes in maxillary sinus mucosa following intramuscular or perioral treatment. *Scand. J. Infect. Dis.,* **1974,** *6,* 187–195.

McCormack, W. M.; Chowdhury, A. M.; Jahangir, N.; Fariduddin Ahmed, A. B.; and Mosley, W. H. Tetracycline prophylaxis in families of cholera patients. *Bull. WHO,* **1968,** *38,* 787–792.

Menon, M. P., and Das, A. K. Tetracycline asthma—a case report. *Clin. Allergy,* **1977,** *7,* 285–290.

Nagao, L., and Mauer, A. M. Concordance for drug-induced aplastic anemia in identical twins. *N. Engl. J. Med.,* **1969,** *281,* 7–11.

Neu, H. C. A symposium on tetracyclines: a major appraisal. Introduction. *Bull. N.Y. Acad. Med.,* **1978,** *54,* 141–155.

Neuvonen, P. J.; Gothoni, G.; Hackman, R.; and Bjorksten, K. Interference of iron with the absorption of tetracyclines in man. *Br. Med. J.,* **1970,** *4,* 532–534.

Neuvonen, P. J., and Penttilä, O. Interaction between doxycycline and barbiturates. *Br. Med. J.,* **1974,** *1,* 535–536.

Orr, L. H., Jr.; Rudisill, E., Jr.; Brodkin, R.; and Hamilton, R. W. Exacerbation of renal failure associated with doxycycline. *Arch. Intern. Med.,* **1978,** *138,* 793–794.

Parker, R. H., and Schmid, F. Antimicrobial activity of synovial fluid during therapy of septic arthritis. *Arthritis Rheum.,* **1971,** *14,* 96–104.

Penttilä, O.; Neuvonen, P. J.; Aho, K.; and Lehtovaara, R. Interaction between doxycycline and some antiepileptic drugs. *Br. Med. J.,* **1974,** *2,* 470–472.

Pickering, L. K.; DuPont, H. L.; and Olarte, J. Single-dose tetracycline therapy for shigellosis in adults. *J.A.M.A.,* **1978,** *239,* 853–854.

Piffaretti, J. C., and Froment, Y. Binding of chloramphenicol and its acetylated derivatives to *Escherichia coli* ribosomal subunits. *Chemotherapy,* **1978,** *24,* 24–28.

Polak, B. C. P.; Wesseling, H.; Herxheimer, A.; and Meyler, L. Blood dyscrasias attributed to chloramphenicol. *Acta Med. Scand.,* **1972,** *192,* 409–414.

Polin, H. B., and Plaut, M. E. Chloramphenicol. *N.Y. State J. Med.,* **1977,** *77,* 378.

Pride, G. L.; Cleary, R. E.; and Hamburger, R. J. Disseminated intravascular coagulation associated with tetracycline-induced hepatorenal failure during pregnancy. *Am. J. Obstet. Gynecol.,* **1973,** *115,* 585–586.

Robertson, R. P.; Wahab, M. F. A.; and Raasch, F. O. Evaluation of chloramphenicol and ampicillin in *Salmonella* enteric fever. *N. Engl. J. Med.,* **1968,** *278,* 171–176.

Rose, J. L.; Choi, H. K.; and Schentag, J. J. Intoxication caused by interaction of chloramphenicol and phenytoin. *J.A.M.A.,* **1977,** *237,* 2630–2631.

Sack, D. A.; Kaminsky, D. C.; Sack, R. B.; Itotja, J. N.; Arthur, R. R.; Kapikian, A. Z.; Orskov, F.; and Orskov, I. Prophylactic doxycycline for travelers' diarrhea. Results of a prospective double-blind study of Peace Corps volunteers in Kenya. *N. Engl. J. Med.,* **1978,** *298,* 758–763.

Salih, S. Y., and Mustafa, D. Louse-borne relapsing fever: II. Combined penicillin and tetracycline therapy in 160 Sudanese patients. *Trans. R. Soc. Trop. Med. Hyg.,* **1977,** *71,* 49–51.

Sanders, C. V.; Saenz, R. E.; and Lopez, M. Splinter hemorrhages and onycholysis: unusual reactions associated with tetracycline hydrochloride therapy. *South. Med. J.,* **1976,** *69,* 1090–1092.

Sanford, J. P. *Guide to Antimicrobial Therapy, 1979.* Sanford, Bethesda, **1979.**

Sauer, G. C. Safety of long-term tetracycline therapy for acne. *Arch. Dermatol.,* **1976,** *112,* 1603–1605.

Scheld, W. M.; Brown, R. S., Jr.; Fletcher, D. D.; and Sande, M. A. Bactericidal versus bacteriostatic antibiotic therapy of experimental pneumococcal meningitis. *Ann. Clin. Res.,* **1979,** *27,* 355a.

Schneider, R. Doxycycline esophageal ulcers. *Am. J. Dig. Dis.,* **1977,** *22,* 805–807.

Schuck, O.; Nadvorn Ikov, A. H.; and Grafnetterov, A. J. The influence of ethacrynic acid, hydrochlorothiazide, and clopamide on the renal excretion of chloramphenicol and its metabolites. *Int. J. Clin. Pharmacol. Biopharm.,* **1978,** *16,* 217–219.

Schultz, J. C.; Adamson, J. S., Jr.; Workman, W. W.; and Norman, T. D. Fatal liver disease after intravenous administration of tetracycline in high dosage. *N. Engl. J. Med.,* **1963,** *269,* 999–1004.

Shaw, W. V. Comparative enzymology of chloramphenicol resistance. *Ann. N.Y. Acad. Sci.,* **1971,** *182,* 234–242.

Shaw, W. V., and Brodsky, R. F. Characterization of chloramphenicol acetyltransferase from chloramphenicol-resistant *Staphylococcus aureus. J. Bacteriol.,* **1968,** *95,* 28–36.

Shils, M. E. Renal disease and the metabolic effects of tetracycline. *Ann. Intern. Med.,* **1963,** *58,* 389–408.

Skinnider, L. F., and Ghadially, F. N. Chloramphenicol-induced mitochondrial and ultrastructural changes in hemopoietic cells. *Arch. Pathol. Lab. Med.,* **1976,** *100,* 601–605.

Smadel, J. E., and Jackson, E. B. CHLOROMYCETIN, an antibiotic with chemotherapeutic activity in experimental rickettsial and viral infections. *Science,* **1947,** *106,* 418–419.

Smith, C. B.; Friedewald, W. T.; and Chanock, R. M. Shedding of *Mycoplasma pneumoniae* after tetracycline and erythromycin therapy. *N. Engl. J. Med.,* **1967,** *276,* 1172–1175.

Snyder, M. J.; Gonzalez, O.; Palomino, C.; Music, S. I.; Hornick, R. B.; Perroni, J.; Woodward, W. E.; Gonzalez, C.; DuPont, H. R.; and Woodward, L. E. Comparative efficacy of chloramphenicol, ampicillin, and co-trimoxazole in the treatment of typhoid fever. *Lancet,* **1976,** *2,* 1155–1157.

Standiford, H. C. The tetracyclines and chloramphenicol. In, *Principles and Practice of Infectious Diseases.* (Mandell, G. L.; Douglas, R. G., Jr.; and Bennett, J. E.; eds.) John Wiley & Sons, Inc., New York, **1979,** pp. 273–289.

Stuart, B. H., and Litt, T. F. Tetracycline-associated intracranial hypertension in an adolescent: a complication of systemic acne therapy. *J. Pediatr.,* **1978,** *92,* 679–680.

Suhrland, L. F., and Weisberger, A. S. Chloramphenicol toxicity in liver and renal disease. *Arch. Intern. Med.,* **1963,** *112,* 747–754.

Sutherland, J. M. Fatal cardiovascular collapse of infants receiving large amounts of chloramphenicol. *Am. J. Dis. Child.,* **1959,** *97,* 761–767.

Turk, D. C. A comparison of chloramphenicol and ampicillin as bactericidal agents for *Haemophilus influenzae* type B. *J. Med. Microbiol.,* **1977,** *10,* 127–131.

van Klingeren, B.; van Embden, J. D. A.; and Dessens-Kroon, M. Plasmid-mediated chloramphenicol resistance in *Haemophilus influenzae. Antimicrob. Agents Chemother.,* **1977,** *11,* 383–387.

Wallerstein, R. O.; Condit, P. K.; Kasper, C. K.; Brown, J. W.; and Morrison, F. R. Statewide study of chloramphenicol therapy and fatal aplastic anemia. *J.A.M.A.,* **1969,** *208,* 2045–2050.

Ward, H. P. The effect of chloramphenicol on RNA and heme synthesis in bone marrow cultures. *J. Lab. Clin. Med.,* **1966,** *68,* 400–410.

Weinstein, L.; Goldfield, M.; and Chang, T. W. Infections

occurring during chemotherapy: a study of their frequency, type and predisposing factors. *N. Engl. J. Med.,* **1954,** *251,* 247–255.

Weiss, C. F.; Glazko, A. J.; and Weston, J. K. Chloramphenicol in the newborn infant: a physiologic explanation of its toxicity when given in excessive dose. *N. Engl. J. Med.,* **1960,** *262,* 787–794.

Werner, R.; Kollak, A.; Nierhaus, D.; Schreiner, G.; and Nierhaus, K. H. Experiments on the binding sites and the action of some antibiotics which inhibit ribosomal functions. In, *Drug Receptor Interactions in Antimicrobial Chemotherapy,* Vol I. (Drews, J., and Hahn, F. E., eds.) Springer-Verlag, New York, **1975,** pp. 217–234.

Weyman, J. Tetracyclines and teeth. *Practitioner,* **1965,** *195,* 661–665.

Wheeldon, L. W., and Lehninger, A. L. Energy-linked synthesis and decay of membrane proteins in isolated rat liver mitochondria. *Biochemistry,* **1966,** *5,* 3533–3545.

Williams, D. N.; Laughlin, L. W.; and Lee, Y.-H. Minocycline: possible vestibular side-effects. *Lancet,* **1974,** *2,* 744–746.

Yunis, A. A. Chloramphenicol-induced bone marrow suppression. *Semin. Hematol.,* **1973,** *10,* 225.

Monographs and Reviews

Bowie, W., and Holmes, K. K. *Chlamydia* trachomatis (trachoma, inclusion conjunctivitis, lymphogranuloma venereum). In, *Principles and Practice of Infectious Diseases.* (Mandell, G. L.; Douglas, R. G., Jr.; and Bennett,

J. E.; eds.) John Wiley & Sons, Inc., New York, **1979,** pp. 1464–1476.

Brock, T. D. Chloramphenicol. *Bacteriol. Rev.,* **1961,** *25,* 32–48.

Chopra, I., and Howe, T. G. B. Bacterial resistance to the tetracyclines. *Microbiol. Rev.,* **1978,** *42,* 707–724.

Dowling, H. F. *Tetracycline.* Medical Encyclopedia, Inc., New York, **1955.**

Kunin, C. M., and Finland, M. Clinical pharmacology of the tetracycline antibiotics. *Clin. Pharmacol. Ther.,* **1961,** *2,* 51–69. (121 references.)

Lepper, M. H. AUREOMYCIN (*Chlortetracycline*). Medical Encyclopedia, Inc., New York, **1956.** (769 references.)

Moser, R. H. Reactions to tetracycline. *Clin. Pharmacol. Ther.,* **1966,** *7,* 117–132.

Musselman, M. M. TERRAMYCIN (*Oxytetracycline*). Medical Encyclopedia, Inc., New York, **1956.** (664 references.)

Pratt, W. B. *Chemotherapy of Infection.* Oxford University Press, New York, **1977,** pp. 128–175.

Reynolds, H. Y. Chronic bronchitis in acute infectious exacerbations. In, *Principles and Practice of Infectious Diseases.* (Mandell, G. L.; Douglas, R. G., Jr.; and Bennett, J. E.; eds.) John Wiley & Sons, Inc., New York, **1979,** pp. 484–489.

Wilson, W. R. Antimicrobial agents—tetracycline, chloramphenicol, erythromycin, and clindamycin. *Mayo Clin. Proc.,* **1977,** *52,* 635–640.

Woodward, T. E., and Wisseman, C. L., Jr. CHLOROMYCETIN (*Chloramphenicol*). Medical Encyclopedia, Inc., New York, **1958.** (738 references.)

53 ANTIMICROBIAL AGENTS

[Continued]

Drugs Used in the Chemotherapy of Tuberculosis and Leprosy

Gerald L. Mandell and Merle A. Sande

The pharmacological characteristics and the therapeutic use of each class of compounds employed in the chemotherapy of tuberculosis and leprosy are discussed in this chapter. The treatment of infections in man caused by mycobacteria is still an important and challenging problem. For years, patients with tuberculosis and leprosy were cared for in specialized hospitals. Physicians who treated these patients developed concepts of therapy that at times seemed discordant with those that pertained to the management of other infections. It is now clear that the basic tenets of antimicrobial therapy also apply to these diseases. However, since the microorganisms grow slowly and the diseases are often chronic, there are special therapeutic problems particularly related to patient compliance, drug toxicity, and the development of microbial resistance.

I. Drugs for Tuberculosis

The introduction in the 1960s of two new drugs for the chemotherapy of tuberculosis—ethambutol and rifampin—changed many of the concepts and practices that were prevalent until that time. Drugs used for this disease may be divided into two major categories. Those of first choice combine the greatest level of efficacy with an acceptable degree of toxicity; these agents include isoniazid, rifampin, ethambutol, and streptomycin. The large majority of patients with tuberculosis can be treated successfully with these drugs. Administration of rifampin in combination with the older but still dominant agent isoniazid may represent optimal therapy for all forms of disease caused by sensitive strains of *Mycobacterium tuberculosis.* Occasionally, however, because of micro-

bial resistance or patient-related factors, it may be necessary to resort to a "second-line" drug; this category of agents includes pyrazinamide, ethionamide, aminosalicylic acid, amikacin, kanamycin, capreomycin, cycloserine, viomycin, and amithiozone.

ISONIAZID

This agent is still considered to be the primary drug for the chemotherapy of tuberculosis, and all patients with disease caused by isoniazid-sensitive strains of the tubercle bacillus should receive the drug if they can tolerate it.

History. The discovery of isoniazid was somewhat fortuitous. In 1945, Chorine reported that nicotinamide possesses tuberculostatic action. Examination of the compounds related to nicotinamide revealed that many pyridine derivatives possess tuberculostatic activity; among these are congeners of isonicotinic acid. Because the thiosemicarbazones were known to inhibit *M. tuberculosis,* the thiosemicarbazone of isonicotinaldehyde was synthesized and studied. The starting material for this synthesis was the methyl ester of isonicotinic acid, and the first intermediate was isonicotinylhydrazide (isoniazid). The interesting history of these chemical studies has been reviewed by Fox (1953).

Chemistry and Structure-Activity Relationship. *Isoniazid* is the hydrazide of isonicotinic acid; the structural formula is as follows:

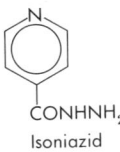

Isoniazid

Only one congener is known that markedly inhibits the multiplication of the tubercle bacillus, the isopropyl derivative *iproniazid* (1-isonicotinyl-2-isopropylhydrazide). This compound, which is a potent inhibitor of monoamine oxidase, is too toxic for use in man, and it is no longer employed, either for tuberculosis or as an antidepressant.

Antibacterial Activity. Isoniazid is both tuberculostatic and tuberculocidal *in vitro;* the minimal tuberculostatic concentration is 0.025 to 0.05 μg/ml. The bacteria undergo one or two divisions before multiplication is arrested. The bactericidal effects of isoniazid are exerted only against actively growing tubercle bacilli; "resting" microorganisms resume normal multiplication when removed from contact with the drug.

Among the various atypical mycobacteria, only *M. kansasii* is usually susceptible to isoniazid. However, sensitivity must always be tested *in vitro*, since the inhibitory concentration required may be rather high.

Isoniazid is highly effective for the treatment of experimental tuberculosis in animals and is strikingly superior to streptomycin. Control of induced infection in guinea pigs is achieved with doses as low as 1 mg per day. Unlike streptomycin, isoniazid penetrates cells with ease and is just as effective against bacilli growing within cells as it is against those growing in culture media (Suter, 1952).

Bacterial Resistance. When tubercle bacilli are grown *in vitro* in increasing concentrations of isoniazid, mutants are readily selected that are resistant to the drug, even when the drug is present in enormous concentrations. However, cross-resistance between isoniazid and other tuberculostatic drugs does not occur. Present evidence suggests that the mechanism of resistance is related to failure of the drug to penetrate or to be taken up by the microorganisms.

As with the other agents described, treatment with isoniazid also leads to the emergence of resistant strains *in vivo.* The shift from primarily sensitive to mainly insensitive microorganisms occasionally occurs within a few weeks after therapy is started; however, there is considerable variation in the time of appearance of this phenomenon from one case to another. Approximately one in 10^6 tubercle bacilli will be genetically resistant to isoniazid; since tuberculous cavities may contain as many as 10^7 to 10^9 microorganisms, it is not surprising that treatment with isoniazid alone results in the selection of these resistant bacteria. The incidence of primary resistance to isoniazid in the United States appears to be fairly stable at 2 to 5% of isolates of *M. tuberculosis,* but it may be much higher in certain populations of patients (Kopanoff *et al.,* 1978).

Mechanism of Action. While the mechanism of action of isoniazid is unknown, there are several hypotheses. These include effects on lipids, nucleic acid biosynthesis, and glycolysis (Davis and Weber, 1977). Takayama and associates (1972) have suggested a primary action of isoniazid to inhibit the biosynthesis of mycolic acids, important constituents of the mycobacterial cell wall. Low concentrations of the drug may prevent elongation of the very-long-chain fatty acid precursor of the molecule (Takayama *et al.,* 1975). Since mycolic acids are unique to mycobacteria, this action would explain the high degree of selectivity of the antimicrobial activity of isonia-

zid. Exposure to isoniazid leads to a loss of acid fastness and a decrease in the quantity of methanol-extractable lipid of the microorganisms. Only isoniazid sensitive tubercle bacilli take up the drug (Wimpenny, 1967; Youatt, 1969). This uptake appears to be an active process, although most of the drug within the bacilli is the isonicotinic acid metabolite (Jenne and Beggs, 1973).

Absorption, Distribution, and Excretion. Isoniazid is readily absorbed when administered either orally or parenterally. Peak plasma concentrations of 3 to 5 μg/ml develop 1 to 2 hours after oral ingestion of usual doses. There is genetic variation in the metabolism of this drug in man, which significantly alters the plasma concentrations achieved and its half-life in the circulation (*see* below). The half-life of the drug may be prolonged in the presence of hepatic insufficiency.

Isoniazid diffuses readily into all body fluids and cells. The drug is detectable in significant quantities in pleural and ascitic fluids; concentrations in the cerebrospinal fluid are about 20% of those in the plasma. Isoniazid penetrates well into caseous material. The concentration of the agent is initially higher in the plasma and muscle than in the infected tissue, but the latter retains the drug for a long time in quantities well above those required for bacteriostasis (*see* Robson and Sullivan, 1963).

From 75 to 95% of a dose of isoniazid is excreted in the urine in 24 hours, entirely as metabolites of the drug (Des Prez and Boone, 1961). The main excretory products in man are the result of enzymatic acetylation, acetylisoniazid, and enzymatic hydrolysis, isonicotinic acid. Small quantities of an isonicotinic acid conjugate, probably isonicotinyl glycine, one or more isonicotinyl hydrazones, and traces of N-methylisoniazid are also detectable in the urine.

Human populations show genetic heterogeneity with regard to the rate of acetylation of isoniazid (Mandel *et al.,* 1959; Evans *et al.,* 1960; Sunahara *et al.,* 1961). There is bimodal distribution of slow and rapid inactivators of the drug due to differences in the activity of an acetyltransferase.

The frequency of the rate of acetylation of isoniazid is dependent upon race but is not influenced by sex or age. Fast acetylation is found in Eskimos and Japanese. Slow acetylation is the predominant phenotype in most Scandanavians, Jews, and North African Caucasians. The incidence of slow inactivators among the various racial types in the United States is 50% (Mattila and Tiitinen, 1967; La Du, 1972). Since high acetyltransferase activity (fast acetylation) is inherited as an autosomal dominant trait, rapid inactivators of isoniazid are either heterozygous or homozygous (Weber, 1973). The average concentration of active isoniazid in the circulation of rapid inactivators is about 30 to 50% of that present in persons who acetylate the drug slowly. In the whole population, the half-life of isoniazid varies from less than 1 to more than 3 hours. The mean half-life in rapid acetylators is approximately 80 minutes, while a value of 3 hours is characteristic of slow inactivators (Tiitinen, 1969). However, it is important to emphasize that there is no conclusive evidence of a difference in therapeutic efficacy or in the incidence of toxicity related to rate of acetylation of isoniazid in patients receiving the drug every day. Fast acetylators may do less well in chemotherapy programs wherein isoniazid is given only weekly (WHO, 1977a).

The clearance of isoniazid is dependent to only a small degree on the status of renal function, but patients who are slow inactivators of the drug may accumulate toxic concentrations if their renal function is impaired. It has been suggested (Bowersox et al., 1973) that 300 mg per day of the drug can be administered safely to individuals in whom the plasma creatinine concentration is less than 12 mg/dl.

Preparations, Routes of Administration, and Dosage. *Isoniazid,* U.S.P. (*isonicotinic acid hydrazide;* HYZYD, NICONYL, NYDRAZID, others), is available in official tablets containing 100 and 300 mg, as a syrup containing 10 mg/ml, and as an injection in a concentration of 100 mg/ml. The commonly used total daily dose of the drug is 5 mg/kg, with a maximum of 300 mg; oral and intramuscular doses are identical. Isoniazid is usually given orally in a single daily dose but may be given in two divided doses. While doses of 10 mg/kg with a maximum of 600 mg are occasionally employed in severely ill patients, there is no evidence that this regimen is more effective. Children under 4 years of age should receive 10 mg/kg per day. Isoniazid may be used as intermittent therapy for tuberculosis. After 1 to 4 months of conventional therapy, patients may be treated with twice-weekly doses of isoniazid (15 mg/kg, orally) plus twice-weekly doses of either streptomycin (25 to 30 mg/kg, intramuscularly) or ethambutol (50 mg/kg, orally) for 18 months after the first negative culture is maintained (Sbarbaro et al., 1974).

Pyridoxine (10 mg per day) should be administered with isoniazid to minimize adverse reactions (*see* below), especially in malnourished patients and those predisposed to neuropathy (*e.g.,* diabetics and alcoholics).

Untoward Effects. The incidence of adverse reactions to isoniazid was estimated to be 5.4% among more than 2000 patients treated with the drug; the most prominent of these reactions were *rash* (2%), *fever* (1.2%), *jaundice* (0.6%), and *peripheral neuritis* (0.2%) (Pitts, 1977). Hypersensitivity to isoniazid may result in *fever,* various *skin eruptions, hepatitis,* and *morbilliform, maculopapular, purpuric,* and *urticarial rashes. Hematological reactions* may also occur (agranulocytosis, eosinophilia, thrombocytopenia, anemia). *Vasculitis* associated with *antinuclear antibodies* may appear during treatment but disappears when it is stopped (Rothfield et al., 1978). *Arthritic symptoms* (*back pain,* bilateral proximal interphalangeal *joint involvement, arthralgia* of the knees, elbows, and wrists, and the *"shoulder-hand" syndrome*) have been attributed to this agent (Good et al., 1965; Doust and Moatamed, 1968).

If pyridoxine is not given concurrently, *peripheral neuritis* is the most common reaction to isoniazid and occurs in nearly 20% of patients receiving 6 mg/kg of the drug daily. The neuropathological changes associated with this untoward effect include disappearance of synaptic vesicles, mitochondrial swelling or condensation, and fragmentation of axon terminals; alterations of the lumbar and sacral spinal ganglia and spinal cord occur occasionally (Schröder, 1970a, 1970b). The prophylactic administration of pyridoxine largely prevents these changes, in keeping with the facts that the excretion of pyridoxine is increased by isoniazid, the concentration of the vitamin in the plasma falls, and the clinical picture resembles that of pyridoxine deficiency. As little as 6 mg per day of pyridoxine is effective. This prevents the development not only of peripheral neuritis but also of most other nervous system dysfunction in practically all instances, even when therapy is carried on for as long as 2 years.

Isoniazid may precipitate *convulsions* in patients with seizure disorders and, rarely, in patients with no prior history of seizures. *Optic neuritis* and atrophy have also occurred during therapy with the drug. *Muscle twitching, dizziness, ataxia, paresthesias, stupor,* and *toxic encephalopathy* that may terminate fatally are among other manifestations of the neurotoxicity of isoniazid. A number of *men-*

tal abnormalities may appear during the use of this drug; among these are *euphoria, transient impairment of memory, separation of ideas and reality, loss of self-control* and *florid psychoses.*

Signs and symptoms of *excessive sedation* or *incoordination* may develop when isoniazid is given to patients with seizure disorders who are simultaneously being treated with phenytoin. Isoniazid is known to inhibit the parahydroxylation of this anticonvulsant, but the effect is usually significant only in patients who acetylate isoniazid slowly (Kutt *et al.,* 1966).

Although jaundice has been known for some time to be an untoward effect of exposure to isoniazid, it was not until 1970 that it became apparent that *severe hepatic injury* leading to death may occur in some individuals receiving this drug (Garibaldi *et al.,* 1972). Additional studies in adults and children have confirmed this observation; the characteristic pathology is bridging and multilobular necrosis. Continuation of the drug after symptoms of hepatic dysfunction have appeared tends to increase the severity of damage. The mechanisms responsible for this toxicity are unknown, although acetylhydrazine, which is a metabolite of isoniazid, causes hepatic damage in adults (Mitchell *et al.,* 1976). Some studies suggest that rapid acetylators (who produce more acetylhydrazine) are more prone to hepatic toxicity; however, others dispute this claim. The contributory role of alcoholic hepatitis has also been questioned. Age appears to be a very important factor in determining the risk of hepatotoxicity due to isoniazid. Hepatic damage is rare in patients less than 20 years old; the complication is observed in 0.3% of those 20 to 34 years old, and the incidence increases to 1.2% and 2.3% in individuals 35 to 49 and greater than 50 years of age, respectively (Public Health Service, 1974). A much larger percentage of patients receiving isoniazid (up to 12%) may have elevated plasma transaminase activities (Bailey *et al.,* 1974). Patients receiving isoniazid should be carefully evaluated at monthly intervals for symptoms of hepatitis (anorexia, malaise, fatigue, nausea, and jaundice). Some also prefer to determine serum glutamic-oxalacetic transaminase (SGOT) activities at monthly intervals (Byrd *et al.,* 1977). They

feel that an elevation greater than three times normal is cause for discontinuation of the drug. Most hepatitis occurs 4 to 8 weeks after the start of therapy. Isoniazid should be administered with great care to those with preexisting hepatic disease. (*See* Maddrey and Boitnott, 1973; Stead and Texter, 1973.)

Among miscellaneous reactions associated with isoniazid therapy are *dryness of the mouth, epigastric distress, methemoglobinemia, tinnitus,* and *urinary retention.* In those with the predisposition to *pyridoxine-deficiency anemia,* the administration of isoniazid may result in its appearance in full-blown form. Treatment with large doses of the vitamin gradually returns the blood picture to normal in such cases (*see* Goldman and Braman, 1972). Overdose of isoniazid, as in attempted suicide, may result in coma, seizures, metabolic acidosis, and hyperglycemia.

Therapeutic Status. Isoniazid is still the most important drug for the treatment of all types of tuberculosis. Toxic effects can be minimized by prophylactic therapy with pyridoxine and careful surveillance of the patient. The drug must be used in combination with another agent for treatment, although it is used alone for prophylaxis.

Details of the use of isoniazid in the chemotherapy of tuberculosis are described below.

RIFAMPIN

The rifamycins are a group of structurally similar, complex macrocyclic antibiotics produced by *Streptomyces mediterranei;* rifampin is a semisynthetic derivative of one of these—rifamycin B.

Chemistry. Rifampin is a zwitterion and is soluble in organic solvents and in water at acidic pH. It has the following structure:

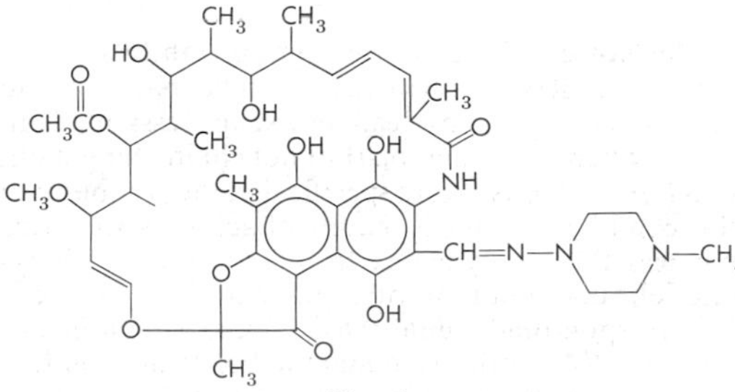

Rifampin

Antibacterial Activity. Rifampin inhibits the growth of most gram-positive bacteria, as well as many gram-negative microorganisms such as *Escherichia coli, Pseudomonas,* indole-positive and -negative *Proteus,* and *Klebsiella* (*see* Atlas and Turck, 1968; Kunin *et al.,* 1969). It is less active than penicillin G but slightly more effective than erythromycin, lincomycin, and cephalothin against gram-positive microorganisms; it is distinctly inferior to tetracycline, chloramphenicol, kanamycin, and colistin against gram-negative bacilli (McCabe and Lorian, 1968). Rifampin is very active against *Staphylococcus aureus;* bactericidal concentrations range from 3 to 12 ng/ml (Tuazon *et al.,* 1978). The drug is also highly active against *Neisseria meningitidis;* minimal inhibitory concentrations range from 0.1 to 0.8 μg/ml (Ivler *et al.,* 1970). Finally, the drug may inhibit the growth of certain types of viruses (Lester, 1972), but this effect has not been useful clinically.

Rifampin in concentrations of 0.005 to 0.2 μg/ml is inhibitory to *M. tuberculosis in vitro* (Verbist and Gyselen, 1968; Lorian and Finland, 1969). Among atypical mycobacteria, *M. kansasii* is inhibited by 0.25 to 1 μg/ml. The majority of strains of *M. scrofulaceum* and *M. intracellulare* are suppressed by concentrations of 4 μg/ml, but certain strains may be resistant to 16 μg/ml. *Mycobacterium fortuitum* is highly resistant to the drug (Molavi and Weinstein, 1971). Rifampin increases the *in-vitro* activity of streptomycin and isoniazid, but not that of ethambutol, against *M. tuberculosis* (Hobby and Lenert, 1972).

Bacterial Resistance. Microorganisms, including mycobacteria, may develop resistance to rifampin rapidly *in vitro* as a one-step process, and one of every 10^7 to 10^8 tubercle bacilli is resistant to the drug. This also appears to be the case *in vivo,* and therefore the antibiotic must not be used alone in the chemotherapy of tuberculosis. When rifampin has been used for eradication of the meningococcal carrier state, failures have been due to the appearance of drug-resistant bacteria after treatment for as short a period as 2 days (Devine *et al.,* 1971). Microbial resistance to rifampin is due to an alteration of the target of this drug, DNA-dependent RNA polymerase (di Mauro *et al.,* 1969). Certain rifampin-resistant bacterial mutants have decreased virulence (Mandell, 1975). Tuberculosis caused by rifampin-resistant mycobacteria has been described in patients who had not received prior chemotherapy, but this is very rare (*see* Stottmeier, 1976).

Mechanism of Action. Rifampin inhibits DNA-dependent RNA polymerase of mycobacteria and other microorganisms, leading to suppression of initiation of chain formation (but not chain elongation) in RNA synthesis. More specifically, the β subunit of this complex enzyme is the site of action of the drug. Nuclear RNA polymerase from a variety of eukaryotic cells does not bind rifampin, and RNA synthesis is correspondingly unaffected. While rifampin can inhibit RNA synthesis in mammalian mitochondria, considerably higher concentrations of the drug are required than for the inhibition of the bacterial enzyme. Rifampin is bactericidal. (*See* Zillig *et al.,* 1970; Konno *et al.,* 1973.)

Absorption, Distribution, and Excretion. The oral administration of rifampin produces peak concentrations in plasma in 2 to 4 hours; after ingestion of 600 mg this value is about 7 μg/ml, but there is considerable variability. Aminosalicylic acid may delay the absorption of rifampin, and adequate plasma concentrations may not be reached. If these agents are used concurrently, they should be given separately at an interval of 8 to 12 hours (*see* Radner, 1973).

Following absorption from the gastrointestinal tract, rifampin is rapidly eliminated in the bile, and an enterohepatic circulation ensues. During this time there is progressive deacetylation of the drug, such that nearly all of the antibiotic in the bile is in the deacetylated form after 6 hours. This metabolite retains essentially full antibacterial activity. Intestinal reabsorption is reduced by deacetylation (as well as by food), and metabolism thus facilitates elimination of the drug. The half-life of rifampin varies from 1.5 to 5 hours and is increased in the presence of hepatic dysfunction; it may be *decreased* in patients receiving isoniazid concurrently who are slow inactivators of this drug. There is a progressive shortening of the half-life of rifampin by about 40% during the first 14 days of treatment, due to increased biliary excretion. Up to 30% of a dose of the drug is excreted in the urine; half of this may be unaltered antibiotic. Adjustment of dosage is *not* necessary in patients with impaired renal function.

Rifampin is distributed throughout the body and is present in effective concentrations in many organs and body fluids, including the cerebrospinal fluid (Sippel *et al.,* 1974). This is perhaps best exemplified by the fact that the drug may impart an orange-red color to the urine, feces, saliva, sputum, tears, and sweat; patients should be so warned. (For various aspects of rifampin metabolism, *see* Furesz *et al.,* 1967; Cohn, 1969; Furesz, 1970; Jenne and Beggs, 1973; Radner, 1973.) Rifampin penetrates into phagocytic cells and kills microorganisms that survive in the intracellular environment (Mandell, 1973).

Untoward Effects. Rifampin does not cause untoward effects with great frequency. When given in usual doses, less than 4% of patients with tuberculosis develop significant adverse reactions; the most common are *rash* (0.8%), *fever* (0.5%), and *nausea and vomiting* (1.5%) (*see* Girling, 1977; Pitts, 1977). However, intermittent administration of higher doses of rifampin has been associated with frequent adverse reactions, including a *flu-like syndrome* and *thrombocytopenia* (Pujet *et al.*, 1974; Singapore Tuberculosis Service/ British Medical Research Council, 1975).

The most notable problem is the development of *jaundice* (Scheuer *et al.*, 1974). Sixteen deaths associated with this reaction have been recorded in 500,000 treated patients. Hepatitis from rifampin rarely occurs in patients with normal hepatic function; likewise, the combination of isoniazid and rifampin appears generally safe in such patients. However, chronic liver disease, alcoholism, and old age appear to increase the incidence of severe hepatic problems when rifampin is given alone or in combination with isoniazid (Gronhagen-Riska *et al.*, 1978).

Intermittent exposure to rifampin has been reported to be associated with the development of the *hepatorenal syndrome* (Flynn *et al.*, 1974). Elevations of plasma SGOT and alkaline phosphatase activities have also been reported; these return to normal when therapy is stopped. Biliary excretion of the drug competes with that of contrast media used for study of the gallbladder and may also cause retention of BSP. There is a significant interaction (of unknown mechanism) between rifampin and oral anticoagulants of the coumarin type that leads to a decrease in efficacy of the latter agents. This appears about 5 to 8 days after rifampin administration is started and persists for 5 to 7 days after it is stopped (O'Reilly, 1975; Romankiewicz and Ehrman, 1975). The drug appears to enhance the catabolism of glucocorticoids and estrogens (Buffington *et al.*, 1976), and for this reason it decreases the effectiveness of oral contraceptives (Skolnick *et al.*, 1976). Methadone metabolism is also increased, and the precipitation of withdrawal syndromes has been reported.

Gastrointestinal disturbances produced by rifampin (*epigastric distress, nausea, vomiting, abdominal cramps, diarrhea*) have occa-

sionally required discontinuation of the drug. Various symptoms related to the nervous system have also been noted, including *fatigue, drowsiness, headache, dizziness, ataxia, confusion, inability to concentrate, generalized numbness, pain in the extremities,* and *muscular weakness.* Among hypersensitivity reactions are *fever, pruritus, urticaria,* various types of *skin eruptions, eosinophilia,* and *soreness of the mouth and tongue. Hemolysis, hemoglobinuria, hematuria, renal insufficiency,* and *acute renal failure* have been observed rarely; these are also thought to be hypersensitivity reactions. *Thrombocytopenia, transient leukopenia,* and *anemia* have occurred during therapy. Since the potential teratogenicity of rifampin is unknown, it is best to avoid the use of this agent during pregnancy; the drug is known to cross the placenta.

Immunoglobulin light-chain proteinurea (either kappa, lambda, or both) has been noted by Graber and associates (1973) in about 85% of patients with tuberculosis treated with rifampin. None of the patients had symptoms or electrophoretic patterns compatible with myeloma. Renal failure has, however, been associated with light-chain proteinuria (Warrington *et al.*, 1977).

Rifampin suppresses the transformation of antigen-sensitized lymphocytes by the antigen. The administration of rifampin in conventional doses has been noted to suppress cutaneous hypersensitivity to tuberculin (Mukerjee *et al.*, 1973) and T-cell function (Gupta *et al.*, 1975). Rifampin also causes immunosuppression in animal models (Bassi *et al.*, 1973); this may be related to inhibition of protein synthesis by cells involved in the immune process (Buss *et al.*, 1978). However, rifampin does not suppress the antibody reponse to influenza vaccine (Albert *et al.*, 1978), and there is no evidence that rifampin-induced immunosuppression causes deleterious effects in patients receiving the drug.

Preparations. *Rifampin*, U.S.P. (RIFADIN, RIMACTANE), is supplied in official capsules containing 300 mg. The dose for therapy of tuberculosis in adults is 600 mg, given once daily, either 1 hour before or 2 hours after a meal. Children should receive 10 to 20 mg/kg, with a daily maximum of 600 mg, given in the same way. To prevent meningococcal disease (*see* below), adults and children may be treated with these same doses once daily for 4 days.

Therapeutic Status. Rifampin and isoniazid are the most effective drugs for the treatment of tuberculosis (*see* Raleigh, 1972). Rifampin (like isoniazid) should never be used alone for this disease because of the rapidity with which resistance may develop. The combination of isoniazid and rifampin is probably as effective, for sensitive microorganisms, as are programs that utilize three or more agents (*see* British Thoracic and Tuberculosis Association, 1975). Despite the long list of untoward effects from rifampin, their incidence is low and treatment seldom has to be interrupted. The drug may find its greatest usefulness in combination with isoniazid in the initial treatment of pulmonary tuberculosis in an outpatient therapeutic regimen (*see* Newman *et al.*, 1974). The use of rifampin in the chemotherapy of tuberculosis is detailed below.

Rifampin is a drug of choice for chemoprophylaxis of meningococcal disease in household contacts of patients with such infections. The drug also shows promise in the treatment of certain nonmycobacterial diseases (*see* Simmons, 1977). Combined with a beta-lactam antibiotic or vancomycin, rifampin may be useful for therapy of selected cases of staphylococcal endocarditis or osteomyelitis, especially those in patients with prosthetic cardiac valves and those caused by penicillin-"tolerant" staphylococci (*see* Chapter 50). Rifampin may be indicated for therapy of infections in patients with inadequate leukocytic bactericidal activity and for eradication of the staphylococcal nasal carrier state in patients with chronic furunculosis. The drug enhances the antifungal activity of amphotericin B *in vitro* and in murine models of fungal infection (Kitahara *et al.*, 1976; Arroyo *et al.*, 1977).

ETHAMBUTOL

History. While screening selected compounds, Thomas and coworkers (1961) found that N,N'-di*iso*propylethylenediamine was effective in the treatment of experimental tuberculous infections in mice. A number of congeners of this compound were examined; the one that eventually proved to be most tuberculostatic was ethylenediimino-di-l-butanol dihydrochloride; *in-vitro* and *in-vivo* studies revealed that the *d* form of this substance (ethambutol) exhibited 200 times more activity than did the *l* isomer.

Chemistry. Ethambutol is a water-soluble and heat-stable compound. The structural formula is as follows:

$$H-\underset{\underset{C_2H_5}{|}}{\overset{\overset{CH_2OH}{|}}{C}}-NH-CH_2-CH_2-HN-\underset{\underset{CH_2OH}{|}}{\overset{\overset{C_2H_5}{|}}{C}}-H$$

Ethambutol

Antibacterial Activity. Nearly all strains of *M. tuberculosis* and *M. kansasii* are sensitive to ethambutol. The sensitivities of other atypical organisms are variable (Karlson, 1961). Ethambutol has no effect on other bacteria. It suppresses the growth of isoniazid- and streptomycin-resistant tubercle bacilli. Resistance to ethambutol develops very slowly and with difficulty *in vitro*.

Mycobacteria take up ethambutol rapidly when the drug is added to cultures that are in the exponential growth phase. However, growth is not significantly inhibited before about 24 hours; the drug is tuberculostatic. The mechanism of action of ethambutol is unknown (*see* Beggs and Ayran, 1972; Jenne and Beggs, 1973).

The therapeutic activity of ethambutol given orally to animals infected with *M. tuberculosis* is similar to that of isoniazid. When given parenterally, it is superior to streptomycin. Bacterial resistance to the drug develops *in vivo* when it is given in the absence of another effective agent.

Absorption, Distribution, and Excretion. About 75 to 80% of an orally administered dose of ethambutol is absorbed from the gastrointestinal tract. Concentrations in plasma are maximal in man 2 to 4 hours after the drug is taken and are proportional to the dose. A single dose of 15 mg/kg produces a plasma concentration of about 5 μg/ml at 2 to 4 hours. The drug has a half-life of 3 to 4 hours; about 50% of the peak concentration is present in the blood at 8 hours and less than 10% at 24 hours. One to two times as much ethambutol is present in the erythrocytes as in the plasma. Red blood cells thereby may serve as a depot from which the drug slowly enters the plasma.

Within 24 hours, 50% of an ingested dose of ethambutol is excreted unchanged in the urine; up to 15% is excreted in the form of two metabolites, an aldehyde and a dicarboxylic acid derivative (Place and Thomas, 1963; Peets *et al.*, 1965). Renal clearance of ethambutol is approximately $7 \text{ ml} \cdot \text{min}^{-1} \cdot \text{kg}^{-1}$, and thus it is evident that the drug is excreted by tubular secretion in addition to glomerular filtration.

Preparations, Route of Administration, and Dosage. *Ethambutol Hydrochloride,* U.S.P. (MYAMBUTOL), is available in official compressed tablets containing 100 or 400 mg of the *d* isomer. The usual adult dose is 15 mg/kg, given once a day. Some physicians prefer to institute therapy with a dose of 25 mg/kg per day for the first 60 days and then to reduce the dose to 15 mg/kg per day.

Ethambutol accumulates in patients with impaired renal function, and adjustment of dosage is necessary (*see* Appendix II). Ethambutol is not recommended for children under 13 years of age.

Untoward Effects. Ethambutol produces very few reactions. Daily doses of 15 mg/kg are minimally toxic. Less than 2% of nearly 2000 patients who received 15 mg/kg of ethambutol developed adverse reactions; of these, 0.8% experienced *diminished visual acuity,* 0.5% had a *rash,* and 0.3% developed *drug fever* (Pitts, 1977). Other side effects that have been observed are *pruritus, joint pain, gastrointestinal upset, abdominal pain, malaise, headache, dizziness, mental confusion, disorientation,* and possible *hallucination. Numbness* and *tingling of the fingers* due to *peripheral neuritis* are infrequent. *Anaphylaxis* and *leukopenia* are rare.

The most important side effect is *optic neuritis,* resulting in *decrease of visual acuity* and *loss of ability to perceive the color green.* The incidence of this reaction is proportional to the dose of ethambutol and is observed in 15% of patients receiving 50 mg/kg per day, 5% of patients receiving 25 mg/kg per day, and less than 1% of patients receiving daily doses of 15 mg/kg. The intensity of the visual difficulty is related to the duration of therapy after decrease in visual acuity first becomes apparent, and it may be unilateral or bilateral. *Tests of visual acuity prior to the start of therapy and periodically thereafter are thus strongly recommended.* Recovery usually occurs when ethambutol is withdrawn; the time required is a function of the degree of visual impairment (Place and Thomas, 1963).

Therapy with ethambutol results in an increased concentration of urate in the blood in about 50% of patients, due to decreased renal excretion of uric acid. The effect may be detectable as early as 24 hours after a single dose or as late as 90 days after treatment is started. This untoward effect is possibly enhanced by isoniazid and pyridoxine (Postlethwaite *et al.,* 1972).

Therapeutic Status. Ethambutol has been used with notable success in the therapy of tuberculosis of various forms in combination with isoniazid. Because of a lower incidence of toxic side effects and better acceptance by patients, it has essentially replaced aminosalicylic acid (*see* Bobrowitz, 1971, 1974).

The use of ethambutol in the chemotherapy of tuberculosis is described below.

STREPTOMYCIN

A discussion of the pharmacology of streptomycin, including its adverse effects and its uses in infections other than tuberculosis, is presented in Chapter 51. Only those features of the drug related to its antibacterial activity and therapeutic effects in the management of diseases caused by mycobacteria are considered here.

History. Streptomycin was the first clinically effective drug to become available for the treatment of tuberculosis, and from 1947 to 1952 it was the only effective agent available to treat the disease. At first, it was given in large doses, but problems related to toxicity and the development of resistant microorganisms seriously limited its usefulness. This led to administration of the antibiotic in smaller quantities, but streptomycin administered alone still proved to be far from the ideal agent for the management of all forms of this disease. However, after the discovery of other tuberculostatic compounds that, given concurrently with the antibiotic, reduced the rate at which microorganisms became drug resistant despite prolonged exposure, streptomycin reached its full potential in the therapy of tuberculosis.

Antibacterial Activity. Streptomycin is bactericidal for the tubercle bacillus *in vitro.* Concentrations as low as 0.4 μg/ml may inhibit growth. The vast majority of strains of *M. tuberculosis* are sensitive to 10 μg/ml. *M. kansasii* is frequently sensitive, but other atypical mycobacteria are only occasionally susceptible.

The activity of streptomycin *in vivo* is essentially suppressive. When the antibiotic is administered to experimental animals prior to inoculation with the tubercle bacillus, the development of disease is not prevented. Infection progresses until the animals' immunological mechanisms respond. The presence of viable microorganisms in nonsloughing abscesses at the sites of injection and in the regional lymph nodes, together with the fact that omission of the drug, after many months of therapy, results in rapid spread of infection, adds support to the concept that the activity of streptomycin *in vivo* is to suppress, not to eradicate, the tubercle bacillus. This may be related to the observation that streptomycin does not readily enter living cells and thus cannot kill intracellular microbes.

Bacterial Resistance. Large populations of all strains of tubercle bacilli include a number of cells that are markedly resistant to the antibiotic because of mutation. However, primary resistance to streptomycin is found in only 1 to 2% of isolates of *M. tuberculosis.*

There is every reason to believe that selection for resistant tubercle bacilli occurs *in vivo* as it does *in vitro.* In general, the longer therapy is continued, the greater is the incidence of resistance to streptomycin. When streptomycin was used alone, as many as 80% of patients harbored insensitive tubercle bacilli after 4 months of treatment; many of these microorganisms were not inhibited by concentrations of drug as high as 1000 μg/ml.

Preparations, Routes of Administration, and Dosage. The preparations and routes of administration of streptomycin are considered in detail in Chapter 51. The dosage schedules used in the treatment of various forms of tuberculosis are discussed below.

Untoward Effects. Untoward effects of streptomycin are considered in detail in Chapter 51. Of 515 patients with tuberculosis who were treated with this aminoglycoside, 8.2% developed adverse reactions; half of these involved the auditory and vestibular functions of the eighth cranial nerve, and other relatively frequent problems included rash (in 2%) and fever (in 1.4%) (Pitts, 1977).

Therapeutic Status. Since other effective agents have become available, the use of streptomycin for the treatment of pulmonary tuberculosis has been sharply reduced. Many clinicians prefer to give three drugs, of which streptomycin may be one, for the most serious forms of tuberculosis, such as disseminated disease or meningitis.

The use of streptomycin in the chemotherapy of tuberculosis is described below.

PYRAZINAMIDE

Chemistry. Pyrazinamide is the synthetic pyrazine analog of nicotinamide. It has the following structural formula:

Pyrazinamide

Antibacterial Activity. Pyrazinamide exhibits tuberculostatic activity *in vitro* only at a slightly acidic pH. The growth of tubercle bacilli within monocytes *in vitro* is completely inhibited by the drug in a concentration of 12.5 μg/ml.

Absorption, Distribution, and Excretion. Pyrazinamide is well absorbed from the gastrointestinal tract, and it is widely distributed throughout the body. The oral administration of 1 g produces plasma concentrations of about 45 μg/ml at 2 hours and 10 μg/ml at 15 hours. The drug is excreted primarily by renal glomerular filtration; urinary concentrations are 50 to 100 μg/ml for several hours after a single dose (Stottmeier *et al.,* 1968). Pyrazinamide is hydrolyzed to pyrazinoic acid and subsequently hydroxylated to 5-hydroxypyrazinoic acid, the major excretory product (Weiner and Tinker, 1972).

Preparations, Route of Administration, and Dosage. *Pyrazinamide,* U.S.P., is marketed in official tablets containing 500 mg. It is available only in hospitals. The daily dosage is 20 to 35 mg/kg orally, given in three or four equally spaced doses. The maximal quantity to be given is 3 g per day, regardless of weight.

Untoward Effects. Injury to the *liver* is the most common and serious side effect of pyrazinamide. When a dose of 3 g per day is administered orally, signs and symptoms of hepatic disease appear in about 15% of patients, jaundice supervenes in 2 to 3%, and death due to *hepatic necrosis* results in rare instances (McDermott *et al.,* 1954). Elevations of the plasma glutamic-oxaloacetic and glutamic-pyruvate transaminases are the earliest abnormalities produced by the drug. All patients who are being treated with pyrazinamide should have studies of hepatic function carried out before the drug is administered; these should be repeated at frequent intervals during the entire period of treatment. If evidence of significant hepatic damage becomes apparent, therapy must be stopped. Pyrazinamide should not be given to individuals with any degree of hepatic dysfunction, unless this is absolutely unavoidable.

The drug inhibits excretion of urate, and acute episodes of gout have occurred. Among other untoward effects that have been observed with pyrazinamide are *arthralgias, anorexia, nausea and vomiting, dysuria, malaise,* and *fever. Diabetes mellitus* may become difficult to control in patients who are receiving the drug. Fatal *hemoptysis* during the treatment of pulmonary tuberculosis with pyrazinamide has been reported.

Therapeutic Status. Pyrazinamide is a secondary agent. It is less effective and considerably more toxic than several of the other drugs discussed above. It has been utilized in daily and intermittent regimens for ambulatory patients in underdeveloped countries where primary resistance to other more effective agents is high (East African/British Medical Research Councils, 1974).

ETHIONAMIDE

Chemistry. Synthesis and study of a variety of congeners of thioisonicotinamide revealed that an alpha-ethyl derivative, ethionamide, is considerably more effective than the parent compound. Ethionamide is a yellow substance, practically insoluble in water, with a faint-to-moderate sulfide odor. It has the following structural formula:

Ethionamide

Antibacterial Activity. The multiplication of human strains of *M. tuberculosis* is suppressed by concentrations of ethionamide ranging from 0.6 to 2.5 µg/ml. Resistance can develop rapidly *in vitro*. Approximately 75% of photochromogenic mycobacteria are inhibited by a concentration of 10 µg/ml or less; the scotochromogens are more resistant. Ethionamide is very effective in the treatment of experimental tuberculosis in animals, although its activity varies greatly with the animal model studied (Rist *et al.*, 1959).

Absorption, Distribution, and Excretion. The oral administration of 1 g of ethionamide yields peak concentrations in plasma of about 20 µg/ml in 3 hours; the concentration at 9 hours is 3 µg/ml. The drug has a shorter half-life than does isoniazid. Because of gastric irritation, about 50% of patients are unable to tolerate a single dose larger than 500 mg.

Ethionamide is rapidly and widely distributed; the concentrations in the blood and various organs are approximately equal. Significant concentrations are present in cerebrospinal fluid. Ethionamide, like aminosalicylic acid, inhibits the acetylation of isoniazid *in vitro*.

Less than 1% of ethionamide is excreted in active form in the urine. Metabolites detected in the urine include three dihydropyridines: carbamoyl, thiocarbamoyl, and S-oxocarbamoyl (Bieder *et al.*, 1966).

Preparations, Route of Administration, and Dosage. *Ethionamide*, U.S.P. (TRECATOR-SC), is administered only by the oral route. Tablets containing 250 mg of the drug are available. The initial dose for adults is 250 mg, given twice a day. This is increased by 125 mg per day every 5 days until 1 g is being given daily; this dose must not be exceeded. The drug is best taken with meals in order to minimize gastric irritation.

Untoward Effects. The most common reactions to ethionamide are *anorexia, nausea,* and *vomiting*. A metallic taste may also be noted. *Severe postural hypotension, mental depression, drowsiness,* and *asthenia* are common. *Convulsions* and *peripheral neuropathy* are rare. Other reactions referable to the nervous system include *olfactory disturbances, blurred vision, diplopia, dizziness, paresthesias, headache, restlessness,* and *tremors*. *Severe allergic skin rashes, purpura, stomatitis, gynecomastia, impotence, menorrhagia, acne,* and *alopecia* have also been observed. *Acute rheumatic symptoms* have been noted. Increased difficulty in the management of *diabetes*

mellitus may become a problem in patients with this disease who are taking ethionamide.

Hepatitis has been associated with the use of the drug in about 5% of cases. This has usually appeared in diabetics and is accompanied by elevated plasma transaminase activities (Simon *et al.*, 1969); liver biopsy has revealed periportal round-cell infiltration, a few swollen and destroyed hepatic cells, areas of fibrosis, and hepatic-cell regeneration. The signs and symptoms of hepatotoxicity clear when treatment is stopped (Phillips and Tashman, 1963). Hepatic function should be assessed at regular intervals in patients receiving ethionamide.

Therapeutic Status. Ethionamide is a secondary agent, to be used in combination with other drugs only when therapy with primary agents is ineffective or contraindicated. (*See* Schwartz, 1966; Lees, 1967.)

AMINOSALICYLIC ACID

History. The demonstration by Bernheim that benzoic and salicyclic acids increase the oxygen consumption of tubercle bacilli, the speculation that similar compounds play a role in the normal metabolism of *M. tuberculosis*, and the theory that related substances might have a reverse effect led to the discovery of the tuberculostatic activity of *aminosalicylic acid* (PAS, para-aminosalicylic acid). The metabolic effect of this acid was found by Lehmann (1946) to be associated with suppression of both growth and multiplication of the microorganisms. When examination of the *in-vivo* effects of the drug in experimental tuberculosis revealed that it altered the course of the disease, aminosalicylic acid was subjected to clinical trial.

Chemistry. The structural formula of aminosalicylic acid is as follows:

Aminosalicylic Acid

Aqueous solutions of the drug are very unstable and undergo decarboxylation. The sodium salt of aminosalicylic acid is much more stable, is highly soluble in water, and forms slightly alkaline solutions that do not decompose at room temperature but are decomposed by heat.

Antibacterial Activity. Aminosalicylic acid is bacteriostatic. *In vitro*, most strains of *M. tuberculosis* are sensitive to a concentration of 1 µg/ml. The antimicrobial activity of aminosalicylic acid is highly specific, and microorganisms other than *M. tuberculosis* are unaffected. Most atypical mycobacteria are not inhibited by the drug.

Studies of the treatment of experimental infections caused by human strains of *M. tuberculosis* indicate that this drug exerts a beneficial effect on the disease. However, the doses of aminosalicylic acid required are relatively large, and the compound must be present continuously. Aminosalicylic acid alone is of little value in the treatment of tuberculosis in man; it is much less effective than either streptomycin, isoniazid, or rifampin.

Bacterial Resistance. Strains of tubercle bacilli insensitive to several hundred times the usual bacteriostatic concentration of aminosalicylic acid can be produced *in vitro*. In general, resistance to aminosalicylic acid is somewhat more difficult to induce *in vitro* than is that to streptomycin.

Resistant strains of tubercle bacilli also emerge in patients treated with aminosalicylic acid, but much more slowly than with streptomycin.

Mechanism of Action. Aminosalicylic acid is a structural analog of para-aminobenzoic acid, and its mechanism of action appears to be very similar to that of the sulfonamides (*see* Chapter 49). Since the sulfonamides are ineffective against *M. tuberculosis* and aminosalicylic acid is inactive against sulfonamide-susceptible bacteria, it is probable that the enzymes responsible for folate biosynthesis in various microorganisms may be quite exacting in their capacity to distinguish various analogs from the true metabolite (*see* Pratt, 1977).

Absorption, Distribution, and Excretion. Aminosalicylic acid is readily absorbed from the gastrointestinal tract. A single oral dose of 4 g of the free acid produces maximal concentrations in plasma of about 75 μg/ml within 1.5 to 2 hours. The sodium salt is absorbed even more rapidly. The drug appears to be distributed throughout the total body water and reaches high concentrations in pleural fluid and caseous tissue. However, values in cerebrospinal fluid are low, perhaps because of active outward transport (Spector and Lorenzo, 1973).

The drug has a half-life of about 1 hour, and concentrations in plasma are negligible within 4 to 5 hours after a single conventional dose. Over 80% of the drug is excreted in the urine; more than 50% is in the form of the acetylated compound in man. The largest portion of the remainder is made up of the free acid; small quantities of free and acetylated para-aminosalicyluric and 2,4-dihydroxybenzoic acids are present in the urine (Way *et al.*, 1948). Excretion of aminosalicylic acid is greatly retarded in the presence of renal dysfunction, and the use of the drug is not recommended in such patients. Probenecid decreases the renal excretion of this agent.

Preparations, Routes of Administration, and Dosage. *Aminosalicylate Sodium*, U.S.P. (PAMISYL SODIUM, PARASAL SODIUM, TEEBACIN, others), is available in official *tablets* containing 500, 690, and 1000 mg. Capsules, enteric-coated tablets, and granules are also supplied. *Aminosalicylate Potassium*, U.S.P. (TEEBACIN KALIUM), *Aminosalicylate Calcium*, U.S.P. (TEEBACIN CALCIUM, PAS CALCIUM), and *Aminosalicylic Acid*, U.S.P. (TEEBACIN ACID, others), are marketed in a variety of preparations for oral use. Aminosalicylic acid is administered orally in a daily

dose of 8 to 12 g. To obtain an equivalent amount of aminosalicyclic acid, the dose of the Na⁺ salt must be increased 38%; the corresponding values for the Ca²⁺ and K⁺ salts are 30% and 24%, respectively. Because it is a gastric irritant, the drug is best administered after meals, the daily intake being divided into three or four equal-sized doses.

Untoward Effects. The incidence of untoward effects associated with the use of aminosalicylic acid is approximately 10%. Gastrointestinal problems, including anorexia, nausea, epigastric pain, abdominal distress, and diarrhea are predominant (Pitts, 1977), and patients with peptic ulcer tolerate the drug poorly. Hypersensitivity reactions to aminosalicylic acid are also common. *High fever* may develop abruptly, with intermittent spiking, or it may appear gradually and be low grade. *Generalized malaise, joint pains,* or *sore throat* may be present at the same time. *Skin eruptions of various types* appear as isolated reactions or accompany the fever. Among the hematological abnormalities that have been observed are *leukopenia, agranulocytosis, eosinophilia, lymphocytosis,* an atypical mononucleosis syndrome, and *thrombocytopenia. Acute hemolytic anemia* may appear in some instances.

Therapeutic Status. The importance of aminosalicylic acid in the management of pulmonary and other forms of tuberculosis has markedly decreased since more active agents, especially rifampin and ethambutol, have been developed (*see* discussion of chemotherapy of tuberculosis, below).

CYCLOSERINE

Cycloserine is a broad-spectrum antibiotic produced by *Streptomyces orchidaceus.* It was first isolated from a fermentation brew in 1955 and was later synthesized.

Chemistry. Cycloserine is D-4-amino-3-isoxazolidone; the structural formula is as follows:

Cycloserine

The drug is stable in alkaline solution but is rapidly destroyed when exposed to neutral or acidic pH.

Antibacterial Activity and Mechanism of Action. Cycloserine is inhibitory for *M. tuberculosis* in concentrations of 5 to 20 μg/ml *in vitro*. There is no cross-resistance between cycloserine and other tuberculostatic agents. While the antibiotic is effective in experimental infections caused by other microorganisms, studies *in vitro* reveal no suppression of growth in cultures made in conventional media. Hoeprich (1963) determined that this is due to the presence of D-alanine in the commonly used culture media and that the amino acid blocks the antibacterial activity of cycloserine. The two compounds are structural analogs, and cycloserine inhibits reactions in which D-alanine is involved in bacterial cell-wall synthesis (*see* Chapter 50). The use of media free of D-alanine reveals that the antibiotic inhibits the growth *in vitro* of enterococci, paracolon strains, *E. coli, Staph. aureus, Nocardia* species, and *Chlamydia.*

Absorption, Distribution, and Excretion. When given orally, cycloserine is rapidly absorbed. Peak concentrations in plasma are reached 3 to 4 hours after a single dose and are in the range of 20 to 35 μg/ml in children who receive 20 mg/kg; only small quantities are present after 12 hours. In adults, doses of 750 mg, given at 6-hour intervals, produce plasma concentrations in excess of 50 μg/ml (*see* Storey and McLean, 1957). Multiple doses lead to accumulation of the drug in the circulation after 3 days.

Cycloserine is distributed throughout body fluids and tissues. There is no appreciable blood-brain barrier to the drug, and cerebrospinal fluid concentrations in all patients are approximately the same as those in plasma.

About 50% of a parenteral dose of cycloserine is excreted, in unchanged form, in the urine in the first 12 hours; a total of 65% is recoverable in the active form over a period of 72 hours. Approximately 35% of the antibiotic is metabolized to an as-yet-unidentified substance. The drug may accumulate to toxic concentrations in patients with renal insufficiency; it may be removed from the circulation by dialysis.

Preparations, Routes of Administration, and Dosage. *Cycloserine,* U.S.P. (SEROMYCIN), is available in official capsules containing 250 mg for oral administration. The usual dose for adults is 250 mg twice a day; this is associated with a small risk of toxic reactions. In more severely ill individuals, 500 mg may be given twice a day for short periods. The dose should be adjusted to yield plasma concentrations no greater than 30 μg/ml in order to minimize toxicity.

Untoward Effects. Reactions to cycloserine most commonly involve the central nervous system (CNS). They tend to appear within the first 2 weeks of therapy and usually disappear when the drug is withdrawn. Among the *central manifestations* are somnolence, headache, tremor, dysarthria, vertigo, confusion, nervousness, irritability, psychotic states with suicidal tendencies, paranoid reactions, catatonic and depressed reactions, twitching, ankle clonus, hyperreflexia, visual disturbances, paresis, and grand mal or absence seizures. Large doses of cycloserine or the ingestion of ethyl alcohol increases the risk of seizures. Cycloserine is contraindicated in individuals with a history of epilepsy and may be dangerous in persons who are depressed or are experiencing severe anxiety.

Therapeutic Status. Cycloserine should be reserved for those cases in which safer and more effective agents are interdicted either because of a history of clinically significant reactions or because of resistance of the responsible strain of tubercle bacillus. When cycloserine is employed to treat tuberculosis, it must be given together with other effective agents.

VIOMYCIN

Source, Chemistry, and Antimicrobial Activity. Viomycin is a strongly basic, complex antibiotic produced by an actinomycete. It is a cyclic peptide with a structure that is very similar to that of capreomycin. Viomycin is most active *in vitro* against *M. tuberculosis.* Practically all strains of this microorganism are inhibited by drug concentrations of 1 to 10 μg/ml. Mycobacteria insensitive to kanamycin are also resistant to viomycin *in vitro.* On the other hand, viomycin-resistant strains may retain their sensitivity to kanamycin. Viomycin inhibits protein synthesis by *M. tuberculosis.*

Absorption, Distribution, and Excretion. The absorption and the excretion of viomycin in man are similar to those of streptomycin. Absorption from the gastrointestinal tract is limited. The intramuscular injection of 25 to 50 mg/kg produces maximal plasma concentrations in 2 hours. A large proportion of a dose of the drug is recoverable in the urine. Penetration into cerebrospinal fluid is poor.

Preparations, Routes of Administration, and Dosage. The usual dose of viomycin is two injections of 1 g each, 12 hours apart, not more often than twice weekly. Viomycin is not available commercially in the United States at the present time.

Untoward Effects. The incidence of untoward effects produced by viomycin is higher than that which follows the administration of streptomycin. *Allergic reactions* include eosinophilia and urticarial, erythematous, or pruritic skin rashes. The most important toxic manifestations involve the *kidney* and *labyrinth.* Patients receiving the drug over extended periods almost invariably exhibit proteinuria, cylindruria, hematuria, and pyuria; these abnormalities most often appear within 2 weeks of initiation of therapy. Nitrogen retention and serious disturbances in electrolyte balance have been observed in a number of instances. Renal function usually recovers quite rapidly when treatment is stopped. *Impairment of vestibular function* is quite common and more frequent than with streptomycin. Partial deafness is also a risk. These usually become manifest within a month or more after the institution of viomycin therapy.

OTHER DRUGS

The agents grouped in this section are similar in several aspects. They are all drugs of second or third choice that are used only for therapy of disease caused by resistant microorganisms or by atypical mycobacteria. They all must be given by intramuscular injection, and they have similar pharmacokinetics and toxicity. Since these agents are potentially ototoxic and nephrotoxic, two drugs in this group should not be used simultaneously, and they should not be used in combination with streptomycin.

Kanamycin, an aminoglycoside that is discussed in detail in Chapter 51, inhibits the growth of *M. tuberculosis in vitro* in a concentration of 10 μg/ml or less. Small groups of patients with tuberculosis have been treated with 1 g of kanamycin daily, and a slight therapeutic effect has been observed; toxic effects have been common.

Amikacin is also an aminoglycoside (*see* Chapter 51). It is extremely active against several mycobacterial species and may become an important drug for treatment of disease caused by atypical mycobacteria (*see* Sanders *et al.,* 1976; Dalovisio and Pankey, 1978).

Capreomycin is an antimycobacterial cyclic peptide elaborated by *Streptomyces capreolus*. It consists of four active components—capreomycins IA, IB, IIA, and IIB—the structures of which have largely been elucidated by Bycroft and associates (1971). Capreomycin and viomycin are members of a closely related family of antibiotics; their chemical and pharmacological properties are similar. The agent used clinically contains primarily IA and IB; the other fractions make up only 10% of the drug. The drug is effective both *in vitro* and in experimental tuberculosis (Wilson, 1967). Bacterial resistance to capreomycin develops when it is given alone; such microorganisms show cross-resistance with kanamycin and viomycin (Tsukamura *et al.,* 1967).

Capreomycin must be given intramuscularly. The recommended daily dose is 20 mg/kg or 1 g for 60 to 120 days, followed by 1 g two to three times a week. Capreomycin should be administered together with another effective tuberculostatic agent. It has proven of value in the therapy of "resistant," or treatment-failure, tuberculosis when given with ethambutol or isoniazid (Wilson, 1967; Donomae, 1968). *Sterile Capreomycin Sulfate,* U.S.P. (capastat), is supplied in ampuls containing 1 g of the drug for solution in 2 ml of sodium chloride injection or sterile water.

The reactions associated with the use of capreomycin are hearing loss, tinnitus, transient proteinuria, cylindruria, and nitrogen retention. Severe renal failure is rare. These effects are similar to those described for viomycin (*see* above). Eosinophilia is common. Leukocytosis, leukopenia, rashes, and fever have also been observed. Injections of the drug may be painful.

CHEMOTHERAPY OF TUBERCULOSIS

The availability of effective tuberculostatic agents has so altered the treatment of tuberculosis that the need for sanatorium care has been strikingly reduced. Patients with tuberculosis are now being admitted to general hospitals. After a period sufficient to establish the diagnosis and to initiate and stabilize therapy, patients may, with uncommon exception, be returned to their homes. Prolonged bed rest is not necessary or even helpful in speeding recovery. Arrangements must be made to minimize the risk of exposure of contacts, especially children, in the home. The patients must be seen at frequent

intervals to follow the course of their disease and treatment.

The vast majority of previously untreated tuberculosis in the United States is caused by microorganisms that are sensitive to isoniazid, rifampin, ethambutol, and streptomycin. To prevent the development of resistance to these agents that frequently occurs *during* the course of therapy of the individual patient, *treatment must include at least two drugs to which the bacteria are sensitive* (*see* Chapter 48, page 1099). Isoniazid should be included in such a regimen if at all possible, and rifampin should be used if isoniazid cannot be given. The combination of isoniazid and rifampin is probably the most effective treatment available. However, in life-threatening disease, large cavitary disease, or renal tuberculosis, three drugs should be used initially to be certain that the mycobacteria are sensitive to at least two of them (*see* Bailey *et al.,* 1977).

Therapy of Specific Types of Tuberculosis. The usual therapy of *pulmonary tuberculosis* consists of isoniazid, 5 mg/kg (up to 300 mg per day), plus ethambutol (15 mg/kg). Pyridoxine, 10 mg per day, should also be included for most adults. The microorganisms should be cultured for the determination of their sensitivity to antimicrobial agents, but results will not be available for several weeks. For more severe disease, the combination of isoniazid and rifampin (600 mg per day) is preferred. Many authorities prefer, in such cases, to add a third drug to assure that the tubercle bacilli are sensitive to at least two drugs until this can be determined. The third agent may be either ethambutol or streptomycin (1 g daily). The dosage of streptomycin is reduced to 1 g twice weekly after 2 months. *Chemotherapy must be continued for 18 months to 2 years.* Treatment of shorter duration (minimum of 9 months) may be effective when both isoniazid and rifampin are used (American Thoracic Society, 1980). Surgery is rarely indicated.

Clinical improvement is readily discernible in the vast majority of patients with pulmonary tuberculosis if the treatment is appropriate. Efficacy usually becomes obvious within the first 2 weeks of therapy and is evidenced by a reduction of fever, decrease in cough, gain in weight, and increase in the sense of well-being. There is also progressive roentgenographic improvement. Over 90% of patients who receive optimal treatment will have negative cultures within 3 to 6 months, depending on the severity of the disease. Cultures that remain positive after 6 months frequently yield resistant microorganisms; the value of using an alternative therapeutic program should then be considered.

Disseminated tuberculosis, including tuberculous meningitis and cases with renal, bone, or joint involvement, is treated initially with isoniazid and rifampin plus either ethambutol or streptomycin. While some clinicians increase the dose of isoniazid to 10 mg/kg in these conditions, this is not of proven benefit. When the microorganisms are found to be susceptible to both isoniazid and rifampin, the third drug may be discontinued.

Failure of chemotherapy may be due to (1) irregular or inadequate therapy (resulting in persistent or resistant mycobacteria) due to poor patient compliance during the protracted therapeutic regimen; (2) the use of a single drug, with interruption necessitated by toxicity or hypersensitivity; (3) an inadequate initial regimen; or (4) the primary resistance of the microorganism.

Problems in Chemotherapy. *Bacterial Resistance to Drugs.* One of the more important problems in the chemotherapy of tuberculosis is bacterial resistance. For this reason concurrent administration of two or more drugs should be employed in the treatment of all active tuberculous disease.

A spate of publications has appeared on the incidence of resistance of bacilli isolated from untreated patients. Results depend on the population studied (*e.g.*, patients in Veterans Administration hospitals harbor more resistant microorganisms than do those in the United States as a whole), geographical location, and ethnic and socioeconomic factors. Most observers believe that the frequency of bacterial resistance is presently not rising at a rate such that the effectiveness of programs of concurrent drug therapy is threatened. However, *the physician must obtain sensitivity data at the beginning of therapy to assure the selection of a proper combination of drugs.* Disease caused by strains of *M. tuberculosis* that are found to be resistant to the drugs being used should be treated with two or three drugs to which the microorganisms are known to be susceptible.

Where drug resistance is suspected but sensitivities are not yet known (such as in patients who have undergone several courses of treatment), therapy should be instituted with five or six drugs, including two or three that the patient has not received in the past. Such a program might include isoniazid, rifampin, ethambutol, streptomycin, pyrazinamide, and ethionamide. Some physicians include isoniazid in the therapeutic regimen even if microorganisms are resistant because of some evidence that disease with isoniazid-resistant mycobacteria does not "progress" during such therapy. Others prefer to discontinue isoniazid to lessen the possibility of toxicity. Therapy should be continued for at least 24 months.

Atypical Mycobacteria. These microorganisms have been recovered from a variety of lesions in man. Because they are frequently resistant to many of the commonly used tuberculostatic agents, they must be examined for sensitivity *in vitro* and drug therapy selected on this basis. In some instances, surgical removal of the infected tissue followed by long-term treatment with effective agents is necessary.

Mycobacterium kansasii causes disease similar to that caused by *M. tuberculosis* but it may be milder.

The microorganisms are often resistant to isoniazid. Therapy with isoniazid, rifampin, and ethambutol has been successful (Davidson, 1976; Nicholson, 1976). *Mycobacterium avium-intracellulare* complex (also known as Battey bacillus) may cause a disease with symptoms that resemble chronic bronchitis. Cavities are found in the lung in most patients. The microorganisms are often highly resistant to drugs *in vitro*. Therapy with isoniazid, rifampin, streptomycin, ethambutol, and cycloserine has been successful (*see* Yaeger, 1979). *Mycobacterium marinum* causes skin lesions. A combination of rifampin and ethambutol is probably effective; minocycline (Loria, 1976) or tetracycline is active *in vitro* and is used by some physicians (Izumi *et al.,* 1977). *Mycobacterium scrofulaceum* causes cervical lymphadenitis, especially in children. Surgical excision still seems to be the therapy of choice (Lincoln and Gilberg, 1972). Microbes of the *M. fortuitum* complex (including *M. chelonei*) are usually saprophytes, but they may cause chronic lung disease and infections of skin and soft tissues. The microorganisms are highly resistant to most drugs, but amikacin and tetracyclines are active *in vitro* (Brosbe *et al.,* 1964; Sanders *et al.,* 1977; Dalovisio and Pankey, 1978).

Chemoprophylaxis of Tuberculosis. Prophylactic therapy can effectively prevent the development of active tuberculosis in certain instances (*see* Farer, 1979). There are three categories of patients for whom prophylactic therapy should be considered: those exposed to tuberculosis but who have no evidence of infection; those with infection (positive tuberculin test; more than 5 mm of induration to 5 units of PPD) and no apparent disease; and those with a history of tuberculosis but in whom the disease is presently "inactive" (*see* Public Health Service, 1974; Edwards, 1977; Snider and Farer, 1978).

Household contacts and other close associates of patients with tuberculosis who have negative tuberculin tests should receive isoniazid for at least 3 months after the contact has been broken. This is especially important for children. If the tuberculin skin test becomes positive, therapy should be modified accordingly.

Persons without apparent disease whose skin test has converted from negative to positive within the preceding 2 years should receive isoniazid for 12 months. These patients are considered to be "infected" but not to have clinical disease. Those with positive skin tests, no matter when they became so, who are under 35 years of age or who are at risk of infection because of such factors as immunosuppressive therapy, leukemia, lymphoma, or silicosis should receive isoniazid for 1 year.

Patients with old "inactive" tuberculosis who have not received adequate chemotherapy in the past should be considered for 1 year of treatment with isoniazid (*see* Bailey *et al.,* 1977).

Prophylaxis with isoniazid is contraindicated for patients who have hepatic disease or who have had reactions to the drug. There are insufficient data on the advisability of prophylaxis with alternative drugs, such as rifampin. In pregnant women, prophylaxis should be delayed until after delivery

(Public Health Service, 1974). For prophylaxis, isoniazid is generally given to adults in a daily dose of
300 mg. Children should receive 10 mg/kg to a maximal daily dose of 300 mg.

II. Drugs for Leprosy

Although leprosy is rarely seen in the
United States, it is estimated that there are
12 million patients with this disease worldwide (WHO, 1977b). Most patients can be
managed outside of hospitals because of the
development of effective chemotherapy for
leprosy.

SULFONES

The sulfones, as a class, are derivatives of 4,4'-
diaminodiphenylsulfone (dapsone, DDS), all of
which have certain pharmacological properties in
common. They are discussed here as a class; only the
two members that have official status in the United
States, *dapsone* and *sulfoxone,* will be considered
individually.

History. The sulfones first attracted interest because of their chemical relationship to the sulfonamides. Dapsone was found in 1937 to be 30 times
more active and only 15 times as toxic as sulfanilamide when used in streptococcal infections in mice.
At that time, the drug was considered too toxic for
administration to man, and attempts were initiated
to find a compound with a better therapeutic index.
None of the sulfones that have since been synthesized has proven of value in the therapy of the
common acute bacterial infections. However, when
Rist and associates (1940) and Feldman and coworkers (1941) noted that dapsone and glucosulfone
(PROMIN), a derivative of dapsone, were effective in
suppressing experimental infections with the tubercle bacillus, attention was attracted to the potential
value of these agents in the treatment of human
tuberculosis. Although dapsone and some of its
congeners eventually proved to be of very limited
usefulness in this disease, the interest stimulated by
the observations that a drug exerted a marked effect
on experimental tuberculosis led to the demonstration that glucosulfone exerted a favorable effect in
rat leprosy (Cowdry and Ruangsiri, 1941). This was
soon followed by successful clinical trials of this agent
in human leprosy. The sulfones are presently the
most important drugs for the treatment of this disease.

Chemistry. All the sulfones of clinical value are
derivatives of dapsone. Despite the study and development of a large variety of sulfones, this drug
remains the agent most useful clinically. The structures of dapsone and sulfoxone sodium are as follows:

Dapsone

Sulfoxone Sodium

Antibacterial Activity. The sulfones are bacteriostatic, not bactericidal, *in vitro* for the tubercle bacillus. Dapsone suppresses the growth of pathogenic
strains of this microorganism in a concentration of
about 10 μg/ml. The tubercle bacillus does not develop resistance to the drug *in vitro*. Because *Mycobacterium leprae* does not grow on artificial media,
conventional methods cannot be applied to determine its susceptibility to potential therapeutic agents
in vitro.

The *in-vivo* activity of dapsone in patients with
leprosy has been studied by Shepard and coworkers
(1968). Using the technic of footpad inoculation in
the mouse as an index, they noted that therapy with
this agent for 28 days reduced the degree of infect-
iousness of leprous material from nasal washings and
skin to about 10% of that present before treatment.
After 90 days, there were so few *M. leprae* left that
they were barely detectable. The drug is bacteriostatic, but not bactericidal, for *M. leprae,* and the
estimated sensitivity to dapsone is between 1 and
10 ng/ml for microorganisms recovered from untreated patients (Shepard *et al.,* 1969; Gelber *et al.,*
1971). *Mycobacterium leprae* may become resistant to
the drug during therapy.

The mechanism of action of the sulfones is probably similar to that of the sulfonamides since both
possess approximately the same range of antibacterial activity and both are antagonized by para-aminobenzoic acid.

Untoward Effects. The reactions induced by various sulfones are very similar. The most common
untoward effect is *hemolysis* of varying degree. This
develops in almost every individual treated with 200
to 300 mg of dapsone per day. Doses of 100 mg or
less in normal healthy persons and 50 mg or less in
healthy individuals with a glucose-6-phosphate dehydrogenase deficiency do not cause hemolysis
(DeGowin, 1967). *Methemoglobinemia* is also common, and Heinz-body formation may occur. While
diminished red-cell survival usually occurs during
the use of sulfones, and is presumed to be a dose-
related effect of their oxidizing activity, *hemolytic
anemia* is unusual unless there is a disorder either of
the erythrocytes or of the bone marrow (Pengelly,
1963). The hemolysis may be so severe that manifestations of hypoxia become striking.

Anorexia, nausea, and *vomiting* may follow the
oral administration of sulfones. Isolated instances of
*headache, nervousness, insomnia, blurred vision, par-
esthesia, reversible peripheral neuropathy* (thought to
be due to axonal degeneration), *drug fever, hema-*

turia, pruritus, psychosis, and a variety of *skin rashes* have been reported (Rapoport and Guss, 1972). An *infectious mononucleosis–like syndrome,* which may be fatal, occurs occasionally (Leiker, 1956). The sulfones may induce an *exacerbation of lepromatous leprosy;* this is thought to be analogous to the Jarisch-Herxheimer reaction. This "sulfone syndrome" may develop 5 to 6 weeks after initiation of treatment in malnourished people. Its manifestations include fever, malaise, exfoliative dermatitis, jaundice with hepatic necrosis, lymphadenopathy, methemoglobinemia, and anemia (DeGowin, 1967).

The sulfones may be given safely for many years in doses adequate for the successful therapy of leprosy if proper precautions are observed. Treatment should be initiated with a small dose and the quantity then increased gradually. Patients must be under consistent and prolonged laboratory and clinical supervision. The reactions induced by the sulfones, especially those related to exacerbation of the leprosy, may be very severe and demand the cessation of treatment as well as the institution of specific measures to reduce the threat to life.

Absorption, Distribution, and Excretion. Dapsone is slowly and nearly completely absorbed from the gastrointestinal tract. The disubstituted sulfones, such as sulfoxone, are incompletely absorbed when administered orally, and large amounts are excreted in the feces. Peak concentrations of dapsone in plasma are reached in 1 to 3 hours after administration, and its half-life of elimination ranges from 10 to 50 hours, with a mean of 28 hours. Twenty-four hours after oral ingestion of 100 mg, plasma concentrations range from 0.4 to 1.2 μg/ml (Shepard *et al.,* 1976), and a dose of 100 mg of dapsone per day produces an average of 2 μg of "free" dapsone per gram of blood or nonhepatic tissue. About 50% of the drug is bound to plasma protein (Riley and Levy, 1973). Concentrations in plasma following conventional doses of sulfoxone sodium are 10 to 15μg/ml. These values fall relatively rapidly; however, appreciable quantities are still present at 8 hours.

The sulfones are distributed throughout the total body water and are present in all tissues. They tend to be retained in skin and muscle, and especially in liver and kidney; traces of the drug are present in these organs up to 3 weeks after therapy is stopped. The sulfones are retained in the circulation for a long time because of intestinal reabsorption from the bile; periodic interruption of treatment is advisable for this reason. Dapsone is acetylated in the liver, and the degree of acetylation is genetically determined.

The urinary excretion of sulfones varies with the type of drug; about 70 to 80% of a dose of dapsone is so excreted. The drug is present in urine as an acid-labile mono-N-glucuronide and mono-N-sulfamate in addition to an unknown number of unidentified metabolites (Shepard, 1969). Probenecid decreases the urinary excretion of the acid-labile dapsone metabolites significantly and that of free dapsone to a lesser extent (Goodwin and Sparell, 1969).

Preparations, Routes of Administration, and Dosage. *Dapsone,* U.S.P. (*DDS;* AVLOSULFON), is available in tablets containing 25 or 100 mg. It is given primarily by the oral route. Several dosage schedules have been recommended (*see* Trautman, 1965; Browne, 1967; Bullock, 1979). Daily therapy with 50 mg has been successful in adults. If the clinical response is not adequate, the daily dose may be increased to 100 mg. Doses of 100 to 400 mg twice weekly have also been effective. Therapy is usually begun with smaller amounts, and dosage is increased to those recommended by 1 to 2 months. Therapy should be continued for at least 2 years and may be necessary for the lifetime of the patient (*see* below).

Sulfoxone Sodium, U.S.P. (DIASONE SODIUM), may be substituted for dapsone in patients in whom the latter drug produces sufficient gastric distress to impede effective therapy. It is available for oral administration as enteric-coated tablets containing 330 mg. The maximal dose is 660 mg daily.

The use of sulfones in *malaria* resistant to the usual antimalarial drugs is discussed in Chapter 45.

RIFAMPIN

This antibiotic has been discussed above with regard to its use in tuberculosis. Rifampin may be used as a companion drug to dapsone for certain patients with leprosy (Peters *et al.,* 1978). Rifampin can rapidly sterilize mouse footpads infected with *M. leprae* and thus appears to be bactericidal (Holmes *et al.,* 1976). However, despite its ability to penetrate cells and nerves (Allen *et al.,* 1975), viable drug-sensitive *M. leprae* may persist after prolonged therapy with rifampin (Rees *et al.,* 1976). There are presently no clinical data to support the superiority of combination therapy with rifampin and dapsone over that with dapsone alone for the treatment of leprosy.

CLOFAZIMINE

Clofazimine is a phenazine congener that is used in patients infected with *M. leprae* that are resistant to the sulfones (Shepard, 1969). Its structural formula is as follows:

Clofazimine

Clofazimine may inhibit the template function of DNA by binding to it (Morrison and Marley, 1976). The drug also exerts an anti-inflammatory effect and prevents the development of erythema nodosum leprosum (Browne, 1967). There is growing evidence that persistent and established exacerbations in lepromatous leprosy are improved and cured by *clofaz-*

imine. This compound is also useful for therapy of chronic skin ulcers (Buruli ulcer) produced by *M. ulcerans.*

The drug is absorbed by the oral route and appears to accumulate in tissues. This makes possible discontinuous therapy with individual doses separated by 2 or more weeks. Human leprosy from which dapsone-resistant bacilli have been recovered has been treated with clofazimine with good results. However, unlike dapsone-sensitive microorganisms in which killing occurs immediately after dapsone is administered, dapsone-resistant strains do not exhibit appreciable effect until 50 days after therapy with clofazimine has been initiated. The dose of clofazimine is 100 to 300 mg; the optimal interval between doses in man remains to be determined, but 100 mg twice weekly is effective. (*See* Convit *et al.,* 1970; Shepard *et al.,* 1971a, 1971b; Levy *et al.,* 1972.) Patients treated with clofazimine may develop red discoloration of the skin; this may be very distressing to light-skinned individuals (Levy and Randall, 1970). Eosinophilic enteritis has also been described as an adverse reaction to the drug (Mason *et al.,* 1977).

Clofazimine (LAMPRENE) is supplied in capsules containing 100 mg and is available only from the National Leprosarium, United States Public Health Service Hospital, Carville, Louisiana, 70721.

AMITHIOZONE

The tuberculostatic activity of thiosemicarbazones and related drugs was first observed by Domagk and coworkers (1946). Study of structure-activity relationship suggested that 4-acetylamino benzaldehyde thiosemicarbazone (amithiozone) was the most promising of these compounds. The structural formula of amithiozone is as follows:

$$H_3C-\underset{\underset{O}{\|}}{C}-NH-\langle C_6H_4\rangle-CH{=}N-NH-\underset{\underset{S}{\|}}{C}-NH_2$$

Amithiozone

Lowe (1954) was the first to discover the effectiveness of amithiozone in leprosy. It appears to exert a greater effect on the tuberculoid than on the lepromatous form of the disease. *Mycobacterium leprae* tends to become resistant to this agent as treatment is continued, as evidenced by a slower rate of improvement in the second year of therapy and the occurrence of relapse in the third year. It has been suggested that amithiozone can be substituted for the sulfones when the latter, for some reason, cannot be administered.

The most common untoward effects of the thiosemicarbazones and derivatives are *anorexia, nausea,* and *vomiting.* The drugs may *depress bone-marrow function.* Some degree of *anemia* is observed in a large percentage of patients receiving amithiozone. *Leukopenia* and *agranulocytosis* occur; the incidence of serious reactions involving the leukocytes is about 0.5%. *Acute hemolytic anemia* may develop when high doses are administered. *Skin rashes* are not infrequent; they may be of any type, but exfoliative dermatitis has not yet been noted. Although mild *albuminuria* has been observed, the drugs are not regarded as nephrotoxic. The fairly high incidence of *jaundice* in patients receiving amithiozone suggests that it is hepatotoxic; the effect on the liver disappears when treatment is stopped.

Amithiozone (*thiacetazone;* PANRONE, TIBIONE) is well absorbed from the gastrointestinal tract, and large amounts are excreted in the urine (Robson and Sullivan, 1963). The initial dose is 50 mg per day for 1 to 2 weeks, after which the daily quantity is gradually increased to a maximum of 200 mg. The drug appears to be as effective when given in a single dose each day as when the daily dose is divided. Amithiozone is also administered daily (150 mg) or twice weekly (450 mg per dose) in underdeveloped countries for treatment of tuberculosis caused by mycobacteria that are resistant to more effective drugs. The drug is not available in the United States.

MISCELLANEOUS AGENTS

The efficacy of a great many agents in the therapy of leprosy has been investigated (*see* International Congress on Leprology, 1963). Browne (1967) has reported considerable enthusiasm for the use of long-acting sulfonamides in this disease in South America and certain areas of Africa. Derivatives of diphenylthiourea such as thiambutosine have also attracted interest. However, exacerbations of the disease have occurred, presumably due to resistance to this agent.

Thalidomide seems to be effective for the treatment of *erythema nodosum leprosum* (Iyer *et al.,* 1971). Doses of 100 to 300 mg per day have been effective. The marked teratogenicity of thalidomide limits its use; it is not available in the United States.

CHEMOTHERAPY OF LEPROSY

Few physicians, other than specialists in the field, are called upon to treat leprosy. Consultation is available with physicians at the National Leprosarium, United States Public Health Service Hospital, Carville, Louisiana, 70721. Therefore, the following discussion will serve mainly to familiarize the reader with the progress that has been made in the treatment of this chronic bacterial disease that has proven very resistant to chemotherapy.

Five clinical types of leprosy are recognized (*see* Ridley and Jopling, 1966). At one end of the spectrum is *tuberculoid leprosy.* This form of the disease is characterized by skin macules with clear centers and well-defined margins; these are invariably anesthetic. *Mycobacterium leprae* is rarely found in smears made from quiescent lesions, but may appear during activity. Virchow cells are not demonstrable. Noncaseating foci with giant cells of the Langhans variety are present. The patient's cell-mediated immune responses are normal, and the lepromin test (intradermal injection of a suspension of heat-killed, bacillus-laden tissue) is invariably positive. The disease is characterized by prolonged remissions with periodic reactivation. At the other end of the spectrum is the widely disseminated *lepromatous* form of the disease. These patients have markedly impaired cell-mediated immunity and are frequently anergic; the lepromin test causes no reaction. *Lepromatous disease* is characterized by diffuse or ill-defined localized infiltration of the skin, which becomes thickened, glossy, and corrugated; areas of decreased sensation may appear. *Mycobacterium leprae* is demonstrable in smears, and granulomas containing bacteria-laden histiocytes (Virchow cells) are present. As the disease progresses, large nerve trunks are involved and anesthesia, atrophy of skin and muscle, absorption of small bones, ulceration, and spontaneous amputations may occur. Three intermediate forms of the disease are recognized: borderline tuberculoid disease, borderline lepromatous disease, and borderline disease.

Patients with tuberculoid leprosy may develop "reversal reactions," which are manifestations of delayed hypersensitivity to antigens of *M. leprae*. Cutaneous ulcerations and deficits of peripheral nerve function may occur. Early therapy with corticosteroids or clofazimine is effective.

Reactions in the lepromatous form of the disease (*erythema nodosum leprosum*) are characterized by the appearance of raised, tender, intracutaneous nodules, severe constitutional symptoms, and high fever. This reaction may be triggered by several conditions but is often associated with therapy. It is thought to be an arthus-type reaction related to release of microbial antigens in patients harboring large numbers of bacilli. Treatment with thalidomide or clofazimine is effective.

The outlook for persons with leprosy has been remarkably altered by successful chemotherapy, surgical procedures that help to restore function and repair disfigurement, and a striking change in the attitude of the public toward patients who have this infection. The social stigma based on ignorance and Biblical castigation of individuals with this affliction is gradually being replaced by the attitude that considers leprosy a disease and not a social stigma. Patients with leprosy can be classified as "infectious" or "noninfectious" on the basis of the type, duration, and effects of therapy. Thus, even "infectious" patients may be discharged from leprosaria, provided adequate medical supervision and therapy are maintained, the home environment meets specific conditions, and the local health officer concurs in the disposition of the case.

Therapy, when effective, heals ulcers and mucosal lesions in months. Cutaneous nodules respond more slowly, and it may take years to eradicate bacteria from mucous membranes, skin, and nerves. The degree of residual pigmentation or depigmentation, atrophy, and scarring depends upon the extent of the initial involvement. Severe ocular lesions show little response to the sulfones. If treatment is initiated before ocular disease is evident, it may be prevented. Keratoconjunctivitis and corneal ulceration may be secondary to nerve involvement. Patients with disease caused by relatively few microorganisms may be treated with dapsone alone for 2 to 4 years. Many patients with tuberculoid and borderline tuberculoid disease fall into this category. All other patients should probably be treated for much longer periods

(10 years to life); this includes those with lepromatous, borderline lepromatous, and borderline disease. Some authorities feel that two drugs should be used initially in such patients to minimize the development of resistance. Clofazimine or rifampin is the agent usually chosen to be given in combination with dapsone. A reasonable program would include dapsone and rifampin for 3 months to 1 year followed by dapsone alone for 10 years to life (Leiker, 1975; Languillon *et al.*, 1979).

Albert, R. K.; Lakshminarayan, S.; and Miller, W. T. Long-term therapy with rifampin and the secondary antibody response to killed influenza vaccine. *Am. Rev. Respir. Dis.*, **1978**, *117*, 605–607.
Allen, B. W.; Ellard, G. A.; Gammon, P. T.; King, R. C.; McDougall, A. C.; Rees, R. J. W.; and Wedell, A. G. M. The penetration of dapsone, rifampicin, isoniazid and pyrazinamide into peripheral nerves. *Br. J. Pharmacol.*, **1975**, *55*, 151–155.
American Thoracic Society. Guidelines for short-course tuberculosis chemotherapy. *Am. Rev. Respir. Dis.*, **1980**, *121*, 611–614.
Arroyo, J.; Medoff, G.; and Kobayashi, G. S. Therapy of murine aspergillosis with amphotericin B in combination with rifampin or 5-fluorocytosine. *Antimicrob. Agents Chemother.*, **1977**, *11*, 21–25.
Atlas, E., and Turck, M. Laboratory and clinical evaluation of rifampicin. *Am. J. Med. Sci.*, **1968**, *256*, 247–254.
Bailey, W. C.; Weill, H.; DeRouen, T. A.; Ziskind, M. M.; Jackson, H. A.; and Greenberg, H. B. The effect of isoniazid on transaminase levels. *Ann. Intern. Med.*, **1974**, *81*, 200–202.
Bassi, L.; DiBerardino, L.; Arioli, V.; Silvestri, L. G.; and Cherie Ligniere, E. L. Conditions for immunosuppression by rifampicin. *J. Infect. Dis.*, **1973**, *128*, 736–744.
Beggs, W. H., and Ayran, N. F. Uptake and binding of ^{14}C-ethambutol by tubercle bacilli and the relation of binding to growth inhibition. *Antimicrob. Agents Chemother.*, **1972**, *2*, 390–394.
Bieder, A.; Brunel, P.; and Mazeau, L. Identification de trois nouveaux métabolites de l'ethionamide: chromatographie, spectrophotométrie, polarographie. *Ann. Pharm. Fr.*, **1966**, *24*, 493–500.
Bobrowitz, I. D. Ethambutol compared to streptomycin in original treatment of advanced pulmonary tuberculosis. *Chest*, **1971**, *60*, 14–21.
———. Ethambutol-isoniazid versus streptomycin-ethambutol-isoniazid in original treatment of cavitary tuberculosis. *Am. Rev. Respir. Dis.*, **1974**, *109*, 548–553.
Bowersox, D. W.; Winterbauer, R. H.; Stewart, G. L.; Orme, B.; and Barron, E. Isoniazid dosage in patients with renal failure. *N. Engl. J. Med.*, **1973**, *289*, 84–87.
British Thoracic and Tuberculosis Association. Short-course chemotherapy in pulmonary tuberculosis. *Lancet*, **1975**, *1*, 119–124.
Brosbe, E. A.; Sugihara, P. T.; Smith, C. R.; and Hyde, L. Experimental drug studies on *Mycobacterium fortuitum*. *Antimicrob. Agents Chemother.*, **1964**, *4*, 733–736.
Buffington, G. A.; Dominguez, J. H.; Piering, W. F.; Hebert, L. A.; Kouffman, H. M.; and Lemann, J. Interaction of rifampin and glucocorticoids. *J.A.M.A.*, **1976**, *236*, 1958–1960.
Buss, W. C.; Morgan, R.; Guttman, J.; Barela, T.; and Stalter, K. Rifampicin inhibition of protein synthesis in mammalian cells. *Science*, **1978**, *200*, 432–434.
Bycroft, B. W.; Cameron, D.; Croft, L. R.; Hassanali-Walji, A.; Johnson, A. W.; and Webb, T. Total structure of capreomycin IB, a tuberculostatic peptide antibiotic. *Nature*, **1971**, *231*, 301–302.
Cohn, H. D. Clinical studies with a new rifamycin derivative. *J. Clin. Pharmacol.*, **1969**, *9*, 118–125.

Convit, J.; Browne, S. G.; Languillon, J.; Pettit, J. H. S.; Ramanujam, K.; Sagher, F.; Sheskin, J.; deSouza Lima, L.; Tarabini, G.; Tolentino, J. G.; Waters, M. F. R.; Bechelli, L. M.; and Martinez Dominguez, V. Therapy of leprosy. *Bull. WHO,* **1970,** *42,* 667–672.

Cowdry, E. V., and Ruangsiri, C. Influence of PROMIN, starch, and heptaldehyde on experimental leprosy in rats. *Arch. Pathol.,* **1941,** *32,* 632–640.

Dalovisio, J. R., and Pankey, G. A. *In vitro* susceptibility of *Mycobacterium fortuitum* and *Mycobacterium chelonei* to amikacin. *J. Infect. Dis.,* **1978,** *137,* 318–321.

Davidson, P. T. Treatment and long-term follow-up of patients with atypical mycobacterial infections. *Bull. Int. Union Tuberc.,* **1976,** *51,* 257–261.

Davis, W. B., and Weber, M. M. Specificity of isoniazid on growth inhibition and competition for an oxidized nicotinamide adenine dinucleotide regulatory site on the electron transport pathway in *Mycobacterium phlei. Antimicrob. Agents Chemother.,* **1977,** *12,* 213–218.

DeGowin, R. L. A review of the therapeutic and hemolytic effects of dapsone. *Arch. Intern. Med.,* **1967,** *120,* 242–248.

Des Prez, R., and Boone, I. U. Metabolism of C^{14} isoniazid in humans. *Am. Rev. Respir. Dis.,* **1961,** *84,* 42–51.

Devine, L. F.; Johnson, D. P.; Rhode, S. L., III; Hagerman, C. R.; Pierce, W. E.; and Peckinpaugh, R. D. Rifampin—effect of two-day treatment on the meningococcal carrier state and the relationship to the levels of the drug in sera and saliva. *Am. J. Med. Sci.,* **1971,** *26,* 74–83.

di Mauro, D.; Snyder, L.; Marino, P.; Lamberti, A.; Coppo, A.; and Tocchini-Valentini, G. P. Rifampicin sensitivity of the components of DNA-dependent RNA polymerase. *Nature,* **1969,** *222,* 533–537.

Domagk, G.; Behnisch, R.; Mietzsch, F.; and Schmidt, H. Über eine neue, gegen Tuberkelbazillen *in vitro* wirksame Verbindungsklasse. *Naturwissenschaften,* **1946,** *33,* 315.

Donomae, I. The combined use of capreomycin and ethambutol in re-treatment of pulmonary tuberculosis. *Am. Rev. Respir. Dis.,* **1968,** *98,* 699–702.

Doust, J. Y., and Moatamed, F. Arthralgia in pulmonary tuberculosis during chemotherapy. *Dis. Chest,* **1968,** *53,* 62–64.

East African/British Medical Research Councils. Controlled clinical trial of four short-course (6-month) regimens of chemotherapy for treatment of pulmonary tuberculosis. *Lancet,* **1974,** *2,* 237–240.

Edwards, P. Q. Tuberculosis, now and the future: short-term therapy, preventive therapy, and bacillus Calmette-Guerin. *Bull. N.Y. Acad. Med.,* **1977,** *53,* 526–531.

Evans, D. A. P.; Manley, K. A.; and McKusick, V. A. Genetic control of isoniazid metabolism in man. *Br. Med. J.,* **1960,** *2,* 485–491.

Feldman, W. H.; Hinshaw, H. C.; and Moses, H. E. Treatment of experimental tuberculosis with PROMIN (sodium salt of *p,p'*-diamino-diphenyl sulfone-N,N'-dextrose sulfonate): preliminary report. *Proc. Staff Meet. Mayo Clin.,* **1941,** *16,* 118–125.

Flynn, C. T.; Rainford, D. J.; and Hope, E. Acute renal failure and rifampicin: danger of unsuspected intermittent dosage. *Br. Med. J.,* **1974,** *2,* 482.

Fox, H. H. The chemical attack on tuberculosis. *Trans. N.Y. Acad. Sci.,* **1953,** *15,* 234–242.

Furesz, S.; Scott, R.; Pallanza, R.; and Mapelli, E. Rifampicin: a new rifamycin. III. Absorption, distribution, and elimination in man. *Arzneim. Forsch.,* **1967,** *17,* 533–537.

Garibaldi, R. A.; Drusin, R. E.; Ferebee, S. H.; and Gregg, M. B. Isoniazid-associated hepatitis. Report of an outbreak. *Am. Rev. Respir. Dis.,* **1972,** *106,* 357–365.

Gelber, R.; Peters, J. H.; Gordon, G. R.; Glazko, A. J.; and Levy, L. The polymorphic acetylation of dapsone in man. *Clin. Pharmacol. Ther.,* **1971,** *12,* 225–238.

Girling, D. J. Adverse reactions to rifampicin in antituberculosis regimens. *J. Antimicrob. Chemother.,* **1977,** *3,* 115–132.

Good, A. E.; Green, R. A.; and Zarafonetis, C. J. D. Rheumatic symptoms during tuberculosis therapy: a manifestation of isoniazid toxicity. *Ann. Intern. Med.,* **1965,** *63,* 800–807.

Goodwin, C. S., and Sparell, G. Inhibition of dapsone excretion by probenecid. *Lancet,* **1969,** *2,* 884–885.

Graber, C. D.; Jebaily, J.; Galphin, R. L.; and Doering, E. Light chain proteinuria and humoral immunocompetence in tuberculous patients treated with rifampin. *Am. Rev. Respir. Dis.,* **1973,** *107,* 713–717.

Gronhagen-Riska, C.; Hellstrom, P. E.; and Froseth, B. Predisposing factors in hepatitis induced by isoniazid-rifampin treatment of tuberculosis. *Am. Rev. Respir. Dis.,* **1978,** *118,* 461–466.

Gupta, S.; Grieco, M. H.; and Siegel, I. Suppression of t-lymphocyte rosettes by rifampin. *Ann. Intern. Med.,* **1975,** *82,* 484–488.

Hobby, G. L., and Lenert, T. F. Observations on the action of rifampin and ethambutol alone and in combination with other antituberculous drugs. *Am. Rev. Respir. Dis.,* **1972,** *105,* 292–295.

Hoeprich, P. D. Alanine:cycloserine antagonism. II. Significance of phenomenon to therapy with cycloserine. *Arch. Intern. Med.,* **1963,** *112,* 405–414. III. Quantitative aspects and relation to heating of culture media. *J. Lab. Clin. Med.,* **1963,** *62,* 657–662.

Holmes, I. B.; Banerjee, D. K.; and Hilson, G. R. F. Effect of rifampin, clofazimine, and B1912 on the viability of *Mycobacterium leprae* in established mouse footpad infection (39276). *Proc. Soc. Exp. Biol. Med.,* **1976,** *151,* 637–641.

Ivler, D.; Leedom, J. M.; and Mathies, A. W., Jr. *In vitro* susceptibility of *Neisseria meningitidis* to rifampin. In, *Antimicrobial Agents and Chemotherapy—1969.* (Hobby, G. L., ed.) American Society for Microbiology, Bethesda, **1970,** pp. 473–478.

Iyer, C. G. S.; Languillon, J.; and Ramanujam, K. WHO coordinated short-term double-blind trial with thalidomide in the treatment of acute lepra reactions in male lepromatous patients. *Bull. WHO,* **1971,** *45,* 719–732.

Izumi, A. K.; Hanke, E. W.; and Higaki, M. *M. marinum* infections treated with tetracycline. *Arch. Dermatol.,* **1977,** *113,* 1067–1068.

Jenne, J. W., and Beggs, W. H. Correlation of *in vitro* and *in vivo* kinetics with clinical use of isoniazid, ethambutol and rifampin. *Am. Rev. Respir. Dis.,* **1973,** *107,* 1013–1021.

Johnson, J. R.; Turk, T. L.; and MacDonald, F. M. Corticosteroids in pulmonary tuberculosis. III. Indications. *Am. Rev. Respir. Dis.,* **1967,** *96,* 62–73.

Karlson, A. G. The *in vitro* activity of ethambutol (dextro-2-2'-[ethylenediimino]-di-l-butanol) against tubercle bacilli and other microorganisms. *Am. Rev. Respir. Dis.,* **1961,** *84,* 905–906.

Kitahara, M.; Kobayashi, G. S.; and Medoff, G. Enhanced efficacy of amphotericin B and rifampicin combined in treatment of murine histoplasmosis and blastomycosis. *J. Infect. Dis.,* **1976,** *133,* 663–668.

Konno, K.; Oizumo, K.; and Oka, S. Mode of action of rifampin on mycobacteria. II. Biosynthetic studies on the inhibition of ribonucleic acid polymerase of *Mycobacterium bovis* BCG by rifampin and uptake of rifampin-^{14}C by *Mycobacterium phlei. Am. Rev. Respir. Dis.,* **1973,** *107,* 1006–1012.

Kopanoff, D. E.; Kilburn, J. O.; Glassroth, J. L.; Snider, D. E.; Farer, L. S.; and Good, R. C. A continuing survey of tuberculosis primary drug resistance in the United States: March 1975 to November 1977. *Am. Rev. Respir. Dis.,* **1978,** *118,* 835–842.

Kunin, C. M.; Brandt, D.; and Wood, H. Bacteriologic studies of rifampin, a new semisynthetic antibiotic. *J. Infect. Dis.,* **1969,** *119,* 132–137.

Kutt, H.; Winters, W.; and McDowell, F. H. Depression of parahydroxylation of diphenylhydantoin by antituberculosis chemotherapy. *Neurology (Minneap.),* **1966,** *16,* 594–602.

La Du, B. N. Isoniazid and pseudocholinesterase polymorphisms. *Fed. Proc.*, **1972**, *31*, 1276–1285.

Languillon, J.; Yawalkar, S. J.; and McDougall, A. C. Therapeutic effects of adding RIMACTANE (rifampicin) 450 milligrams daily or 1200 milligrams once monthly in a single dose to dapsone 50 milligrams daily in patients with lepromatous leprosy. *Int. J. Lepr.*, **1979**, *47*, 37–43.

Lees, A. W. Ethionamide, 500 mg daily, plus isoniazid, 500 mg or 300 mg daily, in previously untreated patients with pulmonary tuberculosis. *Am. Rev. Respir. Dis.*, **1967**, *95*, 109–111.

Lehmann, J. Para-aminosalicylic acid in treatment of tuberculosis: preliminary communication. *Lancet*, **1946**, *1*, 15–16.

Leiker, D. L. The mononuclear syndrome in leprosy patients treated with sulfones. *Int. J. Lepr.*, **1956**, *24*, 402–405.

Levy, L., and Randall, H. P. A study of skin pigmentation by clofazimine. *Int. J. Lepr.*, **1970**, *38*, 404–416.

Levy, L.; Shepard, C. C.; and Fasal, P. Clofazimine therapy of lepromatous leprosy caused by dapsone-resistant *Mycobacterium leprae*. *Am. J. Trop. Med. Hyg.*, **1972**, *21*, 315–321.

Loria, P. R. Minocycline hydrochloride treatment for atypical acid-fast infection. *Arch. Dermatol.*, **1976**, *112*, 517–519.

Lorian, V., and Finland, M. *In vitro* effect of rifampin on mycobacteria. *Appl. Microbiol.*, **1969**, *17*, 202–207.

Lowe, J. The chemotherapy of leprosy: late results of treatment with sulfone and with thiosemicarbazone. *Lancet*, **1954**, *2*, 1065–1068.

McCabe, W. R., and Lorian, V. Comparison of the antibacterial activity of rifampicin and other antibiotics. *Am. J. Med. Sci.*, **1968**, *256*, 255–265.

McDermott, W.; Ormond, L.; Muschenheim, C.; Deuschle, K.; McCune, R. M.; and Tompsett, R. Pyrazinamide-isoniazid in tuberculosis. *Am. Rev. Tuberc.*, **1954**, *69*, 319–333.

Maddrey, W. C., and Boitnott, J. K. Isoniazid hepatitis. *Ann. Intern. Med.*, **1973**, *79*, 1–12.

Mandell, G. L. Interaction of intraleukocytic bacteria and antibiotics. *J. Clin. Invest.*, **1973**, *52*, 1673–1679.

———. Catalase, superoxide dismutase, and virulence of *Staphylococcus aureus*. *Ibid.*, **1975**, *55*, 561–566.

Mandel, W.; Heaton, A. D.; Russell, W. F.; and Middlebrook, G. Combined drug treatment of tuberculosis. II. Studies of antimicrobially active isoniazid and streptomycin serum levels in adult tuberculous patients. *J. Clin. Invest.*, **1959**, *38*, 1356–1365.

Mason, G. H.; Ellis-Pegler, R. B.; and Arthur, J. F. Clofazimine and eosinophilic enteritis. *Lepr. Rev.*, **1977**, *48*, 175–180.

Mattila, M. J., and Tiitinen, H. The rate of isoniazid inactivation in Finnish diabetic and non-diabetic patients. *Ann. Med. Exp. Biol. Fenn.*, **1967**, *45*, 423–427.

Molavi, A., and Weinstein, L. *In vitro* susceptibility of atypical mycobacteria to rifampin. *Appl. Microbiol.*, **1971**, *22*, 23–25.

Morrison, N. E., and Marley, G. M. Clofazimine binding studies with deoxyribonucleic acid. *Int. J. Lepr.*, **1976**, *44*, 475–481.

Mukerjee, P.; Schuldt, S.; and Kasik, J. E. Effect of rifampin on cutaneous hypersensitivity to purified protein derivatives in humans. *Antimicrob. Agents Chemother.*, **1973**, *4*, 607–611.

Newman, R.; Doster, B. E.; Murray, F. J.; and Woolpert, S. F. Rifampin in initial treatment of pulmonary tuberculosis. *Am. Rev. Respir. Dis.*, **1974**, *109*, 216–232.

Nicholson, D. P. Atypical tuberculosis: features and therapy. *Br. J. Dis. Chest*, **1976**, *70*, 217–218.

O'Reilly, R. A. Interaction of chronic daily warfarin therapy and rifampin. *Ann. Intern. Med.*, **1975**, *83*, 506–508.

Peets, E. A.; Sweeney, W. M.; Place, V. A.; and Buyske, D. A. The absorption, excretion and metabolic fate of ethambutol in man. *Am. Rev. Respir. Dis.*, **1965**, *91*, 51–58.

Pengelly, C. D. R. Dapsone-induced hemolysis. *Br. Med. J.*, **1963**, *2*, 662–664.

Peters, J. H.; Murray, J. F., Jr.; Gordon, F. R.; and Jacobson, R. R. Metabolic-bacteriologic relationships in the chemotherapy of lepromatous patients with dapsone or dapsone-rifampin. *Int. J. Lepr.*, **1978**, *46*, 115–116.

Phillips, S., and Tashman, H. Ethionamide jaundice. *Am. Rev. Respir. Dis.*, **1963**, *87*, 896–898.

Place, V. A., and Thomas, J. P. Clinical pharmacology of ethambutol. *Am. Rev. Respir. Dis.*, **1963**, *87*, 901–904.

Postlethwaite, A. E.; Bartel, A. G.; and Kelley, W. N. Hyperuricemia due to ethambutol. *N. Engl. J. Med.*, **1972**, *286*, 761–762.

Public Health Service, U.S. Department of Health, Education, and Welfare. Isoniazid-associated hepatitis: summary of the report of the Tuberculosis Advisory Committee and special consultants to the Director, Center for Disease Control. *Morbidity and Mortality.* (Weekly report.) **1974**, *23*, No. 11, 97–98.

Pujet, J. C.; Homberg, J. C.; and Decroix, G. Sensitivity to rifampicin: incidence, mechanism, and prevention. *Br. Med. J.*, **1974**, *2*, 415–418.

Radner, D. B. Toxicologic and pharmacologic aspects of rifampin. *Chest*, **1973**, *64*, 213–216.

Rapoport, A. M., and Guss, S. B. Dapsone-induced peripheral neuropathy. *Arch Neurol.*, **1972**, *27*, 184–186.

Rees, R. J. W.; Waters, M. F. R.; Pearson, J. M. H.; Helmy, H. S.; and Laing, A. B. G. Long-term treatment of dapsone-resistant leprosy with rifampin: clinical and bacteriological status. *Int. J. Lepr.*, **1976**, *44*, 159–169.

Riley, R. W., and Levy, L. Characteristics of the binding of dapsone and monoacetyldapsone by serum albumin. *Proc. Soc. Exp. Biol. Med.*, **1973**, *142*, 1168–1170.

Rist, N.; Block, F.; and Hamon, V. Action inhibitrice du sulfamide et d'une sulfone sur la multiplication *in vitro* et *in vivo* du bacilli tuberculeux aviaire. *Ann Inst. Pasteur* (*Paris*), **1940**, *64*, 203–237.

Rist, N.; Grumbach, F.; and Libermann, D. Experiments on the antituberculous activity of alpha-ethyl thioisonicotinamide. *Am. Rev. Tuberc.*, **1959**, *79*, 1–5.

Romankiewicz, J. A., and Ehrman, M. Rifampin and warfarin: a drug interaction. *Ann. Intern. Med.*, **1975**, *82*, 224–225.

Rothfield, N. F.; Bierer, W. F.; and Garfield, J. W. Isoniazid induction of antinuclear antibodies. *Ann. Intern. Med.*, **1978**, *88*, 650–652.

Sanders, W. E., Jr.; Cacciatore, R.; Valdez, H.; Schneider, N.; and Hartwig, C. Activity of amikacin against mycobacteria *in vitro* and in experimental infections with *M. tuberculosis. Am. Rev. Respir. Dis.*, **1976**, *113*, 59.

Sanders, W. E., Jr.; Hartwig, E. C.; Schneider, N. J.; Cacciatore, R.; and Valdez, H. Susceptibility of organisms in the *Mycobacterium fortuitum* complex to antituberculous and other antimicrobial agents. *Antimicrob. Agents Chemother.*, **1977**, *12*, 295–297.

Sbarbaro, J. A.; Barlow, P. B.; Craig, M. W.; Johnston, R. F.; Reagan, W. P.; and Reichman, L. B. Intermittent chemotherapy for adults with tuberculosis. *Am. Rev. Respir. Dis.*, **1974**, *110*, 374–376.

Scheuer, P. J.; Summerfield, J. A.; Lal, S.; and Sherlock, S. Rifampin hepatitis. *Lancet*, **1974**, *1*, 421–425.

Schröder, J. M. Zur Pathogenese der Isoniazid-Neuropathie. 1. Eine feinstrukturelle Differenzierung gegenüber der Wallerschen Degeneration. *Acta Neuropathol.* (*Berl.*), **1970a**, *16*, 301–323.

———. Zur Pathogenese der Isoniazid-Neuropathie. II. Phasenkontrast- und elektronenmikroskopische Untersuchungen am Rückenmark, an Spinalganglien und Muskelspindeln. *Ibid.*, **1970b**, *16*, 324–341.

Schwartz, W. S. Comparison of ethionamide with isoniazid in original treatment cases of pulmonary tuberculosis. XIV. A report of the Veterans Administration–Armed

Forces Cooperative Study. *Am. Rev. Respir. Dis.*, **1966**, *93*, 685–692.

Shepard, C. C.; Ellard, G. A.; Levy, L.; Upromolla, V.; Pattyn, S. R.; Peters, J. H.; Rees, R. J. W.; and Waters, M. F. R. Experimental chemotherapy of leprosy. *Bull. WHO*, **1976**, *53*, 425–433.

Shepard, C. C.; Levy, L.; and Fasal, P. The death of *Mycobacterium leprae* during treatment with 4,4′-diaminodiphenylsulfone (DDS): initial rates in patients. *Am. J. Trop. Med. Hyg.*, **1968**, *17*, 769–775.

———. The sensitivity to dapsone (DDS) of *Mycobacterium leprae* from patients with and without previous treatment. *Ibid.*, **1969**, *18*, 258–263.

———. The death rate of *Mycobacterium leprae* during treatment of lepromatous leprosy with acedapsone (DADDS). *Ibid.*, **1972**, *21*, 440–445.

Shepard, C. C.; Walker, L. L.; Van Landingham, R. M.; and Redus, M. A. Discontinuous administration of clofazimine (B663) on *Mycobacterium leprae* infections. *Proc. Soc. Exp. Biol. Med.*, **1971a**, *137*, 725–727.

———. Comparison of B1912 and clofazimine (B663) in *Mycobacterium leprae* infections. *Ibid.*, **1971b**, *137*, 728–729.

Simon, E.; Veres, E.; and Banki, G. Changes in SGOT activity during treatment with ethionamide. *Scand. J. Respir. Dis.*, **1969**, *50*, 314–322.

Singapore Tuberculosis Service/British Medical Research Council. Controlled trial of intermittent regimens of rifampicin plus isoniazid for pulmonary tuberculosis in Singapore. *Lancet*, **1975**, *2*, 1105–1109.

Sippel, J. E.; Mikhail, I. A.; Girgis, N. I.; and Youssef, H. H. Rifampin concentrations in cerebrospinal fluid of patients with tuberculous meningitis. *Am. Rev. Respir. Dis.*, **1974**, *109*, 579–580.

Skolnick, J. L.; Stoler, B. S.; Katz, D. B.; and Anderson, W. H. Rifampin, oral contraceptives, and pregnancy. *J.A.M.A.*, **1976**, *236*, 1382.

Spector, R., and Lorenzo, W. V. The active transport of para-aminosalicylic acid from the cerebrospinal fluid. *J. Pharmacol. Exp. Ther.*, **1973**, *185*, 642–648.

Stead, W. W., and Texter, E. C., Jr. Isoniazid hepatitis: backlash of progress. *Ann. Intern. Med.*, **1973**, *79*, 125–127.

Storey, P. B., and McLean, R. L. A current appraisal of cycloserine. *Antibiotic Med. Clin. Ther.*, **1957**, *4*, 223–232.

Stottmeier, K. D. Emergence of rifampin-resistant *Mycobacterium tuberculosis* in Massachusetts. *J. Infect. Dis.*, **1976**, *133*, 88–90.

Stottmeier, K. D.; Beam, R. E.; and Kubica, G. P. The absorption and excretion of pyrazinamide. I. Preliminary study in laboratory animals and man. *Am. Rev. Respir. Dis.*, **1968**, *98*, 70–74.

Strauss, I., and Erhardt, F. Ethambutol absorption, excretion and dosage in patients with renal tuberculosis. *Chemotherapy*, **1970**, *15*, 148–157.

Sunahara, S.; Urano, M.; and Ogawa, M. Genetical and geographic studies on isoniazid inactivation. *Science*, **1961**, *134*, 1530.

Suter, E. Multiplication of tubercle bacilli within phagocytes cultivated *in vitro*, and the effect of streptomycin and isonicotinic acid hydrazide. *Am. Rev. Respir. Dis.*, **1952**, *65*, 775–776.

Takayama, K.; Schnoes, H. K.; Armstrong, E. L.; and Boyle, R. W. Site of inhibitory action of isoniazid in the synthesis of mycolic acids in *Mycobacterium tuberculosis*. *J. Lipid Res.*, **1975**, *16*, 308–317.

Takayama, K.; Wang, L.; and David, H. L. Effect of isoniazid on the *in vivo* mycolic acid synthesis, cell growth, and variability of *Mycobacterium tuberculosis*. *Antimicrob. Agents Chemother.*, **1972**, *2*, 29–35.

Thomas, J. P.; Baughn, C. O.; Wilkinson, R. G.; and Shepherd, R. G. A new synthetic compound with antituberculous activity in mice: ethambutol (dextro-2-2′-(ethyl-

enediimino)-di-l-butanol). *Am. Rev. Respir. Dis.*, **1961**, *83*, 891–893.

Tiitinen, H. Isoniazid and ethionamide serum levels and inactivation in Finnish subjects. *Scand. J. Respir. Dis.*, **1969**, *50*, 110–124.

Trautman, J. R. The management of leprosy and its complications. *N. Engl. J. Med.*, **1965**, *273*, 756–758.

Tsukamura, M.; Toyama, H.; Mizuno, S.; and Tsukamura, S. Cross resistance relationship among capreomycin, kanamycin, viomycin and streptomycin resistances of *Mycobacterium tuberculosis*. *Kekkaku*, **1967**, *42*, 399–404.

Tuazon, C. U.; Lin, M. Y. C.; and Sheagren, J. N. *In vitro* activity of rifampin alone and in combination with nafcillin and vancomycin against pathogenic strains of *Staphylococcus aureus*. *Antimicrob. Agents Chemother.*, **1978**, *13*, 759–761.

Verbist, L., and Gyselen, A. Antituberculous activity of rifampin *in vitro* and *in vivo* and the concentrations attained in human blood. *Am. Rev. Respir. Dis.*, **1968**, *98*, 923–932.

Warrington, R. J.; Hogg, G. R.; Paraskevas, F.; and Tse, K. S. Insidious rifampin-associated renal failure with light-chain proteinuria. *Arch. Intern. Med.*, **1977**, *137*, 927–930.

Way, E. L.; Smith, P. K.; Howie, D. L.; Weiss, R.; and Swanson, R. The absorption, distribution, excretion and fate of para-aminosalicylic acid. *J. Pharmacol. Exp. Ther.*, **1948**, *93*, 368–382.

Weber, W. W. Acetylation of drugs. In, *Metabolic Conjugation and Metabolic Hydrolysis*. (Fishman, W. W., ed.) Academic Press, Inc., New York, **1973**, pp. 249–296.

Weiner, I. M., and Tinker, J. P. Pharmacology of pyrazinamide: metabolic and renal function studies related to the mechanism of drug-induced urate retention. *J. Pharmacol. Exp. Ther.*, **1972**, *180*, 411–434.

WHO. A study of two twice-weekly and a once-weekly continuation regimens of tuberculosis chemotherapy including a comparison of two durations of treatment. *Tubercle*, **1977a**, *58*, 129–136.

Wilson, T. M. Current therapeutics. CCXL. Capreomycin and ethambutol. *Practitioner*, **1967**, *199*, 817–824.

Wimpenny, J. W. T. The uptake and fate of isoniazid in *Mycobacterium tuberculosis* var. *bovis* BCG. *J. Gen. Microbiol.*, **1967**, *47*, 389–403.

Youatt, J. A review of the action of isoniazid. *Am. Rev. Respir. Dis.*, **1969**, *99*, 729–749.

Zillig, W.; Zechel, K.; Rabussay, D.; Schachner, M.; Sethi, U. S.; Palm, P.; Heil, A.; and Seifert, W. On the role of different subunits of DNA-dependent RNA polymerase from *E. coli* in the transcription process. *Cold Spring Harbor Symp. Quant. Biol.*, **1970**, *35*, 47–58.

Monographs and Reviews

Alford, R. Antimycobacterial agents. In, *Principles and Practice of Infectious Diseases*. (Mandell, G. L.; Douglas, R. G., Jr.; and Bennett, J. E.; eds.) John Wiley & Sons, Inc., New York, **1979**, pp. 328–343.

Arnold, H. L., and Fasal, P. *Leprosy: Diagnosis and Management*, 2nd ed. Charles C Thomas, Pub., Springfield, Ill., **1973**.

Bailey, W. C.; Raleigh, H. W.; and Turner, P. Treatment of mycobacterial disease. *Am. Rev. Respir. Dis.*, **1977**, *115*, 185–187.

Browne, S. G. Advances in the treatment of leprosy. *Practitioner*, **1967**, *199*, 525–531.

Bryceson, A., and Pfaltzgraff, R. E. *Leprosy for Students of Medicine*. Churchill Livingstone, Ltd., Edinburgh, **1973**.

Bullock, W. E. *Mycobacterium leprae* (leprosy). In, *Principles and Practice of Infectious Diseases*. (Mandell, G. L.; Douglas, R. G., Jr.; and Bennett, J. E.; eds.) John Wiley & Sons, Inc., New York, **1979**, pp. 1943–1953.

Byrd, R. B.; Horn, B. R.; Griggs, G. A.; and Solomon,

D. A. Isoniazid chemoprophylaxis. *Arch. Intern. Med.,* **1977,** *137,* 1130–1133.

Farer, L. *Mycobacterium tuberculosis.* In, *Principles and Practice of Infectious Diseases.* (Mandell, G. L.; Douglas, R. G., Jr.; and Bennett, J. E.; eds.) John Wiley & Sons, Inc., New York, **1979,** pp. 1905–1925.

Furesz, S. Chemical and biological properties of rifampicin. *Antibiot. Chemother.,* **1970,** *16,* 316–351.

Goldman, A. L., and Braman, S. S. Isoniazid: a review with emphasis on adverse effects. *Chest,* **1972,** *62,* 71–77.

Grove, D. I.; Warren, K. S.; and Mahmoud, A. A. F. Algorithms in the diagnosis and management of exotic diseases. XV. Leprosy. *J. Infect. Dis.,* **1976,** *134,* 205–210.

International Congress on Leprology. (Various authors.) *Int. J. Lepr.,* **1963,** *31,* 515–610.

Jacobson, R. R., and Trautman, J. R. The diagnosis and treatment of leprosy. *South. Med. J.,* **1976,** *69,* 979–985.

Kucers, A., and Bennett, N. M. (eds.). *The Use of Antibiotics,* 2nd ed. William Heinemann Medical Books, Ltd., London, **1975.**

Leiker, D. L. Chemotherapy in leprosy. *Int. J. Dermatol.,* **1975,** *14,* 254–262.

Lester, W. Rifampin: a semisynthetic derivative of rifamycin—a prototype for the future. *Annu. Rev. Microbiol.,* **1972,** *26,* 85–102.

Lincoln, E. M., and Gilberg, L. A. Disease in children due to mycobacteria other than *M. tuberculosis. Am. Rev. Respir. Dis.,* **1972,** *105,* 683–714.

Mitchell, J. R.; Zimmerman, H. J.; Ishak, K. G.; Thorgeirsson, U. P.; Timbrell, J. A.; Snodgrass, W. R.; and Nelson, S. D. Isoniazid liver injury: clinical spectrum, pathology, and probable pathogenesis. *Ann. Intern. Med.,* **1976,** *84,* 181–192.

Pitts, F. W. Tuberculosis: prevention and therapy. In, *Current Concepts of Infectious Diseases.* (Hook, E. W.; Mandell, G. L.; Gwaltney, J. M., Jr.; and Sande, M. A.; eds.) John Wiley & Sons, Inc., New York, **1977,** pp. 181–194.

Pratt, W. B. *Chemotherapy of Infection.* Oxford University Press, New York, **1977.**

Raleigh, J. W. Rifampin in treatment of advanced pulmonary tuberculosis. *Am. Rev. Respir. Dis.,* **1972,** *105,* 397–409.

Ridley, D. S., and Jopling, W. H. Classification of leprosy according to immunity. *Int. J. Lepr.,* **1966,** *31,* 255.

Robson, J. M., and Sullivan, F. M. Antituberculosis drugs. *Pharmacol. Rev.,* **1963,** *15,* 169–223.

Sanders, W. E., Jr. Rifampin. *Ann. Intern. Med.,* **1976,** *85,* 82–86.

Shepard, C. C. Chemotherapy of leprosy. *Annu. Rev. Pharmacol.,* **1969,** *9,* 37–50.

Simmons, N. A. Synergy and rifampicin. *J. Antimicrob. Chemother.,* **1977,** *3,* 109–111.

Snider, D. E., and Farer, L. S. Preventive therapy with isoniazid for "inactive" tuberculosis. *Chest,* **1978,** *73,* 4–5.

WHO. Technical Report Series, No. 607. World Health Organization, Geneva, **1977b.**

Yaeger, H. Other *Mycobacterium* species. In, *Principles and Practice of Infectious Diseases.* (Mandell, G. L.; Douglas, R. G., Jr.; and Bennett, J. E.; eds.) John Wiley & Sons, Inc., New York, **1979,** pp. 1953–1962.

Miscellaneous Antibacterial Agents; Antifungal and Antiviral Agents

Merle A. Sande and Gerald L. Mandell

I. Miscellaneous Antibacterial Agents

ERYTHROMYCIN

History and Source. *Erythromycin* is an orally effective antibiotic, discovered in 1952 by McGuire and coworkers in the metabolic products of a strain of *Streptomyces erythreus* (Waksman), originally obtained from a soil sample collected in the Philippine Archipelago. These investigators also carried out the initial *in-vitro* observations, determined the range of toxicity, and demonstrated the effectiveness of the drug in experimental and naturally occurring infections due to gram-positive cocci.

Chemistry. Erythromycin is one of the macrolide antibiotics, so named because they contain a many-membered lactone ring to which are attached one or more deoxy sugars. It is a white crystalline compound, soluble in water to the extent of 2 mg/ml. The structural formula of erythromycin is as follows:

Erythromycin

Antibacterial Activity. Erythromycin may be either bacteriostatic or bactericidal, depending on the microorganism and the concentration of the drug. The bactericidal activity is greatest against a small number of rapidly dividing microorganisms and increases markedly as the pH of the medium is raised over the range of 5.5 to 8.5. The antibiotic is most effective *in vitro* against gram-positive cocci such as *Streptococcus pyogenes* and *Strep. pneumoniae,* for which the minimal inhibitory concentration (MIC) is from 0.001 to 0.2 µg/ml (Steigbigel, 1979). Resistant

strains of these bacteria are rare and are usually isolated from populations of people who have been recently exposed to macrolide antibiotics (Sanders *et al.,* 1968). Strains of *Strep. pneumoniae* and *Strep. pyogenes* that have been selected for resistance to erythromycin are often also resistant to lincomycin. Streptococci of the *viridans* group are often inhibited by 0.02 to 3.1 µg/ml. While some staphylococci are sensitive to erythromycin, the range of inhibitory concentrations is great (MIC for *Staphylococcus epidermidis,* 0.2 to 100 µg/ml; for *Staph. aureus,* 0.005 to 100 µg/ml). Erythromycin-resistant strains of *Staph. aureus* are frequently encountered in hospitals, and resistance may emerge during treatment of an individual patient (Griffith and Black, 1970); cross-resistance with other macrolide antibiotics and with lincomycin is common. Many other gram-positive bacilli are also sensitive to erythromycin; values of MIC are from <0.1 to 8 µg/ml for *Clostridium perfringens,* from 0.006 to 3.1 µg/ml for *Corynebacterium diphtheriae,* and from 0.1 to 0.3 µg/ml for *Listeria monocytogenes.*

Erythromycin is not active against most aerobic gram-negative bacilli. It has moderate activity *in vitro* against *Haemophilus influenzae* (MIC, 0.1 to 6 µg/ml) and *Neisseria meningitidis* (MIC, 0.1 to 1.6 µg/ml), and excellent activity against most strains of *N. gonorrhoeae* (MIC, 0.005 to 0.4 µg/ml). Useful antibacterial activity is also observed against *Pasteurella multocida, Borrelia, Bordetella pertussis,* and less than half of the strains of *Bacteroides fragilis* (the MIC ranging from 0.1 to 100 µg/ml). Erythromycin is effective against *Mycoplasma pneumoniae* (MIC, 0.001 to 0.02 µg/ml) and the agent of Legionnaires' disease, *Legionella pneumophila* (MIC, <0.5 µg/ml). It is without effect on viruses, yeasts, and fungi. Some of the atypical mycobacteria are sensitive to erythromycin *in vitro.* Approximately 85% of strains of *Mycobacterium scrofulaceum* and nearly all of *M. kansasii* are sensitive to 0.5 to 2 µg/ml of the drug; the remainder are inhibited by 4 to 16 µg/ml. Nearly all strains of *M. fortuitum* are resistant, while strains of *M. intracellulare* vary in sensitivity (Molavi and Weinstein, 1971).

Mechanism of Action. Erythromycin and other macrolide antibiotics inhibit protein synthesis by binding to 50 S ribosomal subunits of sensitive microorganisms. Erythromycin can interfere with the binding of chloramphenicol, which also acts at this site. Certain resistant microorganisms with mutational changes in components of this subunit of the ribosome fail to bind the drug. The association between erythromycin and the ribosome is reversible and takes place only when the 50 S subunit is free from tRNA molecules bearing nascent peptide chains. The production of small peptides goes on normally in the presence of the antibiotic, but that of highly polymerized homopeptides is suppressed. Gram-positive bacteria accumulate about 100 times more erythromycin than do gram-negative microorganisms. The nonionized form of the drug is considerably more permeable to cells, and this probably explains the increased antimicrobial activity that is observed at alkaline pH (Sabath *et al.,* 1968b). (*See* Mao and Wiegand, 1968; Tanaka *et al.,* 1968; Weisblum and Davies, 1968; Mao and Putterman, 1969; Vogel *et al.,* 1971.)

Absorption, Distribution, and Excretion. *Erythromycin base* is adequately absorbed from the upper part of the small intestine; it is inactivated by gastric juice, and the drug is thus administered as an enteric-coated tablet that dissolves in the duodenum. Food in the stomach delays its ultimate absorption. Peak concentrations in plasma are only 0.3 to 0.5 μg/ml 4 hours after oral administration of 250 mg of the base and are 0.3 to 1.9 μg/ml after ingestion of a 500-mg tablet. Various esters of erythromycin have been prepared to attempt to improve stability and facilitate absorption. However, concentrations of erythromycin in plasma are little different if the *stearate* is given orally. *Erythromycin estolate* is less susceptible to acid than is the parent compound; it is better absorbed than other forms of the drug, and this is not appreciably altered by food. A single, oral 250-mg dose of the estolate produces peak concentrations in plasma of approximately 1.5 μg/ml after 2 hours, and a 500-mg tablet produces peak concentrations of 4 μg/ml. At the peak, this includes both the ester and the free base, with the "active" component comprising 20 to 35% of the total (Tardrew *et al.,* 1969). Thus, the actual concentration of erythromycin base in plasma may be similar for the three preparations. The estolate is hydrolyzed to the active base *in vivo* with a $t_{1/2}$ of approximately 90 minutes.

The actual antibacterial activity of the estolate ester of erythromycin is difficult to measure *in vitro*. Only the free base binds to bacterial ribosomes. However, strains of *Staph. aureus* are more susceptible to the estolate ester than to the base if bacteria are exposed for short periods (10 minutes). This

suggests that the estolate penetrates into the bacterial cell more rapidly and is hydrolyzed by bacterial enzymes to the active component. Such esterases have been isolated from various species of bacteria.

Erythromycin ethylsuccinate is another ester that is adequately absorbed following oral administration, particularly when the stomach is empty. Peak concentrations in plasma are 1.5 μg/ml (0.5 μg/ml of base) 1 to 2 hours after administration of a 500-mg tablet.

High concentrations of erythromycin can be achieved by intravenous administration. Values are approximately 10 μg/ml 1 hour after intravenous administration of 500 to 1000 mg of *erythromycin lactobionate* or *gluceptate.*

Only 2 to 5% of orally administered erythromycin is excreted in active form in the urine; from 12 to 15%, after intravenous infusion. When large doses of erythromycin are given by mouth, the feces may contain as much as 0.5 mg/g. The antibiotic is concentrated in the liver and excreted in active form in the bile, which may contain as much as 250 μg/ml when plasma concentrations are very high. Some of the drug may be inactivated by demethylation in the liver (Mao and Tardrew, 1965). The plasma half-life of erythromycin is approximately 1.4 hours. Although some reports suggest a prolonged half-life in patients with anuria, reduction of dosage is not recommended (Kunin, 1967). The drug is not removed by either peritoneal dialysis or hemodialysis.

Erythromycin diffuses readily into intracellular fluids, and antibacterial activity can be achieved at essentially all sites *except* the brain and cerebrospinal fluid. Erythromycin is one of the few antibiotics that penetrates into prostatic fluid; concentrations are approximately 40% of those in plasma. The extent of binding of erythromycin to plasma proteins varies among the different forms of the drug but probably exceeds 70% in all cases. Erythromycin traverses the placental barrier, and concentrations of the drug in fetal plasma are about 5 to 20% of those in the maternal circulation.

Preparations, Routes of Administration, and Dosage. *Oral Preparations. Erythromycin,* U.S.P. (E-MYCIN, ILOTYCIN), is available in enteric-coated tablets containing 250 mg of the drug or as film-coated tablets containing 500 mg. *Erythromycin Stearate Tablets,* U.S.P. (BRISTAMYCIN, ERYTHROCIN STEARATE, ETHRIL), contain 125, 250, or 500 mg each. *Erythromycin Estolate,* U.S.P. (ILOSONE), is supplied as capsules (125 and 250 mg), tablets (500 mg), chewable tablets (125 and 250 mg), an oral suspension (125 and 250 mg/5 ml), and drops (100 mg/ml). *Erythromycin Ethylsuccinate,* U.S.P. (E.E.S., PEDIAMYCIN), is available as granules or powder for oral suspension (200 or 400 mg/5 ml), chewable tablets (200 mg), film-coated tablets (400 mg), and drops (100 mg/2.5 ml).

Parenteral Preparations. Sterile Erythromycin Gluceptate, U.S.P. (ILOTYCIN GLUCEPTATE), and *Erythromycin Lactobionate for Injection,* U.S.P. (ERYTHROCIN LACTOBIONATE), are available for *intravenous* injection in the form of sterile dry powders (250 or 500 mg or 1 g of antibiotic). *Erythromycin Ethylsuccinate Injection,* U.S.P. (ERYTHROCIN ETHYLSUCCINATE-I.M.), contains 50 mg/ml in 2- and 10-ml containers for intramuscular injection. This preparation includes butyl aminobenzoate (2%) as a local anesthetic.

The usual *oral* dose of erythromycin for *adults* ranges from 1 to 2 g per day, in equally divided and spaced amounts, usually given every 6 hours, depending on the nature and severity of the infection. Daily doses of erythromycin as large as 8 g orally, given for 3 months, have been well tolerated. Food should not be given immediately before or after oral administration of erythromycin base; this precaution need not be taken when the estolate is administered. The *oral* dose of erythromycin for *children* is 30 to 50 mg/kg per day, divided into four portions. *Intramuscular injection* of erythromycin is not recommended because of the pain it causes. *Intravenous administration* is used infrequently and is reserved for the therapy of severe infections. The usual dose is 0.5 to 1 g every 6 hours; 1 g of erythromycin gluceptate has been given intravenously every 6 hours for as long as 4 weeks with no difficulty except for thrombophlebitis at the site of injection.

Untoward Effects. Serious untoward effects are only rarely caused by erythromycin. Among the *allergic reactions* are *fever, eosinophilia,* and *skin eruptions,* which may occur alone or in combination; each disappears shortly after therapy is stopped. *Cholestatic hepatitis* is the most striking side effect. It is caused primarily by *erythromycin estolate* and only rarely by the other preparations (*see* Braun, 1969; Ginsburg and Eichenwald, 1976). The illness starts after about 10 to 20 days of treatment and is characterized initially by nausea, vomiting, and abdominal cramps. The pain often mimics that of acute cholecystitis, and unnecessary surgery has been performed. These symptoms are followed shortly thereafter by jaundice, which may be accompanied by fever, leukocytosis,

eosinophilia, and elevated activities of transaminases in plasma; the cholecystogram is usually negative. Biopsy of the liver reveals cholestasis, periportal infiltration by neutrophils, lymphocytes, and eosinophils, and, occasionally, necrosis of neighboring parenchymal cells. The syndrome resembles acute cholecystitis, extrahepatic biliary obstruction, pancreatitis, viral hepatitis, or the hepatic disturbance produced by androgenic steroids. All manifestations usually disappear within a few days after cessation of drug therapy and rarely are prolonged. No deaths or subsequent chronic hepatic disease have been directly attributed to this adverse drug reaction, and it occurs relatively rarely. The syndrome may represent a hypersensitivity reaction to the estolate ester (*see* Tolman *et al.,* 1974; Cooksley and Powell, 1977). Because of this reaction, the Food and Drug Administration has advocated the removal of erythromycin estolate from the market in the United States.

Artifactual elevation of glutamic oxalacetic transaminase activity may be reported when serum from patients taking erythromycin estolate is assayed by the colorimetric procedure; the enzymatic assay method is not affected (*see* Sabath *et al.,* 1968a; Braun, 1969). However, mild elevations of the SGOT were also noted in 16 of 161 pregnant women who received 250 mg of erythromycin estolate orally four times a day for 3 to 6 weeks during the second trimester. In 4 of the 16 pregnant women, transaminase activities had returned to normal by the last day of treatment. Three of 97 patients treated with erythromycin stearate reacted similarly (McCormack *et al.,* 1977).

Erythromycin often produces *irritative effects.* Oral administration, especially of large doses, is very frequently accompanied by epigastric distress, which may be quite severe. Intramuscular injection of quantities larger than 100 mg produces extremely severe pain that persists for hours. Intravenous infusion of 1-g doses, even when dissolved in a large volume, almost regularly is followed by thrombophlebitis.

Transient auditory impairment is a rare complication of treatment with erythromycin that has been observed to follow intravenous administration of large doses of the lactobionate (4 g per day) or oral ingestion of large doses of the estolate (Eckman *et al.,* 1975; Karmody and Weinstein, 1977). Hypertrophic pyloric stenosis was observed in five infants during administration of erythromycin estolate (Filippo, 1976).

There are no known contraindications to the use of erythromycin except prior allergic reactions to the drug. Patients with hepatic dysfunction should probably not receive the estolate.

Therapeutic Uses. Extensive studies of the clinical application of erythromycin have demonstrated its usefulness in a variety of infections, but it is currently the preferred drug for only a few.

Mycoplasma pneumoniae Infections. Erythromycin (given orally in doses of 500 mg three or four times daily, or, if oral administration is not tolerated, given intravenously) reduces the duration of fever caused by *M. pneumoniae.* In addition, the rate of clearing as noted in the chest x-ray is accelerated (Rasch and Mogabgab, 1965). Tetracycline is just as effective.

Legionnaires' Disease. Erythromycin is currently recommended for the treatment of Legionnaires' disease. The antibiotic may be given orally (0.5 to 1 g four times daily) or intravenously (1 to 4 g per day). Clinical evidence and studies in guinea pigs suggest that erythromycin is the most active antimicrobial agent available (*see* Balows and Fraser, 1979).

Diphtheria. Erythromycin is very effective in eradicating the acute or chronic *diphtheria bacillus carrier state.* Erythromycin estolate (250 mg four times daily for 7 days) was found to be effective in 90% of adults. Most of the failures were due to lack of patient compliance (McClosky *et al.,* 1971). It must be remembered, however, that neither erythromycin nor any other antibiotic alters the course of an acute infection with the diphtheria bacillus or the risk of complications.

Pertussis. If administered early in the course of whooping cough, erythromycin may shorten the duration of illness. The drug has little influence on the disease once the paroxysmal stage is reached, although it may eliminate the microorganisms from the nasopharynx (*see* Bass *et al.,* 1969). Erythromycin can prevent whooping cough in susceptible individuals who are exposed to the disease.

Streptococcal Infections. Pharyngitis, scarlet fever, and *erysipelas* produced by *Strep. pyogenes* respond to erythromycin. The oral administration of 250 to 500 mg every 6 hours or 20 mg/kg per day (of the estolate) or 30 mg/kg per day (for other forms of erythromycin) for 10 days cures these diseases, prevents the appearance of suppurative complications, and suppresses the formation of antistreptococcal antibodies. Treatment with erythromycin appears to produce a rate of cure about equal to that obtained with penicillin G (Shapera *et al.,* 1973). *Pneumococ-*

cal pneumonia responds promptly to oral therapy with 250 to 500 mg of erythromycin every 6 hours. Erythromycin is thus a valuable alternative for the treatment of streptococcal infections in patients who are allergic to penicillin.

Staphylococcal Infections. Erythromycin is an alternative agent for the treatment of relatively minor infections caused by either penicillin-sensitive or penicillin-resistant *Staph. aureus.* However, the emergence of appreciable numbers of strains that are resistant to erythromycin limits the use of the drug. The availability of the penicillinase-resistant penicillins and the cephalosporins has reduced the need to use erythromycin for the treatment of serious staphylococcal disease. The oral administration of 500 mg of erythromycin every 6 hours for 7 to 10 days is effective treatment for staphylococcal infections of the skin or of wounds in patients who are allergic to penicillins and cephalosporins.

Tetanus. Erythromycin (500 mg orally every 6 hours for 10 days) may be given to eradicate *Clostridium tetani* in patients with tetanus who are allergic to penicillin. The mainstays of therapy are debridement, physiological support, tetanus antitoxin, and drug control of convulsions.

Syphilis. Erythromycin in doses of 2 to 4 g per day for 10 to 15 days has been employed successfully in the treatment of early syphilis in the patient who is allergic to penicillin (Schroeter *et al.,* 1972; Sanford, 1979).

Gonorrhea. Both erythromycin estolate and the base have been used in the therapy of gonococcal urethritis. However, the relapse rate is nearly 25% after the oral administration of 9 g over a 4-day period; this is unacceptably high for routine use (Brown *et al.,* 1977). Erythromycin may be useful for disseminated gonococcal disease in the pregnant patient who is allergic to penicillin (since tetracyclines should be avoided during pregnancy). Thirteen patients who were treated with 500 mg of erythromycin estolate or stearate, given orally every 6 hours for 5 days, showed rapid clinical and bacteriological responses.

Prophylactic Uses. Although penicillin is the drug of choice for the *prophylaxis of recurrences of rheumatic fever,* another antistreptococcal agent must be used in individuals who are allergic to this antibiotic. The sulfonamides are cheap and effective for this purpose. In some instances, however, it may be preferable to use erythromycin, which is also efficacious.

LINCOMYCIN

Lincomycin is elaborated by an actinomycete, *Streptomyces lincolnensis,* so named because it was isolated from soil collected near Lincoln, Nebraska; it was the first lincosamide antibiotic to be used clinically. *Clindamycin,* the 7-deoxy, 7-chloro derivative of lincomycin, is more active and causes fewer unwanted effects. There are thus few, if any, valid reasons to use lincomycin (LINCOCIN). Its properties are discussed in the *fifth edition* of this textbook.

CLINDAMYCIN

Chemistry.   *Clindamycin* is a derivative of the amino acid trans-L-4-*n*-propylhygrinic acid, attached to a sulfur-containing derivative of an octose. The structural formula of clindamycin is as follows:

Clindamycin

Mechanism of Action.   Clindamycin and lincomycin bind exclusively to the 50 S subunit of bacterial ribosomes and suppress protein synthesis. Although clindamycin, erythromycin, and chloramphenicol are not structurally related, they all act at this site, and the binding of one of these antibiotics to the ribosome may inhibit the reaction of the other. There are no clinical indications for the concurrent use of these antibiotics.

Antibacterial Activity.   In general, clindamycin is similar to erythromycin in its activity *in vitro* against pneumococci, *Strep. pyogenes,* and *viridans* streptococci. Almost all such bacterial strains are inhibited by concentrations of 0.04 μg/ml (Steigbigel, 1979), although resistant microorganisms are encountered rarely (Sanders *et al.,* 1968). It is also active against many strains of *Staph. aureus* but may not inhibit methicillin-resistant strains (the MIC varies from 0.04 to 100 μg/ml, with a median of 0.1 μg/ml) (Barrett *et al.,* 1968). Strains that are resistant to clindamycin are often also resistant to erythromycin. In some hospitals, such resistance has been found in 20% of isolates (Nunnery and Riley, 1964). Resistance to clindamycin has developed during treatment of experimental staphylococcal endocarditis (Sande and Johnson, 1975). Clindamycin is inactive against enterococci and *Neisseria meningitidis* in concentrations that can be achieved clinically.

Clindamycin is more active than erythromycin against many anaerobic bacteria, especially *B. fragilis* (MIC, 0.03 to 8 μg/ml; median, 0.5 μg/ml). Minimal inhibitory concentrations for other anaerobes are as follows: *Bacteroides melaninogenicus,* 0.1 to 1 μg/ml; *Fusobacterium,* <0.5 μg/ml; *Peptostreptococcus,* <0.1 to 0.5 μg/ml; *Peptococcus,* 1 to 100 μg/ml; and *Cl. perfringens,* <0.1 to 8 μg ml. Occasional isolates of these latter two microorganisms and a significant number of other clostridia are resistant to clindamycin. Strains of *Actinomyces israelii* are sensitive. Essentially all aerobic gram-negative bacilli are resistant. Strains of *Toxoplasma gondii* have been inhibited by clindamycin in experimental ocular infections (Tabbara *et al.,* 1979). (*See* Lerner, 1969; Meyers *et al.,* 1969; Bartlett *et al.,* 1972; Sutter *et al.,* 1973; Wilkins and Thiel, 1973; Steigbigel, 1979.)

Absorption, Fate, and Excretion.   Clindamycin is nearly completely absorbed following oral administration, and peak plasma concentrations of 2 to 3 μg/ml are attained within 1 hour after the ingestion of 150 mg. The presence of food in the stomach does not reduce absorption significantly. The half-life of the antibiotic is about 2.5 hours, and modest accumulation of drug is to be expected if it is given at 6-hour intervals.

Clindamycin palmitate, an oral preparation for pediatric use, is itself inactive, but the ester is hydrolyzed rapidly *in vivo.* Its absorption is similar to that of clindamycin. After several oral doses at 6-hour intervals, children attain plasma concentrations of 2 to 4 μg/ml with the administration of 8 to 16 mg/kg.

The phosphate ester of clindamycin, which is given parenterally, is also rapidly hydrolyzed *in vivo* to the active parent compound. Following intramuscular injection, peak concentrations in plasma are not attained for 3 hours in adults and 1 hour in children. The recommended parenteral dosages provide peak plasma concentrations of 5 to 15 μg/ml and effective antimicrobial activity for approximately 8 hours.

While clindamycin is widely distributed in many fluids and tissues, including bone, significant concentrations are not attained in cerebrospinal fluid, even when the meninges are inflamed. The drug readily crosses the placental barrier. Ninety percent or more of clindamycin is bound to plasma proteins. (*See* Panzer *et al.,* 1972; Vacek *et al.,* 1972; Philipson *et al.,* 1973.)

Only about 10% of administered clindamycin is excreted unaltered in the urine, and small quantities are found in the feces. Most of the drug is inactivated by metabolism to N-demethylclindamycin and clindamycin sulfoxide, which are excreted in the urine and bile. The half-life of clindamycin is lengthened only slightly in patients with markedly impaired renal function, and little adjustment of dosage is required for such individuals. Greater accumulation of drug may occur in patients with severe hepatic failure.

The clinical pharmacology of clindamycin is discussed by Lwin and Collipp (1970), DeHaan and associates (1972, 1973), Fass and Saslaw (1972), Kauffman and coworkers (1972), and Balanchandar and colleagues (1973).

Preparations, Routes of Administration, and Dosage. *Clindamycin Hydrochloride,* U.S.P. (CLEOCIN), is supplied for oral administration in capsules containing 75 or 150 mg. *Clindamycin Palmitate Hydrochloride,* U.S.P. (CLEOCIN PEDIATRIC), is a preparation of flavored granules for suspension to a concentration of 75 mg/5 ml. *Clindamycin Phosphate,* U.S.P. (CLEOCIN PHOSPHATE), is for intramuscular or intravenous use and is supplied as a solution of 150 mg/ml in 2- and 4-ml containers.

The *oral* dose of clindamycin for *adults* is 150 to 300 mg every 6 hours; for severe infections, 300 to 450 mg every 6 hours. *Children* should receive 8 to 12 mg/kg per day in three or four divided doses; for severe infections, 13 to 25 mg/kg per day. However, children weighing less than 10 kg should receive $\frac{1}{2}$ teaspoonful of clindamycin palmitate hydrochloride (37.5 mg) three times daily as a minimal dose.

For serious infections due to aerobic gram-positive cocci and the more sensitive anaerobes (not generally including *B. fragilis, Peptococcus,* and *Clostridium* species other than *Cl. perfringens*), intravenous or intramuscular administration is recommended in dosages of 600 to 1200 mg per day, given in two to four equal portions to adults. For more severe infections, particularly those proven or suspected to be caused by *B. fragilis, Peptococcus,* or *Clostridium* species other than *Cl. perfringens,* parenteral administration of 1200 to 2700 mg per day of clindamycin is suggested. In life-threatening situations due to aerobes or anaerobes, these doses may be increased. Daily doses as high as 4800 mg have been given intravenously to adults. *Children* should receive 10 to 40 mg/kg per day in three or four divided doses; in severe infections, a minimal daily dose of 300 mg is recommended, regardless of body weight.

Untoward Effects. The reported incidence of *diarrhea* associated with the administration of clindamycin ranges from 2 to 20%; the average appears to be about 8%. A number of patients have developed *pseudomembranous colitis,* characterized by diarrhea, abdominal pain, fever, and mucus and blood in the stools. *This syndrome may be lethal.* It is apparently due to the elaboration of an exotoxin by clindamycin-resistant strains of *Clostridium difficile* (Larson and Price, 1977; Rifkin *et al.,* 1977; Bartlett *et al.,* 1978). If significant diarrhea or colitis occurs during therapy with clindamycin, the drug should be discontinued immediately; *vancomycin,* given orally in doses of 2 g per day, is effec-

tive in reducing the frequency of diarrhea (Tedesco, 1977). Cholestyramine (4 g, given three or four times daily) has also proven beneficial, but vancomycin is preferred. Agents that inhibit peristalsis, such as opioids, may prolong and worsen the condition. While the incidence of this problem is unknown, it is clear that the therapeutic indications for clindamycin should be considered very seriously before it is given. The oral administration of this drug should be avoided if possible for the treatment of infections that will respond to less toxic agents.

Skin rashes occur in approximately 10% of patients treated with clindamycin. Other reactions, which are uncommon, include exudative erythema multiforme (Stevens-Johnson syndrome), reversible elevation of SGOT and SGPT, granulocytopenia, thrombocytopenia, and anaphylactic reactions. Local thrombophlebitis may follow intravenous administration of the drug.

Therapeutic Uses. While a number of infections with gram-positive cocci will respond favorably to clindamycin, the high incidence of diarrhea and the occurrence of colitis require limitation of its use to infections in which it is clearly superior to other agents. Infections for which clindamycin is indicated particularly include those produced by *Bacteroides,* especially *B. fragilis.* Some species of this genus are, however, variably or poorly sensitive. Abdominal and pelvic abscesses, bacteremia, pneumonia, lung abscess, empyema, soft-tissue infections, and decubitus ulcers due to *Bacteroides* or *Fusobacterium* respond favorably when parenteral treatment is undertaken and continued for 1 to 2 weeks. In some instances, especially when a mixture of microorganisms is present (*e.g.,* intra-abdominal abscess secondary to rupture of a viscus), adjunct therapy with other antibiotics and particularly surgical drainage are critical in producing cure. (*See* Douglas and Kislak, 1973; Fass *et al.,* 1973; Thadepalli *et al.,* 1973.) Disease due to *Actinomyces israelii* or to anaerobic streptococci has been treated successfully with clindamycin. Chloramphenicol, to which most anaerobes including *Bacteroides* are sensitive, is preferable to clindamycin for the therapy of anaerobic infections of the central nervous system (CNS), such as brain abscess, because clindamycin penetrates the blood-brain barrier poorly.

SPECTINOMYCIN

Source and Chemistry. *Spectinomycin* is an antibiotic produced by *Streptomyces spectabilis.* The drug is an aminocyclitol; its structural formula is as follows:

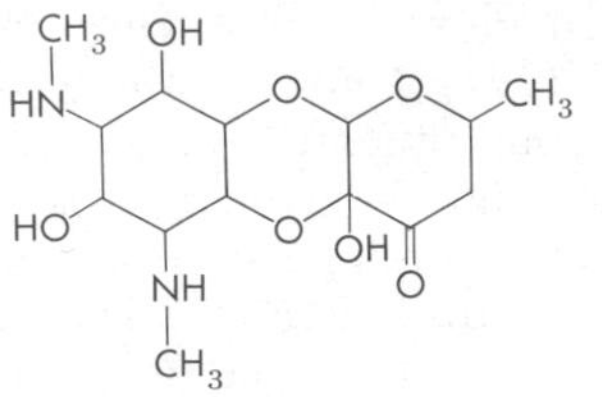

Spectinomycin

Antibacterial Activity and Mechanism. Spectinomycin is active against a number of gram-negative bacterial species, but it is inferior to other drugs to which such microorganisms are susceptible (Schoutens *et al.,* 1972). However, it readily inhibits gonococci at concentrations of 7 to 20 μg/ml, concentrations produced in plasma by the administration of recommended doses.

Spectinomycin selectively inhibits protein synthesis in gram-negative bacteria. The antibiotic binds to and acts on the 30 S ribosomal subunit. There are similarities in its action to that of the aminoglycosides; however, spectinomycin is not bactericidal and does not cause misreading of polyribonucleotides. A high degree of bacterial resistance may develop as a result of mutation (Davies *et al.,* 1965).

Absorption, Distribution, and Excretion. Spectinomycin is rapidly absorbed after intramuscular injection. A single dose of 2 g produces peak concentrations in plasma of 100 μg/ml at 1 hour; a 4-g injection, 160 μg/ml. Eight hours after injection of 2 or 4 g, the concentrations in plasma are 15 μg or 30 μg/ml, respectively. The drug is not significantly bound to plasma protein. Spectinomycin is excreted in biologically active form in the urine; all of an administered dose is recovered within 48 hours after injection.

Preparations. *Sterile Spectinomycin Hydrochloride,* U.S.P. (TROBICIN), is supplied as a sterile powder for reconstitution with water containing 0.9% benzyl alcohol. Vials of 2 and 4 g are available. This solution is for intramuscular injection only.

Untoward Effects. Spectinomycin, when given as a single intramuscular injection, produces few significant untoward effects (Duncan *et al.,* 1972). *Urticaria, chills,* and *fever* have been noted after single doses, as have *dizziness, nausea,* and *insomnia.* The injection may be painful. Ototoxicity and nephrotoxicity have not been reported.

Therapeutic Uses. Spectinomycin is primarily recommended for the treatment of uncomplicated gonococcal infections (*i.e., acute genital and rectal gonorrhea*) in patients who are allergic to penicillin or in those who are infected with penicillinase-producing microorganisms. The recommended dose for both men and women is a single deep intramuscular injection of 2 g. The rate of cure for these forms of gonorrhea is about 95%. Spectinomycin is also the preferred drug for patients with such infections who have not been cured by other treatment regimens. High rates of failure (50%) have followed single-dose

treatment with spectinomycin for gonococcal pharyngitis. Multiple doses of spectinomycin (2 g intramuscularly, twice a day for 3 days) are recommended for the treatment of disseminated gonococcal infections (arthritis-dermatitis syndrome) caused by penicillinase-producing strains of *N. gonorrhoeae* (*see* Center for Disease Control, 1979). It must be emphasized that spectinomycin is without effect on incubating or established syphilis (Reyn *et al.,* 1973).

POLYMYXIN B AND COLISTIN

History and Source. The *polymyxins,* discovered in 1947, are a group of closely related antibiotic substances elaborated by various strains of *Bacillus polymyxa,* an aerobic spore-forming rod found in soil. *Colistin* (polymyxin E) is produced by *Bacillus (Aerobacillus) colistinus,* a microorganism isolated from a soil sample obtained from Fukushima Prefecture, Japan.

Chemistry. The polymyxins, which are cationic detergents, are relatively simple, basic peptides with molecular weights of about 1000. They readily form water-soluble salts with mineral acids. The structural formula for polymyxin B, which is itself a mixture of polymyxins B_1 and B_2, is as follows:

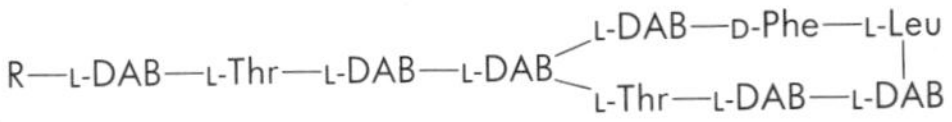

Polymyxin B_1: R = (+)-6-Methyloctanoyl
Polymyxin B_2: R = 6-Methylheptanoyl
DAB = α,γ-Diaminobutyric Acid

Colistin is polymyxin E; polymyxins E_1 and E_2 differ from each other in the same manner as do B_1 and B_2. Colistin is identical to polymyxin B except for the substitution of a residue of D-leucine for that of D-phenylalanine. Solutions of colistin salts are relatively unstable above pH 6.

Colistin is available for clinical use as colistin sulfate, for oral use, and as colistimethate sodium (colistin sodium methanesulfonate), a parenteral preparation. Colistimethate is a sulfamethylated form of polymyxin E and is inactive; however, hydrolysis *in vivo* results in generation of colistin.

Antibacterial Activity. The antimicrobial activity of polymyxin B and colistin are similar and are restricted to gram-negative bacteria. *Enterobacter, Escherichia coli, Klebsiella, Salmonella, Pasteurella, Bordetella,* and *Shigella* are usually sensitive to concentrations of 0.05 to 2.0 μg/ml. Most strains of *Pseudomonas aeruginosa* are inhibited by less than 8 μg/ml *in vitro*. However, *Proteus* and most strains of *Neisseria, Providencia,* and *Serratia* are resistant to these drugs. Synergism against *Pseud. aeruginosa* has been demonstrated between the polymyxins and tetracycline, sulfamethoxazole, chloramphenicol, and carbenicillin (Jawetz, 1961; Barnett *et al.,* 1964; Goodwin, 1970). Polymyxins and sulfonamides may act synergistically against some gram-negative bacilli that are resistant to polymyxins, such as *Proteus* and *Serratia* (Holmgren and Möller, 1970). A synergistic effect has also been achieved against multiple-resistant gram-negative bacilli by the concurrent administration of colistin, sulfamethoxazole, and trimethoprim (Thomas *et al.*, 1976).

Polymyxin B is rapidly bactericidal *in vitro*, and resistance rarely develops during therapy. While development of bacterial resistance to polymyxin B is infrequent in most species and there is no cross-resistance with other types of antibiotics, there is complete cross-resistance between polymyxin B and colistin.

Mechanism of Action. Polymyxins are surface-active agents, containing lipophilic and lipophobic groups separated within the molecule. They interact strongly with phospholipids and penetrate into and disrupt the structure of cell membranes. The permeability of the bacterial membrane changes immediately on contact with the drug. The cell membranes of polymyxin B–sensitive bacteria take up more of the antibiotic than do those of resistant bacteria, and sensitivity to polymyxin B is apparently related to the phospholipid content of the cell wall-membrane complex (Brown and Wood, 1972). The cell wall of certain resistant bacteria may prevent access of the drug to the cell membrane (*see* Pratt, 1977).

Absorption, Distribution, and Excretion. Neither polymyxin B nor colistin is absorbed when given orally. They are also poorly absorbed from mucous membranes and the surface of large burns. After daily intramuscular injection of 4.8 mg/kg of polymyxin B, concentrations in the plasma of children range from 3 to 7 μg/ml. The daily administration of 2 to 4 mg/kg parenterally to adults yields values of 1 to 8 μg/ml, the peak occurring about 2 hours after injection.

Intramuscular injection of 150 mg of colistimethate in adults produces a peak concentration in plasma of 4 to 6 μg/ml at 2 hours; this declines with a half-time of 2 hours. The actual antibacterial activity is less than that measured (approximately 65% at 2 hours and 90% at 4 hours) due to the gradual hydrolysis of the drug to its active form (Sande and Kaye, 1970). The same quantity given intravenously yields a maximal concentration in plasma of 18 μg/ml; this falls to about 0.4 μg/ml at 12 hours. An intravenous dose of 2.5 mg/kg per day diluted in 300 to 500 ml of 5% dextrose in water produces concentrations in plasma of approximately 5 μg/ml when administered as a constant infusion.

Although very little polymyxin B is eliminated by the kidney during the first 12 hours after injection, large amounts are eventually excreted by this route. Concentrations of 20 to 100 μg/ml are found in the urine after continued parenteral therapy with conventional doses. Elimination continues for 1 to 3 days after the drug is stopped. A total of 60% of the administered polymyxin B can be recovered from the urine. Urinary concentrations of colistin exceed 200 μg/ml during the first 2 hours after a usual intramuscular dose. The drug is excreted more rapidly in children than in adults. High concentrations of these antibiotics accumulate in patients with renal

insufficiency. The polymyxins do not gain access to the cerebrospinal fluid from the circulation, even when the meninges are inflamed. Colistin does pass from the maternal to fetal circulation.

Preparations, Routes of Administration, and Dosage. *Polymyxin B Sulfate,* U.S.P. (AEROSPORIN), is available in vials containing 500,000 units for parenteral injection or for ophthalmic use. Pure polymyxin B base contains 10,000 units of polymyxin B activity per milligram. (The official U.S.P. preparation of polymyxin B sulfate contains not less than 6000 units/mg.) The content of a vial of polymyxin B (50 mg) is dissolved in 2 ml of 1% procaine hydrochloride solution for intramuscular injection or in 300 to 500 ml of 5% dextrose solution for intravenous infusion. The intramuscular route is preferred. Dosage by either route is 1.5 to 2.5 mg/kg per day in two or three divided doses, but this *must be reduced* in patients with impaired renal function. Polymyxin B can also be given by mouth, by intrathecal instillation, and topically. An official combination of neomycin and polymyxin is used for irrigation of the urinary bladder.

Colistin Sulfate for Oral Suspension, U.S.P. (COLY-MYCIN S ORAL SUSPENSION), is marketed as a powder (300 mg) to be suspended in distilled water prior to dispensing (5 mg/ml). *Sterile Colistimethate Sodium,* U.S.P. (COLY-MYCIN M PARENTERAL), is marketed for *intravenous* or *intramuscular* injection in vials containing the equivalent of 20 or 150 mg of colistin base to be reconstituted to contain 10 or 75 mg/ml, respectively. The parenteral dose of colistimethate for adults and children is 2.5 to 5 mg/kg per day, in three divided doses. Colistin sulfate has been administered *orally* to infants and children with diarrhea caused by bacteria susceptible to the drug; the dose is 3 to 5 mg/kg daily, in three divided portions.

If colistimethate must be used in patients with renal insufficiency, dosage schedules must be altered radically (*see* manufacturer's instructions). When patients being treated with the drug are subjected to dialysis, the dose must also be adjusted. Curtis and Eastwood (1968) have recommended the injection of 2 to 3 mg/kg intravenously after each hemodialysis, if this is carried out twice a week. The administration of 2 mg/kg daily during peritoneal dialysis has been suggested by Greenberg and Sanford (1967); this produces effective antibacterial blood levels without excessive accumulation of the drug.

Untoward Effects. Polymyxin B applied to intact or denuded skin or mucous membranes produces no systemic reactions because of almost complete lack of absorption of the antibiotic from these sites. *Hypersensitization* is uncommon when the antibiotic is used in this way. Fever and punctate, macular, or urticarial rashes, the primary manifestations of hypersensitivity to the drug, occur infrequently when polymyxin B is administered parenterally. Nausea, vomiting, and diarrhea are produced by large doses (600 mg) taken orally. *Pain* after intramuscular injection is common. A "drawing" or "aching" pain, varying in intensity, may appear about 40 to 60 minutes after an intramuscular injection of polymyxin B and radiate along the peripheral nerve distribution; it cannot be prevented by the addition of a local anesthetic to the antibiotic. Intramuscular administration of colistimethate is less painful. Intrathecal injection of more than 5 mg of polymyxin B may produce the signs of *meningeal irritation, headache, fever,* and *increase in cells and protein in the spinal fluid* in some individuals.

Other untoward effects of polymyxin B and colistin are *facial flushing, dizziness, paresthesias* in a circumoral and "glove-and-stocking" distribution, *diplopia* due to peripheral ophthalmoplegia, *ptosis, generalized weakness, slurred speech, generalized areflexia, increase in weakness in patients with myasthenia gravis, blurred vision, difficulty in speaking,* and *dysphagia.* Seizures and coma have been reported with large doses (Wolinsky and Hines, 1962). In some cases, the drug produces noncompetitive *neuromuscular blockade* that results in respiratory paralysis. Respiratory arrest may occur with the first dose of the drug or only after it has been given for as long as 45 days; it is more common when renal failure is present and when plasma concentrations are high, and is very often preceded by dyspnea and restlessness. It is not antagonized by neostigmine or calcium gluconate, as is the case with the aminoglycoside antibiotics (Lindesmith *et al.,* 1968).

The most significant untoward effect of these drugs is *renal toxicity* (Appel and Neu, 1977). Polymyxin B is more nephrotoxic than is colistin; however, in general, the antibacterial activity of these compounds is proportional to their toxicity. Epithelial cells of the renal tubules are most affected. Damage may be potentiated by other nephrotoxic drugs, such as aminoglycosides and cephaloridine. The daily injection of 2.5 mg/kg of polymyxin often results in *proteinuria, hematuria,* and *cylindruria.* With doses of 3 mg/kg or more, *azotemia* and *decrease in glomerular filtration rate* are common; these effects tend to increase in severity with continued treatment, but are usually reversible if therapy is stopped. Excessively high and sustained concentrations of polymyxin B develop in the plasma of patients with renal insufficiency; neurotoxicity and nephrotoxicity, including anuria and tubular necrosis, occur more frequently and with greater intensity in such individuals. Renal function must be monitored carefully and dosages reduced if there is renal insufficiency. In general, these drugs should not be used in patients with renal disease if alternatives are available.

Therapeutic Uses. The primary use of polymyxin B and colistin is for treatment of infections caused by gram-negative bacteria, especially *Pseudomonas,* that are resistant to the penicillins and aminoglycosides. The present availability of gentamicin and carbenicillin has reduced markedly the clinical use of these drugs.

Polymyxin B and colistin are employed to treat severe urinary tract infections caused by *Pseud. aeruginosa* and other gram-negative bacteria not susceptible to other antibiotics and for the rare *meningeal infections* due to such microorganisms. Since systemically administered polymyxin B does not diffuse into cerebrospinal fluid, treatment of meningitis requires intrathecal injection for 3 weeks. Polymyxins are relatively ineffective for the treatment of

bacteremia, infections of deep tissues, endocarditis, and, especially, infections in granulocytopenic patients. The major potential use of these drugs is in combination with trimethoprim and sulfamethoxazole (or other suitable synergistic antimicrobial agents) in the therapy of gram-negative bacillary infection caused by strains that are resistant to several drugs. Impressive results have been observed in the therapy of infections caused by *Serratia, Pseud. cepacia, Pseud. maltophilia,* and some resistant strains of *Pseud. aeruginosa* (Nord *et al.,* 1974; Rosenblatt and Stewart, 1974; Thomas *et al.,* 1976).

Infections of the skin, mucous membranes, eye, and ear due to polymyxin B–sensitive microorganisms respond to local application of the antibiotic in solution or ointment. *External otitis,* frequently due to *Pseudomonas,* may be cured by the topical use of the drug. *Pseudomonas aeruginosa* is a common cause of infection of *corneal ulcers;* local application or subconjunctival injection (up to 10 mg per day) of polymyxin B is often curative.

NOVOBIOCIN

Novobiocin is a toxic antibiotic with a narrow antibacterial spectrum. A description of the drug is provided in the *fourth edition* of this textbook. There are no current valid indications for its therapeutic use.

VANCOMYCIN

History and Source. *Vancomycin* is an antibiotic produced by *Streptomyces orientalis,* an actinomycete isolated from soil samples obtained in Indonesia and India. Purification of the antibiotic was accomplished and its antimicrobial properties were described within a short time after its discovery (McCormick *et al.,* 1956).

Chemistry. Vancomycin is a complex and unusual glycopeptide with a molecular weight of about 1500. Its structural formula was determined only recently by x-ray analysis (Sheldrick *et al.,* 1978). Vancomycin hydrochloride is a white powder, soluble in water to a concentration of over 100 mg/ml.

Antibacterial Activity. Vancomycin is primarily active against gram-positive bacteria. Strains of *Staph. aureus,* including those resistant to methicillin, are inhibited by concentrations of 0.1 to 2 µg/ml. Rare strains of *Staph. aureus* are resistant to concentrations of the antibiotic that can be achieved clinically, but there has been no increase in the incidence of such resistance during the 20 years that the drug has been used. The minimal inhibitory concentrations of vancomycin for *Staph. epidermidis* range from 0.4 to 1.5 µg/ml; for *Strep. pyogenes,* from 0.15 to 2 µg/ml; for *Strep. pneumoniae,* from 0.1 to 0.3 µg/ml; for the *viridans* streptococci, from 0.3 to 1.5 µg/ml; and for *Strep. faecalis,* from 0.3 to 2.5 µg/ml. Vancomycin is not generally bactericidal for *Strep. faecalis;* however, 40 to 70% of strains are sensitive to a synergistic bactericidal effect when vancomycin and streptomycin are used concurrently (Mandell *et al.,* 1970), and nearly all strains are killed by a combination of vancomycin and genta- micin (Harwick *et al.,* 1973; Watanakunakorn and Bakie, 1973). In experimental endocarditis, vanco- mycin and streptomycin together are more effective in reducing bacterial counts in cardiac vegetations than is vancomycin alone (Hook *et al.,* 1975). *Cory- nebacterium* species (diptheroids) are inhibited by less than 0.04 to 3.1 μg/ml of vancomycin, most species of *Actinomyces* by 5 to 10 μg/ml, and *Clos- tridium* species by 0.39 to 6 μg/ml. Essentially all species of gram-negative bacilli and mycobacteria are resistant.

Mechanism of Action. Vancomycin inhibits the synthesis of the cell wall in sensitive bacteria by binding with high affinity to precursors of this struc- ture. The D-alanyl-D-alanine portion of the cell-wall precursor units appears to be a crucial site of attach- ment (*see* Figure 50–3, page 1129; Nieto and Perkins, 1971a, 1971b). The drug is rapidly bactericidal for dividing microorganisms.

Absorption, Distribution, and Excretion. Vanco- mycin is poorly absorbed after oral administration, and large quantities are excreted in the stool. For parenteral therapy, the drug should be administered intravenously. A single intravenous dose of 500 mg in adults produces plasma concentrations of 6 to 10 μg/ml at the end of 1 to 2 hours, 2 to 4 μg/ml after 6 hours, and 1 to 2 μg/ml after 12 hours; the drug has a half-life in the circulation of about 6 hours. Approximately 10% of vancomycin is bound to plasma protein. Vancomycin appears in various body fluids, including the cerebrospinal fluid when the meninges are inflamed. More than 90% of an injected dose is excreted by the kidney; in the pres- ence of renal insufficiency, dangerously high con- centrations may accumulate in the blood. The drug is not removed from the plasma by hemodialysis (Eykyn *et al.,* 1970).

Preparations, Routes of Administration, and Dos- age. *Sterile Vancomycin Hydrochloride,* U.S.P. (VANCOCIN), is marketed for *intravenous* use, in 10-ml vials containing powder (500 mg) for solution. The desired dose is preferably diluted and injected intravenously over a 30-minute period, every 6 or 12 hours. The dose of vancomycin for adults is 500 mg every 6 to 12 hours or 1 g every 12 hours. The daily dose for children is 44 mg/kg in equally divided and spaced quantities every 8 to 12 hours. The amount administered daily to premature infants and neo- nates ranges from 6 to 15 mg/kg. Because of incom- pletely developed renal function in this age group, the drug must be used with caution. Alteration of dosage is required for patients with impaired renal function (*see* Appendix II). The drug has been used effectively in functionally anephric patients (who are being dialyzed) by the administration of 1 g each week. When 1 g is given intravenously to such pa- tients, the peak concentration in plasma is 40 to 50 μg/ml; this falls to a value of 15 μg/ml in 3 to 5 hours. After 7 days, concentrations in plasma are usually still in the therapeutic range (5 to 7 μg/ml). Measurement of the concentration of antibiotic in plasma is recommended (Eykyn *et al.,* 1970).

Vancomycin can be administered *orally* to patients

with "antibiotic-associated" colitis (*see* discussion of clindamycin, above) or for the treatment of diarrhea due to other toxin-producing microorganisms that are sensitive to vancomycin. The dose for adults is 500 mg every 6 hours; the total daily dose for chil- dren is 44 mg/kg, given in divided doses. *Vanco- mycin Hydrochloride for Oral Solution,* U.S.P., is available for this purpose. The content of a 10-g container of the antibiotic is mixed with 115 ml of distilled water, so that each 6-ml portion provides approximately 500 mg of the drug.

Untoward Effects. Among the *hypersensitivity reactions* produced by vancomycin are *macular skin rashes* and *anaphylaxis. Phlebitis* and *pain* at the site of intravenous injection are relatively uncommon. *Chills* and *fever* may occur, and a *shocklike state* (so-called *red-neck syndrome*) happens rarely during the course of intravenous infusion. The most signifi- cant untoward reactions have been *ototoxicity* and *nephrotoxicity.* Auditory impairment, which is fre- quently although not always permanent, may follow the use of this drug. Ototoxicity is associated with excessively high concentrations of the drug in plasma and is extremely unusual if concentrations are main- tained below 30 μg/ml. In animals, ototoxicity is worsened by simultaneous treatment with aminogly- cosides or high-ceiling diuretics such as ethacrynic acid and furosemide. Nephrotoxicity was formerly quite common but has become an unusual side effect when appropriate doses are used, as judged by renal function and determinations of the concentration of the antibiotic in blood. The drug should not be used concomitantly with other nephrotoxic drugs or in patients with impaired renal function if other effec- tive and less toxic antibiotics are available.

Therapeutic Uses. Vancomycin should be em- ployed only to treat serious infections and is particu- larly useful in the management of infections due to methicillin-resistant staphylococci, including *staphy- lococcal pneumonia, empyema, endocarditis, osteomy- elitis,* and *soft-tissue abscesses.* The drug is also ex- tremely valuable in severe staphylococcal infections in patients who are allergic to penicillins and cepha- losporins (Geraci, 1977). Treatment with vancomycin is effective and convenient when there is dissemi- nated staphylococcal infection or localized infection of a shunt in a patient with irreversible renal disease who is being maintained by hemodialysis.

Administration of vancomycin is an effective al- ternative for the treatment of endocarditis caused by *viridans* streptococci in patients who are allergic to penicillin. In combination with an aminoglycoside, it may also be used for endocarditis caused by *Strep. faecalis.* As an oral agent, vancomycin benefits pa- tients with colitis caused by toxin-producing bacteria such as *Cl. difficile* and *Staph. aureus* (Fekety, 1979).

BACITRACIN

History and Source. *Bacitracin* is an antibiotic produced by the Tracy-I strain of *Bacillus subtilis,* isolated in 1943 from the damaged tissue and street dirt debrided from a compound fracture in a young girl named Tracy; hence the name *bacitracin.* The history, properties, and uses of bacitracin have been reviewed by Meleney and Johnson (1949).

Chemistry. The bacitracins are a group of polypeptide antibiotics; multiple components have been demonstrated in the commercial products. The major constituent is *bacitracin A* (*see* Newton and Abraham, 1953); its probable structural formula is as follows:

Bacitracin

A *unit* of the antibiotic is equivalent to 26 μg of the U.S.P. standard.

Antibacterial Activity. A variety of gram-positive cocci and bacilli, *Neisseria, H. influenzae,* and *Treponema pallidum* are sensitive to 0.1 unit or less of bacitracin per milliliter. *Actinomyces* and *Fusobacterium* are inhibited by concentrations of 0.5 to 5 units/ml. *Enterobacteriaceae, Pseudomonas, Candida, Torula,* and *Nocardia* are resistant to the drug. Bacitracin inhibits bacterial cell-wall synthesis.

Absorption, Fate, and Excretion. While bacitracin has been employed parenterally in the past, current use is essentially restricted to topical application. The reader is referred to *earlier editions* of this textbook for descriptions of the pharmacokinetics of this antibiotic.

Preparations, Routes of Administration, and Dosage. Only information pertinent to topical application will be presented. *Bacitracin,* U.S.P. (BACIQUENT), is available in official *ophthalmic* and *dermatological ointments;* these contain 500 units per gram of suitable base. *Bacitracin Zinc,* U.S.P., is marketed for incorporation in ointments. The antibiotic is also available in the form of a *dry powder* (50,000 units per vial) for the preparation of topical solutions. The ointments are applied directly to the involved surface one or more times daily. A number of topical preparations of bacitracin to which neomycin or polymyxin or both have been added are available, and some contain the three antibiotics plus hydrocortisone.

Untoward Effects. Serious *nephrotoxicity* results from the parenteral use of this antibiotic. *Hypersensitivity reactions* result from topical application, but this is uncommon.

Therapeutic Uses. *Topical* bacitracin alone or in combination with other antimicrobial agents has no established value in the treatment of *furunculosis,*

pyoderma, carbuncle, impetigo, and *superficial and deep abscesses.* For open infections such as *infected eczema* and *infected dermal ulcers,* the local application of the antibiotic may be of some help in eradicating sensitive bacteria. Bacitracin has an advantage over other antibiotics in that topical administration, even in an ointment, rarely produces hypersensitivity. *Suppurative conjunctivitis* and *infected corneal ulcer* respond well to the topical use of bacitracin when they are caused by susceptible bacteria.

II. Antifungal Agents

NYSTATIN

History and Source. *Streptomyces noursei* is the source of *nystatin,* and the name of the antibiotic is derived from *New York State.* Nystatin inhibits the growth of a variety of pathogenic and nonpathogenic yeasts and fungi but not bacteria. The chemical nature and properties of the drug were reported by Dutcher and colleagues (1954).

Chemistry. Nystatin is a polyene antibiotic. Such compounds contain a hydrophilic region (which includes a hydroxylated hydrocarbon backbone) and a sequence of four to seven conjugated double bonds, which is lipophilic. Nystatin and amphotericin B, another polyene antibiotic discussed in this chapter, also contain an aminodeoxyhexose, mycosamine. The structure of nystatin is thus very similar in its general features to that of amphotericin B (*see* below). Nystatin is only slightly soluble in water (10 to 20 units per milliliter). It quickly decomposes in the presence of water or plasma. The potency of commercial preparations of nystatin is expressed in units; 1.0 mg of the drug contains not less than 2000 units, in order to meet U.S.P. standards.

Antifungal Activity. Nystatin is both fungistatic and fungicidal. *Candida, Cryptococcus, Histoplasma, Blastomyces, Trichophyton, Epidermophyton,* and *Microsporum audouini* are sensitive *in vitro* to concentrations ranging from 1.5 to 6.5 μg/ml. It is generally less susceptible to changes in pH than are other antifungal agents. Nystatin is without effect on bacteria, protozoa, or viruses.

Mechanism of Action. Nystatin is bound by drug-sensitive yeasts and fungi but not by resistant microorganisms. The antifungal activity of the antibiotic is dependent on its binding to a sterol moiety, primarily ergosterol, present in the membrane of sensitive fungi. By virtue of their interaction with the sterols of cell membranes, polyenes appear to form pores or channels. The result is an increase in the permeability of the membrane, allowing leakage of a variety of small molecules. (*See* Kinsky, 1962; Weissman and Sessa, 1967; Hamilton-Miller, 1974.)

Fungal Resistance. Repeated subculture of *Candida albicans* in increasing concentrations of nystatin results in little or no development of resistance, but other species of *Candida* (*C. tropicalis, C. guiller-*

mondi, C. krusei, and *C. stellatoides*) become quite resistant and also insensitive to amphotericin at the same time. Resistance does not, as a rule, develop *in vivo.*

Absorption and Excretion. Absorption of nystatin from the gastrointestinal tract is negligible, and the drug appears in the feces. When doses of 8 million units or more are given, individuals with normal renal function may have plasma concentrations of only 1 to 2.5 μg/ml. Persons with renal insufficiency may occasionally develop significant plasma concentrations of nystatin while taking conventional doses by mouth. Parenteral treatment is not employed. Nystatin is not absorbed from the skin or mucous membranes.

Preparations, Routes of Administration, and Dosage. Official preparations of *Nystatin,* U.S.P. (MY-COSTATIN, NILSTAT, OV-STATIN), are *ointments, oral suspensions,* and *oral* and *vaginal tablets. Creams, powders, ointments, suspensions,* and *drops* contain 100,000 units of nystatin per gram or per milliliter; many topical preparations also contain other antibiotics such as neomycin or gramicidin, and hydrocortisone is incorporated in some. Tablets for oral therapy contain 500,000 units; vaginal tablets contain 100,000 units.

The *oral dose for adults* for oral or esophageal candidiasis is 500,000 to 1 million units, three or four times a day; for *children,* 100,000 units, three to four times per day. Some have prescribed vaginal suppositories *per os,* sucked on like a troche three or four times per day, to produce constant bathing of the lesions with drug. Topical application is usually made two or three times a day. Vaginal tablets are inserted once or twice daily for 14 days.

Untoward Effects. Untoward effects of nystatin are uncommon. Mild and transitory nausea, vomiting, and diarrhea may occur after oral administration of the drug. Irritation of the skin and mucous membranes does not result from topical application. Hypersensitivity reactions have not been reported, nor have toxic effects on the blood or blood-forming organs been noted. Since nystatin has no effect on bacteria, suprainfections do not occur even when large doses are used.

Therapeutic Uses. Nystatin is used primarily to treat *Candida* infections of skin, mucous membrane, and intestinal tract. Paronychia, vaginitis, and sto-

matitis (thrush) caused by this microorganism are usually benefited by topical therapy. Oral, esophageal, and gastric candidiasis are common complications in patients with hematological malignancies, especially those receiving immunosuppressive therapy; such infections will frequently respond to oral nystatin. However, if dysphagia is not improved after several days of treatment or if the patient is severely ill, amphotericin B should be administered parenterally. *Intestinal candidiasis* is a rare disease, but it may be a cause of cramps and diarrhea. Its presence is suggested by the recovery of large numbers of *Candida* in the feces after other causes of enteric infection have been ruled out (Kane *et al.,* 1976). The oral ingestion of nystatin appears to produce good results in such cases. It must be stressed that patients receiving antibiotics orally may have overgrowth of yeasts in the intestine without diarrhea. *Vaginal candidiasis* usually responds well to topical application of the drug.

Prophylactic Uses. Nystatin has been administered with the tetracyclines for the purpose of preventing the overgrowth of yeasts and fungi in the bowel of patients predisposed to infections with *Candida.* A controlled study failed to demonstrate a reduction in the incidence of oral candidiasis in patients with acute leukemia who received nystatin orally (Williams *et al.,* 1977).

AMPHOTERICIN B

History and Source. *Streptomyces nodosus,* a soil actinomycete, is the source of two antifungal agents, amphotericins A and B, which are produced together during the fermentation process. The physical and chemical properties of these agents, methods for separating them, and the preparation of an almost pure *amphotericin B* (containing only 1 to 2% amphotericin A) were elucidated by Vandeputte and coworkers (1956). The antibiotic used clinically is amphotericin B.

Chemistry. Amphotericin B, like nystatin, is a polyene antibiotic. The general structural features of the polyenes have been described above. The structural formula of amphotericin B is shown below. Amphotericin B is insoluble in water and is quite unstable. The antifungal effects of the antibiotic are maximal between pH 6.0 and 7.5 and decrease at low pH.

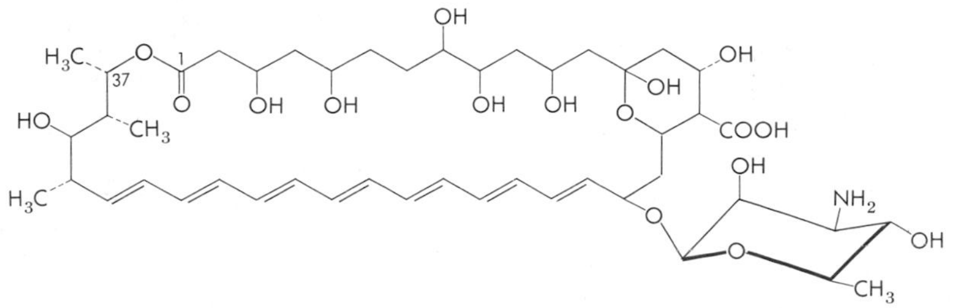

Amphotericin B

Antifungal Activity. *Histoplasma capsulatum, Cryptococcus neoformans, Coccidioides immitis, Candida* species, *Torulopsis glabrata, Rhodotorula, Blastomyces dermatitidis, B. braziliensis,* some strains of *Aspergillus,* and *Sporotrichum schenckii* are sensitive to concentrations of amphotericin B ranging from 0.03 to 1.0 µg/ml *in vitro.* The antibiotic is either fungistatic or fungicidal, depending on the concentration of the drug and the sensitivity of the fungus. It is without effect on bacteria, rickettsiae, or viruses.

The antifungal activity of amphotericin can be enhanced when the drug is combined with certain antimicrobial agents (Bennett, 1979). Rifampin, which has no antifungal activity when used alone, reduces the concentration of amphotericin B required to inhibit the growth of *Aspergillus, Histoplasma,* or *Candida* by fourfold *in vitro* (Kobayashi et al., 1972; Beggs et al., 1976; Kitahara et al., 1976b). Similar effects have also been observed in experimental infections (Kitahara et al., 1976a; Arroyo et al., 1977). Likewise, minocycline enhances the activity of amphotericin B *in vitro* against *Candida, Torulopsis,* and *Cryptococcus* (Lew et al., 1978). Flucytosine also reduces the concentration of amphotericin B necessary to inhibit growth of *Candida* and *Cryptococcus in vitro* (Medoff et al., 1971a); however, these two drugs have no synergistic effect in the treatment of experimental infections caused by *Candida, Cryptococcus,* and *Aspergillus* (see Arroyo et al., 1977; Sande et al., 1977). The mechanism of these synergistic interactions is not completely understood but may involve increased penetration of drug because of damage to the cell membrane caused by amphotericin B.

Mechanism of Action. The mechanism of action of amphotericin B is the same as that of nystatin (*see above*).

Fungal Resistance. Strains of *C. albicans* and *Coccid. immitis* serially subcultured in increasing concentrations of amphotericin B become resistant to the drug. Mutants of *C. albicans* that are resistant to the polyene also have an altered colonial morphology, slower rate of growth, and decreased virulence for animals (Hebeka and Solotorovsky, 1965). There is no evidence at present that resistance develops *in vivo.*

Absorption, Distribution, and Excretion.
Amphotericin B is poorly absorbed from the gastrointestinal tract. The *oral administration* of about 3 g a day produces plasma concentrations of about 0.1 to 0.5 µg/ml. The *intravenous injection* of 1 to 5 mg of amphotericin B per day initially, followed by the gradual increase of the daily dose to 0.4 to 0.6 mg/kg, yields peak values of approximately 0.5 to 2 µg/ml. After a rapid initial fall, the concentration of the drug in plasma approaches a plateau of about 0.5 µg/ml (Bindschalder and Bennett, 1969). It is probable that most

of the antibiotic is bound to cholesterol-containing membranes in many different tissues. However, details of possible pathways of drug metabolism are unknown. Approximately 95% of the drug circulating in plasma is bound to lipoproteins (Block et al., 1974; Bennett, 1977). Concentrations of amphotericin B in fluids from inflamed pleura, peritoneum, synovium, and aqueous humor are approximately two thirds of trough concentrations in plasma. The drug probably crosses the placenta readily (Bennett, 1979). Little amphotericin B penetrates into cerebrospinal fluid, vitreous humor, or normal amniotic fluid.

The antifungal agent is excreted very slowly in the urine, and only a small fraction of a given dose is excreted in active form; when therapy is stopped, the drug can be detected in the urine for at least 7 to 8 weeks. The concentration of amphotericin B in urine roughly parallels that in plasma. Since this represents only a small fraction of the dose administered, there is no further accumulation of the drug in the plasma of patients with impaired renal function (Feldman et al., 1973). Hemodialysis does not alter the concentration of amphotericin B in plasma.

The clinical pharmacology of amphotericin B is discussed by Bindschalder and Bennett (1969), Diamond and Bennett (1973), Feldman and associates (1973), and Bennett (1974, 1979).

Preparations, Routes of Administration, and Dosage. *Amphotericin B,* U.S.P. (FUNGIZONE), is available as an official injection. The sterile, lyophilized *powder* is marketed in vials containing 50 mg of amphotericin B, plus sodium deoxycholate to effect a colloidal dispersion of the insoluble antibiotic, buffers, and diluent. The contents of the vial should be dissolved, with shaking, in 10 ml of sterile water and then added to 5% dextrose in water to make a final concentration of 0.1 mg/ml. *Solutions of electrolytes, acidic solutions, or solutions with preservatives should not be used* because they cause precipitation of the antibiotic. Solutions in which precipitate or foreign material is present must be discarded. Fresh solutions should be prepared for each injection. The addition of 0.7 mg/kg of hydrocortisone may abolish or reduce chills in some but not all patients. Intravenous infusion by means of a pediatric scalp-vein needle and the addition of heparin (1000 units per infusion) minimizes the risk of thrombophlebitis. A cream, lotion, and ointment containing 3% amphotericin B are also marketed.

Opinions vary as to the most effective dosage and schedule for administration of amphotericin B. To a certain extent, this is dependent on the type and severity of infection. Most agree that a small test dose (1 mg dissolved in 20 ml of 5% dextrose solution) should first be administered intravenously over 10 to 30 minutes. The temperature, pulse, respiratory rate, and blood pressure should be recorded every 30 minutes for 4 hours and the size of the next dose determined by the severity of the reaction. Fever, chills, hypotension, and dyspnea are common. A patient with a severe, rapidly progressing fungal infection, good cardiopulmonary function, and a mild reaction to the test dose can immediately receive 0.3 mg/kg of amphotericin B intravenously dissolved in 500 ml of 5% dextrose in water over a period of 2 to 6 hours (Bennett, 1979). If the patient has a severe reaction to the test dose or cardiopulmonary impairment, a smaller second dose is recommended—for example, 5 to 10 mg. This may then be increased by 5 to 10 mg per day to a final daily dosage of 0.5 mg/kg or, at most, 0.7 mg/kg in patients with normal renal function. While daily maintenance doses of 1 to 1.5 mg/kg have been recommended in the past by some investigators, such regimens often cause renal toxicity and have no documented therapeutic advantage. Others have suggested that smaller daily doses (0.3 to 0.5 mg/kg) can be used effectively for the treatment of most mycoses. They recommend that dosage be adjusted to produce a peak concentration in plasma at least twice that required to inhibit growth of the fungus isolated from the patient (see Andrioli and Kravetz, 1962; Drutz et al., 1968; Bindschalder and Bennett, 1969). Still others have suggested that adjustment of dose on the basis of concentrations in plasma and the sensitivity of the microorganism is of little value, since the technic is difficult and of unproven clinical benefit (Bennett, 1974). Unusually small doses of the drug given intravenously (10 to 355 mg over 4 to 18 days) have cured some patients with severe Candida infections (Medoff et al., 1971b).

The febrile reactions associated with the administration of amphotericin B usually subside despite consistent use of the drug, and the concurrent use of hydrocortisone can frequently be stopped. Amphotericin B may be administered every other day by doubling the recommended daily dose without sacrifice of therapeutic efficacy (Bennett, 1979). Although this schedule decreases the number of venipunctures and allows more ambulation, there is no reduction in nephrotoxicity and the severity of febrile reactions may increase.

Intrathecal infusion of amphotericin B may be necessary in patients with meningitis caused by Coccidioides. Up to 0.5 mg of the drug is dissolved in at least 5 ml of spinal fluid and is injected two or three times a week into the lumbar, cisternal, or ventricular cerebrospinal fluid. The addition of hydrocortisone (5 to 15 mg) to the injection may reduce side effects, such as fever, headache, and nausea. Use of an artificial reservoir may be necessary for long-term treatment (Posner, 1973); daily doses of up to 0.3 mg infused intraventricularly over a 1-hour period have been used. The incidence of complications with this technic is high (Diamond and Bennett, 1973). Intra-articular doses of 5 to 15 mg have also been administered.

Untoward Effects. A large number and variety of untoward effects may be associated with the use of amphotericin B. These include *anaphylaxis, thrombopenia, flushing, generalized pain, convulsions, chills, fever, phlebitis, headache, anemia, anorexia,* and *decreased renal function.* About 50% of initial intravenous injections of the drug are associated with chills and about 20% with vomiting; the temperature may rise to as high as 40° C. Fever and chills may develop with every injection in the same individual, but they usually decrease with sequential injections. There is no clear proof that amphotericin B causes hepatic toxicity (Bennett, 1974), although early reports suggested this association.

Renal function becomes impaired in over 80% of persons given amphotericin B, and this should thus be expected as a result of treatment. The degree of azotemia commonly plateaus at a level that correlates with the daily dose. Renal function usually returns toward normal upon completion of therapy, but most patients who receive a complete course will be left with some residual reduction in glomerular filtration (Butler et al., 1964). The degree of damage is dependent on the total dose of drug and does not correlate with the concentration of creatinine in plasma during therapy. However, reduction in dosage is recommended when plasma creatinine increases above 3.5 mg/dl to prevent symptoms of uremia (Bennett, 1979). Adequate hydration remains the most important method of minimizing azotemia. *Mild renal tubular acidosis* and *hypokalemia* are frequent, and supplemental administration of potassium may be required. *Hypomagnesemia* is also observed, but it is not clear if this effect is of renal origin. In general, when a total dose of 4 g is administered over 6 weeks or more, permanent damage may occur. Pathological changes are seen particularly in the renal tubular cells but also may include thickening and fragmentation of the glomerular basement membrane, hypercellularity, fibrosis and hyalinization of the glomeruli, and nephrocalcinosis (McCurdy et al., 1968; Douglas and Healy, 1969).

Amphotericin B frequently produces normochromic, normocytic *anemia;* the bone marrow reveals a decrease in erythrocyte production; the blood picture usually becomes normal after treatment is stopped. Amphotericin-induced anemia is associated with very low concentrations of erythropoietin (MacGregor *et al.*, 1978). *Leukopenia* and *thrombopenia* may occur rarely.

The *intrathecal injection* of amphotericin B may produce *pain along the distribution of lumbar nerves, headache, paresthesias, nerve palsies* (including *footdrop*), *chemical meningitis, difficulty in micturition,* and possibly *impairment of vision.*

The subconjunctival injection of amphotericin B may produce permanent yellow discoloration of the conjunctiva. When the dose exceeds 5 mg, salmon-colored, raised nodules develop on the conjunctiva; these resolve gradually after treatment is stopped (Bell and Ritchey, 1973).

For reviews of the untoward effects of amphotericin B, *see* Utz and coworkers (1964), Bennett (1974, 1979), and Weinstein and Weinstein (1974).

Therapeutic Uses. Amphotericin B is effective in a number of *fungal infections* that, prior to the availability of this drug, were almost invariably fatal (*see* page 1239).

The duration of treatment with amphotericin B varies with the nature, severity, and course of the infection, as well as with the development of untoward effects that may necessitate the temporary cessation of therapy or a reduction in dose; recurrences require another full course of drug. Except for treatment of certain infections caused by *Candida,* the period of therapy is usually about 6 to 10 weeks; it may need to be extended to as long as 3 to 4 months in some cases. *All patients requiring amphotericin B must be hospitalized,* at least for the initiation of therapy, and they must be under close observation throughout a course of systemic administration of the drug. Hemograms and urinalyses, as well as determinations of the concentrations of potassium, magnesium, urea nitrogen, and creatinine in plasma, should be made two to three times a week, especially during the period when the dose is being increased. If evidence of significant renal insufficiency appears, the dose may have to be reduced.

Amphotericin B has been administered simultaneously with tetracyclines to suppress overgrowth of yeasts and fungi that may be induced by the broad-spectrum antibiotics. There is no clinical evidence that this is either necessary or effective.

FLUCYTOSINE

Chemistry. *Flucytosine* is a fluorinated pyrimidine related to fluorouracil and floxuridine. It is 5-fluorocytosine, the formula of which is as follows:

Flucytosine

Antifungal Activity. Flucytosine inhibits the multiplication of *Cryp. neoformans* at concentrations of 0.5 to 4 $\mu g/ml$. In some studies, up to 50% of strains of *C. albicans* are resistant (MIC, $>100\ \mu g/ml$), while susceptible strains of *Candida* are suppressed by concentrations of the drug ranging from 0.4 to 8 $\mu g/ml$. Strains of *Torula glabrata* are inhibited by concentrations of 0.5 to 1 $\mu g/ml$. The minimal fungistatic concentrations for *Aspergillus* species range from 0.5 to greater than 100 $\mu g/ml$, and the majority of isolates are probably resistant (MIC, $>15\ \mu g/ml$). Some species of *Cladosporium*, especially *Cladosporium trichoides* (Block *et al.*, 1973), and *Phialophora* (Vandevelde *et al.*, 1972), the agents responsible for chromoblastomycosis, are sensitive. The combination of flucytosine and amphotericin B results in supra-additive activity *in vitro* against *Cryp. neoformans* and sensitive strains of *C. albicans* and *C. tropicalis.* Flucytosine is without effect on most strains of *Spor. schenckii* and all strains of *B. dermatitidis, H. capsulatum, Coccid. immitis, Rhizopus oryzae,* and *Absidia corymbifer.* Bacteria are resistant. (*See* Marks *et al.*, 1971; Medoff *et al.*, 1971a; Brandsberg and French, 1972; Bennett, 1974, 1979; Lauer *et al.*, 1978.)

Fungal Resistance. Development of resistance to flucytosine *during therapy* has been described in 30% of patients with cryptococcosis (Block *et al.*, 1973), and this has severely restricted its use for the sole treatment of fungal infections. Resistance to flucytosine can also develop during treatment of infections with *C. albicans* (Normark and Schönebeck, 1972). The mechanisms of drug resistance are not completely understood.

Mechanism of Action. Flucytosine is converted in fungal cells to *fluorouracil* by the enzyme cytosine deaminase. Fluorouracil can then be metabolized to 5-fluorodeoxyuridylic acid, an inhibitor of thymidylate synthetase. Synthesis of 5-fluorouridine triphosphate and RNA that contains this analog may also take place. Cells of the host do not convert large amounts of flucytosine to fluorouracil, as do fungi. This is crucial for the selective action of this compound. The cytotoxic activity of fluorinated pyrimidines is discussed in detail in Chapter 55.

Absorption, Distribution, and Excretion. Flucytosine is rapidly and well absorbed from the gastrointestinal tract. It is widely distributed in the body, with a volume of distribution closely approximating the total body water. The drug is minimally bound to plasma proteins. The peak plasma concentration in patients with normal renal function is approximately 70 to 80 $\mu g/ml$ 1 to 2 hours after a dose of 37.5 mg/kg (Bennett *et al.*, 1979). Approximately 80% of a given dose is excreted in the urine by glomerular filtration in unchanged form; concentrations in the urine range from 200 to 500 $\mu g/ml$. The half-life of the drug is 3 to 6 hours in normal individuals. In renal failure, the half-life may be as long as 200 hours. There is a linear relation between the elimination rate constant and creatinine clearance; in normal persons, the renal clearance of flucytosine is about 75% of that for creatinine. Because of the obligate renal excretion of the drug, modification of dosage is necessary in patients with a serum creatinine of 1.7 mg/dl or greater (*see* Appendix II). It is recommended that concentrations of drug in plasma be measured periodically in patients with renal insufficiency. Peak concentrations should range between 50 and 100 μg/ml. Flucytosine is cleared by hemodialysis, and patients undergoing such treatment should receive a single dose of 37.5 mg/kg after dialysis (Bennett, 1979); the drug is also removed by peritoneal dialysis.

Flucytosine is present in cerebrospinal fluid at a concentration about 65 to 90% of that simultaneously present in the plasma. The drug also penetrates into the aqueous humor.

Preparations, Routes of Administration, and Dosage. *Flucytosine,* U.S.P. (ANCOBON), is supplied in capsules containing either 250 or 500 mg for oral administration. There are no parenteral preparations. The usual daily dose is 50 to 150 mg/kg, given at 6-hour intervals. This dosage must be altered, as described above, for patients with renal insufficiency.

Untoward Effects. Flucytosine may depress the function of bone marrow and lead to the development of *anemia, leukopenia,* and *thrombocytopenia;* patients are more prone to the appearance of this complication if they have an underlying hematological disorder, are being treated with radiation or drugs that injure the bone marrow, or have a history of treatment with such agents. Other untoward effects, including *nausea, vomiting, diarrhea,* and severe *enterocolitis,* have been noted. In approximately 5% of patients elevation of the activities of hepatic enzymes in plasma and *hepatomegaly* have occurred, but these are reversible when therapy is stopped (Steer *et al.,* 1972). All of these complications are more frequent in patients with azotemia and are markedly increased when concentrations of the drug in plasma exceed 100 to 125 μg/ml (Kauffman and Frame, 1977). Some toxicity may be the result of conversion of flucytosine to 5-fluorouracil by the host (Diasio *et al.,* 1978).

Therapeutic Uses. Amphotericin B remains the most effective therapeutic agent for the management of infections due to yeasts and fungi; flucytosine is used predominantly in combination with amphotericin B. It is less toxic than amphotericin B and it can be administered orally. However, except in the treatment of chromoblastomycosis, rapid emergence of flucytosine-resistant strains has restricted its use as a single drug (Mauceri *et al.,* 1974). The concurrent administration of amphotericin B (0.3 mg/kg per day) and flucytosine (150 mg/kg per day) has become the treatment of choice for cryptococcal meningitis (*see* page 1239; Utz *et al.,* 1975; Bennett *et al.,* 1979).

GRISEOFULVIN

History and Source. *Griseofulvin* was first isolated from *Penicillium griseofulvum dierckx* by Oxford and coworkers in 1939. Because it was ineffective against bacteria, no further attention was paid to it for some time. In 1946, Brian and associates found a substance in *Penicillium janczewski* that produced shrinking and stunting of fungal hyphae; they named this the *curling factor;* it was later found to be *griseofulvin.* During the next 10 years, the antibiotic was widely employed in the treatment of a variety of fungal diseases in plants and of ringworm of cattle. In the course of a search for potential therapeutic compounds for the management of fungal infections of the feet of Scottish miners, Gentles (1958) observed that griseofulvin cured experimentally produced mycotic disease of guinea pigs. Soon thereafter, the drug was widely subjected to clinical trial and became available for general use.

Chemistry. The structural formula of griseofulvin is as follows:

Griseofulvin

The drug is practically insoluble in water. It is remarkably thermostable.

Antifungal Activity. Griseofulvin is fungistatic *in vitro* for various species of the dermatophytes *Microsporum, Epidermophyton,* and *Trichophyton.* The drug has no effect on bacteria or on other fungi, yeasts, *Actinomyces,* or *Nocardia.* Young, actively metabolizing cells may be killed by the drug, but older, more dormant elements are only inhibited.

Fungal Resistance. *Trichophyton, Epidermophyton,* and *Microsporum* can be made resistant to griseofulvin *in vitro,* and such strains remain fully virulent as infectious agents in animals. Isolates from humans receiving the antibiotic appear, with a few exceptions, to retain their sensitivity to the drug when examined *in vitro.* Dermatophytes concentrate griseofulvin by an energy-dependent process, and such uptake is correlated with the sensitivity of the fungi to the antibiotic (*see* El-Nakeeb and Lampen, 1965).

Mechanism of Action. A prominent morphological manifestation of the action of griseofulvin is the production of multinucleate cells, and the drug thus inhibits fungal mitosis (Gull and Trinci, 1973). An explanation for this phenomenon appears to come from studies of the effects of higher concentrations of the antibiotic on mammalian cells. Griseofulvin causes disruption of the mitotic spindle by interacting with polymerized microtubules. While the effects of the drug are thus similar to those of colchicine and the *Vinca* alkaloids, its binding sites on the microtubular protein are distinct. (*See* Malawista *et al.,* 1968; Wilson, 1970; Grisham *et al.,* 1973.)

Absorption, Distribution, and Excretion. The oral administration of griseofulvin produces peak plasma concentrations at about 4 hours, approximately 1 μg/ml when a single dose of 0.5 g is given. These values are quite variable, perhaps due to difficulty in absorption from the intestine (mainly the upper small intestine), because of the insolubility of griseofulvin in aqueous media. Micronized preparations are much better absorbed. The drug has a half-life in plasma of about 1 day, and approximately 50% of the oral dose can be detected in the urine within 5 days, mostly in the form of metabolites. The primary metabolite is 6-methylgriseofulvin (Lin *et al.,* 1973).

The drug has a greater affinity for diseased skin than for normal skin. It is deposited in keratin precursor cells. The antibiotic present in such cells when they differentiate is tightly bound to, and persists in, *keratin* and makes this substance resistant to fungal invasion. For this reason, the new growth of hair or nails is the first to become free of disease. As the fungus-containing keratin is shed, it is replaced by normal tissue. Griseofulvin is detectable in the stratum corneum of the skin within 4 to 8 hours of oral administration. Sweat and transepidermal fluid loss play an important role in the transfer of the drug in the stratum corneum (Shah *et al.,* 1974). Only a very small fraction of a dose of the drug is present in body fluids and tissues.

Preparations, Routes of Administration, and Dosage. *Griseofulvin,* U.S.P. (FULVICIN U/F, GRIFULVIN V, GRISACTIN), is marketed in *capsules* containing 125 or 250 mg and in *tablets* containing 125, 250, or 500 mg; it is also available as an *oral suspension* (125 mg/5 ml). The daily dose recommended for children is 10 mg/kg; for adults, 500 mg to 1.0 g. Larger doses (1.5 to 2 g per day) may be used for a short time in severe and extensive infections, but the amount should be reduced to 500 mg to 1 g per day when the lesions begin to respond. Best results may be obtained when the calculated dose is divided into four equal parts and given at 6-hour intervals. The length of treatment varies with the location of the infection, as discussed below. Tablets incorporating an ultramicrosized preparation (FULVICIN P/G, GRIS-PEG) contain 125 or 250 mg of griseofulvin (equivalent to 250 or 500 mg of the preparations listed above).

Untoward Effects. The incidence of serious reactions associated with the use of griseofulvin is very low. Among the minor effects, the incidence of which may be as high as 15%, is *headache* that is sometimes severe and usually disappears as therapy is continued. Other *nervous system manifestations* include peripheral neuritis, lethargy, mental confusion, impairment of performance of routine efforts, fatigue, syncope, vertigo, blurred vision, transient macular edema, and augmentation of the effects of alcohol. Among the side effects involving the *alimentary tract* are nausea, vomiting, diarrhea, heartburn, flatulence, dry mouth, and angular stomatitis. *Hepatotoxicity* has also been observed. *Hematological effects* include leukopenia, neutropenia, punctate basophilia, and

monocytosis; these often disappear despite continuation of therapy. Blood studies should be carried out at least once a week during the first month of treatment or longer. Common *renal effects* include albuminuria and cylindruria, without evidence of renal insufficiency. Reactions involving the *skin* are cold and warm urticaria, photosensitivity, lichen planus, erythema, erythema multiforme-like rashes, and vesicular and morbilliform eruptions. *Serum-sickness syndromes* and severe *angioedema* develop rarely during treatment with griseofulvin. *Estrogen-like effects* have been observed in children. A moderate but inconsistent increase of *fecal protoporphyrins* has been noted when the drug is used for a long period of time. *Candida intertrigo* may complicate griseofulvin therapy.

Griseofulvin appears to reduce the activity of warfarin-like anticoagulants, and adjustment of the dosage of the latter agent may be necessary in at least some patients. Barbiturates decrease the absorption of griseofulvin from the gastrointestinal tract; the effect of this interaction on the antifungal response requires further study (Riegelman *et al.,* 1970).

Therapeutic Uses. Mycotic disease of the *skin, hair,* and *nails* due to *Microsporum, Trichophyton,* or *Epidermophyton* respond to griseofulvin therapy. Since other fungal diseases are not affected by the drug, careful mycological study with identification of the responsible organism is critical. Readily treatable with this agent are infections of the *hair* (*tinea capitis*) caused by *M. canis, M. audouini, T. schoenleini,* and *T. verrucosum;* "ringworm" *of the glabrous skin; tinea cruris* and *tinea corporis* caused by *M. canis, T. rubrum, T. verrucosum,* and *Epidermophyton floccosum;* and *tinea of the hands* (*T. rubrum, T. mentagrophytes*) and *beard* (*Trichophyton* species). Griseofulvin is also highly effective in "athlete's foot" or epidermophytosis involving the skin and nails, the vesicular form of which is most commonly due to *T. mentagrophytes,* and the hyperkeratotic type to *T. rubrum.*

Symptomatic relief of disease of the skin usually appears after 48 to 96 hours of griseofulvin therapy. The first change is a decrease in erythema and induration of the lesions, followed by involution of scaling and hyperpigmentation over a period of several weeks. Lesions in non-intertriginous areas usually disappear completely in 2 to 4 weeks. Cultures for fungi become negative in 1 to 2 weeks. Treatment should be continued for about 3 weeks, if the palms, soles, and nails are not involved. Infections of the palms and soles respond more slowly and require therapy for 4 to 8 weeks; cultures become negative in 2 to 6 weeks. Since fingernails grow out completely in 4 months and toenails in about 6 months, fungal infections of these tissues require therapy for long periods—4 to 6 months for fingernails and 6 to 12 months for toenails. *Trichophyton rubrum* and *T. mentagrophytes* infections may require higher-than-conventional doses. It has been suggested that the hair be clipped after 2 to 3 weeks of treatment in cases of *tinea capitis;* the advantage of this has not been proved. (For review of griseofulvin therapy, *see* Symposium, 1960; Goldman, 1970.)

MISCELLANEOUS ANTIFUNGAL AGENTS

Hydroxystilbamidine Isethionate. This drug, an aromatic diamidine, is active against fungi and protozoa. Like its congener, *pentamidine* (Chapter 47), it has a suppressive effect on *B. dermatitidis in vitro* and in experimental infections in mice, and has produced favorable results in cutaneous and pulmonary *human North American blastomycosis;* however, the incidence of relapse has been high. The alarming untoward effects that may be produced by the compound are the same as those caused by pentamidine. *Sterile Hydroxystilbamidine Isethionate,* U.S.P., is available in vials containing 225 mg of dry, sterile powder. A freshly prepared solution of 225 mg of the drug in 200 ml of 5% dextrose in water or isotonic sodium chloride solution is infused over a period of 2 to 3 hours, every 24 hours; rapid infusion may cause hypotension. The solution must be protected from light. The duration of therapy varies with the location and the severity of the disease, but the drug is not usually recommended to treat severe blastomycosis (*see* below). Anorexia, malaise, and nausea are common untoward responses to hydroxystilbamidine; rash and hepatotoxicity also occur.

Miconazole. This drug, an imidazole, is described in Chapter 41, as are its uses as a topical antifungal agent. Miconazole is also used parenterally for the treatment of severe systemic fungal infection (*see* Bennett, 1979); for this purpose it is supplied in 20-ml ampuls that contain 10 mg of miconazole per milliliter (MONISTAT I.V.). Following infusion of 600 to 1000 mg of miconazole to adults, concentrations in plasma exceed 1 μg/ml for only 1 to 2 hours (Stevens *et al.,* 1976); the minimal inhibitory concentrations for most pathogenic fungi range from 2 to 8 μg/ml. This dosage is usually administered every 8 hours. Penetration into cerebrospinal fluid is poor, and intrathecal administration of the drug is necessary in meningitis. Intracisternal doses of 5 to 15 mg have been used successfully to treat coccidioidal meningitis. The drug has also been used with limited success in other forms of coccidioidomycosis, paracoccidioidomycosis, and petriellidiosis (Stevens, 1977; Stevens *et al.,* 1978; Lutwick *et al.,* 1979). There are few data to support its use in the treatment of systemic candidiasis and cryptococcosis.

Adverse reactions are frequent after the intravenous administration of miconazole and include nausea, phlebitis, anemia, thrombocytopenia, and, especially, pruritus. The majority of patients who receive the drug for extended periods develop severe itching (Stevens, 1977). Hyponatremia has been observed in up to 50% of patients. Arthralgias, anaphylaxis, acute psychosis, and hyperlipidemia have also been observed.

THERAPY OF SYSTEMIC FUNGAL INFECTIONS

Therapeutic regimens for the treatment of systemic fungal infections have been reviewed by Bennett (1974, 1979) and by Medoff and Kobayashi (1980).

Cryptococcosis. Cryptococcal infection may primarily involve the lungs or the meninges or be widely disseminated. Meningeal or disseminated infections always require therapy, since mortality without treatment is nearly uniform. Some patients with symptomatic cryptococcal pneumonia may also benefit from treatment with amphotericin B (Scheld *et al.,* 1979). Treatment of cryptococcal meningitis with high doses of amphotericin B (1 mg/kg daily for 6 weeks) results in favorable clinical responses in 75% of patients, but relapse occurs in up to one third of these individuals after treatment is discontinued (Sarosi *et al.,* 1969). In addition, the incidence of toxicity is extremely high. Low doses of amphotericin B (0.3 to 0.4 mg/kg daily for 10 weeks) are equally efficacious and cause less toxicity (Drutz *et al.,* 1968). The concurrent administration of low doses of amphotericin B (20 mg daily) and flucytosine (150 mg/kg per day) for 6 weeks apparently cured 12 patients (Utz *et al.,* 1975), and this report stimulated a multicenter study to compare amphotericin B (0.4 mg/kg per day for 10 weeks) with a regimen of amphotericin B (0.3 mg/kg per day) plus flucytosine (150 mg/kg per day) for 6 weeks. Results suggest that the combination is superior, as measured by a more rapid rate of sterilization of the cerebrospinal fluid and reduced toxicity. The overall rate of cure also favored the two-drug regimen (Bennett, 1979).

Histoplasmosis. *Histoplasma capsulatum* produces a variety of clinical syndromes. Acute pulmonary histoplasmosis is usually self-limited and rarely requires treatment. However, when symptoms are severe or persist beyond 14 days, patients will often respond rapidly to an abbreviated course of amphotericin B (0.4 to 0.7 mg/kg per day for a total dose of 800 to 1000 mg) (Fosson and Wheeler, 1975; Naylor, 1977). Chronic cavitary histoplasmosis is typically a progressive disease, and the mortality rate, if untreated, is 30%. Administration of a total of 1.5 to 2 g of amphotericin B over a period of 10 weeks has been successful therapy (Sutliff, 1972; Goodwin and Des Prez, 1978). Progressive disseminated histoplasmosis has a mortality rate of 80 to 90% if untreated and requires intensive treatment with amphotericin B (Smith and Utz, 1972); the usual course is a total of 2 g of amphotericin B given over a period of 10 weeks (Goodwin and Des Prez, 1978).

Coccidioidomycosis. Amphotericin B has been recommended for treatment of disseminated coccidioidomycosis, although miconazole has also been studied recently. While primary pulmonary coccidioidomycosis usually does not require treatment, amphotericin B may be of benefit when symptoms are severe. Since this microorganism is relatively resistant to amphotericin B (MIC, 1 μg/ml), doses of 1 mg/kg given every other day may be required for prolonged periods. Treatment of meningitis usually requires intrathecal administration of 1 mg of amphotericin B three times per week. As mentioned above, direct intraventricular administration with a reservoir may be used, and treatment should probably be continued for at least 3 months after the cerebrospinal fluid appears sterile (Goldstein et al., 1972).

Relapsing and resistant cases of coccidioidomycosis have responded to immunotherapy with transfer factor plus amphotericin B (Graybill, 1977). Studies are currently under way to evaluate this treatment. Miconazole is indicated in patients who cannot tolerate amphotericin B.

Blastomycosis and Paracoccidioidomycosis. Both of these diseases respond to treatment with amphotericin B. Recommended doses are similar to those for disseminated histoplasmosis—a total dose of 1.5 g, given over 6 to 10 weeks. Sulfonamides have been used to treat patients with paracoccidioidomycosis (South American blastomycosis), and favorable clinical responses occur, but patients invariably relapse when therapy is discontinued (Abernathy, 1973). Hydroxystilbamidine isethionate is effective for cutaneous or localized pulmonary blastomycosis. However, it is less effective than amphotericin B and should not be used in patients with disseminated disease.

Sporotrichosis. Amphotericin B in standard doses (total dose of 1.5 to 2 g over 6 to 10 weeks) has been used successfully in the therapy of systemic sporotrichosis, especially when the disease involves bones and joints (Crout et al., 1977). The cutaneous-lymphatic form of sporotrichosis frequently responds to the oral administration of iodides.

Candidiasis. Amphotericin B is the preferred drug for the treatment of disseminated candidiasis. Most patients with this disease have suppressed immunological responses, are neutropenic, and show evidence of sustained fungemia (multiple positive blood cultures for Candida). Amphotericin B is effective in eradicating the fungus in some instances; total doses have varied from 100 to 2500 mg (Young et al., 1974). A dose of 40 mg, given every other day, to a total dose of 600 to 1000 mg is probably adequate in many instances. Treatment is usually not necessary for transient fungemia associated with infected indwelling intravascular catheters, since the microorganism usually disappears when the foreign body is removed. Very low doses of amphotericin B (20 mg daily for 10 days) have been used to treat esophagitis caused by Candida (Medoff et al., 1972). The response is usually dramatic, with a reduction in symptoms and disappearance of the plaquelike lesions. Endocarditis produced by Candida species that involves natural or prosthetic valves may respond clinically to amphotericin B (with or without concurrent administration of flucytosine), but cure almost always requires surgical removal of the infected valve.

Other Infections. Invasive infections caused by Aspergillus species and Zygomycetes respond erratically to treatment with amphotericin B (Meyer et al., 1973). Addition of flucytosine to the regimen may be useful for patients who are immunologically suppressed (Burton et al., 1972). Primary amebic meningoencephalitis has occasionally responded to the intrathecal administration of amphotericin B (Anderson and Jamieson, 1972) and to a combination of miconazole, rifampin, and intrathecal amphotericin B (Morbidity and Mortality Weekly Report, 1978).

III. Antiviral Agents

The development of compounds useful for the prophylaxis and therapy of viral disease has presented more difficult problems than those encountered in the search for drugs effective in disorders produced by other microorganisms. This is so because, in contrast to most other infectious agents, viruses are obligate intracellular parasites that require the active participation of the metabolic processes of the invaded cell. Thus, agents that may inhibit or cause the death of viruses are also very likely to injure the host cells that harbor them. Although the search for substances that might be of use in the management of viral infections has been long and intensive, very few agents have been found to have clinical applicability. Indeed, even these have exhibited very narrow activity, limited to one or only a few specific viruses. These drugs are described briefly here. (See Weinstein and Chang, 1973; Hayden and Douglas, 1979; Hirsch and Swartz, 1980.)

Idoxuridine. Idoxuridine, U.S.P. (DENDRID, HERPLEX, STOXIL), is 5-iodo-2'-deoxyuridine. It is soluble in water (2 mg/ml) and stable at temperatures up to 65° C but sensitive to light. Official preparations are an ophthalmic ointment (0.5%) and an ophthalmic solution (0.1%).

Idoxuridine is a halogenated pyrimidine that resembles thymidine. Following phosphorylation within cells, the triphosphate derivative is incorporated into both viral and mammalian DNA. Such DNA is more susceptible to breakage, and altered viral proteins may result from faulty transcription (see Pratt, 1977). Thus, the activity of idoxuridine is largely limited to DNA viruses, primarily members of the herpesvirus group. The drug is active in vitro against vaccinia virus, herpes simplex virus, varicella virus, cytomegalovirus, and others at concentrations of 10 μg/ml or less (Prusoff and Goz, 1973; Prusoff and Ward, 1976). The development of resistance of viruses to the drug in vitro occurs readily, but the clinical significance of such resistance is not well documented.

Idoxuridine is rapidly inactivated by nucleotidases; this fact precludes its use by other than intravenous or topical administration. After intravenous injection, most of the active form of the drug disappears from the blood in about 30 minutes. A small amount is excreted in the urine.

The primary clinical use of the drug has been in herpes simplex keratitis. Maxwell (1963) reported on 1500 cases; he noted a correlation between the type of infection and the response to therapy. Epithelial infections, especially initial attacks in which a dendritic figure is present, respond best. The results are less favorable when the stroma is involved. In recurrent episodes, the acute disease is often controlled, but scarring caused by a previous attack is not altered. It is important to stress that total healing or improvement does not occur in all instances, even in those with the most superficial involvement. *Herpes simplex* type 2 does not respond to the drug. When applied topically to the conjunctiva, irritation, pain, pruritus, inflammation or edema of the eyelids, and photophobia may develop. Punctate areas may appear in the cornea; it is difficult to ascertain whether these are related to the disease or to therapy. Topical *vidarabine* is equally effective and probably less irritating and allergenic (Pavan-Langston and Buchanan, 1976).

The *dose* of the official 0.1% solution of idoxuridine is 1 drop in the conjunctival sac every hour during the day and every 2 hours during the night until definite improvement is apparent, after which the same quantity is applied every 2 hours during the day and every 4 hours at night. When the 0.5% ointment is used, it is applied every 4 hours during the day and once before bedtime. Therapy is continued for 3 to 5 days after healing is complete, as demonstrated by fluorescein staining.

Two placebo-controlled double-blind studies of the efficacy of idoxuridine in proven cases of herpes simplex encephalitis have failed to demonstrate any therapeutic value of the drug (100 mg/kg per day for 5 days). Myelosuppression caused by idoxuridine coupled with its failure to prevent death led to the termination of these studies (*see* Boston Interhospital and Cooperative Study, 1975). There are currently no indications for the parenteral use of this drug.

Amantadine. *Amantadine* (*1-adamantanamine*) is a synthetic antiviral agent first described by Davies and associates (1964). It is a water-soluble, tricyclic amine of unusual structure unrelated to that of any of the other antimicrobial agents. Its structural formula is as follows:

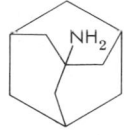

Amantadine

Amantadine inhibits replication of strains of influenza A virus at an early point, probably the stage of uncoating. Attachment of the virus to cells and penetration are not impaired (Skehel *et al.*, 1978). Using a sensitive plaque-reduction assay, Hayden and Douglas (1979) found that most strains of influenza A viruses, including H3N2, Hsw1N1, and H1N1 subtypes, are inhibited by 0.4 µg/ml of amantadine or less. Higher concentrations than can be safely achieved in man are required to inhibit influenza B, parainfluenza, respiratory syncytial, or rubella viruses.

Amantadine is almost completely absorbed from the gastrointestinal tract. Approximately 90% of an orally administered dose is excreted in the urine (50% within 20 hours) in unchanged form; the drug is not metabolized in the body.

A number of studies have demonstrated the effectiveness of this compound in *preventing* infection of tissue cultures and experimental animals by different strains of influenza A viruses. An adequate number of studies have been performed to indicate that amantadine has prophylactic value when administered to humans who have had contact with an active case of influenza A or who have served as experimental subjects for this infection. The drug is valuable in both nosocomial and community settings (*see* Hayden and Douglas, 1979). In double-blind, placebo-controlled studies of amantadine in patients with naturally occurring infections due to influenza A virus, the drug has been found to produce a therapeutic effect even when given within 48 hours after onset of illness. Statistically significant increases in the rates of overall clinical improvement, defervescence, and disappearance of signs and symptoms of illness were observed in the patients who received amantadine, compared to those given a placebo (Little *et al.*, 1976, 1978). A decrease in the frequency and quantity of shedding of virus has also been observed (Rabinovich *et al.*, 1969; Knight *et al.*, 1970). The development of specific antibody is not suppressed (Nafta *et al.*, 1970).

The use of amantadine is recommended in the presence of a documented influenza A virus epidemic in patients of all ages at high risk who have not received vaccine. Prophylactic administration of amantadine to high-risk patients should be initiated as soon as influenza A activity is documented in the community and continued for the duration of the epidemic (usually 5 to 6 weeks). Since the drug does not impair the immune response to influenza vaccine, patients can be vaccinated at the same time and amantadine discontinued after 10 to 14 days. The administration of amantadine to patients with established disease is controversial. Some suggest that treatment is worthwhile if it can be instituted within 48 hours of the onset of symptoms. The dosage is 200 mg per day for 3 to 5 days (Hayden and Douglas, 1979).

The discovery that amantadine is also useful in the treatment of parkinsonism was an act of serendipity. This therapeutic application is discussed in Chapter 21.

Amantadine Hydrochloride, U.S.P. (SYMMETREL), is available in capsules containing 100 mg and as a syrup (50 mg/5 ml). The dose for children 1 to 9 years of age is 4.4 to 8.8 mg/kg, but it should not exceed a total of 150 mg per day. For older children and adults, the dose is 200 mg once daily or 100 mg twice daily. Peak concentrations in plasma are 0.3 to 0.6 µg/ml after ingestion of a 200-mg dose. The drug accumulates in patients with impaired renal function. Plasma concentrations of 1 to 5 µg/ml are associated with CNS toxicity, including nervousness, confusion, hallucinations, seizures, and coma. One to 5% of patients with normal renal function who receive amantadine (200 mg per day) report minor neurological symptoms, including insomnia and difficulty in concentrating (LaMontagne and Galasso, 1979). Symptoms may be reduced by administration of 100 mg twice a day (Monto *et al.*, 1979). Persons with cerebral atherosclerosis, psychiatric disorders, or a history of epilepsy must be observed closely when taking this drug. It should not be given to pregnant women.

Methisazone. The structural formula of *methisazone* is as follows:

Methisazone

It is a synthetic antiviral agent that currently has little clinical use. The activity of this type of thiosemicarbazone against the pox group of viruses was first demonstrated by Hamre and associates (1950). The effectiveness of isatin 3-thiosemicarbazone in mice infected with vaccinia virus was reported by Thompson and coworkers (1953); the N-methyl congener, methisazone, was found by Bauer and Sadler (1960) to be markedly active against variola virus in mice.

The mechanism of action of methisazone is unclear. It does not interfere with the production of viral components during the early phases of the infectious cycle, but it appears to prevent proper translation of "late" viral mRNA. Despite the fact that the drug can inhibit the replication of a number of viruses in tissue culture, methisazone is effective *in vivo* mainly against the pox group of viruses.

Methisazone (MARBORAN) is only slightly soluble. For this reason, it is not administered parenterally. It is given as tablets or as a micronized preparation in syrup. The plasma concentrations achieved are variable. The only important reported *side effect* of methisazone is *vomiting;* this is common and may be severe, requiring the use of phenothiazines or other antiemetic agents.

Methisazone appears to be an effective prophylactic agent for smallpox, but it is without therapeutic effect once smallpox has developed. It has been suggested that it is useful in the treatment of two complications of vaccinia, *vaccinia gangrenosa* and *eczema vaccinatum.* Therapy involves the administration of an initial dose of 200 mg/kg, followed by 50 mg/kg every 6 hours for eight doses. Methisazone is currently not generally available in the United States.

Vidarabine. *Vidarabine* (adenine arabinoside, ara-A) is an analog of adenosine (arabinose is the $2'$-epimer of ribose). Its structural formula is as follows:

Vidarabine

Vidarabine and cytarabine were originally developed as antileukemic agents (*see* Chapter 55). Vidarabine has proven to be more effective in the treatment of *herpes simplex encephalitis* and *keratoconjunctivitis,* and it causes less toxicity than cytarabine. The latter drug is no longer used as an antiviral agent.

Vidarabine is phosphorylated to the corresponding nucleotides within the cell and acts by inhibiting viral DNA polymerase; mammalian DNA synthesis is inhibited to a lesser extent (Muller *et al.,* 1977). Vidarabine is also metabolized to the less active hypoxanthine arabinoside, which may act synergistically with the parent compound to inhibit the replication of large DNA viruses (Bryson and Connor, 1976; Champney *et al.,* 1978). The drug is most active against vaccinia virus (MIC, ~0.5 μg/ml), while most strains of herpes simplex virus, cytomegalovirus, and varicella-zoster virus are inhibited by 3 μg/ml or less (Luby *et al.,* 1975). The drug is not active against other DNA viruses, such as adenoviruses or papovaviruses, nor against RNA viruses.

Preparations and Dosage. The recommended daily dose of vidarabine for treatment of encephalitis caused by herpes simplex virus is 15 mg/kg. Since vidarabine is only slightly soluble in water, large volumes of fluid are needed to dissolve the compound (*e.g.,* 2.5 liters). The drug should be given intravenously at a constant rate over a 12- to 24-hour period daily, for 10 days. Treatment of herpes simplex keratoconjunctivitis is with a 3% ophthalmic ointment, which is administered topically every 3 hours.

Sterile Vidarabine, U.S.P. (VIRA-A), is available for injection in 5-ml vials that contain 200 mg/ml of the monohydrate (equivalent to 187 mg of vidarabine). The drug is also supplied as a 3% ophthalmic ointment (VIRA-A OPHTHALMIC).

Adverse Effects. Vidarabine causes relatively few side effects, but these can include nausea, vomiting, diarrhea, rash, weakness, and thrombophlebitis at the site of drug administration. Effects on the CNS, such as hallucinations, psychoses, ataxia, tremor, and dizziness, have been noted with high doses (20 mg/kg per day). Four patients with renal transplants and renal failure developed coma and died after receiving 10 mg/kg per day (Marker *et al.,* 1978). Although the relationship of treatment with vidarabine to the fatalities was unclear, the dosage should be reduced in patients with renal insufficiency. There is evidence that vidarabine is mutagenic and carcinogenic. It obviously should not be used to treat trivial infections.

Therapeutic Uses. Vidarabine has proven to be effective in the treatment of herpes simplex encephalitis. Mortality of this serious disease was reduced from 70% in controls to 28% in patients who received 15 mg/kg per day (Whitley *et al.,* 1977). There was also a reduction in neurological sequelae, but patients already in coma at the time of initiation of therapy did not benefit from the drug. Recent evidence suggests that severe infections with herpes simplex virus in neonates may also be effectively treated with vidarabine.

In herpes zoster infections in patients with suppressed immunological responses, vidarabine is effective in reducing the formation of new vesicles; it accelerates the clearance of virus from vesicles, and it reduces pain (Whitley *et al.,* 1976). The drug should not be used to treat unimpaired hosts with uncomplicated herpes zoster.

As previously mentioned, vidarabine given topically is as effective for herpes simplex keratoconjunctivitis as idoxuridine and is less irritating (Pavan-Langston and Buchanan, 1976). *Trifluorothymidine,* a new halogenated pyrimidine, is currently being tested and appears to be superior to either agent (Wellings *et al.,* 1972; Pavan-Langston and Langston, 1975).

Vidarabine is ineffective in smallpox (Koplan *et al.,* 1975), cytomegalovirus infections (Marker *et al.,* 1978), and recurrent or primary herpes genitalis (Goodman *et al.,* 1975; Adams *et al.,* 1976).

Human Interferon. Interferons are relatively small glycoproteins that inhibit the multiplication of many viruses. Endogenous production and release of interferon occur in response to viral infection, and synthesis of the protein can be induced by double-stranded RNA. The present availability of modest quantities of human interferon from leukocytes has allowed preliminary investigation of its utility. The material clearly has biological activity in man, but the limited supply still prevents full examination of its clinical potential (*see* Symposium, 1977; Hirsch, 1978).

In a controlled trial in patients with lymphoma, early treatment of herpes zoster with human interferon prevented distant cutaneous and visceral spread of infection and, in addition, stopped the spread of the infection in the primary dermatome (Merigan *et al.,* 1978). Since interferon has a uniquely broad spectrum of antiviral activity *in vitro,* clinical trials have been undertaken in patients infected with exotic agents such as Ebola-Marburg virus and rabies virus and with the ubiquitous hepatitis B virus (Greenberg *et al.,* 1976). In the last-named infection, interferon has shown promising additive effects when used in combination with vidarabine.

Abernathy, R. S. Treatment of systemic mycoses. *Medicine (Baltimore),* 1973, *52,* 385–394.

Adams, H. G.; Benson, E. A.; Alexander, E. R.; Vontver, L. A.; Remington, M. A.; and Holmes, K. K. Genital herpetic infection in men and women: clinical course and effect of topical application of adenine arabinoside. *J. Infect. Dis.,* 1976, *133,* Suppl., A151–159.

Anderson, K., and Jamieson, A. Primary amoebic meningoencephalitis. *Lancet,* 1972, *1,* 902–903.

Andrioli, V. T., and Kravetz, H. M. The use of amphotericin B in man. *J.A.M.A.,* 1962, *180,* 269–272.

Appel, G. B., and Neu, H. C. Nephrotoxicity of antimicrobial agents. *N. Engl. J. Med.,* 1977, *296,* 722–728.

Arroyo, J.; Medoff, G.; and Kobayashi, G. S. Therapy of murine aspergillosis with amphotericin B in combination with rifampin or 5-fluorocytosine. *Antimicrob. Agents Chemother.,* 1977, *11,* 21–25.

Balanchandar, V.; Collipp, P. J.; and Rising, B. J. Intramuscular clindamycin phosphate in children. *Clin. Med.,* 1973, *80,* 24–30.

Balows, A., and Fraser, D. (eds.). International symposium on Legionnaire's disease. *Ann. Intern. Med.,* 1979, *90,* 489–707.

Barnett, N.; Bushby, S. R. M.; and Wilkinson, S. Sodium sulphomethyl derivatives of polymixins. *Br. J. Pharmacol.,* 1964, *23,* 552–574.

Barrett, F. F.; McGehee, R. J., Jr.; and Finland, M. Methicillin-resistant *Staphylococcus aureus* at Boston City Hospital. *N. Engl. J. Med.,* 1968, *279,* 441–450.

Bartlett, J. G.; Chang, T. W.; Gurwith, M.; Gorbach, S. L.; and Onderdonk, A. B. Antibiotic-associated pseudomembranous colitis due to toxin-producing clostridia. *N. Engl. J. Med.,* 1978, *298,* 531–534.

Bartlett, J. G.; Sutter, V. L.; and Finegold, S. M. Treatment of anaerobic infections with lincomycin and clindamycin. *N. Engl. J. Med.,* 1972, *287,* 1006–1010.

Bass, J. W.; Klenk, E. L.; Klotheimer, J. B.; Linnemann, C. C.; and Smith, M. H. D. Antimicrobial treatment of pertussis. *J. Pediatr.,* 1969, *75,* 768–781.

Bauer, D. J., and Sadler, P. W. The structure-activity relationships of the antiviral chemotherapeutic activity of isatin β-thiosemicarbasone. *Br. J. Pharmacol. Chemother.,* 1960, *15,* 101–110.

Beggs, W. H.; Sarosi, G. A.; and Walker, M. I. Synergistic action of amphotericin B and rifampin against *Candida* species. *J. Infect. Dis.,* 1976, *133,* 206–209.

Bell, R. W., and Ritchey, J. P. Medical therapy for *Aspergillus* corneal ulcer. *Arch. Ophthalmol.,* 1973, *90,* 402–404.

Bennett, J. E. Amphotericin B binding to serum beta lipoprotein. In, *Recent Advances in Medical and Veterinary Mycology.* (Iwata, K., ed.) University of Tokyo Press, Tokyo, 1977, pp. 107–109.

Bennett, J. E., and others. A collaborative study. Amphotericin B–flucytosine in cryptococcal meningitis. *N. Engl. J. Med.,* 1979, *301,* 126–131.

Bindschalder, D. D., and Bennett, J. E. A pharmacologic guide to the clinical use of amphotericin B. *J. Infect. Dis.,* 1969, *120,* 427–436.

Block, E. R.; Bennett, J. E.; Livoti, L. G.; Klein, W. J.; Brandriss, M. W.; MacGregor, R. R.; and Henderson, L. Flucytosine and amphotericin B: hemodialysis effects on the plasma concentration and clearance. *Ann. Intern. Med.,* 1974, *80,* 613–617.

Block, E. R.; Jennings, A. E., and Bennett, J. E. Experimental therapy of cladosporiosis and sporotrichosis with 5-fluorocytosine. *Antimicrob. Agents Chemother.,* 1973, *3,* 95–99.

Boston Interhospital and Cooperative Study. Boston Interhospital Virus Study Group and the NIAID-Sponsored Cooperative Antiviral Clinical Study. Failure of high dose 5-iodo-2′-deoxyuridine in the therapy of herpes simplex virus encephalitis. Evidence of unacceptable toxicity. *N. Engl. J. Med.,* 1975, *292,* 599–603.

Brandsberg, J. W., and French, M. *In vitro* susceptibility of isolates of *Aspergillus fumigatus* and *Sporothrix schenkii* to amphotericin B. *Antimicrob. Agents Chemother.,* 1972, *2,* 402–404.

Brown, M. R. W., and Wood, S. M. Relation between cation and lipid content of cell walls of *Pseudomonas aeruginosa, Proteus vulgaris* and *Klebsiella aerogenes* and their sensitivity to polymyxin B and other antibacterial agents. *J. Pharm. Pharmacol.,* 1972, *24,* 215–228.

Brown, S. T.; Pedersen, A. H. B.; and Holmes, K. K. Comparison of erythromycin base and estolate in gonococcal urethritis. *J.A.M.A.,* 1977, *238,* 1371–1373.

Bryson, Y. J., and Connor, J. D. *In vitro* susceptibility of varicella zoster virus to adenine arabinoside and hypoxanthine arabinoside. *Antimicrob. Agents Chemother.,* 1976, *9,* 540–543.

Burton, J. R.; Zachery, J. B.; Bessin, R.; Rathbun, H. K.; Greenough, W. B., III; Sterioff, S.; Wright, J. R.; Slavin, R. E.; and Williams, G. M. Aspergillosis in four renal transplant recipients. *Ann. Intern. Med.,* 1972, *77,* 383–388.

Butler, W. T.; Bennett, J. E.; Alling, D. W.; Wertlake, P. T.; Utz, J. P.; and Hill, G. J. Nephrotoxicity of amphotericin B. Early and late effects in 81 patients. *Ann. Intern. Med.,* 1964, *61,* 175–187.

Center for Disease Control. Gonorrhea. Recommended

treatment schedules, 1979. *Ann. Intern. Med.,* **1979,** *90,* 809–811.

Champney, K. J.; Lauter, C. B.; Bailey, E. J.; and Lerner, A. M. Anti-herpesvirus activity in human sera and urines after administration of adenine arabinoside. *J. Clin. Invest.,* **1978,** *62,* 1142–1153.

Cooksley, W. G. E., and Powell, L. W. Erythromycin jaundice: diagnosis by an *in vitro* challenge test. *Aust. N.Z. J. Med.,* **1977,** *7,* 291–293.

Crout, J. E.; Brewer, N. S.; and Tompkins, R. B. Sporotrichosis arthritis. Clinical features in seven patients. *Ann. Intern. Med.,* **1977,** *86,* 294–297.

Curtis, J. R., and Eastwood, J. B. Colistin sulphomethate sodium administration with presence of severe renal failure and during haemodialysis and peritoneal dialysis. *Br. Med. J.,* **1968,** *1,* 484–485.

Davies, J.; Anderson, P.; and Davis, B. D. Inhibition of protein synthesis by spectinomycin. *Science,* **1965,** *149,* 1096–1098.

Davies, W. L.; Grunert, R. R.; Haff, R. F.; McGahen, J. W.; Neumayer, E. M.; Paulshock, M.; Watts, J. C.; Wood, T. R.; Hermann, E. C.; and Hoffmann, C. E. Antiviral activity of 1-adamantanamine (amantadine). *Science,* **1964,** *144,* 862–863.

DeHaan, R. M.; Metzler, C. M.; Schellenberg, D.; and Vanden Bosch, W. D. Pharmacokinetic studies of clindamycin phosphate. *J. Clin. Pharmacol.,* **1973,** *13,* 190–209.

DeHaan, R. M.; Metzler, C. M.; Schellenberg, D.; Vanden Bosch, W. D.; and Masson, E. L. Pharmacokinetic studies of clindamycin hydrochloride in humans. *Int. J. Clin. Pharmacol.,* **1972,** *6,* 105–119.

Diamond, R. D., and Bennett, J. E. A subcutaneous reservoir for intrathecal therapy for fungal meningitis. *N. Engl. J. Med.,* **1973,** *288,* 186–188.

Diasio, R. B.; Lakings, D. E.; and Bennett, J. E. Evidence for conversion of 5-fluorocytosine to 5-fluorouracil in humans. Possible factor in 5-fluorocytosine clinical toxicity. *Antimicrob. Agents Chemother.,* **1978,** *14,* 903–908.

Douglas, J. B., and Healy, J. K. Nephrotoxic effects of amphotericin B, including renal tubular acidosis. *Am. J. Med.,* **1969,** *46,* 154–162.

Douglas, R. L., and Kislak, J. W. Treatment of *Bacteroides fragilis* bacteremia with clindamycin. *J. Infect. Dis.,* **1973,** *128,* 569–571.

Drutz, D. J.; Spickard, A.; Rogers, D. E.; and Koenig, M. G. Treatment of disseminated mycotic infections: a new approach to amphotericin B therapy. *Am. J. Med.,* **1968,** *45,* 405–418.

Duncan, W. C.; Holder, W. R.; Roberts, D. P.; and Know, J. M. Treatment of gonorrhea with spectinomycin hydrochloride: comparison with standard penicillin schedules. *Antimicrob. Agents Chemother.,* **1972,** *1,* 210–214.

Dutcher, J. D.; Boyak, G.; and Fox, S. The preparation and properties of crystalline fungicidin (nystatin). In, *Antibiotics Annual, 1953–1954.* Medical Encyclopedia, Inc., New York, **1954,** pp. 191–193.

Eckman, M. R.; Johnson, T.; and Riess, R. Partial deafness after erythromycin. (Letter.) *N. Engl. J. Med.,* **1975,** *292,* 649.

El-Nakeeb, M. A., and Lampen, J. O. Uptake of griseofulvin by microorganisms and its correlation with sensitivity to griseofulvin. *J. Gen. Microbiol.,* **1965,** *39,* 285–293.

Eykyn, S.; Phillips, I.; and Evans, J. Vancomycin for staphylococcal shunt site infections in patients on regular haemodialysis. *Br. Med. J.,* **1970,** *3,* 80–82.

Fass, R. J., and Saslaw, S. Clindamycin: clinical and laboratory evaluation of parenteral therapy. *Am. J. Med. Sci.,* **1972,** *263,* 369–382.

Fass, R. J.; Scholand, J. F.; Hodges, G. R.; and Saslaw, S. Clindamycin in the treatment of serious anaerobic infections. *Ann. Intern. Med.,* **1973,** *78,* 853–859.

Feldman, H. A.; Hamilton, J. D.; and Gutman, R. A.

Amphotericin therapy in an anephric patient. *Antimicrob. Agents Chemother.,* **1973,** *4,* 402–405.

Filippo, J. A. Infantile hypertrophic pyloric stenosis related to ingestions of erythromycin estolate: a report of five cases. *J. Pediatr. Surg.,* **1976,** *11,* 177–180.

Fosson, A. R., and Wheeler, W. E. Short-termed amphotericin B treatment of severe childhood histoplasmosis. *J. Pediatr.,* **1975,** *86,* 32–36.

Gentles, J. C. Experimental ringworm in guinea pigs: oral treatment with griseofulvin. *Nature,* **1958,** *182,* 476–477.

Geraci, J. E. Vancomycin. *Mayo Clin. Proc.,* **1977,** *52,* 631–634.

Goldstein, E.; Winship, M. J.; and Pappagianis, D. Ventricular fluid and the management of coccidioidal meningitis. *Ann. Intern. Med.,* **1972,** *77,* 243–246.

Goodman, E. L.; Luby, J. P.; and Johnson, M. T. Prospective double-blind evaluation of topical adenine arabinoside in male herpes progenitalis. *Antimicrob. Agents Chemother.,* **1975,** *8,* 693–697.

Goodwin, N. J. Colistin and sodium colistimethate. *Med. Clin. North Am.,* **1970,** *54,* 1267–1276.

Goodwin, R. A., Jr., and Des Prez, R. M. Histoplasmosis. *Am. Rev. Respir. Dis.,* **1978,** *117,* 929–956.

Graybill, J. R. Clinical course of coccidioidomycosis following transfer factor therapy (for the Coccidioidomycosis Cooperative Treatment Group). In, *Coccidioidomycosis: Current Clinical and Diagnostic Status.* (Libero Ajello, L., ed.) Symposia Specialists, Miami, **1977,** pp. 335–345.

Greenberg, H. B.; Pollard, R. B.; Lutwick, L. I.; Gregory, P. B.; Robinson, W. S.; and Merigan, T. C. Effect of human leukocyte interferon on hepatitis B virus infection in patients with chronic active hepatitis. *N. Engl. J. Med.,* **1976,** *295,* 517–522.

Griffith, R. S., and Black, H. R. Erythromycin. *Med. Clin. North Am.,* **1970,** *54,* 1199–1215.

Grisham, L. M.; Wilson, L.; and Bensch, K. Antimitotic action of griseofulvin does not involve disruption of microtubules. *Nature,* **1973,** *244,* 294–296.

Gull, K., and Trinci, A. P. J. Griseofulvin inhibits fungal mitosis. *Nature,* **1973,** *244,* 292–294.

Hamilton-Miller, J. M. T. Fungal sterols and the mode of action of the polyene antibiotics. *Adv. Appl. Microbiol.,* **1974,** *17,* 109–134.

Hamre, D.; Bernstein, J.; and Donovick, R. Activity of *p*-aminobenzaldehyde 3-thiosemicarbazone on vaccinia virus in the chick embryo and in the mouse. *Proc. Soc. Exp. Biol. Med.,* **1950,** *73,* 275–278.

Harwick, H. J.; Kalmanson, G. M.; and Guze, L. B. *In vitro* activity of ampicillin or vancomycin combined with gentamicin or streptomycin against enterococci. *Antimicrob. Agents Chemother.,* **1973,** *4,* 383–387.

Hebeka, E. K., and Solotorovsky, M. Development of resistance to polyene antibiotics in *Candida albicans.* *J. Bacteriol.,* **1965,** *89,* 1533–1539.

Hirsch, M. S. Interferon—its hour come at last? *N. Engl. J. Med.,* **1978,** *298,* 1022–1023.

Holmgren, J., and Möller, O. Studies on the sensitivity of *Proteus mirabilis* and *Proteus vulgaris* to sulphonamide and colistin alone and in combination. *Scand. J. Infect. Dis.,* **1970,** *2,* 121.

Hook, E. W., III; Roberts, R. B.; and Sande, M. A. Antimicrobial therapy of experimental enterococcal endocarditis. *Antimicrob. Agents Chemother.,* **1975,** *8,* 564–570.

Jawetz, E. Polymyxin, colistin and bacitracin. *Pediatr. Clin. North Am.,* **1961,** *8,* 1057–1071.

Kane, J. G.; Chretien, J. H.; and Garaqusi, V. F. Diarrhoea caused by *Candida. Lancet,* **1976,** *1,* 335–336.

Karmody, C. S., and Weinstein, L. Reversible sensorineural hearing loss with intravenous erythromycin lactobionate. *Ann. Otol. Rhinol. Laryngol.,* **1977,** *86,* 9–11.

Kauffman, C., and Frame, P. T. Bone marrow toxicity associated with 5-fluorocytosine therapy. *Antimicrob. Agents Chemother.,* **1977,** *11,* 244–247.

Kauffman, R. E.; Shoeman, D. W.; Wan, S. H.; and Azarnoff, D. L. Absorption and excretion of clindamycin-2-phosphate in children after intramuscular injection. *Clin. Pharmacol. Ther.*, **1972**, *13*, 704–709.

Kinsky, S. C. Nystatin binding by protoplasts and a particulate fraction of *Neurospora crassa*, and a basis for the selective toxicity of polyene antifungal antibiotics. *Proc. Natl. Acad. Sci. U.S.A.*, **1962**, *48*, 1049–1056.

Kitahara, M.; Kobayashi, G. S.; and Medoff, G. Enhanced efficacy of amphotericin B and rifampin in treatment of murine histoplasmosis and blastomycosis. *J. Infect. Dis.*, **1976a**, *133*, 663–668.

Kitahara, M.; Seth, U. K.; Medoff, G.; and Kobayashi, G. S. Activity of amphotericin B, 5-fluorocytosine and rifampin against six clinical isolates of aspergillus. *Antimicrob. Agents Chemother.*, **1976b**, *9*, 915–919.

Knight, V.; Fedson, D.; Baldini, J.; Douglas, R. G.; and Couch, R. B. Amantadine therapy of epidemic influenza A2 (Hong Kong). *Infect. Immun.*, **1970**, *1*, 200–204.

Kobayashi, G. S.; Medoff, G.; Schlessinger, D.; Kwan, C. N.; and Musser, W. E. Amphotericin B potentiation of rifampin as an antifungal agent against the yeast phase of *Histoplasma capsulatum*. *Science*, **1972**, *177*, 709–710.

Koplan, J. P.; Monsur, K. A.; Foster, S. O.; Huq, F.; Rahaman, M. M.; Huq, S.; Buchanan, R.; and Ward, N. A. Treatment of variola major with adenine arabinoside. *J. Infect. Dis.*, **1975**, *131*, 34–39.

Kunin, C. M. A guide to use of antibiotics in patients with renal disease. *Ann. Intern. Med.*, **1967**, *67*, 151–158.

LaMontagne, J. R., and Galasso, G. J. Report of a workshop on clinical studies of the efficacy of amantadine and rimantadine against influenza virus. *J. Infect. Dis.*, **1979**, *138*, 928–931.

Larson, H. E., and Price, A. B. Pseudomembranous colitis: presence of clostridial toxin. *Lancet*, **1977**, *2*, 1312–1314.

Lauer, B. A.; Reller, L. B.; and Schröter, G. P. J. Susceptibility of *Aspergillus* to 5-fluorocytosine and amphotericin B alone and in combination. *J. Antimicrob. Chemother.*, **1978**, *4*, 375–380.

Lerner, P. I. Susceptibility of *Actinomyces* species to linco mycin and its 7-halogenated analogues. In, *Antimicrobial Agents and Chemotherapy—1968.* (Hobby, G. L., ed.) American Society for Microbiology, Bethesda, **1969**, pp. 461–464.

Lew, M.; Beckett, K. M.; and Levin, M. J. Combined activity of minocycline and amphotericin B *in vitro* against medically important yeasts. *Antimicrob. Agents Chemother.*, **1978**, *14*, 465.

Lin, C.; Magat, J.; Chang, R.; McGlotten, J.; and Symchowicz, S. Absorption, metabolism and excretion of ¹⁴C-griseofulvin in man. *J. Pharmacol. Exp. Ther.*, **1973**, *187*, 415–422.

Lindesmith, L. A.; Baines, R. D.; Bigelow, D. B.; and Petty, T. L. Reversible respiratory paralysis associated with polymyxin therapy. *Ann. Intern. Med.*, **1968**, *68*, 318–327.

Little, J. W.; Hall, W. J.; Douglas, R. G., Jr.; Hyde, R. W.; and Speers, D. M. Amantadine effect on peripheral airways abnormalities in influenza. *Ann. Intern. Med.*, **1976**, *85*, 177–182.

Little, J. W.; Hall, W. J.; Douglas, R. G., Jr.; Mudholkar, G. S.; Speers, D. M.; and Patel, K. Attenuation of airway hyperreactivity by amantadine in natural influenza A infection. *Am. Rev. Respir. Dis.*, **1978**, *118*, 295–303.

Luby, J. P.; Jones, S. R.; Johnson, M. T.; and Mikulec, D. Sensitivities of herpes simplex virus types 1 and 2 and varicella-zoster virus to adenine arabinoside. In, *Arabinoside: An Antiviral Agent.* (Pavan-Langston, D., ed.) Raven Press, New York, **1975**, pp. 171–175.

Lutwick, L. I.; Rytel, M. W.; Yañez, J. P.; Galgiani, J. N.; and Stevens, D. A. Deep infections from *Petriellidum boydii* treated with miconazole. *J.A.M.A.*, **1979**, *241*, 272–273.

Lwin, H., and Collipp, P. J. Absorption and tolerance of clindamycin-2-palmitate in infants below 6 months of age. *Curr. Ther. Res.*, **1970**, *12*, 648–657.

McClosky, R. V.; Eller, J. J.; Green, M.; Mauney, C. U.; and Richards, S. E. M. The 1970 epidemic of diphtheria in San Antonio. *Ann. Intern. Med.*, **1971**, *75*, 495–503.

McCormack, W. M.; Donner, G. H.; Kodgis, L. F.; Alpert, S.; Lower, E. W.; and Kass, E. H. Hepatotoxicity of erythromycin estolate during pregnancy. *Antimicrob. Agents Chemother.*, **1977**, *12*, 630–635.

McCormick, M. H.; Stark, W. M.; Pittenger, G. E.; Pittenger, R. C.; and McGuire, J. M. Vancomycin, a new antibiotic. I. Chemical and biologic properties. In, *Antibiotics Annual, 1955–1956.* Medical Encyclopedia, Inc., New York, **1956**, pp. 606–611.

McCurdy, D. K.; Frederic, M.; and Elkinton, J. R. Renal tubular acidosis due to amphotericin B. *N. Engl. J. Med.*, **1968**, *278*, 124–131.

MacGregor, R. R.; Bennett, J. E.; and Ersley, A. J. Erythropoietin concentration in amphotericin B–induced anemia. *Antimicrob. Agents Chemother.*, **1978**, *14*, 270–273.

Malawista, S. E.; Sato, H.; and Bensch, K. G. Vinblastine and griseofulvin reversibly disrupt the living mitotic spindle. *Science*, **1968**, *160*, 770–772.

Mandell, G. L.; Lindsey, E.; and Hook, E. W. Synergism of vancomycin and streptomycin for enterococci. *Am. J. Med. Sci.*, **1970**, *259*, 346–349.

Mao, J. C.-H., and Putterman, M. The intermolecular complex of erythromycin and ribosome. *J. Mol. Biol.*, **1969**, *44*, 347–361.

Mao, J. C.-H., and Tardrew, P. L. Demethylation of erythromycin by rabbit tissues *in vitro*. *Biochem. Pharmacol.*, **1965**, *14*, 1049–1058.

Mao, J. C.-H., and Wiegand, R. G. Mode of action of macrolides. *Biochim. Biophys. Acta*, **1968**, *157*, 404–413.

Marker, S. C.; Groth, K. E.; Howard, R. J.; Simmons, R. L.; Najarian, J. S.; and Balfour, H. H., Jr. Neurological deterioration and lack of therapeutic efficacy in cytomegalovirus-infected renal transplant patients treated with adenine arabinoside. *Program and Abstracts, 18th Interscience Conference on Antimicrobial Agents and Chemotherapy*, No. 519. American Society for Microbiology, Washington, D. C., **1978**, pp. 1–300.

Marks, M. I.; Steer, P.; and Eickhoff, T. C. *In vitro* sensitivity of *Torulopsis glabrata* to amphotericin B, 5-fluorocytosine, and clotrimazole (Bay 5097). *Appl. Microbiol.*, **1971**, *22*, 93–95.

Mauceri, A. A.; Cullen, F. I.; Vandevelde, A. G.; and Johnson, J. E. Flucytosine in effective oral treatment for chromomycosis. *Arch. Dermatol.*, **1974**, *109*, 873–876.

Maxwell, E. Treatment of herpes keratitis with 5-iodo-2-deoxyuridine (IDU): a clinical evaluation of 1500 cases. *Am. J. Ophthalmol.*, **1963**, *56*, 571–573.

Medoff, G.; Comfort, M.; and Kobayashi, G. S. Synergistic action of amphotericin B and 5-fluorocytosine against yeast-like organisms. *Proc. Soc. Exp. Biol. Med.*, **1971a**, *138*, 571–574.

Medoff, G.; Dismukes, W. E.; Meade, R. H., III; and Moses, J. M. A new therapeutic approach to *Candida* infections. *Arch. Intern. Med.*, **1972**, *130*, 241–245.

———. Therapeutic program for *Candida* infection. In, *Antimicrobial Agents and Chemotherapy—1970.* (Hobby, G. L., ed.) American Society for Microbiology, Bethesda, **1971b**, pp. 286–290.

Merigan, T. C.; Rand, K. H.; Pollard, R. B.; Abdallah, P. S.; Jordan, G. W.; and Fried, R. P. Human leukocyte interferon for the treatment of herpes zoster in patients with cancer. *N. Engl. J. Med.*, **1978**, *298*, 981–987.

Meyer, R. D.; Young, L. S.; Armstrong, D.; and Yu, B. Aspergillosis complicating neoplastic disease. *Am. J. Med.*, **1973**, *54*, 6–15.

Meyers, B. R.; Kaplan, K.; and Weinstein, L. Microbiological and pharmacological behavior of 7-chlorolincomycin. *Appl. Microbiol.*, **1969**, *17*, 653–657.

Molavi, A., and Weinstein, L. *In vitro* activity of erythromycin against atypical mycobacteria. *J. Infect. Dis.,* **1971,** *123,* 216–219.

Monto, A. S.; Gunn, R. A.; Bandy, K. M. G.; and King, C. L. Prevention of Russian influenza by amantadine. *J.A.M.A.,* **1979,** *241,* 1003–1007.

Morbidity and Mortality Weekly Report. Primary amoebic meningoencephalitis in California, Florida, and New York. *Morbid. Mortal. Weekly Rep.,* **1978,** *27,* 343.

Muller, W. E. G.; Zahn, R. K.; Bittlingmaier, K.; and Falke, D. Inhibition of herpes virus DNA synthesis by 9-D-arabinofuranosyladenine in cellular and cell-free systems. *Ann. N.Y. Acad. Sci.,* **1977,** *284,* 34–48.

Nafta, I.; Turcanu, A. G.; Braun, I.; Companetz, W.; Simionescu, A. B. E.; and Florea, V. Administration of amantadine for the prevention of Hong Kong influenza. *Bull. WHO,* **1970,** *42,* 423–427.

Naylor, B. A. Low-dose amphotericin B therapy for acute pulmonary histoplasmosis. *Chest,* **1977,** *71,* 404–406.

Newton, G. G. F., and Abraham, E. P. Observations on the nature of bacitracin A. *Biochem. J.,* **1953,** *53,* 604–613.

Nieto, M., and Perkins, H. R. Physicochemical properties of vancomycin and iodovancomycin and their complexes with diacetyl-L-lysyl-D-alanyl-D-alanine. *Biochem. J.,* **1971a,** *123,* 773–787.

———. The specificity of combination between ristocetins and peptides related to bacterial cell wall mucopeptide precursors. *Biochem. J.,* **1971b,** *124,* 845–852.

Nord, C.; Wadström, T.; and Wretlind, B. Synergistic effects of combinations of sulfamethoxazole, trimethoprim and colistin against *Pseudomonas maltophilia* and *Pseudomonas cepacia. Antimicrob. Agents Chemother.,* **1974,** *6,* 521–523.

Normark, S., and Schönebeck, J. *In vitro* studies of 5-fluorocytosine resistance in *Candida albicans* and *Torulopsis glabrata. Antimicrob. Agents Chemother.,* **1972,** *2,* 114–121.

Nunnery, A. W., and Riley, H. D. Clinical and laboratory studies of lincomycin in children. *Antimicrob. Agents Chemother.,* **1964,** *4,* 142–146.

Panzer, J. D.; Brown, D. C.; Epstein, W. L.; Lipson, R. L.; Mahaffrey, H. W.; and Atkinson, W. H. Clindamycin levels in various body tissues and fluids. *J. Clin. Pharmacol.,* **1972,** *12,* 259–262.

Pavan-Langston, D., and Buchanan, R. A. Vidarabine therapy of simple and IDU- complicated herpetic keratitis. *Trans. Am. Acad. Ophthalmol. Otolaryngol.,* **1976,** *81,* 813–827.

Pavan-Langston, D., and Langston, R. H. S. Recent advances in antiviral therapy. In, *International Ophthalmology Clinics: Ocular Viral Disease.* (Pavan-Langston, D., ed.) Little, Brown & Co., Boston, **1975,** pp. 89–100.

Philipson, A.; Sabath, L. D.; and Charles, D. Transplacental passage of erythromycin and clindamycin. *N. Engl. J. Med.,* **1973,** *288,* 1219–1221.

Posner, J. B. Reservoirs for intraventricular chemotherapy. (Editorial.) *N. Engl. J. Med.,* **1973,** *288,* 212.

Prusoff, W. H., and Goz, B. Potential mechanisms of action of antiviral agents. *Fed. Proc.,* **1973,** *32,* 1679–1687.

Prusoff, W. H., and Ward, D. C. Nucleoside analogs with antiviral agents. *Biochem. Pharmacol.,* **1976,** *25,* 1233–1239.

Rabinovich, S.; Baldine, J. T.; and Bannister, R. Treatment of influenza. The therapeutic efficacy of rimantadine HCl in a naturally occurring influenza A2 outbreak. *Am. J. Med. Sci.,* **1969,** *257,* 328–335.

Rasch, J. R., and Mogabgab, W. J. Therapeutic effect of erythromycin on *Mycoplasma pneumoniae* pneumonia. *Antimicrob. Agents Chemother.,* **1965,** *5,* 693–699.

Reyn, A.; Schmidt, H.; Trier, M.; and Bentzon, M. W. Spectinomycin hydrochloride (TROBICIN) in the treatment of gonorrhea. Observation of resistant strains of *Neisseria gonorrhoeae. Br. J. Vener. Dis.,* **1973,** *49,* 54–59.

Riegelman, S.; Rowland, M.; and Epstein, W. L. Griseofulvin-phenobarbital interaction in man. *J.A.M.A.,* **1970,** *213,* 426–431.

Rifkin, G. D.; Fekety, F. R.; and Silva, J. Antibiotic-induced colitis: implication of a toxin neutralized by *Clostridium sordellii* antitoxin. *Lancet,* **1977,** *2,* 1103–1106.

Rosenblatt, J. E., and Stewart, P. R. Combined activity of sulfamethoxazole, trimethoprim, and polymyxin B against gram-negative bacilli. *Antimicrob. Agents Chemother.,* **1974,** *6,* 84–92.

Sabath, L. D.; Gerstein, D. A.; and Finland, M. Serum glutamic oxalacetic transaminase: false elevations during administration of erythromycin. *N. Engl. J. Med.,* **1968a,** *279,* 1137–1139.

Sabath, L. D.; Gerstein, D. A.; Loder, P. B.; and Finland, M. Excretion of erythromycin and its enhanced activity in urine against gram-negative bacilli with alkalinization. *J. Lab. Clin. Med.,* **1968b,** *72,* 916–923.

Sande, M. A.; Bowman, C. R.; and Calderone, R. A. Experimental *C. albicans* endocarditis. Characterization of the disease and response to therapy. *Infect. Immun.,* **1977,** *17,* 140–147.

Sande, M. A., and Johnson, M. L. Antimicrobial therapy of experimental endocarditis caused by *Staphylococcus aureus. J. Infect. Dis.,* **1975,** *131,* 367–375.

Sande, M. A., and Kaye, D. Evaluation of methods for determining antibacterial activity of serum and urine after colistimethate injection. *Clin. Pharmacol. Ther.,* **1970,** *11,* 873–882.

Sanders, E.; Foster, M. T.; and Scott, D. Group A beta-hemolytic streptococci resistant to erythromycin and lincomycin. *N. Engl. J. Med.,* **1968,** *278,* 538–540.

Sarosi, G. A.; Parker, J. D.; Doto, I. L.; and Tosh, F. E. Amphotericin B in cryptococcal meningitis: long-term results of treatment. *Ann. Intern. Med.,* **1969,** *71,* 1079–1087.

Scheld, W. M.; Brown, R. S., Jr.; Fletcher, D. D.; and Sande, M. A. Bactericidal versus bacteriostatic antibiotic therapy of experimental pneumococcal meningitis. *Clin. Res.,* **1979,** *27,* 355A.

Schoutens, E.; Peromet, M.; and Yourassowsky, E. Microbiological and clinical study of spectinomycin in urinary tract infections: reevaluation with hospital strains. *Curr. Ther. Res.,* **1972,** *14,* 349–357.

Schroeter, A. L.; Lucas, J. B.; Price, E. V.; and Falcone, V. H. Treatment of early syphilis and reactivity of serologic tests. *J.A.M.A.,* **1972,** *221,* 471–476.

Shah, V. P.; Epstein, W. L.; and Riegelman, S. Role of sweat in accumulation of orally administered griseofulvin in skin. *J. Clin. Invest.,* **1974,** *53,* 1673–1678.

Shapera, R. M.; Hable, K. A.; and Matsen, J. M. Erythromycin therapy twice daily for streptococcal pharyngitis. Controlled comparison with erythromycin or penicillin phenoxymethyl four times daily or penicillin G benzathine. *J.A.M.A.,* **1973,** *226,* 531–555.

Sheldrick, G. M.; Jones, P. G.; Kennard, O.; Williams, D. H.; and Smith, G. A. Structure of vancomycin and its complex with acyl-D-alanyl-D-alanine. *Nature,* **1978,** *271,* 223–225.

Skehel, J. J.; Hay, A. J.; and Armstrong, J. A. On the mechanism of inhibition of influenza virus replication by amantadine hydrochloride. *J. Gen. Virol.,* **1978,** *38,* 97–110.

Smith, J. W., and Utz, J. P. Progressive disseminated histoplasmosis. A prospective study of 26 patients. *Ann. Intern. Med.,* **1972,** *76,* 557–566.

Steer, P. O.; Marks, M. I.; Klite, P. D.; and Eickhoff, T. C. 5-Fluorocytosine: an oral antifungal compound. A report on clinical and laboratory experience. *Ann. Intern. Med.,* **1972,** *76,* 15–22.

Stevens, D. A. Miconazole in the treatment of systemic fungal infection. *Am. Rev. Respir. Dis.,* **1977,** *116,* 801–806.

Stevens, D. A.; Levine, H. B.; and Deresinski, S. C. Miconazole in coccidioidomycosis. II. Therapeutic and pharmacologic studies in man. *Am. J. Med.,* **1976,** *60,* 191–202.

Stevens, D. A.; Restrepo, M. A.; Cortes, A.; Betancourt, J.;

Galgiani, J. N.; and Gomez, I. Paracoccidioidomycosis (South American blastomycosis): treatment with miconazole. *Am. J. Trop. Med. Hyg.*, **1978**, *27*, 801–807.

Sutliff, W. D. Histoplasmosis cooperative study. V. Amphotericin B dosage for chronic pulmonary histoplasmosis. *Am. Rev. Respir. Dis.*, **1972**, *105*, 60–67.

Sutter, V. L.; Kwok, Y.-Y.; and Finegold, S. M. Susceptibility of *Bacteroides fragilis* to six antibiotics determined by standardized antimicrobial disc sensitivity testing. *Antimicrob. Agents Chemother.*, **1973**, *3*, 188–193.

Tabbara, K. F.; Dy-Liaco, J.; Nozik, R. A.; O'Connor, G. R.; and Blackman, H. J. Clindamycin in chronic toxoplasmosis. Effect of periocular injections on recoverability of organisms from healed lesions in the rabbit eye. *Arch. Ophthalmol.*, **1979**, *97*, 542–544.

Tanaka, K.; Teraoka, H.; Tamaki, M.; Otaka, E.; and Osawa, S. Erythromycin-resistant mutant of *Escherichia coli* with altered ribosomal protein component. *Science*, **1968**, *162*, 576–578.

Tardrew, P. L.; Mao, J. C. H.; and Kenney, D. Antibacterial activity of 2'-esters of erythromycin. *Appl. Microbiol.*, **1969**, *18*, 159–165.

Thadepalli, H.; Gorbach, S. L.; Broido, P. W.; Norsen, J.; and Nyhus, L. Abdominal trauma, anaerobes, and antibiotics. *Surg. Gynecol. Obstet.*, **1973**, *137*, 270–276.

Thomas, F. E.; Leonard, J. M.; and Alford, R. H. Sulfamethoxazole-trimethoprim-polymyxin therapy of serious multiply drug-resistant *Serratia* infections. *Antimicrob. Agents Chemother.*, **1976**, *9*, 201–207.

Thompson, R. L.; Minton, S. A.; Officer, J. E.; and Hitchings, J. E. The effect of heterocyclic and other thiosemicarbazones on vaccinia infections in the mouse. *J. Immunol.*, **1953**, *70*, 229–234.

Tolman, K. G.; Sannella, J. J.; and Freston, J. W. Chemical structure of erythromycin and hepatotoxicity. *Ann. Intern. Med.*, **1974**, *81*, 58–60.

Utz, J. P.; Bennett, J. E.; Brandriss, M. W.; Butler, W. T.; and Hill, G. J., II. Amphotericin B toxicity: combined clinical staff conference at the National Institutes of Health. *Ann. Intern. Med.*, **1964**, *61*, 334–354.

Utz, J. P.; Garriques, I. L.; Sande, M. A.; Warner, J. F.; Mandell, G. L.; McGehee, R. F.; Duma, R. J.; and Shadomy, S. Therapy of cryptococcosis with a combination of flucytosine and amphotericin B. *J. Infect. Dis.*, **1975**, *132*, 368–373.

Vacek, V.; Heizler, M.; Salvik, M.; and Pavlansky, R. Penetration of clindamycin into bone in man. *Chemotherapy*, **1972**, *17*, 22–25.

Vandeputte, J.; Wachtel, J. L.; and Stiller, E. T. Amphotericins A and B, antifungal antibiotics produced by a streptomyces. II. The isolation and properties of the crystalline amphotericins. In, *Antibiotics Annual, 1955–1956.* Medical Encyclopedia, Inc., New York, **1956**, pp. 587–591.

Vandevelde, A. G.; Mauceri, A. A.; and Johnson, J. E., III. 5-Fluorocytosine in the treatment of mycotic infections. *Ann. Intern. Med.*, **1972**, *77*, 43–51.

Vogel, Z.; Vogel, T.; and Elson, D. The effect of erythromycin on peptide bond formation and the termination reaction. *FEBS Lett.*, **1971**, *15*, 249–253.

Wade, D. N., and Sudlow, G. The kinetics of 5-fluorocytosine elimination in man. *Aust. N.Z. J. Med.*, **1972**, *2*, 153–158.

Watanakunakorn, C., and Bakie, C. Synergism of vancomycin-gentamicin and vancomycin-streptomycin against enterococci. *Antimicrob. Agents Chemother.*, **1973**, *4*, 120–124.

Weissmann, G., and Sessa, G. The action of polyene antibiotics on phospholipid-cholesterol structures. *J. Biol. Chem.*, **1967**, *242*, 616–625.

Wellings, P. C.; Awdry, P. N.; Bors, F. H.; Jones, B. R.; Brown, D. C.; and Kaufman, H. E. Clinical evaluation of trifluorothymidine in the treatment of herpes simplex corneal ulcers. *Am. J. Ophthalmol.*, **1972**, *73*, 932–942.

Whitley, R. J.; Ch'ien, L. T.; Dolin, R.; Galasso, G. J.; and

Alford, C. A. Adenine arabinoside therapy of herpes zoster in the immunosuppressed. *N. Engl. J. Med.*, **1977**, *297*, 289–294.

Whitley, R. J.; Soong, S. L.; Dolin, R.; Galasso, G. J.; and Ch'ien, L. T. Adenine arabinoside therapy of biopsy-proved herpes simplex encephalitis. *N. Engl. J. Med.*, **1976**, *294*, 1193–1199.

Wilkins, T. D., and Thiel, T. Resistance of some species of *Clostridium* to clindamycin. *Antimicrob. Agents Chemother.*, **1973**, *3*, 136–137.

Williams, C. J.; Whitehouse, J. M. A.; Lister, T. A.; and Wrigley, P. F. M. Oral anticandidal prophylaxis in patients undergoing chemotherapy for acute leukemia. *Med. Pediatr. Oncol.*, **1977**, *3*, 275–280.

Wilson, L. Properties of colchicine binding protein from chick embryo brain. Interactions with vinca alkaloids and podophyllotoxin. *Biochemistry*, **1970**, *9*, 4999–5007.

Wolinsky, E., and Hines, J. D. Neurotoxic and nephrotoxic effects of colistin in patients with renal disease. *N. Engl. J. Med.*, **1962**, *266*, 759–764.

Young, R. C.; Bennett, J. E.; Geelhoed, G. W.; and Levine, A. S. Fungemia with compromised host resistance. *Ann. Intern. Med.*, **1974**, *80*, 605–612.

Monographs and Reviews

Bennett, J. E. Chemotherapy of systemic mycoses. *N. Engl. J. Med.*, **1974**, *290*, 30–32, 320–323.

———. Antifungal agents. In, *Principles and Practice of Infectious Diseases.* (Mandell, G. L.; Douglas, R. G., Jr.; and Bennett, J. E.; eds.) John Wiley & Sons, Inc., New York, **1979**, pp. 243–253.

Braun, P. Hepatotoxicity of erythromycin. *J. Infect. Dis.*, **1969**, *119*, 300–306.

Brownlee, G.; Bushby, S. R. M.; and Short, E. I. The chemotherapy and pharmacology of the polymyxins. *Br. J. Pharmacol. Chemother.*, **1952**, *7*, 170–188.

Fekety, R. Vancomycin. In, *Principles and Practice of Infectious Diseases.* (Mandell, G. L.; Douglas, R. G., Jr.; and Bennett, J. E.; eds.) John Wiley & Sons, Inc., New York, **1979**, pp. 304–307.

Ginsburg, C. M., and Eichenwald, H. F. Erythromycin: a review of its uses in pediatric practice. *J. Pediatr.*, **1976**, *86*, 272A.

Goldman, L. Griseofulvin. *Med. Clin. North Am.*, **1970**, *54*, 1339–1345.

Greenberg, P. A., and Sanford, J. P. Removal and absorption of antibiotics in patients with renal failure undergoing peritoneal dialysis: tetracycline, chloramphenicol, kanamycin, and colistimethate. *Ann. Intern. Med.*, **1967**, *66*, 465–479.

Hamilton-Miller, J. M. T. Chemistry and biology of the polyene macrolide antibiotics. *Bacteriol. Rev.*, **1973**, *37*, 166–196.

Hayden, F. G., and Douglas, R. G., Jr. Antiviral agents. In, *Principles and Practice of Infectious Diseases.* (Mandell, G. L.; Douglas, R. G., Jr.; and Bennett, J. E.; eds.) John Wiley & Sons, Inc., New York, **1979**, pp. 353–369.

Hirsch, M. S., and Swartz, M. N. Antiviral agents. *N. Engl. J. Med.*, **1980**, *302*, 903–907, 949–953.

Kucers, A., and Bennett, N. M. (eds.). *The Use of Antibiotics*, 2nd ed. William Heinemann Medical Books, Ltd., London, **1975**.

Medoff, G., and Kobayashi, G. S. Strategies in the treatment of systemic fungal infections. *N. Engl. J. Med.*, **1980**, *302*, 145–155.

Meleney, F. L., and Johnson, B. A. Bacitracin. *Am. J. Med.*, **1949**, *7*, 794–806.

Newton, B. A. The properties and mode of action of the polymyxins. *Bacteriol. Rev.*, **1956**, *20*, 14–27.

———. Surface active bactericides. In, *Strategy of Chemotherapy*, Vol. 8 (Symposium of the Society for General Microbiology). J. & A. Churchill, Ltd., London, **1958**, pp. 62–93.

Pratt, W. B. *Chemotherapy of Infection.* Oxford University Press, New York, **1977**.

Prusoff, W. H. Recent advances in chemotherapy of viral diseases. *Pharmacol. Rev.,* **1967,** *19,* 209–250.

Sanford, J. P. *Guide to Antimicrobial Therapy, 1979.* Sanford, Bethesda, **1979.**

Sawyer, P. R.; Brogden, R. N.; Pinder, R. M.; Speight, T. M.; and Avery, G. S. Miconazole: a review of its antifungal activity and therapeutic efficacy. *Drugs,* **1975,** *9,* 406–423.

Sebek, O. K. Polymyxins and circulin. In, *Antibiotics.* Vol. 1, *Mechanism of Action.* (Gottlieb, D., and Shaw, P. D., eds.) Springer-Verlag, Berlin, **1967,** pp. 142–152.

Steigbigel, N. H. Erythromycin, lincomycin and clindamycin. In, *Principles and Practice of Infectious Diseases.* (Mandell, G. L.; Douglas, R. G., Jr.; and Bennett, J. E.; eds.) John Wiley & Sons, Inc., New York, **1979,** pp. 290–300.

Symposium. (Various authors.) Griseofulvin and dermat-omycoses. *Arch. Dermatol.,* **1960,** *81,* 650–882.

Symposium. (Various authors.) The interferon system: a current review to 1978. *Tex. Rep. Biol. Med.,* **1977,** *35,* 1–573.

Tedesco, F. J. Clindamycin and colitis: a review. *J. Infect. Dis.,* **1977,** *135S,* 95–98.

Van Cutsem, J., and Reyntjens, A. Miconazole treatment of pityriasis versicolor. A review. *Mykosen,* **1978,** *21,* 87–91.

Weinstein, L., and Chang, T. W. The chemotherapy of viral infections. *N. Engl. J. Med.,* **1973,** *289,* 725–730.

Weinstein, L., and Weinstein, A. J. The pathophysiology and pathoanatomy of reactions to antimicrobial agents. *Adv. Intern. Med.,* **1974,** *19,* 109–134.

Weisblum, B., and Davies, J. Antibiotic inhibitors of the bacterial ribosome. *Bacteriol. Rev.,* **1968,** *32,* 493–528.

Chemotherapy of Neoplastic Diseases

INTRODUCTION

Paul Calabresi and Robert E. Parks, Jr.

Fundamental advances continue to be made in the chemotherapy of neoplastic diseases. The greatest progress in the last 5 years has been not in the discovery of large numbers of new, useful chemotherapeutic agents but at the conceptual level: the design of more effective regimens for concurrent administration of drugs; the acquisition of knowledge of the mechanisms of action of many antitumor agents, which facilitates the design of new methods to prevent or minimize drug toxicity; the increased use of adjuvant chemotherapy (*e.g.,* the design of chemotherapeutic approaches to destroy micrometastases and prevent the development of secondary neoplasms after removal or destruction of the primary tumor by surgery or irradiation); and increased knowledge about such vital processes as tumor initiation and the dissemination, implantation, and growth of metastases. Of great importance is recognition of the problems imposed by the heterogeneity of tumors, with the realization that individual tumors may contain many subpopulations of neoplastic cells that differ in crucial characteristics, such as karyotype, morphology, immunogenicity, rate of growth, the capacity to metastasize, and, significantly, responsiveness to antineoplastic agents (Calabresi *et al.,* 1979). Information also continues to accumulate in the fields of molecular and cellular biology, resulting in a greater understanding of cellular division and differentiation, tumor immunology, and viral and chemical carcinogenesis. Particularly significant has been the continued evolution of effective technics for clinical investigation; this often involves large multi-institutional collaborative studies, which have enabled the efficient evaluation and prompt introduction of new drugs or drug combinations into the clinic.

Fifteen years ago, significant palliative results were achieved with chemotherapy for a number of human neoplasms, and the first indications had emerged that choriocarcinoma in women could be cured by treatment with methotrexate. Today, we can list a substantial number of neoplastic diseases that need not shorten life if treated with drugs alone or with drugs in combination with other modalities. These include choriocarcinoma in women; acute leukemia, Wilms' tumor, Ewing's sarcoma, rhabdomyosarcoma, and retinoblastoma in children; and Hodgkin's disease, diffuse histiocytic lymphoma, Burkitt's lymphoma, mycosis fungoides, and testicular carcinoma. Despite these impressive advances, there is the sobering realization that many of the most prevalent forms of human cancer still resist effective chemotherapeutic intervention.

The entire population of neoplastic cells must be eradicated in order to obtain these desired results. The concept of "total cell-kill" applies to chemotherapy as it does to other means of treatment; total excision of tumor is necessary for surgical cure, and complete destruction of all cancer cells is required for a cure with radiation therapy. By investigation of a model tumor system, the L1210 leukemia of mice, Skipper and colleagues have established a number of important principles that have guided and redirected modern cancer chemotherapy. These may be briefly summarized as follows: (1) A single clonogenic malignant cell can give rise to sufficient progeny to kill the host; to achieve cure it is thus necessary to destroy every such cell. Since the doubling-time of most tumors is relatively constant during logarithmic growth, the life-span of the host is inversely related to the number of malignant cells that are inoculated or that survive therapeutic measures. (2) In contrast to antimicrobial chemotherapy where, in most instances, there are major contributions by the immune mechanisms and other host defenses, these play a negligible role in the therapy of neoplastic disease unless only a small number of malignant cells is present. (3) The cell-kill caused by antineoplastic agents follows first-order kinetics; that is, a constant percentage, rather than a constant number, of cells is killed by a given therapeutic maneuver. This finding has had a profound impact on clinical cancer chemotherapy. For example, a patient with advanced acute lymphocytic leukemia might harbor 10^{12} or about 1 kg of malignant cells. A drug capable of killing 99.99% of these cells would reduce the tumor mass to about 100 mg, and this would be apparent as a complete clinical remission. However, 10^8 malignant cells would remain, any of which could cause a relapse in the disease. The logical outgrowth of these concepts has been the attempt to achieve total cell-kill by the use of several chemotherapeutic agents concurrently or in rational sequences. The resulting prolonged survival of patients with acute lymphocytic leukemia through the use of such multiple-drug regimens has encouraged the application of these principles to the treatment of other neoplasms.

An understanding of cell-cycle kinetics is essential for the proper use of the current generation of antineoplastic agents. Many of the most potent cytotoxic agents act at specific phases of the cell cycle and, therefore, have activity only against cells that are in the process of division. Accordingly, human malignancies that are currently most susceptible to chemotherapeutic measures are those with a large growth fraction, that is, a high percentage of cells in the process of division. Similarly, normal tissues that proliferate rapidly (bone marrow, hair follicles, and intestinal epithelium) are often subject to damage by some of these potent antineoplastic drugs, and such toxicity often limits drug utility. On the other hand, slow-growing tumors with a small growth fraction, for example, carcinomas of the colon or lung, are often unresponsive to cytotoxic drugs. Although differences in the duration of the cell cycle occur between cells of various types, all cells display a similar pattern during the division process. This may be characterized as follows: (1) there is a presynthetic phase (G_1); (2) the synthesis of DNA occurs (S); (3) an interval follows the termination of DNA synthesis, the postsynthetic phase (G_2); and (4) mitosis (M) ensues—the G_2 cell, containing a double complement of DNA, divides into two daughter G_1 cells. Each of these may immediately reenter the cell cycle or pass into a nonproliferative stage, referred to as G_0. The cells of certain specialized tissues may differentiate into functional cells that are no longer capable of division. On the other hand, many cells, especially those in slow-growing tumors, may remain in the G_0 state for prolonged periods, only to be recruited into the division cycle again at a much later time. Most antineoplastic agents act specifically on processes such as DNA synthesis, transcription, or the function of the mitotic spindle and, therefore, are regarded as cell-cycle specific. It is obvious that further understanding of the cell cycle and of the factors that regulate the recruitment of G_0 cells into the cycle should prove of great value in future attempts to develop chemotherapeutic measures for slow-growing tumors.

A great variety of compounds has been investigated in experimental animals, and a few have proven sufficiently useful in the clinical treatment of human neoplasms, at acceptable levels of toxicity, to deserve the designation of chemotherapeutic agents. It should be emphasized that the compounds selected for discussion represent, for the most part, those that are generally available and have withstood the test of time, although a few have been included either because they illustrate special circumstances or because they are representative of newer developments. Not discussed are several biologically active alkylating agents, hormones, antibiotics, and other compounds that are not commonly used in clinical practice, either because their structural variations offer no particular advantage over existing drugs or because additional investigation is deemed to be necessary. It is also important, in this rapidly changing field, continually to reappraise the current status of available agents, with respect not only to new additions but also to appropriate deletions of compounds the clinical importance of which has declined. Information concerning drugs in the latter category may be found in *earlier editions* of this textbook. Other compounds, particularly certain antimetabolites that were originally developed as antineoplastic agents, have now assumed such important roles in the management of non-neoplastic disorders that they belong more properly in other chapters. Indeed, this spin-off in cancer chemotherapy research represents an area of increasing interest and practical importance to medicine in general. Illustrative examples of such stimulating developments include the effectiveness of allopurinol in controlling hyperuricemia and gout, the beneficial effects of azaribine and methotrexate in psoriasis, the inhibitory actions of analogs of pyrimidine and purine nucleosides on the proliferation of certain viruses of the DNA type, and the use of various cytotoxic agents for the suppression of immune responses.

The use of cytotoxic drugs to cause immunosuppression has played an essential role in establishing the feasibility of renal transplantation across histocompatibility barriers. Success has been variable with transplantation of other organs, including bone marrow, endocrine glands, heart, and liver. The drugs most commonly used to prevent rejection of a homograft are the purine antimetabolite azathioprine, the alkylating agent cyclophosphamide, and the adrenocorticosteroid prednisone. Other agents with potent immunosuppressive properties include methotrexate, cytarabine, thioguanine, dactinomycin, various alkylating agents, and antilymphocyte globulin. They are not as frequently used, however, because of greater toxicity, difficulty of administration, or lesser efficacy. Encouraged by the immunosuppressive activity of these drugs in experimental systems and their effectiveness in renal transplantation, clinical investigators have explored their utility in a number of diseases that are characterized by altered immunological reactivity and manifestations of autoimmunity. These include various collagen-vascular disorders (*e.g.*, systemic lupus erythematosus, necrotizing vasculitis, scleroderma, polymyositis, rheumatoid arthritis, and related entities such as Wegener's granulomatosis), as well as regional enteritis, ulcerative colitis, chronic active hepatitis, glomerulonephritis, the nephrotic syndrome, Goodpasture's syndrome, autoimmune hemolytic anemia, idiopathic thrombocytopenic purpura, pemphigus, and others. (For detailed reviews and references to the original literature, *see* Kaplan and Calabresi, 1973; Rosman and Bertino, 1973; Reza *et al.*, 1975; Sartorelli and Johns, 1975; Tilney *et al.*, 1978; Fauci *et al.*, 1979.) Although immunosuppressive agents are widely employed and recommended by experienced clinicians for specific clinical situations, such use is not officially approved in the United States and remains largely investigational. Because of the complex and poorly understood etiologies of these conditions, it is not entirely clear whether the beneficial effects of these drugs are exerted through an immunosuppressive, anti-inflammatory, or other mechanism. Recent advances in the understanding of the biochemical properties of lymphocytes, which have stemmed from studies of states of congenital immunodeficiency, may offer the promise of devising important new technics to achieve selective immunosuppression. Deficiencies in the enzymes of purine metabolism, adenosine deaminase and purine nucleoside phosphorylase, are associated with specific impairments of the functions of T and B lymphocytes. Potent inhibitors of adenosine deaminase such as pentostatin (deoxycoformycin) can reproduce many features of the combined immunodeficiency state (Agarwal *et al.*, 1975, 1978).

While desirable results may be achieved with cytotoxic chemotherapy in diseases that are associated with altered immunological reactivity, as well as in neoplastic disorders, severe untoward complications can result from their administration. There may be increased susceptibility to infections caused by pathogenic bacteria or opportunistic microorganisms. Some immune responses, particularly cellular immunity mediated by T lymphocytes, are also thought to play important roles in the natural resistance of the host against malignant tumors; others, however, including humoral "blocking factors" produced by B lymphocytes, may be deleterious to the host by interfering with the capacity of cytotoxic lymphocytes to react against neoplastic cells. Coupled with the possibility of genetic damage, the chronic use of immunosuppressive agents carries an increased risk of neoplasia, usually of histiocytic or lymphoid origin. Since cytotoxic drugs can suppress or enhance these immune responses selectively, depending upon

Table XIII–1. CHEMOTHERAPEUTIC AGENTS USEFUL IN NEOPLASTIC DISEASE

CLASS	TYPE OF AGENT	NONPROPRIETARY NAMES (OTHER NAMES)	DISEASE *
Alkylating Agents	Nitrogen Mustards	Mechlorethamine (HN$_2$)	Hodgkin's disease, non-Hodgkin's lymphomas, breast, ovary
		Cyclophosphamide	Acute and chronic lymphocytic leukemias, Hodgkin's disease, non-Hodgkin's lymphomas, multiple myeloma, neuroblastoma, breast, ovary, lung, Wilms' tumor, rhabdomyosarcoma
		Melphalan (L-sarcolysin)	Plasma-cell myeloma, breast, ovary
		Uracil mustard	Chronic lymphocytic leukemia, non-Hodgkin's lymphomas, Hodgkin's disease, ovary, primary thrombocytosis
		Chlorambucil	Chronic lymphocytic leukemia, primary macroglobulinemia, Hodgkin's disease, non-Hodgkin's lymphomas, breast, ovary, testis
	Ethylenimine Derivatives	Thiotepa (triethylene*thio*phosphoramide)	Hodgkin's disease, non-Hodgkin's lymphomas, retinoblastoma, breast, ovary
	Alkyl Sulfonates	Busulfan	Chronic granulocytic leukemia, polycythemia vera, primary thrombocytosis
	Nitrosoureas	Carmustine (BCNU)	Hodgkin's disease, non-Hodgkin's lymphomas, primary brain tumors, malignant melanoma, renal cell, stomach, myeloma
		Lomustine (CCNU)	Hodgkin's disease, non-Hodgkin's lymphomas, primary brain tumors, renal cell, stomach, colon, "oat cell"
		Semustine (methyl-CCNU)	Hodgkin's disease, non-Hodgkin's lymphomas, primary brain tumors, renal cell, stomach, colon, malignant melanoma
		Streptozocin (streptozotocin)	Malignant pancreatic insulinoma, malignant carcinoid
	Triazenes	Dacarbazine (DTIC; dimethyltriazenoimidazolecarboxamide)	Malignant melanoma, Hodgkin's disease, soft-tissue sarcomas
Antimetabolites	Folic Acid Analogs	Methotrexate (amethopterin)	Acute lymphocytic leukemia, choriocarcinoma, mycosis fungoides, breast, testis, head and neck, lung, osteogenic sarcoma
	Pyrimidine Analogs	Fluorouracil (5-fluorouracil; 5-FU)	Breast, colon, stomach, pancreas, ovary, head and neck, urinary bladder, premalignant skin lesions (topical)
		Cytarabine (cytosine arabinoside)	Acute granulocytic and acute lymphocytic leukemias

* Neoplasms are carcinomas unless otherwise indicated.

CLASS	TYPE OF AGENT	NONPROPRIETARY NAMES (OTHER NAMES)	DISEASE *
Antimetabolites	Pyrimidine Analogs	Azaribine (triacetyl-6-azauridine)	Mycosis fungoides, polycythemia vera
	Purine Analogs	Mercaptopurine (6-mercaptopurine; 6-MP)	Acute lymphocytic, acute granulocytic, and chronic granulocytic leukemias
		Thioguanine (6-thioguanine; TG)	Acute granulocytic, acute lymphocytic, and chronic granulocytic leukemias
Natural Products	Vinca Alkaloids	Vinblastine (VLB)	Hodgkin's disease, non-Hodgkin's lymphomas, breast, renal cell, testis
		Vincristine (VCR)	Acute lymphocytic leukemia, neuroblastoma, Wilms' tumor, rhabdomyosarcoma, Hodgkin's disease, non-Hodgkin's lymphomas, breast, "oat cell"
	Antibiotics	Dactinomycin (actinomycin D)	Choriocarcinoma, Wilms' tumor, rhabdomyosarcoma, testis
		Daunorubicin (daunomycin; rubidomycin)	Acute granulocytic and acute lymphocytic leukemias
		Doxorubicin (adriablastina)	Soft-tissue, osteogenic, and other sarcomas; Hodgkin's disease, non-Hodgkin's lymphomas, acute leukemias, breast, genitourinary, thyroid, lung, stomach, neuroblastoma
		Bleomycin	Testis, head, neck, skin, esophagus, and genitourinary tract; Hodgkin's disease, non-Hodgkin's lymphomas
		Mithramycin	Testis, malignant hypercalcemia
		Mitomycin (mitomycin C)	Stomach, cervix, colon, breast, pancreas, bladder
	Enzymes	L-Asparaginase	Acute lymphocytic leukemia
Miscellaneous Agents	Platinum Coordination Complexes	Cisplatin (*cis*-DDP)	Testis, ovary, bladder, head and neck, thyroid, cervix, endometrium, neuroblastoma, osteogenic sarcoma
	Substituted Urea	Hydroxyurea	Chronic granulocytic leukemia, malignant melanoma
	Methyl Hydrazine Derivative	Procarbazine (N-methylhydrazine, MIH)	Hodgkin's disease
	Adrenocortical Suppressant	Mitotane (*o,p'*-DDD)	Adrenal cortex
Hormones and Antagonists	Adrenocorti-costeroids	Prednisone (several other equivalent preparations available; *see* Chapter 63)	Acute and chronic lymphocytic leukemia, non-Hodgkin's lymphomas, Hodgkin's disease, breast

Table XIII-1. CHEMOTHERAPEUTIC AGENTS USEFUL IN NEOPLASTIC DISEASE (Continued)

CLASS	TYPE OF AGENT	NONPROPRIETARY NAMES (OTHER NAMES)	DISEASE *
Hormones and Antagonists	Progestins	Hydroxyprogesterone caproate Medroprogesterone acetate Megestrol acetate	Endometrium, renal cell, breast, prostate
	Estrogens	Diethylstilbestrol Ethinyl estradiol (other preparations available; *see* Chapter 61)	Breast, prostate
	Antiestrogen	Tamoxifen	Breast
	Androgens	Testosterone propionate Fluoxymesterone (other preparations available; *see* Chapter 62)	Breast
Radioactive Isotopes	Phosphorus	Sodium phosphate P 32	Polycythemia vera, chronic lymphocytic and granulocytic leukemias
	Iodine	Sodium iodide I 131	Thyroid

* Neoplasms are carcinomas unless otherwise indicated.

dosage and schedule of administration, the subtle interactions between these agents and the immunological defenses of the host represent an increasingly important area of investigation (Heppner and Calabresi, 1976).

The emphasis in Chapter 55 is placed upon the drugs themselves. Although this is appropriate in a textbook of pharmacology, it is also essential to point out the importance of the role played by the patient. It is generally agreed that patients in good nutritional state and without severe metabolic disturbances, infections, or other complications are better candidates for significant improvement from antineoplastic therapy than are severely debilitated individuals. Ideally, the patient also should have adequate renal, hepatic, and bone-marrow function, uncompromised by tumor invasion, previous chemotherapy, or radiation (particularly of the spine or pelvis). Occasionally, however, even patients with advanced disease have improved dramatically with chemotherapy. Although methods that would enable accurate prediction of the responsiveness of a particular tumor to a given agent are still investigational (Salmon *et al.*, 1978), efforts are being made to establish better clinical and laboratory criteria for the rational selection of patients prior to therapy. Despite efforts to anticipate the development of complications, anticancer agents, like many other potent drugs with only moderate selectivity, may cause severe toxicity. In such circumstances, the physician must have at his disposal adequate facilities for vigorous supportive therapy; some of these, including platelet transfusions and the administration of allopurinol to prevent the complications of hyperuricemia, have been widely adopted, while others, including better methods to combat or prevent infections, are the subject of intensive investigation.

Drugs currently used in chemotherapy of neoplastic diseases may be divided into several classes, as shown in Table XIII-1. This somewhat arbitrary classification is used in Chapter 55 as a convenient framework for describing the various types of agents; the major clinical indications for the drugs are listed in Table XIII-1 in order to facilitate rapid reference. Dosage regimens, which are often complex, are discussed under the individual drugs.

Mechanistic classification of these agents is increasingly important, particularly as investigators attempt to utilize this information to design "rational" regimens for chemotherapy. A simplified overview of the sites of action of many of the drugs described in Chapter 55 is shown in Figure XIII–1.

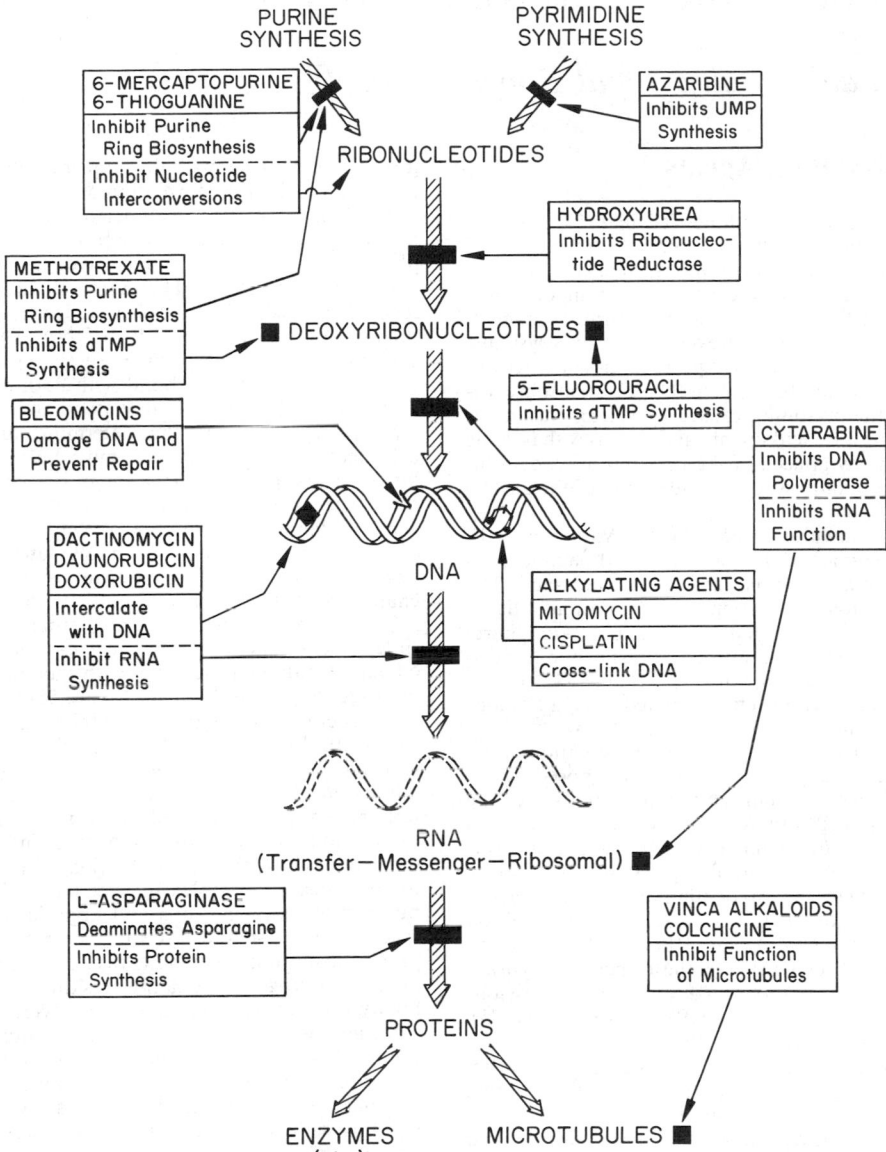

Figure XIII–1. *Summary of the mechanisms and sites of action of chemotherapeutic agents useful in neoplastic disease.*

55 ANTIPROLIFERATIVE AGENTS AND DRUGS USED FOR IMMUNOSUPPRESSION

Paul Calabresi and Robert E. Parks, Jr.

I. Alkylating Agents

History. Although synthesized in 1854, the vesicant properties of *sulfur mustard* were not described until 1887. During World War I, medical attention was first focused on the vesicant action of sulfur mustard on the skin, eyes, and respiratory tract. It was appreciated later, however, that serious systemic intoxication also follows exposure. In 1919, Krumbhaar and Krumbhaar made the pertinent observation that the poisoning caused by sulfur mustard is characterized by leukopenia and, in cases that came to autopsy, by aplasia of the bone marrow, dissolution of lymphoid tissue, and ulceration of the gastrointestinal tract.

In the interval between World Wars I and II, extensive studies of the biological and chemical actions of the *nitrogen mustards* were conducted. The marked cytotoxic action on lymphoid tissue prompted Gilman, Goodman, and T. F. Dougherty to study the effect of nitrogen mustards on transplanted lymphosarcoma in mice, and in 1942 clinical studies were initiated. This launched the era of modern cancer chemotherapy (Gilman, 1963).

In their early phases, all these investigations were conducted under secrecy restrictions imposed by the use of classified chemical-warfare agents. At the termination of World War II, however, the nitrogen mustards were declassified and a general review was presented by Gilman and Philips (1946), and shortly thereafter there appeared summaries of clinical research by Goodman and associates (1946), Jacobson and coworkers (1946), and Rhoads (1946). Many reviews have been written on these agents (*see earlier editions* of this textbook). More recent discussions include those by Wheeler (1973), Connors (1975), Ross (1975), and Ludlum (1977, 1978).

Thousands of variants of the basic chemical structure of the nitrogen mustards have been prepared. However, most attempts at the rational design of "active-site-directed" molecules have failed, and only a few of these agents have proven more useful than the original compound in specific clinical circumstances (*see* below). At the present time five major types of alkylating agents are used in the chemotherapy of neoplastic diseases: (1) the nitrogen mustards, (2) the ethylenimines, (3) the alkyl sulfonates, (4) the nitrosoureas, and (5) the triazenes.

Chemistry. The chemotherapeutic alkylating agents have in common the property of undergoing strongly electrophilic chemical reactions through the formation of carbonium ion intermediates or of transition complexes with the target molecules. These reactions result in the formation of covalent linkages (alkylation) with various nucleophilic substances, including such biologically important moieties as phosphate, amino, sulfhydryl, hydroxyl, carboxyl, and imidazole groups. The cytotoxic and other effects of the alkylating agents are directly related to the alkylation of components of DNA. The 7 nitrogen atom of guanine is particularly susceptible to the formation of a covalent bond with both monofunctional and bifunctional alkylators and may well represent the key target that determines the biological effects of these agents. It must be appreciated, however, that other atoms in the purine and pyrimidine bases of DNA—for example, the 1 or 3 nitrogens of adenine, the 3 nitrogen of cytosine, and the 6 oxygen of guanine—may also be alkylated to a lesser degree, as are the phosphate atoms of the DNA chains and the proteins associated with DNA.

To illustrate the actions of alkylating agents, possible consequences of the reaction of mechlorethamine (nitrogen mustard) with guanine residues in DNA chains are shown in Figure 55–1. First, one 2-chloroethyl side chain undergoes a first-order (S_N1) intramolecular cyclization, with release of a chloride ion and formation of a highly reactive ethylenimonium intermediate. By this reaction the tertiary amine is converted to a quaternary ammonium compound. The ethylenimonium intermediates can react avidly, through formation of a carbonium ion or transition complex intermediate, with a large number of inorganic ions and organic radicals by reactions that resemble a second-order (S_N2) nucleophilic substitution reaction (Price, 1975). Alkylation of the 7 nitrogen of guanine residues in DNA, a highly favored reaction, may exert several effects of considerable biological importance, as illustrated in Figure 55–1. Normally, guanine residues in DNA exist predominantly as the keto tautomers and readily make Watson-Crick base pairs by hydrogen bonding with cytosine residues. However, when the 7 nitrogen of guanine is alkylated (to become a quaternary ammonium nitrogen), the guanine residue is more acidic and the enol tautomer is favored. Guanine in this form can make base pairs with thymine residues, thus leading to possible miscoding and the ultimate substitution of an adenine-thymine base pair for a guanine-cytosine base pair. Second, alkylation of the 7 nitrogen labilizes the imidazole ring, making possible the opening of the imidazole ring or depurination by excision of guanine residues, either of which can result in serious damage to the DNA molecule (Shapiro, 1968). Third, with bifunctional alkylators, such as nitrogen mustard, the second

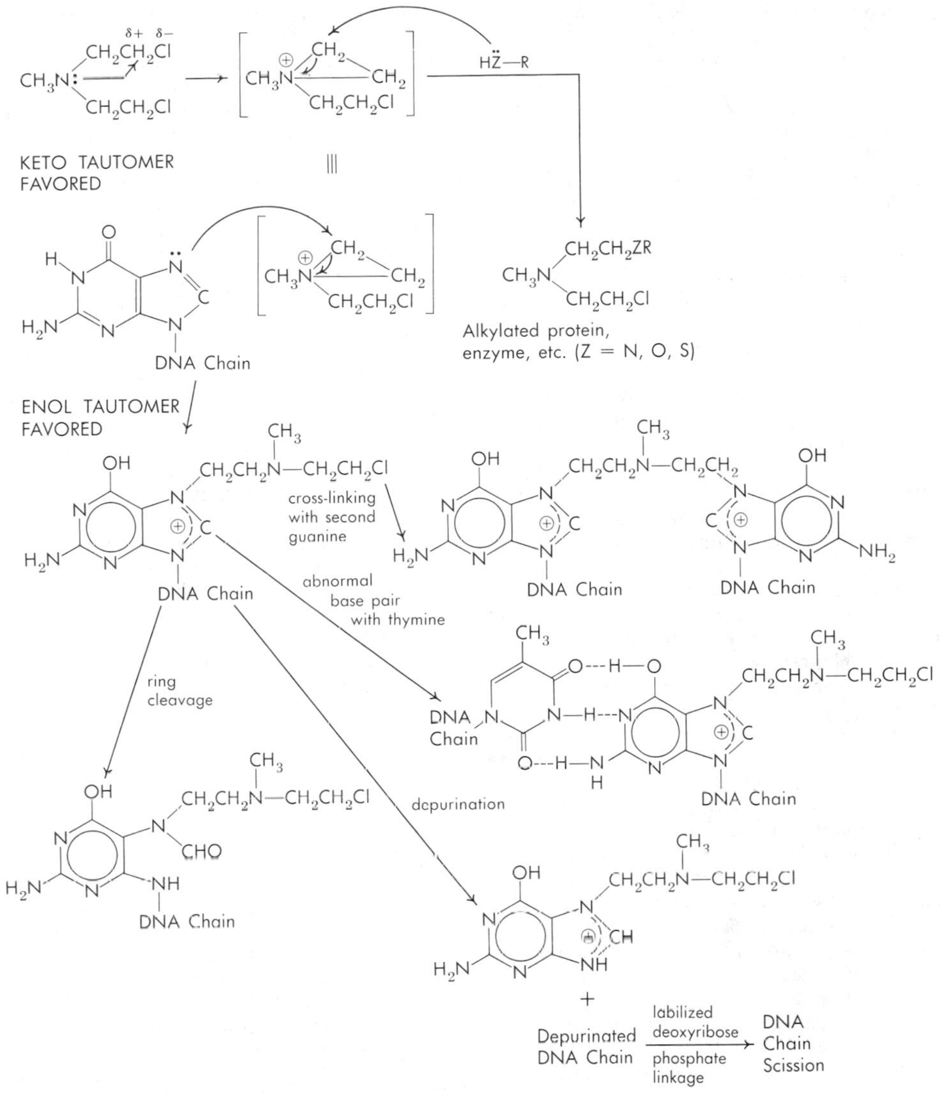

Figure 55-1. *Mechanism of action of alkylating agents.*

2-chloroethyl side chain can undergo a similar cyclization reaction and alkylate a second guanine residue or another nucleophilic moiety, such as an amino group or a sulfhydryl radical of a protein. This can result in the cross-linking of two nucleic acid chains or the linking of a nucleic acid to a protein by very strong covalent bonds, reactions that would cause a major disruption in nucleic acid function. Any of these effects could adequately explain both the mutagenic and the cytotoxic effects of alkylating agents.

In addition to the formation of covalent bonds with purine or pyrimidine residues of DNA, a wide variety of other chemical reactions are possible that can result in a number of other important effects on cellular function and viability.

All nitrogen mustards are chemically unstable but vary greatly in their degree of instability. Therefore, the specific chemical properties of each member of this class of drugs must be considered individually in therapeutic applications. For example, *mechlorethamine* is so hygroscopic and unstable in aqueous form that it is marketed as the dry crystals of the hydrochloride salt. Solutions are prepared immediately prior to injection and, within a few minutes after administration, mechlorethamine reacts almost completely within the body. On the other hand, agents such as *chlorambucil* are sufficiently stable to permit oral administration, and *cyclophosphamide,* which is much less reactive than mechlorethamine, requires biochemical activation by the cytochrome P-450 system of the liver in order to achieve chemotherapeutic effectiveness.

The ethylenimine derivatives react by an S_N2 reaction; however, since the opening of the ethyl-enimine ring is acid catalyzed, they are more reactive at acidic pH. Busulfan is an atypical alkylating agent with unusual biological properties that differ significantly from substituted nitrogen mustards and ethylenimines (Fox, 1975).

Structure-Activity Relationship. The alkylating agents used in chemotherapy encompass a diverse group of chemicals that have in common the capacity to contribute, under physiological conditions, alkyl groups to biologically vital macromolecules such as DNA. In most instances, physical and chemical parameters, such as lipophilicity, capacity to cross biological membranes, acid dissociation constants, stability in aqueous solution, and so forth, rather than similarity to cellular constituents, have proven crucial to biological activity. With several of the most valuable agents, for example, cyclophosphamide and the nitrosoureas, the active alkylating moieties are generated *in vivo* following complex degradative reactions, some of which are enzymatic. Since many of these physicochemical factors and activation reactions are still unclear, most alkylating agents in use today were discovered by empirical rather than by rational approaches. In most instances where clinically useful agents were uncovered by presumably "rational" methods, it was later learned that the original premises were defective, and the biological usefulness resulted from factors not considered in the original design. Therefore, much more information must become available before the structure-activity relationship of the alkylating agents is fully understood and applied.

The nitrogen mustards may be regarded as nitrogen analogs of sulfur mustard. The biological activity of both types of compounds is based upon the presence of the *bis*-(2-chloroethyl) grouping. In sulfur mustard, the two reactive groups are attached to bivalent sulfur; since nitrogen is trivalent, a third substituent must be present on the nitrogen atom. Although a very large number of alkylating agents have been synthesized and evaluated, the methyl derivative, *mechlorethamine,* has received wide clinical use and has been accepted generally as a standard of reference. Various structural modifications

have been made in order to achieve greater selectivity and, therefore, less toxicity. *Bis*-(2-chloroethyl) groups have been linked to (1) amino acids (phenylalanine, glycine, DL-alanine); (2) substituted phenyl groups (aminophenyl butyric acid, as in *chlorambucil*); (3) pyrimidine bases (uracil); (4) benzimidazole; (5) antimalarial agents; (6) sugars (mannitol); and (7) several other substances, including a cyclic phosphamide ester. Although none of these modifications has achieved the goal of producing a highly selective and general cytotoxic action for malignant cells, some of the compounds exhibit notable differences in their secondary pharmacological properties and have attracted much clinical, as well as theoretical, interest.

The structural formulas of some of the more commonly used nitrogen mustards are shown in Table 55–1.

There is no definite evidence that the use of special prosthetic groups, such as phenylalanine, a precursor of melanin, conveys unusual selectivity of action on malignant melanoma. The addition of substituted phenyl groups has produced a series of derivatives that retain the ability to react by an S_N1 mechanism; however, the electron-withdrawing capacity of the aromatic ring greatly reduces the rate of carbonium ion formation, and these compounds can therefore reach distant sites in the body before reacting with components of blood and other tissues. Chlorambucil is the most successful example of such aromatic mustards. These molecular modifications of mechlorethamine have not altered its general spectrum of action; however, by reducing the high reactivity characteristic of the parent compound, the derivatives may be administered orally and are safer and more convenient in the treatment of chronic malignancies of the lymphocytic or plasma-cell series, particularly in the presence of extensive infiltration of the bone marrow.

A classical example of the role of the host metabolism in the activation of an alkylating agent is seen with *cyclophosphamide*—now the most widely used agent of this class. The original rationale that guided design of this molecule was twofold. First, if a cyclic phosphamide group replaced the N-methyl of

Table 55–1. NITROGEN MUSTARDS EMPLOYED IN THERAPY

Mechlorethamine   Cyclophosphamide   Uracil Mustard

Melphalan   Chlorambucil

mechlorethamine, the compound might be relatively inert, presumably because the *bis*-(2-chloroethyl) group of the molecule could not ionize until the cyclic phosphamide was cleaved at the phosphorus-nitrogen linkage. Second, it was hoped that neoplastic tissues might possess high phosphatase or phosphamidase activity capable of accomplishing this cleavage, thus resulting in the selective production of an activated nitrogen mustard in the malignant cells. In accord with these predictions, cyclophosphamide displays only weak cytotoxic, mutagenic, or alkylating activity and is relatively stable in aqueous solution. However, when administered to experimental animals or patients bearing susceptible tumors, marked chemotherapeutic effects, as well as mutagenicity and carcinogenicity, are seen. Although a definite role for phosphatases or phosphamidases in the mechanism of action of cyclophosphamide has not yet been demonstrated, it is clearly established that the drug initially undergoes metabolic activation by the cytochrome P-450 mixed-function oxidase system of the liver, with subsequent transport of the activated intermediate to sites of action, as discussed below. Thus, a crucial factor in the structure-activity relationship of cyclophosphamide concerns its capacity to undergo metabolic activation in the liver, rather than to alkylate malignant cells directly. It also appears that the selectivity of cyclophosphamide against certain malignant tissues may result in part from the capacity of normal tissues, such as liver, to protect themselves against cytotoxicity by further degrading the activated intermediates.

Although initially considered as an antimetabolite, the triazene derivative 5-(3,3-dimethyl-1-triazeno)-imidazole-4-carboxamide, usually referred to as *dacarbazine* or DTIC, is now known to function through alkylation. Its structural formula is as follows:

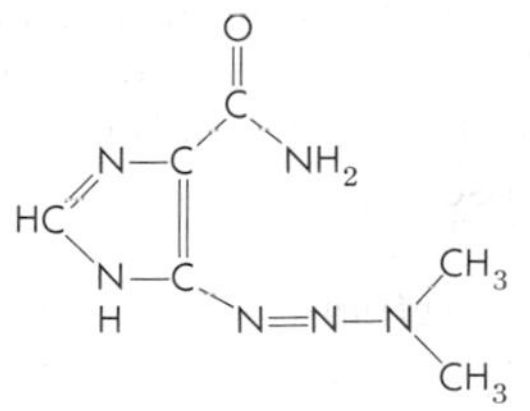

Dacarbazine

This compound bears a striking resemblance to the known metabolite 5-aminoimidazole-4-carboxamide (AIC), which is capable of conversion to inosinic acid by enzymes of purine synthesis. Thus, it was suspected that dacarbazine acts by inhibiting purine metabolism and nucleic acid synthesis. This resemblance to AIC may be fortuitous, since, for chemotherapeutic effectiveness, dacarbazine requires initial activation by the cytochrome P-450 system of the liver through an N-demethylation reaction. In the target cell, there then occurs a spontaneous cleavage liberating AIC and an alkylating moiety, presumably diazomethane (Oliverio, 1973a).

Although the mechanism of action is not yet fully established, it is generally assumed that the *nitro-*

soureas, which include compounds such as 1,3-*bis*-(2-chloroethyl)-1-nitrosourea (carmustine, BCNU), 1-(2-chloroethyl)-3-cyclohexyl-1-nitrosourea (lomustine, CCNU), and its methyl derivative (semustine, methyl-CCNU), as well as the antibiotic *streptozocin* (*streptozotocin*), exert their cytotoxicity through the liberation of alkylating and carbamoylating moieties. Their structural formulas are shown in Table 55-2.

The antineoplastic nitrosoureas have in common the capacity to undergo spontaneous, nonenzymatic degradation with the formation of a variety of products. Of these, the methyl carbonium ion (from MNU compounds) and the 2-chloroethyl carbonium ion (from CNU compounds) are strongly electrophilic and can alkylate a variety of substances, including the purine and pyrimidine bases of DNA. Indeed, when the 2-chloroethyl carbonium ion alkylates an entity such as the 7 nitrogen of guanine, it may then serve as a bifunctional alkylator and cross-link DNA molecules. The occurrence of cross-linking may not become apparent until many hours after exposure of the cells to the drug. As with the nitrogen mustards, it appears likely that this phenomenon is directly related to cytotoxicity (Heal *et al.,* 1979). In addition to the generation of carbonium ions, the spontaneous degradation of nitro-

Table 55-2. CLASSIFICATION AND STRUCTURES OF SOME ANTINEOPLASTIC NITROSOUREAS

METHYLNITROSOUREAS (MNU)

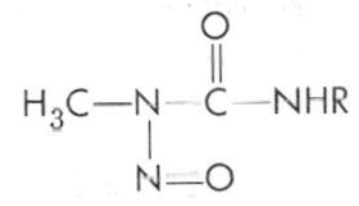

Streptozocin
R — 2-substituted glucose

2-CHLOROETHYLNITROSOUREAS (CNU)

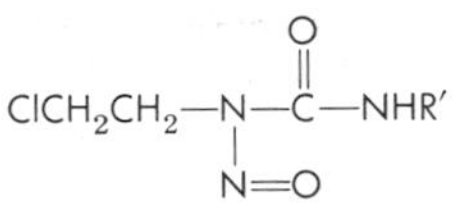

Carmustine (BCNU)
R′ = —CH₂CH₂Cl

Lomustine (CCNU)

R′ =

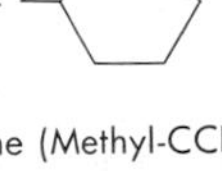

Semustine (Methyl-CCNU)

R′ =

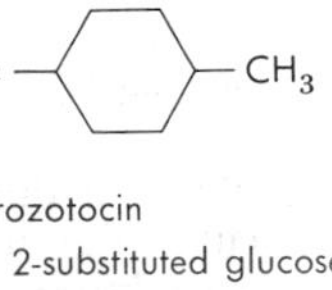

Chlorozotocin
R′ = 2-substituted glucose

soureas liberates organic isocyanates that are capable of carbamoylating lysine residues of proteins. This reaction can apparently inactivate certain of the DNA repair enzymes, and it has been suggested that high carbamoylating activity might be related to myelosuppression. This has, however, been questioned (*see* Heal *et al.,* 1979). The reactions of the nitrosoureas with macromolecules are shown in Figure 55–2. (For recent reviews of the nitrosoureas, *see* Ludlum, 1977, 1978.)

Since the formation of the ethylenimonium ion constitutes the initial reaction of the nitrogen mustards, screening programs have been devised to discover useful ethylenimine derivatives. These studies have yielded several active compounds, including triethylenemelamine (TEM), triethylenephosphoramide (TEPA), and triethylene*thio*phosphoramide (thiotepa), a more stable sulfur-containing derivative. Other chemical relatives of current interest because of their activity against selected human solid tumors are the methylmelamines; hexamethylmelamine (HMM) is available for experimental clinical use, and a more soluble derivative, pentamethylmelamine (PMM), is in the early stages of clinical trial. The structural formulas of these compounds are as follows:

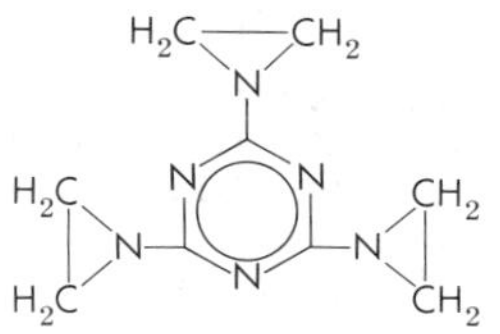

Triethylenemelamine (TEM)

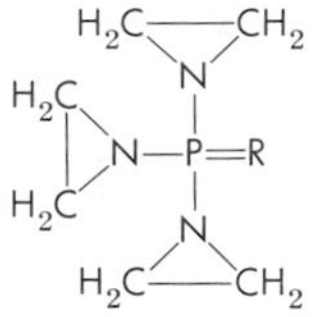

Triethylenephosphoramide (TEPA): R = O
Triethylene*thio*phosphoramide (Thiotepa): R = S

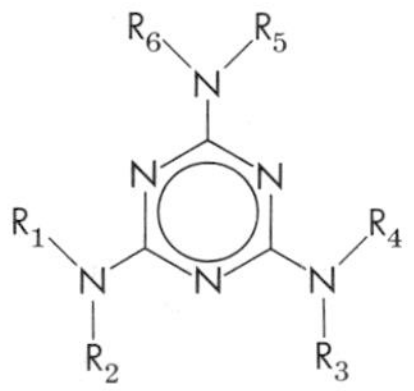

Hexamethylmelamine (HMM)

$R_{1-6} = -CH_3$

Pentamethylmelamine (PMM)

$R_1 = -H$
$R_{2-6} = -CH_3$

While TEM, TEPA, and thiotepa are cytotoxic, they have no particular clinical advantage over the other alkylating agents. Information on their phar-

macological properties may be found in *earlier editions* of this textbook. Although there is no evidence that the methylmelamines function as alkylating agents, HMM and PMM are discussed here because of their chemical similarity to the ethylenimine melamines. The methylmelamines are N-demethylated by hepatic microsomes, with the release of formaldehyde, and there is a relationship between the degree of the demethylation and their activity against murine tumors. HMM requires microsomal activation to display cytotoxicity (*see* Rutty and Connors, 1977).

From a large group of esters of alkanesulfonic acids, synthesized as alkylating agents for chemotherapy of neoplastic disease, several interesting compounds have emerged; one of these, busulfan, is of great value in the treatment of chronic granulocytic leukemia; its structural formula is as follows:

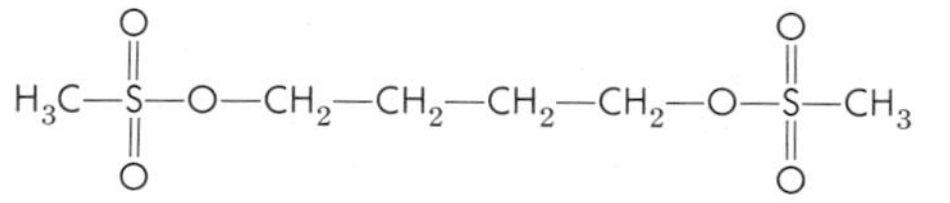

Busulfan

Busulfan is a member of a series of symmetrical methanesulfonic acid esters that permit determination of the effects of altering the length of a bridge of methylene groups ($n = 2$ to 10); the compounds of intermediate length ($n = 4$ or 5) possess the highest activities and therapeutic indices.

PHARMACOLOGICAL ACTIONS

The pharmacological actions of the various groups of alkylating agents are considered together in the following discussion. Although there are many similarities, there are, of course, some notable differences. Primary consideration will be given to the cytotoxic actions that follow the administration of a sublethal dose.

Cytotoxic Actions. The most important pharmacological actions of the alkylating agents are those that disturb the fundamental mechanisms concerned with cell growth, mitotic activity, differentiation, and function. The capacity of these drugs to interfere with normal mitosis and cell division in all rapidly proliferating tissues provides the basis for their therapeutic applications and for many of their toxic properties. Whereas certain alkylating agents may have damaging effects on tissues with normally low mitotic indices, for example, liver, kidney, and mature lymphocytes, they are most cytotoxic to rapidly proliferating tissues in which a large proportion of the cells are in division. These com-

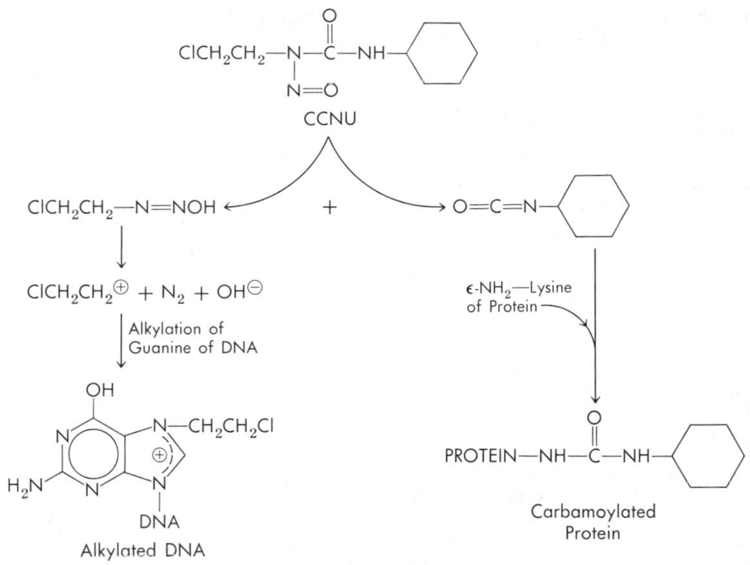

Figure 55-2. *Degradation of lomustine (CCNU) with generation of alkylating and carbamoylating intermediates.*

pounds may readily alkylate nondividing cells, but cytotoxicity is seen only if such cells are stimulated to divide. Thus, the process of alkylation itself may be a relatively nontoxic event, as long as the DNA repair enzymes can correct the lesions in DNA prior to the next cellular division.

In contrast to many other antineoplastic agents, the effects of the alkylating drugs, although dependent on proliferation, are not cell-cycle specific, and the drugs may act on cells at any stage of the cycle. However, the toxicity is usually expressed when the cell enters the S phase and progression through the cycle is blocked at the G_2 (premitotic) phase (*see* Wheeler, 1967). While not strictly cell-cycle specific, quantitative differences may be detected when nitrogen mustards are applied to synchronized cells at different phases of the cycle. Cells appear more sensitive in late G_1 or S than in G_2, mitosis, or early G_1. Polynucleotides are more susceptible to alkylation in the unpaired state than in the helical form. During replication of DNA, portions of the molecule are so unpaired.

The cells accumulating behind the block at G_2 may have a double complement of DNA while continuing to synthesize other cellular components, such as protein and RNA. This can result in unbalanced growth, with the formation of enlarged or giant cells that can continue to synthesize DNA, making as much as four or five times the normal complement. Lethal cytotoxic action may occur by so-called interphase death and mitotic death; on the other hand, relatively undifferentiated cells of mammalian germinal tissues may remain nonproliferative during exposure and later undergo nuclear and cytoplasmic

hypertrophy, differentiating without further mitosis into more adult cell types. Interphase death is generally regarded as the result of damage to many cellular sites. Nevertheless, this may not be the case; certainly it occurs without any evidence of mitotic activity. For a comprehensive review of the cytotoxic and biochemical effects of alkylating agents, *see* Connors (1975).

Biochemical Actions. The great preponderance of evidence indicates that the primary target of pharmacological doses of alkylating agents is the DNA molecule, as illustrated in Figure 55-1. A crucial distinction that must be emphasized is between the bifunctional agents, in which cytotoxic effects predominate, and the monofunctional agents, which have much greater capacity for mutagenesis and carcinogenesis. This suggests that biochemical events such as the cross-linking of DNA strands, only possible with bifunctional agents, represent a much greater threat to cellular survival than do other effects, such as depurination and chain scission. On the other hand, the latter reactions may cause permanent modifications in DNA structure that are compatible with continued life of the cell and transmissible to subsequent generations; such modifications may result in mutagenesis or carcinogenesis. (*See* Ludlum, 1975.)

The remarkable DNA repair systems found in most cells appear to play a key, if not determining, role in the relative resistance of nonproliferating tissues, the selectivity of action against particular cell types, and acquired resistance to alkylating agents. While alkylation of a single strand of DNA may often be repaired with relative ease, interstrand cross-linkages, such as those produced by the bifunctional alkylating agents, are more difficult to repair and involve more complex mechanisms. Many of the cross-links formed in DNA by these agents at low doses may also be corrected; higher doses cause extensive cross-linkage, and DNA breakdown occurs.

Mechanisms of Resistance to Alkylating Agents. Acquired resistance to alkylating agents is a common event, and the acquisition of resistance to one alkylating agent may impart cross-resistance to other alkylators. While definitive information on the biochemical mechanisms of resistance is lacking, several biochemical mechanisms have been implicated in the development of such resistance by tumor cells. In contrast to the development of resistance to antimetabolites, where single-step mutations can result in almost complete resistance to drug effects, the acquisition of resistance to alkylating agents is usually a slower process, not resulting from single biochemical changes. Resistance of this type may represent the summation of a series of biochemical changes, none of which by itself can confer significant resistance. Among the biochemical changes identified in cells resistant to alkylating agents are decreased permeability to the drugs and increased production of nucleophilic substances that can compete with the target DNA for alkylation. For example, the administration of cysteine can considerably reduce the antitumor effects of alkylating agents, and there are several examples of animal tumors with acquired resistance that have greater concentrations of free thiol groups than do the sensitive tumor lines from which they were derived. There has been much speculation about the possibility that increased activity of the DNA repair system may permit cells to acquire resistance to alkylating agents. (*See* Connors, 1974.)

Hematological and Immunosuppressive Actions.

The hematopoietic system is very susceptible to the effects of alkylating agents. Within 6 to 8 hours after administration of a sublethal dose of a nitrogen mustard, cessation of mitosis and disintegration of formed elements may be evident in the marrow and lymphoid tissues of experimental animals. Lymphocytes appear to be more sensitive to the destructive action of the mustards and relatively resistant to the effects of busulfan, an action that is considered responsible for the immunosuppressive effects observed with the former group, particularly cyclophosphamide. Busulfan seems to be more toxic to granulocytes, and it has been shown that suitable combinations of busulfan and chlorambucil, an aromatic mustard, can simulate closely the hematological effects of whole-body x-radiation. The effects of chlorambucil are followed by rapid recovery, except in lymphoid organs, whereas depression of hematopoiesis after busulfan occurs gradually and is more prolonged. In patients treated with mechlorethamine, lymphocytopenia is usually apparent within 24 hours and becomes progressively more severe for 6 to 8 days; within a few days, granulocytopenia becomes evident and lasts for 10 days to 3 weeks. Variable degrees of depression of platelet and erythrocyte counts may occur during the second or third week after therapy; with ensuing regeneration, hematological recovery is complete at the end of 4 to 6 weeks and rebound hyperplasia may be present from the fifth to the seventh week.

Actions on Reproductive Tissues. In women, amenorrhea of several months' duration sometimes follows a course of therapy with alkylating agents. Impairment of spermatogenesis may be noted in man. Interesting differences and similarities have been found between the effects of these agents and x-rays on the stages of spermatogenesis in rodents. Busulfan mimics most closely the effects of radiation by acting on an early stage of spermatogenesis; this results, after 8 weeks, in a systematic sequential depletion of spermatogonia, spermatocytes, spermatids, and spermatozoa. Triethylenemelamine and the aliphatic mustards affect later stages and produce infertility within 4 weeks. On the other hand, cytotoxic doses of phenylalanine mustard and chlorambucil do not interfere with the fertility of male rats.

Actions on Other Epithelial Tissues. The intestinal mucosa can be damaged by the parenteral administration of minimal lethal doses of a nitrogen mustard in experimental animals; mitotic arrest, cellular hypertrophy, pyknosis, disintegration, and desquamation of the epithelium are evident. Damage to the hair follicles is much more pronounced with cyclophosphamide than with other mustards and frequently results in alopecia; this effect is usually reversible, even with continued therapy. An interesting commercial application of this finding involves the administration of this drug to sheep in order to facilitate the harvesting of wool.

Sulfur mustard and the nitrogen mustards are powerful local vesicants. Either direct contact with the compounds or exposure to vapors can lead to serious local reactions. The susceptible tissues are skin, eyes, and respiratory tract. The mustards are not escharotic *per se;* rather, the onset of action is delayed for many hours and the mechanism of tissue injury presumably involves the reaction of their transformation products with essential components of the cell. The vesicant properties of the nitrogen mustards are of concern to the clinician in that local reactions can occur if certain precautions are not observed during the course of administration (*see* below).

Actions on the Nervous System. All nitrogen mustards are powerful stimulants of the central nervous system (CNS). Nausea and vomiting are prominent side effects, particularly of mechlorethamine, and are presumably the result of CNS stimulation. Convulsions, progressive muscular paralysis, and various cholinomimetic effects have been observed. These effects and a poorly understood "delayed-death" syndrome reported in animals indicate that the cytotoxicity of the alkylating agents extends to cellular functions unrelated to proliferative activity. More detailed descriptions and references appear in the *fourth* and *earlier editions* of this textbook.

NITROGEN MUSTARDS

The chemistry and the pharmacological actions of the alkylating agents as a group, and of the nitrogen mustards, have been presented above. Only the unique pharmacological characteristics of the individual agents are considered below.

MECHLORETHAMINE

Mechlorethamine was the first of the nitrogen mustards to be introduced into clinical medicine and is the most rapidly acting of the drugs in this class.

Chemistry. The chemical structure of mechlorethamine has been presented above (*see* Table 55–1).

Absorption and Fate. Severe local reactions of exposed tissues necessitate intravenous injection of mechlorethamine for clinical use. In either water or body fluids, at rates affected markedly by pH, mechlorethamine rapidly undergoes chemical transformation and combines with either water or reactive compounds of cells, so that the drug is no longer present in active form after a few minutes. Indeed, it is possible to protect a given tissue from the effects of the agent by the simple expedient of interrupting the blood supply to the area for a few minutes during and immediately after injection of the drug. Conversely, it is possible, but not always feasible, to localize the action of mechlorethamine or related agents to a large extent in a given tissue by injecting the drug into the arterial blood stream supplying that tissue.

Preparations, Dosage, and Routes of Administration. *Mechlorethamine Hydrochloride for Injection,* U.S.P. (MUSTARGEN), is supplied in rubber-stoppered vials containing 10 mg of mechlorethamine hydrochloride triturated with 100 mg of sodium chloride. The solution for injection must be freshly prepared before each administration by adding 10 ml of sterile distilled water to the contents of the vial by means of a syringe and needle, with the use of surgical gloves for protection of the hands. The contents of the vial are dissolved while the needle is still in the rubber stopper, and the required volume of solution is then withdrawn and injected immediately. The solution should be injected into the tubing of a rapidly flowing intravenous infusion; this not only reduces the possibility of extravasation of the drug but also lowers the concentration of vesicant that comes in contact with the intima of the vein. The exact rate of injection is relatively unimportant, provided it is completed within a few minutes. In patients who have elevated venous pressure in the antebrachial veins because of compression of the great veins by mediastinal tumors, it is advisable to administer the drug through an indwelling catheter inserted into the femoral vein.

A course of therapy with mechlorethamine consists in the injection of a total dose of 0.4 mg/kg of body weight or 10 mg/sq m. Although this total dose may be given in either two or four daily consecutive injections, a single administration is preferable; the therapeutic response is equal, and the patient is spared an additional 2 or 3 days of anorexia, nausea, and vomiting. The recommended total dosage to be given during a single course should be exceeded only by those who are completely familiar with the use of the drug. In the presence of extensive infiltration of bone marrow by neoplastic cells, as is often the case in lymphocytic lymphosarcoma, it is wise to reduce the dose to 0.3 or even 0.2 mg/kg, at least for the first course of therapy.

A course of mechlorethamine may be repeated only after bone-marrow function has recovered. This is best ascertained by study of the peripheral blood or by evaluation of bone-marrow granulocyte reserve. Usually, at least 6 weeks should elapse between courses of this agent.

Direct intracavitary administration of the drug (0.2 to 0.4 mg/kg) for malignant effusions, particularly of pleural origin, provides valuable palliation.

Therapeutic Uses and Clinical Toxicity. The beneficial results of mechlorethamine in *Hodgkin's disease* and, less predictably, in other *lymphomas* have been extensively confirmed. Although the drug has been effective alone, current practice favors its use in combination with other agents. In generalized Hodgkin's disease (stages III and IV), the so-called MOPP regimen (the combination of mechlorethamine, vincristine (ONCOVIN), procarbazine, and prednisone) is considered the treatment of choice (DeVita *et al.,* 1972).

In patients with generalized *mycosis fungoides,* very dilute solutions (0.25%) of mechlorethamine may be painted on the involved cutaneous areas with marked beneficial results.

In the treatment of leukemias and related myeloproliferative disorders, mechlorethamine has been superseded by other agents. Although palliative results have been observed in carcinomas of the bronchus, ovary, breast, and other solid tumors, alkylating agents of intermediate or slower reactivity are preferable. (*See* Table XIII–1, page 1252, and discussion under individual agents; *see also* Calabresi and Welch, 1962; Lanc, 1977.)

The major toxic manifestations of mechlorethamine include nausea and vomiting, as well as myelosuppression. Leukopenia and thrombocytopenia constitute the major limitation on the amount of drug that can be given in a single course. Rarely, hemorrhagic complications of nitrogen mustard therapy may be due to hyperheparinemia; in such a circumstance, specific therapy with protamine corrects the hemorrhagic diathesis (Chapter 58).

On rare occasions, a maculopapular *skin eruption* may follow therapy with mechlorethamine. The reaction apparently is not one of the hypersensitivity type, does not necessarily recur with subsequent administration of the drug, and does not provide a contraindication to further therapy. *Herpes zoster* is another type of skin lesion frequently associated with nitrogen mustard therapy. Apparently a latent viral infection is not uncommonly present in patients with malignant lymphoma, and therapy with either a nitrogen mustard or radiation may be followed by overt manifestations of the viral disease.

Women should be warned that *menstrual irregularities* may be produced by mechlorethamine, and, since *fetal abnormalities* have been induced in experimental animals, the drug should not be used if pregnancy exists or is suspected. After a course of therapy, catamenia may be delayed or several consecutive menstrual periods may be missed. The effect is presumably the result of arrest of maturation of the Graafian follicles, but there appears to be no permanent damage to ovarian function.

Local reactions to extravasation of mechlorethamine into the subcutaneous tissue result in a severe, brawny, tender induration that may persist for a long time. If the local reaction is unusually severe, a slough may result. If it is obvious that extravasation has occurred, the involved area should be promptly infiltrated with an isotonic solution of sodium thiosulfate (⅙ M); an ice compress then should be applied intermittently for 6 to 12 hours. The purpose of the thiosulfate is to provide an ion that reacts avidly with the nitrogen mustard and thereby protects tissue constituents. If thiosulfate solution is not available, prompt injections of isotonic sodium chloride solution may have some value by reducing the local concentration of the vesicant agent.

Thrombophlebitis is a potential complication of therapy with mechlorethamine. It rarely occurs if the drug is injected into the tubing during the course of an intravenous infusion.

CYCLOPHOSPHAMIDE

Efforts to modify the chemical structure of mechlorethamine to achieve greater selectivity for neoplastic tissues led to the development of cyclophosphamide. After studies of the pharmacological activity of cyclophosphamide, clinical investigations by European workers demonstrated its effectiveness in selected malignant neoplasms. (For references to the original literature, *see* Calabresi and Welch, 1962; Symposium, 1967.)

Chemistry. The chemical structure of cyclophosphamide and the interesting rationale that led to its synthesis have been presented above (*see* Table 55–1).

Pharmacological and Cytotoxic Actions. None of the severe acute CNS manifestations reported with the typical nitrogen mustards has been noted with cyclophosphamide. Nausea and vomiting, however, may occur. Although the general cytotoxic action of this drug is similar to that of other alkylating agents, some notable differences have been observed. When compared with mechlorethamine, damage to the megakaryocytes and thrombocytopenia are less common. Another unusual manifestation of selectivity consists in more prominent damage to the hair follicles, resulting frequently in alopecia. The drug is not a vesicant, and local irritation does not occur.

Absorption, Fate, and Excretion. Cyclophosphamide is well absorbed orally. As mentioned above, the drug is activated by metabolism in the liver by the mixed-function oxidase system of the smooth endoplasmic reticulum (Brock, 1967); several toxic metabolites have been identified (Hill *et al.*, 1972a; Sladek, 1973; Connors, 1975). The current view of the metabolism and fate of cyclophosphamide is presented in Figure 55–3. The hepatic cytochrome P-450 mixed-function oxidase system converts cyclophosphamide to 4-hydroxycyclophosphamide, which is in a steady state with the acyclic tautomer, aldophosphamide. These compounds may be oxidized further by hepatic aldehyde oxidase and perhaps by other enzymes, yielding the metabolites carboxyphosphamide and 4-ketocyclophosphamide, neither of which possesses significant biolog-

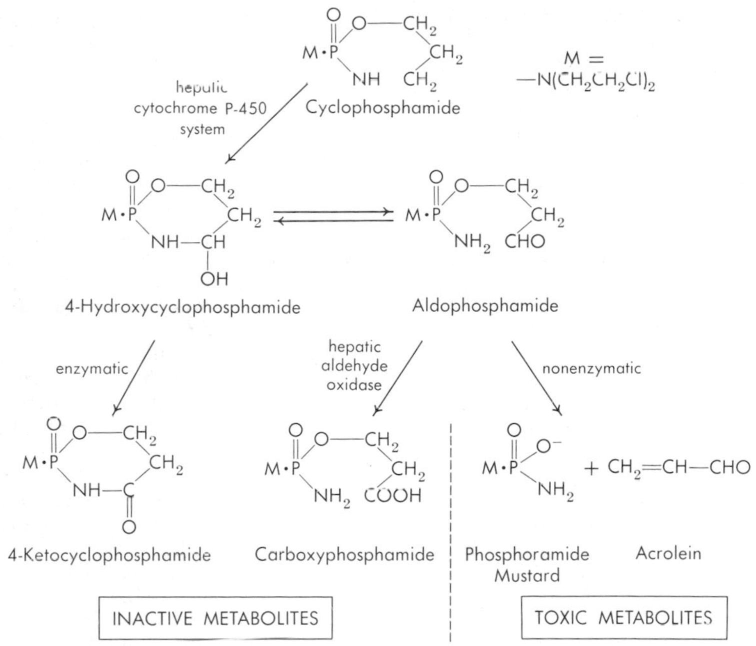

Figure 55–3. *Metabolism of cyclophosphamide.*

ical activity. It appears that hepatic damage is minimized by these secondary reactions, whereas significant amounts of the activated metabolites, such as aldophosphamide, are transported to the target sites by the circulatory system. It has been proposed that, in cells that are susceptible to cytolysis, the aldophosphamide is cleaved by a β-elimination reaction, generating stoichiometric amounts of phosphoramide mustard and acrolein, both of which are highly cytotoxic (Connors, 1975; Ludlum, 1977).

If the cytochrome P-450 system is induced by pretreatment of an animal with phenobarbital or inhibited by administration of proadifen (SK & F 525-A), however, the antitumor activity and therapeutic index of cyclophosphamide are not significantly modified (Sladek, 1972). The explanation proposed for this unexpected finding illustrates several important pharmacological principles. Cyclophosphamide, which is biologically relatively inactive, is eliminated from the body very slowly. The activated metabolites (*e.g.*, aldophosphamide) alkylate the target sites in susceptible cells in an "all-or-none" type of reaction or are detoxicated by formation of inactive metabolites that are rapidly excreted by the kidneys. The cytotoxic effects are related to the total amount rather than to the velocity of generation of the activated metabolites. Thus, it seems likely that the biological actions of cyclophosphamide may be affected more drastically by alterations in the rates of detoxication and elimination than by changes in the rate of generation of the activated metabolites.

Studies with ^{3}H-labeled cyclophosphamide in dogs and humans (Bolt *et al.*, 1961) showed that urinary recovery of unchanged drug was less than 14%, and fecal recovery after intravenous administration was negligible. Maximal concentrations in plasma are achieved 1 hour after oral administration, and a significant amount of unchanged drug is found in the stool when this route is employed. The half-life of cyclophosphamide in plasma is 6 to 7 hours (Bagley *et al.*, 1973). Prior treatment with allopurinol significantly prolongs this value.

Preparations, Dosage, and Routes of Administration. *Cyclophosphamide*, U.S.P. (CYTOXAN), is supplied as 25- and 50-mg tablets and as a powder (100, 200, or 500 mg) in sterile vials. Solutions are prepared by addition of 5 ml of sterile water per 100 mg of drug.

The drug has been administered orally, intravenously, intramuscularly, intrapleurally, and intraperitoneally. A conservative daily dose of 2 to 3 mg/kg, orally or intravenously, has been recommended for patients with more susceptible neoplasms such as lymphomas and leukemias or with compromised bone-marrow function. A higher daily dosage of 4 to 8 mg/kg intravenously for 6 days, followed by an oral maintenance dose of 50 to 300 mg daily, 5 mg/kg intravenously twice weekly, or 10 to 15 mg/kg intravenously every 7 to 10 days, has been used for the treatment of carcinomas and more resistant neoplasms. Large single doses of 30 mg/kg or 750 to 1000 mg/sq m have been very effective in patients with lymphomas and cause a rapid response approaching that seen with mechlorethamine; in patients without complications or previous therapy, the recommended total initial loading dose is 40 to 50 mg/kg, administered orally or intravenously over a period of 2 to 4 days. Careful evaluation of bone-marrow function is imperative, and prolonged therapy is guided by keeping the total leukocyte count between 2500 and 4000 cells per cubic millimeter of blood or by obtaining the desired response of the tumor.

Therapeutic Uses and Clinical Toxicity. The clinical spectrum of activity for cyclophosphamide is very broad and similar to that of nitrogen mustard. It is probably the most commonly used agent for antineoplastic chemotherapy and is an essential component of many effective drug combinations. The initial good results observed in Hodgkin's disease and lymphosarcoma have been confirmed. Complete remissions and presumed cures have been reported in Burkitt's lymphoma and in acute lymphoblastic leukemia of childhood when the drug is used concurrently with other agents (Livingston and Carter, 1970). It is frequently used in combination with methotrexate and fluorouracil as adjuvant therapy after surgery for carcinoma of the breast when there is involvement of axillary nodes; this regimen is particularly effective in premenopausal women (Bonadonna *et al.*, 1978).

Notable advantages of this drug are the availability of oral as well as parenteral routes of administration and the possibility of giving fractionated doses over prolonged periods of time. For these reasons it possesses a versatility of action that allows an intermediate range of use, between that of the highly reactive intravenous mechlorethamine and that of oral chlorambucil. Beneficial results have been obtained in multiple myeloma, chronic lymphocytic leukemia, bronchogenic carcinoma, carcinoma of the breast, carcinoma of the cervix, and ovarian malignancies, as well as in neuroblastoma, retinoblastoma, and other neoplasms of childhood. In addition to the combination mentioned above, it is also often used in combination with doxorubicin, vincristine, and prednisone. (*See* Livingston and Carter, 1970; National Conference on Cancer Chemotherapy, 1972; Holland and Frei, 1973.)

Because of its potent *immunosuppressive* properties, cyclophosphamide has received considerable attention in recent years for the control of organ rejection after transplantation and in nonneoplastic disorders associated with altered immune reactivity, including Wegener's granulomatosis, rheumatoid arthritis, the nephrotic syndrome in children, and autoallergic ocular disease. Appropriate caution is advised when the drug is considered for use in these conditions, not only because of its acute toxic effects but also because of its high potential for inducing

sterility, teratogenic effects, mutations, and cancer. (*See* Kaplan and Calabresi, 1973; Gershwin *et al.*, 1974; Calabresi, 1979.)

The clinical toxicity of cyclophosphamide differs from that of other nitrogen mustards in that significant degrees of thrombocytopenia are much less common, but there is frequent occurrence of alopecia. Patients should be forewarned of this possible event, which is usually reversible even without interruption of therapy. Nausea and vomiting are common and occur with equal frequency whether the drug is given by the oral or the intravenous route. Mucosal ulcerations, dizziness of short duration, transverse ridging of the nails, increased skin pigmentation, interstitial pulmonary fibrosis, and hepatic toxicity have been reported. Extravasation of the drug into subcutaneous tissues does not produce local reactions, and thrombophlebitis does not complicate intravenous administration. The occurrence of sterile, hemorrhagic cystitis has been reported in 5 to 10% of patients. This has been attributed to chemical irritation produced by reactive derivatives of cyclophosphamide, probably carboxyphosphamide and aldophosphamide. Its incidence has been reduced in animals by bladder irrigation with a solution of acetylcysteine (Primack, 1971). For routine clinical use, ample fluid intake and frequent voiding are recommended. Administration of the drug should be interrupted at the first indication of dysuria or hematuria. The syndrome of inappropriate secretion of antidiuretic hormone (ADH) has been observed in patients receiving cyclophosphamide, usually at doses higher than 50 mg/kg (DeFronzo *et al.*, 1973). It is important to be aware of the possibility of water intoxication, since these patients are usually vigorously hydrated.

MELPHALAN

This phenylalanine derivative of nitrogen mustard is also known as L-sarcolysin. Early clinical studies demonstrated a spectrum of activity similar to that of other alkylating agents.

Chemistry. The chemical structure and the rationale for the synthesis of this amino acid derivative of mechlorethamine have been presented above (*see* Table 55-1; *see also* Livingston and Carter, 1970; Greenwald, 1973; Wheeler, 1975).

Pharmacological and Cytotoxic Actions. The general pharmacological and cytotoxic actions of melphalan are similar to those of other nitrogen mustards. The drug is not a vesicant.

Absorption, Fate, and Excretion. Melphalan is well absorbed when given by the oral route and seems to be equally effective whether given by mouth or intravenously. The drug has a half-life in plasma of approximately 90 minutes, and 10 to 15% of an administered dose is excreted unchanged in the urine (Alberts *et al.*, 1979b).

Preparation, Dosage, and Route of Administration. *Melphalan*, U.S.P. (ALKERAN), is available in scored, 2-mg tablets. The usual oral dose is 6 mg daily for a period of 2 to 3 weeks, during which time the blood count should be carefully followed. A rest period of up to 4 weeks should then intervene. When the leukocyte and platelet counts are rising, maintenance therapy, ordinarily 2 to 4 mg daily, is begun. It is usually necessary to maintain a significant degree of bone-marrow depression (total leukocyte count in the range of 3000 to 3500 cells per cubic millimeter) in order to achieve optimal results.

Therapeutic Uses and Clinical Toxicity. Although the general spectrum of action of melphalan seems to resemble that of other nitrogen mustards, the advantages of a gradual but continuous administration by the oral route have made the drug useful in the treatment of *multiple myeloma* (Bergsagel, 1972). Beneficial effects have also been reported in malignant melanoma and in carcinoma of the breast and ovary. Its use as adjuvant therapy after surgery for breast cancer is currently under active study, with indications of promising results in premenopausal women who have involvement of one to three axillary nodes (Fisher *et al.*, 1977). The clinical toxicity of melphalan is mostly hematological and is similar to that of other alkylating agents. Nausea and vomiting are infrequent. Alopecia does not occur, and changes in renal or hepatic function have not been observed.

URACIL MUSTARD

Uracil mustard was synthesized in an unsuccessful attempt to produce an active-site-directed alkylator by linking the *bis*-(2-chloroethyl) group to the pyrimidine base uracil. Its activity in experimental neoplasms was demonstrated shortly thereafter. No relationship has been demonstrated, however, with the biological functions of uracil.

Chemistry. The structural formula of uracil mustard and its chemical relationship to other alkylating agents are presented above (*see* Table 55–1). It is a crystalline compound that is quite unstable in water.

Pharmacological and Cytotoxic Actions. Uracil mustard may cause nausea and vomiting. The drug is not a vesicant. Cytotoxicity characteristic of the nitrogen mustards has been observed in subacute and chronic toxicity studies of uracil mustard in animals.

Absorption, Fate, and Excretion. Uracil mustard is absorbed quickly but not completely after oral administration in dogs. Concentrations in plasma decline rapidly after either oral (2 mg/kg) or intravenous (1 mg/kg) administration, and no evidence of drug is detected at 2 hours. Less than 1% of the administered dose is recovered unchanged in the urine.

Preparation, Dosage, and Route of Administration. *Uracil Mustard,* U.S.P., is available in capsules containing 1 mg. Two oral dosage schedules are recommended: (1) 1 to 2 mg daily for 3 weeks, repeated after an interruption of 1 week; and (2) 3 to 5 mg daily for 7 days, then 1 mg daily for 3 weeks.

Therapeutic Uses and Clinical Toxicity. Uracil mustard can be administered orally and, in contrast to cyclophosphamide, does not cause frank alopecia. Its clinical spectrum of action is similar to that of other related alkylating agents. Hematopoietic depression is the major manifestation of toxicity, and uracil mustard has been considered useful for controlling thrombocytosis. Nausea, vomiting, diarrhea, and dermatitis have also been noted.

CHLORAMBUCIL

This aromatic derivative of mechlorethamine was synthesized first at the Chester Beatty Research Institute in England. Initial clinical studies demonstrated beneficial results primarily in chronic lymphocytic leukemia, as well as in Hodgkin's disease and related malignant lymphomas. (For references to the early reports, *see* Calabresi and Welch, 1962.)

Chemistry. The chemical formula of chlorambucil and its relation to the nitrogen mustards are presented above (*see* Table 55–1).

Pharmacological and Cytotoxic Actions. Although CNS stimulation can occur, this has been observed only with large doses. Nausea and vomiting may result from single oral doses of 20 mg or more. Cytotoxic effects on the bone marrow, lymphoid organs, and epithelial tissues are similar to those observed with the nitrogen mustards.

Absorption, Fate, and Excretion. Oral absorption of chlorambucil is adequate and reliable. The drug has a half-life in plasma of approximately 90 minutes, and it is almost completely metabolized (Alberts *et al.*, 1979a).

Preparations, Dosage, and Route of Administration. *Chlorambucil,* U.S.P. (LEUKERAN), is available in 2-mg tablets for oral administration. The standard initial daily dosage is 0.1 to 0.2 mg/kg, continued for at least 3 to 6 weeks. The total daily dose, usually 4 to 10 mg, is given at one time. With fall in the peripheral total leukocyte count or clinical improvement, the dosage is reduced; maintenance therapy (usually 2 mg daily) is feasible and may be required, depending on the nature of the disease.

Therapeutic Uses and Clinical Toxicity. At the recommended dosages, chlorambucil is the slowest-acting nitrogen mustard in clinical use. It is the treatment of choice in chronic lymphocytic leukemia and in primary (Waldenström's) macroglobulinemia.

In chronic lymphocytic leukemia, chlorambucil may be given orally for long periods of time, achieving its effects gradually and often without toxicity to a precariously compromised bone marrow. Its spectrum of action is similar to that of other alkylating agents, and remissions may be expected in Hodgkin's disease and lymphomas, and sometimes in solid tumors. Clinical improvement comparable to that with melphalan or cyclophosphamide has been observed in some patients with plasma-cell myeloma. In combination with methotrexate and dactinomycin it has been useful in the management of testicular carcinomas. Beneficial results have also been reported in disorders with altered immune reactivity, such as vasculitis associated with rheumatoid arthritis and autoimmune hemolytic anemia with cold agglutinins. (*See* Livingston and Carter, 1970; Gardner, 1972; Knospe *et al.,* 1974.)

Although it is possible to induce marked hypoplasia of the bone marrow with excessive doses of chlorambucil administered over long periods of time, its myelosuppressive action is usually moderate, gradual, and rapidly reversible. Gastrointestinal discomfort, dermatitis, and hepatotoxicity may be encountered occasionally. A marked increase in the incidence of leukemia and other tumors has been noted in a large controlled study of its use for the treatment of polycythemia vera by the National Polycythemia Vera Study Group, as well as in patients with breast cancer receiving long-term adjuvant chemotherapy (Lerner, 1978).

ETHYLENIMINES AND METHYLMELAMINES

TRIETHYLENEMELAMINE (TEM), THIOTEPA (TRIETHYLENETHIOPHOSPHORAMIDE), AND HEXAMETHYLMELAMINE (HMM)

Triethylenemelamine (TEM) was first synthesized by industrial chemists for use in improving the finish of rayon fabrics. Because of the presence of ethylenimine groups in its structure, the cytotoxic and pharmacological actions were studied by various investigators (*see* Calabresi and Welch, 1962). Thiotepa was introduced clinically in 1953.

Chemistry. The chemical structures of TEM, thiotepa, and HMM are discussed above in conjunction with the structure-activity relationship of the alkylating agents.

Status. Although still available for clinical use, ethylenimines are now seldom employed as therapeutic agents, having been replaced by selected nitrogen mustards. Their areas of usefulness are presented in Table XIII-1 (page 1252), and their pharmacological properties are described in the *third edition* of this textbook.

Although hexamethylmelamine (HMM) was introduced for clinical trial in the early 1960s, it has only recently been shown that the drug has significant activity for the treatment of ovarian cancer and is active against human pulmonary and renal tumors grown in athymic mice. A prospective clinical trial of HMM, cyclophosphamide, methotrexate, and fluorouracil has demonstrated that this concurrent use of four drugs is more effective than melphalan in the management of advanced ovarian adenocarcinoma (Young *et al.,* 1978). Hexamethylmelamine is available only for investigational purposes in the United States. It is administered orally but is poorly absorbed, and it causes nausea and vomiting, myelosuppression, and neurotoxicity. A more soluble compound, pentamethylmelamine, which is a major metabolite of HMM, is in the early phases of clinical testing (Rutty and Connors, 1977).

ALKYL SULFONATES

BUSULFAN

During the course of an investigation to determine the antineoplastic properties of a series of alkanesulfonic acid esters, the rather selective action of *busulfan* was detected. This finding led to the use of the drug in patients with chronic granulocytic leukemia.

Chemistry. Busulfan is quite stable in dry form. The chemical formula of this compound is shown on page 1260.

Pharmacological and Cytotoxic Actions. Busulfan is unique in that it exerts virtually no pharmacological action other than myelosuppression. At low doses, selective depression of granulocytopoiesis is evident. Platelets are also affected by relatively small amounts of drug, and erythroid elements may be suppressed as the dosage is raised; eventually, a pancytopenia results. Cytotoxic action does not appear to extend to either the lymphoid tissues or the gastrointestinal epithelium.

Absorption, Fate, and Excretion. Busulfan is well absorbed after oral administration, and it disappears from the blood rapidly after intravenous administration. Almost all of the drug is excreted in the urine as methanesulfonic acid. The metabolism of busulfan has been reviewed in relation to its mechanism of action by Warwick (1963).

Preparation, Dosage, and Route of Administration. *Busulfan,* U.S.P. (MYLERAN), is available in scored, 2-mg tablets. The initial oral dose varies with the total leukocyte count and the severity of the disease; daily doses from 2 to 6 mg are recommended to initiate therapy and are adjusted appropriately to subsequent hematological and clinical responses. It has been reported that reduction of the total leukocyte count to 10,000 or fewer cells per cubic millimeter before discontinuing the drug results in longer remissions. If maintenance doses are required to keep the hematological status under control, 1 to 3 mg may be given daily.

Therapeutic Uses and Clinical Toxicity. The beneficial effects of busulfan in chronic granulocytic leukemia are well established, and remissions may be expected in 85 to 90% of patients after the initial course of therapy. (*See* Galton, 1969; Livingston and Carter, 1970.)

Reduction in morbidity is readily apparent with symptomatic response, characterized by increased appetite and sense of well-being, which may occur within a few days. Reduction of the leukocyte count is noted during the second or third week, and regression of splenomegaly follows. Evidence has been advanced that median longevity in patients receiving busulfan is increased by 9 months, as compared to a control series. The results obtained are considered to be better than those achieved by treatment with either ^{32}P–inorganic phosphate, x-radiation, antimetabolites, or other alkylating agents. Beneficial results have been reported in other myeloproliferative disorders, including polycythemia vera and myelofibrosis with myeloid metaplasia. The drug is of no value in acute leukemia or in the "blastic crisis" of chronic granulocytic leukemia.

The major toxic effects of busulfan are related to its myelosuppressive properties, and thrombocytopenia may be a hazard. Occasional instances of nausea, vomiting, diarrhea, impotence, sterility, amenorrhea, and fetal malformation have been reported. Hyperuricemia, resulting from extensive purine catabolism accompanying the rapid cellular destruction, and renal damage from precipitation of urates have been noted. To avoid this complication, the concurrent use of *allopurinol* is recommended. A number of unusual complications have been observed in patients receiving busulfan, but their relation to the drug is poorly understood; these include generalized skin pigmentation, gynecomastia, cheilosis, glossitis, anhidrosis, and pulmonary fibrosis. (For references, *see* Calabresi and Welch, 1962.)

NITROSOUREAS

The nitrosoureas are important antitumor agents that have demonstrated activity against a wide spectrum of human malignancies; they appear to function chemotherapeutically as bifunctional alkylating agents. Since their introduction by investigators at the Southern Research Institute (Johnston *et al.,* 1963; Schabel, 1973), many nitrosoureas have been synthesized. Certain of these agents, particularly carmustine (BCNU), lomustine (CCNU), and semustine

(methyl-CCNU), have attracted special interest because of their high solubility in lipid and, thus, their capacity to cross the blood-brain barrier; this enables their use in the treatment of meningeal leukemias and brain tumors (Wilson *et al.,* 1970; Walker, 1973). Unfortunately, the nitrosoureas used in the clinic to date, with the exception of streptozocin, cause profound, cumulative myelosuppression that limits their therapeutic value.

Streptozocin, originally discovered as an antibiotic, is of special interest. This compound has a methylnitrosourea (MNU) moiety attached to the 2 carbon of glucose (*see* Table 55–2). It has special affinity for beta cells of the islets of Langerhans and is employed as a diabetogenic agent in experimental animals. Streptozocin has proven to be useful in the treatment of human pancreatic islet-cell carcinoma and malignant carcinoid tumors, as well as other human malignancies (Schein *et al.,* 1973, 1974). Although MNU, the active moiety of streptozocin, is cytotoxic to selected human tumors, it also produces powerful and delayed myelosuppression. Furthermore, MNU is particularly prone to cause carbamoylation of lysine residues of proteins (Figure 55–2). Streptozocin is not myelosuppressive and displays little carbamoylating activity. These observations have suggested that the nitrosourea-type moiety might be attached to various carrier molecules, with possible alterations in crucial properties such as tissue specificity, distribution, and toxicity. Chlorozotocin, an agent in which the 2 carbon of glucose is substituted by the chloronitrosourea group (CNU), has been prepared and is in early stages of clinical testing. This compound, unlike streptozocin, is not diabetogenic and, unlike many other nitrosoureas, causes little myelosuppression or carbamoylation. There is reason for optimism that important new nitrosourea-containing derivatives will be prepared. (*See* reviews by Wheeler, 1973, 1975; Ludlum, 1977, 1978.)

CARMUSTINE (BCNU)

This compound was the first of the nitrosourea series to receive extensive clinical evaluation. It is effective against a wide range of experimental tumors.

Pharmacological and Cytotoxic Actions. Carmustine is capable of inhibiting the synthesis of DNA, RNA, and protein in a manner similar but not identical to that of other alkylating agents (Livingston and Carter, 1970). Although bone-marrow suppression is observed, there is an unusually delayed onset of leukopenia and thrombocytopenia that is characteristic of this drug. The nadir of the leukocyte and platelet counts may not be reached until 6 weeks after treatment. Cytotoxic effects on the liver, kidneys, and CNS have been reported (Oliverio, 1973b).

Absorption, Fate, and Excretion. Although carmustine is rapidly absorbed by the oral route, it is administered intravenously because tissue uptake and metabolism occur very quickly; disappearance from the plasma takes place within 5 to 15 minutes. Approximately 80% of radioactively labeled drug appears in the urine within 24 hours as degradation products of the parent compound. The pharmacokinetic properties of the drug may be affected by the lipid content of the plasma and the other tissues. Active metabolites may be responsible for the delayed bone-marrow toxicity. Entry of these products into the cerebrospinal fluid (CSF) is rapid, and their concentrations in the CSF of man are 15 to 30% of the concurrent plasma values (Oliverio, 1973b, 1976; Levin et al., 1978).

Preparation, Dosage, and Route of Administration. *Carmustine* (BICNU) is a light-yellow powder at 4° C; it melts to an oily liquid at 27° C and is stable in the anhydrous state. It is available in vials containing 100 mg. The half-life of the drug in 0.9% sodium chloride solution at pH 6 is 24 hours at room temperature. Carmustine is usually administered intravenously at doses of 100 to 200 mg/sq m, given by infusion during a period of about 1 hour, and it is not repeated for 6 weeks. When used in combination with other chemotherapeutic agents, the dose is usually reduced by 25 to 50%.

Therapeutic Uses and Clinical Toxicity. The spectrum of activity of carmustine is similar to that of other alkylating agents, with significant responses observed in Hodgkin's disease and to a lesser extent in other lymphomas and myeloma. Because of its ability to cross the blood-brain barrier, it has been used in meningeal leukemia and in primary and metastatic tumors of the brain,

with encouraging results. Beneficial responses have been reported in melanomas, as well as in gastrointestinal, breast, bronchogenic, and renal-cell carcinomas (Young et al., 1971; Carter, 1973; Moertel, 1973; Walker, 1973; Wilson et al., 1976).

The most significant clinical toxicity is the characteristically delayed hematopoietic depression described above. The drug is not a vesicant, but local burning pain has been reported after intravenous administration. Nausea and vomiting occur approximately 2 hours after injection, and flushing of the skin and conjunctiva, CNS toxicity, esophagitis, diarrhea, dyspnea, interstitial pulmonary fibrosis, and renal and hepatic toxicity have been reported (Young et al., 1971; Durant et al., 1979).

LOMUSTINE (CCNU) AND SEMUSTINE (METHYL-CCNU)

Pharmacological and Cytotoxic Actions. Lomustine and its methylated analog, semustine, were selected for clinical studies because of their lipid solubility and superiority to carmustine in the treatment of certain experimental tumors. The cytotoxic effects of these compounds are similar to those of carmustine, as is their clinical toxicity. Delayed bone-marrow depression, reflected by leukopenia and thrombocytopenia, is characteristic and similar to that caused by carmustine (Moertel, 1973; Wasserman et al., 1975; Wasserman, 1976).

Absorption, Fate, and Excretion. Lomustine and semustine are rapidly absorbed from the gastrointestinal tract and are administered orally. Although lomustine is rapidly and completely metabolized, prolonged plasma half-life of its metabolites, ranging from 16 to 48 hours, has been reported. Approximately 50% of the administered dose is detectable in the urine within 24 hours and 75% within 4 days. Radioactively labeled semustine is not detectable in either plasma or urine. The chloroethyl moiety has a half-life of 36 hours, while the cyclohexyl portion has a biphasic disappearance curve with an early half-life of 24 hours and a slower secondary phase with a half-life of 72 hours. Although neither drug can be detected intact in the CSF, active metabolites appear in significant concentrations within 30 minutes (Oliverio, 1973b, 1976; Carter and Slavik, 1974).

Preparation, Dosage, and Route of Administration. *Lomustine* (CEENU) is available in a dosage package that contains two 100-mg, two 40-mg, and two 10-mg capsules. Semustine is available only for investigational use. The usual oral dose of lomustine is 130 mg/sq m, while the recommended oral dose of semustine is 200 mg/sq m. Both drugs are administered as a single dose, which is not repeated for 6 weeks. When used concurrently with other antineoplastic drugs, the dose is usually reduced by 25 to 50% (Wasserman, 1976).

Therapeutic Uses and Clinical Toxicity. These agents have a wide spectrum of activity. Lomustine appears to be more effective than carmustine in Hodgkin's disease. Beneficial results of therapy with lomustine and particularly semustine, alone and concurrently with other agents, have been reported in patients with malignant gliomas, adenocarcinomas of the gastrointestinal tract, Hodgkin's disease and other lymphomas, carcinoma of the breast, malignant melanoma, hypernephromas, multiple myeloma, and various squamous-cell carcinomas (Symposium, 1973; Carter and Slavik, 1974; Wilson *et al.*, 1976; Moertel, 1978).

The clinical toxicity of both drugs is similar, with the characteristically delayed bone-marrow suppression described above being the dose-limiting effect. Nausea and vomiting are frequently encountered.

STREPTOZOCIN

This naturally occurring nitrosourea is an antibiotic derived from *Streptomyces acromogenes*. It has been particularly useful in treating functional, malignant pancreatic islet-cell tumors (Livingston and Carter, 1970). The drug is capable of inhibiting synthesis of DNA in microorganisms and mammalian cells; it affects all stages of the mammalian cell cycle. Biochemical studies have also revealed potent inhibitory effects on pyridine nucleotides and on key enzymes involved in glyconeogenesis.

Absorption, Fate, and Excretion. Streptozocin is administered parenterally. After intravenous infusions of 200 to 1600 mg/sq m, peak concentrations in the plasma are 30 to 40 μg/ml; the half-life of the drug is approximately 15 minutes. Only 10 to 20% of a dose is recovered in the urine (Schein *et al.*, 1973).

Preparation, Dosage, and Route of Administration. Although streptozocin is not commercially available, it can be obtained from the Cancer Therapy Evaluation Branch of the National Cancer Institute, Bethesda, Maryland 20014. The drug is administered intravenously or intra-arterially in doses of 500 to 1500 mg/sq m once a week for 4 weeks. It may be continued if a beneficial response is observed.

Therapeutic Uses and Clinical Toxicity. Streptozocin has been used primarily in patients with meta-

static pancreatic islet-cell carcinoma, and beneficial responses are translated into a significant increase in 1-year survival rate and a doubling of median survival time for the responders. It has also been found to be active in Hodgkin's disease, other lymphomas, and occasionally in melanoma and malignant carcinoid tumors (Schein *et al.*, 1974). Broder and Carter (1973) noted nausea and vomiting in almost all of 52 patients treated for islet-cell carcinoma. Renal or hepatic toxicity occurs in approximately two thirds of cases; although usually reversible, renal toxicity may be fatal, and proximal tubular damage is the most important toxic effect. Serial determinations of urinary protein are most valuable in detecting early renal effects. Hematological toxicity, consisting in anemia, leukopenia, or thrombocytopenia, occurs in 20% of patients.

TRIAZENES

DACARBAZINE (DTIC)

Dacarbazine, the chemistry of which is described above, was originally believed to act as an antimetabolite; more recent evidence indicates that it functions as an alkylating agent after metabolic activation in the liver by microsomal enzymes. Dacarbazine appears to inhibit the synthesis of RNA and protein more than that of DNA. It kills cells slowly, and there appears to be no phase of the cell cycle in which sensitivity is increased (Bono, 1976). Minimal immunosuppressive activity has been noted.

Absorption, Fate, and Excretion. Dacarbazine is administered intravenously; after an initial rapid phase of disappearance ($t_{1/2}$ of about 20 minutes), the drug is removed from plasma with a half-time of about 5 hours (Loo *et al.*, 1976). The half-life is prolonged in the presence of hepatic or renal disease. Almost one half of the compound is excreted intact in the urine by tubular secretion. Elevated urinary concentrations of 5-aminoimidazole-4-carboxamide (AIC) are derived from the catabolism of dacarbazine, rather than by inhibition of *de-novo* purine biosynthesis. Concentrations of dacarbazine in CSF are approximately 14% of those in plasma.

Preparation, Dosage, and Route of Administration. *Dacarbazine* (DTIC-DOME) is available in vials that contain 100 or 200 mg. The recommended regimen is to give 3.5 mg/kg per day, intravenously, for a 10-day period; this is repeated every 28 days. Alternatively, 250 mg/sq m can be given daily for 5 days and repeated every 3 weeks. Extravasation of the drug may cause tissue damage and severe pain.

Therapeutic Uses and Clinical Toxicity. At present, dacarbazine is employed principally for the treatment of malignant melanoma; the overall response rate is about 20%. Beneficial responses have also been reported in patients with Hodgkin's disease, particularly when the drug is used concurrently with doxorubicin, bleomycin, and vinblastine, as well as in various sarcomas when used with doxorubicin (Costanzi, 1976; Gottlieb *et al.*, 1976). Toxicity includes nausea and vomiting in more than 90% of patients, which usually develops 1 to 3 hours after treatment, and myelosuppression, with both leukopenia and thrombocytopenia. Hepatotoxicity, fever, myalgias, malaise, alopecia, facial flushing, neurotoxicity, and dermatological reactions have also been reported.

II. Antimetabolites

FOLIC ACID ANALOGS

METHOTREXATE

This class of antimetabolites not only produced the first striking, although temporary, remissions in leukemia (Farber et al., 1948) but also provided the first drug to cause long-lasting remissions in choriocarcinoma in women, a relatively rare hormone-producing neoplasm (Hertz, 1963). The attainment of a high percentage of permanent remissions in this otherwise-lethal disease has justified the use of the word cure and has given great impetus to chemotherapeutic investigation. However, interpretation of these results must be tempered by the knowledge that choriocarcinoma is a transplanted tumor that arises from fetal membranes and, therefore, may be affected by host defense mechanisms. Interest in folate antagonists has increased greatly with the introduction of "rescue" technics that employ leucovorin (folinic acid, citrovorum factor) and/or thymidine to protect normal tissues against lethal damage. These methods permit the use of very high doses of folate analogs such as methotrexate and extend their utility to tumors such as osteogenic sarcoma that do not respond to lower doses.

Methotrexate has also been used with benefit in the therapy of psoriasis, a nonneoplastic disease of the skin characterized by abnormally rapid proliferation of epidermal cells (Van Scott et al., 1964; McDonald and Bertino, 1968). Additionally, folate antagonists are potent inhibitors of some types of immune reactions and have been employed as immunosuppressive agents, for example, in organ transplantation (Hitchings

and Elion, 1963; Schwartz, 1965). (For recent reviews, see Bertino, 1975, 1979; Chabner and Johns, 1977; Ensminger et al., 1979.)

Structure-Activity Relationship. Folic acid is an essential dietary factor from which is derived a coenzyme, tetrahydrofolic acid, and a group of structurally related derivatives; these are concerned with the metabolic transfer of one-carbon units. A detailed description of the biological functions and therapeutic applications of folic acid appears in Chapter 57.

Although there are many metabolic loci where folate analogs (antifols) might act, the enzyme dihydrofolate reductase is the primary site of action of most analogs studied to date (see Figure 57-1). This enzyme has been purified from a number of species. Important structural differences among the various enzymes have enabled the design of important therapeutic agents for the treatment of bacterial and malarial infections (see discussion of trimethoprim, Chapter 49; pyrimethamine, Chapter 45). Of necessity, these inhibitors have much greater activity against the bacterial and protozoal dihydrofolate reductases than they do against the mammalian enzyme. Such developments have introduced a new level of sophistication into the science of chemotherapy and suggest the possibility of developing new analogs of folate that have unique advantages for the chemotherapy of neoplastic diseases.

A crucial consideration is that folic acid and many of its analogs enter mammalian cells by means of a carrier-mediated membrane transport system, rather than by diffusion. This saturable transport system displays relatively high structural specificity. For example, the rate of influx is increased by about 100-fold if an amino group replaces the hydroxyl group on the 4 carbon of the pteridine ring (as in methotrexate; see structure below); if the glutamate moiety of folic acid has only one free carboxyl group, influx is decreased. This subject is currently under intensive investigation in the hope that detailed understanding of this transport process will permit the design of new and more effective agents (see Sirotnak et al., 1979).

Another important factor is the poor ability of methotrexate to cross the blood-brain barrier, due to its very polar nature. Among numerous new agents under experimental study is 2,4-diamino-5-(3',4'-dichlorophenyl)-6-methylpyrimidine (DDMP). This is a lipid-soluble folate antagonist, and it is fully active against cells that are resistant to methotrexate because of a lack of the specific transport system. DDMP readily penetrates the blood-brain barrier and may concentrate in brain tumors at levels tenfold greater than those found in plasma. For further discussion and references, see Hitchings and

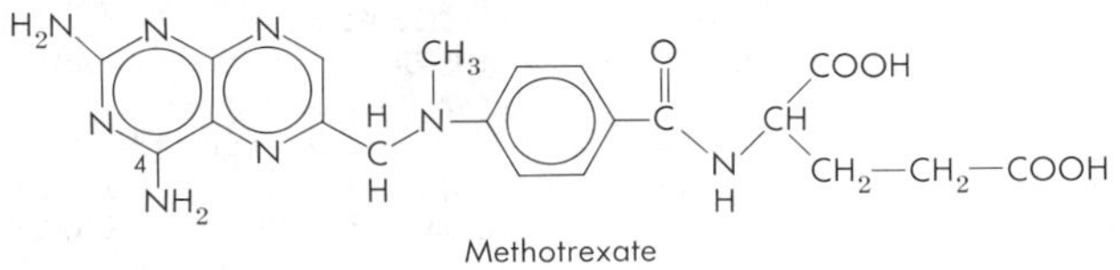

Methotrexate

Burchall (1965), Johns and Bertino (1973), Ensminger and associates (1979), and Sirotnak and coworkers (1979).

Mechanism of Action. To understand the mechanism of action of folate analogs such as methotrexate, it is necessary to appreciate the complexities of the metabolism of folate cofactors and their multiplicity of functions; this is discussed in Chapter 57. To function as a cofactor in one-carbon transfer reactions, folate must first be reduced by dihydrofolate reductase to tetrahydrofolate (FH_4). Single carbon fragments are added enzymatically to FH_4 in various configurations and may then be transferred in specific synthetic reactions. A key metabolic event is catalyzed by thymidylate synthetase and involves the conversion of 2-deoxyuridylate (dUMP) to thymidylate, an essential component of DNA. The methyl group transferred to the uracil moiety of dUMP is donated by N^{5-10}-methylene FH_4. Significantly, this carbon atom is transferred to the pyrimidine ring at the oxidation level of formaldehyde and is reduced to methyl by the pteridine ring of the folate coenzyme; the result is the formation of dihydrofolate (FH_2). Thus, to function again as a cofactor, FH_2 must first be reduced to FH_4 by dihydrofolate reductase. Inhibitors with a high affinity for dihydrofolate reductase prevent the formation of FH_4 and cause major disruptions in cellular metabolism by producing an acute intracellular deficiency of folate coenzymes. The folate coenzymes become trapped as FH_2 polyglutamates, which cannot function metabolically. One-carbon transfer reactions crucial for the *de-novo* synthesis of purine nucleotides and of thymidylate cease, with the subsequent interruption of the synthesis of DNA and RNA (as well as other vital metabolic reactions).

Understanding of these events enables appreciation of the rationale for the use of thymidine and/or leucovorin (N^5-formyl FH_4; folinic acid) in the "rescue" of normal cells from toxicity caused by drugs such as methotrexate. Leucovorin is a fully reduced, metabolically functional folate coenzyme; it enters cells via the specific carrier-mediated transport system and is convertible to other folate cofactors. Thus, it may function directly, without the need for reduction by dihydrofolate reductase, in reactions such as those required for purine biosynthesis. On the other hand, thymidine may be converted to thymidylate by thymidine kinase, thus bypassing the reaction catalyzed by thymidylate synthetase and providing the necessary precursor for DNA synthesis.

An important feature of the binding of active folate antagonists with dihydrofolate reductases is the very low inhibition constants observed (on the order of 1 nM). Covalent bonds are not involved in the enzyme-inhibitor interactions despite the unusually great affinity of the antagonists for dihydrofolate reductase. Huennekens (1968) has pointed out that the negative free-energy change of the binding of aminopterin to chicken liver dihydrofolate reductase is about 3.7 kcal per mole greater than that of dihydrofolate. This is approximately the amount of free energy required for the formation of either a single hydrogen bond or an ionic bond. Recently the structure of the ternary complex formed by dihydrofolate

reductase (from *Lactobacillus casei*), methotrexate, and NADPH has been solved at 2.5 Å resolution by x-ray analysis. The substrate binding sites have been identified, and structural models offer insights into the reaction mechanism and the conformational changes that occur when substrates or inhibitors bind, as well as an explanation for the very high affinity of methotrexate for the enzyme. Studies of this type are landmarks in the history of chemotherapy and hopefully will allow the design of therapeutic agents on the basis of specific and detailed knowledge of the chemical structures of target enzymes or receptors (*see* Matthews *et al.,* 1978).

As with most inhibitors of cellular reproduction, a selective effect on neoplastic cells is obtainable to only a partial extent with methotrexate. Folate antagonists kill cells during the S phase of the cell cycle, and evidence indicates that methotrexate is much more effective when the cellular population is in the logarithmic phase of growth, rather than in the plateau phase. Because it is also capable of inhibiting RNA and protein synthesis, however, methotrexate slows the entry of cells into S phase and its cytotoxic action has been referred to as "self-limiting" (Skipper and Schabel, 1973).

Mechanism of Resistance to Antifolates. Although evidence is incomplete, three biochemical mechanisms of acquired resistance to methotrexate have been clearly demonstrated: (1) impaired transport of methotrexate into cells, (2) production of altered forms of dihydrofolate reductase that have decreased affinity for the inhibitor, and (3) increased concentrations of intracellular dihydrofolate reductase. It has been known for years that blood elements with marked increases in the activity of dihydrofolate reductase appear within days after treatment of patients with leukemia with single doses of methotrexate. This may reflect induction of new enzyme synthesis, temporary elimination from the marrow of cells that are susceptible to the drug because of low enzymatic activity, or protection of dihydrofolate reductase against catabolic degradation by intracellular proteases. It is well established that the enzyme, complexed with methotrexate, undergoes conformational changes that render it remarkably resistant to proteolysis.

Of special interest is the discovery of the phenomenon of gene amplification and its relationship to acquired resistance to methotrexate and perhaps other cytotoxic agents. Increases in dihydrofolate reductase activity can result from increased synthesis of the enzyme because of elevated intracellular concentrations of its specific mRNA. This phenomenon is apparently due to the occurrence in these resistant cells of increased numbers of copies of the gene for dihydrofolate reductase. For further discussion, *see* Schimke and associates (1978) and Bertino (1979).

Various therapeutic tactics have been recommended to avoid selection of resistant cells. The use of high doses of methotrexate with leucovorin "rescue" may permit the intracellular accumulation of methotrexate in concentrations that inactivate dihydrofolate reductase even when the enzyme is present at markedly elevated levels. Alternation of treatment with methotrexate with other active therapeutic agents that function by different mechanisms is another way to attempt to kill cells that are resistant.

General Toxicity and Cytotoxic Action. The actions of 4-amino analogs of folate in animals have been studied extensively. Animals given a minimal lethal dose survive for at least 48 hours and usually die within 3 to 5 days. Anorexia, progressive weight loss, bloody diarrhea, leukopenia, depression, and coma are the outstanding features of fatal intoxication. The major lesions occur in the *intestinal tract* and *bone marrow.* Swelling and cytoplasmic vacuolization of the mucosal cells of the intestinal epithelium are evident within 6 hours. These changes are followed by desquamation of epithelial cells, extrusion of plasma into the lumen of the bowel, and leukocytic infiltration of the submucosa. Terminally, the entire intestinal tract exhibits a severe hemorrhagic desquamating enteritis. Degeneration of bone marrow develops rapidly. Within 24 hours there is evident disturbance in the maturation of erythrocytes. Proliferation of erythroid precursors is inhibited, and significant proportions of primitive erythroid elements have the appearance of megaloblasts. Rapid pathological alteration in myelopoiesis also occurs, and within a few days the bone marrow becomes aplastic. There is diminution in content of lymphoid cells in lymphatic tissue, but there is no evidence of necrosis. The disturbance in hematopoiesis is reflected in the circulating blood by a marked granulocytopenia and reticulocytopenia and a moderate lymphopenia.

Folic acid antagonists seriously interfere with *embryogenesis.* The site of action is on the embryonic mesenchyme. Decidual and placental tissues are unaffected by doses of the drugs that cause fetal death. Young embryos are much more susceptible than are the more developed. The administration of methotrexate during pregnancy obviously is accompanied by great hazards to the fetus.

Absorption, Fate, and Excretion. Methotrexate is readily absorbed from the gastrointestinal tract at doses routinely employed in clinical practice (0.1 mg/kg), but larger doses are incompletely absorbed. The drug is also absorbed from parenteral sites of injection. A direct relationship exists between dose and plasma concentrations. Following intravenous administration, the drug disappears from plasma in a triphasic fashion (Huffman *et al.,* 1973). The first phase, due to the distribution into body fluids, has a half-time of about 45 minutes. The second phase reflects renal clearance ($t_{1/2}$ of 2.0 to 3.5 hours). The final phase has a half-time of about 10 hours and begins when the concentration in plasma approximates 0.1 μM. This terminal half-life, if unduly prolonged, may be responsible for major toxic effects of the drug on the marrow and gastrointestinal tract. Distribution of methotrexate into body spaces, such as the pleural or peritoneal cavities, may occur. If such spaces are expanded (*e.g.,* by ascites or pleural effusion), they may act as a site of storage and release of drug with resultant prolonged elevation of plasma concentrations and more severe toxicity.

Approximately 50% of the drug is bound to plasma proteins. Laboratory studies suggest that it may be displaced from plasma albumin by a number of drugs, including sulfonamides, salicylates, tetracycline, chloramphenicol, and phenytoin; caution should be used if these are given concomitantly. Of the drug absorbed, from 40 to 50% of a small dose (2.5 to 15 μg/kg) to about 90% of a large dose (150 μg/kg) is excreted unchanged in the urine within 48 hours, mostly within the first 8 hours. A small amount of methotrexate is also excreted in the stool, probably through the biliary tract. Metabolism of methotrexate in man does not seem to occur to a significant degree. After high doses, however, a potentially nephrotoxic 7-hydroxylated metabolite has been detected. The portion of each dose of methotrexate that normally is excreted rapidly gains access to the urine by a combination of glomerular filtration and active tubular secretion. Therefore, the concurrent use of drugs that also undergo tubular secretion, as well as impaired renal function, can influence markedly the response to this drug. Particular caution must be exercised in treating patients with renal insufficiency.

The portion of methotrexate that is retained in human tissues remains for long periods, for example, for weeks in the kidneys and for several months in the liver. The data strongly suggest that methotrexate retained within cells is bound primarily by dihydrofolate reductase, which thereby is prevented from functioning. The affinity of methotrexate for the cytoplasmic enzyme protein is so great that the very gradual release of drug may represent only the minute amounts that are gradually displaced by folate and dihydrofolate, as well as that released by cells that die.

It is important to emphasize that methotrexate is very poorly transported across the blood-brain barrier; hence, neoplastic cells that have entered the CNS probably are not affected by usual concentrations of drug in the plasma. When high doses of methotrexate are given, followed by leucovorin "rescue" (see below), substantial concentrations of methotrexate may be attained in the CNS. The pharmacokinetic properties of methotrexate have been discussed by Bleyer (1978); see also Appendix II.

Preparations, Dosage, and Routes of Administration. *Methotrexate*, U.S.P. (*amethopterin*), is provided in scored, 2.5-mg tablets and also as a dry powder (the sodium salt) in vials containing either 2.5, 20, or 25 mg for preparation of sterile injectable solutions.

Although the standard daily oral dosage of methotrexate ordinarily employed in patients with *leukemia* has been 2.5 to 5 mg for children and 2.5 to 10 mg for adults, newer therapeutic concepts have emerged involving revised dosage schedules and the use of multiple drugs sequentially and concurrently. Methotrexate *induces* remission slowly, probably because the cells in advanced leukemia are not in the logarithmic phase of growth. For induction of remission it has been superseded by the more rapid and effective therapy with vincristine plus prednisone, with or without daunorubicin. Methotrexate is of great value in the *maintenance* of remissions, particularly when administered intermittently at high doses of 30 mg/sq m, intramuscularly, twice a week (Acute Leukemia Group B, 1965), or by intensive 2-day "pulses" of 175 to 525 mg/sq m at monthly intervals.

The *intrathecal administration* of methotrexate has been employed, particularly when manifestations of cerebral involvement in either leukemia or choriocarcinoma have appeared, as occurs not infrequently even during systemic remissions. This route of administration achieves high concentrations of methotrexate in the CSF and is effective also in patients whose systemic disease has become resistant to methotrexate, since the leukemic cells in the CNS beyond the blood-brain barrier have survived in a pharmacological sanctuary and retain their original degree of sensitivity to the drug. The recommended intrathecal dose is 0.2 to 0.5 mg/kg, given once or repeated at intervals of 2 to 5 days, depending on the severity of involvement and the response to therapy; another dosage schedule is 12 mg/sq m once weekly for 2 weeks and then monthly. Leucovorin may be administered intramuscularly to counteract the systemic toxicity of methotrexate.

In the treatment of *choriocarcinoma* with methotrexate, intensive treatment is usually employed, for example, 15 mg/sq m (15 to 30 mg) daily for 5 days orally or parenterally. Courses are repeated at 1- to 2-week intervals, toxicity permitting, and urinary gonadotropin titers are used as a guide for persistence of disease.

Methotrexate has been used in the treatment of severe, disabling *psoriasis* in doses of 2.5 to 5 mg orally for 5 days or 25 to 50 mg intravenously weekly. An initial parenteral test dose of 5 to 10 mg is recommended to detect any possible idiosyncrasy. Complete awareness of the pharmacology and toxic potential of methotrexate is a prerequisite for its use in this nonneoplastic disorder (Weinstein, 1977).

Continuous infusion of relatively large amounts of methotrexate may be employed (from 250 mg to 1 g/sq m, or more, weekly), but only when the technic of leucovorin "rescue" is used. The rationale for the administration of high doses is to achieve an excess of intracellular unbound drug, such that DNA synthesis is inhibited almost completely. Extremely high (0.1 to 1 mM) concentrations of drug must be achieved extracellularly in order to overcome any deficiency of the carrier-mediated transport system. After infusion of methotrexate for 6 to 30 hours, leucovorin is injected at a dose of 6 to 16 mg/sq m every 6 hours for 48 to 72 hours; the goal is to rescue normal cells and thereby prevent toxicity. Other technics for rescue, involving carboxypeptidase G, asparaginase, and thymidine, have also been investigated. The administration of methotrexate at these dosages may be extremely dangerous and should be performed only by experienced chemotherapists who are capable of quantification of the concentrations of methotrexate and leucovorin in plasma. With appropriate precautions, these investigational schedules are surprisingly free of toxicity. It is imperative to maintain the output of a large volume of alkaline urine, since methotrexate precipitates in the renal tubules in acidic urine. In the presence of malignant effusions, delayed clearance may cause severe toxicity. Although the use of methotrexate in high doses with leucovorin "rescue" has been studied clinically for several years with very encouraging results, the optimal timing, dose of leucovorin required, and proof of enhanced therapeutic efficacy remain to be established (see Djerassi et al., 1972; Jaffe, 1972; Levitt et al., 1973; Chabner et al., 1975; Bertino, 1977; Bleyer, 1978; Goldin, 1978).

Therapeutic Uses and Clinical Toxicity. Methotrexate is a useful drug in the management of *acute lymphoblastic leukemia* in children. However, methotrexate is of very limited value in the types of leukemia seen in adults. It is of established value in *choriocarcinoma* and related trophoblastic tumors of women, with complete and lasting remissions occurring in approximately 75% of women treated sequentially with methotrexate and dactinomycin, and in over 90% when early diagnosis is accompanied by a low concentration of gonadotropin in the urine. A number of these patients are living without evidence of disease more than 20 years after initiation of therapy. In addition, many women with nonmeta-static trophoblastic disease, *hydatidiform mole,* and *chorioadenoma destruens,* have been treated successfully with methotrexate (Hertz *et al.,* 1963). Beneficial results have also been reported in patients with *mycosis fungoides* and with *carcinomas* of the breast, tongue, pharynx, and testes (in conjunction with chlorambucil and dactinomycin), as well as in occasional patients with other tumors. High-dose methotrexate, with subsequent leucovorin "rescue," can cause substantial tumor regression in at least two tumors highly refractory to most chemotherapeutic agents: carcinoma of the lung (Djerassi *et al.,* 1972) and osteogenic sarcoma (Jaffe, 1972). (For other references, *see* Calabresi and Welch, 1962; Livingston and Carter, 1970; Greenwald, 1973.) Striking improvement has been observed with the use of methotrexate in the treatment of severe *psoriasis.* Furthermore, methotrexate is an effective immunosuppressive agent and has been used for prevention of graft-versus-host reactions that result from marrow transplantation, as well as in the management of dermatomyositis, rheumatoid arthritis, Wegener's granulomatosis, and pityriasis rubra pilaris (*see* Weinstein, 1977; Bleyer, 1978).

Treatment with methotrexate requires constant surveillance of the patient in order to judge dosage properly and to avoid serious toxic reactions. In persons treated with conventional doses or with concomitant leucovorin, it is frequently possible to avoid severe leukopenia or aplasia of the bone marrow. Thrombocytopenia with bleeding can be treated with platelet transfusions, but it may be difficult to control, particularly in the presence of infection. It is imperative that a skilled medical team and sophisticated facilities, particularly abundant platelet transfusions and measures for preventing and combating infections, be available in order to provide the intensive supportive therapy necessary to control the severe toxic manifestations that may result when intensive dosage schedules are used.

Other untoward reactions also may complicate the use of methotrexate. Ulcerative stomatitis and diarrhea are frequent side effects and require interruption of the therapeutic regimen; hemorrhagic enteritis and death from intestinal perforation may occur. Additional toxic manifestations include alopecia, dermatitis, nephrotoxicity, defective oogenesis or spermatogenesis, abortion, teratogenesis, and hepatic dysfunction, usually reversible but sometimes leading to cirrhosis. The long-term complications associated with the use of methotrexate for immunosuppressive therapy are discussed by Schein and Winokur (1975).

PYRIMIDINE ANALOGS

This class of agents encompasses a diverse, interesting, and, in some cases, clinically useful group of drugs that have in common the capacity to impede the biosynthesis of pyrimidine nucleotides or to mimic these natural metabolites to such an extent that they interfere with vital cellular activities, such as the synthesis and functioning of nucleic acids. Certain of the drugs in this group are employed in the treatment of a variety of afflictions, including neoplastic diseases, psoriasis, and infections caused by fungi and DNA-containing viruses. When selected members of the group are used together or concurrently with other antimetabolites, synergistic effects have been demonstrated against various experimental tumors, and some of these treatment schedules are being investigated clinically. (*See* reviews by Calabresi and Welch, 1962; Heidelberger, 1973, 1975; Chabner *et al.,* 1975; Creasey, 1975a; Ho and Freireich, 1975; Prusoff and Goz, 1975; Skoda, 1975; Maley, 1977.)

General Mechanism of Action and Structure-Activity Relationship. The antineoplastic agents fluorouracil (5-FU) and cytarabine (ara-C), the antiviral compound idoxuridine, and the antifungal agent flucytosine (Chapter 54) are the drugs in this group that are established clinically. However, several other compounds are in early stages of clinical investigation. Especially exciting prospects evolve from recent discoveries about the biochemical properties of certain viruses, for example, herpes simplex I and II and related DNA viruses. These viral pathogens induce the synthesis of a highly unusual nucleoside kinase. Thus, if the 5'-hydroxyl group of idoxuridine (*see* Table 55–3) is replaced by an amino group, as in 5'-amino-idoxuridine, this enzyme catalyzes the phosphorylation of the amino group with the ultimate formation in the cells of the highly unstable analog of dTPP (Cheng *et al.,* 1975). Similarly, this enzyme can catalyze the synthesis of nucleotides from purine nucleoside analogs such as acycloguanosine (Schaeffer *et al.,* 1978). These new agents appear to have high antiviral activity but low toxicity to normal cells. Especially intriguing is the prospect of designing agents that are active against the Epstein-Barr virus, a DNA virus closely related to herpes viruses, which is presumed to be the causative agent of infectious mononucleosis; it has also been implicated in the etiology of certain malignancies such as Burkitt's lymphoma, Hodgkin's disease, and nasopharyngeal carcinoma.

Several new agents display potent inhibitory activity at specific points in the pathway of synthesis of pyrimidine nucleotides. Especially interesting is the compound N-phosphonoacetyl L-aspartate (PALA). PALA was originally designed as a "transition-state" inhibitor of the enzyme aspartate transcarbamylase, which catalyzes an early step in pyrimidine biosynthesis (Collins and Stark, 1971). This analog, which is in the early stages of clinical study, has shown high activity in the treatment of certain murine cancers while causing negligible bone-marrow toxicity. Two other agents are potent inhibitors of a later step in pyrimidine nucleotide synthesis, the coupled enzy-

Table 55-3. STRUCTURAL FORMULAS OF PYRIMIDINE ANALOGS

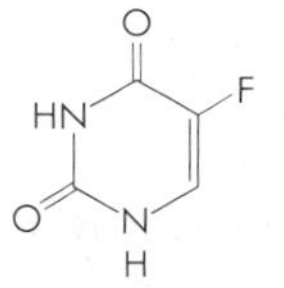

Fluorouracil
(pK$_a$ 8.1)

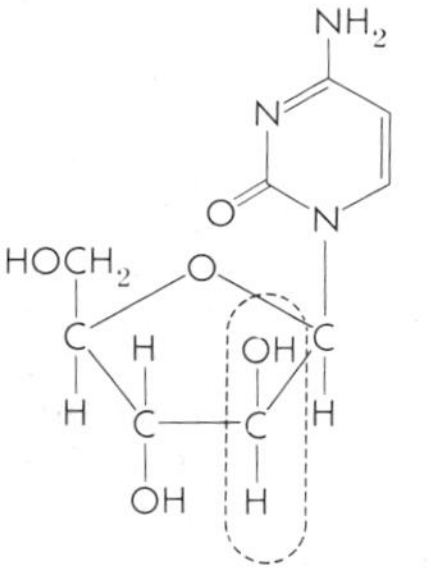

Cytarabine
(Cytosine Arabinoside)
(pK$_a$ 4.5)

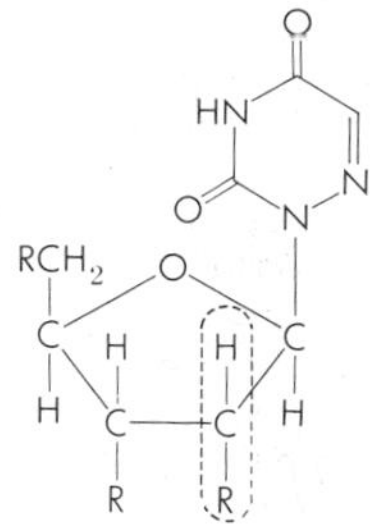

Azauridine: R = —OH

Azaribine: R = —O—C—CH$_3$
(pK$_a$ 6.7)

R	van der Waals Radii ($\overset{\circ}{A}$)	Compound	pK$_a$
H	1.20	Deoxyuridine	9.3
F	1.35	Floxuridine (fluorodeoxyuridine)	7.6
Cl	1.80	Chlorodeoxyuridine	7.9
Br	1.95	Bromodeoxyuridine	7.9
CH$_3$	2.00	Thymidine	9.8
I	2.15	Idoxuridine (iododeoxyuridine)	8.25
CF$_3$	2.44	Trifluoromethyldeoxyuridine	7.35

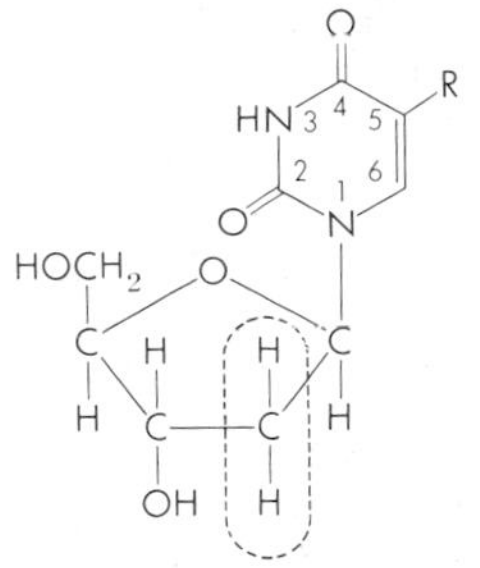

matic reactions by which orotate is first converted to the 5'-monophosphate (orotidylate) and then decarboxylated to form uridylate. The compounds 6-azauridine and pyrazofuran are first themselves converted to the corresponding 5'-monophosphates and then act as potent inhibitors of orotidylate decarboxylase. 6-Azauridine (in the form of the prodrug azaribine; *see* Table 55-3) displays considerable therapeutic activity in patients with severe psoriasis, mycosis fungoides (Calabresi and Turner, 1966), and polycythemia vera (DeConti and Calabresi, 1970). Another new antipyrimidine nucleoside, 3-deazauridine, blocks the metabolism of pyrimidine nucleotides at a still later stage—the formation of cytidine triphosphate (CTP) from uridine triphosphate (UTP).

Among the best-established agents in this class are the halogenated pyrimidines, a group that includes such compounds as fluorouracil and idoxuridine. If one compares the van der Waals radii of the various substituents (Table 55-3), the dimension of the fluorine atom resembles that of hydrogen, whereas the bromine and iodine atoms are close in size to the methyl group. Idoxuridine has relatively little effect on the biosynthesis of thymidylic acid; like thymidine, however, it is converted enzymatically within cells to phosphorylated derivatives; it is also degraded to the corresponding base, iodouracil, which is converted to uracil and iodide. The phosphorylated forms of idoxuridine inhibit competitively the utilization of the analogous derivatives of thymidine and can lead, in appropriate circumstances, to incor-

poration of the analog, as iododeoxyuridylic acid, into DNA in place of thymidylic acid. These activities can suppress temporarily the growth of both experimental and human neoplasms; in addition, incorporation of the iodo- or bromo- analogs into DNA renders the latter more susceptible to the injurious effects of radiation.

If the hydrogen on position 5 of the pyrimidine ring is replaced with fluorine, the chemical reactivity of the ring is significantly altered, although the molecule, fluorouracil, behaves as does uracil with several enzymes. Fluorine has an inductive (electron-withdrawing) effect, which is reflected in a much lower pK$_a$ with fluorouracil-containing compounds than with the natural compounds. The ionization that occurs is as follows:

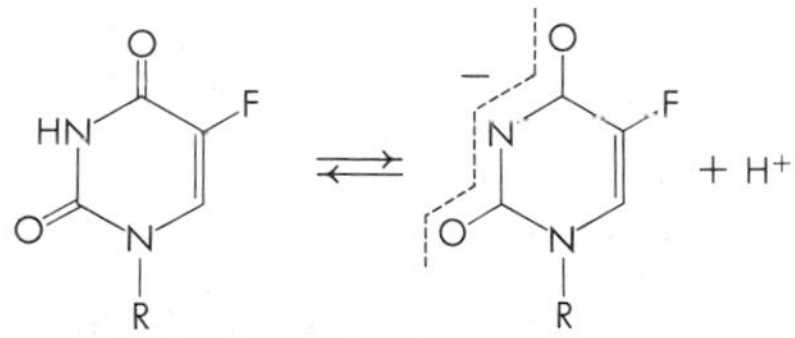

In addition, the carbon-fluorine bond is stronger than the carbon-hydrogen bond and is less susceptible to enzymatic cleavage. Thus, substitution of a halogen atom of the correct dimensions can produce a molecule that sufficiently resembles a natural pyrimidine to interact with enzymes of pyrimidine metabolism and also to interfere drastically with certain other aspects of pyrimidine action.

Among the various modifications of the sugar moiety attempted, the replacement of the ribose of cytidine with arabinose has yielded a useful chemotherapeutic agent, cytarabine. As may be seen in Table 55–3, the deviation from normal in this case involves the 2' carbon of the pentose, in which the hydroxyl group is in the opposite configuration from that of the natural ribonucleoside, cytidine. This yields a molecule that sufficiently resembles a deoxynucleoside to be capable of conversion to the nucleotide level, but which blocks the synthesis of DNA (*see* reviews by Chabner *et al.*, 1975; Creasey, 1975a).

FLUOROURACIL AND FLOXURIDINE (FLUORODEOXYURIDINE)

The chemistry and structure-activity relationship of these analogs are discussed above. The interesting rationale of Heidelberger for the synthesis of these fluorinated pyrimidines is described in the reviews previously cited.

Mechanism of Action. Fluorouracil, as such, is without significant inhibitory activity in mammalian systems, and, in order to inhibit cellular growth, it must first be converted enzymatically to the nucleotide level. Several routes are available for the formation of the 5'-monophosphate nucleotide (F-UMP) in animal cells. Fluorouracil may be converted to fluorouridine by uridine phosphorylase and then to F-UMP by uridine kinase (*see* Heidelberger, 1975), or it may react directly with 5-phosphoribosyl-1-pyrophosphate (PRPP), catalyzed by the enzyme orotate phosphoribosyl transferase, to form F-UMP. The latter enzyme is present in higher concentrations in certain tumors than in liver and reacts with orotate as its natural substrate. Many metabolic pathways are available to F-UMP, including incorporation into RNA. However, the reaction sequence crucial for antineoplastic activity involves reduction of the diphosphate nucleotide by the enzyme ribonucleotide diphosphate reductase to the deoxynucleotide level and the eventual formation of 5-fluoro-2'-deoxyuridine-5'-phosphate (F-dUMP). This complex metabolic pathway for the generation of the actual growth inhibitor, F-dUMP, may be bypassed through use of the deoxyribonucleoside of fluorouracil—floxuridine (fluorodeoxyuridine, FUdR)—which is a substrate for intracellular thymidine kinase. Thus, in a single enzymatic step, the inhibitor of thymidylate synthetase, F-dUMP, can be produced in cells by the use of FUdR. Unfortunately, FUdR is a good substrate for both thymidine and deoxyuridine phosphorylases, and it is rapidly degraded to fluorouracil. The formation of FUdR by the reaction of fluorouracil with deoxyribose-1-phosphate has been demonstrated, but the possible significance of this anabolic reaction in chemotherapy is unclear.

There have been notable advances in our understanding of the interaction between F-dUMP and the enzyme thymidylate synthetase, which is generally regarded as the principal site of cytotoxic action of the drug (Santi and McHenry, 1972). The folate cofactor, $N^{5\text{-}10}$-methylenetetrahydrofolate and F-dUMP form a covalently bound ternary complex with the enzyme, which possibly resembles the transition state formed during the normal enzymatic reaction when dUMP is converted to thymidylate. After incubating purified thymidylate synthetase with F-dUMP and $N^{5\text{-}10}$-methylenetetrahydrofolate, it was possible to isolate from pronase-treated digests short peptides (six to eight amino acids) with both F-dUMP and the folate cofactor attached (Sommer and Santi, 1974). (For details of this mechanism and the nature of the postulated inhibitory ternary complex, *see* Danenberg, 1977.)

Although it has been shown that fluorouracil is much more lethal to logarithmically growing cells than to stationary cells, there is no clearly demonstrated effect at a definite stage of the cell cycle. The phenomenon of "thymineless death" has been invoked to explain the cytotoxic effects of fluorouracil and its derivatives. The blockade of the thymidylate synthetase reaction inhibits DNA synthesis, while cellular production of both RNA and protein continues. An imbalance in growth occurs that is not compatible with cell survival. In accord with this proposal, the administration of thymidine can often reverse the toxicity, presumably through bypass of the block at thymidylate synthetase.

General Toxicity and Cytotoxic Action. The major sites of action of fluorouracil and floxuridine on normal tissues are the bone marrow and the epithelium of the gastrointestinal and oral mucosa. These are described in detail under Therapeutic Uses and Clinical Toxicity (*see* below).

Absorption, Fate, and Excretion. Fluorouracil and floxuridine are usually administered intravenously, since absorption after ingestion of the drugs is unpredictable and incomplete. Metabolic degradation occurs, particularly in the liver. Floxuridine is converted by thymidine or deoxyuridine phosphorylases into fluorouracil, and the latter is catabolized in much the same way as is uracil. Thus, 5-fluoro-5,6-dihydrouracil is formed, the ring of which is opened to give α-fluoro-β-ureidopropionic acid, which may be degraded further to α-fluoro-β-alanine (Heidelberger, 1975). In man, an important product of the metabolism of fluorouracil is urea.

It is of considerable interest that, given as single daily intravenous doses, the effects of neither fluorouracil nor floxuridine can be prevented by large doses of thymidine; in fact, under these conditions this precursor of DNA *increases* the toxicity of the nucleoside. The apparent paradox is explained by the very rapid metabolic conversion of thymidine to the corresponding base, thymine, which competes with the enzyme that can degrade either fluorouracil, uracil, or thymine. In this manner, an increased concentration of fluorouracil is made available for anabolic utilization. On the other hand, when thymidine is given by intravenous infusion, together with floxuridine, the effects of the latter can be nullified, since in this manner enough thymidylate can be provided simultaneously to susceptible cells to circumvent the inhibition of thymidylate synthetase.

Oral absorption of fluorouracil is quite variable and unpredictable (Bruckner and Creasey, 1974). Rapid intravenous administration of fluorouracil produces plasma concentrations of 0.1 to 1.0 mM; plasma clearance is rapid ($t_{1/2} = 10$ to 20 minutes). Urinary excretion of intravenously injected fluorouracil-2-^{14}C, given as a single dose, amounts to only 11% in 24 hours; however, during this period, 63% of the radioactivity is expired as carbon dioxide. Given by continuous intravenous infusion for 24 hours, plasma concentrations in the range of 0.5 to 3.0 μM are obtained and the urinary excretion of fluorouracil is only 4%, while the $^{14}CO_2$ excretion rises to 90% (Mukherjee et al., 1963). These findings probably account for the lower cytotoxicity of fluorouracil administered by infusion, compared to that seen with single doses. Fluorouracil readily enters the CSF, and concentrations of about 7 μM are reached within 30 minutes after intravenous administration; values are sustained for approximately 3 hours and subside slowly during a period of 9 hours (Bourke et al., 1973).

Preparation, Dosage, and Routes of Administration. *Fluorouracil,* U.S.P. *(5-FU),* is available in sterile ampuls containing 500 mg in 10 ml for intravenous administration. The recommended dose for average-risk patients in good nutritional status with adequate hematopoietic, renal, and hepatic function is 12 mg/kg daily for 4 days, by rapid injection, followed by 6 mg/kg on alternate succeeding days for two to four doses if no toxicity is observed. The maximal daily dose has been established arbitrarily at 800 mg. Treatment should be discontinued at the earliest manifestation of toxicity (usually stomatitis or diarrhea) because the maximal effects of bone-marrow suppression will not be evident until the ninth to fourteenth day. The first course of therapy should be administered either in the hospital or under extremely close supervision in order to establish the tolerance of the individual patient. After a period of 4 weeks from the first injection of the preceding course, a new course of therapy is initiated; the dosage is adjusted on the basis of the previous response and is repeated at monthly intervals. Another type of maintenance schedule is 10 to 15 mg/kg or 600 mg/sq m, administered weekly as a single rapid injection. It is usually necessary to produce mild-to-moderate toxicity in order to achieve significant antineoplastic effects.

In the selection of patients, the roles of nutritional deficiencies and protein depletion have been stressed, particularly in relation to surgery. Reduced tolerance of the hematopoietic system may be present in elderly patients or as a result of invasion of the bone marrow by either neoplastic cells or myelofibrosis. Patients with compromised bone-marrow function as a result of previous therapy either with alkylating agents or x-ray to the pelvis or vertebrae are particularly sensitive to the myelosuppressive action of these compounds. In patients with extensive liver metastases, catabolism of the drug may be markedly impaired and therapy may be contraindicated; if treatment is instituted, reduced doses must be administered to prevent the hazards of overdosage.

Fluorouracil has been administered by infusion into the hepatic artery with favorable results in patients with metastases to the liver (Ansfield et al., 1971; Tandon et al., 1973).

Topical fluorouracil as a 1 or 5% cream or a 1 to 5% solution in propylene glycol (EFUDEX, FLUOROPLEX) has been used successfully in dermatology.

Floxuridine, U.S.P., *(fluorodeoxyuridine, FUdR),* is available for injection as a powder, 500 mg in 5-ml containers. It may be administered in schedules identical with those of fluorouracil, except that the individual doses, in milligrams, are twice those used with the latter agent. Continuous infusion of floxuridine has produced objective responses with ⅟₃₀ to ⅟₆₀ the dose necessary with multiple individual doses, but with similar toxicity. Continuous infusion of fluorinated pyrimidines into the arterial blood supply of localized tumors, particularly in the liver or in the head and neck region, may provide beneficial clinical effects (Sullivan et al., 1967). Intra-arterial infusions, at doses of 0.1 to 0.6 mg/kg for 24 hours, are administered continuously until local toxicity is encountered.

Therapeutic Uses and Clinical Toxicity. Clinical use of fluorinated pyrimidines has been concerned primarily with *fluorouracil,* and accumulated experience indicates that the drug can be of palliative value in certain types of carcinoma, particularly of the breast and the gastrointestinal tract; beneficial effects have also been reported in hepatoma, as well as in carcinoma of the ovary, cervix, urinary bladder, prostate, pancreas, and oropharyngeal areas. There is little evidence, however, to encourage the expectation that significant overall prolongation of life can be achieved in the majority of patients. (*See* Calabresi and Welch, 1962; Greenwald, 1973; Heidelberger, 1973.) Fluorouracil is widely used with very favorable results for the topical treatment of premalignant keratoses of the skin and multiple superficial basal-cell carcinomas (Klein *et al.,* 1972).

The clinical manifestations of toxicity caused by fluorouracil and floxuridine are similar and may be difficult to anticipate because of their delayed appearance. The earliest untoward symptoms during a course of therapy are anorexia and nausea; these are followed shortly after by stomatitis and diarrhea, which constitute reliable warning signs that a sufficient dose has been administered. Stomatitis is manifested by formation of a white patchy membrane that ulcerates and becomes necrotic. The occurrence of similar lesions in the stoma of colostomies and at post-mortem examination of the gastrointestinal tract, as well as complaints of dysphagia, retrosternal burning, and proctitis, indicates that enteric injury may occur at any level. The major toxic effects, however, result from the myelosuppressive action of these drugs; clinically, the effects are most frequently manifested as leukopenia, the nadir of which is usually between the ninth and fourteenth day after the first injection of drug. Thrombocytopenia and anemia may complicate the picture. Loss of hair, occasionally progressing to total alopecia, nail changes, dermatitis, and increased pigmentation and atrophy of the skin may be encountered. Neurological manifestations, including an acute cerebellar syndrome, have been reported, and myelopathy has been observed after the intrathecal administration of fluorouracil. The low therapeutic indices of these agents emphasize the need for very skillful supervision by physicians familiar with the action of the fluorinated pyrimidines and the possible hazards of chemotherapy.

CYTARABINE (CYTOSINE ARABINOSIDE)

Among the more interesting antimetabolites is cytarabine (cytosine arabinoside, arabinosylcytosine, ara-C), more properly called 1-β-D-arabinofuranosylcytosine. The profound effects of this agent on the growth of certain experimental tumors (Evans *et al.,* 1961) led to its preliminary investigation in man. Its clinical usefulness in acute leukemia, alone and concurrently with other agents, is well established. (For references,

see Greenwald, 1973; Heidelberger, 1973; Ho and Freireich, 1975; Maley, 1977.)

Mechanism of Action. This compound is an analog of 2'-deoxycytidine with the 2'-hydroxyl in a position *trans* to the 3'-hydroxyl of the sugar, as shown in Table 55–3. The 2'-hydroxyl causes steric hindrance to the rotation of the pyrimidine base around the nucleosidic bond. The bases of polyarabinonucleotides cannot stack normally as do the bases of polydeoxynucleotides. This might lead to nucleic acid dysfunction if arabinosylcytosine residues replace deoxycytidines in a nucleic acid.

As with most purine and pyrimidine antimetabolites, cytarabine must be "activated" by conversion to the 5'-monophosphate nucleotide, in this case catalyzed by deoxycytidine kinase. The nucleotide analog, AraCMP, can react with appropriate nucleotide kinases to form the diphosphate and triphosphate nucleotides (AraCDP and AraCTP).

There is still no agreement on a single site of action to explain the cytotoxicity of cytarabine. Early investigations by Chu and Fischer (1962) suggested a block of ribonucleoside diphosphate reductase by a nucleotide of cytarabine, such as AraCTP, as a crucial effect. Studies with partially purified preparations of the enzyme from Novikoff ascites cells revealed only moderate inhibition by AraCDP and AraCTP (Moore and Cohen, 1967). Several other biochemical effects appear significant. An important observation is that AraCTP, in concentrations achievable in cells, is a potent inhibitor of calf thymus DNA polymerase ($K_i \cong 1\ \mu$M). It has been shown that AraCTP is about 200 times more inhibitory to a virally induced RNA-dependent DNA polymerase (reverse transcriptase) than to the DNA-dependent enzyme. The inhibition of DNA polymerases can adequately account for the marked inhibition of DNA synthesis and the S-phase–specific action of cytarabine, but it has not yet been definitely correlated with cytotoxicity.

In addition to their ability to block nucleic acid polymerases, nucleotides of cytarabine can become incorporated into both the RNA and DNA of the cell. There is no clear evidence, however, that DNA-chain termination occurs, and little correlation is seen between lethality and the degree of incorporation of cytarabine into DNA. On the other hand, acute cell death, not reversible by deoxycytidine administration, has been correlated with the amount of incorporation of antimetabolites into RNA (Chu and Fischer, 1968; Chu, 1971).

Since most of its actions relate closely to DNA biosynthesis and function, cytarabine is regarded as specific for the S phase of the cell cycle (Skipper and Schabel, 1973).

Mechanism of Resistance to Cytarabine. Both natural and acquired resistance to cytarabine occur. Many normal tissues, as well as some tumors not susceptible to cytarabine, have high concentrations of cytidine deaminase, an enzyme capable of converting cytarabine to the noncytotoxic metabolite, arabinosyl uracil. The ratio of deoxycytidine kinase to cytidine deaminase is a key factor in determining susceptibility of tissues to cytarabine (Chabner et al., 1975). A powerful and apparently irreversible inhibitor of this deaminase, tetrahydrouridine, has been identified (Comiener and Smith, 1968), which causes increases in the plasma half-life and excretion of unchanged drug when administered together with cytarabine. It has not been determined, however, whether inhibition of the deamination of cytarabine effects a favorable change in its therapeutic index. It seems probable that tissues normally protected by cytidine deaminase will suffer adverse effects if cytarabine is administered in combination with tetrahydrouridine. Another method for circumventing this mechanism of resistance is the design of analogs of cytarabine with high substrate activity for the kinases required for synthesis of the corresponding nucleotides but with low activity for deoxycytidine and 5'-deoxycytidylate deaminases.

Several probable mutations have been identified that result in acquired resistance to the cytotoxicity of cytarabine. Most frequently seen are deletions or modifications of deoxycytidine kinase, the enzyme required for the "lethal synthesis" of AraCMP (Chu and Fischer, 1965). Less frequent are mutants possessing DNA polymerases with decreased affinity for AraCTP (Creasey, 1975a).

Immunosuppressive Action. In addition to its antineoplastic activity, cytarabine has immunosuppressive properties (Calabresi, 1967; Mitchell et al., 1969a, 1969b). It is of interest that variations in dosage or schedule of administration selectively suppress humoral or cellular immunity (Calabresi, 1967; Griswold et al., 1972). These findings have led to the demonstration that plasma blocking factors (humoral antibodies) can be selectively suppressed by cytarabine, with resultant inhibition of tumor growth by cellular immunity (Heppner and Calabresi, 1972, 1976).

Although cytarabine is capable of inhibiting DNA viruses and has been used clinically to treat viral infections, the use of idoxuridine (iododeoxyuridine, IUdR) or vidarabine (arabinosyladenine, ara-A) is preferred, since these antimetabolites do not demonstrate the potentially deleterious immunosuppressive properties of cytarabine. Adverse effects of cytarabine on disseminated herpes zoster have been reported in a controlled clinical study in which depression of immunological responses was demonstrated (Stevens et al., 1973). Of considerable interest in this respect is the finding that idoxuridine is capable of significantly enhancing production of antibody through mechanisms yet to be explained (Griswold et al., 1975).

Absorption, Fate, and Excretion. Cytarabine is poorly and unpredictably absorbed after oral administration, with less than 20% of the drug reaching the circulation. After intravenous administration of a 5- or 10-mg/kg dose of ^{3}H-labeled drug to patients with neoplastic disease, the blood concentration is no longer measureable after 20 minutes in most patients (Creasey et al., 1966). Other workers describe a biphasic plasma disappearance curve, with an initial rapid phase ($t_{1/2} = 12$ minutes) and a second, slower phase ($t_{1/2} = 110$ minutes) (Ho and Frei, 1971). Only 4 to 10% of the injected dose is excreted unchanged in the urine within 12 to 24 hours, while 86 to 96% of the radioactivity appears as the inactive, deaminated product, arabinosyl uracil. Higher concentrations of cytarabine are found in CSF after continuous infusion than after rapid intravenous injection. After intrathecal administration of the drug at a dose of 50 mg/sq m, relatively little deamination occurs, even after 7 hours (Ho and Frei, 1971; Ho, 1977).

Preparation, Route of Administration, and Dosage. *Cytarabine,* U.S.P. (cytosar), is marketed for the treatment of acute leukemias in children and adults. It is supplied as a lyophilized powder in multidose vials containing either 100 or 500 mg of drug, to be reconstituted for injection by adding 5 or 10 ml, respectively, of water. Two dosage schedules are recommended: (1) rapid intravenous injection of 100 to 200 mg/sq m daily for 5 to 7 days; or (2) continuous intravenous infusion of 5 to 100 mg/sq m daily for 5 to 7 days. In general, children seem to tolerate higher doses than do adults. *Maintenance* therapy with subcutaneous injections of 1 mg/kg, weekly or every other week, can be used, although the drug appears more effective for the *induction* of remissions in acute leukemia. Investigations of its efficacy and safety in the treatment of meningeal leukemia, by intrathecal injection, are in progress.

Therapeutic Use and Clinical Toxicity. Cytarabine is indicated for *induction* of remission in acute leukemia in children and adults. When used alone, remission rates of 20 to 40% have been reported (Greenwald, 1973). The drug is particularly useful in acute granulocytic leukemia in adults, since chemotherapy is generally disappointing in this disorder. Cytarabine is more effective when used with other agents, particularly thioguanine and daunorubicin; complete remission rates of greater than 50% have been reported (Crowther et al., 1970; Clarkson, 1972; Heidelberger, 1973; Kremer, 1975). The drug has been studied in patients with a variety of neoplastic diseases. Beneficial effects have been observed in Hodgkin's disease and related lymphomas but very rarely in patients with carcinomas or other tumors. Cytarabine is primarily a potent myelosuppressive agent capable of producing severe leukopenia, thrombocytopenia, and anemia with striking megaloblastic changes. Other toxic manifestations reported include gastrointestinal disturbances and, less frequently, stomatitis, hepatic dysfunction, thrombophlebitis at the site of injection, fever, and dermatitis.

Azaribine

Azaribine is the triacetyl derivative and prodrug form of azauridine; it was synthesized in order to achieve better absorption following oral administration and to prevent metabolism of azauridine to azauracil by intestinal microorganisms, a factor which contributes to CNS toxicity from azauridine (Handschumacher et al., 1962; Creasey et al., 1963). Azaribine has marked therapeutic activity in psoriasis, mycosis fungoides, and polycythemia vera (Calabresi and Turner, 1966; DeConti and Calabresi, 1970; McDonald and Calabresi, 1971; Skoda, 1975). Unfortunately, when the drug became available for clinical usage, some patients with psoriasis developed thromboembolic disorders; since recent evidence indicates an increased incidence of the complication in psoriasis, it is questionable whether this problem should be attributed to the drug or to the disease (McDonald and Calabresi, 1978; Shubin, 1979).

Chemistry. The structural formulas of azauridine (AzUR) and azaribine (2′,3′,5′-triacetyl-6-azauridine) are shown in Table 55–3, and their chemical relationship to other pyrimidine analogs is discussed above.

Mechanism of Action. Azaribine is deacetylated in the blood to AzUR, and this in turn undergoes intracellular conversion to 6-azauridylic acid (AzUMP). AzUMP inhibits the formation of uridylic acid from its carboxylated precursor, orotidylic acid, by blocking the enzyme orotidylate decarboxylase in the *de-novo* pathway of pyrimidine biosynthesis. Significant amounts of orotic acid and orotidine are excreted in the urine. The drug also has demonstrated uricosuric properties.

General Toxicity and Cytotoxic Action. Normal leukopoiesis and thrombocytopoiesis are not markedly affected by prolonged administration of azaribine. Moderate anemia, characterized by mild megaloblastic changes, reticulocytopenia, and elevated plasma iron concentrations, occurs after chronic use of high doses of drug and constitutes the basis for its use in polycythemia vera. This is readily reversible by discontinuation of drug or by administration of uridine.

Absorption, Fate, and Excretion. Azaribine is well absorbed after oral administration and is almost entirely deacetylated to AzUR in the blood, with some monoacetyl derivative detectable. Peak plasma concentrations of AzUR are usually reached after 2 to 4 hours; the half-time of disappearance from plasma is approximately 6 to 8 hours. Unlike azauracil, AzUR does not cross the blood-brain barrier and is not detectable in the CSF. When neurotoxic manifestations have been encountered, significant concentrations of azauracil have been measured in the CSF (Doolittle *et al.,* 1977). Approximately 95% of an ingested dose of azaribine is excreted in the urine as AzUR within 16 hours.

Preparation, Dosage, and Route of Administration. *Azaribine* (TRIAZURE) is available for investigational purposes as 500-mg tablets for oral administration. It has been utilized for the treatment of severe, recalcitrant, and disabling psoriasis that is not adequately responsive to other forms of therapy. The recommended dosage is 125 mg/kg daily, administered at 8-hour intervals in three equally divided doses. Occasionally, it may be necessary to use doses up to 200 mg/kg daily. Therapy should be continued

until a remission is achieved or moderate anemia intervenes. Clearing of the lesions usually occurs within 8 weeks, after which a remission of several months may ensue. In some patients intermittent maintenance therapy may be required, and reduction of dosage by at least 20% may be necessary if anemia is a significant problem.

At higher dosages in the range of 270 mg/kg daily, administered at 8-hour intervals in three equally divided doses for several weeks, azaribine may result in significant but reversible suppression of erythropoiesis, a finding that prompted its use in the treatment of polycythemia vera (DeConti and Calabresi, 1970). At these dosages the drug has also been effective in the treatment of mycosis fungoides.

Therapeutic Uses and Clinical Toxicity. In *generalized psoriasis,* azaribine has produced remission rates of 70 to 90% (Calabresi and Turner, 1966; Vogler and Olansky, 1970; Crutchler and Moschella, 1975). Although the drug may be of considerable benefit in treating the acute manifestations of psoriatic arthritis (Levine and Paulus, 1976), it has caused unexplained exacerbations in patients with rheumatoid arthritis.

When used at higher doses, azaribine has proven as effective and less toxic than other agents in the treatment of *mycosis fungoides* (McDonald and Calabresi, 1971), and the drug deserves further study in the management of *polycythemia vera;* clinical toxicity is usually minimal or absent. Hematopoietic suppression appears to be relatively selective for erythropoiesis, with very little if any effect noted on normal leukocyte or platelet counts. Signs of mild CNS dysfunction, including drowsiness, lethargy, and dizziness, have been reported with lower doses, while hyperreflexia, tremor, diplopia, expressive aphasia, and dysarthria may occur at higher doses. These effects, caused by the metabolite azauracil, subside promptly upon discontinuation of the medication. Although thromboembolic manifestations have been encountered in patients with psoriasis treated with azaribine, recent evidence indicates that a previously undetected, increased incidence of this complication occurs in psoriasis and is actually reduced by treatment with azaribine (McDonald and Calabresi, 1978).

PURINE ANALOGS

Since the pioneering studies of Hitchings and associates, begun in 1942, many analogs of natural purine bases, nucleosides, and nucleotides have been examined in a wide variety of biological and biochemical systems. These extensive investigations have led to the development of several drugs, not only of use in the treatment of malignant diseases (mercaptopurine, thioguanine) but also for immunosuppressive (azathioprine) and antiviral (arabinosyladenine) therapy. The hypoxanthine analog allopurinol, a potent inhibitor of xanthine oxidase, is an important by-product of this effort (*see* Chapter 29). A recent development of great promise has been the discovery of powerful inhibitors of adenosine deaminase, for example, erythro-hydroxynonyladenine (EHNA) and pentostatin (2'-deoxycoformycin). In experimental systems these inhibitors of adenosine deaminase have produced marked synergistic effects in combination with various analogs of adenosine, such as arabinosyladenine (ara-A); they also show promise as immunosuppressive agents. (*See* reviews by Elion and Hitchings, 1965, 1975; Paterson and Tidd, 1975; Crabtree, 1978.)

Structure-Activity Relationship. Mercaptopurine and thioguanine, both established clinical agents for the therapy of human leukemias, are analogs of the natural purines hypoxanthine and guanine, in which the keto group on carbon 6 of the purine ring is replaced by a sulfur atom. Substitution in this position by chlorine or selenium also yields antineoplastic compounds. Cytotoxicity is also observed with the β-D-ribonucleoside and β-D-2'-deoxyribonucleoside derivatives. Because these nucleoside analogs are excellent substrates for purine nucleoside phosphorylase, a highly active enzyme in many tissues, the analog nucleosides often serve as prodrugs and liberate the respective hypoxanthine or guanine analogs in tissues. With several important exceptions,

analogs of purine bases or nucleosides must undergo enzymatic conversion to the nucleotide level in order to display cytotoxic activity.

Many attempts have been made to modify the structures of such analogs in order to improve their therapeutic indices or tissue selectivity. Azathioprine (Table 55–4) was developed to decrease the rate of inactivation of 6-mercaptopurine by enzymatic S-methylation, nonenzymatic oxidation, or conversion to thiourate by xanthine oxidase. Azathioprine can react with sulfhydryl compounds such as glutathione (apparently nonenzymatically) and thus serves as a prodrug, permitting the slow liberation of mercaptopurine in tissues. Superior immunosuppressive activity is achieved in comparison with mercaptopurine (Elion, 1967).

An important new development has been the discovery of potent inhibitors of adenosine deaminase such as pentostatin (2'-deoxycoformycin; inhibition constant = 2.5 pM). This inhibitor and its close relative coformycin (the ribonucleoside) were discovered as antibiotics. Pentostatin (Table 55–4) may be viewed as an analog of the natural nucleoside 2'-deoxyinosine, in which the six-membered pyrimidine ring is replaced by a seven-membered diazapin ring. This disrupts the natural aromatic and planar purine ring. The keto-enol tautomer of 2'-deoxyinosine is replaced by a secondary alcohol. These structural changes increase the binding of pentostatin to adenosine deaminase by about 10 million-fold compared to that of adenosine. The enzyme-inhibitor complex dissociates with a $t_{1/2}$ of about 25 to 30 hours (Agarwal *et al.,* 1977, 1978; Rogler-Brown *et al.,* 1978). Thus, pentostatin blocks not only the deami-

Table 55–4. STRUCTURAL FORMULAS OF ADENOSINE AND VARIOUS PURINE ANALOGS

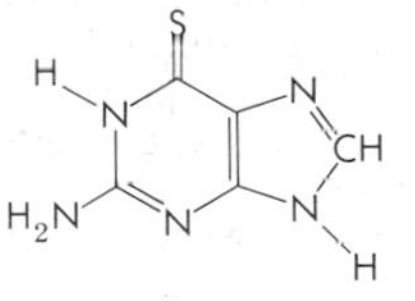

Thioguanine

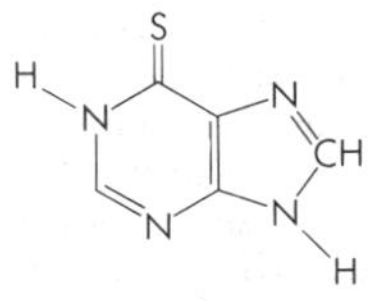

Mercaptopurine

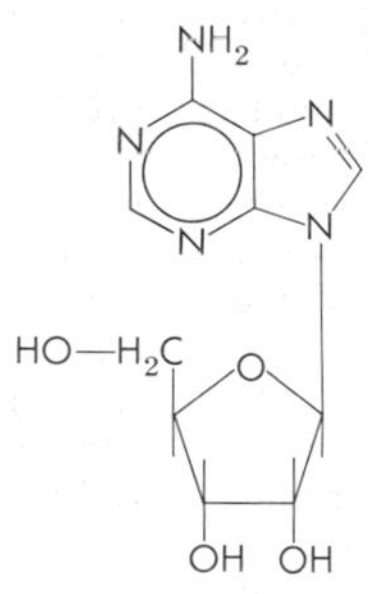

Adenosine

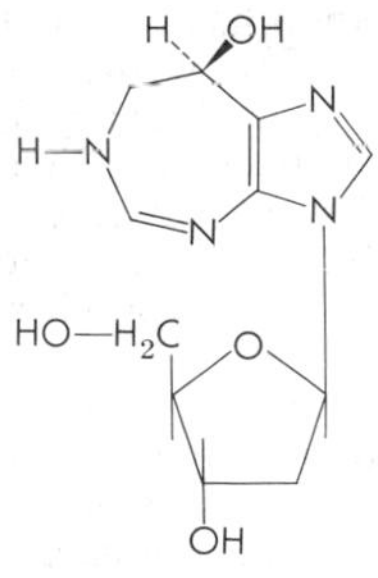

Pentostatin
(Deoxycoformycin)

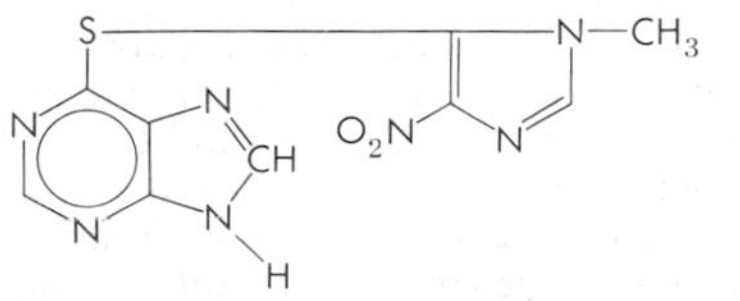

Azathioprine

nation of natural nucleosides but also that of many analogs used in chemotherapy. Since genetic deficiency of adenosine deaminase is associated with malfunction of both T and B lymphocytes with little effect on other normal cells (Giblett et al., 1972), pentostatin is being tested not only as a potentiator of various analogs of adenosine but also as an immunosuppressive agent. Furthermore, since adenosine deaminase activity may be greatly elevated in certain lymphoblastic leukemic cells as compared with normal peripheral lymphocytes, inhibitors of adenosine deaminase may have therapeutic activity when used alone. Also significant is the recent discovery of patients with a deficiency of nucleoside phosphorylase who have normal humoral (B lymphocyte–related) but defective cellular (T lymphocyte–related) immunity. This discovery suggests that potent inhibitors of purine nucleoside phosphorylase specifically interfere with cellular immunity (Giblett et al., 1975).

The glutamine antagonists azaserine (O-diazoacetyl-L-serine), 6-diazo-5-oxo-L-norleucine (DON), and duazomycin, although not purine analogs, are potent inhibitors of the de-novo pathway of purine nucleotide biosynthesis. These glutamine analogs are diazoketones with chemical reactivities resembling those of diazomethane. They inhibit purine biosynthesis through the formation of covalent bonds with a cysteine residue in the active site of a key enzyme in the pathway, formylglycinamide ribotide amidotransferase. Although these compounds have only weak cytostatic activity when used alone, they can produce significant potentiation when administered with purine analogs such as mercaptopurine or thioguanine (Bennett, 1975).

Mechanism of Action. Although purine analogs and their derivatives have been studied intensively, the mechanisms responsible for cell death or selective cytotoxicity are still not established. Considerable information has been obtained regarding many metabolic effects of these compounds, and such studies have contributed greatly to our understanding of metabolism and its regulation. In the following discussion, it is assumed that the reader understands the biosynthesis of nucleic acids; if this is not the case, he should consult an outline of metabolic pathways.

Although animal tissues have deoxynucleoside kinases that are capable of converting the 2'-deoxyribonucleosides of guanine, hypoxanthine, adenine, and many of their analogs to the corresponding 5'-monophosphates, similar reactions do not occur with inosine, guanosine, or their analogs. On the other hand, the synthesis of nucleotides from adenosine and its analogs can be catalyzed by adenosine kinase, an enzyme found in most animal tissues. Inosine, guanosine, and their analogs must first undergo phosphorolysis by purine nucleoside phosphorylase, which is present in high activity in many human tissues. The liberated bases may then be converted to the corresponding nucleotide by hypoxanthine-guanine phosphoribosyltransferase (HGPRT). Similarly, 2'-deoxyguanosine, 2'-deoxyinosine, and many related analogs may react with purine nucleoside phosphorylase, and the product of this reaction, a purine base or analog, is then con-

verted to the corresponding ribonucleoside 5'-monophosphate.

An important relationship exists between the enzymes adenosine kinase and adenosine deaminase. Because ATP and dATP are powerful feedback inhibitors of major metabolic reactions (e.g., glycolysis, PRPP synthesis [inhibited by ATP], ribonucleotide reductase [inhibited by dATP]), it is crucial that the intracellular concentrations of these key nucleotides be strictly regulated. In most tissues the activity of adenosine deaminase is substantially higher than are those of the kinases for adenosine and 2'-deoxyadenosine. Therefore, if adenosine or 2'-deoxyadenosine or their analogs accumulate in cells in high concentration (as when there is breakdown of tissue), most will be deaminated by adenosine deaminase with subsequent phosphorolysis to yield hypoxanthine. If, however, adenosine deaminase activity is absent (due to a genetic disorder or the presence of an inhibitor), these compounds may be phosphorylated by the nucleoside kinases and enter the pools of intracellular nucleotides in high concentrations. Lymphocytes appear to be the most susceptible to deficiency of adenosine deaminase, which can result in severe impairment of both cellular and humoral immunity (Giblett et al., 1972). As mentioned, this discovery offers the hope that inhibitors of adenosine deaminase may be useful immunosuppressive agents. In addition, many analogs of adenosine that can cause marked cytotoxicity are rapidly degraded by adenosine deaminase to inactive analogs of inosine. Striking synergism is observed in rodent tumor systems when pentostatin is administered in conjunction with analogs of adenosine. Such concurrently employed agents may soon be tested in patients with advanced cancer.

Both thioguanine and mercaptopurine are excellent substrates for HGPRT and are converted to the ribonucleotides 6-thioguanosine-5'-phosphate (6-thioGMP) and 6-thioinosine-5'-phosphate (T-IMP), respectively. Because T-IMP is a poor substrate for guanylate kinase, the enzyme that converts GMP to GDP, T-IMP accumulates intracellularly. Careful studies have demonstrated, however, that mercaptopurine can be incorporated into cellular DNA in the form of thioguanine, indicating that slow reactions catalyzed by enzymes of guanine metabolism can operate. The accumulation of T-IMP may inhibit several vital metabolic reactions; examples are the conversion of inosinate (IMP) to adenylosuccinate (AMPS) and then to adenosine-5'-phosphate (AMP) and the oxidation of IMP to xanthylate (XMP) by inosinate dehydrogenase. These reactions are crucial steps in the conversion of IMP to adenine and guanine nucleotides. On the other hand, in cells incubated with thioguanine, 6-thioGMP first accumulates; it is a poor, but definite, substrate for guanylate kinase. Thus, there is slow conversion to 6-thioGDP and 6-thioGTP and entry of thioguanine nucleotides into the nucleic acids of the cell (Parks et al., 1975). In addition, the concentrations of 6-thioGMP achieved are sufficient to cause progressive and irreversible inhibition of inosinate dehydrogenase, presumably through the formation of disulfide bonds. Furthermore, both 6-thioGMP and T-IMP, as well as a number of other 5'-monophosphate derivatives of purine nucleoside analogs, can cause "pseudofeedback inhibition" of the first committed step in the *de-novo* pathway of purine biosynthesis, the reaction of glutamine and PRPP to form ribosylamine-5-phosphate. This enzyme is a major control point in the biosynthesis of purine nucleotides, and its rate of catalysis is highly responsive to the intracellular concentrations of 5'-mononucleotides (natural, as well as analogs). The synthesis of PRPP is also powerfully inhibited by ATP or certain analogs of ATP. In view of the multiplicity of these effects, it can be appreciated that the intracellular accumulation of analogs of various purine nucleotides can produce major metabolic disruptions and, in some instances, may play a key role in cytotoxicity.

Despite extensive investigations, it is still not possible to assess precisely the role of incorporation of thioguanine or mercaptopurine into cellular DNA in the production of either the therapeutic or toxic effects of these drugs. These compounds can cause marked inhibition of the coordinated induction of various enzymes required for DNA synthesis, as well as potentially critical alterations in the synthesis of polyadenylate-containing RNA (Carrico and Sartorelli, 1977). These effects, which are potentially lethal to cellular survival, can occur in model systems at a time before any synthesis of DNA is observed. These observations and others make it impossible to ascribe the cytotoxicity of these agents solely to incorporation of the thiopurines into DNA. It seems likely that this class of drugs acts by multiple mechanisms, including effects on purine nucleotide synthesis and metabolism, as well as alterations in the synthesis and function of RNA and DNA. (*See* Scannell and Hitchings, 1966; Barranco and Humphrey, 1971; Carrico and Sartorelli, 1977; LePage, 1977; Crabtree, 1978.)

Of many adenosine analogs studied experimentally, *vidarabine* (arabinosyladenine, ara-A) has recently been approved for clinical use in the United States for the treatment of herpetic infections (*see* Chapter 54); its testing as an antineoplastic agent in combination with inhibitors of adenosine deaminase has been proposed. Vidarabine is converted enzymatically to ara-ATP. This analog nucleotide can inhibit DNA polymerases by competing with dATP and, in fact, may be incorporated into DNA. In this regard vidarabine resembles the analgous pyrimidine nucleoside antimetabolite cytarabine (ara-C). By contrast, vidarabine, when administered alone, is relatively nontoxic and causes minimal immunosuppression. (*See* Bloch, 1975; Herrmann, 1977.)

Mechanisms of Resistance to Antipurines. As with other tumor-inhibiting antimetabolites, the occurrence of acquired resistance represents perhaps the major obstacle to the successful use of antipurines. Many studies have been performed with experimental systems to determine the mechanisms of resistance to purine analogs, such as mercaptopurine; the most commonly encountered finding is the deficiency or complete lack of the enzyme HGPRT. In addition, resistance can result from decreases in the affinity of this enzyme for its substrates. Since HGPRT is not essential for cell survival but is required for the "lethal" synthesis of fraudulent ribonucleotides of guanine or hypoxanthine analogs, cells deficient in this enzyme would not be damaged by exposure to a drug such as mercaptopurine and would be selected for growth and survival. Cells that are resistant by means of this mechanism usually show cross-resistance between such analogs as mercaptopurine, thioguanine, and azaguanine.

Another mechanism of resistance that has been detected in cells isolated from a number of leukemic patients is an increase in particulate alkaline phosphatase activity. Additional mechanisms include (1) "exclusion" of mercaptopurine from contact with HGPRT in the intact, resistant cell; (2) an increased rate of degradation of the purine base or ribonucleoside analogs; (3) an alteration in the "pseudofeedback inhibition" of ribosylamine 5-phosphate synthesis; and (4) genetic loss of the enzyme adenine phosphoribosyltransferase or adenosine kinase, which makes cells resistant to analogs of adenine or adenosine. (*See* Brockman, 1974.)

MERCAPTOPURINE

The introduction of mercaptopurine by Elion and coworkers represents a landmark in the history of antineoplastic and immunosuppressive therapy. Today this antipurine and its derivative, azathioprine, are among the most important and clinically useful drugs of the class. The structure-activity relationship and the mechanism of action and of drug resistance are discussed above. The structural formula of mercaptopurine is presented in Table 55–4.

Absorption, Fate, and Excretion. Mercaptopurine is readily absorbed after oral ingestion. The intestinal epithelium is not damaged in the process. About one half of an oral dose can be accounted for as urinary excretion products in the first 24 hours. After an intravenous dose, the half-life of the drug in plasma is relatively short (about 90 minutes) due to uptake by cells, renal excretion, and rapid metabolic degradation. There are two main pathways for the metabolism of mercaptopurine. The first involves methylation of the sulfhydryl group and subsequent oxidation of the methylated derivatives. The formation of nucleotides of 6-methylmercaptopurine has been shown to occur following administration of mercaptopurine or mercaptopurine ribonucleoside. Substantial amounts of the mono, di, and triphosphate nucleotides of 6-methylmercaptopurine ribonucleoside (6-MMPR) have been identified in the blood and bone marrow of patients treated with mercaptopurine or azathioprine. Desulfuration of thiopurines can occur, and relatively large percentages of the administered sulfur are excreted as inorganic sulfate.

The second major pathway for mercaptopurine metabolism involves the enzyme xanthine oxidase, which is present in relatively large amounts in the liver. Mercaptopurine is a good substrate for this enzyme, which oxidizes it to 6-thiouric acid, a noncarcinostatic metabolite (Elion, 1967).

An attempt to modify the metabolic inactivation of mercaptopurine by xanthine oxidase led to the development of *allopurinol*. This analog of hypoxanthine is a powerful inhibitor of xanthine oxidase, and not only blocks the conversion of mercaptopurine to 6-thiouric acid but also interferes with the production of uric acid from hypoxanthine and xanthine (*see* Chapter 29). Because of its ability to interfere with the enzymatic oxidation of mercaptopurine and related derivatives, allopurinol increases the exposure of cells to the action of these compounds. Although it greatly potentiates the antineoplastic action of mercaptopurine in tumor-bearing mice, allopurinol increases the toxicity as well, and there is no apparent improvement in the therapeutic index.

Preparation, Dosage, and Route of Administration. *Mercaptopurine,* U.S.P. (*6-mercaptopurine;* PURINETHOL), is marketed as scored, 50-mg tablets. The average daily oral dose is 2.5 mg/kg. Starting doses usually range from 100 to 200 mg a day; with hematological and clinical improvement, the dose is diminished to an appropriate multiple of 25 mg and, in general, maintenance therapy of 50 to 100 mg a day is continued. If beneficial effects have not been noted after 4 weeks, the dose may be increased gradually until evidence of toxicity is encountered. The total dose required to produce depression of the bone marrow in patients with nonhematological malignancies is about 45 mg/kg and may range from 18 to 106 mg/kg.

Hyperuricemia with hyperuricosuria may occur during treatment; the accumulation of uric acid presumably reflects the destruction of cells with release of purines that are oxidized by xanthine oxidase, as well as an inhibition of the conversion of inosinic acid to precursors of nucleic acids. This circumstance may be an indication for the use of *allopurinol.* Special caution must be employed if mercaptopurine or its imidazolyl derivative, azathioprine, is used with allopurinol, for reasons presented above. Patients treated simultaneously with both drugs should receive approximately 25% of the usual dose of mercaptopurine.

Therapeutic Uses and Clinical Toxicity.
In the early studies with mercaptopurine, bone-marrow remissions were described in over 40% of children with *acute leukemia,* and some benefit was obtained in an addi-

tional group (Burchenal, 1954). In adults with acute leukemia, the results have been much less impressive, but occasional remissions have been obtained (Ellison *et al.,* 1972). Cross-resistance does not occur between mercaptopurine and other classes of antileukemic agents.

A review of clinical results with mercaptopurine indicates that in acute leukemia a rapid decrease in the total leukocyte count may begin about 5 or 6 days after the initiation of therapy, although a period of 2 to 4 weeks of continuous daily administration may be necessary before a response is observed. The average time necessary for the appearance of bone-marrow remissions in responsive adults is 7 to 8 weeks. The drug has contributed significantly to the treatment of lymphoblastic leukemia, more by maintaining than by inducing remissions (Frei *et al.,* 1965; Holland and Glidewell, 1972).

In the treatment of chronic granulocytic leukemia, maintenance therapy with mercaptopurine can be useful, but the drug of choice is busulfan. Mercaptopurine has not been of value in chronic lymphocytic leukemia, Hodgkin's disease and related lymphomas, and a wide variety of carcinomas, even at unusually high doses (Esterhay *et al.,* 1978). Although active as an immunosuppressive agent, it has been superseded by its imidazolyl derivative, azathioprine.

The principal toxic effect of mercaptopurine is bone-marrow depression, although, in general, this develops more gradually than with folic acid antagonists; accordingly, thrombocytopenia, granulocytopenia, or anemia may not be encountered for several weeks. When depression of normal bone-marrow elements occurs, cessation of therapy with the drug usually results in prompt recovery. Anorexia, nausea, or vomiting is seen in approximately 25% of adults, but stomatitis and diarrhea are rare; manifestations of gastrointestinal effects are less frequent in children than in adults. The occurrence of jaundice in about one third of adult patients treated with mercaptopurine has been reported; although the pathogenesis of this manifestation is obscure, it usually clears upon discontinuation of therapy. Its appearance has been associated with bile stasis and hepatic necrosis. Dermatological manifestations have been reported. The long-term complications associated with the use of mercaptopurine and its derivative, azathioprine, for immunosuppressive therapy are discussed by Schein and Winokur (1975).

AZATHIOPRINE

Azathioprine, a derivative of 6-mercaptopurine, is used as an immunosuppressive agent. The structural formula is shown in Table 55–4. The rationale that led to its synthesis and its mechanism of action and metabolic degradation have been discussed above.

Azathioprine, U.S.P. (IMURAN), is currently approved for use in the United States only as an adjunct for the prevention of rejection in renal transplantation. All other uses remain investigational. The drug is available in 50-mg tablets and in vials that contain 100 mg of the sodium salt for injection. The oral dose of azathioprine varies from 3 to 5 mg/kg daily. For maintenance therapy the dose may be reduced to 1 to 2 mg/kg daily, unless rejection is threatened. Patients with transplanted kidneys or impaired renal function may have reduced clearance of the drug and its metabolites; unless the dose is reduced appropriately, a dangerous cumulative effect may result. Among the conditions for which treatment with azathioprine is being studied are idiopathic thrombocytopenic purpura, autoimmune hemolytic anemias, systemic lupus erythematosus, and other disorders believed to be associated with altered immunological reactivity. The drug has been used alone or concomitantly with corticosteroids and other antiproliferative agents. If allopurinol is administered concurrently, the dose of azathioprine should be reduced to approximately 25%, since inhibition of xanthine oxidase impairs the conversion of azathioprine to 6-thiouric acid and may result in dangerous enhancement of its myelosuppressive effect. Bone-marrow depression, usually leukopenia, is the most common toxic effect of azathioprine. Infection may be a complication of any immunosuppressive regimen. Toxic hepatitis and biliary stasis have been reported. Infrequent complications include stomatitis, dermatitis, fever, alopecia, and gastrointestinal disturbances.

THIOGUANINE

The synthesis of thioguanine was first described by Elion and Hitchings in 1955. It is of particular value in the treatment of acute granulocytic leukemia when given with cytarabine (Clarkson, 1972). The structural formula of thioguanine is shown in Table 55–4, and its mechanism of action is discussed above.

Absorption, Fate, and Excretion. Peak concentrations in the blood are reached 6 to 8 hours after oral administration of thioguanine, and approximately 40% of the dose is excreted in the urine within 24 hours. When thioguanine is administered to man, the S-methylation product, 2-amino-6-methylthiopurine, rather than free thioguanine appears in the urine. After 8 hours, inorganic sulfate becomes a major urinary metabolite. Lesser amounts of 6-thiouric acid are formed (Elion, 1967), suggesting that deamination catalyzed by the enzyme guanase does not play a major role in the metabolic inactivation of thioguanine. Accordingly, it may be administered concurrently with allopurinol without reduction in dosage, unlike mercaptopurine and azathioprine.

Preparation, Dosage, and Route of Administration. *Thioguanine,* U.S.P. (*6-thioguanine, TG*), is available in scored, 40-mg tablets. The average daily dose is 2 mg/kg. If there is no clinical improvement or toxicity after 4 weeks, the dosage may be cautiously increased to 3 mg/kg daily.

Therapeutic Uses and Clinical Toxicity. Clinically, the compound has been used in the treatment of acute leukemia and, in conjunction with cytarabine, is one of the most effective agents for induction of remissions in acute granulocytic leukemia (Clarkson, 1972); it has not been useful in the treatment of patients with solid tumors. Thioguanine has been used as an immunosuppressive agent, particularly in patients with nephrosis (Wolff and Goodman, 1962) and with collagen-vascular disorders (Demis *et al.,* 1964). Toxic manifestations include bone-marrow depression and gastrointestinal effects, although the latter may be less pronounced than with mercaptopurine.

III. Natural Products

VINCA ALKALOIDS

History. The beneficial properties of the periwinkle plant (*Vinca rosea* Linn.), a species of myrtle, have been described in medicinal folklore for many years in various parts of the world. Working with extracts of the periwinkle, Noble and coworkers (1958) observed granulocytopenia and bone-marrow suppression in rats, effects that led to purification of an active alkaloid. Other investigations by Johnson and associates demonstrated activity of certain alkaloidal fractions against an acute lymphocytic neoplasm in mice. Fractionation of these extracts yielded four active dimeric alkaloids: *vinblastine, vincristine, vinleurosine,* and *vinrosidine.* Two of these, vinblastine and vincristine, are important clinical agents. Comprehensive reviews of the vinca alkaloids have been published (Johnson *et al.,* 1963; Symposium, 1968; Johnson, 1973; Creasey, 1975b, 1977).

Chemistry. The four vinca alkaloids are very similar chemically. They are asymmetrical dimeric compounds; the structures of vincristine and vinblastine are as follows:

Vincristine   Vinblastine

$R = O{=}C{-}H$ $R = CH_3$

No definite information is available regarding metabolic changes that may be necessary for chemical activation or degradative alterations *in vivo.*

Structure-Activity Relationship. The minor differences in structure of these large alkaloidal molecules result in notable differences in toxicity and antitumor spectra of vincristine and vinblastine. Additional minor changes in the structures of the other two active alkaloids apparently are responsible for differences in their experimental antitumor spectra. A number of related dimeric alkaloids are without biological activity. Removal of the acetyl group at C 4 of one portion of vinblastine destroys its antileukemic activity, as does acetylation of the hydroxyl groups. Either hydrogenation of the double bond or reductive formation of carbinols reduces or destroys activity of these compounds.

Mechanism of Action. The vinca alkaloids are cell-cycle–specific agents and, in common with other drugs such as colchicine and podophyllotoxin, block mitosis with metaphase arrest. The biochemical effects of the vinca alkaloids have been explored extensively, and a number of interesting phenomena have been uncovered. It seems likely, however, that most of the biological activities of these drugs can be explained by their ability to bind specifically with the protein tubulin, a key component of cellular microtubules. When cells are incubated with vinblastine, dissolution of the microtubules occurs, and highly regular crystals are formed that contain 1 mole of bound vinblastine per mole of tubulin. Colchicine and podophyllotoxin also can bind specifically with tubulin, but apparently at a site on the protein different from that bound by vinblastine. Through disruption of the microtubules of the mitotic apparatus, cell division is arrested in metaphase. In the absence of an intact mitotic spindle, the chromosomes may disperse throughout the cytoplasm (exploded mitosis) or may occur in unusual groupings, such as balls or stars. Apparently the inability to segregate chromosomes correctly during mitosis leads ultimately to cellular death.

In addition to their key role in the formation of mitotic spindles, microtubules have been associated with many other cellular functions. Therefore, it is not surprising that vinca alkaloids may affect these functions as well. Some types of cellular movements, phagocytosis, and certain functions of the CNS appear to involve microtubules, which may explain some of the other effects of vinca alkaloids. (*See* Creasey, 1975b.)

Despite their structural similarity, a remarkable lack of cross-resistance between individual vinca alkaloids has been noted. It has been proposed that their dissimilarities in antitumor spectra, potencies, and toxic effects may be ascribed to variation in their capacity to enter specific types of cells, since it is difficult to envision a different mechanism of action for each drug.

Cytotoxic Actions. Clinical as well as experimental studies have demonstrated that bone-marrow depression, chiefly manifested by leukopenia, is the most important cytotoxic effect on normal cells. In this respect, vincristine is not nearly as potent as vinblastine; with the latter, this is the effect that limits dosage. The relatively low toxicity of vincristine for normal marrow cells makes this agent unusual among antineoplastic drugs, and it is often included in combination chemotherapy with other myelosuppressive agents. Loss of hair, presumably secondary to effects on the epithelial cells of the hair follicles, appears to occur more frequently with vincristine than with vinblastine. No definite explanation is available for the striking differences in the toxicities of these closely related chemical structures.

Neurological Actions. Although neurotoxicity may occasionally be encountered with vinblastine, particularly at high dosage levels, neuromuscular abnormalities are frequently observed with vincristine. Indeed, it is this type of untoward effect that most frequently proves to be the limiting factor during therapy with vincristine. Several types of manifestations have been recognized. In experimental animals, acute toxicity after large doses is characterized by clonic convulsions, muscular weakness, ataxia, tremors, vomiting, and catalepsy. The development of CNS leukemia in patients receiving vincristine and in hematological remission has been interpreted as evidence that the alkaloid penetrates the blood-brain barrier poorly. Although torpor, hallucinations, and coma were observed during exploratory clinical studies with very high doses of vincristine (75 μg/kg weekly), peripheral neuropathy is the most common manifestation of neurotoxicity at usual clinical doses. Numbness and tingling of the extremities, followed by weakness, loss of reflexes, foot-drop, ataxia, muscular cramps, and neuritic pains, have been observed frequently. Clinical neurophysiological studies have demonstrated that asymptomatic depression of the Achilles reflex is the earliest and most consistent sign of vincristine-induced neuropathies. Muscular weakness involving the larynx and the extrinsic muscles of the eye also has been noted. An effect on the autonomic nervous system may be responsible for severe, and even obstructive, constipation that frequently may develop with prolonged administration of vincristine, but it is seen only rarely with vinblastine. Temporary mental depression, occurring on the second or third day after treatment, especially with vinblastine, may be of clinical significance and is of particular interest because other compounds derived from indole (*e.g.*, lysergic acid diethylamide [LSD], reserpine, and 5-hydroxytryptophan) are known for their effects on mood and behavior.

Absorption, Fate, and Excretion. Unpredictable absorption has been reported after oral administration of vinblastine. The compound is cleared very rapidly from the blood. Within minutes after intravenous injection, radioactively labeled vinblastine is detected mostly in the liver; in less than an hour, significant amounts are no longer present in the circulating blood. Vincristine and vinblastine can be infused into the arterial blood supply of tumors in doses several times larger than those that can be administered intravenously with comparable toxicity; thus, either local uptake or destruction is very rapid. The vinca alkaloids appear to be excreted primarily by the liver into the bile. Radioactively labeled vinblastine has been traced through this route into the intestinal tract, with less than 5% of the label appearing in the urine. Greater toxicity is encountered when vincristine is administered to patients with obstructive jaundice.

VINBLASTINE

Preparations, Route of Administration, and Dosage. *Vinblastine Sulfate,* U.S.P. (VELBAN), is supplied in ampuls containing 10 mg of dry powder for preparation of fresh solutions (10 ml). The drug is given intravenously, either with a needle different from the one employed in filling the syringe or by injection directly into the tubing of an intravenous infusion; special precautions must be taken against subcutaneous extravasation, since this may cause painful irritation and inflammatory changes. The drug should not be injected into an extremity with impaired circulation. After a single dose of 0.1 to 0.15 mg/kg of body weight, hematological responses are observed for 7 to 10 days. If a moderate level of leukopenia (approximately 3000 cells per cubic millimeter) is not attained, the weekly dose may be increased gradually by increments of 0.05 mg/kg of body weight. Beneficial results, however, may occur at lower doses. Once the optimal amount is established, weekly dosage is continued; if the leukocyte count does not return to 4000 cells per cubic millimeter within 10 to 14 days, the treatment schedule is adjusted accordingly.

Therapeutic Uses and Clinical Toxicity. The most important clinical use of vinblastine is with bleomycin and cisplatin (*see* below) in the therapy of metastatic testicular tumors. This regimen is the preferred treatment for these neoplasms, and a substantial number of complete remissions, which are probably cures, have followed its implementation (Einhorn and Donahue, 1977). Beneficial responses have been reported in various lymphomas, particularly Hodgkin's disease, where significant improvement may be noted in 50 to 90% of cases. The effectiveness of vinblastine in a high proportion of lymphomas is not diminished when the disease is refractory to alkylating agents. It is also active in neuroblastoma and Letterer-Siwe disease (histiocytosis X), as well as in carcinoma of the breast and choriocarcinoma in women (Johnson, 1973; Creasey, 1975b).

The nadir of the leukopenia that follows the administration of vinblastine usually occurs within 4 to 10 days, after which recovery ensues within 7 to 14 days; with higher dosage, the total leukocyte counts may not return to normal until 3 weeks have elapsed. Other toxic effects of vinblastine include neurological manifestations, such as temporary mental depression, paresthesias, loss of deep-tendon reflexes, and, more rarely, headache, convulsions, and psychoses; dysfunction of the autonomic nervous system, with marked constipation, paralytic ileus, urinary retention, bilateral pain and tenderness of the parotid glands associated with dryness of the mouth, and sinus tachycardia, has been reported at higher doses. Gastrointestinal disturbances, including nausea, vomiting, anorexia, and diarrhea, may be encountered. Loss of hair, mucositis of the mouth, and dermatitis may occur infrequently. Extravasation during injection may lead to cellulitis and phlebitis. Local injection of hyaluronidase and application of moderate heat to the area may be of help by dispersing the drug.

VINCRISTINE

Preparations, Route of Administration, and Dosage. *Vincristine Sulfate,* U.S.P. (ONCOVIN), is available as a dry powder in ampuls containing either 1 or 5 mg of drug. Vincristine used together with corticosteroids is presently the treatment of choice to induce remissions in childhood leukemia; the optimal dosages for these drugs appear to be vincristine, intravenously, 2 mg/sq m of body surface, weekly, and prednisone, orally, 40 mg/sq m, daily. In adults, the usual method of administration is to start therapy with intravenous doses of 0.01 mg/kg of body weight. After observation of the patient for 1 week, the dose is raised by weekly increments of 0.01 mg/kg until either the desired response is obtained or toxicity is encountered. Adult patients with carcinomas or lymphomas often will respond to weekly doses of 0.02 to 0.05 mg/kg. When used with other drugs, for example, in the MOPP regimen (*see* below), the recommended dose of vincristine is 1 to 1.5 mg/sq m. High doses of vincristine seem to be tolerated better by children with leukemia than by adults, who may experience severe neurological toxicity. Administration of the drug more frequently than every 7 days or at higher doses seems to increase the toxic manifestations without proportional improvement in the response rate. Maintenance therapy with vincristine is not recommended in children with leukemia (*see* below). The same precautions described for vinblastine should be used to avoid extravasation during intravenous administration.

Therapeutic Uses and Clinical Toxicity. Vincristine has a spectrum of clinical activity that is similar to that of vinblastine, but there are some notable differences. An important feature is the lack of cross-resistance between these agents, a remarkable finding in view of the very close similarity of their chemical structures. Vincristine is effective in Hodgkin's disease and other lymphomas. While it appears to be somewhat less beneficial than vinblastine when used alone in Hodgkin's disease, when used with mechlorethamine, prednisone, and procarbazine (the so-called MOPP regimen), it is the preferred treatment for the advanced stages (III and IV) of this disease (DeVita *et al.*, 1972). In non-Hodgkin's lymphomas, vincristine is an important agent, particularly when used with cyclophosphamide, bleomycin, doxorubicin, and prednisone (Luce *et al.*, 1971; Bagley *et al.*, 1972). Vincristine is more useful than vinblastine in lymphocytic leukemia. Another area of difference in clinical response to these drugs is acute leukemia, particularly in children; whereas vinblastine is rarely useful in this disease, vincristine is extremely effective.

The rapidity of action of vincristine and its lesser tendency for myelosuppressive action make it a more desirable agent for therapy in the presence of pancytopenia or in conjunction with other myelotoxic agents. It is particularly useful for the *induction* of remission in acute lymphoblastic leukemia of children when given with prednisone. It is the treatment of choice for this purpose and produces complete remissions in approximately 90% of children on the first course of antileukemic therapy (Symposium, 1968; Holland, 1971; Greenwald, 1973). The approximate rate of second remissions is 70 to 80%. Vincristine and prednisone should be promptly discontinued after remission is induced, since other agents (*e.g.*, methotrexate and mercaptopurine) are more effective for *maintenance.* Vincristine has not prevented the occurrence of leukemia in the CNS; for reasons mentioned previously, it should not be given intrathecally. Beneficial responses have been reported in patients with a variety of other neoplasms, particularly Wilms' tumor, neuroblastoma, brain tumors, rhabdomyosarcoma, and carcinomas of the breast, bladder, and the male and female reproductive systems (*see* Symposium, 1968; Holland *et al.*, 1973; Johnson, 1973; Creasey, 1975b).

The clinical toxicity of vincristine is mostly neurological, with paresthesias, loss of deep-tendon reflexes, neuritic pain, muscle weakness that may be manifested by foot-drop and inability to walk, hoarseness, headache, ptosis, and double vision. The more severe neurological manifestations may be avoided or reversed by either suspending therapy or reducing the dosage upon occurrence of the earliest symptoms, usually tingling and numbness of the extremities. Severe constipation, sometimes resulting in colicky abdominal pain and obstruction, may be prevented by a prophylactic program of laxatives and hydrophilic agents.

Alopecia occurs in about 20% of patients given vincristine; however, it is always reversible, frequently even without cessation of therapy. Although less common than with vinblastine, leukopenia may occur with vincristine, and thrombocytopenia, anemia, polyuria, dysuria, fever, and gastrointestinal symptoms have been reported occasionally. The syndrome of hyponatremia associated with high urinary sodium and inappropriate ADH secretion has been occasionally observed during vincristine therapy. In view of the rapid action of the vinca alkaloids, it is advisable to take appropriate precautions to prevent the complication of hyperuricemia. This can be accomplished by the administration of *allopurinol* (*see* above).

ANTIBIOTICS

DACTINOMYCIN (ACTINOMYCIN D)

History. The first crystalline antibiotic agent to be isolated from a culture broth of a species of *Streptomyces* was actinomycin A (Waksman and Woodruff, 1940). Many related antibiotics, including actinomycin D, have subsequently been obtained (Waksman Conference on Actinomycins, 1974). Dactinomycin has beneficial effects in the treatment of a number of tumors, particularly certain neoplasms of childhood and choriocarcinoma.

Chemistry and Structure-Activity Relationship. The actinomycins are chromopeptides, and most of them contain the same chromophore, the planar phenoxazone *actinocin*, which is responsible for the yellow-red color of the compounds. The differences among naturally occurring actinomycins are confined to the peptide side chains, and the variations are in the structure, but not in the number or in the configuration of the α carbon, of the constituent amino acids. By varying the amino acid content of the growth medium it is possible to alter the types of actinomycins produced. It has been demonstrated that changes in the amino acid composition of both polypeptide chains can influence the biological activity of the molecule and that a number of chemical alterations can abolish activity totally (*see* Waksman Conference on Actinomycins, 1974; Goldberg *et al.*, 1977). The chemical structure of dactinomycin is as follows:

Dactinomycin

$$\left(\begin{array}{l} \text{Sar} = \text{sarcosine} \\ \text{Meval} = \text{N-methylvaline} \end{array} \right)$$

Mechanism of Action. The capacity of actinomycins to bind with double-helical DNA is responsible for their biological activity and cytotoxicity. X-ray studies of a crystalline complex between dactinomycin and deoxyguanosine permitted formulation of a model that appears to explain the binding of the drug to DNA (Sobell, 1973). The planar phenoxazone ring intercalates between adjacent guanine-cytosine base pairs of DNA, where the guanine moieties are on opposite strands of the DNA. The summation of several interactions provides great stability to the dactinomycin-DNA complex, and, as a result of the binding of dactinomycin, the function of RNA polymerase and, thus, the transcription of the DNA molecule are blocked. The DNA-dependent RNA polymerases are much more sensitive to the effects of dactinomycin than are the DNA polymerases. (*See* Waksman Conference on Actinomycins, 1974; Goldberg *et al.*, 1977.)

Cytotoxic Action. The drug inhibits rapidly proliferating cells of normal and neoplastic origin and, on a molar basis, is among the most potent antitumor agents known. Atrophy of thymus, spleen, and other lymphatic tissues occurs in experimental animals. Detailed studies of the hematological, gastrointestinal, and other toxic effects of dactinomycin in animals have been described. It may produce damage to the hair roots and is capable of marked local inflammatory action. Erythema sometimes progressing to necrosis has been noted in areas of the skin exposed to x-radiation either before, during, or after administration of the drug.

Absorption, Fate, and Excretion. Dactinomycin is much less potent when given orally than when administered by parenteral injection. Very little active drug can be detected in the circulating blood 2 minutes after its intravenous injection. In rats, approximately 50% of the compound is excreted unchanged in the bile and 10% in the urine. There is no evidence of metabolic modification of the molecule. The drug appears incapable of crossing the blood-brain barrier. Studies on its clinical pharmacology are lacking and information is incomplete.

Preparation, Dosage, and Route of Administration. *Dactinomycin*, U.S.P. (*actinomycin D;* COS-MEGEN), is supplied as a lyophilized powder (0.5 mg in each vial). Solutions should not be exposed to direct sunlight. The usual daily dose is 15 μg/kg; this is given intravenously for 5 days; if no manifestations of toxicity are encountered, additional courses may be given at intervals of 2 to 4 weeks. Daily injections of 100 to 400 μg have been given to children for 10 to 14 days; in other regimens, 3 to 6 μg/kg, for a total of 125 μg/kg, and weekly maintenance doses of 7.5 μg/kg have been used. Although larger amounts have been given in more prolonged courses, in general the total dose necessary to produce antineoplastic effects has been approximately 2.5 to 5 mg. Although it is safer to administer the drug into the tubing of an intravenous infusion, direct intravenous injections have been given, with the precaution of discarding the needle used to withdraw the drug from the ampul in order to avoid subcutaneous reaction.

Therapeutic Uses and Clinical Toxicity. The most important clinical use of dactinomycin is in the treatment of rhabdomyosarcoma and Wilms' tumor in children. In the latter case, remissions that last for several years and increased survival have been reported in patients with advanced disease, including pulmonary metastases (Farber, 1966; Greenwald, 1973; Waksman Conference on Actinomycins, 1974). Antineoplastic activity has been noted in Ewing's tumor, Kaposi's sarcoma, and soft-tissue sarcomas. Its use together with vincristine and cyclophosphamide has been advocated in children with solid tumors. Dactinomycin can be effective in women with methotrexate-resistant choriocarcinoma. It may also be used with chlorambucil and methotrexate for patients with metastatic testicular carcinomas, but this regimen is not preferable to the concurrent use of vinblastine, cisplatin, and bleomycin. It is of limited value in other neoplastic diseases of adults, although a response may sometimes be observed in patients with Hodgkin's disease and related lymphomas. Dactinomycin has also been used to inhibit immunological responses, particularly the rejection of renal transplants.

Toxic manifestations include anorexia, nausea, and vomiting, usually beginning a few hours after administration. Hematopoietic suppression with pancytopenia may occur from 1 to 7 days after completion of therapy. A decrease in the platelet count is often the first manifestation of bone-marrow depression, and pancytopenia may develop rapidly. Proctitis, diarrhea, glossitis, cheilitis, and ulcerations of the oral mucosa are common; dermatological manifestations include alopecia, as well as erythema, desquamation, and increased pigmentation in areas subjected to x-radiation. Severe injury may occur as a result of local toxic action.

DAUNORUBICIN AND DOXORUBICIN

These anthracycline antibiotics and their derivatives are among the most important of the newer antitumor agents. They are produced by the fungus *Streptomyces peucetius* var. *caesius*. Daunorubicin was isolated independently by DiMarco and by Dubost and their colleagues in 1963. Doxorubicin was identified by Arcamone and coworkers in 1969. Although they differ only slightly in chemical structure, daunorubicin has been used primarily in the acute leukemias, whereas doxorubicin displays activity against a wide range of human neoplasms, including a variety of solid tumors. Unfortunately, the clinical value of both agents is limited by an unusual cardiomyopathy; its occurrence is related to the total dose of the drug, and it is often irreversible. (*See* Chabner *et al.*, 1975; DiMarco, 1975; Goldberg *et al.*, 1977.)

Chemistry. The anthracycline antibiotics have tetracycline ring structures with an unusual sugar, daunosamine, attached by glycosidic linkage. Cytotoxic agents of this class all have quinone and hydroquinone moieties on adjacent rings that permit them to function as electron-accepting and -donating agents. Although there are marked differences in the clinical use of daunorubicin and doxorubicin, their chemical structures differ only by a single hydroxyl group on C 14. The chemical structures of daunorubicin and doxorubicin are as follows:

Daunorubicin: R = H
Doxorubicin: R = OH

Mechanism of Action. Several biochemical actions of the anthracycline antibiotics have been described that may be relevant to their cytotoxic effects. X-ray diffraction and other studies suggest that these agents may intercalate between adjacent base pairs of DNA and that the sugar, daunosamine, plays an essential role in this binding. The DNA helix is untwisted to permit intercalation; this produces a longer, thinner molecule and inhibits the template activity of the nucleic acid (Pigram *et al.*, 1972).

Observations that raise serious questions about the significance of binding of the anthracyclines to DNA have come from studies of a congener of doxorubicin, N-trifluoroacetyl adriamycin-14-valerate (AD-32). This compound is an active antitumor agent but appears not to enter the nucleus nor to bind to DNA (Krishan *et al.*, 1976). There is also evidence for disruptive effects of anthracyclines on cellular membranes (Tritton *et al.*, 1978). A biochemical action of potential importance results from the quinone-hydroquinone structure of the anthracycline aglycone, which permits this molecule to accept electrons to form semiquinones. The addition of either doxorubicin or daunorubicin to hepatic microsomes significantly augments the oxidation of NADPH and the transfer of electrons to molecular oxygen, resulting in the formation of superoxide anion radicals (O_2^-) (*see* Oberly and Buettner, 1979). The enzyme responsible for this effect is probably NADPH–cytochrome P-450 reductase (Bachur *et al.*, 1977).

Strands of DNA undergo cleavage when incubated with doxorubicin, suggesting that intercalation may not only block the function of DNA but also cause chain scission through generation of reactive free radicals in the immediate vicinity of the DNA molecule. The production of free radicals is also shown by the marked accumulation of malonyldial-

dehyde in cardiac tissue after treatment of mice with doxorubicin. This substance is known to be a product of free radical attack on unsaturated fatty acids. Further supportive evidence for a role of free radicals in anthracycline-induced cardiotoxicity is the protective effect afforded by free radical scavengers such as α-tocopherol and coenzyme Q. Manipulations such as this do not alter the antitumor effect of doxorubicin (Myers *et al.*, 1977). These observations and others offer the hope that it will be possible to separate the antitumor from the cardiotoxic effects of this class of drugs.

As with other chemotherapeutic agents, resistance is observed to the anthracyclines. As yet, however, there is no clear biochemical explanation of such resistance. Complete cross-resistance has been reported between daunorubicin and doxorubicin in leukemia L 1210 sublines. Interestingly, cross-resistance has also been described between daunorubicin, dactinomycin, and the vinca alkaloids, which raises the possibility that alteration of cellular permeability may be involved.

As might be expected of the compounds that inhibit the function of DNA, maximal cytotoxic effects are observed during the S phase of the cell cycle, although cytotoxicity is evident during other phases as well.

Absorption, Fate, and Excretion. Daunorubicin and doxorubicin are usually administered intravenously, and they are then cleared from the plasma rapidly. The disappearance curve for doxorubicin is triphasic, with an initial $t_{1/2}$ of about 12 minutes, an intermediate $t_{1/2}$ of about 3.3 hours, and a terminal value of approximately 30 hours. There is rapid uptake of the drugs in the heart, kidneys, lungs, liver, and spleen. They do not appear to cross the blood-brain barrier.

There are notable differences in the metabolism of the two compounds. Daunorubicin is metabolized primarily to daunorubicinol. A significant fraction of doxorubicin is excreted unchanged, and there appear to be multiple metabolites, including, in particular, adriamycinol. Both drugs are metabolized chiefly in the liver and excreted in the bile. The hepatic clearance of doxorubicin has been estimated to be approximately 60% of hepatic blood flow, and severe clinical toxicity may result if the drug is administered to patients with impaired hepatic function (Chabner *et al.*, 1975; Takanashi and Bachur, 1975a, 1975b; Benjamin *et al.*, 1977; Riggs *et al.*, 1977; Ahmed *et al.*, 1978).

Daunorubicin: Preparation, Dosage, and Route of Administration. *Daunorubicin (daunomycin, rubidomycin;* CERUBIDINE, DAUNOBLASTINA) is available for investigational purposes as a lyophilized powder in 20-mg vials. The recommended dosage is 30 to 60 mg/sq m daily for 3 days or once weekly. The drug has also been given in doses of 0.8 to 1 mg/kg daily for 3 to 6 days, and other dosage schedules are being investigated. The agent is administered intravenously with appropriate care to prevent extravasation, since local vesicant action may result. Patients should be advised that the drug may impart a red color to the urine for 1 or 2 days after administration.

Daunorubicin: Therapeutic Uses and Clinical Toxicity. Daunorubicin is very useful in the treatment of acute lymphocytic and acute granulocytic leukemias. It is the single most active drug in acute nonlymphoblastic leukemia in adults and, given with cytarabine, is the treatment of choice in these conditions.

The drug has some activity against solid tumors in children and in lymphomas; its activity against solid tumors in adults appears to be minimal but has not been adequately tested (Samuels *et al.*, 1971; Jones *et al.*, 1972; Sutow *et al.*, 1972; Weil *et al.*, 1973). The toxic manifestations of daunorubicin include bone-marrow depression, stomatitis, alopecia, gastrointestinal disturbances, and dermatological manifestations. Cardiac toxicity is a peculiar adverse effect observed with this agent. It is characterized by tachycardia, arrhythmias, dyspnea, hypotension, and congestive failure unresponsive to digitalis (*see* below).

Doxorubicin: Preparation, Dosage, and Route of Administration. *Doxorubicin Hydrochloride,* U.S.P. (ADRIAMYCIN), is supplied as a red-orange lyophilized powder in 10- and 50-mg vials. The currently recommended dose is 60 to 75 mg/sq m, administered as a single rapid intravenous infusion and repeated after 21 days. The drug has also been given in doses of 0.5 to 1 mg/kg daily for 2 to 6 days or in doses of 20 to 30 mg/sq m daily for 3 days or once weekly. Care should be taken to avoid extravasation, since local vesicant action and tissue necrosis may result. Patients should be advised that the drug may impart a red color to the urine for 1 or 2 days after administration.

Doxorubicin: Therapeutic Uses and Clinical Toxicity. Doxorubicin is effective in acute leukemias and malignant lymphomas; however, in contrast to daunorubicin, it is also extremely active in a number of solid tumors. Used concurrently with cyclophosphamide, vincristine, bleomycin, and prednisone, it is an important ingredient for the successful treatment of non-Hodgkin's lymphomas. Together with cisplatin, it has considerable activity against carcinoma of the ovary. It is a valuable component of various regimens of chemotherapy for carcinoma of the breast and small(oat)-cell carcinoma of the lung. The drug is also particularly beneficial in a wide range of sarcomas, including osteogenic, Ewing's, and soft-tissue sarcomas. It is one of the most active single agents for the treatment of metastatic adenocarcinoma of the breast, carcinoma of the bladder, bronchogenic carcinoma, and neuroblastoma. In metastatic thyroid carcinoma, doxorubicin is proba-

bly the best available agent. The drug has demonstrated activity in carcinomas of the endometrium, testes, prostate, cervix, and head and neck, and plasma-cell myeloma (Blum and Carter, 1974; Gottlieb and Hill, 1974; DiMarco, 1975).

The toxic manifestations of doxorubicin are similar to those of daunorubicin. Myelosuppression is a major dose-limiting complication, with leukopenia usually reaching a nadir during the second week of therapy and recovering by the fourth week; thrombocytopenia and anemia follow a similar pattern but are usually less pronounced. Stomatitis, gastrointestinal disturbances, and alopecia are common but reversible. Cardiomyopathy is a unique characteristic of the anthracycline antibiotics. Two types of cardiomyopathies may occur: (1) An acute form is characterized by abnormal ECG changes, including ST-T wave alterations and arrhythmias. This is brief and rarely a serious problem. Cineangiographic studies have shown an acute, reversible reduction in ejection fraction 24 hours after a single dose. (2) Chronic, cumulative dose-related toxicity is manifested by congestive heart failure that is unresponsive to digitalis. The mortality rate is in excess of 50%. Total dosage of doxorubicin as low as 250 mg/sq m can cause myocardial toxicity, as demonstrated by subendocardial biopsies. Nonspecific alterations, including a decrease in the number of myocardial fibrils, mitochondrial changes, and cellular degeneration, are visible by electron microscopy (LeFrak *et al.*, 1973). Although no practical and reliable predictive tests are available, the frequency of serious cardiomyopathy is negligible at total doses below 500 mg/sq m. The risk increases markedly (to >20% of patients) at total doses higher than 550 mg/sq m, and this total dosage should be exceeded only under exceptional circumstances. Previous cardiac irradiation or prior administration of cyclophosphamide or another anthracycline or related antibiotic increases the risk of cardiotoxicity. Because doxorubicin is primarily metabolized and excreted by the liver, it is important to reduce the dosage in patients with impaired hepatic function (Blum and Carter, 1974; Chabner *et al.*, 1975; Minow *et al.*, 1977; Bristow *et al.*, 1978).

BLEOMYCINS

The bleomycins are an important group of antitumor agents discovered by Umezawa and colleagues as fermentation products of *Streptomyces verticillus.* The drug that is currently employed clinically is a mixture of copper-chelating glycopeptides that consists predominantly of two closely related agents, bleomycin A_2 and bleomycin B_2. The various bleomycins differ only in their terminal-amine moiety (*see* below), and the addition of various amines to fermentation broths have made possible the preparation of more than 200 different congeners. Preliminary evidence indicates that both the toxic effects and the antitumor spectrum can be modified

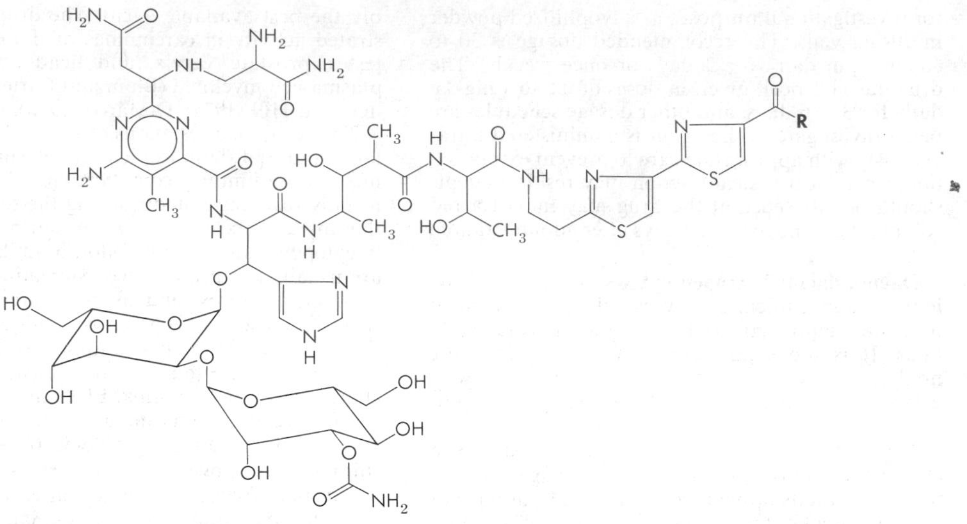

Bleomycinic Acid: **R** = OH

Bleomycin A$_2$: **R** = NHCH$_2$CH$_2$CH$_2$—S$^+$CH$_3$ / CH$_3$

Bleomycin B$_2$: **R** = NHCH$_2$CH$_2$CH$_2$CH$_2$NHC(NH)NH$_2$

by such changes. (*See* Umezawa, 1973a, 1973b, 1979; Chabner *et al.*, 1975; Pietsch, 1975; Goldberg *et al.*, 1977.)

Bleomycins have attracted great interest because of their activity in a variety of human tumors, including squamous carcinomas of skin, head, neck, and lungs, in addition to lymphomas and testicular tumors. In comparison with many other antineoplastic agents, the bleomycins in current use have minimal myelosuppressive and immunosuppressive activities. They do, however, cause unusual cutaneous and pulmonary toxicity. Since the toxic manifestations of the bleomycins do not overlap significantly with those of most other drugs and since their apparent mechanism of action is also unique (*see* below), it seems likely that the bleomycins will find an important place in multidrug chemotherapy.

Chemistry. The bleomycins are water-soluble, basic glycopeptides that differ from one another in their terminal-amine moieties. The structures of bleomycin A$_2$ and B$_2$ are shown above (Oppenheimer *et al.*, 1979). The core of the bleomycin molecule is a complex structure containing a pyrimidine chromophore linked to propionamide, a β-aminoalanine amide side chain, and the sugars L-gulose and 3-O-carbamoyl-D-mannose. It also includes a side chain with the amino acids L-histidine and L-threo-

nine, a methylvalerate residue, and a bithiazole carboxylic acid. The terminal amine is coupled through an amide linkage to this carboxylic acid. The bleomycins form equimolar complexes with cupric ions, with ligands involving the β-aminoalanine amide, the pyrimidine ring, the imidazole of L-histidine, and the carbamoyl group of mannose.

Mechanism of Action. While the bleomycins have a number of interesting biochemical properties, it seems most likely that their cytotoxic action relates to their ability to cause chain scission and fragmentation of DNA molecules. Marked chromosomal abnormalities have also been described that probably are due to the damage to DNA.

Bleomycin appears to cause scission of DNA by interacting with O$_2$ and ferrous iron. Presumably, the chelation of Fe^{2+} is the same as that described for cupric ions. It has been postulated that the bithiazole group of bleomycin intercalates with DNA, bringing the complexed Fe^{2+} close to a deoxyribose moiety. The crucial reaction appears to result from oxidation of the DNA-bound Fe^{2+}-bleomycin complex. The oxidized complex (Fe^{3+}-bleomycin) can dissociate from the DNA, be reduced to Fe^{2+}-bleomycin, and bind again to the DNA. Each cycle of oxidation and reduction may cause the release of one purine or pyrimidine base. The oxidative attack is apparently on the glycosidic linkages, since free bases are liberated. The oxidative attack of the Fe^{2+}-bleomycin complex on DNA may result from the generation of free radicals, possibly superoxide or hydroxyl radicals (Sausville *et al.*, 1978a, 1978b; Povirk, 1979).

Studies *in vitro* indicate that bleomycin causes accumulation of cells in the G$_2$ phase of the cell cycle, and many of these cells are severely injured. Promising results have been reported on the synchronization of tumor cells in patients infused with bleomycin. Of considerable interest is the apparent mechanism of the selective action of the bleomycins against squamous-cell carcinomas and their toxicity to lung and skin. Most tissues, except lung and skin, have relatively high activities of an enzyme, bleomycin hydrolase, that hydrolyzes the amide group of the β-aminoalanine amide of the bleomycin core and thereby inactivates the molecule. The cupric chelate of bleomycin is resistant to such hydrolysis (*see* Umezawa, 1979).

Absorption, Fate, and Excretion. Bleomycin is usually administered parenterally, and data on oral absorption are lacking. Relatively high concentrations of the drug are detected in the skin and lungs of experimental animals, the major sites of toxicity. In man, bleomycin localizes in various tumors, suggesting a lower level of inactivating enzyme at these sites. The average steady-state concentration of bleomycin in plasma of patients receiving continuous intravenous infusions of 30 units daily for 4 to 5 days is approximately 150 ng/ml, and there is little bound to plasma proteins. Bleomycin disappears from plasma in a biphasic fashion; the initial $t_{1/2}$ is about 1.3 hours, and the terminal $t_{1/2}$ is approximately 9 hours. Nearly two thirds of the drug is normally excreted in the urine, probably by glomerular filtration. Concentrations in plasma are greatly elevated if usual doses are given to patients with renal impairment (*see* Broughton *et al.,* 1977).

Preparation, Dosage, and Route of Administration. *Sterile Bleomycin Sulfate,* U.S.P. (BLENOXANE), is available as a lyophilized powder in 15-unit ampuls to be reconstituted with 5 ml of sterile water, saline solution, or 5% dextrose solution. The recommended dose is 10 to 20 units/sq m, weekly or twice weekly, and the drug is most commonly administered intravenously or intramuscularly. It may also be given by subcutaneous or intra-arterial injection. Total courses exceeding 400 units should be given with great caution because of a marked increase in the incidence of pulmonary toxicity; this may occur at lower doses when bleomycin is used concomitantly with other antineoplastic agents.

Therapeutic Uses and Clinical Toxicity. Bleomycin is effective in the treatment of testicular carcinomas. The overall response rate is approximately 30%, and this has increased to 90% when the drug is used with vinblastine. Recently, with the addition of cisplatin to this regimen, impressive numbers of complete remissions have been obtained that have lasted for several years (Einhorn and Donahue, 1977). Bleomycin is also useful in the palliative treatment of squamous-cell carcinomas of the head, neck, esophagus, skin, and the genitourinary tract, including the cervix, vulva, scrotum, and penis. It is active in Hodgkin's disease and in other lymphomas (*see* Carter *et al.,* 1976).

In contrast to most other antineoplastic agents, bleomycin causes minimal bone-marrow toxicity. The most commonly encountered adverse effects are mucocutaneous reactions, including stomatitis and alopecia as well as hyperpigmentation, hyperkeratosis, pruritic erythema, ulceration, and vesiculation of the skin. These changes may begin with swelling and hyperesthesia of the hands or erythematous, ulcerating lesions over the pressure areas of the body. Recrudescence of mucocutaneous complications has been reported when other antineoplastic agents are used within 6 weeks after a course of bleomycin. The most serious adverse reaction to this drug is pulmonary toxicity. This poorly characterized manifestation may begin with decreasing pulmonary function, fine rales, cough, and diffuse basilar infiltrates, progressing to severe, and sometimes fatal, pulmonary fibrosis. Approximately 5 to 10% of patients receiving bleomycin develop this severe complication, and about 1% of all individuals treated with the drug have died of pulmonary toxicity. Pulmonary function studies have not been of predictive value. The risk is related to the total dose, with a significant increase in the incidence of pulmonary fibrosis noted at doses higher than 400 units and in patients over 70 years of age or with underlying pulmonary disease. The use of corticosteroids has been advocated, but their value in reversing or preventing this complication remains to be established. Other toxic manifestations include hyperpyrexia, headache, nausea, and vomiting, as well as a peculiar, acute fulminant reaction observed in patients with lymphomas. This is characterized by profound hyperpyrexia, hypotension, and sustained cardiorespiratory collapse; it does not appear to be a classical anaphylactic reaction and may possibly be related to release of an endogenous pyrogen. Because this reaction has occurred in approximately 1% of patients with lymphomas and has resulted in deaths, it is recommended that patients with lymphomas receive a 1-unit test dose of bleomycin, followed by a 24-hour period of observation, before administration of the drug on standard dosage schedules. Unexplained exacerbations of rheumatoid arthritis have also been reported during bleomycin therapy (Chabner *et al.,* 1975; Carter *et al.,* 1976).

MITHRAMYCIN

This cytotoxic antibiotic was isolated from cultures of *Streptomyces tanashiensis* by Rao and associates in 1962. Although the drug is highly toxic, it has some clinical value in the treatment of advanced embryonal tumors of the testes. Mithramycin appears to have a relatively specific effect on osteoclasts and lowers the plasma calcium concentrations in hypercalcemic patients, including those with various types of cancer and metastatic tumors in bone. The drug has been used experimentally in the treatment of symptomatic Paget's disease, and striking reductions in plasma alkaline phosphatase activity with concomitant relief of bone pain have been observed. For a discussion of the chemistry of mithramycin and related antibiotics, *see* Umezawa (1979). The structural formula of mithramycin is as shown.

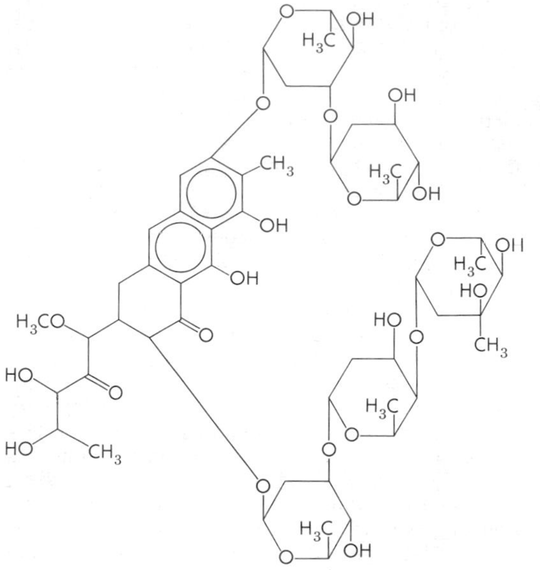

Mithramycin

Mechanism of Action. Mithramycin inhibits the synthesis of RNA in a variety of tissues without affecting directly the synthesis of protein or DNA (Yarbro *et al.,* 1966). It has been postulated that the mechanism of action at the molecular level is similar to that of dactinomycin.

The relatively specific effect of mithramycin on plasma calcium concentrations suggests that the drug may have a direct action on bone (Robins and Jowsey, 1973). Studies with a tissue culture system of embryonic rat bone showed that the release of calcium caused by the addition of parathyroid hormone can be abolished by simultaneous treatment with low concentrations of mithramycin (Cortes *et al.,* 1972). These effects are thought to be the result of a direct action on osteoclasts.

Absorption, Fate, and Excretion. Mithramycin is much less potent when administered orally than when given intravenously. Studies of its clinical pharmacology are lacking, and information on distribution, metabolic fate, and excretion is incomplete.

Preparation, Dosage, and Route of Administration. *Mithramycin,* U.S.P. (MITHRACIN), is available as a freeze-dried powder in vials containing 2.5 mg of drug. The recommended dosage for treatment of testicular tumors is 25 to 30 µg/kg daily or on alternate days for eight to ten doses or until toxicity intervenes. The drug is usually diluted in 1 liter of 5% dextrose in water and administered by slow intravenous infusion over a period of 4 to 6 hours. Extravasation can cause local irritation and cellulitis. For the treatment of hypercalcemia or hypercalci-

uria, 25 µg/kg has been given daily for one to three doses; this is repeated at intervals of 1 week or more.

Therapeutic Uses and Clinical Toxicity. Mithramycin is of limited value in the treatment of neoplastic disease because of its severe toxicity. It has been beneficial in patients with disseminated testicular carcinomas, especially of the embryonal-cell type (Ream *et al.,* 1968; Kennedy, 1970; Hill *et al.,* 1972b). The drug is useful in treating patients with severe hypercalcemia or hypercalciuria, particularly when associated with advanced or metastatic carcinoma that involves bone or produces parathyroid hormone–like substances (Perlia *et al.,* 1970). Its effectiveness in severe Paget's disease is encouraging but still considered investigational (Ryan *et al.,* 1970; Elias and Evans, 1972). Mithramycin is toxic to the bone marrow, liver, and kidneys. It produces a severe hemorrhagic diathesis, which may be the result of impaired synthesis of various clotting factors in addition to thrombocytopenia. Characteristically, this begins with epistaxis and may proceed to generalized hemorrhagic complications and even death. Adverse gastrointestinal, cutaneous, and neurological manifestations are also frequently observed. At the lower total dose recommended above for the treatment of hypercalcemia, toxicity is less severe.

MITOMYCIN

This antibiotic was isolated from *Streptomyces caespitosus* by Wakaki and associates in 1958. Mitomycin contains a urethane and a quinone group in its structure, as well as an aziridine ring, which is essential for antineoplastic activity (*see* Kersten, 1975; Crooke and Bradner, 1976). Its structural formula is as follows:

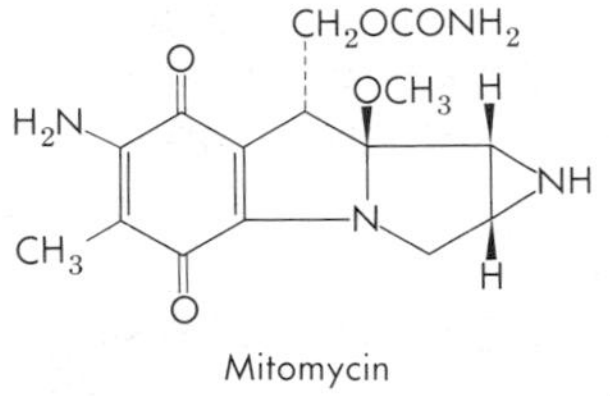

Mitomycin

Mechanism of Action. After intracellular enzymatic reduction of the quinone and loss of the methoxy group, mitomycin becomes a bifunctional or trifunctional alkylating agent. It inhibits DNA synthesis and cross-links DNA to an extent proportional to its content of guanine and cytosine. Its action is most prominent during the late G_1 and early S phases of the cell cycle. Mitomycin is teratogenic and carcinogenic in rodents, but its immunosuppressive properties are relatively weak (Crooke and Bradner, 1976).

Absorption, Fate, and Excretion. Mitomycin is administered intravenously, and it disappears rapidly from the blood after injection. The drug is widely distributed throughout the body but is not detected in the brain. It is metabolized primarily in the liver, and less than 10% of the active drug is excreted in the urine or the bile.

Preparation, Dosage, and Route of Administration. *Mitomycin,* U.S.P. (*mitomycin C;* MUTAMYCIN), is available as deep blue-violet crystals in vials containing 5 or 20 mg. It is soluble in water and is readily reconstituted for administration through a running intravenous infusion. Extravasation may result in severe local injury. The currently recommended dosage is 2 mg/sq m or 50 μg/kg daily for 5 days; this course is repeated after a 2-day interval. The drug may be given again by this schedule after recovery from myelosuppressive toxicity.

Therapeutic Uses and Clinical Toxicity. Mitomycin is useful for the palliative treatment of gastric adenocarcinoma, in conjunction with fluorouracil and doxorubicin. It has produced temporary beneficial effects in carcinomas of the cervix, colon, rectum, pancreas, breast, bladder, head and neck, and lung, and in melanoma. It has also shown activity against lymphomas and leukemia, particularly chronic granulocytic leukemia, but not in myeloma. All responses have been of brief duration and are complicated by severe toxicity. The major toxic effect is myelosuppression, characterized by marked leukopenia and thrombocytopenia; this may be delayed and cumulative. Nausea, vomiting, diarrhea, stomatitis, dermatitis, fever, and malaise have been observed. Interstitial pneumonia and glomerular damage resulting in renal failure are unusual but well-documented complications (Moore *et al.,* 1968; Crooke and Bradner, 1976; Orwoll *et al.,* 1978).

ENZYMES

L-ASPARAGINASE

History. When L-asparaginase (L-asparagine amidohydrolase) was first introduced into cancer chemotherapy, it was believed that a distinct, qualitative biochemical difference had been detected between normal and certain malignant cells. Although this enzyme has found a limited place in the treatment of acute lymphoblastic leukemia, it is now appreciated that many normal tissues are also sensitive to L-asparaginase. Many toxic effects result from its impairment of the synthesis of secreted proteins, such as insulin, prothrombin and other clotting factors, albumin, and parathyroid hormone.

Preparation and Unitage. A virtually limitless source of L-asparaginase became available when Mashburn and Wriston (1964) identified an L-asparaginase with antileukemic activity in *Escherichia coli.* This microorganism produces two L-asparaginase isozymes, only one of which (EC-2) has antileukemic activity. The *E. coli* enzyme has been purified to homogeneity and is available for therapeutic use. *Asparaginase* (ELSPAR) is a dry powder in sealed vials containing 10,000 international units (I.U.) per vial. The molecular weight of the enzyme is about 133,000, and it consists of four equivalent subunits (*see* Patterson, 1975). These preparations of *E. coli* L-asparaginase have weak glutaminase activity that may play a role in certain of the biological effects. Also, it is suspected that certain toxic manifestations seen with earlier, less pure preparations may have been due to contamination by bacterial endotoxin.

Mechanism of Action and Clinical Toxicity. Most normal tissues synthesize L-asparagine in amounts sufficient for their metabolic needs. Certain neoplastic tissues, however, including acute lymphoblastic leukemic cells in children, require an exogenous source of this amino acid. L-Asparaginase, by catalyzing the hydrolysis of asparagine to aspartic acid and ammonia, deprives these malignant cells of the asparagine available from extracellular fluid, resulting in cellular death.

Of considerable importance in chemotherapy is that, in contrast to most other antitumor drugs, L-asparaginase has minimal effects on the bone marrow, and it does not damage oral or intestinal mucosa or the hair follicles. On the other hand, severe toxicity has been observed that affects the liver, kidneys, pancreas, CNS, and the clotting mechanism (Oettgen *et al.,* 1970). Biochemical evidence of hepatic dysfunction is present in more than 50% of those treated, and most patients display a substantial elevation of blood ammonia (as great as 700 to 900 μg/dl). Disorders of pancreatic function, including decreased insulin production, are often seen, and approximately 5% of treated adults develop overt pancreatitis; death has resulted from hemorrhagic pancreatitis. CNS dysfunction, ranging from depression to impaired sensorium and coma, has occurred in adults. It is suggested that all or most of these toxic effects result from inhibition of protein synthesis in various tissues of the body. L-Asparaginase has immunosuppressive activity, as seen by inhibition of antibody synthesis, delayed hypersensitivity, lymphocyte transformation, and graft rejection. Thus, both T- and B-lymphocyte functions are affected. Since L-asparaginase is a relatively large, foreign protein, it is antigenic, and hypersensitivity phenomena ranging from mild allergic reactions to anaphylactic shock have been reported in 5 to 20% of treated patients.

Therapeutic Status and Dosage. Unfortunately, L-asparaginase has not fulfilled its early promise of high tumoricidal activity with minimal toxicity in the treatment of human malignancies. Complete remissions have been observed in acute lymphoblastic leukemia refractory to other antileukemic agents (Tallal *et al.,* 1970; Sutow *et al.,* 1971); the duration of these remissions, however, has been disappointingly short. Transient remissions have been observed in other forms of leukemia, and occasional beneficial responses have been reported in a few patients with malignant melanoma and non-Hodgkin's lymphomas. Objective responses have not been seen with most solid tumors (Clarkson *et al.,* 1970). The role of asparaginase in antineoplastic chemotherapy is currently limited to the treatment of acute lymphoblastic leukemia refractory to standard regimens for induction of remission (*see* Patterson, 1975; Uren and Handschumacher, 1977).

The suggested dosage for the induction of remission in acute lymphoblastic leukemia is 200 I.U./kg daily for 28 days. Higher daily doses (1000 I.U./kg) for periods not exceeding 10 days have also been proposed as a method of avoiding anaphylaxis, which ordinarily appears only after the tenth day.

IV. Miscellaneous Agents

CISPLATIN

The platinum coordination complexes are a new class of cytotoxic agents that were first identified by Rosenberg and coworkers in 1965. Growth inhibition of *E. coli* was observed when electrical current was delivered between platinum electrodes. The inhibitory effects on bacterial replication were subsequently shown to be due to the formation of inorganic platinum-containing compounds in the presence of ammonium and chloride ions (Rosenberg *et al.,* 1965, 1967). *cis*-Diamminedichloroplatinum (II) (cisplatin) was found to be the most active of these substances in experimental tumor systems and is currently available for clinical use (Rosenberg *et al.,* 1969; Rosenberg, 1973). Other platinum-containing compounds have subsequently been synthesized and tested against animal tumors with promising results (Connors *et al.,* 1972; Speer *et al.,* 1975). Despite pronounced nephrotoxicity and ototoxicity, cisplatin is very useful in combination chemotherapy of metastatic testicular and ovarian carcinoma; encouraging effects have also been reported during treatment of tumors of the bladder and of the head and neck (*see* Gale, 1975; Rozencweig *et al.,* 1977).

Chemistry.   *cis*-Diamminedichloroplatinum (II) (cisplatin) is an inorganic water-soluble, platinum-containing complex. The *II* indicates the valence of platinum. The structural formula of cisplatin is relatively simple, as follows:

$$\begin{array}{c} Cl^- \quad NH_3 \\ \diagdown Pt^{2+} \diagup \\ \diagup \qquad \diagdown \\ Cl^- \quad NH_3 \end{array}$$

Cisplatin

The corresponding complex with the ammonia residues in the *trans* configuration lacks antitumor activity.

Mechanism of Action.   Cisplatin appears to enter cells by diffusion; the chloride ions are subsequently lost by hydrolysis, resulting in the formation of two active ligand sites. Interstrand and intrastrand cross-linking of DNA then occurs in a manner similar to that produced by bifunctional alkylating agents (Roberts and Pascoe, 1972; Mansy *et al.,* 1975; Munchausen and Rahn, 1975). The primary binding site appears to be the guanine base. Recent studies of the binding of the platinum complexes to closed circular DNA indicate that both the *cis* and the *trans* compounds can form covalent linkages. The binding of platinum complexes to DNA appar-

ently disrupts and unwinds the double helix. Although differences are seen in the electrophoretic mobilities of DNA complexed with the *cis* and the *trans* isomers, the marked difference in antitumor activity is not yet explained (Cohen *et al.,* 1979). There is no phase specificity in the action of cisplatin on the cell cycle. Cisplatin has mutagenic and teratogenic effects; its carcinogenic potential has not been investigated but is probably similar to that of bifunctional alkylating agents. Immunosuppressive properties have been reported in several experimental systems involving functions of both B and T lymphocytes. (*See* Gale, 1975; Leh and Wolf, 1976; Rozencweig *et al.,* 1977; Williams and Popovich, 1978.)

Absorption, Fate, and Excretion.   Cisplatin is not effective when administered orally. After rapid intravenous administration the drug has an initial half-life in plasma of 25 to 50 minutes; concentrations decline subsequently with a half-life of 58 to 73 hours. More than 90% of the platinum in the blood is bound to plasma proteins. High concentrations of cisplatin are found in the kidney, liver, intestines, and testes, but there is poor penetration into the CNS. Only a portion of the drug is excreted by the kidney; the extent of biliary or intestinal excretion is unknown (Hill *et al.,* 1975).

Preparation, Dosage, and Route of Administration.   *Cisplatin* (PLATINOL) is available as a lyophilized powder in vials that contain 10 mg of drug. When used alone, the usual intravenous dose is 100 mg/sq m, given once every 4 weeks. Cisplatin is frequently used with other drugs in chemotherapy, and the dosage is reduced in such situations. In order to prevent renal toxicity, hydration of the patient is recommended by the infusion of 1 to 2 liters of fluid for 8 to 12 hours prior to treatment. The appropriate amount of cisplatin is then diluted in a solution of dextrose and saline containing 37.5 to 60 g of mannitol and administered intravenously over a period of 6 to 8 hours. Continued hydration to ensure adequate urinary output is recommended for 24 hours thereafter. Some investigators have advocated the concurrent administration of 40 mg of furosemide. Repeat courses of drug should not be given until all tests of renal and hematopoietic function, as well as auditory acuity, are within acceptable normal limits. Since aluminum reacts with and inactivates cisplatin, it is important not to use needles or other equipment that contains aluminum when preparing or administering the drug.

Therapeutic Uses and Clinical Toxicity.   Cisplatin appears to be particularly effective in the treatment of testicular tumors when used alone or, preferably, with bleomycin and vinblastine (Higby *et al.,* 1974; Samson *et al.,* 1976; Einhorn and Donahue, 1977). The drug is also beneficial in carcinoma of the ovary, particularly when used with doxorubicin (Witshaw and Kroner, 1976; Bruckner *et al.,* 1976). Cisplatin may also be useful in the treatment of carcinomas of the bladder, head and neck, and endometrium, as well as for chemotherapy of lymphomas and some neoplasms of childhood (*see* Rozencweig *et al.*, 1977; Sternberg *et al.*, 1977; Randolph *et al.*, 1978; Yagoda *et al.*, 1978; Einhorn and Williams, 1979).

The major toxicity caused by cisplatin is dose-related, cumulative impairment of renal tubular function; this usually occurs during the second week of therapy. When higher doses or repeated courses of the drug are given, irreversible renal damage may occur (Rozencweig *et al.*, 1977; Dentino *et al.*, 1978). Ototoxicity caused by cisplatin is manifested by tinnitus and hearing loss in the high-frequency range (4000 to 8000 Hz) (Merrin *et al.*, 1978). It can be unilateral or bilateral, tends to be more frequent and severe with repeated doses, and may be more pronounced in children. Marked nausea and vomiting occur in almost all patients. Mild-to-moderate myelosuppression may occur with transient leukopenia and thrombocytopenia. Hyperuricemia, peripheral neuropathies, seizures, and cardiac abnormalities have been reported. Anaphylactic-like reactions, characterized by facial edema, bronchoconstriction, tachycardia, and hypotension, may occur within minutes after administration and should be treated by intravenous injection of epinephrine and with corticosteroids or antihistamines (Von Hoff *et al.*, 1976; Cheng *et al.*, 1978).

HYDROXYUREA

First synthesized in 1869 by Dresler and Stein, hydroxyurea was found to produce leukopenia, anemia, and megaloblastic changes in the bone marrow of rabbits (Rosenthal *et al.*, 1928). It was later shown to have antineoplastic activity against sarcoma 180. Studies of its biological activity and the preliminary assessments of clinical efficacy have been reviewed (*see* Symposium, 1964). The structural formula of hydroxyurea is as follows:

$$H_2N-\overset{\overset{\displaystyle O}{\|}}{C}-NH-OH$$

Hydroxyurea

Cytotoxic Action. Hydroxyurea is representative of a group of compounds that have as their primary site of action the enzyme ribonucleoside diphosphate reductase. Other members of this class that have shown promise in the laboratory are guanazole and the α-N-heterocyclic carboxaldehyde thiosemicarbazones (*see* Agarwal and Sartorelli, 1975). A striking correlation has been observed between the relative growth rate of a series of rat hepatomas and the activity of ribonucleoside diphosphate reductase. This enzyme, which catalyses the reductive conversion of ribonucleotides to deoxyribonucleotides, is a crucial and probably rate-limiting step in the biosynthesis of DNA, and it represents a logical target for the design of chemotherapeutic agents. Nonheme iron is an important component of this enzyme, and many of the active inhibitors can chelate or form complexes with iron. These compounds are specific for the S phase of the cell cycle. (*See* Agarwal and Sartorelli, 1975.)

Absorption, Fate, and Excretion. In man, hydroxyurea is readily absorbed from the gastrointestinal tract, and peak plasma concentrations are reached in 2 hours; within 24 hours, it is essentially undetectable in the blood. Approximately 80% of the drug is recovered in the urine within 12 hours after either oral or intravenous administration (Beckloff *et al.*, 1965).

Preparation, Dosage, and Route of Administration. *Hydroxyurea*, U.S.P. (HYDREA), is available for oral use in 500-mg capsules. Two dosage schedules are recommended: (1) intermittent therapy with 80 mg/kg, administered orally as a single dose every third day, and (2) continuous therapy with 20 to 30 mg/kg, administered orally as a single daily dose. Treatment should be continued for a period of 6 weeks in order to determine its effectiveness; if satisfactory antineoplastic results are obtained, therapy can be continued indefinitely, although leukocyte counts at weekly intervals are advisable.

Therapeutic Uses and Clinical Toxicity. At present, the primary role of hydroxyurea in chemotherapy appears to be in the management of chronic granulocytic leukemia, particularly in patients no longer responsive to busulfan (Kennedy and Yarbro, 1966). It has also produced temporary remissions in patients with metastatic malignant melanoma and occasionally in those with other solid tumors (Ariel, 1970). Hematopoietic depression, involving leukopenia, megaloblastic anemia, and occasionally thrombocytopenia, is the major toxic effect; recovery of the bone marrow is usually prompt if the drug is discontinued for a few days. Other adverse reactions include gastrointestinal disturbances and mild dermatological reactions; more rarely, stomatitis, alopecia, and neurological manifestations have been encountered.

PROCARBAZINE

A group of antitumor agents, the methylhydrazine derivatives, was discovered among a large number of substituted hydrazines, which had been originally synthesized as potential monoamine oxidase inhibitors. Antineoplastic effects in experimental tumors have been reported with several compounds in this series (Bollag, 1963), including procarbazine, an agent useful clinically in Hodgkin's disease. Comprehensive and detailed descriptions of the biological effects, immunosuppressive activity, physiological disposition, carcinogenicity, and clinical effectiveness of procarbazine have been published (Symposium, 1965; Oliverio, 1973a; Reed, 1975). The structural formula of procarbazine is as follows:

$$CH_3-NH-NH-CH_2-\underset{\text{Procarbazine}}{\bigcirc}-CONH-\underset{\underset{CH_3}{|}}{\overset{\overset{CH_3}{|}}{CH}}$$

Cytotoxic Action. The mechanism of action of procarbazine has not been determined. Inhibition of DNA, RNA, and protein synthesis has been observed, although the latter is delayed until after nucleic acid synthesis is inhibited. A progressive decrease in viscosity of DNA solutions is caused by the drug in the presence of oxygen, but not if this is replaced by an inert gas or if peroxidase, catalase, or cysteamine is added. Auto-oxidation occurs in aqueous solutions with production of hydrogen peroxide. The reducing substances also formed are capable of participating in the conversion of hydrogen peroxide to hydroxyl radicals, which may be responsible for the degradation of DNA but not necessarily for the cytotoxic action of the drug. Since only the methyl-substituted hydrazines have been found to be active and only these are capable of forming formaldehyde and its derivatives, it has been suggested that this conversion may play an important role. Cytological studies indicate suppression of mitosis as a result of prolongation of interphase. A very high percentage of broken chromatids has been observed; these effects may be responsible for disturbances of cell division, as well as for the induction of pulmonary tumors, mammary adenocarcinomas, and leukemia in experimental animals.

Absorption, Fate, and Excretion. Procarbazine is absorbed almost completely from the gastrointestinal tract. After parenteral administration, the drug is readily equilibrated between the plasma and the CSF. It is rapidly metabolized in man, and its half-life in the blood after intravenous injection is approximately 7 minutes. Oxidation of procarbazine produces the corresponding azo compound and hydrogen peroxide. From 25 to 70% of an oral or parenteral dose given to man is recovered from the urine during the first 24 hours after administration; less than 5% is excreted as the unchanged compound, and the rest is mostly in the form of a metabolite, N-isopropylterephthalanic acid (Bollag, 1965; Oliverio, 1973a).

Preparation, Dosage, and Route of Administration. *Procarbazine Hydrochloride,* U.S.P. (MATU-LANE), is marketed in 50-mg capsules. The recommended oral daily dose ranges from 100 to 200 mg for the first week of therapy; then daily doses of 300 mg are given until maximal response is obtained or toxicity intervenes.

Therapeutic Uses and Clinical Toxicity. The greatest therapeutic effectiveness of procarbazine is in Hodgkin's disease, particularly when given with mechlorethamine, vincristine, and prednisone (the MOPP regimen) (DeVita *et al.,* 1970). Of major importance is the apparent lack of cross-resistance with other antineoplastic agents. When used with various other agents, procarbazine has also demonstrated activity against oat-cell carcinoma of the lung, non-Hodgkin's lymphomas, myeloma, melanoma, and brain tumors (Greenwald, 1973; Oliverio, 1973a; Kreis, 1977).

The most common toxic effects include leukopenia, thrombocytopenia, nausea, and vomiting, which occur in 50 to 70% of patients. Other gastrointestinal symptoms as well as neurological and dermatological manifestations have been noted in 5 to 10% of cases; psychic disturbances have also been reported. Because of augmentation of sedative effects, the concomitant use of CNS depressants should be avoided. The ingestion of alcohol by patients receiving procarbazine may cause intense warmth and reddening of the face, as well as other effects resembling the acetaldehyde syndrome produced by disulfiram. Since procarbazine is a weak monoamine oxidase inhibitor, hypertensive reactions may result from its use concurrently with sympathomimetic agents, tricyclic antidepressants, and foods with high tyramine content.

MITOTANE (*o,p'*-DDD)

The principal application of mitotane, a compound chemically similar to the insecticides DDT and DDD, is in the treatment of neoplasms derived from the adrenal cortex. In studies of the toxicology of related insecticides in dogs, it was noted that the adrenal cortex was severely damaged, an effect caused by the presence of the *o,p'* isomer of DDD. Its structural formula is as follows:

Mitotane

Cytotoxic Action. The mechanism of action of mitotane has not been elucidated, but its relatively selective attack upon adrenocortical cells, normal or neoplastic, is well established. Thus, administration of the drug causes a rapid reduction in the levels of adrenocorticosteroids and their metabolites in blood and urine, a response that is useful both in guiding dosage and in following the course of hyperadrenocorticism (Cushing's syndrome) resulting from an adrenal tumor or hyperplasia. Damage to the liver, kidneys, or bone marrow has not been encountered.

Absorption, Fate, and Excretion. Clinical studies indicate that approximately 40% of the drug is absorbed after oral administration. After daily doses of 5 to 15 g, concentrations of 10 to 90 μg/ml of unchanged drug and 30 to 50 μg/ml of a metabolite are present in the blood. After discontinuation of therapy, plasma concentrations of mitotane are still measurable for 6 to 9 weeks. Although the drug is found in all tissues, fat is the primary site of storage. A water-soluble metabolite of mitotane is found in the urine; approximately 25% of an oral or parenteral dose is recovered in this form. About 60% of an oral dose is excreted unchanged in the stool.

Preparation, Dosage, and Route of Administration. *Mitotane,* U.S.P. (*o,p'*-DDD; LYSODREN), is supplied in 500-mg scored tablets. Initial daily oral doses of 8 to 10 g are usually given in three or four divided portions, but the maximal tolerated dose may vary from 2 to 16 g per day. Treatment should be continued for at least 3 months; if beneficial effects are observed, therapy is maintained indefinitely.

Therapeutic Uses and Clinical Toxicity. Mitotane is indicated in the palliative treatment of inoperable adrenocortical carcinoma. In addition to 138 patients reported by Hutter and Kayhoe (1966), 115 have been studied by Lubitz and associates (1973). Clinical effectiveness has been reported in 34 to 54% of these cases. Apparent cures have been reported in some patients with metastatic disease (Becker and Schumacher, 1975; Ostumi and Roginsky, 1975). Although the administration of mitotane produces anorexia and nausea in approximately 80% of patients, somnolence and lethargy in about 34%, and dermatitis in 15 to 20%, these effects do not contraindicate the use of the drug at lower doses. Since this drug damages the adrenal cortex, administration of adrenocorticosteroids is indicated, particularly in patients with evidence of adrenal insufficiency, shock, or severe trauma (Hogan *et al.*, 1978).

V. Hormones

ADRENOCORTICOSTEROIDS

The pharmacology, major therapeutic uses, and toxic effects of the adrenocorticosteroids are discussed in Chapter 63. Only the applications of the hormones in the treatment of neoplastic disease will be considered here. Because of their lympholytic effects and their ability to suppress mitosis in lymphocytes, the greatest value of these steroids is in the treatment of acute leukemia in children and of malignant lymphoma. They are especially effective in the management of frank hemolytic anemia and the hemorrhagic complications of thrombocytopenia that frequently accompany malignant lymphomas and chronic lymphocytic leukemia.

In acute lymphoblastic or undifferentiated leukemia of childhood, adrenocorticosteroids may produce prompt clinical improvement and objective hematological remissions in 30 to 50% of children. Although these responses frequently are characterized by complete disappearance of all detectable leukemic cells from the peripheral blood and bone marrow, the duration of remission is extremely variable (2 weeks to 9 months) and relapse of the disease invariably occurs; eventually, drug resistance develops. Remissions occur more rapidly with corticosteroids than with antimetabolites, and there is no evidence of cross-resistance to unrelated agents. For these reasons, therapy is often initiated with a steroid and another type of agent, usually vincristine, in order to *induce* remissions. This approach, followed by continuous *maintenance* treatment with various agents, seems to yield more prolonged remissions (*see* section on methotrexate). Adult leukemia seldom responds to induced hypercorticism, but marked constitutional symptoms of the disease and the hemorrhagic manifestations of thrombocytopenia may be controlled effectively, albeit temporarily, without demonstrable changes in platelet counts.

Corticosteroids have been useful in some patients with carcinoma of the breast and other carcinomas; however, palliative effects are of short duration and complications are frequent. Although the overall results in the treatment of carcinoma with these agents have been disappointing, the judicious short-term use of corticosteroids may be indicated for specific complications such as hypercalcemia and intracranial metastases.

The adrenocorticosteroids are used in conjunction with x-ray therapy to reduce the occurrence of radiation edema in critical areas such as the superior mediastinum, brain, and spinal cord. These drugs are particularly useful in the symptomatic palliation of patients with severe hematopoietic depression secondary to bone-marrow involvement or previous radiation or chemotherapy. They may produce rapid symptomatic improvement in critically ill patients by temporarily suppressing fever, sweats, and pain, and by restoring, to some degree, appetite, lost weight, strength, and sense of well-being. The symptoms tend to recur after the hormone is withdrawn, which indicates that the effects of the disease, but not necessarily the disease process itself, have been affected. Therefore, the value of this type of therapy is to provide the patient with a relatively asymptomatic period during which the general physical condition may improve sufficiently to permit further definitive therapy.

Several preparations are available and at appropriate dosages exert similar effects (*see* Chapter 63). Prednisone, for example, is usually administered orally in doses as high as 60 to 100 mg, or even higher, for the first few days and gradually reduced to levels of 20 to 40 mg per day. A continuous attempt should be made to lower the dosage required to control the manifestations of the disease.

PROGESTINS

Progestational agents (*see* Chapter 61) have been found useful in the management of patients with endometrial carcinoma previously treated by surgery and radiotherapy (Kelley and Baker, 1961). These compounds were tried initially because of the concept that carcinoma of the endometrium results from the prolonged, unopposed overstimulation by estrogen (Hertig and Sommers, 1949). This led to the use of progesterone, which would correct this situation because of its physiological effect in producing maturation and secretory activity of the normal endometrium. Apparently a portion of neoplastic cells arising from this tissue is still influenced by normal hormonal controls.

There are several preparations available. Hydroxyprogesterone caproate is usually administered intramuscularly in doses of 500 mg twice weekly; medroprogesterone acetate can be administered orally in doses of 100 to 200 mg daily or intramuscularly in doses of 400 mg twice weekly. An alternative oral agent is megestrol acetate (40 to 320 mg daily, in divided doses). Beneficial effects, usually characterized by regression of pulmonary metastases, have been observed in approximately one third of patients. Responses to progestational agents have also been reported in metastatic carcinomas of the breast (Stoll, 1972) and prostate (Fergusson, 1972), and in hypernephromas (Bloom, 1972).

ESTROGENS AND ANDROGENS

A discussion of the pharmacology of the estrogens and androgens appears in Chapters 61 and 62. Their use in the treatment of certain neoplastic diseases will be discussed here. They are of value in this connection because certain organs that are often the primary site of malignant growth, notably the prostate and the mammary gland, are dependent upon hormones for their growth, function, and morphological integrity. Carcinomas arising from these organs often retain some of the hormonal requirements of their normal counterparts for varying periods of time. By changing the hormonal environment of such tumors it is possible to alter, to some degree, the course of the neoplastic process.

Androgen-Control Therapy of Prostatic Carcinoma. The development of the androgen-control regimen for the treatment of prostatic carcinoma is largely the contribution of Huggins and associates (1941). Their studies are of importance for several reasons: (1) they typify the rational approach to cancer chemotherapy in that the theoretical considerations that led to the trial of the therapeutic regimen were based upon fundamental biochemical concepts; (2) androgen-control therapy represents the first effective chemotherapeutic measure in disseminated carcinomatosis and has provided a great stimulus for research in the field; (3) although no case of prostatic carcinoma has been cured by androgen-control therapy, life expectancy has been increased and thousands of patients have enjoyed the benefit of its ameliorating effects; and (4) approximately 95% of patients with clinical manifestations of carcinoma of the prostate have nonresectable disease and require androgen-control therapy.

History and Rationale. The relationship between the prostate and testicular function was appreciated early in the nineteenth century, when it was noted that regression of the prostate followed orchiectomy. Huggins observed that, in the dog, shrinkage of the gland and cessation of secretion followed castration and that these effects could be reversed by the administration of androgen. Of even greater significance was the observation that the administration of estrogen could block the effects of the androgen. On the basis of these experimental findings, Huggins and associates (1941) postulated that significant clinical improvement should occur after bilateral orchiectomy in patients with advanced prostatic carcinoma, a theory that proved to be correct. It was also demonstrated that similar results could be obtained by the administration of estrogen (Herbst, 1941).

The fundamental mechanism by which the lack of androgen results in regressive changes in normal and malignant prostatic cells is unknown. Relapse eventually occurs in patients on androgen-control therapy, and this constitutes another fundamental problem. The most likely explanation is that survival of progressively undifferentiated cells favors the emergence of cell types that are no longer dependent on androgen.

Therapeutic Regimen. From a statistical analysis of over 1800 cases (Nesbit and Baum, 1950), it appears that 5-year control of prostatic cancer is most effectively obtained by the combined use of orchiectomy and estrogen in patients who, when first treated, are free from metastases. When metastases are already present, orchiectomy seems to be more effective than estrogen therapy, and their combination does not appear to offer any advantage. When either orchiectomy or estrogen alone is employed as a therapeutic measure and the patient relapses, some degree of symptomatic improvement is then obtained by the alternative procedure, but this usually is not outstanding. In view of the fact that orchiectomy is indicated regardless of metastases, and that under certain circumstances further benefit is to be derived from the use of estrogen, it is recommended that both procedures be employed in any case of prostatic carcinoma as soon as the diagnosis is established.

The choice of estrogen is largely determined by cost and convenience. Natural products have no advantage over synthetic preparations, and the oral route of administration causes the least inconvenience to the patient. For these reasons, diethylstilbestrol or a related synthetic compound is the preparation of choice. There is no evidence that survival is improved with excessively large doses. An average dose of diethylstilbestrol is 5 mg three times daily. Indeed, many authorities reduce the daily dose to as little as 1 mg after a few weeks. The dose of other estrogens is in proportion to their potency.

Response to Therapy. Subjective and objective improvements rapidly follow the institution of androgen-control therapy of prostatic carcinoma. From the patient's point of view the most gratifying of these is relief of pain. This is associated with an increase in appetite, weight gain, and a feeling of well-being. Objectively, there are regressions of the primary tumor and soft-tissue metastases. Serial biopsies reveal nuclear and cytoplasmic changes in the malignant tissue; after some months, most of it may be replaced by scar tissue. Malignant cells, however, do not completely disappear. Elevated plasma acid phosphatase activity usually falls to normal. Alkaline phosphatase activity may first rise and then fall. There is often an associated recovery from anemia. Some patients with prostatic carcinoma show no response to androgen-control therapy. Eventually prostatic tumors become insensitive to the lack of androgen or the presence of estrogen; however, it is now well established that effective palliation is afforded by the therapeutic regimen and that the life expectancy of the treated patient is significantly increased.

Androgen-Control Therapy of Carcinoma of the Male Breast. Carcinoma of the male breast is a rare tumor that is seldom diagnosed sufficiently early to permit definitive surgical intervention. The neoplasm regresses in a high proportion of cases in response to androgen-control therapy. Although this may be achieved by either orchiectomy or the administration of estrogen, it is preferable to initiate treatment with orchiectomy; when evidence of exacerbation appears, estrogen therapy is instituted. Remissions of several years can be achieved with this therapeutic regimen (Treves, 1959; Kennedy, 1965).

Untoward Effects of Androgen-Control Therapy. Androgen-control therapy is one of the safest forms of cancer chemotherapy. The psychic trauma of orchiectomy is not inconsequential, but is tempered somewhat by the age of the patient. The same is true of the sexual impotence that usually accompanies either orchiectomy or estrogen therapy. After orchiectomy alone, hot flushes are not uncommon; these can be controlled by the administration of estrogen. Estrogens are capable of producing the untoward responses described in detail in Chapter 61. Mild gastrointestinal disturbances may be noted, occasionally, these may be severe enough to require discontinuation of the drug. There also may be some expansion of extracellular fluid volume in patients with poor cardiac function. There was a significant excess mortality from cardiac and cerebrovascular complications reported when a group of men treated with 5 mg of diethylstilbestrol daily was compared with controls (Veterans Administration Co-Operative Urological Research Group, 1967). Gynecomastia is frequent and may be a disturbing feature in some patients; it is said to be prevented by low-dose radiation of the breasts at the outset of hormonal therapy (Larrson and Sundbom, 1962). In rare instances, carcinoma of the male breast has occurred in patients given estrogen for prolonged periods of time.

Estrogens and Androgens in the Treatment of Mammary Carcinoma. Estrogens and androgens have found application in the treatment of advanced mammary carcinoma. The hormones afford some measure of relief in patients with nonresectable disease in whom the metastatic lesions are too widespread to permit effective radiation.

History and Rationale. Hormonal-control therapy for carcinoma of the breast is by no means a recent development, and late in the nineteenth century castration was recommended. Not long thereafter, radiation of the ovaries was introduced. Both procedures are still practiced. Early experimental work on the relation of ovarian secretions to carcinoma of the breast led to the observation that the incidence of spontaneous breast cancer in female mice could be substantially decreased by castration (Loeb, 1919). Later, Lacassagne (1936) demonstrated that, in a strain of mice in which the females but not the males exhibited a high incidence of spontaneous breast carcinoma, the administration of estrogen to the males resulted in proliferation of the ductal epithelium, from which metastatic adenocarcinoma developed. He was also able, by the injection of estrogen, to increase the incidence of carcinoma of the breast to 100% in a strain of mice that normally had a very low incidence of spontaneous tumors. Among the first reports of the use of testosterone were those of Ulrich in 1939 and Loeser in 1941. In 1944, Haddow and coworkers in Great Britain first reported the results of estrogen therapy. (*See* Kennedy, 1965; Krakoff, 1967; Lippman, 1978.)

Therapeutic Regimen. The therapeutic regimen for the use of androgens and estrogens in the treatment of carcinoma of the breast is largely empirical. The first cardinal principle is that hormonal therapy should be reserved for patients for whom surgical treatment or radiotherapy has been fully considered and deemed no longer of value. Once this qualification has been met, androgen therapy may be employed for patients in any age group. Objective remissions are obtained in approximately 20% of patients (Goldenberg, 1964). Estrogen therapy generally is contraindicated in patients who are not at least 5 years past the menopause, regardless of chronological age. Experience has shown that estro-

gen may accelerate the neoplastic process in women who are still menstruating. In premenopausal women, oophorectomy is the first recommended procedure to institute hormonal control. On the basis of earlier observations, androgen was said to be preferable for the treatment of bone metastases, whereas estrogen was considered to be the preparation of choice for soft-tissue metastases. Subsequent evidence does not entirely substantiate these findings, however, and it is often the practice to change from one type of hormone to the other in unresponsive patients.

Progress in endocrinology has led to the development of methods that are very useful for the selection of patients for ablative or additive hormonal therapy; this may well remove much of the empiricism from this area. Tissues that are responsive to estrogens contain receptors for the hormones that can be detected by ligand binding technics (Hilf and Wittliff, 1975). Strong evidence has accumulated that a breast malignancy lacking specific estrogen-binding capacity rarely responds to hormonal manipulation. The tumors that contain receptors usually do respond and, furthermore, are associated with a better overall prognosis independent of any type of therapy (Jensen *et al.,* 1971; Knight *et al.,* 1977; Young *et al.,* 1977; Kiang *et al.,* 1978; Legha *et al.,* 1978; Lippman, 1978).

Hormonal therapy utilizes doses much larger than those needed for physiological replacement. Androgen therapy is preferably with oral agents; commonly used regimens include fluoxymesterone, 10 mg orally three times a day, or calusterone, 50 mg orally four times daily. Parenteral androgen therapy may be given as dromostanolone propionate, 100 mg intramuscularly three times weekly. The prototypical parenteral androgen preparations, testosterone propionate and testosterone enanthate, while as effective as other androgens, are now rarely employed because of their marked virilizing property.

Compounds with estrogenic activity are numerous. Oral diethylstilbestrol is the most frequently used; it is given initially in doses of 5 mg daily. This dose is gradually increased to a maintenance dose of 5 mg three times daily over a 1- to 2-week period. Ethinyl estradiol is also commonly used, the dosage being gradually increased from 0.5 mg orally once daily to the customary maintenance dose of 3 mg daily, given in three portions. Ethinyl estradiol may be tried if diethylstilbestrol causes intolerable gastrointestinal side effects.

Response to Therapy. The onset of action of the hormones is slow, and it is necessary to continue therapy for 8 to 12 weeks before a decision can be reached as to effectiveness. If a favorable response is obtained, hormonal treatment should be continued until an exacerbation of symptoms occurs. Withdrawal of the hormone at this time may occasionally be followed by another remission.

In a retrospective study of 944 patients with disseminated mammary carcinoma, objective remissions were noted in approximately 20% of patients receiving androgens and in 30 to 40% of postmenopausal women treated with estrogens. Two major factors appear to temper the rate of response: the menopausal age of the patient and the body system most importantly involved by the disease (local, best;

visceral, worst; and osseous, intermediate). It is of interest that, despite regression of the lesions, only rarely is it possible to demonstrate morphological changes in the tumors. The duration of the induced remission averages about 6 months to 1 year; however, some patients may receive benefit for several years. Average survival time in patients who respond to therapy appears to be longer than in untreated controls or in those who do not respond.

Untoward Effects. All the untoward effects that commonly accompany estrogen and androgen therapy have been observed in the use of these agents in the treatment of mammary carcinoma; these effects are described in Chapters 61 and 62. Two toxic manifestations require emphasis. With either hormone, the combined effect of a steroid and osteolytic metastases may result in marked hypercalcemia. The chief dangers are ectopic calcification, particularly in the urinary tract, and the physiological disturbances that may accompany an increase in the concentration of ionized calcium in the extracellular fluid. Patients who show an elevation in plasma calcium should receive a high fluid intake. Severe hypercalcemia, whether spontaneous or drug induced, is a true medical emergency. If an estrogen or androgen is being used, it should be discontinued. Forced hydration, by vein if the patient cannot drink, is mandatory. Further measures may be necessary; these include administration of diuretics, adrenocorticosteroids in large doses, oral or intravenous phosphate supplementation, or the intravenous administration of mithramycin (*see* above; *see also* Chapter 65). When drug-induced hypercalcemia is corrected, further therapy may be cautiously attempted. The incidence of hypercalcemia in patients receiving androgens is approximately 10%; it occurs less frequently with estrogen therapy. Plasma calcium concentrations should be determined routinely in patients receiving hormonal therapy.

Rarely, either estrogen or androgen therapy may cause exacerbation of the malignant process; this occurs more frequently as a result of estrogen administration.

ANTIESTROGENS

TAMOXIFEN

About one third of patients with advanced carcinoma of the breast benefit from either endocrine ablation or hormonal therapy. The growth of certain breast cancer cells depends on the presence of estrogens and, in these cases, oophorectomy may suppress tumor growth. A new development has been the introduction of effective and relatively nontoxic antiestrogenic agents that block the peripheral functions of estrogens on target tissues (*see* Chapter 61). Of various compounds tested, *tamoxifen* has been approved for clinical use in the United States; it is effective, palliative treatment for certain patients with advanced breast cancer. Tumors that contain estrogen receptors and those whose growth was slowed by prior hormonal therapy tend to respond to tamoxifen; others are often insensitive (*see* Tormey *et al.,* 1976; Kiang and Kennedy, 1977; Moseson *et al.,* 1978). The structural formula of tamoxifen is shown in Chapter 61.

Mechanism of Action. Receptors for estrogen are detected in only 15% of breast cancers in premenopausal women, while they are present in approximately two thirds of those in postmenopausal patients. Antiestrogens, such as tamoxifen, bind to estrogen receptors in a fashion similar to that of estradiol. The complex of the receptor and the antiestrogen may bind to nuclear chromatin in an atypical manner and for a longer time than the normal hormone-receptor complex. Furthermore, antiestrogens may deplete the cytoplasm of free receptor. Either or both of these effects could severely impair the continued growth of an estrogen-dependent tumor. These observations offer a sound rationale for the use of antiestrogen therapy in combination with various ablative operations—oophorectomy, adrenalectomy, or hypophysectomy. Although any of these procedures may decrease the concentrations of estrogens in tissues, they do not completely eliminate the synthesis of the hormones. For example, after oophorectomy, androgens produced by the adrenals may be converted to estradiol in peripheral tissues. Three antiestrogens have shown useful actions in the treatment of human breast cancer: *clomiphene, nafoxidine,* and *tamoxifen.* Of these, tamoxifen is favored because of its relative lack of toxicity (*see* Legha *et al.,* 1978).

Absorption, Fate, and Excretion. After oral administration, peak concentrations of tamoxifen are found in blood after 4 to 7 hours. The decline in plasma concentration is biphasic; the initial $t_{1/2}$ is 7 to 14 hours, and the terminal $t_{1/2}$ is longer than 7 days. Studies in animals indicate that tamoxifen undergoes extensive metabolic conversion by hydroxylation and conjugation. The monohydroxylated derivative has more antiestrogenic activity than does the parent compound or the dihydroxylated metabolite. After enterohepatic circulation, glucuronides and other metabolites are excreted in the stool; excretion in the urine is minimal.

Preparation, Dosage, and Route of Administration. *Tamoxifen citrate* (NOLVADEX) is marketed in 10-mg tablets. The recommended dose is 20 to 40 mg daily, administered orally in two divided doses. Objective responses usually occur in 4 to 10 weeks but may be delayed for several months in patients with bone metastases.

Therapeutic Uses and Clinical Toxicity. Tamoxifen is useful in the palliative treatment of advanced carcinoma of the breast in postmenopausal women. Patients who have tumors that contain estrogen receptors are most likely to respond to the drug; those with a recent negative assay for receptor-binding activity are unlikely to benefit. Although a few premenopausal women have responded to this agent, it is more effective in patients who are several years postmenopausal, have metastases to soft tissues rather than to bone, and have derived beneficial effects from previous hormone therapy.

The most frequent adverse reactions include hot flashes, nausea, and vomiting. These may occur in approximately 25% of patients and are rarely severe enough to necessitate discontinuation of therapy. Menstrual irregularities, vaginal bleeding and discharge, pruritus vulvae, and dermatitis have occurred less frequently. The occurrence of pain in tumors, particularly bone metastases, as well as local flare of disease, characterized by increase in size and marked erythema of the lesions, is sometimes associated with good responses. Other infrequent adverse effects include hypercalcemia, peripheral edema, anorexia, depression, pulmonary embolism, lightheadedness, headache, mild-to-moderate thrombocytopenia, and leukopenia. Tamoxifen is said to be carcinogenic and teratogenic in animals. (Further information about tamoxifen may be found in the publications of Lerner *et al.*, 1976; Manni *et al.*, 1976; Tormey *et al.*, 1976; Kiang and Kennedy, 1977; Young *et al.*, 1977; Kiang *et al.*, 1978; Legha *et al.*, 1978; Moseson *et al.*, 1978.)

VI. Radioactive Isotopes

Mechanism of Cytotoxic Action of Ionizing Radiations. It is beyond the scope of this chapter to present a definitive account of present concepts of the mechanism of the cytotoxic actions of ionizing radiations. In view of the highly technical problems associated with the proper use of radioactive isotopes for either metabolic tracing, diagnostic, or therapeutic purposes, reference should be made to a variety of excellent reviews and books on these subjects (*see* Haynie *et al.*, 1973; Hall, 1978).

SODIUM PHOSPHATE-^{32}P

Preparations, Physical Properties, Distribution, and Excretion. *Sodium Phosphate P 32 Solution,* U.S.P. (*sodium phosphate-^{32}P;* PHOSPHOTOPE), is supplied as a solution for oral use, as well as in sterile form for injection. The half-life is 14.3 days. ^{32}P emits an electron with an average energy of about 0.6 million electron volts (mev) (maximum of about 1.7 mev); the other product of its decomposition is nonradioactive sulfur (^{32}S). The emitted beta particle of ^{32}P penetrates to an average depth of about 2 mm (with a maximum of not more than 8 mm) of tissue. The differential uptake of phosphate by cells is dependent upon at least three factors: (1) the total amount of phosphate in exchangeable form in the tissue; (2) the rate of turnover of the phosphate groups; and (3) the rate at which new cells are formed. The material will enter particularly those tissues in which the metabolic turnover of phosphate groups is high, as in neoplastic cells or in normal cells of the bone marrow, spleen, and lymph nodes.

Ultimately, as phosphate-^{32}P leaves the soft tissues through turnover, the bones become the most radioactive tissue, regardless of the initial distribution of the isotope. The renal elimination of absorbed radioactivity, originally rapid (25 to 50% during the first 4 to 6 days), soon becomes very slow (less than 1% per day). If administered orally, about 25% of the radioactivity of sodium phosphate-^{32}P is unabsorbed and is excreted in the feces. Uptake into osseous tissues, in addition to immediate direct utilization by bone-marrow cells, affords opportunities for both early and long-continued bombardment of both bone-marrow and osseous cells; hence, overdosage

can lead to severe depression of bone-marrow function, with resultant leukopenia, thrombocytopenia, and anemia. Indeed, neoplastic changes in these tissues can be produced by large doses of radioactive phosphate.

Therapeutic Uses and Dosage. The high uptake of phosphate-^{32}P by critical normal tissues does not permit a truly selective attack upon malignant tissues. Although the isotope was used at one time for the therapy of chronic leukemias, chemotherapy is now the treatment of choice.

Sodium phosphate-^{32}P has been used for palliation in polycythemia vera because of its capacity to suppress the overproduction of erythrocytes, as well as the accompanying excessive proliferation of platelets and leukocytes. However, its employment in this disorder has been largely discontinued because of a growing awareness that patients treated with this agent have a higher incidence of leukemia. In the future it will probably be completely replaced by chemotherapy. When used in severe and refractory polycythemia vera, the initial intravenous dosage of sodium phosphate-^{32}P is usually about 3 mCi, ranging between 2.5 and 5 mCi. Subsequent ^{32}P therapy, with or without phlebotomy, usually is not given for at least 2 or 3 months, and preferably after longer intervals (Wasserman, 1976).

GOLD-198

This short-lived isotope of gold (half-life, 2.7 days), which emits both beta particles (principally 0.97 mev; 90 to 94%) and gamma rays (principally 0.41 mev; 6 to 10%), is supplied in the form of colloidal material, 25 to 200 mCi/ml, *Gold Au 198 Injection,* U.S.P. (AURCOLOID-198, AUREOTOPE). Since the dosage of ^{198}Au ranges between 35 and 150 mCi, treated patients afford a very significant hazard to nursing and other personnel; in addition, the therapy is costly and offers no therapeutic advantage in the treatment of malignant effusions over the use of alkylating agents, talc, or quinacrine. For these reasons, it has been replaced by these agents.

ISOTOPES OF IODINE

These preparations are discussed in Chapter 60.

Acute Leukemia Group B. New treatment schedule with improved survival in childhood leukemia. *J.A.M.A.,* **1965,** *194,* 187–193.

Agarwal, R. P.; Sagar, S. M.; and Parks, R. E., Jr. Adenosine deaminase from human erythrocytes: purification and effects of adenosine analogs. *Biochem. Pharmacol.,* **1975,** *24,* 693–701.

Agarwal, R. P.; Spector, T.; and Parks, R. E., Jr. Tight-binding inhibitors. IV. Inhibition of adenosine deaminases by various inhibitors. *Biochem. Pharmacol.,* **1977,** *26,* 359–367.

Ahmed, N. K.; Felsted, R. L.; and Bacher, N. R. Heterogeneity of anthracycline antibiotic carbonylreductases in mammalian livers. *Biochem. Pharmacol.,* **1978,** *27,* 2713–2720.

Alberts, D. S.; Chang, S. Y.; Chen, H.-S. G.; Larcom, B. J.; and Jones, S. E. Pharmacokinetics and metabolism of chlorambucil in man: a preliminary report. *Cancer Treat. Rev.,* **1979a,** *6,* 9.

Alberts, D. S.; Chang, S. Y.; Chen, H.-S. G.; Moon, T. E.; Evans, T. L.; Furner, R. L.; Himmelstein, K.; and Gross, J. F. Kinetics of intravenous melphalan. *Clin. Pharmacol. Ther.,* **1979b,** *26,* 73–80.

Ansfield, F. J.; Ramirez, G.; Skibba, J. L.; Bryan, G. T.; Davis, H. L.; and Wirtanen, G. W. Intrahepatic arterial infusion with 5-fluorouracil. *Cancer,* **1971,** *28,* 1147–1151.

Ariel, I. Therapeutic effects of hydroxyurea. Experience with 118 patients with inoperable solid tumors. *Cancer,* **1970,** *25,* 705–714.

Bachur, N. R.; Gordon, S. L.; and Gee, M. V. Anthracycline antibiotic augmentation of microsomal electron transport and free radical formation. *Mol. Pharmacol.,* **1977,** *13,* 901–910.

Bagley, C. M., Jr.; Bostick, F. W.; and DeVita, V. T., Jr. Clinical pharmacology of cyclophosphamide. *Cancer Res.,* **1973,** *33,* 226–233.

Bagley, C. M., Jr.; DeVita, V. T., Jr.; Berard, C. W.; and Canellos, G. P. Advanced lymphosarcoma: intensive cyclical combination chemotherapy with cyclophosphamide, vincristine, and prednisone. *Ann. Intern. Med.,* **1972,** *76,* 227–234.

Barranco, S. C., and Humphrey, R. M. The effects of 2'-deoxythioguanosine on survival and progression in mammalian cells. *Proc. Soc. Exp. Biol. Med.,* **1971,** *31,* 583–586.

Becker, D., and Schumacher, O. P. *o,p'*-DDD therapy in invasive adrenocortical carcinoma. *Ann. Intern. Med.,* **1975,** *82,* 677–679.

Beckloff, G. L.; Lerner, H. J.; Frost, D.; Russo-Alesi, F. M.; and Gitomer, S. Hydroxyurea (NSC-32065) in biological fluids: dose-concentration relationship. *Cancer Chemother. Rep.,* **1965,** *48,* 57–58.

Benjamin, R. S.; Riggs, C. E., Jr.; and Bachur, N. R. Plasma pharmacokinetics of adriamycin and its metabolites in humans with normal hepatic and renal function. *Cancer Res.,* **1977,** *37,* 1416–1420.

Bertino, J. R. Rescue techniques in cancer chemotherapy: use of leucovorin and other rescue agents after methotrexate treatment. *Semin. Oncol.,* **1977,** *4,* 203–216.

Bleyer, W. A. The clinical pharmacology of methotrexate—historical background. *Cancer Treat. Rep.,* **1978,** *62,* 307–312.

Bloch, A. (ed.). Chemistry, biology, and clinical uses of nucleoside analogs. *Ann. N.Y. Acad. Sci.,* **1975,** *255,* 1–610.

Bollag, W. The tumor-inhibitory effects of the methylhydrazine derivative Ro 4-6467/1 (NSC-77213). *Cancer Chemother. Rep.,* **1963,** *33,* 1–4.

————. Experimental studies with a methylhydrazine derivative, ibenzymethyzin. In, *Natulan (Ibenzymethyzin).* (Jelliffe, A. M., and Marks, J., eds.) John Wright & Sons, Ltd., Bristol, **1965,** pp. 1–8.

Bolt, W. von; Ritzl, F.; Toussaint, R.; and Nahrmann, H. Verteilung und Ausscheidung eines cystostatisch wirkenden mit Tritium markierten N-Lost-Derivatives beim krebskranken Menschen. *Arzneim. Forsch.,* **1961,** *11,* 170–175.

Bonadonna, G., and others. Are surgical adjuvant trials altering the course of breast cancer? *Semin. Oncol.,* **1978,** *5,* 450–464.

Bono, V. H., Jr. Studies on the mechanism of action of DTIC (NSC-45388). *Cancer Treat. Rep.,* **1976,** *60,* 141–148.

Bourke, R. S.; West, C. R.; Chheda, G.; and Tower, D. B. Kinetics of entry and distribution of 5-fluorouracil in cerebrospinal fluid and brain following intravenous injection in a primate. *Cancer Res.,* **1973,** *33,* 1735–1746.

Bristow, M. R.; Billingham, M. E.; Mason, J. W.; and Daniels, J. R. Clinical spectrum of anthracycline antibiotic cardiotoxicity. *Cancer Treat. Rep.,* **1978,** *62,* 873–879.

Brock, N. Pharmacologic characterization of cyclophosphamide (NSC-26271) and cyclophosphamide metabolites. *Cancer Chemother. Rep.,* **1967,** *51,* 315–325.

Broder, L. E., and Carter, S. K. Pancreatic islet cell carcinoma. II. Results of therapy with streptozotocin in 52 patients. *Ann. Intern. Med.,* **1973,** *79,* 108–118.

Broughton, A.; Strong, J. E.; Hoyle, P. Y.; and Bedrossian, C. W. M. Clinical pharmacology of bleomycin following intravenous infusion as determined by radioimmunoassay. *Cancer,* **1977,** *40,* 2772–2778.

Bruckner, H. W.; Cohen, C. C.; Deppe, G.; Kabakow, B.; Wallach, R. C.; Greenspan, E. M.; Gusberg, S. B.; and Holland, J. F. Chemotherapy of gynecological tumors with platinum II. *J. Clin. Hematol. Oncol.,* **1976,** *3,* 121–139.

Bruckner, H. W., and Creasey, W. A. The administration of 5-fluorouracil by mouth. *Cancer,* **1974,** *33,* 14–18.

Calabresi, P. New techniques for measuring the effects of chemotherapeutic agents upon neoplastic and normal host cells. *Verlag Wien. Med. Akad.,* **1967,** *7,* 99–111.

————. Principles of oncologic treatment: irradiation, cytotoxic drugs and immunostimulatory procedures. In, *Cecil Textbook of Medicine,* 15th ed. (Beeson, P. B.; McDermott, W.; and Wyngaarden, J. B.; eds.) W. B. Saunders Co., Philadelphia, **1979,** pp. 1922–1941.

Calabresi, P.; Dexter, D. L.; and Heppner, G. H. Clinical and pharmacological implications of cancer cell differentiation and heterogeneity. *Biochem. Pharmacol.,* **1979,** *28,* 1933–1941.

Calabresi, P., and Turner, R. W. Beneficial effects of triacetyl azauridine in psoriasis and mycosis fungoides. *Ann. Intern. Med.,* **1966,** *64,* 352–371.

Carrico, C. K., and Sartorelli, A. C. Effects of 6-thioguanine on macromolecular events in regenerating rat liver. *Cancer Res.,* **1977,** *37,* 1868–1875.

Cheng, E.; Cvitkovic, E.; Wittes, R. E.; and Golbey, R.-B. Germ cell tumors (II). *Cancer,* **1978,** *42,* 2162–2168.

Cheng, Y. C.; Neenan, J. P.; Ward, D. C.; and Prusoff, W. H. Selective inhibition of herpes simplex virus by 5-amino-2',5'-dideoxy-5-iodouridine. *J. Virol.,* **1975,** *15,* 1284–1285.

Chu, M. Y. Incorporation of arabinosyl cytosine into 2-7S ribonucleic acid and cell death. *Biochem. Pharmacol.,* **1971,** *20,* 2057–2063.

Chu, M. Y., and Fischer, G. A. A proposed mechanism of action of 1-β-D-arabinofuranosylcytosine as an inhibitor of the growth of leukemic cells. *Biochem. Pharmacol.,* **1962,** *11,* 423–430.

————. Comparative studies of leukemic cells sensitive and resistant to cytosine arabinoside. *Ibid.,* **1965,** *14,* 333–341.

————. The incorporation of ³H-cytosine arabinoside and its effect on murine leukemic cells (L5178Y). *Ibid.,* **1968,** *17,* 753–767.

Clarkson, B. D. Acute myelocytic leukemia in adults. *Cancer,* **1972,** *30,* 1572–1582.

Clarkson, B. D.; Krakoff, I. H.; Burchenal, J. H.; Karnofsky, D. A.; Golbey, R. B.; Dowling, M. D.; Oettgen, H. F.; and Lipton, A. Clinical results of treatment with E. coli L-asparaginase in adults with leukemia, lymphosarcoma and solid tumors. *Cancer,* **1970,** *25,* 279–305.

Cohen, G. L.; Bauer, W. R.; Barton, J. K.; and Lippard, S. J. Binding of *cis-* and *trans*-dichlorodiammine platinum (II) to DNA: evidence for unwinding and shortening of the double helix. *Science,* **1979,** *203,* 1014–1016.

Collins, K. D., and Stark, G. R. Aspartate transcarbamylase. Interaction with the transition state analog N-(phosphonacetyl)-L-aspartate. *J. Biol. Chem.,* **1971,** *246,* 6599–6606.

Comiener, G. W., and Smith, C. G. Studies of the enzymatic deamination of ara-cytidine. V. Inhibition *in vitro* and *in vivo* by tetrahydrouridine and other reduced pyrimidine nucleosides. *Biochem. Pharmacol.,* **1968,** *17,* 1981–1991.

Connors, T. A.; Jones, M.; Ross, W. C. J.; Braddock, P. D.; Kokhar, A. R.; and Tobe, M. L. New platinum complexes with anti-tumour activity. *Chem. Biol. Interact.,* **1972,** *5,* 415–424.

Cortes, E. P.; Holland, J. F.; Moskowitz, R.; and Depoli, E. Effects of mithramycin on bone resorption *in vitro. Cancer Res.,* **1972,** *32,* 74–76.

Costanzi, J. J. Studies in the Southwest Oncology Group. *Cancer Treat. Rep.,* **1976,** *60,* 189–192.

Creasey, W. A.; Fink, M. E.; Handschumacher, R. E.; and Calabresi, P. Clinical and pharmacological studies with 2′,3′,5′-triacetyl-6-azauridine. *Cancer Res.,* **1963,** *23,* 444–453.

Creasey, W. A.; Papac, R. J.; Markiw, M. E.; Calabresi, P.; and Welch, A. D. Biochemical and pharmacological studies with 1-β-D-arabinofuranosylcytosine in man. *Biochem. Pharmacol.,* **1966,** *15,* 1417–1428.

Crowther, D.; Bateman, C. J.; Vartan, C. P.; Whitehouse, J. M.; Malpas, J. S.; Hamilton-Fairley, G.; and Scott, R. B. Combination chemotherapy using L-asparaginase, daunorubicin, and cytosine arabinoside in adults with acute myelogenous leukemia. *Br. Med. J.,* **1970,** *4,* 513–517.

Crutchler, W. A., and Moschella, S. L. Double-blind controlled crossover high-dose study of azaribine in psoriasis. *Br. J. Dermatol.,* **1975,** *92,* 199–205.

Danenberg, P. V. Thymidylate synthetase—a target enzyme in cancer chemotherapy. *Biochim. Biophys. Acta,* **1977,** *473,* 73–92.

DeConti, R. C., and Calabresi, P. Treatment of polycythemia vera with azauridine and azaribine. *Ann. Intern. Med.,* **1970,** *73,* 575–579.

DeFronzo, R. A.; Braine, H.; and Colvin, O. M. Water intoxication in man after cyclophosphamide therapy. Time course and relation to drug activation. *Ann. Intern. Med.,* **1973,** *78,* 861–869.

Demis, D. J.; Brown, C. S.; and Crosby, W. H. Thioguanine in the treatment of certain autoimmune, immunologic and related diseases. *Am. J. Med.,* **1964,** *37,* 195–205.

Dentino, M.; Luft, F. C.; Yum, M. N.; Williams, S. D.; and Einhorn, L. H. Long term effect of cis-diamminedichloride platinum (CDDP) on renal function and structure in man. *Cancer,* **1978,** *4,* 1274–1281.

Djerassi, I.; Rominger, C. J.; Kim, J. S.; Turchi, J.; Suvansri, U.; and Hughes, D. Phase I study of high doses of methotrexate, with citrovorum factor in patients with lung cancer. *Cancer,* **1972,** *30,* 22–30.

Doolittle, C. H.; McDonald, C. J.; and Calabresi, P. Pharmacological studies of neurotoxicity in patients with psoriasis treated with azaribine, utilizing high-pressure liquid chromatography. *J. Lab. Clin. Med.,* **1977,** *90,* 773–785.

Durant, J. R.; Norgard, M. J.; Murad, T. M.; Bartolucci, A. A.; and Langford, K. H. Pulmonary toxicity associated with bischloroethylnitrosourea (BCNU). *Ann. Intern. Med.,* **1979,** *90,* 191–194.

Einhorn, L. H., and Donahue, J. Cis-diamminedichloroplatinum, vinblastine, and bleomycin: combination chemotherapy in disseminated testicular cancer. *Ann. Intern. Med.,* **1977,** *87,* 293–298.

Einhorn, L. H., and Williams, S. D. The role of cis-platinum in solid tumor therapy. *N. Engl. J. Med.,* **1979,** *300,* 289–291.

Elias, E. G., and Evans, J. T. Mithramycin in the treatment of Paget's disease of bone. *J. Bone Joint Surg. [Am.],* **1972,** *54-A,* 1730–1736.

Ellison, R. R.; Hoogstraten, B.; Holland, J. F.; Levy, R. N.; Lee, S. L.; Silver, R. T.; ten Pas, A.; Blom, J.; Jacquillat, C.; and Haurani, F. Intermittent therapy with 6-mercaptopurine (NSC-755) and methotrexate (NSC-740) given intravenously to adults with acute leukemia. *Cancer Chemother. Rep.,* **1972,** *56,* 535–542.

Esterhay, R. J., Jr.; Aisner, J.; Levi, J. A.; and Wiernik, P. H. High-dose 6-mercaptopurine in advanced refractory cancer. *Cancer Treat. Rep.,* **1978,** *62,* 1229–1231.

Evans, J. S.; Musser, E. A.; Mengel, G. D.; Forsblad, K. R.;

and Hunter, J. H. Antitumor activity of 1-β-D-arabinofuranosylcytosine hydrochloride. *Proc. Soc. Exp. Biol. Med.,* **1961,** *106,* 350–353.

Farber, S. Chemotherapy in the treatment of leukemia and Wilms' tumor. *J.A.M.A.,* **1966,** *198,* 826–836.

Farber, S.; Diamond, L. K.; Mercer, R. D.; Sylvester, R. F.; and Wolff, V. A. Temporary remissions in acute leukemia in children produced by folic antagonist 4-amethopteroylglutamic acid (aminopterin). *N. Engl. J. Med.,* **1948,** *238,* 787–793.

Fauci, A. S.; Katz, P.; Haynes, B. F.; and Wolff, S. M. Cyclophosphamide therapy of severe systemic necrotizing vasculitis. *N. Engl. J. Med.,* **1979,** *301,* 235–238.

Fisher, B., and others. L-Phenylalanine mustard (L-PAM) in the management of primary breast cancer. *Cancer,* **1977,** *39,* 2883–2903.

Frei, E., III, and others. The effectiveness of combinations of anti-leukemic agents in inducing and maintaining remission in children with acute leukemia. *Blood,* **1965,** *26,* 642–656.

Gershwin, M. E.; Goetzl, E. J.; and Steinberg, A. D. Cyclophosphamide: use in practice. *Ann. Intern. Med.,* **1974,** *80,* 531–540.

Giblett, E. R.; Ammann, A. J.; Sandman, R.; Wara, D. W.; and Diamond, L. K. Nucleoside phosphorylase deficiency in a child with severely defective T-cell immunity and normal B-cell immunity. *Lancet,* **1975,** *1,* 1010–1013.

Giblett, E. R.; Anderson, J. E.; Cohen, F.; Pollara, B.; and Meuwissen, H. J. Adenosine-deaminase deficiency in two patients with severely impaired cellular immunity. *Lancet,* **1972,** *2,* 1067–1069.

Gilman, A. The initial clinical trial of nitrogen mustard. *Am. J. Surg.,* **1963,** *105,* 574–578.

Goldenberg, I. S. Testosterone propionate therapy in breast cancer. *J.A.M.A.,* **1964,** *188,* 1069–1072.

Goldin, A. Studies with high-dose methotrexate—historical background. *Cancer Treat. Rep.,* **1978,** *62,* 307–312.

Goodman, L. S.; Wintrobe, M. M.; Dameshek, W.; Goodman, M. J.; Gilman, A.; and McLennan, M. Nitrogen mustard therapy: use of methylbis (β-chlorethyl) amino hydrochloride for Hodgkin's disease, lymphosarcoma, leukemia and certain allied and miscellaneous disorders. *J.A.M.A.,* **1946,** *132,* 126–132.

Gottlieb, J. A., and Hill, C. S., Jr. Treatment of thyroid cancer with adriamycin: experience with 30 patients. *N. Engl. J. Med.,* **1974,** *290,* 193–197.

Gottlieb, J. A., and others. Role of DTIC (NSC-45388) in the chemotherapy of sarcomas. *Cancer Treat. Rep.,* **1976,** *60,* 199–203.

Griswold, D. E.; Heppner, G. H.; and Calabresi, P. Selective suppression of humoral and cellular immunity with cytosine arabinoside. *Cancer Res.,* **1972,** *32,* 298–301.

———. Stimulation of hemolysin plaque-forming cells by idoxuridine. *Ibid.,* **1975,** *35,* 88–92.

Heal, J. M.; Fox, P. A.; and Schein, P. S. Effect of carbamoylation on the repair of nitrosourea-induced DNA alkylation damage in L1210 cells. *Cancer Res.,* **1979,** *39,* 82–89.

Heppner, G. H., and Calabresi, P. Suppression by cytosine arabinoside of serum-blocking factors of cell-mediated immunity to syngeneic transplants of mouse mammary tumors. *J. Natl. Cancer Inst.,* **1972,** *48,* 1161–1167.

———. Selective suppression of humoral immunity by antineoplastic drugs. *Annu. Rev. Pharmacol.,* **1976,** *16,* 367–379.

Herbst, W. P. Effects of estradiol dipropionate and diethyl stilbestrol on malignant prostatic tissue. *Trans. Am. Assoc. Genitourin. Surg.,* **1941,** *34,* 195–202.

Herrmann, C. (ed.). Third conference on antiviral substances. *Ann. N.Y. Acad. Sci.,* **1977,** *284,* 1–197.

Hertig, A. T., and Sommers, S. C. Genesis of endometrial carcinoma. I. A study of prior biopsies. *Cancer,* **1949,** *2,* 946–956.

Hertz, R. Folic acid antagonists: effects on the cell and the patient. Clinical staff conference at N.I.H. *Ann. Intern. Med.,* **1963,** *59,* 931–956.

Hertz, R.; Ross, G. T.; and Lipsett, M. B. Primary chemotherapy of nonmetastatic trophoblastic disease in women. *Am. J. Obstet. Gynecol.,* **1963,** *86,* 808–814.

Higby, D. J.; Wallace, H. J., Jr.; Albert, D.; and Holland, J. F. Diamminodichloroplatinum in the chemotherapy of testicular tumors. *J. Urol.,* **1974,** *112,* 100–104.

Hill, D. L.; Laster, W. R.; and Struck, R. F. Enzymatic metabolism of cyclophosphamide and nicotine and production of a toxic cyclophosphamide metabolite. *Cancer Res.,* **1972a,** *32,* 658–665.

Hill, G. H.; Sedransk, N.; Rochlin, D.; Bisel, H.; Andrews, N. C.; Fletcher, W.; Schroeder, J. M.; and Wilson, W. L. Mithramycin (NSC 24559) therapy of testicular tumors. *Cancer,* **1972b,** *30,* 900–908.

Hill, J. M.; Loeh, E.; MacLellan, A.; Hill, N. O.; Khan, A.; and King, J. J. Clinical studies of platinum coordination compounds in the treatment of various malignant diseases. *Cancer Chemother. Rep.,* **1975,** *59,* 647–659.

Ho, D. H. W. Potential advances in the clinical use of arabinosylcytosine. *Cancer Treat. Rep.,* **1977,** *61,* 717–722.

Ho, D. H. W., and Frei, E., III. Clinical pharmacology of the l-β-D-arabinofuranosyl cytosine. *Clin. Pharmacol. Ther.,* **1971,** *12,* 944–954.

Hogan, T. F.; Citrin, D. L.; Johnson, B. M.; Nakamura, S.; Davis, T. E.; and Borden, E. C. *o,p'*-DDD (mitotane) therapy of adrenal cortical carcinoma. *Cancer,* **1978,** *42,* 2177–2181.

Holland, J. F., and Glidewell, O. Chemotherapy of acute lymphocytic leukemia of childhood. *Cancer,* **1972,** *30,* 1480–1487.

Holland, J. F., and others. Vincristine treatment of advanced cancer: a cooperative study of 392 cases. *Cancer Res.,* **1973,** *33,* 1258–1264.

Huffman, D. H.; Wan, S. H.; Azarnoff, D. L.; and Hoogotraten, B. Pharmacokinetics of methotrexate. *Clin. Pharmacol. Ther.,* **1973,** *14,* 572–579.

Huggins, C.; Stevens, R. E., Jr.; and Hodges, C. V. Studies on prostatic cancer: effects of castration on advanced carcinoma of prostate gland. *Arch. Surg.,* **1941,** *43,* 209–223.

Jacobson, L. O.; Spurr, C. L.; Barron, E. S. G.; Smith, T. R.; Lushbaugh, C.; and Dick, G. F. Nitrogen mustard therapy: studies on the effect of methyl-*bis*(beta-chloroethyl) amine hydrochloride on neoplastic diseases and allied disorders of the hemopoietic system. *J.A.M.A.,* **1946,** *132,* 263–271.

Jaffe, N. Recent advances in the chemotherapy of metastatic osteogenic sarcoma. *Cancer,* **1972,** *30,* 1627–1631.

Johnston, T. P.; McCaleb, G. S.; and Montgomery, J. A. The synthesis of antineoplastic agents. XXXII. N-Nitrosoureas. *J. Med. Chem.,* **1963,** *6,* 669–681.

Jones, B., and others. Daunorubicin (NSC-83142) vs. daunorubicin plus prednisone (NSC-10023) vs. daunorubicin plus vincristine (NSC-67574) plus prednisone in advanced childhood acute lymphocytic leukemia. *Cancer Chemother. Rep.,* **1972,** *56,* 729–737.

Kaplan, S. R., and Calabresi, P. Drug therapy: immunosuppressive agents. Pt. I. *N. Engl. J. Med.,* **1973,** *289,* 952–954.

Kelley, R. M., and Baker, W. H. Progestational agents in the treatment of carcinoma of the endometrium. *N. Engl. J. Med.,* **1961,** *264,* 216–222.

Kennedy, B. J. Hormone therapy for advanced breast cancer. *Cancer,* **1965,** *18,* 1151–1157.

———. Mithramycin therapy in advanced testicular neoplasms. *Ibid.,* **1970,** *26,* 755–766.

Kennedy, B. J., and Yarbro, J. W. Metabolic and therapeutic effects of hydroxyurea in chronic myeloid leukemia. *J.A.M.A.,* **1966,** *195,* 1038–1043.

Kiang, D. T.; Frenning, D. H.; Goldman, A. I.; Ascensao, V. F.; and Kennedy, B. J. Estrogen receptors and re-

sponses to chemotherapy and hormonal therapy in advanced breast cancer. *N. Engl. J. Med.,* **1978,** *299,* 1330–1334.

Kiang, D. T., and Kennedy, B. J. Tamoxifen (antiestrogen) therapy in advanced breast cancer. *Ann. Intern. Med.,* **1977,** *87,* 687–690.

Klein, E.; Milgrom, H.; Stoll, H. L.; Helm, F.; Walker, H. J.; and Holtermann, O. A. Topical 5-fluorouracil chemotherapy for premalignant and malignant epidermal neoplasms. In, *Cancer Chemotherapy II.* (Brodsky, I., and Kahn, S. B., eds.) Grune & Stratton, Inc., New York, **1972,** pp. 147–166.

Knight, W. A.; Livingston, R. B.; and Gregory, E. J. Estrogen receptor as an independent prognostic factor for early recurrence in breast cancer. *Cancer Res.,* **1977,** *31,* 4669–4671.

Knospe, W. H.; Loeb, V.; and Huguley, C. M. Bi-weekly chlorambucil treatment of chronic lymphocytic leukemia. *Cancer,* **1974,** *33,* 555–562.

Krakoff, I. H. Chemotherapy and hormonal therapy of carcinoma of the breast. In, *Cancer Chemotherapy.* (Brodsky, I.; Kahn, S. B.; and Moyer, J. H.; eds.) Grune & Stratton, Inc., New York, **1967,** pp. 77–83.

Kremer, W. B. Cytarabine. *Ann. Intern. Med.,* **1975,** *82,* 684–688.

Krishan, A.; Israel, M.; Modest, E. J.; and Frei, E., III. Difference in cellular uptake and cytofluorescence of adriamycin and N-trifluoroacetyladriamycin-14-valerate. *Cancer Res.,* **1976,** *36,* 2108–2109.

Lacassagne, A. Hormonal pathogenesis of adenocarcinoma of the breast. *Am. J. Cancer,* **1936,** *27,* 217–228.

Larrson, L. G., and Sundbom, C. M. Roentgen irradiation of the male breast. *Acta Radiol. [Diagn.] (Stockh.),* **1962,** *58,* 253–256.

LeFrak, E. A.; Pitha, J.; Rosenheim, S.; and Gottlieb, J. A. A clinicopathologic analysis of adriamycin cardiotoxicity. *Cancer,* **1973,** *32,* 302–314.

Legha, S. S.; Slavik, M.; and Carter, S. K. Hexamethylmelamine. *Cancer,* **1976,** *38,* 27–35.

Lerner, H. J. Acute myelogenous leukemia in patients receiving chlorambucil as long-term adjuvant chemotherapy for stage II breast cancer. *Cancer Treat. Rep.,* **1978,** *62,* 1135–1143.

Lerner, H. J.; Band, P. R.; Israel, L.; and Leung, B. S. Phase II study of tamoxifen: report of 74 patients with stage IV breast cancer. *Cancer Treat. Rep.,* **1976,** *60,* 1431–1435.

Levin, V. A.; Hoffman, W.; and Weinkam, R. J. Pharmacokinetics of BCNU in man: a preliminary study of 20 patients. *Cancer Treat. Rep.,* **1978,** *62,* 1305–1312.

Levine, S., and Paulus, H. E. Treatment of psoriatic arthritis with azarhibine. *Arthritis Rheum.,* **1976,** *19,* 21–28.

Levitt, M.; Mosher, M. B.; DeConti, R. C.; Farber, L. R.; Skeel, R. T.; Marsh, J. C.; Mitchell, M. S.; Papac, R. J.; Thomas, E. D.; and Bertino, J. P. Improved therapeutic index of methotrexate with "leucovorin rescue." *Cancer Res.,* **1973,** *33,* 1729–1734.

Lippman, M. E. (ed.). John F. Fogarty Center Conference on hormones and cancer. *Cancer Res.,* **1978,** *38,* 3981–4376.

Loeb, L. Further investigations on the origin of tumors in mice. VI. Internal secretion as a factor in the origin of tumors. *J. Med. Res.,* **1919,** *40,* 477–496.

Loo, T. L.; Housholder, G. E.; Gerulath, A. H.; Saunders, P. H.; and Farquhar, D. Mechanism of action and pharmacology studies with DTIC (NSC-45388). *Cancer Treat. Rep.,* **1976,** *60,* 149–157.

Lubitz, J. A.; Freeman, L.; and Okun, R. Mitotane use in inoperable adrenal cortical carcinoma. *J.A.M.A.,* **1973,** *223,* 1109–1112.

Luce, J. K.; Gamble, J. F.; Wilson, H. E.; Monto, R. W.; Isaacs, B. L.; Palmer, R. L.; Coltman, C. A., Jr.; Hewlett, J. S.; Gehan, E. A.; and Frei, E., III. Combined cyclophosphamide, vincristine, and prednisone therapy of malignant lymphoma. *Cancer,* **1971,** *28,* 306–317.

McDonald, C. J., and Bertino, J. R. Parenteral methotrexate for psoriasis. *Lancet,* **1968,** *1,* 864.

McDonald, C. J., and Calabresi, P. Azaribine for mycosis fungoides. *Arch. Dermatol.,* **1971,** *103,* 158–167.

———. Psoriasis and occlusive vascular disease. *Br. J. Dermatol.,* **1978,** *99,* 469–475.

Manni, A.; Trujillo, J.; Marshall, J. S.; and Pearson, O. H. Antiestrogen-induced remissions in stage IV breast cancer. *Cancer Treat. Rep.,* **1976,** *60,* 1445–1450.

Mansy, S.; Rosenberg, B.; and Thompson, A. J. Binding of *cis-* and *trans-*dichlorodiammineplatinum (II) (NSC-119875) on DNA. *Cancer Chemother. Rep.,* **1975,** *59,* 643–646.

Mashburn, L. T., and Wriston, J. C. Tumor inhibitory effect of L-asparaginase from *Escherichia coli. Arch. Biochem. Biophys.,* **1964,** *105,* 450–452.

Matthews, D. A., and others. Dihydrofolate reductase from *Lactobacillus casei;* x-ray structure of the enzyme-methotrexate-NADPH complex. *J. Biol. Chem.,* **1978,** *253,* 6946–6954.

Merrin, C.; Beckley, S.; and Takita, H. Multimodal treatment of advanced testicular tumor with radical reductive surgery and multisequential chemotherapy with *cis* platinum, bleomycin, vinblastine, vincristine and actinomycin D. *J. Urol.,* **1978,** *120,* 73–76.

Minow, R. A.; Benjamin, R. S.; Lee, E. T.; and Gottlieb, J. A. Adriamycin cardiomyopathy-risk factors. *Cancer,* **1977,** *39,* 1397–1402.

Mitchell, M. S.; Kaplan, S. R.; and Calabresi, P. Alteration of antibody synthesis in the rat by cytosine arabinoside. *Cancer Res.,* **1969a,** *29,* 896–904.

Mitchell, M. S.; Wade, M. E.; DeConti, R. C.; Bertino, J. R.; and Calabresi, P. Immunosuppressive effects of cytosine arabinoside and methotrexate in man. *Ann. Intern. Med.,* **1969b,** *70,* 535–547.

Moertel, C. G. Therapy of advanced gastrointestinal cancer with the nitrosoureas. *Cancer Chemother. Rep.,* **1973,** *4,* 27–34.

Moore, E. C., and Cohen, S. S. Effects of arabinonucleotides on ribonucleotide reduction by an enzyme system from rat tumor. *J. Biol. Chem.,* **1967,** *242,* 2116–2118.

Moore, G. E.; Bross, I. D. J.; Ausman, R.; Nadler, S.; Jones, R., Jr.; Slack, N.; and Rimm, A. A. Effects of mitomycin C (NSC-26980) in 346 patients with advanced cancer. *Cancer Chemother. Rep.,* **1968,** *52,* 675–684.

Moseson, D. L.; Sasaki, G. H.; Kraybill, W. G.; Leung, B. S.; Davenport, C. E.; and Fletcher, W. S. The use of antiestrogens tamoxifen and nafoxidine in the treatment of human breast cancer in correlation with estrogen receptor values. *Cancer,* **1978,** *41,* 797–800.

Mukherjee, K. L.; Curreri, A. R.; Javid, M.; and Heidelberger, C. Studies on fluorinated pyrimidines. XVII. Tissue distribution of 5-fluorouracil-2-C14 and 5-fluoro-2'-deoxyuridine in cancer patients. *Cancer Res.,* **1963,** *23,* 67–77.

Munchausen, L. L., and Rahn, R. O. Biologic and chemical effects of *cis-*dichlorodiammineplatinum (II) (NSC-119875) on DNA. *Cancer Chemother. Rep.,* **1975,** *59,* 643–646.

Myers, C. E.; McGuire, W. P.; Liss, R. H.; Ifrim, E.; Grotzinger, K.; and Young, R. C. Adriamycin: the role of lipid peroxidation in cardiac toxicity and tumor response. *Science,* **1977,** *197,* 165–167.

Nesbit, R. M., and Baum, W. C. Endocrine control of prostatic carcinoma. *J.A.M.A.,* **1950,** *143,* 1317–1320.

Noble, R. L.; Beer, C. T.; and Cutts, J. H. Further biological activities of vincaleukoblastine—an alkaloid isolated from *Vinca rosea* (L.). *Biochem. Pharmacol.,* **1958,** *1,* 347–348.

Oettgen, H. F., and others. The toxicity of E. coli L-asparaginase in man. *Cancer,* **1970,** *25,* 253–278.

Oppenheimer, N. J.; Rodrigues, L. O.; and Hecht, S. M. Proton nuclear magnetic resonance study of the structure of bleomycin and the zinc bleomycin complex. *Biochemistry,* **1979,** *18,* 3439–3445.

Orwoll, E. S.; Kiessling, P. J.; and Patterson, J. R. Interstitial pneumonia from mitomycin. *Ann. Intern. Med.,* **1978,** *89,* 352–355.

Ostumi, J. A., and Roginsky, M. S. Metastatic adrenal cortical carcinoma. *Arch. Intern. Med.,* **1975,** *139,* 1257–1258.

Perlia, C. P.; Gubisch, N. J.; Wolter, J.; Edelberg, D.; Dederick, M. M.; and Taylor, S. G. Mithramycin treatment of hypercalcemia. *Cancer,* **1970,** *25,* 389–394.

Pigram, W. J.; Fuller, W.; and Hamilton, L. D. Stereochemistry of intercalation: interaction of daunomycin with DNA. *Nature [New Biol.],* **1972,** *235,* 17–19.

Povirk, L. F. Catalytic release of deoxyribonucleic bases by oxidation and reduction of an iron bleomycin complex. *Biochemistry,* **1979,** *18,* 3989–3995.

Primack, A. Amelioration of cyclophosphamide-induced cystitis. *J. Natl. Cancer Inst.,* **1971,** *47,* 223–227.

Randolph, V. L.; Vallejo, A.; Spiro, R. H.; Shah, J.; Strong, E. W.; Huvos, A. G.; and Wittes, R. E. Combination therapy of advanced head and neck cancer. *Cancer,* **1978,** *41,* 460–467.

Ream, N. W.; Perlia, C. P.; Wolter, J.; and Taylor, S. Mithramycin therapy in disseminated germinal testicular cancer. *J.A.M.A.,* **1968,** *204,* 96–102.

Reza, M. J.; Dornfeld, L.; Goldberg, L. S.; Bluestone, R.; and Pearson, C. M. Wegener's granulomatosis. Long-term follow-up of patients treated with cyclophosphamide. *Arthritis Rheum.,* **1975,** *18,* 501–506.

Rhoads, C. P. Nitrogen mustards in treatment of neoplastic disease: official statement. *J.A.M.A.,* **1946,** *131,* 656–658.

Riggs, C. E.; Benjamin, R. S.; Serpick, A. A.; and Bachur, N. R. Biliary disposition of adriamycin. *Clin. Pharmacol. Ther.,* **1977,** *22,* 234–241.

Roberts, J. J., and Pascoe, J. M. Cross-linking of complementary strands of DNA in mammalian cells by antitumor platinum compounds. *Nature,* **1972,** *235,* 282–284.

Rogler-Brown, T.; Agarwal, R. P.; and Parks, R. E., Jr. Tight-binding inhibitors. VI. Interactions of deoxycoformycin and adenosine deaminase in intact human erythrocytes and sarcoma 180 cells. *Biochem. Pharmacol.,* **1978,** *27,* 2289–2296.

Rosenberg, B. Platinum coordination complexes in cancer chemotherapy. *Naturwissenschaften,* **1973,** *60,* 399–406.

Rosenberg, B.; VanCamp, L.; Grimley, E. B.; and Thomson, A. J. The inhibition of growth or cell division in *Escherichia coli* by different ionic species of platinum (IV) complexes. *J. Biol. Chem.,* **1967,** *242,* 1347–1352.

Rosenberg, B.; VanCamp, L.; and Krigas, T. Inhibition of cell division in *Escherichia coli* by electrolysis products from a platinum electrode. *Nature,* **1965,** *205,* 698–699.

Rosenberg, B.; VanCamp, L.; Trosko, J. E.; and Mansour, V. H. Platinum compounds: a new class of potent antitumour agents. *Nature,* **1969,** *222,* 385–386.

Rosenthal, F.; Wislicki, L.; and Kollek, L. Über die Beziehungen von schwersten Blutgiften zu Abbauprodukten des Eiweisses. *Klin. Wochenschr.,* **1928,** *7,* 972.

Rosman, M., and Bertino, J. R. Azathioprine. *Ann. Intern. Med.,* **1973,** *79,* 694–700.

Rutty, C. J., and Connors, T. A. *In vitro* studies with hexamethylmelamine. *Biochem. Pharmacol.,* **1977,** *26,* 2385–2391.

Ryan, W. G.; Schwartz, T. B.; and Northrop, G. Experiences in the treatment of Paget's disease of bone with mithramycin. *J.A.M.A.,* **1970,** *213,* 1153–1157.

Salmon, S. E.; Hamburger, A. W.; Soehnlen, B.; Durie, B. G. M.; Alberts, D. S.; and Moon, T. E. Quantitation of differential sensitivity of human tumor cells to anticancer drugs. *N. Engl. J. Med.,* **1978,** *298,* 1321–1327.

Samson, M. K.; Baker, L. H.; Devos, J. M.; Buroker, T. R.; Izbicki, R. M.; and Vaitkevicius, V. K. Phase I clinical trial of combined therapy with vinblastine (NSC-49842), bleomycin (NSC-125066), and cis-dichlorodiammine-platinum (II) (NSC-119875). Cancer Treat. Rep., 1976, 60, 91–97.

Samuels, L. D.; Newton, W. A., Jr.; and Heyn, R. Daunorubicin therapy in advanced neuroblastoma. Cancer, 1971, 27, 831–834.

Santi, D. V., and McHenry, C. S. 5-Fluoro-2'-deoxyuridylate: covalent complex with thymidylate synthetase. Proc. Natl. Acad. Sci. U.S.A., 1972, 69, 1855–1857.

Sausville, E. A.; Peisach, J.; and Horwitz, S. B. Effect of chelating agents and metal ions on the degradation of DNA by bleomycin. Biochemistry, 1978a, 17, 2740–2745.

Sausville, E. A.; Stein, R. W.; Peisach, J.; and Horwitz, S. B. Properties and products of the degradation of DNA by bleomycin and iron (II). Biochemistry, 1978b, 17, 2746–2754.

Scannell, J. P., and Hitchings, G. H. Thioguanine in deoxyribonucleic acid from tumors of 6-mercaptopurine-treated mice. Proc. Soc. Exp. Biol. Med., 1966, 122, 627–629.

Schaeffer, H. J.; Beauchamp, L.; deMiranda, P.; Elion, G. N.; Bauer, D. J.; and Collins, P. 9-(2-Hydroxyethoxymethyl) guanine activity against viruses of the herpes group. Nature, 1978, 272, 583–585.

Schein, P.; Kahn, R.; Gorden, P.; Wells, S.; and DeVita, V. T. Streptozotocin for malignant insulinomas and carcinoid tumor. Arch. Intern. Med., 1973, 132, 555–561.

Schein, P. S.; O'Connell, M. J.; Blom, J.; Hubbard, S.; Magrath, I. T.; Bergevin, P.; Wiernick, P. H.; Ziegler, J. L.; and DeVita, V. T. Clinical antitumor activity and toxicity of streptozotocin (NCS-86998). Cancer, 1974, 34, 993–1000.

Schein, P. S., and Winokur, S. H. Immunosuppressive and cytotoxic chemotherapy: long-term complications. Ann. Intern. Med., 1975, 82, 84–95.

Schwartz, R. S. Immunosuppressive drugs. Prog. Allergy, 1965, 9, 246–303.

Shubin, S. TRIAZURE and public drug policies. Perspect. Biol. Med., 1979, 22, 185–204.

Sladek, N. E. Therapeutic efficacy of cyclophosphamide as a function of its metabolism. Cancer Res., 1972, 32, 535–542.

———. Evidence for an aldehyde possessing alkylating activity as the primary metabolite of cyclophosphamide. Ibid., 1973, 33, 651–658.

Sommer, H., and Santi, D. V. Purification and amino acid analysis of an active site peptide from thymidylate synthetase containing covalently bound 5-fluoro-2'-deoxyuridylate and methylenetetrahydrofolate. Biochem. Biophys. Res. Commun., 1974, 57, 689–695.

Speer, R. J.; Ridgway, H.; Hall, L. M.; Stewart, D. P.; Howe, K. E.; Lieberman, D. Z.; Newman, A. D.; and Hill, J. M. Coordination complexes of platinum as antitumor agents. Cancer Chemother. Rep., 1975, 59, 629–641.

Sternberg, J. J.; Bracken, B.; Handel, P. B.; and Johnson, D. E. Combination chemotherapy (CISCA) for advanced urinary tract carcinoma. J.A.M.A., 1977, 238, 2282–2287.

Stevens, D. A.; Jordan, G. W.; Waddell, T. F.; and Merigan, T. C. Adverse effect of cytosine arabinoside on disseminated zoster in a controlled trial. N. Engl. J. Med., 1973, 289, 873–878.

Sutow, W. W.; Garcia, F.; Starling, K. A.; Williams, T. E.; Lane, D. M.; and Gehan, E. A. L-Asparaginase therapy in children with advanced leukemia. Cancer, 1971, 28, 819–824.

Sutow, W. W.; Vietti, T. J.; Lonsdale, D.; and Talley, R. W. Daunomycin in the treatment of metastatic soft tissue sarcoma in children. Cancer, 1972, 29, 1293–1297.

Takanashi, S., and Bachur, N. R. Adriamycin metabolism in man. Evidence from urinary metabolites. Drug Metab. Dispos., 1975a, 4, 79–87.

———. Daunorubicin metabolites in human urine. J. Pharmacol. Exp. Ther., 1975b, 195, 41–49.

Tallal, L.; Tan, C.; Oettgen, H.; Wollner, N.; McCarthy, M.; Helson, L.; Burchenal, J.; Karnofsky, D.; and Murphy, M. L. E. coli L-asparaginase in the treatment of leukemia and solid tumors in 131 children. Cancer, 1970, 25, 306–320.

Tandon, R. N.; Bunnell, I. L.; and Cooper, R. G. The treatment of metastatic carcinoma of the liver by the percutaneous selective hepatic artery infusion of 5-fluorouracil. Surgery, 1973, 73, 118–121.

Tilney, N. L.; Strom, T. B.; Vineyard, G. C.; and Merrill, J. P. The declining mortality rate of renal transplantation. N. Engl. J. Med., 1978, 299, 1321–1324.

Tormey, D. C.; Simon, R. M.; Lippman, M. E.; Bull, J. M.; and Myers, C. E. Evaluation of tamoxifen dose in advanced breast cancer: a progress report. Cancer Treat. Rep., 1976, 60, 1451–1459.

Treves, N. The treatment of cancer of the male breast, especially inoperable by ablative surgery (orchiectomy, adrenalectomy, hypophysectomy) and the hormone therapy with estrogens and corticosteroids: an analysis of 42 patients. Acta Un. Int. Cancer, 1959, 15, 1169–1178.

Tritton, T. R.; Murphee, S. A.; and Sartorelli, A. C. Adriamycin: a proposal on the specificity of drug action. Biochem. Biophys. Res. Commun., 1978, 84, 802–808.

Van Scott, E. J.; Auerbach, R.; and Weinstein, G. D. Parenteral methotrexate in psoriasis. Arch. Dermatol., 1964, 89, 550–556.

Veterans Administration Co-Operative Urological Research Group. Treatment and survival of patients with cancer of the prostate. Surgery Gynecol. Obstet., 1967, 124, 1011–1017.

Vogler, W. R., and Olansky, A. A double-blind study of azaribine in the treatment of psoriasis. Ann. Intern. Med., 1970, 73, 951–956.

Von Hoff, D. D.; Slavik, M.; and Muggia, F. M. Allergic reactions to cis-platinum. Lancet, 1976, 1, 90.

Waksman, S. A., and Woodruff, H. B. Bacteriostatic and bactericidal substances produced by a soil actinomyces. Proc. Soc. Exp. Biol. Med., 1940, 45, 609–614.

Wasserman, T. H. The nitrosoureas: an outline of clinical schedules and toxic effects. Cancer Treat. Rep., 1976, 60, 709–711.

Wasserman, T. H.; Slavik, M.; and Carter, S. H. Clinical comparison of the nitrosoureas. Cancer, 1975, 36, 1258–1268.

Weil, M., and others. Daunorubicin in the therapy of acute granulocytic leukemia. Cancer Res., 1973, 33, 921–928.

Weinstein, G. D. Methotrexate. Ann. Intern. Med., 1977, 86, 199–204.

Williams, J. M., and Popovich, N. G. Application of cis-diamminedichloroplatinum in combination antineoplastic therapy of testicular cancer. Drug Intell. Clin. Pharm., 1978, 12, 226–229.

Wilson, C. B.; Boldrey, E. B.; and Enot, K. J. 1,3-bis(2-chloroethyl)-1-nitrosourea (NSC-409962) in the treatment of brain tumors. Cancer Chemother. Rep., 1970, 54, 273–281.

Wilson, C. B.; Gutin, P.; Boldrey, E. B.; Crafts, D.; Levin, V. A.; and Enot, K. J. Single-agent chemotherapy of brain tumors. Arch. Neurol., 1976, 33, 739–744.

Witshaw, E., and Kroner, T. Phase II study of cis-dichlorodiammine-platinum (II) (NSC-119875) in advanced adenocarcinoma of the ovary. Cancer Treat. Rep., 1976, 60, 55–60.

Wolff, S. M., and Goodman, H. C. Hypogammaglobulinemia produced by administration of 6-thioguanine to patients with nephrosis. J. Clin. Invest., 1962, 41, 1413–1420.

Yagoda, A.; Watson, R. C.; Kemeny, N.; Barzell, W. E.; Grabstald, H.; and Whitmore, W. F., Jr. Diamminedichloride platinum II and cyclophosphamide in the treatment of advanced urothelial cancer. *Cancer,* **1978,** *41,* 2121–2130.

Yarbro, J. W.; Kennedy, B. J.; and Barnum, C. P. Mithramycin inhibition of ribonucleic acid synthesis. *Cancer Res.,* **1966,** *26,* 36–39.

Young, R. C.; Chabner, B. A.; Hubbard, S. P.; Fisher, R. I.; Bender, R. A.; Anderson, T.; Simon, R. M.; Canellos, G. P.; and DeVita, V. T., Jr. Advanced ovarian adenocarcinoma. *N. Engl. J. Med.,* **1978,** *299,* 1261–1266.

Young, R. C.; DeVita, V. T., Jr.; Serpick, A. A.; and Canellos, G. P. Treatment of advanced Hodgkin's disease with [1,3 *bis*(2-chloroethyl)-1-nitrosourea] BCNU. *N. Engl. J. Med.,* **1971,** *285,* 475–479.

Monographs and Reviews

Agarwal, K. C., and Sartorelli, A. C. α-(N)-heterocyclic carboxaldehyde thiosemicarbazones. In, *Antineoplastic and Immunosuppressive Agents,* Pt. II. (Sartorelli, A. C., and Johns, D. G., eds.) *Handbuch der Experimentellen Pharmakologie,* Vol. 38. Springer-Verlag, Berlin, **1975,** pp. 793–807.

Agarwal, R. P.; Cha, S.; Crabtree, G. W.; and Parks, R. E., Jr. Coformycin and deoxycoformycin: tight-binding inhibitors of adenosine deaminase. In, *Symposium on Chemistry and Biology of Nucleosides and Nucleotides. American Chemical Society Advances in Chemistry.* (Robins, R. K.; Townsend, L. B.; and Harman, R. E.; eds.) Academic Press, Inc., New York, **1978,** pp. 159–197.

Bennett, L. L. Glutamine antagonists. In, *Antineoplastic and Immunosuppressive Agents,* Pt. II. (Sartorelli, A. C., and Johns, D. G., eds.) *Handbuch der Experimentellen Pharmakologie,* Vol. 38. Springer-Verlag, Berlin, **1975,** pp. 484–511.

Bergsagel, D. E. Plasma cell myeloma. An interpretive review. *Cancer,* **1972,** *30,* 1588–1594.

Bertino, J. R. Folate antagonists. In, *Antineoplastic and Immunosuppressive Agents,* Pt. II. (Sartorelli, A. C., and Johns, D. G., eds.) *Handbuch der Experimentellen Pharmakologie,* Vol. 38. Springer-Verlag, Berlin, **1975,** pp. 468–483.

———. Toward improved selectivity in cancer chemotherapy: The Richard and Hinda Rosenthal Foundation Lecture Award. *Cancer Res.,* **1979,** *39,* 293–340.

Bloom, H. J. G. Renal cancer. In, *Endocrine Therapy in Malignant Disease.* (Stoll, A. A., ed.) W. B. Saunders Co., Philadelphia, **1972,** pp. 339–367.

Blum, R. H., and Carter, S. K. Adriamycin. A new anticancer drug with significant clinical activity. *Ann. Intern. Med.,* **1974,** *80,* 249–259.

Bolt, H. M. Metabolism of estrogens—natural and synthetic. *Pharmacol. Ther.,* **1979,** *4,* 155–181.

Brockman, R. W. Resistance to purine analogs. Clinical Pharmacology Symposium. *Biochem. Pharmacol.,* **1974,** *23,* Suppl. 2, pp. 107–117.

Burchenal, J. H. The treatment of leukemias. *Bull. N.Y. Acad. Med.,* **1954,** *30,* 429–447.

Calabresi, P., and Welch, A. D. Chemotherapy of neoplastic diseases. *Annu. Rev. Med.,* **1962,** *13,* 147–202.

Carter, S. K. An overview of the status of the nitrosoureas in other tumors. *Cancer Chemother. Rep.,* **1973,** *4,* 35–45.

Carter, S. K.; Ichikawa, T.; Mathe, G.; and Umezawa, H. (eds.). *Gann Monograph in Cancer Research.* No. 19, *Fundamental and Clinical Studies of Bleomycin.* University Park Press, Baltimore, **1976.**

Carter, S. K., and Slavik, M. Chemotherapy of cancer. *Annu. Rev. Pharmacol.,* **1974,** *14,* 157–179.

Chabner, B. A., and Johns, D. G. Folate antagonists. In, *Cancer 5: A Comprehensive Treatise.* (Becker, F. F., ed.) Plenum Press, New York, **1977,** pp. 363–377.

Chabner, B. A.; Myers, C. E.; Coleman, C. N.; and Johns, D. G. The clinical pharmacology of antineoplastic agents. *N. Engl. J. Med.,* **1975,** *292,* 1107–1113, 1159–1168.

Connors, T. A. Mechanisms of clinical drug resistance.

Clinical Pharmacology Symposium. *Biochem. Pharmacol.,* **1974,** *23,* Suppl. 2, 89–100.

———. Mechanism of action of 2-chloroethylamine derivatives, sulfur mustards, epoxides, and aziridines. In, *Antineoplastic and Immunosuppressive Agents,* Pt. II. (Sartorelli, A. C., and Johns, D. G., eds.) *Handbuch der Experimentellen Pharmakologie,* Vol. 38. Springer-Verlag, Berlin, **1975,** pp. 18–34.

Crabtree, G. W. Mechanisms of action of pyrimidine and purine analogues. In, *Cancer Chemotherapy III.* (Brodsky, I.; Kahn, S. B.; and Conroy, J. F.; eds.) Grune & Stratton, Inc., New York, **1978,** pp. 35–47.

Creasey, W. A. Arabinosylcytosine. In, *Antineoplastic and Immunosuppressive Agents,* Pt. II. (Sartorelli, A. C., and Johns, D. G., eds.) *Handbuch der Experimentellen Pharmakologie,* Vol. 38. Springer-Verlag, Berlin, **1975a,** pp. 232–256.

———. Vinca alkaloids and colchicine. *Ibid.,* **1975b,** pp. 670–694.

———. Plant alkaloids. In, *Cancer 5: A Comprehensive Treatise.* (Becker, F. F., ed.) Plenum Press, New York, **1977,** pp. 379–425.

Crooke, S. T., and Bradner, W. T. Mitomycin C: a review. *Cancer Treat. Rev.,* **1976,** *3,* 121–139.

DeVita, V. T., Jr.; Canellos, G. P.; and Moxley, J. H., III. A decade of combination chemotherapy of advanced Hodgkin's disease. *Cancer,* **1972,** *30,* 1495–1504.

DeVita, V. T., Jr.; Serpick, A. A.; and Carbone, P. P. Combination chemotherapy in the treatment of advanced Hodgkin's disease. *Ann. Intern. Med.,* **1970,** *73,* 881–895.

DiMarco, A. Daunomycin and adriamycin. In, *Antineoplastic and Immunosuppressive Agents,* Pt. II. (Sartorelli, A. C., and Johns, D. G., eds.) *Handbuch der Experimentellen Pharmakologie,* Vol. 38. Springer-Verlag, Berlin, **1975,** pp. 593–614.

Elion, G. B. Biochemistry and pharmacology of purine analogs. *Fed. Proc.,* **1967,** *26,* 898–904.

Elion, G. B., and Hitchings, G. H. Metabolic basis for the actions of analogs of purines and pyrimidines. *Adv. Chemother.,* **1965,** *2,* 91–177.

———. Azathioprene. In, *Antineoplastic and Immunosuppressive Agents,* Pt. II. (Sartorelli, A. C., and Johns, D. G., eds.) *Handbuch der Experimentellen Pharmakologie,* Vol. 38. Springer-Verlag, Berlin, **1975,** pp. 404–425.

Ensminger, W. D.; Grindley, G. B.; and Hoglind, J. A. Antifolate therapy: experimental approaches using rescue, selective host protection, and drug combinations. *Advances in Cancer Chemotherapy,* Vol. 1. (Rosowsky, A., ed.) Marcel Dekker, Inc., New York, **1979,** pp. 61–109.

Fergusson, J. D. Secondary endocrine therapy. In, *Endocrine Therapy in Malignant Disease.* (Stoll, B. A., ed.) W. B. Saunders Co., Philadelphia, **1972,** pp. 263–272.

Fox, B. W. Mechanism of action of methanesulfonates. In, *Antineoplastic and Immunosuppressive Agents,* Pt. II. (Sartorelli, A. C., and Johns, D. G., eds.) *Handbuch der Experimentellen Pharmakologie,* Vol. 38. Springer-Verlag, Berlin, **1975,** pp. 35–46.

Gale, G. R. Platinum compounds. In, *Antineoplastic and Immunosuppressive Agents,* Pt. II. (Sartorelli, A. C., and Johns, D. G., eds.) *Handbuch der Experimentellen Pharmakologie,* Vol. 38. Springer-Verlag, Berlin, **1975,** pp. 829–840.

Galton, D. A. Chemotherapy of chronic myelocytic leukemia. *Semin. Hematol.,* **1969,** *6,* 323–343.

Gardner, F. H. Treatment of lymphoproliferative disease. In, *Cancer Chemotherapy II.* (Brodsky, I., and Kahn, S. B., eds.) Grune & Stratton, Inc., New York, **1972,** pp. 361–373.

Gilman, A., and Philips, F. S. The biological actions and therapeutic applications of the β-chlorethylamines and sulfides. *Science,* **1946,** *103,* 409–415.

Goldberg, I. H.; Beerman, T. A.; and Poon, R. Antibiotics: nucleic acids as targets in chemotherapy. In, *Cancer 5: A*

Comprehensive Treatise. (Becker, F. F., ed.) Plenum Press, New York, **1977**, pp. 427–456.

Greenwald, E. S. *Cancer Chemotherapy.* Medical Examination Publishing Co., Inc., Flushing, N.Y., **1973**.

Hall, E. *Radiobiology for the Radiobiologist,* 2nd ed. Harper & Row, Pub., Hagerstown, Md., **1978**.

Handschumacher, R. E.; Calabresi, P.; Welch, A. D.; Bono, V.; Fallon, H.; and Frei, E., III. Summary of current information on 6-azauridine. *Cancer Chemother. Rep.,* **1962**, No. 21, 1–18.

Haynie, T. P., III; Johns, M. F.; and Glenn, H. J. Principles of nuclear medicine. In, *Cancer Medicine.* (Holland, J. F., and Frei, E., III, eds.) Lea & Febiger, Philadelphia, **1973**, pp. 567–599.

Heidelberger, C. Pyrimidine and pyrimidine nucleosides. In, *Cancer Medicine.* (Holland, J. F., and Frei, E., III, eds.) Lea & Febiger, Philadelphia, **1973**, pp. 768–791.

————. Fluorinated pyrimidines and their nucleosides. In, *Antineoplastic and Immunosuppressive Agents,* Pt. II. (Sartorelli, A. C., and Johns, D. G., eds.) *Handbuch der Experimentellen Pharmakologie,* Vol. 38. Springer-Verlag, Berlin, **1975**, pp. 193–231.

Hilf, R., and Wittliff, J. L. Mechanisms of actions of hormones: estrogens. In, *Antineoplastic and Immunosuppressive Agents,* Pt. II. (Sartorelli, A. C., and Johns, D. G., eds.) *Handbuch der Experimentellen Pharmakologie,* Vol. 38. Springer-Verlag, Berlin, **1975**, pp. 104–138.

Hitchings, G. H., and Burchall, J. J. Inhibition of folate biosynthesis and function as a basis for chemotherapy. *Adv. Enzymol.,* **1965**, *27,* 417–468.

Hitchings, G. H., and Elion, G. B. Chemical suppression of the immune response. *Pharmacol. Rev.,* **1963**, *15,* 365–405.

Ho, D. H. W., and Freireich, E. J. Clinical pharmacology of arabinosylcytosine. In, *Antineoplastic and Immunosuppressive Agents,* Pt. II. (Sartorelli, A. C., and Johns, D. G., eds.) *Handbuch der Experimentellen Pharmakologie,* Vol. 38. Springer-Verlag, Berlin, **1975**, pp. 257–271.

Holland, J. F. *E pluribus unum:* presidential address. *Cancer Res.,* **1971**, *31,* 1319–1329.

Holland, J. F., and Frei, E., III (eds.). *Cancer Medicine.* Lea & Febiger, Philadelphia, **1973**.

Huennekens, F. M. Folate and B_{12} coenzymes. In, *Biological Oxidations.* (Singer, T. P., ed.) John Wiley & Sons, Inc., New York, **1968**, pp. 439–513.

Hutter, A. M., Jr., and Kayhoe, D. E. Adrenal cortical carcinoma: clinical features of 138 patients. *Am. J. Med.,* **1966**, *41,* 572–592.

Jensen, E. V.; Black, G. E.; Smith, S.; Kuper, K.; and DeSombre, E. R. Estrogen receptors and breast cancer response to adrenalectomy. *Natl. Cancer Inst. Monogr.,* **1971**, *34,* 55–79.

Johns, D. G., and Bertino, J. R. Folate antagonists. In, *Cancer Medicine.* (Holland, J. F., and Frei, E., III, eds.) Lea & Febiger, Philadelphia, **1973**, pp. 739–754.

Johnson, I. S. Plant alkaloids. In, *Cancer Medicine.* (Holland, J. F., and Frei, E., III, eds.) Lea & Febiger, Philadelphia, **1973**, pp. 840–850.

Johnson, I. S.; Armstrong, J. G.; Gorman, M.; and Burnett, J. P. The vinca alkaloids: a new class of oncolytic agents. *Cancer Res.,* **1963**, *23,* 1390–1427.

Kersten, H. Mechanisms of action of mitomycins. In, *Antineoplastic and Immunosuppressive Agents,* Pt. II. (Sartorelli, A. C., and Johns, D. G., eds.) *Handbuch der Experimentellen Pharmakologie,* Vol. 38. Springer-Verlag, Berlin, **1975**, pp. 47–64.

Kreis, W. Hydrazines and triazenes. In, *Cancer 5: A Comprehensive Treatise.* (Becker, F. F., ed.) Plenum Press, New York, **1977**, pp. 489–519.

Lane, M. Chemotherapy of cancer. In, *Cancer,* 5th ed. (del Regato, J. A., and Spjut, H. J., eds.) C. V. Mosby Co., St. Louis, **1977**, pp. 105–130.

Legha, S. S.; Davis, H. L.; and Muggia, F. M. Hormonal

therapy of breast cancer: new approaches and concepts. *Ann. Intern. Med.,* **1978**, *88,* 69–77.

Leh, F. K. V., and Wolf, W. Platinum complexes: a new class of antineoplastic agents. *J. Pharm. Sci.,* **1976**, *65,* 315–327.

LePage, G. A. Purine antagonists. In, *Cancer 5: A Comprehensive Treatise.* (Becker, F. F., ed.) Plenum Press, New York, **1977**, pp. 309–326.

Livingston, R. B., and Carter, S. K. *Single Agents in Cancer Chemotherapy.* Plenum Press, New York, **1970**.

Ludlum, D. B. Molecular biology of alkylation: an overview. In, *Antineoplastic and Immunosuppressive Agents,* Pt. II. (Sartorelli, A. C., and Johns, D. G., eds.) *Handbuch der Experimentellen Pharmakologie,* Vol. 38. Springer-Verlag, Berlin, **1975**, pp. 6–17.

————. Alkylating agents and the nitrosoureas. In, *Cancer 5: A Comprehensive Treatise.* (Becker, F. F., ed.) Plenum Press, New York, **1977**, pp. 285–303.

————. The alkylating agents and nitrosoureas. In, *Cancer Chemotherapy III.* (Brodsky, I.; Kahn, S. B.; and Conroy, J. F.; eds.) Grune & Stratton, Inc., New York, **1978**, pp. 17–24.

Maley, F. Pyrimidine antagonists. In, *Cancer 5: A Comprehensive Treatise.* (Becker, F. F., ed.) Plenum Press, New York, **1977**, pp. 327–353.

Moertel, C. G. Current concepts in chemotherapy of gastrointestinal cancer. *N. Engl. J. Med.,* **1978**, *299,* 1049–1052.

National Conference on Cancer Chemotherapy. *Cancer,* **1972**, *30,* 1473–1661.

North, T. W., and Cohen, S. S. Aranucleosides and aranucleotides in viral chemotherapy. *Pharmacol. Ther.,* **1979**, *4,* 81–108.

Oberly, L. W., and Buettner, G. R. Role of superoxide dimutase in cancer: a review. *Cancer Res.,* **1979**, *39,* 1141–1149.

Oliverio, V. T. Derivatives of triazenes and hydrazines. In, *Cancer Medicine.* (Holland, J. F., and Frei, E., III, eds.) Lea & Febiger, Philadelphia, **1973a**, pp. 806–817.

————. Toxicology and pharmacology of the nitrosoureas. *Cancer Chemother. Rep.,* **1973b**, *4,* Pt. 3, No. 3, 13–20.

————. Pharmacology of the nitrosoureas: an overview. *Cancer Treat. Rep.,* **1976**, *60,* 703–707.

Parks, R. E., Jr.; Crabtree, G. W.; Kong, C. M.; Agarwal, R. P.; Agarwal, K. C.; and Scholar, E. M. Incorporation of analog purine nucleosides into the formed elements of human blood: erythrocytes, platelets, and lymphocytes. *Ann. N.Y. Acad. Sci.,* **1975**, *255,* 412–434.

Paterson, A. R. P., and Tidd, D. M. 6-Thiopurines. In, *Antineoplastic and Immunosuppressive Agents,* Pt. II. (Sartorelli, A. C., and Johns, D. G., eds.) *Handbuch der Experimentellen Pharmakologie,* Vol. 38. Springer-Verlag, Berlin, **1975**, pp. 389–403.

Patterson, M. K., Jr. L-Asparaginase: basic aspects. In, *Antineoplastic and Immunosuppressive Agents,* Pt. II. (Sartorelli, A. C., and Johns, D. G., eds.) *Handbuch der Experimentellen Pharmakologie,* Vol. 38. Springer-Verlag, Berlin, **1975**, pp. 695–722.

Pietsch, P. Phleomycin and bleomycin. In, *Antineoplastic and Immunosuppressive Agents,* Pt. II. (Sartorelli, A. C., and Johns, D. G., eds.) *Handbuch der Experimentellen Pharmakologie,* Vol. 38. Springer-Verlag, Berlin, **1975**, pp. 850–876.

Price, C. C. Chemistry of alkylation. In, *Antineoplastic and Immunosuppressive Agents,* Pt. II. (Sartorelli, A. C., and Johns, D. G., eds.) *Handbuch der Experimentellen Pharmakologie,* Vol. 38. Springer-Verlag, Berlin, **1975**, pp. 1–5.

Prusoff, W. H., and Goz, B. Halogenated pyrimidine deoxyribonucleosides. In, *Antineoplastic and Immunosuppressive Agents,* Pt. II. (Sartorelli, A. C., and Johns, D. G., eds.) *Handbuch der Experimentellen Pharmakologie,* Vol. 38. Springer-Verlag, Berlin, **1975**, pp. 272–347.

Reed, D. J. Procarbazine. In, *Antineoplastic and Immunosuppressive Agents*, Pt. II. (Sartorelli, A. C., and Johns, D. G., eds.) *Handbuch der Experimentellen Pharmakologie,* Vol. 38. Springer-Verlag, Berlin, **1975**, pp. 747–765.

Robins, P. R., and Jowsey, J. Effect of mithramycin on normal and abnormal bone turnover. *J. Lab. Clin. Med.,* **1973**, *82,* 576–586.

Ross, W. C. J. Rational design of alkylating agents. In, *Antineoplastic and Immunosuppressive Agents*, Pt. II. (Sartorelli, A. C., and Johns, D. G., eds.) *Handbuch der Experimentellen Pharmakologie,* Vol. 38. Springer-Verlag, Berlin, **1975**, pp. 33–51.

Rozencweig, M.; Von Hoff, D. D.; Slavik, M.; and Muggia, F. M. *Cis*-diammine dichloroplatinum (II)—a new cancer drug. *Ann. Intern. Med.,* **1977**, *86,* 803–812.

Sartorelli, A. C., and Johns, D. G. (eds.). *Antineoplastic and Immunosuppressive Agents*, Pt. II. *Handbuch der Experimentellen Pharmakologie,* Vol. 38. Springer-Verlag, Berlin, **1975**.

Schabel, F. M., Jr. Historical development and future promise of the nitrosoureas as anticancer agents. *Cancer Chemother. Rep.,* **1973**, *4,* Part 3, No. 3, 3–6.

Schimke, R. T.; Kaufman, R. J.; Alt, F. W.; and Kellems, R. F. Gene amplification and drug resistance in cultured murine cells. *Science,* **1978**, *202,* 1051–1055.

Segal, S. T., and Koide, S. S. Molecular pharmacology of estrogens. *Pharmacol. Ther. [B.]*, **1979**, *4,* 183–220.

Shapiro, R. Chemistry of guanine and its biologically significant derivatives. *Prog. Nucleic Acid Res. Mol. Biol.,* **1968**, *8,* 73–112.

Sirotnak, F. M.; Chello, P. L.; and Brockman, R. W. Potential for exploitation of transport systems in anticancer drug design. In, *Methods in Cancer Research, XVI: Cancer Drug Development*, Pt. A. (DeVita, V. T., Jr., and Busch, H., eds.) Academic Press, Inc., New York, **1979**, pp. 382–447.

Skipper, H. T., and Schabel, F. M., Jr. Quantitative and cytokinetic studies in experimental tumor models. In, *Cancer Medicine*. (Holland, J. F., and Frei, E., III, eds.) Lea & Febiger, Philadelphia, **1973**, pp. 629–650.

Skoda, J. Azapyrimidine nucleosides. In, *Antineoplastic and Immunosuppressive Agents*, Pt. II. (Sartorelli, A. C., and Johns, D. G., eds.) *Handbuch der Experimentellen Pharmakologie,* Vol. 38. Springer-Verlag, Berlin, **1975**, pp. 348–372.

Sobell, H. M. The stereochemistry of actinomycin binding to DNA and its implications in molecular biology. *Prog. Nucleic Acid Res. Mol. Biol.,* **1973**, *13,* 153–190.

Stoll, B. A. Androgen, corticosteroid and progestin therapy. In, *Endocrine Therapy in Malignant Disease.* (Stoll, B. A., ed.) W. B. Saunders Co., Philadelphia, **1972**, pp. 165–191.

Symposium. (Various authors.) Hydroxyurea. (Thurman, W. G., ed.) *Cancer Chemother. Rep.,* **1964**, *40,* 1–78.

Symposium. (Various authors.) *Natulan.* (Jelliffe, A. M., and Marks, J., eds.) John Wright & Sons, Ltd., Bristol, **1965**.

Symposium. (Various authors.) Cyclophosphamide in pediatric neoplasia. (Oernbach, D. J., ed.) *Cancer Chemother. Rep.,* **1967**, *51,* 315–412.

Symposium. (Various authors.) Vincristine. *Cancer Chemother. Rep.,* **1968**, *52,* 455–535.

Symposium. (Various authors.) The nitrosoureas. *Cancer Chemother. Rep.,* **1973**, *4,* Part 3, 1–82.

Umezawa, H. Studies on bleomycin: chemistry and the biological action. *Biomedicine,* **1973a**, *18,* 459–475.

———. Principles of antitumor antibiotic therapy. In, *Cancer Medicine.* (Holland, J. F., and Frei, E., III, eds.) Lea & Febiger, Philadelphia, **1973b**, pp. 817–826.

———. Cancer drugs of microbial origin. In, *Methods in Cancer Research, XVI: Cancer Drug Development*, Pt. A. (DeVita, V. T., Jr., and Busch, H., eds.) Academic Press, Inc., New York, **1979**, pp. 43–72.

Uren, J. R., and Handschumacher, R. E. Enzyme therapy. In, *Cancer 5: A Comprehensive Treatise.* (Becker, F. F., ed.) Plenum Press, New York, **1977**, pp. 457–487.

Waksman Conference on Actinomycins: their potential for cancer chemotherapy. *Cancer Chemother. Rep.,* **1974**, *58,* 1–123.

Walker, M. D. Nitrosoureas in central nervous system tumors. *Cancer Chemother. Rep.,* **1973**, *4,* 21–26.

Warwick, G. P. The mechanism of action of alkylating agents. *Cancer Res.,* **1963**, *23,* 1315–1333.

Wheeler, G. P. Some biochemical effects of alkylating agents. *Fed. Proc.,* **1967**, *26,* 885–892.

———. Alkylating agents. In, *Cancer Medicine.* (Holland, J. F., and Frei, E., III, eds.) Lea & Febiger, Philadelphia, **1973**, pp. 791–806.

———. Mechanism of action of nitrosoureas. In, *Antineoplastic and Immunosuppressive Agents*, Pt. II. (Sartorelli, A. C., and Johns, D. G., eds.) *Handbuch der Experimentellen Pharmakologie,* Vol. 38. Springer-Verlag, Berlin, **1975**, pp. 65–84.

Young, R. C.; Lippman, M.; DeVita, V. T., Jr.; Brell, J.; and Tormey, D. Perspectives in the treatment of breast cancer: 1976. *Ann. Intern. Med.,* **1977**, *86,* 784–798.

Ziegler, J. L. Treatment results of 54 American patients with Burkitt's lymphoma are similar to the African experience. *N. Engl. J. Med.,* **1977**, *297,* 75–80.

Drugs Acting on the Blood and the Blood-Forming Organs

A large number of drugs, including many vitamins and minerals, affect the blood and the blood-forming organs, either directly or indirectly. Agents effective in specific anemias include iron, copper, cobalt, vitamin B_{12}, folic acid, pyridoxine, and riboflavin; these substances are discussed in the following two chapters. In the final chapter of this section, chief attention is devoted to the anticoagulants, heparin and the oral anticoagulants; to thrombolytic agents; and to drugs affecting platelet function.

Many dietary factors are important for normal hematopoiesis, blood coagulation, and the integrity of the vascular wall; some of them are discussed in the section concerning the vitamins. Certain internal secretions can profoundly influence the blood, such as those from the thyroid, the gonads, and the adrenal cortex; these are dealt with in the section devoted to the hormones. A vast array of drugs exert toxic effects on the formed elements of the blood, on hemoglobin, or on the hematopoietic organs. The toxic effects include granulocytopenia, thrombocytopenia, aplastic anemia, hemolytic anemia, and the conversion of hemoglobin into nonfunctional forms. Agents that somewhat selectively depress abnormal proliferation of the cellular elements of the blood are discussed in Chapter 55.

The discovery of liver therapy for pernicious anemia, by Minot and Murphy in 1926, was followed by a marked revival of interest in the field of blood diseases and their therapy. As a result, our knowledge of the mechanisms of blood formation and destruction, the metabolism of iron, the pathological physiology of pernicious and other megaloblastic anemias, and the specificity of hematinic agents is decidedly more complete. The physician now has at his command many reliable procedures for the accurate diagnosis of blood disorders and several drugs for their specific therapy. It is no longer permissible to prescribe these agents without first ascertaining, as nearly as possible, the exact nature of the abnormality. Proper treatment rests upon a clear understanding of the pharmacological properties of the hematopoietic drugs.

The term *nutritional anemias* has been used to indicate the multifactorial nature of anemias that occur in individuals whose diets are inadequate in quantity or quality. Most frequently, deficiencies of iron or protein are responsible; however, in certain geographical areas and in certain individuals with unusual diets, other deficiencies, particularly that of folic acid, are prominent. Each deficiency anemia has its own peculiarities with respect to diet, and more often than not it occurs alone. For the practicing physician, the term *nutritional anemia* now has little value and encourages inappropriate generalization. Possible causes of deficiency need to be considered on an individual basis. All arise from one or more of the following basic causes: inadequate ingestion, absorption, or utilization, or increased requirement, excretion, or metabolic destruction of the nutrient. Knowledge of the food sources and metabolism of nutrients is therefore crucial to determine the causes of such deficiencies; this information is provided in the following two chapters as it relates to iron, folate, vitamin B_{12}, and other nutritional factors that are important for hematopoiesis.

56 DRUGS EFFECTIVE IN IRON-DEFICIENCY AND OTHER HYPOCHROMIC ANEMIAS

Clement A. Finch

IRON AND IRON SALTS

History. Early in civilization man learned to procure iron from the earth and to forge tools of great strength. This *Iron Age* carried with it a belief in the special powers of the metal. For several thousand years legends and early writings described the many medicinal uses to which this "metal from Heaven" could be put (Fairbanks *et al.*, 1971). Iron was used extensively by European physicians through the Middle Ages and the Renaissance, but with little rationale. In the sixteenth century the causative role of iron deficiency in the then-prevalent "green sickness" or chlorosis of adolescent women began to be recognized. It may be that the treatment of this disorder with iron had already enjoyed some vogue in Europe, but Sydenham is properly credited with identifying iron as a specific remedy to take the place of bleedings and purgings. In 1681, he wrote (*see* Latham, 1850): ". . . I comfort the blood and the spirit belonging to it by giving a chalybeate [containing or charged with iron] 30 days running. This is sure to do good. To the worn out or languid blood it gives a spur or fillip, whereby the animal spirits which before lay prostrate and sunken under their own weight are raised and excited. Clear proof of this is found in the effect of steel in chlorosis. The pulse gains strength, the face (no longer pale and deathlike) a fresh ruddy color." In 1713, Lemery and Geoffry provided more direct evidence of the relationship by showing that iron was present in blood (ash) (*see* Christian, 1903). In 1832, the French physician Pierre Blaud wrote that the malady chlorosis ". . . arises from a faulty formation of blood as a result of which the blood is an imperfect fluid or the coloring matter is so defective that it is no longer suitable for stimulating the organism and maintaining the regular exercise of its functions." Blaud recognized that failure in the treatment of chlorosis had been due to the use of too small doses of iron and reported the rapid cure of 30 patients given a mixture of equal parts of ferrous sulfate and potassium carbonate in dosage increasing to as much as 770 mg of elemental iron daily. For many years Blaud's nephew distributed the "veritable pills of Blaud" throughout the world (Neuroth and Lee, 1941). The treatment of anemia with iron followed the principles enunciated by Sydenham and Blaud until the last decade of the nineteenth century and was comparable to modern practice in the amount of iron available for absorption that was prescribed. At that time, however, the teachings of Bunge, Quincke, von Noorden, and others cast doubt on this straightforward approach to the treatment of chlorosis. The dose of iron employed was reduced, and the resulting inefficacy of smaller doses brought discredit on the therapy. It was not until the third and fourth decades of the present century, through the efforts of Faber and Gram (1924), Bloomfield (1932), Heath and associates (1932), Heath and Patek (1937), and Reimann and coworkers (1937), that the lessons taught by the earlier physicians were relearned (*see* Haden, 1939).

The past half century has brought a clearer understanding of many aspects of iron metabolism in man. In 1937, McCance and Widdowson reported on studies of iron balance that suggested a limited daily absorption and excretion of the element. At the same time, Heilmeyer and Plotner (1937) made quantitative measurements of the concentration of iron in plasma and discussed its function in transport. Laurell in 1947 presented similar information concerning the plasma iron transport protein, which he called *transferrin*. In the early 1940s, Hahn (Hahn *et al.*, 1943) introduced the use of radioactive isotopes of iron as a means to quantitate absorption and demonstrated the capacity of the intestinal mucosa to regulate this function. In the next decade, Huff and associates (1950) initiated isotopic studies of internal iron exchange. In the past 20 years practical clinical measurements of the degree of saturation of transferrin and red-cell protoporphyrin have been developed to a point that permits the accurate detection of iron-deficient erythropoiesis, while quantitation of iron in plasma ferritin and in marrow reveals the status of the body's stores (*see* Bothwell *et al.*, 1979). Even more recently, quantitative methods have been developed for evaluation of the absorption of iron in food, and these have explained the high prevalence of iron deficiency in man as a function of the limited availability of iron in the contemporary diet (Cook and Finch, 1975).

Iron and the Environment. Iron is the fourth most abundant element in the earth's crust; only oxygen, silicon, and aluminum are more common. Metallic iron is chemically unstable and is slowly converted to the ferrous or ferric state; the earth's atmosphere favors oxidation to the insoluble ferric form. This is found in crystalline structures in most rocks and soils, and its availability is limited unless solubilized by acid or chelates or converted to organic compounds by microorganisms. While virtually all living matter must procure a certain amount of iron for normal development, this is not always possible. In alkaline or high-phosphate environments, which reduce the availability of iron, plants develop chlorosis, an iron-deficiency disease manifest by yellowness or blanching of normally green parts. Some plants have unique root secretions that mobilize iron from calcareous soils to be transported and incorporated into both nonheme and heme-containing enzymes or stored as phytoferritin. Bacteria too have developed mechanisms for acquiring this crucial nutrient; in some instances they secrete high-affinity siderophores, which can extract iron in the vicinity (Neilands, 1974). The evolution of such adaptive mechanisms reflects the poor availability of most environmental iron. It might be expected that vertebrates would have the greatest problem meeting their needs for iron, since their requirement for the element has been expanded tenfold by the use of the iron-containing protein hemoglobin for oxygen transport. Surprisingly, most mammals have little difficulty in acquiring essential iron. This is probably explained by the greater availability of the iron derived from plants and other animals that comprise their diet. Man, however, is an exception.

Iron Metabolism in Man. The body store of iron is divided between iron-containing compounds that are essential and those in which excess iron is held in storage. From a quantitative standpoint, *hemoglobin* dominates the essential fraction (Table 56–1). This protein, with a molecular weight of 64,500, contains four atoms of iron per molecule, amounting to 1.1 mg of iron per milliliter of red blood cells. Other forms of essential iron include myoglobin and a variety of heme and nonheme iron-dependent enzymes (Dallman,

Table 56–1. THE BODY CONTENT OF IRON

	MALE	FEMALE
	mg/kg of body weight	
Essential iron		
Hemoglobin	31	28
Myoglobin and enzymes	6	5
Storage iron	13	4
Total	50	37

1974; Sigel, 1977). *Ferritin* is the protein of iron storage, and it exists as individual molecules or in an aggregated form. Apoferritin has a molecular weight of about 450,000 and is composed of some 24 polypeptide subunits; these form an outer shell within which there is a storage cavity for polynuclear hydrous ferric oxide phosphate (Harrison, 1977). Over 30% of the weight of ferritin may be iron. Aggregated ferritin, referred to as *hemosiderin* and visible by light microscopy, constitutes about one third of normal stores, a fraction that increases as stores enlarge. The two predominant sites of iron storage are the reticuloendothelial system and the hepatocytes, although some storage also occurs in muscle (Bothwell *et al.*, 1979).

Internal exchange of iron is accomplished by the plasma protein *transferrin* (Aisen and Brown, 1977). This β_1-glycoprotein has a molecular weight of about 76,000 and two binding sites for ferric iron. Iron is delivered from transferrin to specific receptors on tissue cell membranes. The concentration of these receptors for transferrin on a given cell is related to the widely disparate requirement of different tissues for iron. The essential role of transferrin is illustrated by the maldistribution of iron that occurs in congenital atransferrinemia. These patients have iron-deficiency anemia despite excessive concentrations of iron in nonerythroid tissues (Goya *et al.*, 1972).

The flow of iron through the plasma amounts to a total of 30 to 40 mg per day in the adult (about 0.46 mg/kg of body weight) (Finch *et al.*, 1970). The major internal circulation of iron involves the erythron and the reticuloendothelial cell (Figure 56–1). About 80% of the iron in plasma goes to the erythroid marrow to be packaged into new erythrocytes; these normally circulate for about 120 days before being catabolized by the reticuloendothelium. At that time a portion of the iron is immediately returned to the plasma bound to transferrin, while another portion is incorporated into the ferritin stores of the reticuloendothelial cell and is returned to the circulation more gradually. Isotopic studies indicate some degree of iron wastage in this process, wherein defective cells or unused portions of their iron are transferred to the reticuloendothelial cell during maturation, bypassing the circulating blood. In

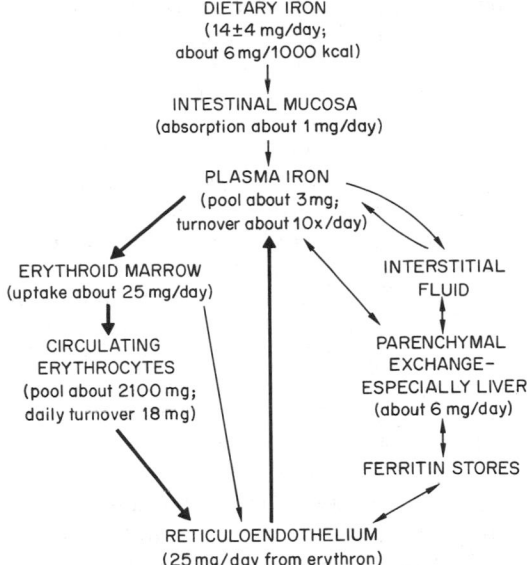

DIETARY IRON
(14±4 mg/day;
about 6 mg/1000 kcal)
↓
INTESTINAL MUCOSA
(absorption about 1 mg/day)
↓
PLASMA IRON
(pool about 3 mg;
turnover about 10x/day)

ERYTHROID MARROW
(uptake about 25 mg/day)

INTERSTITIAL
FLUID

CIRCULATING
ERYTHROCYTES
(pool about 2100 mg;
daily turnover 18 mg)

PARENCHYMAL
EXCHANGE—
ESPECIALLY LIVER
(about 6 mg/day)

FERRITIN STORES

RETICULOENDOTHELIUM
(25 mg/day from erythron)

Figure 56–1. *Pathways of iron metabolism in man (excretion omitted).* (*See* text for explanation.)

hemolytic anemia the uptake of iron by the erythron may increase by as much as eightfold, with a corresponding increase in red-cell breakdown. When there are abnormalities in maturation of red cells, the predominant portion of iron assimilated by the erythroid marrow may be rapidly localized in the reticuloendothelial cell as defective red-cell precursors are broken down, this is termed *ineffective erythropoiesis*. With red-cell aplasia, the rate of turnover of iron in plasma may be reduced by one half or more, with all of the iron now going to the hepatocyte for storage. It should be noted that non-erythroid tissues do not have the ability of the erythron to increase their number of membrane receptors for transferrin; their capacity to take up iron is thus always limited.

The most remarkable feature of iron metabolism in man is the degree to which the body store is conserved. Only 10% of the total is lost per year from normal men, that is, about 1 mg per day (Green *et al.,* 1968). Two thirds of this iron is excreted from the gastrointestinal tract as extravasated red cells, iron in bile, and iron in exfoliated mucosal cells. The other third is accounted for by small amounts of iron in desquamated skin and in the urine. Physiological losses of

iron in the male vary over a relatively narrow range, decreasing to about 0.5 mg in the iron-deficient individual and increasing to as much as 1.5 or possibly 2 mg per day when excessive iron is consumed. Additional losses of iron occur in the female due to menstruation (Hallberg *et al.,* 1966a). While this averages about 0.5 mg per day, 10% of normal menstruating females lose over 2 mg per day. Menstrual losses are influenced by various types of contraceptive therapy. Loss is reduced by about one half when estrogen-containing oral contraceptives are used and is increased by intrauterine devices. Pregnancy imposes a requirement for iron of even greater magnitude (Table 56–2). In addition to these physiological losses, there is a great variety of other causes of iron loss. Examples include the donation of blood, the use of anti-inflammatory drugs that cause bleeding from the gastric mucosa, gastrointestinal disease with associated bleeding, and so forth (Fairbanks *et al.,* 1971). Much rarer is the hemosiderinuria that follows intravascular hemolysis, which may result in urinary losses of iron of as much as 20 mg per day; still rarer is pulmonary siderosis, wherein iron is deposited in the lungs and becomes unavailable to the rest of the body.

The limited physiological losses of iron point to the primary importance of absorption as the determinant of the body's content of iron. Unfortunately, the biochemical nature of the absorptive process is understood only in general terms (Bothwell *et al.,* 1979). After acidification and partial digestion of food in the stomach, its content of iron is

Table 56–2.   IRON REQUIREMENTS FOR PREGNANCY

	AVERAGE *mg*	RANGE *mg*
External iron loss	170	150–200
Expansion of red-blood-cell mass	450	200–600
Fetal iron	270	200–370
Iron in placenta and cord	90	30–170
Blood loss at delivery	150	90–310
Total requirement *	980	580–1340
Cost of pregnancy †	680	440–1050

* Blood loss at delivery not included.

† Iron lost to the mother; expansion of red-cell mass not included.

(After Council on Foods and Nutrition, 1968. Courtesy of the *Journal of the American Medical Association.*)

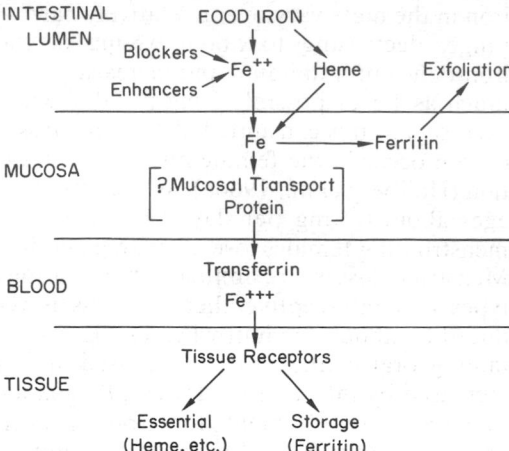

Figure 56–2. *Pathway of iron absorption. (See* text for explanation.)

presented to the intestinal mucosa as either inorganic or heme iron. These fractions are taken up by the absorptive cells of the duodenum and upper small intestine, and the iron is either transported directly into the plasma or is stored as mucosal ferritin (Figure 56–2). Absorption is regulated by the relative activity of these two pathways, which is in some manner determined by the internal state of iron metabolism. Recent work suggests that the amount of a specific transferrin-like mucosal protein regulates absorption (Huebers *et al.,* 1976; Pollack and Lasky, 1976). Normal absorption is about 1 mg per day in the adult male and 1.4 mg per day in the adult female. Increased uptake and delivery of iron into the circulation occur when there is iron deficiency, when iron stores are depleted, or when erythropoiesis is increased (Heinrich, 1970). However, there is a ceiling on the amount that may be absorbed, and this is set not only by the absorptive processes of the intestinal mucosa but also by the amount of available iron in the diet.

Iron Requirements and the Availability of Dietary Iron. Iron requirements are determined by obligatory physiological losses and the needs imposed by growth. Thus, the adult male has a requirement of only 13 μg/kg per day (about 1 mg), whereas the menstruating female requires about 21 μg/kg per day (about 1.4 mg). In the last two trimesters of pregnancy, requirements increase to about 80 μg/kg per day, and there are

similar requirements for the infant due to its rapid growth (Finch, 1976). These requirements (Table 56–3) must be considered in the context of the amount of dietary iron available for absorption.

The dietary content of iron in developed countries is about 6 mg/1000 kcal; this places the average daily iron intake of the adult male between 12 and 20 mg and that of the adult female between 8 and 15 mg. Foods high in iron (greater than 5 mg/100 g) include organ meats such as liver and heart, brewer's yeast, wheat germ, egg yolks, oysters, and certain dried beans and fruits; foods containing intermediate amounts of iron (1 to 5 mg/100 g) include most muscle meats, fish and fowl, most green vegetables, and most cereals; foods low in iron (less than 1 mg/100 g) include milk and milk products and most nongreen vegetables (*see* Sunderman and Boerner, 1949). The general distribution of iron among foods, however, limits the value of manipulation of iron intake by food selection (Wretlind, 1970). The content of iron in food is further affected by the manner of its preparation, since iron may be added through contamination with dirt and from cooking in iron pots.

While the iron content of the diet is obviously important, of greater nutritional significance is the bioavailability of iron in food (Cook and Finch, 1975). Of the two forms of iron that are absorbed, heme iron is by far the more available, and its absorption is independent of the composition of the diet. Its relative absorption is illustrated by the study carried out by Björn-Rasmussen and associates (1974) in which a diet was fed that contained 17.4 mg of iron per day, of which 16.4 mg was nonheme iron and 1 mg was contained in heme; 37% of the heme iron but only 5% of the nonheme iron was absorbed. Thus, heme iron, which constituted only 6% of the dietary iron, represented 30% of that absorbed. Nevertheless, it is the availability of the *nonheme fraction* that deserves the greatest attention, since it represents by far the largest amount of dietary iron and is almost exclusively the form of dietary iron that is ingested by the economically underprivileged. Unfortunately, nonheme iron is usually largely unavailable, and its absorption is profoundly affected by other foods ingested concurrently. In a vegetarian diet,

Table 56-3. DAILY IRON INTAKE AND ABSORPTION *

SUBJECT	WEIGHT kg	CALORIES Intake/kg	IRON REQUIREMENT μg/kg	TOTAL DIETARY IRON mg	AVAILABLE IRON IN POOR DIET μg/kg	AVAILABLE IRON IN GOOD DIET μg/kg	SAFETY FACTOR Available Iron/Requirement
Infant	8	100	67	3	33	66	0.5
Child	20	80	22	9.6	48	96	2
Adolescent (male)	60	50	21	18	30	60	1.5
Adolescent (female)	50	50	20	15	30	60	1.5
Adult (male)	70	40	13	18	26	52	2
Adult (female)	60	30	21	11	18	36	1
Pregnant (female)	60	30	73	11	18	36	0.25

* Food iron content is based on the ratio of 6 mg of iron per 1000 kcal. Low availability of dietary iron is considered to permit 10% and high availability 20% absorption in the iron-deficient subject. The basal requirement (that for the adult male) is assumed to be 13 μg/kg, while that for menstruation 5 μg/kg. Requirement for growth is based on 35 μg of iron for each gram increase in weight. Thus, 54 μg/kg per day in infancy reflects a weight gain of 15 g per day, equivalent to 430 μg of iron divided by 8 kg of body weight. To this was added the 13-μg/kg basal iron requirement. Similarly, calculations of growth requirements in childhood and in the adolescent male and female were based on a weight increase of 5, 15, and 10 g per day, respectively, corresponding to iron requirements of 9, 9, and 7 μg/kg per day. In pregnancy, requirements for the second and third trimester have been estimated at 3 to 5 mg per day. Safety factor is calculated for a dietary iron absorption of 10%.

nonheme iron is absorbed very poorly because of the inhibitory action of a variety of components, particularly phosphates (Layrisse and Martinez-Torres, 1971). Two substances are known to facilitate the absorption of nonheme iron—ascorbic acid and meat. Ascorbate forms complexes with and/or reduces ferric to ferrous iron. While meat facilitates the absorption of iron by stimulating production of gastric acid, it is possible that some other effect, not yet identified, is also involved. Either of these substances can increase availability severalfold. Thus, assessments of available dietary iron should include not only the amount of iron ingested but also an estimate of its availability based on the intake of substances that enhance its absorption (Monsen *et al.,* 1978) (Figure 56–3).

A comparison of iron requirements with available dietary iron is made in Table 56–3. Obviously, pregnancy and infancy represent periods of negative balance (Pritchard and Scott, 1970). The menstruating woman is also at risk, whereas iron balance in the adult male and nonmenstruating female is reasonably secure. The difference between dietary supply and requirements is reflected in the size of iron stores. These will be low or absent when iron balance is precarious and high when iron balance is favorable. Thus, in the infant after the third month of life and in the

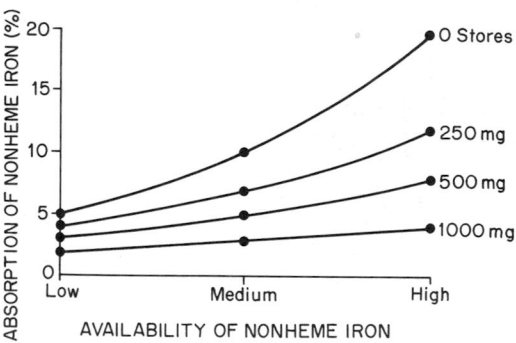

Figure 56–3. *Effect of iron status on the absorption of nonheme iron in food.*

The percentages of iron absorbed from diets of low, medium, and high bioavailability in individuals with iron stores of 0, 250, 500, and 1000 mg are portrayed. (After Monsen, Hallberg, Layrisse, Hegsted, Cook, Mertz, and Finch, 1978. © *American Journal of Clinical Nutrition.* Courtesy of American Society for Clinical Nutrition.)

pregnant woman after the first trimester, stores of iron are negligible (Beaton, 1974). Menstruating females have approximately one third the stored iron found in the adult male, indicative of the extent to which the additional average daily loss of 0.5 mg of iron affects balance (Finch *et al.,* 1977).

Iron Deficiency. Iron deficiency is rampant in human beings, and its victims number in the hundreds of millions (WHO Scientific Group, 1968). The estimate of the prevalence of iron deficiency in the United States and other developed countries depends on the economic status of the population studied and on the methods employed for evaluation. However, most data suggest that some 20 to 40% of individuals who are particularly prone to an unfavorable iron balance, that is, the infant and the pregnant woman, are iron deficient (Beaton, 1974). The prevalence of iron deficiency in the menstruating woman is estimated at 10 to 20%, but is less than 5% in the adult male and the postmenopausal female (American Medical Association, 1968; Cook *et al.,* 1976). The difficulty experienced by a substantial proportion of the population in achieving iron balance is recognized by the current practice of fortification of flour with 13 to 16.5 mg of iron per pound, by the use of iron-fortified formulas for infants, and by the prescription of medicinal iron supplements in pregnancy. There have been proposals to increase the current level of fortification of flour in the United States.

Iron-deficiency anemia is due to a dietary intake of iron that is inadequate to meet normal requirements (nutritional iron deficiency), to some condition that produces an increased requirement for iron because of blood loss, or to interference with iron absorption. Most nutritional iron deficiency in the United States is mild. Severe iron deficiency is usually the result of blood loss, either from the gastrointestinal tract or, in the female, from the uterus. *In such patients, no effort should be spared in determining the cause of the bleeding.* Infrequently, impaired absorption of the iron in food results from partial gastrectomy or sprue.

The recognition of iron deficiency rests on an appreciation of the sequence of events that occur with iron depletion. A negative balance first results in a reduction of iron

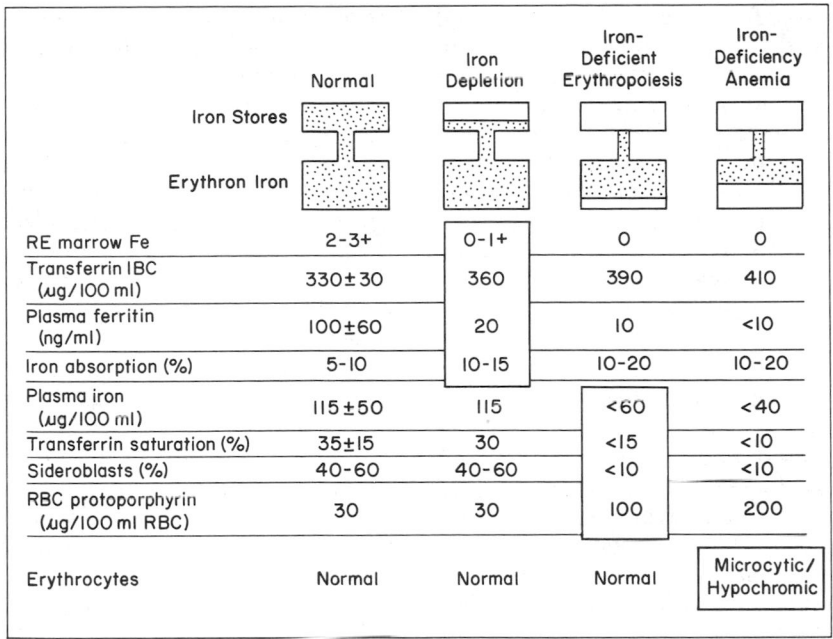

	Normal	Iron Depletion	Iron-Deficient Erythropoiesis	Iron-Deficiency Anemia
RE marrow Fe	2-3+	0-1+	0	0
Transferrin IBC (µg/100 ml)	330±30	360	390	410
Plasma ferritin (ng/ml)	100±60	20	10	<10
Iron absorption (%)	5-10	10-15	10-20	10-20
Plasma iron (µg/100 ml)	115±50	115	<60	<40
Transferrin saturation (%)	35±15	30	<15	<10
Sideroblasts (%)	40-60	40-60	<10	<10
RBC protoporphyrin (µg/100 ml RBC)	30	30	100	200
Erythrocytes	Normal	Normal	Normal	Microcytic/ Hypochromic

Figure 56–4. *Sequential changes (from left to right) in the development of iron deficiency.*

Rectangles enclose the first appearance of the indicated abnormal test results. IBC = iron-binding capacity. (After Hillman and Finch, 1974, as modified from Bothwell and Finch, 1962. Courtesy of F. A. Davis Co.)

stores and, eventually, a parallel decrease in red-cell iron and iron-related enzymes (Figure 56–4). *Depleted stores* may be recognized by a plasma ferritin of less than 12 µg per liter and the absence of reticuloendothelial hemosiderin in the marrow aspirate. *Iron-deficient erythropoiesis,* defined as a suboptimal supply of iron to the erythron, is identified by a decreased saturation of transferrin to less than 16% and/or by an increase above normal in red-cell protoporphyrin. *Iron-deficiency anemia* represents that stage where the depletion of essential body iron is associated with a recognizable decrease in the concentration of hemoglobin in blood. However, the physiological variation in the concentration of hemoglobin is so great that only about half of the individuals with iron-deficient erythropoiesis are identified by recognizable anemia (Cook *et al.,* 1976).

The importance of mild iron deficiency lies more in identifying the underlying cause of the deficiency than in any symptoms related to the deficient state. Because of the frequency of iron deficiency in infancy and in the menstruating or pregnant woman, the need for exhaustive evaluation of such individuals is usually determined by the severity of the anemia. However, in the male and the postmenopausal female, in whom iron balance should be favorable, it becomes important to pursue the search for a site of bleeding whenever iron deficiency is present.

A definite diagnosis of iron deficiency can be more accurately established by laboratory tests than by therapeutic trial, particularly when the deficiency is mild. The presence of *microcytic anemia* is the most commonly recognized indicator of iron deficiency. Other laboratory tests, such as quantitation of *transferrin saturation, red-cell protoporphyrin,* or *plasma ferritin,* are required to distinguish iron deficiency from other causes of microcytosis. Such measurements are particularly useful when circulating red cells are not yet microcytic due to the recent nature of blood loss, but iron supply is nonetheless limiting erythropoiesis. More difficult is the differentiation of true iron deficiency from iron-deficient erythropoiesis due to inflammation (Finch, 1978). In the latter condition, the stores of iron are actually increased, but the release of iron from the reticuloendothelial cell is blocked; the concentration of iron in plasma is decreased, and the supply of iron to the erythroid marrow becomes inadequate. The increased stores of iron in this condition may be demonstrated directly by examination of an aspirate of marrow or may be inferred from determination of an elevated concentration of ferritin in plasma (Lipschitz *et al.,* 1974).

TREATMENT OF IRON DEFICIENCY

General Therapeutic Principles. The administration of medicinal iron is followed by an increased rate of production of red cells, and the increase is proportional to the amount of iron made available to the erythroid marrow. The immediate purpose of treatment is to elevate the concentration of iron in plasma to a normal or even an increased value for a continuous period of time. Some idea of the importance of the concentration of iron in plasma is found in the studies of Hillman and Henderson (1969). After phlebotomy of normal subjects, erythropoiesis was reduced to less than one third the normal rate if the concentration of iron in plasma was below 70 μg/dl, whereas it was increased to four to five times normal if the concentration was between 75 and 150 μg/dl. Even higher rates of erythropoiesis are possible with a consistently elevated concentration of iron in plasma (Hillman and Giblett, 1965).

The most practical way to evaluate response is by monitoring the concentration of hemoglobin or the hematocrit, each of which begins to increase within about 3 days of treatment. If the concentration of hemoglobin before treatment is reduced by more than 3 g/dl, an average increment of hemoglobin of 0.2 g/dl per day is achieved with the usual therapeutic doses of iron, administered either orally or parenterally. It should be noted that this is less than the 0.6 g/dl per day that the erythroid marrow can achieve when the supply of iron is optimal, which simply indicates that either route of administration provides considerably less iron than the erythroid marrow can use. An increase of 2 g/dl or more in the concentration of hemoglobin in blood within 3 weeks is considered to be a positive response to iron, assuming there has been no other change in the patient's clinical status to account for this improvement. If a response does not occur in this interval, the diagnosis must be reconsidered. Laboratory data should be scrutinized, and such factors as the presence of a concurrent infectious disease or poor compliance by the patient must be assessed. Continued bleeding invalidates the use of hemoglobin as the indicator of response. In this event it is necessary to demonstrate an increase in the number of reticulocytes.

There is no justification for the continuation of iron therapy beyond 3 weeks if no favorable response has occurred. Once a response to oral iron is demonstrated, therapy should be continued until the hemoglobin returns to normal; it may be further extended if it is desired to reestablish iron stores.

Therapy with Oral Iron; Preparations, Dosage, and Untoward Effects. Orally administered ferrous sulfate, the least expensive of iron preparations, is the treatment of choice for iron deficiency (Fairbanks *et al.,* 1971; Callender, 1974; Bothwell *et al.,* 1979). Ferrous salts are absorbed about three times as well as ferric salts, and the discrepancy becomes even greater at high dosage (Brise and Hallberg, 1962). Variations in the particular ferrous salt have relatively little effect on bioavailability, and the sulfate, lactate, succinate, glutamate, gluconate, and other ferrous salts are absorbed to approximately the same extent.

Preparations and Dosage. Ferrous Sulfate, U.S.P. (*iron sulfate*), is the hydrated salt, $FeSO_4 \cdot 7H_2O$, which contains 20% iron; it consists of pale, bluish-green crystals or granules, soluble 1:1.5 in water. In moist air, crystals of ferrous sulfate rapidly oxidize and become coated with a brownish-yellow, basic ferric sulfate, and must then not be used for medicinal purposes. The drug is odorless and has a saline, astringent taste. It is usually dispensed as pills or tablets, coated to protect them from moisture. The salt is mixed with glucose or lactose to protect it against oxidation. Ferrous sulfate tablets usually contain 195, 300, or 325 mg of the salt (39, 60, or 65 mg of iron, respectively). *Dried Ferrous Sulfate,* U.S.P., is a grayish-white powder that contains not less than 80% of the anhydrous salt. *Ferrous Sulfate Syrup,* U.S.P., contains 40 mg of the salt (8 mg of iron) in each milliliter. The average adult dose is 2 tsp, thrice daily; for *children* who weigh from 15 to 35 kg, 1 tsp, twice or thrice daily. *Ferrous Sulfate*

Oral Solution, U.S.P., contains 125 mg (25 mg of iron) in each milliliter; the average therapeutic dosage is 2 ml, three or four times daily. Palatable *elixirs* of ferrous sulfate are also available.

Ferrous Fumarate, U.S.P., occurs as an anhydrous, reddish-brown granular powder. It contains 33% iron and is moderately soluble in water, stable, and almost tasteless. Unlike ferrous sulfate, it does not require mixing or coating with glucose to protect it against oxidation. Official ferrous fumarate tablets usually contain 200 mg of the salt; the average adult dosage is 600 to 800 mg daily, in divided portions.

Ferrous Gluconate, U.S.P., and *ferrous lactate* have also been successfully employed in the therapy of iron-deficiency anemia; the gluconate contains 12% metallic iron; the lactate, 19%. Both are tolerated as well as ferrous sulfate. The effective dose of either in terms of iron content is approximately the same as that of the sulfate. The same is true for other compounds of iron.

Other iron compounds have utility in fortification of foods. Reduced iron (metallic iron, elemental iron) is considered as effective as ferrous sulfate, provided that the material employed has a small particle size (Elwood, 1968; Cook *et al.,* 1973). Large-particle *ferrum reductum* and iron phosphate salts have a much lower bioavailability (Cook *et al.,* 1973), and their use for the fortification of foods is undoubtedly responsible for some of the confusion concerning effectiveness. Recently, ferric edetate has been shown to have a suitable bioavailability and to have advantages for maintenance of the normal appearance and taste of food (Viteri *et al.,* 1978).

The amount of iron, rather than the mass of the total salt in iron tablets, is important, since the latter is obviously modified by the mass of the anion and by the degree of hydration of the compound. It is also essential that the coating of the tablet dissolves rapidly in the stomach. Enteric-coated tablets are virtually worthless but are still being marketed. Surprisingly, since iron is usually absorbed in the upper small intestine, certain delayed-release preparations have been reported to be effective (Nielson *et al.,* 1976) and have been said to be even more effective than ferrous sulfate when taken with meals. However, reports of absorption from such preparations vary (Crossland-Taylor *et al.,* 1965; Callender and Warner, 1971; Baird *et al.,* 1974). Because there are a number of different forms of delayed-release preparations on the market and information on their bioavailability is limited, the effectiveness of most such preparations must be considered questionable.

A variety of substances designed to enhance the absorption of iron have been marketed, including surface-acting agents, carbohydrates, inorganic salts, amino acids, and vitamins (Hallberg *et al.,* 1966c; Hallberg and Sölvell, 1966; Medical Letter, 1978). One of the more popular of these is ascorbic acid. When present in an amount of 200 mg or more, ascorbic acid increases the absorption of medicinal iron by at least 30% (Brise, 1962). However, the increased uptake is associated with a significant increase in the incidence of side effects (Hallberg *et al.,* 1966b), and, therefore, the addition of ascorbic acid seems to have little advantage over increasing the amount of iron administered. There is no practical

benefit in employing these compounded preparations. It is particularly undesirable to use preparations that contain other compounds with therapeutic actions of their own, such as vitamin B_{12}, folate, or cobalt, since the patient's response to the combination cannot be easily interpreted. Despite the highly specific response of iron deficiency to the element and the straightforward nature of therapy with iron, it is discouraging to see the frequency with which expensive preparations with worthless additives are prescribed.

Iron therapy might be more quantitative were it not for certain other complicating factors. The principal difficulty is the time at which the medicine is ingested. Absorption is optimal when the ferrous salt is taken by the patient when fasting. As previously noted, food variably reduces the availability of an iron salt, depending on the composition of the diet. Bioavailability of iron ingested with food is probably one half or one third of that in the fasting subject (Brise, 1962; Grebe *et al.,* 1975; Ekenved, 1976). Thus, it is preferable to administer iron in the fasting state, even if the dose must be reduced considerably in response to toxic effects. Antacids also reduce the absorption of iron if given concurrently. Other considerations are patient compliance with the prescribed regimen and individual variation in absorptive capacity among iron-deficient subjects.

The usual therapeutic dose of iron is about 200 mg per day (2 to 3 mg/kg). In selecting the optimal dose for adults, allowance should be made for body size. Children weighing 15 to 30 kg can take half the average adult dose, and smaller children and infants can tolerate relatively larger doses of iron, for example, 5 mg/kg. The dose employed is a practical compromise between the therapeutic action desired and the toxic effects. It is the physician's responsibility to modify dosage to meet the needs of the individual patient. Prophylaxis and mild nutritional iron deficiency may be managed with modest doses. When the object is the prevention of iron deficiency in pregnant patients, for example, doses of 15 to 30 mg of iron per day, if not taken with meals, are adequate to meet the 3- to 6-mg daily requirement of the last two trimesters. When the purpose is to treat iron-deficiency anemia, but the circumstances do not demand haste, a total of about 100 mg (35 mg, three times daily) may be used. The average dose for the treatment of iron-deficiency anemia is about 200 mg of iron per day, given in three equal doses of 65 mg. In the case of continued bleeding, as much as 120 mg may be administered four times a day. As mentioned, the usual therapeutic dose of iron results in an increase of between 0.15 and 0.25 g of hemoglobin per deciliter of whole blood per day, beginning on the third or fourth day of treatment. An estimate of the effects to be expected from different amounts of oral iron are given in Table 56–4, although these effects may be modified by the severity of the iron-deficiency anemia and by the time of ingestion of iron relative to meals. It is well established that the amount of iron absorbed increases progressively with larger doses; however, the percentage absorbed decreases and the therapeutic value of larger doses is offset by an increase in the frequency of undesirable gastrointestinal symptoms.

Table 56-4.   AVERAGE RESPONSE TO ORAL IRON

TOTAL DOSE mg of iron per day	ESTIMATED ABSORPTION %	 mg	INCREASE IN HEMOGLOBIN g/dl of blood per day
35	40	14	0.07
105	24	25	0.14
195	18	35	0.19
390	12	45	0.22

The *duration of treatment* is governed by the recovery of hemoglobin and the desire to create iron stores (Norrby, 1974). The former depends on the severity of the anemia. With a daily rate of repair of 0.2 g of hemoglobin per deciliter of whole blood, the red-cell mass is usually reconstituted within 1 to 2 months. Thus, the individual with 5 g of hemoglobin per deciliter may achieve a normal complement of 15 g/dl in about 50 days, whereas the individual with a hemoglobin of 10 g/dl may take only half that time. The creation of stores of iron is a different matter, requiring many months of oral iron administration. The rate of absorption decreases rapidly after recovery from anemia and, after 3 to 4 months of treatment, stores may be increasing at a rate of not much more than 100 mg per month. Much of the strategy of continued therapy depends on the estimated future iron balance of the individual. The person with an inadequate diet may require continued therapy with low doses of iron. The individual whose bleeding has stopped will require no further therapy after the hemoglobin has returned to normal. For the individual with continued bleeding, chronic therapy is clearly indicated.

Untoward Effects of Oral Preparations of Iron.   Contrary to many advertisements, intolerance to oral preparations of iron is primarily a function of the amount of soluble iron in the upper gastrointestinal tract and of psychological factors. Symptoms include heartburn, nausea, upper gastric discomfort, constipation, and diarrhea. Early studies suggested that most side effects associated with the oral administration of iron were of psychic origin. For example, Girdwood (1952) found that 14 of 16 patients who complained of intolerance to ferrous sulfate in green tablets became asymptomatic when ferrous sulfate in white tablets was substituted. However, more recent studies on some 5000 subjects have established beyond doubt that physical intolerance does occur (Hallberg et al., 1966b; Hallberg and Sölvell, 1966; Sölvell, 1970). With a dose of 200 mg of iron per day divided into three equal portions,

symptoms occurred in approximately 25% of individuals, compared to an incidence of 13% among those receiving placebos; this increased to 42% when the dosage of iron was doubled. Nausea and upper abdominal pain were increasingly common manifestations at high dosage (Sölvell, 1970). Constipation and diarrhea, perhaps related to iron-induced changes in the intestinal bacteria flora, were not more prevalent at higher dosage, nor was heartburn.

There have been many attempts to improve absorption of iron while at the same time reducing gastrointestinal irritation, but this has not been convincingly accomplished. The optimal dose for the individual patient thus depends on the urgency of the clinical situation, the efficiency of absorption of iron, and individual tolerance for the preparation. The higher the dose given, the more rapid is the response but the greater is the likelihood that side effects will be produced. Frequently, the issue of intolerance preempts other considerations in the management of the iron-deficient patient; changing one pill for another of different appearance may permit successful therapy. At other times, the dosage must be reduced or the preparation given with meals with the hope of improving patient compliance. A good policy, particularly if there has been previous intolerance to iron, is to initiate therapy at a small dosage in order to demonstrate freedom from symptoms at that level and then gradually to increase the dosage to that desired. If an elixir is given, one can place the iron solution on the back of the tongue with a dropper to prevent transient staining of teeth.

Toxicity due to the long-continued administration of iron with the resultant production of iron overload (hemochromatosis) has been the subject of a number of case reports (*see* Bothwell et al., 1979); this is the result of inappropriate therapy. Available evidence suggests that the normal individual is able to control absorption of iron despite high intake, and it is only individuals with underlying disorders that augment the absorption of iron who run the hazard of hemochromatosis.

Iron Poisoning.   Large amounts of ferrous salts of iron are toxic but, in adults, fatalities are rare and almost exclusively suicidal. Most deaths occur in childhood and particularly between the ages of 12 and 24 months (Fairbanks et al., 1971; Bothwell et al., 1979). As little as 1 to 2 g of iron may cause death, but 2 to 10 g is usually ingested in fatal cases. The high frequency of iron poisoning obviously relates to its availability in the household, particularly the supply that remains after pregnancy. The colored sugar coating of many of the commercially available tablets gives them the appearance of candy. All such preparations should be kept in child-proof bottles.

Signs and symptoms of severe poisoning may occur within 30 minutes or may be delayed for several hours after ingestion. They are largely those of abdominal pain, diarrhea, or vomiting brown or bloody stomach contents containing pills. Of particular concern are pallor or cyanosis, lassitude, drowsiness, hyperventilation due to acidosis, and cardiovascular collapse. If death does not occur within 6 hours, there may be a transient period of apparent recovery, followed by death in 12 to 24 hours. The corrosive injury to the stomach may result in subsequent pyloric stenosis or gastric scarring. Hemorrhagic gastroenteritis and hepatic damage are prominent findings at autopsy. In the evaluation of the child who is thought to have ingested iron, a color test for iron in the gastric contents and an emergency determination of the concentration of iron in plasma can be performed. If the latter is less than 500 μg/dl, the child is not in immediate danger. However, vomiting should be induced when there is iron in the stomach, and an x-ray should be taken to evaluate the number of pills remaining in the small bowel. Iron in the upper gastrointestinal tract should be precipitated by lavage with sodium bicarbonate or phosphate solution. When the plasma concentration of iron is over 500 μg/dl, deferoxamine should be administered; dosage and routes of administration are detailed in Chapter 69. Shock, dehydration, and acid-base abnormalities should be treated in the conventional manner. Most important is the speed of diagnosis and therapy. With earlier and more effective treatment, the mortality from iron poisoning has been reduced from as high as 45% to about 1% at the present time.

Therapy with Parenteral Iron; Preparations, Dosage, and Untoward Effects. Parenteral administration of iron is the alternative to the use of oral preparations (Fairbanks *et al.*, 1971; Callender, 1974; Bothwell *et al.*, 1979). The rate of response to such parenteral therapy is similar to that which follows usual oral doses (Cope *et al.*, 1956; McCurdy, 1965; Pritchard, 1966; Strickland *et al.*, 1977). One of the advantages is that iron stores may be rapidly created, something that would take months to achieve by the oral route. Its most important indication is when disease such as sprue prevents absorption of iron from the gastrointestinal tract or in patients who are receiving parenteral nutrition. Parenteral iron may also be indicated when oral administration is thought to have an adverse effect on inflammatory disease of the bowel and, on rare occasions, when intolerance to oral iron prevents effective therapy. In such situations, parenteral iron is thought to represent less of a hazard to the iron-deficient subject than does a transfusion of red blood cells. It has also been used in chronic inflammatory states, such as rheumatoid arthritis, where a partial block to the absorption of iron exists, but here an additional block to the utilization of parenteral iron would be expected at the level of the reticuloendothelial cell (*see* above). Other indications have been suggested that do not seem to be soundly based. These include the unsubstantiated beliefs that the response to parenteral iron is faster than that to oral iron, and that patients undergoing dialysis (who absorb oral iron perfectly well) are better managed by the parenteral route. In the occasional patient who presents specific diagnostic problems and who is poorly compliant in taking pills, parenteral iron has been given to ensure the administration of a known amount of iron.

Iron Dextran Injection, U.S.P. (IMFERON), is the parenteral preparation in general use in the United States at the present time. It is a complex of ferric hydroxide with dextrans of 5000 to 7000 daltons in a colloidal solution containing 50 mg/ml of iron. Iron dextran is available in 10-ml vials containing 0.5% phenol for intramuscular use and in 2- and 5-ml ampuls for intramuscular or intravenous administration. When given intramuscularly, a variable portion (10 to 50%) may become fixed locally for many months. The remainder enters the blood, mostly through the lymphatic circulation, and elevates the concentration of iron in plasma for days or 1 or 2 weeks due to the presence of the iron-dextran complex. During this time determination of plasma iron does not indicate the amount of iron present in transferrin. The iron dextran must first be phagocytized by reticuloendothelial cells, and the iron is then split from the sugar molecule of the dextran before it becomes available to the body (Garby and Sjolin, 1957; Karlefors and Norden, 1958). A portion of the processed iron is rapidly returned to the plasma and made available to the erythroid marrow; however, an even greater portion remains temporarily trapped within the reticuloendothelial cell. These iron dextran deposits are very gradually converted into a usable form of iron. While all iron is eventually used (Kernoff *et al.*, 1975), many months are required before this is complete, and, in the interim, iron dextran within the reticuloendothelial cell can confuse the physician who attempts to evaluate the iron status of the patient.

Intramuscular injection of iron dextran has been carried out with an initial dose of 1 or 2 ml, followed by the administration of as much as 10 ml at a time,

5 ml in each buttock. However, local reactions, including long-continued discomfort at the site of injection and local discoloration of the skin, and the concern about malignant change at the site of injection (Weinbren *et al.*, 1978) make the intramuscular route inappropriate except when the intravenous route is inaccessible.

Intravenous administration of iron dextran avoids the deposition of iron in muscle and local reactions at the site of injection. The technic of intravenous administration involves first the injection of 1 or 2 drops of iron dextran over a period of 5 minutes to determine whether any signs or symptoms of anaphylaxis appear. If not, 500 mg of iron may then be injected over a period of 5 to 10 minutes. This dose may be repeated to reach the total amount required. Alternately, the total dose needed to reconstitute red-cell mass and tissue stores may be administered in one infusion over several hours (Basu, 1965). Such a dose (in milligrams) may be calculated from the following formula: $0.66 \times$ body weight in kilograms $\times$ (100 − [patient's hemoglobin in g/dl $\times$ 100 ÷ 14.8]). However, such calculations do not take into consideration the delay in the utilization of the material injected or the possibility of continued loss of iron. In practice, more iron needs to be given than might be calculated if an increase in hemoglobin of 0.2 g/dl of whole blood per day is required.

Reactions to intravenous iron include headache, malaise, fever, generalized lymphadenopathy, arthralgias, urticaria, and, in some patients with rheumatoid arthritis, an exacerbation of the disease. Of greatest concern, however, is the rare anaphylactic reaction, which may be fatal in spite of treatment. While only a few such deaths have been reported, it remains a deterrent to the use of iron dextran. Thus, there must be *specific* indications for the parenteral administration of iron.

Another form of iron available for parenteral use in Europe at the present time, but not in the United States, is iron-poly(sorbitol gluconic acid) complex (Fielding, 1977). This material contains 25 mg of iron per milliliter. It may be given in doses of up to 500 mg intramuscularly but should *not* be given intravenously. It must follow the same pathway to the reticuloendothelial cell for processing before it is available to the marrow. There is more loss of iron in the urine with this preparation than with iron dextran, but it may be utilized somewhat more rapidly. While anaphylactic reactions to this preparation have not yet been described, experience with its use is relatively limited.

COPPER

Deficiency of copper is extremely rare in man (Underwood, 1971; Evans, 1973). The amount present in food is more than adequate to provide the needed body complement of slightly over 100 mg. There is no evidence that copper ever needs to be added to a normal diet, either prophylactically or therapeutically. Even in clinical states associated with hypocupremia (sprue, celiac disease, nephrotic syndrome), effects of copper deficiency are usually not demonstrable. Recently, however, anemia due to copper deficiency has been described in individuals who have undergone intestinal bypass surgery (Zidar *et al.*, 1977), in those who are receiving parenteral nutrition (Karpel and Peden, 1972; Dunlap *et al.*, 1974), in malnourished infants (Holtzman *et al.*, 1970), and in infants taking copper-deficient diets (Cordano *et al.*, 1964; Graham and Cordano, 1976). While an inherited disorder affecting the transport of copper in man (Menkes' disease; steely hair syndrome) is associated with reduced activity of several copper-dependent enzymes, this disease is not associated with hematological abnormalities.

Copper deficiency in experimental animals interferes with the absorption of iron and its release from reticuloendothelial cells (Lee *et al.*, 1976). The associated microcytic anemia is related both to a decrease in the availability of iron to the normoblasts and, perhaps even more importantly, to a decreased mitochondrial production of heme. It may be that the specific defect in the latter case is a decrease in the activity of cytochrome oxidase. There are other pathological effects observed in deficient experimental animals that involve the skeletal, cardiovascular, and nervous systems (O'Dell, 1976). In man, the outstanding findings have been leukopenia, particularly granulocytopenia, and anemia. Concentrations of iron in plasma are variable, and the anemia is not always microcytic. When a low plasma copper concentration is determined in the presence of leukopenia and anemia and in a setting conducive to a deficiency of the element, a therapeutic trial with copper is appropriate. Daily doses up to 0.1 mg/kg of copper sulfate have been given by mouth, or up to half this amount may be added to the solution of nutrients for parenteral administration. (Commercial preparations are not available.) Copper deficiency usually occurs concurrently with multiple nutritional deficiencies, so that its specific role in the production of anemia is usually difficult to ascertain.

COBALT

The administration of cobalt can produce polycythemia in experimental animals and in the human subject without metabolic disease (Berk *et al.*, 1949). The same effect may be observed in patients with hematological disorders where the underlying proliferative capacity of the marrow is unimpaired (sickle-cell anemia, thalassemia, chronic infection, and renal disease) (Symposium, 1955). In the 1950s cobalt was employed in doses of up to 200 to 300 mg of cobaltous chloride daily, given in divided doses by mouth to patients with various types of anemia. While beneficial effects did not occur in those with aplastic anemia, a response was observed in two patients with pure red-cell aplasia (Voyce, 1963). Cobalt deficiency has not been reported in man.

Cobalt stimulates the production of erythropoietin (Symposium, 1962). It is thought that cobalt acts by inhibition of enzymes involved in oxidative metabolism and that the response is the result of tissue hypoxia. More specifically, cobalt blocks the conversion of pyruvate to acetyl coenzyme A and of α-ketoglutarate to succinate (Webb, 1962). Large amounts of cobaltous chloride depress the production of erythrocytes. Accidental intoxication in children may produce cyanosis, coma, and death. Other undesirable effects of doses of cobaltous chloride used clinically include cutaneous flushing, retrosternal chest pain, dermatitides, tinnitus, nausea and vomiting, nerve deafness, thyroid hyperplasia with tracheal compression, myxedema, congestive heart failure, malaise, weakness, anorexia, and fatigue. The only disease in which the clinical use of cobalt is still advocated by some is the normochromic, normocytic anemia associated with severe renal failure (Duckham and Lee, 1976). Unwanted effects, including anorexia, nausea and vomiting, and diarrhea, are frequent in these patients, although such effects are said to be reduced by the use of enteric-coated pills in doses below 50 mg per day. In general, the administration of androgens accomplishes the same end and is considered preferable for those with anemia that is associated with renal disease (*see* Chapter 62).

PYRIDOXINE

Since the first case of pyridoxine-responsive anemia was described in 1956 by Harris and associates, about 100 such cases have been observed (Horrigan and Harris, 1968; Harris and Kellermeyer, 1970). These patients have in common a population of developing red cells that show impairment in hemoglobin synthesis and the accumulation of iron; the disease belongs in the group of so-called sideroblastic anemias. The disorder may be familial or sporadic. It may involve only hemoglobin synthesis, in which case it is microcytic and hypochromic, or it may include a combination of nuclear and cytoplasmic defects, in which case the red-cell population may be slightly macrocytic but hypochromic. There is no way to predict responsiveness to pyridoxine in patients with sideroblastic anemia, so that all should probably be treated with pyridoxine, orally or intramuscularly, for 3 weeks. The usual dose is 50 to 200 mg per day. Response is evaluated by quantitation of reticulocytes at the end of the first week or by a later increase in the concentration of hemoglobin. One patient was reported who responded only when tryptophan was given in addition to pyridoxine (Horrigan, 1973). It has been further reported that some patients lack the enzyme pyridoxine kinase in their red cells and therefore are unable to convert pyridoxine to the active coenzyme, pyridoxal phosphate (Hines and Love, 1975). Accordingly, treatment with pyridoxal phosphate has been advised; however, others have not confirmed the usefulness of this compound (Chillar *et al.*, 1976; Solomon and Hillman, 1979a). A number of diseases and drugs, particularly alcohol and isoniazid, have been associated with sideroblastic changes, although the exact nature of their causative role is unclear (Bottomley, 1977; Solomon and Hillman, 1979b).

Pyridoxine-responsive anemia is probably never due primarily to nutritional deficiency of the vitamin; it cannot be produced in man by a pyridoxine-deficient diet or by antagonists of pyridoxine. Furthermore, those patients who respond to pyridoxine almost invariably do so incompletely, and their red cells may remain somewhat hypochromic. It is probable that pyridoxine acts in its coenzyme role to stimulate the production of heme in these individuals, thereby partially compensating for the deficiency of an unknown enzyme involved in hemoglobin synthesis or for a defect in utilization of pyridoxine (Hines and Grasso, 1970). Since pyridoxine is not toxic for man in the doses used, a therapeutic trial with this agent is indicated in all obscure anemias where there is a deficiency in the synthesis of hemoglobin with accumulation of iron in mitochondria. Pyridoxine is further discussed in Chapter 66.

RIBOFLAVIN

A pure red-cell aplasia that responded to the administration of riboflavin was reported in patients with protein depletion and complicating infections (Foy *et al.*, 1961). Lane and associates (1964) induced riboflavin deficiency in man and demonstrated that a hypoproliferative anemia resulted within a month. To produce the anemia it was necessary not only to restrict dietary riboflavin but also to administer galactoflavin, a riboflavin antagonist. The anemia was corrected by oral or intramuscular riboflavin, 10 mg daily. The spontaneous appearance in man of red-cell aplasia due to riboflavin deficiency is undoubtedly rare, if, in fact, it occurs at all. It has been described in combination with infection and protein deficiency, both of which are capable of producing a hypoproliferative anemia. However, it seems reasonable to include riboflavin in the nutritional management of patients with gross, generalized malnutrition. Riboflavin is further discussed in Chapter 66.

Baird, I. McL.; Walters, R. L.; and Sutton, R. D. Absorption of a slow-release iron and effects of ascorbic acid in normal subjects and after partial gastrectomy. *Br. Med. J.,* **1974,** *4,* 505–508.

Basu, S. K. Administration of iron-dextran complex by continuous intravenous infusion. *J. Obstet. Gynaecol. Br. Commonw.,* **1965,** *72,* 253–258.

Berk, L.; Burchenal, J. H.; and Castle, W. B. Erythropoietic effect of cobalt in patients with or without anemia. *N. Engl. J. Med.,* **1949,** *240,* 754–761.

Björn-Rasmussen, E.; Hallberg, L.; Isaksson, B.; and Arvidsson, B. Food iron absorption in man. Applications of the two-pool extrinsic tag method to measure haem and non-haem iron absorption from the whole diet. *J. Clin. Invest.,* **1974,** *53,* 247–255.

Blaud, P. Sur les maladies chlorotiques, et sur un mode de traitement, spécifique dans ces affections. *Rev. Med. Fr. Etrang.,* **1832,** *1,* 337–367.

Bloomfield, A. L. Relations between primary hypochromic anemia and chlorosis. *Arch. Intern. Med.,* **1932,** *50,* 328–337.

Brise, H. Effect of surface-active agents on iron absorption. *Acta Med. Scand.,* **1962,** *171,* Suppl. 376, 47–50.

Brise, H., and Hallberg, L. Absorbability of different iron compounds. *Acta Med. Scand.,* **1962,** *171,* Suppl. 376, 23–38. (*See also* related articles by these authors, pp. 7–22 and 51–58.)

Callender, S. T., and Warner, G. T. Absorption of "slow Fe" measured with a total body counter. *Curr. Ther. Res.,* **1971,** *13,* 591–594.

Chillar, R. K.; Johnson, C. S.; and Beutler, E. Erythrocyte pyridoxine kinase levels in patients with sideroblastic anemia. *N. Engl. J. Med.,* **1976,** *295,* 881–883.

Christian, H. A. A sketch of the history of the treatment of chlorosis with iron. *Med. Lib. Hist. J.,* **1903,** *1,* 176–180.

Cook, J. D.; Finch, C. A.; and Smith, N. Evaluation of the iron status of a population. *Blood,* **1976,** *48,* 449–455.

Cook, J. D.; Minnich, V.; Moore, C. V.; Rasmussen, A.; Bradley, W. B.; and Finch, C. A. Absorption of fortification iron in bread. *Am. J. Clin. Nutr.,* **1973,** *26,* 861–872.

Cope, E.; Gillhespy, R. O.; and Richardson, R. W. Treatment of iron deficiency anaemia. Comparison of methods. *Br. Med. J.,* **1956,** *2,* 638.

Cordano, A.; Baertl, J. M.; and Graham, G. G. Copper deficiency in the malnourished infant. *Pediatrics,* **1964,** *34,* 324.

Crossland-Taylor, P.; Keeling, D. H.; and Cromie, B. S. A trial of slow-release tablets of ferrous sulphate. *Curr. Ther. Res.,* **1965,** *7,* 244–248.

Duckham, J. M., and Lee, H. A. The treatment of refractory anaemia of chronic renal failure with cobalt chloride. *Q. J. Med.,* **1976,** *45,* 277–294.

Dunlap, W. M.; James, G. W., III; and Hume, D. M. Anemia and neutropenia caused by copper deficiency. *Ann. Intern. Med.,* **1974,** *80,* 470–476.

Ekenved, G. Iron absorption studies: studies on oral iron preparations using serum iron and different radioiron isotope techniques. *Scand. J. Haematol.,* **1976,** Suppl. 28, 7–97.

Faber, K., and Gram, H. C. Relations between gastric achylia and simple and pernicious anemia. *Arch. Intern. Med.,* **1924,** *34,* 658–668.

Fielding, J. (ed.). Ferastral. Iron-poly(sorbitol-gluconic acid) complex. *Scand. J. Haematol.,* **1977,** Suppl. 32, 1–399.

Finch, C. A. Iron metabolism. In, *Nutrition Reviews' Present Knowledge in Nutrition,* 4th ed. (Hegsted, D. M., ed.) The Nutrition Foundation, Inc., New York, **1976,** pp. 280–289.

———. Anemia of chronic disease. *Postgrad. Med.,* **1978,** *64,* 107–113.

Finch, C. A.; Cook, J. D.; Labbe, R. F.; and Culala, M. Effect of blood donation on iron stores as evaluated by serum ferritin. *Blood,* **1977,** *50,* 441–447.

Foy, H.; Kondi, A.; and MacDougall, L. Pure red-cell aplasia in marasmus and kwashiorkor treated with riboflavin. *Br. Med. J.,* **1961,** *1,* 937–941.

Garby, L., and Sjolin, S. Some observations on the distribution kinetics of radioactive colloidal iron (IMFERON and ferric hydroxide). *Acta Med. Scand.,* **1957,** *157,* 310–325.

Girdwood, R. H. Treatment of anaemia. *Br. Med. J.,* **1952,** *1,* 599.

Goya, N.; Miyazaki, S.; Kodate, S.; and Ushio, B. A family of congenital atransferrinemia. *Blood,* **1972,** *40,* 239–245.

Grebe, C.; Martinez-Torres, C.; and Layrisse, M. Effect of meals and ascorbic acid on the absorption of a therapeutic dose of iron as ferrous and ferric salts. *Curr. Ther. Res.,* **1975,** *17,* 382–397.

Green, R.; Charlton, R. W.; Seftel, H.; Bothwell, T.; Mayet, F.; Adams, B.; Finch, C.; and Layrisse, M. Body iron excretion in man. A collaborative study. *Am. J. Med.,* **1968,** *45,* 336–353.

Haden, R. J. Historical aspects of iron therapy in anemia. *J.A.M.A.,* **1939,** *111,* 1059–1061.

Hahn, P. F.; Bale, W. F.; Ross, J. F.; Balfour, W. M.; and Whipple, G. H. Radioactive iron absorption by the gastrointestinal tract: influence of anemia, anoxia and antecedent feeding; distribution in growing dogs. *J. Exp. Med.,* **1943,** *78,* 169–188.

Hallberg, L.; Hogdahl, A. M.; Nilsson, L.; and Rybo, G. Menstrual blood loss and iron deficiency. *Acta Med. Scand.,* **1966a,** *180,* 639–650.

Hallberg, L.; Ryttinger, L.; and Sölvell, L. Side effects of oral iron therapy. A double blind study of different iron compounds in tablet form. *Acta Med. Scand.,* **1966b,** *181,* Suppl. 459, 3–10.

Hallberg, L., and Sölvell, L. Succinic acid as absorption promotor in iron tablets. Absorption and side-effect studies. *Acta Med. Scand.,* **1966,** *181,* Suppl. 459, 23–35.

Hallberg, L.; Sölvell, L.; and Brise, H. Search for substances promoting the absorption of iron. Studies on absorption and side-effects. *Acta Med. Scand.,* **1966c,** *181,* Suppl. 459, 11–21.

Heath, C. W., and Patek, J. J., Jr. The anemia of iron deficiency. *Medicine (Baltimore),* **1937,** *16,* 267–350.

Heath, C. W.; Strauss, M. B.; and Castle, W. B. Quantitative aspects of iron deficiency in hypochromic anemia. (The parenteral administration of iron.) *J. Clin. Invest.,* **1932,** *11,* 1293–1312.

Hillman, R. S., and Giblett, E. R. Red cell membrane alteration associated with marrow stress. *J. Clin. Invest.,* **1965,** *44,* 1730–1736.

Hillman, R. S., and Henderson, P. A. Control of marrow production by relative iron supply. *J. Clin. Invest.,* **1969,** *48,* 454–460.

Hines, J. D., and Love, D. L. Abnormal vitamin B_6 metabolism in sideroblastic anemia: effect of pyridoxal phosphate (PLP) therapy. *Clin. Res.,* **1975,** *23,* 403A.

Holtzman, N. A.; Charache, P.; Cordano, A.; and Graham, G. G. Distribution of serum copper in copper deficiency. *Johns Hopkins Med. J.,* **1970,** *126,* 34–42.

Horrigan, D. L. Pyridoxine-responsive anemia: influence of tryptophan on pyridoxine responsiveness. *Blood,* **1973,** *42,* 187–193.

Huebers, H.; Huebers, E.; Csiba, E.; and Finch, C. A. Iron uptake from rat plasma transferrin by rat reticulocytes. *J. Clin. Invest.,* **1978,** *62,* 944–951.

Huebers, H.; Huebers, E.; Rummel, W.; and Crichton, R. R. Isolation and characterization of iron-binding proteins from rat intestinal mucosa. *Eur. J. Biochem.,* **1976,** *66,* 447–455.

Huff, R. L.; Hennessy, T. G.; Austin, R. E.; Garcia, J. F.; Roberts, B. M.; and Lawrence, J. H. Plasma and red cell iron turnover in normal subjects and in patients having various hematopoietic disorders. *J. Clin. Invest.,* **1950,** *29,* 1041–1052.

Karlefors, T., and Norden, A. Studies on iron-dextran complex. *Acta Med. Scand.,* **1958,** *163,* Suppl. 342, 1–54.

Karpel, J. T., and Peden, V. H. Copper deficiency in long-term parenteral nutrition. *J. Pediatr.,* **1972,** *80,* 32–36.

Kernoff, L. M.; Dommisse, J.; and du Toit, E. D. Utilization of iron dextran in recurrent iron deficiency anaemia. *Br. J. Haematol.,* **1975,** *30,* 419–424.

Kerr, D. N. S., and Davidson, S. Gastrointestinal intolerance to oral iron preparations. *Lancet,* **1958,** *2,* 489–492.

Lane, M.; Alfrey, C. P.; Megel, C. E.; Doherty, M. A.; and Doherty, J. The rapid induction of human riboflavin deficiency with galactoflavin. *J. Clin. Invest.,* **1964,** *43,* 357–373.

Latham, R. G. *The Works of Thomas Sydenham, M.D.,* Vol. 2. C. & J. Adlard, London, **1850,** p. 97.

Lipschitz, D. A.; Cook, J. D.; and Finch, C. A. A clinical evaluation of serum ferritin as an index of iron stores. *N. Engl. J. Med.,* **1974,** *290,* 1213–1216.

McCance, R. A., and Widdowson, E. M. Absorption and excretion of iron. *Lancet,* **1937,** *233,* 680–684.

McCurdy, R. P. Oral and parenteral iron therapy. A comparison. *J.A.M.A.,* **1965,** *191,* 659–862.

Medical Letter. Oral iron. **1978,** *20,* 45–47.

Monsen, E. R.; Hallberg, L.; Layrisse, M.; Hegsted, D. M.; Cook, J. D.; Mertz, W.; and Finch, C. A. Estimation of available dietary iron. *Am. J. Clin. Nutr.,* **1978,** *31,* 134–141.

Neuroth, M. L., and Lee, C. O. A history of Blaud's pills. *J. Am. Pharm. Assoc., Sci. Ed.,* **1941,** *30,* 60–63.

Nielson, J. B.; Ikkala, E.; Sölvell, L.; Björn-Rasmussen, E.; and Ekenved, G. Absorption of iron from slow-release and rapidly-disintegrating tablets—a comparative study in normal subjects, blood donors and subjects with iron deficiency anaemia. *Scand. J. Haematol.,* **1976,** Suppl. 28, 89–97.

Norrby, A. Iron absorption studies in iron deficiency. *Scand. J. Haematol.,* **1974,** Suppl. 20, 5–125.

Pollack, S., and Lasky, F. D. A new iron-binding protein isolated from intestinal mucosa. *J. Lab. Clin. Med.,* **1976,** *87,* 670–679.

Pritchard, J. A. Hemoglobin regeneration in severe iron deficiency anemia. Response to orally and parenterally administered iron preparations. *J.A.M.A.,* **1966,** *195,* 717–720.

Pritchard, J. A., and Scott, D. E. Iron demands during pregnancy. In, *Iron Deficiency: Pathogenesis, Clinical Aspects, Therapy.* (Hallberg, L.; Harwerth, H.-G.; and Vannotti, A.; eds.) Academic Press, Inc., New York, **1970,** pp. 173–182.

Reimann, F.; Fritsch, F.; and Schick, K. Eisenbilanzversuche bei Gesunden und bei Anämischen. II. Untersuchungen über das Wesen der eisenempfindlichen Anämien ("Asiderosen") und der therapeutischen Wirkung des Eisens bei diesen Anämien. *Z. Klin. Med.,* **1936,** *131,* 1–50.

Rybo, G., and Hallberg, L. Influence of heredity and environment on normal menstrual blood loss. *Acta Obstet. Gynecol. Scand.,* **1966,** *45,* Suppl. 7, 25–45.

Rybo, G., and Sölvell, L. Side effect studies on a new sustained release iron preparation. *Scand. J. Haematol.,* **1971,** *8,* 257–264.

Solomon, L. R., and Hillman, R. S. Vitamin B$_6$ metabolism in idiopathic sideroblastic anaemia and related disorders. *Br. J. Haematol.,* **1979a,** *42,* 239–253.

———. Vitamin B$_6$ metabolism in anaemic and alcoholic man. *Ibid.,* **1979b,** *41,* 343–356.

Sölvell, L. Oral iron therapy—side effects. In, *Iron Deficiency: Pathogenesis, Clinical Aspects, Therapy.* (Hallberg, L.; Harwerth, H.-G.; and Vannotti, A.; eds.) Academic Press, Inc., New York, **1970,** pp. 573–583.

Strickland, I. D.; DeSaintouge, C.; Boulton, F. E.; Francis, B.; Ronbikova, J.; and Waters, J. I. The therapeutic equivalence of oral and intravenous iron in renal dialysis patients. *Clin. Nephrol.,* **1977,** *7,* 55–57.

Sunderman, F. W., and Boerner, F. *Normal Values in Clinical Medicine.* W. B. Saunders Co., Philadelphia, **1949.**

Viteri, F. E.; Garcia-Ibanez, R.; and Torun, B. Sodium iron NaFeEDTA as an iron fortification compound in Central America. Absorption studies. *Am. J. Clin. Nutr.,* **1978,** *31,* 961–971.

Voyce, M. A. A case of pure red-cell aplasia successfully treated with cobalt. *Br. J. Haematol.,* **1963,** *9,* 412–418.

Weinbren, K.; Salm, R.; and Greenberg, G. Intramuscular injections of iron compounds and oncogenesis in man. *Br. Med. J.,* **1978,** *1,* 683–685.

Wretlind, A. Food iron supply. In, *Iron Deficiency: Pathogenesis, Clinical Aspects, Therapy.* (Hallberg, L.; Harwerth, H.-G.; and Vannotti, A.; eds.) Academic Press, Inc., New York, **1970,** pp. 39–69.

Zidar, B. L.; Shadduck, R. K.; Zeigler, Z.; and Winkelstein, A. Observations on the anemia and neutropenia of human copper deficiency. *Am. J. Hematol.,* **1977,** *3,* 177–185.

Monographs and Reviews

Aisen, P., and Brown, E. B. The iron-binding function of transferrin in iron metabolism. *Semin. Hematol.,* **1977,** *14,* 31–53.

American Medical Association, Committee on Iron Deficiency. Iron deficiency in the United States. *J.A.M.A.,* **1968,** *203,* 407–412.

Beaton, G. H. Epidemiology of iron deficiency. In, *Iron in Biochemistry and Medicine.* (Jacobs, A., and Worwood, M., eds.) Academic Press, Inc., New York, **1974,** pp. 477–528.

Bothwell, T. H.; Charlton, R. W.; Cook, J. D.; and Finch, C. A. *Iron Metabolism in Man.* Blackwell Scientific Publications, Oxford, **1979.**

Bothwell, T. H., and Finch, C. A. *Iron Metabolism.* Little, Brown & Co., Boston, **1962.**

Bottomley, S. S. Porphyrin and iron metabolism in sideroblastic anemia. *Semin. Hematol.,* **1977,** *14,* 169–185.

Callender, S. T. Treatment of iron deficiency. In, *Iron in Biochemistry and Medicine.* (Jacobs, A., and Worwood, M., eds.) Academic Press, Inc., New York, **1974,** pp. 529–542.

Cook, J. D., and Finch, C. A. Iron nutrition. *West. J. Med.,* **1975,** *122,* 474–481.

Council on Foods and Nutrition. Iron deficiency in the United States. *J.A.M.A.,* **1968,** *203,* 119–124.

Dallman, P. Tissue effects of iron deficiency. In, *Iron in Biochemistry and Medicine.* (Jacobs, A., and Worwood, M., eds.) Academic Press, Inc., New York, **1974,** pp. 437–475.

Elwood, P. A. Radioactive studies of the absorption by human subjects of various iron preparations from bread. In, *Iron in Flour.* Ministry of Health Reports on Public Health and Medicine, Subject 117. Her Majesty's Stationery Office, London, **1968,** pp. 1–50.

Evans, G. W. Copper homeostasis in the mammalian system. *Physiol. Rev.,* **1973,** *53,* 535.

Fairbanks, V. F.; Fahey, J. L.; and Beutler, E. *Clinical Disorders of Iron Metabolism,* 2nd ed. Grune & Stratton, Inc., New York, **1971.**

Finch, C. A., and others. Ferrokinetics in man. *Medicine (Baltimore),* **1970,** *40,* 17–53.

Graham, G. G., and Cordano, A. Copper deficiency in human subjects. In, *Trace Elements in Human Health and Disease.* Vol. 1, *Zinc and Copper.* (Prasad, A. S., and Oberleas, D., eds.) Academic Press, Inc., New York, **1976,** pp. 363–372.

Harris, J. W., and Kellermeyer, R. W. *The Red Cell,* rev. ed. Harvard University Press, Cambridge, Mass., **1970.**

Harrison, P. M. Ferritin: an iron-storage molecule. *Semin. Hematol.,* **1977,** *14,* 55–70.

Heilmeyer, L., and Plotner, K. *Das Serumeisen und die Eisenmangelkrankheit.* Gustav Fischer Verlag, Jena, **1937.**

Heinrich, H. C. Intestinal iron absorption in man—methods of measurement, dose relationship, diagnostic and therapeutic applications. In, *Iron Deficiency: Pathogenesis, Clinical Aspects, Therapy.* (Hallberg, L.; Harwerth, H.-G.; and Vannotti, A.; eds.) Academic Press, Inc., New York, **1970,** pp. 213–296.

Hillman, R. S., and Finch, C. A. *Red Cell Manual,* 4th ed. F. A. Davis Co., Philadelphia, **1974.**

Hines, J. D., and Grasso, J. A. The sideroblastic anemias. *Semin. Hematol.,* **1970,** *7,* 86–106.

Horrigan, D. L., and Harris, J. W. Pyridoxine-responsive anemias in man. *Vitam. Horm.,* **1968,** *26,* 549.

Laurell, C. B. Studies on the transportation and metabolism of iron in the body. *Acta Physiol. Scand.,* **1947,** *14,* Suppl. 46, 1–129.

Layrisse, M., and Martinez-Torres, C. Iron absorption from food. *Prog. Hematol.,* **1971,** *6,* 137–160.

Lee, G. R.; Williams, D. M.; and Cartwright, G. E. Role of copper in iron metabolism and heme biosynthesis. In, *Trace Elements in Human Health and Disease.* Vol. 1, *Zinc and Copper.* (Prasad, A. S., and Oberleas, D., eds.) Academic Press, Inc., New York, **1976,** pp. 373–390.

National Research Council, Committee on Medical and Biologic Effects of Environmental Pollutants, Subcommittee on Iron, Division of Medical Sciences, Assembly of Life Sciences. *Iron.* University Park Press, Baltimore, **1979.**

Neilands, J. B. (ed.).   *Microbial Iron Metabolism: A Comprehensive Treatise.* Academic Press, Inc., New York, **1974.**

O'Dell, B. L.   Biochemistry of copper. *Med. Clin. North Am.,* **1976,** *60,* 687–703.

Sigel, H.   *Metal Ions in Biological Systems.* Vol. 7, *Iron in Model and Natural Compounds.* Marcel Dekker, Inc., New York, **1977,** pp. 1–417.

Symposium. (Various authors.)   The use of cobalt and cobalt-iron preparations in the therapy of anemia. *Blood,* **1955,** *10,* 852–861.

Symposium. (Various authors.)   *Erythropoiesis.* (Jacobson, L. O., and Doyle, M., eds.) Grune & Stratton, Inc., New York, **1962.**

Underwood, E. J.   *Trace Elements in Human and Animal Nutrition,* 3rd ed. Academic Press, Inc., New York, **1971.**

Webb, M.   The biological action of cobalt and other metals. *Biochim. Biophys. Acta,* **1962,** *65,* 47.

WHO Scientific Group.   *Nutritional Anaemias.* World Health Organization Technical Report Series No. 405, WHO, Geneva, **1968.**

CHAPTER

57 VITAMIN B₁₂, FOLIC ACID, AND THE TREATMENT OF MEGALOBLASTIC ANEMIAS

Robert S. Hillman

Vitamin B_{12} and folic acid are dietary essentials for man. A deficiency of either vitamin results in defective synthesis of DNA in any cell that attempts chromosomal replication and division. Since tissues with the greatest rate of cell turnover show the most dramatic changes, the hematopoietic system is especially sensitive to deficiencies of these vitamins. Clinically, the earliest sign of deficiency is a megaloblastic anemia, where the derangement in DNA synthesis results in a characteristic morphological abnormality of the precursor cells in the bone marrow. Abnormal macrocytic red blood cells are the product, and the patient becomes severely anemic. Recognition of this pattern of abnormal hematopoiesis, more than 100 years ago, permitted the initial diagnostic classification of such patients as having "pernicious anemia" and the investigations that subsequently led to the discovery of the clinical value of vitamin B_{12} and folic acid. Even today, the characteristic abnormality in morphology is used both for diagnosis and as a therapeutic guide for administration of the vitamins.

History. The discovery of vitamin B_{12} and folic acid is a dramatic story that starts more than 150 years ago and includes two Nobel prize-winning discoveries (*see* Castle, 1961; Kass, 1976). The first descriptions of what must have been megaloblastic anemias are credited to Combe and Addison, who published several case reports between 1824 and 1855. While Combe suggested that the disorder might have some relationship to digestion, it was Austin Flint who, in 1860, first described the severe gastric atrophy and called attention to its possible relationship to the anemia. The name "progressive pernicious anemia" was coined in 1872 by Biermer. This exceptionally colorful term has persisted, for it is still common practice to describe the condition as Addisonian pernicious anemia.

Following the observation by Whipple in 1925 that liver is a source of a potent hematopoietic substance for iron-deficient dogs, Minot and Murphy carried out their Nobel prize-winning experiments that demonstrated the effectiveness of the feeding of

liver in pernicious anemia. Within a few years, Castle defined the need for both an *intrinsic* factor, a substance secreted by the parietal cells of the gastric mucosa, and an *extrinsic factor,* the vitamin-like material provided by crude liver extracts. However, nearly 20 years passed before Rickes and coworkers and Smith and Parker isolated and crystallized vitamin B_{12}; Dorothy Hodgkin then determined its crystal structure by x-ray diffraction and subsequently received the Nobel prize for this work.

As attempts were being made to purify extrinsic factor, Wills and her associates described a macrocytic anemia in women in India that responded to a factor present in crude liver extracts but not in the purified fractions known to be effective in pernicious anemia (Wills and Bilimoria, 1932; Wills *et al.,* 1937). This factor, first called Wills' factor and later vitamin M, is now known to be folic acid. The actual term *folic acid* was coined by Mitchell and coworkers in 1941, following its isolation from leafy vegetables (Mitchell *et al.,* 1941).

More recent work has shown that neither vitamin B_{12} nor folic acid as purified from liver or various foodstuffs is the active coenzyme for man. During extraction procedures, active, labile forms are converted to stable congeners of vitamin B_{12} and folic acid, cyanocobalamin and pteroylglutamic acid, respectively. These congeners must then be modified *in vivo* to be effective. While much has been learned of the intracellular metabolic pathways in which these vitamins participate, many questions remain to be answered, especially the relationship of vitamin B_{12} deficiency to the neurological abnormalities that occur with this disorder.

Relationships between Vitamin B_{12} and Folic Acid. The known roles of vitamin B_{12} and folic acid in intracellular metabolism are summarized in Figure 57–1. Intracellular vitamin B_{12} is maintained as two active coenzymes, methylcobalamin and deoxyadenosylcobalamin (Stahlberg, 1967; Linnell *et al.,* 1971). The latter is the coenzyme for the isomerization of L-methylmalonyl coenzyme A (CoA) to succinyl CoA, an important reaction in both carbohydrate and lipid metabolism (Huennekens, 1968; Weissbach and Taylor, 1968). Methylcobalamin acts as a methyl-group donor for the conversion of homocysteine to methionine (Weissbach and

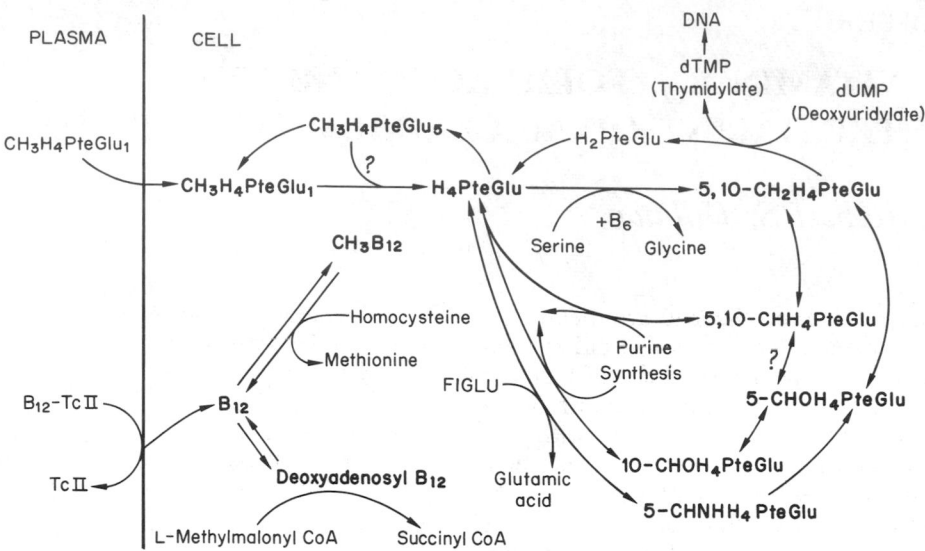

Figure 57–1. *Interrelationships and metabolic roles of vitamin B_{12} and folic acid.*

See text for explanation and Figure 57–5 for structures of the various folate coenzymes. *FIGLU* is formiminoglutamic acid, which arises from the catabolism of histidine.

Taylor, 1970). However, this is not the only source of methionine for the cell, since the amino acid is also available from the diet. Of greater importance is the interaction of vitamin B_{12} with the intracellular metabolic pathways that involve folate.

Methyltetrahydrofolate ($CH_3H_4PteGlu_1$) is the principal folate congener supplied to cells and the primary source of methyl groups for the formation of methylcobalamin. The product of this reaction, tetrahydrofolate ($H_4PteGlu_1$), is a substrate in a number of important metabolic pathways. It is the precursor of methyltetrahydrofolate pentaglutamate ($CH_3H_4PteGlu_5$), the principal form of "stored" methyltetrahydrofolate in the cell. It also is the substrate for the synthesis of several active folate coenzymes that are involved in purine and pyrimidine metabolism. $H_4PteGlu$ acts as the acceptor of a one-carbon unit in the conversion of serine to glycine, with the resultant formation of 5,10-methylenetetrahydrofolate (5,10-$CH_2H_4PteGlu$) (Kisliuck and Sakami, 1954). The latter derivative can then donate the methylene group to deoxyuridylate for the synthesis of thymidylate—an extremely important reaction in DNA synthesis. In the process, the 5,10-$CH_2H_4PteGlu$ is converted to dihydrofolate ($H_2PteGlu$); the completion

of the cycle thus requires reduction of $H_2PteGlu$ to $H_4PteGlu$ by dihydrofolate reductase, a step that can be blocked by "folate antagonists" such as methotrexate (*see* Chapter 55; Friedkin, 1957). Other sources of 5,10-$CH_2H_4PteGlu$ include pathways that generate 10-formyltetrahydrofolate (10-$CHOH_4Pte Glu$) and 5,10-methenyltetrahydrofolate (5,10-$CHH_4PteGlu$). $H_4PteGlu$ also acts as an acceptor of the formimino group donated by formiminoglutamic acid (FIGLU) to form 5-formiminotetrahydrofolate (5-$CHNHH_4PteGlu$), which is then converted to 5-formyltetrahydrofolate (5-$CHOH_4PteGlu$) and finally to 5,10-CH_2H_4-PteGlu (*see* reviews by Herbert and Bertino, 1967; Stokstad and Koch, 1967; Blakely, 1969; Chanarin, 1969; Das and Herbert, 1976; Beck, 1977; Herbert, 1979).

Although a deficiency in $H_4PteGlu$ interferes with all these reactions, the methylation of deoxyuridylate to thymidylate is an important point of control in the cellular synthesis of DNA. Reduction in the rate of this reaction appears to be the major cause for the impairment of DNA synthesis and the resultant megaloblastosis in patients who are deficient in either folic acid or vitamin B_{12} (Herbert and Zalusky, 1962; Noronha and Silverman, 1962). Folic acid deficiency deprives the cell of sufficient CH$_3$H$_4$Pte-Glu$_1$ to maintain the production of 5,10-CH$_2$H$_4$PteGlu; when there is a vitamin B$_{12}$ deficiency, CH$_3$H$_4$PteGlu$_{1-5}$ appears to be metabolically *trapped* by the lack of sufficient B$_{12}$ to accept and transfer methyl groups. All the subsequent steps that require H$_4$PteGlu are then deprived of substrate, even though plasma and intracellular concentrations of CH$_3$H$_4$PteGlu are normal or increased. This is referred to as the *methylfolate-trap hypothesis*. The theory is now supported by a number of observations, including the elevation of concentrations of folate in many although not all patients, the delayed clearance of isotopically labeled CH$_3$H$_4$PteGlu$_1$ from plasma, an impairment in the uptake of CH$_3$H$_4$PteGlu$_1$ by phytohemagglutinin-stimulated lymphocytes and cultured bone-marrow cells, an increase in the excretion of FIGLU, and the reduction in total cellular polyglutamates noted in vitamin B$_{12}$-deficient patients and/or animals (*see* excellent review by Das and Herbert, 1976).

The mechanisms responsible for the neurological lesions of vitamin B$_{12}$ deficiency are less well understood (Herbert and Tisman, 1973; Reynolds, 1976). Damage to the myelin sheath is the most obvious lesion in B$_{12}$-deficiency neuropathy. This has led to the suggestion that the abnormality is related to the role of deoxyadenosyl B$_{12}$ in the isomerization of L-methylmalonyl CoA to succinyl CoA, a step in propionate metabolism. However, children with congenital methylmalonic aciduria also lack the required coenzyme for this conversion but do not have damaged myelin.

VITAMIN B$_{12}$

Chemistry. The structural formula of vitamin B$_{12}$ is shown in Figure 57–2 (Smith, 1965; Skeggs, 1967; Pratt, 1972; Herbert, 1979). The three major portions of the molecule are:

1. A planar group or corrin nucleus—a porphyrin-like ring structure with four reduced pyrrole rings (designated *A* to *D*) linked to a central cobalt atom and extensively substituted with methyl, acetamide, and propionamide residues.

2. A 5,6-dimethylbenzimidazolyl nucleotide, which links almost at right angles to the corrin nucleus with bonds to the cobalt atom and to the propionate side chain of the D ring.

3. A variable R group—the most important of which is found in the stable compounds cyanocobalamin and hydroxocobalamin and the active coenzymes methylcobalamin and 5-deoxyadenosylcobalamin. While there are a number of other cobalamin derivatives in nature, formed by covalent binding of various ligands to the cobalt atom, these are of no apparent value to man.

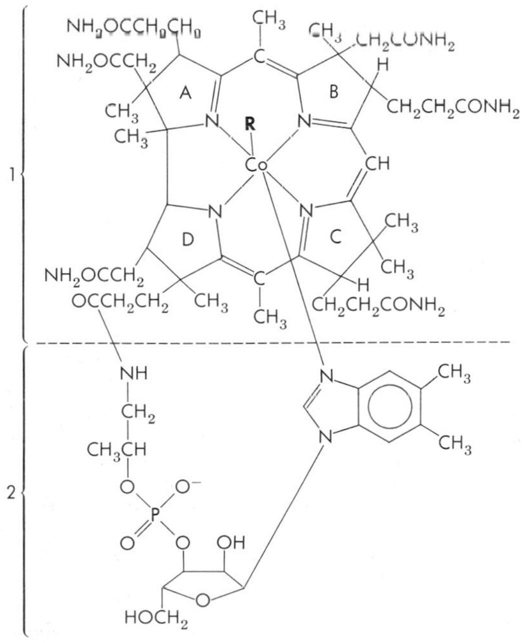

VITAMIN B$_{12}$ CONGENERS	
Permissive Name	**R Group**
Cyanocobalamin (Vitamin B$_{12}$)	—CN
Hydroxocobalamin	—OH
Methylcobalamin	—CH$_3$
5′-Deoxyadenosyl-cobalamin	—5′-Deoxyadenosyl

Figure 57–2. *The structure and nomenclature of vitamin B$_{12}$ congeners. (See text for explanation.)*

The terms *vitamin B₁₂* and *cyanocobalamin* are used interchangeably as generic terms for all the cobamides active in man. Preparations of vitamin B_{12} for therapeutic use contain either cyanocobalamin or hydroxocobalamin, since only these derivatives are stable with storage (Hutchins *et al.*, 1956).

Metabolic Functions.   The active coenzymes, methylcobalamin and 5-deoxyadenosylcobalamin, are essential for cell growth and replication and the maintenance of normal myelin throughout the nervous system. Methylcobalamin is required for the formation of methionine from homocysteine (Weissbach and Taylor, 1970). In addition, when concentrations of vitamin B_{12} are inadequate, folate becomes "trapped" as methyltetrahydrofolate to cause a functional deficiency of other vital intracellular forms of folic acid (*see* Figure 57–1 and discussion above). It is this latter phenomenon that is the most likely cause of the hematological abnormalities that are observed in vitamin B_{12}–deficient patients (Herbert and Zalusky, 1962; Noronha and Silverman, 1962).

5-Deoxyadenosylcobalamin is required for the isomerization of L-methylmalonyl CoA to succinyl CoA. This suggests that vitamin B_{12} is involved in both lipid and carbohydrate metabolism, since utilization of propionic acid by some animal tissues proceeds via the conversion of methylmalonate to succinate. Impairment of this reaction may interfere with the synthesis of the lipid portion of the myelin sheath and contribute to the neurological damage in patients with vitamin B_{12} deficiency. However, it is quite possible that the neurological complications are also related to the concurrent abnormality in folate metabolism (Reynolds, 1976).

Sources in Nature.   Man depends on exogenous sources of vitamin B_{12} (Herbert, 1973). In nature, the only original source is certain microorganisms that grow in soil, sewage, water, or the intestinal lumen, and that synthesize the vitamin. Vegetable products are free of vitamin B_{12} unless they are contaminated with such microorganisms, so that animals are dependent on synthesis in their own alimentary tract or the ingestion of animal products containing vitamin B_{12}. In man, vitamin B_{12} synthesized in the large bowel is unavailable for absorption, and a daily nutritional requirement of 3 to 5 µg

must be obtained from animal by-products in the diet. At the same time, strict vegetarians rarely develop vitamin B_{12} deficiency. A certain amount of vitamin B_{12} is available from legumes, which are contaminated with bacteria capable of synthesizing vitamin B_{12}, and vegetarians generally fortify their diets with a wide range of vitamins and minerals.

Absorption, Distribution, Elimination, and Daily Requirements.   The development of vitamin B_{12} deficiency during adult life does not usually result from a deficient diet; rather, it reflects some defect in gastrointestinal absorption (*see* Figure 57–3). Classical Addisonian pernicious anemia is caused by a failure of gastric parietal-cell function and production of the glycoprotein *gastric intrinsic factor*, often called the intrinsic factor of Castle in recognition of his major contributions to the field (*see* Castle, 1953). Dietary vitamin B_{12}, in the presence of gastric acid, is released from proteins to which it is bound and is then immediately bound to intrinsic

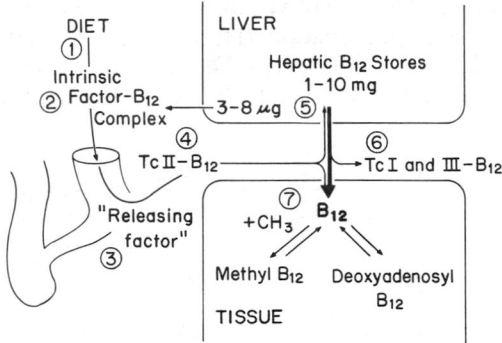

Figure 57–3.   *The absorption and distribution of vitamin B_{12}.*

Deficiency of vitamin B_{12} can result from a congenital or acquired defect in any one of the following: (*1*) inadequate dietary supply; (*2*) inadequate secretion of intrinsic factor (classical pernicious anemia); (*3*) ileal disease; (*4*) congenital absence of transcobalamin II (Tc II); or (*5*) rapid depletion of hepatic stores by interference with reabsorption of vitamin B_{12} excreted in bile. The utility of measurements of the concentration of vitamin B_{12} in plasma to estimate supply available to tissues can be compromised by liver disease and (*6*) the appearance of abnormal amounts of transcobalamins I and III (Tc I and III) in plasma. Finally, the formation of methylcobalamin requires (*7*) normal transport into cells and an adequate supply of folic acid as $CH_3H_4PteGlu_1$.

factor, a glycoprotein with a molecular weight in the range of 60,000. The vitamin B$_{12}$–intrinsic factor complex then reaches the ileum, where it interacts with a specific receptor on ileal mucosal cells and is transported to the circulation. Intrinsic factor is required for ileal transport of vitamin B$_{12}$—both the vitamin in the diet and that which is continuously excreted in the bile (Gräsbeck, 1969; Allen and Mehlman, 1973; Glass, 1974).

Any of a number of intestinal diseases or defects can interfere with the absorption of the intrinsic factor–B$_{12}$ complex. The combination of gastric achlorhydria and decreased secretion of intrinsic factor secondary to gastric atrophy or gastric surgery is a common cause of vitamin B$_{12}$ deficiency in adults. Antibodies to intrinsic factor or to the intrinsic factor–B$_{12}$ complex may also play a role in impaired uptake by ileal cells. Bacterial overgrowth or certain intestinal parasites can prevent an adequate supply of B$_{12}$ from reaching the ileum. Finally, any damage to ileal mucosal cells by disease or surgical procedures can interfere with absorption (Herbert, 1979).

Once absorbed, vitamin B$_{12}$ binds to transcobalamin II, a plasma β-globulin, for transport to tissues (Gräsbeck, 1969; Hall and Finkler, 1971). Two other transcobalamins (I and III) are also present in plasma; their concentrations are related to the rate of turnover of granulocytes. They may represent intracellular storage proteins that are released with cell death (Scott et al., 1974). Vitamin B$_{12}$ bound to transcobalamin II is rapidly cleared from plasma and is preferentially distributed to hepatic parenchymal cells. The liver is thus a storage depot for other tissues. In the normal adult, as much as 90% of the body's stores of vitamin B$_{12}$, from 1 to 10 mg, is in the liver (Chanarin et al., 1966). Vitamin B$_{12}$ is stored as the active coenzyme with a turnover rate of 0.05 to 0.2% per day or 0.5 to 8 μg per day, depending on the size of the body stores (Heyssel et al., 1966; Reizenstein et al., 1966; Adams and Boddy, 1968). The minimal daily requirement of the vitamin is estimated to be as little as 1 μg (Sullivan and Herbert, 1965; FAO/WHO Expert Group, 1970). Recommended dietary allowances are presented in Table XVI–1.

Approximately 3 to 8 μg of vitamin B$_{12}$ is secreted into bile each day, and this is normally reabsorbed in the ileum. This enterohepatic cycle is important, since interference with reabsorption by intestinal disease can result in a continuous depletion of hepatic stores of the vitamin. This explains why patients will develop vitamin B$_{12}$ deficiency within 3 to 4 years following major gastric surgery even though a daily requirement of 1 to 2 μg would not be expected to deplete hepatic stores of more than 2 to 3 mg during this period.

The supply of vitamin B$_{12}$ available for tissues is directly related to the size of the hepatic storage pool and the amount of vitamin B$_{12}$ bound to transcobalamin II. Since vitamin B$_{12}$ in liver cannot be easily measured, the concentration of vitamin B$_{12}$ in plasma is the best routine measure of B$_{12}$ deficiency. Normal individuals have plasma concentrations of the vitamin between 200 and 900 pg/ml, while a deficiency state is usually present whenever the value falls below 200 pg/ml. The correlation is excellent except when the concentrations of transcobalamin I and III in the plasma increase as a result, for example, of hepatic disease or a myeloproliferative disorder. Inasmuch as the vitamin B$_{12}$ bound to these transport proteins has a very slow turnover and, therefore, is relatively unavailable to cells, it is possible for there to be a deficiency within tissues at a time when the concentration of vitamin B$_{12}$ in plasma is normal or even high (Retief et al., 1967). A congenital absence of transcobalamin II has been observed in at least two families (Hakami et al., 1971; Hitzig et al., 1974). In the children, megaloblastic anemia was present despite relatively normal concentrations of vitamin B$_{12}$ in plasma. At the same time, the children were quite responsive to doses of parenteral vitamin B$_{12}$ that were sufficient to exceed renal clearance, allow accumulation of the unbound vitamin in plasma, and thereby provide free vitamin B$_{12}$ to cells.

Defects in intracellular metabolism of vitamin B$_{12}$ have been reported in children with methylmalonic aciduria and homocystinuria. Mechanisms involved may include an incapacity of cells to transport vitamin B$_{12}$ or accumulate the vitamin because of a failure to synthesize an intracellular acceptor, a defect in the formation of deoxyadenosylcobalamin, or a congenital lack of methylmalonyl CoA isomerase (Cooper, 1976). Numerous examples of the last-named defect have been reported under the classification of congenital methylmalonic aciduria. In the above-listed situations, large doses of vitamin B_{12} may have a salutary effect.

Vitamin B_{12} Deficiency. Vitamin B_{12} deficiency is recognized clinically by its impact on both the hematopoietic and the nervous systems. The sensitivity of the hematopoietic system relates to its high rate of turnover of cells. There is nothing else unique about the hematopoietic system in this respect, and other tissues with high rates of cell turnover (*e.g.*, mucosa and cervical epithelium) have similar high requirements for the vitamin.

As a result of an inadaquate supply of vitamin B_{12}, DNA replication becomes highly abnormal. Once a hematopoietic stem cell is committed to enter a programmed series of cell divisions, the defect in chromosomal replication results in an inability of maturing cells to complete nuclear divisions while cytoplasmic maturation continues at a relatively normal rate. This results in the production of morphologically abnormal cells or death of cells during the maturation phase, a phenomenon referred to as ineffective hematopoiesis (Finch *et al.*, 1956). From the clinical viewpoint, these abnormalities are readily identified by examination of the bone marrow and peripheral blood. Usually, the changes are most marked for the red-cell series. The marrow shows proliferation of red-cell precursors that is appropriate to the severity of the anemia, but maturation is highly abnormal (megaloblastic erythropoiesis). A majority of the megaloblastic cells die within the marrow, so that the reticulocyte index, the measure of effective red-cell production, is much less than that expected for the level of proliferation in marrow. Finally, those cells that do leave the marrow are highly abnormal, and many cell fragments, poikilocytes, and hyperchromic macrocytes appear in the peripheral blood. The mean red-cell volume increases to values greater than 110 μm^3. When deficiency is marked, all cell lines may be affected, and a pronounced pancytopenia results.

The diagnosis of a vitamin B_{12}–deficiency state can be made by determination of the concentration of vitamin B_{12} in plasma and by tests of gastric function. Measurements of gastric acidity may provide indirect evidence of a defect in parietal-cell function, while the Schilling test can be used to quantitate ileal absorption of vitamin B_{12}. (Isotopically labeled vitamin B_{12} is administered orally, and the radioactivity in urine is quantified.) In addition, the Schilling test performed after the oral administration of intrinsic factor can help to delineate the mechanism of the abnormality of absorption (Schilling, 1953). A less commonly used index of vitamin B_{12} deficiency is the measurement of urinary methylmalonate. While a normal subject excretes only trace amounts of methylmalonate (0 to 3.5 mg per day), the B_{12}-deficient patient will excrete as much as 300 mg in 24 hours (Cox and White, 1962). Finally, as first used by Minot and Murphy in their discovery of vitamin B_{12} (then called the anti–pernicious anemia principle) and later by Castle in his classical studies of intrinsic factor, the observation of reticulocytosis following a therapeutic trial of vitamin B_{12} confirms the diagnosis.

Vitamin B_{12} deficiency can result in *irreversible* damage to the nervous system. Progressive swelling of myelinated neurons, demyelination, and cell death are seen in the spinal column and cerebral cortex. This causes a wide range of neurological signs and symptoms, including paresthesias of the hands and feet, diminution of sensation of vibration and position with resultant unsteadiness, decreased deep-tendon reflexes, and, in the later stages, loss of memory, confusion, moodiness, and even a loss of central vision. The patient may exhibit delusions, hallucinations, or even an overt psychosis. Since the neurological damage can be dissociated from the changes in the hematopoietic system, especially by the administration of pharmacological doses of folic acid, vitamin B_{12} deficiency must be considered as a possibility in elderly patients with psychosis. However, it is unusual to see patients who are routinely followed by their physicians develop severe neurological complications. The sensitivity of methods for evaluation of the hematopoietic system, the ease of measurement of the concentration of vitamin B$_{12}$ in plasma, and the awareness of the medical profession of the causes of vitamin B$_{12}$ deficiency have made possible an earlier and more accurate diagnosis of B$_{12}$-deficient states, early and adequate therapy, and hence avoidance of neurological complications.

Preparations, Dosage, and Routes of Administration. Vitamin B$_{12}$ is available in pure form for injection or oral administration or in combination with other vitamins and minerals for oral administration. The choice of a preparation must always be made with recognition of the cause of the deficiency. While oral preparations may be used to supplement deficient diets or to prevent vitamin B$_{12}$ deficiency in situations where there is increased utilization, *they are of little value in the treatment of patients with deficiency of intrinsic factor or ileal disease.* Even though small amounts of vitamin B$_{12}$ may be absorbed by simple diffusion, the oral route of administration cannot be relied upon for effective therapy in the patient with a marked deficiency of B$_{12}$ and abnormal hematopoiesis or neurological deficits. Therefore, the preparation of choice for treatment of a vitamin B$_{12}$–deficiency state is cyanocobalamin, and it should be given by intramuscular or deep subcutaneous injection.

Cyanocobalamin Injection, U.S.P. (REDISOL, RUBRAMIN, others), is a clear aqueous solution with a characteristic red color. The purified vitamin is a dark-red crystalline, hygroscopic powder that is sparingly soluble in water. It is very stable at room temperature and can be autoclaved for 15 minutes at 121° C. However, it must be protected from sunlight.

The aqueous solution is available in concentrations of 30, 100, and 1000 μg/ml in vials containing from 1 to 30 ml. One-milliliter single-dose syringes are also available. Cyanocobalamin injection is extremely safe when given by the intramuscular or deep subcutaneous route, but it should never be given intravenously. There have been rare reports of transitory exanthema and anaphylaxis following injection. Therefore, if a patient reports a previous sensitivity to injections of vitamin B$_{12}$, an intradermal skin test should be carried out before the full dose is administered.

Cyanocobalamin is administered in doses of 1 to 100 μg. Tissue uptake, storage, and utilization depend on the availability of transcobalamin II (*see above*). Doses in excess of 100 μg are rapidly cleared from plasma into the urine, and administration of larger amounts of vitamin B$_{12}$ will thus not result in greater retention of the vitamin. Administration of 1000 μg is of value, however, in the performance of the Schilling test. Following oral administration of isotopically labeled vitamin B$_{12}$, the compound that is absorbed can be quantitatively recovered in the urine if 1000 μg of cyanocobalamin is administered intramuscularly. This unlabeled material saturates the transport system and tissue binding sites, so that more than 90% of the labeled and unlabeled vitamin is excreted during the next 24 hours.

A number of multivitamin preparations are marketed either as nutritional supplements or for the treatment of anemia. Many of these contain from 5 to 20 μg of cyanocobalamin without or with intrinsic factor concentrate prepared from the stomachs of hogs or other domestic animals. Purified preparations of intrinsic factor are standardized according to their ability to promote vitamin B$_{12}$ absorption in patients with pernicious anemia. One intrinsic unit of intrinsic factor is defined as that amount of material that will bind and transport 15 μg of cyanocobalamin. Most multivitamin preparations supplemented with intrinsic factor contain 0.5 oral unit per tablet. While the combination of oral vitamin B$_{12}$ and intrinsic factor would appear to be ideal for patients with an intrinsic factor deficiency, *such preparations are not reliable.* Antibodies to human intrinsic factor may effectively counteract absorption of vitamin B$_{12}$. With prolonged therapy, some patients develop refractoriness to oral intrinsic factor, perhaps related to production of an intralumenal antibody against the hog protein (Ramsey and Herbert, 1965). All oral preparations of vitamin B$_{12}$ and intrinsic factor thus carry a warning that patients must be reevaluated at 3-month intervals for recurrence of pernicious anemia.

In the past, vitamin B$_{12}$ deficiency has been treated with various regimens, including injection of crude liver extracts, oral administration of large doses of oral cyanocobalamin (100 to 1000 μg per day), or intramuscular injection of hydroxocobalamin. Crude liver extract has no advantage over purified cyanocobalamin for the treatment of the anemia and can result in local inflammatory reactions. While a small amount of cyanocobalamin can cross the intestinal barrier without intrinsic factor, the oral administration of even very large amounts of cyanocobalamin cannot be relied upon to treat pernicious anemia. In addition, such therapy can be extremely expensive. Finally, hydroxocobalamin given in doses of 100 μg intramuscularly has been reported to have a more sustained effect than cyanocobalamin, a single dose maintaining plasma vitamin B$_{12}$ concentrations in the normal range for up to 3 months. However, a number of patients show reductions of the concentration of B$_{12}$ in plasma within 30 days, similar to that seen after cyanocobalamin. Furthermore, the administration of hydroxocobalamin has resulted in the formation of antibodies to the transcobalamin II–vitamin B$_{12}$ complex (Skouby *et al.,* 1971). *Hydroxocobalamin,* U.S.P. (ALPHAREDISOL, others), is thus not recommended.

General Principles of Therapy. Vitamin B$_{12}$ has an undeserved reputation as a health tonic and has been used for a number of diverse disease states. Effective use of the vitamin depends on accurate diagnosis and an understanding of the following general principles of therapy:

1. Vitamin B_{12} should be given prophylactically only when there is a reasonable indication. Dietary deficiency in the strict vegetarian, the predictable malabsorption of vitamin B_{12} in patients who have had a gastrectomy, and certain diseases of the small intestine constitute such indications. When gastrointestinal function is normal, an oral prophylactic supplement of vitamins and minerals, including vitamin B_{12}, may be indicated. Otherwise, the patient should receive monthly injections of cyanocobalamin.

2. The relative ease of treatment with vitamin B_{12} should not prevent a full investigation of the etiology of the disease. Usually, the initial diagnosis of a deficiency state is made from the characteristic defect in hematopoiesis; a full understanding of the etiology of the disease state involves studies of dietary supply, gastrointestinal absorption, and transport.

3. Therapy should always be as specific as possible. While a large number of multivitamin preparations are available, the use of "shotgun" vitamin therapy in the treatment of vitamin B_{12} deficiency can be dangerous. *With such therapy, there is the danger that sufficient folic acid will be given to result in a hematological recovery; however, this may mask continued vitamin B_{12} deficiency, and neurological damage will develop or progress if already present.*

4. While a classical therapeutic trial with small amounts of vitamin B_{12} can help confirm the diagnosis, the acutely ill, elderly patient may not be able to tolerate the delay in the correction of a severe anemia with resultant tissue hypoxia. Such patients require supplemental blood transfusions and immediate therapy with both folic acid and vitamin B_{12} to guarantee recovery.

5. Long-term therapy with vitamin B_{12} must be evaluated at intervals of 6 to 12 months in patients who are otherwise well. If there is an additional illness or a condition that may increase the requirement for the vitamin (*e.g.*, pregnancy), assessment of treatment should be performed more frequently. The concentration of vitamin B_{12} in plasma should be monitored; peripheral blood counts and parameters of macrocytosis must be evaluated.

Treatment of the Acutely Ill Patient. The therapeutic approach depends on the severity of the patient's illness. The individual with an uncomplicated pernicious anemia, in which the abnormality is restricted to a mild or moderate anemia without leukopenia, thrombocytopenia, or neurological signs or symptoms, will respond quite well to the administration of vitamin B_{12} alone. Moreover, therapy may be delayed until other causes of megaloblastic anemia have been ruled out and sufficient studies of gastrointestinal function have been performed to reveal the underlying etiology of the disease. In this situation, a therapeutic trial with small amounts of parenteral vitamin B_{12} (1 to 10 μg per day) can be extremely valuable in confirming the presence of an uncomplicated vitamin B_{12} deficiency.

In contrast, patients with neurological changes or severe leukopenia or thrombocytopenia associated with infection or bleeding require emergency treatment. The older individual with a severe anemia (hematocrit less than 20%) is likely to have tissue hypoxia, cerebrovascular insufficiency, and congestive heart failure. Effective therapy must not wait for detailed diagnostic tests. Once the megaloblastic erythropoiesis has been confirmed and sufficient blood collected for later measurements of concentrations of vitamin B_{12} and folic acid, the patient should receive intramuscular injections of 100 μg of cyanocobalamin and 1 to 5 mg of folic acid. For the next 1 to 2 weeks the patient should receive daily intramuscular injections of 100 μg of cyanocobalamin, together with a daily oral supplement of 1 to 2 mg of folic acid. Since an effective increase in red-cell mass will not occur for 10 to 20 days, the patient with a markedly depressed hematocrit and tissue hypoxia should also receive a transfusion of 1 to 3 units of packed red cells; if congestive heart failure is present, phlebotomy to remove an equal volume of whole blood can be performed (Duke *et al.*, 1964). Disorders of hemostasis secondary to thrombocytopenia should be treated with platelet transfusions (daily or every other day) until the platelet count has increased, and any ongoing infection should be treated aggressively with appropriate antibiotics. However, such patients should not receive chloramphenicol, since this antibiotic can prevent recovery of granulocytes (*see* Chapter 52).

The therapeutic response to vitamin B_{12} is characterized by a number of subjective and objective changes (Figure 57-4). Patients usually report an increased sense of well-being within the first 24 hours after the initiation of therapy. Objectively, memory and orientation can show dramatic improvement, although full recovery of mental function may take months or, in fact, may never occur. In addition, even before there is an obvious hematological response, the patient may report an increase in strength, a better appetite, and an improvement in the soreness of the mouth and tongue.

The first objective hematological change is the disappearance of the megaloblastic morphology of the bone marrow. As the ineffective erythropoiesis is corrected, the concentration of iron in plasma falls dramatically as the metal is used in the formation of hemoglobin. This usually occurs within the first 48

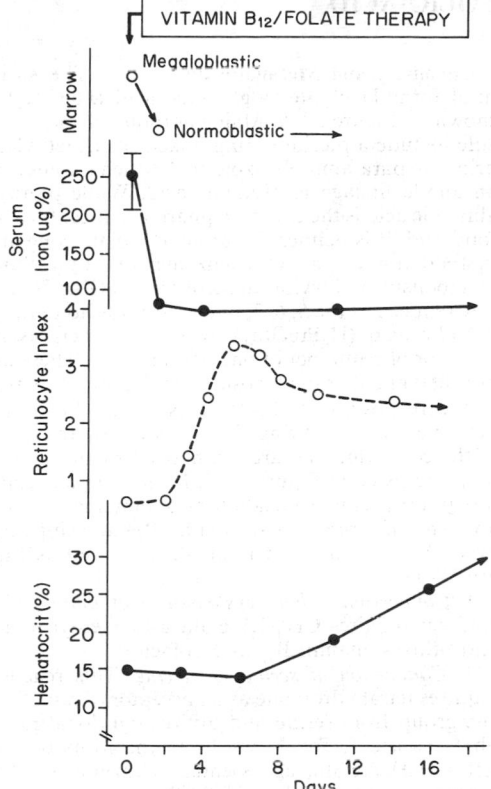

Figure 57-4. *Hematological response to the administration of vitamin B$_{12}$ or folic acid in patients with deficiency of the administered vitamin.*

Appropriate therapy with vitamin B$_{12}$ or folic acid results in a predictable series of subjective and objective changes. For the hematopoietic system, these include: an almost immediate reversion of the megaloblastic marrow to normoblastic morphology; a dramatic fall in the plasma iron as efficient erythropoiesis resumes; a rise in the reticulocyte index to values that are three to five times normal in 5 to 7 days; and a gradual increase in the hematocrit beginning in the second week. This pattern of response has been used as the basis for a therapeutic trial. When a small amount of either vitamin B$_{12}$ (less than 10 μg) or folic acid (less than 100 μg) is administered, the patient will respond only if the appropriate deficiency state is present.

hours. Full correction of precursor maturation in marrow with production of an increased number of reticulocytes begins on or about the second or third day and reaches a peak 3 to 5 days later. When the anemia is moderate to severe, the maximal reticulocyte index will be between three and five times the normal value, that is, a reticulocyte count of 20 to 40% (Hillman *et al.*, 1968). The ability of the marrow

to sustain a high rate of production of reticulocytes determines the rate of recovery of the hematocrit. Patients with complicating iron deficiency, an infection or other inflammatory state, or renal disease may be unable to maintain a sufficient rate of production to correct their anemia. It is important, therefore, to monitor the reticulocyte index over the first several weeks. If it does not continue at levels greater than twice normal for as long as the hematocrit is less than 35%, plasma concentrations of iron and folic acid should again be determined and the patient should be reevaluated for a complicating illness that could inhibit the response of the marrow.

During recovery from a vitamin B$_{12}$-related thrombocytopenia, the platelet count rises within 10 days to values that exceed normal. This overshoot is a typical response to the correction of an ineffective thrombocytopoietic state. The recovery of the white blood cells is less dramatic. In the absence of infection, the granulocyte count reverts to normal within the first 2 weeks, and large multilobed polymorphonuclear leukocytes gradually disappear from the circulation. Even though the turnover of circulating granulocytes is less than 8 to 12 hours, the continued presence of multilobed polymorphonuclear leukocytes in the peripheral blood reflects continued entry of abnormal cells from the granulocytic pool of the marrow.

While patients report an increase in mental well-being almost as soon as therapy has begun, alleviation of other neurological signs and symptoms can require a much longer time. Usually, the degree of improvement depends on the severity and the duration of the neurological abnormalities. Signs or symptoms that have been present for only a few months disappear quite rapidly. When a defect has been present for months or years, it may require several months for objective improvement, or a full return to normal function may never occur.

The incidence of mortality due to deficiency of vitamin B$_{12}$ usually correlates with the patient's hematological status. Severe anemia and hypoxia in the elderly patient can overtax the already-compromised cardiovascular and cerebrovascular systems. Heart failure and cardiac arrhythmias are likely causes of death in the severely anemic patient. With marked leukopenia, a complicating infection can also be life threatening.

However, since the hematopoietic abnormalities are completely reversible, the long-term morbidity of vitamin B$_{12}$ deficiency is restricted to the neurological and gastrointestinal systems. In patients who have had a severe deficiency state with major neurological defects, it is not unusual to see continued difficulties with gait, a loss of position and vibratory sense, and the continued complaint of paresthesias. Chronic problems with gastrointestinal function tend to reflect the etiology of the vitamin B$_{12}$-deficiency state.

Chronic Therapy with Vitamin B$_{12}$. Once begun, *vitamin B$_{12}$ therapy must be maintained for life.* This fact must be impressed upon the patient and family, and a system should be established to guarantee continued monthly injections of cyanocobalamin. An injection of 100 μg of cyanocobalamin, intramuscularly, every 2 to 4 weeks is sufficient to maintain a normal concentration of vitamin B_{12} in plasma and an adequate supply for tissues; administration of larger amounts (e.g., 1000 μg or more as a single injection) has no greater value. More than 90% of such a dose is quickly excreted in the urine, since there is an insufficient number of transcobalamin and tissue binding sites to prevent such excretion. Patients with severe neurological symptoms and signs may be treated with larger doses of vitamin B_{12} in the period immediately following the diagnosis. Doses of 100 μg per day or several times per week may be given for several months with the hope of encouraging faster and more complete recovery. Whether recovery is more rapid has not been proven. While other preparations and regimens described above have been used for maintenance therapy, they cannot be considered to be as reliable as monthly injections of cyncobalamin. Regardless of the method of therapy employed, it is important to monitor vitamin B_{12} concentrations in plasma and to obtain peripheral blood counts at intervals of 3 to 6 months to confirm the adequacy of therapy. Since refractoriness to therapy can develop at any time, evaluation must continue throughout the patient's life.

Other Therapeutic Uses of Vitamin B_{12}. Vitamin B_{12} has been used in the therapy of a number of conditions, including trigeminal neuralgia, multiple sclerosis and other neuropathies, various psychiatric disorders, poor growth or nutrition, and as a "tonic" for patients complaining of tiredness or easy fatigability. There is no evidence for the validity of such therapy in any of these conditions. Maintenance therapy with vitamin B_{12} has been used for the treatment of children with methylmalonic aciduria with some apparent success (Cooper, 1976).

FOLIC ACID

Chemistry and Metabolic Functions. The structural formula of pteroylglutamic acid (PteGlu$_1$) is shown in Figure 57–5. Major portions of the molecule include a pteridine ring linked by a methylene bridge to para-aminobenzoic acid, which is joined by an amide linkage to glutamic acid. While pteroylglutamic acid is the common pharmaceutical form of folic acid, it is neither the principal folate congener in food nor the active coenzyme for intracellular metabolism. Following absorption, PteGlu$_1$ is rapidly reduced at the 5, 6, 7, and 8 positions to tetrahydrofolic acid (H_4PteGlu$_1$), which then acts as an acceptor of a number of one-carbon units. These are attached at either the 5 position of the pteridine ring or the 10 position or bridge these atoms to form a new five-membered ring. The most important forms of the coenzyme that are synthesized by these reactions are listed in Figure 57–5. Each plays a specific role in intracellular metabolism, summarized as follows (see also previous section on Relationships between Vitamin B_{12} and Folic Acid, as well as Figure 57–1):

1. *Conversion of homocysteine to methionine.* This reaction requires CH_3H_4PteGlu as a methyl donor and utilizes vitamin B_{12} as a cofactor.

2. *Conversion of serine to glycine.* This reaction requires tetrahydrofolate as an acceptor of a methylene group from serine and utilizes pyridoxal phosphate as a cofactor. It results in the formation of 5,10-CH_2H_4PteGlu, an essential coenzyme for the synthesis of thymidylate (dTMP).

3. *Synthesis of thymidylate.* CH_3H_4PteGlu donates a methyl group to deoxyuridylate for the synthesis of thymidylate—a rate-limiting step in DNA synthesis.

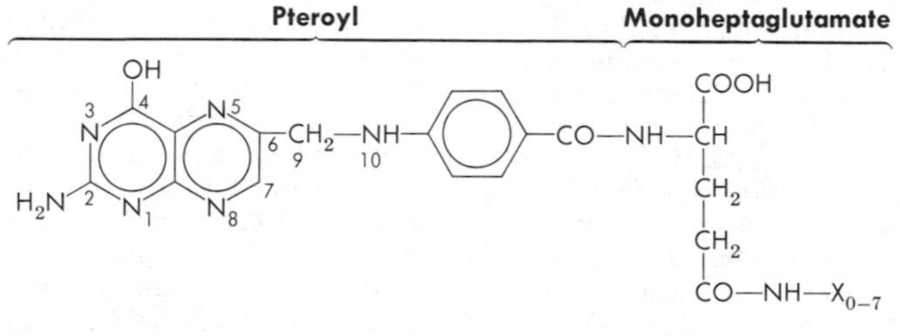

Position	Radical	Congener	
N^5	—CH_3	CH_3H_4PteGlu	Methyltetrahydrofolate
N^5	—CHO	5-$CHOH_4$PteGlu	Folinic acid (Citrovorum Factor)
N^{10}	—CHO	10-$CHOH_4$PteGlu	10-Formyltetrahydrofolate
N^{5-10}	—CH—	5,10-CHH_4PteGlu	5,10-Methenyltetrahydrofolate
N^{5-10}	—CH_2—	5,10-CH_2H_4PteGlu	5,10-Methylenetetrahydrofolate
N^5	—CHNH	$CHNHH_4$PteGlu	Formiminotetrahydrofolate
N^{10}	—CH_2OH	CH_2OHH_4PteGlu	Hydroxymethyltetrahydrofolate

Figure 57–5. *The structures and nomenclature of pteroylglutamic acid (folic acid) and congeners.*

See text for explanation. X represents additional residues of glutamate; polyglutamates are storage forms of the vitamin. The subscript that designates the number of residues of glutamate is frequently omitted because this number is variable.

4. *Histidine metabolism.* $H_4PteGlu$ also acts as an acceptor of a formimino group in the conversion of formiminoglutamic acid to glutamic acid.

5. *Synthesis of purines.* Two steps in the synthesis of purine nucleotides require the participation of derivatives of folic acid. Glycinamide ribonucleotide is formylated by $5,10$-$CHH_4PteGlu$; 5-aminoimidazole-4-carboxamide ribonucleotide is formylated by 10-$CHOH_4PteGlu$. By these reactions carbon atoms at positions 8 and 2, respectively, are incorporated into the growing purine ring.

6. *Utilization or generation of formate.* This reversible reaction utilizes $H_4PteGlu$ and 10-$CHOH_4$-PteGlu.

Daily Requirements. Virtually all food sources are rich in folates, especially fresh green vegetables, liver, yeast, and some fruits. However, protracted cooking can destroy up to 90% of the folate content of such food (Herbert, 1973). Generally, a standard U.S. diet provides 50 to 500 μg of absorbable folate per day, although individuals with high intakes of fresh vegetables and meats will ingest as much as 2 mg per day. In the normal adult, the minimal daily requirement has been estimated at 50 μg, while the pregnant or lactating female and patients with high rates of cell turnover (as in patients with a hemolytic anemia) may require as much as 100 to 200 μg or more per day. Recommended dietary allowances of folate are presented in Table XVI–1.

Absorption, Distribution, and Elimination. As with vitamin B_{12}, diagnosis and management of deficiencies of folic acid depend on an understanding of the transport pathways and intracellular metabolism of the vitamin (Figure 57–6). Folates present in food are largely in the form of reduced polyglutamates (Tamura and Stokstad, 1973). Absorption requires transport and the action of a pteroyl-γ-glutamyl carboxypeptidase associated with mucosal cell membranes (Rosenberg, 1976). The mucosae of the duodenum and upper part of the jejunum are rich in dihydrofolate reductase and are capable of methylating most, if not all, absorbed, reduced folate. Since most folate is absorbed by the proximal portion of the small intestine, it is not unusual for folate deficiency to occur when there is pathology of the jejunum. Nontropical and tropical sprue are common causes of folate deficiency and

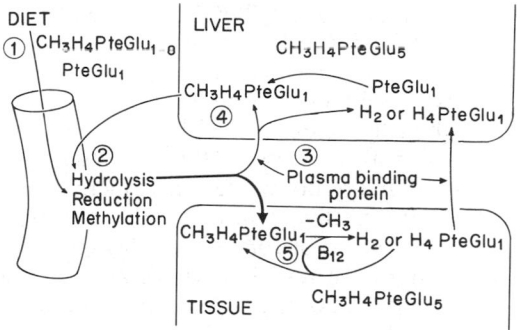

Figure 57-6. *Absorption and distribution of folate derivatives.*

Dietary sources of folate polyglutamates are hydrolyzed to the monoglutamate, reduced, and methylated to $CH_3H_4PteGlu_1$ during gastrointestinal transport. Folate deficiency commonly results from (*1*) inadequate dietary supply and (*2*) small intestinal disease. In patients with uremia, alcoholism, or hepatic disease there may be defects in (*3*) the concentration of folate binding proteins in plasma and (*4*) the flow of $CH_3H_4PteGlu_1$ into bile for reabsorption and transport to tissue (the folate enterohepatic cycle). Finally, vitamin B_{12} deficiency will (*5*) "trap" folate as $CH_3H_4PteGlu$, thereby reducing the availability of $H_4PteGlu_1$ for its essential roles in purine and pyrimidine synthesis.

megaloblastic anemia (Wellcome Trust Collaborative Study, 1971).

Once absorbed, folate is rapidly transported as $CH_3H_4PteGlu_1$ to tissues. While plasma proteins do bind folate derivatives, they have a greater affinity for nonmethylated analogs. The role of binding to plasma protein in folate homeostasis is not well understood (Rothenberg *et al.*, 1977). An increase in such binding capacity is detectable during deficiency of folate and in certain disease states, such as uremia, cancer, and alcoholism. Whether this increase interferes with folate transport and tissue supply requires further investigation.

Following permeation into cells, CH_3H_4-PteGlu acts as a methyl donor for the formation of methylcobalamin and as a source of $H_4PteGlu$ and other folate congeners, as described above. Folate is stored within cells as polyglutamates, which, because of their charge, do not diffuse into the extracellular space (Baugh and Krumdieck, 1969; Hoffbrand *et al.*, 1977).

Supplies of $CH_3H_4PteGlu_1$ are maintained both by food and by an enterohepatic cycle of the vitamin. The liver actively reduces and methylates $PteGlu_1$ (and H_2 or $H_4PteGlu_1$) and then transports the $CH_3H_4PteGlu_1$ into bile for reabsorption by the gut and subsequent delivery to tissues (Steinberg *et al.,* 1979). This pathway may provide as much as 200 μg or more of folate each day for recirculation to tissues. The importance of the enterohepatic cycle is suggested by studies in animals that show a rapid reduction of the concentration of folate in plasma following either drainage of bile or ingestion of alcohol, which apparently block the release of $CH_3H_4PteGlu_1$ from hepatic parenchymal cells (Hillman *et al.,* 1977).

Folate Deficiency. Folate deficiency is a common complication of diseases of the small intestine, which interfere with the absorption of folate from food and the recirculation of folate through the enterohepatic cycle. In acute or chronic alcoholism, daily intake of folate in food may be severely restricted, and the enterohepatic cycle of the vitamin may be impaired by the toxic effect of alcohol on hepatic parenchymal cells; this is perhaps the most common cause of folate-deficient megaloblastic erythropoiesis. However, it is also the most amenable to therapy, inasmuch as the reinstitution of a normal diet is sufficient to overcome the effect of alcohol. Disease states characterized by a high rate of cell turnover, such as congenital hemolytic anemias, are often complicated by deficiency of folate (Lindenbaum, 1977). Additionally, drugs that inhibit dihydrofolate reductase (*e.g.,* methotrexate, trimethoprim) or that interfere with the absorption and storage of folate in tissues (*e.g.,* certain anticonvulsants, oral contraceptives) are capable of lowering the concentration of folate in plasma and at times may cause a megaloblastic anemia (Stebbins *et al.,* 1973; Stebbins and Bertino, 1976).

Folate deficiency is recognized by its impact on the hematopoietic system. As with vitamin B_{12}, this reflects the increased requirement of organ systems with high rates of cell turnover. The megaloblastic anemia that results from folate deficiency cannot be distinguished from that caused by a deficiency of vitamin B_{12}. This is to be expected

from the final common pathway of the major intracellular metabolic roles of the two vitamins. At the same time, folate deficiency is rarely if ever associated with neurological abnormalities. Certainly, the observation of characteristic abnormalities in vibratory and position sense and in motor and sensory pathways rules against the presence of an *isolated* deficiency of folic acid.

The appearance of megaloblastic anemia following deprivation of folate is much more rapid than that caused by the sudden interruption of the absorption of vitamin B_{12} (*e.g.,* gastric surgery). This reflects the fact that stores of folate are quite limited *in vivo.* In Herbert's classical study of a single normal individual maintained on a diet low in folate for several months, megaloblastic erythropoiesis appeared after approximately 10 to 12 weeks (Herbert, 1962). Subsequent studies have shown that the rate of induction of megaloblastic erythropoiesis varies according to the population studied and the dietary background of the individual (Eichner *et al.,* 1971). A folate deficiency state may appear in 1 to 4 weeks, depending on the individual's dietary habits and stores of the vitamin.

Folate deficiency is best diagnosed from measurements of folate in plasma and in cells by use of a microbiological assay or a competitive binding technic. The concentration of folate in plasma is extremely sensitive to changes in dietary intake of the vitamin and the influence of inhibitors of folate metabolism or transport, such as alcohol. Normal folate concentrations in plasma range from 4 to 20 ng/ml. A deficiency state may be considered to be present whenever the value is below 4 ng/ml. In the case of the alcoholic, the plasma folate concentration falls rapidly to values indicative of deficiency within 24 to 48 hours of steady ingestion of alcohol, while megaloblastic erythropoiesis becomes apparent after 1 to 2 weeks (Eichner and Hillman, 1971, 1973). At the same time, the plasma folate concentration will quickly revert to normal once such ingestion is stopped, even while the marrow is still megaloblastic. Such rapid fluctuations are but one example of the dynamic state of the concentration of folate in plasma. Thus, while it is an extremely sensitive measure of the supply of the vitamin available for tissues, it must be determined *before* any therapy is initiated, including the reinstitution of a normal diet. Measurement of folate in red cells or the adequacy of stores in lymphocytes (by use of the deoxyuridine suppression test) may be employed to diagnose a long-standing deficiency of folic acid (Herbert *et al.,* 1973). (In this test, deoxyuridine fails to suppress the synthesis of DNA if normal amounts of folate are present in the cells.) For either test to be positive, a state of deficiency must have existed for a sufficient time to allow the production of a new population of cells with deficient stores of folate.

Preparations. *Folic Acid,* U.S.P. (FOLVITE, others), is a yellow crystalline powder that is quite insoluble in water. It is marketed as oral preparations, alone or in combination with other vitamins or minerals, and as an aqueous solution for injection. Tablets of folic acid contain either 0.1, 0.25, 0.4, 0.8, or 1 mg of pteroylglutamic acid. Folic acid is also available in combination with a number of other vitamins and/or iron in tablets and capsules that contain from 100 μg to 1 mg of the vitamin.

Folic Acid Injection, U.S.P., is an aqueous solution of the sodium salt of pteroylglutamic acid, made soluble by adjusting the pH to 9.0 with sodium hydroxide. It is available in a concentration of 5 mg/ml in 10-ml multidose vials; the vials should be refrigerated and kept in the dark.

Leucovorin Calcium Injection, U.S.P. (*folinic acid, 5-CHOH$_4$PteGlu, citrovorum factor*), is marketed both as a 1-ml ampul containing 3 mg of leucovorin calcium for intramuscular injection and as a vial containing 50 mg of leucovorin calcium cryodesiccated powder, which can be reconstituted with 5 ml of sterile water to make a solution (10 mg/ml) for intramuscular injection. The reconstituted solution must be used as soon as possible, since precipitation occurs on standing.

The principal indication for the use of folinic acid is to circumvent the action of inhibitors of dihydrofolate reductase, such as methotrexate. It is *not* indicated for use in the treatment of folic acid deficiency. Certainly, leucovorin should never be used for the treatment of pernicious anemia or other megaloblastic anemias secondary to a deficiency of vitamin B$_{12}$. Just as with folic acid, its use can result in an apparent response of the hematopoietic system, but neurological damage may occur or progress if already present.

Untoward Effects. There have been rare reports of reactions to parenteral injections of both folic acid and leucovorin. If a patient describes such a reaction before the drug is given, caution should be exercised. Oral folic acid is not toxic for man. Even with doses as high as 15 mg per day, there have been no substantiated reports of side effects. Folic acid in large amounts may counteract the antiepileptic effect of phenobarbital, phenytoin, and primidone and increase the frequency of seizures in susceptible children (Reynolds, 1968). While some studies have not supported these contentions, the U.S. Food and Drug Administration has recommended that oral tablets of folic acid be limited to strengths of 1 mg or less.

General Principles of Therapy. The therapeutic use of folic acid is limited to the prevention and treatment of deficiencies of the vitamin. As with vitamin B$_{12}$ therapy, effective use of the vitamin depends on accurate diagnosis and an understanding of the mechanisms that are operative in a specific disease state. The following general principles of therapy should be respected:

1. Prophylactic administration of folic acid should be undertaken only when there is a clear indication. Dietary supplementation is necessary when there is an increased requirement that is not satisfied by normal dietary sources. Pregnancy, with the increased demands of the fetus, or lactation, where as much as 50 μg of folate is lost each day in the breast milk, are indications for supplementation with folate. The most popular form of supplementation for this situation is a multivitamin preparation that contains 400 to 500 μg of pteroylglutamic acid. Patients with a disease state characterized by high levels of cell turnover (*e.g.,* a hemolytic anemia) should also receive folic acid prophylactically, usually one or two 1-mg tablets of folic acid each day. Finally, any patient who demonstrates folate deficiency because of an undesired effect of a drug (*see* above) may receive supplementation with a preparation of folic acid for oral use.

2. As with vitamin B$_{12}$ deficiency, any patient with folate deficiency and a megaloblastic anemia should be carefully evaluated to determine the underlying etiology of the deficiency state. This should include evaluation of the effects of medications, the amount of alcohol intake, the patient's history of travel, and the function of the gastrointestinal tract.

3. Therapy should always be as specific as possible. Multivitamin preparations should be avoided unless there is good reason to suspect deficiency of several vitamins.

4. The potential complications of mistreating a patient who has vitamin B$_{12}$ deficiency with folic acid must be kept in mind. The administration of large doses of folic acid can result in an apparent improvement of the megaloblastic anemia, inasmuch as PteGlu is converted by dihydrofolate reductase to H$_4$PteGlu$_1$; this circumvents the methylfolate "trap." Such therapy does not prevent or alleviate the neurological defects of vitamin B$_{12}$ deficiency, and these may become irreversible.

Treatment of the Acutely Ill Patient. As described in detail in the section on vitamin B_{12}, treatment of the patient who is *acutely ill* with megaloblastic anemia should begin with intramuscular injections of both vitamin B_{12} and folic acid. Inasmuch as the patient requires therapy before the exact etiology of the disease has been defined, it is important to avoid the potential problem of a combined deficiency of both vitamin B_{12} and folic acid. When both are present, therapy with only one vitamin will not provide an optimal response. Long-standing nontropical sprue is one example of a disease in which combined deficiency of B_{12} and folate is common. When indicated, both vitamin B_{12} (100 μg) and folic acid (1 to 5 mg) should be administered intramuscularly, immediately, and the patient should then be maintained on daily oral supplements of 1 to 2 mg of folic acid for the next 1 to 2 weeks. Indications and recommendations for further administration of vitamin B_{12} are described above.

Oral administration of folate is generally satisfactory for all patients who are not acutely ill, regardless of the etiology of the deficiency state. Even the patient with tropical or nontropical sprue and a demonstrable defect in absorption of folic acid will respond adequately to such therapy. Abnormalities in the activity of pteroyl-γ-glutamyl carboxypeptidase and the function of mucosal cells will not prevent passive diffusion of sufficient amounts of PteGlu across the mucosal barrier if dosage is adequate, and continued ingestion of alcohol or other drugs will also not prevent an adequate therapeutic response. The effect of most inhibitors of folate transport or dihydrofolate reductase is easily overcome by pharmacological doses of the vitamin. Perhaps the only situation in which this is not true is when there is a severe deficiency of vitamin C. The patient with scurvy may suffer from a megaloblastic anemia despite increased intake of folate and normal or high concentrations of the vitamin in plasma and cells.

An oral dose of 1 mg of folate two or at the most three times a day is generally adequate for adults; children should respond to a daily regimen that contains as little as 1 mg of the vitamin. The therapeutic response may be monitored by study of the hematopoietic system in a fashion identical to that described for vitamin B_{12} (*see* Figure 57–4). Within 48 hours of the initiation of appropriate therapy, megaloblastic erythropoiesis disappears and, as efficient erythropoiesis begins, the concentration of iron in plasma falls to normal or below-normal values. The reticulocyte count begins to rise on about the second or third day and reaches a peak by the fifth to seventh day; the reticulocyte index reflects the proliferative state of the marrow. Finally, the hematocrit begins to rise during the second week.

It is possible to use this reliable pattern of recovery as the basis for a therapeutic trial. For this purpose, the patient should receive a daily parenteral injection of 50 to 100 μg of folic acid. Administration of doses in excess of 100 μg per day entails the risk of inducing a hematopoietic response in patients who are deficient in vitamin B_{12}, while oral administration of the vitamin may be unreliable because of intestinal malabsorption. A number of other compli-

cations may also interfere with the therapeutic trial. The patient with sprue and deficiencies of other vitamins or iron may fail to respond because of these inadequacies. In cases of alcoholism, the presence of hepatic disease, inflammation, or iron deficiency can act to blunt the proliferative response of the marrow and to prevent the correction of the anemia. For these reasons the therapeutic trial has not gained great popularity for the evaluation of the patient with a potential deficiency of folic acid.

Adams, J. F., and Boddy, K. Metabolic equilibrium of tracer and natural vitamin B_{12}—an experimental study. *J. Lab. Clin. Med.,* **1968,** *72,* 392–396.

Allen, R. H., and Mehlman, C. S. Isolation of gastric vitamin B_{12}-binding proteins using affinity chromatography. I. Purification and properties of human intrinsic factor. *J. Biol. Chem.,* **1973,** *248,* 3660–3669.

Baugh, C. M., and Krumdieck, C. L. Naturally occurring folates. *Ann. N.Y. Acad. Sci.,* **1969,** *186,* 7–28.

Chanarin, I.; Hutchinson, M.; MacLean, N.; and Moule, M. Hepatic folate in man. *Br. Med. J.,* **1966,** *1,* 396–399.

Cox, E. V., and White, A. M. Methylmalonic acid excretion: an index of vitamin B_{12} deficiency. *Lancet,* **1962,** *2,* 853–861.

Duke, M.; Herbert, V.; and Abelmann, W. H. Hemodynamic effects of blood transfusion in chronic anemia. *N. Engl. J. Med.,* **1964,** *271,* 975–980.

Eichner, E. R., and Hillman, R. S. The evolution of anemia in alcoholic patients. *Am. J. Med.,* **1971,** *50,* 218–232.

————. The effect of alcohol on the serum folate level. *J. Clin. Invest.,* **1973,** *52,* 584–591.

Eichner, E. R.; Pierce, I.; and Hillman, R. S. Folate balance in dietary induced megaloblastic anemia. *N. Engl. J. Med.,* **1971,** *284,* 933–938.

FAO/WHO Expert Group. Requirements of ascorbic acid, vitamin D, vitamin B_{12}, folate and iron. *WHO Tech. Rep. Ser.,* **1970,** *452,* 3–75.

Finch, C. A.; Colman, D. H.; Motulsky, A. G.; Donohue, D. M.; and Reiff, R. H. Erythrokinetics in pernicious anemia. *Blood,* **1956,** *11,* 807–820.

Friedkin, M. Enzymatic conversion of deoxyuridylic acid to thymidylic acid and the participation of tetrahydrofolate. *Fed. Proc.,* **1957,** *16,* 183.

Hakami, N.; Nieman, P. E.; Canellos, G. P.; and Lazerson, J. Neonatal megaloblastic anemia due to inherited transcobalamin II deficiency in two siblings. *N. Engl. J. Med.,* **1971,** *285,* 1163–1170.

Hall, C. A., and Finkler, A. E. Isolation and evaluation of the various B_{12} binding proteins in human plasma. In, *Vitamins and Coenzymes.* (McCormick, D. B., and Wright, L. D., eds.) Academic Press, Inc., New York, **1971,** pp. 108–126.

Herbert, V. Experimental nutritional folate deficiency in man. *Trans. Assoc. Am. Physicians,* **1962,** *75,* 307–320.

Herbert, V.; Tisman, G.; Go, L. T.; and Brenner, L. The dU suppression test using ^{125}I-UdR to define biochemical megaloblastosis. *Br. J. Haematol.,* **1973,** *24,* 713–723.

Herbert, V., and Zalusky, R. Interrelations of vitamin B_{12} and folic acid metabolism: folic acid clearance studies. *J. Clin. Invest.,* **1962,** *41,* 1263–1276.

Heyssel, R. M.; Bozian, R. C.; Darby, W. J.; and Bell, M. C. Vitamin B_{12} turnover in man: the assimilation of vitamin B_{12} from natural foodstuff by man and estimates of minimal daily dietary requirements. *Am. J. Clin. Nutr.,* **1966,** *18,* 176–184.

Hillman, R. S.; Adamson, J.; and Burka, E. Characteristics of B_{12} correction of the abnormal erythropoiesis of pernicious anemia. *Blood,* **1968,** *31,* 419–432.

Hillman, R. S.; McGuffin, R.; and Campbell, C. Alcohol

interference with the folate enterohepatic cycle. *Trans. Assoc. Am. Physicians,* **1977**, *90*, 145–156.

Hitzig, W. H.; Dohmann, U.; Pluss, H. J.; and Vischer, D. Hereditary transcobalamin II deficiency: clinical findings in a new family. *J. Pediatr.,* **1974**, *85*, 622–628.

Hoffbrand, A. V.; Tripp, E.; and Lavoie, A. Folate polyglutamate synthesis and breakdown in cells. In, *Folic Acid: Proceedings of a Workshop on Human Folate Requirements, 1975.* National Academy of Sciences, Washington, D. C., **1977**, pp. 110–121.

Huennekens, F. M. Folate and B_{12} coenzymes. In, *Biological Oxidation.* (Singer, T. P., ed.) John Wiley & Sons, Inc., New York, **1968**, pp. 439–513.

Hutchins, H. H.; Cravioto, P. J.; and Macek, T. J. A comparison of the stability of cyanocobalamin and its analogs in ascorbate solution. *J. Am. Pharm. Assoc., Sci. Ed.,* **1956**, *45*, 806–808.

Kisliuck, R. L., and Sakami, W. The stimulation of serine biosynthesis in pigeon liver extracts by tetrahydrofolate acid. *J. Am. Chem. Soc.,* **1954**, *76*, 1456.

Lindenbaum, J. Folic acid requirement in situations of increased need. In, *Folic Acid: Proceedings of a Workshop on Human Folate Requirements, 1975.* National Academy of Sciences, Washington, D. C., **1977**, pp. 256–276.

Linnell, J. C.; Hoffbrand, A. V.; Peters, T. T.; and Matthews, D. M. Chromatographic and bioautographic estimation of plasma cobalamins in various disturbances of vitamin B_{12} metabolism. *Clin. Sci.,* **1971**, *40*, 1–16.

Mitchell, H. K.; Snell, E. E.; and Williams, R. J. The concentration of "folic acid." *J. Am. Chem. Soc.,* **1941**, *63*, 2284.

Noronha, J. M., and Silverman, M. On folic acid, vitamin B_{12}, methionine and formiminoglutamic acid metabolism. In, *Vitamin B_{12} and Intrinsic Factor: Second European Symposium.* (Heinrich, H. C., ed.) Ferdinand Enke Verlag, Stuttgart, **1962**.

Ramsey, C., and Herbert, V. Dialysis assay for intrinsic factor and its antibody: demonstration of species specificity of antibodies to human and hog intrinsic factor. *J. Lab. Clin. Med.,* **1965**, *65*, 143–152.

Reizenstein, P.; Ek, G., and Matthews, C. M. E. Vitamin B_{12} kinetics in man. Implications of total-body B_{12} determinations, human requirements and normal and pathological cellular B_{12} uptake. *Phys. Med. Biol.,* **1966**, *11*, 295–306.

Retief, F. P.; Gottlieb, C. W.; and Herbert, V. Delivery of $Co^{57}B_{12}$ to erythrocytes from alpha to beta globulin of normal, B_{12}-deficient, and chronic myeloid leukemia serum. *Blood,* **1967**, *29*, 837–851.

Reynolds, E. H. Mental effects of anticonvulsants and folic acid metabolism. *Brain,* **1968**, *91*, 197–214.

Rothenberg, S. P.; DaCosta, M.; and Fischer, C. Use and significance of folate binders. In, *Folic Acid: Proceedings of a Workshop on Human Folate Requirements, 1975.* National Academy of Sciences, Washington, D. C., **1977**, pp. 82–97.

Schilling, R. F. Intrinsic factor studies. II. The effect of gastric juice on the urinary excretion of radioactivity after the oral administration of radioactive vitamin B_{12}. *J. Lab. Clin. Med.,* **1953**, *42*, 860–866.

Scott, J. M.; Bloomfield, F. J.; Stebbins, R.; and Herbert, V. Studies on derivation of transcobalamin III from granulocytes. *J. Clin. Invest.,* **1974**, *53*, 228–239.

Skouby, A. P.; Hippe, E.; and Olesen, H. Antibody to transcobalamin II and B_{12} binding capacity in patients treated with hydroxycobalamin. *Blood,* **1971**, *38*, 769–774.

Stahlberg, K. G. Studies on methyl-B_{12} in man. *Scand. J. Haematol.,* **1967**, Suppl. 1, 3–99.

Stebbins, R.; Scott, J.; and Herbert, V. Drug-induced megaloblastic anemias. *Semin. Hematol.,* **1973**, *10*, 235–251.

Steinberg, S.; Campbell, C.; and Hillman, R. S. Kinetics of the normal folate enterohepatic cycle. *J. Clin. Invest.,* **1979**, *64*, 83–89.

Sullivan, L. W., and Herbert, V. Studies on the minimum daily requirement for vitamin B_{12}: hematopoietic responses to 0.1 microgm. of cyanocobalamin or coenzyme B_{12} and comparison of their relative potency. *N. Engl. J. Med.,* **1965**, *272*, 340–346.

Tamura, T., and Stokstad, E. L. R. The availability of food folate in man. *Br. J. Haematol.,* **1973**, *25*, 513–532.

Weissbach, H., and Taylor, R. T. Metabolic role of vitamin B_{12}. *Vitam. Horm.,* **1968**, *26*, 395–412.

———. Roles of vitamin B_{12} and folic acid in methionine synthesis. *Vitam. Horm.,* **1970**, *28*, 415–440.

Wills, L., and Bilimoria, H. S. Studies in pernicious anaemia of pregnancy: production of macrocytic anaemia in monkeys by deficient feeding. *Indian J. Med. Res.,* **1932**, *20*, 391–402.

Wills, L.; Clutterbuck, P. W.; and Evans, P. D. F. A new factor in the production and cure of macrocytic anaemias and its relation to other haemopoietic principles curative in pernicious anaemia. *Biochem. J.,* **1937**, *31*, 2136–2147.

Monographs and Reviews

Beck, W. S. Erythrocyte disorders—anemias related to disturbance of DNA synthesis (megaloblastic anemias). In, *Hematology,* 2nd ed. (Williams, W. J.; Beutler, E.; Erslev, A. J.; and Rundles, R. W.; eds.) McGraw-Hill Book Co., New York, **1977**, pp. 334–355.

Blakely, R. L. *The Biochemistry of Folic Acid and Related Pteridines.* North-Holland Publishing Co., Amsterdam; John Wiley & Sons, Inc., New York, **1969**.

Castle, W. B. Development of knowledge concerning the gastric intrinsic factor and its relation to pernicious anemia. *N. Engl. J. Med.,* **1953**, *249*, 603–614. (125 references.)

———. A century of curiosity about pernicious anemia. *Trans. Am. Clin. Climatol. Assoc.,* **1961**, *73*, 54–80.

Chanarin, I. *The Megaloblastic Anemias.* Blackwell Scientific Publications, Oxford; F. A. Davis Co., Philadelphia, **1969**.

Cooper, B. A. Folate and vitamin B_{12} in pregnancy. *Clin. Haematol.,* **1973**, *2*, 461–476.

———. Megaloblastic anaemia and disorders affecting utilization of vitamin B_{12} and folate in childhood. *Ibid.,* **1976**, *5*, 631–659.

Das, K. C., and Herbert, V. Vitamin B_{12}-folate interrelations. *Clin. Haematol.,* **1976**, *5*, 697–725.

Glass, G. B. J. *Gastric Intrinsic Factor and Other Vitamin B_{12} Binders: Biochemistry, Physiology, Pathology and Relation to Vitamin B_{12} Metabolism.* George Thieme Verlag, Stuttgart; Intercontinental Medical Book Co., New York, **1974**.

Gräsbeck, R. Intrinsic factor and other vitamin B_{12} transport proteins. *Prog. Hematol.,* **1969**, *6*, 233–260.

Herbert, V. Folic acid and vitamin B_{12}. In, *Modern Nutrition in Health and Disease,* 5th ed. (Goodhart, R. S., and Shils, M. E., eds.) Lea & Febiger, Philadelphia, **1973**, pp. 221–244.

———. Megaloblastic anemias. In, *Cecil-Loeb Textbook of Medicine,* 15th ed. (Beeson, P. B.; McDermott, W.; and Wyngaarden, J. B.; eds.) W. B. Saunders Co., Philadelphia, **1979**, pp. 1719–1729.

Herbert, V., and Bertino, J. R. Folic acid. In, *The Vitamins: Chemistry, Physiology, Pathology, Methods,* 2nd ed., Vol. VII. (Gyorgy, P., and Pearson, W. N., eds.) Academic Press, Inc., New York, **1967**, pp. 243–269.

Herbert, V., and Tisman, G. Effects of deficiencies of folic acid and vitamin B_{12} on central nervous system function and development. In, *Biology of Brain Dysfunction,* Vol. 1. (Gaull, G., ed.) Plenum Press, New York, **1973**, pp. 373–392.

Hoffbrand, A. V.; Ganeshaguru, K.; Hooton, J. W. L.; and Tripp, E. Megaloblastic anaemia: initiation of DNA synthesis in excess of DNA chain elongation as the underlying mechanism. *Clin. Haematol.,* **1976**, *5*, 727–745.

Kass, L. *Pernicious Anemia,* Vol. II. W. B. Saunders Co., Philadelphia, **1976.**

Pratt, J. M. *Inorganic Chemistry of Vitamin B_{12}.* Academic Press, Inc., New York, **1972.**

Reynolds, E. H. Neurological aspects of folate and vitamin B_{12} metabolism. *Clin. Haematol.,* **1976,** *5,* 661-696.

Rosenberg, I. Absorption and malabsorption of folates. *Clin. Haematol.,* **1976,** *5,* 589-618.

Skeggs, H. R. Vitamin B_{12}. In, *The Vitamins: Chemistry, Physiology, Pathology, Methods,* 2nd ed., Vol. VII. (Gyorgy, P., and Pearson, W. N., eds.) Academic Press, Inc., New York, **1967,** pp. 277-301.

Smith, E. L. *Vitamin B_{12},* 3rd ed. Methuen & Co., London; John Wiley & Sons, Inc., New York, **1965.**

Stebbins, R., and Bertino, J. R. Megaloblastic anemia produced by drugs. *Clin. Haematol.,* **1976,** *5,* 619-630.

Stokstad, E. L. R., and Koch, J. Folic acid metabolism. *Physiol. Rev.,* **1967,** *47,* 83-116.

Wellcome Trust Collaborative Study. *Tropical Sprue and Megaloblastic Anaemia.* Churchill Livingston, Ltd., Edinburgh, **1971.**

CHAPTER

58 ANTICOAGULANT, ANTITHROMBOTIC, AND THROMBOLYTIC DRUGS

Robert A. O'Reilly

Therapy with anticoagulant, antithrombotic, and thrombolytic drugs is based on the premise that interference with hemostasis will reduce the morbidity and mortality from thrombotic and thromboembolic disease. Unfortunately, experimental data from laboratory animals have contributed little to the clinical application of these drugs, because the methods used to induce a thrombus are too unlike the natural diseases. Thus, the use of such drugs in patients often is empirical and is based on observations from clinical trials. In addition, secondary prophylactic therapy for established disease is difficult for the physician, because he is apprised more of therapeutic failure, expressed as further thrombosis or as hemorrhage, than of therapeutic success, which can manifest itself only as the absence of thrombosis (Wessler and Gitel, 1979). The disputable good, the potential harm, and the many complexities that the use of anticoagulants entails for both physician and patient may have earned this therapy a dubious reputation. This pessimism is somewhat offset, however, by optimism for the new advances in therapy, particularly with drugs that alter the function of platelets.

MECHANISMS OF THROMBOGENESIS AND BLOOD COAGULATION

Thrombogenesis. *Hemostasis* is the spontaneous arrest of bleeding from damaged blood vessels, which contract immediately when cut. Within seconds, platelets are bound to the exposed collagen of the injured vessel, a process called *platelet adhesion.* Platelets also stick to each other, *platelet aggregation,* and, as they lose their individual membranes, a viscous mass is formed (termed *viscous metamorphosis).* This platelet plug can stop bleeding quickly, but it must be reinforced by fibrin for long-term effectiveness. This reinforcement is initiated by the local stimulation of the coagulation process by the exposed collagen of the cut vessel and the released contents and membranes of platelets. Days later, an ingrowth of fibroblasts along a scaffolding of fibrin repairs the vascular rent permanently upon completion of fibrosis.

Thrombogenesis and hemostasis are similar processes; an intravascular thrombus results from a pathological disturbance of hemostasis. The nineteenth century triad of Virchow that described thrombogenesis in terms of the contributions of stasis, hypercoagulability, and change of the vessel wall is still the basis for current theories. The *white* or *arterial thrombus* is initiated by the adhesion of circulating platelets to a vessel wall. This initial adhesion and the release of adenosine diphosphate (ADP) from platelets is followed by platelet-platelet interaction or aggregation. The thrombus can then grow to occlusive proportions in the areas of slower arterial blood flow. When the thrombus finally occludes the blood vessel, hemostasis occurs locally, and a red thrombus forms around the white thrombus. Thus, when occlusion of the artery is total, a mixed white and red thrombus is present (Mustard, 1977). In contrast, a *red* or *venous thrombus* develops in areas of stagnation or slow blood flow in veins and resembles a blood clot formed *in vitro.* The bulk of it is a fibrin network enmeshed with red blood cells and platelets. A venous thrombus has a long "tail" that can easily detach and result in embolization of the pulmonary arteries. Thus, arterial thrombi cause serious disease by local ischemia, whereas venous thrombi do so primarily by distant embolization.

A platelet plug formed solely by ADP-stimulated platelet interaction is unstable. After the initial aggregation and viscous metamorphosis of platelets, fibrin becomes an important constituent of a thrombus. Production of thrombin (*see* below) occurs by activation of the reactions of blood coagulation at the site of the platelet mass. This thrombin stimulates further platelet aggregation not only by inducing the release of more ADP from the platelets but also by stimulating the synthesis of prostaglandins—aggregating agents that are more powerful then ADP (*see* Chapter 28). Two classes of prostaglandins with opposite effects on platelet aggregation and thrombogenesis are formed. Thromboxane $A_2(TXA_2)$, synthesized by the aggregated platelets, stimulates further aggregation, while prostacyclin (PGI_2), hypothesized to come predominantly from the vessel wall, inhibits thrombosis (Moncada and Vane, 1979).

Blood Coagulation. The coagulation of blood entails the formation of fibrin by the interaction of more than a dozen proteins in a cascading series of

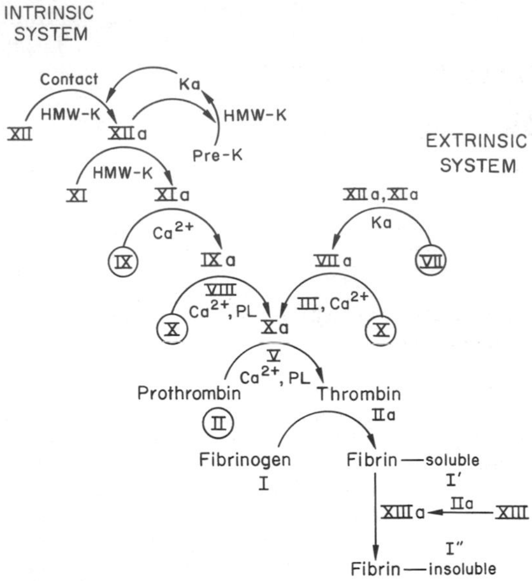

INTRINSIC
SYSTEM

Figure 58-1. *Intrinsic and extrinsic systems of blood coagulation.*

The circled clotting factors are dependent on vitamin K for their synthesis. Hageman factor (XII) undergoes contact activation and becomes bound to surfaces. This surface-bound factor XII undergoes proteolytic activation by kallikrein (Ka) in the presence of high-molecular-weight kininogen (HMW-K) (Ogston and Bennett, 1978). Factor XIIa constitutes an arm of a feedback loop and activates more Ka from prekallikrein (Pre-K or Fletcher factor), in the presence of HMW-K. Factor XIIa in the presence of HMW-K also activates factor XI. Factor XIa in the presence of Ca^{2+} proteolytically activates factor IX to IXa. Factor VIII, factor IXa, Ca^{2+}, and phospholipid micelles (PL) from blood platelets form a lipoprotein complex with factor X and activate it. Factor V, factor Xa, Ca^{2+}, and PL also form a lipoprotein complex with factor II or prothrombin and activate it to IIa or thrombin. In seconds, thrombin splits two small pairs of peptides off the large fibrinogen (I) molecule, followed by rapid noncovalent aggregation of soluble fibrin monomers (I'). Factor XIII, activated by thrombin to XIIIa, cross-links adjacent fibrin monomers (I') covalently to form the insoluble fibrin clot (I'').

In the extrinsic system, factor VII undergoes proteolytic activation by factors XIIa, XIa, and Ka from the intrinsic system. Factor VIIa, Ca^{2+}, tissue thromboplastin (III), and factor X form a lipoprotein complex that results in activation of factor X. From this step onward the extrinsic system is identical to the intrinsic system. Factor Xa is the principal factor that is inhibited by heparin, following the interaction of heparin with its cofactor, antithrombin III.

proteolytic reactions (*see* Figure 58-1). At each step a clotting factor (*e.g.*, XII) undergoes limited proteolysis and itself becomes an active protease (*e.g.*, XIIa)

(Table 58-1). This clotting-factor enzyme activates the next clotting factor (XI) until ultimately an insoluble fibrin clot is formed (Rosenberg, 1978). The soluble precursor of fibrin circulates in the blood as fibrinogen (I). Fibrinogen is a substrate for the enzyme thrombin (IIa), a protease that is formed during the coagulation process by activation of a circulating proenzyme, prothrombin (II). Prothrombin is converted to thrombin by activated factor X in the presence of factor V, Ca^{2+}, and phospholipid.

Two separate pathways lead to the formation of activated factor X and the activation of prothrombin. In the *intrinsic system,* all the protein factors necessary for coagulation are present in the circulating blood. In the *extrinsic system,* unidentified lipoproteins called tissue thromboplastin (factor III), which are not present in the circulating blood, activate blood coagulation at the level of factor X (*see* Figure 58-1). In the intrinsic system the prothrombin-activating principle, factor Xa, requires many minutes for formation, whereas the extrinsic system is activated within seconds because the early time-consuming reactions are bypassed. Both pathways must be intact for adequate hemostasis (*see* Esnouf, 1977; Ogston and Bennett, 1978).

I. Anticoagulants

HEPARIN

History. In 1916, the medical student McLean, while investigating the nature of ether-soluble procoagulants, made the serendipitous finding of a phospholipid anticoagulant. Soon thereafter, a water-soluble mucopolysaccharide, named *heparin* because of its abundance in liver, was discovered by Howell (1922), in whose laboratory McLean had been working (*see* Jaques, 1978). The use of heparin *in vitro* to prevent the clotting of shed blood led to its use *in vivo* to treat venous thrombosis. Improved purification of the tissue extracts in Canada and in Sweden permitted clinical trials with large doses of

Table 58-1. BLOOD CLOTTING FACTORS

FACTOR	COMMON SYNONYMS
I	Fibrinogen
I'	Fibrin monomer
I''	Fibrin polymer
II	Prothrombin
III	Tissue thromboplastin
IV	Calcium, Ca^{2+}
V	Labile factor
VII	Proconvertin
VIII	Antihemophilic globulin, AHG
IX	Christmas factor, PTC
X	Stuart factor
XI	Plasma thromboplastin antecedent, PTA
XII	Hageman factor
XIII	Fibrin-stabilizing factor
HMW-K	High-molecular-weight kininogen, Fitzgerald factor
Pre-K	Prekallikrein, Fletcher factor
Ka	Kallikrein
PL	Platelet phospholipid

heparin in 1938. While Best's suggestion in 1948—that endogenous inhibitors that keep blood fluid might be useful clinically—presaged the possibility of therapy with *low doses* of heparin, the efficacy of this procedure was not demonstrated for more than 20 years. Studies *in vitro* by Wessler and Yin in 1970 and clinical trials by Kakkar and colleagues in 1973 led the way for this important improvement in the use of heparin for anticoagulant therapy.

Chemistry and Source. Heparin is a heterogeneous group of straight-chain anionic mucopolysaccharides, called glycosaminoglycans, of molecular weights that average 15,000 daltons (Jaques, 1977). Less than 1% of the native glycosaminoglycans obtained by alkaline hydrolysis from a covalently conjugated protein core is heparin. Commercial heparin consists of polymers of two repeating disaccharide units: D-glucosamine-L-iduronic acid and D-glucosamine-D-glucuronic acid. In the structure that appears below, the upper disaccharide unit is composed of an iduronic acid and a glucosamine residue, while the lower unit contains residues of glucuronic acid and glucosamine. Most samples of heparin sodium contain 8 to 15 sequences of each disaccharide unit, but not necessarily in equal proportions. Heparin is strongly acidic because of its content of covalently linked sulfate and carboxylic acid groups. Sulfamides and sulfate esters are formed at positions 2 and 6, respectively, of glucosamine, and a sulfate ester is also found at the 2-OH group of iduronic acid (Kiss, 1976).

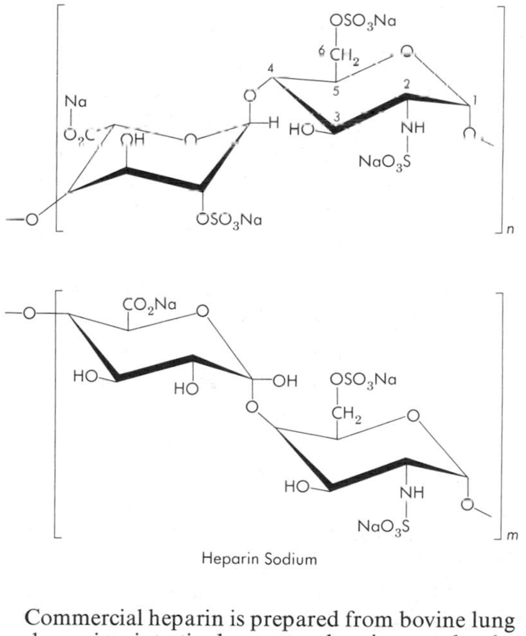

Heparin Sodium

Commercial heparin is prepared from bovine lung and porcine intestinal mucosa, but it can also be obtained from sheep and whales. Although porcine mucosal heparin is more potent in its antifactor Xa activity and plasma lipolytic activity (*see* below) than is that from bovine lung, all heparins are biologically equivalent. However, the incidence of thrombocytopenia is lower with porcine mucosal heparin (Powers

et al., 1979). Since heparin from mammalian-tissue sources is in limited supply, semisynthetic sulfated polymers have been prepared from disaccharides composed of D-glucosamine and D-glucuronic acid. These "heparinoids" have high anticoagulant and lipolytic activities, but their clinical utility has not been tested.

Occurrence and Physiological Function. Heparin occurs intracellularly in mammalian tissues that contain mast cells, but only in a macromolecular form of at least 750,000 daltons. This "big" heparin has only 10 to 20% of the anticoagulant activity of commercial heparin. *Heparan sulfate,* a compound similar to heparin sulfate (in name and chemistry) but with less anticoagulant activity, is a ubiquitous component at the mammalian cell surface (Lindahl *et al.,* 1977). When native heparin is released from its bound and inactive state in the metachromatic granules of mast cells, it is ingested and rapidly destroyed by macrophages (Weiler *et al.,* 1978). Because heparin cannot be detected in the circulating blood and is inactive in its tissue form, its physiological function is still unknown.

PHARMACOLOGICAL PROPERTIES

When injected intravenously, heparin has two major pharmacological effects—impairment of blood coagulation and reduction of the concentration of triglycerides in plasma.

Action on Blood Coagulation and Antithrombin III. The anticoagulant effect of heparin is essentially immediate, and it occurs both *in vitro* and *in vivo*. Heparin acts indirectly by means of a plasma cofactor. The heparin cofactor, or antithrombin III, is an α_2-globulin and a protease inhibitor that neutralizes several activated clotting factors, that is, XIIa, kallikrein (activated Fletcher factor), XIa, IXa, Xa, IIa, and XIIIa. Although antithrombin III was thought to be the only macromolecule able to inactivate thrombin, other plasma proteins are now known to possess this activity. These include the general protease inhibitors, α_1-antitrypsin and α_2-macroglobulin. Antithrombin III forms irreversible complexes with thrombin, and, as a result, both proteins are inactivated (Seegers, 1978). Heparin markedly accelerates the velocity, but not the extent, of this reaction (Barrowcliffe *et al.,* 1978). A ternary complex is apparently formed between heparin, antithrombin III, and the clotting factors (Pomerantz and Owen, 1978). Low concentrations of heparin increase the activity of antithrombin III, particularly against factor Xa and thrombin; this forms the basis for the administration of *low doses of heparin* as a therapeutic regimen.

Patients who receive intermittent or continuous therapy with heparin have a progressive reduction of antithrombin-III activity to values that approximate one third of normal (Marciniak and Gockerman, 1977). Thus, a heparin-induced reduction of the activity of antithrombin III may paradoxically increase the thrombotic tendency in man. The standard regimens for treatment of thromboembolic diseases may require modification to minimize depletion of antithrombin III during therapy with conventional or high doses of heparin (Kakkar *et al.,* 1980). Estrogen-containing contraceptives also reduce the apparent concentrations of antithrombin III. The thrombotic symptoms that characterize familial deficiency of antithrombin III often are first seen during pregnancy. Because the oral anticoagulants (*see* below) *increase* antithrombin-III activity, they are the treatment of choice for patients with this inherited disorder.

Platelet factor 4 is a cationic, low-molecular-weight protein that is associated with a chondroitin sulfate carrier; this factor is released from aggregated platelets during coagulation, and it binds to and neutralizes heparin (Okuno and Crockatt, 1977). Although its physiological function is unknown, platelet factor 4 may bind heparin locally and thereby facilitate the accumulation of thrombin and clot formation. Since the activity of platelet factor 4 reflects both blood clotting and the consumption of platelets, this activity has been measured in many patients with thromboembolic diseases in an effort to detect those at risk from thrombosis.

Lipoprotein Lipase. The effect of injected heparin on plasma lipids, the well-known "clearing" effect of heparin on turbid, lipemic plasma, results from the release into the blood of tissue-bound, lipid-hydrolyzing enzymes. One of these enzymes, lipoprotein lipase, hydrolyzes the triglycerides of chylomicrons and very-low-density lipoproteins bound to capillary endothelial cells into fatty acids and partial glycerides. These products are then metabolized by extrahepatic tissues (Olivecrona *et al.,* 1977). Heparin is thought not to activate these enzymes but to release them from tissues and stabilize them. Lipoprotein lipase activity is high in adipose tissue and skeletal muscle, where the fatty acids released from the catabolism of plasma triglycerides are oxidized aerobically.

Miscellaneous Actions. When added to blood, heparin does not alter routine chemical determinations, but it does distort the morphology of red and white blood cells. Heparinized blood is unsuitable for tests that involve complement, isoagglutinins, or erythrocyte fragility, unless the heparin is removed or neutralized *in vitro* by protamine (*see* below), but it may be used for determination of hematocrit, white-blood-cell count, and erythrocyte sedimentation rate. Blood that is sampled from indwelling venous cannulas "flushed" intermittently with heparinized saline solution contains increased concentrations of free fatty acids; these can inhibit the binding to plasma proteins of lipophilic drugs such as propranolol, quinidine, phenytoin, and digoxin and thus interfere with quantification of this parameter (Wood *et al.,* 1979).

Heparin has been reported to suppress the secretory rate of aldosterone, increase free concentration of thyroxine in plasma, inhibit fibrinolytic activators, retard wound healing, depress cell-mediated immunity, suppress graft-versus-host reactions, and accelerate the healing of thermal burns (Saliba, 1978).

Absorption, Fate, and Excretion. Heparin crosses membranes poorly because of its polarity and large molecular size. It is thus not absorbed from gastrointestinal and sublingual sites; fortunately, its passage both across the placenta and into maternal milk is also hindered. The deep subcutaneous or intrafat injection site is used when therapy with low doses of heparin is chosen and for treatment of ambulatory patients. Intramuscular injection of heparin should be avoided because large hematomas can form at the site of injection. Administration of high doses of heparin is accomplished by continuous or intermittent intravenous injection. The anticoagulant activity of heparin disappears from the blood by *apparent* first-order kinetics; nevertheless, the half-life is dependent on the dose. When 100, 400, or 800 units/kg of heparin is injected intravenously, the approximate half-life of the anticoagulant activity is approximately 1, 2, and 3 hours, respectively (*see* Appendix II). Surprisingly, steady-state concentrations of heparin may not be reached even after 48 hours of continuous infusion because of dose-dependent kinetics and uptake by the reticuloendothelial system (McAvoy, 1979). Heparin is metabolized in the liver by an enzyme termed *heparinase,* and the inactive metabolic products are excreted in the urine. Heparin itself appears in the urine only after administration of large doses intravenously. In patients with renal failure or hepatic cirrhosis, the half-life of the anticoagulant activity of heparin is significantly longer than in normal subjects (Teien, 1977). Patients with pulmonary embolism require higher doses of heparin because of more rapid clearance of the drug (Simon *et al.,* 1978).

Unitage and Preparations. In the absence of a suitable chemical assay, standardization of a sample of heparin is based on comparison *in vitro* with a known standard in a nonspecific assay of anticoagulant activity. The U.S.P. unit of heparin is the quantity that will prevent 1.0 ml of citrated sheep plasma from clotting for 1 hour after the addition of 0.2 ml of 1:100 $CaCl_2$ solution. *Heparin Sodium,* U.S.P., must contain at least 120 U.S.P. units/mg. Because the potency (and chain lengths) of different preparations may vary widely, heparin should always be prescribed on a unit basis. The drug is available as *Heparin Sodium Injection,* U.S.P. (HEPATHROM, LIPO-HEPIN, LIQUAEMIN, PANHEPRIN, others), in sterile water in concentrations of 250 to 40,000 U.S.P. units/ml. *Calcium heparin injection* (CALCIPARINE), widely used in European clinical trials to evaluate low doses of heparin, is reported to cause a significantly lower incidence of local hematoma.

Routes of Administration and Dosage. As mentioned, heparin must be administered parenterally. Blood clotting *in vitro* is fully prevented by a concentration of 1 unit/ml of whole blood. A 10,000-unit bolus of heparin administered intravenously to a 70-kg patient results in an initial plasma concentration of heparin of about 3 units/ml, and anticoagulant activity disappears with a half-life of 1.5 hours. *Intermittent intravenous therapy* is best performed by means of an indwelling, rubber-capped needle (or heparin-lock); a dose of 10,000 units initially, followed by doses of 5000 to 10,000 units every 4 or 6 hours, is administered. The size and frequency of the maintenance dose depend on the weight of the patient and especially on the response to previous doses of the anticoagulant. This response should be measured 1 hour before the next dose. For children, the initial dose is 100 units/kg, the maintenance dose is 50 to 100 units/kg every 4 hours, adjusted according to the anticoagulant response, and the total daily dose is as much as 500 units/kg of body weight or 20,000 units/m² of body surface area. Administration of *low doses* of heparin preoperatively for primary prophylaxis of deep venous thrombosis is begun 2 hours before surgery with 5000 units of heparin administered *subcutaneously;* this dose is repeated every 8 to 12 hours until the patient is discharged from the hospital (Council on Thrombosis, American Heart Association, 1977).

Continuous intravenous infusion is initiated with a loading dose of 5000 to 10,000 units of heparin injected directly into the infusion tubing. A constant infusion pump or a mechanical syringe pump controls the flow rate and fluid volume (Prupas, 1977). A solution sufficient for only 6 hours is prepared to avoid accidental overdose. For a 70-kg patient, 6000 units of heparin is added to 100 ml of 5% dextrose or 100 ml of 0.5% saline solution, and this is infused at a rate of 1000 units every hour. The rate of infusion and the amount of heparin added to each 6-hour aliquot are adjusted to keep a measure of blood clotting, the activated partial thromboplastin time, at least twice that of the patient's pretreatment value.

Thus, the average-sized patient in 24 hours receives 24,000 units of heparin and 400 ml of fluid and requires four changes of the volume-control unit. The site of heparin-lock needles should be rotated every 2 to 3 days, especially in patients who are neutropenic or otherwise susceptible to infections. *Implantable pumps* for continuous intravenous infusion of heparin have been used successfully for as long as 18 months in patients with recurrent venous thromboembolic disease.

Deep subcutaneous (intrafat) injection of heparin has been used to slow the rate of absorption and thereby prolong the therapeutic concentration of this evanescent drug in blood. Technics that are helpful to minimize local ecchymoses include use of a very small (#26), 1.25-cm (½-in.) needle; a 1-ml tuberculin syringe; heparin in high concentrations to reduce the injected volume; gentle grasping of a 2.5- to 5-cm (1- to 2-in.) area of iliac or abdominal fat away from the deeper tissues; rotating the sites of injection; cleaning the needle of any heparin solution before injection; positioning the needle perpendicular to the skin surface; clearing the needle with 0.1 ml of air kept at the plunger end of the syringe, which is injected last; and application of firm pressure over the site for 1 to 2 minutes after injection.

Jet-injected subcutaneous administration of low doses of heparin is less painful and faster than needle injection (Black *et al.,* 1978). *Intrapulmonary administration* of aerosolized heparin to human volunteers results in an anticoagulant effect that lasts for days; this technic warrants further study (Wright and Jaques, 1979). When heparin is administered *intraperitoneally* during peritoneal dialysis, it often loses its anticoagulant activity locally because of the disappearance of antithrombin-III activity (Furman *et al.,* 1978). Heparin may also be inactivated when it is added to the *artificial kidney* because of the influx of calcium, magnesium, and acetate ions from the dialysate.

Side Effects, Toxicity, and Contraindications. Purified commercial preparations of heparin are relatively nontoxic, and side effects from the drug are infrequent. Because heparin is obtained from animal tissue, it should be used cautiously in patients with any history of allergy. A trial dose of 1000 units should precede usual therapeutic doses. Hypersensitivity reactions include chills, fever, urticaria, or anaphylactic shock. Local and systemic allergic reactions to the preservative used in multidose rubber-capped vials have been reported. Heparin intended for use in heart-lung machines is free of preservatives. Increased loss of hair and reversible, transient alopecia have been reported. Osteoporosis and spontaneous fractures occur in patients who have received 15,000 units or more of heparin daily for over 6 months (Avioli, 1975).

Hemorrhage. The chief complication of therapy with heparin is hemorrhage. Bleeding may be reduced to a minimum by careful control of dosage. The anticoagulant effect should be monitored by a test of blood clotting, such as the partial thromboplastin time. Significant gastrointestinal or genitourinary bleeding may be indicative of an underlying occult pathological lesion. Elderly women in particular develop hemorrhagic complications. Increased bleeding by patients in renal failure occurs during therapy with heparin.

Thrombocytopenia. Heparin causes transient mild thrombocytopenia in about 25% of patients and severe thrombocytopenia in a few. The mild reaction results from heparin-induced platelet aggregation, while severe thrombocytopenia follows the formation of heparin-dependent antiplatelet antibodies. The latter is characterized by its delayed occurrence (the eighth to twelfth day of treatment), tolerance to the anticoagulant action of heparin, recurrent thromboembolic disease, a platelet count as low as $5000/mm^3$, elevated fibrin degradation products in plasma, reduced plasma fibrinogen, adequate megakaryocytes in bone-marrow specimens (consistent with peripheral consumption of platelets), and improvement of thrombocytopenia after discontinuation of the heparin. An immunoglobulin G directed against an antigen common to several preparations of heparin has been detected in the plasma of heparinized patients with thrombocytopenia (Trowbridge *et al.,* 1978). It reacts with the heparin-platelet complex to trigger the release reaction of platelets, which results in platelet aggregation and thrombocytopenia. The following considerations apply to all patients given heparin: platelet counts should be done frequently; any new thrombus might be the *result* of the heparin therapy; thrombocytopenia sufficient to cause hemorrhage should be considered to be heparin induced; and thromboembolism thought to result from heparin should be treated by discontinuation of heparin and substitution of an oral anticoagulant, if clinically warranted (Duffy, 1979). Severe thrombocytopenia, hemorrhage, and death have occurred even in patients receiving "low-dose" heparin therapy.

Contraindications. Heparin therapy is contraindicated in patients who are hyper-sensitive to the drug, who are actively bleeding, or who have hemophilia, purpura, thrombocytopenia, intracranial hemorrhage, bacterial endocarditis, active tuberculosis, increased capillary permeability, ulcerative lesions of the gastrointestinal tract, severe hypertension, threatened abortion, or visceral carcinoma. Heparin should be withheld during and after surgery of the brain, eye, or spinal cord and should not be administered to patients undergoing lumbar puncture or regional anesthetic block. The drug should be used only when clearly indicated in pregnant women, despite its apparent lack of transfer across the placenta.

Antagonists of Heparin. Mildly excessive anticoagulant effects of heparin are treated by discontinuation of the drug. If the effects are severe and bleeding occurs, administration of a specific antagonist may be indicated. Protamine is available for this purpose.

Protamine Sulfate. The protamines are proteins of low molecular weight that are found in the sperm or mature testes of fish of the family Salmonidae. They are strongly basic because of their high content of arginine. *In vitro,* protamine sulfate combines ionically with heparin to form a stable complex that is devoid of anticoagulant activity. Protamine administered intravenously in the absence of heparin interacts with platelets and with many proteins, including fibrinogen; these interactions may account for its own anticoagulant activity and toxicity. *In vivo,* protamine inhibits the anticoagulant effect of heparin, but the effect of heparin on platelet aggregation may persist; this persistence may be particularly prominent after open-heart surgery (Ellison *et al.,* 1978). The amount of protamine required to antagonize heparin can be estimated; 1 mg of protamine should be administered for every 100 units of heparin *remaining* in the patient. Alternatively, the requirement for protamine can be determined directly *in vitro* by titration of the patient's blood with the protein.

Protamine Sulfate Injection, U.S.P., is available in 5-ml ampuls and in 25-ml vials as a solution containing 10 mg/ml, and in vials containing 50 mg of the powder. It must be given only by the intravenous route and then slowly (not more than 20 mg/minute, or up to 50 mg in a 10-minute period). Rapid injection may cause dyspnea, flushing, bradycardia, and hypotension, perhaps as a result of the release of histamine. Hypersensitivity reactions have been reported, especially in patients allergic to fish.

Therapeutic Uses. The therapeutic uses of heparin are discussed later in this chapter.

ORAL ANTICOAGULANTS

History. Sweet clover was planted in the Dakota plains and Canada at the turn of the century because it flourished on poor soil and substituted for corn in silage. Schofield (1924) reported a previously undescribed hemorrhagic disorder in cattle that resulted from the ingestion of spoiled sweet clover silage. After Roderick traced the cause to a toxic reduction of plasma prothrombin, Campbell and Link, in 1939, identified the hemorrhagic agent as bishydroxycoumarin (dicumarol) (Link, 1944). Many congeners of dicumarol were synthesized in Link's laboratories, the most useful of which, racemic warfarin, was prepared by Ikawa and associates (1944). (*Warfarin* is an acronym for the patent holder, Wisconsin Alumni Research Foundation, plus the coum*arin*-derived suffix.) Initially it was thought to be too toxic for man, but it became the

world's most useful rodenticide. In 1951, a man survived an attempted suicide with large and repeated doses of a warfarin-containing rodenticide; this event quickly led to clinical trials that established the safety of its use in humans (Link, 1959). The large multicenter clinical trial of the American Heart Association resulted in a report, in 1954, of seemingly favorable responses of patients with myocardial infarction to dicumarol. This unfortunately led to the overuse of the drug. The oral anticoagulants have since become heuristic models in clinical pharmacology for the study of pharmacokinetics and its correlation with biological effects, genetic control of drug metabolism, and the elucidation of mechanisms of drug interactions.

Chemistry. The structure of the hemorrhagic agent of sweet clover disease was found to be bishydroxycoumarin, a derivative of 4-hydroxycoumarin. Many anticoagulant drugs have been synthesized as derivatives of 4-hydroxycoumarin or indan-1,3-dione (Table 58–2). The essential chemical characteristics of the coumarin derivatives for anticoagulant activity are an intact 4-hydroxycoumarin residue with a carbon substituent at the 3 position (Kralt and Claassen, 1972). Acenocoumarol, phenprocoumon, and warfarin all have an asymmetrical carbon atom

Table 58-2. STRUCTURAL FORMULAS OF THE ORAL ANTICOAGULANTS *

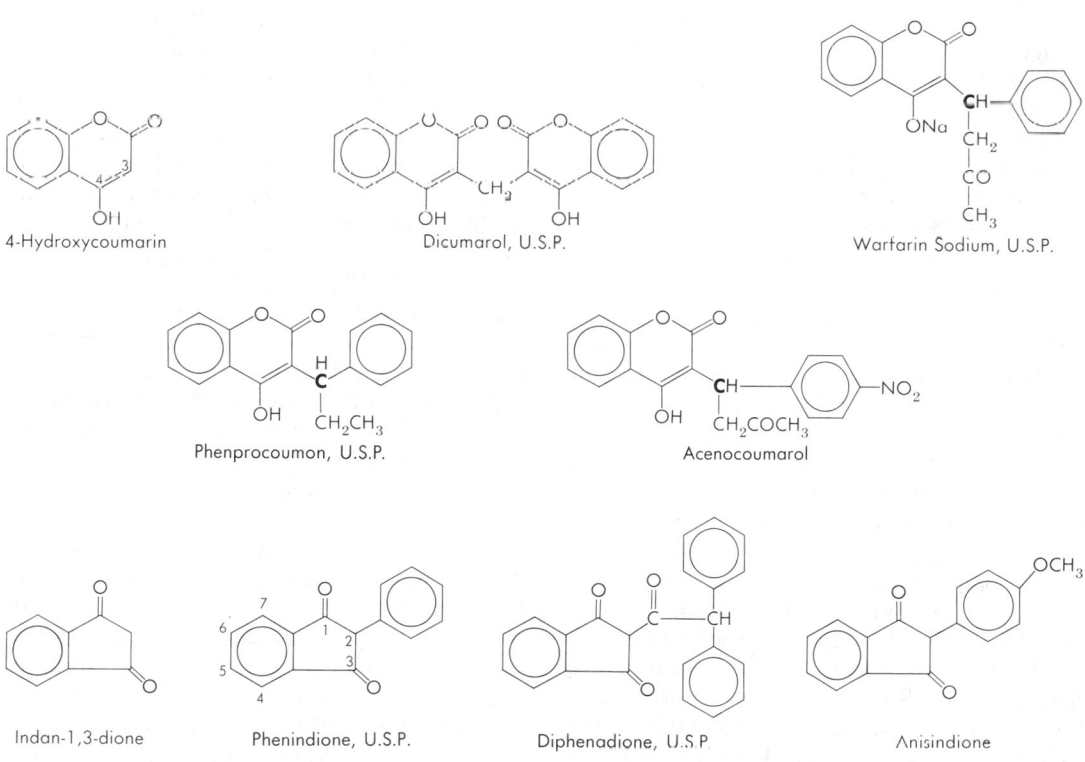

4-Hydroxycoumarin

Dicumarol, U.S.P.

Warfarin Sodium, U.S.P.

Phenprocoumon, U.S.P.

Acenocoumarol

Indan-1,3-dione

Phenindione, U.S.P.

Diphenadione, U.S.P.

Anisindione

* 4-Hydroxycoumarin and indan-1,3-dione are included to indicate the parent molecules from which the oral anticoagulants are derived. Asymmetrical carbon atoms in warfarin, phenprocoumon, and acenocoumarol are indicated in boldface type.

in the substituent at the 3 position, and the available preparations of the drugs are mixtures of the two optical isomers (Renk and Stoll, 1968). The levorotatory or S-(−)-enantiomorphs of warfarin and phenprocoumon are more potent anticoagulants than are the dextrorotatory or R-(+)-enantiomorphs, but the converse has been reported for acenocoumarol (Meinertz *et al.*, 1978). Some of the drug interactions that have been reported for racemic warfarin are more prominent with the S-(−)-enantiomorph (O'Reilly, 1976a).

PHARMACOLOGICAL PROPERTIES

The anticoagulant effects of the various oral agents that are available for clinical use differ only quantitatively. However, there are differences in pharmacokinetic properties and toxicity that make racemic warfarin sodium the drug of choice, the prototype, and by far the most widely used oral anticoagulant in the United States (Hull *et al.*, 1978).

Effects on Blood Coagulation. The major pharmacological effect of oral anticoagulants is inhibition of blood clotting by interference with the hepatic synthesis of the vitamin K–dependent clotting factors (II, VII, IX, and X). These drugs are often called indirect anticoagulants because they act only *in vivo*, whereas heparin is termed a direct anticoagulant because it acts *in vitro* as well. The therapeutic effect is delayed for 8 to 12 hours after oral or intravenous administration of racemic warfarin, because it results from an altered balance between the partially inhibited rates of synthesis and unaltered rates of degradation of the four proteins. The kinetics of the pharmacological effect is thus dependent on the half-lives of these clotting factors in the circulation, which are 6, 24, 40, and 60 hours for factors VII, IX, X, and II, respectively. Larger initial doses of drug (about 0.75 mg/kg of racemic warfarin) hasten the onset of hypoprothrombinemia only to a certain limited extent; beyond this, the rate of onset is independent of the size of the dose. The principal effect of a large loading dose is to prolong the time that the concentration of drug in plasma remains above that required for suppression of synthesis of clotting factors. The 1- to 3-day delay between the peak concentration of drug in plasma and its maximal hypoprothrombinemic effect is consistent with a kinetic model in which a linear relationship is assumed between the logarithm of the concentration of drug in plasma and the reduction of the *rate of synthesis* of the vitamin K–dependent clotting factors (Nagashima *et al.*, 1969). The only significant difference that exists in the inherent ability of various oral anticoagulant drugs to produce and maintain hypoprothrombinemia is their half-life (O'Reilly and Aggeler, 1970).

Mechanism of Action. The oral anticoagulants are antagonists of vitamin K (*see* Chapter 67). Their administration to man or other animals leads to the appearance of precursors of the four vitamin K–dependent clotting factors in plasma and liver. These precursor proteins are antigenically active but are biologically inactive in tests of coagulation (Hauschka *et al.*, 1978). The precursor protein to prothrombin can be activated to thrombin nonphysiologically by several snake venoms, demonstrating that the portion of the molecule necessary for this activity is intact. However, the precursor proteins cannot bind divalent cations such as calcium, and they cannot interact with phospholipid-containing membranes, which are their normal sites of activation. The vitamin K–sensitive step in the synthesis of clotting factors is the postribosomal carboxylation of ten or more glutamic acid residues at the amino-terminal end of the precursor protein to form a unique amino acid, γ-carboxyglutamate. These amino acid residues chelate calcium, which is apparently necessary for the binding of the four vitamin K–dependent clotting factors to phospholipid-containing membranes (*see* Olson and Suttie, 1977). Both oral anticoagulants and deficiency of vitamin K reduce the γ-carboxyglutamate content of *osteocalcin,* a protein of bone. This suggests a mechanism for the production of *chondrodysplasia punctata* in infants born of mothers taking oral anticoagulants during the first trimester of pregnancy (Pettifor and Benson, 1975).

In hepatic microsomes, the reduction of vitamin K to its hydroquinone form (vitamin KH_2) precedes the bicarbonate-dependent carboxylation of precursor prothrombin, descarboxyprothrombin, to prothrombin (Figure 58–2). This carboxylase activity for the synthesis of prothrombin is linked to an epoxidase activity for vitamin KH_2, which oxidizes the vitamin to vitamin K epoxide (KO). An epoxide reductase, which requires

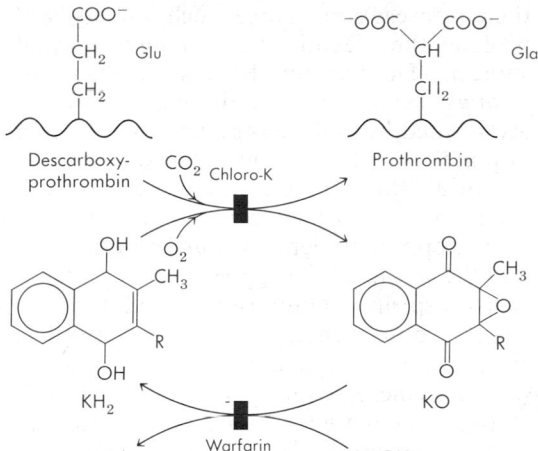

Figure 58–2. *Vitamin K cycle: metabolic interconversions of vitamin K associated with the synthesis of vitamin K–dependent clotting factors.*

Vitamin K_1 or K_2 is reduced to the hydroquinone form (KH_2). Stepwise oxidation to vitamin K epoxide (KO) is coupled to protein carboxylation, wherein descarboxyprothrombin (descarboxy-II) is converted to prothrombin (II) by carboxylation of glutamate residues (*Glu*) to γ-carboxyglutamate (*Gla*). Enzymatic reduction of the epoxide with reduced nicotinamide adenine dinucleotide (*NADH*) as a cofactor regenerates vitamin KH_2. The oxidation of vitamin K is inhibited by the chloro analog of vitamin K (*Chloro-K*), whereas the reduction of vitamin K epoxide is the warfarin-sensitive step (*Warfarin*). The R on the vitamin K molecule represents a 20-carbon phytyl side chain in vitamin K_1 and a 5- to 65-carbon prenyl side chain in vitamin K_2.

reduced nicotinamide adenine dinucleotide, converts vitamin K epoxide back to vitamin KH_2. This reaction is probably the site of action of warfarin (Whitlon *et al.*, 1978) and the site of genetic resistance to warfarin, which is characterized by an increased requirement for vitamin K (O'Reilly, 1971). The vitamin K analog chloro-K_1 (in which the 2-methyl group of vitamin K_1 is replaced by a chloro group) directly inhibits the carboxylase and epoxidase reactions, which are not sensitive to warfarin.

Factors That Affect Activity. Physiological and pathological factors can increase or decrease the response to oral anticoagulant drugs. These factors seldom affect the kinetics of accumulation of the anticoagulant drug, but they do influence its biological effect.

Factors That Increase the Hypoprothrombinemic Response. Inadequate diet, disease of the small bowel, and diseases that hinder the delivery of bile to the small intestine all cause *vitamin K deficiency* and increase the response to oral anticoagulants. Although vitamin K is synthesized by enteric bacteria, antimicrobial agents have little effect on anticoagulant therapy unless both dietary and intestinal sources of vitamin K are simultaneously reduced.

Administration of oral anticoagulants to patients with *hepatic disease* of diverse etiologies results in greater hypoprothrombinemia than when the drugs are given to normal subjects. The effect is ascribable to impaired hepatic synthesis of the clotting factors (Williams *et al.*, 1976). Patients in congestive heart failure who are given oral anticoagulants also have an augmented hypoprothrombinemic response; this lessens as myocardial function improves. Variable results have followed the administration of vitamin K to patients with hepatic disease, apparently because many hemostatic abnormalities can occur in such patients, including alterations of platelets and blood vessels and deficiencies of clotting factors I, II, V, VII, IX, X, XI, and XIII. Because of the sporadic unreliability of alcoholic patients, *chronic alcoholism* may be the most common proximate cause of bleeding in subjects taking oral anticoagulants. When compliant subjects receive warfarin, 10 to 20 oz of wine at mealtime has no significant effect on the steady-state concentration of prothrombin (O'Reilly, 1979).

Hypermetabolic states, such as fever and hyperthyroidism, increase the responsiveness to oral anticoagulants, whereas myxedematous patients require larger doses of these drugs. The reduced dose requirement for oral anticoagulants in patients with hypermetabolic states results from increased catabolism of the vitamin K–dependent clotting factors. There is also a positive correlation between *patient age* and the degree of response to oral anticoagulants; this effect is independent of body weight, and the pharmacokinetics of warfarin is unaltered (Shepherd *et al.*, 1977).

Factors That Decrease the Hypoprothrombinemic Response. During *pregnancy* a state of decreased responsiveness to oral anticoagulants results from increased activity of factors VII, VIII, IX, and X. However, this affects only the mother, and the fetus is highly susceptible to oral anticoagulants because these drugs cross the placenta freely and the fetus has a limited capacity to synthesize clotting factors. As noted above, heparin does not cross the placenta and its use is thus safer for the fetus, but the many injections required and the hemorrhagic complications for the mother remain as formidable problems. Two patients with the *nephrotic syndrome* have been observed to have a high requirement for warfarin; this may be caused by a shortened half-life of the anticoagulant resulting from proteinuria and the excretion of drug bound to albumin. *Uremia* has little or no effect on the hypoprothrombinemic response of patients receiving warfarin chronically, but it does significantly increase both the fraction of the drug in plasma that is free and the clearance of warfarin from the circulation (Bachmann *et al.*, 1977). *Hereditary resistance* to oral anticoagulants, which has been observed in two human kindreds and in rats in many geographic loci, is an autosomal dominant trait. The metabolism of the drug is normal, but the requirement for vitamin K is markedly increased in both species (O'Reilly, 1971).

Drug Interactions. Chronic treatment with oral anticoagulants is frequently necessary in patients who must also take other drugs for serious disease. Drug interactions with oral anticoagulants are all too common, and the ready occurrence of bleeding renders them indelibly obvious and frequently ominous. Drugs most commonly taken that interact with oral anticoagulants are *barbiturates, salicylates,* and *phenylbutazone.* These and other interactions have been studied extensively because of their importance and because interactions of the oral anticoagulants have come to be regarded as a model for understanding the intricacies of this subject. Interactions of both pharmacokinetic and pharmacodynamic types have been revealed.

Drugs That Increase the Response to Oral Anticoagulants. It is hazardous to administer any drug containing *acetylsalicylic acid* during anticoagulant therapy. Even one 325-mg tablet of aspirin can reduce the release of ADP by platelets and thereby impair their aggregation. Three such tablets will prolong the bleeding time of most normal subjects. The bleeding time is a measure of *primary hemostasis,* wherein platelet "plugs" are formed by collagen-induced aggregation of platelets and thrombin-induced formation of fibrin. When there is impairment of both functions—that is, the formation of fibrin (as in hemophilic patients or during anticoagulant therapy) and the aggregation of platelets (when aspirin is administered)—the hemorrhagic consequences can be catastrophic. Furthermore, large daily doses of aspirin (over 3 g) increase the hypoprothrombinemic response of patients taking oral anticoagulants. *Acetaminophen* and *sodium salicylate* are alternatives to aspirin for analgesia and antipyresis in such patients. These drugs do not interact adversely with oral anticoagulants, nor do they affect platelet function. However, there is no good alternative to aspirin for its anti-inflammatory effects in these patients, because other salicylates and even the newer nonsteroidal agents can cause gastrointestinal bleeding and may affect platelet function, even though they do not alter the hypoprothrombinemic response significantly.

Phenylbutazone and *oxyphenbutazone* can cause severe hemorrhage during anticoagulant therapy by impairment of platelet aggregation, induction of peptic ulceration, and augmentation of the hypoprothrombinemia. Phenylbutazone displaces warfarin from albumin and thereby transiently increases the concentration of free warfarin in plasma; chloral hydrate also has this effect. In addition, phenylbutazone interacts stereoselectively with racemic warfarin by inhibiting the metabolism of levowarfarin—the more potent isomer (Lewis *et al.*, 1974). It has little or no effect on the hypoprothrombinemic action of dextrowarfarin (O'Reilly *et al.*, 1980a). Other drugs that increase the hypoprothrombinemic effect of warfarin by alteration of its pharmacokinetic parameters include *disulfiram,* which inhibits drug metabolism, and *metronidazole* and *trimethoprim-sulfamethoxazole,* which selectively prolong the half-life of levowarfarin and thus enhance the efficacy of the racemic drug mixture (O'Reilly and Motley, 1979). *Sulfonamides* and other antimicrobial agents have little effect on anticoagulant therapy unless both intestinal and dietary sources of vitamin K are reduced simultaneously. *Cimetidine* prolongs the prothrombin time by an unknown mechanism (Flind, 1978); this has also been reported for *sulfinpyrazone.*

Clofibrate reduces adhesiveness of platelets and their epinephrine-induced aggregation; it augments the one-stage prothrombin activity; it increases the turnover rate of clotting factors II and X; but it does not affect the steady-state concentration or half-life of racemic warfarin or its enantiomorphs (Bjornsson *et al.,* 1977). Thus, the hemorrhagic complications that occur when therapy with clofibrate and warfarin is concurrent result from an additive hemostatic defect of reduced platelet function and more rapid turnover of the vitamin K–dependent clotting factors. Increased responsiveness to oral anticoagulants occurs with other hypolipidemic drugs, such as D-*thyroxine,* and also with *anabolic steroids.* The administration of heparin obviously complicates oral anticoagulant therapy because of the combined effect of both drugs on the one-stage prothrombin time. If *heparin* is discontinued and the oral anticoagulant continued at the usual dose (*e.g.,* when a patient leaves the hospital), the prothrombin time may be reduced to the normal range of values of the test.

Drugs That Decrease the Response to Oral Anticoagulants. Induction of hepatic microsomal enzymes by *barbiturates* increases the clearance of oral anticoagulants, which correlates with a decrease in the degree of hypoprothrombinemia (Levy *et al.,* 1970). *Glutethimide* has similar effects. The reduced response to oral anticoagulants is exaggerated when dicumarol is administered, because it is absorbed poorly and barbiturates further interfere with this process. *Benzodiazepines* and *chloral hydrate* have little or no effect during chronic concurrent administration of oral anticoagulants.

Rifampin markedly reduces both the concentrations of drug in the blood and the hypoprothrombinemia produced by oral anticoagulants (O'Reilly, 1975). *Diuretics* either have no effect or decrease the response to oral anticoagulants (Nilsson *et al.,* 1978). The latter effect may be due to concentration of clotting factors in plasma subsequent to diuresis, as reported for *chlorthalidone* and *spironolactone* (O'Reilly, 1980b). *Cholestyra-mine* reduces the hypoprothrombinemia and enhances the plasma clearance of oral anticoagulants by increasing the elimination of unchanged drug in the stool. *Antacids* have no effect on the absorption of warfarin or its hypoprothrombinemic effect, although they may impair the absorption of dicumarol. *Vitamin C* in massive doses reduces the hypoprothrombinemic response of some patients on long-term therapy with oral anticoagulants.

Other Concurrent Drug Effects. Case reports of accumulation of *oral hypoglycemic* agents in patients receiving dicumarol have not been substantiated. Intoxication with *phenytoin* may occur with concurrent administration of dicumarol, but not when warfarin or phenindione is used.

Absorption, Fate, and Excretion. Racemic warfarin sodium is rapidly and completely absorbed, and peak concentrations in plasma are reached within 1 hour after ingestion. The bioavailability of warfarin potassium in man is significantly less than that of warfarin sodium (McGilveray *et al.,* 1978). Food decreases the rate but not the extent of absorption of warfarin.

Racemic warfarin in the circulation is almost totally bound (99%) to plasma albumin during long-term therapy, which largely prevents its diffusion into red blood cells, cerebrospinal fluid, urine, and breast milk (Orme *et al.,* 1977). The half-life of racemic warfarin administered by intravenous bolus is 35 hours, and the volume of distribution is that of the albumin space, 11 to 12% of body weight (Wagner *et al.,* 1977).

In man, the dextrowarfarin enantiomorph is metabolized by side chain reduction to a secondary alcohol, whereas levowarfarin is metabolized by oxidation of the ring, primarily to 7-hydroxywarfarin (Lewis and Trager, 1971). These inactive metabolic products are to some extent conjugated with glucuronic acid, undergo an enterohepatic circulation, and are ultimately excreted in the urine and stool.

Preparations, Routes of Administration, and Dosage. *Warfarin Sodium,* U.S.P. (COUMADIN, PAN-WARFIN), is available in tablets containing 2, 2.5, 5, 7.5, 10, and 25 mg of drug. Although the manufacturer still recommends an initial dose of 40 to 60 mg, most physicians avoid a large loading dose in order to reduce the danger of hemorrhage in sick patients who may be particularly sensitive to the drug

(O'Reilly and Aggeler, 1968). Therapy can be initiated with a daily dose of 10 to 15 mg *without* a large loading dose; a daily maintenance dose in the range of 2 to 15 mg is then determined by observation of the one-stage prothrombin activity. Initially, this test is performed daily until the result is stable at about 25% of normal activity. The time between tests may then be lengthened gradually to weekly and later to monthly intervals for patients on long-term therapy in whom the results of the test are stable. *Warfarin Potassium,* U.S.P. (ATHROMBIN-K), is available in tablets containing 5 and 10 mg of drug. *Warfarin Sodium for Injection,* U.S.P., containing sodium chloride and thiomerosal, is available in vials of 50 mg with ampuls of sterile water, but parenteral administration is seldom needed and does not alter the kinetics of response.

Toxic Effects. *Hemorrhage* is the main unwanted effect caused by therapy with oral anticoagulants. *Anticoagulant therapy must always be monitored by determination of one-stage prothrombin times, and the patient must be observed carefully for development of bleeding. Bleeding often occurs even when the prothrombin time is within the expected therapeutic range.* In order of decreasing frequency, complications include ecchymoses, hematuria, uterine bleeding, melena or hematochezia, epistaxis, hematoma, gingival bleeding, hemoptysis, and hematemesis (O'Reilly, 1976b). Particularly *serious bleeding episodes* in patients who are chronically receiving either heparin or oral anticoagulants include compression neuropathy following brachial artery puncture for arteriographic or blood-gas studies, intraperitoneal hemorrhage resulting from rupture of a corpus luteum, retroperitoneal hemorrhage with compression femoral neuropathy, hemopericardium even in the absence of myocardial infarction or pericarditis, intracranial hemorrhage, adrenal hemorrhage, and necrosis of skin and breasts. Identified factors that increase the risk of hemorrhagic complications during long-term therapy include poor supervision of the patient, use of the drug despite medical contraindications, poor control of the drug in relation to laboratory values, administration of large loading doses, administration of therapy that is too intensive for the patient, concomitant administration of interacting drugs, or therapy of the elderly or post-partum patient or those with disorders of the gastrointestinal or genitourinary systems.

The *treatment of hemorrhage* caused by therapy with oral anticoagulants consists in immediate withdrawal of the drug and the oral administration of 10 to 20 mg of vitamin K_1 (*phytonadione*). This regimen will stop minor bleeding and return the prothrombin time to the normal range within 24 hours. Vitamin K_3, or menadione, is *ineffective* as an antidote for hemorrhage from oral anticoagulants. For hemorrhage that is either severe or in a closed body space (*e.g.,* the pericardium or central nervous system), at least 50 mg of vitamin K_1 must be administered intravenously (*see* Chapter 67). If the hemorrhage is not reduced significantly within a few hours, additional vitamin K_1 should be given intravenously and transfusion should be initiated with fresh whole blood, frozen plasma, or plasma concentrates of the vitamin K–dependent clotting factors. After treatment with vitamin K_1, the patient may require higher-than-usual doses of oral anticoagulants when and if such therapy is resumed.

When *elective surgery* is to be performed, the anticoagulant drug may be continued daily, even parenterally, and its hypoprothrombinemic effect partially reversed with one 5-mg tablet of phytonadione the day before surgery or 2.5 mg of phytonadione per day orally for 2 days before surgery. The former method will bring the prothrombin activity from the so-called therapeutic range of 25% of normal to the normal range of 90 to 100% activity; the latter method will bring the value to 50 to 60% of normal activity. The prothrombin activity will return to its previous level of 25% in about 4 days. Alternatively, warfarin may be discontinued and low doses of heparin substituted during the perioperative period for 5 to 7 days, followed by reinstitution of the oral anticoagulant regimen.

Precautions and Contraindications. Long-term anticoagulant therapy of nonhospitalized patients should not be undertaken unless the patient or someone in residence is willing and able to take responsibility for his/her care, has sufficient literacy and visual acuity to read instructions, and is intelligent enough to understand the serious nature of the therapy and the necessity for close control and supervision. Suitable laboratory facilities must be available and used for accurate control of therapy, and the patient must be consistent in keeping appointments. Oral and parenteral preparations of vitamin K_1 should be readily available, as well as fresh whole blood, frozen plasma, and concentrates of the vitamin K–dependent clotting factors for emergency transfusion.

All of the contraindications listed above for heparin apply to the oral anticoagulants as well. In addition, severe hepatic or renal disease, vitamin K deficiency, chronic alcoholism, and a requirement for intensive salicylate therapy are relative contraindications to the use of oral anticoagulant therapy. Physicians experienced with this therapy give their patients detailed verbal and written instructions about the nature of the therapy (Scalley et al., 1979). They point out the danger signs of bleeding and symptoms of recurring thromboembolic disease, the times to contact the physician, the danger of relying on memory for the frequency and size of the drug dose, and the value of keeping a calendar or daily diary of the amount of drug actually taken; they instruct the patient to carry on his person a MEDALERT bracelet, "dog tag," or wallet card to alert medical and paramedical personnel in an emergency. They also order a supply of vitamin K_1 tablets for the patient for emergency use.

Therapeutic Uses. The clinical uses of the oral anticoagulant drugs are discussed later in this chapter.

OTHER ORAL ANTICOAGULANTS

Oral anticoagulants other than racemic warfarin are seldom used in the United States because of their less favorable pharmacological properties.

Dicumarol. Dicumarol, U.S.P. (bishydroxycoumarin), is the agent formed in spoiled silage that causes hemorrhagic sweet clover disease in cattle; it is now prepared synthetically. Dicumarol is slowly and incompletely absorbed by man. The drug has a half-life in plasma that is dependent on dose. It frequently causes mild gastrointestinal side effects, such as nausea, flatulence, crampy abdominal pain, and diarrhea. The recommended dosage schedule is 300 mg the first day, 200 mg the second day, and a maintenance dose of 25 to 150 mg based on the therapeutic response measured by the one-stage prothrombin time. Dicumarol is available in 25-, 50-, and 100-mg tablets and 25- and 50-mg capsules.

Acenocoumarol. This drug is a racemic mixture, of which the dextrorotatory enantiomorph is apparently the more potent anticoagulant. The half-life of the unchanged drug is short in man, about 8 hours, but the anticoagulant activity of its reduced metabolites prolongs the hypoprothrombinemic effect of acenocoumarol (Dieterle et al., 1977). This finding may account for its satisfactory long-term control of prothrombin activity when a 2- to 10-mg maintenance dose is administered just once daily. Loading doses are still recommended for the initiation of therapy: 16 to 28 mg the first day, 8 to 16 mg the second day, and then the maintenance dose as guided by the one-stage prothrombin activity. Gastrointestinal irritation, dermatitis, urticaria, and alopecia have been reported as side effects and may limit the utility of this drug. It is available in 4-mg tablets (SINTROM).

Phenindione. Phenindione, U.S.P. (HEDULIN), which contains an indanedione nucleus also has antivitamin-K activity. Unfortunately, phenindione causes serious side effects, many of which have been fatal, and the clinical use of the drug has thus been sharply curtailed. These toxic effects include renal damage with tubular necrosis, hepatitis, agranulocytosis, and exfoliative dermatitis (Hargreaves and Howell, 1965). A red- to orange-appearing urinary metabolite of the drug can be distinguished from hematuria by its disappearance on acidification. Phenindione cannot be recommended for clinical usage.

Diphenadione. Diphenadione, U.S.P. (DIPAXIN), is also an indanedione derivative and, although it is much less toxic than phenindione, its use has been limited. It has a half-life in man of 2 to 3 weeks, and its duration of action is thus very long. Vampire-bat parasitism of cattle in Latin America has been controlled by injection of diphenadione into the cattle's rumen. After absorption into the circulation, it is ingested by the bats drinking the cattle's blood. The resultant internal bleeding by secondary poisoning with the unchanged anticoagulant is fatal to the bats (Elias et al., 1978). The only side effects reported in man are mild gastrointestinal disorders. Loading doses are recommended for the initiation of therapy: 20 to 30 mg the first day, 10 to 15 mg the second day, and a maintenance dose of 2.5 to 5 mg daily as dictated by the one-stage prothrombin activity. This agent is available in 5-mg tablets.

Phenprocoumon. Phenprocoumon, U.S.P. (LIQUAMAR), is used widely in continental Europe as MARCUMAR. Phenprocoumon is a racemic mixture wherein, like warfarin, the levorotatory enantiomorph is a more potent hypoprothrombinemic agent (Hewick and Shepherd, 1976). Its half-life in plasma is long—6 days. Only nausea, diarrhea, and dermatitis have been reported as relatively frequent side effects. Large loading doses are still recommended for the initiation of therapy because of the long half-life: 21 mg the first day, 9 mg the second day, and a maintenance dose of 0.5 to 6 mg according to the one-stage prothrombin activity; it is available in 3-mg tablets.

Anisindione. This indanedione derivative has a half-life in man of 4 days. Although the drug is far less toxic than phenindione, its use has been limited. It is available in 50-mg tablets (MIRADON).

LABORATORY CONTROL OF ANTICOAGULANT MEDICATION

The goal of laboratory evaluation of anti-coagulant activity in patients is to reduce the frequency of both bleeding episodes and in-effective treatment. The physician should ask the patient about any previous bleeding history, use laboratory tests before treatment to detect defects of hemostasis, be familiar with regimens for the proper administration of an anticoagulant drug, and monitor the antico-agulant effect of therapy in order to optimize its use.

Heparin. The *partial thromboplastin time* (PTT) has replaced the whole-blood clotting time because it is more reproducible, more sensitive to the effect of the drug, and less costly. Even "low-dose" heparin can prolong the PTT of those who are particularly sensitive, prolong the bleeding time of patients who also are given aspirin, and increase the bleeding of wounds and the size of postoperative hematomas (Gurewich *et al.,* 1978). The PTT should be kept as close as possible to twice the patient's pretreatment baseline time (of 30 to 35 seconds) and should be used to modulate both the continuous and intermit-tent methods for administration of heparin. For the intermittent method, the PTT should be performed daily about 1 hour before a scheduled dose. An unexpected test result in a patient is easily adjusted. A PTT that is too long (over 120 seconds) is readily shortened by omitting a dose, since heparin has a short half-life; a PTT that is too short (less than 50 seconds) is readily prolonged by increasing the dose, since the onset of heparin's action is rapid. When "low-dose" heparin therapy is utilized, laboratory tests are generally not necessary to monitor treat-ment; the dosage and schedule are fixed and hemor-rhage rarely occurs.

Heparin and oral anticoagulant drugs often are used together in the acute treatment of thromboem-bolic disease. The problem in the regulation of such concurrent medication is the *combined effect* of the two drugs on the one-stage prothrombin time. Thus, when heparin is discontinued, the prothrombin time will shorten toward normal because the dosage of the oral agent by itself is insufficient. (Heparin has less effect on the P & P and THROMBOTEST methods of the one-stage test because of the tenfold dilution of the patient's plasma [O'Reilly and Aggeler, 1970].) The impact of an infusion of heparin on the prothrombin time can be ascertained by serial performance of the test: before the heparin infusion, during the infusion before the initiation of treatment with the oral anti-coagulant, and during the combined therapy. The effect of heparin on therapy with an oral agent can be minimized by replacing the infusion with inter-mittent intravenous injections and by determination of the prothrombin time just before the next dose of heparin. The dosage of the oral anticoagulant may need to be increased as the heparin is discontinued.

Oral Anticoagulants. Therapy with oral anti-coagulants is best regulated with the original one-stage prothrombin time, by use of a preparation of tissue thromboplastin that has been standardized and a reference plasma from selected patients to form a standard curve (*see* International Committee, 1980). The conversion of the prothrombin time in seconds to percent of normal prothrombin activity partially compensates for variations between different labora-tories, but each physician must determine the thera-peutic and toxic range for the laboratory he uses. The physician should instruct the patient to use the same laboratory and to notify him when this is not possible. The test is sensitive to the presence of sev-eral clotting factors, particularly three of the four that are dependent on vitamin K: II, VII, and X. The prothrombin time should be determined daily when administration of oral anticoagulants is begun and at least once a month in well-controlled patients re-ceiving long-term therapy.

Patients on chronic therapy usually should be maintained at a one-stage prothrombin activity of about 25%, which, expressed in seconds, is about twice the normal baseline of 12 seconds. However, the so-called therapeutic range is based more on the avoidance of bleeding than on the achievement of a proven therapeutic effect. Furthermore, achievement of the therapeutic range during the first few days results primarily from a reduction of the activity of factor VII, which is not involved in intravascular clotting and probably not involved in thrombo-genesis (O'Reilly and Aggeler, 1968, 1970). An un-expected laboratory test result is not easily adjusted. A prothrombin time that is too long (over 30 sec-onds) is not readily shortened by omitting a dose because of the long half-life of oral anticoagulants; a test result that is too short (less than 15 seconds) is not readily lengthened by increasing the daily dose because of the delayed effect of the therapy. A new "plateau" of therapeutic effect is not achieved for 1 to 2 weeks. Wide fluctuations in the patient's pro-thrombin time are usually the result of poor compli-ance by the patient or excessive changes of the daily dose of drug by the physician. Often, a graph of the doses of drug and the results of the determinations of prothrombin time may help one to diagnose the difficulty or may reveal a change that can be traced to the administration or discontinuation of an inter-acting drug.

II. Antithrombotic and Thrombolytic Drugs

ANTITHROMBOTIC DRUGS

The antithrombotic drugs suppress platelet function and are used primarily for arterial thrombotic disease, whereas anticoagulant drugs, such as warfarin and heparin, sup-press the synthesis or function of clotting factors and are used to control venous thromboembolic disorders. The antithrombotic efficacy of the drugs that prevent platelet aggregation has been inferred from tests of platelet function *in vitro, ex vivo* (platelets obtained from the blood of subjects who have received the drug), and from models in experimental animals. Because platelet plugs form the bulk of arterial thrombi, the best therapeutic strategies may be to utilize agents that interfere with the adherence of platelets to vessel walls and to each other. Nevertheless, the proof of efficacy of any agent will come only from extensive clinical trials, which are only now being conducted.

Aspirin. Acetylsalicylic acid inhibits the release of ADP by platelets and their aggregation by acetylating the enzymes of the platelet that synthesize the precursors of prostaglandins and thromboxane A$_2$ (TXA$_2$) that stimulate these reactions (*see* Chapters 28 and 29). Although aspirin is cleared from the body within hours, its effects on platelets are irreversible and thus last for the life of the platelet. Doses (0.325 to 1.3 g) used in studies of the antithrombotic effect may prolong the bleeding time for several days after the drug is discontinued (Weiss, 1978). However, aspirin may neither reduce platelet adhesion to subendothelium nor prolong the reduced survival of platelets that is characteristic of thromboembolic disorders. The inhibition of prostacyclin (PGI$_2$) synthesis in the vessel wall by aspirin may account for these results and reduce its effectiveness as an antithrombotic agent (Moncada and Vane, 1979). Because the results of long-term studies of the efficacy of aspirin in the prevention of cerebral or myocardial infarction are not yet conclusive, these clinical uses must be held in abeyance (*see* Fields *et al.*, 1977; Hennekens *et al.*, 1978; Aspirin Myocardial Infarction Study Group, 1980).

Sulfinpyrazone. This drug is used for its uricosuric properties (*see* Chapters 29 and 38). It also prolongs the survival of platelets in patients with various thromboembolic disorders. The drug inhibits a number of platelet functions, including the release reaction and adherence to subendothelial cells, and inhibits synthesis of prostaglandins. In large, randomized clinical trials in which 200 mg of sulfinpyrazone was taken four times a day, a reduction in the incidence of sudden death after myocardial infarction was described (Anturane Reinfarction Trial Research Group, 1978, 1980); however, no reduction was observed in ischemic stroke or the incidence of death from cardiac ischemia (Canadian Cooperative Study Group, 1978). More definitive data must be obtained before sulfinpyrazone can be recommended as an antithrombotic agent.

Dipyridamole. This drug is a vasodilator that, in combination with warfarin, inhibits embolization from prosthetic heart valves and, in combination with aspirin, prolongs the survival of platelets in patients with thrombotic diseases. Dipyridamole by itself has little or no clinical effect. It may interfere with platelet function by potentiating the effect of prostacyclin (PGI$_2$) or by inhibiting cyclic nucleotide phosphodiesterase activity, thereby increasing the intracellular concentration of cyclic adenosine 3',5'-monophosphate (cyclic AMP) (Moncada and Korbut, 1978). A large study of recurrent myocardial infarction called *PARIS* is evaluating the use of three regimens. These include daily doses of dipyridamole (225 mg) plus aspirin (1 g), aspirin (1 g), and placebo. The only current recommended use of dipyridamole is for primary prophylaxis of thromboemboli in patients with prosthetic heart valves; the drug is given in combination with warfarin. Dipyridamole is available in 25-mg tablets (PERSANTINE).

Dextran 70 and Dextran 75. These substances, which are used as plasma expanders, are partially hydrolyzed polymers of glucose that are obtained from the bacterium *Leuconostoc mesenteroides* (*see* Chapter 35). Dextran added to blood *in vitro* has no effect on platelet function; however, the bleeding time, polymerization of fibrin, and platelet function may be impaired *in vivo*. Infusions of dextran increase the colloidal osmotic pressure, which necessitates care in their use in patients with pulmonary edema, congestive heart failure, and decreased renal function. Dextran-induced formation of rouleaux interferes with blood typing, cross matching, and Rh testing, which requires the performance of those tests on blood obtained before dextran infusion. Dextran is contraindicated in patients with significant anemia, severe thrombocytopenia, and reduced concentrations of fibrinogen in plasma. Side effects include occasional urticaria, wheezing, a feeling of tightness in the chest, mild hypotension, and, rarely, severe anaphylaxis. Dextran continues to be studied in randomized double-blind trials for efficacy in the prevention of postoperative thromboembolic disease in surgical patients (Davies, 1978). *Dextran 70* is available as a 6% injection with 5% dextrose solution in 500-ml bottles (MACRODEX) or as a 6% injection with 0.9% sodium chloride solution in 250- and 500-ml bottles. *Dextran 75* is available as a 6% injection with 5% dextrose solution in 500-ml bottles, a 6% injection with 10% invert sugar solution in 500-ml bottles (GENTRAN 75 AND 10% TRAVERT), and a 6% injection with 0.9% sodium chloride solution in 500-ml bottles and plastic containers.

Clofibrate. Clofibrate is a hypolipidemic drug that may reduce platelet adhesiveness *in vitro* and increase abnormally short survival of platelets in some patients with coronary artery disease. Previous favorable results with clofibrate in patients with angina pectoris have not been confirmed in a large, randomized clinical trial in patients who had suffered a myocardial infarction (Coronary Drug Project Research Group, 1975). Its use as an antithrombotic agent cannot be recommended. Clofibrate is discussed further in Chapter 34.

THROMBOLYTIC DRUGS

Streptokinase and urokinase are proteins that have demonstrated efficacy for the treatment of acute thromboembolic disease. They promote the dissolution of thrombi by stimulating the conversion of endogenous plasminogen to *plasmin* (fibrinolysin), a proteolytic enzyme that hydrolyzes fibrin. Because these drugs can profoundly alter hemostasis, they should be used only by physicians who have had extensive experience in the management of thromboembolic disease. Thrombolytic therapy is indicated in patients with extensive pulmonary emboli and in severe iliofemoral thrombophlebitis (*see* Bell and Meek, 1979).

Streptokinase (STREPTASE) is a protein without known enzymatic activity that is obtained from group-C beta-hemolytic streptococci. It interacts with the proactivator of plasminogen. This complex, which has protease activity, catalyzes the conversion of plasminogen to plasmin. Following the administration of streptokinase there is a high incidence of bleeding from sites of percutaneous trauma and in wounds, because plasmin lyses fibrin in hemostatic plugs and degrades fibrinogen and factors V and VII. Thus, concurrent use of an anticoagulant or a drug that prevents agglutination of platelets should be avoided when streptokinase (or urokinase) is being given. Fever is common, and allergic reactions and even anaphylaxis result from the formation of antibodies, which may interfere with prolonged or future treatment. Furthermore, naturally occurring antistreptococcal antibodies cross-react with streptokinase and reduce its ability to prolong the thrombin time (Verstraete, 1978). Streptokinase has been used successfully to treat acute pulmonary embolism and deep-vein thrombosis, but randomized, controlled trials are needed to determine whether mortality is lowered. The usual loading dose of streptokinase is 250,000 international units (I.U.), given intravenously over a 30-minute period, followed by 100,000 I.U. per hour, adjusted according to the thrombin time. Therapy is continued for 24 to 72 hours and must be monitored by the thrombin time, which should be prolonged by two to five times the control value. A 24-hour course of treatment with streptokinase is currently expensive (about $250). Heparin and oral anticoagulants should be administered after treatment with streptokinase has been completed. Streptokinase is available as lyophilized powder in vials of 100,000, 250,000, and 750,000 I.U. for reconstitution in 0.9% saline or 5% dextrose solution. Streptokinase is also under study for its potential value in the therapy of acute myocardial infarction (*see* European Cooperative Study Group, 1979).

Urokinase (ABBOKINASE) is a proteolytic enzyme, and its only known natural substrate, plasminogen, is activated by urokinase to the fibrinolytic enzyme plasmin. Urokinase, originally isolated from human urine, is prepared from cultures of human renal cells. A controlled study to evaluate urokinase resulted in the observation of accelerated resolution of pulmonary emboli, but the incidence of bleeding was twofold higher than in heparin-treated patients. Urokinase is contraindicated in children or in patients with any kind of healing wound, recent trauma, visceral or intracranial malignancy, pregnancy, or recent cerebrovascular accident, in addition to *all* of the contraindications listed for heparin and oral anticoagulants. Febrile episodes occasionally occur, but serious allergic reactions are rare. The usual intravenous loading dose of urokinase is 4400 I.U./kg, given over a period of 10 minutes, followed by a continuous infusion of 4400 I.U./kg per hour for 12 hours and then by heparin or oral anticoagulants (Sasahara *et al.*, 1979). It is not necessary to monitor the thrombin time during treatment with urokinase, but it should be evaluated before heparin is given. A course of therapy is currently very expensive, about $3000. It should be used when indicated for patients who are allergic to streptokinase. It is available as a lyophilized powder in vials of 250,000 I.U. for reconstitution by the aseptic addition of sterile water; the solution is further diluted with 0.9% saline just prior to intravenous infusion.

Aminocaproic Acid, U.S.P. (AMICAR), is a specific antidote for an overdose of a fibrinolytic agent. It is available as an injection (250 mg/ml), a syrup (250 mg/ml), and tablets (500 mg). The usual dose is 5 g initially (orally or intravenously), followed by 1.25 g per hour until bleeding is under control. The dosage should not exceed 30 g in 24 hours. Rapid intravenous administration should be avoided to prevent hypotension, bradycardia, and other arrhythmias (*see* Griffen and Ellman, 1978).

III. Therapeutic Uses of Anticoagulant, Antithrombotic, and Thrombolytic Drugs

The anticoagulant model for prevention of thromboembolic disease suggests that slowing the rate of formation of fibrin should have therapeutic efficacy. Because fibrin thrombi occur primarily in the venous system, anticoagulant drugs are used in the prophylaxis of venous thrombosis. Low doses of heparin have been used for primary prophylaxis in patients who are undergoing elective surgery, to prevent postoperative venous thrombosis. Heparin in conventional doses and oral anticoagulants have been used as secondary prophylaxis to prevent the extension or recurrence of venous thrombi, thrombophlebitis, or pulmonary emboli.

The antithrombotic model for treatment of thromboembolic disease suggests that inhibition of platelet function should have therapeutic efficacy. Because platelet thrombi occur primarily in the arterial system, antithrombotic drugs are used in patients with arterial thrombi in the heart and brain. Several antithrombotic drugs are being evaluated as secondary prophylactic agents to prevent recurrence of myocardial infarctions and strokes. Oral anticoagulant drugs have no effect on platelets and, therefore, no place in the treatment of thrombotic disease in the arterial system.

The thrombolytic model suggests that activation of the fibrinolytic mechanism by the formation of plasmin will dissolve thrombi that have already formed. Fibrinolytic agents are now available for the treatment of patients with established pulmonary emboli or with proximal venous thrombi, such as occur in iliofemoral thrombosis.

Myocardial Infarction. The acute phase of myocardial infarction was one of the earliest disorders in which therapy with oral anticoagulants was employed. The hope was that anticoagulant therapy would at least reduce the incidence of secondary thromboembolism. While there have been a large number of conflicting studies over several decades, many of the discrepant findings are explained by failure, at that time, to understand the elements of the randomized, controlled clinical trial (*see* Selzer, 1978). Recent studies with oral anticoagulants have indicated short-term efficacy only in women and long-term efficacy only when results from the patients in multiple studies were pooled (Chalmers *et al.,* 1977). Low doses of heparin provide primary prophylaxis against thromboembolism after myocardial infarction, and drugs that prevent aggregation of platelets increase platelet survival and improve the patency of surgically implanted bypass grafts in patients with coronary artery disease (Steele *et al.,* 1978). Three large-scale, controlled studies on the effects of antiplatelet drugs on mortality after myocardial infarction have recently been completed. The Aspirin in Myocardial Infarction Study (AMIS) showed little evidence of a beneficial effect of aspirin (Aspirin Myocardial Infarction Study Group, 1980); the study on sulfinpyrazone in myocardial reinfarction demonstrated a beneficial effect that lacked statistical significance, although the incidence of sudden death was lowered (Anturane Reinfarction Trial Research Group, 1980); and the combined use of dipyridamole and aspirin in the Persantine Aspirin Reinfarction Study (PARIS) also showed an insignificant effect (Marx, 1980). Thus, no antithrombotic agent can be recommended unequivocally at this time in the prevention of myocardial reinfarction (Mackie and Douglas, 1978).

Cerebrovascular Disease. Treatment of completed strokes with oral anticoagulants declined because of the high incidence of intracranial bleeding apparently caused by the drugs. Treatment of a stroke-in-progress is contraindicated because the stroke can result from hemorrhage or from proximal arterial stenosis; surgery is indicated in the latter case. Multiple episodes of transient ischemic attacks are treated with anticoagulants, and the use of inhibitors of platelet aggregation in this condition is under investigation (*see* Olsson *et al.,* 1980). The high incidence of deep-vein thrombosis in hemiplegics and quadriplegics has been reduced significantly by the use of low doses of heparin as primary prophylaxis after an acute stroke.

Rheumatic Heart Disease. Thromboembolism occurs in rheumatic heart disease typically as a result of disease of the mitral valve with atrial fibrillation. Primary therapy of these disorders is valvular surgery and conversion of the atrial fibrillation to sinus rhythm; this reduces the thromboembolic risk factor of atrial stasis. When such therapy cannot be used or is not successful in eliminating thromboembolic disease, the administration of oral anticoagulants can reduce the number of embolic episodes. Oral anticoagulants, often in combination with an inhibitor of platelet aggregation like dipyridamole, are also useful in long-term reduction of the incidence of thromboembolism associated with surgical placement of a prosthetic valve, even when the valves are made with the newer, less thrombogenic materials. Some cardiologists advocate the administration of oral anticoagulants for 1 to 2 weeks to patients with atrial fibrillation before attempted conversion to sinus rhythm.

Venous Thrombosis and Pulmonary Embolism. *Secondary prophylactic treatment* of these diseases with heparin and the oral anticoagulants is the oldest use of these drugs. The recent demonstration of marked antifactor-X activity as a result of heparin-induced antithrombin-III hyperactivity led to the successful application of low doses of heparin for *primary prophylaxis* of deep-vein thrombosis and of pulmonary embolism after surgery. This regimen consists of a dose of 5000 units of heparin administered subcutaneously, once 2 hours prior to the elective surgery and then every 8 to 12 hours thereafter for at least 7 days. A highly significant reduction in the occurrence of deep-vein thrombosis, with no appreciable increase in the requirement for transfusions or in the incidence of hematoma, has been reported, even for neurosurgical patients (Cerrato *et al.,* 1978). This form of prophylaxis was ineffective, however, in surgical patients who underwent total hip replacement, except when used in combination with *dihydroergotamine mesylate,* a drug that increases venous return from the limbs by constricting capacitance vessels (Kakkar *et al.,* 1979). The many *mechanical means* of preventing venous stasis in the legs include early ambulation, elastic stockings, leg elevation and exercises, intermittent pneumatic compression devices applied to the legs, intermittent galvanic stimulation of the calf muscles, and graduated compression diminishing from the ankle proximally. However, these devices and technics, designed to prevent stasis, have seldom been evaluated by randomized, clinical trials (Turpie *et al.,* 1979).

The best "treatment" of pulmonary embolus is its prevention by primary prophylaxis of deep-vein thrombosis in the proximal iliofemoral venous system. Such primary prophylaxis with low doses of heparin has been correlated with prevention of deep-vein thrombosis in the distal venous system of the calf in patients at high risk for formation of thrombi, as detected with [^{125}I] fibrinogen. Known *risk factors* include injury; surgery, especially in patients over the age of 40 years; malignancy; congestive heart failure; varicose veins; obesity; pregnancy; the use of oral contraceptives; immobilization from strokes, paraplegia, or heart attacks; and previous venous thromboembolic disease (Morris and Mitchell, 1978).

The treatment of pulmonary emboli and deep-vein thrombi is more established by practice than by randomized, control trials. Conventional doses of heparin in the hospital, followed by chronic administration of oral anticoagulants, is the traditional therapy for the prevention of recurrence or extension of these lesions. Dissolution of massive pulmonary emboli by thrombolytic drugs can be lifesaving.

Miscellaneous Uses. Heparin may be of value in selected cases of *disseminated intravascular coagulation* (DIC), a syndrome in which the blood is incoagulable and extensive intravascular fibrin thrombi are present. DIC occurs in patients desperately ill from a variety of serious causes, including obstetrical, infectious, and malignant disorders. The widespread development of thrombi consumes clotting factors, and the resultant bleeding becomes an additional grave problem. Heparin sometimes arrests the intravascular coagulation and thereby allows accumulation of normal amounts of coagulation factors and cessation of bleeding. However, bleeding may sometimes be aggravated by heparin, or DIC may occur during the course of heparin therapy. The administration of protamine may then be necessary. It is difficult to select patients with DIC who should be treated with heparin and to forecast the outcome (Hamilton *et al.*, 1978).

To avoid thrombus formation in a cannula used for an intravenous infusion, heparin can be added to the solution or can be bound ionically to the surface of the cannula when manufactured (Larsson *et al.*, 1977). Heparinization of the patient or the extracorporeal device is mandatory for cardiovascular surgery and hemodialysis, to prevent blood coagulation and deposition of thrombotic material in heart-lung machines and dialyzers.

Anturane Reinfarction Trial Research Group. Sulfinpyrazone in the prevention of cardiac death after myocardial infarction. *N. Engl. J. Med.*, **1978**, *298*, 289–295.

——. Sulfinpyrazone in the prevention of sudden death after myocardial infarction. *Ibid.*, **1980**, *302*, 250–256.

Aspirin Myocardial Infarction Study Group. A randomized, controlled trial of aspirin in persons recovered from myocardial infarction. *J.A.M.A.*, **1980**, *243*, 661–669.

Avioli, L. V. Heparin-induced osteopenia: an appraisal. *Adv. Exp. Med. Biol.*, **1975**, *52*, 375–387.

Bachmann, K.; Shapiro, R.; and Mackiewicz, J. Warfarin elimination and responsiveness in patients with renal dysfunction. *J. Clin. Pharmacol.*, **1977**, *17*, 292–299.

Bjornsson, T. D.; Meffin, P. J.; and Blaschke, T. F. Inter-

action of clofibrate with warfarin. I. Effect of clofibrate on the disposition of the optical enantiomorphs of warfarin. *J. Pharmacokinet. Biopharm.*, **1977**, *5*, 495–505.

Black, J.; Nagle, C. J.; and Strachan, C. J. L. Prophylactic low-dose heparin by jet injection. *Br. Med. J.*, **1978**, *2*, 95.

Canadian Cooperative Study Group. A randomized trial of aspirin and sulfinpyrazone in threatened stroke. *N. Engl. J. Med.*, **1978**, *299*, 53–59.

Cerrato, D.; Ariano, C.; and Fiacchino, F. Deep vein thrombosis and low-dose heparin prophylaxis in neurosurgical patients. *J. Neurosurg.*, **1978**, *49*, 378–381.

Chalmers, T. C.; Matta, R. J.; Smith, H., Jr.; and Kunzler, A. M. Evidence favoring the use of anticoagulants in the hospital phase of acute myocardial infarction. *N. Engl. J. Med.*, **1977**, *297*, 1091–1096.

Coronary Drug Project Research Group. Clofibrate and niacin in coronary heart disease. *J.A.M.A.*, **1975**, *231*, 360–381.

Council on Thrombosis, American Heart Association. Special report: prevention of venous thromboembolism in surgical patients by low-dose heparin. *Circulation*, **1977**, *55*, 423A–426A.

Davies, W. T. Dextran or heparin? *Lancet*, **1978**, *2*, 732.

Dieterle, V.; Faigle, J. W.; Montigel, C.; Sulc, M.; and Theobald, W. Biotransformation and pharmacokinetics of acenocoumarol (SINTROM) in man. *Eur. J. Clin. Pharmacol.*, **1977**, *11*, 367–375.

Duffy, T. P. Heparin-induced thrombocytopenia. (Editorial.) *J.A.M.A.*, **1979**, *241*, 2424.

Elias, D. J.; Thompson, R. D.; and Savarie, P. J. Effects of the anticoagulant diphenadione on suckling calves. *Bull. Environ. Contam. Toxicol.*, **1978**, *20*, 71–78.

Ellison, N.; Edmunds, L. H., Jr.; and Colman, R. W. Platelet aggregation following heparin and protamine administration. *Anesthesiology*, **1978**, *48*, 65–68.

European Cooperative Study Group for Streptokinase Treatment of Acute Myocardial Infarction. Streptokinase in acute myocardial infarction. *N. Engl. J. Med.*, **1979**, *301*, 797–802.

Fields, W. S.; Lemak, N. A.; Frankowski, R. F.; and Hardy, R. J. Controlled trial of aspirin in cerebral ischemia. *Stroke*, **1977**, *8*, 301–314.

Flind, A. C. Cimetidine and oral anticoagulants. *Br. Med. J.*, **1978**, *2*, 1367.

Furman, K. I.; Gomperts, E. D.; and Hockley, J. Activity of intraperitoneal heparin during peritoneal dialysis. *Clin. Nephrol.*, **1978**, *9*, 15–18.

Gurewich, V.; Nunn, T.; Kuriakose, T. T. X.; and Hume, M. Hemostatic effects of uniform, low-dose subcutaneous heparin in surgical patients. *Arch. Intern. Med.*, **1978**, *138*, 41–44.

Hargreaves, T., and Howell, M. Phenindione jaundice. *Br. Heart J.*, **1965**, *27*, 932–936.

Hauschka, P. V.; Lian, J. B.; and Gallop, P. M. Vitamin K and mineralization. *Trends Biochem. Sci.*, **1978**, *3*, 75–78.

Hennekens, C. H.; Karlson, L. K.; and Rosner, B. A case-control study of regular aspirin use and coronary deaths. *Circulation*, **1978**, *58*, 35–38.

Hewick, D. S., and Shepherd, A. M. M. The plasma elimination of the enantiomers of phenprocoumon in man. *J. Pharm. Pharmacol.*, **1976**, *28*, 257–258.

Howell, W. H. Heparin, an anticoagulant. Preliminary communication. *Am. J. Physiol.*, **1922**, *63*, 434–435.

Hull, J. H.; Murray, W. J.; Brown, H. S.; Williams, B. O.; Chi, S. L.; and Koch, G. G. Potential anticoagulant drug interactions in ambulatory patients. *Clin. Pharmacol. Ther.*, **1978**, *24*, 644–649.

Ikawa, M.; Stahmann, M. A.; and Link, K. P. Studies on 4-hydroxycoumarins. V. Condensation of alpha, beta-unsaturated ketones with 4-hydroxycoumarin. *J. Am. Chem. Soc.*, **1944**, *66*, 902–906.

International Committee on Thrombosis and Haemostasis/International Committee for Standardization in Hematology. Prothrombin time standardization: report of the expert panel on oral anticoagulant control. *Thromb. Haemostas.,* **1980,** *42,* 1073–1114.

Jaques, L. B. Addendum: the discovery of heparin. *Semin. Thromb. Hemostas.,* **1978,** *4,* 350–353.

Kakkar, V. V.; Bentley, P. G.; Scully, M. F.; MacGregor, I. R.; Jones, N. A. G.; and Webb, P. J. Antithrombin III and heparin. *Lancet,* **1980,** *1,* 103–104.

Kakkar, V. V.; Stamatakis, J. D.; Bentley, P. G.; Lawrence, D.; DeHaas, H. A.; and Ward, V. P. Prophylaxis for postoperative deep-vein thrombosis. Synergistic effect of heparin and dihydroergotamine. *J.A.M.A.,* **1979,** *241,* 39–42.

Kiss, J. Chemical structure of heparin. In, *Heparin: Chemistry and Clinical Usage.* (Kakkar, V. V., and Thomas, D. P., eds.) Academic Press, Inc., New York, **1976,** pp. 3–20.

Larsson, R. L.; Hjelte, M. B.; Eriksson, J. C.; Lagergren, H. R.; and Olsson, P. The stability of glutardialdehyde-stabilized S^{35}-heparinized surfaces in contact with blood. *Thromb. Haemostas.,* **1977,** *37,* 262–273.

Levy, G.; O'Reilly, R. A.; Aggeler, P. M.; and Keech, G. M. Pharmacokinetic analysis of the effect of barbiturate on the anticoagulant action of warfarin in man. *Clin. Pharmacol. Ther.,* **1970,** *11,* 372–377.

Lewis, R. J., and Trager, W. F. The metabolic fate of warfarin: studies on the metabolites in plasma. *Ann. N.Y. Acad. Sci.,* **1971,** *179,* 205–212.

Lewis, R. J.; Trager, W. F.; Chan, K. K.; Breckenridge, A.; Orme, M.; Roland, M.; and Schary, W. Warfarin. Stereochemical aspects of its metabolism and the interaction with phenylbutazone. *J. Clin. Invest.,* **1974,** *53,* 1607–1617.

Lindahl, U.; Höök, M.; Bäckström, G.; Jacobsson, I.; Riesenfeld, J.; Malmström, A.; Rodén, L.; and Feingold, D. S. Structure and biosynthesis of heparin-like polysaccharides. *Fed. Proc.,* **1977,** *36,* 20–24.

McAvoy, T. J. Pharmacokinetic modeling of heparin and its clinical implications. *J. Pharmacokinet. Biopharm.,* **1979,** *7,* 331–354.

McGilveray, I. J.; Midha, K. K.; and Cooper, J. K. Bioavailability of Canadian tablet formulations of warfarin sodium and potassium. *Can. J. Pharm. Sci.,* **1978,** *13,* 9–11.

Marciniak, E., and Gockerman, J. P. Heparin-induced decrease in circulating antithrombin-III. *Lancet,* **1977,** *2,* 581–584.

Markwardt, F.; Nowak, G.; and Hoffman, J. The influence of drugs on disseminated intravascular coagulation (DIC). II. Effects of naturally occurring and synthetic thrombin inhibitors. *Thromb. Res.,* **1977,** *11,* 275–283.

Marx, J. AMIS negative on aspirin and heart attacks. *Science,* **1980,** *207,* 859–860.

Meinertz, T.; Kasper, W.; Kahl, C.; and Jähnchen, E. Anticoagulant activity of the enantiomers of acenocoumarol. *Br. J. Clin. Pharmacol.,* **1978,** *5,* 187–188.

Moncada, S., and Korbut, R. Dipyridamole and other phosphodiesterase inhibitors act as antithrombotic agents by potentiating endogenous prostacyclin. *Lancet,* **1978,** *1,* 1286–1289.

Nagashima, R.; O'Reilly, R. A.; and Levy, G. Kinetics of pharmacologic effects in man: anticoagulant action of warfarin. *Clin. Pharmacol. Ther.,* **1969,** *10,* 22–35.

Nilsson, C. M.; Horton, E. S.; and Robinson, D. S. The effect of furosemide and bumetanide on warfarin metabolism and anticoagulant response. *J. Clin. Pharmacol.,* **1978,** *18,* 91–94.

Okuno, T., and Crockatt, D. Platelet factor 4 activity and thromboembolic episodes. *Am. J. Clin. Pathol.,* **1977,** *67,* 351–355.

Olivecrona, T.; Bengtsson, G.; Marklund, S. E.; Lindahl, U.; and Hook, M. Heparin-lipoprotein lipase interactions. *Fed. Proc.,* **1977,** *36,* 60–65.

Olsson, J.-E.; Brechter, C.; Bäcklund, H.; Krook, H.; Muller, R.; Nitelius, E.; Olsson, O.; and Tornberg, A. Anti-coagulant vs anti-platelet therapy as prophylactic against cerebral infarction in transient ischemic attacks. *Stroke,* **1980,** *11,* 4–9.

O'Reilly, R. A. Vitamin K in hereditary resistance to oral anticoagulant drugs. *Am. J. Physiol.,* **1971,** *221,* 1327–1330.

———. Interaction of chronic daily warfarin therapy and rifampin. *Ann. Intern. Med.,* **1975,** *83,* 506–508.

———. Stereoselective interaction of warfarin and metronidazole (FLAGYL) in man. *N. Engl. J. Med.,* **1976a,** *295,* 354–357.

———. Lack of effect of mealtime wine on the hypoprothrombinemia of oral anticoagulants. *Am. J. Med. Sci.,* **1979,** *277,* 189–194.

———. Stereoselective interaction of trimethoprim-sulfamethoxazole with the separated enantiomorphs of racemic warfarin in man. *N. Engl. J. Med.,* **1980a,** *302,* 33–35.

———. Interaction of spironolactone and racemic warfarin in man. *Clin. Pharmacol. Ther.,* **1980b,** *27,* 198–201.

O'Reilly, R. A., and Aggeler, P. M. Studies on coumarin anticoagulant drugs: initiation of therapy without a loading dose. *Circulation,* **1968,** *38,* 169–177.

———. Covert anticoagulant ingestion: study of 25 patients and review of world literature. *Medicine (Baltimore),* **1976,** *55,* 389–399.

O'Reilly, R. A., and Motley, C. H. Interaction of racemic warfarin and trimethoprim-sulfamethoxazole in man. *Ann. Intern. Med.,* **1979,** *91,* 34–36.

O'Reilly, R. A.; Trager, W. F.; Motley, C. H.; and Howald, W. Stereoselective interaction of phenylbutazone with $^{12}C/^{13}C$-warfarin pseudoracemates in man. *J. Clin. Invest.,* **1980,** *65,* 746–753.

Orme, M. L'E.; Lewis, P. J.; DeSwiet, M.; Serlin, M. F.; Sibeon, R.; Baty, J. D.; and Breckenridge, A. M. May mothers given warfarin breast-feed their infants? *Br. Med. J.,* **1977,** *1,* 1564–1565.

Pettifor, J. M., and Benson, R. Congenital malformations associated with the administration of oral anticoagulants during pregnancy. *J. Pediatr.,* **1975,** *86,* 459–462.

Pomerantz, M. W., and Owen, W. G. A catalytic role for heparin. Evidence for a ternary complex of heparin cofactor thrombin and heparin. *Biochim. Biophys. Acta,* **1978,** *535,* 66–77.

Powers, P. J.; Cuthbert, D.; and Hirsh, J. Thrombocytopenia found uncommonly during heparin therapy. *J.A.M.A.,* **1979,** *241,* 2396–2397.

Prupas, H. M. Therapeutics: guidelines for heparin administration in thromboembolic disease. *Postgrad. Med.,* **1977,** *62,* 157–161.

Rosenberg, R. D.; Armand, G.; and Lam, L. Structure-function relationships of heparin species. *Proc. Natl. Acad. Sci. U.S.A.,* **1978,** *75,* 3065–3069.

Saliba, M. J., Jr. Heparin's endogenous function, primarily anticellular-destructive, incidentally anticoagulant, is dose-, source-, and pH-dependent. *Thromb. Haemostas.,* **1978,** *40,* 200–202.

Sasahara, A. A.; Ho, D. D.; and Sharma, G. V. R. K. When and how to use fibrinolytic agents. *Drug Ther.,* **1979,** *9,* 111–128.

Scalley, R. D.; Kearney, E.; and Jakobs, E. Interdisciplinary inpatient warfarin education program. *Am. J. Hosp. Pharm.,* **1979,** *36,* 219–220.

Schofield, F. W. Damaged sweet clover: cause of a new disease in cattle simulating hemorrhagic septicemia and blackleg. *J. Am. Vet. Med. Assoc.,* **1924,** *64,* 553–575.

Selzer, A. Use of anticoagulant agents in acute myocardial infarction: statistics or clinical judgment? (Editorial.) *Am. J. Cardiol.,* **1978,** *41,* 1315–1317.

Shepherd, A. M. M.; Hewick, D. S.; Moreland, T. A.; and Stevenson, I. H. Age as a determinant of sensitivity to warfarin. *Br. J. Clin. Pharmacol.,* **1977,** *4,* 315–320.

Simon, T. L.; Hyers, T. M.; Gaston, J. P.; and Harker, L. A. Heparin pharmacokinetics: increased requirements in pulmonary embolism. *Br. J. Haematol.,* **1978,** *39,* 111–120.

Steele, P.; Rainwater, J.; Vogel, R.; and Genton, E. Platelet-suppressant therapy in patients with coronary artery disease. *J.A.M.A.,* **1978,** *240,* 228–231.

Teien, A. N. Heparin elimination in patients with liver cirrhosis. *Thrombo. Haemostas.,* **1977,** *38,* 701–706.

Trowbridge, A. A.; Caraveo, J.; Green, J. B., III; Amaral, B.; and Stone, M. J. Heparin-related immune thrombocytopenia: studies of antibody-heparin specificity. *Am. J. Med.,* **1978,** *65,* 277–283.

Turpie, A. G. G.; Delmore, T.; Hirsh, J.; Hull, R.; Genton, E.; Hiscoe, C.; and Gent, M. Prevention of venous thrombosis by intermittent sequential calf compression in patients with intracranial disease. *Thromb. Res.,* **1979,** *15,* 611–616.

Wagner, J. G. Pharmacokinetic data: pharmacokinetic parameters estimated from intravenous data by uniform methods and some of their uses. *J. Pharmacokinet. Biopharm.,* **1977,** *5,* 161–182.

Weiler, J. M.; Yurt, R. W.; Fearon, D. T.; and Austen, K. F. Modulation of the formation of the amplification convertase of complement, C3b, Bb, by native and commercial heparin. *J. Exp. Med.,* **1978,** *147,* 409–421.

Whitlon, D. S.; Sadowski, J. A.; and Suttie, J. W. Mechanism of coumarin action: significance of vitamin K epoxide reductase inhibition. *Biochemistry,* **1978,** *17,* 1371–1377.

Williams, R. L.; Schary, W. L.; Blaschke, T. F.; Meffin, P. J.; Melmon, K. L.; and Rowland, M. Influence of acute viral hepatitis on disposition and pharmacologic effect of warfarin. *Clin. Pharmacol. Ther.,* **1976,** *20,* 90–97.

Wood, M.; Shand, D. G.; and Wood, A. J. J. Altered drug binding due to the use of indwelling heparinized cannulas (heparin lock) for sampling. *Clin. Pharmacol. Ther.,* **1979,** *25,* 103–107.

Wright, C. J., and Jaques, L. B. Heparin via the lung. *Can. J. Surg.,* **1979,** *22,* 317–319.

Monographs and Reviews

Barrowcliffe, T. W.; Johnson, E. A.; and Thomas, D. Antithrombin III and heparin. *Br. Med. Bull.,* **1978,** *34,* 143–150.

Bell, W. R., and Meek, A. G. Guidelines for the use of thrombolytic agents. *N. Engl. J. Med.,* **1979,** *301,* 1266–1270.

Clagett, G. P., and Collins, G. J. Platelets, thromboembolism and the clinical utility of antiplatelet drugs. *Surg. Gynecol. Obstet.,* **1978,** *147,* 257–272.

Coon, W. W. Some recent developments in the pharmacology of heparin. *J. Clin. Pharmacol.,* **1979,** *19,* 337–349. (101 references.)

Coon, W. W., and Willis, P. W., III. Some aspects of the pharmacology of oral anticoagulants. *Clin. Pharmacol. Ther.,* **1970,** *11,* 312–336. (192 references.)

Esnouf, M. P. Biochemistry of blood coagulation. *Br. Med. Bull.,* **1977,** *33,* 213–218.

Griffin, J. D., and Ellman, L. Epsilon-aminocaproic acid (EACA). *Semin. Thromb. Hemostas.,* **1978,** *5,* 27–40.

Hamilton, P. J.; Stalker, A. L.; and Douglas, A. S. Disseminated intravascular coagulation: a review. *J. Clin. Pathol.,* **1978,** *31,* 609–619.

Jaques, L. B. Determination of heparin and related sulfated mucopolysaccharides. *Methods Biochem. Anal.,* **1977,** *24,* 203–312. (186 references.)

———. Heparin: an old drug with a new paradigm. *Science,* **1979,** *206,* 528–533.

Kralt, T., and Claassen, V. Anticoagulants structurally and functionally related to vitamin K. In, *Drug Design,* Vol 3. (Ariëns, E. J., ed.) Academic Press, Inc., New York, **1972,** pp. 189–203.

Link, K. P. Anticoagulant from spoiled sweet clover hay. *Harvey Lect.,* **1944,** *39,* 162–216.

———. Discovery of dicumarol and its sequels. *Circulation,* **1959,** *19,* 97–107.

Mackie, M. J., and Douglas, A. S. Oral anticoagulants in arterial disease. *Br. Med. Bull.,* **1978,** *34,* 177–182.

Moncada, S., and Vane, J. R. Arachidonic acid metabolites and the interactions between platelets and blood vessel walls. *N. Engl. J. Med.,* **1979,** *300,* 1142–1147.

Morris, G. K., and Mitchell, J. R. A. Clinical management of venous thromboembolism. *Br. Med. Bull.,* **1978,** *34,* 169–175.

Mustard, J. F. Atherosclerosis, thrombosis and clinical complications. In, *Thromboembolism: A New Approach to Therapy.* (Mitchell, J. R. A., and Domenet, J. G., eds.) Academic Press, Inc., New York, **1977,** pp. 3–25.

Ogston, D., and Bennett, B. Surface-mediated reactions in the formation of thrombin, plasmin and kallikrein. *Br. Med. Bull.,* **1978,** *34,* 107–112.

Olson, R. E., and Suttie, J. W. Vitamin K and γ-carboxyglutamate biosynthesis. *Vitam. Horm.,* **1977,** *35,* 59–108.

O'Reilly, R. A. The binding of sodium warfarin to plasma albumin and its displacement by phenylbutazone. *Ann. N.Y. Acad. Sci.,* **1973,** *226,* 293–308.

———. Vitamin K and the oral anticoagulant drugs. *Annu. Rev. Med.,* **1976b,** *27,* 245–261.

O'Reilly, R. A., and Aggeler, P. M. Determinants of the response to oral anticoagulant drugs in man. *Pharmacol. Rev.,* **1970,** *22,* 35–96. (703 references.)

Renk, E., and Stoll, W. G. Orale Antikoagulantien. *Prog. Drug Res.,* **1968,** *22,* 226–355. (899 references.)

Rosenberg, R. D. Heparin, antithrombin, and abnormal clotting. *Annu. Rev. Med.,* **1978,** *29,* 367–378.

Schafer, A. I., and Handin, R. I. The role of platelets in thrombotic and vascular disease. *Prog. Cardiovasc. Dis.,* **1979,** *22,* 31–52. (189 references.)

Seegers, W. H. Antithrombin III. Theory and clinical applications. H. P. Smith Memorial Lecture. *Am. J. Clin. Pathol.,* **1978,** *69,* 367–374.

Turpie, A. G. G., and Hirsh, J. Prophylaxis and therapy of venous thromboembolism. *CRC Crit. Rev. Clin. Lab. Sci.,* **1979,** *10,* 247–274.

Verstraete, M. Biochemical and clinical aspects of thrombolysis. *Semin. Hematol.,* **1978,** *15,* 35–54.

Weiss, H. J. Drug therapy. Antiplatelet therapy. *N. Engl. J. Med.,* **1978,** *298,* 1344–1347, 1403–1406.

Wessler, S., and Gilel, S. N. Review. Heparin: new concepts relevant to clinical use. *Blood,* **1979,** *53,* 525–544.

SECTION
XV

Hormones and Hormone Antagonists

INTRODUCTION

Ferid Murad and Robert C. Haynes, Jr.

Preparations that contain the active principles of the endocrine glands may be classified from the pharmacological viewpoint as drugs. Whereas most drugs are considered to be substances foreign to the body, the hormones are natural secretions of the endocrine glands and exert important functional effects upon other tissues. Consequently, there has been a tendency to place hormones in a different category, although there is really no valid reason for doing so; indeed, some endocrine preparations have unobtrusively broken down this arbitrary distinction. For example, epinephrine is much more frequently viewed as a powerful sympathomimetic drug than as a hormone of the adrenal medulla.

Pharmacological studies on the actions of drugs of endocrine origin have contributed greatly to an understanding of the normal functions of the endocrine glands. Conversely, much can be learned about the effects of a hormonally active drug by observing the consequences of a deficiency or an excess of the hormone in question. The diverse actions of cortisol and its congeners, for instance, are strikingly illustrated by the changes from the normal shown by patients suffering from adrenal deficiency on the one hand and by patients with oversecretion on the other.

It is useful to preserve the distinction between hormones and other active substances of animal origin. By definition, a hormone is a substance secreted by a specific tissue and transported to a distance where it exerts its effect upon other specific tissues. One can quibble with the details of this definition in some instances; for example, growth hormone seems to act upon so many tissues that the term *specific* becomes imprecise, and the distance traveled by the hypothalamic releasing hormones is rather short. But there are many active substances derived from tissues or body fluids that may not serve any important regulatory function or that may act predominantly at the immediate site of release and thus do not meet the definition of a hormone. The latter compounds are designated as *autacoids* and are discussed in an earlier section (Chapters 26, 27, and 28).

Analogs of the hormones, synthetic compounds resembling the natural products but differing from them in some important respects, have often proven more useful in therapeutics than have the hormones themselves. One aim in endocrinology is the isolation, identification, and synthesis of the active principles of each of the endocrine glands. Sometimes, when these formidable efforts have been successful, the product has been found to be of little use in therapy. It may prove inactive when given by mouth, as are the catecholamines, or it may also be so rapidly degraded that unless injected frequently little effect can be achieved, as in the case of the natural sex hormones. The design of synthetic analogs, compounds altered enough to outwit degradative enzymes but not enough to confuse the receptor sites, is one of the major contributions to endocrine therapy. A striking example was the discovery, 45 years ago, of

1367

diethylstilbestrol, a cheap synthetic substance that duplicates the actions of estrogen when given orally. In a number of instances the synthetic analogs, by their more desirable properties, represent striking improvements upon nature. Innovative systems for the delivery of drugs can also influence the therapeutic efficacy of a hormone or analog by allowing control of its site or rate of delivery or its metabolism.

A number of useful drugs can influence the synthesis or secretion of hormones or antagonize their cellular actions. Most endocrine tissues store their hormones or precursors thereof intracellularly, often in granules that contain a prohormone or the biologically active compound itself. Secretion is frequently accomplished by exocytosis of the packaged products, and this process, stimulus-secretion coupling, generally requires calcium ion. Synthesis, storage, and secretion of hormones are regulated at numerous steps. The antithyroid drugs provided the initial example of drugs that inhibit hormone synthesis; they selectively inhibit the synthesis of thyroid hormone, and this action makes them effective in the treatment of hyperthyroidism. More recently, equally specific substances have been developed to block one or another step in the synthesis of the hormones of the adrenal cortex.

Direct inhibition of the action of a hormone upon its receptor sites has been achieved experimentally in several instances and has been put to good use in isolated cases. Inhibition of the action of estrogen seems to account for the therapeutic efficacy of clomiphene in reproductive disorders in women. By relieving the inhibitory influence of estrogen upon the pituitary, the substance acts to promote the secretion of gonadotropins.

Usually, when considering the clinical applications of the hormones, one thinks first of their use in replacement therapy—treatment of Addison's disease, myxedema, and so forth, with the appropriate drug. However, if the normal regulatory interactions of an endocrine system are understood, hormones and their antagonists can be exploited for a variety of additional therapeutic and diagnostic purposes. Regulation of the endocrine systems characteristically takes place on a multitude of levels. Many systems are ultimately responsive to neural or neuroendocrine control of either a stimulatory or inhibitory nature or both. A change in the magnitude of such control results in an appropriate alteration of secretion in a dependent target, and this secretion may serve as the immediate regulator of yet another endocrine organ. Any of the intermediate products, but more commonly the final hormonal secretion in such a chain, may "feed back" at any level to regulate the intensity of a controlling signal. Such feedback is predominantly negative; thus, a hormone can inhibit its own synthesis and secretion when its critical concentration is exceeded. Positive feedback systems are, however, occasionally utilized. Blood-borne chemicals the concentrations of which are subject to hormonal regulation are also used extensively as feedback regulators in such control systems. This knowledge is useful clinically, and it must be applied in the interpretation of a patient's basal laboratory data and in the performance of a variety of provocative tests of endocrine function. Similarly, therapeutic maneuvers also depend on these regulatory interactions. For example, the activity of the adrenal cortex can be suppressed by an adrenocorticosteroid through inhibition of the secretion of corticotropin; ovulation, if unwanted, can be abolished by ovarian hormones that suppress the secretion of hypophyseal gonadotropins.

The last 20 years have witnessed an explosive increase in knowledge of the mechanisms of hormone action, and this is understood in detail for some endocrine secretions. In a number of cases, hormones interact with specific receptors in cellular plasma membranes that are linked to the enzyme adenylate cyclase, discovered by Sutherland and Rall. This enzyme is stimulated or inhibited in some way by the hormone-receptor complex, and the result is an altered rate of synthesis of cyclic adenosine 3′,5′-monophosphate (cyclic AMP) from adenosine triphosphate (ATP) (*see* Figure 4–7, page 79). Cyclic AMP then acts as an intracellular mediator for the hormone, and the system thus functions as a mechanism for transferring and amplifying the information inherent in the extracellular hormone. Cyclic AMP regulates a variety of intracellular processes, and the ultimate effects are dependent on the cell's capacity to respond—its differentiated repertoire. The mechanism of cyclic AMP action in many cases involves the activation of protein kinases that phosphorylate cellular constituents and alter the rates at which processes involving these constituents proceed. Cyclic AMP is metabolized to 5′-AMP by specific phosphodiesterases, and inhibitors of these enzymes, such as methylxanthines, can sometimes exert hormone-like effects. The hormones discussed in the following chapters that appear to use this mechanism include the trophic hormones of the adenohypophysis, the melanocyte-stimulating hormones, some of the hypothalamic releasing hormones, glucagon, parathyroid hormone, and calcitonin. Many hormones appear to act by altering the uptake, release, and intracellular distribution of calcium ion; calcium, like cyclic AMP, may thus be viewed as an intracellular messenger. There are also situations in which cyclic AMP can influence the distribution and actions of calcium and *vice versa*. These systems are thus frequently interactive.

The steroid hormones utilize a different mechanism of information transfer. They gain access to the intracellular compartment and bind to cytoplasmic receptor proteins. Following this interaction the hormone-receptor complex, without or with some modification, is transported to sites of action within the nucleus. The remaining hormones, which in many ways appear to constitute a group, include growth hormone, somatomedins, prolactin, insulin, and other proteins (not discussed here) such as nerve growth factor. Their mechanisms of action remain more obscure; however, in view of their protein nature, it is appealing to envision interaction with the plasma membrane and the subsequent generation of "second messengers" analogous to cyclic AMP.

Finally, mention should be made of recent methodological advances that have greatly facilitated research and clinical applications in endocrine pharmacology. Foremost, perhaps, is radioimmunoassay, pioneered by Berson and Yalow. Using this sensitive and specific technic, the physician now has rapid access to a wealth of analytical information about his patient. Advances in peptide and protein chemistry are also outstanding. The technics for determination of amino acid sequences developed by Edman and for automated peptide synthesis developed by Merrifield are making the clinical use of various peptides a practical possibility. The last several years have also witnessed remarkable advances in molecular biology. Recombinant DNA technology has permitted the incorporation of purified or *synthetic* genes that code for the synthesis of specific human hormones into the bacterial genome. The objective is large-scale microbial synthesis of the human protein. This technic should have a major impact upon the availability of scarce hormones, such as human growth hormone, and should overcome the immunological difficulties that are encountered with the clinical use of animal products such as insulin.

CHAPTER
59 ADENOHYPOPHYSEAL HORMONES AND RELATED SUBSTANCES

Ferid Murad and Robert C. Haynes, Jr.

The hormones of the adenohypophysis regulate many important processes in the body; additionally, they are the mediators of various disturbances in the endocrine system and are themselves sensitive to the aberrations of systemic disease. Their secretion is profoundly influenced by many hormones of the peripheral endocrine glands as well as by stimulatory and inhibitory hormones of hypothalamic origin. Similarly striking effects on their secretion are exerted by many drugs, including natural hormones, hormonal analogs, and inhibitors of hormone synthesis and action.

The endocrine systems are dependent upon the adenohypophysis, not only for the delicate regulation of their secretions but also for the trophic effect necessary for their maintenance. Without the gonadotropins the entire reproductive system fails, and, consequently, the capacity of higher forms of life to perpetuate themselves is lost. Normal growth and development are impossible without growth hormone and thyrotropin; these hormones with those from the adrenal cortex are essential for energy metabolism—the assimilation, storage, and combustion of fuel.

Among the vertebrates, ten adenohypophyseal hormones are recognized: growth hormone, prolactin, two gonadotropins, thyrotropin, corticotropin, two melanocyte-stimulating hormones, and two lipotropins. Of these, the first six are demonstrably important in man. However, it would be premature to deny the possibility that there may be others. Since the pituitary gland is rich in polypeptides and small proteins, as might be expected of an organ devoted to the synthesis of such a profusion of peptide hormones, the isolation of pure compounds can be a formidable undertaking. While some of these peptides doubtless represent degraded or unfinished precursors of the hormones, it would perhaps be surprising if some of them did not have biological properties of physiological importance.

Elucidation of the amino acid sequences of the recognized hormones of the adenohypophysis has shed light on the amazing diversity of the organ. Three groups of hormones are apparent (Table 59-1). The members of the first group, growth hormone and prolactin, show considerable sequence homology, a fact that accounts for both the lactogenic activity of growth hormone and the delay in recognizing human prolactin as a distinct entity. Amino acid sequences are said to be homologous if the corresponding amino acid residues are either identical or replaced with similar amino acids. It is hypothesized that both proteins evolved from a single, perhaps prolactin-like molecule. The gonadotropins and thyrotropin (TSH) constitute the second group, closely related glycoprotein hormones. These complex proteins are each composed of two different noncovalently linked subunits (α and β). Remarkably, the α subunits of the group are nearly identical, while biological specificity resides

in unique β subunits. Thus, hybrid hormones can be formed; for example, the α subunit of luteinizing hormone (LH) can be combined with the β subunit of TSH to yield a molecule with thyroid-stimulating activity. Since the β subunits of LH and TSH also show significant homology with the α subunits, all of these peptide chains may have evolved from a common α subunit-like ancestor. The remaining group comprises corticotropin, the melanocyte-stimulating hormones, and the so-called lipotropins. As part of their sequence, these hormones all share a common heptapeptide (Table 59-1).

Hormones of the first two groups are not unique to the adenohypophysis, since at least one representative of each group is also produced by the placenta. The placental lactogen is very similar to growth hormone, and chorionic gonadotropin resembles LH. A chorionic thyrotropin (CTSH) and a chorionic follicle-stimulating hormone (CFSH) have also been described.

History. The name *pituitary* comes from the Latin *pituita,* meaning "phlegm." The gland was first thought to be a source of phlegm to moisten the membranes of the nose. In 1887, Minkowski associated the features of acromegaly with a tumor of the gland. Although the cause-and-effect relationship was by no means clear at first, by 1900 Hutchinson was able to conclude that ". . . in the pituitary body we appear to have a sort of growth-regulating centre for the entire body, the disturbance of which in early life will produce the phenomena of gigantism, and in later life those of acromegaly."

The induction of growth by the injection of pituitary extract was first accomplished in rats by Evans and Long in 1921; concurrently they noted for the first time the gonadotropic effect. Hypophysectomy as an experimental approach was introduced by Aschner in 1909. However, it was not until 1927 that the true consequences of hypophysectomy in mammals were clarified by Smith's classical experiments in the rat (Smith, 1927, 1930). The failure of growth and the atrophy of the gonads, thyroid, and adrenals that followed hypophysectomy were correctable by hypophyseal implants. This work had been anticipated 10 years earlier by parallel studies on the hypophysectomized tadpole wherein the several functions of the three parts of the pituitary were correctly assigned (*see* Allen, 1917). Smith's work in the rat was quickly followed by the definition of a thyrotropic hormone by Aron and by Loeb and Bassett in 1929, the preparation of an adrenotropic extract by Collip and coworkers in 1933, and the preparation and naming of prolactin by Riddle and associates in the same year. The year 1933 was further notable for the publication by Fevold and coworkers of the separate identity of a follicle-stimulating and a luteinizing hormone.

During the 1950s and 1960s, the development of sophisticated technics of protein purification and analysis (countercurrent distribution, ion-exchange chromatography, gel filtration, electrophoresis) greatly facilitated research in this area. Such purification of the hormones provided better products for biological investigation, and the great importance of species specificity came to be recognized. It was most strikingly shown in the case of growth hormone, only the product from the pituitaries of primates being active in monkeys and man (Knobil and Greep, 1959; Raben, 1959). This reopened the field of clinical investigation to the development of effective and new therapeutic applications. Of immense, recent significance in this regard are technics and instruments for automated amino acid sequence analysis and solid-phase peptide synthesis. These capabilities are now making the clinical use of synthetic peptides feasible.

When it was recognized in the early 1940s that the major vascular supply to the anterior pituitary was made up of blood that had already traversed the capillaries of the median eminence of the hypothalamus, the proper setting for the neurohumoral control of the gland was evident. It has now come to be generally recognized that hypothalamic cells transmit to the anterior lobe individual factors that regulate the secretion of each of its hormones, and this is presently an area of intense research activity (*see* page 1389).

Hypopituitarism. Typically in endocrinology the functions of a gland and its secretions can be surmised from alterations that occur when it is congenitally absent or when the gland is destroyed or removed. A great deal has been learned from the consequences of pituitary deficiency.

Hypopituitarism in the Adult. Post-partum pitui-

Table 59–1. PROPERTIES OF THE PROTEIN HORMONES OF THE HUMAN ADENOHYPOPHYSIS AND PLACENTA

HORMONE	MOLECULAR WEIGHT	PEPTIDE CHAINS	AMINO ACID RESIDUES	CARBO-HYDRATE	COMMENTS
Group 1					
Growth hormone (GH)	22,000	1	191	0	Human GH, Prl, and PL have considerably less homology of amino acid sequence, in contrast to the striking degree that is observed in other species
Prolactin (Prl)	23,000	1	198	0	
Placental lactogen (PL)	22,000	1	191	0	
Group 2					
Luteinizing hormone (LH)	30,000	2	α-89 β-115	16%	Glycoproteins with nonidentical subunits (α and β); biological specificity is in β subunit
Follicle-stimulating hormone (FSH)	32,000	2	α 89 β-115	18%	The α subunits of LH, FSH, TSH, and CG are nearly identical and interchangeable
Thyrotropin (TSH)	28,000	2	α-89 β-112	13%	FSH-α and FSH-β are similar in amino acid composition
Chorionic gonadotropin (CG)	38,000	2	α-92 β-145	31%	FSH-β and TSH-β share a sequence of 49 amino acid residues, while FSH-β and LH-β share a sequence of 39 residues
Chorionic thyrotropin (CTSH)	28,000	?	?	3.5%	Residues 1 to 115 of CG-β have about 80% homology with the β subunits of LH, FSH, and TSH. CTSH is physicochemically and antigenically different from TSH. CFSH is antigenically similar to FSH
Group 3					
Corticotropin (ACTH)	4500	1	39	0	Group shares a common heptapeptide: Met-Glu-His-Phe-Arg-Trp-Gly
α-Melanocyte-stimulating hormone (α-MSH)	1650	1	13	0	ACTH (1-13) = α-MSH
β-Melanocyte-stimulating hormone (β-MSH)	2100	1	18	0	β-LPH (1-58) = γ-Lipotropin β-LPH (41-58) = β-MSH
β-Lipotropin (β-LPH)	9500	1	91	0	
γ-Lipotropin (γ-LPH)	5800	1	58	0	

tary necrosis, described by Sheehan (*see* Sheehan and Summers, 1949), can amount to complete destruction of the anterior lobe, and the patient may die, presumably from adrenal deficiency. If she survives, recovery of strength and well-being is slow and incomplete. The infant cannot be nursed, as there is no milk; the pubic hair, if shaved, does not grow back, and axillary and other body hair later falls out; the menstrual periods do not resume, and the genital tract atrophies. The skin becomes thin, soft, and finely wrinkled, assuming a waxy pallor from the mild anemia and the loss of dermal pigment. Libido is lost. There is reduced thyroid function with sensitivity to cold, lack of sweating, low rate of metabolism, poor accumulation of radioiodine by the thyroid, and increased plasma cholesterol. Various indices of adrenocortical function also show a profound deficit. There is sensitivity to physical stress and to the stress of infection, and there may be frequent episodes of collapse or severe illnesses. Body weight is not grossly altered, but there is a tendency toward plumpness. Survival for 30 years or longer without diagnosis or specific treatment is not unusual. Sometimes one or more of the clinical features are not present, presumably because destruction of the pituitary is not complete.

Hypopituitarism from local tumors often seems to affect the secretion of some hormones before others. The menstrual cycle may stop several years before the thyroid or adrenals are affected, or failure of growth may be the first manifestation. There may be features of advanced hypopituitarism at a time when the thyroid seems still to be normal. By contrast, the consequences of hypophysectomy in man resemble the complete picture of Sheehan's syndrome. In recent years, this operation has been carried out extensively for the palliative treatment of cancer and for the amelioration of some of the concomitants of diabetes mellitus.

When hypopituitarism in the adult is treated by replacement with a glucocorticoid, thyroid hormone, and the appropriate sex hormone, complete clinical recovery is apparently achieved. The individual still lacks growth hormone, melanocyte-stimulating hormone, prolactin, and all other factors that have been detected in the adenohypophysis. However, such patients look like normal people, and they feel well and are capable of normal activities. Gametogenesis is lacking, but in isolated cases this has been shown to be correctable with human gonadotropins. Other deficits are by no means obvious. There may be a tendency to excess fat, sparse body and scalp hair, somewhat reduced dermal pigment, and the eyes may seem a bit sunken—little else.

Hypopituitary Dwarfism. Failure of the pituitary to develop during embryogenesis is, surprisingly, compatible with almost normal longevity; the manifestations are ascribable to the lack of the adenohypophyseal hormones, especially growth hormone. The most striking feature of the condition is, as the name implies, failure to grow normally. At the age of earliest recognition the child is small, with the deviation from the normal becoming more pronounced with advancing years. The dwarfism affects all parts of the body, and the individual comes to resemble a very small version of a normal child. Although growth is very slow, it does not cease; indeed, because it is not arrested by puberty as it is in the normal case, it continues throughout life and almost normal stature may eventually be achieved.

During the years of childhood, the defect in gonadotropic function cannot be recognized clinically, although it can be detected by sensitive immunoassays of the blood for *gonadotropic hormones*. In the absence of these hormones there is no sexual development in later years. Although there may be no *thyrotropin* or *corticotropin*, there is a small but important amount of activity on the part of the thyroid gland and the adrenal cortex. The dwarfing and retarded osseous development are not as extreme as in cretinism, nor does the hypopituitary dwarf show the mental retardation, the changes of the skin, or the facies of the cretin. However, thyroid function tests indicate hypoactivity, and the thyroid is easily stimulated by thyrotropin. The adrenal cortex is presumed to be usefully functional also, for quite apart from secretion of aldosterone, which does not require corticotropin, some capacity to make a glucocorticoid is presumed because so many bodily functions are not recognizably abnormal. Addisonian crises are not a feature of the condition, and the subjects withstand the stresses of life and of illness rather well. However, it can again be shown that adrenocortical secretions are deficient. The detection of such thyroid and adrenal deficiency helps to differentiate hypopituitarism from the host of other causes of dwarfism, including the isolated deficiency of secretion of growth hormone by the adenohypophysis.

Hypersecretion of Pituitary Hormones. In acromegaly and in gigantism, the most prominent features are those of excessive action of growth hormone, but it is possible that other hormones are also secreted in excess. Thyrotropin in the blood has been found to be increased, and there is a higher incidence of goiter and enlargement of the adrenal cortex; sometimes lactation is noted. One form of Cushing's syndrome is caused by an oversecretion of corticotropin, and in this condition, as in acromegaly, a tumor of the pituitary is often responsible. Precocious sexual development in association with tumors at the base of the brain appears to be due to isolated hypersecretion of the gonadotropins. Pituitary tumors that secrete one or both gonadotropins or thyrotropin are extremely rare. Excessive secretion of the several trophic hormones follows impaired function of the individual target glands, owing to the operation of the normal servomechanism. For example, with ovarian failure of the menopause, concentrations of the gonadotropins are markedly elevated. Similarly, primary disorders of the adrenal or thyroid result in decreased "feedback inhibition" of the pituitary and increases in the rates of secretion of the corresponding trophic hormones.

GROWTH HORMONE

Chemistry. Of all the active principles of the anterior pituitary, growth hormone is easily the most abundant. In the human gland, up to 10% of the dry weight is growth hormone, and current methods of extraction obtain a high percentage of the hormone from the glands in a form suitable for human use.

Growth hormone is a simple protein made up of a single chain of 191 amino acids. There are two intrachain disulfide bonds, and the complete amino acid sequence of the human hormone is known (Li *et al.*, 1966; Niall *et al.*, 1971). While the bovine and ovine hormones are very similar to the human protein in their general features, there are significant differences in primary structure. There is approximately 60% identity of their amino acid sequence with that of human growth hormone. The differences presumably account for their relative inability to bind to putative receptors for growth hormone in human liver (Carr and Friesen, 1976) and, thus, for their relative inactivity in man.

"Big" and "little" forms of growth hormone have been studied in pituitary extracts and plasma (Goodman *et al.*, 1972; Gordon *et al.*, 1973, 1976). The larger form is about twice the size of the smaller, which has a molecular weight of 22,000. While both forms are readily detected in radioimmunoassays for the hormone, the smaller form is more active in a radioreceptor assay, which is thought to be a better reflection of biological activity than is the radioimmunoassay. The larger form is readily converted to the smaller and may represent a precursor or progrowth hormone. Large and small species of other hormones, such as insulin, corticotropin, luteinizing hormone, gastrin, and parathyroid hormone, have also been reported, which suggests that many and perhaps most peptide hormones may be synthesized and stored in granules in a larger precursor form. About 70 to 90% of the immunoreactive growth hormone in plasma in normal individuals and those with acromegaly is the smaller, biologically active species (Gordon *et al.*, 1976).

Recurring regions of amino acid sequence homology within the growth hormone molecule have led to the hypothesis that growth hormone (and the lactogenic hormones) have evolved from smaller ancestors by processes involving the tandem linkage of reduplicated genes (Niall *et al.*, 1971). This concept also suggests the possibility of an "active core" in these hormones. The identification of such an "active core" would be particularly worthwhile, since intact nonprimate growth hormones are poorly active in man. Active fragments of growth hormone have been described. It remains unresolved whether the "little" growth hormone is also a prohormone that is cleaved *in vivo* to still smaller but active fragments (Lewis *et al.*, 1975; Baumann and Hodgen, 1976). A relatively small active fragment should prove clinically useful, and synthesis might be practical.

Physiological Actions. The concept of a growth hormone sprang from clinical observations on gigantism and acromegaly and was strengthened by the finding that crude extracts of the pituitary gland of the ox, when injected into dogs and rats, elicited increased growth.

Growth. The stimulus to growth provided by growth hormone administered to the rat affects nearly every organ and tissue of the body, the possible exceptions being the brain and the eye. The rat has been the favored experimental animal for such studies because it is exceptional in several ways. The epiphyses of almost all the long bones remain open throughout life, and growth continues for as long as good nutrition and good health prevail. Maximal sensitivity to growth hormone is manifested when growth in young animals is arrested by hypophysectomy. The rat is also peculiar in responding indiscriminately to the growth hormone of all other mammals thus far explored. Hypophysectomy during the early days of life in the rat is eventually fatal, seemingly because the growing brain cannot be accommodated in the dwarfed cranium. The other organs and tissues of the body respond to growth hormone by a proportional increase in size that is in keeping with the total increase in body weight. The growth of bones is reflected in increased body length; the skin and its appendages grow, and the skeletal muscles enlarge. The thoracic and abdominal viscera also grow, sometimes to a greater extent than does the rest of the body. Growth of the thymus is a sensitive index of the action of growth hormone; like that of the lymph nodes, it can be countered by a direct action of the corticosteroids. Enlargement of the liver and increased cellular proliferation therein follow brief treatment with growth hormone, and accumulation of fat may augment somewhat the increase in weight. Effects on the size of the spleen are usually obscured by other factors that affect this organ, but the heart, lungs, kidneys, and gastrointestinal tract enlarge in response to growth hormone. There is also slight enlargement of the gonads, adrenals, and thyroid, probably attributable to growth hormone itself rather than to specific trophic hormones that contaminate some preparations.

Studies on the growth effects in other species have not been nearly as detailed as those in the rat; indeed, the animal that has been next best studied is the human being. Such investigation in man represents the first thorough exploration of the effects of growth hormone in the same species from which it was derived. Growth in the human being in response to human growth hormone has been studied largely in dwarfs, and particularly in hypopituitary dwarfs, in whom striking effects, amounting to therapeutic triumphs, have been achieved. The growth is normally proportioned, but there is no sexual maturation, splanchnomegaly, or disproportionate growth of skin or flat bones. No features of gigantism or acromegaly have yet been described, but the results of prolonged treatment with large doses have not been reported.

Effects on the Metabolism of Nitrogen. Growth connotes increased protoplasm and thus protein, the most abundant nitrogen-containing component of the body. It is to be expected that growth is associated with the accumulation of nitrogen in the organism; indeed, a positive nitrogen balance is the classical biochemical expression of growth. In several species, and under a variety of conditions, growth hormone has been shown to cause a retention of nitrogen, and this property has come to be equated with its anabolic effect.

However, it is difficult to measure growth by measuring the retention of nitrogen. Protein contains about 16% nitrogen and most tissue about 10 to 15% protein. The building-up of a kilogram of tissue, then, requires the retention of about 20 g of nitrogen. A rapidly growing boy during the peak of the puberal growth spurt gains, on the average, 7 kg a year. If one third of this is bone and fat, he acquires about 4.5 kg of tissue containing about 100 g of nitrogen. To accomplish this, he need retain only 0.3 g of nitrogen per day. In careful metabolic studies in man, a positive balance of this magnitude is of borderline significance and would probably be obscured by many inevitable variables. For example, several hundred milligrams of nitrogen are lost each day by desquamation of the skin, sweating, attrition of hair and nails, and possibly exhalation of N_2. These cannot be readily measured and would cause an error in the calculation of balance. When growth hormone is given to human subjects in doses of 5 to 10 mg a day, a total of 3 to 5 g of nitrogen is retained daily—many times the amount needed for a normal rate of growth. Although prolonged balances have not been measured, evidently the effect is evanescent, and the site of storage of this extra nitrogen is unknown.

Along with the retained nitrogen there is accretion of other constituents of tissue—sodium, chloride, potassium, phosphorus, calcium, and other elements. In the case of calcium, there is a paradoxical increase in the urinary loss of the element that is balanced by an augmented absorption from the intestinal tract.

Animal experiments have shown that treatment with growth hormone increases the transport of amino acids into tissues and accelerates their incorporation into protein. Thus, in man, one of the early effects of growth hormone is a decrease in the concentration of urea in the blood, evidently because of diversion of amino acids into anabolic pathways. A variety of anabolic effects can also be observed with isolated tissues incubated *in vitro,* and in this respect the hormone mimics the action of insulin. These anabolic effects likely reflect a hormonal action to increase selectively the rate of information flow from specific regions of DNA to RNA to protein. However, this statement must be made without prejudgment about the number and location of such controlled sites. Their understanding will await far more detailed analysis of the molecular biology of eukaryotic cells.

Effects on Metabolism of Carbohydrate and Lipid. Growth hormone has a number of important and complex effects on carbohydrate and lipid metabolism (*see* Symposium, 1973; Frantz, 1976). A large number of hormones, notably growth hormone, insulin, glucocorticoids, catecholamines, and glucagon, play important roles in lipid, carbohydrate, and nitrogen homeostasis. As a first important approximation, insulin and growth hormone can be viewed as the major anabolic influences, with the glucocorticoids and catecholamines as their catabolic antagonists. However, the details are not that simple. Each hormone in fact exerts a number of effects at different sites. Although an oversimplification of the facts, it might be said that growth hormone seems to switch over the source of fuel for the body from carbohydrate to fat. Thus, while insulin favors the use of sugar and its conversion to fat, growth hormone has just the opposite effect.

Houssay's important observation that hypophysectomy relieves the diabetes consequent upon removal of the pancreas did not establish that growth hormone is the responsible agent. Indeed, the work of Long and coworkers later proved that the adrenocorticosteroids are essential to the full expression of diabetes. But Houssay showed that crude extracts of the pituitary given to his animals caused the diabetic state to return in full intensity (Houssay, 1942). Later work made it seem highly likely that the responsible agent in his extracts was growth hormone. Thus, from the earliest experiments in this area in the completely depancreatized animal it was clear that the *diabetogenic* action of growth hormone was not *just* an antagonism of insulin. However, in a great many experimental situations, growth hormone opposes certain of the actions of insulin. Thus, treatment with growth hormone renders certain species of animals insensitive to insulin, reduces tolerance to glucose, and corrects the hypersensitivity of the hypophysectomized animal to insulin.

In patients suffering from diabetes mellitus, growth hormone does exert a clear-cut diabetogenic effect that can be offset by a larger dose of insulin. Some patients with severe diabetes, hypophysectomized for the palliation of ocular or renal lesions and treated with small doses of insulin, have been found to be exquisitely sensitive to growth hormone. A small fraction of the therapeutic dose for promotion of growth can lead to severe intensification of hyperglycemia and ketosis. In the nondiabetic subject, on the other hand, large doses can be given without detectable effects upon tolerance to carbohydrate.

The antagonism of insulin by growth hormone is, however, not always apparent. Following hypophysectomy there is a tendency toward hypoglycemia that is corrected by the dual administration of glucocorticoids and growth hormone. However, the acute administration of growth hormone does not cause prominent hyperglycemia and may in fact cause a paradoxical and transient insulin-like hypoglycemia. Another insulin-like action of growth hormone involves enhanced uptake of glucose by muscle *in vitro*. Perhaps similarly, hepatic and muscular glycogen stores are depleted after hypophysectomy, and glucocorticoids and growth hormone again suffice to promote glycogen deposition. Thus, growth hormone, glucocorticoids, and insulin all facilitate the storage of carbohydrate in the form of glycogen.

The prominent metabolic actions of growth hormone resemble those brought about by fasting, and during fasting increased secretion of the hormone may be of central importance in adaptation to lack of food. With fasting there is increasing intolerance to carbohydrate (hunger diabetes), inhibited lipogenesis, mobilization of fat, and

ketosis—responses that can be evoked by growth hormone. Circulating growth hormone also increases with exercise, and hypoglycemia is a particularly potent stimulus. In teleological terms it is difficult to understand this response. Growth, in the sense of building of protoplasm, cannot take place without food, and one is led to imagine that, without growth hormone, tissue might be broken down during fasting and used indiscriminately for fuel. Growth hormone might hinder this and thereby enforce the use of fat instead.

The first, as well as a most consistent, effect of human growth hormone in man is an increase in free fatty acids in the blood. The response begins about 2 hours after the injection and reflects enhanced mobilization of fatty acids from adipose tissue. Within a few hours of giving growth hormone to normal rats or mice, there is an increase in fat in the liver and it can be shown that this is derived from the depots. Other lipolytic agents, such as epinephrine, corticotropin, and thyrotropin, share this action, but only in the case of epinephrine does the effect seem to have physiological relevance.

Detailed studies have been carried out on the actions of hormones upon adipose tissue and upon isolated fat cells incubated *in vitro*. Insulin is antilipolytic and strongly stimulates the accumulation of glucose by adipose tissue, the conversion of glucose to fat and glycogen, and its oxidation to CO_2. Epinephrine and several adenohypophyseal hormones promote the hydrolysis of fat and the liberation of free fatty acid, actions that are inhibited in part by insulin and glucose. These lipolytic hormones have a rapid effect that is due to their ability to enhance the synthesis of cyclic adenosine 3',5'-monophosphate (cyclic AMP) (*see* Chapter 4). Cyclic AMP, in turn, activates a protein kinase that phosphorylates and stimulates a triglyceride lipase—the rate-limiting enzyme in the lipolytic pathway (Huttunen *et al.*, 1970). Growth hormone may also promote lipolysis by influencing the cyclic AMP system, but the nature of its effect is less well understood.

Although the effects of fasting mimic some of the actions of growth hormone and may in fact be thus mediated, the analogy by itself cannot be indefinitely extrapolated. On the one hand, growth hormone causes retention of nitrogen, increased assimilation of amino acids by tissue, and growth, whereas starvation has the reverse effects; on the other, growth hormone intensifies those very manifestations of the diabetic state that are ameliorated by fasting. It is difficult to escape the conclusion that the action of growth hormone is closely tied to the action of insulin and that the two hormones work against one another as well as together. When they work together, anabolic effects are dominant; in the fasting state, insulin is inconspicuous but not entirely lacking, and growth hormone then further depresses the use of carbohydrate and promotes the mobilization of fat and mild ketosis; in diabetes, when insulin is lacking or has decreased effectiveness, anabolism is impossible and growth hormone assumes the role of a diabetogenic agent. When growth hormone is lacking, insulin acts unopposed, carbohydrate is burned or converted to fat too quickly, and fasting becomes a major stress because, among other defects, there is difficulty in mobilizing fat for fuel.

The adrenocorticosteroids of the glucocorticoid type influence the action of growth hormone. They are inhibitory to most anabolic actions but augmentative to the others. In physiological doses, they play a permissive role in numerous processes, such as the mobilization of fat, while in large doses they are strongly catabolic and intensify the diabetic state. Growth ceases when children or young animals are given excessive doses of corticosteroids, and, in hypophysectomized animals, the opposing actions of growth hormone and the corticosteroids can be titrated against one another by the use of some index of growth such as gain in body weight, the size of the thymus, the width of a growing cartilage, or nitrogen balance. Some of the effects of high doses of glucocorticoids and estrogens to retard growth in children may relate to depressed formation of somatomedins, which are discussed below.

Somatomedin (Sulfation Factor). Serum from normal rats increases the incorporation of sulfate into the constituents of cartilage incubated *in vitro*, while serum from hypophysectomized animals is ineffective (Daughaday *et al.*, 1959). However, if growth hormone is injected into the hypophysectomized animals, their sera become endowed with the stimulating property. Added directly to the cartilage or admixed with serum, growth hormone is ineffectual. Normal human serum is also active, that from acromegalic patients more so, and that from patients suffering from hypopituitarism inert. The activity in serum appearing in response to the action of growth hormone is referred to as *sulfation factor*, or *somatomedin*. The concept has thus emerged that growth hormone acts predominantly by means of stimulation of the accumulation of somatomedin, although

certain of the effects of the hormone may result from other actions.

It is now apparent that a number of peptides in plasma have somatomedin activity in various biological or protein-binding assays (Daughaday, 1977). These peptides are heat stable and have molecular weights of 5000 to 8000. Several somatomedins have now been purified, and they are similar or identical to other growth factors that have been characterized in recent years, such as nonsuppressible insulin-like activity (NSILA-S, also called insulin-like growth factor, or IGF) and multiplication stimulatory activity (MSA). Somatomedins have regions of homology with insulin, which explains some of the similarities of their effects and their cross-reactivity in radioreceptor and protein-binding assays (*see* Chapter 64; Rinderknecht and Humbel, 1976). The number and nature of plasma materials that fulfill the definition of sulfation factor or somatomedin are unknown. Other growth-promoting factors have been described in plasma that have some of the properties of somatomedins. These include nerve growth factor (NGF), epidermal growth factor (EGF), fibroblast growth factor (FGF), and erythropoietin.

The half-life of growth hormone in the circulation is only about 20 minutes, but its effects are much longer lasting. In the treatment of hypopituitary dwarfism, human growth hormone is effective even when injected at weekly intervals. Several hours after the administration of growth hormone, somatomedins appear in the plasma, where they are bound to larger proteins; such binding probably accounts for their relatively long half-life of 3 to 4 hours. Experiments in hypophysectomized rats suggest that the liver is the major source of somatomedins. While controversial, it has been suggested that somatomedins are also produced by kidney, muscle, and perhaps other tissues. In the form of familial dwarfism described by Laron, there is an abundance of circulating growth hormone that is biologically active, but somatomedin activity is lacking and injection of growth hormone fails to stimulate its appearance (Daughaday *et al.*, 1969). This genetic resistance to growth hormone may be due to a deficiency of receptors for growth hormone or to an inability to generate somatomedins in response to the hormone (Jacobs *et al.*, 1976).

Somatomedins from different species can be distinguished immunologically, and there is species specificity in their action in radioreceptor assays; plasma from man and monkeys demonstrates cross-reactivity, but plasma obtained from primates and subprimate species does not. The specificity is thus similar to that for growth hormone. The effects of somatomedins are quite diverse and encompass many of the effects of growth hormone. These include enhanced sulfate incorporation into proteoglycans, increased protein, RNA, and DNA synthesis, and increased amino acid and glucose transport into muscle; in adipose tissue increased glucose oxidation, increased lipid synthesis, and decreased lipolysis are observed. Similar to the effects of insulin, somatomedin inhibits epinephrine-induced increases in cyclic AMP concentrations in fat and liver (Tell *et al.*, 1973). For a review of recent information on the somatomedins, *see* Phillips and Vassilopoulou-Sellin (1980).

Regulation of the Secretion of Growth Hormone. Growth hormone is synthesized and stored in granules of specific acidophilic cells of the anterior pituitary referred to as *somatotrophs*. These growth hormone–containing cells are probably derived from common stem cells that are also precursors for prolactin-containing cells, or *lactotrophs*. Conventional staining and immunohistochemical technics have been used to identify these and other types of cells in the pituitary (Doniach, 1977).

Detailed information on the secretion of growth hormone has become available since the development of sensitive radioimmunoassays for the protein (*see* Reichlin, 1974; Goldfine, 1978). Such measurements of plasma growth hormone concentration have shown surprisingly large and rapid fluctuations in response to metabolic alterations that are due to changes in the rate of secretion of the hormone from the pituitary. In the resting subject before breakfast, the plasma growth hormone concentration is 1 to 2 ng/ml (range 0 to 3). With continued fasting, the value slowly rises to about 8 ng/ml in 60 hours. After a meal or the drinking of a solution of glucose, the concentration falls rapidly to normal. Hypoglycemia induced by insulin is a particularly potent stimulus, the value rising to 25 to 50 ng/ml in 30 minutes. Hypoglycemia from other causes, as well as interference with the utilization of glucose by 2-deoxyglucose, evokes a similar response. Physical exertion, stress, and emotional excitement are normal stimuli to enhanced secretion of growth hormone. After section of the pituitary stalk, there is no change in the plasma concentration of growth hormone in response to hypoglycemia or to glucose, although the basal concentration of growth hormone is normal. Obesity causes reduction or absence of responses of growth hormone to fasting and other stimuli. Inhibitory influences on secretion of growth hormone are exerted by free fatty acids and perhaps, by way of a negative-feedback loop, by growth hormone itself.

Several provocative tests have been devised to evaluate the capacity of the pituitary to secrete growth hormone. The intravenous infusion of arginine in a dose of 30 g in 30 minutes in adults or 0.5 g/kg in children is safer and just as useful as the induction of hypoglycemia with insulin (Parker *et al.,*

1967). Three to 5 hours after a dose of glucose, as used in the glucose tolerance test, there is normally a rise in the concentration of growth hormone in plasma. In this test, excessively obese subjects often do not respond (Theodoridis *et al.,* 1969). The administration of levodopa, apomorphine, antagonists of 5-hydroxytryptamine (5-HT), and methylphenidate can also be used to evoke secretion of growth hormone, but there is a relatively high incidence of false-negative responses in these tests.

A consistent finding and probably a most important one is the rise in the concentration of growth hormone in the plasma shortly after the onset of deep sleep. This is not just a reflection of a circadian rhythm; if the subject is kept awake all night or fitfully naps often, the rise does not take place until after he falls fast asleep the next day. In fact, prepubertal children may secrete growth hormone primarily during sleep, while secretion of growth hormone during waking hours becomes more significant in adolescents. Both prepubertal and pubertal boys have higher concentrations of plasma growth hormone than do adult males. Unlike the responses to hypoglycemia and to the other adverse influences mentioned above, this response to sleep makes physiological sense; that is, it fits with one's preconceived notion of how the secretion of growth hormone should be ordered. The old adage to the effect that one grows in his sleep may be right after all.

The increased secretion of growth hormone in response to fasting, hypoglycemia, excitement, and exercise is harder to understand. Under these conditions it seems that it is released when there is a need for fuel. If it caused a rapid release of free fatty acids from adipose tissue, it would accomplish this purpose; however, the time course of these events is such that a more complex explanation seems to be required (*see* Zierler, 1968).

Normally, secretion of growth hormone is controlled by two hypothalamic factors—growth hormone–releasing factor and growth hormone release-inhibiting hormone (somatostatin) (*see* below). A variety of drugs can influence the secretion of growth hormone, presumably by altering the secretion or activity of these regulators. For example, large doses of glucocorticoids suppress secretion of growth hormone in normal subjects, and this may contribute to their inhibitory effects on the growth of children. However, steroids may also influence the synthesis or secretion of somatomedin. Dopaminergic agonists acutely increase the secretion of growth hormone in normal subjects, and this is the basis of the levodopa test for growth hormone reserve. In contrast, in most acromegalic patients both levodopa and dopaminergic agonists decrease growth hormone secretion and may be used therapeutically. This area and the role of hypothalamic stimulatory and inhibitory hormones in the regulation of the secretion of growth hormone are discussed below.

Assays. The most commonly used bioassays for growth hormone utilize young hypophysectomized rats. *Gain in weight* during 10 days of daily, subcutaneous injection is roughly proportional to the dose. In the *tibia test,* which is more sensitive, the increase in width of the epiphyseal cartilage is measured microscopically. The substances under test are injected subcutaneously daily for 4 days.

Radioimmunoassays for growth hormone are far more sensitive. These methods depend upon competition for binding sites on a limited quantity of antibody between pure, radioactive hormone and an unknown quantity of unlabeled hormone. The various methods differ principally in the way in which the bound and the free hormone are separated.

Radioreceptor assays for growth hormone have also been described (Carr and Friesen, 1976). This technic is conceptually analogous to that of radioimmunoassay. However, a tissue-binding protein is substituted for the antibody. With this method, sensitivity is usually high, and the technic will detect hormonal derivatives with biological activity that may have lost immunoreactivity.

Therapeutic Uses. The previously limited supply of human growth hormone restricted its therapeutic use almost exclusively to hypopituitary dwarfism. While recent improvements in the extraction and purification of the human hormone from cadaver pituitaries have alleviated this situation, the protein remains rather precious and very expensive. Exciting advances in recombinant DNA technology may soon allow the mass production of the human hormone by bacteria (*see* Seeburg *et al.,* 1978; Martial *et al.,* 1979).

The first patient to receive prolonged therapy showed the uninterrupted response depicted in Figure 59–1 (Raben, 1962a, 1962b). At age 17, he was 4 ft 2½ in. tall, weighed 68 lb, and exhibited all the features of hypopituitarism. Treatment with thyroid did not promote growth, and cortisone had little clinical effect. Growth hormone was given subcutaneously in a dose of 2 mg three times weekly for the first 14 months, and over the ensuing years the dose was increased by increments to a maximum of 5 mg three times a week. When he had been treated for 3 years, he had grown to a height of 4 ft 9 in.; although 20 years old, he showed no signs of sexual maturation and, therefore, treatment with androgen was begun. Although he received only 60 mg of testosterone cypionate every 2 weeks, in 4 years there was full development of the penis, growth of axillary and pubic hair, increased body hair, more prominent musculature, and a beginning growth of beard. The bone age, which had advanced slowly with growth hormone, reached 15½ years with androgen therapy. This value is associated with nearly complete closure of the epiphyses of the long bones, implying that growth in height was nearly at an end. As there was an insignificant increase in height during a further 7½ months of treatment, growth hormone was discontinued without stopping the other replacement therapy. He had grown a total of 14 in. in 7 years and had reached the height of 5 ft 4½ in. at the age of 24.

In the majority of cases pituitary dwarfs respond satisfactorily by an increased rate of growth over many years of treatment. Usually the gain in height declines with succeeding years, and sometimes this is correctable by increasing the dose. Restoration of responsiveness has also been noted after a 3-month interruption of therapy (Rudman *et al.,* 1973). Antibodies can frequently be detected during treatment, but they do not usually influence the effectiveness of the hormone and a declining response might not correlate with the development of antibodies.

When there is a poor response or none at all, the diagnosis of hypopituitarism or of isolated deficiency of growth hormone may come into question. Normal children and children with short stature from other causes are much less sensitive to growth hormone than are those who are deficient. However, patients with partial deficiency and intermediate concentrations of plasma growth hormone may respond and should be treated.

To select those cases of short stature that are caused by deficient growth hormone, it is necessary to measure the growth hormone in the plasma and to determine whether there is an appropriate response to a provocative stimulus. Requirements for therapy with growth hormone include documentation of the failure to grow and a deficiency of the hormone. Once initiated, therapy should be evaluated for 8 to 12 months for the expected acceleration of growth. If growth hormone deficiency is the cause and therapy is successful, growth of 5 cm or more in 8 to 12 months can be expected. Evaluation of the response to shorter periods of therapy is frequently not possible. Treatment should ideally be continued throughout childhood, and sex hormones, if needed, should be given at the age of puberty to promote normal sexual development (*see* Chapters 61 and 62).

Undesirable side effects and complications are notably lacking; pain and swelling at sites of injection, allergic reactions, and chronic ill effects do not occur, even when serum antibodies can be shown.

Most of the growth hormone utilized in the United States is for treatment programs that include research studies and is obtained from the National Pituitary Agency of the National Institutes of Health, Bethesda, Maryland, upon approval of its Medical Advisory Committee. Hormone is supplied for a

TREATMENT OF A MALE PITUITARY DWARF

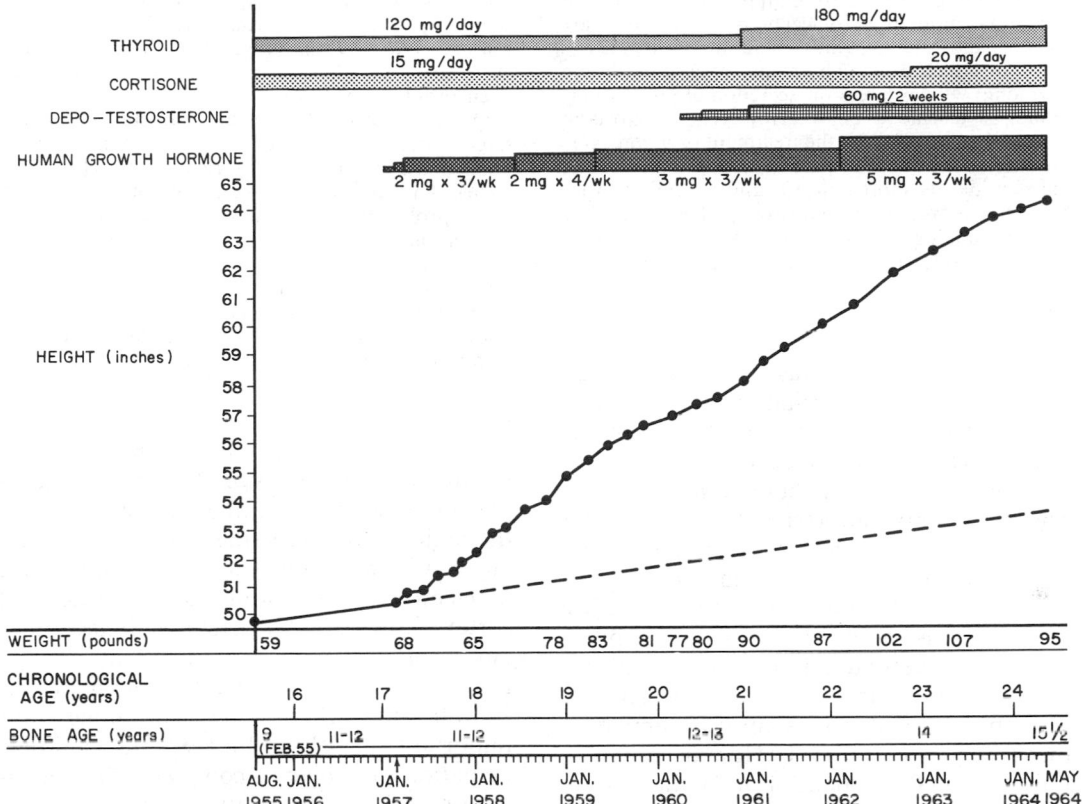

Figure 59-1. *Treatment of a patient with pituitary dwarfism with human growth hormone during replacement therapy with thyroid, cortisone, and testosterone.* (Modified from Raben, 1962b. Courtesy of the *New England Journal of Medicine.*)

specific patient, and with yearly reapplication the supply is usually committed until the patient attains a height of 5 ft. All pathologists should cooperate by sending human pituitaries obtained at post-mortem examination to the National Pituitary Agency. Growth hormone is also available commercially, as ASELLACRIN, for patients with documented clinical and laboratory evidence of deficiency.

Acromegaly. In acromegaly, the causative hypersecretion of growth hormone is from a pituitary tumor. These tumors can display a spectrum of independence from normal physiological and even pharmacological factors with respect to their secretion. Tumors that secrete growth hormone can be removed surgically or they can be treated with irradiation. While levodopa increases the secretion of growth hormone in normal subjects, it exerts a paradoxical inhibitory effect in patients with acromegaly. This observation has led to the effective therapeutic use of dopaminergic agonists for the management of acromegaly. Secretion of growth hormone by these tumors can be suppressed successfully with *bromocriptine* (2-bromo-α-ergokryptine) (Wass *et al.,* 1977;

Goldfine, 1978). This therapy should be reserved for tumors without suprasellar extension and alterations in visual fields. Oral administration of 2.5 to 40 mg a day in divided doses is frequently effective. The initial dose of 1.25 to 2.5 mg per day should be increased every few days, if necessary, in order to minimize side effects; these include nausea, vomiting, constipation, and perhaps hypotension. Failure of bromocriptine to lower concentrations of growth hormone in plasma acutely does not necessarily imply that the drug will not be effective during chronic administration. Withdrawal of the drug leads to a resurgence of growth hormone secretion. Increased secretion of prolactin may also occur with acromegaly or other pituitary tumors, due to the removal of inhibitory control from the hypothalamus. Bromocriptine will effectively inhibit prolactin secretion, as discussed below. The dose required for suppression of prolactin is somewhat smaller. While bromocriptine is approved in the United States for use in hyperprolactinemia, its employment in acromegaly is experimental. Bromocriptine is further discussed in Chapters 21 and 39.

Antagonists of 5-HT such as cyproheptadine and metergoline, as well as α-adrenergic antagonists (*e.g.,* phentolamine), can also inhibit the secretion of growth hormone in acromegaly, but their effects are weaker and inconsistent (Feldman *et al.,* 1976). Somatostatin (growth hormone release-inhibiting hormone) will suppress the secretion of growth hormone, as discussed below. However, somatostatin has not been useful for the treatment of acromegaly because of the need for parenteral administration of the peptide, its short half-life, and its ability to inhibit the secretion of numerous other hormones. Selective analogs of somatostatin with long half-lives might be useful if such could be developed.

PROLACTIN

Although prolactin was discovered in 1928 and a wealth of information was obtained about its role in a wide variety of species, unequivocal evidence for the existence of the hormone in man was obtained relatively recently. It is now appreciated, however, that prolactin plays an important role in normal human function and in certain pathophysiological states (Thorner, 1977; Frantz, 1978).

Prolactin is widely distributed in the pituitaries of vertebrates. It is synthesized and stored in pituitary lactotrophs, which are probably derived from stem cells similar to those for somatotrophs. Human amniotic fluid has concentrations of prolactin that are severalfold higher than those in plasma, and placental tissue can synthesize and secrete the hormone (Golander *et al.,* 1978).

The term *prolactin* was coined for the hormone responsible for the secretion of milk by the crop glands of the pigeon (Riddle *et al.,* 1933). In this bird there is a bilateral outpouching of the esophagus and, prompted by the psychological concomitants of brooding, a glandular structure grows within each pouch so that by the time of hatching a thick secretion, the crop milk, becomes available to each parent for regurgitating down the throats of the young. The response of the bird is a sensitive one; it is sufficient for one partner to see his mate sitting on the eggs for his pituitary to secrete prolactin and provoke the growth of the crop glands. In so naming the hormone, the tenuous analogy between the mammary gland and the crop sac was correctly drawn because it later was clear that prolactin is also of importance in initiating secretion from the breast.

Chemistry. The difficulty in isolating human prolactin is attributable to the facts that growth hormone is very similar in structure, possesses significant lactogenic activity in conventional bioassays for the hormone, and is present in human pituitaries in quantities about 100-fold greater than is prolactin. However, refined bioassay technics permitted verification of the existence of human prolactin (Frantz

and Kleinberg, 1970), and the technic of affinity chromatography permitted purification of a primate prolactin and subsequent development of a specific radioimmunoassay (Guyda and Friesen, 1971; Hwang *et al.,* 1971). Progress in the purification, chemistry, and physiology of human prolactin has been rapid since these advances.

Ovine prolactin has been characterized extensively, since the pituitaries of sheep are readily available and constitute a very rich source (Li *et al.,* 1970). The amino acid sequences of human and ovine prolactin are now known to be quite similar (Shome and Parlow, 1977). The general structural features are very similar to those of the growth hormones (Table 59–1), and the proposed evolutionary relationship of these molecules has been discussed above. As with the growth hormones, large and small forms of prolactin have been described (Suh and Frantz, 1974).

Physiological Actions. *Breast.* The mammary gland is a site of immensely complex interactions; a number of hormones and the majority of endocrine organs participate vigorously in the initiation and maintenance of lactation. The hormones of the adrenal cortex, thyroid, and ovaries are all necessary, and their presence is dependent on the trophic hormones of the adenohypophysis. Insulin and perhaps growth hormone exert important anabolic influences. The vital participation of prolactin completes the contribution of the anterior pituitary, with all of its major secretions at work. The role of oxytocin is considered in Chapter 39.

The actions of prolactin on the mammary gland have been studied particularly in explanted rodent tissue. However, investigations of normal and aberrant prolactin secretion assure the existence of comparable functions in the human female. The increasing concentration of prolactin during pregnancy is required for growth and development of the breast in preparation for breast feeding post partum. In systems *in vitro,* prolactin in the proper hormonal milieu binds to specific receptors and promotes proliferation and subsequent differentiation of mammary ductal and alveolar epithelium. There is a rapid increase in RNA synthesis and induction of the synthesis of milk proteins and of enzymes necessary for lactose synthesis (Topper, 1970; Turkington *et al.,* 1973). At the subcellular level, activation of the development of rough endoplasmic reticulum, Golgi apparatus, and secretory granules is prominent.

These "mammotrophic" actions of prolactin suggest a possible role of prolactin in mammary tumorigenesis (Smithline *et al.*, 1975). Prolonged prolactin administration, the grafting of extra pituitaries, or experimental lesions in the median eminence that cause increased prolactin secretion all result in a high percentage of mammary tumors in susceptible rats and mice. Furthermore, estrogen will not produce tumors in the absence of the pituitary; however, in rats treated with carcinogens, prolactin promotes tumorigenesis in the absence of estrogens or progestins. Furthermore, drugs that enhance prolactin secretion (*e.g.*, reserpine, haloperidol—*see* below) facilitate experimental tumor growth, while those that inhibit secretion (*e.g.*, ergot derivatives) impede growth and reduce the incidence of spontaneous tumors in rodent models. Extrapolation between highly susceptible strains of rodents and man is obviously of questionable value, but these observations may provide additional explanations for the effectiveness of hormonal therapy of breast tumors. They may also relate to some of the conflicting reports of the increased incidence of breast cancer among women who have been treated with reserpine for hypertension (*see* Frantz, 1978). However, most studies have shown normal concentrations of prolactin in patients with breast tumors, and there is thus no reason to believe that disorders of prolactin metabolism have etiological significance in mammary carcinogenesis in the human female. The hormone may, however, play a permissive role.

Gonads. The effects of prolactin on the ovary are species dependent. While the hormone has in the past also been referred to as *luteotropin,* this description was based on observations on rats and mice. In these species prolactin can prolong the life of the functioning corpus luteum, but it probably does not fulfill the role of a true luteotropic hormone. Notably, prolactin will not stimulate progesterone biosynthesis by corpora lutea in a variety of species, including rats (*see* Dorfman, 1972). It may, however, function to promote the luteal synthesis of cholesterol, the steroidal precursor. In contrast, luteinizing hormone is uniformly effective in stimulating progesterone synthesis. Surprisingly, evidence suggests that the sharp rise in prolactin secretion seen during proestrus in the rat may be responsible for luteolysis of corpora lutea formed during the previous cycle (Meites *et al.*, 1972).

In human subjects prolactin may inhibit the secretion of gonadotropins or their effects on the gonads (Thorner, 1977). Suckling is a potent stimulus to prolactin secretion for several months post partum. The elevation of prolactin with breast feeding and its inhibitory effects on ovarian function can explain the usual lack of ovulation and infertility during breast feeding. This natural mechanism of contraception becomes ineffective several months post partum as the suckling stimulus to the secretion of prolactin declines. Prolactin-secreting tumors frequently lead to galactorrhea, amenorrhea, anovulatory cycles, and infertility in women, while hyperprolactinemia in men may cause loss of libido and impotence (Thorner, 1977; Franz, 1978). Paradoxically prolactin may also directly stimulate testicular synthesis of testosterone (Rubin *et al.*, 1976).

Other Effects. Sexual behavior of lower animals and birds is thought to be influenced by gonadotropins and steroids, while parental behavior involving the care, feeding, and protection of offspring may be regulated by prolactin. There is no evidence that similar functions of prolactin occur in man. Although prolactin has effects on salt and water metabolism in lower forms, the consensus is that comparable effects do not occur in man, despite several reports to the contrary; these may be attributable to contaminants in the hormonal preparations used (Baumann and Loriaux, 1976).

Prolactin Secretion. Refined assay technics not only have been instrumental in the identification and purification of human prolactin but also have allowed exploration of physiological, pathological, and pharmacological influences on prolactin secretion (*see* Friesen, 1973; Thorner, 1977; Frantz, 1978). Concentrations in plasma are high in newborns but decrease to low levels until puberty, when they begin to increase in girls. The normal adult human plasma concentration of prolactin approximates 5 to 10 ng/ml and is somewhat less in males than in females. Prolactin concentrations rise markedly during pregnancy, reaching a maximum at term. Prolactin, in concert with placental lactogen, steroids, and probably other hormones, is responsible for growth and development of the breasts during pregnancy and the formation of the milk. After delivery the concentrations of prolactin decline unless the mother breast-feeds. In nursing mothers prolactin secretion is critically controlled by the sucking stimulus or breast manipulation. Prolactin concentration can rise 10- to 100-fold within 30 minutes of stimulation. This response becomes less prominent after several months of breast feeding, and prolactin concentrations decline. Exceptions are noted in some primitive cultures where the response of prolactin to suckling may persist for longer times. In some normal menstruating women, but not in men, breast manipulation may produce small increases in the rate of secretion of prolactin.

Many of the physiological factors that influence the secretion of growth hormone have similar effects on prolactin. These include sleep, stress, hypoglycemia, fluctuations of the concentrations of estrogen, and exercise, which increase the secretion of both hormones. Prolactin shows a circadian rhythm, with peaks during sleep; superimposed on this pattern are minute-to-minute fluctuations due to pulsatile secretion. The half-life of prolactin in plasma is 15 to 20 minutes. A variety of endogenous factors and drugs can alter the secretion of prolactin and are discussed below.

Secretion of prolactin by the pituitary is under predominantly negative control by the hypothalamus, and in this respect it is unique among the pituitary hormones. A prolactin release-inhibiting hormone (PRIH) is secreted by the hypothalamus and is carried by the hypothalamicoadenohypophyseal portal system to the adenohypophysis, where it inhibits prolactin secretion. There is considerable evidence that the release of prolactin is under adrenergic (dopaminergic) control, and PRIH may in fact be dopamine (MacLeod, 1976). Thus, the administration of levodopa *in vivo* inhibits prolactin secretion, and dopamine is a highly effective inhibitor when instilled into the third ventricle or when applied to the isolated pituitary *in vitro*. Predictably, the phenothiazine and butyrophenone antipsychotics (*e.g.*, chlorpromazine, haloperidol), which are dopamine antagonists, enhance prolactin secretion, as can reserpine and α-methyldopa (*see* Chapter 19). The antipsychotic agents can cause significant galactorrhea associated with elevated concentrations of prolactin in plasma.

While thyrotropin-releasing hormone (TRH) can stimulate prolactin secretion, the physiological significance of this effect is not known. Another factor, designated prolactin-releasing factor (PRF), which is of hypothalamic origin, is thought to play a stimulatory role in the regulation of prolactin secretion, but the nature of this material is not known (Boyd *et al.*, 1976).

Hyperprolactinemia. This disorder may be associated with various drugs such as dopaminergic antagonists, infiltrative disorders of the hypothalamus or pituitary that interfere with regulation of prolactin secretion by PRIH, hypothyroidism with accompanying increases in TRH, and the use of oral contraceptives. Prolactin-secreting tumors are another cause, and these may become apparent because of galactorrhea, amenorrhea, and infertility. These tumors usually are treated with irradiation or by surgical removal. When the tumors are microadenomata that are not associated with suprasellar extension or alterations in visual fields, pharmacological suppression of prolactin secretion is effective and should be considered. Suppression of galactorrhea by administration of levodopa has been attempted with variable success (Turkington, 1972). Some patients who respond initially become refractory to the drug. More promising clinical results have been achieved with ergot derivatives (Floss *et al.*, 1973). Inhibition of lactation in women suffering from ergotism was observed centuries ago. This phenomenon has gained scientific credence with the discovery that ergot derivatives profoundly inhibit prolactin secretion *in vivo* and in isolated pituitary preparations *in vitro*. Since the inhibitory effect *in vitro* is antagonized by haloperidol, it is likely that ergot

alkaloids activate the dopaminergic receptors that inhibit prolactin release. The compound that has shown significant clinical promise is *bromocriptine,* which is now available as bromocriptine mesylate in 2.5-mg tablets (PARLODEL). The dosage and side effects of this drug are discussed above. Other ergot derivatives are also effective, but experience with them has been limited (*see* Parkes, 1977). When bromocriptine is used to suppress prolactin secretion by such functional tumors, the galactorrhea and amenorrhea usually cease within several weeks and pregnancy becomes possible. Pregnancies and offspring have been normal, but it is recommended that bromocriptine be discontinued during pregnancy. Generally galactorrhea, amenorrhea, and infertility will recur in the nonpregnant patient when the drug is stopped. The use of bromocriptine to induce fertility has yet to be approved in the United States.

Assays. The classical procedure for bioassay of prolactin is based on the original work of Riddle and associates (1933), namely, the increase in weight of the crop sacs of doves and pigeons. Other methods are based on the induction of secretory changes in the suitably prepared mammary glands of guinea pigs and rabbits. As mentioned above, radioimmunoassays have proven invaluable. A radioreceptor assay that utilizes a membrane receptor preparation isolated from rabbit mammary glands is also useful to assess biological activity (Shiu *et al.*, 1973).

Human Placental Lactogen. Preparations from the human placenta contain growth-promoting and lactogenic activity (*see* Fukushima, 1961); Josimovich and MacLaren (1962) showed that such extracts cross-reacted with antisera to human growth hormone. Purified preparations caused a local response in the crop sac of the pigeon and maintained the function of the corpora lutea of rats but caused little growth in hypophysectomized animals; the active principle was named *placental lactogen.* Friesen (1966) purified the protein to homogeneity and demonstrated that it was strikingly lactogenic in pseudopregnant rabbits.

The chemical similarity of the substance to human growth hormone was shown by Sherwood (1967), and the complete amino acid sequence has been elucidated by Niall and associates (1971) and Li and coworkers (1973). The resemblance to growth hormone was amply confirmed by these studies, since both hormones contain 191 amino acids that differ in only 32 positions. The greater similarity of amino acid sequence of human placental lactogen and human growth hormone than of human and bovine growth hormones suggests a later evolutionary appearance of the placental lactogen. Because of its resemblance to growth hormone, the unwieldy name *chorionic somatomammotropin* is also in use.

The functions of human placental lactogen have not been clearly defined. It is produced by the syncytiotrophoblasts of the placenta, and concentrations in maternal plasma increase progressively during pregnancy. In addition to promoting growth and development of the mammary gland, it is luteotropic and may stimulate production of steroids by the corpus luteum during pregnancy. The metabolic effects of placental lactogen resemble those of growth hormone, and it is postulated that these effects may be important for fetal nutrition, growth, and development (Chatterjee and Munro, 1977).

GONADOTROPIC HORMONES

The pituitary gland plays an important part in the regulation of gonadal function throughout the vertebrate phylum, but the fullest understanding of the mechanisms involved has been achieved among mammals. The adenohypophysis is physiologically and anatomically so situated that it can mediate neural messages that arise from the environment as well as intercept humoral signals from within. It can regulate such diverse phenomena as the annual growth and regression of the gonads of monestrous mammals in response to the changing length of daylight, the release of ova in the rabbit 10 hours after mating, and the reinitiation of follicular growth when a corpus luteum fails for lack of successful impregnation.

For over 45 years it has been known that two gonadotropins are involved, and it seems a general rule among mammals that follicular growth and development on the one hand and ovulation and the formation of a corpus luteum on the other are separately controlled. These same substances stimulate, respectively, the germinal elements of the testis and the androgen-secreting Leydig cells of the interstitial tissue. In the regulation of the function of the corpus luteum, several adaptations have arisen. In some species luteinizing hormone serves as the luteotropin, in others prolactin plays such a role, while in several species the uterus is somehow involved. During pregnancy the pituitary seems essential in some animals, while in most it is dispensable; luteal function may be autonomous, as in the herbivora, or regulated in part by a placental luteotropin, as in man.

Until recently the functions of the gonadotropins in man were largely inferred from information derived from other mammals. Direct observations on human beings of the effects of gonadal hormones and their analogs and human gonadotropins have given better understanding and have opened new therapeutic approaches to the disturbances of human reproductive function.

Chemistry. The five gonadotropins considered here (two of pituitary and three of placental origin) are follicle-stimulating hormone (FSH), luteinizing hormone (LH), chorionic gonadotropin (CG), chorionic follicle-stimulating hormone (CFSH), and the gonadotropin of pregnant mares' serum. The gonadotropins, with thyrotropin (TSH), constitute the glycoprotein group of hormones, and their similarities and general chemical features have been mentioned above (*see* Table 59-1).

FSH, LH, CG, and TSH have been purified and characterized from several sources, including man. These hormones have two nonidentical and noncovalently linked peptide subunits, designated α and β. The α subunits of each hormone are nearly identical; the biological specificity resides in the β subunits. The α subunit of one hormone can be combined with the β subunit of another to yield a hybrid molecule with biological activity of the β-subunit donor. The β subunits also have a great deal of similarity. For example, the β subunit of human chorionic gonadotropin consists of 145 amino acid residues, and residues 1 to 115 are about 80% homologous with the β subunits of LH, FSH, and TSH. The carbohydrate content of each of these glycoproteins is however quite different (Shome and Parlow, 1973, 1974; Lipsett and Ross, 1978). While a large form of LH with a molecular weight of about 140,000 is present in plasma, it is not known if this is merely an aggregate of the more common monomer or if it represents a prohormone (Graesslin *et al.,* 1976).

Less is known about the chemistry of another glycoprotein hormone included in this class, chorionic follicle-stimulating hormone (CFSH). This glycoprotein is synthesized by the placenta and contains 32% carbohydrate; its properties are quite different from chorionic gonadotropin (CG). Since it readily reacts with antisera to human FSH, they are presumably quite similar. The function of CFSH is unknown (*see* Chatterjee and Munro, 1977).

The gonadotropin of pregnant mare's serum has an exceedingly high carbohydrate content (47%). This glycoprotein is also composed of two subunits.

Secretion and Physiological Actions. Despite an extraordinarily large number of experimental observations of the secretion and actions of gonadotropins, understanding of these areas is far from complete. Most studies have been carried out in species different from that of origin of the hormone, and in some instances impure preparations have been used, which may account for some anomalous responses. Observations on the responses of the normal human gonads to human gonadotropins are still fragmentary.

Secretion. LH and FSH are produced and secreted by the same cell type in the pituitary. In infancy and prepuberty their concentrations in plasma are measurable, but quite low. At puberty gonadotropin secretion increases, probably due to diminished feedback inhibition of secretion by sex steroids (*see* Franchimont, 1977). In men, concentrations are relatively constant, while rates of secretion in women are somewhat higher and vary according to the phases of the menstrual cycle (*see* below). In some gonadal disorders, in postmenopausal women, and to some extent in elderly men, concentrations of gonadotropins increase due to diminished concentrations of sex steroids and a resultant loss of their feedback inhibition on the pituitary. Gonadotropins are secreted in a pulsatile manner, which accounts for the minute-to-minute oscillations in plasma concentrations. Pituitary tumors may rarely secrete one or both gonadotropins (Friend *et al.,* 1976; Snyder and Sterling, 1976).

Actions on the Ovary. During the follicular phase of the ovarian cycle successive groups of small follicles start to grow, and by the time ovulation is imminent follicles in all stages of development are found. This ovarian response represents the predominant action of FSH, and it is during this phase that estrogen is the main ovarian secretory product (*see* Figure 61–2, page 1424). Since some highly purified preparations of FSH induce follicular growth in hypophysectomized rats without evoking the secretion of estrogen, it is believed that small amounts of LH are required for the secretion of estrogen (Mills *et al.,* 1971). However, since the hypophysectomized animal suffers multiple deficiencies, further experiments are needed to establish the point.

Shortly before ovulation is to take place, a series of ovarian changes follow in rapid succession, presumably mediated by a burst of LH secretion at this time. The largest follicles expand quickly; those in just the right stage of development to ovulate undergo cytological changes in the granulosa in the direction of luteinization and show intense hyperemia of the theca interna. One area on the surface of the follicle thins and then undergoes dissolution, leaving an aperture through which the viscous follicular fluid oozes, carrying desquamated granulosa cells

and the cumulus and its contained ovum with it. Those large follicles not destined to ovulate, perhaps for reasons of improper stage of development, remain avascular and begin to show regressive changes. While ovulation is in progress, widespread atresia involves all the other follicles that shortly before had been flourishing under the influence of FSH, and in certain species the atresic process extends also to the residual corpora lutea of antecedent cycles. It is tempting to attribute the regressive changes in the ovary, which parallel so closely ovulation and luteinization, to an action of LH, but it must be admitted that experimental evidence in support of this concept is not entirely uniform.

With the earliest stages of preovulatory follicular swelling there is evidence of the first secretion of progesterone. This has been shown in species that require the luteotropic action of prolactin as well as in those that do not. The critical influence is exerted by LH.

Measurements of the gonadotropins in plasma throughout the menstrual cycle show that FSH is elevated during the follicular phase and slowly falls before it rises again at midcycle; it is lowest during the luteal phase. LH shows a striking peak at midcycle, usually on the same day that the FSH is highest (*see* Figure 61–2, page 1424). This surge in the secretion of LH is an immediately preovulatory event (*see* Faiman and Ryan, 1967; Midgley and Jaffe, 1968). Further interactions between the gonadotropins and the sex steroids are discussed in Chapters 61 and 62.

Actions on the Testis. Whereas in the ovary both gonadotropins are involved in the secretion of hormones, LH plays a predominant role in the testis. FSH is primarily a gametogenic hormone in males; it is responsible for the anatomical integrity of the seminiferous tubules and only under its influence are the complex stages of gametogenesis carried through to the production of spermatozoa. In the hypophysectomized animal, the major effect of FSH is stimulation of the seminiferous tubules. As the tubules make up the bulk of the testis, tubular growth is accurately reflected by an increase in testicular weight. Possible effects of FSH on testosterone secretion from the Leydig cells are controversial and are discussed in Chapter 62.

LH stimulates the interstitial cells to secrete androgen, but the androgen, in turn, exerts a direct effect upon the tubules so that both components of the testis appear to be stimulated. These effects of LH have led to its alternate designation as interstitial cell–stimulating hormone (ICSH).

Mechanism of Action. LH and FSH bind with apparent specificity to various particulate fractions derived from testis and ovary. Furthermore, both gonadotropins are known to stimulate cyclic AMP synthesis in appropriate gonadal preparations (Marsh *et al.*, 1966; Murad *et al.*, 1969). Cyclic AMP then stimulates sex steroid biosynthesis by mechanisms apparently analogous to those operative in the adrenal cortex. The nucleotide also induces luteinization of cultured granulosa cells (Channing and Seymour, 1970) and transplanted ovarian follicles (Ellsworth and Armstrong, 1973). It has been suggested that prostaglandins play a role in the stimulation of cyclic AMP synthesis by LH (Kuehl *et al.*, 1970), and similar observations have been made with TSH, a structural cousin (Zor *et al.*, 1969).

Chorionic Gonadotropin (CG). Chorionic gonadotropin is a hormone of human pregnancy; it is secreted by the syncytiotrophoblasts of fetal placenta as early as 7 days after ovulation, and it is absorbed into the blood in sufficient quantity to sustain luteal function and forestall the next menstrual period; the secretion of LH remains suppressed because of the rising concentrations of estrogen and progesterone (Lipsett and Ross, 1978).

Chorionic gonadotropin is detectable in the urine by immunoassay several days before the first missed period, and this is the basis of the most commonly used test of pregnancy. The quantity excreted increases rapidly thereafter to a maximum about 6 weeks after ovulation. The urinary content then declines over the next month or so and stabilizes at a lower level for the remainder of pregnancy.

The changes in the corpus luteum in early pregnancy reflect the intense stimulation provided by the LH-like action of chorionic gonadotropin. Furthermore, as noted above, concentrations of placental lactogen increase progressively during pregnancy; it also is luteotropic and may play some role in concert with chorionic gonadotropin to stimulate steroid production by the corpus luteum. With the increasing secretion of estrogen and progesterone by the placenta during the third month, the ovaries and the corpus luteum become unessential to the maintenance of gestation, but the corpus luteum does not undergo a pronounced change at this time. Instead, there is a slow regression that, histologically, is not complete even at the time of delivery. In the presence of the flood of chorionic gonadotropin during pregnancy, the rest of the ovary remains quiescent; there is no growth or maturation of follicles and no changes suggesting luteinization either of the granulosa or of thecal or stromal elements.

Assays of chorionic gonadotropin and its subunits are also used to diagnose and to evaluate the treatment of trophoblastic tumors (Vaitukaitis *et al.*, 1976). Quantification of the secretion of the hormone by choriocarcinomas and hydatidiform moles can provide an accurate index of tumor regression or recurrence. This ability has contributed to the high rate of successful treatment of these tumors.

The action of chorionic gonadotropin on the testis can hardly be regarded as physiological, for the hormone gains access to the male only *in utero*, when it does cause minimal gonadal stimulation; otherwise the hormone is found in the male only in the rare event of a teratomatous tumor containing chorionic elements. Injected into men, however, chorionic gonadotropin stimulates the interstitial cells of the testis to secrete androgen. Activation of the seminiferous epithelium is minimal and may be mediated entirely by the androgen of Leydig-cell origin.

Chorionic gonadotropin also has some thyrotropic activity, which is thought to be unimportant except in some trophoblastic tumors where the large amounts of hormone can lead to hyperthyroidism (Cave and Dunn, 1976; Morley *et al.*, 1976).

The mechanism of action of chorionic gonadotropin appears to be identical to that of LH.

Absorption, Fate, and Excretion. The gonadotropins of either pituitary or placental origin are effective only if given by injection. The length of survival of the injected and presumably of the endogenously secreted hormones is determined largely by the rate of degradation in the body, because little is excreted in the urine except in the case of chorionic gonadotropin. Studies on the rate of disappearance of endogenous human LH, FSH, and chorionic gonadotropin indicate removal from the plasma with at least two distinct half-times. The shorter half-lives for these three hormones approximate 20 minutes, 4 hours, and 11 hours, respectively, while the longer half-lives appear to be 4, 70, and 23 hours (Yen *et al.*, 1968, 1970). Removal of sialic acid from chorionic gonadotropin greatly decreases its half-life, but this may not be important in its normal metabolism. While appreciable amounts of chorionic gonadotropin are excreted in the urine, it has been estimated that only 5% of secreted FSH is found in the urine in an active form (Coble *et al.*, 1969). During the latter part of pregnancy, material reacting immunologically like chorionic gonadotropin appears in the urine in quantities several times greater than the quantity of biologically active hormone (Hobson and Wide, 1964), suggesting that there is partial degradation before excretion, and this mechanism may be involved in the rapid clearance of the active hormone from the body after delivery of the placenta.

The gonadotropin of pregnant mares' serum does not appear in the urine of the mare, and it has not been detected in the urine of other animals after injection. In the rat, the duration of action of a single dose is very long; with a moderate dose the maximal ovarian weight is reached about 5 days after the injection, so the substance may have a very long survival in the body.

Assays. Bioassay remains a necessary technic for evaluation of functional activity, which often bears no relationship to immunoreactivity. The gonadotropins pose a special problem because many responses to one hormone are modified by the concurrent action of others, and special conditions must be chosen to minimize this influence. References and descriptions of several technics can be found in the *third* and *fourth editions* of this textbook.

For many purposes, particularly the measurement of gonadotropins in blood and urine, radioimmunoassays are more accurate and far simpler than bioassays. References have been cited by Vande Wiele and Dyrenfurth (1973).

Preparations and Dosages. Currently no purified gonadotropins prepared from human pituitaries are available commercially. For clinical purposes, quite crude preparations are suitable, even though they contain both FSH and LH as well as other active principles. The limiting factor is the scarcity of human pituitary glands and not the preparation of suitable extracts.

Menotropins for Injection, U.S.P. (PERGONAL), is a preparation of gonadotropins from the urine of postmenopausal women. While FSH and LH activities are present in equal unitage, chorionic gonadotropin is usually required in conjunction with menotropins to induce ovulation. The recommended initial dose is 75 I.U. of each gonadotropin intramuscularly daily for 9 to 12 days. This is followed by 10,000 I.U. of chorionic gonadotropin. If there is no evidence of ovulation, several treatment cycles may be necessary and the dosage may be increased. In some cases large quantities may be needed. Menotropins for injection is supplied in ampuls containing 75 I.U. of FSH and 75 I.U. of LH. The powder is dissolved in 2 ml of sterile 0.9% sodium chloride solution and is administered intramuscularly, immediately.

Chorionic Gonadotropin for Injection, U.S.P., is a preparation derived from the urine of pregnant women, which is sold under various trade names (ANTUITRIN-S, A.P.L. SECULES, FOLLUTEIN, LIBIGEN, PREGNYL, others). It is usually given intramuscularly in doses of 1000 to 4000 I.U. two or three times weekly for several weeks for the treatment of cryptorchism or hypogonadism in men, and in doses of 8000 to 10,000 I.U. one day following treatment with menotropins to evoke ovulation. It is available in vials containing 1000, 5000, 10,000, or 20,000 I.U. of powder with an ampul of suitable diluent.

Gonadotropin of pregnant mares' serum has been used clinically to a limited extent for 4 decades; however, no clear-cut indications have emerged and there are few guidelines to dosage.

Purified human LH and FSH are available for investigational use only from the National Pituitary Agency of the National Institutes of Health, Bethesda, Maryland.

Therapeutic Uses. The gonadotropins are used in therapy primarily for the treatment of infertility and cryptorchism.

Infertility. The widest potential usefulness of the gonadotropins is in the induction of ovulation in women who are infertile because of pituitary insufficiency. Extensive clinical experience with menotropins and human chorionic gonadotropin, summarized by Thompson and Hansen (1970), indicated the occurrence of ovulation in 75% of appropriately selected patients treated with the drugs. While ovulation was occasionally seen during administration of menotropins before human chorionic gonadotropin was given, it usually took place about 18 hours after administration of the latter hormone. Pregnancy resulted in approximately 25% of the patients; of these, the abortion rate was 25% and fetal abnormalities occurred in 2%. Twenty percent of pregnancies resulted in multiple births (15% twins and 5% with three or more concepti). Interestingly, in another series the male-to-female sex ratio in single births was 0.88, but only 0.43 for births of twins. The growth and development of children born of mothers receiving gonadotropin treatment have been normal (Hack *et al.*, 1970).

The only complications reported for this therapy have been excessive ovarian enlargement as a result of the maturation of many follicles; this, in turn, may lead to the release of multiple ova and to multiple births. Ovarian hyperstimulation may be seen several days after the administration of chorionic gonadotropin in a few percent of patients. In this condition the enlarged ovaries give rise to pain in the lower abdomen, and, if there is bleeding into the peritoneal cavity, the pain is severe. Under the latter circumstance, hospitalization and observation for ovarian rupture are required. Methods have been devised to avoid these complications (Brown *et al.*,

1969). For example, one can test ovarian responsiveness by measuring the excretion of estrogens in the urine in a preliminary trial and thereby be guided in the dosage appropriate for a therapeutic attempt. If the urinary estrogens exceed 150 μg/24 hours, chorionic gonadotropin should be withheld. Alternatively, several trials may be made with small doses before the larger recommended amounts are used.

It is remarkable how closely the experience with human gonadotropins parallels that following the use of clomiphene (*see* Chapter 61). Further experience will be needed to determine which types of ovarian disorders are best treated with gonadotropin and which with clomiphene; currently clomiphene would seem the better agent in the syndrome of polycystic ovaries whereas gonadotropin would be indicated when the pituitary is primarily at fault.

While the use of human gonadotropin, either from the pituitary gland or from menopausal urine, to promote fertility in the male is a field that has not been extensively explored, men with hypopituitarism have been rendered fertile by this means (Gemzell and Kjessler, 1964; Mancini *et al.,* 1971). As the process of germinal maturation in the tubules requires 10 weeks and the transit of the spermatozoa through the vas deferens several weeks more, investigation of this form of treatment is time consuming. The effectiveness of therapy with gonadotropins when more subtle forms of gametogenic failure are under study is more difficult to evaluate and more extensive experience is required. Often testicular failure appears to be due to an intrinsic fault of the testis itself, and additional gonadotropin would not be expected to be beneficial.

Cryptorchism. Failure of the descent of one testis or both is sometimes noted in childhood; it is most frequent in infancy and is less prevalent with advancing age until it becomes a rare finding in the adult. In the majority of cases, testes undescended in childhood assume their normal position at the time of puberty, a sequence of events that is normal in monkeys. In rare cases, cryptorchism denotes an abnormality of testicular development and in this event descent at puberty does not take place. There is also some indication that testicular development is quite normal if descent is achieved before age seven (Lattimer, 1973). This can often be accomplished by the administration of an androgen or chorionic gonadotropin. Such treatment is more effective when failure of testicular descent is bilateral, in contrast to the unilateral condition. Chorionic gonadotropin is usually used and is customarily given intramuscularly in doses of 1000 to 4000 I.U. two or three times weekly for several weeks, but therapy is stopped as soon as the desired result has been achieved. If such treatment is not successful, the undescended testis should be placed in the scrotum surgically or removed, since the incidence of testicular tumors is markedly increased in cryptorchism.

THYROTROPIN (TSH)

The regulatory effects of thyrotropin on the thyroid gland are considered in Chapter 60. The essential chemical features of human thyrotropin are summarized in Table 59–1 (*see also* Pierce, 1971; Burger and Patel, 1977).

Assays. A widely used bioassay is that described by McKenzie (1961). Thyroid stimulation is reflected in increased circulating radioactivity in mice with thyroids prelabeled with radioiodine. Radioimmunoassays for human thyrotropin now permit diagnostic studies of the circulating hormone. In primary hypothyroidism, the feedback inhibition of thyroid hormone to regulate the secretion of TSH is reduced or absent, resulting in increased secretion of the trophic hormone. Thus, hypothyroidism with elevated concentrations of TSH in plasma indicates thyroid failure, whereas the occurrence of normal or low concentrations of both thyroid hormone and TSH points to a hypothalamic or pituitary defect. As discussed below and in Chapter 60, the use of thyrotropin-releasing hormone (TRH) is useful to distinguish between the latter two possibilities.

Clinical Application. *Thyrotropin* (THYTROPAR) is not used as a therapeutic agent but to diagnose thyroid disorders. The single clinical application of this bovine preparation is in the evaluation of thyroid function in conjunction with the use of radioiodine. Hypopituitarism can be differentiated from primary myxedema by the stimulation of thyroid accumulation of radioiodine by thyrotropin in the former condition but not in the latter. In the usual procedure, a dose of 10 units is given as a single intramuscular injection followed by a tracer dose of radioiodine 18 to 24 hours later. Twenty-four hours after the tracer, the accumulation in hypopituitarism is usually substantially higher than it was before thyrotropin, whereas it usually remains low in spontaneous myxedema. Since thyrotropin concentrations in plasma are elevated in primary myxedema, the increasing availability of radioimmunoassays for thyrotropin should reduce the need for administration of thyrotropin for diagnostic purposes.

OTHER THYROID STIMULATORS

Three other proteins with varying resemblance to pituitary thyrotropin have been described.

Chorionic Thyrotropin. This glycoprotein has a molecular weight of 28,000, of which 3.5% is carbohydrate. It is produced by the human placenta and stimulates the secretion of thyroid hormone much as does TSH. However, the physicochemical and antigenic properties of chorionic thyrotropin are quite different from those of the pituitary hormone. Its significance, if any, is unknown, and its secretion is not influenced by thyrotropin-releasing hormone (TRH) (Hershman, 1972; Chatterjee and Munro, 1977).

Molar Thyrotropin. This material derives its name from its detection in benign and malignant hydatidiform moles, and both *chorionic* and *molar* thyrotropins are thus *trophoblastic* thyrotropins. Molar thyrotropin has also been detected in normal placenta. It appears to have approximately twice the molecular weight of TSH or chorionic thyrotropin (Hershman, 1972). This thyroid stimulator has been responsible for thyrotoxicosis in several patients with hydatidiform mole or choriocarcinoma. In some patients with choriocarcinoma, hyperthyroidism may exist because of marked elevation of the concentration of chorionic gonadotropin, which also possesses some thyrotropic activity (Cave and Dunn, 1976; Morley *et al.,* 1976).

Long-Acting Thyroid Stimulator. In the blood of most patients suffering from Graves' disease (hyperthyroidism) substances have been found that exert a prolonged stimulatory action upon the thyroids of animals used in the assay of thyrotropin. These substances are called *long-acting thyroid stimulators* (LATS) and *long-acting thyroid stimulator-protector* (LATS-P), to distinguish them from thyrotropin. These proteins are immunoglobulins of the IgG class and can bind to antigenic sites on the plasma membrane of thyroid follicular cells (Adams and Purves, 1957; Adams and Kennedy, 1967; McKenzie and Zakarija, 1977). Presumably the binding of these and perhaps other thyroid-stimulating antibodies can mimic the effects of thyrotropin and account for the hyperthyroidism (*see* Kriss, 1970; Volpe, 1978). However the precise role of thyroid-stimulating immunoglobulins in the pathogenesis of Graves' disease remains obscure. Their actions on the thyroid gland are essentially identical to those of thyrotropin, and this may be logical since both TSH and LATS can stimulate the synthesis of cyclic AMP (Yamashita and Field, 1972). The proteins evidently can traverse the placenta and thereby account for hyperthyroidism of the newborn infants of some hyperthyroid mothers.

EXOPHTHALMOS-PRODUCING SUBSTANCE

Injection of pituitary extract into animals can cause protrusion of the eyeballs. The phenomenon, first noted in the duck (Shockaert, 1931), has been studied in the guinea pig and several species of fish. It was thought to be caused by thyrotropin, and this seemed logical at a time when thyrotropin was assumed to be an etiological factor in Graves' disease, which is often associated with exophthalmos. However, it is now known that thyrotropin concentrations are very low in Graves' disease. Furthermore, clinical conditions in which secretion of thyrotropin is elevated are not characterized by such ocular changes. While apparent dissociation of thyroid-stimulating activity and exophthalmos-producing activity was obtained in the past, homogeneous thyrotropin indeed possesses both activities and certain proteolytic fragments of the molecule retain exophthalmos-producing activity after loss of most thyroid-stimulating activity (Kohn and Winand, 1971). It is of course possible that there are other substances that can also cause exophthalmos, and certain reports suggest that exophthalmos is mediated by immunological mech-

anisms (*see* Volpe, 1978). The etiology of the condition in man is even more obscure than is the etiology of Graves' disease.

CORTICOTROPIN

The essential features of the chemistry of corticotropin (ACTH) are included in Table 59-1, and the structure of the hormone is shown in Figure 63-1. While the discussion of ACTH appears in Chapter 63, the polypeptide precursor of the hormone contains the sequences of several other important peptides, as shown in Figure 59-2; these will be considered here. Corticotropin-like intermediate lobe peptide (CLIP) is a 22 amino acid peptide that is identical to residues 18 to 39 of ACTH (Figure 59-2) and is found in the intermediate lobe of the pituitary. The functions of CLIP, if any exist, are unknown.

LIPOTROPINS

It has long been known that the injection of certain pituitary extracts into animals causes ketosis, lowering of the respiratory quotient, and increased fat in the liver. Subsequent studies have shown increased circulating free fatty acids and a direct lipolytic action on isolated adipose tissue *in vitro*, suggesting that mobilization of depot fat is the primary action concerned. As already noted, this is an important part of the action of growth hormone. While TSH, LH, and ACTH have a similar effect, only the response to TSH is thought to be of possible physiological consequence. However, the pituitary does contain lipolytic factors that differ from the hormones discussed above. Two such ovine proteins have been purified and analyzed (Li *et al.,* 1965; Chrétien and Li, 1968), and they are included in Table 59-1 and Figure 59-2. Despite their designation as β- and γ-lipotropins, they are potent lipolytic

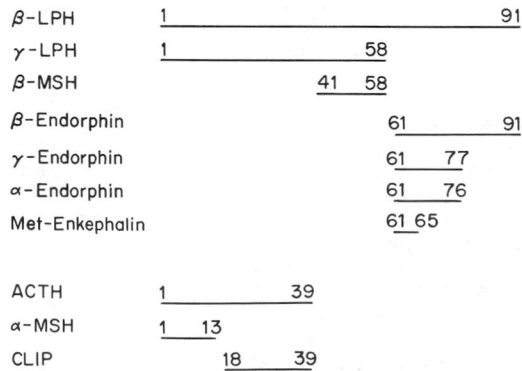

Figure 59-2. *Some structural relationships of certain pituitary peptides.* (After Daughaday, 1978. Courtesy of Plenum Medical Book Co.)

agents in certain species, particularly the rabbit. In view of their structural relationship to corticotropin and melanocyte-stimulating hormone, it is likely that these materials stimulate lipolysis by a cyclic AMP–dependent mechanism. There is some evidence to favor this hypothesis (Lis *et al.,* 1972). These factors are not lipolytic in the rat, and neither they nor their counterparts from human pituitaries are active in man. The possibility of the presence of additional lipolytic substances in human pituitary remains open.

ENDORPHINS AND ENKEPHALINS

Oligopeptides have been isolated from extracts of brain and pituitary that possess pharmacological properties similar to those of opioids (Hughes *et al.,* 1975). These morphinomimetic peptides are called *endorphins* and *enkephalins,* and their structural relationship to β-lipotropin is summarized in Figure 59–2. The pentapeptide methionine-enkephalin is identical to the sequence that extends from amino acids 61 through 65 of β-lipotropin (Tyr-Gly-Gly-Phe-Met), while α-endorphin, β-endorphin, and γ-endorphin are identical to amino acids 61 to 76, 61 to 91, and 61 to 77, respectively, in β-lipotropin (Lazarus *et al.,* 1976; Terenius, 1978). These studies suggest that β-lipotropin may serve as a precursor for these morphinomimetic peptides. This topic is also discussed in Chapters 12 and 22.

MELANOCYTE-STIMULATING HORMONE (MSH)

The intermediate lobe of the pituitary is a part of the adenohypophysis, but in most mammals it is separated from the anterior lobe by the hypophyseal cleft and is composed of a sheet of tissue firmly attached to the contiguous surface of the neurohypophysis.

The term *intermedin* was coined by Zondek for the hormone of the intermediate lobe that mediates various pigmentary responses in the lower vertebrates (*see* Zondek and Krohn, 1932). More recently, the term *melanocyte-stimulating hormone* (MSH) has been adopted, a designation that would embrace an action upon the melanocytes of mammalian skin, in keeping with the finding of a darkening of human skin in response to hormone (Lerner and McGuire, 1964). Two compounds have thus far been isolated from pituitary extracts and designated α-MSH and β-MSH (Thody, 1977).

Chemistry. When strong concentrates of ACTH were first prepared, they were found to be highly active in causing darkening of the skin of frogs. The confusion that arose as a result of this finding was finally resolved when first one component and later two were separated from ACTH. The relationships of α-MSH and β-MSH to corticotropin and the lipotropins are summarized in Figure 59–2. The sequence of 13 amino acids making up the molecule of α-MSH is identical with the first 13 residues of ACTH, and the terminal serine amino group is acetylated. While mammalian α-MSH appears to have a constant amino acid sequence in the species examined, β-MSH is variable between species and is larger than α-MSH. A peptide that is analogous to the β-MSH of other species can be found in the pituitary of man, and its structure is identical to amino acid residues 41 to 58 of the lipotropins. Pure ACTH does have inherent MSH activity, being about 1/40 as active as α-MSH on a molar basis. The bioassays used are based on hormone-induced darkening of the skin of the frog, chameleon, and related species.

Physiological Actions. Melanocyte-stimulating hormones regulate the pigmentation of fish and amphibian skin by causing dispersal of the pigment granules of the melanophores, thus making the cells appear darker. However, the role of MSH in pigmentation in man is debatable. In primary adrenal insufficiency (Addison's disease) and in syndromes characterized by ectopic production of ACTH, increased pigmentation of the skin may be prominent; this is due to the activity of ACTH itself and possibly to lipotropins, rather than to α- or β-MSH. MSH can cause hyperpigmentation when given in large doses (Lerner and McGuire, 1964). While it has been suggested that changes in skin pigmentation during the menstrual cycle and pregnancy may be due to altered secretion of MSH, the hormone has not been detected in human plasma. It is possible that MSH has no function in man and may represent an evolutionary vestige. The MSH-like radioimmunoassayable activity in plasma probably represents β-lipotropin. In lower animals, MSH has natriuretic and lipolytic effects and may increase heart rate, fetal and placental weight, and sebaceous secretions (*see* Thody, 1977). In keeping with the proposed evolutionary relationship of MSH and ACTH, these peptides increase cyclic AMP formation in appropriate tissues (Abe *et al.,* 1969).

HYPOTHALAMIC CONTROL OF THE ANTERIOR PITUITARY

It is now well established that the influence of the central nervous system upon adenohypophyseal function is mediated by neurohumoral substances transported to the gland by the hypothalamicoadenohypophyseal-portal system from a capillary network in the region of the median eminence. These substances are referred to as either releasing hormones, releasing factors, or regulatory hormones. At least some have been shown to meet the commonly accepted definition of a hormone and also to influence both the synthesis and release of adenohypophyseal hormones (Schally *et al.,* 1973). There is great current interest in the identification of hypothalamic regulatory hormones and in their potential use as therapeutic and diagnostic agents. Only a brief summary can be pro-

Table 59–2.   HYPOTHALAMIC ACTIVITIES THAT CONTROL THE RELEASE OF PITUITARY HORMONES

RELEASING HORMONE OR FACTOR	ABBREVIATION	STRUCTURE
Corticotropin-releasing factor	CRF	Unknown
Thyrotropin-releasing hormone	TRH	Tripeptide
Luteinizing hormone–releasing hormone and follicle-stimulating hormone–releasing hormone (gonadotropin-releasing hormone)	LH-RH/FSH-RH; Gn-RH	Decapeptide
Growth hormone release-inhibiting hormone	GH-RIH; somatostatin	Tetradecapeptide
Growth hormone–releasing factor	GH-RF	Unknown
Prolactin release-inhibiting hormone	PRIH	Probably dopamine
Prolactin-releasing factor	PRF	Unknown
Melanocyte-stimulating hormone release-inhibiting factor	MIF	Unknown
Melanocyte-stimulating hormone–releasing factor	MRF	Unknown

vided here, and several reviews are recommended for detailed discussion and references (Blackwell and Guillemin, 1973; Schally *et al.*, 1973; Guillemin, 1978; Krieger, 1978; Schally, 1978).

There is evidence to suggest the existence of at least nine regulatory *activities* in the secretions of the hypothalamus. These activities and the abbreviations used to designate them are listed in Table 59–2. For at least three adenohypophyseal hormones (prolactin, growth hormone, and MSH), there appears to be dual (stimulatory and inhibitory) regulation. ACTH, TSH, LH, and FSH are perhaps subject only to stimulatory control by this mechanism.

The successful isolation and identification of these hormones have required herculean efforts. Tons of hypothalamic starting material containing hundreds of thousands of hypothalami have been required to purify milligram quantities of these substances.

Regulation of Thyrotropin. Thyrotropin-releasing hormone (TRH) was the first to be identified chemically, in 1970. The porcine, ovine, bovine, and human hormones are identical in structure. TRH is a tripeptide with both terminal amino and carboxyl groups blocked: L-pyroglutamyl-L-histidyl-L-proline amide. Pyroglutamate is derived from the cyclization of glutamic acid. Synthetic TRH is now available in quantity for clinical diagnostic use. Derivatives of TRH have also been synthesized and studied; 3-methyl-His-TRH is eight to ten times more potent than the naturally occurring hormone. These studies have prompted the search for other analogs that possess even greater activity or that act as antagonists.

An extremely small quantity of TRH is effective at its site of action; picogram amounts are sufficient to release thyrotropin *in vitro*. Human subjects respond to 50 μg administered intravenously, while a dose of 5 mg or more is required orally. In normal man, intravenous TRH provokes a maximal secretion of thyrotropin within 15 to 30 minutes. Plasma concentrations of thyrotropin remain elevated for 2 to 4 hours, although TRH is inactivated rapidly by human plasma and has a half-life *in vivo* of approximately 5 minutes. There is evidence that TRH stimulates the synthesis as well as the secretion of thyrotropin, although it is not known if this is a primary effect of TRH. In addition, prolactin secretion is also enhanced (*see* below). Specific binding of TRH to pituitary membrane receptors has been demonstrated, as has an associated stimulation of cyclic AMP synthesis. Since cyclic AMP can mimic the actions of TRH *in vitro*, it seems likely that the cyclic nucleotide "second messenger" system is operative here.

The pituitary is the site of negative feedback exerted by the thyroid hormones to inhibit thyrotropin secretion. The action of TRH is antagonized at a molecular site distal to its initial interaction with the plasma membrane. Sites of thyroid hormone feedback may also exist in the central nervous system. Clinical use is made of TRH in the diagnosis of thyroid disease; with TRH it can be determined whether secondary hypothyroidism is of pituitary or hypothalamic origin, and patients with primary and secondary hypothyroidism can also be distinguished. Patients with hyperthyroidism fail to respond. Testing involves the intravenous administration of TRH (200 to 500 μg), followed by serial determinations of thyroid hormones and of plasma thyrotropin by immunoassay. Additional discussion of the use of TRH appears in Chapter 60.

Regulation of Gonadotropins. Predictably, this subject is more complex. Convincing evidence indicates that the secretion of luteinizing hormone is regulated by a hypothalamic hormone, LH-RH, and this material has been purified, identified, and synthesized. Porcine and ovine LH-RH is a decapeptide and has the amino acid sequence pyroGlu-His-Trp-Ser-Tyr-Gly-Leu-Arg-Pro-Gly-NH$_2$. No species specificity for the effect of LH-RH has been demonstrated, suggesting that the decapeptide is similar or identical in a number of species. The major difficulty is that LH-RH stimulates the release of both luteinizing hormone and follicle-stimulating hormone, and it has been proposed that there is but a single gonadotropin-releasing hormone (LH-RH/FSH-RH, also designated Gn-RH).

Synthetic LH-RH is highly active in man. Intravenous administration of 10 to 100 μg causes rapid elevation of plasma gonadotropins; the release of LH is faster than that of FSH. Prolonged or repeated administration results in characteristic and predictable alterations in gonadal function. Ovulation and stimulation of spermatogenesis have been induced in both experimental animals and human subjects. Again, the hormone also stimulates the synthesis of gonadotropin in addition to its release. LH-RH has been used alone or in combination with human menopausal gonadotropin to induce ovulation and promote pregnancy in some amenorrheic women. The use of LH-RH for this purpose may offer an advantage in that superovulation and multiple births have not been observed in the few patients treated to date.

While variations in secretion of luteinizing hormone and follicle-stimulating hormone may be simultaneous, normal divergent patterns of secretion are also well known (*see* Figure 61–2, page 1424). Attempts to explain this in the face of but one gonadotropin-releasing hormone invoke, among other observations, the "feedback" effects of sex hormones, gonadal products such as *inhibin,* and other endogenous regulators on responses to the regulatory decapeptide. While important regulatory effects are thought to occur at neuronal sites in the hypothalamus and elsewhere, direct effects on the pituitary seem probable. Estrogens inhibit the secretion of FSH but have a biphasic effect on the secretion of LH. Inhibin, a peptide with a molecular weight of 15,000 to 30,000 that is derived from the testis or ovary, can feed back and suppress the secretion of both FSH and LH (*see* Franchimont, 1977). Dopamine has been observed to inhibit LH secretion without effect on the secretion of FSH (Leblanc *et al.,* 1976). These interactions are highly complex, and it is impossible at this time to state whether the combined effects of sex hormones, other gonadal products, and one gonadotropin-releasing hormone will supply the necessary controls.

The question of paramount importance involves the existence of a separate FSH-RH. Experimental difficulties with follicle-stimulating hormone itself add to the problem. The fact that LH-RH is also a FSH-RH does not exclude the possibility that an additional regulatory hormone is present.

The obvious clinical implications of regulation of gonadotropins have already prompted the synthesis and evaluation of hundreds of analogs of LH-RH. LH-RH is rapidly hydrolyzed in plasma and excreted in urine with a half-life of about 4 minutes. Unfortunately, no smaller active fragments of LH-RH have been obtained. A variety of amino acid substitutions at positions 6 and 10 of the peptide chain have produced analogs with potency increased as much as 10-fold to 60-fold and a prolonged duration of activity. Some very active analogs have been used successfully to treat cryptorchism and have been effective after oral, intranasal, or rectal administration (Saito *et al.,* 1977). Paradoxically, prolonged use of high concentrations of LH-RH has caused reversible ovarian and uterine atrophy in animals and has prevented implantation of ova and gestation. In males, high concentrations of LH-RH can inhibit testicular synthesis of testosterone. Some LH-RH analogs also have inhibitory activity and may prove to be effective contraceptives (De La Cruz *et al.,* 1976). In these and other experimental studies, significant untoward effects have not been observed.

Regulation of Corticotropin. Corticotropin-releasing factor (CRF) was the first to be demonstrated by physiological technics, and these early *in-vitro* studies prompted the purification and characterization of this and other hypothalamic releasing hormones. However, experimental difficulties have prevented the identification of CRF. While antidiuretic hormone and fragments thereof have significant CRF activity, the true hormone is probably an unrelated peptide.

Regulation of Growth Hormone. Growth hormone is subject to regulation by both a GH-RF and a release-inhibiting hormone (GH-RIH). Characterization of the GH-RF awaits further work. Since cyclic nucleotides are effective stimulators of growth hormone secretion *in vitro,* GH-RF may also utilize this mechanism.

Brazeau and associates (1973) have isolated a tetradecapeptide from the ovine hypothalamus that markedly inhibits the secretion of immunoreactive growth hormone *in vivo* and *in vitro.* The same peptide has also been isolated from porcine hypothalami. Its structure is shown at the bottom of the page. This peptide is thought to represent a GH-RIH, and for simplicity of nomenclature it has been called *somatostatin.* Somatostatin inhibits secretion of growth hormone that is induced by most stimuli, including arginine, insulin, levodopa, exercise, sleep, and meals (Guillemin and Gerich, 1976). The effect is rapid and immediately reversible when infusion of somatostatin is terminated. Larger peptides with several additional amino acids at the amino terminus have also been isolated and may represent precursors of the tetradecapeptide. With immunohistochemical technics somatostatin has been found in other regions of the brain, and in the spinal cord, D cells of the pancreatic islets, and gastric and duodenal mucosae, as well as in the hypothalamus (Hökfelt *et al.,* 1975).

Surprisingly, somatostatin also inhibits the secretion of TSH, ACTH, insulin, glucagon, gastrin, secretin, pancreozymin or cholecystokinin, pepsin, and renin (Lucke *et al.,* 1975; Fehm *et al.,* 1976; Konturek *et al.,* 1976). In addition, the peptide inhibits the *effects* of pentagastrin and histamine on gastric acid production (Barros D'Sa *et al.,* 1975).

Ala—Gly—Cys—Lys—Asn—Phe—Phe—Trp—Lys—Thr—Phe—Thr—Ser—Cys

Thus, somatostatin can inhibit secretion from a variety of endocrine and exocrine tissues and also the action of some hormones; the full significance of this is unknown. Current evidence suggests that somatostatin does have local effects in regional tissues where it is stored and released. While these divergent effects are somewhat perplexing, potential clinical applications of somatostatin have been explored. For example, infusion of somatostatin can prevent the development of ketoacidosis in patients with juvenile-type diabetes deprived of insulin for 18 hours; this was attributed to inhibition of glucagon secretion (Gerich et al., 1975). Somatostatin can also decrease the secretion of insulin and gastrin that results from pancreatic tumors (Curnow et al., 1975). However, the short half-life of somatostatin (several minutes) has precluded potential therapeutic uses. Analogs are being prepared that have greater potency and that are eliminated more slowly. Some analogs have also shown selective inhibition of the secretion of one hormone with lesser effects on others. Perhaps such studies could provide materials that are useful in the therapy of pituitary disease, diabetes mellitus, acid-pepsin disorders, and syndromes associated with hormone-secreting tumors. Administration of somatostatin to baboons and human subjects has resulted in abnormalities of platelets (Besser et al., 1975; Koerker et al., 1975). Other side effects have included nausea, diarrhea, and abdominal cramps.

Regulation of Prolactin. Several aspects of hypothalamic regulation of prolactin secretion have been discussed above. The inhibitory influence of a prolactin release–inhibiting hormone (PRIH) appears to predominate. Such a material is probably dopamine, and this provides an explanation of the effects of dopaminergic agonists and antagonists on prolactin secretion. TRH has prolactin-releasing activity. It is not known if TRH serves physiologically as a prolactin-releasing factor (PRF). However, a rare syndrome characterized by primary hypothyroidism and high circulating prolactin concentration with associated galactorrhea is at least suggestive of a pathological function of TRH in the regulation of prolactin secretion. Another material in hypothalamic extracts can also stimulate the secretion of prolactin. While this material may be a physiologically important PRF, it has not yet been purified or characterized (Boyd et al., 1976).

Regulation of Melanocyte-Stimulating Hormone. MSH secretion in animals is probably controlled by MSH-releasing factor (MRF) and MSH release-inhibiting factor (MIF), which are thought to originate in the hypothalamus (see Thody, 1977). While several small peptides have MIF and MRF activity, the structures of MIF and MRF are unknown. It has been suggested that both MIF and MRF are derived from oxytocin and represent small fragments of this peptide. Sex steroids and light can increase MSH secretion. The effects of light appear to be mediated through the pineal by means of activation of the biosynthesis of melatonin, which increases the secretion of MSH.

Neurotensin. This is a tridecapeptide isolated from bovine hypothalami, the structure of which is Glu-Leu-Tyr-Glu-Asn-Lys-Pro-Arg-Arg-Pro-Tyr-Ile-Leu. Immunoreactive material has also been demonstrated in other species, including man. This peptide increases secretion of ACTH, gonadotropins, and glucagon and decreases the secretion of insulin. It can elevate plasma glucose concentrations, lower blood pressure, decrease body temperature, contract smooth muscle in guinea pig ileum, and relax rat duodenum. The effects of neurotensin on insulin, glucagon, and plasma glucose (Carraway et al., 1976) are qualitatively similar but greater than the effects of substance P, an undecapeptide also isolated from hypothalamus (see Chapters 12 and 27). The physiological significance of these peptides is not clear.

Regulation of Regulatory Hormones. Although any significant discussion of this important area of neuroendocrinology is beyond the scope of this text, a few points should be made. There is ample evidence to indicate important neural control of regulatory hormone release. Evidence exists for adrenergic, dopaminergic, and tryptaminergic mechanisms that regulate the formation and secretion of various hypothalamic releasing factors (see Weiner and Ganong, 1978). This has been discussed above in regard to the inhibitor of prolactin secretion. Similar evidence implicates adrenergic mechanisms in the secretion of growth hormone, thyrotropin, and gonadotropins. Drugs that alter central adrenergic mechanisms exert significant influences on the secretion of the adenohypophyseal hormones, and these are discussed under the individual agents involved.

Abe, K.; Robison, G. A.; Liddle, G. W.; Butcher, R. W.; Nicholson, W. E.; and Baird, C. E. Role of cyclic AMP in mediating the effects of MSH, norepinephrine, and melatonin on frog skin color. Endocrinology, 1969, 85, 674–682.

Adams, D. D., and Kennedy, T. H. Occurrence in thyrotoxicosis of a gamma globulin which protects LATS from neutralization by an extract of thyroid gland. J. Clin. Endocrinol. Metab., 1967, 27, 173–177.

Adams, D. D., and Purves, H. D. The role of thyrotropin in hyperthyroidism and exophthalmos. Metabolism, 1957, 6, 26–35.

Allen, B. M. Effects of extirpation of the anterior lobe of the hypophysis of Rana pipiens. Biol. Bull. Mar. Biol. Lab., Woods Hole, 1917, 32, 117–130.

Aron, M. Action de la préhypophyse sur la thyroide chez le cobaye. C. R. Soc. Biol. (Paris), 1929, 102, 682–684.

Aschner, B. Demonstration von Hunden nach Extirpation der Hypophyse. Wien. Klin. Wochenschr., 1909, 22, 1730–1731.

Barros D'Sa, A. A. J.; Bloom, S. R.; and Baron, J. H. Direct inhibition of gastric acid by growth-hormone releasing-inhibiting hormone in dogs. Lancet, 1975, 1, 886–887.

Baumann, G., and Hodgen, G. Lack of in vivo transformation of human growth hormone to its "activated" isohormones in peripheral tissues of the rhesus monkey. J. Clin. Endocrinol. Metab., 1976, 43, 1009–1014.

Baumann, G., and Loriaux, D. L. Failure of endogenous prolactin to alter renal salt and water excretion and adrenal function in man. J. Clin. Endocrinol. Metab., 1976, 43, 643–649.

Besser, G. M.; Paxton, A. M.; Johnson, S. A. N.; Hall, R.;

Gomez-Pan, A.; Schally, A. V.; Kastin, A. J.; and Coy, D. H. Impairment of platelet function by growth-hormone release-inhibiting hormone. *Lancet,* **1975,** *1,* 1166–1168.

Boyd, A. E.; Spencer, E.; Jackson, I. M. D.; and Reichlin, S. Prolactin-releasing factor (PRF) in porcine hypothalamic extract distinct from TRH. *Endocrinology,* **1976,** *99,* 861–871.

Brazeau, P.; Vale, W.; Burgus, R.; Ling, N.; Butcher, M.; Rivier, J.; and Guillemin, R. Hypothalamic polypeptide that inhibits the secretion of immunoreactive pituitary growth hormone. *Science,* **1973,** *179,* 77–79.

Brown, T. B.; Evans, J. H.; Adey, F. D.; Taft, H. P.; and Townsend, L. Factors involved in the induction of fertile ovulation and human gonadotropins. *J. Obstet. Gynaecol. Br. Commonw.,* **1969,** *76,* 289–307.

Carr, D., and Friesen, H. G. Growth hormone and insulin binding to human liver. *J. Clin. Endocrinol. Metab.,* **1976,** *42,* 484–493.

Carraway, R. E.; Demers, L. M.; and Leeman, S. E. Hyperglycemic effect of neurotensin, a hypothalamic peptide. *Endocrinology,* **1976,** *99,* 1452–1462.

Cave, W. T., and Dunn, J. T. Choriocarcinoma with hyperthyroidism: probable identity of the thyrotropin with human chorionic gonadotropin. *Ann. Intern. Med.,* **1976,** *85,* 60–63.

Channing, C. P., and Seymour, J. F. Effects of dibutyryl cyclic-3′,5′-AMP and other agents upon luteinization of porcine granulosa cells in culture. *Endocrinology,* **1970,** *87,* 165–169.

Chrétien, M., and Li, C. H. Isolation, purification, and characterization of γ-lipotropic hormone from sheep pituitary gland. *Can. J. Biochem.,* **1968,** *45,* 1163–1174.

Coble, Y. D., Jr.; Kohler, P. O.; Cargille, C. M.; and Ross, G. T. Production rates and metabolic clearance rates of human follicle-stimulating hormone in premenopausal and postmenopausal women. *J. Clin. Invest.,* **1969,** *48,* 359–363.

Collip, J. B.; Anderson, E. M.; and Thomson, D. L. The adrenotropic hormone of the anterior pituitary lobe. *Lancet,* **1933,** *2,* 341–348.

Curnow, R. T.; Carey, R. C.; Taylor, A.; Johansson, A.; and Murad, F. Somatostatin inhibition of insulin and gastrin hypersecretion in pancreatic islet cell carcinoma. *N. Engl. J. Med.,* **1975,** *292,* 1385–1386.

Daughaday, W. H.; Laron, Z.; Pertzelan, A.; and Heins, J. N. Defective sulfation factor generation: a possible etiological link in dwarfism. *Trans. Assoc. Am. Physicians,* **1969,** *82,* 129–140.

Daughaday, W. H.; Salmon, W. D., Jr.; and Alexander, F. Sulfation factor activity of sera from patients with pituitary disorders. *J. Clin. Endocrinol. Metab.,* **1959,** *19,* 743–758.

De La Cruz, A.; Coy, D. H.; and Vilchez-Martinez, J. A. Blockade of ovulation in rats by inhibitory analogs of luteinizing hormone–releasing hormone. *Science,* **1976,** *191,* 195–197.

Ellsworth, L. R., and Armstrong, D. T. Luteinization of transplanted ovarian follicles in the rat induced by dibutyryl cyclic AMP. *Endocrinology,* **1973,** *92,* 840–846.

Evans, H. M., and Long, J. A. The effect of the anterior lobe administered intraperitoneally upon growth, maturity, and oestrous cycles of the rat. *Anat. Rec.,* **1921,** *21,* 62–63.

Faiman, C., and Ryan, R. J. Serum follicle-stimulating hormone and luteinizing hormone concentrations during the menstrual cycle as determined by radioimmunoassays. *J. Clin. Endocrinol. Metab.,* **1967,** *27,* 1711–1716.

Fehm, H. L.; Voigt, K. H.; Lang, R.; Beinert, K. E.; Raptis, S.; and Pfeiffer, E. F. Somatostatin: a potent inhibitor of ACTH—hypersecretion in adrenal insufficiency. *Klin. Wochenschr.,* **1976,** *54,* 173–175.

Feldman, J. M.; Plonk, J. W.; and Bivens, C. H. Inhibitory

effect of serotonin antagonists on growth hormone release in acromegalic patients. *Clin. Endocrinol. (Oxf.),* **1976,** *5,* 71–78.

Fevold, H. L.; Hisaw, F. L.; Hellbaum, A.; and Hertz, A. Sex hormones of the anterior lobe of the hypophysis: further purification of a follicular stimulating factor and the physiological effects in immature rats and rabbits. *Am. J. Physiol.,* **1933,** *104,* 710–723.

Frantz, A. G., and Kleinberg, D. L. Prolactin: evidence that it is separate from growth hormone in human blood. *Science,* **1970,** *170,* 745–747.

Friend, J. N.; Judge, D. M.; Sherman, B. M.; and Santen, R. J. FSH-secreting pituitary adenomas: stimulation and suppression studies in two patients. *J. Clin. Endocrinol. Metab.,* **1976,** *43,* 650–657.

Friesen, H. Lactation induced by human placental lactogen and cortisone acetate in rabbits. *Endocrinology,* **1966,** *79,* 212–215.

———. Human prolactin in clinical endocrinology: the impact of radioimmunoassays. *Metabolism,* **1973,** *22,* 1039–1045.

Fukushima, M. Studies on somatotropic hormone secretion in gynecology and obstetrics. *Tohoku J. Exp. Med.,* **1961,** *74,* 161–174.

Gemzell, C., and Kjessler, B. Treatment of infertility after partial hypophysectomy with human pituitary gonadotropins. *Lancet,* **1964,** *1,* 644.

Gerich, J. E.; Lorenzi, M.; Bier, D. M.; Schneider, V.; Tsalikian, E.; Karam, J. H.; and Forsham, P. H. Prevention of human diabetic ketoacidosis by somatostatin. Evidence for an essential role of glucagon. *N. Engl. J. Med.,* **1975,** *292,* 985–989.

Golander, A.; Hurley, T.; Barrett, J.; Hizi, A.; and Handwerger, S. Prolactin synthesis by human chorion-decidual tissue: a possible source of prolactin in the amniotic fluid. *Science,* **1978,** *202,* 311–313.

Goodman, A. D.; Tanenbaum, R.; and Rabinowitz, D. Existence of two forms of immunoreactive growth hormone in human plasma. *J. Clin. Endocrinol. Metab.,* **1972,** *35,* 868–878.

Gordon, P.; Lesniak, M. A.; Eastman, R.; Hendricks, C. M.; and Roth, J. Evidence for higher portion of "little" growth hormone with increased radioreceptor activity in acromegalic plasma. *J. Clin. Endocrinol. Metab.,* **1976,** *43,* 364–373.

Gordon, P.; Lesniak, M. A.; Hendricks, C. M.; and Roth, J. "Big" growth hormone components from human plasma: decreased reactivity demonstrated by radioreceptor assay. *Science,* **1973,** *182,* 829–831.

Graesslin, D.; Leidenberger, F. A.; Lichtenberg, V.; Glinsmann, D.; Hess, N.; Czygan, P. J.; and Betlendorf, G. Existence of big and little forms of luteinizing hormone in human serum. *Acta Endocrinol. (Kbh.),* **1976,** *83,* 466–482.

Guyda, H. J., and Friesen, H. G. The separation of monkey prolactin from monkey growth hormone by affinity chromatography. *Biochem. Biophys. Res. Commun.,* **1971,** *42,* 1068–1075.

Hack, M.; Brish, M.; Serr, D. M.; Inster, V.; and Lunenfeld, B. Outcome of pregnancies after induced ovulation. Follow-up of pregnancies and children born after gonadotropin therapy. *J.A.M.A.,* **1970,** *211,* 791–797.

Hershman, J. M. Hyperthyroidism induced by trophoblastic thyrotropin. *Mayo Clin. Proc.,* **1972,** *47,* 913–918.

Hobson, B., and Wide, L. The immunological and biological activity of human chorionic gonadotropin in urine. *Acta Endocrinol. (Kbh.),* **1964,** *46,* 632–638.

Hökfelt, T.; Efendic, S.; Hellerström, C.; Johansson, O.; Luft, R.; and Arimura, A. Cellular localization of somatostatin in endocrine-like cells and neurons of the rat with special references to the A₁-cells of the pancreatic islets and to the hypothalamus. *Acta Endocrinol. (Kbh.),* **1975,** *80,* Suppl. 200, 5–41.

Houssay, B. A. Advancement of knowledge of the role of

the hypophysis in carbohydrate metabolism during the last twenty-five years. *Endocrinology,* **1942,** *30,* 884–897.

Hughes, J.; Smith, T. W.; Kosterlitz, H. W.; Fathergill, L. H.; Morgan, B. A.; and Morris, H. R. Identification of two related pentapeptides from the brain with potent opiate agonist activity. *Nature,* **1975,** *258,* 577–579.

Huttunen, J. K.; Steinberg, D.; and Mayer, S. E. ATP-dependent and cyclic AMP–dependent activation of rat adipose tissue lipase by protein kinase from rabbit skeletal muscle. *Proc. Natl. Acad. Sci. U.S.A.,* **1970,** *67,* 290–295.

Hwang, P.; Guyda, H.; and Friesen, H. A radioimmunoassay for human prolactin. *Proc. Natl. Acad. Sci. U.S.A.,* **1971,** *68,* 1902–1906.

Jacobs, L. S.; Sneid, D. S.; Garland, J. T.; Laron, Z.; and Daughaday, W. H. Receptor-active growth hormone in Laron dwarfism. *J. Clin. Endocrinol. Metab.,* **1976,** *42,* 403–406.

Josimovich, J. B., and MacLaren, J. A. Presence in the human placenta and term serum of a highly lactogenic substance immunologically related to pituitary growth hormone. *Endocrinology,* **1962,** *71,* 209–220.

Koerker, D. J.; Harker, L. A.; and Goodner, C. J. Effects of somatostatin on hemostasis in baboons. *N. Engl. J. Med.,* **1975,** *293,* 476–479.

Kohn, L. D., and Winand, R. J. Relationship of thyrotropin to exophthalmos-producing substance. Formation of an exophthalmos-producing substance by pepsin digestion of pituitary glycoproteins containing both thyrotropic and exophthalmogenic activity. *J. Biol. Chem.,* **1971,** *246,* 6570–6575.

Konturek, S. J.; Tasler, J.; Cieszkowski, M.; Coy, D. H.; and Schally, A. V. Effect of growth hormone release-inhibiting hormone on gastrin secretion, mucosal blood flow and serum gastrin. *Gastroenterology,* **1976,** *70,* 737–741.

Kriss, J. P. The long-acting thyroid stimulator and thyroid disease. *Adv. Intern. Med.,* **1970,** *16,* 135–154.

Kuehl, F. A.; Humes, J. L.; Tarnoff, J.; Cirillo, V. J.; and Ham, E. A. Prostaglandin receptor site: evidence for an essential role in the action of luteinizing hormone. *Science,* **1970,** *169,* 883–886.

Lattimer, J. K. The optimum treatment for undescended testis. *Med. Coll. Va. Q.,* **1973,** *9,* 270–274.

Lazarus, L. H.; Ling, N.; and Guillemin, R. β-Lipotropin as a prohormone for the morphinomimetic peptides endorphins and enkephalins. *Proc. Natl. Acad. Sci. U.S.A.,* **1976,** *73,* 2156–2159.

Leblanc, H.; Lachelin, G. C. L.; Abu-Fadil, S.; and Yen, S. S. C. Effects of dopamine infusion on pituitary hormone secretion in humans. *J. Clin. Endocrinol. Metab.,* **1976,** *43,* 668–674.

Lerner, A. B., and McGuire, J. S. Melanocyte-stimulating hormone and adrenocorticotrophic hormone: their relation to pigmentation. *N. Engl. J. Med.,* **1964,** *270,* 539–546.

Lewis, V. J.; Pence, S. J.; Singh, R. N. P.; and VanderLaan, S. P. Enhancement of the growth promoting activity of human growth hormone. *Biochem. Biophys. Res. Commun.,* **1975,** *67,* 617–624.

Li, C. H.; Barnafi, L.; Chrétien, M.; and Chung, D. Isolation and amino-acid sequence of β-LPH from sheep pituitary glands. *Nature,* **1965,** *208,* 1093–1094.

Li, C. H.; Dixon, J. S.; and Chung, D. Amino acid sequence of human chorionic somatomammotropin. *Arch. Biochem. Biophys.,* **1973,** *155,* 95–110.

Li, C. H.; Dixon, J. S.; Lo, T.-B.; Schmidt, K. D.; and Pankov, Y. A. Studies on pituitary lactogenic hormone. XXX. The primary structure of the sheep hormone. *Arch. Biochem. Biophys.,* **1970,** *141,* 705–737.

Li, C. H.; Liu, W. K.; and Dixon, J. S. Human pituitary growth hormone. XII. The amino acid sequence of the hormone. *J. Am. Chem. Soc.,* **1966,** *88,* 2050–2051.

Lis, M.; Gilardeau, C.; and Chrétien, M. Fat cell adenyl-

ate cyclase activation by sheep β-lipotropic hormone. *Proc. Soc. Exp. Biol. Med.,* **1972,** *139,* 680–683.

Liu, W.-K.; Nahm, H. S.; Sweeney, C. M.; Holcomb, G. N.; and Ward, D. N. The primary structure of ovine luteinizing hormone. II. The amino acid sequence of the reduced, S-carboxymethylated A-subunit (LH-β). *J. Biol. Chem.,* **1972,** *247,* 4365–4381.

Loeb, L., and Bassett, R. B. Effect of hormones of anterior pituitary on thyroid gland in the guinea pig. *Proc. Soc. Exp. Biol. Med.,* **1929,** *26,* 860–862.

Lucke, C.; Höffken, B.; and Vonzur Mühlen, A. The effect of somatostatin on TSH levels in patients with primary hypothyroidism. *J. Clin. Endocrinol. Metab.,* **1975,** *41,* 1082–1084.

McKenzie, J. M. Studies on the thyroid activator of hyperthyroidism. *J. Clin. Endocrinol. Metab.,* **1961,** *21,* 635–647.

Mancini, R. E.; Vilar, O.; Donini, P.; and Pérez Lloret, A. Effect of human urinary FSH and LH on the recovery of spermatogenesis in hypophysectomized patients. *J. Clin. Endocrinol. Metab.,* **1971,** *33,* 888–895.

Marsh, J. M.; Butcher, R. W.; Savard, K.; and Sutherland, E. W. The stimulatory effect of luteinizing hormone on adenosine 3′,5′-monophosphate accumulation in corpus luteum slices. *J. Biol. Chem.,* **1966,** *241,* 5436–5440.

Midgley, A. R., and Jaffe, R. B. Regulation of human gonadotropins. IV. Correlation of serum concentrations of follicle stimulating and luteinizing hormones during the menstrual cycle. *J. Clin. Endocrinol. Metab.,* **1968,** *28,* 1699–1703.

Mills, T. M.; Davies, P. J. A.; and Savard, K. Stimulation of estrogen synthesis in rabbit follicles by luteinizing hormone. *Endocrinology,* **1971,** *88,* 857–862.

Morley, J. E.; Jacobson, R. J.; Melamed, J.; and Hershman, J. M. Choriocarcinoma as a cause of thyrotoxicosis. *Am. J. Med.,* **1976,** *60,* 1036–1040.

Murad, F.; Strauch, B. S.; and Vaughan, M. The effect of gonadotropins on testicular adenyl cyclase. *Biochim. Biophys. Acta,* **1969,** *177,* 591–598.

Niall, H. D.; Hogan, M. L.; Sauer, R.; Rosenblum, I. Y.; and Greenwood, F. C. Sequences of pituitary and placental lactogenic and growth hormones: evolution from a primordial peptide by gene reduplication. *Proc. Natl. Acad. Sci. U.S.A.,* **1971,** *68,* 866–869.

Parker, M. L.; Hammond, J. M.; and Daughaday, W. H. The arginine provocative test: an aid in the diagnosis of hyposomatotropism. *J. Clin. Endocrinol. Metab.,* **1967,** *27,* 1129–1136.

Pierce, J. G. The subunits of pituitary thyrotropin—their relationship to other glycoprotein hormones. *Endocrinology,* **1971,** *89,* 1331–1344.

Raben, M. S. Growth hormone. 1. Physiologic aspects. *N. Engl. J. Med.,* **1962a,** *266,* 31–35. 2. Clinical use of human growth hormone. *Ibid.,* **1962b,** *266,* 82–86.

Raben, M. S., and Hollenberg, C. H. Effect of growth hormone on plasma fatty acids. *J. Clin. Invest.,* **1959,** *38,* 484–488.

Reichlin, S. Regulation of somatotropic hormone secretion. In, *The Pituitary Gland and Its Neuroendocrine Control,* Vol. 4, Pt. 2. Sect. 7, *Endocrinology. Handbook of Physiology.* (Knobil, E., and Sawyer, W. H., eds.) American Physiological Society, Washington, D. C., **1974,** pp. 405–447.

Riddle, O.; Bates, R. W.; and Dykshorn, S. W. The preparation, identification and assay of prolactin—a hormone of the anterior pituitary. *Am. J. Physiol.,* **1933,** *105,* 191–216.

Rinderknecht, E., and Humbel, R. E. Amino terminal sequences of two polypeptides from human serum with nonsuppressible insulin-like and cell-growth-promoting activities: evidence for structural homology with insulin β chain. *Proc. Natl. Acad. Sci. U.S.A.,* **1976,** *73,* 4379–4381.

Rubin, R. T.; Poland, R. E.; and Tower, B. B. Prolactin-related testosterone secretion in normal adult man. *J. Clin. Endocrinol. Metab.,* **1976,** *42,* 112–116.

Rudman, D.; Patterson, J. H.; and Gibbas, D. L. Responsiveness of growth hormone–deficient children to human growth hormone. *J. Clin. Invest.,* **1973,** *52,* 1108–1112.

Saito, M.; Kumasaka, T.; Yaoi, Y.; Nishi, N.; Arimura, A.; Coy, D. H.; and Schally, A. V. Stimulation of luteinizing hormone (LH) and follicle stimulating hormone by [D-Leu[6], Des-Gly[10]-NH$_2$]-LH-releasing hormone ethylamide after subcutaneous, intravaginal and intrarectal administration to women. *Fertil. Steril.,* **1977,** *28,* 240–245.

Seeburg, P. H.; Shine, J.; Martial, J. A.; Ivarie, R. D.; Morris, J. A.; Ullrich, A.; Baxter, J. D.; and Goodman, H. M. Synthesis of growth hormone by bacteria. *Nature,* **1978,** *276,* 795–798.

Sheehan, H. L., and Summers, V. K. The syndrome of hypopituitarism. *Q. J. Med.,* **1949,** *18,* 319–379.

Sherwood, L. M. Similarities in the chemical structure of human placental lactogen and pituitary growth hormone. *Proc. Natl. Acad. Sci. U.S.A.,* **1967,** *58,* 2307–2314.

Shiu, R. P. C.; Kelly, P. A.; and Friesen, H. G. Radioreceptor assay for prolactin and other lactogenic hormones. *Science,* **1973,** *180,* 968–971.

Shockaert, J. A. Hyperplasia of thyroid and exophthalmos in treatment with anterior pituitary in young ducks. *Proc. Soc. Exp. Biol. Med.,* **1931,** *29,* 306–308.

Shome, B., and Parlow, A. F. The primary structure of the hormone-specific, beta subunit of human pituitary luteinizing hormone (hLH). *J. Clin. Endocrinol. Metab.,* **1973,** *36,* 618–621.

———. Human follicle stimulating hormone. *Ibid.,* **1974,** *39,* 199–202, 203–205.

———. Human pituitary prolactin (hPrl), the entire amino acid sequence. *Ibid.,* **1977,** *45,* 1112–1115.

Smith, P. E. The disabilities caused by hypophysectomy and their repair. *J.A.M.A.,* **1927,** *88,* 158–161.

———. Hypophysectomy and a replacement therapy. *Am. J. Anat.,* **1930,** *45,* 205–256.

Snyder, P. J., and Sterling, F. H. Hypersecretion of LH and FSH by a pituitary adenoma. *J. Clin. Endocrinol. Metab.,* **1976,** *42,* 544–550.

Suh, H. K., and Frantz, A. G. Size heterogeneity of human prolactin in plasma and pituitary extracts. *J. Clin. Endocrinol. Metab.,* **1974,** *39,* 928–935.

Tell, G. P. E.; Cuatrecasas, P.; Van Wyk, J. J.; and Hintz, R. L. Somatomedin inhibition of adenylate cyclase activity in subcellular membranes of various tissues. *Science,* **1973,** *180,* 312–315.

Theodoridis, C. G.; Brown, G. A.; Chance, G. W.; and Rayner, P. H. W. Growth-hormone response to oral glucose in children with simple obesity. *Lancet,* **1969,** *1,* 1068–1069.

Thompson, C. R., and Hansen, L. M. PERGONAL (menotropins): a summary of clinical experience in the induction of ovulation and pregnancy. *Fertil. Steril.,* **1970,** *21,* 844–853.

Turkington, R. W. Inhibition of prolactin secretion and successful therapy of the Forbes-Albright syndrome with L-dopa. *J. Clin. Endocrinol. Metab.,* **1972,** *34,* 306–311.

Wass, J. A. H.; Thorner, M. O.; Morris, D. V.; Rees, L. H.; Stuart, M. A.; Jones, A. E.; and Besser, G. M. Long-term treatment of acromegaly with bromocriptine. *Br. Med. J.,* **1977,** *1,* 875–878.

Yamashita, K., and Field, J. B. Effects of long-acting thyroid stimulator on thyrotropin stimulation of adenyl cyclase activity in thyroid plasma membranes. *J. Clin. Invest.,* **1972,** *51,* 463–472.

Yen, S. S. C.; Llerena, O.; Little, B.; and Pearson, O. H. Disappearance rates of endogenous luteinizing hormone and chorionic gonadotropin in man. *J. Clin. Endocrinol. Metab.,* **1968,** *28,* 1763–1767.

Yen, S. S. C.; Llerena, L. A.; Pearson, O. H.; and Littell, A. S. Disappearance rates of endogenous follicle-stimulating hormone in serum following surgical hypophysectomy in man. *J. Clin. Endocrinol. Metab.,* **1970,** *30,* 325–329.

Zierler, K. L. Effects of growth hormone on metabolism of muscle and adipose tissue of the forearm of man. In, *Clinical Endocrinology II.* (Astwood, E. B., and Cassidy, C. E., eds.) Grune & Stratton, Inc., New York, **1968,** pp. 55–68.

Zondek, B., and Krohn, H. Hormon des Zwischenlappens der Hypophyse (Intermedin). *Naturwissenschaften,* **1932,** *8,* 134–136.

Zor, U.; Kaneko, T.; Lowe, I. P.; Bloom, G.; and Field, J. B. Effect of thyroid-stimulating hormone and prostaglandins on thyroid adenyl cyclase activation and cyclic adenosine 3′,5′-monophosphate. *J. Biol. Chem.,* **1969,** *244,* 5189–5195.

Monographs and Reviews

Blackwell, R. E., and Guillemin, R. Hypothalamic control of adenohypophysial secretions. *Annu. Rev. Physiol.,* **1973,** *35,* 357–390.

Burger, H. G., and Patel, Y. C. Thyrotropin releasing hormone—TSH. *Clin. Endocrinol. Metab.,* **1977,** *6,* 83–100.

Chatterjee, M., and Munro, H. N. Structure and biosynthesis of human placental peptide hormones. *Vitam. Horm.,* **1977,** *35,* 149–208.

Daughaday, W. H. Hormonal regulation of growth by somatomedin and other tissue growth factors. *Clin. Endocrinol. Metab.,* **1977,** *6,* 117–135.

———. Anterior pituitary. In, *The Year in Endocrinology: 1977.* (Ingbar, S. H., ed.) Plenum Medical Book Co., New York, **1978,** pp. 27–71.

Doniach, I. Histopathology of the anterior pituitary. *Clin. Endocrinol. Metab.,* **1977,** *6,* 21–52.

Dorfman, R. I. Mechanism of action of gonadotropins and prolactin. In, *Biochemical Actions of Hormones,* Vol. II. (Litwack, G., ed.) Academic Press, Inc., New York, **1972,** pp. 295–316.

Floss, H. G.; Cassady, J. M.; and Robbers, J. E. Influence of ergot alkaloids on pituitary prolactin and prolactin-dependent processes. *J. Pharm. Sci.,* **1973,** *62,* 699–715.

Franchimont, P. Pituitary gonadotropins. *Clin. Endocrinol. Metab.,* **1977,** *6,* 101–116.

Frantz, A. G. Prolactin, growth hormone and human placental lactogen. In, *Peptide Hormones.* (Parsons, J. A., ed.) University Park Press, Baltimore, **1976,** pp. 199–230.

———. Prolactin. *N. Engl. J. Med.,* **1978,** *298,* 201–207.

Goldfine, I. D. Medical treatment of acromegaly. *Annu. Rev. Med.,* **1978,** *29,* 407–415.

Guillemin, R. Peptides in the brain: the new endocrinology of the neuron. *Science,* **1978,** *202,* 390–401.

Guillemin, R., and Gerich, J. E. Somatostatin: physiological and clinical significance. *Annu. Rev. Med.,* **1976,** *27,* 379–388.

Knobil, E., and Greep, R. O. Physiology of growth hormone with particular reference to its action in rhesus monkey and "species specificity" problem. *Recent Prog. Horm. Res.,* **1959,** *15,* 1–69.

Krieger, D. T. Hypothalamus. In, *The Year in Endocrinology: 1977.* (Ingbar, S. H., ed.) Plenum Medical Book Co., New York, **1978,** pp. 1–26.

Lipsett, M. B., and Ross, G. T. The ovary. In, *The Year in Endocrinology: 1977.* (Ingbar, S. H., ed.) Plenum Medical Book Co., New York, **1978,** pp. 233–254.

McKenzie, J. M., and Zakarija, M. LATS in Graves's disease. *Recent Prog. Horm. Res.,* **1977,** *33,* 29–57.

MacLeod, R. M. Regulation of prolactin secretion. In, *Frontiers in Neuroendocrinology,* Vol. 4. (Martini, L., and Ganong, F., eds.) Raven Press, New York, **1976,** pp. 169–194.

Martial, J. A.; Hallewell, R. A.; Baxter, J. D.; and Goodman, H. M. Human growth hormone: complementary

DNA cloning and expression in bacteria. *Science,* **1979,** *205,* 602–606.

Meites, J.; Lu, K. H.; Wuttke, W.; Welsch, C. W.; Nagasawa, H.; and Quadri, S. K. Recent studies on functions and control of prolactin secretion in rats. *Recent Prog. Horm. Res.,* **1972,** *28,* 471–516.

Parkes, D. Bromocriptine. *Adv. Drug Res.,* **1977,** *12,* 247–344.

Phillips, L. S., and Vassilopoulou-Sellin, R. Somatomedins. *N. Engl. J. Med.,* **1980,** *302,* 371–379, 438–446.

Raben, M. S. Human growth hormone. *Recent Prog. Horm. Res.,* **1959,** *15,* 71–114.

Schally, A. V. Aspects of hypothalamic regulation of the pituitary gland: its implications for the control of reproductive functions. *Science,* **1978,** *202,* 18–28.

Schally, A. V.; Arimura, A.; and Kastin, A. J. Hypothalamic regulatory hormones. *Science,* **1973,** *179,* 341–350.

Smithline, F.; Sherman, L.; and Kolodny, H. D. Prolactin and breast carcinoma. *N. Engl. J. Med.,* **1975,** *292,* 784–792.

Symposium. (Various authors.) *Advances in Human Growth Hormone Research.* (Raiti, S., ed.) Department of Health, Education, and Welfare Publication No. (NH)74-612, U.S. Government Printing Office, Washington, D. C., **1973.**

Terenius, L. Endogenous peptides and analgesia. *Annu. Rev. Pharmacol. Toxicol.,* **1978,** *18,* 189–204.

Thody, A. J. The significance of melanocyte-stimulating hormone (MSH) and control of its secretion in the mammal. *Adv. Drug Res.,* **1977,** *11,* 23–74.

Thorner, M. O. Prolactin. *Clin. Endocrinol. Metab.,* **1977,** *6,* 201–222.

Topper, Y. J. Multiple hormone interactions in the development of mammary gland *in vitro. Recent Prog. Horm. Res.,* **1970,** *26,* 287–303.

Turkington, R. W.; Majumder, G. C.; Kadohama, N.; MacIndoe, J. H.; and Frantz, W. L. Hormonal regulation of gene expression in mammary cells. *Recent Prog. Horm. Res.,* **1973,** *29,* 417–449.

Vaitukaitis, J. L.; Ross, G. T.; Braunstein, G. D.; and Rayford, P. L. Gonadotropins and their subunits: basic and clinical studies. *Recent Prog. Horm. Res.,* **1976,** *32,* 289–331.

Vande Wiele, R. L., and Dyrenfurth, I. Gonadotropin-steroid interrelationships. *Pharmacol. Rev.,* **1973,** *25,* 189–207.

Volpe, R. The pathogenesis of Graves's disease: an overview. *Clin. Endocrinol. Metab.,* **1978,** *7,* 3–29.

Weiner, R. I., and Ganong, W. F. Role of brain monoamines and histamine in regulation of anterior pituitary secretion. *Physiol. Rev.,* **1978,** *58,* 905–976.

CHAPTER

60 THYROID AND ANTITHYROID DRUGS

Robert C. Haynes, Jr., and Ferid Murad

THYROID

The thyroid gland is the source of two fundamentally different types of hormones. *Thyroxine* and *triiodothyronine* are vital for normal growth and development and play an important role in energy metabolism. The other known glandular secretion, *calcitonin*, is considered in Chapter 65.

History. The thyroid gland was first described in 1656 by Wharton. Harington (1935) reviewed the many older and often amusing opinions concerning the function of this gland. Wharton thought, for example, that the viscous fluid within the follicles lubricated the trachea. He also believed that the gland was larger in women to serve a cosmetic function in giving grace to the contour of the neck. Later observers, influenced by the liberal blood supply of the gland, believed that it provided a vascular shunt for the brain. With this function in mind, Rush in 1820 expressed the belief that the larger size of the gland in women was "necessary to guard the female system from the influence of the more numerous causes of irritation and vexation of mind to which they are exposed than the male sex." However, Hofrichter (1820) cleverly opposed this theory by pointing out that, "If it were indeed true that the thyroid contains more blood at some times than at others, this effect would be visible to the naked eye; in this case women would certainly have long ceased to go about with bare necks, for husbands would have learned to recognize the swelling of this gland as a danger signal of threatening trouble from their better halves."

Numerous other theories of thyroid function were advanced, based upon little or no experimental evidence. The belief ultimately became prevalent that the gland served no important physiological role. The thyroid was first recognized as an organ of importance when enlargement was observed to be associated with changes in the eyes and in the heart in the condition we now call hyperthyroidism. It is of interest that this condition, the manifestations of which can on occasion be as striking as any in medicine, escaped description until Parry saw his first case in 1786. Parry's account was not published until 1825 (*see* Parry, 1895) and was followed in 1835 and 1840 by those of Graves and Basedow, whose names became applied to the disorder. It was not until 1874 that Gull first associated atrophy of the gland with the symptoms now known to be characteristic of thyroid deficiency. Hypofunction of the thyroid in adults is still known as *Gull's disease*. The term *myxedema* was applied to the clinical syndrome by Ord (1878) in the belief that the characteristic thickening of the subcutaneous tissues was due to excessive formation of mucus.

Extirpation experiments to elucidate the function of the thyroid were at first misinterpreted because of the simultaneous removal of the parathyroids. However, the pioneer research on the latter organs by Gley (1891) allowed the functional differentiation of these two endocrine glands. It was not until after calcitonin was discovered in 1961 that it was realized that the thyroid itself was also concerned with the regulation of calcium. Murray (1891) was the first to treat a case of hypothyroidism by injecting an extract of the thyroid gland; in the following year, Howitz, Mackenzie, and Fox independently discovered that thyroid tissue was fully effective when given by mouth.

Magnus-Levy (1895) discovered the effect of the thyroid on metabolic rate; he found that Gull's disease was characterized by a low rate of metabolism and that the administration of thyroid to hypothyroid or normal individuals increased oxygen consumption.

Chemistry. The active principles of the thyroid gland are the iodine-containing amino acid derivatives of thyronine thyroxine and triiodothyronine (Table 60–1). Thyroxine was first isolated in crystalline form from a hydrolysate of thyroid by Kendall (1915), who found that the crystalline product exerted the same physiological effects as the extract from which it was obtained. It was not until 1926, however, that the structural formula of thyroxine was elucidated by Harington, and in the following year Harington and Barger (1927) synthesized the hormone.

Following the isolation and the chemical identification of thyroxine, it was generally believed that all the hormonal activity of thyroid tissue could be accounted for by its content of thyroxine. However, careful studies revealed that crude thyroid preparations possessed greater calorigenic activity than could be accounted for by their thyroxine content. The enigma was resolved with the detection, isolation, and synthesis of triiodothyronine (Gross and Pitt-Rivers, 1952; Roche *et al.*, 1952a, 1952b). Further studies revealed that triiodothyronine is qualitatively similar to thyroxine in its biological action but that it is much more potent on a molar basis (Gross and Pitt-Rivers, 1953a, 1953b).

Structure-Activity Relationship. A great many structural analogs of thyroxine have been synthesized in order to define the structure-activity relationship, to detect antagonists of thyroid hormones, or to find

Table 60-1.   THYRONINE, THYROID HORMONES, AND PRECURSORS

Thyronine

Thyroxine

3,5,3'-Triiodothyronine

Diiodotyrosine

Iodotyrosine

compounds exhibiting one desirable type of activity while not showing unwanted effects. The only significant success has been the partial separation of the cholesterol-lowering action of thyroxine analogs from their calorigenic effect. The D isomer of thyroxine is sometimes employed clinically to lower the level of plasma cholesterol (*see* Chapter 34). A listing of the compounds tested has been made by Pittman and Pittman (1974).

The structural requirements for a significant degree of thyroid hormone activity have been defined (Jorgensen, 1964). The two aromatic rings should be connected by an ether or thioether linkage. However, potent methylene-bridged analogs have been synthesized (Psychoyos *et al.*, 1973). A carboxyl-containing aliphatic side chain in position 1 is important, with L-alanine being the best. Halogen or methyl groups are necessary on positions 3 and 5. Position 4' should be occupied by a hydroxyl group, an amino group, or a group capable of metabolic conversion to a hydroxyl. For maximal activity, halogen atoms, alkyl, or aromatic substituents are necessary at the 3' position or at the 3' and 5' positions. The 3'-monosubstituted compounds are more active than the

3',5'-disubstituted molecules. Thus, triiodothyronine is four times more potent than thyroxine, while 3'-isopropyl-3,5-diiodothyronine has seven times the activity.

While the chemical nature of the 3, 5, 3', and 5' substituents is important, their effects on the conformation of the molecule are apparently even more so. In thyronine, the two rings are angulated at about 120° at the ether oxygen and are free to rotate on their axes. As depicted schematically in Figure 60-1, when the 3,5 iodines are in place there is some restriction to rotation of the two rings, and they tend to take up positions perpendicular to one another; now positions 2' and 3' are no longer equivalent to positions 5' and 6'. Substituents at the 3' position can be either distal (on the convex side, as in Figure 60-1) or proximal to the phenylalanine ring, depending on the rotation. Substitution at the more hindered 2' position probably requires the distal conformation. Much biological evidence indicates that this distal conformation is necessary for activity. Thus, bulky and lipophilic groups in the 3' position enhance activity, and 2' substituents are tolerated. As mentioned, substitutions in the 5' position detract from activity. While not potent, even halogen-free derivatives possess some activity if the proper conformation is possible (Pittman *et al.*, 1973).

While analogs that antagonize the actions of the thyroid hormones have been evaluated, none has yet proven clinically useful.

Synthesis of Thyroid Hormones. The synthesis of the thyroid hormones is unique, complex, and seemingly grossly inefficient. The thyroid hormones are synthesized and stored as amino acid residues of thyroglobulin, a protein constituting the vast majority of the thyroid follicular colloid. The thyroid gland is unique in storing great quantities of potential hormone in this way, and extracellular thyroglobulin can represent a large portion of the mass of the gland. It is a complex glycoprotein made up of several nonidentical subunits. The molecular weight

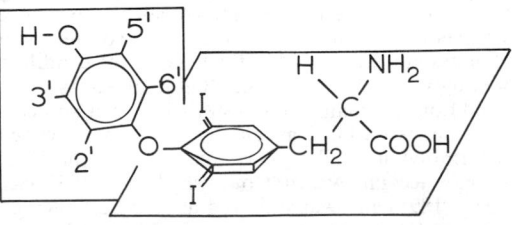

Figure 60-1. *Structural formula of 3,5-diiodothyronine, drawn to show the conformation in which the planes of the aromatic rings are perpendicular to each other. (After Jorgensen, 1964. Courtesy of The Mayo Association. See also Cody and Duax, 1973.)*

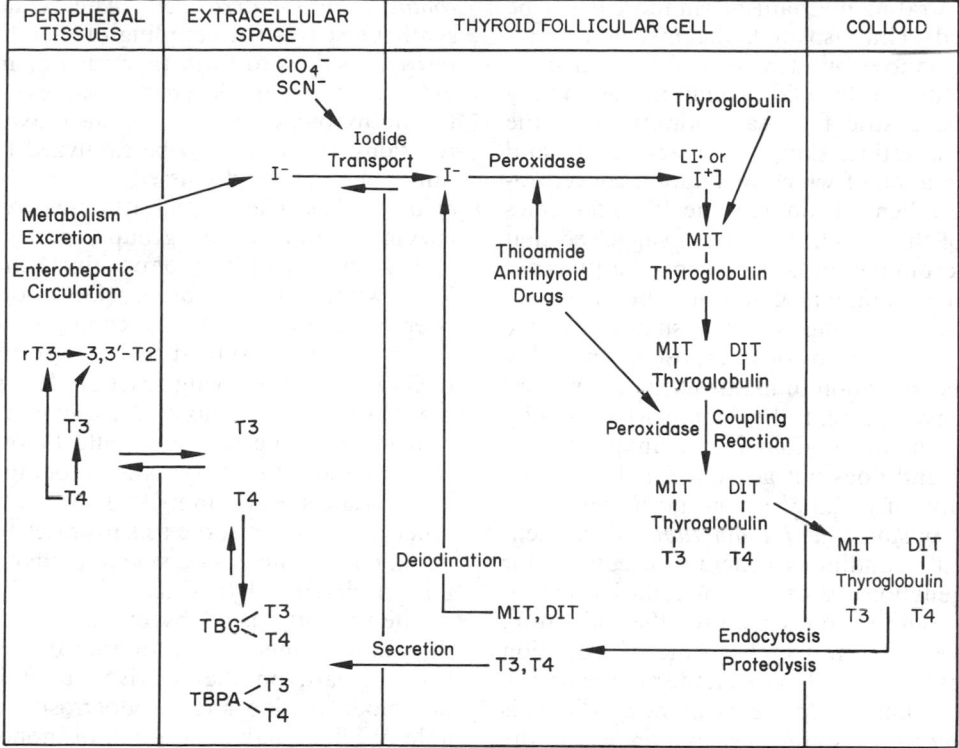

Figure 60-2. *The major pathways of iodine metabolism.*

Abbreviations are as follows: *T3* = triiodothyronine; *T4* = thyroxine; *rT3* = 3,3′,5′-triiodo-thyronine; *3,3′-T2* = 3,3′-diiodothyronine; *MIT* = monoiodotyrosine, *DIT* = diiodotyrosine; *TBG* = thyroxine-binding globulin; *TBPA* = thyroxine-binding prealbumin.

is 660,000 (19 S), and it contains 10% carbohydrate.

The major steps in the synthesis, storage, release, and interconversion of thyroid hormones are the following: (1) the uptake of iodide ion by the gland, (2) the oxidation of iodide and the iodination of tyrosyl groups of thyroglobulin, (3) the conversion of iodotyrosyl residues to iodothyronyl residues in this protein, (4) the proteolysis of thyroglobulin and the release of thyroxine and triiodothyronine into the blood, and (5) the conversion of thyroxine to triiodothyronine in peripheral tissues. These processes are summarized in Figure 60-2.

1. *Uptake of Iodide.* Iodine ingested in the diet reaches the circulation in the form of iodide. Under normal circumstances the concentration in the blood is very low, 0.2 to 0.4 μg/dl, but the thyroid efficiently and actively transports the ion. As a result, the ratio

of thyroid to plasma iodide concentration is usually between 20 and 50 and can far exceed 100 when the gland is stimulated. The iodide transport mechanism is inhibited by a number of ions such as thiocyanate and perchlorate (*see* below), appears to require concurrent transport of potassium, and is depressed by cardiac glycosides that inhibit the accumulation of potassium by cells (*see* Wolff, 1964).

The transport system is stimulated by thyrotropin (*see* below) and is also controlled by an autoregulatory mechanism. Thus, decreased stores of thyroid iodine enhance iodide uptake, and the administration of iodide can reverse this situation. Some incorporation of iodide into organic form must occur, however, for the inhibitory effect of excess iodide to become apparent (Vander-Laan, 1955).

If the further metabolism of iodide is blocked by antithyroid drugs, the iodide-concentrating mechanism can more easily be studied. Thus isolated, the mechanism resembles those found in other bodily structures that concentrate iodide, including the salivary glands, gastric mucosa, midportion of the small intestine, skin, mammary gland, and placenta, all of which maintain a concentration gradient of iodide some 10 to 50 times that of the blood. It has been suggested that the accumulation of iodide by the placenta and the mammary gland may be of importance in providing adequate supplies for the young, but no obvious purpose is served by the accumulation of iodide at the other sites. It is evident that the iodide-accumulating system of the thyroid is not unique to the gland and does not account for the specific function of making thyroid hormone.

2. *Oxidation and Iodination.* Consistent with the conditions generally necessary for halogenation of aromatic rings, the iodination of tyrosine residues requires the iodinating species to be in a higher state of oxidation than is the anion. However, the precise nature of the iodinating species is unknown. There is evidence against the participation of I_2 in the reaction. Possibly the reaction sequence involves the combination of oxidized free radicals of iodine and the tyrosyl acceptor, or the active species may be the iodinium ion (I^+) (DeGroot and Niepomniszcze, 1977). Whatever it may be, the requisite state of oxidation is produced by a peroxidase-catalyzed reaction. The H_2O_2 that serves as a substrate for the peroxidase is presumed to be formed in close proximity to its site of utilization, and the reactions probably involve the oxidation of NADPH by NADPH-cytochrome *c* reductase, the oxidation of NADH by NADH–cytochrome b_5 reductase, and the subsequent reduction of O_2 to H_2O_2 (*see* DeGroot and Niepomniszcze, 1977).

Taurog and associates (1970) have purified and characterized a heme-containing peroxidase from thyroid particulate fractions that catalyzes the iodination of tyrosyl residues in protein in the presence of H_2O_2. This enzyme appears to be concentrated in membranes at or near the apical surface of the thyroid cell and to catalyze the iodination of thyroglobulin just prior to its storage in the lumen of the thyroid follicle. The initial products of the reaction are monoiodotyrosyl and diiodotyrosyl residues in thyroglobulin.

3. *Formation of Thyroxine and Triiodothy-ronine from Iodotyrosines.* The remaining synthetic step is the coupling of two diiodotyrosyl residues to form thyroxine or monoiodotyrosyl and diiodotyrosyl residues to form triiodothyronine. These are also oxidative reactions and appear to be catalyzed by the same peroxidase discussed above (Lamas *et al.,* 1972). The mechanism involves the enzymatic transfer of groups, perhaps as iodotyrosyl free radicals or positively charged ions, within thyroglobulin (DeGroot and Niepomniszcze, 1977). The configuration of the protein is presumed to be important in facilitating this coupling reaction. It is possible that specific amino acid sequences adjacent to thyroxine residues could favor such conformation and enzymatic recognition of appropriate sites (Dunn, 1970). While many other proteins can serve as substrates for the peroxidase, none is as efficient as thyroglobulin in yielding thyroxine.

The proportions of thyroxine and triiodothyronine formed in the thyroid depend, at least in part, on the relative quantities of monoiodotyrosine and diiodotyrosine available. While a high proportion of monoiodotyrosine seems to favor the formation of triiodothyronine over thyroxine, deficient diiodotyrosine can impair the formation of both thyronines. Thyroxine predominates by a factor of severalfold under most circumstances, and about one fourth of the iodine in the thyroid of most species is in the form of thyroxine. When there is a deficiency of iodine in rat thyroid, however, the ratio of thyroxine to triiodothyronine decreases from 4:1 to 1:3 (Greer *et al.,* 1968). Since triiodothyronine is four times as active as thyroxine and contains only three fourths as much iodine, this change could provide a sixfold increase in hormonal effect from a given quantity of available iodine.

4. *Secretion of Thyroid Hormone.* Since thyroxine and triiodothyronine are synthesized and stored as parts of the molecule of thyroglobulin, proteolysis is an important part of the secretory process. It is generally believed that thyroglobulin must be completely broken down into its constituent amino acids in order for the hormones to be released. As the molecular weight of thyroglobulin is 660,000 and the protein is made up of about 300 carbohydrate residues and 5500 amino acid residues, only two to five of which are thyroxine (Rall *et al.,* 1964), this is a profligate

process indeed. Evidently evolution has not brought economy to the thyroid or perhaps sufficient intelligence to the scientist to understand the rationale of the process utilized. When thyroglobulin is hydrolyzed, monoiodotyrosine and diiodotyrosine are liberated also, but they usually do not leave the thyroid. Instead, they are selectively metabolized, and the iodine, liberated in the form of iodide, is reincorporated into protein (Roche *et al.,* 1952c). Normally, all this iodide is reused; however, when the process is activated intensely by thyrotropin (TSH), some of the iodide reaches the circulation, at times accompanied by trace amounts of the iodotyrosines.

The secretory process is initiated by endocytosis of colloid from the follicular lumen at the apical surface of the cell. This "ingested" thyroglobulin appears as intracellular colloid droplets, which apparently then fuse with lysosomes containing the requisite proteolytic enzymes (Wollman *et al.,* 1964). The liberated hormones presumably exit from the cell at its basal membrane.

5. *Conversion of Thyroxine to Triiodothyronine.* The normal daily production of thyroxine has been estimated to range between 70 and 90 μg, while that of triiodothyronine is between 15 and 30 μg. It is less certain what fraction of the triiodothyronine is secreted by the thyroid and how much results from the metabolism of thyroxine in peripheral tissues. When thyroxine is given to hypothyroid patients in doses that produce normal concentrations of thyroxine in plasma, the plasma concentration of triiodothyronine also reaches the normal range. Thus, peripheral production of triiodothyronine from thyroxine is apparently the major source of the hormone (*see* Utiger, 1974). This metabolic step has been demonstrated in preparations of a number of different tissues *in vitro* (Nakagawa and Ruegamer, 1967) and in athyrotic and normal man (Braverman *et al.,* 1970; Sterling *et al.,* 1970). The estimation of the total amount of thyroxine eventually converted to triiodothyronine is a difficult one, but it has been calculated to be in the range of 35% (*see* Schimmel and Utiger, 1977).

Transport of Thyroid Hormone in the Blood. Iodine in the circulation is normally present in several forms, with 95% as organic iodine and approximately 5% as iodide. Most of the organic iodine is thyroxine (90 to 95%), while triiodothyronine represents a relatively minor fraction (about 5%). The thyroid hormones are transported in the blood in strong but noncovalent association with certain plasma proteins.

Thyroxine-binding globulin is the major carrier of thyroid hormones. It is an acidic glycoprotein with a molecular weight of approximately 40,000, and it binds one molecule of thyroxine per molecule of protein with a very high association constant (about 10^{10}). Triiodothyronine is bound less avidly (Sterling *et al.,* 1971). Thyroid hormones are also found associated with *thyroxine-binding prealbumin.* This protein is present in higher concentration than is the thyroxine-binding globulin, but it binds thyroxine and triiodothyronine with association constants near 10^7 and 10^6, respectively (Nilsson and Peterson, 1971). Despite the fact that the prealbumin has four apparently identical subunits, it has a single high-affinity binding site. Albumin can also serve as a carrier for thyroxine when the more avid carriers are saturated. It is difficult, however, to estimate its quantitative or physiological importance.

Protein binding of thyroid hormones protects them from metabolism and excretion, resulting in their long half-life in the circulation. Only about 0.03% of the total thyroxine in plasma is free (*see* Utiger, 1974). While triiodothyronine is much less firmly bound, the quantity that is free, 0.2 to 0.5%, is still a small percentage of the total. However, the unbound thyroid hormones constitute the fractions available for action, and their concentrations thus assume particular importance.

Certain drugs and a variety of pathological and physiological conditions can alter the binding of thyroid hormones to proteins or the amounts of these proteins. Thus, the total amounts of thyroid hormones in the plasma and the quantities of *free* hormones can vary somewhat independently. For example, pregnancy or the administration of estrogen causes elevation of the concentration of thyroxine-binding globulin. This leads to increased thyroxine binding and could lower the concentration of free hormone. Feedback mechanisms compensate, however, and increased thyroid secretion returns the concentration of free hormone to normal. The result is elevated total and bound thyroxine in plasma and a normal concentration of free thyroxine. Laboratory tests measuring total thyroxine alone, therefore, would be subject to misinterpretation. Appropriate tests of thyroid function are discussed below.

Degradation and Excretion. Thyroxine is eliminated slowly from the body; it has a half-life of 6 to 7 days. In hyperthyroidism the half-life is shortened to 3 or 4 days, whereas in myxedema it may be 9 to 10 days. These changes are probably due to altered rates of metabolism of the hormone. In conditions associated with increased binding to the proteins of plasma, as in pregnancy, elimination is retarded; the reverse is observed when there is reduced protein in plasma, as in nephrosis or hepatic cirrhosis, or when binding to protein is inhibited by certain drugs, such as salicylate or dicumarol. Triiodothyronine, which is less avidly bound to protein, has a half-life of 2 days or less.

The liver is the major site of degradation of thyroid hormones; thyroxine and triiodothyronine are conjugated with glucuronic and sulfuric acids through the phenolic hydroxyl group and excreted in the bile. There is an enterohepatic circulation of the thyroid hormones, since they are liberated by hydrolysis in the intestine and reabsorbed. A portion of the conjugated material reaches the colon unchanged, is hydrolyzed there, and is eliminated as the free compounds in the feces. In man, approximately 20 to 40% of thyroxine is eliminated in the stool.

As discussed above, an important route of metabolism of thyroxine is to triiodothyronine. Another compound formed by peripheral metabolism of thyroxine is 3,3',5'-triiodothyronine, often referred to as reverse T_3. While the concentration of this inactive metabolite in plasma varies with diet and disease states, the significance of this is not currently understood. However, there is some evidence that the compound is secreted by the thyroid as well as being a product of the metabolism of thyroxine (*see* Burman, 1978). Triiodothyronine and reverse T_3 are deiiodinated to 3,3'-diiodothyronine, an inactive metabolite that is a normal constituent of human plasma (Wu *et al.,* 1976; Burman, 1978). Additional metabolites in which the diphenyl ether linkage is either intact (Pittman *et al.,* 1972) or broken (Wynn and Gibbs, 1962) have been detected both *in vitro* and *in vivo*.

Regulation of Thyroid Function. During the last century, it was appreciated that cellular changes occur in the anterior pituitary in association with endemic goiter or following thyroidectomy. The classical experimental observations of Cushing (1912) and the clini-

cal observations of Simmonds (1914) established that ablation or disease of the pituitary causes thyroid hypoplasia. It was eventually determined that the anterior pituitary secretes the specific hormone, thyrotropin (TSH) (Chapter 59).

Although there was evidence that thyroid hormone or lack of it causes cellular changes in the pituitary, the control of secretion of thyrotropin by the negative-feedback action of thyroid hormone was not appreciated fully until its central role in the pathogenesis of goiter was elucidated in the early 1940s. It is now recognized that the rate of secretion of thyrotropin is delicately controlled by the quantity of thyroid hormone in the circulation. If extra hormone is given, the secretion of thyrotropin is suppressed and the thyroid becomes inactive and regresses, whereas any decrease in the normal rate of secretion of the thyroid evokes an enhanced secretion of thyrotropin and the thyroid is stimulated to increased growth and function. The mechanism of this effect of thyroid hormone on thyrotropin secretion and the role of the hypothalamic thyrotropin-releasing hormone (TRH) are discussed in Chapter 59.

Actions of Thyrotropin on the Thyroid. When thyrotropin is given to experimental animals, the first effect on thyroid hormone metabolism that can be measured is an increased secretion. This can be monitored by detecting the radioactivity in the blood leaving the gland that has been prelabeled with radioactive iodine. Under these circumstances, the response can be seen within minutes. All phases of hormone synthesis and release are eventually stimulated: iodide uptake and organification, hormone synthesis, endocytosis, and proteolysis of colloid. There is increased vascularity of the gland and hypertrophy and hyperplasia of thyroid cells.

A primary action of thyrotropin is to activate thyroid adenylate cyclase and to increase the glandular concentration of cyclic adenosine 3',5'-monophosphate (cyclic AMP) (Gilman and Rall, 1968). Cyclic AMP, acting as the intracellular mediator of thyrotropin, appears to be able to reproduce the important actions of the hormone. Thus, iodide uptake and hormone synthesis are stimulated by the cyclic nucleotide, as are endocytosis and secretion of hormone. Protein and nucleic acid synthesis are increased; in fact, cyclic AMP has been shown to be goitrogenic (Pisarev *et al.,* 1970). Several actions of thyrotropin on the intermediary metabolism of thyroid tissue may also be mediated by cyclic AMP, although their immediate importance to hormone metabolism is uncertain. The relationship of cyclic AMP to control of thyroid function has been reviewed by Dumont and associates (1978).

Prostaglandin E_1 is also capable of stimulating accumulation of cyclic AMP in the thyroid (Zor *et al.,* 1969). Predictably, therefore, it too has thyrotropin-like effects on thyroid function.

Relation of Iodine to Thyroid Function. Normal thyroid function obviously requires an adequate intake of iodine; without it, normal amounts of hormone cannot be made, thyrotropin is secreted in excess, and the thyroid hypertrophies. The enlarged and stimulated thyroid becomes remarkably efficient in extracting the residual traces of iodide from the blood. The iodide-concentrating mechanism develops a gradient for the ion that may be ten times the normal, and the vascularity may increase to the point that a bruit is heard. The rush of blood can sometimes be felt by the hand. In this hypertrophied state the thyroid usually succeeds in making sufficient hormone, unless the iodine deficiency is severe.

In some areas of the world *simple* or *nontoxic goiter* is quite prevalent, because iodine is not abundant in most foods. The only rich natural sources commonly eaten are those derived from marine life. Sea fish contain 200 to 1000 µg/kg, shellfish a similar or slightly larger amount, and dried kelp 0.1 to 0.2%, but for those who do not eat marine fish the element can be scarce indeed. To ensure an adequate intake, which is usually taken to be about 100 µg daily, one would have to eat about 5 kg of vegetables or fruit, or 3 kg of meat or fresh-water fish. Milk and eggs are somewhat better sources, but most potable waters contain a negligible amount. However, unnatural sources of iodine in the environment are becoming prevalent and perhaps of concern. A slice of bread may contain 150 µg of iodate, added as a "conditioner" (London *et al.,* 1965). Other sources are as diverse as food colorings and automobile exhaust.

Iodine has been used empirically for the treatment of goiter for 150 years. However, its modern use was the outgrowth of the extensive studies of Marine, which culminated in the use of iodine to prevent goiter in school children in Akron, Ohio, a region where endemic goiter was prevalent (Marine and Kimball, 1917). The success of these experiments led to the adoption of this form of prophylaxis in many regions of endemic goiter thoughout the world.

The most practicable method yet found for providing small supplements of iodine for large segments of the population is the addition of an iodide to table salt, although iodate is now preferred. In some countries, the use of iodine in salt is required by law; in others, including the United States, the use is optional; in some regions, including vast areas of endemic goiter, injection of iodized oil has been used (Thilly *et al.,* 1973); in Japan, supplementation is not needed because kelp is a national delicacy. The quantity of iodide added to table salt varies in different countries; the 100-µg supplement is provided by 1 g of salt in the United States.

Actions of Thyroid Hormones. The actions of the thyroid hormones are considered under the categories of (1) regulation of growth and development, (2) calorigenic effect, (3) metabolic effects, and (4) inhibition of the secretion of thyrotropin by the pituitary. This last-named action on the pituitary is discussed in Chapter 59.

Growth and Development. It is generally believed that the thyroid hormones exert most if not all of their effects through control of protein synthesis. This is certainly true for the actions of the hormones on the normal growth and development of the organism. Perhaps the most dramatic example is found in the tadpole, which is almost magically transformed into a frog by thyroxine. Not only does the animal grow limbs, lungs, and other terrestrial accouterments, but also the hormone stimulates the synthesis of a host of enzymes and at the same time so influences the tail that it is digested away and used to build new tissue elsewhere.

There is a critically important role of thyroid hormone in the development of the nervous system. Examination of the brain of hypothyroid animals reveals deficient development, particularly of axonal and dendritic networks. Myelinization is severely impaired, and several other deficits in biochemical development are also notable. It has thus been hypothesized that the effect of thyroid hormone is to initiate a series of reactions that lead to differentiation and to terminate the phase of cell proliferation (Hamburgh, 1969). However, the effects of thyroid hormones on protein synthesis and enzymatic activity are certainly not limited to the brain, and a large number of tissues are altered by the administration of thyroid hormone or by its deficiency. The extensive defects in growth and development that are found in cretins provide a vivid reminder of the pervasive effects of thyroid hormones in normal individuals.

Cretinism is usually classified as endemic or sporadic. *Endemic cretinism* is encountered in regions of endemic goiter and is usually due to extreme deficiency of iodine. Goiter may or may not be present. There is a high incidence of nerve deafness in *endemic* but not in *sporadic* cretinism. The latter disease is a consequence of failure of the thyroid to develop normally or the result of a defect in the synthesis of thyroid hormone. Goiter is present if a synthetic defect is at fault.

While detectable at birth, cretinism is often not recognized until 3 to 5 months of age. When untreated, the condition eventually leads to such gross changes as to be unmistakable. The child is dwarfed and the extremities are short, and he is mentally retarded, inactive, uncomplaining, and listless. The face is puffy and expressionless, and the enlarged tongue may protrude through the thickened lips of the half-opened mouth. The skin may have a yellowish hue and feel doughy, and it is dry and cool to the touch. The heart rate is slow, the body temperature may be low, closure of the fontanels is delayed, and the teeth erupt late. Appetite is poor, feeding is slow and interrupted by choking, constipation is frequent, and there may be an umbilical hernia.

For treatment to be fully effective, the diagnosis must be made long before these obvious changes have come about. Screening of newborn infants for deficient function of the thyroid has been established in a number of centers. Measurements of the concentrations of thyrotropin and thyroxine in umbilical cord blood are performed. The incidence of congenital dysfunction of the thyroid is about one per 6000 births (Fisher, 1977).

It is thus clear that thyroid hormones are important determinants of genetically coded developmental programs. While the precise biochemical mechanisms through which the thyroid controls growth and development are unknown, the thyroid hormones are bound to a limited number of high-affinity sites in the nuclei of many cells. There is no convincing evidence that the hormones bind first to a cytoplasmic receptor, as is thought to be the case with steroid hormones. Both thyroxine and triiodothyronine are bound in nuclei, although thyroxine is bound with lower affinity. Based on the assumption that binding of the hormones represents initiation of their action, it has been calculated that thyroxine accounts for approximately 15% of the total activity of the thyroid hormones. Beyond this identification of the initial

site of interaction of thyroid hormones with the genetic apparatus, few other details are known (*see* Schwartz and Oppenheimer, 1978).

Calorigenic Effect. Thyroid hormones increase the resting or basal metabolic rate of the whole organism, but only certain tissues seem to be affected when their oxygen consumption is measured *in vitro.* Heart, diaphragm, liver, and kidney are markedly stimulated by thyroxine, while, for example, the ovaries and uterus seem unresponsive. The calorigenic response is important in regulation of temperature in homeotherms. Thyroid secretion, as regulated by the hypothalamus and pituitary, is stimulated by exposure to cold. The calorigenic action is dependent upon protein synthesis. Much of it may be secondary to increased cellular work such as protein synthesis; increased sodium transport probably accounts for a significant portion of thyroxine-induced energy utilization (Ismail-Beigi and Edelman, 1971). While extremely high doses of thyroxine can uncouple oxidative phosphorylation in mitochondria, this does not account for the calorigenic response to moderate doses of thyroid hormones. High-affinity binding sites for thyroid hormones have been described in mitochondria (Sterling, 1979); however, their significance is uncertain (*see* Schwartz and Oppenheimer, 1978).

Hyperactivity of the cardiovascular system is striking in hyperthyroidism, and several factors are probably important (*see* DeGroot, 1972). Cardiac output is undoubtedly augmented secondary to increased peripheral oxygen consumption, but these compensatory mechanisms can explain only a portion of the alterations seen. Chronic treatment with thyroid hormones augments the contractile state of isolated cardiac preparations by mechanisms thought not to involve catecholamines (Buccino *et al.,* 1967). However, it has often been stated that the heart is supersensitive to catecholamines in hyperthyroidism, and several reports indicate that the number of myocardial β-adrenergic receptors is increased (*see* Sterling, 1979). While mechanisms remain in doubt, the stimulatory effects of catecholamines on the stressed hyperthyroid myocardium may be devastating in a clinical setting; there is little doubt of the therapeutic efficacy of drugs that reduce adrenergic function in this condition.

Metabolic Effects. Thyroid hormones appear to stimulate metabolism of cholesterol to bile acids, and hypercholesterolemia is a characteristic feature of hypothyroid states. Some separation of actions has been observed between the effects of thyroxine analogs on cholesterol and on calorigenesis, and D-thyroxine is sometimes used to lower the concentration of cholesterol in plasma (Chapter 34).

Thyroid hormones enhance the lipolytic responses of fat cells to other hormones, for example, catecholamines, and elevated plasma free fatty acid concentrations are seen in hyperthyroidism. In contrast to other lipolytic hormones, thyroid hormones do not directly stimulate the accumulation of cyclic AMP. They may, however, regulate the capacity of other hormones to enhance the synthesis of the cyclic nucleotide (*see* Malbon *et al.,* 1978).

The effects of the thyroid hormones on carbohydrate metabolism are generally consistent with an accelerated utilization of carbohydrate, presumably secondary to increased caloric demand. There is an increased rate of intestinal absorption of glucose that results in higher concentrations of the sugar in plasma during the early phase of an *oral* glucose tolerance test. In contrast, the increased rate of metabolism of carbohydrate results in a flattened response to *intravenous* glucose.

In rats, thyroid hormones enhance the hepatic synthesis of glucose (Menahan and Wieland, 1969). The mechanism appears to involve induction of the hepatic mitochondrial enzyme pyruvate carboxylase and the cytosolic enzyme phosphoenolpyruvate carboxykinase; these proteins are responsible for catalyzing the initial reactions of gluconeogenesis from pyruvate.

Thyroid Hyperfunction. Excessive secretion of thyroid hormones may lead to such striking changes that the diagnosis of hyperthyroidism is obvious to the casual observer, or the effects may cause distressing or subtle symptoms that give no clue to their origin. Two major forms of thyroid hyperfunction are recognized. Diffuse toxic goiter (Graves' disease) is characterized by thyrotoxicosis and ophthalmopathy. This disease is now generally considered to be a disorder of the immune response. Antibodies of the IgG type appear to stimulate the thyroid gland by activating receptors for thyrotropin; other antibodies affect retro-orbital tissue and the eye muscles, leading to the characteristic ophthalmological changes (Volpe, 1978; *see also* Chapter 59). The disease occurs most commonly in young adults. Toxic nodular goiter (Plummer's disease) occurs primarily in older patients and usually arises from long-standing nontoxic goiter; infiltrative ophthalmopathy is uncommon. At times, however, the distinction between these conditions can be difficult.

Most of the signs and symptoms of hyperthyroidism stem from the excessive production of heat and from increased motor activity and increased activity of the sympathetic nervous system. The skin is flushed, warm, and moist; the muscles are weak and tremulous; the heart rate is rapid, and the heart beat is forceful; and the arterial pulses are prominent and bounding. The increased expenditure of energy gives rise to increased appetite and, if intake is insufficient, to loss of weight. There may also be insomnia, difficulty in remaining still, anxiety and apprehension, intolerance to heat, and increased frequency of bowel movements. Angina, arrhythmias, and heart failure are frequently present in older patients. Some individuals may show extensive muscular wasting, suggestive of myopathy. Others have osteoporosis from excessive loss of calcium.

Thyroid Hypofunction. Deficiency of thyroid hormone can be manifested at any age. In the adult, the condition is referred to simply as hypothyroidism or, particularly when severe, as myxedema. If the gland fails to develop or is congenitally incompetent, the deficiency may be noted soon after birth by the signs of cretinism (*see* above). Later in childhood, failure of growth and development added to the features of the adult counterpart is recognized as juvenile myxedema.

Myxedema. In its fully developed, classical form, myxedema is associated with degeneration and atrophy of the thyroid gland. The same condition follows surgical removal of the thyroid or its destruction by radioactive iodine. Myxedema is sometimes associated with goiter when there is a severe defect in synthesis of thyroid hormone, when the gland is extensively involved in chronic thyroiditis (Hashimoto's disease), or when antithyroid drugs have been given. When the disease is mild, it may be subtle in its presentation. By the time it has become severe, however, all of the signs are overt. The appearance of the patient is pathognomonic. The face is quite expressionless, puffy, and pallid. The skin is cold and dry, the scalp is scaly, and the hair is coarse, brittle, and sparse. The fingernails are thickened and brittle, the subcutaneous tissue appears to be thickened, and there may be true edema. The voice is husky and low pitched, speech is slow, the hearing is often faulty, and mentality is impaired. The appetite is poor, the gastric juice contains little free hydrochloric acid, gastrointestinal activity is diminished, and abdominal distention and constipation are common. Atony of the urinary bladder suggests that the function of other smooth muscles may also be impaired. The voluntary muscles are weak and flabby, and deep-tendon reflexes are slowed. The heart is often dilated, and cardiac output is diminished. There may also be hydropericardium, hydrothorax, and ascites. Refractory anemia, occasionally hyperchromic and macrocytic in character, is often associated with the disease. Menstrual irregularities are prominent. The patient is prone to be drowsy and to sleep a great deal, and he complains of the cold in winter but not of the heat in summer.

Thyroid Function Tests. The laboratory diagnosis of thyroid disease is complicated by the extremely low quantities of thyroid hormones in plasma; by problems of specificity, particularly when analytical technics are directed at iodine; and by variations in the extent of protein binding of the hormones. The availability of protein-binding assays and radioimmunoassays for the thyroid hormones has greatly improved the laboratory diagnosis of disorders of the thyroid. These specific assays, together with the resin-triiodothyronine-uptake (RT3U) test, which estimates the extent of saturation of thyroid-binding globulin, provide a valuable approach to an accurate diagnosis. Their use permits the estimation of the concentration of free thyroxine in plasma, an excellent index of the activity of the thyroid gland.

As mentioned above, the total concentration of thyroxine in plasma changes with alterations in the concentration of the thyroid-binding globulin, so that, for example, it is high in pregnancy and low in nephrosis even though the patient is euthyroid. From the estimates of the extent of saturation of the thyroid-binding globulin and the measurement of the total concentration of thyroxine in plasma, a free-thyroxine index can be calculated. The measurement of plasma triiodothyronine by radioimmunoassay is useful for the diagnosis of hyperthyroidism when this hormone is elevated predominantly.

The radioimmunoassay of thyrotropin (TSH) is also helpful. Determination of an elevated concentration of this hormone in the plasma can provide confirmation of suspected failure of the thyroid gland. Patients with frank hypothyroidism who have normal or decreased concentrations of TSH in plasma are likely to have hypothyroidism secondary to pituitary or hypothalamic dysfunction. The response of plasma TSH to an injection of thyrotropin-releasing hormone may also be useful in this regard (*see* Chapter 59).

Measurement of the accumulation of radioactive iodine by the thyroid gland as a diagnostic technic is discussed below. The use of laboratory tests in the diagnosis of thyroid disease has been reviewed by Feldman (1977) and Merimee (1978).

Preparations. Thyroid as well as thyroxine and triiodothyronine are official preparations. *Thyroid,* U.S.P., is a fine powder made from the thyroids of animals, usually pigs, by defatting and drying with acetone. The U.S.P. specifies that the content of iodine be between 0.17 and 0.23%, and, as most thyroid powders are stronger than this, they are diluted by an inert material. Although neither bioassay nor chemical analyses for thyroxine or triiodothyronine are specified, the product is remarkably uniform. *Thyroid Tablets,* U.S.P. (available as THYRAR, THYROCRINE, and preparations marketed under the nonproprietary name), are made from the compressed powder in numerous sizes from 15 to 300 mg. *Thyroglobulin,* U.S.P. (PROLOID), is a purified extract of pig thyroid available in tablets containing from 15 to 300 mg. It conforms to the U.S.P. standard for iodine content and is subjected to bioassay. Its potency is adjusted to be equivalent to *Thyroid,* U.S.P., and it is about twice as expensive. *Levothyroxine Sodium,* U.S.P. (SYNTHROID, LETTER, and nonproprietary preparations), is the sodium salt of the natural isomer of thyroxine and is dispensed in the form of tablets containing 25 to 500 μg and as a powder for reconstitution for injection. *Liothyronine Sodium,* U.S.P. (CYTOMEL), is the somewhat uninformative designation for the salt of L-triiodothyronine. It also is marketed as tablets containing 5, 25, and 50 μg. Mixtures of the sodium salts of thyroxine and triiodothyronine in a ratio of 4 : 1 are also marketed as *Liotrix,* U.S.P. (EUTHROID, THYROLAR). Their dubious advantage is replacement therapy with a pure mixture resembling the normal secretion of the gland.

Certain bizarre combinations of thyroid and other drugs (especially amphetamines) are still available. The use of thyroid or such mixtures for the purpose of weight reduction is dangerous, and sudden deaths from cardiac arrhythmias have occurred. *Obesity is not an acceptable indication for thyroid hormone therapy.*

Thyrotropin (THYTROPAR) is a preparation made from bovine pituitaries. It is available in ampuls containing 10 I.U. of powdered hormone to be reconstituted for injection. This is used only to test the ability of the thyroid to respond to exogenous stimulation. Synthetic *thyrotropin-releasing hormone* (*protirelin;* THYPINONE) is available in ampuls containing 500 μg in 1 ml.

Choice of Preparation. The pure compounds carry the attraction of single, reproducible substances of known and constant composition. There is some evidence that absorption of levothyroxine sodium is variable and incomplete, as much as 30 to 40% being recoverable in the stool (Van Middlesworth, 1960). Depending upon the form in which it is given, the proportion of a single oral dose absorbed may vary from 42 to 74%; this fraction is rapidly absorbed, while the rest traverses the intestine in a bound unabsorbable form. Nevertheless, levothyroxine sodium has been extensively used with satisfaction and is widely held to be superior to thyroid because of better standardization and stability. Variability of absorption also occurs with dessicated thyroid. The two preparations are about the same price.

Liothyronine sodium may occasionally be preferred to levothyroxine sodium when a quicker action is desired. It may be useful, therefore, when hypothyroidism has recently supervened from overtreatment with an antithyroid drug or following treatment with radioiodine or thyroidectomy, and in the rare event of coma due to myxedema. It is perhaps less desirable than the other preparations for prolonged therapy because its briefer action might require more frequent doses for steady response. Other disadvantages include altered normal values for thyroid function tests and high cost.

Comparative Responses to Thyroid Preparations. There is no significant difference in the qualitative response of the patient with myxedema to triiodothyronine, thyroxine, or thyroid. However, there are obvious quantitative differences. Following the subcutaneous administration of a large experimental dose of 1 mg of L-triiodothyronine, a metabolic response can be detected within 4 to 6 hours, at which time the skin becomes detectably warmer and the pulse rate and the temperature increase. With this dose, a metabolic rate of −40% can be raised to normal within 24 hours. The maximal response occurs in 2 days or less, and the effects subside with a half-life of about 8 days. The same single dose of thyroxine exerts much less effect. However, if thyroxine is given in approximately four times the dose of triiodothyronine, a comparable elevation in metabolic rate can be achieved. The peak effect of a single dose is evident in about 9 days, and this declines to half the maximum in 11 to 15 days. In both cases the effects outlast the presence of detectable amounts of hormone; these disappear from the blood with mean half-lives of approximately 2 and 6 days, respectively. Equivalent clinical responses are obtained from the daily administration of approximately 60 mg of thyroid, 60 mg of thyroglobulin, 100 μg of levothyroxine, or 25 μg of liothyronine.

Therapeutic Uses of Thyroid Hormone.
The two major indications for the therapeutic use of thyroid hormone are *hypothyroidism* or *myxedema* and *simple goiter.* Inasmuch as they result from thyroid hypofunction, these uses represent true replacement therapy.

Hypothyroidism. It has been said that treatment of adult myxedema is as perfect a form of therapy as any known to medicine. The main objective is to arrive at the proper dose of a suitable thyroid preparation. The dose varies somewhat according to complications, especially those involving the heart. The object of therapy is to restore the patient to normal. Often the patient may think he is well when the astute observer can see that he is still hypothyroid. The reverse may also be true; the patient can know that he is ill, but the doctor does not recognize the insidious onset of the signs and symptoms of myxedema. Because long-standing hypothyroidism may have undesirable effects, including a predisposition to atherosclerosis, a full replacement dose should be given if possible.

A reasonable therapeutic regimen for adults is to give a daily dose of 50 μg of thyroxine for 1 to 2 weeks, a daily dose of 100 μg for the next 1 to 2 weeks, then a permanent daily dose of 150 μg, depending on the response of the patient. Medication should be taken on an empty stomach to minimize irregular absorption. The patient should be carefully observed during the institution of treatment for untoward reactions such as cardiac pain or palpitations. If angina occurs, care should be exercised but therapy should not necessarily be withheld. Cardiac symptoms are the only serious complications of treatment. Arrhythmias have caused death during the initiation of thyroid therapy in myxedema.

In childhood, treatment is the same as in adults, and every attempt should be made to give a fully therapeutic dose without causing symptoms or failure to gain weight normally, in order to ensure normal growth and development. Usually a full adult dose is needed, and the schedule above can be used.

Myxedema Coma. A large number of dosage regimens have been advocated for this emergency, and the following serve as examples. Levothyroxine (500 μg, intravenously) or liothyronine (25 μg, intravenously, every 6 to 12 hours, or 100 μg immediately) is preferred initially. Thyroid (120 to 240 mg) may be given by gastric tube if necessary. Treatment with cortisol is also recommended because of the likelihood of adrenal insufficiency. Further therapy is dictated by the initial clinical response.

Cretinism. Success in the treatment of cretinism depends upon the age at which therapy is started. Unfortunately, many cases do not come to the attention of physicians until the retardation in development has become so obvious as to be alarming to the parents. In such cases, the detrimental effects of the deficiency on mental development will not be completely overcome. If, on the other hand, therapy is started soon after birth, normal physical and mental development may be achieved. Prognosis also depends on the age of onset of the deficiency. If no thyroid develops in the fetus, deficiency probably dates from the fetal age of 3 months, because little hormone is provided from the mother. It is felt, however, that the most critical need for thyroid hormone is the period of central nervous system (CNS) myelination that occurs about the time of birth. Recommended daily doses of levothyroxine are 10 μg/kg for infants under 6 months of age, 8 μg/kg from 6 to 12 months, 6 μg/kg from 1 to 5 years, and 4 μg/kg from 5 to 10 years. Therapy is monitored by determination of the concentrations of thyroxine and TSH and, occasionally, triiodothyronine in the plasma (*see* Fisher, 1978). Intellectual and physical development are also guides for therapy in this condition, and error, if unavoidable, should be made on the side of higher dosage. Excessive dosage will, however, advance the bone age inappropriately.

Mild Hypothyroidism. Hypothyroidism with few of the manifestations of myxedema is a condition that some years ago would have been denied existence by certain physicians. Its reality was firmly established by its similarity to the artificially induced condition in patients in the early stages of their approach to myxedema from overdosage with antithyroid drugs or radioiodine, and by employment of thyroid function tests. In both kinds, the response to treatment provides convincing confirmation. Mild hypothyroidism is frequently encountered among patients with simple goiter. The symptoms may be those of myxedema in mild form, but they may be limited to one or more symptoms such as fatigue, muscle cramps, paresthesias, and intolerance to cold. The treatment for mild hypothyroidism is the same as for myxedema and with the same doses.

Simple Goiter. In simple goiter, or thyroid enlargement without hyperthyroidism, the usual problem is deficient secretion of thyroid hormone, causing an excessive output of thyrotropin. The exceptions are unrecognized cases of subacute thyroiditis, Hashimoto's thyroiditis, and autonomous thyroid tumors. As the cause of the condition is frequently some defect in the production of thyroid hormone, treatment with thyroid can properly be regarded as replacement therapy.

The aim in treatment is to give full replacement doses of thyroid hormone to suppress the secretion of thyrotropin. Usually, this amounts to 100 to 200 μg of levothyroxine daily, but some patients may require 300 μg. The effectiveness of treatment can be judged by the return of the concentration of thyrotropin in plasma to normal values and by the clinical response in the decrease in size of the goiter.

There have been wide differences in the experience of competent observers as to the proportion of cases of goiter that respond to treatment with a decrease in the size of the thyroid. Some have observed that only in a minority of the cases is a worthwhile regression achieved. In several large series, however, there has been an appreciable regression in the goiter in about two thirds of the cases and a complete disappearance in half of these. In other series, almost every case showed some response (*see* Doniach *et al.*, 1958; Starr and Goodwin, 1958; Astwood *et al.*, 1960; Higgins *et al.*, 1964). The degree of response is greatly affected by the duration of the goiter, its cause, and the degree of nodularity. In areas of endemic goiter where deficiency of iodine is the likely cause, Stanbury and associates have found thyroid medication to be prompt and effective unless the goiter had advanced to the stage of nodular degeneration (*see* Means *et al.*, 1963). However, correction of the iodine deficiency is a more direct approach and is advocated for most cases.

Response to treatment of goiter commonly seen in the United States with thyroid hormone may be noticed within a few days; usually, however, it is counted in weeks, and the maximal response may not be seen for many months. Observations on the incidence of relapse when treatment is stopped are insufficient to provide a meaningful figure, but the observation that all do not recur has not been explained.

Nodular Goiter. The transition of diffuse to nodular goiter is much more important than the cosmetic aspect or the infrequent symptoms of compression with difficulty in swallowing. In some instances nodules may secrete hormone and cause hyperthyroidism (*toxic nodular goiter*); however, they are frequently not functional. Herein lies a controversial area of thyroid therapy, since it is necessary to determine if the nonfunctional nodule is malignant. While some advocate excision or biopsy, many prefer to administer replacement doses of thyroid hormone for several months to determine if the nodule

will diminish in size—an unlikely occurrence with nonfunctional malignant nodules. Since there is some evidence that nonfunctional nodules are responsive to thyrotropin, there is logic in such efforts; however, it is more difficult to shrink a nodule than to decrease the size of a diffusely enlarged gland.

Thyrotropin-Dependent Carcinoma. Certain carcinomas of the thyroid gland, particularly those of the papillary type, may remain sensitive to the growth-promoting effects of TSH. If such tumors are not treatable by more definitive technics, the administration of thyroid hormone to suppress the secretion of TSH may cause regression of malignant lesions.

ANTITHYROID DRUGS AND OTHER THYROID INHIBITORS

A large number of compounds are capable of interfering, directly or indirectly, with the synthesis of thyroid hormones. Several are of great clinical value for the temporary or extended control of hyperthyroid states. These will be discussed in detail. Others are primarily of research or toxicological interest and can only be mentioned. The major inhibitors may be classified into four categories: (1) antithyroid drugs, which interfere directly with the synthesis of thyroid hormones; (2) ionic inhibitors, which block the iodide transport mechanism; (3) iodide itself, which in high concentrations suppresses the thyroid; and (4) radioactive iodine, which damages the gland with ionizing radiations.

ANTITHYROID DRUGS

The antithyroid drugs that have clinical utility are thioamides; propylthiouracil may be considered as the prototype.

History. Regulatory feedback mechanisms are now well appreciated. Thus, a deficient concentration of circulating thyroid hormone evokes increased secretion of thyrotropin, and the result is thyroid hypertrophy—a goiter. It was studies on the mechanism of the development of goiter that first established the importance of this system of control.

In 1928, Chesney described goiter in rabbits fed a diet composed largely of cabbage (Chesney *et al.*, 1928). This result was probably due to the presence of precursors of the thiocyanate ion in cabbage leaves (*see* below). These experiments led to the work of Hercus and Purves (1936), who showed a goitrogenic effect from feeding the seeds of the cabbage family of plants. A few years later two pure compounds were shown to produce goiter. Sulfaguanidine, used by the Mackenzies and McCollum (1941) to inhibit intestinal flora for nutritional studies, and phenylthiourea, used by Richter and Clisby (1942) for tests on taste, caused goiter in rats.

A study of thiourea derivatives in rats revealed that their thyroid glands underwent hyperplastic changes characteristic of intense thyrotropic stimulation. However, it was soon established that the animals were hypothyroid. The first measurable effect in young rats was a loss of organic iodine from the thyroid; after treatment was begun, no new hormone could be made. It was evident, therefore, that the primary action was an inhibition of the formation of thyroid hormone. Furthermore, following hypophysectomy or the administration of thyroid hormone, the goitrogen had no visible effect upon the thyroid gland. This suggested that the goiter was a compensatory change resulting from the induced state of hypothyroidism (Astwood, 1945).

When it became clear from experimental studies in the 1940s that the primary action of the compounds was to inhibit the formation of thyroid hormone, the therapeutic possibilities in hyperthyroidism were evident and the substances so used became known as *antithyroid drugs.*

Structure-Activity Relationship. The two goitrogens found in the early 1940s proved to be prototypes of two different classes of antithyroid drugs. These two, with one later addition, make up three general categories into which the majority of the agents can be assigned: (1) *thioamides,* of which thiourea is the simplest member, include all the compounds currently used clinically (Table 60-2); (2) *aniline derivatives,* of which the sulfonamides make up the largest number, embrace a few substances that have been found to inhibit the human thyroid; and (3) *polyhydric phenols,* such as resorcinol, which have caused goiter in man when applied to the abraded skin. A few other compounds, mentioned briefly below, do not fit into any of these categories.

Thioamides. Thiourea and its simpler aliphatic derivatives and heterocyclic compounds containing a thioureylene group make up the majority of the known antithyroid agents that are also effective in man. Although most of them incorporate the entire thioureylene group, in some a nitrogen atom is replaced by oxygen or sulfur so that only the thioamide group is common to all. Among the heterocyclic compounds, the sulfur derivatives that are active are representatives of imidazole, oxazole, hydantoin, thiazole, thiadiazole, uracil, and barbituric acid.

Aniline Derivatives. In this group, optimal antithyroid activity in the rat is associated with a para-substituted aminobenzene grouping with or without aliphatic substitution on the amino nitrogen. While sulfathiazole and sulfadiazine possess significant activity, the sulfonamides are not detectably antithyroid in man in doses used clinically. However, aminosalicylic acid, which formerly was given in doses of many grams daily for months, has caused hypothyroidism and goiter.

Polyhydric Phenols. Hypothyroidism and goiter have followed the use of resorcinol in the form of an ointment for the treatment of leg ulcers. Antithyroid activity seems to be associated with meta substitution

on the benzene ring with two polar groups (Arnott and Doniach, 1952; Rosenberg, 1952).

Individual Compounds of Interest. L-5-Vinyl-2-thiooxazolidone (goitrin) is responsible for the goiter that results from consuming turnips or the seeds or green parts of cruciferous plants. These plants are eaten by cows, and the compound is found in cow's milk in areas of endemic goiter in Finland (Arstica *et al.,* 1969); it is about as active as propylthiouracil in man. Van Etten (1969) has reviewed the chemistry of naturally occurring goitrogens.

As the result of industrial exposure, toxicological studies, or clinical trials for various purposes, several other compounds have been noted to possess antithyroid activity. Among compounds used clinically, phenylbutazone and thiopental are weakly antithyroid in experimental animals. This is not significant at usual doses in man. However, antithyroid effects in man have been observed from dimercaprol and from lithium salts (Schou *et al.,* 1968; Temple *et al.,* 1972).

Mechanism of Action. Antithyroid drugs inhibit the formation of thyroid hormones by interfering with the incorporation of iodine into tyrosyl residues of thyroglobulin; they also inhibit the coupling of these iodotyrosyl residues to form iodothyronines. This implies that they interfere with the oxidation of iodide ion and iodotyrosyl groups, but the elucidation of the detailed mechanism has not yet been completed. Taurog (1970, 1976) has proposed that the drugs inhibit the peroxidase enzyme, thereby preventing oxidation

Table 60-2.   ANTITHYROID DRUGS OF THE THIOAMIDE TYPE

Propylthiouracil

Methimazole

Carbimazole

of iodide or iodotyrosyl groups to the required active state. Another mechanism, the reduction of oxidized iodine (and presumably the reduction of activated iodotyrosyl groups) at a stage in which the oxidized entity is still bound to the peroxidase, has been supported by the experiments of Morris and Hager (1966) and Davidson and associates (1978). Whatever the precise mechanism, inhibition of hormone synthesis results, over a period of time, in the depletion of stores of iodinated thyroglobulin as the protein is hydrolyzed and the hormones are released into the circulation. Only when the preformed hormone is depleted and the concentrations of circulating thyroid hormones begin to decline do clinical effects become noticeable.

There is some evidence that the coupling reaction may be more sensitive to an antithyroid drug, such as propylthiouracil, than is the iodination reaction (Taurog, 1970). This may explain why patients with hyperthyroidism respond well to doses of the drug that only partially suppress organification.

In addition to blocking hormone synthesis, propylthiouracil also inhibits the peripheral deiodination of thyroxine to triiodothyronine (Geffner et al., 1975; Saberi et al., 1975). Methimazole does not have this effect. Although the quantitative significance of this inhibition has not been established, it does provide a theoretical rationale for the choice of propylthiouracil over other antithyroid drugs in the treatment of thyroid storm. In this acute situation, a decreased rate of conversion of circulating thyroxine to triiodothyronine would be beneficial.

Absorption, Metabolism, and Excretion. Measurements of the course of organification of radioiodine by the thyroid show that absorption of *effective* amounts of propylthiouracil follows within 20 or 30 minutes after an oral dose. They also show that the duration of action of the compounds used clinically is brief. The effect of a dose of 100 mg of propylthiouracil begins to wane in 2 to 3 hours, and even a 500-mg dose is completely inhibitory for only 6 or 8 hours. As little as 0.5 mg of methimazole similarly stops the organification of radioiodine in the thyroid gland, but a single dose of 10 to 25 mg is needed to extend the inhibition to 24 hours.

Studies with radioactive drugs also reveal rapid absorption of the compounds. The half-life of propylthiouracil in plasma approximates 2 hours, while that for methimazole has been estimated to be between 6 and 13 hours (Marchant et al., 1978). All the useful drugs appear to be concentrated in the thyroid, and methimazole, derived from the metabolism of carbimazole, accumulates after carbimazole is administered (Marchant et al., 1978). Radioactive drugs and metabolites appear largely in the urine.

The antithyroid drugs cross the placenta and can also be found in milk. The use of these drugs during pregnancy is discussed below; women taking these agents should not breast-feed their infants.

Untoward Reactions. The incidence of side effects from propylthiouracil and methimazole as currently used is relatively low. The overall incidence as compiled by VanderLaan and Storrie (1955) from published cases was 3% for propylthiouracil and 7% for methimazole, with 0.44 and 0.12% of cases, respectively, developing the most serious reaction, agranulocytosis. Further observation suggests that there is little, if any, difference in side effects between these two agents, and that an incidence of agranulocytosis of 1 in 500 is a maximal figure. This reaction usually occurs during the first few months of therapy. Since agranulocytosis can develop rapidly, periodic white-cell counts are of little help. Patients should immediately report the development of sore throat or fever, which usually heralds the onset of this reaction. If the drug is discontinued rapidly, recovery is the rule. Mild granulocytopenia, if noted, may be due to thyrotoxicosis or may be the first sign of this dangerous drug reaction. Caution and frequent leukocyte counts are then required.

The most common reaction is a mild, sometimes purpuric, papular rash. It often subsides spontaneously without interrupting treatment but sometimes calls for changing to another drug, since cross-sensitivity is uncommon. Other less frequent complications are pain and stiffness in the joints, paresthesias, headache, nausea, and loss or depigmentation of the hair. Drug fever, hepatitis, and nephritis are very rare.

Preparations and Dosage. The compounds in current use are *Propylthiouracil*, U.S.P. (6-*n*-propylthiouracil), in the form of 50-mg tablets that can be broken in half, and *Methimazole*, U.S.P. (1-methyl-2-mercaptoimidazole; TAPAZOLE), marketed in 5- and 10-mg tablets. *Methylthiouracil*, U.S.P., is not available commercially in the United States at the present time. *Carbimazole* (NEOMERCAZOLE) is a carbethoxy derivative of methimazole, which it closely resembles and into which it is converted in the body; it is widely used in Great Britain, where it is available in 5- and 10-mg tablets.

There are no commercial preparations available for parenteral use in the rare event that treatment cannot be given by mouth. For this eventuality and for experimental purposes, the freely water-soluble compound, methimazole, can be dissolved in saline solution and sterilized.

The usual dose of propylthiouracil for the treatment of hyperthyroidism is 75 to 100 mg every 8 hours. In some cases larger doses, up to 900 mg daily, may be required. Failures of response to treatment with 300 mg daily are sometimes attributable to improper spacing of the doses, since the drug is fully effective for only a few hours. Delayed responses are also sometimes noted when the thyroid is unusually large and when iodine in any form has been given beforehand. When doses larger than 300 mg daily are needed, further subdivision of the time of administration of the daily dose into 4- or 6-hour intervals is perhaps advisable. After the patient is euthyroid, dosage can usually be reduced to one third for maintenance.

The corresponding initial dose of methimazole or carbimazole for the majority of cases is 5 or 10 mg every 8 hours. Because the half-life of methimazole is 6 to 13 hours, this dosage regimen should produce an uninterrupted suppression of the thyroid gland. Methylthiouracil is usually given in a daily dose of 200 mg, divided into two or four equally spaced doses. When a complete response has been achieved, the dose is reduced but the total daily dose is still subdivided. Only when very small amounts are needed is the frequency of dosage reduced to two or even one dose per day.

Therapeutic Uses. The antithyroid drugs are used in the treatment of *hyperthyroidism* in the following three ways: (1) as definitive treatment, to control the disorder in anticipation of a spontaneous remission; (2) in conjunction with radioiodine, to hasten recovery while awaiting the effects of radiation; and (3) to control the disorder in preparation for surgical treatment. There is no uniformity of opinion as to which form of treatment is the most desirable.

Response to Treatment. Hyperthyroidism may be of two kinds, Graves' disease and hyperthyroidism from one or more overfunctioning thyroid nodules; whichever the cause, the hyperthyroidism seems to respond to antithyroid drugs in the same way. After treatment is instituted, there is usually a latent period of a few days to 2 or more weeks before improvement is clearly manifest; however, in a few cases, and particularly when the hyperthyroidism is severe, definite improvement may be seen in 1 or 2 days. In patients with large goiters and particularly if nodular, the response may be slower. When iodine was commonly used for therapy, it was frequently observed that prior treatment with iodine delayed the response to antithyroid drugs for many weeks. Thus, it would appear that the rate of response is determined by the quantity of stored hormone, the rate of turnover of hormone in the thyroid, and the completeness of the block in synthesis imposed by the dosage given. When large doses are continued, and sometimes with the usual dose, recovery is followed by the development of hypothyroidism. The earliest signs of hypothyroidism call for a reduction in dose; if by chance they have advanced to the point of discomfort, thyroid hormone can be given to hasten recovery. A full dose of 120 to 180 mg daily of thyroid or the equivalent of thyroxine or triiodothyronine for a week will usually suffice. The lower maintenance dose of antithyroid drug discussed above is instituted for continued suppression.

In most cases, treatment with an antithyroid drug requires medical attention only at monthly or bimonthly intervals and adjustment of dosage can be made entirely upon the basis of symptoms and simple clinical signs. If confirmatory tests are desirable, those reflecting the concentration of circulating hormones are the most helpful.

Control of the hyperthyroidism is not associated with further enlargement of the goiter unless hypothyroidism is induced. When this happens, the new enlargement is quickly reversed by giving thyroid hormone. The presumption is, therefore, that thyrotropin is secreted in excessive amounts in response to the hypothyroidism and can be suppressed by thyroid hormone.

Remissions. The antithyroid drugs have been used in many patients to control the hyperthyroidism of Graves' disease until a spontaneous remission occurs. Solomon and associates (1953) reported that 50% of patients so treated for 1 year remained well without further therapy for long periods, perhaps indefinitely. More recent reports have indicated that a much smaller percentage of patients sustain remissions after such treatment (Wartofsky, 1973; Greer et al., 1977).

Unfortunately, there is no way of predicting before treatment is begun which patients will eventually achieve a lasting remission and which will relapse. It is clear that a favorable outcome is unlikely when the disorder is of long standing and when various forms of treatment have failed. To complicate the issue further, it is thought that remission and eventual hypothyroidism may represent the natural history of Graves' disease.

During treatment, a fairly certain sign that a remission may have taken place is a reduction in the size of the goiter. The persistence of goiter usually indicates failure, unless the patient becomes hypothyroid. Another favorable indication is continued freedom from all signs of hyperthyroidism when the maintenance dose is small. A helpful test to determine whether treatment may safely be discontinued involves measuring the accumulation of radioiodine by the thyroid gland after giving 180 mg of thyroid powder or its equivalent daily for 3 weeks. Pronounced suppression of accumulation implies the reestablishment of the normal feedback mechanism, and a state of remission usually can be correctly inferred (Cassidy and VanderLaan, 1960).

The Therapeutic Choice. Because of the low rates of permanent remission of Graves' disease that can be achieved with antithyroid drugs, the majority of patients will eventually require surgery or treatment with radioactive iodine; a 1-year trial of antithyroid agents is not advisable. It may be worthwhile to try prolonged therapy with antithyroid drugs in patients who have minimal enlargement of the thyroid or very mild hyperthyroidism.

Radioiodine or surgery is indicated for definitive therapy in toxic nodular goiter, since spontaneous remissions are not characteristic of this condition.

There is considerable disagreement about the therapy of thyrotoxicosis during *pregnancy.* The antithyroid drugs cross the placenta and can cause fetal hypothyroidism and goiter. Knowledge of thyroid hormone transport to the fetus is poor. There are three choices of therapy, each with its advocates: minimal doses of antithyroid drugs, full doses of antithyroid drugs with thyroid hormone supplementation, or surgery. Radioiodine is clearly contraindicated.

Preoperative Preparation. An important use of antithyroid drugs is in the preparation of the hyperthyroid patient for subtotal thyroidectomy. It is possible to bring virtually 100% of patients to a euthyroid state; as a consequence, the operative mortality for a single-stage thyroidectomy in expert hands is now very low. The treatment is continued until the patient is judged to be normal or nearly so, and then iodide is added to the regimen for the 7 to 10 days immediately before the operation. Iodide reduces the vascularity of the gland and makes it less friable, which lessen the difficulties for the surgeon.

Propranolol. This β-adrenergic antagonist does not inhibit the function of the thyroid, but it is useful for the temporary suppression of the signs and symptoms of thyrotoxicosis. As mentioned above, some of the cardiovascular manifestations of hyperthyroidism may be reinforced by the cardiac effects of catecholamines. Adrenergic antagonists also reduce the heart rate, tremor, and stare in hyperthyroidism and relieve palpitation, anxiety, and tension. The control of these manifestations is unmistakable and rapid (*see* Shanks *et al.*, 1969). It is thus valuable in controlling symptoms while awaiting the response to antithyroid drugs or radioiodine, and it is very useful in the rare but potentially lethal complication, thyroid storm (Das and Krieger, 1969). A usual oral dose of propranolol is 20 to 40 mg every 6 hours, but the amount should be adjusted according to the response; the heart rate is a reliable indicator.

IONIC INHIBITORS

The term *ionic inhibitors* serves to designate the substances that interfere with the concentration of iodide ion by the thyroid gland. The effective agents are themselves anions that in some ways resemble iodide ion; they are all monovalent, hydrated anions of a size similar to that of iodide. The most studied example, *thiocyanate,* differs from the others qualitatively; it is not concentrated by the thyroid gland, and in large amounts it inhibits the organification of iodine. Thiocyanate ion is produced following the enzymatic hydrolysis of certain plant glycosides. Thus, the eating of some foods (*e.g.,* cabbage) results in an increased concentration of thiocyanate in the blood and urine. Dietary precursors of thiocyanate may be a contributing factor in endemic goiter in certain parts of the world, particularly when the intake of iodine is very low (Delange and Ermans, 1971).

Wyngaarden and associates (1952) found a number of inorganic ions to be effective in rats; *perchlorate* (ClO_4^-) is ten times as active as thiocyanate and *nitrate* about $\frac{1}{30}$ as active. While perchlorate can be used to control hyperthyroidism, it may cause fatal aplastic anemia and has been abandoned except in very unusual circumstances. Perchlorate can be used to "discharge" inorganic iodide from the thyroid gland in a diagnostic test of organification.

Other ions, selected on the basis of their size, have also been found to be active; fluoborate (BF_4^-) is as effective as perchlorate, whereas fluosulfonate (SO_3F^-) and difluophosphate ($PO_2F_2^-$) are less so (Anbar *et al.*, 1960). Wolff and Maurey (1963) have related the inhibitory properties of a series of anions to their partial molal ionic volumes. A linear relationship was found in the range of 25 to 46 ml per mole, with bromide (Br^-) the smallest and least effective and pertechnetate (TcO_4^-) the largest and most potent.

IODIDE

Iodide is the oldest remedy for disorders of the thyroid gland. Before the antithyroid drugs were used, it was the only substance available for the control of the signs and symptoms of hyperthyroidism. Its use in this way is indeed paradoxical, and the explanation for this paradox is still incomplete.

Response to Iodide in Hyperthyroidism. The response of the patient with hyperthyroidism to iodide is often striking and rapid. The effect is usually discernible within 24 hours, and the basal metabolic rate may fall at a rate comparable to that following thyroidectomy. This provides evidence that the release of hormone into the circulation is quickly interrupted. The maximal effect is attained after 10 to 15 days of continuous therapy when the signs and symptoms of hyperthyroidism may have greatly improved.

The changes in the thyroid gland have been studied in detail; vascularity is reduced, the gland becomes much firmer and even hard to the touch, the cells become smaller, colloid reaccumulates in the follicles, and the quantity of bound iodine increases. The changes are those that would be expected if the excessive stimulus to the gland had somehow been removed or antagonized.

Unfortunately, iodide therapy usually does not completely control the manifestations of hyperthyroidism, and after a variable period of time the beneficial effect disappears. With continued treatment, the hyperthyroidism may return in its initial intensity or may become even more severe than it was at first. It is for this reason that, when iodide was the only agent available for the treatment of hyperthyroidism, its use was usually restricted to preoperative preparation of the patient for thyroidectomy.

Mechanism of Action.   High concentrations of iodide appear to influence all important aspects of iodine metabolism by the thyroid gland (*see* Ingbar, 1972). The capacity of iodide to limit its own transport has been mentioned above. Acute inhibition of the synthesis of iodotyrosine and iodothyronine by iodide is also well known (the *Wolff-Chaikoff effect*) (Wolff and Chaikoff, 1948). This inhibition is observed only above critical concentrations of iodide, and the intracellular rather than the extracellular concentration of the anion appears to be the major determinant. With time there is "escape" from this inhibition that is associated with an adaptive decrease in iodide transport and a lowered intracellular iodide concentration. The mechanism of the Wolff-Chaikoff effect is not understood. DeGroot and Niepomniszcze (1977) have reviewed the numerous hypotheses that have been proposed as explanations.

The most important clinical effect of high iodide concentration is an inhibition of the release of thyroid hormone. This action is rapid and efficacious in severe thyrotoxicosis. The effect is exerted directly on the thyroid gland, and it can be demonstrated in the euthyroid subject and experimental animals as well as in the hyperthyroid patient.

Iodide antagonizes the ability of both thyrotropin and cyclic AMP to stimulate endocytosis of colloid, proteolysis, and hormone secretion (Pisarev *et al.*, 1971). Several groups of investigators have reported that iodide attenuates the effect of TSH on cyclic AMP *in vivo* and in isolated tissues (Sherwin and Tong, 1975; Van Sande *et al.*, 1975). Because of the likelihood that cyclic AMP mediates many, if not all, of the effects of TSH (and presumably the effects of

the TSH-imitative immunoglobulins as well), this may help to explain the action of iodide.

Preparations and Dosage.   The dosage or form in which iodide is administered bears little relationship to the response achieved in hyperthyroidism, provided not less than the minimal effective amount is given; this dose is 6 mg per day in most, but not all, patients. Lugol's solution (*Strong Iodine Solution,* U.S.P.) is widely used and consists of 5% iodine and 10% potassium iodide. The iodine is reduced to iodide in the intestine before absorption. *Sodium Iodide,* U.S.P., and *Potassium Iodide,* U.S.P., are available in solid form, as is *Potassium Iodide Oral Solution,* U.S.P., for oral administration. While a dosage of 500 mg of iodide per day is often used, 50 to 100 mg per day seems more reasonable.

Other preparations that contain iodine include several designed for use as antiseptics (*see* Chapter 41) and a large number of compounds that are employed as radiographic contrast media.

Therapeutic Uses.   The uses of iodide in the treatment of *hyperthyroidism* are in the immediate preoperative period in preparation for thyroidectomy and, in conjunction with antithyroid drugs and propranolol, in the treatment of thyrotoxic crisis. Prior to surgery, iodine is sometimes employed alone, but more frequently it is used after the hyperthyroidism has been controlled by an antithyroid drug. It is then given during the 10 days that immediately antedate the operation. Optimal control of hyperthyroidism is achieved if antithyroid drugs are first given alone. If iodine is also given from the beginning, variable responses are observed; sometimes the effect of iodide predominates, storage of hormone is promoted, and prolonged antithyroid treatment is required before the hyperthyroidism is controlled. Recent data indicate that the combination of potassium iodide and propranolol may prove to be a superior regimen for preparation of patients with Graves' disease for surgery (Feek *et al.*, 1980).

Iodide salts are also useful *expectorants* when it is desired to liquefy tenacious bronchial secretions, for example, in the later stages of bronchitis, bronchiectasis, and asthma. Sodium or potassium iodide is commonly used in a dose of 0.3 g in aqueous solution every 6 hours. Gastrointestinal irritation, anorexia, and vomiting are frequent side effects. The drug should not be administered longer than is actually necessary to "loosen" the cough. However, in some patients with chronic bronchitis or asthma, iodide may be prescribed more or less continuously if it appears to afford relief.

Iodide sometimes aids in the resolution of the granulomatous lesions of tuberculosis, leprosy, syphilis, and various fungal diseases. This does not depend on the effect of iodide on the responsible microorganism. With the advent of more efficacious drugs for the treatment of these diseases, iodide is rarely employed, except in the treatment of sporotrichosis (*see* Seabury and Dascomb, 1964).

Untoward Reactions.   Occasional individuals show marked sensitivity to iodide or to organic preparations that contain iodine when they are administered intravenously. The onset of an *acute reaction* may occur immediately or several hours after administration. Angioedema is the outstanding symptom, and swelling of the larynx may lead to suffocation. Multiple cutaneous hemorrhages may be present. Also, manifestations of the serum-sickness type of hypersensitivity, such as fever, arthralgia, lymph node enlargement, and eosinophilia, may appear. Thrombotic thrombocytopenic purpura and fatal periarteritis nodosa attributed to hypersensitivity to iodide have also been described.

The severity of symptoms of *chronic intoxication* with iodide (*iodism*) is related to the dose. The symptoms start with an unpleasant brassy taste and burning in the mouth and throat, as well as soreness of the teeth and gums. Increased salivation is noted. Coryza, sneezing, and irritation of the eyes with swelling of the eyelids are commonly observed. Mild iodism simulates a "head cold." The patient often complains of a severe headache that originates in the frontal sinuses. Irritation of the mucous glands of the respiratory tract causes a productive cough. Excess transudation into the bronchial tree may lead to pulmonary edema. In addition, the parotid and submaxillary glands may become enlarged and tender, and the syndrome may be mistaken for mumps parotitis. There also may be inflammation of the pharynx, larynx, and tonsils. Skin lesions are common, and vary in type and intensity. They usually are mildly acneform and distributed in the seborrheic areas. Rarely, severe and sometimes fatal eruptions (*ioderma*) may occur after the prolonged use of iodides. The lesions are bizarre, resemble those caused by bromide, and, as a rule, involute quickly when iodide is withdrawn. Symptoms of gastric irritation are common; and diarrhea, which is sometimes bloody, may occur. Fever is occasionally observed, and anorexia and depression may be present. The mechanisms involved in the production of these derangements remain unknown.

Fortunately, the symptoms of iodism disappear spontaneously within a few days after stopping the administration of iodide. The renal excretion of I⁻ can be increased by procedures that promote Cl⁻ excretion (*e.g.*, osmotic diuresis, chloruretic diuretics, and salt loading). These procedures may be useful when the symptoms of iodism are severe.

Iodide-Induced Goiter and Myxedema. In a small proportion of individuals given large doses of iodide for long periods, as in the treatment of asthma or chronic bronchitis, goiter and hypothyroidism supervene. The thyroid gland shows hyperplasia and is depleted of stores of iodine. Thyroid hormone corrects the hypothyroidism and causes the goiter to subside, and the same result follows the withdrawal of the iodide.

RADIOACTIVE IODINE

Chemical and Physical Properties. While there are several radioactive isotopes of iodine, greatest use has been made of ^{131}I, ^{125}I, and ^{123}I. ^{131}I has been the most widely employed for biological purposes. It has a half-

life of 8 days, and, therefore, over 99% of its radiant energy is expended within 56 days. Its radioactive emissions include both x-rays and β particles. ^{125}I is made by bombarding ^{124}Xe with neutrons; its 60-day half-life and its soft radiation made up of x-rays, conversion electrons, and Auger electrons make it highly suitable for many applications (Myers and Vanderleeden, 1960). It has been suggested, on theoretical grounds, that ^{125}I might impair hormone synthesis with less permanent damage to thyroid-cell nuclei (Greig *et al.*, 1970). The short-lived radionuclide of iodine, ^{123}I, is produced from ^{123}Xe, and it emits x-rays with a half-life of only 13 hours. This permits relatively brief exposure to radiation during thyroid scans.

Effects on the Thyroid Gland. The chemical behavior of the radioactive isotopes of iodine is identical to that of the stable isotope, ^{127}I. ^{131}I is rapidly and efficiently trapped by the thyroid, incorporated into the iodoamino acids, and deposited in the colloid of the follicles, from which it is slowly liberated. Thus, the destructive beta rays originate within the follicle and act almost exclusively upon the parenchymal cells of the thyroid with little or no damage to surrounding tissue. The x-rays pass through the tissue and can be quantified by external detection. The effects of the radiation depend upon the dosage. When small tracer doses of ^{131}I are administered, thyroid function is not disturbed. However, when large amounts of radioactive iodine gain access to the gland, the characteristic cytotoxic actions of ionizing radiation are observed. Pyknosis and necrosis of the follicular cells are followed by disappearance of colloid and fibrosis of the gland. With properly selected doses of ^{131}I, it is possible to destroy the thyroid gland completely without detectable injury to adjacent tissues. After smaller doses, some of the follicles, usually in the periphery of the gland, retain their function.

Preparations. *Sodium Iodide I 131*, U.S.P. (IODOTOPE I-131, ORIODIDE-131, THERIODIDE-131, and preparations marketed under the nonproprietary name), is available as a solution or in capsules containing ^{131}I suitable for either oral or intravenous administration. *Sodium Iodide I 125*, U.S.P., is available in capsules, as a solution for oral administration, and as an injection for intravenous use. The radioactive nuclides are processed in the form of sodium iodide in such a manner that they are essentially carrier free. Other chemical forms of radioactivity are absent. The information on the label includes the activity at a given hour and date, the name and quantity of any added substance (preservative, dye, or stabilizing agent), the intended use, whether oral or intravenous and whether diagnostic or therapeutic, and the recommended dosage. *Sodium Iodide I 123*, U.S.P., is available only as an investigational drug.

Therapeutic Uses. Radioactive iodine finds its widest use in the treatment of *hyperthyroidism* and in the *diagnosis of disorders of thyroid function.* Discussion will be limited to the uses of [131]I.

Hyperthyroidism. Radioactive iodine is highly useful in the treatment of hyperthyroidism, and in many circumstances it is regarded as the therapeutic procedure of choice for this condition.

Dosage and Technic. [131]I is administered orally, either dissolved in half a glass of water or as a capsule. The amount given is so small that it cannot be detected by taste or odor. The effective dose of ^{131}I differs for individual patients. It depends primarily upon the size of the thyroid, the iodine uptake of the gland, and the rate of release of radioactive iodine from the gland subsequent to its deposition in the colloid. To determine these variables insofar as possible, many investigators administer a tracer dose of ^{131}I and calculate the iodine uptake by the gland and the rate of loss therefrom. The weight of the gland is estimated by palpation. From these data, the dose of isotope necessary to provide from 7000 to 10,000 rads per gram of thyroid tissue is determined. Even when dosage is controlled in this manner, it is difficult to predict the response of an individual to a given amount of the isotope. For these reasons, the optimal dose of ^{131}I, expressed in terms of microcuries taken up per gram of thyroid tissue, varies in different laboratories from 80 to 150 μCi. The usual total dose is 4 to 10 mCi. Lower-dosage ^{131}I therapy (80 μCi/g thyroid) has been advocated to reduce the incidence of subsequent hypothyroidism (Cevallos et al., 1974). While the incidence of hypothyroidism in the early years after such therapy is lower, the ultimate number of patients with this complication may be the same. Since long-term surveillance is difficult, more patients with late hypothyroidism may go undetected (Glennon et al., 1972).

Course of Disease. The course of Graves' disease in a patient who has received an optimal dose of ^{131}I is characterized by progressive recovery. It is very unusual for any tenderness to be noted in the thyroid region, and most observers have failed to detect any exacerbation of hyperthyroidism from loss of hormone from the damaged gland. Beginning after a variable interval of a few days to a few weeks, the symptoms of hyperthyroidism gradually abate over a period of 2 to 3 months. If therapy has been inadequate, the necessity for further treatment is apparent within 3 months.

Depending to some extent upon the dosage schedule adopted, one half to two thirds of patients are cured by a single dose, one third to one fifth require two doses, and in the remainder three or more doses are needed before the disorder is controlled. Although it is usual to allow only about 3 months to elapse before concluding that an incomplete response calls for another dose, late effects of the radiation make it desirable to wait much longer. But, again, this further delays the recovery.

Propranolol or antithyroid drugs or both can be used to hasten the control of hyperthyroidism while awaiting the full effects of the radioiodine. However, the antithyroid drugs should be withheld for a few days or a week after the therapeutic dose of [131]I.

Advantages. The advantages of radioactive iodine in the treatment of Graves' disease are many. No death as a direct result of the use of the isotope has been reported, and only by a gross miscalculation of dose could such an event conceivably occur. In the nonpregnant patient, no tissue other than the thyroid is exposed to sufficient ionizing radiation to be detectably altered. (Nevertheless, the continuing concern about potential effects of radiation on germ cells prompts a choice for surgery in younger patients who are acceptable operative risks.) The patient is spared the risks and discomfort of surgery. The incidence of progressive exophthalmos appears to be no different than after surgical treatment. Finally, the cost is low, hospitalization usually is not required, and the patient can indulge in his customary activities during the entire procedure.

Disadvantages. The chief disadvantage of the use of radioactive iodine is the high incidence of delayed hypothyroidism that is induced. Even when elaborate procedures are employed to estimate iodine uptake and gland size, a certain percentage of patients will be overtreated. A distressing feature of this complication is its rising prevalence with the passage of time; the longer the interval after treatment, the higher the incidence. Several analyses of groups of patients treated 10 or more years previously suggest that the eventual rate may exceed 50% (Dunn and Chapman, 1964; Green and Wilson, 1964). However, it now appears that the incidence of hypothyroidism also increases progressively after subtotal thyroidectomy, and such failure of glandular function is suspected to be part of the natural progression of Graves' disease, no matter what the therapy.

Although it is often said that hypothyroidism is not a serious complication because it can so easily be treated with thyroid hormone, its onset may be quite insidious and overlooked for some time. Also, once diagnosed it is difficult to ensure that patients who need the hormone actually take it. Hypothyroidism is obviously a serious complication deserving of painstaking care to make certain that optimal replacement therapy is provided.

Another disadvantage is the long period of time that is sometimes required before the hyperthyroidism is controlled. When a single dose is effective, the response is most satisfactory; however, when multiple doses are needed, it may be many months or a year or more before the patient is well.

Indications. The clearest indication for this form of treatment is hyperthyroidism in older patients and in those with heart disease. Here hyperthyroidism is such a serious disorder that myxedema, as a complication, is of lesser consequence. Furthermore, hypothyroidism is not a common sequela following treatment with radioiodine for toxic nodular goiter, the usual cause of hyperthyroidism in the older age group. Radioiodine is also the best form of treatment when hyperthyroidism has persisted or recurred after subtotal thyroidectomy and when prolonged treatment with antithyroid drugs has not led to remission. Other aspects of this problem have been discussed above.

Contraindications. If for no other reason, the risk of hypothyroidism makes radioiodine an unsuitable treatment for hyperthyroidism in childhood. The risk of causing neoplastic changes in the gland has been constantly under consideration since radioiodine was first introduced, and only small numbers of children have been treated in this way. Indeed, many clinics have declined to treat younger patients for fear of causing cancer and have reserved radioiodine for patients over some arbitrary age, such as 25 to 30 years. Since there is now vast experience with ^{131}I, these age limits are lower than they were in the past. There is no evidence that radioiodine therapy has caused thyroid or other forms of cancer in adults. The use of radioiodine during pregnancy is contraindicated; after the first trimester the fetal thyroid would concentrate the isotope and thus suffer damage, but even during the first trimester radioiodine is best avoided because there may be adverse effects of radiation on fetal tissues.

Hyperthyroidism with Nodular Goiter. It is thought that the risk of inducing hypothyroidism is less in nodular goiter than in Graves' disease, perhaps because of the natural progression of the latter.

Metastatic Thyroid Cancer. Most thyroid carcinomas accumulate very little iodine. However, follicular carcinomas, which comprise 25% of thyroid malignancies, often do so, although they rarely synthesize sufficient hormone to cause thyrotoxicosis. If metastases accumulate iodine, therapy with large doses of ^{131}I may prolong life, particularly in younger patients (Leeper, 1973). In an attempt to stimulate uptake, thyrotropin has been given or secretion of endogenous thyrotropin has been evoked by inducing hypothyroidism by removal or radiation of the thyroid, or by prolonged treatment with antithyroid drugs. The increased uptake thus achieved is usually not large and may be negligible. Moreover, it has been noted by a number of observers that growth of the metastases may be stimulated by these maneuvers, and they have therefore questioned their advisability (Maloof *et al.*, 1956; Crile, 1957; Thomas, 1958).

Papillary carcinoma is the most common type of thyroid cancer and may be partially dependent on thyrotropin. Metastatic lesions occasionally regress when thyrotropin secretion is suppressed by administration of thyroid hormone.

Diagnostic Uses. Tracer studies with radioiodine have found wide application in studies of disorders of the thyroid gland. Measurement of the thyroidal accumulation of a tracer dose is helpful in the diagnosis of hyperthyroidism, hypothyroidism, and goiter, and the response of the thyroid to thyrotropin or to suppression by thyroid hormone can be evaluated in this way. Following the administration of a tracer dose, the pattern of localization in the thyroid gland can be depicted by special scanning apparatus, and this technic is sometimes useful in finding ectopic thyroid tissue and occasionally metastatic thyroid tumors.

Anbar, M.; Guttmann, S.; and Lewitus, Z. The mode of action of perchlorate ions on the iodine uptake of the thyroid gland. *Int. J. Appl. Radiat. Isot.,* **1960,** *7,* 87–96.

Aranow, H., and Day, R. M. Management of thyrotoxicosis in patients with ophthalmopathy: antithyroid regimen determined primarily by ocular manifestations. *J. Clin. Endocrinol. Metab.,* **1965,** *25,* 1–10.

Arnott, D. G., and Doniach, J. The effect of compounds allied to resorcinol upon the uptake of radioactive iodine (^{131}I) by the thyroid of the rat. *Biochem. J.,* **1952,** *50,* 473–479.

Arstica, A.; Krusius, F.-E.; and Peltola, P. Studies on transfer of thio-oxazolidone-type goitrogens into cow's milk in goiter endemic districts of Finland and in experimental conditions. *Acta Endocrinol. (Kbh.),* **1969,** *60,* 712–718.

Astwood, E. B. Chemotherapy of hyperthyroidism. *Harvey Lect.,* **1945,** *40,* 195–235.

Astwood, E. B.; Cassidy, C. E.; and Aurbach, G. D. Treatment of goiter and thyroid nodules with thyroid. *J.A.M.A.,* **1960,** *174,* 459–464.

Braverman, L. E.; Ingbar, S. H.; and Sterling, K. Conversion of thyroxine (T4) to triiodothyronine (T3) in athyreotic human subjects. *J. Clin. Invest.,* **1970,** *49,* 855–864.

Buccino, R. A.; Spann, J. F., Jr.; Pool, P. E.; Sonnenblick, E. B.; and Braunwald, E. Influence of thyroid state on the intrinsic contractile properties and energy stores of the myocardium. *J. Clin. Invest.,* **1967,** *46,* 1669–1682.

Cassidy, C. E., and VanderLaan, W. P. Thyroid-suppression test in the prognosis of hyperthyroidism treated by antithyroid drugs. *N. Engl. J. Med.,* **1960,** *262,* 1228–1229.

Cevallos, J. L.; Hagen, G. A.; Maloof, F.; and Chapman, E. M. Low-dosage ^{131}I therapy of thyrotoxicosis (diffuse goiters). A five-year follow-up study. *N. Engl. J. Med.,* **1974,** *290,* 141–143.

Chesney, A. M.; Clawson, T. A.; and Webster, B. Endemic goitre in rabbits. I. Incidence and characteristics. *Bull. Johns Hopkins Hosp.,* **1928,** *43,* 261–277.

Chopra, I. J. A radioimmunoassay for measurement of thyroxine in unextracted serum. *J. Clin. Endocrinol. Metab.,* **1972,** *34,* 938–947.

Cody, V., and Duax, W. L. Distal conformation of the thyroid hormone 3,5,3'-triiodo-L-thyronine. *Science,* **1973,** *181,* 757–758.

Crile, G., Jr. The endocrine dependency of certain thyroid cancers and the danger that hypothyroidism may stimulate their growth. *Cancer,* **1957,** *10,* 1119–1137.

Cushing, H. *The Pituitary Body and Its Disorders.* J. B. Lippincott Co., Philadelphia, **1912.**

Das, G., and Krieger, M. Treatment of thyrotoxic storm with intravenous administration of propranolol. *Ann. Intern. Med.,* **1969,** *70,* 985–988.

Davidson, B.; Soodak, M.; Neary, J. T.; Strout, H. V.; Kieffer, J. D.; Mover, H.; and Maloof, F. The irreversible inactivation of thyroid peroxidase by methylmercaptoimidazole, thiouracil, and propylthiouracil *in vitro* and its relationship to *in vivo* findings. *Endocrinology,* **1978,** *103,* 871–882.

DeGroot, L. J. Thyroid and the heart. *Mayo Clin. Proc.,* **1972,** *47,* 864–871.

Delange, F., and Ermans, A. M. Role of a dietary goitrogen in the etiology of endemic goiter on Idjwi Island. *Am. J. Clin. Nutr.,* **1971,** *24,* 1354–1360.

Doniach, D.; Hudson, R. V.; Trotter, W. R.; and Waddams, A. Effects of thyroxine, triiodothyronine and TRIAC on metabolic rate, blood lipids and thyroid size and function in subjects with nontoxic goitre. *Clin. Sci.,* **1958,** *17,* 519–529.

Dunn, J. T. The amino acid neighbors of thyroxine in thyroglobulin. *J. Biol. Chem.,* **1970,** *245,* 5954–5961.

Dunn, J. T., and Chapman, E. M. Rising incidence of hypothyroidism after radioactive-iodine therapy in thyrotoxicosis. *N. Engl. J. Med.,* **1964,** *271,* 1037–1042.

Feek, C. M.; Stewart, J.; Sawers, A.; Irvine, W. J.; Beckett, J.; Ratcliffe, W. A.; and Toft, A. D. Combination of potassium iodide and propranolol in preparation of patients with Graves' disease for thyroid surgery. *N. Engl. J. Med.,* **1980,** *302,* 883–885.

Fisher, D. A. Screening for congenital hypothyroidism. *Hosp. Pract.,* **1977,** *12,* 73–78.

———. Pediatric aspects. In, *The Thyroid,* 4th ed. (Werner, S. G., and Ingbar, S. H., eds.) Harper & Row, Pub., Inc., Hagerstown, Md., **1978,** pp. 947–764.

Geffner, D. L.; Azukizawa, M.; and Hershman, J. M. Propylthiouracil blocks extrathyroidal conversion of thyroxine to triiodothyronine and augments thyrotropin secretion in man. *J. Clin. Invest.,* **1975,** *55,* 224–229.

Gilman, A. G., and Rall, T. W. Factors influencing adenosine 3′,5′-phosphate accumulation in bovine thyroid slices. *J. Biol. Chem.,* **1968,** *243,* 5867–5871.

Glennon, J. A.; Gordon, E. S.; and Sawin, C. T. Hypothyroidism after low-dose ^{131}I treatment of hyperthyroidism. *Ann. Intern. Med.,* **1972,** *76,* 721–723.

Gley, E. Sur les effets de l'extirpation du corps thyroide. *C. R. Soc. Biol.* (*Paris*), **1891,** *43,* 551–554.

Green, M., and Wilson, G. M. Thyrotoxicosis treated by surgery or iodine-131, with special reference to development of hypothyroidism. *Br. Med. J.,* **1964,** *1,* 1005–1010.

Greer, M. A.; Grimm, Y.; and Studer, H. Qualitative changes in the secretion of thyroid hormones induced by iodine deficiency. *Endocrinology,* **1968,** *83,* 1193–1198.

Greer, M. A.; Kammer, H.; and Bouma, D. J. Short-term antithyroid drug therapy for the thyrotoxicosis of Graves's disease. *N. Engl. J. Med.,* **1977,** *297,* 1973–1976.

Greig, W. R.; Smith, J. F. B.; and Orr, J. S. Comparative survivals of rat thyroid cells *in vivo* after ^{131}I, ^{125}I, and X irradiations. *Br. J. Radiol.,* **1970,** *43,* 542–548.

Gross, J., and Pitt-Rivers, R. The identification of 3·5:3′ L-triiodothyronine in human plasma. *Lancet,* **1952,** *1,* 439–441.

———. 3:5:3′-Triiodothyronine. 1. Isolation from thyroid gland and synthesis. *Biochem. J.,* **1953a,** *53,* 645–652. 2. Physiological activity. *Ibid.,* **1953b,** *53,* 652–657.

Harington, C. R. Chemistry of thyroxine: isolation of thyroxine from thyroid gland. *Biochem. J.,* **1926,** *20,* 293–299.

———. Biochemical basis of thyroid function. *Lancet,* **1935,** *1,* 1199–1204, 1261–1266.

Harington, C. R., and Barger, G. Thyroxine. III. Constitution and synthesis of thyroxine. *Biochem. J.,* **1927,** *21,* 169–183.

Hercus, C. E., and Purves, H. D. Studies on endemic and experimental goitre. *J. Hyg.* (*Camb.*), **1936,** *36,* 182–203.

Higgins, H. P.; Elkan, I.; Diosy, A.; Bayley, T. A.; and Buckley, G. C. Prognostic value of high 10-minute ^{131}I uptake in non-toxic goiters. *Can. Med. Assoc. J.,* **1964,** *91,* 689–693.

Ingbar, S. H. Autoregulation of the thyroid response to iodide excess and depletion. *Mayo Clin. Proc.,* **1972,** *47,* 814–823.

Ismail-Beigi, F., and Edelman, I. S. Mechanism of the calorigenic action of thyroid hormone. *J. Gen. Physiol.,* **1971,** *57,* 710–722.

Jorgensen, E. C. Stereochemistry of thyroxine and analogues. *Mayo Clin. Proc.,* **1964,** *39,* 560–568.

Kendall, E. C. The isolation in crystalline form of the compound containing iodine which occurs in the thyroid: its chemical nature and physiological activity. *Trans. Assoc. Am. Physicians,* **1915,** *30,* 420–449.

Lamas, L.; Dorris, M. L.; and Taurog, A. Evidence for a catalytic role for thyroid peroxidase in the conversion of diiodotyrosine to thyroxine. *Endocrinology,* **1972,** *90,* 1417–1426.

Leeper, R. D. The effect of ^{131}I therapy on survival of patients with metastatic papillary or follicular thyroid carcinoma. *J. Clin. Endocrinol. Metab.,* **1973,** *36,* 1143–1152.

Levey, G. S., and Epstein, S. E. Myocardial adenyl cyclase: activation by thyroid hormones and evidence for two adenyl cyclase systems. *J. Clin. Invest.,* **1969,** *48,* 1663–1669.

London, W. T.; Vought, R. L.; and Brown, F. A. Bread—a dietary source of large quantities of iodine. *N. Engl. J. Med.,* **1965,** *273,* 381.

Mackenzie, J. B.; Mackenzie, C. G.; and McCollum, E. V. Effect of sulfanilylguanidine on thyroid of rat. *Science,* **1941,** *94,* 518–519.

Magnus-Levy, A. Über den respiratorischen Gaswechsel unter den Einfluss der Thyroidea sowie unter verschiedenen pathologischen Zustanden. *Berl. Klin. Wochenschr.,* **1895,** *32,* 650–652.

Malbon, C. C.; Moreno, F. J.; Cabelli, R. J.; and Fain, J. N. Fat cell adenylate cyclase and β-adrenergic receptors in altered thyroid states. *J. Biol. Chem.,* **1978,** *253,* 671–677.

Maloof, F.; Vickery, A. L.; and Rapp, B. An evaluation of various factors influencing the treatment of metastatic thyroid carcinoma with ^{131}I. *J. Clin. Endocrinol. Metab.,* **1956,** *16,* 1–27.

Marine, D., and Kimball, O. P. The prevention of simple goiter in man: a survey of the incidence and types of thyroid enlargements in the schoolgirls of Akron, Ohio, from the 5th to the 12th grades, inclusive; the plan of prevention proposed. *J. Lab. Clin. Med.,* **1917,** *3,* 40–48.

Menahan, L. A., and Wieland, O. The role of thyroid function in the metabolism of perfused rat liver with particular reference to gluconeogenesis. *Eur. J. Biochem.,* **1969,** *10,* 188–194.

Morris, D. R., and Hager, L. P. Mechanism of the inhibition of enzymatic halogenation by the antithyroid agents. *J. Biol. Chem.,* **1966,** *241,* 3582–3589.

Murray, G. R. Note on the treatment of myxedema by hypodermic injection of an extract of the thyroid gland of a sheep. *Br. Med. J.,* **1891,** *2,* 796–797.

Myers, W. G., and Vanderleeden, J. C. Radioiodine-125. *J. Nucl. Med.,* **1960,** *1,* 149–164.

Nakagawa, S., and Ruegamer, W. R. Properties of a rat tissue iodothyronine deiodinase and its natural inhibitor. *Biochemistry,* **1967,** *6,* 1249–1261.

Nilsson, S. F., and Peterson, P. A. Evidence for multiple thyroxine-binding sites in human prealbumin. *J. Biol. Chem.,* **1971,** *246,* 6098–6105.

Oppenheimer, J. H. Thyroid hormones in liver. *Mayo Clin. Proc.,* **1972,** *47,* 854–863.

Ord, W. M. On myxoedema, a term proposed to be applied to an essential condition in the "cretinoid" affection occasionally observed in middle-aged women. *Med. Chir. Trans.* (*Lond.*), **1878,** *61,* 57–78.

Parry, C. H. *Collections from the Unpublished Medical Writings of Dr. C. H. Parry.* Underwood, London, **1895.**

Pisarev, M. A.; DeGroot, L. J.; and Hati, R. KI and imidazole inhibition of TSH and c-AMP induced thyroidal iodine secretion. *Endocrinology,* **1971,** *88,* 1217–1221.

Pisarev, M. A.; DeGroot, L. J.; and Wieber, J. F. Cyclic-AMP production of goiter. *Endocrinology,* **1970,** *87,* 339–342.

Pittman, C. S.; Buck, M. W.; and Chambers, J. B., Jr. Urinary metabolites of ^{14}C-labeled thyroxine in man. *J. Clin. Invest.,* **1972,** *51,* 1759–1766.

Pittman, J. A.; Beschi, R. J.; Block, P., Jr.; and Lindsay,

R. H. Thyromimetic activity of 3,5,3′,5′-tetramethyl-thyronine. *Endocrinology,* **1973,** *93,* 201–204.

Psychoyos, S.; Ma, D. S.; Czernik, A. J.; Bowers, H. S.; Atkins, C. D.; Malicki, C. A.; and Cash, W. D. Thyromimetic activity of methylene-bridged thyroid hormone analogs. *Endocrinology,* **1973,** *92,* 243–250.

Rappoport, B.; West, M. N.; and Ingbar, S. H. Inhibitory effect of dietary iodine on the thyroid adenylate cyclase response to thyrotropin in the hypophysectomized rat. *J. Clin. Invest.,* **1975,** *56,* 516–519.

Richter, C. P., and Clisby, K. H. Toxic effects of bitter-tasting phenylthiocarbamide. *Arch. Pathol.,* **1942,** *33,* 46–57.

Roche, J.; Lissitzky, S.; and Michel, R. Sur la triiodothyronine, produit intermédiare de la transformation de la diiodothyronine en thyroxine. *C. R. Acad. Sci.* [*D*] (*Paris*), **1952a,** *234,* 997–998.

———. Sur la présence de triiodothyronine dans la thyroglobuline. *Ibid.,* **1952b,** *234,* 1228–1230.

Roche, J.; Michel, R.; Michel, O.; and Lissitzky, S. Sur la déshalogénation enzymatique des iodotyrosine par la corps thyroide et sur son rôle physiologique. *Biochim. Biophys. Acta,* **1952c,** *9,* 161–169.

Rosenberg, I. N. The antithyroid activity of some compounds that inhibit peroxidase. *Science,* **1952,** *116,* 503–505.

Saberi, M.; Sterling, F. H.; and Utiger, R. D. Reduction in extrathyroidal triiodothyronine production by propylthiouracil in man. *J. Clin. Invest.,* **1975,** *55,* 218–223.

Schou, M.; Amdisen, A.; Jensen, S. E.; and Olsen, T. Occurrence of goitre during lithium treatment. *Br. Med. J.,* **1968,** *3,* 710–713.

Seabury, J. H., and Dascomb, H. E. Results of the treatment of systemic mycoses. *J.A.M.A.,* **1964,** *188,* 509–513.

Shanks, R. G.; Hadden, D. R.; Lowe, D. C.; McDevitt, D. G.; and Montgomery, D. A. D. Controlled trial of propranolol in thyrotoxicosis. *Lancet,* **1969,** *1,* 993–994.

Sherwin, J. R., and Tong, W. Thyroidal autoregulation. Iodide-induced suppression of thyrotropin-stimulated cyclic AMP production and iodinating activity in thyroid cells. *Biochim. Biophys. Acta,* **1975,** *404,* 30–39.

Simmonds, M. Ueber Hypophysisschwund mit todlichem Ausang. *Dtsch. Med. Wochenschr.,* **1914,** *40,* 322–323.

Solomon, D. H.; Beck, J. C.; VanderLaan, W. P.; and Astwood, E. B. Prognosis of hyperthyroidism treated by antithyroid drugs. *J.A.M.A.,* **1953,** *152,* 201–205.

Starr, P., and Goodwin, W. Use of triiodothyronine for reduction of goiter and detection of thyroid cancer. *Metabolism,* **1958,** *7,* 287–292.

Sterling, K.; Brenner, M. A.; and Newman, E. S. Conversion of thyroxine to triiodothyronine in normal human subjects. *Science,* **1970,** *169,* 1099–1100.

Sterling, K.; Hamada, S.; Takemura, Y.; Brenner, M. A.; Newman, E. S.; and Inada, M. Preparation and properties of thyroxine-binding alpha globulin (TBG). *J. Clin. Invest.,* **1971,** *50,* 1758–1771.

Taurog, A. The mechanism of action of thioureylene antithyroid drugs. *Endocrinology,* **1976,** *98,* 1031–1046.

Taurog, A.; Lothrop, M. L.; and Estabrook, R. W. Improvements in the isolation procedure for thyroid peroxidase: nature of the heme prosthetic group. *Arch. Biochem. Biophys.,* **1970,** *139,* 221–229.

Temple, R.; Berman, M.; Carlson, H. E.; Robbins, J.; and Wolff, J. The use of lithium in Graves' disease. *Mayo Clin. Proc.,* **1972,** *47,* 872–878.

Thilly, C. H.; Delange, F.; Goldstein-Golaire, J.; and Ermans, A. M. Endemic goiter prevention of iodized oil: a reassessment. *J. Clin. Endocrinol. Metab.,* **1973,** *36,* 1196–1204.

Thomas, C. C., Jr. The use of L-triiodothyronine as a pituitary depressant in the management of thyroid cancer. *Surg. Gynecol. Obstet.,* **1958,** *106,* 137–144.

VanderLaan, W. P. The biological significance of the iodide-concentrating mechanism of the thyroid gland. *Brookhaven Symp. Biol.,* **1955,** *7,* 30–37.

Van Middlesworth, L. Thyroxine requirement and the excretion of thyroxine metabolites. In, *Clinical Endocrinology I.* (Astwood, E. B., ed.) Grune & Stratton, Inc., New York, **1960,** pp. 103–111.

Van Sande, J.; Grenier, G.; Willems, C.; and Dumont, J. E. Inhibition by iodide of the activation of the thyroid cyclic 3′,5′-AMP system. *Endocrinology,* **1975,** *96,* 781–786.

Wartofsky, L. Low remission after therapy for Graves' disease: possible relation of dietary iodine with antithyroid therapy results. *J.A.M.A.,* **1973,** *226,* 1083–1088.

Wolff, J., and Chaikoff, I. L. Plasma inorganic iodide as a homeostatic regulator of thyroid function. *J. Biol. Chem.,* **1948,** *174,* 555–564.

Wolff, J., and Maurey, J. R. Thyroidal iodide transport. IV. The role of ion size. *Biochim. Biophys. Acta,* **1963,** *69,* 58–67.

Wollman, S. H.; Spicer, S. S.; and Burstone, M. S. Localization of esterase and acid phosphatase in granules and colloid droplets in rat thyroid epithelium. *J. Cell Biol.,* **1964,** *21,* 191–201.

Wu, S. Y.; Chopra, I. J.; Nakamura, Y.; Solomon, D. H.; and Bennett, L. R. A radioimmunoassay for measurement of 3,3′-L-diiodothyronine (T$_2$). *J. Clin. Endocrinol. Metab.,* **1976,** *43,* 682–685.

Wyngaarden, J. B.; Wright, B. M.; and Ways, P. The effect of certain anions upon the accumulation and retention of iodide by the thyroid gland. *Endocrinology,* **1952,** *50,* 537–549.

Wynn, J., and Gibbs, R. Thyroxine degradation. II. Products of thyroxine degradation by rat liver microsomes. *J. Biol. Chem.,* **1962,** *237,* 3499–3505.

Zor, U.; Kaneko, T.; Lowe, I. P.; Bloom, G.; and Field, J. B. Effect of thyroid-stimulating hormone and prostaglandins on thyroid adenyl cyclase activation and cyclic adenosine 3′,5′-monophosphate. *J. Biol. Chem.,* **1969,** *244,* 5189–5195.

Monographs and Reviews

Burman, K. D. Recent developments in thyroid hormone metabolism: interpretation and significance of measurements of reverse T$_3$, 3,3′T$_2$, and thyroglobulin. *Metabolism,* **1978,** *27,* 615–630.

DeGroot, L. J., and Niepomniszcze, H. Biosynthesis of thyroid hormone: basic and clinical aspects. *Metabolism,* **1977,** *26,* 665–718. (248 references.)

Dumont, J. E.; Boeynaems, J. M.; Decoster, C.; Erneux, C.; Lamy, F.; Lecocq, R.; Mockel, J.; Unger, J.; and Van Sande, J. Biochemical mechanisms in the control of thyroid function and growth. *Adv. Cyclic Nucleotide Res.,* **1978,** *9,* 723–734.

Fain, J. N. Biochemical aspects of drug and hormone action on adipose tissue. *Pharmacol. Rev.,* **1973,** *25,* 67–118.

Feldman, J. M. The practical use of thyroid function tests. *Am. Family Physician,* **1977,** *16,* 159–165.

Hamburgh, M. The role of thyroid and growth hormones in neurogenesis. *Curr. Top. Dev. Biol.,* **1969,** *4,* 109–148.

Marchant, B.; Lees, J. F. H.; and Alexander, W. D. Antithyroid drugs. *Pharmacol. Ther.* [*B*], **1978,** *3,* 305–348.

Means, J. H.; DeGroot, L. J.; and Stanbury, J. B. *The Thyroid and Its Diseases,* 3rd ed. McGraw-Hill Book Co., New York, **1963.**

Merimee, T. J. Thyroid function tests: what they do and do not measure. *Postgrad. Med.,* **1978,** *63,* 113–117.

Pittman, C. S., and Pittman, J. A. Relation of chemical structure to the action and metabolism of thyroactive substances. In, *Thyroid,* Vol. 3. Sect. 7, *Endocrinology. Handbook of Physiology.* (Greer, M. A., and Solomon, D. H., eds.) American Physiological Society, Washington, D. C., **1974,** pp. 233–253. (134 references.)

Rall, J. E.; Robbins, J.; and Lewallen, C. G. The thyroid. In, *The Hormones,* Vol. 5. (Pincus, G.; Thimann, K. V.; and Astwood, E. B.; eds.) Academic Press, Inc., New York, **1964,** pp. 159–439.

Schimmel, M., and Utiger, R. D. Thyroidal and peripheral production of thyroid hormones. *Ann. Intern. Med.,* **1977,** *87,* 760–768.

Schwartz, H. L., and Oppenheimer, J. H. Physiologic and biochemical actions of thyroid hormone. *Pharmacol. Ther.* [B], **1978,** *3,* 349–376.

Sterling, K. Thyroid hormone action at the cell level. *N. Engl. J. Med.,* **1979,** *300,* 117–123, 173–177.

Taurog, A. Thyroid peroxidase and thyroxine biosynthesis. *Recent Prog. Horm. Res.,* **1970,** *26,* 189–241.

Utiger, R. D. Serum triiodothyronine in man. *Annu. Rev. Med.,* **1974,** *25,* 289–302.

VanderLaan, W. P., and Storrie, V. M. A survey of the factors controlling thyroid function, with especial reference to newer views on antithyroid substances. *Pharmacol. Rev.,* **1955,** *7,* 301–334.

VanEtten, C. H. Goitrogens. In, *Toxic Constituents of Plant Foodstuffs.* (Liener, I. E., ed.) Academic Press, Inc., New York, **1969,** pp. 103–142.

Volpe, R. The pathogenesis of Graves' disease: an overview. *Clin. Endocrinol. Metab.,* **1978,** *7,* 3–29.

Wolff, J. Transport of iodide and other anions in the thyroid gland. *Physiol. Rev.,* **1964,** *44,* 45–90.

Ferid Murad and Robert C. Haynes, Jr.

The controlled and cyclic formation of estrogens and progesterone is unique to the ovary. These hormones play a vital role in preparing the female reproductive tract for the reception of sperm and implantation of a fertilized ovum. However, it is recognized and appreciated that many attributes of the female habitus are also influenced by these agents. Current knowledge of the synthesis and action of the ovarian hormones has permitted rational therapeutic intervention in certain diseases. Much more clinical use, however, has been made of agents that can mimic the effects of these hormones and that act as contraceptives.

History. It has long been known that removal of the ovaries results in uterine atrophy and a loss of sexual functions. The hormonal nature of the ovarian control of the female reproductive system was established in 1900 by Knauer when he found that ovarian transplants prevented the symptoms of gonadectomy. This observation was extended by Halban (1900), who showed that, if the glands were transplanted even in immature animals, normal sexual development and function were assured. In 1923, Allen and Doisy devised a simple, quantitative bioassay method for ovarian extracts based upon changes produced in the vaginal smear of the rat. Loewe (1925) first reported a female sex hormone in the blood of various species and, shortly thereafter, Frank and associates (1925) detected an active sex principle in the blood of sows in estrus. Of even greater significance was the discovery by Loewe and Lange (1926) of a female sex hormone in the urine of menstruating women and the observation that the concentration of the hormone in the urine varied with the phase of the menstrual cycle. The excretion of large amounts of estrogen in the urine during pregnancy was also reported (Zondek, 1928). This finding was a boon to the chemists, who soon isolated an active substance in crystalline form (Butenandt, 1929; Doisy *et al.*, 1929, 1930). A few years later its chemical structure was elucidated.

The results of early investigations indicated that the ovary secretes two substances. Beard (1897) had postulated that the corpus luteum serves a necessary function during pregnancy, and supporting evidence was offered by Fraenkel (1903), who showed that destruction of the corpora lutea in pregnant rabbits causes abortion. The contributions of Corner and Allen (1929) firmly established the hormonal function of the corpus luteum. These investigators showed that the abortion following extirpation of the corpora lutea in pregnant rabbits can be prevented by the injection of luteal extracts.

ESTROGENS

Biosynthesis and Chemistry. The ovary is capable of converting acetate to cholesterol and subsequently to other steroids, as summarized in Figure 61–1. The formation of estrogens by ovarian follicles is regulated by follicle-stimulating hormone (FSH). The effects of this gonadotropin are mediated through the formation and subsequent action of cyclic adenosine 3′,5′-monophosphate (cyclic AMP) (Fontaine *et al.*, 1971). However, the precise mechanism of the action of cyclic AMP to stimulate the synthesis of estrogen, as well as other steroids, is unknown. In men, the testis can also produce and secrete small amounts of estradiol and estrone (*see* Chapter 62).

The estrogens are ultimately formed from either androstenedione or testosterone as immediate precursors. The reaction of central importance is the aromatization of ring A. The first step in this reaction involves hydroxylation of C 19, the angular methyl group residing on C 10 of the precursor. Then the newly formed hydroxymethyl group is lost from the nucleus, and ring A is aromatized to yield a phenolic hydroxyl at C 3 (*see* Ryan, 1959). In certain pathological conditions, this reaction appears to be defective and the androgenic precursor escapes into the circulation. Some cases of hirsutism and virilism are thought to be caused by this defect, and at least one of the features of the Stein-Leventhal syndrome associated with large polycystic ovaries is attributable to the same biosynthetic difficulty (Mahesh and Greenblatt, 1964).

Of the three main estrogens of human beings, *estradiol-17β* is the most potent and the major secretory product of the ovary; it is

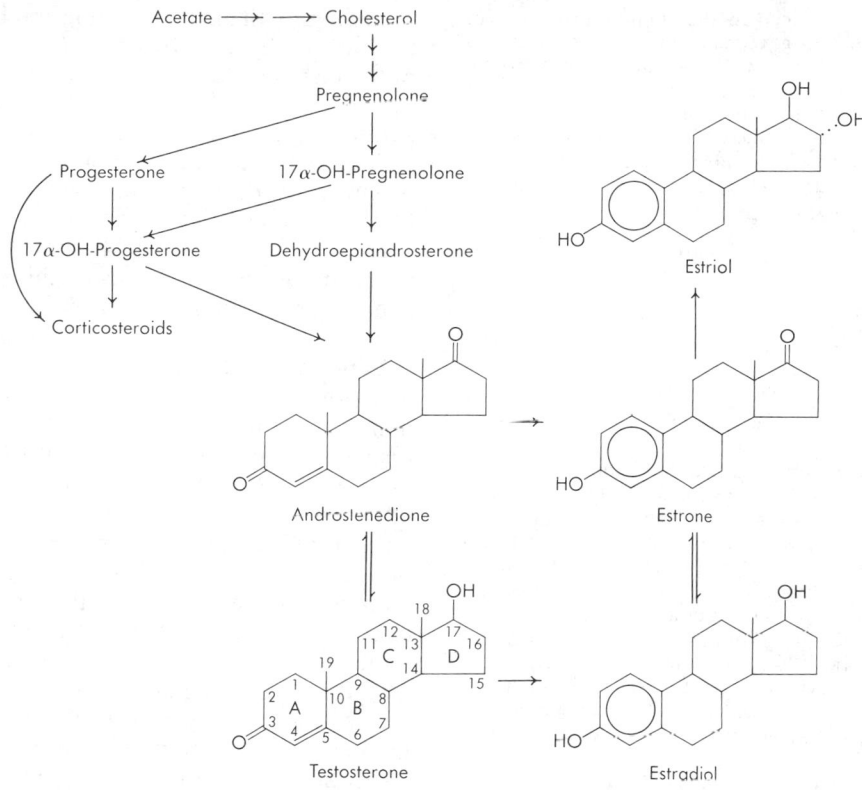

Figure 61-1. *The biosynthetic pathway for the estrogens.* Additional details and structures are shown in Figure 63-3 (page 1472).

readily oxidized to *estrone,* which in turn can be hydrated to *estriol.* These transformations take place mainly in the liver, where there is free interconversion between estrone and estradiol (Ryan and Engel, 1953). All three estrogens are excreted in the urine as glucuronides and sulfates, along with a host of related, minor products in water-soluble complexes. During pregnancy, estrogens are synthesized in large quantities by the placenta and apparently by the same enzymatic reactions as occur in the ovary. However, there are complex interactions with the fetus, and the fetal adrenal cortex is required for some synthetic steps that are deficient in the placenta (*see* Kellie, 1971). Human urine of pregnancy is thus an abundant source of natural estrogens. Animals of the genus *Equus,* including the horse, are remarkable estrogen factories. The pregnant mare excretes over 100 mg daily, a record exceeded only by the stallion, who, despite clear manifestations of virility, excretes into his environment more estrogen than any other living creature.

The formation of estrogens is not limited to the gonads, placenta, and adrenal since peripheral tissues such as liver, fat, skeletal muscle, and hair follicles can form significant quantities of estrogens from steroid precursors. These tissues can aromatize the A ring of androstenedione and testosterone to form estrogens, particularly estrone (*see* Marcus and Korenman, 1976). This reaction is thought to provide a major source of estrogen in males and postmenopausal females, and its contribution to the pool of estrogens is regulated by the availability of the androgenic precursors.

Estrogenic activity is a property shared by a great number of steroidal and nonsteroidal compounds. The wide distribution of estrogenic activity among natural compounds has sometimes proven to be of economic importance. Sterility in sheep noted in Australia when flocks were allowed to graze on pastures populated by the so-called subterranean clover was eventually traced to the abundant quantity of the weak estrogen *genistein,* an isoflavone contained in this plant (Curnow, 1954). Many nonsteroidal materials with estrogenic activity have since been described in a variety of plants.

Among the first nonsteroidal estrogens to be encountered and still the most potent is *diethylstilbestrol* (Dodds *et al.,* 1938), the *trans* configuration of which is as follows:

Diethylstilbestrol

In this active *trans* configuration, diethylstilbestrol can be seen to be related structurally to the steroidal compounds. Its estrogenic potency in animals varies somewhat with the assay used, but in most tests it is fully as active as estradiol. In contrast to the natural estrogens, it is highly active when given by mouth and the duration of action of a single dose is longer, properties in keeping with its slower rate of degradation in the body. The introduction of a cheap, plentiful, orally active estrogen at a time when the natural products were scarce and expensive was a milestone in the development of effective endocrine therapy.

Certain chemical alterations of the natural estrogens render them effective by mouth, largely through protection from inactivation by the liver. One of the most highly potent estrogens known, *ethinyl estradiol,* is an example of this type wherein the elements of acetylene are attached at C 17. As little as 20 μg daily serves as replacement therapy in the menopause, and 50 μg may be sufficient to cause withdrawal bleeding. This estrogen and some of its derivatives are widely used and are also incorporated with progesterone-like compounds for regulation of the menstrual cycle and for the control of fertility.

Physiological and Pharmacological Actions. The estrogens are largely responsible for the changes that take place at puberty in girls, and they go a long way toward accounting for the tangible and intangible attributes of femininity. By a direct action, they cause growth and development of the vagina, uterus, and Fallopian tubes. They cause enlargement of the breasts through promotion of ductal growth, stromal development, and the accretion of fat, effects in which pituitary hormones also play a part; they also contribute in a poorly understood manner to molding the body contours, shaping the skeleton, and bringing about changes in the epiphyses of the long bones that condition the puberal

spurt in growth and its culmination by fusion of the epiphyses. Growth of axillary and pubic hair and regional pigmentation of the skin of the nipples and areolae and of the genital region are also effects of estrogen.

Psychological and emotional effects, so prominently displayed in lower animals in the form of sexual behavior, estrus, or heat, are partially obscured in human beings by other influences, but presumably estrogen conditions feminine behavior in important ways.

Superimposed upon the feminizing influences of the estrogens is the cyclical component in the intensity of their action, which is responsible for many features of the normal menstrual cycle. During the follicular phase of the cycle, there is proliferation of the vaginal and uterine mucosae, increased secretion of the glands of the uterine cervix, and perhaps noticeable fullness of the breasts. Decline in estrogenic activity at the end of the cycle can bring about menstruation and its attendant phenomena. In the mature cycle with ovulation, progesterone further modifies the genital tract and mammary gland in the direction of pregnancy, and it is the cessation of secretion of progesterone that is the more forceful determinant of menstruation (Erickson, 1978; Naftolin and Tolis, 1978).

Androgens from the Ovary. A question long of interest is whether the androgens secreted by the normal ovary are physiologically important. Measurements of steroid synthesis by ovarian slices *in vitro* and fractionation of steroids contained in venous ovarian blood indicate that both testosterone and androstenedione, precursors of estrogens, are normal ovarian secretions. The daily production rates of testosterone and androstenedione in women are about 0.5 and 1.5 mg, respectively (Rosenfield, 1972). Furthermore, studies with rabbit ovary have demonstrated that luteinizing hormone (LH) increases ovarian incorporation of radioactive acetate into testosterone as well as testosterone secretion (Hilliard *et al.,* 1974).

The remarkably complete sexual development that can be brought about by the administration of estrogen alone and the faithful reproduction of all the features of the menstrual cycle (except the ovarian changes) that can be achieved with estrogen and progesterone seem to leave little place for an androgen in the feminine economy. And yet there may be certain features missing when estrogen-progestin therapy replaces ovarian function. The rapid rate of growth at puberty is hard to explain in view of the limited anabolic and growth-promoting properties of estrogen. The development of axillary and pubic hair under the influence of estrogen alone may not be as complete as it is in the normal girl, and it may be lacking altogether following therapy with estrogen in patients with hypopituitarism. When small doses of androgen are added to the estrogen, growth and distribution of hair on the body are normal even without the pituitary. The apparent effects of estrogen on the growth of hair may be attributable in part to their effects upon adrenal synthesis of androgens (Sabrinho *et al.*, 1971).

Acne, so common during puberty in girls, is closely related to the growth and secretion of the sebaceous glands. The normal development and function of these structures cannot be brought about by estrogen or progesterone, but both can be induced by the administration of small amounts of androgen (*e.g.*, 2.5 mg of methyltestosterone daily; *see* Chapter 62). Furthermore, while other treatments are preferred, acne can be effectively treated and the sebaceous glands caused to regress by suppressing gonadotropin secretion and ovarian function with estrogen or with a preparation of an estrogen and a progestin (Briggs, 1976; Kay, 1977).

Although estrogen alone is effective replacement therapy in the menopause, some observers believe that a more normal result is achieved when small amounts of androgen are given as well. The small quantities of testosterone and androstenedione secreted by the ovary are probably sufficient to account for the aforementioned observations without being virilizing in the usual sense of that term.

Actions on the Pituitary. The precise actions of estrogens on the secretory activity of the adenohypophysis have been very difficult to define. In the normal sexual cycle of mammals, the structural and the secretory changes in the ovary are brought about by the precisely timed and sequential secretion of gonadotropins from the hypophysis (*see* Franchimont, 1977; Erickson, 1978; Naftolin and Tolis, 1978). The central mechanisms

and events that lead to the cyclic secretion of gonadotropins and thereby initiate the onset of puberty and gonadal development are unknown (Boyer, 1978). However, the improvements in technics available to measure sex steroids and gonadotropins have led to a greater understanding during recent years and have provided critical confirmations of certain earlier studies.

One major difficulty has been the demonstration of a single gonadotropin-releasing hormone (RH), LH-RH/FSH-RH, which increases the pituitary secretion of both LH and FSH (*see* Chapter 59). The varying blood concentrations of each gonadotropin during the menstrual cycle (Figure 61–2) suggest that another regulatory hormone might exist to explain the apparent independence of their secretion. However, complex feedback effects of sex steroids and perhaps other gonadal factors on the pituitary and hypothalamus influence the secretion and action of LH-RH/FSH-RH, and this could explain the divergent patterns of release of each gonadotropin. This question is still open (*see* Schally, 1978).

While generalization is premature, certain interrelations seem definite. As the ovarian follicle grows under the influence of FSH, the increasing titer of estrogen that is produced decreases the release of LH-RH and thereby suppresses FSH secretion. Under the influence of FSH the Graafian follicle may also secrete *inhibin* or an analogous material that feeds back to decrease the secretion of FSH (Baker *et al.*, 1975). Inhibin, a peptide with a molecular weight of approximately 20,000, was first described in the testis (McCullogh, 1932); more recently it has been characterized in cultures of testicular Sertoli cells (Steinberger and Steinberger, 1976) and in ovarian follicular fluid (DeJong and Sharpe, 1976). Inhibin suppresses the secretion of FSH more than it does the secretion of LH. While estrogens can decrease FSH secretion, they have a biphasic effect on LH. The rapid swelling of the follicle, culminating in ovulation, is brought about by the midcycle surge in LH (Figure 61–2), probably due to increased LH-RH release as well as to greater estrogen-induced sensitivity of the pituitary to the regulatory hormone. It is not known why just one of the many follicles that develop under the influence of FSH in primates

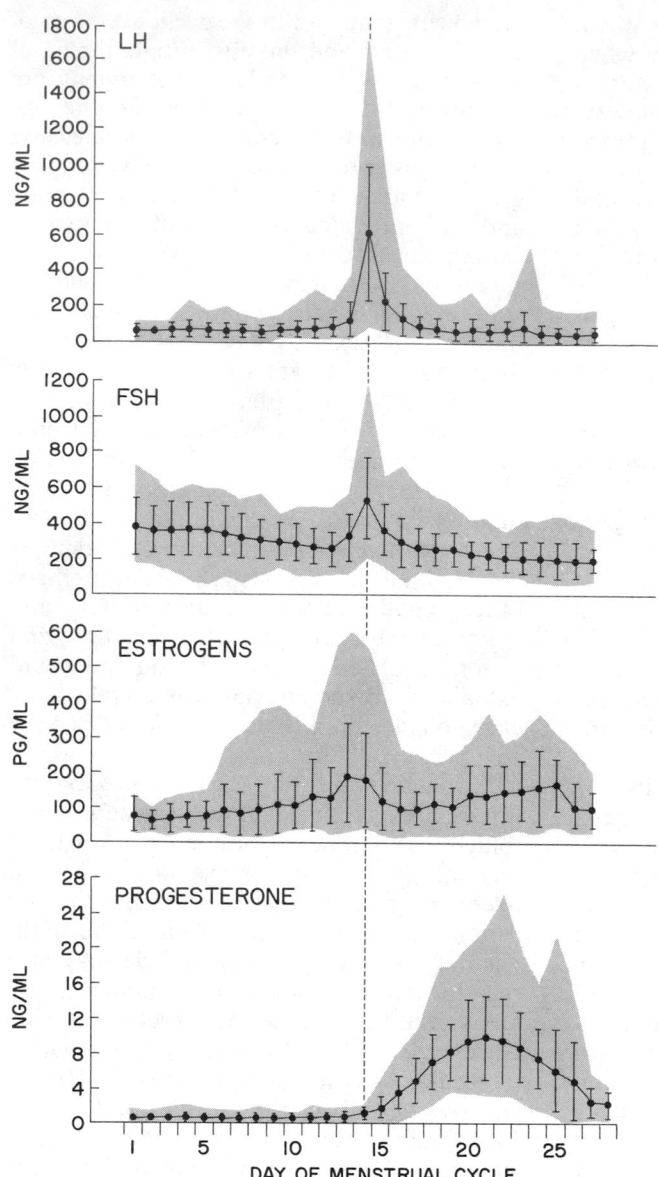

Figure 61-2. *Plasma concentrations of ovarian hormones and gonadotropins in women during normal menstrual cycles.*

Values are the mean ± standard deviation of 40 women. The shaded areas indicate the entire range of observations. Day 1 is the onset of menses. Ovulation on day 14 of the menstrual cycle occurs with the midcycle peak of LH, represented by the dash line. (After Vande Wiele and Dyrenfurth, 1973. Courtesy of *Pharmacological Reviews.* © 1973 The Williams & Wilkins Co., Baltimore.)

is selected for rupture and ovulation (Linder *et al.,* 1977; Erickson, 1978).

Progesterone begins to be secreted during the formation of the corpus luteum, and secretion continues throughout its functional life. The control of the secretion of the corpus luteum is managed by various species in quite different ways. In woman it is under the predominant control of LH.

The major mystery in the pituitary secretion of gonadotropins and thus ovarian secretion of estrogens and progesterone is the

relatively precise cyclic nature with which this takes place. In addition to the more prolonged and larger oscillations in gonadotropins during the menstrual cycle, smaller short-term variations in concentrations of gonadotropins in plasma have been observed in normal women (Midgley and Jaffe, 1968). The significance of the pulsatile secretion that causes these variations is not known.

In contrast, total daily secretion of gonadotropins in men is quite stable, while secretion during the course of the day is variable

(Franchimont, 1977). In the male the secretion of both FSH and LH can be inhibited by estrogen and inhibin; as a result, spermatogenesis is arrested, the testicular tubules become atrophic, and the regressive changes in the genital tract show that the secretion of androgen is reduced (see Chapter 62).

When the ovaries or testes are removed or cease to function, there is overproduction of FSH and LH, which are excreted in the urine. Measurements of urinary or plasma gonadotropins are valuable clinical tests and can be used to show the effectiveness of replacement doses of estrogen or testosterone, which, in amounts that might be considered physiological, specifically inhibit overproduction.

Estrogens and Menstruation. When the ovaries are not functional or have been removed, menstrual flow can be induced by the administration and subsequent withdrawal of estrogen. Both the size of the dose and the duration of treatment are involved in determining whether bleeding will follow, and, within limits, the two determinants can be varied reciprocally with a similar outcome. Bleeding can be induced by a single large dose or by treatment for several weeks with a much smaller amount. When doses within a certain range are given, menstrual flow may ensue even when the treatment is not interrupted. This range lies between the dose that is too small to cause bleeding upon withdrawal and the dose that is large enough to prevent menstrual flow even when continued for a long time. By way of explanation, it is assumed that the longer a certain dose is given, the more sensitive the endometrium becomes to the breakdown that causes bleeding. In the spayed rhesus monkey, Zuckerman (1941) showed that what he termed the "threshold dose" for this kind of bleeding was about 10 μg of estrone injected in oil once daily. With continued treatment for as long as 18 months, periodic bleeding was noted at irregular intervals, averaging 6 weeks in length. It is tempting to relate this type of irregular cycle to the clinical condition called functional uterine bleeding.

The action of progesterone upon the estrogen-treated uterus in causing menstruation is quite unrelated to its action in causing the secretory changes seen microscopically. When estrogen is given without interruption in amounts well above the threshold dose, brief treatment with progesterone is followed by menstruation a few days later; as little as 1 mg given in a single dose may be enough, whereas the histological changes in the endometrium require many days to develop.

Menstrual bleeding during continuous treatment with threshold doses of estrogen can be prevented by increasing the dose; however, when a brief treatment with progesterone is introduced, estrogen, even in large doses, will not prevent the ensuing menstruation.

Metabolic Actions. The similarity of the estrogens to the androgens in causing retention of salt and water as well as nitrogen and the elements required for the building of protoplasm is discussed in Chapter 62. Estrogens are weaker anabolic agents than the androgens. Retention of salt and water to the point of causing edema is not a common feature of therapy with estrogen. However, edema may be troublesome when estrogen is given in large doses and particularly if an associated condition predisposes to retention of fluid. Thus, the edema of heart failure or renal disease may be accentuated, and excessive fluid retention may complicate therapy with estrogen in older patients and in patients who are bedridden or malnourished. While the edema responds well to diuretics, one should discontinue the estrogen if possible. The moderate fluid retention common in the latter half of the menstrual cycle is a result of the action of estrogen.

Although estrogens have no effect on fasting plasma glucose concentration, alterations in oral and intravenous glucose tolerance tests may be seen when oral contraceptive combinations containing "high" doses of estrogens are given to some patients with what may be preclinical diabetes mellitus or with a family history of diabetes mellitus (Kalkoff, 1972; Briggs, 1976). The precise mechanism for the altered glucose tolerance is not known. While it is generally reversible when the estrogen is discontinued, the physician should alert the patient to the possible development of overt diabetes mellitus at a future date.

Estrogen, in therapeutic doses or in larger amounts, can cause alterations in the composition of circulating lipids. The increase in lipoproteins and triglycerides and the decrease in cholesterol that may result from the administration of estrogen or oral contraceptives are discussed in Chapter 34.

Carcinogenic Action. In several mammalian species, the administration of estrogens is followed by the development of certain tumors. Since the early studies of Lacassagne (1936), it has been known that estrogens can induce tumors of the breast, uterus, testis, bone, kidney, and several other tissues in various animal species. These early studies disseminated a fear of cancer resulting from estrogen use. Until 1971, however, no evidence of a carcinogenic action of estrogens in human subjects had been reported. Since that time there have been many clinical reports of tumors that may be related to estrogens. In the earliest studies (Greenwald *et al.,* 1971; Herbst *et al.,* 1971), an increased incidence of vaginal and cervical adenocarcinoma was noted in female offspring of mothers who had taken diethylstilbestrol or other synthetic estrogens during the first trimester of pregnancy. This has been amply confirmed, and the incidence of clear-cell vaginal and cervical adenocarcinoma in women who were exposed to estrogens *in utero* is estimated to be 0.01 to 0.1% (FDA Drug Bulletin, 1978c). Although most of the affected women have been about 20 to 25 years of age at the time of detection of disease, it is not known if a longer latency is also possible for these and other problems. Estrogen use during pregnancy can also cause vaginal adenosis (a nonmalignant proliferation of glandular tissue) in female offspring. While males exposed to exogenous estrogens during intrauterine development have an increased incidence of genital abnormalities, tumors have apparently not resulted from such exposure.

Pregnant patients should not be given estrogens, particularly during the first trimester—a time when the fetal reproductive tract is developing and may be influenced by exogenous estrogens.

Data from epidemiological studies have indicated that the use of estrogen by postmenopausal women is associated with the development of endometrial carcinoma (Smith *et al.,* 1975; Ziel and Finkle, 1975, 1976; Antunes *et al.,* 1979; Jick *et al.,* 1979). The risk is estimated to be increased as much as 5- to 15-fold by estrogen and is related to duration of use. However, other investigators have calculated the risk to be increased about two-fold (Horwitz and Feinstein, 1978). An apparent association of endometrial carcinoma in premenopausal women with the use of oral contraceptives was suggested in preliminary studies (Silverberg and Makowski, 1975). However, this has not been confirmed.

While several reports have aroused the suspicion that estrogens or oral contraceptives may increase the incidence of breast tumors, most studies have not demonstrated this association (*see* Leis *et al.,* 1976; Kay, 1977). The fact that has clearly emerged, however, is that estrogens do not protect patients from the development of premalignant or malignant changes of the breast.

After a report that the use of oral contraceptives by young women was associated with the occurrence of benign hepatomas (Baum *et al.,* 1973), a number of similar studies have confirmed this relationship. The frequency with which these rare adenomas appear in such individuals is unknown.

Thus, while estrogens have been in use for decades and an increased incidence of tumors was feared on the basis of animal experiments, the demonstrations of such a correlation have been relatively few and have taken many years to be noted. Estrogens can, indeed, increase the incidence of various tumors, but it seems likely that a long latent period is frequently required. This latent period and the fact that the increase in the incidence of certain tumors is small explain why few definitive studies are available.

Mechanism of Action. Considerable progress has been made in the elucidation of the mechanism of action of estrogens (*see* Gorski and Gannon, 1976). Putative receptor proteins for the hormone have been detected in estrogen-responsive tissues (female reproductive tract, breast, pituitary, and hypothalamus). Estrogens are first bound with very high affinity to a cytoplasmic receptor protein. Following modification, the estrogen-protein complex is converted to a species that is translocated to the nucleus, where ultimate binding of the estrogen-containing complex occurs. As a result of such binding characteristic metabolic alterations ensue. Specific mRNA and certain specific but unknown proteins are apparently synthesized rapidly, perhaps because of unmasking of restricted regions of DNA. A more general increase in the synthesis of various types of RNA and protein becomes obvious a few hours later, and stimulation of DNA synthesis is an even later event. These effects of estrogens can be blocked by inhibitors of RNA synthesis (dactinomycin) or protein synthesis (cycloheximide). It is not clear whether the prominent general stimulation of RNA synthesis is a result of increased RNA polymerase activity, increased chromatin template activity, altered nuclear transport phenomena, or combinations thereof. The presence of cytoplasmic receptors for estrogens greatly increases the likelihood of a palliative response to estrogen therapy in women with metastatic breast cancer (*see* below and Chapter 55).

Absorption, Fate, and Excretion. Estrogens used in therapy are, in general, readily absorbed through the skin, mucous membranes, and gastrointestinal tract. When they are applied for a local action, absorption is often sufficient to cause systemic effects, and in factory workers gynecomastia has followed handling of diethylstilbestrol without gloves. The absorption of most natural estrogens and their derivatives from the gastrointestinal tract is prompt and quite complete. Thus, the limited oral effectiveness of the natural estrogens and their esters is due to their metabolism, as discussed below.

The natural estrogens are practically insoluble in water. When injected dissolved in oil, they are rapidly absorbed and quickly metabolized. The aryl and alkyl esters of estradiol become less and less polar as the size of the substituents increases; correspondingly, the rate of absorption of oily preparations is progressively slowed and the duration of action prolonged. Therapeutic doses of estradiol benzoate are effective for several days; estradiol dipropionate is absorbed over several weeks.

The natural estrogens and their esters are handled in the body in much the same way as are the endogenous hormones (*see* Fotherby and James, 1972). Inactivation of estrogen in the body is carried out mainly in the liver. A certain proportion of the estrogen reaching that organ is excreted into the bile, only to be reabsorbed from the intestine. During this enterohepatic circulation, degradation of estrogen occurs through conversion to less active products such as estriol and numerous other estrogens, through oxidation to nonestrogenic substances, and through conjugation with sulfuric and glucuronic acids.

The course of metabolism of *ethinyl estradiol* is different. This compound is active by mouth since its inactivation in the liver and other tissues is very slow. This accounts for the high intrinsic potency of the analog. Similarly the nonsteroidal estrogens are slowly degraded in the body.

The natural estrogens circulate in the blood in association with sex hormone–binding globulin and albumin (Heyns, 1977). A significant proportion of the estrogen is in the form of conjugates, particularly sulfate. These water-soluble conjugates are strong acids and are thus fully ionized in the body fluids; penetration into cells is therefore limited, and excretion by the kidney is favored because little tubular reabsorption is possible.

As mentioned above, endogenous estrogens appear in the urine as glucuronides and sulfates of estradiol, estrone, and estriol. Small quantities of a great many other derivatives have also been identified. In the normal menstrual cycle the mean daily excretion of estrogens at the midcycle ovulatory maximum is 25 to 100 μg; the second rise during the luteal phase is more prolonged, but the maximal rates of excretion are somewhat smaller (10 to 80 μg). After the menopause the average excretion of estrogens in normal women totals about 5 to 10 μg daily. The values for normal men average 2 to 25 μg per day, quantities about equal to the urinary estrogens of women during the first week of the menstrual cycle. In young children none is detectable. During the first trimester of pregnancy the placenta becomes the primary source of the urinary estrogens, which continue to increase and reach levels of about 30 mg per day near term. Their serial determination can be used to assess placental and fetal function.

Assays. Most biological assays for estrogen are based upon the original method of Allen and Doisy, vaginal cornification in the spayed rat or mouse, or upon growth of the uterus in these species. The vaginal response is highly specific, and almost by definition a substance giving rise to a cornified vaginal smear is an estrogen. The test is influenced by other factors, however, and it is inhibited by progesterone and androgen; for this reason, tests on compounds of mixed activity may be difficult to interpret. Most tests based upon the increased weight of the uterus are less specific than the vaginal smear.

Local application of substances to the vagina of spayed animals also provides a very sensitive test for estrogen. With the natural estrogens the test is several hundred times more sensitive than tests based on subcutaneous injection, and the method is especially valuable for the assay of biological materials.

The development of competitive protein-binding and radioimmunoassay methods has accelerated investigation in this and other areas (*see* Vande Wiele and Dyrenfurth, 1973). Compared to various bioassay methods, these technics are generally simpler and faster. Since they also usually offer a high degree of sensitivity and specificity, such methods are rapidly becoming routine procedures in many clinical laboratories. However, the immunoassay methods are not useful for studying structure-activity relationship, and it is unlikely that bioassay and sensitive receptor-protein methods will be displaced in research laboratories.

Preparations. Several widely used, orally active nonsteroidal estrogens are available. The most popular have been preparations of *Diethylstilbestrol,* U.S.P., available in tablets containing from 0.1 to 5 mg; suppositories containing 0.1, 0.5, or 1 mg are also marketed. *Diethylstilbestrol Diphosphate,* U.S.P. (STILPHOSTROL), is available as an injection (250 mg/5-ml ampul) and in 50-mg tablets. A number of chemically related compounds for oral or topical use include *Benzestrol,* U.S.P. (CHEMESTROGEN), *Dienestrol,* U.S.P. (DIENSTROL, SYNESTROL), *hexestrol, methallenestril* (VALLESTRIL), and *promethestrol dipropionate* (MEPRANE).

Estradiol, U.S.P. (AQUADIOL, PROGYNON, others), is available in aqueous suspension containing 0.5 or 1 mg/ml for intramuscular injection and as 25-mg pellets for subcutaneous implantation. Various esters of estradiol (benzoate, cypionate, enanthate, propionate, undecylate, and valerate) are prepared in aqueous suspensions or oily solution for slow release after intramuscular injection. These preparations contain 0.5 to 40 mg/ml and are sold under various trade names (DELESTROGEN, DEPO-ESTRADIOL, OVOCYLIN, many others). *Polyestradiol phosphate* (ESTRADURIN) is also available for intramuscular use in prostatic carcinoma.

Various sulfate esters of *Estrone,* U.S.P., are available in tablets containing 0.75 to 6 mg (OGEN, others). These esters and estrone are also supplied under various trade names in aqueous suspension and oily solution containing 1 to 5 mg/ml for intramuscular injection.

Ethinyl Estradiol, U.S.P. (ESTINYL, FEMINONE, others), is the most active oral preparation known, and the tablets contain 0.02 to 0.5 mg. It is roughly 20 times as potent as diethylstilbestrol. The 3-methyl ester of ethinyl estradiol, *Mestranol,* U.S.P., is nearly as active and is widely used in the combination oral contraceptives (*see* below).

Conjugated Estrogens, U.S.P. (OVEST, PREMARIN, many others), contains 50 to 65% sodium estrone sulfate and 20 to 35% sodium equilin sulfate; it is available in oral (0.3 to 2.5 mg) and injectable (5 mg/ml) preparations, and as a vaginal cream containing 0.625 mg/g.

Esterified Estrogens, U.S.P. (AMNESTROGEN, EVEX, SK-ESTROGENS, ZESTE, others), contains 75 to 85% sodium estrone sulfate and 6.5 to 15% equilin sodium sulfate in tablets of 0.3 to 2.5 mg. Other mixtures of estrogens available in tablet and injectable forms are also marketed under various trade names.

Chlorotrianisene, U.S.P. (TACE), is a long-acting oral preparation because of sequestration in adipose tissue and, therefore, is not widely used. It is available in 12-, 25-, and 72-mg capsules and has about one eighth the activity of diethylstilbestrol.

A number of preparations in which estrogen is combined with another agent are also available. Oral contraceptives containing an estrogen and a progestin are discussed later in the chapter. There are no compelling reasons to use formulations of estrogens combined with androgens or antianxiety preparations.

A variety of topical preparations in creams and suppositories are no longer widely used. However, *senile vaginitis* and *kraurosis vulvae* may be effectively treated with such topical preparations. Many of the "over-the-counter" cosmetics and creams that contained estrogens have been removed from the United States market in recent years. However, several are still available that do not require a prescription. While their frequent and excessive use can cause systemic effects, these are minimal when they are used as directed. Intravaginal use of some preparations can lead to significant concentrations of estrogen in blood, since the estrogen is readily absorbed and the initial circulation through the liver is bypassed with this route of administration (Rigg *et al.,* 1978).

Choice of Preparations. Claims have been made that some preparations of estrogen cause fewer side effects than others. However, the prevailing information suggests that all estrogenic materials can cause the more serious cardiovascular and perhaps tumorigenic effects. The following dosages of some estrogens are approximately equivalent: estradiol, 50 μg; mestranol, 80 μg; diethylstilbestrol, 1 mg; conjugated estrogens, 5 mg. The choice of preparation is largely determined by cost and convenience to the patient. By all odds oral therapy is the best; the action begins promptly and treatment can be terminated at will. With substances such as diethylstilbestrol or ethinyl estradiol, which are not quickly inactivated, a single dose each day is usually sufficient. Conjugated natural estrogens are less effective and if used are given in divided doses. Several doses per day may be needed when high dosage is required. Parenteral therapy has little to recommend it; frequent injections can be avoided by the use of a long-acting preparation, but then the onset and cessation of action are slow, gradual, and uncertain. Conceivably, the long-acting esters given by injection may be useful for long-continued treatment with large doses in the therapy of patients with cancer. The esters are unsuitable in the management of menstrual disorders or as replacement therapy in menopause when cyclic therapy is desirable; the action slowly declines in a way that is quite unlike the prompt cessation of secretion characteristic of the normal menstrual cycle. Cyclic therapy can be accomplished with various schedules; therapy can be interrupted for 1 week per month or, less commonly, for several days per week. Few disorders require continuous therapy or long-acting preparations.

Untoward Responses. The most frequent unpleasant symptom attending the use of estrogen is *nausea*. With large doses there may also be anorexia and even vomiting and mild diarrhea. The nausea is of a peculiar type that seldom interferes with eating and does not cause a loss of weight; it may be noted at various times of the day but, like the "morning sickness" of early pregnancy, it is often troublesome at breakfast time. With continued treatment the symptom usually disappears, and only rarely is it so distressful that treatment must be stopped. Even when very large doses are given, as in the treatment of cancer of the breast, nausea is generally troublesome only for the first 1 or 2 weeks. The symptom can usually be avoided by starting with a small dose and gradually increasing it. Statements that certain preparations are less apt to cause nausea than others may be viewed with skepticism. Other untoward responses are discussed below, under oral contraceptives.

Therapeutic Uses. *Oral Contraception.* A major use of estrogens is in combination with progestins as oral contraceptives; such use is discussed in a separate section later in this chapter.
Menopause. At a variable age, but usually in the late 40s, the functions of the ovaries decline. Ovulation is lost first, and anovulatory cycles may continue for 1 or 2 years before menstruation ceases altogether. Irregular menstrual cycles are particularly prevalent at this time due to deficient or poorly cycling estrogen and diminished progesterone soon thereafter. Lack of appreciation of the endocrine basis of the menstrual disturbance usually leads to the conclusion that some mechanical factor, such as fibroid tumors, is at fault.

The decline in the secretion of estrogen by the ovary is a slow and gradual process that continues for some years after menstruation has ceased (see Eskin, 1978). It is a frequent observation that menopausal symptoms are more severe following abrupt removal of estrogen, such as with oophorectomy, than with the natural menopause. Sometimes hot flashes appear for the first time or become more intense if the ovaries are removed after the menopause. The formation of small quantities of estrogens from androgenic precursors by nonovarian tissues may be important in slowing the estrogen withdrawal and the onset of menopausal symptoms in some patients (*see* above).

Frequently the decline in ovarian function at the menopause is associated with symptoms that are clearly due to deficiency of estrogen. The characteristic hot flashes may alternate with chilly sensations, inappropriate sweating, and paresthesias, including formication. A variety of other symptoms often occur during menopause and include muscle cramps, myalgias, arthralgias, anxiety, overbreathing, palpitation, dizziness, faintness, and syncope. These symptoms may or may not be associated with estrogen deficiency. A few women become chronic invalids and experience years of ill health; some feel genuinely miserable and lack vigor and initiative; many, obviously, tolerate the event quite well. About 15 to 25% of menopausal women will seek medical advice or treatment.

Treatment with estrogen is specific and effective. Replacement therapy clearly relieves the hot flashes and other vasomotor symptoms and atrophic vaginitis. The lowest dose needed varies somewhat but can easily be determined by trial. The dose of diethylstilbestrol is about 0.2 to 1 mg once daily by mouth; 0.5 mg is seldom sufficient to cause withdrawal bleeding, 1 mg daily for several weeks sometimes causes bleeding when stopped, and 2 mg often does. Comparable doses of ethinyl estradiol are 0.01 to 0.05 mg; conjugated estrogens may be used in doses of 0.6 to 5 mg daily. Therapy with estrogen is best given in a cyclic manner, 3 or 4 weeks of treatment followed by 1 week without treatment. If withdrawal bleeding is going to occur, it will begin toward the end of the week of no treatment and the estrogen can be resumed before this induced menstrual period ceases. Menopausal symptoms usually do not return in full intensity during the week without treatment. A less widely used alternative procedure is to give an effective dose of estrogen without interruption and to evoke a menstrual period every 4 to 6 weeks with a progestin. Occasionally during cyclic therapy with estrogen alone uterine bleeding may continue in an irregular manner after estrogen is resumed. Larger doses of estrogen have been employed to control this bleeding, but the use of a progestin is more uniformly effective. Once a progesterone-withdrawal period has been induced, there may be no further trouble from the use of estrogen alone for many months.

While some physicians prescribe a small dose of androgen along with estrogen, many prefer not to administer any androgen. Androgen enhances strength and imparts a sense of well-being. Withdrawal bleeding from estrogen is said to be reduced when androgen is given concurrently. Large doses of androgen in women may increase libido, but in the small doses used in the menopause the effect is seen

only in some cases. Excessive dosage leads to undesirable masculinizing effects and the danger of hepatic injury (*see* Chapter 62), but the usual dose of 5
or 10 mg of methyltestosterone daily, interrupted
when the estrogen is stopped, does not usually cause
detectable virilization. Some observers believe that
the estrogen counteracts the masculinizing influence.

Senile or *atrophic vaginitis,* often associated with
chronic infection of the atrophic structures, responds
well to estrogen. Estrogens are more effective in
preventing than in reversing atrophic changes of the
vagina and the decrease in skin turgor (*see* Eskin,
1978). *Kraurosis vulvae,* a distressingly itchy condition due in part to deficiency in estrogen and in part
to scratching and other as-yet-unknown factors, is
favorably influenced by estrogen supplemented by
local treatment, including the application of adrenocorticosteroids.

Some physicians are disinclined to prescribe estrogens in the menopause; they feel that the symptoms are largely emotional in origin and are better
managed by reassurance and psychotherapy and
with the use of small doses of a sedative. Others
prescribe estrogens for periods of months or a few
years only. Physicians with these views are undoubtedly concerned about the possible minor and serious
side effects of estrogens in light of very little strong
evidence to demonstrate their efficacy in preventing
the more serious physical disorders accompanying
menopause, such as atherosclerosis and osteoporosis.
However, indefinite systemic replacement in all
menopausal patients, advocated by some, is certainly
controversial and may introduce more undesirable
effects than the symptomatic improvement warrants
(*see* Medical Letter, 1976). Patients receiving estrogens should be examined every 6 to 12 months for
possible side effects, and abnormal uterine bleeding
should be investigated. Most agree that the risk-to-
benefit ratio for estrogen therapy needs to be evaluated for each patient and should be reconsidered
periodically; when used, estrogens should be administered in the lowest effective dose for the shortest
possible time.

Pregnancy. In the past, large doses of estrogens
have been given during pregnancy in attempts to
prevent threatened or habitual abortion or because
of abnormalities of urinary estrogen excretion in
toxemia of pregnancy. There is no evidence that such
uses are of any value. Because of this and the risk of
producing vaginal tumors in female offspring and
possible teratogenic effects in male offspring (*see*
above), *the use of estrogens in pregnancy is not indicated.* The use of progestins in this condition is discussed subsequently.

Dysmenorrhea. Sturgis and Albright (1940) reported the relief of dysmenorrhea by inhibiting ovulation with estrogen, and such treatment has since
been widely used. Oral dosage can be taken, for
example, in the form of diethylstilbestrol in a daily
dose of about 2 mg, starting 5 days after the onset of
a menstrual period and continuing for 15 to 20 days.
Indeed, treatment can be continued for several weeks
longer, if desired, so that the artificial periods are less
frequent. Cyclic therapy can often be used successfully month after month if too long an interval is not
permitted to elapse between courses. The additional

use of an orally active progesterone-like steroid facilitates management, as it does when the method is
used as a contraceptive measure, and combined oral
contraceptive agents are now preferred (*see* below).
It is not known why dysmenorrhea is relieved when
cycles are anovulatory.

The use of estrogens in the treatment of *endometriosis* is discussed in connection with the therapeutic
uses of the progestins.

Dysfunctional Uterine Bleeding. This disorder
usually occurs at the time of menarche or menopause
and results from anovulatory cycles, with continuous
secretion of estrogen and endometrial hyperplasia.
Insufficient secretion of progesterone results in incomplete sloughing of the proliferative endometrium
and excessive bleeding. While estrogen can be used
with some success, the cyclic use of a progestin is
logically preferred (*see* below).

Failure of Ovarian Development. There are several unusual conditions wherein the ovaries do not
develop and, in consequence, puberty does not
occur. In *ovarian dysgenesis* with dwarfism (Turner's
syndrome) diagnosis can often be made before the
age of puberty by the associated congenital anomalies and the stature. Therapy with estrogen at the
appropriate time brings about a perfect replica of the
events of puberty, except for the spurt in growth and,
of course, the changes in the ovary. The genital
structures grow to normal size. The breasts develop,
there is growth of axillary and pubic hair, and the
body assumes the normal feminine contour. Also,
androgens have been used successfully to promote
growth (*see* Chapter 62). It is common practice to
start with small doses of estrogen, such as 0.5 mg of
diethylstilbestrol or 0.02 mg of ethinyl estradiol, and
then increase the dose slowly over a year or so before
initiating menstrual periods by cyclic treatment with
larger doses. It is felt that there may be some merit in
thus imitating the normal sequence of events at
puberty.

Failure of ovarian development is also a part of
the picture of *hypopituitarism* in childhood. Deficiency of the thyroid and the adrenal cortex is easily
corrected with replacement therapy, and the failure
of sexual development is treated with estrogen as
outlined just above. If human growth hormone is
used, these girls can achieve a normal adult stature
(*see* Chapter 59). Treatment with estrogen at the
normal age of puberty can be expected to cause a
small acceleration of growth, but the addition of
small doses of androgen has a greater growth-promoting effect, as noted in Chapter 62. While estrogens and androgens promote bone growth, they also
accelerate epiphyseal fusion, and their premature use
can thus result in a shorter ultimate height. Indeed,
estrogens have been used in high doses to accelerate
epiphyseal closure in tall girls; to be effective, estrogen must be given prior to menarche. This use of
estrogen is rarely, if ever, indicated (*see* Wentz,
1977).

Acne. The common form of acne is a feature of
puberty in both sexes, and androgen seems to be the
essential factor, operating through stimulation of
sebaceous glands. Treatment with estrogen is effective in both sexes by suppressing gonadotropins and
gonadal androgen secretion, but its usefulness in the

male is limited by gynecomastia, suppression of the testis, uncertain effects on skeletal growth, and danger of hastening epiphyseal closure. In young women estrogen is effective therapy in doses designed to suppress the ovary and may be continued with benefit for many months in cyclic fashion. One of the combined oral contraceptive agents is more convenient. It may be given in the same manner as when used to prevent ovulation, and the preparations with larger amounts of estrogen are used. However, tretinoin (all *trans*-retinoic acid) and antibiotics (tetracyclines or erythromycin) are preferred (*see* Chapters 67 and 52).

Hirsutism. In most instances, excessive growth of body hair in women cannot be traced to an endocrine cause, but occasionally a mild androgenic influence of ovarian or adrenal origin is suspected. When suppression of the adrenal cortex by the administration of a corticosteroid is ineffectual, suppression of the ovary with an estrogen may be worthwhile. If it is to be tried, suppression of the ovary for about a year with continuous therapy may be needed before it can be ascertained whether the maneuver is successful. Doses of about 2 mg daily of diethylstilbestrol or its equivalent are sufficient. Menstrual periods during this time can be evoked at intervals by cyclic use of an oral progestin, with preference for a progestin that is devoid of androgenic activity.

Prevention of Heart Attacks. In view of the favored position of women in the incidence of fatal myocardial infarction, estrogen therapy has been tried as a prophylactic measure in men. A large-scale study was conducted by the Coronary Drug Project Research Group. The administration of conjugated estrogens daily led to an *increased* incidence of cardiac and thromboembolic complications (Coronary Drug Project Research Group, 1970, 1973). Although the use of estrogen in the form of combination oral contraceptives also apparently increases the incidence of morbidity and mortality from myocardial infarction in premenopausal women (*see* below), the administration of estrogen to postmenopausal women has not been associated with an increased incidence of complications from coronary artery disease (Rosenberg *et al.,* 1976). There is thus no evidence that administration of estrogen delays the progression of atherosclerosis, a previous notion that contributed to their excessive use in postmenopausal women.

Osteoporosis. Osteoporosis is a disorder of the skeleton associated with the loss of both hydroxyapatite (calcium phosphate complexes) and protein matrix (colloid). The result is thinning and weakening of the bones and an increased incidence of fractures, particularly compression fractures of the vertebrae. In older patients it is called *senile osteoporosis* and affects both sexes. Coming after menopause it is referred to as *postmenopausal osteoporosis* and occurs in about one fourth of such women. Many different methods of treatment have been tried with the aim of increasing bone density and substance. Several groups (Riggs *et al.,* 1972; Lindsay *et al.,* 1976; Recker *et al.,* 1977) have demonstrated that, after several months of estrogen replacement in postmenopausal patients, calcium balance becomes positive and bone resorption decreases to normal. The benefits of estrogen replacement, however, may last only 9 to 14 months in spite of continued estrogen treatment. It is not known whether periodic long courses of estrogen therapy would continue to be effective if interrupted by periods of withdrawal.

The prophylactic effect of estrogen in this condition appears greatest if hormone is given before significant osteoporosis occurs (*see* Gordon, 1978). However, since only 25% of postmenopausal patients develop osteoporosis and treatment with calcium salts is as or more effective, the routine prophylactic use of estrogen is difficult to justify. In women who have undergone oophorectomy and hysterectomy, such use of an estrogen is more defensible, since one of the possible toxicities, endometrial carcinoma, is no longer an issue. Androgens are less effective than estrogens in the treatment of postmenopausal osteoporosis, but they are probably more effective in preventing osteoporosis induced by glucocorticoids (*see* Gordon, 1978). The use of androgens is discussed in Chapter 62.

Breast Cancer. Many carcinomas of the breast are dependent upon the proper hormonal environment for their growth. About 50 to 65% of all breast cancers possess cytosolic estrogen receptor; this frequency is somewhat greater in tumors in postmenopausal patients than in those that occur in premenopausal women. Alteration of the hormonal environment can be used as a palliative measure in the therapy of metastatic breast cancer. Removal of estrogen by oophorectomy or the administration of antiestrogens (*see* below) or the administration of estrogens themselves can prolong both the quality and duration of life. Favorable responses can be obtained in about 60 to 70% of patients if estrogen receptors are present in the tumor, while such responses are observed in only 10 to 20% if receptors are absent (McGuire, 1975; Kiang *et al.,* 1978; Legha *et al.,* 1978). This subject is discussed in more detail in Chapter 55.

Suppression of Post-Partum Lactation. Estrogens, progestins, and androgens are used to decrease milk production in the post-partum period. Estrogens probably inhibit the action of prolactin and are more effective in the immediate post-partum period than after lactation is established. Doses of 0.1 to 0.15 mg of ethinyl estradiol daily for 5 to 7 days or 5 mg of diethylstilbestrol daily for 5 days followed by tapered doses for several days are effective. Androgens are also widely used for this purpose (*see* Chapter 62).

ANTIESTROGENS

The term *antiestrogen* has been rather broadly applied to several different types of compounds that inhibit or modify the action of estrogen. Progestins and androgens have been described as antiestrogenic; some weak estrogens are antiestrogenic by some criteria, and certain compounds are antiestrogenic when applied locally to the responsive tissue.

Two compounds with prominent antiestrogenic activity are currently available for clinical use in the United States—*clomiphene* and *tamoxifen.*

These highly effective inhibitors of estrogen came from an unexpected direction. The weakly estrogenic compound *chlorotrianisene* (Table 61–1), unlike most estrogens, was noted not to cause enlargement of the pituitary when given to rats in large doses. Estradiol normally causes pronounced enlargement of the pituitary, but when chlorotrianisene was given concurrently the effect was greatly reduced (Segal and Thompson, 1956). The related, nonestrogenic compound *ethamoxytriphetol* (Table 61–1) was found to be strikingly antiestrogenic. It inhibited endogenous estrogen as well as estrogen given in the form of the natural compounds, diethylstilbestrol, or chlorotrianisene. More extensive human studies have been carried out with the related compounds *clomiphene, tamoxifen,* and *nafoxidine.*

Pharmacological Effects.   Initial animal tests with clomiphene showed very slight estrogenic activity and moderate antiestrogenic activity. The striking effect was inhibition of the pituitary's gonadotropic function. Thus, in both sexes the compound was a potent contraceptive. When given to human beings, however, the most prominent effect was impressive enlargement of the ovaries. Properly applied, the compound has proven to be a most remarkable and useful agent for the treatment of infertility. Greenblatt and coworkers (1962) made extensive and careful studies and found that ovulation could be induced in a high proportion of patients with amenorrhea, the Stein-Leventhal syndrome, and dysfunctional uterine bleeding with anovulatory cycles. Pregnancy followed in a significant number of cases when infertility had been the problem. Excessive enlargement of the ovaries and the formation of ovarian cysts were common features of the treatment when doses of 100 to 200 mg daily were given for 2 or 3 weeks, but with doses of 50 or 75 mg daily this complication was less frequent and the ovaries returned to normal size after treatment had been completed. The substance gave evidence of antiestrogenic effects. Hot flashes were experienced by some patients, vaginal cornification in precocious puberty in young girls was inhibited, and in one case suppression of ovulation with ethinyl estradiol was prevented by clomiphene. There was no clinical evidence of progestational or androgenic effects.

Mechanism of Action.   The nonsteroidal compounds in Table 61–1 have some structural similarities to estrogens, which may explain their actions. Clomiphene and related antiestrogens bind to cytoplasmic estrogen receptors, and the modified complex is translocated to the nucleus. Such competition for estrogen binding sites and the resultant diminished amount of estrogen receptor

Table 61-1.   STRUCTURAL RELATIONSHIP OF CHLOROTRIANISENE AND THE ANTIESTROGENS

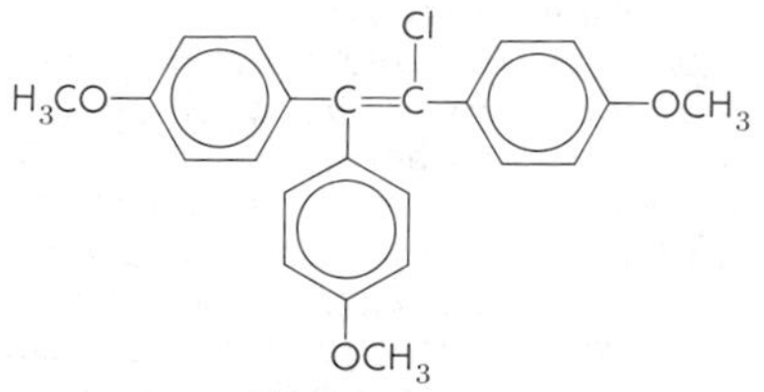

Chlorotrianisene

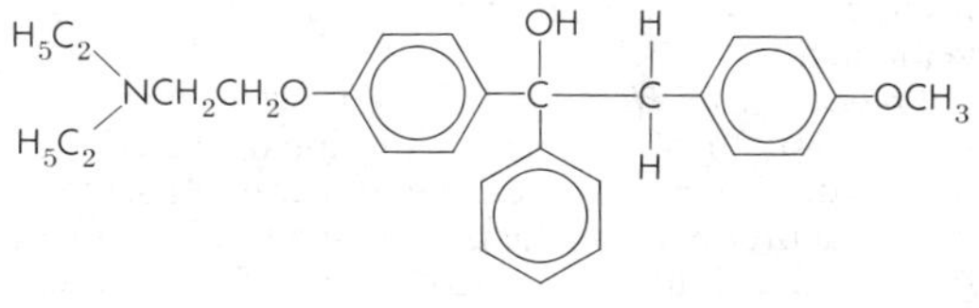

Ethamoxytriphetol

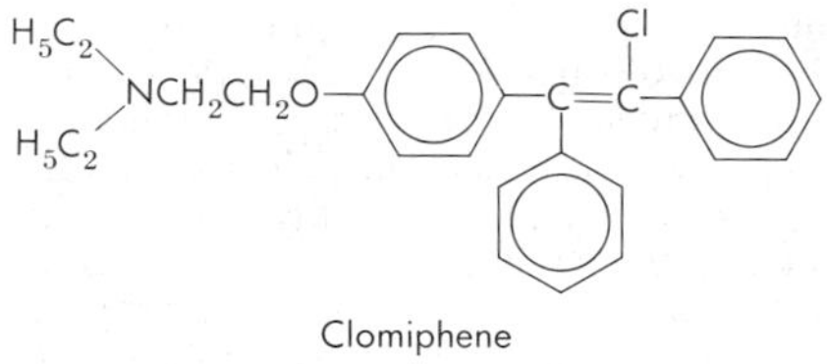

Clomiphene

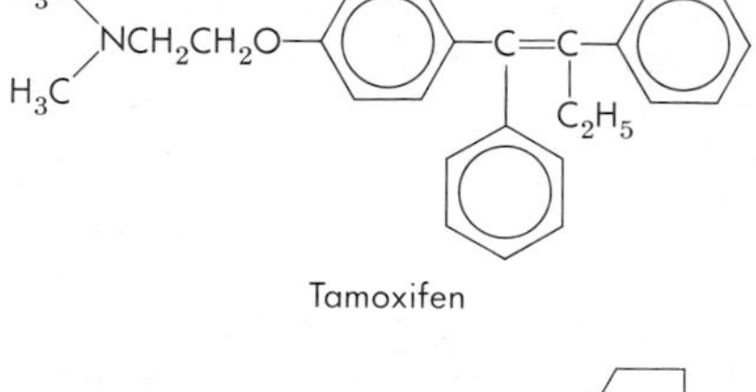

Tamoxifen

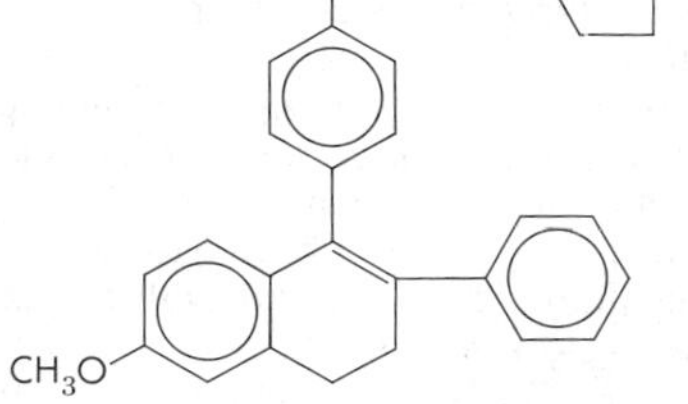

Nafoxidine

that is available for endogenous hormone are presumed to explain and have been used to predict their antiestrogenic activity (Kato *et al.,* 1968; Legha *et al.,* 1978; Marshall, 1978). Antiestrogens prevent the normal "feedback inhibition" of control of estrogen synthesis in the hypothalamus and pituitary, and this causes an increased secretion of LH-RH/FSH-RH and gonadotropins. The formation of large and cystic ovaries is the result of increased concentrations of gonadotropins, leading to ovarian stimulation, ovulation, and sustained function of corpora lutea.

Malignant mammary cells from human subjects with breast cancer have been successfully cloned and propagated in tissue culture for prolonged periods. These cell lines possess estrogen receptors, and their survival and growth in culture are dependent upon the presence of estrogen in the medium (*see* Strobel and Lippman, 1978). The addition of antiestrogens prevents the effects of estrogen and results in cell death. The effects of antiestrogens on the growth of estrogen-responsive tumors are discussed further in Chapter 55.

Therapeutic Uses and Preparations. *Clomiphene Citrate,* U.S.P. (CLOMID), has been used clinically for the treatment of infertility in women in doses varying between 25 and 200 mg daily by mouth, for periods of a few days to a few weeks. It is available in 50-mg tablets. In view of the development of enlarged ovaries with higher doses, a dose of 50 mg daily for 5 days is recommended initially. This is started on the fifth day of the menstrual cycle except in patients who have not menstruated recently. In infertility and menstrual disorders, treatment has been repeated at monthly intervals with success. If ovulation and fertility are not achieved, the dose may be increased to 100 mg or even 150 mg per day for 5 days (*see* Marshall, 1978). Ovulation is achieved in most patients whose pituitary and ovaries are capable of stimulated function, and pregnancy occurs in 40 to 50% of such women. The use of clomiphene and gonadotropins in infertility is also discussed in Chapter 59. As with gonadotropins, hyperstimulation of the ovaries with the formation of multiple cysts and a high incidence of multiple births is seen. The incidence of multiple births with clomiphene is about 6 to 8%, compared to an incidence of 15 to 25% when gonadotropins are used to induce ovulation and fertility. About 75% of the multiple births that follow the use of clomiphene are twins. It has not been resolved whether the incidence of abortion, premature deliveries, or congenital malformations is altered when either clomiphene or gonadotropin is used. In addition to the undesirable effects already noted, there have been instances of gastric upset, skin rashes, and visual disturbances. The latter are reversible after withdrawal of the drug.

Clomiphene in doses of 200 to 300 mg per day is effective for the palliation of disseminated breast cancer in selected patients. However, it is not approved for this use in the United States. *Tamoxifen,* which is also used for this purpose, is discussed in Chapter 55. *Nafoxidine* is another antiestrogen that is not yet available in the United States.

PROGESTINS

For some years after Corner and Allen had isolated progesterone from the corpora lutea of sows, the small amounts of the hormone available, at first from natural sources and later from synthesis, hampered experimental work and therapeutic application. The hormone had to be given by injection, and the duration of action was brief. With the introduction during the 1950s of new classes of progestational agents with prolonged activity and enhanced oral effectiveness, the structures associated with activity were found to be quite diverse. The number of progestins has proliferated abundantly, and some have had wide clinical use as contraceptive agents.

Chemistry. Some of the progestins have inherent estrogenic or androgenic effects, some show dissociations of effectiveness in various tests, and some have properties that resemble progesterone very closely. The compounds of greatest interest in therapeutics are those that are effective when given by mouth. Some representative progestins are shown in Table 61–2.

The first progestin that was reasonably effective orally was 17α-ethinyltestosterone (*ethisterone*). Derivatives of testosterone lacking the angular methyl group (C 19) attached to C 10, the 19-nortestosterones, were much more effective orally. The parent compound, 19-nortestosterone, is inactive, but a number of 17α-alkyl derivatives are effective. The 17α-methyl derivative is progestational and androgenic. 17α-Ethyl-19-nortestosterone (*norethandrolone*) is also progestational and androgenic and is used clinically as an anabolic agent. Its structural formula is given in Table 62–4. 17α-Ethinyl-19-nortestosterone, or *norethindrone* (*norethisterone*), is a potent oral progestin in man and is only mildly androgenic. Shift of the double bond in norethindrone yields the isomer *norethynodrel*, one of the first compounds to be widely used as a contraceptive. Reduction of the 3-keto group of norethindrone yields a partially reduced derivative of ethinyl estradiol termed *ethynodiol,* the diacetate of which is a particularly potent progestational agent in man. Removal of the oxygen function at position 3 gives rise to an interesting series of compounds, the *estrenols,* the biological activity of which is critically dependent upon the substituent grouping on C 17.

Table 61–2. STRUCTURAL RELATIONSHIP OF VARIOUS PROGESTINS TO PROGESTERONE

Progesterone   Ethisterone   Medroxyprogesterone Acetate

Hydroxyprogesterone Caproate   Norethindrone   Norethynodrel

Ethynodiol Diacetate   Dydrogesterone   Dimethisterone

Ethinylestrenol   Megestrol Acetate   Norgestrel

Thus, *ethinylestrenol* is a powerful progestational agent free of androgenic and anabolic effects, *allylestrenol* has progestational and other actions, and *ethylestrenol* (Table 62–4) is used as an anabolic agent. The 13-ethyl analog of norethindrone, or 18-homonorethisterone (*norgestrel*), was found to be 100 times as progestational as norethindrone in the Clauberg test, which is based upon the endometrial changes in immature rabbits pretreated with estrogen.

Another series of orally active progestins is typified by the compound *chlormadinone acetate,* which is 6α-chloro-Δ^6-17α-acetoxy progesterone, a purely progestational agent of high potency previously used in contraceptive formulations. The 6-methyl analog has similar properties and is referred to as *megestrol.*

Additional progestational compounds took origin from a different line of investigation. 17α-Hydroxyprogesterone, first isolated from the adrenal glands in 1940, was virtually inert. On the other hand, the acetic acid ester had appreciable activity and could be taken by mouth, although very large doses were required. When the compound was given by injection in oil, activity was prolonged, a property shared by other esters such as the *valerate* and *caproate*. The caproate has been used extensively as a long-acting progestin, but it is virtually inactive by mouth. Other derivatives of 17α-hydroxyprogesterone were found to be effective orally, and the one most widely studied is the 6-methyl analog, *medroxyprogesterone acetate*. The 16α, 17α-dihydroxy derivative of progesterone in the form of the *acetophenone* is moderately active by mouth but has the property of extremely long action when given parenterally.

Perhaps the most potent progestin yet encountered is *cyproterone acetate*. It has had only limited use as a progestin, perhaps because of a greater interest in its use as an antiandrogen (Chapter 62).

Synthesis and Secretion. Progesterone is secreted by the ovary mainly from the corpus luteum during the second half of the menstrual cycle. Secretion actually begins just before ovulation from the follicle that is destined to release an ovum. The formation of progesterone from steroid precursors is summarized in Figure 61-1 and occurs in the ovary, testis, adrenal cortex, and placenta. The stimulatory effect of LH on progesterone synthesis and secretion by the corpus luteum is mediated by an increased synthesis of cyclic AMP (Marsh *et al.*, 1966; Linder *et al.*, 1977).

If the ovum is fertilized, implantation takes place about 7 days later in the human being and almost at once the developing trophoblast secretes its luteotropic hormone, chorionic gonadotropin, into the maternal circulation, and the functional life of the corpus luteum is sustained. Chorionic gonadotropin, detectable in urine several days before the expected time of the next menstrual period, is excreted in progressively increasing amounts for the next 5 weeks or so, and in reduced quantities thereafter throughout pregnancy. During the second or third month of pregnancy the developing placenta begins to secrete estrogen and progesterone, and thereafter the corpus luteum is not essential to continued gestation. Estrogen and progesterone continue to be secreted in large amounts by the placenta up to the time of delivery.

Measurements of the rate of secretion of progesterone suggest that, from a few milligrams a day secreted during the follicular phase of the cycle, the rate increases to 10 to 20 mg during the luteal phase and to several hundred milligrams during the latter part of pregnancy (Vande Wiele *et al.*, 1960). Rates of from 1 to 5 mg per day have been measured in men, and are comparable to the values in women during the follicular phase of the cycle.

Physiological and Pharmacological Actions. Progesterone released during the luteal phase of the cycle leads to the development of a secretory endometrium. Abrupt decline in the release of progesterone from the corpus luteum at the end of the cycle is the main determinant of the onset of menstruation. If the duration of the luteal phase is artificially lengthened, either by sustaining luteal function or by treatment with progesterone, decidual changes in the endometrial stroma similar to those seen in early pregnancy can be induced. Under normal circumstances, estrogen antecedes and accompanies progesterone in its action upon the endometrium and is essential to the development of the normal pattern. When the orally active progestins were first tested and given from day 5 of the cycle for 20 days, the endometrial stroma showed intense luteal action while the glands, stimulated at first, actually became atrophic. It turned out that these patterns were caused by progestins with little or no intrinsic estrogenic activity; if estrogen was given as well, the response closely resembled the normal.

The endocervical glands are also influenced by progesterone, and the abundant watery secretion of the estrogen-stimulated structures is changed to a scant viscid material. When the estrogen-stimulated secretion dries on a glass slide, sodium chloride crystallizes to form a dendritic pattern called "ferning." Progestins inhibit this pattern.

The estrogen-induced maturation of the human vaginal epithelium is modified toward the condition of pregnancy by the action of progesterone, a change that can be detected in cytological alterations in the vaginal smear. If the quantity of estrogen concurrently acting is known to be adequate, or if it is assured by giving estrogen, the cytological response to a progestin can be used to evaluate its progestational potency.

Pregnancy. The increasing concentrations of progesterone that are present during the course of pregnancy have been discussed above. While progesterone is very important for the maintenance of pregnancy, in part because it suppresses uterine contractility, other effects may be equally important. For example, progesterone may contribute to a state of "transplantation immunity" and prevent immunological rejection of the fetus (Siiteri *et al.,* 1977). While chorionic gonadotropin was thought to play such a role by inhibiting the functions of T lymphocytes, this action is now ascribed to progesterone. The effects of progesterone to maintain pregnancy have led to the use of progestins to prevent threatened abortion. However, administration of progestins is of questionable benefit, probably because diminished progesterone is rarely the cause of spontaneous abortion (*see* below).

Mammary Gland. During pregnancy and to a minor degree during the luteal phase of the cycle, progesterone, acting with estrogen, brings about a proliferation of the acini of the mammary gland. Toward the end of pregnancy the acini fill with secretion and the vasculature of the gland is notably increased; however, only after the influences of estrogen and progesterone are withdrawn by the event of parturition does lactation begin. The action of estrogen or estrogen and progesterone, when used post partum for relieving the sensation of engorgement, is probably largely a direct one upon the mammary tissue to inhibit the effects of prolactin and the secretion of milk.

Thermogenic Action. If the body temperature is measured each day throughout the normal menstrual cycle, preferably at the same time before arising each morning, an increase of about 1° F may be noted at midcycle; this correlates with the event of ovulation. The temperature rise persists for the remainder of the cycle until the onset of menstrual flow. The phenomenon is caused by progesterone, as can be shown by giving the hormone to nonovulating women or to men. The minimal detectably effective dose of progesterone is about 5 mg once daily, and a dose of 10 or 20 mg daily is fully effective. These doses also span the range of effectiveness on the changes in the endometrium, cervix, and vagina, as discussed above. Certain progestational compounds, such as ethisterone and dydrogesterone, are not thermogenic.

Mechanism of Action. Many studies of the action of progesterone have been performed with the chick oviduct as a model tissue (*see* Chan and O'Malley, 1976). In this tissue progesterone binds to a specific cytosolic receptor with a molecular weight of 225,000 (Schrader *et al.,* 1977). The amount of this receptor protein is increased following pretreatment of animals with estrogen. Following translocation of the progesterone-receptor complex to the nucleus, the synthesis of mRNA for ovalbumin, avidin, and other proteins is markedly stimulated. The complex structure of the gene for ovalbumin has been elucidated in detail (Dugaiczyk *et al.,* 1979), and further study should reveal just how its expression is regulated.

Absorption, Fate, and Excretion. Progesterone injected in oily solution is readily absorbed but at a rate that is too rapid for optimal therapeutic efficiency. In animal tests several doses per day are more effective than the same dose once daily, and less frequent dosage is quite inefficient. Inactivation takes place largely in the liver. Many pregnane derivatives and isomers conjugated with glucuronide or sulfate are found in the urine. One of the major urinary products is the glucuronide of pregnane-3α,20α-diol. The rate of turnover of endogenous progesterone is unusually rapid, the half-life in blood being a few minutes, and doubtless exogenous material is handled in the same way. A small amount of progesterone is stored in body fat, but this is generally regarded as quantitatively unimportant. Although it is quickly disposed of, progesterone given at daily intervals in sufficient dose is thoroughly effective; its actions upon tissue continue after it has disappeared from the plasma. When progesterone is given by mouth, it is much less effective, but a similar proportion is eliminated in the urine as pregnanediol. Absorption from the intestinal tract is prompt, but the compound is rapidly transformed during passage through the liver and possibly also during absorption through the intestinal mucosa.

About 50 to 60% of administered radioactive progesterone appears in the urine and about 10% in feces. Pregnanediol in urine accounts for 12 to 15% of the progesterone metabolized. When progesterone is given for a prolonged period, during the luteal phase of the cycle or during pregnancy, a larger proportion (25 to 30%) appears in the urine as pregnanediol (*see* Fotherby and James, 1972). Pregnanediol is a notably specific product, and measurements of urinary pregnanediol provide a valuable index of the secretion and metabolism of progesterone. Approximately 1 mg per day is excreted during the follicular phase of the cycle, after menopause, and by men. During the luteal phase of the cycle 2- to 4-mg amounts are excreted daily, and during pregnancy the values increase to 50 to 70 mg before term.

Assays. Many of the new steroids are not purely estrogenic, progestational, androgenic, or anabolic but show several types of activity. No one bioassay for progesterone-like action adequately characterizes a compound, and each is modified in one way or another by the estrogenic and androgenic potencies of the material being tested; some bioassays are influenced differently from others. A great deal has been learned about the characteristics and limitations of these tests, but none yields an unequivocal estimate of progestational potency of new compounds.

Some bioassay methods are based on changes in the microscopic appearance or carbonic anhydrase activity of the endometrium of animals. Other methods are based upon the maintenance of pregnancy in oophorectomized animals or inhibition of ovulation. The reader is referred to the *fourth edition* of this textbook for a more complete description of bioassay methods used and for references. Various chemical assays for progesterone and pregnanediol are also available. As discussed earlier for estrogens, protein-binding assays and immunoassays are also available, specific, and sensitive (*see* Vande Wiele and Dyrenfurth, 1973).

Preparations. Currently, many orally active and parenteral preparations of progestational agents are available (Table 61-2). Some of these substances in combination with estrogens are used widely as oral contraceptives, which are discussed below.

Progesterone Injection, U.S.P. (GESTEROL LIPO-LUTIN, PROLUTON), contains 50 mg of progesterone per milliliter of vegetable oil. Progesterone is peculiar among the commonly used steroids in being locally irritating, and not more than about 50 mg can be given intramuscularly in a single injection; *Sterile Progesterone Suspension*, U.S.P. (GESTEROL AQUEOUS), is particularly painful and is seldom used. Progesterone is also available in a T-shaped intrauterine contraceptive device that provides continuous delivery of progesterone in the uterine cavity over 1 year. This is marketed under the name of PROGESTASERT and contains 38 mg of progesterone.

Medroxyprogesterone Acetate, U.S.P. (DEPOPROVERA), contains 100 or 400 mg/ml in aqueous medium for intramuscular injection, and *Medroxyprogesterone Acetate Tablets*, U.S.P. (PROVERA), contain 2.5 or 10 mg each.

Hydroxyprogesterone Caproate Injection, U.S.P. (DELALUTIN), is provided as an oily solution of 125 mg/ml (in sesame oil) or 250 mg/ml (in castor oil) for intramuscular injection.

Megestrol Acetate (MEGACE) is available in 20- and 40-mg tablets.

Dydrogesterone, U.S.P. (DUPHASTON, GYNOREST), is marketed as 5- and 10-mg tablets.

Norethindrone, U.S.P. (MICRONOR, NOR-Q.D., NOR-LUTIN), and *Norethindrone Acetate*, U.S.P. (NORLUTATE), are available alone in 0.35- and 5-mg tablets

and in combination with estrogens as oral contraceptives (*see* below).

A variety of other oral progestin preparations are also combined with estrogens (ethinyl estradiol or mestranol) as oral contraceptives (*see* Table 61-3, page 1440).

It is not possible to give accurate values for the relative clinical effectiveness of the several compounds because careful comparisons are limited in number and different responses have been used in the published studies. In various tests in women, as with different bioassays in animals, the relative potencies of the progestins are not the same. Furthermore, some progestins possess more or less estrogenic and androgenic activities than do others.

Therapeutic Uses. Application of physiological principles in the management of ovarian disorders and contraception has made it possible to use these new agents with notable therapeutic success.

Contraception. This undoubtedly represents the major use of these agents and is discussed later in this chapter.

Dysfunctional Uterine Bleeding. This is a common disorder, characterized by grossly irregular cycles and episodes of prolonged and sometimes exsanguinating hemorrhage. The condition may arise at any time during menstrual life, but is more frequent in young girls before regular ovulatory cycles are established and again with the approach of menopause. The condition usually results from the continuous action of estrogen, which causes endometrial hyperplasia, combined with an insufficient amount and poor cycling of progesterone. Other causes for uterine bleeding must be excluded before initiating cyclic therapy with progestins.

The immediate goal is to stop the bleeding, and the long-range aim is to regulate the cycle. Both estrogens and androgens have been used effectively, but a progestin is specific. The condition can be treated with small doses of a progestin for a few days with the aim of inducing progesterone-withdrawal bleeding and counting on the termination of this to stop the bleeding. As little as 5 mg of progesterone, injected once daily for 4 days, or a single dose of 50 mg is effective. It is much better to give an orally active progestin in full doses to stop the bleeding. Five to 10 mg of norethindrone every 4 to 6 hours will usually be effective in 24 hours, and then 5 mg twice daily can be continued for 1 or 2 weeks to give a respite from bleeding. Withdrawal bleeding at the end of treatment will, in effect, be a normal menstrual flow, usually accompanied by cramps; however, it will be self-limited in duration and, if nothing further is done, there will be a free interval of several weeks. Other progestins may also be used, but those without inherent estrogenic activity are more effective if combined with an estrogen such as 2 mg of diethylstilbestrol or 0.1 mg of ethinyl estradiol daily. To prevent a recurrence of bleeding, cyclic therapy is called for; an oral progestin, such as norethindrone, in a dose of 5 to 10 mg daily is given for 5 days at monthly intervals, beginning 20 to 25 days after the induced period. Regular menstrual periods can thus be induced for as long as one chooses. This allows time to elapse for the young patient to mature, for the premenopausal patient to age, and for many of the other patients to recover spontaneously from whatever caused the upset. There is some evidence to suggest, moreover, that cyclic therapy may exert a favorable effect upon the establishment of a normal interplay between ovary and pituitary.

Dysmenorrhea. Relief of dysmenorrhea by inhibiting ovulation is discussed under estrogen. A progestin can be used to advantage either with the estrogen from days 5 to 25 of the cycle or added to the estrogen during the last 5 days. In either case menstruation is prompt, the treatment can be resumed 5 days later, and the cycle can be repeated indefinitely. Such cycles are entirely physiological, lacking only the ovarian components and ovulation, and fertility is not usually a consideration when dysmenorrhea is the problem.

Premenstrual Tension. This is an ill-defined condition of uncertain etiology. Changes in concentrations of hormones and electrolytes are probably responsible for the irritability, breast tenderness, headache, and weight gain during the luteal phase of the cycle. Progesterone or an oral progestin may be effective when given during the last week or 10 days of the cycle. Sometimes this is not effective, and the symptoms are sufficiently distressing to warrant inhibition of ovulation with combined progestin-estrogen therapy.

Endometriosis. The severe dysmenorrhea of this condition is not completely understood. In many instances, suppression of ovulation with estrogen is followed by a painless, estrogen-withdrawal period; this suggests that the pain in the two conditions is of similar origin. Treatment of this form of endometriosis thus becomes the treatment of dysmenorrhea. In certain severe cases of endometriosis, the major problem is the development of painful extrauterine masses and infertility. Treatment is aimed at causing regression of the ectopic endometrial growths. Prolonged treatment, designed to prevent menstruation for many months, relieves a major difficulty by preventing bleeding into the endometrial masses or peritoneal cavity. Favorable effects have been achieved even with the continuous use of estrogen alone for this purpose. Better results have been described from the continuous use of oral progestins, and actual regression of the endometrial growths has been observed. In women with normal cycles, Ferin (1962) induced amenorrhea for intervals of as long as 30 months by continuous treatment with progestins. There was ovarian and pronounced endometrial regression but no adverse effects upon subsequent cycles and ovulation. Medroxyprogesterone acetate may be used in doses of 2.5 mg daily for 2 to 3 weeks, after which the dose is increased to 10 to 15 mg daily. Symptomatic relief can be expected in about 80% of patients and return of fertility in about 50% of patients (Wentz, 1977). Danazol, which is a weak androgen, is also effective for the treatment of endometriosis (*see* Chapter 62).

Threatened and Habitual Abortion. Progestins have been used extensively in attempts to prevent abortion, but there is no evidence that the treatment is effective in the majority of patients. Although the side effects from the administration of progestational agents are usually quite minimal, this does not pertain to the fetus. These agents can cause a variety of fetal anomalies, including virilization and genital deformities of male and female fetuses (Jacobson, 1962; Wentz, 1977; Aarskog, 1979). These effects should be avoided by discontinuation of progestins during pregnancy.

There are thought to be a few patients who have an inadequate luteal response to gonadotropins with deficient secretion of progesterone; such women may benefit from treatment with a progestin during the first trimester of pregnancy. To identify such patients, urinary metabolites of progesterone must be determined. The potential risks to the fetus must also be considered.

Suppression of Post-Partum Lactation. The administration of estrogens and/or progestins is effective in suppressing lactation in the immediate postpartum period as mentioned above. Significant reduction in milk secretion is seen with concentrations of estrogens and progestins contained in oral contraceptive preparations.

Endometrial Carcinoma. Progestins may be used as a palliative measure in recurrent or metastatic endometrial carcinoma. When used in this manner, megestrol acetate may be given in oral doses of 40 mg daily for several months as a trial. Alternative therapy is the weekly intramuscular administration of 400 mg of medroxyprogesterone acetate. Improvement can be expected in about one half of the patients treated (*see* Wentz, 1977).

ORAL CONTRACEPTIVES

Of drugs requiring a prescription, oral contraceptives are among the most widely used agents. It is estimated that 8 million women in the United States and 50 million worldwide are currently taking these agents. The lives of approximately half of the women in the United States between the ages of 15 and 29 are punctuated daily by the taking of a medicine for a condition from which they do not suffer—a prophylaxis for a contingency that may not materialize.

History. The incredible growth of the world population stands out as one of the fundamental events of our era. The Old Testament dictum "Be fruitful, and multiply" (Genesis 9:1) has been religiously followed by readers and nonreaders of the Bible alike. In 1798, Thomas Robert Malthus started a great controversy by opposing the prevailing view of unlimited progress for man by making two postulates and a conclusion. He postulated that "food is necessary to the existence of man," and that sexual attraction between woman and man is necessary and likely to persist, since "towards the extinction of the passion between the sexes, no progress whatever has hitherto been made," barring ". . . individual exceptions." Malthus concluded that "the power of population is infinitely greater than the power in the earth to produce subsistence for man," a "natural inequality" that would someday loom "insurmountable in the way to the perfectibility of society." Malthus' essay sparked great controversy and inquiry into the principle governing the growth of population. In seeking to discover the causes of population increase, T. R. Edmonds in 1832 suggested that "a deterioration in the condition of the English labourers . . . , the destruction of the feeling of self-respect" was such a great distress that "among the great body of the people . . . , sexual intercourse is the only gratification. . . . When they are better fed they will have other enjoyments at command than sexual intercourse, and their numbers . . . will not increase in the same proportion as at present." Today we realize that our sheer numbers have increased so much that they are straining Earth's capacity to supply food, energy, and raw materials. We also know, perhaps better than T. R. Edmonds, where some of the blame for this growth lies. Advances in medicine and public health have led to a significant decline in mortality and an increased life expectancy. Thus, medical science has begun to assume a portion of the responsibility for overpopulation. To this end, drugs in the form of hormones and their analogs have been developed to control human fertility.

A comprehensive investigation of the inhibition of ovulation by the use of progestational agents was initiated by Rock, Pincus, and Garcia in women who seemed normal in every way but who had failed to conceive. There was some basis for the rationale of inducing a kind of pseudopregnant condition in the expectation that, when treatment was stopped, fertility might be enhanced by the operation of compensatory mechanisms. That this aspect of the study met with some success was of passing interest; that the study showed that ovulation could be abolished at will for as long as desired and with great regularity was a fundamental contribution (*see* Rock *et al.,* 1957; Pincus, 1960). The compounds used were derivatives of 19-nortestosterone, given by mouth in an arbitrarily adopted schedule from day 5 to day 25 of the menstrual cycle (the first day of menses is day 1). Withdrawal bleeding occurred within a few days of completing the course, and treatment was begun again 4 days after the first day of flow. Extensive field studies were started in San Juan, Puerto Rico, in 1955, under the direction of Pincus and associates at the Puerto Rico Family Planning Center. The tablet used was ENOVID, containing 10 mg of the progestin norethynodrel and 0.15 mg of the estrogen mestranol, and it was taken daily on the same schedule. It was soon found that, when the schedule was followed, no pregnancies occurred; when tablets were allegedly missed for 1 to 5 days, some pregnancies followed but the rate was only 4% of that to be expected if no contraception were practiced. When 6 to 19 days of tablet-taking were missed, the pregnancy rate was 25% of expectation. The success of these studies prompted many others, and the results of broad, almost worldwide, experience followed (Pincus, 1965; Kistner, 1969).

Among the first of the orally active steroids to be used in inhibiting ovulation, some had inherent estrogenic activity and some preparations of the progestins were later found to be contaminated with estrogen. In a way this was a happy chance, because it served to show that estrogen enhanced the suppressive effect of the progestin and led to the general use of a mixture of the two. The substance considered to be the most likely estrogenic contaminant of norethynodrel was the 3-methyl ether of ethinyl estradiol, *mestranol,* which was therefore incorporated in ENOVID. As experience was gained, the dose of the progestin was reduced and that of the estrogen was increased without loss of contraceptive efficiency.

Types of Oral Contraceptives. The most common type of oral contraceptive is the combination preparation, which contains both an estrogen and a progestin. Experience with these preparations shows them to be so near to 100% effective that a closer estimate cannot be made. This method of reversible contraception is, then, the most effective yet devised. Other modifications of steroidal contraception have also been tried with success. *Sequential* preparations, in which an estrogen is taken for 14 to 16 days and a combination of an estrogen and a progestin is then taken for 5 or 6 days, have been about 98 to 99% successful as oral contraceptives. However, because of reports suggesting an increased incidence of endometrial tumors and a lower efficacy, sequential preparations have been removed from the market.

Single-entity preparations are also available. A progestin alone has come to be called the "minipill," while an estrogen alone is a postcoital or "morning-after pill." The "minipills" were introduced in order to eliminate the estrogen, the agent in *combined* preparations that is thought to be responsible for most if not all of the minor and major side effects of oral contraceptives. The contraceptive efficacy of the "minipill" is about 97 to 98%, which is somewhat less than that of the combined preparations, and the menstrual cycles are more irregular. The intramuscular injection of medroxyprogesterone every few months has been effective but is not approved for use as a contraceptive in the United States (FDA Drug Bulletin, 1978b). Diethylstilbestrol is effective as a postcoital contraceptive. Although its *general* use for this purpose is unpleasant and may be dangerous, postcoital contraception with an estrogen can be useful when the desirability of avoiding pregnancy is obvious, as in cases of rape or incest.

Preparations and Dosage. Some of the formulations used as oral contraceptives are listed in Table

Table 61–3. COMPOSITION AND DOSES OF SOME ORAL CONTRACEPTIVES

MG—ESTROGEN	MG—PROGESTIN	TRADE NAME
Combinations *		
0.02 Ethinyl estradiol	1 Norethindrone	LOESTRIN 1/20; ZORANE 1/20
0.03 Ethinyl estradiol	0.3 Norgestrel	LO/OVRAL
0.03 Ethinyl estradiol	1.5 Norethindrone	LOESTRIN 1.5/30; ZORANE 1.5/30
0.035 Ethinyl estradiol	0.4 Norethindrone	OVCON-35
0.035 Ethinyl estradiol	0.5 Norethindrone	BREVICON; MODICON
0.05 Mestranol	1 Norethindrone	NORINYL 1+50; ORTHO-NOVUM 1/50
0.05 Ethinyl estradiol	0.5 Norgestrel	OVRAL
0.05 Ethinyl estradiol	1 Ethynodiol diacetate	DEMULEN
0.05 Ethinyl estradiol	1 Norethindrone	OVCON-50; ZORANE 1/50
0.05 Ethinyl estradiol	1 Norethindrone acetate	NORLESTRIN, 1
0.05 Ethinyl estradiol	2.5 Norethindrone acetate	NORLESTRIN, 2.5
0.06 Mestranol	10 Norethindrone	ORTHO-NOVUM, 10 MG
0.075 Mestranol	5 Norethynodrel	ENOVID 5 MG
0.08 Mestranol	1 Norethindrone	NORINYL 1+80; ORTHO-NOVUM 1/80
0.10 Mestranol	1 Ethynodiol diacetate	OVULEN
0.10 Mestranol	2 Norethindrone	NORINYL, 2 MG; ORTHO-NOVUM, 2 MG
0.10 Mestranol	2.5 Norethynodrel	ENOVID-E
0.15 Mestranol	9.85 Norethynodrel	ENOVID 10 MG
"Minipills" †		
———	0.35 Norethindrone	MICRONOR; NOR-Q.D.
———	0.075 Norgestrel	OVRETTE
Postcoital ‡		
25 Diethylstilbestrol	———	———

* Combination tablets are taken for 20 or 21 days and off for 7 or 8 days. These preparations are listed in order of increasing content of estrogen.

† "Minipills" are taken daily continually.

‡ 25 mg twice daily for 5 days within 72 hours after sexual intercourse; *see* text for indications.

61–3. The *combined* preparations contain 0.02 to 0.15 mg of ethinyl estradiol or mestranol and various amounts of a progestin and are taken for 20 or 21 days. The next course is started 7 days after the last dose or 5 days after the onset of the menstrual flow.

Many contraceptive preparations are dispensed in convenient calendar-like containers that help the user to count the days. Some obviate the need of counting by incorporating seven blank pills in the package to provide 3 weeks of treatment and 1 week off. A pill is taken every day, regardless of when menstruation starts or stops.

The "minipills" (MICRONOR and NOR-Q.D., containing 0.35 mg of norethindrone, and OVRETTE, containing 75 µg of norgestrel) are taken daily continually. Since they are less effective and pregnancy is possible during their administration, patients should discontinue the "minipill" if they have amenorrhea for more than 60 days, and they should be examined for pregnancy. Likewise, if patients have missed one or more pills and have amenorrhea for more than 45 days, they should be similarly evaluated.

Medroxyprogesterone Acetate, U.S.P. (DEPOPRO-

VERA), is injected intramuscularly in a dose of 150 mg every 3 months but should be used only if the possibility of permanent infertility is acceptable to the patient. *Norethindrone (norethisterone) enanthate,* when administered intramuscularly in oil in a dose of 200 mg every 3 months, is also effective for contraception. Although long-acting preparations of a progestin are employed in a number of countries for contraception (*see* Vecchio, 1976), such use remains investigational in the United States.

The postcoital contraceptive diethylstilbestrol is started within 72 hours after sexual intercourse at a dose of 25 mg twice daily for 5 days. To be effective the tablets must be continued for 5 consecutive days in spite of nausea and vomiting, which commonly occur. Since estrogens are not advised in pregnancy because of the possibility of vaginal carcinoma in female offspring (*see* above), abortion should be performed if diethylstilbestrol is not effective.

Effects on Laboratory Tests. A substantial number of laboratory results may be altered by the use of oral contraceptives. These changes are, in general, due to physiological alterations in the patient, rather than to interference with the analysis. A tabulation has appeared in the Medical Letter (1979).

Mechanism of Action. The administration of estrogen and a progestin, as contained in combination preparations, could interfere with fertility in any of several ways. However, it is clear that, as currently used, the mixture inhibits ovulation. The questions then are how is ovulation prevented and what other mechanisms might interfere with impregnation. The effects of ovarian hormones upon the gonadotropic functions of the pituitary are discussed earlier in this chapter; the predominant effect of estrogen is to inhibit the secretion of FSH, while continued action of progesterone serves to inhibit the release of LH. It is clear that ovulation could be prevented either by inhibiting the ovulatory stimulus or by preventing the growth of follicles, and this accords with the experimental observations that follicular growth and ovulation can be prevented by either estrogen or progesterone given singly. The orally active progestins cannot be equated as a group with progesterone because some are inherently estrogenic, some slightly androgenic, and some purely progestational; correspondingly, their ovulation-inhibiting potentialities may be mediated in somewhat different ways.

Measurements of circulating FSH and LH show that estrogen-progestin combinations suppress both hormones. The plasma concentrations of FSH and LH are stable; early follicular FSH and midcycle FSH and LH peaks are not seen (Swerdloff and Odell, 1969; Briggs, 1976). When estrogen and progesterone are given sequentially, estrogen alone suppresses FSH but causes an irregular increase in LH; when a progestin is then given, there is a brief rise in LH followed by a sustained decline.

One might reasonably conclude that the most widely used preparations to date owe their effectiveness in inhibiting ovulation to the estrogenic component and that the progestin serves the major purpose of ensuring that withdrawal bleeding will be prompt, brief, and essentially physiological.

Even if ovulation were not prevented, it is easy to imagine that the contraceptive agents could interfere with impregnation by their direct actions upon the genital tract. It is abundantly clear from animal experiments that the endometrium must be just in the right stage of development under estrogen and progesterone for nidation to take place. It seems unlikely that implantation would be possible in the altered endometrium developed under the influence of most of the suppressants. Similarly, the abundant watery secretion of the cervix at the time of ovulation has always been regarded as essential to the well-being of the sperm and the thick tenacious mucus secreted under the influence of progesterone to be a hostile environment. Little is known of the coordinated contractions of the cervix, uterus, and Fallopian tubes that are presumed to be essential for the transport of spermatozoa to the egg and the precisely timed conveyance of the blastocyst to the uterine lumen, but probably the correct hormonal environment is essential for the execution of these important maneuvers. Although it can easily be imagined that estrogen-progestin mixtures could interfere with impregnation in these ways, there has been no opportunity to find out, because ovulation is almost always prevented when the agents are used in the usual way.

The fear that estrogen may have deleterious effects prompted the use of a *progestin alone* in various ways. Continuous administration of a progestin in sufficient dose abolishes the cycle for as long as it is given and leads to ovarian and endometrial atrophy (Ferin, 1962). Very small doses may alter the structure of the endometrium and the consistency of the cervical mucus without disrupting the cycle or inhibiting ovulation. In seeking a dose sufficient to be contraceptive but too small to inhibit the ovary, Martinez-Manautou and coworkers (1967) established that 0.5 mg of chlormadinone acetate, when given without interruption, was fully effective as a contraceptive, with some women showing evidence of ovulation. As currently administered, oral contraceptives that contain only a progestin cause variable suppression of FSH, LH, and ovulation, which may explain their lower degree of efficacy (*see* Briggs, 1976). With continued daily administration, menstruation occurs but the length of the cycle and the duration of bleeding are quite variable, factors that have influenced their popularity.

Long-acting progestins, given by intramuscular injection, are also effective, as noted above. For example, 150 mg of medroxyprogesterone acetate, administered every 3 months starting just after parturition, prevents pregnancy in all; irregular bleeding, troublesome at first, gives way to amenorrhea and an atrophic endometrium in most cases (Mishell *et al.*, 1968). This form of contraception also utilizes the highly active, purely progestational compounds by incorporating them in pessaries to provide vaginal absorption, in intrauterine devices, or in plastic capsules for subcutaneous application. An intrauterine device containing a reservoir of 38 mg of progesterone is available (*see* above) and releases progesterone continuously into the uterine cavity for 1 year. It is about as effective as other intrauterine devices (97 to 98%), and the side effects are also similar except that the incidence of ectopic pregnancies may be greater (FDA Drug Bulletin, 1978a).

The development of *postcoital* contraceptives is an intriguing subject but, unfortunately, a most difficult problem to approach. A vast number of hormones and other agents are effective in this regard in animals, but controlled experiments in women are difficult to design and still more difficult to carry out. It has long been known that the use of large doses of estrogen in women is effective in preventing implantation, but such doses are tolerated only in cases of single or very infrequent exposure. There is a rough correlation between the contraceptive potency of these substances and their estrogenic activity.

Large doses of estrogens used as postcoital contraceptives may act by inhibiting fertilization and nidation in several ways. The motility of the oviduct may be altered, the endometrium is changed, and withdrawal from the large doses of estrogens induces bleeding.

The use of prostaglandins to promote abortion is discussed in Chapter 39.

Undesirable Effects. A variety of major and minor side effects have been attributed to the use of oral contraceptives. In some instances the undesirable effects are well documented and their incidence has been determined. Of most concern are cardiovascular side effects and the induction or promotion of tumors. However, a number of possible side effects are not well substantiated. Furthermore, the incidence of some

disorders has been lowered by the use of oral contraceptives. An assessment of the risk-to-benefit ratio is essential for each patient in order to provide the most efficacious method of contraception with the least possible risk (*see* Koide and Ch'iu Lyle, 1975; Briggs, 1976; Kay, 1977).

Cardiovascular Disorders. Clinical trials in sizable groups of women had been under way for 5 years or so before side effects of any consequence were described. Instances of *thrombophlebitis,* a rare disorder in healthy young women, then began to be noted, and several reports of *thromboembolism* appeared from England (Inman and Vessey, 1968; Vessey and Doll, 1968). In the latter report it was estimated that the incidence of thrombophlebitis in young women was increased sixfold to tenfold with oral contraceptives.

These retrospective studies suffered from a statistical dilemma, because what was really studied was the incidence of medication among those with complications versus those without. Retrospective studies are also generally criticized since cause-and-effect relationships cannot be established and because biases are introduced due to the means by which information is obtained.

Because of the British reports, numerous retrospective and prospective studies have since been conducted. Although an increased incidence of thrombophlebitis was not observed by some (*see* Drill, 1972), the consensus of most reports is that the incidence of thrombophlebitis and thromboembolism is increased significantly. While there have been no differences between users of *combined* and *sequential* preparations, the incidence of thromboembolism is greater with preparations containing higher doses of estrogens (*see* Kaplan, 1978). The Coronary Drug Project Research Group (1973) also found a twofold increase in the incidence of thrombophlebitis and pulmonary embolism in *men* who received conjugated estrogens daily for 4 to 5 years.

The increase in the incidence of thromboembolism is also supported by studies with various clotting factors. Patients taking estrogens or combined oral contraceptives have been found to have accelerated blood clotting and increased blood concentrations of some clotting factors, as well as increased platelet aggregation. These effects have not been observed with preparations containing only progestin.

The incidence of cerebral and coronary thrombosis is also increased in "pill" users (Inman *et al.*, 1970). The Collaborative Group for the Study of Stroke in Young Women (1973, 1975) found an increased incidence of thrombotic and hemorrhagic strokes among women taking oral contraceptives. Similarly, in men with prostatic carcinoma the administration of diethylstilbestrol daily was associated with an increased incidence of myocardial infarction and strokes (Veterans Administration, 1967). Users of the "pill" appear to have a twofold to fivefold greater incidence of nonfatal and fatal myocardial infarction and a twofold to tenfold increase in the frequency of strokes (Mann and Inman, 1975; Mann *et al.*, 1975; Kaplan, 1978). The increased risk of myocardial infarction with use of oral contraceptives appears to be additive to other risk factors, such as age, smoking, and hypertension; this information has recently been added to oral contraceptive package inserts.

While the amalgamation and interpretation of these numerous studies are somewhat risky and mortality figures are quite variable in the age groups utilizing oral contraceptives, most agree that the morbidity and mortality from cardiovascular diseases are increased with the use of *combined* oral contraceptives (*see* Kaplan, 1978). The magnitude of the increased mortality is probably about threefold. Low-dose estrogen preparations reduce the risk but do not eliminate it.

It is widely believed that the incidence of thrombophlebitis and its complications rises during pregnancy and the post-partum period. Furthermore, increased mortality from various causes during pregnancy supports the view that the increased incidence of thromboembolic disorders with oral contraceptives is probably a comparatively minor and acceptable risk, since pregnancy is effectively prevented. Serious complications of pregnancy are perhaps so much more frequent than are those resulting from the use of oral contraceptives that the incidence of difficulties from unwanted pregnancies might be still higher if all couples switched to other methods of contraception, all of which are less effective.

Hypertension has been observed in about 5% of oral contraceptive users (Laragh, 1976). While the increase in blood pressure is usually gradual, it may be quite severe. Generally the hypertension is reversible within several months of discontinuation of medication (Weir *et al.*, 1974). These effects are also attributable to estrogen in the preparations and result from the retention of sodium and water secondary to increases in circulating concentrations of renin and angiotensin.

Cancer. Because of the numerous animal studies that demonstrate an increased incidence of several different types of tumors with estrogen, there has also been much concern that similar problems would occur in users of oral contraceptives.

As discussed above, vaginal and uterine carcinomas have apparently been caused by the use of estrogens. In addition, a number of cases of benign hepatomas have been associated with the use of oral contraceptives. While an increased incidence of endometrial carcinoma in premenopausal women receiving oral contraceptives has been suggested (Silverberg and Makowski, 1975), this preliminary report has not been confirmed. A few studies have suggested an increased incidence of breast tumors, but most have found no association of this disease with the use of oral contraceptives (*see* Leis *et al.*, 1976; Kay, 1977). The relatively few incriminating reports, despite the vast use of these agents, may reflect the latent period needed for cellular transformation. Future studies will be particularly important to resolve these questions.

Other Effects. The frequent, mild side effects—nausea, occasional vomiting, dizziness, headache, discomfort in the breasts, and gain in weight—are manifestations of early pregnancy and are attributable entirely, or nearly so, to the estrogen in the preparations. These symptoms are more frequent and may be more troublesome than the side effects in menopausal women given estrogen, probably because the contraceptives are not taken for the relief of symptoms. However, most of them are short lived or are noted only in the first cycle or two. Irregular menstrual bleeding, the so-called breakthrough bleeding, is also more frequent at first; it seems to be less troublesome with the preparations containing the larger doses of estrogen.

Many other minor disturbances have been attributed to the oral contraceptives (Koide and Ch'iu Lyle, 1975). Some symptoms, including depression of mood, easy fatigue, and lack of initiative, have been attributed to the progestin in the tablets and are less troublesome or even unnoticed with the newer preparations containing smaller amounts. An increase in female-initiated sexual activity that is said to be present at the time of ovulation is suppressed or absent in women using oral contraceptives (Adams *et al.,* 1978).

Various ocular conditions have also been reported, including corneal sensitivity, retinal thrombosis, optic neuritis, diplopia, and others. However, it has not been determined that these are in fact related to oral contraceptives. Skin rashes, photosensitivity, alopecia, and hirsutism seldom occur, but chloasma (brownish macules of the face) frequently occurs with prolonged use of most preparations. Cholestatic jaundice due to the 17-alkyl-substituted steroids in all of the preparations is rare; an increased incidence of gallbladder disease with estrogens has been reported by the Boston Collaborative Drug Surveillance Program (1974). Oral contraceptives increase the concentration of cholesterol in bile, which may provide the biochemical explanation for the increased incidence of cholelithiasis (Bennion *et al.,* 1976). Folate absorption may be decreased, but few patients develop anemia or other signs of deficiency (*see* Briggs, 1976). The impairment in glucose tolerance in some patients was discussed earlier. The resumption of spontaneous menses usually requires about 6 to 10 weeks after oral contraceptives have been discontinued. However, some patients have prolonged periods of anovulation and amenorrhea (sometimes associated with galactorrhea), requiring therapy with clomiphene, gonadotropin, or bromocriptine (*see* Chapter 59). The use of oral contraceptives may in some way provide a setting for the subsequent development of hyperprolactinemia when discontinued. Continuation of intake of oral contraceptives during pregnancy has been reported to increase congenital limb deformation, masculinization, and cryptorchism in offspring (Janerich *et al.,* 1974; Koide and Ch'iu Lyle, 1975; Rothman and Louik, 1978). Administration of oral contraceptives soon after delivery will decrease lactation and interfere with breast feeding.

In view of these considerations, it seems highly prudent to continue to evaluate each patient and her need for oral contraceptives. Clearly in some patients pregnancy is either very undesirable or contraindicated due to preexisting disease; the additional risks from oral contraceptives seem minor. However, in most patients the decision is more difficult. There are many alternative means of contraception, but none is quite as effective as oral contraceptives. For extensive population control, these agents are extremely useful and a low incidence of complications is to be expected. With the United States Supreme Court decision on abortion, the future need for a *totally* effective contraceptive method may be less urgent for some individuals.

If oral contraceptives are prescribed, preparations with lower estrogen content are generally preferred, and patients require periodic evaluation for side effects. The United States Food and Drug Administration exercises strict control over the labeling of estrogens and oral contraceptives. Contraindications to their use are thromboembolic disorders or a past history of these conditions, markedly impaired hepatic function, known or suspected carcinoma of the breast or other estrogen-dependent neoplasia, and undiagnosed genital bleeding. In addition, various warnings and precautions, as well as the possible adverse reactions outlined above, must be listed. The extent to which these possible adverse reactions should be discussed with the patient at first was left to the discretion of the physician, but now a brief description of the hazards of this form of contraception is included in each package dispensed to the patient.

Aarskog, D. Maternal progestins as a possible cause of hypospadias. *N. Engl. J. Med.,* **1979,** *300,* 75–78.

Adams, D. B.; Gold, A. R.; and Burt, A. D. Rise in female-initiated sexual activity at ovulation and its suppression by oral contraceptives. *N. Engl. J. Med.,* **1978,** *299,* 1145–1150.

Allen, E., and Doisy, E. A. An ovarian hormone: a preliminary report on its localization, extraction, and partial purification, and action in test animals. *J.A.M.A.,* **1923,** *81,* 819–821.

Antunes, C. M.; Stolley, P. D.; Rosenshein, N. B.; Davies, J. L.; Tonascia, J. A.; Brown, C.; Burnett, L.; Rutledge, A.; Pokempner, M.; and Garcia, R. Endometrial cancer and estrogen use—report of a large case-control study. *N. Engl. J. Med.,* **1979,** *300,* 9–13.

Baum, J. K.; Bookstein, J. J.; Holtz, F.; and Klein, E. W. Possible association between benign hepatomas and oral contraceptives. *Lancet,* **1973,** *2,* 926–929.

Beard, J. *The Span of Gestation and the Cause of Birth.* Gustav Fischer Verlag, Jena, **1897.**

Bennion, L. J.; Ginsberg, R. L.; Garnick, M. B.; and Bennett, P. H. Effects of oral contraceptives on the gallbladder bile of normal women. *N. Engl. J. Med.,* **1976,** *294,* 189-192.

Boston Collaborative Drug Surveillance Program. Surgically confirmed gall bladder disease, venous thromboembolism, and breast tumors in relation to postmenopausal estrogen therapy. *N. Engl. J. Med.,* **1974,** *290,* 15-18.

Butenandt, A. Über "PROGYNON," ein crystallisiertes, weibliches Sexualhormon. *Naturwissenschaften,* **1929,** *17,* 879.

Collaborative Group for the Study of Stroke in Young Women. Oral contraception and increased risk of cerebral ischemia or thrombosis. *N. Engl. J. Med.,* **1973,** *288,* 871-878.

————. Oral contraceptives and stroke in young women; associated risk factors. *J.A.M.A.,* **1975,** *231,* 718-722.

Corner, G. W., and Allen, W. M. Physiology of the corpus luteum. II. Production of a special uterine reaction (progestational proliferation) by extracts of the corpus luteum. *Am. J. Physiol.,* **1929,** *88,* 326-346.

Coronary Drug Project Research Group. The coronary drug project. Initial findings leading to modifications of its research protocol. *J.A.M.A.,* **1970,** *214,* 1303-1313.

————. The coronary drug project. Findings leading to discontinuation of the 2.5-mg/day estrogen group. *Ibid.,* **1973,** *226,* 652-657.

Curnow, D. H. Oestrogenic activity of subterranean clover. II. Isolation of genistein from subterranean clover and methods of quantitative estimation. *Biochem. J.,* **1954,** *58,* 283-287.

DeJong, F. H., and Sharpe, R. M. Evidence for inhibin-like activity in bovine follicular fluid. *Nature,* **1976,** *263,* 71-72.

Dodds, E. C.; Goldberg, L.; Lawson, W.; and Robinson, R. Oestrogenic activity of alkylated stilboestrols. *Nature,* **1938,** *142,* 34.

Doisy, E. A.; Veler, C. D.; and Thayer, S. A. Folliculin from the urine of pregnant women. *Am. J. Physiol.,* **1929,** *90,* 329-330.

————. The preparation of the crystalline ovarian hormone from the urine of pregnant women. *J. Biol. Chem.,* **1930,** *86,* 499-509.

Drill, V, A. Oral contraceptives and thromboembolic disease. I. Prospective and retrospective studies. *J.A.M.A.,* **1972,** *219,* 583-592.

Dugaiczyk, A.; Woo, S. L. C.; Colbert, D. A.; Lai, E. C.; Mace, M. L., Jr.; and O'Malley, B. W. The ovalbumin gene: cloning and molecular organization of the entire natural gene. *Proc. Natl. Acad. Sci. U.S.A.,* **1979,** *76,* 2253-2257.

FDA Drug Bulletin. PROGESTASERT IUD and ectopic pregnancy. **1978a,** *8,* 10.

————. Approval of DEPO-PROVERA for contraception denied. **1978b,** *8,* 10-11.

————. HEW recommends follow-up on DES patients. **1978c,** *8,* 31.

Ferin, J. Artificial induction of hypo-oestrogenic amenorrhea with methylestrenolone or with lynestrenol. *Acta Endocrinol. (Kbh.),* **1962,** *39,* 47-67.

Fontaine, Y.-A.; Fontaine-Bertrand, E.; Salmon, C.; and Delerue-Lebelle, N. Stimulation *in vitro* par les deux hormones gonadotropes hypophysaires (LH et FSH) de l'activité adénylcyclasique de l'ovaire chez la ratte prépubère. *C. R. Acad. Sci. [D] (Paris),* **1971,** *272,* 1137-1140.

Fraenkel, L. Die Funktion des Corpus Luteum. *Arch. Gynaekol.,* **1903,** *68,* 483-545.

Frank, R. T.; Frank, M. L.; Gustavson, R. G.; and Weyerts, W. W. Demonstration of the female sex hormone in the circulating blood. I. Preliminary report. *J.A.M.A.,* **1925,** *85,* 510.

Greenblatt, R. B.; Roy, S.; Mahesh, V. B.; Barfield, W. E.; and Jungck, E. C. Induction of ovulation. *Am. J. Obstet. Gynecol.,* **1962,** *84,* 900-909.

Greenwald, P.; Barlow, J. J.; Nasca, P. C.; and Burnett, W. S. Vaginal cancer after maternal treatment with synthetic estrogens. *N. Engl. J. Med.,* **1971,** *285,* 390-392.

Halban, J. Ueber den Einfluss der Ovarien auf die Entwicklung des Genitales. *Monatsschr. Geburtshilfe Gynäkol.,* **1900,** *12,* 496-503.

Herbst, A. L.; Ulfelder, H.; and Poskanzer, D. C. Adenocarcinoma of the vagina. Association of maternal stilbestrol therapy with tumor appearance in young women. *N. Engl. J. Med.,* **1971,** *284,* 878-881.

Hilliard, J.; Scaramuzzi, R. J.; Pang, C.-N.; Penardi, R.; and Sawyer, C. H. Testosterone secretion by rabbit ovary *in vivo. Endocrinology,* **1974,** *94,* 267-271.

Horwitz, R. I., and Feinstein, A. R. Alternative analytic methods for case-control studies of estrogens and endometrial cancer. *N. Engl. J. Med.,* **1978,** *299,* 1089-1094.

Inman, W. H. W., and Vessey, M. P. Investigation of deaths from pulmonary, coronary and cerebral thrombosis and embolism in women of childbearing age. *Br. Med. J.,* **1968,** *2,* 193-199.

Inman, W. H. W.; Vessey, M. P.; Westerholm, B.; and Engelund, A. Thromboembolic disease and the steroidal content of oral contraceptives. *Br. Med. J.,* **1970,** *2,* 203-209.

Jacobson, B. D. Hazards of norethindrone therapy during pregnancy. *Am. J. Obstet. Gynecol.,* **1962,** *84,* 962-968.

Janerich, D. T.; Piper, J. M.; and Glebatis, D. M. Oral contraceptives and congenital limb-reduction defects. *N. Engl. J. Med.,* **1974,** *291,* 697-700.

Jick, H.; Watkins, R. N.; Hunter, J. R.; Dinan, B. J.; Madsen, S.; Rothman, K. J.; and Walker, A. M. Replacement estrogens and endometrial cancer. *N. Engl. J. Med.,* **1979,** *300,* 218-222.

Kato, J.; Kobayashi, T.; and Villee, C. A. Effect of clomiphene on the uptake of estradiol by the anterior hypothalamus and hypophysis. *Endocrinology,* **1968,** *82,* 1049-1052.

Kiang, D. T.; Frenning, D. H.; Goldman, A. I.; Ascensao, V. F.; and Kennedy, B. J. Estrogen receptors and responses to chemotherapy and hormonal therapy in advanced breast cancer. *N. Engl. J. Med.,* **1978,** *299,* 1330-1334.

Kiang, D. T., and Kennedy, B. J. Tamoxifen (antiestrogen) therapy in advanced breast cancer. *Ann. Intern. Med.,* **1977,** *87,* 687-690.

Knauer, E. Die Ovarien-Transplantation. *Arch. Gynaekol.,* **1900,** *60,* 322-376.

Knowles, D. M.; Casarella, W. J.; Johnson, P. M.; and Wolff, M. The clinical, radiologic and pathologic characterization of benign hepatic neoplasms: alleged association with oral contraceptives. *Medicine (Baltimore),* **1978,** *57,* 223-237.

Lacassagne, A. Tumeurs malignes, apparues au cours d'un traitement hormonal combiné, chez des souris appartenant a'des lignées réfractaires au cancer spontané. *C. R. Soc. Biol. (Paris),* **1936,** *121,* 607-609.

Lindsay, R.; Aitken, J.; Anderson, J. B.; Hart, D. M.; MacDonald, E. B.; and Clarke, A. C. Long-term prevention of postmenopausal osteoporosis by estrogen. *Lancet,* **1976,** *1,* 1038-1040.

Loewe, S. Nachweis brunsterzeugender Stoffe im weiblichen Blute. *Klin. Wochenschr.,* **1925,** *4,* 1407-1408.

Loewe, S., and Lange, F. Der Gehalt des Frauenharns an brunsterzeugenden Stoffen in Abhängigkeit von ovariellen Zyklus. *Klin. Wochenschr.,* **1926,** *5,* 1038-1039.

McCullogh, D. R. Dual endocrine activity of the testes. *Science,* **1932,** *76,* 19-20.

Mann, J. I., and Inman, W. H. W. Oral contraceptives and death from myocardial infarction. *Br. Med. J.,* **1975,** *2,* 245-248.

Mann, J. I.; Inman, W. H. W.; and Thorogood, M. Oral

contraceptive use in older women and fatal myocardial infarction. *Br. Med. J.*, **1976**, *2*, 445–447.

Mann, J. I.; Vessey, M. P.; Thorogood, M.; and Doll, R. Myocardial infarction in young women with special reference to oral contraceptive practice. *Br. Med. J.*, **1975**, *2*, 241–245.

Marsh, J. M.; Butcher, R. W.; Savard, K.; and Sutherland, E. W. The stimulatory effect of luteinizing hormone on adenosine 3′,5′-monophosphate accumulation in corpus luteum slices. *J. Biol. Chem.*, **1966**, *241*, 5436–5440.

Martinez-Manautou, J.; Giner-Velasquez, J.; and Rudel, H. Continuous progestogen contraception: a dose relationship study with chlormadinone acetate. *Fertil. Steril.*, **1967**, *18*, 57–62.

Medical Letter. The "new" estrogens: are they safer? **1976**, *18*, 45–46.

———. Effects of oral contraceptives on laboratory test results. **1979**, *21*, 54–56.

Midgley, A. R., and Jaffe, R. B. Regulation of human gonadotropins. IV. Correlation of serum concentrations of follicle stimulating and luteinizing hormones during the menstrual cycle. *J. Clin. Endocrinol. Metab.*, **1968**, *28*, 1699–1703.

Mishell, D. R., Jr.; El-Habashy, M. A.; Good, R. G.; and Moyer, D. L. Contraception with an injectable progestin: a study of its use in postpartum women. *Am. J. Obstet. Gynecol.*, **1968**, *101*, 1046–1053.

Patterson, J. S., and Baum, M. Safety of tamoxifen. *Lancet*, **1978**, *1*, 105.

Pincus, G. Clinical effects of new progestational compounds. In, *Clinical Endocrinology I*. (Astwood, E. B., ed.) Grune & Stratton, Inc., New York, **1960**, pp. 526–531.

Recker, R. R.; Saville, P. D.; and Heaney, R. P. Effect of estrogens and calcium carbonate on bone loss in postmenopausal women. *Ann. Intern. Med.*, **1977**, *87*, 649–655.

Rigg, L. A.; Hermann, H.; and Yen, S. S. C. Absorption of estrogens from vaginal creams. *N. Engl. J. Med.*, **1978**, *298*, 195–197.

Riggs, B. L.; Jowsey, J.; Goldsmith, R. S.; Kelly, P. J.; Hoffman, D. L.; and Arnaud, C. D. Short- and long-term effects of estrogen and synthetic anabolic hormone in postmenopausal osteoporosis. *J. Clin. Invest.*, **1972**, *51*, 1659–1663.

Rosenberg, L.; Armstrong, B.; and Jick, H. Myocardial infarction and estrogen therapy in postmenopausal women. *N. Engl. J. Med.*, **1976**, *294*, 1256–1259.

Rothman, K. J., and Louik, C. Oral contraceptives and birth defects. *N. Engl. J. Med.*, **1978**, *299*, 522–524.

Ryan, K. J. Biological aromatization of steroids. *J. Biol. Chem.*, **1959**, *234*, 268–272.

Ryan, K. J., and Engel, L. L. The interconversion of estrone and estradiol by human tissue slices. *Endocrinology*, **1953**, *52*, 287–291.

Sabrinho, L. G.; Kase, N. G.; and Grint, J. A. Changes in adrenocortical function of patients with gonadal dysgenesis after treatment with estrogen. *J. Clin. Endocrinol. Metab.*, **1971**, *33*, 110–114.

Schrader, W. T.; Kuhn, R. W.; and O'Malley, B. W. Progesterone binding components of chick oviduct. Receptor subunit protein purified to apparent homogeneity from laying hen oviducts. *J. Biol. Chem.*, **1977**, *252*, 299–307.

Segal, S. J., and Thompson, C. R. Inhibition of estradiol-induced pituitary hypertrophy in rats. *Proc. Soc. Exp. Biol. Med.*, **1956**, *91*, 623–625.

Siiteri, P. K.; Febres, F.; Clemens, L. E.; Chang, R. J.; Gondos, B.; and Stites, D. Progesterone and maintenance of pregnancy: is progesterone nature's immunosuppressant? *Ann. N.Y. Acad. Sci.*, **1977**, *286*, 384–397.

Silverberg, S. G., and Makowski, E. L. Endometrial carcinoma in young women taking oral contraceptive agents. *Obstet. Gynecol.*, **1975**, *46*, 503–506.

Smith, D. C.; Prentice, R.; Thompson, D. J.; and Hermann, W. L. Association of exogenous estrogens and endometrial carcinoma. *N. Engl. J. Med.*, **1975**, *293*, 1164–1167.

Steinberger, A., and Steinberger, E. Secretion of an FSH-inhibiting factor by cultured Sertoli cells. *Endocrinology*, **1976**, *99*, 918–921.

Strobel, J. S., and Lippman, M. E. Studies of steroid hormone effects on human breast cancer cells in long-term tissue culture. In, *Hormones, Receptors, and Breast Cancer*. (McGuire, W. L., ed.) Raven Press, New York, **1978**, pp. 85–106.

Sturgis, S. H., and Albright, F. The mechanism of estrin therapy in the relief of dysmenorrhea. *Endocrinology*, **1940**, *26*, 68–72.

Swerdloff, R. S., and Odell, W. D. Serum luteinizing and follicle stimulating hormone levels during sequential and nonsequential contraceptive treatment of eugonadal women. *J. Clin. Endocrinol. Metab.*, **1969**, *29*, 157–163.

Vande Wiele, R. L.; Gurpide, E.; Kelly, W. G.; Laragh, J. H.; and Lieberman, S. The secretory rate of progesterone and aldosterone in normal and abnormal late pregnancy. *Acta Endocrinol. (Kbh.)*, **1960**, *34*, Suppl. 51, 159.

Vessey, M. P., and Doll, R. Investigation of relation between use of oral contraceptives and thromboembolic disease. *Br. Med. J.*, **1968**, *2*, 199–205.

Veterans Administration. The Veterans Administration co-operative urological research group: treatment and survival of patients with cancer of the prostate. *Surg. Gynecol. Obstet.*, **1967**, *124*, 1011–1017.

Weir, R. J.; Briggs, E.; Mack, A.; Naismith, L.; Taylor, L.; and Wilson, E. Blood pressure in women taking oral contraceptives. *Br. Med. J.*, **1974**, *1*, 533–535.

Ziel, H. K., and Finkle, W. D. Increased risk of endometrial carcinoma among users of conjugated estrogens. *N. Engl. J. Med.*, **1975**, *293*, 1167–1170.

———. Association of estrone with the development of endometrial carcinoma. *Am. J. Obstet. Gynecol.*, **1976**, *124*, 735–740.

Zondek, B. Darstellung des weiblichen Sexualhormon aus dem Harn, insbesondere dem Harn von Schwageren. *Klin. Wochenschr.*, **1928**, *7*, 485–486.

Zuckerman, S. Periodic uterine bleeding in spayed rhesus monkeys injected daily with a constant dose of oestrone. *J. Endocrinol.*, **1941**, *2*, 263–267.

Monographs and Reviews

Baker, H. W. G.; Bremner, W. J.; Burger, H. G.; deKretser, D. M.; Dulmonis, A.; Eddie, L. W.; Hudson, B.; Keogh, L. J.; Lee, V. W. K.; and Rennie, G. C. Testicular control of FSH secretion. *Recent Prog. Horm. Res.*, **1975**, *32*, 429–444.

Berendes, H. W. Association of liver tumors and cancer of the endometrium with oral contraceptive use. In, *Pharmacology of Steroid Contraceptive Drugs*. (Garattini, S., and Berendes, H. W., eds.) Raven Press, New York, **1977**, pp. 219–224.

Boyer, R. M. Control of the onset of puberty. *Annu. Rev. Med.*, **1978**, *29*, 509–520.

Briggs, M. Biochemical effects of oral contraceptives. *Adv. Steroid Biochem. Pharmacol.*, **1976**, *5*, 66–160.

Chan, L., and O'Malley, B. W. Mechanism of action of sex steroid hormones. *N. Engl. J. Med.*, **1976**, *294*, 1322–1328, 1372–1381, 1430–1437.

Erickson, G. F. Normal ovarian function. *Clin. Obstet. Gynecol.*, **1978**, *21*, 31–52.

Eskin, B. A. Sex hormones and aging. *Adv. Exp. Med. Biol.*, **1978**, *97*, 207–224.

Fotherby, K., and James, F. Metabolism of synthetic steroids. *Adv. Steroid Biochem. Pharmacol.*, **1972**, *3*, 67–165.

Franchimont, P. Pituitary gonadotropins. *Clin. Endocrinol. Metab.*, **1977**, *6*, 101–116.

Gordon, G. S. Drug treatment of osteoporosis. *Annu. Rev. Pharmacol. Toxicol.*, **1978**, *18*, 253–268.

Gorski, J., and Gannon, F. Current models of steroid hormone action: a critique. *Annu. Rev. Physiol.,* **1976,** *38,* 425–450.

Heyns, W. The steroid-binding β-globulin of human plasma *Adv. Steroid Biochem. Pharmacol.,* **1977,** *6,* 59–79.

Kalkhoff, R. K. Effects of oral contraceptive agents and sex steroids on carbohydrate metabolism. *Annu. Rev. Med.,* **1972,** *23,* 429–438.

Kaplan, N. M. Cardiovascular complications of oral contraceptives. *Annu. Rev. Med.,* **1978,** *29,* 31–40.

Kay, C. R. Oral contraceptives—the clinical perspective. In, *Pharmacology of Steroid Contraceptive Drugs.* (Garattini, S., and Berendes, H. W., eds.) Raven Press, New York, **1977,** pp. 1–24.

Kellie, A. E. The pharmacology of the estrogens. *Annu. Rev. Pharmacol.,* **1971,** *11,* 97–112.

Kistner, R. W. *The Pill: Facts and Fallacies about Today's Oral Contraceptives.* Delacorte Press, Dell Publishing Co., Inc., New York, **1969.**

Koide, S. S., and Ch'iu Lyle, K. Unusual signs and symptoms associated with oral contraceptive medication. *J. Reprod. Med.,* **1975,** *15,* 214–224.

Laragh, J. H. Oral contraceptive-induced hypertension—nine years later. *Am. J. Obstet. Gynecol.,* **1976,** *126,* 141–147.

Legha, S. S.; Davis, H. L.; and Muggia, F. M. Hormonal therapy of breast cancer: new approaches and concepts. *Ann. Intern. Med.,* **1978,** *88,* 69–77.

Leis, H. P.; Black, M. M.; and Sall, S. The pill and the breast. *J. Reprod. Med.,* **1976,** *16,* 5–9.

Linder, H. R.; Amsterdam, A.; Solomon, Y.; Tsafriri, A.; Nimrod, A.; Lamprecht, S. A.; Zor, U.; and Koch, Y. Intraovarian factors in ovulation: determinants of follicular response to gonadotropins. *J. Reprod. Fertil.,* **1977,** *51,* 215–235.

McGuire, W. L. Endocrine therapy of breast cancer. *Annu. Rev. Med.,* **1975,** *26,* 353–363.

Mahesh, V. B., and Greenblatt, R. B. Steroid secretions of the normal and polycystic ovary. *Recent Prog. Horm. Res.,* **1964,** *20,* 341–394.

Marcus, R., and Korenman, S. G. Estrogens and the human male. *Annu. Rev. Med.,* **1976,** *27,* 357–370.

Marshall, J. R. Induction of ovulation. *Clin. Obstet. Gynecol.,* **1978,** *21,* 147–162.

Naftolin, F., and Tolis, G. Neuroendocrine regulation of the menstrual cycle. *Clin. Obstet. Gynecol.,* **1978,** *21,* 17–29.

Pincus, G. *The Control of Fertility.* Academic Press, Inc., New York, **1965.**

Rock, J.; Garcia, C. M.; and Pincus, G. Synthetic progestins in the normal human menstrual cycle. *Recent Prog. Horm. Res.,* **1957,** *13,* 323–339.

Rosenfield, R. L. Role of androgens in growth and development of the fetus, child, and adolescent. *Adv. Pediatr.,* **1972,** *19,* 172–213.

Schally, A. V. Aspects of hypothalamic regulation of the pituitary gland: its implications for the control of reproductive functions. *Science,* **1978,** *202,* 18–28.

Vande Wiele, R. L., and Dyrenfurth, I. Gonadotropin-steroid interrelationships. *Pharmacol. Rev.,* **1973,** *25,* 189–207.

Vecchio, T. J. Long-acting injectable contraceptives. *Adv. Steroid Biochem. Pharmacol.,* **1976,** *5,* 1–64.

Wentz, A. C. Assessment of estrogen and progestin therapy in gynecology and obstetrics. *Clin. Obstet. Gynecol.,* **1977,** *20,* 461–482.

62 ANDROGENS AND ANABOLIC STEROIDS

Ferid Murad and Robert C. Haynes, Jr.

ANDROGENS

The testis, ovary, and adrenal cortex are responsible for the normal synthesis of androgens. An understanding of the regulation of the synthesis and secretion of androgens and of the effects of these compounds has led to their clinical use, primarily in hypogonadal conditions in men and to promote anabolism in both sexes. Additional knowledge of gonadotropic and androgenic regulation of spermatogenesis may permit the general use of these agents and their analogs as contraceptives in men in the foreseeable future.

History. The observation that castration makes the eunuch, properly credited to primitive man, ushered in the dawn of endocrinology. By the year 1771, John Hunter had induced male characteristics in the hen by transplanting testes from the cock (*see* Forbes, 1947); however, credit for the discovery that the testis is a gland of internal secretion is usually ascribed to Berthold, who in 1849 showed that the transplantation of gonads into castrated roosters prevented the typical signs of castration. This was the first published experimental evidence for the effect of an endocrine gland. However, it was not this observation but the popular belief that failure of testicular function was the cause of the symptoms of old age in men that stimulated many attempts to isolate an active testicular principle. As an example of the wide acceptance of this belief may be cited the experiments of Brown-Séquard (1889), the renowned French physiologist, who prepared a testicular extract and administered it to himself. He was convinced that he had gained in vigor and capacity for work from the treatment, but it is now known that his aqueous extract was devoid of any significant quantity of hormone.

Chemistry. The elucidation of the chemistry of the male sex hormones was made possible by the development of methods of assay. The procedure of Koch and coworkers for the determination of androgenic activity utilizing the growth response of the capon's comb was employed in the isolation of active androgenic substances from urine. The isolation of the urinary principle was first accomplished by Butenandt (1931), who by herculean effort obtained 15 mg of crystalline *androsterone* from 15,000 liters of male urine.

Following the isolation of another androgenic principle from urine (dehydroepiandrosterone—later shown to be of adrenal origin), attention next focused on the testes as the real source of male sex hormone. Active testicular extracts were first prepared as early as 1927 by Loewe, using the mammalian seminal vesicle for assay (*see* Loewe and Voss, 1930). The testicular principle was isolated in crystalline form by Laqueur and associates (*see* David *et al.*, 1935), and soon its chemical structure was elucidated and the hormone synthesized (Ruzicka and Wettstein, 1935); this substance was called *testosterone*.

Testosterone is 10 times as active as androsterone in promoting comb growth in the capon, and about 70 times as potent in its action on the seminal vesicles of castrated rats. Testosterone is the true testicular hormone, and androsterone and its androgenically inert isomer, etiocholanolone or 5β-androsterone, are its major metabolites that appear in the urine. *Androstenedione,* an intermediary metabolite, is likewise intermediate in potency between testosterone and androsterone (*see* Table 62–1).

A great many other steroids with androgenic activity soon became known; some were isolated from ovarian and adrenal tissue as well as from the testis, and numerous analogs and derivatives were prepared. Several structural modifications of the basic steroid nucleus are required for or enhance androgenic activity (*see* Mainwaring, 1977). An oxygen atom at the C 3 position and a 17-hydroxy group are required for activity. The androgenic activity of 17-ketosteroids may be a result of their conversion to 17β-hydroxysteroids in tissues. Additional methyl groups at positions 1, 7, or 17 increase biological activity significantly. X-ray crystallographic analysis indicates that the most active compounds are relatively planar, which offers an explanation for the effects of some functional groups in determination of the structure-activity relationship.

17α-Methyltestosterone is unique among 17α-substituted alkyl derivatives in retaining androgenic potency while at the same time being active when given orally. The 17α-ethyl and higher derivatives are almost inert and the 17α-ethinyl is a weak androgen but is active as a progestin. Efforts to improve upon methyltestosterone as an orally active androgen have been vigorously pursued. Fluoxymesterone, the 9α-fluoro-11β-hydroxy derivative of methyltestosterone, is more active than the parent compound in animal tests, and mesterolone, the 1-methyl derivative of dihydrotestosterone, is a potent, orally active androgen in man. Thus far, no nonsteroid androgen has been discovered.

The acetic acid ester of testosterone was found to

Table 62–1. METABOLISM OF ANDROGENS

Testosterone   Androstenedione   Androsterone   Etiocholanolone

be more potent than testosterone and to have a greatly prolonged action. As the size of the ester substituent increased, so did the duration of action. Testosterone propionate was found to be particularly potent and is still widely used in therapeutics; the cypionate (cyclopentylpropionate) and enanthate (heptanoate) esters are other long-acting preparations that are currently in use.

A great many derivatives of testosterone have also been prepared and tested in the search for compounds that might promote general body growth without having masculinizing effects. Such compounds are often called *anabolic steroids*. The degree of dissociation of the androgenic and anabolic effects with various compounds is dependent upon the bioassays used and is often a matter of debate. Testosterone itself is one of the most potent anabolic steroids, and it may be impossible to separate the two activities totally. However, it would be highly desirable to have anabolic compounds that are not androgenic, for this would permit their use in women without inducing masculinization and in children without causing undesirable effects on sexual and osseous development.

Synthesis and Secretion of Testosterone. The concentrations of testosterone are relatively high in male infants and fall to typical prepubertal levels within several months after birth (Forest *et al.*, 1973). Through poorly understood mechanisms, the pituitary begins to secrete increased amounts of luteinizing hormone (LH) and follicle-stimulating hormone (FSH) at the time of puberty. The increase in the secretion of gonadotropins begins in a cyclic fashion that is synchronized with the sleep cycle. As puberty progresses, however, pulsatile secretion of gonadotropins is observed during both sleep and waking periods (Franchimont, 1977; Boyar, 1978). At this stage of development the hypothalamus and pituitary also become less sensitive to feedback inhibition by sex hormones. The initiating event for these effects is unknown.

Prior to puberty, concentrations of testosterone in plasma are very low (0 to 20 ng/dl), although the immature testes are capable of synthesizing androgens if challenged. In the adult male, plasma testosterone concentrations rise to 0.2 to 1 μg/dl, and the rate of production is 2.5 to 11 mg per day (Rosenfield, 1972). Pathways of androgen biosynthesis are shown in Figure 61–1 (page 1421). In plasma, about 98% of testosterone is bound to sex hormone–binding globulin, cortisol-binding protein, and albumin. About 1% of the steroid is free, and this concentration correlates with the magnitude of androgenic effects (*see* Fotherby and James, 1972; Heyns, 1977; Givens, 1978).

Androgen-Gonadotropin Relationships. As mentioned, gonadotropins are secreted in a pulsatile manner. In adult men, the concentrations of LH, FSH, and testosterone in plasma fluctuate during the course of the day, while integrated daily values are constant (Naftolin *et al.*, 1973). Similar pulsations in gonadotropins are observed in women, superimposed upon the daily alterations that occur during the menstrual cycle (*see* Figure 61–2, page 1424).

LH and FSH together are responsible for increasing testicular growth, spermatogenesis, and steroidogenesis. Prolactin can also stimulate the synthesis and secretion of testosterone (Rubin *et al.*, 1976; Bartke *et al.*, 1978), but the significance of this observation is not known. All of the actions of the gonadotropins are probably mediated through cyclic adenosine 3′,5′-monophosphate (cyclic AMP) (Murad *et al.*, 1969; *see* Eik-Nes, 1971). LH, also called interstitial cell–stimulating hormone (ICSH), interacts with the interstitial (Leydig) cells of the testes to increase the synthesis of cyclic AMP and subsequently the formation of androgens from acetate and cholesterol (*see* Catt and Dufau, 1976). The precise site of stimulation of steroidogenesis by cyclic AMP in this and other tissues is unknown. While the major effects of FSH are thought to be on spermatogenesis in the seminiferous tubules and that of LH on testosterone synthesis by Leydig cells, complex interactions exist in the testis. Some studies have indicated that FSH can also enhance testosterone synthesis and can augment the activity of LH (*see* Bartke *et al.,* 1978; Ewing and Robaire, 1978). Furthermore, testosterone is required for spermatogenesis and maturation of sperm. With immunohistochemical technics, LH has been localized to Leydig and peritubular cells and FSH to tubular Sertoli cells (Castro *et al.,* 1972). The Sertoli cells of the seminiferous tubules may also produce testosterone (Lacy and Pettit, 1970). It has been speculated that the testosterone from the Sertoli cells may act locally and be particularly important for spermatogenesis, and that the hormone produced by the Leydig cells is released into the circulation. However, both LH and FSH have growth-promoting effects on the testes, and both probably regulate the synthesis of testosterone. The nonphysiological effects of human chorionic gonadotropin in the male to increase testosterone synthesis appear identical to those of LH (Dufau *et al.,* 1973).

The nature of the mechanism of feedback of the testicular secretions upon the gonadotropic function of the pituitary is a problem of continuing uncertainty. Testosterone suppresses the secretion of gonadotropins and thereby causes atrophy of both the interstitial tissue and the tubules of the normal testis. The administration of testosterone also suppresses the excessive secretion of gonadotropins in the urine in eunuchism. However, the doses of testosterone that are required to inhibit gonadotropin secretion seem to be larger than one might expect. Implantation of testosterone in the median eminence of rats inhibits pituitary gonadotropin secretion (*see* Davidson, 1969) by decreasing the level of gonadotropin-releasing hormone (LH-RH/FSH-RH) (Schally, 1978).

Other work has shown that certain testicular extracts devoid of androgenic activity also suppress gonadotropin, suggesting that there are other testicular products that serve a regulatory function. Because estrogens are produced in the testis and are potent inhibitors of gonadotropin secretion (*see* Chapter 61), an estrogen is a candidate. In normal men, the concentrations of estradiol and estrone in the spermatic vein exceed those in peripheral plasma

(Kelch *et al.,* 1972; Longcope, 1972). Indeed, other studies have indicated that the testis is the major source of estradiol in men (Saez *et al.,* 1972; Armstrong and Dorrington, 1977). However, estrogens are also synthesized from testosterone elsewhere in the body (*see* Marcus and Korenman, 1976), and experimental evidence suggests that estrogens formed from *administered* or *endogenous* androgen may be responsible for the inhibition of gonadotropin secretion that results. Mesterolone is a potent androgen that is methylated at C 1 on the saturated A ring and thus cannot be aromatized to an estrogen. Mesterolone does not suppress the secretion of gonadotropins in men unless very large amounts are given. Oral doses of 30 mg daily are androgenically effective, but doses as high as 150 mg daily influence neither the size nor the microscopic appearance of the testis (Laschet *et al.,* 1967b; Petry *et al.,* 1968). Similarly, oxandrolone (Table 62–3, page 1458), given to normal men in high doses, does not reduce the seminal volume or the sperm count; this compound also cannot be aromatized to an estrogen. Findings such as these suggest that the feedback effect of the testicular secretion on the gonadotropic function of the pituitary is not mediated as much by androgen as by one of its metabolites, estrogen.

A nonsteroidal substance that inhibits the secretion of FSH has also been isolated from testicular extracts (McCullagh, 1932; Keogh *et al.,* 1976). This material, called *inhibin,* has a molecular weight of approximately 20,000. Inhibin has also been detected in extracts from cultures of Sertoli cells and in ovarian follicular fluid (DeJong and Sharpe, 1976; Steinberger and Steinberger, 1976). The physiological significance of inhibin as a feedback regulator of the secretion of gonadotropins is currently unknown.

Ovarian and Adrenal Androgens. Androgens and androgenic precursors are also normally secreted by the ovary and the adrenal cortex. Dehydroepiandrosterone is a weak androgen and a precursor for estrogen that is secreted by the ovary and adrenal. However, androstenedione, which is also produced by the ovary and adrenal, is converted in peripheral tissues to testosterone. The daily rate of production of testosterone in women is about 0.5 mg, and about one half of this is derived from the metabolic conversion of androstenedione to testosterone (*see* Sommerville and Collins, 1970; Rosenfield, 1972; Givens, 1978). However, the remainder is derived from testosterone produced and secreted by the ovary. Studies with rabbit ovary *in vivo* and *in vitro* have demonstrated synthesis and secretion of testosterone, which are enhanced by the administration of LH (Mills and Savard, 1972; Hilliard *et al.,* 1974).

Alterations in plasma concentrations of

testosterone and androstenedione are observed in women during the menstrual cycle. The concentration of testosterone in plasma of women is about 15 to 65 ng/dl. Two peaks of androgen concentration are seen that are qualitatively similar to those of the estrogens at the preovulatory and luteal phases of the cycle (Judd and Yen, 1973). In some ovarian disorders, such as the Stein-Leventhal syndrome, ovarian secretion of androgens may be markedly increased, resulting in virilization.

In men about 10% of the androgen production is from the adrenal cortex. This amount is not sufficient to maintain spermatogenesis or secondary sexual features of the adult male. However, as discussed in Chapter 61, the androgens secreted by the ovary and adrenal cortex probably have physiological significance in women. In abnormal conditions such as the adrenogenital syndrome, the adrenal cortex can secrete large quantities of steroids and androgenic precursors due to a defect in steroid hydroxylation.

Physiological and Pharmacological Actions. The normal function of androgen in man is familiar to everyone in the remarkable changes of *puberty* that transform the boy into a man. Minimal androgen secretion from the infantile-sized prepuberal testis and adrenal cortex suppresses secretion of gonadotropins until, at a variable age, secretion of gonadotropins breaks out of restraints and the testis starts to enlarge (*see* Franchimont, 1977; Boyar, 1978). Shortly thereafter the penis and scrotum begin to grow and pubic hair appears. Early in puberty penile erections and masturbation become frequent in most individuals. Almost simultaneously the remarkable growth-promoting property of androgen is revealed in rapid increase in height and the development of the skeletal musculature, which contributes to a rapid increase in body weight. As the muscles grow there is increased physical vigor, which probably becomes maximal at the end of puberty or shortly thereafter. The testes reach adult proportions before all the changes of puberty are completed. As a result of the actions of androgens, the skin becomes thicker and tends to be oily because of a proliferation of sebaceous glands; the latter are prone to infection, leading to acne

in some individuals. Subcutaneous fat is lost, and the veins are prominent under the skin. Axillary hair grows, and hair on the trunk and limbs develops into a pattern typical of the male. Growth of the larynx causes difficulty at first in adjusting the tone of speech and later brings about a permanent deepening of the voice. Growth of beard lags well behind the other events of puberty and is the last of the secondary sex characteristics to develop. Concurrently, those whose inheritance so dictates show the first signs of growing bald, with recession of the hairline at the temples and thinning of the hair at the crown. At about this time the major spurt in growth comes to an end as the epiphyses of the larger long bones begin to unite, and over the next few years only 1 to 2 cm of additional growth is usual.

It is also thought that androgens are responsible for the aggressive and sexual behavior of males (*see* Lunde and Hamburg, 1972; Horn, 1977). However, this is an area of controversy, and some believe that behavior is predominantly acquired and not biologically determined. While this is a difficult matter to resolve, the differential behavioral patterns of many male and female animals suggest that sex hormones play an important role. Further, the sexual behavior of female rats is changed to that characteristic of males after treatment with testosterone, either as neonates or as adults (Sachs *et al.*, 1973).

When androgen is given before puberty or to a young eunuchoid man, its actions begin almost at once. The skin darkens, and there is also a dusky reddening of the scrotum and adjoining genital region. Within 1 or 2 days of the start of treatment erections appear, which become embarrassingly inappropriate and frequent even to the point of discomfort; with continued treatment at the same dose this response subsides. Increased muscular strength and physical vigor are noted within a few days, and a general feeling of well-being prevails. Within a few weeks a distinct change in the voice can be noted, and soon thereafter the penis begins to grow and traces of axillary and pubic hair appear. The striking effects on growth are expressed. The rapidity of growth is impressive; the height may increase 10 cm or more during the first year and continue at a somewhat diminished rate for 2 or 3 years. With continued treatment, development follows the course of normal puberty with the growth of a beard as the final expression of therapy.

Hypogonadism Due to Failure of Puberty. The normal actions of androgens are also displayed by the consequences of deficiency. If the testes fail to function or are removed in boyhood, there is no puberty. Failure of testicular development may result from the deficiency of gonadotropins or may represent a primary testicular defect. A boy so afflicted continues to grow and becomes abnormally tall; the hands and feet become especially large and the limbs unduly long. The childish appearance and demeanor are in striking contrast to the stature; the larynx does not grow, leaving the voice high pitched. The skeletal musculature is underdeveloped and is made still more inconspicuous by a layer of subcutaneous fat. Accumulation of fat is especially prominent around the shoulders and breasts and over the upper thighs, hips, and abdomen, the whole giving the mistaken impression of femininity. Familial baldness does not appear, the beard is scant or nonexistent, the axillary and pubic hair is very sparse, and the body hair is short and fine. The genitalia are those of a child, and there is no sexual drive.

Hypogonadism after Puberty. Some of the sexual characteristics developed during puberty are self-sustaining, while others must be supported by the continued action of androgen. Hypogonadism in the adult is typified by castration after puberty. The general bodily proportions remain the same, the penis does not shrink, the voice does not change, and the beard and body hair remain unchanged for a long time. Libido and potency are greatly reduced or annihilated, and the oft-quoted exceptions to this generalization are misleading. The prostate and seminal vesicles are atrophic, and the volume of the semen is very small or there is none at all.

Complete failure of the endocrine function of the testis in adult life is not a common event; a partial deficiency is more usual, and it often originates from incomplete development at puberty (*see* Odell and Swerdloff, 1978). As mentioned earlier, testicular function commonly decreases with age; generally this occurs at a slow rate after the sixth or seventh decade, and alterations in sexual characteristics are minimal or unapparent. The decrease in libido in some men after age 40 or 50 usually cannot be attributed to altered testicular function.

Actions on the Testis and Accessory Structures. As early as fetal life, testicular androgens begin to be secreted and express their important role in the differentiation and development of the reproductive tract. Lack of androgens in the male fetus results in the acquisition of female sex structures (Jost, 1971). In the genotypic male, the Y chromosome is crucial for testicular development, which in turn determines that of accessory features of the male phenotype. In the pres-

ence of the developing testes and a protein that they produce (Müllerian regression factor), the Müllerian ducts of the fetus degenerate (Josso *et al.*, 1975). Subsequently, under the influence of testosterone, each of the Wolffian ducts differentiates into the epididymis, vas deferens, and seminal vesicle; the penis and scrotum also develop. While differentiation of the external genitalia can be influenced by exogenous androgens, local endogenous testosterone appears to be important for differentiation of the Wolffian ducts. During the latter part of pregnancy fetal androgens begin to decline, and several months after birth they become essentially undetectable (*see* Rosenfield, 1972).

At puberty and thereafter androgens exert a direct effect upon the testis, at least in certain species. Following hypophysectomy in the rat, shrinkage of the testis is slowed by the injection of androgen and spermatogenesis is maintained for a long time. This peculiar effect is also revealed by the biphasic response of the normal animal to androgen; moderate doses produce atrophy of the testis through suppression of gonadotropins, while with larger doses the atrophy is less because of the direct sustaining effect upon the seminiferous tubules.

Androgens are required not only for spermatogenesis in the seminiferous tubules but also for the maturation of sperm in their passage through the epididymis and vas deferens. These processes are highly ordered and complex, and the nature of the effects of testosterone thereon is unknown. Studies of these events are obviously complicated by the 10 weeks required for spermatogenesis in men and the several weeks needed for passage of sperm through the vas deferens and for maturation.

In fetal, prepuberal, and puberal life the actions of testosterone result in growth of the clitoris or penis. Androgens are also required for the growth and function of the seminal vesicle and prostate. At the least these structures act as a reservoir for and sources of secretions that are added to semen.

Anabolic Effects. The nitrogen-retaining effect was first measured in castrated dogs injected with androgen-containing extracts from the urine of normal men (Kochakian and Murlin, 1935). Papanicolaou and Falk (1938) showed that the skeletal muscles of male guinea pigs are much larger than those of the female, and that the difference is abolished by removal of the testes. Injection of testosterone propionate into the female or the castrated male caused pronounced muscular development. The large muscles of the male represent a sexual character dependent upon androgen for its expression, and these agents are sometimes abused by athletes for this purpose. If this is done during adolescence, premature closure of epiphyses and ultimate short stature are likely (*see* below). Hypertrophy of the musculature in response to testosterone obviously requires retention of nitrogen and other elements; protein synthesis is increased.

The anabolic effects of androgen were carefully investigated by Kenyon and associates (*see* Knowlton *et al.,* 1942). The effects were more pronounced in hypogonadal men, in boys before puberty, and in women than in normal men. A maximally effective dose of 25 mg of testosterone propionate daily caused an average retention of nitrogen of 63 mg/kg daily in hypogonadal men. There was also retention of potassium, sodium, phosphorus, sulfur, and chloride associated with a gain in weight, which could be accounted for by the water held in association with the retained salts and protein. When the administration of androgen was stopped, sodium, chloride, and water were quickly lost from the body, phosphorus and potassium were lost less rapidly and completely, and the stored nitrogen was retained for weeks. The relatively small dose of 5 mg of testosterone propionate daily also was effective. The nitrogen retained was about half that observed after 25 mg daily. The daily dose of 5 mg was not accompanied by conspicuous effects on sexual development.

Estradiol benzoate in the large dose of 5 mg daily exerts anabolic effects similar to those observed after an equal dose of testosterone propionate (*see* Chapter 61). Progesterone, on the other hand, is mildly *catabolic;* daily doses of 50 or 100 mg, given intramuscularly, cause a slightly negative balance of nitrogen and a loss of salt in normal men and women (Landau *et al.,* 1955).

While many of the newer steroids used for their anabolic effects have been carefully studied in animals, their anabolic potency compared to testosterone in man is largely unknown. Furthermore, their androgenic activity in man has not been determined with any degree of accuracy. The problem would be simplified if there were some rapid and simple indicators of the actions of androgens.

Effects on Sebaceous Glands. The preva-

lence of acne at puberty and during treatment with androgens is related to the growth and secretion of the sebaceous glands. The effect is specific for androgens. Methyltestosterone is active in doses as small as 5 mg daily, while a dose of 2.5 mg daily of fluoxymesterone has variable effects. However, these effects are not seen in adult males, whose glands are apparently maximally stimulated. When acne results from endogenous androgenic stimulation, estrogens will ameliorate this condition, probably by decreasing the secretion of gonadotropins and androgen (*see* Ebling, 1970; Chapter 61).

Mechanism of Action. At most sites of action, testosterone is not the active form of the hormone. It is converted by a 5α-reductase in most target tissues to the more active dihydrotestosterone (*see* Liao and Fang, 1969; Wilson and Gloyna, 1970). In one form of male pseudohermaphroditism the target tissues are deficient in the reductase. In this disorder the genotypic male secretes normal amounts of testosterone from the testes, but the hormone is not converted to dihydrotestosterone and the external genitalia fail to develop (Walsh *et al.,* 1974; Imperato-McGinley *et al.,* 1979).

Not all target tissues require the conversion of testosterone to dihydrotestosterone for activity. Androgenic and anabolic effects in skeletal muscle, bone marrow, and some other tissues are mediated by either testosterone or some metabolite other than dihydrotestosterone (*see* Mainwaring, 1977; Givens, 1978; Odell and Swerdloff, 1978). The effects of testosterone to suppress the secretion of gonadotropin-releasing hormone and gonadotropins may result from its conversion to estrogen or perhaps dihydrotestosterone (Naftolin *et al.,* 1975; Juneja *et al.,* 1977).

Dihydrotestosterone binds to a cytoplasmic protein receptor and is transferred to the nucleus; increased RNA polymerase activity and increased synthesis of specific RNA and protein result. As in other steroid-sensitive cells, the modification and translocation of the steroid-receptor complex and the alterations in the synthesis of nucleic acids and protein that occur are complex and incompletely understood (*see* Mainwaring, 1977). In another type of male pseudohermaphroditism, the genotypic male with normal amounts of testosterone undergoes feminine development because of an absence of the receptor protein for dihydrotestosterone (Wilson *et al.*, 1974).

Since skeletal muscle does not contain specific receptors for androgens, it has been proposed that the anabolic effects of androgens in muscle may result from their competition for cytosolic receptor for glucocorticoids (Mayer and Rosen, 1975). If this is true, the catabolic effects of glucocorticoids in muscle could be prevented with androgens without the need for conversion of the latter to active metabolites. Such studies suggest that it may be possible to develop anabolic agents with little ability to cause virilization.

Absorption, Metabolism, and Excretion. Testosterone injected as a solution in oil is so quickly absorbed, metabolized, and excreted that the androgenic effect is small. Testosterone given by mouth is readily absorbed, but is even less effective, since most of the hormone is metabolized by the liver before reaching the systemic circulation. The testosterone esters are much less polar and, when injected intramuscularly in oil, greatly favor the lipid phase and are absorbed much more slowly. Testosterone propionate is much more active than testosterone even when each is injected every day, and the ester produces a steady effect when injected at 2- or 3-day intervals. The cypionate and enanthate esters are fully effective when given at 1- or 2-week intervals in proportionately larger doses. Suspensions of testosterone esters in aqueous media are effective and long acting, but they sometimes cause local irritation and the rate of absorption may not always be uniform. Densely compacted pellets of testosterone implanted under the skin are an efficient source from which a steady rate of absorption continues for a long time; the last remnants may not disappear for 6 to 8 months. Some success in clinical trials has also been gained with subcutaneous implantation of silicone-rubber (SILASTIC) capsules containing testosterone to provide prolonged, continuous release of the hormone (*see* Segal, 1973).

As mentioned earlier, about 99% of testosterone in plasma is bound to protein—mostly to sex hormone–binding globulin (testosterone-estradiol–binding globulin) and smaller amounts to albumin and cortisol-binding protein (transcortin) (*see* Marcus and Korenman, 1976; Heyns, 1977; Givens, 1978). Thus, the concentration of the sex hormone–binding globulin determines the concentration of free testosterone in plasma and thereby its half-life, which is generally 10 to 20 minutes. Testosterone decreases the rate of hepatic synthesis of sex hormone–binding globulin, while estrogens increase its synthesis. For this reason the concentration of the globulin in females is about twice that in males. In disorders characterized by excess synthesis of androgens, the free concentration of the hormone may be increased disproportionately as a result of diminished synthesis of sex hormone–binding globulin.

Testosterone is inactivated primarily in the liver. Metabolism to androstenedione involves oxidation of the 17-OH group; reduction of ring A leads to formation of androstanedione, with markedly reduced activity. The 3-keto group is reduced to form androsterone and its isomer etiocholanolone (Table 62–1); the 17-keto group is further reduced to form androstanediol (*see* Fotherby and James, 1972, and references therein).

Alkylation of androgens at the 17 position markedly retards their hepatic metabolism and permits such analogs to be effective orally. However, they are generally less efficacious than parenteral preparations. Another disadvantage is that the 17-α-alkyl androgens can cause hepatotoxicity (*see* below).

After the administration of radioactive testosterone, about 90% of the radioactivity appears in the urine; 6% appears in the feces after undergoing enterohepatic circulation. Urinary products include primarily androsterone and etiocholanolone. Small amounts of androstanediol and estrogens are also excreted. These steroids are in the form of glucuronide and sulfate conjugates.

Androsterone and etiocholanolone, among many other compounds, are measured as *17-ketosteroids* in the usual clinical tests, but the major fraction of the ketosteroids of urine consists of metabolic products of secretions of the adrenal cortex. About 30% of urinary 17-ketosteroids are derived from metabolism of testicular hormones. Thus, measurement of the excretion of 17-ketosteroids is a poor test for the functional activity of the testis and is a much better index of adrenocortical function. Low values point to adrenal insufficiency rather than to hypogonadism, and high values almost always are indicative of adrenocortical hyperactivity or tumor. Without the testes, the human male is nearly depleted of androgen even though the urinary 17-ketosteroids may be within the normal range. In women, if pronounced virilization is associated with normal or nearly normal excretion of ketosteroids, an ovarian tumor producing testosterone is likely, whereas high values point to an adrenocortical origin of the disorder.

The esters of testosterone are metabolized in much the same way as is testosterone itself, but other changes in the molecule (as in methyltestosterone and fluoxymesterone) alter the course of metabolic degradation. Such synthetic androgens are metabolized to a lesser degree than is testosterone and have longer half-lives. Unaltered compounds, metabolites, and conjugates are excreted in the urine and feces (Fotherby and James, 1972).

Assays. Androgens used in therapeutics are pure substances, and the doses are measured by weight. Bioassay is used in the evaluation of androgenic potency of new compounds and of compounds used primarily as progestins or for their anabolic effect. The classical assay based upon the growth of the comb of the capon is still used.

Better correlation with clinical effectiveness is given by bioassays in mammals, and the most widely used test depends upon the growth of the seminal vesicles or ventral prostate of the castrated rat.

In clinical laboratories, the use of sex hormone–binding globulin as well as sensitive and specific radioimmunoassays (*see* James *et al.*, 1977) offers several advantages over bioassay methods; the more notable are simplicity, sensitivity, and lower cost.

Bioassay for Anabolic Potency. The search for nonandrogenic anabolic steroids has made use of assays employing the growth of the kidney or levator ani muscle of castrated animals. Another test for anabolic activity involves examination of nitrogen excretion and the nitrogen-retaining effects of agents given to animals on controlled diets (*see earlier editions* of this textbook for references). Unfortunately, none of these assays is totally satisfactory and able to predict the results obtained in clinical trials.

Preparations and Dosage. Some of the preparations of androgens available for clinical use are summarized in Table 62–2. Additional, little-used esters of testosterone (phenylacetate, ketolaurate) are also available.

Androgen therapy is used primarily in androgen-deficient males for the development or maintenance of secondary sexual characteristics. When full replacement therapy with androgen is required, the intramuscular preparations are the most effective. Dosage should provide at least 10 mg per day; with testosterone propionate this is met by giving 25 mg three times weekly. With the longer-acting esters, which may be somewhat less efficient, the dose is about 200 mg every 2 weeks. Long-term treatment

with these doses may not cause full masculine development; there may still be remnants of a eunuchoid habitus, poorly developed muscles, and a sparse beard.

Preparations Used for Their Anabolic Effects. Some of these preparations are summarized in Table 62–3. These compounds have been introduced primarily for use as anabolic agents with the expectation that they would be relatively less androgenic than testosterone and its close relatives. None is free of androgenic activity in man. Some have come to be used primarily as androgens, and many have been applied in the palliative treatment of carcinoma of the breast. The small doses recommended for some of the compounds have detectable anabolic activity without noticeable androgenic effects.

Various mixtures of androgenic and anabolic steroids with estrogens, vitamins, and other agents are also available. However, the use of these fixed-dose combinations is to be discouraged. In particular, their prolonged use in postmenopausal women and geriatric patients is costly and usually irrational.

Untoward Effects. When used in women, all the androgens carry the risk of causing masculinization. Among the earliest of the undesirable manifestations are acne, the growth of facial hair, and hoarsening or deepening of the voice. Menstrual irregularities will occur if gonadotropin secretion is suppressed. If treatment is discontinued as soon as these are noticed, they slowly subside. With continued treatment, as in the use of androgen in mammary carcinoma, there may also develop the male pattern of baldness, excessive body hair, prominent musculature and veins, and hypertrophy of the clitoris. With prolonged treatment many of these effects, including the deepening of the voice, are irreversible. During initial androgen-replacement therapy in hypogonadal males, sustained and painful erections (*priapism*) are commonly seen. This effect subsides with continued therapy at the same or lower doses of androgen.

Serious disturbances of growth and of sexual and osseous development can occur when androgens are given to children. The effects of androgens to enhance epiphyseal closure in children may persist for as long as several months after discontinuation of the drug. Anabolic agents should be used with great care in children.

Edema. Retention of water in association with sodium chloride appears to be a constant sequel to the administration of androgen and accounts for a portion of the gain in weight, at least in short-term treatment. In

Table 62-2. SOME ANDROGENIC STEROIDS USED IN THERAPY

NONPROPRIETARY NAME AND SOME TRADE NAMES	CHEMICAL STRUCTURE	DOSAGE FORMS (*Usual Dosage for Androgen Deficiency*) *
Testosterone, U.S.P. ANDROID-T ORETON		Aqueous suspension: 25, 50, and 100 mg/ml for i.m. use (50 mg three times weekly) Pellets: 75 mg for s.c. use (300 mg every 4 to 6 months)
Testosterone Propionate, U.S.P. ORETON PROPIONATE	$O-COCH_2CH_3$	Tablets: 10 mg (buccal; 10 to 20 mg daily) Oily solution: 25, 50, and 100 mg/ml for i.m. use (25 mg two to four times weekly)
Testosterone Enanthate, U.S.P. DELATESTRYL	$O-CO(CH_2)_5CH_3$	Oily solution: 100 and 200 mg/ml for i.m. use (100 to 400 mg every 2 to 4 weeks)
Testosterone Cypionate, U.S.P. DEPO-TESTOSTERONE	$O-COCH_2CH_2-$	Oily solution: 50, 100, and 200 mg/ml for i.m. use (100 to 400 mg every 2 to 4 weeks)
Methyltestosterone, U.S.P. METANDREN ORETON METHYL	OH CH_3	Tablets: 5, 10, and 25 mg (buccal: 5 to 25 mg daily) Capsules: 10 mg (10 to 50 mg daily)
Fluoxymesterone, U.S.P. HALOTESTIN ORA-TESTRYL	OH CH_3 HO F	Tablets: 2, 5, and 10 mg (2 to 30 mg daily)
Danazol, U.S.P. DANOCRINE	OH $C\equiv CH$	Capsules: 200 mg (200 to 800 mg daily)

* Dosage schedules for breast carcinoma in females are generally two to three times those for androgen replacement.

1456

Table 62-3. SOME ANABOLIC STEROIDS USED IN THERAPY

NONPROPRIETARY NAME AND SOME TRADE NAMES	CHEMICAL STRUCTURE	DOSAGE FORMS (*Usual Dosage for Anabolic Effects*)
Calusterone METHOSARB		Tablets: 50 mg (200 mg daily for breast carcinoma)
Dromostanolone Propionate, U.S.P. DROLBAN		Oily solution: 50 mg/ml for i.m. use (100 mg three times weekly for breast carcinoma)
Ethylestrenol MAXIBOLIN		Elixir: 2 mg/5 ml Tablets: 2 mg (4 to 8 mg daily)
Methandriol ANABOL		Aqueous and oily solutions: 50 mg/ml for i.m. use (50 to 100 mg once or twice weekly)
Methandrostenolone, U.S.P. DIANABOL		Tablets: 2.5 and 5 mg (5 mg daily)
Nandrolone Decanoate, U.S.P. DECA-DURABOLIN		Oily solution: 50 and 100 mg/ml for i.m. use (50 to 100 mg every 3 to 4 weeks)
Nandrolone Phenpropionate, U.S.P. DURABOLIN		Oily solution: 25 and 50 mg/ml for i.m. use (25 to 50 mg weekly)

Table 62–3. SOME ANABOLIC STEROIDS USED IN THERAPY (Continued)

NONPROPRIETARY NAME AND SOME TRADE NAMES	CHEMICAL STRUCTURE	DOSAGE FORMS (*Usual Dosage for Anabolic Effects*)
Oxandrolone, U.S.P. ANAVAR		Tablets: 2.5 mg (5 to 10 mg daily)
Oxymetholone, U.S.P. ADROYD ANADROL		Tablets: 5, 10, and 50 mg (5 to 15 mg daily; as much as 50 to 100 mg daily for anemia)
Stanozolol, U.S.P. WINSTROL		Tablets: 2 mg (6 mg daily)
Testolactone, U.S.P. TESLAC		Tablets: 50 and 250 mg (150 mg daily) Aqueous suspension: 100 mg/ml for i.m. use (100 mg three times weekly for breast carcinoma)

the doses used to treat hypogonadism, retention of fluid usually does not lead to detectable edema, but edema may become troublesome when large doses are given in the treatment of neoplastic diseases. Water and electrolyte retention is undesirable in patients with heart failure or in patients prone to edema from some other cause, such as cirrhosis of the liver, renal disease, or hypoproteinemia. Edema may limit the use of large doses of androgen for their anabolic effects in states of malnutrition. Salt and water retention from androgens responds to the administration of natriuretics.

Jaundice. Methyltestosterone was the first of a number of therapeutic agents discovered to cause cholestatic hepatitis. Jaundice is the prominent clinical feature, and the underlying disturbance is stasis and accumulation of bile in the biliary capillaries of the central portion of the hepatic lobules, without obstruction in the larger ducts. The contiguous hepatic cells exhibit only minor histological changes and remain viable. Steroids with a 17α-methyl substituent are particularly apt to cause it, but other androgens do not cause jaundice (*see* Tables 62–2 and 62–3). Alterations in various tests of hepatic function can occur, including increases in the concentration of bilirubin and the activities of glutamic-oxaloacetic transaminase and alkaline phosphatase in the plasma and reduced elimination of sulfobromophthalein. The response is clearly dependent on dose and becomes a frequent complication when very large amounts are given, as for palliation in neoplastic diseases. With 17α-methyl-19-nortestosterone, for example, given in doses of 30 mg daily, some increase in circulating bilirubin is an almost constant finding. Since these derivatives have long half-lives, it has become common practice in the use of the 17α-substituted steroids to give short courses of treatment of 3 or 4 weeks each, interrupted by drug-free intervals of similar length. If possible, their use should be avoided in patients with liver disease.

Hepatic Carcinoma. Patients who have received androgens and anabolic steroids for prolonged periods may develop hepatic adenocarcinoma (Bernstein *et al.,* 1971; Johnson *et al.,* 1972; Henderson *et al.,* 1973). All the patients described had received 17-alkyl derivatives for aplastic anemia for 1 to 7 years.

Impotence and Azoospermia. While androgens are required for spermatogenesis and may maintain spermatogenesis for prolonged periods in animals after hypophysectomy, continued use of androgens may result in azoospermia due to inhibition of gonadotropin secretion and conversion of androgens to estrogens. After administration of 25 mg of testosterone propionate daily for 6 weeks, spermatogenesis declines. Anabolic steroids may produce the same effect, and since they can also suppress endogenous production of testosterone, they can lead to impotence after their withdrawal.

Local Irritation. Buccal and sublingual preparations may result in stomatitis, and implantation of androgen-containing pellets may produce localized inflammation.

Urinary Obstruction. In some adult men who have been androgen deficient for a long time, the administration of androgens may increase the size of the prostate and cause urinary obstruction. However, this effect is uncommon. The use of androgens in patients with prostatic carcinoma is contraindicated.

Steroid Fever. The increase in body temperature that follows intramuscular administration of etiocholanolone, a major metabolite of testosterone, is probably the result of an intense local inflammatory reaction. This effect is less prominent in females because of antagonism by estrogen (Wolff *et al.,* 1973) and can be diminished by administration of hydrocortisone, which decreases the local inflammation, at the same site. The part played by etiocholanolone and other steroids in various febrile states is unsettled.

Effects on Laboratory Tests. Androgens can decrease the concentration of thyroid-binding globulin in plasma and thereby influence thyroid function tests, increase the excretion of 17-ketosteroids, alter plasma cholesterol, and increase the hematocrit. Alterations in tests of hepatic function are discussed above.

Therapeutic Uses. The clearest therapeutic indication for the androgens is deficient endocrine function of the testes. Their use as anabolic agents, although of much wider potential application, is fraught with uncertainties and difficulties.

Hypogonadism. Failure of the testis to secrete androgen usually cannot be recognized in childhood and is first to be seriously considered when the changes of puberty seem to be delayed. However, there is some evidence that cryptorchism may be associated with primary testicular defects and eventual androgen deficiency.

The age of onset of puberty varies widely among individuals, and, when there is no evidence of maturation at age 15 to 17, there may be great concern on the part of the patient and his parents. There is a good deal of debate about the use of androgen to hasten the changes of puberty in normal boys with delayed sexual maturation. Most physicians would agree that androgens should be withheld if parental pressures can be overcome.

Patients with delayed puberty should be evaluated for pituitary as well as gonadal function. If growth hormone deficiency is also present, androgens should be withheld until acceptable height is achieved with human growth hormone (*see* below and Chapter 59). If puberal changes are to be induced with an androgen, it can be given in courses of 4 to 6 months at a time, and stopped for like periods to ascertain whether the testes are enlarging and development is progressing spontaneously. The secretion of gonadotropins must also be reevaluated after discontinuation of androgens.

When there is complete testicular failure and puberty cannot occur, prolonged therapy is required. One of the long-acting esters of testosterone, such as the cypionate or the enanthate, may be given intramuscularly. To prevent a period of rapid growth and epiphyseal closure, it is recommended that initial doses of about one half of the eventual maintenance dose be given for 1 year; the eventual maintenance dose of the long-acting esters of testosterone is about 200 mg monthly. The oral preparations are also satisfactory for this purpose, particularly if the patient is reliable. Methyltestosterone in the recommended dose of 30 to 50 mg daily or fluoxymesterone in a 10- to 20-mg dose daily has been used, but the androgenic response is limited in patients with gonadotropin deficiency and even larger doses fail to bring about complete sexual development (*see* Paulsen, 1974). This does not appear to be the case with patients with primary testicular failure.

When hypogonadism starts in adult life and the maturation of puberty has already come about, it is customary to use somewhat smaller doses as replacement therapy than are used in the undeveloped adolescent. Long-acting esters of testosterone in doses of 200-mg every month may be sufficient, and even methyltestosterone or fluoxymesterone in full doses may be effective.

Hypopituitarism. As discussed in Chapter 59, growth hormone is used to promote growth in children with hypopituitarism and dwarfism. Such children are also given replacement doses of thyroid and a corticosteroid if these deficiencies exist (*see* Chapters 60 and 63). *After* human growth hormone is used (or in the event that it is not available), androgens may be administered to promote growth in children with hypopituitarism. Treatment with androgen is not given until the age of puberty, so that the time of sexual development will be appropriate. Therapy should be deferred even longer if possible in the hope of achieving a maximal increase in height. The growth response attained is highly variable and may range from 5 to 30 cm. Obviously less growth is achieved in those individuals with advanced radiological bone age. In boys, the same schedule of treatment as that in hypogonadism has been used, and acceleration of growth has been recorded that is just as rapid as in individuals with normal pituitaries. In girls, large doses of androgen cannot be given and treatment with estrogen induces only a slight acceleration of growth. It is reasonable to give only small doses of androgens to both sexes during the first year or so of treatment in the hope that a greater increment of growth may be achieved before the epiphyses unite.

To Accelerate Growth in Childhood. The advisability of using anabolic-androgenic steroids in children is a much-debated question, and no authoritative answer can yet be given. There are many causes of dwarfism, and a few of these can be remedied. Androgens have been used successfully to promote growth in girls with Turner's syndrome (gonadal dysgenesis) (Johanson et al., 1969). In many instances no cause can be found for short stature, and it is here that the question of the advisability of treatment with androgenic-anabolic steroids arises.

Some children with short stature are diagnosed as having *constitutional delay of growth and development* and will eventually attain normal height and sexual development. While treatment should be delayed or withheld if possible, patients and parents may request therapy. Androgens given before puberty reproduce not only the normal puberal spurt in growth but also the inevitable closure of the epiphyses that puts an end to linear growth. It is possible that doses may be found that promote growth without closing the epiphyses, or perhaps favorable results will be obtained with courses of treatment extending over a few months and alternating with like intervals without treatment. Some compounds, for example, oxandrolone, have been observed to favor growth over epiphyseal maturation (Ray et al., 1965), suggesting that useful effects may be achieved with proper dosage.

The younger the child the greater is the risk of compromising the final mature height. In teen-agers in whom delayed puberty is the reason for short stature, careful treatment with androgen is probably justified, particularly in males. Treatment for a 6-month period might be given with the following drugs, in the indicated daily doses: oxandrolone, 0.1 mg/kg; methandrostenolone, 0.04 mg/kg; ethylestrenol, 0.1 to 0.2 mg/kg; or methyltestosterone, in a total daily dose of 5 mg or less (Sobel, 1968). If positive effects, such as growth or sexual maturation, are seen, treatment might be discontinued for 6 months to observe whether spontaneous puberty has supervened; if it has not, further courses could be given. In younger children, the decision to use this form of treatment is more difficult to make; it is usually undertaken as a last resort and always with awareness of the risk of limiting mature stature.

Use in Aging Men. There is a good deal of continuing debate about the question of a male counterpart to the menopause of women. It is clear that castration in the adult is frequently followed by symptoms typical of the menopause that can be relieved by androgen. It is also well established that the various indices of testicular function show a very gradual decline with advancing years. These include reduced libido, reduced sexual activity, and lessened muscular size and strength. There is a rise in urinary gonadotropin with age, and a decline in the volume of the semen and the total number of spermatozoa (Eskin, 1978). At about the age of 50 the mean concentration of testosterone in plasma is reduced, while estrogens in plasma increase somewhat due to increased peripheral conversion of androgens to estrogens (Siiteri and MacDonald, 1973; Marcus and Korenman, 1976). By the age of 80 to 90, plasma testosterone is decreased by about 60%. Although there is normally no sharp decline in the endocrine function of the testes to justify the term *climacteric* and the increase in gonadotropins is less than that which occurs in women, reduction of testicular function does seem to be a normal process in older men. If the concentration of testosterone in plasma is clearly lower than expected, replacement of androgen can increase libido and maintain secondary sexual characteristics in aging males; otherwise, androgen replacement is not convincingly beneficial (*see* Eskin, 1978).

Osteoporosis. As discussed in Chapter 61, androgens and estrogens can improve calcium balance and decrease bone resorption when given to patients with osteoporosis. Because of the side effects of androgens, estrogens are preferred when steroid therapy is selected for female patients with postmenopausal osteoporosis. Androgens appear to be more effective in preventing glucocorticoid-induced osteoporosis (*see* Gordon, 1978; Chapter 63). Riggs and coworkers (1972) demonstrated that after 1 or 2 years of therapy bone formation declines, and this counteracts the beneficial effects of androgens. It is not known if this apparent refractoriness to therapy can be overcome with interrupted courses of steroids. Calcium carbonate is also effective in osteoporosis and can be used alone or in conjunction with steroid therapy (*see* Chapter 65).

Endometriosis. In this disorder endometrial tissue is found outside the uterus in the peritoneal cavity. This may result in dysmenorrhea, dyspareunia, and even sterility. Endometriosis can be treated effectively with androgens such as danazol in doses of 200 to 800 mg daily for several months. However, progestins or combined oral contraceptives are equally effective and considerably less expensive (*see* Chapter 61).

Anemia. McCullagh and Jones (1942) were the first to show that the mild anemia of hypogonadal individuals can be corrected by replacement therapy with androgen. It was later noted that large doses of androgen sometimes caused excessive erythropoiesis, leading to moderate polycythemia, and advantage was taken of this effect by Gardner and Pringle (1961) in the treatment of hypoplastic anemia and the anemia of neoplastic disease. Doses as high as 1.2 g per week of testosterone enanthate and 200 mg per day of methyltestosterone were used. There was a slight reticulocytosis and an increase in erythrocytes and hemoglobin. There was, of course, intense virilization but no other untoward effect except jaundice from methyltestosterone. The effects of androgens on erythrocyte formation explain the normally higher hematocrit in males.

Androgenic-anabolic steroids are now widely used in the treatment of aplastic anemia, red-cell aplasia, hemolytic anemias, and the anemias associated with renal failure, myeloid metaplasia, lymphoma, leukemia, and various other disorders. Androgens are the most useful nonspecific stimulants of erythropoiesis (*see* Shahidi, 1973). Although the response of the bone marrow varies in different conditions, erythropoiesis is stimulated first and most consistently, leukopenia is ameliorated later, and improvement in thrombocytopenia occurs last. Androgens and anabolic steroids are effective in less than half of the patients treated, and up to 3 months may be needed to see an increase in red blood cells and longer for increases in neutrophils and platelets (Li *et al.*, 1972). The consensus is that these agents are beneficial in milder cases and probably of little or no benefit in severe anemia. Beneficial effects are seen more commonly in children. Since the prognosis of many of these disorders is poor, most agree that a therapeutic trial is appropriate.

The doses of androgenic-anabolic steroids used have been large, and it is not known if smaller doses are effective. Weekly injections of esters of testosterone in doses of 600 mg to 1 g are used. Many other agents, including nandrolone decanoate and oxymetholone, have also been used in variable amounts with success.

The mechanism of action has been sought in the stimulation of secretion of erythropoietin by the kidney. Although such an action can be shown under some circumstances, androgens have also been found to stimulate directly the synthesis of heme, an action potentiated by erythropoietin. The response of the other elements of the bone marrow suggests a direct effect thereon of the androgenic-anabolic agents.

The use of 17-alkyl androgens for these disorders for the prolonged periods that are frequently necessary has resulted in hepatic carcinoma in some individuals (*see* above).

Promotion of Anabolism. Androgenic-anabolic steroids have been used in a wide assortment of conditions, ranging from postoperative recovery to chronic debilitating diseases. Studies of various designs have shown that the androgens reduce the negative nitrogen balance and may convert a mildly negative balance to a positive one. The effects are intimately related to the intake of protein and calories, and, depending upon the conditions, a small increase in either one of these may have a greater effect than the administration of the anabolic agent. While few would disagree that these agents are anabolic and may induce short-term effects, it seems unlikely that their use has altered the outcome of, or shortened the recovery from, the underlying illness. However, they promote a feeling of well-being and improve appetite, and their use in terminal diseases cannot be criticized.

Suppression of Lactation. As discussed in Chapter 61, estrogens and progestins are used when it is advisable to decrease post-partum lactation. Androgens have also proven very effective. Side effects are not seen or are minimal with the administration of 50 to 100 mg of esters of testosterone for 1 to 4 days post partum. Oral preparations are used for 4 to 6 days. These agents should be started at the time of delivery.

Carcinoma of the Breast. Androgens are used as a palliative measure for recurrent and metastatic carcinoma of the breast in women (*see* Chapter 55). The use of endocrine organ ablation and hormonal therapy for breast carcinoma was initially prompted by studies of an altered incidence of mammary tumors in rodents after castration or treatment with estrogens and androgens. The presence of receptors for estrogen and/or progesterone in extracts of breast tumors has proven to be useful for the prediction of responses to endocrine ablative procedures and hormonal therapy (*see* Chapter 61). These receptors are present in about one half of breast tumors and, when present, alterations in the hormonal environment may produce beneficial responses in 60 to 70% of patients (*see* McGuire, 1975; Kiang *et al.*, 1978). Remissions may take 3 months to develop and may last 6 to 12 months. If androgens are used, they are given in large doses such as 50 to 100 mg of testosterone propionate three times a week. In addition to side effects discussed above, some patients with metastases to bone develop hypercalcemia during therapy, an indication to withdraw the androgen. Androgens are contraindicated in men with carcinoma of the breast as well as carcinoma of the prostate.

ANTIANDROGENS

A search for compounds that might inhibit the synthesis or action of androgen was doubtless prompted by clinical considerations. Treatment of cancer of the prostate was one of the earlier aims; however, the uses of potent antagonists might range from virilization in women to precocious puberty in boys, and from acne to satyriasis. These compounds might also be valuable as male contraceptives. Recent developments suggest that some of these aspirations can be fulfilled.

Estrogens, in a restricted sense, may be regarded as antiandrogenic. They may have actions of their own upon genital tissues, which differ from those of androgens and in this way seem to antagonize androgen.

Progesterone comes nearer to being an antiandrogen, albeit a very weak one, and some of the more potent antiandrogens now known are derivatives of progesterone. Two other weak antiandrogens with no known hormonal activity of any other kind are the derivatives dodecahydrophenanthrene (Randall and Selitto, 1958) and A-norprogesterone; the former somewhat resembles progesterone lacking a D ring; the latter is progesterone with one carbon atom missing from ring A (Lerner, 1964). Several other steroids also have weak antiandrogenic activity, although most studies have been confined to animals.

Nonsteroidal antiandrogens have also been studied in animals and in systems *in vitro*. These compounds block the action or synthesis of testosterone and include dimethanesulfonate derivatives, N-(3,5-dimethyl-4-isoxazolylmethyl) phthalimide (DIMP), 4'-nitro-3'-trifluoromethylisobutyranilide (flutamide), and cyanoketone (*see* Neri, 1976; Mainwaring, 1977).

Cyproterone Acetate. In the search for orally active progestins, steroids with a 1,2-α-methylene substitution were found to be antiandrogenic. Cyproterone acetate is among the most potent, and its structure is as follows:

Cyproterone Acetate

While it is a potent antiandrogen, it also possesses progestational activity and suppresses the secretion of gonadotropins (Neri, 1976; Neumann, 1977). In androgen-dependent target tissues cyproterone acetate competes with dihydrotestosterone for its receptor site. Treatment of the pregnant rat with 1 or 10 mg daily led to the remarkable finding that the male fetuses were "feminized," the penis was underdeveloped and resembled a clitoris, the prostate was missing, and the testes were small and undescended. These changes were permanent (Hamada *et al.,* 1963).

In the mature rat, the compound causes atrophy of the seminal vesicles, prostate, levator ani muscle, and other androgen-responsive organs, as well as cellular changes in the pituitary typical of castration with increased gonadotropin secretion (Neumann, 1966). This latter effect is not observed in men (Jackson and Jones, 1972). The testes are unaffected by small or moderate doses, although larger doses can decrease Leydig-cell function and spermatogenesis. In the castrated animal, only about five times as much antagonist as testosterone is needed to reduce the androgenic response by 50%. With large doses of cyproterone acetate the antagonism is almost complete (Neumann *et al.,* 1970).

Laschet and associates (1967a) gave doses of cyproterone of 100 to 200 mg daily to men with severe deviations in sexual behavior and noted that male sexuality virtually disappeared in 10 to 14 days. The effect was gone within 2 weeks after discontinuing treatment; no gynecomastia or other side effects were noted. This loss of libido when the drug is given to males obviously precludes its general use as a male contraceptive. Furthermore, its efficacy as a contraceptive in men has not been consistent in several studies. Because of its antigonadotropic effect, it has been used in combination with estrogen as an oral

contraceptive in women. Some success has been reported with the use of cyproterone acetate in the treatment of hirsutism and virilization in women and acne and baldness in both sexes (*see* Neri, 1976; Neumann, 1977).

Cyproterone has also been used effectively in the therapy of precocious puberty (Kauli *et al.,* 1976). It delays the onset of puberty, decreases breast, testicular, and hair growth, stops menstruation if present, and delays the premature closure of epiphyses. However, in animals, cyproterone acetate can also prevent the anabolic effects of androgens and retard growth. Thus, its efficacy in precocious puberty may be offset by potential side effects.

Several studies have been encouraging with regard to the use of cyproterone, in daily doses of 200 to 300 mg, in prostatic carcinoma (*see* Wein and Murphy, 1973). Although cyproterone acetate is the most active antiandrogen so far encountered, closely related analogs are also active. Antiandrogenic drugs are still in the investigational stage and are not yet generally available.

MALE CONTRACEPTIVES

There are many requirements of the ideal contraceptive drug: simplicity, acceptability, reversibility, lack of toxicity, and, of course, efficacy. Although all these criteria have not been attained in the oral contraceptives for women, the agents discussed in Chapter 61 come relatively close. In this respect, women have been liberated long before men. The neglect of the development of analogous contraceptives for men undoubtedly reflects many biological and sociological factors (*see* Diller and Hembree, 1977).

The highly ordered and precise processes that occur during the genesis and maturation of sperm should allow numerous approaches to their regulation and thus to contraception. A variety of compounds, in addition to the antiandrogens discussed above, can inhibit spermatogenesis. These include antineoplastic agents, cadmium, nitrofuranes, α-chlorhydrin, and dinitropyrrole (*see* Jackson and Jones, 1972; Bremner and DeKretser, 1976; Ewing and Robaire, 1978). However, the irreversible effects of some and the toxicity of many preclude their clinical use. Studies in animals, including man, have resulted in a rational approach to this problem with androgens, estrogens, progestins, and their combinations.

Sex steroids can suppress secretion of FSH and LH, which are required for spermatogenesis and the synthesis of testosterone by the testes (*see* Chapters 59 and 61). While estrogens and progestins are effective contraceptives in males, suppression of testosterone decreases both libido and potency; gynecomastia may also occur. These unacceptable side effects can be overcome by utilizing androgens to inhibit secretion of gonadotropins and spermatogenesis. Although androgens can be used successfully as contraceptives, the high doses required are associated with other effects, including jaundice, edema, and hypercholesterolemia. The use of androgens alone is thus not encouraging. Estrogens in combination with androgens are also effective (Briggs and Briggs, 1974). Again, however, the side effects of estrogens in men (*e.g.*, gynecomastia and thrombotic disorders) limit the utility of this approach.

Perhaps the most promising regimen to date involves the dual administration of an androgen and progestin (Brenner *et al.*, 1975). Clinical trials in which patients received continuous testosterone and a progestin (usually administered in the form of silicone-rubber capsule implants) have resulted in sterility with minimal side effects. The rationale for this combination is to suppress gonadotropin secretion and spermatogenesis with a progestin and to prevent alteration of accessory sexual structures by the simultaneous administration of testosterone (*see* Segal, 1973; Bremner and DeKretser, 1976; Ewing and Robaire, 1978). Sperm counts are suppressed only after several months of treatment. A similar amount of time is required for the recovery of spermatogenesis when the drugs are stopped.

All the methods described above for contraception in the male remain investigational. However, some of the clinical studies provide indications that reversible, pharmacological control of fertility in men will become available in the foreseeable future.

Bernstein, M. S.; Hunter, R. L.; and Yachnin, S. Hepatoma and peliosis hepatitis in Fanconi's anemia. *N. Engl. J. Med.,* **1971,** *284,* 1135–1136.

Brenner, P. F.; Bernstein, G. S.; Roy, S.; Jeckt, E. W.; and Mischell, D. R. Administration of norethandrolone and testosterone as a contraceptive agent for men. *Contraception,* **1975,** *11,* 193–207.

Briggs, M., and Briggs, M. Oral contraceptive for men. *Nature,* **1974,** *252,* 585–586.

Brown-Séquard, C. E. Des effets produits chez l'homme par des injections souscutanées d'un liquide retiré des testicules frais de cobaye et de chien. *C. R. Soc. Biol. (Paris),* **1889,** *1,* 420–430.

Butenandt, A. Über die chemische Untersuchung der Sexualhormons. *Z. Angew. Chem.,* **1931,** *44,* 905–908.

Castro, A. E.; Alonso, A.; and Mancini, R. E. Localization of follicle stimulating and luteinizing hormones in the rat testis using immunohistological tests. *J. Endocrinol.,* **1972,** *52,* 129–136.

David, K.; Dingemanse, E.; Freud, J.; and Laquer, E. Über krystallinisches männliches Hormon aus Hoden (Testosteron), wirksamer als aus Harn oder aus Cholesterin bereitetes Androsteron. *Hoppe Seylers Z. Physiol. Chem.,* **1935,** *233,* 281–282.

DeJong, F. H., and Sharpe, R. M. Evidence for inhibin-like activity in bovine follicular fluid. *Nature,* **1976,** *263,* 71–72.

Diller, L., and Hembree, W. Male contraception and family planning: a social and historical review. *Fertil. Steril.,* **1977,** *28,* 1271–1279.

Dufau, M. L.; Watanabe, K.; and Catt, K. J. Stimulation of cyclic AMP production by the rat testis during incubation with hCG *in vitro. Endocrinology,* **1973,** *92,* 6–11.

Forbes, T. R. Crowing hen: early observations on spontaneous sex reversal in birds. *Yale J. Biol. Med.,* **1947,** *19,* 955–970.

Forest, M.; Cathiard, A.; and Bertrand, J. Total and unbound testosterone levels in the newborn and in normal and hypogonadal children: use of a sensitive radio-

immunoassay for testosterone. *J. Clin. Endocrinol. Metab.,* **1973,** *36,* 1132–1142.

Gardner, F. H., and Pringle, J. C. Androgens and erythropoiesis. I. Preliminary clinical observations. *Arch. Intern. Med.,* **1961,** *107,* 846–862.

Hamada, H.; Neumann, F.; and Junkmann, K. Intrauterine antimaskuline Beinflüssung von Rattenfeten durch ein stark Gestagen wirksames Steroid. *Acta Endocrinol. (Kbh.),* **1963,** *44,* 380–388.

Henderson, J. T.; Richmond, J.; and Sumerling, M. D. Androgenic-anabolic steroid therapy and hepatocellular carcinoma. *Lancet,* **1973,** *1,* 934.

Hilliard, J.; Scaramuzzi, R. J.; Pang, C.-N.; Penardi, R.; and Sawyer, C. H. Testosterone secretion by rabbit ovary *in vivo. Endocrinology,* **1974,** *94,* 267–271.

Imperato-McGinley, J.; Peterson, R. E.; Gautier, T.; and Sturla, E. Androgens and the evaluation of male gender identity among male pseudohermaphrodites with 5α-reductase deficiency. *N. Engl. J. Med.,* **1979,** *300,* 1233–1237.

Johanson, A. J.; Brasel, J. A.; and Blizzard, R. M. Growth in patients with gonadal dysgenesis receiving fluoxymesterone. *J. Pediatr.,* **1969,** *75,* 1015–1021.

Johnson, F. L.; Feagler, J. R.; Lerner, K. G.; Majerus, P. W.; Siegel, M.; Hartmann, J. R.; and Thomas, E. D. Association of androgenic-anabolic steroid therapy with development of hepatocellular carcinoma. *Lancet,* **1972,** *2,* 1273–1276.

Josso, N.; Forest, M. G.; and Picard, J. Y. Müllerian-inhibiting activity of calf fetal testes: relationship to testosterone and protein synthesis. *Biol. Reprod.,* **1975,** *13,* 163–167.

Judd, H. L., and Yen, S. S. C. Serum adrenostenedione and testosterone levels during the menstrual cycle. *J. Clin. Endocrinol. Metab.,* **1973,** *36,* 475–481.

Kauli, R.; Pertzelan, A.; Prager-Lewin, R.; Grunebaum, M.; and Laron, Z. Cyproterone acetate in treatment of precocious puberty. *Arch. Dis. Child.,* **1976,** *51,* 202–208.

Kelch, R. P.; Jenner, M. R.; Weinstein, R.; Kaplan, S. L.; and Grumbach, M. M. Estradiol and testosterone secretion by human, simian, and canine testes in males with hypogonadism and in male pseudohermaphrodites with the feminizing testes syndrome. *J. Clin. Invest.,* **1972,** *51,* 824–830.

Keogh, E. J.; Lee, V. W. K.; Rennie, G. C.; Burger, H. G.; Hudson, B.; and DeKretser, D. M. Selective suppression of FSH by testicular extracts. *Endocrinology,* **1976,** *98,* 997–1004.

Kiang, D. T.; Frenning, D. H.; Goldman, A. I.; Ascensao, V. F.; and Kennedy, B. J. Estrogen receptors and responses to chemotherapy and hormonal therapy in advanced breast cancer. *N. Engl. J. Med.,* **1978,** *289,* 1330–1334.

Knowlton, K.; Kenyon, A. T.; Sandiford, I.; Lotwin, G.; and Fricker, R. Comparative study of metabolic effects of estradiol benzoate and testosterone propionate in man. *J. Clin. Endocrinol. Metab.,* **1942,** *2,* 671–684.

Kochakian, C. D., and Murlin, J. R. The effect of male hormone on the protein and energy metabolism of castrate dogs. *J. Nutr.,* **1935,** *10,* 437–459.

Lacy, D., and Pettit, A. J. Sites of hormone production in the mammalian testis, and their significance in the control of male fertility. *Br. Med. Bull.,* **1970,** *26,* 87–91.

Landau, R. L.; Bergenstal, D. M.; Lugibihl, K.; and Kascht, M. E. The metabolic effects of progesterone in man. *J. Clin. Endocrinol. Metab.,* **1955,** *15,* 1194–1215.

Laschet, U.; Laschet, L.; Felzner, H.-R.; Glaesel, H.-U.; Mall, G.; and Naab, M. Results in the treatment of hyper- and abnormal sexuality of men with antiandrogens. *Acta Endocrinol. (Kbh.),* **1967a,** *56,* Suppl. 119, 54.

Laschet, U.; Nierman, H.; Laschet, L.; and Paarmann, H. F. Mesterolone, a potent oral active androgen without gonadotropin inhibition. *Acta Endocrinol. (Kbh.)*, **1967b,** *56,* Suppl. 119, 55.

Li, F. P.; Alter, B. P.; and Nathan, D. G. The mortality of acquired aplastic anemia in children. *Blood,* **1972,** *40,* 153–162.

Loewe, S., and Voss, H. E. Der Stand der Erfassung des männlichen Sexualhormons (Androkinins). *Klin. Wochenschr.,* **1930,** *9,* 481–487.

Longcope, C. The metabolism of estrone sulfate in normal males. *J. Clin. Endocrinol. Metab.,* **1972,** *34,* 113–122.

McCullagh, D. R. Dual endocrine activity of the testes. *Science,* **1932,** *76,* 19–20.

McCullagh, E. P., and Jones, R. Effect of androgens on the blood count of men. *J. Clin. Endocrinol. Metab.,* **1942,** *2,* 243–251.

Mayer, M., and Rosen, F. Interaction of anabolic steroids with glucocorticoid receptor sites in rat muscle cytosol. *Am. J. Physiol.,* **1975,** *229,* 1381–1386.

Mills, T. M., and Savard, K. *In vitro* steroid synthesis by follicles isolated from the rabbit ovary. *Steroids,* **1972,** *20,* 247–262.

Murad, F.; Strauch, B. S.; and Vaughan, M. The effect of gonadotropins on testicular adenyl cyclase. *Biochim. Biophys. Acta,* **1969,** *177,* 591–598.

Naftolin, F.; Judd, H. L.; and Yen, S. S. C. Pulsatile patterns of gonadotropins and testosterone in man: the effects of clomiphene with and without testosterone. *J. Clin. Endocrinol. Metab.,* **1973,** *36,* 285–288.

Neumann, H. Auftreton von Kastrationszellen im Hypophysenvorderlappen männlicher Ratten nach Behandlung mit einem Antiandrogen. *Acta Endocrinol. (Kbh.),* **1966,** *53,* 53–60.

Papanicolaou, G. N., and Falk, E. A. General muscular hypertrophy induced by androgenic hormones. *Science,* **1938,** *87,* 238–239.

Petry, R.; Rausch-Strooman, J.-G.; Heinz, H. A.; Senge, T.; and Mauss, J. Androgen treatment without inhibiting effect on hypophysis and male gonads. *Acta Endocrinol. (Kbh.),* **1968,** *59,* 497–507.

Randall, L. O., and Selitto, J. J. Anti-androgenic activity of a synthetic phenanthrene. *Endocrinology,* **1958,** *62,* 693–695.

Ray, C. G.; Kirschvink, J. F.; Waxman, S. H.; and Kelley, V. C. Studies of anabolic steroids. III. The effect of oxandrolone on height and skeletal maturation in mongoloid children. *Am. J. Dis. Child.,* **1965,** *110,* 618–623.

Riggs, L.; Jowsey, J.; Goldsmith, R. S.; Kelly, P. J.; Hoffman, D. L.; and Arnaud, C. D. Short- and long-term effects of estrogen and synthetic anabolic hormone in postmenopausal osteoporosis. *J. Clin. Invest.,* **1972,** *51,* 1659–1663.

Rubin, R. T.; Poland, R. E.; and Tower, B. B. Prolactin-related testosterone secretion in normal adult men. *J. Clin. Endocrinol. Metab.,* **1976,** *42,* 112–116.

Ruzicka, L., and Wettstein, A. Synthetische Darstellung des Testishormons, Testosteron (Androsten-3-on-17-ol). *Helv. Chim. Acta,* **1935,** *18,* 1264–1275.

Sachs, B. D.; Pollak, E. I.; Kreiger, M. S.; and Barfield, R. J. Sexual behavior: normal male patterning in androgenized female rats. *Science,* **1973,** *181,* 770–772.

Saez, J. M.; Morera, A. M.; Dazard, A.; and Bertrand, J. Adrenal and testicular contribution to plasma estrogens. *J. Endocrinol.,* **1972,** *55,* 41–49.

Segal, S. Male fertility control studies: an editorial comment. *Contraception,* **1973,** *8,* 187–188.

Shahidi, N. T. Androgens and erythropoiesis. *N. Engl. J. Med.,* **1973,** *289,* 72–80.

Sobel, E. H. Anabolic steroids. In, *Clinical Endocrinology II.* (Astwood, E. B., and Cassidy, C. E., eds.) Grune & Stratton, Inc., New York, **1968.**

Steinberger, A., and Steinberger, E. Secretion of an FSH-inhibiting factor by cultured Sertoli cells. *Endocrinology,* **1976,** *99,* 918–921.

Walsh, P. C.; Madden, J. D.; Harrod, M. J.; Goldstein, J. L.; MacDonald, P. C.; and Wilson, J. D. Familial incomplete male pseudohermaphroditism. Type 2. Decreased dihydrotestosterone formation in pseudovaginal perineoscrotal hypospadias. *N. Engl. J. Med.,* **1974,** *291,* 944–949.

Wein, A. J., and Murphy, J. J. Experience in the treatment of prostatic carcinoma with cyproterone acetate. *J. Urol.,* **1973,** *109,* 68–70.

Wilson, J. D.; Harrod, M. J.; Goldstein, J. L.; Hemsell, D. L.; and MacDonald, P. C. Familial incomplete male pseudohermaphroditism. Type 1. Evidence for androgen resistance and variable clinical manifestations in a family with the Reifenstein syndrome. *N. Engl. J. Med.,* **1974,** *290,* 1097–1103.

Wolff, S. M.; Kimball, H. R.; and Marshall, J. R. The effects of hydrocortisone and estrogen on experimental fever induced by etiocholanolone. *J. Infect. Dis.,* **1973,** *128,* 243–247.

Monographs and Reviews

Armstrong, D. T., and Dorrington, J. H. Estrogen biosynthesis in the ovaries and testes. *Adv. Sex Horm. Res.,* **1977,** *3,* 217–258.

Bartke, A.; Hafiez, A. A.; Bex, F. J.; and Dalterio, S. Hormonal interactions in regulation of androgen secretion. *Biol. Reprod.,* **1978,** *18,* 44–54.

Boyar, R. M. Control of the onset of puberty. *Annu. Rev. Med.,* **1978,** *29,* 509–520.

Bremner, W. J., and DeKretser, D. M. The prospects for new reversible male contraceptives. *N. Engl. J. Med.,* **1976,** *295,* 1111–1116.

Catt, K. J., and Dufau, M. L. Basic concepts of the mechanism of action of peptide hormones. *Biol. Reprod.,* **1976,** *14,* 1–15.

Davidson, J. M. Feedback control of gonadotropin secretion. In, *Frontiers in Neuroendocrinology.* (Ganong, W. F., and Martini, L., eds.) Oxford University Press, New York, **1969,** pp. 343–388.

Ebling, F. J. Steroids, hormones and sebaceous secretion. *Adv. Steroid Biochem. Pharmacol.,* **1970,** *2,* 1–39.

Eik-Nes, K. B. Production and secretion of testicular steroids. *Recent Prog. Horm. Res.,* **1971,** *27,* 517–535.

Eskin, B. A. Sex hormones and aging. *Adv. Exp. Med. Biol.,* **1978,** *97,* 207–224.

Ewing, L. L., and Robaire, B. Endogenous antispermatogenic agents: prospects for male contraception. *Annu. Rev. Pharmacol. Toxicol.,* **1978,** *18,* 167–187.

Fotherby, K., and James, F. Metabolism of synthetic steroids. *Adv. Steroid Biochem. Pharmacol.,* **1972,** *3,* 67–165.

Franchimont, P. Pituitary gonadotropins. *Clin. Endocrinol. Metab.,* **1977,** *6,* 101–116.

Givens, J. R. Normal and abnormal androgen metabolism. *Clin. Obstet. Gynecol.,* **1978,** *21,* 115–123.

Gordon, G. S. Drug treatment of osteoporosis. *Annu. Rev. Pharmacol. Toxicol.,* **1978,** *18,* 253–268.

Heyns, W. The steroid-binding β-globulin of human plasma. *Adv. Steroid Biochem. Pharmacol.,* **1977,** *6,* 59–79.

Horn, H. J. Role of antiandrogens in psychiatry. In, *Androgens and Antiandrogens.* (Martini, L., and Motta, M., eds.) Raven Press, New York, **1977,** pp. 351–355.

Jackson, H., and Jones, A. R. The effects of steroids and their antagonists on spermatogenesis. *Adv. Steroid Biochem. Pharmacol.,* **1972,** *3,* 167–192.

James, V. H. T.; Braunsberg, H.; Rippon, A. E.; and Parker, V. Measurement of androgens in biological fluids. In, *Androgens and Antiandrogens.* (Martini, L., and Motta, M., eds.) Raven Press, New York, **1977,** pp. 19–35.

Jost, A. Embryonic sexual differentiation. In, *Hermaphroditism, Genital Anomalies and Related Endocrine Disorders,* 2nd ed. (Jones, H. W., and Scott, W. W., eds.) The Williams & Wilkins Co., Baltimore, **1971,** pp. 16–64.

Juneja, H. S.; Motta, M.; Vasconi, F.; and Martini, L. Negative and positive effects of androgens on gonadotropin release. In, *Androgens and Antiandrogens.* (Martini, L., and Motta, M., eds.) Raven Press, New York, **1977**, pp. 127–135.

Lerner, L. J. Hormone antagonists: inhibitors of specific activities of estrogen and androgen. *Recent Prog. Horm. Res.,* **1964,** *20,* 435–476.

Liao, S., and Fang, S. Receptor-proteins for androgens and the mode of action of androgens on gene transcription in ventral prostate. *Vitam. Horm.,* **1969,** *27,* 17–90.

Lunde, D. T., and Hamburg, D. A. Techniques for assessing the effects of sex steroids on affect, arousal, and aggression in humans. *Recent Prog. Horm. Res.,* **1972,** *28,* 627–663.

McGuire, W. L. Endocrine therapy of breast cancer. *Annu. Rev. Med.,* **1975,** *26,* 353–363.

Mainwaring, W. I. P. (ed.). The mechanism of action of androgens. *Monogr. Endocrinol.,* **1977,** *10,* 1–178.

Marcus, R., and Korenman, S. G. Estrogens and the human male. *Annu. Rev. Med.,* **1976,** *27,* 357–370.

Naftolin, F.; Ryan, K. J.; Davies, I. J.; Reddy, V. V.; Flores, F.; Petro, Z.; and Kuhn, M. The formation of estrogens by central neuroendocrine tissues. *Recent Prog. Horm. Res.,* **1975,** *31,* 295–319.

Neri, R. O. Antiandrogens. *Adv. Sex Horm. Res.,* **1976,** *2,* 233–262.

Neumann, F. Pharmacology and potential use of cyproterone acetate. *Horm. Metab. Res.,* **1977,** *9,* 1–13.

Neumann, F.; Berswordt-Wallrabe, R. von; Elger, W.; Steinbeck, H.; Hahn, J.; and Kramer, M. Aspects of androgen-dependent events as studied by antiandrogens. *Recent Prog. Horm. Res.,* **1970,** *26,* 337–405.

Odell, W. D., and Swerdloff, R. S. Abnormalities of gonadal function in men. *Clin. Endocrinol. (Oxf.),* **1978,** *8,* 149–180.

Paulsen, C. A. The testes. In, *Textbook of Endocrinology,* 5th ed. (Williams, R. H., ed.) W. B. Saunders Co., Philadelphia, **1974,** pp. 323–367.

Rosenfield, R. L. Role of androgens in growth and development of the fetus, child, and adolescent. *Adv. Pediatr.,* **1972,** *19,* 172–213.

Schally, A. V. Aspects of hypothalamic regulation of the pituitary gland: its implications for the control of reproductive processes. *Science,* **1978,** *202,* 18–28.

Siiteri, P. K., and MacDonald, P. C. Role of extraglandular estrogen in human endocrinology. In, *Female Reproductive System,* Vol. 2, Pt. 1. Sect. 7, *Endocrinology. Handbook of Physiology.* (Greep, R. O., and Astwood, E. B., eds.) American Physiological Society, Washington, D. C., **1973,** pp. 615–629.

Sommerville, I. F., and Collins, W. P. Indices of androgen production in women. *Adv. Steroid Biochem. Pharmacol.,* **1970,** *2,* 267–314.

Wilson, J. D., and Gloyna, R. E. The intranuclear metabolism of testosterone in the accessory organs of reproduction. *Recent Prog. Horm. Res.,* **1970,** *26,* 309–336.

63 ADRENOCORTICOTROPIC HORMONE; ADRENOCORTICAL STEROIDS AND THEIR SYNTHETIC ANALOGS; INHIBITORS OF ADRENOCORTICAL STEROID BIOSYNTHESIS

Robert C. Haynes, Jr., and Ferid Murad

Adrenocorticotropic hormone (ACTH, corticotropin) and the steroids of the adrenal cortex are considered together in this chapter because the primary physiological and pharmacological effects of ACTH result from the secretion of adrenocortical steroids. Biologically active synthetic analogs of the adrenocorticosteroids and those nonsteroidal substances that alter the pattern of secretion of the adrenal cortex by inhibiting certain biosynthetic pathways are also included. Synthetic steroids and other compounds that inhibit the action of aldosterone on the renal tubule are discussed in Chapter 36.

History. The physiological significance of the adrenals began to be appreciated as a consequence of the description by Addison (1855) of the clinical syndrome resulting from destructive disease of the adrenal glands. His observations interested the physiologist Brown-Séquard (1856), who did the pioneer experiments on the effects of adrenalectomy and concluded that the adrenal glands are essential to life.

By the third decade of this century it was generally recognized that the cortex rather than the medulla is the life-maintaining portion of the gland. Soon the literature was replete with descriptions of the numerous physiological abnormalities exhibited by adrenalectomized animals. The complex nature of adrenocortical deficiency was dramatized in the 1930s by the partisan character of research groups oriented to study either the imbalance of electrolytes or the defects in carbohydrate metabolism present in the deficient state. Renal loss of sodium was convincingly demonstrated to be a characteristic of adrenocortical insufficiency by Harrop and associates (1933) as well as by Loeb and coworkers (1933). Equally convincing was the demonstration of a depletion of carbohydrate stores (Cori and Cori, 1927). Furthermore, hypoglycemia could be corrected by adrenocortical extracts (Britton and Silvette, 1931). Glucose and glycogen, formed under the influence of the adrenal cortex during fasting, appeared to be derived

from tissue protein (Long *et al.*, 1940). From these studies there emerged the concepts of two types of adrenocortical hormones. The mineralocorticoids primarily regulate electrolyte homeostasis, and the glucocorticoids are hormones concerned with carbohydrate metabolism. This concept of the dichotomy of "salt" and "sugar" hormones (mineralocorticoids and glucocorticoids) has proven useful and survives at the present time in a modified form.

In 1932, the neurosurgeon Cushing described the syndrome of hypercorticism, which bears his name (Cushing, 1932). The cases Cushing described were those of "pituitary basophilism," recognized subsequently as being a condition characterized by hypersecretion of ACTH. The symptom complex is now known to result from excessive plasma concentrations of adrenocortical hormones, regardless of whether they originate endogenously or as the consequence of therapeutic intervention.

The preparation of adrenocortical extracts with a reasonable degree of activity was first accomplished by Swingle and Pfiffner (1930a, 1930b) as well as by Hartman and associates (1930). The existence of biologically active tissue extracts presented a challenge to organic chemists, who by 1942 had isolated, crystallized, and elucidated the structures of 28 steroids from the adrenal cortex (Reichstein and Shoppee, 1943). Five of these compounds—cortisol, cortisone, corticosterone, 11-dehydrocorticosterone, and 11-desoxycorticosterone—were demonstrated to be biologically active. Another decade passed before the principal mineralocorticoid was discovered. Stimulus for the search for this elusive material was provided by the work of Deming and Luetscher (1950), who isolated from the urine of patients with edema a substance that induced sodium retention and potassium excretion in adrenalectomized rats. The definitive evidence for its source was provided by Tait and coworkers (1952), who purified the compound from adrenocortical extracts. The substance was crystallized, the structure was established, and the hormone was eventually named *aldosterone* (Simpson *et al.*, 1954).

Meanwhile, other investigators had turned their attention to the adenohypophysis. The classical studies of Foster and Smith (1926) established the fact that hypophysectomy results in atrophy of the adrenal cortex. Not long thereafter, it was demonstrated that cell-free extracts of the anterior pituitary had a stimulating effect upon the adrenal cortex of the hypophysectomized animal (Collip et al., 1933; Evans, 1933; Houssay et al., 1933). Further chemical fractionation of such extracts led to the isolation of a hormone, ACTH, that acted selectively to cause chemical and morphological changes in the adrenal cortex (Li et al., 1943; Sayers et al., 1943; Astwood et al., 1952). The structure of ACTH was established by Bell and coworkers (1956). Further brilliant chemistry culminated in the synthesis of biologically active peptides (Hofmann et al., 1961) and of an ACTH of 39 amino acid residues (Schwyzer and Sieber, 1963). The rate of release of ACTH from the adenohypophysis was shown to be determined by the balance of inhibitory effects of the secretions of the adrenal cortex (Ingle et al., 1938) and the excitatory effects of the nervous system. The hypothalamus was established as the "final common path" for the variety of stimuli impinging on the adenohypophysis (see Harris, 1955).

A detailed analysis of the morphology of the adrenal cortex had suggested to Swann (1940) and to Deane and Greep (1946) that the zona glomerulosa of the adrenal cortex functions relatively independently of the pituitary. Following hypophysectomy, the zona glomerulosa thickens, whereas the fasciculata shrinks markedly and the reticularis disappears almost entirely. These morphological observations, together with the fact that the hypophysectomized rat, in contrast to the adrenalectomized animal, can survive without salt therapy, prompted Swann as well as Deane and Greep to assign to the zona glomerulosa the specific function of autonomously elaborating a hormone regulating electrolyte balance. This hormone is now known to be aldosterone. Subsequent experimental studies have shown that the rate of secretion of aldosterone is regulated by a complex system, of which the pituitary is a relatively unimportant element.

Throughout the 1940s there was intense interest in the physiological roles of ACTH and adrenocortical steroids, stimulated by the appreciation that many physiological and biochemical responses to noxious stimuli are dependent upon the integrity of the adenohypophyseal-adrenocortical system. The most ardent exponent of the relationship between the adrenal cortex and "stress" was Selye (see Selye, 1946).

It was upon such a background that Hench and coworkers in 1949 announced the dramatic effects of cortisone and ACTH in diseases other than adrenocortical insufficiency. As early as 1929, Hench was impressed by the fact that arthritic patients, when pregnant or jaundiced, experienced a temporary remission; he believed that a metabolite was responsible for the remission. The possibility that the antirheumatic substance might be an adrenocortical hormone was actively entertained, and as soon as cortisone was available in sufficient quantity it was tested in a case of acute rheumatoid arthritis. Fortunately, an adequate dose was employed and the response was dramatic. Thereafter, the salutary effects of ACTH were also demonstrated. The observations (Hench et al., 1949) immediately evoked wide interest. Soon, therapeutic applications were extended to other fields, with results to be presented later in this chapter. The impact upon the medical world can be gained from the fact that, in the year following the first published report of the efficacy of cortisone in the treatment of rheumatoid arthritis, the Nobel Prize in Medicine was jointly awarded to Kendall and Reichstein, who were responsible for much of the basic chemical research that led to the synthesis of the steroid, and to Hench, whose contribution has just been described.

In addition to a surge of clinical investigation, the therapeutic success of cortisone stimulated a wave of basic research in the 1950s. In that decade knowledge of the biochemistry of adrenal steroid synthesis and metabolism was brought close to its present level. As noted above, aldosterone was discovered; it was established that ACTH controls the reaction of cholesterol side chain scission (Stone and Hechter, 1954) and acts through the intermediacy of cyclic adenosine 3',5'-monophosphate (cyclic AMP) (Haynes et al., 1959); most synthetic analogs of cortisol used today were introduced, and practical technics for determination of cortisol became available to the clinician.

Effective clinical use of the corticosteroids has become possible because of their isolation, elucidation of structure, and economical synthesis. Manipulation of structure has yielded a variety of synthetic analogs, a few of which represent significant therapeutic gains in terms of the ratio of anti-inflammatory potency to effects on electrolyte metabolism. However, high hopes for elimination of toxicity have not been fulfilled. For this reason, it cannot be overemphasized that the corticosteroids, in pharmacological doses, are powerful drugs with slow cumulative toxic effects on many tissues, which may be inapparent until made manifest by a catastrophe.

ADRENOCORTICOTROPIC HORMONE

Chemistry. The structure of human ACTH, a peptide of 39 amino acid residues, is shown in Figure 63–1. Loss of one amino acid from the N-terminal end of the molecule by hydrolytic cleavage results in complete loss of biological activity. In contrast, a number of amino acids may be split off the C-terminal end with no effect on potency. A 24–amino acid peptide (sequence 1 through 24, Figure 63–1) retains the activity of the parent hormone, and the eicosopeptide (sequence 1 through 20) likewise is fully active. The structure-activity relationship of ACTH has been reviewed by Otsuka and Inouye (1975). Potency and duration of action can be enhanced by making substitutions in the amino acid chain, for example, D-serine for L-serine in position 1; this and other substitutions increase resistance of the peptide to the action of proteolytic enzymes. However, no advantages have yet been gained in clinical practice by such manipulations. The structural relationships between ACTH, the lipotropins, and the melanocyte-stimulating hormones are discussed in Chapter 59.

<0.1%   30% 100%
  ↓   ↓   ↓
Ser—Tyr—Ser—Met—Glu—His—Phe—Arg—Try—Gly—Lys—Pro—Val—Gly—Lys—Lys—Arg—Arg—Pro—Val—Lys—Val—
  1   2   3   4   5   6   7   8   9   10   11   12   13   14   15   16   17   18   19   20   21   22

                              NH₂
                               |
Tyr—Pro—Asp—Gly—Ala—Glu—Asp—Glu—Leu—Ala—Glu—Ala—Phe—Pro—Leu—Glu—Phe
 23   24   25   26   27   28   29   30   31   32   33   34   35   36   37   38   39

Figure 63–1. *Amino acid sequence of human ACTH.*

Ovine, porcine, and bovine ACTHs differ from human ACTH only at amino acid positions 25, 31, and 33 (Li, 1972). Synthetic peptides with amino acid sequences represented by the structures to the left of the arrows have been prepared and assayed (Hofmann, 1962). Full biological activity is retained as the chain is shortened until 19 is reached, at which length a significant reduction in potency occurs.

Actions on Adrenal Cortex. ACTH stimulates the human adrenal cortex to secrete cortisol, corticosterone, aldosterone, and a number of weakly androgenic substances. In the absence of the adenohypophysis, the adrenal cortex undergoes atrophy and the rates of secretion of cortisol and corticosterone are markedly reduced and remain virtually unchanged in response to otherwise-effective stimuli. Although ACTH can stimulate secretion of aldosterone, the rate of secretion is relatively independent of the adenohypophysis, and this explains the nearly normal electrolyte balance in the hypophysectomized animal. The zona glomerulosa is the least affected by atrophic changes that follow hypophysectomy, and it is the glomerulosa that is mainly responsible for the elaboration of aldosterone.

Prolonged administration of large doses of ACTH induces hyperplasia and hypertrophy of the adrenal cortex with continuous high output of cortisol, corticosterone, and weak androgens.

Mechanism of Action. ACTH acts to stimulate the *synthesis* of adrenocortical hormones; if it facilitates the release of preformed steroids from the adrenal cortex at all, this effect is overshadowed by the greater effect on synthesis. ACTH, as many other hormones, controls its target tissue through the agency of cyclic AMP. Thus, treatment with ACTH causes an increase in concentration of the cyclic nucleotide within adrenocortical cells (Haynes, 1958); cyclic AMP mimics ACTH in stimulating steroidogenesis (Haynes *et al.,* 1959) and in maintaining the weight of the adrenal after hypophysectomy (Ney, 1969). ACTH reacts with a specific hormone receptor in the adrenal-cell plasma membrane, and the result is a stimulation of adenylate cyclase activity and the formation of cyclic AMP.

The principal metabolic site at which steroidogenesis is regulated by the cyclic nucleotide is the oxidative cleavage of the side chain of cholesterol, the reaction that results in the formation of pregnenolone (*see* Figure 63-3, page 1472). This step is rate limiting in the sequence of reactions that leads to the formation of adrenal steroid hormones (Stone and Hechter, 1954). Exposure of adrenocortical cells to ACTH together with aminoglutethimide (to block side chain cleavage; *see* below) leads to increased amounts of cholesterol within the adrenal mitochondria, the locus of the side chain–cleaving enzyme (Mahaffee *et al.,* 1974). Furthermore, cholesterol bound to cytochrome P-450 is increased by ACTH (Bell and Harding, 1974; Paul *et al.,* 1976). These findings, together with evidence that the availability of cholesterol is the factor that limits the rate of the cleavage reaction in intact mitochondria (Kahnt *et al.,* 1974), suggest that ACTH, via cyclic AMP, stimulates the initial reaction in steroidogenesis from cholesterol by making the substrate available in increased concentration to the enzyme within the mitochondria. ACTH stimulates the formation of free cholesterol in the gland by activating cholesterol esterase, and this activation is apparently accomplished by phosphorylation of the enzyme (Beckett and Boyd, 1975; Pittman and Steinberg, 1977). ACTH also acts to increase the availability of cholesterol by stimulating its uptake from plasma lipoproteins (Gwynne *et al.,* 1976).

The trophic effects of ACTH on the adrenal cortex are little understood beyond the fact that they, like stimulation of steroidogenesis, appear to be mediated by cyclic AMP (Ney, 1969). The regulation of the adrenal cortex by ACTH has been reviewed by Gill (1976).

Extra-adrenal Effects of ACTH. Large doses of ACTH given to adrenalectomized animals cause a number of metabolic changes, including ketosis, lipolysis, hypoglycemia (early after administration), and resistance to insulin (late after administration). These extra-adrenal effects are of doubtful physiological significance, particularly since large doses are needed to induce them (Engel, 1961). Intravenous administration of ACTH (synthetic or porcine, but not bovine) leads to a transient elevation of the concentration of growth hormone in the plasma of adults but not children (Lee *et al.*, 1973).

Natural and synthetic corticotropins darken the isolated skin of the frog; this is not surprising since the amino acid sequence, 1 through 13, is identical with that of the melanocyte-stimulating hormone, α-MSH. Large doses of highly purified α-MSH and ACTH have been demonstrated to darken the skin of adrenalectomized human subjects. The hyperpigmentation of the skin that occurs in Addison's disease is thought to result from the high concentrations of ACTH that circulate in this condition. Previous reports of elevated concentrations of β-MSH in the plasma of Addisonian patients are probably the consequence of analytical artifacts. Evidence suggests that β-MSH is not present in man (Thody, 1977).

Regulation of the Secretion of ACTH. The fluctuations in the rates of secretion of cortisol, corticosterone, and, to some extent, aldosterone are determined by the fluctuations in the release of ACTH from the adenohypophysis. The adenohypophysis, in turn, is under the influence of the *nervous system* and *negative-feedback control* exerted by *corticosteroids*.

Nervous System: The Final Common Path. Stimuli that induce release of ACTH are subserved by neural paths converging on the median eminence of the hypothalamus. The functional link between the median eminence and the adenohypophysis, the final common path, is vascular, not neural. In response to an appropriate stimulus, corticotropin-releasing factor (CRF) is elaborated at neuronal endings in the median eminence and transported in the hypophyseal-portal vessels to the adenohypophysis, where it stimulates the secretion of ACTH. CRF itself has not yet been characterized (*see* Chapter 59).

ACTH is synthesized in basophilic cells of the adenohypophysis and, like many other peptide hormones, it is derived from a larger precursor. "Big ACTH" is a glycoprotein of about 30,000 molecular weight. Its conversion to ACTH, with a molecular weight of 4500, has been studied in mouse pituitary tumors (Eipper and Mains, 1978; Roberts *et al.*, 1978). As indicated in Figure 59–2 (page 1388), the precursor of ACTH includes the sequences of MSH, the lipotropins, and the endorphins. In man, the role of these three groups of active peptides remains conjectural and a subject of active investigation.

Negative Feedback of the Corticosteroids (Cortisol and Corticosterone). Administration of certain corticosteroids suppresses the secretion of ACTH, reduces the store of ACTH in the adenohypophysis, and induces morphological changes (hyalinization of the basophilic cells) suggestive of functional impairment of the adenohypophysis. The adrenal cortex itself undergoes atrophy. In contrast, adrenalectomized animals and patients with Addison's disease have abnormally high concentrations of ACTH in the blood even under optimal environmental conditions. When a stimulus is applied to an adrenalectomized animal, the concentration of ACTH reaches even higher levels. These observations point out the important inhibitory role of the corticosteroids and clearly demonstrate that ACTH release remains under control of the nervous system in the absence of corticosteroid feedback. Secretion of ACTH at any instant is determined by the balance of neural excitatory and corticosteroid inhibitory effects.

Mechanism of Feedback by Corticosteroids. The sites of control of ACTH secretion by adrenocortical hormones have not been established. Binding of glucocorticoids has been detected in the pituitary, hypothalamus, and other areas of the brain (McEwen, 1977); however, the link between such binding and inhibition of the secretion of ACTH has not been elucidated. Glucocorticoids cause a decrease in the activity of mRNA for ACTH in the pituitary, indicating that the effect may be at the transcriptional level, at least in part (Nakanishi *et al.*, 1977).

Examples of Effective Stimuli of Secretion. A number of conditions have been demonstrated to stimulate adrenocortical secretion in man. These include the agonal state, severe infections, surgery, parturition, cold, exercise, and emotional stress. Stressful stimuli override the normal negative-feedback control mechanisms, and plasma concentrations of adrenocortical steroids can be elevated within a few minutes of the initiation of an appropriate stimulus.

Diurnal Cycles in Adrenocortical Activity. The rate of secretion of cortisol by the adrenal cortex of a normal human subject under optimal conditions is about 20 mg per day. However, the rate is not steady and exhibits rhythmic fluctuations; concentrations of adrenocortical steroids in plasma are relatively high in the early morning hours, decline during the day, and reach a minimum about midnight. Plasma concentrations of ACTH are higher at 6 A.M. than at 6 P.M. The diurnal patterns of glucocorticoids and ACTH are not observed in patients with Cushing's disease, and this factor is considered in the diagnosis of the disorder.

Absorption, Fate, and Excretion. ACTH is readily absorbed from parenteral sites, and is usually administered by intramuscular injection and occasionally by intravenous infusion. The hormone rapidly disappears from the circulation following its intravenous administration; in man, the half-life in plasma is about 15 minutes.

Bioassay. The U.S.P. has adopted the *Third International Standard for Corticotropin* (Bangham *et al.,* 1962) as the reference standard in the United States. Potency is based on an assay in hypophysectomized rats in which depletion of adrenal ascorbic acid is measured after subcutaneous administration of the ACTH. All commercial preparations are now described in these units only.

Preparations, Dosage, and Routes of Administration. *Corticotropin Injection,* U.S.P. (ACTH), is available as a sterile solution or as a lyophilized powder (ACTHAR) for intramuscular or intravenous use. The preparation is derived from the pituitaries of mammals used for food. Maximal adrenocortical secretion is obtained in adults with a total dose of 25 U.S.P. units infused for 8 hours.

Repository Corticotropin Injection, U.S.P. (H.P. ACTHAR GEL, CORTROPHIN GEL, others), is administered either intramuscularly or subcutaneously. It is a highly purified ACTH in gelatin solution. A typical dose is 40 units, given once daily.

Some gel preparations of ACTH have been approved for intravenous administration. However, it is preferable to utilize the purer *Corticotropin for Injection,* U.S.P., for intravenous therapy and *cosyntropin* (*see* below) for diagnostic use, in order to minimize the possibility of allergic reactions.

Sterile Corticotropin Zinc Hydroxide Suspension, U.S.P. (CORTROPHIN-ZINC), is a preparation of purified corticotropin adsorbed on zinc hydroxide, intended for intramuscular injection. A typical dose is 40 units, given once daily.

Cosyntropin for injection (CORTROSYN) is a synthetic peptide corresponding to amino acid residues 1 to 24 of human ACTH. This preparation, approved for diagnostic purposes, is given intramuscularly or intravenously in a dose of 0.25 mg (equivalent to 25 units).

Therapeutic and Diagnostic Applications of ACTH. At the present time, the most important use of ACTH is as a *diagnostic agent* in adrenal insufficiency. For this purpose, ACTH is administered and the concentration of cortisol in plasma is determined. A normal increase in plasma cortisol rules out primary adrenocortical failure. If there is no acute response, prolonged administration of ACTH is carried out. In cases of pituitary insufficiency, prolonged treatment can be expected to elicit a rise in plasma cortisol concentration.

Therapeutic uses of ACTH have included the treatment of adrenocortical insufficiency and nonendocrine disorders that are responsive to glucocorticoids. However, therapy with ACTH is less predictable and much less convenient than is that with appropriate steroids. Furthermore, ACTH stimulates secretion of mineralocorticoids and, therefore, may cause acute retention of salt and water. While this generally does not persist with continuing therapy, it is a potentially serious problem in patients who have cardiac insufficiency. ACTH would obviously be of

no value in the treatment of primary adrenocortical failure. Furthermore, there is no substantial evidence that therapeutic goals can be attained with ACTH in secondary adrenocortical insufficiency that cannot be attained with appropriate doses of currently available steroids. It must be kept in mind, however, that ACTH and corticosteroids are not pharmacologically equivalent. Treatment with ACTH exposes the tissues to a mixture of glucocorticoids, mineralocorticoids, and androgens, in contrast to the conventional, contemporary practice of administering a single glucocorticoid. It is possible that the steroid mixture resulting from adrenal stimulation by ACTH has effects that differ significantly from those of a single, synthetic glucocorticoid. Thus, Grahame (1969) reported the absence of dermal atrophy in patients treated for prolonged periods of time with ACTH, in contrast to that found with corticosteroid treatment. This has been tentatively attributed to a protective action of androgens against the inhibitory effects of glucocorticoids on fibroblasts (Harvey and Grahame, 1973).

Clinical Toxicity of ACTH. The toxicity of ACTH, aside from rare hypersensitivity reactions, is entirely attributable to the increased rate of secretion of adrenocorticosteroids (*see* below). Hypersensitivity reactions, ranging from mild fever to anaphylaxis and death, have been reported. The synthetic ACTH peptides are thought to be less antigenic than is the parent molecule. Nevertheless, hypersensitivity to them does occur (Forssman and Mulder, 1973). Because it stimulates synthesis and secretion of mineralocorticoids and androgens, ACTH causes more sodium retention, a greater degree of hypokalemic alkalosis, and more acne than do the synthetic congeners of cortisol.

ADRENOCORTICAL STEROIDS

The adrenal cortex synthesizes two classes of steroids: the corticosteroids with 21 carbons and the adrenal androgens with 19 carbons. A typical corticosteroid, *cortisol,* is shown in Figure 63–2; a typical adrenal androgen, *dehydroepiandrosterone,* is shown in Figure 63–3 (page 1472).

Adrenocorticosteroid Biosynthesis. Cholesterol is an obligatory intermediate in the biosynthesis of corticosteroids. Although the adrenal cortex synthesizes cholesterol from acetate by processes similar to those in liver, the greater part of the cholesterol (60 to 80%) utilized for corticosteroidogenesis comes from exogenous sources, both at rest and following administration of ACTH. Cholesterol is enzymatically converted to 21-carbon corticosteroids and 19-carbon weak androgens by a series of steps presented in simplified form in Figure 63–3. Most of the reactions are catalyzed by mixed-function oxidases that contain cytochrome P-450 and require NADPH and molecular oxygen.

In addition to other androgens, the adrenal cortex

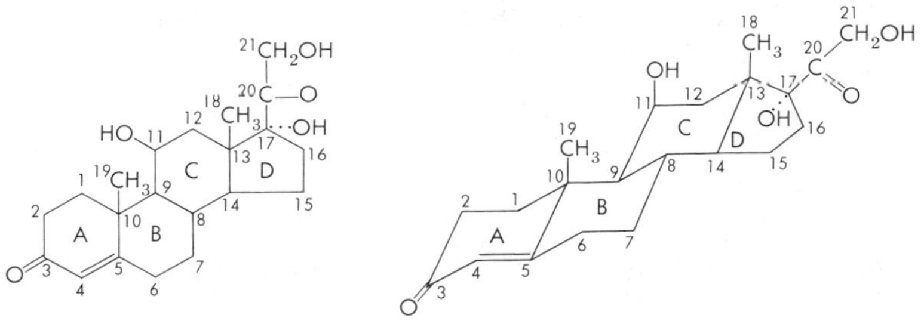

Figure 63-2. *Structure, stereochemistry, and nomenclature of adrenocorticosteroids, as typified by cortisol (hydrocortisone).*

The four rings—A, B, C, and D—are not in a flat plane, as conventionally represented in *I,* but have the approximate configuration shown in *II.* (The planarity of the valence angles about the double bond between C 4 and C 5 prevents the chair form of ring A, as shown, from being an energetically probable conformational state. As a result, ring A is in a half-chair conformation, not easily represented in two dimensions.) Orientation of the groups attached to the steroid ring system is importantly related to biological activity. The methyl groups at C 18 and C 19, the hydroxyl group at C 11, and the two-carbon ketol side chain at C 17 project above the plane of the steroid and are designated β. Their connection to the ring system is shown by full-line bonds. The hydroxy at C 17 projects below the plane and is designated α, and the connection to the ring is shown by a dotted bond. The ketone at C 3 in association with the double bond between C 4 and C 5 in ring A is an important structural feature of the biologically active corticosteroids. Reduction of the ketone at C 3 leads to the formation of two isomers: one, 3β-hydroxy; the other, 3α-hydroxy. Saturation of the 4,5 double bond leads to the formation of two isomers: 5α and 5β. Reduction of the ketone at C 20 creates an asymmetrical carbon at this site, the two possible isomers being designated α and β.

In formal chemical nomenclature, the adrenocortical hormones are described as derivatives of androstane or of pregnane. Double bonds are indicated by the symbol Δ with superscripts to indicate the position of the double bond. In this convention, cortisol is designated 11β,-17α,21-trihydroxy-Δ^4-pregnene-3,20-dione. Dehydroepiandrosterone is designated 3β-hydroxy-Δ^5-androsten-17-one.

secretes testosterone; however, about half the plasma testosterone of normal women is derived from androstenedione at an extra-adrenal site.

Adrenocorticosteroids are not stored in the adrenal. The amounts of corticosteroids found in adrenal tissue are insufficient to maintain normal rates of secretion for more than a few minutes in the absence of continuing biosynthesis. For this reason, the rate of biosynthesis is tantamount to the rate of secretion. Table 63-1 shows typical rates of secretion of the physiologically most important corticosteroids in man—cortisol and aldosterone—and also their approximate concentrations in peripheral plasma. The mechanism of control of steroidogenesis by ACTH has been discussed above, and the regulation of aldosterone synthesis by renin and angiotensin is described in Chapter 27.

PHYSIOLOGICAL FUNCTIONS AND PHARMACOLOGICAL EFFECTS

The effects of the corticosteroids are numerous and widespread. They influence carbohydrate, protein, fat, and purine metabolism; electrolyte and water balance; and the functions of the cardiovascular system, the kidney, skeletal muscle, the nervous system, and other organs and tissues. Furthermore, the corticosteroids endow the organism with the capacity to resist many types of noxious stimuli and environmental change. The adrenal cortex is the organ, *par excellence,* of homeostasis, being responsible to a large extent for the relative freedom that higher organisms exhibit in a constantly changing environment. In the absence of the adrenal cortex, survival is possible but only under the most rigidly prescribed conditions; for example, food must be available regularly, sodium chloride ingested in relatively large quantities, and environmental temperature maintained within a suitably narrow range.

A given dose of corticosteroid may be *physiological* or *pharmacological,* depending on the environment and the activities of the organism. Under favorable conditions, a small dose of corticosteroid maintains the adrenalectomized animal in a state of well-being. Under adverse conditions a relatively

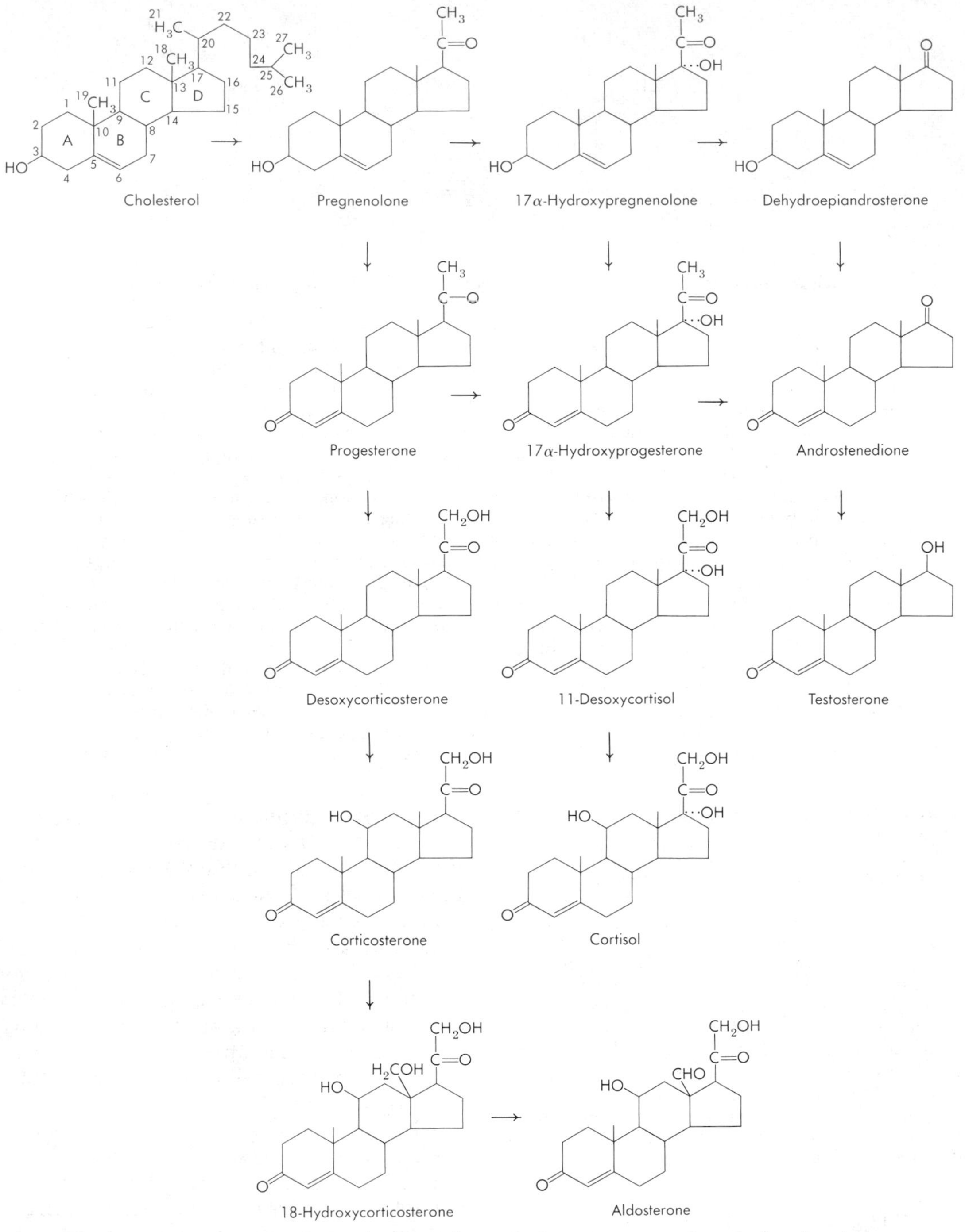

Figure 63–3. *Principal pathways for biosynthesis of adrenocorticosteroids and adrenal androgens.*

large dose is needed if the animal is to survive. This same large dose given repetitively under optimal conditions induces hypercorticism, that is, signs of excess of corticosteroid. The fluctuations in the secretory activity of a normal subject are presumed to reflect the varying needs of the organism for corticosteroids.

The regulatory actions of corticosteroids are often complexly related to the regulatory

Table 63-1. RATES OF SECRETION AND TYPICAL PLASMA CONCENTRATIONS OF THE MAJOR BIOLOGICALLY ACTIVE CORTICOSTEROIDS IN MAN

	CORTISOL	ALDOSTERONE
Rate of secretion under optimal conditions, mg/day	20	0.125
Concentrations in peripheral plasma of man, μg/dl	8 A.M. 16 4 P.M. 4	0.01

actions of other hormones. For example, in the absence of lipolytic hormones, cortisol even in large concentrations has virtually no effect on the rate of lipolysis in adipose tissue *in vitro*. Likewise, a sympathomimetic amine has only slight effect on the rate of lipolysis if there is a deficiency of glucocorticoids. However, if a necessary minimal amount of cortisol is added, the lipolytic effect of the sympathomimetic amine becomes evident. The necessary but not sufficient role of corticosteroids acting in concert with other regulatory forces has been termed "permissive" by Ingle (1954).

Certain of the biological actions of the corticosteroids lend themselves to quantitative measurement. Estimates of the potencies of naturally occurring and synthetic corticosteroids in the categories of *sodium retention* (reduction of sodium excretion by the kidney of the adrenalectomized animal), *hepatic deposition of glycogen*, and *anti-inflammatory effect* (inhibition of the action of an agent that induces inflammation) are presented in Table 63–2. It should be noted that such values are not fixed ratios but vary considerably with the conditions of the bioassays used. Potencies of steroids as judged by ability to maintain the adrenalectomized animal in a state of well-being closely parallel those determined for sodium retention. Potencies based on liver glycogen deposition, anti-inflammatory effect, work capacity of skeletal muscle, and involution of lymphoid tissue closely parallel one another. Dissociations exist between potencies based on sodium retention and on liver glycogen deposition; traditionally the corticosteroids have thus been classified into *mineralocorticoids* and *glucocorticoids*, according to potencies in the two categories. Desoxycorticosterone, the prototype of the mineralocorticoids, is highly

potent in regard to sodium retention but without effect on hepatic glycogen deposition. Cortisol, the prototype of the glucocorticoids, is highly potent in regard to liver glycogen deposition but weak in regard to sodium retention. The naturally occurring corticosteroids cortisol and cortisone as well as synthetic corticosteroids such as prednisolone and triamcinolone are glucocorticoids. However, corticosterone is a steroid that has modest but significant activities in both categories. Finally, aldosterone is exceedingly potent with respect to sodium retention, with modest but appreciable potency for liver glycogen deposition. At rates secreted by the adrenal cortex or in doses that exert maximal effects on electrolyte balance, aldosterone has no significant effect on carbohydrate metabolism; it is thus classified as a mineralocorticoid.

In the descriptions of the physiological functions and the pharmacological effects of the corticosteroids to follow, the terms *mineralocorticoid* and *glucocorticoid* will be employed for convenience. It is to be emphasized that the biological characteristics of the corticosteroids range over a spectrum from that of a strictly mineralocorticoid type at the one end to that of a strictly glucocorticoid type at the other. A comprehensive review of the actions of the glucocorticoids is that of Baxter (1976).

Mechanism of Action. Corticosteroids, like other steroid hormones, are thought to act by controlling the rate of synthesis of proteins. As is true with estrogens (Chapter 61), the corticosteroids react with receptor proteins in the cytoplasm of sensitive cells to form a steroid-receptor complex. Such receptors

Table 63-2. RELATIVE POTENCIES OF CORTICOSTEROIDS

	SODIUM RETENTION	LIVER GLYCOGEN DEPOSITION	ANTI-INFLAMMATORY EFFECT
Natural Steroids			
Cortisol	1 *	1	1
Cortisone	0.8 *	0.8	0.8
Corticosterone	15	0.35	0.3
11-Desoxycorticosterone	100	0	0
Aldosterone	3000	0.3	?
Synthetic Steroids			
Prednisolone	<1 *	4	4
Triamcinolone	0	5	5

* Promotes sodium excretion under certain circumstances.

have been identified in many tissues (Ballard *et al.,* 1974). The steroid-receptor complex undergoes a conformational change, as noted by an increase in the sedimentation constant; following this, the complex moves into the nucleus, where it binds to chromatin. Information carried by the steroid or more likely by the receptor protein directs the genetic apparatus to transcribe RNA. In recent years there have been direct demonstrations that glucocorticoids, in appropriate tissues, increase the quantity of mRNA that codes for enzymes whose synthesis is stimulated by these hormones (Schutz *et al.,* 1975; Iynedjian and Hanson, 1977).

Steroid hormones thus stimulate transcription and ultimately the synthesis of specific proteins. While this is true for corticosteroids in some tissues, such as the liver, in other tissues, for example, lymphoid cells and fibroblasts, the overall effect of the hormones is a catabolic one. This suggests that the steroid-receptor complex may inhibit rather than stimulate transcription in these instances. However, Makman and co-workers (1971) presented evidence suggesting that steroids act in lymphatic cells to stimulate the synthesis of an inhibitory protein, which presumably causes the catabolic effects.

Carbohydrate and Protein Metabolism.

The effects of adrenocortical hormones on carbohydrate and protein metabolism are epitomized in the teleological view that these steroids have evolved to protect glucose-dependent cerebral functions by stimulating the formation of glucose, diminishing its peripheral utilization, and promoting its storage as glycogen. Adrenalectomized animals exhibit no marked abnormality in carbohydrate metabolism if food is regularly available. Under such circumstances, normal concentrations of glucose in the plasma are maintained and glycogen is stored in the liver. However, a brief period of starvation rapidly depletes carbohydrate reserves. The concentration of glycogen in the liver, and to a lesser extent that in muscle, decreases and hypoglycemia develops. In light of these facts, it is not surprising that the adrenalectomized animal is hypersensitive to insulin. Patients with Addison's disease have similar abnormalities in carbohydrate metabolism.

Administration of a glucocorticoid such as cortisol corrects the defect in carbohydrate metabolism of the adrenalectomized animal; glycogen stores, particularly in the liver, are increased; concentrations of glucose in plasma remain normal during fasting; sensitivity to insulin returns to normal. Increased excretion of nitrogen accompanies the increased production of glucose, indicating that protein is converted to carbohydrate (Long *et al.,* 1940). Prolonged exposure to large doses of glucocorticoids leads to an exaggeration of these changes in glucose metabolism, so that a diabetic-like state is produced: glucose in the plasma tends to be elevated in the fasting subject, there is increased resistance to insulin, glucose tolerance is decreased, and glucosuria may be present.

The mechanism by which the glucocorticoids inhibit utilization of glucose in peripheral tissues is not understood. Decreased uptake of glucose has been demonstrated in adipose tissue, skin, fibroblasts, and thymocytes as a result of glucocorticoid action.

Glucocorticoids promote gluconeogenesis by both peripheral and hepatic actions. Peripherally these steroids act to mobilize amino acids from a number of tissues. This catabolic action of the glucocorticoids is reflected in the atrophy of lymphatic tissues, reduced mass of muscle, osteoporosis (reduction in protein matrix of bone followed by calcium loss), thinning of the skin, and a negative nitrogen balance. Amino acids funnel into the liver, where they serve as substrates for enzymes involved in the production of glucose and glycogen.

In the liver the glucocorticoids induce *de-novo* synthesis of a number of enzymes involved in gluconeogenesis and amino acid metabolism. For example, the hepatic enzymes phosphoenolpyruvate carboxykinase, fructose-1,6-diphosphatase, and glucose-6-phosphatase, which catalyze reactions of glucose synthesis, are increased in concentration. However, induction of these enzymes requires a matter of hours and cannot account for the earliest effects of the hormones on gluconeogenesis. More rapid effects of glucocorticoids are apparent on hepatic mitochondria, such that they carboxylate pyruvate to form oxaloacetate at an accelerated rate (Adam and Haynes, 1969). This is the first reaction in the synthesis of glucose from pyruvate.

Prolonged, but not acute, treatment with glucocorticoids has been found to elevate the concentration of glucagon in the plasma (Marco *et al.,* 1973; Wise *et al.,* 1973). Inasmuch as glucagon itself stimulates gluconeogenesis, the rise in glucagon should also contribute to the enhanced synthesis of glucose. The deposition of glycogen in the liver found after treatment with glucocorticoids is thought to be at least in part secondary to the rise in plasma insulin concentration elicited by the elevated plasma glucose (Kreutner and Goldberg, 1967).

Lipid Metabolism.

Two effects of corticosteroids on lipid metabolism are firmly established. The first is the dramatic redistribution of body fat that occurs in the hypercorticoid state. The other is the facilitation of the effect of adipokinetic agents in eliciting lipolysis of the triglycerides of adipose tissue. A number of other effects of corticosteroids on lipids have been reported, but in few, if any, instances have they turned out to be direct actions of the corticosteroids themselves.

Administration of large doses of glucocorticoids to human subjects over a long period of time or the hypersecretion of cortisol that occurs in Cushing's syndrome leads to a peculiar alteration in fat distribution. There is a gain of fat in depots in the back of the neck ("buffalo hump"), supraclavicular area, and face ("moon face") and a loss of fat from the extremities. The mode of action of the corticosteroids in bringing about abnormal fat distribution is unknown; the phenomenon illustrates the complexity of the effects of steroids on fat metabolism, for it is apparent that the fat depots are heterogeneous and differ from area to area in their responses to the same hormone.

The mobilization of fat from peripheral fat depots by epinephrine, norepinephrine, or adipokinetic peptides of the adenohypophysis is markedly blunted in the absence of the adrenal cortex or the adenohypophysis. It appears that cortisol acts in adipose tissue to facilitate the lipolytic response to cyclic AMP, rather than to enhance its accumulation. Hypophysectomy in rats has only a slight effect on the accumulation of cyclic AMP after exposure of adipose tissue to graded doses of epinephrine (Birnbaum and Goodman, 1973); however, hypophysectomy greatly decreases the lipolytic response of adipose tissue to the cyclic nucleotide. Treatment with cortisol restores the normal response to lipolytic hormones and to cyclic AMP (Goodman, 1968). Plasma lipids are not changed consistently in either hypocorticism or hypercorticism.

Electrolyte and Water Balance. Mineralocorticoids act on the distal tubules of the kidney to enhance the reabsorption of sodium ions from the tubular fluid into the plasma; they increase the urinary excretion of both potassium and hydrogen ions. The consequences of these three primary effects in concert with similar actions on cation transport in other tissues appear to account for the entire spectrum of physiological and pharmacological activities that are characteristic of the mineralocorticoids. Thus, the primary features of *hypercorticism* are positive sodium balance and expansion of the extracellular fluid volume, normal or slight increase in the concentration of sodium in the plasma, hypokalemia, and alkalosis. In contrast, those of the deficient state, *hypo-*

corticism, are sodium loss, hyponatremia, hyperkalemia, contraction of the extracellular fluid volume, and cellular hydration. The classical studies of Harrop and Loeb and their associates (*see* Harrop *et al.,* 1933; Loeb, 1933; Loeb *et al.,* 1933) revealed a defect of major consequence in adrenocortical insufficiency, namely, the renal loss of sodium. The renal tubules normally reabsorb practically all the sodium filtered at the glomerulus. For example, on an ordinary diet, 99.5% may be reabsorbed to maintain sodium balance. Typically, in a patient with Addison's disease under the same circumstances of dietary intake, maximal reabsorption attainable is 98.5%. Since approximately 24,000 mEq of sodium is filtered per day, the 1% difference between reabsorption in the normal subject and reabsorption in the patient with Addison's disease amounts to a loss of 240 mEq of sodium per day. The gravity of the situation is obvious when one considers that this amount of sodium is normally present in 1.7 liters of extracellular fluid. Proportionately more sodium than water is lost through the kidney and the concentration of extracellular sodium decreases; extracellular fluid becomes hypoosmotic, and water shifts from the extracellular into the intracellular compartment. This shift, together with the renal loss of water, results in a marked reduction in the volume of the extracellular fluid. Cells are hydrated, and the increase in the hematocrit value is due not only to a shrinkage of the plasma volume but also to the swelling of the erythrocytes. Hyperkalemia and the tendency toward acid-base disturbances are a result of impairments in the excretion of potassium and of hydrogen ions. Without administration of mineralocorticoids or sodium chloride solution or both, a rapid downhill course ensues in adrenocortical insufficiency. The shrinkage of extracellular fluid volume, the cellular hydration, and the hypodynamic state of the cardiovascular system combine to cause circulatory collapse, renal failure, and death.

In adrenocortical insufficiency, a basic defect in ion transport occurs in a variety of secretory cells. Not only the kidney but also the salivary glands, the sweat glands, the exocrine pancreas, and the mucosa of the gastrointestinal tract elaborate fluids abnormally high in the concentration of sodium and abnormally low in the concentration of potassium. In the patient with Addison's disease, sweating may contribute significantly to the negative balance of sodium.

Aldosterone is by far the most potent of the naturally occurring corticosteroids with regard to electrolyte balance and plays an important role in the regulation of sodium and potassium balance. Evidence of this is the relatively normal electrolyte balance exhibited by the hypophysectomized animal as a result of the secretion of aldosterone by the adrenal cortex. The increased rate of secretion of aldosterone that occurs in man when dietary salt is severely limited would appear to be a compensatory adjustment of physiological importance. However, *changes* in the rate of secretion of aldosterone are not the cause of *rapid* changes that may occur in sodium excretion. The latent period of action of the steroid is too long.

The intravenous administration of aldosterone to a normal subject is followed, after a delay of about an hour, by a decrease in the rate of renal sodium ion excretion and an increase in the rate of potassium ion and hydrogen ion excretion. If the administration of relatively large amounts of aldosterone is continued over a period of more than 2 or 3 days, sodium excretion again equals sodium intake. However, potassium ion and hydrogen ion excretion continues at an accelerated rate, resulting in hypokalemic hypochloremic alkalosis. The mechanism of "escape" from acute sodium retention is not understood. The effects of the mineralocorticoids have been reviewed by Mulrow and Forman (1972).

The morphological complexity of the mammalian kidney presents a formidable obstacle to an attack on the question as to how aldosterone increases sodium reabsorption. Aldosterone stimulates sodium transport by the toad bladder, and it is understandable that investigators have turned to this structurally simple organ as an experimental system.

Studies with the toad bladder have indicated that aldosterone, like other steroids, probably acts to initiate transcription of RNA that serves as template for the synthesis of a protein or proteins. This hypothetical "aldosterone-induced protein" is thought to facilitate the transport of sodium ions. Two major hypotheses have been developed from experiments with toad bladders to explain the actions of aldosterone in the kidney. Both use the following model of renal sodium ion reabsorption. The sodium ions of the tubular filtrate enter the cells of the distal tubules down a concentration gradient through the cell membrane facing the tubular lumen (apical or mucosal surface). They diffuse through the cell to the serosal surface, which is in contact with extracellular fluid. At this interface the ions are pumped out of the cell against a concentration gradient by an energy-requiring pump that has the operational characteristics of a Na^+,K^+-activated adenosine triphosphatase (Na,K-ATPase). The "permease" hypothesis proposes that mineralocorticoids increase the permeability of the mucosal surface to sodium ions. Sodium ions therefore enter the cells at an accelerated rate and are pumped out into the extracellular space by the sodium ion pump at the serosal surface. The alternative or "pump" hypothesis proposes that the mucosal surface of the tubular cells is freely permeable to sodium ions. Aldosterone increases the sodium-pumping activity at the serosal surface by activating the pump enzyme(s) or by providing additional energy to drive the pump (Feldman *et al.,* 1972).

The mechanisms of the enhanced excretion of potassium and hydrogen ions are less well understood. For practical purposes one may visualize these ions as being "exchanged" for the additional sodium ions reabsorbed under the influence of the steroids, because the sum of the equivalents of the additional potassium and hydrogen ions excreted is equal to that of the additional sodium ions retained.

The *glucocorticoids* decrease the absorption of calcium from the intestine and increase its renal excretion, thus producing a negative balance of the cation. These effects are considered to be the basis of the favorable therapeutic response to glucocorticoids seen in hypercalcemia (*see* Chapter 65).

Desoxycorticosterone is a natural mineralocorticoid of some historical interest for it was the first corticosteroid to be synthesized and made available for the treatment of Addison's disease. Desoxycorticosterone is practically devoid of glucocorticoid effects. Qualitatively, it is identical to aldosterone in its effects on electrolytes; quantitatively, it is about 3% as potent (*see* Table 63–2). Thus, despite the fact that the concentration of desoxycorticosterone in plasma is approximately the same as that of aldosterone, it apparently is of little physiological significance in the normal individual (Biglieri, 1978).

Cortisol induces sodium retention and potassium excretion, but much less effectively than does aldosterone. Acute treatment with cortisol, unlike that with aldosterone, does not increase net acid secretion (Lemann *et al.,* 1970). In striking contrast to aldosterone, cortisol, under certain circumstances, especially sodium loading, enhances sodium excretion. This may be accounted for by the capacity of cortisol to increase the glomerular filtration rate (GFR). Aldosterone and desoxycorticosterone are ineffective in this regard. Furthermore, cortisol has a significant stimulatory influence on tubular secretory activity.

Impaired water diuresis in response to an administered water load is sufficiently characteristic of adrenal insufficiency to have been used as a diagnostic criterion. In adrenal insufficiency, GFR is reduced and plasma antidiuretic hormone (ADH) concentration is increased; these factors account for failure to excrete a water load (Ahmed *et al.*, 1967). Administration of cortisol, but not of aldosterone, increases GFR and restores water diuresis. The influence of cortisol on the concentration of ADH in plasma has not been settled (Gill *et al.*, 1962).

Hypercorticism due to administration of large doses of cortisol (or related glucocorticoids) or to excessive secretion of cortisol by the adrenals is sometimes associated with a hypokalemic hypochloremic alkalosis. However, the changes, particularly the degree of hypokalemia, are moderate in severity and reflect the relatively weak effect of cortisol as compared to aldosterone on electrolyte balance. Muscular weakness associated with glucocorticoid treatment is usually due to a loss of muscle mass rather than of potassium.

Cardiovascular System. The most striking effects of corticosteroids on the cardiovascular system are those that are the consequence of regulation of renal sodium ion excretion. These are seen most vividly in hypocorticism when reduction in blood volume accompanied by increased viscosity can lead to hypotension and cardiovascular collapse. However, the impairment of the cardiovascular system in adrenocortical insufficiency obviously involves additional, poorly understood processes The corticosteroids exert important actions on the various elements of the circulatory system, including the capillaries, the arterioles, and the myocardium. In the absence of the corticosteroids, there is increased capillary permeability, inadequate vasomotor response of the small vessels, and reduction in cardiac size and output.

An excess of mineralocorticoids occurs in its purest form in *primary aldosteronism,* the result of excessive secretion of this steroid. In this disease the major clinical findings are hypertension and hypokalemia. The hypokalemia is an obvious consequence of the renal effects of aldosterone, but the genesis of the hypertension has not been clarified. Development of hypertension requires a prolonged excess of mineralocorticoid and increased sodium intake (Mulrow and Forman, 1972). Hypertension occurs in most cases of Cushing's syndrome but rarely, if at all, as the result of administration of synthetic glucocorticoids lacking mineralocorticoid activity. Steroid-induced hypertension may be the result of prolonged, excessive sodium retention; one hypothesis proposes that this leads to edema within the walls of arterioles, thereby reducing their lumina and increasing peripheral vascular resistance (Tobian, 1960). Another possibility is that salt retention or mineralocorticoids themselves sensitize blood vessels to pressor agents, in particular angiotensin and catecholamines (Brunner *et al.*, 1972; Yard and Kadowitz,

1972). The concentration of renin substrate is elevated in Cushing's syndrome, and this too may play a role (Krakoff *et al.*, 1975).

Skeletal Muscle. The maintenance of normal function of skeletal muscle requires adequate concentrations of corticosteroids, but excessive amounts of either mineralocorticoids or glucocorticoids lead to abnormalities.

It is well known that one of the outstanding signs of adrenocortical insufficiency is a diminished work capacity of striated muscle. This is manifested in patients with Addison's disease by weakness and fatigue. The most important single factor responsible for this dysfunction appears to be the inadequacy of the circulatory system. Abnormalities in electrolyte balance and carbohydrate metabolism in adrenocortical insufficiency contribute only in small measure to the impairment in skeletal muscle function.

Muscle weakness in primary aldosteronism is in large measure a result of the hypokalemia characteristic of this disease. Glucocorticoids given for prolonged periods in high doses or secreted in abnormal amounts in Cushing's syndrome tend to cause a wasting of skeletal muscle. The mechanism of this is not known. This steroid myopathy is responsible, at least in part, for the weakness and fatigue noted in the syndrome.

Central Nervous System. The corticosteroids affect the central nervous system (CNS) in a number of indirect ways; in particular, they maintain normal concentrations of glucose in plasma, an adequate circulation, and the normal balance of electrolytes in the body. The steroids may also have direct effects, but these are as yet poorly defined. An influence of the corticosteroids can be observed on mood, behavior, the EEG, and brain excitability.

Patients with Addison's disease exhibit apathy, depression, and irritability, and some are frankly psychotic. Desoxycorticosterone is ineffective but cortisol is very effective in correcting these abnormalities of psyche and behavior. An array of reactions, varying in degree and kind, is seen in patients to whom glucocorticoids are administered for therapeutic purposes. Most patients respond with elevation in mood, which may be explained in part by the relief of the symptoms of the disease being treated. In some, more definite mood changes occur, characterized by euphoria, insomnia, restlessness, and increased motor activity. A smaller but significant percentage of patients treated with high doses of cortisol become anxious or depressed, and a still smaller percentage exhibit psychotic reactions. There is a high incidence of neuroses and psychoses among patients with Cushing's syndrome. The abnormalities of behavior usually disappear when the corticosteroids are withdrawn or the Cushing's syndrome is effectively treated.

There is usually an increase in the excitability of neural tissue in hypocorticism and a decrease in animals given large doses of desoxycorticosterone; these alterations appear to be related to changes in the concentrations of electrolytes in the brain. The ratios of extracellular to intracellular sodium and intracellular to extracellular potassium are decreased in hypocorticism and increased with excess desoxycorticosterone. Furthermore, the administration of sodium chloride in excess to adrenalectomized animals maintains ion concentrations and neuronal excitability at normal levels. In contrast, chronic administration of cortisol increases brain excitability without influencing the concentrations of sodium and potassium in the brain. It is concluded that the influence of desoxycorticosterone on excitability is mediated through its influence on sodium transport, whereas cortisol acts by a different and as-yet-unknown mechanism. That cortisol may act directly on the brain is suggested by the report that there are cortisol-binding proteins possessing the characteristics of steroid receptors in the brain (Ballard *et al.*, 1974).

Thresholds for the perception of taste, smell, and sound stimuli are reduced in adrenocortical insufficiency and elevated in hypercorticism. Glucocorticoids restore thresholds to normal, but desoxycorticosterone is without effect (Henkin, 1970).

Formed Elements of Blood. Glucocorticoids tend to increase the hemoglobin and red-cell content of the blood, as evidenced by the frequent occurrence of polycythemia in Cushing's syndrome and a mild, normochromic, normocytic anemia in Addison's disease.

The corticosteroids also affect circulating white cells. Administration of glucocorticoids leads to an increase in the number of polymorphonuclear leukocytes in the blood, while the numbers of lymphocytes, eosinophils, monocytes, and basophils decrease. The response of platelets is unclear, as both thrombocytosis and thrombocytopenia have been reported to follow glucocorticoid administration.

There is evidence that glucocorticoids retard erythrophagocytosis (Greendyke *et al.*, 1965). A stimulation of erythropoiesis has not been convincingly demonstrated in the healthy individual. However, the steroids do elicit a normoblastic response in the marrow of patients with megaloblastic anemia (Doig *et al.*, 1957).

Steroid-induced granulocytosis is thought to result from the combination of an increased rate of entrance of polymorphonuclear leukocytes into the blood from the marrow and a diminished rate of their removal (Bishop *et al.*, 1968).

The lymphocytopenia that results from the actions of the corticosteroids is presumably related to the widespread effects of the glucocorticoids on lymphoid tissue (*see* following section). A single dose of cortisol in man produces a decline of about 70% in circulating lymphocytes and a decline of over 90% in monocytes in 4 to 6 hours. The thymus-derived lymphocytes are decreased proportionately more than those that are derived from the bone marrow. The profile of cellular responses of the lymphocytes remaining in the blood to various mitogens and antigens is altered when contrasted to that of lymphocytes of untreated subjects. This presumably indicates that subpopulations of lymphocytes are differentially affected by the steroids. It is currently thought that, at least in man, the lymphocytopenia is the result of redistribution rather than of destruction of cells (Fauci and Dale, 1974).

Monocytes from volunteers who received glucocorticoids display an impaired ability to kill microorganisms, although the process of phagocytosis is not defective (Rinehart *et al.*, 1975).

Lymphoid Tissue. Addison was the first to observe the increase in mass of lymphoid tissue that accompanies adrenocortical insufficiency; there is also a lymphocytosis. In contrast, Cushing's syndrome is characterized by lymphocytopenia and decreased mass of lymphoid tissue.

In a number of laboratory animals glucocorticoids cause a rapid lysis of lymphatic tissue, especially striking in cells of the thymus (Dougherty and White, 1944, 1947). Man is much more resistant to this lympholytic effect of the steroids, and some investigators doubt that the glucocorticoids have a comparable effect in man (Claman, 1972). This implies that the changes in lymphoid tissue seen in man in chronic hypercorticosteroid or hypocorticosteroid states must result from changes in rates of cellular formation or destruction that become manifest over a prolonged period of time. As noted above, the acute effects of steroids on circulating lymphocytes may be due to sequestration from the blood, rather than to lymphocytolysis.

Within 1 to 3 hours following the administration of glucocorticoids to rats or mice, dissolution of lymphocytes in lymphoid tissue becomes apparent. The nuclei become pyknotic and disintegrate, or the cells may shed their cytoplasm. The cellular debris is phagocytized. Dissolution continues during the period of steroid administration. Thereafter, there is a return to normal lymphoid structure, characterized by differentiation of lymphocytes from reticulum cells and resumption of mitosis.

The mechanism of the dramatic lympholytic effects of the glucocorticoids in rodents has been the subject of many investigations. The presence of a glucocorticoid receptor protein in rat thymus suggests that these effects are mediated by an interaction between a steroid-receptor complex and the chromatin of the nucleus. Early changes in biochemical functions produced in the thymus by glucocorticoids include decreased transport of amino acids, nucleotides, and ions and decreased glucose utilization, synthesis of RNA, and phosphorylation.

The addition of an inhibitor of protein synthesis, cycloheximide, after the effects of the steroids are established reverses the inhibitions. This strongly suggests that the steroids induce the synthesis of a protein that, in turn, acts to inhibit various cellular functions. In addition, it appears that the synthesis of this protein must continue for the steroids to be effective (Makman *et al.*, 1971).

Immune Responses. Corticosteroids and ACTH modify the clinical course of a variety of diseases in which hypersensitivity is believed to play an important role. Although massive doses of methylprednisolone have been shown to cause a fall in the concentration of IgG in the plasma of human volunteers, these same subjects produced antibody normally in response to antigenic stimuli (Butler, 1975). On the whole, there is no convincing evidence that the therapeutic use of the corticosteroids has a significant effect on the titer of circulating antibodies, either IgG or IgE, that play a major role in allergic and autoimmune states (David *et al.*, 1970). Metabolism of complement is likewise probably not significantly affected (Claman, 1975). This is true in spite of the fact that the symptoms of the diseases are often alleviated dramatically by the steroids. It is also now believed that in clinical situations in which the glucocorticoids are used to prevent the consequences of cell-mediated (delayed hypersensitivity) immune reactions, for example, graft rejection, the steroids do not interfere with the normal processes in the development of cell-mediated immunity. Rather, they prevent or suppress the inflammatory responses that take place as a consequence of the hypersensitivity reactions (Cohen, 1971; Balow and Rosenthal, 1973; Weston *et al.*, 1973).

In delayed sensitivity reactions, lymphocytes previously sensitized to a particular antigen encounter the antigen within a tissue at a site destined to be the location of the inflammatory response. These lymphocytes, activated by the antigen, begin production of a number of soluble factors, *lymphokines*, that control the cellular response. Among the lymphokines is the macrophage migration inhibitory factor (MIF), which causes an accumulation of nonsensitized macrophages in the area by inhibiting their mobility (Bloom and Bennett, 1966). Glucocorticoids do not affect the production of MIF by lymphocytes that have been activated by an appropriate antigen,

but the steroids do block the effect of MIF on macrophages; that is, the movement of these cells is no longer impeded, and they do not accumulate locally (Balow and Rosenthal, 1973).

The dramatic lympholysis in steroid-treated rodents has possibly proved to be misleading in developing an understanding of the effects of glucocorticoids in suppressing immune reactions. The assumption has been that the steroids act by destroying or damaging lymphoid cells critical to the development of immune reactions. The demonstration that the small number of cells remaining in the thymus of the mouse after treatment with cortisol have an undiminished capacity to establish cell-mediated immune responses has made this concept untenable (Cohen *et al.*, 1970).

Anti-inflammatory Properties. Cortisol and the synthetic analogs of cortisol have the capacity to prevent or suppress the development of the local heat, redness, swelling, and tenderness by which inflammation is recognized. At the microscopic level, they inhibit not only the early phenomena of the inflammatory process (edema, fibrin deposition, capillary dilatation, migration of leukocytes into the inflamed area, and phagocytic activity) but also the later manifestations (capillary proliferation, fibroblast proliferation, deposition of collagen, and, still later, cicatrization).

Although understanding of these effects is unsatisfactory, many observations have been made that have therapeutic relevance and that must be taken into account in explanatory formulations. Perhaps the most important of these for the physician is that corticosteroids inhibit the inflammatory response whether the inciting agent is radiant, mechanical, chemical, infectious, or immunological. In clinical terms, the administration of corticosteroids for their anti-inflammatory effects is palliative therapy; the underlying cause of the disease remains; the inflammatory manifestations are merely suppressed. It is this suppression of inflammation and its consequences that has made the corticosteroids such valuable therapeutic agents—indeed, at times lifesaving. It is also this property that gives them a nearly unique potential for therapeutic disaster. The signs and symptoms of inflammation are expressions of the disease process that are often used by the physician in diagnosis and in evaluating the effectiveness of treatment. These may be missing in patients treated with glucocorticoids. For example, an infection may continue to progress while the patient superficially appears to improve, and a peptic ulcer may perforate without producing clinical signs. This situation has been epitomized in the grimly facetious remark that the corticosteroids, misused, permit a patient to walk all the way to the autopsy room!

Cortisol and presumably other anti-inflammatory steroids are to be found in inflamed tissues, although they are not selectively concentrated there. Anti-inflammatory effects depend upon the direct local action of the steroids, since those that do not require metabolic modification for activity are very effective on topical application to skin or eye.

Several discrete effects of the steroids relevant to their anti-inflammatory properties are beginnning to be understood. For example, a considerable amount is known about the inhibitory effects of the glucocorticoids on fibroblasts, phenomena that are of undoubted importance in the suppression of later phases of inflammation (Gray *et al.,* 1971). The mechanism by which glucocorticoids inhibit accumulation of macrophages is discussed in the preceding section. It has also been found that cortisol, when added to a mixture of cultured lymphocytes and monocytes, causes the appearance of a factor in the culture medium that stimulates the migration of polymorphonuclear leukocytes (Stevenson, 1973). This may account for suppression of infiltration by polymorphonuclear cells. The effects of glucocorticoids on neutrophils have been reviewed by Mishler (1977). Low concentrations of glucocorticoids inhibit the formation by macrophages of an activator of plasminogen (Vassalli *et al.,* 1976), an effect that may contribute to their anti-inflammatory properties. There is also substantial evidence that the glucocorticoids inhibit release of arachidonic acid from phospholipids and thereby decrease formation of prostaglandins and related compounds, such as prostaglandin endoperoxides and thromboxane, which may play an important role in inflammation (*see* Gryglewski *et al.,* 1975; Hong and Levine, 1976; Blackwell *et al.,* 1978; Chapters 28 and 29).

Growth and Cell Division. Pharmacological doses of glucocorticoids retard or interrupt the growth of children, indicating an adverse effect on the epiphyseal cartilage. Inhibition of growth is a rather widespread effect of the glucocorticoids. For example, they inhibit cell division or the synthesis of DNA in thymocytes (Dougherty and White, 1945); fibroblasts (Pratt and Aronow, 1966); normal, developing, and regenerating liver (Howard, 1964; Loeb and Sternschein, 1973); gastric mucosa (Loeb and Sternschein, 1973); developing brain (Howard, 1964); developing lung (Carson *et al.,* 1973); and epidermis (Fisher and Malbach, 1971). Nevertheless, this effect is somewhat selective, and corticosteroids do not characteristically produce the bone-marrow depression or the enteritis that follows exposure to nonspecific antimitotic agents. The mechanism of this effect of the steroids is not known.

ABSORPTION, TRANSPORT, METABOLISM, AND EXCRETION

Absorption. Cortisol and numerous congeners, including synthetic analogs, are effective when given by mouth. Desoxycorticosterone acetate is unusual in that it is ineffective by this route.

Water-soluble esters of cortisol and its synthetic congeners are administered intravenously in order to achieve high concentrations in body fluids rapidly. More prolonged effects are obtained by intramuscular injection of suspensions of cortisol, congeners, and esters. Minor changes in chemical structure may result in large changes in the rate of absorption, time of onset of effect, and duration of action.

Glucocorticoids are absorbed from sites of local application such as synovial spaces, the conjunctival sac, and the skin. The absorption may be sufficient, when administration is chronic or large areas of skin are involved, to cause systemic effects, including adrenocortical suppression.

Transport, Metabolism, and Excretion. In the plasma, 90% or more of the cortisol is reversibly bound to protein under normal circumstances. The binding is accounted for by two protein fractions. One, corticosteroid-binding globulin, is a glycoprotein; the other is albumin. The globulin has high affinity but low total binding capacity, while albumin has low affinity but relatively large binding capacity. Consequently, at low or normal concentrations of corticosteroids most of the hormone is bound to globulin. When the amount of corticosteroid is increased, concentrations of both free and albumin-bound steroid increase with little change in the concentration of that bound to the globulin. Corticosteroids compete with each other for binding sites on the corticosteroid-binding globulin. Cortisol has high affinity; glucuronide-conjugated steroid metabolites and aldosterone have low affinities.

During pregnancy and during estrogen treatment in both sexes, corticosteroid-binding globulin, total plasma cortisol, and free cortisol increase severalfold. The physiological significance of these facts is not known. The free hormone as opposed to the protein-bound steroid is biologically active, available for hepatic metabolism, and may be excreted by the kidney.

All the biologically active adrenocortical steroids and their synthetic congeners have a double bond in the 4,5 position and a ketone group at C 3. Reduction of the 4,5 double bond can occur at both hepatic and extrahepatic sites and yields an inactive substance. Subsequent reduction of the 3-ketone substituent to a 3-hydroxyl to form tetrahydrocortisol has been demonstrated only in liver. Most of the ring-A–reduced metabolites are enzymatically coupled through the 3-hydroxyl with sulfate or with glucuronic acid to form water-soluble sulfate esters or glucuronides, and they are excreted as such. These conjugation reactions occur principally in liver and to some extent in kidney.

Reversible oxidation of the 11-hydroxyl group has been demonstrated to occur slowly in a variety of extrahepatic tissues and rapidly in liver. Corticosteroids with an 11-ketone substituent require reduction to 11-hydroxyl compounds for their biological activity (Sweat and Bryson, 1960). Reduction of the 20-ketone group to a 20-hydroxyl configuration yields a substance having little, if any, biological activity. Corticosteroids with a hydroxyl group at C 17 undergo an oxidation that yields 17-ketosteroids and a two-carbon fragment. These 17-ketosteroids are totally lacking in corticosteroid activity but, in a few instances, have weak androgenic properties.

When radioactive-carbon, ring-labeled steroids are injected intravenously in man, most of the radioisotope is recovered in the urine within 72 hours. Neither biliary nor fecal excretion is of any quantitative importance in man. Tait and Burstein (1964) have estimated that the liver metabolizes at least 70% of the cortisol secreted.

The metabolism of cortisol has been studied more extensively than that of all other corticosteroids, and it is generally assumed that the metabolism of its congeners and synthetic derivatives is qualitatively similar. Cortisol has a plasma half-life of about 1.5 hours. The metabolism of corticosteroids is greatly slowed by introduction of the 1,2 double bond or a fluorine atom into the molecule, and the half-life is correspondingly prolonged.

Clinical laboratories measure urinary cortisol and metabolites with reduced ring A as "17-hydroxycorticosteroids." These compounds and those where the ketone at carbon 20 has been reduced are included in the group referred to as "17-ketogenic steroids." The urinary metabolites that have lost their side chain contribute to the "17-ketosteroids."

STRUCTURE-ACTIVITY RELATIONSHIP

Cortisone was the first corticosteroid used for its anti-inflammatory effect. Modifications of structure have led to increases in the ratio of anti-inflammatory to sodium-retaining potency, such that in a number of presently available compounds electrolyte effects are of no serious consequence, even at the highest doses used. However, in all compounds studied to date, effects on inflammation and on carbohydrate and protein metabolism have paralleled one another. It seems likely that effects on inflammation and on organic metabolism are mediated by the same type of receptor.

Changes in molecular structure may bring about changes in biological potency as a result of changes in absorption, protein binding, rate of metabolic transformation, rate of excretion, ability to traverse membranes, and intrinsic effectiveness of the molecule at its site of action. In the following paragraphs, modifications of the pregnane nucleus that have been of value in therapeutic agents are described. The molecular sites of alteration are shown in Figure 63–4 in bold lines and letters. Table 63–3 lists the effects of the modifications discussed relative to cortisol. As indicated above, relative potencies vary to some extent with different conditions of bioassay.

Ring A. The 4,5 double bond and the 3-ketone are both necessary for typical adrenocorticosteroid activity. Introduction of a 1,2 double bond, as in prednisone or prednisolone, enhances the ratio of carbohydrate-regulating potency to sodium-retaining potency by selectively increasing the former. In addition, prednisolone is metabolized more slowly than cortisol.

Ring B. 6α-Substitution has unpredictable effects. In the particular instance of cortisol, 6α-methylation increases anti-inflammatory, nitrogen-wasting, and sodium-retaining effects in man. In contrast, 6α-methylprednisolone has slightly greater anti-inflammatory potency and less electrolyte-regulating potency than prednisolone. Fluorination in the 9α position enhances all biological activities of the cor-

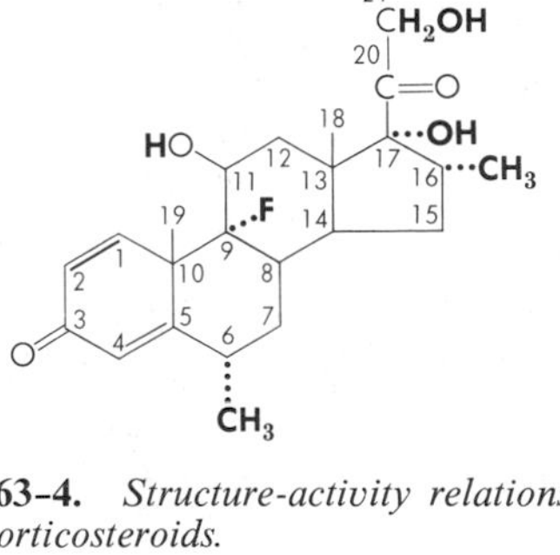

Figure 63–4. *Structure-activity relationship of adrenocorticosteroids.*

Light lines and letters indicate structural features common to compounds having anti-inflammatory action. Bold lines and letters indicate modifications that enhance or suppress characteristic activities. (After Liddle, 1961. Courtesy of *Clinical Pharmacology and Therapeutics.*)

Table 63-3. RELATIVE POTENCIES AND EQUIVALENT DOSES OF CORTICOSTEROIDS

COMPOUND	RELATIVE ANTI-INFLAMMATORY POTENCY	RELATIVE SODIUM-RETAINING POTENCY	DURATION OF ACTION *	APPROXIMATE EQUIVALENT DOSE † (mg)
Cortisol				
(Hydrocortisone)	1	1	S	20
Tetrahydrocortisol	0	0	—	—
Prednisone				
(Δ^1-Cortisone)	4	0.8	I	5
Prednisolone				
(Δ^1-Cortisol)	4	0.8	I	5
6α-Methylprednisolone	5	0.5	I	4
Fludrocortisone				
(9α-Fluorocortisol)	10	125	S	—
11-Desoxycortisol	0	0	—	—
Cortisone				
(11-Dehydrocortisol)	0.8	0.8	S	25
Corticosterone	0.35	15	S	—
Triamcinolone				
(9α-Fluoro-16α-hydroxyprednisolone)	5	0	I	4
Paramethasone				
(6α-Fluoro-16α-methylprednisolone)	10	0	L	2
Betamethasone				
(9α-Fluoro-16β-methylprednisolone)	25	0	L	0.75
Dexamethasone				
(9α-Fluoro-16α-methylprednisolone)	25	0	L	0.75

* S = Short or 8- to 12-hour biological half-life; I = intermediate or 12- to 36-hour biological half-life; L = long or 36- to 72-hour biological half-life (see Rose and Saccar, 1978).

† These dose relationships apply only to oral or intravenous administration; relative potencies may differ greatly when injected intramuscularly or into joint spaces.

ticosteroids, apparently by its electron-withdrawing effect on the 11β-hydroxy group.

Ring C. The presence of an oxygen function at C 11 is indispensable for significant anti-inflammatory and carbohydrate-regulating potency (cortisol versus 11-desoxycortisol) but is not necessary for high sodium-retaining potency, as demonstrated by desoxycorticosterone.

Ring D. 16-Methylation or hydroxylation eliminates the sodium-retaining effect but only slightly modifies potency with respect to effects on organic metabolism and inflammation.

All presently used anti-inflammatory steroids are 17α-hydroxy compounds. Although some carbohydrate-regulating and anti-inflammatory effects may occur in 17-desoxy compounds (cortisol versus corticosterone), the fullest expression of these activities requires the presence of the 17α-hydroxy substituent.

All natural corticosteroids and most of the active synthetic analogs have a 21-hydroxy group. While some glycogenic and anti-inflammatory activities may occur in its absence, its presence is required for significant sodium-retaining activity.

PREPARATIONS AND ROUTES OF ADMINISTRATION

Organic chemists have synthesized a bewildering number of modified adrenocorticosteroids, many of which share the same properties and differ only with respect to absolute dosage. At the outset it should be reemphasized that, whereas a clear separation has

been made between mineralocorticoids and glucocorticoids, there is no member of the latter group that is unique with respect to a separation of therapeutic and toxic effects. A working knowledge of a small number of preparations is sufficient for nearly every clinical purpose.

Corticosteroids are administered orally, parenterally (intravenous, intramuscular, intrasynovial, and intralesional routes), and topically (dermal ointments, creams, and lotions; ophthalmic ointments and solutions; respiratory aerosols; enemas). Some absorption into the systemic circulation occurs with all forms of topical administration. In the case of most aerosols, absorption is virtually equivalent to that from parenteral or oral administration. Adrenocortical suppression can occur with applications of steroids to the conjunctival sac and to the skin. Absorption from the skin is especially marked when the steroid is applied under plastic film over a large surface area.

Information on available steroid preparations is presented in Table 63-4 (pages 1484-1486).

TOXICITY OF ADRENOCORTICAL STEROIDS

Two categories of toxic effects are observed in the therapeutic use of adrenocorticosteroids: those resulting from *withdrawal* and those resulting from *continued use of large doses.* Acute adrenal insufficiency results from too rapid withdrawal of corticosteroids after prolonged therapy. Protocols for discontinuing corticosteroid therapy in patients who have been subjected to suppressive therapy for long periods have been described by Harter and associates (1963) and Byyny (1976). There is a characteristic corticosteroid withdrawal syndrome, consisting in fever, myalgia, arthralgia, and malaise, which may be extremely difficult to distinguish from "reactivation" of rheumatoid arthritis or rheumatic fever (Amatruda *et al.*, 1960). Pseudotumor cerebri with papilledema is a rare reaction that follows reduction or withdrawal of corticosteroid therapy (Levine and Leopold, 1973).

The use of corticosteroids for days or a few weeks does not lead to adrenal insufficiency upon cessation of treatment, but prolonged therapy with corticosteroids may result in suppression of pituitary-adrenal function that can be slow in returning to normal. Graber and coworkers (1965) found that the processes of recovery of normal pituitary and adrenal function required 9 months in some patients. During this recovery period and for an additional 1 to 2 years, the patient may need to be protected during stressful situations, such as surgery or severe infections, by the administration of corticosteroids.

In addition to pituitary-adrenal suppression, the principal complications resulting from prolonged therapy with corticosteroids are fluid and electrolyte disturbances; hyperglycemia and glycosuria; increased susceptibility to infections, including tuberculosis; peptic ulcers, which may bleed or perforate; osteoporosis; a characteristic myopathy; behavioral disturbances; posterior subcapsular cataracts; arrest of growth; and Cushing's habitus, consisting in "moon face," "buffalo hump," enlargement of supraclavicular fat pads, "central obesity," striae, ecchymoses, acne, and hirsutism.

Hypokalemic alkalosis and *edema* are infrequently encountered in patients being treated with synthetic corticosteroid congeners and almost never in patients taking the 16-substituted compounds. *Glycosuria* can usually be managed with diet and/or insulin, and its occurrence should not be an important factor in the decision to continue corticosteroid therapy or to initiate it in diabetic patients.

Increased susceptibility to infection in patients treated with corticosteroids is not specific for any particular bacterial or fungal pathogen. If infection develops in a patient treated with corticosteroids, the dose should be maintained or increased and the best available treatment for the infection vigorously administered. Corticosteroid therapy may be initiated in patients having known infections of some consequence if effective, specific chemotherapy can be administered concomitantly with the hormones.

Peptic ulceration is an occasional complication of corticosteroid therapy. The high incidence of hemorrhage and perforation in these ulcers and the insidious nature of their development make them severe therapeutic problems. Some investigators believe the available evidence does not support the conclusion that steroids cause ulcers (Conn and Blitzer, 1976). Others feel that only patients with rheumatoid arthritis have an increased incidence of ulcers. In this disease the nearly universal administration of aspirin or other ulcerogenic drugs makes it difficult to evaluate the evidence. It has been proposed that the glucocorticoids alter the mucosal defense mechanisms. The problem of steroid-associated ulcers is reviewed by Fenster (1973).

Myopathy, characterized by weakness of the proximal musculature of arms and legs and of their associated shoulder and pelvic muscles, is occasionally seen in patients taking large doses of corticosteroids. It may occur soon after treatment is begun and be sufficiently severe to prevent ambulation. It is not specific for synthetic corticosteroid congeners, for it is found in endogenous Cushing's syndrome. It is a serious complication and an indication for withdrawal of therapy. Recovery may be slow and incomplete.

Behavioral disturbances may take various forms, for example, nervousness, insomnia, changes in mood or psyche, and psychopathies of the manic-depressive or schizophrenic type. Suicidal tendencies are not uncommon. It is no longer believed that previous psychiatric problems predispose to behavioral disturbances during therapy with glucocorticoids. Conversely, the absence of a history of psychiatric illness is no guarantee against the occurrence of psychosis during hormonal therapy.

Table 63–4. PREPARATIONS OF ADRENOCORTICAL STEROIDS AND THEIR SYNTHETIC ANALOGS *

NONPROPRIETARY NAME AND TRADE NAMES	ORAL FORMS	INJECTABLE FORMS	TOPICAL FORMS
Desoxycorticosterone Acetate, U.S.P. [1] (DOCA ACETATE, PERCORTEN ACETATE)	—	5 mg/ml (oil) 125 mg (pellets)	—
Desoxycorticosterone Pivalate, U.S.P. (PERCORTEN PIVALATE)	—	25 mg/ml (susp.)	—
Fludrocortisone Acetate, U.S.P. [2] (FLORINEF ACETATE)	0.1 mg	—	—
Cortisol, U.S.P. [1] (Hydrocortisone) (CORTEF, HYDROCORTONE, others)	5, 10, 20 mg	25, 50 mg/ml (susp.)	0.125–2.5% cream 0.25, 2.5% ointment 0.125, 2.5% lotion 0.5, 1.5% gel 0.5% aerosol 100-mg/60 ml enema 0.2% suspension †
Cortisol Acetate, U.S.P. (CORTEF ACETATE, HYDROCORTONE ACETATE, others)	—	25, 50 mg/ml (susp.)	1, 2.5% ointment 15-, 25-mg supposi- tories 10% rectal foam 2.5% suspension † 1.5% ointment †
Cortisol Cypionate, U.S.P. (CORTEF FLUID)	2 mg/ml (susp.)	—	—
Cortisol Sodium Phosphate, U.S.P. (HYDROCORTONE PHOSPHATE)	—	50 mg/ml	—
Cortisol Sodium Succinate, U.S.P. (SOLU-CORTEF)	—	100, 250, 500 mg 1 g (powder)	—
Beclomethasone Dipropionate, U.S.P. [3] (VANCERIL)	—	—	10-mg inhaler
Betamethasone, U.S.P. [2] (CELESTONE)	0.6 mg 0.6 mg/5 ml (syrup)	4 mg/ml	0.2% cream
Betamethasone Sodium Phosphate and Acetate, U.S.P. (CELESTONE SOLUSPAN)	—	6 mg/ml (susp.)	—
Betamethasone Dipropionate, U.S.P. (DIPROSONE)	—	—	0.05% cream, oint- ment, or lotion 0.1% aerosol
Betamethasone Valerate, U.S.P. (VALISONE)	—	—	0.01, 0.1% cream 0.1% ointment 0.1% lotion 0.15% aerosol
Betamethasone Benzoate, U.S.P. (BENISONE, FLUROBATE)	—	—	0.025% cream, gel, or lotion
Cortisone Acetate, U.S.P. [2] (CORTONE ACETATE)	5, 10, 25 mg	25, 50 mg/ml (susp.)	1.5, 2.5% suspen- sion †
Dexamethasone, U.S.P. [2] (DECADRON, GAMMACORTEN, others)	0.25–4.0 mg 0.5 mg/5 ml (elixir)	—	0.04% cream 0.1% gel 0.011% aerosol (topical) 0.1% suspension †

NONPROPRIETARY NAME AND TRADE NAMES	ORAL FORMS	INJECTABLE FORMS	TOPICAL FORMS
Dexamethasone Sodium Phosphate, U.S.P. (DECADRON PHOSPHATE, HEXADROL PHOSPHATE)	—	4, 10, 24 mg/ml	0.1% cream 0.1% solution † 0.05% ointment †
Dexamethasone Acetate, U.S.P. (DECADRON-L.A.)	—	8 mg/ml	—
Fluprednisolone [3] (ALPHADROL)	1.5 mg	—	—
Meprednisone, U.S.P. [3] (BETAPAR)	4 mg	—	—
Methylprednisolone, U.S.P. [2] (MEDROL)	2-32 mg	—	—
Methylprednisolone Acetate, U.S.P. (DEPO-MEDROL, MEDROL ACETATE)	—	20, 40, 80 mg/ml (susp.)	0.25, 1% ointment 40-mg/unit enema
Methylprednisolone Sodium Succinate, U.S.P. (SOLU-MEDROL)	—	40, 125, 500 mg 1 g (powder)	
Paramethasone Acetate, U.S.P. [2] (HALDRONE)	1, 2 mg	—	—
Prednisolone, U.S.P. [2] (DELTA-CORTEF, others)	1, 2.5, 5 mg	—	0.5% aerosol 0.5% cream
Prednisolone Acetate, U.S.P. (METICORTELONE ACETATE, others)	—	25, 50, 100 mg/ml (susp.)	0.12, 1% suspension †
Prednisolone Sodium Phosphate, U.S.P. (HYDELTRASOL, others)	—	20 mg/ml	0.125, 0.5, 1% solution † 0.25% ointment †
Prednisolone Sodium Succinate, U.S.P. (METICORTELONE SOLUBLE)	—	50 mg (powder)	
Prednisolone Tebutate, U.S.P. (HYDELTA-T.B.A.)	—	20 mg/ml (susp.)	—
Prednisone, U.S.P. [2] (DELTASONE, PARACORT, others)	1-50 mg	—	—
Triamcinolone, U.S.P. [2] (ARISTOCORT, KENACORT)	1, 2, 4, 8, 16 mg	—	—
Triamcinolone Acetonide, U.S.P. (ARISTODERM, KENALOG)	—	40 mg/ml (susp.)	0.025, 0.1, 0.5% cream 0.025, 0.5% ointment 0.1% foam 0.025, 0.1% lotion 0.1% gel 0.1% spray 0.1% dental paste

* Preparations above the double line are intended for use as mineralocorticoids.

† Topical ophthalmic preparation; other preparations of certain steroid derivatives are available for subconjunctival injection.

[1] *See* Figure 63-3 for structure.

[2] *See* Table 63-3 for chemical name.

[3] Beclomethasone, 9α-chloro,16β-methylprednisolone,17,21-dipropionate; desonide, 16α-hydroxyprednisolone,16,17-acetal with acetone; fluprednisolone, 6α-fluoroprednisolone; meprednisone, 16β-methylprednisone; desoxymetasone, Δ',9α-fluoro,16α-methyl-corticosterone; flumethasone, 6α,9α-difluoro,16α-methylprednisolone; fluocinolone, 6α,9α-difluoro,16α-hydroxyprednisolone,16,17-acetal with acetone; fluocinonide, 6α,9α-difluoro,16α-hydroxyprednisolone,16,17-acetal with acetone,21-acetate; fluorometholone, Δ'-9α-fluoro,6α-methyl-11β,17-dihydroxyprogesterone; fluorandrenolide, 6α-fluoro,16α-hydroxycortisol,16,17-acetal with acetone; halcinonide, 21-chloro,9-fluoro,11β,16α,17-trihydroxypregn-4-ene-3,20-dione,16,17-acetal with acetone; medrysone, 11β-hydroxy,6α-methylprogesterone.

Table 63–4.   **PREPARATIONS OF ADRENOCORTICAL STEROIDS AND
THEIR SYNTHETIC ANALOGS** * (Continued)

NONPROPRIETARY NAME AND TRADE NAMES	ORAL FORMS	INJECTABLE FORMS	TOPICAL FORMS
Triamcinolone Diacetate, U.S.P. (ARISTOCORT DIACETATE, KENACORT DIACETATE)	2, 4 mg/5 ml (syrup)	40 mg/ml (susp.)	—
Triamcinolone Hexacetonide, U.S.P. (ARISTOSPAN)	—	5, 20 mg/ml (susp.)	—
Desonide [3] (TRIDESILON)	—	—	0.05% cream or ointment
Desoximetasone, U.S.P. [3] (TOPICORT)	—	—	0.25% cream
Flumethasone Pivalate, U.S.P. [3] (LOCORTEN)	—	—	0.025% cream
Fluocinolone Acetonide, U.S.P. [3] (FLUONID, SYNALAR)	—	—	0.01, 0.025, 0.2% cream 0.025% ointment 0.01% solution
Fluocinonide, U.S.P. [3] (LIDEX, TOPSYN GEL)	—	—	0.05% cream, gel, or ointment
Fluorometholone, U.S.P. [3] (OXYLONE)	—	—	0.025% cream 0.1% suspension †
Flurandrenolide, U.S.P. [3] (CORDRAN)	—	—	0.025, 0.05% cream or ointment 0.05% lotion 4-µg/sq cm tape
Halcinonide [3] (HALOG)	—	—	0.025, 0.1% cream 0.1% ointment 0.1% solution
Medrysone, U.S.P. [3] (HMS LIQUIFILM, MEDROCORT)	—	—	1% suspension †

* Preparations above the double line are intended for use as mineralocorticoids.
† Topical ophthalmic preparation; other preparations of certain steroid derivatives are available for subconjunctival injection.
[1] See Figure 63–3 for structure.
[2] See Table 63–3 for chemical name.
[3] Beclomethasone, 9α-chloro,16β-methylprednisolone,17,21-dipropionate; desonide, 16α-hydroxyprednisolone,16,17-acetal with acetone; fluprednisolone, 6α-fluoroprednisolone; meprednisone, 16β-methylprednisone; desoxymetasone, Δ',9α-fluoro,16α-methyl-corticosterone; flumethasone, 6α,9α-difluoro,16α-methylprednisolone; fluocinolone, 6α,9α-difluoro,16α-hydroxyprednisolone,16,17-acetal with acetone; fluocinonide, 6α,9α-difluoro,16α-hydroxyprednisolone,16,17-acetal with acetone,21-acetate; fluorometholone, Δ'-9α-fluoro,6α-methyl-11β,17-dihydroxyprogesterone; flurandrenolide, 6α-fluoro,16α-hydroxycortisol,16,17-acetal with acetone; halcinonide, 21-chloro,9-fluoro,11β,16α,17-trihydroxypregn-4-ene-3,20-dione,16,17-acetal with acetone; medrysone, 11β-hydroxy,6α-methylprogesterone.

Posterior subcapsular cataracts have been reported in children receiving corticosteroid therapy. Nearly all patients with rheumatoid arthritis who receive 20 mg of prednisone per day for 4 years develop cataracts (Levine and Leopold, 1973); it is possible that patients with this disease are particularly susceptible to this complication. The problem of corticosteroid-induced cataracts has been reviewed by Lubkin (1977).

Osteoporosis and *vertebral compression*

fractures are frequent serious complications of corticosteroid therapy in patients of all ages. Ribs and vertebrae, bones with a high degree of trabecular structure, are generally most severely affected. Glucocorticoids appear to inhibit the activities of osteoblasts directly, and, because of their inhibition of calcium absorption by the intestine, glucocorticoids cause an increased secretion of parathyroid hormone (PTH). PTH stimulates the activity of osteoclasts (Hahn, 1978); thus there is both decreased formation and increased resorption of bone. Osteoporosis is an indication for withdrawal of therapy and should be looked for regularly in radiographs of the spine in patients taking glucocorticoids for longer than a few months. The possibility of development of osteoporosis should be an important consideration in initiating and managing corticosteroid therapy, especially in postmenopausal women.

Inhibition or arrest of growth can result from the administration of relatively small doses of glucocorticoids to children. This cannot be overcome with exogenous human growth hormone (Morris *et al.*, 1968). The widespread inhibitory effect of the glucocorticoids on DNA synthesis and cell division discussed above is apparently responsible. Inhibition of growth by glucocorticoids has been reviewed by Loeb (1976).

THERAPEUTIC USES

With the exception of substitution therapy in deficiency states, the use of corticosteroids and their congeners in disease is empirical. From the experience accumulated since the introduction of glucocorticoids for clinical use, at least six therapeutic principles may be abstracted, as follows: (1) for any disease, in any patient, the appropriate dose to achieve a given therapeutic effect must be determined by trial and error and must be reevaluated from time to time as the stage and the activity of the disease alter; (2) a *single* dose of corticosteroid, even a large one, is virtually without harmful effects; (3) a few days of corticosteroid therapy, in the absence of specific contraindications, is unlikely to produce harmful results except at the most extreme dosages; (4) as corticosteroid therapy is prolonged over periods of months, and to the extent that the dose exceeds the equivalent of substitution therapy, the incidence of disabling and potentially lethal effects increases; (5) except in adrenal insufficiency, the administration of corticosteroids is neither etiological nor curative therapy but only palliative by virtue of the anti-inflammatory effects; and (6) abrupt cessation of prolonged, high-dosage corticosteroid therapy is associated with a significant risk of adrenal insufficiency of sufficient severity to be threatening to life.

Translated into the terms of clinical practice, these general principles are equivalent to the following rules. When corticosteroids are to be administered over long periods, the dose must be the smallest one that will achieve a desired effect. This dose must be found by trial and error. Where the goal of therapy is relief of painful or distressing symptoms not associated with an immediately life-threatening disease, for example, rheumatoid arthritis, the initial dose should be small and gradually increased until pain or distress has been reduced to tolerable levels. Complete relief is not sought. At frequent intervals the dose should be gradually reduced until the development of more severe symptoms signals that the minimal acceptable dose has been found. When therapy is directed at an immediately life-threatening state, for example, pemphigus, the initial dose should be a large one, estimated to achieve, almost with certainty, control of the crisis. If some benefit is not observed in a short time, the dose should be doubled or tripled. When potentially lethal disease is controlled by large amounts of corticosteroid, reduction of the dose should be carried out under conditions that permit frequent, accurate observations of the patient. Under these circumstances it is essential to assess constantly the relative dangers of therapy and of the disease being treated.

The apparently innocuous character of a single administration of corticosteroid in amounts within the conventional therapeutic range justifies its use without a definite diagnosis for crises in which there exists some probability that life is threatened by primary adrenal or pituitary insufficiency. If one of these conditions is present, a single intravenous injection of a soluble corticosteroid may prevent immediate death and allow time for diagnostic procedures.

Short courses of systemic corticosteroids in large doses may properly be given for diseases that do not threaten life, in the absence of specific contraindications. The general rule is that long courses of therapy at high dosage should be reserved for life-threatening disease. On occasion, and for definite cause, when the patient is threatened with permanent disability, this rule is justifiably violated.

It is not possible to define the precise dose of glucocorticoids that will produce pituitary and adrenocortical suppression in a given patient, since there is considerable variation. In general, the higher the dose and the more prolonged the therapy, the greater is the likelihood of suppression.

Harter and associates (1963) suggested that some dissociation of therapeutic effects from certain undesirable metabolic effects can be achieved by the administration of a single large dose of corticosteroid every other day, in contrast to the usual daily multiple-dose schedule. A single dose every other day or at even longer intervals is acceptable therapy for some, but not all, patients with a variety of diseases modified by corticosteroid therapy. When this therapeutic regimen is possible, the degree of suppression of the pituitary and adrenal cortex can be minimized. Steroids that are long acting are not suitable for use by this dosage schedule.

Substitution Therapy. Insufficiency of secretion of the adrenal cortex results from structural or functional lesions of the adrenal cortex itself or from structural or functional lesions of the anterior pituitary. In either case, the patient may present with acute, catastrophic adrenal insufficiency (adrenal crisis) or chronic adrenal insufficiency. When the adrenal itself is the site of the lesion, all elements of normal adrenal secretion may be reduced or absent or the deficiency may be selective for one or more components of secretion.

Acute Adrenal Insufficiency. This disease is characterized by gastrointestinal symptoms, dehydration, weakness, lethargy, and hypotension. It is usually associated with disorders of the adrenal, rather than the pituitary, although exceptions occur. It frequently follows abrupt withdrawal of high doses of corticosteroids.

The immediate needs of such patients are water, sodium, chloride, glucose, cortisol, and appropriate therapy for precipitating causes, for example, infection, trauma, or hemorrhage. Inasmuch as these patients have a diminished capacity for a water diuresis and have often undergone some degree of cellular hydration, they are susceptible to water intoxication. The principal intravenous fluid should be isotonic sodium chloride solution. Glucose is required for nutrition and to prevent or treat hypoglycemia, but it should be given intravenously in isotonic sodium chloride solution. The total amount of intravenous fluid administered during the first 24 hours should not, in most instances, exceed 5% of ideal body weight. The patient should be monitored for evidences of rising venous pressure and pulmonary edema, because the functional capacity of the cardiovascular system is reduced by adrenocortical insufficiency. Cortisol hemisuccinate or sodium phosphate must be given in the intravenous fluids at a rate of 100 mg every 8 hours, following an initial intravenous injection of 100 mg. In the period of

transition from intravenous fluid therapy to normal diet and activity, intramuscular cortisol hemisuccinate or sodium phosphate may be used in a dose of 25 mg every 6 or 8 hours.

For the treatment of suspected but unconfirmed acute adrenal insufficiency, 4 mg of dexamethasone sodium phosphate should be substituted for cortisol. In addition, ACTH (5 units per hour) should be given. Concentrations of cortisol in plasma and 17-hydroxycorticosteroids in urine are determined at the outset and at intervals during the course of treatment. A failure to obtain a response to ACTH (stimulation of steroid secretion) is diagnostic of adrenal insufficiency.

Chronic Adrenal Insufficiency. This disease results from adrenal surgery or destructive lesions of the adrenal cortex. It requires the administration of cortisone acetate, 25 to 37.5 mg per day or equivalent, in single or divided doses. A common dose schedule is 25 mg on arising and 12.5 mg in the late afternoon. Most patients will also require a potent mineralocorticoid. The most convenient drug to use for this purpose is fludrocortisone acetate. The usual adult dose is 0.1 to 0.3 mg daily. Some patients do not need a mineralocorticoid and are adequately treated with cortisone and generous dietary salt. Therapy is guided by the patient's sense of well-being, alertness, appetite, weight, muscular strength, pigmentation, blood pressure, and freedom from orthostatic hypotension.

Congenital Adrenal Hyperplasia. This is a familial disorder in which activity of one of several enzymes required for biosynthesis of corticosteroids is deficient. With diminished or absent production of cortisol, aldosterone, or both, and consequent lack of inhibitory feedback, the adrenal cortex is stimulated to the overproduction of other hormonally active steroids. The clinical presentation, laboratory findings, and treatment depend on which of the six enzyme deficiencies thus far described is responsible. Only the syndrome of 21-hydroxylase deficiency will be described here.

In about 90% of the patients with congenital adrenal hyperplasia there is a deficiency of 21-hydroxylase activity. When the deficiency is only partial, the usual case, cortisol is secreted at normal rates as a result of continuous hypersecretion of ACTH, with consequent overproduction of adrenal androgens and their precursors. Aldosterone secretion is approximately normal. Female children undergo virilization, female "pseudohermaphroditism," and male children show precocious development of secondary sexual characteristics, "macrogenitosomia." Linear growth is accelerated in childhood, but the height at maturity is reduced by premature closure of the epiphyses.

In about 30% of patients with 21-hydroxylase deficiency, the enzymatic defect is sufficiently severe to compromise increased aldosterone secretion in response to a hypovolemic stimulus. Such patients are unable to conserve sodium normally, in addition to manifesting androgenic effects (Bongiovanni et al., 1967).

All patients with congenital adrenal hyperplasia resulting from a 21-hydroxylase deficiency require substitution therapy with cortisol or a suitable congener, and those with a salt-losing tendency require, in addition, a sodium-retaining steroid. The usual oral dose of cortisol is about 0.6 mg/kg daily in four divided doses, the last one being given as late as possible in order to maintain pituitary suppression overnight. When parenteral substitution therapy is desired, cortisone acetate may be given intramuscularly every other day. The mineralocorticoid usually given is fludrocortisone acetate, 0.05 to 0.2 mg per day. Therapy is guided by gain in weight and height, by excretion of urinary 17-ketosteroids, and by blood pressure. Sudden spurts of linear growth may indicate inadequate pituitary suppression and excessive androgen secretion, whereas growth failure suggests overtreatment.

A number of rare forms of congenital adrenal hyperplasia are known in which enzyme deficiencies of the adrenal cortex, with similar defects of the gonads, result in clinical and laboratory findings very different from those described above for 21-hydroxylase deficiency. The types described thus far are: "desmolase" deficiency (Camacho et al., 1968), 3β-hydroxysteroid dehydrogenase deficiency (Bongiovanni et al., 1967), 17α-hydroxylase deficiency (Goldsmith et al., 1968), 11β-hydroxylase deficiency (Bongiovanni et al., 1967), and 18-hydroxylase deficiency (David et al., 1968). The clinical and laboratory findings and the treatment in these rare forms are quite different from those in 21-hydroxylase deficiency. The publications cited should be consulted for details.

Adrenal Insufficiency Secondary to Anterior Pituitary Insufficiency. This condition is not usually associated with the dramatic signs and symptoms characteristic of adrenal insufficiency resulting from disease of the adrenal cortex unless there are complicating circumstances, for example, unusual fluid losses, trauma, or starvation. Hypoglycemia is the most frequent cause of symptoms. Quantitation of the electrolytes in plasma often reveals a dilutional hyponatremia. The administration of 25 mg of cortisone acetate on arising and 12.5 mg in late afternoon is adequate replacement therapy for most patients with anterior pituitary insufficiency. This schedule mimics, to some extent, the normal diurnal cycle of adrenal secretion. When initiating treatment, it is customary to begin cortisol first and to add thyroid replacement therapy after adrenal insufficiency is under some degree of control, on the grounds that the administration of thyroid to a hypopituitary patient may precipitate acute adrenal insufficiency. Additional treatment is necessary during periods of stress. Cortisol, 300 to 400 mg per day, should be given to approximate the normal response to severe stress.

Therapeutic Uses in Nonendocrine Diseases. Brief outlines of important uses of corticosteroids in diseases other than those involving the pituitary-adrenal complex are set forth below.

The dosage of glucocorticoids varies greatly with the condition being treated. In the following discussion approximate doses of a representative corticosteroid congener, usually prednisone, are suggested. It is not meant to imply that prednisone has peculiar

merit in general or for any particular disease over the other congeners. For comparison of doses of glucocorticoids, *see* Table 63-3.

Arthritis. In *rheumatoid arthritis,* the criterion for initiating corticosteroid therapy is progressive disease with consequent disability, despite intensive treatment with rest, physical therapy, aspirin-like drugs, gold, and other agents. The decision to embark upon a program of hormone therapy must be made with due consideration for the fact that corticosteroid therapy, once started, may have to be continued for many years or for life, with the attendant risks of serious complications. The initial dose should be small and increased slowly until the desired degree of control is attained. The symptomatic effect of small reductions should be frequently tested in order to maintain the dose as low as possible. Complete relief is not sought. A regimen of rest, physical therapy, and salicylates is continued. The usual initial dose is about 10 mg of prednisone (or equivalent) per day in divided doses. Optimal therapy for some patients with painful symptoms confined to one or a few joints may be intra-articular injection of the steroid into the affected joints. Typical doses are 5 to 20 mg of triamcinolone acetonide or the equivalent, depending upon the size of the joint cavity.

In *osteoarthritis,* intra-articular injection of corticosteroids is recommended for treatment of episodic manifestations of acute inflammation: local heat, swelling, and pain. Injections for this purpose should be infrequent because, in both rheumatoid arthritis and osteoarthritis, a significant incidence of painless destruction of the joint, reminiscent of Charcot's arthropathy, may be associated with repeated intra-articular injections of corticosteroids (Rheumatism Review Committee, 1963).

Rheumatic Carditis. Corticosteroids are reserved for patients failing to respond to salicylates and as initial therapy for patients severely ill with fever, acute congestive heart failure, arrhythmia, and pericarditis; acute manifestations are more rapidly suppressed by corticosteroids than by salicylates, a possibly lifesaving difference in a moribund patient. A dose of approximately 40 mg of prednisone or equivalent is usually given daily, in divided amounts, although much larger doses may on occasion be required. Reactivation of the disease occurs in a number of instances following withdrawal of steroid therapy. For this reason it has been suggested that salicylates be given concurrently with corticosteroids and be continued through and after the period of withdrawal of hormone therapy.

Renal Diseases. Corticosteroids do not modify the course of acute or chronic glomerulonephritis. However, patients with some forms of the *nephrotic syndrome* attributable to systemic lupus erythematosus or to primary renal disease, except renal amyloidosis, may be benefited by corticosteroid therapy. A typical therapeutic regimen consists in the daily administration, in divided doses, of 60 mg of prednisone or equivalent (2 mg/kg of edema-free body weight in children) for 3 or 4 weeks. If a remission with a diuresis and decreased proteinuria occurs during this period, maintenance treatment is continued for as long as a year. For this, the daily dose of prednisone is given only for the first 3 days of each week (Bacon and Spencer, 1973).

Collagen Diseases. The manifestations of most of the diseases in this group are controlled by glucocorticoids. An exception is *scleroderma,* which is generally considered refractory to these agents. It is important to distinguish between scleroderma and *mixed connective disease syndrome,* which is responsive to steroids (Yount *et al.,* 1973). *Polymyositis, polyarteritis nodosa,* and the granulomatous-polyarteritis group (*Wegener's granulomatosis, temporalcranial arteritis,* and *polymyalgia rheumatica*) are treated with daily doses of prednisone, approximately 1 mg/kg or equivalent, to induce a remission. The dose is then tapered down to the minimally effective level. Glucocorticoids decrease morbidity in all these diseases and prolong the survival times of patients with polyarteritis nodosa and Wegener's granulomatosis. *In temporal (giant-cell) arteritis, adequate steroid therapy is necessary to prevent the blindness that occurs in about 20% of untreated cases.* Fulminating systemic lupus erythematosus is a life-threatening condition, the manifestations of which should be suppressed by adrenocorticosteroid therapy with doses large enough to produce a prompt effect. Treatment usually consists in a 1-mg/kg daily dose of prednisone or equivalent. Within 48 hours, reduction of fever and improvement in the signs and symptoms of arthritis, pleuritis, or pericarditis should be observed. If not, the dose should be increased in 20-mg increments daily until a favorable response occurs. After the acute episode has been brought under control, corticosteroid therapy should be reduced by small steps, for example, 5 mg of prednisone per week, until signs or symptoms warn against further reductions. Salicylate or related drugs are then introduced and may permit a further reduction of corticosteroid dosage (Robinson, 1962). There have been favorable reports on the treatment of systemic lupus erythematosus with a combination of glucocorticoids and antimetabolites, such as azathioprine, or the alkylating agent cyclophosphamide. This combination therapy is still experimental and not recommended for general use (Yount *et al.,* 1973).

Allergic Diseases. The manifestations of allergic disease that are of limited duration, such as *hay fever, serum sickness, urticaria, contact dermatitis, drug reactions, bee stings, angioneurotic edema,* and *anaphylaxis,* can, if necessary, be suppressed by adequate doses of glucocorticoids given as a supplement to the primary therapy. It must be emphasized, however, that the effects of the steroids require some time to develop, and *severe reactions such as anaphylaxis and angioneurotic edema of the glottis require immediate therapy with epinephrine, 0.5 to 1.0 ml of a 1:1000 solution (0.5 to 1.0 mg) subcutaneously.* In life-threatening situations steroids may be given intravenously; dexamethasone sodium phosphate (8 to 12 mg or equivalent) is appropriate. In less severe diseases, such as serum sickness or hay fever, antihistaminic compounds are the drugs of first choice.

Bronchial Asthma. The corticosteroids should *not* be used in the treatment of any asthmatic condition, acute or chronic, that can promptly be brought under moderate control with other measures. In *status asthmaticus,* cortisol (50 to 100 mg) is adminis-

tered by intravenous infusion over 8 hours. The procedure is repeated daily until the acute attack is under control, following which the patient is given 10 mg of prednisone twice daily for 4 or 5 days. The dose is then reduced in steps and withdrawal planned for about the tenth day after initiation of the prednisone therapy. Under favorable circumstances, the patient can subsequently be managed once again with his prior medication.

In the treatment of *severe chronic bronchial asthma,* uncontrolled by other measures, the administration of a corticosteroid may be considered. The decision must be made with great care since the majority of patients, once started on corticosteroid therapy, remain indefinitely on such therapy. Many such patients are effectively managed with inhalation of beclomethasone valerate. A dose of 400 μg per day (two inhalations four times daily) is often adequate for chronic suppression of symptoms. Aerosol therapy is ineffective in acute attacks, in which airways may be plugged with mucus. *Ordinary doses of beclomethasone administered by inhalation have little systemic effects, and patients given this therapy obtain little or no protection against adrenal insufficiency should it occur as a result of previous treatment with a glucocorticoid.* Patients who have been taking a glucocorticoid orally must continue this medication in slowly decreasing dosage when inhalation therapy with beclomethasone is begun. Asymptomatic oropharyngeal candidiasis develops in a high percentage of patients using beclomethasone (Webb-Johnson and Andrews, 1977).

Ocular Diseases. Corticosteroids are frequently used to suppress inflammation in the eye, and employed properly they are often responsible for preservation of sight. Levine and Leopold (1973) list 28 disorders of the eye that respond to corticosteroids. They are administered locally for disease of the outer eye and anterior segment. Both natural and synthetic corticosteroids attain therapeutic concentrations in the aqueous humor following instillation into the conjunctival cul-de-sac. For disease of the posterior segment, systemic administration is required.

A typical prescription is 0.1% dexamethasone sodium phosphate solution (ophthalmic), 2 drops in the conjunctival sac every 4 hours while awake, and 0.05% dexamethasone phosphate ointment (ophthalmic) at bedtime. For inflammations of the posterior segment of the eye, usual daily doses are approximately 30 mg of prednisone or equivalent, administered orally in divided doses.

It has been convincingly demonstrated that topical corticosteroid therapy *frequently induces intraocular hypertension* in normal eyes and further increases pressure in eyes with initially elevated pressure. The glaucoma has not always been reversible on cessation of corticosteroid treatment. It has been recommended that intraocular pressure be monitored when corticosteroids are applied to the eye for more than 2 weeks.

The local administration of corticosteroids to patients with bacterial, viral, or fungal conjunctivitis *may mask evidences of progression of the infection until sight is lost.* Corticosteroids are *contraindicated in herpes simplex* (dendritic keratitis) of the eye, because progression of the disease and irreversible clouding of the cornea may occur. Topical steroids should not be used in the treatment of mechanical lacerations and abrasions of the eye. They delay healing and promote the development and spread of infection.

Skin Diseases. The development of corticosteroid preparations suitable for topical administration has revolutionized the therapy of the more common varieties of skin disease. Maibach and Stoughton (1973) have divided 20 dermatological disorders that respond to topical corticosteroids into those that are very responsive and those that require higher concentrations of steroids, occlusion of the drug under a plastic film, or intralesional administration. Attention must be paid to the concentration of steroid used, and there are a large number of preparations of various concentrations available for topical use (Table 63–4). A typical prescription for an eczematous eruption is 1% cortisol ointment applied locally twice daily. Effectiveness is enhanced by application of the cream or ointment under a transparent plastic wrapping. Unfortunately, systemic absorption is also enhanced, occasionally sufficiently to suppress the pituitary-adrenal axis or to produce Cushing's syndrome. Adrenocorticosteroids are administered systemically for severe episodes of acute skin disorders and exacerbations of chronic disorders. The dose is usually 40 mg per day of prednisone or equivalent. Systemically administered corticosteroids may be lifesaving in *pemphigus.* Up to 120 mg of prednisone or equivalent per day may be required to control the disease.

Diseases of the Intestinal Tract. Patients severely ill with untreated *celiac sprue* can often benefit from a course of glucocorticoid therapy given at the same time that management with a gluten-free diet is begun. Prednisolone, 30 mg per day or equivalent, is continued for 3 to 4 weeks. Patients who fail to respond to a gluten-free diet are helped by lower doses of prednisolone (7 to 12 mg per day or equivalent) for an indefinite period (Wall, 1973).

Corticosteroid therapy is indicated in selected patients with *chronic ulcerative colitis.* Mildly ill patients with bowel symptoms but without disabling systemic symptoms usually can and should be managed with rest, diet, sedation, anticholinergic agents, and chemotherapy. However, patients who do not improve should have a trial of methylprednisolone acetate, 40 mg or equivalent, in a nightly retention enema, in an attempt to induce remission. Alternate-day therapy may be effective. Severely ill patients with fever, anorexia, anemia, and malnutrition often improve dramatically when given systemic corticosteroid therapy. Large doses, 60 to 120 mg per day of prednisone, or the equivalent, are recommended. Major complications of ulcerative colitis may occur despite corticosteroid therapy. Signs and symptoms of intestinal perforation and peritonitis may be difficult to detect during corticosteroid treatment (Korelitz and Lindner, 1964).

Cerebral Edema. Corticosteroids are of value in the reduction or prevention of cerebral edema associated with neoplasms, especially those that are metastatic. In spite of widespread use of glucocorticoids for treatment of the cerebral edema due to trauma or cerebrovascular accidents, there is no convincing evidence of their value in these conditions (Nelson and Dick, 1975).

Malignancies. The chemotherapy of *acute lymphocytic leukemia* and *lymphomas* has been greatly improved by the introduction of therapy with multiple agents, and glucocorticoids are used because of their antilymphocytic effects. At the present time these diseases are treated in a complex fashion with rigidly scheduled sequences of combined drug therapy. Prednisone is commonly used in conjunction with an alkylating agent such as cyclophosphamide, an antimetabolite, and a vinca alkaloid (*see* Chapter 55). These therapeutic regimens are only suitable for use in medical centers under the supervision of oncologists.

Objective tumor regression in *carcinoma of the breast* can be induced by glucocorticoids in about 15% of patients; prednisolone (30 mg per day) has been the usual treatment. The presumed mechanism by which the corticosteroids act in these patients is through adrenocortical suppression, with an accompanying decrease in production of androgens, which are precursors of tumor-stimulating estrogens (Brennan, 1973). Similar therapy has been suggested to suppress adrenal androgens in the castrated patient with carcinoma of the prostate.

Diseases of the Liver. The use of glucocorticoids in the treatment of hepatic diseases has been the subject of controversy. Careful studies have now indicated several diseases of the liver in which therapy with steroids significantly improves survival rates; these are *subacute hepatic necrosis* and *chronic active hepatitis, alcoholic hepatitis,* and *nonalcoholic cirrhosis in females* (Lesesne and Fallon, 1973; Copenhagen Study Group for Liver Diseases, 1974). Only certain patients with chronic active hepatitis should receive steroid therapy. Those who benefit have symptomatic disease, histological evidence of severe disease, and a negative reaction for hepatitis B surface antigen (Berk *et al.,* 1976). Treatment of *subacute hepatic necrosis* and *chronic active hepatitis* includes prednisolone, 60 to 100 mg per day; the dose is tapered as the disease improves. Treatment of *alcoholic hepatitis* with corticosteroids is reserved for patients who are severely ill, with evidence of hepatic encephalopathy. Prednisone (40 mg per day) is given for 1 month, followed by withdrawal over a period of 2 to 4 weeks. *Nonalcoholic cirrhosis in women* should be treated with glucocorticoids if the patient does not have ascites. Daily dosages average 15 to 20 mg of prednisone or equivalent when they are adjusted to the needs of the individual patients. The data indicate that *steroid treatment lowers survival rates when ascites is present.* Treatment of cirrhotic male patients with steroids has not been shown to be beneficial.

Shock. While corticosteroids are often administered to patients in shock, there is no convincing evidence to indicate that such therapy is efficacious (Reichgott and Melmon, 1975).

Miscellaneous Diseases. Sarcoidosis is treated with prednisone, approximately 1 mg/kg per day or equivalent, to induce a remission. Maintenance doses, which are often required for long periods of time, may be 10 mg of prednisone per day or less. In this, as in other diseases treated by prolonged steroid therapy, patients with positive tuberculin reactions or other evidence of tuberculosis should receive prophylactic antituberculosis therapy. In *thrombocytopenia,* prednisone, 0.5 mg/kg or equivalent, is used to decrease the bleeding tendency. In severe cases and for initiation of treatment of *idiopathic thrombocytopenia,* daily doses of prednisone, 1 to 1.5 mg/kg, are employed. *Hemolytic anemias* with a positive Coombs' test are treated with prednisone, 1 mg/kg per day or equivalent. If hemolysis is severe, therapy is initiated with 100 mg of hydrocortisone intravenously; as the disease improves, the dose is decreased. Small maintenance doses may be needed for several months if a positive response is obtained. In *organ transplantation,* high doses of prednisone (50 to 100 mg) are given at the time of the transplant surgery. Smaller maintenance doses (10 to 20 mg per day) are continued indefinitely, and the dosage is increased if rejection is threatened. In *aspiration of gastric contents,* prednisone (50 to 100 mg) is given for 2 to 3 days to suppress the inflammatory reaction in the lung and to prevent development of pulmonary abscess.

DIAGNOSTIC APPLICATIONS OF ADRENOCORTICAL STEROIDS

Potent synthetic congeners of cortisol reduce urinary excretion of cortisol metabolites by inhibition of pituitary ACTH release. The dose required is so small, in gravimetric terms, that it contributes only negligibly to the urinary steroids. Liddle (1960) reported that the administration of 0.5 mg of dexamethasone every 6 hours for a total of eight doses results in a marked suppression of excretion of cortisol metabolites in normal persons, but has almost no effect on the urinary steroids of persons with pituitary-dependent hypercorticism. This test is useful in distinguishing persons with some nonspecific elevation of steroid excretion, for example, that due to obesity or stress, from patients with Cushing's syndrome. The administration of 2 mg of dexamethasone every 6 hours for a total of eight doses usually causes a suppression of cortisol secretion in patients with pituitary-dependent hypercorticism, but ordinarily has little if any effect on the urinary steroids of patients with adrenal neoplasms or ACTH-producing tumors (Meador *et al.,* 1962). However, "suppressible" tumors have been reported. The results of these tests are likely to be most definite if the urinary steroids are measured daily for 2 days before and for at least 2 days during administration of the suppressing agent. Variations of this procedure (shorter test period and measurement of plasma cortisol rather than urinary metabolites) have been described (Sawin *et al.,* 1968).

INHIBITORS OF THE BIOSYNTHESIS OF ADRENOCORTICAL STEROIDS

Three pharmacological agents have proven most useful as inhibitors of adrenocortical secretion. *Mitotane* (*o,p'*-DDD), an adrenocorticolytic agent, is discussed in Chapter 55. *Metyrapone* and *aminoglutethimide* are discussed here. The subject has been reviewed by Temple and Liddle (1970).

Metyrapone. Metyrapone reduces cortisol production by inhibition of the 11β-hydroxylation reaction. Metyrapone also inhibits side chain cleavage to some degree (Cheng *et al.,* 1974), but this block is largely overcome when ACTH stimulates the gland. The biosynthetic process is terminated at 11-desoxycortisol (Figure 63–3), a compound that has practically no inhibitory influence on the secretion of ACTH. In the normal person, a compensatory increase in ACTH secretion follows, and the secretion of 11-desoxycortisol, a "17-hydroxycorticoid," is markedly accelerated. Consequently, in normal persons, administration of metyrapone induces increased renal excretion of "17-hydroxycorticoids."

Metyrapone is used to test the capacity of the pituitary to respond to a decreased concentration of plasma cortisol. A response that is greater than normal is usually found in patients with Cushing's syndrome of pituitary origin. In most cases of Cushing's syndrome due to ectopic production of ACTH there is no response to the drug. Administration of metyrapone to patients with disease of the hypothalamico-pituitary complex who are unable to achieve a compensatory increase in the rate of secretion of ACTH is, of course, not followed by increased renal excretion of 17-hydroxycorticoids.

The ability of the adrenal to respond to ACTH should be demonstrated before metyrapone is employed, for two reasons: (1) administration of metyrapone can be used as a test for normal hypothalamico-pituitary function only if the adrenal glands are capable of responding to ACTH, and (2) the drug may induce acute adrenal insufficiency in patients with reduced adrenal secretory capacity. Metyrapone also inhibits synthesis of aldosterone, which, like cortisol, is an 11β-hydroxylated compound. However, metyrapone does not typically cause a deficiency of mineralocorticoids, with a consequent loss of sodium and retention of potassium, because the inhibition of the 11β-hydroxylation reaction results in an increased production of 11-desoxycorticosterone, a mineralocorticoid.

Metyrapone has been used successfully to treat the hypercortisolism that results from adrenal neoplasms that function autonomously and from ectopic ACTH production by tumors. Its use in treatment of Cushing's syndrome resulting from hypersecretion of ACTH by the pituitary is controversial (Orth, 1978; Gold, 1979). Metyrapone has been used experimentally in patients with Cushing's syndrome during the period of time required for radiation treatment to become effective (Orth, 1978).

Metyrapone, U.S.P. (METOPIRONE), is 2-methyl-1,2-di-3-pyridyl-1-propanone. The drug is marketed as 250-mg oral tablets and as a solution of the ditartrate salt (100 mg/ml equivalent to 43.8 mg/ml of the base) in 10-ml ampuls for intravenous administration. Following two 24-hour control periods, the drug is given orally in the dose of 750 mg every 4 hours for six doses, or intravenously (30 mg/kg), infused over a period of 4 hours. Maximal urinary excretion of 11-desoxycorticosteroids is observed on the next day following oral administration and on the same day following intravenous infusion.

Aminoglutethimide. This compound, α-ethyl-*p*-aminophenyl-glutarimide, inhibits the conversion of cholesterol to 20α-hydroxycholesterol. This inhibition of the first reaction of steroidogenesis from cholesterol interrupts production of both cortisol and aldosterone.

Aminoglutethimide has been used successfully to decrease the hypersecretion of cortisol in autonomously functioning adrenal tumors and in hypersecretion resulting from ectopic production of ACTH. It has also been used in combination with metyrapone in the treatment of Cushing's syndrome that results from hypersecretion of ACTH by the pituitary (*see* Gold, 1979).

Aminoglutethimide is available only for investigational studies.

Adam, P. A. J., and Haynes, R. C., Jr. Control of hepatic mitochondrial CO_2 fixation by glucagon, epinephrine, and cortisol. *J. Biol. Chem.*, **1969**, *244*, 6444–6450.

Addison, T. *On the Constitutional and Local Effects of Disease of the Suprarenal Capsules.* Samuel Highley, London, **1855**.

Ahmed, A. B. J.; George, B. C.; Gonzalez-Auvert, C.; and Dingman, J. F. Increased plasma arginine vasopressin in clinical adrenocortical insufficiency and its inhibition by glucosteroids. *J. Clin. Invest.*, **1967**, *46*, 111–123.

Amatruda, T. T., Jr.; Hollingsworth, D. R.; D'Esopo, N. D.; Upton, G. V.; and Bondy, P. K. A study of the mechanism of the steroid withdrawal syndrome. *J. Clin. Endocrinol. Metab.*, **1960**, *20*, 339–354.

Astwood, E. B.; Raben, M. S.; and Payne, R. W. Chemistry of corticotrophin. *Recent Prog. Horm. Res.*, **1952**, *7*, 1–57.

Bacon, G. E., and Spencer, M. L. Pediatric uses of steroids. *Med. Clin. North Am.*, **1973**, *57*, 1265–1276.

Ballard, P. L.; Baxter, J. D.; Higgins, S. J.; Rousseau, G. C.; and Tomkins, G. M. General presence of glucocorticoid receptors in mammalian tissues. *Endocrinology*, **1974**, *94*, 998–1002.

Balow, J. E., and Rosenthal, A. S. Glucocorticoid suppression of macrophage migration inhibitory factor. *J. Exp. Med.*, **1973**, *137*, 1031–1039.

Bangham, D. R.; Mussett, M. V.; and Stack-Dunne, M. P. The third international standard for corticotrophin. *Bull. WHO*, **1962**, *27*, 395–408.

Barger, A. C.; Berlin, R. D.; and Tulenko, J. F. Infusion of aldosterone, 9-α-fluorohydrocortisone and antidiuretic hormone into the renal artery of normal and adrenalectomized, unanesthetized dogs: effect on electrolyte and water excretion. *Endocrinology*, **1958**, *62*, 804–815.

Beckett, G. J., and Boyd, G. S. Evidence for the activation of bovine cholesterol ester hydrolase by a phosphorylation involving an adenosine 3′:5′-monophosphate-dependent protein kinase. *Biochem. Soc. Trans.*, **1975**, *3*, 892–894.

Bell, J. J., and Harding, B. W. The acute action of adrenocorticotropic hormone on adrenal steroidogenesis. *Biochim. Biophys. Acta*, **1974**, *348*, 285–298.

Bell, P. H.; Howard, K. S.; Shepherd, R. G.; Finn, B. M.; and Meisenhelder, J. H. Studies with corticotropin. II. Pepsin degradation of β-corticotropin. *J. Am. Chem. Soc.*, **1956**, *78*, 5059–5066.

Berk, P. D.; Jones, E. A.; Plotz, P. H.; Seeff, L. B.; and Wright, E. C. Corticosteroid therapy for chronic active hepatitis. *Ann. Intern. Med.*, **1976**, *85*, 523–525.

Biglieri, E. G. Aldosterone and the renin-angiotensin system. In, *The Year in Endocrinology: 1977.* (Ingbar, S. H., ed.) Plenum Medical Book Co., New York, **1978**, pp. 191–204.

Birnbaum, R. S., and Goodman, H. M. Effects of hypophysectomy on cyclic AMP accumulation and action in adipose tissue. *Fed. Proc.*, **1973**, *32*, 535.

Bishop, C. R.; Athens, J. W.; Boggs, D. R.; Warner, H. R.; Cartwright, G. E.; and Wintrobe, M. M. Leukokinetic

studies. XIII. A non-steady-state kinetic evaluation of the mechanism of cortisone-induced granulocytosis. *J. Clin. Invest.*, **1968**, *47*, 249–260.

Blackwell, G. J.; Flower, R. J.; Nijkamp, F. P.; and Vane, J. R. Phospholipase A_2 activity of guinea pig isolated perfused lungs: stimulation and inhibition by anti-inflammatory steroids. *Br. J. Pharmacol.*, **1978**, *62*, 79–89.

Bloom, B. R., and Bennett, B. Mechanism of a reaction *in vitro* associated with delayed hypersensitivity. *Science*, **1966**, *153*, 80–82.

Brennan, M. J. Corticosteroids in the treatment of solid tumors. *Med. Clin. North Am.*, **1973**, *57*, 1225–1239.

Britton, S. W., and Silvette, H. Some effects of corticoadrenal extract and other substances on adrenalectomized animals. *Am. J. Physiol.*, **1931**, *99*, 15–32.

Brown-Séquard, C. E. Recherches expérimentales sur la physiologie et la pathologie des capsules surrenales. *C. R. Acad. Sci.* [D] (Paris), **1856**, *43*, 422–425.

Brunner, H. R.; Chang, P.; Wallace, R.; Sealey, J. E.; and Laragh, J. H. Angiotensin II vascular receptors. *J. Clin. Invest.*, **1972**, *51*, 58–67.

Bush, I. E. Species differences in adrenocortical secretion. *J. Endocrinol.*, **1953**, *9*, 95–100.

Butler, W. T. Corticosteroids and immunoglobulin synthesis. *Transplant. Proc.*, **1975**, *7*, 49–53.

Byyny, R. L. Withdrawal from glucocorticoid therapy. *N. Engl. J. Med.*, **1976**, *295*, 30–32.

Camacho, A. M.; Kowarski, A.; Migeon, C. J.; and Brough, A. J. Congenital adrenal hyperplasia due to a deficiency of one of the enzymes involved in the biosynthesis of pregnenolone. *J. Clin. Endocrinol. Metab.*, **1968**, *28*, 153–161.

Carson, S. H.; Taeusch, W. H., Jr.; and Avery, M. E. Inhibition of lung cell division after hydrocortisone injection into fetal rabbits. *J. Appl. Physiol.*, **1973**, *34*, 660–663.

Cheng, S. C.; Harding, B. W.; and Carballeira, A. Effects of metyrapone on pregnenolone biosynthesis and on cholesterol–cytochrome P-450 interaction in the adrenal. *Endocrinology*, **1974**, *94*, 1451–1458.

Claman, H. N. Corticosteroids and lymphoid cells. *N. Engl. J. Med.*, **1972**, *287*, 388–397.

———. How corticosteroids work. *J. Allergy Clin. Immunol.*, **1975**, *55*, 145–151.

Cohen, J. J. The effects of hydrocortisone on the immune response. *Ann. Allergy*, **1971**, *29*, 358–361.

Cohen, J. J.; Fischbach, M.; and Claman, H. N. Hydrocortisone resistance of graft *vs* host activity in mouse thymus, spleen and bone marrow. *J. Immunol.*, **1970**, *105*, 1146–1150.

Collip, J. B.; Anderson, E. M.; and Thompson, D. L. The adrenotropic hormone of the anterior pituitary lobe. *Lancet*, **1933**, *2*, 347–348.

Conn, H. O., and Blitzer, B. L. Nonassociation of adrenocorticosteroid therapy and peptic ulcer. *N. Engl. J. Med.*, **1976**, *294*, 473–479.

Copenhagen Study Group for Liver Diseases. Sex, ascites, and alcoholism in survival of patients with cirrhosis. Effect of prednisone. *N. Engl. J. Med.*, **1974**, *293*, 271–273.

Cori, C. F., and Cori, G. T. The fate of sugar in the animal body. VII. The carbohydrate metabolism of adrenalectomized rats and mice. *J. Biol. Chem.*, **1927**, *74*, 473–494.

Cushing, H. The basophil adenomas of the pituitary body and their clinical manifestations. *Bull. Johns Hopkins Hosp.*, **1932**, *50*, 137–195.

David, R.; Golon, S.; and Drucker, W. Familial aldosterone deficiency: enzyme defect, diagnosis and clinical course. *Pediatrics*, **1968**, *41*, 403–414.

Deane, H., and Greep, R. O. A morphological and histochemical study of the rat's adrenal cortex after hypophysectomy, with comments on the liver. *Am. J. Anat.*, **1946**, *79*, 117–146.

Deming, Q. B., and Luetscher, J. A., Jr. Bioassay of desoxycorticosterone-like material in urine. *Proc. Soc. Exp. Biol. Med.*, **1950**, *73*, 171–175.

Doig, A.; Girdwood, R. H.; Duthie, J. J. R.; and Knox, J. D. E. Response of megaloblastic anaemia to prednisolone. *Lancet,* **1957,** *2,* 966–972.

Dougherty, T. F., and White, A. Influence of hormones on lymphoid tissue structure and function: role of pituitary adrenotrophic hormone in regulation of lymphocytes and other cellular elements of the blood. *Endocrinology,* **1944,** *35,* 1–14.

———. Functional alterations in lymphoid tissue induced by adrenal cortical secretion. *Am. J. Anat.,* **1945,** *77,* 81–115.

———. Evaluation of alterations produced in lymphoid tissue by pituitary adrenal cortical secretion. *J. Lab. Clin. Med.,* **1947,** *32,* 584–605.

Eipper, B. A., and Mains, R. E. Analysis of the common precursor to corticotropin and endorphin. *J. Biol. Chem.,* **1978,** *253,* 5732–5744.

Engel, F. L. Extra-adrenal actions of adrenocorticotropin. *Vitam. Horm.,* **1961,** *19,* 189–227.

Evans, H. M. Present position of our knowledge of anterior pituitary function. *J.A.M.A.,* **1933,** *101,* 425–432.

Farrell, G. L.; Rauschkolb, E. W.; and Royce, P. C. Secretion of aldosterone by the adrenal of the dog: effects of hypophysectomy and ACTH. *Am. J. Physiol.,* **1955,** *182,* 269–272.

Fauci, A. S., and Dale, D. C. The effect of *in vivo* hydrocortisone on subpopulations of human lymphocytes. *J. Clin. Invest.,* **1974,** *53,* 240–246.

Feldman, D.; Funder, J. W.; and Edelman, I. S. Subcellular mechanisms in the action of the adrenal steroids. *Am. J. Med.,* **1972,** *53,* 545–560.

Fenster, L. F. The ulcerogenic potential of glucocorticoids and possible prophylactic measures. *Med. Clin. North Am.,* **1973,** *57,* 1289–1294.

Fisher, L. B., and Maibach, H. I. The effect of corticosteroids on human epidermal mitotic activity. *Arch. Dermatol.,* **1971,** *103,* 39–44.

Forssman, O., and Mulder, J. Hypersensitivity to different ACTH peptides. *Acta Med. Scand.,* **1973,** *193,* 557–559.

Foster, G. L., and Smith, P. E. Hypophysectomy and replacement therapy in relation to basal metabolism and specific dynamic action in the rat. *J.A.M.A.,* **1926,** *87,* 2151–2153.

Gill, G. N. ACTH regulation of the adrenal cortex. *Pharmacol. Ther. [B],* **1976,** *2,* 313–338.

Gill, J. R., Jr.; Gann, D. S.; and Bartter, F. C. Restoration of water diuresis in Addisonian patients by expansion of the volume of extracellular fluid. *J. Clin. Invest.,* **1962,** *41,* 1078–1085.

Goldsmith, O.; Solomon, D. H.; and Horton, E. Hypogonadism and mineralocorticoid excess: the 17-hydroxylase deficiency syndrome. *N. Engl. J. Med.,* **1968,** *277,* 673–677.

Goodman, H. M. Endocrine control of lipolysis. In, *Progress in Endocrinology: Proceedings of the Third International Congress of Endocrinology, Mexico.* (Gual, C., and Ebling, F. J. G., eds.) Excerpta Medica, Amsterdam, **1968,** pp. 115–123.

Graber, A. L.; Ney, R. E.; Nicholson, W. E.; Island, D. P.; and Liddle, G. W. Natural history of pituitary-adrenal recovery following long term suppression with corticosteroids. *J. Clin. Endocrinol. Metab.,* **1965,** *25,* 11–16.

Grahame, R. Elasticity of human skin *in vivo.* A study of the physical properties of the skin in rheumatoid arthritis and the effect of corticosteroids. *Ann. Phys. Med.,* **1969,** *10,* 130–136.

Gray, J. G.; Pratt, W. B.; and Aronow, L. Effect of glucocorticoids on hexose uptake by mouse fibroblasts *in vitro.* *Biochemistry,* **1971,** *10,* 277–284.

Greendyke, R. M.; Bradley, E. M.; and Swisher, S. N. Studies on the effects of administration of ACTH and adrenal corticosteroids on erythrophagocytosis. *J. Clin. Invest.,* **1965,** *44,* 746–753.

Gryglewski, R. J.; Panczenko, B.; Korbut, R.; Grodzinska, L.; and Ocetkiewicz, A. Corticosteroids inhibit prostaglandin release from perfused mesenteric blood vessels of rabbit and from perfused lungs of sensitized guinea pig. *Prostaglandins,* **1975,** *10,* 343–355.

Gwynne, J. T.; Mahaffee, D.; Brewer, H. B.; and Ney, R. L. Adrenal cholesterol uptake from plasma lipoproteins: regulation by corticotropin. *Proc. Natl. Acad. Sci. U.S.A.,* **1976,** *73,* 4329–4333.

Hammarstrom, S.; Hamburg, M.; Duell, E. A.; Stawiski, M. A.; Anderson, T. F.; and Voorhees, J. J. Glucocorticoid in inflammatory proliferative skin disease reduces arachidonic and hydroxyeicosotetraenoic acids. *Science,* **1977,** *197,* 994–995.

Harris, G. W. *Neural Control of the Pituitary Gland.* Edward Arnold, London, **1955.**

Harrop, G. A.; Soffer, L. J.; Ellsworth, R.; and Trescher, J. H. Studies on the suprarenal cortex. III. Plasma electrolytes and electrolyte excretion during suprarenal insufficiency in the dog. *J. Exp. Med.,* **1933,** *58,* 17–38.

Harter, J. G.; Reddy, W. J.; and Thorn, G. W. Studies on an intermittent corticosteroid dosage regimen. *N. Engl. J. Med.,* **1963,** *269,* 591–596.

Hartman, F. A.; Brownell, K. A.; and Hartman, W. E. A further study of the hormone of the adrenal cortex. *Am. J. Physiol.,* **1930,** *95,* 670–680.

Harvey, W., and Grahame, R. Effect of some adrenal steroid hormones on skin fibroblast replication *in vitro.* *Ann. Rheum. Dis.,* **1973,** *32,* 272.

Haynes, R. C., Jr. The activation of adrenal phosphorylase by the adrenocorticotropic hormone. *J. Biol. Chem.,* **1958,** *233,* 1220–1222.

Haynes, R. C., Jr.; Koritz, S. B.; and Péron, F. G. Influence of adenosine 3',5'-monophosphate on corticoid production by rat adrenal glands. *J. Biol. Chem.,* **1959,** *234,* 1421–1423.

Hench, P. S.; Kendall, E. C.; Slocumb, C. H.; and Polley, H. F. The effect of a hormone of the adrenal cortex (17-hydroxy-11-dehydrocorticosterone; compound E) and of pituitary adrenocorticotropic hormone on rheumatoid arthritis. *Proc. Staff Meet. Mayo Clin.,* **1949,** *24,* 181–197.

Henkin, R. I. The effects of corticosteroids and ACTH on sensory systems. *Prog. Brain Res.,* **1970,** *32,* 270–294.

Hofmann, K. Chemistry and function of polypeptide hormones. *Annu. Rev. Biochem.,* **1962,** *31,* 213–246.

Hofmann, K.; Montibeller, J. A.; and Finn, F. M. ACTH antagonists. *Proc. Natl. Acad. Sci. U.S.A.,* **1974,** *71,* 80–83.

Hofmann, K.; Yajima, H.; Yanaihara, N.; Liu, T.; and Lande, S. Studies on polypeptides. XIII. The synthesis of a tricosapeptide possessing essentially the full biological activity of natural ACTH. *J. Am. Chem. Soc.,* **1961,** *83,* 487–489.

Hong, S. L., and Levine, L. Inhibition of arachidonic acid release from cells as the biochemical action of anti-inflammatory corticosteroids. *Proc. Natl. Acad. Sci. U.S.A.,* **1976,** *73,* 1730–1734.

Houssay, B. A.; Biasotti, A.; Mazzoco, P.; and Sammartino, R. Acción del extracto antero-hipofisario sobre las glandulas adrenales. *Rev. Soc. Argent. Biol.,* **1933,** *9,* 262–268.

Howard, E. Effects of corticosterone and food restriction on growth and on DNA, RNA, and cholesterol contents of the brain and liver in infant mice. *J. Neurochem.,* **1964,** *12,* 181–191.

Ingle, D. J. Permissive action of hormones. *J. Clin. Endocrinol. Metab.,* **1954,** *14,* 1272–1274.

Ingle, D. J.; Higgins, G. M.; and Kendall, E. C. Atrophy of the adrenal cortex in the rat produced by administration of large amounts of cortin. *Anat. Rec.,* **1938,** *71,* 363–372.

Iynedjian, P. B., and Hanson, R. W. Messenger RNA for renal phosphoenolpyruvate carboxykinase and its regulation by glucocorticoids and by changes in acid base balance. *J. Biol. Chem.,* **1977,** *252,* 8398–8403.

Kahnt, F. W.; Milani, A.; Steffen, H.; and Neher, R. The rate-limiting step of adrenal steroidogenesis and adenosine 3':5'-monophosphate. *Eur. J. Biochem.*, **1974**, *44*, 243–250.

Korelitz, B. I., and Lindner, A. E. The influence of corticotrophin and adrenal steroids on the course of ulcerative colitis: a comparison with the presteroid era. *Gastroenterology*, **1964**, *46*, 671–679.

Krakoff, L.; Nicolis, G.; and Amsel, B. Pathogenesis of hypertension in Cushing's syndrome. *Am. J. Med.*, **1975**, *58*, 216–220.

Kreutner, W., and Goldberg, N. D. Dependence on insulin of the apparent hydrocortisone activation of hepatic glycogen synthetase. *Proc. Natl. Acad. Sci. U.S.A.*, **1967**, *58*, 1515–1519.

Lee, P. A.; Keenan, B. S.; Migeon, C. J.; and Blizzard, R. M. Effect of various ACTH preparations on the secretion of growth hormone in normal subjects and in hypopituitary patients. *J. Clin. Endocrinol. Metab.*, **1973**, *37*, 389–396.

Lemann, J., Jr.; Piering, W. F.; and Lennon, E. J. Studies of the acute effects of aldosterone and cortisol on the interrelationship between renal sodium, calcium, and magnesium excretion in normal man. *Nephron*, **1970**, *7*, 117–130.

Lesesne, H. R., and Fallon, H. J. Treatment of liver disease with corticosteroids. *Med. Clin. North Am.*, **1973**, *57*, 1191–1201.

Levine, S. B., and Leopold, I. H. Advances in ocular corticosteroid therapy. *Med. Clin. North Am.*, **1973**, *57*, 1167–1177.

Li, C. H. Adrenocorticotropin 45. Revised amino acid sequences for sheep and bovine hormones. *Biochem. Biophys. Res. Commun.*, **1972**, *49*, 835–839.

Li, C. H.; Evans, H. M.; and Simpson, M. E. Adrenocorticotropic hormone. *J. Biol. Chem.*, **1943**, *149*, 413–424.

Liddle, G. W. Tests of pituitary-adrenal suppressibility in the diagnosis of Cushing's syndrome. *J. Clin. Endocrinol. Metab.*, **1960**, *20*, 1539–1560.

Loeb, J. N., and Sternschein, M. J. Suppression of thymidine incorporation into the gastric mucosa of cortisone-treated rats: possible relation to glucocorticoid-induced gastric ulceration. *Endocrinology*, **1973**, *92*, 1322–1377.

Loeb, R. F. Effect of sodium chloride in the treatment of a patient with Addison's disease. *Proc. Soc. Exp. Biol. Med.*, **1933**, *30*, 808–812.

Loeb, R. F.; Atchley, D. W.; Benedict, E. M.; and Leland, J. Electrolyte balance studies in adrenalectomized dogs with particular reference to the excretion of sodium. *J. Exp. Med.*, **1933**, *57*, 775–792.

Long, C. N. H.; Katzin, B.; and Fry, E. G. Adrenal cortex and carbohydrate metabolism. *Endocrinology*, **1940**, *26*, 309–344.

Lubkin, V. L. Steroid cataract—a review and conclusion. *J. Asthma Res.*, **1977**, *14*, 55–59.

McEwen, B. S. Adrenal steroid feedback on neuroendocrine tissues. *Ann. N.Y. Acad. Sci.*, **1977**, *297*, 568–579.

Mahaffee, D.; Reitz, R. C.; and Ney, R. L. The mechanism of action of adrenocorticotropic hormone. The role of mitochondrial cholesterol accumulation in the regulation of steroidogenesis. *J. Biol. Chem.*, **1974**, *249*, 227–233.

Maibach, H. I., and Stoughton, R. B. Topical corticosteroids. *Med. Clin. North Am.*, **1973**, *57*, 1253–1264.

Makman, M. H.; Dvorkin, B.; and White, A. Evidence for induction by cortisol *in vitro* of a protein inhibitor of transport and phosphorylation in rat thymocytes. *Proc. Natl. Acad. Sci. U.S.A.*, **1971**, *68*, 1269–1273.

Marco, J.; Calle, C.; Román, D.; Diaz-Ferros, M.; Villanueva, M. L.; and Valverde, I. Hyperglucagonism induced by glucocorticoid treatment in man. *N. Engl. J. Med.*, **1973**, *288*, 128–131.

Meador, C. K.; Liddle, G. W.; Island, D. P.; Nicholson, W. E.; Lucas, C. P.; Nuckton, J. G.; and Luetscher, J. A. Cause of Cushing's syndrome in patients with tumors arising from "nonendocrine" tissue. *J. Clin. Endocrinol. Metab.*, **1962**, *22*, 693–703.

Mishler, J. M. The effects of corticosteroids on mobilization and function of neutrophils. *Exp. Hematol.*, **1977**, *5*, Suppl., 15–32.

Morris, H. G.; Jorgensen, J. R.; Elrick, H.; and Goldsmith, R. E. Metabolic effects of human growth hormone in corticosteroid-treated children. *J. Clin. Invest.*, **1968**, *47*, 436–451.

Nakanishi, S.; Kita, T.; Taii, S.; Imura, H.; and Numa, S. Glucocorticoid effect on the level of corticotropin messenger RNA activity in rat pituitary. *Proc. Natl. Acad. Sci. U.S.A.*, **1977**, *74*, 3283–3286.

Nelson, S. R., and Dick, A. R. Steroids in the treatment of brain edema. In, *Steroid Therapy.* (Azarnoff, D. L., ed.) W. B. Saunders Co., Philadelphia, **1975**, pp. 313–324.

Ney, R. L. Effects of dibutyryl cyclic AMP on adrenal growth and steroidogenic capacity. *Endocrinology*, **1969**, *84*, 168–170.

Orth, D. N. Metyrapone is useful only as adjunctive therapy in Cushing's disease. *Ann. Intern. Med.*, **1978**, *89*, 128–130.

Otsuka, H., and Inouye, L. K. Structure-activity relationships of adrenocorticotropin. *Pharmacol. Ther. [B]*, **1975**, *1*, 501–527.

Paul, D. P.; Gallant, S.; Orme-Johnson, N. R.; Orme-Johnson, W. H.; and Brownie, H. C. Temperature dependence of cholesterol binding to cytochrome P-450 of the rat adrenal. Effect of adrenocorticotropic hormone and cycloheximide. *J. Biol. Chem.*, **1976**, *251*, 7120–7126.

Pittman, R. C., and Steinberg, D. Activatable cholesterol esterase and triacylglycerol lipase activities of rat adrenal and their relationship. *Biochim. Biophys. Acta*, **1977**, *487*, 431–444.

Pratt, W. B., and Aronow, L. The effect of glucocorticoids on protein and nucleic acid synthesis in mouse fibroblasts growing *in vitro. J. Biol. Chem.*, **1966**, *241*, 5244–5250.

Reichgott, M. J., and Melmon, K. L. The role of corticosteroids in the treatment of shock. In, *Steroid Therapy.* (Azarnoff, D. L., ed.) W. B. Saunders Co., Philadelphia, **1975**, pp. 118–133.

Rinehart, J. J.; Sagone, A. L.; Balcerzak, S. P.; Ackerman, G. A.; and LoBuglio, A. L. Effects of corticosteroid therapy on human monocyte function. *N. Engl. J. Med.*, **1975**, *292*, 236–241.

Roberts, J. L.; Phillips, M.; Rosa, P. A.; and Herbert, E. Steps involved in processing of common precursor forms of adrenocorticotropin and endorphin in cultures of mouse pituitary cells. *Biochemistry*, **1978**, *17*, 3609–3618.

Robinson, W. D. Management of systemic lupus erythematosus. *Arthritis Rheum.*, **1962**, *5*, 521–528.

Sawin, C. T.; Bray, G. A.; and Idelson, B. A. Overnight suppression test with dexamethasone in Cushing's syndrome. *J. Clin. Endocrinol. Metab.*, **1968**, *28*, 422–424.

Sayers, G.; White, A.; and Long, C. N. H. Preparation and properties of pituitary adrenotropic hormone. *J. Biol. Chem.*, **1943**, *149*, 425–436.

Scherrer, K. Messenger RNA in eukaryotic cells: the life history of duck globin messenger RNA. *Acta Endocrinol. (Kbh.)*, **1973**, *180*, Suppl., 95–129.

Schutz, G.; Killewich, L.; Chen, G.; and Feigelson, P. Control of the mRNA for hepatic tryptophan oxygenase during hormonal and substrate induction. *Proc. Natl. Acad. Sci. U.S.A.*, **1975**, *72*, 1017–1020.

Schwyzer, R., and Sieber, P. Total synthesis of adrenocorticotropic hormone. *Nature*, **1963**, *199*, 172–174.

Selye, H. General adaptation syndrome and diseases of adaptation. *J. Clin. Endocrinol. Metab.*, **1946**, *6*, 117–230.

Simpson, S. A.; Tait, J. F.; Wettstein, A.; Neher, R.; Euw, J. V.; Schindler, O.; and Reichstein, T. Konstitution des Aldosterons des neuen Mineralocorticoids. *Experientia*, **1954**, *10*, 132–133.

Steiger, M., and Reichstein, T. Desoxy-cortico-steron (21-Oxy-progesteron) aus Δ^5-3-Oxy-ätio-cholensäure. *Helv. Chim. Acta*, **1937**, *20*, 1164–1179.

Stevenson, R. D. Hydrocortisone and the migration of

human leukocytes: an indirect effect mediated by mononuclear cells. *Clin. Exp. Immunol.,* **1973,** *14,* 417–426.

Stone, D., and Hechter, O.   Studies on ACTH action in perfused bovine adrenals: the site of action of ACTH in corticosteroidogenesis. *Arch. Biochem. Biophys.,* **1954,** *51,* 457–469.

Swann, H. G.   The pituitary-adrenocortical relationship. *Physiol. Rev.,* **1940,** *20,* 493–521.

Sweat, M. L., and Bryson, M. J.   The role of phosphopyridinenucleotides in the metabolism of cortisol by peripheral tissue. *Biochim. Biophys. Acta,* **1960,** *44,* 217–223.

Swingle, W. W., and Pfiffner, J. J.   Experiments with an active extract of the suprarenal cortex. *Anat. Rec.,* **1930a,** *44,* 225–226.

———.   An aqueous extract of the suprarenal cortex which maintains the life of bilaterally adrenalectomized cats. *Science,* **1930b,** *71,* 321–322.

Tait, J. F.; Simpson, S. A.; and Grundy, H. M.   The effect of adrenal extract on mineral metabolism. *Lancet,* **1952,** *1,* 122–124.

Thody, A. J.   The significance of melanocyte-stimulating hormone (MSH) and the control of its secretion in the mammal. *Adv. Drug Res.,* **1977,** *11,* 23–74.

Tobian, L.   Interrelationship of electrolytes, juxtaglomerular cells and hypertension. *Physiol. Rev.,* **1960,** *40,* 280–312.

Vassalli, J.-D.; Hamilton, J.; and Reich, E.   Macrophage plasminogen activator: modulation of enzyme production by anti-inflammatory steroids, mitotic inhibitors, and cyclic nucleotides. *Cell,* **1976,** *8,* 271–281.

Wall, A. J.   The use of glucocorticoids in intestinal disease. *Med. Clin. North Am.,* **1973,** *57,* 1241–1252.

Webb-Johnson, D. C., and Andrews, J. L.   Bronchodilator therapy. *N. Engl. J. Med.,* **1977,** *297,* 476–482, 758–764.

Weston, W. L.; Claman, H. N.; and Krueger, G. G.   Site of action of cortisol in cellular immunity. *J. Immunol.,* **1973,** *110,* 880–883.

Wise, J. K.; Hendler, R.; and Felig, P.   Influence of glucocorticoids on glucagon secretion and plasma amino acid concentrations in man. *J. Clin. Invest.,* **1973,** *52,* 2774–2782.

Yard, A. C., and Kadowitz, P. J.   Studies on the mechanism of hydrocortisone potentiation of vasoconstrictor responses to epinephrine in the anesthetized animal. *Eur. J. Pharmacol.,* **1972,** *20,* 1–9.

Yount, W. J.; Utsinger, P. D.; Puritz, E. M.; and Ortbals, D. W.   Corticosteroid therapy of the collagen vascular disorders. *Med. Clin. North Am.,* **1973,** *57,* 1343–1355.

Monographs and Reviews

Baxter, J. D.   Glucocorticoid hormone action. *Pharmacol. Ther.* [B], **1976,** *2,* 605–659. (267 references.)

Bongiovanni, A. M.; Eberlein, W. R.; Goldman, A. S.; and New, M.   Disorders of adrenal steroid biogenesis. *Recent Prog. Horm. Res.,* **1967,** *23,* 375–449.

David, D. S.; Grieco, M. H.; and Cushman, P., Jr.   Adrenal glucocorticoids after twenty years. A review of their clinically relevant consequences. *J. Chronic Dis.,* **1970,** *22,* 637–711.

Gold, E. M.   The Cushing's syndromes: changing views of diagnosis and treatment. *Ann. Intern. Med.,* **1979,** *90,* 829–844.

Hahn, T. J.   Corticosteroid-induced osteopenia. *Arch. Intern. Med.,* **1978,** *138,* 882–885.

Liddle, G. W.   Clinical pharmacology of the anti-inflammatory steroids. *Clin. Pharmacol. Ther.,* **1961,** *2,* 615–635.

Loeb, J. N.   Corticosteroids and growth. *N. Engl. J. Med.,* **1976,** *295,* 547–552.

Mulrow, P. J., and Forman, B. H.   The tissue effects of mineralocorticoids. *Am. J. Med.,* **1972,** *53,* 561–572.

Reichstein, T., and Shoppee, C. W.   The hormones of the adrenal cortex. *Vitam. Horm.,* **1943,** *1,* 346–413.

Rheumatism Review Committee.   Rheumatism and arthritis. *Ann. Intern. Med.,* **1963,** *59,* 1–125.

Rose, L. I., and Saccar, C.   Choosing corticosteroid preparations. *Am. Fam. Physician,* **1978,** *17,* 198–204.

Tait, J. F., and Burstein, S.   *In vivo* studies of steroid dynamics in man. In, *The Hormones,* Vol. 5. (Pincus, G.; Thimann, K. V.; and Astwood, E. B.; eds.) Academic Press, Inc., New York, **1964,** pp. 441–557.

Temple, T. E., and Liddle, G. W.   Inhibitors of adrenal steroid biosynthesis. *Annu. Rev. Pharmacol. Toxicol.,* **1970,** *10,* 199–218.

CHAPTER

64 INSULIN AND ORAL HYPOGLYCEMIC DRUGS; GLUCAGON

Joseph Larner

INSULIN

History. Credit for the discovery of insulin is given to Banting and Best, who extracted the active principle from the pancreas and demonstrated its therapeutic effects in diabetic dogs and human subjects in the years 1921 and 1922 (*see* Best, 1963). However, many investigators had paved the way for the discovery, including E. L. Scott, who in 1911 had extracted an active principle from the pancreas with acid ethanol (*see* Magner, 1977). Paulesco (1921) also demonstrated the presence of a pancreatic material that was capable of producing hypoglycemia in animals. Probably of greatest earlier import was the demonstration by von Mering and Minkowski in 1889 that pancreatectomized dogs exhibit a syndrome similar to diabetes mellitus in man, with polyuria, polyphagia, wasting, ketosis, poor wound healing, and infection. They also demonstrated that deprivation of the exocrine function of the pancreas by ligation of the pancreatic duct did not cause diabetes, despite marked atrophy of the gland. The suggestion was made that diabetes occurred in the absence of a factor from the pancreas. Banting approached the problem with two working hypotheses: (1) the islet tissue secreted insulin, and (2) previous difficulties in isolating the active principle had been due in many instances to the proteolytic destruction of insulin by the digestive enzymes of the pancreas during the course of extraction. He devised elegantly simple approaches to circumvent the difficulty. He tied the pancreatic ducts so that the acinar tissue degenerated and left the islet tissue undisturbed, and from the remaining tissue extracted the active principle in relatively high concentration. He also used fetal pancreas as starting material, tissue with functional islets but lacking proteolytic digestive activity. Later on, normal pancreas was used as a commercial source when it was rediscovered that acid alcohol not only extracted insulin but also prevented proteolytic destruction.

The first patient to receive the active extracts prepared by Banting and Best was Leonard Thompson, aged 14 (Banting *et al.,* 1922). He appeared at the Toronto General Hospital with a blood glucose of 500 mg/dl, and he was excreting 3 to 5 liters of urine per day. Despite rigid control of diet (450 kcal per day), he continued to excrete large quantities of glucose, and, without insulin, the most likely course was death after a few months. Extracts were first administered on January 11, 1922, and they induced a reduction in the concentration and excretion of blood glucose. Daily injections were then begun, and

there was immediate improvement. The excretion of glucose was reduced from over 100 to as little as 7.5 g per day. Furthermore, ". . . the boy became brighter, looked better and said he felt stronger." Here was as dramatic an interruption of a fatal metabolic disorder as one will find in the annals of the history of medical science.

Immediately after the discovery of insulin there was justifiable excitement and then unfortunate relaxation, an attitude that the problems of treatment and of etiology of diabetes mellitus had been solved. True, the discovery of insulin was a momentous advance, but as time went by it became apparent that treatment was more than simply injection of insulin, that the etiology was more complex in many instances than mere destruction of islet tissue, and that the explanation of the action of the hormone was an exceedingly complex problem involving the elucidation of the intermediary metabolism not only of carbohydrate but also of protein and fat.

The chemistry of insulin has progressed from the preparation of active extracts to the preparation of insulin in crystalline form (Abel, 1926), to the establishment of the amino acid sequence of the polypeptide hormone (Sanger, 1960), and, eventually, to the complete synthesis of the molecule (Katsoyannis *et al.,* 1963; Meienhofer *et al.,* 1963) Of great practical importance in treatment has been the preparation of insulin in a variety of forms that exhibit a wide range in rate of absorption.

The studies on the etiology of diabetes mellitus took an interesting turn when Houssay (1936a, 1936b) reported that hypophysectomy ameliorated diabetes in the dog and that extracts of the anterior pituitary exacerbated the condition. Soon thereafter, Young (1937) induced permanent diabetes in dogs by prolonged administration of anterior pituitary extract. Long and Lukens (1936) provided convincing evidence that the adrenal cortex, as well as the adenohypophysis, exerts effects antagonistic to insulin. A new attitude developed. Diabetes could be caused not only by a deficiency of insulin but also by an excess of certain hormones, for example, growth hormone, glucocorticoids, and, more recently, glucagon. While hypersecretion of these hormones probably does not occur in the vast majority of diabetic patients, there may be exceptions. Both growth hormone and an adenohypophyseal "diabetogenic peptide" have been suggested to play etiological roles in the generation of at least certain forms of the disease (Louis *et al.,* 1966; Bornstein, 1978; Lostroh and Krahl, 1978; *see also* Chapter 59). Furthermore, the concentrations of glucagon in plasma are elevated in

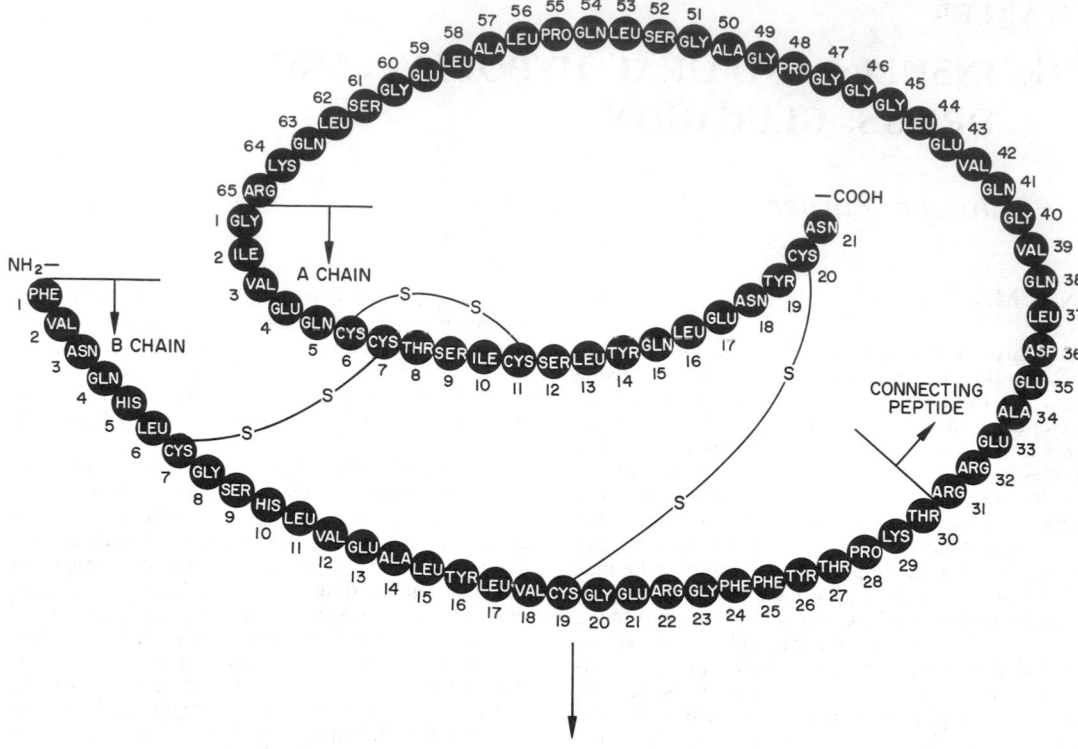

Figure 64-1. *Human proinsulin and its conversion to insulin.*

The amino acid sequence of human proinsulin is shown. By proteolytic cleavage, four basic amino acids (31, 32, 64, 65) and the connecting peptide are removed and proinsulin is converted to insulin. (For details, *see* the text.)

many patients with diabetes (Unger and Orci, 1976). The search for the etiology of diabetes mellitus has recently turned from strictly endocrine to immunological, infectious, and genetic factors (*see* below).

Chemistry and Biosynthesis. Insulin, with a molecular weight of about 6000, is made up of two chains of amino acids joined together by disulfide linkages (*see* Figure 64-1). The sequence of amino acids in the two chains (termed A for acidic and B for basic) and the arrangement of the three disulfide bridges were worked out in a brilliant series of investigations by Sanger and associates in the period 1945-1955 (*see* Sanger, 1960). The efforts of the chemists culminated in the complete synthesis of both ovine and human insulin (Katsoyannis *et al.*, 1963; Meienhofer *et al.*, 1963).

While it had been assumed that the A and B chains were synthesized separately and then joined together in the β cells of the pancreatic islets, Steiner and colleagues and Chance and associates (*see* Steiner, 1977) demonstrated that the β cells form insulin from a single-chain precursor termed *proinsulin* (Figure 64-1). On conversion of human proinsulin to insulin, four basic amino acids (arginine 31, arginine 32, lysine 64, and arginine 65) and the remaining connector or C-peptide (residues 33

through 63) are removed. The resultant insulin molecule has two chains, the A chain with glycine at the amino-terminal residue and the B chain with phenylalanine at the amino terminus. In many commercial preparations of insulin it is possible to detect small amounts of proinsulin and other related molecules resulting from incomplete conversion of the prohormone.

An even larger molecule termed *preproinsulin* has now been identified as a precursor of proinsulin. Preproinsulin is extended at the N terminus of the B chain by at least 23 amino acids, many of which are hydrophobic (Chan *et al.*, 1976). It is cleaved to proinsulin in the endoplasmic reticulum, where it is synthesized, and is therefore not a product that accumulates in the β cell.

Hodgkin and associates (*see* Hodgkin and Mercola, 1972) have determined the three-dimensional structure of insulin by x-ray analysis of single crystals. Insulin can exist as a monomer, a dimer, or a hexamer composed of three such dimers. Two molecules of Zn^{2+} are coordinated in the hexamer, which is presumably the form stored in the granules of the β cell. The biologically active form of the hormone is thought to be the monomer. X-ray analysis has also shown that the two chains are compactly arranged, with the A chain positioned above the central helical portion of the B chain. From each end of this helical region the terminal portions of the B chain extend as arms, and the A chain is enclosed between them.

Many species variations are known, and some are of clinical significance. For example, the major sites of chemical difference among porcine, ovine, equine, and cetacean insulins are in positions 8, 9, and 10 of the A chain. The porcine hormone is most similar to that of man and differs only by the substitution of an alanine residue at the carboxy terminus of the B chain (Steiner *et al.*, 1972). By the use of porcine insulin as the starting material, human insulin can now be synthesized with relative ease (Ruttenberg, 1972). Production of human insulin by cloning of chemically synthesized DNA in bacteria has also now been reported (Goeddel *et al.*, 1979). It seems likely that this exciting new technology will allow the production of human insulin on a commercial scale.

The specific activities of various mammalian insulins are very similar (22 to 27 units/mg). Proinsulin has only slight biological activity, while the separated A and B chains are essentially inactive.

The Assay of Insulin in Plasma. In addition to the older *in-vivo* bioassays, which depend on the lowering of blood glucose in rabbits or the production of convulsions in mice (*see* Humbel *et al.*, 1972), several *in-vitro* methods have attained popularity because of their high degree of sensitivity and their relative simplicity of execution. One method is based on the capacity of insulin to increase the glycogen content or the glucose uptake of the rat diaphragm. Adipose tissue assays are based on the capacity of insulin to stimulate glucose metabolism by the epididymal fat pad of the rat or by suspensions of isolated fat cells. Measured end points are CO_2 production from glucose, incorporation of the ^{14}C of labeled glucose into fat, or glucose uptake from the medium.

The radioimmunoassay of insulin in human plasma is based on the capacity of human insulin to compete with porcine or bovine insulin (labeled with ^{131}I or ^{125}I) for binding sites on an antibody derived from the serum of guinea pigs that have been injected with porcine or bovine insulin. This type of method, originally described by Yalow and Berson (1960), has now been applied to many hormones and other molecules. The sensitivity of the radioimmunoassay for insulin is an order of magnitude greater than the *in-vitro* bioassays and two or more orders of magnitude greater than the *in-vivo* bioassays.

Types of Plasma Insulin. Plasma insulin estimated by bioassay is called *insulin-like activity* (ILA), and plasma insulin estimated by immunoassay is called *immunoreactive insulin* (IRI). IRI and ILA differ both quantitatively and qualitatively. The concentration of plasma IRI of normal persons after an overnight fast is under 20 microunits/ml.

When insulin antibody is added to plasma, a decrease in ILA is observed (suppressible ILA); however, a considerable portion (sometimes over 90%) of the ILA may persist, and this is termed nonsuppressible ILA or NSILA. The amount of suppressible ILA corresponds to the amount of IRI (Oelz *et al.*, 1972). Thus, estimates of plasma ILA are invariably higher than are those of IRI. NSILA has been intensively studied. Although it is not increased in plasma after the administration of glucose and persists in plasma after pancreatectomy, there is evidence that growth hormone, insulin, thyroxine, and nutritional status regulate its concentration (*see* Chochinov and Daughaday, 1976). It behaves like insulin metabolically and, also like insulin, promotes the growth of cells in culture (*see* Schoenle *et al.*, 1977). It consists of at least two components: NSILA-S (soluble in acid ethanol, molecular weight 5000) (Rinderknecht and Humbel, 1976) and NSILA-P (precipitated in acid ethanol, molecular weight 85,000) (Leichter and Poffenbarger, 1978). NSILA-S is itself composed of two peptides, is structurally related to the B chain of insulin, and may be related to somatomedin (*see* Chapter 59; Rinderknecht and Humbel, 1976).

Secretion of Insulin: Morphological and Chemical Events. The islet is composed of four recognizable cell types, and each synthesizes a distinct polypeptide: insulin in the β cell, glucagon in the α cell, somatostatin in the D cell, and pancreatic polypeptide in the D_1 or F cell. Each cell type has a characteristic distribution within the islet (Orci, 1976; Orci *et al.*, 1976), and specialized connections between the cells have been described. Thus, with the neural and vascular elements, the islets of Langerhans appear to represent complex functional entities. Of interest are changes in islet morphology that accompany experimental or pathological hypoinsulinemic and hyperinsulinemic states. Alterations in apparent numbers of cells are seen in D and D_1 cells in addition to β cells (*see* Unger and Orci, 1977a; Gepts and DeMey, 1978).

Preproinsulin is synthesized in the membrane-associated polyribosomes of the rough endoplasmic reticulum of the β cells and is converted at this site to proinsulin. Proinsulin is first transferred to the cisternae of the reticulum and then via transitional elements (vesicles) to the Golgi complex, where it is concentrated within immature granules. Here the conversion of proinsulin to insulin begins. Eventually proinsulin- and insulin-containing storage granules bud off from the Golgi apparatus, and the enzymatic conversion of proinsulin to insulin plus C-peptide is completed. The granules may be either stored, destroyed (by lysosomes), or released by emiocytosis (exocytosis). (*See* Ostlund, 1977; Steiner, 1977.)

Regulation of Insulin Secretion. Gastrointestinal Mechanisms. Insulin release appears to be controlled by the coordinated interplay of the availability of food products, gastrointestinal hormones, and other hormonal and neural stimuli. In the last-named category, both the autonomic nervous system and the central nervous system (CNS) are of major importance.

In keeping with insulin's role to promote the storage of all fuels, it is not surprising that, in addition to glucose, amino acids, fatty acids of all chain lengths, and ketone bodies will call forth its secretion. In man, glucose is most probably the principal stimulus. But in other animals, depending on diet, amino acids or fatty acids may be of primary importance.

It has been known for over 70 years that glucose is more effective in provoking glycosuria when injected intravenously than when administered orally. However, it was recognized only relatively recently that this difference is due to a greater capacity of oral glucose to evoke the secretion of insulin (McIntyre et al., 1964); the same may also be true for other nutrients (Renold et al., 1978). This strongly suggests the presence of an anticipatory signal from the gastrointestinal tract to the pancreas. Several of the gastrointestinal hormones, including secretin, pancreozymin-cholecystokinin, gastrin, and gastrointestinal or "gut" glucagon, have now been shown to stimulate insulin secretion *in vitro* and *in vivo* (Renold et al., 1978). More recently a new polypeptide (43 amino acid residues) termed GIP (gastric inhibitory polypeptide) has been purified and its amino acid sequence determined. It is structurally homologous with glucagon and secretin and may be an extremely important β-cell stimulant whose secretion is sensitive to glucose, fat, and amino acids (Brown and Otte, 1978). Pancreozymin-cholecystokinin may also play a similar role as a protein- and amino acid–sensitive signal (*see* Unger and Lefebvre, 1972; Buchanan, 1973). It is thus believed that the upper gastrointestinal tract and the pancreas form an enteropancreatic axis responsible not only for digestion and absorption of foods but also for their effective and controlled utilization. (For a review of this rapidly developing field, *see* Bloom and Grossman, 1978; Hedeskov, 1980.)

Autonomic Mechanisms. The predominant effect of norepinephrine or epinephrine is to inhibit insulin secretion, a response mediated by α-adrenergic receptors. In addition, *selective* activation of β₂-adrenergic receptors results in stimulation of the secretion of insulin. Exercise and pathological states associated with activation of the autonomic nervous system, including hypoxia, hypothermia, surgery, and severe burns, all lead to a suppression of insulin secretion via the α-receptor mechanism (Smith et al., 1979). Cholinomimetic drugs and vagal-nerve stimulation enhance insulin release (*see* Smith et al., 1979).

The adrenergic and cholinergic systems, which richly innervate the islets, may control the basal rate of secretion of insulin as well as the reaction to stress. Thus, α-receptor blockade raises and muscarinic or β-receptor blockade lowers the basal concentration of insulin in plasma.

Control by Other Hormones. It is now recognized that the secretory activity of the pancreatic β cell is affected by a wide variety of hormones. An unexpected finding was the demonstration that glucagon stimulates insulin release (*see* Marks and Samols, 1970). In addition, a variety of hormones (including thyroxine, growth hormone, and glucocorticoids) and autacoids can either stimulate or inhibit insulin release and modify the secretory response of the β cell to nutrients and drugs (Kipnis, 1971). While certain prostaglandins can enhance secretion of insulin *in vitro* (Johnson et al., 1973), the infusion of PGE₁ *in vivo* inhibits the release of the hormone (Robertson and Chen, 1977). Somatostatin, a tetradecapeptide of hypothalamic and other origins, inhibits the secretion of insulin and glucagon in addition to that of growth hormone. Its potential usefulness as an adjunct to insulin in the treatment of diabetes is also of considerable interest (*see* Chapter 59; Gerich, 1977).

Biochemical Mechanisms and Kinetics. In man, glucose is the only nutrient that stimulates both insulin *secretion* and *biosynthesis* at physiological concentrations, and this action has been studied extensively. While carbohydrate utilization is an important feature of the glucose-induced release of insulin, evidence indicates that it is the hexose molecule itself that is the secretagogue. Thus, α-D-glucose is a more potent secretagogue than the β-D isomer, which differs only in the configuration of the hydroxyl on C 1 (Rossini et al., 1974). While concentrations of glycolytic intermediates measured in islets after exposure to glucose do not change in a manner sufficient to explain secretion, there are significant changes in glycolytic flux that can be related to secretion. In general, there is a correlation between the capacity of sugars to undergo glycolysis and their ability to stimulate insulin release. Furthermore, inhibition of glycolysis also inhibits secretion of insulin (Zawalich and Matschinsky, 1977). Glucose thus appears to serve several roles; it is hypothesized to act as a secretagogue by means of interaction with a glucoreceptor on the cell membrane, and it serves, of course, as an energy source and possibly as the source of another signal within the β cell. Other potential signals that have been suggested include adenosine triphosphate (ATP), glucose-6-phosphate, NADH or NADPH, and phosphoenolpyruvate (Sugden and Ashcroft, 1977).

The fact that β-adrenergic agonists and glucagon stimulate insulin secretion suggests that cyclic adenosine 3',5'-monophosphate (cyclic AMP) has a role in mediating the response. Glucagon and glucose can also increase the concentration of cyclic AMP in islets (Goldfine et al., 1972; Charles et al., 1973). The exact role of cyclic AMP is not clear, but it may be related to the requirement for Ca^{2+}. Insulinotropic agents act only in the presence of extracellular Ca^{2+}, facilitating its influx and decreasing its efflux. Cyclic AMP and Ca^{2+} may activate the microtubule-microfilament system that is hypothetically involved in the migration and emiocytosis of the insulin-containing granules (see Devis et al., 1977).

Of great importance has been the discovery of the biphasic kinetics of the glucose-induced insulin release from the β cell. Both in vitro and in vivo, there occurs an initial burst of secretion that reaches a peak in minutes and rapidly declines, followed by a second, longer-lasting peak that may duplicate the initial peak value after an hour or longer. The concept of two pools of stored insulin, one more rapidly released than the other, has emerged. The rapidly secreted insulin may be a more important determinant of the rate at which glucose is utilized in the body, and selective hypersecretion or impairment of the early phase of secretion is noted in many "prediabetic" and diabetic patients (see below). Secretion of insulin during the second phase may depend in part on protein synthesis, the availability of Ca^{2+} within the cell, or the assembly of microtubules (Sando and Grodsky, 1973; Malaisse et al., 1974; Naber et al., 1977). A kinetic model that involves feedback control by insulin itself has also been proposed to explain the biphasic pattern of secretion.

Effects of Alloxan, Streptozotocin, and Other Toxins. Agents that rather selectively destroy the β cells induce hypoinsulinemic diabetes mellitus. These compounds include alloxan, uric acid, dialuric acid, dehydroascorbic acid, dehydroisoascorbic acid, some quinolones, streptozotocin, and magnesium. Of these, alloxan (mesoxalylurea) attained great importance in research because its administration is a convenient means for the production of insulin-deficiency diabetes in otherwise-normal experimental animals. Mechanistic studies suggest that alloxan and α-D-glucose are structurally similar and therefore may interact with a common receptor on the β cell (Weaver et al., 1978). Unfortunately, alloxan has not been of value in the treatment of insulin-secreting tumors of the pancreas. When streptozotocin, the N-nitroso derivative of glucosamine produced by *Streptomyces achromogenes,* is injected into rats, degeneration of pancreatic β cells follows. In recent years streptozotocin has replaced alloxan as the preferred agent to produce a diabetic state in

experimental animals (see Rerup, 1970), and it is useful clinically to treat insulin-secreting tumors (see Chapter 55).

Distribution, Excretion, and Fate. While a fraction of the endogenous or exogenous insulin in plasma may be associated with certain proteins, there is doubt that these associations are of importance for the transport of insulin, the bulk of which appears to circulate in blood and lymph as the free hormone. The volume of distribution of insulin approximates the volume of extracellular fluid. Under fasting conditions, the pancreas secretes 20 μg of insulin per hour into the portal vein; the concentration of insulin in portal blood is 2 to 4 ng/ml (50 to 100 microunits/ml) and that in the peripheral circulation is 500 pg/ml (12 microunits/ml).

The plasma half-life of insulin injected intravenously is less than 9 minutes in man, and there is no detectable difference between normal and diabetic subjects. The main sites of destruction are the liver and kidney, and about 50% of the insulin that reaches the liver via the portal vein is destroyed in a single passage, never reaching the general circulation. Insulin is filtered by the renal glomeruli and is reabsorbed by the tubules, which also degrade it. Severe impairment of renal function appears to affect the rate of disappearance of circulating insulin to a greater extent than does hepatic disease, since the liver operates closer to its capacity to destroy the hormone and cannot compensate for such loss of renal catabolic function. Although peripheral tissues such as muscle and fat bind and inactivate insulin, this is of minor quantitative significance.

In-vitro experiments suggest that two systems are involved in the degradation of insulin by the liver: (1) a proteolytic enzyme(s) that cleaves the intact molecule or the reduced chains to peptides and amino acids; and (2) an enzyme termed glutathione-insulin transhydrogenase, which utilizes reduced glutathione to reduce the disulfide bridges of insulin and produce separate chains. A highly purified glutathione-insulin transhydrogenase enzyme without proteolytic activity has been isolated from liver by Varandani and Nafz (1976). Presumably because of the reductive separation of the two chains of insulin, free A chains have been demonstrated in the plasma and urine of normal individuals and diabetic patients (Varandani, 1970).

A proteolytic enzyme that degrades insulin, glucagon, and secretin has been extensively purified from rat skeletal muscle (Duckworth and Kitabchi, 1974).

This enzyme is interesting, because its K_m for insulin is within the physiological range of hormone concentrations. The initial site of cleavage of intact insulin is between residues 16 and 17 of the B chain (Duckworth *et al.*, 1979).

Insulin seems to be internalized by hepatic and other cells (Schlessinger *et al.*, 1978) and appears finally in lysosomes, where it is destroyed. Other evidence suggests that there may be specific destruction of insulin at the cell membrane related to hormone binding and action at receptors (Terris and Steiner, 1975).

Insulin and Diabetes Mellitus. Progress has been made in the classification of diabetes mellitus into separate categories. While several schemes have been proposed, only one is described herein: (1) insulin-dependent (previously termed juvenile-onset) diabetes mellitus; (2) insulin-independent (previously termed maturity-onset) diabetes mellitus; (3) maturity-onset or insulin-independent diabetes in the young—a rare dominantly inherited, mild type of disease; (4) diabetes mellitus or carbohydrate intolerance associated with certain genetic syndromes; (5) secondary diabetes mellitus (drug-induced, pancreatic disease, hormonal, receptor abnormalities, etc.); and (6) gestational diabetes mellitus. The first two forms of the disease account for the great majority of patients.

Insulin-dependent and insulin-independent forms of diabetes mellitus have been recognized clinically for years. Both types of disease have genetic components, particularly the latter, and studies of identical twins have indicated a very high degree of concordance for insulin-independent diabetes (*see* Pyke, 1977). There is also a high prevalence of such disease among the offspring of diabetic couples and among first-degree relatives. The genetic mechanism is not completely understood because insulin-independent diabetes probably consists of a group of related diseases and can occur with or without obesity (note type 3 above). Studies of identical twins reveal a lower degree of concordance for insulin-dependent diabetes, suggesting environmental as well as genetic influences. Autoimmune and viral etiologies have been proposed. Antibodies to components of islet cells can be detected in a high proportion of cases if patients are examined early in the onset of the disease, in contrast to insulin-independent disease where they are rarely found. Patients who have antibodies to islet cells tend to have immunoglobulins that react with preparations of adrenal, parathyroid, and thyroid gland as well. There is an association of insulin-dependent diabetes with specific histocompatibility leukocyte antigens (HLA), especially at the B locus (B8 and B15) and at the D locus

(Dw3 and Dw4) on human chromosome 6; this presumably indicates that humoral and cell-mediated immune mechanisms are involved in the etiology of the disease. Direct evidence for a viral etiology in animals (Yoon *et al.*, 1976) and suggestive evidence in man (MacLaren, 1977; Yoon *et al.*, 1979) have also been obtained. Whatever the cause or causes, the final result in insulin-dependent diabetes is a hypoinsulinemic state with an extensive loss of β cells of the islets; there is no such loss of cells in insulin-independent disease.

Numerous studies have demonstrated the absence of insulin in the circulation and in the pancreas in insulin-dependent diabetics (*see* Rastogi *et al.*, 1973). An independent estimate of β-cell function has been devised, based on plasma concentrations of the connector or C-peptide. Its absence from the plasma of patients with insulin-dependent diabetes again indicates failure of β-cell function (Rubenstein *et al.*, 1977). This form of the disease usually begins with marked hyperglycemia or an episode of ketoacidosis associated with extremely low concentrations of immunoreactive insulin and C-peptide in the plasma. A period of clinical remission usually follows, accompanied by improvement in carbohydrate tolerance and a reduction in the requirement for insulin administration. During this time β-cell function returns, as evidenced by restoration of plasma immunoreactive insulin and C-peptide. However, in the fully established disease that follows, the function of the β cell appears to be lost totally.

Individuals with insulin-independent diabetes have functional β cells, as evidenced by the presence of both immunoreactive insulin and C-peptide in plasma. However, there are abnormalities in the initial secretion of insulin when stimulated by glucose, even in the mildest forms of the disease; these may consist in either increased or decreased secretion. Impaired β-cell function is also revealed by the fact that less insulin is secreted at any given glucose concentration in both diabetic subjects and those with latent disease. The defect may be in the glucoreceptor of the β-cell membrane (*see* Robertson and Porte, 1973; Cerasi, 1975). However, there is not complete agreement on this point; Reaven and coworkers (1972), for example, described increased concentrations of insulin in plasma associated with resistance to insulin in patients in early stages of this form of diabetes (*see also* Olefsky, 1976).

The secretory function of α cells of pancreatic islets is also compromised in diabetes mellitus. Concentrations of immunoreactive glucagon in plasma are elevated in diabetic patients, particularly during ketoacidosis, and the normal suppression of plasma glucagon by hyperglycemia is impaired. Instead, glucagon concentrations may rise paradoxically following an oral glucose load. In addition, the α cells respond excessively to arginine or to a protein meal (Unger and Orci, 1977b). Glucagon concentrations are lowered in most diabetic subjects when insulin is administered in higher doses (Raskin and Unger, 1978).

A vitally important and pathognomonic feature of diabetes mellitus is the capillary basement-membrane thickening that occurs early in the course of the disease. This pathological change may be responsible for the major vascular complications of diabetes, including premature atherosclerosis, intercapillary glomerulosclerosis, retinopathy, neuropathy, and ulceration and gangrene of the extremities. While considerable progress is being made in the chemical characterization of basement membranes from normal and diabetic subjects (Miller, 1978), it is not known whether the lesion is a consequence of insulin deficiency or if it is more primary and perhaps of etiological significance. An early sign of abnormal vascular permeability is the appearance of detectable protein in the urine (*see* Cahill, 1978).

Of considerable interest is the fact that glucose or phosphorylated glucose is able to react covalently with the amino-terminal valine residue of hemoglobin to form a glucosylated protein; the major species that can be quantitated is termed hemoglobin A_1C. Since the rate of formation of hemoglobin A_1C is proportional to the concentration of glucose in blood and the half-life of the derivatized protein is long, its measurement is considered to provide an *integrated index* of the glycemic state and thus an estimate of the long-term effectiveness of the control of the blood glucose concentration. It has been suggested that the nerve lesions and cataracts that are characteristic of diabetes may be caused by the covalent reaction of glucose with endogenous proteins in nerve and crystalline lens, in a manner analogous to the reaction of the hexose with hemoglobin (Peterson and Jones, 1977). It has also been hypothesized that the accumulation of sorbitol and resultant osmotic swelling are significant in the etiology of these lesions.

It is well established that insulin receptors are altered in diabetes. In general, the number of receptors for the hormone seems to be inversely related to the plasma insulin concentration, perhaps because insulin itself may be able to "down-regulate" the number of its own receptors. In obesity and in insulin-independent diabetes there appears to be a decrease in the number of receptors associated with the hyperinsulinemia. In some rare cases (termed type B) of insulin-resistant diabetes associated with *acanthosis nigricans,* antibodies to the receptors are found, while in other cases (termed type A) the cause of the resistance is thought to be distal to the receptor and in the metabolic machinery of the cell (*see* Bar and Roth, 1977).

Insulin Deficiency: How Insulin Corrects the Metabolic Aberrations of the Diabetic State.

Diabetes mellitus due to inadequate insulin secretion by the β cells of the pancreas is characterized by hyperglycemia, hyperlipemia, ketonemia, and azoturia. When deficiency is severe, there may be *diabetic ketoacidosis.* The purpose of the following discussion is to explain these metabolic aberrations in terms of the effects of insulin and glucagon on various tissues and organs. The steps described refer to Figure 64–2.

Hyperglycemia. The hyperglycemia of insulin deficiency and glucagon excess is a consequence of underutilization and overproduction of glucose.

In the absence of insulin there is a marked reduction in the rate of transport of glucose across certain cell membranes. Lundsgaard (1939) first suggested that insulin acted to enhance glucose transport, and Levine and associates (1949) demonstrated that insulin increased the volume of distribution of galactose (which is not metabolized) in the nephrectomized, eviscerated dog. They reasoned that the hormone accelerates transport of certain hexoses, including glucose, across cell membranes (steps Muscle-①[M-①] and Adipocyte-① [A-①], Figure 64–2); the exclusion of glucose from the intracellular compartment by a relatively "impermeable" plasma membrane explained the underutilization of glucose in the diabetic state. However, it could also be explained as an effect on the rate of glucose phosphorylation, the obligatory first step in metabolism. That insulin acts to increase transport of glucose independent of rate of phosphorylation was demonstrated in the isolated rat diaphragm preparation by Park and associates (1955). Normally the concentration of glucose is virtually zero within skeletal muscle cells in the presence or the absence of insulin. Once glucose enters the cell, it is quickly phosphorylated to glucose-6-phosphate (steps Liver-② [L-②], M-②, and A-②, Figure 64–2). Park and coworkers showed that at low temperatures, even though the conversion of glucose to glucose-6-phosphate was slowed, insulin

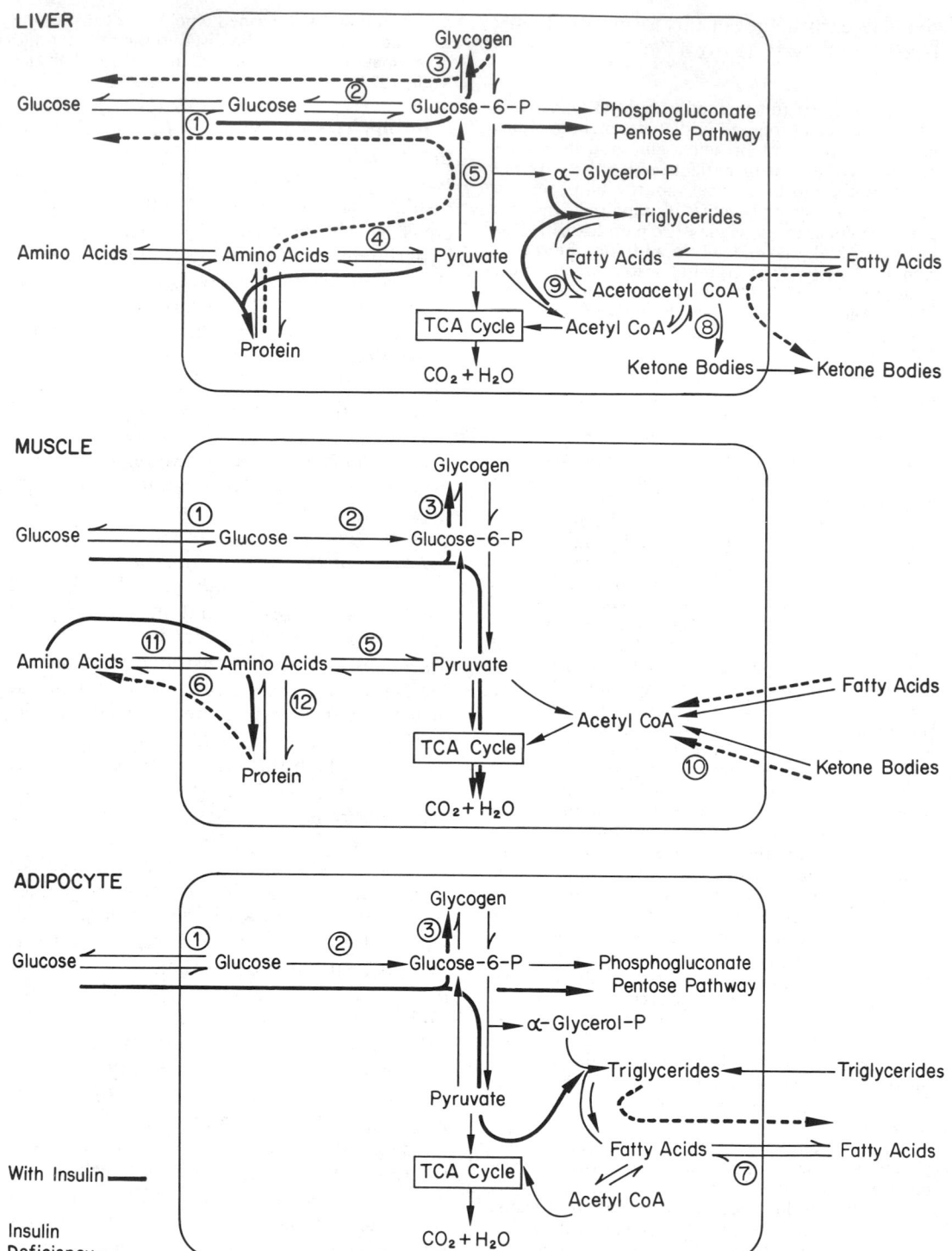

Figure 64-2. *Major metabolic effects of insulin deficiency.*

Thick solid arrows (──►) show the pathways that are favored in the presence of insulin, while thick broken arrows (┅┅►) depict those that predominate when the action of the hormone is insufficient. (For explanation, *see* the text.)

clearly increased the transfer of glucose from the medium into the cells. Likewise, it can be shown that insulin accelerates the transfer of glucose into the fat cell, wherein it is transformed to fat or glycogen or oxidized to CO_2.

Obviously, underutilization of glucose is to an important degree the consequence of a reduced rate of entrance of the sugar into cells. Because of this inability to gain entrance to the metabolic machinery, the oxidation of glucose to CO_2 and its conversion to glycogen and fat are slowed. It is of practical importance to note that exercise increases the rate of transport of glucose into muscle cells, even in the absence of insulin. Vigorous exercise will induce hypoglycemia in the diabetic subject, and the dose and site of insulin injection must be adjusted accordingly. This response may be due to the release of bound insulin from the injection site or from within the muscle itself or its vasculature (Dieterle et al., 1973; Koivisto and Felig, 1978).

Insulin does not influence the rate of transfer of glucose across all cell membranes. In insulin deficiency, transport of glucose into the hepatic cell (step L-①) is not significantly reduced; this is not a factor of importance in the development of the metabolic aberrations of the hepatic cell. In diabetes, rate of entry of glucose into the brain is unaffected and function of the nervous system remains normal unless a state of ketoacidosis develops. However, certain nuclei in the hypothalamus may be sensitive to insulin (Szabo and Szabo, 1975) and the brain may contain the hormone as well (Havrankova et al., 1978). Erythrocytes, leukocytes, and cells of the renal medulla take up glucose at a rate designed to meet their needs quite independently of insulin. As expected, the rate of glucose oxidation is reduced but by no means to zero in insulin deficiency. This point is illustrated by experiments in which the conversion of labeled glucose to CO_2 is compared in normal and diabetic subjects. A significant reduction characterizes diabetes, but in quantitative terms the reduction may not be dramatic.

In the absence of insulin there is a marked reduction in the activity of the enzyme system that catalyzes the conversion of glucose to glycogen. Insulin added to isolated rat diaphragm or injected into the dog increases the activity of the enzyme (glycogen synthase) that is involved in the conversion of glucose to glycogen in skeletal muscle (step M-③), in liver (step L-③), and in the adipocyte (step A-③) (*see* Lawrence and Larner, 1978).

In the absence of insulin there is an abnormally high rate of conversion of protein to glucose. In insulin deficiency the quantity of glucose excreted in the urine can far exceed the quantity ingested. One can immediately dismiss fat as a source of the excess glucose, since *net* production of glucose from fat cannot occur. However, proteins and amino acids are converted to glucose at an abnormally high rate when there is a deficiency of insulin and an excess of glucagon. The liver is the site of such conversion (steps L-④ and L-⑤). Protein and amino acids are mobilized from peripheral tissues (*see* the section on azoturia, below). For example, in muscle the branched-chain amino acids are oxidized to pyruvate, which is transaminated to alanine. This amino acid is released into the blood and is converted in the liver back to pyruvate and to glucose. In addition to alanine, large amounts of glutamine are also released by muscle into the blood. In Figure 64–2, a net loss of amino acid is shown for muscle (step M-⑥); the amino acids so mobilized in insulin deficiency are converted in the liver to glucose (steps L-④ and L-⑤) and to urea.

Hyperlipemia, Ketonemia, and Acidosis. The abnormally high concentration of free fatty acids in the plasma of the diabetic subject is due, in large measure, to their increased mobilization from the peripheral fat depots (step A-⑦). Insulin inhibits the hormone-sensitive lipase concerned with the mobilization of fatty acids, while glucagon, growth hormone, glucocorticoids, thyroid hormones, and catecholamines enhance lipolysis. The marked hyperlipemia that characterizes the diabetic state may be regarded as a consequence of the uninhibited actions of the above hormones on the fat depots. The antilipolytic and the antigluconeogenic effects of insulin are among the most sensitive actions of the hormone.

The source of the ketone bodies in the diabetic subject or the fasting normal subject is the liver (step L-⑧). In the absence of insulin, lipolysis, facilitated by various counterregulatory hormones, proceeds unchecked. The liver takes up large quantities of the free fatty acids thus liberated and oxidizes them to acetyl coenzyme A (CoA) (step L-⑨). The reduced capacity of the insulin-deficient liver to synthesize fatty acids from acetyl CoA results in the increased diversion of this substrate to ketone bodies (acetone, acetoacetate, and β-hydroxybutyrate; step L-⑧), which appear in the blood in large quantities. Glucagon and perhaps other counterregulatory hormones appear to be necessary for ketone body formation in liver. Some of the ketone bodies are utilized as a source of energy by skeletal muscle, cardiac muscle, and other tissues (step M-⑩).

The production of large amounts of acetoacetate and β-hydroxybutyrate, which are relatively strong acids, causes the acidosis of severe insulin deficiency. Urinary excretion of these anions is in part responsible for the loss of fixed cation and contributes to the depletion of electrolytes characteristic of diabetic ketoacidosis; the loss of potassium may be particularly severe and averages 5 mEq/kg of body weight in patients with ketoacidosis. Concentrations of potassium in plasma are not usually depressed, however, since intracellular potassium is exchanged for extracellular protons to compensate for the acidosis. Cations are also excreted in combination with phosphate and sulfate, which are lost in the urine in excessive quantities, and as a result of osmotic diuresis due to hyperglycemia.

Azoturia. Insulin deficiency and glucagon excess result in conversion of large amounts of protein to glucose with consequent increased production and excretion of urea and ammonia. Increased excretion of ammonia is a renal homeostatic mechanism stimulated by ketoacidosis. In the absence of insulin there is reduced movement of amino acids into muscle and possibly other cells (step M-⑪) and reduced incorporation of amino acids into protein (step M-⑫). Both effects are independent of glucose transport since they can be demonstrated *in vitro* in the absence of glucose in the medium. In insulin deficiency, amino acids do enter the hepatic cell, where they are deaminated and oxidized to yield pyruvate and contribute importantly to the hepatic overproduction of glucose. Hepatic gluconeogenesis from pyruvate and lactate is markedly accelerated by insulin deficiency. Furthermore, the protein catabolic actions of glucagon, adrenocortico-

steroids, and thyroid hormones are unopposed in insulin deficiency, thus tilting the protein anabolic-catabolic balance toward catabolism.

Mechanism of Insulin Action. While certain aspects of the action of insulin are rather well understood, much remains to be done to understand the mechanisms in molecular terms. In general, the actions of the hormone are to stimulate transport of metabolites and ions through cell membranes, biosynthesis of various molecules and macromolecules, and cell growth; this has been termed the pleiotypic response (Hershko *et al.,* 1971). Principally through the work of Cuatrecasas (1973) and of Kono (1969), the putative receptor for insulin from the cell membrane has been characterized as an insulin-binding protein and purified partially (*see* Jacobs *et al.,* 1977). The interaction of the hormone with the receptor is highly specific, and the kinetics of the process has been defined. This binding reaction is clearly different from any that results in degradation of insulin. Further evidence that the initial action of the hormone is at the cell surface is the fact that the action of insulin is competitively inhibited by a large "diabetogenic peptide" (Miller and Larner, 1972), and the demonstration that human antireceptor antibody both blocks insulin binding to the receptor and exhibits striking insulin-like effects, even on intracellular enzyme systems (Lawrence *et al.,* 1978).

The relationship of insulin action to cyclic nucleotide metabolism is of great interest but is still not clear. Decreased intracellular concentrations of cyclic AMP (or, perhaps, increased concentrations of cyclic GMP) could explain some of the metabolic effects of insulin. While insulin can cause a lowering of the cyclic AMP concentration in some tissues, this has been observed convincingly only when cyclic AMP synthesis is first stimulated by counterregulatory hormones (Jefferson *et al.,* 1968). Basal concentrations of the cyclic nucleotide are not demonstrably depressed when insulin acts alone (Larner *et al.,* 1979). This has been the main argument against a direct relationship between the action of insulin and cyclic AMP. Effects of insulin on the enzymes that catalyze the synthesis and destruction of cyclic AMP have been investigated. Inhibition of adenylate cyclase (Hepp, 1977) and stimulation of cyclic nucleotide phosphodiesterase (Solomon *et al.,* 1977) have been observed. While the biochemical mechanisms and the physiological significance of these observations are unclear, they may explain the ability of insulin to depress elevated cyclic AMP concentrations (Hepp, 1977).

As described in Chapter 4 (*see* Figure 4–7, page 79), glycogen synthesis and glycogenolysis are controlled by a cascading series of protein phosphorylation reactions. In the presence of cyclic AMP, a protein kinase is activated, and the eventual result is a stimulation of glycogen breakdown and an inhibition of glycogen synthesis. Insulin acts to tip the balance in the other direction—toward glycogen synthesis. The hormone appears to reduce the sensitivity of the protein kinase to cyclic AMP, in effect inhibiting the action of the cyclic nucleotide without the need to lower its concentration (Larner et al., 1979). Glycogen synthase is activated, since a phosphoprotein phosphatase is less opposed and acts to dephosphorylate the enzyme (conversion of the D to the I form); indeed, the phosphatase may also be activated under certain conditions. By analogous mechanisms, the action of insulin results in dephosphorylation of phosphorylase and of a triglyceride lipase (Huttunen et al., 1970; Steinberg et al., 1975); the metabolic sequelae are inhibition of glycogenolysis and lipolysis, respectively.

Pyruvate dehydrogenase, an important mitochondrial enzyme, is also controlled by insulin (and other hormones) by phosphorylation and dephosphorylation reactions (see review by Randle, 1976). The active form of the enzyme is the dephosphorylated one, and it is increased after insulin treatment by an unknown mechanism. As a result, pyruvate is oxidized or converted to fat and is unavailable for glucose formation. A similar control of acetyl CoA carboxylase by phosphorylation and dephosphorylation has been demonstrated (Hardie and Cohen, 1978).

In addition to the enhanced synthesis of fat, insulin increases the activity of membrane-bound lipoprotein lipase, which makes fatty acids derived from circulating lipoproteins available to the cell (Hollenberg, 1962).

In protein metabolism, insulin promotes amino acid uptake, enhances protein synthesis, and inhibits protein degradation (see Manchester, 1972; Morgan et al.,1972). In general, the effects on protein synthesis have been localized to translational events, including polyribosome formation (Wool et al., 1972; Evans et al., 1974) and peptide chain initiation (Morgan et al., 1971). However, there may also be a control at the transcriptional level, since albumin mRNA is increased in liver following the administration of insulin (Peavy et al., 1978). Stabilization of lysosomes has been suggested as a mechanism to explain the ability of insulin to inhibit proteolysis (Mortimore and Mondon, 1970).

The mechanisms of the important actions of insulin to enhance the facilitated diffusion of glucose and the active transport of amino acids are not known. Membrane vesicles that are altered in a stable manner to transport glucose at an enhanced rate can be prepared from fat cells treated with insulin. Advances have been made in the reconstitution of the glucose transport system in artificial lipid vesicles. Such systems should allow elucidation of mechanisms of control in molecular terms (see Shanahan and Czech, 1977). It is possible that alterations of the state of phosphorylation of membrane proteins following exposure to insulin may be relevant to its effects on transport (Benjamin and Singer, 1975; Avruch et al., 1978).

The action of insulin to promote K^+ uptake into cells, even in the absence of glucose, is classical; a similar effect on Mg^{2+} accumulation has also been demonstrated (Aikawa, 1960). Since K^+ and Mg^{2+} are important in metabolism, for example, in protein biosynthesis, it has been suggested that these cations may play roles as "second messengers" to mediate the actions of insulin (Krahl, 1972). While many have sought such second-messenger systems to mediate the actions of insulin within the cell, clear demonstrations of a system analogous, for example, to hormone-sensitive adenylate cyclase have not yet appeared.

Insulin Unitage. Insulin preparations must be bioassayed as described above in order to ascertain their physiological activity. The assay described in the U.S.P. is based on the capacity of samples to lower the blood glucose concentration. The potency is expressed in U.S.P. units, and the standard of comparison is the U.S.P. *Insulin Reference Standard.* The potency of the reference-standard crystals is indicated on the label of each preparation. It is of the order of 22 units/mg. Newer, more pure preparations of the hormone (see below) have potencies of 26 to 30 units/mg.

Preparations. Significant advances and changes have been made in the United States and Europe in the purity and formulation of insulin preparations. These have been summarized by Rosenbloom (1974) and by Schlichtkrull and coworkers (1975).

As a result of a recommendation of the American Diabetes Association's Committee on the Use of Therapeutic Agents, U-40 and U-80 insulins (40 and 80 units/ml) are being eliminated in favor of a single U-100 dosage form for all types of insulin (see Committee, 1972). The objective is to reduce the chance of patient error, which is greater with the multiple dosage forms and dually calibrated syringes than with a single dosage form (see McKinley and Farquar, 1976). Concentrated preparations of regular insulin (U-500) are available for patients who are resistant to the hormone (see below).

Prior to 1973, insulin preparations available for therapeutic use contained, as potentially antigenic components, significant amounts of proinsulin and its incompletely converted products as well as other pancreatic hormones (Bloom et al., 1978). New procedures have been devised to prepare purer preparations of the hormone. Two such preparations are "single-peak" insulin (essentially one protein peak obtained by fractionation on SEPHADEX G50 chromatography) and "single-component" insulin, in which the hormone is subjected to ion-exchange chromatography (Schlichtkrull et al., 1975; Chance et al., 1976). The purity of most commercial insulin in the United States is now that of "single-peak" insulin (99%). While greatly improved in purity over previous products, "single-peak" insulin appears still to contain antigenic components (Chance et al., 1976). However, antibody production is markedly reduced with "single-component" insulin (purity greater than 99%). Such highly purified preparations of pork insulin are now available commercially (ILETIN II); because these products are expensive and their supply is limited, their use should be restricted to those patients with specific indications, such as persistent allergy to less purified insulin or to bovine insulin.

Most regular insulin preparations (and all regular U-100 preparations) in the United States are now supplied at neutral pH. This has resulted in improved stability of the hormone, and patients need no longer refrigerate the vial of insulin in use. However, excessive heat and sunlight should be avoided.

Furthermore, neutral regular insulin can be mixed in any desired proportion with other, modified insulin preparations since all marketed insulin preparations will be at the same pH.

Preparations of insulin are divided into three categories according to promptness, duration, and intensity of action following subcutaneous administration. They are classified as fast-, intermediate-, and long-acting types (*see* Table 64–1). However, it is recognized that a particular insulin preparation can show wide variations of activity in a population of patients and even in a single individual, especially one with labile diabetes. Insulin precipitated from solution in the amorphous (noncrystalline) form and then prepared for subcutaneous injection by solution in water at either neutral or acidic pH (about 3.2) (*Insulin Injection,* U.S.P.) is rapidly absorbed; action is prompt in onset, intense, and short in duration. The term *amorphous* applies to the noncrystalline physical state of the insulin. Crystalline insulin is prepared by the precipitation of the hormone in the presence of zinc (as zinc chloride) in a suitable buffer medium. Crystalline insulin when dissolved in water at neutral or acidic pH is also known as *Insulin Injection,* U.S.P., but may bear the additional label

"insulin made from zinc-insulin crystals." Following subcutaneous injection it has a slightly slower onset and a slightly longer duration of action than does amorphous insulin.

By permitting insulin and zinc to react with the basic protein protamine, Hagedorn and associates (1936) prepared a protein complex, *protamine zinc insulin.* When the complex is injected subcutaneously in an aqueous suspension, it dissolves only slowly at the site of deposition, and the insulin is absorbed at a retarded but steady rate. The objective of therapy with protamine zinc insulin suspension is to provide the daily requirement of hormone in a single injection. In the severely diabetic patient, however, the onset of action of protamine zinc insulin suspension is too slow, and if large doses are employed the duration of action is too prolonged for adequate control. To obviate this difficulty, combination therapy with regular insulin and protamine zinc insulin suspension was introduced. The two insulins can be given either as separate injections or mixed in the proper proportion immediately prior to injection.

The search has continued for a stable solution of insulin that possesses the desirable properties of

Table 64–1. **PROPERTIES OF VARIOUS PREPARATIONS OF INSULIN**

TYPE	PREPARATION	APPEARANCE	PROTEIN MODIFIER	APPROX-IMATE TIME OF ONSET * (*hours*)	APPROX-IMATE DURA-TION OF ACTION * (*hours*)	COMPATIBLE MIXED WITH
Fast-Acting	*Insulin Injection,* U.S.P. (regular insulin)	Clear solution	None	1	6	All preparations
	Insulin Injection, U.S.P. "Insulin made from zinc-insulin crystals" (regular insulin)	Clear solution	None	1	8	All preparations
	Prompt Insulin Zinc Suspension, U.S.P. (SEMILENTE insulin)	Cloudy suspension	None	1	14	LENTE preparations
Intermediate-Acting	*Isophane Insulin Suspension,* U.S.P. (NPH insulin, isophane insulin)	Cloudy suspension	Protamine	2	24	Insulin injection
	Insulin Zinc Suspension, U.S.P. (LENTE insulin)	Cloudy suspension	None	2	24	Insulin injection, SEMILENTE
	Globin Zinc Insulin Injection, U.S.P.	Clear solution	Globin	2	18	—
Long-Acting	*Protamine Zinc Insulin Suspension,* U.S.P.	Cloudy suspension	Protamine	7	36	Insulin injection
	Extended Insulin Zinc Suspension, U.S.P. (ULTRALENTE insulin)	Cloudy suspension	None	7	36	Insulin injection, SEMILENTE

* These figures are representative. The values may be expected to vary over a relatively wide range, depending on the dose and the individual patient.

fairly rapid onset and moderately prolonged duration of action. Three preparations of this type are *Globin Zinc Insulin Injection,* U.S.P., *Isophane Insulin Suspension,* U.S.P., and LENTE *insulins.*

Globin Zinc Insulin Injection, U.S.P., is a mixture of insulin and the protein globin (derived from beef hemoglobin) and zinc chloride. The time of onset and the duration of action of this preparation are intermediate between those of regular insulin and protamine zinc insulin suspension. Globin zinc insulin injection is now rarely used.

Isophane Insulin Suspension, U.S.P., is also known as NPH-50 insulin; the *N* denotes a neutral solution (pH 7.2), the *P* refers to the protamine zinc insulin content, the *H* signifies the origin in Hagedorn's laboratory, and the *50* refers to the content of 0.50 mg of protamine per 100 U.S.P. units of insulin. It is a modified protamine zinc insulin suspension that is crystalline. The concentrations of insulin, protamine, and zinc are so arranged that the preparation has an onset and a duration of action intermediate between those of regular insulin and protamine zinc insulin suspension. The advantage of this mixture is its stability in regard to the ratio of "free" to "bound" insulin. Its effects on blood sugar are indistinguishable from those of an extemporaneous mixture of 2 to 3 units of regular insulin and 1 unit of protamine zinc insulin suspension.

Chemical studies have revealed that the solubility of insulin is determined in important measure by its physical state (amorphous, crystalline, size of the crystals) and by the zinc content and the nature of the buffer in which it is suspended. Insulin can thus be prepared in a slowly absorbed, slow-acting form without the use of other proteins, such as protamine or globin, to bind it. Large crystals of insulin with high zinc content, when collected and resuspended in a solution of sodium acetate–sodium chloride (pII 7.1 to 7.5), are slowly absorbed after subcutaneous injection and exert an action of long duration. This preparation is named *Extended Insulin Zinc Suspension,* U.S.P. (ULTRALENTE insulin). Amorphous insulin precipitated at high pH is almost as rapid in onset and as short in duration of action as regular insulin. The preparation is named *Prompt Insulin Zinc Suspension,* U.S.P. (SEMILENTE insulin). The two forms of insulin may be mixed to yield a stable mixture of crystalline (7 parts) and amorphous (3 parts) insulin—*Insulin Zinc Suspension,* U.S.P. (LENTE insulin)—that is intermediate in onset and duration of action between SEMILENTE and ULTRALENTE preparations.

The properties of the various official insulin preparations are presented in Table 64–1. Most commercial insulin preparations in the United States are mixtures of the bovine and porcine hormones. Pure porcine or pure bovine insulin is also available. The LENTE insulins contain methylparaben as a preservative; the other preparations contain either phenol or cresol. All preparations are usually given by subcutaneous injection. *Only Insulin Injection can be given by the intravenous route.* The insulins are marketed in 10-ml vials.

Hypoglycemia Associated with Hyperinsulinism. Hypoglycemic reactions may

occur in any diabetic subject treated with insulin or with an oral hypoglycemic agent. Reactions are seen frequently in the labile form of the disease, a form characterized by unpredictable spontaneous reductions in insulin requirement. In other instances, precipitating causes are usually responsible, for example, failure to eat, unaccustomed exercise, and inadvertent administration of too large a dose of insulin (*see* Tattersall, 1977).

The reaction pattern associated with hypoglycemia has been fully described in connection with insulin shock therapy for schizophrenia (long since outmoded) and in carefully controlled clinical studies in normal and diabetic volunteers (Sussman *et al.,* 1963). The pattern and the temporal sequence of signs and symptoms are fairly, but by no means absolutely, constant. When the rate of fall in blood glucose is rapid, the early symptoms are those brought on by the compensating secretion of epinephrine; these include sweating, weakness, hunger, tachycardia, and "inner trembling." When the concentration of glucose falls slowly, the symptoms and signs are referable to the brain and include headache, blurred vision, diplopia, mental confusion, incoherent speech, coma, and convulsions. If the fall in blood glucose is rapid, profound, and persistent, all such symptoms may be present. In only a few patients, the onset is heralded by hunger or nausea; bradycardia and mild hypotension may occur in association with the gastrointestinal discomfort.

From a practical point of view, about half of the patients may be expected to call for help; nevertheless, another large fraction will not, presumably because of the confusion attending hypoglycemia or because the reaction may occur during sleep. Fortunately, the patients who have neither signs nor symptoms preceding convulsions and coma are few in number, but they present one of the most difficult problems in the management of diabetes.

The majority of the signs and symptoms of insulin hypoglycemia are the result of functional abnormalities of the CNS, since hypoglycemia deprives the brain of the substrate (glucose) upon which it is almost exclusively dependent for its oxidative metabolism. During insulin coma, oxygen consumption in human brain decreases by nearly half. The reduction in glucose consumption is proportionately greater, which indicates that the brain is utilizing some other substrate. After prolonged fasting in man the brain adapts, and the bulk of the fuel utilized is made up of ketone bodies (Owen et al., 1967).

Hypoglycemic convulsions appear to be markedly influenced by the degree of cerebral hydration. However, this finding is not unique for hypoglycemic convulsions; the convulsive threshold for other types of stimuli is also reduced by cellular hydration.

A prolonged period of hypoglycemia causes irreversible damage to the brain, as evidenced in experimental animals by histological changes in the cortex, basal ganglia, and rostral parts of the medulla. There are isolated reports of neurological or mental changes in man following insulin-induced convulsions and coma, including mental retardation, hemiparesis, ataxia, incontinence, aphasia, choreiform movements, parkinsonism, and epilepsy.

Although the signs and the symptoms of insulin hypoglycemia seem well defined, it is often difficult clinically to distinguish this condition from severe diabetic ketoacidosis (diabetic coma). Unfortunately, many cases of insulin coma have been treated with insulin. The symptoms of hypoglycemia yield almost immediately to the intravenous injection of glucose unless hypoglycemia has been sufficiently prolonged to induce organic changes in the brain. If the patient is not able to take soluble carbohydrate or fruit juice orally and if glucose is not available for intravenous injection, 0.5 to 1 mg of glucagon is given (see below). It is important to note that insulin-dependent diabetics who are also receiving β-adrenergic antagonists such as propranolol may have delayed recovery from hypoglycemic episodes; propranolol also masks many of the signs and symptoms of hypoglycemia (see Editorial, 1977; Chapter 9).

Every diabetic patient taking insulin should carry an identification card or bracelet containing pertinent medical information.

Other Adverse Reactions. Local or systemic allergic reactions are often seen in patients receiving insulin for the first time or when insulin treatment is reinstituted. The local reactions that result from skin sensitivity usually subside spontaneously. Allergic

urticaria, angioedema, and anaphylactic reactions occur infrequently and usually can be avoided by changing to insulin obtained from a different species or by utilizing single-component insulin. Rarely, desensitization may be required; insulin-allergy desensitization kits are available (Wentworth et al., 1976).

Patients who experience atrophy of subcutaneous fat at the site of injection (insulin lipoatrophy) should inject the insulin in areas that are usually covered by clothing; the problem may be minimized by changing the site of injection frequently. There have been reports of decreased incidence of lipoatrophy with the newer, more highly purified insulins (see Chance et al., 1976), and injection of these preparations directly into sites of lipoatrophy may facilitate reversal of the process.

Visual disturbances in uncontrolled diabetes that are due to refractive changes are reversed during the early treatment phase. However, since several weeks may be required to stabilize the osmotic equilibrium in the eye, alterations of prescriptions for corrective lenses should be postponed for 3 to 6 weeks.

ORAL HYPOGLYCEMIC AGENTS

History. Janbon and coworkers (1942), in the course of clinical studies on the treatment of typhoid fever, discovered that a sulfonamide (*p*-amino-benzene-sulfonamido-isopropylthiadiazole) induced hypoglycemia. Janbon's colleague, Loubatières (1957), then made the fundamental discovery that the compound exerted no hypoglycemic effect in the completely pancreatectomized animal and suggested that the action was the result of stimulation of the pancreas to secrete insulin. There was no practical application of these findings until Franke and Fuchs capitalized on the discovery that the antibacterial agent *carbutamide* lowered the blood sugar in patients treated for infectious diseases. These workers demonstrated the apparent usefulness of carbutamide in the treatment of diabetes mellitus. Soon thereafter, the compound *tolbutamide* was introduced. This substance is not antibacterial, is less toxic than carbutamide, and soon became popular for the management of certain diabetic patients. Tolbutamide is a member of the class of oral hypoglycemic agents designated as *sulfonylureas*.

Another group of compounds, the *biguanides*, was developed independently of the sulfonylureas. Historically, the development began with the discovery in 1918 by Watanabe that guanidine causes hypoglycemia in rats. While the compound *phenformin* was introduced into clinical practice and was utilized for several years, it has now been removed from the markct in thc United States, particularly because of its tendency to cause severe lactic acidosis. Further information on phenformin can be found in the *fifth edition* of this textbook.

SULFONYLUREAS

Chemistry. A number of sulfonylurea compounds exert hypoglycemic activity. The commercially available preparations are *tolbutamide, acetohexamide, tolazamide,* and *chlorpropamide,* which have the following structural formulas:

$$H_3C-\text{(benzene ring)}-SO_2-NH-\overset{\displaystyle O}{\overset{\|}{C}}-NH-(CH_2)_3CH_3$$

Tolbutamide

$$H_3C-CO-\text{(benzene ring)}-SO_2-NH-\overset{\displaystyle O}{\overset{\|}{C}}-NH-\text{(cyclohexyl)}$$

Acetohexamide

$$H_3C-\text{(benzene ring)}-SO_2-NH-\overset{\displaystyle O}{\overset{\|}{C}}-NH-N\begin{matrix}CH_2-CH_2-CH_2\\CH_2-CH_2-CH_2\end{matrix}$$

Tolazamide

$$Cl-\text{(benzene ring)}-SO_2-NH-\overset{\displaystyle O}{\overset{\|}{C}}-NH-(CH_2)_2CH_3$$

Chlorpropamide

All the effective compounds are arylsulfonylureas with substitutions on the benzene and the urea groups. In the case of tolbutamide, the aryl group is tolyl and the urea substitution is butyl. Tolbutamide differs from the antibacterial compound carbutamide in having methyl instead of amino on the benzene ring. This substitution accounts for the loss of antibacterial properties and for the reduction of toxicity.

Mechanism of Action.

The sulfonylureas stimulate the islet tissue to secrete insulin. The evidence, coming as it does from a variety of experimental and clinical studies, unequivocally supports such a conclusion. Administration of sulfonylureas increases the concentration of insulin in the pancreatic vein in cross-circulation experiments. Recipient animals, diabetic or nondiabetic, exhibit hypoglycemia in response to the infusion of pancreatic vein blood from donor animals treated with sulfonylureas but not to the infusion of mesenteric or femoral vein blood from the same animals. Sulfonylureas cause degranulation of the β cells, a phenomenon

associated with increased rate of secretion of insulin. Clinical studies demonstrate that the sulfonylureas are ineffective in completely pancreatectomized patients and in insulin-dependent diabetic subjects. On the other hand, they are effective in insulin-independent diabetic patients in whom the pancreas retains the capacity to secrete insulin. There may also be some effect of sulfonylureas on adrenergic control of insulin secretion, since these agents can inhibit the release of catecholamines (Hsu *et al.,* 1975).

Although the molecular mechanism of action of these agents is not understood, pertinent observations have been made. Hellman and associates (1971) concluded that labeled tolbutamide is restricted in its action to the extracellular space and does not need to enter the β cell. The invoked release of insulin is immediate and is intimately related to thc action of glucose; the drug may sensitize the cell to the normal secretagogue (Cerasi, 1975).

In experimental animals and in diabetic patients, conflicting results have been obtained on the effects of sulfonylureas on plasma concentrations of glucagon. Samols and Harrison (1978) have suggested that tolbutamide can enhance glucagon secretion from the α cell, although this may be masked by the effect of the sulfonylurea to stimulate the secretion of insulin. Local actions of insulin within the islet may cause a reduction in the secretion of glucagon; the nct effect could be either stimulation or suppression of glucagon secretion.

During chronic administration, a significant portion of the hypoglycemic action of the sulfonylureas may be due to extrapancreatic actions. Insulin biosynthesis may actually decrease, and peripheral tissues become more sensitive to a fixed dose of administered hormone, due, possibly, to an increase in the number of insulin receptors (Lebovitz and Feinglos, 1978). Other extrapancreatic effects of the sulfonylureas have been noted in various organs, and certain of these may potentiate the effects of insulin. A reduction in the hepatic uptake of endogenous insulin has been described (Marshall *et al.,* 1970). Tolbutamide enhances the antilipolytic action of insulin in adipose tissue. This appears to be related to an altered effectiveness of cyclic AMP rather than to any change in metabolism of the cyclic nucleotide (Brown *et al.,* 1972; Fain *et al.,* 1972), and an inhibitory effect of the drug on cyclic AMP–dependent protein kinase has been observed (Wray and Harris, 1973). Other reports indicate a variety of influences on cyclic AMP metabolism in different tissues (Brooker and Fichman, 1971; Kuo *et al.,* 1972; Lasseter *et al.,* 1972).

Duration of Action, Fate, and Excretion.

The sulfonylureas are readily absorbed from the gastrointestinal tract. The most important difference among the sulfonylureas, for clinical purposes, is in their duration of action; in increasing order they are tolbutamide, acetohexamide, tolazamide, and chlorpropamide.

Tolbutamide can be detected in the blood within 30 minutes after oral administration; peak concentrations are reached within 3 to 5 hours. The drug is bound to plasma proteins. Tolbutamide is oxidized in the body to butyl-*p*-carboxyphenylsulfonylurea, which is a major excretory product. The half-life of tolbutamide is about 6 hours. Two or occasionally three doses are required daily.

Acetohexamide is rapidly absorbed, and maximal hypoglycemic activity is observed about 3 hours after ingestion. The total duration of action is 12 to 24 hours. Much of the activity is ascribable to a metabolite, *hydroxyhexamide,* which has a plasma half-life of about 6 hours; the parent compound, acetohexamide, has a plasma half-life of 1.3 hours. In persons with normal renal and hepatic function, more than 80% is excreted, largely as metabolites, in 24 hours. Two doses are usually required daily.

Tolazamide is slowly absorbed; the onset of hypoglycemic action occurs at 4 to 6 hours and persists at a significant level up to 15 hours after a single dose. Tolazamide is metabolized to a number of hypoglycemic substances that are largely excreted by the kidney. For most patients controlled by tolazamide, a single daily dose is sufficient; a few patients require administration of the drug twice daily.

Chlorpropamide is also rapidly absorbed from the gastrointestinal tract and is bound to plasma proteins. In contrast to tolbutamide, chlorpropamide is not metabolically altered to any significant degree and is excreted very slowly in unchanged form. The half-life of a single dose is about 36 hours, or six times as long as that of tolbutamide. With daily doses of 250 to 500 mg, concentrations in blood may not be expected to reach a plateau before 3 or more days. Chlorpropamide is administered in a single daily dose.

Toxicity. O'Donovan (1959) analyzed the incidence of side effects to *tolbutamide* in 9168 cases. The total incidence of side effects was 3.2%; the drug was withdrawn in 1.5% of the patients. The reactions have been classified as hematological (0.24%), cutaneous (1.1%), and gastrointestinal (1.4%). Of the 22 subjects exhibiting hematological abnormalities, 19 had a transient leukopenia; in 9 instances, the leukocyte count returned to normal despite continuation of the drug. Paresthesia, tinnitus, and headache may also occur.

The total incidence of untoward reactions is about 6% for *chlorpropamide* (hematological, 0.6; cutaneous, 3; gastrointestinal, 2; and jaundice, 0.4%). The jaundice is of the cholestatic type and is usually transient. Hyponatremia occurs in a small number of patients treated with tolbutamide and chlorpropamide. Inappropriate secretion of antidiuretic hormone has been observed, and chlorpropamide potentiates the renal tubular effects of the hormone.

The frequency and the kinds of toxic reactions produced by *acetohexamide* and *tolazamide* are similar to those encountered with tolbutamide and chlorpropamide. Hematological (leukopenia, agranulocytosis, thrombocytopenia, pancytopenia, and hemolytic anemia), cutaneous (rashes, photosensitivity), gastrointestinal (nausea, vomiting, rarely hemorrhage), and hepatic (increased serum alkaline phosphatase, cholestatic jaundice) reactions have been reported.

Hypoglycemic reactions, including coma, may occur (Seltzer, 1972). While they are usually not severe, several fatalities have been reported. Hypoglycemic episodes may last for several days so that prolonged or repeated glucose administration is required. Reactions have occurred after one dose, after several days of treatment, or after months of drug administration. Most reactions are observed in patients over 50 years of age, and they are more likely to occur in patients with impaired hepatic or renal function. Overdosage or inadequate or irregular food intake may initiate hypoglycemia. Drugs that may increase the risk of hypoglycemia from sulfonylureas include other hypoglycemic agents, sulfonamides, propranolol, salicylates, clofibrate, phenylbutazone, probenecid, dicumarol, chloramphenicol, monoamine oxidase inhibitors, and alcohol.

Sulfonylureas should not be used in a patient with hepatic or renal insufficiency because of the important role of the liver in their metabolism and of the kidney in the excretion of the drugs and their metabolites. Intolerance to alcohol reminiscent of the disulfiram reaction, with flushing, palpitations, and nausea, occurs occasionally in patients taking sulfonylureas.

These agents are also not recommended for use in pregnancy, but only sparse data have been reported on this point. Teratogenesis in animals has been observed to follow the administration of large doses.

A cooperative clinical trial in 12 university-based clinics (University Group Diabetes Program; UGDP) was established in 1961 to determine if the control of blood glucose concentration helps to prevent or delay vascular disease in insulin-independent diabetic patients. About 200 subjects in each of five therapeutic regimens were treated with diet and either placebo, a standard dose of tolbutamide, a standard dose of insulin, a variable dose of insulin, or a standard dose of phenformin. This large multicenter study was one of the first such attempts to evaluate long-term effects of drug therapy, and difficulties inherent in this type of investigation were thus encountered.

During a period of over 8 years of observation, there were 120 deaths, including 87 from cardiovascular causes; while 10 to 12 cardiovascular deaths occurred in each of the placebo or insulin-treated groups, 26 such deaths (a significantly higher number) were recorded among the patients in each group taking oral hypoglycemic agents. The overall mortality rate was correspondingly higher in these two groups of diabetic patients. Some of the conclusions of this study were that the combination of diet and either tolbutamide or phenformin was no more effective in prolonging life than diet alone; furthermore, it was felt that diet and either tolbutamide or phenformin may be *less* effective than diet alone or diet together with insulin in preventing cardiovascular mortality. (*See* University Group Diabetes Program, 1970, 1976; Knatterud *et al.,* 1971.)

During the decade that has followed the appearance of the UGDP report, a flood of comments and reports has appeared, both critical and supportive of the study. In response to this, at the instigation of the Director of the National Institutes of Health, the Biometric Society appointed a committee to review the UGDP report. The committee concluded that the shortcomings of the study do not invalidate its observations and conclusions. (*See* Chalmers, 1975; Report of the Committee, 1975.) Despite this, debate has continued, fueled most recently by some opportunities to review the original data and patient records. These have revealed deficiencies in patient compliance and selection, among other problems, and have prompted the American Diabetes Association to withdraw its endorsement of the UGDP study. (*See* Feinstein, 1976; Kilo *et al.,* 1979; Kolata, 1979.)

Throughout the controversy, many physicians have maintained an invariant approach to the use of oral hypoglycemic agents, based on cogent arguments. Despite uncertainties about the incidence of serious toxicity caused by these drugs, there *never* has been any proof that their use is beneficial in the prevention of the long-term complications of diabetes. They are capable of controlling mild hyperglycemia and its associated signs and symptoms, but there are more conservative and rational approaches to the management of these problems. Furthermore, if rigorous control of hyperglycemia is proven to be worthwhile for the prevention of long-term complications of diabetes, dietary management and the administration of insulin, as necessary, are more effective. It is thus possible to formulate recommendations for the appropriate therapeutic use of these drugs (*see* below).

Preparations and Dosage. *Tolbutamide,* U.S.P. (ORINASE), is marketed in the form of 500-mg tablets. The sodium salt (1 g) is also available for administration intravenously for diagnostic use. *Acetohexamide,* U.S.P. (DYMELOR), is available in 250- and 500-mg tablets. *Tolazamide,* U.S.P. (TOLINASE), is supplied in 100-, 250-, and 500-mg tablets. *Chlorpropamide,* U.S.P. (DIABINESE), is marketed as 100- and 250-mg tablets.

The usual daily dose of tolbutamide is 1000 mg, while 2000 mg is the maximally effective total dose; corresponding dosages are 500 and 1500 mg for acetohexamide. Tolazamide and chlorpropamide are usually administered in a daily dosage of 250 mg, while 750 to 1000 mg is maximal.

Therapeutic Uses. *The sulfonylureas should be used only in patients with diabetes of the insulin-independent type who cannot be treated with diet alone and who are unwilling or unable to take insulin if weight reduction and dietary control fail.* The physician must realize that he is most likely using these agents only to control symptoms associated with hyperglycemia, and that dietary control with or without insulin is more effective for this purpose. There is no evidence that the oral hypoglycemic agents prevent cardiovascular complications from diabetes, and the best data available, even though controversial, suggest that the incidence of such complications may be increased in patients taking these drugs. This risk is too high a price for the convenience of an oral agent, unless *all* other measures have been exhausted.

In general, the likelihood of adequate control with an oral hypoglycemic agent is inversely proportional to the dose of insulin required to maintain the patient. When the insulin requirement is in excess of 40 units per day, the chances of success are relatively low. The sulfonylureas are of no value in the insulin-dependent type of diabetes, in which the pancreas has lost all or nearly all of its capacity to secrete insulin. *Such patients require insulin, and attempts to control them with oral therapy are dangerous and doomed to failure.* Deaths from acidosis and dehydration have occurred in patients with unstable ketotic diabetes in whom regulation was attempted with sulfonylureas.

There is no fixed dosage of sulfonylurea to be used in diabetes mellitus. Treatment is guided by the individual patient's response, which must be frequently monitored with chemical determinations, because the requirements change from time to time.

The mildly diabetic patient, whose insulin requirement is fewer than 20 units daily, can be started on the usual dose of the agent chosen, and at the same time all insulin should be discontinued. The dose is then adjusted up or down, depending on the patient's response. In the instance of chlorpropamide, about 3 days is required to attain steady-state concentrations in blood. Consequently, upward adjustments of dose should be made at 3-day intervals. Patients of advanced age should begin with about half the usual daily dose, for some are very responsive to sulfonylureas and may develop severe hypoglycemia after usual doses. During the period of initiating treatment, all patients should test their urine four times daily and communicate the results to the physician daily.

The patient who requires more than 20 and fewer than 40 units of insulin daily should be started on the usual dose of the chosen agent and his insulin dosage should simultaneously be reduced by 50%. Thereafter, guided by the patient's response, insulin dosage is progressively reduced and finally discontinued. Sulfonylurea dosage may need adjustment.

The patient requiring more than 40 units of insulin daily should be given the usual dose of the agent chosen and his insulin dosage should be reduced by 25%. Insulin is then cautiously withdrawn and eventually discontinued, and sulfonylurea is adjusted according to the observed response. It is to be emphasized that the chance of success is relatively poor.

Stimulation of the pancreas of the insulin-independent diabetic can often maintain these subjects under ordinary circumstances. However, when insulin requirements are increased, as in fever, surgical interventions, or trauma, the sulfonylureas are inadequate and the patient must be given insulin to carry him through such critical situations.

Weight reduction is of the greatest importance in the treatment of diabetes. A vigorous effort must be made by the patient and the physician to reduce the patient's weight as an integral part of diabetic treatment, irrespective of the drug chosen.

Patients whose diabetes is not controlled by sufonylureas from the initiation of treatment are said to experience "primary failure." Patients whose diabetes is regulated for a month or more after beginning sulfonylurea treatment, following which inability to maintain control develops, are said to experience "secondary failure." The incidence of this type of failure may be very high, regardless of the agent chosen.

In patients with pancreatic islet-cell tumors, the concentration of glucose in blood drops rapidly after intravenous injection of tolbutamide and remains low for about 3 hours. A similar effect is not observed in other hypoglycemic states, and administration of tolbutamide can thus be used as a diagnostic test. Determinations of immunoreactive insulin in serum should also be performed. Care is necessary, since fatal hypoglycemia has occurred.

TREATMENT OF DIABETES MELLITUS

The Ambulatory Patient. The objectives of therapy are maintenance of health and a symptom-free, productively active life. These are attained by attention to diet, body weight, and activity and, if necessary, by the use of insulin. Inability to use insulin in a given patient with insulin-independent diabetes may necessitate the administration of an oral hypoglycemic agent.

Insulin is required for control of diabetes in most persons in whom the disease has its onset before attainment of adult stature (insulin-dependent diabetes), in most underweight persons in whom it appears after cessation of growth, and in pregnant women whose disorder is not controlled by diet. Insulin will be temporarily required in the treatment of ketoacidosis in the obese patient whose diabetes is otherwise controlled by dietary regulation with or without an oral hypoglycemic agent. Insulin is effective in all forms of diabetes. It is the only effective agent for severe manifestations of diabetes and should be used when these are present or threatened, for example, during surgery or infection or following vascular occlusions, irrespective of previous therapy.

Most patients with onset of diabetes in middle or late life are obese. *A serious effort should be made to regulate their diabetes by diet and weight reduction alone.* In doing so, it is important to avoid confusing weight loss resulting from restricted caloric intake with that resulting from uncontrolled diabetes. Weekly determination of weight and 24-hour urine glucose values will prevent this error. A program of graded physical exercise is also important. Weight, glycosuria, and requirement for insulin or oral hypoglycemic agent should diminish.

Insulin therapy can be satisfactorily initiated on an ambulatory basis in an asymptomatic or mildly symptomatic patient with newly discovered diabetes. However, a short period of hospitalization offers superior opportunities for accurate evaluation of the patient, for the rapid attainment of control, and for education of the patient and his family. A novel, automated closed-loop device that senses glucose and delivers insulin has been developed; its use materially shortens the time required in the hospital to obtain control (Albisser and Leibel, 1977).

Whether insulin therapy is begun at home or in the hospital, urine should be collected from bedtime to breakfast, from breakfast to lunch, from lunch to supper, and from supper to bedtime. A diet calculated for the patient's needs is begun. Many physicians prefer to use regular insulin in multiple daily doses 20 minutes before meals and at bedtime for the first few days. The usual first dose of regular insulin in the nonketotic patient is 10 units. Subsequent doses are determined by the glycosuria, glycemia, and response to preceding doses. After control is achieved, a single dose of modified insulin given before breakfast may be substituted for multiple doses of regular insulin. The total dose of modified insulin is initially equal to 80% of the total daily dose of regular insulin. The basic ingredient of nearly all insulin regimens is an intermediate-acting preparation—isophane insulin suspension or insulin zinc suspension. By adjustment of dose, diet, and exercise, many patients with insulin-independent diabetes can be satisfactorily regulated with a single prebreakfast injection of intermediate-acting insulin. In other patients, persistence of morning glycosuria, despite afternoon and evening aglycosuria, is an indication for addition of a fast-acting insulin (Table 64–1) to the program. In other patients, persistence of nocturnal glycosuria, despite afternoon and evening aglycosuria, is an indication for the addition of long-acting insulin—extended zinc insulin suspension or protamine zinc insulin suspension. A number of patients with severe, labile diabetes must receive supplementary injections of a fast-acting insulin, before meals or before bedtime. An alternative that is often effective is injection of intermediate-acting insulin in two doses, about three fourths of the total requirement before breakfast and the remainder before supper or before retiring. It has been shown recently that patients are able to achieve true normalization of the concentration of glucose in blood by monitoring its value at home with a portable reflectance meter; doses of insulin are then adjusted accordingly. This is a potentially important therapeutic advance (*see* Sonksen *et al.*, 1978; Walford *et al.*, 1978).

Diabetic Ketoacidosis. Diabetic ketoacidosis is a continuum, ranging in severity from slight ketonuria without readily detectable ketonemia (ketosis) to the syndrome of diabetic coma, which is characterized by glycosuria, hypovolemia, ketonuria, ketonemia, metabolic acidosis, and coma, and which may progress to circulatory collapse, anuria, and death. Representative treatment protocols for the more severe form of diabetic ketoacidosis are presented below, but the principles upon which these recommendations are based also govern the treatment of less severe forms of diabetic acidosis. *It is of paramount importance for the patient to be hospitalized and for the physician to remain with the patient until the crisis is past; an accurate running record of all medications, clinical observations, and laboratory tests is essential.*

Traditional therapy of diabetic ketoacidosis has involved the administration of large doses of insulin, for example, 2 units/kg initially (divided intravenously and subcutaneously), followed by 1 unit/kg every 2 hours; this regimen is continued until the concentration of glucose in plasma approaches values of approximately 300 mg/dl. Such treatment results in concentrations of insulin in plasma of approximately 1000 microunits/ml, which are presumably far in excess of those usually required to produce a maximal biological response.

Doses of insulin in the range of 2 to 10 units per hour given by continuous intravenous infusion produce concentrations of the hormone in plasma that are nearly maximally effective (∼100 microunits/ml). When patients with diabetic ketoacidosis are treated with such doses of insulin, the plasma glucose concentration declines at a rate of approximately 75 to 100 mg/dl each hour and usually reaches values of 200 to 300 mg/dl in 4 to 6 hours. This rate is essentially the same as that achieved with higher doses of the hormone. The advantage of such regimens is that high concentrations of insulin do not persist in the plasma when administration is stopped; complications of hypoglycemia and hypokalemia are thus minimized (*see* Alberti and Hockaday, 1977; Kreisberg, 1978).

While most patients with diabetic ketoacidosis respond to low-dose regimens, a few patients are resistant to insulin and require much higher doses. A rare patient may require thousands of units of insulin during the first few hours of treatment. The results of therapy must therefore be monitored carefully, no matter what the regimen, and the dosage of insulin adjusted to the needs of the individual patient.

Appropriate fluid therapy is an essential element in the successful treatment of ketoacidosis and should be started immediately. The first fluid administered to a patient with diabetic coma is usually 0.9% sodium chloride solution, approximately 1 liter for an adult. Subsequently, 0.45% sodium chloride solution is administered. Central venous pressure should be monitored in patients with congestive heart failure, renal insufficiency, or shock. In order to restore the volume of body fluids, most patients with diabetic coma will need to retain an amount of fluid approximating at least 5% of body weight. This should be largely achieved in the first 12 hours of treatment. In the presence of a brisk diuresis resulting from glycosuria, it may be necessary to give intravenous fluids at a rate of 20 ml or more per minute in order to achieve a satisfactory rate of rehydration. Observation of the central venous pressure, the hematocrit, and the cumulative hourly difference between fluid intake and urine volume permits avoidance of overhydration. Reduction in plasma glucose and ketone concentrations signals the need for reduction in the rate of administration of insulin. At this time 0.45% sodium chloride solution containing 5% glucose is administered. Patients who require exceptionally large doses of insulin for control of the critical phase of their acidosis are particularly subject to hypoglycemia for a day or more after the treatment of the critical phase of acidosis, even though insulin may have been completely withdrawn. It is better to tolerate mild glycosuria for 1 or 2 days following treatment of severe acidosis than to risk hypoglycemia.

The administration of alkali is usually not necessary in the treatment of diabetic acidosis and may lead to development of alkalosis as insulin corrects the ketoacidosis. However, severe exhausting hyperpnea justifies the administration of 50 mEq of sodium bicarbonate added to the 0.45% solution of sodium chloride.

Patients with diabetic ketoacidosis usually have a normal or moderately elevated plasma concentration of potassium on admission to the hospital, as a consequence of cellular buffering of metabolic acids. At the same time, there exists an intracellular depletion of potassium that may be of the order of hundreds of milliequivalents in patients with severe or prolonged acidosis (average 5 mEq/kg). During treatment, as the rate of production of ketoacids diminishes, as potassium moves from the extracellular space to the intracellular space under the influence of insulin, and as the patient is rehydrated, hypokalemia may develop, usually beginning after the fourth hour of therapy. When this occurs, there is danger of progressive flaccid paralysis, which may eventually involve muscles of respiration.

Potassium salts usually should not be administered until it is established that the urine flow is at least of the order of 1 ml per minute and that hyperkalemia is absent; otherwise, cardiotoxic concentrations of potassium can readily accumulate in the extracellular fluid. If these conditions are met, potassium chloride should be given. For adults, the administration of 10 to 20 mEq of potassium per hour (added to the saline infusion) is a reasonable initial regimen. The deficit of potassium can, in general, be replaced during the first 24 hours. If the patient is hypokalemic, *cautious* administration of potassium may be necessary despite oliguria.

Deficiency of phosphorus in diabetic ketoacidosis has been known for decades. As a result of such deficiency, there may be lowered concentrations of 2,3-diphosphoglycerate in erythrocytes, with consequent changes in the affinity of hemoglobin for oxygen (*see* Chapter 16). While replacement of phosphate has occasionally been advocated, its efficacy is not known. As with potassium, concentrations of phosphate in plasma may at first be nearly normal despite significant depletion of total stores of the anion. Concentrations in extracellular fluid appear to fall markedly during treatment of ketoacidosis (*see* Kreisberg, 1978). The deficit of phosphorus in ketoacidosis probably averages 1 mmol/kg of body weight. It is often replaced in part by the administration of potassium phosphate rather than potassium chloride. Data are needed to establish the value of this procedure.

After 6 to 8 hours of treatment, most patients are able to tolerate a liquid diet. In patients treated for uncomplicated ketoacidosis, the usual diet can be resumed in 24 hours. Modified insulin should not be given until the patient is eating regularly.

Hyperosmolar Coma. Hyperosmolar coma is a variant form of diabetic ketoacidosis, but it differs in several important respects. Whereas ketoacidosis almost invariably occurs in patients with insulin-dependent diabetes, hyperosmolar coma usually occurs in elderly and obese diabetic patients who often have only moderate hyperglycemia and who do not ordinarily require therapy with insulin. The reason for the absence of severe ketosis in hyperosmolar coma is not known with certainty; however, concentrations of insulin in plasma are low to normal in this type of diabetes and may be adequate to inhibit ketogenesis. Typically, infection or other stress causes a worsening of hyperglycemia, followed by glycosuria and osmotic diuresis. In the absence of hyperpnea, vomiting, and other signs of ketoacidosis, the diuresis may be unnoticed and proceed for several days, leading to severe dehydration and decreased renal blood flow. The urinary route for the disposal of glucose is then lost, and the concentration of glucose in plasma increases dramatically, often exceeding 1500 mg/dl; osmolality of the plasma is often greater than 350 mOsm per liter. Coma and death follow quickly unless vigorous treatment is begun. The general principles of treatment are the same as for ketoacidosis. However, it is important to recognize that dehydration is usually much more severe. The fluid deficit may be 8 to 12 liters. Although some patients with hyperosmolar coma appear to be very sensitive to insulin, treatment can be initiated with the same dosages employed for the management of ketoacidosis; concentrations of glucose and potassium in plasma should of course be monitored carefully. The incidence of hyperosmolar coma is probably as great as is that of ketoacidosis. Because of the age of the patient, severity of dehydration, and coincidental illness, the mortality rate is high (*see* Arieff and Carroll, 1972).

Insulin Resistance. Traditionally, patients requiring more than 200 units of insulin daily are said to be insulin resistant. Insulin resistance is usually defined as a condition in which the daily requirement for insulin is in excess of the amount normally secreted. A useful point of reference is the daily insulin requirement of pancreatectomized man, frequently as low as 30 units. The figure of 200 units per day arbitrarily dividing resistance from nonresistance is undoubtedly too high.

Insulin resistance can be acute or chronic. Acute insulin resistance is associated with surgical or other trauma, emotional disturbances, and many infections (especially staphylococcal). It is reasonable to postulate that increased blood concentrations of adrenocortical hormones in response to trauma, anxiety, and infection may be contributory. The treatment of acute insulin resistance is the treatment of the precipitating cause and the administration of large doses of insulin together with needed water and electrolytes.

Chronic insulin resistance is frequently, but not always, associated with large amounts of insulin-binding antibodies in plasma. Insulin resistance often appears after resumption of insulin therapy following a period of discontinuance. Identifiable endocrine disturbances (acromegaly, adrenal hypercorticism, and pheochromocytoma) are rarely the cause of chronic insulin resistance and almost never the cause of extreme insulin resistance (daily insulin requirements in excess of 500 units). A rare and readily recognizable condition associated with chronic insulin resistance is lipoatrophic diabetes, a disorder characterized by absence of normal body fat depots, hyperlipemia and cutaneous xanthomata, hepatomegaly, and cirrhosis, and by insulin-resistant, nonketotic diabetes mellitus (*see* Renold *et al.*, 1978). Other rare forms of chronic insulin resistance are associated with increased degradation of insulin, antibodies to insulin receptors, and postreceptor defects (*see* above).

In order to supply adequate insulin to those with chronic insulin resistance, it may be convenient to use the preparation containing 500 units/ml. Some patients may be selectively resistant to bovine insulin while remaining sensitive to porcine insulin. The rationale for using porcine insulin is based on its chemical similarity to the human hormone.

Chemical alterations have been made to diminish the antigenic properties of porcine insulin. One such modification is dealaninated porcine insulin, where the carboxy-terminal alanine of the B chain is selectively cleaved by enzymatic (carboxypeptidase) action; there is no loss in biological activity. Antibodies to mixed porcine-bovine insulin or to porcine insulin do not react with dealaninated porcine insulin. Reports have appeared of the effectiveness of dealaninated porcine insulin in treating insulin-resistant diabetic patients who failed to respond to the porcine or bovine hormone (Burman *et al.*, 1973). Sulfonylureas reduce the insulin requirement in some insulin-resistant patients, presumably as a consequence of release of endogenous insulin, which has less affinity for circulating antibody than does exogenous bovine or porcine insulin. Sulfated bovine insulin has also been used, with some success, to treat immunologically related insulin resistance (Davidson and DeBra, 1978).

GLUCAGON

History. Glucagon was discovered by Murlin and coworkers in 1923—2 years after the discovery of insulin. The contrast between the subsequent history of insulin and glucagon, each secreted by adjoining cells in the islets, could hardly be more striking. Because of its immediate therapeutic importance, insulin was well accepted as a hormone and hailed as a major medical advance. Glucagon was of little interest, its discoverers received little recognition, and the

hormone was not purified extensively until over 30 years had passed (Staub *et al.*, 1955).

Chemistry. Glucagon is a single-chain polypeptide with a molecular weight of nearly 3500. In contrast to insulin, it contains no cysteine and, consequently, no disulfide linkages; the sequence of its 29 amino acids has been determined by Bromer and associates (1956) (*see* Figure 64–3). Of interest is a striking structural analogy between glucagon and the hormone *secretin,* suggesting a common genetic origin. The structure of human glucagon is identical to porcine and bovine glucagon and probably to the rat and rabbit hormone as well (Unger and Orci, 1976). Glucagon is synthesized *in vivo* as a prohormone (Noe *et al.*, 1977). The total chemical synthesis of glucagon has been accomplished (*see* Wunsch and Weinges, 1972).

Bioassay and Radioimmunoassay of Glucagon in Plasma. A number of bioassays for glucagon have been developed, based on the ability of the hormone to cause hyperglycemia *in vivo* or to stimulate cyclic AMP production, phosphorylase activity, or glucose production *in vitro*. With the advent of radioimmunoassay, this has become the most widely used method to determine the concentration of glucagon. The chief problem has been cross-reaction of antisera with a related peptide from the gastrointestinal tract—gut glucagon. Since it is becoming increasingly clear that pancreatic and gut glucagons differ chemically and biologically, it is of greatest importance to use specific antisera. The best current methodology yields values for basal plasma pancreatic glucagon concentrations in the range of 50 to 60 pg/ml

Regulation of Glucagon Secretion. Glucagon secretion, like that of insulin, is controlled by the interplay of gastrointestinal food products and hormones. Glucose is the most potent and important regulator. A rise in plasma glucose concentration leads to an inhibition of glucagon secretion and *vice versa* (*see* Unger and Orci, 1976). As with insulin secretion, glucose given orally is a more effective signal than glucose administered intravenously. A gastrointestinal signal is thus suggested, and, although the evidence is not complete, secretin may play an inhibitory role. Other gut hormones, including gastrin, pancreozymin-cholecystokinin, and gastric inhibitory polypeptide, stimulate the secretion of glucagon. The suppression of glucagon secretion by glucose is malfunctional in certain diabetic patients (*see* above). It is not clear whether this is a primary defect in the α cell or if it is secondary to β-cell failure and hyperglycemia.

In experimental animals, free fatty acids of various

$$
\begin{array}{c}
\overset{\displaystyle NH_2}{|}\\
H-His-Ser-Glu-Gly-Thr-Phe-Thr-Ser-Asp-Tyr-Ser-Lys-Tyr-Leu-Asp-
\end{array}
$$

$$
\begin{array}{c}
\quad\ \ \overset{\displaystyle NH_2}{|}\qquad\qquad \overset{\displaystyle NH_2}{|}\qquad\qquad \overset{\displaystyle NH_2}{|}\\
Ser-Arg-Arg-Ala-Glu-Asp-Phe-Val-Glu-Tyr-Leu-Met-Asp-Thr-OH
\end{array}
$$

Figure 64–3. *The structure of glucagon.*

chain lengths and ketones suppress glucagon secretion in a manner analogous to that of glucose; the effects are opposite to those on insulin secretion.

Of the three primary energy sources, amino acids have a unique effect. Their administration leads to an immediate rise in the concentrations of *both* glucagon and insulin in plasma. It has been argued teleologically that the purpose is to promote gluconeogenesis in the liver. This sugar can then replace that which disappears from the plasma as a result of insulin secretion and action, thus preventing hypoglycemia. If sufficient glucose is administered with amino acids to prevent hypoglycemia, enhanced glucagon secretion is not observed. As in the case of glucose, oral amino acids appear to be more potent secretagogues for glucagon than do those given intravenously. The stimulatory gastrointestinal hormones listed above may again play an important role (*see* Unger and Orci, 1976).

Glucagon secretion is also controlled by autonomic neural mechanisms; both sympathetic nerve stimulation and sympathomimetic amines, including levodopa, enhance the secretion of the hormone. Conflicting data have accumulated on the effects of acetylcholine.

Distribution and Inactivation. Pancreatic glucagon circulating in plasma is the same as that extracted from the organ, although a fraction of the immunoreactive material in plasma is contained in a biologically inactive fraction of higher molecular weight (Kuku *et al.,* 1976). Glucagon is extensively degraded in the liver and kidney, as well as in plasma, and at its tissue receptor sites in plasma membranes (Pohl *et al.,* 1972). Its half-life in plasma is approximately 3 to 6 minutes, which is similar to that of insulin (Alberti and Nattrass, 1977). Enzymatic destruction of glucagon is by proteolysis, and the removal of the amino-terminal histidine leads to loss of biological activity. Cathepsin C inactivates the hormone, as does a proteolytic enzyme purified from rat skeletal muscle that acts on both insulin and glucagon (Duckworth and Kitabchi, 1974)

Physiological and Pharmacological Actions. The hormonal role of glucagon is now well established, and, in general, its actions are antagonistic to those of insulin. Insulin serves as a hormone of fuel storage, while glucagon serves as a hormone of fuel mobilization. Following a meal, β-cell secretion of insulin and suppression of α-cell secretion of glucagon serve to store fuels in liver, muscle, and adipose tissue. Conversely, during starvation, stimulation of glucagon secretion and suppression of insulin secretion direct the breakdown of fuels stored intracellularly to meet the energy needs of the brain and other tissues. A related role for glucagon as the hormone of injury and insult (catabolic illness) has been proposed. For example, impaired glucose tolerance and hyperglycemia

noted with infection are associated with increased concentrations of plasma glucagon (Rayfield *et al.,* 1973). Similar increases are seen in patients with burns and after major trauma (Thorner and Bloom, 1974). Here, glucagon acts to stimulate gluconeogenesis and provide the glucose needed under conditions of insult.

The known actions of glucagon appear to result from stimulation of the synthesis of cyclic AMP. This is particularly true in liver and adipose tissue, and its metabolic effects at these sites are essentially the same as those of epinephrine (*see* Chapter 4). It is worth noting that studies of the mechanism of the hyperglycemic action of glucagon and epinephrine led to the discovery of cyclic AMP (Rall and Sutherland, 1958). In high concentrations, glucagon has a positive cardiac inotropic effect, also perhaps related to its ability to stimulate the synthesis of the cyclic nucleotide in the heart.

Therapeutic Use and Preparations. Glucagon hydrochloride is useful in the treatment of insulin-induced hypoglycemia when dextrose solution is not available. It may be given intravenously, intramuscularly, or subcutaneously in a dose of 1 mg. When it is given subcutaneously for hypoglycemic coma induced by either insulin or oral hypoglycemic agents, a return to consciousness should be observed within 20 minutes; otherwise, intravenous glucose must be administered as soon as possible. Failure of glucagon to relieve the coma may be due to irreversible brain damage as a consequence of prolonged hypoglycemia or due to marked depletion of glycogen stores in the liver. Nausea and vomiting have been the most frequent adverse effects.

Clinical investigations have been conducted to explore the use of large doses of glucagon in cardiac disorders as an inotropic and chronotropic agent. Unfortunately, it is not very effective. The hormone has also been used experimentally in the diagnosis and treatment of hypoglycemic disorders and as a stimulus for growth hormone secretion (Galloway, 1972). Although the mechanism is unclear, glucagon is also used to relax the intestines for x-ray visualization (Bertrand *et al.,* 1977).

Glucagon for Injection, U.S.P., the hydrochloride of glucagon, is dispensed as a dry powder in 1- or 10-mg ampuls, packaged with sufficient diluent to make a 1-mg/ml solution.

Miscellaneous Hyperglycemic Agents. *Diazoxide,* a nondiuretic thiazide with antihypertensive activity (*see* Chapter 32), causes hyperglycemia. This effect is usually transitory (maximum of 8 hours) and is apparently due to both decreased insulin secretion and decreased peripheral utilization of glucose (*see* Altszuler *et al.,* 1977). Diazoxide appears to exert α-adrenergic-like actions on the islet β cell (Culbert *et al.,* 1974), and it also stimulates the release of endogenous catecholamines. Propranolol may potentiate the action of diazoxide, while α-adrenergic blocking agents and sulfonylureas can overcome its effect. The drug may be used to control hypoglycemia, including that caused by insulin-secreting islet-cell tumors (Balsam *et al.,* 1972). *Streptozotocin* has sometimes been employed concurrently (Harell *et al.,* 1972). *Diazoxide* (PROGLYCEM) is available in 50- and 100-mg capsules and in an oral suspension (50 mg/ml). The usual daily dose for adults and children is 3 to 8 mg/kg, divided into two or three equal portions; for neonates and infants, the usual daily dose is 8 to 15 mg/kg. *Phenytoin* can induce hyperglycemia in man and in experimental animals (Levin *et al.,* 1970). The drug inhibits the secretion of insulin, possibly by an effect to decrease intracellular Na^+ (Kizer *et al.,* 1970); it has been used to ameliorate hypoglycemia due to insulin-secreting tumors in adults and children (Hofeldt *et al.,* 1974).

Abel, J. J. Crystalline insulin. *Proc. Natl. Acad. Sci. U.S.A.,* **1926,** 12, 132–136.

Aikawa, J. K. Effect of glucose and insulin on magnesium metabolism in rabbits. A study with Mg^{28}. *Proc. Soc. Exp. Biol. Med.,* **1960,** 103, 363–366.

Alberti, K. G. M. M., and Nattrass, M. The physiological function of glucagon. (Editorial.) *Eur. J. Clin. Invest.,* **1977,** 7, 151–154.

Altszuler, N.; Hampshire, J.; and Morarv, E. On the mechanism of diazoxide-induced hyperglycemia. *Diabetes,* **1977,** 26, 931–935.

Avruch, J.; Witters, L. A.; Alexander, M. C.; and Bush, M. A. Effects of glucagon and insulin on cytoplasmic protein phosphorylation of hepatocytes. *J. Biol. Chem.,* **1978,** 253, 4754–4761.

Balsam, M. J.; Baker, L.; Bishop, H. C.; Hummeler, K.; Yakovac, W. C.; and Kaye, R. Beta cell adenoma in a child with hypoglycemia controlled with diazoxide. *J. Pediatr.,* **1972,** 80, 788–795.

Banting, F. G.; Best, C. H.; Collip, J. B.; Campbell, W. R.; and Fletcher, A. A. Pancreatic extracts in the treatment of diabetes mellitus. *Can. Med. Assoc. J.,* **1922,** 12, 141–146.

Benjamin, W. B., and Singer, I. Actions of insulin, epinephrine, and dibutyryl cyclic adenosine 5'-monophosphate on fat cell protein phosphorylations. Cyclic adenosine 5'-monophosphate dependent and independent mechanisms. *Biochemistry,* **1975,** 14, 3301–3309.

Bertrand, G.; Linscheer, W. G.; Raheja, K. L.; and Woods, R. E. Double blind evaluation of glucagon and propantheline bromide (PRO-BANTHINE) for hypotonic duodenography. *Am. J. Roentgenol.,* **1977,** 128, 197–200.

Bornstein, J. Biological actions of synthetic part sequences of human growth hormone. *Trends Biochem. Sci.,* **1978,** 3, 83–86.

Bromer, W. W.; Sinn, L. G.; Staub, A.; and Behrens, O. K. The amino acid sequence of glucagon. *J. Am. Chem. Soc.,* **1956,** 78, 3858–3860.

Brooker, G., and Fichman, M. Chlorpropamide and tolbutamide inhibition of adenosine 3',5' cyclic monophosphate phosphodiesterase. *Biochem. Biophys. Res. Commun.,* **1971,** 42, 824–828.

Brown, J. D.; Steele, A. A.; Stone, D. B.; and Steele, F. A. The effect of tolbutamide on lipolysis and cyclic AMP concentration in white fat cells. *Endocrinology,* **1972,** 90, 47–59.

Buchanan, K. D. Gut and islet hormones in diabetes. *Postgrad. Med. J.,* **1973,** 49, 117–121.

Burman, K. D.; Cunningham, E. H.; Klachko, D. M.; and

Burns, T. W. Successful treatment of insulin resistance with dealaninated pork insulin (DPI). *Mo. Med.,* **1973,** 70, 363–366.

Chalmers, T. C. Settling the UGDP controversy. *J.A.M.A.,* **1975,** 231, 624–625.

Chan, S. J.; Keim, P.; and Steiner, D. F. Cell-free synthesis of rat preproinsulins: characterization and partial amino acid sequence determination. *Proc. Natl. Acad. Sci. U.S.A.,* **1976,** 73, 1964–1968.

Charles, M. A.; Fanska, R.; Schmid, F. G.; Forsham, P. A.; and Grodsky, G. M. Adenosine 3',5'-monophosphate in pancreatic islets: glucose-induced insulin release. *Science,* **1973,** 179, 569–571.

Committee on the Use of Therapeutic Agents of the American Diabetes Association. U100 insulin: a new era in diabetes mellitus therapy. *Diabetes,* **1972,** 21, 832.

Cuatrecasas, P. Insulin receptor of liver and fat cell membranes. *Fed. Proc.,* **1973,** 32, 1838–1846.

Culbert, S.; Sharp, R.; Rogers, M.; Felts, P.; and Burr, I. M. Diazoxide modification of streptozotocin-induced diabetes in rats. *Diabetes,* **1974,** 23, 282–286.

Davidson, J. K., and DeBra, D. W. Immunologic insulin resistance. *Diabetes,* **1978,** 27, 307–318.

Devis, G.; Somers, G.; and Malaisse, W. J. Dynamics of calcium-induced insulin release. *Diabetologia,* **1977,** 13, 531–536.

Dieterle, P.; Birkner, B.; Gmeiner, K.-H.; Wagner, P.; Erhardt, F.; Henner, J.; and Dieterle, C. Release of peripherally stored insulin during acute muscular work in man. *Horm. Metab. Res.,* **1973,** 5, 316–322.

Duckworth, W. C., and Kitabchi, A. E. Insulin and glucagon degradation by the same enzyme. *Diabetes,* **1974,** 23, 536–543.

Duckworth, W. C.; Stentz, F. B.; Heinemann, M.; and Kitabchi, A. E. Initial site of insulin cleavage by insulin protease. *Proc. Natl. Acad. Sci. U.S.A.,* **1979,** 76, 635–639.

Editorial. Beta blockers for diabetics. *Lancet,* **1977,** 1, 843.

Editorial. Policy statement: the UGDP controversy. *Diabetes Care,* **1979,** 2, 1.

Evans, R. B.; Morhenn, V.; Jones, A. L.; and Tomkins, G. M. Concomitant effects of insulin on surface membrane conformation and polysome profiles of serum-starved BALB-C 3T3 fibroblasts. *J. Cell Biol.,* **1974,** 61, 95–106.

Fain, J. N.; Rosenthal, J. W.; and Ward, W. F. Antilipolytic action of tolbutamide on brown fat cells. *Endocrinology,* **1972,** 90, 52–59.

Feinstein, A. R. Clinical biostatistic 36. The persistent biometric problems of the UGDP study. *Clin. Pharmacol. Ther.,* **1976,** 19, 472–485.

Goeddel, D. V.; Kleid, D. G.; Bolivar, F.; Heyneker, H. L.; Yansura, D. G.; Crea, R.; Hirose, T.; Kraszewski, A.; Itakura, K.; and Riggs, A. D. Expression in *Escherichia coli* of chemically synthesized genes for human insulin. *Proc. Natl. Acad. Sci. U.S.A.,* **1979,** 76, 106–110.

Goldfine, I. D.; Roth, J.; and Birnbaumer, L. Glucagon receptors in β-cells. *J. Biol. Chem.,* **1972,** 247, 1211–1218.

Hagedorn, H. C.; Jensen, B. N.; Krarup, N. B.; and Wodstrup, I. Protamine insulinate. *J.A.M.A.,* **1936,** 106, 177–180.

Hardie, D. G., and Cohen, P. The regulation of fatty acid biosynthesis: simple procedure for the purification of acetyl CoA carboxylase from lactating rabbit mammary gland and its phosphorylation by endogenous cyclic AMP dependent and independent protein kinase activities. *FEBS Lett.,* **1978,** 91, 1–7.

Harell, A.; Laurian, L.; Ayalon, D.; Kisch, E.; and Cordova, T. Hypoglycemia due to hyperinsulinism treated by streptozotocin and diazoxide. *Isr. J. Med. Sci.,* **1972,** 8, 895–896.

Havrankova, J.; Schmechel, D.; Roth, J.; and Brownstein, M. Identification of insulin in rat brain. *Proc. Natl. Acad. Sci. U.S.A.,* **1978,** 75, 5737–5741.

Hellman, B.; Sehlin, J.; and Taljedal, I.-B. The pancreatic

β-cell recognition of insulin secretogogues. II. Site of action of tolbutamide. *Biochem. Biophys. Res. Commun.,* **1971,** *45,* 1384–1388.

———. Ionic effects on the uptake of sulfonylurea (glibenclamide) by pancreatic islets. *Horm. Metab. Res.,* **1976,** *8,* 427–429.

Hershko, A.; Mamont, P.; Shields, R.; and Tomkins, G. M. Pleiotypic response. *Nature [New Biol.],* **1971,** *232,* 206–211.

Hofeldt, F. D.; Dippe, S. E.; Levin, S. R.; Karam, J. H.; Blum, M. R.; and Forsham, P. H. Effects of diphenylhydantoin upon glucose-induced insulin secretion in three patients with insulinoma. *Diabetes,* **1974,** *23,* 192–198.

Hollenberg, C. H. The effect of incubation on the characteristics of the lipolytic activity of rat adipose tissue. *Can. J. Biochem. Physiol.,* **1962,** *40,* 703–707

Houssay, B. A. The hypophysis and metabolism. *N. Engl. J. Med.,* **1936a,** *214,* 961–971.

———. Carbohydrate metabolism. *Ibid.,* **1936b,** *214,* 971–982.

Hsu, C.-Y.; Brooker, G.; Peach, M. J.; and Westfall, T. C. Inhibition of catecholamine release by tolbutamide and other sulfonylureas. *Science,* **1975,** *187,* 1086–1087.

Huttunen, J. K.; Steinberg, D.; and Mayer, S. E. Protein kinase activation and phosphorylation of a purified hormone-sensitive lipase. *Biochem. Biophys. Res. Commun.,* **1970,** *41,* 1350–1356.

Jacobs, S.; Shechter, Y.; Bissell, K.; and Cuatrecasas, P. Purification and properties of insulin receptors from rat liver membranes. *Biochem. Biophys. Res. Commun.,* **1977,** *77,* 981–988.

Janbon, M.; Chaptal, J.; Vedel, A.; and Schaap, J. Accidents hypoglycemiques graves par un sulfamidothiadiazol (le VK57 ou 2254RP). *Montpell. Méd.,* **1942,** *21–22,* 441–444.

Jefferson, L. S.; Exton, J. H.; Butcher, R. W.; Sutherland, E. W.; and Park, C. R. Role of adenosine 3′,5′-monophosphate in the effects of insulin and anti-insulin serum on liver metabolism. *J. Biol. Chem.,* **1968,** *243,* 1031–1038.

Johnson, D. G.; Fujimoto, W. Y.; and Williams, R. H. Enhanced release of insulin by prostaglandins in isolated pancreatic islets. *Diabetes,* **1973,** *22,* 658–663.

Katsoyannis, P. G.; Tometsko, A.; and Fukuda, K. Insulin peptides IX: the synthesis of the A-chain of insulin and its combination with natural B-chain to generate insulin activity. *J. Am. Chem. Soc.,* **1963,** *85,* 2863–2865.

Kilo, C.; Williamson, J. R.; Choi, S. C.; and Miller, J. P. Insulin treatment and diabetic vascular complications. *J.A.M.A.,* **1979,** *241,* 26–27.

Kipnis, D. M. Nutrient regulation of insulin secretion in human subjects. *Diabetes,* **1971,** *21,* Suppl. 2, 606–616.

Kizer, S.; Vargas-Cordon, M.; Brendel, K.; and Bressler, R. Studies on the mechanism of diphenylhydantoin-induced inhibition of insulin secretion. *J. Clin. Invest.,* **1970,** *49,* 52a.

Knatterud, G. L.; Meinert, C. L.; Klimt, C. R.; Osborne, R. K.; and Martin, D. B. Effects of hypoglycemic agents on vascular complications in patients with adult-onset diabetes. *J.A.M.A.,* **1971,** *217,* 777–784.

Koivisto, V. A., and Felig, P. Effects of leg exercise on insulin absorption in diabetic patients. *N. Engl. J. Med.,* **1978,** *298,* 79–83.

Kolata, G. B. Controversy over study of diabetes drugs continues for nearly a decade. *Science,* **1979,** *203,* 986–990.

Kono, T. Destruction of insulin effector systems of adipose tissue cells by proteolytic enzymes. *J. Biol. Chem.,* **1969,** *244,* 1772–1778.

Krahl, M. E. Insulin action at the molecular level; facts and speculations. *Diabetes,* **1972,** *21,* 695–702.

Kuku, S. F.; Jaspan, J. B.; Emmanouel, D. S.; Zeidler, A.; Katz, A. I.; and Rubenstein, A. H. Heterogeneity of plasma glucagon. Circulating components in normal

subjects and patients with chronic renal failure. *J. Clin. Invest.,* **1976,** *58,* 742–750.

Kuo, W.-N.; Hodgins, D. S.; and Kuo, J. F. Adenylate cyclase in islets of Langerhans: isolation of islets and regulation of adenylate cyclase activity by various hormones and agents. *J. Biol. Chem.,* **1972,** *248,* 2705–2711.

Lasseter, K. C.; Levey, G. S.; Palmer, R. F.; and McCarthey, J. S. The effect of sulonylurea drugs on rabbit myocardial contractility, canine Purkinje fiber automaticity and adenyl cyclase activity from rabbit and human hearts. *J. Clin. Invest.,* **1972,** *51,* 2429–2434.

Lawrence, J. C., and Larner, J. Activation of glycogen synthase in rat adipocytes by insulin and glucose involves increased glucose transport and phosphorylation. *J. Biol. Chem.,* **1978,** *253,* 2104–2113.

Lawrence, J. C.; Larner, J.; Kahn, C. R.; and Roth, J. Autoantibodies to the insulin receptor activate glycogen synthase in rat adipocytes. *Mol. Cell. Biochem.,* **1978,** *22,* 153–157.

Lebovitz, H. E., and Feinglos, M. N. Sulfonylurea drugs: mechanism of antidiabetic action and therapeutic usefulness. *Diabetes Care,* **1978,** *1,* 189–198.

Leichter, S. B., and Poffenbarger, P. L. The effects of nonsuppressible insulin-like protein (NSILP) on cyclic nucleotide metabolism in rat liver. *Biochem. Biophys. Res. Commun.,* **1978,** *84,* 403–410.

Levey, G. S.; Prindle, K. H., Jr.; and Epstein, S. E. Effects of glucagon on adenyl cyclase activity in the left and right ventricles and liver in experimentally-produced isolated right ventricular failure. *J. Mol. Cell. Cardiol.,* **1970,** *1,* 403–410.

Levin, S. R.; Booker, J., Jr.; Smith, D. F.; and Grodsky, G. M. Inhibition of insulin secretion by dipenylhydantoin in the isolated perfused pancreas. *J. Clin. Endocrinol. Metab.,* **1970,** *30,* 400–401.

Levine, R.; Goldstein, M.; Klein, S.; and Huddlestun, B. The action of insulin on the distribution of galactose in eviscerated nephrectomized dogs. *J. Biol. Chem.,* **1949,** *179,* 985–986.

Long, C. N. H., and Lukens, F. D. W. The effects of adrenalectomy and hypophysectomy upon experimental diabetes in the cat. *J. Exp. Med.,* **1936,** *63,* 465–490.

Lostroh, A. J., and Krahl, M. E. Synthetic fragment of human growth hormone with hyperglycemic properties: residues 44–77. *Diabetes,* **1978,** *27,* 597–598.

Loubatières, A. The hypoglycemic sulfonamides: history and development of the problem from 1942 to 1955. *Ann. N.Y. Acad. Sci.,* **1957,** *71,* 4–11.

Louis, L. H.; Conn, J. W.; and Minick, M. C. A diabetogenic polypeptide from bovine adenohypophysis similar to that excreted in lipoatrophic diabetes. *Metabolism,* **1966,** *15,* 309–324.

Lundsgaard, E. On mode of action of insulin. *Ups. Läkför. Förh.,* **1939,** *45,* 143–152.

McIntyre, N.; Holdsworth, C. D.; and Turner, D. S. New interpretation of oral glucose tolerance. *Lancet,* **1964,** *2,* 20–21.

McKinley, I., and Farquar, J. W. Use of 100 units/ml insulin in treatment of diabetic children. *Arch. Dis. Child.,* **1976,** *51,* 796–798.

Magner, L. N. Ernest Lyman Scott's work with insulin: a reappraisal. *Pharm. Hist.,* **1977,** *19,* 103–108.

Malaisse, W. J.; Van Obberghen, E.; Devis, G.; Somers, G.; and Ravazzola, M. Dynamics of insulin release and microtubular-microfilamentous system. *Eur. J. Clin. Invest.,* **1974,** *4,* 313–318.

Manchester, K. L. Effect of insulin on protein synthesis. *Diabetes,* **1972,** *21,* Suppl. 2, 447–452.

Marks, V., and Samols, E. Intestinal factors in the regulation of insulin secretion. *Adv. Metab. Disord.,* **1970,** *4,* 1–38.

Marshall, A.; Gingerich, R. L.; and Wright, P. H. Hepatic effect of sulfonylureas. *Metabolism,* **1970,** *19,* 1046–1052.

Meienhofer, J.; Schnabel, E.; Brinkoff, O.; Zabel, R.; Sroka, W.; Klostermeyer, H.; Brandenburg, D.; Okuda, T.; and Zahn, H. Synthese der Insulin Ketten und ihre Kombination zu Insulin-aktiven Präparaten. *Z. Naturforsch.* [C], **1963**, *18b*, 1120.

Miller, T. B., and Larner, J. Anti-insulin actions of a bovine pituitary diabetogenic peptide on glycogen synthesis. *Proc. Natl. Acad. Sci. U.S.A.*, **1972**, *69*, 2774-2777.

Morgan, H. E.; Jefferson, L. S.; Wolpert, E. B.; and Rannels, D. E. Regulation of protein synthesis in heart muscle. *J. Biol. Chem.*, **1971**, *246*, 2163-2170.

Mortimore, G. E., and Mondon, C. E. Inhibition by insulin of valine turnover in liver. Evidence for a general control of proteolysis. *J. Biol. Chem.*, **1970**, *245*, 2375-2383.

Murlin, J. E.; Clough, H. D.; Gibbs, C. B. F.; and Stakes, A. M. Aqueous extracts of pancreas. I. Influence on the carbohydrate metabolism of depancreatized animals. *J. Biol. Chem.*, **1923**, *56*, 253-296.

Naber, S. P.; McDaniel, M. L.; and Lacy, P. E. The effect of glucose on the acute uptake and efflux of calcium-45 in isolated rat islets. *Endocrinology*, **1977**, *101*, 686-693.

Noe, B. D.; Baste, C. A.; and Bauer, G. E. Studies on proinsulin and proglucagon biosynthesis and conversion at the subcellular level. *J. Cell Biol.*, **1977**, *74*, 589-604.

O'Donovan, C. J. Analysis of long-term experience with tolbutamide (ORINASE) in the management of diabetes. *Curr. Ther. Res.*, **1959**, *1*, 69-87.

Orci, L.; Baetens, D.; Ravazzola, M.; Stefan, Y.; and Malaisse-Lagae, F. Pancreatic polypeptide and glucagon: non-random distribution in pancreatic islets. *Life Sci.*, **1976**, *19*, 1811-1816.

Owen, O. E.; Morgan, A. P.; Kemp, H. G.; Sullivan, J. M.; Herrera, M. G.; and Cahill, G. F., Jr. Brain metabolism during fasting. *J. Clin. Invest.*, **1967**, *46*, 1589-1595.

Park, C. R.; Bornstein, J.; and Post, R. L. Effect of insulin on free glucose content of rat diaphragm *in vitro*. *Am. J. Physiol.*, **1955**, *182*, 12-16.

Paulesco, N. C. Action de l'extrait pancréatique injecté dans le sang, chez un animal diabétique. *C. R. Soc. Biol.* (*Paris*), **1921**, *85*, 555-557.

Peavy, D. E.; Taylor, J. M.; and Jefferson, L. S. Correlation of albumin production rates and albumin in RNA levels in livers of normal, diabetic and insulin-treated diabetic rats. *Proc. Natl. Acad. Sci. U.S.A.*, **1978**, *75*, 5879-5883.

Pohl, S. L.; Michiel, H.; Krans, J.; Birnbaumer, L.; and Rodbell, M. Inactivation of glucagon by plasma membranes of rat liver. *J. Biol. Chem.*, **1972**, *247*, 2295-2301.

Rall, T. W., and Sutherland, F. W. Formation of a cyclic adenine ribonucleotide by tissue particles. *J. Biol. Chem.*, **1958**, *232*, 1065-1076.

Raskin, P., and Unger, R. H. Effect of insulin therapy on the profiles of plasma immunoreactive glucagon in juvenile-type and adult-type diabetes. *Diabetes*, **1978**, *27*, 411-419.

Rastogi, G. K.; Sinha, M. K.; and Dash, R. J. Insulin and proinsulin content of pancreases from diabetic and nondiabetic subjects. *Diabetes*, **1973**, *22*, 804-807.

Rayfield, E. J.; Curnow, R. T.; George, D. T.; and Beisel, W. R. Impaired carbohydrate metabolism during a mild viral illness. *N. Engl. J. Med.*, **1973**, *289*, 618-620.

Reaven, G. M.; Olefsky, J.; and Farquhar, J. W. Does hyperglycaemia or hyperinsulinaemia characterize the patient with chemical diabetes? *Lancet*, **1972**, *1*, 1247-1249.

Report of the Committee for the Assessment of Biometric Aspects of Controlled Trials of Hypoglycemic Agents. *J.A.M.A.*, **1975**, *231*, 583-608.

Rerup, C. C. Drugs producing diabetes through damage of the insulin secreting cells. *Pharmacol. Rev.*, **1970**, *22*, 485-518.

Rinderknecht, L. E., and Humbel, R. E. Amino-terminal sequences of two polypeptides from human serum with nonsuppressible insulin-like and cell-growth-promoting activities: evidence for structural homology with insulin B chain. *Proc. Natl. Acad. Sci. U.S.A.*, **1976**, *73*, 4379-4381.

Robertson, R. P., and Chen, M. A role for prostaglandin E in defective insulin secretion and carbohydrate intolerance in diabetes mellitus. *J. Clin. Invest.*, **1977**, *60*, 747-753.

Robertson, R. P., and Porte, D., Jr. The glucose receptor. A defective mechanism in diabetes mellitus distinct from the beta adrenergic receptor. *J. Clin. Invest.*, **1973**, *52*, 870-876.

Rosenbloom, A. L. Advances in commercial insulin preparations. *Am. J. Dis. Child.*, **1974**, *128*, 631-633.

Rossini, A. A.; Soeldner, J. S.; Hiebert, J. M.; Weir, G. C.; and Gleason, R. E. The effect of glucose anomers upon insulin and glucagon secretion. *Diabetologia*, **1974**, *10*, 795-799.

Ruttenberg, M. A. Human insulin: facile synthesis by modification of porcine insulin. *Science*, **1972**, *177*, 623-626.

Sando, H., and Grodsky, G. M. Dynamic synthesis and release of insulin and proinsulin from perfused islets. *Diabetes*, **1973**, *22*, 354-360.

Sanger, F. Chemistry of insulin. *Br. Med. Bull.*, **1960**, *16*, 183-188.

Schlessinger, J.; Schechter, Y.; Willingham, M. C.; and Pastan, I. Direct visualization of binding, aggregation, and internalization of insulin and epidermal growth factor on living fibroblastic cells. *Proc. Natl. Acad. Sci. U.S.A.*, **1978**, *75*, 2659-2663.

Schoenle, E.; Zapf, J.; and Froesch, E. R. Effects of insulin and NSILA on adipocytes of normal and diabetic rats: receptor binding, glucose transport and glucose metabolism. *Diabetologia*, **1977**, *13*, 243-249.

Seltzer, H. S. Drug-induced hypoglycemia. A review based on 473 cases. *Diabetes*, **1972**, *21*, 955-966.

Shanahan, M. F., and Czech, M. P. Purification and reconstitution of the adipocyte plasma membrane D-glucose transport system. *J. Biol. Chem.*, **1977**, *252*, 8341-8343.

Solomon, S. S.; Palazzo, M.; and King, L. F., Jr. Cyclic nucleotide phosphodiesterase: insulin activation detected in adipose tissue by gel electrophoresis. *Diabetes*, **1977**, *26*, 967-972.

Sonksen, P. H.; Judd, S. L.; and Lowry, C. Home monitoring of blood-glucose, method for improving diabetic control. *Lancet*, **1978**, *1*, 729-732.

Staub, A.; Sinn, L.; and Behrens, O. K. Purification and crystallization of glucagon. *J. Biol. Chem.*, **1955**, *214*, 619-632.

Steinberg, D.; Mayer, S. E.; Khoo, J. C.; Miller, E. A.; Miller, R. E.; Fredholm, B.; and Eichner, R. Hormonal regulation of lipase, phosphorylase, and glycogen synthase in adipose tissue. *Adv. Cyclic Nucleotide Res.*, **1975**, *5*, 549-568.

Steiner, D. F. Insulin today. *Diabetes*, **1977**, *26*, 322-340.

Sugden, M. C., and Ashcroft, S. J. H. Phosphoenolpyruvate in rat pancreatic islets: a possible intracellular trigger. *Diabetologia*, **1977**, *13*, 481-486.

Sussman, K. E.; Crout, J. R.; and Marble, A. Failure of warning in insulin-induced hypoglycemic reactions. *Diabetes*, **1963**, *12*, 38-45.

Szabo, O., and Szabo, A. Studies on the nature and mode of action of the insulin-sensitive glucoregulator receptor in the central nervous system. *Diabetes*, **1975**, *24*, 328-336.

Terris, S., and Steiner, D. F. Binding and degradation of ^{125}I-insulin by rat hepatocytes. *J. Biol. Chem.*, **1975**, *250*, 8389-8398.

Thorner, M. O., and Bloom, S. R. Rapid glucagon release in artificial fever. *Lancet*, **1974**, *2*, 654.

University Group Diabetes Program. A study of the effects

of hypoglycemic agents on vascular complications in patients with adult-onset diabetes. *Diabetes,* **1970,** *19,* Suppl. 2, 747–830.

———. Supplementary report on nonfatal events in patients treated with tolbutamide. *Ibid.,* **1976,** *25,* Suppl. 6, 1129–1153.

Varandani, P. T. Urinary excretion of insulin A chain by normal and diabetic subjects. *Diabetes,* **1970,** *19,* 98–101.

Varandani, P. T., and Nafz, M. A. Insulin degradation XVIII: on the regulation of glutathione-insulin transhydrogenase in the hyperglycemic obese (ob/ob) mouse. *Biochim. Biophys. Acta,* **1976,** *451,* 382–392.

Walford, S.; Glae, E. A. M.; Allison, S. P.; and Tattersall, R. B. Self-monitoring of blood-glucose, improvement of diabetic control. *Lancet,* **1978,** *1,* 732–735.

Weaver, D. C.; McDaniel, M. L.; Naber, S. P.; Barry, C. D.; and Lacy, P. E. Alloxan stimulation and inhibition of insulin release from isolated rat islets of Langerhans. *Diabetes,* **1978,** *27,* 1205–1214.

Wentworth, S. M.; Galloway, J. A.; Davidson, J. A.; Root, M. A.; Chance, R. E.; and Haunz, E. A. An update of results of the use of "single peak" (SP) and "single component" (SC) insulin in patients with complications of insulin therapy. *Diabetes,* **1976,** *25,* 326.

Wray, H. L., and Harris, A. W. Adenosine 3′,5′-monophosphate-dependent protein kinase in adipose tissue: inhibition by tolbutamide. *Biochem. Biophys. Res. Commun.,* **1973,** *53,* 291–294.

Yalow, R. S., and Berson, S. A. Immunoassay of endogenous plasma insulin in man. *J. Clin. Invest.,* **1960,** *39,* 1157–1175.

Yoon, J. W.; Austin, M.; Onodera, T.; and Notkins, A. L. Virus-induced diabetes mellitus: isolation of a virus from the pancreas of a child with diabetic ketoacidosis. *N. Engl. J. Med.,* **1979,** *300,* 1173–1179.

Yoon, J. W.; Lesniak, M. A.; Fussganger, E.; and Notkins, A. L. Genetic differences in susceptibility of pancreatic β cells to virus-induced diabetes mellitus. *Nature,* **1976,** *264,* 178–180.

Young, F. G. Permanent experimental diabetes produced by pituitary (anterior lobe) injections. *Lancet,* **1937,** *2,* 372–374.

Zawalich, W. S., and Matschinsky, F. M. Sequential analysis of the releasing and fuel function of glucose in isolated perfused pancreatic islets. *Endocrinology,* **1977,** *100,* 1–8.

Monographs and Reviews

Alberti, K. G. M. M., and Hockaday, T. D. R. Diabetic coma: a reappraisal after five years. *Clin. Endocrinol. Metab.,* **1977,** *6,* 421–455.

Albisser, A. M., and Leibel, B. S. The artificial pancreas. *Clin. Endocrinol. Metab.,* **1977,** *6,* 457–479.

Arieff, A. I., and Carroll, H. U. Nonketotic coma with hyperglycemia. *Medicine (Baltimore),* **1972,** *51,* 73–94.

Bar, R. S., and Roth, J. Insulin receptor status in disease states in man. *Arch. Intern. Med.,* **1977,** *137,* 474–481.

Best, C. H. *Selected Papers of Charles H. Best.* University of Toronto Press, Toronto, **1963.**

Bloom, S. R., and Grossman, M. I. (eds.). *Gut Hormones.* Churchill-Livingstone, Ltd., Edinburgh, **1978.**

Bloom, S. R.; West, A. M.; Polak, J. M.; Barnes, A. J.; and Adrian, T. E. Hormonal contaminants of insulin. In, *Gut Hormones.* (Bloom, S. R., and Grossman, M. I., eds.) Churchill-Livingstone, Ltd., Edinburgh, **1978,** pp. 318–322.

Brown, J. C., and Otte, S. C. Gastrointestinal hormones and the control of insulin secretion. *Diabetes,* **1978,** *27,* 782–787.

Cahill, G. F., Jr. Diabetes mellitus: a brief overview. *Johns Hopkins Med. J.,* **1978,** *143,* 155–159.

Cerasi, E. Insulin secretion: mechanism of the stimulation by glucose. *Q. Rev. Biophys.,* **1975,** *8,* 1–41.

Chance, R. E.; Root, M. A.; and Galloway, J. A. The immunogenicity of insulin preparations. *Acta Endocrinol. (Kbh.),* **1976,** *205,* 185–196.

Chochinov, R. H., and Daughaday, W. H. Current concepts of somatomedin and other biologically related growth factors. *Diabetes,* **1976,** *25,* 994–1004.

Clements, R. S., Jr., and Vourganti, B. Fatal diabetic ketoacidosis: major causes and approaches to their prevention. *Diabetes Care,* **1978,** *1,* 314–325.

Galloway, J. A. The pharmacology and clinical use of glucagon. In, *Glucagon: Molecular Physiology, Clinical and Therapeutic Implications.* (Lefebvre, P. J., and Unger, R. H., eds.) Pergamon Press, Ltd., Oxford, **1972,** pp. 299–318.

Gepts, W., and DeMey, J. Islet cell survival determined by morphology. *Diabetes,* **1978,** *27,* Suppl. 1, 251–261.

Gerich, J. E. Somatostatin: its possible role in carbohydrate homeostasis and the treatment of diabetes mellitus. *Arch. Intern. Med.,* **1977,** *137,* 659–666.

Hedeskov, C. J. Mechanism of glucose-induced insulin secretion. *Physiol. Rev.,* **1980,** *60,* 442–509.

Hepp, K. D. Studies on the mechanism of insulin action: basic concepts and clinical implications. *Diabetologia,* **1977,** *13,* 177–186.

Herberg, L., and Coleman, D. L. Laboratory animals exhibiting obesity and diabetes syndromes. *Metabolism,* **1977,** *26,* 59–99.

Hodgkin, D. C., and Mercola, D. The secondary and tertiary structure of insulin. In, *Endocrine Pancreas,* Vol. 1. Sect. 7, *Endocrinology. Handbook of Physiology.* (Steiner, D. F., and Freinkel, N., eds.) American Physiological Society, Washington, D. C., **1972,** pp. 139–157.

Humbel, R. E.; Bosshard, H. R.; and Zahn, H. Chemistry of insulin. In, *Endocrine Pancreas,* Vol. 1. Sect. 7, *Endocrinology. Handbook of Physiology.* (Steiner, D. F., and Freinkel, N., eds.) American Physiological Society, Washington, D. C., **1972,** pp. 111–132.

Kreisberg, R. A. Diabetic ketoacidosis: new concepts and trends in pathogenesis and treatment. *Ann. Intern. Med.,* **1978,** *88,* 681–695.

Larner, J.; Lawrence, J. C.; Roach, P. J.; DePaoli-Roach, A. A.; Walkenbach, R. J.; and Guinovart, J. About insulin and glycogen. In, *Cold Spring Harbor Symposium on Cell Proliferation.* Cold Spring Harbor, N.Y., **1979,** pp. 95–112.

MacLaren, N. K. Viral and immunological bases of beta cell failure in insulin-dependent diabetes. *Am. J. Dis. Child.,* **1977,** *131,* 1149–1154.

Miller, E. J. Comparison of basement membrane collagens with interstitial collagens. In, *Biology and Chemistry of Basement Membranes.* (Kefalides, N. A., ed.) Academic Press, Inc., New York, **1978,** 265–278.

Morgan, H. E.; Rannels, D. E.; Wolpert, E. B.; Giger, K. E.; Robertson, J. W.; and Jefferson, L. S. Effect of insulin on protein turnover in heart and skeletal muscle. In, *Insulin Action.* (Fritz, I. B., ed.) Academic Press, Inc., New York, **1972,** pp. 437–449.

Oelz, O.; Froesch, E. R.; Bunzli, H. R.; Humbel, R. E.; and Ritschard, W. J. Antibody-suppressible and non-suppressible insulin-like activities. In, *Endocrine Pancreas,* Vol. 1. Sect. 7, *Endocrinology. Handbook of Physiology.* (Steiner, D. F., and Freinkel, N., eds.) American Physiological Society, Washington, D. C., **1972,** pp. 685–702.

Olefsky, J. M. The insulin receptor: its role in insulin resistance of obesity and diabetes. *Diabetes,* **1976,** *25,* 1154–1162.

Orci, L. The microanatomy of the islets of Langerhans. *Metabolism,* **1976,** *25,* Suppl. 1, 1303–1313.

Ostlund, R. E., Jr. Contractile proteins and pancreatic beta-cell secretion. *Diabetes,* **1977,** *26,* 245–252.

Peck, F. B. Therapy: insulin types. In, *Diabetes Mellitus: Diagnosis and Treatment.* (Danowski, T. S., ed.) American Diabetes Association, Inc., New York, **1964,** pp. 83–86.

Peterson, C. M., and Jones, R. L.   Minor hemoglobins, diabetic "control" and diseases of postsynthetic protein modification. *Ann. Intern. Med.,* **1977,** *87,* 489–491.

Pyke, D. A.   Genetics of diabetes. *Clin. Endocrinol. Metab.,* **1977,** *6,* 285–303.

Randle, P. J.   Phosphorylation and dephosphorylation of enzymes in the regulation of enzyme activity. In, *Polypeptide Hormones: Molecular and Cellular Aspects.* Ciba Foundation Symposium, Vol. 41. Elsevier/Excerpta Medica/North Holland, Amsterdam; **1976,** pp. 353–361.

Renold, A. E.; Mintz, D. H.; Muller, W. A.; and Cahill, G. F., Jr.   Diabetes mellitus. In, *Metabolic Basis of Inherited Disease,* 4th ed. (Stanbury, J. B.; Wyngaarden, J. B.; and Fredrickson, D. S.; eds.) McGraw-Hill Book Co., New York, **1978,** pp. 80–110.

Rubenstein, A. H.; Steiner, D. F.; Horwitz, D. L.; Mako, M. E.; Block, M. B.; Starr, J. I.; Kazuya, H.; and Melani, F.   Clinical significance of circulating proinsulin and C-peptide. *Recent Prog. Horm. Res.,* **1977,** *33,* 435–468.

Samols, E., and Harrison, J.   Tolbutamide: stimulator and suppressor of glucagon secretion. In, *Glucagon and Its Role in Physiology and Clinical Medicine.* (Foa, P. P.; Bajaj, J. S.; and Foa, N. L.; eds.) Springer-Verlag, Berlin, **1978,** pp. 699–710.

Schlichtkrull, J.; Pingel, M.; Heding, L. G.; Brange, J.; and Jorgensen, K. H.   Insulin preparations with prolonged effect. In, *Insulin.* (Dörzbach, H. E., ed.) *Handbuch der Experimentellen Pharmakologie,* Vol. 32. Springer-Verlag, Berlin, **1975,** pp. 729–777.

Smith, P. H.; Pork, D., Jr.; and Robertson, R. P.   Neural regulation of the endocrine pancreas. In, *Proceedings of the First International Symposium on the Endocrinology of the Pancreas and Diabetes.* (Pierluissi, J., ed.) Excerpta Medica International Congress Series. Elsevier Publishing Co., Amsterdam, **1979,** pp. 64–95.

Steiner, D. F.; Kemmler, W.; Clark, J. L.; Oyer, P. E.; and Rubenstein, A. H.   The biosynthesis of insulin. In, *Endocrine Pancreas,* Vol. 1. Sect. 7, *Endocrinology. Handbook of Physiology.* (Steiner, D. F., and Freinkel, N., eds.) American Physiological Society, Washington, D. C., **1972,** pp. 175–198.

Tattersall, R.   Brittle diabetes. *Clin. Endocrinol. Metab.,* **1977,** *6,* 403–419.

Unger, R. H., and Lefebvre, P. J.   Glucagon physiology. In, *Glucagon: Molecular Physiology, Clinical and Therapeutic Implications.* (Lefebvre, P. J., and Unger, R. H., eds.) Pergamon Press, Ltd., Oxford, **1972,** pp. 213–244.

Unger, R. H., and Orci, L.   Physiology and pathophysiology of glucagon. *Physiol. Rev.,* **1976,** *56,* 778–826.

———.   Possible roles of the pancreatic D-cell in the normal and diabetic states. *Diabetes,* **1977a,** *26,* 241–244.

———.   Role of glucagon in diabetes. *Arch. Intern. Med.,* **1977b,** *137,* 482–491.

Wool, I. G.; Castles, J. J.; Leader, D. P.; and Fox, A.   Insulin and the function of muscle ribosomes. In, *Endocrine Pancreas,* Vol. 1. Sect. 7, *Endocrinology. Handbook of Physiology.* (Steiner, D. F., and Freinkel, N., eds.) American Physiological Society, Washington, D. C., **1972,** pp. 385–394.

Wunsch, E., and Weinges, K. F.   The synthesis of glucagon. Properties of synthetic glucagon. In, *Glucagon: Molecular Physiology, Clinical and Therapeutic Implications.* (Lefebvre, P. J., and Unger, R. H., eds.) Pergamon Press, Ltd., Oxford, **1972,** pp. 31–46.

CHAPTER

65 AGENTS AFFECTING CALCIFICATION: CALCIUM, PARATHYROID HORMONE, CALCITONIN, VITAMIN D, AND OTHER COMPOUNDS

Robert C. Haynes, Jr., and Ferid Murad

CALCIUM

Calcium is the fifth most abundant element in the body, and the major portion is in bone. It is present in small quantities in the extracellular fluid and to a minor extent in the structure and cytoplasm of cells of soft tissue. Calcium plays important physiological roles, many of which are only poorly understood. It is essential for the functional integrity of nerve and muscle, where it has a major influence on excitability. It is necessary for cardiac function, for maintenance of the integrity of membranes, and for coagulation of the blood.

To carry out these various roles, ionized calcium must be available to the appropriate tissues in the proper concentration. As is the case for other essential constituents of the body, an endocrine control system has evolved that ordinarily keeps the plasma concentration of ionized calcium within narrow limits. This is accomplished in the case of calcium by placing controls at the site of entry of calcium into the system (intestinal absorption) and at a site of exit (the kidney), and by keeping a large store (the skeleton) accessible for deposits or withdrawals depending upon peripheral demand. Intracellular concentrations of ionized calcium are also strictly regulated, in part by control of the exchange of the ion between the cell and its environment.

This chapter will describe the roles of calcium and the three endocrine factors that control its metabolism: parathyroid hormone (PTH), calcitonin, and vitamin D. The actions of these hormones can be summarized as follows.

PTH is secreted in response to a fall in plasma calcium ion concentration, and the hormone acts to increase this concentration by accelerating transfer of calcium from the bone compartment, enhancing intestinal absorption of calcium, and increasing reabsorption of calcium by the kidney. In addition, PTH promotes phosphate excretion in the urine. The secretion of calcitonin can be stimulated by a rise in the concentration of calcium ion in plasma; the hormone may lower this concentration by decreasing calcium resorption from bone and by increasing the renal excretion of the ion. Vitamin D, now recognized as a hormone, stimulates intestinal absorption of calcium and phosphate and decreases their renal excretion; it also enhances resorption of bone.

Calcium Requirements and Body Stores. The calcium intake varies from 200 to 2500 mg per day, and, in the United States, the predominant source is dairy products. Calcium requirements are presented in Table XVI–1 (page 1553). The skeleton contains more than 90% of the calcium of the body. The inorganic salts of bone resemble the mineral hydroxyapatite $[Ca_{10}(PO_4)_6(OH)_2]$. Bone crystals are not pure, however, and contain additional ions in the crystal lattice and in association with the crystals. These include sodium, potassium, magnesium, carbonate, and fluoride (Raisz, 1977). The steady-state content of calcium in the skeleton is a consequence of the net effect of bone resorption and new-bone formation, and the calcium of bone is in a constant exchange with the calcium of the interstitial fluids. The rates of exchange are modifiable by drugs, hormones, vitamins, and other factors that may influence the level of calcium in the interstitial fluids and also the forms in which the cation is present.

The calcium in plasma is maintained at a fairly constant concentration of about 2.5 mM (5.0 mEq/l; 10 mg/dl). However, this represents the total of three different components: (1) about 40% of the plasma calcium is bound to proteins, primarily albumin; (2) about one tenth is diffusible but complexed with anions (*e.g.,* citrate and phosphate); (3) the remaining fraction represents diffusible ionic calcium. The ionized calcium is the fraction that exerts physiological effects, and symptoms of hypocalcemia occur with its reduction. It is clear that hypocalcemia due to hypoproteinemia and a reduced concentration of protein-bound calcium is not likely to be accompanied by the symptoms and signs of hypocalcemia, unless there is a reduction in the concentration of ionized calcium as well. Hence, the interpretation of the significance of any given value of plasma calcium is impossible without knowledge of the coincident concentration of plasma proteins, and nomograms are available for this purpose. As an approximation, an alteration in plasma albumin of 1 g/dl (from a normal value of 4.0 to 4.4 g/dl) can be expected to change total calcium by 0.8 mg/dl.

Absorption and Excretion. In general, the major portion of intestinal absorption takes place in the more proximal segments of the small bowel; in man, approximately one third of the ingested calcium is absorbed. Intestinal absorption involves the soluble ionized form of calcium and reflects at least two separate steps: (1) calcium uptake at the mucosal pole and (2) efflux at the serosal pole of the intestinal epithelium. Mucosal uptake of calcium is presumably carrier mediated, and a calcium-binding protein under study is a candidate for the transmucosal carrier. However, the role of this calcium-binding protein in transport has recently been questioned (*see* below).

The factors that clearly augment absorption of calcium—vitamin D and PTH—are discussed below. It is also generally accepted that a diet low in calcium results in increased fractional absorption of the ion.

Glucocorticoids and other factors depress calcium transport across the small intestine. For example, phytate, oxalate, and probably phosphate in the bowel promote the formation of a complex or insoluble salt of calcium that is not absorbed through the wall of the gut. Disease states such as steatorrhea may result in decreased absorption of calcium. Other diarrheas with chronic gastrointestinal malabsorption may promote increased fecal losses of calcium as well.

Calcium is secreted into the gastrointestinal tract in saliva, bile, and pancreatic juice. This endogenous calcium and the unabsorbed dietary calcium constitute the sources of the cation excreted in the feces. There is significant loss of calcium in milk during lactation, and also daily losses in sweat.

The *urinary excretion* of calcium is the net result of the quantity filtered and the amount reabsorbed. There is no evidence of renal tubular secretion of calcium. The mechanisms for the renal reabsorption of calcium are unknown, and for unexplained reasons there is, in general, a correlation between the urinary excretion of sodium and calcium. This is true when natriuresis is increased by loading with salt, and it also is noted with diuretics that act at the ascending limb of the loop of Henle and the distal tubule (Davis and Murdaugh, 1970).

In animal studies approximately two thirds of the filtered calcium is reabsorbed in the proximal convolution, 20 to 25% in the loop of Henle, and 10% in the distal convolution (Murayama *et al.,* 1972; Massry and Coburn, 1973).

PTH stimulates the reabsorption of calcium by the kidney apparently by means of an effect on the distal tubule, whereas the active metabolites of vitamin D stimulate proximal tubular reabsorption of calcium (Puschett *et al.,* 1972). Calcitonin inhibits the proximal tubular reabsorption of calcium, thus facilitating excretion of the cation (Paillard *et al.,* 1972).

The influence of renal disease on urinary calcium excretion is variable. In chronic renal failure due primarily to glomerular disease, calcium excretion diminishes as filtration rate falls. However, in those instances where filtration is only minimally depressed and the secretion of hydrogen ions is deficient due to an inability to attain a high concentration gradient for hydrogen ions between tubular cell and lumen (renal tubular acidosis), the excretion of calcium may be enhanced. This hypercalciuria may be diminished by the correction of the systemic acidosis.

PHYSIOLOGICAL AND PHARMACOLOGICAL ACTIONS

The cytoplasmic concentration of ionized calcium is normally maintained at very low values ($\sim$0.1 to 1 μM) by the extrusion of the ion from the cell and by its sequestration within cellular organelles, particularly mitochondria and, in muscle, sarcoplasmic reticulum. The provocative hypothesis has been offered that the need for such transport systems arose in evolution when cells accumulated high concentrations of phosphate for use in energy metabolism (*see* Kretsinger, 1976). (The solubility product of calcium phosphate is very low.) Given this high gradient of calcium, use can be made of the ion in mechanisms for transmembrane signaling. Thus, in response to various electrical or chemical stimuli, calcium influx across the plasma membrane or release from internal stores is triggered. This calcium interacts with high-affinity binding sites on specific intracellular proteins (such as troponin or calmodulin) and thereby regulates a number of functional and metabolic processes of the cell.

Local Actions.   Certain salts of calcium, notably the chloride, are intensely irritating to tissue and will cause painful sloughing if injected subcutaneously. Therefore, whenever calcium chloride is administered parenterally, it must be given intravenously and every effort should be made to prevent extravasation. Calcium chloride is also somewhat irritating to the gastrointestinal tract and is usually administered with a demulcent.

Neuromuscular System.   Moderate elevations of the concentration of calcium in the extracellular fluid may have no clinically detectable influences on the neuromuscular apparatus. However, when hypercalcemia becomes extreme, the threshold for excitation of nerve and muscle is increased. This is manifested clinically by muscle weakness, lethargy, and eventually coma. In contrast, modest diminution in the level of ionized calcium may decrease the thresholds of excitation in a striking fashion, leading to positive Chvostek and Trousseau signs and tetanic seizures. The role played by calcium in regulating the excitability of tissues is not completely elucidated. Calcium influx across the plasma membrane is thought to be by means of carrier-mediated facilitated diffusion and by exchange of calcium for sodium, which participates both in excitation and in the maintenance of the steady state. However, in nerve and skeletal muscle, the concentration of cytoplasmic ionic calcium is not controlled by cellular influx and efflux to nearly the same extent that it is by the mitochondria and sarcoplasmic reticulum, which sequester intracellular calcium. Calcium causes relatively small changes in resting membrane potentials but modifies the time-voltage relationships during the action potential in nerve and muscle. In addition, calcium appears to play an important role in the regulation of cell-membrane permeability to sodium and potassium. Increased concentrations of calcium diminish the permeability of the cell, while decreased calcium concentrations augment permeability.

Calcium plays additional roles both in coupling excitation with muscle contraction and in the release of neurohumoral transmitters. The action potential in muscle stimulates the release of calcium ions from the sarcoplasmic reticulum, and the divalent cation activates contraction. The binding of calcium to troponin abolishes the inhibitory effect of troponin on the interaction of actin and myosin. Muscle relaxation occurs when ionic sarcoplasmic calcium is pumped back into the sarcoplasmic reticulum, permitting the inhibitory effect of troponin on actin and myosin.

Calcium also plays an important role in stimulus-secretion coupling in most exocrine and endocrine glands. The release of catecholamines from the adrenal medulla, neurotransmitters at synapses, and autacoids from various sites is dependent on calcium ions. Calcium is necessary for exocytosis (Douglas, 1968).

There is an interesting interrelation between calcium and potassium. A potassium deficiency coincident with hypocalcemia appears to protect against hypocalcemic tetany. Correction of the potassium deficit without attention to the level of calcium may provoke tetany without a change in the concentration of calcium in plasma.

Cardiovascular System. It is probable that the above-described processes relating to nerve and skeletal muscle apply to cardiac muscle as well. In the myocardium, a slow inward current occurs during the plateau of the action potential and is dependent on ionic calcium (New and Trautwein, 1972). This slow channel probably carries inward calcium current and may initiate excitation-contraction coupling. It has long been recognized that there are certain similarities in the effect of calcium and the cardiac glycosides on cardiac muscle. This subject is discussed in Chapter 30.

Miscellaneous Effects. Calcium salts may play a role in maintaining the integrity of mucosal membranes, cell adhesion, and functions of individual cell membranes as well. The use of calcium salts to prevent effusions across capillary endothelial membranes is, however, without demonstrated benefit. Calcium is involved in blood coagulation, but the ion is not used to treat disorders of coagulation. Calcium chloride is an acidifying salt and will promote diuresis; however, ammonium salts are much more effective acidifying agents.

ABNORMALITIES OF CALCIUM METABOLISM

It should be clear from the discussion of some of the factors involved in maintaining calcium homeostasis that there are many ways in which significant alterations in calcium metabolism can occur. Some of these alterations may be accompanied by hypocalcemia and others by hypercalcemia.

Hypocalcemic States. The prominent signs and symptoms of hypocalcemia include tetany and related phenomena such as paresthesias, increased neuromuscular excitability, laryngospasm, muscle cramps, and convulsions (usually grand mal). The hypocalcemic states are as follows:
Deprivation of calcium and vitamin D may readily promote hypocalcemia. This combination of events is observed in the various malabsorption states and also occurs from inadequate diets. When due to malabsorption, the hypocalcemia is accompanied by a depressed level of phosphorus, the total proteins are usually low, and hypomagnesemia is common. During magnesium deficiency, hypocalcemia may be accentuated by diminished secretion and action of PTH (*see* below). In adults, hypocalcemia stimulates the release of PTH, which causes the mobilization of calcium from bone. This leads to demineralization, principally affecting the spine, rib cage, and long bones. In infants with malabsorption or inadequate calcium intake, the calcium concentration is usually depressed, there is hypophosphatemia, and the resultant bone disease is *rickets* (*see* section on vitamin D).

Hypoparathyroidism may occur spontaneously as a result of a genetic disorder or as a consequence of thyroid or other neck surgery. In these disorders there is distinct hypocalcemia but *hyper*phosphatemia. Although other conditions of hypocalcemia may be associated with opacity of the lens, papilledema, and calcification of the basal ganglia, these occur more commonly with hypoparathyroidism. Other changes include trophic alterations and fungal infections of the skin. Pseudohypoparathyroidism is probably a group of genetic diseases characterized by multiple structural defects and a failure to respond to exogenous PTH. The structural changes are manifested by a round face, short, thick figure, shortening of some of the metacarpal and metatarsal bones, and soft-tissue calcifications. As discussed below, at least one variety of this disease results from a deficiency of calcitriol (1,25-dihydroxycholecalciferol).

In the period (1 to 4 days) following *removal of a parathyroid adenoma,* hypocalcemia is not unusual, especially if there is bone disease.

Neonatal tetany may result from a temporary hypoparathyroidism that occurs in the newborn of mothers with hyperparathyroidism; indeed, it may be the infant's tetany that provides the clue to the mother's disorder. This is usually transient in the infant and disappears as soon as its own parathyroid glands respond appropriately. Other situations in which neonatal hypocalcemia may supervene include hypernatremia and acute infections.

Hypocalcemia is frequently associated with advanced *renal insufficiency accompanied by hyperphosphatemia.* For reasons that are not clear, many of these patients do not develop tetany unless the severe accompanying acidosis is improved with treatment. High concentrations of phosphate in plasma appear to inhibit the conversion of 25-hydroxycholecalciferol to 1,25-dihydroxycholecalciferol (Haussler and McCain, 1977).

Sodium fluoride forms an insoluble salt with calcium and, if ingested in large enough quantities, may induce hypocalcemia and tetany.

Hypocalcemia can also occur following massive *transfusions with citrated blood.*

Preparations and Routes of Administration in the Treatment of Hypocalcemia. There are several preparations available if the systemic action of calcium is desired. These differ in calcium content and permissible routes of administration.

Calcium Chloride, U.S.P. ($CaCl_2 \cdot 2H_2O$), contains 27% calcium and consists of white granules freely soluble in water. It is valuable in the treatment of hypocalcemic tetany. The salt can be given either by mouth or intravenously. *It must never be injected into tissues.* It is somewhat irritating to the gastrointestinal tract and should be administered in some demulcent vehicle, such as milk. It should never be given by gavage to infants, as necrosis and ulceration of the gastrointestinal tract may result. *Calcium*

Chloride Injection, U.S.P., is irritating to veins. Injections are accompanied by peripheral vasodilatation and a cutaneous burning sensation. The salt is usually given intravenously in a concentration of 5 to 10% (equivalent to 0.68 to 1.36 mEq Ca^{2+}/ml). Injection rate should be slow (not over 1 to 2 ml per minute) to prevent a high concentration of calcium from reaching the heart and causing syncope. A moderate fall in blood pressure due to vasodilatation may attend the injection. Since calcium chloride is an acidifying salt, it is usually undesirable in the treatment of the hypocalcemia caused by renal insufficiency.

Calcium Gluceptate Injection, U.S.P., is a 23% solution (18 mg or 0.9 mEq Ca^{2+}/ml) that is provided in 5-ml ampuls. It is administered intravenously in a dose of 5 to 20 ml (4.5 to 18 mEq Ca^{2+}) for the treatment of severe hypocalcemic tetany; the injection may produce a transient tingling sensation. When the intravenous route is not possible, the injection may be given intramuscularly in a dose up to 5 ml, which may produce a mild local reaction.

Calcium Gluconate, U.S.P. ($[CH_2OH\{CHOH\}_4$-$COO]_2Ca \cdot H_2O$), contains 9% calcium. It is available as *Calcium Gluconate Tablets,* U.S.P., containing 325, 500, 650, or 1000 mg of the salt (equivalent to 1.5, 2.3, 3.0, or 4.6 mEq Ca^{2+}, respectively). It is nonirritating to the gastrointestinal tract. For intramuscular and intravenous injection, *Calcium Gluconate Injection,* U.S.P., is administered as a 10% solution (0.45 mEq Ca^{2+}/ml). It is a readily available source of calcium ions, and the intravenous administration of this salt is the treatment of choice for severe hypocalcemic tetany. The intramuscular route should not be employed in infants, as abscess formation at the site of injection may result.

Calcium Lactate, U.S.P. ($[CH_3CHOHCOO]_2Ca \cdot 5H_2O$), contains 13% calcium. Its physical properties are similar to those of the gluconate. The official tablets are given by the oral route. In the treatment of tetany, its absorption is apparently enhanced by the simultaneous administration of lactose.

Precipitated Calcium Carbonate, U.S.P., is an insoluble, fine, white microcrystalline powder containing 40% calcium. Calcium carbonate is also available as *Calcium Carbonate Tablets,* U.S.P., containing 650 mg. After ingestion, it is converted to soluble calcium salts in the bowel, and calcium is thereby made available for absorption. Patients with achlorhydria may not solubilize calcium from this preparation. It is also used as an antacid.

Dibasic Calcium Phosphate, U.S.P., and *tribasic calcium phosphate,* although chiefly used as gastric antacids, are valuable sources of the calcium ion, especially when it is desired to supply both calcium and phosphorus. They are insoluble, tasteless white powders that must be given orally. *Calcium phosphate* is a mixture of normal, basic, and acidic calcium phosphate salts.

Calcium Levulinate, U.S.P., contains 13% calcium. It may be administered orally or parenterally. It is available in powder form or as a 10% solution (0.69 mEq Ca^{2+}/ml), as *Calcium Levulinate Injection,* U.S.P. It has a bitter, saline taste.

Other calcium preparations are described in connection with gastric antacids.

Therapeutic Uses. Calcium salts are specific in the immediate treatment of *low-calcium tetany* regardless of etiology. In severe manifest tetany, the symptoms are best brought under control by intravenous medication. Five to 20 ml of either 10% calcium gluconate or 23% calcium gluceptate solution is injected slowly. For the control of milder symptoms or latent tetany, oral medication suffices. Average doses are *calcium chloride,* 6 to 8 g daily in divided doses, best given in milk; *calcium gluconate,* 15 g daily in divided doses; *calcium lactate,* 4 g, plus lactose, 8 g, with each meal; *calcium carbonate* or *calcium phosphate,* 1 to 2 g with meals, as a watery suspension or sprinkled on food; and *calcium levulinate,* 4 to 5 g with each meal.

Hypercalcemic States. Hypercalcemia occurs in a number of diverse clinical conditions and requires differential diagnosis and appropriate corrective measures.

Ingestion of large quantities of a calcium salt is unlikely by itself to cause hypercalcemia except in patients who have hypothyroidism.

Hyperparathyroidism is classically associated with hypercalcemia accompanied by significant hypophosphatemia; the latter is due to the diminished ability of the renal tubules to reabsorb phosphorus, owing to the excessive quantities of PTH. Some patients have renal calculi and peptic ulceration, and a few have mental aberrations with psychotic components. In more advanced stages, characteristic bone lesions are present and the condition can be diagnosed by radiography.

Although very uncommon now, there is the hypercalcemic disorder known as the *milk-alkali syndrome,* caused by the ingestion of large quantities of milk and alkalinizing powders.

Vitamin D excess is a cause of hypercalcemia (*see* below).

Sarcoidosis is associated with about a 20% incidence of hypercalcemia. Increased intestinal absorption of calcium has been attributed to a hypersensitivity to vitamin D. Hypercalcemia peaks during summer months with increased exposure to sunlight.

Neoplasms with or without metastases to the bones may be accompanied by hypercalcemia. Some tumors secrete PTH-like peptides; others appear to secrete an osteoclast-stimulating factor; still others produce prostaglandins that stimulate bone resorption (Odell and Wolfsen, 1978). The hypercalcemia associated with these tumors is usually heralded by lethargy, weakness, nausea, and vomiting and not by renal stones or bone disease.

Occasionally, patients with *hyperthyroidism* have hypercalcemia. This is presumably due to an increased rate of bone resorption.

Disuse atrophy, as may occur when a patient must lie relatively immobile for a long period of time, may lead to hypercalcemia. This is most common after trauma that has involved large areas of the body and when extensive splinting with casts is necessary.

Idiopathic hypercalcemia of infants is an unusual disease of unknown etiology. There are many similarities to intoxication with vitamin D.

Hypercalcemia is uncommonly noted in *adreno-cortical deficiency states*, as in Addison's disease or during the period following operation for a hyperfunctioning tumor of the adrenal cortex or removal of bilateral hyperplastic adrenal glands.

Hypercalcemia occurs occasionally following successful *renal transplantation*. This is due to secondary hyperparathyroidism resulting from the previous chronic renal failure.

The *differential diagnosis* of the various causes of hypercalcemia may be difficult. In contrast to former belief, hypophosphatemia is quite common with hypercalcemia of origins other than hyperparathyroidism. Many cases of hypercalcemia are discovered as a result of routine determination of serum calcium. The differential diagnosis of hypercalcemia entails the use of many tests, none of which is completely conclusive. Immunoassay of parathyroid hormone in plasma is quite useful, but there are limitations (*see* below). The excretion of cyclic adenosine 3′,5′-monophosphate (cyclic AMP) in the urine is increased in hyperparathyroidism, and evaluation of this parameter can facilitate diagnosis. Renal reabsorption of filtered phosphate is diminished in hyperparathyroidism, and this measurement can also be of diagnostic value.

Hypercalcemia of any etiology can have dire consequences. The predominant and most devastating lesion usually occurs in the kidney with reduction of renal function. Pathological changes are prominent in the collecting ducts and distal tubules. Painful bone cysts, osteoporosis, and fractures may also occur if hypercalcemia is due to hyperparathyroidism.

There are occasions when hypercalcemia is in itself a life-threatening situation. The use of agents that augment the excretion of calcium, such as the administration of saline and diuretics, is the treatment of first choice. The employment of steroids to reduce hypercalcemia is of benefit in those situations where the hypercalcemia is a consequence of diseases such as sarcoid. Administration of calcitonin, mithramycin, or phosphate may be necessary and helpful (*see* below). The use of sodium phosphate intravenously, as described by Massry and coworkers (1968), is clearly effective in reducing the concentration of calcium in plasma. The mode of action is presumably by promoting the deposition of calcium in bone and decreasing bone resorption. Unfortunately, deposition of calcium in soft tissues is also common.

Preparations Used for the Reduction of Hypercalcemia. *Edetate Disodium*, U.S.P., is a chelating agent that forms soluble complexes with calcium. Chelation occurs in the blood and results in a rapid decrease in the concentration of ionized calcium in plasma before excretion of the complex occurs. Because of potential toxicities this agent is now used only rarely. Among the dangers of such therapy is the possibility that the concentration of calcium may be reduced too quickly and to hypocalcemic levels, thus resulting in tetany, convulsions, severe cardiac arrhythmias, and respiratory arrest. The slow intravenous administration of dilute solutions of the drug minimizes the risk of hypocalcemia. The chelator is usually dissolved in 500 ml of 0.9% saline solution or in 5% dextrose and water and administered intravenously (15 to 50 mg/kg) over a period of 4 hours. This procedure should be undertaken only when the severity of the hypercalcemia justifies the risk. The drug should be used with caution in patients with hypokalemia or congestive heart failure, and it is contraindicated in patients with significant renal disease.

Sodium phosphate has been employed intravenously in solutions prepared to contain 0.081 M Na_2HPO_4 and 0.019 M KH_2PO_4 (11.5 and 2.6 g per liter, respectively). Although hypercalcemia may be reduced, the hazards are significant in terms of extraskeletal precipitation of calcium phosphate salts.

Prednisone and other steroids with similar characteristics are capable of reducing hypercalcemic concentrations to normal values, particularly when the abnormality is a consequence of sarcoid. Patients with nonmetastatic carcinomas or hyperparathyroidism are less responsive. Frequently, large doses of 30 to 50 mg of prednisone a day may be necessary initially. The response to glucocorticoid therapy is slow, and 1 to 2 weeks may be required before a fall in serum calcium occurs. A low-calcium intake (virtual elimination of all milk and derivative dairy products) permits the use of the lowest dose of steroid possible to maintain normocalcemia. The complications of the chronic use of steroids must be recalled, and the osteoporosis that results with prolonged administration of glucocorticoid can limit the duration of therapy.

Mithramycin, U.S.P. (MITHRACIN), is a cytotoxic antibiotic that can be very useful in decreasing plasma calcium concentration in hypercalcemia (Perlia *et al.,* 1970). This agent probably acts directly on bone and blocks calcium resorption. Reduction in plasma calcium concentration occurs within 24 to 48 hours with low doses of this agent (one tenth the antineoplastic dose), and its toxicity is thus less severe (*see* Chapter 55).

Calcitonin (CALCIMAR) may be useful for the treatment of hypercalcemia (*see* below); its administration for this purpose is investigational.

Indomethacin, U.S.P. (INDOCIN) (*see* Chapter 29), can be valuable for the treatment of hypercalcemia that results from certain tumors that produce prostaglandins (Odell and Wolfsen, 1978). Its use in this condition is experimental.

PHOSPHATE

In addition to its roles as a dynamic constituent of intermediary and energy metabolism, it is well known that phosphate plays important roles in modifying concentrations of calcium in tissues. Furthermore, the acid-base equilibrium may be modified because phosphate ions are buffers of the intracellular fluid and also play a primary role in the renal excretion of hydrogen ion.

Absorption, Distribution, and Excretion. Phosphate is absorbed from, and to a limited extent secreted into, the gastrointestinal tract. The transport of phosphate from the lumen of the gut is an active, energy-dependent process, and there are factors that appear to modify the degree of its intestinal absorption. The presence of large quantities of calcium or aluminum may lead to the formation of large amounts of insoluble phosphate and may therefore diminish the net absorption of phosphate from the bowel. Vitamin D stimulates phosphate absorption, and this effect precedes the action of the vitamin on transport of calcium (Birge and Miller, 1977). In general, in adults, about two thirds of the ingested phosphate is absorbed from the bowel, and that which is absorbed from the gut is almost entirely excreted into the urine. In growing children, there is a positive balance of phosphate. Concentrations of phosphate in plasma are higher in children than in adults. This "hyperphosphatemia" decreases the affinity of hemoglobin for oxygen and is hypothesized to explain the physiological "anemia" of childhood (Card and Brain, 1973).

Phosphate is present in plasma and extracellular fluid, in cell membranes and intracellular fluid, and in collagen and bone tissue. In the extracellular fluid, phosphate is primarily in inorganic form and only a small component of esterified phosphate is present. Plasma phosphate concentration is inversely related to the rate of renal hydroxylation of 25-hydroxycholecalciferol. A reduction of the plasma phosphate concentration permits the presence of more calcium in the blood and inhibits deposition of new bone salt. An increased concentration of the phosphate anion in plasma facilitates the effect of calcitonin on deposition of calcium in bone (Werner et al., 1972). The concentration of plasma inorganic phosphate may vary with age, and the range has been recorded in great detail by Greenberg and coworkers (1960). The ratio of disodium phosphate and monosodium phosphate in extracellular fluid is 4:1 at a pH of 7.40. The buffer ratio varies, of course, with pH; however, owing to the relatively low concentration, phosphate contributes relatively little to buffering capacity of extracellular fluid. Cell phosphate plays a more important role in intracellular buffering owing to the quantities that are available.

The renal excretion of phosphate has been studied quite extensively. More than 90% of the phosphate in plasma is filterable, and the bulk is then actively reabsorbed by the initial segment of the proximal tubule. Phosphate reabsorption takes place to a smaller extent in the pars recta and/or the loop of Henle, in the distal convoluted tubule, and possibly in the collecting duct (Kuntziger et al., 1974; Lechene et al., 1978). Expansion of plasma volume causes increased urinary phosphate excretion (Steele, 1970). Phosphate excreted in the urine probably represents the net difference between the amount filtered and that reabsorbed. The occurrence of renal tubular secretion of phosphate is still debatable. Parathyroid hormone increases the urinary excretion of phosphate by blocking reabsorption in all segments proximal to the collecting duct (Lechene et al., 1978). Vitamin D_3 and its metabolites directly stimulate proximal tubular reabsorption of phosphate (Puschett et al., 1972).

Role of Phosphate in the Acidification of the Urine. The interrelations that exist between the rates of excretion of phosphate and titratable acid are referred to in Chapter 35 and in the Introduction to Section VIII. Although the concentration of phosphate is low in the extracellular fluid, the anion is progressively concentrated in the renal tubule and represents the most abundant buffer system in the distal tubule. At this site, the secretion of H^+ by the tubular cell in exchange for Na^+ in the tubular urine converts disodium hydrogen phosphate to sodium dihydrogen phosphate. In this manner, large amounts of acid can be excreted without lowering the pH of the urine to a degree that would block H^+ transport by a high concentration gradient between the tubular cell and luminal fluid.

Actions of the Phosphate Ion. Once phosphate gains access to the body fluids and tissues, it exerts little pharmacological effect. If the ion is introduced into the gastrointestinal tract, the absorbed phosphate is rapidly excreted. If large amounts are given by this route, much of it may escape absorption. This leads to a cathartic action, and, therefore, the phosphate salts are employed as mild laxatives. Inorganic phosphate poisoning following ingestion of laxatives that contain phosphate salts has been reported in adults and children (McConnell, 1971; Levitt et al., 1973). The ingestion of large amounts of sodium dihydrogen phosphate lowers the pH of the urine. If phosphate salts are introduced intravenously in high concentration, they may prove toxic. Toxicity results from reducing the concentration of Ca^{2+} in the circulation, and the symptoms are those of hypocalcemia.

Phosphate Depletion. There has been a question for some time concerning the possibility of clinical consequences of phosphate depletion. Familial hypophosphatemia is an X-linked dominant trait apparently due to defective intestinal absorption and/or renal reabsorption of inorganic phosphate that results in rickets and dwarfism. In a report by Lichtman and coworkers (1969), a patient with striking hypophosphatemia is described who had a significant depression in the steady-state concentration of erythrocyte adenosine triphosphate (ATP). Certain minimal concentrations of ATP are required for the viability of red cells in the circulation. In addition to reduced ATP, hypophosphatemia causes a marked decrease in concentrations of 2,3-diphosphoglycerate in erythrocytes. Acute hemolytic anemia and impaired oxygenation of tissues can occur in severe hypophosphatemia (Jacob and Amsden, 1971). This raises the possibility that other cellular stores of ATP and other critical organic phosphate compounds may be depleted. These biochemical abnormalities, in turn, could well be responsible for certain features of the clinical syndrome.

In general, the phosphorus present in ordinary foods is an adequate source of the ion. The use of expensive preparations of organic phosphates as "tonics" has no validity.

Pathological Conditions Associated with a Disturbance in Phosphate Metabolism. A defect in phosphate metabolism occurs in a variety of diseases, as briefly mentioned below.

Osteoporosis. This condition is considered to be a primary disorder in the formation of bone matrix. There is no primary defect in phosphate metabolism, and plasma concentrations of phosphorus are within usual limits.

Rickets. The consequences of deficiency of vitamin D with regard to the metabolism of both phosphate and calcium are described below, as are other forms of rickets. *Familial hypophosphatemia* is due to defective absorption and/or excretion of inorganic phosphate and has been mentioned above.

Osteomalacia. The loss of calcium in stools (due to malabsorption) or the loss from body fluids by way of the kidney (essential hypercalciuria or renal tubular acidosis with augmented calcium excretion) promotes a negative balance of calcium. Such loss deprives the body of calcium stores, and the calcium concentration in plasma falls slightly. This, in turn, stimulates the secretion of PTH, which restores the calcium concentration to normal but tends to promote some depression of plasma phosphorus.

Osteitis Fibrosa Cystica. In this disorder, there is a primary increase in the secretion of PTH that is usually accompanied by an increase in plasma calcium, some reduction of plasma phosphorus, and a decreased renal tubular reabsorption of phosphate.

Secondary Hyperparathyroidism. This condition may be seen in patients with chronic renal insuffi-

ciency. The sequence of events probably starts with a high plasma concentration of phosphorus and a low value for calcium; this situation stimulates parathyroid secretion. Since the elevated plasma phosphorus is a consequence of renal insufficiency, it persists. The continuing hyperphosphatemia may be modified by the administration of aluminum hydroxide gel, which tends to inhibit the absorption of phosphate from the bowel, owing to the formation of insoluble aluminum phosphates.

Hypoparathyroidism. In this disorder, characterized by deficient parathyroid secretion, there is a rise in plasma phosphorus and a decreased concentration of calcium. This condition can be readily treated with vitamin D.

Preparations. Only certain of the preparations of *inorganic phosphates* are mentioned here; *calcium phosphates* are described elsewhere.

Sodium Phosphate, U.S.P., is available as *Dried Sodium Phosphate,* U.S.P., and as *Effervescent Sodium Phosphate,* U.S.P. (a dry, effervescent powder). It is also available in combination with *Sodium Biphosphate,* U.S.P., as *Sodium Phosphates Oral Solution,* U.S.P., and *Sodium Phosphates Enema,* U.S.P. *Phosphoric Acid,* N.F., is a colorless, syrupy liquid that is prescribed in the form of *Diluted Phosphoric Acid,* N.F., a solution containing 10% phosphoric acid by weight; it should be further diluted before administration.

Therapeutic Uses. The phosphates are of limited therapeutic usefulness. Sodium phosphate has been employed to diminish hypercalcemia. The phosphates have a role in the management of the phosphate-depletion syndrome. Phosphate salts are also effective saline cathartics (*see* Chapter 43).

PARATHYROID HORMONE

History. Although there were many earlier references to the yellow glandular bodies attached to the thyroid, credit for the discovery of the parathyroid gland is usually given to Sandstrom, who in 1880 published an anatomical report that attracted little attention among physiologists. The glands were rediscovered by Gley (1891), who determined the effects of their extirpation with the thyroid. Vassale and Generali (1900) successfully removed the parathyroids without interfering with the thyroid and noted that tetany, convulsions, and death quickly followed. They thereby demonstrated that this syndrome was specifically due to parathyroid removal. However, the symptoms following parathyroidectomy varied so greatly in different species that the importance of the organs was not appreciated, and controversies continued as to whether they were essential to life. The subsequent discovery of internal and accessory parathyroids accounted for the discrepancies in experimental results and paved the way to the elucidation of the important physiological role played by this endocrine gland.

MacCallum and Voegtlin (1909) first noted the effect of parathyroidectomy on the concentration of plasma calcium. Since Howell (1899) and Loeb

(1901) had previously established the physiological importance of the calcium ion, the relation of low plasma calcium to parathyroprivic symptoms was quickly appreciated and a comprehensive picture of parathyroid function began to form. After various attempts to obtain active extracts of the gland, success was finally attained (Berman, 1924; Collip, 1925; Hanson, 1925). It was readily demonstrated that active extracts could alleviate hypocalcemic tetany in parathyroidectomized animals and raise the concentration of calcium in the plasma of normal animals. For the first time, the relation of certain definite clinical abnormalities to parathyroid hyperfunction was appreciated.

While investigators in the United States, Canada, and England were utilizing the physiological approach to solve the problem of the function of the parathyroid glands, German and Austrian pathologists were associating the skeletal changes of osteitis fibrosa cystica with the presence of parathyroid tumors. In a delightful historical review, Albright (1948) traced the manner in which these two diverse types of investigations finally arrived at the same conclusion.

Chemistry. Human, bovine, and porcine parathyroid hormones are all single polypeptide chains of 84 amino acid residues. Their molecular weights are approximately 9500, and the entire amino acid sequence has been established for each. Biological activity is particularly associated with the N-terminal portion of the peptide. Bovine and porcine PTH differ by only seven amino acid residues, and the amino-terminal segment of the human hormone differs from the equivalent portion of the bovine and porcine molecules by only four and three amino acid residues, respectively. The three differ little in biological activity, but they are immunologically distinguishable; however, they cross-react with a single antibody and this facilitates an immunoassay for PTH, as discussed below. The sequence comprised of the first 34 amino acids of human and bovine PTH has been synthesized and shown to have characteristic biological activity. (*See* Brewer *et al.,* 1974.)

Synthesis, Secretion, and Immunoassay. PTH is now known to be synthesized initially in a prehormone form. The product of translation that is destined to become PTH is called preproparathyroid hormone, an unfortunate name that grew by accretion in an adaptation to new knowledge of PTH synthesis. This single-chain peptide of 115 amino acids is rapidly converted to proparathyroid hormone by cleavage of a 25 amino-acid peptide fragment from the amino terminus. This reaction is thought to take place within the intracisternal space of the endoplasmic reticulum, and it has been postulated that the N-terminal peptide, which is strongly hydrophobic, functions in the transport of the nascent hormone into this space. The proparathyroid hormone, which persists somewhat longer than its precursor (15 to 20 minutes, compared to 1 to 2 minutes), moves to the Golgi apparatus and is converted to PTH, again by the cleavage of an N-terminal fragment of six predominantly basic amino acids. The PTH is enclosed within secretory granules, where it remains until released into the circulation. Neither preproparathyroid hormone nor proparathyroid hormone appears in plasma (Habener and Potts, 1978).

After secretion, PTH is cleaved further, notably between amino acid residues 33 and 34, into at least two major fragments; the site in the body of this reaction has not been established, but it may occur in the plasma. The larger fragment (molecular weight about 6000) from the carboxy terminus is biologically inactive but is reactive with antibody to the intact hormone. The biologically active fragment(s) unfortunately shows relatively poor immunoreactivity with such antibody. PTH fragments may also be secreted from the parathyroid glands after proteolysis of the hormone within the cells of the gland. Cleavage into small fragments also takes place, at least in part, in tissues such as liver and kidney.

Biological, chemical, and immunological heterogeneity of circulating "PTH" and fragments thereof obviously compounds the difficulties encountered in the immunoassay of plasma PTH, an important procedure in the evaluation of clinical disorders of bone and of calcium metabolism. Present immunoassays measure primarily biologically inactive fragments of PTH, but they are nevertheless useful for the diagnosis of parathyroid disease because the immunoreactive cleavage products are derived predominantly from intact secreted PTH. Antibodies made to smaller biologically active fragments of the human hormone should add considerably to the value of these assay technics, particularly because the half-life of the larger fragment may be considerably longer than that of the biologically active moiety (*see* DiBella *et al.,* 1978; Segre *et al.,* 1978; Yalow, 1978).

Physiological Functions. The primary function of PTH is to elicit adaptive changes that serve to maintain a constant concentration of calcium ion in the extracellular fluid. Processes that are regulated include the absorption of calcium from the gastrointestinal tract, the deposition of calcium in bone and its mobilization therefrom, and the excretion of the ion in urine, feces, sweat, and milk. There is evidence that PTH accomplishes its functions by directly or indirectly influencing all of these mechanisms, but its most prominent effect is to promote the mobilization of calcium from bone.

Regulation of Secretion. The concentration of ionized calcium in the blood (or, more likely, the concentration of ionized calcium in parathyroid cells) is the primary factor that regulates the secretory activity of the parathyroid gland. When the concentration of ionized calcium is low, the secretion of PTH is increased, and hypertrophy and hyperplasia of the gland result if the hypocalcemia is sustained. If the concentration of ionized calcium is high, the secretion of PTH is decreased, and hypoplasia may result if the hypercalcemia is sustained. *In-vitro* studies show that amino acid uptake, nucleic acid and protein synthesis, cytoplasmic growth, and secretion of PTH are stimulated by exposure to low concentrations of calcium and suppressed by exposure to high concentrations. Thus, the calcium ion *per se* appears to regulate growth of the parathyroid gland and its synthesis and secretion of hormone (Roth and Raisz, 1964). The mechanism by which calcium controls the biosynthesis of PTH is not known, but the regulated site does not appear to be the cleavage reactions required to convert preproparathyroid hormone to PTH. Degradation of PTH stored within the gland is stimulated by high concentrations of calcium and inhibited by low concentrations of the ion. This provides rapid adjustment of the rate of secretion of the hormone independently of slower changes in the rate of biosynthesis that are controlled by calcium (Habener and Potts, 1978).

Catecholamines may play a role in secretion of PTH. Both epinephrine (Fischer *et al.*, 1973) and dopamine (Brown *et al.*, 1977) can stimulate release of PTH. Calcitriol (*see* below) inhibits secretion of PTH, but whether this is a direct effect of this vitamin D analog or the result of increasd calcium in plasma is not certain (Haussler and McCain, 1977). There appears to be no direct relation between extracellular concentrations of phosphate and the secretion of PTH, except indirectly as changes in phosphate values affect the concentration of calcium. Both hypermagnesemia and hypomagnesemia can inhibit the secretion of PTH (Rude *et al.*, 1976).

Thus, the extracellular concentration of ionized calcium is controlled on a minute-to-minute basis by a feedback system, the afferent limb of which is sensitive to the concentration of calcium and the efferent limb of which releases PTH. The hormone acts on various peripheral tissues to mobilize calcium into the extracellular fluid and thus restores the concentration to normal (Arnaud, 1978).

Effects on Bone. PTH acts on bone to increase the rate of resorption of calcium and phosphate. The site of the resorptive effect appears to be on the stable, older portion of bone mineral and not on the labile fraction.

Resorption of bone is brought about by osteolytic cells—osteoclasts and osteocytes. PTH stimulates the rate of bone resorption by these cells, increases the rate of conversion (differentiation) of mesenchymal cells to osteoclasts, and prolongs the half-life of these latter cells. Twenty minutes after the administration of PTH to some species, activation of osteoclasts is evident by the appearance of ruffled borders on the cells adjacent to bone surfaces (Miller, 1978). With prolonged action of PTH the number of bone-forming osteoblasts is also increased; thus, the rate of bone turnover and remodeling is enhanced. However, individual osteoblasts appear to be less active than normal, and PTH acts to inhibit their synthesis of collagen, a major component of bone matrix.

Biochemical correlates of PTH action have also been studied extensively in bone cultures. PTH causes resorption of cultured bone, and a number of biochemical effects of PTH have been described. A difficulty with this approach is that bone resorption *per se* leads to biochemical changes that may have no relation to specific actions of PTH. PTH stimulates the release of collagenase and other hydrolytic enzymes into the culture medium, stimulates glycolysis, and inhibits the oxidation of citrate—responses that may only reflect the breakdown of bone. Consequently, no satisfactory hypothesis has yet been offered to explain the action of PTH at the biochemical level. Some effects that may be of fundamental importance to the action of PTH include activation of adenylate cyclase with resulting accumulation of cyclic AMP, increased entry of calcium into the cells, change in membrane potential of osteoclasts, and increased incorporation of uridine into osteoclast RNA. How these observations relate to the action of PTH in bone remains to be clarified (*see* Raisz, 1977).

Effects on the Kidney. PTH acts on the kidney to increase tubular reabsorption of calcium and to inhibit tubular reabsorption of phosphate. As a result, calcium is retained and its concentration tends to increase in the plasma; phosphate is excreted and the plasma concentration tends to fall.

Calcium. PTH increases tubular calcium reabsorption at a distal site (Agus *et al.*, 1973). Therefore, when the concentration of calcium in plasma is in the normal range, extirpation of the gland decreases tubular reabsorption of calcium and thereby increases calcium excretion in the urine. When the plasma concentration falls significantly (to less than 7 mg/dl), a decrease in calcium excretion occurs because the amount of calcium filtered through the glomeruli is lowered to the point that the cation is almost completely reabsorbed despite the reduced tubular reabsorptive capacity. However, when parathyroidectomized animals are kept on a high-calcium diet and plasma calcium remains higher than 7 mg/dl, the hypercalciuria persists. If PTH is administered to such hypoparathyroid animals or man, tubular reabsorption of calcium is increased and there is initially a decrease in the excretion of calcium. This, along with mobilization of calcium from bone and increased absorption from the gut, results in increased concentration of calcium in plasma. When the value rises above normal, the hypercalciuria so characteristic of hyperparathyroidism ensues.

Phosphate. It is now well established that PTH increases the renal excretion of inorganic phosphate. PTH decreases the reabsorption of phosphate in all or most segments of the nephron proximal to the collecting duct (Lechene *et al.*, 1978).

Cyclic AMP appears to mediate the effects of PTH on the kidney. Adenylate cyclase that stimulated by PTH is located in the renal cortex, and cyclic AMP synthesized in response to the hormone affects tubular transport mechanisms. A portion of the cyclic nucleotide synthesized at this site escapes into the urine, and its assay serves as a measure of parathyroid activity (*see* Chase *et al.*, 1969; *see also* below). Cyclic AMP may inhibit proximal tubular reabsorption of calcium, phosphate, bicarbonate, and sodium. The final effect on calcium excretion is, however, inhibitory, since it stimulates distal calcium reabsorption out of proportion to that of sodium (Agus *et al.*, 1973).

Other Ions. PTH also influences the excretion of other ions, most of which are constituents of bone. Renal excretion of magnesium is reduced by the hormone, and the plasma concentration is elevated; in parathyroidectomized animals, magnesium excretion is usually increased and the plasma concentration is reduced. The hormonal effect on magnesium is probably due, as in the case for calcium, to both increased renal tubular reabsorption of magnesium and its mobilization from the exchangeable compartment of bone (MacIntyre *et al.*, 1963). The excretion of water, amino acids, citrate, potassium, bicarbonate, sodium, chloride, and sulfate is increased, whereas the excretion of hydrogen ion is decreased by PTH. The increased excretion of bicarbonate ion appears to be mainly due to inhibition of proximal tubular reabsorption of this anion; it is antagonized by calcium. Although the effects of PTH on regulation of acid-base metabolism by the kidney are similar to those of acetazolamide, they are independent of the carbonic anhydrase system. The effects of PTH on other ions involve actions on both proximal and distal tubules.

Effects on the Gastrointestinal Tract. PTH acts indirectly to increase intestinal absorption of calcium and phosphate. This effect is now believed to be mediated entirely through the hormone's enhancement of the conversion of calcifediol to calcitriol in the kidney, and the effects of PTH on absorption are the consequence of increased concentrations of calcitriol (*see* section on vitamin D below).

Miscellaneous Effects. PTH decreases the concentration of calcium in milk and saliva. These effects are the opposite from those that would be expected from the concurrent changes in plasma calcium concentration. It appears likely, therefore, that the hormone can conserve calcium in the extracellular fluid not only by its effects on bone, kidney, and gut but also by reducing the rate of calcium transport from extracellular fluid to milk and saliva.

PTH also reduces the calcium concentration in the lens, a fact that explains the prevalence of cataracts in patients with hypoparathyroidism and the increased content of calcium in the lens in hormone-deficient animals.

Hypoparathyroidism. Extirpation or hypofunction of the parathyroids leads to a characteristic syndrome. Symptoms are the direct result of hypocalcemia and the consequent reduction in the threshold of excitability of polarized membranes. After removal of the parathyroids in dogs, appetite is gradually lost. Fine fibrillary twitchings of skeletal muscles develop and soon become coarser. The animal shows a characteristic awkward gait. Neuromuscular disturbance becomes progressively worse and culminates in convulsions, which may follow in rapid succession or occur at intervals of several days. Death follows respiratory failure, probably resulting from spasm of the muscles of the larynx and diaphragm.

Clinical Hypoparathyroidism. Hypoparathyroidism is only one of the many causes of hypocalcemia and occurs relatively rarely. The deficiency syndrome most commonly follows operative procedures on either the thyroid gland or the parathyroids themselves. Less frequently, disease of the parathyroids is the cause (*idiopathic hypoparathyroidism*). Also uncommon is a genetic disorder in which the target organs do not respond to PTH, despite adequate concentrations of the hormone (*pseudohypoparathyroidism*).

In all varieties of hypoparathyroidism, hypocalcemia and its associated symptoms are encountered clinically. The earliest prodromal symptoms of hypocalcemia are paresthesias in the extremities. Mechanical stimulation of peripheral nerves during physical examination usually produces contraction of the appropriate skeletal muscles. These signs and symptoms may be followed by manifest tetany, consisting in muscle spasms, especially carpopedal spasm and laryngospasm. Eventually, generalized convulsions and other central nervous system (CNS) manifestations occur. It is highly probable that smooth muscle is also affected. For example, hypocalcemia may be followed by spasm of the ciliary muscle, iris, esophagus, intestine, urinary bladder, and bronchi. ECG changes and a marked tachycardia indicate that the heart is involved. Vascular spasm in the fingers and toes is also commonly observed. In *chronic hypoparathyroidism,* ectodermal changes, consisting in loss of hair, grooved and brittle fingernails, defects of the dental enamel, and cataracts, are frequently encountered; there is also calcification in the basal ganglia and perhaps other soft tissues. Psychiatric symptoms such as emotional lability, anxiety, depression, and delusions are often present. The EEG may be abnormal (*see* Rasmussen, 1974).

Hypoparathyroidism is treated primarily with vitamin D (*see* below). Dietary supplementation with calcium may also be necessary.

Hyperparathyroidism. The administration of PTH to an experimental animal can cause the changes in blood chemistry that are characteristic of hyperparathyroidism. The concentration of calcium in the plasma increases markedly, reaching values as high as 18 to 20 mg/dl (4.5 to 5.0 mM) in 12 to 18 hours. This is accompanied by a variable decrease in the concentration of plasma phosphate. Chronic administration of the hormone leads to decalcification of bone and the development of bone cysts, deformities, and spontaneous fractures. The calcium mobilized from bone is precipitated in the soft tissues. Metastatic calcification is observed especially in the kidney, the wall of the stomach, the bronchi, the interstitial connective tissue, the heart muscle, and the tunica media of the smaller arteries. The animals exhibit anorexia, vomiting, diarrhea, and muscle atony. They die eventually as a result of renal insufficiency due to diffuse nephrocalcinosis and nephrolithiasis.

Clinical Hyperparathyroidism. *Primary hyperparathyroidism* results either from hypersecretion of the parathyroid glands (due to hyperplasia, adenoma, or, rarely, carcinoma) or from secretion of PTH-like polypeptides from tumors arising at other sites. In some cases such polypeptides may be distinguished from PTH by immunological technics. Plasma calcium concentrations may be normal with primary hyperparathyroidism, but they are usually elevated and plasma phosphate values are usually decreased. Hyperparathyroidism may also be *secondary* to conditions causing negative calcium balance, such as malabsorption and renal disease; in these cases the concentration of calcium in plasma is low and provides the stimulus for increased secretion of PTH. Hypersecretion of PTH from any cause may lead to a bone disorder known as *osteitis fibrosa generalisata.* However, only one third of cases of hyperparathyroidism exhibit advanced bone changes; another third show minor degrees of decalcification; and the remaining cases present no obvious skeletal abnormalities. However, metabolic studies indicate that resorption of bone is actively occurring in the last-named group; the calcium intake may be sufficient to maintain calcium balance. The symptoms of early decalcification are aching and pain in the bones and joints.

Uncomplicated primary hyperparathyroidism is invariably associated with hypercalciuria and hyperphosphaturia, and is sometimes accompanied by polyuria and polydipsia. The excretion of excessive amounts of calcium and phosphate results in a high incidence of renal calculi, which often cause the presenting symptoms. An equally serious complication is a diffuse nephrocalcinosis, which may progress to a stage of extreme renal insufficiency. It is well to keep in mind that renal insufficiency secondary to nephrocalcinosis or to sequelae of urolithiasis may mask some of the cardinal biochemical features of hyperparathyroidism, namely, hyperphosphaturia, hypercalciuria, and hypophosphatemia.

Hypercalcemia *per se* can be the cause of some of the signs and symptoms of hyperparathyroidism. These include hypotonicity of muscle, with general skeletal muscle weakness and smooth muscle dysfunction leading to constipation, flatulence, anorexia, nausea, and vomiting. Occasionally, cardiac irregularities are observed. A higher-than-normal incidence of peptic ulcers and pancreatitis has been reported in patients with the disease. Neuropsychiatric manifestations also occur in many cases. Advanced cases of osteitis fibrosa generalisata may exhibit anemia and leukopenia.

In addition to laboratory study of calcium and phosphorus, there are certain more specific tests for hyperparathyroidism. The most widely used is the radioimmunoassay of PTH in plasma. However, as discussed above, this test is dependent on the preparation of antibody used. Another method involves determination of the concentration of cyclic AMP in urine, which is elevated by the action of PTH on the kidney (Murad and Pak, 1972).

Treatment. Surgical resection of the hyperplastic or adenomatous glands is almost always required for the treatment of primary hyperparathyroidism. Surgery can return the patient to a euparathyroid state and prevent continued renal damage and bone dissolution. As discussed earlier, transient hypocalcemia often occurs following surgery, particularly when bone disease is present; this requires brief therapy with calcium. If an excessive amount of parathyroid tissue is removed, permanent hypoparathyroidism may ensue. In this case vitamin D therapy and/or supplementation of the diet with calcium is required. Chronic treatment with oral neutral phosphate, a low-calcium diet, and liberal amounts of fluids is used to lower the plasma calcium concentration in selected patients in whom surgery is contraindicated (Purnell *et al.,* in Symposium, 1974). (For details of clinical hyperparathyroidism and its classification, diagnosis, and treatment, *see* Rasmussen and Bordier, 1974; Symposium, 1974.)

Preparations, Bioassay, and Unitage. *Parathyroid Injection,* U.S.P., is made from bovine parathyroid glands. Bioassay to determine its activity is performed on healthy mature dogs. One unit of hormone is $\frac{1}{100}$ the amount necessary to raise the concentration of calcium in plasma 1 mg/dl within 16 to 18 hours after subcutaneous injection. Preparations are adjusted to contain approximately 100 units/ml. Bioassays for the hormone based on immunochemical procedures have been developed, as described above (*see* Symposium, 1974). Some batches of commercial parathyroid extract also contain a hypocalcemic factor, probably calcitonin (*see* below; *see also* Copp, 1964). *Synthetic parathyroid hormone* (bovine) is also available for investigational purposes as the (1-34 amino acid) tetratriacontapeptide in 5-ml bottles, 1000 to 1200 units in each.

Absorption, Fate, and Excretion. PTH must be given parenterally. The usual route of administration is subcutaneous or intravenous. The maximal effect is obtained approximately 18 hours after a single subcutaneous injection; the response may last for 36 hours. The peak effect of hormone given intravenously is seen considerably sooner. Studies in animals with radioiodinated PTH and with the endogenous hormone bioassayed by the immunological method demonstrate that its half-life in the body is about 20 minutes, a value considerably shorter than previously thought. The hormone appears to be transported in the blood, at least in part, in the α-globulin fraction of plasma protein. Excretion in the urine is minimal (less than 1%). The sites of degradation of PTH are still unknown, but they appear to include both the kidney and liver.

Clinical Uses. There are currently no valid therapeutic uses of PTH; while it was formerly employed to elevate the concentration of calcium in plasma, this can be accomplished with greater safety by the administration of calcium and/or vitamin D.

PTH is used for the *diagnosis* of pseudohypoparathyroidism. Since this disease is characterized by target-organ resistance to the hormone, these patients fail to show an increased concentration of calcium in plasma and fail to excrete increased amounts of phosphate and cyclic AMP after the administration of PTH (200 units, intravenously) (*see* Chase *et al.,* 1969).

CALCITONIN

History and Source. A hypocalcemic hormone, the effects of which are generally opposite to those of the parathyroid hormone, was discovered and named *calcitonin* by Copp in 1962 (*see* Copp, 1964). It was demonstrated as a result of perfusion of dogs' parathyroid and thyroid glands with hypercalcemic blood. This caused an immediate transitory hypocalcemic effect in the systemic blood that occurred significantly earlier than does the hypocalcemia observed after total parathyroidectomy. The observations led Copp to conclude that the parathyroid glands secreted calcitonin in response to hypercalcemia and in this way reduced the elevated plasma calcium concentration to normal. Munson and colleagues (Hirsch *et al.,* 1963) noted that parathyroid-

ectomy in rats performed by cauterization caused more severe hypocalcemia than did thyroparathyroidectomy. They thus suspected the existence of a hypocalcemic principle in the thyroid gland. They found that extracts of thyroid produced a hypocalcemic response and named the thyroid factor *thyrocalcitonin*. It is now known that the two factors are the same and that the hormone does originate from the thyroid; however, calcitonin is the name that is generally used.

The parafollicular "C" cells from the thyroid, which are embryologically derived from the ultimobranchial body, are the site of production and secretion of calcitonin. In nonmammalian vertebrates, calcitonin is found only in ultimobranchial bodies, which are separate organs from the thyroid gland. The hormone from both sources, thyroid and ultimobranchial bodies, is the same. In man, calcitonin is present in the thyroid, parathyroid, and thymus, an indication that the "C" cells are widely distributed.

Chemistry and Immunoreactivity. The calcitonins from the thyroid of the pig and a number of other species, including salmon and man, have been isolated, characterized chemically, and totally synthesized. They are all single-chain polypeptides with a molecular weight of 3600, and contain 32 amino acids. A cystine disulfide bridge exists in the 1-7 position at the amino end of the chain; it is essential for biological activity. The carboxyl-terminal amino acid is prolinamide. Calcitonin isolated from human "C"-cell tumors differs from the porcine hormone in 18 of its amino acid residues. Thus, the immunoassay of human tissues and fluids based on antibodies to porcine material has been unreliable because of poor cross-reactivity. However, specific radioimmunoassay for the human hormone has now been developed with calcitonin derived from medullary carcinoma of the human thyroid as the antigen (*see* Tashjian *et al.,* 1974).

Regulation of Secretion. The secretion and biosynthesis of calcitonin in both animals and man are regulated by the concentration of calcium in plasma. When the calcium concentration is high, the amount of the hormone in plasma increases. When the concentration is low, the amount of the hormone decreases markedly and may be undetectable. Normal basal concentrations of calcitonin in plasma as measured by the radioimmunoassay method are <100 pg/ml in more than 75% of subjects. Calcium infusion increases the basal concentration twofold to threefold (Tashjian *et al.,* 1974). The mean concentration of calcitonin in the plasma of women is significantly lower than in men and is less responsive to hypercalcemia (Heath and Sizemore, 1977). The half-life of calcitonin is short (about 10 minutes);

hence the hormone most likely is secreted at a fairly continuous rate at normal plasma calcium concentrations. A role of cyclic AMP in the release of calcitonin from "C" cells of the thyroid is indicated by the fact that the dibutyryl derivative of cyclic AMP, epinephrine, and glucagon stimulate its release, as do gastrin and cholecystokinin. The effects of the gastrointestinal hormones could constitute a mechanism for regulation of calcitonin secretion following the ingestion of calcium salts (Deftos, 1978).

While it is clear that calcitonin secretion can be modulated by several different agents under experimental conditions, it is not known to what extent normal physiological variations in secretion occur or if calcitonin plays a significant role in calcium homeostasis. High concentrations of calcitonin have been found in plasma, urine, and tumor tissue (50 to 5000 times normal) in patients with medullary carcinoma of the thyroid gland. The tumor cells originate from the parafollicular cells of the thyroid, and this disease represents a true calcitonin-excess syndrome. The radioimmunoassay of calcitonin appears to be a valuable procedure for detection of thyroid medullary carcinoma, particularly because one form of this disease is inherited as a dominant trait. Relatives of patients must therefore be examined repeatedly (Tashjian et al., 1974).

Mechanism and Actions. There is general agreement from both acute and chronic experiments *in vivo* and culture of bone *in vitro* that the hypocalcemic and hypophosphatemic effects of calcitonin are due predominantly to *direct inhibition of bone resorption* by altering osteoclastic and osteocytic activity. This effect on bone resorption is elicited in parathyroidectomized, nephrectomized, and eviscerated animals. Calcitonin enhances bone formation by an effect on osteoblasts. However, the effect is short lived, and osteoclastic as well as osteoblastic activity is decreased during chronic administration of the hormone; hence its use is contraindicated in osteoporosis. In addition, calcitonin negates the effects of PTH on osteolysis mediated by osteocytic and osteoclastic activity.

The intimate biochemical and cellular effects of calcitonin are not yet known, but it does not act as an antiparathyroid hormone. Thus, it does not block the

activation of bone-cell adenylate cyclase by PTH and does not inhibit the initial PTH-induced uptake of calcium into bone. The actions of calcitonin are not blocked by inhibitors of RNA and protein synthesis. The hormone produces a decrease in the amount of ruffled border of osteoclasts, indicating their diminished activity in bone resorption (Raisz, 1977). Part of the effect of calcitonin appears to be mediated through increasing the cyclic AMP concentration in bone cells, presumably in cells different from those so activated by PTH (Murad et al., 1970).

Calcitonin also antagonizes the inhibitory effects of PTH on pyrophosphatase activity in isolated Ehrlich ascites tumor cells. Pyrophosphate and pyrophosphatase are intimately involved in the processes of bone formation and resorption. Calcitonin decreases glucose utilization and lactate production in bone, effects opposite to those of PTH. As a result of depressed bone resorption, the urinary excretion of calcium, magnesium, and hydroxyproline is decreased by calcitonin. Plasma phosphate concentration is also lowered, due mainly to decreased resorption of bone and also to increased urinary phosphate excretion. The direct effects of calcitonin on the kidney are dependent on species. In man, calcitonin increases the excretion of calcium, phosphate, and sodium, effects also mediated in part by cyclic AMP (Murad et al., 1970; Pak, 1971; Paillard et al., 1972). Calcitonin may act physiologically to decrease intestinal absorption of calcium as well as other salts; however, this remains controversial (see Corradino, 1976).

Bioassay, Preparations, and Dosage. Bioassay of calcitonin preparations is performed by assessing their ability to lower plasma calcium concentration in the rat. The results are compared with a British Medical Research Council (MRC) Standard and expressed in MRC units. One unit is equivalent to approximately 4 μg of pure porcine calcitonin. (For summaries, see Rasmussen and Bordier, 1974; Symposium, 1974.)

Salmon, porcine, and human calcitonins have been studied experimentally. The hormone from salmon is considerably more potent in man than are the other two, perhaps because it is cleared from the circulation more slowly. Salmon calcitonin is available for clinical use as *calcitonin* (CALCIMAR), a synthetic preparation supplied in vials of 400 MRC units with 4 ml of a diluent containing 16% gelatin. The recommended dosage is 100 units per day, administered subcutaneously or intramuscularly. The drug is expensive.

Therapeutic Uses. Calcitonin is effective in diminishing hypercalcemia and decreasing concentrations of phosphate in the plasma of patients with hyperparathyroidism, idiopathic hypercalcemia of infancy, vitamin D intoxication, and osteolytic bone metastases. The effect of a single dose lasts for 6 to 10 hours. The decrease in plasma calcium and phosphate is the result of their decreased resorption from bone. Although calcitonin is effective in the initial treatment of hypercalcemia from various causes, other measures are recommended and are generally more practical (see section above on hypercalcemia).

Calcitonin is effective in diseases characterized by increased skeletal remodeling (increased bone resorption and bone formation), such as occurs in Paget's disease (Deftos, 1978). In this disease, calcitonin given chronically produces symptomatic relief and reduction in alkaline phosphatase activity in plasma, urinary hydroxyproline, and blood flow through the affected area. However, patients may become resistant to therapy after several months. Development of antibodies to porcine or salmon calcitonin does occur with long-term therapy in many patients; this is more common with the porcine preparation and may explain the development of resistance. While optimal dosage has not been established, favorable results were obtained in one study with 100 MRC units of salmon calcitonin given daily or three times a week by subcutaneous injection. The minimal dose for long-term therapy appeared to be 50 MRC units injected three times weekly. Side effects include nausea and swelling and tenderness of the hands; urticaria has also been observed (DeRose *et al.*, 1974).

SODIUM ETIDRONATE

This drug has recently been made available for the treatment of Paget's disease of bone. It is structurally related to pyrophosphate, which may have a role in bone mineralization, and has the following formula:

$$\text{HO}-\overset{\overset{\displaystyle\text{ONa}}{|}}{\underset{\underset{\displaystyle\text{O}}{\|}}{\text{P}}}-\overset{\overset{\displaystyle\text{OH}}{|}}{\underset{\underset{\displaystyle\text{CH}_3}{|}}{\text{C}}}-\overset{\overset{\displaystyle\text{ONa}}{|}}{\underset{\underset{\displaystyle\text{O}}{\|}}{\text{P}}}-\text{OH}$$

Sodium Etidronate

This compound (and other diphosphonates), when added to appropriate solutions and suspensions of calcium phosphate, slows the formation and dissolution of crystals of hydroxyapatite. Diphosphonates can protect experimental animals against calcification of soft tissues in vitamin D intoxication (Francis *et al.*, 1969).

The physicochemical action of this drug on the dynamics of crystal formation and dissolution are thought to be responsible for its favorable effects in patients with Paget's disease. In this disease there are foci of increased turnover of bone; these lead to the characteristic alterations of bone structure, which in turn may produce secondary problems, including deafness, spinal cord injuries, high-output cardiac failure, and disabling pain. Sodium etidronate may decrease the elevated plasma alkaline phosphatase activity and the urinary excretion of hydroxyproline that are characteristic of this disease. Most patients experience a decrease in bone pain, but worsening of bone pain has also been reported. There is an increase in the amount of nonmineralized osteoid, especially after treatment with higher doses; this may increase the risk of fractures (Altman *et al.*, 1973; Canfield *et al.*, 1977). The drug is effective orally. It is excreted without metabolic alteration by the kidney; dosage must therefore be reduced when there is renal insufficiency (Russell and Fleisch, 1975).

Advantages of this agent over calcitonin include its oral efficacy, lower cost, and lack of antigenicity. The relative merits of these two agents or a combination of the two are as yet undetermined.

Etidronate disodium (DIDRONEL) is available in tablets containing 200 mg. The usual dose is 5 mg/kg, given once daily in courses that should be given for no more than 6 months. Such treatment may induce a remission of Paget's disease that can last for years. If symptoms recur, additional courses of therapy may be effective.

VITAMIN D

Traditionally, vitamin D was assigned a passive role in calcium metabolism in that its presence in adequate concentrations was thought to permit proper absorption of dietary calcium and to allow full expression of the actions of parathyroid hormone. Recent findings indicate a much more active role of vitamin D in the homeostatic mechanisms that control calcium metabolism. It now appears that vitamin D (or its active metabolite) may be considered to be a hormone that plays a major role in the precise control of the concentration of calcium ion in plasma. The following characteristics of vitamin D are consistent with hormonal activity: vitamin D is synthesized in the skin and under ideal conditions probably is not required in the diet; it is transported by the blood to distant sites in the body, where it is activated; its active form then affects target tissues, resulting in increased plasma calcium concentration; and the conversion of vitamin D to its active form is a reaction that is regulated in a negative-feedback system by plasma calcium.

History. Vitamin D is the name applied to two related fat-soluble substances, cholecalciferol and calciferol, that have in common the ability to prevent or cure rickets. Prior to the discovery of vitamin D a high percentage of urban children, especially in the temperate zones, developed rickets. Some thought that the disease was due to lack of fresh air and sunshine; others claimed a dietary factor caused the disease. By 1920 the work of Mellanby and Huldschinsky had shown both of these notions to be correct; the addition of cod liver oil to the diet or exposure to sunlight would either prevent or cure the disease. In 1924 it was found that irradiation of animal rations was as efficacious in curing rickets as was irradiation of the animal itself (Hess and Weinstock, 1924; Steenbock and Black, 1924). These observations led to the elucidation of the structures of cholecalciferol and calciferol and eventually to the discovery that these compounds are further metabolized in the body to active compounds. This latter discovery of metabolic activation is primarily attributable to studies conducted in the laboratories of DeLuca in the United States and Kodicek in England (*see* DeLuca and Schnoes, 1976).

Chemistry and Occurrence. Ultraviolet irradiation of a variety of animal and plant sterols results in their conversion to compounds with vitamin D (antirachitic) activity. Cleavage of the carbon-to-carbon bond between C 9 and C 10 is the essential alteration produced by the photochemical process, but not all sterols that undergo this cleavage possess antirachitic activity. The principal provitamin found in animal tissues is 7-dehydrocholesterol, which is synthesized in the skin. Exposure of the skin to sunlight converts 7-dehydrocholesterol to cholecalciferol (vitamin D_3) (*see* Figure 65–1). Holick and Clark (1978) have found an intermediate in the photolysis reaction, previtamin D_3, a 6,7-*cis* isomer that accumulates in the skin after exposure to ultraviolet radiation. This slowly converts spontaneously to vitamin D_3 and may provide a sustained source of D_3 for some time after exposure to ultraviolet light. The active form of vitamin D is now thought to be

calcitriol [1,25-$(OH)_2$ cholecalciferol], which is formed by two successive hydroxylations of vitamin D_3.

Ergosterol, which is present in yeasts and fungi, is the provitamin for vitamin D_2 (calciferol). Ergosterol and vitamin D_2 differ from 7-dehydrocholesterol and vitamin D_3, respectively, only by each having a double bond between C 22 and C 23 and a methyl group at C 24. Vitamin D_2 is the active constituent in a number of commercial vitamin preparations as well as in irradiated bread and irradiated milk. The material historically designated as vitamin D_1 was later shown to be a mixture of antirachitic substances.

In some species the antirachitic potencies of vitamin D_2 and vitamin D_3 differ greatly from each other. In man there is no practical difference between the two, and in the following discussion vitamin D will be used as the collective term for vitamins D_2 and D_3.

A glycoside of calcitriol has recently been found in a South American plant, *Solanum malacoxylon* (Haussler *et al.*, 1977). It has been recognized for some time that animals poisoned by grazing on this plant experience hypercalcemia, hyperphosphatemia, and soft-tissue calcification.

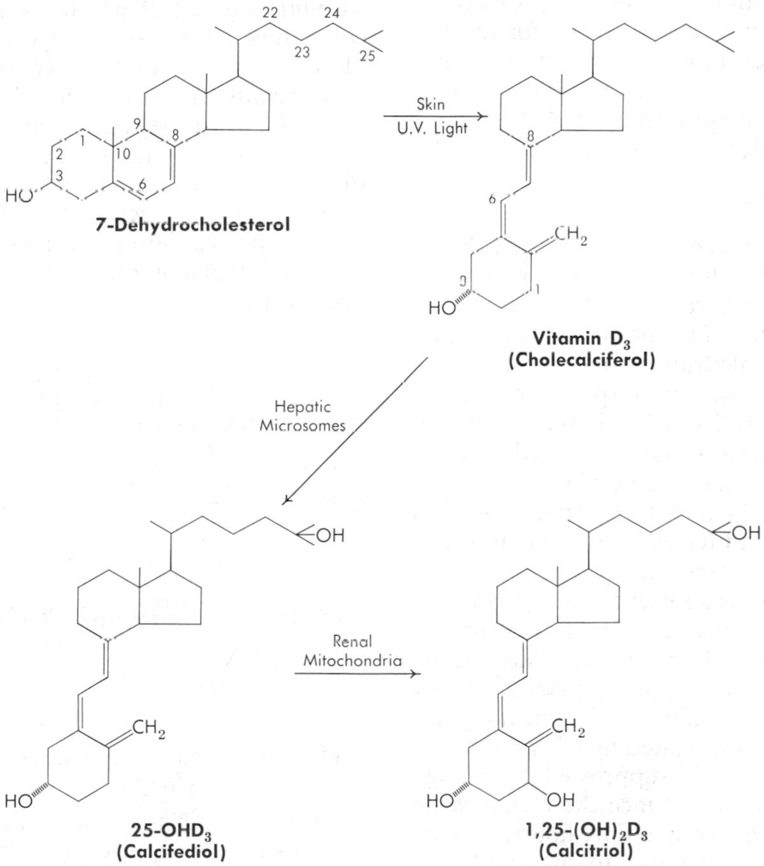

Figure 65–1. *Metabolic activation of vitamin D. (See* text for explanation and abbreviations.)

METABOLIC ACTIVATION

Dietary vitamin D, or that which is synthesized intrinsically, requires metabolic activation in order to exert its characteristic actions on target tissues. It is now believed that the active form of the vitamin is calcitriol, the product of two successive hydroxylations of D_3. The pathway of activation is shown in Figure 65–1. This subject has been reviewed by DeLuca and Schnoes (1976), Haussler and McCain (1977), and DeLuca (1978).

25-Hydroxylation of Vitamin D. In man the initial step in the activation of vitamin D_3 occurs predominantly in the liver, and the product is 25-hydroxycholecalciferol (or calcifediol). The hepatic enzyme system responsible for 25-hydroxylation of vitamin D has not been fully characterized, but it is associated with the microsomal fraction of liver homogenates and requires the presence of NADPH and molecular oxygen for the hydroxylation reaction. This reaction is not inhibited by carbon monoxide and therefore differs from the cytochrome P-450–containing drug-metabolizing enzyme system of the liver.

1-Hydroxylation of 25-OHD₃. After being produced in the liver, 25-OHD₃ enters the blood stream, where it circulates in association with vitamin D–binding globulin. Final activation to calcitriol occurs in the kidney. The enzyme system responsible for 1-hydroxylation of 25-OHD₃ is associated with the mitochondria. It too is a mixed-function oxidase and requires molecular oxygen and NADPH as cofactors. Cytochrome P-450, a flavoprotein, and ferredoxin are components of the enzyme complex.

This enzyme is subject to dietary and endocrine regulations that are of great importance for calcium homeostasis. Thus, the activity of the hydroxylase increases in dietary deficiencies of vitamin D, calcium, and phosphate, and it is stimulated by PTH, prolactin, and estrogens. It is suppressed by a high intake of vitamin D. Since these changes in activity of the enzyme require hours, they are not responsible for rapid adaptations.

The detailed mechanisms by which the various dietary and endocrine factors regulate the concentration of calcitriol in plasma by modifying the 25-OHD₃-1α-hydroxylase activity in the kidney remain under active investigation. The slowness of the responses and their sensitivity to metabolic inhibitors strongly suggest that the variations in enzymatic activity represent changes in the quantity of enzyme protein in the kidney. The model presented by Haussler and McCain (1977) encompasses the major concepts that have developed in this area during the past few years, although there is still controversy over the role of phosphate (Edelstein *et al.,* 1978). Variations of concentrations of calcium and phosphate in plasma are thought to be the primary regulators of the hydroxylase of the kidney. A low concentration of calcium in plasma stimulates the secretion of PTH, and the hormone enhances the activity of the renal enzyme (*see* Figure 65–2). Similarly, a low concentration of phosphate stimulates the enzyme, although probably through a direct effect on the renal tubular cells; thus, PTH may also act on the hydroxylase by means of the hypophosphatemia that results from its phosphaturic effect. Calcitriol exerts negative-feedback control of the enzyme that may be a consequence of a direct action on the renal tissue or by an inhibition of the secretion of PTH. The nature of the regulatory mechanisms of estrogens and prolactin on the 1α-hydroxylase is not known.

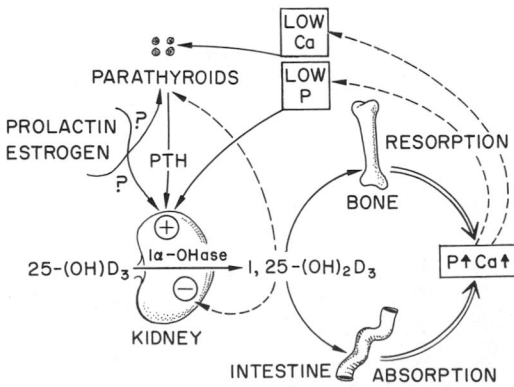

Figure 65–2. *Model for regulation of the biosynthesis of 1,25-(OH)₂D₃.*

Solid arrows indicate a positive effect; dashed arrows refer to negative feedback (*see* text for explanation). (Modified from Haussler and McCain, 1977. Courtesy of the *New England Journal of Medicine.*)

Physiological Functions, Mechanism of Action, and Pharmacological Properties of Vitamin D

The physiological role of vitamin D is best characterized as that of a positive regulator in calcium homeostasis. Phosphate metabolism is affected by the vitamin in a parallel manner to that of calcium.

The two most important mechanisms by which vitamin D acts to maintain normal concentrations of calcium and phosphate in plasma are to facilitate their absorption by the small intestine and to enhance their mobilization from bone. In addition, there is evidence of a direct effect of the vitamin on the kidney that results in increased retention of calcium and phosphate by enhancing their proximal tubular reabsorption (Puschett et al., 1972; Costanzo et al., 1974; Harris et al., 1976).

These processes serve to maintain calcium and phosphate ions at concentrations in plasma that are essential for normal neuromuscular activity, mineralization of bone, and a number of other calcium-dependent functions. A direct role of the vitamin in the mineralization of bone has not been demonstrated; rather, it is thought that normal rates of bone formation occur when calcium and phosphate concentrations in the plasma are adequate.

Intestinal Absorption of Calcium. A defect in intestinal absorption of calcium in vitamin D–deficient rats was demonstrated in the late 1930s (Nicolaysen, 1937). More recently, movement of calcium from the mucosal to the serosal surface of the intestine has been shown to be a process involving a carrier and active transport against an electrochemical gradient (Adams and Norman, 1970). The active-transport mechanism is present in the microvilli of the brush border (luminal side) of the intestinal epithelial cells.

Calcitriol appears to act on the intestine in a manner that is analogous to the way steroid hormones such as estrogens act on target tissues. For example, the cytosol of chicken intestinal cells contains a 3.7 S protein that binds calcitriol specifically and with high affinity. Formation of a complex with this receptor facilitates the transfer of calcitriol to the nuclear chromatin (Brumbaugh and Haussler, 1974). When given in vivo, labeled calcitriol can be shown by autoradiographic technics to be located in the nuclei of cells of the intestinal villi and crypts (Zile et al., 1978). Calcitriol stimulates synthesis of RNA and at least two proteins in the intestinal mucosa, alkaline phosphatase and a calcium-binding protein.

The latter is absent from vitamin D–deficient animals, and it was thought to appear before the onset of increased transport of calcium when calcitriol is administered. On this basis it was proposed that the calcium-binding protein is involved in the transport of calcium. Further examination of the sequence of events that follow the administration of calcitriol has shown, however, that stimulation of calcium transport is demonstrable 1 hour after calcitriol is given, but synthesis of the calcium-binding protein does not begin for 2 hours (Spencer et al., 1978). Furthermore, cycloheximide blocks calcitriol-stimulated synthesis of intestinal proteins, including alkaline phosphatase and calcium-binding protein, but it does not prevent stimulation of calcium transport (Bikle et al., 1978). Thus, the events that link the binding of calcitriol in the cytoplasm and nucleus of the intestinal cells to the stimulation of calcium and phosphate transport remain obscure.

It has been reported that calcitriol-induced stimulation of intestinal transport of phosphate precedes that of calcium, and it is possible that the primary effect of the vitamin is on phosphate rather than calcium transport (Birge and Miller, 1977). Neither parathyroidectomy nor administration of PTH modifies the response of the intestine to calcitriol (Garabedian et al., 1974).

Mobilization of Bone Salts. Large doses of vitamin D cause decalcification of bone. In 1952, Carlsson demonstrated that physiological doses of vitamin D promote mobilization of calcium from bone. In 1963, Rasmussen and coworkers showed that small doses of vitamin D are required for PTH to promote such mobilization. However, the requirement for PTH for stimulation of decalcification by vitamin D remains controversial. Calcitriol stimulates resorption of bone in tissue culture in the absence of PTH (Raisz et al., 1972), and dihydrotachysterol, a derivitive of vitamin D_2, will promote bone resorption in vivo in hypoparathyroid individuals (see below). Experimental studies of vitamin D in vivo, however, are contradictory with regard to the obligatory role of PTH. It has been reported that administration of calcitriol to thyroparathyroidectomized rats increases bone resorption as in normal animals (Reynolds et al., 1976), whereas Garabedian and associates (1974) concluded that calcitriol has a diminished action on bone after removal of the parathyroids.

The molecular mechanisms responsible for mobilization of bone salts are unclear. Active translocation of calcium across osteocytes (Talmage, 1972) or across a hypothetical bone membrane (Neuman and Ramp, 1971) has been proposed as the mechanism by which plasma calcium is maintained as a supersaturated solution that is not in chemical equilibrium with calcium in bone fluid. In such a scheme, mobilization of calcium from the bone compartment occurs when active transport of calcium from bone fluid to extracellular fluid is enhanced. Thus, vitamin D could promote mobilization of calcium from bone by stimulating active transport of calcium in osteocytes, perhaps by the same mechanisms that stimulate intestinal absorption of calcium. In bone cells maintained in tissue culture, calcitriol stimulates phosphatase and hyaluronate synthesis in osteoclast-like cells and decreases alkaline phosphatase, citrate decarboxylation, and collagen synthesis in osteoblast-like cells (Wong *et al.,* 1977). The relationship between these effects and demineralization is not clear.

Signs and Symptoms of Deficiency. A deficiency of vitamin D results in inadequate absorption of calcium and phosphate. The consequent decrease in plasma calcium stimulates PTH secretion, which acts to restore plasma calcium at the expense of bone calcium; plasma concentrations of phosphate remain subnormal. In infants and children, this results in a failure to mineralize newly formed osteoid tissue and cartilage matrix, causing the defect in bone growth known as *rickets.* As a consequence of inadequate calcification, the bones of individuals suffering from rickets are unusually soft, and the stress and strain of weight bearing give rise to the characteristic deformities of the disease.

In adults, vitamin D deficiency results in *osteomalacia* or adult rickets, which is most likely to occur during times of increased need for calcium, such as during pregnancy or lactation. The disease is characterized by a generalized decrease in bone density. Unlike osteoporosis, the remaining bone is abnormal in that it contains excessive amounts of uncalcified matrix. Gross deformities of bone occur only in advanced stages of the disease.

Hypervitaminosis. The acute or chronic administration of excessive amounts of vitamin D or enhanced responsiveness to normal amounts of the vitamin leads to a number of clinical syndromes that are probably the result of deranged calcium metabolism. The physiological or pathological responses to vitamin D are a function of endogenous production of vitamin D, tissue reactivity to the vitamin, and particularly vitamin D intake. Some infants seem to be hyperreactive to relatively small doses of vitamin D. Certain cases of hypervitaminosis D in adults result from the administration of large doses of the vitamin in the attempt to treat conditions that have been wrongly purported to benefit from vitamin D therapy. Other cases are the consequence of excessive doses used in the treatment of hypoparathyroidism. More commonly, toxicity is seen in children as a result of accidental ingestion or excessive administration of the vitamin by parents.

There is wide individual variation in the amount of vitamin D that causes hypervitaminosis. As a rough approximation, it may be stated that the continued ingestion of 50,000 units or more daily by a person with normal sensitivity to vitamin D may result in poisoning. Hypercalcemia is particularly dangerous in patients who are receiving digitalis because the toxic effects of the cardiac glycosides are enhanced (*see* Chapter 30).

Signs and Symptoms. The initial signs and symptoms of vitamin D toxicity are those associated with hypercalcemia and consist in weakness, fatigue, lassitude, headache, nausea, vomiting, and diarrhea. Early impairment of renal function from hypercalcemia is manifest by polyuria, polydipsia, nocturia, decreased urinary concentrating ability, and proteinuria. Some of these effects are due to inhibition of the action of antidiuretic hormone by calcium. With prolonged hypercalcemia there may be deposition of calcium salts in soft tissues, most significantly within the kidney; this results in nephrolithiasis, diffuse nephrocalcinosis, or both. Other sites of calcification may include blood vessels, heart, lungs, and skin. Some individuals exhibit hypertension. The characteristic changes in blood chemistry are elevated concentrations of plasma calcium and nonprotein nitrogen; phosphate concentrations are variable. Mobilization of calcium from bone contributes to the hypercalcemia and is also responsible for the roentgenographic finding of localized or generalized osteoporosis in a significant percentage of cases of hypervitaminosis D (Holman, 1952).

In children, a single episode of moderately severe hypercalcemia may arrest growth completely for 6 months or more, and the deficit in height may never be fully corrected (Parfitt, 1972).

Vitamin D toxicity may be manifested in the fetus. There is a relationship between excess maternal vitamin D intake or extreme sensitivity to the vitamin and nonfamilial congenital supravalvular aortic stenosis. In infants, this anomaly is often found in association with other stigmata of hypercalcemia. Similar lesions have been produced experimentally in offspring of rabbits treated with large doses of vitamin D during pregnancy (Friedman and Roberts, 1966; Taussig, 1966). Maternal hypercalcemia may also result in suppression of parathyroid function in the newborn, with resultant hypocalcemia, tetany, and seizures.

An occasional sequela resulting from an acute episode of hypercalcemia in patients treated for hypoparathyroidism is a marked increase in response to vitamin D after the disappearance of the hypercalcemia (Leeson and Fourman, 1966).

Treatment of hypervitaminosis D consists in immediate withdrawal of the vitamin, a low-calcium diet, administration of glucocorticoids, and a generous intake of fluid. With this regimen the plasma calcium falls to normal and the calcium in the soft tissue tends to be mobilized. A conspicuous improvement in renal function is often noted with return of the plasma calcium to normal, but this may not occur if renal damage has been severe.

Absorption, Fate, and Excretion. Vitamin D is usually given by mouth, and gastrointestinal absorption is adequate under most conditions. Both vitamin D_2 and vitamin D_3 are absorbed from the small intestine, although vitamin D_3 may be absorbed more completely and more rapidly. The exact portion of the gut that is most effective in vitamin D absorption may be a function of the vehicle in which the vitamin is suspended or dissolved. Most of the vitamin appears first in lymph and primarily in the chylomicron fraction as a lipoprotein complex.

In animals and man, bile is essential for adequate intestinal absorption and deoxycholic acid is the most important constituent of bile in this regard. Thus, hepatic or biliary dysfunction may seriously impair absorption of vitamin D. Likewise, other abnormalities of gastrointestinal function, especially those associated with steatorrhea, may interfere with proper absorption of orally administered vitamin D.

Absorbed vitamin D circulates in the blood in association with vitamin D–binding protein, which is a specific α-globulin (Smith and Goodman, 1971). Vitamin D disappears from plasma with a half-life of 19 to 25 hours, but it is stored in the body for prolonged periods (6 months or longer in the rat), apparently in fat deposits throughout the body (Rosenstreich et al., 1971).

As discussed above, the liver is the site of conversion of vitamin D to its 25-hydroxy derivative, which also circulates in association with vitamin D–binding protein. In fact, calcifediol has a higher affinity for the binding protein than does the parent compound (Belsey et al., 1971). The 25-hydroxy derivative has a biological half-life of 19 days and constitutes the major circulating form of vitamin D (Smith and Goodman, 1971). The plasma half-life of calcitriol is estimated to be between 3 and 5 days in man, and 40% of an administered dose is excreted within 10 days (Mawer et al., 1976). Calcitriol is hydroxylated to $1,24,25\text{-}(OH)_3D_3$ by a renal hydroxylase that is induced by calcitriol and suppressed by those factors that stimulate the $25\text{-}OHD_3\text{-}1\alpha$-hydroxylase. This enzyme also hydroxylates calcifediol to form $24,25\text{-}$ $(OH)_2D_3$. Both 24-hydroxylated compounds are less active than calcitriol and presumably represent metabolites destined for excretion (DeLuca, 1978). Side chain oxidation of calcitriol also occurs (DeLuca, 1977).

The primary route of excretion of vitamin D is in the bile, and only a small percentage of an administered dose is found in the urine.

An important interaction has been demonstrated between vitamin D and phenytoin or phenobarbital. Patients receiving the anticonvulsant agents for a prolonged time have a high incidence of rickets and osteomalacia (Dent et al., 1970; Hunter et al., 1971). Plasma concentrations of calcifediol are decreased in patients receiving these drugs, and it was proposed that phenytoin and phenobarbital accelerate the metabolism of vitamin D to inactive products (Hahn et al., 1972a, 1972b). Furthermore, these drugs protect rats against the toxic effects of high doses of vitamin D (Gascon-Barré and Côte, 1978). However, concentrations of calcitriol in plasma are normal, despite the depression of the concentration of calcifediol, in patients receiving anticonvulsant therapy (Jubiz et al., 1977). A normal concentration of calcitriol in the plasma after such treatment is consistent with the findings of several groups of investigators that anticonvulsant therapy increases target organ resistance to vitamin D and that this is the basis for the interaction. The effects of vitamin D on intestinal absorption of calcium and on bone resorption are diminished by the drugs (see Habener and Mahaffey, 1978). There have been some indications that therapy with glucocorticoids may alter the metabolism of vitamin D. The data relative to this are contradictory, and the issue remains unresolved (Habener and Mahaffey, 1978). The regulation of the metabolism of vitamin D has been reviewed by Fraser (1980).

Human Requirements and Unitage. An exhaustive and critical summary of the prophylactic requirements for vitamin D has been compiled by the Committee on Nutrition of the American Academy of Pediatrics (see Committee on Nutrition, 1963). In the more than 50 years that have elapsed since Mellanby (1921) demonstrated the efficacy of cod liver oil in the prevention of rickets, the disease has become a clinical rarity in the United States. Although sunlight provides adequate antirachitic prophylaxis in the equatorial belt, in the temperate climates insufficient cutaneous solar radiation may necessitate dietary vitamin D supplementation.

Previously the recommended allowance of vitamin D could be achieved only by the addition of oral vitamin D supplements to a normal diet. Since the advent of the addition of the vitamin to foodstuffs (especially milk, milk products, cereals, and candy), individuals of all ages receive variable and even excessive vitamin D without its special addition to the diet. Thus, the supplemental requirements vary not only with age, pregnancy, and lactation but also with the quality of the diet. According to the Committee on Nutrition (1963), hypothetical average and high vitamin D diets at various ages would lead to the intake of the following amounts of the vitamin per day without any special vitamin supplements: 6 months, average 400 units; 3 years, average 600 units, high 1600 units; 8 years, average 800 units, high 1900 units. Serious toxicity may result from excessive ingestion of the vitamin, and even as little as 1800 U.S.P. units per day in infants may lead to possible inhibition of growth (Jeans and Stearns, 1938). It is clear, therefore, that any recommendation for vitamin D supplementation must be made only after careful scrutiny of the diet.

In both the premature and the normal infant, a total of 400 units per day of vitamin D ensures full antirachitic prophylaxis and optimal growth. Whether this is obtained by way of the diet, by vitamin D supplementation, or by a combination of both is of no consequence. During adolescence and adulthood this amount is probably also sufficient. There is some evidence that vitamin D requirements are greater than normal during pregnancy and lactation, although a daily intake of 400 units is sufficient in these conditions as well (*see* Table XVI–1, page 1553).

The U.S.P. unit is identical with the international unit and is equivalent to the specific biological activity of 0.025 μg of vitamin D_3 (*i.e.,* 1 mg equals 40,000 units).

Bioassay procedures have been used in the past and depend upon evidence of alleviation of the rachitic state. They are still in use for experimental purposes.

Modified Forms of Vitamin D. Two derivatives of vitamin D are of considerable experimental and therapeutic interest.

Dihydrotachysterol (DHT) is an analog of vitamin D that may be regarded as the reduction product of vitamin D_2 (and is sometimes referred to as DHT_2). Although DHT is the compound available for therapeutic use, the corresponding derivative of vitamin D_3 (DHT_3) has been used in experimental studies. Presumably DHT behaves in a manner analogous to that described for DHT_3. DHT is about $1/450$ as active as vitamin D in the usual antirachitic assay, but at high doses it is much more effective than vitamin D in mobilizing calcium from bone (Suda *et al.*, 1970). The latter effect is the basis for the use of DHT to maintain normal concentrations of calcium in plasma in hypoparathyroidism.

Studies describing the metabolic activation of DHT_3 provide an explanation for the above findings. DHT_3 undergoes 25-hydroxylation to yield 25-

Dihydrotachysterol (DHT)

hydroxydihydrotachysterol$_3$ (25-OHDHT$_3$), which appears to be the active form of DHT in both intestine and bone (Hallick and DeLuca, 1972). Both DHT_3 and 25-OHDHT$_3$ are active in nephrectomized rats (Omdahl and DeLuca, 1973), indicating that DHT_3 does not require 1-hydroxylation in the kidney. A comparison of the structures of DHT and 1,25-$(OH)_2D_3$ shows that ring A of DHT is rotated so as to place its 3-hydroxyl group in approximately the same geometrical position as the 1-hydroxyl group of 1,25-$(OH)_2D_3$. It seems reasonable, therefore, that 25-OHDHT$_3$ could interact with receptor sites for 1,25-$(OH)_2D_3$ without undergoing 1-hydroxylation in the kidney. Thus, DHT bypasses the renal mechanisms of metabolic control.

1α-*Hydroxycholecalciferol,* 1-OHD$_3$, is a synthetic derivative of vitamin D_3 that is hydroxylated in the 1α position. It is readily hydroxylated in the 25 position by the hepatic microsomal system to form 1,25-$(OH)_2D_3$ and was therefore introduced as a substitute for this compound. In the chick assays for stimulation of intestinal absorption of calcium and bone mineralization it is essentially equal in activity to calcitriol (Boris, 1977). Because it does not require renal hydroxylation it has been used to treat renal osteodystrophy. Although in theory it should be equivalent to calcitriol, unlike the natural metabolite it has been found at certain dosages to cause a progressive increase in absorption of calcium, leading to hypercalcemia that sometimes persists for weeks after therapy is discontinued (David, 1977).

Preparations. Although many preparations containing vitamin D are marketed, official U.S.P. preparations are primarily listed below.

Ergocalciferol, U.S.P.(*calciferol;* DRISDOL, GELTABS), is pure vitamin D_2. *Ergocalciferol Capsules,* U.S.P., consists of ergocalciferol in edible vegetable oil solution, encapsulated with gelatin. Capsules usually contain 625 μg (25,000 U.S.P. units) or 1.25 mg (50,000 U.S.P. units) each. *Ergocalciferol Oral Solution,* U.S.P., is a solution of the vitamin in an edible vegetable oil, polysorbate 80, or propylene glycol. Each gram of solution must contain at least 250 μg (10,000 U.S.P. units) of ergocalciferol. *Ergocalciferol Tablets,* U.S.P., contain 1.25 mg (50,000 U.S.P. units).

Cholecalciferol, U.S.P., is pure vitamin D_3.

Decavitamin Capsules, U.S.P., and *Decavitamin Tablets,* U.S.P., contain at least 400 U.S.P. vitamin D units (10 μg of vitamin D as ergocalciferol or chole-calciferol) per capsule or tablet. The vitamin can be from natural sources, or as vitamin D_2 or vitamin D_3, or as the irradiation products of ergosterol or 7-dehydrocholesterol.

Dihydrotachysterol, U.S.P. (HYTAKEROL), is the pure crystalline compound obtained by reduction of vitamin D_2 and is available as tablets (0.2 mg), capsules (0.125 mg), and solution in oil (0.25 mg/ml). These preparations are all for oral administration.

Calcitriol (1,25-dihydroxycholecalciferol; ROCAL-TROL) is marketed in capsules for oral administration that contain 0.25 or 0.5 μg. Dosage must be individualized but is often effective at 0.5 to 1 μg per day. This preparation is considerably more expensive than those listed above and is rarely required.

THERAPEUTIC USES

The major therapeutic uses of vitamin D may be divided into three categories: (1) prophylaxis and cure of nutritional rickets, (2) treatment of metabolic rickets and osteomalacia, and (3) treatment of hypo-parathyroidism.

Nutritional Rickets. Nutritional rickets results from inadequate exposure to sunlight or a deficiency of vitamin D in the diet. The condition is extremely rare in the United States and other countries where milk and other foods contain added vitamin D. Infants and children receiving adequate amounts of vitamin D-fortified food do not require additional vitamin D; however, breast-fed infants or those fed unfortified formula should receive 400 units of vitamin D daily as a supplement. The usual practice is to administer vitamin A in combination with vitamin D. A number of well-balanced vitamin A and D preparations are available for this purpose. Premature infants are especially susceptible to rickets and may require supplemental vitamin D, since the fetus acquires more than 85% of its calcium stores during the third trimester.

The curative dose of vitamin D for the treatment of *fully developed rickets* is larger than the prophylactic dose. One thousand units daily will produce normal calcium and phosphate concentrations in plasma in approximately 10 days and roentgeno-graphic evidence of healing within about 3 weeks. However, a daily dose of 3000 to 4000 units is often prescribed for more rapid healing; this is of particular importance in severe cases of thoracic rickets when respiration is embarrassed.

There are certain conditions that are known to lead to *poor absorption of vitamin D.* If untreated by vitamin supplementation, a frank deficiency may develop. Therefore, vitamin D may be of definite prophylactic value in such disorders as diarrhea, steatorrhea, biliary obstruction, and any other abnormality in gastrointestinal function in which absorption is appreciably diminished. Parenteral administration may be used in such cases.

Metabolic Rickets and Osteomalacia. This group of diseases, which presents as rickets in infants and children and osteomalacia in adults, is characterized by a failure to respond to physiological doses of vitamin D. Three types of metabolic rickets are discussed below, and the reader is referred to articles by Parfitt (1972), Smith (1972), and Scriver and co-workers (1978) for more complete discussions of other forms of the disease.

Hypophosphatemic vitamin D–resistant rickets is an X-linked inherited disorder of calcium and phosphate metabolism. It is *not* characterized by a defect in vitamin D metabolism, but treatment with large doses of calcitriol in combination with phosphate salts may lead to clinical improvement (Brickman *et al.,* 1973).

Vitamin D–dependent rickets (pseudo-vitamin D deficiency rickets) is an inherited, autosomal recessive disease that appears to be due to an inborn error of vitamin D metabolism involving defective conversion of 25-OHD$_3$ to 1,25-(OH)$_2$D$_3$ (Fraser *et al.,* 1973). The condition responds to physiological doses of calcitriol (Fraser *et al.,* 1973).

Renal osteodystrophy (renal rickets) is associated with chronic renal failure, and it also is characterized by a decreased ability of the kidney to convert 25-OHD$_3$ to 1,25-(OH)$_2$D$_3$. The use of calcitriol in this condition can lower the concentrations of PTH and raise the concentration of calcium in plasma and help maintain bone mineralization and growth in children (Berl *et al.,* 1978; Chesney *et al.,* 1978). DHT and 1-OHD$_3$ can also be used effectively, since renal hydroxylation is not required for their activity.

Hypoparathyroidism. Hypoparathyroidism is characterized by hypocalcemia and hyperphosphatemia (*see* above). Dihydrotachysterol has long been used to treat this condition, since it has a more rapid onset of action, a shorter duration of action, and, as noted above, a greater effect on mobilization of bone salts than does vitamin D. Calcitriol is reported to be effective in the management of hypoparathyroidism (Rosen *et al.,* 1977) and at least certain forms of pseudohypoparathyroidism in which an abnormally low concentration of calcitriol is present in plasma (Metz *et al.,* 1977). However, with the exception of the latter rare form of pseudohypoparathyroidism where the hydroxylase is deficient, most hypoparathyroid patients respond to any of the forms of vitamin D.

Miscellaneous Uses of Vitamin D. Miscellaneous uses of vitamin D include treatment of the hypophosphatemia seen in the *Fanconi syndrome.* The use of large doses of vitamin D in patients with osteoporosis is of doubtful value and can be dangerous. Furthermore, the indiscriminate use of "over-the-counter" vitamin D preparations for conditions other than the aforementioned is irrational, can be dangerous, and should not be condoned.

FLUORIDE

Fluoride is of interest because of its toxic properties and its effect on dental enamel and bone. Fluoride is widely distributed in nature, and the soils of different regions of the world vary greatly in their fluoride content. Fluoride gains access to plants from the soil as well as from atmospheric sources. The sources of atmospheric fluoride include the burning of soft coal and the manufacturing of superphosphate, aluminum, steel, lead, copper, and nickel. Man obtains fluoride from the ingestion of plants and water. Incidental sources include food additives (*e.g.,* baking powder) that are contaminated with fluoride, and the ingestion of rodenticides and insecticides that contain fluoride compounds.

Absorption, Distribution, and Excretion. Fluorides are absorbed from the gastrointestinal tract, the lungs, and the skin. The gastrointestinal tract is the major site of absorption. The degree of absorption of a fluoride compound is best correlated with its solubility. The relatively soluble compounds, such as sodium fluoride, are almost completely absorbed, whereas relatively insoluble compounds, such as cryolite (Na_3AlF_6) and the fluoride found in bone meal (fluoroapatite), are poorly absorbed. Certain dietary cations (*e.g.,* calcium and iron) retard absorption of fluoride ion by forming low-solubility complexes in the gastrointestinal tract. The second most common route of absorption is by way of the lungs. Pulmonary inhalation of fluoride present in dusts and gases constitutes the major route of industrial exposure. A third, and relatively rare, route of absorption is through the skin (Burke *et al.,* 1973).

Fluoride has been detected in all organs and tissues examined; however, there is no evidence that it is concentrated in any tissues except bone, thyroid, aorta, and perhaps kidney (Armstrong, 1967). Fluoride is preponderantly deposited in the skeleton and teeth, and the degree of skeletal storage is related to intake and age. This is thought to be a function of the turnover rate of skeletal components, with growing bone showing a greater fluoride deposition than bone in mature animals. Prolonged periods of time are required for mobilization of fluoride from bone. Fluoride is accumulated by the aorta, and concentrations increase with age, probably reflecting the calcification that occurs in this artery.

The major route of fluoride excretion is by way of the kidneys; however, fluoride is also excreted in small amounts by the sweat glands, the lactating breast, and the gastrointestinal tract. Under conditions of excessive sweating, the fraction of total fluoride excretion contributed by sweating can reach nearly one half. About 90% of the fluoride filtered by the glomerulus is reabsorbed by the renal tubules. Whether tubular secretion of fluoride occurs is unknown.

Pharmacological Actions. The pharmacological actions of fluoride, with the possible exception of its effect on bone and teeth, can be classified as toxic. Fluoride is an inhibitor of several enzyme systems and diminishes tissue respiration and anaerobic glycolysis. Fluoride is also a useful anticoagulant *in vitro* due to its binding of calcium ions. It also inhibits the glycolytic utilization of glucose by erythrocytes, and for this reason is added to specimen tubes that receive blood for glucose determinations.

Fluoride has been used in treating Paget's disease of bone, but more effective therapeutic agents are now available. Fluoride has also been used to treat otosclerosis and osteogenesis imperfecta (Castells, 1973; Daniel *et al.,* 1973). Further studies are re-

quired to establish the efficacy of the anion in these disorders. The radioactive nuclide ^{18}F has proven useful in bone imaging and the detection of bone metastases (Jones *et al.,* 1973).

Acute Poisoning. Acute fluoride poisoning is not rare. It usually results from the accidental ingestion of insecticides or rodenticides containing fluoride salts.

Initial symptoms are secondary to the local action of fluoride on the mucosa of the gastrointestinal tract. Salivation, nausea, abdominal pain, vomiting, and diarrhea are frequent. Systemic symptoms are varied and severe. The patient shows signs of increasing irritability of the nervous system, including paresthesias, a positive Chvostek sign, hyperactive reflexes, and tonic and clonic convulsions. These signs are related to the calcium-binding effect of fluoride. Hypocalcemia and hypoglycemia are frequent laboratory findings. The signs may be delayed for several hours. Pain in various muscle groups may occur. The blood pressure falls, presumably due to central vasomotor depression as well as direct toxic action on cardiac muscle. The respiratory center is first stimulated and later depressed. Death usually results from either respiratory paralysis or cardiac failure. It is stated that the lethal dose of sodium fluoride for man is about 5 g; however, recovery has been reported in patients ingesting much larger doses, whereas a dose as low as 2 g has been fatal. In children, as little as 0.5 g of sodium fluoride may be fatal. *Treatment* includes the intravenous administration of glucose in saline and gastric lavage with limewater (0.15% calcium hydroxide solution) to precipitate the fluoride. Calcium gluconate is given intravenously for tetany; urine volume is kept high with parenteral fluid.

Chronic Poisoning. In man, the major manifestations of chronic ingestion of excessive amounts of fluoride are osteosclerosis and mottled enamel. Chronic exposure to excess fluoride causes increased osteoblastic activity. Osteosclerosis is a phenomenon wherein the density and calcification of bone are increased; in the case of fluoride intoxication, it is thought to represent the replacement of hydroxyapatite by the denser fluoroapatite. However, the mechanism of its development remains unknown. The degree of skeletal involvement varies from changes that are barely detectable radiologically to marked thickening of the cortex of long bones, numerous exostoses scattered throughout the skeleton, and calcification of ligaments, tendons, and muscle attachments to bone. In its severest form it is a disabling disease and is designated as *crippling fluorosis*.

Mottled enamel or dental fluorosis is a well-recognized entity that was first described over 50 years ago. The gross changes in very mild mottling consist in small, opaque, paper-white areas scattered irregularly over the tooth surface. In severe cases, discrete or confluent, deep brown- to black-stained pits give the tooth a corroded appearance. Mottled enamel is the result of a partial failure of the enamel-forming cells properly to elaborate and lay down enamel. It is a nonspecific response to a variety of stimuli, one of which is the ingestion of excessive amounts of fluoride.

Since mottled enamel is a developmental injury, the ingestion of fluoride following the eruption of the tooth has no effect. Mottling is one of the first visible signs of an excessive intake of fluoride during childhood. A quantitative relationship between the fluoride concentration of drinking water and mottling has been demonstrated. Continuous use of water containing about 1.0 ppm of fluoride may result in the very mildest form of mottled enamel in 10% of children. The incidence rises to 40 to 50% at about 1.7 ppm; at 2.5 ppm, it is as high as 80%, with 25% classified as moderate or severe; between 4.0 and 6.0 ppm, the incidence approaches 100%, with marked increase in severity.

Some concern has been expressed that fluoridation of public water supplies may result in an increased frequency of cancer or other diseases. Recent studies carried out by the National Cancer Institute and by the Bureau of Epidemiology of the United States Public Health Service indicate that mortality from cancer and mortality from all causes do not significantly differ between cities with fluoridated and those with nonfluoridated water (Hoover et al., 1976; Erickson, 1978).

Fluoride and Dental Caries. Experiments in controlling the fluoride content of water took an unexpected and significant turn when it was observed that children born at Bauxite, Arkansas, after a new water supply had been obtained, showed a much higher incidence of caries than those who had been exposed to the former fluoride-containing water. This led to extensive studies on the part of the United States Public Health Service to ascertain whether the fluoridation of water could be employed as a practical measure to reduce the incidence of tooth decay. It has now been definitely established on the basis of large-scale studies in a number of communities that the fluoridation of water to a concentration of 1.0 ppm is a safe and practical public health measure that results in substantial reduction in the incidence of caries in permanent teeth.

There are partial benefits for children who begin drinking fluoridated water at any age; however, optimal benefits are obtained at ages before permanent teeth erupt. Topical applications of fluoride solutions by dental personnel appear to be particularly effective on newly erupted teeth and can reduce the incidence of caries by 30 to 40%. The prescription of dietary fluoride supplements should be considered for children whose drinking water contains less than 0.7 ppm of fluoride. Conflicting results have been reported from studies of the effectiveness of fluoride-containing toothpastes.

Adequate incorporation of fluoride into teeth causes the outer layers of enamel to be harder and more resistant to demineralization. The deposition of fluoride ion appears to be an anion-exchange process with hydroxyl or citrate ions. Fluoride occupies the anionic spaces in the enamel apatite crystal surface. The mechanism of prevention of caries exerted by the deposition of minute amounts of fluoride in surface enamel is not completely understood. There is no convincing evidence that fluoride from any source reduces the development of caries after the permanent teeth are completely formed (usually about age 14).

Preparations and Uses. *Sodium Fluoride,* U.S.P., *Sodium Fluoride Oral Solution,* U.S.P., *Sodium Fluoride Tablets,* U.S.P., and *Stannous Fluoride,* U.S.P., are official fluoride preparations. The fluoride salts presently employed in dentifrices are sodium fluoride, stannous fluoride, and *Sodium Fluoride and Phosphoric Acid Topical Solution,* U.S.P. Sodium fluoride, sodium fluosilicate (Na_2SiF_6), and cryolite are the salts commonly used for insecticides.

Adams, T. H., and Norman, A. W. Studies on the mechanism of action of calciferol. I. Basic parameters of vitamin D–mediated calcium transport. *J. Biol. Chem.,* **1970,** *245,* 4421–4431.

Agus, Z. S.; Gardner, L. B.; Beck, L. H.; and Goldberg, M. Effects of parathyroid hormone on renal tubular reabsorption of calcium, sodium, and phosphate. *Am. J. Physiol.,* **1973,** *224,* 1143–1148.

Altman, R. D.; Johnston, C. C.; Khairi, M. R. A.; Wellman, H.; Seratin, A. N.; and Sankey, R. R. Influence of disodium etidronate on clinical and laboratory manifestations of Paget's disease of bone (osteitis deformans). *N. Engl. J. Med.,* **1973,** *289,* 1379–1384.

Armstrong, W. D. Body fluid fluoride distribution. *J. Dent. Res.,* **1967,** *46,* 60–62.

Arnaud, C. D. Calcium homeostasis: regulatory elements and their integration. *Fed. Proc.,* **1978,** *37,* 2557–2560.

Belsey, R.; DeLuca, H. F.; and Potts, J. T., Jr. Competitive binding assay for vitamin D and 25-OH vitamin D. *J. Clin. Endocrinol. Metab.,* **1971,** *33,* 554–557.

Berl, T.; Berns, A. S.; Huffer, W. E.; Hammil, K.; Alfrey, A. C.; Arnaud, C. D.; and Schrier, R. W. 1,25 Dihydroxycholecalciferol effects in chronic dialysis. *Ann. Intern. Med.,* **1978,** *88,* 774–780.

Berman, L. A. Crystalline substance from the parathyroid glands that influences the calcium content of the blood. *Proc. Soc. Exp. Biol. Med.,* **1924,** *21,* 465.

Bikle, D. D.; Zolook, D. T.; Morrissey, R. L.; and Herman, R. H. Independence of 1,25-dihydroxyvitamin D–mediated calcium transport from *de novo* RNA and protein synthesis. *J. Biol. Chem.,* **1978,** *253,* 484–488.

Birge, S. J., and Miller, R. The role of phosphate in the action of vitamin D on the intestine. *J. Clin. Invest.,* **1977,** *60,* 980–988.

Blaustein, M. P., and Hodgkin, A. L. The effect of cyanide on the efflux of calcium from squid axons. *J. Physiol. (Lond.),* **1969,** *200,* 497–528.

Boris, A. Structure-activity relationships of vitamin D analogues. *Am. J. Med.,* **1977,** *62,* 543–544.

Brewer, H. B.; Fairwell, T.; Rittel, W.; Littledike, T.; and Arnaud, C. D. Recent studies on the chemistry of human, bovine and porcine parathyroid hormones. *Am. J. Med.,* **1974,** *56,* 759–766.

Brickman, A. S.; Coburn, J. W.; Kurokawa, K.; Bethune, J. E.; Harrison, H. E.; and Norman, A. W. Actions of 1,25-dihydroxycholecalciferol in patients with hypophosphatemic, vitamin-D-resistant rickets. *N. Engl. J. Med.,* **1973,** *289,* 495–498.

Brown, E. M.; Carroll, R. J.; and Aurbach, G. D. Dopaminergic stimulation of cyclic AMP accumulation and parathyroid hormone release from dispersed bovine parathyroid cells. *Proc. Natl. Acad. Sci. U.S.A.,* **1977,** *74,* 4210–4213.

Brumbaugh, P. F., and Haussler, M. R. 1α,25-Dihydroxycholecalciferol receptors in intestine. II. Temperature-dependent transfer of hormone to chromatin via a specific cytosol receptor. *J. Biol. Chem.,* **1974,** *249,* 1258–1262.

Burke, W. J.; Hoegg, U. R.; and Phillips, R. E. Systemic fluoride poisoning resulting from a fluoride skin burn. *J. Occup. Med.,* **1973,** *15,* 39–41.

Canfield, R.; Rosner, W.; Skinner, J.; McWhorter, J.; Resnick, L.; Feldman, F.; Kammerman, S.; Ryan, K.; Kunigonis, M.; and Bohne, W. Diphosphonate therapy of Paget's disease of bone. *J. Clin. Endocrinol. Metab.,* **1977,** *44,* 96–106.

Card, R. T., and Brain, M. C. The "anemia" of childhood: evidence for a physiologic response to hyperphosphatemia. *N. Engl. J. Med.,* **1973,** *288,* 388–392.

Carlsson, A. Tracer experiments on the effect of vitamin D on skeletal metabolism of calcium and phosphorus. *Acta Physiol. Scand.,* **1952,** *26,* 212–222.

Castells, S. New approaches to treatment of osteogenesis imperfecta. *Clin. Orthop.,* **1973,** *93,* 239–249.

Chase, L. R.; Melson, G. L.; and Aurbach, G. D. Pseudohypoparathyroidism: defective excretion of 3′,5′-AMP in response to parathyroid hormone. *J. Clin. Invest.,* **1969,** *48,* 1823–1844.

Chesney, R. W.; Moorthy, A. V.; Eisman, J. A.; Jax, D. K.; Mazess, R. B.; and DeLuca, H. F. Increased growth after long-term oral $1\alpha,25$-vitamin D_3 in childhood renal osteodystrophy. *N. Engl. J. Med.,* **1978,** *298,* 238–242.

Collip, J. B. The extraction of a parathyroid hormone which will prevent or control parathyroid tetany and which regulates the level of blood calcium. *J. Biol. Chem.,* **1925,** *63,* 395–438.

Committee on Nutrition. The prophylactic requirement and toxicity of vitamin D. *Pediatrics,* **1963,** *31,* 512–523.

Corradino, R. A. Parathyroid hormone and calcitonin: no direct effect on vitamin D_3-mediated, intestinal calcium absorptive mechanism. *Horm. Metab. Res.,* **1976,** *8,* 485–488.

Costanzo, L. S.; Sheehe, P. R.; and Weiner, I. M. Renal actions of vitamin D in vitamin D deficient rats. *Am. J. Physiol.,* **1974,** *226,* 1490–1495.

Daniel, H. J.; Shambaugh, G. E.; and Fisch, U. Fluoride and clinical otosclerosis. *Arch. Otolaryngol.,* **1973,** *98,* 327–329.

David, D. S. Clinical studies of vitamin D analogues in renal failure. *Am. J. Med.,* **1977,** *62,* 544–546.

Davis, B. B., and Murdaugh, H. V. Evaluation of interrelationship between calcium and sodium excretion by canine kidney. *Metabolism,* **1970,** *19,* 439–444.

DeLuca, H. F. Vitamin D as a prohormone. *Biochem. Pharmacol.,* **1977,** *26,* 563–566.

Dent, C. E.; Richens, A.; Rowle, D. J. F.; and Stamp, T. C. B. Osteomalacia with long-term anticonvulsant therapy in epilepsy. *Br. Med. J.,* **1970,** *4,* 69–72.

DeRose, J.; Singer, F. R.; Avramides, A.; Flores, A.; Dziadiw, R.; Baker, R. K.; and Wallach, S. Response of Paget's disease to porcine and salmon calcitonins. Effects of long-term treatment. *Am. J. Med.,* **1974,** *56,* 858–866.

DiBella, E. P.; Flueck, J. A.; von Lilienfeld-Toal, H.; and Arnaud, C. D. Hyperfunctioning parathyroid glands: a major source of immunoheterogeneity of parathyroid hormone in serum. In, *Endocrinology of Calcium Metabolism.* (Copp, D. H., and Talmage, R. V., eds.) Excerpta Medica, Amsterdam, **1978,** pp. 338–341.

Edelstein, S.; Noff, D.; Sinai, L.; Harell, A.; Puschett, J. B.; Golub, E. E.; and Bronner, F. Vitamin D metabolism and expression in rats fed on low-calcium and low-phosphorus diets. *Biochem. J.,* **1978,** *170,* 227–233.

Erickson, J. D. Mortality in selected cities with fluoridated and non-fluoridated water supplies. *N. Engl. J. Med.,* **1978,** *298,* 1112–1116.

Fischer, J. A.; Blum, J. W.; and Binswanger, U. Acute parathyroid hormone response to epinephrine *in vivo. J. Clin. Invest.,* **1973,** *52,* 2434–2440.

Francis, M. D.; Russell, R. G. G.; and Fleisch, H. Diphosphonates inhibit formation of calcium phosphate crystals *in vitro* and pathological calcification *in vivo. Science,* **1969,** *165,* 1264–1266.

Fraser, D.; Kooh, S. W.; Kind, H. P.; Holick, M. F.;

Tanaka, Y.; and DeLuca, H. F. Pathogenesis of hereditary vitamin-D-dependent rickets: an inborn error of vitamin D metabolism involving defective conversion of 25-hydroxyvitamin D to $1\alpha,25$-dihydroxyvitamin D. *N. Engl. J. Med.,* **1973,** *289,* 817–822.

Friedman, W. R., and Roberts, W. C. Vitamin D and the supravalvular aortic stenosis syndrome. *Circulation,* **1966,** *34,* 77–86.

Garabedian, M.; Tanaka, Y.; Holick, M. F.; and DeLuca, H. F. Response of intestinal calcium transport and bone mobilization to 1,25-dihydroxyvitamin D_3 in thyroparathyroidectomized rats. *Endocrinology,* **1974,** *94,* 1022–1027.

Gascon-Barré, M., and Côte, M. G. Effects of phenobarbital and diphenylhydantoin on acute vitamin D toxicity in the rat. *Toxicol. Appl. Pharmacol.,* **1978,** *43,* 125–135.

Gley, M. E. Sur les effets de l'extirpation du corps thyroide. *C. R. Soc. Biol. (Paris),* **1891,** *43,* 551–554.

Greenberg, B. G.; Winters, R. W.; and Graham, J. B. The normal range of serum inorganic phosphorus and its utility as a discriminant in the diagnosis of congenital hypophosphatemia. *J. Clin. Endocrinol. Metab.,* **1960,** *20,* 364–379.

Hahn, T. J.; Birge, S. J.; Scharp, C. R.; and Avioli, L. V. Phenobarbital-induced alterations in vitamin D metabolism. *J. Clin. Invest.,* **1972a,** *51,* 741–748.

Hahn, T. J.; Hendin, B. A.; Scharp, C. R.; and Haddad, J. G., Jr. Effect of chronic anticonvulsant therapy on serum 25-hydroxycalciferol levels in adults. *N. Engl. J. Med.,* **1972b,** *287,* 900–904.

Hallick, R. B., and DeLuca, H. F. Metabolites of dihydrotachysterol$_3$ in target tissues. *J. Biol. Chem.,* **1972,** *247,* 91–97.

Hanson, A. M. The hormone of the parathyroid gland. *Proc. Soc. Exp. Biol. Med.,* **1925,** *22,* 560–561.

Harris, C. A.; Sutton, R. A. L.; and Seeley, J. F. Effect of 1,25-(OH)$_2$-vitamin D_3 on renal electrolyte handling in the vitamin deficient rat: dissociation of calcium and sodium excretion. *Clin. Res.,* **1976,** *24,* 685A.

Haussler, M. R.; Hughes, M. R.; McCain, T. A.; Zerwekh, J. E.; Brumbaugh, P. F.; Jubiz, W.; and Wasserman, R. H. 1,25-Dihydroxy D_3: mode of action in intestine and parathyroid glands, assay in humans and isolation of its glycoside from *Solanum malacoxylon. Calcif. Tissue Res.,* **1977,** *22,* Suppl., 1–17.

Heath, H., iii, and Sizemore, G. W. Plasma calcitonin in normal man. Differences between men and women. *J. Clin. Invest.,* **1977,** *60,* 1135–1140.

Hess, A. F., and Weinstock, M. Antirachitic properties imparted to inert fluids and to green vegetables by ultraviolet irradiation. *J. Biol. Chem.,* **1924,** *62,* 301–313.

Hirsch, P. F.; Gauthier, G. F.; and Munson, P. C. Thyroid hypocalcemic principle and recurrent laryngeal nerve injury as factors affecting the response to parathyroidectomy in rats. *Endocrinology,* **1963,** *73,* 244–252.

Holick, M. F., and Clark, M. B. The photobiogenesis and metabolism of vitamin D. *Fed. Proc.,* **1978,** *37,* 2561–2574.

Holman, C. B. Roentgenologic manifestations of vitamin D intoxication. *Radiology,* **1952,** *59,* 805–816.

Hoover, R. N.; McKay, F. W.; and Fraumeni, J. F., Jr. Fluoridated drinking water and the occurrence of cancer. *J. Natl. Cancer Inst.,* **1976,** *57,* 757–768.

Howell, W. H. On the relation of the blood to the automaticity and sequence of the heartbeat. *Am. J. Physiol.,* **1899,** *2,* 47–81.

Hunter, J.; Maxwell, J. D.; Stewart, D. A.; Parsons, V.; and Williams, R. Altered calcium metabolism in epileptic children on anticonvulsants. *Br. Med. J.,* **1971,** *4,* 202–204.

Jacob, H. S., and Amsden, T. Acute hemolytic anemia with rigid red cells in hypophosphatemia. *N. Engl. J. Med.,* **1971,** *285,* 1446–1450.

Jeans, P. C., and Stearns, G. Effect of vitamin D on linear growth in infancy: effect of intakes above 1,800 U.S.P. units daily. *J. Pediatr.,* **1938,** *13,* 730–740.

Jones, A. E.; Ghaed, N.; Dunson, G. L.; and Hosain, F.

Clinical evaluation of orally administered fluorine 18 for bone scanning. *Radiology,* **1973,** *107,* 129–131.

Jubiz, W.; Haussler, M. R.; McCain, T. A.; and Tolman, K. G. Plasma 1,25-dihydroxyvitamin D levels in patients receiving anticonvulsant drugs. *J. Clin. Endocrinol. Metab.,* **1977,** *44,* 617–621.

Kuntziger, H.; Amiel, C.; Roinel, N.; and Morel, F. Effect of parathyroidectomy and cyclic AMP on renal transport of phosphate, calcium, and magnesium. *Am. J. Physiol.,* **1974,** *227,* 905–911.

Lechene, C.; Colindres, R. E.; and Knox, F. G. Electron probe microanalysis of the renal effect of parathyroid hormone. In, *Endocrinology of Calcium Metabolism.* (Copp, D. H., and Talmage, R. V., eds.) Excerpta Medica, Amsterdam, **1978,** pp. 230–233.

Leeson, P. M., and Fourman, P. Increased sensitivity to vitamin D after vitamin D poisoning. *Lancet,* **1966,** *1,* 1182–1185.

Levitt, M.; Gessert, C.; and Finberg, L. Inorganic phosphate (laxative) poisoning resulting in tetany in an infant. *J. Pediatr.,* **1973,** *82,* 479–481.

Lichtman, M. A.; Miller, D. R.; and Freeman, R. B. Erythrocyte adenosine triphosphate depletion during hypophosphatemia. *N. Engl. J. Med.,* **1969,** *280,* 240–244.

Loeb, J. On an apparently new form of muscular irritability (contact irritability?) produced by solutions of salts (preferably sodium salts) whose anions are liable to form insoluble calcium compounds. *Am. J. Physiol.,* **1901,** *5,* 362–373.

MacCallum, S. G., and Voegtlin, C. On the relation of tetany to the parathyroid glands and to calcium metabolism. *J. Exp. Med.,* **1909,** *11,* 118–151.

McConnell, T. H. Fatal hypocalcemia from phosphate absorption from laxative preparations. *J.A.M.A.,* **1971,** *216,* 147–148.

MacIntyre, I.; Boss, S.; and Troughton, V. A. Parathyroid hormone and magnesium homoeostasis. *Nature,* **1963,** *198,* 1058–1060.

Massry, S. G., and Coburn, J. W. The hormonal and nonhormonal control of renal excretion of calcium and magnesium. *Nephron,* **1973,** *10,* 66–112.

Massry, S. G.; Muella, E.; Silverman, A. G.; and Kleeman, C. R. Inorganic phosphate treatment of hypercalcemia. *Arch. Intern. Med.,* **1968,** *12,* 307–312.

Mawer, E. B.; Backhouse, J.; Davies, M.; Hill, C. F.; and Taylor, C. M. Metabolic fate of administered 1,25-dihydroxycholecalciferol in controls and in patients with hypoparathyroidism. *Lancet,* **1976,** *1,* 1203–1206.

Mellanby, E. Experimental rickets. *Spec. Rep. Ser. Med. Res. Coun.,* **1921,** Series 61, 1–78.

Metz, S. A.; Baylink, D. J.; Hughes, M. R.; Haussler, M. R.; and Robertson, R. P. Selective deficiency of 1,25-dihydroxycholecalciferol. *N. Engl. J. Med.,* **1977,** *297,* 1084–1090.

Miller, S. C. Rapid activation of the medullary bone osteoclast cell surface by parathyroid hormone. *J. Cell Biol.,* **1978,** *76,* 615–618.

Murad, F.; Brewer, H. B.; and Vaughan, M. Effect of thyrocalcitonin on adenosine 3',5'-cyclic phosphate formation by rat kidney and bone. *Proc. Natl. Acad. Sci. U.S.A.,* **1970,** *65,* 446–453.

Murad, F., and Pak, C. Y. C. Urinary excretion of adenosine 3',5'-monophosphate and guanosine 3',5'-monophosphate. *N. Engl. J. Med.,* **1972,** *286,* 1382–1387.

Murayama, Y.; Morel, F.; and Le Grimellec, C. Phosphate, calcium and magnesium transfers in proximal tubules and loops of Henle, as measured by single nephron microperfusion experiments in the rat. *Pfluegers Arch.,* **1972,** *333,* 1–16.

Neuman, W. F., and Ramp, W. K. The concept of a bone membrane: some implications. In, *Cellular Mechanisms for Calcium Transfer and Homeostasis.* (Nichols, G., Jr., and Wasserman, R. H., eds.) Academic Press, Inc., New York, **1971,** pp. 197–206.

New, W., and Trautwein, W. Inward membrane currents in mammalian myocardium. *Pfluegers Arch.,* **1972,** *334,* 1–23.

Nicolaysen, R. Studies upon the mode of action of vitamin D. III. The influence of vitamin D on the absorption of calcium and phosphorus in the rat. *Biochem. J.,* **1937,** *31,* 122–129.

Odell, W. D., and Wolfsen, A. R. Humoral syndromes associated with cancer. *Annu. Rev. Med.,* **1978,** *29,* 379–406.

Paillard, F.; Ardaillou, R.; Malendin, H.; Fillastre, J. P.; and Prier, S. Renal effects on salmon calcitonin in man. *J. Lab. Clin. Med.,* **1972,** *80,* 200–216.

Parfitt, A. M. Hypophosphatemic vitamin D refractory rickets and osteomalacia. *Orthop. Clin. North Am.,* **1972,** *3,* 653–680.

Perlia, C. P.; Gubisch, N. J.; Wolter, J.; Edelberg, D.; Dederick, M. M.; and Taylor, S. G., III. Mithramycin treatment of hypercalcemia. *Cancer,* **1970,** *25,* 389–394.

Puschett, J. B.; Moranz, J.; and Kurnick, W. S. Evidence for a direct action of cholecalciferol and 25-hydroxycholecalciferol on the renal transport of phosphate, sodium, and calcium. *J. Clin. Invest.,* **1972,** *51,* 373–385.

Raisz, L. G. Bone metabolism and calcium regulation. In, *Metabolic Bone Disease,* Vol. I. (Avioli, L. V., and Krane, S. M., eds.) Academic Press, Inc., New York, **1977,** pp. 1–48.

Raisz, L. G.; Trummel, C. L.; Holick, M. F.; and DeLuca, H. F. 1,25-Dihydroxycholecalciferol: a potent stimulator of bone resorption in tissue culture. *Science,* **1972,** *175,* 768–769.

Rasmussen, H.; DeLuca, H.; Arnaud, C.; Hawker, C.; and Stedingk, M. von. The relationship between vitamin D and parathyroid hormone. *J. Clin. Invest.,* **1963,** *42,* 1940–1946.

Reynolds, J. J.; Pavlovitch, H.; and Balsan, S. 1,25-Dihydroxycholecalciferol increases bone resorption in thyroparathyroidectomized rats. *Calcif. Tissue Res.,* **1976,** *21,* 207–212.

Rosen, J. F.; Fleischman, A. R.; Finberg, L.; Eisman, J.; and DeLuca, H. F. 1,25-Dihydroxycholecalciferol: its use in the long-term management of idiopathic hypoparathyroidism in children. *J. Clin. Endocrinol. Metab.,* **1977,** *45,* 457–468.

Rosenstreich, S. J.; Rich, C.; and Volwiler, W. Deposition in and release of vitamin D_3 from body fat; evidence for a storage site in the rat. *J. Clin. Invest.,* **1971,** *50,* 679–687.

Roth, S. I., and Raisz, L. G. Effect of calcium concentration on the ultrastructure of rat parathyroid in organ culture. *Lab. Invest.,* **1964,** *13,* 331–345.

Rude, R. K.; Oldham, S. B.; and Singer, F. R. Functional hypoparathyroidism and parathyroid hormone end-organ resistance in human magnesium deficiency. *Clin. Endocrinol. (Oxf.),* **1976,** *5,* 209–224.

Russell, R. G. G., and Fleisch, H. Pyrophosphate and diphosphonates in skeletal metabolism. *Clin. Orthop.,* **1975,** *108,* 241–263.

Scriver, C. R.; Reade, T. M.; DeLuca, H. F.; and Hamstra, A. J. Serum 1,25-hydroxyvitamin D levels in normal subjects and in patients with hereditary rickets or bone disease. *N. Engl. J. Med.,* **1978,** *299,* 976–979.

Segre, G. V.; D'Amour, P.; Rosenblatt, M.; and Potts, J. T., Jr. Heterogeneity and metabolism of parathyroid hormone. In, *Endocrinology of Calcium Metabolism.* (Copp, D. H., and Talmage, R. V., eds.) Excerpta Medica, Amsterdam, **1978,** pp. 329–331.

Smith, J. E., and Goodman, DeW. S. The turnover and transport of vitamin D and of a polar metabolite with the properties of 25-hydroxycholecalciferol in human plasma. *J. Clin. Invest.,* **1971,** *50,* 2159–2167.

Smith, R. The pathophysiology and management of rickets. *Orthop. Clin. North Am.,* **1972,** *3,* 601–621.

Spencer, R.; Charman, M.; Wilson, P. W.; and Lawson, D. E. M. The relationship between vitamin D–stimulated calcium transport and intestinal calcium–

binding protein in the chicken. *Biochem. J.,* **1978,** *170,* 93–101.

Steele, T. H. Increased urinary phosphate excretion following volume expansion in normal man. *Metabolism,* **1970,** *19,* 29–39.

Steenbock, H., and Black, A. Fat-soluble vitamins. XVII. The induction of growth-promoting and calcifying properties in a ration by exposure to ultraviolet light. *J. Biol. Chem.,* **1924,** *61,* 405–422.

Suda, T.; Hallick, R. B.; DeLuca, H. F.; and Schnoes, H. K. 25-Hydroxydihydrotachysterol₃. Synthesis and biological activity. *Biochemistry,* **1970,** *9,* 1651–1657.

Talmage, R. V. Further studies on the control of calcium homeostasis by parathyroid hormone. In, *Calcium, Parathyroid Hormone, and the Calcitonins.* (Talmage, R. V., and Munson, P. L., eds.) Excerpta Medica, Amsterdam, **1972,** pp. 422–429.

Tashjian, A. H.; Wolfe, H. J.; and Voelkel, E. F. Human calcitonin. Immunologic assay, cytochemical localization and studies on medullary thyroid carcinoma. *Am. J. Med.,* **1974,** *56,* 840–849.

Taussig, H. B. Possible injury to the cardiovascular system from vitamin D. *Ann. Intern. Med.,* **1966,** *65,* 1195–1200.

Vassale, G., and Generali, F. Fonction parathyroidienne et fonction thyroidienne. *Arch. Ital. Biol.,* **1900,** *33,* 154–156.

Werner, J. A.; Gorton, S. J.; and Raisz, L. G. Escape from inhibition of resorption in cultures of fetal bone treated with calcitonin and parathyroid hormone. *Endocrinology,* **1972,** *90,* 752–759.

Wong, G. L.; Luben, R. A.; and Cohn, D. V. 1,25-Dihydroxycholecalciferol and parathormone: effects on isolated osteoclast-like cells. *Science,* **1977,** *197,* 663–665.

Yalow, R. S. Significance of the heterogeneity of parathyroid hormone. In, *Endocrinology of Calcium Metabolism.* (Copp, D. H., and Talmage, R. V., eds.) Excerpta Medica, Amsterdam, **1978,** pp. 308–312.

Zile, M.; Bunge, E. C.; Barsness, L.; Yamada, S.; Schnoes, H. K.; and DeLuca, H. F. Localization of 1,25-dihydroxyvitamin D in intestinal nuclei *in vivo. Arch. Biochem. Biophys.,* **1978,** *186,* 15–24.

Monographs and Reviews

Albright, F. A page out of the history of hyperparathyroidism. *J. Clin. Endocrinol. Metab.,* **1948,** *8,* 637–657.

Arena, J. M. *Poisoning: Toxicology-Symptoms-Treatments,* 3rd ed. Charles C Thomas, Pub., Springfield, Ill., **1973.**

Copp, D. H. Parathyroids, calcitonin, and control of plasma calcium. *Recent Prog. Horm. Res.,* **1964,** *20,* 59–88.

Deftos, L. J. Calcitonin in clinical medicine. *Adv. Intern. Med.,* **1978,** *23,* 159–193.

DeLuca, H. F. Vitamin D metabolism and function. *Arch. Intern. Med.,* **1978,** *138,* 836–847.

DeLuca, H. F., and Schnoes, H. K. Metabolism and mechanism of action of vitamin D. *Annu. Rev. Biochem.,* **1976,** *45,* 631–666.

Douglas, W. W. Stimulus-secretion coupling: the concept and clues from chromaffin and other cells. (The First Gaddum Memorial Lecture.) *Br. J. Pharmacol.,* **1968,** *34,* 451–474.

Fraser, D. R. Regulation of the metabolism of vitamin D. *Physiol. Rev.,* **1980,** *60,* 551–613.

Habener, J. F., and Mahaffey, J. E. Osteomalacia and disorders of vitamin D metabolism. *Annu. Rev. Med.,* **1978,** *29,* 327–342.

Habener, J. F., and Potts, J. T. Biosynthesis of parathyroid hormone. *N. Engl. J. Med.,* **1978,** *299,* 580–585, 635–644.

Haussler, M. R., and McCain, T. A. Basis and clinical concepts related to vitamin D metabolism and action. *N. Engl. J. Med.,* **1977,** *297,* 974–983.

Kretsinger, R. H. Evolution and function of calcium-binding proteins. *Int. Rev. Cytol.,* **1976,** *46,* 323–393. (313 references.)

Omdahl, J. L., and DeLuca, H. F. Regulation of vitamin D metabolism and function. *Physiol. Rev.,* **1973,** *53,* 327–372. (231 references.)

Pak, C. Y. C. Parathyroid hormone and thyrocalcitonin: their mode of action and regulation. *Ann. N.Y. Acad. Sci.,* **1971,** *179,* 450–474.

Rasmussen, H. Parathyroid hormone, calcitonin, and the calciferols. In, *Textbook of Endocrinology,* 5th ed. (Williams, R. H., ed.) W. B. Saunders Co., Philadelphia, **1974,** pp. 660–773.

Rasmussen, H., and Bordier, P. *The Physiological and Cellular Basis of Metabolic Bone Disease.* The Williams & Wilkins Co., Baltimore, **1974.**

Symposium. (Various authors.) Parathyroid hormone, calcitonin and vitamin D: clinical considerations. (Forscher, B. K., and Arnaud, C. D., eds.) *Am. J. Med.,* **1974,** *56,* 743–870; *57,* 1–62.

Symposium. (Various authors.) *Calcium-Regulating Hormones.* (Talmage, R. V.; Owen, M.; and Parsons, J. A.; eds.) Excerpta Medica, Amsterdam, **1975.**

Symposium. (Various authors.) *Phosphate Metabolism.* (Massry, S. G., and Ritz, E., eds.) *Adv. Exp. Med. Biol.,* **1977,** *81,* 3–636.

Symposium. (Various authors.) *Endocrinology of Calcium Metabolism.* (Copp, D. H., and Talmage, R. V., eds.) Excerpta Medica, Amsterdam, **1978.**

SECTION
XVI

The Vitamins

INTRODUCTION

Darla Erhard Danford and Hamish N. Munro

The diet is the source of some 40 nutrients for man. These are classically divided into energy-yielding dietary components (carbohydrates, fats, and proteins), sources of essential and nonessential amino acids (proteins), minerals (including trace minerals), and vitamins (water-soluble and fat-soluble organic compounds). In this section, the subject is vitamins.

Centuries ago, physicians described many of the diseases now recognized as vitamin deficiencies, notably night blindness (vitamin A deficiency), beriberi (thiamine deficiency), pellagra (niacin deficiency), scurvy (ascorbic acid deficiency), and rickets (vitamin D deficiency). Long before the era of vitamins, dietary factors were considered to be involved in all these conditions. However, the eventual identification of the active factor in the diet usually required reproduction of the disease in an experimental animal by feeding it a diet similar to that presumed to cause the condition in man, followed by prevention or cure of the disease by addition of certain foods or extracts of foods to the experimental diet. For example, scurvy was identified as a disease in the Middle Ages, and in 1747 Lind showed that citrus fruits could cure scurvy. However, the demonstration in 1907 that a diet of oats and bran causes scurvy in guinea pigs allowed tests for antiscorbutic activity in fractions from citrus fruits; this culminated in the identification of ascorbic acid in 1932. Similarly, beriberi, a form of polyneuritis, has been known for centuries to occur in populations eating polished (refined) rice. In 1897, Eijkman showed that fowl fed polished rice developed a polyneuritis similar to beriberi that could be cured by adding the husks or an extract of the husks back to the polished rice from which they had been derived. This animal model allowed Funk, in 1911, to isolate from the extract an antiberiberi substance, which he believed to be an amine. Being vital for life, he called the substance a *vitamine* and suggested that not only beriberi but also scurvy, pellagra, and possibly rickets were due to the lack of similar organic bases in the diet. The name was shortened to *vitamin* when it was subsequently recognized that dietary factors in this class are not necessarily amines and, indeed, have unrelated structures.

In the meantime, Osborne and Mendel (1911 to 1913) had demonstrated the presence in butter of a factor necessary for the growth of rats. In 1915, McCollum and Davis confirmed its presence in several dietary fats and named it *fat-soluble A*, which they distinguished from *water-soluble B*, another dietary factor necessary for the growth of rats; the latter was subsequently identified as Funk's antiberiberi factor. It soon became apparent that both the fat-soluble and the water-soluble factors (vitamins) consisted of several active components. Fats were shown to contain a factor (vitamin D) that prevented rickets and could be distinguished from the rat growth factor, vitamin A. Subsequent work has identified other fat-soluble factors (vitamins E and K) as essential dietary components. The water-soluble B fraction also proved to contain several components needed by man, namely thiamine, riboflavin, nicotinic acid, pyridoxine, pantothenic acid, biotin, folic acid, and cyanocobalamin (vitamin B_{12}). These were originally grouped together because they could be extracted in high concentration from certain foods, notably liver and yeast, in which the antiberiberi factor B had been identified. When active constituents were separately recognized in factor B, they were assigned the names vitamin B_1, vitamin B_2, and so forth; these have subsequently been replaced by chemical names. The members of the vitamin B complex are quite dissimilar in chemical structure, and they also differ in function. However, their continued classification together is justified by the similarity of their dietary sources and the consequent tendency for deficiency diseases to involve inadequate intakes of more than one member of the group. Finally, the water-soluble, antiscorbutic factor was named vitamin C, or ascorbic acid.

Vitamins are thus a group of substances of diverse chemical composition. They can be defined as *organic* substances that must be provided in small quantities in the diet for the synthesis, by tissues, of cofactors that are essential for various metabolic reactions. This definition differentiates vitamins from essential trace minerals, which are *inorganic* nutrients needed in small quantities. It also excludes the essential amino acids, which are organic substances needed preformed in the diet in much larger quantities. The Nomenclature Committee of the American Institute of Nutrition recommends that the term *vitamin* be restricted to include only organic substances required for the nutrition of mammals; substances required only by microorganisms and cells in culture should be defined as *growth factors,* in order to prevent scientifically unsound claims for their therapeutic benefit as vitamins for man. When the vitamin occurs in more than one chemical form (*e.g.,* pyridoxine, pyridoxal, pyridoxamine) or as a precursor (*e.g.,* carotene for vitamin A), these analogs are sometimes referred to as *vitamers.*

Appropriate Uses of Vitamins. The intelligent use of vitamins is part of a general appreciation of the current status of our knowledge of nutrition. Interest in the role of nutrition in the causation and treatment of disease has recently increased greatly. United States Congressional hearings have resulted in a proposal for a National Nutrition Policy (Select Committee on Nutrition and Human Needs, 1977) and identification of a need for more research into the role of nutrition in the etiology of obesity, cardiovascular disease, and other chronic conditions.

The United States Food and Drug Administration (FDA), under the authority of the Federal Food, Drug, and Cosmetic Act, regulates the labeling of vitamin and mineral products sold as foods and as drugs. In 1973, the FDA introduced labeling of the nutrient content of conventional foods ("nutrition labeling") and also proposed a regulation to govern the composition of dietary supplements of vitamins and minerals (Food and Drug Administration, 1976). These regulations have subsequently been reviewed (Food and Drug Administration, 1979). Dietary supplements, by definition, are for use by healthy people to supplement the diet and are subject to regulation as foods, whereas vitamins and minerals marketed for the prevention or treatment of disease are controlled either as "over-the-counter" or prescription drugs. All vitamin and mineral preparations designed for *parenteral* administration are regulated as prescription drugs. The current status of such regulations is discussed later in this introductory section. The physician who wants a standard for the intelligent use of vitamin and mineral supplements should refer to the ninth edition of the handbook entitled *Recommended Dietary Allowances* (Food and Nutrition Board, National Research Council, 1979). These standards (Table XVI–1) are the basis on which national policies, including those of the FDA, are based.

Recommended Dietary Allowances. In many countries throughout the world, scientific committees periodically assess the evidence about the requirements of the population for individual nutrients. In the United States, the National Academy of Sciences has a Food and Nutrition Board, one of whose functions is to recommend allowances of nutrients that will serve as a goal for good nutrition and will "encourage patterns of food consumption in the United States that will maintain and promote health" (Food and Nutrition Board, 1979). Recommended dietary allowances (RDA) for nutrients to ensure health were first published in 1941 and are periodically revised to incorporate new knowledge by the Dietary Allowances Committee of the Food and Nutrition Board. In 1979, the Ninth Edition of *Recommended Dietary Allowances* was issued. Its recommendations for males and females of different ages are summarized in Table XVI–1. With the exception of the recommended intakes of energy, these

Table XVI-1. RECOMMENDED DAILY DIETARY ALLOWANCES [a]

	Age	Weight	Height	Energy	Protein	FAT-SOLUBLE VITAMINS			WATER-SOLUBLE VITAMINS							MINERALS					
						Vita-min A	Vita-min D	Vita-min E	Vita-min C	Thia-mine	Ribo-flavin	Nia-cin [e]	Vita-min B_6	Fola-cin [f]	Vita-min B_{12}	Cal-cium	Phos-phorus	Magne-sium	Iron	Zinc	Io-dine
	(years)	(kg)	(cm)	(kcal)	(g)	(µg R.E.) [b]	(µg) [c]	(mg α-T.E.) [d]	(mg)	(mg)	(mg)	(mg)	(mg)	(µg)	(µg)	(mg)	(mg)	(mg)	(mg)	(mg)	(µg)
Infants	0.0–0.5	6	60	kg × 115	kg × 2.2	420	10	3	35	0.3	0.4	6	0.3	30	0.5 [g]	360	240	50	10	3	40
	0.5–1.0	9	71	kg × 105	kg × 2.0	400	10	4	35	0.5	0.6	8	0.6	45	1.5	540	360	70	15	5	50
Children	1–3	13	90	1300	23	400	10	5	45	0.7	0.8	9	0.9	100	2.0	800	800	150	15	10	70
	4–6	20	112	1700	30	500	10	6	45	0.9	1.0	11	1.3	200	2.5	800	800	200	10	10	90
	7–10	28	132	2400	34	700	10	7	45	1.2	1.4	16	1.6	300	3.0	800	800	250	10	10	120
Males	11–14	45	157	2700	45	1000	10	8	50	1.4	1.6	18	1.8	400	3.0	1200	1200	350	18	15	150
	15–18	66	176	2800	56	1000	10	10	60	1.4	1.7	18	2.0	400	3.0	1200	1200	400	18	15	150
	19–22	70	177	2900	56	1000	7.5	10	60	1.5	1.7	19	2.2	400	3.0	800	800	350	10	15	150
	23–50	70	178	2700	56	1000	5	10	60	1.4	1.6	18	2.2	400	3.0	800	800	350	10	15	150
	51+	70	178	2400	56	1000	5	10	60	1.2	1.4	16	2.2	400	3.0	800	800	350	10	15	150
Females	11–14	46	157	2200	46	800	10	8	50	1.1	1.3	15	1.8	400	3.0	1200	1200	300	18	15	150
	15–18	55	163	2100	46	800	10	8	60	1.1	1.3	14	2.0	400	3.0	1200	1200	300	18	15	150
	19–22	55	163	2100	44	800	7.5	8	60	1.1	1.3	14	2.0	400	3.0	800	800	300	18	15	150
	23–50	55	163	2000	44	800	5	8	60	1.0	1.2	13	2.0	400	3.0	800	800	300	18	15	150
	51+	55	163	1800	44	800	5	8	60	1.0	1.2	13	2.0	400	3.0	800	800	300	10	15	150
Pregnant				+300	+30	+200	+5	+2	+20	+0.4	+0.3	+2	+0.6	+400	+1.0	+400	+400	+150	[h]	+5	+25
Lactating				+500	+20	+400	+5	+3	+40	+0.5	+0.5	+5	+0.5	+100	+1.0	+400	+400	+150	[h]	+10	+50

[a] The allowances are intended to provide for individual variations among most normal persons as they live in the United States under usual environmental stresses. Diets should be based on a variety of common foods in order to provide other nutrients for which human requirements have been less well defined.

[b] Retinol equivalents. 1 retinol equivalent = 1 µg of retinol or 6 µg of β-carotene

[c] As cholecalciferol. 10 µg of cholecalciferol = 400 I.U. of vitamin D.

[d] α-Tocopherol equivalents. 1 mg of d-α-tocopherol = 1 α-T.E.

[e] 1 N.E. (niacin equivalent) is equal to 1 mg of niacin or 60 mg of dietary tryptophan.

[f] The folacin allowances refer to dietary sources as determined by *Lactobacillus casei* assay after treatment with enzymes ("conjugases") to make polyglutamyl forms of the vitamin available to the test microorganism.

[g] The RDA for vitamin B_{12} in infants is based on the average concentration of the vitamin in human milk. The allowances after weaning are based on energy intake (as recommended by the American Academy of Pediatrics) and consideration of other factors such as intestinal absorption.

[h] The increased requirement during pregnancy cannot be met by the iron content of habitual American diets nor by the existing iron stores of many women; therefore, the use of 30 to 60 mg of supplemental iron is recommended. Iron needs during lactation are not substantially different from those of nonpregnant women, but continued supplementation of the mother for 2 to 3 months after parturition is advisable in order to replenish stores depleted by pregnancy.

(Modified from Food and Nutrition Board, National Research Council, 1979.)

allowances are set at levels sufficiently high to cover the needs of almost all healthy individuals in that age and sex category. This is done because the exact amounts of nutrients needed by each individual in the population are not known, and estimates are made from experiments on a limited number of subjects. If the upper limit of this range is taken as the recommended allowance, it is unlikely that a deficiency will occur in the population. Those with intakes below the recommended allowance will not necessarily develop a deficiency, but the risk of becoming deficient increases in proportion to the extent to which intake is less than the amount recommended.

An exception is the allowance for energy, for which the table provides the *average* requirement of the population. To recommend the upper extreme of the range of energy requirements would result in most of the population consuming too much energy-yielding nutrients, and this would encourage obesity. Energy needs also emphasize another aspect of the RDA, namely, that adults need to consume progressively less food as they grow older due to reduction in active tissue (lean body mass), accompanied by less physical activity. This is reflected in the ninth edition of *Recommended Dietary Allowances* by the subdivision of the allowance for energy into three categories of adults—23 to 50, 51 to 75, and 76 years and older; the allowances for other nutrients are only divided into two age groups of adults—23 to 50 and 51 years and older (Table XVI-1).

Another novel feature of the ninth edition of *Recommended Dietary Allowances* is the introduction of *provisional allowances* for some nutrients not previously given RDA. Table XVI-1 lists allowances for only 18 out of the 40 or so known essential nutrients consumed by man. In previous editions of the RDA text a mixed diet was advised in order to include unrecognized nutritional needs and to ensure an adequate intake of essential nutrients for which no allowance could be provided. However, rising consumption of formulated foods, other highly processed foods, and supplements of vitamins and trace elements has increased the risk of imbalances between nutrients, of deficiencies from underconsumption by some members of the population, and of toxicity from overdosage in others. The current RDA text therefore provides allowances for certain additional nutrients in the form of ranges within which adequate intakes are likely to be achieved (Table XVI-2). These provisional allowances include two water-soluble vitamins (pantothenic acid and biotin) and one fat-soluble vitamin (vitamin K), as well as sodium, potassium, chloride, and several trace elements (copper, manganese, fluorine, chromium, selenium, and molybdenum). Although these provisional allowances are presented as recommended ranges of intakes, it is to be emphasized that an intake at one end of the range should not be construed as more desirable than one at the other. Thus, all intakes within the recommended range are considered safe and effective, but consumption of greater or smaller amounts over extended periods of time will increase the risk of marginal toxicity or deficiency, respectively.

In addition to nutrients with well-documented requirements for which RDA are appropriate and those where there is less secure quantitative information for which only provisional allowances can be provided at present, there are a number of other constituents in food that have been claimed to be needed by man. As described in the 1979 RDA text, these substances fall into four classes: (1) those known to be essential for some animals but not shown to be needed by man, such as nickel, vanadium, and silicon; (2) substances in foods that are said to be vitamins but whose actions are probably pharmacological or nonexistent, such as "vitamin P" substances (*e.g.,* rutin and hesperidin), for which claims of antihemorrhagic and other actions have been made but are unsubstantiated (*see* Munro *et al.,* 1947); (3) substances that act as growth factors only for lower forms of life, such as para-aminobenzoic acid, carnitine, and pimelic acid; and (4) substances for which scientific proof of a nutrient action has not been provided, such as pangamic acid (erroneously designated vitamin B_{15}), laetrile (misnamed vitamin B_{17}), and others promoted in the health-food literature and commercial outlets. Herbert (1979a, 1979b) has written detailed factual reviews of the controversies over laetrile and pangamic acid.

Federal Regulations on Vitamins and Minerals.   Early attempts to regulate the safety and usefulness of vitamins in dietary supplements or added to foods for the purpose of enrichment

Table XVI-2. ESTIMATED SAFE AND ADEQUATE DAILY DIETARY INTAKES OF ADDITIONAL SELECTED VITAMINS AND MINERALS *

	Age (years)	VITAMINS			TRACE ELEMENTS						ELECTROLYTES		
		Vitamin K (µg)	Biotin (µg)	Pantothenic Acid (mg)	Copper (mg)	Manganese (mg)	Fluoride (mg)	Chromium (mg)	Selenium (mg)	Molybdenum (mg)	Sodium (mg)	Potassium (mg)	Chloride (mg)
Infants	0–0.5	12	35	2	0.5–0.7	0.5–0.7	0.1–0.5	0.01–0.04	0.01–0.04	0.03–0.06	115–350	350–925	275–700
	0.5–1	10–20	50	3	0.7–1.0	0.7–1.0	0.2–1.0	0.02–0.06	0.02–0.06	0.04–0.08	250–750	425–1275	400–1200
Children and Adolescents	1–3	15–30	65	3	1.0–1.5	1.0–1.5	0.5–1.5	0.02–0.08	0.02–0.08	0.05–0.1	325–975	550–1650	500–1500
	4–6	20–40	85	3–4	1.5–2.0	1.5–2.0	1.0–2.5	0.03–0.12	0.03–0.12	0.06–0.15	450–1350	775–2350	700–2100
	7–10	30–60	120	4–5	2.0–2.5	2.0–3.0	1.5–2.5	0.05–0.2	0.05–0.2	0.1–0.3	600–1800	1000–3000	925–2775
	11+	50–100	100–200	4–7	2.0–3.0	2.5–5.0	1.5–2.5	0.05–0.2	0.05–0.2	0.15–0.5	900–2700	1525–4575	1400–4200
Adults		70–140	100–200	4–7	2.0–3.0	2.5–5.0	1.5–4.0	0.05–0.2	0.05–0.2	0.15–0.5	1100–3300	1875–5625	1700–5100

* Because there is less information on which to base an allowance, these are not given in the main table of dietary allowances but are provided here in the form of ranges of recommended intakes. Since the toxic levels for many trace elements may be only several times usual intakes, the upper levels for the trace elements given in this table should not be habitually exceeded. (Modified from Food and Nutrition Board, National Research Council, 1979.)

resulted in the formulation of minimal daily requirements (MDR) for six vitamins and four minerals. These values were replaced and expanded to include recommendations for 20 nutrients as the United States Recommended Daily Allowances (U.S. RDA), developed in 1973 by the Food and Drug Administration. The U.S. RDA are a set of values derived by the Food and Drug Administration from the RDA of the Food and Nutrition Board. While the MDR were based on somewhat arbitrary minimal intakes needed to prevent deficiency disease, the U.S. RDA for adults and children 4 or more years of age generally represent the highest daily allowance for each nutrient for males and nonpregnant, nonlactating females over the age of 4 years given in the seventh (1968) edition of *Recommended Dietary Allowances.* Additional U.S. RDA were developed for infants, children less than 4 years of age, and for pregnant and lactating women. Some revision and further expansion of the U.S. RDA may be expected as a result of the appearance of the ninth edition of the RDA text in 1979.

Through the development of the U.S. RDA the FDA has modified and simplified the RDA to facilitate the labeling of conventional foods and thus to provide the public with information about their nutrient content. Thus, the purchaser can determine what proportion of his daily allowance of each nutrient is provided by a given amount of the food. In addition, the U.S. RDA are used to label the amounts of vitamins and minerals relative to needs in supplements sold to the public. Although the FDA has limited authority to control the nutrient content of supplements, except those intended for use by children under 12 years of age and by pregnant or lactating women, the label does provide the user with explicit information on content, thus permitting judgment of whether the product purchased contains reasonable amounts, too little, or an excess of each nutrient relative to daily allowances. The Food and Drug Administration attempted in 1973 to classify *all* vitamin and mineral preparations in which the dosages exceeded 150% of the U.S. RDA as drugs rather than as special foods, but the regulation was struck by court order. Regulations also developed in 1973 prevented sale to the public of *vitamins A* and *D* in doses exceeding 10,000 international units (I.U.) of the former and 400 I.U. of the latter without a prescription. This was done because of the concern that higher doses of these fat-soluble vitamins can cause toxicity. The regulation was revoked in 1978 because of a court determination that dosages in excess of those amounts could not be *uniquely* classified as drugs by the FDA. Also, an amendment of the Federal Food, Drug, and Cosmetic Act passed by Congress in 1976 limits FDA control of supplements for adult use to cases of demonstrated toxicity but retains the Agency's authority over dietary supplements for children under 12 years and for pregnant or lactating women.

The uses of vitamins and other nutrients to treat disease come under FDA review, either as foods for special dietary use, including food supplements, or as "over-the-counter" or prescription drugs, depending on the purposes for which the product is intended and the claims made for it. Nutrient products designed specifically for special application in medical treatment, such as parenteral solutions for hyperalimentation and so-called medical foods (such as defined formula diets), are evaluated for safety and efficacy, as are "over-the-counter" drugs containing vitamins and minerals. An FDA Over-the-Counter Vitamin, Mineral, and Hematinics Review Panel has recently recommended appropriate formulations for these preparations (Food and Drug Administration, 1979). In the near future, it is reasonable to assume that FDA will proceed to finalize regulations governing the composition and labeling of "over-the-counter" preparations containing vitamins and minerals.

Range of Intakes of Vitamins and Minerals. The practicing physician is exposed to pressures from different types of extremists in the area of vitaminology. One group, with representatives in medical practice, in a few pharmaceutical houses, and also in the general public, recommends large intakes of vitamins both for prophylactic purposes and for the treatment of an enormous variety of illnesses for which evidence of therapeutic efficacy of the vitamins is lacking. Many millions of individuals living in the United States regularly ingest quantities of vitamins vastly in excess of the RDA. In 1972, a Study of Health Practices and Opinions (National Analysts, 1972) reinforced previous concern of the FDA that vast numbers of Americans hold some inflated concepts regarding the benefits of taking supplemental vitamins and minerals. Thus, a survey found that more than half the adults interviewed had at one time used vitamin pills and some 20% were using them at the time of interview; many were under a physician's care. The primary reason for taking vitamin supplements was the erroneous belief that such supplements provide extra energy and made one "feel better," and two thirds of those holding this belief did indeed claim to feel better.

This evidence of widespread nutritional self-medication, which is confirmed by other surveys, indicates that vigilance should be maintained by the physician when he interviews patients. It is not uncommon for the physician to elicit a history of extensive drug taking but to fail to uncover intake of vitamins and/or minerals in large amounts.

Excessive intake of the fat-soluble vitamins is much more liable to cause serious toxicity than is ingestion of the water-soluble vitamins. The latter are readily excreted in the urine, whereas fat-soluble vitamins must be either metabolized or stored. For example, excessive intake of vitamin A, such as used in the treatment of acne, has led to unnecessary brain surgery when, in fact, the underlying lesion was the vitamin-induced hydrocephalus (Muenter *et al.*, 1971). Similarly, vitamin A intoxication due to megavitamin therapy for hyperactivity has caused thickening of leg bones (Shaywitz *et al.*, 1977), and excessive intake of vitamin D leads to hypercalcinosis (NAS Committee, 1974). While water-soluble vitamins are generally less toxic, some undesirable effects of megadosage have been recorded. For example, a high intake of ascorbic acid can elevate blood concentrations of administered salicylates (Loh and Wilson, 1975) and interfere with the anticoagulant action of warfarin (Rosenthal, 1971).

The use of dietary supplements of vitamins is medically advisable in a variety of circumstances where *vitamin deficiencies* are likely to occur. Such situations may arise from inadequate intake, malabsorption, increased tissue needs, or inborn errors of metabolism. In practice, these causes may overlap, as in the case of the alcoholic, who usually has an inadequate food intake and also impaired absorption (Leevy and Baker, 1968).

Vitamin deficiency due primarily to *inadequate intake* occurs under a variety of circumstances. While gross vitamin deficiencies due to inadequate intakes are still encountered in underdeveloped areas of the world, few florid cases can be seen in the United States; however, a degree of subclinical deficiency of nutrients due to inadequate intake has been documented. The Ten-State Nutrition Survey (1972) evaluated the nutritional status of 40,000 individuals, mostly within low-income families. The highest prevalence of unsatisfactory nutritional status occurred among adolescents, especially males, and elderly persons (who were not necessarily too poor to purchase adequate amounts of food). On the basis of biochemical tests and dietary evaluations, the most common deficiency disease was anemia due to iron deficiency, also associated in some cases with low concentrations of folic acid in blood. Iron-deficiency anemia not only was prevalent in women of child-bearing age but also was found in adolescent and adult males. The major inadequacies in vitamin status encountered in the Ten-State Nutrition Survey were of vitamin A, vitamin C, and riboflavin. Low intake of vitamin A and low plasma concentrations were found particularly among the low-income Spanish-speaking American population. Recent reinterpretation of the data suggests that the intake of folic acid may be low in both Spanish and black populations. Inadequate concentrations of vitamin C in plasma were observed in many of the elderly. Finally, evaluation of urinary excretion of riboflavin suggested inadequate intake among many blacks and in young people. In none of these populations did a significant incidence of overt vitamin deficiency accompany the subnormal biochemical values.

Certain individuals are exposed to deficient intakes of vitamins as a result of eccentric diets, such as food faddism, and the avoidance of food because of anorexia. Intakes of vitamins less than those recommended can also occur in subjects on reducing diets and among elderly people who eat little food for economic or social reasons. The consumption of excessive amounts of alcohol can also lead to inadequate intakes of vitamins and other nutrients.

A *disturbance in absorption* of vitamins is also seen in a variety of conditions. Examples are diseases of the liver and biliary tract, prolonged diarrhea from any cause, hyperthyroidism, pernicious anemia, sprue, surgical bypass of the small intestine for the treatment of obesity, and a variety of other disorders of the digestive system, including those related to alcoholism (Leevy and Baker, 1968). Moreover, since a substantial proportion of vitamin K and biotin is synthesized by the bacteria of the gastrointestinal tract, treatment with antimicrobial agents that alter the intestinal bacterial flora inevitably leads to decreased availability of these vitamins.

Increased tissue requirements for vitamins may cause a nutritional deficiency to develop despite the ingestion of a diet that had previously been adequate. There is good evidence that requirements for some vitamins increase during stress. Special losses of vitamins can occur from patients undergoing dialysis. During parenteral alimentation, excessive urinary losses of water-soluble vitamins can occur, especially when excessive doses are given. Requirements for some vitamins such as pyridoxine may also be increased by the use of oral contraceptives and by certain antivitamin drugs (Roe, 1976a, 1976b). Diseases associated with an increased metabolic rate, such as hyperthyroidism and conditions accompanied by fever or tissue wasting, also increase the body's requirements for vitamins.

Finally, an increasing number of cases are recorded in which *genetic abnormalities* lead to an increased need for a vitamin. This is usually due to an abnormality in the structure of an enzyme for which the vitamin provides a cofactor, leading to a decreased affinity of the abnormal enzyme protein for the cofactor (Scriver, 1973).

Role of Vitamins in Therapeutics. Specific diseases caused by vitamin deficiency are relatively rare in the United States, but oral supplements of vitamins are indicated for the conditions listed above that do lead to deficiency. Descriptions of official preparations are given in *The United States Pharmacopeia* (1980) and in the relevant chapters of this textbook. *Decavitamin Tablets and Capsules,* U.S.P., each provide the approximate equivalent of the adult RDA for vitamins A and D, ascorbic acid, thiamine, riboflavin, nicotinamide, pyridoxine, and pantothenate, with somewhat lower levels of folate and vitamin B_{12}. These tablets and capsules contain no minerals.

For patients who cannot consume sufficient regular food for their needs, a number of specially defined formula diets are available (Shils, 1977). The vitamin content of these is regulated as *medical foods* by the FDA. Some patients require a complete supply of nutrients by the parenteral route. For this purpose, the dosage of water-soluble vitamins may have to be higher because of excessive losses in the urine (Vanamee, 1976; Nichoalds *et al.,* 1977; Moran and Greene, 1979).

In addition to the fact that individual diseases vary in their effects on nutritional requirements, the same disease will make varying demands on nutrients according to its phase and intensity. The need for therapy with vitamins may thus change throughout the course of the illness and, eventually, cure should be associated with cessation of this therapy; this point sometimes escapes the physician, who does not remind the patient to abandon the vitamin supplement.

Cook, J. D.; Finch, C. A.; and Smith, N. J. Evaluation of the iron status of a population. *Blood,* **1976,** *48,* 449–455.

Food and Drug Administration. Food labeling. *Federal Register,* **1973,** *38,* No. 13, 2126–2128, 2131, 2144–2150, 2155–2162.

———. Vitamin and mineral products. *Ibid.,* **1976,** *41,* No. 203, 46157–46158, 46166–46176.

———. Over-the-counter vitamin and mineral drug products for human use. *Ibid.,* **1979,** *44,* No. 53, 16126–16201.

Herbert, V. Laetrile: the cult of cyanide—promoting poison for profit. *Am. J. Clin. Nutr.,* **1979a,** *32,* 1121–1158.

———. Pangamic acid ("vitamin B_{15}"). *Ibid.,* **1979b,** *32,* 1534–1540.

Leevy, C. M., and Baker, H. Vitamins and alcoholism: introduction. *Am. J. Clin. Nutr.,* **1968,** *21,* 1325–1328.

Loh, H. S., and Wilson, C. M. The interactions of aspirin and ascorbic acid in normal men. *J. Clin. Pharmacol.,* **1975,** *15,* 36–45.

Moran, J. R., and Greene, H. L. The B vitamins and vitamin C in human nutrition. II. "Conditional" B vitamins and vitamin C. *Am. J. Dis. Child.,* **1979,** *133,* 308–314.

Muenter, M. D.; Perry, H. O.; and Ludwig, J. Chronic vitamin A intoxication in adults—hepatic, neurologic and dermatologic complications. *Am. J. Med.,* **1971,** *50,* 129–136.

Munro, H. N.; Lazarus, S.; and Bell, G. H. The value of capillary strength tests in the diagnosis of vitamin C and vitamin P deficiency in man. *Nutr. Abstr. Rev.,* **1947,** *17,* 291–309.

NAS Committee on Nutritional Misinformation. *Hazards of Overuse of Vitamin D.* National Academy of Sciences, Washington, D. C., **1974.**

National Analysts, Inc. *A Study of Health Practices and Opinions.* National Technical Information Service, Springfield, Va., **1972,** pp. 9–26.

Nichoalds, G. E.; Meng, H. C.; and Caldwell, M. D. Vitamin requirements in patients receiving total parenteral nutrition. *Arch. Surg.,* **1977,** *112,* 1061–1064.

Roe, D. A. Antivitamins. In, *Drug Induced Nutritional Deficiencies.* The AVI Publishing Co., Inc., Westport, Conn., **1976a,** pp. 154–185.

———. Nutritional effects of oral contraceptives. *Ibid.,* **1976b,** pp. 222–238.

Rosenthal, G. Interaction of ascorbic acid and warfarin. *J.A.M.A.,* **1971,** *215,* 1671.

Scriver, C. R. Vitamin-responsive inborn error of metabolism. *Metabolism,* **1973,** *22,* 1319–1344.

Select Committee on Nutrition and Human Needs, United States Senate. *Dietary Goals for the United States.* U.S. Government Printing Office, Washington, D. C., **1977.**

Shaywitz, B. A.; Seigel, N. J.; and Pearson, H. A. Megavitamins for minimal brain dysfunction: a potentially dangerous therapy. *J.A.M.A.,* **1977,** *238,* 1749–1750.

Shils, M. E. (ed.). *Defined Formula Diets for Medical Purposes.* American Medical Association, Chicago, Ill., **1977.**

Ten-State Nutrition Survey, 1968–1970. Center for Disease Control, Department of Health, Education, and Welfare Publication Nos. (HSM) 72-8130-8134. U.S. Government Printing Office, Washington, D. C., **1972.**

United States Department of Health, Education, and Welfare. *Preliminary Findings of the First Health and Nutrition Examination Survey, United States 1971–1972. Dietary Intake and Biochemical Findings.* Department of Health, Education, and Welfare Publication No. (HRA) 74-1219-1. U.S. Government Printing Office, Washington, D. C., **1974.**

The United States Pharmacopeia, 20th rev. (The United States Pharmacopeial Convention, Inc.) Mack Printing Co., Easton, Pa., published **1980,** became official **1980.**

Vanamee, P. Parenteral nutrition. In, *Present Knowledge of Nutrition,* 4th ed. (Hegsted, D. M.; Chichester, C. O.; Darby, W. J.; McNutt, K. W.; Stalvey, R. M.; and Stotz, F. H; eds.) The Nutrition Foundation, Washington, D. C., **1976,** pp. 415–427.

Monographs and Reviews

Food and Nutrition Board, National Research Council. *Recommended Dietary Allowances,* 9th ed. National Academy of Sciences, Washington, D. C., **1979.**

Goodhart, R. S., and Shils, M. E. (eds.). *Modern Nutrition in Health and Disease,* 6th ed. Lea & Febiger, Philadelphia, **1979.**

Hegsted, D. M.; Chichester, C. O.; Darby, W. J.; McNutt, K. W.; Stalvey, R. M.; and Stotz, E. H. (eds.). *Present Knowledge of Nutrition,* 4th ed. The Nutrition Foundation, Washington, D. C., **1976.**

Roe, D. A. *Drug Induced Nutritional Deficiencies.* The AVI Publishing Co., Inc., Westport, Conn., **1976.**

Schneider, H. A.; Anderson, C. E.; and Coursin, D. B. (eds.). *Nutritional Support of Medical Practice.* Harper & Row, Pub., Inc., New York, **1977.**

White, P. L. (ed.). Nutrition misinformation and food faddism. *Nutr. Rev., 1974, 32,* Suppl. 1, 1–73.

CHAPTER

66 WATER-SOLUBLE VITAMINS

The Vitamin B Complex and Ascorbic Acid

Darla Erhard Danford and Hamish N. Munro

As discussed in the introductory section preceding this chapter, the water-soluble vitamins consist of members of the vitamin B complex and vitamin C (ascorbic acid).

The vitamin B complex comprises a large number of compounds that differ extensively in chemical structure and biological action. The reason for grouping them in a single class was their original isolation from the same sources, notably liver and yeast. Because of their somewhat similar distribution in foods, there is a tendency for dietary deficiency to involve several members of the vitamin B complex in the same patient.

There are traditionally 11 members of the vitamin B complex, namely, thiamine, riboflavin, nicotinic acid, pyridoxine, pantothenic acid, biotin, folic acid, cyanocobalamin (vitamin B_{12}), choline, inositol, and para-aminobenzoic acid. Folic acid and cyanocobalamin are considered in Chapter 57 because of their special function in hematopoiesis. Para-aminobenzoic acid (PABA) is not a true vitamin for any mammalian species but is a growth factor for certain bacteria, where it is a precursor in the synthesis of folic acid (*see* Chapter 57). The vitamins of the B complex function in intermediary metabolism in many essential reactions; some of these functions are shown in Figure 66-1, which serves to illustrate their prevalence and importance.

In addition to the vitamin B complex, this chapter also considers ascorbic acid (vitamin C). This water-soluble vitamin is especially concentrated in citrus fruits and is thus obtained mostly from sources differing from those of members of the vitamin B complex. A further series of water-soluble compounds, the flavonoids (*e.g.*, rutin and hesperidin), has been claimed in the past to have vitamin activity beneficial for certain types of hemorrhagic disease. This claim is unsubstantiated and, therefore, the actions of these compounds will not be described here.

Table 66-1 summarizes the chemical properties, dietary sources, symptoms of deficiency, tests for deficiency, and effects of overdosage for each of the vitamins of the B complex and for vitamin C.

I. The Vitamin B Complex

THIAMINE

History. Thiamine was the first member of the vitamin B complex to be identified. Lack of thiamine produces a form of polyneuritis known as beriberi; this disease became widespread in East Asia in the nineteenth century due to the introduction of steam-powered rice mills, which produced polished rice lacking the vitamin-rich husk. A dietary cause for the disease was first indicated in 1880, when Admiral Takaki greatly reduced the incidence of beriberi in the Japanese Navy by adding fish, meat, barley, and vegetables to the sailors' diet of polished rice. In 1897, Eijkman, a Dutch physician working in Java where beriberi was also common, showed that fowl fed polished rice develop a polyneuritis similar to beriberi and that this could be cured by adding the rice polishings (husks) or an aqueous extract of the polishings back to the diet. He also demonstrated that rice polishings could cure beriberi in humans.

In 1911, Funk isolated a highly concentrated form of the active factor and recognized that it belonged to a new class of food factors, which he called *vitamines,* later shortened to *vitamins.* The active factor was subsequently named vitamin B_1; in 1926 it was isolated in crystalline form by Jansen and Donath, and in 1936 its structure was determined by Williams. The Council on Pharmacy and Chemistry adopted the name *thiamine* to designate crystalline vitamin B_1, and this is now the official U.S.P. name of the vitamin. Similarly, other members of the vitamin B complex were given official names following their chemical identification.

Chemistry. Thiamine is an organic molecule containing a pyrimidine and a thiazole nucleus. Thiamine functions in the body in the form of the coenzyme thiamine pyrophosphate (TPP). The structures of thiamine and thiamine pyrophosphate are as follows:

Thiamine

Thiamine Pyrophosphate

The conversion of thiamine to its coenzyme form is carried out with adenosine triphosphate (ATP) as a pyrophosphate (PP) donor. Antimetabolites to thiamine have been synthesized. The most important of these are neopyrithiamine (pyrithiamine) and oxythiamine.

Pharmacological Actions. Thiamine is practically devoid of pharmacodynamic actions when given in usual therapeutic doses. Even large doses have no effect on the blood glucose concentration despite the physiological role of the vitamin in the intermediary metabolism of carbohydrate. Isolated clinical reports of toxic reactions to the parenteral administration of thiamine probably represent rare instances of hypersensitivity.

Physiological Functions. Thiamine pyrophosphate, the physiologically active form of thiamine, functions in carbohydrate metabolism as a coenzyme in the decarboxylation of α-keto acids such as pyruvate and α-ketoglutarate and in the utilization of pentose in the hexose monophosphate shunt; the latter function involves the thiamine pyrophosphate–dependent enzyme transketolase. Several metabolic changes of clinical importance can be related directly to the biochemical action of thiamine. In thiamine deficiency, the oxidation of α-keto acids is impaired, and an increase in the concentration of pyruvate in the blood has been used as one of the diagnostic signs of the deficiency state. A more specific diagnostic test for thiamine deficiency is based upon measurement of transketolase activity in erythrocytes (Brin, 1968). The requirement for thiamine is related to metabolic rate and is greatest when carbohydrate is the source of energy. This is of practical significance for patients who are maintained by parenteral alimentation and who thereby receive practically all their calories in the form of dextrose. Such patients should be given a *generous* allowance of the vitamin.

Symptoms of Deficiency. Severe thiamine deficiency leads to the condition known as beriberi. In the East, this is due to consumption of diets of polished rice, which are deficient in the vitamin. In Western countries, thiamine deficiency is most commonly seen in alcoholics. A severe form of acute thiamine deficiency can also occur in infants.

The major symptoms of thiamine deficiency are related to the nervous system (*dry beriberi*) and to the cardiovascular system (*wet beriberi*). Many of the neurological signs and symptoms are characteristic of peripheral neuritis, with sensory disturbances in the extremities, including localized areas of hyperesthesia or anesthesia. Muscle strength is gradually lost and may result in wrist-drop or complete paralysis of a limb. Personality disturbances, depression, lack of initiative, and poor memory may also result from lack of the vitamin.

Cardiovascular symptoms can be prominent and include dyspnea on exertion, palpitation, tachycardia, and other cardiac abnormalities characterized by an abnormal ECG (chiefly flattening or inversion of the T wave and prolongation of the Q-T interval) and cardiac failure of the high-output type. Such failure has been termed *wet beriberi;* there is extensive edema, largely as a result of hypoproteinemia from an inadequate intake of protein together with failing ventricular function.

Symptoms referable to the gastrointestinal tract are also observed in severe cases of deficiency. Loss of appetite occurs early and is followed by constipation.

Human Requirements. Because thiamine is essential for energy metabolism, especially of carbohydrate, requirement for thiamine is commonly related to caloric intake. The minimal thiamine requirement in man approximates 0.3 mg/1000 kcal. To provide a margin of safety, the Dietary Allowances Committee of the National Research Council recommends a daily intake of 0.5 mg/1000 kcal (*see* Table XVI–1, page 1553). There is evidence that older people utilize thiamine less efficiently and, in consequence, not less than 1 mg daily is recommended for adults of all ages, no matter how low their caloric intake. During pregnancy and lactation, an additional intake of 0.6 mg/1000 kcal is recommended.

Absorption, Fate, and Excretion. Absorption of the usual dietary amounts of thiamine from the gastrointestinal tract occurs by sodium-dependent active transport; at higher concentrations, passive diffusion is also significant (Rindi and Ventura, 1972). Absorption is usually limited to a maximal daily amount of 8 to 15 mg, but this can be exceeded by oral administration in divided doses with food.

In adults, approximately 1 mg of thiamine per day is completely degraded by the tissues, and this is roughly the minimal daily requirement. When intake is at this low level,

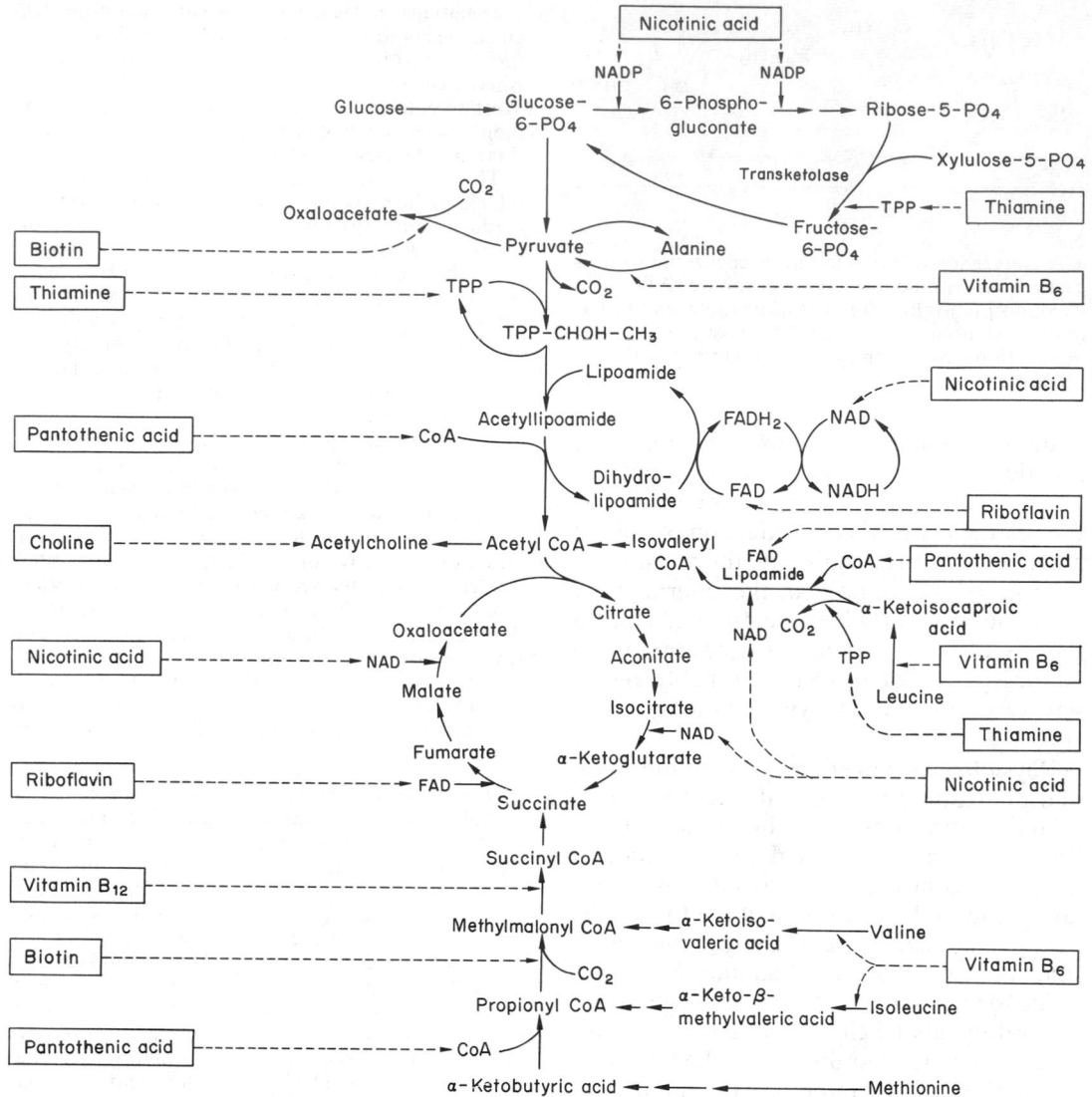

Figure 66–1. *Some major metabolic pathways involving coenzymes formed from water-soluble vitamins.* (Abbreviations are defined in the text.)

little or no thiamine is excreted in the urine. When intake exceeds the minimal requirement, tissue stores are first saturated. Thereafter, the excess appears quantitatively in the urine as intact thiamine or as pyrimidine, which arises from degradation of the thiamine molecule. As the intake of thiamine is further increased, more of the excess is excreted unchanged, indicating that the capacity of tissues to split thiamine to pyrimidine is limited.

Preparations. Thiamine can be prescribed as the pure vitamin, in mixtures of pure vitamins, or in the form of vitamin-rich concentrates.

Thiamine Hydrochloride, U.S.P. (*vitamin B$_1$ hydrochloride*), occurs as small, white crystals or as a crystalline powder. *Thiamine Hydrochloride Tablets,* U.S.P., can usually be obtained in amounts ranging from 5 to 500 mg each. *Thiamine Hydrochloride Injection,* U.S.P., is a sterile solution of thiamine hydrochloride in water. Preparations available usually contain 100 mg/ml. Thiamine is also available as *thiamine hydrochloride elixir,* containing 2.25 mg/ 5ml. The mononitrate salt, *Thiamine Mononitrate,* U.S.P., is an additional formulation.

Therapeutic Uses. The only established therapeutic use of thiamine is in the treatment or the prophylaxis of thiamine deficiency. To correct the disorder as rapidly as possible, parenteral doses as large as 30 mg three times daily are justified. Once thiamine deficiency has been corrected, there is no need for parenteral injection or the administration of amounts in excess of daily requirements except in instances when gastrointestinal disturbances preclude the ingestion or absorption of adequate amounts of vitamin.

The syndromes of thiamine deficiency seen clinically can range from beriberi through Wernicke's encephalopathy and Korsakoff's syndrome to alcoholic polyneuropathy. The type appears to depend on the amount of deprivation (McLaren, 1978). Encephalopathy and Korsakoff's syndrome result from severe deprivation, whereas beriberi heart disease occurs in less deficient subjects; polyneuritis is observed in milder deprivation. The following discussion describes briefly the varieties of thiamine deficiency and their treatment.

Alcoholic Neuritis. Alcoholism is the most common cause of thiamine deficiency in the United States. Alcoholic neuritis is basically a nutritional deficiency due to an inadequate intake of thiamine. Two factors contribute to such inadequate intake in the chronic alcoholic. Appetite is usually poor. Food consumption drops, and a large portion of the caloric intake is in the form of alcohol. The symptoms of neurological involvement in alcoholics are those of a polyneuritis with motor and sensory defects. Wernicke's syndrome is an additional serious consequence of alcoholism and thiamine deficiency. Certain characteristic signs of this disease, notably ophthalmoplegia, nystagmus, and ataxia, respond rapidly to the administration of thiamine but to no other vitamin. However, Wernicke's encephalopathy is usually accompanied by signs of Korsakoff's psychosis, characterized by a striking impairment of retentive memory, inability to acquire new information, and confabulation (Platt, 1967); once florid, these changes are usually irreversible.

Chronic alcoholics with polyneuritis and motor or sensory defects should receive 40 mg of oral thiamine daily. The Wernicke-Korsakoff syndrome represents an *acute emergency* that should be treated with daily doses of 100 mg of the vitamin, intravenously (McLaren, 1978).

Infantile Beriberi. Thiamine deficiency also occurs as an acute disease in infancy and may run a rapid and fulminating course. The onset consists in loss of appetite, vomiting, and greenish stools followed by paroxysmal attacks of muscular rigidity. Aphonia due to loss of laryngeal nerve function is a diagnostic feature. Signs of cardiac involvement are also prominent. The pulse becomes weak and rapid, the face is cyanotic, and the neck veins are engorged. Death may follow the initial signs within 12 to 24 hours unless vigorous treatment is instituted. Infants with mild forms of this condition respond to oral therapy with 10 mg of thiamine daily. If acute col-

lapse occurs, doses of 25 mg intravenously can be given cautiously, but the prognosis remains poor (McLaren, 1978).

Subacute Necrotizing Encephalomyelopathy. This is a fatal genetic disease of children, with brain lesions very similar to those characteristic of Wernicke's encephalopathy. The brains of such patients at autopsy are essentially devoid of phosphorylated thiamine derivatives. When patients with this syndrome are treated daily with large doses of thiamine, most exhibit marked temporary improvement (Pincus *et al.,* 1973). Other inborn errors of metabolism that are sensitive to the administration of thiamine have also been described (Scriver, 1973).

Cardiovascular Disease. Cardiovascular disease of nutritional origin is observed in chronic alcoholics, pregnant women, persons with gastrointestinal disorders, and those whose diet is deficient for other reasons. When the diagnosis of cardiovascular disease due to thiamine deficiency has been correctly made, the response to the administration of thiamine is striking. One of the pathognomonic features of the syndrome is an increased blood flow due to arteriolar dilatation. Within a few hours after the administration of thiamine, the rate of blood flow is reduced and the utilization of oxygen begins to return to normal. If edema is present and due to myocardial insufficiency, diuresis results after proper therapy. The rate of improvement is seemingly inversely proportional to the rate of onset and duration of the disease, and individuals suffering from a chronic deficiency may require protracted treatment. The usual dose of thiamine is 10 to 30 mg three times daily, given parenterally. The dosage can be reduced and the patient maintained on oral medication or by dietary management after signs of the deficiency state have been reversed.

Gastrointestinal Disorders. In experimental and clinical beriberi, certain symptoms occur that are referable to the gastrointestinal tract. On this basis, thiamine has been used uncritically as a therapeutic agent for such unrelated conditions as ulcerative colitis, gastrointestinal hypotonia, and chronic diarrhea. Unless the disease being treated is the direct result of a deficiency of thiamine, there is no reason to expect the vitamin to be efficacious.

Neuritis of Pregnancy. Pregnancy increases the thiamine requirement slightly. The neuritis of pregnancy takes the form of multiple peripheral nerve involvement, and the signs and symptoms in well-developed cases resemble those described in patients with beriberi. The problem occurs when the diet is poor or in patients with hyperemesis gravidarum. Proof that the neuritis is due to a thiamine deficiency is gained in those cases in which dramatic clinical improvement is observed after thiamine therapy. The dose employed is from 5 to 10 mg daily, given parenterally if vomiting is severe.

Mild Thiamine Deficiency. This condition is probably not rare in the United States and may easily escape detection. The symptoms include loss of appetite, muscular weakness, pain and paresthesias in the extremities, a tendency to edema, decreased blood pressure, and low body temperature. The diagnosis may be confirmed by a careful study of the dietary history and by determination of erythrocyte transketolase activity. Thiamine deficiency

Table 66–1. MAJOR PROPERTIES OF THE WATER-SOLUBLE VITAMINS *

VITAMIN	STABILITY	FOOD SOURCES	HUMAN DEFICIENCY SYMPTOMS	TESTS OF DEFICIENCY	TOXICITY FROM OVERDOSE
Thiamine (B₁)	Stable in acidic solution; rapidly destroyed by heat in neutral or alkaline solution	Pork, organ meats, wheat germ, whole grain, enriched cereals and bread	*Adults:* anorexia, GI atony, constipation, beriberi (including polyneuritis and cardiac failure) *Alcoholics:* Wernicke-Korsakoff encephalopathy *Infants:* aphonia, convulsions, and acute cardiac failure	Erythrocyte transketolase Blood lactate and pyruvate concentrations Red-blood-cell thiamine pyrophosphate concentrations	Sensitivity of individuals to injection of 1000 x RDA (thiamine shock)
Riboflavin (B₂)	Rapidly decomposed by UV light and by alkali; resists heat in acid	Milk, organ meats, eggs, green leafy vegetables, dried yeast, enriched bread and flour	Angular stomatitis, chilosis, magenta tongue, seborrheic dermatitis of face, and certain functional and organic eye disorders, including vascularization	Erythrocyte glutathione reductase Urinary B₂ excretion	None known
Nicotinic acid (niacin)	Stable to heat, oxidation, and light	Liver, kidney, meat, fish, poultry, whole grain, enriched flour and cereal, and coffee; also sources of tryptophan (protein)	Pellagra with dermatitis, diarrhea, and dementia (neurological signs and symptoms)	Urinary methylnicotinamide and pyridone excretion	Vasodilatation, flushing, itching, and increased peristalsis (not with nicotinamide)
Pyridoxine (B₆)	Substantial losses during cooking; sensitive to UV light and oxidation	Meat, liver, kidney, whole-grain cereals, wheat germ, and soybeans	*Adults:* hypochromic anemia and CNS lesions *Infants:* epileptiform seizures and EEG changes	Tryptophan loading test (urinary xanthurenic acid) Plasma and erythrocyte transaminase Plasma pyridoxal phosphate concentration	None known
Pantothenic acid	Easily destroyed by heat and alkali	Organ meats, beef, egg yolk, peanuts, broccoli, cauliflower, cabbage, and whole grains	Fatigue, headache, nausea, vomiting, paresthesias, and incoordination; "burning foot" syndrome	Plasma pantothenic acid concentration Urinary pantothenic acid excretion	None known

	Stability	Dietary Sources	Deficiency	Assessment	Toxicity
Biotin	Stable to cooking, but less so in alkali	Organ meats and peanuts; synthesis by GI bacteria	Nausea, depression, muscle pain, anemia, dermatitis, atrophic glossitis, and hyperesthesia	Plasma biotin concentration Urinary biotin excretion	None known
Choline	Stable to acid and heat	Egg yolk and vegetable and animal fat (mostly as lecithin)	*Animals:* fatty liver, hemorrhagic kidney, motor incoordination *Humans:* no deficiency observed	None known	None known
Inositol	Stable to acid and heat	Fruits, plants, and whole-grain cereals (as phytic acid)	No known deficiency syndrome; needed for human cell growth in tissue culture	None known	None known
Ascorbic acid (vitamin C)	Easily destroyed by heat, oxygen, oxidases, and alkali	Citrus fruits, tomatoes, strawberries, cabbage, greens, and potatoes	*Adults:* scurvy with petechial hemorrhages, bleeding gums, poor wound healing, and anemia *Infants:* lassitude, anemia, and subperiosteal hematomas	Plasma ascorbic acid concentration White cell ascorbic acid concentration	Megadoses increase oxalate excretion; can cause rebound scurvy in newborn infant

* The status of inositol as a vitamin is uncertain; choline does not meet the definition of a vitamin but is discussed in the chapter (*see* text).

may, however, occur in association with an apparently adequate diet, since the vitamin is not stored in the body to a great extent. Thus, an increase in metabolic rate or a gastrointestinal disturbance, such as diarrhea of fairly long duration, may necessitate an increased intake of thiamine. Thiamine deficiency can also occur from the consumption of large amounts of raw fish containing thiaminase (Murata, 1965) or large quantities of tea, which contains a thiamine antagonist (Vimokesant *et al.*, 1974).

RIBOFLAVIN

History. At various times from 1879 onward, series of yellow pigmented compounds have been isolated from a variety of sources and designated as flavins, prefixed to indicate the source (*e.g.*, lacto-, ovo-, and hepato-). It was then demonstrated that these various flavins are identical in chemical composition.

In the meantime, water-soluble vitamin B had been separated into a heat-labile antiberiberi factor (B_1) and a heat-stable growth-promoting factor (B_2), and it was eventually appreciated that concentrates of so-called vitamin B_2 had a yellow color, the intensity of which was related to vitamin activity. In 1932, Warburg and Christian described a yellow respiratory enzyme in yeast, and in 1933 the yellow pigment portion of the enzyme was identified as vitamin B_2. All doubt as to the identity of vitamin B_2 and the naturally occurring flavins was removed when lactoflavin was synthesized and the synthetic product was shown to possess full biological activity. The vitamin was designated as *riboflavin* by the Council on Pharmacy and Chemistry because of the presence of ribose in its structure. The term later became official in the U.S.P.

Chemistry. Riboflavin carries out its functions in the body in the form of one or the other of two coenzymes, riboflavin phosphate, commonly called flavin mononucleotide (FMN), and flavin adenine dinucleotide (FAD). The structures of riboflavin,

FMN, and FAD are shown below. Riboflavin is converted to FMN and FAD by two enzyme-catalyzed reactions (*see* Wagner-Jauregg, 1972; McCormick, 1975):

1. Riboflavin + ATP $\longrightarrow$ FMN + ADP
2. FMN + ATP $\longrightarrow$ FAD + PP

Pharmacological Actions. No overt pharmacological effects follow the oral or parenteral administration of riboflavin.

Physiological Functions. FMN and FAD, the physiologically active forms of riboflavin, serve a vital role in metabolism as coenzymes for a wide variety of respiratory flavoproteins, some of which contain metals (*e.g.*, xanthine oxidase).

Symptoms of Deficiency. The signs and symptoms of spontaneous or experimentally produced riboflavin deficiency have been reviewed by Rivlin (1970) and by Lane and colleagues (1975). Sore throat and angular stomatitis generally appear first. Later, glossitis, chilosis (red denuded lips), seborrheic dermatitis of the face, and dermatitis over the trunk and extremities occur, followed by anemia and neuropathy. In some subjects corneal vascularization and cataract formation are prominent.

The anemia that develops in riboflavin deficiency is normochromic and normocytic and is associated with reticulocytopenia; the leukocytes and platelets are generally normal. Administration of riboflavin to deficient patients causes reticulocytosis, and the concentration of hemoglobin returns to normal. Anemia in patients with riboflavin deficiency may be related, at least in part, to disturbances in folic acid metabolism.

The problem in the clinical recognition of riboflavin deficiency is that certain features, such as glossitis

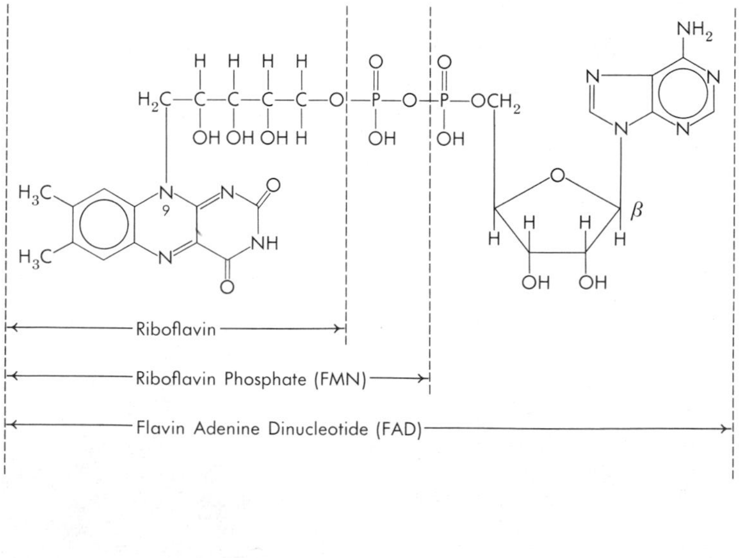

Riboflavin

Riboflavin Phosphate (FMN)

Flavin Adenine Dinucleotide (FAD)

and dermatitis, are common signs, both in deficiencies of other vitamins and as manifestations of other diseases. Recognition of riboflavin deficiency is also difficult because it rarely occurs in isolation. In nutritional surveys of children in an urban area and of randomly selected hospitalized patients, deficiency of riboflavin was frequently observed, but almost invariably in conjunction with other vitamin deficiencies. Riboflavin deficiency has likewise been observed in association with deficiencies of other vitamins in a large proportion of urban alcoholics of low economic status (Rivlin, 1979). Assessment of the adequacy of stores of riboflavin can only be made by correlating dietary history with clinical and laboratory findings (Goldsmith, 1964). Biochemical tests include evaluation of urinary excretion of the vitamin (excretion of less than 50 µg of riboflavin daily is indicative of deficiency). Although concentrations of riboflavin and FMN in blood are not of much diagnostic value, the concentrations of glutathione reductase in the red blood cells can be correlated with the intake of riboflavin; in deficiency, the activity of this enzyme is increased following the administration of riboflavin.

Human Requirements. The minimal requirement for riboflavin to prevent clinical signs of deficiency appears to be less than 0.35 mg/1000 kcal. To provide a margin of safety, the Dietary Allowances Committee of the National Research Council recommends a somewhat higher intake of riboflavin of 0.6 mg/1000 kcal. This is equivalent to 1.6 mg daily for young adult males and 1.2 mg daily for young adult females. It is recommended that intake for elderly adults should not be less than 1.2 mg daily, even when caloric intake falls below 2000 kcal.

Absorption, Fate, and Excretion. Riboflavin is readily absorbed from the upper gastrointestinal tract by a specific transport mechanism involving phosphorylation of the vitamin to FMN (Jusko and Levy, 1975). Here and in other tissues, riboflavin is converted to FMN by flavokinase, a reaction that is sensitive to thyroid-hormone status and is inhibited by chlorpromazine and by tricyclic antidepressants (Rivlin, 1979). Riboflavin is distributed to all tissues, but concentrations are uniformly low and little is stored. The relationship of riboflavin intake to urinary excretion has been studied extensively (Horwitt et al., 1956). When riboflavin is ingested in amounts that approximate the minimal daily requirement, only about 9% appears in the urine. As the intake of riboflavin is increased above the minimal requirement, a larger proportion is excreted unchanged.

Riboflavin is present in the feces. This probably represents vitamin synthesized by intestinal microorganisms, since, on low intakes of riboflavin, the amount excreted in the feces exceeds that ingested. There is no evidence that riboflavin synthesized by the bacteria in the colon can be absorbed.

Preparations. *Riboflavin,* U.S.P. (*vitamin B₂*), is a yellow to orange-yellow crystalline powder with a slight odor. While the vitamin is sparingly soluble in water, it is more so in isotonic sodium chloride solution. When dry, riboflavin is not affected appreciably by light; however, when it is in solution, light induces quite rapid deterioration, especially at alkaline pH. *Riboflavin Tablets,* U.S.P., are usually available in amounts ranging from 5 to 50 mg. *Riboflavin Injection,* U.S.P., is a sterile solution of riboflavin in water. For purposes of increasing the solubility of the vitamin, official preparations may contain solubilizing agents. Available preparations for injection usually contain 50 mg/ml.

Therapeutic Uses. The only established therapeutic application of riboflavin is to treat or prevent disease caused by deficiency. Ariboflavinosis seldom occurs in the United States as a discrete deficiency but usually accompanies other nutritional diseases, particularly pellagra. Therefore, therapy of ariboflavinosis should include other members of the B complex in addition to riboflavin. Specific therapy with riboflavin usually consists in the oral administration of 5 to 10 mg daily.

NICOTINIC ACID

History. Pellagra (Italian for *pelle agra,* or "rough skin") has been known for centuries in countries where maize is eaten in quantity, notably Italy and North America. In 1914, Funk postulated that the disease was due to a deficiency in the diet, and this was confirmed by the classical work of Goldberger and coworkers of the United States Public Health Service. Goldberger fed deficient diets to dogs and produced the condition known as "black tongue," analogous to human pellagra. In rats, the same diet caused a marked dermatitis that could be cured by dietary measures. The next step was the discovery that black tongue could also be cured by appropriate alterations of diet.

In 1935, Warburg and associates obtained nicotinic acid amide (nicotinamide) from a coenzyme isolated from the red blood cells of the horse. This finding stimulated further studies on the nutritional value of nicotinic acid. Liver extracts were known to be highly effective in curing human pellagra and canine black tongue. Elvehjem and associates prepared concentrates of liver that were highly effective in the treatment of canine black tongue, and, in 1937, they identified the active substance as nicotinamide. Proof was established by the demonstration that synthetic nicotinic acid derivatives were also effective in alleviating the symptoms of black tongue and curing human pellagra. Goldberger and Tanner had previously shown that tryptophan could cure human pellagra; this effect was later determined to be due to the conversion of tryptophan to nicotinic acid. Goldsmith (1958) produced pellagra experimentally in man by feeding a diet deficient in nicotinic acid and tryptophan.

With the recognition of nicotinic acid as the pellagra-preventing vitamin, the compound soon became an official drug. Nicotinic acid is also known as *niacin,* a term introduced to avoid confusion between the vitamin and the alkaloid nicotine.

Chemistry. Nicotinic acid functions in the body after conversion to either nicotinamide adenine dinucleotide (NAD) or nicotinamide adenine dinucleotide phosphate (NADP). It is to be noted that nicotinic acid occurs in these two nucleotides in the form of its amide, nicotinamide. The structures of nicotinic acid, nicotinamide, NAD, and NADP are shown below, where $R = H$ in NAD and $R = PO_3H_2$ in NADP.

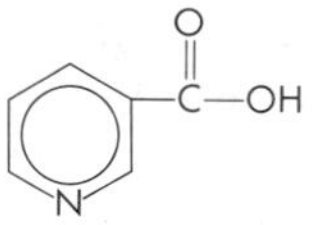

Nicotinic Acid

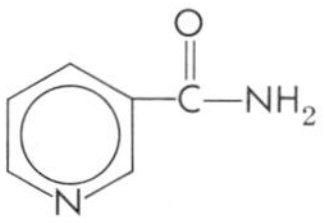

Nicotinamide

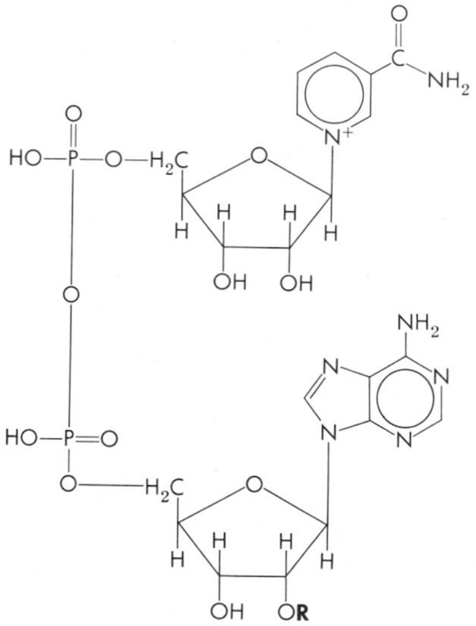

NAD and NADP

Pharmacological Actions. The pharmacological effects and toxicity of nicotinic acid in man have been reviewed by Mosher (1970). These include flushing, pruritus, gastrointestinal distress, hepatotoxicity, and activation of peptic ulcer disease. The compound has been used as a vasodilator and for

its effects to lower plasma cholesterol (*see* Chapter 34). Nicotinamide has no such cardiovascular effects.

Physiological Functions. NAD and NADP, the physiologically active forms of nicotinic acid, serve a vital role in metabolism as coenzymes for a wide variety of proteins that catalyze oxidation-reduction reactions essential for tissue respiration. The coenzymes, bound to appropriate dehydrogenases, function as oxidants accepting electrons and hydrogen from substrates and thus becoming reduced. The reduced pyridine nucleotides, in turn, are reoxidized by flavoproteins.

The metabolic pathway by which nicotinic acid is converted into NAD has been elucidated for a variety of tissues, including human erythrocytes (Preiss and Handler, 1958). The conversion is carried out by three consecutive enzyme-catalyzed reactions (1 to 3 on page 1569, where PRPP is 5-phosphoribosyl-1-pyrophosphate). NADP is synthesized from NAD according to reaction 4. The biosynthesis of NAD from tryptophan is more complicated. Tryptophan is converted to quinolinic acid by a series of enzymatic reactions; quinolinic acid is converted to nicotinic acid ribonucleotide (Nishizuka and Hayaishi, 1963), which enters the pathway at reaction 2.

Symptoms of Deficiency. Nicotinic acid is an essential dietary constituent, the lack of which leads to the clinical condition known as pellagra. Pellagra is characterized by signs and symptoms referable especially to the skin, gastrointestinal tract, and central nervous system (CNS), a triad frequently referred to as dermatitis, diarrhea, and dementia, or the "three Ds." An erythematous eruption resembling sunburn first appears on the back of the hands. Other areas exposed to light (forehead, neck, and feet) are later involved, and eventually the lesions may be more widespread. The cutaneous manifestations are characteristically symmetrical and may darken, desquamate, and scar.

The chief symptoms referable to the digestive tract are stomatitis, enteritis, and diarrhea. The tongue becomes very red and swollen and may ulcerate. There is also excessive salivary secretion, and the salivary glands may be enlarged. Diarrhea is recurrent. The stools are watery and may occasionally be bloody. Nausea and vomiting are also common. Gastric achylia is observed in about 50% of cases.

Symptoms referable to the CNS are headache, dizziness, insomnia, depression, and impairment of memory. In severe cases, delusions, hallucinations, and dementia may appear. Motor and sensory disturbances of the peripheral nerves also occur. In

1. Nicotinic Acid + PRPP $\longrightarrow$ Nicotinic Acid Ribonucleotide + PP

2. Nicotinic Acid Ribonucleotide + ATP $\longrightarrow$ Desamido-NAD + PP

3. Desamido-NAD + Glutamine + ATP $\longrightarrow$ NAD + Glutamate + ADP + P

4. NAD + ATP $\longrightarrow$ NADP + ADP

addition, certain cases of pellagra manifest a macrocytic anemia. A milder degree of deficiency has been termed *subclinical pellagra.*

Biochemical assessment of deficiency is accomplished by the measurement of urinary excretion of methylated metabolites of nicotinic acid (*e.g.,* N-methylnicotinamide). These tests do not as yet provide unequivocal evidence of deficiency.

Human Requirements. As indicated above, the dietary requirement for this vitamin can be satisfied not only by nicotinic acid but also by nicotinamide and the amino acid tryptophan. Therefore, the nicotinic acid requirement is influenced by the quantity and the quality of dietary protein. Administration of tryptophan to normal human subjects, as well as to patients with pellagra, and analysis of urinary metabolites indicate that an average of 60 mg of dietary tryptophan is equivalent to 1 mg of nicotinic acid. This conversion rate is reduced in women taking oral contraceptives. The minimal requirement of nicotinic acid (including that formed from tryptophan) to prevent pellagra averages 4.4 mg/1000 kcal. The recommended allowance of the Dietary Allowances Committee of the National Research Council, expressed in nicotinic acid equivalents, is 6.6 mg/1000 kcal (*see* Table XVI–1, page 1553). For people who consume few calories (*e.g.,* the elderly), daily intake should not fall below 13 mg of nicotinic acid or the equivalent.

The relationship between the nicotinic acid requirement and the intake of tryptophan has helped to explain the historical association between the incidence of pellagra and the presence of large amounts of corn in the diet. Corn protein is low in tryptophan, and the nicotinic acid in corn and other cereals is largely unavailable. When cornmeal provides the major portion of dietary protein, pellagra will develop at levels of intake of nicotinic acid that would be adequate if the dietary protein contained more tryptophan.

The *carcinoid syndrome* in man may be manifested as pellagra, despite intakes of tryptophan and nicotinic acid that would normally be adequate. Carcinoid tumors synthesize large amounts of 5-hydroxytryptophan and 5-hydroxytryptamine, thus diverting significant quantities of tryptophan from the pathway utilized to synthesize nicotinic acid ribonucleotide. Metabolites of 5-hydroxytryptophan (*e.g.,* 5-hydroxyindoleacetic acid) that are excreted in the urine can be measured in patients who are suspected of having pellagra to evaluate the possible contribution of such a tumor.

Absorption, Fate, and Excretion. Both nicotinic acid and nicotinamide are readily absorbed from all portions of the intestinal tract, and the vitamin is distributed to all tissues. When therapeutic doses of nicotinic acid or its amide are administered, only small amounts of the unchanged vitamin appear in the urine. When extremely high doses of these vitamins are given, the unchanged vitamin represents the major urinary component. The principal route of metabolism of nicotinic acid and nicotinamide is by the formation of N-methylnicotinamide, which in turn is further metabolized to N-methyl-2-pyridone-5-carboxamide and N-methyl-4-pyridone-3-carboxamide. Nicotinuric acid, the glycine peptide of nicotinic acid, is an additional metabolite.

Preparations. *Niacin,* U.S.P. (*nicotinic acid, 3-pyridinecarboxylic acid*), occurs as white crystals or as a crystalline powder. *Niacin Tablets,* U.S.P., are usually available in 25-, 50-, 100-, 250-, and 500-mg amounts. Several oral preparations containing considerably greater quantities, intended for use as cholesterol-lowering agents, are also available. *Niacin Injection,* U.S.P., is a sterile solution of nicotinic acid prepared with the aid of sodium carbonate or sodium hydroxide. Preparations available for injection usually contain 50 or 100 mg/ml.

Niacinamide, U.S.P. (*nicotinamide, nicotinic acid amide*), occurs as a white crystalline, odorless powder with a bitter taste. *Niacinamide Tablets,* U.S.P., are usually available in 25-, 50-, 100-, and 500-mg amounts. *Niacinamide Injection,* U.S.P., is a sterile solution in water. Preparations available usually contain 100 mg/ml.

Therapeutic Uses. Nicotinic acid, nicotinamide, and their derivatives are used for prophylaxis and treatment of pellagra. In the acute exacerbations of the disease, therapy must be intensive. The recommended oral dose is 50 mg, given up to ten times daily. If oral medication is impossible, intravenous injection of 25 mg is given two or more times daily. Pellagra is now quite uncommon in the United States, probably as a direct result of supplementation of flour with nicotinic acid since 1939. When observed, it is usually secondary to chronic gastrointestinal disease or to alcoholism and, in these cases, multiple nutritional deficiencies often exist. Pellagra also occurs in Hartnup's disease, in which there is a defect in the absorption of tryptophan (Darby, *et al.,* 1976) and, as mentioned above, in some patients with a carcinoid tumor.

The response to nicotinic acid or its derivatives is dramatic. Within 24 hours, the fiery redness and swelling of the tongue disappear and sialorrhea diminishes. Associated oral infections heal rapidly. Other infections of mucous membranes, notably those involving the pharynx, urethra, vagina, and rectum, also disappear. Nausea, vomiting, and diarrhea may stop within 24 hours, and at the same time the patient is relieved of epigastric distress, abdominal pain, and distention. Appetite also improves. Mental symptoms are quickly relieved, sometimes overnight. Confused patients become mentally clear, and those who are delirious become calm, adjusted to their environment, and remember with insight the events of their psychotic state. So specific are nicotinic acid and its derivatives in this regard that they can be used as diagnostic agents in patients with frank psychoses but with questionable additional evidence of pellagra. Large doses of niacin are recommended, especially when the psychosis is associated with encephalopathy; the syndrome is particularly prone to occur in chronic alcoholics deficient in nicotinic acid. The dermal lesions blanch and heal, but this occurs more slowly. The vitamin has less effect on cutaneous lesions that are moist, ulcerated, or pigmented. The porphyrinuria associated with pellagra also disappears.

Pellagra may be complicated by thiamine deficiency with associated peripheral neuritis. This complication does not respond to nicotinic acid or its congeners and must be treated with thiamine. Many pellagrins are also benefited by additional therapy with riboflavin and pyridoxine.

PYRIDOXINE

History. In 1926, dermatitis was produced in rats by feeding a diet deficient in vitamin B_2. However, in 1936 György distinguished the water-soluble factor whose deficiency was responsible for the dermatitis from vitamin B_2 and named it vitamin B_6. The structure of the vitamin was elucidated in 1939. Several related natural compounds (pyridoxine, pyridoxal, pyridoxamine) have been shown to possess the same biological properties, and therefore all should be called vitamin B_6. However, the Council on Pharmacy and Chemistry has assigned the name *pyridoxine* to the vitamin.

Chemistry. The structures of the three forms of vitamin B_6—that is, pyridoxine, pyridoxal, and pyridoxamine—are shown at the top of the next column. The compounds differ in the nature of the substituent on the carbon atom in position 4 of the pyridine nucleus: pyridoxine is a primary alcohol, pyridoxal is the corresponding aldehyde, and pyridoxamine contains an aminomethyl group in this position. Each of the three forms of the vitamin can be readily utilized by the mammalian organism. The physiologically active forms of vitamin B_6 are pyridoxal phosphate and pyridoxamine phosphate, where the

Pyridoxine

Pyridoxal

Pyridoxamine

phosphate is esterified with the alcohol at position 5 of the pyridine ring.

All three forms of vitamin B_6 are converted in the body to pyridoxal phosphate; pyridoxal is converted to pyridoxal phosphate by the enzyme pyridoxal kinase.

Antimetabolites to pyridoxine have been synthesized and are capable of blocking the action of the vitamin and producing signs and symptoms of deficiency. The most active is 4-deoxypyridoxine, in which the substituent on the carbon atom in position 4 is a methyl group. The anti–vitamin B_6 activity of 4-deoxypyridoxine has been attributed to the formation *in vivo* of 4-deoxypyridoxine-5-phosphate, which is a competitive inhibitor of several pyridoxal phosphate–dependent enzymes.

Isonicotinic acid hydrazide (*isoniazid; see* Chapter 53) combines with pyridoxal or pyridoxal phosphate to form hydrazones; as a result, it is a potent inhibitor of pyridoxal kinase. Enzymatic reactions in which pyridoxal phosphate participates as a coenzyme are also inhibited, but only by concentrations about 1000 times as great as that required to inhibit the formation of pyridoxal phosphate. Isoniazid thus appears to exert its anti–vitamin B_6 effect primarily by inhibiting the formation of the coenzyme form of the vitamin.

Pharmacological Actions. Pyridoxine has low toxicity and elicits no outstanding pharmacodynamic actions after either oral or intravenous administration. Extremely large oral doses (in the range of 2 to 6 g/kg) produce convulsions and death in rats and mice (Brin, 1978), but lower doses can be given daily without any obvious effects. In man, oral doses up to 1000 mg daily have not caused adverse reactions (Bauernfeind and Miller, 1978), but symptoms of dependency have been noted in adults given only 200 mg daily followed by withdrawal (Canham *et al.*, 1964).

Physiological Functions. Pyridoxal phosphate serves an important role in metabolism as a coenzyme for a wide variety of metabolic transformations of amino acids, including decarboxylation, transamination, and racemization, as well as for enzymatic steps in the metabolism of tryptophan, sulfur-containing amino acids, and hydroxy-amino acids. In the case of transamination, enzyme-bound pyridoxal phosphate is aminated to pyridoxamine phosphate by the donor amino acid, and the bound pyridoxamine phosphate is then deaminated to pyridoxal phosphate by the acceptor α-keto acid. In the metabolism of tryptophan, vitamin B_6 is involved in a number of enzymatic reactions (Henderson and Hulse, 1978). In vitamin B_6-deficient man and animals a number of metabolites of tryptophan are excreted in abnormally large quantities. The measurement of these metabolites, particularly xanthurenic acid, in urine following tryptophan loading tests has been used to test for vitamin B_6 deficiency (Gershoff, 1976). Vitamin B_6 is a cofactor in the conversion of tryptophan to 5-hydroxytryptamine. The conversion of methionine to cysteine is also dependent on the vitamin (Sturman, 1978).

Biochemical interactions occur between pyridoxal phosphate and certain drugs and toxins (Bauernfeind and Miller, 1978). Thus, isoniazid increases urinary excretion of vitamin B_6, and prolonged use of penicillamine has caused deficiency of vitamin B_6. The drugs cycloserine and hydralazine are also antagonists of vitamin B_6. Administration of the vitamin reduces the neurological side effects associated with the use of these compounds. Vitamin B_6 enhances the peripheral decarboxylation of levodopa and reduces its effectiveness for the treatment of Parkinson's disease. Vitamin B_6 and multivitamin preparations should thus be avoided in patients receiving levodopa (*see* Chapter 21).

Symptoms of Deficiency. Symptoms referable to pyridoxine deficiency have been produced in all mammalian species that have been studied, including man. It is claimed that the incidence of vitamin B_6 deficiency among alcoholics is 20 to 30% (Li, 1978). Important features of the deficiency observed in more than one species relate to the skin, the nervous system, and erythropoiesis.

Skin. In the rat, a florid dermatitis occurs; this consists in hyperkeratosis and acanthosis of the ears, paws, and snout as well as edema of the corium. In man, seborrhea-like skin lesions about the eyes, nose, and mouth accompanied by glossitis and stomatitis can be produced within a few weeks by feeding a diet poor in vitamin B complex plus daily doses of the vitamin antagonist 4-deoxypyridoxine. The lesions clear rapidly after the administration of pyridoxine but do not respond to other members of the B complex (Mueller and Vilter, 1950).

Nervous System. Rats, pigs, dogs, and man may have convulsive seizures when maintained on a diet deficient in pyridoxine. These seizures can be prevented or cured by the vitamin. In the pig, degenerative changes in peripheral nerves, dorsal root ganglion cells, and posterior columns of the spinal cord have been described. In man, a peripheral neuritis associated with synovial swelling and tenderness, especially of the carpal synovia (*carpal tunnel disease*), has been attributed to deficiency of pyridoxine; the syndrome is reversible upon treatment with high dosage of the vitamin (Ellis *et al.*, 1979).

The electroshock threshold for producing clonic seizures in rats is substantially lowered by pyridoxine deficiency and can be raised to normal by the administration of pyridoxine. The induction of convulsive seizures by pyridoxine deficiency may be the result of a lowered concentration of γ-aminobutyric acid, an inhibitory CNS neurotransmitter, the synthesis of which is carried out by glutamic acid decarboxylase, a pyridoxal phosphate–requiring enzyme (Roberts, 1963).

Erythropoiesis. In the dog, pig, and monkey, pyridoxine deficiency results in microcytic, hypochromic anemia. While dietary deficiency of pyridoxine in man may rarely cause anemia, the usual pyridoxine-responsive anemia of man is apparently not due to inadequate supplies of the vitamin as judged by normal standards. This type of anemia is described in Chapter 56.

Human Requirements. The requirement for pyridoxine increases with the amount of protein in the diet (Linkswiler, 1978). The average adult minimal requirement for pyridoxine is about 1.5 mg per day in individuals ingesting 100 g of protein per day. To provide a reasonable margin of safety and to allow for daily intakes of more than 100 g of protein, a level of 2.2 mg per day is recommended for adult males and 2.0 mg per day for adult females (*see* Table XVI-1, page 1553).

Absorption, Fate, and Excretion. Pyridoxine, pyridoxal, and pyridoxamine are readily absorbed from the gastrointestinal tract. The principal excretory product when any of the three forms of the vitamin is fed to man is 4-pyridoxic acid, formed by the action of hepatic aldehyde oxidase on free pyridoxal. Administration of pyridoxine and pyridoxamine also results in an increased excretion of pyridoxal in man, indicating that both compounds may be first transformed, directly or indirectly, to pyridoxal, which is then oxidized to 4-pyridoxic acid (for review, *see* Brin, 1978).

Preparations. *Pyridoxine Hydrochloride*, U.S.P., occurs as colorless or white crystals or as a white crystalline powder. *Pyridoxine Hydrochloride Tablets,* U.S.P., are available in sizes ranging from 5 to 500 mg. *Pyridoxine Hydrochloride Injection,* U.S.P., is a sterile solution of pyridoxine hydrochloride in water, usually containing 50 or 100 mg/ml.

Therapeutic Uses. Although there is no doubt that pyridoxine is essential in human nutrition, the clinical syndrome of pyridoxine deficiency has not been well defined. Nevertheless, it may be presumed that an individual with a deficiency of other members of the B complex may also have a relative deficiency of pyridoxine. Therefore, pyridoxine therapy may be advantageous in individuals suffering from a deficiency of other members of the B complex. On the basis that pyridoxine is essential in human nutrition, it is incorporated into many multivitamin preparations for prophylactic use. It has already been pointed out that 30% or more of alcoholics have biochemically demonstrable deficiency of vitamin B_6 (Li, 1978).

As indicated above, vitamin B_6 influences the metabolism of certain drugs and *vice versa.* With considerable justification, vitamin B_6 is given prophylactically to patients receiving isoniazid or hydralazine to prevent the development of peripheral neuritis. Biochemical evidence of pyridoxine deficiency has been obtained in a fraction of women taking oral contraceptives containing estrogen (Rose, 1978). As in pregnancy, the administration of estrogen can cause increased urinary excretion of tryptophan metabolites, such as xanthurenic acid, especially following a tryptophan load. There is a reduction in the pyridoxal phosphate concentration in the blood of those who take oral contraceptives, and Rose (1978) considers that 15 to 20% of such women have direct biochemical evidence of vitamin B_6 deficiency. However, the *recommended intakes* of vitamin B_6 appear to be sufficient to meet the requirements of such individuals (Bossé and Donald, 1979; Donald and Bossé, 1979).

Pyridoxine-responsive anemia is a well-documented but uncommon condition. The use of the vitamin in this disease is discussed in Chapter 56. Such anemias in patients without apparent pyridoxine deficiency, as well as a seizure disorder in infants that responds to the administration of pyridoxine, and the abnormalities characterized by xanthurenic aciduria, primary cystathioninuria, or homocystinuria appear to constitute a group of genetically determined clinical states of "pyridoxine dependency," manifested by a requirement for large amounts of the vitamin (*see* Mudd, 1971).

PANTOTHENIC ACID

History. Pantothenic acid was first identified by Williams and associates in 1933 as a substance essential for the growth of yeast. Its name, derived from Greek words signifying "from everywhere," is indicative of the wide distribution of the vitamin in nature. The role of pantothenic acid in animal nutrition was first defined in chicks, in which a deficiency disease characterized by skin lesions was known to be cured by fractions prepared from liver extract. Although first thought to be a form of "chick pellagra," it was not cured by nicotinic acid. Shortly thereafter, in 1939, Woolley and coworkers and also Jukes demonstrated that the chick antidermatitis factor was pantothenic acid. This compound also cured graying of the hair of black rats that was produced by feeding certain diets. One must hasten to note, however, that the graying of human hair is not due to a deficiency of pantothenic acid.

Chemistry. Pantothenic acid is an optically active organic acid, and biological activity is characteristic only of the *d* isomer. The vitamin functions in the body following its incorporation into coenzyme A. Their chemical structures are as follows:

Pantothenic Acid

Coenzyme A

The metabolic pathway by which pantothenic acid is converted into coenzyme A involves five consecutive enzyme-catalyzed reactions.

Many analogs of pantothenic acid have been studied in an attempt to find an antimetabolite. Although active antagonists have been synthesized and are of value as research tools, they are not therapeutic agents.

Pharmacological Actions. Pantothenic acid has no outstanding pharmacological actions when it is administered to experimental animals or normal man. The vitamin is essentially nontoxic; as much as 10 g can be given daily to man without producing symptoms (Ralli and Dumm, 1953).

Physiological Functions. Coenzyme A, the physiologically active form of panto-

---

thenic acid, serves as a cofactor for a variety of enzyme-catalyzed reactions involving transfer of acetyl (two-carbon) groups; the precursor fragments of various lengths are bound to the sulfhydryl group of coenzyme A. Such reactions are important in the oxidative metabolism of carbohydrates, gluconeogenesis, synthesis and degradation of fatty acids, and the synthesis of sterols, steroid hormones, and porphyrins (Wright, 1976).

Symptoms of Deficiency. Pantothenic acid is essential for the growth of various microorganisms. In animals, deficiency of pantothenic acid is manifested by symptoms of neuromuscular degeneration, adrenocortical insufficiency, and death. By administering a semisynthetic diet low in the vitamin together with a pantothenic acid antagonist, ω-methylpantothenic acid, a syndrome in man is produced that is characterized by fatigue, headache, sleep disturbances, nausea, abdominal cramps, occasional vomiting, and flatulence (Hodges *et al.,* 1959). The subjects complain of paresthesias in the extremities, muscle cramps, and impaired coordination. The eosinopenic response to ACTH is lost and increased sensitivity to insulin develops, but there is no change in the concentration of 17-keto steroids in urine or in the concentration of sodium in blood or urine. Fry and coworkers (1976) have produced the same syndrome by giving human subjects a diet devoid of pantothenic acid for 10 weeks. Pantothenic acid deficiency has not been recognized in man consuming a normal diet, presumably because of the ubiquitous occurrence of the vitamin in ordinary foods. However, a "burning foot" syndrome associated with paresthesia in the legs and seen in malnourished persons may be a form of pantothenic acid deficiency, since there is a favorable response to the vitamin (Glusman, 1947).

Human Requirements. Pantothenic acid is a required nutrient, but the magnitude of need is not precisely known. Accordingly, the Committee on Dietary Allowances provides provisional amounts in the form of ranges of intakes (Table XVI–2, page 1555). For adults, the provisional allowance is 4 to 7 mg per day. Intakes for other groups are proportional to caloric consumption. In view of the widespread distribution of pantothenic acid in foods, dietary deficiency is very unlikely.

Absorption, Fate, and Excretion. Pantothenic acid is readily absorbed from the gastrointestinal tract. It is present in all tissues, in concentrations ranging from 2 to 45 μg/g. Pantothenic acid apparently is not metabolized in the human body since the intake and the excretion of the vitamin are approximately equal. About 70% of the absorbed pantothenic acid is excreted unchanged in the urine.

Preparations. *Calcium Pantothenate,* U.S.P., is available as official tablets containing from 10 to 250 mg. *Racemic Calcium Pantothenate* is also official in the U.S.P.

Therapeutic Uses. No clearly defined uses for pantothenic acid exist, although it is commonly included in multivitamin preparations and in products for enteral and parenteral alimentation.

BIOTIN

History. The discovery of biotin resulted from two different experimental approaches: one, the study of a toxic syndrome, which eventually was proven to be due to a substance *antagonistic* to biotin; the other, a study of the growth requirements of yeast. In 1916, Bateman observed that rats fed a diet containing raw egg white as the sole source of protein developed a syndrome characterized by neuromuscular disorders, severe dermatitis, and loss of hair (*egg-white injury*). The syndrome could be prevented by cooking the protein or by administering yeast, liver, or extracts of these. In 1936, Kögl and Tönnis isolated a factor in crystalline form from egg yolk that was essential for growth of yeast, which they called *biotin*. It was then demonstrated that biotin and the factor that protected against egg-white toxicity were the same substance (György, 1940). In 1942, duVigneaud established the structural formula of biotin, and shortly thereafter the vitamin was synthesized.

In the meantime, the nature of the antagonist to biotin in egg white received extensive study. The compound is a protein, first isolated by Eakin and associates in 1940 and called *avidin*. Avidin is a glycoprotein that binds biotin with great affinity and thus prevents its absorption.

Chemistry. Biotin is an optically active organic acid, and the active form is the *d* isomer. The vitamin has the following structural formula:

Biotin

Three forms of biotin, apart from free biotin itself, have been found in natural materials. These derivatives are biocytin (ε-biotinyl-L-lysine) and the D and L sulfoxides of biotin. The derived forms of biotin are active in supporting growth of some microorganisms. Their efficacy as substitutes for biotin in human nutrition has not been studied. Biocytin may represent a degradation product of a biotin-protein complex, since, in its role as a coenzyme, the vitamin is covalently linked to an ϵ-amino group of a lysine residue of the apoenzyme involved.

A number of compounds antagonize the actions of biotin. Among them are biotin sulfone, desthiobiotin, and certain imidazolidone carboxylic acids. The antagonism between avidin and biotin is described above.

Pharmacological Actions. Relatively large amounts of biotin have been administered to both animals and man with impunity (Wright, 1956).

Physiological Functions. Biotin is a coenzyme for several enzyme-catalyzed carboxylation reactions and, as such, plays an important role in CO_2 fixation. The CO_2 fixation occurs in a two-step reaction, the first involving binding of CO_2 to the biotin moiety of the biotin enzyme, and the second involving transfer of the biotin-bound CO_2 to an appropriate acceptor (*see* McCormick, 1976). As a cofactor for both pyruvate carboxylase and acetyl coenzyme A (acetyl-CoA) carboxylase, biotin plays an important role in both carbohydrate and fat metabolism.

Symptoms of Deficiency. The ease of producing biotin deficiency varies with the animal species. In a few species, a deficiency state can be produced merely by feeding a synthetic diet deficient in this nutrient. In most, however, presumably owing to synthesis of the vitamin by intestinal bacteria, it is necessary to eliminate bacteria from the intestinal tract, feed raw egg white, or administer antimetabolites of biotin in order to produce the deficiency. The symptoms of deficiency vary with the species and include failure of growth, loss of hair, dermatitis, poor lactation, and loss of muscular control with a spastic gait. Syndenstricker and associates (1942) produced a deficiency syndrome in man by the feeding of egg white that responded to the administration of small doses of biotin. Signs and symptoms included dermatitis, atrophic glossitis, hyperesthesia, muscle pain, lassitude, anorexia, slight anemia, and changes in the ECG. These disappeared on administering biotin. Spontaneous deficiency in man has been observed in some subjects who have consumed raw eggs over long periods (Bonjour, 1977). Seborrheic dermatitis of infancy is probably a form of biotin deficiency, since it can be cured by giving biotin parenterally in 5-mg daily doses. Inborn errors of biotin-dependent enzyme systems are known; these conditions respond to the administration of massive doses of biotin (Bonjour, 1977).

Human Requirements. The daily requirement of adults for biotin has been assigned a provisional value of 100 to 200 μg by the Committee on Dietary Allowances (Table XVI-2, page 1555). The average American diet provides some 100 to 300 μg of the vitamin. Part of the biotin synthesized by the bacterial flora is also available for absorption.

Absorption, Fate, and Excretion. Ingested biotin is rapidly absorbed from the gastrointestinal tract and appears in the urine predominantly in the form of intact biotin and in lesser amounts as the metabo-

lites *bis*-norbiotin and biotin sulfoxide. Mammals are unable to degrade the ring system of biotin.

Preparations. Although there is no official preparation of biotin, it is available commercially.

Therapeutic Uses. Large doses of biotin (5 to 10 mg daily) are administered to babies with infantile seborrhea and to individuals with genetic alterations of biotin-dependent enzymes.

CHOLINE

History. In 1932, Best and associates observed that pancreatectomized dogs maintained on insulin developed fatty livers; this could be prevented by inclusion in the diet of crude egg-yolk lecithin or beef pancreas. The substance responsible for this effect was shown to be choline. These studies marked the beginning of an extensive literature on the role of lipotropic substances, especially choline, in animal nutrition. Choline has other important functions in addition to those related to lipid metabolism. For example, it is a precursor of the neurochemical transmitter acetylcholine.

For reasons given below, however, choline should *not* be considered as a vitamin for man.

Chemistry. Choline (trimethylethanolamine) has the following structural formula:

$$H_3C-\overset{\overset{\displaystyle CH_3}{|}}{\underset{\underset{\displaystyle CH_3}{|}}{N^+}}-CH_2CH_2OH$$

Choline

Pharmacological Actions. Qualitatively, choline has the same pharmacological actions as does acetylcholine, but it is far less active. The acute toxicity of choline, especially by mouth, is relatively low (about 5 g/kg for rats) in comparison with that of some of its esters and many other quaternary ammonium compounds. The oral LD50 for man is estimated to be of the order of 200 to 400 g. Single oral doses of 10 g produce no obvious pharmacodynamic response.

Physiological Functions. Choline has several roles in the body. It is an important component of phospholipids, affects the mobilization of fat from the liver (lipotropic action), acts as a methyl donor, and is essential for the formation of the neurotransmitter acetylcholine.

Phospholipid Constituent. Choline is a component of the major phospholipid, lecithin, and is also a constituent of plasmalogens, which are abundant in mitochondria, and sphingomyelin, which is found particularly in brain. Choline thus provides an essential structural component of many biological membranes and also of the plasma lipoproteins.

Lipotropic Action. As mentioned, the initial recognition of choline as a significant dietary factor depended on its capacity to reduce the fat content of the livers of diabetic dogs. Substances that stimulate removal of excess fat from the liver are known as lipotropic agents and include choline, inositol, methionine, vitamin B_{12}, and folic acid. Certain of these compounds appear to act by providing methyl groups for the synthesis of choline in the body. Formation of the lipid components of plasma lipoproteins is thus permitted, and this facilitates transport of fat from the liver.

Methyl Donor. Choline can donate methyl groups necessary for the synthesis of other compounds. The first step in transfer is the formation of betaine, which is the immediate donor of the methyl group. Thus, choline can transfer a methyl group to homocysteine to form methionine. The roles of cyanocobalamin and folic acid in the metabolism of one-carbon compounds are discussed in Chapter 57.

Acetylcholine Formation. Acetylcholine is synthesized from choline and acetyl-CoA by choline acetyltransferase and is broken down by acetlycholinesterase (*see* Chapter 4). Choline is transported between the brain and the plasma by a bidirectional system localized in the endothelium of brain capillaries. This system operates by facilitated diffusion, and the amount of choline available to central neurons thus varies as a function of the concentration of choline in the plasma. When rats are given choline chloride, there is a sequential increase in the concentrations of plasma choline, brain choline, and brain acetylcholine. Consumption of lecithin, which contains choline, also causes these changes (Growdon and Wurtman, 1979). These findings are relevant to the treatment of diseases involving reduced capacity to synthesize acetylcholine (*see* below).

Symptoms of Deficiency. The effects of choline deficiency on animals are discussed in two reviews (Griffith and Nye, 1971; Kuksis and Mookerjea, 1978). The deficiency state is really one of available methyl groups, and consequently can only be produced as a result of a combined deficiency of choline and other methyl donors. In animals, the amount of choline needed is affected by growth rate, age, quantity of dietary fat, and quality of dietary protein, as well as by species differences in the capacity to synthesize choline from methyl donors. Some species, such as the guinea pig, have such a low capacity for synthesis that choline is a dietary essential. In such species it is possible to induce choline deficiency with a suitable diet. Not only is there accumulation of fat in the liver, followed by cirrhosis, but hemorrhagic renal lesions and motor incoordination from nerve degeneration have also been observed. Newberne and Chandra (1977) describe damage to the fetus, including atrophy of the thymus, when the pregnant rat is fed a diet with marginal contents of choline, methionine, folate, and vitamin B_{12}. None of these symptoms of deficiency has been identified in man (Kuksis and Mookerjea, 1978).

Human Requirements. The needs of the tissues for choline are met from both exogenous (dietary) and endogenous (metabolic) sources. Biosynthesis of choline occurs by transmethylation of ethanolamine with the methyl group of methionine or by a series of reactions requiring vitamin B_{12} and folate as cofactors. Thus, an adequate supply of methyl-group donors in the diet is desirable to protect against the hepatic accumulation of lipid. In addition, large amounts of choline appear to have a therapeutic effect on certain diseases of the nervous system, by means of stimulation of the synthesis of acetylcholine. However, none of the functions of choline justifies its classification as a vitamin. It has not been shown to act as a cofactor in any enzymatic reaction, and the doses needed to produce therapeutic effects (several grams) are much greater than those of any vitamin.

Because of the lack of evidence of a choline deficiency syndrome in human subjects, choline cannot be considered an essential dietary constituent for man. In addition, the American diet provides 400 to 900 mg per day of choline as a constituent of lecithin; it is thus difficult to consume a diet that is low in choline. Since human breast milk contains 7 mg choline/100 kcal, the Committee on Nutrition of the American Academy of Pediatrics (1976) recommends the fortification of infant formulas to this level.

Absorption, Fate, and Excretion. Choline is absorbed from the diet as such or as lecithin. The latter is hydrolyzed by the intestinal mucosa to glycerophosphoryl choline, which either passes to the liver to liberate choline or to the peripheral tissues via the intestinal lymphatics. Free choline is not fully absorbed, especially after large doses, and intestinal bacteria metabolize choline to trimethylamine. Since this compound imparts a strong odor of decaying fish to the feces, lecithin is the clearly preferred oral vehicle for the administration of choline.

Preparations. Choline is not at present an official drug. However, preparations of choline bitartrate, choline dihydrogen citrate, and choline chloride are available. In addition, preparations of lecithin are available, although many of them consist mainly of other phosphatides (Wurtman, 1979).

Therapeutic Uses. The use of choline to treat fatty liver and cirrhosis, usually alcoholic in etiology, has not proven to be consistently effective (Griffith and Nye, 1971). Because of the synthesis of choline from other methyl donors, provision of a well-balanced diet is just as effective in alleviating the symptoms of hepatic damage.

The use of choline in large doses for the treatment of certain disorders of the nervous system has also been advocated (Growdon and Wurtman, 1979). Five such diseases are candidates for treatment with choline (Barbeau, 1978). They include tardive dyskinesia, a disease characterized by choreiform movements that are caused by chronic treatment with some neuroleptic drugs (*see* Growdon, 1978; Chapter 19). Some clinical improvement with choline treatment has also been reported in Huntington's chorea (Growdon, 1978), in which impaired mental function and voluntary muscle contractions are probably associated with reduced acetylcholine synthesis, in Gilles de la Tourette's disease, in Friedreich's ataxia, and in presenile dementia (Barbeau, 1978). Doses of 150 to 300 mg/kg of choline chloride and of 350 mg/kg of lecithin have been administered in these various studies. However, the status of choline as a therapeutic agent for these diseases is still not well established. The hypothesis that the basic defect is in synthesis of the neurotransmitter, acetylcholine, also requires further experimental evaluation.

INOSITOL

History. Although inositol was identified more than 100 years ago in the urine of diabetic patients, a role for this substance in animal nutrition was not suspected until 1941, when Gavin and McHenry found that inositol had a lipotropic action in rats. Inositol was subsequently observed to cure alopecia induced in rats and mice by dietary means. A nutritional role for inositol was considerably strengthened when Eagle and colleagues showed in 1957 that this substance is essential for the growth of all human and other animal cells in tissue culture. However, its status as a vitamin for man remains uncertain, for reasons given below.

Chemistry. Inositol (hexahydroxycyclohexane) is an isomer of glucose. There are seven optically inactive and one pair of optically active stereoisomeric forms of inositol possible, of which only one, the optically inactive *myo*-inositol, is nutritionally active. It has the following structural formula:

Myo-Inositol

Pharmacological Actions. Inositol possesses no significant pharmacological actions when given parenterally in doses of 1 to 2 g to human subjects.

Physiological Functions. The physiological role of inositol remains obscure but appears in part to resemble that of choline (Kuksis and Mookerjea, 1978). Thus, inositol is present in the form of phosphatidylinositol in the phospholipids of cell membranes and plasma lipoproteins. Furthermore, inositol has a lipotropic action on fatty livers, and, in the case of the gerbil, will prevent fat accumulation in the intestine (Hegsted *et al.*, 1974). These effects on the transport of fat out of the cells of the liver and intestine appear to be dependent on the need for inositol in order to complete the fat-carrying lipoprotein molecule in the plasma.

Symptoms of Deficiency. Variable reserves of inositol, its production by gut bacteria, and possibly its synthesis in the cells of the body have made the demonstration of a dietary need for inositol difficult to achieve. However, certain animals can be made

deficient; alopecia and fatty infiltration of the liver result. There has been no demonstration of a dietary need by man, but the studies of Eagle and colleagues (1957) showed that 18 human cell lines all needed *myo*-inositol for growth, probably because of its structural role in the formation of cell membranes. In view of the absence of a demonstrable human need for inositol, Eagle and coworkers suggest that it may be synthesized in only a few organs, which then make it available for use by all cells. Experiments with labeled glucose show that the growing rat can synthesize inositol, although this does not exclude a partial dependence on dietary inositol during periods of rapid growth.

Human Requirements. Although there has been no demonstration of a human need for inositol, a high concentration is present in human milk (Committee on Nutrition, Academy of Pediatrics, 1976). As with choline, it may be desirable to add inositol to infant formulas to mimic more closely the content of human milk. The normal daily intake of inositol is about 1 g, mostly from plant sources. Inositol is present in cereals as the hexaphosphate, phytic acid. Inositol in this form is partly available for absorption because of hydrolysis by the enzyme phytase in the intestinal mucosa. Inositol also occurs in vegetable and animal foods in other forms.

Absorption, Fate, and Excretion. The consumption of inositol by man is about 1 g per day. The compound is easily absorbed from the gastrointestinal tract. Inositol is readily metabolized to glucose and is about one third as effective as glucose in alleviating starvation ketosis. The concentration of inositol in normal human plasma is about 0.5 mg/dl. Within the tissues, the concentration of inositol is particularly high in heart muscle, brain, and skeletal muscle (1.6, 0.9, and 0.4 g/100 g dry weight, respectively). Urine normally contains only small amounts of inositol, but in diabetic humans and animals the amount is markedly increased, probably because of competition between inositol and glucose for reabsorption by the renal tubule.

Preparations. There is no official preparation of inositol.

Therapeutic Uses. Inositol has been given for the management of diseases associated with disturbances in the transport and metabolism of fat. There is no persuasive evidence that it has therapeutic efficacy.

II. Ascorbic Acid (Vitamin C)

History. Scurvy, the deficiency disease caused by lack of vitamin C, has been known since the time of the Crusades, especially among northern European populations who subsisted on diets lacking fresh fruits and vegetables over extensive periods of the year (Sharman, 1974). The incidence of scurvy was reduced by the introduction to Europe in the seventeenth century of the potato, an additional source of vitamin C. However, the long sea voyages of exploration in the sixteenth to eighteenth centuries, which were undertaken without a supply of fresh fruits and vegetables, resulted in large numbers of the crew dying from scurvy.

A dietary cause for scurvy had long been suspected. In 1535, Jacques Cartier learned from the Indians of Canada how to cure the scurvy in his crew by making a decoction from spruce leaves, and several subsequent ship captains prevented or cured scurvy by administration of lemon juice. However, a systematic study of the relationship of diet to scurvy had to wait until 1747 when Lind, a physician in the British Royal Navy, carried out a clinical trial on cases of frank scurvy who were given either cider, vitriol, vinegar, sea water, oranges and lemons, or garlic and mustard. Those who received citrus fruits recovered rapidly. The consequent introduction of lemon juice into the British Navy in 1800 resulted in a dramatic reduction in the incidence of scurvy; whereas the Royal Naval Hospital at Portsmouth admitted 1457 cases in 1780, only 2 cases were seen there in 1806. At the present time, frank scurvy is occasionally seen in infants, in older people on restricted diets, and in alcoholics.

The next significant episode in the history of vitamin C was the identification in 1907 of a suitable experimental animal by Holst and Fröhlich, who found that guinea pigs develop scurvy on a diet of oats and bran that is not supplemented with fresh vegetables. It was subsequently shown that most mammals synthesize ascorbic acid; man, the monkey, and the guinea pig are exceptions. The demonstration of scurvy in the guinea pig allowed testing of fractions from citrus fruits for antiscorbutic potency. In 1928, Szent-Györgyi isolated a reducing agent in pure form from cabbage and from adrenal glands; in 1932, Waugh and King identified Szent-Györgyi's compound as the active antiscorbutic factor in lemon juice. The chemical structure of this substance was then soon established in several laboratories, and the trivial chemical name *ascorbic acid* was assigned to designate its function in preventing scurvy. The term *vitamin C* should be used as a generic descriptor for all compounds that exhibit qualitatively the biological activity of ascorbic acid; the latter name should be restricted to that specific substance.

Chemistry. Ascorbic acid is a six-carbon compound structurally related to glucose and other hexoses. It is reversibly oxidized in the body to dehydroascorbic acid. The latter compound possesses full vitamin C activity. The structural formulas of ascorbic acid and dehydroascorbic acid are as follows:

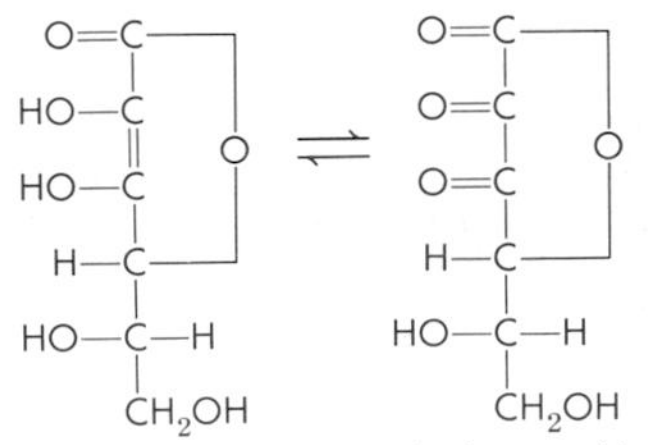

Ascorbic acid has an optically active carbon atom, and antiscorbutic activity resides almost totally in the L isomer. Another isomer, erythorbic acid (D-isoascorbic acid, D-araboascorbic acid), has very weak antiscorbutic action but has a similar redox potential. Both compounds have therefore been used to prevent nitrosoamine formation from nitrites in cured meats such as bacon. The reason for the lack of a stronger antiscorbutic action of erythorbic acid is probably the incapacity of the tissues to retain it in the quantities that ascorbic acid is stored (Hughes *et al.*, 1971). One consequence of the facile oxidation of ascorbic acid is the readiness with which it can be destroyed by exposure to air, especially in an alkaline medium and if copper is present as a catalyst. Ascorbic acid-2-sulfate is a derivative that is present in tissues and urine; it has no antiscorbutic activity in guinea pigs or monkeys, which may also be correlated with the low capacity of tissues to concentrate this form of ascorbate (Hornig, 1974).

Pharmacological Actions. In the strict sense of the word, vitamin C may be said to possess few pharmacological actions. Administration of the compound in amounts greatly in excess of the physiological requirements causes few demonstrable effects except in the scorbutic individual, whose symptoms are rapidly alleviated. Secondary symptoms accompanying the deficiency disease (scurvy) are likely to be varied and may include anemia, infections, metabolic disturbances, and other symptoms. As a result, an extensive literature has accumulated concerning the effect of vitamin C on practically every function of the body.

Physiological Functions. Ascorbic acid functions in a number of biochemical reactions, mostly involving oxidation. Thus, it is required for or facilitates the conversion of certain proline residues in collagen to hydroxyproline in the course of collagen synthesis (Myllylä *et al.*, 1978), the oxidation of lysine side chains in proteins to provide hydroxytrimethyllysine for carnitine synthesis (Hulse *et al.*, 1978), the synthesis of steroids by the adrenal cortex (Deana *et al.*, 1975), the conversion of folic acid to folinic acid (Stokes *et al.*, 1975), microsomal drug metabolism (Zannoni and Sato, 1975), and tyrosine metabolism. Instead of acting as a cofactor for an enzyme, ascorbic acid has the capacity to protect an enzyme, *p*-hydroxyphenylpyruvic acid oxidase, from inhibition by its substrate. The protection is apparently necessary only after ingestion of large amounts of tyrosine; it does not seem to be required under ordinary dietary conditions. This role of ascorbic acid in tyrosine metabolism is not specific, since various analogs of ascorbic acid and even a dye, 2,6-dichlorophenolindophenol, which has a similar redox potential, can replace the vitamin (La Du and Zannoni, 1961).

At the tissue level, a major function of ascorbic acid is related to the synthesis of intercellular substances, including collagen, the matrix of tooth and bone, and the intercellular cement of the capillary endothelium (Sebrell and Harris, 1967). In consequence, scurvy is associated with a defect in collagen synthesis that is apparent by the failure of wounds to heal, in defects in tooth formation, and in the rupture of capillaries, which leads to numerous petechiae and their coalescence to form ecchymoses. While this last has been attributed to leakage from capillaries because of inadequate adhesion of the endothelial cells, it is also thought that the pericapillary fibrous tissue is defective in scurvy, leading to inadequate support of the capillary and its rupture under pressure.

Absorption, Distribution, and Excretion.
Ascorbic acid is readily absorbed from the intestine, and absorption of dietary ascorbate is nearly (80 to 90%) complete (Kallner *et al.,* 1977). Ascorbic acid is present in the plasma and is ubiquitously distributed in the cells of the body. Concentrations of the vitamin in leukocytes are sometimes taken to represent those in tissue and are less susceptible to depletion than is the plasma. The white blood cells of healthy adults have concentrations of about 27 μg of ascorbic acid per 10^8 cells. Nursing-home patients in Great Britain often have only half this concentration, and values rise after the oral administration of ascorbic acid (Andrews *et al.,* 1969). Concentrations in plasma also vary with intake. Adequate ingestion is associated with concentrations over 0.5 mg/dl, whereas concentrations of 0.15 mg/dl are seen in individuals with frank scurvy.

When the diet contains essentially no ascorbate, concentrations in plasma fall and, as mentioned, symptoms of scurvy are obvious when a value of 0.15 mg/dl is reached; the total body store of the vitamin at this time approximates 300 mg. When the intake of ascorbate is raised, the concentration in

plasma also increases—at first linearly. The daily ingestion of 5 to 10 mg provides a total body store of 600 to 1000 mg of ascorbate. When 60 mg of vitamin C is consumed per day (the recommended dietary allowance for adults), the concentration in plasma reaches about 0.8 mg/dl and the body store is around 1500 mg. If intake is raised beyond 200 mg daily, the body store tends to level off at 2500 mg and the concentration in plasma at 2 mg/dl. However, the renal threshold for ascorbic acid is about 1.5 mg/dl of plasma, and increasing amounts of the ingested ascorbic acid are excreted when the daily intake exceeds 100 mg.

Studies with isotopically labeled L-ascorbic acid have shown that the vitamin is oxidized to CO_2 in rats and guinea pigs, but considerably less conversion can be detected in man. One route of metabolism of L-ascorbate in man involves its conversion to oxalate and eventual excretion in the urine; dehydroascorbate is presumably an intermediate. Ascorbic acid–2–sulfate has also been identified as a metabolite of vitamin C in human urine.

Biosynthesis of Ascorbic Acid. Man and other primates as well as the guinea pig are the only mammals known to be unable to synthesize ascorbic acid; consequently, they require dietary vitamin C for the prevention of scurvy. An explanation for this has come from biochemical studies (*see* Burns, 1959). The rat, a typical species that does not require dietary vitamin C, synthesizes ascorbic acid from glucose through the intermediate formation of D-glucuronic acid, L-gulonic acid, and L-gulonolactone. Man, monkey, and guinea pig lack the hepatic enzyme required to carry out the last reaction, that is, the conversion of L-gulonolactone to L-ascorbic acid. This reaction is presumably missing because of a genetically controlled enzyme "deficiency."

Symptoms of Deficiency. A deficiency in the intake of vitamin C can lead to scurvy. Cases of scurvy are encountered among elderly people (often men living alone), alcoholics, drug addicts, and others with inadequate diets, including infants.

Experimental scurvy has been produced in man in a number of studies (Crandon *et al.,* 1940; Krebs *et al.,* 1948; Hodges *et al.,* 1969). For example, the surgeon Crandon submitted himself to a diet devoid of vitamin C for 161 days, during which the concentration of ascorbic acid in his plasma fell to negligible values within 41 days, while the concentration in his white blood cells became undetectable after 121 days. Perifollicular hyperkeratosis (an accumulation of epidermal cells around the hair follicles) occurred at 120 days; hemorrhages appeared under his skin (petechiae and ecchymoses) at 161 days, and a wound made into the back failed to heal. In spontaneous cases of scurvy, there is usually loosening of the teeth, gingivitis, and anemia, which may be due to a specific function of ascorbic acid in hemoglobin synthesis. The picture of spontaneous scurvy in clinical practice is often complicated by insufficiencies of other nutrients as well.

Scurvy occurs in infants receiving formula diets with inadequate concentrations of ascorbic acid. The infant is irritable and resents being touched because of pain. This is due to hemorrhages under the periosteum of the long bones, and the resulting hematomas are often visible as swellings on the shafts of these bones.

Human Requirements. The daily intake of ascorbic acid must equal the amount that is destroyed by oxidation or excreted. Studies on healthy adult human subjects given [^{14}C] ascorbic acid show an average daily removal rate of 3% of the body store; values of 4% were observed in some subjects (Baker *et al.,* 1971). To maintain a body store of 1500 mg of ascorbic acid or more in an adult man, it would thus be necessary to absorb approximately 60 mg daily (4% of 1500 mg). Values for vitamin C requirements of other age groups are based on similar reasoning (Table XVI–1, page 1553).

Under special circumstances, more ascorbic acid appears to be required to achieve normal concentrations in the plasma. Thus, South African miners have been observed to require 200 to 250 mg of vitamin C daily to maintain a plasma concentration of 0.75 mg/dl (Visagie *et al.,* 1975). Concentrations of ascorbate in plasma are lowered by the use of cigarettes (Pelletier, 1977) and of oral contraceptive agents (Rivers, 1975), but the significance of these changes is unclear. Requirements can increase in certain diseases, particularly infectious diseases, and also following surgery (Irvin *et al.,* 1978).

Preparations. *Ascorbic Acid,* U.S.P., consists of white or slightly yellow crystals or powder. The vitamin is reasonably stable in the dry state, but solutions deteriorate rapidly if exposed to air. *Ascorbic Acid Tablets,* U.S.P. (CEVALIN, several nonproprietary preparations), usually contain 25, 50, 100, 250, 500, or 1000 mg of the vitamin. Solutions for oral use are also available in various concentrations. *Ascorbic Acid Injection,* U.S.P., is a sterile neutral solution of the vitamin designed for parenteral injection. The currently available preparations contain 50, 100, 200, 250, or 500 mg/ml. Most multivitamin preparations contain ascorbic acid.

There are many foods that have a high content of vitamin C. Orange and lemon juices are outstanding in this respect and contain approximately 0.5 mg/ml. This high vitamin content permits the use of fruit juices in therapy in place of pure preparations of the vitamin.

Apart from its role in nutrition, ascorbic acid is commonly used as an antioxidant to protect natural flavor and color of many foods (*e.g.,* processed fruit, vegetables, and dairy products).

Routes of Administration. Vitamin C is usually administered by the oral route; however, in conditions that prevent adequate absorption from the gastrointestinal tract, solutions of the sodium salt may be given by intramuscular or intravenous injection. In addition, ascorbic acid should be given to patients receiving parenteral hyperalimentation. Because of the loss of much of the infused ascorbic acid in the urine, daily doses of 200 mg are needed to maintain normal concentrations in plasma of 1 mg/dl (Nichoalds *et al.,* 1977).

Therapeutic Uses. Vitamin C is used for the treatment of ascorbic acid deficiency, especially frank scurvy, which occurs rather infrequently in infants and in adults.

Human breast milk contains 30 to 55 mg of ascorbic acid per liter, depending on the mother's intake (Irwin and Hutchins, 1976). Consequently, the infant consuming 850 ml of breast milk will receive about 35 mg of ascorbic acid, which has been set as the recommended dietary allowance (Table XVI–1, page 1553). However, during the first week of life, the newborn infant, especially the premature, may have an increased requirement for ascorbic acid to meet the demands of metabolizing large amounts of tyrosine in the diet (Irwin and Hutchins, 1976). To prevent transient accumulation of tyrosine, daily intake of 100 mg of ascorbic acid is recommended. Orange juice is customarily given to infants to meet such requirements, especially to infants who are receiving formulas based on cow's milk. Many commercial formulas are, however, fortified to provide ascorbic acid at these levels. In the rare cases of infantile scurvy, much larger therapeutic doses are used. Adults with scurvy should receive 1 g of ascorbic acid daily. This dose will cause a rapid disappearance of the subcutaneous hemorrhages.

The reducing properties of vitamin C have also been employed to control *idiopathic methemoglobinemia,* although it is less effective than methylene blue. Doses of at least 150 mg of ascorbic acid are needed to be effective in this condition.

In addition to these specific uses of vitamin C, extensive literature has appeared on the application of this vitamin to a wide variety of diseases. Many such claims are associated with megadosage practices, which are stated to prevent or cure viral respiratory infections (Pauling, 1970) and to be beneficial in cancer (Cameron and Pauling, 1978) and other diseases. Creagan and associates (1979) were unable to demonstrate any beneficial effect of high doses of ascorbic acid given to patients with advanced cancer. Anderson (1977) has carried out a series of three carefully designed studies in Canada to test whether vitamin C plays any role in the prevention and treatment of the common cold. No obvious effect on the incidence of headcolds was seen from the administration of ascorbic acid, although there was a slight reduction in the number of days of missed work. Many other studies have yielded negative or inconsistent results (*see* Pitt and Costrini, 1979). Any benefit that might be derived from such use of ascorbic acid seems small when weighed against the expense and the risks of the megadosage treatment. The latter include formation of kidney stones resulting from the excessive excretion of oxalate, rebound scurvy in the offspring of mothers taking high doses (Herbert, 1975), and a similar phenomenon when subjects who are consuming large amounts of vitamin C suddenly stop; a precipitous reduction in ascorbic acid concentration in plasma follows (Anderson, 1977). These rebound phenomena are presumably due to induction of pathways of ascorbic acid metabolism as a result of the preceding high dosage. Excessive doses of ascorbic acid can also enhance the absorption of iron (Cook and Monsen, 1977) and interfere with anticoagulant therapy (Rosenthal, 1971).

Anderson, T. W. Large scale studies with vitamin C. *Acta Vitaminol. Enzymol.* (*Milano*), **1977**, *31*, 43–50.

Andrews, J.; Letcher, M.; and Brook, M. Vitamin C supplementation in the elderly: a 17-month trial in an old persons' home. *Br. Med. J.*, **1969**, *2*, 416–418.

Baker, E. M.; Hodges, R. E.; Hood, J.; Sauberlich, H. E.; March, S. C.; and Canham, J. E. Metabolism of 14C and 3H-labeled L-ascorbic acid in human scurvy. *Am. J. Clin. Nutr.*, **1971**, *24*, 444–454.

Barbeau, A. Emerging treatments: replacement therapy with choline or lecithin in neurological diseases. *Can. J. Neurol. Sci.*, **1978**, *5*, 157–160.

Bauernfeind, J. C., and Miller, O. N. Vitamin B_6: nutritional and pharmaceutical usage, stability, bioavailability, antagonists, and safety. In, *Human Vitamin B_6 Requirements*. National Academy of Sciences, Washington, D. C., **1978**, pp. 78–110.

Bonjour, J. P. Biotin in man's nutrition and therapy—a review. *Int. J. Vitam. Nutr. Res.*, **1977**, *47*, 107–118.

Bossé, T. R., and Donald, E. A. The vitamin B_6 requirement in oral contraceptive users. I. Assessment by pyridoxal level and transferase activity in erythrocytes. *Am. J. Clin. Nutr.*, **1979**, *32*, 1015–1023.

Brin, M. Blood transketolase determination in the diagnosis of thiamine deficiency. *Heart Bull.*, **1968**, *17*, 86–89.

———. Vitamin B_6: chemistry, absorption, metabolism, catabolism and toxicity. In, *Human Vitamin B_6 Requirements*. National Academy of Sciences, Washington, D. C., **1978**, pp. 1–20.

Burns, J. J. Biosynthesis of L-ascorbic acid: basic defect in scurvy. *Am. J. Med.*, **1959**, *26*, 740–748.

Cameron, E., and Pauling, L. Supplemental ascorbate in the supportive treatment of cancer: prolongation of survival times in terminal human cancer. *Proc. Natl. Acad. Sci. U.S.A.*, **1978**, *73*, 3685–3689.

Canham, J. E.; Nunes, W. T.; and Eberlin, E. W. Electroencephalographic and central nervous system manifestations of B_6 deficiency and induced B_6 dependency in normal human adults. In, *Proceedings of the Sixth International Congress of Nutrition.* E. & S. Livingstone, Ltd., Edinburgh, **1964**, p. 537.

Committee on Nutrition, Academy of Pediatrics. Commentary on breast-feeding and infant formulas, including proposed standards for formulas. *Pediatrics*, **1976**, *57*, 278–285.

Cook, J. D., and Monsen, E. R. Vitamin C, the common cold and iron absorption. *Am. J. Clin. Nutr.*, **1977**, *30*, 235–241.

Crandon, J. H.; Lund, C. C.; and Dill, D. B. Experimental human scurvy. *N. Engl. J. Med.*, **1940**, *223*, 353–369.

Creagan, E. T.; Moertel, C. C.; O'Fallon, J. R.; Schutt, A. J.; O'Connell, M. J.; Rubin, J.; and Frytak, S. Failure of high-dose vitamin C to benefit patients with advanced cancer. *N. Engl. J. Med.*, **1979**, *301*, 687–690.

Darby, W. J.; McNutt, K. W.; and Todhunter, E. N. Niacin. In, *Present Knowledge in Nutrition.* (Hegsted, D. M.; Chichester, C. O.; Darby, W. J.; McNutt, K. W.; Stalvey, R. M.; and Stotz, E. H.; eds.) The Nutrition Foundation, Washington, D. C., **1976**, pp. 162–174.

Deana, R.; Bharaj, B. S.; Verjee, Z. H.; and Galzigna, L. Changes relevant to catecholamine metabolism in liver and brain of ascorbic acid deficient guinea pigs. *Int. J. Vitam. Nutr. Res.*, **1975**, *45*, 175–182.

Dodge, P. R.; Prensky, A. L.; and Feigin, R. D. Effect of vitamin deficiencies and excesses on the nervous system. In, *Nutrition and the Developing Nervous System.* (Holmes, S. J., ed.) C. V. Mosby Co., St. Louis, **1975**, pp. 429–437.

Donald, E. A., and Bossé, T. R. The vitamin B_6 requirement in oral contraceptive users. II. Assessment by tryptophan metabolites, vitamin B_6, and pyridoxic acid levels in urine. *Am. J. Clin. Nutr.*, **1979**, *32*, 1024–1032.

Eagle, H.; Oyama, V.; Levy, M.; and Freeman, A. Myoinositol as an essential growth factor for normal and malignant human cells in tissue culture. *J. Biol. Chem.*, **1957**, *229*, 191–205.

Ellis, J.; Folkers, K.; Watanabe, T.; Kaji, M.; Saji, S.; Caldwell, J. W.; Temple, C. A.; and Wood, F. S. Clinical results of a cross-over treatment with pyridoxine and placebo of the carpal tunnel syndrome. *Am. J. Physiol.*, **1979**, *32*, 2040–2046.

Fry, P. C.; Fox, H. M.; and Tao, H. G. Metabolic response to a pantothenic acid deficient diet in humans. *J. Nutr. Sci. Vitaminol.* (*Tokyo*), **1976**, *22*, 339–346.

Gershoff, S. N. Vitamin B_6. In, *Present Knowledge in Nutrition.* (Hegsted, D. M.; Chichester, C. O.; Darby, W. J.; McNutt, K. W.; Stalvey, R. M.; and Stotz, E. H.; eds.) The Nutrition Foundation, Washington, D. C., **1976**, pp. 149–161.

Glusman, M. The syndrome of "burning feet" (nutritional melalgia) as a manifestation of nutritional deficiency. *Am. J. Med.*, **1947**, *3*, 211–223.

Goldsmith, G. A. Niacin-tryptophan relationship in man and niacin requirement. *Am. J. Clin. Nutr.*, **1958**, *6*, 479–486.

———. Vitamins and avitaminosis. In, *Diseases of Metabolism: Detailed Methods of Diagnosis and Treatment.* (Duncan, G. G., ed.) W. B. Saunders Co., Philadelphia, **1964**, pp. 567–663.

Griffith, W. H., and Nye, J. F. Choline. In, *The Vitamins*, 2nd ed., Vol. III. (Sebrell, W. H., and Harris, R. S., eds.) Academic Press, Inc., New York, **1971**, pp. 3–154.

Growdon, J. H. Effects of choline on tardive dyskinesia and other movement disorders. *Psychopharmacol. Bull.*, **1978**, *14*, 55–56.

Growdon, J. H., and Wurtman, R. J. Dietary influences on the synthesis of neurotransmitters in the brain. *Nutr. Rev.*, **1979**, *37*, 129–136.

György, P. A further note on the identity of vitamin H with biotin. *Science*, **1940**, *92*, 609.

Hegsted, D. M.; Gallagher, A.; and Hanford, H. Inositol requirement of the gerbil. *J. Nutr.*, **1974**, *104*, 588–592.

Henderson, L. M., and Hulse, J. D. Vitamin B_6: relationship in tryptophan metabolism. In, *Human Vitamin B_6 Requirements.* National Academy of Sciences, Washington, D. C., **1978**, pp. 21–36.

Herbert, V. The rationale of massive-dose vitamin therapy. In, *Proceedings, Western Hemisphere Nutrition Congress IV.* Publishing Sciences Group, Inc., Acton, Mass., **1975**, pp. 84–91.

Hodges, R. E.; Baker, E. M.; Hood, J.; Sauberlich, H. E.; and March, S. C. Experimental scurvy in man. *Am. J. Clin. Nutr.*, **1969**, *22*, 535–548.

Hodges, R. E.; Bean, W. B.; Ohlson, M. A.; and Bleiler, R. Human pantothenic acid deficiency produced by omega-methyl pantothenic acid. *J. Clin. Invest.*, **1959**, *38*, 1421–1425.

Hornig, D. Recent advances in vitamin C metabolism. In, *Vitamin C: Recent Aspects of Its Physiological and Technological Importance.* (Birch, G. G., and Parker, K. J., eds.) Applied Science Publishers, Ltd., London, **1974**, pp. 91–103.

Horwitt, M. K.; Harvey, C. C.; Rothwell, W. S.; Cutler, J. L.; and Haffron, D. Tryptophan-niacin relationships in man. *J. Nutr.*, **1956**, *60*, Suppl. 1, 1–43.

Hughes, R. E.; Hurley, R. J.; and Jones, P. R. The retention of ascorbic acid by guinea-pig tissues. *Br. J. Nutr.*, **1971**, *26*, 433–438.

Hulse, J. D.; Ellis, S. R.; and Henderson, L. M. Carnitine biosynthesis. *J. Biol. Chem.*, **1978**, *253*, 1654–1659.

Irvin, T. T.; Chattopadhyay, D. K.; and Smythe, A. Ascorbic acid requirements in postoperative patients *Surg Gynecol. Obstet.*, **1978**, *147*, 49–55.

Jusko, W. J., and Levy, G. Absorption, protein binding, and elimination of riboflavin. In, *Riboflavin.* (Rivlin, R. S., ed.) Plenum Press, New York, **1975**, pp. 99–152.

Kallner, A.; Hartman, D.; and Hornig, D. On the absorption of ascorbic acid in man. *Int. J. Vitam. Nutr. Res.*, **1977**, *47*, 383–388.

Krebs, H. A.; Peters, R. A.; Coward, K. H.; Mapson, L. W.; Parsons, L. G.; Platt, B. S.; Spence, J. C.; and O'Brien, J. R. P. Vitamin-C requirement of human adults: experimental study of vitamin-C deprivation in man. *Lancet*, **1948**, *1*, 853–858.

Kuksis, A., and Mookerjea, S. Choline. *Nutr. Rev.*, **1978**, *36*, 201–207.

———. Inositol. *Ibid.*, **1978**, *36*, 233–238.

La Du, B. N., and Zannoni, U. G. The role of ascorbic acid in tyrosine metabolism. *Ann. N.Y. Acad. Sci.*, **1961**, *92*, 175–191.

Lane, M.; Smith, F. E.; and Alfrey, C. P. Experimental dietary and antagonist-induced human riboflavin deficiency. In, *Riboflavin.* (Rivlin, R. S., ed.) Plenum Press, New York, **1975**, pp. 245–277.

Li, T. Factors influencing vitamin B_6 requirement in alcoholism. In, *Human B_6 Requirements.* National Academy of Sciences, Washington, D. C., **1978**, pp. 210–225.

Linkswiler, H. M. Vitamin B_6 requirements of men. In, *Human B_6 Requirements.* National Academy of Sciences, Washington, D. C., **1978**, pp. 279–290.

McCormick, D. B. Metabolism of riboflavin. In, *Riboflavin.* (Rivlin, R. S., ed.) Plenum Press, New York, **1975**, pp. 153–198.

———. Biotin. In, *Present Knowledge in Nutrition.* (Hegsted, D. M.; Chichester, C. O.; Darby, W. J.; McNutt, K. W.; Stalvey, R. M.; and Stotz, E. H.; eds.) The Nutrition Foundation, Washington, D. C., **1976**, pp. 217–225.

McLaren, D. Metabolic disorders. In, *Current Therapy.* (Conn, H. F., ed.) W. B. Saunders Co., Philadelphia, **1978**, pp. 409–410.

Mosher, L. R. Nicotinic acid side effects and toxicity. a review. *Am. J. Psychiatry*, **1970**, *126*, 1290–1296.

Mudd, S. H. Pyridoxine-responsive genetic disease. *Fed. Proc.*, **1971**, *30*, 970–976.

Mueller, J. F., and Vilter, R. W. Pyridoxine deficiency in human beings induced with desoxypyridoxine. *J. Clin. Invest.*, **1950**, *29*, 193–201.

Munro, H. N.; Lazarus, S.; and Bell, G. H. The value of capillary strength tests in the diagnosis of vitamin C and vitamin P deficiency in man. *Nutr. Abstr. Rev.*, **1947**, *17*, 291–309.

Murata, K. Thiaminase. In, *Review of Japanese Literature on Beriberi and Thiamine.* (Shimazono, N., and Katsura, E., eds.) Igaku Shoin, Ltd., Tokyo, **1965**, pp. 220–254.

Myllylä, R.; Kuutti-Savolainen, E. R.; and Kivirikko, K. I. The role of ascorbate in the prolyl hydroxylase reaction. *Biochem. Biophys. Res. Commun.*, **1978**, *33*, 441–448.

Newberne, P. M., and Chandra, R. K. *Nutrition, Immunity and Infection: Mechanisms of Interactions.* Plenum Press, New York, **1977**.

Nicholads, G. E.; Meng, H. C.; and Caldwell, M. D. Vitamin requirements in patients receiving total parenteral nutrition. *Arch. Surg.*, **1977**, *112*, 1061–1064.

Nishizuka, Y., and Hayaishi, O. Studies on the biosynthesis of nicotinamide adenine dinucleotide. I. Enzymic synthesis of niacin ribonucleotides from 3-hydroxyanthranilic acid in mammalian tissues. *J. Biol. Chem.*, **1963**, *238*, 3369–3377.

Pauling, L. Evolution and the need for ascorbic acid. *Proc. Natl. Acad. Sci. U.S.A.*, **1970**, *67*, 1643–1648.

Pelletier, O. Vitamin C and tobacco. *Int. J. Vitam. Nutr. Res.*, **1977**, *16*, 147–169.

Pincus, J. H.; Cooper, J. R.; Murphy, J. V.; Rabe, E. F.; Lonsdale, D.; and Dunn, H. G. Thiamine derivatives in subacute necrotizing encephalomyelopathy: a preliminary report. *Pediatrics*, **1973**, *51*, 716–721.

Pitt, H. A., and Costrini, A. M. Vitamin C prophylaxis in marine recruits. *J.A.M.A.*, **1979**, *241*, 908–911.

Platt, S. Thiamine deficiency in human beriberi and in Wernicke's encephalopathy. In, *Thiamine Deficiency.* (Wolstenholm, G. W., and O'Connor, M., eds.) Little, Brown, & Co., Boston, **1967**, pp. 135–143.

Preiss, J., and Handler, P. Biosynthesis of diphosphopyridine nucleotide. II. Enzymatic aspects. *J. Biol. Chem.*, **1958**, *233*, 493–500.

Ralli, E. P., and Dumm, M. E. Relation of pantothenic acid to adrenal cortical function. *Vitam. Horm.*, **1953**, *11*, 133–158.

Rindi, G., and Ventura, U. Thiamine intestinal transport. *Physiol. Rev.*, **1972**, *52*, 821–827.

Rivers, J. M. Oral contraceptives and ascorbic acid. *Am. J. Clin. Nutr.*, **1975**, *28*, 550–554.

Rivlin, R. S. Riboflavin metabolism. *N. Engl. J. Med.*, **1970**, *283*, 463–472.

———. Hormones, drugs and riboflavin. *Nutr. Rev.*, **1979**, *37*, 241–246.

Roberts, E. Some thoughts about the γ-aminobutyric acid system in nervous tissue. *Nutr. Rev.*, **1963**, *21*, 161–165.

Rose, D. P. Oral contraceptives and vitamin B_6. In, *Human B_6 Requirements.* National Academy of Sciences, Washington, D. C., **1978**, pp. 193–201.

Rosenthal, G. Interaction of ascorbic acid and warfarin. *J.A.M.A.*, **1971**, *215*, 1671.

Scriver, C. R. Vitamin-responsive inborn errors of metabolism. *Metabolism*, **1973**, *22*, 1319–1344.

Sebrell, W. H., and Harris, R. S. (eds.). *The Vitamins: Chemistry, Physiology, Pathology, Methods,* Vol. I. Academic Press, Inc., New York, **1967**.

Sharman, I. M. Vitamin C: historical aspects. In, *Vitamin C: Recent Aspects of Its Physiological and Technological Importance.* (Birch, G. G., and Parker, K. J., eds.) Applied Science Publishers, Ltd., London, **1974**, pp. 1–14.

Stokes, P. L.; Melikian, V.; Leeming, R. L.; Portman-Graham, H.; Blair, J. A.; and Cooke, W. T. Folate metabolism in scurvy. *Am. J. Clin. Nutr.*, **1975**, *28*, 126–129.

Sturman, J. A. Vitamin B_6 and the metabolism of sulfur amino acids. In, *Human Vitamin B_6 Requirements.* National Academy of Sciences, Washington, D. C., **1978**, pp. 37–60.

Sydenstricker, V. P.; Singal, S. A.; Briggs, A. P.; DeVaughn, N. M.; and Isbell, H. Observations on the "egg white injury" in man. *J.A.M.A.*, **1942**, *118*, 1199–1200.

Vimokesant, S. L.; Nakornchi, S.; Dhanamitta, S.; and Hilker, D. M. Effect of tea consumption on thiamine status in man. *Nutr. Rep. Int.*, **1974**, *9*, 371–374.

Visagie, M. E.; DuPlessis, J. P.; and Laubsher, N. Effect of vitamin C supplementation on black mine-workers. *S. Afr. Med. J.*, **1975**, *49*, 889–892.

Wagner-Jauregg, T. Riboflavin. II. Chemistry. In, *The Vitamins,* 2nd ed., Vol. V. (Sebrell, W. H., and Harris, R. S., eds.) Academic Press, Inc., New York, **1972**, pp. 3–43.

Wittenborn, J. R.; Weber, E. S. P.; and Brown, M. Niacin in long-term treatment of schizophrenia. *Arch. Gen. Psychiatry*, **1973**, *28*, 308–315.

Wright, L. D. The metabolism of biotin. In, *Symposium on Vitamin Metabolism.* Nutrition Symposium Series, No. 13. National Vitamin Foundation, New York, **1956**, pp. 104–115.

———. Pantothenic acid. In, *Present Knowledge in Nutrition.* (Hegsted, D. M.; Chichester, C. O.; Darby, W. J.; McNutt, K. W.; Stalvey, R. M.; and Stotz, E. H.; eds.) The Nutrition Foundation, Washington, D. C., **1976**, pp. 226–231.

Wurtman, J. J. Sources of choline and lecithin in the diet. In, *Nutrition and the Brain,* Vol. 5. (Barbeau, A.; Growdon, J. H.; and Wurtman, R. J.; eds.) Raven Press, New York, **1979,** pp. 73–81.

Zannoni, V. G., and Sato, P. H. Effects of ascorbic acid on microsomal drug metabolism. *Ann. N.Y. Acad. Sci.,* **1975,** *258,* 119–131.

Monographs and Reviews

American Medical Association Report. *Guidelines for Multivitamin Preparations for Parenteral Use.* Department of Foods and Nutrition, American Medical Association, Chicago, **1975,** pp. 1–27.

Bicknell, R., and Prescott, F. *The Vitamins in Medicine,* 2nd ed. White Friars Press, London, **1946.**

Birch, G. G., and Parker, K. J. (eds.). *Vitamin C: Recent Aspects of Its Physiological and Technological Importance.* Applied Science Publishers, Ltd., London, **1974.**

Dakshinamurti, K. B_6 vitamins and nervous system function. In, *Nutrition and the Brain,* Vol. I. (Wurtman, R. J., and Wurtman, J. J., eds.) Raven Press, New York, **1977,** pp. 250–318.

Dodge, P. R.; Prensky, A. L.; and Feigin, R. D. (eds.). *Nutrition and the Developing Nervous System.* C. V. Mosby Co., St. Louis, **1975.**

Food and Nutrition Board, National Research Council. *Human Vitamin B_6 Requirements.* National Academy of Sciences, Washington, D. C., **1978.**

Food and Nutrition Board, National Research Council.

Recommended Dietary Allowances, 9th ed. National Academy of Sciences, Washington, D. C., **1979.**

Goldsmith, G. A. Vitamins and avitaminosis. In, *Diseases of Metabolism.* (Duncan, G. G., ed.) W. B. Saunders Co., Philadelphia, **1964,** pp. 567–642.

Goodhart, R. S., and Shils, M. E. (eds.). *Modern Nutrition in Health and Disease,* 6th ed. Lea & Febiger, Philadelphia, **1979.**

Hanck, A., and Ritzel, G. (eds.). Re-evaluation of vitamin C. *Int. J. Vitam. Nutr. Res.,* **1977,** *16,* 1–310.

Hegsted, D. M.; Chichester, C. O.; Darby, W. J.; McNutt, K. W.; Stalvey, R. M.; and Stotz, E. H. (eds.). *Present Knowledge in Nutrition,* 4th ed. The Nutrition Foundation, Washington, D. C., **1976.**

Irwin, M. I., and Hutchins, B. K. A conspectus of research on vitamin C requirements of man. *J. Nutr.,* **1976,** *106,* 823–879.

Moran, J. R., and Greene, H. L. The B vitamins and vitamin C in human nutrition. I. General considerations and 'obligatory' B vitamins. II. 'Conditional' B vitamins and vitamin C. *Am. J. Dis. Child.,* **1979,** *133,* 192–199, 308–314.

Rechcigl, M. Effect of nutrient deficiencies in man. In, *CRC Handbook Series in Nutrition and Food,* Sect. E. *Nutritional Disorders,* Vol. III. CRC Press, Inc., West Palm Beach, Fla., **1978.**

Scriver, C. R. Vitamin-responsive inborn errors of metabolism. *Metabolism,* **1973,** *22,* 1319–1344.

Sebrell, W. H., and Harris, R. S. (eds.). *The Vitamins,* 2nd ed., Vols. I, II, III, IV, V. Academic Press, Inc., New York, **1971–1974.**

CHAPTER

67 FAT-SOLUBLE VITAMINS

Vitamins A, K, and E

H. George Mandel and Victor H. Cohn

VITAMIN A

History. Night blindness was apparently first described in Egypt around 1500 B.C. Although this disease was not then linked to dietary deficiency, topical treatment with roasted or fried liver was wisely recommended, and Hippocrates later suggested eating beef liver as a cure for the affliction. The relationship to nutritional deficiency was definitively recognized in the last century. Ophthalmia Brasiliana, a disease of the eyes that primarily afflicted poorly nourished slaves, was first described in 1865. In 1887, endemic night blindness was reported to occur among the orthodox Russian Catholics who fasted during the Lenten period. More pertinent was the observation that the nurslings of mothers who fasted were prone to develop spontaneous sloughing of the cornea. Many other reports of nutritional keratomalacia soon followed from all parts of the world, including the United States.

Experimental rather than clinical observations, however, led to the discovery of vitamin A. In 1913, two groups (McCollum and Davis, Osborne and Mendel) independently reported that animals fed on artificial diets with lard as a sole source of fat developed a nutritional deficiency that could be corrected by the addition of a factor contained in butter, egg yolk, and cod liver oil to the diet. An outstanding symptom of this experimental nutritional deficiency was xerophthalmia (dryness and thickening of the conjunctiva). Clinical and experimental vitamin A deficiencies were recognized as related during World War I, when it became apparent that xerophthalmia in human beings was a result of a decrease in the content of butterfat in the diet.

Chemistry and Occurrence. The simple observation of Steenbock (1919) that the vitamin A content of vegetables varies with the degree of pigmentation paved the way for the isolation and discovery of the chemical nature of the vitamin. Subsequently, Euler and associates (1929) and Moore (1929) demon-

strated that the purified plant pigment carotene (provitamin A) is a remarkably potent source of vitamin A. β-Carotene, the most active carotenoid found in plants, has the structural formula shown below. In the United States, the average adult receives about half of his daily intake of vitamin A as the preformed vitamin and the rest as carotenoids. Major dietary sources of vitamin A are liver, butter, cheese, whole milk, egg yolk, certain fish, and various yellow or green fruits and vegetables.

Vitamin A exists in a variety of forms, and the term is frequently used to represent the various compounds. *Retinol* (vitamin A_1), a primary alcohol, is present in esterified form in the tissues of animals and salt-water fishes, mainly in the liver. Its structural formula, established by Karrer and associates (1931), is as follows:

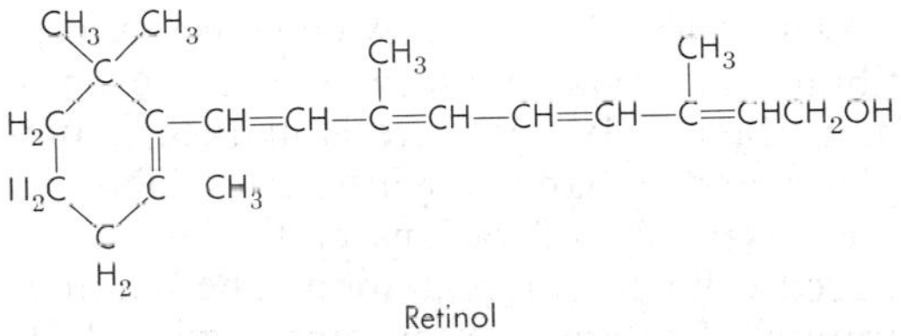

Retinol

A closely related compound, 3-dehydroretinol (vitamin A_2), is obtained from the tissues of fresh-water fishes and usually occurs mixed with retinol.

A number of geometric isomers of retinol exist because of the possible *cis-trans* configurations of the side chain containing double bonds. Fish liver oils contain mixtures of the stereoisomers; synthetic retinol is the all-*trans* isomer. Interconversion between isomers readily takes place in the body. In the visual cycle, the reaction between retinal (vitamin A aldehyde) and opsin to form rhodopsin only occurs with the 11-*cis* isomer.

Certain structural modifications of retinol are possible without destroying its activity. Retinoic acid

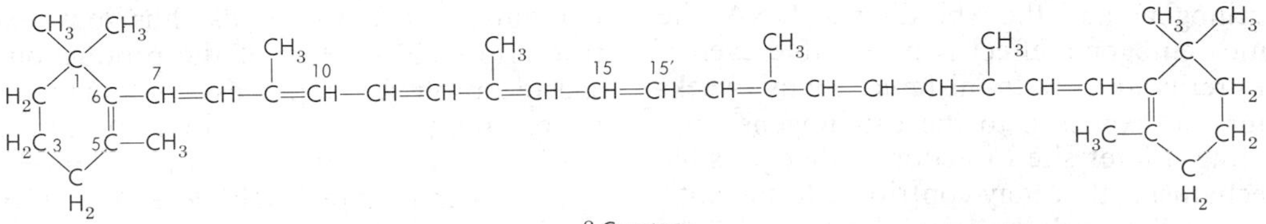

β-Carotene

1583

(vitamin A acid), in which the alcohol group has been oxidized, shares some but not all of the actions of retinol. Retinoic acid is very potent in promoting growth and controlling differentiation and maintenance of epithelial tissue in vitamin A–deficient animals, but it is ineffective in restoring visual, auditory, or reproductive function in certain species where retinol is effective.

Ethers and esters derived from the alcohol also show activity. The ring structure of retinol (β-ionone), or the more unsaturated ring in 3-dehydroretinol (dehydro-β-ionone), is essential for activity; hydrogenation destroys biological activity. Of all known derivatives, *trans*-retinol and its aldehyde, retinal, exhibit the greatest biological potency.

Pharmacological Actions. Vitamin A plays an essential role in various biochemical and physiological processes. As a pharmacological agent, the vitamin or preferably synthetic derivatives known as "retinoids" are useful in the treatment of certain dermatitides (*see* below). There has also been considerable interest in the apparent ability of these compounds to interfere with carcinogenesis. However, significant toxicity is associated with administration of excessive quantities of the vitamin (*see* below).

Deficiency of vitamin A enhances susceptibility to carcinogenesis, apparently even in man (Bjelke, 1975); there is marked hyperplasia and enhanced synthesis of DNA by the basal cells of various epithelia and reduced cellular differentiation. The administration of vitamin A or other retinoids to animals reverses these changes in the epithelium of the respiratory tract, mammary gland, urinary bladder, and skin. The compounds also prevent the development of epithelial cancer of the tissues mentioned. Thus, the progression of premalignant cells to cells with invasive, malignant characteristics is slowed, arrested, or even reversed in experimental animals.

The exact mechanism of the anticarcinogenic effect remains unclear, but obviously it is of enormous interest (Bollag, 1975; Sporn et al., 1976). Although the retinoids may interfere with the metabolic activation of carcinogens and their binding to DNA, the anticarcinogenic effect is observable even if the retinoid is administered many weeks after the exposure to the carcinogens, suggesting a later site of action. Other possible mechanisms that may contribute to the antitumor effect include destabilization of lyso-

somes, enhancement of antitumor immunity, or a direct cytotoxic action of the retinoid.

Present limitations to the therapeutic application of the retinoids are their toxicity to the liver and their failure to distribute to specific organs as desired. Newer derivatives, such as 13-*cis*-retinoic acid, are being tested in man for their antitumor properties. It must be noted, however, that retinoids can also increase the incidence of certain tumors in animals.

Physiological Functions. Vitamin A has a number of important functions in the body. It plays an essential role in the function of the retina. It is apparently essential for growth and differentiation of epithelial tissue. The vitamin is required for growth of bone, reproduction, and embryonic development. It also has a stabilizing effect on various membranes and acts to regulate membrane permeability (*see* Wasserman and Corradino, 1971).

The functions of vitamin A are mediated by different forms of the molecule. In vision, the functional vitamin is retinal; retinol is apparently responsible for the actions of the vitamin in reproductive processes, and retinoic acid or a metabolite is important in other roles. The major recognized reactions are as follows:

Retinol (transport) ⇌ Retinal → Retinoic Acid

Retinol Esters (tissue storage) / (Visual Pigments) light opsin / Inactive Products / Active Metabolite? (growth, tissue maintenance)

It appears that in vitamin A–deficient animals nuclear RNA synthesis is diminished, and that retinol or retinoic acid stimulates RNA synthesis in specific organs to a degree proportional to the ability of the retinoid to overcome the deficiency (Jayaram and Ganguly, 1977). Retinoids thus may exert transcriptional control of the production of specific proteins, a process that may have far-reaching implications with respect to regulation of cellular differentiation and development of malignancies (Blalock and Gifford, 1977).

Retinol appears to have a specific biochemical function in the synthesis of mannose- and galactose-containing glycoproteins and glycolipids. Retinol is converted to retinyl phosphate in epithelial tissues, and this intermediate is in turn metabolized to mannosylretinylphosphate in a reaction that is catalyzed by a microsomal enzyme and requires guanosine diphosphomannose as a glycosyl donor (Rosso *et al.,* 1975). The glycosylated derivative of the vitamin mediates the transfer of mannose to specific glycoproteins. Thus, the formation of such proteins is sharply curtailed when there is deficiency of vitamin A. Reactions of this type may explain the function of the vitamin in the maintenance of epithelia, the regulation of cellular adhesiveness, and the restoration of density-dependent growth in transformed cells in culture (De Luca, 1977; Hassell *et al.,* 1978).

There are numerous reports that vitamin A acts as a cofactor in various biochemical reactions, such as mucopolysaccharide synthesis, sulfate activation, hydroxysteroid dehydrogenation, cholesterol synthesis, and hepatic microsomal demethylation and hydroxylation of drugs. Although these reactions are diminished in vitamin A deficiency, it now appears more likely that, instead of being produced directly by lack of vitamin A, the effects are caused by the inanition and other perturbations that follow reduced food consumption (and the depletion of vitamin C) (Rogers, 1969).

Vitamin A and the Visual Cycle. It has long been known that vitamin A deficiency interferes with vision in dim light, a condition known as night blindness (nyctalopia). The fundamental observations of Hecht (1937), carefully elaborated by Wald and Brown (1965) and Hubbard and colleagues (1965), have contributed greatly to an understanding of this phenomenon (*see* Wald, 1968; Fisher *et al.,* 1970).

Adaptation to dark is a function of both the rods and the cones. Primary adaptation is accomplished by the cones, and the process is completed in a few minutes. Secondary adaptation is a function of the rods, and is not completed for 30 minutes or longer. The process of adaptation is a chemical one, and consists in the formation of photosensitive pigments in the retina that, upon exposure to light of low intensity, are bleached and undergo chemical reactions that result in the initiation of a receptor potential. After breakdown, the pigment is resynthesized. The photosensitive pigment of the rods of land vertebrates is known as rhodopsin—a combination of the protein, opsin, and a prosthetic group, 11-*cis*-retinal. The known photosensitive pigment of the cones is iodopsin, and it is probable that many other pigments exist to account for color vision. Iodopsin is a combination of retinal with a protein very similar to opsin, called photopsin. Both photosensitive pigments react similarly but to light of different wavelengths.

In the synthesis of rhodopsin, *cis*-retinol is converted to *cis*-retinal in a reversible reaction that requires nicotinamide adenine dinucleotide (NAD) or nicotinamide adenine dinucleotide phosphate (NADP). *Cis*-retinal then combines with the ε-amino group of lysine in opsin to form rhodopsin. Most rhodopsin is located in the membranes of the discs situated in the outer segments of the rods. Photodecomposition begins upon absorption of a photon of light. Although the exact reaction sequence is still disputed, the initial reaction probably involves a conformational change of the protein to form bathorhodopsin, which is followed by the isomerization of 11-*cis*-retinal to the *trans* configuration (Lewis, 1978). These reactions may trigger the liberation of a transmitter that moves from the discs to the plasma membrane of the rod, where the electrical photoreceptor is generated. *Trans*-retinal can be reconverted to *cis*-retinal directly and recombine with opsin again to form rhodopsin. Alternatively, *trans*-retinal can be reduced to *trans*-retinol, which is first converted to *cis*-retinol and then to rhodopsin in the manner described above. The overall sequence of events in the visual cycle is depicted in Figure 67–1.

When human beings are fed diets deficient in vitamin A, their ability for dark adaptation is gradually diminished. Rod vision is affected more than cone vision. Upon depletion of the vitamin from liver and blood (usually at concentrations less than 20 μg of retinol per deciliter of plasma), the concen-

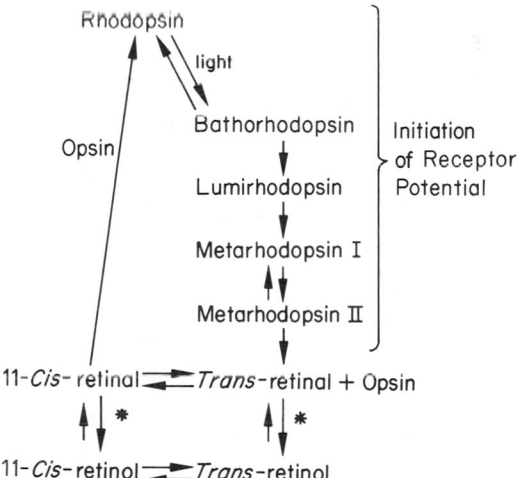

Figure 67–1. *The visual cycle.*

The asterisks (*) refer to the reactions in which retinol dehydrogenase and NAD or NADP are involved. For explanation, *see* the text.

tration of retinol and of rhodopsin in the retina falls. Unless the deficiency is overcome, opsin, lacking the stabilizing effect of retinal, decays and anatomical deterioration of the rods' outer segments takes place. Irreversible ultrastructural changes in the photoreceptor leading to blindness then supervene in rats maintained on a vitamin A–deficient diet, a process that takes 10 months.

Following short-term deprivation of vitamin A, dark adaptation can be restored to normal by the addition of vitamin A to the diet. However, vision does not return to normal for several weeks after adequate amounts of the vitamin have been added to the diet. The cause for this delay is unknown.

Vitamin A and Epithelial Structures. The functional and structural integrity of epithelial cells throughout the body is dependent upon an adequate supply of vitamin A. The vitamin plays a major role in the induction and control of epithelial differentiation in mucus-secreting or keratinizing tissues. In the presence of retinol, basal epithelial cells are stimulated to produce mucus. Excessive retinol leads to the production of a thick layer of mucin, the inhibition of keratinization, and the display of goblet cells.

In the absence of retinol, goblet mucous cells disappear and atrophy of epithelium occurs, followed by a proliferation of basal cells at the expense of mucous cells. The new cells, by their continued growth, undermine and replace the original epithelium with a stratifed, keratinizing epithelium. The suppression of normal secretions leads to irritation and infection.

Signs and Symptoms of Deficiency. As is the case with all dietary essentials, a deficiency of retinol retards normal growth and development. Indeed, the bioassay of vitamin A is based upon the ability of the vitamin to restore normal growth in rats fed a diet deficient in vitamin A but complete in all other respects.

Tissue reserves of vitamin A in the normal adult are sufficiently large to require long-term dietary deprivation in order to induce deficiency. Vitamin A deficiency occurs more commonly, therefore, in chronic diseases affecting fat absorption, such as biliary tract or pancreatic disease, sprue, colitis, and portal cirrhosis; following partial gastrectomy; or during extreme, chronic dietary inadequacy.

The deficiency is quite widespread in Southeast Asia, the Middle East, Africa, and Central and South America, particularly in children, and is associated with general malnutrition (*see* McLaren, 1966). Vitamin A deficiency and protein malnutrition are the two most serious nutritional deficiency diseases in the world today. Deficiency of vitamin A may be fatal, especially in infants and young children suffering from kwashiorkor or marasmus. It is estimated that tens of thousands of children in the world go blind every year because of inadequate intake of vitamin A. In the United States, about 15% of the population has concentrations of vitamin A in plasma or liver below the accepted lower limits of normal (20 μg/dl or 40 μg/g, respectively), indicating a risk of deficiency. Most of these individuals are infants or children (*see* Roels, 1970), and a dispro-

portionate percentage are Mexican-American or black children.

Signs and symptoms of mild vitamin A deficiency are easily overlooked. Skin lesions, such as follicular hyperkeratosis and infections, are among the earliest signs of deficiency, but the most recognizable manifestation is night blindness, even though its onset occurs only when vitamin A depletion is severe. A quantitative assessment of retinal function would be useful in the evaluation of patients with suspected vitamin A deficiency.

Eye. Keratomalacia, characterized by desiccation, ulceration, and xerosis of the cornea and conjunctiva, is occasionally seen as an acute symptom in the very young who are ingesting severely deficient diets. It is foreshadowed, usually, by xerophthalmia and "Bitot's spot" and ultimately leads to severe visual impairment and even blindness (McLaren, 1966).

Bronchorespiratory Tract. Changes in the bronchorespiratory epithelium from mucus secretion to keratinization lead to increased incidence of respiratory infections in the deficiency state. There is also a decrease in elasticity of the lung and other tissues.

Skin. Keratinization and drying of the epidermis occur and papular eruptions, involving the pilosebaceous follicles, may be found, especially on the extremities.

Genitourinary System. Urinary calculi are frequent concomitants of vitamin A deficiency. The epithelium of the urinary tract shares in the general pathological changes of all epithelial structures. Epithelial debris may thus provide the nidus around which a calculus is formed. Abnormalities of reproduction include impairment of spermatogenesis, degeneration of testes, abortion, resorption of fetuses, and production of malformed offspring.

Gastrointestinal Tract. The intestinal mucosa shows a reduction in the number of goblet cells but no keratinization. Alterations in intestinal epithelium and metaplasia of pancreatic ductal epithelium are common. They may be responsible for the diarrhea occasionally seen in vitamin A deficiency.

Sweat Glands. These glands may undergo atrophy and keratinizing squamous-cell metaplasia.

Bone. In animals, vitamin A deficiency is associated with faulty modeling of bone (with production of thick, cancellous bone instead of thinner, more compact bone).

Miscellaneous. Often there is an impairment of both taste and smell in vitamin A–deficient individuals, which undoubtedly results from a keratinizing effect. Hearing may also become decreased. Vitamin A deficiency can interfere with erythropoiesis, which may be masked by abnormal losses of fluid. Nerve lesions, increased cerebrospinal fluid pressure, and hydrocephalus have been reported.

Hypervitaminosis A. An intake of vitamin A greatly in excess of requirement results in a toxic syndrome known as hypervitaminosis A. Several cases in children have been reported (Oliver, 1958); the syndrome has also been detected in a few adults. Excess vitamin

E appears to protect against hypervitaminosis A.

All the reported cases in children have been associated with the chronic ingestion of retinol. Usually, high intakes have resulted from overzealous prophylactic vitamin therapy on the part of parents, from extended self-medication, or from food fads. Retinoids used for the therapy of acne or other skin lesions have produced toxicity when administered in high doses orally. The daily intake of 3 to 6 mg of vitamin A for 2 years has led to hypervitaminosis in an adult, although most patients with hypervitaminosis have consumed higher doses for a shorter period (Bauernfeind *et al.*, 1974; Vollbracht and Gilroy, 1976).

Early signs and symptoms of *chronic* vitamin A intoxication include irritability, vomiting, loss of appetite, headache, dry and pruritic skin, skin desquamation, and erythematous dermatitis. Fatigue, pain in ankles and feet, myalgia, loss of body hair, papilledema, nystagmus, gingivitis, mouth fissures, and lymph node enlargement have been observed. In addition to hepatosplenomegaly, pathological changes in the liver include hypertrophy of fat-storing cells, fibrosis, sclerosis of central veins, and cirrhosis, with resultant portal hypertension and ascites. Intracranial pressure may be increased, and neurological symptoms may mimic those of a brain tumor. The diagnosis is usually made following the appearance of tender, deep, hard swellings on the extremities and the occipital region of the head. Hyperostoses in the underlying bone are easily demonstrated roentgenographically. The activity of alkaline phosphatase in plasma rises because of the increased osteoblastic activity, and a number of cases of hypercalcemia have been reported.

Concentrations of vitamin A in plasma ranging from 300 to 2000 μg/dl are diagnostic of hypervitaminosis A. Treatment consists in withdrawal of the vitamin. Most signs and symptoms disappear within a week, but the hyperostoses remain evident for several months after clinical recovery has occurred.

Acute poisoning in man is known to follow the ingestion of polar bear liver. Signs and symptoms include drowsiness, sluggishness, irritability or irresistible desire to sleep, severe headache, vomiting, papilledema, and, after 24 hours, generalized peeling of the skin. The high content of vitamin A in polar bear liver, up to 12 mg of retinol per gram (Russell, 1967), is responsible for the syndrome. The acute consumption of more than 500 mg or a daily intake exceeding 50 mg of retinol frequently results in toxic effects in adults.

In infants acute poisoning has been noted following ingestion of lesser amounts. Increased intracranial pressure, a bulging fontanel, and vomiting are seen early and usually disappear within 36 hours after cessation of ingestion of the vitamin. As little as 7.5 to 15 mg of retinol daily for 30 days has induced such toxicity in infants (Yaffe and Filer, 1971). The toxicity of the vitamin depends on the age of the patient, the dose, and the duration of administration.

Congenital abnormalities can apparently occur in human infants whose mothers have consumed excessive amounts of vitamin A during pregnancy (Bernhardt and Dorsey, 1974; Stånge *et al.*, 1978). Obviously, pregnant women should not ingest quantities of this vitamin in excess of those recommended. Congenital abnormalities have also been reported in the offspring of hypervitaminotic animals; these include hydrocephalus, encephalocele, urinary tract anomalies, and skeletal deformities.

Hypervitaminosis A has been studied extensively in experimental animals. The most characteristic lesions occur in the bones and result from accelerated resorption of bone and cartilage and formation of new bone. Bones continue to grow in length but not in thickness, with increased susceptibility to fractures. In young animals, premature closure of epiphyses inhibits growth of bones. Other manifestations of hypervitaminosis A are anorexia, cutaneous lesions, temporary thickening of skin, exophthalmos, hypoprothrombinemia, and eventually death. The hypoprothrombinemia observed may be successfully treated with vitamin K.

Large amounts of vitamin A activate the lysosomes to release a protease, cathepsin D, that degrades the structural protein component of bone and cartilage matrix and results in a loss of mucopolysaccharide (Fell and Dingle, 1963; Dingle and Lucy, 1965). Lipoprotein membranes exhibit increased permeability and decreased stability in the presence of excessive concentrations of vitamin A, leading to mitochondrial swelling, lysosomal rupture, and probably the decreased cohesiveness of keratin. Such effects may stimulate mitosis, the proliferation of lower epidermis, and the synthesis or release of prostaglandins, but this area is still controversial (Logan, 1972). Aspirin, which inhibits prostaglandin synthesis, can protect mice against lethal doses of retinoic acid.

In cell culture, vitamin A inhibits the synthesis of chondroitin sulfate by chondrocytes and cartilage rudiments, and the inhibition of chondrogenesis in the developing embryo may result in malformations of the limb (Lewis *et al.,* 1978).

Table 67–1 compares the effects of hypervitaminosis A and hypovitaminosis A.

Human Requirement. Human requirements for vitamin A have been approximated from studies that have attempted to correct experimentally produced deficiency states. The present recommendations of the Food and Nutrition Board of the National Research Council are based upon the amount of vitamin necessary to maintain normal dark adaptation plus an additional factor of safety to cover variations in absorption and utilization of the vitamin. The recommended daily allowances for the normal male and female adult are 1000 and 800 retinol equivalents per day, respectively (5000 and 4000 units, assuming that 50% of dietary vitamin A is derived from retinol and 50% from β-carotene). For the requirements of infants and children, *see* Table XVI–1 (page 1553) and below.

Absorption, Distribution to Target Cells, Fate, and Excretion. Much of this information has been derived from animal experiments, but it is likely that similar considerations are true for man. More than 90% of the intake of preformed vitamin A is in the form of retinol esters, usually as retinyl palmitate.

Vitamin A is readily absorbed from the normal gastrointestinal tract. If the amount ingested is not much greater than the requirement, absorption is complete; however, when a large excess is taken, some of the vitamin escapes in the feces. Inasmuch as vitamin A is fat soluble, it is not unexpected to find that the absorption of the vitamin is related to that of lipid and is enhanced by bile; nevertheless, aqueous dispersions of retinol or its ester are absorbed more rapidly than are oily solutions.

In the presence of abnormalities of fat absorption, the absorption of vitamin A is reduced. In such patients water-miscible preparations should be used. Intestinal absorption of vitamin A is reduced when diets are low in protein. The absorption of vitamin A is also disturbed in patients with intestinal infections, cystic fibrosis, and hepatic disease.

Intestinal absorption apparently occurs by a carrier-mediated process and is sensitive to metabolic inhibitors. Retinol esters are hydrolyzed in the lumen of the intestine by pancreatic enzymes and within the brush border of the intestinal cell before absorption, followed by reesterification, mainly to the palmitate (Ganguly, 1969); there may be several cycles of hydrolysis and reesterification. Significant quantities of vitamin A are also absorbed directly into the circulation.

The long-chain fatty acid ester enters the circulation by transport in the chylomicron fraction of lymph (Goodman *et al.,* 1966), and concentrations of esterified retinol reach a peak in plasma about 4 hours after the administration of the vitamin. Most of the

Table 67–1.   GENERAL CONSEQUENCES OF VITAMIN A DEFICIENCY AND EXCESS *

SITE	HYPOVITAMINOSIS A	HYPERVITAMINOSIS A
General	Growth retardation; susceptibility to infection; death	Malaise; lethargy; deposition of carotenoids; labilization of membranes; release of lysosomal enzymes; death
Skin and mucous membranes	Xerosis; keratinizing metaplasia; xerophthalmia; keratomalacia	Mucous cell formation, desquamation
Skeletal tissues and bone	Cancellous structure; defective remodeling	Decalcification, fractures, early epiphyseal closure; cortical thickening and bone tenderness
Reproductive system	Degeneration of testes; gonadal resorption; congenital malformation	Resorption; congenital malformation
Nervous system	Compression by bone, increased intracranial pressure, atrophy and ataxia	Increased intracranial pressure
Retina	Night blindness	

* After Fisher, Carr, Huff, and Huber, 1970, as modified from McLaren, 1966. Courtesy of *Federation Proceedings.*

vitamin is stored in the liver, mainly in parenchymal hepatocytes as the palmitate ester. The vitamin is associated with the components of hepatic cell membranes, mainly in the Golgi fraction and the endoplasmic reticulum (Glover *et al.*, 1974). There are several pools of vitamin A in the liver, one of which is filled by newly absorbed vitamin, which supplies other tissues preferentially; another serves for storage.

The median concentration of vitamin A in man is about 100 μg/g of liver, and the normal range in plasma is 30 to 70 μg/dl. Other tissues, such as kidney, lung, adrenal, and intraperitoneal fat, contain about 1 μg of vitamin A per gram. There is also selective localization of the vitamin in the retina of the eye. Administration of low doses of vitamin E markedly increases the tissue storage of vitamin A. Until hepatic saturation takes place, the administration of vitamin A leads mainly to its accumulation in the liver rather than in blood.

Prior to entering the circulation from the liver, the hepatic retinol ester is hydrolyzed, and almost all the retinol is associated with an α_1-globulin, which has a single binding site for the vitamin. This retinol-binding protein (RBP) circulates in the blood in man complexed with and stabilized by a pre-albumin protein that also functions in the transport of thyroxine. The formation of this complex protects the circulating RBP (and retinol) from glomerular filtration and excretion by the kidney. Normally less than 5% of the total vitamin in the blood is present as the retinyl ester, which is associated with lipoprotein (Goodman, 1974; Peterson *et al.*, 1974).

When hepatic stores of the vitamin and the RBP carrier system become saturated because of excessive intake of the vitamin or hepatic damage, up to 65% of the vitamin in plasma may be present as retinyl esters associated with lipoprotein. Since retinol is biologically inert while bound to RBP, these retinyl esters, which are surfactants, may be responsible for at least some of the toxicity that is observed (Mallia *et al.*, 1975).

If an individual ingests a diet free of vitamin A or its precursors, plasma concentrations are maintained over many months at the expense of hepatic reserves. Blood concentrations, therefore, are not an accurate guide to an individual's vitamin A status, but low plasma values of vitamin A imply that hepatic storage of the vitamin may be exhausted. Signs and symptoms of vitamin A deficiency appear when the plasma concentration falls below 10 to 20 μg/dl. Hepatic reserves of vitamin A decrease with a half-life of about 50 days in animals; signs of deficiency thus develop only after a prolonged period of inadequate intake.

Retinol bound to RBP is delivered to the various target organs, where the vitamin is released, permeates the cell, and interacts with another specific protein, the cellular retinol-binding protein (CRBP) (Bashor *et al.*, 1973). All organs except heart and skeletal muscle contain the apparent receptor protein, which may function analogously to those for estrogens and other steroids. The interaction is restricted to retinol and closely related derivatives, and their affinity for CRBP parallels their physiological activity. Retinoic acid does not bind to CRBP but has its own specific receptor (*see* below). In the fetal rat, the distribution of CRBP reflects the apparent needs of the organ for retinol for proper development.

The concentration of RBP in plasma is crucial for the regulation of vitamin A in plasma and its transport to tissues (Smith and Goodman, 1976). In vitamin A deficiency, the hepatic content of RBP rises and its concentration in plasma falls, apparently because the secretion of RBP from the liver is blocked. Once the vitamin again becomes available, the liver rapidly releases RBP into the plasma for transport of the vitamin to the tissues. When there is protein deficiency (*e.g.*, caused by malnutrition, kwashiorkor, or parenchymal liver disease), the concentration of RBP becomes insufficient, and concentrations of vitamin A in plasma fall despite normal stores in the liver. Replenishment with calories and protein is then required. Deficiency of both RBP and vitamin A cannot be corrected by the administration of the vitamin alone.

Other pathological conditions also alter plasma concentrations of vitamin A and RBP in plasma. Synthesis or release of RBP from the liver is depressed and plasma vitamin A concentrations are reduced in cystic fibrosis. The opposite is true during administration of estrogens or oral contraceptives. In renal disease or infections with fever, such as pneumonia, the concentration of vitamin A in the blood may be reduced drastically, partially because of increased urinary excretion.

Pregnancy also alters the concentration of vitamin A in blood. During the first trimester there is a fall in the mean content of vitamin A in plasma, followed by a slow rise, and another fall at parturition. It is likely that the increased demands for vitamin A lead to the withdrawal of the vitamin from the blood at a rate exceeding that of mobilization from the hepatic reserve. The placental barrier prevents the extensive transfer of vitamin A or carotenoids (Gal and Parkinson, 1974). Studies in animals suggest that there is transplacental transport of RBP during early pregnancy; thereafter the fetus begins to synthesize its own RBP. The concentration of the vitamin in fetal blood is thus less than in maternal blood. Both colostrum and milk offer the newborn an adequate supply of vitamin A. The concentration of vitamin A in the milk is maintained at a fixed maximal concentration if the dietary intake of the vitamin is adequate to permit storage in the liver.

Retinol is in part conjugated to form a β-glucuronide, which undergoes enterohepatic circulation and is oxidized to retinal and retinoic acid. Several other water-soluble metabolites are also excreted in urine and feces (Rietz et al., 1974). Normally no vitamin A can be recovered unchanged from human urine.

Retinoic Acid.   After oral administration, retinoic acid reaches the circulation by the portal vein and is transported in plasma as a complex with albumin. Unlike retinol, retinoic acid is not stored in the liver but is rapidly excreted. It is metabolized in the liver, and various degradation products are secreted into bile and excreted in urine and feces. Retinoic acid binds to a specific cellular retinoic acid–binding protein (CRABP), which is distinct from CRBP (Ong and Chytil, 1975). The affinity of a series of retinoids for CRABP parallels their growth-promoting ability and their capacity to promote mucous metaplasia of keratinized epithelia in vitamin A–deficient animals. In adult rats, CRABP is located mainly in brain, skin, eye, testis, uterus, and ovary; it is not found in liver or most other organs. In the retina CRBP (but not CRABP) is located predominantly in the region of the photoreceptors (Wiggert et al., 1978). This is consistent with the inability of retinoic acid to substitute for retinol in the visual cycle or to be converted to retinal (Chen and Heller, 1978). Following the binding of retinoic acid to CRABP in the cytosol of target tissues, the complex migrates to the nucleus, where it presumably initiates a cascade of specific biochemical events (Sani and Hill, 1976).

Carotenoids.   Unlike the extensive absorption of retinol, only about one third of β-carotene or other carotenoids is absorbed by man. Absorption depends upon the presence of bile and absorbable fat in the intestinal tract and is greatly decreased by steatorrhea and chronic diarrhea. The ingestion of mineral oil decreases the absorption of carotene, whereas water-soluble dispersing agents enhance absorption. The conversion of carotene to vitamin A occurs in the wall of the small intestine. Two molecules of retinal are produced by cleavage of the 15,15′ double bond. This reaction is mediated by the dioxygenase system, requires molecular oxygen, and is influenced by the amount of dietary protein. Some of the retinal is further oxidized to retinoic acid; about one half is reduced to retinol, which is then esterified and transported in the lymph, as described above. Carotene is biologically active only following conversion to retinol. Some carotene gains access to the circulation. If very large amounts of carotene are ingested, very high concentrations may be achieved in blood, and the hypercarotenemia results in a yellow discoloration of the skin, which is reversible; this can be distinguished from jaundice by the absence of scleral pigmentation. Hypervitaminosis does not develop, however.

Bioassay and Unitage.   Most commercial preparations are synthetic retinol esters, which have largely replaced natural vitamin A obtained from fish liver oils. Preparations from animal sources must be biologically assayed to establish their activity. This assay depends upon the ability of the vitamin to support growth in vitamin-depleted rats of specified age and weight and fed a standard vitamin A–deficient diet over a given period of time. The concentration of suitably purified preparations can be determined by spectrophotometric analysis. One U.S.P. vitamin A unit is the specific biological activity of 0.3 μg of retinol, 0.34 μg of retinyl acetate, or 0.6 μg of β-carotene. Because of the relatively inefficient dietary utilization of β-carotene compared to retinol, the new nomenclature is in terms of the retinol equivalent, which represents 1 μg of retinol, 6 μg of dietary β-carotene, or 12 μg of other provitamin A carotenoids. Thus, 1 retinol equivalent equals 3.3 units of vitamin A activity as supplied by retinol or 10 units of vitamin A activity as supplied by β-carotene (Bieri, 1974). The methods for standardizing vitamin A have been reviewed recently (Parrish, 1977).

Preparations.   There are many types of preparations that contain vitamin A. These range from solutions of pure synthetic vitamin A in oil to numerous fish liver oils and concentrates that contain both vitamin A and vitamin D in various proportions. In the United States, commercial production of synthetic vitamin A is about 1000 tons per year. Absorption is greatest for aqueous preparations, intermediate for emulsions, and slowest for oil solutions. Whereas oil-soluble preparations may lead to greater hepatic storage of the vitamin, water-miscible preparations usually provide higher concentrations in plasma (Srikantia and Reddy, 1970).

Vitamin A Capsules, U.S.P., contain 1.5 to 15 mg of retinol (5000 to 50,000 U.S.P. vitamin A units) per capsule. There are also many multivitamin preparations that include vitamin A, such as *Decavitamin Capsules,* U.S.P., and *Decavitamin Tablets,* U.S.P.

Tretinoin, U.S.P. (*all*-trans-*retinoic acid*; RETIN-A), is available for topical use as a solution (0.05%), a cream (0.05 and 0.1%), and a gel (0.025 and 0.01%); it is also available in 0.05% saturated swabs. It is an irritant, causes skin peeling, and is used for the treatment of acne and other skin diseases.

Therapeutic Uses. The normal requirement of vitamin A for adults is supplied by an adequate diet. The rational uses of vitamin A are in the treatment of deficiency of vitamin A and as prophylaxis during periods of increased requirement, such as infancy, pregnancy, and lactation. However, limitation in diet due to economic stress or food fads can give rise to the symptoms of deficiency. In addition, the ingestion of large doses of vitamin E or C may alter the vitamin A status of an individual, judging from animal experiments. Once a vitamin A deficiency has been diagnosed, intensive therapy should be instituted. The patient should then be maintained on a proper diet.

During infancy, pregnancy, or lactation, it is best to supply supplemental vitamin A rather than to rely solely upon the diet. Infants usually receive vitamin A in conjunction with vitamin D. A daily intake of 400 to 700 retinol equivalents of vitamin A (400 to 700 μg of retinol) should be provided for infants and growing children. However, ingestion of 6000 retinol equivalents or more per day for 1 to 2 months by healthy infants or children on good diets is likely to produce signs and symptoms of overdosage. During pregnancy (especially the second and third trimesters) and lactation, the intake of vitamin A should be maintained at approximately 1000 and 1200 retinol equivalents per day, respectively.

Rarely, the absorption, mobilization, or the storage of vitamin A may be adversely affected, and under such circumstances long-continued therapy with the vitamin may be indicated, as, for example, in an individual with steatorrhea, severe biliary obstruction, cirrhosis of the liver, or following a total gastrectomy. In other disease states where considerable vitamin A is lost from the body, replacement therapy may be necessary. In various infections in which mucous-cell turnover is accelerated and urinary excretion of the vitamin is increased, the need for retinol is further enhanced. Individuals already suffering from vitamin A deficiency who develop infections, especially of the respiratory tract, will benefit from the inclusion of adequate amounts of vitamin A in the diet. There is no evidence, however, that an excessive intake of vitamin A will influence the incidence of infections in an individual whose intake of vitamin A is adequate. However, moderate amounts of vitamin A apparently do no harm. If vitamin A is prescribed as a dietary supplement, intake of 1500 μg of retinol represents one and one-half times the recommended daily allowance. Long-term ingestion of much larger amounts may lead to hypervitaminosis.

In kwashiorkor and other severe vitamin A deficiencies in children, a single intramuscular injection of 30 mg of retinol as the water-miscible palmitate has been advocated, followed by intermittent oral treatment with vitamin A in oil (*see* Bauernfeind *et al.,* 1974). In areas of the world where protein malnutrition and vitamin A deficiencies abound, 60 to 120 mg of retinol in oil should be administered to children every 3 to 6 months, depending on the age. Vitamin E should be coadministered, since it apparently increases the efficacy of vitamin A and also protects against vitamin A toxicity by increasing storage in the liver.

Vitamin A may be helpful in certain diseases of the skin, such as acne, psoriasis, Darier's disease, and ichthyosis. The use of tretinoin (retinoic acid) in these conditions has largely replaced that of vitamin A, and various newer retinoids such as 13-*cis*-retinoic acid are currently being evaluated.

The topical use of tretinoin for *acne vulgaris* is efficacious (*see* Heel *et al.,* 1977). The drug prevents the formation of comedones, suppresses the synthesis of keratin without altering bacterial skin counts, and produces improvement in most patients. Its efficacy is similar to that of regimens that include methylprednisolone and neomycin, and it may surpass that of benzoyl peroxide. For more severe cases, topical application of tretinoin may be combined with the oral administration of antibiotic, such as a tetracycline or erythromycin. Treatment with tretinoin should be continued for about 3 months. When applied to human skin, about 5% of the compound is recovered in the urine, indicating some absorption; this is increased when there is acne or psoriasis.

Although many patients tolerate the topical application of tretinoin without undue side effects, erythema and desquamation occur frequently. These adverse effects are not necessary for therapeutic benefit and may be avoided with a less concentrated preparation. The drug sensitizes the skin to sunlight, and individuals who are particularly susceptible to skin damage from sunlight should be especially careful. Alterations in hepatic function after tretinoin are minor and reversible. Allergic contact dermatitis and decreased pigmentation have occurred. The drug irritates the mucous membranes of the eyes, nose, and mouth. Temporary exacerbation of the acne may occur during the first weeks of treatment, but therapy should be continued. The oral administration of tretinoin is associated with a greater risk of toxicity and has limited application. Symptoms from oral overdosage more commonly include hypervitaminosis, dizziness, hepatic damage, thirst, and petechiae.

Preliminary results with 13-*cis*-retinoic acid, given orally in an average dose of 2 mg/kg per day to patients with severe cystic and conglobate acne, are very encouraging (Peck *et al.*, 1979). Remissions in these patients have been prolonged after a 4-month course of therapy.

VITAMIN K

History. Vitamin K is a dietary principle essential for the normal biosynthesis of several factors required for clotting of blood. In 1929, Dam observed that chickens fed on inadequate diets developed a deficiency disease in which the outstanding symptom was spontaneous bleeding, apparently due to a low content of prothrombin in the blood. In subsequent publications, Dam and coworkers (1935, 1936) reported that, although the condition was not cured by any of the known vitamins, it could be rapidly alleviated by feeding an unidentified fat-soluble substance. To this substance Dam gave the name *vitamin K* (*Koagulation* vitamin). Independently, Almquist and Stokstad (1935) described the same hemorrhagic disease in chickens and the method for its prevention.

The investigations of Dam and Almquist and their respective associates were reported at a time when the attention of several groups of workers was centered on the cause of the hemorrhagic tendency in patients with obstructive jaundice and diseases of the liver. For example, Quick and coworkers (1935) made the pertinent observation that the coagulation defect in jaundiced individuals was due to a decrease in the concentration of prothrombin in the blood. In the same year, Hawkins and Whipple reported that animals with biliary fistulas were likely to develop excessive bleeding. Hawkins and Brinkhous (1936) subsequently showed that this was due to a deficiency in prothrombin and that the condition could be relieved by the feeding of bile salts.

The culmination of these experimental studies came with the demonstration of Butt and coworkers (1938) as well as Warner and associates (1938) that combination therapy with vitamin K and bile salts was effective in the treatment of the hemorrhagic diathesis in cases of jaundice. Thus, the relationship between vitamin K, adequate hepatic function, and the physiological mechanisms operating in the normal clotting of blood was established.

Occurrence and Chemistry. The early investigations described above showed that vitamin K is a fat-soluble substance present in hog liver fat and in alfalfa. Subsequently, it has been demonstrated that the vitamin is concentrated in the chloroplasts of plant leaves and in many vegetable oils. The feces of most species of animals contain large amounts of the vitamin, which is synthesized by the bacteria in the intestinal tract (*see* Pennock, 1966).

The isolation and the elucidation of the chemical structure of vitamin K were carried out concurrently and independently by several groups of investigators. It was soon appreciated that vitamin K activity was associated with at least two distinct substances, designated as vitamin K_1 and vitamin K_2. Vitamin K_1, or phytonadione (phylloquinone), is 2-methyl-3-phytyl-1,4-naphthoquinone; vitamin K_2 represents a series of compounds (the menaquinones) in which

the phytyl side chain of phytonadione has been replaced by a side chain built up of 2 to 13 prenyl units (*see* Isler and Wiss, 1959). Phytonadione is found in plants; it is the only natural vitamin K available for therapeutic use. The menaquinones are synthesized, in particular, by gram-positive bacteria.

Phytonadione (Vitamin K_1)

Menaquinone (Vitamin K_2) Series

A large number of natural and synthetic quinone derivatives have been tested for their vitamin K activity (*see* review by Isler and Wiss, 1959). Among those that possess activity approaching that of the natural vitamin is 2-methyl-1,4-naphthoquinone, commonly known as menadione or vitamin K_3, which is, depending on the bioassay system used, at least as active on a molar basis as phytonadione.

Menadione

The natural vitamins K and menadione are lipid soluble. It is possible to make active water-soluble derivatives of menadione by forming the sodium bisulfite salt or the tetrasodium salt of the diphosphoric acid ester. These compounds are converted in the body to menadione.

Pharmacological Actions and Physiological Function. In normal animals and man, phytonadione and the menaquinones are virtually devoid of pharmacodynamic activity. In animals and man deficient in vitamin K, the pharmacological action of vitamin K is identical to its normal physiological function, that is, to promote the hepatic biosynthesis of prothrombin (factor II), proconvertin (factor VII), plasma thromboplastin component (PTC, Christmas factor, factor IX), and the Stuart factor (factor X). The role of these factors in blood clotting is discussed in Chapter 58.

The vitamin K–dependent blood clotting

factors, in the absence of vitamin K (or in the presence of the coumarin type of anticoagulant), are biologically inactive precursor proteins in the liver. Vitamin K functions as an essential cofactor for a microsomal enzyme system that activates these precursors by the conversion of multiple, peptide-bound residues of glutamic acid in each precursor to γ-carboxyglutamyl residues in the completed protein. The formation of this new amino acid, γ-carboxyglutamic acid, allows the protein to bind calcium ions and in turn to be bound to a phospholipid surface, both of which are necessary in the cascade of events that lead to clot formation (*see* Chapter 58; Nelsestuen, 1978). The exact role and mechanism of involvement of vitamin K in this carboxylation reaction have not yet been elucidated, but carboxylation is apparently linked to the cyclic interconversion of vitamin K, vitamin K hydroquinone, and vitamin K-2,3-epoxide (*see* Figure 58-2, page 1355; *see also* Stenflo, 1978; Suttie *et al.*, 1978). γ-Carboxyglutamate has also been found in proteins in bone (osteocalcin), blood (protein S and protein C), and kidney. The functions of these newly discovered vitamin K–dependent proteins have yet to be elucidated, but they may share an involvement in calcium metabolism (*see* Lian *et al.*, 1978).

Human Requirement. There is no generally accepted figure for the human requirement of vitamin K; it appears to be extremely small. Frick and associates (1967) estimated the minimal daily requirement, in patients made vitamin K deficient by a starvation diet and antibiotic therapy for 3 to 4 weeks, to be a minimum of 0.03 μg/kg of body weight; others place the daily requirement at 0.5 to 1 μg/kg (*see* Suttie, 1978). In the infant, 10 μg/kg of body weight of phytonadione is sufficient to prevent hypoprothrombinemia. Needs are satisfied by the average diet, and, in addition, the vitamin synthesized by intestinal bacteria is also available to the host. Recommendations of the Food and Nutrition Board, National Research Council, are presented in Table XVI-2 (page 1555).

Symptoms of Deficiency. The chief clinical manifestation of vitamin K deficiency is an increased tendency to bleed. Ecchymoses, epistaxis, hematuria, gastrointestinal bleeding, and postoperative hemorrhage are common; intracranial hemorrhage may occur. Hemoptysis is uncommon. A further discussion of hypoprothrombinemia is presented in the section on oral anticoagulants (Chapter 58). The discovery of a γ-carboxyglutamate-containing protein in bone that is dependent upon vitamin K for its synthesis suggests that the fetal bone abnormalities

associated with the administration of oral anticoagulants during the first trimester of pregnancy may be related to a deficiency of the vitamin.

Toxicity. Phytonadione and the menaquinones are nontoxic to animals, even when given in huge amounts. In man, rapid intravenous administration of phytonadione has produced flushing, dyspnea, chest pains, and rarely death. Whether these reactions were due to the vitamin itself or to the agents used to disperse and emulsify the preparation is not clear.

The administration of large doses of menadione and its derivatives to animals has resulted in the production of anemia, polycythemia, splenomegaly, renal and hepatic damage, and death (*see* Finkel, 1961). In man, menadione is irritating to the skin and the respiratory tract. Its solutions have vesicant properties. Menadione and its derivatives have been implicated in producing hemolytic anemia, hyperbilirubinemia, and kernicterus in the newborn, especially premature infants (*see* below). Menadione also can induce hemolysis in individuals who are genetically deficient in glucose-6-phosphate dehydrogenase (Zinkham and Childs, 1957). In patients who have severe hepatic disease, the administration of large doses of menadione or phytonadione may further depress function of the liver (*see* below).

Absorption, Fate, and Excretion. The mechanism of intestinal absorption of compounds with vitamin K activity varies with their solubility. Phytonadione and the menaquinones are adequately absorbed from the gastrointestinal tract only if bile salts are present. Menadione and its water-soluble derivatives, however, are absorbed even in the absence of bile (Shearer *et al.*, 1974). Phytonadione and the menaquinones are absorbed almost entirely by way of the lymph; menadione and its water-soluble derivatives enter the blood stream directly (*see* Woolf and Babior, 1972). Phytonadione is absorbed by an energy-dependent, saturable process in proximal portions of the small intestine (Hollander, 1973); menaquinone and menadione are absorbed by diffusion in the distal portions of the small intestine and in the colon (Hollander and Rim, 1976; Hollander *et al.*, 1976). Following intramuscular injection, both natural and synthetic vitamin K preparations are readily absorbed. After absorption, phytonadione is initially concentrated in the liver, but the concentration declines rapidly. Very little vitamin K accumulates in other tissues.

Phytonadione is rapidly metabolized to more polar metabolites that are excreted in the bile and urine. The major urinary metabolites result from shortening of the side chain to five or seven carbon atoms, yielding carboxylic acids that are conjugated with glucuronate prior to excretion. Treatment with a coumarin-type anticoagulant results in a marked increase in the amount of phytonadione-2,3-epoxide in liver and blood (Matschiner et al., 1970). Such treatment also increases the urinary excretion of phytonadione metabolites, primarily degradative products of phytonadione-2,3-epoxide. The biliary metabolites of phytonadione have not been identified (see Shearer et al., 1974). Menadione is apparently reduced to the diol (hydroquinone) form and excreted as glucuronide and sulfate conjugates.

Apparently there is little storage of vitamin K in the body. The limited stores of the vitamin present in tissue are slowly destroyed. Under circumstances where lack of bile interferes with absorption of vitamin K, for example, hypoprothrombinemia develops slowly over a period of several weeks.

Assay and Unitage. Drugs with vitamin K activity may be chemically assayed and do not require bioassay. For the determination of the vitamin K content of foods, an assay based upon the ability of the preparation to increase the prothrombin level of deficient chicks is employed.

Preparations. *Phytonadione,* U.S.P. (*vitamin K₁, phylloquinone;* AQUAMEPHYTON, KONAKION, MEPHYTON), is a viscous liquid that is insoluble in water. It is marketed in 5-mg tablets, and in ampuls containing an emulsion of 2 or 10 mg/ml of phytonadione dispersed in a solution of buffered polysorbate and propylene glycol (KONAKION) or polyethylated fatty acid derivatives and dextrose (AQUAMEPHYTON). KONAKION is administered only intramuscularly; AQUAMEPHYTON may be given by any parenteral route.

Menadione, U.S.P. (*vitamin K₃*), is a bright-yellow crystalline powder that is practically insoluble in water. Menadione is available for oral administration in tablets containing 5 mg, and as a sterile solution of menadione in oil (usually 25 mg/ml) designed for intramuscular administration. *Menadione Sodium Bisulfite,* U.S.P. (HYKINONE), occurs as a white crystalline, hygroscopic powder. It is highly soluble in water and is marketed in 1-ml ampuls containing 5 to 10 mg/ml. *Menadiol Sodium Diphosphate Injection,* U.S.P. (KAPPADIONE, SYNKAVITE), is marketed in ampuls containing 5, 10, or 37.5 mg/ml. *Menadiol Sodium Diphosphate Tablets,* U.S.P., contain 5 mg of the salt for oral use.

THERAPEUTIC USES

The rational therapeutic use of vitamin K is based on its ability to correct the bleeding tendency or hemorrhage associated with its deficiency. A deficiency of vitamin K and its attendant deficiency of prothrombin and related clotting factors can result from inadequate intake, absorption, or utilization of the vitamin, or as a consequence of the action of a vitamin K antagonist.

Inadequate Intake. After infancy, hypoprothrombinemia arising from a dietary deficiency of vitamin K is extremely rare, because not only is the vitamin present in many foods but also it is synthesized by intestinal bacteria. The combination of an inadequate diet and the prolonged use of drugs that inhibit intestinal bacterial growth may lead, however, to vitamin K deficiency (see Frick et al., 1967). Occasionally, the use of a poorly absorbed sulfonamide or a broad-spectrum antibiotic may of itself produce a hypoprothrombinemia that responds readily to small doses of vitamin K and reestablishment of normal bowel flora. The use of such antibiotics in patients who have other causes for hypoprothrombinemia or a deficiency of vitamin K may have profound consequences. Hypoprothrombinemia can occur in patients receiving prolonged intravenous alimentation (Ham, 1971).

Hypoprothrombinemia of the Newborn. Newborn infants have a hypoprothrombinemia due to vitamin K deficiency for the few days after birth, the time required to obtain an adequate dietary intake of the vitamin and to establish a normal intestinal bacterial flora. At birth, the normal infant has only 20 to 40% of the adult plasma concentrations of clotting factors II, VII, IX, and X. These concentrations decline even further during the first 2 or 3 days after birth, before they begin to rise toward the adult values. In premature infants and in infants with hemorrhagic disease of the newborn, these concentrations are depressed even further (see Aballi and deLamerens, 1962). Hemorrhagic disease of the newborn has been associated with breast feeding; human milk has low concentrations of vitamin K (see Sutherland et al., 1967), and, in addition, the intestinal flora of breast-fed infants apparently lacks microorganisms that synthesize the vitamin (Keenan et al., 1971).

Administration of vitamin K to the normal newborn infant prevents the decline in concentration of the clotting factors on the days following birth; it does not, however, raise these concentrations to the adult level. Premature infants usually display less of a response to the administration of vitamin K. In the infant with hemorrhagic disease of the newborn, the administration of vitamin K raises the concentration of these clotting factors to the level normal for the newborn infant and controls the bleeding tendency within about 6 hours (Wefring, 1962).

Although small doses of menadione and its derivatives are considered safe, moderate doses have produced hemolytic anemia, hyperbilirubinemia, and kernicterus in newborn, especially premature, infants, even when administered to the mother prior to delivery. Menadione is excreted in part as a glucuronide and competes with bilirubin for a detoxication mechanism of limited capacity in the newborn. Moreover, menadione may induce some hemolysis, especially in the newborn infant with a congenital defect in erythrocyte glucose-6-phosphate dehydrogenase or with a low concentration of alpha-tocopherol in blood; this causes a further increase in the concentration of bilirubin (*see* Finkel, 1961; Wynn, 1963).

The routine prophylactic administration of a small dose of phytonadione to the newborn infant is now recommended (*see* below). Phytonadione is the drug of choice since it appears to be nontoxic. A single dose of 0.5 to 1 mg should be administered parenterally to the infant immediately after delivery. This dose may have to be increased or repeated if the mother has received anticoagulant or anticonvulsant drug therapy, or if the infant develops bleeding tendencies.

Infants 1 to 5 months old seem to be quite vulnerable to vitamin K deficiency, especially if they have not received prophylactic administration of the vitamin at birth. Infant formulas that do not contain cows' milk are frequently inadequate in vitamin K. Inadequate intake may be exacerbated by diarrhea, antibiotics that reduce intestinal flora, or any of the malabsorption syndromes (*see* below; *see also* Committee on Nutrition, 1971; Lukens, 1972).

Inadequate Absorption. Hypoprothrombinemia may be associated with either intrahepatic or extrahepatic biliary obstruction, because the lipid-soluble vitamin is poorly absorbed in the absence of bile. A severe defect in the intestinal absorption of fat from other causes can also interfere with absorption of the vitamin.

Biliary Obstruction or Fistula. Bleeding that accompanies obstructive jaundice or biliary fistula responds promptly to the administration of vitamin K. Oral phytonadione administered with bile salts is both safe and effective and should be used in the care of the jaundiced patient, both preoperatively and postoperatively. In the absence of significant hepatocellular disease, the prothrombin activity of the blood rapidly returns to normal. If for some reason oral administration is not feasible, a parenteral preparation should be employed. The usual dose is 10 mg of vitamin K or menadione per day.

The treatment of a patient during hemorrhage is more difficult. Significant hemorrhage will obviously require replacement of blood. In such cases transfusion of fresh blood or reconstituted fresh plasma accomplishes the dual purposes of combating shock and furnishing an immediate supply of prothrombin. Vitamin K should also be given. If biliary obstruction has caused injury to hepatic cells, the response to vitamin K therapy may be poor. Under these circumstances, bleeding associated with hypopro-

thrombinemia may require continuing administration of fresh blood or reconstituted plasma.

Malabsorption Syndromes. Various disorders that result in inadequate absorption from the intestinal tract may lead to a deficiency of vitamin K and hypoprothrombinemia. These include mucoviscidosis, sprue, regional enteritis and enterocolitis, ulcerative colitis, dysentery, and extensive resection of bowel. Since drugs that greatly reduce the bacterial population of the bowel are frequently used in many of these disorders, the availability of the vitamin may be further reduced. Moreover, dietary restrictions may also limit the availability of the vitamin. For immediate correction of the deficiency, parenteral therapy should be given.

Inadequate Utilization. *Hepatocellular Disease.* Hypoprothrombinemia may accompany or follow hepatocellular disease, for example, toxic or infectious hepatitis, or advanced cirrhosis. Hepatocellular damage may also be secondary to long-lasting obstruction of bile ducts. In these conditions the damaged parenchymal cells may not be able to produce the vitamin K–dependent clotting factors, even if excess vitamin is available. Thus, hypoprothrombinemia under these circumstances is usually not favorably influenced by the administration of vitamin K. However, in some instances an inadequate secretion of bile salts may contribute to the syndrome and some benefit may be obtained from the parenteral administration of 10 mg of phytonadione daily. Paradoxically, the administration of large doses of vitamin K or its analogs in an attempt to correct the hypoprothrombinemia associated with severe hepatitis or cirrhosis may actually result in a further depression of the concentration of prothrombin. The mechanism for this is unknown. The vitamin does not, apparently, further depress hepatic function.

The response of hypoprothrombinemia to parenteral administration of vitamin K has been used as a test to distinguish between jaundice due to obstruction and that due to hepatocellular disease (Deutsch, 1966).

Drug-Induced Hypoprothrombinemia. Anticoagulant drugs such as dicumarol and its congeners act as competitive antagonists of vitamin K and interfere with the hepatic biosynthesis of prothrombin and factors VII, IX, and X (*see* Chapter 58). These proteins then disappear from the blood at rates dependent on their individual turnover rates: factor VII declines first, followed by factor IX, factor X, and prothrombin.

Excessive hypoprothrombinemia or bleeding produced by the administration of coumarin or indanedione anticoagulants can be corrected in a period of a few hours by the administration of vitamin K. Phytonadione is much more effective than menadione or its derivatives (*see* Griminger, 1966) and should be used to counteract the effects of overdosage or overresponse to these anticoagulants. Mild overdosage may be treated simply by drug withdrawal or reduction of the dose, or by the administration of a single dose of 1 to 5 mg of phytonadione. Larger doses of the vitamin may interfere with subsequent oral anticoagulant therapy for several days. If bleeding is severe, the immediate administration of 20 to 40 mg of phytonadione is indicated. Additional doses at 4-hour intervals may be necessary to return the prothrombin time to normal. Transfusion of fresh whole blood, frozen plasma, or concentrates of the vitamin K–dependent clotting factors may also be needed.

If severe hypoprothrombinemia should occur as a result of the administration of large amounts of salicylate, the treatment is the same as that outlined for dicumarol-induced hypoprothrombinemia, after withdrawal of the salicylate.

Vitamin K may be of help in combating the bleeding and hypoprothrombinemia following the bite of the tropical American pit viper or other species whose venom destroys or inactivates prothrombin.

Hypoprothrombinemia is also associated with excessive intake of vitamin A. Two mechanisms appear to be involved: an inhibition of intestinal bacterial biosynthesis of menaquinone and a direct antagonism of the hepatic actions of vitamin K (*see* Green, 1966).

VITAMIN E

In animals, the signs of deficiency of vitamin E include structural and functional abnormalities of many organs and organ systems. Attending these morphological alterations are biochemical defects that appear to involve fatty acid metabolism and numerous other enzyme systems. Notable is the fact that many signs and symptoms of vitamin E deficiency in animals superficially resemble disease states in humans; however, there is little unequivocal evidence that vitamin E is of nutritional significance in man or is of any value in therapy.

History. The existence of vitamin E was first demonstrated in 1922 by Evans and Bishop, who found that female rats required a then-unrecognized dietary principle in order to sustain a normal pregnancy. Deficient animals were found to ovulate and conceive normally, but at some time during the period of gestation death and resorption of the fetuses occurred. Lesions in the testes were also described, and for a while vitamin E was referred to as the "antisterility vitamin." Further studies, however, revealed the more widespread effects of deficiency of the vitamin (*see* below). Some experiments seem to indicate that vitamin E is not an essential dietary constituent in animals; at present, the significance of these reports must still be evaluated, but they add further complexities to an already complex and sometimes confusing picture (*see* Wagner and Folkers, 1963).

Chemistry. The vitamin was isolated by Evans and coworkers (1936) from wheat germ oil. Eight naturally occurring tocopherols with vitamin E activity are now known. Alpha-tocopherol (5,7,8-trimethyl tocol) is considered to be the most important tocopherol since it comprises about 90% of the tocopherols in animal tissues and displays the greatest biological activity in most bioassay systems. It was identified chemically by Fernholtz (1938) and synthesized by Karrer and associates (1938). Optical

isomerism affects activity; *d* forms are more active than *l* forms.

Alpha-tocopherol

Alpha-tocopherol bears a striking structural similarity to the 6-chromanol form of coenzyme Q_4, with which it shares biological activity in several systems (*see* Smith *et al.*, 1963).

One of the important chemical features of the tocopherols is that they are antioxidants. Furthermore, the compounds form reversible oxidation-reduction systems (*see* Dam, 1957). The tocopherols deteriorate slowly when exposed to air or ultraviolet light.

Pharmacological Actions and Physiological Functions. Aside from relieving symptoms of its deficiency in animals, vitamin E displays no notable pharmacological effects or toxicity. There is, as yet, no unifying concept to explain its mode of action. Numerous contradictory findings and claims for the actions and mechanisms of action characterize the literature on vitamin E. A major part of the nutritive or therapeutic value of vitamin E in animals appears to be related to its properties as an antioxidant (*see* Dam, 1957; Horwitt, 1965; Molenaar *et al.*, 1972; Hafeman and Hoekstra, 1977). In acting as an antioxidant, vitamin E presumably prevents oxidation of essential cellular constituents, or prevents the formation of toxic oxidation products such as the peroxidation products formed from unsaturated fatty acids that have been detected in its absence. Diets high in polyunsaturated fatty acids increase an animal's requirement for vitamin E (*see* Witting, 1972). However, other chemically unrelated substances, such as synthetic antioxidants, selenium, some sulfur-containing amino acids, and the coenzyme Q group, are able to prevent or reverse symptoms of vitamin E deficiency in animal species (*see* Wasserman and Taylor, 1972).

Some symptoms of vitamin E deficiency in animals are not relieved by other antioxidants, and it is presumed in these cases that the vitamin is acting in a more specific manner (*see* Schwarz, 1965; Diplock *et al.*, 1968; Green, 1972). Olsen and Carpenter (1967) suggested that vitamin E functions as a repressor that regulates the synthesis of specific proteins and enzymes required in differentiation or adaptation of tissues.

Wagner and Folkers (1963) have cited experiments that question the essential nature of vitamin E. By dietary manipulations, animals have been raised that are capable of producing normal offspring in the absence of vitamin E or other antioxidants in their diet. Tissues of these animals appear to be devoid of the vitamin. Wagner and Folkers have further questioned whether vitamin E may not merely be mimicking the actions of a member of the coenzyme Q group, which is almost identical in structure to alpha-tocopherol, possesses similar biological activities, and is present normally in tissues. (*See also* Symposium, 1965.)

There is an apparent relationship between vitamins A and E. Vitamin E may facilitate the absorption, hepatic storage, and utilization of vitamin A. In addition, it seems to protect against various effects of hypervitaminosis A (*see* Bauernfeind *et al.,* 1974).

Symptoms of Deficiency. Although manifestations of vitamin E deficiency in experimental animals are protean, various effects on the reproductive, muscular, cardiovascular, and hematopoietic systems are most important because they bear the closest resemblance to the clinical syndromes alleged to be benefited by vitamin E therapy.

Reproductive System. With the exception of the work cited by Wagner and Folkers (1963), evidence indicates that vitamin E is essential for normal reproduction in several mammalian species below the primate level. The most complete observations have been made on rats. In the male rat, prolonged deficiency produces irreversible sterility due to degeneration of the germinal epithelium. In the vitamin E–deficient female, pregnancy terminates in about 10 days with fetal death and resorption of the uterine contents. The fundamental mechanism by which vitamin E deficiency interferes with reproduction is obscure. Fat metabolism and the antioxidant properties of the vitamin appear to be involved and probably are interrelated, at least in the rat. As mentioned above, the amounts of vitamin E and unsaturated fatty acids in the diet affect reproduction, and antioxidants incorporated into the diet can completely obviate the need for vitamin E for normal growth and reproduction in the rat (Crider *et al.,* 1961). Thus, the essential nature of vitamin E in pregnancy is unclear.

On the basis of such animal studies, vitamin E has been used in man for the treatment of recurrent abortion and for sterility in the male and female. It has also been used in toxemia of pregnancy, disorders of menstruation, vaginitis, and menopausal symptoms. In spite of early enthusiastic usage of vitamin E, there is no conclusive evidence that the vitamin is beneficial in any of these conditions.

Muscular System. In many species a vitamin E–deficient diet leads to the development of muscular dystrophy. In addition to well-defined anatomical lesions, metabolic abnormalities, including creatinuria, increased oxygen uptake of affected muscles, and changes in the activity of numerous enzyme systems, are also seen (*see* Mason, 1973). The anatomical and biochemical changes can be prevented, reversed, or ameliorated with alpha-tocopherol or other lipid-soluble antioxidants, including coenzyme Q. The pathogenesis of the dystrophy is unknown. Tappel and associates (1963) attributed tissue damage to the release of cathepsin, ribonuclease, β-galactosidase, and sulfatase from lysosomes damaged by the action of fatty acid peroxidation products. Even though muscular dystrophy accompanies vitamin E deficiency in the monkey (Dinning and Day, 1957), there is no evidence of a vitamin E deficiency or a therapeutic response to the administration of the vitamin in muscular dystrophy in man (*see* Pappenheimer, 1943; Berneske *et al.,* 1960).

Cardiovascular System. The lesions produced in skeletal muscle by a deficiency of vitamin E apparently are also found in cardiac muscle of several species, although involvement of the heart is generally less common and less severe. The cardiac lesions are sometimes associated with ECG alteration, pathological changes, and even heart failure. On this basis, vitamin E has been used in many types of cardiac disorder and in peripheral vascular disease in man. Carefully controlled clinical studies have failed to demonstrate any benefit from the vitamin (*see* Report of the Council, 1950; Olsen, 1973).

Hematopoietic System. In several animal species a deficiency of vitamin E is associated with an anemia that has features of both abnormal hematopoiesis and decreased lifetime of erythrocytes. Erythrocytes from such animals have increased susceptibility to hemolysis by oxidizing agents. Indeed, in man this *in-vitro* laboratory test is the only consistent finding associated with low levels of tocopherol in plasma (*see* Leonard and Losowsky, 1967). Presumably, tocopherol protects the lipids in the erythrocyte membrane from peroxidation, which results in membrane destruction and hemolysis.

Four clinical situations have been reported to include alpha-tocopherol–responsive anemia (*see* Darby, 1968; Symposium, 1968). (1) A macrocytic, megaloblastic anemia observed in children with severe protein-calorie malnutrition, while unresponsive to treatment with iron, cyanocobalamin, folic acid, or ascorbic acid, was successfully reversed with large doses of alpha-tocopherol acetate (Majaj *et al.,* 1963; Whitaker *et al.,* 1967). However, subsequent controlled studies have attributed the defective hematopoiesis to deficiency of protein and/or iron rather than to vitamin E (*see* Bieri and Farrell, 1976). (2) Premature infants may develop a hemolytic anemia that is sometimes associated with increased erythrocyte susceptibility to peroxide hemolysis and low concentrations of tocopherol in plasma. This anemia, while not responsive to iron, cyanocobalamin, or folic acid, has been reported to respond to 200 to 800 mg of alpha-tocopherol acetate (Oski and Barness, 1967). In addition to the hematological response, alpha-tocopherol was also reported to relieve the edema and skin lesions accompanying vitamin E deficiency and a diet high in polyunsaturated fatty acids (Hassan *et al.,* 1966). Others, however, have not been able to confirm these results (*see* Bieri and Farrell, 1976). (3) Erythrocytes that hemolyze spontaneously *in vitro* constitute one characteristic of the acanthocytosis syndrome. Patients with this rare genetic disease lack plasma β-lipoprotein and, therefore, have little or no circulating alpha-tocopherol. Further, they have impaired intestinal absorption of the vitamin. Parenteral administration of 100 mg of alpha-tocopherol acetate raised the plasma alpha-tocopherol concentrations and apparently corrected the autohemolytic feature of the disease for several weeks (Kayden *et al.,* 1965). (4) In malabsorption syndromes characterized by steatorrhea (*e.g.,* sprue, mucoviscidosis, chronic pancreatitis), alpha-tocopherol is not absorbed. Here, too, decreased erythrocyte lifetime and increased erythrocyte sensitivity to hydrogen peroxide are coincident with low concentrations of alpha-tocopherol in plasma. These patients after long-term deprivation may develop other abnormalities associated with vitamin E deficiency in animals, such as muscle weakness and necrosis, creatinuria, and deposition of ceroid pigment in intestinal smooth muscle. Only the creatinuria and hematological abnormalities are responsive to administration of alpha-tocopherol. Adult man, intentionally deprived of vitamin E over an extended period of time, has similar hematological lesions and responds to alpha-tocopherol (Horwitt et al., 1963).

While the evidence outlined above seems to implicate vitamin E in normal hematopoiesis, other factors must also be considered. Patients with each of the above syndromes have multiple deficiencies. Furthermore, the ability of the coenzymes Q, selenium, and the sulfur-amino acids to relieve "tocopherol-deficient" syndromes to varying degrees provides further complications for a definitive interpretation. (See Symposium, 1965, 1968; Whitaker et al., 1967; Bieri and Farrell, 1976.)

Human Requirement. In a long-term controlled study of vitamin E depletion in man, Horwitt and coworkers (see Horwitt, 1962) found that vitamin E concentration in plasma declined significantly only after months on a deficient diet. There were no clinical manifestations of the depletion. From these studies, Horwitt estimated that a daily intake of 10 to 30 mg of vitamin E is sufficient to maintain vitamin E concentrations in blood within the normal range. Diets containing large amounts of unsaturated fatty acids increase the daily requirement (Harris and Embree, 1963; Witting, 1972); diets containing selenium, sulfur-amino acids, chromenols, or antioxidants decrease the requirement.

The 1979 recommendations of the Food and Nutrition Board of the National Research Council include 10 alpha-tocopherol equivalents per day for adult men and 8 alpha-tocopherol equivalents per day for adult women. (See Table XVI–1, page 1553.) Human milk (in contrast to cows' milk) has sufficient alpha-tocopherol to meet normal requirements of infants. Tocopherols are present in adequate amounts in the normal adult diet. Indeed, vitamin E deficiency has not been detected as a primary deficiency disease in otherwise-healthy children or adults.

Absorption, Fate, and Excretion. Vitamin E is absorbed from the gastrointestinal tract by a mechanism probably similar to that for the other fat-soluble vitamins (MacMahon and Neale, 1970). Vitamin E enters the blood stream by way of the lymph. It appears first in chylomicrons and then is primarily associated with plasma β-lipoproteins (McCormick et al., 1960). Vitamin E is distributed to all tissues. However, newborn infants have plasma tocopherol concentrations only about one fifth those of their mothers, suggesting poor placental transfer. Tissue stores can provide a source of the vitamin for long periods of time, as evidenced by the long time animals must be kept on a vitamin E–deficient diet before signs of deficiency appear.

Seventy to 80% of an intravenously administered dose of radioactive vitamin E is excreted by the liver over a period of a week; the balance appears as metabolites in the urine. The urinary metabolites are glucuronides of tocopheronic acid and its γ-lactone.

Several other metabolites with quinone structures have been found in tissues: one of these is very similar in structure to ubiquinone and may be related to an active form of the vitamin (see Green and McHale, 1965); dimer and trimer forms of the vitamin are believed to result from reaction with lipid peroxides (see Draper and Csallany, 1970).

Plasma concentrations vary widely among normal individuals. Many attempts have been made to correlate the plasma tocopherol values with disease states. In general, tocopherol concentrations in plasma appear to be related more closely to dietary intake and defects in intestinal absorption of fat than to the presence or absence of disease. Low tocopherol values are generally associated, however, with an increased susceptibility of erythrocytes to hemolysis by oxidizing agents (Leonard and Losowsky, 1967).

Assay and Unitage. The vitamin E activity of foods may be determined chemically, or bioassayed for the protection afforded pregnant female rats against death of the fetus. One international unit (I.U.) is equivalent to the activity of 1 mg of dl-alpha-tocopheryl acetate. d-Alpha-tocopheryl acetate has a potency of 1.36 I.U./mg; d-alpha-tocopherol, 1.49 I.U./mg; d-alpha-tocopheryl succinate, 1.21 I.U./mg. The activity of 1 mg of d-alpha-tocopherol is equal to 1 alpha-tocopherol equivalent.

Preparations. Vitamin E, U.S.P. (AQUASOL E, E-FEROL, others), is a form of alpha-tocopherol that includes the d or the d and l isomers of alpha-tocopherol, alpha-tocopheryl acetate, or alpha-tocopheryl succinate. Official capsules contain 30 to 1000 I.U. of the vitamin. Tablets of many sizes and injectable forms (100 or 200 I.U./ml) are also available. Several multivitamin tablets, capsules, and drops contain small amounts of vitamin E.

Therapeutic Uses. The lack of efficacy of vitamin E in treatment of those diseases in man that bear some resemblance to vitamin E deficiency in animals, namely, recurrent abortion, progressive muscular dystrophy, and cardiovascular disease, has been discussed. These are by no means the only disorders in which vitamin E therapy has been studied. The list extends from minor skin ailments to schizophrenia. With the possible exception of its potential value in treating the anemias associated with extreme protein-calorie malnutrition, prematurity, or acanthocytosis (see above), results with alpha-tocopherol have in general been so disappointing that the conclusion seems justified that, at present, there is no persuasive evidence that vitamin E has any therapeutic use.

Aballi, A. J., and deLamerens, S. Coagulation changes in the neonatal period and in early infancy. *Pediatr. Clin. North Am.,* **1962,** *9,* 785–815.

Almquist, H. J., and Stokstad, C. L. R. Hemorrhagic chick disease of dietary origin. *J. Biol. Chem.,* **1935,** *111,* 105–113.

Bashor, M. M.; Toft, D. O.; and Chytil, F. *In vitro* binding of retinol to rat-tissue components. *Proc. Natl. Acad. Sci. U.S.A.,* **1973,** *70,* 3483–3487.

Bauernfeind, J. C.; Newmark, H.; and Brin, M. Vitamin A and E nutrition via intramuscular or oral route. *Am. J. Clin. Nutr.*, **1974**, *27*, 234–253.

Berneske, G. M.; Butson, A. R. C.; Gauld, E. N.; and Levy, D. Clinical trial of high dosage vitamin E in human muscular dystrophy. *Can. Med. Assoc. J.*, **1960**, *82*, 418–421.

Bernhardt, I. B., and Dorsey, D. J. Hypervitaminosis A and congenital renal anomalies in a human infant. *Obstet. Gynecol.*, **1974,-43**, 750–755.

Bieri, J. G. Fat-soluble vitamins in the eighth revision of the Recommended Daily Allowances. *J. Am. Diet. Assoc.*, **1974**, *64*, 171–174.

Bjelke, E. Dietary vitamin A and human lung cancer. *Int. J. Cancer*, **1975**, *15*, 561–565.

Blalock, J. E., and Gifford, G. E. Retinoic acid (vitamin A acid) induced transcriptional control of interferon production. *Proc. Natl. Acad. Sci. U.S.A.*, **1977**, *74*, 5382–5386.

Bollag, W. Therapy of epithelial tumors with an aromatic retinoic acid analog. *Chemotherapy*, **1975**, *21*, 236–247.

Butt, H. R.; Snell, A. M.; and Osterberg, A. E. The use of vitamin K and bile in treatment of hemorrhagic diathesis in cases of jaundice. *Proc. Staff Meet. Mayo Clin.*, **1938**, *13*, 74–80.

Chen, C.-C., and Heller, J. Transport and utilization of retinoic acid by the retina: intravascular injection of retinoic acid as a complex with retinol binding protein. *Exp. Eye Res.*, **1978**, *26*, 561–565.

Committee on Nutrition, American Academy of Pediatrics. Vitamin K supplementation for infants receiving milk substitute infant formulas and for those with fat malabsorption. *Pediatrics*, **1971**, *48*, 483–487.

Crider, Q.; Alaupovic, P.; and Johnson, B. C. Function and metabolism of vitamin E. III. Vitamin E and antioxidants in the nutrition of the rat. *J. Nutr.*, **1961**, *73*, 64–70.

Dam, H. Cholesterinstoffwechsel in Hühnereiern und Hühnchen. *Biochem. Z.*, **1929**, *215*, 475–492.

Dam, H., and Schønheyder, F. The antihaemorrhagic vitamin of the chick. *Nature*, **1935**, *135*, 652–653.

Dam, H.; Schønheyder, F.; and Tage-Hansen, E. Studies on the mode of action of vitamin K. *Biochem. J.*, **1936**, *30*, 1075–1079.

Dinning, J. S., and Day, P. L. Vitamin E deficiency in the monkey. *J. Exp. Med.*, **1957**, *105*, 395–402.

Dinning, J. S.; Fitch, C. D.; Shunk, C. H.; and Folkers, K. The response of the anemic and dystrophic monkey to treatment with coenzyme Q. *J. Am. Chem. Soc.*, **1962**, *84*, 2007–2008.

Dinning, J. S.; Majaj, A. S.; Azzam, S. A.; Darby, W. J.; Shunk, C. H.; and Folkers, K. Response of macrocytic anemia in children to the coenzyme Q_4-chromanol. *Am. J. Clin. Nutr.*, **1963**, *13*, 169–172.

Diplock, A. T.; Cawthorne, M. A.; Murrell, E. A.; Green, J.; and Bunyan, J. Measurement of lipid peroxidation and α-tocopherol destruction *in vitro* and *in vivo* and their significance in connection with the biological function of vitamin E. *Br. J. Nutr.*, **1968**, *22*, 465–472.

Draper, H. H., and Csallany, A. S. Metabolism of vitamin E. In, *The Fat Soluble Vitamins*. (DeLuca, H. F., and Suttie, J. W., eds.) University of Wisconsin Press, Madison, **1970**, pp. 347–353.

Euler, B. von; Euler, H. von; and Karrer, P. Zur Biochemie der Carotinoide. *Helv. Chim. Acta*, **1929**, *12*, 278–285.

Evans, H. M., and Bishop, K. S. On the relationship between fertility and nutrition. II. The ovulation rhythm in the rat on inadequate nutritional regimes. *J. Metab. Res.*, **1922**, *1*, 319–356.

Evans, H. M.; Emerson, O. H.; and Emerson, G. A. The isolation from wheat germ oil of an alcohol, α-tocopherol, having properties of vitamin E. *J. Biol. Chem.*, **1936**, *113*, 329–332.

Fell, H. B., and Dingle, J. T. Studies on the mode of action of excess vitamin A. 6. Lysosomal protease and the deg-

radation of cartilage matrix. *Biochem. J.*, **1963**, *87*, 403–408.

Fernholtz, E. On the constitution of α-tocopherol. *J. Am. Chem. Soc.*, **1938**, *60*, 700–705.

Fisher, K. D.; Carr, C. J.; Huff, J. E.; and Huber, T. E. Dark adaptation and night vision. *Fed. Proc.*, **1970**, *29*, 1605–1638.

Frick, P.G.; Riedler, G.; and Brögli, H. Dose response and minimal daily requirement for vitamin K in man. *J. Appl. Physiol.*, **1967**, *23*, 387–389.

Gal, I., and Parkinson, C. E. Effects of nutrition and other factors on pregnant women's serum vitamin A levels. *Am. J. Clin. Nutr.*, **1974**, *27*, 688–695.

Ganguly, J. Absorption of vitamin A. *Am. J. Clin. Nutr.*, **1969**, *22*, 923–933.

Goodman, DeW. S.; Blomstrand, R.; Werner, B.; Huang, H. S.; and Shiratori, T. The intestinal absorption and metabolism of vitamin A and β-carotene in man. *J. Clin. Invest.*, **1966**, *45*, 1615–1623.

Green, J. Vitamin E and the biological antioxidant theory. *Ann. N.Y. Acad. Sci.*, **1972**, *203*, 29–44.

Griminger, P. Biological activity of the various vitamin K forms. *Vitam. Horm.*, **1966**, *24*, 605–618.

Hafeman, D. G., and Hoekstra, W. G. Lipid peroxidation *in vivo* during vitamin E and selenium deficiency in the rat as monitored by ethane evolution. *J. Nutr.*, **1977**, *107*, 666–672.

Ham, J. M. Hypoprothrombinemia in patients undergoing prolonged intensive care. *Med. J. Aust.*, **1971**, *2*, 716–718.

Harris, P.L., and Embree, N. D. Quantitative consideration of the effect of polyunsaturated fatty acid content of the diet upon the requirement for vitamin E. *Am. J. Clin. Nutr.*, **1963**, *13*, 385–392.

Hassan, H.; Hashim, S. A.; Van Itallie, T. B.; and Sebrell, W. H. Syndrome in premature infants associated with low plasma vitamin E levels and high polyunsaturated fatty acid diet. *Am. J. Clin. Nutr.*, **1966**, *19*, 147–157.

Hassell, J. R.; Silverman-Jones, C. S.; and DeLuca, L. M. The *in vitro* stimulation of mannose incorporation into mannosylretinylphosphate, dolichylmannosylphosphate and specific glycopeptides of rat liver by high doses of retinylpalmitate. *J. Biol. Chem.*, **1978**, *253*, 1627–1631.

Hawkins, W. B., and Brinkhous, K. M. Prothrombin deficiency the cause of bleeding in bile fistula dogs. *J. Exp. Med.*, **1936**, *63*, 795–801.

Hecht, S. Rods, cones, and chemical basis of vision. *Physiol. Rev.*, **1937**, *17*, 239–290.

Hollander, D. Vitamin K, absorption by everted intestinal sacs of the rat. *Am. J. Physiol.*, **1973**, *225*, 360–364.

Hollander, D.; Muralidhara, K. S.; and Rim, E. Colonic absorption of bacterially synthesized vitamin K_2 in the rat. *Am. J. Physiol.*, **1976**, *230*, 251–255.

Hollander, D., and Rim, E. Vitamin K_2 absorption by rat everted small intestine sacs. *Am. J. Physiol.*, **1976**, *231*, 415–419.

Horwitt, M. K. Interrelations between vitamin E and polyunsaturated fatty acids in adult men. *Vitam. Horm.*, **1962**, *20*, 541–558.

———. Role of vitamin E, selenium, and polyunsaturated fatty acids in clinical and experimental muscle disease. *Fed. Proc.*, **1965**, *24*, 68–72.

Horwitt, M. K.; Century, B.; and Zeman, A. A. Erythrocyte survival time and reticulocyte level after tocopherol depletion in man. *Am. J. Clin. Nutr.*, **1963**, *12*, 99–106.

Hubbard, R.; Bownds, D.; and Yoshizawa, T. The chemistry of visual photoreception. *Cold Spring Harbor Symp. Quant. Biol.*, **1965**, *30*, 301–315.

Jayaram, M., and Ganguly, J. The effect of vitamin A nutritional status on the ribonucleic acids of liver, intestinal mucosa and testes of rats. *Biochem. J.*, **1977**, *166*, 339–346.

Karrer, P.; Fritzsche, H.; Ringier, B. H.; and Salomon, H. α-Tocopherol. *Helv. Chim. Acta*, **1938**, *21*, 520–525.

Karrer, P.; Morf, R.; and Schöpp, K. Zur Kenntnis des

Vitamins A aus Fischtranen. *Helv. Chim. Acta,* **1931,** *14,* 1431–1436.

Kayden, H. J.; Silber, R.; and Kossman, C. E. The role of vitamin E deficiency in the abnormal autohemolysis of acanthocytosis. *Trans. Assoc. Am. Physicians,* **1965,** *78,* 334–342.

Keenan, W. J.; Jewett, T.; and Glueck, H. I. Role of feeding and vitamin K in hypoprothrombinemia of the newborn. *Am. J. Dis. Child.,* **1971,** *121,* 271–277.

Leonard, P. J., and Losowsky, M. S. Relationship between plasma vitamin E level and peroxide hemolysis test in human subjects. *Am. J. Clin. Nutr.,* **1967,** *20,* 795–798.

Levin, S.; Gordon, M. H.; Nitowsky, H. M.; Goldman, C.; di Sant'Agnese, P.; and Gordon, H. H. Studies of tocopherol deficiency in infants and children. VI. Evaluation of muscle strength and effect of tocopherol administration in children with cystic fibrosis. *Pediatrics,* **1961,** *27,* 578–588.

Lewis, A. A molecular mechanism of excitation in visual transduction and bacteriorhodopsin. *Proc. Natl. Acad. Sci. U.S.A.,* **1978,** *75,* 549–553.

Lewis, C. A.; Pratt, R. M.; Pennypacker, J. P.; and Hassell, J. R. Inhibition of limb chondrogenesis *in vitro* by vitamin A: alterations in cell surface characteristics. *Dev. Biol.,* **1978,** *64,* 31–47.

Lian, J. B.; Hanschka, P. V.; and Gallop, P. M. Properties and biosynthesis of a vitamin K–dependent calcium binding protein in bone. *Fed. Proc.,* **1978,** *37,* 2615–2620.

Logan, W. S. Vitamin A and keratinization. *Arch. Dermatol.,* **1972,** *105,* 748–753.

Lukens, J. H. Vitamin K and the older infant. *Am. J. Dis. Child.,* **1972,** *124,* 639–640.

McCollum, E. V., and Davis, M. The necessity of certain lipins in the diet during growth. *J. Biol. Chem.,* **1913,** *15,* 167–175.

McCormick, E. C.; Cornwell, D. G.; and Brown, J. B. Studies on the distribution of tocopherol in human serum. *J. Lipid Res.,* **1960,** *1,* 221–228.

McLaren, D. S. Present knowledge of the role of vitamin A in health and disease. *Trans. R. Soc. Trop. Med. Hyg.,* **1966,** *60,* 436–462.

MacMahon, M. T., and Neale, E. The absorption of α-tocopherol in control subjects and in patients with intestinal malabsorption. *Clin. Sci.,* **1970,** *38,* 197–210.

Majaj, A. S.; Dinning, J. S.; Azzam, S. A.; and Darby, W. J. Vitamin E responsive megaloblastic anemia in infants with protein-calorie malnutrition. *Am. J. Clin. Nutr.,* **1963,** *12,* 374–379.

Mallia, A. K.; Smith, J. E.; and Goodman, D. S. Metabolism of retinol-binding protein and vitamin A during hypervitaminosis in the rat. *J. Lipid Res.,* **1975,** *16,* 180–188.

Matschiner, J. T.; Bell, R. G.; Amelotti, J. M.; and Knauer, T. E. Isolation and characterization of a new metabolite of phylloquinone in the rat. *Biochim. Biophys. Acta,* **1970,** *201,* 309–315.

Moore, T. Relation of carotin to vitamin A. *Lancet,* **1929,** *2,* 380–381.

Nelsestuen, G. L. Interaction of vitamin K–dependent proteins with calcium ions and phospholipid membranes. *Fed. Proc.,* **1978,** *37,* 2621–2625.

Oliver, T. K., Jr. Chronic vitamin A intoxication: report of a case in an older child and review of the literature. *Am. J. Dis. Child.,* **1958,** *95,* 57–68.

Olsen, R. E. Vitamin E and its relation to heart disease. *Circulation,* **1973,** *48,* 179–184.

Olsen, R. E., and Carpenter, P. C. The regulatory function of vitamin E. *Adv. Enzyme Regul.,* **1967,** *5,* 325–334.

Ong, D. E., and Chytil, F. Retinoic acid binding protein in rat tissue. Partial purification and comparison to rat tissue retinol-binding protein. *J. Biol. Chem.,* **1975,** *250,* 6113–6117.

Osborne, T. B., and Mendel, L. B. The relation of growth

to the chemical constituents of the diet. *J. Biol. Chem.,* **1913,** *15,* 311–326.

Oski, F. A., and Barness, L. A. Vitamin E deficiency: a previously unrecognized cause of hemolytic anemia in the premature infant. *J. Pediatr.,* **1967,** *70,* 211–220.

Quick, A. J.; Stanley-Brown, M.; and Bancroft, F. W. A study of the coagulation defect in hemophilia and in jaundice. *Am. J. Med. Sci.,* **1935,** *190,* 501–511.

Report of the Council on Foods and Nutrition. Deficiencies of the fat-soluble vitamins. *J.A.M.A.,* **1950,** *144,* 34–45.

Roels, O. A. Vitamin A physiology. *J.A.M.A.,* **1970,** *214,* 1097–1102.

Rogers, W. E., Jr. Reexamination of enzyme activities thought to show evidence of a coenzyme role for vitamin A. *Am. J. Clin. Nutr.,* **1969,** *22,* 1003–1013.

Rosso, G. C.; DeLuca, L.; Warren, C. D.; and Wolf, G. Enzymatic synthesis of mannosyl retinyl phosphate from retinyl phosphate and guanosine diphosphate mannose. *J. Lipid Res.,* **1975,** *16,* 235–243.

Russell, F. E. Vitamin A content of polar bear liver. *Toxicon,* **1967,** *5,* 61–62.

Sani, B. P., and Hill, D. L. A retinoic acid–binding protein from chick embryo skin. *Cancer Res.,* **1976,** *36,* 409–413.

Schwarz, K. Role of vitamin E, selenium, and related factors in experimental nutritional liver disease. *Fed. Proc.,* **1965,** *24,* 58–67.

Simon, E. J.; Gross, C. S.; and Milhorat, A. T. The metabolism of vitamin E. *J. Biol. Chem.,* **1956,** *221,* 797–817.

Smith, F. R., and Goodman, D. S. Vitamin A transport in human vitamin A toxicity. *N. Engl. J. Med.,* **1976,** *294,* 805–808.

Smith, J. L.; Bhagavan, H. N.; Hill, R. B.; Gaetani, S.; RamaRao, P. B.; Crider, Q. E.; Johnson, B. C.; Shunk, C H.; Wagner, A F.; and Folkers, K. Biological activities of compounds in the vitamin E, vitamin K and coenzyme Q groups in chicks, rabbits and rats. *Arch. Biochem. Biophys.,* **1963,** *101,* 388–395.

Sporn, M. B.; Dunlop, N. M.; Newton, D. L.; and Smith, J. M. Prevention of chemical carcinogenesis by vitamin A and its synthetic analogs (retinoids). *Fed. Proc.,* **1976,** *35,* 1332–1338.

Srikantia, S. G., and Reddy, V. Effect of a single massive dose of vitamin A on serum and liver levels of the vitamin. *Am. J. Clin. Nutr.,* **1970,** *23,* 114–118.

Stånge, L.; Carlström, K.; and Eriksson, M. Hypervitaminosis A in early human pregnancy and malformations of the central nervous system. *Acta Obstet. Gynecol. Scand.,* **1978,** *57,* 289–291.

Steenbock, H. White corn vs. yellow corn, and a probable relation between the fat-soluble vitamin and yellow plant pigments. *Science,* **1919,** *50,* 352–353.

Sutherland, J. M.; Glueck, H. I.; and Glaser, G. Hemorrhagic disease of the newborn. Breast feeding as a necessary factor in the pathogenesis. *Am. J. Dis. Child.,* **1967,** *113,* 524–533.

Suttie, J. W.; Larson, A. E.; Canfield, L. M.; and Carlisle, T. L. Relationship between vitamin K–dependent carboxylation and vitamin K epoxidation. *Fed. Proc.,* **1978,** *37,* 2605–2614.

Tappel, A. L.; Savant, P. L.; and Shibko, S. Lysosomes: distribution in animals, hydrolytic capacity and other properties. In, *Lysosomes* (a Ciba Foundation symposium). (de Reuck, A. V. S., and Cameron, M. P., eds.) Little, Brown & Co., Boston; J. & A. Churchill, Ltd., London, **1963.**

Vollbracht, R., and Gilroy, J. Vitamin A induced benign intracranial hypertension. *Can. J. Neurol. Sci.,* **1976,** *3,* 59–61.

Wagner, A. F., and Folkers, K. Considerations of veristic and quasi-biological activities for coenzyme Q and vitamins E and K. *Perspect. Biol. Med.,* **1963,** *6,* 347–356.

Wald, G. The molecular basis of visual excitation. *Nature,* **1968,** *219,* 800–807.

Wald, G., and Brown, P. K. Human color vision and color blindness. *Cold Spring Harbor Symp. Quant. Biol.,* **1965,** *30,* 345–361.

Warner, E. D.; Brinkhous, K. M.; and Smith, H. P. Bleeding tendency of obstructive jaundice: prothrombin deficiency and dietary factors. *Proc. Soc. Exp. Biol. Med.,* **1938,** *37,* 628–630.

Wefring, K. W. Hemorrhage in the newborn and vitamin K prophylaxis. *J. Pediatr.,* **1962,** *61,* 686–692.

Whitaker, J.; Fort, E. G.; Vimokesant, S.; and Dinning, J. S. Hematologic response to vitamin E in the anemia associated with protein-calorie malnutrition. *Am. J. Clin. Nutr.,* **1967,** *20,* 783–789.

Wiggert, B.; Bergsma, D. R.; Helmsen, R.; and Chader, G. J. Vitamin A receptors. Retinoic acid binding in ocular tissue. *Biochem. J.,* **1978,** *169,* 87–94.

Witting, L. A. The role of polyunsaturated fatty acids in determining vitamin E requirements. *Ann. N.Y. Acad. Sci.,* **1972,** *203,* 192–198.

Woolf, I. L., and Babior, B. M. Vitamin K and warfarin. Metabolism, function, and interaction. *Am. J. Med.,* **1972,** *53,* 261–267.

Wynn, R. M. The obstetrical significance of factors affecting the metabolism of bilirubin, with particular reference to the role of vitamin K. *Obstet. Gynecol. Surv.,* **1963,** *18,* 333–354.

Yaffe, S. J., and Filer, L. J. The use and abuse of vitamin A. American Academy of Pediatrics, Joint Committee Statement, Committee on Drugs and Nutrition. *Pediatrics,* **1971,** *48,* 655–656.

Zinkham, W. H., and Childs, B. Effect of vitamin K and naphthalene metabolites on glutathione metabolism of erythrocytes from normal newborns and patients with naphthalene hemolytic anemia. *Am. J. Dis. Child.,* **1957,** *94,* 420–423.

Monographs and Reviews

Bieri, J. G., and Farrell, P. M. Vitamin E. *Vitam. Horm.,* **1976,** *34,* 31–75.

Dam, H. Influence of antioxidants and redox substances on signs of vitamin E deficiency. *Pharmacol. Rev.,* **1957,** *9,* 1–16.

Dam, H., and Søndergaard, E. Vitamin K. In, *The Enzymes,* 2nd ed., Vol. 3. (Boyer, P. D., Lardy, H.; and Myrbäck, K.; eds.) Academic Press, Inc., New York, **1960,** pp. 329–352.

Darby, W. J. Tocopherol-responsive anemias in man. *Vitam. Horm.,* **1968,** *26,* 685–699.

De Luca, L. M. The direct involvement of vitamin A in glycosyl transfer reactions of mammalian membranes. *Vitam. Horm.,* **1977,** *35,* 1–57.

———. Vitamin A. In, *The Fat Soluble Vitamins.* (DeLuca, H. F., ed.) *Handbook of Lipid Research,* Vol. 2. Plenum Press, New York, **1978,** pp. 1–67.

Deutsch, E. Vitamin K in medical practice: adults. *Vitam. Horm.,* **1966,** *24,* 665–680.

Dingle, J. T., and Lucy, J. A. Vitamin A, carotenoids, and cell function. *Biol. Rev.,* **1965,** *40,* 422–461.

Finkel, M. J. Vitamin K_1 and vitamin K analogues. *Clin. Pharmacol. Ther.,* **1961,** *2,* 794–814.

Fitch, C. D. Experimental anemias in primates due to vitamin E deficiency. *Vitam. Horm.,* **1968,** *26,* 501–514.

Glover, J.; Jay, C.; and White, G. H. Distribution of retinol-binding protein in tissues. *Vitam. Horm.,* **1974,** *32,* 215–236.

Goodman, DeW. Vitamin A transport and retinol-binding protein in tissues. *Vitam. Horm.,* **1974,** *32,* 167–180.

Green, J. Antagonists of vitamin K. *Vitam. Horm.,* **1966,** *24,* 619–631.

Green, J., and McHale, D. Quinones related to vitamin E. In, *Biochemistry of Quinones.* (Morton, R. A., ed.) Academic Press, Inc., New York, **1965,** pp. 261–285.

Heel, R. C.; Brogden, R. N.; Speight, T. M.; and Avery, G. S. Vitamin A acid: a review of its pharmacological properties and therapeutic use in the topical treatment of acne vulgaris. *Drugs,* **1977,** *14,* 401–419.

Isler, O., and Wiss, O. Chemistry and biochemistry of the K vitamins. *Vitam. Horm.,* **1959,** *17,* 54–92.

Martius, C. Chemistry and function of vitamin K. In, *Blood Clotting Enzymology.* (Seeger, W. H., ed.) Academic Press, Inc., New York, **1967,** pp. 557–575.

Mason, K. E. Effects of nutritional deficiencies on muscle. In, *The Structure and Function of Muscle,* 2nd ed., Vol. 4. (Bourne, G. H., ed.) Academic Press, Inc., New York, **1973,** pp. 155–206.

Molenaar, I.; Vos, J.; and Hommes, F. A. Effect of vitamin E deficiency on cellular membranes. *Vitam. Horm.,* **1972,** *30,* 45–82.

Moore, T. *Vitamin A,* 2nd ed. American Elsevier Publishing Co., New York, **1957.**

Oski, F. A., and Naiman, J. L. *Hematological Problems in the Newborn.* W. B. Saunders Co., Philadelphia, **1966.**

Pappenheimer, A. M. Muscular disorders associated with deficiency of vitamin E. *Physiol. Rev.,* **1943,** *23,* 37–50.

Parrish, D. B. Determination of vitamin A in foods—a review. *CRC Crit. Rev. Food Sci. Nutr.,* **1977,** *9,* 375–394.

Peck, G. L.; Olsen, T. G.; Yoder, F. W.; Strauss, J. S.; Downing, D. T.; Pandya, M.; Butkus, D.; and Arnaud-Battandier, J. Prolonged remissions of cystic and conglobate acne with 13-*cis*-retinoic acid. *N. Engl. J. Med.,* **1979,** *300,* 329–333.

Pennock, J. F. Occurrence of vitamins K and related quinones. *Vitam. Horm.,* **1966,** *24,* 307–329.

Peterson, P.; Nilsson, S.; Ostberg, L.; Rask, L.; and Vahlquist, A. Aspects of the metabolism of retinol-binding protein and retinol. *Vitam. Horm.,* **1974,** *32,* 181–214.

Rietz, P.; Weiss, O.; and Weber, F. Metabolism of vitamin A and the determination of vitamin A status. *Vitam. Horm.,* **1974,** *32,* 237–250.

Stenflo, J. Vitamin K, prothrombin, and gamma-carboxyglutamic acid. *Adv. Enzymol.,* **1978,** *46,* 1–31.

Shearer, M. J.; McBurney, A.; and Barkham, P. Studies on the absorption and metabolism of phylloquinone (vitamin K_1) in man. *Vitam. Horm.,* **1974,** *32,* 513–542.

Stüttgen, G. (ed.). The therapeutic use of vitamin A in glycosyl transfer reactions of mammalian membranes. *Vitam. Horm.,* **1975,** *35,* 1–57.

Suttie, J. W. Vitamin K. In, *Handbook of Lipid Research,* Vol. 2. (DeLuca, H. F., ed.) Plenum Press, New York, **1978,** pp. 211–277.

Symposium. (Various authors.) Interrelationships among vitamin E, coenzyme Q, and selenium. *Fed. Proc.,* **1965,** *24,* 55–92.

Symposium. (Various authors.) Hematological aspects of vitamin E. *Am. J. Clin. Nutr.,* **1968,** *21,* 1–56.

Symposium. (Various authors.) Vitamin E. Biochemistry, nutritional requirements, and clinical studies. *Am. J. Clin. Nutr.,* **1974,** *27,* 937–1037.

Wasserman, R. H., and Corradino, R. A. Metabolic role of vitamins A and D. *Annu. Rev. Biochem.,* **1971,** *40,* 501–532.

Wasserman, R. H., and Taylor, A. N. Metabolic roles of fat-soluble vitamins D, E, and K. *Annu. Rev. Biochem.,* **1972,** *41,* 179–201.

Wolf, G. International symposium on the metabolic function of vitamin A. *Am. J. Clin. Nutr.,* **1969,** *22,* 897–1138.

SECTION XVII
Toxicology

CHAPTER

68 PRINCIPLES OF TOXICOLOGY

Curtis D. Klaassen

Toxicology is the science of the adverse effects of chemicals on living organisms. The discipline is often divided into several major areas. The *descriptive toxicologist* performs toxicity tests (described below) to obtain information that can be used to evaluate the risk that exposure to a chemical poses to man and the environment. The *mechanistic toxicologist* attempts to determine how chemicals exert deleterious effects on living organisms. Such studies are useful for the development of tests for the prediction of risks, to facilitate the search for safer chemicals, and for rational treatment of the manifestations of toxicity. The *regulatory toxicologist* judges if a drug or other chemical has a low enough risk to be made available for its intended purpose. The Food and Drug Administration (FDA) regulates drugs, cosmetics, and food additives in interstate commerce. The Environmental Protection Agency (EPA) regulates most other chemicals.

Two specialized areas of toxicology are particularly important for medicine. *Forensic toxicology,* wherein analytical chemistry and fundamental toxicological principles are hybridized, is concerned with the medicolegal aspects of the use of chemicals that are harmful to animals and man. Forensic toxicologists assist in post-mortem investigations to establish the cause or circumstances of death. *Clinical toxicology* focuses on diseases that are caused by or are uniquely associated with toxic substances. Clinical toxicologists treat patients who are poisoned by drugs and other chemicals and develop new technics for the diagnosis and treatment of such intoxications.

The physician must evaluate the possibility that a patient's signs and symptoms might be caused by toxic chemicals present in the environment or administered as therapeutic agents. Many of the adverse effects of drugs mimic those of disease. Appreciation of the principles of toxicology is necessary for the recognition and management of such problems.

DOSE-EFFECT RELATIONSHIP

Evaluation of the dose-response or the dose-effect relationship is crucially important to toxicologists (*see* Chapter 2). There is both a graded dose-response relationship in an *individual* and a quantal dose-response relationship in the *population*. Graded doses of a drug given to an individual usually result in a greater magnitude of response as the dose is increased. In a quantal dose-effect relationship, the percentage of the population affected increases as the dose is raised; the relationship is quantal in that the effect is specified to be either present or absent in a given individual. This quantal dose-effect phenomonen is extremely important in toxicology and is used to determine the *median lethal dose* (LD50) of drugs and other chemicals.

The LD50 is determined experimentally. The chemical is usually administered to mice or rats orally or intraperitoneally, using several doses (usually four or five) in the lethal range (*see* Figure 2–5, page 37). To linearize such data, the response (deaths) can be converted to units of *deviation from the mean*, or *probits* (from the contraction of *probability units*). The probit designates the deviation from the median; a probit of 5 corresponds to a 50% response, and, since each probit equals one standard deviation, a probit of 4 equals 16% and a probit of 6 equals 84% (Litchfield and Wilcoxon, 1949; Bliss, 1957; Finney, 1971). A plot of percent of population responding, in probit units, against log dose yields a straight line (Figure 68–1). The LD50 is determined by drawing a vertical line from the point where the probit unit = 5 (50% mortality). The slope of the dose-effect is also important. The LD50 for both compounds depicted in Figure 68–1 is the same (10 mg/kg). However, the slopes of the dose-response curves are quite different. At a dose equal to one half of the LD50 (5 mg/kg), less than 5% of the animals exposed to compound B would die, but 30% of the animals given compound A would die.

The quantal or "all-or-none" response is not limited to lethality. Similar dose-effect curves can be constructed for chemicals that produce cancer, hepatic injury, or any other toxic response.

TOXIC OR SAFE VERSUS RISK OR HAZARD

There obviously are marked differences in the LD50 of various chemicals. Some produce death in doses of a fraction of a microgram (LD50 for botulinus toxin = 10 pg/kg);

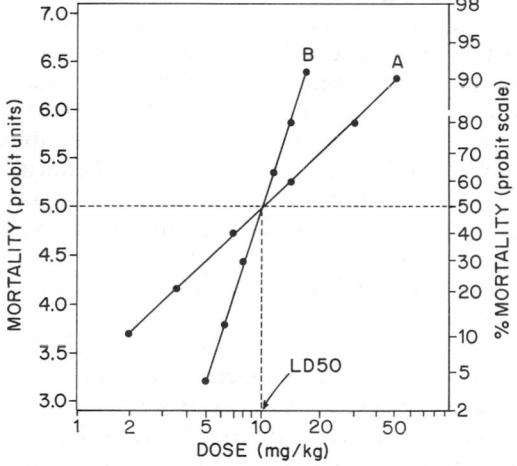

Figure 68–1. *Dose-response relationships.*

The logarithm of the dose is plotted versus the percentage of the population killed by two toxicants in probit units (*see* text).

others may be relatively harmless in doses of several grams or more. While categories of toxicity that are of some practicality have been devised, based on the amount required to produce death, it often is not easy to distinguish between toxic and nontoxic chemicals. Paracelsus (1493–1541) noted . . . "All substances are poisons; there is none which is not a poison. The right dose differentiates a poison and a remedy." *While society wants the toxicologist to categorize all chemicals as either safe or toxic, this is not possible.* The real concern is the *risk* or *hazard* associated with use of the chemical, not whether a chemical is toxic or safe. In the assessment of risk one must also consider the harmful effects of the chemical accrued directly or indirectly through adverse effects on the environment when used in the quantity and in the manner proposed. Depending on the use and disposition of a chemical, a very toxic compound may be less harmful, ultimately, than a relatively nontoxic one.

Assessment of *benefits* to individuals, society, and the environment clearly influences the acceptability of the risks of the use of a chemical. High risks may be acceptable with lifesaving drugs but cannot be tolerated for food additives. The level of acceptable risk depends on a number of factors: (1) the need met by the substance in question, (2) alternatives to the use of the compound, (3) anticipated extent of use by or exposure of the public, (4) economic considerations, (5) effects on the quality of the environment, and (6) conservation of natural resources.

Acute versus Chronic Exposure. Effects of acute exposure to a chemical often differ from those that follow subacute or chronic exposure. Acute exposure occurs when a dose is delivered as a single event. Intravenous and oral doses are usually exposures of short duration, but exposure by inhalation of a volatile substance may be prolonged and repeated, such as throughout an 8-hour work day. Chronic exposure is likely to be to small quantities of a toxic substance over a long period of time, which often results in the slow accumulation of toxic concentrations of the compound in the body. Evaluation of *cumulative* toxic effects is receiving increased attention because of chronic exposure to low concentrations of various natural and synthetic chemical substances in the environment.

SPECTRUM OF UNDESIRED EFFECTS

The spectrum of undesired effects of chemicals may be broad and ill defined. In therapeutics, a drug typically produces numerous effects, but only one is usually sought as the primary goal of treatment; most of the other effects are referred to as *undesirable* or *side effects* of that drug for that therapeutic indication. Mechanistic categorization of such effects is a necessary prelude to their avoidance or, if they occur, to their rational and successful management.

Allergic Reactions. *Chemical allergy* is an adverse reaction that results from previous sensitization to a particular chemical or to one that is structurally similar; such reactions are mediated by the immune systems. Although the term *hypersensitivity* is often used to describe the allergic state, this term (or *hyperreactivity*) is more appropriately used to describe the response of subjects at the lower end of the frequency distribution of the quantal dose-response curve.

For a low-molecular-weight chemical to cause an allergic reaction, it or its metabolic product usually acts as a hapten, combining with an endogenous protein to form an antigenic complex. Such antigens induce the synthesis of antibodies, usually after a latent period of at least 1 or 2 weeks. Subsequent exposure of the organism to the chemical results in an antigen-antibody interaction that provokes the typical manifestations of allergy. Dose-response relationships are usually not apparent for the provocation of allergic reactions because of the nature of the humoral and cellular responses to antigens. Extremely small quantities of an allergen can provoke a reaction, often serious, and the consequences of such a reaction are amplified by the liberation of a variety of potent autacoids (*see* Section IV).

The manifestations of allergy to drugs and other chemicals are numerous and include the full spectrum of immediate and delayed types of reactions produced by foreign macromolecules. Skin reactions extend from mild rash to severe exfoliative dermatitis. Those of blood vessels range from acute urticaria and angioedema to severe arteritis with localized medial degeneration. Drug fever is an allergic phenomenon that very closely resembles serum sickness; it is manifested by fever, leukocytosis, arthralgia, and dermatitis. Rhinitis, asthma, and even anaphylactic shock are other familiar allergic responses that can be precipitated by drugs.

Idiosyncratic Reactions. *Idiosyncracy* is defined as a genetically determined abnormal reactivity to a chemical (Goldstein *et al.,* 1974). The observed response is qualitatively similar in all individuals, but it may take the form of extreme sensitivity to low doses or extreme insensitivity to high doses of the agent. For example, many black males (about 10%) develop a serious hemolytic anemia when they receive primaquine. Such individuals have a deficiency of erythrocytic glucose-6-phosphate dehydrogenase (*see* Chapter 45). Genetically determined resistance to the anticoagulant action of warfarin is due to an alteration in the receptor for the drug (*see* Chapter 58).

Delayed Toxicity. Most toxic effects of drugs occur at a predictable, usually short, time after administration. However, such is not always the case. For example, aplastic anemia caused by chloramphenicol may appear weeks after the drug has been discontinued. Carcinogenic effects of chemicals usually have a long latency period, and 20 to 30 years often must pass before tumors are observed. Such delayed effects obviously cannot be assessed during any reasonable period of initial evaluation of a chemical; there is an urgent need for reliably predictive, short-term tests for such toxicity as well as for systematic surveillance of the long-term effects of marketed drugs and other chemicals.

Chemical carcinogenesis is a multistep process. Most carcinogens are themselves unreactive (*procarcinogens* or *secondary carcinogens*) but are converted to *primary carcinogens* in the body. The cytochrome P-450 monooxygenases of the endoplasmic reticulum often convert the procarcinogens to reactive electron-deficient intermediates (electrophiles). These reactive intermediates can interact with electron-rich (nucleophilic) centers in DNA to produce a mutation. Such interaction of the primary carcinogen with specific receptors of the cell is called initiation. The transformed cells may revert to normal if DNA repair mechanisms operate successfully; if not, the transformed cell may grow into a tumor that becomes apparent clinically. A *cocarcinogen* or *promoter* is not a carcinogen by itself, but it potentiates the effects of a carcinogen. Promotion involves facilitation of the growth and development of so-called dormant or latent tumor cells. The time from initiation to the development of a tumor probably depends on the presence of such promoters; for many human tumors the latent period is usually 15 to 45 years.

Reversible and Irreversible Toxic Effects. The effects of drugs on man must, insofar as possible, be reversible; otherwise the drugs would be prohibitively toxic. If a chemical produces injury to a tissue, the capacity of the tissue to regenerate or recover will largely determine the reversibility of the effect. Many injuries to a tissue such as liver, which has a high capacity to regenerate, are reversible; injury to the central nervous system (CNS) is largely irreversible because the highly differentiated neurons of the brain cannot divide and regenerate.

Local versus Systemic Toxicity. Effects of chemicals can also be classified by their site of action. Local effects are those that occur at the site of first contact between the biological system and the toxicant. Examples of local effects are ingestion of caustic substances or inhalation of irritant materials. Systemic effects require absorption and distribution of the toxicant; most substances, with the exception of chemically highly reactive species, produce such effects. The two categories are not mutually exclusive. Tetraethyl lead, for example, injures skin at the site of contact and is absorbed into the circulation to affect the CNS.

Most systemic toxicants affect one or a few organs predominantly. The target organ of toxicity is not necessarily the site of accumulation of the chemical. For example, lead is concentrated in bone, but its primary toxic action is on soft tissues; DDT is concentrated in adipose tissue but produces no known toxic effects there.

The CNS is most frequently involved in systemic toxicity. Many compounds having prominent effects elsewhere also affect the brain. Next in order of frequency of involvement in systemic toxicity are the circulatory system; the blood and hematopoietic system; visceral organs such as liver, kidney, and lung; and the skin. Muscle and bone are least often affected. With substances that have a predominant local effect, the frequency of tissue reaction depends largely on the portal of entry (skin, gastrointestinal tract, or respiratory tract).

Phototoxic and Photoallergic Reactions. Some drugs and chemicals can induce photosensitivity reactions in individuals who ingest the agents or use them topically and then expose their skin to sunlight. The same drugs are generally innocuous to skin in the absence of exposure to light. The list of offenders includes selected sulfonamides, tetracyclines, nalidixic acid, sulfonylureas, thiazides, phenothiazines, furocoumarins, and coal tars. Photosensitizing chemicals usually have a low molecular weight (200 to 500) and planar, tricyclic, or polycyclic configurations with resonating structures. All absorb ultraviolet or visible radiation.

Photosensitivity reactions may include an acute and abnormal sunburn (erythema), edema, papules, macules, bullae or vesicles, and acute eczematous or urticarial reactions. They may result in telangiectasia, desquamation, and hyperpigmentation. These reactions are classified into two broad categories—phototoxic reactions and photoallergic reactions. Phototoxic reactions are dose related and can be elicited in most individuals who are exposed to adequate amounts of the chemical and radiation of the appropriate wavelength. The action spectrum for most drug-induced photosensitivity reactions is generally in the long-wave ultraviolet range (320 to 400 nm). The reaction can occur within 5 to 18 hours after exposure to the sun and is usually maximal by 36 to 72 hours.

Photoallergic reactions to drugs involve the immune system. Light may promote a photochemical reaction between the drug and cutaneous proteins with resultant formation of a photoantigen. The clinical manifestations may range from acute urticarial reactions, which develop a few minutes after exposure to sunlight, to eczematous or papular lesions, which appear after 24 hours or more.

Interactions between Chemicals. The existence of numerous toxicants requires consideration of their potential interactions (*see also* Chapters 1 to 3 and Appendix III). Substances can interact with each other chemically, which usually results in a decreased toxic response. Concurrent exposures may alter rates of absorption, change the degree of protein binding, or alter the rates of metabolism or excretion of one or both interacting compounds. Effects that result from the combined actions of multiple chemicals may also be altered. The response to combined toxicants may thus be equal to, greater than, or less than the sum of the effects of the individual agents.

Numerous terms describe pharmacological and toxicological interactions. An *additive* effect describes the combined effect of two chemicals that is equal to the sum of the effect of each agent given alone; the additive effect is the most common. A *synergistic* effect is one in which the combined effect of two chemicals is greater than the sum of the effect of each agent given alone. For example, both carbon tetrachloride and ethanol are hepatotoxins, but together they produce much more injury to the liver than expected from the mathematical sum of their individual effects. *Potentiation* is the increased effect of a toxic agent acting simultaneously with a nontoxic one. Isopropanol alone, for example, is not hepatotoxic; however, it greatly increases the hepatotoxicity of carbon tetrachloride. *Antagonism* is the interference of one chemical with the action of another. An antagonistic agent is often desirable as an antidote. *Functional or physiological antagonism* occurs when two chemicals produce opposite effects on the same physiological function. This principle is applied to maintain perfusion of vital organs during certain severe intoxications characterized by marked hypotension and hypoxia, by intravenous administration of dopamine; convulsions can often be controlled by the administration of benzodiazepines (*see* Chapter 20). *Chemical antagonism* or *inactivation* is a reaction between two chemicals to neutralize their effects. For example, dimercaprol (BAL) chelates with various metals to decrease their toxicity; protamine sulfate, a basic low-molecular-weight protein, forms a stable complex with heparin, an anticoagulant. *Dispositional antagonism* is the alteration of the disposition of a substance (its absorption, metabolism, distribution, or excretion) so that less of the agent reaches the target organ or its persistence there is reduced (*see* below). *Antagonism* at the *receptor* for the chemical entails the blockade of the effect of an agonist with an appropriate antagonist that competes for the same site. The antagonist naloxone is used to treat the respiratory depressant effects of opioids; atropine, used to treat poisoning by organic phosphate insecticides, blocks muscarinic cholinergic receptors.

DESCRIPTIVE TOXICITY TESTS IN ANIMALS

Two main principles underlie all descriptive toxicity tests that are performed in animals. First, effects of chemicals produced in laboratory animals, when properly qualified, apply to toxicity in man. When calculated on the basis of dose per unit of body surface, toxic effects in man are usually encountered in the same range of concentrations as are those in experimental animals. On the basis of body weight, man is generally more vulnerable than experimental animals by a fac-

tor of about ten. Such information is used to select dosages for clinical trials of candidate therapeutic agents and to attempt to set limits on permissible exposure to environmental toxicants.

The second main principle is that exposure of experimental animals to toxic agents in high doses is a necessary and valid method to discover possible hazards to humans. This principle is based on the quantal dose-response concept. As a matter of practicality, the number of animals used in experiments on toxic materials will usually be small compared with the size of human populations potentially at risk. For example, 0.01% incidence of a serious toxic effect (such as cancer) represents 20,000 people in a population of 200 million. Such an incidence is unacceptably high. Yet, detecting it directly might require a minimum of 30,000 animals. To estimate risk at low dosage, large doses must be given to relatively small groups. The validity of the necessary extrapolation is clearly a crucial question.

Chemicals are first tested for toxicity by determination of the LD50 in four animal species by two routes of administration; one of these is the expected route of exposure. Animals most often used are mice, rats, rabbits, and dogs. In mice and rats the LD50 is usually determined as described above. In larger species the LD50 is approximated by increasing the dose until serious toxic effects are demonstrated. The number of animals that die in a 7- or 14-day period after a single dose is tabulated. The animals are also examined for signs of intoxication, lethargy, behavioral modification, and morbidity.

The chemical is next tested for toxicity by subacute exposure, usually for 90 days. The subacute study is most often performed in two species (rat and dog) by the route of intended use or exposure, and at least three doses are employed. A variety of parameters are monitored during this period, and, at the end of the study, organs and tissues are examined by a pathologist.

Long-term or chronic studies are carried out in animals at the same time that clinical trials are undertaken (*see* Chapter 3). The length of exposure depends somewhat on the intended use in man. If the drug would normally be used for short periods under medical supervision, as would an antimicrobial agent, a chronic exposure of animals for 6 months might suffice. If the drug would be used in man for longer periods, a chronic study of 2 years might be required.

Study of chronic exposure is often used to determine the carcinogenic potential of chemicals. These studies are usually performed in rats and mice and cover the average lifetime of the species. Other tests are designed to evaluate teratogenicity, perinatal and postnatal toxicity, and effects on fertility. In addition, drugs are often tested for *mutagenic* potential. The most popular such test currently available, the reverse mutation test developed by Ames and colleagues (Ames *et al.,* 1975), uses a strain of *Salmonella typhimurium* that has a mutant gene for the enzyme phosphoribosyl adenosine triphosphate (ATP) synthetase. This enzyme is required for histidine synthesis, and the bacterial strain is unable to grow in a histidine-deficient medium unless a reverse mutation is induced. Since many chemicals are not mutagenic or carcinogenic unless metabolized by the endoplasmic reticulum, rat hepatic microsomes are usually added to the medium containing the mutant bacteria and the drug. The Ames test is rapid and sensitive. However, its usefulness for the prediction of the carcinogenic potential of chemicals for man is controversial, and the subject is currently receiving considerable attention.

SELECTIVE TOXICITY

Selective toxicity is the capacity of a chemical to injure one kind of living matter without harming another, even though the two may be in intimate contact (Albert, 1965, 1973). Drugs and other chemical agents that are used for such a purpose are selective for one of two reasons. Either the chemical is equitoxic to both species but accumulates to higher concentrations in one or the agent reacts fairly specifically with receptors that are unique to or more important to one of the organisms. Selectivity in distribution is usually due to differences in absorption, biotransformation, or excretion of the toxicant. The selective toxicity of an insecticide, for example, is partially due to the large surface area (per unit weight) of an insect, compared to that of a mammal. Carbon tetrachloride is toxic to the liver because this tissue has a high capacity to metabolize CCl_4 to the trichloromethyl free radical ($\cdot CCl_3$).

INCIDENCE OF ACUTE POISONING

The true incidence of poisoning in the United States is not known, but, in 1976, about 150,000 cases were voluntarily reported to the National Clearinghouse for Poison Control Centers. The number of real or potential poisonings is probably at least tenfold greater than the number reported.

Deaths in the United States due to poisoning by liquid and solid substances number over 4000 per year (Table 68–1); more than 5000 people (many fire victims) die each year in the United States from exposure to carbon monoxide. The incidence of poisoning in the United States is increasing; however, the incidence of poisoning in children (under 5 years of age) has decreased dramatically over the last few years. This favorable trend (a

Table 68-1. DEATHS FROM POISONINGS IN 1976 *

TOXICANT	NUMBER
Antibiotics and other antimicrobial agents	20
Hormones and synthetic substitutes	26
Hematological agents	58
Analgesics and antipyretics	1067
Sedatives and hypnotics	508
Autonomic nervous system and psychotherapeutic drugs	190
Central nervous system depressants and stimulants	36
Cardiovascular drugs	138
Gastrointestinal drugs	4
Other and unspecified drugs	792
Total Drugs	2839
Alcohol	337
Cleaning and polishing agents	14
Disinfectants	6
Petroleum products and other solvents	45
Pesticides, fertilizers, or plant foods	31
Heavy metals	15
Corrosives and caustics	22
Noxious foodstuffs and poisonous plants	6
Other and unspecified solid and liquid substances	846
Total Other Substances	1322
Total	4161

* Individual poison reports submitted to the National Clearinghouse for Poison Control Centers.

60% decrease over an 8-year period) is probably due to safety packaging of aspirin, prescription drugs, drain cleaners, turpentine, and other household chemicals, as well as increased public awareness of potential poisons. Of the deaths caused by liquid and solid substances, about 60% are caused by drugs and the rest by other chemicals.

Marked differences in the incidence of poisoning are seen at different ages. Children under 5 years account for about 60% of the poisoning, but their mortality rate is much less; these cases account for only 2.5% of the total deaths from poisons. About 50% of accidental poisoning occurs in children 1 to 2 years old, the age at which they actively explore the environment. The agent responsible for poisoning also differs in various age groups. In toddlers, the agents are usually chemicals other than drugs. In 1976, plants were the category most frequently implicated, followed by cleaning agents. As the age of the patient increases, drugs are more frequent causes of poisoning. In people over 15 years of age, about 75% of cases of poisoning are due to drugs.

MAJOR SOURCES OF INFORMATION ON TOXICOLOGY

Pharmacology textbooks are a good source of information on treatment of poisoning by drugs, but they usually say little about other chemicals. Additional information on drugs and other chemicals can be found in various books on poisoning. (*See* Moeschlin, 1965; Deichmann and Gerarde, 1969; Arena, 1973; Sax, 1975; Dreisbach, 1977; Doull *et al.,* 1980.)

An extremely useful source of information on the treatment of acute poisoning by commercial products is *Clinical Toxicology of Commercial Products* by Gosselin and associates (1976). This book contains seven major sections. One section lists over 17,500 trade names of products that might be ingested accidentally or suicidally. It lists the manufacturer and ingredients of each commercial product and notes components believed responsible for harmful effects.

There are about 600 poison control centers in the United States, coordinated and served by the Food and Drug Administration's National Clearinghouse for Poison Control Centers. Each center has a card index with information on composition, toxicity, symptoms of poisoning, and recommended treatment for many products sold in the United States. Two microfiche systems for information on toxic substances are TOXFILE (Chicago-Micro Corporation, Chicago, Illinois) and POISINDEX (Micromedex, Inc., Denver, Colorado).

PREVENTION AND TREATMENT OF POISONING

Many acute poisonings can be prevented if physicians provide and parents accept commonsense instructions about the storage of drugs and other chemicals. These are so widely publicized that they need not be repeated here.

For clinical purposes all toxic agents can be divided into two classes: those for which a specific treatment and antidote exists and those for which there is no specific treatment. For the vast majority of drugs and other chemicals, there is no specific treatment and symptomatic medical care that supports vital functions is the only approach.

Supportive therapy, as in other medical emergencies, is the most important aspect of the treatment of drug poisoning. The adage, "Treat the patient, not the poison," remains the most basic and important principle of clinical toxicology. Maintenance of respiration and circulation takes precedence. Serial measurement and charting of vital signs and important reflexes help to judge progress of intoxication, response to therapy, and the need for additional treatment. This usually requires hospitalization. The classification in Table 68–2 is often used to indicate the severity of CNS intoxication (Henderson and Merrill, 1966; Espelin and Done, 1968). Treatment with large doses of stimulants and sedatives can often cause more harm than the poison. Chemical antidotes should be used judiciously; heroic measures are seldom necessary.

Treatment of acute poisoning must be prompt. The first goal is to keep the concentration of poison in the crucial tissues as low as possible; the second goal is to combat the pharmacological and toxicological effects at the effector sites.

Table 68–2. SIGNS AND SYMPTOMS OF CNS INTOXICATION

DEGREE OF SEVERITY	CHARACTERISTICS
	Depressants
0	Asleep, but can be aroused and can answer questions
I	Semicomatose, withdraws from painful stimuli, reflexes intact
II	Comatose, does not withdraw from painful stimuli, no respiratory or circulatory depression, most reflexes intact
III	Comatose, most or all reflexes absent, but without depression of respiration or circulation
IV	Comatose, reflexes absent, respiratory depression with cyanosis or circulatory failure and shock or both
	Stimulants
I	Restlessness, irritability, insomnia, tremor, hyperreflexia, sweating, mydriasis, flushing
II	Confusion, hyperactivity, hypertension, tachypnea, tachycardia, extrasystoles, sweating, mydriasis, flushing, mild hyperpyrexia
III	Delirium, mania, self-injury, marked hypertension, tachycardia, arrhythmias, hyperpyrexia
IV	As in III, plus convulsions, coma, and circulatory collapse

PREVENTION OF FURTHER ABSORPTION OF POISON

Emesis. Although emesis is indicated after poisoning by oral ingestion of most chemicals, it is contraindicated in certain situations. (1) If the patient has ingested a corrosive poison, such as strong acids or alkalis (*e.g.*, drain cleaners), emesis increases the likelihood of gastric perforation and further necrosis of the esophagus. (2) If the patient is comatose or in a state of stupor or delirium, emesis may cause aspiration of the gastric contents. (3) If the patient has ingested a CNS stimulant, further stimulation associated with vomiting may precipitate convulsions. (4) If the patient has ingested a petroleum distillate (*e.g.*, kerosene, gasoline, or petroleum-based liquid furniture polish), regurgitated hydrocarbons can be aspirated readily and cause chemical pneumonitis.

In the past, emesis was absolutely contraindicated after oral ingestion of petroleum distillates. However, there are marked differences in the capabilities of various petroleum distillates to produce hydrocarbon pneumonia, which is an acute, hemorrhagic necrotizing disease. In general, the ability of various hydrocarbons to produce pneumonitis is inversely proportional to the viscosity of the agent: if the viscosity is high, as with oils and greases, the risk is limited; if viscosity is low, as with mineral seal oil found in liquid furniture polishes, the risk of aspiration is high. Emesis is still contraindicated for patients who have ingested such low-viscosity petroleum distillates. Although controversial, emesis is now advocated for some cases of hydrocarbon ingestion (Rumack, 1977). All petroleum distillates produce depression of the CNS, and doses as low as 10 ml have produced fatalities; emesis is indicated when such volumes have been ingested. Emesis should also be considered after the consumption of petroleum distillates that contain potentially dangerous compounds, such as pesticides.

Vomiting can be induced mechanically by stroking the posterior pharynx or by the administration of powdered mustard in warm water. However, neither technic is entirely satisfactory.

Ipecac. The most useful household emetic is syrup of ipecac (not ipecac fluidextract, which is 14 times more potent). It is available in 1-fluidounce containers (approximately 30 ml), which may be purchased without prescription. The drug can be given orally, but it takes 15 to 30 minutes to produce emesis; this compares favorably with the time usually required for adequate gastric lavage. Furthermore, emesis is more effective in emptying the stomach than is gastric lavage (Arnold *et al.*, 1959; Abdallah and Tye, 1967; Corby *et al.*, 1967). The dose is 15 to 20 ml, and this may be repeated after 20 to 30 minutes if vomiting has not occurred. To obtain maximal results, a glass of water should be given after administration of ipecac; emesis may not occur if the stomach is empty.

Ipecac acts as an emetic because of its local irritant effect on the enteric tract (Allport, 1959) and its effect on the chemoreceptor trigger zone (CTZ) in the area postrema of the medulla (Borison and Wang, 1953). Syrup of ipecac should not be used when antiemetic drugs (such as phenothiazines) have been ingested; nor should activated charcoal be administered with ipecac, because charcoal can absorb the ipecac and reduce the emetic effect. Ipecac does produce toxic effects on the heart because of its content of emetine (*see* Chapter 46), but this is usually not a problem with the usual dose used for emesis (Manno and Manno, 1977). If emesis does not occur, these effects should be remembered and the ipecac removed by gastric lavage.

Apomorphine. Apomorphine stimulates the CTZ and causes emesis. Its advantage over ipecac is the rapidity of its action, and vomiting usually occurs within 3 to 5 minutes. However, it is not effective orally and must be given parenterally, usually by the subcutaneous route—6 mg for adults and 1 to 2 mg for children (Arena, 1975b). Additionally, the drug is often not readily available. Since apomorphine is a respiratory depressant, it should not be used if the patient has been poisoned by a CNS depressant or if the patient's respiration is slow and labored. Respiratory depression and emesis produced by apomorphine can be reversed by an opioid antagonist such as naloxone, but this usually is not necessary.

Gastric Lavage. Gastric lavage is accomplished by inserting a tube into the stomach and washing the stomach with water or a harmless solvent to remove the unabsorbed poison. The procedure should be performed only if vital functions are adequate or supportive procedures have been implemented, but it should be performed as soon as possible. Lavage may be useful for as long as 3 hours after ingestion of a poison and, if gastric emptying has been delayed, lavage may be useful for as long as 12 hours after inges-tion. The contraindications to this procedure are the same as for emesis. Unlike emesis, gastric lavage can be used for patients who are hysterical, comatose, or otherwise unco-operative.

The only equipment needed for gastric lavage is a tube and a large syringe. The tube should be as large as possible so that the wash solution, food, and the poison, whether in the form of a capsule, pill, or liquid, will flow freely and lavage can be accom-plished quickly. In children a common urethral catheter (8–12 F) and in adults a tube with an inter-nal diameter between 0.8 and 1.25 cm ($\frac{5}{16}$ and $\frac{1}{2}$ in.) is usually satisfactory (Arena, 1973). A double-lumen tube allows one to deliver fluid and aspirate simultaneously. A tracheal catheter with an inflata-ble cuff can be used to minimize or prevent aspira-tion.

During gastric lavage the patient should be placed on his left side, due to the anatomical asymmetry of the stomach, with the head hanging over the edge of the examining table and with the face down. If possible, the foot of the table should be elevated. This technic is particularly important if the patient is drowsy or comatose, because it minimizes chances of aspiration from reflex gagging (Arena, 1973).

The contents of the stomach should be aspirated with an irrigating syringe and saved for chemical analysis. The stomach may then be washed with water, saline solution, or some special solution for a specific poison (such as potassium permanganate, 1:5000, which is active against many alkaloids). Sodium chloride solution (0.45 or 0.9%) is much safer than water in young children because of the risk of water intoxication, manifested by tonic and clonic seizures and coma (Arena, 1975b). Only small volumes (120 to 300 ml) of lavage solution should be instilled into the stomach at one time so that the poison is not pushed into the intestine. Lavage should be repeated until the returns are clear, which usually requires 10 to 12 washings and a total of 1.5 to 4 liters of lavage fluid. When the lavage is com-plete, the stomach may be left empty or an antidote may be instilled through the tube. If no specific antidote is known for the poison, a thin aqueous suspension of activated charcoal or a cathartic is sometimes given.

Chemical Adsorption. Activated charcoal rapidly inactivates many poisons by adsorp-tion (*see* Holt and Holz, 1963; Corby *et al.*, 1970). It must be administered rapidly after oral ingestion of a poison; charcoal can only bind drug that is not yet absorbed from the gastrointestinal tract.

Activated charcoal is usually prepared as a mixture of two tablespoons in a glass of water (or 50 g in 400 ml of water). Then 5 ml/kg is administered ei-ther orally or via a gastric tube. Since most poisons do not appear to desorb from the charcoal, the ad-

sorbed poison need not be removed from the gastro-intestinal tract. However, the effectiveness of acti-vated charcoal can be enhanced by emesis (Corby *et al.*, 1970). As mentioned, activated charcoal should not be used simultaneously with ipecac.

A variety of adsorbents have been evaluated as alternatives to charcoal. These include cation-exchange resins (Edwards and McCredie, 1967), cholestyramine (Dordoni *et al.*, 1973), kaolin (Sorby and Plein, 1961), talc (Sorby and Plein, 1961), Alas-kan montmorillonite (Smith *et al.*, 1967), evaporated milk (Chin *et al.*, 1969), and "universal antidote" (Holt and Holz, 1963; Picchioni *et al.*, 1966). Al-though some of these substances may be useful for a specific poison, none has the general utility of acti-vated charcoal. The "universal antidote" is a mixture of 2 parts of activated charcoal, 1 part of magnesium oxide, and 1 part of tannic acid; it is available com-mercially. In practice, the "universal antidote" is less effective than activated charcoal alone in detoxifying common drugs (Sorby and Plein, 1961; Holt and Holz, 1963; Picchioni *et al.*, 1966). Some of the tannic acid is adsorbed by the charcoal, and less charcoal is thus available for adsorption of the poi-son (Daly and Cooney, 1978).

If a compound is excreted into the bile in an active form, the presence of an adsorbent in the intestine may interrupt enterohepatic circulation of the toxicant, thus enhancing its excretion. Poisoning by methylmercury can be treated with a nonabsorbable polythiol resin, which binds mercury excreted into the bile (Bakir *et al.*, 1973). Similarly, cholestyr-amine hastens the elimination of cardiac gly-cosides (Caldwell *et al.*, 1971; Chapter 30).

Chemical Inactivation. Antidotes can change the chemical nature of a poison to render it less toxic or prevent its absorption. Intoxication due to alkaloids such as atropine and morphine can be treated by gastric lavage with solutions of potassium perman-ganate, 1:5000, or tannic acid, 4% (Arena, 1975b). Formaldehyde poisoning can be treated with ammo-nia to form hexamethylenetetramine (Goldstein *et al.*, 1974); sodium formaldehyde sulfoxylate can convert mercuric ion to the less soluble metallic mercury (Gosselin *et al.*, 1976). However, these tech-nics are seldom used today because valuable time may be lost. Emetics and gastric lavage are rapid and effective.

In the past, neutralization was the usual treatment of poisoning with acids or bases. Many current books prescribe vinegar, orange juice, or lemon juice for the patient who has ingested alkali, and labels often advocate the use of basic substances for treatment of burns with acids. The use of neutralizing agents is controversial, since they may produce excessive heat when used. Carbon dioxide gas produced from car-bonates used to treat oral poisoning with acids can cause gastric distention and even perforation. The treatment of choice for poisoning with either acids or alkalis is water or milk; neither causes an exothermic chemical reaction (Rumack and Burrington, 1977). Burns on the skin should be treated with copious amounts of water.

Purgation. The rationale for using an osmotic cathartic is to minimize absorption by hastening the passage of the toxicant through the gastrointestinal tract. Few, if any, controlled clinical data are available on the effectiveness of cathartics in the treatment of poisoning. Cathartics are generally considered harmless unless the poison has injured the gastrointestinal tract. Cathartics are indicated after the ingestion of enteric-coated tablets, when the time after ingestion is greater than 1 hour, and for poisoning by volatile hydrocarbons (Rumack, 1980). Preferred agents are the saline cathartics (sodium sulfate and magnesium sulfate), which act promptly and usually have minimal toxicity.

Inhalation and Dermal Exposure to Poisons. When a poison has been inhaled, the first priority is to remove the patient from the source of exposure. Similarly, the skin should be thoroughly washed with water if it has come in contact with a poison. Even if the poison is a strong acid or base, irrigation with large volumes of water is preferred to neutralization with a base or acid. Contaminated clothing should be removed. Initial treatment of all types of chemical injuries to the eye must be rapid; thorough irrigation of the eye with water for 5 minutes should be immediately performed.

ENHANCED BIOTRANSFORMATION
AND EXCRETION OF THE POISON

Biotransformation. Many drugs are me tabolized by the cytochrome P-450 system in the endoplasmic reticulum of the liver, and this system can be induced by an array of different compounds (see Chapter 1). However, induction of these oxidative enzymes is too slow (days) to be valuable in the treatment of acute poisoning by most chemical agents.

Some poisons are conjugated with glucuronic acid, glycine, sulfate, or glutathione before elimination from the body, and the availability of the endogenous compound for conjugation may limit the rate of elimination. For example, the rate-limiting step in the elimination of salicylate is its conjugation with glycine; however, administration of the amino acid does not enhance the rate of conjugation and excretion (Yaffe et al., 1970). Detoxication of cyanide by conversion to thiocyanate can be accelerated by the administration of thiosulfate (see Chapter 70). Conversion of methanol to its highly toxic metabolite, formic acid, can be *inhibited* by administration of ethyl alcohol, a competitive

substrate for alcohol dehydrogenase (see Chapter 18). The accumulation of highly reactive electrophilic intermediates during the metabolism of drugs such as acetaminophen is a consequence of depletion of nucleophils (e.g., glutathione), which normally act as scavengers for such metabolites (see Chapter 1; Jollow et al., 1973, 1974, 1977; Mitchell et al., 1973). Administration of acetylcysteine (N-acetylcysteine) or cysteamine appears to be useful for the prevention of hepatotoxicity due to overdosage with acetaminophen (see Chapter 29; Prescott et al., 1974, 1977).

Biliary Excretion. The liver excretes many drugs and other foreign chemicals into the bile (Klaassen, 1977), but little is known about efficient ways to enhance biliary excretion of xenobiotics for the treatment of acute poisoning. Inducers of microsomal enzyme activity enhance biliary excretion of some xenobiotics (Klaassen, 1970, 1974), but the effect is slow in onset. Eventually, the procedure may be useful to enhance the elimination of certain compounds with long biological half-lives (Magos and Clarkson, 1973; Klaassen, 1975).

Urinary Excretion. Drugs and poisons are excreted into the urine by glomerular filtration and active tubular secretion (Chapter 1); they can be reabsorbed into the blood if they are in a lipid-soluble form that will penetrate the tubule or if there is an active mechanism for their transport.

There are no methods known to accelerate the active transport of poisons into urine, and enhancement of glomerular filtration is not a practical means to facilitate elimination of toxicants. However, passive reabsorption from the tubular lumen can be altered. Diuretics decrease reabsorption by decreasing the concentration gradient of the drug from the lumen to the tubular cell and by increasing flow through the tubule. Osmotic diuretics are well suited for this purpose, and mannitol is the most widely used such agent (Chapter 36). Since nonionized compounds are reabsorbed far more rapidly than ionized, polar molecules, a shift from the nonionized to the ionized species of the toxicant by alteration of the pH of the tubular fluid may hasten elimination (Chapter 1).

Acidic compounds such as phenobarbital and salicylates are cleared much more rapidly in an alkaline than in an acidic urine. The effect of increasing urine flow and alkalinization of the urine on the clearance of phenobarbital is shown in Figure 68–2. Agents used to alkalinize urine include sodium bicarbonate, sodium lactate, and inhibitors of carbonic anhydrase. Renal excretion of basic drugs such as amphetamine can be enhanced by acidification of the urine. Ammonium chloride and ascorbic acid can be used to acidify urine. Urinary excretion of an acidic compound is particularly sensitive to changes in urinary pH if its pK_a is within the range of 3.0 to 7.5; for bases the corresponding range is 7.5 to 10.5 (Milne *et al.*, 1958).

Dialysis. Procedures such as peritoneal dialysis or hemodialysis have limited use in the treatment of intoxication with chemicals; however, under certain circumstances, such procedures can be lifesaving. The efficiency of dialysis depends on the concentration gradient of the poison between the blood and the dialysis fluid. Thus, if a poison has a large volume of distribution, the plasma will contain too little of the compound for effective dialysis. Extensive binding of the compound to plasma proteins also impairs dialysis greatly. The kinetics of elimination of a toxicant by dialysis is dependent on the rate of dissociation of the compound from binding sites in plasma and tissues, and, for some chemicals, this may be too slow (*see* Maher, 1977; Gwilt and Perrier, 1978). It is important to keep the concentration of the diffusible form of the poison in the dialysate as low as possible. It may be feasible to add "traps" for the agent in question—for example, albumin for compounds that bind to the protein or an oil for lipid-soluble materials.

Peritoneal Dialysis. Peritoneal dialysis is performed by the introduction of dialysis fluid into the peritoneal cavity by means of a catheter placed through a small incision in the right section of the mesogastric region. Outflow is accomplished by making an incision in the left hypogastrium and inserting two catheters with several openings near the tip (Arena, 1975a). Up to 2000 ml of dialysis fluid can be introduced into the peritoneal cavity of an adult (about 75 to 100 ml/kg is used for infants). The fluid is usually infused over an interval of 15 to 20 minutes, and it is drained about 90 minutes later. The procedure can be repeated every 2 hours. Peritoneal dialysis requires a minimum of personnel and can be started as soon as the patient is admitted to the hospital.

Hemodialysis, Hemoperfusion, and Exchange Transfusion. Hemodialysis (extracorporeal dialysis) is being used more frequently in the treatment of acute intoxication. It is usually much more effective than peritoneal dialysis and may be essential in life-threatening intoxications. Passage of blood through a column of charcoal or adsorbent resin (hemoperfusion) is a technic for the extracorporeal removal of a poison (*see* Winchester and Gilfand, 1978). Due to the high adsorptive capacity and affinity of the material in the column, some chemicals that are bound to plasma proteins can be removed; however, at the present time, controlled studies with specific poisons are not available (Rumack, 1980). Blood-exchange transfusions can be an efficient way to remove poisons that have a small volume of distribution but that are eliminated only slowly by dialysis because, for example, of extensive and avid binding to plasma proteins.

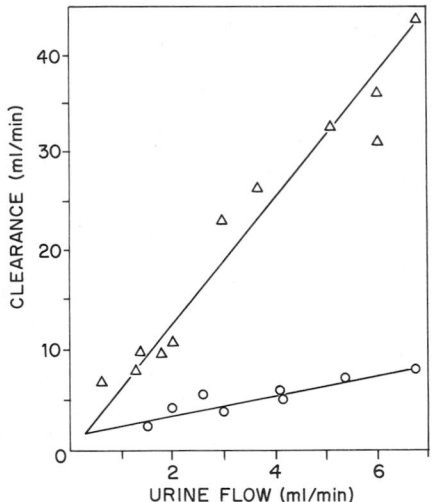

Figure 68–2. *Renal clearance of phenobarbital in the dog as it is related to rate of urine flow.*

The values designated by circles are from experiments in which diuresis was induced by administration of water orally or Na_2SO_4 intravenously and the urinary pH was below 7.0. The values designated by triangles are from experiments in which $NaHCO_3$ was administered intravenously and in which the urinary pH was 7.8 to 8.0. (After Waddell and Butler, 1957. Courtesy of *Journal of Clinical Investigation*.)

ANTAGONISM OR CHEMICAL INACTIVATION OF AN ABSORBED POISON

Functional and pharmacological antagonism of the effects of absorbed toxicants has been discussed above. If a patient is poisoned with a compound that acts as an agonist at a receptor for which a specific blocking agent is available, administration of the antagonist may be highly effective. Functional antagonism is also a cornerstone of treatment in that support of the patient's vital functions is imperative. However, drugs that stimulate antagonistic physiological mechanisms may be of little clinical value or worse. It is often difficult to titrate the effect of one drug against another when the two act on opposing systems. An example of such difficulty is the use of CNS stimulants to attempt to reverse respiratory depression. Convulsions are a typical complication of such therapy, and mechanical support of respiration is much preferred if necessary. In addition, the duration of action of the poison and the antidote may differ, sometimes leading to poisoning with the antidote.

Specific chemical antagonists of a toxicant are valuable but unfortunately rare. Chelating agents with high selectivity for certain metallic ions provide such examples (see Chapter 69). Antibodies offer the potential for the production of specific antidotes for a host of common poisons and for drugs that are frequently abused or misused. A notable example of the successful reversal of severe intoxication is by the administration of digoxin-specific antibody (see Chapter 30). There are, however, numerous difficulties to be overcome before such treatment can be generally applicable or economically feasible. The quantity of antibody required is large, populations of antibodies raised in animals are heterogeneous, and such antibodies are foreign proteins that are capable of causing severe immunological reactions. Many of these difficulties may be solved by the application of exciting new technics of cell biology. Antibodies can now be raised in tissue culture in large quantities and as the secretory product of a single clone of cells (monoclonal antibodies). Because of their monoclonal nature, the population of immunoglobulins is homogeneous and has reproducible characteristics. It should be possible to apply these technics to human cells in vitro and thus obtain products with little immunogenicity (see Melchers et al., 1978).

Abdallah, A. H., and Tye, A. A comparison of the efficacy of emetic drugs and stomach lavage. Am. J. Dis. Child., **1967,** 113, 571–575.

Albert, A. Fundamental aspects of selective toxicity. Ann. N.Y. Acad. Sci., **1965,** 123, 5–18.

Allport, R. B. Ipecac is not innocuous. J. Dis. Child., **1959,** 98, 786 787.

Ames, B. N.; McCann, J.; and Yamasaki, E. Methods for detecting carcinogens and mutagens with the Salmonella/mammalian microsome mutagenicity test. Mutat. Res., **1975,** 31, 347–364.

Arena, J. M. Poisoning—treatment and prevention. J.A.M.A., **1975a,** 232, 1272–1275; 233, 358–363, 900–903.

Arnold, F. J.; Hodges, J. B.; Barta, R. A.; Spector, S.; Sunshine, I.; and Wedgwood, R. J. Evaluation of the efficacy of lavage and induced emesis in treatment of salicylate poisoning. Pediatrics, **1959,** 23, 286–301.

Bakir, F.; Damluji, S. F.; Amin-Zaki, L.; Murtada, M.; Khalidi, A.; Al-Rawi, N. Y.; Tikriti, S.; Dhahir, H. I.; Clarkson, T. W.; Smith, J. C.; and Doherty, R. A. Methylmercury poisoning in Iraq. Science, **1973,** 181, 230–241.

Beckett, A. H.; Salmon, J. A.; and Mitchard, M. The relationship between blood levels and urinary excretion of amphetamine under controlled acidic and under fluctuating urinary pH values using [^{14}C]amphetamine. J. Pharm. Pharmacol., **1969,** 21, 251–258.

Bliss, C. I. Some principles of bioassay. Am. Sci., **1957,** 45, 449 466.

Boyd, L. J., and Scherf, D. The electrocardiogram in acute emetine intoxication. J. Pharmacol. Exp. Ther., **1941,** 71, 362–372.

Brem, T. II., and Konwaller, B. E. Fatal myocarditis due to emetine hydrochloride. Am. Heart J., **1955,** 50, 476–481.

Butler, V. P.; Watson, J. F.; Schmidt, D. H.; Gardner, J. D.; Mandel, W. J.; and Skelton, C. L. Reversal of the pharmacological and toxic effects of cardiac glycosides by specific antibodies. Pharmacol. Rev., **1973,** 25, 239–247.

Caldwell, J. H.; Bush, C. A.; and Greenberger, N. J. Interruption of the enterohepatic circulation of digitoxin by cholestyramine. II. Effect on metabolic disposition of tritium-labeled digitoxin and cardiac systolic intervals in man. J. Clin. Invest., **1971,** 50, 2638–2644.

Cera, L. J. Emetine toxicity with electrocardiographic abnormalities. Circulation, **1956,** 14, 33–37.

Chin, L.; Picchioni, A. L.; and Duplisse, B. R. Comparative antidotal effectiveness of activated charcoal, Arizona montmorillonite, and evaporated milk. J. Pharm. Sci., **1969,** 58, 1353–1356.

Clemmesen, C., and Nilsson, E. Therapeutic trends in the treatment of barbiturate poisoning: the Scandinavian method. Clin. Pharmacol. Ther., **1961,** 2, 220–229.

Corby, D. G.; Fiser, R. H.; and Decker, W. J. Re-evaluation of the use of activated charcoal in the treatment of acute poisoning. Pediatr. Clin. North Am., **1970,** 17, 545–556.

Corby, D. G.; Lisciandro, R. C.; Lehman, R. H.; and Decker, W. J. The efficiency of methods used to evacuate the stomach after acute ingestions. Pediatrics, **1967,** 40, 871–874.

Daly, J. S., and Cooney, D. O. Interference by tannic acid with the effectiveness of activated charcoal in "universal antidote." Clin. Toxicol., **1978,** 12, 512–522.

Decker, W. J.; Combs, H. F.; and Corby, D. G. Absorption of drugs and poisons by activated charcoal. Toxicol. Appl. Pharmacol., **1968,** 13, 454–460.

Dordoni, B.; Willson, R. A.; Thompson, R. P. H.; and Williams, R. Reduction of absorption of paracetamol by activated charcoal and cholestyramine: a possible therapeutic measure. Br. Med. J., **1973,** 3, 86–87.

Edwards, K. D. G., and McCredie, M. Studies on the binding properties of acidic, basic and neutral drugs to anion and cation exchange resins and charcoal in vitro. Med. J. Aust., **1967,** 1, 534–539.

Espelin, D., and Done, A. Amphetamine poisoning. N. Engl. J. Med., **1968,** 278, 1361–1365.

Gosselin, R. E., and Smith, R. P. Trends in the therapy of acute poisonings. *Clin. Pharmacol. Ther.,* **1966,** *7,* 279–299.

Gwilt, P. R., and Perrier, D. Plasma protein binding and distribution characteristics of drugs as indices of their hemodialyzability. *Clin. Pharmacol. Ther.,* **1978,** *24,* 154–161.

Hayden, J. W., and Comstock, E. G. Use of activated charcoal in acute poisoning. *Clin. Toxicol.,* **1975,** *8,* 515–533.

Henderson, L. W., and Merrill, J. P. Treatment of barbiturate intoxication with a report of recent experience at Peter Bent Brigham Hospital. *Ann. Intern. Med.,* **1966,** *64,* 876–891.

Holt, L. E., and Holz, P. H. The black bottle; a consideration of the role of charcoal in the treatment of poisoning in children. *J. Pediatr.,* **1963,** *63,* 306–314.

Jollow, D. J.; Mitchell, J. R.; Potter, W. Z.; Davis, D. C.; Gillette, J. R.; and Brodie, B. B. Acetaminophen-induced hepatic necrosis. II. Role of covalent binding *in vivo. J. Pharmacol. Exp. Ther.,* **1973,** *187,* 195–202.

Jollow, D. J.; Mitchell, J. R.; Zampaglione, N.; and Gillette, J. R. Bromobenzene-induced liver necrosis. Protective role of glutathione and evidence for 3,4-bromobenzene oxide as the hepatotoxic metabolite. *Pharmacology,* **1974,** *11,* 151–169.

Klaassen, C. D. Effects of phenobarbital on the plasma disappearance and biliary excretion of drugs in rats. *J. Pharmacol. Exp. Ther.,* **1970,** *175,* 289–300.

———. Effect of microsomal enzyme inducers on the biliary excretion of cardiac glycosides. *Ibid.,* **1974,** *191,* 201–211.

———. Biliary excretion of mercury compounds. *Toxicol. Appl. Pharmacol.,* **1975,** *33,* 356–365.

———. Biliary excretion. In, Sect. 9, *Reactions to Environmental Agents. Handbook of Physiology.* (Lee, D. H. K., ed.) American Physiological Society, Washington, D. C., **1977,** pp. 537–553.

Levy, G., and Tsuchiya, T. Effect of activated charcoal on aspirin absorption in man. *Clin. Pharmacol. Ther.,* **1972,** *13,* 317–322.

Litchfield, J. T., and Wilcoxon, F. A simplified method of evaluating dose-effect experiments. *J. Pharmacol. Exp. Ther.,* **1949,** *96,* 99–113.

Magos, L., and Clarkson, T. W. Effect of phenobarbitone on the biliary excretion of methylmercury in rats and mice. *Nature* [*New Biol.*], **1973,** *246,* 152.

Maher, J. F. Principles of dialysis and dialysis of drugs. *Am. J. Med.,* **1977,** *62,* 475–481.

Marino, A. Electrocardiographic and behavioral effects of emetine. *Science,* **1961,** *133,* 385–386.

Milne, M. D.; Schribner, B. H.; and Crawford, M. A. Non-ionic diffusion and the excretion of weak acids and bases. *Am. J. Med.,* **1958,** *24,* 709–729.

Mitchell, J. R.; Jollow, D. J.; Potter, W. Z.; Gillette, J. R.; and Brodie, B. B. Acetaminophen-induced hepatic necrosis. IV. Protective role of glutathione. *J. Pharmacol. Exp. Ther.,* **1973,** *187,* 211–217.

Picchioni, A. L.; Chin, L.; Verhulst, H. L.; and Dieterle, B. Activated charcoal vs "universal antidote" as an antidote for poisons. *Toxicol. Appl. Pharmacol.,* **1966,** *8,* 447–454.

Prescott, L. F.; Ballantyne, A.; Park, J.; Adriaenssens, P.; and Proudfoot, A. T. Treatment of paracetamol (acetaminophen) poisoning with N-acetylcysteine. *Lancet,* **1977,** *2,* 432–434.

Prescott, L. F.; Swainson, C. P.; Forrest, A. R. W.; Newton, R. W.; Wright, N.; and Matthew, H. Successful treatment of severe paracetamol overdosage with cysteamine. *Lancet,* **1974,** *1,* 588–592.

Rumack, B. H. Hydrocarbon ingestions in perspective. *J. Am. Coll. Emerg. Physicians,* **1977,** *6,* 4.

Rumack, B. H., and Burrington, J. P. Caustic ingestions: a rational look at diluents. *Clin. Toxicol.,* **1977,** *11,* 27–34.

Sayid, I. A. Auricular fibrillation after emetine injection. *Lancet,* **1935,** *2,* 556.

Smith, R. P., and Gosselin, R. E. Current concepts about the treatment of selected poisonings: nitrite, cyanide, sulfide, barium, and quinidine. *Annu. Rev. Pharmacol. Toxicol.,* **1976,** *16,* 189–199.

Smith, R. P.; Gosselin, R. E.; Henderson, J. A.; and Anderson, D. M. Comparison of the absorptive properties of activated charcoal and Alaskan montmorillonite for some common poisons. *Toxicol. Appl. Pharmacol.,* **1967,** *10,* 95–104.

Smith, R. P., and Smith, D. M. Acute ipecac poisoning: report of a fatal case and review of the literature. *N. Engl. J. Med.,* **1961,** *265,* 523–525.

Sorby, D. L., and Plein, E. M. Absorption of phenothiazine derivatives by kaolin, talc, and norit. *J. Pharm. Sci.,* **1961,** *50,* 355.

Waddell, W. J., and Butler, T. C. The distribution and excretion of phenobarbital. *J. Clin. Invest.,* **1957,** *36,* 1217–1226.

Winchester, J. F., and Gilfand, M. C. Hemoperfusion in drug intoxication: chemical and laboratory aspects. *Drug Metab. Rev.,* **1978,** *8,* 69–104.

Monographs and Reviews

Albert, A. *Selective Toxicity.* Chapman & Hall, London, **1973.**

Arena, J. M. *Poisoning: Toxicology, Symptoms, Treatments,* 3rd ed. Charles C Thomas, Pub., Springfield, Ill., **1973.**

———. Poisoning and its treatment. In, *Pediatric Therapy,* 5th ed. (Shirkey, H. C., ed.) C. V. Mosby Co., St. Louis, **1975b,** pp. 101–136.

Bochner, F.; Carruthers, G.; Kampmann, J.; and Steiner, J. *Handbook of Clinical Pharmacology.* Little, Brown & Co., Boston, **1978.**

Borison, H. L., and Wang, S. C. Physiology and pharmacology of vomiting. *Pharmacol. Rev.,* **1953,** *5,* 193–230. (194 references.)

Deichman, W. B., and Gerarde, H. W. *Toxicology of Drugs and Chemicals.* Academic Press, Inc., New York, **1969.**

Doull, J.; Klaassen, C. D.; and Amdur, M. O. (eds.). *Casarett and Doull's Toxicology: The Basic Science of Poisons,* 2nd ed. Macmillan Publishing Co., Inc., New York, **1980.**

Dreisbach, R. H. *Handbook of Poisoning,* 9th ed. Lange Medical Publications, Los Altos, Calif., **1977.**

Finney, D. J. *Probit Analysis,* 3rd ed. Cambridge University Press, Cambridge, **1971.**

Goldstein, A.; Aronow, L.; and Kalman, S. M. *Principles of Drug Action: The Basis of Pharmacology,* 2nd ed. John Wiley & Sons, Inc., New York, **1974.**

Gosselin, R. E.; Hodge, H. C.; Smith, R. P.; and Gleason, M. N. *Clinical Toxicology of Commercial Products,* 4th ed. The Williams & Wilkins Co., Baltimore, **1976.**

Jollow, D. J.; Kocsis, J. J.; Snyder, R.; and Vainio, H. *Biological Reactive Intermediates.* Plenum Press, New York, **1977.**

Levine, R. R. *Pharmacology: Drug Actions and Reactions,* 2nd ed. Little, Brown & Co., Boston, **1978.**

Loomis, T. A. *Essentials of Toxicology,* 2nd ed. Lea & Febiger, Philadelphia, **1974.**

Manno, B. R., and Manno, J. E. Toxicology of ipecac: a review. *Clin. Toxicol.,* **1977,** *10,* 221–242.

Melchers, F.; Potter, M.; and Warner, N. L. (eds.). *Lymphocyte Hybridomas,* Vol. 81. *Current Topics in Microbiology and Immunology.* Springer-Verlag, Berlin, **1978.**

Moeschlin, S. *Poisoning: Diagnosis and Treatment.* Grune & Stratton, Inc., New York, **1965.**

Rumack, B. H. Clinical toxicology. In, *Casarett and Doull's Toxicology: The Basic Science of Poisons,* 2nd ed. (Doull, J.; Klaassen, C. D.; and Amdur, M. O.; eds.) Macmillan Publishing Co., Inc., New York, **1980.**

Sax, I. N. *Dangerous Properties of Industrial Materials.* Van Nostrand Reinhold Co., New York, **1975.**

Yaffee, S. J.; Sjoqvist, F.; and Alvan, G. Pharmacological principles in the management of accidental poisoning. *Pediatr. Clin. North Am.,* **1970,** *17,* 495–507.

CHAPTER

69 HEAVY METALS AND HEAVY-METAL ANTAGONISTS

Curtis D. Klaassen

Man has always been exposed to heavy metals through natural concentrations in soil and water; in areas with high concentrations, metallic contamination of food and water probably led to the first poisonings. Metals leached from eating utensils and cookware increased the risk. The emergence of the industrial age and large-scale mining brought occupational diseases caused by various toxic metals. Metallic constituents of pesticides and therapeutic agents (*e.g.,* antimicrobials) were additional sources of hazardous exposure. The burning of fossil fuels containing heavy metals and the addition of tetraethyllead to gasoline have now made environmental pollution the major source of heavy-metal poisoning.

Heavy metals, which, of course, cannot be metabolized, persist in the body and exert their toxic effects by combining with one or more reactive groups essential for normal physiological functions (ligands). Heavy-metal antagonists (chelating agents) are designed specifically to compete with these groups for the metals, and thereby prevent or reverse toxic effects and enhance the excretion of the metals. Heavy metals, particularly those in the transition series, may react with O, S, and N ligands, which in the body take the form of $-OH$, $-COO^-$, $-OPO_3H^-$, $>C=O$, $-SH$, $-S-S-$, $-NH_2$, and $>NH$. The resultant metal complex (or coordination compound) is formed by a coordinate bond—one in which both electrons are contributed by the ligand.

The heavy-metal antagonists discussed in this chapter possess the common property of forming complexes with heavy metals and preventing or reversing the binding of metallic cations to body ligands; these drugs are all *chelating agents.* A *chelate* is a complex formed between a metal and a compound that contains two or more potential ligands. The product of such a reaction contains a heterocyclic ring. Such a chelate is usually far more stable than the nonchelate complex of the same metal with only one ligand. Five- and six-membered chelate rings are the most stable, and a polydentate (multiligand) chelator is typically designed to form such a highly stable complex. Chelates are generally less stable at low pH, and control of the pH of body fluids may be an important consideration during treatment with chelating agents.

Naturally, the stability of chelates varies with the metal and the ligand atoms. For example, lead and mercury have greater affinities for sulfur and nitrogen than for oxygen ligands; calcium behaves in the opposite manner. These differences afford selectivity of action of a chelating agent in the body, and the degree of such selectivity is, in certain circumstances, high.

The effectiveness of a chelating agent for the treatment of poisoning by a heavy metal depends on its relative affinity for that metal compared to essential metals such as calcium. However, disposition of a chelating agent in the body is also crucial. Some may not be useful because of rapid elimination by metabolism or excretion or because of a distribution that differs from that of the toxic metal. Others may form a stable complex with a toxic metal but remain immobilized at the site of such reaction by formation of ternary complexes with fixed ligand acceptors in the tissues.

An ideal chelating agent would have the following properties: high solubility in water, resistance to metabolic degradation, ability to penetrate to sites of metal storage, ready excretion of the chelate, ability to retain chelating activity at the pH of body fluids, and the property of forming complexes with metals that are less toxic than the free metallic ion. A low affinity for calcium is desirable, since calcium in plasma is readily available

1615

for chelation; a drug might serve primarily as a hypocalcemic agent despite high affinity for heavy metals. The most important property is greater affinity for the metal atom than that possessed by the endogenous ligands. The large number of available ligands in the body is a formidable barrier to the effectiveness of a chelating agent. Observations *in vitro* on chelator-metal interactions provide only a rough guide to the treatment of heavy-metal poisoning. Empirical observations *in vivo* are necessary to determine the clinical utility of a chelating agent.

LEAD

Lead enters the air, water, and soil as a result of numerous human activities. Notably, the combustion of gasoline containing tetraethyllead as an "antiknock" ingredient (about 1 ml per liter) has added large quantities of inorganic lead to the atmosphere. Lead poisoning in children with pica is clearly associated with paints applied to dwellings before World War II, when lead carbonate (white) and lead oxide (red) were common constituents of both interior and exterior house paint. In such paint, lead may constitute 5 to 40% of dried solids. Young children are poisoned most often by nibbling lead-painted windowsills and frames. The American Standards Association specified in 1955 that paints for toys, furniture, and the interior of dwellings should not contain more than 1% of lead in the final dried solids of fresh paint (National Academy of Sciences, 1972).

Acidic foods and beverages, including tomato juice, fruit juice, cola drinks, cider, and pickles, can dissolve the lead in improperly glazed containers. Food and beverage thus contaminated have caused fatal human lead poisoning. Lead is also a common contaminant of illicitly distilled whisky ("moonshine") made in the United States, since automobile radiators are frequently used as condensers and other components are connected by lead solder. Discarded automobile-battery casings made of wood and vulcanite and used as fuel during times of economic distress have caused intoxication. Sporadic cases of lead poisoning have been traced to miscellaneous sources such as lead toys, lead dust in shooting galleries, soluble lead compounds conveyed in lead pipes, artists' paint pigments, ashes and fumes of painted wood, jewelers' wastes, home battery manufacture, and lead type.

Occupational exposure to lead has decreased markedly over the last 50 years because of appropri-

ate regulations and programs of medical surveillance. Workers in lead smelters have the highest potential for exposure, since fumes are generated and dust containing lead oxide is deposited in their environment. Workers in storage-battery factories face similar risks.

Absorption, Distribution, and Excretion. The major routes of absorption of lead are from the gastrointestinal tract and the respiratory system. About 40 μg of lead is inhaled daily and, of this, 15 μg is retained by the lung and absorbed. The average daily dietary intake of lead in the United States is 120 to 350 μg, but only about 25 μg is absorbed (Kehoe *et al.,* 1933; Kehoe, 1961a, 1961b). However, children absorb a substantially greater portion (40%) of dietary lead than do adults. Little is known about lead transport across the gastrointestinal mucosa. It has been speculated that lead and calcium may compete for a common transport mechanism, since there is a reciprocal relationship between the dietary content of calcium and lead absorption.

After absorption, inorganic lead is distributed initially in the soft tissues, particularly in the tubular epithelium of the kidney (Murakami and Hirosawa, 1973) and in the liver. In time, lead is redistributed and deposited in bone, teeth, and hair. About 95% of the body burden of the metal is concentrated in bone. Only small quantities of inorganic lead accumulate in the brain, with most of that in gray matter and the basal ganglia (Task Group, 1973). Nearly all circulating inorganic lead is associated with erythrocytes; only when lead is present in relatively high concentrations does a significant portion remain in the plasma.

The deposition of lead in bone closely resembles that of calcium (Cantarow and Trumper, 1944), but it is deposited as tertiary lead phosphate. Lead in the bone salts does not contribute to toxicity. After a recent exposure, the concentration of lead is often higher in the flat bones than in the long bones (Kehoe, 1961a, 1961b), although, as a general rule, the long bones contain more lead. In the early period of deposition, the concentration of lead is highest in the epiphyseal portion of the long bones. This is especially true in growing bones, where deposits may be detected by x-ray examination as rings of increased density in the ossification centers of the epiphyseal cartilage and as a series of transverse lines in the diaphyses. Such findings are of diagnostic significance in children.

Factors that affect the distribution of calcium similarly affect that of lead. Thus, a high intake of phosphate favors skeletal storage of lead and a lower concentration in soft tissues. Conversely, a low phosphate intake mobilizes lead in bone and elevates its content in soft tissues. High intake of calcium in the absence of elevated intake of phosphate has a similar effect, owing to competition with lead for available phosphate. Vitamin D tends to promote the deposition of lead in bone if a sufficient amount of phosphate is available; otherwise, deposition of calcium preempts that of lead. Parathyroid hormone and dihydrotachysterol mobilize lead from the skeleton and augment the concentration of lead in blood and its rate of urinary excretion.

In experimental animals, lead is excreted into the bile, and much more lead is excreted into the feces than into the urine (Klaassen and Shoeman, 1974). In man, urinary excretion is a more important route (Kehoe, 1961a, 1961b), and the concentration of lead in urine is directly proportional to that in plasma (Zielhuis, 1971). However, since most lead in blood is in the erythrocytes, very little is filtered. Lead is also excreted in milk and sweat and deposited in hair and nails.

The half-life of lead in blood is about 1 month, and a steady state is thus achieved in about 5 months. After establishment of a steady state early in human life, the daily intake of lead approximates the output, under normal conditions, and concentrations of lead in soft tissues change little. However, the concentration of lead in bone appears to increase (Barry, 1975; Gross et al., 1975). Because the rate of excretion of lead is limited, even a slight increase in daily intake may produce a positive lead balance. The normal daily intake of lead is approximately 0.3 mg, while positive lead balance begins at a daily intake of about 0.6 mg. This amount will not ordinarily produce overt toxicity within a lifetime. However, the time to accumulate toxic amounts shortens disproportionately as the amount ingested rises; whereas a daily intake of 2.5 mg of lead requires nearly 4 years for the accumulation of a toxic burden, a daily intake of 3.5 mg requires but a few months, since deposition in bone is too slow to protect the soft tissues during rapid accumulation.

Acute Lead Poisoning. Acute lead poisoning is rare and occurs from ingestion of acid-soluble lead compounds. Local actions in the mouth produce marked astringency, thirst, and a metallic taste. Nausea, abdominal pain, and vomiting ensue, and the vomitus may be milky from the presence of lead chloride. Although the abdominal pain is severe, it is unlike that of chronic poisoning. Stools may be black from lead sulfide, and there may be diarrhea or constipation. If large amounts of lead are absorbed rapidly, a shock syndrome may develop. Acute central nervous system (CNS) symptoms include paresthesias, pain, and muscle weakness. An acute hemolytic crisis sometimes occurs and causes severe anemia and hemoglobinuria. The kidneys are damaged, and oliguria and urinary changes are evident. Death may occur in 1 or 2 days. If the patient survives the acute episode, characteristic signs and symptoms of chronic lead poisoning are likely to appear.

Emergency therapy includes copious gastric lavage and magnesium sulfate–induced catharsis to speed passage of lead through the intestinal tract. Although morphine may be needed for pain, atropine or other antispasmodics should be tried initially. Therapy of shock may be necessary. Chelating agents should be employed as described below.

Chronic Lead Poisoning. Signs and symptoms of chronic lead poisoning (plumbism) can be divided into six categories: gastrointestinal, neuromuscular, CNS, hematological, renal, and other. They may occur separately or in combination. The neuromuscular and CNS syndromes tend to result from intense exposure, while the abdominal syndrome is a more common manifestation of a very slowly and insidiously developing intoxication. In the United States, the CNS syndrome is the most common among children and the gastrointestinal syndrome among adults.

Gastrointestinal Effects. Lead affects the smooth muscle of the gut, producing intestinal symptoms that are an important, early sign of exposure to the metal. The abdominal syndrome often begins with vague symptoms, such as anorexia, muscle discomfort, malaise, and headache. Constipation is usually an early sign, especially in adults, but diarrhea occasionally occurs. A persistent metallic taste appears early in the course of the syndrome. As intoxication advances, anorexia and constipation become more marked. Intestinal spasm, which causes severe abdominal pain, or *lead colic,* is the most distressing feature of the advanced abdominal syndrome. The attacks are paroxysmal and generally excruciating. The abdominal muscles become rigid, and tenderness is especially manifested in the region of the umbilicus. In cases where colic is not severe, removal of the patient from the environment in which he was exposed may be sufficient for relief of symptoms. Calcium gluconate administered intravenously is recommended for relief of pain.

Neuromuscular Effects. The neuromuscular syndrome, or *lead palsy,* is now rare in the United States. It is a manifestation of advanced subacute poisoning. Muscle weakness and easy fatigue occur long before actual paralysis and may be the only symptoms. Weakness or palsy may not become evident until after extended muscle activity. The muscle groups involved are usually the most active ones (extensors of the forearm, wrist, and fingers and extraocular muscles), and the palsy often occurs only on the dominant side. Wrist-drop and, to a lesser extent, foot-drop have been considered almost pathognomonic for lead poisoning. There is no sensory involvement. Degenerative changes in the motoneurons and their axons have been described (Fullerton, 1966; Catton et al., 1970).

CNS Effects. The CNS syndrome has been termed *lead encephalopathy.* It is the most serious manifestation of lead poisoning. It occurs rarely in adults and only as a consequence of rapid, intense absorption of the metal, but the syndrome is common in children. The first clues to the development of the syndrome may be clumsiness, vertigo, ataxia, falling, headache, insomnia, restlessness, and irritability. As the encephalopathy develops, the patient may first become excited and confused; delirium with repetitive grand mal convulsions or lethargy and coma follow. Vomiting, a common sign, is usually projectile. Visual disturbances are also present. Although the signs and symptoms are characteristic of increased intracranial pressure, flap craniotomy to relieve intracranial pressure is not beneficial (Greengard *et al.,* 1962). There may be a proliferative meningitis, intense edema, punctate hemorrhages, gliosis, and areas of focal necrosis. Demyelination has been observed in nonhuman primates. The mortality rate among patients developing cerebral involvement is about 25%. Approximately 40% of survivors have neurological sequelae, such as mental retardation, EEG abnormalities or frank seizures, cerebral palsy, optic atrophy, or dystonia musculorum deformans (Sanford,·1955; Popoff *et al.,* 1963; Smith *et al.,* 1963).

Exposure to lead occasionally produces clear-cut, progressive mental deterioration in children. The history of these children indicates normal development during the first 12 to 18 months of life or longer, followed by a steady loss of motor skills and speech. They may have severe hyperkinetic and aggressive behavior disorders and a poorly controlled convulsive disorder. The lack of sensory perception severely impairs learning. Concentrations of lead in blood exceed 60 μg/dl of whole blood, and x-rays may show heavy, multiple bands of increased density in the growing long bones (*see* above). Until recently it was thought that such exposure to lead was largely restricted to those in inner-city slums. However, all children are exposed chronically to low levels of lead in their diets, in the air they breathe, and in the dirt and dust in their play areas. This is reflected in elevated concentrations of lead in blood of many children (30 to 60 μg/dl) and may be a cause of subtle CNS toxicity.

Hematological Effects. A widely known hematological manifestation of plumbism is the formation of aggregates of ribonucleic acid in erythrocytes, which produce punctate basophilic stippling. This is not unique to nor pathognomonic of lead poisoning.

Microcytic hypochromic anemia is more common than stippling and is an almost invariable finding in affected children. The anemia may result, in part, from the destruction of erythrocytes. The type of hemoglobin (HbA$_3$) found in erythrocytes of anemic children with elevated concentrations of lead in blood is characteristic of prematurely senescent erythrocytes, but the life-span of the majority of the erythrocytes is normal (Berk *et al.,* 1970). Anemia caused by lead poisoning is seldom severe.

Very low concentrations of lead influence the synthesis of heme. The enzymes necessary for heme synthesis are widely distributed in mammalian tissues, and it is highly probable that each cell synthesizes its own heme for incorporation into such proteins as hemoglobin, myoglobin, cytochromes, and catalases. Lead clearly inhibits heme formation at several points, as shown in Figure 69–1. Inhibition

of δ-aminolevulinate (δ-ALA) dehydratase and ferrochelatase, which are sulfhydryl-dependent enzymes, is well documented. Lead poisoning in both man and experimental animals is characterized by accumulation of protoporphyrin IX and nonheme iron in red blood cells, by accumulation of δ-ALA in plasma, and by increased urinary excretion of δ-ALA. There is also increased urinary excretion of coproporphyrin III (the oxidation product of coproporphyrinogen III), but it is not clear whether this is due to inhibition of enzymatic activity or other factors. Increased excretion of porphobilinogen and uroporphyrin has been reported only in severe cases. The pattern of excretion of pyrroles found in lead poisoning differs from that characteristic of acute intermittent porphyria and other hepatocellular disorders, as shown in Table 69–1. The increase in δ-ALA synthase activity is due to the reduction of the cellular concentration of heme, which regulates the synthesis of δ-ALA synthase by feedback inhibition.

Measurement of heme precursors provides a sensitive index of recent absorption of inorganic lead salts. δ-ALA dehydratase activity in hemolysates and δ-ALA in urine are sensitive indicators of exposure to lead, and abnormalities of these parameters precede the appearance of symptoms (National Academy of Sciences, 1972). Because they are early signs of abnormal exposure to lead and can be detected by relatively simple laboratory procedures, these measurements are used routinely in diagnosis.

Renal Effects. Although the renal effects of lead are less dramatic than those in the CNS and gastrointestinal tract, nephropathy does occur. Amino acids, glucose, and phosphate cannot be reabsorbed

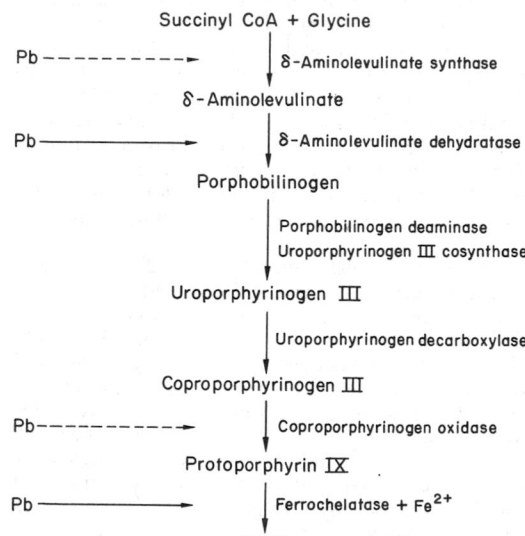

Figure 69–1. *Lead interferes with the biosynthesis of heme at several enzymatic steps.*

Steps that are definitely inhibited by lead are indicated by ——; steps at which lead is thought to act but evidence is inconclusive are indicated by – – –.

Table 69-1.   PATTERNS OF INCREASED EXCRETION OF PYRROLES IN URINE OF ACUTELY SYMPTOMATIC PATIENTS *

DISEASE	PYRROLES †			
	ALA	*PBG*	*URO*	*COPRO*
Lead poisoning	+ + +	o	±	+ + +
Acute intermittent porphyria	+ + + +	+ + + +	+ to + + + +	+ to + + +
Acute hepatitis	o	o	o	+ to + + +
Acute alcoholism	o	o	±	+ to + + +

* Modified from Chisolm, 1967.

† o = normal; + to + + + + = degree of increase; ALA = δ-aminolevulinic acid; PBG = porphobilinogen; URO = uroporphyrin; COPRO = coproporphyrin.

normally (Fanconi syndrome), and hypophosphatemia may occur. Albumin, erythrocytes, and casts are frequently found in the urine. In some patients, hyperuricemia, with or without manifest gout, may be associated with renal insufficiency (Ball and Sorensen, 1969).

Renal injury is most often observed after prolonged exposure to large amounts of lead. The resultant insufficiency is progressive and apparently irreversible. Renal biopsies and specimens obtained at autopsy show nonspecific interstitial fibrosis, tubular degeneration, and glomerular and vascular changes in small arteries and arterioles (Richet et al., 1964; Morgan et al., 1966).

Other Effects.   Other signs and symptoms of plumbism are an ashen color of the face and pallor of the lips; retinal stippling; appearance of "premature aging," with stooped posture, poor muscle tone, and emaciation; and a black or grayish so-called lead line along the gingival margin. The lead line, a result of periodontal deposition of lead sulfide, may be removed by good dental hygiene and is usually absent. Similar pigmentation may result from the absorption of mercury, bismuth, silver, thallium, or iron.

Diagnosis of Lead Poisoning.   In the absence of a positive history of abnormal exposure to lead, the clinical diagnosis of lead poisoning is easily missed. Furthermore, the signs and symptoms of lead poisoning are shared by other diseases. For example, the signs of encephalopathy may resemble those of various degenerative conditions. Physical examination does not easily distinguish lead colic from peptic ulcer, pancreatitis, or acute intermittent porphyria.

The concentration of lead in blood is the best indication of recent absorption of the metal. In normal children and adults, this value ranges from 10 to 40 μg/dl of whole blood. People with concentrations of 40 to 60 μg/dl exhibit no known functional injury or symptoms; however, they may have a definite decrease in δ-ALA dehydratase activity and a slight increase in urinary excretion of δ-ALA. Patients with a blood lead concentration of 60 to 80 μg/dl have a decrease in δ-ALA dehydratase activity in erythrocytes, an increased urinary excretion of δ-ALA and coproporphyrin, and some nonspecific, mild symptoms of lead poisoning. Clear symptoms of lead poisoning are associated with a concentration of 80 μg/dl of whole blood (Kehoe, 1961a, 1961b), and

lead encephalopathy is almost always apparent when lead concentrations are greater than 120 μg/dl (National Academy of Sciences, 1972). In persons with moderate-to-severe anemia, interpretation of the significance of concentrations of lead in blood may be improved by correcting the observed value to approximate that which would be expected if the patient's hematocrit were within the normal range.

Urinary excretion of lead in normal adults is generally less than 80 μg per liter (Kehoe, 1961a, 1961b; Goldwater and Hoover, 1967). Most patients with lead poisoning show concentrations of lead in urine of 150 to 300 μg per liter. However, in persons with chronic lead nephropathy or other forms of renal insufficiency, urinary excretion of lead may be within the normal range.

Because the onset of lead poisoning is usually insidious, it is often desirable to estimate the body burden of lead of individuals who are exposed to an environment that is contaminated with the metal. Use of the calcium disodium edetate ($CaNa_2EDTA$) mobilization test helps determine whether there is an increased body burden of lead in those in whom exposure occurred much earlier (Emmerson, 1963). This test is performed by intravenous infusion over 1 hour of 1 g of $CaNa_2EDTA$ in 250 ml of a 5% solution of dextrose. All urine is collected for 4 days. The upper limit of excretion of lead by normal adults is 600 μg under these conditions. This test is not used in symptomatic patients or in those whose concentration of lead in blood is greater than 100 μg/dl because the dose of $CaNa_2EDTA$ may be insufficient to meet therapeutic needs.

Organic Lead Poisoning.   Tetraethyllead and tetramethyllead are lipid-soluble compounds used as "antiknock" additives in gasoline. They are readily absorbed from the skin or the gastrointestinal tract, and they may also be inhaled. Nevertheless, the hazard from contact with leaded gasoline is minimal, and, because of vigorous industrial health measures, intoxication by organic lead is rare.

The major symptoms of intoxication with tetraethyllead are referable to the CNS (Sanders, 1964; Gething, 1975; Seshia et al., 1978). The victim suffers from insomnia, nightmares, anorexia, nausea and vomiting, diarrhea, headache, muscular weakness, and emotional instability. Subjective CNS symptoms such as irritability, restlessness, and anxiety are next evident. At this time there is usually hypothermia, bradycardia, and hypotension. With continued exposure, or in the case of intense acute exposure, CNS manifestations progress to delusions, ataxia, exaggerated muscular movements, and, finally, a maniacal state.

The diagnosis of poisoning by tetraethyllead is established by relating these signs and symptoms to a history of exposure. The urinary excretion of lead may increase markedly, but the concentration of lead in blood remains nearly normal. There is no effect on the metabolism of porphyrins. Basophilic stippling of erythrocytes is uncommon. In the case of severe exposure, death may occur within a few hours or may be delayed for several weeks. If death does not occur within this time, recovery is usually complete; however, instances of residual CNS damage have been reported.

CALCIUM DISODIUM EDETATE AND THE THERAPY OF LEAD POISONING

Ethylenediaminetetraacetic acid (EDTA), its sodium salt (*disodium edetate, Na$_2$EDTA*), and a number of closely related compounds have been used for years as industrial and analytical reagents because they chelate many divalent and trivalent metals. Although the first studies in animals had shown that Na$_2$EDTA causes hypocalcemic tetany, the relatively nontoxic nature of the calcium chelate (*calcium disodium edetate, CaNa$_2$EDTA*) was soon established (Popovici *et al.*, 1950). Subsequently, it was determined that CaNa$_2$EDTA could be utilized for treatment of poisoning by metals that have higher affinity for the chelating agent than does Ca^{2+}; its principal clinical use now is in lead poisoning.

The structure of calcium disodium edetate is as follows:

Calcium Disodium Edetate

Mechanism of Action. All known pharmacological effects of EDTA are due to formation of chelates with divalent and trivalent metals. CaNa$_2$EDTA will bind any available metals *in vivo* that have a greater affinity for EDTA than has calcium. Next to calcium, zinc seems to be most accessible to EDTA in the body. Intravenous administration of CaNa$_2$EDTA considerably increases the urinary excretion of zinc (Perry and Perry, 1959). There is also a slight enhancement of urinary excretion of cadmium, manganese, lead, iron, and copper.

The successful use of CaNa$_2$EDTA in the treatment of lead poisoning is due, in part, to the capacity of lead to displace calcium from the chelate. Enhanced mobilization and excretion of lead indicate that the metal is accessible to EDTA. Mercury poisoning, by contrast, does not respond to the drug, despite the fact that mercury displaces calcium from CaNa$_2$EDTA *in vitro*. Mercury is unavailable to the chelate, perhaps because it is too tightly bound by body ligands (—SH) or sequestered in body compartments that are not penetrated by CaNa$_2$EDTA. Due to its ionic character, it is unlikely that CaNa$_2$EDTA penetrates cells significantly.

Bone provides the primary source of lead that is chelated by CaNa$_2$EDTA (Hammond *et al.*, 1967; Hammond, 1971). After such chelation, lead is redistributed from soft tissues to the skeleton.

Absorption, Fate, and Excretion. CaNa$_2$-EDTA is poorly absorbed from the gastrointestinal tract (Foreman *et al.*, 1953; Foreman and Trujillo, 1954) and, when administered orally, it does not increase urinary excretion of calcium (Spencer, 1960). After intravenous administration, CaNa$_2$-EDTA disappears exponentially from the circulation with a half-life of 20 to 60 minutes. In blood, all of the drug is found in the plasma. About 50% is excreted in the urine in 1 hour and over 95% in 24 hours. For this reason, adequate renal function is necessary for successful therapy. Renal clearance of the compound in dogs equals that of inulin; glomerular filtration accounts entirely for urinary excretion (Forland *et al.*, 1966). Altering either the pH or the rate of flow of urine has no effect on the rate of excretion. Almost none of the compound is metabolized. The drug is distributed mainly in the extracellular fluids, but very little gains access to the spinal fluid (5% of the plasma concentration). The concentration of Ca^{2+} in the spinal fluid remains unchanged after injection of Na$_2$EDTA (Soffer and Toribara, 1961).

Toxicity. Rapid intravenous administration of Na$_2$EDTA causes hypocalcemic tetany. However, a slow infusion (less than 15 mg per minute) administered to a normal individual elicits no symptoms of hypocalcemia because of the ready availability of extracirculatory stores of calcium (Spencer et al., 1952). In contrast, CaNa$_2$EDTA can be administered intravenously in relatively large quantities with no untoward effects because the change in the concentration of calcium in the plasma and total body is negligible.

The principal toxic effect of CaNa$_2$EDTA is on the kidney. Death from lower-nephron nephrosis has occurred during its use in the treatment of metal poisoning. Tubular destruction can be produced by large doses of either CaNa$_2$EDTA or Na$_2$EDTA. Severe hydropic degeneration of proximal tubules has been observed in rats and man, in some cases with almost total destruction of the proximal tubular epithelium (Dudley et al., 1955; Foreman et al., 1956; Altman et al., 1962). Changes in distal tubules and glomeruli are less conspicuous. The renal effects are usually reversible, and urinary abnormalities disappear rapidly upon cessation of treatment.

Renal toxicity may be related to the large amounts of chelated metals that pass through the renal tubule in a relatively short period of time during drug therapy. Some dissociation of chelates may occur because of competition for the metal by physiological ligands or because of pH changes in the cell or the lumen of the tubule (Johnson and Seven, 1960). However, raising the pH of urine with bicarbonate does not diminish the renal toxicity of CaNa$_2$EDTA in rats (Foreman et al., 1956). Removal of essential metals from the tubular cells may also be a factor in toxicity, although tubular vacuolization during administration of CaNa$_2$EDTA has been observed in the absence of any discernible change in renal content of metal (Doolan et al., 1967). Schwartz and coworkers (1970) suggested that vacuolization reflects an induction of pinocytosis by the chelate.

A febrile systemic reaction has been observed in patients 4 to 8 hours after infusion of the drug. The reaction is characterized by a rapid onset of malaise, fatigue, and excessive thirst, followed by the sudden appearance of chills and fever. This, in turn, is followed by severe myalgia, frontal headache, anorexia, occasional nausea and vomiting, and, rarely, increased urinary frequency and urgency. Other toxic effects include a histamine-like reaction, with sneezing, nasal congestion, and lacrimation; glycosuria; anemia; dermatitis, with lesions strikingly similar to those of vitamin B$_6$ deficiency; transitory lowering of systolic and diastolic blood pressures; prolonged prothrombin time; and inversion of the T wave of the ECG.

Preparation, Routes of Administration, and Dosage. CaNa$_2$EDTA is available as *Edetate Calcium Disodium*, U.S.P. (CALCIUM DISODIUM VERSENATE). It is marketed as 500-mg tablets but is not usually given orally because of poor oral absorption. For parenteral use, *Edetate Calcium Disodium Injection*, U.S.P., a 20% solution, is employed.

For therapeutic use, 1 g (5 ml) in 250 to 500 ml of 5% glucose in water or isotonic saline solution is administered slowly by intravenous drip over a 1-hour period. A dilute solution is necessary to avoid thrombophlebitis. Two such infusions are administered daily for 3 to 5 days. The drug is then withheld for several days, after which the course may be repeated if necessary. The total daily dose should not exceed 50 mg/kg of body weight in order to avoid toxic symptoms. For children, maximal daily dosage is 70 mg/kg of body weight, divided into two doses. In patients with lead encephalopathy and increased intracranial pressure, excess fluids must be avoided. In such cases a 20% solution in 0.5 to 1.5% procaine hydrochloride solution is administered intramuscularly. Further details on the treatment of lead poisoning in children are presented below.

Edetate Disodium, U.S.P., is available as *Edetate Disodium Injection*, U.S.P. (ENDRATE, SODIUM VERSENATE). The drug is utilized for the emergency treatment of hypercalcemia and, under certain circumstances, to control arrhythmias associated with digitalis intoxication. It is marketed in 20-ml ampuls that contain 150 mg/ml or 15-ml ampuls containing 200 mg/ml. The usual dose is 50 mg/kg. The appropriate amount of the solution is diluted in 500 ml of 5% dextrose solution and is infused over a period of 2.5 to 4 hours.

Treatment of Lead Poisoning. Treatment consists in supportive measures and the use of chelating agents. Adequate urine flow must first be restored. In patients with acute lead encephalopathy, excitement, mania, and convulsions are controlled quickly by administration of diazepam. When an acute episode is over, barbiturates or phenytoin can be utilized.

The objective of therapy with chelating agents is to mobilize lead from the tissues and promote its excretion. Adults are given 1 g of CaNa$_2$EDTA by intravenous drip over a 1-hour period. Two such courses are administered each day for 3 to 5 days. The drug is then withheld for 2 days before further courses of therapy are given, if necessary. This period without drug allows redistribution of the lead, thus increasing the amount of metal available for chelation. The administration of CaNa$_2$EDTA alleviates symptoms quickly. Colic may disappear within 2 hours; muscular weakness and tremors disappear after 4 or 5 days. Coproporphyrinuria, stippled red blood cells, and gingival lead lines tend to decrease in 4 to 9 days. Urinary excretion of lead is greatest after the first infusion; it decreases with subsequent treatment due to depletion of readily accessible lead.

Lead poisoning in small children is far more dangerous than in adults. Severe lead encephalopathy has a mortality rate of up to 65% if untreated, and survivors have residual brain damage such as ataxia, impaired mental capacity, and, in very severe cases, blindness, idiocy, and hemiplegia. Early diagnosis, prompt removal of the child from exposure, and careful supportive management during the first 48 to 72 hours of CaNa$_2$EDTA administration are essential. In view of the unpredictable and fulminating course of lead encephalopathy, it is advisable to assume that all patients have potentially severe poisoning. Unfortunately, CaNa$_2$EDTA alone is less effective than is desired in the treatment of severe lead poisoning in children. Chisolm (1967, 1970) recommends that all children with lead poisoning be treated with both CaNa$_2$EDTA and *dimercaprol,* with the following dosage schedule: first dose, dimercaprol only, 4 mg/kg intramuscularly; every 4 hours thereafter, in addition to dimercaprol, CaNa$_2$EDTA, 12.5 mg/kg intramuscularly. This regimen is continued for 5 days. In this way toxic effects are minimized, urinary excretion of lead is accelerated, and there is a more rapid decrease in blood lead and urinary δ-ALA levels than during therapy with either drug alone. Of great importance is the decreased incidence of residual neurological symptoms so often seen after lead encephalopathy.

A course of dimercaprol and CaNa$_2$EDTA or CaNa$_2$EDTA alone is often followed by administration of *penicillamine.* Even though it is inferior to CaNa$_2$EDTA in accelerating excretion of lead, penicillamine is effective orally and the other two chelators are not. The daily dose is 30 to 40 mg/kg for 3 to 6 months in children who previously manifested encephalopathy, whose concentration of lead in blood exceeds 60 μg/dl, and in whom there is prominent radiographic evidence of deposition of lead in bone. In adults, the daily dose of penicillamine is 500 to 750 mg for 2 months or until the urinary excretion of lead falls below 500 μg per day. When penicillamine is given for long-term prophylactic chelation, it must be remembered that the drug can promote absorption of lead from the gut and thus favor intoxication; every effort must be made to prevent further ingestion of lead.

Lead is present in tetraethyllead in the nonionic form and is thereby inaccessible to CaNa$_2$EDTA. Symptomatic relief from administration of the chelator is slight, and the urinary excretion of lead, although increased somewhat, is not dramatic (Boyd, 1957).

DIETHYLENETRIAMINEPENTAACETIC
ACID (DTPA)

DTPA is structurally similar to EDTA, but it has a somewhat greater affinity for most heavy metals (Chaberek and Martell, 1959; Dwyer and Mellor, 1964). DTPA has thus been tried in cases of heavy-metal poisoning that do not respond to EDTA, particularly poisoning by radioactive metals. Unfortunately, success has been limited.

Like EDTA, DTPA rapidly binds calcium. For this reason, the calcium chelate, CaNa$_2$DTPA, is employed. Lack of much clinical success with DTPA is not surprising, because EDTA has a very high affinity for many of these heavy metals, and the accessibility of this class of chelators to sites of metal storage is presumably a major factor.

MERCURY

Mercury was an important constituent of drugs for centuries—as an ingredient in many diuretics, antibacterials, antiseptics, skin ointments, and laxatives. More specific and effective modes of therapy have largely replaced the mercurials, in recent decades, and drug-induced signs of mercury poisoning have become rare. Mercury poisoning from environmental pollution has, however, become a problem. Concentrations of mercury in air, soil, and water have increased because of greater use of fossil fuels, which contain mercury, and of more use of mercury in industry and agriculture. There have been epidemics of mercury poisoning among wildlife and human populations in many countries. With very few exceptions and for numerous reasons, such outbreaks were misdiagnosed for months or even years. Factors in these tragic delays included the insidious onset of the affliction, vagueness of early clinical signs, and the medical profession's unfamiliarity with the disease (Gerstner and Huff, 1977).

Chemical Forms and Sources of Mercury. With regard to the toxicity of mercury, three major chemical forms of the metal must be distinguished: mercury vapor (elemental mercury), salts of mercury, and organic mercurials.

Elemental mercury is the most volatile of the inorganic forms of the metal. Human exposure to mercury vapor is mainly occupational and has been known since antiquity. Chronic exposure to mercury in ambient air after inadvertent spills in poorly ventilated rooms, often scientific laboratories, can produce toxic effects.

Salts of mercury exist in two states of oxidation—as monovalent mercurous salts and as divalent mercuric salts. Mercurous chloride or calomel, the best-known mercurous compound, is still used in some skin creams as an antiseptic and was employed as a diuretic and cathartic. Mercuric salts are the most irritating and acutely toxic form of the metal. Mercuric nitrate was a common industrial hazard in the felt-hat industry more than 400 years ago. Occupational exposure produced neurological and behavioral changes depicted by the Mad Hatter in Lewis Carroll's *Alice's Adventures in Wonderland.* Mercuric chloride, once a widely used antiseptic, was also commonly used for suicidal purposes. Mercuric salts are still widely employed in industry, and industrial discharge of mercury into rivers has polluted many parts of the world.

The organomercurials in use today contain mercury with one covalent link to a carbon atom. This is a heterogeneous group of compounds, and its members have varying abilities to produce toxic effects. The alkylmercury salts are by far the most dangerous of these compounds; methylmercury is the most common. Alkylmercury salts have been widely used as fungicides and, as such, have produced toxic effects in man. Major incidents of human poisoning from the inadvertent consumption of mercury-treated seed grain have occurred in Iraq, Pakistan, and Guatemala. The most catastrophic outbreak occurred in Iraq in 1972. During the fall of 1971, Iraq imported large quantities of seed (wheat and barley) treated with methylmercury and distributed the grain for spring planting. Despite official warnings, the grain was ground into flour and made into bread. As a result, 6530 victims were hospitalized and 500 died (Bakir *et al.*, 1973).

Minamata disease was also due to methylmercury. Minamata is a small town in Japan, and its major industry is a chemical plant that empties its effluent directly into Minamata Bay. The chemical plant used inorganic mercury as a catalyst, and some of it was methylated before it entered the bay. In addition, microorganisms convert inorganic mercury to methylmercury; the compound is then taken up rapidly by plankton algae and is concentrated in fish via the food chain. Residents of Minamata who consumed fish as a large portion of their diet were the first to be poisoned. Eventually 121 persons were poisoned and 46 died (McAlpine and Shukuro, 1958; Smith and Smith, 1975).

Chemistry and Mechanism of Action. Mercury readily forms covalent bonds with sulfur, and it is this property that accounts for most of the biological properties of the metal. When the sulfur is in the form of sulfhydryl groups, divalent mercury replaces the hydrogen atom to form mercaptides, X—Hg—SR and Hg(SR)$_2$, where X is an electronegative radical and R is protein. Organic mercurials form mercaptides of the type RHg—SR'. Mercurials even in low concentrations are capable of inactivating sulfhydryl enzymes and thus of interfering with cellular metabolism and function. The affinity of mercury for thiols provides the basis for treatment of mercury poisoning by such agents as dimercaprol and penicillamine. Mercury also combines with other ligands of physiological importance, such as phosphoryl, carboxyl, amide, and amine groups.

The various therapeutic and toxic actions of the mercurials are associated with chemical substituents that affect solubility, dissociation, relative affinity for various cellular receptors, distribution, and excretion.

Absorption, Biotransformation, Distribution, and Excretion. *Elemental Mercury.* Elemental mercury is not particularly toxic when ingested, since the metal in this form cannot react with biologically important molecules. Furthermore, it occurs as large globular particles in the gastrointestinal tract and is absorbed very poorly. However, the vapor of elemental mercury crosses cell membranes easily and is readily absorbed through the lungs. After absorption, the dissolved vapor is rapidly oxidized in erythrocytes to produce a divalent mercuric cation (Clarkson, 1972a). Within a few hours the deposition of inhaled mercury vapor resembles that after ingestion of mercuric salts, with one important difference. Since mercury vapor crosses membranes much more readily than does divalent mercury, a significant amount of the vapor enters the brain before it is oxidized. CNS toxicity is thus more prominent after exposure to mercury vapor than to divalent forms of the metal.

Inorganic Salts of Mercury. The soluble inorganic mercuric salts (Hg^{2+}) gain access to the circulation when taken orally. The extent of absorption (about 10%) is not known with certainty; a considerable portion of the ingested Hg^{2+} may remain bound to the alimentary mucosa and the intestinal contents. Insoluble inorganic mercurous compounds, such as calomel (Hg$_2$Cl$_2$), may undergo some oxidation to soluble, absorbable compounds. Inorganic mercury has a markedly nonuniform distribution after absorption. The highest concentration of Hg^{2+} is found in the kidneys, where the metal is retained longer than in other tissues. Concentrations of inorganic mercury are similar in whole blood and plasma. Inorganic mercurials do not readily pass the blood-brain barrier or the placenta. The metal is excreted in the urine and feces; studies in laboratory animals indicate that fecal excretion is quantitatively more important (Norseth and Clarkson, 1971; Klaassen, 1976). In general, the body burden of mercury in man has a half-life of about 60 days (Friberg and Vostal, 1972).

Organic Mercurials. Organic mercurials are more completely absorbed from the gastrointestinal tract than are the inorganic salts because they are more lipid soluble and less corrosive to the intestinal mucosa. Over 90% of methylmercury is absorbed from the human gastrointestinal tract. The organic mercurials cross the blood-brain barrier and the placenta and thus produce more neurological and teratogenic effects than do the inorganic salts. Organic mercurials are also distributed more evenly to the various tissues than are the inorganic salts (Klaassen, 1975). A significant portion of the body burden of organic mercurials is in the red blood cells (Swensson and Ulfarsson, 1963); its concentration in erythrocytes is usually about five times higher than that in plasma (Bakir *et al.*, 1973). Since inorganic mercury is equally distributed between red blood cells and plasma, this difference in distribution can be used to distinguish between poisoning with inorganic and organic mercury. The carbon-mercury bond of organic mercurials is cleaved after absorption; with methylmercury the cleavage is quite slow and the inorganic mercury formed is not thought to play a major role in methylmercury toxicity (Norseth and Clarkson, 1970).

Excretion of methylmercury by man is mainly in the feces; less than 10% of a dose appears in urine (Eckman *et al.*, 1968). The biological half-life of methylmercury in man is about 65 days (Eckman *et al.*, 1968; Bakir *et al.*, 1973).

Acute Mercury Poisoning. Acute poisoning usually results from oral ingestion of highly dissociated inorganic preparations, but it may also be caused by inhalation of vapors of elemental mercury, by organic mercurials, or even by mercurial ointments applied topically. When mercuric chloride is ingested, the precipitation of proteins of the mucous membranes rapidly causes as ashen-gray appearance of the mouth, pharynx, and gastric mucosa. Intense pain in the affected tissues is aggravated by vomiting. However, vomiting is protective; if the stomach is quickly and effectively emptied, the patient's chance for survival is much greater. A high concentration of the poison may reach the epithelium of the small intestine. The local effect on the bowel soon results in severe, profuse, bloody diarrhea, and shreds of intestinal mucosa are present in the stool. Profound shock and death may result. The patient commonly recovers from the local symptoms, especially if vomiting has been extensive or chemical antidotes have been administered. If the poisoning occurs by inhalation of fumes of metallic mercury or organic mercurials, the syndrome is characterized by pneumonitis, lethargy or restlessness, fever, tachypnea, cough, chest pain, cyanosis, diarrhea, and vomiting; atelectasis, emphysema, hemorrhage, and pneumothorax often follow.

Systemic effects of the poison start within a few hours and may last for days; death may ensue. Inorganic mercury and phenylmercuric compounds act diffusely on capillary endothelium and specifically at the sites of excretion—the kidney, colon, and mouth. There is first a strong metallic taste; within 24 to 36 hours, a stomatitis develops, characterized by foul breath, sore gums, and excessive salivation. Discoloration of the gingival margins, similar to the lead line, appears later, and local infection, loosening of the teeth, and necrosis of the alveolar processes may follow. Systemic signs of acute poisoning by elemental mercury and ethylmercuric or methylmercuric compounds include those referable to the CNS, such as lethargy, excitement, hyperreflexia, and tremor.

Renal lesions produced by mercury are largely confined to the tubular epithelium, but the glomeruli are also injured. Renal function may be disturbed within a few minutes after the poison reaches the circulation. If the circulation is adequate, the first response of the kidney may be a diuresis caused by inhibition of tubular reabsorptive function. Soon, renal damage is so extensive that oliguria and finally anuria result (*see* Hammond and Beliles, 1980).

Vomiting, diarrhea, and diuresis cause hypovolemia and, usually, acidosis. In severe cases, widespread capillary damage causes capillary dilatation and shock. Protein and fluid are lost through the vessel walls, and the circulatory volume is markedly diminished. The concentration of protein in plasma is also reduced as a result of albuminuria. The excretion of mercury into the colon results in colitis, which intensifies and prolongs the diarrhea.

Chronic Mercury Poisoning. *Central Neural Effects.* The most consistent and pronounced effects of exposure to both elemental mercury vapor and short-chain alkylmercury compounds such as methylmercury are on the CNS. The effects of exposure to mercury vapor are both neurological and psychiatric. Common symptoms include depression, irritability, exaggerated response to stimulation (erethism), excessive shyness, insomnia, emotional instability, forgetfulness, confusion, and vasomotor disturbances such as excessive perspiration and uncontrolled blushing. Tremors are also common in individuals exposed to mercury vapor. These are exaggerated when a task is required but are minimal when the patient is at rest or asleep. A fine trembling of fingers, eyelids, lips, and tongue may be interrupted intermittently by coarse shaking movements. Both the erethism and the tremors are reversible (Clarkson, 1977).

Tremors also follow intoxication with methylmercury; however, sensory effects, which are not characteristic of exposure to mercury vapor, occur more consistently and at lower levels of exposure. The earliest sign is paresthesia. At somewhat higher levels of exposure other effects occur, such as ataxia, constriction of the visual field, dysarthria, and hearing defects (Table 69-2). These alterations are irreversible when poisoning is severe. Neuropsychiatric effects, so prominent after exposure to elemental mercury, occur less consistently. They are likely to involve spontaneous fits of laughing and crying and intellectual deterioration.

The CNS of the fetus appears to be especially sensitive to the toxic effects of methylmercury. Pregnant women who have been exposed to doses of methylmercury without apparent effect have given birth to children who developed cerebral palsy.

Table 69-2. FREQUENCY OF SYMPTOMS OF METHYLMERCURY POISONING IN RELATION TO CONCENTRATION OF MERCURY IN BLOOD *

CONCENTRATION OF MERCURY IN BLOOD ($\mu g/ml$)	Paresthesias	Ataxia	Visual Defects	Dysarthria	Hearing Defects	Death
0.1–0.5	5	0	0	5	0	0
0.5–1.0	42	11	21	5	5	0
1–2	60	47	53	24	5	0
2–3	79	60	56	25	13	0
3–4	82	100	58	75	36	17
4–5	100	100	83	85	66	28

* Based on data in Bakir *et al.,* 1973.

Other manifestations of neurological damage have included chorea, ataxia, tremors, seizures, and mental retardation (Koos and Longo, 1976).

Renal Effects. The kidney is the primary target of inorganic mercury, probably because the metal is most concentrated in that organ, and chronic industrial exposure to inorganic mercury salts results in nephrotoxicity. Proteinuria is often observed and, if the loss of protein is sufficient, hypoproteinemia and edema result. Exposure to inorganic mercury at levels sufficient to cause proteinuria does not increase excretion of free amino acids. Renal function is seldom affected by methylmercury, even when severe neurological effects are evident.

Other Effects. Chronic poisoning with inorganic mercury causes gingivitis, stomatitis, and excessive salivation. Mercurialentis (a colored reflex from the lens) is also observed but does not indicate intoxication. A number of nonspecific symptoms, such as anorexia, weight loss, anemia, and muscular weakness, are also associated with chronic exposure to inorganic salts of mercury.

Diagnosis of Mercury Poisoning. The upper limit of a normal concentration of mercury in blood is 0.01 to 0.03 μg/ml. Since methylmercury is concentrated in erythrocytes and inorganic mercury is not, the distribution of total mercury between red blood cells and plasma indicates whether the patient has been poisoned with inorganic or organic mercury. Measurement of total mercury in red blood cells gives a better estimate of the body burden of methylmercury. The relationship between concentrations of mercury in blood and the frequency of symptoms that result from exposure to methylmercury is shown in Table 69–2. Concentrations of mercury in plasma provide a better index of the body burden of inorganic mercury; however, the relationship between body burden and the concentration of inorganic mercury in plasma is not well documented. The relationship between the concentration of inorganic mercury in blood and toxicity depends on the form of exposure. For example, exposure to vapor results in concentrations in brain about ten times higher than those that follow an equivalent dose of inorganic mercuric salts.

The concentration of mercury in the urine has also been used as a measure of the body burden of the metal. The upper limit for excretion of mercury into urine in the normal population is 25 μg per liter. There is a linear relationship between plasma concentration and urinary excretion of mercury after exposure to vapor; workers in a chloralkali plant exhibited tremors when the concentrations of mercury in urine reached 500 μg per liter (Langolf *et al.,* 1977). In contrast, the excretion of mercury in urine is a poor indicator of the amount of methylmercury in the blood (Bakir *et al.,* 1973).

Hair is rich in sulfhydryl groups, and the concentration of mercury in hair is thus about 300 times that in blood. Furthermore, the most recent growth of hair reflects the current concentration of mercury in blood. Human hair grows about 20 cm a year, and a history of exposure may be obtained by analysis of different segments of hair.

DIMERCAPROL AND THE THERAPY OF MERCURY POISONING

History. During World War II, an intensive effort was made to develop an antidote to *lewisite,* a vesicant arsenical war gas. Knowing that arsenicals reacted with SH-containing molecules, Stocken and Thompson, at Oxford University, initiated a systematic study of thiol compounds to find one that would successfully compete with the tissue SH groups for the arsenicals (Stocken and Thompson, 1949). Their investigations indicated that the arsenicals would form a very stable and relatively nontoxic chelate ring with the dithiol compound, dimercaprol (2,3-dimercaptopropanol). When scientists in the United States joined their British colleagues in these studies, they designated dimercaprol as British antilewisite (BAL). Pharmacological investigations revealed that this compound would protect against the toxic effects of other heavy metals as well. At the end of the war, when the results of the work were published, dimercaprol was recognized as effective against poisoning by many heavy metals; such an antidote was a long-sought goal.

Chemistry. Dimercaprol has the following structure:

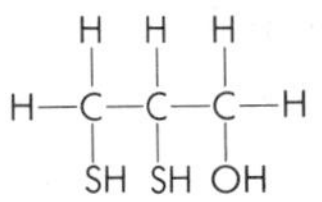

$$\begin{array}{c c c}
H & H & H \\
| & | & | \\
H-C-C-C-H \\
| & | & | \\
SH & SH & OH
\end{array}$$

Dimercaprol

It is a clear, colorless, viscous, oily fluid with a pungent, disagreeable odor typical of mercaptans. It is soluble in water (7 g/dl) and is also soluble in vegetable oils, alcohol, and various other organic solvents. Because of its instability in aqueous solution, peanut oil is the solvent employed in pharmaceutical preparations.

Dimercaprol and related thiols are readily oxidized *in vitro* in the presence of a number of catalysts. Presumably, oxidation to a cyclic S—S compound can occur *in vivo.*

Mechanism of Action. The molecular properties of the dimercaprol-metal chelate have considerable practical significance. With mercury (also with cadmium, arsenic, and possibly other heavy metals), the strategy is to maintain a complex that consists of two molecules of dimercaprol to one metal atom. The 1:1 complex is insoluble, whereas the 2:1 complex is soluble in water; moreover, the 2:1 complex is more stable. Nevertheless, dissociation of the complex and oxidation of dimercaprol can occur *in vivo.* Thus, animals injected with the preformed complex will die of mercury poisoning unless treated with dimercaprol for a period of time (Gilman *et al.,* 1946a, 1946b; Peters and Stocken, 1947). The dosage regimen is therefore designed to maintain a concentration of dimercaprol in plasma adequate to favor the continuous formation of the 2:1 complex and its rapid excretion. However, because of pronounced and dose-related side effects, excessive plasma concentrations must be avoided. The concentration in plasma must therefore be maintained by repeated fractional dosage until the offending metal can be excreted.

Dimercaprol is much more effective if given as soon as possible after exposure to mercury (Longcope and Leutscher, 1946), because it is more effective in preventing inhibition of sulfhydryl enzymes than in reactivating them. This therapeutic principle applies to the use of all chelating agents.

Dimercaprol antagonizes the biological actions of metals that form mercaptides with essential cellular sulfhydryl groups, principally arsenic, mercury, and cadmium. Intoxication by selenites, which oxidize sulfhydryl enzymes, is not influenced by dimercaprol. Other metals occupy an intermediate position.

Absorption, Fate, and Excretion. Dimercaprol cannot be administered orally; it is given intramuscularly as a 10% solution in oil. Peak concentrations in blood are attained in 30 to 60 minutes. The half-life is short, and metabolic degradation and excretion are essentially complete within 4 hours. Following injection of dimercaprol into experimental animals, there is a sharp rise in urinary excretion of neutral sulfur, which accounts for approximately 50% of the sulfur adminis-

tered as dimercaprol. There is no increase in ethereal sulfur. A rise in urinary glucuronic acid suggests that a portion of dimercaprol may be excreted as glucuronide.

Toxicity. In man, the administration of dimercaprol produces a variety of side effects that are more alarming than serious; nevertheless, they limit the amount of dithiol that can be administered. Reactions to dimercaprol occur in approximately 50% of subjects receiving 5 mg/kg intramuscularly. The effects of repeated administration of this dose are not cumulative if an interval of at least 4 hours elapses between injections. One of the most consistent responses to dimercaprol is a rise in systolic and diastolic arterial pressures, accompanied by tachycardia. The rise in pressure is roughly proportional to the dose administered and may be as great as 50 mm Hg in response to the second of two doses (5 mg/kg) given 2 hours apart. The pressure rises immediately but returns to normal within 2 hours. Other signs and symptoms, many of which tend to parallel the change in blood pressure in time and intensity, are the following, listed in approximate order of frequency: (1) nausea and, in some instances, vomiting; (2) headache; (3) a burning sensation in the lips, mouth, and throat and a feeling of constriction, sometimes pain, in the throat, chest, or hands; (4) conjunctivitis, lacrimation, rhinorrhea, and salivation; (5) tingling of the hands; (6) a burning sensation in the penis; (7) sweating of the forehead, hands, and other areas; (8) abdominal pain; and (9) occasional appearance of painful sterile abscesses at the injection site. Symptoms are often accompanied by a feeling of anxiety and unrest. Because the dimercaprol-metal complex breaks down easily in an acidic medium, production of an alkaline urine protects the kidney during therapy.

Children react as do adults, although approximately 30% may also experience a fever that disappears upon withdrawal of the drug. A transient reduction of the percentage of polymorphonuclear leukocytes may also be observed. Two children who, through an error in dosage, received inordinately large amounts of dimercaprol (one, 40 mg/kg; the other, 25 mg/kg, repeated in 4 hours) exhibited vasomotor changes, hypertension, convulsions, and coma. Recovery appeared to be complete within an hour after the onset of brief convulsions.

Preparations. *Dimercaprol, U.S.P.* (*2,3-dimercaptopropanol, BAL*), is available in the form of *Dimercaprol Injection, U.S.P.*, a solution of 10% dimercaprol (w/v) and benzyl benzoate in vegetable oil. Each milliliter contains 100 mg of dimercaprol. The preparation is marketed in 3-ml ampuls.

Use of Dimercaprol in the Treatment of Mercury Poisoning. The recommended dose of dimercaprol for treatment of mercury poisoning is 5 mg/kg given once, intramuscularly, and 2.5 mg/kg given every 8 or 12 hours during the first day of therapy and every 12 or 24 hours thereafter for 10 days or until recovery. Children tolerate dimercaprol as well as do adults if the dosage is calculated on the basis of body weight.

Experimental observations indicate that dimercaprol, even at high doses, is unable to reduce concentrations of mercury in brain (Berlin and Rylander, 1964; Berlin and Lewander, 1965; Magos, 1968). Dimercaprol cannot alleviate neurological disorders caused by exposure to mercury vapor. It is also ineffective in protecting experimental animals against lethal doses of methylmercury (Glomme and Gustavson, 1959) and has not been effective in treating symptoms of human brain damage from methylmercury (Hays *et al.*, 1963). Thus, dimercaprol should not be regarded as a useful therapeutic agent for all cases of mercury poisoning. It is most effective in protection against renal damage due to acute exposure to inorganic mercury salts.

2,3-DIMERCAPTOSUCCINIC ACID

2,3-Dimercaptosuccinic acid has the following structure:

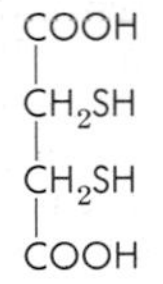

COOH
|
CH$_2$SH
|
CH$_2$SH
|
COOH

2,3-Dimercaptosuccinic Acid

It is a disulfhydryl compound and is thus similar to dimercaprol. However, it is about 30 times less toxic than dimercaprol and is effective orally (Graziano *et al.*, 1978b). While its use is still experimental, 2,3-dimercaptosuccinic acid is a promising, orally effective, relatively nontoxic chelator for the treatment of not only mercury poisoning (Friedheim and Corvi, 1975; Magos, 1976) but also poisoning with arsenic (Graziano *et al.*, 1978a) and lead (Friedheim *et al.*, 1976; Graziano *et al.*, 1978b).

PENICILLAMINE AND THE THERAPY OF MERCURY POISONING

Penicillamine is D-β,β-dimethylcysteine. Its structure is as follows:

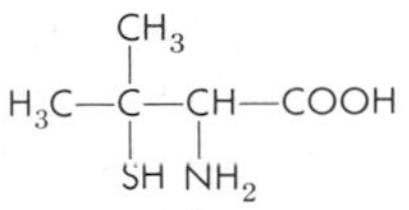

CH$_3$
|
H$_3$C—C—CH—COOH
| |
SH NH$_2$
Penicillamine

It is prepared by the hydrolytic degradation of penicillin. Penicillamine is an effective chelator of copper, mercury, zinc, and lead and promotes the excretion of these metals in the urine.

Absorption, Fate, and Excretion. Penicillamine is well absorbed from the gastrointestinal tract and, therefore, has a decided advantage over other chelating agents. It is rapidly excreted in the urine. Unlike cysteine, the nonmethylated parent compound, it is somewhat resistant to attack by cysteine desulfhydrase or L-amino acid oxidase (Aposhian, 1961). As a result, penicillamine is relatively stable *in vivo*. This probably explains the effectiveness of penicillamine and the lack of effectiveness of cysteine in promoting excretion of metals, although *in vitro* both compounds form stable metal chelates. This explanation is further substantiated by the fact that N-acetylpenicillamine is even more effective than penicillamine in protecting against the toxic effects of mercury (Aposhian and Aposhian, 1959), because the acetylated derivative is more resistant to metabolic degradation than is the parent compound.

Toxicity. D-Penicillamine is relatively nontoxic, and much of the toxicity reported is attributable to use of the L or D,L forms. L-Penicillamine inhibits enzymes that are dependent on pyridoxal (Aposhian, 1961). The toxic effects in rats given high doses of penicillamine resemble those seen in pyridoxine deficiency and are reversed by feeding the vitamin (Heddle *et al.*, 1963). In human beings, pyridoxine antagonism is readily demonstrated with the L and the D,L forms, but rarely with the D form.

Acute allergic reactions, manifested by fever, rashes (pruritic, morbilliform, and urticarial), leukopenia, eosinophilia, and thrombocytopenia, have been encountered early in the course of therapy. These reactions require prompt discontinuation of the drug. Desensitization with small doses of the drug or administration of corticosteroids may overcome these reactions. Rarely, one or more of these side effects prevent the use of penicillamine. Anorexia, nausea, and vomiting occur infrequently. Loss of taste for salt and sweet has been observed (Knudsen and Weismann, 1978). Several cases of nephrotoxicity have been reported, even in patients given only D-penicillamine (Adams et al., 1964; Sternlieb and Scheinberg, 1964; Rosenberg and Hayslett, 1967; Elsas et al., 1971). A case of optic neuritis, assumed to be drug related, has also occurred. It responded to treatment with pyridoxine (Tu et al., 1963). After therapy for 1 to 2 years' duration a systemic lupus erythematosus–like syndrome has been observed. Extravasation of blood into the skin over pressure points (elbows, knees, toes) occurs in some patients after prolonged administration of high doses of penicillamine. Plasma proteins and tests of coagulation remain normal. Individuals who are allergic to penicillin may have a similar reaction to penicillamine.

Preparations and Dosage. *Penicillamine,* U.S.P., the D-isomer, is a white crystalline, water-soluble powder. In aqueous solution, it is comparatively stable at pH 2 to 4. The drug is dispensed as 125- or 250-mg capsules, *Penicillamine Capsules,* U.S.P. (CUPRIMINE). It is administered orally, 1 to 4 g per day, in four divided doses. It is given while the stomach is empty to avoid interference by metals in food. Potassium sulfide, 40 mg, is also given with each meal to minimize absorption of copper when the drug is used to treat hepatolenticular degeneration.

Use of Penicillamine in the Treatment of Mercury Poisoning. The original observation that D-penicillamine increased the urinary excretion of copper (Walshe, 1956) led to its use in the treatment of heavy-metal poisoning (Boulding and Baker, 1957; Aposhian, 1958). Increased urinary excretion of mercury after administration of penicillamine has been demonstrated in people exposed to mercury vapor (Smith and Miller, 1961; Parameshvara, 1967; Goldblatt et al., 1971), and penicillamine appears to be the agent of choice for such intoxication. Penicillamine also facilitates the removal of methylmercury from the body; however, clinical efficacy in the treatment of intoxication with methylmercury is not impressive (Bakir et al., 1976). The dose of penicillamine normally used in the treatment of poisoning with inorganic mercury (1 g per day) produces only a small reduction in the concentration of methylmercury in the blood; larger doses (2 g per day) are needed. During the initial 1 to 3 days of administration of penicillamine the concentration of mercury in the blood increases before it decreases. This is prob-

ably due to the mobilization of metal from tissues to blood at a rate more rapid than that at which mercury is excreted into urine and feces.

Other Uses. As mentioned, penicillamine is an effective chelator *in vivo* not only of mercury but also of copper, zinc, and lead. The use of penicillamine in the treatment of lead poisoning has been described earlier in this chapter. Since the drug is effective orally, it can be given for the long periods of "de-leading" that are often required.

Penicillamine is effective in the treatment of *hepatolenticular degeneration* (Wilson's disease) (Sternlieb and Scheinberg, 1964). The disease is due to deposition of toxic amounts of copper in various tissues and is associated with a deficiency of ceruloplasmin, a copper-containing plasma protein. Therefore, promotion of copper excretion, coupled with a reduction in copper intake, is a rational approach to therapy. Patients treated in this way with penicillamine exhibit marked clinical improvement, particularly in the neurological manifestations. Patients who are originally asymptomatic do not develop clinical symptoms if treated prophylactically. Occasionally it is desirable to use both dimercaprol and penicillamine to treat patients with Wilson's disease.

Penicillamine is of value in the treatment of *cystinuria* and the associated nephrolithiasis. In a dose of 30 mg/kg per day, it lowers or eliminates urinary cystine and prevents further development of stones (MacDonald and Fellers, 1966). In some cases it reduces the size of stones and finally dissolves them after 6 to 12 months of therapy. The mechanism of action is believed to involve the formation of penicillamine-cysteine disulfide, which is 50 times more soluble in water than is the cysteine-cysteine disulfide (cystine).

Penicillamine treatment of *rheumatoid arthritis* is promising (Multicentre Trial Group, 1973). Patients who would be considered suitable for gold therapy also respond well to penicillamine. As with gold therapy, a beneficial effect is seen only after several weeks of treatment, and arthritic symptoms return if the drug is withdrawn prematurely. Its use in rheumatoid arthritis does not appear to be related to its metal-binding properties.

POLYTHIOL RESINS AND HEMODIALYSIS IN THE THERAPY OF METHYLMERCURY POISONING

Methylmercury compounds undergo extensive enterohepatic recirculation in experimental animals (Norseth and Clarkson, 1971). Therefore, introduction of a nonabsorbable mercury-binding substance into the intestinal tract should facilitate their removal from the body. A polythiol resin has been used for this purpose in man and appears to be effective (Bakir et al., 1973). The resin has certain advantages over penicillamine. It does not cause redistribution of mercury in the body with a subsequent increase in the concentration of mercury in blood, and it has fewer adverse effects than do sulfhydryl agents that are absorbed.

While a considerable amount of methylmercury concentrates in erythrocytes, little is contained in the plasma; conventional hemodialysis is thus of little value. However, it has been shown that L-cysteine can be infused into the arterial blood entering the dialyzer to convert methylmercury into a diffusible form (Al-Abbasi *et al.*, 1978). Both free cysteine and the methylmercury-cysteine complex formed in the blood then diffuse across the membrane into the dialysate.

ARSENIC

Arsenic was known more than 2400 years ago in Greece and Rome as a therapeutic agent and poison. The history and folklore of arsenic prompted intensive studies by early pharmacologists. Indeed, the foundations of many modern concepts of chemotherapy derive from Ehrlich's early work with organic arsenicals. The advent of penicillin disposed of antiluetic arsenicals, and newer drugs have nearly eclipsed the use of other organic arsenicals. In current therapeutics, arsenicals are important only in the treatment of certain tropical diseases (*see* Chapter 47). In the United States the impact of arsenic on health is currently more from industrial and environmental exposures than from medicinal exposure.

Arsenic is found in soil, water, and air as a common environmental toxicant. The element is usually not mined as such but is recovered as a by-product from the smelting of copper, lead, zinc, and other ores. This can lead to the release of arsenic into the environment. Mineral-spring waters and the effluent from geothermal power plants leach arsenic from soils and rocks containing high concentrations of the metal (Fowler, 1977). Arsenic has been found in some sources of drinking water. It is also present in coal at variable concentrations and is released into the environment during combustion. Application of pesticides and herbicides containing arsenic has increased its environmental dispersion. Fruits and vegetables sprayed with arsenicals may also be a source of this element, and it is concentrated in many species of fish and shellfish. Arsenicals are sometimes used as feed additives for poultry and other livestock to promote growth.

The average daily human intake of arsenic is about 900 μg (Lisella *et al.*, 1972). Almost all of this is ingested with food and water. The normal body burden in adults is about 20 mg.

Chemical Forms of Arsenic. The arsenic atom exists in the elemental form and in trivalent and pentavalent oxidation states. The toxicity of a given arsenical is related to the rate of its clearance from the body and, therefore, to its degree of accumulation in tissues. In general, toxicity increases in the sequence of $RAs—X < As^{5+} < As^{3+} <$ arsine (AsH_3).

The organic arsenicals contain arsenic linked to a carbon atom by a covalent bond, where arsenic exists in the trivalent or pentavalent state. Arsphenamine contains trivalent arsenic; sodium arsanilate contains arsenic in the pentavalent form.

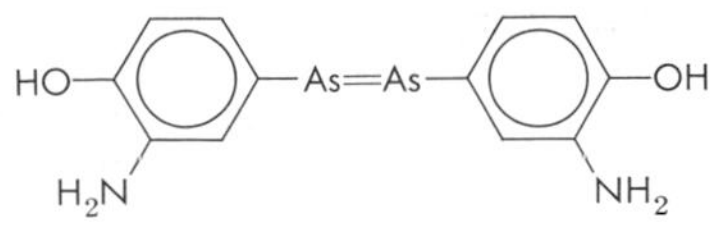

Arsphenamine

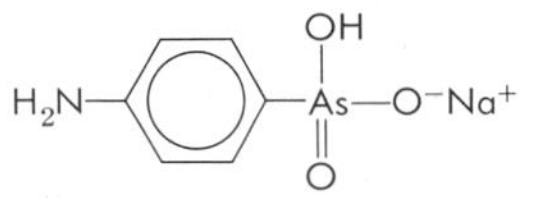

Sodium Arsanilate

The organic arsenicals are usually excreted more rapidly than are the inorganic forms.

The pentavalent oxidation state is found in arsenates (such as lead arsenate, $PbHAsO_4$), which are salts of arsenic acid, H_3AsO_4. The pentavalent arsenicals have very low affinity for thiol groups, in contrast to the trivalent compounds, and are much less toxic. The arsenites, for example, potassium arsenite $(KAsO_2)$, and salts of arsenious acid $(H_2As_2O_3)$ contain trivalent arsenic. Arsine (AsH_3) is a gaseous hydride of trivalent arsenic; it produces toxic effects that are distinct from those of the other arsenic compounds.

Mechanism of Action. Arsenate has long been known to uncouple mitochondrial oxidative phosphorylation. The mechanism is thought to be related to competitive substitution of arsenate for inorganic phosphate, with subsequent formation of an unstable arsenate ester that is rapidly hydrolyzed. This process is termed *arsenolysis*.

Trivalent arsenicals, including inorganic arsenite, are regarded primarily as sulfhydryl reagents. As such, they inhibit many enzymes. The pyruvate dehydrogenase system is especially sensitive to trivalent arsenicals because of their interaction with two sulfhydryl groups of lipoic acid to form a stable six-membered ring, as shown below.

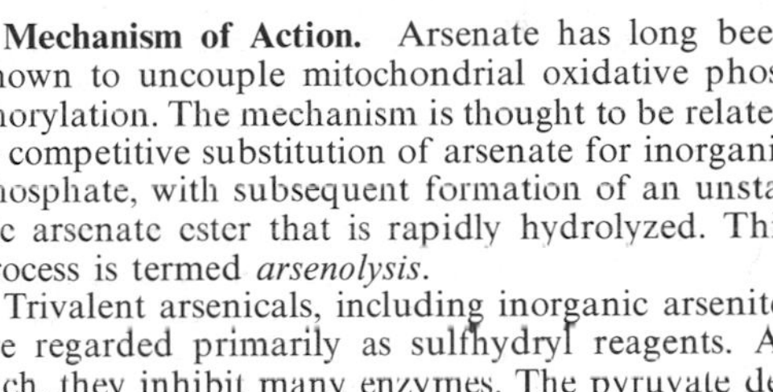

Absorption, Distribution, and Excretion. The absorption of poorly water-soluble arsenicals, such as As_2O_3, greatly depends upon the physical state of the compound. Coarsely powdered material is less toxic because it can be eliminated in feces before it dissolves. The arsenite salts are more soluble in water and are better absorbed than the oxide. The pentavalent inorganic arsenicals are better absorbed than the trivalent compounds, probably because they react less with the intestinal contents and mucosa.

The trivalent organic arsenicals are also generally poorly absorbed from the gastrointestinal tract. Pentavalent organic compounds are absorbed to varying extents. Some have been given orally in the treatment of systemic infections; others are poorly absorbed and can be effective against intraintestinal parasites.

The distribution of arsenic depends upon the duration of administration and the particular arsenical involved. Arsenic is stored mainly in liver, kidney, wall of the gastrointestinal tract, spleen, and lung. Much smaller amounts are found in muscle and neural tissue. Because of the high sulfhydryl content of keratin, high concentrations of arsenic are found in the hair and nails. Deposition in the hair starts within 2 weeks after administration, and arsenic stays fixed at this site for years. It is also deposited in bone and retained there for long peroids. Arsenic readily crosses the placental barrier, and fetal damage has been reported in animals and human beings (Ferm and Carpenter, 1968; Lugo *et al.*, 1969).

Little is known about the biotransformations of arsenicals in man. Some pentavalent arsenicals are partly reduced *in vivo* to the trivalent form. However, the redox equilibria *in vivo* favor oxidation, and trivalent arsenic is slowly oxidized in the body to the pentavalent state. The low toxicity and high recovery of pentavalent arsenicals in urine and excreta indicate that very little reduction takes place. It seems probable that both trivalent and pentavalent forms are partly converted to methylarsenates.

The fraction of a dose of trivalent arsenical that is absorbed is excreted slowly. While arsenic is eliminated by many routes (feces, urine, sweat, milk, hair, skin, lungs), most is excreted in urine and feces. Arsenite salts are excreted mainly in the feces, while arsenates are predominantly eliminated in the urine. It may take 10 days for complete elimination of arsenite after a single dose and up to 70 days after repeated administration. This slow excretion is the basis for the cumulative toxic action of arsenic. The pentavalent forms are so rapidly excreted by man that very little accumulates unless very large doses are given over a period of time.

Pharmacological and Toxicological Effects of Arsenic. Arsenicals have vesicant effects on the skin, causing necrosis and sloughing. They also have a number of systemic effects.

Circulation. Small doses of inorganic arsenic induce mild vasodilatation. Larger doses evoke capillary dilatation; increased capillary permeability may occur in all capillary beds, but it is most pronounced in the splanchnic area. Transudation of plasma and a sharp diminution in blood volume result. Arteriolar and myocardial damage appears later, and the blood pressure falls profoundly. ECG abnormalities may persist for months after recovery from acute intoxication.

Gastrointestinal Tract. Small doses of inorganic arsenicals, especially the trivalent compounds, cause mild splanchnic hyperemia. Capillary transudation of plasma, resulting from larger doses, produces vesicles under the gastrointestinal mucosa. These eventually rupture, epithelial fragments slough off, and plasma is discharged into the lumen of the intestine, where it coagulates. Tissue damage and the bulk cathartic action of the increased fluid in the lumen lead to increased peristalsis and characteristic "rice-water" stools. Normal proliferation of the epithelium is suppressed, which accentuates the damage. Soon the feces become bloody. Vomiting frequently occurs, and the vomitus may be bloody. Stomatitis may also be evident. The onset of gastrointestinal symptoms may be so gradual that the possibility of arsenic poisoning may be overlooked.

Kidneys. The action of arsenic on the renal capillaries, tubules, and glomeruli may cause severe renal damage. The initial effect is on the glomeruli. The vessels dilate, allow the escape of protein, and swell to fill the glomerular capsule. There are varying degrees of tubular necrosis and degeneration. The urine is scant and contains protein, red blood cells, and casts.

Skin. Chronic ingestion of low doses of inorganic arsenicals causes cutaneous vasodilatation and a "milk and roses" complexion. Prolonged use of arsenic, however, also causes hyperkeratosis and hyperpigmentation. Eventually these actions proceed to atrophy and degeneration, and possibly to cancer. Skin eruptions are common after inorganic arsenic medication.

Central Nervous System. Chronic exposure to inorganic but rarely to organic arsenicals may cause peripheral neuritis. In severe cases, the spinal cord may also be involved. After acute ingestion of toxic doses of inorganic arsenic, approximately 5% of the patients have central depression without gastrointestinal symptoms. Encephalopathy is the most common type of toxic response to trivalent organic arsenicals. Symptoms include severe headache, high fever, convulsions, and coma. Premonitory signs are increases in the cell count and protein content of the spinal fluid. The cerebral lesions are mainly vascular in origin and occur in both the gray and white matter; characteristic multiple, symmetrical foci of hemorrhagic necrosis occur. In addition to dimercaprol, treatment consists in anticonvulsant therapy and measures designed to reduce cerebral edema, such as intravenous injection of hypertonic mannitol solution.

Blood. Inorganic arsenicals affect the bone marrow and alter the cellular composition of the blood. The vascularity of the bone marrow is increased. Moderate doses of arsenic lower the erythrocyte count, and large doses cause morphological changes with the appearance of megalocytes and microcytes. Inorganic arsenicals also suppress production of leukocytes. Some of the chronic hematological effects may result from impaired absorption of folic acid (Van Tongeren *et al.*, 1965). Arsenites also interfere with the synthesis of porphyrins. Blood and bone-marrow disturbances from organic arsenicals are extremely serious, but they are rare. A few cases of agranulocytosis have reportedly been caused by glycobiarsol.

Liver. Inorganic arsenicals and a number of now-obsolete organic arsenicals are particularly toxic to the liver and produce fatty infiltration, central necrosis, and cirrhosis; tryparsamide may induce hepatic damage in therapeutic doses. The damage may be mild or so severe that acute yellow atrophy and death ensue. The injury is generally to the hepatic parenchyma, but in some cases the clinical picture may closely resemble occlusion of the common bile duct, the principal lesions being pericholangiitis and bile thrombi in the finer biliary radicles.

Metabolic Effects. The early toxic actions of inorganic arsenicals give rise to occult edema due to capillary damage and may be mistaken for a gain in weight, which was once misinterpreted as a "tonic" effect. In arsenic poisoning, elimination of nitrogen is increased because of extensive damage to tissues.

Carcinogenesis and Teratogenesis. Arsenic causes chromosomal breaks in cultured human leukocytes and teratogenic effects in hamsters, but whether such effects occur in man is unknown. There is overwhelming epidemiological evidence that chronic ingestion of arsenic in drinking water or chronic exposure from the use of inorganic arsenicals in sheep-dip or vineyard sprays predisposes to intraepidermal squamous-cell and superficial basal-cell carcinomas of the skin. Evidence has also accumulated that the chronic use of Fowler's solution (potassium arsenite) for psoriasis or other disorders causes skin cancer (Fierz, 1965; Novey and Martel, 1969). Among metal workers, there is a strong correlation between the intensity and duration of exposure to arsenic and lung cancer (Lee and Fraumeni, 1969). The carcinogenicity of arsenic has been reviewed by Buchanan (1962) and Black (1967).

Acute Arsenic Poisoning. Federal restrictions on the allowable content of arsenic in food and in the occupational environment not only have improved safety procedures and decreased the number of intoxications but also have decreased the amount of arsenic in use; only the annual production of arsenic-containing herbicides is increasing.

The incidence of accidental, homicidal, and suicidal arsenic poisoning has greatly diminished in recent decades. Arsenic in the form of As_2O_3 used to be a common cause of poisoning because it is readily available, is practically tasteless, and has the appearance of sugar.

Gastrointestinal discomfort is usually experienced within an hour after intake of an arsenical, although it may be delayed as much as 12 hours after oral ingestion if food is in the stomach. Burning lips, constriction of the throat, and difficulty in swallowing may be the first symptoms, followed by excruciating gastric pain, projectile vomiting, and severe diarrhea. The urine is scanty, albuminous, and bloody; eventually anuria may occur. The patient often complains of marked skeletal muscle cramps and severe thirst. As the loss of fluid proceeds, symptoms of shock appear. Hypoxic convulsions may occur terminally, and coma and death ensue. In severe poisoning, death can occur within an hour, but the usual interval is 24 hours.

Because of vigorous therapy, patients who previously would have died from the effects of fluid loss during the acute phase of arsenic poisoning now often survive, only to develop neuropathies and other disorders. In a series of 57 such patients, 37 had peripheral neuropathy and 5 had encephalopathy. The motor system appears to be spared only in the mildest cases; severe crippling is common (Jenkins, 1966).

Chronic Arsenic Poisoning. The most common early signs of chronic arsenic poisoning are diarrhea, skin pigmentation (especially of the neck, eyelids, nipples, and axillae), hyperkeratosis, and circumscribed edema, especially of the lower eyelids, face, and ankles. Other signs and symptoms that should arouse suspicion of arsenic poisoning include garlic odor of the breath and perspiration, excessive salivation and sweating, stomatitis, generalized itching, sore throat, coryza, lacrimation, numbness, burning or tingling of the extremities, dermatitis, vitiligo, and alopecia. Poisoning may begin insidiously with symptoms of weakness, languor, anorexia, occasional nausea and vomiting, and diarrhea or constipation. Subsequent symptoms may simulate acute coryza. Dermatitis and keratosis of the palms and soles are common features. Desquamation and scaling of the skin may initiate an exfoliative process involving many epithelial structures of the body. The liver may enlarge, and obstruction of the bile ducts may result in jaundice. Eventually cirrhosis may occur from the hepatotoxic action. The renal glomeruli and tubules are damaged.

As intoxication advances, encephalopathy may develop. Peripheral neuritis results in motor and sensory paralysis of the extremities; usually the legs are more severely affected than the arms, in contrast to lead palsy.

The bone marrow is seriously injured by arsenic. All elements of the myeloid tissue may be depressed, and aplastic anemia is the hematopoietic disorder most often encountered.

Therapy of Arsenic Poisoning. In the event of *acute arsenic poisoning,* dimercaprol in oil should be administered intramuscularly at the earliest possible opportunity. If poisoning is severe, single doses of 3 mg/kg should be given at 4-hour intervals during the first 48 hours. On the third day, the interval between injections should be increased to 6 hours; thereafter, the dosage interval can be increased to every 12 hours for an additional 10 days or until recovery. Because treatment with dimercaprol is relatively innocuous, a short course (six doses of 2.5 mg/kg at 4-hour intervals) can be given whenever arsenic poisoning is suspected. In addition to dimercaprol, copious gastric lavage and saline cathartics should be given if the poison was taken orally, particularly if powdered arsenic was ingested, because this material may remain in the stomach for some time. Efforts should be directed as soon as possible toward repair of fluid and electrolyte deficits. Morphine is of great value in controlling pain. Further symptomatic treatment is instituted as indicated but is usually unnecessary if therapy with dimercaprol is prompt and adequate.

Dimercaprol is also generally effective in the treatment of *chronic poisoning* by either inorganic or organic arsenicals. Clinical improvement may occur in 1 to 3 days, and recovery is the rule within 1 to 3 weeks, depending on the organ or system involved. However, if damage has become irreversible, as with aplastic anemia, advanced encephalopathy, and most cases of jaundice, the removal of arsenic from the body is of little help. Chronic intoxication should be treated with prolonged courses of dimercaprol. An exacerbation of symptoms following an initial course of therapy demands prompt initiation of a second course. Glucocorticoids may be indicated if dermatitis or conjunctivitis exists.

Arsine. Arsine gas, generated by electrolytic or metallic reduction of arsenic in metal products, is a rare cause of industrial intoxication. Arsine is bound to erythrocytes, rendering the red blood cells exceedingly fragile; massive hemolysis occurs if the exposure is sufficient. A few hours after exposure, headache, anorexia, vomiting, paresthesia, abdominal pain, chills, hematemesis, hemoglobinuria, bilirubinemia, and anuria occur. Jaundice appears after 24 hours. A coppery skin pigmentation is frequently observed and is thought to be due to methemoglobin (Macaulay and Stanley, 1956). Kidneys of persons poisoned by arsine characteristically contain casts of hemoglobin, and there is cloudy swelling and necrosis of the cells of the proximal tubule (Hocken and Bradshaw, 1970; Uldall *et al.*, 1970). Death results from renal failure. Treatment is that for an acute massive hemolysis. Dimercaprol is not effective.

CADMIUM

Cadmium ranks close to lead and mercury as a metal of current toxicological concern. It occurs in nature in association with zinc and lead. Extraction of these ores also pollutes the environment with cadmium. Before the beginning of this century, the use of cadmium was infrequent. However, recognition of its valuable metallurgical properties, such as resistance to corrosion, has increased its use markedly, for example, in the manufacture of alloys and as an electroplated coating on steel. It is widely used in nickel cadmium batteries. Coal and other fossil fuels contain cadmium, and their combustion releases the element into the environment.

Workers in smelters and other metal-processing plants may be exposed to high concentrations of cadmium in the air; however, for most of the population, exposure from contamination of food is most important. Uncontaminated foodstuffs contain less than 0.05 μg of cadmium per gram wet weight, and the average daily intake is about 50 μg. Drinking water normally does not significantly contribute to cadmium intake; cigarette smoking does. Shellfish and animal liver and kidney are among the foods that may have concentrations higher than 0.05 μg/g, even under normal circumstances. When foods such as rice and wheat are contaminated by cadmium in soil and water, the concentration of the metal may increase considerably (1 μg/g).

In Fuchu, Japan, shortly after World War II, numerous patients, mainly multiparous women, complained of rheumatic and myalgic pains; the disease was named *itai-itai* ("ouch-ouch"). It was determined that cadmium in the local rice played an

etiological role. The source of the metal was the effluent from a Pb-Zn-Cd mine located upstream from the rice fields.

Absorption, Distribution, and Excretion. Cadmium occurs only in one valence state, 2 +, and does not form stable alkyl compounds or other organometallic compounds of known toxicological significance.

Cadmium is poorly absorbed from the gastrointestinal tract. Studies in laboratory animals indicate the extent of absorption to be only about 1.5% (Decker *et al.*, 1957; Klaassen and Kotsonis, 1977), and limited studies in man indicate a value of about 5% (Rahola *et al.*, 1972). Absorption from the respiratory tract appears to be more complete; cigarette smokers may absorb 10 to 40% of inhaled cadmium (Friberg *et al.*, 1974).

After absorption, cadmium has a strong preferential affinity for liver and kidney. About 50% of the total body burden is found in these two organs. Liver and kidney also contain a low-molecular-weight protein that is called metallothionein because it has a high affinity for metals such as cadmium and zinc; one third of its amino acid residues are cysteine (Kägi and Vallee, 1960, 1961). This metal-binding protein may act as a scavenging agent and lower the concentration of cadmium at more critical sites within the cell. Cadmium also appears to induce the synthesis of this protein.

The half-life of cadmium in the body is 10 to 30 years, and concentrations of the metal in tissues thus increase throughout life. The body burden of cadmium in a 50-year-old adult in the United States is about 30 mg (Friberg *et al.*, 1974). Cadmium is probably the environmental poison most prone to accumulation. After a single intravenous injection of cadmium into laboratory animals, the biliary route of excretion is quantitatively more important than the urinary route (Klaassen and Kotsonis, 1977). After multiple exposures the biliary excretion of cadmium is almost abolished because of binding to metallothionein (Klaassen, 1978).

Acute Cadmium Poisoning. Acute poisoning may result from inhalation of cadmium dusts and fumes (usually cadmium oxide) and from the ingestion of cadmium salts. The major toxic effects are due to local irritation. In the case of oral intake, these include nausea, vomiting, salivation, diarrhea, and abdominal cramps. Cadmium is more toxic when inhaled. Signs and symptoms, which appear after a few hours, include irritation of the upper respiratory tract, chest pains, nausea, dizziness, and diarrhea. Permanent lung damage may occur in the form of emphysema and peribronchial and perivascular fibrosis (Beton *et al.*, 1966; Blejer *et al.*, 1966; Zavon and Meadow, 1970). Death is usually due to massive pulmonary edema.

Chronic Cadmium Poisoning. The toxic effects of chronic exposure to cadmium differ somewhat with the route of exposure. The kidney is affected following either pulmonary or gastrointestinal exposure; marked effects are observed in the lungs only after exposure by inhalation.

Kidney. When the concentration of cadmium in the kidney reaches a level of 200 $\mu g/g$, there is renal injury. It seems probable that binding of the metal by metallothionein protects the organ when concentrations are lower (Kotsonis and Klaassen, 1978). Proteinuria is due to decreased tubular reabsorption of low-molecular-weight proteins that are present in the glomerular filtrate (Piscator, 1962, 1966; Kazantzis *et al.*, 1963). The quantitation of β_2-microglobulin in urine appears to be the most sensitive index of cadmium-induced nephrotoxicity (Piscator and Pettersson, 1977). In severe cases the rate of glomerular filtration is decreased and there is glycosuria and amino aciduria (Kazantzis *et al.*, 1963; Piscator, 1966).

Lung. The consequence of excessive inhalation of cadmium fumes and dusts is loss of ventilatory capacity, with a corresponding increase in residual lung volume. The disease thus has the cardinal features of emphysema.

The pathogenesis of cadmium-induced emphysema and pulmonary fibrosis is not well understood. However, cadmium specifically inhibits plasma α_1-antitrypsin (Chowdhury and Louria, 1976), and there is an association between severe α_1-antitrypsin deficiency of genetic origin and emphysema in man.

Cardiovascular System. Perhaps the most controversial issue concerning the effects of cadmium on man is the suggestion that the metal plays a significant role in the etiology of hypertension (Schroeder, 1965). The initial study was epidemiological. People dying from hypertension were found to have significantly higher concentrations of cadmium and higher cadmium-to-zinc ratios in their kidneys than people dying of other causes. Others have found similar correlations (Thind and Fischer, 1976; Voors and Shuman, 1977). Cadmium-induced hypertension has been reported in female rats after prolonged exposure to the metal in their drinking water (Schroeder and Vinton, 1962; Perry and Erlanger, 1974). This finding has not, however, been uniform (Porter *et al.*, 1974; Doyle *et al.*, 1975; Kotsonis and Klaassen, 1977, 1978). Hypertension is not prominent in either industrial cadmium poisoning or *itai itai*.

Bone. One of the hallmarks of *itai-itai* was osteomalacia. However, studies in Sweden and the United Kingdom have failed to corroborate this effect of cadmium poisoning (Friberg, 1950; Kazantzis *et al.*, 1963; Adams *et al.*, 1969). The intake of calcium and fat-soluble vitamins such as vitamin D is much higher in these countries than in Japan. The Japanese victims were mostly women, and the average had been pregnant six times. Thus, there appears to be an interaction between cadmium, nutrition, and bone disease. The effect of cadmium may be due to interference with renal regulation of calcium and phosphate balance.

Testis. Testicular necrosis, a common characteristic of acute exposure to cadmium in experimental animals, is uncommon when exposure has been chronic and at low concentrations (Kotsonis and Klaassen, 1978). Cadmium-induced testicular necrosis has not been observed in man.

Therapy of Cadmium Poisoning. Little is known about the management of cadmium poisoning, but several chelating agents have been studied with regard to mobilization of the metal. Dimercaprol chelates and markedly increases urinary excretion of cadmium in rabbits; however, it also increases mortality from renal injury produced by cadmium (Gilman *et al.*, 1946b). Apparently some cadmium-dimercaprol chelate dissociates in the kidney and thereby increases the cadmium concentration and subsequent renal injury. CaNa$_2$EDTA has been shown to be an effective chelator in some studies (Sivjakov, 1959; Eybl and Sykora, 1966), but others have observed increased renal injury (Friberg, 1956). Chelating agents are thus generally contraindicated for the treatment of cadmium poisoning.

IRON

Although iron is not an environmental poison, accidental intoxication with ferrous salts used to treat iron-deficiency anemias has made iron a frequent toxicological problem in young children. Acute iron poisoning is discussed in Chapter 56.

DEFEROXAMINE AND THE THERAPY OF IRON POISONING

The structure of deferoxamine is below. It is isolated as the iron chelate from *Streptomyces pilosus* and is treated chemically to obtain the metal-free ligand. Deferoxamine has the desirable properties of a remarkably high affinity for ferric iron ($K_a = 10^{31}$) coupled with a very low affinity for calcium ($K_a = 10^2$). It readily competes for the iron of ferritin and hemosiderin, but it removes only a small amount of the iron of transferrin. The iron in cytochromes and hemoglobin is inaccessible to deferoxamine. Less than 15% of an oral dose is absorbed, and parenteral administration is required in most cases. Given orally, deferoxamine binds iron in the lumen of the bowel and renders the metal nonabsorbable. Deferoxamine is metabolized principally by plasma enzymes, but the pathways have not yet been defined. The drug is also readily excreted in the urine.

$$H_2N—(CH_2)_5—N—C—(CH_2)_2—C—N—(CH_2)_5—N—C—(CH_2)_2—C—N—(CH_2)_5—N—C—CH_3$$

Deferoxamine

Deferoxamine causes a number of toxic effects. Reactions have included hypotension, probably due to release of histamine (especially during intravenous administration), skin rashes, and gastrointestinal irritation. Occasional cases of cataract formation in man have been reported, and similar effects have been seen experimentally in dogs. Although chronic renal infection may be exacerbated in some patients, renal damage in otherwise-normal individuals has not been demonstrated, even after 2 years of deferoxamine therapy.

Preparations, Dosage, and Uses. *Sterile Deferoxamine Mesylate,* U.S.P. (DESFERAL MESYLATE), is available in ampuls containing 500 mg of the drug. The recommended dose in acute oral iron poisoning is 8 g by nasogastric tube, followed by the parenteral procedures described below. For the mobilization of iron from storage sites the intramuscular route is preferred, unless the patient is in shock. Initially, for adults and children, 1 g is given, followed by 500 mg every 4 hours for two doses. The 500-mg injections may be continued at 4- or 12-hour intervals, depending on the clinical response, but the total amount of drug administered should not exceed 6 g in 24 hours. The intravenous route is required when a patient is in shock. The dosage schedule and limitations are the same as those indicated for the intramuscular route. However, the infusion rate must never exceed 15 mg/kg per hour. As soon as the clinical situation permits, intravenous administration should be discontinued and the drug given intramuscularly. Other aspects of the treatment of acute iron poisoning are discussed in Chapter 56.

Although results of deferoxamine therapy in primary hemochromatosis and hemosiderosis secondary to hepatic cirrhosis are disappointing, some patients with transfusion siderosis respond well to deferoxamine therapy. The dosage and frequency of administration must be tailored to the individual patient according to the severity of the disease and the rate of urinary iron excretion.

RADIOACTIVE HEAVY METALS

The widespread production and use of radioactive heavy metals for nuclear generation of electricity, nuclear weapons, laboratory research, and medical diagnosis have generated unique problems in dealing with accidental poisoning by such metals. The toxicity of radiation energy became apparent when many of the pioneer radiologists and nuclear physicists died of skin or bone cancer and when Muller demonstrated in 1929 that such energy produced somatic and inheritable mutations. Since the toxicity of radioactive metals is almost entirely a consequence of ionizing radiation, the therapeutic objective following exposure is not just the chelation of the metals but their removal from the body as rapidly and completely as possible.

Treatment of the acute radiation syndrome is largely symptomatic. Attempts have been made to investigate the effectiveness of organic reducing agents (such as cysteamine), administered in an attempt to prevent the formation of free radicals. Success has been limited.

Major products of a nuclear accident or the use of weapons include ^{239}Pu and ^{90}Sr. The latter and isotopes of Ra have proven to be extremely difficult to remove from the body with chelating agents. This is due to two factors. One is that their affinity for calcium chelates is no greater than that of calcium itself, so that little replacement takes place when, for example, CaNa$_2$EDTA is administered. The second, more insidious factor is that radiations from strontium and radium in bone destroy nearby capillaries; blood flow in bone is thereby compromised, and the radioisotopes become imprisoned. ^{239}Pu exerts its toxic effects in bone mainly as soluble salts and in the lungs and gastrointestinal tract as insoluble salts. Diethylenetriaminepentaacetate (DTPA) has been shown to be an effective chelating agent for promoting the excretion of ^{239}Pu (Bair and Thompson, 1974). One gram of DTPA, administered by slow intravenous drip on alternate days, three times per week, has enhanced excretion 50- to 100-fold in animals and in human subjects exposed in accidents. As is seen commonly with heavy-metal poisoning, effectiveness of treatment diminishes very rapidly with an increased time between exposure and the initiation of therapy.

Adams, D. A.; Goodman, R.; Maxwell, M. H.; and Latta, H.   Nephrotic syndrome associated with penicillamine therapy of Wilson's disease. *Am. J. Med.,* **1964,** *36,* 330–336.

Adams, R. G.; Harrison, J. F.; and Scott, P.   The development of cadmium-induced proteinuria, impaired renal function and osteomalacia in alkaline battery workers. *Q. J. Med.,* **1969,** *38,* 425–443.

Al-Abbasi, A. H.; Kostyniak, P. J.; and Clarkson, T. W.   An extracorporeal complexing hemodialysis system for the treatment of methylmercury poisoning. III. Clinical applications. *J. Pharmacol. Exp. Ther.,* **1978,** *207,* 249–254.

Altman, J.; Watkim, K. G.; and Winkelmann, R. K.   Effects of edathamil disodium on the kidney. *J. Invest. Dermatol.,* **1962,** *38,* 215–218.

Aposhian, H. V.   Protection by D-penicillamine against the lethal effects of mercuric chloride. *Science,* **1958,** *128,* 93.
——— .   Biochemical and pharmacological properties of the metal-binding agent penicillamine. *Fed. Proc.,* **1961,** *20,* Suppl. 10, 185–188.

Aposhian, H. V., and Aposhian, M. M.   N-acetyl-DL-penicillamine, a new oral protective agent against the lethal effects of mercuric chloride. *J. Pharmacol. Exp. Ther.,* **1959,** *126,* 131–135.

Bakir, F.; Al-Khalidi, A.; Clarkson, T. W.; and Greenwood, R.   Clinical observations on treatment of alkylmercury poisoning in hospital patients. *Bull. WHO,* **1976,** *53,* Suppl., 87–92.

Bakir, F.; Damluji, S. F.; Amin-Zaki, L.; Mortadha, M.; Khalidi, A.; Al-Rawi, N. Y.; Tikriti, S.; Dhahir, H. I.; Clarkson, T. W.; Smith, J. C.; and Doherty, R. A.   Methylmercury poisoning in Iraq. An interuniversity report. *Science,* **1973,** *181,* 230–241.

Ball, G. V., and Sorensen, L. B.   Pathogenesis of hyperuricemia in saturnine gout. *N. Engl. J. Med.,* **1969,** *280,* 1199–1202.

Barry, P. S. I. A comparison of concentrations of lead in human tissues. *Br. J. Ind. Med.,* **1975,** *32,* 119–139.

Berk, P. D.; Tschudy, D. P.; Shepley, L. A.; Waggnoner, J. G.; and Berlin, N. I. Hematologic and biochemical studies in a case of lead poisoning. *Am. J. Med.,* **1970,** *48,* 137–144.

Berlin, M., and Lewander, T. Increased brain uptake of mercury caused by 2,3-dimercaptopropanol (BAL) in mice given mercuric chloride. *Acta Pharmacol. Toxicol. (Kbh.),* **1965,** *22,* 1–7.

Berlin, M., and Rylander, R. Increased brain uptake induced by 2,3-dimercaptopropanol (BAL) in mice exposed to phenylmercuric acetate. *J. Pharmacol. Exp. Ther.,* **1964,** *146,* 236–240.

Beton, D. C.; Andrews, G. S.; Davies, H. J.; Howells, L.; and Smith, G. F. Acute cadmium fume poisoning, five cases with one death from renal necrosis. *Br. J. Ind. Med.,* **1966,** *23,* 292–301.

Black, M. M. Prolonged ingestion of arsenic. *Pharm. J.,* **1967,** *199,* 593–597.

Blejer, H. P.; Caplan, P. E.; and Alcocer, A. E. Acute cadmium fume poisoning in welders—a fatal and a non-fatal case in California. *Calif. Med.,* **1966,** *105,* 290–296.

Boulding, J. E., and Baker, R. A. The treatment of metal poisoning with penicillamine. *Lancet,* **1957,** *2,* 985.

Boyd, P. R. The treatment of tetraethyl lead poisoning. *Lancet,* **1957,** *1,* 181–185.

Catton, M. J.; Harrison, M. J. G.; Fullerton, P. M.; and Kazantzis, G. Subclinical neuropathy in lead workers. *Br. Med. J.,* **1970,** *2,* 80–82.

Chisolm, J. J., Jr. Treatment of acute lead intoxication—choice of chelating agents and supportive therapeutic measures. *Clin. Toxicol.,* **1970,** *3,* 527–540.

Chowdhury, P., and Louria, D. B. Influence of cadmium and other trace metals on human α_1-antitrypsin; an *in vitro* study. *Science,* **1976,** *191,* 480–481.

Decker, C. F.; Byerrum, R. V.; and Hoppert, C. A. A study of the distribution and retention of cadmium-115 in the albino rat. *Arch. Biochem. Biophys.,* **1957,** *66,* 140–145.

Doolan, P. D.; Schwartz, S. L.; Hayes, J. R.; Mullen, J. C.; and Cummings, N. B. An evaluation of the nephrotoxicity of ethylenediaminetetraacetate and diethylenetriaminepentaacctate in the rat. *Toxicol. Appl. Pharmacol.,* **1967,** *10,* 481–500.

Doyle, J. J.; Bernhoft, R. A.; and Sanstead, H. H. The effects of a low level of dietary cadmium on blood pressure, ^{22}Na, ^{42}K, and water retention in growing rats. *J. Lab. Clin. Med.,* **1975,** *86,* 57–63.

Dudley, H. R.; Ritchie, A. C.; Schilling, A.; and Baker, W. H. Pathologic changes associated with the use of sodium ethylenediaminetetraacetate in the treatment of hypercalcemia. *N. Engl. J. Med.,* **1955,** *252,* 331–337.

Eckman, L.; Greitz, V.; Magi, A.; Snihs, J. O.; and Aberg, B. Metabolism and retention of methyl-203-mercury nitrate in man. *Nord. Med.,* **1968,** *79,* 450–456.

Elsas, L. J.; Hayslett, J. P.; Spargo, B. H.; Durant, J. L.; and Rosenberg, L. E. Wilson's disease with reversible renal tubular dysfunction. Correlation with proximal tubular ultrastructure. *Ann. Intern. Med.,* **1971,** *75,* 427–433.

Emmerson, B. T. Chronic lead neuropathy: the diagnostic use of calcium EDTA and the association with gout. *Aust. Ann. Med.,* **1963,** *12,* 310–324.

Eybl, V., and Sykora, J. Die Schutzwirkung von Chelatbildnern bei der akuten Kadmiumchloridvergiftung. *Acta Biol. Med. Ger.,* **1966,** *16,* 61–64.

Ferm, V. H., and Carpenter, S. J. Malformation induced by sodium arsenate. *J. Reprod. Fertil.,* **1968,** *17,* 199–201.

Fierz, V. Katamnestische Untersuchungen über die Nebenwirkungen der Therapie mit anorganischem Arsen bei Hautkrankheiten. *Dermatologica,* **1965,** *131,* 41–58.

Foreman, H.; Finnegan, C.; and Lushbaugh, C. C. Nephrotoxic hazards from uncontrolled edathamil calcium disodium therapy. *J.A.M.A.,* **1956,** *160,* 1042–1046.

Foreman, H., and Trujillo, T. T. The metabolism of C^{14} labeled ethylenediaminetetraacetic acid in human beings. *J. Lab. Clin. Med.,* **1954,** *43,* 566–571.

Foreman, H.; Vier, M.; and Magee, M. The metabolism of C^{14}-labeled ethylenediaminetetraacetic acid in the rat. *J. Biol. Chem.,* **1953,** *203,* 1045–1053.

Forland, M.; Pullman, T. N.; Lavender, A. R.; and Aho, I. The renal excretion of ethylenediaminetetraacetate in the dog. *J. Pharmacol. Exp. Ther.,* **1966,** *153,* 142–147.

Fowler, B. A. Toxicology of environmental arsenic. In, *Advances in Modern Toxicology.* Vol. 2, *Toxicology of Trace Elements.* (Goyer, R. A., and Mehlman, M. A., eds.) Hemisphere Publishing Co., Washington, D. C., 1977, pp. 79–122.

Friberg, L. Health hazards in the manufacture of alkaline accumulators with special reference to chronic cadmium poisoning. *Acta Med. Scand.,* **1950,** *138,* Suppl. 240, 1–24.

————. Edathamil calcium-disodium in cadmium poisoning. *Arch. Ind. Health,* **1956,** *13,* 13–23.

Friedheim, E., and Corvi, C. Meso-dimercaptosuccinic acid: a chelating agent for the treatment of mercury poisoning. *J. Pharm. Pharmacol.,* **1975,** *27,* 624–626.

Friedheim, E.; Corvi, C.; and Walker, C. J. Meso-dimercaptosuccinic acid: a chelating agent for the treatment of mercury and lead poisoning. *J. Pharm. Pharmacol.,* **1976,** *28,* 711–712.

Fullerton, P. M. Chronic peripheral neuropathy produced by lead poisoning in guinea pigs. *J. Neuropathol. Exp. Neurol.,* **1966,** *25,* 214–236.

Gerstner, H., and Huff, J. Clinical toxicology of mercury. *J. Toxicol. Environ. Health,* **1977,** *2,* 491–526.

Gething, J. Tetramethyl lead absorption: a report of human exposure to a high level of tetramethyl lead. *Br. J. Ind. Med.,* **1975,** *32,* 329–333.

Gilman, A.; Allen, R. P.; Philips, F. S.; and St. John, E. The treatment of acute systemic mercury poisoning in experimental animals with BAL, thiosorbitol and BAL glucoside. *J. Clin. Invest.,* **1946a,** *25,* 549–556.

Gilman, A.; Philips, F. S.; Allen, R. P.; and Koelle, E. The treatment of acute cadmium intoxication in rabbits with 2,3-dimercaptopropanol (BAL) and other mercaptans. *J. Pharmacol. Exp. Ther.,* **1946b,** *87,* Suppl., 85–101.

Glomme, J., and Gustavson, K. H. Treatment of experimental acute mercury poisoning by chelating agents BAL and EDTA. *Acta Med. Scand.,* **1959,** *164,* 175–182.

Goldblatt, D.; Greenwood, M. R.; and Clarkson, T. W. Chronic metallic mercury poisoning treated with N-acetyl-penicillamine. *Neurology (Minneap.),* **1971,** *21,* 439.

Goldwater, L. J., and Hoover, A. W. An international study of "normal" levels of lead in blood and urine. *Arch. Environ. Health,* **1967,** *15,* 60–63.

Graziano, J. H.; Cuccia, D.; and Friedheim, C. Potential usefulness of 2,3-dimercaptosuccinic acid for the treatment of arsenic poisoning. *J. Pharmacol. Exp. Ther.,* **1978a,** *207,* 1051–1055.

Graziano, J. H.; Leong, J. K.; and Friedheim, E. 2,3-Dimercaptosuccinic acid: a new agent for the treatment of lead poisoning. *Ibid.,* **1978b,** *206,* 696–700.

Greengard, J.; Voris, D. C.; and Hayden, R. The surgical therapy of acute lead encephalopathy. *J.A.M.A.,* **1962,** *180,* 660–664.

Gross, J. B.; Pfitzer, E. A.; Yeager, D. W.; and Kehoe, R. A. Lead in human tissues. *Toxicol. Appl. Pharmacol.,* **1975,** *32,* 638–651.

Hammond, P. B. The effects of chelating agents on the tissue distribution and excretion of lead. *Toxicol. Appl. Pharmacol.,* **1971,** *18,* 296–310.

Hammond, P. B.; Aronson, A. L.; and Olson, W. C. The mechanism of mobilization of lead by ethylenediaminetetraacetate. *J. Pharmacol. Exp. Ther.,* **1967,** *157,* 196–206.

Hay, W. J.; Richards, A. G.; McMenemey, W. H.; and Cummings, J. N. Organic mercurial encephalopathy. *J. Neurol. Neurosurg. Psychiatry,* **1963,** *26,* 199–202.

Heddle, J. G.; McHenery, E. W.; and Beaton, G. H. Penicillamine and vitamin B_6 interrelationships in the rat. *Can. J. Biochem. Physiol.*, **1963**, *41*, 1215–1222.

Hocken, A. G., and Bradshaw, G. Arsine poisoning. *Br. J. Ind. Med.*, **1970**, *27*, 56–60.

Jenkins, R. B. Inorganic arsenic and the nervous system. *Brain*, **1966**, *89*, 479–498.

Johnson, L. A., and Seven, M. J. Observations on the *in vivo* stability of metal chelates. In, *Metal-Binding in Medicine*. (Seven, M. J., ed.) J. B. Lippincott Co., Philadelphia, **1960**, pp. 225–229.

Kägi, J., and Vallee, B. Metallothionein: a cadmium- and zinc-containing protein from equine renal cortex. *J. Biol. Chem.*, **1960**, *235*, 3460–3465.

———. Metallothionein: a cadmium- and zinc-containing protein from equine renal cortex. II. Physicochemical properties. *Ibid.*, **1961**, *236*, 2435–2442.

Kazantzis, G.; Flynn, F. V.; Spowage, J.; and Trott, D. G. Renal tubular malfunction and pulmonary emphysema in cadmium pigment workers. *Q. J. Med.*, **1963**, *32*, 165–192.

Kehoe, R. A. The metabolism of lead in man in health and disease. *Arch. Environ. Health*, **1961a**, *2*, 418–422.

———. The metabolism of lead in man in health and disease: The Harben Lectures, 1960. *J. R. Inst. Public Health Hyg.*, **1961b**, *24*, 81–97, 101–120, 129–143.

Kehoe, R. A.; Thamann, F.; and Cholak, J. On the normal absorption and excretion of lead. II. Lead absorption and lead excretion in modern American life. *J. Ind. Hyg.*, **1933**, *15*, 273–288.

Klaassen, C. D. Biliary excretion of mercury compounds. *Toxicol. Appl. Pharmacol.*, **1975**, *33*, 356–365.

———. Effect of metallothionein on the hepatic disposition of metals. *Am. J. Physiol.*, **1978**, *234*, E47–E53.

Klaassen, C. D., and Kotsonis, F. N. Biliary excretion of cadmium in the rat, rabbit and dog. *Toxicol. Appl. Pharmacol.*, **1977**, *41*, 101–112.

Klaassen, C. D., and Shoeman, D. W. Biliary excretion of lead in rats, rabbits, and dogs. *Toxicol. Appl. Pharmacol.*, **1974**, *29*, 447–457.

Knudsen, L., and Weismann, K. Taste dysfunction and changes in zinc and copper metabolism during penicillamine therapy for generalized scleroderma. *Acta Med. Scand.*, **1978**, *204*, 75–79.

Koos, B. J., and Longo, L. Mercury toxicity in pregnant women, fetus and newborn infant. *Am. J. Obstet. Gynecol.*, **1976**, *126*, 390–409.

Kotsonis, F. N., and Klaassen, C. D. Toxicity and distribution of cadmium administered to rats at sublethal doses. *Toxicol. Appl. Pharmacol.*, **1977**, *41*, 667–680.

———. The relationship of metallothionen to the toxicity of cadmium after prolonged oral administration to rats. *Ibid.*, **1978**, *46*, 39–54.

Langolf, G. D.; Chaffin, D. B.; Whittle, H. P.; and Henderson, R. Effects of industrial mercury exposure on urinary mercury, EMG and psychomotor functions. In, *Clinical Chemistry and Chemical Toxicology of Metals*. (Brown, S. S., ed.) Elsevier/North Holland Biomedical Press, Amsterdam, **1977**, pp. 213–220.

Lee, A. M., and Fraumeni, J. F. Arsenic and respiratory cancer in man: an occupational study. *J. Natl. Cancer Inst.*, **1969**, *42*, 1045–1052.

Lisella, F. S.; Long, K. R.; and Scott, H. G. Health aspects of arsenicals in the environment. *J. Environ. Health*, **1972**, *34*, 511–518.

Longcope, W. T., and Leutscher, J. A., Jr. Clinical uses of 2,3-dimercaptopropanol (BAL). XI. The treatment of acute mercury poisoning by BAL. *J. Clin. Invest.*, **1946**, *25*, 557–567.

Lugo, G.; Cassady, G.; and Palmisano, P. Acute maternal arsenic intoxication with neonatal death. *Am. J. Dis. Child.*, **1969**, *117*, 328.

McAlpine, D., and Shukuro, A. Minimata disease. An unusual neurological disorder caused by contaminated fish. *Lancet*, **1958**, *2*, 629–631.

Macaulay, D. G., and Stanley, D. A. Arsine poisoning. *Br. J. Ind. Med.*, **1956**, *13*, 217–221.

MacDonald, W. B., and Fellers, F. X. Penicillamine in the treatment of patients with cystinuria. *J.A.M.A.*, **1966**, *197*, 396–402.

Magos, L. Effect of 2,3-dimercaptopropanol (BAL) on urinary excretion and brain content of mercury. *Br. J. Ind. Med.*, **1968**, *25*, 152–154.

Morgan, J. M.; Hartley, M. W.; and Miller, R. E. Neuropathy in chronic lead poisoning. *Arch. Intern. Med.*, **1966**, *118*, 17–29.

Multicentre Trial Group. Controlled trial of D-(−)penicillamine in severe rheumatoid arthritis. *Lancet*, **1973**, *1*, 275–280.

Murakami, M., and Hirosawa, K. Electron microscope autoradiography of kidney after administration of ^{210}Pb in mice. *Nature*, **1973**, *245*, 153–154.

Norseth, T., and Clarkson, T. W. Studies on the biotransformation of ^{203}Hg-labeled methylmercury chloride in rats. *Arch. Environ. Health*, **1970**, *21*, 717–727.

———. Intestinal transport of ^{203}Hg-labeled methyl mercury chloride. Role of biotransformation in rats. *Ibid.*, **1971**, *22*, 568–577.

Novey, H. S., and Martel, S. H. Asthma, arsenic, and cancer. *J. Allergy*, **1969**, *44*, 315–319.

Parameshvara, V. Mercury poisoning and its treatment with N-acetyl-D,L-penicillamine. *Br. J. Ind. Med.*, **1967**, *24*, 73–76.

Perry, H. M., Jr., and Erlanger, M. W. Metal-induced hypertension following chronic feeding of low doses of cadmium and mercury. *J. Lab. Clin. Med.*, **1974**, *83*, 541–547.

Perry, H. M., and Perry, E. F. Normal concentrations of some trace metals in human urine: change produced by ethylenediaminetetraacetate. *J. Clin. Invest.*, **1959**, *38*, 1452–1463.

Peters, R. A., and Stocken, L. A. Preparation and pharmacological properties of 4-hydroxymethyl-2-(3′-amino-4′-hydroxyphenyl)-1:3-dithia-2-arsacyclopentane (mapharside-BAL compound). *Biochem. J.*, **1947**, *41*, 53–56.

Piscator, M. Proteinuria in chronic cadmium poisoning. I. An electrophoretic and chemical study of urinary and serum proteins from workers with chronic cadmium poisoning. *Arch. Environ. Health*, **1962**, *4*, 607–622.

———. Proteinuria in chronic cadmium poisoning. III. Electrophoretic and immunoelectrophoretic studies on urinary proteins from cadmium workers, with special reference to the excretion of low molecular weight proteins. *Ibid.*, **1966**, *12*, 335–344.

Piscator, M., and Pettersson, B. Plenary lecture. Chronic cadmium poisoning: diagnosis and prevention. In, *Clinical Chemistry and Chemical Toxicology of Metals*. (Brown, S. S., ed.) Elsevier/North Holland Biomedical Press, Amsterdam, **1977**, pp. 143–155.

Popoff, N.; Weinberg, S.; and Feigin, I. Pathologic observations in lead encephalopathy. *Neurology (Minneap.)*, **1963**, *13*, 101–112.

Popovici, A.; Geshickter, C. F.; Reinosky, A.; and Rubin, M. Experimental control of serum calcium levels *in vivo*. *Proc. Soc. Exp. Biol. Med.*, **1950**, *74*, 415–417.

Porter, M. C.; Miya, T. S.; and Bousquest, W. F. Cadmium: inability to induce hypertension in the rat. *Toxicol. Appl. Pharmacol.*, **1974**, *27*, 692–695.

Rahola, T.; Aaran, R. K.; and Mietinen, J. K. Half-time studies of mercury and cadmium by whole body counting. International Atomic Energy Agency symposium on the assessment of radioactive organ and body burdens. In, *Assessment of Radioactive Contamination in Man*. The Agency, Vienna, **1972**.

Richet, G.; Albahary, C.; Ardaillou, R.; Sultan, C.; and

Morel-Maroger, A. Le rein du saturnisme chronique. *Rev. Fr. Etud. Clin. Biol.*, **1964,** *9,* 188–196.

Rosenberg, L. E., and Hayslett, J. P. Nephrotoxic effect of penicillamine in cystinuria. *J.A.M.A.*, **1967,** *201,* 698–699.

Sanders, L. W. Tetraethyllead intoxication. *Arch. Environ. Health*, **1964,** *8,* 270–277.

Sanford, H. N. Lead poisoning in young children. *Postgrad. Med.*, **1955,** *17,* 162–169.

Schroeder, H. A. Cadmium as a factor in hypertension. *J. Chronic Dis.*, **1965,** *18,* 217–228.

Schroeder, H. A., and Vinton, W. H., Jr. Hypertension induced in rats by small doses of cadmium. *Am. J. Physiol.*, **1962,** *202,* 515–518.

Schwartz, S. L.; Johnson, C. B.; and Doolan, P. D. Studies on the mechanism of renal vaculogenesis induced in the rat by ethylenediaminetetraacetate. Comparison of the cellular activities of calcium and chromium chelates. *Mol. Pharmacol.*, **1970,** *6,* 54–60.

Seshia, S. S.; Rajani, K. R.; Boeckx, R. L.; and Chow, P. N. The neurological manifestations of chronic inhalation of leaded gasoline. *Dev. Med. Child Neurol.*, **1978,** *20,* 323–334.

Sivjakov, K. J. The treatment of acute selenium, cadmium and tungsten intoxication in rats with cadmium disodium ethylenediaminetetraacetate. *Toxicol. Appl. Pharmacol.*, **1959,** *1,* 602–607.

Smith, A. D. M., and Miller, J. W. Treatment of inorganic mercury poisoning with N-acetyl-D,L-penicillamine. *Lancet*, **1961,** *640,* 642.

Smith, H. D.; Boehner, R. L.; Carney, T.; and Majors, W. J. The sequelae of pica with and without lead poisoning. *Am. J. Dis. Child.*, **1963,** *105,* 609–616.

Soffer, A., and Toribara, T. Changes in serum and spinal fluid calcium effected by disodium ethylenediaminetetraacetate. *J. Lab. Clin. Med.*, **1961,** *58,* 542–547.

Spencer, H. Studies on the effect of chelating agents in man. *Ann. N.Y. Acad. Sci.*, **1960,** *88,* 435–449.

Spencer, H.; Vankinscott, V.; Lewin, I.; and Laszlo, D. Removal of calcium in man by ethylenediaminetetraacetic acid. A metabolic study. *J. Clin. Invest.*, **1952,** *31,* 1023–1027.

Sternlieb, I., and Scheinberg, I. H. Penicillamine therapy for hepatolenticular degeneration. *J.A.M.A.*, **1964,** *189,* 748–754.

Thind, G. S., and Fischer, G. Plasma cadmium and zinc in human hypertension. *Clin. Sci. Mol. Med.*, **1976,** *51,* 483–486.

Tu, J.; Blackwell, R. Q.; and Lee, P. DL-Penicillamine as a cause of optic axial neuritis. *J.A.M.A.*, **1963,** *185,* 83–86.

Uldall, P. R.; Khan, H. A.; Ennis, J. E.; McCallum, R. I.; and Grimson, T. A. Renal damage from industrial arsine poisoning. *Br. J. Ind. Med.*, **1970,** *27,* 372–377.

Van Tongeren, J. H. M.; Kunst, A.; Majoor, C. L. H.; and Schilling, P. H. M. Folic acid deficiency in chronic arsenic poisoning. *Lancet*, **1965,** *1,* 784–786.

Voors, A. W., and Shuman, M. S. Liver cadmium levels in North Carolina residents who died of heart disease. *Bull. Environ. Contam. Toxicol.*, **1977,** *17,* 692–696.

Walshe, J. M. Penicillamine, a new oral therapy for Wilson's disease. *Am. J. Med.*, **1956,** *21,* 487–495.

Zavon, M. R., and Meadow, C. D. Vascular sequelae to cadmium fume exposure. *Am. Ind. Hyg. Assoc. J.*, **1970,** *31,* 180–182.

Zielhuis, R. L. Interrelationship of biochemical responses to the absorption of inorganic lead. *Arch. Environ. Health,* **1971,** *23,* 299–311.

Monographs and Reviews

Bair, W. J., and Thompson, R. C. Plutonium: biomedical research. *Science*, **1974,** *183,* 715–722.

Buchanan, W. D. *Toxicity of Arsenic Compounds.* Elsevier Publishing Co., Amsterdam, **1962.**

Byers, R. K. Lead poisoning. Review of literature and report on 45 cases. *Pediatrics*, **1959,** *23,* 585–603.

Cantarow, A., and Trumper, M. *Lead Poisoning.* The Williams & Wilkins Co., Baltimore, **1944.**

Chaberek, S., and Martell, A. E. *Organic Sequestering Agents.* John Wiley & Sons, Inc., New York, **1959.**

Chang, L. W. Neurotoxic effects of mercury—a review. *Environ. Res.*, **1977,** *14,* 329–373.

Chisholm, J. J., Jr. Treatment of lead poisoning. *Mod. Treat.*, **1967,** *4,* 710–727.

Clarkson, T. W. The pharmacology of mercury compounds. *Annu. Rev. Pharmacol.*, **1972a,** *12,* 375–406.

———. Recent advances in the toxicology of mercury with emphasis on the alkylmercurials. *CRC Crit. Rev. Toxicol.*, **1972b,** *1,* 203–234.

———. Mercury poisoning. In, *Clinical Chemistry and Chemical Toxicology of Metals.* (Brown, S. S., ed.) Elsevier/North-Holland Biomedical Press, Amsterdam, **1977,** pp. 189–200.

Dwyer, F. P., and Mellor, D. P. (eds.). *Chelating Agents and Metal Chelates.* Academic Press, Inc., New York, **1964.**

Friberg, L.; Piscator, M.; Norberg, G. F.; and Kjellstrom, T. *Cadmium in the Environment,* 2nd ed. CRC Press, Inc., Cleveland, **1974.**

Friberg, L., and Vostal, J. *Mercury in the Environment: An Epidemiological and Toxicological Appraisal.* CRC Press, Inc., Cleveland, **1972.**

Gosselin, R. E.; Hodge, H. C.; Smith, R. P.; and Gleason, M. *Clinical Toxicology of Commercial Products: Acute Poisoning,* 4th ed. The Williams & Wilkins Co., Baltimore, **1976.**

Hammond, P. B., and Beliles, R. P. Metals. In, *Casarett and Doull's Toxicology: The Basic Science of Poisons,* 2nd ed. (Doull, J.; Klaassen, C. D.; and Amdur, M. O.; eds.) Macmillan Publishing Co., Inc., New York, **1980,** pp. 409–467.

Klaassen, C. D. Biliary excretion of metals. *Drug Metab. Rev.*, **1976,** *5,* 165–196.

National Academy of Sciences. *Lead: Airborne Lead in Perspective.* National Research Council, Washington, D. C., **1972.**

Smith, W. E., and Smith, A. M. *Minamata.* Holt, Rinehart & Winston, New York, **1975.**

Stocken, L. A., and Thompson, R. H. S. Reactions of British antilewisite with arsenic and other metals in living systems. *Physiol. Rev.*, **1949,** *29,* 168–194.

Swensson, A., and Ulfarsson, V. Toxicology of organic mercury compounds used as fungicides. *Occup. Health Rev.*, **1963,** *15,* 5–11.

Task Group on Metal Accumulation. Accumulation of toxic metals with specific reference to their absorption, excretion, and biological half-times. *Environ. Physiol. Biochem.*, **1973,** *3,* 65–107.

70 NONMETALLIC ENVIRONMENTAL TOXICANTS: AIR POLLUTANTS, SOLVENTS AND VAPORS, AND PESTICIDES

Curtis D. Klaassen

Environmental pollution, an undesired spin-off of human activity, was relatively insignificant until urbanization. People dug coal from the ground, used it to heat homes, and thus created an atmosphere of sulfurous smoke above the cities. From the thirteenth century onward, periodic efforts were made to forbid the burning of coal in London, but, on the whole, people have accepted a polluted atmosphere as part of urban life. Power plants burn fossil fuels to generate electricity; steel mills have grown along river banks and lake shores; oil refineries have risen near ports and oil fields; smelters roast and refine metals near great mineral deposits; the automobile is all-prevalent. All these operations pollute the air, water, and soil around them.

When synthetic materials came of age, factories were built to produce them. Little thought was given to the toxicity of chemicals not intended for use in man. Only a few of the three million known chemicals have been tested for toxic effects; many have been indiscriminately disseminated throughout the environment.

AIR POLLUTION

Air pollutants enter the body predominantly through the lungs. Some of these chemicals are absorbed into the blood, while the lungs clear substances that are not absorbed.

Absorption and Deposition of Toxicants by the Lungs

The site of deposition of aerosols in the respiratory tract depends on the size of the particle. Particles of 5 μm or larger in diameter are usually deposited in the upper airway. Those deposited in the unciliated anterior portion of the nose remain until removed by wiping, blowing, or sneezing. In the posterior portion of the nose, a mucus blanket propelled by cilia carries insoluble particles to the pharynx in minutes. These particles are swallowed and pass to the gastrointesinal tract. Soluble particles dissolved in the mucus may be carried to the pharynx or absorbed through the epithelium into the blood.

Particles of 2 to 5 μm are deposited in the tracheobronchial tree and cleared by the cilia's upward movement of mucus. Although the rate of ciliary movement varies in different parts of the respiratory tract, it is rapid and efficient. Rates of transport are between 0.1 and 1 mm per minute, resulting in half-lives for the particles that range from 30 to 300 minutes. Coughing and sneezing move mucus and particles rapidly toward the glottis. The particles may also be swallowed.

Particles less than 2 μm in diameter remain suspended in the inhaled air and reach the alveolar zone of the lung, where they may be readily absorbed. The surface area is large (50 to 100 sq m); the rate of blood flow is high; and the blood is in close proximity to the alveolar air (10 μm). The alveoli are often a site for absorption of liquid aerosols and particles, as well as of gases. The factors that govern the rate of absorption of gases are discussed in Chapter 13. Liquid aerosols pass the alveolar cell membranes by passive diffusion in proportion to their lipid solubility. Mechanisms for removal or absorption of particulate matter (usually less than 1 μm in diameter) from the alveolus are less clearly defined and are less efficient than those that remove particles from the tracheobronchial tree. Three processes are apparently operative. The first is physical removal; particles deposited on the fluid layer of the alveoli are believed to be aspirated onto the mucociliary escalator of the bronchotracheal tree. The second is phagocytosis, usually by mononuclear phagocytes or alveolar macrophages. The third is by absorption into the lymphatic system. Particles can remain in lymphatic tissue for long periods of time, and, for this reason, the tissue has been called the dust store of the lungs.

Overall, removal of particulates from the alveolus is relatively inefficient. Only about 20% of such matter is removed during the first day after deposition; that which remains longer than 24 hours is often removed very slowly. The rate of this clearance can be predicted from the solubility of the substance in lung fluids. The least soluble compounds are removed at a slower rate. Such removal is apparently largely due to dissolution and absorption into the blood. Some particles may remain in the alveoli indefinitely if the cells that phagocytize them proliferate and join the reticular network to form an alveolar dust plaque or nodule.

TYPES AND SOURCES OF AIR POLLUTANTS

Five pollutants account for nearly 98% of air pollution. These are carbon monoxide (52%), sulfur oxides (18%), hydrocarbons (12%), particulate matter (10%), and nitrogen oxides (6%) (Amdur, 1980). A distinction is often made between two kinds of pollution. The first is characterized by sulfur dioxide and smoke from incomplete combustion of coal and by conditions of fog and cool temperatures. Because of its chemical nature, it is termed a *reducing type of pollution*. The second is characterized by hydrocarbons, oxides of nitrogen, and photochemical oxidants. It is caused by automobile exhaust and occurs especially in areas such as the Los Angeles basin, where intense sunlight causes photochemical reactions in polluted air masses that are trapped by a meteorological inversion layer. Because of its nature, it is described as an *oxidizing type of pollution* or *photochemical air pollution*.

Five major sources account for 90% of the tons of pollutants that are emitted annually (Amdur, 1980): transportation (particularly automobiles) (60%), industry (18%), electric power generation (13%), space heating (6%), and refuse disposal (3%).

HEALTH EFFECTS OF AIR POLLUTION

Acute episodes of high pollution cause mortality and morbidity. There are three classical examples: 65 people died in the Meuse Valley, Belgium in 1930; 20 people died in Donora, Pennsylvania in 1948; 4000 people died in London in 1952. Each of these incidents occurred during an atmospheric temperature inversion that lasted for 3 to 4 days. During this time the concentration of pollutants surpassed the normal levels for these already heavily polluted areas, where coal was the main fuel; the pollution was the reducing kind. Most of the people who became ill or died were elderly; some had either cardiac or respiratory diseases or both; none could cope with the added stress of breathing heavily polluted air.

Acute effects on health are thus clearly associated with the reducing type of pollution. While there is less evidence to associate photochemical oxidant pollution with such effects on human health, there are significant correlations between levels of oxidants in the air and hospital admissions for allergic disorders, inflammatory disease of the eye, acute upper respiratory infections, influenza, and bronchitis.

TOXICOLOGY OF AIR POLLUTANTS

The National Air Pollution Control Administration of the United States (now under the Environmental Protection Agency) issued six documents that review knowledge about various pollutants. These are: *Air Quality Criteria for Particulate Matter* (USDHEW, 1969a), *for Sulfur Oxides* (USDHEW, 1969b), *for Carbon Monoxide* (USDHEW, 1970a), *for Photochemical Oxidants* (USDHEW, 1970b), *for Hydrocarbons* (USDHEW, 1970c), and *for Nitrogen Oxides* (USDHEW, 1971). These documents established criteria that were legal prerequisites for the Air Quality Standards.

Sulfur Dioxide. Sulfur dioxide gas is generated primarily by the burning of fossil fuels that contain sulfur. The concentration of sulfur dioxide required to kill laboratory animals is so high that it has little relevance to problems of air pollution. However, daily exposure of rats to 10 ppm of sulfur dioxide for 1 to 2 months thickens the mucus layer in the trachea from 5 μm to about 25 μm (Dalhamn, 1956). Although the cilia beat with normal frequency, the thick mucus slows clearance. The abnormal mucus layer is caused by increased numbers of mucus-secreting cells in the main bronchi, where such cells are common, and in the peripheral airways, where they are normally absent (Reid, 1963; Hirsch et al., 1975).

A basic physiological response to inhalation of sulfur dioxide is a mild degree of bronchial constriction (Frank and Speizer, 1965). The constriction appears to be due to changes in smooth muscle tone and is dependent on intact parasympathetic innervation (Nadel et al., 1965). When exposed to 5 ppm of sulfur dioxide for 10 minutes, most human subjects show increased resistance to the flow of air (Frank et al., 1962).

Sulfuric Acid. A portion of sulfur dioxide in the atmosphere is converted to sulfuric acid, ammonium sulfate, and other sulfates. The conversion to sulfuric acid can be initiated by soot or by trace metals such as vanadium or manganese. Recent evidence indicates that stable sulfite complexes may be formed in the presence of metals such as copper or iron.

Sulfuric acid increases airway resistance in relation to both concentration and particle size (Amdur et al., 1978b). Particles of 1 μm (1 mg/m^3) produce a rapid and marked increase in resistance to flow, while particles of 7 μm produce only a slight increase because they cannot penetrate beyond the upper respiratory tract. Sulfuric acid produces a greater increase in resistance to flow than does sulfur dioxide after either an acute (Amdur et al., 1978b) or a chronic exposure (Alarie et al., 1975).

Particulate Sulfates. Sulfates vary greatly in their effects on respiration, and the sulfate ion per se does not alter respiratory function (Amdur et al., 1978a). Zinc ammonium sulfate, a reported constituent of the Donora fog, increases respiratory resistance at a concentration of 0.25 mg/m^3 (Amdur and Corn, 1963); it produces a greater increase in resistance to flow than does sulfur dioxide.

Ozone. The oxidant found in the highest concentrations in polluted atmosphere is ozone (O_3). Several miles above the earth's surface there is sufficient short-wave ultraviolet light to convert O_2 to O_3 by direct absorption. Of the major atmospheric pollutants, nitrogen dioxide is the most efficient in absorbing ultraviolet light. Such absorption leads to a complex series of reactions, which may be simplified as follows:

$$NO_2 \xrightarrow{\text{UV}} NO + O$$
$$O + O_2 \longrightarrow O_3$$
$$O_3 + NO \longrightarrow NO_2 + O_2$$

Since NO_2 is regenerated by the reaction of NO and O_3, the result is cyclical. Simultaneously, oxygen atoms react with hydrocarbons in the atmosphere, especially olefins and substituted aromatics, resulting in oxidized compounds and free radicals that react with NO to produce more NO_2. The result is accu-

mulation of NO_2 and O_3, while concentrations of NO are depleted.

Ozone is a lung irritant that is capable of causing death from pulmonary edema (Stokinger, 1965). The LC50 (lethal concentration 50) following exposure for 3 hours varies from about 50 ppm for guinea pigs to about 20 ppm for mice. Gross pulmonary edema is evident in mice exposed to concentrations above 2 ppm. Ozone causes desquamation of the epithelium throughout the ciliated airways (Boatman et al., 1974) and produces degenerative changes in type-I cells and swelling or rupture of the capillary endothelium in the alveoli (Boatman et al., 1974; Stephens et al., 1974). The type-I cells are later replaced by type-II cells It is important to note that pulmonary pathology has been observed in experimental animals after relatively short exposures to concentrations of ozone that occasionally exist for short periods in polluted urban areas.

Long-term exposure to ozone damages peripheral areas of the lung. It may cause a morphological lesion—a thickening of the terminal respiratory bronchioles (Stephens et al., 1973). Chronic bronchitis, fibrosis, and emphysematous changes are observed in a variety of species exposed to ozone at concentrations slightly above 1 ppm (Amdur, 1980).

Ozone causes shallow, rapid breathing and a decrease in pulmonary compliance, which can be oberved at about 0.3 ppm. Ozone also increases the sensitivity of the lung to bronchoconstrictors such as histamine, acetylcholine, and allergens (Easton and Murphy, 1967; Lee et al., 1977). It increases the incidence of infection in laboratory animals exposed to an aerosol of infectious microorganisms, which is thought to result from inhibition of clearance mechanisms (Coffin and Blommer, 1967).

The biochemical mechanism of pulmonary injury produced by ozone may be due to the formation of reactive free-radical intermediates (Stokinger, 1965; Menzel, 1970). Ozone-induced free radicals may be derived from interaction with sulfhydryl groups, from oxidative decomposition of unsaturated fatty acids, or both. Several lines of evidence indicate that one of the biological actions of ozone is reaction with unsaturated fatty acids (Menzel, 1970). The ozonization of these fatty acids is essentially equivalent to lipid peroxidation. Decreases in concentrations of glutathione in lung occur after exposure to ozone (DeLucia et al., 1975), and sulfhydryl compounds and reducing agents (such as ascorbic acid and α-tocopherol) protect against ozone toxicity.

Nitrogen Dioxide. Nitrogen dioxide, like ozone, is a lung irritant that is capable of producing pulmonary edema. This is a risk to farmers, because sufficient amounts can be liberated from ensilage to produce the symptoms of pulmonary damage known as silo-filler's disease. The LC50 for a 4-hour exposure to nitrogen dioxide is about 90 ppm. As with ozone, nitrogen dioxide damages type-I cells of the alveoli, which are replaced by cuboidal cells that have some characteristics of type-II cells. Chronic exposure of animals to nitrogen dioxide results in emphysematous lesions (Riddick et al., 1968; Freeman et al., 1972).

Experimental exposure of animals or human subjects to nitrogen dioxide causes measurable alterations in pulmonary function. The pattern of changes resembles that produced by ozone—increased respiratory frequency and decreased compliance. Pulmonary resistance to air flow is minimally altered. The changes in pulmonary function occur when healthy subjects are exposed to 2 to 3 ppm and may happen at far lower concentrations in some asthmatic subjects (Orehek *et al.*, 1976). Short-term or long-term exposure to nitrogen dioxide can increase the susceptibility of experimental animals to respiratory infection (Coffin *et al.*, 1976).

Aldehydes. Aldehydes are major products of the photooxidation of hydrocarbons and of the reactions of hydrocarbons with ozone, oxygen atoms, or free radicals. About 50% of the total aldehyde in polluted air is *formaldehyde* (H_2CO), and about 5% is *acrolein* ($H_2C{=}CHCHO$). These materials probably contribute to the odor of photochemical smog and the ocular irritation that it causes.

Formaldehyde irritates mucous membranes of the nose, upper respiratory tract, and eyes. Concentrations of 0.5 to 1 ppm are detectable by odor, 2 to 3 ppm produce mild irritation, and 4 to 5 ppm are intolerable to most people. The overall pattern of respiratory response to formaldehyde resembles that to sulfur dioxide; exposure of guinea pigs to 0.3 ppm increases airway resistance and decreases pulmonary compliance (Amdur, 1960).

Acrolein is much more irritating than formaldehyde. It increases airway resistance and tidal volume and decreases respiratory frequency (Murphy *et al.*, 1963). Aldehydes increase resistance to air flow at concentrations below those that decrease respiratory frequency.

Carbon Monoxide. Carbon monoxide (CO) is a colorless, odorless, tasteless, and nonirritating gas resulting from incomplete combustion of organic matter. CO is the most abundant pollutant in the lower atmosphere, and a large number of accidental and suicidal deaths occur yearly from its inhalation.

The average concentration of CO in the atmosphere is about 0.1 ppm. Natural sources, such as atmospheric oxidation of methane, forest fires, terpine oxidation, and the ocean (where microorganisms produce CO), are responsible for about 90% of the atmospheric CO; human activity produces about 10%. Acute poisoning from CO results from high local concentrations of the gas, usually due to the burning of fossil fuels.

Inadequate venting of furnaces and automobiles results in many deaths each year. Most victims of fires die from acute CO poisoning rather than from burns. The automobile is the greatest source of CO; concentrations can reach 115 ppm in heavy traffic, 75 ppm in vehicles on expressways, and 23 ppm in residential areas. In underground garages and tunnels, CO levels have been found to exceed 100 ppm for extended periods. The installation of pollution control devices, including catalytic converters in automobile exhaust systems, has reduced CO emissions from about 90 to 3.4 g per mile of automobile travel

and should decrease concentrations of CO in urban atmospheres (National Research Council, 1977).

The average concentration of CO in the atmosphere appears to be stabilized by efficient natural means of removal (sinks). The most important sink seems to be the reaction of CO with ambient hydroxyl radicals to form carbon dioxide; the upper atmosphere and the soil also are sinks.

Another source of exposure to CO is smoking. Goldsmith and Landaw (1968) reported a median carboxyhemoglobin (COHb) level of 5.9% in heavy smokers (two packs of cigarettes per day) who inhale. Chronic exposure to CO under various natural conditions results in mean COHb levels in smokers two to three times those in nonsmokers (Lawther and Commins, 1970; Stewart *et al.*, 1973).

Reaction of CO with Hemoglobin. CO owes its toxicity to its combination with hemoglobin to form COHb. Hemoglobin in this form cannot carry oxygen, since both gases react with the same group in the hemoglobin molecule. However, CO combines with hemoglobin at a rate about 1/10 that of oxygen and it dissociates from hemoglobin at a rate about 1/2200 that of oxygen (Rodkey *et al.*, 1974). Therefore, the affinity of hemoglobin for CO is approximately 220 times greater than for oxygen. This high affinity makes it dangerous at very low concentrations. Since air contains 21% oxygen by volume, exposure to a gas mixture of 0.1% CO (1000 ppm) in air would result in approximately 50% carboxyhemoglobinemia.

The reduction in the oxygen-carrying *capacity* of blood is proportional to the amount of COHb present. However, the amount of oxygen *available* to the tissues is still further reduced by the inhibitory influence of COHb on the dissociation of any oxyhemoglobin (O_2Hb) still available. This can be understood best by comparing an anemic individual having a hemoglobin value of 8.0 g/dl with a person having a hemoglobin value of 16.0 g/dl but with half of it in the form of COHb (*see* Figure 70–1). In each instance the oxygen-carrying *capacity* is the same. The anemic individual may show few, if any, symptoms whereas the person suffering from CO poisoning will be near collapse. This is because the presence of COHb interferes with the *release* of oxygen carried by unaltered O_2Hb.

Factors Governing CO Toxicity. Factors that govern the toxicity of CO include the concentration of the gas in the inspired air, the duration of exposure, the respiratory minute volume, the cardiac output, the oxygen demand of the tissues, and the concentration of hemoglobin in the blood. Anemic persons are more susceptible to CO than are individuals with normal amounts of hemoglobin. Increased metabolic rate enhances the severity of symptoms in CO poisoning; this is why children succumb earlier than adults when exposed to a given concentration of the gas. The same principle underlies the use of small animals with high metabolic rates for the detection of toxic quantities of CO. Canaries are used for this purpose in mines. The test animals die before toxic symptoms are noted in man.

Change in barometric pressure does not affect the relative affinities of hemoglobin for O_2 and CO.

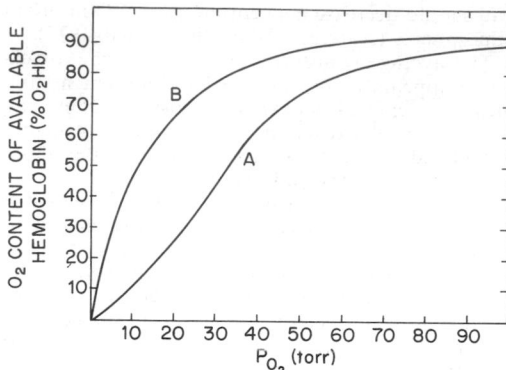

Figure 70-1. *The effect of carboxyhemoglobin (COHb) on the dissociation curve of oxyhemoglobin.*

Curve A represents the normal oxygen dissociation curve, which is unaffected by the presence of anemia (*e.g.*, 8 g hemoglobin/dl blood). Curve B represents the situation when there is 50% COHb and a normal concentration of hemoglobin (16 g hemoglobin/dl blood and half of the binding sites occupied by CO). The oxygen-carrying capacity is the same in both cases; however, when COHb is present, oxygen dissociates from hemoglobin at lower values of P_{O_2}. This effect results from interactions between binding sites for O_2 or CO; there are four such sites per molecule of hemoglobin.

However, at high altitudes and in other situations where oxygen tension is low, the effects of a given concentration of CO will be correspondingly more severe.

Signs and Symptoms of CO Toxicity. The signs and symptoms of CO poisoning are characteristic of hypoxia. They have been correlated with the COHb content of the blood. The relation between symptomatology and COHb concentration is shown in Table 70-1. It should not be inferred that all these symptoms are experienced by any one individual. Although inhalation of a high concentration may produce warning signs (transient weakness and dizziness) before consciousness is lost, there may be no warning at all. The intensity of symptoms is greatly modified by the oxygen demands of the tissues.

Moderate concentrations of COHb have little effect on vital functions in the human subject at rest. As mentioned previously, the presence of COHb reduces the oxygen-carrying capacity but not the P_{O_2} of arterial blood. As a result, there is no stimulation of the carotid and aortic chemoreceptor mechanism. For example, Apthrop and coworkers (1958) gave four normal men subjected to steady-state exercise sufficient CO to raise their COHb to between 30 and 50%. No change was observed in respiratory rate or respiratory minute volume. Cardiac rate, on the other hand, was significantly increased in all subjects when COHb reached 30%, probably to compensate for peripheral vasodilatation caused by hypoxia.

The clinical findings in patients acutely poisoned

by CO are varied. Many patients exhibit symptoms not usually associated with CO poisoning: skin lesions, excessive sweating, hepatic enlargement, bleeding tendency, pyrexia, leukocytosis, albuminuria, and glycosuria (Meigs and Hughes, 1952).

Pathology of Acute CO Poisoning. The severity of pathological changes is directly related to the duration and degree of hypoxia. The tissues most affected are those most sensitive to oxygen deprivation, such as the brain and the heart. The severe headache following exposure to CO is believed to be caused by cerebral edema and increased intracranial pressure resulting from excessive transudation across hypoxic capillaries.

A study of 351 fatal cases of accidental CO poisoning (Finck, 1966) revealed three major types of gross pathological changes. These changes and their percentage of occurrence in critical tissues are as follows: (1) congestion and/or edema in lungs (66%), brain (25%), heart (2%), and viscera (7%); (2) petechiae in brain (10%) and heart (33%); and (3) hemorrhage in lungs (7%), pleura (1%), and brain (2%). Rapidly fatal cases of CO poisoning are characterized by congestion and hemorrhages in all organs. In less acutely fatal cases, the hypoxic lesions observed are related to the duration of posthypoxic unconsciousness.

Bokonjić (1963) has shown that the maximal period of CO-induced posthypoxic unconsciousness compatible with complete neurological recovery is 21 hours in patients under 48 years of age and 11 hours in older patients. Complete recovery of mental function was not observed when the CO-induced unconsciousness exceeded 15 hours in the older group or 64 hours in the younger group. Prolonged posthypoxic unconsciousness may damage vital organs severely. In man, histological studies of the brain have shown extensive demyelination of the white

Table 70-1. CORRELATION BETWEEN % COHb AND SIGNS AND SYMPTOMS OF CO POISONING *

% OF BLOOD SATURATION	SIGNS AND SYMPTOMS
0–10	No symptoms
10–20	Tightness across forehead; possibly slight headache, dilatation of cutaneous blood vessels
20–30	Headache; throbbing in temples
30–40	Severe headache, weakness, dizziness, dimness of vision, nausea and vomiting, collapse
40–50	Same as previous item with greater possibility of collapse or syncope; increased respiration and pulse
50–60	Syncope, increased respiration and pulse; coma with intermittent convulsions; Cheyne-Stokes respiration
60–70	Coma with intermittent convulsions, depressed cardiac function and respiration, possible death
70–80	Weak pulse and slowed respiration; respiratory failure and death

* Modified from Sayers and Davenport, 1930.

matter, bilateral necrosis of the globus pallidus, and necrotic lesions of Ammon's horn (Brucher, 1967; Lapresle and Fardeau, 1967). The heart is also sensitive to hypoxia and may be permanently damaged by the presence of COHb in the blood. Cosby and Bergeron (1963) reported that nine of ten patients with severe CO poisoning exhibited one or more of the following abnormal ECG changes: sinus tachycardia, T-wave abnormalities, S-T segment depression, and atrial fibrillation. Evidence of ischemic changes and subendocardial infarction also has been observed (Anderson *et al.*, 1967). Severe CO poisoning can produce skin lesions varying from areas of erythema and edema to marked blister and bulla formation (Long, 1968). The pathological lesions that occur in brain, heart, skin, and other organs are primarily vascular, and they consist of small hemorrhages and perivascular infiltration with focal necrosis.

Diagnosis of Acute CO Poisoning. The presumptive diagnosis of acute CO poisoning is usually facilitated by circumstantial evidence, since the victim is commonly found under circumstances that leave little doubt as to the cause of his condition. COHb is cherry-red in color, and its presence in high concentrations in capillary blood may impart an abnormal red color to the skin, mucous membranes, and fingernails. However, Matthew (1971) has emphasized that the living patient is commonly cyanotic and pale and that "cherry-red cyanosis" is seen only at necropsy. A final diagnosis depends upon the demonstration of COHb in the blood. Therapy is not delayed to perform such a test in a severely poisoned individual, but the demonstration of COHb often has a forensic significance. If a person succumbs in an atmosphere containing CO, a post-mortem blood sample usually contains 60% COHb; however, death sometimes occurs at lower concentrations. If the patient is removed from such an atmosphere while still breathing, the concentration of COHb rapidly declines, and, if respiratory exchange continues to be adequate, the blood is freed of this form of hemoglobin over a course of hours.

Fate and Excretion of CO. COHb is fully dissociable and, once acute exposure is terminated, the CO will be excreted via the lungs (Roughton and Root, 1945; Roughton, 1963). Only a very small amount is oxidized to CO_2.

There is no excretion of CO without active respiration. Furthermore, COHb is extremely stable and is little affected by putrefaction. Therefore, valid measurements of COHb concentrations in the body can be made long after death. Conversely, little or no CO is absorbed post mortem and analysis of the blood in the heart provides an accurate measurement of the concentration of COHb in the blood at death. These factors have great medicolegal importance.

When room air is breathed by a resting subject, the CO content of blood decreases with a half-time of 320 minutes. If 100% oxygen is substituted for air, the equilibrium of the reaction $CO + O_2Hb \rightleftarrows O_2 + COHb$ is shifted toward the left so that the time for halving the concentration of COHb in the blood is reduced to 80 minutes. If 100% oxygen is administered under hyperbaric conditions, the half-time is decreased to about 23 minutes (Peterson and Stew-

art, 1970). These facts provide the basic principles for treatment of CO poisoning.

Treatment of CO Poisoning. The first essential is to transfer the patient to fresh air. If respiration has failed, artificial respiration must be instituted immediately. Treatment is then directed toward providing an adequate supply of oxygen to the body cells and hastening elimination of the CO. Administration of 100% oxygen is the preferred treatment; this not only provides oxygen in solution for the tissues but also hastens the dissociation of COHb. In severe CO poisoning with loss of consciousness, the best treatment is oxygen at 2 to 3 atmospheres pressure (*see* Chapter 16; Smith *et al.*, 1962; Norman and Ledingham, 1967). Complete rest and supportive treatment are also essential. The patient should not be allowed to become hypothermic. It is especially important to keep the patient quiet in order to keep tissue demands for oxygen at a minimum. Clinical or ECG evidence of myocardial damage indicates the need for a period of bed rest (Anderson *et al.*, 1967).

Toxicity of Prolonged and Low-Level Exposure to CO. The cardiovascular system, particularly the heart, is susceptible to adverse effects of low concentrations of COHb. At 6 to 12% COHb there is a shift from aerobic to anaerobic metabolism (Ayres *et al.*, 1970). Experimental and clinical studies have suggested that chronic exposure to CO can facilitate the development of atherosclerosis (Webster *et al.*, 1970; Thomsen, 1974). CO also seems to affect human behavior. Performance on tests of vigilance is impaired when there is only 2 to 5% COHb (Beard and Grandstaff, 1975; O'Hanlon, 1975). However, these low levels of COHb probably have no effect on other behaviors, such as driving, reaction time, temporal discriminations, coordination, sensory processes, and complex intellectual tasks (National Research Council, 1977).

The fetus may be extremely susceptible to effects of CO, and the gas readily crosses the placenta. Infants born to women who have survived acute exposure to a high concentration of the gas while pregnant often display neurological sequelae, and there may be gross damage to the brain (Longo, 1977). Persistent low levels of COHb in the fetus of a woman who smokes may also reduce the infant's mental abilities.

Polycythemia develops in the course of chronic exposure to CO. Other compensatory mechanisms are likely, but they have not been demonstrated. Stewart (1975) has concluded that the primary chronic effect of CO on man results from hypoxic stress secondary to the reduced oxygen-carrying capacity of blood. Healthy human subjects are exquisitely responsive to any hypoxic stress; they immediately compensate by increasing cardiac output and flow to critical organs. Those with significant cardiovascular disease are more vulnerable to the toxicity of CO because they may be unable to compensate for the hypoxia.

Particulate Material. *Pneumoconiosis* is a category of disease caused by inhalation of dusts. The most common condition of this type is *silicosis*. Next to oxygen, silicon is the most abundant element. Approximately 60% of the rocks in the earth's crust contain silica, and silica dusts are prevalent in many industries, particularly in the mining of gold, iron, and coal; in stonework; and in sandblasting. Particles larger than 10 μm are of little clinical significance, because they seldom reach the alveoli. Particles less than 2 to 3 μm are phagocytized by alveolar macrophages, and these cells are eventually destroyed (Schlipkoeter and Lindner, 1961; Bruch, 1967). Other macrophages proliferate and migrate to sites of reaction, where they may release a soluble substance that stimulates the accumulation of collagen (Heppleston and Styles, 1967). The silicotic nodules that result from such reactions are scattered uniformly throughout both lungs. The disease usually requires 10 to 25 years to develop. As the mass of fibrotic tissue increases, vital capacity decreases and the afflicted individual experiences shortness of breath.

Other pulmonary diseases develop concurrently with silicosis, and their pathogenesis may be facilitated by silica. Long known to enhance susceptibility to tuberculosis (Kettle, 1930), silicosis also increases the risk of infection by other microorganisms.

Asbestosis results from chronic inhalation of asbestos dust. Asbestos is a fibrous substance composed of hydrated silicate minerals. It is widely used in industry because it is nonflammable and flexible, and has high tensile strength, low density, resistance to acids and alkalies, and high electrical resistivity. It is often used for insulation, brake linings, shingles, and draperies.

Asbestosis (a form of pulmonary fibrosis) develops first in areas adjacent to the bronchioles, where there seems to be preferential deposition of longer asbestos fibers. There is also a fibrous pleuritis in which the pleural membrane thickens to encase the lung in a rigid fibrous capsule. Clinical symptoms of asbestosis resemble those of silicosis: dyspnea, tachypnea, and cough. However, tuberculosis is not a prominent complication (Casarett, 1975).

Bronchial cancer associated with inhalation of asbestos occurs some 20 to 30 years after initial exposure. Inhalation of asbestos combined with cigarette smoking significantly increases the incidence of lung cancer over that caused by exposure to either factor alone. *Mesothelioma*, a rapidly fatal malignancy, is also associated with exposure to asbestos fibers. It may appear in the pleura or the peritoneum, usually 25 to 40 years after initial exposure (Selikoff *et al.*, 1968; Selikoff, 1969).

Many other occupational pulmonary diseases are caused by chronic inhalation of dusts containing minerals or organic matter. These include coal workers' pneumoconiosis (black lung disease), aluminosis (bauxite lung), baritosis, beryllium disease, byssinosis, and others (*see* Bouhuys and Gee, 1977).

SOLVENTS AND VAPORS

Organic solvents and their vapors are a common part of our environment. Short, incidental exposures to low concentrations of solvent vapors, such as gasoline, lighter fluids, aerosol sprays, and spot removers, may be relatively harmless; however, exposures to paint removers, floor and tile cleaners, and other solvents in home or industry may be dangerous. Because so many industrial workers are exposed to toxic solvents and vapors, considerable effort has gone into determining safe levels of exposure. Threshold limit values (TLV) or maximum allowable concentrations (MAC) have been established for the airborne poisons; a TLV represents the concentration to which most workers may be safely exposed for an 8-hour period.

A variety of anesthetic gases, solvents, and fluorohydrocarbons (used as propellants in aerosol products) cause subjective effects when inhaled and are frequently abused in this way. This dangerous practice, which has caused many deaths, is discussed in Chapter 23.

ALIPHATIC HYDROCARBONS

C_1-C_4 **Aliphatic Hydrocarbons.** The straight-chain hydrocarbons with less than four carbon atoms are present in natural gas (methane, ethane) and in bottled gas (propane, butane). Methane and ethane produce no general systemic effects. They are "simple asphyxiants"; their toxic action is the lowering of the partial pressure of oxygen.

C_5-C_8 **Aliphatic Hydrocarbons.** The higher-molecular-weight aliphatic hydrocarbons, like most organic solvents, depress the central nervous system (CNS) and cause dizziness and incoordination. *n*-Hexane also produces a slowly reversible polyneuropathy. This was observed first in Japan, where 93 workers engaged in the production of sandals were afflicted by the use of a glue that contained at least 60% *n*-hexane (Yamamura, 1969; Iida *et al.*, 1973). Methyl *n*-butyl ketone produces neurological changes similar to those of *n*-hexane. Because both of these agents are metabolized to 5-hydroxy-2-hexanone and 2,5-hexanediol, it is postulated that one of these chemicals is responsible for this toxic effect (DeVincenzo *et al.*, 1976).

Gasoline and Kerosene. Gasoline and kerosene, petroleum distillates prepared by the fractionation of crude petroleum oil, contain aliphatic, aromatic, and a variety of branched and unsaturated hydrocarbons. They are used as illuminating fuels, heating fuels, motor fuels, vehicles for many pesticides, cleaning agents, and paint thinners. Because they are often stored in containers previously used for milk, carbonated drinks, and other beverages, they are a common cause of accidental poisoning in children.

Intoxication by ingestion of gasoline and kerosene resembles that from ethyl alcohol (Machle, 1941). Signs and symptoms include incoordination, restlessness, excitement, confusion, disorientation, ataxia, delirium, and finally coma, which may last for a few hours or several days. Inhalation of high concentrations of gasoline vapors, as by workmen cleaning storage tanks, can cause immediate death. Chenoweth (1946) observed that gasoline vapors sensitize the myocardium such that small amounts of circulating epinephrine may precipitate ventricular fibrillation; many hydrocarbons have this action. High concentrations of gasoline vapor may also lead to rapid depression of the CNS and death from respiratory failure.

Poisoning from these hydrocarbons results either from inhalation of the vapors or from ingestion of the liquid. Ingestion is more hazardous, because the liquids have a low surface tension and can be easily aspirated into the respiratory tract by vomiting or eructation. Morbidity is attributed to aspiration, whether it occurs at the time of ingestion or during treatment. Chemical pneumonitis, complicated by secondary bacterial pneumonia and pulmonary edema, is the most serious sequel to aspiration (Lawton and Malmquist, 1961; Press and Done, 1967). Death caused by hemorrhagic pulmonary edema usually occurs in 16 to 18 hours and seldom later than 24 hours after aspiration.

Examination of tissues from fatal cases reveals heavy, edematous, and hemorrhagic lungs. The alveoli are filled with an exudate that is rich in proteins, cells, and fibrin, often in a pattern resembling that of hyaline membrane disease. Alveolar walls are weakened and may rupture, leading to less frequent sequelae, such as emphysema and pneumothorax. Pulmonary lymph nodes are inflamed, and bronchopneumonia and atelectasis have been noted.

Symptomatic and supportive care is probably the best treatment for intoxication by gasoline or kerosene (Gosselin et al., 1976). Because of the danger of aspiration, emesis or gastric lavage should not be employed unless the risks are justified by the excessive quantity ingested, the presence of additional toxic substances in the petroleum, or the condition of the patient. If gastric lavage is felt to be indicated, great care should be taken to prevent leakage into the lungs as the catheter passes the pharynx. An endotracheal tube with an inflatable balloon may be useful; a lavage tube with a balloon that can be inflated within the esophagus has been recommended. An oil may be administered to decrease absorption and act as a cathartic. The oil will also mix with the kerosene; the mixture will have a higher viscosity, and this makes aspiration less likely should vomiting occur (Gerarde, 1963).

Antibiotics are sometimes given to prevent secondary bacterial pneumonia, and corticosteroids have been used to attempt to prevent pulmonary edema and necrotizing pneumonitis; however, the efficacy of such prophylactic therapy is not supported by experimental studies in dogs (Steele et al., 1972). Epinephrine and related substances should be avoided because they may induce cardiac arrhythmias. Treatment should include correction of imbalances of fluid and electrolytes.

HALOGENATED HYDROCARBONS

The excellent solvent properties and low flammability of halogenated hydrocarbons have placed them among the most widely used industrial solvents. Since the halogenated hydrocarbons are extremely soluble in lipid, they are readily absorbed after inhalation or ingestion. Like most other organic solvents, halogenated hydrocarbons depress the CNS.

Carbon Tetrachloride. Carbon tetrachloride (CCl_4) has been used for medical purposes and was once commonly employed as a spot remover and carpet cleaner; however, its use has now been abandoned because there are safer alternatives.

Transient exposure to toxic concentrations of CCl_4 vapor results in the following symptoms: irritation of the eyes, nose, and throat; nausea and vomiting; a sense of fullness in the head; dizziness, and headache. If the exposure is soon terminated, symptoms usually disappear within a few hours. Continued exposure or absorption of larger quantities of the chemical may cause stupor, convulsions, coma, or death from CNS depression. Sudden death may occur from ventricular fibrillation or depression of vital medullary centers.

Delayed toxic effects of CCl_4 include nausea, vomiting, abdominal pain, diarrhea, and hematemesis. The most serious delayed toxic effects of CCl_4 result from its hepatotoxic and nephrotoxic actions. Signs and symptoms of hepatic injury may appear after a delay of several hours or 2 to 3 days and may occur in the absence of earlier severe effects on the CNS. Biochemical evidence of hepatic injury often includes greatly elevated activities of transaminases and a variety of other enzymes in plasma. Alkaline phosphatase activity is, however, only slightly elevated. The chief histological abnormalities include hepatic steatosis and hepatic centralobular necrosis.

The mechanism of CCl_4-induced hepatic injury has interested many investigators, and the compound has become the reference substance for all hepatotoxic compounds. Injury produced by CCl_4 seems to be mediated through a reactive metabolite—trichloromethyl free radical ($\cdot CCl_3$)—formed by the homolytic cleavage of CCl_4 (Slater, 1966). This biotransformation occurs by oxidation in the endoplasmic reticulum. Thus, agents such as DDT (McLean and McLean, 1966) and phenobarbital (Garner and McLean, 1969), which stimulate such drug metabolism, enhance the hepatotoxic effects of CCl_4 strikingly. Conversely, agents that inhibit the drug-metabolizing activity diminish the hepatotoxicity of CCl_4. The toxicity produced by CCl_4 is thought to be due to the reaction of the free radical with the lipids and proteins; however, the relative importance of each in producing injury is controversial. Recknagel and Glende (1973) have proposed that the free radical causes the peroxidation of the polycnoic lipids of the endoplasmic reticulum and the generation of secondary free radicals derived from these lipids—a chain reaction. This destructive lipid peroxidation leads to breakdown of membrane structure and function, and, if a sufficient quantity of CCl_4 has been consumed, damage extends to all cellular membranes. Detailed reviews of the hepatotoxic actions of CCl_4 have been written by Recknagel (1967), Recknagel and Glende (1973), Plaa and Witschi (1976), Zimmerman (1978), and Plaa (1980).

Individuals recovering from acute ingestion of ethanol seem more susceptible to the hepatotoxic properties of halogenated hydrocarbons (Von Oettingen, 1964). Other alcohols, such as isopropanol, have an even greater ability to potentiate such effects of CCl_4 (Cornish and Adefuin, 1967; Plaa et al., 1975). This interaction between isopropanol and CCl_4 was highlighted by an industrial accident in an isopropanol packaging plant, where workers exposed to both agents were affected (Folland et al., 1976).

As hepatic injury develops, signs of renal damage may also be observed and may dominate the clinical picture. Experimental studies in rats indicate that CCl_4 produces an early, reversible lesion of the proximal tubule; initial changes occur in the mitochondria and are followed by cellular swelling, proliferation of the smooth endoplasmic reticulum, and a simultaneous increase in the excretion of sodium salts and water (Striker et al., 1968). Mild poisoning in man may be characterized by a reversible oliguria lasting only a few days. In nonfatal poisoning, recovery of renal function occurs in three phases (Sirota, 1949). In the first, after 1 to 3 days, oliguria stops, but concentrations of creatinine and urea in plasma remain elevated. The second phase starts with a rapid decline in these concentrations. In the third phase, about 1 month after the initial injury, renal blood flow and glomerular filtration begin to improve, and renal function is recovered after 100 to 200 days. In more severe intoxication the oliguria may progress in a week or so to near anuria, with red blood cells and albumin in the scanty urine. Hypertension, acidosis, and terminal uremia develop if renal function is not restored.

Emergency *treatment* of CCl_4 poisoning should be initiated promptly in any person suspected of having absorbed toxic quantities of the compound. The individual exposed to toxic vapor should be moved to fresh air. If the patient is seen shortly after oral ingestion of CCl_4, the stomach should be emptied immediately, by inducing vomiting if the patient is conscious or by gastric lavage, and a saline laxative should be administered to minimize absorption. If the patient is first seen in the stage of advanced CNS depression, every effort should be made to prevent hypoxia. Oxygen and artificial respiration should be administered if necessary. Under no circumstances should an attempt be made to elevate the blood pressure by the use of sympathomimetic drugs because of the danger of producing serious arrhythmias in the sensitized myocardium.

Treatment of the acute hepatic and renal insufficiency caused by CCl_4 is difficult. Although hepatic insufficiency is a very prominent feature of CCl_4 poisoning, renal failure is the most frequent cause of death. Even though the presenting signs and symptoms may be associated with functional impairment of the liver, renal function should be observed closely and oliguria or anuria anticipated. Fortunately, the basic measures employed in the conservative treatment of acute renal insufficiency—administration of glucose to provide calories and careful maintenance of the volume and composition of the body fluids—apply equally to management of acute hepatic insufficiency.

Other Halogenated Hydrocarbons. Chloroform, dichloromethane (methylene chloride), trichloroeth-ylene, tetrachloroethylene, 1,1,1-trichloroethane, and 1,1,2-trichloroethane produce many of the same toxic effects as does CCl_4 (Von Oettingen, 1964). All these compounds produce CNS depression, and some have been used as inhalational anesthetics. They also have the potential to sensitize the heart to arrhythmias produced by catecholamines (Reinhardt et al., 1973). The hepatotoxic potential is highest with chloroform and 1,1,2-trichloroethane, and least with trichloroethylene, tetrachloroethylene, 1,1,1-trichloroethane, and dichloromethane (Klaassen and Plaa, 1966, 1967); chloroform may be hepatotoxic because it is metabolized to phosgene (Krishna et al., 1978). Chloroform, 1,1,2-trichloroethane, and tetrachlorocthylene are also nephrotoxic (Klaassen and Plaa, 1966, 1967, 1969). Since they produce less organ damage than CCl_4 and chloroform, 1,1,1-trichloroethane and trichloroethylene are widely used as dry-cleaning agents and dichloromethane is employed as a paint stripper. Dichloromethane has an additional toxic effect because it is metabolized to CO by cytochrome P-450 (Kubic and Anders, 1975).

ALIPHATIC ALCOHOLS

The toxicological properties of ethanol and methanol are discussed in Chapter 18.

Isopropanol. Isopropanol, used for rubbing alcohol, hand lotions, and in deicing and antifreeze preparations, is occasionally the cause of accidental poisoning. Like ethanol and methanol it is a CNS depressant, but it does not produce retinal damage or acidosis as does methanol.

The probable lethal dose of isopropanol is about 250 ml; it is thus more toxic than ethanol. While the signs and symptoms of isopropanol toxicity resemble those of ethanol, there are notable exceptions. Isopropanol produces a more prominent gastritis, with pain, nausea, vomiting, and hemorrhage. Vomiting with aspiration is a serious threat and dangerous complication. Isopropanol intoxication lasts longer because the compound is oxidized more slowly than ethanol (Gosselin et al., 1976) and because its major metabolite, acetone, is also a CNS depressant. As with the other alcohols, hemodialysis is a useful procedure for removing isopropanol from the body (Freireich et al., 1967; King et al., 1970).

GLYCOLS

In addition to their use as heat exchangers, antifreeze formulations, hydraulic fluids, or chemical intermediates, glycols are also employed as solvents for pharmaceuticals, food additives, cosmetics, and lacquers.

Ethylene Glycol. Ethylene glycol ($HOCH_2CH_2$-OH) is widely used as antifreeze for automobile radiators, and such products are the usual cause of ethylene glycol poisonings. Like ethanol, ethylene glycol produces CNS depression. Patients who ingest large quantities develop narcosis, which leads to coma and death. In addition to the CNS depression, ethylene glycol produces severe renal injury; most victims experience acute renal failure. Those who die from uremia exhibit marked renal pathology, including destruction of epithelial cells, interstitial edema, focal hemorrhagic necrosis in the cortex, extensive hydropic degeneration, numerous cellular casts, and oxalate crystals in the convoluted tubules (Gosselin et al., 1976).

Initial steps in the oxidation of ethylene glycol to the dialdehyde (glyoxal) and to glyoxylic acid (HCOCOOH) seem to be mediated by alcohol dehydrogenase; decarboxylation of glyoxylic acid yields carbon dioxide and formic acid. Glyoxylic acid is also oxidized to oxalic acid (HOOCCOOH). The glycol probably causes the initial CNS depression; oxalate and the other intermediates seem to be responsible for nephrotoxicity. Formic acid produces the metabolic acidosis of ethylene glycol poisoning, as it does in poisoning with methanol.

The specific treatment of poisoning with ethylene glycol is similar to that for methanol (Gosselin et al., 1976). Metabolic acidosis must be treated with a base such as sodium bicarbonate. Ethanol may be used as a competitive substrate for alcohol dehydrogenase to decrease the rate of formation of metabolites (Wacker et al., 1965). As with other alcohols, dialysis is effective. Parenteral administration of calcium is recommended for muscle spasms, which may develop because of chelation of calcium by the oxalate formed in the biotransformation of ethylene glycol.

Diethylene Glycol. Diethylene glycol ($HOCH_2$-$CH_2OCH_2CH_2OH$) is used in lacquer, cosmetics, antifreeze, and lubricants, and as a softening agent and plasticizer. Its toxicity was a major problem only when the compound was used in the 1930s as a solvent in a preparation of sulfanilamide (Leech, 1937; Geiling and Cannon, 1938). In that incident, 105 of 353 people who ingested the sulfanilamide-diethylene glycol preparation died from renal damage. Effects of diethylene glycol resemble those of ethylene glycol, and intoxication should be treated similarly.

Propylene Glycol. The physical properties of propylene glycol ($CH_3CHOHCH_2OH$) are similar to those of ethylene glycol, but it is much less toxic. For this reason propylene glycol is used as a solvent for drugs, cosmetics, lotions, and ointments; in food materials; as a plasticizer; in antifreeze formulations; as a heat exchanger; and in hydraulic fluids. Like ethanol, its primary pharmacological action is to produce CNS depression; however, its elimination is slower and its actions are thus prolonged.

AROMATIC HYDROCARBONS

Benzene. Benzene is an excellent solvent and is widely used for chemical syntheses; it is a natural constituent of auto fuels. However, it is very toxic.

After acute exposure to a large amount of benzene, by ingestion or by breathing concentrated vapors, the major toxic effect is on the CNS. Symptoms from mild exposure include dizziness, weakness, euphoria, headache, nausea, vomiting, tightness in the chest, and staggering. If exposure is more severe, symptoms progress to blurred vision, tremors, shallow and rapid respiration, ventricular irregularities, paralysis, and unconsciousness.

Chronic exposure to benzene is usually due to inhalation of vapor. Signs and symptoms include effects on the CNS and the gastrointestinal tract (headache, loss of appetite, drowsiness, nervousness, and pallor), but the major manifestation of toxicity is aplastic anemia. Bone-marrow cells in early stages of development are the most sensitive to benzene (Snyder et al., 1977), and arrest of maturation leads to gradual depletion of circulating cells. Savilahti (1956) has documented the relative frequency of the various blood abnormalities that occur in chronic benzene poisoning.

A major concern is the relationship between chronic exposure to benzene and leukemia. Epidemiological studies have been conducted on workers in the tire industry (McMichael et al., 1975) and in shoe factories (Aksoy et al., 1974), where benzene is used extensively. Among workers who died from exposure to benzene, death was caused by either leukemia or aplastic anemia, in approximately equal proportions.

The first product of the metabolic oxidation of benzene is postulated to be a highly unstable compound, benzene oxide (Jerina and Daley, 1974). Benzene oxide, formed by introduction of oxygen into the molecule by the mixed-function oxidase system, rapidly rearranges to form phenol. The sulfate ester of phenol is the major metabolite in the urine, and the level of exposure of workers to benzene can be estimated by determination of the increase in organic sulfate excreted in the urine (Elkins, 1959). Benzene oxide, an electrophil, may also bind covalently to nucleophilic sites on proteins and nucleic acids. Such binding is suspected as the cause of aplastic anemia and leukemia resulting from benzene toxicity.

Toluene. Toluene ($C_6H_5CH_3$) is widely used as a solvent in paints, varnishes, glues, enamels, and lacquers and as a chemical intermediate in the synthesis of organic compounds. Toluene is a CNS depressant, and low concentrations produce fatigue, weakness, and confusion. It is for the CNS effects of solvents such as toluene that "glue sniffers" inhale the vapors of glue. Unlike benzene, toluene produces neither aplastic anemia nor leukemia. However, the solvents in glue are often mixed, and the "glue sniffer" is usually exposed to others beside toluene.

PESTICIDES

Pesticide is a general classification that includes insecticides, rodenticides, fungicides, herbicides, and fumigants. These compounds, manufactured for the sole purpose of destroying some form of life, are classified as pesticides because they are directed against organisms that society deems undesirable. While selective toxicity of pesticides is extremely desirable, all can produce at least some toxicity in man.

Mortality attributed to accidental poisoning by pesticides in the United States seems to have declined in the past 2 decades. Hayes and Vaughn (1977) reported that there were only 52 fatal accidental poisonings with pesticides in 1974, compared to 152 in 1956. During this period the proportion of fatal poisonings in children declined from 61% to 31%. This decline was attributed to increased awareness by poison control centers, pediatricians, and parents of the hazards of pesticides to children.

INSECTICIDES

The use of insecticides in agriculture has grown tremendously since World War II, and there is a great potential for occupational exposure to these chemicals, both in production and in use. However, exposure to insecticides is not limited to occupational incidents; residues often remain on produce, and man is exposed to low levels of the chemicals in food. Numerous incidents of acute poisoning from pesticides have resulted from eating food that was grossly contaminated during storage or shipping. Insecticides used in homes and gardens cause accidental poisoning in young children.

Organochlorine Insecticides. Organochlorine insecticides include chlorinated ethane derivatives, of which DDT is the best known; cyclodienes, including chlordane, aldrin, dieldrin, heptachlor, and endrin; and other hydrocarbons, including such hexachlorocyclohexanes as lindane, toxaphene, mirex, and chlordecone (KEPONE). From the mid-1940s to the mid-1960s, organochlorine insecticides were widely used in agriculture and in programs for the control of malaria.

DDT. DDT, the most common of the chlorinated ethane derivatives, is also known as *chlorophenothane.*

Prior to placement of major restrictions on its use in many countries, DDT was the best-known, least-expensive, and probably one of the most effective synthetic insecticides. It was thus widely used after its introduction in the mid-1940s.

DDT has an extremely low solubility in water and very high solubility in fat. It is readily absorbed when dissolved in oils, fats, or lipid solvents but is poorly absorbed as a dry powder or an aqueous suspension. Once absorbed, DDT concentrates in adipose tissue. Storage of DDT in the fat is protective, because it decreases the amount of the chemical at its site of toxic action—the brain.

Since DDT is degraded very slowly in the environment and is stored in the fat of animals, it is a prime candidate for biomagnification; that is, a series of organisms in a food chain accumulate increasingly greater quantities in their fat at each higher trophic level. Ultimately, a species at the top of a food chain is adversely affected. For example, the population of fish-eating birds has declined. The decline is attributed to thinning of the eggshell, a demonstrated result of ingesting DDT and related chlorinated hydrocarbon insecticides.

Due to the ubiquity of DDT, everyone born since the mid-1940s has had a lifetime of exposure to this insecticide and storage of it in fatty tissues. At a constant rate of intake, the concentration of DDT in adipose tissue reaches a steady-state value and remains relatively constant. The concentration of DDT and its metabolites in the fat of man is about 7 ppm (National Academy of Sciences, 1977). When exposure ceases, DDT is eliminated from the body slowly. Elimination has been estimated to be at a rate of approximately 1% of stored DDT excreted per day. Prior to excretion it is slowly dehalogenated and oxidized by mixed-function oxidases; one of the major excretory products is DDA (*bis*[*p*-chlorophenyl] acetic acid) (Peterson and Robison, 1964; Pinto *et al.*, 1965).

DDT has a wide margin of safety and, despite its widespread use and availability, there is no documented, unequivocal report of a fatal human poisoning from DDT. The few human deaths associated with excess exposure to DDT probably resulted from the kerosene solvent rather than the insecticide. The most prominent acute effect of DDT is stimulation of the CNS; in rats, there is a good correlation between concentrations of DDT in brain and signs of toxicity (Dale *et al.*, 1963).

Signs and symptoms of poisoning from high doses of DDT in man include paresthesias of the tongue, lips, and face; apprehension; hypersusceptibility to stimuli; irritability; dizziness; tremor; and tonic and clonic convulsions (Murphy, 1980). The mechanism of DDT's action on the CNS is not completely known. The compound is capable of altering the transport of sodium and potassium ions across axonal membranes, resulting in an increased negative afterpotential (O'Brien, 1967), prolonged action potentials, repetitive firing after a single stimulus, and spontaneous trains of action potentials (Narahashi and Hass, 1967). Specifically, DDT seems to inhibit the inactivation of sodium channels and the activation of potassium conductance (Narahashi, 1969).

In laboratory animals, intravenous administration of DDT causes death by ventricular fibrillation (Philips *et al.*, 1946). Apparently, DDT shares with other chlorinated hydrocarbons a tendency to sensitize the myocardium, and, through its action on the CNS and adrenal medulla, it may produce the stimulus necessary for ventricular fibrillation.

Relatively low doses of DDT induce the mixed-function oxidase system of the hepatic endoplasmic reticulum. This has been demonstrated in exterminators (Kolmodin *et al.*, 1969) and in workers in a DDT factory (Poland *et al.*, 1970). The result is altered metabolism of drugs, xenobiotics, and steroid hormones. The last-named effect is reflected in increased excretion of 6β-hydroxycortisol in the urine (Poland *et al.,* 1970). It is probably also responsible for the increased frequency of breakage of eggs and the status of the breeding population in the peregrine falcon, sparrow hawk, and golden eagle (e.g., *see* Radcliffe, 1967). Induction of the mixed-function oxidase seems to increase metabolism of estrogens in the birds. This creates an endocrine imbalance that probably affects calcium metabolism, egg laying, and nesting in such a way that total reproductive success and survival of the young may be reduced.

Human volunteers have consumed 35 mg of DDT daily, about 1000 times higher than the average human intake, for as long as 25 months without obvious ill effects (Hayes, 1963). However, there is concern that DDT might be carcinogenic following exposure to small amounts of the chemical over a long period. Extensive use of DDT in industrial countries has not been associated with increased hepatic cancer in man. Innes and associates (1969) reported a statistically significant increase in hepatomas in two strains of mice exposed to DDT, and this finding has been confirmed by additional studies sponsored by the International Agency of Research in Cancer (IARC, 1974a). Interpretation of such data is, however, extremely difficult.

DDT was banned in the United States in 1972 for all but essential public health use and for a few minor uses to protect crops for which there were no effective alternatives. The decision was prompted by the prospect of ecological imbalance from continued use of DDT, the uncertainty of the effect, if any, of continued prolonged exposure and storage of low concentrations of DDT in man, and the development of resistant strains of insects. Several other countries have taken similar actions. As a result, other pesticides have replaced DDT, but many of them are more toxic to man.

Methoxychlor. The structural formula of methoxychlor, a chlorinated ethane derivative, is as follows:

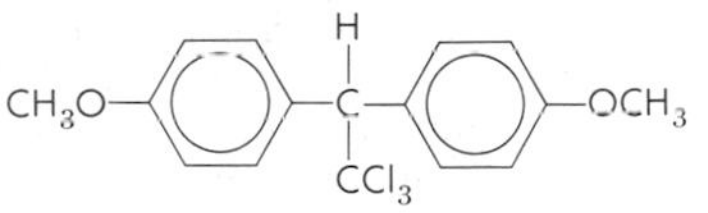

Methoxychlor

The compound is used increasingly as a replacement for DDT. The attractiveness of methoxychlor is that it is much less toxic to mammals than DDT (LD50 in rats is 6000 mg/kg compared to 250 mg/kg for DDT) and does not persist in the body for as long. Methoxychlor is stored in adipose tissue to about 0.2% of the extent of DDT, and its half-life in rats is only about 2 weeks, compared to 6 months for DDT (Murphy, 1980). The shorter half-life is a reflection of more rapid metabolism by O-demethylation (Kapoor *et al.,* 1970); it is then conjugated and excreted in the urine.

Chlorinated Cyclodienes. Structures of the more common chlorinated cyclodienes are shown in Table 70–2. These compounds stimulate the CNS, and many signs and symptoms of poisoning thus resemble those of DDT. Unlike DDT, however, these

Table 70–2. CHEMICAL STRUCTURES OF SOME CHLORINATED CYCLODIENES

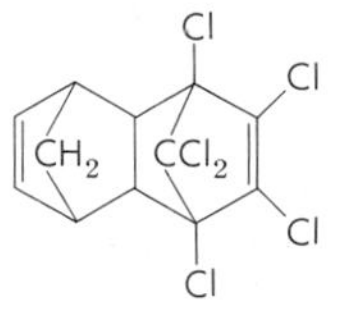

Aldrin

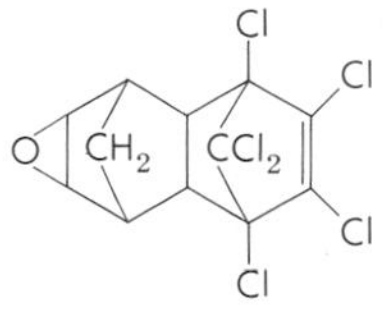

Dieldrin *

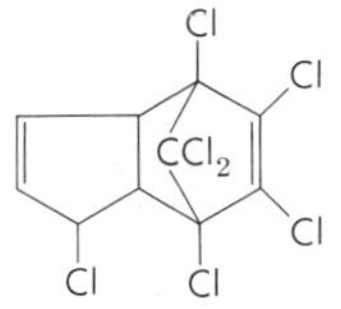

Heptachlor

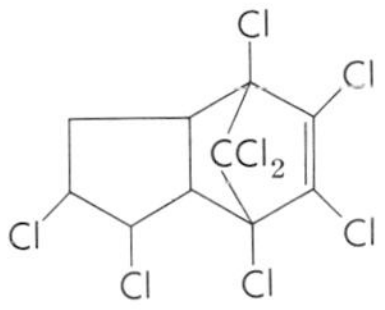

Chlordane

* Endrin is a stereoisomer of dieldrin.

compounds tend to produce convulsions before other, less serious signs of illness have appeared. Persons poisoned by cyclodiene insecticides have reported headache and nausea, vomiting, dizziness, and mild clonic jerking, but some patients have convulsions without warning symptoms (Hayes, 1963). Electroencephalographic abnormalities are seen in patients without clinical illness, both before and after convulsions (Kazantzis *et al.,* 1964). Unlike DDT, cyclodiene insecticides have caused numerous fatalities as a result of acute poisoning.

An important difference between DDT and the chlorinated cyclodienes is that the latter are readily absorbed from intact skin. Cyclodienes may not pose an appreciably greater risk than DDT to the general population exposed to small quantities in food, but manipulation of concentrated solutions of a cyclodiene is more hazardous.

Like DDT, chlorinated cyclodiene insecticides are highly soluble in lipid and are stored in adipose tissue; they induce the mixed-function oxidase system of the liver, are degraded slowly, persist in the environment, and undergo biomagnification through the food chain of animals. This class of insecticides has produced dose-related hepatomas in mice and has the greatest carcinogenic potential among the insecticides (National Academy of Sciences, 1977). For these reasons aldrin and dieldrin were banned in the United States in 1974, and the use of chlordane and heptachlor for agricultural crops was suspended in 1976.

Other Chlorinated Hydrocarbons. This group of insecticides includes lindane, toxaphene, mirex, and chlordecone. These chemicals share many properties with DDT.

Benzene Hexachloride (BHC) and Lindane. Benzene hexachloride (more properly called hexachlorocyclohexane) has the following structural formula:

Benzene Hexachloride

It is a mixture of eight isomers, and the γ isomer is referred to as *lindane*. The γ isomer is the most toxic, and virtually all insecticidal activity of BHC resides in lindane. The compound is used clinically as an ectoparasiticide (*see* Chapter 41). Lindane causes signs of poisoning that resemble those produced by DDT: tremors, ataxia, convulsions, and prostration. Violent tonic and clonic convulsions occur in severe cases of acute poisoning. The α and γ isomers are CNS stimulants, but the β and δ isomers are depressants. Lindane induces hepatic microsomal enzymes. Lindane and BHC have been implicated in numerous cases of aplastic anemia (Loge, 1965; West, 1967); however, evidence for a causal relationship is inconclusive. The α and β isomers of BHC produce hepatomas when fed to rodents, but lindane has not been shown to be tumorigenic.

Biotransformation of the isomers of BHC involves the formation of chlorophenols (Freal and Chadwick, 1973; Chadwick *et al.*, 1975). Compared to DDT, lindane has a relatively low persistence in the environment.

Toxaphene. In recent years this insecticide has ranked first in quantity used in the United States (Von Rumker *et al.*, 1975). Toxaphene is a complex mixture of more than 175 C_{10} polychlorinated hydrocarbons, of which only a few are known (*e.g.*, heptachlorobornane) (Saleh *et al.*, 1977; Turner *et al.*, 1977). Like the other chlorinated hydrocarbon insecticides, the major toxicity of toxaphene is stimulation of the CNS. Toxaphene seems to be metabolized quite readily, and this probably accounts for the low persistence of this preparation in comparison to other chlorinated hydrocarbon insecticides. Very recently carcinogenic action has been reported for toxaphene. Further assessment of this observation is essential.

Mirex and Chlordecone. Mirex and chlordecone (KEPONE) are extremely persistent chlorinated hydrocarbon insecticides, and they are concentrated several thousandfold in the food chain (Hansen *et al.*, 1976; Waters *et al.*, 1977). Their structural formulas are as follows:

Mirex

Chlordecone

Chlordecone does not appear to be biodegradable; mirex is probably oxidized to chlordecone (Carlson *et al.*, 1976). Similar to the other chlorinated hydrocarbon insecticides, mirex and chlordecone produce stimulation of the CNS, hepatic injury, and induction of the mixed-function oxidase system. Both can be carcinogenic in laboratory animals (Cueto *et al.*, 1976; Waters *et al.*, 1977).

Gross negligence in industrial hygiene resulted in poisoning of 76 of 148 exposed workers engaged in the manufacture of chlordecone in Hopewell, Virginia (Taylor *et al.*, 1978). These workers suffered neurological effects, characterized by tremors, ocular flutter (opsoclonus), hepatomegaly, splenomegaly, rashes, mental changes, and widened gaits. Laboratory tests showed reduced sperm counts and reduced motility of sperm. Contamination of the area surrounding the manufacturing plant resulted in curtailment of fishing and the procurement of shellfish in the James river and threatened portions of the Chesapeake Bay.

Cholestyramine (*see* Chapter 34) can be used to hasten excretion of chlordecone by interrupting its enterohepatic recirculation. When given orally to patients, cholestyramine enhances the fecal excretion of chlordecone by 3- to 18-fold, reduces the half-life of the insecticide dramatically, and enhances the rate of recovery from toxic manifestations (Cohn *et al.*, 1978).

Organophosphorus Insecticides. Organophosphorus insecticides have largely replaced the chlorinated hydrocarbons. The organophosphates do not persist in the environment and have an extremely low carcinogenic potential; however, they have a much higher acute toxicity in man. In fact, parathion is the pesticide most frequently involved in fatal poisoning. The pharmacology and toxicology of these agents are discussed in Chapter 6.

Carbamate Insecticides. The carbamate insecticides resemble the organophosphates in many ways. The most common of these agents is carbaryl; since carbaryl and related compounds are inhibitors of cholinesterase, they too are discussed in Chapter 6.

Botanical Insecticides. *Pyrethrums* are obtained from flowers of the pyrethrum plant, *Chrysanthemum cincerariaefolium.* The insecticidal activity and toxicity of this group of chemicals reside in a number of structurally similar compounds, and the greatest insecticidal activity resides in *pyrethrin I.* Its structural formula is as follows:

Pyrethrin I

Pyrethrum extract is used in many household insecticides because of its rapid action. Pyrethrum is generally rated as the safest insecticide because its primary toxicity is low; however, its allergenic properties are marked in comparison with other pesticides. Many cases of contact dermatitis and respiratory allergy have been reported. Persons sensitive to ragweed pollen are particularly prone to such reactions.

Rotenone is obtained from the roots of plants such as *Derris* and *Lonchocarpus.* It was first used to paralyze fish before being used as an insecticide. Rotenone has the following structural formula:

Rotenone

Human poisoning by rotenone is rare. The compound has been applied directly to treat head lice, scabies, and other ectoparasites. Local effects include conjunctivitis, dermatitis, pharyngitis, and rhinitis. Oral ingestion of rotenone produces gastrointestinal irritation, nausea, and vomiting. Inhalation of the dust is more hazardous; it can cause respiratory stimulation followed by depression and convulsions. Rotenone inhibits the oxidation of NADH to NAD. Consequently, it blocks the oxidation by NAD of substrates such as glutamate, α-ketoglutarate, and pyruvate.

Nicotine is one of the most toxic insecticides (*see* Chapter 10). Poisoning is followed by salivation and vomiting (from ganglionic stimulation), muscular weakness (from stimulation followed by depression at the neuromuscular junction), and, ultimately, clonic convulsions and cessation of respiration (effects on the CNS).

FUMIGANTS

Fumigants are used to control insects, rodents, and soil nematodes. They exert pesticidal action in gaseous form and are used because they will penetrate otherwise-inaccessible areas. Agents used to protect stored foodstuffs include hydrogen cyanide, acrylonitrile (an organic cyanide, CH_2=CHCN), carbon disulfide, carbon tetrachloride, chloropicrin, ethylene dibromide, ethylene oxide, methyl bromide, and phosphine.

Cyanide. Cyanide (*hydrocyanic acid, prussic acid*) is one of the most rapidly acting poisons. Victims may die within minutes of exposure. Hydrogen cyanide gas is used to fumigate ships and buildings and to sterilize soil. Because of their ability to form complexes with metals, cyanides are used in metallurgy, electroplating, and metal cleaning. In the home, cyanides are present in silver polish, insecticides, rodenticides, and fruit seeds. The major toxicity of *laetrile* is due to its cyanogenic glycoside. Cyanide is also used for executions in so-called gas chambers and was recently used for more than 900 religious "suicide-murders" in Guyana.

Cyanide has a very high affinity for iron in the ferric state. When absorbed, it reacts readily with the trivalent iron of cytochrome oxidase in mitochondria; cellular respiration is thus inhibited and cytotoxic hypoxia results. Since utilization of oxygen is blocked, venous blood is oxygenated and is almost as bright red as arterial blood. Respiration is stimulated because chemoreceptive cells respond as they do to decreased oxygen. A transient stage of CNS stimulation with hyperpnea and headache is observed, finally there are hypoxic convulsions and death due to respiratory arrest.

Treatment of cyanide poisoning must be rapid to be effective. Diagnosis may be aided by the characteristic odor of cyanide (oil of bitter almonds). Since toxicity results from binding to the ferric form of cytochrome oxidase, treatment is aimed at prevention or reversal of such binding by providing a large pool of ferric iron to compete for cyanide. An effective mechanism is to administer substances, such as nitrite, that oxidize hemoglobin to methemoglobin. Amyl nitrite is usually administered by inhalation, while a solution of sodium nitrite is prepared for intravenous administration (10 ml of a 3% solution). Methemoglobin competes with cytochrome oxidase for the cyanide ion; the reaction favors methemoglobin because of mass action. Cyanmethemoglobin is formed, and cytochrome oxidase is restored.

The major mechanism for removing cyanide from the body is its enzymatic conversion, by the mitochondrial enzyme rhodanese (transsulfurase), to thiocyanate, which is relatively nontoxic. To accelerate detoxication, thiosulfate is administered intravenously (50 ml of a 25% aqueous solution), and the thiocyanate formed is readily excreted in the urine.

$$Na_2S_2O_3 + CN^- \xrightarrow{Rhodanese} SCN^- + Na_2SO_3$$

Way and associates (1972) demonstrated that nitrite increases the LD50 of potassium cyanide in mice from 11 mg/kg to 21 mg/kg; administration of thiosulfate increases the value to 35 mg/kg, while with nitrite followed by thiosulfate the LD50 is 52 mg/kg. Chen and Rose (1956) reported that 48 of 49 cases of acute poisoning by cyanide in man were treated successfully with such therapy.

Oxygen alone, even at hyperbaric pressures, has only a slight protective effect in cyanide poisoning; however, it dramatically potentiates the protective effects of thiosulfate or of nitrite and thiosulfate (Way et al., 1966, 1972; Sheehy and Way, 1968). The mechanism for this action is not clear, but the intracellular oxygen tension may be high enough to cause nonenzymatic oxidation of reduced cytochromes or oxygen may displace cyanide from cytochrome oxidase by mass action.

If cyanide has been ingested, gastric lavage should follow, not precede, initiation of more specific treatment.

Methyl Bromide. Methyl bromide is used as an insecticidal fumigant and in some fire extinguishers. It is said to have been responsible for more deaths in California in recent years among occupationally exposed persons than all the organophosphate-insecticides (Hine, 1969). Because methyl bromide is so toxic, chloropicrin (CCl_3NO_2), a powerful stimulator of lacrimation, is added as a warning.

Major signs and symptoms of intoxication with methyl bromide are referable to the CNS. These include malaise, headache, visual disturbances, nausea, and vomiting. Death usually occurs during a convulsion. After severe respiratory exposure, pulmonary edema may prove fatal.

Dibromochloropropane and Ethylene Dibromide. Dibromochloropropane ($ClCH_2CHBrCH_2Br$) and ethylene dibromide (1,2-dibromoethane) are soil fumigants used to control nematodes. In man, they produce moderate depression of the CNS and pulmonary congestion after exposure by inhalation, and they cause acute gastrointestinal distress and pulmonary edema after ingestion. Both agents cause gastric carcinoma in rats and mice (Olson et al., 1973; Powers et al., 1975; IARC, 1977). Dibromochloropropane is highly suspected of causing sterility and/or abnormally low sperm counts in workmen engaged in its manufacture. Future use of both agents will likely be curtailed because of their carcinogenicity and their adverse effect on reproductive function.

Phosphine. Phosphine (PH_3), a fumigant for grain, is released gradually, in the presence of atmospheric moisture, from tablets of aluminum phosphide. Phosphine is more toxic than methyl bromide; however, since less is required to fumigate a given volume of grain, it has proven to be safer.

RODENTICIDES

Some rodenticides are quite toxic to man, but the toxicity of others is more selective. In some cases,

selectivity is based on a unique aspect of the physiology of rodents; in others, advantage is taken of the habits of these animals. Since rodenticides can be used in baits and placed in inaccessible places, the likelihood of their contaminating the environment is much less than that of insecticides. The toxicological problem posed by rodenticides, therefore, is primarily one of acute accidental or suicidal ingestion.

Warfarin. Warfarin, one of the most frequently used rodenticides, is considered safe because its toxicity depends on repeated ingestion. However, daily intake by man of 1 to 2 mg/kg for 6 days has produced severe illness in an attempted suicide. Warfarin, an oral anticoagulant, is discussed in Chapter 58.

Red Squill. The bulbs of red squill (*Urginea maritima*) have been used for many years as a relatively safe rodenticide. The active principles are scillaren glycosides. These glycosides, like the digitalis glycosides, have cardiotonic actions (*see* Chapter 30). Signs and symptoms associated with ingestion of large doses of red squill include vomiting and abdominal pain, blurred vision, cardiac irregularities, convulsions, and death from ventricular fibrillation. The selective rodenticidal usefulness of squill is due to the inability of rats to vomit (Lisella et al., 1971). Treatment of ingestion in man, if indicated, is the same as for overdosage of digitalis (*see* Chapter 30).

Sodium Fluoroacetate. Sodium fluoroacetate and fluoroacetamide are among the most potent rodenticides. Because they are also highly toxic to other animals, their use is restricted to licensed pest-control operators. Fluoroacetate produces its toxic action by inhibiting the citric acid cycle. The compound is incorporated into fluoroacetyl coenzyme A, which condenses with oxaloacetate to form fluorocitrate. Fluorocitrate inhibits the enzyme aconitase and thereby inhibits conversion of citrate to isocitrate. As might be expected, the heart and CNS are the tissues most critically involved by a general inhibition of oxidative energy metabolism. Thus, the signs and symptoms of fluoroacetate poisoning, in addition to nonspecific signs of nausea and vomiting, include cardiac irregularities, cyanosis, generalized convulsions, and death from ventricular fibrillation or respiratory failure (Brockmann et al., 1955). Provision of large quantities of acetate appears to antagonize fluoroacetate in a competitive manner; monkeys have been successfully protected from fluoroacetate poisoning by the administration of glycerol monoacetate (Chenoweth et al., 1951).

Phosphorus. White or yellow elemental phosphorus has poisoned man when it was spread in paste on bread to bait rodents. Shortly after ingestion, phosphorus produces severe gastrointestinal irritation, and, if the dose is sufficient, hemorrhage and cardiovascular failure may prove fatal within 24 hours. The vomitus is luminescent and has a characteristic garlic odor. If the patient survives the initial phase of gastrointestinal injury, secondary systemic poisoning and hepatic necrosis may ensue. Severe acute yellow atrophy of liver is a delayed sequela that may prove fatal.

Chronic poisoning from phosphorus is characterized by cachexia, anemia, bronchitis, and necrosis of the mandible, the so-called phossy jaw.

Zinc Phosphide. Zinc phosphide reacts with water and HCl in the gastrointestinal tract to produce the gas phosphine (PH_3), which causes severe gastrointestinal irritation. Apparent insensitivity of dogs and cats has been attributed to the emetic qualities of zinc in animals other than rodents. Later phases of toxicity resemble poisoning by yellow elemental phosphorus.

α-Naphthylthiourea. The structural formula of α-naphthylthiourea is as follows:

α-Naphthylthiourea

Its selective rodenticidal properties are due to different susceptibilities of various species. The LD50 in rats is about 3 mg/kg, in dogs 10 mg/kg, in guinea pigs 400 mg/kg, and in monkeys 4 g/kg. The principal toxic effect in susceptible species is massive pulmonary edema and pleural effusion, apparently the result of an action on pulmonary capillaries (Lillie, 1945; McClosky and Smith, 1945). Sulfhydryl blocking agents are effective antidotes for rats in some experimental conditions (DuBois et al., 1946; Koch and Schwarze, 1955).

Thallium. Thallium sulfate is very hazardous. Since it is not selectively toxic for rodents and many people have been poisoned by thallium, its use is now strictly regulated in many countries. Acute poisoning is accompanied by gastrointestinal irritation, motor paralysis, and death from respiratory failure. Sublethal doses, taken over a period of time, redden the skin and cause alopecia, characteristic signs of thallium poisoning. Pathological changes include perivascular cuffing and degenerative changes in the brain, liver, and kidney. Neurological symptoms are prominent and include tremors, leg pains, paresthesias of hands and feet, and polyneuritis, especially in the legs. Psychoses, delirium, convulsions, and other types of encephalopathy may also be noted. Diethyldithiocarbamate and diphenylthiocarbazone have been used as chelators for thallium. Dimercaprol (BAL) is of little benefit. Limited clinical experience has resulted in no consensus on the effectiveness of these agents in the treatment of thallium toxicity (Gosselin et al., 1976).

HERBICIDES

The production and use of chemicals for destruction of noxious weeds have increased markedly in the last decade. Herbicides now exceed insecticides in quantities used and values of sales. Although some herbicidal compounds have very low toxicity in mammals, others are highly toxic and have caused human fatalities.

Chlorophenoxy Compounds. The compounds *2,4-dichlorophenoxyacetic acid* (2,4-D) and *2,4,5-trichlorophenoxyacetic acid.* (2,4,5-T), as their salts and esters, are probably the most familiar herbicides. Their structural formulas are as follows:

2,4-D   2,4,5-T

They are used to control broad-leaf weeds in fields and to control woody plants along highways and rights-of-way; the compounds act as growth hormones in plants. Animals killed by massive doses of 2,4-D are believed to die of ventricular fibrillation (Hill and Carlisle, 1947). At lower doses, when death is delayed, there are various signs of neuromuscular involvement, including stiffness of the extremities, ataxia, paralysis, and, eventually, coma. Clinical reports of poisoning from chlorophenoxy herbicides are rare.

These herbicides do not accumulate in animals. They are not extensively metabolized but are actively excreted into the urine (Berndt and Koschier, 1973); their plasma half-life in man is about 1 day (Gehring et al., 1973).

Chorophenoxy herbicides have produced contact dermatitis in man, and a rather severe type of dermatitis, chloracne, has been observed in workers involved in the manufacture of 2,4,5-T (Poland et al., 1971). The dermatitis seems due primarily to the action of a contaminant, 2,3,7,8-tetrachlorodibenzo-*p*-dioxin (TCDD), the structure of which is as follows:

TCDD

TCDD is considered to be the most toxic chemical manufactured. It has an LD50 of 0.6 μg/kg in guinea pigs. The mechanism of death is not known, but morphological changes in the liver, thymus, and reproductive organs are observed. TCDD is a potent inducer of aryl hydrocarbon hydroxylase, a microsomal mixed-function oxidase (*see* Chapter 1; Poland and Glover, 1974). It is also a very potent teratogen (Neubert et al., 1973) and has been demonstrated to be a carcinogen (Van Miller et al., 1977; Kociba et al., 1978). Hence, there is considerable concern about the contamination of 2,4,5-T with TCDD, and its content is regulated at 0.1 ppm or less in the herbicide.

Dinitrophenols. Several substituted dinitrophenols, alone or as salts of aliphatic amines or alkalies, are used in weed control. Human poisonings by dinitroorthocresol (DNOC) have been reported (Bidstrup and Payne, 1951). The acute toxicity of dinitrophenols is due to the uncoupling of oxidative phosphorylation. The metabolic rate of the poisoned individual can increase markedly, and the body temperature is elevated. Signs and symptoms of acute poisoning in man include nausea, restlessness, flushed skin, sweating, rapid respiration, tachycardia, fever, cyanosis, and, finally, collapse and coma. The illness runs a rapid course; there is death or recovery within 24 to 48 hours. If production of heat exceeds the capacity for its dissipation, fatal hyperthermia may result. Specific treatment consists in ice baths to reduce fever; oxygen is administered, and fluid and electrolyte imbalances should be corrected.

Bipyridyl Compounds. Paraquat is the best-known compound in this class of herbicides, and its use is increasing. The structural formula of paraquat is as follows:

Paraquat

More than 200 cases of accidental or suicidal fatalities from paraquat poisoning have been reported during the past few years (Campbell, 1968; Davies *et al.*, 1977). Pathological changes observed at autopsy are indicative of damage to the lungs, liver, and kidneys; myocarditis is sometimes present. The most striking pathological change is a widespread proliferation of cells in the lungs, an effect that is not dependent on the route of administration. Although ingestion of paraquat causes gastrointestinal upset within a few hours, the onset of respiratory symptoms and eventual death by respiratory distress may be delayed for several days.

A biochemical mechanism for paraquat-induced pulmonary injury has been proposed by Bus and associates (1976). Paraquat is believed to undergo a single-electron, cyclic reduction-oxidation, with subsequent formation of superoxide anions (O_2^-). Superoxide is nonenzymatically transformed to singlet oxygen, which attacks polyunsaturated lipids associated with cell membranes to form lipid hydroperoxides. The lipid hydroperoxides are unstable in the presence of trace amounts of transition metal ions and decompose to lipid-free radicals. The chain reaction of lipid peroxidation thus initiated is somewhat similar to that described above for CCl_4.

Due to the serious, delayed pulmonary toxicity produced by paraquat, prompt treatment is important. This involves removal of paraquat from the alimentary tract by gastric lavage and the use of cathartics, prevention of further absorption by oral administration of Fuller's earth, and removal of absorbed paraquat by hemodialysis or hemoperfusion (Cavalli and Fletcher, 1977; Davies *et al.*, 1977).

Public interest in the toxicology of paraquat was recently stimulated by revelation of its use in a herbicide spray program to control illicit production of marihuana and heroin in Mexico. High concentrations of paraquat were found in some marihuana cigarettes. It was estimated that 0.3 μg of paraquat could be inhaled by smoking a marihuana cigarette contaminated with 1000 ppm of the herbicide, and it was suggested that a slow accumulation of lung "scarring" might occur in persons who inhaled even these small quantities (Smith, 1978). There is at this time little or no documentation to support these suggestions.

Other Herbicides. There are a large number of other herbicides that, for the most part, have relatively low acute toxicities for mammals. These include carbamates (*e.g., propham* and *barban*), substituted ureas (*e.g., monuron* and *diuron*), triazines (*e.g., atrazine* and the related compound *aminotriazole*), aniline derivatives (*e.g., alachlor, propachlor,* and *propanil*), dinitroaniline derivatives (*e.g., trifalin*), and benzoic acid derivatives (*e.g., amiben*).

FUNGICIDES

Fungicides, like other classes of pesticides, comprise a heterogeneous group of chemical compounds. With few exceptions, the fungicides have not been the subject of detailed toxicological research. Although many compounds used to control fungal diseases on plants, seeds, and produce are rather nontoxic acutely, there are some notable exceptions; the mercury-containing fungicides have caused the greatest concern. They have been responsible for many deaths or permanent neurological disabilities resulting from the misdirection of treated seed grains into human and animal food. The toxicities of mercury and its compounds are discussed in Chapter 69.

Dithiocarbamates. Fungicides of this group are commonly used in agriculture. They have a low order of acute toxicity, and values of the oral LD50 in rats range from several hundred milligrams to several grams per kilogram. There is little evidence of human injury from exposure to these compounds; however, they may have some teratogenic and/or carcinogenic potential (World Health Organization, 1975). Two groups of dithiocarbamates that have been used, the dimethyldithiocarbamates and the ethylenebisdithiocarbamates, have the following general formulas:

Dimethyldithiocarbamates

Ethylenebisdithiocarbamates

The names of the fungicides are derived from the metallic cations. For example, when the cation is zinc or iron, the respective dimethyldithiocarbamates are *ziram* or *ferbam*. With manganese, zinc, or sodium as the cation in the diethyldithiocarbamate series, the respective fungicides are *maneb, zineb,* or *nabam*. Some dimethyldithiocarbamates are reported to be teratogenic in animals, and they can form nitrosamines *in vitro* and *in vivo* (IARC, 1974b; World Health Organization, 1975). The ethylenebisdithiocarbamates are also reported to be teratogenic (Petrova-Vergieva and Ivanova-Tchemishanska, 1973). Furthermore, this group of compounds breaks down to form ethylenethiourea (ETU) *in vivo,* in the environment, and during cooking of foods containing their residues. ETU is carcinogenic, mutagenic, and teratogenic, as well as an antithyroid agent (IARC, 1974b, 1976). Dithiocarbamate fungicides are analogs of disulfiram, and they can produce a disulfiram-like response when ethanol is ingested (*see* Chapter 18).

Hexachlorobenzene. Exposure to hexachlorobenzene results in an increase in hepatic weight, in the quantity of smooth endoplasmic reticulum and cytochrome P-450, and in the activities of mixed-function oxidases (Carlson and Tardiff, 1976). Between 1955 and 1959, more than 300 human poisonings occurred in Turkey as a result of the use of hexachlorobenzene-treated wheat (Schmid, 1960). Some deaths resulted; the major syndrome was cutaneous porphyria with skin lesions, porphyrinuria, and photosensitization.

Pentachlorophenol. Pentachlorophenol is used as an insecticide and a herbicide, as well as a fungicide, with major application as a wood preservative. Several cases of human poisoning have been associated with its use. The acute toxic action of pentachlorophenol in man and experimental animals resembles that of the nitrophenolic herbicides—a marked increase in metabolic rate as the result of uncoupling of oxidative phosphorylation. Pentachlorophenol is readily absorbed through the skin. Two cases of fatal poisonings and several nonfatal cases occurred in a hospital nursery; pentachlorophenol had been used as a fungicide in the laundry room and ultimately came in contact with infants through their diapers (Armstrong *et al.,* 1969).

In recent years it has become apparent that many commercial samples of pentachlorophenol are contaminated with polychlorinated dibenzodioxins and dibenzofuran (Buser, 1975). These contaminants are generally less toxic than the tetrachlorodioxin contaminant (TCDD) in 2,4,5-T. Although pentachlorophenol is highly toxic in its own right, some studies suggest that the contaminants may be responsible for some of the untoward effects of the technical-grade product (Johnson *et al.,* 1973; Goldstein *et al.,* 1976).

Aksoy, M.; Erdem, S.; and Dincol, G. Leukemia in shoeworkers exposed to chronic benzene. *Blood,* **1974,** *44,* 837–841.

Alarie, Y. C.; Krumm, A. A.; Busey, W. M.; Ulrich, C. E.; and Kantz, R. J., Jr. Long-term exposure to sulfur dioxide, sulfuric acid mist, fly ash, and their mixtures. Results of studies in monkeys and guinea pigs. *Arch. Environ. Health,* **1975,** *30,* 254–262.

Amdur, M. O. The response of guinea pigs to inhalation of formaldehyde and formic acid alone and with a sodium chloride aerosol. *Int. J. Air Pollut.,* **1960,** *3,* 201–220.

Amdur, M. O.; Bayles, J.; Ugro, V.; and Underhill, D. W. Comparative irritant potency of sulfate salts. *Environ. Res.,* **1978a,** *16,* 1–8.

Amdur, M. O., and Corn, M. The irritant potency of zinc ammonium sulfate of different particle sizes. *Am. Ind. Hyg. Assoc. J.,* **1963,** *24,* 326–333.

Amdur, M. O.; Dubriel, M.; and Creasia, D. A. Respiratory response of guinea pigs to low levels of sulfuric acid. *Environ. Res.,* **1978b,** *15,* 418–423.

Anderson, R. F.; Allensworth, D. C.; and de Groot, W. J. Myocardial toxicity from carbon monoxide poisoning. *Ann. Intern. Med.,* **1967,** *67,* 1172–1182.

Apthrop, G. H.; Bates, D. V.; Marshall, R.; and Mendel, D. Effect of acute carbon monoxide on work capacity. *Br. Med. J.,* **1958,** *2,* 476–478.

Armstrong, R. W.; Eichner, E. R.; Klein, D. E.; Barthel, W. F.; Bennett, J. V.; Jonsson, V.; Bruce, H.; and Loveless, L. E. Pentachlorophenol poisoning in a nursery for newborn infants. II. Epidemiologic and toxicologic studies. *J. Pediatr.,* **1969,** *75,* 317–325.

Ayres, S. M.; Giammelli, S., Jr.; and Mueller, H. Effects of low concentrations of carbon monoxide. Part IV. Myocardial and systemic responses to carboxyhemoglobin. *Ann. N.Y. Acad. Sci.,* **1970,** *174,* 268–293.

Beard, R. R., and Grandstaff, N. Carbon monoxide and human functions. In, *Behavioral Toxicology.* (Weiss, B., and Laties, V. G., eds.) Plenum Press, New York, **1975,** pp. 1–26.

Berndt, W. O., and Koschier, F. *In vitro* uptake of 2,4-dichlorophenoxyacetic acid (2,4,-D) and 2,4,5-trichlorophenoxyacetic acid (2,4,5-T) by renal cortical tissue of rabbits and rats. *Toxicol. Appl. Pharmacol.,* **1973,** *26,* 1114–1117.

Bidstrup, P. I., and Payne, D. J. H. Poisoning by dinitroorthocresol: report of eight fatal cases occurring in Great Britain. *Br. Med. J.,* **1951,** *2,* 16–19.

Boatman, E. S.; Sato, S.; and Frank, R. Acute effects of ozone on cat lungs. II. Structural. *Am. Rev. Respir. Dis.,* **1974,** *110,* 157–169.

Bokonjić, N. Stagnant anoxia and carbon monoxide poisoning. *Electroencephalogr. Clin. Neurophysiol.,* **1963,** Suppl. 21, 1–102.

Brockmann, J. L.; McDowell, A. V.; and Leeds, W. G. Fatal poisoning with sodium fluoroacetate. *J.A.M.A.,* **1955,** *159,* 1529–1532.

Bruch, J. Ein elektronemikroskopischer Beitrag zum Fruhstadium der Silikose. *Fortschr. Stanbulgensforsch,* **1967,** *2,* 249.

Brucher, J. M. Neuropathological problems posed by carbon monoxide poisoning and anoxia. *Prog. Brain Res.,* **1967,** *24,* 75–100.

Bus, J. S.; Cagen, S. Z.; Olgaard, M.; and Gibson, J. E. A mechanism of paraquat toxicity in mice and rats. *Toxicol. Appl. Pharmacol.,* **1976,** *35,* 501–513.

Buser, H. R. Analysis of polychlorinated dibenzo-*p*-dioxins and dibenzofurans in chlorinated phenols by mass fragmentography. *J. Chromatogr.,* **1975,** *107,* 295–310.

Campbell, S. Paraquat poisoning. *Clin. Toxicol.,* **1968,** *1,* 245–249.

Carlson, D. A.; Konyhu, K. D.; Wheeler, W. B.; Marshall, G. P.; and Zaylskie, R. G. Mirex in the environment: its degradation to KEPONE and related compounds. *Science,* **1976,** *94,* 939–941.

Carlson, G. P., and Tardiff, R. G. Effect of chlorinated benzenes on the metabolism of foreign organic compounds. *Toxicol. Appl. Pharmacol.,* **1976,** *36,* 383–394.

Cavalli, R. D., and Fletcher, K. An effective treatment for paraquat poisoning. In, *Biochemical Mechanism of*

Paraquat Toxicity. (Autor, A. P., ed.) Academic Press, Inc., New York, **1977**, pp. 213–228.

Chadwick, R. W.; Choang, L. T.; and Williams, K. Dehydrogenation: a previously unreported pathway of lindane metabolism in mammals. *Pesticide Biochem. Physiol.,* **1975,** *5,* 575–586.

Chen, K. K., and Rose, C. L. Treatment of acute cyanide poisoning. *J.A.M.A.,* **1956,** *162,* 1154–1156.

Chenoweth, M. B. Ventricular fibrillation induced by hydrocarbons and epinephrine. *J. Ind. Hyg. Toxicol.,* **1946,** *28,* 151–158.

Chenoweth, M. B.; Kandel, A.; Johnson, L. B.; and Bennett, D. R. Factors influencing fluroacetate poisoning: practical treatment with glycerol monoacetate. *J. Pharmacol. Exp. Ther.,* **1951,** *102,* 31–49.

Coffin, D. L., and Blommer, E. J. Acute toxicity of irradiated auto exhaust. Its indication by enhancement of mortality from streptococcal pneumonia. *Arch. Environ. Health,* **1967,** *15,* 36–38.

Coffin, D. L.; Gardiner, D. E.; and Blommer, E. J. Time-dose response for nitrogen dioxide exposure in an infectivity model system. *Environ. Health Perspect.,* **1976,** *13,* 11–15.

Cohn, W. J.; Boylan, J. J.; Blanke, R. V.; Furiss, M. W.; Howell, J. R.; and Guzelian, P. S. Treatment of chlordecone (KEPONE) toxicity with cholestyramine. *N. Engl. J. Med.,* **1978,** *298,* 243–248.

Cornish, H. H., and Adefuin, J. Potentiation of carbon tetrachloride toxicity by aliphatic alcohols. *Arch. Environ. Health,* **1967,** *14,* 447–449.

Cosby, R. S., and Bergeron, M. Electrocardiographic changes in carbon monoxide poisoning. *Am. J. Cardiol.,* **1963,** *11,* 93–96.

Cueto, C.; Page, N.; and Saffiott, V. *Report of Carcinogenesis, Bioassay of Technical Grade Chlordecone* (KEPONE). National Cancer Institute, Bethesda, **1976.**

Dale, W. E.; Gaines, T. B.; Hayes, W. J., Jr.; and Pearce, G. W. Poisoning by DDT: relation between clinical signs and concentration in rat brain. *Science,* **1963,** *142,* 1474–1476.

Dalhamn, T. Mucous flow and ciliary activity in the trachea of healthy rats and rats exposed to respiratory irritant gases (SO_2, H_3N, HCHO). A functional and morphologic (light microscopic and electron microscopic) study, with special reference to technique. *Acta Physiol. Scand.,* **1956,** *36,* Suppl. 123, 1–161.

Davies, D. S.; Hawksworth, G. M.; and Bennett, P. N. Paraquat poisoning. *Proc. Eur. Soc. Toxicol.,* **1977,** *18,* 21–26.

DeLucia, A. J.; Mustaffa, M. G.; Hussain, M. Z.; and Cross, C. E. Ozone interaction with rodent lung. III. Oxidation of reduced glutathione and formation of mixed disulfides between protein and nonprotein sulfhydryls. *J. Clin. Invest.,* **1975,** *55,* 794–802.

DeVincenzo, G.; Kaplan, C.; and Dedinas, J. Characterization of the metabolites of methyl N-butyl ketone, methyl isobutyl ketone, methyl ethyl ketone in guinea pig serum and their clearance. *Toxicol. Appl. Pharmacol.,* **1976,** *36,* 511–522.

DiazGomez, M. I.; deCastro, C. R.; DiAcosta, N.; de Fenos, O. M.; Deferreya, E. C.; and Castro, A. J. Species differences in carbon tetrachloride–induced hepatotoxicity: the role of CCl_4 activation and of lipid preoxidation. *Toxicol. Appl. Pharmacol.,* **1975,** *34,* 102–114.

DuBois, K. P.; Holm, L. W.; and Doyle, W. L. Biochemical changes following poisoning of rats by alpha-naphthylthiourea. *Proc. Soc. Exp. Biol. Med.,* **1946,** *61,* 102–104.

Easton, R. E., and Murphy, S. D. Experimental ozone pre-exposure and histamine. Effect on the acute toxicity and respiratory function effects of histamine in guinea pigs. *Arch. Environ. Health,* **1967,** *15,* 160–166.

Folland, D. S.; Schaffner, W.; Grinn, H. E.; Crofford, O. B.; and McMurray, D. R. Carbon tetrachloride toxicity

potentiated by isopropyl alcohol. *J.A.M.A.,* **1976,** *236,* 1853–1856.

Frank, N. R.; Amdur, M. O.; Worchester, J.; and Whittenberger, J. L. Effects of acute controlled exposure to SO_2 on respiratory mechanics in healthy male adults. *J. Appl. Physiol.,* **1962,** *17,* 252–258.

Frank, N. R., and Speizer, F. E. SO_2 effects on the respiratory system in dogs. Changes in mechanical behavior at different levels of the respiratory system during acute exposure to the gas. *Arch. Environ. Health,* **1965,** *11,* 624–634.

Freal, J. J., and Chadwick, R. W. Metabolism of hexachlorocyclohexane to chlorophenols and effects of isomer pretreatment on lindane metabolism in rat. *J. Agric. Food Chem.,* **1973,** *21,* 424–427.

Freeman, G.; Crane, S. C.; Furiosi, N. J.; Stephens, R. J.; Evans, M. J.; and Moore, W. D. Covert reduction in ventilatory surface in rats during prolonged exposure to subacute nitrogen dioxide. *Am. Rev. Respir. Dis.,* **1972,** *106,* 563–579.

Freireich, A. W.; Cinque, T. J.; Xanthaky, G.; and Landau, D. Hemodialysis for isopropanol poisoning. *N. Engl. J. Med.,* **1967,** *277,* 699–700.

Garner, R. C., and McLean, A. E. M. Increased susceptibility to carbon tetrachloride poisoning in the rat liver after pretreatment with oral phenobarbitone. *Biochem. Pharmacol.,* **1969,** *18,* 645.

Gehring, P. J.; Kramer, C. G.; Schwetz, B. A.; Rose, J. Q.; and Rowe, V. K. The fate of 2,4,5-trichlorophenoxyacetic acid (2,4,5-T) following oral administration to man. *Toxicol. Appl. Pharmacol.,* **1973,** *26,* 352–361.

Geiling, E. M. K., and Cannon, P. R. Pathologic effects of elixir sulfanilamide (diethylene glycol) poisoning; clinical and experimental correlations: final report. *J.A.M.A.,* **1938,** *111,* 919–926.

Gerarde, H. W. Toxicological studies on hydrocarbons. IX. The aspiration hazard and toxicity of hydrocarbons and hydrocarbon mixtures. *Arch. Environ. Health,* **1963,** *6,* 329–391.

Goldsmith, J. R., and Landaw, S. A. Carbon monoxide and human health. *Science,* **1968,** *162,* 1352–1359.

Goldstein, J. A.; Linder, R. E.; Hickman, P.; and Bergman, H. Effects of pentachlorophenol on hepatic drug metabolism and porphyria related to contamination with chlorinated dibenzo-p-dioxins. *Toxicol. Appl. Pharmacol.,* **1976,** *37,* 145–146.

Hansen, D. J.; Wilson, A. J.; Nimmo, D. R.; Schimmel, S. C.; Bahner, L. H.; and Huggett, R. KEPONE: hazard to aquatic organisms. *Science,* **1976,** *193,* 528.

Hayes, W. J., Jr., and Vaughn, W. K. Mortality from pesticides in the United States in 1973 and 1974. *Toxicol. Appl. Pharmacol.,* **1977,** *42,* 235–252.

Heppleston, A. G., and Styles, J. A. Activity of a macrophage factor in collagen formation by silica. *Nature,* **1967,** *214,* 521–522.

Hill, E. C., and Carlisle, H. Toxicity of 2,4-dichlorophenoxyacetic acid for experimental animals. *J. Ind. Hyg. Toxicol.,* **1947,** *29,* 85–95.

Hine, C. H. Methyl bromide poisoning: a review of ten cases. *J. Occup. Med.,* **1969,** *11,* 1–10.

Hirsch, J. A.; Swenson, E. W.; and Wanner, A. Tracheal mucous transport in beagles after long-term exposure to 1 ppm sulfur dioxide. *Arch. Environ. Health,* **1975,** *30,* 249–253.

Iida, M.; Yamamoto, H.; and Sobue, I. Prognosis of *n*-hexane polyneuropathy: follow-up studies on mass outbreak in F district of Mie prefecture. *Igaku No Ayumi,* **1973,** *84,* 199–201.

Innes, J. R. M., and others. Bioassay of pesticides and industrial chemicals for tumorigenicity in mice: a preliminary note. *J. Natl. Cancer Inst.,* **1969,** *42,* 1101–1114.

Jerina, D. M., and Daley, J. R. Arene oxides: a new aspect of drug metabolism. *Science,* **1974,** *185,* 573–582.

Johnson, R. L.; Gehring, P. J.; Kociba, R. J.; and Schwetz, B. A. Chlorinated dibenzodioxins and pentachlorophenol. *Environ. Health Perspect.*, **1973**, *5,* 171–175.

Kapoor, I. P.; Metcalf, R. L.; Nystrom, R. F.; and Sangha, G. H. Comparative metabolism of methoxchlor, methioclor, and DDT in mouse, insects and in a model ecosystem. *J. Agric. Food Chem.*, **1970**, *18,* 1145–1152.

Kazantzis, G.; McLaughlin, A. I. G.; and Prior, P. F. Poisoning in industrial workers by the insecticide aldrin. *Br. J. Ind. Med.*, **1964**, *21,* 46–51.

Kettle, E. H. The relation of dust to infection. *Proc. R. Soc. Med.*, **1930**, *24,* 79–94.

King, L. H.; Bradley, K. P.; and Shires, D. L. Hemodialysis for isopropyl alcohol poisoning. *J.A.M.A.*, **1970**, *211,* 1855.

Klaassen, C. D., and Plaa, G. L. Relative effect of various chlorinated hydrocarbons on liver and kidney function in mice. *Toxicol. Appl. Pharmacol.*, **1966**, *9,* 139–151.

————. Relative effects of various chlorinated hydrocarbons on liver and kidney functions in dogs. *Ibid.*, **1967**, *10,* 199–134.

————. Comparison of the biochemical alterations elicited in livers from rats treated with carbon tetrachloride, chloroform, 1,1,2-trichloroethane, and 1,1,1-trichloroethane. *Biochem. Pharmacol.*, **1969**, *18,* 2019–2027.

Koch, R., and Schwarze, W. Die Hemmung der α-Naphthylthioharnstoffvergiftung durch Cysteamin und seine Derivate. (Zugleich ein Beitrag zur Toxikologie und Strahlenschutzwirkung dieser Sulfhydrylkorper). *Naunyn Schmiedebergs Arch. Exp. Pathol. Pharmakol.*, **1955**, *225,* 428–411.

Kociba, R. J., and others. Result of a 2-year chronic toxicity and oncogenicity study of 2,3,7,8-tetrachlorodibenzo-p-dioxin in rats. *Toxicol. Appl. Pharmacol.*, **1978**, *46,* 279–303.

Kolmodin, B.; Azarnoff, D. L.; and Sjoqvist, F. Effect of environmental factors on drug metabolism: decreased plasma half-live of antipyrine in workers exposed to chlorinated hydrocarbon insecticides. *Clin. Pharmacol. Ther.*, **1969**, *10,* 638–642.

Krishna, G.; Pohl, I. R.; and Bhooshan, B. Mechanism of the metabolic activation of chloroform. *Toxicol. Appl. Pharmacol.*, **1978**, *45,* 238.

Kubic, V., and Anders, M. Metabolism of dihalomethanes to carbon monoxide. II. In vitro studies. *Drug Metab. Dispos.*, **1975**, *3,* 104–112.

Lapresle, J., and Fardeau, M. The central nervous system and carbon monoxide poisoning. II. Anatomical study of brain lesions following intoxication with carbon monoxide (22 cases). *Prog. Brain Res.*, **1967**, *24,* 31–74.

Lawther, P. J., and Commins, B. T. Cigarette smoking and exposure to carbon monoxide. *Ann. N.Y. Acad. Sci.*, **1970**, *174,* 135–147.

Lawton, J. J., Jr., and Malmquist, C. P. Gasoline addiction in children. *Psychiatr. Q.*, **1961**, *35,* 555–561.

Lee, L. Y.; Bleeker, E.; and Nadel, J. A. Ozone-induced airway hyperirritability in dogs. *Fed. Proc.*, **1977**, *36,* 616.

Leech, P. N. Elixir of sulfanilamide-Massengill. Chemical, pharmacologic, pathologic and necropsy reports; preliminary toxicity reports on diethylene glycol and sulfanilamide. *J.A.M.A.*, **1937**, *109,* 1531–1539.

Lillie, R. D. Studies on the pharmacologic action and the pathology of alpha-naphthylthiourea. II. Pathology. *Public Health Rep.*, **1945**, *60,* 1108–1113.

Lisella, F. S.; Long, K. R.; and Scott, H. G. Toxicology of rodenticides and their relation to human health. *J. Environ. Health*, **1971**, *33,* 231–237, 361–365.

Loge, J. P. Aplastic anemia following exposure to benzene hexachloride (LINDANE). *J.A.M.A.*, **1965**, *193,* 110–114.

Long, P. I. Dermal changes associated with carbon monoxide intoxication. *J.A.M.A.*, **1968**, *205,* 51–52.

Longo, L. D. The biological effects of carbon monoxide on the pregnant woman, fetus, and newborn infant. *Am. J. Obstet. Gynecol.*, **1977**, *129,* 69–103.

McClosky, W. T., and Smith, M. I. Studies of the pharmacologic action and the pathology of alpha-naphthyl-thiourea. 1. Pharmacology. *Public Health Rep.*, **1945**, *60,* 1101–1108.

Machle, W. Gasoline intoxication. *J.A.M.A.*, **1941**, *117,* 1965–1971.

McLean, A. E. M., and McLean, E. K. The effect of diet and 1,1,1,-trichloro 2,2-*bis*-(p-chlorphenyl) ethane (DDT) on microsomal hydroxylating enzymes and on the sensitivity of rats to carbon tetrachloride poisoning. *Biochem. J.*, **1966**, *100,* 564–571.

McMichael, A.; Spirtas, R.; Kupper, L.; and Gamble, J. Solvent exposure and leukemia among rubber workers: an epidemiological study. *J. Occup. Med.*, **1975**, *17,* 234–239.

Matthew, H. Acute poisoning: some myths and misconceptions. *Br. Med. J.*, **1971**, *1,* 519–522.

Meigs, J. W., and Hughes, J. P. W. Acute carbon monoxide poisoning: an analysis of one hundred five cases. *A.M.A. Arch. Ind. Hyg. Occup. Med.*, **1952**, *6,* 344–356.

Murphy, S. D.; Klingshirn, D. A.; and Ulrich, C. E. Respiratory response of guinea pigs during acrolein inhalation and its modification by drugs. *J. Pharmacol. Exp. Ther.*, **1963**, *141,* 79–83.

Nadel, J. A.; Salem, H.; Tamplin, B.; and Tokiwa, Y. Mechanism of bronchoconstriction during inhalation of sulfur dioxide. *J. Appl. Physiol.*, **1965**, *20,* 164–167.

Narahashi, T. Mode of action of DDT and allethrin on nerve: cellular and molecular mechanisms. *Residue Rev.*, **1969**, *25,* 275–288.

Narahashi, T., and Hass, H. G. DDT: interaction with nerve membrane conductance changes. *Science*, **1967**, *157,* 1438–1440.

National Academy of Sciences. *Drinking Water and Health.* The Academy, Washington, D. C., **1977**, p. 939.

Neubert, D.; Zens, P.; Rothenwallner, A.; and Merker, H. J. A survey of the embryotoxic effects of TCDD in mammalian species. *Environ. Health Perspect.*, **1973**, *5,* 67–79.

Norman, J. N., and Ledingham, I. McA. Carbon monoxide poisoning: investigations and treatment. *Prog. Brain Res.*, **1967**, *24,* 101–122.

O'Hanlon, J. F. Preliminary studies of the effects of carbon monoxide on vigilance in man. In, *Behavioral Toxicology.* (Weiss, B., and Laties, V. G., eds.) Plenum Press, New York, **1975**, pp. 593–602.

Olson, W. A.; Hubermann, R. T.; Weisburger, E. K.; Ward, J. M.; and Weisburger, J. H. Induction of stomach cancer in rats and mice by halogenated aliphatic fumigants. *J. Natl. Cancer Inst.*, **1973**, *51,* 1933–1955.

Orehek, J.; Massar, J. P.; Gayrard, P.; Grimaud, C.; and Charpin, J. Effect of short-term, low-level nitrogen dioxide exposure on bronchial sensitivity of asthmatic patients. *J. Clin. Invest.*, **1976**, *57,* 301–307.

Peterson, J. E., and Robison, W. H. Metabolic products of *p,p′*-DDT in the rat. *Toxicol. Appl. Pharmacol.*, **1964**, *6,* 321–327.

Peterson, J. E., and Stewart, R. D. Absorption and elimination of carbon monoxide by inactive young men. *Arch. Environ. Health*, **1970**, *21,* 165–171.

Petrova-Vergieva, T., and Ivanova-Tchemishanska, L. Assessment of the teratogenic activity of dithiocarbamate fungicides. *Food Cosmet. Toxicol.*, **1973**, *11,* 239–244.

Philips, F. S.; Gilman, A.; and Crescitelli, F. N. Studies on the pharmacology of DDT (2,2-*bis*(parachlorophenyl)-l,l,l-trichloroethane). II. The sensitization of the myocardium to sympathetic stimulation during acute DDT intoxication. *J. Pharmacol. Exp. Ther.*, **1946**, *86,* 213–221.

Pinto, J. D.; Camien, M. N.; and Dunn, M. S. Metabolic fate of *p,p′*-DDT. [1,1,1,-trichloro-2,2-*bis*(p-chlorophenyl) ethane] in rats. *J. Biol. Chem.*, **1965**, *240,* 2148–2154.

Plaa, G. L.; Traiger, G. J.; Hanusono, G. K.; and Witschi, H. P. Effect of alcohols on various forms of chemically induced liver injury. In, *Alcoholic Liver Pathology.* (Khanna, J. M.; Israel, Y.; and Kalant, H.; eds.) Addiction Research Foundation, Toronto, **1975**, pp. 225–244.

Poland, A. P., and Glover, E. Comparison of 2,3,7,8-tetrachlorodibenzo-*p*-dioxin, a potent inducer of aryl hydrocarbon hydroxylase, with 3-methylcholanthrene. *Mol. Pharmacol.,* **1974**, *10,* 349–359.

Poland, A. P.; Smith, D.; Kuntzman, R.; Jacobson, M.; and Conney, A. H. Effect of extensive occupational exposure to DDT on phenylbutazone and cortisol metabolism in human beings. *Clin. Pharmacol. Ther.,* **1970**, *11,* 724–732.

Poland, A. P.; Smith, D.; Metter, G.; and Possiek, P. A health survey of workers in a 2,4-D and 2,4,5-T plant with special attention to chloracne, porphyria cutaneatarda and psychologic parameters. *Arch. Eviron. Health,* **1971**, *22,* 759–768.

Powers, M. B.; Voelker, R. W.; Page, N. P.; Weisburger, E. K.; and Kraybill, H. F. Carcinogenicity of ethylene dibromide (EDB) and 1,2-dibromo-3 chloropropane (DBCP) after oral administration in rats and mice. *Toxicol. Appl. Pharmacol.,* **1975**, *33,* 171–172.

Press, E., and Done, A. K. Solvent sniffing. *Pediatrics,* **1967**, *39,* 451–461, 611–622.

Radcliffe, D. A. Decrease in eggshell weight in certain birds of prey. *Nature,* **1967**, *215,* 208–210.

Reid, L. An experimental study of hypersecretion of mucus in the bronchial tree. *Br. J. Exp. Pathol.,* **1963**, *44,* 437–445.

Reinhardt, C.; Mullin, L.; and Maxfield, M. Epinephrine-induced cardiac arrhythmia potential of some common industrial solvents. *J. Occup. Med.,* **1973**, *15,* 953–955.

Riddick, J. H., Jr.; Campbell, K. I.; and Coffin, D. L. Histopathologic changes secondary to nitrogen dioxide exposure in dog lungs. *Am. J. Clin. Pathol.,* **1968**, *49,* 239.

Rodkey, F. L.; O'Nea, J. D.; Collison, H. A.; and Uddin, D. E. Relative affinity of hemoglobin S and hemoglobin A for carbon monoxide and oxygen. *Clin. Chem.,* **1974**, *20,* 83–84.

Roughton, F. J. W. Kinetics of gas transport in the blood. *Br. Med. Bull.,* **1963**, *19,* 80–89.

Roughton, F. J. W., and Root, W. S. The fate of CO in the body during recovery from mild carbon monoxide poisoning in man. *Am. J. Physiol.,* **1945**, *145,* 239–252.

Saleh, M. A.; Turner, W. V.; and Casida, J. E. Polychlorobornane components of toxaphene: structure-toxicity relations and metabolic reductive dechlorination. *Science,* **1977**, *198,* 1256–1258.

Savilahti, M. Mehr als 100 Vergiftungstalle durch Benzol in einer Schuhfabrik. *Arch. Gewerbepathol. Gewerbehyg.,* **1956**, *15,* 147–157.

Schlipkoeter, H. W., and Lindner, E. Electron microscopic study of quartz granuloma in experimental silicosis in white rats. *Z. Hyg. Infektionskr.,* **1961**, *147,* 287–318.

Schmid, R. Cutaneous porphyria in Turkey. *N. Engl. J. Med.,* **1960**, *263,* 397–398.

Selikoff, I. J. Asbestos. *Environment,* **1969**, *11,* 3–7.

Selikoff, I. J.; Hammond, E. C.; and Churg, J. Asbestos exposure, smoking and neoplasia. *J.A.M.A.,* **1968**, *204,* 106–112.

Sheehy, M., and Way, J. L. Effect of oxygen on cyanide intoxication. III. Mithridate. *J. Pharmacol. Exp. Ther.,* **1968**, *161,* 163–168.

Slater, T. F. Necrogenic action of carbon tetrachloride in the rat: a speculative mechanism based on activation. *Nature,* **1966**, *209,* 36–40.

Smith, G.; Ledingham, I. McA.; Sharb, G. R.; Norman, J. N.; and Bates, E. H. Treatment of coal-gas poisoning with oxygen at 2 atmospheres pressure. *Lancet,* **1962**, *1,* 816–818.

Smith, R. J. Poisoned pot becomes burning issue in high places. *Science,* **1978**, *200,* 417–418.

Snyder, R.; Lee, E. W.; Kocsis, J. J.; and Witmer, C. M. Bone marrow depressant and leukemogenic actions of benzene. *Life Sci.,* **1977**, *21,* 1709–1722.

Steele, R. W.; Conklin, R. H.; and Mark, H. M. Corticosteroids and antibiotics for the treatment of fulminant hydrocarbons aspiration. *J.A.M.A.,* **1972**, *219,* 1434–1437.

Stephens, R. J.; Freeman, G.; Stara, J. F.; and Coffin, D. L. Cytologic changes in dog lungs induced by chronic exposure to ozone. *Am. J. Pathol.,* **1973**, *73,* 711–718.

Stephens, R. J.; Sloan, M. F.; Evans, M. J.; and Freeman, G. Early response of lung to low levels of ozone. *Am. J. Pathol.,* **1974**, *74,* 31–57.

Stewart, R. D.; Baretta, E. D.; Platte, L. R.; Stewart, E. B.; Kalbfleisch, J. H.; Yserlo, B. V.; and Rimm, A. A. Carboxyhemoglobin concentrations in blood from donors in Chicago, Milwaukee, New York and Los Angeles. *Science,* **1973**, *182,* 1362–1364.

Striker, G. E.; Smuckler, E. A.; Kohnen, P. W.; and Nagle, R. B. Structural and functional changes in rat kidney during CCl_4 intoxication. *Am. J. Pathol.,* **1968**, *53,* 769–789.

Taylor, J. R.; Selhorst, J. B.; Houff, S. A.; and Martinez, A. J. Chlordecone intoxication in man. 1. Clinical observations. *Neurology (Minneap.),* **1978**, *28,* 626–635.

Thomsen, H. K. Carbon monoxide–induced atherosclerosis in primates. An electron-microscopic study on the coronary arteries of *Macaca irus* monkeys. *Atherosclerosis,* **1974**, *20,* 233–240.

Turner, W. A.; Engel, J. L.; and Casida, J. E. Toxaphene components and related compounds: preparation and toxicity of some hepta-, octa-, and nonachlorobornanes, hexa-, and heptachlorobornenes and a hexachlorobornadiene. *J. Agric. Food Chem.,* **1977**, *25,* 1394–1401.

Van Miller, J. P.; Lalich, J. J.; and Allen, J. R. Increased incidence of neoplasms in rats exposed to low levels of 2,3,7,8-tetrachlorodibenzo-*o*-dioxin. *Chemosphere,* **1977**, *9,* 537–544.

Wacker, W. E. C.; Haynes, H.; Druyan, R.; Fisher, W.; and Coleman, J. E. Treatment of ethylene glycol poisoning with ethyl alcohol. *J.A.M.A.,* **1965**, *194,* 1231–1233.

Waters, E. M.; Huff, J. E.; and Gerstner, H. B. Mirex, an overview. *Environ. Res.,* **1977**, *14,* 212–222.

Way, J. L.; End, E.; Sheehy, M. H.; DeMiranda, P.; Feitknecht, O. F.; Bachand, R.; Gibbson, S. L.; and Burrows, G. E. Effects of oxygen on cyanide intoxication. IV. Hyperbaric oxygen. *Toxicol. Appl. Pharmacol.,* **1972**, *22,* 415–421.

Way, J. L.; Gibbson, S. L.; and Sheehy, M. Effect of oxygen on cyanide intoxication. I. Prophylactic protection. *J. Pharmacol. Exp. Ther.,* **1966**, *153,* 381–385.

Webster, W. S.; Clarkson, T. B.; and Lofland, H. B. Carbon monoxide–aggravated atherosclerosis in the squirrel monkey. *Exp. Mol. Pathol.,* **1970**, *13,* 36–50.

West, I. Lindane and hematologic reactions. *Arch. Environ. Health,* **1967**, *15,* 97–101.

Yamamura, Y. N-hexane polyneuropathy. *Folia Psychiatr. Neurol. Jpn.,* **1969**, *23,* 45–57.

Monographs and Reviews

Amdur, M. O. Air pollutants. In, *Casarett and Doull's Toxicology: The Basic Science of Poisons,* 2nd ed. (Doull, J.; Klaassen, C. D.; and Amdur, M. O.; eds.) Macmillan Publishing Co., Inc., New York, **1980**, pp. 608–631.

Bouhuys, A., and Gee, J. B. L. Environmental lung disease. In, *Harrison's Principles of Internal Medicine,* 8th ed. (Thorn, G. W.; Adams, R. D.; Braunwald, E.; Isselbacher, K. J.; and Petersdorf, R. G.; eds.) McGraw-Hill Book Co., New York, **1977**, pp. 1378–1388.

Casarett, L. J. Toxicology of the respiratory system. In, *Toxicology: The Basic Science of Poisons.* (Casarett, L. J., and Doull, J., eds.) Macmillan Publishing Co., Inc., New York, **1975**, pp. 201–224.

Elkins, H. B. *The Chemistry of Industrial Toxicology,* 2nd ed. John Wiley & Sons, Inc., New York, **1959**.

Finck, P. A. Exposure to carbon monoxide: review of the literature and 567 autopsies. *Milit. Med.,* **1966,** *131,* 1513–1539.

Gosselin, R. E.; Hodge, H. C.; Smith, R. P.; and Gleason, M. N. *Clinical Toxicology of Commercial Products,* 4th ed. The Williams & Wilkins Co., Baltimore, **1976.**

Hayes, W. J., Jr. *Clinical Handbook on Economic Poisons.* Public Health Service Publication No. 476, U.S. Government Printing Office, Washington, D. C., **1963.**

IARC. *Monographs on the Evaluation of the Carcinogenic Risk of Chemicals to Man.* Vol. 5, *Some Organochlorine Pesticides.* International Agency for Research on Cancer, Lyon, France, **1974a.**

————. *Monographs on the Evaluation of the Carcinogenic Risk of Chemicals to Man.* Vol. 7, *Some Antithyroid and Related Substances, Nitrofurans and Industrial Chemicals.* International Agency for Research on Cancer, Lyon, France, **1974b.**

————. *Monographs on the Evaluation of Carcinogenic Risk of Chemicals to Man.* Vol. 12, *Some Carbamates, Thiocarbamates and Carbazides.* International Agency for Research on Cancer, Lyon, France, **1976.**

————. *Monographs on the Evaluation of the Carcinogenic Risk of Chemicals to Man.* Vol. 15, *Some Fumigants, the Herbicides 2,4-D and 2,4,5-T, Chlorinated Dibenzodioxins and Miscellaneous Industrial Chemicals.* International Agency for Research on Cancer, Lyon, France, **1977.**

Menzel, D. B. Toxicity of ozone, oxygen, and radiation. *Annu. Rev. Pharmacol.,* **1970,** *10,* 379–394.

Murphy, S. D. Pesticides. In, *Casarett and Doull's Toxicology: The Basic Science of Poisons,* 2nd ed. (Doull, J.; Klaassen, C. D.; and Amdur, M. O.; eds.) Macmillan Publishing Co., Inc., New York, **1980,** pp. 357–408

National Research Council. Committee on Medical and Biologic Effects of Environmental Pollutants. *Carbon Monoxide.* National Academy of Sciences, Washington, D. C., **1977.**

O'Brien, R. D. *Insecticides, Action and Metabolism.* Academic Press, Inc., New York, **1967.**

Plaa, G. L. Toxic responses of the liver. In, *Casarett and Doull's Toxicology: The Basic Science of Poisons,* 2nd ed. (Doull, J.; Klaassen, C. D.; and Amdur, M. O.; eds.) Macmillan Publishing Co., Inc., New York, **1980,** pp. 206–231.

Plaa, G. L., and Witschi, H. P. Chemicals, drugs, and lipid peroxidation. *Annu. Rev. Pharmacol. Toxicol.,* **1976,** *16,* 125–141.

Recknagel, R. O. Carbon tetrachloride hepatotoxicity. *Pharmacol. Rev.,* **1967,** *19,* 145–208.

Recknagel, R. O., and Glende, E. H., Jr. Carbon tetrachloride hepatotoxicity: an example of lethal cleavage. *CRC Crit. Rev. Toxicol.,* **1973,** *2,* 263–297.

Sayers, P. R., and Davenport, S. J. *Review of Carbon Monoxide Poisoning.* Public Health Bulletin No. 195, U.S. Government Printing Office, Washington, D. C., **1930.**

Stewart, R. D. The effects of carbon monoxide on humans. *Annu. Rev. Pharmacol.,* **1975,** *15,* 409–423.

Stokinger, H. E. Ozone toxicology. A review of research and industrial experience: 1954–1964. *Arch. Environ. Health,* **1965,** *10,* 719–731.

United States Department of Health, Education, and Welfare. *Air Quality Criteria for Particulate Matter.* National Air Pollution Control Administration Publication AP-49, Washington, D. C., **1969a.**

————. *Air Quality Criteria for Sulfur Oxides.* National Air Pollution Control Administration Publication AP-50, Washington, D. C., **1969b.**

————. *Air Quality Criteria for Carbon Monoxide.* National Air Pollution Control Administration Publication AP-62, Washington, D. C., **1970a.**

————. *Air Quality Criteria for Photochemical Oxidants.* National Air Pollution Control Administration Publication AP-63, Washington, D. C., **1970b.**

————. *Air Quality Criteria for Hydrocarbons.* National Air Pollution Control Administration Publication AP-64, Washington, D. C., **1970c.**

————. *Air Quality Criteria for Nitrogen Oxides.* National Air Pollution Control Administration Publication AP-84, Washington, D. C., **1971.**

Von Oettingen, W. F. *The Halogenated Hydrocarbons of Industrial and Toxicological Significance.* Elsevier Publishing Co., New York, **1964.**

Von Rumker, R.; Lawless, E. W.; Meiners, A. F.; Lawrence, K. A.; Kelso, G. L.; and Horay, F. *Production, Distribution, Use, and Environmental Impact Potential of Selected Pesticides.* EPA Publication 540/1-74-001, Environmental Protection Agency, Washington, D. C., **1975.**

World Health Organization. *1974 Evaluations of Some Pesticide Residue in Food.* World Health Organization Pesticide Residue Series, No. 4. Geneva, Switzerland, **1975,** pp. 261–263.

Zimmerman, H. J. *Hepatotoxicity: The Adverse Effects of Drugs and Other Chemicals on the Liver.* Appleton-Century-Crofts, New York, **1978.**

APPENDIX

I PRINCIPLES OF PRESCRIPTION ORDER WRITING AND PATIENT COMPLIANCE INSTRUCTION

Ewart A. Swinyard

The prescription order is an important therapeutic transaction between the physician and his patient. It represents a summary of the physician's diagnosis, prognosis, and treatment of the patient's illness. It brings to focus on one slip of paper the diagnostic acumen and therapeutic proficiency of the physician with instructions for palliation or restoration of the patient's health. The most carefully conceived prescription order may become therapeutically useless, however, unless it communicates clearly with the pharmacist and adequately instructs the patient on how to take the prescribed medication.

The importance of clarity in the physician's communication with the pharmacist cannot be overemphasized. Some drugs look alike when they are written or sound alike when spoken. Over 1000 pairs of such drugs have been identified by Teplitsky (1975). When these like-appearing names are written unclearly, or when like-sounding names are garbled over the telephone, the burden of avoiding misinterpretation falls mainly on the pharmacist who fills the prescription order. This problem can be avoided by indicating clearly the complete name of the drug.

Numerous studies suggest that too many physicians fail to instruct patients adequately on how to take their prescription medication. Reviews of such studies indicate that 25 to 50% of patients in a variety of clinical situations failed to take their prescription medication as directed (Blackwell, 1976; Sackett, 1976). Most errors were related to the prescription order directions; the patient took the medication either in the wrong dose, for the wrong purpose, or at the wrong time. Also, some patients either missed doses or failed to complete the treatment regimen. Data of this kind emphasize the physician's need to understand the basic principles of prescription order writing and how to instruct the patient about his medication.

PRESCRIPTION ORDER WRITING

The teaching of prescription order writing is often neglected in the medical school curriculum. This is largely because the practice of writing

long, complicated prescription orders containing many active ingredients, adjuvants, correctives, and elegant vehicles has been abandoned in favor of single drugs and mixtures of drugs compounded by pharmaceutical companies. Even when two or more active ingredients are desired for oral administration, they are preferably prescribed separately so that the physician may adjust the dose of each to the individual requirements of the patient.

The National Prescription Audit (1978) reveals that virtually all (99%) prescription orders are for precompounded drugs. Only a few (1%) require compounding. This is desirable in most instances, but such simplicity has its drawbacks. Many physicians rely upon fixed-dose combinations rather than adjust the doses of the agents to the particular needs of the patient. For example, the prescription audit referred to above shows that 70 of the 200 most frequently prescribed drugs are combination products. Other forms of irrational prescribing (Task Force on Prescription Drugs, 1969) include "the use of drugs without demonstrated efficacy; the use of drugs with an inherent hazard not justified by the seriousness of the illness; the use of drugs in excessive amounts, or for excessive periods of time, or inadequate amounts for inadequate periods; the simultaneous use of two or more drugs without appropriate consideration of their possible interaction; [and] the multiple prescribing, by one or several physicians for the same patient, of drugs which may be unnecessary, cumulative, interacting, or needlessly expensive." Certainly such conditions can be corrected if as much careful thought is given to treatment as is given to diagnosis.

To be able accurately and speedily to write prescription orders requires considerable practice. The prescription order should be written legibly. If one has poor handwriting, the prescription order should be printed or typewritten. It is convenient and the accepted form to have one's name, address, telephone number, office hours, and Drug Enforcement Administration (DEA) registry number printed on the prescription order blank. Because prescription orders are medicolegal documents, they should be written in ink, although this is compulsory only for controlled substances in schedule II. It is also an excellent custom, too infrequently followed, for the doctor to keep an exact or carbon copy for his files. This copy protects him and serves to complete the record of treatment.

Helpful suggestions on prescription order writing may be found in "Prescription Writing and Prescription Labeling," developed by the American Pharmaceutical Association and the American Society of Internal Medicine (1974).

Choice of Language. Prescription orders should be written with proper grammar. Abbreviations and empirical jargon, whether in Latin or English, should *not* be employed.

Choice of Drug Name. Most drugs can be prescribed by their official names (*United States Pharmacopeia;* U.S.P.), by their nonproprietary names (United States Adopted Names; USAN), or by the manufacturers' proprietary (trade) names. The nonproprietary name is often referred to as the generic name. The latter term, based on strict definition, is properly used to designate a chemical relationship among drugs, such as sulfonamides, barbiturates, and so forth. However, the distinction has been overlooked, and the term *generic* is used almost to the exclusion of *nonproprietary.* When the proprietary name is used, the pharmacist filling the prescription order must dispense only the drug of the specified manufacturer. In the other cases he may select any of the available preparations. However, federal enabling legislation (in the United States) is under consideration that, if adopted by a state, would compel physicians to prescribe by the nonproprietary name. Therefore, physicians and pharmacists should be alert for legislative changes that may restrict the physician's freedom to prescribe a particular manufacturer's product and the pharmacist's privilege to dispense that product.

There is much discussion concerning the relative advantages of prescribing by nonproprietary versus proprietary name. Arguments in favor of the use of nonproprietary names are based, for the most part, on the elimination of duplication of drug products and the possibility of an economic benefit to the patient. Arguments against such practice usually include the lack of quality control, variability in the formulation and, consequently, in the biological availability of the drug (*see* Chapter 1), and the fact that many nonproprietary names are difficult to remember and to spell. An argument against prescribing by nonproprietary name is provided by the list of 110 drugs identified as having bioavailability problems (Food and Drug Administration, 1977) and the required package insert for phenytoin, which

advises physicians to keep patients on one dosage form and one manufacturer's product (Food and Drug Administration, 1978). An excellent review of the problems associated with bioavailability and its regulation was published by the United States Office of Technology Assessment (Drug Bioequivalence, 1974).

Nonproprietary names are now selected by the United States Adopted Name (USAN) Council. The USAN Council is sponsored jointly by the American Medical Association, the United States Pharmacopeial Convention, Inc., and the American Pharmaceutical Association. Provision was made in 1967 for a liaison representative of the United States Food and Drug Administration also to serve on the Council. For details relative to how the USAN Council functions, *see* Jerome and Sagan (1975).

In writing prescription orders it is *best to use the nonproprietary name followed by the name of the manufacturer in parentheses if a specific manufacturer's product has distinct advantages.* This not only eliminates the necessity for memorizing multiple drug names but also assures the physician that the product of a particular manufacturer will be dispensed. Furthermore, the nonproprietary name is commonly used in teaching pharmacology to medical students. For these reasons, nonproprietary names will be used exclusively in this appendix. For purposes of identification, proprietary names, designated by SMALL-CAP TYPE, appear throughout the text in chapter sections dealing with preparations as well as in the Index. This does not imply a complete listing of proprietary names, since the number for a single drug may be large and since proprietary names differ from country to country.

Choice of a System of Weights and Measures. Prescription orders should always be written in the metric system. It is a self-explanatory decimal system, employed throughout the scientific world and official in the U.S.P. Most medical publications give quantities and doses exclusively in the metric system.

The Metric System. In the metric system, only Arabic numbers are used. In the United States, fluids are measured and solids are weighed, and ordinarily no attention is paid to differences in specific gravity of fluids. It is necessary, therefore, only to designate amounts of drug by numbers without writing "g" or "ml" to indicate that the metric system was employed.

In the prescription order itself, the Arabic number is placed after the official name of the drug and, if several ingredients are prescribed, the decimal points are placed in the same vertical line. Many physicians substitute a vertical line for decimal points, and this "decimal line" may be printed on the prescription order pad. Above this line one may place "g or ml," although this is not necessary inasmuch as the decimal line presupposes the metric system. It should be emphasized, however, that when the decimal line is used all ingredient quantities must be expressed in the basic units of the metric system (g or ml) and this line cannot be used to express decimal fractions of *milligrams*.

Apothecaries' System. Since doses in older publications may appear in units of the apothecaries' system, metric and apothecaries' equivalents are presented in Table A–1.

Household Measures. Unfortunately, the drugs prescribed so carefully by the physician in milligrams and milliliters are usually measured by the patient with convenient kitchen utensils. The advantages gained by the use of liquid preparations are thus often lost because of the inaccuracy of the devices used to measure and to administer them. The "drop," which varies in size, presents a special problem. Its size depends on the particular fluid being dropped—its specific gravity, temperature, and viscosity—as well as on the orifice of the dropper and the angle at which the dropper is held (Hirschorn and Silverman, 1968). The U.S.P. does not sanction the prescribing of doses in drops but provides an official standardized dropper for those who wish to use it. This official dropper, when held vertically, delivers drops of water, each of which weighs between 45 and 55 mg. Most commercial products provide a calibrated dropper for this type of preparation.

The size of the household teaspoon also varies considerably, and a given teaspoon will yield volumes of medicine ranging from 2.5 to 7.8 ml depending on the technic of measuring the liquid. Moreover, the same spoon when used by different persons may deliver from 3 to 7 ml (Committee on Drugs, American Academy of Pediatrics, 1975). For household purposes, an American Standard Teaspoon has been established by the American National Standards Institute, containing 4.93 ± 0.24 ml. The U.S.P. specifies that this teaspoon may be regarded as containing 5 ml. Therefore, a prescription order calling for 120 ml

Table A–1. METRIC AND APOTHECARIES' EQUIVALENTS

1 milligram	=	$1/65$	grain
1 gram	=	15.43	grains
1 kilogram	=	2.20	pounds
1 milliliter	=	16.23	minims
1 grain	=	0.065	gram
1 ounce	=	31.1	grams
1 minim	=	0.062	ml
1 fluid ounce	=	29.57	ml
1 pint	=	473.2	ml
1 quart	=	946.4	ml

should be considered as containing 24, not 30, teaspoonful doses. A tablespoon is said to contain 15 ml. Its use suffers from the same type of variability described for the teaspoon.

Other devices, such as calibrated droppers, molded plastic cylinders, and measuring caps, have been developed for measuring and administering liquid medications. A novel oral syringe may be used to measure and administer drugs to children; these syringes (both glass and plastic) are available in a variety of sizes to assure accurate administration of drugs. Such devices have been strongly recommended by the Committee on Drugs, American Academy of Pediatrics (1975), to replace the usual household utensils. Physicians who find it necessary to prescribe liquid medicines for oral administration should request the pharmacist to supply the appropriate device with the medication in order to assure that the patient can conveniently take the prescribed dose.

Construction of the Prescription Order. Traditionally, a prescription order follows a definite pattern that facilitates its interpretation. This pattern is essentially the same whether the prescription order is for a single drug or a mixture of two or more drugs. *Only one prescription should be written on an order blank.* The major elements of a model order are illustrated in example No. 1. The numbers at the left call attention to the several parts of a prescription order, which are explained below. (These numbers do not appear on the prescription order itself.)

1. *Date.* The date when the prescription order is written is important. Federal law requires that prescription orders for drugs listed in schedules II, III, and IV of the Controlled Substances Act of 1970 be dated; orders for substances in schedules III and IV cannot be filled or refilled more than 6 months after date of issuance.

2. *Name and Address of the Patient.* These are necessary in order to expedite the handling of the prescription order and to avoid possible confusion with medications intended for someone else. The age should also be included; newborn, pediatric, adult, and geriatric patients differ markedly in ability to absorb, distribute, and excrete various drugs (*see* Chapter 1). Moreover, the pharmacist has no reliable way to monitor the prescribed dose without such information. The pharmacist should place the name of the patient on the bottle or container exactly as the doctor has written it. Therefore, it is important that the physician write the full name of the patient on the prescription order and that it be spelled correctly. Prescription orders for schedule-II drugs are required to contain the full name and address of the patient, and the pharmacist must transfer this

(No. 1)

1.	May 28, 1980
2.	John Jones, Age 6
	596 South Main Street
	Salt Lake City, Utah 84101
3.	℞
4.	Ampicillin Oral Suspension (Pfizer) 250 mg/5 ml
5.	Dispense 200 ml (with oral syringe).
6.	Label: Take 5 ml orally at 8 A.M., 12 noon, 4 P.M., and 8 P.M. daily for 10 days for infection.
	Ampicillin 250 mg/5 ml.
7.	Do not refill.
8.	Thomas A. Brown, M.D.
	DEA No. AB1234321
	508 South Main Street
	Salt Lake City, Utah 84101

information to the label that is placed on the container of the completed prescription.

3. *Superscription.* The superscription consists of the symbol ℞ (not "Rx"), an abbreviation for *recipe,* the Latin for "take thou."

4. *Inscription.* The inscription is the body of the prescription order and contains the name and strength (dose) of the desired drug. Drugs are prescribed in the United States by official English names. Abbreviations should be avoided since their use frequently results in error. For example, "sulf." may be mistaken for sulfide or sulfonate, and "chlor." may be mistaken for chlorate or chloral. When two or more drugs are desired in the same prescription order, the name and amount of each drug are placed together on a separate line directly under the preceding one. The names of the drugs are capitalized. Traditionally, the order of ingredients, should there be more than one, is as follows:

Basis. The basis is the principal drug and gives the prescription its chief action.

Adjuvant. As the name suggests, the adjuvant is a drug that aids or increases the action of the principal ingredient.

Corrective. The corrective modifies or corrects undesirable effects of the basis or adjuvant.

Vehicle. The vehicle is the agent used as the solvent in the solution, to increase the bulk, or to dilute the mixture.

In practice, prescription orders seldom contain more than one drug name. However, when three agents are prescribed, the most potent or principal drug is listed first, the other ingredient second, and the vehicle last, as shown below.

5. *Subscription.* The subscription contains the directions to the pharmacist. In prescription orders for a single drug this usually consists in "Dispense 10 tablets," "Dispense 200 ml," "Dispense with oral syringe," and so forth; in the case of prescription orders for two or more drugs it usually consists in either a short sentence such as "Make a solution" or "Mix and place into 10 capsules" or a word such as "Mix." The latter is commonly written as the letter "M," from the Latin *misce* ("mix"), which the pharmacist proceeds to do according to his art.

6. *Signature.* The signature of the prescription order consists in the directions to the patient. The term *signature* does not refer to the physician's name; rather, it is derived from the Latin *signa,* meaning "write," "mark," or "label." Since English is the preferred language, the directions are preceded by the word *Label;* antiquated terms, such as the Latin *Signa* or the abbreviation "Sig." or "S," should not be used. Occasionally, this part of the prescription order is called the *transcription* and the term *signature* is then reserved for the physician's name.

The directions to the patient should always be written in English. The use of Latin abbreviations, such as "1 cap. q.d." or "1 cap. t.i.d.a.c.," serves no useful purpose; indeed, the little dots in "q.d." may look like "q.i.d." or the "a.c." like "p.c." to the reader. Since the pharmacist *always* writes the label in English, the use of such abbreviations or symbols should be discouraged.

The directions to the patient contain instructions as to the amount of drug to be taken, the time and frequency of the dose, and other factors such as dilution and route of administration. If the drug is to be used externally only, or to be shaken well before using, or if it is a poison, such facts are included. The pharmacist has printed labels, covering many of these points, which he attaches to the container, and often he affixes them at his own discretion, except for a poison label.

Expressions such as "take as directed" and "take as necessary" are *never* satisfactory and should be avoided. Whenever possible, exact times of the day should be specified. If it is therapeutically important to take the medication at specific intervals around the clock or for a specific period of time, this should be stated in the directions to the patient. An ill patient or a distracted and worried parent or relative cannot always be relied upon to remember clearly the verbal directions given by the physician, or he may remember them incorrectly. If the directions are too lengthy or too complicated to be placed in the prescription order, they should be written on a separate instruction sheet and left with the patient. To avoid possible error, the first word of the directions to the patient should be employed as a reminder of the correct route of administration. Thus, the directions for a preparation for internal use should start with the word *take;* for an ointment or lotion, the word *apply;* for suppositories, the word *insert;* and for drops to be placed in the conjunctival sac, external auditory canal, or nostril, the word *place.* The directions to the patient should also be employed as a reminder of the intended purpose of the prescription, by including such phrases as "for relief of pain," "for relief of headache," or "to relieve itching." However, directions that would be embarrassing to the patient if placed on the prescription order or label should be given in private.

There are many cogent reasons why prescription medication should be identified on the label. For example, the rapid identification of a drug can help with the initiation of appropriate therapy in the case of adverse drug reactions, or accidental or deliberate overdosage. Therefore, many states require that the name, strength, and quantity of drug dispensed be indicated on the label. When appropriate, the pharmacist should also indicate the expiration date and special storage instructions on the prescription label.

The pharmacist always should be on the alert to detect overdoses of potent drugs in the prescriptions he dispenses. This serves as an added check for the safety of the patient. If it is desirable to administer a drug in a larger amount than is customarily employed, it is best for the prescriber to underline the dose, and to write "correct amount" or "correct dose" and his initials at the side. This notation informs the pharmacist that a mistake has not been made, and saves time otherwise lost in verifying the physician's dosage.

7. *Refill Information.* Under the Durham-Humphrey Amendment to the Federal Food, Drug, and Cosmetic Act (*see* page 1670), prescription orders for drugs that bear the caution legend, "Federal law prohibits dispensing without prescription," may not be refilled without the consent of the prescriber. Under the Drug Abuse Control Amendments to the above act (*see* page 1670), prescription orders for schedule-III and schedule-IV drugs cannot be refilled *more than five times* and the prescription order is invalid 6 months from date of issue. For these reasons, the physician should indicate his wishes with respect to refills on each original prescription order. This may be indicated by instruction to refill a certain number of times or not to refill. Statements such as "Refill prn" and "Refill ad lib" are never appropriate. Such information need not be written on narcotic prescription orders for schedule-II substances, since by law these cannot be refilled.

8. *Prescriber's Signature.* The prescription order is completed by the practitioner writing his signature at the bottom of the blank, with the appropriate professional degree following it. Federal law requires that the physician's address and DEA registry number also appear on every prescription order for schedule-II drugs and that such an order be signed (last name in full) with ink or indelible pencil.

Classes of Prescription Orders. On the basis of the availability of the prescribed medication, prescription orders may be divided into two classes, *precompounded* and *extemporaneous.* A *precompounded* prescription order is one that calls for a drug or mixture of drugs supplied by the pharmaceutical company by its official or proprietary name and in a form that the pharmacist dispenses without pharmaceutical alteration. An *extemporaneous* prescription order, also called *magistral* or *compounded,* is the type in which the physician selects the drugs, doses, and pharmaceutical form that he desires and the pharmacist prepares the medication. The extemporaneous prescription order is considerably more difficult to construct and to write; hence, many physicians avoid this type of order by writing for a precompounded official or proprietary preparation. Examples of prescription orders for precompounded and extemporaneous preparations are given below and will serve to illustrate the principles of prescription order writing.

Examples of Prescription Orders for Precompounded Preparations. Practically all the official preparations in the United States, that is, those formulations included in the U.S.P., are available in precompounded form. Thus, such remedies are prescribed by their official names and, if they contain more than one substance, the specific ingredients need not be listed. A survey of the U.S.P. will acquaint the physician with the wide scope of the official preparations. Innumerable precompounded nonofficial preparations are also available under various proprietary names.

When writing a prescription order for a precompounded preparation, it is necessary to know the name of the preparation desired, the pharmaceutical form in which it is available (*i.e.,* ointment, tablet, etc.), the single dose, the route and the frequency of administration, and the approximate number of days of therapy. Suppose one wishes to renew a prescription order for a 3-month supply of digoxin for an adult with congestive heart failure, who is well stabilized and has been thoroughly instructed regarding compliance. Since digoxin is available under ten different trade names and is marketed by over 50 different companies, it is good practice to prescribe the drug by its USAN, but to indicate a manufacturer's product that will ensure adequate, dependable bioavailability, as shown below.

(No. 2)

℞

Digoxin Tablets
(Burroughs Wellcome Co.)   0|00025
Dispense 100 such tablets.

Label: Take 1 tablet at 9:00 A.M. each morning.
Digoxin, 0.25 mg.

When the decimal line is used, the unit dose *must* be expressed in grams or decimal fractions thereof. When the decimal line is not used, the unit dose *must be clearly stated.* For example, the above prescription could also be written as follows:

℞

Digoxin Tablets
(Burroughs Wellcome Co.)   0.25 mg

or

℞

Digoxin Tablets
(Burroughs Wellcome Co.)   250 μg

Precompounded prescription orders for orally administered liquid preparations are constructed in a similar manner. It is necessary, however, to know the concentration of the active ingredient(s) in the preparation. Suppose one desires to prescribe the official U.S.P. phenobarbital elixir (4 mg/ml) as prophylactic therapy (4 mg/kg/day) for a 15-kg infant with a history of a previous febrile seizure. A prescription order providing 6 days of medication may be written as follows:

(No. 3)

℞

Phenobarbital Elixir, U.S.P.   90|0
Label: Give ½ teaspoonful at the onset of fever and every 4 hours until fever subsides. Phenobarbital Elixir.

Do not refill.

Prescription orders for other orally administered precompounded remedies, such as solutions, syrups, suspensions, and tinctures, are written as illustrated in the previous example, as are those for preparations that are intended for local application. If special instructions to the pharmacist are necessary, these may be indicated. For example, physicians should remember that the 1970 Poison Prevention Packaging Act was extended in 1974 to require child-resistant containers for *all oral* prescriptions, although several exceptions are permitted (*e.g.,* oral contraceptives). Many patients have difficulty in using the special containers. In such cases the prescriber or patient may request the use of a conventional container.

Examples of Prescription Orders for Extemporaneous Preparations. In writing prescription orders for an extemporaneous preparation for oral administration, it is of course necessary to know the single dose of each ingredient, the number of doses to be taken each day, and the number of days of medication. This knowledge allows the calculation of the total dosage of each ingredient in the prescription. Suppose it is desired to prescribe an antitussive-expectorant mixture to be taken orally every 4 hours for a nonproductive, exhausting cough. This means that at least four doses will be taken daily. If teaspoonful doses (5 ml) are used and enough medicine is dispensed to last 6 days, approximately 24 doses or a 120-ml total volume will be needed. Calculations are shown below for a mixture of codeine phosphate (antitussive), ammonium chloride (expectorant), and terpin hydrate elixir (vehicle). (*Obviously, these calculations should not appear on the completed prescription order.*)

			Single dose × No. of doses
Codeine Phosphate	0|24	⟷	10 mg × 24
Ammonium Chloride	7|2	⟷	0.3 g × 24
Terpin Hydrate Elixir, to make	120|0	⟷	5.0 ml × 24

Extemporaneous prescription orders for other liquid preparations for oral administration, such as syrups, suspensions, and drop medication, are constructed similarly.

The principles of calculation of dosage illustrated above apply also to prescription orders for dry forms of medication to be taken internally. Since pharmacists are not equipped to compound compressed tablets, dry forms of medication are commonly prescribed in capsule form. Whereas it is fairly easy to ingest liquid medicines, it may be difficult to swallow capsules that are too large. Therefore, these are limited to approximately 0.5 g in bulk (for adults) for most medicines. If a larger amount is required for the single dose, then the drug must be divided into 2 or more capsules for each dose. If the ingredients make too small a bulk to be dispensed conveniently in solid form, an inert powder may be added. There are many such powders and excipients (licorice, lactose, etc.), and the pharmacist often selects and adds them at his own discretion.

Suppose it is desired to prescribe in capsule form an analgesic mixture containing aspirin, phenacetin, and amobarbital for a patient with painful myositis. The medicine is to be taken every 4 hours during waking hours (*i.e.,* four doses per day) and enough is to be prescribed to last 5 days. The construction of the prescription order is as follows:

(No. 4)

July 29, 1980

Mary Thomas, Age 54
606 Constitution Avenue, N.W.
Washington, D. C. 20001

℞   Single dose × No. of doses
    Aspirin   6│0 ⟷ 0.3 g × 20
    Phenacetin   6│0 ⟷ 0.3 g × 20
    Amobarbital 1│0 ⟷ 0.05 g × 20
    Mix and divide into 40 capsules.

Label: Take 2 capsules at 8:00 A.M., 12 noon, 4:00 P.M., and 8:00 P.M. for muscle pain. Aspirin, Phenacetin, and Amobarbital.

Do not refill.

Prescription orders for medicines to be taken internally may also be written by the *single-dose method.* The pharmacist is then instructed to prepare a given number of doses, and he must carry out the calculations illustrated above. For example, prescription order No. 4, if written by the single-dose method, would appear as follows:

(No. 5)

℞
    Aspirin   0│3
    Phenacetin   0│3
    Amobarbital   0│05
    Make 20 such doses and place in 40 capsules.

Label: etc.

Prescription orders for ointments are usually fairly simple to construct because the ingredients may be calculated on a *percentage basis* rather than by absolute doses. Suppose that it is desired to prescribe an ointment for a fungal infection of the feet, and that benzoic acid (6%) and salicylic acid (3%) are to be incorporated in a base of hydrophilic petrolatum and white petrolatum. If a

60-g amount of ointment is to be dispensed, the order appears as follows:

(No. 6)

℞
    Benzoic Acid   3│6
    Salicylic Acid   1│8
    Hydrophilic Petrolatum
    White Petrolatum, of each an equal
        amount to make   60│0
    Make an ointment.

Label: Apply a thin film to the affected parts night and morning. Benzoic Acid and Salicylic Acid.

When prescribing locally acting drugs, the *percentage form may be used as such* rather than as a basis for calculating absolute amounts of ingredients. Prescription order No. 6 thus may be written as follows:

(No. 7)

℞
    Benzoic Acid   6%
    Salicylic Acid   3%
    Hydrophilic Petrolatum
    White Petrolatum, of each an equal
        amount to make   60│0
    Make an ointment.

Label: etc.

One may desire to prescribe an ointment containing 5% sulfur. The U.S.P. includes an official *Sulfur Ointment,* which contains 10% precipitated sulfur in mineral oil (10%) and white ointment (80%). This prescription order may be written as follows:

(No. 8)

℞
    Sulfur Ointment   5%   60│0

Label: Apply to affected skin at 8:00 A.M. and 8:00 P.M. daily. Sulfur Ointment.

Although this order does not call for the U.S.P. percentage of sulfur, the use of the official title indicates to the pharmacist that the physician wishes the U.S.P. preparation diluted to a 5% sulfur content by addition of the proper ointment base.

A prescription order for a lotion for external use on the skin is similar in construction to that for an ointment in that only the approximate percentages of the ingredients and not absolute doses need be ordered. An order for a simple lotion incorporating 8% calamine (essentially a pink insoluble powder of zinc oxide), 8% zinc oxide, 2% glycerin in 25% bentonite magma (native, colloidal, hydrated aluminum silicate) and limewater is written as follows:

(No. 9)

R

Calamine	19	2
Zinc Oxide	19	2
Glycerin	4	8
Bentonite Magma	60	0
Calcium Hydroxide Solution,		
to make	240	0

M.

Label: Shake well and apply to sunburned areas as needed. Calamine Lotion.

This lotion is identical with *Calamine Lotion, U.S.P.* It is often modified to suit the specific needs of the patient. A pleasant odor can be obtained by the substitution of rose water for the limewater. If the skin lesion itches, phenol may be added to the lotion in 1 or 2% concentration. Olive oil to the extent of 30% may be substituted for bentonite magma.

Prescription orders for many liquid preparations for local administration, such as ophthalmic solutions, nasal sprays, inhalants, gargles, and douches, are constructed similarly to those cited above. For example, a sterile ophthalmic solution of zinc sulfate and phenylephrine hydrochloride for use in mild conjunctivitis may be prescribed as follows:

(No. 10)

R

Zinc Sulfate	0	08
Phenylephrine Hydrochloride	0	04
Purified Water, to make	30	00

Make a sterile solution.

Label: Place 2 or 3 drops in affected eye every 3 hours. Zinc Sulfate and Phenylephrine Hydrochloride.

Aqueous solutions prepared for use in the eye are less irritating if they are adjusted to isotonicity with the lacrimal fluid. If it is desired to prescribe an isotonic ophthalmic solution, this fact can be indicated by inserting the phrase, "Sodium Chloride, to make isotonic." The pharmacist will then add sufficient sodium chloride to make the solution isotonic with the fluids of the eye. The above order should then be written as follows:

R

Zinc Sulfate	0	08
Phenylephrine Hydrochloride	0	04
Sodium Chloride, to make isotonic		
Purified Water, to make	30	00

Make a sterile solution.

Label: etc.

Nasal and otic prescription orders follow the same general form, it being necessary to know only the approximate concentration of each in-

gredient. Solutions to be used in the nose can also be employed with much greater comfort if made approximately isotonic. The physician can instruct the pharmacist to make nasal solutions isotonic with the body fluids by inserting the phrase, "Dextrose, to make isotonic" or "Sodium Chloride, to make isotonic." The pharmacist will then add the requisite quantity of dextrose or sodium chloride to adjust the tonicity of the preparation to that of the nasal fluid.

Dosage. Instructions about dosage are an extremely important part of prescription order writing. One must know the method of calculating doses (*see* above) and the factors influencing the amount of drug to be prescribed (*see* Chapters 1 and 3).

Factors Influencing the Total Bulk of the Prescription. The number of days for which medication is contemplated, the number of doses per day, and the size of each dose determine the bulk of the prescription. There is *no minimal limit* to the total quantity of prescribed medication, and as little as a single dose may be ordered, if this is all that is required. On the other hand, a *maximal limit* is indicated for most prescriptions, even when medication is to continue for an indefinite period; this limit is influenced by the stability and cost of the drug and the possible necessity for alteration of the treatment. A major factor that should be a determinant of the quantity of the drug dispensed is the mental state of the patient and the potential toxicity of the drug. If a patient is depressed or potentially suicidal, do not prescribe total quantities of drug that would prove lethal if taken all at one time. If there are no such problems, a convenient rule of thumb is to prescribe only enough medication for 7 to 14 days. *Storage* of unused portions of a prescription and *sharing* of prescriptions with others who were not intended to receive them should be explicitly discussed with any patient who receives an important prescription. If a disease is self-limited or if the prescription drug is likely to be curative, the patient should be instructed to discard any unused portion. Accidental poisonings and suicides have resulted from stockpiled drugs. This may also lead to the sharing of drugs with relatives or friends. Blackwell (1972) reported that 9 of 75 patients used drugs that were prescribed for other individuals.

Size and Form of Unit-Dose Medication. The upper limit of the bulk of unit-dose medication (capsules, tablets, etc.) is usually *0.5 g total,* for adults. However, this arbitrary limit based on what the patient can comfortably swallow may be exceeded when the drug product is dense. Conversely, even a smaller unit dosage may be indicated for light, bulky medication or for certain patients, especially the very young or old.

Many drugs are commercially available only in a limited variety of dose forms (*e.g.,* only capsules of a single weight). For obvious reasons of convenience and economy, these "standard" forms of medication should be preferred, except under unusual circumstances. Until knowledge of the unit-dose forms available for the various drugs is acquired through experience, the physician is well advised to rely upon his pharmacist for this information. Other useful sources of information include the sections on preparations in this textbook; *AMA Drug Evaluations (AMA–DE),* a publication of the American Medical Association; *Remington's Pharmaceutical Sciences; Hospital Formulary,* published by the American Society of Hospital Pharmacists; and the *Physicians' Desk Reference* (PDR).

Accuracy of Dosage. Extreme accuracy of dosage is unnecessary except when very potent drugs are prescribed. In calculating the total amount of a drug to be ordered in a prescription, a "rounding-off" process is employed. For example, 0.52 g may be taken as 0.5 g, 0.68 g as 0.7 g, and so forth. In general, a variation of about 10% in dosage is usually permissible.

Official Doses. Official doses in the United States are those listed in the U.S.P. These represent the *Usual Adult Doses* and *Usual Pediatric Doses* that should produce the recognized therapeutic effects in adults and children following oral administration unless otherwise specified. The *Usual Dose* is intended to serve only as a guide to the physician, who very frequently must give more or less than what is usual in order to optimize therapy. This official compendium also gives the *Usual Adult Prescribing Limits,* intended primarily to guide the pharmacist with respect to confirmation of prescription orders calling for unusually large dosages. Dose information can also be obtained from package inserts or the references listed above. Doses of drugs given in this textbook are taken from the above sources and ordinarily represent the *Usual Dose.* It should be kept in mind that these doses may not be safe or sufficient in any given patient. Drug therapy must be individualized.

Latin Phrases and Abbreviations. Although the use of Latin in writing prescription orders has largely been abandoned, there are a number of phrases and abbreviations that stubbornly persist despite the fact that their use is not recommended. These may be found in *earlier editions* of this textbook.

Vehicles, Flavors, and Coloring Agents. The oral route of administration of drugs is more widely accepted by patients than is any other route. Oral medication should be in the form of tablets and capsules, if at all possible. Children and aged patients, however, usually find the liquid forms of oral medication more acceptable; indeed, if bitter, salty, or other objectionable-tasting drugs could be disguised in a liquid preparation, this would be one of the most useful forms of drug administration for such patients. It is therefore necessary for the physician to know how to prescribe medicines in a form sufficiently palatable so that they will be taken by the patient.

The effective flavoring and coloring of a drug formulation often present formidable problems. Pharmaceutical manufacturers spend considerable sums of money and devote much time and effort to assure that an otherwise distasteful drug is marketed in an acceptable, elegant form. In such cases, it is probably best to prescribe the drug in a proprietary formulation. Nevertheless, acceptable extemporaneous liquid medications can be obtained by the careful selection of coloring, flavoring, and diluting agents. The physician is well advised to enlist a pharmacist's aid in demonstrating the use of available agents.

Vehicles. The many vehicles available to the physician for flavoring and diluting drugs may conveniently be divided into three groups: elixirs, syrups, and aromatic waters. Elixirs, sweetened hydroalcoholic solutions that contain approximately 25% alcohol, are suitable vehicles for drugs soluble in either water or dilute alcohol. Syrups, concentrated aqueous solutions of sugar, are useful as vehicles for water-soluble drugs. Aromatic waters, saturated aqueous solutions of volatile oils, are used as vehicles for water-soluble substances and salts. Their use is largely governed by flavor, color, and solubility characteristics of the active medicinal agent. Table A–2 lists the more commonly employed official vehicles.

The following illustrations will show how these vehicles and flavoring agents may be used in extemporaneous prescription orders. Suppose that it is desired to prescribe an antibiotic in liquid form for oral administration. The prescription order may be written as follows:

(No. 11)

℞

| Tetracycline Hydrochloride | 3|0 |
| Cherry Syrup, to make | 60|0 |

Label: Shake well and take 1 teaspoonful orally 1 hour before each meal and at bedtime. Tetracycline Hydrochloride.

Because of its flexibility, iso-alcoholic elixir can be used to advantage in numerous extemporaneous prescription orders. It consists of two formulas, designated as *low-alcoholic elixir* (8 to 10% alcohol) and *high-alcoholic elixir* (73 to 78% alco-

Table A-2. SELECTED VEHICLES FOR EXTEMPORANEOUS PRESCRIPTIONS

VEHICLE	FLAVOR	COLOR	ACID-BASE PROPERTIES	PERCENT ALCOHOL	USE
Elixirs, N.F.					
Aromatic	Orange	Colorless	Neutral	21–23	General
Compound Benzaldehyde	Bitter almond	Colorless	Acid	3–5	Bromides and chlorides
Iso-Alcoholic	Orange	Colorless	Neutral	9–75	Alcohol-soluble drugs
Syrups, N.F.					
Acacia	Vanilla	Colorless	Acid	0	Insoluble drugs
Aromatic Eriodictyon	Aromatic	Brown	Neutral	6–8	Bitter drugs and alkaloids
Cherry	Cherry	Red	Acid	1–2	Bitter and salty drugs
Cocoa	Chocolate	Brown	Neutral	0	Children
Orange	Orange	Straw	Acid	2–5	Salty drugs
Tolu Balsam	Aromatic	Red	Alkaline	3–5	Children
Aromatic Waters, N.F.					
Orange Flower	Orange	Colorless	Neutral	0	General
Peppermint	Peppermint	Colorless	Neutral	0	General

hol). *Iso-alcoholic elixir* represents a mixture of the two formulas adjusted by the pharmacist to meet the alcoholic requirements of the drugs for which it serves as a vehicle or diluent. For example, if the physician wishes to prescribe an elixir, tincture, or fluidextract in a vehicle in order to increase the volume and thus make the dose more convenient to measure, it is important that the alcoholic strength of the vehicle be approximately the same as that of the preparation to be diluted; otherwise, the active principles may be precipitated. The physician need not remember the particular alcohol concentration required but should merely prescribe the iso-alcoholic elixir. The pharmacist then ascertains how much of the elixirs of low and high alcohol content to mix in order to obtain the same alcohol concentration as the solution of drug that is being prescribed. Thus, if phenobarbital elixir is ordered in iso-alcoholic elixir, the alcohol content is adjusted to 15%, which is the alcoholic concentration of the phenobarbital elixir, and the barbiturate will not be precipitated out of solution.

(No. 12)

℞

Phenobarbital Elixir	45|0
Iso-Alcoholic Elixir, to make	90|0
M.	

Label: Take 1 teaspoonful in water every 4 hours, as necessary for restlessness. Phenobarbital Elixir.

By diluting the phenobarbital elixir with the isoalcoholic elixir, fractional teaspoonful doses or "drop dosages" are avoided, since a teaspoonful dose can be adjusted to contain the desired quantity of the barbiturate.

Paregoric, U.S.P., is an example of a medicated tincture that is frequently used as both a vehicle and a therapeutic agent. Suppose it is desired to prescribe paregoric and bismuth subcarbonate for the treatment of diarrhea. The prescription order may be written as follows:

(No. 13)

℞

Bismuth Subcarbonate	8|0
Paregoric, to make	60|0
M.	

Label: Shake well and take ½ teaspoonful every 2 hours, for diarrhea. Bismuth Subcarbonate and Paregoric.

Incompatibilities. This term is applied when physical, chemical, or therapeutic problems arise during the compounding, dispensing, or administration of the prescribed medication. A *physical* incompatibility occurs when liquefaction, deliquescence, precipitation, incomplete solution, or other change in physical state takes place. A *chemical* incompatibility occurs when two ingredients in a prescription react chemically to form new compounds. *Therapeutic* incompatibilities or adverse drug interactions are discussed in Chapter 3 and Appendix III.

The avoidance and prevention of physical and chemical incompatibilities are largely the responsibility of the pharmacist and the industrial pharmaceutical research scientist. A physician who writes extemporaneous prescription orders can avoid physical and chemical incompatibilities, provided he keeps in mind the few broad concepts given in the *fifth edition* of this textbook. The avoidance of therapeutic incompatibilities is largely the responsibility of the physician and requires a thorough knowledge of pharmacology and therapeutics.

Prescription Refills. Prescription drugs were formerly controlled by several federal laws, including the Federal Food, Drug, and Cosmetic Act, the Federal Narcotic–Internal Revenue Regulations (historically known as the Harrison Narcotic Act), and the Federal Marihuana Regulations. On May 1, 1971, the *Comprehensive Drug Abuse Prevention and Control Act* of 1970 became fully effective and, except for the Durham-Humphrey Amendment (Section 503B), repealed all the aforementioned laws controlling prescription drugs.

The Durham-Humphrey Amendment defines certain types of drugs that may be sold by the pharmacist only on the prescription order of a practitioner licensed by law to administer such drugs. These drugs are required to bear the label, *"Caution: Federal law prohibits dispensing without prescription."* Under the Durham-Humphrey Amendment, a prescription order cannot be refilled unless authorized by the prescriber. The prescriber may indicate the number of times a prescription order may be refilled, in the blank space in the statement, "Refill _____ times"; this statement may be printed on the prescription order blank.

The Comprehensive Drug Abuse Prevention and Control Act, commonly referred to as the Controlled Substances Act (*see* below), is designed to control the distribution of all depressant and stimulant drugs (*e.g.,* narcotics, barbiturates, and amphetamines) and other drugs with abuse potential as designated by the Drug Enforcement Administration, Department of Justice. This act requires the pharmacist to keep a record of the receipt and the disposition of all Controlled Substances; such drugs are identified on the label of the *original* container by a symbol, consisting of either the Roman numeral of the schedule within a large letter "C" or the letter "C" followed by the schedule (*e.g.,* C-II). The records must be maintained for a period of at least 2 years and be available for inspection by authorized persons. Prescription orders for Controlled Substances in schedule II must be typewritten, or written in ink or indelible pencil, and signed by the practitioner; such prescription orders *cannot be refilled.* The physician must write a new prescription if administration of the drug is to be continued. Prescription orders for drugs covered by schedule III or IV may be issued either orally or in writing by a practitioner and may be refilled, *if so authorized, not more than five times* and may *not* be filled or refilled *more than 6 months* after date of issue. After five refills or after 6 months, the prescribing practitioner may write or authorize a new prescription order. Drugs in schedule V may be prescribed the same as drugs in schedules III and IV, and, under certain conditions, may be dispensed without a prescription.

Physicians should do all they can to prevent abuses of prescription orders. It is a good practice to write out the number of refills desired on every prescription order; Arabic numerals may easily be altered and, if not indicated, instructions may easily be forged. Furthermore, when an authorization for refill is not given on the prescription order, it cannot be refilled without *personal* authorization by the prescriber.

Controlled Substances Act. Various federal, state, and city laws exist to control the standard of purity of drugs and their manufacture, sale, and dispensing. These laws must be known and observed by the practitioner. The most stringent law takes precedence, whether it be federal, state, or local. The most important laws are embodied in the *Comprehensive Drug Abuse Prevention and Control Act of 1970* (*see* Federal Regulations, April 24, 1971). This act divides narcotic and other drugs into five schedules.

Schedule I. Drugs in this schedule have a high potential for abuse and *no* currently accepted medical use in the United States. Examples of such drugs include heroin, marihuana, peyote, mescaline, psilocybin, tetrahydrocannabinols, LSD, ketobemidone, levomoramide, racemoramide, benzylmorphine, dihydromorphine, morphine methylsulfonate, nicocodeine, nicomorphine, and others. Substances listed in this schedule are not for prescription use but may be obtained for research and instructional use or for chemical analysis by application to the Drug Enforcement Administration, Department of Justice (Form 225), supported by a protocol of the proposed use.

Schedule II. Drugs in this schedule have a high potential for abuse with severe liability to cause psychic or physical dependence. Schedule-II controlled substances consist of certain opioid drugs and drugs containing amphetamines or methamphetamines as the single active ingredient or in combination with each other. Examples of substances included in this schedule are opium, morphine, codeine, hydromorphone (DILAUDID), methadone (DOLOPHINE), meperidine (DEMEROL), cocaine, oxycodone (PERCODAN), anileridine (LERITINE), oxymorphone (NUMORPHAN), dextroamphetamine (DEXEDRINE), and methamphetamine (DESOXYN). Also included in schedule II are phenmetrazine (PRELUDIN), methylphenidate (RITALIN), methaqualone (PAREST, QUAALUDE, SOMNAFAC, SOPOR), amobarbital (AMYTAL), pentobarbital (NEMBUTAL), secobarbital (SECONAL), etorphine hydrochloride, and diphenoxylate.

Schedule III. The drugs in this schedule have

a potential for abuse that is less than for those in schedules I and II; their abuse may lead to moderate or low physical dependence or high psychological dependence. This schedule includes compounds containing limited quantities of certain opioid drugs and also certain nonopioid drugs, such as chlorhexadol, glutethimide (DORIDEN), methyprylon (NOLUDAR), sulfondiethylmethane, sulfonmethane, nalorphine, benzphetamine, chlorphentermine, clortermine, mazindol, phendimetrazine, paregoric, and certain barbiturates (except those listed in another schedule).

Schedule IV. The drugs in this schedule have a low potential for abuse that leads only to limited physical dependence or psychological dependence relative to drugs in schedule III. In this schedule are barbital, phenobarbital, methylphenobarbital, chloral betaine (BETA-CHLOR), chloral hydrate, ethchlorvynol (PLACIDYL), ethinamate (VALMID), meprobamate (EQUANIL, MILTOWN), paraldehyde, pentaerythritol chloral (PETRICHLORAL), methohexital, fenfluramine, diethylpropion, phentermine, chlordiazepoxide (LIBRIUM), diazepam (VALIUM), clorazepate (TRANXENE), flurazepam (DALMANE), oxazepam (SERAX), clonazepam (CLONOPIN), prazepam (VERSTRAN), lorazepam (ATIVAN), mebutamate, and propoxyphene (DARVON).

Schedule V. The drugs in this schedule have a potential for abuse that is less than those listed in schedule IV and consist of preparations containing moderate quantities of certain opioid drugs, generally for antitussive or antidiarrheal purposes, which may be distributed without a prescription order. One drug that is unique to this schedule is loperamide, which is an opioid. Substances in this schedule may be prescribed the same as those in schedules III and IV. In addition, drugs in schedule V may be dispensed without a prescription order provided (1) such distribution is made only by a pharmacist; (2) not more than 240 ml of any schedule-V substance containing opium, nor more than 120 ml or more than 24 solid dosage units of any other controlled substance, is sold to the same consumer in any given 48-hour period without a valid prescription order; (3) the purchaser at retail is at least 18 years of age; (4) the pharmacist obtains suitable identification; (5) a record book is maintained that contains the name and address of the purchaser, name and quantity of Controlled Substance purchased, date of sale, and initials of the pharmacist; and (6) other federal, state, or local law does not require a prescription order.

The label of any Controlled Substance in schedule II, III, or IV, when dispensed to or for a patient pursuant to a prescription order, must contain the following warning; *"Caution: Federal law prohibits the transfer of this drug to any person other than the patient for whom it was prescribed."*

In order to prescribe Controlled Substances, a physician must register with the Drug Enforcement Administration, Registration Section, Department of Justice. If a physician has more than one office in which he administers and/or dispenses any of the drugs listed in the five schedules, he then is required to register at each office. The registration must be renewed annually. The number on the certificate of registration must be indicated on all prescription orders for Controlled Substances. The physician must also file an inventory of the Controlled Substances on hand every 2 years; file a revised form if his location is changed; keep a record of controlled substances listed in schedules II through V that he dispenses, if he regularly charges patients either separately or together with professional services for such medication; and *order his supplies of controlled substances listed in schedule II for dispensing or administration on special order forms,* obtainable from the Drug Enforcement Administration, Registration Section, P.O. Box 28083, Central Station, Washington, D. C. 20005.

Both the physician and the pharmacist are legally responsible for the proper prescribing and dispensing of drugs covered by the Controlled Substances Act. There are many technical details in the regulations and, as a result, the physician may innocently violate the law in his professional use of Controlled Substances, especially as related to the use of opioids for patients with incurable diseases or in the management of drug addiction. An informational outline of the Controlled Substances Act of 1970, entitled *A Manual for the Medical Practitioner,* is especially informative on these problems. Copies may be obtained from the Drug Enforcement Administration at the address indicated in the previous paragraph.

PATIENT COMPLIANCE INSTRUCTION

Most physicians assume that once the diagnosis is made and the prescription order is written the patient will benefit from his diagnostic and therapeutic acumen. Unfortunately, drug treatment of any kind is often compromised by lack of full compliance by the patient. Common errors of compliance to a regimen by a patient may be of omission, purpose (taking medicines for the wrong reasons), dosage, timing or sequence, adding medications not prescribed, or premature termination of drug therapy. In addition, from 3 to 18% of patients fail to have their prescription orders "filled" within 10 days (Hammel and Williams, 1964; Boyd *et al.,* 1974). Observations of this kind suggest that attention should be directed to some of the basic principles of instruction of the patient about the importance of compliance.

Factors Associated with Noncompliance. The drug defaulter, like the placebo reactor, is not a readily identifiable individual (Caron and Roth, 1968; Blackwell, 1973). Patients who are unreliable under one treatment regimen may not be under another. Porter (1969), after a detailed study of this problem, concluded that ". . . it has not proved possible to identify an uncooperative type. Every patient is a potential defaulter; compliance can never be assumed." Nevertheless, Gillum and Barsky (1974), based on a critical review of the literature, reported that psychological, environmental, and social factors, characteristics of the drug regimen, and the nature of the physician-patient interaction were most consistently related to noncompliance. Some of these factors are briefly reviewed here in order to indicate some of the steps that the physician can take to improve patient compliance. For a more detailed analysis, the reader is referred to several excellent articles and reviews (Blackwell, 1972; Stewart and Cluff, 1972; Hulka *et al.,* 1975; Hussar, 1975; Blackwell, 1976; Lasagna, 1976; Sackett and Haynes, 1976; Christensen, 1978; Melmon and Morrelli, 1978; Roth and Caron, 1978).

The Patient's Illness. After the prescription order has been written, the physician should make sure the patient understands the nature and prognosis of his illness, what he may expect from his medication (both acceptable and unacceptable unwanted effects, as well as signs of efficacy that may help to enforce his compliance). The physician should explain how the medication alters the disease process. Patients frequently discontinue taking a medication such as penicillin for streptococcal pharyngitis because they have not been told the necessity for continuing the drug after the acute symptoms have subsided. Similarly, patients taking antidepressant medication frequently discontinue treatment because the physician failed to mention the untoward effects that might appear or to advise the patient that 10 days or more may elapse before he notices any improvement. Patients with chronic illnesses are prone to lapse in compliance, especially if the treatment is prophylactic or suppressive, the condition is associated with only mild or no symptoms, or the consequences of missing a dose or two are not immediate. In contrast, when relapse is immediate or severe, the patient is much less likely to deviate from the prescribed regimen.

The Patient. Errors and noncompliance occur more frequently at the extremes of age and in patients who live alone. Geriatric patients present problems because of lapses in memory or self-neglect. Poor compliance among children is related to problems of taste and swallowing, although the mother's impression of the severity of the illness has a marked influence on compliance in pediatric patients (Becker *et al.,* 1972). The physician must explore in some detail the patient's eating, sleeping, and working habits. Otherwise, he might prescribe a drug to be taken three times a day with meals for a patient who either eats only twice a day or sleeps all day and works at night. Educational, economic, ethnic, and personality factors may also influence patient compliance. According to Blackwell (1973), the less educated, poor patient with a risk-prone personality is more likely to be a drug defaulter. In the United States the problem is severe with patients whose primary language is not English, and who may require carefully worded written and oral instructions in that language.

The Physician. Studies by Mazzullo and associates (1974) suggest that physicians who do not explain the reasons for their decisions may be a major determinant of the patient's noncompliance. The physician's relationship with the patient and how clearly he explains the treatment regimen have a powerful impact on compliance. Thus, the physician-patient relationship should be viewed as a process of instruction and motivation for both parties as they enter into a health-related contract. The effectiveness of physician-patient communication is inversely related to the error rate in the taking of drugs. Directions on prescription orders should include all the details necessary for a patient to know how, with what, when, and how long to take the medication. For example, directions for a patient about tetracycline capsules might read as follows: "Swallow one capsule with a half glass of water 1 hour before each meal and at bedtime for 10 days." The prescription order should be proofread aloud, and an additional note should be given to the patient cautioning him not to take the medication with milk or antacids. Finally, the patient should be asked if he understands the directions, why the medication should not be taken with milk, why the medication should be taken for 10 days, and what the treatment is expected to accomplish.

The Medication Prescribed. Multiple medications, frequent-dose regimens, and the physical features of the medication itself often foster poor compliance. Patients taking three or more medications are less likely to use them as directed. Likewise, the more frequently a medication is directed to be taken, the less likely it will be taken as prescribed. Hulka and associates (1976) reported that omission rates doubled when the number of medications prescribed was increased from one to four. Likewise, the rates doubled when administration was increased from once daily to four times daily. Considerable confusion may also develop when multiple drugs of similar appearance are prescribed for the same patient, as has been emphasized by Mazzullo (1972) and Mazzullo and Lasagna (1972). They have also stressed the desirability of providing the patient with an identifying name for each medication prescribed, for example, "heart pill" or "water pill," assuming he has been told what each medication is designed to accomplish. The color plates in the *Physicians' Desk Reference* can be used to show patients what their medication will look like.

Patients frequently discontinue medication upon the appearance of minor untoward effects because they have not been told that such reactions are common and not to be feared. Special instruction should be given the patient relative to symptoms that indicate overdosage, such as dizziness from antihypertensive agents. Before this is done, however, the doctor should determine (by taking a nonleading history) whether the patient already has the symptoms that could later be misinterpreted as drug related. Such a misunderstanding could lead to an unjustifiable discontinuation of a very useful drug.

The Treatment Environment. The setting in which the prescribed medication is to be taken has a marked influence on compliance. A series of studies in the same psychiatric hospital revealed that noncompliance increased progressively from 19% in inpatients to 37% in day patients and 48% in outpatients (Hare and Wilcox, 1967). This emphasizes the need to teach the principles of self-medication before the patient leaves the hospital and the added responsibility the physician must assume if he is to achieve satisfactory compliance with patients he sees in clinics and in his private office.

Consequences of Noncompliance. The consequences of noncompliance, although quite apparent, are often not fully appreciated by either the physician or the patient. *Underutilization of the prescribed drug* deprives the patient of the intended therapeutic benefits. This may result in a recurrence or worsening of the illness, emergence of antibiotic-resistant microorganisms, or the prescribing of a larger dose or a more potent agent that could lead to toxicity if compliance is improved. Before a patient is judged to be unresponsive or not optimally controlled with initial therapy, some effort should be made to determine whether the medication is being taken according to instructions. Thus, 75% of patients referred for

evaluation of "refractoriness" to phenytoin were found not to be taking the drug as prescribed (Borofsky *et al.*, 1972). The compliance rates of some groups of patients on digoxin, hydrochlorothiazide, and potassium chloride were 92%, 83%, and 60%, respectively (Brook *et al.*, 1971). Hussar (1975) has suggested that the latter illustration indicates that noncompliance is a contributing factor to the frequent cases of hypokalemia and toxicity to cardiac glycosides.

Overutilization of the prescribed drug places the patient at increased risk of adverse reactions. Such problems may develop rather innocently; frequently the patient either forgets a dose and hence doubles the next one or adopts an attitude that if one tablet is good, two must be better. A study of the profile of medications indicates that overutilization of drugs accounts for 65% of problems with compliance (Solomon *et al.*, 1974).

The prevalence of noncompliance has raised questions relative to the effect of this variable on clinical trials of new drugs. Although numerous controls are built into such studies, the difficulties associated with noncompliance must, to some extent, compromise the ability to establish true rates of efficacy and toxicity of any given agent.

The Pharmacist and Patient Compliance. The pharmacist is usually the last professional to be in contact with the ambulatory private patient (or his representative) before medication is started. Pharmacists can effectively cooperate with the physician in education about compliance and can counsel the patient on how to take his medication. Cooperation between physician and pharmacist is in the interest of optimal drug therapy, especially with patients who are likely to make errors in taking drugs. Unfortunately, in certain states such cooperation may be in conflict with laws designed to prevent collusion beween pharmacists and physicians.

American Pharmaceutical Association and American Society of Internal Medicine. Prescription writing and prescription labeling. *J. Am. Pharm. Assoc.,* **1974,** *NS 14,* 654.
Becker, M. H.; Drachman, R. H.; and Kirscht, J. P. Predicting mother's compliance with pediatric medical regimens. *J. Pediatr.,* **1972,** *81,* 843–854.
Blackwell, B. The drug defaulter. *Clin. Pharmacol. Ther.,* **1972,** *13,* 841–848.
———. Patient compliance. *N. Engl. J. Med.,* **1973,** *289,* 249–252.
———. Treatment adherence. *Br. J. Psychiatry,* **1976,** *129,* 513–531.
Borofsky, L. G.; Louis, S.; Kutt, H.; and Roginsky, M. Diphenylhydantoin: efficacy, toxicity, and dose-serum level relationships in children. *J. Pediatr.,* **1972,** *81,* 995–1002.
Boyd, J. R.; Covington, T. R.; Stanaszek, W. F.; and Coussons, R. T. Drug defaulting—Part II: Analysis of noncompliance patterns. *Am. J. Hosp. Pharm.,* **1974,** *31,* 485–491.

Brook, R. H.; Appel, F. A.; Avery, C.; Orman, M.; and Stevenson, R. I. Effectiveness of inpatient follow-up care. *N. Engl. J. Med.,* **1971,** *285,* 1509–1514.

Caron, H. S., and Roth, H. P. Patients' cooperation with a medical regimen: difficulties in identifying the non-cooperator. *J.A.M.A.,* **1968,** *203,* 922–926.

Christensen, D. B. Drug-taking compliance: a review and synthesis. *Health Serv. Res.,* **1978,** *13,* 171–186.

Committee on Drugs, American Academy of Pediatrics. Inaccuracies in administering liquid medication. *Pediatrics,* **1975,** *56,* 327–328.

Drug Bioequivalence: A Report of the Office of Technology Assessment, Drug Bioequivalence Study Panel. U.S Government Printing Office, Washington, D. C., **1974.**

Food and Drug Administration. Drug products, bioequivalence requirements and *in vivo* bioavailability procedures. *Federal Register,* **1977,** *42,* No. 5, 1649.

————. New prescribing directions for phenytoin. *FDA Drug Bull.,* **1978,** *8,* 27.

Gillum, R. F., and Barsky, J. Diagnosis and management of patient noncompliance. *J.A.M.A.,* **1974,** *228,* 1563–1567.

Hammel, R. W., and Williams, P. O. Do patients receive prescribed medication? *J. Am. Pharm. Assoc.,* **1964,** *NS 4,* 331–333, 337.

Hare, E. H., and Wilcox, D. R. C. Do psychiatric inpatients take their pills? *Br. J. Psychiatry,* **1967,** *113,* 1435–1439.

Hirschorn, J. O., and Silverman, H. I. The ubiquitous medicine dropper. *Am. J. Pharm.,* **1968,** *140,* 1–6.

Hulka, B. S.; Cassel, J. C.; and Kupper, L. L. Disparities between medications prescribed and consumed among chronic disease patients. In, *Patient Compliance.* (Lasagna, L., ed.) Futura Publishing Co., Mount Kisco, N.Y., **1976,** pp. 123–152.

Hulka, B. S.; Kupper, L. L.; Cassel, J. C.; Efird, R. L.; and Burdette, J. A. Medication use and misuse: physician-patient discrepancies. *J. Chronic Dis.,* **1975,** *28,* 7–21.

Hussar, D. A. Patient noncompliance. *J. Am. Pharm. Assoc.,* **1975,** *NS 15,* 183–190, 201.

Jerome, J. B., and Sagan, P. The USAN nomenclature system. *J.A.M.A.,* **1975,** *232,* 294–299.

Lasagna, L. (ed.). *Patient Compliance.* Futura Publishing Co., Mount Kisco, N. Y., **1976.**

Mazzullo, J. The nonpharmacologic basis of therapeutics. *Clin. Pharmacol. Ther.,* **1972,** *13,* 157–158.

Mazzullo, J.; Cohn, K.; Lasagna, L.; and Griner, P. Variations in interpretation of prescription instructions. *J.A.M.A.,* **1974,** *227,* 929–931.

Mazzullo, J. M., and Lasagna, L. Take thou . . . but is your patient really taking what you prescribed? *Drug Ther.,* **1972,** *2,* 11–15.

Melmon, K. L., and Morrelli, H. F. (eds.). *Clinical Pharmacology: Basic Principles in Therapeutics,* 2nd ed. Macmillan Publishing Co., Inc., New York, **1978.**

National Prescription Audit: General Information Report, 17th ed. IMS America, Ltd., Ambler, Pa., **1978.**

Porter, A. M. W. Drug defaulting in general practice. *Br. Med. J.,* **1969,** *1,* 218–222.

Roth, H. P., and Caron, H. S. Accuracy of doctors' estimates and patient statements on adherence to a drug regimen. *Clin. Pharmacol. Ther.,* **1978,** *23,* 361–370.

Sackett, D. L. The magnitude of compliance and noncompliance. In, *Compliance with Therapeutic Regimens.* (Sackett, D. L., and Haynes, R. B., eds.) Johns Hopkins University Press, Baltimore, **1976,** pp. 9–25.

Sackett, D. L., and Haynes, R. B. (eds.). *Compliance with Therapeutic Regimens.* Johns Hopkins University Press, Baltimore, **1976.**

Solomon, D. K.; Baumgartner, R. P.; Glascock, L. M.; Briscoe, M. E.; and Billups, N. F. Use of medication profiles to detect potential therapeutic problems in ambulatory patients. *Am. J. Hosp. Pharm.,* **1974,** *31,* 348–354.

Stewart, R. B., and Cluff, L. E. A review of medication errors and compliance in ambulant patients. *Clin. Pharmacol. Ther.,* **1972,** *13,* 463–468.

Task Force on Prescription Drugs. *Final Report.* U.S. Department of Health, Education, and Welfare, Washington, D. C., **1969.**

Teplitsky, B. Caution! 1,000 drugs whose names look-alike or sound-alike. *Pharm. Times,* **1975,** *41,* 75–77.

The United States Pharmacopeia, 20th rev. (The United States Pharmacopeial Convention, Inc.) Mack Printing Co., Easton, Pa., published **1980,** became official **1980.**

II DESIGN AND OPTIMIZATION OF DOSAGE REGIMENS; PHARMACOKINETIC DATA

Leslie Z. Benet and Lewis B. Sheiner

The objective of this appendix is to present pharmacokinetic data in a format that allows the clinician to make rational choices of doses of drugs. The tables contain quantitative information about the absorption, distribution, and elimination of drugs and the effects of disease states on these processes, as well as information concerning the correlation of efficacy and toxicity with measured concentrations of drugs in plasma. In this compilation emphasis is placed on the relationship between pharmacokinetic parameters and physiological variables, rather than on the use of compartmental models to define pharmacokinetic concepts.

To utilize the data that are presented, one must understand clearance concepts and their application for the computation of drug-dosage regimens. One must also know average values of clearance for a number of drugs, as well as some measures of the extent and kinetics of drug absorption and distribution. The text that follows defines the eight basic parameters that are listed in the tabular material for each drug, as well as some factors that influence these values in both normal subjects and in patients with particular diseases. The remainder of the text discusses the dosage strategies available to the clinician and the planning of such regimens. Finally, comments are made on the practical use of measurements of concentrations of drugs, as well as the pitfalls inherent in such usage.

It would obviously be most useful if there was a consensus about the correct value for a given pharmacokinetic parameter, rather than being faced with 10 or 20 separate (and often disparate) estimates of that parameter. Although a standard approach has recently been proposed for the compilation of clinical pharmacokinetic data and for reaching such a consensus (Sheiner *et al.*, 1980), this has been done for only a very limited number of drugs. In the present tables a single value from the literature ($\pm$ standard deviation) has usually been selected for each parameter, based on the scientific judgment of the authors; the reference is identified in each case. Values in the tables are those determined in healthy normal adults, unless otherwise indicated by footnotes. The direction of change for these values in par-

ticular disease states is noted next to the average value, again with a specific reference to the literature.

PHARMACOKINETIC PARAMETERS

Availability. The extent of availability of the drug following oral administration is expressed as a percentage of the dose. This value represents the percentage of an oral dose that is available to produce pharmacological actions—the fraction of the oral dose that reaches the left ventricle in an active form. A drug that is absorbed but inactivated by the gastrointestinal mucosa or metabolized and/or excreted in the bile during initial passage through the liver is not considered to be available. *Fractional availability* (F) is a similar parameter used elsewhere in this appendix; this value varies from 0 to 1. Measures of the *rate* of availability are not provided in the tables. Since pharmacokinetic concepts are most useful in the design of multiple dosage regimens, the *extent* rather than the rate of availability is more critical to obtain an appropriate concentration of drug in the body (as will be discussed subsequently).

Urinary Excretion of Unchanged Drug. The second parameter in the tabular section is the amount of drug eventually excreted unchanged in the urine, expressed as a percentage of the administered dose. Values represent the percentage expected in a healthy young adult (creatinine clearance greater than 100 ml/min). When possible, the value listed is that determined after bolus intravenous administration of the drug, where availability is assumed to be 100%. If the drug is given orally, this parameter may also reflect loss of drug due to low availability; such values are indicated by a footnote.

Binding to Plasma Proteins. The tabulated value is the percentage of drug in the plasma that is bound to plasma proteins at concentrations of the drug that are achieved clinically. In almost all cases the values are from measurements performed *in vitro* (rather than from measurements of binding to the proteins in plasma that was obtained from patients to whom drug had been administered). When a single mean value is presented, there is no apparent change in this percentage over the range of concentrations normally found in the patient population taking the drug. In cases where saturation of binding is approached at usual plasma concentrations, values are provided at concentrations that correspond to the lower and higher limits of the usual range.

Clearance. Total clearance of drug from plasma (CLp) is the volume of plasma that would have to lose *all* the drug it contains per unit time in order to account for the observed rate of loss of the compound by all routes of elimination (excretion and metabolic disposition); values are usually reported in units of $ml \cdot min^{-1} \cdot kg^{-1}$.

$$Rate\ of\ elimination = CLp \cdot Cp$$

where Cp is the concentration of the drug in plasma. In some cases, separate values for renal and nonrenal clearance are also provided. For some drugs, particularly those that are predominantly excreted unchanged in the urine, equations are given that relate total or renal clearance to creatinine clearance (also expressed as $ml \cdot min^{-1} \cdot kg^{-1}$). For drugs that follow first-order kinetics over the range of plasma concentrations usually observed, clearance should be constant. However, for those drugs that exhibit saturation kinetics, total clearance from plasma changes as a function of the concentration of drug in plasma:

$$Total\ plasma\ clearance = V_m/(K_m + Cp)$$

where K_m and V_m represent, respectively, the plasma concentration at which half of the maximal rate of elimination is reached (in units of mass/volume) and the maximal rate of elimination (in units of $mass \cdot time^{-1} \cdot kg$ of body weight^{-1}). Cp must, of course, be in the same units as K_m.

Rowland and associates (1973) and Wilkinson and Shand (1975) have discussed clearance from *blood* for drugs that follow first-order kinetics in terms of the blood flow to the eliminating organ (Q) and the intrinsic ability of the organ to eliminate the drug (CL_{int}):

$$Blood\ clearance = Q \cdot CL_{int}/(Q + CL_{int})$$

The intrinsic clearance is the maximal possible clearance by the organ when blood flow (delivery of drug) is not limiting. Intrinsic clearance is tabulated for a few drugs. Note that the above definition is in terms of *clearance from blood*, rather than clearance from plasma, and that one may only estimate intrinsic clearance of an organ easily when *all* elimination or clearance is by that organ. If one wishes to relate changes in elimina-

tion of drug to pathological changes either in the organ itself or to blood flow to the organ, it is necessary to express clearance with respect to concentrations of drug in blood rather than those in plasma. This requires measurement of concentrations in whole blood or knowledge of the distribution of drug between plasma and red blood cells; such information is currently limited. Clearances from plasma are presented in the tables, since these are most useful to relate dosage of drug to concentrations of drugs in plasma that have been determined previously to be effective or toxic.

Clearance can be determined only when the fractional availability of the drug, F, is known. Therefore, to be accurate, clearances must be determined following intravenous dosage. When such data are not available, the ratio CL/F is given; values of this kind are indicated by a footnote.

Total plasma clearance for a drug that follows first-order kinetics may be determined independently of any particular pharmacokinetic model, since:

$$CLp = dose/AUC_{0\to\infty}$$

where $AUC_{0\to\infty}$ is the total area under the curve that describes the concentration of the drug in plasma as a function of time (from zero to infinity).

Volume of Distribution. The total body volume of distribution at steady state (Vd_{ss}) is expressed in units of liters/kg. A number of pharmacokinetic parameters have been used to indicate the total space for distribution of a drug in the body. The particular definition chosen here is similar to that in Chapter 1—the volume in which a drug would appear to be distributed during the steady state if the drug existed throughout that volume at the same concentration as in the plasma. Direct measurement of this quantity is usually impossible or very inconvenient. Until recently, the only methods reported for calculating Vd_{ss} following an intravenous bolus dose required a prior determination of pharmacokinetic parameters for a particular model or at least a multiexponential fit of the data. However, in a manner analogous to the determination of clearance by the use of areas, Benet and Galeazzi (1979) have described a noncompartmental method for determination of Vd_{ss}.

$$Vd_{ss} = \frac{dose\left[\int_0^\infty t\ Cpdt\right]}{\left[\int_0^\infty Cpdt\right]^2} = \frac{dose\left[AUMC_{0\to\infty}\right]}{\left[AUC_{0\to\infty}\right]^2}$$

where $AUC_{0\to\infty}$ is as defined above and $AUMC_{0\to\infty}$ is the area under the first moment of the plasma concentration curve, that is, the area under the curve of the product of time, t, and plasma concentration, Cp, over the time span zero to infinity.

When Vd_{ss} has not been determined, values for Vd_{area} are provided. These values are obtained by dividing clearance by the terminal rate constant for elimination. Vd_{area} is a convenient and easily calculated parameter. However, unlike Vd_{ss}, this volume term varies when the rate constant for drug elimination changes, even though there has been no change in the distribution space. As the rate constant for elimination decreases, Vd_{area} approaches Vd_{ss}. Since the clinician may wish to know whether a particular disease state influences either clearance or the distribution of the drug within the body independently, it is preferable to define volume in terms of a parameter that is theoretically independent of changes in the rate of elimination.

As is the case for clearance, Vd_{ss} is usually defined in the tables in terms of the concentrations in plasma, rather than in blood. If data were not obtained after intravenous administration of the drug, a footnote will make clear that the parameter determined, Vd_{ss}/F, contains a measure of availability.

Half-life. The time required for one half of the amount of drug in the body to be eliminated is provided. However, drug concentrations in plasma usually follow a multiexponential pattern of decline when this value is measured as a function of time. The single number listed in each table corresponds to the rate of elimination that describes the major fraction of total clearance of drug from the body. In many cases this half-life may correspond to the terminal log-linear rate of elimination. For some drugs, however, a more prolonged half-life may be observed at very low plasma concentrations when extremely sensitive assay technics are used. If this component accounts for only 10% of drug clearance, predictions of steady-state concentrations of drug in plasma will be in error by only 10% if this longer half-life is ignored, no matter how large its value. This is true because half-life is a function of both elimination and distribution, as will be further discussed below.

Effective and Toxic Concentrations. There is no general agreement about the best way to describe the relationship between the concentration of drug in plasma and its effect. Many different kinds of data are presented in the literature, and extraction of a single parameter or even a set of parameters is difficult. Furthermore, there may not be agreement as to which measures are most relevant. Footnotes are common in the tables to indicate the meaning and relevance of these values; in many cases reference is made to a chapter in the text for discussion.

INFLUENCES ON AND DETERMINANTS OF THE PARAMETERS

The following discussion details the factors that may influence or modify the parameters listed in the tables. These modifications may result from physiological or biochemical events that occur in normal individuals, as well as pathological conditions that may exist only in particular disease states.

Availability. It is important to keep in mind that poor patient compliance may be mistaken for decreased bioavailablity. A true decrease in bioavailability may result from a poorly formulated dosage form that fails to disintegrate or dissolve in the gastrointestinal fluids, interactions between drugs in the gastrointestinal tract, metabolism of the drug in the gastrointestinal tract, and/or first-pass hepatic metabolism or biliary excretion (*see* Chapter 1). For drugs such as lidocaine (*see* Chapter 31), hepatic disease may cause increased availability either because hepatic metabolic capacity decreases or because of the development of vascular shunts around the liver.

Urinary Excretion of Unchanged Drug. Renal disease is the primary factor that causes changes in this parameter. This is especially true when alternate pathways of elimination are available; thus, as renal function decreases, a greater fraction of the dose is available for elimination by other routes. Since renal function decreases as a function of age, the percentage of drug excreted unchanged also usually decreases with age when alternate pathways of elimination are available. For a number of acidic and basic drugs with values of pK_a in the range of the usual pH of urine, changes in the latter will affect the rate or extent of urinary excretion (*see* Chapter 1).

Binding to Plasma Proteins. This parameter is primarily affected by disease states (such as hepatic disease) that alter the concentration of albumin or other proteins in plasma that bind drugs. Some metabolic states and conditions such as uremia also change the affinity of binding for some drugs. Such changes in protein binding as a function of disease can dramatically affect the volume of distribution of a drug.

Clearance. Total clearance of a drug from the body may be defined as the sum of the clearances by the individual organs that participate for that drug. In general, three factors may alter the clearance by an organ: blood flow to the organ, Q_O; the fraction of drug unbound in the blood, α; and the maximal ability of the organ to remove unbound drug, CL'_{int}.

When the intrinsic clearance of an organ is very high compared to blood flow (such that $\alpha CL'_{int} \gg Q_O$), $CL_{organ} \approx Q_O$. In such a situation clearance by the organ will be very sensitive to changes in blood flow and essentially independent of binding (provided that the rate of dissociation from binding sites is fast compared to the transit time through the organ).

However, in many cases clearance by the organ is limited by capacity; that is, blood flow is significantly greater than the intrinsic organ clearance ($Q_O \gg \alpha CL'_{int}$), and the equation reduces to $CL_{organ} = \alpha CL'_{int}$, indicating that clearance is directly related to the degree of protein binding. This applies for the renal clearance of drugs that are eliminated solely by glomerular filtration. In such cases, if a drug is neither protein bound nor reabsorbed, CL'_{int} is approximately the rate of glomerular filtration (120 ml/min); renal clearance of drug will be less than this depending on the extent of protein binding.

When clearance by the organ is limited by capacity, a drug may exhibit nonlinear kinetics of elimination, which may be described by the Michaelis-Menten equation:

$$CL_{organ} = \alpha CL'_{int} = CL_{int} = V_m/(K_m + Cp)$$

where $K_m = K'_m/\alpha$, and K'_m is the concentration of free drug at which metabolism is half-saturated. For such drugs (e.g., phenytoin), clearance by the organ will vary as a function of the concentration of drug in plasma or blood, as well as of the fraction bound.

Clearance varies as a function of body size and, therefore, is presented in the tables in units of $ml \cdot min^{-1} \cdot kg$ of body weight^{-1}. Although normalization to measures of size other than weight may sometimes be appropriate, weight is so convenient that this offsets any small loss in accuracy, especially when dealing with adults.

Volume of Distribution. The apparent volume of distribution is a function of four major factors: the volume of the tissues into which the drug distributes, the partition coefficient of the drug between the various tissues and the circulating blood, the blood flow to the tissues, and the extent of binding of the drug both to proteins in the plasma and to components in the various tissues (see Chapter 1). All of the factors can be affected by total body size, age, sex, and disease. The blood flow per unit volume of tissue determines how fast the drug can be delivered and is one of the determinants of the rate at which tissue may

be expected to come into steady state with the blood. The other major determinant is how much drug can be stored or distributed in a tissue. This will depend on the size of the tissue and the ability of the drug to concentrate in the tissue—a function of the partition coefficient between the organ and blood and the extent of binding to the constituents of the tissue.

Volume of distribution is, of course, a function of body size, and values in the tables are in liters/kg. As mentioned for clearance, normalization to measures of size other than weight may sometimes be appropriate.

Half-life. Historically, when drug kinetics was compared in diseased patients and normal subjects, half-life was the measure most often used. Only recently has it been appreciated that half-life is a derived parameter that changes as a function of both clearance and volume of distribution. A useful approximate relationship between the terminal log-linear half-life, clearance, and volume of distribution is given by:

$$t_{1/2} \cong 0.693 \, Vd/CL$$

As clearance decreases due, for example, to a disease process, half-life increases. However, this reciprocal relationship is exact only when the disease does not change the volume of distribution. For example, the half-life of diazepam increases with increasing age; however, it is not clearance that changes as a function of age, but the volume of distribution (Klotz et al., 1975). Similarly, changes in protein binding of the drug may affect its clearance as well as its volume of distribution, leading to unpredictable changes in half-life as a function of disease. The half-life of tolbutamide, for example, decreases in patients with acute viral hepatitis, exactly the opposite from what one might expect. The disease appears to modify protein binding in both plasma and tissues, causing no change in volume of distribution but an *increase* in total clearance because higher concentrations of free drug are present (Williams et al., 1977).

Half-life is usually independent of body size since, as noted above, it is a function of the ratio of two parameters, each of which is proportional to body size.

Effective and Toxic Concentrations. The relationships between the concentration of drug in plasma and the effect of the drug are imperfect, as might be expected (see Chapter 2). Little information is available about the variation between individuals of receptor number or affinity or subsequent coupling to a response, or about the effects of disease states on these factors. For many drugs, the form of the relationship between effect and plasma concentration is unknown. Because the concentration of free drug determines the degree of effect, changes in protein binding due to disease may be expected to cause changes in the *total* concentration of drug associated with a desired or an unwanted effect. It is also important to realize that concentration-effect relationships are only meaningful at steady state or during the terminal log-linear phase of the concentration versus time curve, when the ratio of the drug concentration at sites of action to that in the plasma can be expected to remain constant over time. Thus, when attempting to correlate pharmacokinetics with pharmacodynamics, the time of distribution of drug to its site of action must be taken into account.

PHARMACOKINETIC PRINCIPLES AND DOSAGE REGIMENS

Dosage describes both the route and the rate of administration of drugs, and knowledge of pharmacokinetic principles is important in making such decisions. The choice of route of administration has been discussed in Chapter 1. In principle, the clinician may wish to follow a complex time course of drug administration. In reality, most desired patterns of administration fall into two classes—continuous input by intravenous infusion or a series of bolus doses, usually of equal size and given at approximately equally spaced intervals.

Clearly, there may be other desirable dosage patterns. When a hypnotic is used to induce sleep, a rapid rise and then fall of drug concentration is desirable; intermittent dosage and rapid absorption of the drug are thus desirable. Usually, however, a relatively constant effect is desired. When the margin of safety is small, continuous intravenous infusion or an alternative strategy that results in small fluctuations of concentration is desirable. Unfortunately, for many drugs, the most desirable dosage pattern is not known. For many, a wide variety of patterns is probably equally efficacious. For some drugs, however, such as the aminoglycoside antibiotics or certain cancer chemotherapeutic agents, considerable research effort is being expended to determine optimal patterns of administration that will maximize the ratio of benefit to harm.

Maintenance Dose. It is simpler to consider first the decisions about dosage to be made after a steady state has been achieved. All that is needed is to maintain the status quo, and drug input thus must balance losses. Whether administration of drug is continuous or intermittent, one may think of the average concentration of drug at steady state as a primary determinant of the choice of maintenance dosage.

$$\text{Maintenance dosage} = Cp_{ss}(CL/F)$$

Thus, the average maintenance dosage is determined by the desired concentration at steady state (Cp_{ss}), given a particular set of values for F, the fraction of the dose absorbed by the chosen route, and clearance, CL. When the drug is given by continuous intravenous infusion, the choice of the average (continuous) rate of administration is the only one to be made. When doses are to be administered intermittently, the interval between doses must also be chosen. The factors to be considered in making a rational choice about dosage interval are discussed in Chapter 1 (page 24) and below; the half-life of the drug is a principal determinant.

Loading Dose. When the time to reach steady state is appreciable, as it is for drugs with long half-lives, the physician may wish to administer a loading dose that promptly raises the concentration of drug in plasma to the projected steady-state value (*see* Chapter 1). In theory, only the amount of the loading dose need be computed, not the rate of its administration; to a first approximation, this is so. The amount of drug required to achieve a given steady-state concentration is the amount that will eventually be in the body when the desired steady state is reached. (For intermittent dosage, the amount is that at the mean steady-state concentration.) The volume of distribution (Vd_{ss}) is the proportionality factor that relates the total amount of drug in the body to the plasma concentration at steady state. In theory:

$$\text{Loading dose} = Cp_{ss} \cdot Vd_{ss}$$

For most drugs this can be given as a single dose by the chosen (usually oral) route. However, there is an important caution that depends on the relative rates of drug absorption and distribution. If the rate of absorption is rapid relative to distribution (this is always true for intravenous bolus administration), the concentration of drug in plasma that results from even an appropriate loading dose can initially be considerably higher than desired. Unwanted effects may occur transiently, but these can be severe nonetheless. Thus, while only the amount of a loading dose usually need be calculated, the rate of administration can sometimes be crucial, and slow administration of an intravenous drug (over minutes rather than seconds) is almost always wise.

PLANNING A DOSAGE REGIMEN

Adjustment of Usual Doses. Beginning again with maintenance dosage, how might one choose the desired mean steady-state concentration of drug? There are two approaches. The first, and simplest, is to trust past experience. One may assume that the usual or standard dose of a drug has evolved from appropriate experience with the typical case. If the patient at hand is not expected to differ from the usual one with respect to *sensitivity* to the drug, then one may work with the usual maintenance dosage regimen, rather than with concentrations. All that is required is to compute clearance for the patient (and *F*, if it will differ from usual) and choose a maintenance dosage rate for the patient (R_{pt}) that equals the usual maintenance dosage rate in a normal individual (R_{nl}) times the ratio of the patient's clearance to the normal value and the ratio of the normal *F* to that of the patient.

$$R_{pt} = R_{nl} \left(\frac{CL_{pt}}{CL_{nl}} \cdot \frac{F_{nl}}{F_{pt}} \right)$$

If this is done, the patient's mean steady-state concentration of drug will be identical to whatever it is in the presumably successful treatment of a typical patient.

When an intermittent regimen is adjusted for an individual patient, one may choose to alter the dose given per dosing interval, the dosing interval, or both. The mean steady-state concentration will be the same as long as dose/time is held constant. When the amount of each dose is altered and the interval is held constant, fluctuations about the mean will be less or more than usual, depending on whether the patient's clearance is less or more, respectively, than that of the typical patient. Maximal and minimal concentrations will thus differ from the usual. When the dose interval is altered and the size of the individual dose is held constant, the maximal, minimal, and mean concentrations in the patient match the usual case. This apparently greater similarity to the usual regimen has caused this means of modifying dosage regimens to become popular, and it is often recommended. However, although the three named concentrations do match, the total time course of the concentration does not. If clearance in a given patient is one third of normal and the dosing interval is lengthened threefold to compensate, the absolute amount of time spent below the mean concentration will triple. If the drug is an antibiotic and the mean concentration happens to be the minimal inhibitory concentration for the infecting microorganism, the patient is exposed to subtherapeutic concentrations for longer continuous periods of time than is usual. This simply stresses again that the desired temporal pattern of concentrations is not the same for every drug. Whether to adjust the amount of a dose, the dosing interval, or both is a matter to be decided with knowledge of the desirable characteristics of the total profile of the plasma concentration in time.

As a rule of thumb, the authors recommend adjustment of the amount of each dose, not the interval. Most adjustments of dosage are made to compensate for smaller-than-usual clearances, not the opposite. If the amount of each dose is adjusted, fluctuations about the mean steady-state concentration will be less; the maximal concentration will be smaller and the minimal greater. For most drugs, a more constant concentration-time profile is not only acceptable but preferable.

When there is reason to believe that a particular patient may differ in his requirement for drug (*e.g.*, because of supersensitivity or tolerance), appropriate adjustments must be made. This is obviously done by the choice of a different relative or absolute concentration to be achieved at steady state (*see* below).

Targeting Drug Concentrations. An alternative method for choosing a desired steady-state concentration of drug requires knowledge of the quantitative relationship between concentration and effect for the particular drug. This kind of knowledge currently exists for only a few drugs, notably those for which it is a reasonable practice to measure concentrations of drugs and to use these to plan or adjust therapy. Sheiner and co-workers (1974) have called such an approach to planning a dosage regimen the "target level strategy."

This strategy is simple in theory. It merely asserts that for some drugs it is rational to use the measured concentration of the drug in plasma as an *indirect* or *intermediate therapeutic end point.* Intermediate end points are observable events that tell the clinician something about the consequences of his therapeutic decisions and help improve future decisions through feedback. When antihypertensive therapy is regulated by measurement of blood pressure, this value is an intermediate end point. It is intermediate in that the true or ultimate goal of antihypertensive therapy is to prevent stroke, blindness, renal failure, cardiac failure, and the other ravages of the unchecked disease, rather than to control blood pressure *per se*. Failure can ultimately be measured only by events that are delayed, disastrous, and may be nongraded in severity. When ultimate end points are difficult to measure, delayed, or dangerous, when a drug has a low therapeutic index, when the steady-state concentration of the drug in plasma is known to correlate directly with pharmacological and clinical effects, and when no better intermediate end point (such as blood pressure) is readily available, it is rational to use the measured concentration of drug itself as an indirect therapeutic end point for planning and regulating therapy. Although this concept is inapplicable to many drugs, it does apply to a number of important and widely used agents: digitalis glycosides, theophylline, most antiepileptics, many antiarrhythmic agents, many antibiotics, certain psychiatric drugs, some anti-inflammatory drugs, and some agents used in cancer chemotherapy.

Study of such drugs has served to establish usual "therapeutic ranges." At the low end of the range, substantial numbers of patients will experience appreciable efficacy; at the high end, a few patients will experience significant toxicity. It must be stressed, however, that the therapeutic range is a statistical concept. Individuals differ as much in sensitivity to drugs as they do in the kinetics of drug absorption, distribution, and elimination. Careful regulation of the concentration of drug, when appropriate, guarantees neither the presence of efficacy nor the absence of toxicity, although it does increase the odds.

The tables in this appendix offer approximate therapeutic ranges for several drugs. When a target concentration is chosen, the physician has the opportunity and obligation to use measurements of the concentration to revise the maintenance dosage. When elimination of the drug follows first-order kinetics and steady state has been attained, the adjustment of the maintenance dose is proportional to the ratio of the desired concentration to that which has been measured. Unusual or unexpected measurements should be checked carefully, and perhaps repeated, before major changes in the regimen are undertaken. This does not, of course, mean that an unexpectedly high drug concentration should be ignored until repeated. Prudent, short-term action (holding dosage) should usually be taken while awaiting confirmation.

There is an important complication in the above approach. When clearance becomes limited by capacity (nonlinear or saturation kinetics), the plasma concentration is not linearly related to dosage. Although there are a number of approaches to adjustment of dosage in such situations, perhaps the simplest is to use the average values of K_m and V_m (given for some drugs in the tables) to choose an initial dosage rate (R) that will achieve the desired concentration.

$$R = \frac{V_m \cdot Cp_{ss}}{K_m + Cp_{ss}}$$

When just one steady-state concentration has been measured, an individualized value of V_m is calculated by using the average K_m. A new adjusted dosage rate can thus be obtained. When two or more pairs of values for R and Cp_{ss} are available (assuming the dosage is different for each), one can plot the dosage rate on the ordinate versus the ratio of the dosage rate to the concentration (an estimate of clearance) on the abscissa and fit a straight line to the points. The slope approximates negative K_m and the y-intercept estimates V_m. These refined estimates can then be used to compute a new dosage. While such adjustment can be valuable, the approach is misleading and inappropriate if the dosage history is incorrect, if sampling time is inappropriate, or if protein binding of the drug is unusual. These factors will be discussed further below. Nonlinear kinetics can thus be the cause of confusing situations. If the patient's value of K_m is well below the target concentration of the drug, almost insurmountable problems are often encountered in adjustment of dosage. When this appears to be the case, use of an alternative drug may be the most attractive option.

Knowledge of the status of the binding of the drug to plasma proteins is important to the choice of the desired steady-state concentration. The free-drug concentration in plasma often determines not only the magnitude of drug action but also the rate of metabolism or excretion. These shifts sometimes cancel each other, and no modification of dosage is required. For example, when both effect and elimination depend solely on the concentration of free drug in plasma, steady state will be reached (for any given dosage) at the same free-drug concentration as when binding is normal, and this concentration will also have the usual effect. However, the measured (total) concentration of drug in plasma will be changed, such that the target concentration, expressed (as it usually is) as the total concentration, must be altered. Assuming that the total desired concentration at normal degrees of binding is known ($Cp_{ss\,nl}$), the following equation gives the adjusted target for an altered fraction of free drug:

$$Cp_{ss\,pt} = \frac{\alpha_{nl}}{\alpha_{pt}} \cdot Cp_{ss\,nl}$$

where α_{nl} and α_{pt} are normal and altered fractions of free drug, respectively.

If the rate of elimination of the drug is proportional to the concentration of free drug, rather than total drug, an adjustment for altered binding will have to be made in most of the other equations. In particular, wherever the patient's clearance or K_m appears, it must be multiplied by the ratio of the usual α to that expected in the patient, just as the target concentration is so multiplied above. In contrast, when drug elimination is proportional to the total concentration in plasma, all dosage rate equations remain unaltered. (However, the target concentration must still be changed if effect is proportional to the free concentration.) If one does not know which is the case, it is usually safer to assume that elimination is proportional to total, rather than free, drug concentrations. When clearance of drug from blood (not plasma) approaches the rate of blood flow to the clearing organ, yet binding to plasma proteins is extensive (more than 50%), it is almost certain that clearance is proportional to total plasma concentration. When clearance is low (less than 10% of blood flow), the opposite is usually the case. Unfortunately, as mentioned above, one needs to know the ratio of the concentration of drug in blood to that in plasma at steady state in order to compute clearance from blood.

Adjusting Mean Parameters for the Individual Patient.

The values in the tables represent mean values for populations of normal adults, and their modification may thus be required for individual patients. To compute a desired steady-state concentration, the patient's free fraction (α) must be known; to compute a maintenance dosage rate, the fraction absorbed (F) and clearance must be estimated as well; and to calculate the loading dose and to estimate half-life and dosing interval, knowledge of the volume of distribution is needed. The figures in the tables and the adjustments apply *only to adults* unless specifically designated otherwise. Although the values may sometimes, with caution, be applied to children in excess of about 30 kg (after proper adjustment for size; *see* below), it is best to consult a textbook of pediatrics or other source for definitive advice.

The tables note the changes in the parameters occasioned by certain disease states. In most cases, a qualitative statement is made, such as "clearance decreased in hepatic disease." A reasonable quantitative translation is to multiply the value of the parameter by 0.5 for each applicable condition that is noted to decrease the parameter and to multiply it by 2 for each condition that is noted to increase the parameter. Such an adjustment can only be approximate, yet, since reliable data are limited, no better approach may be possible. The relevant literature should be consulted for more definitive quantitative information.

Protein Binding. Most acidic drugs that are extensively bound to plasma proteins are bound to albumin. The same is true of basic drugs, such as propranolol, which are often bound to other plasma proteins (*e.g.*, α-glycoprotein). The degree of drug binding to proteins will differ in states that cause changes in the concentration of the binding proteins. Unfortunately, only albumin, among binding proteins, is commonly measured. For drugs that are bound to albumin (*alb*), a patient's fraction of free drug (α_{pt}) can be approximated from the following relationship:

$$\alpha_{pt} = 1 \Big/ \left[\left(\frac{alb_{pt}}{alb_{nl}}\right)\left(\frac{1 - \alpha_{nl}}{\alpha_{nl}}\right) + 1 \right]$$

Use of this equation assumes that the molar concentration of drug is far less than that of albumin, that only one type of drug binding site is present on albumin, and that there are no cooperative binding interactions. It cannot, therefore, be exact. However, it is a reasonable approximation and, in the absence of actual measurement of the patient's fraction of free drug, can prove quite useful.

Clearance. Clearance must often be adjusted for alterations in renal function. The quantities required for this adjustment are the fraction of normal renal function remaining and the fraction of drug usually excreted unchanged in the urine. The latter quantity appears in the tables; the former can be estimated as the ratio of the patient's creatinine clearance to a normal value (100–120 ml/min per 70 kg). If creatinine clearance has not been measured, it may be estimated from measurements of the concentration of creatinine in serum, using a number of different equations or nomograms. One such is to estimate the fraction of normal renal function present (rfx) as the reciprocal of the patient's serum creatinine concentration, minus 0.01 for each year of age over 40. This is a crude estimate, but more accurate ones are seldom justified or necessary, since the whole process of adjustment of clearance is already approximate because of considerable unpredictable interindividual variation in clearance, which is independent of renal function. An equation for adjustment of clearance that uses the quantities just discussed is presented in Chapter 1 (page 26). The same relationship is presented here as:

$$rf_{pt} = 1 - fe_{nl}(1 - rfx_{pt})$$

where fe_{nl} is the fraction of drug excreted unchanged in normal individuals (*see* tables). The renal factor (rf_{pt}) is the value that, when multiplied by normal total clearance, gives the total clearance of the drug adjusted for disturbances of renal function.

Adjustment of clearance must also be made for the size of the patient. For convenience, the figures in the tables are normalized to weight. However, clearance of drug often varies in proportion to metabolic rate, which is best related to weight to the 0.75 power. To take this into account, the clearance figure in the tables can be multiplied by the factor *wf*, instead of by weight:

$$wf = Wt_{nl}(Wt_{pt}/Wt_{nl})^{0.75}$$

which for weight in kg (where $Wt_{nl} = 70$ kg) becomes:

$$wf = 2.9(Wt_{pt})^{0.75}$$

Calculation of the weight factor seldom pays for itself by yielding significantly more accurate estimates. It should be done, however, for patients at extremes of size, especially the very obese.

Recall that if drug elimination is proportional to the free (rather than the total) concentration of drug in plasma, clearance is then further adjusted by multiplying it by the ratio of the normal free fraction to the free fraction of the patient, calculated as indicated previously.

All the adjustments to clearance should be applied simultaneously. That is, the figure in the table is multiplied by a weight factor (usually weight itself), *and* multiplied by the binding correction, if applicable, *and* multiplied by the renal correction factor, if applicable, *and,* finally, multiplied by the appropriate values of 0.5 and/or 2 for other factors that are present and qualitatively indicated to modify clearance. Obviously, if a quantitative correction is made for renal function, a qualitative one (multiplication by 0.5) should not also be made for this same factor.

Volume of Distribution. Volume of distribution should be adjusted for the modifying factors indicated in the tables, as well as for size. The figures in the tables are normalized to weight. Unlike clearance, volume of distribution is probably most often proportional to weight itself. Whether or not this is so, however, depends on the actual sites of distribution of drug, and no absolute rule applies.

Whether to adjust volume of distribution for changes in binding to plasma proteins cannot be decided in general, since the decision critically depends on whether the factors that alter binding to plasma proteins also alter binding to tissues. In such cases the qualitative changes in volume of distribution are indicated in the tables. Again, each adjustment to volume of distribution should be made independently of any other, and the final estimate should reflect all adjustments simultaneously.

Half-life. Finally, half-life may be estimated from the adjusted estimates of clearance and volume of distribution. Since, historically, half-life has been the parameter most often measured, qualitative changes for this parameter are almost always given in the tables.

Measurement of Drug Concentrations and Revision of Dosage Regimens. The relevant theory and equations have already been given. It remains only to discuss certain practical details and pitfalls. The first of these concerns the time of sampling for measurement of the drug concentration. If intermittent dosing is utilized, when, during a dosing interval, should samples be taken? It is necessary to distinguish between two possible uses of measured drug concentrations in order to understand the possible answers. A concentration of drug measured in a sample taken at

virtually any time during the dosing interval will provide information that may aid in the assessment of drug toxicity. This is one possible use of a measured concentration. It should be stressed, however, that such use of a measured concentration of drug is fraught with difficulties caused by interindividual variability in sensitivity to the drug. When there is a question of toxicity, the drug concentration can be no more than just one of many items that serve to inform the physician.

Changes in the effects of drugs may be delayed relative to changes in plasma concentration because of relatively poor perfusion of the active site or because of marked concentration of the drug in the tissue in which it acts. Concentrations of digoxin, for example, regularly exceed 2 ng/ml (a potentially toxic value) shortly after an oral dose, yet these peak concentrations do not cause toxicity; indeed, they occur well before peak effects. Thus, concentrations of drugs in samples obtained shortly after administration can be uninformative or even misleading.

When concentrations of drugs are used for purposes of adjusting dosage regimens, samples obtained shortly after administration of a dose are almost invariably misleading. The point of sampling during supposed steady state is to modify one's estimate of clearance and thus one's choice of dosage. Early postabsorptive concentrations do not reflect clearance; they are determined primarily by the rate of absorption, the initial (rather than the steady-state) volume of distribution, and the rate of distribution, all of which are pharmacokinetic parameters of virtually no relevance to long-term, steady-state dosage. When the goal of measurement is adjustment of dosage, the sample should be taken well after the previous dose—as a rule of thumb just before the next planned dose, when the concentration is at its minimum. There is an exception to this approach. Some drugs are nearly completely eliminated between doses and act only during the initial portion of each dosage interval. If, for such drugs, it is questionable whether efficacious concentrations are being achieved, a sample taken shortly after a dose may be helpful. Yet, if another concern is that low clearance (as in renal failure) may cause accumulation of drug, concentrations measured just before the next dose will reveal such accumulation and are considerably more useful for this purpose than is knowledge of the maximal concentration. For such drugs, determination of both maximal and minimal concentrations is thus recommended.

A second important aspect of the timing of sampling is its relationship to the beginning of the maintenance dosage regimen. When constant dosage is given, steady state is reached only after four or five half-lives have passed. (This simple relationship is incorrect for drugs with nonlinear kinetics, which may take very long times to achieve steady state.) If a sample is obtained too soon after dosage is begun, it will not accurately reflect clearance. Yet, for toxic drugs, if one waits until steady state is assured, the damage may have been done. Some simple guidelines can be offered. When it is important to maintain careful control of concentrations, one may take the first sample after two half-lives (as calculated and expected for the patient), assuming no loading dose has been given. If the concentration already exceeds 90% of the eventual expected mean steady-state concentration, the dosage rate should be halved, another sample obtained in another two (supposed) half-lives, and the dosage halved again if this sample exceeds the target. If the first concentration is not too high, one proceeds with the initial rate of dosage; even if the concentration is lower than expected, one can usually await the attainment of steady state in another two to three estimated half-lives and then proceed to adjust dosage as described above.

If dosage is intermittent, there is a third concern with the time at which samples are obtained for determination of drug concentrations. If the sample has been obtained just prior to the next dose, as recommended, concentration will be a minimal value, not the mean. If absorption is rapid and the dosing interval is equal to the half-life of the drug, the minimal concentration will be about 70% of the mean concentration. It will be closer to the mean if absorption is slow (*see* Chapter 1). For all practical purposes the minimal concentration can be regarded as an estimate of the mean when absorption is known to be slow or when the interval between doses is about 50% of one half-life or less. When this is not so and it is important to estimate the mean concentration (as in the situation discussed above,

when samples are drawn prior to steady state), the target or expected steady-state concentration should be adjusted downward by 25 to 30%; the minimal concentration itself can then be used in all subsequent calculations and adjustments.

Other difficulties of interpretation of drug concentrations arise from problems with specificity of assays. Some assays for drugs measure not only the active compound but other substances or metabolites as well. When this is so, the usual relationship of concentration to effect may appear to change over time (*e.g.*, as metabolites that are devoid of pharmacological activity accumulate). This may be especially noticeable in patients with renal failure. The opposite results from accumulation of active metabolites that are not measured by a specific assay. As specific and sensitive assays for drugs and metabolites are developed, such problems should decrease.

Benet, L. Z., and Galeazzi, R. L.   Noncompartmental determination of the steady-state volume of distribution. *J. Pharm. Sci.*, **1979**, *68*, 1971–1974.

Klotz, U.; Avant, G. R.; Hoyumpa, A.; Schenker, S.; and Wilkinson, G. R.   The effects of age and liver disease on the disposition and elimination of diazepam in adult man. *J. Clin. Invest.*, **1975**, *55*, 347–359.

Rowland, M.; Benet, L. Z.; and Graham, G. G.   Clearance concepts in pharmacokinetics. *J. Pharmacokinet. Biopharm.*, **1973**, *1*, 123–136.

Sheiner, L. B.; Benet, L. Z.; and Pagliaro, L. A.   Standard approach to compiling pharmacokinetic data. *J. Pharmacokinet. Biopharm.*, **1980**, *8*.

Sheiner, L. B.; Melmon, K. L.; and Rosenberg, B.   Instructional goals for physicians in the use of blood level data—and the contribution of computers. *Clin. Pharmacol. Ther.*, **1974**, *16*, 260–271.

Wilkinson, G. R., and Shand, D. G.   A physiologic approach to hepatic drug clearance. *Clin. Pharmacol. Ther.*, **1975**, *18*, 377–390.

Williams, R. L.; Blaschke, T. F.; Meffin, P. J.; Melmon, K. L.; and Rowland, M.   Influence of acute viral hepatitis on disposition and plasma binding of tolbutamide. *Clin. Pharmacol. Ther.*, **1977**, *21*, 301–309.

ACEBUTOLOL (Chapter 9)

AVAILABILITY (ORAL) (%)	URINARY EXCRETION (%)	BOUND IN PLASMA (%)	CLEARANCE $(ml \cdot min^{-1} \cdot kg^{-1})$
37 ± 12 [a] (1)	40 ± 11 (2)	26 ± 3 (2)	6.8 ± 0.8 (2)

VOL. DIST. (*liters/kg*)	HALF-LIFE (*hours*)	EFFECTIVE CONCENTRATIONS	TOXIC CONCENTRATIONS
1.2 ± 0.3 (2)	2.7 ± 0.4 (2)	[b]	—

[a] Some increase in availability (perhaps to 50%) occurs at higher doses and at steady state (1).
[b] An acetylated metabolite, which may have pharmacological activity, is present at steady state at concentrations 2.7 times those of acebutolol (3).

1. Meffin, P. J.; Winkle, R. A.; Peters, F. A.; and Harrison, D. C. Dose-dependent acebutolol disposition after oral administration. *Clin. Pharmacol. Ther.*, **1978**, *24*, 542–547.
2. Meffin, P. J.; Winkle, R. A.; Peters, F. A.; and Harrison, D. C. Acebutolol disposition after intravenous administra-
tion. *Clin. Pharmacol. Ther.*, **1977**, *22*, 557–567.
3. Winkle, R. A.; Meffin, P. J.; Kochs, W. B.; and Harrison, D. C. Acebutolol metabolite plasma concentration during chronic oral therapy. *Br. J. Clin. Pharmacol.*, **1977**, *4*, 519–522.

ACETAMINOPHEN [a,b] (Chapter 29)

AVAILABILITY (ORAL) (%)	URINARY EXCRETION (%)	BOUND IN PLASMA (%)	CLEARANCE $(ml \cdot min^{-1} \cdot kg^{-1})$
63 ± 5 89 ± 10 (2) [c] 87 ± 20	3 ± 1 (3) ↔ Neo (4,5), Child (5)	0 at <60 ng/ml (6) 15–20% at 280 ng/ml (6)	5.0 ± 1.4 [d] (2) ↓ Hep [e] (7) ↔ Aged (8)

VOL. DIST. (*liters/kg*)	HALF-LIFE (*hours*)	EFFECTIVE CONCENTRATIONS	TOXIC CONCENTRATIONS
0.95 ± 0.12 [d] (2) ↔ Aged (8), Hep [e] (7)	2.0 ± 0.4 (10) ↔ Urem (9) ↑ Neo (4), Hep [e] (7,10)	10–20 μg/ml [f] (11)	>300 μg/ml [g] (10,12)

[a] Acetaminophen exhibits dose-dependent kinetics for doses greater than 2 g. *See* (1) for predictive kinetic model for doses greater than 2 g.

[b] Values reported are calculated with a linear kinetic model for doses less than 2 g.

[c] Values are for 0.5-, 1-, and 2-g doses.

[d] Assuming 70-kg weight; reported range, 65–72 kg.

[e] Acetaminophen-induced hepatic damage.

[f] Analgesia, antipyresis.

[g] Hepatic toxicity for these concentrations 4 hours after ingestion; no hepatic toxicity if concentrations <120 μg/ml 4 hours after ingestion.

1. Slattery, J. T., and Levy, G. Acetaminophen kinetics in acutely poisoned patients. *Clin. Pharmacol. Ther.*, **1979**, *25*, 184–195.
2. Rawlins, M. D.; Henderson, D. B.; and Hijab, A. R. Pharmacokinetics of paracetamol (acetaminophen) after intravenous and oral administration. *Eur. J. Clin. Pharmacol.*, **1977**, *11*, 283–286.
3. Levy, G., and Yamada, H. Drug biotransformation interactions in man. III. Acetaminophen and salicylamide. *J. Pharm. Sci.*, **1971**, *60*, 215–221.
4. Levy, G.; Khanna, N. N.; Soda, D. M.; Tsuzuki, O.; and Stern, L. Pharmacokinetics of acetaminophen in the human neonate: formation of acetaminophen glucuronide and sulfate in relation to plasma bilirubin concentration and d-glucaric acid excretion. *Pediatrics*, **1975**, *55*, 818–825.
5. Miller, R. P.; Roberts, R. J.; and Fischer, L. J. Acetaminophen elimination kinetics in neonates, children and adults. *Clin. Pharmacol. Ther.*, **1975**, *19*, 284–294.
6. Gazzard, B. G.; Ford-Hutchinson, A. W.; Smith, M. J. H.; and Williams, R. The binding of paracetamol to plasma of

man and pig. *J. Pharm. Pharmacol.*, **1973**, *25*, 964–967.
7. Prescott, L. F., and Wright, N. The effects of hepatic and renal damage on paracetamol metabolism and excretion following overdosage. A pharmacokinetic study. *Br. J. Pharmacol.*, **1973**, *49*, 602–613.
8. Triggs, E. J.; Nation, R. L.; Long, A.; and Ashley, J. J. Pharmacokinetics in the elderly. *Eur. J. Clin. Pharmacol.*, **1975**, *8*, 55–62.
9. Prescott, L. F. The metabolism of phenacetin in patients with renal disease. *Clin. Pharmacol. Ther.*, **1969**, *10*, 383–394.
10. Prescott, L. F.; Wright, N.; Roscoe, P.; and Brown, S. S. Plasma-paracetamol half-life and hepatic necrosis in patients with paracetamol overdosage. *Lancet*, **1971**, *1*, 519–522.
11. Rumack, B. H. Aspirin versus acetaminophen: a comparative view. *Pediatrics*, **1978**, *62*, 943–946.
12. Rumack, B. H., and Matthew, H. Acetaminophen poisoning and toxicity. *Pediatrics*, **1975**, *55*, 871–876.

Key: Adult = adults; Aged = aged; Alb = hypoalbuminemia; AVH = acute viral hepatitis; CF = cystic fibrosis; CHF = congestive heart failure; Child = children; Cirr = cirrhosis; COPD = chronic obstructive pulmonary disease; CP = cor pulmonale; CPBS = cardiopulmonary bypass surgery; CRI = chronic respiratory insufficiency; Cush = cushingoid; Epilep = epilepsy; Fem = females; Hep = hepatitis; HL = hyperlipoproteinemia; HTh = hyperthyroid; Inflam = inflammation; LTh = hypothyroid; MI = myocardial infarction; Neo = neonates; NS = nephrotic syndrome; Obes = obesity; Pneu = pneumonia; Preg = pregnant; Prem = premature infants; RA = rheumatoid arthritis; Smk = smoking; Tach = ventricular tachycardia; Urem = uremia.

N-ACETYLPROCAINAMIDE (Chapter 31)

AVAILABILITY (ORAL) (%)	URINARY EXCRETION (%)	BOUND IN PLASMA (%)	CLEARANCE $(ml \cdot min^{-1} \cdot kg^{-1})$
83 ± 12 (1)	81 ± 4 (2)	10 ± 9 (3)	3.1 ± 0.4 (2) ↓ Urem (4)

VOL. DIST. (liters/kg)	HALF-LIFE (hours)	EFFECTIVE CONCENTRATIONS	TOXIC CONCENTRATIONS
1.4 ± 0.2 (2) ↔ Urem (4)	6.0 ± 0.2 (2) ↑ Urem (4)	12 μg/ml [a] (5)	—

[a] Significant decrease in frequency of premature ventricular contractions in six of nine patients.

1. Strong, J. M.; Dutcher, J. S.; Lee, W.-K.; and Atkinson, A. J., Jr. Absolute bioavailability in man of N-acetylprocainamide determined by a novel stable isotope method. *Clin. Pharmacol. Ther.*, **1975**, *18*, 613–622.
2. ———. Pharmacokinetics in man of the N-acetylated metabolite of procainamide. *J. Pharmacokinet. Biopharm.*, **1975**, *3*, 223–235.
3. Reidenberg, M. M.; Drayer, D. E.; Levy, M.; and Warner, H. Polymorphic acetylation of procainamide in man. *Clin. Pharmacol. Ther.*, **1975**, *17*, 722–730.
4. Stec, G. P.; Atkinson, A. J.; Nevin, M. J.; Thenot, J.-P.; Ruo, T. I.; Gibson, T. P.; Ivanovich, P.; and del Greco, F. N-acetylprocainamide pharmacokinetics in functionally anephric patients before and after perturbation by hemodialysis. *Clin. Pharmacol. Ther.*, **1979**, *26*, 618–628.
5. Lee, W.-K.; Strong, J. M.; Kehoe, R. F.; Dutcher, J. S.; and Atkinson, A. J., Jr. Antiarrhythmic efficacy of N-acetylprocainamide in patients with premature ventricular contractions. *Clin. Pharmacol. Ther.*, **1976**, *19*, 508–514.

ACETYLSALICYLIC ACID [a] (Chapter 29)

AVAILABILITY (ORAL) (%)	URINARY EXCRETION (%)	BOUND IN PLASMA (%)	CLEARANCE $(ml \cdot min^{-1} \cdot kg^{-1})$
68 ± 3 [a] (1)	1.4 ± 1.2 (2)	49 (3) ↓ Urem (3)	9.3 ± 1.1 (4)

VOL. DIST. (liters/kg)	HALF-LIFE (hours)	EFFECTIVE CONCENTRATIONS	TOXIC CONCENTRATIONS
0.15 ± 0.03 (4)	0.25 ± 0.03 (4)	*See* Salicylic Acid	*See* Salicylic Acid

[a] Values given are for unchanged acetylsalicylic acid. Acetylsalicylic acid is converted to salicylic acid during and after absorption. *See* Salicylic Acid for parameters for that compound.

1. Rowland, M.; Riegelman, S.; Harris, P. A.; and Sholkoff, S. D. Absorption kinetics of aspirin in man following oral administration of an aqueous solution. *J. Pharm. Sci.*, **1972**, *61*, 379–385.
2. Cummings, A. J., and King, M. L. Urinary excretion of acetylsalicylic acid in man. *Nature*, **1966**, *209*, 620–621.
3. Andreasen, F. Protein binding of drugs in plasma from patients with renal failure. *Acta Pharmacol. Toxicol. (Kbh.)*, **1973**, *32*, 417–429.
4. Rowland, M., and Riegelman, S. Pharmacokinetics of acetylsalicylic acid and salicylic acid after intravenous administration in man. *J. Pharm. Sci.*, **1968**, *57*, 1313–1319.

Key: Adult = adults; Aged = aged; Alb = hypoalbuminemia; AVH = acute viral hepatitis; CF = cystic fibrosis; CHF = congestive heart failure; Child = children; Cirr = cirrhosis; COPD = chronic obstructive pulmonary disease; CP = cor pulmonale; CPBS = cardiopulmonary bypass surgery; CRI = chronic respiratory insufficiency; Cush = cushingoid; Epilep = epilepsy; Fem = females; Hep = hepatitis; HL = hyperlipoproteinemia; HTh = hyperthyroid; Inflam = inflammation; LTh = hypothyroid; MI = myocardial infarction; Neo = neonates; NS = nephrotic syndrome; Obes = obesity; Pneu = pneumonia; Preg = pregnant; Prem = premature infants; RA = rheumatoid arthritis; Smk = smoking; Tach = ventricular tachycardia; Urem = uremia.

ALPRENOLOL [a] (Chapter 9)

AVAILABILITY (ORAL) (%)	URINARY EXCRETION (%)	BOUND IN PLASMA (%)	CLEARANCE ($ml \cdot min^{-1} \cdot kg^{-1}$)
8.6 ± 5.5 [b] (2)	0.5 (3)	85 ± 3 (4)	15 ± 9 (2) CL_{int} = 117 ± 62 (5)

VOL. DIST. (liters/kg)	HALF-LIFE (hours)	EFFECTIVE CONCENTRATIONS	TOXIC CONCENTRATIONS
3.4 ± 1.2 [c] (2)	3.1 ± 1.2 (2)	30 ng/ml [d] (6)	—

[a] For review, see (1).
[b] Measured at a dose of 200 mg. First-pass hepatic metabolism, which is extensive, may be saturable (2).
[c] Vd_{area}.
[d] To achieve a 50% decrease in exercise-induced cardioacceleration.

1. Johnsson, G., and Regårdh, C. G. Clinical pharmacokinetics of β-adrenoreceptor blocking drugs. *Clin. Pharmacokinet.*, **1976**, *1*, 233–263.
2. Alvan, G.; Lind, M.; Mellström, B.; and von Bahr, C. Importance of "first-pass elimination" for interindividual differences in steady-state concentrations of the adrenergic β-receptor antagonist alprenolol. *J. Pharmacokinet. Biopharm.*, **1977**, *5*, 193–205.
3. Rawlins, M. D.; Collste, P.; Frisk-Holmberg, M.; Lind, M.; Ostman, J.; and Sjöqvist, F. Steady-state plasma concentrations of alprenolol in man. *Eur. J. Clin. Pharmacol.*, **1974**, *7*, 353–356.
4. Borga, O.; Piafsky, K. M.; and Nilsen, O. G. Plasma protein binding of basic drugs. I. Selective displacement from α-acid glycoprotein by *tris* (2-hydroxyethyl) phosphate. *Clin. Pharmacol. Ther.*, **1977**, *22*, 539–544.
5. Johansson, R.; Regårdh, C. G.; and Sjögren, J. Absorption of alprenolol in man from tablets with different rates of release. *Acta Pharm. Suec.*, **1971**, *8*, 59–70.
6. Frisk-Holmberg, M.; Jorfeldt, L.; and Juhlin-Dannfeldt, A. Influence of alprenolol on hemodynamics and metabolic responses to prolonged exercise in subjects with hypertension. *Clin. Pharmacol. Ther.*, **1977**, *21*, 675–684.

AMIKACIN (Chapter 51)

AVAILABILITY (ORAL) (%)	URINARY EXCRETION (%)	BOUND IN PLASMA (%)	CLEARANCE ($ml \cdot min^{-1} \cdot kg^{-1}$)
—	98 (1)	4 ± 8 [a] (1)	1.1 ± 0.2 (2) [b] $CL = 0.6\ CL_{cr} + 0.14$ (2) [b]

VOL. DIST. (liters/kg)	HALF-LIFE (hours)	EFFECTIVE CONCENTRATIONS	TOXIC CONCENTRATIONS
0.21 ± 0.08 (2)	2.3 ± 0.4 (1) 1.4 ± 0.4 (2) ↑ Urem (2)	*See* Chapter 51	*See* Chapter 51

[a] Concentration in serum = 15 μg/ml.
[b] Values reported per 1.73 m²; calculated assuming 70 kg.

1. Clarke, J. T.; Libke, R. D.; Regamey, C.; and Kirby, W. M. M. Comparative pharmacokinetics of amikacin and kanamycin. *Clin. Pharmacol. Ther.*, **1974**, *15*, 610–616.
2. Plantier, J.; Forrey, A. W.; O'Neill, M. A.; Blair, A. D.; Christopher, T. G.; and Cutler, R. E. Pharmacokinetics of amikacin in patients with normal or impaired renal function: radioenzymatic acetylation assay. *J. Infect. Dis.*, **1976**, *134*, Suppl., 5323–5330.

AMITRIPTYLINE (Chapter 19)

AVAILABILITY (ORAL) (%)	URINARY EXCRETION (%)	BOUND IN PLASMA (%)	CLEARANCE $(ml \cdot min^{-1} \cdot kg^{-1})$
—	—	96.4 ± 0.8 [a] (1)	6.1 ± 1.7 (2) ↓ Aged (3)

VOL. DIST. (liters/kg)	HALF-LIFE (hours)	EFFECTIVE CONCENTRATIONS	TOXIC CONCENTRATIONS
8.3 ± 2.0 (2)	15 ± 5 [b] (4) 57 [b] (5)	160–240 ng/ml [c] (7)	>1 µg/ml [d] (8,9)

[a] Determined at 24–26° C in heparinized human plasma.
[b] Conflicting reports in the literature suggest a half-life of from 9 to 25 hours (2,4) or from 32 to 161 hours (5,6).
[c] Optimal range of amitriptyline plus nortriptyline.
[d] Combined data for toxic effects of tricyclic antidepressants.

1. Borga, O.; Azarnoff, D. L.; Plym Forsell, G.; and Sjöqvist, F. Plasma protein binding of tricyclic antidepressants in man. *Biochem. Pharmacol.,* **1969,** *18,* 2135–2143.
2. Jørgensen, A., and Hansen, V. Pharmacokinetics of amitriptyline infused intravenously in man. *Eur. J. Clin. Pharmacol.,* **1976,** *10,* 337–341.
3. Nies, A.; Robinson, D. S.; Friedman, M. J.; Green, R.; Cooper, T. B.; Ravaris, C. L.; and Ives, J. O. Relationship between age and tricyclic antidepressant plasma levels. *Am. J. Psychiatry,* **1977,** *134,* 790–793.
4. Jørgensen, A., and Staer, P. On the biological half-life of amitriptyline. *J. Pharm. Pharmacol.,* **1976,** *28,* 62–64.
5. Gupta, R., and Molnar, G. Measurement of therapeutic concentrations. *Drug Metab. Rev.,* **1979,** *9,* 79–97.
6. Braithwaite, R. A., and Widdop, B. A specific gas chromatographic method for the measurement of "steady-state" plasma levels of amitriptyline and nortriptyline in patients. *Clin. Chim. Acta,* **1971,** *35,* 461–472.
7. Ziegler, V. E.; Co, B. T.; Taylor, J. R.; Clayton, P. J.; and Biggs, J. T. Amitriptyline plasma levels and therapeutic response. *Clin. Pharmacol. Ther.,* **1976,** *19,* 795–801.
8. Petit, J. M.; Spiker, D. G.; Ruwitch, J. F.; Ziegler, V. E.; Weiss, A. N.; and Biggs, J. T. Tricyclic antidepressant plasma levels and adverse effects after overdose. *Clin. Pharmacol. Ther.,* **1977,** *21,* 47–51.
9. Braithwaite, R. A.; Crome, P.; and Dawling, S. Amitriptyline overdosage: plasma concentrations and clinical features. *Br. J. Clin. Pharmacol.,* **1979,** *8,* 388P–389P.

AMOXICILLIN (Chapter 50)

AVAILABILITY (ORAL) (%)	URINARY EXCRETION (%)	BOUND IN PLASMA (%)	CLEARANCE $(ml \cdot min^{-1} \cdot kg^{-1})$
93 ± 10 (1)	52 ± 15 (2)	18 (3)	5.3 ± 1.3 (1) ↓ Urem (4,5)

VOL. DIST. (liters/kg)	HALF-LIFE (hours)	EFFECTIVE CONCENTRATIONS	TOXIC CONCENTRATIONS
0.41 ± 0.18 (1) ↔ Urem (4)	1.0 ± 0.1 (6) ↑ Urem (4,5)	*See* Chapter 50	*See* Chapter 50

1. Spyker, D. A.; Rugloski, R. J.; Vann, R. L.; and O'Brien, W. M. Pharmacokinetics of amoxicillin: dose dependence after intravenous, oral, and intramuscular administration. *Antimicrob. Agents Chemother.,* **1977,** *11,* 132–139.
2. Fiegel, P.; Hoffler, D.; Kohler, H.; and Werner, H. J. Amoxicillin: Pharmakokinetik und Erfahrungen bei der Behandlung von Harnwegsinfektionin. *Chemotherapy,* **1973,** *18,* Suppl., 57–58.
3. Rolinson, G. N. Laboratory evaluation of amoxycillin. *Chemotherapy,* **1973,** *18,* Suppl., 1–10.
4. Humbert, G.; Spyker, D. A.; Fillastre, J. P.; and Leroy, A. Pharmacokinetics of amoxicillin: dosage nomogram for patients with impaired renal function. *Antimicrob. Agents Chemother.,* **1979,** *15,* 28–33.
5. Francke, E. L.; Appel, G. B.; and Neu, H. C. Kinetics of intravenous amoxicillin in patients on long-term dialysis. *Clin. Pharmacol. Ther.,* **1979,** *26,* 31–35.
6. Zarowny, D.; Ogilvie, R.; Tamblyn, D.; MacLeod, C.; and Ruedy, J. Pharmacokinetics of amoxicillin. *Clin. Pharmacol. Ther.,* **1974,** *16,* 1045–1051.

AMPHOTERICIN B (Chapter 54)

AVAILABILITY (ORAL) (%)	URINARY EXCRETION (%)	BOUND IN PLASMA (%)	CLEARANCE $(ml \cdot min^{-1} \cdot kg^{-1})$
—	3 [a] (1)	>90 (2)	0.43 ± 0.08 [a] (1)

VOL. DIST. (liters/kg)	HALF-LIFE (days)	EFFECTIVE CONCENTRATIONS	TOXIC CONCENTRATIONS
4.0 ± 0.4 [a] (1)	15 ± 2 [a] (1)	See Chapter 54	—

[a] Two patients with CL_{cr} of 28 and 37 ml/min.

1. Atkinson, A. J., Jr., and Bennett, J. E. Amphotericin B pharmacokinetics in humans. *Antimicrob. Agents Chemother.,* **1978,** *13,* 271–276.
2. Block, E. R.; Bennett, J. E.; Livoti, L. G.; Klein, W. J., Jr.; MacGregor, R. R.; and Henderson, L. Flucytosine and amphotericin B: hemodialysis effects on the plasma concentration and clearance. *Ann. Intern. Med.,* **1974,** *80,* 613–617.

AMPICILLIN (Chapter 50)

AVAILABILITY (ORAL) (%)	URINARY EXCRETION (%)	BOUND IN PLASMA (%)	CLEARANCE $(ml \cdot min^{-1} \cdot kg^{-1})$
29 ± 3 [a] (1) 62 ± 17 [a] (2)	90 ± 8 (1)	18 ± 2 (2,3) ↓ Neo (4)	3.9 ± 0.7 (2) ↓ Urem (5) ↔ Cirr (6)

VOL. DIST. (liters/kg)	HALF-LIFE (hours)	EFFECTIVE CONCENTRATIONS	TOXIC CONCENTRATIONS
0.28 ± 0.07 (6) ↔ Urem (5) ↑ Cirr (6)	1.3 ± 0.2 (5,6) ↑ Urem (5), Cirr (6), Neo (7)	See Chapter 50	See Chapter 50

[a] Results are highly variable from study to study.

1. Jusko, W. J., and Lewis, G. P. Comparison of ampicillin and hetacillin pharmacokinetics in man. *J. Pharm. Sci.,* **1973,** *62,* 69–76.
2. Ehrnebo, M.; Nilsson, S.-O.; and Boreus, L. O. Pharmacokinetics of ampicillin and its prodrugs, bacampicillin and pivampicillin, in man. *J. Pharmacokinet. Biopharm.,* **1979,** *7,* 429–451.
3. Ehrnebo, M. Distribution of ampicillin in human whole blood. *J. Pharm. Pharmacol.,* **1978,** *30,* 730–731.
4. Ehrnebo, M.; Agurell, S.; Jalling, B.; and Boreus, L. O. Age differences in drug binding by plasma proteins: studies on human foetuses, neonates, and adults. *Eur. J. Clin. Pharmacol.,* **1971,** *3,* 189–193.
5. Jusko, W. J.; Lewis, G. P.; and Schmitt, G. W. Ampicillin and hetacillin pharmacokinetics in normal and anephric subjects. *Clin. Pharmacol. Ther.,* **1972,** *14,* 90–99.
6. Lewis, G. P., and Jusko, W. J. Pharmacokinetics of ampicillin in cirrhosis. *Clin. Pharmacol. Ther.,* **1975,** *18,* 475–484.
7. Colburn, W. A.; Gibaldi, M.; Yoshioka, H.; Takimoto, M.; and Riley, H. D. Pharmacokinetic model for serum concentrations of ampicillin in the newborn infant. *J. Infect. Dis.,* **1976,** *134,* 67–69.

Key: Adult = adults; Aged = aged; Alb = hypoalbuminemia; AVH = acute viral hepatitis; CF = cystic fibrosis; CHF = congestive heart failure; Child = children; Cirr = cirrhosis; COPD = chronic obstructive pulmonary disease; CP = cor pulmonale; CPBS = cardiopulmonary bypass surgery; CRI = chronic respiratory insufficiency; Cush = cushingoid; Epilep = epilepsy; Fem = females; Hep = hepatitis; HL = hyperlipoproteinemia; HTh = hyperthyroid; Inflam = inflammation; LTh = hypothyroid; MI = myocardial infarction; Neo = neonates; NS = nephrotic syndrome; Obes = obesity; Pneu = pneumonia; Preg = pregnant; Prem = premature infants; RA = rheumatoid arthritis; Smk = smoking; Tach = ventricular tachycardia; Urem = uremia.

ATENOLOL (Chapter 9)

AVAILABILITY (ORAL) (%)	URINARY EXCRETION (%)	BOUND IN PLASMA (%)	CLEARANCE ($ml \cdot min^{-1} \cdot kg^{-1}$)
57 (1)	85 (1)	—	1.3 (2) ↓ Urem (3)

VOL. DIST. ($liters/kg$)	HALF-LIFE ($hours$)	EFFECTIVE CONCENTRATIONS	TOXIC CONCENTRATIONS
0.7 [a] (2)	6.3 ± 1.8 (2) ↑ Urem (3)	1.3 μg/ml [b]	—

[a] Vd_{area}.
[b] To achieve a 50% decrease in exercise-induced cardioacceleration (4).

1. Fitzgerald, J. D.; Ruffin, R.; Smedstad, K. G.; Roberts, R.; and McAinsh, J. Studies on the pharmacokinetics and pharmacodynamics of atenolol in man. *Eur. J. Clin. Pharmacol.*, **1978**, *13*, 81–89.
2. Brown, H. C.; Carruthers, G. S.; Johnston, G. D.; Kelly, J. G.; McAinsh, J.; McDevitt, D. G.; and Shanks, R. G. Clinical pharmacologic observations on atenolol, a beta-adrenoreceptor blocker. *Clin. Pharmacol. Ther.*, **1976**, *20*, 524–534.
3. Sassard, J.; Pozet, N.; McAinsh, J.; Legheard, J.; and Zeck, P. Pharmacokinetics of atenolol in patients with renal impairment. *Eur. J. Clin. Pharmacol.*, **1977**, *12*, 175–180.
4. Conway, F. J.; Fitzgerald, J. D.; McArnot, J.; Rowlands, D. J.; and Smyson, W. T. Human pharmacokinetics and pharmacodynamic studies on atenolol (ICI 66082), a new cardioselective β-adrenergic blocking drug. *Br. J. Clin. Pharmacol.*, **1976**, *3*, 267–272.

CARBAMAZEPINE [a] (Chapter 20)

AVAILABILITY (ORAL) (%)	URINARY EXCRETION (%)	BOUND IN PLASMA (%)	CLEARANCE ($ml \cdot min^{-1} \cdot kg^{-1}$)
>70 (2)	<1 (3)	82 ± 5 (4) ↔ Urem (4), Hep (4), Cirr (4), Preg (5)	0.58 ± 0.12 [b,c] (6) 1.3 ± 0.5 [b] (8) ↑ Preg (5)

VOL. DIST. ($liters/kg$)	HALF-LIFE ($hours$)	EFFECTIVE CONCENTRATIONS	TOXIC CONCENTRATIONS
1.4 ± 0.2 [b,d] (6)	27 ± 4 [c] (6) 15 ± 5 (8)	5–10 μg/ml [e] (1) 6.5 ± 3.0 μg/ml [e,f] (9)	12 ± 4 μg/ml [e] (9) >9 μg/ml [e,g] (9)

[a] For review, *see* (1).
[b] Data from oral, multiple-dose regimen; values are CL/F and Vd_{area}/F.
[c] Values for a multiple-dose regimen (200 mg per day for 17 days). Carbamazepine induces its own metabolism; for a single dose, $CL/F = 0.36 ± 0.07$ ml · min⁻¹ · kg⁻¹, half-life = 36 ± 5 hours (6). At daily doses of 6 mg/kg, $t_{1/2}$ decreased from 34 ± 4 hours to 20 ± 4 hours (7).
[d] Single-dose value: 1.1 ± 0.1 liters/kg (6).
[e] A metabolite (the 10,11 epoxide) may contribute to therapeutic and toxic effects (1).
[f] To achieve control of psychomotor seizures.
[g] Threshold concentration for prominent side effects, such as distinct drowsiness, ataxia, and diplopia.

1. Bertilsson, L. Clinical pharmacokinetics of carbamazepine. *Clin. Pharmacokinet.*, **1978**, *3*, 128–143.
2. Faigle, J. W., and Feldmann, K. F. Pharmacokinetic data of carbamazepine and its major metabolites in man. In, *Clinical Pharmacology of Anti-Epileptic Drugs.* (Schneider, H.; Janz, D.; Gardner-Thorpe, C.; Meinardi, H.; and Sherwin, A. L.; eds.) Springer-Verlag, Berlin, **1975**, pp. 159–165.
3. Levy, R. H.; Pitlick, W. H.; Troupin, A. S.; Green, J. R.; and Neal, J. M. Pharmacokinetics of carbamazepine in normal man. *Clin. Pharmacol. Ther.*, **1975**, *17*, 657–668.
4. Hooper, W. D.; Dubetz, D. K.; Bochner, F.; Cother, L. M.; Smith, G. A.; Eadie, M. J.; and Tyrer, J. H. Plasma protein binding of carbamazepine. *Clin. Pharmacol. Ther.*, **1975**, *17*, 433–440.
5. Dam, M.; Christiansen, J.; Munch, O.; and Mygind, K. I. Antiepileptic drugs: metabolism in pregnancy. *Clin. Pharmacokinet.*, **1979**, *4*, 53–62.
6. Gerardin, A. P.; Abadie, F. V.; Campestrini, J. A.; and Theobald, W. Pharmacokinetics of carbamazepine in normal humans after single and repeated oral doses. *J. Pharmacokinet. Biopharm.*, **1976**, *4*, 521–535.
7. Pitlick, W. H.; Levy, R. H.; Troupin, A. S.; and Green, J. R. Pharmacokinetic model to describe self-induced decreases in steady-state concentrations of carbamazepine. *J. Pharm. Sci.*, **1976**, *65*, 462–463.
8. Westenberg, H. G. M.; van der Kleijn, E.; Oei, T. T.; and de Zeeuw, R. A. Kinetics of carbamazepine and carbamazepine-epoxide determined by use of plasma and saliva. *Clin. Pharmacol. Ther.*, **1978**, *23*, 320–328.
9. Schneider, H. Carbamazepine: an attempt to correlate serum levels with antiepileptic and side effects. In, *Clinical Pharmacology of Anti-Epileptic Drugs.* (Schneider, H.; Janz, D.; Gardner-Thorpe, C.; Meinardi, H.; and Sherwin, A. L.; eds.) Springer-Verlag, Berlin, **1975**, pp. 151–158.

CARBENICILLIN (Chapter 50)

AVAILABILITY (ORAL) (%)	URINARY EXCRETION (%)	BOUND IN PLASMA (%)	CLEARANCE $(ml \cdot min^{-1} \cdot kg^{-1})$
—	82 ± 9 (1)	50 (2)	$CL = 0.68\ CL_{cr} + 0.15$ (3)

VOL. DIST. (liters/kg)	HALF-LIFE (hours)	EFFECTIVE CONCENTRATIONS	TOXIC CONCENTRATIONS
0.18 [a] (2)	1.0 ± 0.2 (3) ↑ Urem (3,4), Hep [b] (4)	See Chapter 50	See Chapter 50

[a] Assuming 70-kg body weight.
[b] Half-life is markedly prolonged in oliguric patients with concomitant hepatic dysfunction.

1. Cole, M.; Kenig, M. D.; and Hewitt, W. A. Metabolism of penicillins to penicilloic acids and 6-aminopenicillanic acid in man and its significance in assessing penicillin absorption. Antimicrob. Agents Chemother., 1973, 5, 463–486.
2. Libke, R. D.; Clarke, J. T.; Ralph, E. D.; Luthy, R. P.; and Kirby, W. M. M. Ticarcillin vs carbenicillin: clinical pharmacokinetics. Clin. Pharmacol. Ther., 1975, 17, 441–446.
3. Latos, D. L.; Bryan, C. S.; and Stone, W. J. Carbenicillin therapy in patients with normal and impaired renal function. Clin. Pharmacol. Ther., 1975, 17, 692–700.
4. Hoffman, T. A.; Cestero, R.; and Bullock, W. E. Pharmacodynamics of carbenicillin in hepatic and renal failure. Ann. Intern. Med., 1970, 73, 173–178.

CEFAMANDOLE (Chapter 50)

AVAILABILITY (ORAL) (%)	URINARY EXCRETION (%)	BOUND IN PLASMA (%)	CLEARANCE $(ml \cdot min^{-1} \cdot kg^{-1})$
—	96 ± 3 (1)	74 (2) ↔ Urem [a] (3)	2.8 ± 1.0 (1) ↓ Urem (4)

VOL. DIST. (liters/kg)	HALF-LIFE (hours)	EFFECTIVE CONCENTRATIONS	TOXIC CONCENTRATIONS
0.16 ± 0.05 (1) ↔ Urem (4)	0.77 [b] (1) ↑ Urem (4), Neo (5), CPBS (6)	See Chapter 50	—

[a] No difference between patients with normal and impaired renal function, but percent bound reported as 32% (range 17–58%).
[b] One-compartment model; three compartments are evident with values of 0.08, 0.50, and 1.6 hours.

1. Aziz, N. S.; Gambertoglio, J. G.; Lin, E. T.; Grausz, H.; and Benet, L. Z. Pharmacokinetics of cefamandole using a HPLC assay. J. Pharmacokinet. Biopharm., 1978, 6, 153–164.
2. Fong, I. W.; Ralph, E. D.; Engelking, E. R.; and Kirby, W. M. M. Clinical pharmacology of cefamandole as compared with cephalothin. Antimicrob. Agents Chemother., 1976, 9, 65–69.
3. Mellin, H.-E.; Welling, P. G.; and Madsen, P. O. Pharmacokinetics of cefamandole in patients with normal and impaired renal function. Antimicrob. Agents Chemother., 1977, 11, 262–266.
4. Gambertoglio, J. G.; Aziz, N. S.; Lin, E. T.; Grausz, H.; Naughton, J. L.; and Benet, L. Z. Cefamandole kinetics in uremic patients undergoing hemodialysis. Clin. Pharmacol. Ther., 1979, 26, 592–599.
5. Agbayani, M. M.; Khan, A. J.; Kemawikasit, P.; Rosenfeld, W.; Salazar, D.; Kumar, K.; Glass, L.; and Evans, H. E. Pharmacokinetics and safety of cefamandole in newborn infants. Antimicrob. Agents Chemother., 1979, 15, 674–676.
6. Polk, R. E.; Archer, G. L.; and Lower, R. Cefamandole kinetics during cardiopulmonary bypass. Clin. Pharmacol. Ther., 1978, 23, 473–480.

Key: Adult = adults; Aged = aged; Alb = hypoalbuminemia; AVH = acute viral hepatitis; CF = cystic fibrosis; CHF = congestive heart failure; Child = children; Cirr = cirrhosis; COPD = chronic obstructive pulmonary disease; CP = cor pulmonale; CPBS = cardiopulmonary bypass surgery; CRI = chronic respiratory insufficiency; Cush = cushingoid; Epilep = epilepsy; Fem = females; Hep = hepatitis; HL = hyperlipoproteinemia; HTh = hyperthyroid; Inflam = inflammation; LTh = hypothyroid; MI = myocardial infarction; Neo = neonates; NS = nephrotic syndrome; Obes = obesity; Pneu = pneumonia; Preg = pregnant; Prem = premature infants; RA = rheumatoid arthritis; Smk = smoking; Tach = ventricular tachycardia; Urem = uremia.

CEFAZOLIN [a] (Chapter 50)

AVAILABILITY (ORAL) (%)	URINARY EXCRETION (%)	BOUND IN PLASMA (%)	CLEARANCE $(ml \cdot min^{-1} \cdot kg^{-1})$
—	80 (68–97) (2)	84 ± 1 (3) ↓ Urem [b] (3)	0.95 ± 0.17 [a,c] (1) ↓ Urem (1)

VOL. DIST. (*liters/kg*)	HALF-LIFE (*hours*)	EFFECTIVE CONCENTRATIONS	TOXIC CONCENTRATIONS
0.12 ± 0.03 [a,c] (1) ↑ Urem (3,5)	1.8 ± 0.4 [a] (1) ↑ Urem (1)	*See* Chapter 50	—

[a] For review, *see* (1). Values represent mean ± S.D. for seven different studies.
[b] For patients undergoing dialysis, binding before dialysis was 73 ± 13%; after dialysis the value was 22 ± 21% (4).
[c] Assuming 70-kg weight.

1. Nightingale, C. H.; Greene, D. S.; and Quintiliani, R. Pharmacokinetics and clinical use of cephalosporin antibiotics. *J. Pharm. Sci.,* **1975,** *64,* 1899–1927.
2. Naumann, P., and Reintjens, E. Antibacterial activity and pharmacokinetic behavior of cefazolin as compared with five other cephalosporin antibiotics. *Infection,* **1974,** *2,* 19–24.
3. Craig, W. A.; Welling, P. G.; Jackson, T. C.; and Kunin, C. M. Pharmacology of cefazolin and other cephalosporins in patients with renal insufficiency. *J. Infect. Dis.,* **1973,** *128,* Suppl., 5347–5353.

4. Greene, D. S., and Tice, A. D. Effect of hemodialysis on cefazolin protein binding. *J. Pharm. Sci.,* **1977,** *66,* 1508–1510.
5. Czerwinski, A. W.; Pederson, J. A.; and Barry, J. P. Cefazolin plasma concentrations and urinary excretion in patients with renal impairment. *J. Clin. Pharmacol.,* **1974,** *14,* 560–566.

CEFOXITIN (Chapter 50)

AVAILABILITY (ORAL) (%)	URINARY EXCRETION (%)	BOUND IN PLASMA (%)	CLEARANCE $(ml \cdot min^{-1} \cdot kg^{-1})$
—	78 (1)	73 (2) ↓ Urem (2)	5.6 [a,b] (1) ↓ Urem (2)

VOL. DIST. (*liters/kg*)	HALF-LIFE (*hours*)	EFFECTIVE CONCENTRATIONS	TOXIC CONCENTRATIONS
0.16 (2) ↑ Urem (2)	0.70 ± 0.13 [c] (1) ↑ Urem (2)	*See* Chapter 50	—

[a] Dose of 500 mg; CL = 4.9 and 4.4 ml · min^{-1} · kg^{-1} for 1-g and 2-g doses, respectively.
[b] Calculated from means of parameters and subject weights.
[c] Dose of 500 mg; $t_{1/2}$ = 1.0 and 0.93 hours for 1-g and 2-g doses, respectively.

1. Sonneville, P. F.; Kartodirdjo, R. R.; Skeggs, H.; Till, A. E.; and Martin, C. M. Comparative clinical pharmacokinetics of intravenous cefoxitin and cephalothin. *Eur. J. Clin. Pharmacol.,* **1976,** *9,* 397–403.

2. Garcia, M. J.; Dominguez-Gil, A.; Tabernero, J. M.; and Tomero, J. A. S. Pharmacokinetics of cefoxitin in patients with normal or impaired renal function. *Eur. J. Clin. Pharmacol.,* **1979,** *16,* 119–124.

Key: Adult = adults;   Aged = aged;   Alb = hypoalbuminemia;   AVH = acute viral hepatitis;   CF = cystic fibrosis;   CHF = congestive heart failure;   Child = children;   Cirr = cirrhosis;   COPD = chronic obstructive pulmonary disease;   CP = cor pulmonale;   CPBS = cardiopulmonary bypass surgery;   CRI = chronic respiratory insufficiency;   Cush = cushingoid;   Epilep = epilepsy;   Fem = females;   Hep = hepatitis;   HL = hyperlipoproteinemia;   HTh = hyperthyroid;   Inflam = inflammation;   LTh = hypothyroid;   MI = myocardial infarction;   Neo = neonates;   NS = nephrotic syndrome;   Obes = obesity;   Pneu = pneumonia;   Preg = pregnant;   Prem = premature infants;   RA = rheumatoid arthritis;   Smk = smoking;   Tach = ventricular tachycardia;   Urem = uremia.

CEPHALEXIN [a] (Chapter 50)

AVAILABILITY (ORAL) (%)	URINARY EXCRETION (%)	BOUND IN PLASMA (%)	CLEARANCE $(ml \cdot min^{-1} \cdot kg^{-1})$
90 ± 9 (2)	96 (3)	14 ± 3 (4)	4.3 ± 1.1 [b,c] (5)

VOL. DIST. (*liters/kg*)	HALF-LIFE (*hours*)	EFFECTIVE CONCENTRATIONS	TOXIC CONCENTRATIONS
0.26 ± 0.03 [b,c] (5) ↔ Urem (6)	0.90 ± 0.18 [b] (5) ↑ Urem (6)	*See* Chapter 50	—

[a] For review, *see* (1).
[b] Values represent mean ± standard deviation for five studies.
[c] Assuming 70-kg weight.

1. Nightingale, C. H.; Greene, D. S.; and Quintiliani, R. Pharmacokinetics and clinical use of cephalosporin antibiotics. *J. Pharm. Sci.,* **1975,** *64,* 1899–1927.
2. Finkelstein, E.; Quintiliani, R.; Lee, R.; Bracci, A.; and Nightingale, C. H. Pharmacokinetics of oral cephalosporins: cephradine and cephalexin. *J. Pharm. Sci.,* **1978,** *67,* 1447–1450.
3. Kirby, W. M. M., and Regamey, C. Pharmacokinetics of cefazolin compared with four other cephalosporins. *J. Infect. Dis.,* **1973,** *128,* Suppl., 5341–5346.
4. Singhvi, S. M.; Heald, A. F.; Gadebusch, H. H.; Resnick, M. E.; Difazio, L. T.; and Leitz, M. A. Human serum protein binding of cephalosporin antibiotics *in vitro. J. Lab. Clin. Med.,* **1977,** *89,* 414–420.
5. Greene, D. S.; Flanagan, D. E.; Quintiliani, R.; and Nightingale, C. H. Pharmacokinetics of cephalexin: an evaluation of one- and two-compartment model pharmacokinetics. *J. Clin. Pharmacol.,* **1976,** *16,* 257–264.
6. Spyker, D. A.; Thomas, B. L.; Sande, M. A.; and Bolton, W. K. Pharmacokinetics of cefaclor and cephalexin: dosage nomograms for impaired renal function. *Antimicrob. Agents Chemother.,* **1978,** *14,* 172–177.

CEPHALOTHIN [a] (Chapter 50)

AVAILABILITY (ORAL) (%)	URINARY EXCRETION (%)	BOUND IN PLASMA (%)	CLEARANCE $(ml \cdot min^{-1} \cdot kg^{-1})$
	52 (2,3)	71 ± 3 (4)	6.7 ± 1.7 [b] (5) ↓ CPBS (6)

VOL. DIST. (*liters/kg*)	HALF-LIFE (*hours*)	EFFECTIVE CONCENTRATIONS	TOXIC CONCENTRATIONS
0.26 ± 0.11 [b] (5) ↑ Child (7)	0.57 ± 0.32 (8) ↑ Urem (8), CPBS (6)	*See* Chapter 50	—

[a] For review, *see* (1).
[b] Assuming 70-kg weight; one-compartment model.

1. Nightingale, C. H.; Greene, D. S.; and Quintiliani, R. Pharmacokinetics and clinical use of cephalosporin antibiotics. *J. Pharm. Sci.,* **1975,** *64,* 1899–1927.
2. Kirby, W. M. M., and Regamey, C. Pharmacokinetics of cefazolin compared with four other cephalosporins. *J. Infect. Dis.,* **1973,** *128,* Suppl., 5341–5346.
3. Sonneville, P. F.; Kartodirdjo, R. R.; Skeggs, H.; Till, A. E.; and Martin, C. M. Comparative clinical pharmacokinetics of intravenous cefoxitin and cephalothin. *Eur. J. Clin. Pharmacol.,* **1976,** *9,* 397–403.
4. Singhvi, S. M.; Heald, A. F.; Gadebusch, H. H.; Resnick, M. E.; Difazio, L. T.; and Leitz, M. A. Human serum protein binding of cephalosporin antibiotics *in vitro. J. Lab. Clin. Med.,* **1977,** *89,* 414–420.
5. Kirby, W. M. M.; DeMaine, J. B.; and Serril, W. S. Pharmacokinetics of the cephalosporins in healthy volunteers and uremic patients. *Postgrad. Med. J.,* **1971,** *47,* Suppl., 41–46.
6. Miller, K. W.; Chan, K. K. H.; McCow, H. G.; Fischer, R. P.; Lindsay, W. G.; and Zaske, D. E. Cephalothin kinetics: before, during, and after cardiopulmonary bypass surgery. *Clin. Pharmacol. Ther.,* **1979,** *26,* 54–62.
7. Rolewicz, T. F.; Mirkin, B. L.; Cooper, M. J.; and Anders, M. W. Metabolic disposition of cephalothin and desacetyl-cephalothin in children and adults: comparison of high-performance liquid chromatographic and microbial assay procedures. *Clin. Pharmacol. Ther.,* **1977,** *22,* 928–935.
8. Kabins, S. A., and Cohen, S. Cephalothin serum levels in the azotemic patient. In, *Proceedings of the 4th Interscience Conference on Antimicrobial Agents and Chemotherapy.* (Sylvester, J. C., ed.) American Society for Microbiology, Ann Arbor, **1964,** pp. 207–214.

CEPHAPIRIN [a] (Chapter 50)

AVAILABILITY (ORAL) (%)	URINARY EXCRETION (%)	BOUND IN PLASMA (%)	CLEARANCE $(ml \cdot min^{-1} \cdot kg^{-1})$
—	49 [b] (2)	62 ± 4 (3)	4.3 ± 1.6 [c] (4)

VOL. DIST. (liters/kg)	HALF-LIFE (hours)	EFFECTIVE CONCENTRATIONS	TOXIC CONCENTRATIONS
0.13 ± 0.05 [c] (4)	1.2 ± 0.3 (4) ↑ Urem (5)	See Chapter 50	—

[a] For review, see (1).
[b] Cabana and associates (2) suggest that higher values reported by others result from measurement of desacetyl metabolite.
[c] Assuming 70-kg weight.

1. Nightingale, C. H.; Greene, D. S.; and Quintiliani, R. Pharmacokinetics and clinical use of cephalosporin antibiotics. *J. Pharm. Sci.*, **1975**, *64*, 1899–1927.
2. Cabana, B. E.; Van Harken, D. R.; and Hottendorf, G. H. Comparative pharmacokinetics and metabolism of cephapirin in laboratory animals and humans. *Antimicrob. Agents Chemother.*, **1976**, *10*, 307–317.
3. Arvidsson, A.; Borgå, O.; and Alván, G. Renal excretion of cephapirin and cephaloridine: evidence for saturable tubular reabsorption. *Clin. Pharmacol. Ther.*, **1979**, *25*, 870–876.
4. Bergan, T. Comparative pharmacokinetics of cefazolin, cephalothin, cephacetril, and cephapirin after intravenous administration. *Chemotherapy*, **1977**, *23*, 389–404.
5. McCloskey, R. V.; Terry, E. E.; McCracken, A. W.; Sweeney, M. J.; and Forland, M. E. Effect of hemodialysis and renal failure on serum and urine concentrations of cephapirin sodium. *Antimicrob. Agents Chemother.*, **1972**, *1*, 90–93.

CEPHRADINE [a] (Chapter 50)

AVAILABILITY (ORAL) (%)	URINARY EXCRETION (%)	BOUND IN PLASMA (%)	CLEARANCE $(ml \cdot min^{-1} \cdot kg^{-1})$
>90 (2)	86 ± 10 [b] (3)	14 ± 3 (4)	5.1 ± 1.2 [a,c] (1) ↓ Urem (5)

VOL. DIST. (liters/kg)	HALF-LIFE (hours)	EFFECTIVE CONCENTRATIONS	TOXIC CONCENTRATIONS
0.25 ± 0.01 [a,c] (1)	0.77 ± 0.30 [a] (1) ↑ Urem (5)	See Chapter 50	—

[a] For review, see (1); values represent mean ± standard deviation for two studies.
[b] Oral dose.
[c] Assuming 70-kg weight.

1. Nightingale, C. H.; Greene, D. S.; and Quintiliani, R. Pharmacokinetics and clinical use of cephalosporin antibiotics. *J. Pharm. Sci.*, **1975**, *64*, 1899–1927.
2. Rattie, E. S.; Bernardo, P. D.; and Ravin, L. J. Pharmacokinetic interpretation of cephradine levels in serum after intravenous and extravascular administration in humans. *Antimicrob. Agents Chemother.*, **1976**, *10*, 283–287.
3. Finkelstein, E.; Quintiliani, R.; Lee, R.; Bracci, A.; and Nightingale, C. H. Pharmacokinetics of oral cephalosporins: cephradine and cephalexin. *J. Pharm. Sci.*, **1978**, *67*, 1447–1450.
4. Singhvi, S. M.; Heald, A. F.; Gadebusch, H. H.; Resnick, M. E.; Difazio, L. T.; and Leitz, M. A. Human serum protein binding of cephalosporin antibiotics *in vitro*. *J. Lab. Clin. Med.*, **1977**, *89*, 414–420.
5. Solomon, A. E.; Briggs, J. D.; McGleachy, R.; and Sleigh, J. D. The administration of cephradine to patients in renal failure. *Br. J. Clin. Pharmacol.*, **1975**, *2*, 443–448.

CHLORAMPHENICOL (Chapter 52)

AVAILABILITY (ORAL) (%)	URINARY EXCRETION (%)	BOUND IN PLASMA (%)	CLEARANCE $(ml \cdot min^{-1} \cdot kg^{-1})$
75–90 (1)	5 ± 1 [a] (2)	53 ± 5 (3) ↓ Cirr (3), Prem (3)	3.6 ± 1.7 [b] (3) ↓ Cirr (3,4) ↔ Urem (2)

VOL. DIST. (liters/kg)	HALF-LIFE (hours)	EFFECTIVE CONCENTRATIONS	TOXIC CONCENTRATIONS
0.92 (3,4) ↔ Cirr (3,4)	2.7 ± 0.8 (5) ↔ Urem (5) ↑ Cirr (4)	See Chapter 52	See Chapter 52

[a] Oral dose.
[b] CL/F; after intravenous administration, clearance estimated to be 4.7 ± 1.1 ml·min⁻¹·kg⁻¹ (see 3,4).

1. Glazko, A. J.; Wolf, L. M.; Dill, W. A.; and Bratton, A. C. Biochemical studies on chloramphenicol (CHLOROMYCETIN). II. Tissue distribution and excretion studies. *J. Pharmacol. Exp. Ther.*, 1949, 96, 445–459.
2. Schück, O.; Prát, V.; Grafnetterová, J.; David, I.; Kotanová, E.; and Reitschlägerová, V. Excretion of chloramphenicol and its metabolites by the chronically diseased kidney (with respect to the theory of adaptive nephrons). *Int. J. Clin. Pharmacol.*, 1974, 10, 33–43.
3. Koup, J. R.; Lau, A. H.; Brodsky, B.; and Slaughter, R. L. Chloramphenicol pharmacokinetics in hospitalized patients. *Antimicrob. Agents Chemother.*, 1979, 15, 651–657.
4. Azzollini, F.; Gazzaniga, A.; Lodola, E.; and Natangelo, R. Elimination of chloramphenicol and thiamphenicol in subjects with cirrhosis of the liver. *Int. J. Clin. Pharmacol.*, 1972, 6, 130–134.
5. Kunin, C. M.; Glazko, A. J.; and Finland, M. Persistence of antibiotics in blood of patients with acute renal failure. II. Chloramphenicol and its metabolic products in the blood of patients with severe renal disease or hepatic cirrhosis. *J. Clin. Invest.*, 1959, 38, 1498–1508.

CHLORDIAZEPOXIDE [a] (Chapters 17, 19)

AVAILABILITY (ORAL) (%)	URINARY EXCRETION (%)	BOUND IN PLASMA (%)	CLEARANCE $(ml \cdot min^{-1} \cdot kg^{-1})$
100 (2,3)	<1 (2)	96.5 ± 1.8 (4) ↓ AVH (4), Cirr (4) ↔ Aged (4)	0.37 ± 0.06 (2) ↓ Aged (4,5), AVH (4), Cirr (4) ↑ Fem (6)

VOL. DIST. (liters/kg)	HALF-LIFE (hours)	EFFECTIVE CONCENTRATIONS	TOXIC CONCENTRATIONS
0.30 ± 0.03 (2) ↑ Aged (4,5), AVH [b] (4), Cirr [b] (4), Fem (6)	9.9 ± 2.5 (2) ↑ Aged (4,5), AVH (4), Cirr (4)	>0.7 µg/ml [c] (7)(8) [d]	—

[a] For review, see (1).
[b] Due to decreased protein binding, Vd_{ss} for the free drug is unchanged.
[c] Decrease in anxiety and hostility.
[d] Reduction in anxiety correlated with steady-state concentrations of metabolites (desmethylchlordiazepoxide and demoxepam) but not with chlordiazepoxide.

Key: Adult = adults; Aged = aged; Alb = hypoalbuminemia; AVH = acute viral hepatitis; CF = cystic fibrosis; CHF = congestive heart failure; Child = children; Cirr = cirrhosis; COPD = chronic obstructive pulmonary disease; CP = cor pulmonale; CPBS = cardiopulmonary bypass surgery; CRI = chronic respiratory insufficiency; Cush = cushingoid; Epilep = epilepsy; Fem = females; Hep = hepatitis; HL = hyperlipoproteinemia; HTh = hyperthyroid; Inflam = inflammation; LTh = hypothyroid; MI = myocardial infarction; Neo = neonates; NS = nephrotic syndrome; Obes = obesity; Pneu = pneumonia; Preg = pregnant; Prem = premature infants; RA = rheumatoid arthritis; Smk = smoking; Tach = ventricular tachycardia; Urem = uremia.

CHLORDIAZEPOXIDE (*Cont.*)

1. Greenblatt, D. J.; Shader, R. I.; MacLeod, S. M.; and Sellers, E. M. Clinical pharmacokinetics of chlordiazepoxide. *Clin. Pharmacokinet.,* **1978,** *3,* 381–394.
2. Boxenbaum, H. G.; Geitner, K. A.; Jack, M. L.; Dixon, W. R.; Speigel, H. E.; Symington, J.; Christian, R.; Moore, J. D.; Weissman, L.; and Kaplan, S. A. Pharmacokinetic and biopharmaceutic profile of chlordiazepoxide HCl in healthy subjects: single-dose studies by the intravenous, intramuscular, and oral routes. *J. Pharmacokinet. Biopharm.,* **1977,** *5,* 3–23.
3. Greenblatt, D. J.; Shader, R. I.; MacLeod, S. M.; Sellers, E. M.; Franke, K.; and Giles, H. G. Absorption of oral and intramuscular chlordiazepoxide. *Eur. J. Clin. Pharmacol.,* **1978,** *13,* 267–274.
4. Roberts, R. K.; Wilkinson, G. R.; Branch, R. A.; and Schenker, S. Effect of age and cirrhosis on the disposition and elimination of chlordiazepoxide (LIBRIUM). *Gastroenterology,* **1978,** *75,* 479–485.

5. Shader, R. I.; Greenblatt, D. J.; Harmatz, J. S.; Franke, K.; and Koch-Weser, J. Absorption and disposition of chlordiazepoxide in young and elderly male volunteers. *J. Clin. Pharmacol.,* **1977,** *17,* 709–718.
6. Greenblatt, D. J.; Shader, R. I.; Franke, K.; MacLaughlin, D. S.; Ransil, B. J.; and Koch-Weser, J. Kinetics of intravenous chlordiazepoxide: sex differences in drug distribution. *Clin. Pharmacol. Ther.,* **1977,** *22,* 893–903.
7. Gottschalk, L. A.; Noble, E. P.; Stolzoff, G. E.; Bates, D. E.; Cable, C. G.; Uliana, R. L.; Birch, H.; and Fleming, E. W. Relationships of chlordiazepoxide blood levels to psychological and biochemical responses. In, *The Benzodiazepines.* (Garattini, S.; Mussini, E.; and Randall, L. O.; eds.) Raven Press, New York, **1973,** pp. 257–280.
8. Lin, K. M., and Friedel, R. O. Relationship of plasma levels of chlordiazepoxide and metabolites to clinical response. *Am. J. Psychiatry,* **1979,** *136,* 18–23.

CHLOROTHIAZIDE [a] (Chapter 36)

AVAILABILITY (ORAL) (%)	URINARY EXCRETION (%)	BOUND IN PLASMA (%)	CLEARANCE ($ml \cdot min^{-1} \cdot kg^{-1}$)
8.7 ± 4.1 [b] (1)	92 ± 5 (1)	94.6 ± 1.3 (2)	4.5 ± 1.7 (1)

VOL. DIST. (*liters/kg*)	HALF-LIFE (*hours*)	EFFECTIVE CONCENTRATIONS	TOXIC CONCENTRATIONS
0.20 ± 0.08 (1)	1.5 ± 0.2 (1) ↑ Urem (3), CHF (3)	—	—

[a] Data in (1) for ten normal subjects who received 1-g oral and intravenous doses.
[b] Wide range of values reported previously probably due to difficulties with assay (1).

1. Gee, W. L.; Lin, E. T.; Brater, D. C.; Gustafson, J. H.; and Benet, L. Z. Chlorothiazide pharmacokinetics following oral and i.v. dosing in man. *J. Pharmacokinet. Biopharm.,* **1980,** *8.*
2. Hucker, H. B.; Stauffer, S. C.; and White, S. E. Effect of halofenate on binding of various drugs to human plasma

proteins and on the plasma half-life of antipyrine in monkeys. *J. Pharm. Sci.,* **1972,** *61,* 1490–1492.
3. Brettell, H. R.; Aikawa, J. K.; and Gordon, G. S. Studies with chlorothiazide tagged with radioactive carbon (C^{14}) in human beings. *Arch. Intern. Med.,* **1960,** *106,* 109–115.

CHLORPROMAZINE [a] (Chapter 19)

AVAILABILITY (ORAL) (%)	URINARY EXCRETION (%)	BOUND IN PLASMA (%)	CLEARANCE ($ml \cdot min^{-1} \cdot kg^{-1}$)
32 ± 19 [b] (2)	<1 (3)	95–98 (4)	8.6 ± 2.9 [c] (2) ↓ Child [d] (5)

VOL. DIST. (*liters/kg*)	HALF-LIFE (*hours*)	EFFECTIVE CONCENTRATIONS	TOXIC CONCENTRATIONS
21 ± 9 [c] (2)	30 ± 7 [e] (2) ↔ Cirr (6)	30–350 ng/ml [f] (7–9) Children: 40–80 ng/ml (5)	750–1000 ng/ml [g] (7)

[a] For review, *see* (1).

[b] After single dose. First-pass metabolism is marked, and availability may decrease to about 20% with repeated administration.

[c] $CL/F_{intramuscular}$ and $Vd_{area}/F_{intramuscular}$.

[d] CL/F_{oral}; there may be induction of metabolism and dose-dependent kinetics.

[e] After multiple oral doses. Similar mean values found after single oral or intramuscular doses, but variability is greater (14–103 hours) (2).

[f] Values are controversial, and there are a large number of active and inactive metabolites (1).

[g] Neurotoxicity, manifested by tremors and convulsions.

1. Cooper, T. B. Plasma level monitoring of antipsychotic drugs. *Clin. Pharmacokinet.*, **1978**, *3*, 14–38.
2. Dahl, S. G., and Strandjord, R. E. Pharmacokinetics of chlorpromazine after single and chronic dosage. *Clin. Pharmacol. Ther.*, **1977**, *21*, 437–448.
3. Whitfield, L. R.; Kaul, P. N.; and Clark, M. L. Chlorpromazine metabolism. IX. Pharmacokinetics of chlorpromazine following oral administration in man. *J. Pharmacokinet. Biopharm.*, **1978**, *6*, 187–196.
4. Curry, S. H.; Davis, J. M.; Janowsky, D. S.; and Marshall, J. H. L. Factors affecting chlorpromazine plasma levels in psychiatric patients. *Arch. Gen. Psychiatry*, **1970**, *22*, 209–215.
5. Rivera-Calimlim, L.; Griesbach, P. H.; and Perlmutter, R. Plasma chlorpromazine concentrations in children with behavioral disorders and mental illness. *Clin. Pharmacol. Ther.*, **1979**, *26*, 114–121.
6. Maxwell, J. D.; Carrella, M.; Parkes, J. D.; Williams, R.; Mould, G. P.; and Curry, S. H. Plasma disappearance and cerebral effects of chlorpromazine in cirrhosis. *Clin. Sci.*, **1972**, *43*, 143–151.
7. Rivera-Calimlim, L.; Castaneda, L.; and Lasagna, L. Effect of mode of management on plasma chlorpromazine in psychiatric patients. *Clin. Pharmacol. Ther.*, **1973**, *14*, 978–986.
8. Rivera-Calimlim, L.; Masrallah, H.; Strass, J.; and Lasagna, L. Clinical response and plasma levels: effect of dose, dosage schedules, and drug interactions on plasma chlorpromazine levels. *Am. J. Psychiatry*, **1976**, *133*, 646–652.
9. Curry, S. H. Gas-chromatographic methods for the study of chlorpromazine and some of its metabolites in human plasma. *Psychopharmacol. Commun.*, **1976**, *2*, 1–15.

CHLORTHALIDONE (Chapter 36)

AVAILABILITY (ORAL) (%)	URINARY EXCRETION (%)	BOUND IN PLASMA (%)	CLEARANCE $(ml \cdot min^{-1} \cdot kg^{-1})$
64 ± 10 (1)	65 ± 9 [a] (1)	75 ± 1 (3)	1.6 ± 0.3 (1)

VOL. DIST. *(liters/kg)*	HALF-LIFE *(hours)*	EFFECTIVE CONCENTRATIONS	TOXIC CONCENTRATIONS
3.9 ± 0.8 (1)	44 ± 10 [b] (1)	—	—

[a] Value is for 50- and 100-mg doses; renal clearance is decreased at an oral dose of 200 mg, and there is a concomitant decrease in the percentage excreted unchanged (2).

[b] Chlorthalidone is sequestered in erythrocytes; the half-life is longer if blood is analyzed, rather than plasma (4).

1. Fleuren, H. L. J.; Thien, Th. A.; Verwey-van Wissen, C. P. W.; and van Rossum, J. M. Absolute bioavailability of chlorthalidone in man: a cross-over study after intravenous and oral administration. *Eur. J. Clin. Pharmacol.*, **1979**, *15*, 35–50.
2. Fleuren, H. L. J.; Verwey-van Wissen, C.; and van Rossum, J. M. Dose-dependent urinary excretion of chlorthalidone. *Clin. Pharmacol. Ther.*, **1979**, *25*, 806–812.
3. Collste, P.; Garle, M.; Rawlins, M. D.; and Sjöqvist, F. Interindividual differences in chlorthalidone concentration in plasma and red cells of man after single and multiple doses. *Eur. J. Clin. Pharmacol.*, **1976**, *9*, 319–325.
4. Fleuren, H. L. J., and van Rossum, J. M. Nonlinear relationship between plasma and red blood cell pharmacokinetics of chlorthalidone in man. *J. Pharmacokinet. Biopharm.*, **1977**, *5*, 359–375.

Key: Adult = adults;   Aged = aged;   Alb = hypoalbuminemia;   AVH = acute viral hepatitis;   CF = cystic fibrosis;   CHF = congestive heart failure;   Child = children;   Cirr = cirrhosis;   COPD = chronic obstructive pulmonary disease;   CP = cor pulmonale;   CPBS = cardiopulmonary bypass surgery;   CRI = chronic respiratory insufficiency;   Cush = cushingoid;   Epilep = epilepsy;   Fem = females;   Hep = hepatitis;   HL = hyperlipoproteinemia;   HTh = hyperthyroid;   Inflam = inflammation;   LTh = hypothyroid;   MI = myocardial infarction;   Neo = neonates;   NS = nephrotic syndrome;   Obes = obesity;   Pneu = pneumonia;   Preg = pregnant;   Prem = premature infants;   RA = rheumatoid arthritis;   Smk = smoking;   Tach = ventricular tachycardia;   Urem = uremia.

CIMETIDINE (Chapter 26)

AVAILABILITY (ORAL) (%)	URINARY EXCRETION (%)	BOUND IN PLASMA (%)	CLEARANCE $(ml \cdot min^{-1} \cdot kg^{-1})$
62 ± 6 [a] (1)	77 ± 6 (1)	19 (2)	12 ± 3 (3) ↓ Urem (4), Aged [b] (2,5)

VOL. DIST. (liters/kg)	HALF-LIFE (hours)	EFFECTIVE CONCENTRATIONS	TOXIC CONCENTRATIONS
2.1 ± 1.0 [c] (3) ↓ Aged [b] (2)	2.1 ± 1.1 (3) ↔ Ulcer (2) ↑ Urem (4)	$1.0\ \mu g/ml$ [d] (6)	—

[a] Oral liquid and tablets are equivalent; value is the same in patients with ulcers (2).
[b] Determined in patients with ulcers.
[c] Vd_{area}.
[d] Inhibition by 50% of stimulated acid secretion in patients with peptic ulcer; for normal subjects, see (7,8).

1. Walkenstein, S. S.; Dubb, J. W.; Randolph, W. C.; Westlake, W. J.; Stote, R. M.; and Intoccia, A. P. Bioavailability of cimetidine in man. *Gastroenterology,* **1978,** *74,* 360–365.
2. Somogyi, A.; Rohner, H.-G.; and Gugler, R. Pharmacokinetics and bioavailability of cimetidine in gastric and duodenal ulcer patients. *Clin. Pharmacokinet.,* **1980,** *5,* 84–94.
3. Grahnén, A.; von Bahr, C.; Lindström, B.; and Rosén, A. Bioavailability and pharmacokinetics of cimetidine. *Eur. J. Clin. Pharmacol.,* **1979,** *16,* 335–340.
4. Larsson, R.; Bodemar, G.; and Norlander, B. Oral absorption of cimetidine and its clearance in patients with renal failure. *Eur. J. Clin. Pharmacol.,* **1979,** *15,* 153–157.
5. Redolfi, A.; Borgogelli, E.; and Lodola, E. Blood level of cimetidine in relation to age. *Eur. J. Clin. Pharmacol.,* **1979,** *15,* 257–261.
6. Bodemar, G.; Norlander, B.; and Walan, A. Cimetidine in the treatment of active peptic ulcer disease. In, *Cimetidine.* (Burland, W. L., and Simikins, M. A., eds.) Excerpta Medica, Amsterdam, **1977,** pp. 224–239.
7. Burland, W. L.; Duncan, W. A. M.; Hesselbo, T.; Mills, J. G.; Sharpe, P. C.; Haggie, S. J.; and Wyllie, J. H. Pharmacological evaluation of cimetidine, a new histamine H_2-receptor antagonist, in healthy man. *Br. J. Clin. Pharmacol.,* **1975,** *2,* 481–486.
8. Pounder, R. E.; Williams, J. G.; Hunt, R. H.; Vincent, S. H.; Milton-Thompson, G. J.; and Misiewicz, J. J. The effects of oral cimetidine on food-stimulated gastric acid secretion and 24-hour intragastric acidity. In, *Cimetidine.* (Burland, W. L., and Simikins, M. A., eds.) Excerpta Medica, Amsterdam, **1977,** pp. 189–204.

CLINDAMYCIN (Chapter 54)

AVAILABILITY (ORAL) (%)	URINARY EXCRETION (%)	BOUND IN PLASMA (%)	CLEARANCE $(ml \cdot min^{-1} \cdot kg^{-1})$
~87 [a] (1)	9–14 [b] (2)	93.6 ± 0.2 (3)	3.5 ± 0.8 [c] (4) ↔ Child (2)

VOL. DIST. (liters/kg)	HALF-LIFE (hours)	EFFECTIVE CONCENTRATIONS	TOXIC CONCENTRATIONS
0.66 ± 0.10 [d] (2) ↔ Urem (5,6)	2.7 ± 0.4 [c] (4) ↔ Child (2), Urem (7), Preg (8)	*See* Chapter 54	—

[a] Clindamycin hydrochloride.
[b] Microbiological assay, which includes active metabolites.
[c] Calculated from data in six studies.
[d] Vd/F; calculated from data in six studies. Average value in children, 0.86 liters/kg.

1. Forist, A. A.; DeHaan, R. M.; and Metzler, C. M. Clinda-mycin bioavailability from clindamycin-2-palmitate and clindamycin-2-hexadecylcarbonate in man. *J. Pharmacokinet. Biopharm.*, **1973**, *1*, 89–98
2. DeHaan, R. M.; Metzler, C. M.; Schellenberg, D.; Vanden-Bosch, W. D.; and Masson, E. L. Pharmacokinetic studies of clindamycin hydrochloride in humans. *Int. J. Clin. Pharmacol.*, **1972**, *6*, 105–119.
3. Gordon, R. C.; Regamey, C.; and Kirby, W. M. M. Serum protein binding of erythromycin, lincomycin, and clindamy-cin. *J. Pharm. Sci.*, **1973**, *62*, 1074–1077.
4. DeHaan, R. M.; Metzler, C. M.; Schellenberg, D.; and VandenBosch, W. D. Pharmacokinetic studies of clindamy-cin phosphate. *J. Clin. Pharmacol.*, **1973**, *13*, 190–209.
5. Joshi, A. M., and Stein, R. M. Altered serum clearance of intravenously administered clindamycin phosphate in pa-tients with uremia. *J. Clin. Pharmacol.*, **1974**, *14*, 140–144.
6. Wagner, J. G. Pharmacokinetic parameters estimated from intravenous data by uniform methods and some of their uses. *J. Pharmacokinet. Biopharm.*, **1977**, *5*, 161–182.
7. Peddie, B. A.; Dann, E.; and Bailey, R. R. The effect of impairment of renal function and dialysis on the serum and urine levels of clindamycin. *Aust. N.Z. J. Med.*, **1975**, *5*, 198–202.
8. Philipson, A.; Sabath, L. D.; and Charles, D. Erythromycin and clindamycin absorption and elimination in pregnant women. *Clin. Pharmacol. Ther.*, **1976**, *19*, 68–77.

CLOFIBRATE [a] (Chapter 34)

AVAILABILITY (ORAL) (%)	URINARY EXCRETION (%)	BOUND IN PLASMA (%)	CLEARANCE ($ml \cdot min^{-1} \cdot kg^{-1}$)
95 ± 10 (2)	11 ± 3 [b] (4) 32 ± 14 [b] (2)	96.5 ± 2.0 [c] (3) ↓ NS (3), Cirr (4), Urem (4) ↔ AVH (4)	0.18 ± 0.03 [b] (5) ↓ Urem (4,6) ↔ AVH (4), Cirr (4) ↑ NS (3)

VOL. DIST. (liters/kg)	HALF-LIFE (hours)	EFFECTIVE CONCENTRATIONS	TOXIC CONCENTRATIONS
0.11 ± 0.02 [d] (4) ↑ Cirr (4), Urem (4)	13 ± 3 (2) ↑ Urem (4,6)	—	—

[a] Clofibrate is the ethyl ester of *p*-chlorophenoxyisobutyric acid (CPIB). All values are for CPIB, since clofibrate is rapidly deesterified upon absorption (1).

[b] Assuming availability = 100%; oral administration.

[c] Binding may decrease at high concentrations of CPIB (>200 μg/ml).

[d] Vd_{area}.

1. Thorp, J. M. Experimental evaluation of an orally active combination of androsterone with ethyl chlorphenoxyiso-butyrate. *Lancet*, **1962**, *2*, 1323–1326.
2. Houin, G.; Thebault, J. J.; d'Athis, Ph.; Tillement, J.-P.; and Beaumont, J.-L. A GLC method for estimation of chlor-phenoxyisobutyric acid in plasma. Pharmacokinetics of a sin-gle oral dose of clofibrate in man. *Eur. J. Clin. Pharmacol.*, **1975**, *8*, 433–437.
3. Gugler, R.; Shoeman, D. W.; Huffman, D. H.; Cohlmia, J. B.; and Azarnoff, D. L. Pharmacokinetics of drugs in patients with the nephrotic syndrome. *J. Clin. Invest.*, **1975**, *55*, 1182–1189.
4. Gugler, R.; Kurten, J. W.; Jensen, C. J.; Klehr, U.; and Hartlapp, J. Clofibrate disposition in renal failure and acute and chronic liver disease. *Eur. J. Clin. Pharmacol.*, **1979**, *15*, 341–347.
5. Sedeghat, A., and Ahrens, E. H., Jr. Lack of effect of cholestyramine on the pharmacokinetics of clofibrate in man. *Eur. J. Clin. Invest.*, **1975**, *5*, 177–185.
6. Goldberg, A. P.; Sherrard, D. J.; Haas, L. B.; and Brunzell, J. D. Control of clofibrate toxicity in uremic hypertri-glyceridemia. *Clin. Pharmacol. Ther.*, **1977**, *21*, 317–325.

Key: Adult = adults; Aged = aged; Alb = hypoalbuminemia; AVH = acute viral hepatitis; CF = cystic fibrosis; CHF = congestive heart failure; Child = children; Cirr = cirrhosis; COPD = chronic obstructive pulmonary disease; CP = cor pulmonale; CPBS = cardiopulmonary bypass surgery; CRI = chronic respiratory insufficiency; Cush = cushingoid; Epilep = epilepsy; Fem = females; Hep = hepatitis; HL = hyperlipoproteinemia; HTh = hyperthyroid; Inflam = inflammation; LTh = hypothyroid; MI = myocardial infarction; Neo = neonates; NS = nephrotic syndrome; Obes = obesity; Pneu = pneumonia; Preg = pregnant; Prem = premature infants; RA = rheumatoid arthritis; Smk = smoking; Tach = ventricular tachycardia; Urem = uremia.

CLONAZEPAM (Chapter 20)

AVAILABILITY (ORAL) (%)	URINARY EXCRETION (%)	BOUND IN PLASMA (%)	CLEARANCE $(ml \cdot min^{-1} \cdot kg^{-1})$
98 ± 31 (1)	<1 (2)	47 (3)	0.92 ± 0.25 [a,b] (1)

VOL. DIST. (liters/kg)	HALF-LIFE (hours)	EFFECTIVE CONCENTRATIONS	TOXIC CONCENTRATIONS
3.2 ± 1.1 [a] (1)	39 ± 12 [b,c] (1)	5–70 ng/ml [d] (6)	[e]

[a] Calculated from data given.

[b] Increased clearance and decreased half-life when carbamazepine is given concomitantly (4).

[c] Range in children is reported to be 22–33 hours (5).

[d] Most patients, including children (5), whose seizures are controlled by clonazepam have concentrations of the drug in plasma in this range. However, patients who do not respond and those with side effects display similar values.

[e] Occurrence of side effects is apparently not correlated with concentrations of clonazepam or its 7-amino metabolite (7).

1. Berlin, A., and Dahlstrom, H. Pharmacokinetics of the anticonvulsant drug clonazepam evaluated from single oral and intravenous doses and by repeated oral administration. *Eur. J. Clin. Pharmacol.*, **1975**, *9*, 155–159.
2. Kaplan, S. A.; Alexander, K.; Jack, M. L.; Puglisi, C. V.; deSilva, J. A. F.; Lee, T. L.; and Weinfeld, R. E. Pharmacokinetic profile of clonazepam in dog and humans and of flunitrazepam in dog. *J. Pharm. Sci.*, **1974**, *63*, 527–532.
3. Müller, W., and Wollert, U. Characterization of the binding of benzodiazepines to human serum albumin. *Naunyn Schmiedebergs Arch. Pharmacol.*, **1973**, *280*, 229–237.
4. Lai, A. A.; Levy, R. H.; and Cutler, R. E. Time-course of interaction between carbamazepine and clonazepam in normal man. *Clin. Pharmacol. Ther.*, **1978**, *24*, 316–323.
5. Dreifuss, F. E.; Penry, J. K.; Rose, S. W.; Kupferberg, H. J.; Dyken, P.; and Sato, S. Serum clonazepam concentration in children with absence seizures. *Neurology (Minneap.)*, **1975**, *25*, 255–258.
6. Browne, T. R. Clonazepam: a review of a new anticonvulsant drug. *Arch. Neurol.*, **1976**, *33*, 326–332.
7. Sjö, O.; Hvidberg, E. F.; Naestoft, J.; and Lund, M. Pharmacokinetics and side-effects of clonazepam and its 7-amino metabolite. *Eur. J. Clin. Pharmacol.*, **1975**, *8*, 249–254.

CLONIDINE (Chapters 9, 32)

AVAILABILITY (ORAL) (%)	URINARY EXCRETION (%)	BOUND IN PLASMA (%)	CLEARANCE $(ml \cdot min^{-1} \cdot kg^{-1})$
75 ± 4 (1)	62 ± 11 (1)	—	3.1 ± 1.2 (1)

VOL. DIST. (liters/kg)	HALF-LIFE (hours)	EFFECTIVE CONCENTRATIONS	TOXIC CONCENTRATIONS
2.1 ± 0.4 (1)	8.5 ± 2.0 [a] (1)	1 ng/ml [b]	1 ng/ml [c] (1)

[a] While data are not conclusive, half-life may be a function of dose and be 50% longer with intravenous doses of 275 μg of the drug (2).

[b] Concentration to achieve a 15% reduction in mean blood pressure in normal subjects (1) or a 20% decrease in hypertensive patients (2).

[c] Sedation and decrease in rate of flow of saliva.

1. Davies, D. S.; Wing, L. M. H.; Reid, J. L.; Neill, E.; Tippett, P.; and Dollery, C. T. Pharmacokinetics and concentration-effect relationships of intravenous and oral clonidine. *Clin. Pharmacol. Ther.*, **1977**, *21*, 593–601.
2. Frisk-Holmberg, M.; Edlind, P. O.; and Paalzow, L. Pharmacokinetics of clonidine and its relation to the hypotensive effect in patients. *Br. J. Clin. Pharmacol.*, **1978**, *6*, 227–232.

DESIPRAMINE (Chapter 19)

AVAILABILITY (ORAL) (%)	URINARY EXCRETION (%)	BOUND IN PLASMA (%)	CLEARANCE $(ml \cdot min^{-1} \cdot kg^{-1})$
68 [a]	—	92 $\pm$ 1 [b] (1) $\leftrightarrow$ Urem (2)	24 $\pm$ 12 [c] (3)

VOL. DIST. (*liters/kg*)	HALF-LIFE (*hours*)	EFFECTIVE CONCENTRATIONS	TOXIC CONCENTRATIONS
34 $\pm$ 8 [c] (3)	18 $\pm$ 5 (3) $\uparrow$ Aged (4)	>225 ng/ml [d] (5,6)	>1 μg/ml [e] (7)

[a] Estimated assuming erythrocyte: plasma partition of 2.0, hematocrit of 0.45, hepatic blood flow of 1500 ml/min, and complete absorption of the drug.

[b] Determined at 24–26° C in heparinized human plasma.

[c] CL/F and Vd_{ss}/F. Since F is probably significantly less than 1, actual values may be lower.

[d] Combination of imipramine and desipramine. It is implied but not proven that similar concentrations of desipramine alone are equally effective.

[e] Combined data for toxic effects of tricyclic antidepressants.

1. Borgå, O.; Azarnoff, D. L.; Plym Forshell, G.; and Sjöqvist, F. Plasma protein binding of tricyclic antidepressants in man. *Biochem. Pharmacol.,* **1969**, *18,* 2135–2143.

2. Reidenberg, M. M.; Ingegerd, O.-C.; von Bahr, C.; Borga, O.; and Sjöqvist, F. Protein binding of diphenylhydantoin and desmethylimipramine in plasma from patients with poor renal function. *N. Engl. J. Med.,* **1971**, *285,* 264–267.

3. Alexanderson, B. Pharmacokinetics of desmethylimipramine and nortriptyline in man after single and multiple oral doses. *Eur. J. Clin. Pharmacol.,* **1972**, *5,* 1–10.

4. Nies, A.; Robinson, D. S.; Friedman, M. J.; Green, R.; Cooper, T. B.; Ravaris, C. L.; and Ives, J. O. Relationship between age and tricyclic antidepressant plasma levels. *Am. J. Psychiatry,* **1977**, *134,* 790–793.

5. Glassman, A. H.; Perel, J. M.; Shostak, M.; Kantor, S. J.; and Fleiss, J. L. Clinical implications of imipramine plasma levels for depressive illness. *Arch. Gen. Psychiatry,* **1977**, *34,* 197–204.

6. Reisby, N.; Gram, L. F.; Bech, P.; Nagy, A.; Petersen, G. O.; Ortmann, J.; Ibsen, I.; Dencker, S. J.; Jacobsen, O.; Krautwald, O.; Sondergaard, I.; and Christiansen, J. Imipramine: clinical effects and pharmacokinetic variability. *Psychopharmacology,* **1977**, *54,* 263–272.

7. Petit, J. M.; Spiker, D. G.; Ruwitch, J. F.; Ziegler, V. E.; Weiss, A. N.; and Biggs, J. T. Tricyclic antidepressant plasma levels and adverse effects after overdose. *Clin. Pharmacol. Ther.,* **1977**, *21,* 45–51.

Key: Adult = adults; Aged = aged; Alb = hypoalbuminemia; AVH = acute viral hepatitis; CF = cystic fibrosis; CHF = congestive heart failure; Child = children; Cirr = cirrhosis; COPD = chronic obstructive pulmonary disease; CP = cor pulmonale; CPBS = cardiopulmonary bypass surgery; CRI = chronic respiratory insufficiency; Cush = cushingoid; Epilep = epilepsy; Fem = females; Hep = hepatitis; HL = hyperlipoproteinemia; HTh = hyperthyroid; Inflam = inflammation; LTh = hypothyroid; MI = myocardial infarction; Neo = neonates; NS = nephrotic syndrome; Obes = obesity; Pneu = pneumonia; Preg = pregnant; Prem = premature infants; RA = rheumatoid arthritis; Smk = smoking; Tach = ventricular tachycardia; Urem = uremia.

DIAZEPAM [a] (Chapters 17, 19, 20)

AVAILABILITY (ORAL) (%)	URINARY EXCRETION (%)	BOUND IN PLASMA (%)	CLEARANCE $(ml \cdot min^{-1} \cdot kg^{-1})$
100 ± 14 (2)	<1 (2)	98.7 ± 0.2 (3) ↓ Urem (3), Cirr (4), Neo (5), Alb [b] (6) ↔ Aged (3,4)	0.38 ± 0.06 [c] (4) ↓ Cirr (4,8), Hep (4) ↔ Aged (4), Smk (4) ↑ Alb (9)

VOL. DIST. (liters/kg)	HALF-LIFE (hours)	EFFECTIVE CONCENTRATIONS	TOXIC CONCENTRATIONS
1.1 ± 0.3 (4) ↑ Cirr (4,8), Aged (4), Alb (9)	20–90 [d] (4) ↑ Aged (4), Cirr (4,8), Hep (4)	>600 ng/ml [e] (10)	—

[a] For review, see (1). Diazepam is metabolized primarily to the active compound, desmethyldiazepam.

[b] Alcoholics.

[c] Calculated assuming 70 kg. Essentially identical values were obtained after oral dosage by Eatman and associates (7), assuming $F = 1$.

[d] Dependent on age.

[e] For control of seizures. There is a poor correlation between concentrations of diazepam in plasma and its anxiolytic effect (11), but such effects are likely at concentrations of 400–600 ng/ml.

1. Mandelli, M.; Tognoni, G.; and Garattini, S. Clinical pharmacokinetics of diazepam. *Clin. Pharmacokinet.,* **1978,** *3,* 72–91.
2. Kaplan, S. A.; Jack, M. L.; Alexander, K.; and Weinfeld, R. E. Pharmacokinetic profile of diazepam in man following single intravenous and oral and chronic oral administrations. *J. Pharm. Sci.,* **1973,** *62,* 1789–1796.
3. Abel, J. G.; Sellers, E. M.; Naranjo, C. A.; Shaw, J.; Kadar, D.; and Romach, M. K. Inter- and intrasubject variation in diazepam free fraction. *Clin. Pharmacol. Ther.,* **1979,** *26,* 247–255.
4. Klotz, U.; Avant, G. R.; Hoyumpa, A.; Schenker, S.; and Wilkinson, G. R. The effects of age and liver disease on the disposition and elimination of diazepam in adult man. *J. Clin. Invest.,* **1975,** *55,* 347–359.
5. Kanto, J.; Erkkola, R.; and Sellman, R. Distribution and metabolism of diazepam in early and late human pregnancy. Postnatal metabolism of diazepam. *Acta Pharmacol. Toxicol. (Kbh.),* **1974,** *35,* Suppl. I, 36.
6. Thiessen, J. J.; Sellers, E. M.; Denbeigh, P.; and Dolman, L. Plasma protein binding of diazepam and tolbutamide in chronic alcoholics. *J. Clin. Pharmacol.,* **1976,** *16,* 345–351.
7. Eatman, F. B., and others. Pharmacokinetics of diazepam following multiple-dose oral administration to healthy human subjects. *J. Pharmacokinet. Biopharm.,* **1977,** *5,* 481–494.
8. Andreasen, P. B.; Hendel, J.; Greisen, G.; and Hvidberg, E. F. Pharmacokinetics of diazepam in disordered liver function. *Eur. J. Clin. Pharmacol.,* **1976,** *10,* 115–120.
9. Klotz, U.; Antonin, K.-H.; and Bieck, P. R. Pharmacokinetics and plasma binding of diazepam in man, dog, rabbit, guinea pig, and rat. *J. Pharmacol. Exp. Ther.,* **1976,** *199,* 67–73.
10. Booker, H. E., and Celesia, G. G. Serum concentrations of diazepam in subjects with epilepsy. *Arch. Neurol.,* **1973,** *29,* 191–194.
11. Tansella, M.; Zimmermann-Tansella, C.; Ferrario, L.; Preziati, L.; Tognoni, G.; and Lader, M. Plasma concentrations of diazepam, nordiazepam and amylobarbitone after short-term treatment in anxious patients. *Pharmakopsychiatr. Neuropsychopharmakol.,* **1978,** *11,* 68–75.

Key: Adult = adults; Aged = aged; Alb = hypoalbuminemia; AVH = acute viral hepatitis; CF = cystic fibrosis; CHF = congestive heart failure; Child = children; Cirr = cirrhosis; COPD = chronic obstructive pulmonary disease; CP = cor pulmonale; CPBS = cardiopulmonary bypass surgery; CRI = chronic respiratory insufficiency; Cush = cushingoid; Epilep = epilepsy; Fem = females; Hep = hepatitis; HL = hyperlipoproteinemia; HTh = hyperthyroid; Inflam = inflammation; LTh = hypothyroid; MI = myocardial infarction; Neo = neonates; NS = nephrotic syndrome; Obes = obesity; Pneu = pneumonia; Preg = pregnant; Prem = premature infants; RA = rheumatoid arthritis; Smk = smoking; Tach = ventricular tachycardia; Urem = uremia.

DICLOXACILLIN (Chapter 50)

AVAILABILITY (ORAL) (%)	URINARY EXCRETION (%)	BOUND IN PLASMA (%)	CLEARANCE $(ml \cdot min^{-1} \cdot kg^{-1})$
50–85 (1,2)	60 ± 7 (1)	94.4 ± 1.9 (3) ↓ Urem (4) ↔ CF (3)	1.6 ± 0.3 [a,b] (1) ↓ Urem (1) ↑ CF [c] (3)

VOL. DIST. (liters/kg)	HALF-LIFE (hours)	EFFECTIVE CONCENTRATIONS	TOXIC CONCENTRATIONS
0.09 ± 0.02 [a] (1) ↑ Urem (1)	0.70 ± 0.07 (1) ↑ Urem (1)	*See* Chapter 50	*See* Chapter 50

[a] Assuming 70-kg body weight.
[b] Possible saturation of renal clearance at doses of 1–2 g (1).
[c] Concomitant increase in clearance of both drug and creatinine.

1. Nauta, E. H., and Mattie, H. Dicloxacillin and cloxacillin: pharmacokinetics in healthy and hemodialysis subjects. *Clin. Pharmacol. Ther.,* **1976,** *20,* 98–108.
2. Doluisio, J. T.; LaPiana, J. C.; Wilkinson, G. R.; and Dittert, L. W. Pharmacokinetic interpretation of dicloxacillin levels in serum after extravascular administration. *Antimicrob. Agents Chemother.,* **1969,** 49–55.
3. Jusko, W. J.; Mosovich, L. L.; Gerbracht, L. M.; Mattar, M. E.; and Yaffe, S. J. Enhanced renal excretion of dicloxacillin in patients with cystic fibrosis. *Pediatrics,* **1975,** *56,* 1038–1044.
4. Craig, W. A.; Evenson, M. A.; Sarver, K. P.; and Wagnild, J. P. Correction of protein binding defect in uremic sera by charcoal treatment. *J. Lab. Clin. Med.,* **1976,** *87,* 637–647.

DIGITOXIN [a] (Chapter 30)

AVAILABILITY (ORAL) (%)	URINARY EXCRETION (%)	BOUND IN PLASMA (%)	CLEARANCE $(ml \cdot min^{-1} \cdot kg^{-1})$
>90 (2)	33 ± 15 [b,c] (3)	90 ± 2 (5) ↓ Urem (5)	0.046 ± 0.023 [b] (3)

VOL. DIST. (liters/kg)	HALF-LIFE (days)	EFFECTIVE CONCENTRATIONS	TOXIC CONCENTRATIONS
0.51 ± 0.18 (6)	6.9 ± 2.7 (7) ↔ Urem (8)	>10 ng/ml [d]	>35 ng/ml [e]

[a] For review, *see* (1). Because availability is probably 100%, parameters listed may be derived from data obtained after oral administration, assuming $F = 1$.
[b] Digitoxin and cardioactive metabolites.
[c] A value of 16% was reported when only digitoxin itself was measured (4).
[d] Concensus of studies.
[e] Probability of toxicity is 50% at this concentration; recalculated from data in (9).

1. Perrier, D.; Mayersohn, M.; and Marcus, F. I. Clinical pharmacokinetics of digitoxin. *Clin. Pharmacokinet.,* **1977,** *2,* 292–311.
2. Beermann, B.; Hellstrom, K.; and Rosen, A. Fate of orally administered ³H-digitoxin in man with special reference to the absorption. *Circulation,* **1971,** *43,* 852–861.
3. Storstein, L. Studies on digitalis. I. Renal excretion of digitoxin and its cardioactive metabolites. *Clin. Pharmacol. Ther.,* **1974,** *16,* 14–24.
4. Lukas, D. S., and Peterson, R. E. Double isotope dilution derivative assay of digitoxin in plasma, urine and stools of patients maintained on the drug. *J. Clin. Invest.,* **1966,** *45,* 782–796.
5. Shoeman, D. W., and Azarnoff, D. L. The alterations of plasma proteins in uremia as reflected in their ability to bind digitoxin and diphenylhydantoin. *Pharmacology,* **1972,** *7,* 169–177.
6. Faust-Tinnefeldt, G. von, and Gilfrich, H. J. Digitoxin-Kinetik unter antirheumatischer Therapie mit Azapropazon. *Arzneim. Forsch.,* **1977,** *27,* 2009–2011.
7. Gjerdrum, K. Digitoxin studies. *Acta Med. Scand.,* **1972,** *191,* 25–34.
8. Rasmussen, K.; Jervell, J.; Storstein, L.; and Gjerdrum, K. Digitoxin kinetics in patients with impaired renal function. *Clin. Pharmacol. Ther.,* **1972,** *13,* 6–14.
9. Storstein, O.; Hansteen, V.; Hatle, L.; Hillestad, L.; and Storstein, L. Studies on digitalis. XIII. A prospective study of 649 patients on maintenance treatment with digitoxin. *Am. Heart J.,* **1977,** *93,* 434–443.

DIGOXIN (Chapter 30)

AVAILABILITY (ORAL) (%)	URINARY EXCRETION (%)	BOUND IN PLASMA (%)	CLEARANCE $(ml \cdot min^{-1} \cdot kg^{-1})$
75 ± 11 [a] (1)	72 ± 9 (2)	25 ± 5 (3) $\downarrow$ Urem (3)	$(0.88\ CL_{cr} + 0.33) \pm 52\%$ [b,c] (4) $\downarrow$ LTh (6) $\uparrow$ HTh (6)

VOL. DIST. (liters/kg)	HALF-LIFE (hours)	EFFECTIVE CONCENTRATIONS	TOXIC CONCENTRATIONS
$(3.12\ CL_{cr} + 3.84) \pm 30\%$ (4) $\downarrow$ LTh (6) $\uparrow$ HTh (6)	42 ± 19 [c] (4) $\downarrow$ HTh (6) $\uparrow$ Urem (4), CHF (4), LTh (6)	>0.8 ng/ml [d] (7)	1.8, 2.6, 3.4 ng/ml [e] (7)

[a] LANOXIN tablets; digoxin solutions, elixirs, and capsules may be absorbed more completely.

[b] Equation applies to patients with some degree of heart failure. If heart failure is not present, the coefficient of CL_{cr} is 1.0. Units of CL_{cr} must be ml · min⁻¹ · kg⁻¹.

[c] Occasional individuals metabolize digoxin very rapidly to an inactive metabolite, dihydrodigoxin (5).

[d] Inotropic effect.

[e] Concentrations at which the probability of digoxin-induced arrhythmias are 10, 50, and 90%, respectively.

1. Johnson, B. F.; Bye, C.; Jones, G.; and Sobey, G. A. A completely absorbed oral preparation of digoxin. *Clin. Pharmacol. Ther.*, **1976**, *19*, 746–751.
2. Koup, J. R.; Greenblatt, D. J.; Jusko, W. J.; Smith, T. W.; and Koch-Weser, J. Pharmacokinetics of digoxin in normal subjects after intravenous bolus and infusion doses. *J. Pharmacokinet. Biopharm.*, **1975**, *3*, 181–192.
3. Koup, J. R.; Jusko, W. J.; Elwood, C. M.; and Kobli, R. K. Digoxin pharmacokinetics: role of renal failure in dosage regimen design. *Clin. Pharmacol. Ther.*, **1975**, *18*, 9–21.
4. Sheiner, L. B.; Rosenberg, B. G.; and Marathe, V. V.

Estimation of population characteristics of pharmacokinetic parameters from routine clinical data. *J. Pharmacokinet. Biopharm.*, **1977**, *5*, 445–479.
5. Peters, U.; Falk, L. C.; and Kalman, S. M. Digoxin metabolism in patients. *Arch. Intern. Med.*, **1978**, *138*, 1074–1076.
6. Lawrence, J. R.; Sumner, D. J.; Kalk, W. J.; Ratcliffe, W. A.; Whiting, B.; Gray, K.; and Lindsay, M. Digoxin kinetics in patients with thyroid dysfunction. *Clin. Pharmacol. Ther.*, **1977**, *22*, 7–13.
7. Iisalo, E.; Dahl, M.; and Sundquist, H. Serum digoxin in adults and children. *Int. J. Clin. Pharmacol.*, **1973**, *7*, 219–222.

DISOPYRAMIDE (Chapter 31)

AVAILABILITY (ORAL) (%)	URINARY EXCRETION (%)	BOUND IN PLASMA (%)	CLEARANCE $(ml \cdot min^{-1} \cdot kg^{-1})$
83 ± 11 [a] (1)	55 ± 6 [b] (1)	68% at 0.38 µg/ml 28% at 3.8 µg/ml (4)	1.3 ± 0.7 [c] (5) $\downarrow$ MI (2), Tach (6)

VOL. DIST. (liters/kg)	HALF-LIFE (hours)	EFFECTIVE CONCENTRATIONS	TOXIC CONCENTRATIONS
0.78 ± 0.26 [c] (5)	7.8 ± 1.6 (5) $\leftrightarrow$ MI [d] (2)	Atrial arrhythmias: 2.8–3.2 µg/ml (7) Ventricular arrhythmias: 3.3–7.5 µg/ml (7) 3 ± 1 µg/ml (8)	—

[a] Plasma concentrations are lower after oral administration of disopyramide to patients who have had a myocardial infarction (2).

[b] No effect of urinary pH (3,4).

[c] Values calculated by dividing by mean weight.

[d] Others indicate that half-life is increased in a dose-dependent manner (9).

1. Hinderling, P. H., and Garrett, E. R. Pharmacokinetics of the antiarrhythymic disopyramide in healthy humans. *J. Pharmacokinet. Biopharm.*, **1976**, *4*, 199–230.
2. Ward, J. W., and Kinghorn, G. R. The pharmacokinetics of disopyramide following myocardial infarction with special reference to oral and intravenous dose regimens. *J. Int. Med. Res.*, **1976**, *4*, Suppl. 1, 49–53.
3. Ankier, S. I., and Kaye, C. M. The influence of pH on the buccal absorption and renal excretion of disopyramide in man. *Br. J. Clin. Pharmacol.*, **1976**, *3*, 672–673.
4. Cunningham, J. L.; Shen, D. D.; Shudo, J.; and Azarnoff, D. L. The effects of urine pH and plasma protein binding on the renal clearance of disopyramide. *Clin. Pharmacokinet.*, **1977**, *2*, 373–383.
5. Bryson, S. M.; Whiting, B.; and Lawrence, J. R. Diso-

pyramide serum and pharmacologic effect kinetics applied to the assessment of bioavailability. *Br. J. Clin. Pharmacol.*, **1978**, *6*, 409–419.
6. Rangno, R. E.; Warnica, W.; Ogilvie, R. I.; Kreeft, J.; and Bridger, E. Correlation of disopyramide pharmacokinetics with efficacy in ventricular tachyarrhythmia. *J. Int. Med. Res.*, **1976**, *4*, Suppl. 1, 54–58.
7. Niarchos, A. P. Disopyramide: serum level and arrhythmia conversion. *Am. Heart J.*, **1976**, *92*, 57–64.
8. Mizgala, H. F., and Huvelle, P. R. Acute termination of cardiac arrhythmias with intravenous disopyramide. *J. Int. Med. Res.*, **1976**, *4*, Suppl. 1, 82–85.
9. Ilett, K.; Madsen, B. W.; and Woods, J. D. Disopyramide kinetics in patients with acute myocardial infarction. *Clin. Pharmacol. Ther.*, **1979**, *26*, 1–7.

DOXEPIN (Chapter 19)

AVAILABILITY (ORAL) (%)	URINARY EXCRETION (%)	BOUND IN PLASMA (%)	CLEARANCE $(ml \cdot min^{-1} \cdot kg^{-1})$
27 ± 10 [a] (1)	~0 (1)	—	14 ± 3 [b] (1)

VOL. DIST. (liters/kg)	HALF-LIFE (hours)	EFFECTIVE CONCENTRATIONS	TOXIC CONCENTRATIONS
20 ± 8 [b,c] (1)	17 ± 6 [d] (1)	30–150 ng/ml [e] (2)	—

[a] Calculated from results of oral administration only, assuming complete absorption, elimination only by the liver, hepatic blood flow of 1500 ml/min, and equal partition between plasma and erythrocytes.
[b] Calculated assuming $F = 0.27$.
[c] Vd_{area}.
[d] Active metabolite desmethyldoxepin has a longer half-life (51 ± 17 hours) (1).
[e] Doxepin + desmethyldoxepin; optimal concentrations have not been defined.

1. Ziegler, V. E.; Biggs, J. T.; Wylie, L. T.; Rosen, S. H.; Hawt, D. J.; and Coryell, W. H. Doxepin kinetics. *Clin. Pharmacol. Ther.*, **1978**, *23*, 573–579.

2. Biggs, J. T.; Preskorn, S. H.; Ziegler, V. E.; Rosen, S. H.; and Meyer, D. A. Dosage schedule and plasma levels of doxepin and desmethyldoxepin. *J. Clin. Psychiatry*, **1978**, *39*, 740–742.

DOXYCYCLINE (Chapter 52)

AVAILABILITY (ORAL) (%)	URINARY EXCRETION (%)	BOUND IN PLASMA (%)	CLEARANCE $(ml \cdot min^{-1} \cdot kg^{-1})$
93 (1)	40 ± 4 (2)	82–93 (3,4)	—

VOL. DIST. (liters/kg)	HALF-LIFE (hours)	EFFECTIVE CONCENTRATIONS	TOXIC CONCENTRATIONS
0.9–1.8 [a] (5)	20 ± 4 (2) ↔ Urem (2)	*See* Chapter 52	—

[a] Value in children; Vd/F.

1. Fabre, J.; Milek, E.; Kalfopoulos, P.; and Mérier, G. La cinétique des tétracyclines chez l'homme. *Schweiz. Med. Wochenschr.*, **1971**, *101*, 593–598.
2. Mérier, G.; Laurencet, F. L.; Rudhardt, M.; Chuit, A.; and Fabre, J. Behaviour of doxycycline in renal insufficiency. *Helv. Med. Acta*, **1969/70**, *35*, 124–134.
3. Rosenblatt, J. E.; Barrett, J. E.; Brodie, J. L.; and Kirby, W. M. M. Comparison of *in vitro* activity and clinical pharmacology of doxycycline with other tetracyclines.

Antimicrob. Agents Chemother., **1966**, 134–141.
4. Schach von Wittenau, M., and Yeary, R. The excretion and distribution in body fluids of tetracyclines after intravenous administration to dogs. *J. Pharmacol. Exp. Ther.*, **1963**, *140*, 258–266.
5. Ceccarelli, G.; Rossoni, R.; Romita, F.; and Naddeo, A. Pharmacokinetic study of doxycycline in children. *Chemotherapy*, **1971**, *16*, 1–10.

Key: Adult = adults; Aged = aged; Alb = hypoalbuminemia; AVH = acute viral hepatitis; CF = cystic fibrosis; CHF = congestive heart failure; Child = children; Cirr = cirrhosis; COPD = chronic obstructive pulmonary disease; CP = cor pulmonale; CPBS = cardiopulmonary bypass surgery; CRI = chronic respiratory insufficiency; Cush = cushingoid; Epilep = epilepsy; Fem = females; Hep = hepatitis; HL = hyperlipoproteinemia; HTh = hyperthyroid; Inflam = inflammation; LTh = hypothyroid; MI = myocardial infarction; Neo = neonates; NS = nephrotic syndrome; Obes = obesity; Pneu = pneumonia; Preg = pregnant; Prem = premature infants; RA = rheumatoid arthritis; Smk = smoking; Tach = ventricular tachycardia; Urem = uremia.

ERYTHROMYCIN (Chapter 54)

AVAILABILITY (ORAL) (%)	URINARY EXCRETION (%)	BOUND IN PLASMA (%)	CLEARANCE $(ml \cdot min^{-1} \cdot kg^{-1})$
18–45 [a] (1)	10–15 (3)	72 ± 3 [b] (4)	6.0 ± 2.5 (5) ↔ Urem (5)

VOL. DIST. (liters/kg)	HALF-LIFE (hours)	EFFECTIVE CONCENTRATIONS	TOXIC CONCENTRATIONS
0.72 ± 0.20 (5) ↑ Urem (5)	1.1–3.5 (2,3,5–7) ↔, ↑ Urem (5,8)	See Chapter 54	—

[a] Range of values after administration of erythromycin stearate film-coated tablets in the presence of carbohydrate, protein, and fat meals or to fasted subjects; calculated assuming $Vd = 0.7$ liters/kg (1). After administration of erythromycin estolate, total concentrations of the antibiotic in plasma are higher than with the stearate, but concentrations of the free base are lower (2).

[b] Erythromycin base. Values for the propionate ester range from 90–99% (2,3).

1. Welling, P. G.; Huang, H.; Hewitt, P. F.; and Lyons, L. L. Bioavailability of erythromycin stearate: influence of food and fluid volume. *J. Pharm. Sci.,* **1978,** *67,* 764–766.
2. Welling, P. G.; Elliott, R. L.; Pitterle, M. E.; Corrick-West, H. P.; and Lyons, L. L. Plasma levels following single and repeated doses of erythromycin estolate and erythromycin stearate. *J. Pharm. Sci.,* **1979,** *68,* 150–155.
3. Griffith, R. S.; Johnstone, D. M.; and Smith, J. W. The distribution and excretion of erythromycin following intravenous injection. *Antibiot. Ann.,* **1953–1954,** 496–499.
4. Gordon, R. C.; Regamey, C.; and Kirby, W. M. M. Serum protein binding of erythromycin, lincomycin, and clindamycin. *J. Pharm. Sci.,* **1973,** *62,* 1074–1076.
5. Welling, P. G., and Craig, W. A. Pharmacokinetics of intravenous erythromycin. *J. Pharm. Sci.,* **1978,** *67,* 1057–1059.
6. Wiegand, R. G., and Chun, A. H. C. Serum protein binding of erythromycin and erythromycin 2′-propionate ester. *J. Pharm. Sci.,* **1972,** *61,* 425–428.
7. Colburn, W. A.; DiSanto, A. R.; and Gibaldi, M. Pharmacokinetics of erythromycin on repetitive dosing. *J. Clin. Pharmacol.,* **1977,** *17,* 592–600.
8. Kunin, C. M., and Finland, M. Persistence of antibiotics in blood of patients with acute renal failure. III. Penicillin, streptomycin, erythromycin, and kanamycin. *J. Clin. Invest.,* **1959,** *38,* 1509–1519.

ETHAMBUTOL (Chapter 53)

AVAILABILITY (ORAL) (%)	URINARY EXCRETION (%)	BOUND IN PLASMA (%)	CLEARANCE $(ml \cdot min^{-1} \cdot kg^{-1})$
77 ± 8 (1)	79 ± 3 (1)	20–30 (2)	8.6 ± 0.8 (1)

VOL. DIST. (liters/kg)	HALF-LIFE (hours)	EFFECTIVE CONCENTRATIONS	TOXIC CONCENTRATIONS
1.6 ± 0.2 [a] (1)	3.1 ± 0.4 [a,b] (1) ↑ Urem (3)	—	>10 μg/ml [c]

[a] Two-compartment model.
[b] Over 72 hours, three exponentials are required (1).
[c] Estimated from kinetics and dosage at which visual toxicity occurs.

1. Lee, C. S.; Brater, D. C.; Gambertoglio, J. G.; and Benet, L. Z. Disposition kinetics of ethambutol. *J. Pharmacokinet. Biopharm.,* **1980,** *8.*
2. Lee, C. S.; Gambertoglio, J. G.; Brater, D. C.; and Benet, L. Z. Kinetics of oral ethambutol in the normal subject. *Clin. Pharmacol. Ther.,* **1977,** *22,* 615–621.
3. Dume, Th.; Wagner, Cl.; and Wetzels, E. Zur Pharmakokinetik von Ethambutol bei Gesunden und Patients mit terminaler Niereninsuffizienz. *Dtsch. Med. Wochenschr.,* **1971,** *96,* 1430–1434.

ETHANOL (Chapter 18)

AVAILABILITY (ORAL) (%)	URINARY EXCRETION (%)	BOUND IN PLASMA (%)	CLEARANCE
100 (1)	<3 (2)	—	$V_m = 124 \pm 10 \text{ mg} \cdot \text{kg}^{-1} \cdot \text{hr}^{-1}$ $K_m = 82 \pm 29 \text{ mg/l}$ [a] (3)

VOL. DIST. (*liters/kg*)	HALF-LIFE (*hours*)	EFFECTIVE CONCENTRATIONS	TOXIC CONCENTRATIONS
0.54 ± 0.05 (3)	0.24 ± 0.08 [a] (3)	—	1000–1500 mg/l [b]

[a] Ethanol is eliminated by a saturable (Michaelis-Menten) process; the half-life given is the fastest possible—that theoretically present at zero concentration.

[b] Legal basis for intoxication in many states of the United States.

1. Wilkinson, P. K.; Sedman, A. J.; Sakmar, E.; Kay, D. R.; and Wagner, J. G. Pharmacokinetics of ethanol after oral administration in the fasting state. *J. Pharmacokinet. Biopharm.*, **1977**, *5*, 207–224.
2. Vestal, R. E.; McGuire, E. A.; Tobin, J. D.; Andres, R.; Norris, A. H.; and Mezey, E. Aging and ethanol metabolism. *Clin. Pharmacol. Ther.*, **1977**, *19*, 343–354.
3. Wilkinson, P. K.; Sedman, A. J.; Sakmar, E.; Earhart, R. H.; Weidler, D. J.; and Wagner, J. G. Blood ethanol concentrations during and following constant-rate intravenous infusion of alcohol. *Clin. Pharmacol. Ther.*, **1976**, *19*, 213–223.

ETHOSUXIMIDE [a] (Chapter 20)

AVAILABILITY (ORAL) (%)	URINARY EXCRETION (%)	BOUND IN PLASMA (%)	CLEARANCE ($ml \cdot min^{-1} \cdot kg^{-1}$)
—	19 (1)	0 (2)	0.26 ± 0.05 [b,c] (3) ↓ Adult (1)

VOL. DIST. (*liters/kg*)	HALF-LIFE (*hours*)	EFFECTIVE CONCENTRATIONS	TOXIC CONCENTRATIONS
0.72 ± 0.07 [b] (3) ↔ Adult (1)	33 ± 6 (3) ↑ Adult (1)	40–100 μg/ml (5)	

[a] All values are for children.

[b] Data from oral, multiple-dose regimen; values are CL/F and Vd_{area}/F.

[c] Clearance may decrease as dose is increased (4).

1. Buchanan, R. A.; Kinkel, A. W.; and Smith, T. C. The absorption and excretion of ethosuximide. *Int. J. Clin. Pharmacol.*, **1973**, *7*, 213–218.
2. Chang, T.; Dill, W. A.; and Glazko, A. J. Ethosuximide— absorption, distribution and excretion. In, *Antiepileptic Drugs.* (Woodbury, D. M.; Penry, J. K.; and Schmidt, R. P.; eds.) Raven Press, New York, **1972**, pp. 417–423.
3. Buchanan, R. A.; Fernandez, L.; and Kinkel, A. W. Absorption and elimination of ethosuximide in children. *J. Clin. Pharmacol.*, **1969**, *9*, 393–398.
4. Smith, G. A.; McKauge, L.; Dubetz, D.; Tyrer, J. H.; and Eadie, M. J. Factors influencing plasma concentrations of ethosuximide. *Clin. Pharmacokinet.*, **1979**, *4*, 38–52.
5. Browne, T. R.; Dreifuss, F. E.; Dryken, P. R.; Goode, D. J.; Penry, J. K.; Porter, R. J.; White, B. G.; and White, P. T. Ethosuximide in the treatment of absence (petit mal) seizures. *Neurology (Minneap.)*, **1975**, *25*, 515–524.

Key: Adult = adults; Aged = aged; Alb = hypoalbuminemia; AVH = acute viral hepatitis; CF = cystic fibrosis; CHF = congestive heart failure; Child = children; Cirr = cirrhosis; COPD = chronic obstructive pulmonary disease; CP = cor pulmonale; CPBS = cardiopulmonary bypass surgery; CRI = chronic respiratory insufficiency; Cush = cushingoid; Epilep = epilepsy; Fem = females; Hep = hepatitis; HL = hyperlipoproteinemia; HTh = hyperthyroid; Inflam = inflammation; LTh = hypothyroid; MI = myocardial infarction; Neo = neonates; NS = nephrotic syndrome; Obes = obesity; Pneu = pneumonia; Preg = pregnant; Prem = premature infants; RA = rheumatoid arthritis; Smk = smoking; Tach = ventricular tachycardia; Urem = uremia.

FLUCYTOSINE (Chapter 54)

AVAILABILITY (ORAL) (%)	URINARY EXCRETION (%)	BOUND IN PLASMA (%)	CLEARANCE ($ml \cdot min^{-1} \cdot kg^{-1}$)
High	63–84 [a] (1)	4 (2)	$CL_{renal} = 0.75\, CL_{cr}$ (1)

VOL. DIST. (liters/kg)	HALF-LIFE (hours)	EFFECTIVE CONCENTRATIONS	TOXIC CONCENTRATIONS
0.57 ± 0.02 [b] (1)	5.3 ± 0.7 (1) ↑ Urem (1)	See Chapter 54	See Chapter 54

[a] Oral dose.
[b] Assumes $F = 1$.

1. Dawborn, J. K.; Page, M. D.; and Schiavone, D. J. Use of 5-fluorocytosine in patients with impaired renal function. *Br. Med. J.,* **1973,** *3,* 382–384.
2. Block, E. R.; Bennett, J. E.; Livoti, L. G.; Klein, W. J., Jr.; MacGregor, R. R.; and Henderson, L. Flucytosine and amphotericin B; hemodialysis effects on the plasma concentration and clearance. *Ann. Intern. Med.,* **1974,** *80,* 613–617.

FLUNITRAZEPAM (Chapter 17)

AVAILABILITY (ORAL) (%)	URINARY EXCRETION (%)	BOUND IN PLASMA (%)	CLEARANCE ($ml \cdot min^{-1} \cdot kg^{-1}$)
~85 (1)	<1 (2)	77–79 (1)	1.9 (3) 3.5 ± 0.4 [a] (1)

VOL. DIST. (liters/kg)	HALF-LIFE (hours)	EFFECTIVE CONCENTRATIONS	TOXIC CONCENTRATIONS
2.5 (3) 3.3 ± 0.6 [a] (1)	15 ± 5 (1) 21 (3)	—	—

[a] CL/F and Vd_{ss}/F.

1. Boxenbaum, H. G.; Posmanter, H. N.; Macasieb, T.; Geitner, K. A.; Weinfeld, R. E.; Moore, J. D.; Darragh, A.; O'Kelly, D. A.; Weissman, L.; and Kaplan, S. A. Pharmacokinetics of flunitrazepam following single- and multiple-dose oral administration to healthy human subjects. *J. Pharmacokinet. Biopharm.,* **1978,** *6,* 283–293.
2. Wendt, G. Schicksal des Hypnotikums Flunitrazepam in menschlichen Organismus. In, *Bisherige Erfahrungen mit* ROHYPNOL *(Flunitrazepam) in der Anästhesiologie und Intensivtherapie.* (Hügin, W.; Hossli, G.; and Gemperle, M.; eds.) F. Hoffmann–La Roche & Co., A.G., Basel, **1976,** pp. 27–38.
3. Amrein, R.; Cano, J.-P.; and Hügin, W. Pharmakokinetische und pharmakodynamische Befunde nach einmaliger intravenöser, intramuskulärer und oraler Applikation von "ROHYPNOL." In, *Bisherige Erfahrungen mit* ROHYPNOL *(Flunitrazepam) in der Anästhesiologie und Intensivtherapie.* (Hügin, W.; Hossli, G.; and Gemperle, M.; eds.) F. Hoffmann–La Roche & Co., A. G., Basel, **1976,** pp. 39–56.

Key: Adult = adults; Aged = aged; Alb = hypoalbuminemia; AVH = acute viral hepatitis; CF = cystic fibrosis; CHF = congestive heart failure; Child = children; Cirr = cirrhosis; COPD = chronic obstructive pulmonary disease; CP = cor pulmonale; CPBS = cardiopulmonary bypass surgery; CRI = chronic respiratory insufficiency; Cush = cushingoid; Epilep = epilepsy; Fem = females; Hep = hepatitis; HL = hyperlipoproteinemia; HTh = hyperthyroid; Inflam = inflammation; LTh = hypothyroid; MI = myocardial infarction; Neo = neonates; NS = nephrotic syndrome; Obes = obesity; Pneu = pneumonia; Preg = pregnant; Prem = premature infants; RA = rheumatoid arthritis; Smk = smoking; Tach = ventricular tachycardia; Urem = uremia.

FUROSEMIDE [a] (Chapter 36)

AVAILABILITY (ORAL) (%)	URINARY EXCRETION (%)	BOUND IN PLASMA (%)	CLEARANCE $(ml \cdot min^{-1} \cdot kg^{-1})$
63 ± 9 (2)	74 ± 7 (3)	95.9 ± 2.0 (2) ↓ Urem (2), NS (2) ↔ CHF (4)	2.2 ± 0.3 (2) ↓ Urem (2), CHF (4), Neo (5)

VOL. DIST. (liters/kg)	HALF-LIFE (hours)	EFFECTIVE CONCENTRATIONS	TOXIC CONCENTRATIONS
0.11 ± 0.02 (2) ↔ Urem (2), CHF (4) ↑ NS (2), Neo (5)	0.85 ± 0.17 (2) ↔ NS (2) ↑ Urem (2), CHF (4), Neo (5)	—	—

[a] For review, see (1).

1. Benet, L. Z. Pharmacokinetics/pharmacodynamics of furosemide in man: a review. *J. Pharmacokinet. Biopharm.,* **1979,** *7,* 1–27.
2. Rane, A.; Villeneuve, J. P.; Stone, W. J.; Nies, A. S.; Wilkinson, G. R.; and Branch, R. A. Plasma binding and disposition of furosemide in the nephrotic syndrome and in uremia. *Clin. Pharmacol. Ther.,* **1978,** *24,* 199–207.
3. Smith, D. E.; Brater, D. C.; Lin, E. T.; and Benet, L. Z. Attenuation of furosemide's diuretic effect by indomethacin:

pharmacokinetic evaluation. *J. Pharmacokinet. Biopharm.,* **1979,** *7,* 265–274.
4. Andreasen, F., and Mikkelsen, E. Distribution, elimination and effect of furosemide in normal subjects and in patients with heart failure. *Eur. J. Clin. Pharmacol.,* **1977,** *12,*15–22.
5. Aranda, J. V.; Perez, J.; Sitar, D. S.; Collinge, J.; Portuguez-Malavasi, A.; Duffy, B.; and Dupont, C. Pharmacokinetic disposition and protein binding of furosemide in newborn infants. *J. Pediatr.,* **1978,** *93,* 507–511.

GENTAMICIN (Chapter 51)

AVAILABILITY (ORAL) (%)	URINARY EXCRETION (%)	BOUND IN PLASMA (%)	CLEARANCE $(ml \cdot min^{-1} \cdot kg^{-1})$
—	>90 (1)	<10 (2)	$CL = 0.73\ CL_{cr} + 0.06$ [a] (3–7)

VOL. DIST. (liters/kg)	HALF-LIFE (hours)	EFFECTIVE CONCENTRATIONS	TOXIC CONCENTRATIONS
0.25 [a] (3–7) ↔ Urem (6)	2–3 [a] (3–7) ↑ Urem (3–8) 53 ± 25 [b] (8)	See Chapter 51	See Chapter 51

[a] Calculated by combination of data from various studies (3–7).

[b] Gentamicin has a very long terminal half-life, which accounts for urinary excretion for up to 3 weeks (see Chapter 51).

1. Schentag, J. J.; Jusko, W. J.; Plant, M. E.; Cumbo, T. J.; Vance, J. W.; and Abrutyn, E. Tissue persistence of gentamicin in man. *J.A.M.A.,* **1977,** *238,* 327–329.
2. Christopher, T. G.; Blair, A. D.; Forrey, A. W.; and Cutler, R. E. Hemodialyzer clearances of gentamicin, kanamycin, tobramycin, amikacin, ethambutol, procainamide, and flucytosine, with a technique for planning therapy. *J. Pharmacokinet. Biopharm.,* **1976,** *4,* 427–441.
3. Hull, H. J., and Sarubbi, F. A. Gentamicin serum concentrations: pharmacokinetic parameters. *Ann. Intern. Med.,* **1976,** *85,* 183–189.
4. Cutler, R. E.; Gyselynck, A. M.; Fleet, W. P.; and Forrey, A. W. Correlation of serum creatinine concentration and gentamicin half-life. *J.A.M.A.,* **1972,** *219,* 1037–1041.

5. Chan, R.; Benner, E.; and Hoeprich, P. Gentamicin therapy in renal failure: a nomogram for dosage. *Ann. Intern. Med.,* **1972,** *76,* 773–778.
6. Barza, M.; Brown, R. B.; Shen, D.; Gibaldi, M.; and Weinstein, L. Predictability of blood levels of gentamicin in man. *J. Infect. Dis.,* **1975,** *132,* 165–174.
7. Gyselynck, A. M.; Forrey, A.; and Cutler, R. E. Pharmacokinetics of gentamicin: distribution and plasma and renal clearance. *J. Infect. Dis.,* **1971,** *124,* Suppl., 570–576.
8. Schentag, J. J.; Jusko, W. J.; Vance, J. W.; Cumbo, T. J.; Abrutyn, E.; DeLattre, M.; and Gerbracht, L. M. Gentamicin disposition and tissue accumulation on multiple dosing. *J. Pharmacokinet. Biopharm.,* **1977,** *5,* 559–577.

HEPARIN (Chapter 58)

AVAILABILITY (ORAL) (%)	URINARY EXCRETION (%)	BOUND IN PLASMA (%)	CLEARANCE ($ml \cdot min^{-1} \cdot kg^{-1}$)
—	Negligible (1)	Extensive (2)	0.73 ± 0.17 0.45 ± 0.05 (3) [a] 0.28 ± 0.05

VOL. DIST. (liters/kg)	HALF-LIFE (hours)	EFFECTIVE CONCENTRATIONS	TOXIC CONCENTRATIONS
0.06 ± 0.01 [b] (3)	1.0 ± 0.2 1.6 ± 0.2 (3) [a] 2.5 ± 0.2	*See* Chapter 58	—

[a] Although elimination is apparently first order at any single dose, clearance and half-life are dependent on dose. The values given are for doses of 100 I.U./kg, 200 I.U./kg, and 400 I.U./kg, respectively. This behavior can be explained by assuming saturable metabolism with end-product inhibition (4).

[b] Vd_{area}.

1. Estes, J. W. The fate of heparin in the body. *Curr. Ther. Res.*, **1975**, *18*, 45–57.
2. Estes, J. W., and Poulem, P. F. Pharmacokinetics of heparin. *Thromb. Diath. Haemorrh.*, **1974**, *33*, 26–37.
3. Olsson, P.; Lagergren, H.; and Ek, S. The elimination from plasma of intravenous heparin. *Acta Med. Scand.*, **1963**, *173*, 619–630.
4. McAvoy, T. J. Pharmacokinetic modeling of heparin and its clinical implications. *J. Pharmacokinet. Biopharm.*, **1979**, *7*, 331–354.

HEXOBARBITAL (Chapter 17)

AVAILABILITY (ORAL) (%)	URINARY EXCRETION (%)	BOUND IN PLASMA (%)	CLEARANCE ($ml \cdot min^{-1} \cdot kg^{-1}$)
—	<1 (1)	42–52 (1) $\leftrightarrow$ Cirr (1)	3.6 ± 0.8 (2) $\downarrow$ Cirr (1), AVH (3)

VOL. DIST. (liters/kg)	HALF-LIFE (hours)	EFFECTIVE CONCENTRATIONS	TOXIC CONCENTRATIONS
1.1 ± 0.1 (2) $\leftrightarrow$ Cirr (1), AVH (3)	4.4 ± 1.2 (2) $\uparrow$ Cirr (1), AVH (3)	—	—

1. Zilly, W.; Breimer, D. D.; and Richter, E. Hexobarbital disposition in compensated and decompensated cirrhosis of the liver. *Clin. Pharmacol. Ther.*, **1978**, *23*, 525–534.
2. Breimer, D. D.; Honhoff, C.; Zilly, W.; Richter, E.; and van Rossum, J. M. Pharmacokinetics of hexobarbital in man after intravenous infusion. *J. Pharmacokinet. Biopharm.*, **1975**, *3*, 1–11.
3. Breimer, D. D.; Zilly, W.; and Richter, E. Pharmacokinetics of hexobarbital in acute hepatitis and after apparent recovery. *Clin. Pharmacol. Ther.*, **1975**, *18*, 433–440.

HYDRALAZINE [a,b] (Chapter 32)

AVAILABILITY (ORAL) (%)	URINARY EXCRETION (%)	BOUND IN PLASMA (%)	CLEARANCE ($ml \cdot min^{-1} \cdot kg^{-1}$)
31 ± 7 [b,c,d] (3) 50 ± 7 [e] (3)	12 ± 0.4 [c] (3) 14 ± 0.1 [e] (3)	87 (5)	10 ± 6 [c] (3) 8 ± 2 [e] (3)

VOL. DIST. (liters/kg)	HALF-LIFE (hours)	EFFECTIVE CONCENTRATIONS	TOXIC CONCENTRATIONS
1.6 ± 0.3 (3)	2.2 ± 0.4 [c] (6) 2.6 ± 0.4 [e] (6) $\uparrow$ Urem (7)	$1~\mu g/ml$ [f] (8)	—

a For review, *see* (1). All values for hydralazine may be inaccurate because of poor specificity of the assays used and because of instability of hydralazine and its metabolites (2).

b Hydralazine is metabolized by N-acetylation; slow and fast acetylators exhibit different rates of inactivation.

c Fast acetylators.

d Rapid absorption of large doses (>100 mg) may saturate first-pass metabolism, and availability may increase (3); availability may also increase when taken with meals (4).

e Slow acetylators.

f To achieve a reduction in mean arterial pressure of 20 mm Hg in moderate or severe hypertension when given concurrently with hydrochlorothiazide and propranolol.

1. Talseth, T. Clinical pharmacokinetics of hydralazine. *Clin. Pharmacokinet.*, **1977**, *2*, 317–329.
2. Reece, P. A.; Stanely, P. E.; and Zacest, R. Interference in assays for hydralazine in humans by a major plasma metabolite, hydralazine pyruvic acid hydrazone. *J. Pharm. Sci.*, **1978**, *67*, 1150–1153.
3. Talseth, T. Studies on hydralazine. III. Bioavailability of hydralazine in man. *Eur. J. Clin. Pharmacol.*, **1976**, *10*, 395–401.
4. Melander, A.; Danielson, K.; Hanson, A.; Rudell, B.; Schersten, B.; Tholin, T.; and Wahlin, E. Enhancement of hydralazine bioavailability by food. *Clin. Pharmacol. Ther.*, **1977**, *22*, 104–107.

5. Lesser, J. M.; Israili, Z. H.; Davis, D. C.; and Dayton, P. G. Metabolism and disposition of hydralazine-^{14}C in man and dog. *Drug Metab. Dispos.*, **1974**, *2*, 351–360.
6. Talseth, T. Studies on hydralazine. I. Serum concentrations of hydralazine in man after a single dose and at steady state. *Eur. J. Clin. Pharmacol.*, **1976**, *10*, 183–187.
7. Talseth, T. Studies on hydralazine. II. Elimination rate and steady-state concentration in patients with impaired renal function. *Eur. J. Clin. Pharmacol.*, **1976**, *10*, 311–317.
8. Zacest, R., and Koch-Weser, J. Relation of hydralazine plasma concentration to dosage and hypotensive action. *Clin. Pharmacol. Ther.*, **1972**, *13*, 420–425.

HYDROCHLOROTHIAZIDE (Chapter 36)

AVAILABILITY (ORAL) (%)	URINARY EXCRETION (%)	BOUND IN PLASMA (%)	CLEARANCE $(ml \cdot min^{-1} \cdot kg^{-1})$
71 ± 15 (1)	>95 (2)	64 (3)	4.9 ± 1.1 a (4) ↓CHF (5,6), Urem (6)

VOL. DIST. (*liters/kg*)	HALF-LIFE (*hours*)	EFFECTIVE CONCENTRATIONS	TOXIC CONCENTRATIONS
0.83 ± 0.31 b (4)	2.5 ± 0.2 (7) ↑CHF (5)	—	—

a Renal clearance, which should approximate total plasma clearance; calculated assuming 70 kg.

b Calculated from individual values of renal clearance, terminal half-life, and fraction of drug excreted unchanged, 70-kg body weight assumed.

1. Beermann, B.; Groschinsky-Grind, M.; and Lindstrom, B. Bioavailability of two hydrochlorothiazide preparations. *Eur. J. Clin. Pharmacol.*, **1977**, *11*, 203–205.
2. Beermann, B.; Groschinsky-Grind, M.; and Rosen, A. Absorption, metabolism, and excretion of hydrochlorothiazide. *Clin. Pharmacol. Ther.*, **1976**, *19*, 531–537.
3. Data supplied by Merck, Sharp and Dohme Research Laboratories, West Point, Pennsylvania.
4. Beermann, B., and Groschinsky-Grind, M. Pharmacokinetics of hydrochlorothiazide in man. *Eur. J. Clin. Pharmacol.*, **1977**, *12*, 297–303.

5. ———. Pharmacokinetics of hydrochlorothiazide in patients with congestive heart failure. *Br. J. Clin. Pharmacol.*, **1979**, *8*, 579–583.
6. Anderson, K. V.; Brettell, H. R.; and Aikawa, J. K. C^{14}-Labeled hydrochlorothiazide in human beings. *Arch. Intern. Med.*, **1961**, *107*, 168–174.
7. Jordo, L.; Johnsson, G.; Lundborg, P.; Persson, B. A.; Regårdh, C. G.; and Ronn, O. Bioavailability and disposition of metoprolol and hydrochlorothiazide combined in one tablet and of separate doses of hydrochlorothiazide. *Br. J. Clin. Pharmacol.*, **1979**, *7*, 563–567.

Key: Adult = adults; Aged = aged; Alb = hypoalbuminemia; AVH = acute viral hepatitis; CF = cystic fibrosis; CHF = congestive heart failure; Child = children; Cirr = cirrhosis; COPD = chronic obstructive pulmonary disease; CP = cor pulmonale; CPBS = cardiopulmonary bypass surgery; CRI = chronic respiratory insufficiency; Cush = cushingoid; Epilep = epilepsy; Fem = females; Hep = hepatitis; HL = hyperlipoproteinemia; HTh = hyperthyroid; Inflam = inflammation; LTh = hypothyroid; MI = myocardial infarction; Neo = neonates; NS = nephrotic syndrome; Obes = obesity; Pneu = pneumonia; Preg = pregnant; Prem = premature infants; RA = rheumatoid arthritis; Smk = smoking; Tach = ventricular tachycardia; Urem = uremia.

IMIPRAMINE (Chapter 19)

AVAILABILITY (ORAL) (%)	URINARY EXCRETION (%)	BOUND IN PLASMA (%)	CLEARANCE $(ml \cdot min^{-1} \cdot kg^{-1})$
47 ± 21 [a] (1)	0–1.7 (2)	89–94 (3) ↑ HL (4)	20 ± 10 (5) ↓ Aged (6) ↑ Smk (7,8)

VOL. DIST. (*liters/kg*)	HALF-LIFE (*hours*)	EFFECTIVE CONCENTRATIONS	TOXIC CONCENTRATIONS
15 ± 6 [b] (5)	13 ± 3 [c] (1)	>225 ng/ml [d] (9,10)	>1 μg/ml [e] (11)

[a] Extensive first-pass metabolism causes wide variability in availability.
[b] Vd_{area}.
[c] Metabolized to desipramine (*see* kinetic description).
[d] Antidepressant effect; combination of imipramine and desipramine.
[e] Concentration of imipramine plus desipramine; combined data for toxic effects of tricyclic antidepressants.

1. Gram, L. F., and Christiansen, J. First-pass metabolism of imipramine in man. *Clin. Pharmacol. Ther.,* 1975, *17,* 555–563.
2. Christiansen, J.; Gram, L. F.; Kofod, B.; and Rafaelsen, O.J. Imipramine metabolism in man. *Psychopharmacologia (Berl.),* 1967, *11,* 255–264.
3. Piafsky, K. M., and Borgå, O. Plasma protein binding of basic drugs. II. Importance of α_1-acid glycoprotein for inter-individual variation. *Clin. Pharmacol. Ther.,* 1977, *22,* 545–549.
4. Danon, A., and Chen, Z. Binding of imipramine to plasma proteins: effect of hyperlipoproteinemia. *Clin. Pharmacol. Ther.,* 1979, *25,* 316–321.
5. Nagy, A., and Johansson, R. Plasma levels of imipramine and desipramine in man after different routes of administration. *Naunyn Schmiedebergs Arch. Pharmacol.,* 1975, *290,* 145–160.
6. Nies, A.; Robinson, D. S.; Friedman, M. J.; Green, R.; Cooper, T. B.; Ravaris, C. L.; and Ives, J. O. Relationship between age and tricyclic antidepressant plasma levels. *Am. J. Psychiatry,* 1977, *134,* 790–793.
7. Perel, J. M.; Hurvic, M. J.; and Kanzler, M. B. Pharmacodynamics of imipramine in depressed patients. *Psychopharmacol. Bull.,* 1975, *11,* 16–18.
8. Perel, J. M.; Shostak, M.; Gann, E.; Kantor, S. J.; and Glassman, A. H. Pharmacodynamics of imipramine and clinical outcome in depressed patients. In, *Pharmacokinetics of Psychoactive Drugs.* (Gottschalk, L. A., and Merlis, S., eds.) Spectrum Publications, Inc., New York, 1976, pp. 229–241.
9. Glassman, A. H.; Perel, J. M.; Shostak, M.; Kantor, S. J.; and Fleiss, J. L. Clinical implications of imipramine plasma levels for depressive illness. *Arch. Gen. Psychiatry,* 1977, *34,* 197–204.
10. Reisby, N.; Gram, L. F.; Bech, P.; Nagy, A.; Petersen, G. O.; Ortmann, J.; Ibsen, I.; Dencker, S. J.; Jacobsen, O.; Krautwald, O.; Sondergaard, I.; and Christiansen, J. Imipramine: clinical effects and pharmacokinetic variability. *Psychopharmacology,* 1977, *54,* 263–272.
11. Petit, J. M.; Spiker, D. G.; Ruwitch, J. F.; Ziegler, V. E.; Weiss, A. N.; and Biggs, J. T. Tricyclic antidepressant plasma levels and adverse effects after overdose. *Clin. Pharmacol. Ther.,* 1977, *21,* 47–51.

INDOMETHACIN (Chapter 29)

AVAILABILITY (ORAL) (%)	URINARY EXCRETION (%)	BOUND IN PLASMA (%)	CLEARANCE $(ml \cdot min^{-1} \cdot kg^{-1})$
98 (1)	15 ± 8 (2)	90 (3) ↔ Alb (3)	1.6 ± 0.2 [a] (4) 2.0 ± 0.4 [a,b] (2)

VOL. DIST. (*liters/kg*)	HALF-LIFE (*hours*)	EFFECTIVE CONCENTRATIONS	TOXIC CONCENTRATIONS
0.93 ± 0.53 [a,c] (4) 0.26 ± 0.07 [a,b] (2)	2.6–11.2 [a] (4) 2.4 ± 0.4 [a] (2) ↔ RA (4), Urem (5) ↑ Neo (6), Prem (7)	0.5–3 μg/ml	>6 μg/ml (4)

Key: Adult = adults; Aged = aged; Alb = hypoalbuminemia; AVH = acute viral hepatitis; CF = cystic fibrosis; CHF = congestive heart failure; Child = children; Cirr = cirrhosis; COPD = chronic obstructive pulmonary disease; CP = cor pulmonale; CPBS = cardiopulmonary bypass surgery; CRI = chronic respiratory insufficiency; Cush = cushingoid; Epilep = epilepsy; Fem = females; Hep = hepatitis; HL = hyperlipoproteinemia; HTh = hyperthyroid; Inflam = inflammation; LTh = hypothyroid; MI = myocardial infarction; Neo = neonates; NS = nephrotic syndrome; Obes = obesity; Pneu = pneumonia; Preg = pregnant; Prem = premature infants; RA = rheumatoid arthritis; Smk = smoking; Tach = ventricular tachycardia; Urem = uremia.

[a] Significantly different values reported by Kwan and coworkers (1,2) and Alvan and associates (4). The former group made measurements for 8 hours, the latter for 32 hours. The longer measurements may reflect enterohepatic recirculation of the drug, which may average 50% after intravenous administration (2). However, using single-dose data to calculate parameters, Alvan and coworkers predict steady-state concentrations quite accurately.

[b] Assuming 70 kg.

[c] Vd_{area}.

1. Kwan, K. C.; Breault, G. O.; Davis, R. L.; Lei, B. W.; Czerwinski, A. W.; Besselaar, G. H.; and Duggan, D. E. Effects of concomitant aspirin administration on the pharmacokinetics of indomethacin in man. *J. Pharmacokinet. Biopharm.*, **1978**, *6*, 451–476.

2. Kwan, K. C.; Breault, G. O.; Umbenhauer, E. R.; McMahon, F. G.; and Duggan, D. E. Kinetics of indomethacin absorption, elimination and enterohepatic circulation in man. *J. Pharmacokinet. Biopharm.*, **1976**, *4*, 255–280.

3. Hvidberg, E.; Lausen, H. H.; and Jansen, J. A. Indomethacin: plasma concentration and protein binding in man. *Eur. J. Clin. Pharmacol.*, **1972**, *4*, 119–124.

4. Alvan, G.; Orme, M.; Bertilsson, L.; Ekstrand, R.; and Palmer, L. Pharmacokinetics of indomethacin. *Clin. Pharmacol. Ther.*, **1975**, *18*, 364–373.

5. Stein, G.; Kunze, M.; Zaumseil, J.; and Traeger, A. Zur Pharmakokinetik von Indomethazin und Indomethazinmetaboliten bei wiederholter Applikation an neirengesunden und nierengeschädigten Patienten. *Int. J. Clin. Pharmacol.*, **1977**, *15*, 470–473.

6. Traeger, A.; Nöschel, H.; and Zaumseil, J. Zur Pharmakokinetic von Indomethazin bei Schwangeren, Kreissenden und deren Neugeborenen. *Zentralbl. Gynaekol.*, **1973**, *95*, 635–641.

7. Friedman, Z.; Whitman, V.; Maisels, M. J.; Berman, W., Jr.; Marks, K. H.; and Vesell, E. S. Indomethacin disposition and indomethacin-induced platelet dysfunction in premature infants. *J. Clin. Pharmacol.*, **1978**, *18*, 272–279.

ISONIAZID [a] (Chapter 53)

AVAILABILITY (ORAL) (%)	URINARY EXCRETION (%)	BOUND IN PLASMA (%)	CLEARANCE ($ml \cdot min^{-1} \cdot kg^{-1}$)
[b]	29 ± 5 [c,d] (4) 7 ± 2 [c,e] (4)	~ 0 (6)	2.5 [d,f] (7) 7.0 [e,f] (7)

VOL. DIST. (*liters/kg*)	HALF-LIFE (*hours*)	EFFECTIVE CONCENTRATIONS	TOXIC CONCENTRATIONS
0.61 ± 0.11 [d,e] (8)	3.0 ± 0.8 [d] (9) 1.1 ± 0.2 [e] (9) $\leftrightarrow$ Aged (10), Obes (11) $\uparrow$ AVH (12), Urem [g] (13,14)	*See* Chapter 53	—

[a] For review, *see* (1).

[b] It is usually stated that isoniazid is completely absorbed; however, good estimates of possible loss due to first-pass metabolism are not available. Absorption is decreased in the presence of food (2) or antacids (3).

[c] After oral administration; assay includes unchanged drug and its acid-labile hydrazones. Higher percentages have been noted after intravenous administration, suggesting significant first-pass metabolism (5).

[d] Slow acetylators.

[e] Fast acetylators.

[f] Values calculated from average-rate constants for elimination and mean volume of distribution.

[g] No apparent correlation with degree of renal impairment.

1. Weber, W. W., and Hein, D. W. Clinical pharmacokinetics of isoniazid. *Clin. Pharmacokinet.*, **1979**, *4*, 401–422.

2. Melander, A.; Danielson, K.; and Hanson, A. Reduction of isoniazid bioavailability in normal men by concomitant intake of food. *Acta Med. Scand.*, **1976**, *200*, 93–97.

3. Hurwitz, A., and Schlozman, D. L. Effects of antacids on gastrointestinal absorption of isoniazid in rat and man. *Am. Rev. Respir. Dis.*, **1974**, *109*, 41–47.

4. Ellard, G. A., and Gammon, P. T. Pharmacokinetics of isoniazid metabolism in man. *J. Pharmacokinet. Biopharm.*, **1976**, *4*, 83–113.

5. Boxenbaum, H. G., and Riegelman, S. Pharmacokinetics of isoniazid and some metabolites in man. *J. Pharmacokinet. Biopharm.*, **1976**, *4*, 287–325.

6. Boxenbaum, H. G.; Bekersky, I.; Mattaliano, V.; and Kaplan, S. A. Plasma and salivary concentrations of isoniazid in man: preliminary findings in two slow acetylator subjects. *J. Pharmacokinet. Biopharm.*, **1975**, *3*, 443–456.

7. Jenne, J. W. Pharmacokinetics and dose of isoniazid and *p*-aminosalicylic acid in the treatment of tuberculosis. *Antibiot. Chemother. (Basel)*, **1964**, *12*, 407–432.

8. Jenne, J. W.; MacDonald, F. M.; and Mendoza, E. A study of the renal clearances, metabolic inactivation rates, and serum fall-off interaction of isoniazid and para-aminosalicylic acid in man. *Am. Rev. Respir. Dis.*, **1961**, *84*, 371–378.

9. Jenne, J. W. Studies of human patterns of isoniazid metabolism using an intravenous fall-off technique with a chemical method. *Am. Rev. Respir. Dis.*, **1960**, *81*, 1–8.

10. Farah, F.; Taylor, W.; Rawlins, M. D.; and James, O. Hepatic drug acetylation and oxidation: effects of aging in man. *Br. Med. J.*, **1977**, *2*, 155–156.

11. Reidenberg, M. M. Obesity and fasting: effects on drug metabolism and drug action in man. *Clin. Pharmacol. Ther.*, **1977**, *22*, 729–734.

12. Levi, A. J.; Sherlock, S.; and Walker, D. Phenylbutazone and isoniazid metabolism in patients with liver disease in relation to previous drug therapy. *Lancet*, **1968**, *1*, 1275–1279.

13. Gold, C. H.; Buchanan, N.; Tringham, V.; Viljoen, M.; Struckwold, B.; and Moodley, G. P. Isoniazid pharmacokinetics in patients in chronic renal failure. *Clin. Nephrol.*, **1976**, *6*, 365–369.

14. Bowersox, D. W.; Winterbauer, R. H.; Stewart, C. L.; Orme, B.; and Barron, E. Isoniazid dosage in patients with renal failure. *N. Engl. J. Med.*, **1973**, *289*, 84–87.

ISOSORBIDE DINITRATE (Chapter 33)

AVAILABILITY (ORAL) (%)	URINARY EXCRETION (%)	BOUND IN PLASMA (%)	CLEARANCE ($ml \cdot min^{-1} \cdot kg^{-1}$)
58 ± 21 [a] (1)	0 (2)	—	25 [b] (3) $CL_{int} = 94 \pm 54$ (4)

VOL. DIST. (liters/kg)	HALF-LIFE (hours)	EFFECTIVE CONCENTRATIONS	TOXIC CONCENTRATIONS
1.8 [b] (3)	0.5 (1)	—	—

[a] Isosorbide dinitrate is metabolized extensively to mononitrates, which are pharmacologically active. The value for availability is the *relative availability* (as isosorbide dinitrate) for oral versus sublingual administration. Availability is assumed to be nearly 100% after sublingual administration.

[b] Values are $CL/F_{sublingual}$ and $Vd_{area}/F_{sublingual}$.

1. Assinder, D. F.; Chasseaud, L. F.; and Taylor, T. Plasma isosorbide dinitrate concentrations in human subjects after administration of standard and sustained-release formulations. *J. Pharm. Sci.,* **1977**, *66,* 775–778.
2. Down, W. H.; Chasseaud, L. F.; and Grundy, R. X. Biotransformation of isosorbide dinitrate in humans. *J. Pharm. Sci.,* **1974**, *63,* 1147–1149.
3. Rosseel, M. T., and Bogaert, M. G. GLC determination of nitroglycerin and isosorbide dinitrate in human plasma. *J. Pharm. Sci.,* **1973**, *62,* 754–778.
4. Shane, S. J.; Iazetta, J. J.; Chrisholm, A. W.; Berka, J. F.; and Leung, D. Plasma concentrations of isosorbide dinitrate and its metabolites after chronic high oral dosage in man. *Br. J. Clin. Pharmacol.,* **1978**, *6,* 37–41.

KANAMYCIN (Chapter 51)

AVAILABILITY (ORAL) (%)	URINARY EXCRETION (%)	BOUND IN PLASMA (%)	CLEARANCE ($ml \cdot min^{-1} \cdot kg^{-1}$)
—	90 (1)	0 (2,3)	1.4 ± 0.2 [a] (1) $CL = 0.62\ CL_{cr} + 0.03$ (3)

VOL. DIST. (liters/kg)	HALF-LIFE (hours)	EFFECTIVE CONCENTRATIONS	TOXIC CONCENTRATIONS
0.26 ± 0.05 (1)	2.1 ± 0.2 (1) ↑ Urem (3)	*See* Chapter 51	*See* Chapter 51

[a] Values reported per 1.73 m^2; calculated assuming 70 kg.

1. Clarke, J. T.; Libke, R. K.; Regamey, C.; and Kirby, W. M. M. Comparative pharmacokinetics of amikacin and kanamycin. *Clin. Pharmacol. Ther.,* **1974**, *15,* 610–616.
2. Gordon, R. C.; Regamey, C.; and Kirby, W. M. M. Serum protein binding of the aminoglycoside antibiotics. *Antimicrob. Agents Chemother.,* **1972**, *2,* 214–216.
3. Orme, B. M., and Cutler, R. E. The relationship between kanamycin pharmacokinetics: distribution and renal function. *Clin. Pharmacol. Ther.,* **1969**, *10,* 543–550.

LIDOCAINE (Chapter 31)

AVAILABILITY (ORAL) (%)	URINARY EXCRETION (%)	BOUND IN PLASMA (%)	CLEARANCE ($ml \cdot min^{-1} \cdot kg^{-1}$)
35 ± 11 [a] (1)	2 ± 1 (2) ↑ Neo (3)	51 ± 8 [b] (4) ↓ Neo (3)	9.2 ± 2.4 (5) ↓ CHF (6,7), Cirr (6) ↔ Urem (6,8), AVH [c] (9), Neo (3), Aged (2)

VOL. DIST. (liters/kg)	HALF-LIFE (hours)	EFFECTIVE CONCENTRATIONS	TOXIC CONCENTRATIONS
1.1 ± 0.4 (5) ↓ CHF (6) ↔ Urem (6,8), Aged (2) ↑ Cirr (6), Neo (3)	1.8 ± 0.4 (2) ↔ Urem (6,8), CHF [d] (6) ↑ Cirr (6), MI [e] (2,10), Neo (3)	2–5 µg/ml (12) 1.2–6 µg/ml (13)	Occasional: 6–10 µg/ml (13) Frequent: >10 µg/ml (13)

[a] Preparations available commercially are for parenteral administration.
[b] Value is as high as 75% at 0.4 μg/ml and as low as 30% at 20 μg/ml.
[c] During acute phase, blood clearance was 13 ± 4 ml $\cdot$ min^{-1} $\cdot$ kg^{-1}, which increased to 20 ± 4 ml $\cdot$ min^{-1} $\cdot$ kg^{-1} after recovery.
[d] Short-term studies indicate no change; long-term studies indicate marked increase (11).
[e] Half-life increased in patients with myocardial infarction when infusion longer than 24 hours (10).

1. Boyes, R. M.; Scott, D. B.; Jebson, P. J.; Godman, M. J.; and Julian, D. G. Pharmacokinetics of lidocaine in man. *Clin. Pharmacol. Ther.*, **1971**, *12,* 105–116.
2. Nation, R. L.; Triggs, E. J.; and Selig, M. Lignocaine kinetics in cardiac patients and aged subjects. *Br. J. Clin. Pharmacol.*, **1977**, *4,* 439–448.
3. Mihaly, G. W.; Moore, R. G.; Thomas, J.; Triggs, E. J.; Thomas, D.; and Shanks, C. A. The pharmacokinetics and metabolism of the anilide local anesthetics in neonates. I. Lignocaine. *Eur. J. Clin. Pharmacol.*, **1978**, *13,* 143–152.
4. Tucker, G. T.; Boyes, R. N.; Bridenbaugh, P. O.; and Moore, D. C. Binding of anilide-type local anesthetics in human plasma. I. Relationships between binding, physicochemical properties, and anesthetic activity. *Anesthesiology*, **1970**, *33,* 287–303.
5. Rowland, M.; Thomson, P. D.; Guichard, A.; and Melmon, K. L. Disposition kinetics of lidocaine in normal subjects. *Ann. N.Y. Acad. Sci.*, **1971**, *179,* 383–398.
6. Thomson, P. D.; Melmon, K. L.; Richardson, J. A.; Cohn, K.; Steinbrunn, W.; Cudihee, M. D.; and Rowland, M. Lidocaine pharmacokinetics in advanced heart failure, liver disease and renal failure in humans. *Ann. Intern. Med.*, **1973**, *78,* 499–508.
7. Zito, R. A., and Reid, P. R. Lidocaine kinetics predicted by indocyanine green clearance. *N. Engl. J. Med.*, **1978**, *298,* 1160–1163.
8. Collinsworth, K. A.; Strong, J. M.; Atkinson, A. J., Jr.; Winkle, R. A.; Perlroth, F.; and Harrison, D. C. Pharmacokinetics and metabolism of lidocaine in patients with renal failure. *Clin. Pharmacol. Ther.*, **1975**, *18,* 59–64.
9. Williams, R. L.; Blaschke, T. F.; Meffin, P. J.; Melmon, K. L.; and Rowland, M. Influence of viral hepatitis on the disposition of two compounds with high hepatic clearance: lidocaine and indocyanine green. *Clin. Pharmacol. Ther.*, **1976**, *20,* 290–299.
10. LeLorier, J.; Grenon, D.; Latour, Y.; Caillé, G.; Dumont, G.; Brosseau, A.; and Solignac, A. Pharmacokinetics of lidocaine after prolonged intravenous infusions in uncomplicated myocardial infarction. *Ann. Intern. Med.*, **1977**, *87,* 700–702.
11. Prescott, L. F.; Adjepon-Yamoah, K. K.; and Talbot, R. G. Impaired lignocaine metabolism in patients with myocardial infarction and cardiac failure. *Br. Med. J.*, **1976**, *1,* 939–941.
12. Gianelly, R.; von der Groeben, J. O.; Spivack, A. P.; and Harrison, D. C. Effect of lidocaine on ventricular arrhythmias in patients with coronary heart disease. *N. Engl. J. Med.*, **1967**, *277,* 1215–1219.
13. Harrison, D. C.; Stenson, R. E.; and Constantino, R. T. The relationship of blood levels, infusion rates and metabolism of lidocaine to its antiarrhythmic action. In, *Symposium on Cardiac Arrhythmias*. (Sandøe, E.; Flensted-Jensen, E.; and Olesen, K. H.; eds.) A. B. Astra, Sweden, **1970**, pp. 427–447.

LITHIUM (Chapter 19)

AVAILABILITY (ORAL) (%)	URINARY EXCRETION (%)	BOUND IN PLASMA (%)	CLEARANCE ($ml \cdot min^{-1} \cdot kg^{-1}$)
100 (1)	95 ± 15 (1)	0 (2)	0.35 ± 0.11 [a] (3) $\downarrow$ Urem (4), Aged (4)

VOL. DIST. (*liters/kg*)	HALF-LIFE (*hours*)	EFFECTIVE CONCENTRATIONS	TOXIC CONCENTRATIONS
$0.79 + 0.34$ [b] (3)	22 ± 8 [c] (4) $\uparrow$ Urem (4)	>0.7 mEq/l (5)	>2.0 mEq/l (6)

[a] Renal clearance of Li$^+$ parallels that of Na$^+$. The ratio of clearances of Li$^+$ and creatinine is about 0.2 ± 0.03; clearance of Li$^+$ is thus reduced in older subjects and when there is renal disease (2–4).
[b] Vd_{area}.
[c] A shorter half-life of 5.6 ± 0.5 hours is due to distribution, and this influences drug concentrations for at least 12 hours (1).

1. Groth, V.; Prellwitz, W.; and Jahnchen, E. Estimation of pharmacokinetic parameters of lithium from saliva and urine. *Clin. Pharmacol. Ther.*, **1974**, *16,* 490–498.
2. Thomsen, K., and Schou, M. Renal lithium excretion in man. *Am. J. Physiol.*, **1968**, *215,* 823–827.
3. Mason, R. W.; McQueen, E. G.; Keary, P. J.; and James, N. McL. Pharmacokinetics of lithium: elimination half-time, renal clearance and apparent volume of distribution in schizophrenia. *Clin. Pharmacokinet.*, **1978**, *3,* 241–246.
4. Lehmann, K., and Merten, K. Die Elimination von Lithium in Abhängigkeit vom Lebensalter bei Gesunden und Niereninsuffizienten. *Int. J. Clin. Pharmacol.*, **1974**, *10,* 292–298.
5. Prien, R. F., and Coffey, E. M. Relationship between dosage and response to lithium prophylaxis in recurrent depression. *Am. J. Psychiatry*, **1976**, *133,* 567–569.
6. Allgen, L. G. Laboratory experience with lithium toxicity in man. *Acta Psychiatr. Scand.*, **1969**, *207,* 98–104.

Key: Adult = adults; Aged = aged; Alb = hypoalbuminemia; AVH = acute viral hepatitis; CF = cystic fibrosis; CHF = congestive heart failure; Child = children; Cirr = cirrhosis; COPD = chronic obstructive pulmonary disease; CP = cor pulmonale; CPBS = cardiopulmonary bypass surgery; CRI = chronic respiratory insufficiency; Cush = cushingoid; Epilep = epilepsy; Fem = females; Hep = hepatitis; HL = hyperlipoproteinemia; HTh = hyperthyroid; Inflam = inflammation; LTh = hypothyroid; MI = myocardial infarction; Neo = neonates; NS = nephrotic syndrome; Obes = obesity; Pneu = pneumonia; Preg = pregnant; Prem = premature infants; RA = rheumatoid arthritis; Smk = smoking; Tach = ventricular tachycardia; Urem = uremia.

LORAZEPAM [a] (Chapters 17, 19)

AVAILABILITY (ORAL) (%)	URINARY EXCRETION (%)	BOUND IN PLASMA (%)	CLEARANCE $(ml \cdot min^{-1} \cdot kg^{-1})$
93 ± 10 (2)	<1 (2)	93 ± 2 (3) ↓ Cirr (3)	1.1 ± 0.4 (2) ↔ Aged [b] (3,4), Cirr (3), AVH (3)

VOL. DIST. (liters/kg)	HALF-LIFE (hours)	EFFECTIVE CONCENTRATIONS	TOXIC CONCENTRATIONS
1.3 ± 0.2 [c] (2) ↔ Aged [b] (3) ↑ Ciɪɪ (3)	14 ± 5 (2) ↔ Aged (3), Urem (6) ↑ Cirr (3)	—	—

[a] For review, see (1).
[b] A more recent report (5) shows slight but significant decreases in clearance and volume of distribution in the elderly.
[c] Vd_{area}.

1. Kyriakopoulos, A. A.; Greenblatt, D. J.; and Shader, R. I. Clinical pharmacokinetics of lorazepam: a review. *J. Clin. Psychiatry,* **1978,** *39,* 16–23.
2. Greenblatt, D. J.; Shader, R. I.; Franke, K.; MacLaughlin, D. S.; Harmatz, J. S.; Allen, M. D.; Werner, A.; and Woo, E. Pharmacokinetics and bioavailability of intravenous, intramuscular, and oral lorazepam in humans. *J. Pharm. Sci.,* **1979,** *68,* 57–63.
3. Kraus, J. W.; Desmond, P. V.; Marshall, J. P.; Johnson, R. F.; Schenker, S.; and Wilkinson, G. R. Effects of aging and liver disease on disposition of lorazepam. *Clin. Pharmacol. Ther.,* **1978,** *24,* 411–419.
4. Greenblatt, D. J.; Knowles, J. A.; Comer, W. H.; Shader, R. I.; Harmatz, J. S.; and Ruelius, H. W. Clinical pharmacokinetics of lorazepam. IV. Long-term oral administration. *J. Clin. Pharmacol.,* **1977,** *17,* 495–500.
5. Greenblatt, D. J.; Allen, M. D.; Locniskar, A.; Harmatz, J. S.; and Shader, R. I. Lorazepam kinetics in the elderly. *Clin. Pharmacol. Ther.,* **1979,** *26,* 103–113.
6. Verbeeck, R.; Tjandramaga, T. B.; Verberckmoes, R.; and de Schepper, P. J. Biotransformation and excretion of lorazepam in patients with chronic renal failure. *Br. J. Clin. Pharmacol.,* **1976,** *3,* 1033–1039.

MEPERIDINE (Chapter 22)

AVAILABILITY (ORAL) (%)	URINARY EXCRETION (%)	BOUND IN PLASMA (%)	CLEARANCE $(ml \cdot min^{-1} \cdot kg^{-1})$
52 ± 3 (1)	4–22 [a] (2)	58 ± 9 (3) ↓ Aged (4) ↔ Cirr (5)	17 ± 5 (5) ↓ AVH (3), Cirr (5)

VOL. DIST. (liters/kg)	HALF-LIFE (hours)	EFFECTIVE CONCENTRATIONS	TOXIC CONCENTRATIONS
4.2 ± 1.3 (5) ↔ Cirr (5)	3.2 ± 0.8 (5) ↑ AVH (3), Cirr (5)	—	—

[a] Meperidine is a weak acid ($pK_a = 9.6$) and is excreted to a greater extent in the urine at low urinary pH and to a lesser extent at high pH.

1. Mather, L. E., and Tucker, G. T. Systemic availability of orally administered meperidine. *Clin. Pharmacol. Ther.,* **1976,** *20,* 535–540.
2. Asatoor, A. M.; London, D. R.; Milne, M. D.; and Simerhoff, M. L. The excretion of pethidine and its derivatives. *Br. J. Pharmacol.,* **1963,** *20,* 285–298.
3. McHorse, T. S.; Wilkinson, G. R.; Johnson, R. F.; and Schenker, S. Effect of acute viral hepatitis in man on the disposition and elimination of meperidine. *Gastroenterology,* **1975,** *68,* 775–780.
4. Mather, L. E.; Tucker, G. T.; Pflug, A. E.; Lindop, M. J.; and Wilkerson, C. Meperidine kinetics in man. Intravenous injection in surgical patients and volunteers. *Clin. Pharmacol. Ther.,* **1975,** *17,* 21–30.
5. Klotz, U.; McHorse, T. S.; Wilkinson, G. R.; and Schenker, S. The effect of cirrhosis on the disposition and elimination of meperidine in man. *Clin. Pharmacol. Ther.,* **1974,** *16,* 667–675.

METHICILLIN (Chapter 50)

AVAILABILITY (ORAL) (%)	URINARY EXCRETION (%)	BOUND IN PLASMA (%)	CLEARANCE $(ml \cdot min^{-1} \cdot kg^{-1})$
—	88 ± 17 (1)	28–49 [a] (2)	6.1 ± 1.3 (1) ↓ Urem (3) ↑ CF (1)

VOL. DIST. (liters/kg)	HALF-LIFE (hours)	EFFECTIVE CONCENTRATIONS	TOXIC CONCENTRATIONS
0.43 ± 0.10 (1)	0.85 ± 0.23 (1) ↑ Urem (3)	*See* Chapter 50	*See* Chapter 50

[a] Range of published values.

1. Yaffe, S. J.; Gerbracht, L. M.; Mosovich, L. L.; Mattar, M. E.; Danish, M.; and Jusko, W. J. Pharmacokinetics of methicillin in patients with cystic fibrosis. *J. Infect. Dis.*, **1977**, *135*, 828–831.
2. Warren, G. H. The prognostic significance of penicillin serum levels and protein binding in clinical medicine. A review of current studies. *Chemotherapia*, **1965/1966**, *10*, 339–358.
3. Bulger, R. J.; Lindholm, D. D.; Murray, J. S.; and Kirby, W. M. M. Effect of uremia on methicillin and oxacillin blood levels. *J.A.M.A.*, **1964**, *187*, 319–322.

METHOTREXATE [a] (Chapter 55)

AVAILABILITY (ORAL) (%)	URINARY EXCRETION (%)	BOUND IN PLASMA (%)	CLEARANCE $(ml \cdot min^{-1} \cdot kg^{-1})$
65 [b] (2)	94 [c] (2)	45 ± 14 (2)	1.5 (3) ↓ Urem (4)

VOL. DIST. (liters/kg)	HALF-LIFE (hours)	EFFECTIVE CONCENTRATIONS	TOXIC CONCENTRATIONS
0.40 (5)	8.4 [d] (3) ↑ Urem (4)	—	0.9 μM [e] (6) (0.9 μg/ml)

[a] For review, *see* (1).

[b] Doses greater than 80 ng/m² may be absorbed less completely (2).

[c] After intravenous administration; after oral administration, value is 65% (2).

[d] A shorter half-life is seen initially (1.8 hours) (3).

[e] Bone-marrow toxicity is common if the concentration exceeds this value 48 hours after initiation of the high-dose methotrexate regimen with citrovorum rescue described in (7).

1. Shen, D. D., and Azarnoff, D. L. Clinical pharmacokinetics of methotrexate. *Clin. Pharmacokinet.*, **1978**, *3*, 1–13.
2. Wan, S. H.; Hoffman, D. H.; Azarnoff, D. L.; Stephens, R.; and Hoogstraten, B. Effect of route of administration and effusions on methotrexate pharmacokinetics. *Cancer Res.*, **1974**, *34*, 3487–3491.
3. Isacoff, W. H.; Morrison, P. F.; Aroesty, J.; Willis, K. L.; Bloch, J. B.; and Lincoln, T. L. Pharmacokinetics of high-dose methotrexate with citrovorum factor rescue. *Cancer Treat. Rep.*, **1977**, *61*, 1665–1674.
4. Kristensen, L. O.; Weismann, K.; and Huiters, L. Renal function and the role of disappearance of methotrexate from serum. *Eur. J. Clin. Pharmacol.*, **1975**, *8*, 439–444.
5. Leme, P. R.; Creaven, P. J.; Allen, L. M.; and Berman, M. Kinetic model for the disposition and metabolism of moderate and high-dose methotrexate (NSC-740) in man. *Cancer Chemother. Rep.*, **1974**, *59*, 811–817.
6. Stoller, R. G.; Hard, K. R.; Jacobs, S. A.; Rosenberg, S. A.; and Chabner, B. A. Use of plasma pharmacokinetics to predict and prevent methotrexate toxicity. *N. Engl. J. Med.*, **1977**, *297*, 630–634.
7. Jaffe, N.; Frei, E., III; Traggis, D.; and Bishop, Y. Adjuvant methotrexate and citrovorum factor treatment of osteogenic sarcoma. *N. Engl. J. Med.*, **1974**, *291*, 994–997.

Key: Adult = adults; Aged = aged; Alb = hypoalbuminemia; AVH = acute viral hepatitis; CF = cystic fibrosis; CHF = congestive heart failure; Child = children; Cirr = cirrhosis; COPD = chronic obstructive pulmonary disease; CP = cor pulmonale; CPBS = cardiopulmonary bypass surgery; CRI = chronic respiratory insufficiency; Cush = cushingoid; Epilep = epilepsy; Fem = females; Hep = hepatitis; HL = hyperlipoproteinemia; HTh = hyperthyroid; Inflam = inflammation; LTh = hypothyroid; MI = myocardial infarction; Neo = neonates; NS = nephrotic syndrome; Obes = obesity; Pneu = pneumonia; Preg = pregnant; Prem = premature infants; RA = rheumatoid arthritis; Smk = smoking; Tach = ventricular tachycardia; Urem = uremia.

METHYLDOPA (Chapters 9, 32)

AVAILABILITY (ORAL) (%)	URINARY EXCRETION (%)	BOUND IN PLASMA (%)	CLEARANCE $(ml \cdot min^{-1} \cdot kg^{-1})$
25 ± 16 (1)	63 ± 10 (1)	—	3.1 ± 0.9 (1) $\downarrow$ Urem [a] (2,3)

VOL. DIST. (*liters/kg*)	HALF-LIFE (*hours*)	EFFECTIVE CONCENTRATIONS	TOXIC CONCENTRATIONS
0.37 ± 0.10 (1)	1.8 ± 0.2 (1) $\uparrow$ Urem (4)	—	—

[a] Clearance of unchanged drug and active metabolites is reduced.

1. Kwan, K. C.; Foltz, E. L.; Breault, G. O.; Baer, J. E.; and Totaro, J. A. Pharmacokinetics of methyldopa in man. *J. Pharmacol. Exp. Ther.,* **1976,** *198,* 264–276.
2. Myhre, E.; Brodwall, E. K.; Stenback, Ø.; and Hansen, T. The renal excretion of methyldopa. *Scand. J. Clin. Lab. Invest.,* **1972,** *29,* 201–204.
3. O'Dea, R. F., and Mirkin, B. L. Metabolic disposition of methyldopa in hypertensive and renal-insufficient children. *Clin. Pharmacol. Ther.,* **1980,** *27,* 37–43.
4. Myhre, E.; Brodwall, E. K.; Stenback, Ø.; and Hansen, T. Plasma turnover of methyldopa in advanced renal failure. *Acta Med. Scand.,* **1972,** *191,* 343–347.

METOPROLOL (Chapter 9)

AVAILABILITY (ORAL) (%)	URINARY EXCRETION (%)	BOUND IN PLASMA (%)	CLEARANCE $(ml \cdot min^{-1} \cdot kg^{-1})$
38 ± 14 (1)	10 ± 3 (1)	13 (1)	15 ± 3 (1)

VOL. DIST. (*liters/kg*)	HALF-LIFE (*hours*)	EFFECTIVE CONCENTRATIONS	TOXIC CONCENTRATIONS
4.2 ± 0.7 (1)	3.2 ± 0.2 (1)	25 ng/ml [a] (2)	—

[a] To achieve a 10% decrease in resting heart rate.

1. Regårdh, C. G.; Borg, K. O.; Johansson, R.; Johnsson, G.; and Palmer, L. Pharmacokinetic studies on the selective β_1-receptor antagonist metoprolol in man. *J. Pharmacokinet. Biopharm.,* **1974,** *2,* 347–364.
2. Bengtsson, C.; Johnsson, G.; and Regårdh, C. G. Plasma levels and effects of metoprolol on blood pressure and heart rate in hypertensive patients after an acute dose and between two doses during long-term treatment. *Clin. Pharmacol. Ther.,* **1975,** *17,* 400–408.

MINOCYCLINE (Chapter 52)

AVAILABILITY (ORAL) (%)	URINARY EXCRETION (%)	BOUND IN PLASMA (%)	CLEARANCE $(ml \cdot min^{-1} \cdot kg^{-1})$
100 (1)	11 ± 2 (2)	76 (1)	0.30 ± 0.12 (3) $\leftrightarrow$, $\uparrow$ Urem [a] (3)

VOL. DIST. (*liters/kg*)	HALF-LIFE (*hours*)	EFFECTIVE CONCENTRATIONS	TOXIC CONCENTRATIONS
0.40 ± 0.12 (3) $\uparrow$ Urem (3)	18 ± 4 (3) $\leftrightarrow$ Urem (3)	*See* Chapter 52	—

[a] In patients with reduced CL_{cr}, single-dose infusion studies indicate that clearance is increased, which is consistent with the increased Vd and unchanged $t_{1/2}$. However, there is no accumulation of drug beyond that seen in normal subjects during repeated administration of minocycline to patients with CL_{cr} between 18 and 45 ml/min.

1. Macdonald, H.; Kelly, R. G.; Allen, E. S.; Noble, J. F.; and Kanegis, L. A. Pharmacokinetic studies on minocycline in man. *Clin. Pharmacol. Ther.,* **1973,** *14,* 852–861.
2. Heaney, D., and Eknoyan, G. Minocycline and doxycycline kinetics in chronic renal failure. *Clin. Pharmacol. Ther.,* **1978,** *24,* 233–239.
3. Welling, P. G.; Shaw, W. R.; Uman, S. W.; Tse, F. L. S.; and Craig, W. A. Pharmacokinetics of minocycline in renal failure. *Antimicrob. Agents Chemother.,* **1975,** *8,* 532–537.

MORPHINE [a] (Chapter 22)

AVAILABILITY (ORAL) (%)	URINARY EXCRETION (%)	BOUND IN PLASMA (%)	CLEARANCE $(ml \cdot min^{-1} \cdot kg^{-1})$
20–33 (2)	6–10 (2)	35 ± 2 (3) ↓ Hep (3), Alb (3)	15 ± 2 (4)

VOL. DIST. (liters/kg)	HALF-LIFE (hours)	EFFECTIVE CONCENTRATIONS	TOXIC CONCENTRATIONS
3.2 ± 0.7 [b] (4)	3.0 ± 1.2 (4)	65 ± 80 ng/ml [c] (5)	—

[a] For review, *see* (1).
[b] Vd_{area}.
[c] To achieve surgical analgesia.

1. Berkowitz, B. A. The relationship of pharmacokinetics to pharmacologic activity: morphine, methadone and naloxone. *Clin. Pharmacokinet.*, **1976**, *1*, 219–230.
2. Brunk, S. F., and Delle, M. Morphine metabolism in man. *Clin. Pharmacol. Ther.*, **1974**, *16*, 51–57.
3. Olsen, G. D.; Bennett, W. M.; and Porter, G. A. Morphine and phenytoin binding to plasma proteins in renal and hepatic failure. *Clin. Pharmacol. Ther.*, **1975**, *17*, 677–684.
4. Stanski, D. R.; Greenblatt, D. J.; and Lowenstein, E. Kinetics of intravenous and intramuscular morphine. *Clin. Pharmacol. Ther.*, **1978**, *24*, 52–59.
5. Dahlström, B.; Bolme, P.; Feychting, H.; Noack, G.; and Paalzow, L. Morphine kinetics in children. *Clin. Pharmacol. Ther.*, **1979**, *26*, 354–365.

NADOLOL [a] (Chapter 9)

AVAILABILITY (ORAL) (%)	URINARY EXCRETION (%)	BOUND IN PLASMA (%)	CLEARANCE $(ml \cdot min^{-1} \cdot kg^{-1})$
34 ± 5 (1)	73 ± 4 (1)	20 ± 4 (2)	2.9 ± 0.6 (1)

VOL. DIST. (liters/kg)	HALF-LIFE (hours)	EFFECTIVE CONCENTRATIONS	TOXIC CONCENTRATIONS
2.1 ± 1.0 [b] (1)	16 ± 2 (2) ↑ Urem (3)	—	—

[a] Data in (1) and (2) are from patients with mild essential hypertension.
[b] Vd_{area}.

1. Dreyfuss, J.; Brannick, L. J.; Vukovich, R. A.; Shaw, J. M.; and Willard, D. A. Metabolic studies in patients with nadolol: oral and intravenous administration. *J. Clin. Pharmacol.*, **1977**, *17*, 300–307.
2. Dreyfuss, J.; Griffith, D. L.; Singhvi, S. M.; Shaw, J. M.; Ross, J. J.; Vukovich, R. A.; and Willard, D. A. Pharmacokinetics of nadolol, a beta-receptor antagonist: administration of therapeutic single- and multiple-dosage regimens to hypertensive patients. *J. Clin. Pharmacol.*, **1979**, *19*, 712–721.
3. Frishman, W. Clinical pharmacology of the new beta-adrenergic blocking drugs. Part 9. Nadolol: A new long-acting beta-adrenoceptor blocking drug. *Am. Heart J.*, **1980**, *99*, 124–128.

Key: Adult = adults; Aged = aged; Alb = hypoalbuminemia; AVH = acute viral hepatitis; CF = cystic fibrosis; CHF = congestive heart failure; Child = children; Cirr = cirrhosis; COPD = chronic obstructive pulmonary disease; CP = cor pulmonale; CPBS = cardiopulmonary bypass surgery; CRI = chronic respiratory insufficiency; Cush = cushingoid; Epilep = epilepsy; Fem = females; Hep = hepatitis; HL = hyperlipoproteinemia; HTh = hyperthyroid; Inflam = inflammation; LTh = hypothyroid; MI = myocardial infarction; Neo = neonates; NS = nephrotic syndrome; Obes = obesity; Pneu = pneumonia; Preg = pregnant; Prem = premature infants; RA = rheumatoid arthritis; Smk = smoking; Tach = ventricular tachycardia; Urem = uremia.

NAFCILLIN (Chapter 50)

AVAILABILITY (ORAL) (%)	URINARY EXCRETION (%)	BOUND IN PLASMA (%)	CLEARANCE $(ml \cdot min^{-1} \cdot kg^{-1})$
36 [a] (1)	27 ± 5 (2)	84–90 (2) ↓ Neo (3)	5.9 [b] (4)

VOL. DIST. (liters/kg)	HALF-LIFE (hours)	EFFECTIVE CONCENTRATIONS	TOXIC CONCENTRATIONS
1.1 ± 0.3 [c] (2)	0.9–22 (2) ↑ Urem (4)	See Chapter 50	See Chapter 50

[a] Calculated from mean values of excretion after oral versus intramuscular administration.
[b] Assuming 1.73 m² equivalent to 70 kg.
[c] Vd_{area}.

1. Klein, J. O., and Finland, M. Nafcillin, antibacterial action *in vitro* and absorption and excretion in normal young men. *Am. J. Med. Sci.*, **1963**, *246*, 10–26.
2. Rudnick, M.; Morrison, G.; Walker, B.; and Singer, I. Renal failure, hemodialysis, and nafcillin kinetics. *Clin. Pharmacol. Ther.*, **1976**, *20*, 413–423.
3. Krasner, J.; Giacoia, G. P.; and Yaffe, S. J. Drug-protein binding in the newborn infant. *Ann. N.Y. Acad. Sci.*, **1973**, *226*, 101–114.
4. Kind, A. C.; Tupase, T. E.; Standiford, H. C.; and Kirby, W. M. Mechanisms responsible for plasma levels of nafcillin lower than those of oxacillin. *Arch. Intern. Med.*, **1970**, *125*, 685–690.

NEOSTIGMINE (Chapter 6)

AVAILABILITY (ORAL) (%)	URINARY EXCRETION (%)	BOUND IN PLASMA (%)	CLEARANCE $(ml \cdot min^{-1} \cdot kg^{-1})$
[a]	67 (1)	—	8.4 ± 2.7 (2) ↓ Urem (2)

VOL. DIST. (liters/kg)	HALF-LIFE (hours)	EFFECTIVE CONCENTRATIONS	TOXIC CONCENTRATIONS
0.7 ± 0.3 (2)	1.3 ± 0.8 (2) ↑ Urem (2)	—	—

[a] Absorption is presumed to be less than complete, since oral dosage must greatly exceed intravenous to achieve a similar effect.

1. Nowell, P. T.; Scott, C. A.; and Wilson, A. Determination of neostigmine and pyridostigmine in the urine of patients with myasthenia gravis. *Br. J. Pharmacol.*, **1962**, *18*, 617–624.
2. Cronnelly, R.; Stanski, D. R.; Miller, R. D.; Sheiner, L. B.; and Sohn, Y. J. Renal function and the pharmacokinetics of neostigmine in anesthetized man. *Anesthesiology*, **1979**, *51*, 222–226.

NITRAZEPAM (Chapter 17)

AVAILABILITY (ORAL) (%)	URINARY EXCRETION (%)	BOUND IN PLASMA (%)	CLEARANCE $(ml \cdot min^{-1} \cdot kg^{-1})$
78 ± 16 (1)	<1 (1)	87 (2)	1.0 ± 0.5 [a] (3) ↔ Aged (3)

VOL. DIST. (liters/kg)	HALF-LIFE (hours)	EFFECTIVE CONCENTRATIONS	TOXIC CONCENTRATIONS
2.4 ± 0.8 [a] (3) ↑ Aged (3)	29 ± 7 (3) ↑ Aged (3)	—	>200 ng/ml [b] (3)

[a] CL/F and Vd_{area}/F.
[b] Sedation and drowsiness.

1. Rieder, J. Plasma levels and derived pharmacokinetic characteristics of unchanged nitrazepam in man. *Arzneim. Forsch.*, **1978**, *23*, 212–218.
2. Greenblatt, D. J., and Shader, R. I. *Benzodiazepines in Clinical Practice.* Raven Press, New York, **1974**.

3. Kangas, L.; Iisalo, E.; Kanto, J.; Lehitnen, V.; Pynnönen, S.; Ruikka, I.; Salminen, J.; Sillanpää, M.; and Syvälahti, E. Human pharmacokinetics of nitrazepam: effect of age and diseases. *Eur. J. Clin. Pharmacol.*, **1979**, *15*, 163–170.

NITROGLYCERIN [a] (Chapter 33)

AVAILABILITY (ORAL) (%)	URINARY EXCRETION (%)	BOUND IN PLASMA (%)	CLEARANCE $(ml \cdot min^{-1} \cdot kg^{-1})$
40 (1)	<1 [b] (1)	—	2.2 [b] (1)

VOL. DIST. (*liters/kg*)	HALF-LIFE (*hours*)	EFFECTIVE CONCENTRATIONS	TOXIC CONCENTRATIONS
0.34 [b,c] (1)	1.8 [b] (1)	—	—

[a] Nitroglycerin (glyceryl trinitrate) is metabolized very rapidly to dinitrates and mononitrates. Pharmacokinetic values are for nitroglycerin plus the dinitrates, since the latter are pharmacologically active.
[b] Refers to dinitrates when nitroglycerin is given sublingually.
[c] Vd_{area}.

1. Neurath, G. B., and Dünger, M. Blood levels of the metabolites of glyceryl trinitrate and pentaerythritol tetranitrate after administration of a two-step preparation. *Arzneim. Forsch.*, **1977**, *27*, 416–519.

NORTRIPTYLINE (Chapter 19)

AVAILABILITY (ORAL) (%)	URINARY EXCRETION (%)	BOUND IN PLASMA (%)	CLEARANCE $(ml \cdot min^{-1} \cdot kg^{-1})$
51 ± 5 (1)	2 ± 1 (2)	94.5 ± 0.6 [a] (3)	7.2 ± 1.8 (1)

VOL. DIST. (*liters/kg*)	HALF-LIFE (*hours*)	EFFECTIVE CONCENTRATIONS	TOXIC CONCENTRATIONS
18 ± 4 [b] (1)	31 ± 13 (1)	50–139 ng/ml [c] (4)	—

[a] Determined at 24–26° C in heparinized plasma.
[b] Vd_{area}.
[c] At concentrations in plasma above 140 ng/ml, the antidepressant effect appears to be less (4,5).

1. Gram, L. F., and Overø, K. F. First-pass metabolism of nortriptyline in man. *Clin. Pharmacol. Ther.*, **1974**, *18*, 305–314.
2. Alexanderson, B., and Borga, O. Urinary excretion of nortriptyline and five of its metabolites in man after single and multiple oral dose. *Eur. J. Clin. Pharmacol.*, **1973**, *5*, 174–180.
3. Borgå, O.; Azarnoff, D. L.; Plym Forshell, G.; and Sjöqvist, F. Plasma protein binding of tricyclic antidepressants in man. *Biochem. Pharmacol.*, **1969**, *18*, 2135–2143.
4. Åsberg, M.; Crönholm, B.; Sjöqvist, F.; and Tuck, D. Relationship between plasma level and therapeutic effect of nortriptyline. *Br. Med. J.*, **1971**, *3*, 331–334.
5. Kragh-Sørensen, P.; Åsberg, M.; and Eggert-Hansen, C. Plasma nortriptyline levels in endogenous depression. *Lancet*, **1973**, *1*, 113–115.

Key: Adult = adults; Aged = aged; Alb = hypoalbuminemia; AVH = acute viral hepatitis; CF = cystic fibrosis; CHF = congestive heart failure; Child = children; Cirr = cirrhosis; COPD = chronic obstructive pulmonary disease; CP = cor pulmonale; CPBS = cardiopulmonary bypass surgery; CRI = chronic respiratory insufficiency; Cush = cushingoid; Epilep = epilepsy; Fem = females; Hep = hepatitis; HL = hyperlipoproteinemia; HTh = hyperthyroid; Inflam = inflammation; LTh = hypothyroid; MI = myocardial infarction; Neo = neonates; NS = nephrotic syndrome; Obes = obesity; Pneu = pneumonia; Preg = pregnant; Prem = premature infants; RA = rheumatoid arthritis; Smk = smoking; Tach = ventricular tachycardia; Urem = uremia.

PHENOBARBITAL (Chapters 17, 20)

AVAILABILITY (ORAL) (%)	URINARY EXCRETION (%)	BOUND IN PLASMA (%)	CLEARANCE $(ml \cdot min^{-1} \cdot kg^{-1})$
— [a]	24 ± 5 [b] (2)	51 (3) ↓ Neo (3)	0.093 ± 0.044 [c] (4) ↑ Preg (5), Child (6) ↔ Neo [d] (7)

VOL. DIST. (liters/kg)	HALF-LIFE (hours)	EFFECTIVE CONCENTRATIONS	TOXIC CONCENTRATIONS
0.88 ± 0.33 [c] (4) ↔ Neo (8)	86 ± 7 (2) ↓ Child (9) ↑ Cirr (?), Aged (10)	10–25 µg/ml [e] (11) 15 µg/ml [f] (12)	>30 µg/ml (12) 65–117 µg/ml [g] (13) 100–134 µg/ml [h] (13)

[a] A value of >80% has been calculated from plasma concentrations and assumptions of a value for Vd (1).

[b] Increased when urine is alkaline; decreased with decreased urine flow; no change in Cirr or AVH (2).

[c] Data from oral, multiple-dose regimen; values are CL/F and Vd_{area}/F.

[d] Average clearance following daily intravenous dosage: week 1, 0.10; week 4, 0.17. Insufficient information to determine whether change is due to natural maturation or induction of metabolism by drug.

[e] Grand mal seizures.

[f] Febrile convulsions in children.

[g] Stage III—comatose, reflexes present.

[h] Stage IV—no deep-tendon reflexes.

1. Svensmark, O., and Buchthal, F. Accumulation of phenobarbital in man. *Epilepsia,* **1963,** *4,* 199–206.
2. Alvin, J.; McHorse, T.; Hoyumpa, A.; Bush, M. T.; and Schenker, S. The effect of liver disease in man on the disposition of phenobarbital. *J. Pharmacol. Exp. Ther.,* **1975,** *192,* 224–235.
3. Ehrnebo, M.; Agurell, S.; Jalling, B.; and Boreus, L. O. Age differences in drug binding by plasma proteins: studies on human foetuses, neonates and adults. *Eur. J. Clin. Pharmacol.,* **1971,** *3,* 189–193.
4. Butler, T. C.; Makaffee, C.; and Waddell, W. J. Phenobarbital: studies of elimination, accumulation, tolerance and dosage schedules. *J. Pharmacol. Exp. Ther.,* **1954,** *111,* 425–435.
5. Dam, M.; Christiansen, J.; Munck, O.; and Mygind, K. I. Antiepileptic drugs: metabolism in pregnancy. *Clin. Pharmacokinet.,* **1979,** *4,* 53–62.
6. Svensmark, O., and Buchthal, F. Diphenylhydantoin and phenobarbital serum levels in children. *Am. J. Dis. Child.,* **1964,** *108,* 82–87.
7. Pitlick, W.; Painter, M.; and Pippenger, C. Phenobarbital pharmacokinetics in neonates. *Clin. Pharmacol. Ther.,* **1978,** *23,* 346–350.
8. Painter, M. J.; Pippenger, C.; MacDonald, H.; and Pitlick, W. Phenobarbital and diphenylhydantoin levels in neonates with seizures. *J. Pediatr.,* **1978,** *92,* 315–319.
9. Garrettson, L. K., and Dayton, P. G. Disappearance of phenobarbital and diphenylhydantoin from serum of children. *Clin. Pharmacol. Ther.,* **1970,** *11,* 674–679.
10. Traeger, A.; Kieswetter, R.; and Kunze, M. Zur Pharmakokinetik von Phenobarbital bei Erwachsenen und Griesen. *Dtsch. Ges. Wesen.,* **1974,** *29,* 1040–1042.
11. Buchthal, F.; Svensmark, O.; and Simonsen, H. Relation of EEG and seizure to phenobarbital in serum. *Arch. Neurol.,* **1968,** *19,* 567–572.
12. Buchthal, F., and Lennox-Buchthal, M. A. Phenobarbital. Relation of serum concentration to control of seizures. In, *Antiepileptic Drugs.* (Woodbury, D. M.; Penry, J. K.; and Schmidt, R. P.; eds.) Raven Press, New York, **1972,** pp. 335–343.
13. Sunshine, I. Chemical evidence of tolerance to phenobarbital. *J. Lab. Clin. Med.,* **1957,** *50,* 127–133.

Key: Adult = adults; Aged = aged; Alb = hypoalbuminemia; AVH = acute viral hepatitis; CF = cystic fibrosis; CHF = congestive heart failure; Child = children; Cirr = cirrhosis; COPD = chronic obstructive pulmonary disease; CP = cor pulmonale; CPBS = cardiopulmonary bypass surgery; CRI = chronic respiratory insufficiency; Cush = cushingoid; Epilep = epilepsy; Fem = females; Hep = hepatitis; HL = hyperlipoproteinemia; HTh = hyperthyroid; Inflam = inflammation; LTh = hypothyroid; MI = myocardial infarction; Neo = neonates; NS = nephrotic syndrome; Obes = obesity; Pneu = pneumonia; Preg = pregnant; Prem = premature infants; RA = rheumatoid arthritis; Smk = smoking; Tach = ventricular tachycardia; Urem = uremia.

PHENYTOIN (Chapters 20, 31)

AVAILABILITY (ORAL) (%)	URINARY EXCRETION (%)	BOUND IN PLASMA (%)	CLEARANCE
98 ± 7 (1)	2 ± 8 (2)	89 ± 23 (3) ↓ Urem (3), Hep (3), Alb (3)	$V_m = 8.4 ± 4.6$ mg·kg^{-1}·day^{-1} $K_m = 8.5 ± 1.9$ mg/l (4)

VOL. DIST. (liters/kg)	HALF-LIFE (hours)	EFFECTIVE CONCENTRATIONS	TOXIC CONCENTRATIONS
0.64 ± 0.04 [a] (1)	[b]	>10 µg/ml [c] (5)	>20 µg/ml [d] (5)

[a] Vd_{area}.
[b] Apparent half-life is dependent on plasma concentration (4).
[c] To achieve suppression of grand mal seizures.
[d] Nystagmus; ataxia may not occur until concentrations exceed 30 µg/ml.

1. Jusko, W. J.; Koup, J. R.; and Alvan, G. Nonlinear assessment of phenytoin bioavailability. *J. Pharmacokinet. Biopharm.,* **1976,** *4,* 327-336.
2. Wilder, B. J.; Streiff, R. R.; and Hammer, R. H. Diphenylhydantoin. In, *Antiepileptic Drugs.* (Woodbury, D. M.; Penry, J. K.; and Schmidt, R. P.; eds.) Raven Press, New York, **1972,** 137-148.
3. Hooper, W. D.; Bochner, F.; Eadie, M. J.; and Tyrer, J. H. Plasma protein binding of diphenylhydantoin. Effects of sex hormones, renal and hepatic disease. *Clin. Pharmacol. Ther.,* **1974,** *15,* 276-282.
4. Ludden, T. M.; Allen, J. P.; Valutsky, W. A.; Vicuna, A. V.; Nappi, J. M.; Hoffman, S. F.; Wallace, J. E.; Lalka, D.; and McNay, J. L. Individualization of phenytoin dosage regimens. *Clin. Pharmacol. Ther.,* **1977,** *21,* 287-293.
5. Lund, L. Anticonvulsant effect of diphenylhydantoin relative to plasma levels. *Arch. Neurol.,* **1974,** *31,* 289-294.

PINDOLOL [a] (Chapter 9)

AVAILABILITY (ORAL) (%)	URINARY EXCRETION (%)	BOUND IN PLASMA (%)	CLEARANCE (ml·min^{-1}·kg^{-1})
86 ± 21 [b] (2)	41 (3)	51 ± 3 (2)	6.2 ± 2.4 (3) ↓ Urem (2)

VOL. DIST. (liters/kg)	HALF-LIFE (hours)	EFFECTIVE CONCENTRATIONS	TOXIC CONCENTRATIONS
2.0 ± 0.3 (3) ↓ Urem [c] (3)	3.4 ± 0.2 (5) ↔ Urem (4) ↑ Urem (2)	58 ng/ml [d] (6)	—

[a] For review, *see* (1).
[b] Decreased in renal failure.
[c] The data in (4) can be used to derive the following equation:

$$Vd_{ss}(\text{l/kg}) = 0.58 \, CL_{cr} \, (\text{ml·min}^{-1}\text{·kg}^{-1}) + 1.14$$

[d] To achieve a 50% decrease in exercise-induced cardioacceleration.

1. Johnsson, G., and Regårdh, C. G. Clinical pharmacokinetics of β-adrenoreceptor blocking drugs. *Clin. Pharmacokinet.,* **1976,** *1,* 233-268.
2. Chau, N. P.; Weiss, Y. A.; Safar, M. E.; Lavene, D. E.; Georges, D. R.; and Milliez, P. L. Pindolol availability in hypertensive patients with normal and impaired renal function. *Clin. Pharmacol. Ther.,* **1977,** *22,* 505-510.
3. Gugler, R.; Herold, W.; and Dengler, H. J. Pharmacokinetics of pindolol in man. *Eur. J. Clin. Pharmacol.,* **1974,** *7,* 17-24.
4. Ohnhaus, E. E.; Nüesch, E.; Meier, J.; and Kalberer, F. Pharmacokinetics of unlabelled and ^{14}C-labelled pindolol in uremia. *Eur. J. Clin. Pharmacol.,* **1974,** *7,* 25-29.
5. Hicks, D. C.; Arbab, A. G.; Turner, P.; and Hills, M. A comparison of intravenous pindolol and propranolol in normal man. *J. Clin. Pharmacol.,* **1972,** *12,* 212-216.
6. Gugler, R.; Höbel, W.; Bodem, G.; and Dengler, H. J. The effect of pindolol on exercise-induced cardiac acceleration in relation to plasma levels in man. *Clin. Pharmacol. Ther.,* **1975,** *17,* 127-132.

PRAZOSIN (Chapter 32)

AVAILABILITY (ORAL) (%)	URINARY EXCRETION (%)	BOUND IN PLASMA (%)	CLEARANCE $(ml \cdot min^{-1} \cdot kg^{-1})$
57 ± 10 (1)	<1 (1)	93 ± 2 (2)	3.0 ± 0.3 [a] (1) $\downarrow$ CHF (3,4)

VOL. DIST. (liters/kg)	HALF-LIFE (hours)	EFFECTIVE CONCENTRATIONS	TOXIC CONCENTRATIONS
0.60 ± 0.13 [a] (1)	2.9 ± 0.8 (1) $\uparrow$ CHF (3,4)	—	—

[a] Assuming 70-kg body weight

1. Bateman, D. N.; Hobbs, D. C.; Twomey, T. M.; Stevens, E. A.; and Rawlins, M. D. Prazosin, pharmacokinetics and concentration effect. *Eur. J. Clin. Pharmacol.,* **1979,** *16,* 177–181.
2. Hobbs, D. C., and Twomey, T. M. Protein binding properties of prazosin. *Res. Commun. Chem. Pathol. Pharmacol.,* **1979,** *25,* 189–192.
3. Jaillon, P.; Rubin, P.; Yee, Y.-G.; Ball, R.; Kates, R.; Harrison, D.; and Blaschke, T. Influence of congestive heart failure on prazosin kinetics. *Clin. Pharmacol. Ther.,* **1979,** *25,* 790–794.
4. Baughman, R. A., Jr.; Arnold, S.; Benet, L. Z.; Lin, E. T.; Chatterjee, K.; and Williams, R. L. Altered prazosin pharmacokinetics in congestive heart failure. *Eur. J. Clin. Pharmacol.,* **1980,** *17.*

PREDNISOLONE [a] (Chapter 63)

AVAILABILITY (ORAL) (%)	URINARY EXCRETION (%)	BOUND IN PLASMA (%)	CLEARANCE $(ml \cdot min^{-1} \cdot kg^{-1})$
82 ± 13 (3)	Little	90–95 (<200 ng/ml) [b] (4) $\sim$70 (>1 μg/ml) (4) $\downarrow$ Alb (4) $\leftrightarrow$ Hep (5)	1.4 ± 0.3 [c,d,e] (6) $\downarrow$ Cush (1,7) $\leftrightarrow$ Hep (5)

VOL. DIST. (liters/kg)	HALF-LIFE (hours)	EFFECTIVE CONCENTRATIONS	TOXIC CONCENTRATIONS
0.48 ± 0.08 [c,d] (6) $\downarrow$ Cush (1,7) $\leftrightarrow$ Hep (5)	2.1–4.0 [d,e] (3,6,8) $\leftrightarrow$ Cush (1,7), Hep (5) $\uparrow$ Hep (9)	—	—

[a] For reviews, *see* (1,2).
[b] Extent of binding to plasma proteins is dependent on concentration over range encountered (4).
[c] Values reported per m²; calculated assuming 70-kg weight.
[d] Values for 12-mg intravenous dose; with increasing dose, CL, $t_{1/2}$, and Vd_{ss} increase (6).
[e] More rapid elimination in patients treated previously with prednisolone (5).

1. Gambertoglio, J. G.; Amend, W. J. C.; and Benet, L. Z. Pharmacokinetics and bioavailability of prednisone and prednisolone in healthy volunteers and patients: a review. *J. Pharmacokinet. Biopharm.,* **1980,** *8,* 1–52.
2. Pickup, M. E. Clinical pharmacokinetics of prednisone and prednisolone. *Clin. Pharmacokinet.,* **1979,** *4,* 111–128.
3. Petereit, L. B., and Meikle, A. W. Effectiveness of prednisolone during phenytoin therapy. *Clin. Pharmacol. Ther.,* **1977,** *22,* 912–916.
4. Lewis, G. P.; Burke, C. W.; Graves, L.; and Jusko, W. J. Prednisone side effects and serum protein levels. *Lancet,* **1971,** *2,* 778–781.
5. Schalm, S. W.; Summerskill, W. H. J.; and Go, V. L. W. Prednisone for chronic active liver disease: pharmacokinetics, including conversion to prednisolone. *Gastroenterology,* **1977,** *72,* 910–913.
6. Meikle, A. W.; Weed, J. A.; and Tyler, F. H. Kinetics and interconversion of prednisolone and prednisone studied with new radioimmunoassays. *J. Clin. Endocrinol. Metab.,* **1975,** *41,* 717–721.
7. Gambertoglio, J.; Amend, W.; Vincenti, F.; Feduska, N.; Birnbaum, J.; and Salvatierra, O. The pharmacokinetics of prednisone in cushingoid and noncushingoid kidney transplant patients. *Clin. Res.,* **1979,** *27,* 231A.
8. Sullivan, T. J.; Stoll, R. G.; Sakamar, E.; Blair, D. C.; and Wagner, J. G. *In vitro* and *in vivo* availability of some commercial prednisolone tablets. *J. Pharmacokinet. Biopharm.,* **1974,** *2,* 29–41.
9. Davis, M.; William, R.; Chakraborty, J.; English, J.; Marks, V.; Ideo, G.; and Tempini, S. Prednisone or prednisolone for the treatment of chronic active hepatitis? A comparison of plasma availability. *Br. J. Clin. Pharmacol.,* **1978,** *5,* 501–505.

PREDNISONE [a] (Chapter 63)

AVAILABILITY (ORAL) (%)	URINARY EXCRETION (%)	BOUND IN PLASMA (%)	CLEARANCE $(ml \cdot min^{-1} \cdot kg^{-1})$
78 (range 22–127) [b] (4)	Little	—	3.6 ± 0.8 (3)

VOL. DIST. (*liters/kg*)	HALF-LIFE (*hours*)	EFFECTIVE CONCENTRATIONS	TOXIC CONCENTRATIONS
0.97 ± 0.11 (3)	3.6 ± 0.4 (3)	—	—

[a] For reviews, *see* (1,2). The kinetics of prednisone is often reported in terms of the parameters for prednisolone. However, values in (3) were determined by measurement of prednisone.

[b] Measured relative to equivalent intravenous dose of prednisolone.

1. Gambertoglio, J. G.; Amend, W. J. C.; and Benet, L. Z. Pharmacokinetics and bioavailability of prednisone and prednisolone in healthy volunteers and patients: a review. *J. Pharmacokinet. Biopharm.*, **1980**, *8*, 1–52.
2. Pickup, M. E. Clinical pharmacokinetics of prednisone and prednisolone. *Clin. Pharmacokinet.*, **1979**, *4*, 111–128.
3. Schalm, S. W.; Summerskill, W. H. J.; and Go, V. L. W. Prednisone for chronic active liver disease: pharmacokinetics, including conversion to prednisolone. *Gastroenterology*, **1977**, *72*, 910–913.
4. Davis, M.; William, R.; Chakraborty, J.; English, J.; Marks, V.; Ideo, G.; and Tempini, S. Prednisone or prednisolone for the treatment of chronic active hepatitis? A comparison of plasma availability. *Br. J. Clin. Pharmacol.*, **1978**, *5*, 501–505.

PRIMIDONE (Chapter 20)

AVAILABILITY (ORAL) (%)	URINARY EXCRETION (%)	BOUND IN PLASMA (%)	CLEARANCE $(ml \cdot min^{-1} \cdot kg^{-1})$
92 ± 18 [a,b] (1)	42 ± 15 [a] (1)	19 [c] (2)	0.78 ± 0.62 [a,d] (1)

VOL. DIST. (*liters/kg*)	HALF-LIFE (*hours*)	EFFECTIVE CONCENTRATIONS	TOXIC CONCENTRATIONS
0.59 ± 0.47 [a,d] (1)	8.0 ± 4.8 (3) ↔ Child (1)	5–10 µg/ml [e] (4)	>10 µg/ml (4)

[a] Value in children.

[b] Based on percentage of dose recovered in urine as primidone and its metabolites, phenylethylmalonamide and phenobarbital.

[c] Based on ratio of drug concentrations in cerebrospinal fluid and plasma.

[d] Data from oral, multiple-dose regimen; values are CL/F and Vd_{area}/F.

[e] Concentrations observed in patients with seizures who are improved or controlled by primidone. Concentrations of phenobarbital, a metabolite, are considered to be more relevant (5).

1. Kauffman, R. E.; Habersang, R.; and Lansky, L. Kinetics of primidone metabolism and excretion in children. *Clin. Pharmacol. Ther.*, **1977**, *22*, 200–205.
2. Houghton, G. W.; Richens, A.; Toseland, P. A.; Davidson, S.; and Falconer, M. A. Brain concentrations of phenytoin, phenobarbitone and primidone in epileptic patients. *Eur. J. Clin. Pharmacol.*, **1975**, *9*, 73–78.
3. Gallagher, B. B.; Baumel, I. P.; and Mattson, R. H. Metabolic disposition of primidone and its metabolites in epileptic subjects after single and repeated administration. *Neurology (Minneap.)*, **1972**, *22*, 1186–1192.
4. Kutt, H. Pharmacodynamic and pharmacokinetic measures of antiepileptic drugs. *Clin. Pharmacol. Ther.*, **1974**, *16*, 243–250.
5. Booker, H. E.; Hosokowa, K.; Burdette, R. D.; and Darcy, B. A clinical study of serum primidone levels. *Epilepsia*, **1970**, *11*, 395–402.

Key: Adult = adults; Aged = aged; Alb = hypoalbuminemia; AVH = acute viral hepatitis; CF = cystic fibrosis; CHF = congestive heart failure; Child = children; Cirr = cirrhosis; COPD = chronic obstructive pulmonary disease; CP = cor pulmonale; CPBS = cardiopulmonary bypass surgery; CRI = chronic respiratory insufficiency; Cush = cushingoid; Epilep = epilepsy; Fem = females; Hep = hepatitis; HL = hyperlipoproteinemia; HTh = hyperthyroid; Inflam = inflammation; LTh = hypothyroid; MI = myocardial infarction; Neo = neonates; NS = nephrotic syndrome; Obes = obesity; Pneu = pneumonia; Preg = pregnant; Prem = premature infants; RA = rheumatoid arthritis; Smk = smoking; Tach = ventricular tachycardia; Urem = uremia.

PROCAINAMIDE [a] (Chapter 31)

AVAILABILITY (ORAL) (%)	URINARY EXCRETION (%)	BOUND IN PLASMA (%)	CLEARANCE $(ml \cdot min^{-1} \cdot kg^{-1})$	
75–95 (2) 83 ± 16 (3)	67 ± 8 [b] (4) ↓ CHF (6), COPD (6), CP (6), Cirr (7)	16 ± 5 (8)	Plasma (9): 9.8 ± 2.3 [c] 8.6 ± 3.1 [d] Renal (9): 5.2 ± 1.7 [b,e]	Nonrenal (9): 4.7 ± 0.4 [c] 3.4 ± 0.9 [d] ↓ Urem (9)

VOL. DIST. (*liters/kg*)	HALF-LIFE (*hours*)	EFFECTIVE CONCENTRATIONS	TOXIC CONCENTRATIONS
1.9 ± 0.3 (9) ↓ CHF (2) ↔ Urem (9)	2.9 ± 0.6 [c] (11) 3.0 ± 0.6 [d] (11) ↑ Urem (9), MI (12)	3, 5 μg/ml [f,g] (2)	Minor: 9 μg/ml [g,h] (2) Major: 14 μg/ml [g,h] (2)

[a] For review, *see* (1). *See also* data for N-acetylprocainamide (NAPA), an active metabolite.
[b] No significant difference between slow and fast acetylators (5).
[c] Fast acetylators.
[d] Slow acetylators.
[e] Independent of urine pH and rate of flow (10).
[f] Effective concentrations in 50% and 90% of patients, respectively.
[g] Assay used did not measure NAPA.
[h] Concentrations to produce toxicity in 10% of patients.

1. Karlsson, E.   Clinical pharmacokinetics of procainamide. *Clin. Pharmacokinet.,* **1978,** *3,* 97–107.
2. Koch-Weser, J., and Klein, S. W.   Procainamide dosage schedules, plasma concentrations and clinical effects. *J.A.M.A.,* **1971,** *215,* 1454–1460.
3. Manion, C. V.; Lalka, D.; Baer, D. T.; and Meyer, M. B.   Absorption kinetics of procainamide in humans. *J. Pharm. Sci.,* **1977,** *66,* 981–984.
4. Graffner, C.; Johnsson, G.; and Sjögren, J.   Pharmacokinetics of procainamide intravenously and orally as conventional and slow-release tablets. *Clin. Pharmacol. Ther.,* **1975,** *17,* 414–423.
5. Gibson, T. P.; Matusik, J.; Matusik, E.; Nelson, H. A.; Wilkinson, J.; and Briggs, W. A.   Acetylation of procainamide in man and its relationship to isonicotinic acid hydrazide acetylation phenotype. *Clin. Pharmacol. Ther.,* **1975,** *17,* 395–399.
6. du Souich, P., and Erill, S.   Metabolism of procainamide in patients with chronic heart failure, chronic respiratory failure and chronic renal disease. *Eur. J. Clin. Pharmacol.,* **1978,** *14,* 21–27.
7. du Souich, P., and Erill, S.   Metabolism of procainamide and *p*-aminobenzoic acid in patients with chronic liver disease. *Clin. Pharmacol. Ther.,* **1977,** *22,* 588–595.
8. Reidenberg, M. M.; Drayer, D. E.; Levy, M.; and Warner, H.   Polymorphic acetylation of procainamide in man. *Clin. Pharmacol. Ther.,* **1975,** *17,* 722–730.
9. Gibson, T. P.; Atkinson, A. J., Jr.; Matusik, E.; Nelson, L. D.; and Briggs, W. A.   Kinetics of procainamide and N-acetylprocainamide in renal failure. *Kidney Int.,* **1977,** *12,* 422–429.
10. Galeazzi, R. L.; Sheiner, L. B.; Lockwood, T.; and Benet, L. Z.   The renal elimination of procainamide. *Clin. Pharmacol. Ther.,* **1976,** *19,* 55–62.
11. Karlsson, E., and Molin, L.   Polymorphic acetylation of procaineamide in healthy subjects. *Acta Med. Scand.,* **1975,** *197,* 299–302.
12. Giardina, E.-G.V.; Dreyfuss, J.; Bigger, J. T., Jr.; Shaw, J. M.; and Schreiber, E. C.   Metabolism of procainamide in normal and cardiac subjects. *Clin. Pharmacol. Ther.,* **1976,** *19,* 339–351.

Key: Adult = adults;   Aged = aged;   Alb = hypoalbuminemia;   AVH = acute viral hepatitis;   CF = cystic fibrosis;   CHF = congestive heart failure;   Child = children;   Cirr = cirrhosis;   COPD = chronic obstructive pulmonary disease;   CP = cor pulmonale;   CPBS = cardiopulmonary bypass surgery;   CRI = chronic respiratory insufficiency;   Cush = cushingoid;   Epilep = epilepsy;   Fem = females;   Hep = hepatitis;   HL = hyperlipoproteinemia;   HTh = hyperthyroid;   Inflam = inflammation;   LTh = hypothyroid;   MI = myocardial infarction;   Neo = neonates;   NS = nephrotic syndrome;   Obes = obesity;   Pneu = pneumonia;   Preg = pregnant;   Prem = premature infants;   RA = rheumatoid arthritis;   Smk = smoking;   Tach = ventricular tachycardia;   Urem = uremia.

PROPRANOLOL [a] (Chapters 9, 31–33)

AVAILABILITY (ORAL) (%)	URINARY EXCRETION (%)	BOUND IN PLASMA (%)	CLEARANCE $(ml \cdot min^{-1} \cdot kg^{-1})$
36 ± 10 [b] (2)	<0.5	93.3 ± 1.2 (2) ↑ Inflam [c] (3)	12 ± 3 [b] (2) $CL_{int} = 37 \pm 16$ [b] (2) ↓ Hep (4)

VOL. DIST. (liters/kg)	HALF-LIFE (hours)	EFFECTIVE CONCENTRATIONS	TOXIC CONCENTRATIONS
3.9 ± 0.6 [b,d] (2) ↑ Hep (4)	3.9 ± 0.4 [b] (2) ↑ Hep (4)	20 ng/ml [e] (5)	—

[a] For review, see (1).

[b] Hepatic metabolism (responsible for the low availability) has a saturable component. Data given are for "large" doses at steady state when the component is saturated (2). Measurements were made on whole blood.

[c] The concentration of α_1-acid glycoprotein, a plasma protein that binds propranolol, is elevated in a variety of inflammatory conditions.

[d] Vd_{area}.

[e] To achieve 50% decrease in exercise-induced cardioacceleration. Antianginal effects are manifest at 15–90 ng/ml (6). Concentrations up to 1000 ng/ml may be required to control resistant ventricular arrhythmias (see Chapter 31).

1. Johnsson, G., and Regårdh, C. G. Clinical pharmacokinetics of β-adrenergic blocking drugs. Clin. Pharmacokinet., 1976, 1, 233–263.
2. Kornhauser, D. M.; Wood, J. J.; Vestal, R. E.; Wilkinson, G. R.; Branch, R. A.; and Shand, D. G. Biological determinants of propranolol disposition in man. Clin. Pharmacol. Ther., 1978, 23, 165–174.
3. Piafsky, K. M.; Borgå, O.; Odar-Cederlöf, I.; Johansson, C.; and Sjöqvist, F. Increased plasma protein binding of propranolol and chlorpromazine mediated by disease-induced elevations of plasma α₁ acid glycoproteins. N. Engl. J. Med., 1978, 299, 1435–1438.
4. Branch, R. A.; James, J.; and Read, A. E. A study of factors influencing drug disposition in chronic liver disease, using the model drug (+)-propranolol. Br. J. Clin. Pharmacol., 1976, 3, 243–249.
5. McAinsh, J.; Baker, N. S.; Smith, R.; and Young, J. Pharmacokinetic and pharmacodynamic studies with long-acting propranolol. Br. J. Clin. Pharmacol., 1978, 6, 115–121.
6. Chidsey, C.; Pine, M.; Farrot, L.; Smith, S.; Leonetti, G.; Morselli, P.; and Zanchetti, A. The use of drug concentration measurements in studies of the therapeutic responses to propranolol. Postgrad. Med. J., 1976, 52, Suppl. 4, 26–32.

PROTRIPTYLINE (Chapter 19)

AVAILABILITY (ORAL) (%)	URINARY EXCRETION (%)	BOUND IN PLASMA (%)	CLEARANCE $(ml \cdot min^{-1} \cdot kg^{-1})$
77–93 [a]	—	92 ± 0.6 [b] (1)	3.6 ± 0.6 [c] (2)

VOL. DIST. (liters/kg)	HALF-LIFE (hours)	EFFECTIVE CONCENTRATIONS	TOXIC CONCENTRATIONS
22 ± 1 [d] (2)	78 ± 11 (2)	70–250 ng/ml [e] (3,4)	—

[a] Estimated from reported values of CL/F, assuming erythrocyte-to-plasma ratio ranges from 0 to 2, complete absorption, hepatic blood flow of 1500 ml/min, and hematocrit of 0.45.

[b] Determined at 24–26° C in heparinized plasma.

[c] CL/F.

[d] Vd_{area}/F.

[e] Antidepressant effect; lower limit determined with more specific assay (3). Upper limit of 170 ng/ml may be consistent with the more specific assay (3).

1. Nies, A.; Robinson, D. S.; Friedman, M. J.; Green, R.; Cooper, T. B.; Ravaris, C. L.; and Ives, J. O. Relationship between age and tricyclic antidepressant plasma levels. Am. J. Psychiatry, 1977, 134, 790–793.
2. Moody, J. P.; Whyte, S. F.; MacDonald, A. J.; and Naylor, G. J. Pharmacokinetic aspects of protriptyline plasma levels. Eur. J. Clin. Pharmacol., 1977, 11, 51–56.
3. Biggs, J. T., and Ziegler, V. E. Protriptyline plasma levels and antidepressant response. Clin. Pharmacol. Ther., 1977, 22, 269–273.
4. Whyte, S. F.; MacDonald, A. J.; Naylor, G. J.; and Moody, J. P. Plasma concentrations of protriptyline and clinical effects in depressed women. Br. J. Psychiatry, 1976, 128, 384–390.

PYRIDOSTIGMINE (Chapter 6)

AVAILABILITY (ORAL) (%)	URINARY EXCRETION (%)	BOUND IN PLASMA (%)	CLEARANCE $(ml \cdot min^{-1} \cdot kg^{-1})$
[a]	80–90 (1)	—	8.5 ± 1.7 (2) ↓ Urem (2)

VOL. DIST. (liters/kg)	HALF-LIFE (hours)	EFFECTIVE CONCENTRATIONS	TOXIC CONCENTRATIONS
1.1 ± 0.3 (2)	1.9 ± 0.2 (2) ↑ Urem (2)	50–100 ng/ml [b] (3)	—

[a] Absorption is presumed to be less than complete, since oral dosage must greatly exceed intravenous to achieve a similar effect.
[b] Restoration of neuromuscular transmission in myasthenic patients.

1. Kornfeld, P.; Samuels, A. J.; Wolf, R. L.; and Osserman, K. E. Metabolism of ^{14}C-labeled pyridostigmine in myasthenia gravis. *Neurology (Minneap.)*, **1970**, *20*, 634–641.
2. Cronnelly, R.; Stanski, D. R.; Miller, R. D.; and Sheiner, L. B. Pharmacokinetics of pyridostigmine in patients with and without renal function. *Clin. Pharmacol. Ther.*, **1980**, *27*.
3. Chan, K., and Calvey, T. N. Plasma concentration of pyridostigmine and effects in myasthenia gravis. *Clin. Pharmacol. Ther.*, **1977**, *22*, 596–601.

QUINIDINE (Chapter 31)

AVAILABILITY (ORAL) (%)	URINARY EXCRETION (%)	BOUND IN PLASMA (%)	CLEARANCE $(ml \cdot min^{-1} \cdot kg^{-1})$
Gluconate: 71 ± 17 (1,2) Sulfate: 80 ± 15 (2)	18 ± 5 (1) ↔ CHF (3)	71 ± 11 (4) ↓ Cirr (5), Hep (6) ↔ Urem (6), CRI (6), HL (4), Aged (7)	4.7 ± 1.8 (8) ↓ CHF (3,9), Aged (7), Cirr [a] (9)

VOL. DIST. (liters/kg)	HALF-LIFE (hours)	EFFECTIVE CONCENTRATIONS	TOXIC CONCENTRATIONS
2.7 ± 1.2 (3) ↓ CHF (3) ↔ Aged (7) ↑ Cirr [a] (9)	6.2 ± 1.8 (3) ↔ CHF (3), Urem (10) ↑ Aged (7), Cirr [a] (9)	2–5 µg/ml [b] (10) 3–7 µg/ml (12)	6, 9, 14 µg/ml [b,c] (13)

[a] Only one patient studied.
[b] A number of metabolites of quinidine, some of which are active, have been included in values obtained by older assay methods (11).
[c] Determined by a nonspecific assay. Concentrations that cause toxic effects in 10, 30, and 50% of patients, respectively.

1. Ueda, C. T.; Williamson, B. J.; and Dzindzio, B. S. Absolute quinidine bioavailability. *Clin. Pharmacol. Ther.*, **1976**, *20*, 260–265.
2. Greenblatt, D. J.; Pfeifer, N. J.; Ochs, H. R.; Franke, K.; MacLaughlin, D. S.; Smith, T. W.; and Koch-Weser, J. Pharmacokinetics of quinidine in humans after intravenous, intramuscular and oral administration. *J. Pharmacol. Exp. Ther.*, **1977**, *202*, 365–378.
3. Ueda, C. T., and Dzindzio, B. S. Quinidine kinetics in congestive heart failure. *Clin. Pharmacol. Ther.*, **1978**, *23*, 158–164.
4. Kates, R. E.; Sokoloski, T. D.; and Comstock, T. J. Binding of quinidine to plasma proteins in normal subjects and in patients with hyperlipoproteinemias. *Clin. Pharmacol. Ther.*, **1978**, *23*, 30–35.
5. Affrime, M., and Reidenberg, M. M. The protein binding of some drugs in plasma from patients with alcoholic liver disease. *Eur. J. Clin. Pharmacol.*, **1975**, *8*, 267–269.
6. Pérez-Mateo, M., and Erill, S. Protein binding of salicylate and quinidine in plasma from patients with renal failure, chronic liver disease and chronic respiratory insufficiency. *Eur. J. Clin. Pharmacol.*, **1977**, *11*, 225–231.
7. Ochs, H. R.; Greenblatt, D. J.; Woo, E.; and Smith, T. W. Reduced quinidine clearance in elderly persons. *Am. J. Cardiol.*, **1978**, *42*, 481–485.
8. Ueda, C. T.; Hirschfeld, D. S.; Scheinman, M. M.; Rowland, M.; Williamson, B. J.; and Dzindzio, B. S. Disposition kinetics of quinidine. *Clin. Pharmacol. Ther.*, **1976**, *19*, 30–36.
9. Conrad, K. A.; Molk, B. L.; and Chidsey, C. A. Pharmacokinetic studies of quinidine in patients with arrhythmias. *Circulation*, **1977**, *55*, 1–7.
10. Kessler, K. M.; Lowenthal, D. T.; Warner, H.; Gibson, T.; Briggs, W.; and Reidenberg, M. M. Quinidine elimination in patients with congestive heart failure or poor renal function. *N. Engl. J. Med.*, **1974**, *290*, 706–709.
11. Guentert, T. W.; Upton, R. A.; Holford, N. H. G.; and Riegelman, S. Divergence in pharmacokinetic parameters of quinidine obtained by specific and nonspecific assay methods. *J. Pharmacokinet. Biopharm.*, **1979**, *7*, 303–311.
12. Hirschfeld, D. S.; Ueda, C. T.; Rowland, M.; and Scheinman, M. M. Clinical and electrophysiological effects of intravenous quinidine in man. *Br. Heart J.*, **1977**, *39*, 309–316.
13. Sokolow, M., and Ball, R. E. Factors influencing conversion of chronic atrial fibrillation with special reference to serum quinidine concentration. *Circulation*, **1956**, *14*, 568–583.

RIFAMPIN [a] (Chapter 53)

AVAILABILITY (ORAL) (%)	URINARY EXCRETION (%)	BOUND IN PLASMA (%)	CLEARANCE ($ml \cdot min^{-1} \cdot kg^{-1}$)
[b]	16 ± 4 [c] (4)	89 ± 1 (5)	8.8 ± 0.9 (3) ↑ Neo (1,6)

VOL. DIST. (liters/kg)	HALF-LIFE (hours)	EFFECTIVE CONCENTRATIONS	TOXIC CONCENTRATIONS
1.6 ± 0.2 (3) ↑ Neo (1,6)	2.1 ± 0.3 [d] (3) ↔ Child (1) ↑ Hep (8), Cirr (9), AVH (9)	*See* Chapter 53	—

[a] For review, *see* (1). A high fraction of an oral dose is converted into an active, deacetylated metabolite (2).

[b] Although some studies indicate complete absorption (3), data are insufficient. Such reports presumably refer to rifampin plus its desacetyl metabolite, since considerable first-pass metabolism would be expected.

[c] Microbiological assay, which includes rifampin and active metabolites.

[d] Half-life is longer with high single doses and is shorter after repeated administration (7).

1. Acocella, G. Clinical pharmacokinetics of rifampicin. *Clin. Pharmacokinet.*, **1978**, *3*, 108–127.
2. Acocella, G.; Mattiussi, R.; and Segre, G. Multicompartmental analysis of serum, urine, and bile concentrations of rifampicin and desacetyl-rifampicin in subjects treated for one week. *Pharmacol. Res. Commun.*, **1978**, *10*, 271–288.
3. Furesz, S.; Scotti, R.; Pallanza, R.; and Mapelli, E. Rifampicin: a new rifamycin. *Arzneim. Forsch.*, **1967**, *17*, 534–537.
4. Nitti, V.; Virgilio, R.; Patricolo, M. R.; and Iuliano, A. Pharmacokinetic study of intravenous rifampicin. *Chemotherapy*, **1977**, *23*, 1–6.
5. Boman, G., and Ringberger, V. A. Binding of rifampicin by human plasma proteins. *Eur. J. Clin. Pharmacol.*, **1974**, *7*, 369–373.
6. Acocella, G.; Buniva, G.; Flauto, V.; and Nicolis, F. B. Absorption and elimination of the antibiotic rifampicin in newborns and children. In, *Progress in Antimicrobial and Anticancer Chemotherapy*. University Park Press, Baltimore, **1970**, *2*, 755–760.
7. Acocella, G.; Pagani, V.; Marchetti, M.; Baroni, G. C.; and Nicolis, F. B. Kinetic studies of rifampicin. *Chemotherapy*, **1971**, *16*, 356–370.
8. Acocella, G.; Bonollo, L.; Garimoldi, M.; Mainardi, M.; Tenconi, L. T.; and Nicolis, F. B. Kinetics of rifampicin and isoniazid administered alone and in combination to normal subjects and patients with liver disease. *Gut*, **1973**, *13*, 47–53.
9. Jeanes, C. W. L.; Jessamine, A. G.; and Eidus, L. Treatment of chronic drug-resistant pulmonary tuberculosis with rifampin and ethambutol. *Can. Med. Assoc. J.*, **1972**, *106*, 884–888.

Key: Adult = adults; Aged = aged; Alb = hypoalbuminemia; AVH = acute viral hepatitis; CF = cystic fibrosis; CHF = congestive heart failure; Child = children; Cirr = cirrhosis; COPD = chronic obstructive pulmonary disease; CP = cor pulmonale; CPBS = cardiopulmonary bypass surgery; CRI = chronic respiratory insufficiency; Cush = cushingoid; Epilep = epilepsy; Fem = females; Hep = hepatitis; HL = hyperlipoproteinemia; HTh = hyperthyroid; Inflam = inflammation; LTh = hypothyroid; MI = myocardial infarction; Neo = neonates; NS = nephrotic syndrome; Obes = obesity; Pneu = pneumonia; Preg = pregnant; Prem = premature infants; RA = rheumatoid arthritis; Smk = smoking; Tach = ventricular tachycardia; Urem = uremia.

SALICYLIC ACID [a] (Chapter 29)

AVAILABILITY (ORAL) (%)	URINARY EXCRETION (%)	BOUND IN PLASMA (%)	CLEARANCE $(ml \cdot min^{-1} \cdot kg^{-1})$
100 (2)	[b]	Dose dependent [c] (4) ↓ Urem (4,5), Alb (5), Neo (6), Preg (6)	0.88 ± 0.16 at 11–16 µg/ml 0.20 ± 0.01 at 134–157 µg/ml 0.18 ± 0.02 at 254–312 µg/ml (7) [d] ↓ Neo (8)

VOL. DIST. (liters/kg)	HALF-LIFE (hours)	EFFECTIVE CONCENTRATIONS	TOXIC CONCENTRATIONS
0.17 ± 0.03 [e] (9)	Dose dependent [f] (1,11) ↑ Neo (8)	150–300 µg/ml [g] (12)	>200 µg/ml [h] (13)

[a] Drug displays dose-dependent kinetics. For review, *see* (1).

[b] Dependent on urinary pH (3) and dose (1).

[c] 95% at 14 µg/ml; 80% at 300 µg/ml; decreases further at higher concentrations (4).

[d] Note that total clearance does not decrease over therapeutic range in steady-state studies in normals (urine pH <6) due to inversely related changes in protein binding and clearance of unbound drug (7).

[e] At a dose of 1.2 g per day; *Vd* increases with increasing dose due to changes in protein binding (10).

[f] Ranges from 2.4 hours at 300-mg dose to 19 hours and longer where there is intoxication.

[g] Anti-inflammatory effects.

[h] Tinnitus.

1. Levy, G. Pharmacokinetics of salicylate in man. *Drug Metab. Rev.,* **1979,** *9,* 3–19.
2. Rowland, M.; Riegelman, S.; Harris, P. A.; and Sholkoff, S. D. Absorption kinetics of aspirin in man following oral administration of an aqueous solution. *J. Pharm. Sci.,* **1972,** *61,* 379–385.
3. Smith, P. K.; Gleason, H. L.; Stoll, C. G.; and Ogorzalek, S. Studies on the pharmacology of salicylates. *J. Pharmacol. Exp. Ther.,* **1946,** *87,* 237–255.
4. Borgå, O.; Odar-Cederlöf, I.; Ringberger, V.; and Norlin, A. Protein binding of salicylate in uremic and normal plasma. *Clin. Pharmacol. Ther.,* **1976,** *20,* 464–475.
5. Yacobi, A., and Levy, G. Intraindividual relationships between serum protein binding of drugs in normal human subjects, patients with impaired renal function, and rats. *J. Pharm. Sci.,* **1977,** *66,* 1285–1288.
6. Levy, G.; Procknal, J. A.; and Garrettson, L. K. Distribution of salicylate between neonatal and maternal serum at diffusion equilibrium. *Clin. Pharmacol. Ther.,* **1975,** *18,* 210–214.
7. Furst, D. E.; Tozer, T. N.; and Melmon, K. L. Salicylate clearance, the resultant of protein binding and metabolism. *Clin. Pharmacol. Ther.,* **1979,** *26,* 380–389.
8. Levy, G., and Garrettson, L. K. Kinetics of salicylate elimination by newborn infants of mothers who ingested aspirin before delivery. *Pediatrics,* **1974,** *53,* 201–210.
9. Graham, G. G.; Champion, G. D.; Day, R. O.; and Paull, P. D. Patterns of plasma concentrations and urinary excretion of salicylate in rheumatoid arthritis. *Clin. Pharmacol. Ther.,* **1977,** *22,* 410–420.
10. Levy, G., and Yaffe, S. J. Relationship between dose and apparent volume of distribution of salicylate in children. *Pediatrics,* **1974,** *54,* 713–717.
11. Levy, G. Pharmacokinetics of salicylate elimination in man. *J. Pharm. Sci.,* **1965,** *54,* 959–967.
12. Koch-Weser, J. Serum drug concentrations as therapeutic guides. *N. Engl. J. Med.,* **1972,** *287,* 227–231.
13. Mongan, E.; Kelly, P.; Nies, K.; Porter, W. W.; and Paulus, H. E. Tinnitus as an indication of therapeutic serum salicylate levels. *J.A.M.A.,* **1973,** *226,* 142–145.

SULFAMETHOXAZOLE (Chapter 49)

AVAILABILITY (ORAL) (%)	URINARY EXCRETION (%)	BOUND IN PLASMA (%)	CLEARANCE $(ml \cdot min^{-1} \cdot kg^{-1})$
~100 (1)	30 ± 1 (2)	62 ± 5 (2) ↓ Urem (2), Alb (2)	0.32 ± 0.04 [a] (3)

VOL. DIST. (liters/kg)	HALF-LIFE (hours)	EFFECTIVE CONCENTRATIONS	TOXIC CONCENTRATIONS
0.21 ± 0.02 [a] (3) ↑ Urem (4)	8.6 ± 0.3 [b] (4) ↑ Urem (4)	*See* Chapter 49	—

[a] Assuming 70-kg weight.

[b] Average of five studies, which included concurrent administration of trimethoprim and variation in urinary pH; these factors had no marked effect on the clearance of sulfamethoxazole.

1. Kaplan, S. A.; Weinfeld, R. E.; Abruzzo, C. W.; McFaden, K.; Jack, M. L.; and Weissman, L. Pharmacokinetic profile of trimethoprim-sulfamethoxazole in man. *J. Infect. Dis.,* **1973,** *128,* Suppl., S547–S555.
2. Craig, W. A., and Kunin, C. M. Trimethoprim-sulfamethoxazole: pharmacodynamic effects of urinary pH and impaired renal function. *Ann. Intern. Med.,* **1973,** *78,* 491–497.
3. Morgan, D. J., and Raymond, K. Evaluation of slow infusions of co-trimoxazole by using predictive pharmacokinetics. *Antimicrob. Agents Chemother.,* **1980,** *17,* 132–137.
4. Welling, P. G.; Craig, W. A.; Amidon, G. L.; and Kunin, C. M. Pharmacokinetics of trimethoprim and sulfamethoxazole in normal subjects and in patients with renal failure. *J. Infect. Dis.,* **1973,** *128,* Suppl., S556–S566.

SULFISOXAZOLE (Chapter 49)

AVAILABILITY (ORAL) (%)	URINARY EXCRETION (%)	BOUND IN PLASMA (%)	CLEARANCE $(ml \cdot min^{-1} \cdot kg^{-1})$
100 (1)	53 ± 9 (1)	88–92 (2) ↓ Urem (3)	0.33 ± 0.05 (1)

VOL. DIST. (liters/kg)	HALF-LIFE (hours)	EFFECTIVE CONCENTRATIONS	TOXIC CONCENTRATIONS
0.15 ± 0.02 (1)	5.9 ± 0.9 (1) ↑ Urem (4)	*See* Chapter 49	—

1. Kaplan, S. A.; Weinfeld, R. E.; Abruzzo, C. W.; and Lewis, M. Pharmacokinetic profile of sulfisoxazole following intravenous, intramuscular, and oral administration to man. *J. Pharm. Sci.,* **1972,** *61,* 773–778.
2. Yacobi, A., and Levy, G. Intraindividual relationships between serum protein binding of drugs in normal human subjects, patients with impaired renal function, and rats. *J. Pharm. Sci.,* **1977,** *66,* 1285–1288.
3. Levy, G.; Baliah, T.; and Procknal, J. A. Effect of renal transplantation on protein binding of drugs in serum of donor and recipient. *Clin. Pharmacol. Ther.,* **1976,** *20,* 512–516.
4. Reidenberg, M. M.; Kostenbauder, H.; and Adams, W. P. Rate of drug metabolism in obese volunteers before and during starvation and in azotemic patients. *Metabolism,* **1969,** *18,* 209–213.

TETRACYCLINE (Chapter 52)

AVAILABILITY (ORAL) (%)	URINARY EXCRETION (%)	BOUND IN PLASMA (%)	CLEARANCE $(ml \cdot min^{-1} \cdot kg^{-1})$
77 (1)	48 (1)	65 ± 3 (1)	1.9 (1) $CL_{renal} = 1.1 \pm 0.4$ [a] (2)

VOL. DIST. (liters/kg)	HALF-LIFE (hours)	EFFECTIVE CONCENTRATIONS	TOXIC CONCENTRATIONS
1.3 (1)	9.9 ± 1.5 (3) ↑ Urem (4)	*See* Chapter 52	—

[a] Acidic urine; value is approximately 20% higher when urine is alkaline.

1. Bennett, J. V.; Mickelwait, J. S.; Barrett, J. E.; Brodie, J. L.; and Kirby, W. M. M. Comparative serum binding of four tetracyclines under simulated *in vivo* conditions. *Antimicrob. Agents Chemother.,* **1965,** 180–182.
2. Jaffe, J. M.; Colaizzi, J. L.; Poust, R. I.; and McDonald, R. H. Effect of altered urinary pH on tetracycline and doxycycline excretion in humans. *J. Pharmacokinet. Biopharm.,* **1973,** *1,* 267–282.
3. Doluisio, J. T., and Dittert, L. W. Influence of repetitive dosing of tetracyclines on biologic half-life in serum. *Clin. Pharmacol. Ther.,* **1969,** *10,* 690–701.
4. Kunin, C. M.; Rees, S. B.; Merrill, J. P.; and Finland, M. Persistence of antibiotics in blood of patients with acute renal failure. I. Tetracycline and chlortetracycline. *J. Clin. Invest.,* **1959,** *38,* 1487–1497.

Key: Adult = adults; Aged = aged; Alb = hypoalbuminemia; AVH = acute viral hepatitis; CF = cystic fibrosis; CHF = congestive heart failure; Child = children; Cirr = cirrhosis; COPD = chronic obstructive pulmonary disease; CP = cor pulmonale; CPBS = cardiopulmonary bypass surgery; CRI = chronic respiratory insufficiency; Cush = cushingoid; Epilep = epilepsy; Fem = females; Hep = hepatitis; HL = hyperlipoproteinemia; HTh = hyperthyroid; Inflam = inflammation; LTh = hypothyroid; MI = myocardial infarction; Neo = neonates; NS = nephrotic syndrome; Obes = obesity; Pneu = pneumonia; Preg = pregnant; Prem = premature infants; RA = rheumatoid arthritis; Smk = smoking; Tach = ventricular tachycardia; Urem = uremia.

THEOPHYLLINE [a] (Chapter 25)

AVAILABILITY (ORAL) (%)	URINARY EXCRETION (%)	BOUND IN PLASMA (%)	CLEARANCE ($ml \cdot min^{-1} \cdot kg^{-1}$)
96 ± 8 (2)	8 (3)	56 ± 4 (4) ↓ Neo (4), Cirr (5)	0.69 ± 0.30 (6) ↓ Neo (4), Prem (4), Cirr (5), CHF (6), Pneu (6) ↑ Smk (6)

VOL. DIST. (liters/kg)	HALF-LIFE (hours)	EFFECTIVE CONCENTRATIONS	TOXIC CONCENTRATIONS
0.50 ± 0.16 [b] (6) ↓ Obes (7) ↑ Prem (4), Cirr (5)	9.0 ± 2.1 (7) ↓ Smk (6) ↑ Prem (4), Cirr (5)	>5 µg/ml (8)	>20 µg/ml (3)

[a] For review, see (1).
[b] Vd_{area}.

1. Ogilvie, R. I. Clinical pharmacokinetics of theophylline. *Clin. Pharmacokinet.,* **1978,** *3,* 267–293.
2. Hendeles, L.; Weinberger, M.; and Bighley, L. Absolute bioavailability of oral theophylline. *Am. J. Hosp. Pharm.,* **1977,** *34,* 525–527.
3. Jenne, J. W.; Wyze, E.; Rood, F. S.; and MacDonald, F. M. Pharmacokinetics of theophylline. *Clin. Pharmacol. Ther.,* **1972,** *13,* 349–360.
4. Aranda, J. V.; Sitar, D. S.; Parsons, W. D.; Loughman, P. M.; and Neims, A. H. Pharmacokinetic aspects of theophylline in premature newborns. *N. Engl. J. Med.,* **1976,** *295,* 413–416.
5. Piafsky, K. M.; Sitar, D. S.; Rangno, R. E.; and Ogilvie, R. I. Theophylline disposition in patients with hepatic cirrhosis. *N. Engl. J. Med.,* **1977,** *296,* 1495–1497.
6. Powell, J. R.; Vozeh, S.; Hopewell, P.; Costello, J.; Sheiner, L. B.; and Riegelman, S. Theophylline disposition in acutely ill hospitalized patients. *Am. Rev. Respir. Dis.,* **1978,** *11,* 229–237.
7. Gal, P.; Jusko, W. J.; Yurichak, A. M.; and Franklin, B. A. Theophylline disposition in obesity. *Clin. Pharmacol. Ther.,* **1978,** *23,* 438–444.
8. Mitenko, P. A., and Ogilvie, R. I. Rational intravenous doses of theophylline. *N. Engl. J. Med.,* **1973,** *289,* 600–603.

TICARCILLIN (Chapter 50)

AVAILABILITY (ORAL) (%)	URINARY EXCRETION (%)	BOUND IN PLASMA (%)	CLEARANCE ($ml \cdot min^{-1} \cdot kg^{-1}$)
—	86 (1)	65 (1)	1.9 [a] (1) ↓ Urem (2)

VOL. DIST. (liters/kg)	HALF-LIFE (hours)	EFFECTIVE CONCENTRATIONS	TOXIC CONCENTRATIONS
0.22 [a] (1)	1.2 (1) ↑ Urem (2)	*See* Chapter 50	*See* Chapter 50

[a] Assuming 70-kg weight.

1. Libke, R. D.; Clarke, J. T.; Ralph, E. D.; Luthy, R. P.; and Kirby, W. M. M. Ticarcillin vs carbenicillin: clinical pharmacokinetics. *Clin. Pharmacol. Ther.,* **1975,** *17,* 441–446.
2. Davies, M.; Morgan, J. R.; and Anand, C. Administration of ticarcillin to patients with severe renal failure. *Chemotherapy,* **1974,** *20,* 339–341.

Key: Adult = adults; Aged = aged; Alb = hypoalbuminemia; AVH = acute viral hepatitis; CF = cystic fibrosis; CHF = congestive heart failure; Child = children; Cirr = cirrhosis; COPD = chronic obstructive pulmonary disease; CP = cor pulmonale; CPBS = cardiopulmonary bypass surgery; CRI = chronic respiratory insufficiency; Cush = cushingoid; Epilep = epilepsy; Fem = females; Hep = hepatitis; HL = hyperlipoproteinemia; HTh = hyperthyroid; Inflam = inflammation; LTh = hypothyroid; MI = myocardial infarction; Neo = neonates; NS = nephrotic syndrome; Obes = obesity; Pneu = pneumonia; Preg = pregnant; Prem = premature infants; RA = rheumatoid arthritis; Smk = smoking; Tach = ventricular tachycardia; Urem = uremia.

TOBRAMYCIN [a] (Chapter 51)

AVAILABILITY (ORAL) (%)	URINARY EXCRETION (%)	BOUND IN PLASMA (%)	CLEARANCE $(ml \cdot min^{-1} \cdot kg^{-1})$
—	90 [b] (2)	<10 (3)	$CL = 0.66\ CL_{cr}$ (4)

VOL. DIST. (*liters/kg*)	HALF-LIFE (*hours*)	EFFECTIVE CONCENTRATIONS	TOXIC CONCENTRATIONS
0.26 ± 0.09 (4) $\leftrightarrow$ Urem (4)	2.2 ± 0.1 (2) 100 ± 57 [c] (4) $\uparrow$ Urem (2–4)	*See* Chapter 51	*See* Chapter 51

[a] For reviews, *see* (1).
[b] Possibly higher, since drug persists in tissues for long periods of time.
[c] Tobramycin has a very long terminal half-life, which accounts for prolonged urinary excretion (*see* Chapter 51).

1. Symposium. (Various authors.) Tobramycin: comparative toxicity of aminoglycoside antibiotics. *J. Antimicrob. Chemother.*, **1978**, *4*, Suppl. A, 1–101.
2. Regamey, C.; Gordon, R. C.; and Kirby, W. M. M. Comparative pharmacokinetics of tobramycin and gentamicin. *Clin. Pharmacol. Ther.*, **1973**, *14*, 396–403.
3. Christopher, T. G.; Blair, A. D.; Forrey, A. W.; and Cutler,

R. E. Hemodialyzer clearances of gentamicin, kanamycin, tobramycin, amikacin, ethambutol, procainamide, and flucytosine, with a technique for planning therapy. *J. Pharmacokinet. Biopharm.*, **1976**, *4*, 427–441.
4. Schentag, J. J.; Lasezkay, G.; Cumbo, T. J.; Plaut, M. E.; and Jusko, W. J. Accumulation pharmacokinetics of tobramycin. *Antimicrob. Agents Chemother.*, **1978**, *13*, 649–656.

TOLBUTAMIDE (Chapter 64)

AVAILABILITY (ORAL) (%)	URINARY EXCRETION (%)	BOUND IN PLASMA (%)	CLEARANCE $(ml \cdot min^{-1} \cdot kg^{-1})$
93 ± 10 (1)	0 (2)	93 ± 1 (3) $\downarrow$ AVH (3)	0.30 ± 0.05 (3) $\uparrow$ AVH (3)

VOL. DIST. (*liters/kg*)	HALF-LIFE (*hours*)	EFFECTIVE CONCENTRATIONS	TOXIC CONCENTRATIONS
0.15 ± 0.03 (3) $\leftrightarrow$ AVH (3)	5.9 ± 1.4 (3) $\downarrow$ AVII (3), CRI (4) $\leftrightarrow$ Aged (5), Urem (6)	80–240 µg/ml [a] (7,8)	—

[a] Decrease in blood glucose concentration of greater than 25%.

1. Nelson, E., and O'Reilly, I. Kinetics of carboxytolbutamide excretion following tolbutamide and carboxytolbutamide administration. *J. Pharmacol. Exp. Ther.*, **1961**, *132*, 103–109.
2. Thomas, R. C., and Ikeda, G. J. The metabolic fate of tolbutamide in man and in the rat. *J. Med. Chem.*, **1966**, *9*, 507–512.
3. Williams, R. L.; Blaschke, T. F.; Meffin, P. J.; Melmon, K. L.; and Rowland, M. Influence of acute viral hepatitis on disposition and plasma binding of tolbutamide. *Clin. Pharmacol. Ther.*, **1977**, *21*, 301–309.
4. Sotaniemi, E.; Arvela, P.; Huhti, E.; and Koivisto, O. Half-life of tolbutamide in patients with chronic respiratory failure. *Eur. J. Clin. Pharmacol.*, **1971**, *4*, 29–31.

5. Sotaniemi, E. A., and Huhti, E. Half life of intravenous tolbutamide in the serum of patients in medical wards. *Ann. Clin. Res.*, **1974**, *6*, 146–154.
6. Glogner, P.; Lange, H.; and Pfab, R. Tolbutamidstoffwechsel bei Niereninsuffizienz. *Med. Welt*, **1968**, 2876–2878.
7. Stowers, J. M.; Mahler, R. F.; and Hunter, R. B. Pharmacology and mode of action of the sulfonylureas in man. *Lancet*, **1958**, *1*, 278–283.
8. Mortimore, G. E.; DiRaimondo, V. C.; and Forsham, P. H. Metabolic effects of ORINASE in diabetes including two cases complicated by other endocrinopathies. *Metabolism*, **1956**, *5*, 840–846.

TRIAMTERENE [a] (Chapter 36)

AVAILABILITY (ORAL) (%)	URINARY EXCRETION (%)	BOUND IN PLASMA (%)	CLEARANCE ($ml \cdot min^{-1} \cdot kg^{-1}$)
30–70 (2)	3.9 ± 1.2 [b] (3)	43–53 (2) ↓ Urem (4), Alb (4) ↑ HL (2)	14 ± 7 (2) ↓ Urem [c] (1)

VOL. DIST. (*liters/kg*)	HALF-LIFE (*hours*)	EFFECTIVE CONCENTRATIONS	TOXIC CONCENTRATIONS
2.5 ± 0.8 (2)	2.8 ± 0.9 (5) ↑ Urem [c] (1)	—	—

[a] Values reported are for unchanged drug. However, recent studies indicate that the hydroxy metabolite and its sulfate conjugate are also active (1).

[b] After oral dosage.

[c] For active metabolite (sulfate conjugate); half-life of conjugate in normal subjects is 2.6 ± 0.5 hours (5).

1. Grebian, B.; Geissler, H. E.; Knauf, H.; Mutschler, E.; Schnippenkoetter, I.; Völger, K.-D.; and Wais, U. Zur Pharmakokinetik von Triamteren und seinen wirksamen Metaboliten bei eigeschränkter Nierenfunktion. *Arzneim. Forsch.,* 1978, *28,* 1420–1425.
2. Pruitt, A. W.; Winkel, J. S.; and Dayton, P. G. Variations in the fate of triamterene. *Clin. Pharmacol. Ther.,* 1977, *21,* 610–619.
3. Gundert-Remy, U.; von Kenne, D.; Weber, E.; Geissler, H. E.; Grebian, B.; and Mutschler, E. Plasma and urinary levels of triamterene and certain metabolites after oral administration to man. *Eur. J. Clin. Pharmacol.,* 1979, *16,* 39–44.
4. Reidenberg, M. M., and Affrime, M. Influence of disease on binding of drugs to plasma proteins. *Ann. N.Y. Acad. Sci.,* 1973, *266,* 115–126.
5. Felder, K.; Geissler, H. E.; Hiemstra, S.; Mutschler, E.; Schafer, M.; and Ziegler, E. Pharmacokinetics of a fixed combination with propranolol, hydrochlorothiazide, and triamterene. *Arzneim. Forsch.,* 1979, *29,* 1746–1752.

TRIMETHOPRIM (Chapter 49)

AVAILABILITY (ORAL) (%)	URINARY EXCRETION (%)	BOUND IN PLASMA (%)	CLEARANCE ($ml \cdot min^{-1} \cdot kg^{-1}$)
~100 (1)	53 ± 2 (2)	70 ± 5 (2) ↔ Urem (2), Alb (2)	2.2 ± 0.6 [a] (3)

VOL. DIST. (*liters/kg*)	HALF-LIFE (*hours*)	EFFECTIVE CONCENTRATIONS	TOXIC CONCENTRATIONS
1.8 ± 0.2 [a] (3) ↔ Urem (4)	11 ± 1.4 [b] (4) ↑ Urem (4)	*See* Chapter 49	—

[a] Assuming 70-kg weight.

[b] Average of five studies, which included concurrent administration of sulfamethoxazole and variation in urinary pH; these factors had no marked effect on the clearance of trimethoprim.

1. Kaplan, S. A.; Weinfeld, R. E.; Cotler, S.; Abruzzo, C. W.; and Alexander, K. Pharmacokinetic profile of trimethoprim in dog and man. *J. Pharm. Sci.,* 1970, *59,* 358–363.
2. Craig, W. A., and Kunin, C. M. Trimethoprim-sulfamethoxazole: pharmacokinetic effects of urinary pH and impaired renal function. *Ann. Intern. Med.,* 1973, *78,* 491–497.
3. Morgan, D. J., and Raymond, K. Evaluation of slow infusions of co-trimoxazole by using predictive pharmacokinetics. *Antimicrob. Agents Chemother.,* 1980, *17,* 132–137.
4. Welling, P. G.; Craig, W. A.; Amidon, G. L.; and Kunin, C. M. Pharmacokinetics of trimethoprim and sulfamethoxazole in normal subjects and in patients with renal failure. *J. Infect. Dis.,* 1973, *128,* Suppl., S556–S566.

TUBOCURARINE (Chapter 11)

AVAILABILITY (ORAL) (%)	URINARY EXCRETION (%)	BOUND IN PLASMA (%)	CLEARANCE $(ml \cdot min^{-1} \cdot kg^{-1})$
—	43 ± 8 (1)	40 ± 2 (2) ↔ Urem (3), Cirr (3)	2.3 ± 0.7 (4) ↓ Urem (1)

VOL. DIST. (liters/kg)	HALF-LIFE (hours)	EFFECTIVE CONCENTRATIONS	TOXIC CONCENTRATIONS
0.30 ± 0.11 (4)	2.0 ± 1.1 [a] (4) ↑ Urem (1)	0.6 ± 0.2 μg/ml [b] (4)	—

[a] Calculated from two-compartment analysis. Three-compartment analysis suggests a terminal half-life of 3.9 hours (5).

[b] To achieve 50% reduction in twitch tension in adductor pollicis; this value is less in the presence of halothane at concentrations greater than 0.5% (end tidal).

1. Miller, R. D.; Matteo, R. S.; Benet, L. Z.; and Sohn, Y. J. The pharmacokinetics of *d*-tubocurarine in man with and without renal failure. *J. Pharmacol. Exp. Ther.,* **1977,** *202,* 1–7.
2. Ghoneim, M. M., and Pandya, H. Binding of tubocurarine to specific serum protein fractions. *Br. J. Anaesth.,* **1975,** *47,* 853–856.
3. Ghoneim, M. M.; Kramer, E.; Bannow, R.; Pandya, H.; and Routh, J. I. Binding of *d*-tubocurarine to plasma proteins in normal man and in patients with hepatic or renal disease. *Anesthesiology,* **1973,** *39,* 410–415.
4. Stanski, D. R.; Ham, J.; Miller, R. D.; and Sheiner, L. B. Pharmacokinetics and pharmacodynamics of *d*-tubocurarine during nitrous oxide–narcotic and halothane anesthesia in man. *Anesthesiology,* **1979,** *51,* 235–241.
5. Gibaldi, M.; Levy, G.; and Hayton, W. Kinetics of elimination and neuromuscular blocking effect of *d*-tubocurarine in man. *Anesthesiology,* **1972,** *36,* 213–218.

VALPROIC ACID [a] (Chapter 20)

AVAILABILITY (ORAL) (%)	URINARY EXCRETION (%)	BOUND IN PLASMA (%)	CLEARANCE $(ml \cdot min^{-1} \cdot kg^{-1})$
100 ± 10 (2)	1.8 ± 2.4 (3)	93 ± 4 [b] (3,4) ↓ Urem (6), Cirr (7)	0.12 ± 0.04 [c] (8) ↔ Cirr (7) ↑ Epilep [d] (9,10)

VOL. DIST. (liters/kg)	HALF-LIFE (hours)	EFFECTIVE CONCENTRATIONS	TOXIC CONCENTRATIONS
0.13 ± 0.04 (8) ↑ Epilep [e] (10), Cirr (7)	16 ± 3 (3) ↓ Epilep (11) ↑ Cirr (7), Neo (12)	55–100 μg/ml [f] (11)	—

[a] For review, *see* (1).

[b] For concentrations that prevail after doses of 500 mg per day (average 47 μg/ml). Binding is decreased at higher concentrations (4,5).

[c] Blood clearance 0.47 ± 0.18 ml · min⁻¹ · kg⁻¹ in same subjects.

[d] Increased clearance possibly due to enzyme induction due to concomitant administration of other antiepileptic drugs.

[e] Possibly due to decreased binding.

[f] For control of seizures. Others report no correlation of concentrations in plasma with efficacy or toxicity (13), but these authors also suggest that concentrations of 50–55 μg/ml are more effective than lower values (14).

Key: Adult = adults; Aged = aged; Alb = hypoalbuminemia; AVH = acute viral hepatitis; CF = cystic fibrosis; CHF = congestive heart failure; Child = children; Cirr = cirrhosis; COPD = chronic obstructive pulmonary disease; CP = cor pulmonale; CPBS = cardiopulmonary bypass surgery; CRI = chronic respiratory insufficiency; Cush = cushingoid; Epilep = epilepsy; Fem = females; Hep = hepatitis; HL = hyperlipoproteinemia; HTh = hyperthyroid; Inflam = inflammation; LTh = hypothyroid; MI = myocardial infarction; Neo = neonates; NS = nephrotic syndrome; Obes = obesity; Pneu = pneumonia; Preg = pregnant; Prem = premature infants; RA = rheumatoid arthritis; Smk = smoking; Tach = ventricular tachycardia; Urem = uremia.

VALPROIC ACID (Cont.)

1. Gugler, R., and von Unruh, G. E.   Clinical pharmacokinetics of valproic acid. *Clin. Pharmacokinet.,* **1980,** *5,* 67–83.
2. Perucca, E.; Gatti, G.; Frigo, G. M.; and Crema, A.   Pharmacokinetics of valproic acid after oral and intravenous administration. *Br. J. Clin. Pharmacol.,* **1978,** *5,* 313–318.
3. Gugler, R.; Schell, A.; Eichelbaum, M.; Frocher, W.; and Schulz, H.-U.   Disposition of valproic acid in man. *Eur. J. Clin. Pharmacol.,* **1977,** *12,* 125–132.
4. Bowdle, T. A.; Patel, I. H.; Levy, R. H.; and Wilensky, A. J.   Dose dependent valproate clearance. (Abstracts.) Academy of Pharmaceutical Sciences, Washington, D. C., **1979,** *9,* 98.
5. Cramer, J. A., and Mattson, R. H.   Valproic acid: *in vitro* plasma protein binding and interactions with phenytoin. *Ther. Drug Monitoring,* **1979,** *1,* 105–116.
6. Gugler, R., and Muller, G.   Plasma protein binding of valproic acid in healthy subjects and in patients with renal disease. *Br. J. Clin. Pharmacol.,* **1978,** *5,* 441–446.
7. Klotz, U.; Rapp, T.; and Muller, W. A.   Disposition of valproic acid in patients with liver disease. *Eur. J. Clin. Pharmacol.,* **1978,** *13,* 55–60.
8. Klotz, U., and Antonin, K. H.   Pharmacokinetics and bioavailability of sodium valproate. *Clin. Pharmacol. Ther.,* **1977,** *21,* 736–743.
9. Bowdle, T. A.; Levy, R. H.; and Cutler, R. E.   Effects of carbamazepine on valproic acid kinetics in normal subjects. *Clin. Pharmacol. Ther.,* **1979,** *26,* 629–634.
10. Perucca, E.; Gatti, G.; Frigo, G. M.; and Crema, A.   Disposition of sodium valproate in epileptic patients. *Br. J. Clin. Pharmacol.,* **1978,** *5,* 495–499.
11. Bruni, J.; Wilder, B. J.; Willmore, L. J.; Perchalski, R. J.; and Villarreal, H. J.   Steady-state kinetics of valproic acid in epileptic patients. *Clin. Pharmacol. Ther.,* **1978,** *24,* 324–332.
12. Brachet-Liermain, A., and Demarquez, J. L.   Pharmacokinetics of dipropyl acetate in infants and young children. *Pharm. Weekblad,* **1977,** *112,* 293–297.
13. Wulff, K.; Flachs, H.; Würtz-Jørgensen, A.; and Gram, L.   Clinical pharmacological aspects of valproate sodium. *Epilepsia,* **1977,** *18,* 149–157.
14. Gram, L.; Flachs, H.; Würtz-Jørgensen, A.; Parnas, J.; and Andersen, B.   Sodium valproate, serum level and clinical effect in epilepsy: a controlled study. *Epilepsia,* **1979,** *20,* 303–312.

VANCOMYCIN (Chapter 54)

AVAILABILITY (ORAL) (%)	URINARY EXCRETION (%)	BOUND IN PLASMA (%)	CLEARANCE $(ml \cdot min^{-1} \cdot kg^{-1})$
—	>90 (1)	<10 (2)	$CL = 0.45\ CL_{cr} + 0.03$ [a]

VOL. DIST. *(liters/kg)*	HALF-LIFE *(hours)*	EFFECTIVE CONCENTRATIONS	TOXIC CONCENTRATIONS
0.43 [b] (1)	5–6 (1) ↑ Urem (3)	*See* Chapter 54	*See* Chapter 54

[a] Calculated from data in (3).
[b] Assuming 70-kg weight; Vd_{area}.

1. Kirby, W. M. M., and Divelbiss, C. L.   Vancomycin: clinical and laboratory studies. *Antibiot. Ann.,* **1956/1957,** 107–117.
2. Lindholm, D. D., and Murray, J. S.   Persistence of vancomycin in the blood during renal failure and its treatment by hemodialysis. *N. Engl. J. Med.,* **1966,** *274,* 1047–1051.
3. Nielsen, H. E.; Hansen, H. E.; Korsager, B.; and Skov, P. E.   Renal excretion of vancomycin in kidney disease. *Acta Med. Scand.,* **1975,** *197,* 261–264.

Key: Adult = adults;   Aged = aged;   Alb = hypoalbuminemia;   AVH = acute viral hepatitis;   CF = cystic fibrosis;   CHF = congestive heart failure;   Child = children;   Cirr = cirrhosis;   COPD = chronic obstructive pulmonary disease;   CP = cor pulmonale;   CPBS = cardiopulmonary bypass surgery;   CRI = chronic respiratory insufficiency;   Cush = cushingoid;   Epilep = epilepsy;   Fem = females;   Hep = hepatitis;   HL = hyperlipoproteinemia;   HTh = hyperthyroid;   Inflam = inflammation;   LTh = hypothyroid;   MI = myocardial infarction;   Neo = neonates;   NS = nephrotic syndrome;   Obes = obesity;   Pneu = pneumonia;   Preg = pregnant;   Prem = premature infants;   RA = rheumatoid arthritis;   Smk = smoking;   Tach = ventricular tachycardia;   Urem = uremia.

WARFARIN [a] (Chapter 58)

AVAILABILITY (ORAL) (%)	URINARY EXCRETION (%)	BOUND IN PLASMA (%)	CLEARANCE $(ml \cdot min^{-1} \cdot kg^{-1})$
100 (2)	0 (2)	99 (3) ↓ Urem (4)	0.045 ± 0.024 [b,c] (5)

VOL. DIST. (*liters/kg*)	HALF-LIFE (*hours*)	EFFECTIVE CONCENTRATIONS	TOXIC CONCENTRATIONS
0.11 ± 0.01 [c] (5)	37 ± 15 [d] (2)	2.2 ± 0.4 µg/ml [e]	—

[a] For review, *see* (1). Values are for racemic warfarin.

[b] The kinetics of the S(−) and R(+) enantiomers differ; clearance of the R(+) form is about one third that of the S(−) enantiomer (7).

[c] Conditions leading to decreased binding (*e.g.*, uremia) presumably increase clearance and volume of distribution; *see* (6).

[d] Half-life of the R(+) enantiomer is longer than that of the S(−) form (7).

[e] The S(−) enantiomer is three to five times more potent than the R(+) form (7).

1. Kelly, J. G., and O'Malley, K. Clinical pharmacokinetics of oral anticoagulants. *Clin. Pharmacokinet.*, **1979,** *4,* 1–15.
2. O'Reilly, R. A.; Aggeler, P. M.; and Leong, L. S. Studies on the coumarin anticoagulant drugs: the pharmacodynamics of warfarin in man. *J. Clin. Invest.*, **1963,** *42,* 1542–1551.
3. Bachmann, K. Rapid determination of the concentration of unbound warfarin in human plasma. *Res. Commun. Chem. Pathol. Pharmacol.*, **1974,** *9,* 379–382.
4. Bachmann, K.; Shapiro, R.; and Mackiewicz, J. Influence of renal dysfunction on warfarin plasma protein binding. *J. Clin. Pharmacol.*, **1976,** *16,* 468–472.
5. O'Reilly, R. A.; Welling, P. G.; and Wagner, J. G. Pharmacokinetics of warfarin following intravenous administration in man. *Thromb. Diath. Haemorrh.*, **1971,** *25,* 178–186.
6. Bachmann, K., and Shapiro, R. Protein binding of coumarin anticoagulants in disease states. *Clin. Pharmacokinet.*, **1977,** *2,* 110–126.
7. Breckenridge, A.; Orme, M.; Wesseling, H.; Lewis, R. J.; and Gibbons, R. Pharmacokinetics and pharmacodynamics of the enantiomers of warfarin in man. *Clin. Pharmacol. Ther.*, **1974,** *15,* 424–430.

III DRUG INTERACTIONS

Kenneth L. Melmon and Alfred G. Gilman

Over the last decade, it has become increasingly clear that the effects of many drugs, when given concurrently, are not necessarily predictable on the basis of knowledge of their effects when given alone. The subject of drug interactions interests pharmacologists, and it is now important to clinical therapists. Although the original observations about such interactions stemmed from fundamental research (examination of the effects of agonists and antagonists that act at a common receptor), subsequent knowledge of drug interactions, acquired from experiments on animals, has been used to therapeutic advantage in man (e.g., the use of combinations of antihypertensive agents that act by complementary mechanisms). Later, it became clear that interactions could also be detrimental. For example, when barbiturates were given to patients who were also receiving an oral anticoagulant, the effectiveness of the latter drug was diminished.

There is now some perspective on the clinical values and liabilities of drug interactions. It is understood that interactions of multiple types can occur with the same pair of chemicals. When an interaction occurs, the net pharmacological response may result from enhancement of the effects of one or the other drug, the development of totally new effects that are not seen when either drug is used alone, the inhibition of the effect of one drug by another, or no change whatever in the net effect despite the fact that the kinetics and metabolism of one or both of the drugs may be altered substantially. In any therapeutic situation, the physician must have expectations of the effects of a drug before it is given and set limits of toxicity beyond which the drug will be discontinued. These requirements are particularly pertinent when multiple drugs are given concurrently.

Knowledge of drug interactions enables a physician to minimize or prevent drug toxicity by adjustment of the dosage or schedule of drug administration or by choice of an alternative agent. A physician should find it useful to categorize the multiple mechanisms by which an interaction may occur. The introductory pages of this appendix provide such categorization and thus a framework for the analysis of unanticipated interactions. A list then follows of a large number of drug interactions that are described elsewhere in the textbook. This list is intended to be an

index of these interactions and nothing more. It is by no means a complete list of all drug interactions that have been hypothesized or described, or even a complete list of interactions discussed in the textbook. The intention is to focus on those interactions that result in unwanted or adverse effects. Many of the beneficial effects that result from interactions between drugs have become integral factors in the optimal therapy of some diseases, and they are not included in this appendix.

Direct Chemical or Physical Interactions. Two drugs may interact directly, particularly under conditions where their concentrations are high. As a result of such association, which is usually not covalent, the effects of each drug can obviously be modified. For example, heparin is an acidic mucopolysaccharide with anticoagulant activities that can be inhibited or nullified by a basic compound, such as protamine. This electrostatic interaction is used for therapeutic intent to neutralize excessive effects of heparin. It is useful for the physician to have some knowledge of the chemical nature of drugs so that he will use his observational powers in settings where such interactions could occur. For example, lidocaine is a basic drug. One could be alert to the possible failure of lidocaine as an antiarrhythmic agent when it is administered concurrently with heparin, even though such an interaction has not been described. Similar examples entail the chelating action of tetracyclines, the adsorbent capacities of resins such as cholestyramine, the ionic properties of the aminoglycoside antibiotics, and others. One must also realize that not all of the physicochemical interactions between drugs will be revealed by the formation of precipitates in bottles used for solutions for intravenous injection. Furthermore, important physicochemical interactions may occur by the adsorption of drugs to the glass or plastic surfaces of such bottles or associated equipment.

Interactions in Gastrointestinal Absorption. Interactions between drugs frequently occur prior to absorption from the intestine. Thus, interaction of a tetracycline with calcium or another metallic cation in the gut prevents absorption of the antibiotic. Barbiturates provide examples of a class of drugs that is involved in multiple mechanisms of interaction with a single agent. For instance, barbiturates interfere with both the absorption and the metabolism of dicumarol. Most physicians remember the latter phenomenon but forget that the decreased effect of the anticoagulant can also depend on inhibition of its absorption. Drugs that alter gastric or intestinal motility can inhibit or enhance the rate or extent of absorption of a drug administered concurrently by alteration of the time allowed for its transit through different portions of the gastrointestinal tract. Timing of the administration of two drugs can thus become a crucial determinant of the degree of expression of the drug interaction.

Interactions at the site of absorption can be complex and indirect. For example, antibiotics can alter the gastrointestinal flora, and may thus inhibit the rate of synthesis of vitamin K by intestinal microorganisms. If an oral anticoagulant (vitamin K antagonist) is administered concurrently, the antibiotic will increase its effectiveness. When antibiotics deplete the gut of microorganisms that can conjugate drugs within the intestine, absorption of active drug may increase.

Interactions Due to Protein Binding. Many drugs, particularly those that are acidic, are reversibly bound to plasma proteins, and the extent of competition between drugs for such binding sites depends on the affinity of each for the site and its concentration (*see* Chapter 1). In general, only unbound drug is free to leave the vascular compartment and exert its pharmacological effect. These facts set the stage for an important class of drug interactions, which are most significant for those agents that are extensively bound to plasma proteins at therapeutic concentrations. Tolbutamide and warfarin provide examples of such agents, and their free concentration can be increased significantly in the presence of effective competitors, such as many of the nonsteroidal anti-inflammatory agents. Even a minor percentage change of the extent of binding of drugs that are usually more than 90% bound to plasma proteins may result in a large change in the concentration of the free drug.

Obvious displacement of a bound drug may not occur immediately after initiation of administration of a potential competitor. If the displacing drug has a long half-life and does not reach a plateau concentration for several days after maintenance dosage is started, it may not be present initially in sufficient concentration to cause significant displacement. The pharmacokinetics may be further complicated by enhanced clearance of the displaced drug because of less extensive binding. The intensity of the interaction

may thus wane, despite constant dosage. These types of changes may be particularly difficult to recognize, and their kinetics must be understood to avoid undercompensation, overcompensation, or both at different times.

Interactions at the Receptor Site. Interactions between agonists and antagonists at specific receptor sites are described throughout the text, and many pharmacological agents are obviously valued because of such actions and interactions. What is frequently overlooked, in part because of the convenience of classification, is the lack of specificity of many such drugs. Thus, phenothiazines are effective α-adrenergic antagonists; many antihistamines and tricyclic antidepressants are potent antimuscarinic agents. Such agents have unwanted effects because of their lack of specificity, and these may be most noticeable and troublesome when other drugs are given concurrently and are expected to have their usual efficacy.

Other interactions of an apparent pharmacodynamic nature are poorly understood or are mediated indirectly. Halogenated hydrocarbons, including many general anesthetics, sensitize the myocardium to the arrhythmogenic actions of catecholamines. This effect presumably results from some action on the pathway leading from receptor to effector, but details are unclear. Many signs and symptoms of hypoglycemia are mediated through the adrenergic nervous system and are masked by β-adrenergic blocking agents. Patients taking propranolol may thus fail to note reactions to insulin or oral hypoglycemic agents in time to prevent dangerous consequences, and, furthermore, compensatory mechanisms, such as glycogenolysis, may be blocked by the β-adrenergic antagonist.

Interactions Due to Accelerated Metabolism. Interactions between drugs occur during their metabolism or elimination. Many drugs and a variety of chemicals that are present in the environment, especially insecticides and herbicides, are capable of inducing the synthesis of drug-metabolizing enzymes, particularly those of the hepatic endoplasmic reticulum (*see* Chapter 1). Such induction can enhance the metabolism not only of the inducing agent but also of a variety of drugs administered concurrently and of some endogenous compounds, such as cortisol, bilirubin, and the sex steroids.

Lists of more than 200 agents known to induce their own metabolism and the metabolism of other drugs have been compiled. Much of the data has been obtained from studies of experimental animals and may not be applicable to man. Genetic differences in man also play an important role in determining an individual's response to such enzyme inducers. Despite these variables, which make attempts at prediction imprecise, interactions of this sort are unquestionably important in man. Phenobarbital can dramatically reduce the half-life of quinidine. Rifampin decreases the half-life of estrogens and methadone; the consequences may be an unwanted pregnancy or precipitation of withdrawal from opioids. Enhancement of the rate of metabolism can also result in higher concentrations of active metabolites or of metabolites with unique toxic effects (*see* Chapter 1).

Interactions Due to Inhibition of Metabolism. A number of drug interactions are based on inhibition of metabolism of one drug by another (or by its metabolites). An important example is provided by allopurinol, an inhibitor of xanthine oxidase, which prolongs the half-life and thereby intensifies the effects of 6-mercaptopurine and azathioprine. Profound bone-marrow toxicity will occur if cognizance is not taken of these interactions. The monoamine oxidase inhibitors also provide striking and classical examples of such effects (*see* Chapter 19). Unfortunately, there are few, if any, guidelines to permit predictions of which drugs will inhibit the metabolism of other agents.

Interactions Due to Alteration of pH or Electrolyte Concentrations. Several drugs, particularly including the diuretics, influence the concentrations of electrolytes and the pH of body fluids. Such changes in pH may produce major alterations in the absorption, distribution, or renal clearance of therapeutic agents. Interactions of this type may be unwanted, or they may be sought deliberately, particularly to enhance the elimination of a toxicant (*see* Chapters 1 and 68). The same type of effect may alter the activities of a second drug that is given concurrently. A classical example of such is hypokalemia, resulting from the administration of diuretics, which potentiates the activity of digitalis glycosides, often dangerously.

Summary. Although classification of mechanisms of drug interactions should be helpful to the physician, it must be recalled that a single drug may be involved in multiple types of interactions with the same or different drugs. The major task of the physician is to judge whether an interaction has occurred and the magnitude of the change. Many patients see more than one physician for the same purpose. When they do, the physicians do not always know of each other's therapeutic regimens. Likewise, many patients consume drugs that have been prescribed for other diseases or for another patient. In addition, patients may be erratic in their smoking and drinking habits, which can affect a drug's pharmacokinetic or pharmacodynamic properties. There is no easy way to anticipate such problems. There is, therefore, the requirement that an unanticipated turn of events in a patient's course, whether it be accelerated efficacy or the appearance of unusual and untoward events, be considered as a possible consequence of an interaction between drugs.

Acetaminophen
    anticoagulants, oral, 703
    antidiuretic hormone, 921
    ethanol, 703
Acetazolamide. *See also* Diuretics
    methenamine, 899
    phenytoin, 899
    quinidine, 771
Acetohexamide. *See* Hypoglycemic agents—oral
Acetophenazine. *See* Antipsychotic agents
Acetylcholine. *See also* Cholinergic agonists
    anticholinesterase agents, 94
N-Acetylcysteine
    gold, 715
Acetylsalicylic acid. *See* Salicylates
α-Adrenergic blocking agents. *See also* Phenoxybenzamine
    opioids, 183
    vasodilators, 183
β-Adrenergic blocking agents. *See also* Propranolol

    anesthetics, general, 284
    digitalis glycosides, 193
    hypoglycemic agents, oral, 194, 196
    insulin, 194, 196
    lidocaine, 17, 781
    neuromuscular blocking agents, 229
Adrenocorticosteroids
    barbiturates, 356, 358
    calcium salts, 1486
    neuromuscular blocking agents, 229
    phenytoin, 455
    rifampin, 1205
    vitamin D, 1543
Alcohol, ethyl. *See* Ethanol
Allopurinol
    ampicillin, 721, 1148
    anticoagulants, oral, 721
    azathioprine, 721, 722, 1286, 1287
    cyclophosphamide, 722, 1265
    iron salts, 721

mercaptopurine, 721, 722, 1286
probenecid, 721, 722
uricosuric agents, 722
Aluminum hydroxide. *See also* Antacids
antimuscarinic agents, 990
barbiturates, 990
benzodiazepines, 990
chlorpromazine, 990
dicumarol, 990
digoxin, 990
indomethacin, 990
isoniazid, 990
propranolol, 990
sulfadiazine, 990
tetracyclines, 990, 1184
Amantadine
antimuscarinic agents, 483
Amikacin. *See* Aminoglycoside antibiotics
Aminoglycoside antibiotics
amphotericin B, 1171, 1174
anesthetics, general, 1171
capreomycin, 1211
cephalosporins, 1157
colistin, 1230
cyanocobalamin, 1177
digitalis glycosides, 746
diuretics, 1170
ethacrynic acid, 906
furosemide, 906
heparin, 1174
iron salts, 1177
neuromuscular blocking agents, 229, 1171
penicillins, 1174
polymyxin B, 1171, 1230
vancomycin, 1097, 1171, 1231
Aminophylline. *See* Theophylline
Aminopyrine
antidepressants, tricyclic, 426
Aminosalicylic acid
isoniazid, 1209
probenecid, 1210
rifampin, 1204
salicylates, 698
Amitriptyline. *See* Antidepressants—tricyclic
Amobarbital. *See* Barbiturates
Amodiaquine
chloroquine, 1044
Amphetamine. *See also* Sympathomimetic amines
antacids, 990
barbiturates, 550
opioids, 508, 516
Amphotericin B
aminoglycoside antibiotics, 1171, 1174
digitalis glycosides, 756
Ampicillin. *See also* Penicillins
allopurinol, 721, 1148
Anabolic steroids. *See* Androgens
Androgens. *See also* Methandrostenolone; Testosterone
anticoagulants, oral, 1357
barbiturates, 356, 358
Anesthetics—general. *See also* Methoxyflurane

β-adrenergic blocking agents, 284
aminoglycoside antibiotics, 1171
barbiturates, 353
monoamine oxidase inhibitors, 430
neuromuscular blocking agents, 107, 226, 228, 229, 281, 285, 287, 288
sympathomimetic amines, 147, 151, 280, 287, 311
Anesthetics—local
neuromuscular blocking agents, 229
sulfonamides, 308, 1108
sympathomimetic amines, 304, 311, 318
Antacids. *See also* individual agents
amphetamine, 990
anticoagulants, oral, 1357
antimuscarinic agents, 954
dicumarol, 990
indomethacin, 990
iron salts, 990, 1323
naproxen, 990
phenothiazines, 405
phenylbutazone, 990
pseudoephedrine, 990
quinidine, 990
quinine, 990
salicylates, 990
sulfadiazine, 990
tetracyclines, 954, 990, 1184
Anticholinergic agents. *See* Antimuscarinic agents; Ganglionic blocking agents; Neuromuscular blocking agents
Anticholinesterase agents
acetylcholine, 94
methacholine, 94
neuromuscular blocking agents, 107, 114, 229
quinine, 1056
Anticoagulants
streptokinase, 1362
urokinase, 1362
Anticoagulants—oral. *See also* Dicumarol; Warfarin
acetaminophen, 703
allopurinol, 721
androgens, 1357
antacids, 1357
anti-inflammatory agents, 1356
antimicrobial agents, 1355, 1356
ascorbic acid, 1357, 1580
barbiturates, 358, 1357
chloral hydrate, 362, 1356
cholestyramine, 843, 1357
cimetidine, 1357
clofibrate, 841, 1357
colestipol, 843
dextrothyroxine, 844, 1357
disulfiram, 1356
diuretics, 1357
ethanol, 382
ethchlorvynol, 363
fenoprofen, 711
flurbiprofen, 711
glutethimide, 364, 1357
griseofulvin, 1238
heparin, 1357, 1360

Anticoagulants (*Cont.*)
  hypoglycemic agents, oral, 1357, 1512
  indomethacin, 706
  ketoprofen, 711
  mefenamic acid, 709
  metronidazole, 1356
  naproxen, 711
  oxyphenbutazone, 1356
  phenylbutazone, 700, 1356
  phenytoin, 455, 1357
  quinidine, 774
  rifampin, 1205, 1357
  salicylates, 692, 1356
  spironolactone, 1357
  sulfinpyrazone, 1357
  sulfonamides, 1114, 1356
  thyroid hormones, 1355
  trimethoprim, 1356
Anticonvulsants
  ethanol, 382
Antidepressants—tricyclic. *See also* Imipramine
  aminopyrine, 426
  antimuscarinic agents, 426
  antipsychotic agents, 414, 426
  barbiturates, 358, 426
  bretylium, 201
  chloral hydrate, 362
  clonidine, 427, 798, 799, 813
  contraceptives, oral, 426
  dopamine, 155
  ethanol, 382, 426
  ethchlorvynol, 363
  guanethidine, 198, 200, 201, 427, 813
  lithium, 434
  meprobamate, 366
  methadone, 519
  methaqualone, 367
  methylphenidate, 426
  monoamine oxidase inhibitors, 427, 430
  opioids, 508, 516
  phenylbutazone, 426
  phenytoin, 426
  procarbazine, 1300
  riboflavin, 1567
  salicylates, 426
  sympathomimetic amines, 421, 427
Antidiuretic hormone. *See also* Desmopressin
  acetaminophen, 921
  chlorpropamide, 921, 1512
  demeclocycline, 922
  indomethacin, 921
  lithium, 433, 922
Antihistamines
  antipsychotic agents, 414
  barbiturates, 358
  central nervous system depressants, 626
  ethanol, 626
  monoamine oxidase inhibitors, 430
Antihypertensive agents
  nicotinic acid, 839
Anti-inflammatory agents. *See also* individual agents
  anticoagulants, oral, 1356

Antimicrobial agents
  anticoagulants, oral, 1355, 1356
Antimuscarinic agents
  aluminum hydroxide, 990
  amantadine, 483
  antacids, 954
  antidepressants, tricyclic, 426
  antipsychotic agents, 414
  chlorpromazine, 405
  digitalis glycosides, 746
  levodopa, 479, 481
  magnesium trisilicate, 990
  monoamine oxidase inhibitors, 430
Antipsychotic agents. *See also* Chlorpromazine;
    Phenothiazines; Thioridazine
  antidepressants, tricyclic, 414, 426
  antihistamines, 414
  antimuscarinic agents, 414
  barbiturates, 400, 414, 418
  central nervous system depressants, 400, 414, 418
  clonidine, 813
  dopaminergic agonists, 414
  ethanol, 400, 414, 418
  guanethidine, 198, 199, 200, 414, 813
  levodopa, 414, 480, 481
  lithium, 434
  opioids, 414, 503, 508, 516
  riboflavin, 1567
Antipyrine
  marihuana, 562
  smoking, 559
Antithrombotic agents
  streptokinase, 1362
  urokinase, 1362
Ascorbic acid
  anticoagulants, oral, 1357, 1580
  contraceptives, oral, 1579
  iron salts, 1323, 1580
  salicylates, 1557
  smoking, 1579
  vitamin A, 1591
Aspirin. *See* Salicylates
Atropine. *See* Antimuscarinic agents
Azathioprine
  allopurinol, 721, 722, 1286, 1287

Barbiturates. *See also* Phenobarbital; Thiopental
  adrenocorticosteroids, 356, 358
  aluminum hydroxide, 990
  amphetamine, 550
  androgens, 356, 358
  anesthetics, general, 353
  anticoagulants, oral, 358, 1357
  antidepressants, tricyclic, 358, 426
  antihistamines, 358
  antipsychotic agents, 400, 414, 418
  benzodiazepines, 349, 353
  central nervous system depressants, 353, 358
  contraceptives, oral, 356, 358
  digitoxin, 358
  doxycycline, 358, 1185

ethanol, 356, 358, 359, 382, 383
glutethimide, 353, 364
griseofulvin, 358, 1238
isoniazid, 358
marihuana, 562
meprobamate, 353
methaqualone, 353
methylphenidate, 358
monoamine oxidase inhibitors, 358
neuromuscular blocking agents, 354
opioids, 353
phencyclidine, 353
phenytoin, 358
pilocarpine, 354
salicylates, 356
theophylline, 601
thyroid hormones, 358
vitamin D, 356, 358
vitamin K, 356, 358
warfarin, 18, 356
Benzbromarone. See also Diuretics; Uricosuric agents
pyrazinamide, 933
salicylates, 933
sulfinpyrazone, 933
Benzodiazepines. See also Clonazepam; Diazepam
aluminum hydroxide, 990
barbiturates, 349, 353
central nervous system depressants, 346, 349, 440
ethanol, 346, 348, 349, 382
magnesium trisilicate, 990
methaqualone, 349
opioids, 346
smoking, 559
valproic acid, 349
Bicarbonate
quinidine, 771
tetracyclines, 1184
Bretylium
antidepressants, tricyclic, 201
sympathomimetic amines, 201
Bupivacaine. See Anesthetics—local
Buprenorphine. See Opioids
Butabarbital. See Barbiturates
Butalbital. See Barbiturates
Butorphanol. See Opioids

Caffeine
cholinergic agonists, 597
ergot alkaloids, 945
histamine, 597
pentagastrin, 597
smoking, 559
Calcitriol. See Vitamin D
Calcium carbonate. See Antacids
Calcium salts
adrenocorticosteroids, 1486
digitalis glycosides, 754
tetracyclines, 1184
Capreomycin
aminoglycoside antibiotics, 1211
Carbamazepine

phenobarbital, 460
phenytoin, 455, 460
Carbenoxolone
diuretics, 876
Central nervous system depressants. See also individual agents
antihistamines, 626
antipsychotic agents, 400, 414, 418
barbiturates, 353, 358
benzodiazepines, 346, 349, 440
clonidine, 798
ethanol, 382, 552
levallorphan, 510
meprobamate, 366
methalqualone, 367
monoamine oxidase inhibitors, 430
nalorphine, 510
procarbazine, 1300
propoxyphene, 520
Cephalosporins
aminoglycoside antibiotics, 1157, 1171, 1174
colistin, 1230
ethacrynic acid, 906
furosemide, 906
polymyxin B, 1230
probenecid, 1153
Chloral hydrate. See also Central nervous system depressants
anticoagulants, oral, 362, 1356
antidepressants, tricyclic, 362
ethanol, 362, 363
furosemide, 362
Chloramphenicol
dicumarol, 1195
diuretics, 1195
hypoglycemic agents, oral, 1195, 1512
methotrexate, 1274
phenobarbital, 1195
phenytoin, 455, 1195
Chlordiazepoxide. See Benzodiazepines
Chloroprocaine. See Anesthetics—local
Chloroquine
amodiaquine, 1044
gold, 1045
hydroxychloroquine, 1044
neuromuscular blocking agents, 229
phenylbutazone, 1045
Chlorothiazide. See also Diuretics; Thiazide diuretics
cholestyramine, 843
colestipol, 843
Chlorpromazine. See also Antipsychotic agents; Phenothiazines
aluminum hydroxide, 990
antimuscarinic agents, 405
Chlorpropamide. See also Hypoglycemic agents—oral
antidiuretic hormone, 921, 1512
Chlorprothixene. See Antipsychotic agents
Chlortetracycline. See Tetracyclines
Chlorthalidone. See Diuretics
Cholecalciferol. See also Vitamin D
glutethimide, 364

Cholestyramine
  anticoagulants, oral, 843, 1357
  chlorothiazide, 843
  digitalis glycosides, 746, 755, 843
  phenobarbital, 843
  phenylbutazone, 700, 843
  thyroid hormones, 843
  vitamin D, 843
  vitamin K, 843
Cholinergic agonists. *See also* individual agents
  caffeine, 597
  theophylline, 597
Cholinesterase inhibitors. *See* Anticholinesterase agents
Cimetidine
  anticoagulants, oral, 1357
Clindamycin
  neuromuscular blocking agents, 229
  opioids, 1227
Clofibrate
  anticoagulants, oral, 841, 1357
  desmopressin, 924
  ethacrynic acid, 906
  furosemide, 906
  hypoglycemic agents, oral, 841, 1512
  phenytoin, 841
Clonazepam. *See also* Benzodiazepines
  valproic acid, 463
Clonidine
  antidepressants, tricyclic, 427, 798, 799, 813
  antipsychotic agents, 813
  central nervous system depressants, 798
  ganglionic blocking agents, 797
Clorazepate. *See* Benzodiazepines
Cocaine
  guanethidine, 198
  sympathomimetic amines, 307, 308
Codeine. *See* Opioids
Colestipol
  anticoagulants, oral, 843
  chlorothiazide, 843
  digitalis glycosides, 746, 755, 843
  phenobarbital, 843
  phenylbutazone, 843
  thyroid hormones, 843
  vitamin D, 843
  vitamin K, 843
Colistin
  aminoglycoside antibiotics, 1230
  cephalosporins, 1230
  neuromuscular blocking agents, 229
Contraceptives—oral. *See also* Estrogens
  antidepressants, tricyclic, 426
  ascorbic acid, 1579
  barbiturates, 356, 358
  folic acid, 1342, 1444
  meprobamate, 367
  rifampin, 1205
Corticosteroids. *See* Adrenocorticosteroids
Cortisone. *See* Adrenocorticosteroids
Cyanocobalamin
  aminoglycoside antibiotics, 1177

Cyclobenzaprine
  monoamine oxidase inhibitors, 490
Cyclophosphamide
  allopurinol, 722, 1265
  daunorubicin, 1293
  doxorubicin, 1293
Cycloserine
  pyridoxine, 1571

Dapsone
  probenecid, 1215
Daunorubicin
  cyclophosphamide, 1293
Decamethonium. *See* Neuromuscular blocking agents
Demeclocycline. *See also* Tetracyclines
  antidiuretic hormone, 922
Desipramine. *See* Antidepressants—tricyclic
Desmopressin. *See also* Antidiuretic hormone
  clofibrate, 924
Dexamethasone. *See* Adrenocorticosteroids
Dextroamphetamine. *See* Sympathomimetic amines
Dextrothyroxine
  anticoagulants, oral, 844, 1357
Diazepam. *See also* Benzodiazepines
  methadone, 519
Dicumarol. *See also* Anticoagulants—oral
  aluminum hydroxide, 990
  antacids, 990
  chloramphenicol, 1195
  thyroid hormones, 1402
Diethylstilbestrol. *See* Estrogens
Digitalis glycosides. *See also* Digitoxin; Digoxin
  β-adrenergic blocking agents, 193
  aminoglycoside antibiotics, 746
  amphotericin B, 756
  antimuscarinic agents, 746
  calcium salts, 754
  cholestyramine, 746, 755, 843
  colestipol, 746, 755, 843
  diuretics, 750, 751, 754
  neuromuscular blocking agents, 228, 229, 756
  phenobarbital, 747
  phenylbutazone, 747
  phenytoin, 747
  procainamide, 776
  quinidine, 751, 755, 774
  rifampin, 747
  sympathomimetic amines, 756
  thioridazine, 414
  thyroid hormones, 754
Digitoxin. *See also* Digitalis glycosides
  barbiturates, 358
Digoxin. *See also* Digitalis glycosides
  aluminum hydroxide, 990
  magnesium salts, 990
Dihydrotachysterol. *See* Vitamin D
Dimercaprol
  gold, 715, 716
Disulfiram
  anticoagulants, oral, 1356

ethanol, 387
phenytoin, 455
Diuretics. *See also* individual agents
aminoglycoside antibiotics, 1170
anticoagulants, oral, 1357
carbenoxolone, 876
chloramphenicol, 1195
digitalis glycosides, 750, 751, 754
lithium, 432
neuromuscular blocking agents, 228, 229
trimethoprim-sulfamethoxazole, 1118
Dobutamine. *See* Sympathomimetic amines
Dopamine. *See also* Dopaminergic agonists; Sympathomimetic amines
antidepressants, tricyclic, 155
monoamine oxidase inhibitors, 155
Dopaminergic agonists
antipsychotic agents, 414
Doxepin. *See* Antidepressants—tricyclic
Doxorubicin
cyclophosphamide, 1293
Doxycycline. *See also* Tetracyclines
barbiturates, 358, 1185
phenytoin, 1185

Edrophonium. *See* Anticholinesterase agents
Enflurane. *See* Anesthetics—general
Ephedrine. *See* Sympathomimetic amines
Epinephrine. *See* Sympathomimetic amines
Ergocalciferol. *See* Vitamin D
Ergot alkaloids
caffeine, 945
Erythrityl tetranitrate. *See* Nitrates—organic
Erythromycin
theophylline, 601
Estrogens. *See also* Contraceptives—oral
meprobamate, 367
pyridoxine, 1572
rifampin, 1205
thyroid hormones, 1401
Ethacrynic acid. *See also* Diuretics
aminoglycoside antibiotics, 906
cephalosporins, 906
clofibrate, 906
lithium, 906
vancomycin, 1231
warfarin, 906
Ethambutol
isoniazid, 1207
pyridoxine, 1207
Ethanol
acetaminophen, 703
anticoagulants, oral, 382
anticonvulsants, 382
antidepressants, tricyclic, 382, 426
antihistamines, 626
antipsychotic agents, 400, 414, 418
barbiturates, 356, 358, 359, 382, 383
benzodiazepines, 346, 348, 349, 382
central nervous system depressants, 382, 552
chloral hydrate, 362, 363

disulfiram, 387
folic acid, 1342
griseofulvin, 1238
guanethidine, 200
hypoglycemic agents, oral, 382, 387, 1512
marihuana, 562
meperidine, 515
meprobamate, 366
methaqualone, 367
metronidazole, 387, 1076
monoamine oxidase inhibitors, 430
nifurtimox, 1077
nitrates, organic, 825
opioids, 382
phenytoin, 455
procarbazine, 1300
propoxyphene, 382, 520
salicylates, 379, 382, 691
testosterone, 381
Ethchlorvynol. *See also* Central nervous system depressants
anticoagulants, oral, 363
antidepressants, tricyclic, 363
Ethinyl estradiol. *See* Estrogens
Ethionamide
isoniazid, 1209
Etidocaine. *See* Anesthetics—local

Fenoprofen
anticoagulants, oral, 711
salicylates, 698
Ferrous salts. *See* Iron salts
Flufenamic acid
salicylates, 694
Fluphenazine. *See* Antipsychotic agents
Flurazepam. *See* Benzodiazepines
Flurbiprofen
anticoagulants, oral, 711
Folic acid
contraceptives, oral, 1342, 1444
ethanol, 1342
phenobarbital, 457, 1343
phenytoin, 454, 455, 1343
primidone, 1343
trimethoprim, 1342
Furosemide. *See also* Diuretics
aminoglycoside antibiotics, 906
cephalosporins, 906
chloral hydrate, 362
clofibrate, 906
indomethacin, 706, 905
lithium, 906
vancomycin, 1231
warfarin, 906

Gallamine. *See* Neuromuscular blocking agents
Ganglionic blocking agents
clonidine, 797
neuromuscular blocking agents, 229
Gentamicin. *See* Aminoglycoside antibiotics

Glutethimide. *See also* Central nervous system depressants
  anticoagulants, oral, 364, 1357
  barbiturates, 353, 364
  cholecalciferol, 364
Gold
  N-acetylcysteine, 715
  chloroquine, 1045
  dimercaprol, 715, 716
  penicillamine, 715
Griseofulvin
  anticoagulants, oral, 1238
  barbiturates, 358, 1238
  ethanol, 1238
Guanethidine
  antidepressants, tricyclic, 198, 200, 201, 427, 813
  antipsychotic agents, 198, 199, 200, 414, 813
  cocaine, 198, 199
  ethanol, 200
  monoamine oxidase inhibitors, 430
  phenoxybenzamine, 198, 199
  sympathomimetic amines, 198, 199, 200, 201

Haloperidol. *See* Antipsychotic agents
Halothane. *See* Anesthetics—general
Heparin
  aminoglycoside antibiotics, 1174
  anticoagulants, oral, 1357, 1360
Hexafluorenium bromide
  succinylcholine, 227
Hexobarbital. *See* Barbiturates
Histamine
  caffeine, 597
  theophylline, 597
Histamine H$_1$ receptor blockers. *See* Antihistamines
Hycanthone
  phenothiazines, 1017
Hydralazine
  pyridoxine, 1571
Hydrochlorothiazide. *See* Diuretics; Thiazide diuretics
Hydrocortisone. *See* Adrenocorticosteroids
Hydroxychloroquine
  chloroquine, 1044
Hydroxyzine
  opioids, 509
Hypoglycemic agents—oral. *See also* Chlorpropamide
  β-adrenergic blocking agents, 194, 196, 1512
  anticoagulants, oral, 1357, 1512
  chloramphenicol, 1512
  clofibrate, 841, 1512
  ethanol, 382, 387, 1512
  monoamine oxidase inhibitors, 1512
  phenylbutazone, 700, 1512
  probenecid, 1512
  salicylates, 687, 1512
  sulfinpyrazone, 933
  sulfonamides, 1114, 1512

Imipramine. *See also* Antidepressants—tricyclic
  smoking, 559
Indomethacin
  aluminum hydroxide, 990
  antacids, 990
  anticoagulants, oral, 706
  antidiuretic hormone, 921
  furosemide, 706, 905
  probenecid, 706, 931
  salicylates, 698
  sulfonamides, 1114
Insulin
  β-adrenergic blocking agents, 194, 196, 1510
  phenylbutazone, 700
Iron salts
  allopurinol, 721
  aminoglycoside antibiotics, 1177
  antacids, 990, 1323
  ascorbic acid, 1323, 1580
  magnesium trisilicate, 990
  tetracyclines, 1184
Isocarboxazid. *See* Monoamine oxidase inhibitors
Isoflurane. *See* Anesthetics—general
Isoniazid
  aluminum hydroxide, 990
  aminosalicylic acid, 1209
  barbiturates, 358
  ethambutol, 1207
  ethionamide, 1209
  phenytoin, 455, 1203
  primidone, 459
  pyridoxine, 1571
  rifampin, 1204
Isoproterenol. *See* Sympathomimetic amines
Isosorbide dinitrate. *See* Nitrates—organic

Kanamycin. *See* Aminoglycoside antibiotics
Ketoprofen
  anticoagulants, oral, 711

Levallorphan
  central nervous system depressants, 510
Levodopa
  antimuscarinic agents, 479, 481
  antipsychotic agents, 414, 480, 481
  monoamine oxidase inhibitors, 429, 481
  pyridoxine, 481, 1571
  reserpine, 481
Lidocaine. *See* Anesthetics—local
  β-adrenergic blocking agents, 17, 781
Lincomycin
  neuromuscular blocking agents, 229
Lithium
  antidepressants, tricyclic, 434
  antidiuretic hormone, 433, 922
  antipsychotic agents, 434
  diuretics, 432
  ethacrynic acid, 906
  furosemide, 906

sympathomimetic amines, 434
  theophylline, 437
Local anesthetics. *See* Anesthetics—local
Lorazepam. *See* Benzodiazepines
Loxapine. *See* Antipsychotic agents
Lypressin. *See* Antidiuretic hormone

Magnesium hydroxide. *See also* Antacids; Magnesium trisilicate
  digoxin, 990
  tetracyclines, 990, 1184
Magnesium salts
  neuromuscular blocking agents, 229, 880
Magnesium trisilicate. *See also* Antacids; Magnesium hydroxide
  antimuscarinic agents, 990
  benzodiazepines, 990
  digoxin, 990
  iron salts, 990
Mannitol. *See* Diuretics
Marihuana
  antipyrine, 562
  barbiturates, 562
  ethanol, 562
Mecamylamine. *See* Ganglionic blocking agents
Mefenamic acid
  anticoagulants, oral, 709
Menadione. *See* Vitamin K
Meperidine. *See also* Opioids
  ethanol, 515
  monoamine oxidase inhibitors, 516
Mepivacaine. *See* Anesthetics—local
Meprobamate. *See also* Central nervous system depressants
  antidepressants, tricyclic, 366
  barbiturates, 353
  central nervous system depressants, 366
  contraceptives, oral, 367
  estrogens, 367
  ethanol, 366
  monoamine oxidase inhibitors, 366
  warfarin, 367
Mercaptopurine
  allopurinol, 721, 722, 1286
Mesoridazine. *See* Antipsychotic agents
Metaproterenol. *See* Sympathomimetic amines
Methacholine. *See also* Cholinergic agonists
  anticholinesterase agents, 94
Methacycline. *See* Tetracyclines
Methadone. *See also* Opioids
  antidepressants, tricyclic, 519
  diazepam, 519
  rifampin, 519, 1205
Methamphetamine. *See* Sympathomimetic amines
Methandrostenolone. *See also* Androgens
  oxyphenbutazone, 700
Methantheline. *See* Antimuscarinic agents
Methaqualone. *See also* Central nervous system depressants
  antidepressants, tricyclic, 367

barbiturates, 353
  benzodiazepines, 349
  central nervous system depressants, 367
  ethanol, 367
  monoamine oxidase inhibitors, 367
  phenothiazines, 367
Methenamine
  acetazolamide, 899
  sulfonamides, 1120
Methotrexate
  chloramphenicol, 1274
  phenytoin, 1274
  probenecid, 931
  salicylates, 687, 1274
  sulfonamides, 1114, 1274
  tetracyclines, 1274
Methoxamine. *See* Sympathomimetic amines
Methoxyflurane. *See also* Anesthetics—general
  tetracyclines, 1187
Methyldopa
  monoamine oxidase inhibitors, 430
Methylphenidate
  antidepressants, tricyclic, 426
  barbiturates, 358
Methylxanthines. *See* Caffeine; Theophylline
Metocurine. *See* Neuromuscular blocking agents
Metoprolol. *See* β-Adrenergic blocking agents
Metrifonate
  neuromuscular blocking agents, 1019
Metronidazole
  anticoagulants, oral, 1356
  ethanol, 387, 1076
Minocycline. *See* Tetracyclines
Molindone. *See* Antipsychotic agents
Monoamine oxidase inhibitors
  anesthetics, general, 430
  antidepressants, tricyclic, 427, 430
  antihistamines, 430
  antimuscarinic agents, 430
  barbiturates, 358
  central nervous system depressants, 430
  cyclobenzaprine, 490
  dopamine, 155
  ethanol, 430
  guanethidine, 430
  hypoglycemic agents, oral, 1512
  levodopa, 429, 481
  meperidine, 516
  meprobamate, 366
  methaqualone, 367
  methyldopa, 430
  opioids, 430, 508
  reserpine, 430
  sympathomimetic amines, 159, 429, 430
Morphine. *See* Opioids

Nadolol. *See* β-Adrenergic blocking agents
Nalbuphine. *See* Opioids
Nalidixic acid
  nitrofurantoin, 1121

Nalorphine
    central nervous system depressants, 510
Naproxen
    antacids, 990
    anticoagulants, oral, 711
    salicylates, 694, 698, 711
Narcotics. See Opioids
Neomycin. See Aminoglycoside antibiotics
Neostigmine. See Anticholinesterase agents
Neuromuscular blocking agents
    β-adrenergic blocking agents, 229
    adrenocorticosteroids, 229
    aminoglycoside antibiotics, 229, 1171
    anesthetics, general, 107, 226, 228, 229, 281, 285,
        287, 288
    anesthetics, local, 229
    anticholinesterase agents, 107, 114, 229
    barbiturates, 354
    chloroquine, 229
    clindamycin, 229
    colistin, 229
    digitalis glycosides, 228, 229, 756
    diuretics, 228, 229
    ganglionic blocking agents, 229
    lincomycin, 229
    magnesium salts, 229, 880
    metrifonate, 1019
    opioids, 229
    phenelzine, 229
    polymyxin B, 229
    quinidine, 229
    sympathomimetic amines, 229
    tetracyclines, 229
Nicotinic acid
    antihypertensive agents, 839
Nifurtimox
    ethanol, 1077
Nitrates—organic
    ethanol, 825
Nitrofurantoin
    nalidixic acid, 1121
    probenecid, 931
Nitroglycerin. See Nitrates—organic
Nitrous oxide. See Anesthetics—general
Nortriptyline. See Antidepressants—tricyclic

Opioids. See also Meperidine; Methadone; Propoxy-
        phene
    α-adrenergic blocking agents, 183
    amphetamine, 508, 516
    antidepressants, tricyclic, 508, 516
    antipsychotic agents, 414, 503, 508, 516
    barbiturates, 353
    benzodiazepines, 346
    clindamycin, 1227
    ethanol, 382
    hydroxyzine, 509
    monoamine oxidase inhibitors, 430, 508
    neuromuscular blocking agents, 229
    smoking, 520, 559
    theophylline, 596

Oxazepam. See Benzodiazepines
Oxyphenbutazone. See also Phenylbutazone
    anticoagulants, oral, 1356
    methandrostenolone, 700
Oxytetracycline. See Tetracyclines

Pancuronium. See Neuromuscular blocking agents
Penicillamine
    gold, 715
    pyridoxine, 1571, 1627
Penicillins. See also Ampicillin
    aminoglycoside antibiotics, 1174
    probenecid, 931
    salicylates, 694, 698
Pentaerythritol tetranitrate. See Nitrates—organic
Pentagastrin
    caffeine, 597
    theophylline, 597
Pentazocine. See Opioids
Pentobarbital. See Barbiturates
Pentolinium. See Ganglionic blocking agents
Perphenazine. See Antipsychotic agents
Phenacetin
    smoking, 559
Phencyclidine
    barbiturates, 353
    phenothiazines, 568
Phenelzine. See also Monoamine oxidase inhibitors
    neuromuscular blocking agents, 229
Phenobarbital. See also Barbiturates; Central nerv-
        ous system depressants
    carbamazepine, 460
    chloramphenicol, 1195
    cholestyramine, 843
    colestipol, 843
    digitalis glycosides, 747
    folic acid, 457, 1343
    phenytoin, 455
    quinidine, 774
    valproic acid, 457, 463
    vitamin D, 457, 1543
Phenothiazines. See also Antipsychotic agents;
        Chlorpromazine
    antacids, 405
    hycanthone, 1017
    methaqualone, 367
    phencyclidine, 568
Phenoxybenzamine. See also α-Adrenergic blocking
        agents
    guanethidine, 198, 199
Phentolamine. See α-Adrenergic blocking agents
Phenylbutazone
    antacids, 990
    anticoagulants, oral, 700, 1356
    antidepressants, tricyclic, 426
    chloroquine, 1045
    cholestyramine, 700, 843
    colestipol, 843
    digitalis glycosides, 747
    hypoglycemic agents, oral, 700, 1512
    insulin, 700

phenytoin, 455
salicylates, 694
sulfonamides, 700
thyroid hormones, 700
Phenylephrine. *See* Sympathomimetic amines
Phenytoin
acetazolamide, 899
adrenocorticosteroids, 455
anticoagulants, oral, 455, 1357
antidepressants, tricyclic, 426
barbiturates, 358
carbamazepine, 455, 460
chloramphenicol, 455, 1195
clofibrate, 841
digitalis glycosides, 747
disulfiram, 455
doxycycline, 1185
ethanol, 455
folic acid, 454, 455, 1343
isoniazid, 455, 1203
methotrexate, 1274
phenobarbital, 455
phenylbutazone, 455
primidone, 459
quinidine, 774
salicylates, 455, 694
sulfonamides, 455
valproic acid, 463
vitamin D, 454, 1543
Physostigmine. *See* Anticholinesterase agents
Phytonadione. *See* Vitamin D
Pilocarpine
barbiturates, 354
Piperacetazine. *See* Antipsychotic agents
Piperazine
pyrantel, 1023, 1024
Polymyxin B
aminoglycoside antibiotics, 1171, 1230
cephalosporins, 1230
neuromuscular blocking agents, 229
Potassium salts
procainamide, 777
quinidine, 774
spironolactone, 908
triamterene, 909
Prazepam. *See* Benzodiazepines
Prednisolone. *See* Adrenocorticosteroids
Prednisone. *See* Adrenocorticosteroids
Primaquine
quinacrine, 1078
Primidone. *See also* Phenobarbital
folic acid, 1343
isoniazid, 459
phenytoin, 459
Probenecid. *See also* Uricosuric agents
allopurinol, 721, 722
aminosalicylic acid, 1210
cephalosporins, 1153
dapsone, 1215
hypoglycemic agents, oral, 1512
indomethacin, 706, 931
methotrexate, 931

nitrofurantoin, 931
penicillins, 931
rifampin, 931
salicylates, 694, 931
sulfonamides, 932, 1114
thiazide diuretics, 899
Procainamide
digitalis glycosides, 776
potassium salts, 777
Procaine. *See* Anesthetics—local
Procarbazine
antidepressants, tricyclic, 1300
central nervous system depressants, 1300
ethanol, 1300
sympathomimetic amines, 1300
Progestins. *See* Contraceptives—oral
Propantheline. *See* Antimuscarinic agents
Propoxyphene. *See also* Opioids
central nervous system depressants, 520
ethanol, 382, 520
Propranolol. *See also* β-Adrenergic blocking agents
aluminum hydroxide, 990
smoking, 559
Protriptyline. *See* Antidepressants—tricyclic
Pseudoephedrine. *See also* Sympathomimetic amines
antacids, 990
Pyrantel
piperazine, 1023, 1024
Pyrazinamide
benzbromarone, 933
Pyridostigmine. *See* Anticholinesterase agents
Pyridoxine
cycloserine, 1571
estrogens, 1572
ethambutol, 1207
hydralazine, 1571
isoniazid, 1571
levodopa, 481, 1571
penicillamine, 1571, 1627

Quinacrine
primaquine, 1078
Quinidine
acetazolamide, 771
antacids, 990
anticoagulants, oral, 774
bicarbonate, 771
digitalis glycosides, 751, 755, 774
neuromuscular blocking agents, 229
phenobarbital, 774
phenytoin, 774
potassium salts, 774
vasodilators, 774
Quinine
antacids, 990
anticholinesterase agents, 1056

Reserpine
levodopa, 481
monoamine oxidase inhibitors, 430

Retinol. *See* Vitamin A
Riboflavin
    antidepressants, tricyclic, 1567
    antipsychotic agents, 1567
    thyroid hormones, 1567
Rifampin
    adrenocorticosteroids, 1205
    aminosalicylic acid, 1204
    anticoagulants, oral, 1205, 1357
    contraceptives, oral, 1205
    digitalis glycosides, 747
    estrogens, 1205
    isoniazid, 1204
    methadone, 519, 1205
    probenecid, 931

Salicylates
    aminosalicylic acid, 698
    antacids, 990
    anticoagulants, oral, 692, 1356
    antidepressants, tricyclic, 426
    ascorbic acid, 1557
    barbiturates, 356
    benzbromarone, 933
    ethanol, 379, 382, 691
    fenoprofen, 698
    flufenamic acid, 694
    hypoglycemic agents, oral, 687, 1512
    indomethacin, 698
    methotrexate, 687, 1274
    naproxen, 694, 698, 711
    penicillins, 694, 698
    phenylbutazone, 694
    phenytoin, 455, 694
    probenecid, 694, 931
    spironolactone, 698
    sulfinpyrazone, 694, 933
    sulfonamides, 1114
    thiopental, 694
    thyroid hormones, 694, 1402
    uricosuric agents, 691
    warfarin, 687
Scopolamine. *See* Antimuscarinic agents
Secobarbital. *See* Barbiturates
Smoking
    antipyrine, 559
    ascorbic acid, 1579
    benzodiazepines, 559
    caffeine, 559
    imipramine, 559
    opioids, 520, 559
    phenacetin, 559
    propranolol, 559
    theophylline, 559, 601
    warfarin, 559
Spironolactone. *See also* Diuretics
    anticoagulants, oral, 1357
    potassium salts, 908
    salicylates, 698
    triamterene, 909

Steroids. *See* Adrenocorticosteroids; Contraceptives—oral; Estrogens; Progestins
Streptokinase
    anticoagulants, 1362
    antithrombotic agents, 1362
Streptomycin. *See* Aminoglycoside antibiotics
Succinylcholine. *See also* Neuromuscular blocking agents
    hexafluorenium bromide, 227
Sulfadiazine. *See also* Sulfonamides
    aluminum hydroxide, 990
    antacids, 990
Sulfamethoxazole. *See* Sulfonamides
Sulfinpyrazone. *See also* Uricosuric agents
    anticoagulants, oral, 1357
    benzbromarone, 933
    hypoglycemic agents, oral, 933
    salicylates, 694, 933
Sulfisoxazole. *See* Sulfonamides
Sulfonamides. *See also* Sulfadiazine; Trimethoprim-sulfamethoxazole
    anesthetics, local, 308, 1108
    anticoagulants, oral, 1114, 1356
    hypoglycemic agents, oral, 1114, 1512
    indomethacin, 1114
    methenamine, 1120
    methotrexate, 1114, 1274
    phenylbutazone, 700
    phenytoin, 455
    probenecid, 932, 1114
    salicylates, 1114
    thiazide diuretics, 1114
    uricosuric agents, 1114
Sympathomimetic amines. *See also* individual agents
    anesthetics, general, 147, 151, 280, 287, 311
    anesthetics, local, 304, 311, 318
    antidepressants, tricyclic, 421, 427
    bretylium, 201
    cocaine, 307, 308
    digitalis glycosides, 756
    guanethidine, 198, 199, 200, 201
    lithium, 434
    monoamine oxidase inhibitors, 159, 429, 430
    neuromuscular blocking agents, 229
    procarbazine, 1300

Talbutal. *See* Barbiturates
Terbutaline. *See* Sympathomimetic amines
Testosterone. *See also* Androgens
    ethanol, 381
Tetracaine. *See* Anesthetics—local
Tetracyclines. *See also* Demeclocycline; Doxycycline
    aluminum hydroxide, 990, 1184
    antacids, 954, 990, 1184
    bicarbonate, 1184
    calcium salts, 1184
    iron salts, 1184
    magnesium salts, 1184
    methotrexate, 1274
    methoxyflurane, 1187
    neuromuscular blocking agents, 229

Theophylline
   barbiturates, 601
   cholinergic agonists, 597
   erythromycin, 601
   histamine, 597
   lithium, 437
   opioids, 596
   pentagastrin, 597
   smoking, 559, 601
Thiazide diuretics. *See also* Chlorothiazide; Diuretics
   probenecid, 899
   sulfonamides, 1114
Thiopental. *See also* Barbiturates
   salicyclates, 694
Thioridazine. *See also* Antipsychotic agents
   digitalis glycosides, 414
Thiothixene. *See* Antipsychotic agents
Thyroid hormones
   anticoagulants, oral, 1355
   barbiturates, 358
   cholestyramine, 843
   colestipol, 843
   dicumarol, 1402
   digitalis glycosides, 754
   estrogens, 1401
   phenylbutazone, 700
   riboflavin, 1567
   salicylates, 694, 1402
Timolol. *See* β-Adrenergic blocking agents
Tobramycin. *See* Aminoglycoside antibiotics
α-Tocopherol. *See* Vitamin E
Tolazamide. *See* Hypoglycemic agents—oral
Tolbutamide. *See* Hypoglycemic agents—oral
Tranylcypromine. *See* Monoamine oxidase inhibitors
Triamcinolone. *See* Adrenocorticosteroids
Triamterene. *See also* Diuretics
   potassium salts, 909
   spironolactone, 909
Tricyclic antidepressants. *See* Antidepressants—tricyclic
Trifluoperazine. *See* Antipsychotic agents
Triflupromazine. *See* Antipsychotic agents
Trimethaphan. *See* Ganglionic blocking agents
Trimethoprim
   anticoagulants, oral, 1356
   folic acid, 1342
Trimethoprim-sulfamethoxazole
   diuretics, 1118
d-Tubocurarine. *See* Neuromuscular blocking agents

Uricosuric agents
   allopurinol, 722
   salicylates, 691
   sulfonamides, 1114
Urokinase
   anticoagulants, 1362
   antithrombotic agents, 1362

Valproic acid
   benzodiazepines, 349
   clonazepam, 463
   phenobarbital, 457, 463
   phenytoin, 463
Vancomycin
   aminoglycoside antibiotics, 1097, 1171, 1231
   ethacrynic acid, 1231
   furosemide, 1231
Vasodilators
   α-adrenergic blocking agents, 183
   quinidine, 774
Vasopressin. *See* Antidiuretic hormone
Vitamin A
   ascorbic acid, 1591
   vitamin E, 1589, 1591
   vitamin K, 1596
Vitamin C. *See* Ascorbic acid
Vitamin D. *See also* Cholecalciferol
   adrenocorticosteroids, 1543
   barbiturates, 356, 358
   cholestyramine, 843
   colestipol, 843
   phenobarbital, 457, 1543
   phenytoin, 454, 1543
Vitamin E
   vitamin A, 1589, 1591
Vitamin K
   vitamin A, 1596
   barbiturates, 356, 358
   cholestyramine, 843
   colestipol, 843

Warfarin. *See also* Anticoagulants—oral
   barbiturates, 18, 356
   ethacrynic acid, 906
   furosemide, 906
   meprobamate, 367
   salicylates, 687
   smoking, 559

INDEX

AAT (parathion), 104
ABBOKINASE (urokinase), 1362
Abdominal distention, oxygen in, 330
Abortion, prostaglandins in, 678, 949
  threatened and habitual, progestins in, 1438
Abscesses, choice of drugs in, 1086
Absence seizures. *See* Epilepsy
Absorbable dusting powder, 953
Absorbable gelatin sponge, 955
Absorbable hemostatics, 955
Acacia, 951
Acacia syrup, 951
Acebutolol, 188, 196
  pharmacokinetics, 1684
Aceclidine, pharmacological properties, 98
  structural formula, 97
  use in glaucoma, 98
Acedapsone, 1047, 1058
Acenocoumarol, 1359. *See also* Anticoagulants, oral
Acetaminophen, 701–705. *See also* Aspirin-like
      drugs
  absorption, fate, and excretion, 702–703
  chemistry, 701–702
  hepatotoxicity, 703–704
  history, 701
  interactions with other drugs, 703
  pharmacokinetics, 1685
  pharmacological effects, 702
  poisoning, treatment, 704
  potentiation of effect of ADH, 921
  preparations and dosage, 704–705
  toxicity, 703–704
  uses, 705
Acetanilid, 701
Acetazolamide. *See also* Carbonic anhydrase inhibi-
      tors
  anticonvulsant properties, 468
  preparations, 898
  properties and dosage as diuretic, 896–899
  uses, alkalinization of urine, 868
    epilepsy, 468
    glaucoma, 113
Acetic acid, 971
Acetohexamide, 1510–1514. *See also* Sulfonylureas
  duration of action, fate, and excretion, 1512
  preparations, 1513
Acetone, 980
Acetophenazine maleate. *See also* Antipsychotic
      agents
  chemistry, 409
  dosage forms, 409
  dose as antipsychotic, 409
  side effects, 409
Acetophenetidin. *See* Phenacetin
Acetophenone, 1435

Acetyl-β-methylcholine. *See* Methacholine
Acetylcholine. *See also* Autonomic nervous system
  actions/effects on, autonomic effectors, 70
    cardiovascular system, 93–94
    ganglionic transmission, 70–71
    gastrointestinal system, 94
    glands, 94
    insulin secretion, 1500
    membrane permeability, 70
    prejunctional sites, 71
    skeletal neuromuscular transmission, 69–70
    urinary tract, 94
  biosynthesis, 67–68
  history, 91
  hydrolysis, 68
  mechanisms of action, 91–92
  miscellaneous effects, 94
  preparations and dosage, 95
  role as CNS transmitter, 247–248, 250
  storage and release, 68–69
  structural formula, 92
  structure-activity relationship, 92
  synergists and antagonists, 94–95
  use, ocular, 96
Acetylcholinesterase, 68, 101–103
Acetylcholinesterase inhibitors. *See* Anticholines-
      terases
Acetylcysteine, 1266
  actions and uses, 960
  use in acetaminophen poisoning, 704
Acetyldigitoxin. *See also* Digitalis
  preparation and administration, 749
Acetylmethadol, use in compulsive opioid users, 519,
      574
Acetylpenicillamine, 1627
N-Acetylprocainamide, pharmacokinetics, 1686
Acetylsalicylic acid, 688. *See also* Aspirin; Aspirin-
      like drugs; Salicylates
  pharmacokinetics, 1686
Acetylstrophanthidin, 730
ACHROMYCIN (tetracycline hydrochloride), 1185
Acid-base disturbances, 863–869. *See also* Body
      fluids
  dilution acidosis and subtraction alkalosis, 868
  laboratory diagnosis, 865
  mechanisms of compensation, 864–865
  metabolic acidosis, 866–867
  metabolic alkalosis, 867–868
  plasma values in, 864
  respiratory acidosis, 866
  respiratory alkalosis, 866
Acid-forming salts, 869–870
ACIDULIN (glutamic acid hydrochloride), 998
Acinetobacter infections, choice of drugs in, 1090
Acne, benzoyl peroxide in, 974

Acne (*Cont.*)
13-*cis*-retinoic acid in, 1591
estrogens in, 1436
resorcinol in, 968
tetracyclines in, 1191
tretinoin in, 1591
zinc sulfate in, 977
Acridanes, 396
Acrisorcin, 984
Acrocyanosis, alpha-adrenergic blocking agents in, 187
Acrodermatitis enteropathica, clioquinol in, 1065
iodoquinol in, 1065
zinc sulfatc in, 1065
Acrolein, toxicology, 1641
Acromegaly, 1379
ACTAMER (bithional), 1035
ACTH. *See* Adrenocorticotropic hormone
ACTHAR (corticotropin injection), 1470
Actinomyces israelii infections. *See* Actinomycosis
Actinomycin D. *See* Dactinomycin
Actinomycosis, choice of drugs in, 1092
clindamycin in, 1227
penicillin G in, 1140
tetracyclines in, 1191
Activated charcoal, use in drug poisoning, 954, 1610
ACTIVATED CHARCOAL–MERCK, 954
Acycloguanosine, 1276
ACYLANID (acetyldigitoxin), 749
Adamantanamine, 1241
ADAPIN (doxepin hydrochloride), 424
Addiction to drugs. *See* Drug addiction
Addisonian anemia. *See* Anemia—megaloblastic
Addison's disease. *See* Adrenal insufficiency
Adenohypophyseal hormones, 1369–1396. *See also* individual hormones
general consideration of functions and chemistry, 1369–1372
history, 1370–1371
hypersecretion, 1372
hyposecretion, 1371–1372
hypothalamic control, 1389–1392
Adenosine, antagonism of actions by xanthines, 598–599
effect on cyclic AMP synthesis, 251
physiological actions, 598–599
Adenosine 3′,5′-monophosphate. *See* Cyclic adenosine 3′,5′-monophosphate
Adenylate cyclase. *See also* Cyclic adenosine 3′,5′-monophosphate
relation to receptors, 29
ADH. *See* Antidiuretic hormone
Adrenal corticosteroids. *See* Adrenocorticosteroids
Adrenal hyperplasia, adrenocorticosteroids in, 1488–1489
Adrenal insufficiency, adrenocorticosteroids in, 1488
Adrenal neoplasia, aminoglutethimide in, 1492–1493
metyrapone in, 1492
mitotane in, 1301
Adrenaline. *See* Epinephrine

Adrenergic blocking drugs, 178–197. *See also* Adrenergic neuron blocking drugs; Alpha-adrenergic blocking drugs; Beta-adrenergic blocking drugs; individual agents
common side effects, 176–178
side effects limited to alpha-blocking agents, 177
side effects limited to beta-blocking agents, 177–178
terminology, 176
uses, 186–188, 194, 197
Adrenergic nervous system. *See* Autonomic nervous system
Adrenergic neuron blocking drugs, 198–205. *See also* individual agents
definition and mechanism of action, 176, 198
Adrenergic receptors, types, 77–78, 139–140
Adrenergic stimulating drugs, 138–175. *See also* Sympathomimetic drugs; individual agents
Adrenergic transmission, 71–80
Adrenocortical carcinoma, mitotane in, 1301
Adrenocorticosteroids, 1470–1492. *See also* individual steroids
absorption, transport, metabolism, and excretion, 1480–1481
actions/effects on, ACTH secretion, 1469
carbohydrate metabolism, 1474
cardiovascular system, 1477
central nervous system, 1477–1478
electrolyte and water balance, 1475–1477
epinephrine synthesis, 73
eye, 1490
formed elements of blood, 1478
growth and cell division, 1480
immune responses, 1479
inflammation, 1479–1480
lipid metabolism, 1474–1475
lymphoid tissue, 1478
protein metabolism, 1474
skeletal muscle, 1477
biosynthesis, 1470–1471
chemistry, 1471, 1481–1482
comparative dosages, 1482
history, 1466–1467
inhibitors of synthesis, 1492–1493
mechanism of action, 1473–1474
permissive effects, 1473
physiological functions, 1471–1480
plasma concentrations, 1473
preparations and routes of administration, 1482, 1484–1486
rates of secretion, 1473
relative potencies, 1473, 1482
structure-activity relationship, 1481–1482
toxicity, 1482–1483, 1486–1487
uses, acute adrenal insufficiency, 1488
acute lymphocytic leukemia, 1301, 1491
adrenal hyperplasia, 1488–1489
adrenal insufficiency secondary to anterior pituitary insufficiency, 1489
allergic diseases, 1490
anterior pituitary insufficiency, 1489

aspiration pneumonitis, 1492
bronchial asthma, 1490
carcinoma of the breast, 1491
cerebral edema, 1491
chronic adrenal insufficiency, 1488
cirrhosis, 1491
collagen diseases, 1490
congenital adrenal hyperplasia, 1488–1489
diagnostic agents, 1492
filariasis, 1033
general principles, 1487
hemolytic anemias, 1492
hepatic necrosis, 1491
hepatitis, 1491
hypercalcemia, 1529
immunosuppression, 1492
infantile myoclonic spasms, 470
leukemia, 1491
lymphomas, 1491
myasthenia gravis, 116
neoplastic diseases, 1253, 1301, 1491
nephrotic syndrome, 1489
ocular diseases, 1490
osteoarthritis, 1489
renal diseases, 1489
rheumatic carditis, 1489
rheumatoid arthritis, 1489
sarcoidosis, 1491
shock, 1491
skin diseases, 1491
sprue, 1491
thrombocytopenia, 1491
trichinosis, 1032
ulcerative colitis, 1491
Adrenocorticotropic hormone, 1467–1470
absorption, fate, and excretion, 1469
actions/effects on, adrenal cortex, 1468
activation of adenylate cyclase, 1468
bioassay, 1470
chemical properties, 1371
chemistry, 1467
extra-adrenal effects, 1468–1469
history, 1466–1467
hypothalamic regulation, 1391
mechanism of action, 1468
preparations, dosage, and routes of administration, 1470
regulation of secretion, 1469
toxicity, 1470
uses, diagnostic agent in adrenal insufficiency, 1470
infantile myoclonic spasms, 470
ADRIAMYCIN (doxorubicin hydrochloride), 1293
ADROYD (oxymetholone), 1458
Adsorbents, 953–954. See also individual agents
AEROSPORIN (polymyxin B sulfate), 1229
Affective disorders, 418–436. See also Depression; Mania
treatment, 434–436
AFRIN (oxymetazoline hydrochloride), 168
Agar, 951

Air embolism, oxygen in, 331
Air pollution, 1638–1644. See also individual pollutants
absorption and deposition of toxicants by the lungs, 1638–1639
health effects, 1639
toxicology, 1639–1644
types and sources, 1639
Akathisia, from antipsychotic drugs, 407, 412
AKINETON (biperiden hydrochloride), 486
AKRINOL (acrisorcin), 984
Alachlor, toxicology, 1654
β-Alanine, 246–248
Albumin, drug binding, 10–11
Albumin human, 862
ALBUMINAR (albumin human), 862
ALBUMISOL (albumin human) 862
ALBUSPAN (albumin human), 862
ALBUTEIN (albumin human), 862
Albuterol, 166, 168
receptor-type activity, 142
structural formula, 142
use in premature labor, 172
ALCAINE (proparacaine hydrochloride), 310
Alclofenac, 710. See also Aspirin-like drugs
Alcohol, abuse. See Alcoholism; Ethyl alcohol
Alcoholic neuritis, thiamine in, 1563
Alcoholics Anonymous, 573
Alcoholism, benzodiazepines in, 440
complications, 552–553
conditioned aversion therapy, 575
disulfiram in, 388, 575
folic acid in, 1341, 1342, 1343
hospitalization and psychotherapy, 573
phenothiazines in, 418
role of physician, 575–577
tricyclic antidepressants in, 427
withdrawal symptoms, 552 553
withdrawal technics, 572
ALCOPARA (bephenium hydroxynaphthoate), 1014
Alcuronium. See also Neuromuscular blocking agents
preparations and dosage, 231
structural formula, 221
ALDACTAZIDE (spironolactone-hydrochlorothiazide), 908
ALDACTONE (spironolactone), 908
Aldehyde dehydrogenase, 479
Aldehydes, toxicology, 1641
ALDOMET (methyldopa), 796
ALDOMET ESTER HYDROCHLORIDE (methyldopate hydrochloride), 796
Aldosterone. See also Adrenocorticosteroids
actions/effects on, kidney, 871
water and electrolyte metabolism, 1475–1476
antagonists, 907–908
relative potency, duration of action, and equivalent dose, 1482
Aldrin, toxicology, 1649
Alginic acid, 995
ALIDASE (hyaluronidase for injection), 960

ALKERAN (melphalan), 1266
Alkylating agents, 1256–1272. *See also* individual
　　agents
　　actions/effects on, epithelial tissues, 1260, 1262
　　　hematopoietic system, 1262
　　　nervous system, 1263
　　　reproductive tissues, 1262
　　biochemical actions, 1261
　　chemistry, 1256–1260
　　cytotoxic actions, 1260–1262
　　history, 1256
　　immunosuppressive actions, 1262
　　mechanism of resistance, 1262
　　structure-activity relationship, 1258–1260
　　use in neoplastic diseases, 1252
Alkyl sulfonates, use in neoplastic diseases, 1252
Allergic disorders, adrenocorticosteroids in, 1490
　　cromolyn in, 622
　　H_1-receptor blockers in, 627–629
　　sympathomimetic drugs in, 170–171
Allergic reactions to drugs, 1604
ALLERTOC (pyrilamine maleate), 628
ALLOFERIN (alcuronium chloride), 231
Allopurinol, 720–722
　　absorption, fate, and excretion, 721
　　chemistry, 720
　　conversion to alloxanthine, 720, 721
　　history, 720
　　interactions with other drugs, 721
　　mechanism of action, 720
　　pharmacological effects, 720
　　preparations and dosage, 721
　　structural formula, 720
　　toxicity, 721
　　uses, gout, 722
　　　hyperuricemia, 722, 1286
Alloxan, 1501
Alloxanthine, 720, 721
Allylestrenol, 1434
Almond oil, 952
Alpha-adrenergic blocking drugs, 178–188. *See also*
　　individual agents
　　effects on α_1 versus α_2 receptors, 178
　　uses, 186–188
Alpha-chloralose, 361
ALPHA-CHYMAR (chymotrypsin), 961
ALPHADROL (fluprednisolone), 1485
Alpha-lobeline, 212–213
Alpha-methyldopa. *See* Methyldopa
Alpha-methylnorepinephrine, 81
Alpha-methyltyrosine, pharmacological properties,
　　81, 82, 204
　　use in pheochromocytoma, 187
Alphaprodine, dosage, 507
　　duration of analgesic effect, 507
　　preparations, routes of administration, and dos-
　　　age, 516
　　structural formula, 514
ALPHAREDISOL (hydroxocobalamin), 1337
Alpha-tocopherol, 1596. *See also* Vitamin E
Alprazolam, 340
Alprenolol, 188, 196

hypnotic effect, 369
　　pharmacokinetics, 1687
ALRHEUMAT (ketoprofen), 713
ALTACITE (hydrotalcite), 995
ALUDROX, 991
Alum, 956
Alumina and magnesia oral suspension, preparation
　　and dosage, 995
Alumina and magnesia tablets, 995
Aluminum carbonate, basic, use and dosage as gas-
　　tric antacid, 992
Aluminum chloride, 954
Aluminum hydroxide, 954
　　gastric antacid properties, 990
　　preparations and dosage, 991
　　untoward reactions, 991
　　uses, calcinosis universalis, 991
　　　nephrolithiasis, 991
Aluminum hydroxide gel, 954
Aluminum hydroxychloride, 954
Aluminum nicotinate, 839
Aluminum phenylsulfonate, 954
Aluminum phosphate, preparations and dosage, 992
Aluminum phosphate gel, 954
Aluminum phosphide, toxicology, 1652
Aluminum sulfate, 954
ALUPENT (metaproterenol sulfate), 167
ALURATE (aprobarbital), 350
Amanitin, 98
Amantadine, antiviral properties, 1241
　　effects on central nervous system, 483
　　mechanism of action on central nervous system,
　　　483
　　preparations and dosage, 483, 1241
　　structural formula, 1241
　　untoward effects, 483
　　uses, influenza, 1241
　　　parkinsonism, 483
Ambenonium. *See also* Anticholinesterases
　　preparations, 112
　　structural formula, 104
　　use in myasthenia gravis, 115
AMBERLITE XAD-4, 360
AMBILHAR (niridazole), 1021
AMCILL (ampicillin), 1144
Amebiasis, chloroquine in, 1067
　　clioquinol in, 1064
　　dehydroemetine in, 1066
　　diloxanide furoate in, 1068
　　emetine in, 1066
　　erythromycin in, 1068
　　general considerations, 1061
　　iodoquinol in, 1064
　　metronidazole in, 1063
　　paromomycin in, 1068
　　principles of chemotherapy, 1062–1063
　　tetracyclines in, 1068, 1191
Amebic meningoencephalitis, amphotericin B in,
　　1240
　　miconazole in, 1240
　　rifampin in, 1240
Amebicides, 1061–1069. *See also* individual agents

Ames' test, 1607
AMETHOCAINE (tetracaine hydrochloride), 309
Amethopterin. *See* Methotrexate
Amiben, toxicology, 1654
AMICAR (aminocaproic acid), 1362
AMIGEN (protein hydrolysate injection), 863
Amikacin, 1176. *See also* Aminoglycoside antibiotics; Antimicrobial agents
    pharmacokinetics, 1687
    uses, 1176, 1212
AMIKIN (amikacin), 1176
Amiloride, 909–910
Aminacrine hydrochloride, 980
Amino acids, preparations, 863
Aminocaproic acid, 1362
7-Aminocephalosporanic acid, 1151
    structural formula, 1152
Aminocyclitol, 1163
Aminoglutethimide, 1492–1493
Aminoglycoside antibiotics, 1162–1180. *See also* individual agents
    absorption, 1167
    antibacterial activity, 1165–1167
    chemistry, 1163–1164
    distribution, 1167–1168
    elimination, 1168–1169
    general considerations, 1162
    history and source, 1162–1163
    mechanism of action, 1164–1165
    microbial resistance, 1165
    untoward effects, nephrotoxicity, 1170–1171
        neuromuscular blockade, 1171
        ototoxicity, 1169–1170
Amino-idoxuridine, 1276
Aminooxyacetic acid, 248
6-Aminopenicillanic acid, structural formula, 1128
Aminophylline, 592, 601. *See also* Xanthines
Aminopyrine, status, 701
Aminosalicylic acid, 1209–1210
    absorption, distribution, and excretion, 1210
    action on plasma lipids, 845
    antibacterial activity, 1209
    bacterial resistance, 1210
    chemistry, 1209
    history, 1209
    mechanism of action, 1210
    preparations, routes of administration, and dosage, 1210
    untoward effects, 1210
    use in tuberculosis, 1210
AMINOSOL (protein hydrolysate injection), 863
AMINOSYN (amino acid injection), 863
Aminotriazole, toxicology, 1654
Amithiozone, 1216
AMITRIL (amitriptyline hydrochloride), 424
Amitriptyline. *See also* Tricyclic antidepressants
    pharmacokinetics, 1688
    preparations and dosage, 424
    structural formula, 419
Ammonia, 869–870
Ammoniated mercury, 976
Ammoniated mercury ointment, 976

Ammonium, endogenous metabolism, 869
    pharmacological actions, 870
    preparations, 870
    renal excretion, 869
    reversal of intoxication, 870
    toxicity, 869–870
Ammonium carbonate, 870
Ammonium chloride, 870
AMNESTROGEN (esterified estrogens), 1428
Amobarbital. *See also* Barbiturates
    chemistry, 351
    dosage, half-life, and preparations, 350
    legal regulations, 1670
AMOCO GRADE PX-21 (activated charcoal), 954
Amodiaquine hydrochloride, 1046
Amoxicillin, 1144–1145. *See also* Ampicillin; Penicillins
    pharmacokinetics, 1688
AMOXIL (amoxicillin), 1145
Amphetamine, 159–162. *See also* Dextroamphetamine; Sympathomimetic drugs
    absorption, distribution, and fate, 159
    abuse, 553–557, 1670
    actions/effects on, appetite, 161
        cardiovascular system, 160
        central nervous system, 160–161
        EEG, 160–161
        fatigue, 160
        metabolism, 161
        psyche, 160
        respiration, 161
        smooth muscle, 160
    dependence and tolerance, 162
    history, 159–160
    mechanism of adrenergic action, 81–82
    physical dependence, 556–557
    poisoning, treatment, 162
    precautions and contraindications, 162
    preparations, administration, and dosage, 161
    psychosis from, 556
    receptor-type activity, 142
    structural formula, 142
    tolerance, 556
    toxicity and side effects, 161–162, 556–557
    uses, 162
        motion sickness, 529
        narcolepsy, 171
        pain, 512
    withdrawal symptoms, 556–557
AMPHOJEL, 991, 996
Amphotericin B, 1233–1236. *See also* Antifungal drugs
    absorption, distribution, and excretion, 1234
    antifungal activity, 1234
    chemistry, 1233
    dosage, 1234–1235
    fungal resistance, 1234
    history and source, 1233
    pharmacokinetics, 1689
    preparations and administration, 1234–1235
    toxicity, 1235–1236
    uses, amebic meningoencephalitis, 1240

Amphotericin B (*Cont.*)
  aspergillosis, 1240
  blastomycosis, 1240
  Candida infections, 1240
  coccidioidomycosis, 1239
  cryptococcosis, 1239
  histoplasmosis, 1239
  leishmaniasis, 1075
  Naegleria infections, 1061
  paracoccidioidomycosis, 1240
  sporotrichosis, 1240
  Zygomycetes infections, 1240
Ampicillin, 1143–1145. *See also* Penicillins
  pharmacokinetics, 1689
Amrinone, 756
A-M-T, 991, 996
Amyl nitrite. *See also* Nitrates
  preparations, route of administration, and dosage,
    826
  structural formula, 826
  uses, 825
    cyanide poisoning, 1651
AMYTAL (amobarbital), 350, 1670
AMYTAL SODIUM (amobarbital sodium), 350
ANABOL (methandriol), 1457
Anabolic steroids, 1448–1463. *See also* Androgens;
    individual agents
  structural formulas, preparations, and dosage,
    1457–1458
ANADROL (oxymetholone), 1458
Anaerobic infections, cephalosporins in, 1157
  chloramphenicol in, 1195
  clindamycin in, 1227
  hyperbaric oxygen in, 331
  metronidazole in, 1077
  penicillin in, 1139
Analgesic-antipyretics, 682–713. *See also* Aspirin-
    like drugs; individual agents
Analgesic nephropathy, 686
Anaphylaxis, adrenocorticosteroids in, 1490
  antihistamines in, 627
  epinephrine in, 171
ANAVAR (oxandrolone), 1458
ANCEF (sterile cefazolin sodium), 1154
ANCOBON (flucytosine), 1237
Ancylostomiasis, occurrence and treatment, 1031
Androgen-control therapy, of carcinoma of the male
    breast, 1302
  of prostatic carcinoma, 1302
  untoward effects, 1302–1303
Androgens, 1448–1463. *See also* individual agents
  absorption, metabolism, and excretion, 1454–1455
  actions/effects on, anabolism, 1452–1453
    sebaceous glands, 1453
    testis and accessory structures, 1452
  antagonists, 1461–1462
  assays, 1455
  chemistry, 1448–1449
  deficiency, 1452
  history, 1448
  mechanism of action, 1453–1454
  pharmacological actions, 1451–1453

  physiological functions, 1451–1453
  preparations and dosage, 1455, 1456
    for anabolic effects, 1457–1458
  relationship to gonadotropins, 1449–1450
  secretion by ovary, 1422–1423
  structural formulas, 1449, 1456–1458
  synthesis and secretion, 1449–1451
  synthesis by, adrenal cortex, 1450–1451
    ovary, 1450–1451
  untoward effects, 1455, 1458–1459
  uses, aging men, 1460
    anabolism promotion, 1461
    anemia, 1460–1461
    breast carcinoma, 1461
    endometriosis, 1460
    growth acceleration, 1460
    hypogonadism, 1450
    hypopituitarism, 1459–1460
    male contraception, 1462–1463
    menopause, 1429
    neoplastic diseases, 1254
    osteoporosis, 1460
    suppression of lactation, 1461
Androstenedione, relative androgenic activity, 1448
Androsterone, 1448, 1449
ANDROID T (testosterone), 1456
ANDROYD (oxymetholone), 1458
ANECTINE (succinylcholine chloride), 231
Anemia, oxygen in, 330
Anemia—hemolytic, adrenocorticosteroids in, 1492
  mechanism of drug induction, 1053–1054
Anemia—hypochromic, 1315–1330. *See also* Iron;
    Iron-deficiency anemias
  iron therapy, 1322–1326
  pyridoxine-responsive, 1327
  riboflavin-responsive, 1327
Anemia—megaloblastic, 1331–1346. *See also* Cya-
    nocobalamin; Folic acid
  cyanocobalamin in, 1337–1340
  folic acid in, 1343–1344
  historical aspects, 1331
Anemia—nutritional, 1314
Anemia—refractory, androgens in, 1460–1461
Anesthesia. *See also* individual agents
  analgesic stage, 268
  carbon dioxide in, 334
  curarimimetic agents in, 231
  delerium stage, 268
  depth, 267–269
  EEG as index of depth, 269
  estimate of depth, 268–269
  history, 258–260
  inhalational anesthetics, abuse, 568–569
    administration, 265–267
    anesthetic machines, 265
    atropine premedication, 135
    breathing circuits, 265–267
    concentration effect, 264
    curariform drugs as adjuvants, 231
    diffusion hypoxia, 264–265
    dosage, 267
    elimination, 263–264

gas, heat, and water transfer in, 266–267
induction of anesthesia, 277
intertissue diffusion, 265
metabolism, 264
partial pressure in blood, 261–263
partial pressure in inspired gas, 260
partial pressure in tissues, 262–264
physical properties, 277
potency, 267, 276
pulmonary blood flow, 262
pulmonary ventilation, 261
second-gas effect, 264
solubility in blood, 262
solubility in tissues, 262–263
structural formulas, 277
technics of administration, 265–267
tissue blood flow and, 263
tissue tensions, 263
transfer from alveoli to blood, 261–262
uptake and distribution, 260–263
vaporization, 276–277
intravenous anesthetics, 292–297
barbiturates, 292–295
diazepam, 296
droperidol, 295–296
history, 260
INNOVAR, 295
ketamine, 296–297
neurolept analgesia, 295–296
opioids, 295–296
mechanisms of action, 271–272
medullary depression stage, 268
muscular relaxation, 269
oxygen in, 331
planes, 268
practical considerations in judging depth, 268–269
preanesthetic medication, 269–271
signs and stages, 267–268
surgical stage, 268
ANESTHESIN (benzocaine), 310
Angina pectoris, amyl nitrite in, 825
dipyridamole in, 830
nadolol in, 195
organic nitrates in, 825
perhexiline in, 829
propranolol in, 190, 194, 828
therapeutic considerations, 825
variant, alpha-adrenergic blocking agents in, 828
ergonovine in diagnosis, 828
nifedipine in, 828
nitroglycerin in, 828
perhexilene in, 828
verapamil in, 828
Angioedema, adrenocorticosteroids in, 1490
antihistamines in, 627
epinephrine in, 171
Angiotensin, 647–659
actions/effects on, ADH secretion, 919
adrenal cortex and aldosterone secretion, 650–651
adrenal medulla, 650
autonomic nervous system, 650

cardiovascular system, 649–650
central nervous system, 650
kidney, 651
antagonists, 656–657. *See also* Saralasin
chemistry, 647–648
endogenous, 652–655
central nervous system functions, 654–655
circulatory responses and homeostasis, 654
functions of the renin-angiotensin system, 653–655
in hypertensive states, 654
intrarenal functions, 654
metabolism *in vivo,* 652–653
role in aldosterone secretion, 654
formation *in vivo,* 652
history, 647
mechanism of action, 651
peptides blocking angiotensin receptors, 656
precautions and untoward effects, 655
preparation, 655
renin-angiotensin system, antagonists, 656–659
inhibitors of peptidyl dipeptidase, 657–659
role as CNS transmitter, 253
role in ganglionic transmission, 215
uses, hypotensive states, 655
shock, 655
Angiotensin I, 647–648, 651, 652, 657. *See also* Angiotensin
Angiotensin III, 647–648, 651, 652, 655, 656, 657. *See also* Angiotensin
Angiotensinase, 648, 652
Angiotensinogens, 647–648, 652
ANHYDRON (cyclothiazide), 900
Anhydrous lanolin, 952
Anileridine, dosage, 507
duration of analgesic effect, 507
legal regulations, 1670
preparations and routes of administration, 516
structural formula, 514
withdrawal symptoms, 507
Aniline, structural formula, 702
Animal fats, 952
Anisindione, 1359. *See also* Anticoagulants, oral
Anisotropine, 130
Ankylosing spondylitis, indomethacin in, 706
propionic acid derivatives in, 713
sulindac in, 708
tolmetin in, 710
Anorectic drugs. *See also* Sympathomimetic drugs; individual agents
actions and uses, 171–172
ANSPOR (cephradine), 1155
ANTABUSE (disulfiram), 388
Antacids. *See* Gastric antacids
Antazoline phosphate, preparations and dosage, 628. *See also* H_1-receptor blockers
ANTEPAR CITRATE (piperazine citrate), 1023
ANTEPAR PHOSPHATE (piperazine phosphate), 1023
Anterior pituitary hormones. *See* Adenohypophyseal hormones
Anthelmintics, 1013–1037. *See also* individual agents
definition, 1013

ANTHELVET (tetramisole), 1026

Anthiomaline, 1074

ANTHIPHEN (dichlorophen), 1014

Anthralin, 981

Anthrax, penicillin G in, 1140

Antiandrogens, 1461–1462

Antianxiety drugs, 436–442. *See also* individual
agents

Antiarrhythmic drugs, 761–792. *See also* Cardiac
arrhythmias; individual agents

Antibacterial agents. *See* Antimicrobial agents; individual antibiotics

Antibiotics. *See* Antimicrobial agents; individual
antibiotics

Antibodies, use in drug poisoning, 1613

Anticholinergic drugs. *See* Antimuscarinic drugs;
Belladonna alkaloids; Ganglionic blocking
agents; Neuromuscular blocking agents; individual agents

Anticholinesterases, 100–116. *See also* individual
agents

  absorption, fate, and excretion, 108–109

  actions/effects on, autonomic ganglia, 108

    cardiovascular system, 107–108

    central nervous system, 108

    effector organs, 103

    eye, 106

    gastrointestinal tract, 106–107

    secretory glands, 107

    skeletal neuromuscular junction, 107

    smooth muscle, 107

  chemistry, 103–104

  history, 100–101

  irreversible inhibition of acetylcholinesterase, 101–
  103

  mechanisms of action, 101–103

  pharmacological properties, 104–109

  poisoning, acute signs and symptoms, 109

    atropine in, 136

    chronic neurotoxicity, 111–112

    diagnosis and treatment, 109–110

    pralidoxime in, 110

  preparations, 112

  structure-activity relationship, 103–104

  uses, atony of urinary bladder, 113

    atropine intoxication, 116

    glaucoma, 113–114

    ileus, 113

    myasthenia gravis, 114–116

    ocular, 113–114

Anticoagulants, 1348–1360. *See also* individual
agents

  oral, 1353–1360

    absorption, fate, and excretion, 1357

    chemistry, 1353–1354

    drug interactions, 1356 1357

    effect on blood coagulation, 1354–1355

    factors influencing activity, 1355–1356

    history, 1353

    laboratory control, 1360

    mechanism of action, 1354–1355

    precautions and contraindications, 1358–1359

    preparations, route of administration, and dos-
    age, 1357–1358

    toxicity, 1358

  uses, cerebrovascular disease, 1363

    myocardial infarction, 1363

    pulmonary embolism, 1363–1364

    rheumatic heart disease, 1363

    venous thrombosis, 1363–1364

Anticonvulsants, 448–471. *See also* Epilepsy; individual agents

Antidepressants. *See* Tricyclic antidepressants;
Monoamine oxidase inhibitors

Antidiuretic hormone, 916–925

  absorption, fate, and excretion, 923

  actions/effects on, ACTH secretion, 923

    blood coagulation, 922

    cardiovascular system, 922

    central nervous system, 923

    cyclic AMP formation, 921

    kidney, 920–921

    smooth muscle, 922

  antagonists, 926

  chemistry, 916–917

  evolutionary considerations, 916

  mechanism of renal action, 921

  physiological and pathophysiological considerations, 918–920

  preparations, bioassay, and unitage, 923–924

  role as CNS transmitter, 253

  secretion, pharmacological regulation, 920

    physiological regulation, 918–920

  syndrome of inappropriate secretion, 920

  untoward reactions and contraindications, 924–
  925

  uses, bleeding disorders, 924

    diabetes insipidus, 924

    esophageal varices, 924

    pressor action, 924

Antidotes, use in drug poisoning, 1608–1613

Antiepileptics, 448–471. *See also* Epilepsy; individual agents

  status in pregnancy, 471

Antiestrogens, 1304–1305, 1431–1433. *See also* individual agents

  mechanisms of action, 1304, 1432–1433

  pharmacological effects, 1432

  preparations, 1304, 1433

  uses, carcinoma of the breast, 1304–1305

    infertility, 1433

Antifebrin, 701

Antifungal drugs, 981–984. 1232–1240. *See also* Antimicrobial agents; individual agents

  mechanisms of action, 981–982

  miscellaneous agents, 984

Antihistamines, 622 632. *See also* H_1-receptor
blockers; H_2-receptor blockers

  history, 622

  mechanism of action, 623

  poisoning, physostigmine in, 116

  terminology, 622

Antihypertensive drugs, 793–818. *See also* individual agents
  classification, 793
Anti-inflammatory drugs, 682–720. *See also* Aspirin-like drugs; individual agents
Antileprotic drugs, 1214–1217. *See also* Sulfones
ANTILIRIUM (physostigmine salicylate), 112
Antimalarial drugs, 1038–1060. *See also* Malaria; individual agents
  acquired resistance, 1041–1042
  mechanisms of action, 1040–1041
Antimetabolites, in neoplastic diseases, 1252–1253, 1272–1287
Antimicrobial agents. *See also* Antifungal drugs; Antiseptics; Antiviral agents; Disinfectants; Sulfonamides; individual antibiotics
  age factor in response, 1096
  choice for therapy of infections, 1085–1096
    host factors, 1095–1096
    pharmacokinetic factors, 1094–1095
  classification and mechanism of action, 1081–1082
  clinical aspects of resistance, 1083–1084
  combination therapy, 1097–1100
    to delay bacterial resistance, 1099–1100
    disadvantages and dangers, 1100
    to enhance efficacy, 1099
    evaluation *in vitro*, 1097–1098
    in mixed bacterial infections, 1098
    in severe infections of unknown etiology, 1098–1099
  definition and characteristics, 1081
  determination of bacterial sensitivity, 1085
  general considerations, 1080–1105
  genetic factors in response, 1096
  hepatic and renal functions, effects on dosage, 1094–1095
  historical aspects, 1080
  host defense mechanisms, 1095
  host factors in response, 1095–1096
  misuses, 1103–1104
  pregnancy as factor in use, 1096
  prophylaxis of infections, 1100–1102
  resistance of bacteria, 1082–1084
  suprainfections, 1102
ANTIMINTH (pyrantel pamoate), 1025
Antimony, absorption, distribution, and excretion, 1028–1029
  anthelmintic properties, 1028
  toxicity, 1029
Antimony potassium tartrate, 1029, 1074
Antimony sodium-α,α′-dimercaptosuccinate, 1029–1030
Antimony sodium tartrate, 1029, 1074
Antimuscarinic drugs, 120–137. *See also* individual agents
  classification and terminology, 120
  locus and mechanism of action, 122
  pharmacological properties, 122–132
  selectivity of antagonism, 122
  source and chemistry, 121, 130–132
  structure-activity relationship, 121

uses, 133–136
  parkinsonism, 484–485, 487
Antiparkinsonism drugs, 475–488. *See also* individual agents
Antiperspirants, 954
Antipsychotic agents. *See also* individual agents
  absorption, fate, and excretion, 404–406
  actions/effects on, autonomic nervous system, 403
    basal ganglia, 400–401
    behavior, 397–399
    brain stem, 402
    cardiovascular system, 403–404
    cerebral cortex, 400
    chemoreceptor trigger zone, 402
    complex behavior, 399
    conditioned responses, 399
    dopamine-sensitive adenylate cyclase, 401
    EEG, 400
    endocrine system, 403
    hypothalamus, 402
    kidney, 403
    limbic system, 401 402
    liver, 404
    motor activity, 398–399
    peripheral nerves, 402–403
    seizure threshold, 400
    sleep, 399
    spinal cord, 402
  chemistry, 396–397, 408–411
  history, 392, 395–396
  interactions with other drugs, 414
  neurological side effects, 407–413
  pharmacological properties, 397–414
  preparations and dosage, 406, 408–411
  structure activity relationship, 396 397
  tolerance and physical dependence, 406
  toxic reactions and side effects, 406–414
  uses, alcoholism, 418
    antiemetic, 417–418
    anxiety, 416
    childhood psychosis, 416–417
    Gilles de la Tourette's syndrome, 418
    hiccough, 418
    Huntington's disease, 418
    mania and depression, 416
    nausea and vomiting, 417–418
    organic mental syndrome, 416
    preanesthetic medication, 270
    psychoses, 414–416
    schizophrenia, 414–416
Antipyretic-analgesics, 682–713. *See also* Aspirin-like drugs; individual agents
Antipyrine, status, 701
Antirheumatic agents, 682–717. *See also* Aspirin-like drugs; individual agents
Antiseborrheics, action and uses, 956
Antiseptics, 964–981. *See also* individual agents
  antimicrobial spectra, 966
  desirable properties, 965
  evaluation of activity, 965–966
  germicidal kinetics, 966

Antiseptics (*Cont.*)
  history, 964
  mechanisms of antimicrobial action, 966
  terminology, 964–965
Antithrombin III, 1348, 1349–1350
Antithrombotic drugs, 1360–1361. *See also* individual agents
  uses, 1362–1363
Antithyroid drugs, 1408–1412. *See also* individual agents
  absorption, metabolism, and excretion, 1410
  classification, 1409
  history, 1408–1409
  ionic inhibitors, 1412
  mechanism of action, 1409–1410
  preparations and dosage, 1410–1411
  structure-activity relationship, 1409
  untoward reactions, 1410
  uses, hyperthyroidism, 1411–1412
    preoperative preparation in hyperthyroidism, 1412
Antitubercular drugs, 1200–1214. *See also* Tuberculosis; individual agents
Antitussives, nonopioid, 528–530
ANTIVERT (meclizine hydrochloride), 628
Antiviral agents, 1240–1243. *See also* Antimicrobial agents; individual agents
  general considerations, 1240
ANTRENYL (oxyphenonium bromide), 131
ANTUITRIN-S (chorionic gonadotropin for injection), 1386
ANTURANE (sulfinpyrazone), 933
Anxiety, benzodiazepines in, 441–442
  drugs in treatment, 441–442
  propranolol in, 194
Apazone, 701. *See also* Aspirin-like drugs
A.P.L. SECULES (chorionic gonadotropin for injection), 1386
Apnea, xanthines in, 603
Apomorphine, emetic effect, 496, 502, 509
  preparations and dosage, 509
  structural formula, 484
  uses, drug abuse, 575
    drug poisoning, 575, 1609
    parkinsonism, 483
Aporphines, 483
Apothecaries' system of weights and measures, 1662
A-POXIDE (chlordiazepoxide hydrochloride), 440
APRESOLINE (hydralazine hydrochloride), 800
Aprobarbital. *See also* Barbiturates
  chemistry, 351
  dosage, half-life, and preparations, 350
Aprotinin, 663
AQUADIOL (estradiol), 1428
AQUAMEPHYTON (phytonadione, vitamin K_1), 1594
AQUAPHOR, 953
AQUASOL E (alpha-tocopherol), 1598
Arachidonic acid, 669–671
ARALEN HYDROCHLORIDE (chloroquine hydrochloride), 1044
ARALEN PHOSPHATE (chloroquine phosphate), 1044

ARAMINE (metaraminol bitartrate), 165
Arecoline, history and sources, 96
  structural formula, 97
ARFONAD (trimethaphan camsylate), 217
Arginine, use in ammonia intoxication, 870
Arginine[8] vasopressin, 916, 917
ARISTOCORT (triamcinolone), 1485
ARISTOCORT DIACETATE (triamcinolone diacetate), 1486
ARISTODERM (triamcinolone acetonide), 1485
ARISTOSPAN (triamcinolone hexacetonide), 1486
ARLIDIN (nylidrin hydrochloride), 831
Aromatic amino acid decarboxylase, 71–72
Aromatic L-amino acid decarboxylase, inhibitors, 482–483
Aromatic ammonia spirit, 870
Aromatic waters, 1669
Arrhythmias. *See* Cardiac arrhythmias
Arsenates, 1629
Arsenic, 1629–1632
  absorption, distribution, and excretion, 1629–1630
  actions/effects on, blood, 1630
    carcinogenesis/teratogenesis, 1631
    central nervous system, 1630
    circulation, 1630
    gastrointestinal tract, 1630
    kidney, 1630
    liver, 1630
    metabolism, 1631
    skin, 1630
  chemistry, 1629
  mechanism of action, 1629
  poisoning, acute, 1631
    chronic, 1631
    dimercaprol in, 1631
    dimercaptosuccinic acid in, 1627
    treatment, 1631
  sources of exposure, 1629
Arsenites, 1629
Arsine, 1629, 1632
ARSOBAL (melarsoprol), 1073
ARTANE (trihexyphenidyl hydrochloride), 486
Arteriosclerosis. *See* Atherosclerosis
Arthritis, adrenocorticosteroids in, 1489
  apazone in, 701
  bacterial, choice of drugs in, 1087, 1091
  chloroquine in, 1043
  cyclophosphamide in, 1266
  fenamates in, 709
  gold in, 716
  indomethacin in, 706
  oxyphenbutazone in, 700
  penicillamine in, 1628
  phenylbutazone in, 700
  propionic acid derivatives in, 713
  salicylates in, 698
  sulindac in, 708
  tolmetin in, 710
ARTHROCINE (sulindac), 707
ARTRIBID (sulindac), 707
Asbestosis, 1644

Ascariasis, occurrence and treatment, 1031
Ascites, diuretics in, 911
Ascorbic acid, 1576–1580
  absorption, distribution, fate, and excretion, 1578
  biosynthesis, 1578
  chemistry, 1577
  effect on iron absorption, 1320, 1323
  history, 1576–1577
  human requirement, 1579
  pharmacological actions, 1577
  physiological function, 1577–1578
  preparations, 1579
  recommended dietary allowance, 1553
  symptoms of deficiency, 1578
  untoward effects, 1579–1580
  uses, methemoglobinemia, 1579
    scurvy, 1579
    upper respiratory infections, 1579
ASELLACRIN (growth hormone), 1379
L-Asparaginase, 1297
  clinical toxicity, 1297
  history, 1297
  mechanism of action, 1297
  preparation and unitage, 1297
  therapeutic status, 1297
  use in acute lymphoblastic leukemia, 1253, 1297
Aspartate, role as CNS transmitter, 247–248
Aspergillus infections, amphotericin B in, 1240
  choice of drugs in, 1093
  flucytosine in, 1240
Aspiration pneumonitis, adrenocorticosteroids in, 1492
Aspirin, 688–698. See also Aspirin-like drugs; Salicylates
  effect on platelet aggregation, 1361
  pharmacokinetics, 1686
  preparations and dosage, 695
  structural formula, 689
Aspirin-like drugs, 682–713. See also Salicylates; individual agents
  actions/effects on, Bartter's syndrome, 687, 698, 707
    ductus arteriosus, 687, 698, 707
    fever, 684, 686, 689
    gastrointestinal mucosa, 691
    gestation, 686
    inflammation, 683–684, 686, 692
    kidney, 686, 691
    male fertility, 687
    pain, 684, 686, 689
    platelet function, 686, 691–692
  choice of drug, 687–688
  inhibition of prostaglandin synthetase, 684–685
  mechanism of action, 683–685
  side effects, 686–687, 695–697
  therapeutic activities, 686–687, 697–698
Asthma, adrenocorticosteroids in, 1490
  antihistamines in, 627
  beta-adrenergic stimulants in, 170–171
  cromolyn sodium in, 622
  iodide in, 1413

oxygen in, 329
prostaglandins in, 678
xanthines in, 602–603
ASTIBAN (stibocaptate), 1030
Astringents, 955
ATABRINE (quinacrine hydrochloride), 1078
Atenolol, 188, 196
  pharmacokinetics, 1690
Atherosclerosis, drugs in, 834–846
  relationship to lipid metabolism, 834–835
ATHROMBIN-K (warfarin potassium), 1358
Atrazine, toxicology, 1654
ATIVAN (lorazepam), 350, 440, 1671
Atrial fibrillation, digitalis in, 750
  disopyramide in, 778
  procainamide in, 776
  propranolol in, 785
  quinidine in, 770, 772
  treatment, 769
Atrial flutter, digitalis in, 750
  procainamide in, 776
  propranolol in, 785
  quinidine in, 770, 772
  treatment, 769
ATROMID-S (clofibrate), 841
Atrophic vaginitis, 1430
Atropine, 121–128
  absorption, fate, and excretion, 126–127
  actions/effects on, biliary tract, 126
    body temperature, 126
    cardiovascular system, 124–125
    central nervous system, 122–123
    EEG, 123
    eye, 123–124
    gastrointestinal tract, 125–126
    respiration, 124
    secretory glands, 126
    urinary tract, 126
  chemistry, 121
  history, 121
  mechanism of action, 122
  pharmacological properties, 122–128
  poisoning, 127–128
    physostigmine in, 116
    treatment, 128
  preparations, dosage, and administration, 128
  selectivity of antagonism, 122
  synthetic and semisynthetic substitutes, 128–132
  uses, 133–136
    anticholinesterase poisoning, 110, 136
    cardiac arrhythmias, 135
    common cold, 134
    digitalis intoxication, 755
    gastrointestinal disorders, 133
    genitourinary disorders, 135–136
    mushroom poisoning, 98, 136
    myocardial infarction, 135
    ophthalmological, 133–134
    parkinsonism, 135
    peptic ulcer, 133
    preanesthetic medication, 135, 271

Atropine (*Cont.*)
   rhinitis, 134
Atropinic drugs, *See* Antimuscarinic drugs
Atypical mycobacteria, treatment of infections, 1213
"Atypical pneumonia," choice of drugs in, 1092
Auranofin, 715
AURCOLOID-198 (gold-198), 1305
AUREOMYCIN (chlortetracycline hydrochloride), 1185
AUREOTOPE (gold-198), 1305
Aurothioglucose, 714, 715. *See also* Gold
Autacoids, 608–681. *See also* individual agents
   inhibition of allergic release, 620–621
   involvement in hypersensitivity reactions, 616
Autonomic hyperreflexia, alpha-adrenergic blocking
       drugs in, 188
   ganglionic blocking agents in, 217
   guanethidine in, 201
Autonomic nervous system, 56–90
   acetylcholine, storage and release, 68–69
   acetylcholinesterase in, 68
   adrenal medulla and, 58
   adrenergic transmission, 71–80
      alpha and beta receptors, 77–78
      metabolic disposition of mediators, 76–77
      norepinephrine, 71
      responses of effector organs, 60–61
   alpha-adrenergic effects, 60–61
   anatomy, 56–61
   beta-adrenergic effects, 60–61
   catecholamine synthesis, storage, and release,
      71–75
   central connections, 57
   choline acetyltransferase in, 67–68
   cholinergic transmission, 67–71
      responses of effector organs, 60–61
      various sites, 69–71
   divisions, 57–59
   dopamine in, 71
   effector organ responses, 60–61
   epinephrine in, 71
   functions, 61–62
   ganglionic transmission, 70–71, 211–212, 420
   hypothalamic nuclei, 57
   innervation of neurons and effector organs, 59
   junctional transmission, 65–67
   mechanisms of drug actions on, 82
   muscarinic effects of drugs, 83–84
   neurohumoral transmission, 62–80
      evidence, 64
      historical aspects, 62–64
      steps involved, 64–67
   nicotinic effects of drugs, 83–84
   norepinephrine in, 71
   parasympathetic division, 57–59
      functions, 61–62
   pharmacological considerations, 80–85
      drug interference with transmitter destruction or
         dissipation, 85
      drug interference with transmitter synthesis or
         release, 81
      drug promotion of transmitter release, 81
      muscarinic drug effects, 83–84

      nicotinic drug effects, 83–84
      specificity of action of cholinergic drugs, 83
   relation to endocrine system, 80
   responses of effector organs to nerve impulses,
      60–61
   sympathetic division, 57–58
      functions, 61–62
   visceral afferent fibers in, 57
AVAZYME (chymotrypsin), 961
AVENTYL HYDROCHLORIDE (nortriptyline hydrochlo-
     ride), 424
Avidin, 1573
AVLOCLOR (chloroquine phosphate), 1044
AVLOSULFON (dapsone), 1215
AZAPEN (methicillin sodium), 1142
Azapetine, 186
Azapropazone. *See* Apazone
Azaribine, 1281–1282. *See also* Pyrimidine analogs
   absorption, fate, and excretion, 1282
   chemistry, 1282
   clinical toxicity, 1282
   general toxicity and cytotoxic action, 1282
   mechanism of action, 1282
   preparation, dosage, and route of administration,
     1282
   use in neoplastic diseases, 1253, 1282
   use in psoriasis, 1282
Azaserine, 1284
Azathioprine, 1283, 1286–1287. *See also* Purine ana-
     logs
Azauridine, 1277, 1282
AZENE (clorazepate monopotassium), 440
Azlocillin, 1147
AZO GANTANOL (sulfamethoxazole-phenazopyri-
     dine), 1111, 1122
AZO GANTRISIN (sulfisoxazole-phenazopyridine),
     1111, 1122
AZULFIDINE (sulfasalazine), 1112

Babesia infections, chloroquine in, 1045
   pentamidine in, 1072
Bacampicillin, 1145
Bacillus anthracis infections, choice of drugs in, 1088
BACIQUENT (bacitracin), 1232
Bacitracin, 1231–1232. *See also* Antimicrobial agents
Baclofen, 488–490
   chemistry, preparations, and dosage, 489
Bacteremia, choice of drugs in, 1086
Bacteroides infections, chloramphenicol in, 1195
   choice of drugs in, 1091
   clindamycin in, 1227
   metronidazole in, 1077
   penicillin in, 1139
BACTOCILL (oxacillin sodium), 1143
BACTRIM (trimethoprim-sulfamethoxazole), 1118
BAL. *See* Dimercaprol
Balantidiasis, iodoquinol in, 1065
BANOCIDE (diethylcarbamazine citrate), 1015
BANTHINE (methantheline bromide), 131
Barban, toxicology, 1654
Barbital. *See also* Barbiturates

chemistry, 351
legal regulations, 1671
Barbiturates, 349–361. *See also* individual agents
absorption, 356
abuse, legal regulations, 1671
prevalence and patterns, 549–550
signs and symptoms, 550
actions/effects on, autonomic ganglia, 354
cardiovascular system, 355
central nervous system, 352–354
central synapses, 354
drug-metabolizing enzymes, 355–356
EEG, 352
gastrointestinal tract, 355
hepatic functions, 355–356
kidney, 356
neuromuscular junctions, 354
peripheral nerves, 354
respiration, 355
sleep stages, 352–353
uterus, 356
addiction, treatment, 571
aftereffects, 358
binding by plasma protein, 356
chemistry, 292, 351–352
cross-dependence, 541
dependence, 353–354
distribution, 356–357
dosage, 350
drug interactions, 358
duration of action, 357 358
excretion, 357
general anesthetic action, 292–293
half-lives, 350, 357
hangover from, 358
hyperalgesia, 352
lethal dosage, 359
mechanism and sites of action, 354
metabolic degradation and products, 357
physical dependence, 540, 550–551
poisoning, 359–360
signs and symptoms, 359
treatment, 359–360
porphyria, 294, 358
preparations, 292, 350, 361
redistribution in tissues, 357
renal clearance, 357
routes of administration, 356
sleep induced by, 352–353
structural formula, 351
structure-activity relationship, 351–352
termination of activity, 357
tolerance, 353, 538–539, 550–551
untoward effects, 358
uses, 360–361
alcohol withdrawal, 572
anticonvulsant, 360–361
cerebral edema, 361
cholestasis, 361
diagnostic, 361
hyperbilirubinemia, 361
hypnosis, 361

intravenous anesthesia, 292–295
narcoanalysis and narcotherapy, 361
preanesthetic medication, 269
sedation, 360
withdrawal symptoms, 353, 550–551
withdrawal technics, 571
BARC (isobornyl thiocyanoacetate), 985
Bartter's syndrome, aspirin-like drugs in, 687, 698
indomethacin in, 707
Basal-cell carcinomas, fluorouracil in, 1280
BASALJEL, 991, 992
BASALJEL XS, 991
Batrachotoxin, 65
BAYGON, 101
BCNU. *See* Carmustine
Beclomethasone, 1490. *See also* Adrenocorticosteroids
preparations, 1484
Bee stings, adrenocorticosteroids in, 1490
epinephrine in, 171
Beeswax, 953
Belladonna alkaloids, 121 128. *See also* Antimuscarinic drugs; individual agents
mechanism of action in parkinsonism, 476, 484–485
preparations, dosage, and administration, 128
sources and members, 121
structure-activity relationship, 121
BENADRYL (diphenhydramine hydrochloride), 486, 628
BENDOPA (levodopa), 481
Bendroflumethiazide. *See also* Benzothiadiazides
structural formula, properties, and dosage, 900
Bends, helium in, 335
oxygen in, 331
BENEMID (probenecid), 932
BENISONE (betamethasone benzoate), 1484
BENOQUIN (monobenzone), 959
Benoxinate hydrochloride, 310
Benserazide, 482
BENTYL (dicyclomine hydrochloride), 132
Benzalkonium chloride, 954, 978
Benzathine penicillin G. *See* Penicillin G benzathine
Benzbromarone, 722, 933
uses, gout, 722–723
hyperuricemia, 723
BENZEDREX (propylhexedrine), 168
BENZEDRINE (amphetamine sulfate), 161
Benzene, toxicology, 1647
Benzene hexachloride, toxicology, 1650
Benzestrol, 1428
Benzethonium chloride, 978
Benzocaine, 310
Benzoctamine, 369
Benzodiazepines, 339–349, 437–442. *See also* individual agents
absorption, fate, and elimination, 346–348, 438–439
abuse, 349
actions/effects on, behavior, 341, 437–438
cardiovascular system, 346, 438
central nervous system, 340–346, 437–438

Benzodiazepines (*Cont.*)
  EEG, 342–344, 438
  gastrointestinal tract, 346
  muscle tone, 341
  respiration, 346, 438
  skeletal muscle, 438
  sleep stages, 342–344, 438
  anticonvulsant compounds, 466–467
  chemistry and structure-activity relationship, 340,
    437
  drug interactions, 440
  history, 339, 437
  mechanism of CNS action, 345–346
  pharmacological properties, 340–349
  preparations and dosage, 349–350, 440
  tolerance and physical dependence, 349, 439
  toxic reactions and side effects, 348–349, 439–440
  uses, alcohol withdrawal, 440, 572
    anxiety, 441–442
    cerebral palsy, 441
    epilepsy, 467
    hypnotic, 349, 369–371
    during labor, 440
    preanesthetic medication, 270
    sedative, 349, 369–371
    skeletal muscle relaxation, 488
    tetanus, 441
    upper motoneuron disorders, 441
Benzodioxans, 186
Benzoic acid, 971
  keratolytic effect, 956
Benzoic and salicylic acids ointment, 695, 971, 984
Benzonatate, dosage for cough, 530
Benzophenones, 960
Benzoquinamide, poisoning, physostigmine in, 116
Benzoquinonium. *See also* Neuromuscular blocking
    agents
  structural formula, 221
Benzothiadiazides, 899–903. *See also* Diuretics; indi-
    vidual agents
  absorption, fate, and distribution, 902
  actions/effects on, blood pressure, 803–804
    composition of extracellular fluid, 901
    renal function, 901
  chemistry and structure-activity relationship, 899
  clinical toxicity, 902
  history, 899
  mechanism of diuretic action, 899–900
  preparations and dosage, 900, 902
  uses, antihypertensive, 810, 811, 813
    diabetes insipidus, 902
    diuretic, 902
    hypercalciuria, 902
    nephrogenic diabetes insipidus, 925
Benzoyl metronidazole, 1076
Benzoyl peroxide, 974
Benzphetamine, legal regulations, 1671
  receptor-type activity, 142
  structural formula, 142
  use in obesity, 172
Benzquinamide, use in preanesthetic medication,
    270

Benzthiazide. *See also* Benzothiadiazides
  structural formula, properties, and dosage, 900
Benztropine, 248
  structural formula, preparations, and dosage, 486
  use in parkinsonism, 484–485
Benzyl benzoate, 985
Benzylmorphine, legal regulations, 1670
Benzyl-*p*-chlorophenol, 969
Benzylpenicilloyl-polylysine, 1149
Bephenium hydroxynaphthoate, 1013–1014
Beriberi, thiamine in, 1563
Beta-adrenergic blocking drugs, 188–197. *See also*
    individual agents
  chemistry, 188–189
  classification, 188
  pharmacological properties, 189–197
  uses, 194–196
    angina pectoris, 828–829
    anxiety, 369, 441
    hypertension, 809–813
BETA-CHLOR (chloral betaine), 350, 1671
BETADINE (povidone-iodine), 973
Beta-lactamase, 1130, 1151
Betamethasone. *See also* Adrenocorticosteroids
  preparations, 1484
  relative potency, duration of action, and equiva-
    lent dose, 1482
BETAPAR (meprednisone), 1485
Betazole, 619–620
Betel nut, 96
Bethanechol, actions/effects on, cardiovascular sys-
    tem, 93–94
    gastrointestinal tract, 94
    urinary tract, 94
  history, 91
  mechanism of action, 91–92
  miscellaneous effects, 94
  precautions, toxicity, and contraindications, 95
  preparations and dosage, 95
  structural formula, 92
  structure-activity relationship, 92
  synergists and antagonists, 94–95
  uses, diagnostic, 96
    gastrointestinal disorders, 95
    urinary bladder disorders, 95–96
Bethanidine, 201
Betula oil, 695
Bhang, 560
BICILLIN (sterile penicillin G benzathine suspen-
    sion), 1137
BICNU (carmustine), 1270
Bicuculline, 247–248
BILARCIL (metrifonate), 1018
Bile-acid sequestering resins, 842–843. *See also* indi-
    vidual agents
Bile acids, 998–999
  laxative properties, 1009
  pharmacological and toxic effects, 998
  preparations and dosage, 999
Bile salts, 998–999
  pharmacological and toxic effects, 998
  uses, 999

Biliary colic, belladonna alkaloids in, 133
  opioid analgesics in, 512
Biliary fistula or obstruction, vitamin K in, 1595
Biliary tract infections, choice of drugs in, 1086
Biocytin, 1573
BIO-SORB (absorbable dusting powder), 953
Biotin, 1573–1574
  absorption, fate, and excretion, 1574
  chemistry, 1573
  history, 1573
  human requirement, 1574
  pharmacological actions, 1574
  physiological function, 1574
  provisional dietary allowance, 1555
  symptoms of deficiency, 1574
Biotin sulfone, 1574
Biperidin, chemistry, preparations, and dosage, 486
  use in parkinsonism, 484–485
Bisacodyl, 1007. See also Cathartics, diphenyl-
    methanes
Bishydroxycoumarin. See Dicumarol
Bismuth, 953
Bismuth subnitrate, 997
Bithional, 1035
BITIN (bithional), 1035
Black widow spider poisoning, curariform drugs in,
    232
Black widow spider toxin, 69
Blastomycosis, amphotericin B in, 1240
  choice of drugs in, 1093
  hydroxystilbamidine in, 1240
Blennorrhea, choice of drugs in, 1093
BLENOXANE (bleomycin sulfate), 1295
Bleomycin, 1293–1295
  absorption, fate, and excretion, 1295
  chemistry, 1294
  clinical toxicity, 1295
  mechanism of action, 1294
  preparation, dosage, and route of administration,
    1295
  use in neoplastic diseases, 1253, 1295
BLEPH (sulfacetamide sodium), 1112
Blind-loop syndrome, tetracyclines in, 1191
Blood clotting factors, 1348
Blood coagulation, mechanisms, 1347–1348
Blood-brain barrier, 10, 244
Body fluids, agents affecting volume and composi-
    tion, 848–884
  basal requirements, 853–854
  bicarbonate-carbonic acid system, 864–865
  cellular mechanisms of electrolyte control, 850
  clinical disturbances of volume and osmolality,
    854–862
  composition, 849–850
  correction of disturbances of osmolality, 857–859
  correction of plasma volume, 857–861
  desirable properties of a plasma expander, 860
  dialysis disequilibrium syndrome, 859
  distribution, 849
  evaluation of intensity of dehydration, 857
  external exchanges of water and solute, 852–854
    balance principle, 852–853

normal values of fluid and electrolyte intake
    and output, 852
  fixed and labile ions and solutes, 853
  fluids available for the repair of dehydration, 859
  hypertonic contraction, 856
  hypertonic expansion, 857
  hypotonic contraction, 856
  hypotonic expansion, 857
  internal exchanges of water and solute, 850–852
  interstitial and plasma fluid volumes, 851–852
  intracellular and extracellular fluid volume, 850–
    851
  isotonic contraction, 855–856
  isotonic expansion, 856
  laboratory diagnosis of acid-base disturbances,
    865
  measurement, 849
  mechanisms of compensation for acid-base dis-
    orders, 864–865
  metabolic acidosis, 866–867
  metabolic alkalosis, 867–868
  osmotic pressure, 850
  plasma values in acid-base disorders, 864
  preparations for treatment of acid-base disturb-
    ances, 869
  production rate and composition, 855
  regulation of cell volume, 857
  respiratory acidosis, 866
  respiratory alkalosis, 866
  sodium concentration as an index of plasma os-
    molality, 854 855
  technics of administration, 859
  treatment of fluid and electrolyte deficits, 857–858
BONINE (meclizine hydrochloride), 628
Boric acid, 953, 971
Borrelia recurrentis infections, choice of drugs in,
    1092
Botulinus toxin, 69, 81
  mechanism of anticholinergic action, 69, 82
BRADOSOL BROMIDE (domiphen bromide), 978
Bradykinin. See also Kinins
  history, 659
  synthesis and catabolism, 660–661
Brain tumors, adrenocorticosteroids in, 1491
  carmustine in, 1270
  lomustine in, 1271
  procarbazine in, 1300
  semustine in, 1271
  vincristine in, 1290
Bran, 1004. See also Cathartics, bulk-forming laxa-
    tives
BRETHINE (terbutaline sulfate), 167
Bretylium, 201
  absorption, distribution, and elimination, 787
  actions/effects on, autonomic nervous system, 787
    cardiac electrophysiology, 768, 786–787
    circulation, 787
    electrocardiogram, 768, 787
  chemistry and preparations, 786
  dosage and administration, 787
  mechanism of antiadrenergic action, 74, 81–82
  toxicity, 787

Bretylium (*Cont.*)
  uses, 787
BRETYLOL (bretylium tosylate), 786
BREVICON, 1440
BREVITAL (methohexital), 292
BRICANYL (terbutaline sulfate), 167
Brill's disease, chloramphenicol in, 1196
  choice of drugs in, 1092
  tetracyclines in, 1189
BRISTAMYCIN (erythromycin stearate), 1224
Bromazepam. *See also* Benzodiazepines
  dosage and half-life, 350
Bromide, 369
Bromisovalum, 369
Bromlysergic acid diethylamide, 564
Bromocriptine, 483–484, 941, 942, 943
  structural formula, 484
  use in acromegaly, 1379
  use in hyperprolactinemia, 1382
Bromocriptine mesylate, preparation, 946
Brompheniramine maleate, preparations and dosage, 628. *See also* H_1-receptor blockers
"Brompton's mixture," 512
Bronchial asthma. *See* Asthma
Bronchitis, antimuscarinic drugs in, 135
  choice of drugs in, 1086
  iodide in, 1413
  tetracyclines in, 1191
  trimethoprim-sulfamethoxazole in, 1118
BRONKEPHRINE (ethylnorepinephrine hydrochloride), 154
BRONKOMETER (isoetharine mesylate aerosol), 168
BRONKOSOL (isoetharine solution for nebulization), 168
Broxyquinoline, 1063
Brucellosis, chloramphenicol in, 1196
  choice of drugs in, 1090
  streptomycin in, 1173, 1190
  tetracyclines in, 1190
  trimethoprim-sulfamethoxazole in, 1119
Brucine, 585
BRUFEN (ibuprofen), 711
Bubonic plague, chloramphenicol in, 1196
  streptomycin in, 1173
Buerger's disease. *See* Peripheral vascular disease
Bufotenine, 564, 633
Bumetanide, 903, 904
BUMINATE (albumin human), 862
Bunolol, 196
Bupivacaine, structural formula, 301
Bupivacaine hydrochloride, 309. *See also* Local anesthetics
Buprenorphine, 528
  actions at opioid receptor subtypes, 522
  pharmacological effects, 528
  preparations and dosage, 528
  structural formula, 496
  tolerance, physical dependence, and abuse liability, 528
  uses, 528
Burimamide, 630
Burns, gentamicin in, 1175

mafenide in, 1112
  nitrofurazone in, 979
  silver sulfadiazine in, 977, 1112
Busulfan, 1268–1269. *See also* Alkylating agents
  structural formula, 1260
  use in neoplastic diseases, 1252, 1269
Butabarbital. *See also* Barbiturates
  chemistry, 351
  dosage, half-life, and preparations, 350
Butaclamol, 397
Butalbital. *See also* Barbiturates
  chemistry, 351
  dosage and preparations, 350
Butamben, 310
Butaperazine, 406
BUTAZOLIDIN (phenylbutazone), 700
BUTESIN (butamben), 310
BUTISOL SODIUM (butabarbital sodium), 350
Butorphanol, 527
  pharmacological actions, 527
  preparations and dosage, 527
  structural formula, 496
  tolerance, physical dependence, and abuse liability, 527
  uses, 527
Butoxamine, 188
Butyl aminobenzoate. *See* Butamben
Butylparaben, 969
Butylpiperidines, 395
Butyrocholinesterase, 68
Butyrophenones. *See* Antipsychotic agents; Haloperidol

Cacao butter, 952
Cadmium, 1632–1633
  absorption, distribution, and excretion, 1632
  poisoning, acute, 1632
    chronic, 1632–1633
    treatment, 1633
  sources of exposure, 1632
CAFERGOT (ergotamine tartrate–caffeine tablets), 946
Caffeine, 592–604. *See also* Xanthines
  abuse, 569
  interaction with ergot alkaloids, 947
  preparations, 601
  use in migraine, 947
Caffeine and sodium benzoate injection, 601
Calamine lotion, 977
Calcifediol, 1539, 1540
Calciferol, 1539, 1544
CALCIMAR (salmon calcitonin), 1529, 1537
CALCIPARINE (calcium heparin injection), 1351
Calcitonin, 1536–1538
  chemistry and immunoreactivity, 1536
  history and source, 1536
  mechanism of action, 1537
  physiological actions, 1537
  preparations, bioassay, and dosage, 1537
  regulation of secretion, 1536–1537
  uses, hypercalcemic states, 1537
    Paget's disease, 1538

Calcitriol, 1539, 1540, 1545
Calcium, 1524–1529
  abnormalities in metabolism, 1527–1529
    hypercalcemic states, 1528–1529
    hypocalcemic states, 1527–1528
  absorption and excretion, 1525
  actions/effects on, cardiovascular system, 1527
    cell membranes, 1527
    neuromuscular system, 1526
  digitalis and, 732–734, 735–736
  distribution, 1524–1525
  local actions, 1526
  metabolism, effects of calcitonin, 1537
    effects of parathyroid hormone, 1532–1534
    effects of vitamin D, 1541
  plasma concentrations, 1525
  preparations, 1527–1528
  recommended dietary allowance, 1553
  requirements, 1524–1525
  role in action of autacoids, 614
  routes of administration, 1527–1528
  use in calcium deficiency states, 1528
Calcium carbonate, gastric antacid properties, 992–993
  preparations and dosage, 993
  untoward effects, 993
Calcium carbonate tablets, 1528
Calcium chloride, 1527
Calcium chloride injection, 1528
CALCIUM DISODIUM VERSENATE (edetate calcium disodium), 1621
Calcium gluceptate injection, 1528
Calcium gluconate, use in hyperkalemia, 879
Calcium lactate, 1528
Calcium levulinate, 1528
Calcium levulinate injection, 1528
Calcium phosphate, 1528
Calcium undecylenate, 982
Calusterone, 1457
Calymmatobacterium granulomatis infections, choice of drugs in, 1091
CAMALOX, 991
CAMOLAR (cycloguanil pamoate), 1047
CAMOQUIN (amodiaquine hydrochloride), 1046
Camphor, 955–956
Camphor spirit, 956
Camphorated opium tincture, 509
Camphorated parachlorophenol, 956, 969
Campylobacter fetus infections, choice of drugs in, 1090
Cancer. *See* Neoplastic diseases; individual diseases
CANDEPTIN (candicidin), 984
Candicidin, 984
Candida infections, amphotericin B in, 1240
  candicidin in, 984
  chlordantoin in, 984
  choice of drugs in, 1093
  clotrimazole in, 983
  flucytosine in, 1240
  haloprogin in, 983–984
  miconazole in, 982–983
  nystatin in, 1233

Cannabinoids, 560–563
Cannabis, 560–563
  absorption, fate, and excretion, 562
  abuse, legal regulations, 1670
    patterns, 563
  chemistry, 560
  history and source, 560
  pharmacological effects, 560–562
  physical dependence, 563
  psychological effects in man, 561–562
  tolerance, 563
  uses, 563
Cantharides, 956
Cantharidin, chemistry, actions, and uses, 956
CANTHARONE (cantharidin collodion), 956
CANTIL (mepenzolate bromide), 131
CAPASTAT SULFATE (sterile capreomycin sulfate), 1212
Capreomycin, 1212
Caprylic acid, 982
Captopril, chemistry 657
  clinical applications, 658–659
  pharmacological properties, 657–658
  untoward effects, 659
  uses, antihypertensive, 807
Capuride, 369
Caramiphen, use in cough, 530
CARBACEL OPHTHALMIC (carbachol ophthalmic solution), 95
Carbachol, actions/effects on, cardiovascular system, 93–94
    gastrointestinal tract, 94
    urinary tract, 94
  history, 91
  mechanism of cholinergic action, 81–82, 91–92
  miscellaneous effects, 94
  precautions, toxicity, and contraindications, 95
  preparations and dosage, 95
  structural formula, 92
  structure-activity relationship, 92
  synergists and antagonists, 94–95
  use in glaucoma, 96
Carbamazepine, anticonvulsant effects, 459
  chemistry, 459
  interactions with other drugs, 460
  pharmacokinetics, 459–460, 1690
  plasma concentration, 460
  preparations and dosage, 460
  structural formula, 459
  toxicity, 460
  uses, epilepsy, 460
    neuralgia, 460
Carbamylcholine. *See* Carbachol
Carbanilides, 981
Carbaryl, history, 101
  mechanism of action, 103
  structural formula, 103
Carbenicillin, 1146–1147. *See also* Penicillins
  pharmacokinetics, 1691
  uses, combined with gentamicin, 1174–1175
Carbenicillin indanyl, 1146–1147. *See also* Carbenicillin; Penicillins

Carbenicillin phenyl, 1147
Carbenoxolone sodium, 997
Carbetapentane, use in cough, 530
Carbidopa, chemistry, 482
    combined use with levodopa, 482–483
    mechanism of action, 482
    preparations and dosage, 482–483
    use in parkinsonism, 482, 485
Carbimazole, 1409, 1411. *See also* Antithyroid drugs
Carbinoxamine maleate, preparations and dosage,
        628. *See also* H_1-receptor blockers
CARBOCAINE (mepivacaine hydrochloride), 309
Carbol-fuchsin, 984
Carbon dioxide, 331–334
    actions/effects on, central nervous system, 333
        circulation, 332–333
        respiration, 332
    methods of administration, 333
    preparations, 333
    transfer and elimination, 332
    untoward effects, 333
    uses, anesthesia, 334
        carbon monoxide poisoning, 334
        hiccough, 334
        petit mal, 334
        respiratory depression, 334
Carbon monoxide, acute poisoning, treatment, 330,
        331, 334, 1643
    chronic toxicity, 1643
    diagnosis of poisoning, 1643
    factors governing toxicity, 1641
    fate and excretion, 1643
    pathology of acute poisoning, 1642
    reaction with hemoglobin, 1641
    signs and symptoms of toxicity, 1642
    toxicology, 1641–1643
Carbon tetrachloride, toxicology, 1645–1646
Carbonic anhydrase inhibitors, 896–899. *See also* in-
        dividual agents
    absorption, fate, and excretion, 898
    actions/effects on, central nervous system, 898
        eye, 897
        gastrointestinal tract, 898
        kidney, 897
        plasma composition, 897
        respiration, 898
        urinary electrolyte composition, 898
    chemistry and structure-activity relationship, 897
    clinical toxicity, 899
    history, 896
    mechanism of action, 897
    preparations and dosage, 898
    uses, alkalinization of urine, 899
        diuretic, 899
        epilepsy, 468, 899
        familial periodic paralysis, 899
        glaucoma, 899
        mountain sickness, 899
Carboxymethylcellulose, 1004. *See also* Cathartics,
        bulk-forming laxatives
Carboxymethylcellulose sodium, 951

Carbromal, 369
Carbuterol, 166
Carcinogens, 1604–1605
Carcinoid disease, cyproheptadine in, 639
    effect on nicotinic acid requirement, 1569
    methyldopa in, 797
    methysergide in, 639
    role of 5-hydroxytryptamine, 637
    streptozocin in, 1271
Carcinomas, adrenocorticosteroids in, 1301, 1491
    androgens in, 1461
    bleomycin in, 1295
    carmustine in, 1270
    chlorambucil in, 1268
    choice of drugs in, 1252–1254
    cisplatin in, 1298–1299
    cyclophosphamide in, 1266
    dactinomycin in, 1291
    doxorubicin in, 1293
    estrogens in, 1431
    fluorouracil in, 1279–1280
    hexamethylmelamine in, 1268
    lomustine in, 1271
    mammary, androgens in, 1303–1304, 1461
        estrogens in, 1303–1304
        tamoxifen in, 1304
    mechlorethamine in, 1264
    melphalan in, 1267
    methotrexate in, 1275–1276
    mithramycin in, 1296
    mitomycin in, 1297
    procarbazine in, 1300
    progestins in, 1301, 1438
    prostatic, androgen-control therapy in, 1302
    semustine in, 1271
    tamoxifen in, 1304
    vinblastine in, 1289
    vincristine in, 1290
Cardiac arrest, sympathomimetic drugs in, 170
Cardiac arrhythmias. *See also* individual arrhyth-
        mias
    atropine in, 135
    bretylium in, 769, 787
    digitalis in, 750–751
    disopyramide in, 769, 778
    edetate disodium in, 1621
    lidocaine in, 769, 781
    pathological physiology, 764–767
        abnormalities of automaticity, 764–766
        reentrant arrhythmias, 766–767
    phenytoin in, 769, 783
    procainamide in, 769, 776
    propranolol in, 194, 769, 785
    quinidine in, 769, 771–772
    summary of drug treatment, 769
    sympathomimetic drugs in, 170
Cardiac electrophysiology, 761–764
    action potentials, 761–763
    excitability and refractoriness, 763
    ionic currents, 763
    responsiveness and conduction, 763–764

resting potential, 761

Cardiac failure. *See also* Digitalis; Diuretics; Edema
  digitalis glycosides in, 749–750
  digitalis in prevention, 750
  diuretics in, 911
  dobutamine in, 169
  dopamine in, 169
  hydralazine in, 827
  nitroglycerine in, 825–827
  nitroprusside in, 827
  opioids in, 513
  oxygen in, 330
  phenoxybenzamine in, 188
  phentolamine in, 827
  prazosin in, 827
  thiamine in, 1563
  xanthines in, 602

Cardiac glycosides, 729–756. *See also* individual
  agents

CARDILATE (crythrityl tetranitrate), 826

CARDIOQUIN (quinidine polygalacturonate), 771

Cardiospasm, belladonna alkaloids in, 133

Cardioversion, diazepam in, 441

CARDRASE (ethoxzolamide), 898

CARINAMIDE, 931

Carisoprodol, 366
  chemistry, preparations, and dosage, 489

Carmustine, 1269–1270. *See also* Alkylating agents
  structural formula, 1259
  use in neoplastic diseases, 1252, 1270

Carotene, 1583

Carotenoids, absorption, distribution, and metabolism, 1590

Carphenazine, 406

Casanthranol, 1008

Cascara sagrada, 1007–1008. *See also* Cathartics,
  anthraquinones

Castle's intrinsic gastric factor, 1331, 1334–1335

Castor oil, cathartic properties, 1008
  preparations and dosage, 1008

CATAPRES (clonidine hydrochloride), 798

Cataract, chymotrypsin in extraction, 961

CATARASE (chymotrypsin for ophthalmic solution),
  961

Catecholamines, 144–157. *See also* Sympathomimetic drugs; individual agents
  mechanism of action, 78–80
  role in ganglionic transmission, 212, 215

Catechol-O-methyltransferase, 76–77, 479

Cathartics, 1002–1012. *See also* individual agents
  anthraquinones, 1007–1008
  bulk-forming laxatives, 1003–1005
    toxicity, 1004
  classification and choice, 1003
  contact, 1005–1009
    mechanism of action, 1006
    pharmacological properties, 1005
  dangers of abuse, 1011
  diphenylmethanes, 1006–1007
  habitual use, 1011
  mechanisms of action, 1002–1003

saline, 1005
  systemic effects, 1005
  uses and abuses, 1010–1011

Cathine, 569

Cathinone, 569

Cation-exchange resins, 879

Caudal anesthesia, 317

Caustics, actions and uses, 956

CCNU. *See* Lomustine

CECLOR (cefaclor), 1156

CEDILANID (lanatoside C), 749

CEDILANID-D (deslanoside), 749

CEENU (lomustine), 1271

CEEPRYN (cetylpyridinium chloride), 978

Cefaclor, 1155–1156

Cefadroxil, 1156

CEFADYL (sterile cephapirin sodium), 1154

Cefamandole, 1154. *See also* Cephalosporins
  pharmacokinetics, 1691

Cefatrizine, 1156

Cefazolin, 1154. *See also* Cephalosporins
  pharmacokinetics, 1692

Ceforanide, 1156

Cefotaxime, 1156

Cefoxitin, 1154–1155. *See also* Cephalosporins
  pharmacokinetics, 1692

Cefuroxime, 1156

CELBENIN (methicillin sodium), 1142

CELESTONE (betamethasone), 1484

CELESTONE SOLUSPAN (betamethasone sodium phosphate and acetate), 1484

Cell membranes, structure and composition, 3

Cellulitis, choice of drugs in, 1086

Cellulose, oxidized, 955

CELONTIN (methsuximide), 462

Central nervous system, actions of drugs, 242–246
  cell biology of neurons, 238
  cellular organization of the brain, 237–238
  drugs that modify selectively, 243
  factors that alter drug effects, 243–244
  general characteristics of CNS drugs, 244–245
  general CNS depressants, 243
  general CNS stimulants, 243
  macrofunctions of brain regions, brain stem, 236
    cerebellum, 236–237
    cerebral cortex, 236
    limbic system, 236
    midbrain, 236
    spinal cord, 237
  neurohormones, 241
  neuromediators, 242
  neuromodulators, 241–242
  neurotransmitters, 241. *See also* individual agents
    acetylcholine, 247–248, 250
    amino acids, 246–248
    aspartate, 247, 248
    catecholamines, 248–251
    dopamine, 248, 250–251
    epinephrine, 249–251
    gamma-aminobutyrate, 246–248
    glutamate, 247–248

Central nervous system (*Cont.*)
　glycine, 247–248
　histamine, 252
　5-hydroxytryptamine, 249, 251–252
　identification, 238–241
　norepinephrine, 249–251
　overview of pharmacology, 248–249
　peptides, 252–253
　organization of CNS-drug interactions, 245–246
　organizational principles of the brain, 235–238
　perspectives for future development, 253–254
　synaptic relationships, 238
Central nervous system depressants. *See* Ethyl alcohol; Hypnotics; Sedatives; individual agents
Central nervous system stimulants, 585–607. *See also* individual agents
CEPACOL (cetylpyridinium chloride), 978
Cephacetrile, 1156
Cephalexin, 1151. *See also* Cephalosporins
　pharmacokinetics, 1693
Cephaloglycin, 1156. *See also* Cephalosporins
Cephaloridine, 1155. *See also* Cephalosporins
Cephalosporin C, 1151
Cephalosporin N, 1151
Cephalosporin P, 1151
Cephalosporinase, 1151
Cephalosporins, 1150–1157. *See also* Antimicrobial agents; individual agents
　absorption, distribution, fate, and excretion, 1152–1153
　antimicrobial activity, 1151
　chemistry, 1151
　effect of beta-lactamase on, 1151–1152
　history and source, 1150
　mechanism of action, 1129, 1151
　mechanisms of bacterial resistance, 1151–1152
　toxicity and precautions, 1156–1157
　uses, 1157
Cephalothin, 1153–1154. *See also* Cephalosporins
　pharmacokinetics, 1693
Cephamycins, 1151
Cephapirin, 1154. *See also* Cephalosporins
　pharmacokinetics, 1694
Cephradine, 1155. *See also* Cephalosporins
　pharmacokinetics, 1694
CEPHULAC (lactulose), 1010
Cerate, 953
Cerebral edema, adrenocorticosteroids in, 1491
　barbiturates in, 361
　mannitol in, 896
Cerebral palsy, dantrolene in, 491
　diazepam in, 441
　levodopa in, 487
　skeletal muscle relaxants in, 491
Cerebrovascular disease. *See also* Atherosclerosis
　anticoagulants in, 1363
　antithrombotic drugs in, 1363
　oxygen in, 330–331
　vasodilators in, 830
CEREPAX (temazepam), 350
CERUBIDINE (daunorubicin), 1292
Cestodiasis, occurrence and treatment, 1033–1034

CETAPHIL, 952
Cetylpyridinium chloride, 978
CEVALIN (ascorbic acid), 1579
Chancroid, choice of drugs in, 1090
　streptomycin in, 1173
　sulfonamides in, 1116
　tetracyclines in, 1190
Charas, 560
Charcoal, 954
　use in drug poisoning, 954, 1610
Chelating agents, 1615–1637. *See also* individual agents
CHEMESTROGEN (benzestrol), 1428
Chemotherapeutic agents. *See* Antimicrobial agents; individual antimicrobial and antineoplastic agents
Chenodeoxycholic acid, effect on gallstones, 998–999
Childhood psychoses, antipsychotic drugs in, 416
Chiniofon, 1063
Chlamydia infections, tetracyclines in, 1189
Chlamydia psittaci infections, choice of drugs in, 1092
Chlamydia trachomatis infections, choice of drugs in, 1093
Chlomocran, 396
Chloral, chemistry, 361
Chloral alcoholate, 361
Chloral betaine, 361–363
　dosage, half-life, and preparations, 350
　legal regulations, 1671
Chloral derivatives, 361–363
Chloral hydrate, acute intoxication, 363
　chemistry, 361
　chronic intoxication, 363
　distribution and fate, 362
　dosage, half-life, and preparations, 350
　legal regulations, 1671
　local actions, 361
　systemic actions, 361–362
　untoward effects, 362–363
　use in alcohol withdrawal, 572
Chlorambucil, 1267–1268. *See also* Alkylating agents
　chemistry, 1257, 1258
　use in neoplastic diseases, 1252, 1267
Chloramines, 974
Chloramphenicol, 1191–1196. *See also* Antimicrobial agents
　absorption, distribution, fate, and excretion, 1192–1193
　antimicrobial properties, 1192
　aplastic anemia and, 1193–1194
　dosage, 1193
　drug interactions, 1195
　gray syndrome and, 1194
　history and source, 1191
　mechanism of action, 1192
　microbial resistance, 1192
　pharmacokinetics, 1695
　preparations and administration, 1193
　structural formula, 1191
　suprainfections, 1195

toxicity, 1193–1195
uses, 1195–1196
  brucellosis, 1196
  Haemophilus influenzae meningitis, 1195
  infections caused by anaerobes, 1195
  Klebsiella pneumoniae infections, 1196
  lymphogranuloma venereum, 1196
  meningitis, 1145, 1195
  Mycoplasma infections, 1196
  plague, 1196
  psittacosis, 1196
  Q fever, 1196
  rickettsial infections, 1196
  typhoid fever, 1195
  typhus, 1196
  urinary tract infections, 1196
  Yersinia infections, 1196
Chlorcyclizine, 627. *See also* H$_1$-receptor blockers
  structural formula, 623
Chlordane, toxicology, 1649
Chlordantoin, 984
Chlordecone, toxicology, 1650
Chlordiazepoxide, 437–442. *See also* Benzodiazepines
  dosage, half-life, and preparations, 350
  legal regulations, 1671
  pharmacokinetics, 1695
  preparations and dosage, 440
Chlordiazepoxide hydrochloride, preparations and dosage, 440
Chlorhexadol, legal regulations, 1671
Chlorhexidine, 975
Chloride, provisional dietary allowance, 1555
Chlorinated lime, 974
Chlorine, 973
Chlorisondamine, 215, 217
Chlormadinone acetate, 1434
Chloroamphetamine, 638
Chloroform, 291–292
  history, 259
  toxicology, 1646
Chloroguanide, 1046–1047
  absorption, fate, and excretion, 1046
  antimalarial actions, 1046
  chemistry, 1046
  history, 1046
  mechanism of antimalarial action, 1041, 1046
  preparations, route of administration, and dosage, 1047
  resistance, 1041
  toxicity and side effects, 1047
  use in malaria, 1047
Chloroguanide triazine pamoate, 1047
CHLOROMYCETIN (chloramphenicol), 1193
Chlorophenothane. *See* DDT
Chlorophenylalanine, 249, 638
Chlorophors, 974
Chloroprocaine, structural formula, 301
Chloroprocaine hydrochloride, 309. *See also* Local anesthetics
Chloroproguanil, 1044
Chloroquine, 1042–1045

absorption, fate, and excretion, 1044
amebicidal actions and uses, 1067
antimalarial actions, 1043
chemistry, 1042–1043
history, 1042
mechanism of antimalarial action, 1041, 1043–1044
precautions and contraindications, 1045
preparations, 1044
resistance, 1042
routes of administration and dosage, 1044
toxicity and side effects, 1045
uses, amebiasis, 1045, 1062, 1067
  Babesia infection, 1045
  clonorchiasis, 1035
  discoid lupus erythematosus, 1043
  giardiasis, 1045
  malaria, 1045
  paragonimiasis, 1035
  photoallergic reactions, 1043
  porphyria cutanea tarda, 1043
  rheumatoid arthritis, 1043
  systemic lupus erythematosus, 1043
8-Chlorotheophylline, 623
Chlorothiazide. *See also* Benzothiadiazides
  effect on blood pressure, 803–804
  pharmacokinetics, 1696
  structural formula, properties, and dosage, 900
  use as antihypertensive, 810, 811, 813
Chlorothymol, 969
Chlorotrianisene, 1428, 1432
Chlorphenesin, chemistry, preparations, and dosage, 489
Chlorpheniramine, 627. *See also* H$_1$-receptor blockers
  structural formula, 623
Chlorpheniramine maleate, preparations and dosage, 628
Chlorphenoxamine, chemistry, preparations, and dosage, 487
  use in parkinsonism, 484–485
Chlorphentermine, legal regulations, 1671
  receptor-type activity, 142
  structural formula, 142
  use in obesity, 172
Chlorpromazine hydrochloride. *See also* Antipsychotic agents
  chemistry, 396–397, 408
  dosage forms, 408, 417
  dose as antiemetic, 417
  dose as antipsychotic, 408
  pharmacokinetics, 405, 1696
  side effects, 408
Chlorpropamide, 1510–1514. *See also* Sulfonylureas
  duration of action, fate, and excretion, 1512
  effect on renal function, 926
  potentiation of effect of ADH, 921
  preparations, 1513
  use in nephrogenic diabetes insipidus, 926
Chlorprothixene. *See also* Antipsychotic agents
  chemistry, 396, 410
  dosage forms, 410

Chlorprothixene (Cont.)
  dose as antipsychotic, 410
  side effects, 410
Chlorquinaldol, 1063
Chlortetracycline. See also Tetracyclines
  absorption, distribution, and excretion, 1184
  dosage, 1185, 1186
  preparations and administration, 1185, 1186
  structural formula, 1181
Chlorthalidone. See also Benzothiadiazides
  effect on blood pressure, 803
  pharmacokinetics, 1697
  properties and dosage, 900
  structural formula, 899
  use as antihypertensive, 810, 811, 813
CHLOR-TRIMETON (chlorpheniramine maleate), 628
Chlorzotocin, 1259, 1269
Chlorzoxazone, chemistry, preparations, and dosage,
  489
Cholanic acid, structural formula, 998
Cholecalciferol, 1539, 1544
Cholecystokinin, role as CNS transmitter, 253
Cholecystokinin-pancreozymin, 663
Cholera, choice of drugs in, 1090
  tetracyclines in, 1190
Choleretics, 998
Cholestasis, phenobarbital in, 361
Cholesterol, reduction of blood levels, 838–845
Cholestyramine, 997
  chemistry, 842
  effects on plasma lipids, 842
  preparations, dosage, and uses, 843
  untoward effects and drug interactions, 843
  uses, chlordecone poisoning, 1650
    digitalis intoxication, 755
    hyperlipoproteinemias, 843
    pseudomembranous colitis, 1227
Cholic acid, 998
Choline, 1574–1576
  absorption, fate, and excretion, 1575
  chemistry, 1574
  history, 1574
  human requirement, 1575
  pharmacological actions, 1574
  physiological function, 67–68, 1574–1575
  preparations, 1575
  structural formula, 92
  symptoms of deficiency, 1575
  uses, 1575–1576
Choline acetyltransferase, 67–68
Choline esters, 91–96. See also individual agents
Choline theophyllinate, 592, 601
Cholinergic agonists, 91–98. See also individual
  agents
Cholinergic muscarinic receptors, 91–92
Cholinergic nervous system. See Autonomic nervous
  system
Cholinergic nicotinic receptors, 29, 222–223
Cholinergic receptors, types, 83–84
Cholinesterase reactivators, chemistry and mecha-
  nism of action, 110–111

pharmacology, toxicology, and disposition, 111
Cholinomimetic alkaloids, 96–98. See also individ-
  ual agents
CHOLOXIN (dextrothyroxine sodium), 845
Chorioadenoma destruens, methotrexate in, 1276
Choriocarcinoma, dactinomycin in, 1291
  methotrexate in, 1275
  vinblastine in, 1289
Chorionic follicle-stimulating hormone, 1383
  chemical properties, 1371
Chorionic gonadotropin, 1383–1387
  chemical properties, 1371
Chorionic gonadotropin for injection, 1386
Chorionic somatomammotropin, 1382
Chorionic thyrotropin, 1387
  chemical properties, 1371
Chromium, provisional dietary allowance, 1555
Chromogranin, 73–75
Chronic obstructive pulmonary disease, theophyl-
  line in, 603
Chymotrypsin, 961
Cimetidine, 629–632, 997. See also H$_2$-receptor
  blockers
  absorption, fate, and excretion, 631
  chemistry, 629–630
  pharmacokinetics, 1698
  pharmacological effects, 630–631
  preparations, routes of administration, and dos-
    age, 632
  toxicity, 631
  uses, 632, 997
Cinchona alkaloids, 1054–1057. See also individual
  agents
Cinchonidine, 1055
Cinchonine, 1055
Cinchonism, 1056
Cinnamates, 960
CIN-QUIN (quinidine sulfate), 771
CIRCANOL (ergot alkaloids, dihydrogenated), 946
Cirrhosis, adrenocorticosteroids in, 1491
  diuretics in, 911
Cisplatin, 1298–1299
  absorption, fate, and excretion, 1298
  chemistry, 1298
  mechanism of action, 1298
  preparation, dosage, and route of administration,
    1298
  therapeutic uses and clinical toxicity, 1298–1299
  use in neoplastic disease, 1253, 1298–1299
CITANEST (prilocaine hydrochloride), 309
Citric acid, 869
Citrovorum factor, 1343
Clavine alkaloids, 942
Clavulanic acid, 1130
CLEOCIN (clindamycin hydrochloride), 1227
CLEOCIN PEDIATRIC (clindamycin palmitate hydro-
  chloride), 1227
CLEOCIN PHOSPHATE (clindamycin phosphate), 1227
Clidinium, preparations and structural formula, 130
Climacteric, female, estrogens in, 1429
  male, androgens in, 1460

Clindamycin, 1226–1227. *See also* Antimicrobial agents
  absorption, fate, and excretion, 1226
  antibacterial activity, 1226
  chemistry, 1226
  colitis from, 1227
  dosage, 1227
  mechanism of action, 1226
  pharmacokinetics, 1698–1699
  preparations and administration, 1227
  toxicity, 1227
  uses, *Actinomyces israelii* infections, 1227
    Bacteroides infections, 1227
    Fusobacterium infections, 1227
CLINORIL (sulindac), 707
Clioquinol, 984, 1063–1065
  absorption, fate, and excretion, 1064
  actions on amebae, 1064
  chemistry, 1063
  preparations, 1064
  route of administration and dosage, 1064
  toxicity and side effects, 1064
  uses, 1062, 1064
CLISTIN (carbinoxamine maleate), 628
Clofazimine, 1215–1216
Clofibrate, 840–842
  absorption, fate, and excretion, 841
  actions/effects on, kidney, 920
    plasma lipids, 840–841
    platelet adhesion, 1361
  chemistry, 840
  mechanism of action, 841
  pharmacokinetics, 1699
  preparations, dosage, and uses, 841
  untoward effects and drug interactions, 841
  use in diabetes insipidus, 924
Cloflucarban, 981
Clomethiazole, 369
CLOMID (clomiphene citrate), 1433
Clomiphene, 1304
  action as antiestrogen, 1432
  preparations, 1433
  use in female infertility, 1433
Clomipramine, 249, 419
Clonazepam, absorption, distribution, biotransformation, and excretion, 466
  anticonvulsant properties, 466
  interactions with other drugs, 467
  legal regulations, 1671
  pharmacokinetics, 1700
  plasma concentrations, 467
  preparations and dosage, 467
  structural formula, 466
  toxicity, 466–467
  use in epilepsy, 467
Clonidine, 197–198, 797–799
  absorption and elimination, 798
  effects on opioid withdrawal, 571
  pharmacokinetics, 1700
  pharmacological properties, 797–798
  preparations, administration, and dosage, 798
  structural formula, 797
  toxicity and precautions, 798–799
  uses, hypertension, 811–813
    migraine, 799
CLONOPIN (clonazepam), 467, 1671
Clonorchiasis, occurrence and treatment, 1035
Clopenthixol, 396
Clorazepate, 437–440. *See also* Benzodiazepines
  legal regulations, 1671
Clorazepate potassium, preparations and dosage, 440
Clorgyline, 204, 428
Clormethiazole, use in alcohol withdrawal, 572
CLORPACTIN (oxychlorosene), 974
Clortermine, legal regulations, 1671
Clostridial infections, penicillin in, 1140
Clostridium perfringens infections, choice of drugs in, 1088
Clostridium tetani infections, choice of drugs in, 1088
Clotrimazole, 983
Cloxacillin, 1142–1143. *See also* Penicillins
CLOXAPEN (cloxacillin sodium), 1143
Clozapine, 397
Coal tar, 970
Cobalamin, 1333. *See also* Cyanocobalamin
Cobalt, status in anemias, 1326–1327
  toxicity, 1327
Cobaltous chloride, 1326
Cocaine, 307–308. *See also* Local anesthetics
  absorption, fate, and excretion, 307–308
  abuse, 553–557
    incidence and patterns, 554–556
    legal regulations, 1670
  actions/effects on, body temperature, 307
    cardiovascular system, 307
    central nervous system, 307
    eye, 307
    skeletal muscle, 307
    sympathetic nervous system, 307
  acute poisoning, 308
  addiction, 554
  chemistry, 307
  local anesthetic actions, 307
  physical dependence, 556–557
  preparations and dosage, 308
  source, 300, 307
  structural formula, 301
  tolerance and abuse, 308, 556–557
Coccidioides immitis infections, choice of drugs in, 1093
Coccidioidomycosis, amphotericin B in, 1239
  miconazole in, 1239, 1240
Cocoa, 592, 603
Cocoa butter, 952
Codeine. *See also* Opioids
  absorption, fate, and excretion, 506
  actions/effects on, cough reflex, 502, 513, 529
    respiration, 502
  dosage, 507
  duration of analgesic effect, 507
  legal regulations, 1670

Codeine (*Cont.*)
  preparations, 509
  source, 496
  structural formula, 496
  uses, 511–513
    cough, 513
    pain relief, 511–512
  withdrawal symptoms, 556–557
Coffee, 592, 603
Coformycin, 1283
COGENTIN (benztropine mesylate), 486
COLACE (dioctyl sodium sulfosuccinate), 1009
Colchicine, 718–720
  absorption, fate, and excretion, 719
  actions/effects on, kidney, 922
  history, 718
  mechanism of action, 718
  pharmacological properties, 718
  preparations, 719
  structural formula, 718
  toxicity, 719
  uses, gout, 719
    prevention of Mediterranean fever episodes, 720
Cold. *See* Common cold; Rhinitis
Cold cream, 953
COLESTID (colestipol hydrochloride), 843
Colestipol, chemistry, 842
  effects on plasma lipids, 842
  mechanism of action, 842
  preparations and dosage, 843
  untoward effects and drug interactions, 843
  uses, 843
Colistimethate, dosage, 1229
  preparations, 1229
Colistin, 1228–1230
  absorption and excretion, 1229
  antibacterial activity, 1228
  chemistry, 1228
  history and source, 1228
  preparations, administration, and dosage, 1229
  toxicity, 1229–1230
  uses, *Pseudomonas* infections, 1230
    Serratia infections, 1230
Colitis. *See also* Diarrhea; Dysentery
  adrenocorticosteroids in, 1491
  belladonna alkaloids in, 133
  sulfasalazine in, 1112
  vancomycin in, 1227, 1231
Collagen diseases, adrenocorticosteroids in, 1490
Collagenase, actions and uses, 961–962
Collodion, 953
Colloidal sulfur, 980
COLY-MYCIN M PARENTERAL (sterile colistimethate sodium), 1229
COLY-MYCIN S ORAL SUSPENSION (colistin sulfate for oral suspension), 1229
COMBANTRIN (pyrantel pamoate), 1025
Common cold, belladonna alkaloids in, 134
  H_1-receptor blockers in, 629
  sympathomimetic drugs in, 168

COMPAZINE (prochlorperazine), 406, 417
COMPAZINE EDISYLATE (prochlorperazine edisylate), 417
COMPAZINE MALEATE (prochlorperazine maleate), 417
Compliance. *See* Patient compliance
COMPOCILLIN-V K (penicillin V potassium), 1137
Compound 48/80, 616–617
COMPOUND 3422 (parathion), 104
Compound undecylenic acid ointment, 982
Comprehensive Drug Abuse Prevention and Control Act of 1970, 1670
Condylomata, caustics in, 956
Congestive heart failure. *See* Cardiac failure
Conjugated estrogens, 1428
Conjunctivitis, bacitracin in, 1232
  choice of drugs in, 1093
  sulfacetamide in, 1112
  sulfonamides in, 1115
  tetracyclines in, 1189
  zinc sulfate in, 977
Constipation, laxatives and cathartics in, 1011
Contraceptives. *See also* Oral contraceptives
  male, 1462–1463
Controlled Substances Act, 1670–1671
Convallatoxin, 730
Converting enzyme. *See* Angiotensin; Peptidyl dipeptidase
Convulsions, barbiturates in, 360–361
  drug therapy, 468–471
  emergency therapy, 470–471
Copper, metabolism, 1326
  provisional dietary allowance, 1555
  status in anemias, 1326
CORAMINE (nikethamide), 589
CORDRAN (flurandrenolide), 1486
Corn oil, 952
Coronary thrombosis. *See* Angina pectoris; Myocardial infarction
CORTEF (cortisol), 1484
CORTEF ACETATE (cortisol acetate), 1484
CORTEF FLUID (cortisol cypionate), 1484
Corticosteroids. *See* Adrenocorticosteroids
Corticosterone. *See also* Adrenocorticosteroids
  relative potency, duration of action, and equivalent dose, 1482
Corticotropin. *See* Adrenocorticotropic hormone
Corticotropin-like intermediate lobe peptide, 1388
Corticotropin-releasing factor, 1390, 1391, 1469
Cortisol. *See also* Adrenocorticosteroids
  effect on water and electrolyte metabolism, 1476
  preparations 1484
  relative potency, duration of action, and equivalent dose, 1482
Cortisone. *See also* Adrenocorticosteroids
  preparations, 1484
  relative potency, duration of action, and equivalent dose, 1482
CORTONE ACETATE (cortisone acetate), 1484
CORTROPHIN GEL (repository corticotropin injection), 1470

CORTROPHIN-ZINC (sterile corticotropin zinc hydroxide suspension), 1470

CORTROSYN (cosyntropin for injection), 1470

Corynanthine, 188

Corynebacterium infections, choice of drugs in, 1088

Coryza. *See* Common cold; Rhinitis

COSMEGEN (dactinomycin), 1291

Cosyntropin for injection, 1470

Cottonseed oil, 952

Cough, benzonatate in, 530
   caramiphen in, 530
   carbetapentane in, 530
   codeine in, 513
   dextromethorphan in, 529
   diphenhydramine in, 530
   levopropoxyphene in, 529
   mechanism, 528–529
   noscapine in, 529–530

COUMADIN (warfarin sodium), 1357

CPH (protein hydrolysate injection), 863

CREAMALIN, 991

Cresols, 967

Cretinism, 1404
   thyroid hormones in, 1407

Cromolyn sodium, 621–622
   absorption, fate, and excretion, 621
   chemistry, 621
   history, 621
   pharmacological effects, 621
   preparations and dosage, 622
   toxicity, 621
   uses, 622

Crotamiton, 985

Cryptococcus neoformans infections, amphotericin B in, 1239
   choice of drugs in, 1093
   flucytosine in, 1239

Cryptorchism, gonadotropic hormones in, 1387

Crystal violet, 979, 984

CRYSTICILLIN (sterile penicillin G procaine suspension), 1137

CRYSTODIGEN (digitoxin), 749

CUPREX (tetrahydronaphthalene-cupric oleate), 985

Cupric oleate, 985

CUPRIMINE (penicillamine capsules), 1628

Curare, 220–232. *See also* Tubocurarine
   absorption, fate, and excretion, 230
   actions/effects on, autonomic ganglia, 227–228
      cardiovascular system, 228
      central nervous system, 227
      cholinergic receptor sites, 222–225
      skeletal muscle, 223–227
   histamine release, 228
   history, sources, and chemistry, 220
   mechanism of action, 223–226
   paralytic sequence in man, 226–227
   pharmacological properties, 223–230
   preparations, routes of administration, and dosage, 230
   synergisms and antagonisms, 228–229
   toxicology, 229–230

uses, 231–232

Curariform drugs, 220–232

Cyanide, generation from nitroprusside, 806
   toxicology, 1651–1652

Cyanocobalamin, 1331–1340. *See also* Anemia—megaloblastic
   absorption, 1334–1336
   chemistry, 1333–1334
   deficiency, 1336–1337
   distribution, storage, and fate, 1334–1336
   excretion, 1334–1336
   history, 1331
   human daily requirement, 1335
   interrelations with folic acid, 1331–1333
   metabolic functions, 1334
   plasma concentration and binding capacity, 1335
   preparations, administration, and dosage, 1337
   recommended dietary allowance, 1553
   sources in nature, 1334
   structural formula, 1333
   terminology, 1333
   toxic reactions, 1337
   transport in body, 1335
   uses, 1337–1340

Cyclacillin, 1145

CYCLAINE (hexylcaine hydrochloride), 310

Cyclandelate, 831

CYCLAPEN (cyclacillin), 1145

Cyclazocine, 521–522. *See also* Opioid antagonists
   absorption and duration of action, 524
   pharmacological effects, 524
   use in opioid addiction, 575
   withdrawal syndrome, 524

Cyclic adenosine 3',5'-monophosphate, relationship to, actions of ACTH, 1468
   actions of antidiuretic hormone, 921
   actions of antipsychotic agents, 401
   actions of calcitonin, 1537
   actions of dopamine in basal ganglia, 478
   actions of glucagon, 1518
   actions of opioids, 498
   actions of parathyroid hormone, 1533, 1534
   androgen biosynthesis, 1449–1450
   calcitonin secretion, 1537
   effects of catecholamines and glucagon on carbohydrate metabolism, 78–80
   effects of prostaglandins, 675–676
   estrogen biosynthesis, 1420
   gonadotropin action, 1385
   histamine actions, 614
   hormone action, 1368–1369
   insulin secretion and action, 1501, 1506
   lipolytic action of catecholamines, 149
   lipolytic action of growth hormone, 1375
   lipotropin action, 1389
   MSH action, 1389
   myocardial effects of epinephrine, 79–80
   opioid dependence, 542
   progesterone biosynthesis, 1435
   somatomedin action, 1376

Cyclic adenosine 3′,5′-monophosphate (*Cont.*)
  thyrotropin action, 1388, 1402–1403
  TRH action, 1390
  xanthine actions, 597–598
  role in ganglionic transmission, 212
Cyclic AMP. *See* Cyclic adenosine 3′5′-monophosphate
Cyclizine, structural formula, 623. *See also* H$_1$-receptor blockers
  use in preanesthetic medication, 270
Cyclizine hydrochloride, preparations and dosage, 628
Cyclizine lactate, preparations and dosage, 628
Cyclobenzaprine, 490
  chemistry, preparations, and dosage, 489
Cyclodienes, toxicology, 1649
Cycloguanil pamoate, 1047
  use in leishmaniasis, 1075
CYCLOGYL (cyclopentolate hydrochloride), 132
Cyclomethycaine sulfate, 310
Cyclooxygenase, role in prostaglandin synthesis, 669–670
Cyclopentolate, ocular effects and uses, 134
  preparations and structural formula, 132
Cyclophosphamide, 1264–1266. *See also* Alkylating agents
  absorption, fate, and excretion, 1264–1265
  chemistry, 1257, 1258
  clinical toxicity, 1266
  pharmacological and cytotoxic actions, 1264
  preparations, dosage, and routes of administration, 1265
  use in neoplastic diseases, 1252, 1266
Cyclopropane, 291
  history, 259
Cycloserine, 1210–1211
  mechanism of action, 1129
CYCLOSPASMOL (cyclandelate), 831
Cyclothiazide. *See also* Benzothiadiazides
  structural formula, properties, and dosage, 900
Cycrimine, chemistry, preparations, and dosage, 486
  use in parkinsonism, 484–485
CYLERT (pemoline), 590
Cyproheptadine, 639
Cyproterone acetate, 1435, 1462
Cystinuria, penicillamine in, 1628
Cytarabine, 1280–1281. *See also* Pyrimidine analogs
  absorption, fate, and excretion, 1281
  antiviral properties, 1242
  clinical toxicity, 1281
  immunosuppressive action, 1281
  mechanism of action, 1280
  mechanism of resistance, 1280–1281
  preparations, administration, and dosage, 1281
  use in neoplastic diseases, 1252, 1281
CYTELLIN (sitosterols), 845
Cytochrome P-450, 14–18
CYTOMEL (liothyronine sodium), 1406
CYTOSAR (cytarabine), 1281
Cytosine arabinoside. *See* Cytarabine
CYTOXAN (cyclophosphamide), 1265

2,4-D, toxicology, 1653
Dacarbazine. *See also* Alkylating agents
  structural formula, 1259
  use in neoplastic diseases, 1252, 1271
DACTIL (piperidolate hydrochloride), 132
Dactinomycin, 1290–1291
  absorption, fate, and excretion, 1291
  chemistry and structure-activity relationship, 1290
  clinical toxicity, 1291
  cytotoxic action, 1291
  history, 1290
  mechanism of action, 1290
  preparation, dosage, and route of administration, 1291
  use in neoplastic diseases, 1253, 1291
DADDS. *See* Acedapsone
Dagga, 560
Dakin-Carrel solution, 974
Dakin's solution, 974
DALMANE (flurazepam), 350, 1671
DAM. *See* Diacetylmonoxime
Danazol, 1438, 1456
DANEX (zinc pyrithione), 957
DANOCRINE (danazol), 1456
Danthron, 1008. *See also* Cathartics, anthraquinones
DANTRIUM (dantrolene sodium), 490
Dantrolene, chemistry and pharmacological properties, 490
  preparations and dosage, 490
  toxicity and precautions, 490
  uses, malignant hyperthermia, 490–491
    spasticity, 491
DAPOLAR (cycloguanil pamoate–acedapsone), 1047
Dapsone. *See also* Sulfones
  structural formula, 1214
  uses, dermatitis herpetiformis, 1116
    malaria, 1049, 1058
DARACLOR (chloroquine-pyrimethamine), 1044
DARANIDE (dichlorphenamide), 898
DARAPRIM (pyrimethamine), 1049
DARBID (isopropamide iodide), 130
DARICON (oxyphencyclimine hydrochloride), 132
DARTAL (thiopropazate), 406
DARVON (propoxyphene), 521, 1671
DARVON-N (propoxyphene napsylate), 521
DAUNOBLASTINA (daunorubicin), 1292
Daunomycin. *See* Daunorubicin
Daunorubicin, 1291–1293
  absorption, fate, and excretion, 1292
  chemistry, 1291–1292
  clinical toxicity, 1293
  mechanism of action, 1292
  preparation, dosage, and route of administration, 1292
  use in neoplastic diseases, 1253, 1293
DAXOLIN (loxapine succinate), 411
Daytop Village, 573
dDAVP. *See* Desmopressin
DDAVP. (desmopressin acetate), 923
DDT, toxicology, 1648–1649
1-Deaminopenicillamine oxytocin, 917

1-Deamino-4-valine-8-D-arginine vasopressin, 917
DEAPRIL-ST (ergot alkaloids, dihydrogenated), 946
Deazauridine, 1277
DEBRISAN (dextranomer), 953
Debrisoquin, 201
DECADRON (dexamethasone), 1484
DECADRON-L.A. (dexamethasone acetate), 1485
DECADRON PHOSPHATE (dexamethasone sodium phosphate), 1485
DECA-DURABOLIN (nandrolone decanoate), 1457
Decamethonium. *See also* Neuromuscular blocking agents
  mechanism of action, 225–226
  paralytic sequence in man, 226–227
  pharmacological actions, 225–228
  preparations and dosage, 231
  structural formula, 221
DECHOLIN (dehydrocholic acid), 999
DECHOLIN SODIUM (dehydrocholate sodium injection), 999
DECLOMYCIN (demeclocycline hydrochloride), 1185
Decompression sickness, helium in, 335
Deferoxamine, 1633–1634
  preparations and dosage, 1634
  uses, acute iron poisoning, 1325, 1634
    iron-storage diseases, 1634
    transfusion siderosis, 1634
7-Dehydrocholesterol, 1539
Dehydrocholic acid, laxative properties, 1009
  preparations and dosage, 999
Dehydroemetine, 1062, 1066–1067
Dehydroepiandrosterone, 1448
DELALUTIN (hydroxyprogesterone caproate injection), 1437
DELATESTRYL (testosterone enanthate), 1456
DELCID, 991, 996
DELESTROGEN (estradiol esters), 1428
Delirium tremens, 553, 572
DELTA-CORTEF (prednisolone), 1485
DELTASONE (prednisone), 1485
Demecarium. *See also* Anticholinesterases
  preparations, 112
  structural formula, 104
  use in glaucoma, 113
Demeclocycline. *See also* Tetracyclines
  absorption, distribution, and excretion, 1184
  actions/effects on kidney, 922
  dosage, 1185
  preparations and administration, 1185
  structural formula, 1181
  use in inappropriate ADH secretion, 922, 926
Demelanizing agents, 957–959
DEMEROL (meperidine), 507, 1670
Demulcents, 951–952
DEMULEN, 1440
DENDRID (idoxuridine), 1240
Deodorants, 954–955
Deoxyadenosylcobalamin, 1333
Deoxybarbiturates, 458–459
Deoxycoformycin, 1283
Deoxypyridoxine, 1570

DEPAKENE (valproic acid), 463
DEPO-ESTRADIOL (estradiol esters), 1428
DEPO-MEDROL (methylprednisolone acetate), 1485
DEPO-PROVERA (medroxyprogesterone acetate), 1437, 1440
DEPO-TESTOSTERONE (testosterone cypionate), 1456
Deprenyl, 204, 428, 484
Depression, antipsychotic agents in, 416
  definition, 418
  electroconvulsive therapy in, 425, 427, 435
  monoamine oxidase inhibitors in, 427, 430, 435–436
  treatment, 434–436
  tricyclic antidepressants in, 434–436
DERMABASE, 952
DERMA-CLEAN, 970
Dermatitis. *See also* Eczema; Seborrhea
  adrenocorticosteroids in, 1491
  anthralin in, 981
  antihistamines in, 629
  antiseborrheics in, 956–957
  keratolytics in, 956
  permanganates in, 974
  resorcinol in, 968
  tars in, 970
Dermatitis herpetiformis, dapsone in, 1116
  sulfapyridine in, 1116
Dermatomycoses. *See* Mycotic infections; Tinea infections
[Des-Asp¹] angiotensin I, 647, 648. *See also* Angiotensin
DESFERAL MESYLATE (sterile deferoxamine mesylate), 1631
Desipramine. *See also* Tricyclic antidepressants
  pharmacokinetics, 1701
  structural formula, 419
Desipramine hydrocholoride, preparations and dosage, 424
Deslanoside. *See also* Digitalis
  preparation and administration, 749
Desmopressin, 917
  absorption, fate, and excretion, 923
  use in diabetes insipidus, 924
Desmopressin acetate, 923
Desonide. *See also* Adrenocorticosteroids
  preparations, 1486
Desoximetasone. *See also* Adrenocorticosteroids
  preparations, 1486
Desoxycorticosterone. *See also* Adrenocorticosteroids
  effect on water and electrolyte metabolism, 1476
  preparations, 1484
  relative potency, duration of action, and equivalent dose, 1482
11-Desoxycortisol, relative potency, duration of action, and equivalent dose, 1482
DESOXYN (methamphetamine), 163, 1670
Desthiobiotin, 1574
DET. *See* Diethyltryptamine
Dexamethasone. *See also* Adrenocorticosteroids
  preparations, 1484–1485

Dexamethasone (*Cont.*)
  relative potency, duration of action, and equivalent dose, 1482
DEXEDRINE (dextroamphetamine), 161, 1670
Dextran, 860–861
  effect on platelet aggregation, 1361
Dextran 40 injection, 862
Dextran 70 injection, 862
Dextran 75 injection, 862
Dextranomer, 953
Dextroamphetamine, 159–162. *See also* Amphetamine; Sympathomimetic drugs
  abuse, 553–557
    legal regulations, 1670
  preparations and dosage, 161
  uses, 162
    enuresis, 172
    epilepsy, 172
    hyperkinetic syndrome, 172
    narcolepsy, 171
    obesity, 171–172
    parkinsonism, 171
    psychogenic disorders, 172
Dextromethorphan, chemistry and antitussive action, 529
  preparations and uses, 529
Dextromoramide, dosage, 507
  duration of analgesic effect, 507
Dextrorphan, 513
Dextrose, 861
Dextrose and sodium chloride injection, 861
Dextrothyroxine sodium, use in hyperlipoproteinemia, 844–845
DFP. *See* Di*iso*propyl phosphorofluoridate
D.H.E. 45 (dihydroergotamine mesylate), 946
Diabetes insipidus, antidiuretic hormone in, 924
  benzothiadiazides in, 902, 925
  chlorpropamide in, 926
  clofibrate in, 926
  pathophysiology, 920
Diabetes mellitus, classification, 1502
  insulin in, 1502–1506, 1514–1517
  metabolic abnormalities, 1503–1506
  sulfonylureas in, 1513–1514
  treatment, 1514–1517
Diabetic ketoacidosis, treatment, 1515–1516
DIABINESE (chlorpropamide), 1513
Diacetylmonoxime, dosage, 112
DIAL soap, 981
Diallylbisnortoxiferine, 220
Dialysis, use in drug poisoning, 1612
Dialysis disequilibrium syndrome, 859
Diamine oxidase, 618–619
2,4-Diaminobutyrate, 247
DIAMOX (acetazolamide), 468, 898, 900
DIANABOL (methandrostenolone), 1457
DIAPARENE (methylbenzethonium), 978
DIAPID (lypressin), 923
Diarrhea. *See also* Colitis; Dysentery
  antimuscarinic drugs in, 133
  bulk-forming laxatives in, 1004
  diphenoxylate in, 517

  infections, choice of drugs in, 1086
  kaolin in, 954
  opioids in, 513
  pectin in, 954
  tetracyclines in, 1190, 1191
DIASONE SODIUM (sulfoxone sodium), 1215
Diazepam, 437–441. *See also* Benzodiazepines
  absorption, distribution, biotransformation, and excretion, 466
  action on skeletal muscle tone, 488
  anticonvulsant properties and mechanism of action, 466
  dosage, half-life, and preparations, 350
  drug interactions, 467
  legal regulations, 1671
  pharmacokinetics, 466, 1702
  preparations and dosage, 440, 467
  toxicity, 466–467
  uses, cardioversion, 441
    cerebral palsy, 441
    epilepsy, 467, 470–471
    intravenous anesthesia, 296
    labor, 440
    poisoning by belladonna alkaloids, 128
    preanesthetic medication, 270
    status epilepticus, 470
    strychnine poisoning, 587
    tetanus, 441
    upper motoneuron disorders, 441
Diazoxide, antihypertensive actions, 801–802
  disposition and elimination, 802
  hyperglycemic action, 1518–1519
  pharmacological properties, 801–802
  preparations, administration, and dosage, 802
  structural formula, 801
  side effects and precautions, 802
  use in hypertensive emergencies, 812–813
Dibenamine, 178–183. *See also* Alpha-adrenergic blocking drugs
  structural formula, 178
Dibenzodiazepines, 397. *See also* Antipsychotic agents
Dibenzoxazepines, 397. *See also* Antipsychotic agents
DIBENZYLINE (phenoxybenzamine hydrochloride), 182
Dibozane, 186
Dibromochloropropane, toxicology, 1652
Dibromsalan, 981
Dibucaine hydrochloride, 309
Dichloralphenazone, 361
Dichloroisoproterenol, 188
  structural formula, 188
Dichloromethane, toxicology, 1646
Dichlorophen, 1014
Dichlorophenoxyacetic acid. *See* 2,4-D
Dichlorphenamide, 897, 898
Dicloxacillin, 1142–1143. *See also* Penicillins
  pharmacokinetics, 1703
Dicumarol, 1359. *See also* Anticoagulants, oral
Dicyclomine, pharmacological properties, 129
  preparations and structural formula, 132

DIDREX (benzphetamine hydrochloride), 172
DIDRONEL (etidronate disodium), 1538
Dieldrin, toxicology, 1649
Dienestrol, 1428
DIENSTROL (dienestrol), 1428
Diethazine, 397
Diethylcarbamazine, 1015–1016
  absorption, fate, and excretion, 1015
  anthelmintic action, 1015
  chemistry, 1015
  preparations, route of administration, and dosage, 1015
  toxicity and precautions, 1015–1016
  uses, 1016
Diethyldithiocarbamate, 249
Diethylene glycol, 952
  toxicology, 1647
Diethylenetriaminepentaacetic acid, 1622
  use in radioactive metal poisoning, 1634
Diethylether, 291
  history, 258–259
Diethylpropion, legal regulations, 1671
  receptor-type activity, 142
  structural formula, 142
  use in obesity, 172
Diethylstilbestrol. See also Estrogens
  chemistry, 1422
  preparations, 1428
Diethyltryptamine, 564
Difenoxin, 517
Diflunisal, 689
4,4′-Diformamidodiphenylsulfone, 1058
Digestants, 998–999. See also individual agents
Digitalis, 729–756
  absorption, distribution, and elimination, 746
  actions/effects on, adenosine triphosphatase, 732–733
    atrial fibrillation, 738, 741
    atrial flutter, 738, 741
    automaticity, 734–741
    autonomic control of heart, 737–739
    blood coagulation, 753
    blood pressure, 742–746
    cardiac contractility, 731–732, 739
    cardiac energy metabolism, 732
    cardiac excitability, 734–741
    cardiac output, 742–746
    cardiac rate, 742–746
    cardiovascular system, 730–746
    circulation in heart failure, 743–746
    conduction velocity, 734–741
    coronary circulation, 746
    ECG, 741–742
    electrical activity of atrial and ventricular muscle, 736, 738–739
    electrical activity of the heart in situ, 739–741
    electrical activity mediated indirectly, 737–739
    electrical activity of Purkinje fibers, 734–736
    electrical activity of S-A and A-V nodes, 736
    kidney, 745
    refractory periods, 734–741
    Starling curves, 744–745
    vascular resistance, 742–745
    veins, 743, 745
    Wolff-Parkinson-White syndrome, 741
  aglycones, 730
  assay, 749
  calcium and, 732–734, 735–736
  chemistry, 730
  choice of preparations, 748–749
  dosage, initial digitalization, 747
  dosage and administration, 747–748
  history, 729
  interactions with other drugs, 755–756
  intoxication, 751–755
    atropine in, 755
    cardiac effects, 751–753
    cholestyramine in, 755
    diagnosis and treatment, 754–755
    factors influencing, 753–754
    gastrointestinal effects, 753
    lidocaine in, 755
    neurological effects, 753
    phenytoin in, 755, 783
    potassium in, 755
    propranolol in, 786
    visual effects, 753
  mechanism of inotropic action, 732–734
  onset and duration of action, 748
  plasma concentrations, 748
  potassium and, 732, 734, 736, 753–754, 755
  preparations, 749
  routes of administration, 748–749
  source and composition, 729–730
  unitage, 749
  uses, atrial fibrillation, 750
    atrial flutter, 750–751
    congestive heart failure, 749–750
    paroxysmal tachycardia, 751
    in patients with the sick sinus syndrome, 751
    prevention of heart failure, 750
Digitalis-induced arrhythmias, antiarrhythmic agents in, 769
Digitoxigenin, 730
  structural formula, 730
Digitoxin. See also Digitalis
  absorption and onset of action, 746, 748
  bioavailability, 746
  distribution, 747
  dosage and routes of administration, 747–748
  excretion, 747
  peak effect and half-life, 747–748
  pharmacokinetics, 746–748, 1703
  plasma concentrations, 748
  preparations and administration, 749
Digitoxose, 730
Digoxigenin, 730
Digoxin. See also Digitalis
  absorption and onset of action, 746, 748
  bioavailability, 746
  distribution, 746
  dosage and routes of administration, 747–748
  excretion, 747
  peak effect and half-life, 747–748

Digoxin (*Cont.*)
  pharmacokinetics, 746–748, 1704
  plasma concentrations, 748
  preparations and administration, 749
Dihydrocodeine, dosage, 507
  duration of analgesic effect, 507
Dihydroergocornine, 946
Dihydroergocristine, 942, 946
Dihydroergokryptine, 946
Dihydroergotamine. *See also* Ergot alkaloids
  pharmacological actions, 943
  preparations, 946
Dihydroergotamine mesylate, use to prevent thrombosis, 1363
Dihydro-β-erythroidine, 220–222
Dihydrofolate reductase, 1273
Dihydromorphine, legal regulations, 1670
Dihydrostreptomycin, 1164
Dihydrotachysterol, 1544, 1545
  use in hypoparathyroidism, 1545
Dihydrotestosterone, 1453
Dihydroxyaluminum aminoacetate, 992
Dihydroxyaluminum sodium carbonate, 992
1,25-Dihydroxycholecalciferol, 1539, 1545
Dihydroxytryptamine, 249, 251, 638
Diiodohydroxyquin. *See* Iodoquinol
Di*iso*propyl phosphorofluoridate. *See also* Anticholinesterases; Isoflurophate
  history, 101
  preparations, 112
  structural formula, 105
DILANTIN (phenytoin sodium), 454
DILAUDID (hydromorphone), 507, 509, 1670
Diloxanide furoate, 1067–1068
  use in amebiasis, 1062, 1068
Dimaprit, 610, 620
Dimenhydrinate, preparations and dosage, 628. *See also* H$_1$-receptor blockers
  structural formula, 623
Dimercaprol, 1625–1627
  absorption, fate, and excretion, 1626
  chemistry and physical properties, 1625
  dosage and routes of administration, 1627
  history, 1625
  mechanism of action, 1626
  preparations, 1627
  side effects and toxicity, 1626
  uses, arsenic poisoning, 1631
    cadmium poisoning, 1633
    lead poisoning, 1622
    mercury poisoning, 1627
Dimercaptosuccinic acid, 1627
DIMETANE (brompheniramine maleate), 628
Dimethicone, 953
Dimethisoquin hydrochloride, 310
Dimethisterone, chemistry, 1434
Dimethoxyamphetamine, 564–565
2,5-Dimethoxy-4-ethylamphetamine, 564, 566
2,5-Dimethoxy-4-methylamphetamine, 564, 566
Dimethyl tubocurarine. *See* Metocurine
2,6-Dimethyl-4-chlorophenol, 970
Dimethyldithiocarbamates, toxicology, 1654

Dimethyl-4-phenylpiperazinium, 213–214
  structural formula, 213
Dimethyltryptamine, 252, 564–566, 633
Dinitroorthocresol, 1654
Dinitrophenols, toxicology, 1654
Dinoprost tromethamine, 939
Dinoprostone, 939
Dioctyl calcium sulfosuccinate, 1009
Dioctyl potassium sulfosuccinate, 1009
Dioctyl sodium sulfosuccinate, 1009
Dioctyl sulfosuccinates. *See* Docusates
DIODRAST (iodopyracet), 931
Dioxyline phosphate, 830
DIPAXIN (diphenadione), 1359
Diphemanil, preparations and structural formula, 130
Diphenadione, 1359. *See also* Anticoagulants, oral
Diphenhydramine, 441, 486
  622, 627. *See also* H$_1$-receptor blockers
  absorption, fate, and elimination, 625
  structural formula, 623
  uses, cough, 530
    parkinsonism, 485
    sedation, 369
Diphenhydramine hydrochloride, preparations and dosage, 628
Diphenoxylate, legal regulations, 1670
  pharmacological properties, preparations, and dosage, 517
  structural formula, 514
  use in diarrhea, 517
Diphenylbutylpiperidines, 397. *See also* Antipsychotic agents
Diphenylhydantoin. *See* Phenytoin
Diphtheria, choice of drugs in, 1088
  erythromycin in, 1140, 1225
  penicillin G in, 1140
Diphtheroid infections, choice of drugs in, 1088
Dipipanone, dosage, 507
  duration of analgesic effect, 507
Dipropylacetic acid, 462
DIPROSONE (betamethasone dipropionate), 1484
Dipyridamole, 830
  effect on platelet aggregation, 1361
Dipyrone, status, 701
Disinfectants, 964–981. *See also* individual agents
  antimicrobial spectra, 966
  desirable properties, 965
  evaluation of activity, 965
  germicidal kinetics, 966
  history, 964
  mechanisms of antimicrobial action, 966
  terminology, 964–965
DISIPAL (orphenadrine hydrochloride), 487
DISOMER (brompheniramine maleate), 628
Disopyramide, 777–779
  absorption, fate, and excretion, 778
  actions/effects on, autonomic nervous system, 778
    cardiac electrophysiology, 768, 778
    electrocardiogram, 768, 778
  chemistry and preparations, 778
  dosage and administration, 778

pharmacokinetics, 1704
toxicity, 779
uses, 778
Disseminated intravascular coagulation, heparin in, 1364
Disulfiram, 387–388
  absorption, fate, and excretion, 388
  administration and dosage, 388
  chemistry and preparation, 388
  history, 387
  mechanism of action, 387–388
  toxic reactions and contraindications, 388
  use in chronic alcoholism, 388, 575
Dithiocarbamates, toxicology, 1654
DIULO (metolazone), 900
Diuretics, 892–915. *See also* Kidney; individual agents
  actions/effects on potassium, 876–877
  antihypertensive action, 803–805
  complications of therapy, 912
  extrarenal sites of action, 893
  high-ceiling, 903–907. *See also* Ethacrynic acid; Furosemide
  localization of site of action, 892–893
  urinary electrolyte composition during diuresis, 898
  use of multiple diuretics and adjuvant agents, 912–913
  uses, antihypertensive, 809–813
    ascites, 911
    cardiac edema, 911
    refractory edema, 912
    renal disease, 912
DIURIL (chlorothiazide), 900
DIURNAL-PENICILLIN (sterile penicillin G procaine suspension), 1137
Diuron, toxicology, 1654
Diverticulitis, bulk-forming laxatives in, 1004, 1011
DMA. *See* Dimethoxyamphetamine
DMPP, 213
DMT. *See* Dimethyltryptamine
Dobutamine, 156–157. *See also* Sympathomimetic drugs
  pharmacological effects, 156
  preparations and dosage, 156
  receptor-type activity, 142
  structural formula, 142
  toxicity and precautions, 156
  uses, 156–157
    shock, 156–157, 169
DOBUTREX (dobutamine hydrochloride), 156
DOCA ACETATE (desoxycorticosterone acetate), 1484
Docusates, 1008–1009
DOET. *See* 2,5-Dimethoxy-4-ethylamphetamine
DOLENE (propoxyphene hydrochloride), 521
DOLOPHINE (methadone), 507, 1670
DOM. *See* 2,5-Dimethoxy-4-methylamphetamine
Domiphen bromide, 978
Dopa, in biosynthetic pathway to norepinephrine, 72
Dopa decarboxylase. *See* Aromatic amino acid decarboxylase

Dopamine, 154–155. *See also* Sympathomimetic drugs
  actions/effects on prolactin secretion, 1382, 1392
  activation of adenylate cyclase in caudate nucleus and limbic system, 401, 402
    blockade by antipsychotic agents, 401, 402
  adrenergic transmitter function, 71
  in biosynthetic pathway to norepinephrine, 72
  metabolic disposition, 479
  pharmacological actions, 154–155
  precautions and contraindications, 155
  preparations and dosage, 155
  receptor-type activity, 142
  role as CNS transmitter, 248, 250–251
  role of deficiency in parkinsonism, 476
  role in ganglionic transmission, 212, 215
  structural formula, 142, 479, 484
  uses, 155
    pheochromocytoma, 155
    refractory congestive heart failure, 155, 169
    shock, 155, 169–170
Dopamine-β-hydroxylase, 72–73, 75, 479
Dopaminergic agonists, use in parkinsonism, 483–484
DOPAR (levodopa), 481
DOPRAM (doxapram hydrochloride), 589
DORBANE (danthron), 1008
DORIDEN (glutethimide), 351, 1671
DORSACAINE (benoxinate hydrochloride), 310
Doxapram, chemistry and actions, 589
  preparations, dosage, and uses, 589
Doxepin. *See also* Tricyclic antidepressants
  pharmacokinetics, 1705
  structural formula, 419
Doxepin hydrochloride, preparations and dosage, 424
DOXINATE (docusate sodium), 1009
Doxorubicin, 1291–1293
  absorption, fate, and excretion, 1292
  chemistry, 1291–1292
  clinical toxicity, 1293
  mechanism of action, 1292
  preparation, dosage, and route of administration, 1293
  use in neoplastic diseases, 1253, 1293
Doxycycline. *See also* Tetracyclines
  absorption, distribution, and excretion, 1184
  dosage, 1185
  pharmacokinetics, 1705
  preparations and administration, 1185
  structural formula, 1181
Doxylamine, use as sedative, 369
Dracontiasis, metronidazole in, 1077
  occurrence and treatment, 1033
DRAMAMINE (dimenhydrinate), 628
Dried aluminum hydroxide gel, 954
DRISDOL (ergocalciferol), 1544
DROLBAN (dromostanolone propionate), 1457
Dromostanolone propionate, 1457
Droperidol, 397, 518
  uses, neurolept analgesia, 295–296
    preanesthetic medication, 270

Drug abuse, 535–578. *See also* individual agents
  alcohol, 551–553, 572, 575
  amphetamine, 553–557
  assessment of abuse potential of drugs, 576
  barbiturates, 549–551, 571, 575
  behavioral modification in management, 573–575
  cannabis, 560–563
  clinical characteristics, 544–569
  CNS sympathomimetics, 553–557
  cocaine, 553–557
  compulsive, 535–536
  definition, 535
  drugs as reinforcers, 537
  genesis, 536–544
  hospitalization and psychotherapy, 573
  hypnotics, 549–551, 571, 575
  learning, conditioning, and relapse, 542–543
  legislation, 577, 1670–1671
  miscellaneous substances, 569
  nicotine, 557–560
  opioids, 544–549, 570–571, 574–575
  phencyclidine, 567–568
  physical dependence, 537–542
    cross-dependence, 541
    theories, 541–542
  psychedelics, 563–567
  risks, 536
  role of medical profession in prevention, 575–577
  sociological factors, 544
  tobacco, 557–560
  tolerance, 537–539
    to alcohol, 538–539
    to hypnotics, 538–539
    to opioids, 538
  treatment, 569–577
  types, 535
  voluntary groups and communities for management, 573
  vulnerability, 543–544
  withdrawal technics, 569–573
Drug addiction, 535–578. *See also* individual agents
  definition, 536
Drug interactions, 1738–1751
  direct chemical, 1738
  direct physical, 1738
  gastrointestinal absorption, 1738–1739
  protein binding, 1739
  receptor site, 1739
  resulting from, accelerated metabolism, 1739–1740
    alteration of pH or electrolyte concentrations, 1740
    inhibition of metabolism, 1740
Drugs. *See also* Therapeutics; Toxicology
  absorption, 5–9
    after oral ingestion, 5–7
    after parenteral injection, 5, 7–8
    after rectal administration, 7
    after sublingual administration, 7
    after timed-release preparations, 7
    after topical application, 8
    factors that modify, 5

  attitude toward new drugs, 53
  binding to plasma proteins, 10–11
  bioavailability, 8–9
  biotransformation, 12–20
    first-pass effect, 13
    hepatic microsomal drug-metabolizing systems, 13–19
    in the neonate, 19
    nonmicrosomal, 19–20
    patterns, 12–13
    relation to toxicity, 18–19
  cellular sites of action, 34–35
  choice of names, 1661
  clearance, 22
  clinical trials, 41–43
  concentrations in plasma, 21–26
  design and optimization of dosage regimens, 1679–1684
    adjusting mean parameters for individual patients, 1682–1683
    drug concentrations and revision of regimens, 1683–1684
    targeting drug concentrations, 1680–1682
  development and evaluation of new drugs, 48–50
  distribution, 9–12
    drug reservoirs, 10–12
    passage into central nervous system, 10
    placental transfer, 12
    protein binding, 10–11
  dose-effect relationship, 35–39, 1602–1603
    biological variation, 37–38
    maximal efficacy, 36
    potency, 36
    probit analysis, 1603
  excretion, 20–21
    biliary and fecal, 20–21
    miscellaneous routes, 21
    renal, 20
  factors modifying effects and/or dosage, 43–48
  half-time of elimination, 22–25
  individualization of therapy, 43–48
  interactions, 45–46, 1605–1606
  mechanisms of action, 28–35. *See also* Receptors
    antagonists, 31–32
    drug receptors, 28–35
    nonreceptor-mediated actions, 35
    quantitative description of drug action, 30–33
  median effective dose, 28
  median lethal dose, 38
  nomenclature, 51–52
  official compendia, 53–54
  official doses, 1668
  pharmacokinetic data, 1684–1737
  pharmacokinetics, 2–26, 1675–1737
    basic concepts, 21–22
    choice of dosage interval, 24–26
    factors influencing, 1677–1679
    impaired elimination, 25–26
    initial loading dose, 25
    parameters, 1675–1677
    repeated doses, 22–24
    single doses, 22

placebo effects, 46–47
poisoning. *See also* Toxicology
  activated charcoal in, 954
  alteration of metabolism or excretion in, 1611–1612
  antagonism or inactivation in, 1612–1613
  antidotes in, 1608–1613
  apomorphine in, 509, 1609
  charcoal in, 1610
  dialysis, hemoperfusion, and exchange transfusion in, 1612
  emesis in, 1609
  gastric lavage in, 1609–1610
  incidence, 1607
  ipecac in, 1609
  prevention and treatment, 1608–1613
  purgation in, 1611
prototypes, 52
receptors, chemical properties, 28 29
  classification, 33–34
  drug-receptor interactions, 30–33
  functional properties, 29–30
  ligand-binding assays, 34
  regulation, 30
regulations, 48
routes of administration, 5–8
  inhalation, 8
  intra-arterial, 8
  intramuscular, 8
  intraperitoneal, 8
  intrathecal, 8
  intravenous, 7
  oral, 6–7
  rectal, 7
  subcutaneous, 8
  sublingual, 7
selectivity, 38–39
sources of information, 53–54
structure-activity relationship, 33
therapy as a science, 40–43
timed-release preparations, 7
tolerance, 47
toxicity, 50–51, 1602–1614
transfer across membranes, 2–5
  carrier-mediated transport, 4–5
  influence of pH, 4
  passive processes, 3–4
United States Adopted Name (USAN), 51, 1661
variation in response, 43–47
  disposition, 43–45
  genetic factors, 47
  interactions, 45–46
  pharmacodynamic factors, 45
  placebo effects, 46–47
  tolerance, 47
volume of distribution, 21–24
DTIC. *See* Dacarbazine
DTIC-DOME (dacarbazine), 1271
Duazomycin, 1284
Ductus arteriosus, closure with aspirin-like drugs, 687, 698
  closure with indomethacin, 707

Duhring's disease, sulfapyridine in, 1116
DULCOLAX (bisacodyl), 1007
DUOTRATE (pentaerythritol tetranitrate), 826
DUPHALAC (lactulose), 1010
DUPHASTON (dydrogesterone), 1437
DURABOLIN (nandrolone phenpropionate), 1457
DURACILLIN A.S. (sterile penicillin G procaine suspension), 1137
DURANEST (etidocaine hydrochloride), 309
Durham-Humphrey Law, 1670
DURICEF (cefadroxil), 1156
Dusting powders, 953
dVDAVP. *See* 1-Deamino-4-valine-8-D-arginine vasopressin
Dwarfism, androgens in, 1459–1460
  growth hormone in, 1378–1379
DYAZIDE (triamterene-hydrochlorothiazide), 909
DYCILL (dicloxacillin sodium), 1143
DYCLONE (diclonine hydrochloride), 310
Dyclonine hydrochloride, 310
Dydrogesterone, 1437
  chemistry, 1434
DYMELOR (acetohexamide), 1513
DYNAPEN (dicloxacillin sodium), 1143
Dyphylline, 592, 601
DYRENIUM (triamterene), 909
Dysentery. *See also* Amebiasis; Colitis; Diarrhea; *Salmonella* infections; *Shigella* infections
  diphenoxylate in, 517
  iodoquinol in, 1065
  opioids in, 513
  sulfonamides in, 1115
Dysmenorrhea, estrogen in, 1430
  ibuprofen in, 713
  indomethacin in, 707
  mefenamic acid in, 709
  progestins in, 1438
  salicylates in, 697
Dystonic reactions, from antipsychotic drugs, 407, 412

E-605 (parathion), 104
ECHODIDE (echothiophate iodide for ophthalmic solution), 112
Echothiophate. *See also* Anticholinesterases
  preparations, 112
  structural formula, 105
  use in glaucoma, 113
Eclampsia, antihypertensive drugs in, 812
  magnesium sulfate in, 882
  paraldehyde in, 368
Ectoparasiticides, 985. *See also* individual agents
Eczema, permanganates in, 974
  resorcinol in, 968
  sulfur in, 981
  tars in, 970
  zinc oxide in, 977
Eczema vaccinatum, methisazone in, 1242
EDECRIN (ethacrynic acid), 906
EDECRIN SODIUM (ethacrynic sodium for injection), 906

Edema. *See also* Cardiac failure; Diuretics
  diuretics in, 911–913
  pathological physiology, 911
Edetate calcium disodium, absorption, fate, and ex-
    cretion, 1620
  mechanism of action, 1620
  preparations, routes of administration, and dos-
    age, 1621
  toxicity, 1621
  uses, cadmium poisoning, 1633
    diagnosis of lead poisoning, 1619
    treatment of lead poisoning, 1621–1622
Edetate disodium, 1529, 1621
  uses, cardiac arrhythmias, 1621
    hypercalcemia, 1621
Edrophonium. *See also* Anticholinesterases
  preparations, 112
  structural formula, 104
  uses, diagnosis of myasthenia gravis, 115
    paroxysmal tachycardia, 112
E.E.S. (erythromycin ethylsuccinate), 1224
E-FEROL (alpha-tocopherol), 1598
EFUDEX (topical fluorouracil), 1279
Eicosatetraynoic acid, 670, 671
ELASE (fibrinolysin-deoxyribonuclease), 962
ELAVIL (amitriptyline hydrochloride), 424
ELDOPAQUE (hydroquinone ointment), 959
ELDOQUIN (hydroquinone cream), 959
Electroconvulsive therapy, curarimimetic drugs in,
    231–232
Electrolytes. *See* Body fluids; individual electrolytes
Elixirs, 1668–1669
ELSPAR (asparaginase), 1297
Elymoclavine, 942
Emesis, phenothiazines in, 417–418
  use in drug poisoning, 1609
Emetics. *See* individual agents
Emetine, 1065–1066
  absorption, fate, and excretion, 1065
  chemistry and preparations, 1065
  history, 1065
  mechanism of amebicidal action, 1065
  routes of administration and dosage, 1066
  toxicity and side effects, 1065–1066
  uses, amebiasis, 1062, 1066
    fluke infections, 1035
Emetine hydrochloride, use in fluke infections, 1035
Emollients, 952–953
Emphysema, tetracyclines in, 1191
Empyema, choice of drugs in, 1086
  streptokinase-streptodornase in, 961
E-MYCIN (erythromycin), 1223
Encephalitis, levodopa in, 487
  viral, choice of drugs in, 1093
Encephalomyelopathy, thiamine in, 1563
ENDEP (amitriptyline hydrochloride), 424
Endocarditis, choice of drugs in, 1086
  gentamicin in, 1175
  penicillin in, 1138
  prevention, penicillin G in, 1141
  streptomycin in, 1173
  trimethoprim-sulfamethoxazole in, 1119

Endometrial carcinoma, progestins in, 1301
Endometriosis, androgens in, 1460
  progestins in, 1438
Endorphins, 495, 497–498, 1388, 1389
  role as CNS transmitter, 253
ENDRATE (edetate disodium), 1621
Endrin, toxicology, 1649
ENDURON (methyclothiazide), 900
Enflurane, 283–286. *See also* Anesthesia
  actions/effects on, heart and circulation, 284
    kidney, 285
    liver, 285
    muscle, 285
    nervous system, 284–285
    respiration, 284
    uterus, 285
  advantages, uses, and status, 286
  chemistry and preparations, 283
  disadvantages and limitations, 286
  general anesthetic actions, 283–284
  metabolism and excretion, 285
  pharmacological properties, 283–286
  physical properties, 277, 283
  structural formula, 277
  tension in arterial blood, 261
Enkephalins, 495, 497–498, 663, 1388, 1389
  role as CNS transmitter, 253
ENOVID-E, 1440
ENOVID 5 MG, 1440
ENOVID 10 MG, 1440
ENTAMIDE (diloxanide), 1067
Entamoeba infections. *See* Amebiasis
Enterobacter aerogenes infections, amikacin in, 1176
  carbenicillin in, 1147
  choice of drugs in, 1089
  gentamicin in, 1174
  kanamycin in, 1176
  tetracyclines in, 1190
Enterobiasis, occurrence and treatment, 1032
Enterococcal infections. *See also Streptococcus fae-
    calis* infections
  choice of drugs in, 1086
  gentamicin in, 1175
  penicillin G in, 1138
Enuresis, belladonna alkaloids in, 136
  sympathomimetic drugs in, 172
  tricyclic antidepressants in, 427
Ephedrine, 163–164. *See also* Sympathomimetic
    drugs
  history, 163
  pharmacological actions, 163
  preparations, administration, and dosage, 163–164
  receptor-type activity, 142
  structural formula, 142
  toxic reactions, 164
  uses, 164
    bronchial asthma, 170–171
    enuresis, 172
    hypotensive states, 169
    motion sickness, 629
    narcolepsy, 171
    nasal decongestion, 168

ophthalmic, 171
Epicillin, 1145
Epidermal growth factor, 1376
Epidermophyton infections. *See* Tinea infections
Epididymitis, tetracyclines in, 1190
Epiglottitis, choice of drugs in, 1090
Epilepsy, 448–471. *See also* Status epilepticus
  acetazolamide in, 468
  adrenocorticosteroids in, 470
  carbamazepine in, 460, 469–470
  carbon dioxide in, 334
  carbonic anhydrase inhibitors in, 899
  classification, 448–449
  clonazepam in, 467, 470
  corticotropin in, 470
  definition, 448
  dextroamphetamine in, 172
  diazepam in, 467, 470–471
  drug therapy, 468–471
    in pregnancy, 471
  duration of drug therapy, 469
  ethosuximide in, 462, 470
  ethotoin in, 456
  mechanism of anticonvulsant drug actions, 450–451
  mephenytoin in, 456, 469
  mephobarbital in, 458
  metharbital in, 458
  methsuximide in, 462
  nature and mechanism of seizures, 448, 450
  paramethadione in, 465
  pentylenetetrazol in diagnosis, 588
  phenacemide in, 467
  phenobarbital in, 457, 469–470
  phensuximide in, 462
  phenytoin in, 455, 469–470
  plasma drug concentrations in, 452, 469
  primidone in, 459, 469–470
  principles of therapy, 451, 468–469
  relation of chemical structure to antiepileptic selectivity, 451
  seizure types and characteristics, 449
  trimethadione in, 465, 469
  valproic acid in, 464, 469–470
Epinephrine, 144–151. *See also* Autonomic nervous system; Sympathomimetic drugs
  absorption, fate, and excretion, 150
  actions/effects on, blood pressure, 144–145
    cardiac rhythm, 147–148
    central nervous system, 149
    cerebral circulation, 146
    coronary circulation, 146–147
    ECG, 148
    eye, 150
    heart, 147–148
    metabolism, 78–80, 149–150
    neuromuscular junction, 150
    respiration, 149
    secretory glands, 150
    smooth muscle, 148
    uterus, 148
    vascular beds, 145–147
  adrenergic transmitter function, 71
  arrhythmias from, 147–148, 151
  biosynthetic pathway, 72
  contraindications, 151
  cyclic AMP and, 78–80
  hyperglycemia, 78–80
  metabolic disposition, 76–77
  preparations, dosage, and administration, 151
  receptor-type activity, 142
  role as CNS transmitter, 249–251
  structural formula, 142
  synthesis, storage, and release, 71–75
  toxicity and side effects, 151
  uses, 151
    allergic disorders, 170–171
    bronchial asthma, 170–171
    cardiac arrest, 170
    glaucoma, 113, 171
    local anesthesia, 169
    shock, 169–170
    Stokes-Adams syndrome, 170
    superficial hemorrhage, 168
Epinine, 143
  structural formula, 142
EPN, 105
Epsom salt, 1005
EQUANIL (meprobamate), 351, 1671
Ergocalciferol, 1539, 1544
Ergocornine, structural formula, 941
Ergocristine, structural formula, 941
Ergokryptine, structural formula, 941
Ergolines, 483–484
ERGOMAR (ergotamine tartrate), 946
Ergometrine, structural formula, 941
Ergonovine. *See also* Ergot alkaloids
  actions/effects on, cardiovascular system, 944
    uterus, 944
  preparations, 946
  structural formula, 941
Ergonovine maleate, uses, diagnosis of variant angina, 828
Ergopeptines, 942
Ergosine, structural formula, 941
ERGOSTAT (ergotamine tartrate), 946
Ergosterol, 1539
Ergostine, 941
Ergot. *See also* Ergot alkaloids
  constituents, 940
  history, 940
  poisoning, 945–946
  source, 939–940
Ergot alkaloids, 185, 939–947. *See also* individual agents
  absorption, fate, and excretion, 945
  actions/effects on, cardiovascular system, 185, 944
    metabolism, 185
    uterus, 944
  chemistry, 185, 940–942
  comparative actions, 942–943
  contraindications, 947
  dihydrogenated, preparations, 946
  pharmacological properties, 185

Ergot alkaloids (*Cont.*)
  preparations, dosage, and administration, 946
  toxicity and side effects, 185, 945–946
  uses, migraine, 946–947
    senile dementia, 947
    third stage of labor and puerperium, 948–949
Ergotamine. *See also* Ergot alkaloids
  actions/effects on, cardiovascular system, 944
    uterus, 944
  preparations, 946
  structural formula, 941
Ergotoxine, 941, 942
ERGOTRATE (ergonovine maleate), 946
Erysipelas, choice of drugs in, 1086
Erysipeloid, choice of drugs in, 1088
  penicillin G in, 1140
Erysipelothrix rhusiopathiae infections, choice of
    drugs in, 1088
Erythrityl tetranitrate. *See also* Nitrates
  preparations, routes of administration, and dos-
    age, 826
  structural formula, 826
ERYTHROCIN ETHYL SUCCINATE-I.M. (erythromycin
    ethylsuccinate injection), 1224
ERYTHROCIN LACTOBIONATE (erythromycin lactobio-
    nate for injection), 1224
ERYTHROCIN STEARATE (erythromycin stearate), 1224
Erythrohydroxynonyladenine, 1283
Erythroidine, structural formula, 221
Erythromycin, 1222–1225. *See also* Antimicrobial
    agents
  absorption, distribution, and excretion, 1223
  antibacterial activity, 1222
  dosage, 1224
  history and source, 1222
  mechanism of action, 1222–1223
  pharmacokinetics, 1706
  preparations and administration, 1223–1224
  structural formula, 1222
  toxicity, 1224
  uses, amebiasis, 1068
    diphtheria, 1140, 1225
    gonorrhea, 1225
    Legionnaires' disease, 1225
    Mycoplasma pneumoniae pneumonia, 1225
    pertussis, 1225
    pneumococcal infections, 1225
    rheumatic fever prophylaxis, 1225
    staphylococcal infections, 1225
    streptococcal infections, 1225
    syphilis, 1225
    tetanus, 1225
Escharotics, actions and uses, 956
Escherichia coli infections, amikacin in, 1176
  ampicillin in, 1145
  carbenicillin in, 1147
  choice of drugs in, 1088
  gentamicin in, 1174–1175
  kanamycin in, 1176
  sulfonamides in, 1114
  tetracyclines in, 1190
  trimethoprim-sulfamethoxazole in, 1118

Eserine. *See* Physostigmine
ESIDREX (hydrochlorothiazide), 900
ESKALITH (lithium carbonate), 433
Esophageal varices, antidiuretic hormone in, 924
Esophagitis, antacids in, 997
Esterified estrogens, 1428
ESTINYL (ethinyl estradiol), 1428
Estradiol. *See also* Estrogens
  preparations, 1428
Estradiol-17β, 1420
ESTRADURIN (polyestradiol phosphate), 1428
Estriol, 1420
Estrogens, 1420–1431. *See also* individual agents
  absorption, fate, and excretion, 1427
  actions/effects on, adenohypophysis, 1423–1425
    antithrombin III activity, 1350
    menstruation, 1425
    plasma lipids, 845
  assay, 1427
  biosynthesis, 1420–1421
    relationship to cyclic AMP, 1420
    role in men, 1450
  carcinogenic action, 1426
  chemistry, 1420–1422
  choice of preparations, 1428–1429
  history, 1420
  mechanism of action, 1426
  metabolic actions, 1425
  physiological functions, 1422–1426
  preparations, 1428
  untoward responses, 1429
  uses, acne, 1430
    atrophic vaginitis, 1430
    carcinoma of the breast, 1431
    contraception, 1438–1444
    coronary atherosclerosis, 1431
    dysfunctional uterine bleeding, 1430
    dysmenorrhea, 1430
    failure of ovarian development, 1430
    hirsutism, 1431
    kraurosis vulvae, 1430
    menopause, 1429
    neoplastic diseases, 1254, 1303–1304
    osteoporosis, 1431
    suppression of lactation, 1431
Estrone, 1421. *See also* Estrogens
  preparations, 1428
Ethacrynic acid, 903–907
  absorption, distribution, and excretion, 903
  chemistry and structure-activity relationship, 903
  clinical toxicity, 905–906
  comparative diuretic action, 905
  effect on composition of extracellular fluid, 905
  extrarenal sites of action, 905
  mechanism of diuretic action, 904–905
  preparations, 906
  uses, acute pulmonary edema, 906
    diuretic, 906–907
    hypercalcemia, 907
Ethambutol, 1206–1207
  absorption, distribution, and excretion, 1206
  antibacterial activity, 1206

chemistry, 1206
dosage, 1207
history, 1206
pharmacokinetics, 1706
preparations and routes of administration, 1207
untoward effects, 1207
use in tuberculosis, 1207, 1212–1213
ETHAMIDE (ethoxzolamide), 898
Ethamivan, chemistry and actions, 589
Ethamoxytriphetol, 1432
Ethanol. See Ethyl alcohol
Ethaverine, 830
Ethchlorvynol, 363–364
absorption and fate, 363
central effects, 363
chemistry, 363
dosage, half-life, and preparations, 350
legal regulations, 1671
side effects, intoxication, and abuse, 363–364
Ether. See Diethylether
Ethinamate, dosage, half-life, and preparations, 350
legal regulations, 1671
properties, 368–369
Ethinyl estradiol, 1422, 1428. See also Estrogens
in oral contraceptives, 1440
use in neoplastic diseases, 1254, 1303–1304
Ethinylestrenol, chemistry, 1434
Ethionamide, 1208–1209
Ethisterone, 1433
chemistry, 1434
ETHNINE (pholcodine), 507
Ethoheptazine, actions, preparations, dosage, and use, 517–518
Ethopropazine, 397
chemistry, preparations, and dosage, 486
use in parkinsonism, 484–485
Ethosuximide, absorption, distribution, biotransformation, and excretion, 461
anticonvulsant properties, 461
dosage, 461
pharmacokinetics, 1707
plasma concentrations, 461–462
preparations, 461
structural formula, 460
toxicity, 461
use in epilepsy, 462, 470
Ethotoin, 456
Ethoxzolamide, 897–898
ETHRANE (enflurane), 283
ETHRIL (erythromycin stearate), 1224
Ethyl alcohol, 376–386
absorption, fate, and excretion, 382–384
abuse, complications, 552–553
prevalence and patterns, 551–552
actions/effects on, blood, 381
body temperature, 379
brain metabolism, 377–378
cardiovascular system, 378
central nervous system, 376–378, 552–553
EEG, 377
endocrine glands, 381
fetal development, 380

gastrointestinal tract, 379–380
incidence of cancer, 381
kidney, 381
liver, 380
longevity and heredity, 380–381
mucous membranes, 376
peripheral nerves, 376
plasma lipoproteins, 378
respiration, 377
sexual functions, 381
skeletal muscle, 378–379
skin, 376
acute hallucinosis, 553
acute intoxication, 384–385
treatment, 384
addiction, 551–553. See also Alcoholism
disulfiram therapy, 575
treatment, 572, 575
concentration in body fluids in relation to intoxication, 384
contraindications to use, 385
cross-dependence, 541
cross-tolerance, 538
delirium tremens, 553, 572
diagnosis of intoxication, 384–385
distribution, 382–383
effects on methanol metabolism, 386
food value, 383
germicidal action, 970
interaction with other drugs, 381–382
metabolism, 383
pharmacokinetics, 1707
physical dependence, 540, 552–553
preparations, 385
tolerance, 384, 538–539, 552–553
uses, antipyretic, 385
external, 385
"head colds," 386
hypnotic, 386
relief of pain, 386
withdrawal symptoms, 553, 572
Ethyl aminobenzoate. See Benzocaine
Ethyl chloride, 291
Ethyl yohimbine, 186
Ethylene, 291
Ethylene dibromide, toxicology, 1652
Ethylene glycol, 952
toxicology, 1646
Ethylene oxide, 981
Ethylenebisdithiocarbamates, toxicology, 1654
Ethylenediaminetetraacetate. See Edetate calcium disodium; Edetate disodium
Ethylenethiourea, toxicology, 1655
Ethylenimine derivatives, use in neoplastic diseases, 1252, 1268
Ethylestrenol, 1434, 1457
Ethylketocyclazocine, 521
Ethylnorepinephrine, pharmacological properties, 154
receptor-type activity, 142
structural formula, 142
Ethylparaben, 969

Ethynodiol diacetate, chemistry, 1434
  in oral contraceptives, 1440
Etidocaine, structural formula, 301
Etidocaine hydrochloride, 309. *See also* Local anesthetics
Etidronate sodium, 1538
ETILON (parathion), 104
Etiocholanolone, 1448, 1449
Etofenamic acid, 708. *See also* Fenamates
Etomidate, 369
Etorphine, 496, 509
  legal regulations, 1670
ETRAFON (perphenazine–amitriptyline hydrochloride), 424
ETRENOL (hycanthone mesylate), 1017
Etryptamine, 428
EURAX (crotamiton), 985
EUTHROID (liotrix), 1406
EVEX (esterified estrogens), 1428
Ewing's tumor, dactinomycin in, 1291
  doxorubicin in, 1293
EXCEL (selenium sulfide lotion), 957
EXNA (benzthiazide), 900
Exophthalmos-producing substance, 1388
Extended insulin zinc suspension, 1508, 1509
EXURATE (benzbromarone), 933
EZON (absorbable dusting powder), 953

False-transmitter concept, 158–159
Familial periodic paralysis, carbonic anhydrase inhibitors in, 899
Fanconi syndrome, from degraded tetracyclines, 1187
  vitamin D in, 1545
FANSIDAR (pyrimethamine-sulfadoxine), 1049
FANZIL (sulfadoxine), 1057
FASIGYN (tinidazole), 1075
Fat emulsion, preparations, 863
Fazadinium, 221, 231. *See also* Neuromuscular blocking agents
Federal Food, Drug, and Cosmetic Act, 48, 1670
Federal Narcotic–Internal Revenue Regulations, 1670
Federal Pure Food and Drug Act, 48
Felypressin, 917
FEMINONE (ethinyl estradiol), 1428
Fenamates, 708–709. *See also* Aspirin-like drugs; individual agents
  absorption, fate, and excretion, 708
  chemistry, 708
  interactions with other drugs, 709
  pharmacological properties, 708
  preparations and dosage, 708
  toxic effects, 708–709
  uses, 709
Fenfluramine, effect on 5-hydroxytryptamine storage, 638
  legal regulations, 1671
  receptor-type activity, 142
  structural formula, 142

use in obesity, 172
Fenoprofen, 712. *See also* Propionic acid derivatives
Fenoterol, 166
Fentanyl, actions, preparations, dosage, and uses, 518
  structural formula, 514
  uses, anesthesia, 295
    neurolept analgesia, 295–296
    preanesthetic medication, 270
Ferbam, toxicology, 1655
Ferric edetate, 1323
Ferritin, 1315, 1316, 1318, 1321
Ferrous fumarate, 1323
Ferrous gluconate, 1323
Ferrous glutamate, 1322
Ferrous lactate, 1323
Ferrous succinate, 1322
Ferrous sulfate, 1322
Ferrum reductum, 1323
Fetal alcohol syndrome, 380
FETAMIN (methamphetamine hydrochloride), 163
Fever, acetaminophen in, 705
  aspirin-like drugs in, 684, 686, 697
  phenacetin in, 705
  role of prostaglandins, 684
  salicylates in, 697
Fibrinolysin-deoxyribonuclease, 962
Fibroblast growth factor, 1376
Filarial worm infections. *See* Filariasis; Onchocerciasis
Filariasis, occurrence and treatment, 1032–1033
FLAGYL (metronidazole), 1076
Flavobacterium meningosepticum infections, choice of drugs in, 1090
Flavonoids, 1560
FLAXEDIL (gallamine triethiodide), 231
FLEXERIL (cyclobenzaprine hydrochloride), 489
Flexible collodion, 953
FLORINEF ACETATE (fludrocortisone), 1484
FLOROPRYL (isoflurophate), 112
Floxacillin, 1142–1143. *See also* Penicillins
Floxuridine, 1278–1280. *See also* Pyrimidine analogs
  absorption, fate, and excretion, 1278–1279
  clinical toxicity, 1279–1280
  general toxicity and cytotoxic action, 1278
  mechanism of action, 1278
  preparations, dosage, and routes of administration, 1279
  use in neoplastic diseases, 1279
Flubendazole, 1018
Flucytosine, 1236–1237
  absorption, distribution, and excretion, 1236–1237
  antifungal activity, 1236
  chemistry, 1236
  dosage, 1237
  pharmacokinetics, 1708
  preparations and administration, 1237
  toxicity, 1237
  use in yeast and fungal infections, 1237, 1239–1240
Fludrocortisone. *See also* Adrenocorticosteroids
  preparations, 1484

relative potency, duration of action, and equivalent dose, 1482
Flufenamic acid, 708. *See also* Fenamates
Fluids. *See* Body fluids
Fluke infections, 1034–1035
other than schistosomiasis, treatment, 1035
Flumethasone. *See also* Adrenocorticosteroids
preparations, 1486
Flunitrazepam. *See also* Benzodiazepines
dosage and half-life, 350
pharmacokinetics, 348, 1708
Fluocinolone. *See also* Adrenocorticosteroids
preparations, 1486
Fluocinonide. *See also* Adrenocorticosteroids
preparations, 1486
FLUONID (fluocinolone acetonide), 1486
Fluoride, 1545–1547
absorption, distribution, and excretion, 1546
acute poisoning, 1546
chronic poisoning, 1546–1547
pharmacological actions, 1546
preparations, 1547
provisional dietary allowance, 1555
use in prevention of dental caries, 1547
Fluoroacetamide, toxicology, 1652
Fluoroacetate, toxicology, 1652
Fluorodeoxyuridine. *See* Floxuridine
Fluorometholone. *See also* Adrenocorticosteroids
preparations, 1486
FLUOROPLEX (topical fluorouracil), 1279
6-Fluorotryptophan, 638
Fluorouracil, 1278–1280. *See also* Pyrimidine analogs
absorption, fate, and excretion, 1278–1279
clinical toxicity, 1279–1280
general toxicity and cytotoxic action, 1278
mechanism of action, 1278
preparations, dosage, and routes of administration, 1279
use in neoplastic diseases, 1252, 1279
FLUOTHANE (halothane), 277
Fluoxetine, 249
Fluoxymesterone, 1456
Flupentixol, 396
Fluphenazine. *See also* Antipsychotic agents
side effects, 409
structural formula, 409
Fluphenazine decanoate, dosage forms, 409
dose as antipsychotic, 409
Fluphenazine enanthate, dosage forms, 409
dose as antipsychotic, 409
Fluphenazine hydrochloride, dosage forms, 409
dose as antipsychotic, 409
Fluprednisolone. *See also* Adrenocorticosteroids
preparations, 1485
Flurandrenolide. *See also* Adrenocorticosteroids
preparations, 1486
Flurazepam. *See also* Benzodiazepines
dosage, half-life, and preparations, 350
legal regulations, 1671
pharmacokinetics, 348
structural formula, 340

Flurbiprofen, 712–713. *See also* Propionic acid derivatives
FLUROBATE (betamethasone benzoate), 1484
Fluroxene, 291
Fluspirilene, 397
Fly agaric, 569
Folic acid, 1340–1344. *See also* Anemia—megaloblastic
absorption, distribution, and elimination, 1341–1342
administration and dosage, 1343–1344
chemistry, 1340
deficiency, 1342
history, 1331
human requirements, 1341
interrelations with cyanocobalamin, 1331–1333
metabolic functions, 1340–1341
plasma concentrations, 1342
preparations, 1343
recommended dietary allowance, 1553
role in sulfonamide action, 1108
sources in nature, 1341
structural formula, 1340
terminology, 1340
toxicity, 1343
uses, 1343–1344
Folic acid analogs, use in neoplastic diseases, 1252, 1272–1276
FOLIDOL (parathion), 104
Folinic acid, 1343
uses, leucovorin "rescue" in methotrexate therapy, 1273, 1275
Follicle-stimulating hormone, 1383–1387. *See also* Gonadotropic hormones
chemical properties, 1371
concentration during menstrual cycle, 1424
relationship with estrogens and progestins, 1423–1425
FOLLUTEIN (chorionic gonadotropin for injection), 1386
FOLVITE (folic acid), 1343
FORANE (isoflurane), 288
Formaldehyde, 970–971
toxicology, 1641
Francisella tularensis infections, choice of drugs in, 1090
FREAMINE (amino acid injection), 863
FROBEN (flurbiprofen), 712
Fructose injection, 861
Fructose and sodium chloride injection, 861
FSH. *See* Follicle-stimulating hormone
FUADIN (stibophen), 1030
FULVICIN P/G (griseofulvin), 1238
FULVICIN U/F (griseofulvin), 1238
Fumigants, toxicology, 1651–1652
Fungal infections. *See* Mycotic infections
Fungicides, toxicology, 1654–1655
FUNGIZONE (amphotericin B), 1234
FURACIN (nitrofurazone), 979
FURADANTIN (nitrofurantoin), 1122
Furaltadone, use in trypanosomiasis, 1074
FURAMIDE (diloxanide furoate), 1067

Furosemide, 903–907
    absorption, distribution, and excretion, 903
    antihypertensive action, 805
    chemistry and structure-activity relationship, 903
    clinical toxicity, 905–906
    comparative diuretic action, 905
    effect on composition of extracellular fluid, 905
    effect on renal blood flow, 905
    extrarenal sites of action, 905
    mechanism of diuretic action, 904–905
    pharmacokinetics, 1709
    preparations, 906
    uses, acute pulmonary edema, 906
        antihypertensive, 810, 812
        diuretic, 906–907
        hypercalcemia, 907
Furunculosis, bacitracin in, 1232
Fusobacterium infections, clindamycin in, 1227
Fusobacterium nucleatum infections, choice of drugs in, 1091
Fusospirochetal infections, penicillin G in, 1140

GABA. *See* Gamma-aminobutyrate.
Gallamine. *See also* Neuromuscular blocking agents
    preparations and dosage, 231
    structural formula, 221
Gallstones, hydrocholeretics for, 999
Gamma-aminobutyrate (GABA), role as CNS transmitter, 246–248. *See also* Central nervous system, neurotransmitters
    role in ganglionic transmission, 215
Gamma benzene hexachloride. *See* Lindane
GAMMACORTEN (dexamethasone), 1484
Ganglionic blocking agents, 215–217
    absorption, fate, and excretion, 217
    chemistry and structure-activity relationship, 215–216
    drug classes, 212
    history, 215
    pharmacological properties, 216–217
    preparations, administration, and dosage, 217
    untoward effects and toxicity, 217
    uses, 217
Ganglionic stimulating agents, 212–215. *See also* individual agents
Ganglionic transmission, 211–212
Ganja, 560
GANTANOL (sulfamethoxazole), 1111
GANTRISIN (sulfisoxazole), 1111
GARAMYCIN (gentamicin sulfate), 1173
Gas emboli, hyperbaric oxygen in, 331
Gas gangrene, choice of drugs in, 1088
    hyperbaric oxygen in, 331
    penicillin G in, 1140
Gasoline, toxicology, 1644–1645
Gastric achlorhydria, glutamic acid hydrochloride in, 998
    hydrochloric acid in, 998
Gastric antacids, 988–998. *See also* individual agents
    actions and effects, 988–990
    choice of preparations, 996–997

    dosage and dose intervals, 996
    drug interactions, 989–990
    mixtures, preparations and dosage, 991, 995
        status, 995
    nonsystemic, 989
    pH-related adverse effects, 989
    systemic, 989
    use in peptic ulcer, 995–997
Gastric hypersecretion, cimetidine in, 632
Gastric inhibitory polypeptide, effect on insulin secretion, 1500
Gastric lavage, use in drug poisoning, 1609–1610
Gastrin, 663
    effect on insulin secretion, 1500
    role as CNS transmitter, 253
Gastroenteritis, acute infections, choice of drugs in, 1089
Gastrointestinal atony, bethanechol in, 95
    neostigmine in, 113
GAVISCON, 995, 997
Gelatin, 953
Gelatin sponge, 955
GELFOAM (absorbable gelatin sponge), 955
GELTABS (ergocalciferol), 1544
GELUSIL, 991
GELUSIL-II, 991
GEMONIL (metharbital), 458
General anesthesia. *See* Anesthesia; individual agents
Genital infections, choice of drugs in, 1087, 1090, 1091, 1092
Gentamicin, 1173–1175. *See also* Aminoglycoside antibiotics; Antimicrobial agents
    pharmacokinetics, 1709
    preparations, administration, and dosage, 1173
    structural formula, 1163
    untoward effects, 1174
    uses, combined with carbenicillin, 1174–1175
        enterococcal infections, 1175
        gram-negative microbial infections, 1174–1175
        infected burns, 1175
        meningitis, 1175
        methicillin-resistant staphylococcal infections, 1175
        peritonitis, 1175
        pneumonia, 1174
        sepsis, 1174, 1175
        urinary tract infections, 1174
Gentian violet, 979
Gentisic acid, 694
GENTRAN (dextran 75 injection), 862
GENTRAN 40 (dextran 40 injection), 862
GENTRAN 75 AND 10% TRAVERT (6% dextran 75–10% invert sugar), 1361
GEOCILLIN (carbenicillin indanyl sodium), 1146
GEOPEN (carbenicillin disodium), 1146
GERMANIN (suramin sodium), 1070
GESTEROL (progesterone injection), 1437
GESTEROL AQUEOUS (progesterone suspension), 1437
Giardiasis, chloroquine in, 1045
    iodoquinol in, 1065
    metronidazole in, 1077

quinacrine in, 1070
Gilles de la Tourette's syndrome, haloperidol in, 418
Gingivitis, choice of drugs in, 1091
Glacial acetic acid, 956
Glanders, choice of drugs in, 1090
Glauber's salt, 1005
Glaucoma, aceclidine in, 98
  acetazolamide in, 113
  carbachol in, 96
  carbonic anhydrase inhibitors in, 899
  demecarium in, 113
  echothiophate in, 113
  epinephrine in, 113, 171
  glycerol in, 113
  guanethidine in, 201
  isoflurophate in, 113–114
  mannitol in, 113, 896
  methacholine in, 96
  phenylephrine in, 113, 171
  physostigmine in, 113
  pilocarpine in, 98, 113
  precipitation by belladonna alkaloids, 123–124, 134
  timolol in, 113–114, 195
  types, 113
  untoward effects of drug therapy, 114
GLAUCOSTAT (aceclidine), 98
Gliomas, nitrosoureas in, 1270, 1271
Globin zinc insulin injection, 1508, 1509
Glossopharyngeal neuralgia, carbamazepine in, 460
Glucagon, 1517–1518
  assay, 1517
  chemistry, 1517
  distribution and inactivation, 1518
  effect on insulin secretion, 1500
  history, 1517
  physiological and pharmacological actions, 78–79, 1518
  preparations, 1518
  regulation of secretion, 1517–1518
  uses, cardiac disorders, 1518
    hypoglycemia, 1518
    intestinal relaxation, 1518
    shock, 169
GLUCANTIME (meglumine antimonate), 1074
Glucose-6-phosphate dehydrogenase, role in drug-induced hemolytic anemias, 1053
Glucosulfone, 1214
Glue sniffing, 568
Glutamate, role as CNS transmitter, 247–248
Glutamic acid, use in ammonia intoxication, 870
Glutamic acid decarboxylase, 247
Glutamic acid diethylester, 247, 248
Glutamic acid hydrochloride, 998
Glutaraldehyde, 971
Glutethimide, 364–365
  absorption and fate, 364
  abuse, 365
  chemistry, 364
  dosage, half-life, and preparations, 351
  legal regulations, 1671
  pharmacological actions, 364

toxicity, 364–365
Glycerin, 895, 896, 951–952
  diuretic action, 895
  preparations and dosage, 896
  toxicity, 896
  uses, 896
    glaucoma, 113
Glycerin oral solution, 952
Glycerin suppositories, 952
Glycerol, 951
Glyceryl trinitrate. See Nitroglycerin
Glycine, role as CNS transmitter, 247–248
Glycols, toxicology, 1646–1647
Glycopyrrolate, preparations and structural formula, 130
  uses, preanesthetic medication, 271
Glycyrrhiza, 951
GLYROL (glycerin), 896
GLYSENNID (sennosides A and B), 1007
Goiter, nodular, thyroid hormones in, 1408
  nontoxic, iodide in prophylaxis, 1403
    thyroid hormones in, 1408
Gold, 713–717
  absorption, distribution, and excretion, 714–715
  chemistry, 714
  contraindications, 717
  pharmacological actions, 714
  preparations and dosage, 715
  toxicity, 715–716
  uses, 716–717
    pruritus, 713
    rheumatoid arthritis, 716–717
Gold-198, 1305
Gold sodium thiomalate, 714, 715. See also Gold
Gonadotropic hormones, 1383–1387. See also individual gonadotropins
  absorption, fate, and excretion, 1385–1386
  actions/effects on, ovary, 1384
    testis, 1384–1385
  assays, 1386
  chemistry, 1371, 1383
  general considerations, 1383
  hypothalamic regulation, 1390–1391
  mechanism of action, 1385
  preparations and dosage, 1386
  role in, androgen synthesis, 1449–1450
    spermatogenesis, 1449–1450
  secretion, 1383–1384
  uses, cryptorchism, 1387
    infertility, 1386–1387
Gonadotropin of pregnant mares' serum, 1383, 1386
Gonadotropin-releasing hormone, 1391, 1423
Gonococcal infections. See also Neisseria gonorrhoeae infections
  choice of drugs in, 1087
  erythromycin in, 1225
  penicillins in, 1139
  prophylaxis, penicillin G in, 1141
  spectinomycin in, 1228
  tetracyclines in, 1190
  trimethoprim-sulfamethoxazole in, 1119
Gout, allopurinol in, 722, 723

Gout (*Cont.*)
  benzbromarone in, 722–723
  colchicine in, 719–720, 723
  general considerations, 717–718
  indomethacin in, 706, 723
  oxyphenbutazone in, 700
  phenylbutazone in, 700, 723
  probenecid in, 722–723
  salicylates in, 691
  selection of drugs for, 723
  sulfinpyrazone in, 722–723
Grand mal. *See* Epilepsy
Granulocytic leukemia, busulfan in, 1269
  cytarabine in, 1281
  daunorubicin in, 1293
  doxorubicin in, 1293
  hydroxyurea in, 1299
  mercaptopurine in, 1286
  mitomycin in, 1297
  thioguanine in, 1287
Granuloma inguinale, choice of drugs in, 1091
  streptomycin in, 1173
  tetracyclines in, 1190
Granulomatous colitis, sulfasalazine in, 1112
GRIFULVIN V (griseofulvin), 1238
GRISACTIN (griseofulvin), 1238
Griseofulvin, 1237–1238. *See also* Antifungal drugs
  absorption, distribution, and excretion, 1238
  antifungal properties, 1237
  history and source, 1237
  preparations, administration, and dosage, 1238
  structural formula, 1237
  toxicity, 1238
  use in mycotic infections, 1238
GRIS-PEG (griseofulvin), 1238
Growth hormone, 1372–1380
  actions/effects on, carbohydrate metabolism, 1374–1376
    growth, 1373–1374
    lipid metabolism, 1374–1376
    nitrogen metabolism, 1374
  assays, 1378
  chemical properties, 1371, 1372–1373
  hypothalamic regulation, 1391–1392
  regulation of secretion, 1377–1378
  use, 1378–1380
Growth hormone release-inhibiting hormone, 1391
Growth hormone–releasing factor, 1391
Guanethidine, 198–201
  absorption, fate, and excretion, 200
  actions/effects on, cardiovascular system, 199–200
    gastrointestinal tract, 200
  mechanism of antiadrenergic action, 74–75, 82, 198–199
  pharmacological properties, 199–201
  preparations, routes of administration, and dosage, 200
  structural formula, 198
  toxicity, side effects, and precautions, 200
  uses, antihypertensive, 811
    glaucoma, 201
Guinea worm infections. *See* Dracontiasis

Gum arabic, 951
Gum tragacanth, 951
Guvacine, 247, 248
GYNE-LOTRIMIN (clotrimazole), 983
GYNERGEN (ergotamine tartrate), 946
GYNOREST (dydrogesterone), 1437

Haemophilus ducreyi infections, choice of drugs in, 1090
Haemophilus influenzae infections, ampicillin in, 1145
  cephalosporins in, 1157
  chloramphenicol in, 1195
  choice of drugs in, 1090
  trimethoprim-sulfamethoxazole in, 1119
Hageman factor, role in kinin synthesis, 660–661
Hairs, giant, 1169
Halazone, 974
Halcinonide. *See also* Adrenocorticosteroids
  preparations, 1486
HALCION (triazolam), 350
HALDOL (haloperidol), 410
HALDRONE (paramethasone acetate), 1485
HALOG (halcinonide), 1486
Haloperidol. *See also* Antipsychotic agents
  dose as antipsychotic, 410
  preparations and dosage, 410
  side effects, 410
  structural formula, 410
Haloprogin, 983–984
HALOTESTIN (fluoxymesterone), 1456
HALOTEX (haloprogin), 984
Halothane, 277–283. *See also* Anesthesia
  actions/effects on, cardiovascular system, 278–280
    kidney, 281–282
    liver, 282
    muscle, 281
    nervous system, 281
    respiration, 280–281
    uterus, 281
  advantages, uses, and status, 283
  anesthetic actions, 278
  chemistry and preparations, 277–278
  disadvantages and limitations, 283
  history, 259
  metabolism and excretion, 282–283
  pharmacological properties, 278–283
  physical properties, 277–278
  structural formula, 277
  tension in arterial blood, 261
HANSOLAR (acedapsone), 1047
Hashish, 560
Hay fever, antihistamines in, 627
  belladonna alkaloids in, 134
  sympathomimetic drugs in, 168
Headache. *See also* Migraine
  acetaminophen in, 705
  methysergide in, 639
  phenacetin in, 705
  salicylates in, 697
  xanthines in, 603

Heart block. *See also* Cardiac arrhythmias
  sympathomimetic drugs in, 170
Heart failure. *See* Cardiac failure
Heavy-metal antagonists, 1615–1637. *See also* individual agents
Heavy metals, 1615–1637. *See also* individual metals
  general considerations, 1615–1616
HEDULIN (phenindione), 1359
Helium, 334–335
Helminthiasis, 1031–1035. *See also* individual infections
Hematoma, streptokinase-streptodornase in, 961
Hemicholinium, 81–82
  mechanism of action, 81
Hemiplegia, dantrolene in, 489
Hemoglobin, iron content of, 1316
Hemoglobin A₁C, 1503
Hemolytic anemia. *See* Anemia—hemolytic
Hemoperfusion, use in drug poisoning, 1612
Hemorrhage, albumin in, 870
  dextran in, 860, 861
  plasma in, 860
  surface, epinephrine in, 168
Hemorrhoids, sclerosing agents in, 956
Hemosiderin, 1316
Hemostasis, 1347
Hemostatics, absorbable, 955
Hemothorax, streptokinase-streptodornase in, 961
Heparan sulfate, 1349
Heparin, 1348–1353. *See also* Anticoagulants
  absorption, fate, and excretion, 1350
  actions/effects on, blood cells, 1350
    blood coagulation, 1349–1350
    lipoprotein lipase, 1350
    miscellaneous systems, 1350
  antagonists, 1352
  chemistry, 1349
  dosage, 1351
    for prophylaxis of thrombosis and embolism, 1351, 1363
  history, 1348–1349
  laboratory control, 1360
  occurrence and physiological function, 1349
  pharmacokinetics, 1710
  routes of administration, 1351
  side effects, toxicity, and contraindications, 1351–1352
  unitage and preparations, 1351
  uses, 1362–1364
Heparinoids, 1349
HEPATHROM (heparin sodium injection), 1351
Hepatic coma, kanamycin in, 1177
  lactulose in, 1010
  levodopa in, 487
  neomycin in, 1010, 1178
Hepatic microsomal drug-metabolizing systems, glucuronide synthesis, 14, 16
  induction, 17–18
  inhibition, 16–17
  oxidation, 14, 16
Hepatic necrosis, adrenocorticosteroids in, 1491
Hepatitis, adrenocorticosteroids in, 1491

Hepatolenticular degeneration, penicillamine in, 1628
Hepatoma, fluorouracil in, 1280
Heptachlor, toxicology, 1649
HEPTALGIN (phenadoxone), 507
Herbicides, toxicology, 1653–1654
Heroin. *See also* Opioids
  abuse, legal regulations, 1670
  acute poisoning, narcotic antagonists in, 510, 525
  addiction, treatment, 570–571, 574–575
  dosage, 507
  duration of analgesic effect, 507
  fate and excretion, 506–507
  physical dependence, 539, 546–549
  structural formula, 496
  tolerance, 538, 546–549
  withdrawal symptoms, 546–549
Herpes simplex virus infections, choice of drugs in, 1093
  cytarabine in, 1242
  idoxuridine in, 1240
  vidarabine in, 1242
Herpes zoster virus infections, vidarabine in, 1242
HERPLEX (idoxuridine), 1240
Hetacillin, 1145. *See also* Ampicillin; Penicillins
Hetastarch, 861
Hetastarch injection, 862
HETRAZAN (diethylcarbamazine citrate), 1015
Hexachlorobenzene, toxicology, 1655
Hexacholorophene, 968–969
HEXADROL PHOSPHATE (dexamethasone sodium phosphate), 1485
Hexafluorenium, interaction with succinylcholine, 231
  preparation, dosage, and use, 231
Hexamethonium, 215–217. *See also* Ganglionic blocking agents
  structural formula, 213
Hexamethylmelamine, 1268
Hexestrol, 1428
Hexobarbital. *See also* Barbiturates
  chemistry, 351
  dosage, half-life, and preparations, 350
  pharmacokinetics, 1710
Hexocyclium, preparations and structural formula, 130
Hexylcaine hydrochloride, 310
Hexylresorcinol, 968
HIBICLENS (chlorhexidine gluconate), 975
HIBITANE (chlorhexidine gluconate), 975
Hiccough, carbon dioxide in, 334
  phenothiazines in, 418
High-ceiling diuretics, 903–907
HIPREX (methenamine hippurate), 1120
Hirsutism, estrogens in, 1431
HISTALOG (betazole hydrochloride), 620
Histamine, 609–619
  absorption, fate, and excretion, 618–619
  actions/effects on, adrenal medulla and ganglia, 613
    blood pressure, 612
    capillaries, 611

Histamine (*Cont.*)
  cardiovascular system, 611–612
  central nervous system, 613–614
  exocrine glands, 613
  extravascular smooth muscle, 612–613
  heart, 612
  leukocytes, 614
  nerve endings, 613
  regional circulation, 612
  vascular tissue *in vitro,* 612
 activation of adenylate cyclase, 614
 chemistry, 609–610
 endogenous, 615–618
  distribution, 615
  functions, 615–618
  inhibition of allergic release, 620–621
  mechanism of release, 615–617
  origin, synthesis, and storage, 615
  release in anaphylaxis and allergy, 615–616
  release by drugs, peptides, and venoms, 616–617
  release by physical or chemical insult, 617
  role in gastric secretion, 617
  role in growths of mast cells and basophils, 618
  role in headache, 618
  role in microcirculation, 617
  role in nervous system, 618
  role in tissue growth and repair, 617
 H_1 and H_2 receptors, 610
 headache, 619
 history, 609
 inhibition of allergic release, 620
 mechanism of action, at the cellular level, 614
  H_1 and H_2 receptors, 610, 614
 pharmacological effects, general considerations, 610
 preparations, 619
 role as CNS transmitter, 252
 shock, 612
 toxicity, 619
 triple response, 611–612
 uses, 619
Histamine antagonists. *See* Antihistamines; H_1-receptor blockers; H_2-receptor blockers
Histamine-N-methyltransferase, 618
Histiocytosis X, vinblastine in, 1289
Histoplasma capsulatum infections, choice of drugs in, 1093
Histoplasmosis, amphotericin B in, 1239
HMS LIQUIFILM (medrysone), 1486
Hodgkin's disease, bleomycin in, 1295
  chlorambucil in, 1268
  cyclophosphamide in, 1266
  cytarabine in, 1281
  dacarbazine in, 1271
  dactinomycin in, 1291
  indomethacin in, 706
  lomustine in, 1271
  mechlorethamine in, 1263
  MOPP regimen in, 1263, 1289, 1300
  nitrosoureas in, 1270, 1271
  procarbazine in, 1300
  semustine in, 1271

  streptozocin in, 1271
  vinblastine in, 1289
  vincristine in, 1289
Homatropine, ocular effects and uses, 134
  preparations and dosage, 129
  structural formula, 121
Homatropine methylbromide, chemistry, 121
  pharmacological properties, 129
Homocysteic acid, 248
Homovanillic acid, 76–77
Hookworm infections. *See* Ancylostomiasis; Necatoriasis
Hormones, 1367–1550. *See also* individual hormones
H.P. ACTHAR GEL (repository corticotropin injection), 1470
H_1-receptor agonists, 610
H_2-receptor agonists, 610, 619–620
H_1-receptor blockers, 622–629. *See also* Antihistamines; individual agents
  absorption, fate, and excretion, 625
  actions/effects on, autonomic nervous system, 624, 625
   cardiovascular system, 624, 625
   central nervous system, 624–625
   nerve conduction, 625
  acute poisoning, 626
  antagonism of histamine action, 623–625
   on adrenal medulla and ganglia, 624
   on capillary permeability, 624
   on exocrine glands, 624
   on "flare" and itch, 624
   on hypersensitivity phenomena, 624
   on responses to histamine-releasing drugs, 624
   on smooth muscle, 623–624
  preparations, 626–628
  side effects, 625–626
  structure-activity relationship, 623
  uses, common cold, 629
   diseases of allergy, 627–629
   drug reactions, 629
   hypnotic, 629
   Ménière's disease, 629
   motion sickness, 629
   parkinsonism, 485
   preanesthetic medication, 269
H_2-receptor blockers, 622–623, 629–632. *See also* Antihistamines; individual agents
  chemistry, 629–630
  effect on gastric secretion, 630–631
Human chorionic gonadotropic hormone, 1386. *See also* Gonadotropic hormones
Human placental lactogen, 1382
HUMATIN (paromomycin sulfate), 1066
HUMORSOL (demecarium bromide ophthalmic solution), 112
Huntington's disease, haloperidol in, 418
Hyaluronidase, actions, preparations, and uses, 960–961
HYAZYME (hyaluronidase for injection), 960
Hycanthone, 1016–1017
  absorption, fate, and excretion, 1017
  anthelmintic action, 1016

chemistry, 1016
preparations, route of administration, and dosage, 1017
toxicity and precautions, 1017
uses, 1017
HYCODAN (hydrocodone bitartrate–homatropine methylbromide), 507, 509
Hydantoins, 452–456. *See also* individual agents
Hydatidiform mole, methotrexate in, 1276
HYDELTA-T.B.A. (prednisolone tebutate), 1485
HYDELTRASOL (prednisolone sodium phosphate), 1485
HYDERGINE (ergot alkaloids, dihydrogenated), 946
Hydralazine, 799–801
absorption and elimination, 800
mechanism of action, 799
pharmacokinetics, 1710–1711
pharmacological properties, 799–801
preparations, administration, and dosage, 800
structural formula, 799
toxicity and precautions, 800–801
uses, congestive heart failure, 827
hypertension, 801, 811
HYDREA (hydroxyurea), 1299
Hydroalcoholic vehicles, 1668–1669
Hydrocarbons, 952
aliphatic, toxicology, 1644–1645
aromatic, toxicology, 1647
halogenated, toxicology, 1645–1646
Hydrochloric acid, 998
Hydrochloroquine sulfate, 1046
Hydrochlorothiazide. *See also* Benzothiadiazides
action as antihypertensive, 803–804
pharmacokinetics, 1711
structural formula, properties, and dosage, 900
use as antihypertensive, 809–813
Hydrocholeretics, 998
Hydrocodone, dosage, 507
duration of analgesic effect, 507
preparations, 509
structural formula, 496
Hydrocortisone. *See* Cortisol
HYDROCORTONE (cortisol), 1484
HYDROCORTONE ACETATE (cortisol acetate), 1484
HYDROCORTONE PHOSPHATE (cortisol sodium phosphate), 1484
Hydrocyanic acid. *See* Cyanide
HYDRODIURIL (hydrochlorothiazide), 900
Hydroflumethiazide. *See also* Benzothiadiazides
structural formula, properties, and dosage, 900
Hydrogen peroxide, 974
Hydromorphone, dosage, 507
duration of analgesic effect, 507
legal regulations, 1670
preparations, 509
stuctural formula, 496
HYDROMOX (quinethazone), 900
HYDRONOL (isosorbide), 896
12-Hydroperoxyarachidonic acid, 670, 671. *See also* Prostaglandins
Hydrophilic ointment, 952
Hydrophilic petrolatum, 952

Hydroquinone, chemistry, actions, and toxicity, 959
preparations and uses, 959
HYDROSORB, 953
Hydrotalcite, 995
Hydroxocobalamin, preparation, 1337
structural formula, 1333
Hydroxyamphetamine, 164. *See also* Sympathomimetic drugs
receptor-type activity, 142
structural formula, 142
uses, ophthalmic, 171
12-Hydroxyarachidonic acid, 670, 671, 684. *See also* Prostaglandins
1α-Hydroxycholecalciferol, 1544
25-Hydroxycholecalciferol, 1539, 1540
6-Hydroxydopamine, pharmacological properties, 205
Hydroxy-GABA, 248
Hydroxyphenyl mercuric chloride, 976
Hydroxyprogesterone caproate. *See also* Progestins
chemistry, 1434
preparation, 1437
use in neoplastic diseases, 1254, 1301
8-Hydroxyquinolines, 1063–1065. *See also* individual agents
Hydroxystilbamidine, 1071
antifungal properties and dosage, 1239
uses, 1239
5-Hydroxytryptamine, 632–638
absorption, fate, and excretion, 637
actions/effects on, adrenal medulla, 635
autonomic ganglia, 635
cardiovascular system, 633–634
central nervous system, 635
endocrine glands, 635
exocrine glands, 634–635
nerve endings, 635
respiratory system, 633
smooth muscle, 634
cellular mechanisms of action, 635
endogenous, 635–637
distribution, 635
effects of drugs, 638
origin, synthesis, uptake, and storage, 636
role in carcinoid tumors, 637
role in central nervous system, 636
role in endocrine system, 636
role in enterochromaffin system, 636–637
role in hypothalamic-anterior pituitary function, 636
role in peripheral nervous system, 636
role in pineal gland and melatonin formation, 637
role in platelet function, 637
turnover, 636
history, 632–633
mechanism of action, 635
preparation and use, 638
role as CNS transmitter, 249, 251–252
role in ganglionic transmission, 215
source and chemistry, 633
tryptaminergic neurons, 636

5-Hydroxytryptamine antagonists, 638–639
5-Hydroxytryptophan, 564
Hydroxyurea, 1299
  use in neoplastic diseases, 1253
Hydroxyzine, uses, preanesthetic medication, 269
HYGROTON (chlorthalidone), 900
HYKINONE (menadione sodium bisulfite), 1594
Hyoscine, 121
Hyperalimentation, intravenous, 862–863
Hyperbilirubinemia, phenobarbital in, 361
Hypercalcemia, 1528–1529
  adrenocorticosteroids in, 1301
  calcitonin in, 1537
  disodium edetate in, 1621
  ethacrynic acid in, 907
  furosemide in, 907
  mithramycin in, 1296
Hyperglycinemia, strychnine in, 587
Hyperhidrosis, locally acting drugs in, 954
Hyperkinetic syndrome, caffeine in, 603
  methylphenidate in, 172, 590
  pemoline in, 590
  sympathomimetic drugs in, 172
Hyperlipidemias. See Hyperlipoproteinemias
Hyperlipoproteinemias, aminosalicylic acid in, 845
  benefits of treatment, 845–846
  biochemical and clinical features, 836
  cholestyramine in, 842–843
  classification, 838
  clofibrate in, 840–842
  colestipol hydrochloride in, 842–843
  dextrothyroxine sodium in, 844–845
  estrogens in, 845
  evaluation, 838
  lipoprotein metabolism, 835–838
    chylomicrons, 837
    high-density lipoprotein, 837
    intermediate-density lipoprotein, 837
    lipoprotein apoproteins, 837–838
    low-density lipoprotein, 837
    very-low-density lipoprotein, 837
  neomycin in, 845
  nicotinic acid in, 839–840
  norethindrone in, 845
  probucol in, 843–844
  relationship between blood lipids and vascular disease, 834–835
  sitosterol in, 845
  thyroid hormones in, 844–845
  translating hypercholesterolemia into hyperlipoproteinemia, 835
  treatment, 838–846
Hypernephromas, nitrosoureas in, 1271
Hyperosmolar coma, treatment, 1516
Hyperparathyroidism, clinical features, 1535
  treatment, 1535
Hyperpyrexia, 281
Hypersensitivity reactions, role of autacoids, 615–616, 620, 624
  role of histamine, 615–616
HYPERSTAT I.V. (diazoxide), 802

Hypertension, alpha-adrenergic blocking agents in, 186
  approach to the patient, 808–809
  benzothiadiazides in, 809–813
  captopril in, 807
  chlorthalidone in, 809–813
  clonidine in, 799, 811–813
  diazoxide in, 812–813
  drug therapy, 808–814
    emergency treatment, 812–813
  furosemide in, 810, 812
  ganglionic blocking drugs in, 217
  guanethidine in, 201, 811
  hydralazine in, 801, 811
  methyldopa in, 811
  metoprolol in, 197, 810–812
  minoxidil in, 803
  monoamine oxidase inhibitors in, 807–808
  nadolol in, 195, 810–812
  nitroprusside in, 806, 812–813
  pathophysiology and classification, 808
  prazosin in, 807, 811
  propranolol in, 194, 810–813
  reserpine in, 204, 811
  saralasin in, 807
  spironolactone in, 804–805, 810
  therapeutic regimens, hypertensive emergencies, 812–813
    mild hypertension, 809–811
    moderate-to-severe hypertension, 811–812
    refractory hypertension, 813–814
  trimethaphan in, 813
  veratrum alkaloids in, 808
Hyperthyroidism, 1405
  antithyroid drugs in, 1411–1412
  choice of therapy, 1412
  iodide in, 1413
  propranolol in, 194, 1412
  radioactive iodine in, 1415–1416
Hypertrophic obstructive cardiomyopathy, propranolol in, 194
Hyperuricemia, allopurinol in, 722
  benzbromarone in, 723
  probenecid in, 723
  selection of drugs for, 723
  sulfinpyrazone in, 723
Hypnotics, 339–375. See also individual agents
  abuse, legal regulations, 1670–1671
    prevalence and patterns, 549–550
    signs and symptoms, 550
  addiction, treatment, 571
  cross-dependence, 541
  general considerations, 339
  history, 339
  nonprescription drugs, 369
  physical dependence, 539–540, 550–551
  tolerance, 550–551
  withdrawal symptoms, 550–551
Hypochlorite, 974
Hypochromic anemia. See Anemia—hypochromic
Hypoglycemia, diazoxide in, 1518–1519
  glucagon in, 1518

phenytoin in, 1519
Hypoglycemic agents, oral, 1510–1514. *See also* Sulfonylureas; individual agents
Hypogonadism, female, estrogens in, 1430
male, androgens in, 1459
Hypoparathyroidism, clinical features, 1534–1535
dihydrotachysterol in, 1545
vitamin D in, 1545
Hypopituitarism, adult, 1371–1372
androgens in, 1459–1460
dwarfism, growth hormone in, 1378–1379
Hypoprothrombinemia, vitamin K in, 1594–1596
Hypotension. *See also* Cardiac failure; Hemorrhage; Shock
angiotensin in, 655
sympathomimetic drugs in, 169–170
Hypothalamic releasing hormones, 1389–1392
regulation of, corticotropin, 1391
gonadotropins, 1390–1391
growth hormone, 1391–1392
melanocyte-stimulating hormone, 1392
prolactin, 1392
thyrotropin, 1390
role of adrenergic control, 1392
Hypothyroidism, 1405
thyroid hormones in, 1407–1408
Hypoxia, 321–324. *See also* Oxygen, deprivation
oxygen in, 329–330
HYPROTIGEN (protein hydrolysate injection), 863
Hypsarhythmia. *See also* Epilepsy
adrenocorticosteroids in, 470
benzodiazepines in, 470
corticotropin in, 470
HYTAKEROL (dihydrotachysterol), 1545
HYZYD (isoniazid), 1202

Ibuprofen, 711–712. *See also* Propionic acid derivatives
Ichthammol, 981
Ichthyosis, propylene glycol in, 952
Idiosyncratic reactions to drugs, 1604
Idoxuridine, antiviral properties, 1240
dosage and administration, 1241
uses, herpes infections, 1240
ILETIN II (purified pork insulin), 1507
Ileus, anticholinesterases in, 113
choline esters in, 95
ILOSONE (erythromycin estolate), 1224
ILOTYCIN (erythromycin), 1223
ILOTYCIN GLUCEPTATE (sterile erythromycin gluceptate), 1224
IMFERON (iron dextran injection), 1325
Iminostilbenes, 459–460
Imipramine, 418–427. *See also* Tricyclic antidepressants
mechanism of adrenergic action, 82
pharmacokinetics, 1712
preparations and dosage, 424
IMAVATE (imipramine hydrochloride), 424
IMMOBILON (etorphine hydrochloride), 509
Immunosuppression, adrenocorticosteroids in, 1492
azathioprine in, 1286–1287
chlorambucil in, 1268
cyclophosphamide in, 1266
dactinomycin in, 1291
general principles, 1251
mercaptopurine in, 1286
methotrexate in, 1276
thioguanine in, 1287
Impetigo, bacitracin in, 1232
zinc oxide in, 977
zinc sulfate in, 977
IMURAN (azathioprine), 1286
INAPSINE (droperidol), 295
Inclusion conjunctivitis, choice of drugs in, 1093
erythromycin in, 1189
sulfonamides in, 1115, 1189
tetracyclines in, 1189
IND, 48
Indacrynic acid, 910, 911
INDERAL (propranolol hydrochloride), 193
INDOCIN (indomethacin), 706, 1529
Indolones, 395, 397. *See also* Antipsychotic agents
Indomethacin, 705–707. *See also* Aspirin-like drugs
absorption, fate, and excretion, 705
interaction with other drugs, 705–706
pharmacokinetics, 1712–1713
pharmacological properties, 705
potentiation of effect of ADH, 921
preparations and dosage, 706
structural formula, 705
toxicity, 706
uses, 706–707
hypercalcemia, 1529
Infertility, gonadotropic hormones in, 1386–1387
in women, clomiphene in, 1433
Inflammation, pathogenesis, 683–684
Influenza, viral, amantadine in, 1241
choice of drugs in, 1093
Inhalants, 568–569
Inhalational anesthetics. *See* Anesthesia; individual agents
Inhibin, 1391, 1423, 1450
INNOVAR, 295
Inositol, 1576
Insecticides, toxicology, 1648–1651. *See also* Anticholinesterases
Insomnia, management, 369–371
Insulin, 1497–1510. *See also* Diabetes mellitus
adverse reactions, 1509–1510
assay in plasma, 1499
chemistry and biosynthesis, 1498–1499
dealaninated porcine, 1517
deficiency states, 1502–1506
correction by insulin, 1503–1506
distribution, excretion, and fate, 1501
history, 1497
hypoglycemic syndrome, 1509–1510
mechanism of action, 1506–1507
preparations, 1507–1509
resistance, 1516–1517
secretion, 1499–1501
action of alloxan and other toxins, 1501

Insulin (*Cont.*)
    autonomic mechanisms, 1500
    control by other hormones, 1500
    morphological and chemical events, 1499
    regulation, 1499–1501
    sulfated bovine, 1517
    types of plasma insulin, 1499
    unitage, 1507
    uses, diabetes mellitus, 1514–1516
        diabetic ketoacidosis, 1515–1516
        hyperosmolar coma, 1516
Insulin injection, 1508
Insulin zinc suspension, 1508, 1509
Insulin zinc suspension prompt, 1508, 1509
Insulin-like activity, 1499
Insulin-like growth factor, 1376
INTAL (cromolyn sodium), 622
Interactions of drugs. *See* Drug interactions; individual agents
Interferon, 1243
Intermittent claudication, alpha-adrenergic blocking drugs in, 187
Interstitial cell–stimulating hormone. *See* Luteinizing hormone
Interstitial fluid, composition, 849
INTRALIPID 10% (intravenous fat emulsion), 863
Intravenous anesthetics. *See* Anesthesia; individual agents
Intrinsic gastric factor of Castle, 1331, 1334–1335
INTROPIN (dopamine hydrochloride), 155
INVERSINE (mecamylamine hydrochloride), 217
Iodide, dosage for thyroid disorders, 1413
    effect on thyroid function, 1412–1413
    preparations, 1413
    toxicity, 1413–1414
    transport by thyroid, 1399–1400
    uses, 1413
        hyperthyroidism, 1413
        prophylaxis of simple goiter, 1403
        sporotricosis, 1240
Iodine, 972
    radioactive, 1414–1416
        chemical and physical properties, 1414
        effects on thyroid gland, 1414
        preparations, 1414
        use in diagnosis, 1416
        use in hyperthyroidism, 1415–1416
        use in thyroid cancer, 1416
    recommended dietary allowance, 1553
    relation to thyroid function, 1403
Iodochlorhydroxyquin. *See* Clioquinol
Iodophors, 973
Iodopsin, 1585
Iodoquinol, 984, 1063–1065
    absorption, fate, and excretion, 1064
    actions on amebae, 1064
    chemistry, 1063
    preparations, 1064
    route of administration and dosage, 1064
    toxicity and side effects, 1064
    uses, acrodermatitis enteropathica, 1065
        amebiasis, 1062, 1064

    balantiasis, 1065
    dysentery, 1065
    giardiasis, 1065
IODOTOPE I-131 (sodium iodide I 131), 1414
IONAMIN (phentermine hydrochloride), 172
Ionizing radiations, cytotoxic action, 1305
IOSEL 250 (selenium sulfide lotion), 957
Ipecac, 1065
    use in drug poisoning, 1609
Ipratropium bromide, 135
Iproniazid, 427–428
IRGASAN CF3, 981
IRGASAN DP300, 970, 975, 981
Iridocyclitis, belladonna alkaloids in, 133
Iron, 1315–1326
    absorption, 1317–1318
    availability from diet, 1318–1320
    body content, 1316
    deficiency, 1320–1322
        treatment, 1322–1326
    distribution and types in nature, 1315–1316
    excretion, 1317
    fate, 1317
    in food, 1318–1320
    history, 1315
    metabolism, 1316–1318
    parenteral preparations and dosage, 1325–1326
    plasma concentrations, 1321
    poisoning, 1324–1325
        deferoxamine in, 1325, 1634
    preparations and dosage, 1322–1323, 1325–1326
    recommended dietary allowance, 1553
    requirements, adults, 1318–1320
        infants and children, 1318–1320
        pregnancy, 1317
    stores, 1316
    toxicity and side effects, oral preparations, 1324
        parenteral preparations, 1326
    transport, 1316–1318
    uses, iron-deficiency anemias, 1322–1326
        supplement in pregnancy, 1317, 1323
Iron-deficiency anemias, 1315–1326. *See also* Anemia—hypochromic
Iron dextran, dosage and response to therapy, 1325–1326
Iron-poly (sorbitol gluconic acid) complex, 1326
Iron sulfate, 1322
Irritable colon syndrome, antimuscarinic drugs in, 133
Irritants, classification and uses, 955–956
ISMELIN (guanethidine sulfate), 200
Iso-alcoholic elixir, 1669
Isobornyl thiocyanoacetate, 985
Isocarboxazid. *See also* Monoamine oxidase inhibitors
    preparations and dosage, 424
ISODINE (povidone-iodine), 973
Isoetharine, receptor-type activity, 142
    structural formula, 142
    use in bronchial asthma, 168
Isoflurane, 288–289. *See also* Anesthesia
    physical properties, 277

structural formula, 277
Isoflurophate. *See also* Anticholinesterases
  preparations, 112
  use in glaucoma, 113–114
Isolysergic acid, 941
Isoniazid, 1200–1203
  absorption, distribution, and excretion, 1201–1202
  antibacterial activity, 1201
  bacterial resistance, 1201
  chemistry, 1200
  dosage, 1202
  history, 1200
  inhibition of pyridoxine, 1570
  mechanism of action, 1201
  pharmacokinetics, 1713
  preparation and routes of administration, 1202
  untoward effects, 1202–1203
  use in tuberculosis, 1203, 1212–1213
ISONOL (isosorbide), 896
Isopentaquine, 1051
Isophane insulin suspension, 1508, 1509
ISOPHRIN (phenylephrine hydrochloride), 165
Isoprenaline. *See* Isoproterenol
Isopropamide, preparations and structural formula, 130
Isopropanol, 970
  toxicology, 1646
Isopropyl alcohol, 970
Isopropylarterenol. *See* Isoproterenol
Isopropylnoradrenaline. *See* Isoproterenol
Isopropylnorepinephrine. *See* Isoproterenol
Isoproterenol, 153–154. *See also* Sympathomimetic drugs
  absorption, fate, and excretion, 154
  actions/effects on, cardiovascular system, 145, 153
    metabolism, 153–154
    smooth muscle, 153
  pharmacological actions, 153–154
  preparations, 154
  receptor-type activity, 142
  structural formula, 142
  toxicity and side effects, 154
  uses, 154
    bronchial asthma, 170–171
    shock, 169–170
    Stokes-Adams syndrome, 170
ISOPTO CARBACHOL (carbachol ophthalmic solution), 95
ISOPTO CETAMIDE (sulfacetamide sodium), 1112
ISORDIL (isosorbide dinitrate), 826
Isosorbide, 895–896
  diuretic action, 895
  preparations and dosage, 896
  uses, 896
Isosorbide dinitrate. *See also* Nitrates
  absorption, fate, and excretion, 822–823
  pharmacokinetics, 1714
  preparations, routes of administration, and dosage, 826
  structural formula, 826
Isoxazolyl penicillins, 1142–1143. *See also* individual agents

Isoxsuprine, 831
ISUPREL (isoproterenol hydrochloride), 154
ISUPREL MISTOMETER (isoproterenol hydrochloride inhalation), 154
Itai-itai, 1632, 1633
Ivy poisoning, zinc sulfate in, 977

JANIMINE (imipramine hydrochloride), 424
Jarisch-Herxheimer reaction, 1140
Jimson weed, poisoning, 127
Juniper tar, 970

KAFOCIN (cephaloglycin dihydrate), 1156
Kainic acid, 247, 248
Kala-azar. *See* Leishmaniasis
Kallidin. *See also* Kinins
  history, 659
  synthesis and catabolism, 660–661
Kallikreins, 659, 660
Kanamycin, 1176–1177. *See also* Aminoglycoside antibiotics; Antimicrobial agents
  pharmacokinetics, 1714
  preparations, administration, and dosage, 1176
  structural formula, 1163
  untoward effects, 1176
  uses, gram-negative microbial infections, 1176
    preparation of bowel for surgery, 1176
    prevention of hepatic coma, 1177
    tuberculosis, 1211
KANTREX (kanamycin sulfate), 1176
Kaolin, 954
KAPPADIONE (menadiol sodium diphosphate injection), 1594
Karaya gum, 1005
KASOF (docusate potassium), 1009
Kava, 569
KAYEXALATE (sodium polystyrene sulfonate), 879
KEFLEX (cephalexin), 1155
KEFLIN (cephalothin sodium), 1154
KEFZOL (sterile cefazolin sodium), 1154
KELFIZINA (sulfalene), 1058
KEMADRIN (procyclidine hydrochloride), 486
KENACORT (triamcinolone), 1485
KENACORT DIACETATE (triamcinolone diacetate), 1486
KENALOG (triamcinolone acetonide), 1485
KEPONE (chlordecone), 1650
KERALYT (propylene glycol–salicylic acid), 956
Keratitis, belladonna alkaloids in, 133
Keratoconjunctivitis, choice of drugs in, 1093
Keratolytics, actions and uses, 956
Keratoses, fluorouracil in, 1280
Kernicterus, phenobarbital in, 361
Kerosene, toxicology, 1644–1645
KETAJECT (ketamine hydrochloride), 296
KETALAR (ketamine hydrochloride), 296
Ketamine, use in intravenous anesthesia, 296–297
Ketobemidone, legal regulations, 1670
Ketoprofen, 713. *See also* Propionic acid derivatives

17-Ketosteroids, urinary, from adrenocorticosteroids, 1481
 from androgens, 1454
KETRAX (levamisole), 1026
Khat leaves, 569
Kidney. *See also* Diuretics
 physiological considerations in relation to drug action, 885–892, 929–931
  free-water production, 888–890
  glomerular filtration, 885–886
  hydrogen ion secretion, 890–891
  potassium reabsorption and secretion, 891
  tubular transport of inorganic compounds, 886–891
  tubular transport of organic compounds, 891–892, 929–931
Kininase I, 660–661
Kininase II. *See* Peptidyl dipeptidase
Kininogens, 660
Kinins, 659–663. *See also* Bradykinin; Kallidin
 actions/effects on, autonomic ganglia and chromaffin cells, 662
  cardiovascular system, 661
  central nervous system, 662
  extravascular smooth muscle, 661
  nerve endings and production of pain, 661
 history, 659
 mechanism of action, 662
 proposed endogenous functions, 662
 synthesis and catabolism, 660–661
 therapeutic considerations, 662–663
Klebsiella infections, amikacin in, 1176
 cephalosporins in, 1157
 chloramphenicol in, 1196
 choice of drugs in, 1089
 gentamicin in, 1174
 kanamycin in, 1176
KOLANTYL GEL, 991
KONAKION (phytonadione, vitamin K$_1$), 1594
KONSYL (plantago ovata coating), 1004
Korsakoff's psychosis, 553
 thiamine in, 1563
Kraurosis vulvae, estrogens in, 1430
KWELL (lindane), 985

L.A. FORMULA (psyllium hydrophilic mucilloid), 1004
Labarraque's solution, 974
Labetalol, 197
Labor. *See also* Premature labor
 augmentation, 948
 diazepam in, 440
 dysfunctional, oxytocin in, 948
 induction, 947–948
 meperidine in, 517
 opioids in, 512
 scopolamine in, 135
 third stage, uterine-stimulating agents in, 948–949
Lactation, oxytocin in, 938
 suppression by androgens, 1461
 suppression by estrogens, 1431
 suppression by progestins, 1438

Lactic acid, 972
Lactulose, 1009–1010
 use in ammonia intoxication, 870
Laetrile, toxicology, 1651
LAMPIT (nifurtimox), 1077
LAMPRENE (clofazimine), 1216
Lanatoside C. *See also* Digitalis
 preparation and administration, 749
Lanolin, 952
LANOXIN (digoxin), 749
LAPAQUIN (chloroquine-chloroproguanil), 1044
LARODOPA (levodopa), 481
LAROTID (amoxicillin), 1145
Larva migrans, thiabendazole in, 1031
LASERDIL (isosorbide dinitrate), 826
LASIX (furosemide), 906
Laudanum, 509
Laxatives. *See* Cathartics
L-Dopa. *See* Levodopa
Lead, 1616–1620
 absorption, distribution, and excretion, 1616–1617
 actions/effects on, blood, 1618
  central nervous system, 1617–1618
  gastrointestinal tract, 1617
  heme synthesis, 1618
  kidney, 1618–1619
  neuromuscular system, 1617
  pyrrole excretion, 1619
 organic, poisoning, 1619–1620
 poisoning, acute, 1617
  chronic, 1617–1619
  diagnosis, 1619
  dimercaprol in, 1622
  dimercaptosuccinic acid in, 1627
  edetate calcium disodium in diagnosis, 1619
  edetate calcium disodium in treatment, 1621–1622
  penicillamine in, 1622
  treatment, 1621–1622
 sources of exposure, 1616
LECTOPAM (bromazepam), 350
Legionnaires' disease, choice of drugs in, 1091
 erythromycin in, 1225
Leishmaniasis, amphotericin B in, 1075
 cycloguanil in, 1047. 1075
 pentamidine in, 1072
 sodium stibogluconate in, 1075
LENTE insulin (insulin zinc suspension), 1508, 1509
Leprosy, amithiazone in, 1216
 chemotherapy, 1216–1217
 choice of drugs in, 1091
 clofazimine in, 1215–1216
 rifampin in, 1215
 sulfonamides in, 1216
 sulfones in, 1214–1215
 thalidomide in, 1216
 thiambutosine in, 1216
Leptospira infections, choice of drugs in, 1092
 tetracyclines in, 1191
Lergotrile, 483, 942
LERITINE (anileridine), 507, 516, 1670
LETTER (levothyroxine sodium), 1406

Leucovorin, 1343
    preparations, 1343
    "rescue" in methotrexate therapy, 1273, 1275
Leukemia. *See* Granulocytic leukemia; Lymphocytic
    leukemia; Meningeal leukemia
LEUKERAN (chlorambucil), 1267
Leukotrienes, 671. *See also* Prostaglandins
Levallorphan. *See also* Opioid antagonists
    onset and duration of action, 524
    preparations, 525
Levamisole, 1026–1027
LEVANXOL (temazepam), 350
Levarterenol. *See* Norepinephrine
Levodopa, 477–482
    absorption, fate, and excretion, 479–480
    actions/effects on, cardiovascular system, 477–478
        central nervous system, 477
        metabolic and endocrine functions, 478, 1378
        psyche, 477
    antagonism by pyridoxine, 481
    chemistry, 477
    decarboxylase inhibitors, 482–483
    drug interactions, 481
    history, 476
    mechanism of action, 478
    metabolic pathways, 479
    pharmacological properties, 477–482
    preparations and dosage, 481–482
    side effects and toxicity, 480–481
    uses, cerebral palsy, 487
        encephalitis, 487
        hepatic coma, 487
        parkinsonism, 485, 487
        Reye's syndrome, 487
        torsion dystonias, 487
LEVO-DROMORAN (levorphanol tartrate), 507, 513
Levomoramide, legal regulations, 1670
Levonordefrin, 309
LEVOPHED (norepinephrine), 152
Levopropoxyphene, preparations and use for cough,
    529
Levorphanol, dosage, 507, 513
    duration of analgesic effect, 507, 513
    pharmacological properties, 513
    preparations and dosage, 513
    structural formula, 496
Levothyroxine sodium, 1406
LH. *See* Luteinizing hormone
LIBIGEN (chorionic gonadotropin for injection), 1386
LIBRITABS (chlordiazepoxide), 350, 440
LIBRIUM (chlordiazepoxide), 350, 440, 1671
LIDEX (fluocinonide), 1486
Lidocaine, 308–309. *See also* Local anesthetics
    absorption, distribution, and elimination, 308,
        780–781
    actions/effects on, autonomic nervous system, 780
        cardiac electrophysiology, 768, 779–780
        electrocardiogram, 768, 780
    dosage and administration in cardiac arrhythmias,
        781
    pharmacokinetics, 1714–1715
    plasma concentrations, 781

preparations, 309, 779
structural formula, 301
toxicity, 308, 781
uses, cardiac arrhythmias, 781
    digitalis intoxication, 755
LIDONE (molindone hydrochloride), 411
Light mineral oil, 952
Lignocaine. *See* Lidocaine
Limbic system, anatomy and general functions, 57
LIMBITROL (chlordiazepoxide–amitriptyline hydro-
    chloride), 424
LINCOCIN (lincomycin hydrochloride), 1225
Lincomycin, 1225. *See also* Antimicrobial agents
Lindane, 985
    toxicology, 1650
LIORESAL (baclofen), 489
Liothyronine sodium, 1406
Lipids, in plasma, 834–838
LIPO GANTRISIN (sulfisoxazole acetyl), 1111
LIPO-HEPIN (heparin sodium injection), 1351
LIPOLUTIN (progesterone injection), 1437
Lipoproteins, in plasma, 834–838. *See also* Hyper-
    lipoproteinemias
    properties and composition, 835–838
β-Lipotropin, 497, 498
    chemical properties, 1371, 1388
γ-Lipotropin, chemical properties, 1371, 1388
Lipotropins, 1388–1389
Lipoxygenase, 670, 671
LIQUAEMIN (heparin sodium injection), 1351
LIQUAMAR (phenprocoumon), 1359
Liquefied phenol, 967
Liquid petrolatum, 1009
Listeria infections, penicillin G in, 1140
Listeria monocytogenes infections, choice of drugs in,
    1088
Lisuride, 483, 942
LITHANE (lithium carbonate), 433
Lithium, pharmacokinetics, 1715
    uses, depression, 434–435
Lithium salts, 430–434
    absorption, distribution, and excretion, 432–433
    actions/effects on, central nervous system, 431–432
        water balance, 922
    chemistry, 431
    history, 431
    interactions with other drugs, 434
    pharmacological properties, 431–434
    plasma concentrations and therapeutic response,
        433
    preparations and dosage, 433
    toxicity, 433–434
    uses, mania, 434–435
        manic-depressive psychosis, 434–435
LITHONATE (lithium carbonate), 433
LITHOTABS (lithium carbonate), 433
Lividomycin, 1163
LMD 10% (dextran 40 injection), 862
Lobeline, 212–213
    structural formula, 213
Local anesthetics, 300–320. *See also* individual
    agents

Local anesthetics (*Cont.*)
actions/effects on, cardiovascular system, 305–306
central nervous system, 304–305
ganglionic synapse, 305
neuromuscular junction, 305
smooth muscle, 306
chemistry, 301
clinical uses, 311–319
desirable properties, 300–301
differential sensitivity of nerve fibers, 302–303
effects of, pH, 303
epidural anesthesia, 317–319
caudal anesthesia, 317
field block anesthesia, 312
frequency dependence and use dependence, 304
history, 300
hypersensitivity, 306
infiltration anesthesia, 311–312
intravenous regional anesthesia, 313–314
mechanism of action, 301–302
metabolic disposition, 306–307
nerve block anesthesia, 312–313
prolongation of action by vasoconstrictors, 169, 304
spinal anesthesia, 314–317
cardiovascular consequences, 314–316
dosage and duration, 317
effects on liver, 316
evaluation, 317
neurological complications, 316–317
respiratory complications, 316
structure-activity relationship, 301
surface anesthesia, 311
LOCORTEN (flumethasone pivalate), 1486
LODOSYN (carbidopa), 483
LOESTRIN 1/20, 1440
LOESTRIN 1.5/30, 1440
Loiasis, treatment, 1033
LOMIDINE (pentamidine), 1071
LOMOTIL (diphenoxylate hydrochloride–atropine sulfate), 517
Lomustine, 1270–1271. *See also* Alkylating agents
structural formula, 1259
use in neoplastic diseases, 1252, 1271
Long-acting thyroid stimulator, 1388
LONITEN (minoxidil), 803
LO-OVRAL, 1440
Loperamide, 517
legal regulations, 1671
LOPRESSOR (metoprolol tartrate), 196
Lorazepam, 437–441. *See also* Benzodiazepines
dosage, half-life, and preparations, 350
legal regulations, 1671
pharmacokinetics, 1716
preparations and dosage, 440
use in preanesthetic medication, 270
LORELCO (probucol), 844
LORFAN (levallorphan tartrate injection), 525
LORIDINE (sterile cephaloridine), 1155
LOTRIMIN (clotrimazole), 983
LOTUSATE (talbutal), 350
Loxapine, 394, 411. *See also* Antipsychotic agents

LOXITANE (loxapine succinate), 411
LSD. *See* Lysergic acid diethylamide
Lugol's solution, 972
Lupus erythematosus, adrenocorticosteroids in, 1490
chloroquine in, 1043
gold in, 716, 717
zinc sulfate in, 977
Luteinizing hormone, 1383–1387. *See also* Gonadotropic hormones
chemical properties, 1371, 1383
concentration during menstrual cycle, 1424
relationship with estrogens and progestins, 1423–1425
Luteinizing hormone–releasing hormone, 1390 1391
role as CNS transmitter, 253
Lymphocytic leukemia, adrenocorticosteroids in, 1301, 1491
L-asparaginase in, 1297
chlorambucil in, 1267
cyclophosphamide in, 1266
cytarabine in, 1281
daunorubicin in, 1293
doxorubicin in, 1293
mercaptopurine in, 1286
methotrexate in, 1275
pyrimethamine in, 1050
vinblastine in, 1289
vincristine in, 1289–1290
Lymphogranuloma venereum, chloramphenicol in, 1196
choice of drugs in, 1093
sulfonamides in, 1116
tetracyclines in, 1189
Lymphomas, adrenocorticosteroids in, 1491
L-asparaginase in, 1297
bleomycin in, 1295
chlorambucil in, 1268
cisplatin in, 1299
cyclophosphamide in, 1266
cytarabine in, 1281
dactinomycin in, 1291
daunorubicin in, 1293
doxorubicin in, 1293
lomustine in, 1271
mechlorethamine in, 1263–1264
mitomycin in, 1297
nitrosoureas in, 1270, 1271
procarbazine in, 1300
semustine in, 1271
streptozocin in, 1271
vinblastine in, 1289
vincristine in, 1289–1290
Lymphosarcoma, cyclophosphamide in, 1266. *See also* Lymphomas
Lypressin, 917, 923
use in diabetes insipidus, 924
Lysergic acid, structural formula, 941
Lysergic acid diethylamide, 249, 252
abuse, legal regulations, 1670
patterns and incidence, 566
chemistry, 564–565
history, 564

mechanism of action, 564–565
pharmacological effects, 565–566
relationship to 5-hydroxytryptamine, 633, 634, 636, 638
structural formula, 941
tolerance and physical dependence, 566–567
toxicity, 566–567
uses, 567
Lysergol, 942
Lysine[8] vasopressin, 917
LYSODREN (mitotane), 1300

MAALOX, 991, 996
MAALOX PLUS, 991
MAC (minimal alveolar concentration), 267, 271–272
    correlation with olive oil:gas partition coefficient, 271–272
MACRODANTIN (nitrofurantoin), 1122
MACRODEX (dextran 70 injection), 862, 1361
Macroglobulinemia, chlorambucil in, 1267
Mafenide, pharmacological properties, toxicity, and uses, 1112. See also Sulfonamides
Magaldrate, 994
"Magic mushroom," 569
Magnesia and alumina oral suspension, preparations and dosage, 995
Magnesia and alumina tablets, 995
Magnesium, 879–882
    abnormalities of metabolism, hypermagnesemia, 881–882
        hypomagnesemia, 881
    absorption and excretion, 879–880
    actions/effects on, cardiovascular system, 880–881
        central nervous system, 880
        enzyme systems, 880
        neuromuscular system, 880
    physiological functions, 880–881
    preparations, 882
    recommended dietary allowance, 1553
    uses, deficiency states, 882
        eclampsia, 882
Magnesium carbonate, 993
Magnesium citrate 1005. See also Cathartics, saline
Magnesium hydroxide, 993–994, 1005. See also Cathartics, saline
Magnesium oxide, 994
Magnesium stearate, 953
Magnesium sulfate, 1005. See also Cathartics, saline
Magnesium sulfate injection, 882
Magnesium trisilicate, 953, 994
Malabsorption disorders, tetracyclines in, 1191
    thiamine in, 1563
    vitamin K in, 1595
Malaria, acedapsone in, 1058
    acquired resistance to antimalarial drugs, 1041–1042
    biology of infection, 1038–1039
    causal prophylaxis, 1039

chloramphenicol in, 1057
chloroguanide in, 1047
chloroquine in, 1045
clinical cure, 1040
cycloguanil pamoate in, 1047
dapsone in, 1058
gametocytocidal therapy, 1040
hydroxychloroquine in, 1046
mechanism of action of antimalarial drugs, 1040–1041
mefloquine in, 1051
plasmodia infecting man, 1038
primaquine in, 1054
pyrimethamine in, 1050
quinacrine in, 1042
quinine in, 1057
radical cure, 1040
sulfonamides in, 1057
sulfones in, 1057
suppressive cure, 1040
suppressive treatment, 1039
tetracyclines in, 1058
therapy in relation to biology of infection, 1039–1040
Malathion, metabolism, 104
    structural formula, 105
Malignant hyperpyrexia, 281
Malignant hyperthermia, dantrolene in, 490–491
MALOPRIM (pyrimethamine-dapsone), 1049
MANDELAMINE (methenamine mandelate), 1120
MANDOL (cefamandole nafate), 1154
Maneb, toxicology, 1655
Manganese, provisional dietary allowance, 1555
Mania, antipsychotic agents in, 416
    definition, 418
    lithium carbonate in, 434–435
    treatment, 434–435
Manic-depressive psychosis, antidepressants in, 433
    lithium carbonate in, 434–435
Mannitol, diuretic action, 894–895
    preparations and dosage, 896
    toxicity, 896
    uses, 895–896
        glaucoma, 113
Mannitol hexanitrate. See also Nitrates
    preparations, 826
    structural formula, 826
MANSIL (oxamniquine), 1022
MAOLATE (chlorphenesin carbamate), 489
MARBLEN, 991
MARBORAN (methisazone), 1242
MARCAINE (bupivacaine hydrochloride), 309
MARCUMAR (phenprocoumon), 1359
MAREZINE (cyclizine), 628
Marihuana. See Cannabis
MARPLAN (isocarboxazid), 424
MATULANE (procarbazine), 1300
MAXIBOLIN (ethylestrenol), 1457
MAXIPEN (phenethicillin potassium), 1137
Mazindol, legal regulations, 1671
MDA. See 3,4-Methylenedioxyamphetamine
MEBARAL (mephobarbital), 458

Mebendazole, 1017–1018
Mebutamate, 369
  legal regulations, 1671
Mecamylamine, 215–217. *See also* Ganglionic block-
    ing agents
  structural formula, 215
Mechlorethamine, 1263–1264. *See also* Alkylating
    agents
  absorption and fate, 1263
  chemistry, 1256–1258
  clinical toxicity, 1263–1264
  preparations, dosage, and routes of administra-
    tion, 1263
  use in neoplastic diseases, 1252, 1263–1264
Mecillinam, 1099, 1147
Meclizine hydrochloride, preparations and dosage,
    628. *See also* H$_1$-receptor blockers
Meclofenamic acid, 708. *See also* Fenamates
MEDIHALER-EPI (epinephrine aerosol), 151
MEDIHALER-ERGOTAMINE (ergotamine aerosol), 946
Mediterranean fever, colchicine for prevention of
    attacks, 720
MEDROCORT (medrysone), 1486
MEDROL (methylprednisolone), 1485
MEDROL ACETATE (methylprednisolone acetate), 1485
Medroxyprogesterone acetate, 1437
  chemistry, 1434
Medrysone. *See also* Adrenocorticosteroids
  preparations, 1486
Mefenamic acid, 708. *See also* Fenamates
Mefloquine, 1050–1051
  absorption, fate, and excretion, 1051
  antimalarial actions, 1050
  chemistry, 1050
  preparations and dosage, 1051
  toxicity, 1051
  uses, 1051
MEFOXIN (cefoxitin), 1155
MEGACE (megestrol acetate), 1437
Megestrol acetate, 1437
  chemistry, 1434
  use in neoplastic diseases, 1254
Meglumine antimonate, 1074
Melanizing agents, 957–959
Melanocyte-stimulating hormone, 1389
  hypothalamic regulation, 1392
α-Melanocyte-stimulating hormone, chemical prop-
    erties, 1371, 1389
β-Melanocyte-stimulating hormone, chemical prop-
    erties, 1371, 1389
Melanocyte-stimulating hormone release-inhibiting
    factor, 1392
Melanocyte-stimulating hormone–releasing factor,
    1392
Melanoma, dacarbazine in, 1271
  hydroxyurea in, 1299
  lomustine in, 1271
  melphalan in, 1267
  mitomycin in, 1297
  nitrosoureas in, 1270, 1271
  procarbazine in, 1300
  semustine in, 1271

streptozocin in, 1271
Melarsoprol, 1072–1074
  absorption, fate, and excretion, 1073
  chemistry and preparations, 1072–1073
  route of administration and dosage, 1073
  toxicity and precautions, 1073
  trypanocidal action, 1073
  use in trypanosomiasis, 1073
Mel B (melarsoprol), 1073
Melasma, hydroquinone in, 959
  retinoic acid in, 959
Melatonin, 637
Melioidosis, choice of drugs in, 1090
MELLARIL (thioridazine hydrochloride), 409
Melphalan, 1266–1267. *See also* Alkylating agents
  chemistry, 1258
  use in neoplastic diseases, 1252, 1267
Menadiol sodium diphosphate injection, 1594
Menadiol sodium diphosphate tablets, 1594
Menadione, 1592, 1594
Menadione sodium bisulfite, 1594
Menaquinones, 1592
Menétrièr's disease, antimuscarinic drugs in, 125
Ménière's disease, H$_1$-receptor blockers in, 629
Meningeal leukemia, carmustine in, 1270
  pyrimethamine in, 1050
Meningitis. *See also* Meningococcal infections
  amphotericin B in, 1239–1240
  chloramphenicol in, 1145, 1195
  choice of drugs in, 1086
  flucytosine in, 1237, 1239
  gentamicin in, 1175
  penicillins in, 1138, 1139
  polymyxin B in, 1230
  sulfonamides in, 1115
Meningococcal infections. *See also* Meningitis
  chemoprophylaxis, 1115
  choice of drugs in, 1087
  penicillins in, 1139
  prevention, minocycline in, 1190
    rifampin in, 1206
  sulfonamides in, 1115
Menopause, androgens in, 1429
  estrogens in, 1429
Menotropins for injection, 1386
Mepacrine hydrochloride, 1078
Mepazine, 406
Mepenzolate, preparation and structural formula,
    131
Meperidine, 513–517. *See also* Opioids
  absorption, fate, and excretion, 515–516
  abstinence syndrome, 548
  actions/effects on, cardiovascular system, 515
    central nervous system, 514–515
    EEG, 515
    pain, 514
    respiration, 514–515
    smooth muscle, 515
    uterus, 515
  addiction, treatment, 570
  dosage, 507, 516
  duration of analgesic effect, 507, 514

history, 513
interactions with other drugs, 516
legal regulations, 1670
pharmacokinetics, 1716
preparations and routes of administration, 516
structural formula, 514
tolerance, physical dependence, and liability for abuse, 516-517
untoward effects, precautions, and contraindications, 516
uses, analgesia, 517
obstetrical analgesia, 517
preanesthetic medication, 270
Mephenesin, chemistry, preparations, and dosage, 489
mechanism of action, 488
Mephentermine. See also Sympathomimetic drugs
pharmacological properties, 164
preparations and dosage, 164
receptor-type activity, 142
structural formula, 142
uses, 164
hypotensive states, 169
nasal decongestion, 168
Mephenytoin, 455-456
Mephobarbital. See also Barbiturates
chemistry, 351
properties and status as antiepileptic, 458
MEPHYTON (phytonadione), 1594
Mepivacaine, structural formula, 301
Mepivacaine hydrochloride, 309. See also Local anesthetics
MEPRANE (promethestrol dipropionate), 1428
Meprednisone. See also Adrenocorticosteroids
preparations, 1485
Meprobamate, 441
absorption, fate, and excretion, 366
adverse effects, 366-367
dosage, half-life, and preparations, 351
intoxication, 366-367
legal regulations, 1671
neuropharmacological properties, 365-366
structural formula, 365
uses, 367
Merbromin, 976
Mercaptopurine, 1282-1286. See also Purine analogs
absorption, fate, and excretion, 1285-1286
clinical toxicity, 1286
preparation, dosage, and route of administration, 1286
use in neoplastic diseases, 1253, 1286
Mercurial antiseptics and germicides, 975-976
Mercurial diuretics, 896. See also Diuretics
MERCUROCHROME (merbromin), 976
Mercury, 1622-1625
absorption, distribution, and excretion, 1623
chemistry and mechanism of action, 1622-1623
poisoning, acute, 1624
chronic, 1624-1625
diagnosis, 1625
dimercaprol in, 1627
dimercaptosuccinic acid in, 1627

hemodialysis in, 1628-1629
penicillamine in, 1628
polythiol resins in, 1628-1629
treatment, 1627, 1628-1629
sources of exposure, 1622-1623
MERTHIOLATE (thimerosal), 976
MESANTOIN (mephenytoin), 455
Mescaline, 564-566
legal regulations, 1670
Mesoridazine. See also Antipsychotic agents
chemistry, 408
Mesterolone, 1450
MESTINON (pyridostigmine bromide), 112
Mestranol, 1428
in oral contraceptives, 1440
METAHYDRIN (trichlormethiazide), 900
Metallic iron, 1323
Metallothionein, 1632
Metals, heavy. See Heavy metals
METAMUCIL (psyllium hydrophilic muciloid), 1004
METANDREN (methyltestosterone), 1456
Metanephrine, structural formula, 77
METAPHEN (nitromersol), 976
METAPREL (metaproterenol sulfate), 167
Metaproterenol, 166-167. See also Sympathomimetic drugs
pharmacological properties, 166-167
preparations and dosage, 167
receptor-type activity, 142
structural formula, 142
toxicity and precautions, 167
uses, 167
bronchial asthma, 170-171
premature labor, 172
Metaraminol, 164-165. See also Sympathomimetic drugs
pharmacological actions, 164
preparations and dosage, 165
receptor-type activity, 142
structural formula, 142
uses, 165
hypotensive states, 169
shock, 169
Metaxalone, chemistry, preparations, and dosage, 489
Methacholine, actions/effects on, cardiovascular system, 93-94
gastrointestinal tract, 94
urinary tract, 94
history, 91
mechanism of action, 91-92
miscellaneous effects, 94
precautions, toxicity, and contraindications, 95
preparations and dosage, 95
structural formula, 92
structure-activity relationship, 92
synergists and antagonists, 94-95
uses, diagnostic, 96
glaucoma, 96
Methacycline. See also Tetracyclines
absorption, distribution, and excretion, 1184
dosage, 1185

Methacycline (*Cont.*)
preparations and administration, 1185
structural formula, 1181
Methadone, 518–520. *See also* Opioids
absorption, fate, and excretion, 518–519
actions/effects on, central nervous system, 518
smooth muscle, 518
chemistry, 518
dosage, 507, 519
drug interactions, 519
duration of analgesic effects, 507, 518
legal regulations, 1670
maintenance therapy of opioid addicts, 574
preparations and routes of administration, 519
tolerance, physical dependence, and liability for
abuse, 519
toxicity, side effects, and precautions, 519
uses, 519–520
opioid addiction, 570, 574
withdrawal symptoms, 548
Methadyl acetate, 519
Methallenestril, 1428
Methamphetamine. *See also* Amphetamine; Sympathomimetic drugs
abuse, 553–557
legal regulations, 1670
pharmacological actions, 162–163
preparations and dosage, 163
receptor-type activity, 142
structural formula, 142
uses, 163
narcolepsy, 171
obesity, 171–172
Methandriol, 1457
Methandrostenolone, 1457
Methantheline, pharmacological properties, 129
preparations and structural formula, 131
Methapyrilene, 369
Methaqualone, 367–368
absorption and fate, 367
abuse, legal regulations, 1670
chemistry, 367
dosage, half-life, and preparations, 351
pharmacological properties, 367–368
side effects, intoxication, and dependence, 367–368
Metharbital. *See also* Barbiturates
chemistry, 351
properties and status as antiepileptic, 458
Methazolamide, 897–898
Methemoglobinemia, ascorbic acid in, 1579
methylene blue in, 980
Methenamine, 1119–1120
Methenamine hippurate, 1120
Methenamine mandelate, 1120
Methenamine and sodium biphosphate, 1120
METHERGINE (methylergonovine maleate), 946
Methergoline, 942
Methicillin, 1142. *See also* Penicillins
pharmacokinetics, 1717
Methimazole. *See also* Antithyroid drugs
preparations and dosage, 1411
Methisazone, 1242

Methixene, 131
Methocarbamol, chemistry, preparations, and dosage, 489
Methohexital. *See also* Barbiturates
chemistry, 351
legal regulations, 1671
use in intravenous anesthesia, 292
METHOSARB (calusterone), 1457
Methotrexate, 1272–1276
absorption, fate, and excretion, 1274–1275
chemistry, 1272
clinical toxicity, 1275–1276
cytotoxic action, 1274
mechanism of action, 1273
mechanism of resistance, 1273
pharmacokinetics, 1717
preparations, dosage, and routes of administration, 1275
structure-activity relationship, 1272
uses, 1252, 1275–1276
Methoxamine, 165–166. *See also* Sympathomimetic
drugs
pharmacological actions, 165–166
preparations, administration, and dosage, 166
receptor-type activity, 142
structural formula, 142
uses, 166
hypotensive states, 169
myocardial infarction, 827
paroxysmal atrial or nodal tachycardia, 170
Methoxsalen, chemistry, actions, and toxicity, 958
preparations and uses, 958
Methoxyamphetamine, 564–565
Methoxychlor, toxicology, 1649
Methoxyflurane, 286–288. *See also* Anesthesia
actions/effects on, heart and circulation, 286–287
kidney, 287–288, 922
liver, 287
muscle, 287
nervous system, 287
respiration, 287
uterus, 287
anesthetic actions, 286
chemistry and preparations, 286
evaluation, 288
metabolism, 288
pharmacological properties, 286–288
physical properties, 277, 286
structural formula, 277
tension in arterial blood, 261
5-Methoxy-3,4-methylenedioxyamphetamine, 564–
565
Methoxyphenamine, 166. *See also* Sympathomimetic drugs
receptor-type activity, 142
structural formula, 142
uses, 166
Methscopolamine bromide, chemistry, 121
preparation and dosage, 129
Methsuximide, use in epilepsy, 462
Methyclothiazide, structural formula, properties,
and dosage, 900

Methyl alcohol, 386–387
  metabolism, 386
    relation to ethanol oxidation, 386
  poisoning, 386–387
    treatment and prognosis, 387
Methyl bromide, toxicology, 1652
Methylatropine nitrate, chemistry, 121
Methylbenzethonium chloride, 954, 978
Methyl-CCNU. *See* Semustine
Methylcellulose, 951, 1004. *See also* Cathartics,
    bulk-forming laxatives
Methylcobalamin, 1333
Methyldopa, 198, 793–797
  absorption, fate, and excretion, 795–796
  chemistry, 793
  mechanism of action, 81–82, 794–795
  pharmacokinetics, 1718
  pharmacological properties, 795
  preparations, administration, and dosage, 796
  toxicity and precautions, 796
  uses, carcinoid disease, 797
    hypertension, 811
Methyldopate, conversion to methyldopa, 796
  preparations, administration, and dosage, 796
Methylene blue, 980
Methylene chloride, toxicology, 1646
3,4-Methylenedioxyamphetamine, 564–565
Methylergonovine. *See also* Ergot alkaloids
  preparations, 946
  structural formula, 941
2-Methylhistamine, 610
4-Methylhistamine, 610
Methylmalonic aciduria, cyanocobalamin in, 1340
Methylmelamines, 1268
Methylpantothenic acid, 1573
Methylparaben, 969
Methylphenidate, abuse, 553
  chemistry and actions, 589–590
  legal regulations, 1670
  preparations and dosage, 590
  uses, 590
    hyperkinetic syndrome, 172, 590
    narcolepsy, 590
Methylphenobarbital, legal regulations, 1671
Methylprednisolone. *See also* Adrenocorticosteroids
  preparations, 1485
  relative potency, duration of action, and equiva-
    lent dose, 1482
Methylsalicylate, 698
  poisoning, 695
  structural formula, 689
Methyltestosterone, 1456
Methylthiouracil. *See also* Antithyroid drugs
  preparations and dosage, 1411
Methyltyrosine. *See* Alpha-methyltyrosine
Methylxanthines. *See* Xanthines
Methyprylon, chemistry, 365
  dosage and preparations, 351
  legal regulations, 1671
  pharmacological properties, 365
Methysergide, antagonism of 5-hydroxytryptamine,
    638–639

preparations and dosage, 639, 946
  structural formula, 941
  untoward effects, 639
  use in migraine, 947
Metiamide, 630
METICORTELONE ACETATE (prednisolone acetate),
    1485
METICORTELONE SOLUBLE (prednisolone sodium suc-
    cinate), 1485
Metoclopramide, 997
Metocurine, 220, 231. *See also* Neuromuscular
    blocking agents
Metolazone, properties and dosage, 899, 900
METOPIRONE (metyrapone), 1492
Metopon, dosage, 507
  duration of analgesic effect, 507
Metoprolol, 195–197
  absorption, distribution, and excretion, 195–196
  pharmacokinetics, 1718
  preparations, route of administration, and dosage,
    196–197
  structural formula, 189
  toxicity and precautions, 196
  uses, 197
    antihypertensive, 810–812
METRAZOL (pentylenetetrazol), 588
Metric system of weights and measures, 1661
Metrifonate, 1018–1019
Metronidazole, 1063, 1075–1077
  absorption, fate, and excretion, 1075–1076
  actions on amebae, 1063
  antimicrobial effects, 1075
  chemistry, 1075
  history, 1075
  preparations, 1076
  reactions with alcohol, 387
  routes of administration and dosage, 1076
  toxicity, 1076
  uses, amebiasis, 1062–1063
    bacterial infections, 1077
    dracontiasis, 1077
    giardiasis, 1077
    trichomoniasis, 1077
METUBINE IODIDE (metocurine iodide), 231
Metyrapone, 1492
Metyrosine. *See* Alpha-methyltytosine
Mezlocillin, 1147
MICATIN (miconazole nitrate), 983
Mickey Finn, 363
Miconazole, 982–983
  uses, amebic meningoencephalitis, 1240
    systemic fungal infections, 1239
MICRONOR (norethindrone), 1437, 1440
Microsomal drug metabolism, 13–19
Microsporum infections. *See* Tinea infections
MIDAMOR (amiloride hydrochloride), 910
Migraine, caffeine in, 947
  clonidine in, 799
  ergot alkaloids in, 946–947
  methysergide in, 947
  propranolol in, 194, 947
Mild silver protein, 977

Milk of magnesia, 993, 1005
MILONTIN (phensuximide), 462
MILTOWN (meprobamate), 351, 1671
Minamata disease, 1623
Mineral oil, 952
  laxative properties, 1009
  preparations and dosage, 1009
  toxicity, 1009
Minimal brain dysfunction, methylphenidate in, 590
  pemoline in, 590
  treatment, 416
MINIPRESS (prazosin hydrochloride), 807
MINOCIN (minocycline hydrochloride), 1185
Minocycline. *See also* Tetracyclines
  absorption, distribution, and excretion, 1184
  antifungal activity, 1234
  dosage, 1185
  pharmacokinetics, 1718
  preparations and administration, 1185
  structural formula, 1181
Minoxidil, 803
MINTEZOL (thiabendazole), 1026
MIOCHOL (acetylcholine chloride for ophthalmic solution), 95
MIOSTAT INTRAOCULAR (carbachol intraocular solution), 95
MIRACIL D (lucanthone), 1016
MIRADON (anisindione), 1359
Mirex, toxicology, 1650
MITHRACIN (mithramycin), 1296, 1529
Mithramycin, 1295–1296, 1529
  uses, hypercalcemia, 1529
    neoplastic diseases, 1253, 1296
Mitomycin, 1296–1297
  use in neoplastic disease, 1253, 1297
Mitotane, 1300–1301
  use in neoplastic diseases, 1253, 1300
MMDA. *See* 5-Methoxy-3,4-methylenedioxyamphetamine
MOBAN (molindone hydrochloride), 411
MODICON, 1440
MOGADON (nitrazepam), 350
Molar thyrotropin, 1387–1388
Molindone, 397, 411. *See also* Antipsychotic agents
Molybdenum, provisional dietary allowance, 1555
MONISTAT-7 (miconazole nitrate), 983
MONISTAT I.V. (miconazole), 1239
Monoamine oxidase, 76–77, 479
  isozymes, 159, 204–205
  role in histamine metabolism, 618–619
  role in 5-hydroxytryptamine metabolism, 637–638
  selective inhibitors, 204–205
Monoamine oxidase inhibitors, 204–205, 427–430.
  See also individual agents
  absorption, fate, and excretion, 429
  actions/effects on, animal behavior, 429
    cardiovascular system, 429
    EEG, 428–429
    sleep, 428–429
  chemistry, 428
  history, 427–428
  hypertensive crisis from, 159

  interaction with other drugs, 429–430
  mechanism of hypotensive effect, 158
  pharmacological properties, 428–430
  preparations and dosage, 424
  selective, 159
  specificity, 428
  status as antihypertensives, 807–808
  structure-activity relationship, 428
  toxic reactions and side effects, 429
  uses, depression, 435–436
    narcolepsy, 428, 430
    parkinsonism, 484
    phobic-anxiety states, 430
Monobenzone, chemistry and actions, 959
  preparations and uses, 959
Monoureides, 369
Monuron, toxicology, 1654
MOPP regimen, use in Hodgkin's disease, 1263, 1289, 1300
Morphine. *See also* Opioids
  absorption, distribution, fate, and excretion, 505–506
  actions at opioid receptor subtypes, 522
  actions/effects on, biliary tract, 504–505
    cardiovascular system, 503
    central nervous system, 499–503
    cough reflex, 502
    EEG, 501
    endocrine system, 501
    excitatory thresholds, 501
    gastrointestinal tract, 503–505
    hypothalamus, 501
    nausea and vomiting, 502–503
    pain, 499–500
    pituitary hormones, 501
    pupil, 501
    respiration, 502
    skin, 505
    spinal cord, 498, 500
    ureter and urinary bladder, 505
    uterus, 505
  acute poisoning, 510–511
    opioid antagonists in, 510–511, 525
  addiction, treatment, 570–571, 574–575
  dosage, 507, 509
  duration of analgesic effect, 506–507
  history and source, 494–496
  idiosyncrasy and precautions, 507–508
  interactions with other drugs, 508
  legal regulations, 1670
  mechanism of action, 497–499
  pharmacokinetics, 1719
  pharmacological properties, 497–509
  physical dependence, 546–549
    and liability for abuse, 505
  preparations and administration, 509
  sites of analgesic action, 500
  structural formula, 496
  tolerance, 505, 546–549
  uses, 511–513
    for constipating effect, 513
    dyspnea, 513

obstetrical analgesia, 512
  pain relief, 511–512
  preanesthetic medication, 270
  sedation and sleep, 512–513
  variations in response, 507–508
Morphine methylsulfonate, legal regulations, 1670
Morrhuate sodium injection, 956
Motilin, 637
Motion sickness, amphetamine in, 629
  ephedrine in, 629
  H₁-receptor blockers in, 629
  scopolamine in, 135, 629
MOTRIN (ibuprofen), 711
Mountain sickness, carbonic anhydrase inhibitors in, 899
Moxalactam, 1156
Mucolytics, actions and uses, 960
MUCOMYST (acetylcysteine), 704, 960
Mucor infections, choice of drugs in, 1093
Mucoviscidosis, pancreatic enzymes in, 998
MULTIBASE, 952
MULTIFUGE (piperazine citrate), 1023
Multiple myeloma, cyclophosphamide in, 1266
  lomustine in, 1271
  melphalan in, 1267
  nitrosoureas in, 1270, 1271
  semustine in, 1271
Multiple sclerosis, baclofen in, 489
  dantrolene in, 491
Multiplication stimulatory activity, 1376
Murine typhus, choice of drugs in, 1092
Muscarine, history and sources, 96
  mechanism of action, 96
  pharmacological properties, 96–97
  structural formula, 97
Muscarinic cholinergic receptors, definition, 83–84
Muscimol, 247–248
Muscle relaxants. *See* Skeletal muscle relaxants
Muscle spasm, relaxant drugs in, 491
  status of curariform drugs in, 232
Mushroom poisoning, atropine in, 98, 136
  causes, 98
  thioctic acid in, 98
MUSTARGEN (mechlorethamine), 1263
MUTAMYCIN (mitomycin), 1297
Muzolimine, 903
Myalgia, acetaminophen in, 705
  phenacetin in, 705
  salicylates in, 697
MYAMBUTOL (ethambutol hydrochloride), 1207
Myasthenia gravis, adrenocorticosteroids in, 116
  ambenonium in, 115
  cholinergic crisis, 115
  diagnosis, 115
  immunosuppressive agents in, 116
  myasthenic crisis, 115
  neostigmine in, 115–116
  pathophysiology, 114–115
  plasmapheresis in, 116
  pyridostigmine in, 115–116
  thymectomy in, 116
  treatment, 115–116

Mycetismus, 98
MYCHEL (chloramphenicol), 1193
MYCIFRADIN (neomycin sulfate), 1177
MYCIQUENT (neomycin sulfate for topical use), 1177
Mycobacterial infections, atypical, 1213. *See also* Tuberculosis
  choice of drugs in, 1091
  tetracyclines in, 1191
Mycobacterium leprae infections, choice of drugs in, 1091
Mycobacterium tuberculosis infections, choice of drugs in, 1091
MYCOLOG, 1177
Mycoplasma pneumoniae infections, chloramphenicol in, 1196
  choice of drugs in, 1092
  erythromycin in, 1225
  tetracycline in, 1190
Mycosis fungoides, azaribine in, 1282
  mechlorethamine in, 1263
  methotrexate in, 1276
MYCOSTATIN (nystatin), 1233
Mycotic infections. *See also* individual infections
  amphotericin B in, 1236, 1239–1240
  benzoic and salicylic acids in, 698, 984
  choice of drugs in, 1093
  clotrimazole in, 983
  flucytosine in, 1237, 1239–1240
  griseofulvin in, 1238
  haloprogin in, 983–984
  hydroxystilbamidine in, 1239
  miconazole in, 982, 1239
  miscellaneous agents in, 984
  nystatin in, 1233
  tolnaftate in, 983
  topical agents in, 981–984
  undecylenic acid in, 982
MYDRIACYL (tropicamide), 132
Myelofibrosis, busulfan in, 1269
Myeloma, chlorambucil in, 1268
  doxorubicin in, 1293
  procarbazine in, 1300
MYLANTA, 991
MYLANTA-II, 991, 996
MYLAXEN (hexafluorenium bromide), 231
MYLERAN (busulfan), 1268
MYLICON (simethicone), 954
Myocardial infarction. *See also* Cardiac arrhythmias; Cardiac failure; Shock
  anticoagulants in, 1363
  antithrombotic drugs in, 1363
  atropine in, 135
  beta-adrenergic blocking drugs in, 194
  estrogens in, 1431
  hyaluronidase in, 961
  methoxamine in, 827
  nitroglycerin in, 827
  nitroprusside in, 827
  opioids in, 503
  oxygen in, 330
  phentolamine in, 827
  phenylephrine in, 827

MYOCHRYSINE (gold sodium thiomalate), 715
Myoclonic seizures. *See also* Epilepsy
 drug therapy, 470
MYOTONACHOL (bethanechol chloride), 95
Myotonia congenita, quinine in, 1056
MYPROZINE (natamycin), 984
MYSOLINE (primidone), 458
MYTELASE (ambenonium chloride), 112
Myxedema, 1405–1406
 thyroid hormones in, 1407

Nabam, toxicology, 1655
Nabilone, 563
Nadolol, 195, 196
 pharmacokinetics, 1719
 structural formula, 189
Naegleria infections, amphotericin B in, 1061
NAFCIL (nafcillin sodium), 1143
Nafcillin, 1143. *See also* Penicillins
 pharmacokinetics, 1720
Nafoxidine, 1304, 1433. *See also* Antiestrogens
Nalbuphine, pharmacological effects, 527
 preparations and dosage, 528
 structural formula, 496
 tolerance, physical dependence, and abuse liability, 527–528
 uses, 528
NALFON (fenoprofen calcium), 712
Nalidixic acid, 1120–1121
NALLINE (nalorphine hydrochloride injection), 524–
 525
N-allylnormetazocine, 522
Nalorphine. *See also* Opioid antagonists
 absorption, fate, and excretion, 524
 abuse potential, 524
 actions at opioid receptor subtypes, 522
 antagonism to opioids, 523
 legal regulations, 1671
 pharmacological effects, 523
 precipitation of opioid withdrawal syndrome, 524
 preparations, 524–525
 structural formula, 496
 withdrawal syndrome, 524
Naloxone, 521–525. *See also* Opioid antagonists
 absorption, fate, and excretion, 524
 abuse potential, 524
 actions at opioid receptor subtypes, 522
 antagonism to opioids, 523
 pharmacological effects, 522
 precipitation of opioid withdrawal syndrome,
  523–524
 preparations, 524
 structural formula, 496
 uses, acute opioid poisoning, 510, 525
  opioid addiction, 575
Naltrexone. *See also* Opioid antagonists
 absorption and duration of action, 524
 pharmacological effects, 522
 structural formula, 496
 use in opioid addiction, 575
 withdrawal syndrome, 524

Nandrolone decanoate, 1457
Nandrolone phenpropionate, 1457
Naphazoline, dosage and preparations, 168
 structural formula, 144
 use in nasal congestion, 168
α-Naphthylthiourea, toxicology, 1653
NAPROSYN (naproxen), 712
Naproxen, 712. *See also* Propionic acid derivatives
NAQUA (trichloromethiazide), 900
NARCAN (naloxone hydrochloride injection), 524
NARCAN NEONATAL (naloxone hydrochloride injec-
 tion for use in neonates), 524
Narcolepsy, methylphenidate in, 590
 monoamine oxidase inhibitors in, 428, 430
 sympathomimetic drugs in, 171
Narcotherapy, barbiturates in, 361
Narcotics. *See* Opioids
Narcotics Anonymous, 573
NARDIL (phenelzine sulfate), 424
Nasal decongestion, belladonna alkaloids in, 134
 sympathomimetic amines in, 168
NATACYN (natamycin), 984
Natamycin, 984
National Formulary, 54
NATURETIN (bendroflumethiazide), 900
Nausea and vomiting, phenothiazines in, 417–
 418
NAVANE (thiothixene hydrochloride), 410
NAXOGIN (nimorazole), 1075
NDA, 48
NEBCIN (tobramycin), 1175
Necatoriasis, occurrence and treatment, 1031
NEGGRAM (nalidixic acid), 1121
Neisseria gonorrhoeae infections, choice of drugs in,
 1087
Neisseria infections, cephalosporins in, 1155
 penicillins in, 1139
Neisseria meningitidis infections, choice of drugs in,
 1087
NEMBUTAL (pentobarbital), 350, 1670
NEMBUTAL SODIUM (pentobarbital sodium), 350
NEO-ANTERGAN (pyrilamine maleate), 628
NEOBASE, 952
NEOBIOTIC (neomycin sulfate), 1177
NEOMERCAZOLE (carbimazole), 1411
Neomycin, 1177–1178. *See also* Aminoglycoside antibiotics; Antimicrobial agents
 absorption and excretion, 1177
 antibacterial activity, 1177
 effect on plasma lipids, 845
 preparations, administration, and dosage, 1177
 structural formula, 1164
 untoward effects, 1177–1178
 uses, ammonia intoxication, 870
  cutaneous deodorant, 954
  hepatic coma, 1178
  preparation of bowel for surgery, 1178
  topical, 1178
Neomycin and polymyxin B sulfates and bacitracin
 zinc ointment, 1177
Neomycin and polymyxin B sulfates solution for irrigation, 1177

Neoplastic diseases, 1256–1313. *See also* individual
  diseases
  cell-cycle kinetics, 1250
  chemotherapeutic agents, classification and indi-
    cations, 1252–1254
  principles of therapy, 1249–1255
Neopyrithiamine, 1561
NEOSPORIN (neomycin and polymyxin B sulfates),
  1177
Neostigmine. *See also* Anticholinesterases
  absorption, fate, and excretion, 108
  history, 100
  pharmacokinetics, 1720
  preparations, 112
  structural formula, 104
  uses, ileus, 113
    myasthenia gravis, 115–116
    urinary bladder atony, 113
NEO-SYNEPHRINE (phenylephrine hydrochloride),
  165
NEPHRAMINE (essential amino acid injection), 863
Nephrogenic diabetes insipidus, benzothiadiazides
  in, 925
  pathophysiology, 920
Nephrotic syndrome, adrenocorticosteroids in, 1489
NEPTAZANE (methazolamide), 898
Nerve growth factor, 1376
NESACAINE (chloroprocaine hydrochloride), 309
Netilmicin, 1164
Neuralgia, carbamazepine in, 460
  salicylates in, 697
Neuritis of pregnancy, thiamine in, 1563
Neuroblastoma, cyclophosphamide in, 1266
  doxorubicin in, 1293
  vinblastine in, 1289
  vincristine in, 1290
Neurohumoral transmission, 56–85. *See also* Auto-
  nomic nervous system
Neurolept analgesia, 295–296
  uses and status, 295–296
Neuroleptic drugs, 395–418. *See also* Antipsychotic
  agents
Neuromuscular blocking agents, 220–232. *See also*
  Autonomic nervous system; individual agents
  absorption, fate, and excretion, 230
  actions/effects on, autonomic ganglia, 227–228
    cardiovascular system, 228
    central nervous system, 227
    cholinergic receptor sites, 222–226
    histamine release, 228
    miscellaneous systems, 228
    skeletal muscle, 223–227
  competitive type, 220, 225
  depolarizing type, 220, 225
  history, sources, and chemistry, 220–221
  mechanisms of action, 223–226
  pharmacological properties, 223–231
  preparations, routes of administration, and dos-
    age, 230–231
  structure-activity relationship, 221–222
  synergisms and antagonisms, 228–229
  toxicology, 229–230

  uses, 231–232
Neurophysin, 918
Neuroses, diagnostic terminology, 393
  tricyclic antidepressants in, 427
Neurotensin, 1392
NEUTRAPEN (penicillinase), 1130
Niacin, 1567–1570. *See also* Nicotinic acid
  recommended dietary allowance, 1553
  vasodilator properties, 831
Niacinamide, 1569
Nialamide, 428
  mechanism of adrenergic action, 82
NICALEX (aluminum nicotinate), 839
Niclosamide, 1019–1020
  anthelmintic action, 1019
  chemistry, 1019
  preparations, route of administration, and dosage,
    1019
  toxicity and precautions, 1020
  uses, 1020
Nicocodeine, legal regulations, 1670
Nicomorphine, legal regulations, 1670
NICONYL (isoniazid), 1202
Nicotine, absorption, fate, and excretion, 214
  absorption from smoke, 558
  abuse, 557–560
  acute poisoning and treatment, 214
  chemistry, 213
  effects on the CNS, 558
  history and source, 212–213
  pharmacological actions, 213–214
  physical dependence, 559–560
  structural formula, 213
  tolerance, 559–560
  withdrawal symptoms, 559–560
Nicotinic acid, 839–840, 1567–1570
  absorption, fate, and excretion, 1569
  chemistry, 1568
  effects on plasma lipids, 839
  history, 1567–1568
  human requirement, 1569
    relationship to carcinoid syndrome, 1569
    relationship to tryptophan intake, 1569
  pharmacological actions, 1568
  physiological function, 1568
  preparations and dosage, 839, 1569
  symptoms of deficiency, 1568–1569
  untoward effects, 839
  uses, hyperlipoproteinemias, 840
    pellagra, 1569–1570
    vasodilatation, 831
Nicotinic cholinergic receptors, definition, 83–84
  properties, 29, 222–223
Nicotinyl alcohol, vasodilator properties, 831
Nifedipine, 828
Nifurtimox, 1077–1078
  use in trypanosomiasis, 1078
Nikethamide, chemistry and actions, 589
  preparations, dosage, and uses, 589
NIKORIN (nikethamide), 589
Nilidrin, 831
NILSTAT (nystatin), 1233

Nimorazole, 1075
NIORIC (pentylenetetrazol), 588
Nipecotic acid, 247, 248
NIPRIDE (sodium nitroprusside), 806
NIRAN (parathion), 104
Niridazole, 1020–1022
  absorption, fate, and excretion, 1021
  anthelmintic action, 1020
  chemistry, 1020
  pharmacological effects, 1020–1021
  preparations, route of administration, and dosage, 1021
  toxicity and precautions, 1021
  uses, 1022
NIRVANOL, 455
NISENTIL (alphaprodine hydrochloride), 507, 516
NITRANITOL (mannitol hexanitrate), 826
Nitrates, 819–828. *See also* individual agents
  absorption, fate, and excretion, 822–823
  actions/effects on, cardiovascular system, 820–822
    coronary circulation, 820–821
    heart, 820–822
    smooth muscle, 822
  chemistry, 819–820
  correlation of plasma concentrations and biological activity, 823
  history, 819
  mechanism of action, 821–822
  pharmacological properties, 820–825
  preparations and dosage, 825, 826
  routes of administration, 823–824
  tolerance, 824
  toxicity and untoward responses, 824–825
  uses, angina pectoris, 825
    congestive heart failure, 825–827
    myocardial infarction, 827
    variant angina, 828
Nitrazepam. *See also* Benzodiazepines
  dosage and half-life, 350
  pharmacokinetics, 348, 1720
Nitrites, use in cyanide poisoning, 1651
NITRO-BID (nitroglycerin), 826
Nitrofurantoin, 1121–1122
Nitrofurazone, 979
  use in trypanosomiasis, 1074
Nitrogen, elimination in anesthesia, 266
Nitrogen dioxide, toxicology, 1640
Nitrogen mustards, 1263–1268. *See also* Alkylating agents; individual agents
  use in neoplastic diseases, 1252
Nitroglycerin. *See also* Nitrates
  absorption, fate, and excretion, 822
  dependence, 824
  pharmacokinetics, 1721
  preparations, administration, and dosage, 825, 826
  structural formula, 826
  uses, angina pectoris, 825
    congestive heart failure, 825–827
    myocardial infarction, 827
    variant (Prinzmetal's) angina, 828
NITROL (nitroglycerin), 826
Nitromersol, 976

Nitroprusside, cardiovascular properties, 805
  preparations, administration, and dosage, 806
  toxicity and contraindications, 805–806
  uses, congestive heart failure, 827
    ergot-induced gangrene, 185
    hypertensive emergencies, 812–813
    myocardial infarction, 827
Nitrosoureas, 1269–1271. *See also* Alkylating agents; individual agents
  classification and structures, 1259
  reactions with nucleic acids and proteins, 1259–1261
  use in neoplastic diseases, 1252
NITROSTAT (nitroglycerin), 826
Nitrous oxide, 289–291. *See also* Anesthesia
  actions/effects on, circulation, 290
    miscellaneous systems, 290–291
    respiration, 290
  chemistry, preparations, and properties, 277, 289
  diffusion hypoxia, 264–265
  elimination, 291
  evaluation, 291
  general anesthetic actions, 289–290
  history, 258
  pharmacological properties, 289–291
  physical properties, 277, 289
  tension in arterial blood, 261
  tissue tensions, 264
Nocardia infections, choice of drugs in, 1092
  minocycline in, 1191
  sulfonamides in, 1115
Nocturnal leg cramps, quinine in, 1057
NOLUDAR (methyprylon), 351, 1671
NOLVADEX (tamoxifen citrate), 1304
Noncatecholamines, 157–166. *See also* Sympathomimetic drugs; individual agents
  absorption, distribution, and fate, 159
  locus and mechanism of action, 157–158
Nonketotic hyperglycinemia, strychnine in, 587
Nonsuppressible insulin-like activity, 1376
Noradrenaline. *See* Norepinephrine
Nordefrin, receptor-type activity, 142
  structural formula, 142
Nordiazepam, 439
Norephedrine, 569
Norepinephrine, 71–80, 151–153. *See also* Autonomic nervous system; Sympathomimetic drugs
  absorption, fate, and excretion, 152
  actions/effects on, cardiovascular system, 145–146, 152
    central nervous system, 152
    metabolism, 152
  adrenergic transmitter function, 71
  biosynthetic pathway, 72
  drugs influencing storage and release, 74
  metabolic disposition, 76–77
  preparations, dosage, and administration, 152–153
  receptor-type activity, 142
  release by sympathomimetic drugs, 157–158
  role as CNS transmitter, 249–251
  storage, 140

structural formula, 142
synthesis, uptake, storage, and release, 71–75
toxicity, side effects, and precautions, 153
uses, 153, 169
Norethandrolone, 1433
Norethindrone, 1437
chemistry, 1433, 1434
in oral contraceptives, 1440
Norethynodrel, chemistry, 1434
in oral contraceptives, 1440
NORFLEX (orphenadrine citrate), 489
Norgestrel, chemistry, 1434
in oral contraceptives, 1440
NORINYL 1 + 50, 1440
NORINYL 1 + 80, 1440
NORINYL, 2 MG, 1440
NORISODRINE AEROTROL (isoproterenol hydrochloride inhalation), 154
NORIT A (activated charcoal), 954
NORLESTRIN, 1, 1440
NORLESTRIN 2.5, 1440
NORLUTATE (norethindrone acetate), 1437
NORLUTIN (norethindrone), 1437
Normeperidine, 516
Normetanephrine, structural formula, 77
NORPACE (disopyramide phosphate), 778
NORPRAMIN (desipramine hydrochloride), 424
NOR-Q.D. (norethindrone), 1437, 1440
Nortriptyline. *See also* Tricyclic antidepressants
pharmacokinetics, 1721
structural formula, 419
Nortriptyline hydrochloride, preparations and dosage, 424
Noscapine, dosage and use in cough, 529–530
Novobiocin, 1230
NOVOCAIN (procaine hydrochloride), 308
NOVRAD (levopropoxyphene napsylate), 529
NUBAIN (nalbuphine hydrochloride), 528
NUCHAR C (activated charcoal), 954
NULOGYL (nimorazole), 1075
NUMORPHAN (oxymorphone), 507, 509, 1670
NUPERCAINE (dibucaine hydrochloride), 309
Nutmeg, abuse, 569
Nutrients, dietary recommendations, 1553, 1555
NYDRAZID (isoniazid), 1202
Nystatin, 1232–1233. *See also* Antifungal drugs
absorption and excretion, 1233
antifungal activity, 1232
chemistry, 1232
fungal resistance and mechanism of action, 1232
history and source, 1232
preparations, administration, and dosage, 1233
toxicity, 1233
uses, *Candida* infections, 1233

Obesity, anoretic drugs in, 171–172
Obidoxime, dosage, 112
structural formula, 110
Obsessive-compulsive neurosis, tricyclic antidepressants in, 427
Obstetrical analgesia. *See* Labor

Octyl *p*-dimethylaminobenzoate, 960
Ocular diseases, adrenocorticosteroids in, 1489
antimuscarinic drugs in, 133–134
OCUSERT (sustained-release pilocarpine), 97
OGEN (estrone), 1428
Oil of gaultheria, 682, 695
Oil of wintergreen, 695
Olive oil, 952
Ololiuqui, 569
OMNIPEN (ampicillin), 1144
OMPA, metabolic conversion, 104
structural formula, 105
Onchocerciasis, occurrence and treatment, 1033
suramin in, 1071
ONCOVIN (vincristine sulfate), 1289
OPHTHAINE (proparacaine hydrochloride), 310
Ophthalmia neonatorum, penicillin G in, 1139, 1141
Ophthalmic infections, sulfacetamide in, 1112
OPHTHETIC (proparacaine hydrochloride), 310
Opioid agonist-antagonists, 521–528. *See also* individual agents
effects in physical dependence, 521–522
mechanism of action, 521–522
pharmacological properties, 521–522
Opioid antagonists, 521–525. *See also* individual agents
absorption, fate, and excretion, 524
classification, 521–522
mechanism of action, 521–522
pharmacological properties, 522–525
preparations, 524–525
structure-activity relationship, 522
tolerance, physical dependence, and abuse potential, 524
uses, acute opioid poisoning, 510, 525
opioid addiction, 574–575
Opioids, 494–530. *See also* individual agents
absorption, distribution, fate, and excretion, 505–507
abuse, legal regulations, 1670–1671
actions/effects on, adenylate cyclase, 498
biliary tract, 504–505
cardiovascular system, 503
central nervous system, 499–503
cough, 502
gastrointestinal tract, 503–505
hypothalamus, 501
pain, 499–500
pituitary hormones, 501
respiration, 502
acute poisoning, 510–511
opioid antagonists in, 510, 525
addiction, assessment of potential, 576
incidence and patterns, 544–545
methadone maintenance, 574
opioid antagonist therapy, 574–575
symptoms and effects, 545–546
withdrawal in the newborn, 548–549
withdrawal symptoms, 547–548
withdrawal treatment, 570–571
antagonists, 521–525
chemistry, 496–497

Opioids (*Cont.*)
cross-dependence, 541
idiosyncrasy and variations in response, 507–508
interactions with other drugs, 508
mechanism of action, 497–499
pharmacological properties, 497–509
physical dependence, 539–542, 546–549
and abuse liability, 505
receptors, 497–498, 521–522
sites of analgesic action, 500
structure-activity relationship, 496–497
tolerance, 505, 538, 546–547
toxicity, 507–508, 510–511
uses, 511–513
for constipating effect, 513
cough, 513
dyspnea, 513
intravenous anesthesia, 295–296
obstetrical analgesia, 512
pain relief, 511–512
preanesthetic medication, 270
sedation and sleep, 512
withdrawal symptoms, 570–571
Opium. *See also* Opioids
legal regulations, 1670
preparations and dosage, 509
source and composition, 495–496
OP-THAL-ZIN (zinc sulfate ophthalmic solution), 977
Oral contraceptives, 1438–1444. *See also* Estrogens; Progestins
effects on laboratory tests, 1440
history, 1438–1439
mechanism of action, 1441–1442
preparations and dosage, 1439–1440
types, 1439
undesirable effects, 1442–1444
ORA-TESTRYL (fluoxymesterone), 1456
ORENZYME (chymotrypsin-trypsin), 961
ORETIC (hydrochlorothiazide), 900
ORETON (testosterone), 1456
ORETON METHYL (methyltestosterone), 1456
ORETON PROPIONATE (testosterone propionate), 1456
Organic mental syndrome, antipsychotic agents in, 416
Organophosphates. *See* Anticholinesterases
ORINASE (tolbutamide), 1513
ORIODIDE-131 (sodium iodide I 131), 1414
Ornithosis, choice of drugs in, 1092
Orphenadrine, chemistry, preparations, and dosage, 487, 489
use in parkinsonism, 485
Orthochlormercuriphenol, 984
ORTHO-NOVUM 1/50, 1440
ORTHO-NOVUM 1/80, 1440
ORTHO-NOVUM 2 MG, 1440
ORTHO-NOVUM 10 MG, 1440
Orthophenylphenol, 969
Orthostatic hypotension. *See* Hypotension
ORTHOXINE (methoxyphenamine hydrochloride), 166
ORUDIS (ketoprofen), 713
OSMITROL (mannitol), 896

OSMOGLYN (glycerin), 896
Osmotic diuretics, 894–896
mechanism of action, 894–895
uses, 895–896
Osmotic pressure, role in net movement of water, 850
Osteoarthritis. *See* Arthritis
Osteomalacia, vitamin D in, 1545
Osteomyelitis, choice of drugs in, 1086
Osteoporosis, androgens in, 1460
estrogens in, 1431
Otitis media, choice of drugs in, 1086
trimethoprim-sulfamethoxazole in, 1119
OTRIVIN (xylometazoline hydrochloride), 168
Ouabain. *See also* Digitalis
preparation and administration, 749
Ouch-ouch. *See* Itai-itai
Ovarian dysgenesis, estrogens in, 1430
OVCON-35, 1440
OVCON-50, 1440
OVEST (conjugated estrogens), 1428
OVOCYLIN (estradiol ester), 1428
OVRAL, 1440
OVRETTE (norgestrel), 1440
OV-STATIN (nystatin), 1233
OVULEN, 1440
Ox bile extract, preparations and dosage, 999
Oxacillin, 1142–1143. *See also* Penicillins
OXALID (oxyphenbutazone), 700
Oxamniquine, 1022
Oxandrolone, 1458
Oxantel, 1024
Oxazepam, 437–441. *See also* Benzodiazepines
dosage, half-life, and preparations, 350, 440
legal regulations, 1671
Oxazolam. *See also* Benzodiazepines
dosage and half-life, 350
Oxazolidinediones, 464–466
Oxidized cellulose, 955
Oxolinic acid, 1121
Oxotremorine, pharmacological properties, 96
structural formula, 97
Oxprenolol, hypnotic effect, 369
pharmacological properties, 188, 196
OXSORALEN (methoxalen), 958
Oxtriphylline, 592, 601
OXYCEL SURGICEL (oxidized cellulose), 955
Oxychlorosene, 974
Oxycodone, dosage, 507
duration of analgesic effect, 507
legal regulations, 1670
preparations, 509
structural formula, 496
Oxygen, 321–331
administration, 329
apnea, 327
effects on blood gases, 325–326
effects on cardiovascular system, 325
effects on respiration, 325
methods, 329
pulmonary atelectasis, 327
retrolental fibroplasia, 327
untoward effects, 327–328

carriage and transfer in blood, 322–323, 326
deprivation, effects on cardiovascular system, 323–324
  effects on central nervous system, 324
  effects on individual organs and tissues, 324
  effects on metabolism, 324
  effects on oxygen saturation and tension of blood, 322
  effects on respiration, 322–323
  etiology, 321–322
dissociation curve from hemoglobin, 323
history, 321
hyperbaric, uses, 331
poisoning, 327–328
preparations, 328–329
uses, abdominal distention, 330
  air embolism, 331
  anemia, 330
  anesthesia, 331
  bronchoconstriction, 329
  carbon monoxide poisoning, 330–331, 1643
  cardiac decompensation, 330
  cerebrovascular accidents, 330
  cyanide poisoning, 1652
  diffusion barriers, 330
  high altitudes, 329
  myocardial infarction, 330
  pneumonia, 330
  pneumothorax, 331
  pulmonary edema, 330
  pulmonary emphysema, 330
  pulmonary fibrosis, 330
  shock, 330
  venous-arterial shunts, 330
  ventilation-perfusion inequalities, 330
OXYLONE (fluorometholone), 1486
Oxymetazoline, dosage and preparations, 168
  structural formula, 144
  use in nasal congestion, 168
Oxymetholone, 1458
Oxymorphone, dosage, 507
  duration of analgesic effect, 507
  legal regulations, 1670
  preparations, 509
  structural formula, 496
Oxypertine, 397
Oxyphenbutazone, 700. See also Phenylbutazone
Oxyphencyclimine, preparations and structural formula, 132
Oxyphenisatin acetate, status as cathartic, 1007
Oxyphenonium, preparations and structural formula, 131
Oxytetracycline. See also Tetracyclines
  absorption, distribution, and excretion, 1184
  dosage, 1185
  preparations and administration, 1185
  structural formula, 1181
Oxythiamine, 1561
Oxytocics, 935–949. See also individual agents
Oxytocin, 936–938
  absorption, fate, and excretion, 937–938
  actions/effects on, cardiovascular system, 937

  mammary gland, 937
  uterus, 936–937
  water and electrolyte excretion, 937
bioassay and unitage, 938
mechanism of action, 937
physiological role, 936
preparations, 938
role as CNS transmitter, 253
structural formula, 917
uses, induction of labor at term, 947–948
  during lactation, 938
  third stage of labor and puerperium, 948–949
  uterine inertia, 948
Oxytocin-challenge test, 949
Oxytocin citrate buccal tablets, 938
Oxytocin injection, 938
Oxytocin nasal spray, 938
Oxyuriasis. See Enterobiasis
Ozone, toxicology, 1640

PACATAL (mepazine), 406
Paget's disease, calcitonin in, 1538
  etidronate sodium in, 1538
  mithramycin in, 1296
PAGITANE (cycrimine hydrochloride), 486
Pain, acetaminophen in, 705
  amphetamine in, 512
  aspirin-like drugs in, 686
  Brompton's mixture in, 512
  ibuprofen in, 713
  mefenamic acid in, 709
  opioids in, 499–500, 511–512
  phenacetin in, 705
  role of prostaglandins, 684
  salicylates in, 697
PALFIUM (dextromoramide), 507
PALUDRINE (chloroguanide hydrochloride), 1047
2-PAM. See Pralidoxime
Pamaquine, 1043
PAMELOR (nortriptyline hydrochloride), 424
PAMINE (methscopolamine bromide), 129
PAMISYL SODIUM (aminosalicylate sodium), 1210
Pancreatic enzymes, 998
Pancreatic islet-cell carcinoma, streptozocin in, 1271
Pancreatin, 998
Pancreatitis, antimuscarinic drugs in, 133
  pancreatic enzymes in, 998
Pancreozymin-cholecystokinin, effect on insulin secretion, 1500
Pancuronium. See also Neuromuscular blocking agents
  preparations and dosage, 231
  structural formula, 221
PANHEPRIN (heparin sodium injection), 1351
PANRONE (amithiozone), 1216
PANTOPON (purified opium alkaloids), 509
Pantothenic acid, 1572–1573
  absorption, fate, and excretion, 1573
  chemistry, 1572
  history, 1572
  human requirement, 1573

Pantothenic acid (*Cont.*)
  pharmacological actions, 1572
  physiological function, 1572–1573
  preparations, 1573
  provisional dietary allowance, 1555
  symptoms of deficiency, 1573
PANWARFIN (warfarin sodium), 1357
Papaverine, 495–496, 830
Para-aminobenzoic acid, 960
  status as vitamin, 1560
Para-aminophenol derivatives, 701–705. *See also* individual agents
Parabens, 969
Paracetamol. *See* Acetaminophen
Parachlorometacresol, 968, 969
Parachlorometaxylenol, 968, 969
Parachlorophenol, 969
Paracoccidioidomycosis, amphotericin B in, 1240
  miconazole in, 1239
  sulfonamides in, 1240
PARACODIN (dihydrocodeine), 507
PARACORT (prednisone), 1485
PARADIONE (paramethadione), 465–466
Paraffin, 952
PARAFLEX (chlorzoxazone), 489
Paraldehyde, 368
  dosage and preparations, 351, 368
  legal regulations, 1671
  uses, alcohol withdrawal, 572
Paralytic ileus. *See* Ileus
Paramethadione, use in epilepsy, 465
Paramethasone. *See also* Adrenocorticosteroids
  preparations, 1485
  relative potency, duration of action, and equivalent dose, 1482
Paraoxon, 104
  structural formula, 105
Paraplegia, dantrolene in, 491
Paraquat, toxicology, 1654
PARASAL SODIUM (aminosalicylate sodium), 1210
Parasympathetic nervous system. *See* Autonomic nervous system
Parasympathomimetic drugs, 91–98. *See also* individual agents
Parathion, history, 101
  metabolism, 104
  structural formula, 105
  uses, 104
Parathyroid hormone, 1531–1536
  absorption, fate, and excretion, 1536
  actions/effects on, bone, 1533
    intestinal calcium absorption, 1534
    magnesium metabolism, 881
    renal calcium and phosphate excretion, 1533–1534
  chemistry, 1532
  history, 1531–1532
  hypersecretion, 1535
  hyposecretion, 1534–1535
  physiological function, 1532–1534
  preparations, bioassay, and unitage, 1535–1536
  synthesis and immunoassay, 1532
  use in diagnosis of pseudohypoparathyroidism, 1536
Paratyphoid fever, choice of drugs in, 1089
PAREDRINE (hydroxyamphetamine hydrobromide), 164
Paregoric, legal regulations, 1671
  preparation and dosage, 509
PARENAMINE (protein hydrolysate injection), 863
PAREST (methaqualone), 351, 1670
Pargyline, mechanism of adrenergic action, 82
Parkinsonian syndrome, from antipsychotic drugs, 407, 412
Parkinsonism, amantadine in, 483
  anticholinergic drugs in, 135, 484–485
  antihistamines in, 485
  benztropine in, 484–485
  biperidine in, 484–485
  carbidopa in, 482–483
  chlorphenoxamine in, 485
  clinical features, 475–476
  cycrimine in, 484–485
  decarboxylase inhibitors in, 482–483
  dopaminergic mechanisms, 476
  drugs in, 475–488
  ethopropazine in, 484–485
  etiology, 475
  levodopa in, 485, 487
  orphenadrine in, 485
  procyclidine in, 484–485
  sympathomimetic drugs in, 171
  trihexyphenidyl in, 484–485
PARLODEL (bromocriptine mesylate), 946, 1382
PARNATE (tranylcypromine sulfate), 424
Paromomycin, 1068, 1163
  use in, amebiasis, 1062, 1068
    cestodiasis, 1033, 1034, 1068
Paroxysmal nocturnal dyspnea, morphine in, 513
Paroxysmal tachycardia. *See also* Cardiac arrhythmias
  digitalis in, 751
  edrophonium in, 112
  methoxamine in, 170
  phenylephrine in, 170
  procainamide in, 776
  propranolol in, 785
  quinidine in, 772
  treatment, 769
PARSIDOL (ethopropazine hydrochloride), 486
Particulates, toxicology, 1643–1644
PAS CALCIUM (aminosalicylate calcium), 1210
PAS-C (para-aminosalicylic acid recrystallized in vitamin C), 845
Pasteurella multocida infections, choice of drugs in, 1090
  penicillin G in, 1140
PATHILON (tridihexethyl chloride), 131
PATHOCIL (dicloxacillin sodium), 1143
Patient compliance, 1671–1673
  factors causing noncompliance, 1672–1673
  role of the pharmacist, 1673
PAVULON (pancuronium bromide), 231
PBZ (tripelennamine), 628

Peanut oil, 952
Pectin, 954
PEDIAMYCIN (erythromycin ethylsuccinate), 1224
Pediculosis, benzyl benzoate in, 985
    isobornyl thiocyanoacetate in, 985
    lindane in, 985
    pyrethrins in, 985
    sulfur ointment in, 985
PEGANONE (ethotoin), 456
Pellagra, nicotinic acid in, 1569–1570
PEMA. See Phenylethylmalonamide
Pemoline, 590
Pemphigus, adrenocorticosteroids in, 1491
    gold in, 716
Pempidine, 216–217. See also Ganglionic blocking
        agents
PENBRITIN (ampicillin), 1144
Penbutolol, 188, 196
Penfluridol, 397
Penicillamine, 1627–1628
    absorption, fate, and excretion, 1627
    preparations and dosage, 1628
    side effects and toxicity, 1627–1628
    uses, cystinuria, 1628
        heavy-metal poisoning, 1628
        lead poisoning, 1622, 1628
        mercury poisoning, 1628
        rheumatoid arthritis, 1628
        Wilson's disease, 1628
Penicillinase, effects on, cephalosporins, 1151–1152
        penicillins, 1130
    preparations, 1130
Penicillin F, 1128
Penicillin G. See also Penicillins
    absorption, fate, and excretion, 1132–1136
    antagonism to tetracyclines, 1183
    antimicrobial activity, 1131–1132
    cerebrospinal fluid concentrations, 1135
    chemistry, 1128
    dosage, 1136–1141. See also individual infections
    plasma concentration, 1132–1133, 1135
    preparations and routes of administration, 1136–
        1137
    structural formula, 1134
    toxic and untoward reactions, 1147–1150
    urine concentrations, 1136
Penicillin G benzathine, absorption and plasma con-
        centrations, 1135
    preparations, 1137
Penicillin G procaine, absorption and plasma con-
        centrations, 1135
    preparations, 1137
Penicillin K, 1128
Penicillin N, 1151
Penicillin V. See also Penicillins
    pharmacological and antimicrobial properties,
        1131–1136
    preparations and route of administration, 1137
Penicillin X, 1128
Penicillins, 1126–1150. See also Antimicrobial
        agents; individual agents
    anaphylactic reactions, 1148

antibody production, 1148
antimicrobial activity, factors affecting, 1130–1131
assay, 1128
chemistry, 1128
classification, 1131
history, 1126
hypersensitivity reactions, 1147–1150
mechanism of acquired resistance, 1130
mechanism of action, 1129
microbial resistance, 1130
penicillinase-resistant, 1141–1143
semisynthetic, 1128
source, 1127
suprainfection, 1150
toxic and untoward reactions, 1147–1150
unitage, 1128
uses, 1138–1141, 1145, 1147
    actinomycosis, 1140
    anthrax, 1140
    clostridial infections, 1140
    diphtheria, 1140
    Enterobacter infections, 1147
    enterococcal infections, 1138, 1145
    erysipeloid, 1140
    fusospirochetal infections, 1140
    gonococcal infections, 1139
    Listeria infections, 1140
    meningococcal infections, 1139
    Pasteurella infections, 1140
    pneumococcal infections, 1138
    prophylaxis of endocarditis, 1141
    prophylaxis of gonococcal infections, 1141
    prophylaxis of rheumatic fever, 1141
    prophylaxis of streptococcal infections, 1140
    prophylaxis of syphilis, 1141
    Proteus infections, 1147
    Pseudomonas infections, 1147
    rat-bite fever, 1140
    Salmonella infections, 1145
    scarlet fever, 1138
    sepsis, 1145, 1147
    staphylococcal infections, 1139, 1142
    streptococcal infections, 1138
    subacute endocarditis, 1138
    syphilis, 1139–1140
    urinary tract infections, 1145, 1147
Penicilloic acid, structural formula, 1128
Penicilloyl-polylysine, 1148
Pentachlorophenol, toxicology, 1655
Pentaerythritol chloral, legal regulations, 1671
Pentaerythritol tetranitrate. See also Nitrates
    preparations and dosage, 826
    structural formula, 826
Pentagastrin, 620
Pentamethylmelamine, 1268
Pentamidine, 1071–1072
    absorption, fate, and excretion, 1072
    antifungal activity, 1071
    antiprotozoal activity, 1071
    chemistry and preparations, 1071
    routes of administration and dosage, 1072
    toxicity and side effects, 1072

Pentamidine (*Cont.*)
  uses, *Babesia* infections, 1072
    leishmaniasis, 1072
    pneumonia (*Pneumocystis carinii*), 1072
    trypanosomiasis, 1072
Pentaquine, 1043, 1051, 1052
Pentazocine, 525–527
  absorption, fate, and excretion, 526
  actions at opioid receptor subtypes, 522
  pharmacological effects, 525
  preparations, routes of administration, and dosage, 526
  side effects, toxicity, and precautions, 526
  structural formula, 525
  tolerance, physical dependence, and liability for abuse, 526
  uses, 527
  withdrawal syndrome, 526
PENTHRANE (methoxyflurane), 286
Pentobarbital. *See also* Barbiturates
  chemistry, 351
  dosage, half-life, and preparations, 350
  legal regulations, 1670
Pentolinium, 215–217. *See also* Ganglionic blocking agents
  structural formula, 215
PENTOSTAM (sodium stibogluconate), 1074
Pentostatin, 1283
PENTOTHAL (thiopental sodium), 292
PENTRITOL (pentaerythritol tetranitrate), 826
Pentylenetetrazol, 243, 588
PEN-VEE K (penicillin V potassium), 1137
Pepsin, 998
PEPTAVLON (pentagastrin), 620
Peptic ulcer, antimuscarinic drugs in, 133, 997
  bismuth in, 997
  carbenoxolone sodium in, 997
  cimetidine in, 632, 997
  gastric antacids in, 995–997
  H_2-receptor blockers in, 632
  metoclopramide in, 997
  pathophysiology, 996
  prostaglandins in, 678, 997
Peptidyl dipeptidase, 647, 648, 652, 657, 660, 661
  inhibitors, 657–659
    chemistry, 657
    clinical applications, 658–659
    pharmacological properties, 657–658
    untoward effects, 659
Perchlorate, effects on thyroid function, 1412
PERCODAN (oxycodone), 507, 1670
PERCORTEN ACETATE (desoxycorticosterone acetate), 1484
PERCORTEN PIVALATE (desoxycorticosterone pivalate), 1484
PERGONAL (menotropins for injection), 1386
Perhexiline, 829
PERIACTIN (cyproheptadine hydrochloride), 639
Pericarditis, indomethacin in, 706
Periodic paralysis, carbonic anhydrase inhibitors in, 899
  potassium in, 878

Perioral tremor, 412
Peripheral vascular disease, alpha-adrenergic blocking agents in, 187
  vasodilators in, 830
Peritonitis, gentamicin in, 1175
PERITRATE (pentaerythritol tetranitrate), 826
Permanganates, 974
PERMAPEN (sterile penicillin G benzathine suspension), 1137
PERMITIL HYDROCHLORIDE (fluphenazine hydrochloride), 409
Pernicious anemia. *See* Anemia—megaloblastic
Perphenazine. *See also* Antipsychotic agents
  chemistry, 409
  dosage forms, 409
  dose as antiemetic, 417
  dose as antipsychotic, 409
  side effects, 409
PERSANTINE (dipyridamole), 830, 1361
Persic oil, 952
PERTOFRANE (desipramine hydrochloride), 424
Pertussis, erythromycin in, 1225
Pesticides, toxicology, 1647–1655
PETHADOL (meperidine), 516
Pethidine. *See* Meperidine
Petit mal. *See* Epilepsy
PETRICHLORAL (pentaerythritol chloral), 1671
Petriellidiosis, miconazole in, 1239
Petrolatum, 952
PEXID (perhexiline maleate), 829
Peyote, 569
  legal regulations, 1670
PGI_2. *See* Prostacyclin
Phalloidins, 98
Pharmacist, and patient compliance, 1673
Pharmacodynamics, 28–39. *See also* Drugs
  definition, 2
Pharmacognosy, definition, 1
Pharmacokinetics, 2–26, 1675–1737. *See also* Drugs
  definition, 2
Pharmacology, definition and scope, 1–2
Pharmacotherapeutics, definition, 2
Pharyngitis, choice of drugs in, 1086
PHEMEROL CHLORIDE (benzethonium chloride), 978
Phenacemide, use in epilepsy, 467–468
Phenacetin, 701–705. *See also* Aspirin-like drugs
  absorption, fate, and excretion, 702–703
  abuse liability, 702
  chemistry, 701–702
  hemolytic anemia, 704
  history, 701
  interactions with other drugs, 703
  methemoglobinemia, 704
  nephropathy, 686–687, 703
  pharmacological effects, 702
  preparations and dosage, 705
  toxicity, 703–704
  uses, 705
Phenadoxone, dosage, 507
  duration of analgesic effect, 507
Phenazone. *See* Antipyrine
Phenazopyridine, 1111, 1122

Phencyclidine, 296, 567–568
    absorption, fate, and excretion, 568
    chemistry, 567
    history, 567
    patterns of abuse, 568
    pharmacological actions, 567
    tolerance and physical dependence, 568
    toxicity, 568
Phendimetrazine, legal regulations, 1671
    receptor-type activity, 142
    structural formula, 142
    use in obesity, 172
Phenelzine sulfate. *See also* Monoamine oxidase
        inhibitors
    preparations and dosage, 424
PHENERGAN (promethazine hydrochloride), 417, 628
Phenethicillin. *See also* Penicillins
    pharmacological properties, 1133, 1134
    preparations and routes of administration, 1137
Phenethylamine, 564
Phenformin, 1510
Phenindione, 1359. *See also* Anticoagulants, oral
Pheniprazine, 428
Pheniramine, structural formula, 623. *See also* H_1-
        receptor blockers
Phenmetrazine, legal regulations, 1670
    receptor-type activity, 142
    structural formula, 142
    use in obesity, 172
Phenobarbital. *See also* Barbiturates
    absorption, biotransformation, and excretion, 457
    anticonvulsant properties, 456
    chemistry, 351
    choleresis from, 356
    interactions with other drugs, 457
    legal regulations, 1671
    pharmacokinetics, 1722
    plasma concentrations, 457
    preparations and dosage, for sedation and hypno-
        sis, 350
        in epilepsy, 457
    toxicity, 457
    uses, cholestasis, 361
        epilepsy, 457, 469–470
        hyperbilirubinemia, 361
        hypnotic and sedative, 360
        kernicterus, 361
Phenol, 956, 967
Phenolated calamine lotion, 967
Phenolphthalein, 1006–1007. *See also* Cathartics,
        diphenylmethanes
Phenothiazines. *See also* Antipsychotic agents;
        Chlorpromazine; other agents
    poisoning, physostigmine in, 116
    uses, alcohol withdrawal, 572
        preanesthetic medication, 270
PHENOXENE (chlorphenoxamine hydrochloride), 487
Phenoxybenzamine, 178–183
    absorption, fate, and excretion, 182
    actions/effects on, cardiovascular system, 180–182
        central nervous system, 182
        gastrointestinal tract, 182

    metabolism, 182
    miscellaneous systems, 182
    antihypertensive action, 793
    chemistry, 178
    locus and mechanism of action, 178–179
    pharmacological properties, 179–183
    preparations, routes of administration, and dos-
        age, 182–183
    structural formula, 178
    toxicity, side effects, and precautions, 183
    uses, 186–188
Phenoxyethyl penicillin. *See* Phenethicillin
Phenoxymethyl penicillin. *See* Penicillin V
Phenprocoumon, 1359. *See also* Anticoagulants, oral
Phensuximide, use in epilepsy, 462
Phentermine, legal regulations, 1671
    receptor-type activity, 142
    structural formula, 142
    use in obesity, 172
Phentolamine, 183–184
    absorption, fate, and excretion, 184
    antihypertensive action, 793, 812
    pharmacological properties, 183–184
    preparations, routes of administration, and dos-
        age, 184
    structural formula, 183
    toxicity, side effects, and precautions, 184
    uses, 184
        congestive heart failure, 827
        hypertensive emergencies, 812
        myocardial infarction, 827
        variant (Prinzmetal's) angina, 828
PHENURONE (phenacemide), 467
Phenyl salicylate, 696
Phenylalanine²-lysine⁸ vasopressin, 917
Phenylbutazone, 698–700. *See also* Aspirin-like
        drugs
    absorption, fate, and excretion, 699
    actions/effects on, fever and pain, 699
        inflammation, 699
        uric acid, 699
        water and electrolytes, 699
    interactions with other drugs, 700
    preparations and dosage, 700
    structural formula, 699
    toxicity and contraindications, 700
    uses, 700
Phenylephrine, 165. *See also* Sympathomimetic
        drugs
    pharmacological actions, 165
    preparations, administration, and dosage, 165
    receptor-type activity, 142
    structural formula, 142
    uses, 165
        glaucoma, 113
        hypotensive states, 169
        myocardial infarction, 827
        nasal decongestion, 168
        ophthalmic, 171
        paroxysmal atrial or nodal tachycardia, 170
Phenylethanolamine-N-methyltransferase, 72–73
Phenylethylamine, structural formula, 142

Phenylethylmalonamide, 458

Phenylmercuric acetate, 976

Phenylmercuric nitrate, 976

Phenylpropanolamine, actions, preparations, and dosage, 168
  receptor-type activity, 142
  structural formula, 142
  use in nasal congestion, 168

Phenytoin, 452–455, 781–783. *See also* Epilepsy
  absorption, distribution, biotransformation, and excretion, 453–454, 782
  actions/effects on, autonomic nervous system, 782
    cardiac electrophysiology 768, 782
    electrocardiogram, 768, 782
  dosage, 455, 783
  effects on fetus, 471
  history, 452
  hyperglycemic action, 1519
  interactions with other drugs, 455
  mechanism of action, 453
  pharmacokinetics, 1723
  plasma concentrations, 455
  preparations, 454
  structural formula, 452
  structure-activity relationship, 452
  toxic effects, 454, 783
  uses, digitalis intoxication, 755, 783
    epilepsy, 455, 469–470
    paroxysmal atrial arrhythmias, 783
    trigeminal neuralgia, 455

Pheochromocytoma, alpha-adrenergic blocking agents in, 186–187
  alpha-methyltyrosine in, 187
  dopamine in, 155
  histamine in diagnosis, 619
  norepinephrine in, 169
  propranolol in, 187, 194

Phetharbital, 361

Phobic-anxiety states, monoamine oxidase inhibitors in, 430
  tricyclic antidepressants in, 427

Pholcodine, dosage, 507
  duration of analgesic effect, 507

PHOLDINE (pholcodine), 507

PHOSPHALJEL (aluminum phosphate gel), 992

Phosphate, 1529–1531
  absorption, distribution, and excretion, 1529–1530
  depletion, 1531
  disturbance in metabolism, 1531
  pharmacological actions, 1530
  preparations, 1531
  role in acidification of urine, 1530
  uses, 1531

Phosphate-^{32}P, 1305

Phosphine, toxicology, 1652

PHOSPHOLINE (echothiophate iodide for ophthalmic solution), 112

N-Phosphonoacetyl L-aspartate, 1276

Phosphorus, recommended dietary allowance, 1553
  toxicology, 1652

PHOSPHOTOPE (sodium phosphate P 32 solution), 1305

Photoallergic reactions, chloroquine in, 1043

Phototoxic and photoallergic reactions, 1605

Phthalylsulfathiazole, pharmacological properties, dosage, and uses, 1112. *See also* Sulfonamides·

Phylloquinone, 1592

Physical dependence on drugs, 535–578. *See also* Drug abuse; individual agents
  theories, 541–542

Physostigmine. *See also* Anticholinesterases
  absorption, fate, and excretion, 108
  history, 100
  preparations, 112
  structural formula, 104
  uses, belladonna alkaloid poisoning, 116, 128
    glaucoma, 113
    tricyclic antidepressant poisoning, 426

Phytonadione, 1592, 1594. *See also* Vitamin K
  uses, oral anticoagulant overdosage, 1358, 1359

Picrotoxin, 247–248, 587–588

Picrotoxinin, 587

Pilocarpine, actions/effects on, cardiovascular system, 97
  central nervous system, 97
  glands, 97
  smooth muscle, 96–97
  history and sources, 96
  mechanism of action, 96
  preparations and dosage, 97–98
  structural formula, 97
  toxicity, 97
  use in glaucoma, 98, 113

Pimozide, 397

Pindolol, 188, 196
  pharmacokinetics, 1723

Pinworm infections. *See* Enterobiasis

PIPADONE (dipipanone), 507

Piperacetazine, 396, 408. *See also* Antipsychotic agents

Piperacillin, 1147

Piperazine, 1023–1024
  absorption, fate, and excretion, 1023
  anthelmintic action, 1023
  chemistry, 1023
  preparations, route of administration, and dosage, 1023
  toxicity and precautions, 1023–1024
  uses, 1024

Piperidolate, preparations and structural formula, 132

Piperoxan, 186

PIPIZAN CITRATE (piperazine citrate), 1023

PITOCIN (oxytocin injection), 938

PITOCIN CITRATE (oxytocin citrate buccal tablets), 938

PITRESSIN (vasopressin injection), 923

PITRESSIN TANNATE (vasopressin tannate), 924

Pituitary dwarfism. *See* Dwarfism

PITUITRIN (posterior pituitary injection), 923

PITUITRIN-S (posterior pituitary injection), 923

Pivampicillin, 1145. *See also* Ampicillin; Penicillins

Placebo effects, 46–47

Placental lactogen, 1382

chemical properties, 1371
PLACIDYL (ethchlorvynol), 350, 1671
Plague, choice of drugs in, 1090
    streptomycin in, 1173
Plantago seed, 1004. *See also* Cathartics, bulk-forming laxatives
PLAQUENIL (hydroxychloroquine sulfate), 1046
Plasma expanders, 859–861. *See also* individual agents
Plasma protein fraction, 862
PLASMANATE (plasma protein fraction), 862
PLASMA-PLEX (plasma protein fraction), 862
PLASMATEIN (plasma protein fraction), 862
PLASTIBASE, 953
Platelet factor 4, 1350
Platelet function, drugs affecting, 1360–1361
PLATINOL (cisplatin), 1298
PLEGINE (phendimetrazine tartrate), 172
Pleurisy, indomethacin in, 706
PLURONIC F68, 973
Plutonium, 1634
Pneumococcal infections. *See also Streptococcus pneumoniae* infections
    cephalosporins in, 1157
    choice of drugs in, 1087
    erythromycin in, 1225
    penicillins in, 1138
    tetracyclines in, 1190
Pneumocystis carinii infections, choice of drugs in, 1093
    pentamidine in, 1072
    trimethoprim-sulfamethoxazole in, 1072, 1119
Pneumonia. *See also* causative microorganisms
    choice of drugs in, 1086
    oxygen in, 330
Pneumothorax, oxygen in, 331
Podophyllum, local uses, 956
Podophyllum resin, 956
POISINDEX (microfiche system for information on toxic substances), 1608
Poison Control Centers, 1608
Poisoning. *See* Drugs, poisoning; Toxicology
Pollinosis, antihistamines in, 627
Poloxamer-iodine, 973
Polyarteritis nodosa, adrenocorticosteroids in, 1490
Polycarbophil, 1005
POLYCILLIN (ampicillin), 1144
Polycythemia vera, azaribine in, 1282
    busulfan in, 1269
    chlorambucil in, 1268
    pyrimethamine in, 1050
    sodium phosphate-^{32}P in, 1305
Polyestradiol phosphate, 1428
Polyethylene glycol, 952
Polyethylene glycol ointment, 952
Polyethylene glycols, 951, 952
Polymyalgia rheumatica, adrenocorticosteroids in, 1490
Polymyositis, adrenocorticosteroids in, 1490
Polymyxin B, 1228–1230. *See also* Antimicrobial agents
    absorption, distribution, and excretion, 1229

antibacterial activity, 1228
    chemistry, 1228
    history and source, 1228
    mechanism of action, 1229
    preparations, administration, and dosage, 1229
    toxicity, 1229–1230
    uses, *Pseudomonas* infections, 1230
        Serratia infections, 1230
POLYSORB, 953
Polythiazide. *See also* Benzothiadiazides
    structural formula, properties, and dosage, 900
Polythiol resins, use in mercury poisoning, 1628
PONDIMIN (fenfluramine hydrochloride), 172
PONSTEL (mefenamic acid), 708
PONTOCAINE (tetracaine hydrochloride), 309
Porphyria, from barbiturates, 294, 358
Porphyria cutanea tarda, chloroquine in, 1043
Posterior pituitary injection, 923
Posterior pituitary powder, 923
Postgastrectomy dumping syndrome, cyproheptadine in, 639
    methysergide in, 639
Potassium, 870–879
    absorption and distribution, 870–871
    adaptation to loads, 871–872
    depletion, 874–877
        effects, 874–875
        effects of diuretics, 876–877
        estimation of deficit, 874
        etiology, 874, 875
        preparations for repair, 879
        relationship to metabolic alkalosis, 875–876
        signs and symptoms, 874–875
        treatment, 877–879
    digitalis and, 732, 734, 736, 753–754, 755
    dose, route, and rate of administration, 878
    excess, 874
        treatment, 879
    excretion, 871
    measurement of extracellular concentration, 873
    measurement of intracellular concentration, 874
    provisional dietary allowance, 1555
    relationship to acid-base balance, 872–873
    transient volume of distribution, 877
    uses, 877–879
        digitalis intoxication, 755
        periodic paralysis, 878
        potassium deficit, 877–878
Potassium chloride injection, 879
Potassium chloride oral solution, 879
Potassium chloride tablets, 879
Potassium permanganate, 974
Potassium sodium tartrate, 1005. *See also* Cathartics, saline
POVAN (pyrvinium pamoate), 1026
Povidone-iodine, 973
Practolol, pharmacological properties, 188
Pralidoxime, effect on acetylcholinesterase reactivation, 110–111
    pharmacological properties, 111
    preparations, 112
    structural formula, 111

Pralidoxime (*Cont.*)
  use in anticholinesterase poisoning, 110
Pramoxine hydrochloride, 310
PRANTAL (diphemanil methylsulfate), 130
Prazepam, 437–441. *See also* Benzodiazepines
  dosage, half-life, and preparations, 350, 440
  legal regulations, 1671
Praziquantel, 1024
Prazosin, 184, 806–807
  pharmacokinetics, 1724
  pharmacological properties, 806–807
  preparations, 807
  structural formula, 806
  uses, 807
    congestive heart failure, 827
Preanesthetic medication, 269–271
  antiemetics in, 270
  antihistamines in, 269
  atropine in, 69, 135, 271
  barbiturates in, 269
  benzodiazepines in, 270
  butyrophenones in, 270
  definition and objectives, 269
  fentanyl in, 270
  glycopyrrolate in, 271
  meperidine in, 270
  morphine in, 270
  nonbarbiturate sedatives in, 269–270
  opioids in, 270
  phenothiazines in, 270
  scopolamine in, 69, 135, 271
Precipitated sulfur, 980
Prednisolone. *See also* Adrenocorticosteroids
  pharmacokinetics, 1724
  preparations, 1485
  relative potency, duration of action, and equiva-
    lent dose, 1482
Prednisone. *See also* Adrenocorticosteroids
  pharmacokinetics, 1725
  preparations, 1485
  relative potency, duration of action, and equiva-
    lent dose, 1482
  use in neoplastic diseases, 1253, 1301
Pregnancy, iron supplements in, 1317, 1323
  toxemia. *See* Eclampsia
  vitamin and mineral requirements during, 1553
PREGNYL (chorionic gonadotropin for injection),
    1386
PRELUDIN (phenmetrazine), 172, 1670
PREMARIN (conjugated estrogens), 1428
Premature labor. *See also* Labor
  delay of delivery, albuterol in, 172
    indomethacin in, 707
    metaproterenol in, 172
    terbutaline in, 168, 172
  prevention, 949
Premenstrual tension, progestins in, 1438
PRE-PEN (benzylpenicilloyl-polylysine), 1149
PREPODYNE (poloxamer-iodine), 973
Preproinsulin, 1498, 1499
PRESAMINE (imipramine hydrochloride), 424

PRE-SATE (chlorphentermine hydrochloride), 172
Prescription order, classes, 1664
  construction, 1662–1664
  extemporaneous, 1665–1667
  precompounded preparations, 1664–1665
  refills, 1664, 1670
Prescription order writing, 1660–1671
  choice of drug name, 1661
  choice of language, 1661
  choice of weights and measures, 1661–1662
  dosage considerations, 1667–1668
  incompatibilities of drugs, 1669
  Latin phrases and abbreviations, 1661, 1663, 1668
  vehicles, flavors, and coloring agents, 1668–1669
Prilocaine hydrochloride, 309
Primaquine, 1051–1054
  absorption, fate, and excretion, 1052
  acquired resistance of plasmodia, 1052
  antimalarial actions and efficacy, 1052
  chemistry, 1051
  history, 1051
  mechanism of antimalarial action, 1041, 1052
  mechanism of hemolysis, 1053
  precautions and contraindications, 1054
  preparations, route of administration, and dosage,
    1053
  toxicity and side effects, 1053–1054
  use in malaria, 1054
Primidone, 458–459
  absorption, distribution, biotransformation, and
    excretion, 458
  anticonvulsant effects, 458
  dosage, 458–459
  interactions with other drugs, 459
  pharmacokinetics, 1725
  plasma concentrations, 459
  preparations, 458
  structural formula, 458
  toxicity, 458
  use in epilepsy, 459, 469–470
PRISCOLINE (tolazoline hydrochloride), 184
PRIVINE (naphazoline hydrochloride), 168
Proadifen, 17
PRO-BANTHINE (propantheline bromide), 131
Probenecid, 722–723, 931–932, 1135, 1139
  absorption, fate, and excretion, 932
  actions/effects on, biliary excretion, 931
    cerebrospinal fluid, 931
    renal transport, 931
  chemistry, 931
  history, 931
  preparations and dosage, 932
  untoward reactions and precautions, 932
  uses, adjunct in penicillin therapy, 932
    gout, 722
    hyperuricemia, 723
Probucol, 843–844
Procainamide, 774–777. *See also* Cardiac arrhyth-
    mias
  absorption, fate, and excretion, 775
  actions/effects on, autonomic nervous system, 775

cardiac electrophysiology, 768, 775
electrocardiogram, 768
chemistry and preparations, 774
dosage and administration, 776
history, 774
pharmacokinetics, 1726
toxicity and precautions, 777
uses, 776
Procaine, 308. *See also* Local anesthetics
structural formula, 301
PROCAMIDE (procainamide hydrochloride), 774
PROCAPAN (procainamide hydrochloride), 774
Procarbazine, 1299–1300
use in neoplastic diseases, 1253, 1300
Prochlorperazine, use and dosage as antiemetic, 417
Procyclidine, chemistry, preparations, and dosage, 486
use in parkinsonism, 484–485
Prodrug, definition, 12
PROGESTASERT (intrauterine contraceptive device containing progesterone), 1437
Progesterone, chemistry, 1434
Progesterone injection, 1437
Progestins, 1433–1438. *See also* individual agents
absorption, fate, and excretion, 1436
actions/effects on, male fertility, 1462–1463
mammary gland, 1436
plasma lipids, 845
uterus, 1435
assays, 1437
chemistry, 1433–1435
history, 1420
mechanism of action, 1436
physiological functions, 1435–1436
preparations, 1437
synthesis and secretion, 1435
thermogenic action, 1436
uses, carcinomas, 1254, 1301
contraception, 1438–1444, 1462–1463
dysfunctional uterine bleeding, 1437
dysmenorrhea, 1438
endometrial carcinoma, 1438
endometriosis, 1438
premenstrual tension, 1438
suppression of post-partum lactation, 1438
threatened and habitual abortion, 1438
PROGLYCEM (diazoxide), 1519
PROGYNON (estradiol), 1428
Proinsulin, 1498, 1499
PROKETAZINE (carphenazine), 406
Prolactin, 1380–1383
actions/effects on, breast, 1380–1381
ovary, 1381
assays, 1382
chemical properties, 1371, 1380
hypersecretion, 1382
hypothalamic regulation, 1392
secretion, 1381–1382
effect of levodopa, 478
Prolactin release-inhibiting hormone, 1382, 1392
Prolactin-releasing factor, 1392

PROLIXIN DECANOATE (fluphenazine decanoate), 409
PROLIXIN ETHANATE (fluphenazine ethanate), 409
PROLIXIN HYDROCHLORIDE (fluphenazine hydrochloride), 409
PROLOID (thyroglobulin), 1406
PROLUTON (progesterone injection), 1437
Promazine, 406
Promethazine, 627. *See also* H_1-receptor blockers
structural formula, 623
uses, antiemetic, 417
sedative, 369
Promethazine hydrochloride, dosage, 628
antiemetic use, 417
preparations, 628
Promethestrol dipropionate, 1428
PROMIN (glucosulfone sodium), 1214
PRONESTYL (procainamide hydrochloride), 774
PRONTOSIL, 1106
Pro-opiocortin, 498
Propachlor, toxicology, 1654
PROPADRINE (phenylpropanolamine hydrochloride), 168
Propamidine, 1071
Propanediol carbamates, 441
Propanil, toxicology, 1654
Propantheline, pharmacological properties, 129
preparations and structural formula, 131
Proparacaine hydrochloride, 310
Propham, toxicology, 1654
Propionates, 982
Propionic acid derivatives, 710–713. *See also* Aspirin-like drugs; individual agents
chemistry, 711
interactions with other drugs, 711
pharmacological properties, 710
uses, 713
Propiram, actions at opioid receptor subtypes, 522
Propoxyphene, 520–521
absorption, fate, and excretion, 520
legal regulations, 1671
liability for abuse, 520–521
pharmacological actions, 520
preparations, dosage, and uses, 521
structural formula, 520
toxicity, 520
Propranolol, 188–194
absorption, fate, and excretion, 192–193
actions/effects on, cardiac electrophysiology, 768, 783–785
cardiovascular system, 190–191
central nervous system, 192
electrocardiogram, 768, 785
metabolism, 192
smooth muscle, 192
dosage and administration, as antiarrhythmic agent, 785
pharmacokinetics, 1727
preparations, routes of administration, and dosage, 193
structural formula, 189
toxicity, side effects, and precautions, 193–194, 786

Propranolol (*Cont.*)
  uses, angina pectoris, 194, 828
    anxiety, 194
    cardiac arrhythmias, 194, 785–786
    hypertension, 810–813
    hyperthyroidism, 194, 1412
    hypertrophic obstructive cardiomyopathy, 194
    migraine, 194, 947
    pheochromocytoma, 187, 194
Propylene glycol, 951, 952
  toxicology, 1647
Propylene oxide, 981
Propylhexedrine, dosage and preparations, 168
  receptor-type activity, 142
  structural formula, 142
  use in nasal decongestion, 168
Propylparaben, 969
Propylthiouracil, 1409. *See also* Antithyroid drugs
  preparations and dosage, 1410–1411
PROSERUM (albumin human), 862
Prostacyclin (PGI$_2$), 669, 670. *See also* Prosta-
  glandins
Prostacyclin synthetase, 669
Prostaglandins, 668–681
  actions/effects on, afferent nerves and pain, 675
    autonomic nervous system, 675
    blood, 673
    bronchial and tracheal muscle, 674
    cardiovascular system, 673
    central nervous system, 674–675
    cyclic AMP, 675
    endocrine system, 675
    gastric, pancreatic, and intestinal secretions,
      674, 997
    gastrointestinal muscle, 674
    kidney, 674
    metabolism, 675
    reproduction, 938–939
    thyroid, 1403
    uterus, 674, 939
  biosynthesis and catabolism, 669–673
  chemistry, 668–669
  endogenous role in, endocrine system, 676–677
    inflammatory and immune responses, 677–678,
      683–684
    kidney, 677
    platelets, 676
    smooth muscle, 677
  history, 668
  inhibitors of responses, 676
  inhibitors of synthesis, 671, 684–685
  mechanism of action, 675–676
  preparations and routes of administration, 939
  uses, abortion, 678, 949
    bronchial asthma, 678
    gastric hyperacidity, 678
    induction of labor at term, 947–948
PROSTAPHLIN (oxacillin sodium), 1143
Prostatic carcinoma, androgen-control therapy in,
  1302
PROSTIGMIN (neostigmine bromide), 112
PROSTIN E2 (dinoprostone), 939

PROSTIN F2 ALPHA (dinoprost tromethamine), 939
Protamine sulfate, 1352
Protamine zinc insulin suspension, 1508
Protectives, actions and uses, 953–954
Protein hydrolysate injection, 863
PROTENATE (plasma protein fraction), 862
Proteus infections, amikacin in, 1176
  carbenicillin in, 1147
  choice of drugs in, 1089
  gentamicin in, 1174
  kanamycin in, 1176
  ticarcillin in, 1147
Proteus mirabilis infections, choice of drugs in, 1089
Protirelin, 1406
Protokylol, 154
  receptor-type activity, 142
  structural formula, 142
PROTOPAM (pralidoxime chloride), 112
Protriptyline hydrochloride. *See also* Tricyclic antidepressants
  pharmacokinetics, 1727
  preparations and dosage, 424
  structural formula, 419
PROVERA (medroxyprogesterone acetate tablets),
  1437
Pruritus, gold in, 713
  H$_1$-receptor blockers in, 629
  local anesthetics in, 310
  phenol in, 967
  zinc oxide in, 977
Pseudoephedrine, use as decongestant, 168
Pseudomembranous colitis, from tetracyclines, 1189
  cholestyramine in, 1227
  vancomycin in, 1227, 1231
Pseudomonas aeruginosa infections, amikacin in,
  1176
  carbenicillin in, 1147
  choice of drugs in, 1089
  colistin in, 1230
  gentamicin in, 1174–1175
  polymyxin in, 1230
  ticarcillin in, 1147
  tobramycin in, 1175
Pseudomonas mallei infections, choice of drugs in,
  1090
Pseudomonas pseudomallei infections, choice of
  drugs in, 1090
Psilocin, 564–566
Psilocine, 633
Psilocybin, 564, 566, 633
  legal regulations, 1670
Psittacosis, chloramphenicol in, 1196
  choice of drugs in, 1092
  tetracyclines in, 1189
Psoriasis, anthralin in, 981
  azaribine in, 1282
  methotrexate in, 1276
  methoxsalen in, 958
  resorcinol in, 968
  sulfur in, 981
  tars in, 970
  zinc oxide in, 977

Psychedelic drugs, abuse, 563–567
  chemistry, 564–565
  classification, 564
  general considerations, 563–564
  incidence and patterns of use, 566
  mechanism of action, 564–565
  pharmacological effects, 565–566
  tolerance, toxicity, and physical dependence, 566–567
Psychiatric disorders, biological hypotheses of etiology, 393–394
  drug therapy, 391–442
  nosology, 392–393
Psychoactive drugs, definition, 391
Psychomotor epilepsy. See Epilepsy
Psychoses, biological theories of schizophrenia, 393–394
  biological theory of affective disorders, 393–394
  diagnostic terminology, 392–393
  treatment, 414–417
Psychotherapeutic drugs, 391–442. See also individual agents
  animal evaluation, 394
  classification, 391
  clinical evaluation, 394
  history, 392
Psychotogenic drugs, abuse, 563–567
Psychotomimetic drugs, abuse, 563–567
Psychotoxic drugs, definition, 391
Psychotropic drugs, definition, 391
Psyllium, 1004. See also Cathartics, bulk-forming laxatives
Pteroylglutamic acid, 1340. See also Folic acid
Puerperium, oxytocics in, 948–949
Pulmonary disease, oxygen in, 329–330
Pulmonary edema. See also Cardiac failure
  alpha-adrenergic blocking drugs in, 188
  high-ceiling diuretics in, 906
  opioids in, 513
  oxygen in, 330
Pulmonary embolism, anticoagulants in, 1363–1364
  streptokinase in, 1362, 1364
  urokinase in, 1362, 1364
Purgation, use in drug poisoning, 1611
Purine analogs, 1282–1287. See also individual agents
  mechanism of action, 1284–1285
  mechanism of resistance, 1285
  structure-activity relationship, 1283–1284
  use in neoplastic diseases, 1253
PURINETHOL (mercaptopurine), 1286
PURODIGIN (digitoxin), 749
Pustulants, 955
Pylorospasm, belladonna alkaloids in, 133
Pyoderma, bacitracin in, 1232
PYOPEN (carbenicillin disodium), 1146
Pyrantel pamoate, 1024–1025
Pyrazinamide, 1208
Pyrazofuran, 1277
Pyrazolon derivatives, 698–701. See also individual agents
Pyrethrins, 985

Pyrethrums, toxicology, 1651
PYRIDIUM (phenazopyridine hydrochloride), 1122
Pyridostigmine, absorption, fate, and excretion, 108
  pharmacokinetics, 1728
  preparations, 112
  structural formula, 104
  use in myasthenia gravis, 115–116
Pyridoxal, 1570
Pyridoxamine, 1570
Pyridoxine, 1570–1572
  absorption, fate, and excretion, 1571
  administration with isoniazid, 1202, 1212, 1570
  antagonism of levodopa, 481
  chemistry, 1570
  dependency, 1572
  history, 1570
  human requirement, 1571
  pharmacological actions, 1570
  physiological function, 1570–1571
  preparations, 1571–1572
  recommended dietary allowance, 1553
  status in anemias, 1327
  symptoms of deficiency, 1571
  uses, anemia, 1572
    prophylaxis during hydralazine therapy, 1572
    prophylaxis during isoniazid therapy, 1572
    pyridoxine deficiency, 1572
2-(2-Pyridyl)ethylamine, 610
Pyrilamine, 627. See also H_1-receptor blockers
  structural formula, 623
  use as sedative, 369
Pyrilamine maleate, preparations and dosage, 628
Pyrimethamine, 1048–1050
  absorption, fate, and excretion, 1049
  antimalarial actions and efficacy, 1048–1049
  chemistry, 1048
  dihydrofolate reductase inhibition, 1049
  history, 1048
  potentiation by sulfonamides, 1049
  precautions and contraindications, 1050
  preparations, route of administration, and dosage, 1049
  resistance, 1041
  toxicity, 1050
  uses, malaria, 1050
    meningeal leukemia, 1050
    polycythemia vera, 1050
    toxoplasmosis, 1050
Pyrimidine analogs, 1276–1282. See also individual agents
  mechanism of action, 1276–1278
  structure-activity relationship, 1276–1278
Pyrithiamine, 1561
Pyroxylon, 953
Pyrvinium pamoate, 1025–1026

Q fever, chloramphenicol in, 1196
  choice of drugs in, 1092
  tetracyclines in, 1189
QUAALUDE (methaqualone), 351, 1670
QUALATUM, 953

QUARZAN (clidinium bromide), 130
QUELICIN (succinylcholine chloride), 231
QUESTRAN (cholestyramine resin), 843
QUIDE (piperacetazine), 408
Quinacrine, 1042, 1078
QUINAGLUTE (quinidine gluconate), 771
Quinethazone, properties and dosage, 899, 900
QUINIDEX (sustained-release quinidine sulfate), 771
Quinidine, 768–774
  absorption, fate, and excretion, 770–771
  actions/effects on, atrial fibrillation and flutter, 770
    autonomic nervous system, 770
    cardiac electrophysiology, 768, 769–770
    electrocardiogram, 768, 770
  chemistry, 768, 1055
  dosage, 771
  drug interactions, 774
  history, 768
  pharmacokinetics, 1728
  preparations and routes of administration, 771
  toxic reactions, 772–774
  uses, digitalis-induced arrhythmias, 772
    supraventricular arrhythmias, 772
    ventricular arrhythmias, 772
Quinine, 1054–1057
  absorption, fate, and excretion, 1056
  actions/effects on, cardiovascular system, 1056
    central nervous system, 1055
    gastrointestinal tract, 1056
    plasmodia, 1055
    skeletal muscle, 1056
  chemistry, 1055
  contraindications, 1057
  history, 1054
  local effects, 1055
  preparations, routes of administration, and dosage, 1057
  structure-activity relationship, 1055
  toxicity, 1056
  uses, malaria, 1057
    nocturnal leg cramps, 1057
Quinine and urea hydrochloride, uses, 956
Quinine and urea hydrochloride injection, 956
Quinocide, 1051
QUINORA (quinidine sulfate), 771
Quinterenol, 166
Quinuclidinyl benzoate, 248
QUOTANE (dimethisoquin hydrochloride), 310

"Rabbit" syndrome, 412
Racemoramide, legal regulations, 1670
Radioactive metals, mobilization by chelating agents, 1634
Radium, 1634
Rat-bite fever, penicillin G in, 1140
RAUDIXIN (rauwolfia serpentina), 203
Rauwolfia alkaloids, 202–204. See also individual agents
Raynaud's disease, alpha-adrenergic blocking agents in, 187

Receptors, 28–39. See also Drugs, mechanisms of action; Drugs, receptors
  alpha-adrenergic, 179
  beta-adrenergic, 29, 189–190
  cholinergic muscarinic, 92, 122
  cholinergic nicotinic, 29, 222–223
  insulin, 1506
  opioid, 497–498, 521–522
  progesterone, 1436
Recommended dietary allowances, 1553
Red squill, toxicology, 1652
REDISOL (cyanocobalamin injection), 1337
Reduced iron, 1323
Regional enteritis, sulfasalazine in, 1112
REGITINE (phentolamine hydrochloride), 184
REGITINE MESYLATE (phentolamine mesylate), 184
RELA (carisoprodol), 489
Relapsing fever, choice of drugs in, 1092
  tetracyclines in, 1191
Renal colic, atropine in, 135–136
  opioids in, 499
Renal disease, diuretics in, 912
Renal insufficiency, 882
RENESE (polythiazide), 900
Renin, 647–648, 652. See also Angiotensin
  control of secretion, 653
  extrarenal sources, 655
RENOQUID (sulfacytine), 1111
REPOISE (butaperazine), 406
Repository corticotropin injection, 1470
Reserpine, 202–204
  carcinogenic potential, 204
  effect on norepinephrine uptake, storage, and release, 202–203
  history, 202
  locus and mechanism of action, 202–203
  pharmacological properties, 203
  preparations, routes of administration, and dosage, 203
  source, 202
  structural formula, 202
  toxicity, side effects, and precautions, 203–204
  uses, 204
    hypertension, 811
RESOCHIN (chloroquine phosphate), 1044
Resorcinol, 968
  keratolytic effect, 956
Respiratory depression, carbon dioxide in, 334
  stimulants in, status, 585
  xanthines in, 603
Respiratory obstruction, helium in, 334
RETIN-A (tretinoin), 1591
Retinal, 1584, 1585
Retinoblastoma, cyclophosphamide in, 1266
Retinoic acid, 1583–1584, 1591
  absorption, distribution, and metabolism, 1590
Retinol, 1583. See also Vitamin A
Reye's syndrome, levodopa in, 487
Rhabdomyosarcoma, dactinomycin in, 1291
  vincristine in, 1290
RHEOMACRODEX (dextran 40 injection), 862
Rheumatic fever, adrenocorticosteroids in, 1489

prophylaxis, erythromycin in, 1225
    penicillin G in, 1141
    sulfonamides in, 1116
  salicylates in, 697
Rheumatic heart disease, anticoagulants, in, 1363
  antithrombotic drugs in, 1363
Rheumatoid arthritis. *See* Arthritis
RHEUMOX (azapropazone), 701
Rhinitis, belladonna alkaloids in, 134
  H_1-receptor blockers in, 627–628
  sympathomimetic drugs in, 168
Rhodopsin, 1585
Riboflavin, 1566–1567
  absorption, fate, and excretion, 1567
  chemistry, 1566
  history, 1566
  human requirement, 1567
  pharmacological actions, 1566
  physiological function, 1566
  preparations, 1567
  recommended dietary allowance, 1553
  status in anemias, 1327
  symptoms of deficiency, 1566–1567
  uses, ariboflavinosis, 1567
Ribostamycin, 1163
Rickets, vitamin D in, 1545
Rickettsia infections, chloramphenicol in, 1196
  choice of drugs in, 1092
  tetracyclines in, 1189
Rickettsialpox, choice of drugs in, 1092
  tetracyclines in, 1189
RIFADIN (rifampin), 1205
Rifampin, 1203–1206. *See also* Antimicrobial agents
  absorption, distribution, and excretion, 1204
  antibacterial activity, 1204
  antifungal activity, 1234
  bacterial resistance, 1204
  chemistry, 1203
  dosage, 1205
  mechanism of action, 1204
  pharmacokinetics, 1729
  preparations, 1205
  untoward effects, 1205
  uses, amebic meningoencephalitis, 1240
    chemoprophylaxis of meningococcal disease, 1206
    leprosy, 1215, 1217
    staphylococcal infections, 1206
    tuberculosis, 1206, 1212–1213
RIMACTANE (rifampin), 1205
Rimiterol, 166
Ringworm, griseofulvin in, 1238
  miconazole in, 982
  resorcinol in, 968
  zinc oxide in, 977
RIOPAN (magaldrate), 991, 994
RIOPAN PLUS, 991
RIPERCOL (tetramisole), 1026
RITALIN (methylphenidate), 590, 1670
ROBALATE (dihydroxyaluminum aminoacetate), 992
ROBAXIN (methocarbamol), 489
ROBINUL (glycopyrrolate), 130

ROCALTROL (calcitriol), 1545
Rochelle salt, 1005
Rocky Mountain spotted fever, chloramphenicol in, 1196
  choice of drugs in, 1092
  tetracyclines in, 1189
Rodenticides, toxicology, 1652–1653
ROHYPNOL (flunitrazepam), 350
ROLAIDS (dihydroxyaluminum sodium carbonate), 992
RONDOMYCIN (methacycline hydrochloride), 1185
Rose water ointment, 953
Rotenone, toxicology, 1651
Roundworm infections. *See* Ascariasis; Trichinosis
Rubbing alcohol, 970
Rubefacients, 955
Rubidomycin. *See* Daunorubicin
RUBRAMIN (cyanocobalamin injection), 1337
RU-SPAS (homatropine methylbromide), 129
Russian flies, 956

Salbutamol. *See* Albuterol
Salicin, 682
Salicylamide, 695
  use as sedative, 369
Salicylanilides, 981
Salicylates, 688–698. *See also* Aspirin-like drugs; individual agents
  absorption and distribution, 693
  actions/effects on, acid-base balance, 690
    blood, 691–692
    body temperature, 689, 692
    cardiovascular system, 691
    central nervous system, 689–690
    connective tissue metabolism, 692
    electrolyte pattern, 690
    endocrine system, 693
    gastrointestinal tract, 691
    immune processes, 692
    inflammation, 692
    inhibition of prostaglandin synthesis, 676, 684–685
    kidney, 691
    liver, 691
    metabolism, 692–693
    pain, 689
    platelets, 691–692
    pregnancy, 686, 693
    respiration, 689–690
    rheumatoid states, 692
    uric acid metabolism, 691
  biotransformation and excretion, 694
  chemistry, 688–689
  history, 682–683
  hypersensitivity reactions, 696–697
  local irritation, 693
  mechanism of action, 684–685
  pharmacological effects, 689–693
  plasma concentrations, 694, 698
  poisoning, 695–696
    treatment, 696

Salicylates (*Cont.*)
    preparations, dosage, and administration, 695
    structure-activity relationship, 688
    uses, 697-698
        analgesia, 697
        antipyresis, 697
        Bartter's syndrome, 698
        dysmenorrhea, 697
        epidermophytosis, 698
        local, 698
        myalgia, 697
        neuralgia, 697
        patent ductus arteriosus, 698
        rheumatic fever, 697
        rheumatoid arthritis, 698
Salicylic acid, 682, 695, 698, 984
    keratolytic effect, 956
    pharmacokinetics, 1730
    structural formula, 689
Salicylic alcohol, 682
Salicyluric acid, 694
Saligenin, 682
Salmefamol, 166
Salmonella infections, chloramphenicol in, 1195
    choice of drugs in, 1089
    penicillins in, 1145
    tetracyclines in, 1190
SALURON (hydroflumethiazide), 900
SANDOPTAL (butalbital), 350
SANDRIL (reserpine), 203
SANSERT (methysergide maleate), 639, 946
SANTYL OINTMENT (collagenase ointment), 962
Saralasin, chemistry 648, 656
    clinical applications, 658-659
    pharmacological properties, 656-657
    untoward effects, 659
    uses, antihypertensive, 807
Sarcoidosis, adrenocorticosteroids in, 1491
Sarcolysin. *See* Melphalan
Sarcomas, choice of drugs in, 1252-1254
    dacarbazine in, 1271
    dactinomycin in, 1291
    doxorubicin in, 1293
    methotrexate in, 1276
    vincristine in, 1290
Sarin, history, 101
    structural formula, 105
Saxitoxin, 310-311
Scabies, benzyl benzoate in, 985
    crotamiton in, 985
    lindane in, 985
    sulfur ointment in, 985
    thiabendazole in, 985
Scarlet fever, choice of drugs in, 1086
    penicillins in, 1138
Schistosomiasis, occurrence and treatment, 1034-1035
Schizophrenia, drug treatment, 414-417. *See also* Psychoses
Sclerosing agents, actions and uses, 956
Scopine, 121
Scopolamine, 121-128, 564
    absorption, fate, and excretion, 126-127
    actions/effects on, cardiovascular system, 124-125
        central nervous system, 122-123
        EEG, 123
        eye, 123-124
        respiration, 124
    history, 121
    mechanism of action, 122
    pharmacological properties, 122-128
    poisoning, 127-128
        treatment, 128
    preparations, dosage, and administration, 128
    structural formula, 121
    uses, 133-136
        labor, 135
        motion sickness, 135, 629
        ophthalmological, 133-134
        parkinsonism, 135
        preanesthetic medication, 135, 271
        sedative, 369
Scopolamine-N-oxide, use as sedative, 369
Scurvy, ascorbic acid in, 1579
Seborrhea, resorcinol in, 968
    selenium sulfide in, 957
    sulfur in, 981
    zinc pyrithione in, 977
Secobarbital. *See also* Barbiturates
    chemistry, 351
    dosage, half-life, and preparations, 350
    legal regulations, 1670
SECONAL (secobarbital), 350, 1670
SECONAL SODIUM (secobarbital sodium), 350
Secretin, effect on insulin secretion, 1500
Sedatives, 339-375. *See also* individual agents
    nonprescription drugs, 369
SED-TENS SE (homatropine methylbromide), 129
Seizures. *See* Epilepsy
Selenium, provisional dietary allowance, 1555
Selenium sulfide, 984
    action and uses, 956-957
Selenium sulfide detergent suspension, 957
SELSUN (selenium sulfide lotion), 957
SELSUN BLUE (selenium sulfide shampoo), 957
SEMILENTE insulin (prompt insulin zinc suspension), 1508, 1509
Semustine, 1270-1271. *See also* Alkylating agents
    structural formula, 1259
    use in neoplastic disease, 1252, 1271
Senile dementia, ergot alkaloids in, 947
Senna, 1007. *See also* Cathartics, anthraquinones
Septicemia, amikacin in, 1176
    cephalosporins in, 1157
    choice of drugs in, 1086
    gentamicin in, 1174
    penicillins in, 1145, 1147
    tobramycin in, 1175
SEPTODYNE (poloxamer-iodine), 973
SEPTRA (trimethoprim-sulfamethoxazole), 1118
SERAX (oxazepam), 350, 440, 1671
SERENAL (oxazolam), 350
SERENTIL (mesoridazine besylate), 408
SERNYLAN (phencyclidine hydrochloride), 567

SEROMYCIN (cycloserine), 1211
Serotonin. *See* 5-Hydroxytryptamine
SERPASIL (reserpine), 203
Serratia infections, amikacin in, 1176
   choice of drugs in, 1089
   colistin in, 1230
   gentamicin in, 1174
   polymyxin B in, 1230
   trimethoprim-sulfamethoxazole in, 1230
Serum sickness, adrenocorticosteroids in, 1490
   H_1-receptor blockers in, 629
SEVIN, 101
Shigella infections, choice of drugs in, 1089
   sulfonamides in, 1115
   tetracyclines in, 1190
   trimethoprim-sulfamethoxazole in, 1119
Shock, adrenocorticosteroids in, 170, 1491
   alpha-adrenergic blocking drugs in, 169–170, 187
   angiotensin in, 655
   dobutamine in, 169
   dopamine in, 169
   drug therapy, 187
   glucagon in, 169
   oxygen in, 330
   sympathomimetic drugs in, 169
   vasodilators in, 170
Shohl's solution, 869
Sialorrhea, belladonna alkaloids in, 133
Sideroblastic anemia, 1327
SILAIN-GEL, 991
Silicosis, 1643
SILICOTE (dimethicone), 953
SILVADENE (silver sulfadiazine), 1112
Silver, actions, as an antiseptic, 976
Silver allantoinate, 977
Silver nitrate, 976–977
Silver sulfadiazine, 977
   pharmacological properties and use in burns, 1112. *See also* Sulfonamides
Silver uracil, 977
Simethicone, 954, 991, 995, 997
SINEMET (carbidopa-levodopa), 483
SINEQUAN (doxepin hydrochloride), 424
SINTROM (acenocoumarol), 1359
Sinusitis, choice of drugs in, 1086
   sympathomimetic drugs in, 168
   trimethoprim-sulfamethoxazole in, 1119
Sisomicin, 1164
Sitosterol, 845
SKELAXIN (metaxalone), 489
Skeletal muscle relaxants. *See also* individual agents
   centrally acting, 488–491
   pharmacological actions, 488–491
   therapeutic status, 491
SK-ESTROGENS (esterified estrogens), 1428
SKF 525A. *See* Proadifen
Skin diseases. *See* individual diseases
SK-LYGEN (chlordiazepoxide hydrochloride), 440
SK-PRAMINE (imipramine hydrochloride), 424
SK-SOXAZOLE (sulfisoxazole), 1111
Sleep stages, 343
Slow-reacting substance, 671

Smallpox prevention, methisazone in, 1242
SNP (parathion), 104
Sodium, provisional dietary allowance, 1555
Sodium alginate, 951
Sodium bicarbonate, gastric antacid properties, 994
   uses, alkalinization of urine, 868, 894
      gastric antacid, 995
      metabolic acidosis, 869
      topical, 995
Sodium bicarbonate injection, 862
Sodium bicarbonate tablets, 862
Sodium chloride injection, 862
Sodium citrate, 869
Sodium hypochlorite, 974
Sodium iodide, 1413
Sodium iodide I 131, use in neoplastic diseases, 1254
Sodium lactate injection, 869
Sodium nitrite, 825
Sodium phosphate, 1005. *See also* Cathartics, saline
Sodium phosphate-^{32}P, 1305
   use in neoplastic diseases, 1254
Sodium polystyrene sulfonate, 879
   use in hyperkalemia, 879
Sodium salicylate, 695
   structural formula, 689
Sodium salts, renal excretion, 893–894
Sodium stibogluconate, 1074–1075
   antiprotozoal effects, 1074
   chemistry, 1074
   history, 1074
   preparations, 1074
   routes of administration and dosage, 1074–1075
   uses, leishmaniasis, 1075
Sodium sulfate, 1005. *See also* Cathartics, saline
Sodium tetradecyl sulfate, 956
Sodium thiosulfate, 984
SODIUM VERSENATE (edetate disodium), 1621
SOLGANAL (aurothioglucose), 715
SOLU-CORTEF (cortisol sodium succinate), 1484
SOLU-MEDROL (methylprednisolone sodium succinate), 1485
Solvents, abuse, 568–569
   toxicology, 1644–1647
SOMA (carisoprodol), 489
Soman, history, 101
   structural formula, 105
Somatomedin, 1376
Somatostatin, 663, 1391–1392
   effect on insulin secretion, 1500
   role as CNS transmitter, 253
SOMBULEX (hexobarbital), 350
SOMNAFAC (methaqualone), 351, 1670
SOPOR (methaqualone), 351, 1670
SORBITRATE (isosorbide dinitrate), 826
Sotalol, pharmacological properties, 188, 196
Soterenol, 166
SOTRADECOL (sodium tetradecyl sulfate), 956
Spanish fly, 956
SPARINE (promazine), 406
Spasticity, diazepam in, 441
   muscle relaxants in, 491

Spectinomycin, absorption, distribution, and excretion, 1228
  antibacterial activity and mechanism, 1228
  preparations, 1228
  source and chemistry, 1227
  toxicity, 1228
  use in gonorrhea, 1228
Spermaceti, 953
Spironolactone, 907–908
  antihypertensive action, 804–805
  chemistry, 907
  mechanism of diuretic action, 907
  preparations, 908
  uses, edema, 908
    hypertension, 810
Spiroperidol, 397
Spondylitis, ankylosing. *See* Arthritis
SPOROSTACIN (chlordantoin), 984
Sporothrix schenckii infections, choice of drugs in, 1093
Sporotrichosis, amphotericin B in, 1240
  iodides in, 1240, 1413
Sprue, adrenocorticosteroids in, 1491
  tetracyclines in, 1191
Squill, source and composition, 730
  toxicology, 1652
STADOL (butorphanol tartrate), 527
Stamonium, poisoning, 127
Stanozolol, 1458
STAPHCILLIN (methicillin sodium), 1142
Staphylococcal enteritis, from chloramphenicol, 1195
  from neomycin, 1177
  from tetracyclines, 1188
Staphylococcal infections, cephalosporins in, 1157
  choice of drugs in, 1086
  erythromycin in, 1225
  gentamicin in, 1174, 1175
  penicillins in, 1139
  rifampin in, 1206
  tetracyclines in, 1190
  vancomycin in, 1231
Starch, 953
Starch glycerite, 951
Status epilepticus, barbiturates in, 360–361
  diazepam in, 470
  paraldehyde in, 368
  phenobarbital in, 470
  phenytoin in, 470
STELAZINE (trifluoperazine hydrochloride), 409
Sterile corticotropin zinc hydroxide suspension, 1470
Stibocaptate, 1029
Stibophen, 1030–1031, 1074
Stilbamidine, 1071
STILPHOSTROL (diethylstilbestrol diphosphate), 1428
Stokes-Adams syndrome. *See* Cardiac arrhythmias; Heart block
STOXIL (idoxuridine), 1240
STP. *See* 2,5-Dimethoxy-4-methylamphetamine
STREPTASE (streptokinase), 961, 1362
Streptobacillus moniliformis infections, choice of drugs in, 1091

Streptococcal infections, cephalosporins in, 1157
  erythromycin in, 1225
  penicillins in, 1138
  prophylaxis, penicillin G in, 1140
    sulfonamides in, 1116, 1141
  tetracyclines in, 1190
  trimethoprim-sulfamethoxazole in, 1119
  vancomycin in, 1231
Streptococcus (anaerobic species) infections, choice of drugs in, 1087
Streptococcus agalactae infections, choice of drugs in, 1086
Streptococcus bovis infections, choice of drugs in, 1087
Streptococcus faecalis infections, choice of drugs in, 1086
Streptococcus pneumoniae infections, choice of drugs in, 1087
Streptococcus pyogenes infections, choice of drugs in, 1086
Streptococcus (*viridans* group) infections, choice of drugs in, 1086
Streptodornase, 961
Streptokinase, 1362
  actions and preparations, 961
  uses, 961
Streptokinase-streptodornase, preparations, dosage, and uses, 961
Streptomycin, 1171–1173. *See also* Aminoglycoside antibiotics; Antimicrobial agents
  preparations, administration, and dosage, 1171
  structural formula, 1164
  in tuberculosis, antibacterial activity, 1207
    bacterial resistance, 1208
    history, 1207
    therapeutic status, 1208
  untoward effects, 1172
  uses, brucellosis, 1173
    chancroid, 1173
    endocarditis, 1173
    granuloma inguinale, 1173
    plague, 1173
    tuberculosis, 1208, 1212–1213
    tularemia, 1173
Streptozocin (streptozotocin), chemistry, 1259
  effect on insulin secretion, 1501
  uses, hyperglycemic agent, 1519
    neoplastic diseases, 1252, 1271
Strongyloidiasis, occurrence and treatment, 1032
Strontium, 1634
Strophanthus, sources and composition, 730
Strychnine, 247–248, 585–587
  absorption, fate, and excretion, 586
  mechanism of action, 586
  pharmacological actions, 585–586
  poisoning, symptoms, and treatment, 586–587
  source and chemistry, 585
  uses, 587
Subacute bacterial endocarditis. *See* Endocarditis
SUBLIMAZE (fentanyl citrate injection), 518
Sublimed sulfur, 980
Substance P, 663

role as CNS transmitter, 253
role in ganglionic transmission, 215
Succinic dialdehyde, 971
Succinimides, 460–462
Succinylcholine, actions/effects on, autonomic ganglia, 227–228
　neuromuscular junction, 225–226
　mechanism of action, 223–226
　metabolic fate, 230
　paralytic sequence in man, 226–227
　pharmacological actions, 225–228
　preparations and dosage, 231
　structural formula, 221
Succinylmonocholine, 230
SUCOSTRIN (succinylcholine chloride), 231
Sucrose, diuretic action, 895
SULAMYD SODIUM (sulfacetamide sodium), 1112
Sulfacetamide, pharmacological properties, dosage, and uses, 1112. *See also* Sulfonamides
　structural formula, 1107
Sulfacytine, 1111. *See also* Sulfonamides
Sulfadiazine, pharmacological properties, 1111. *See also* Sulfonamides
　preparations and dosage, 1111
　structural formula, 1107
Sulfadoxine, use in malaria, 1049, 1057
Sulfalene, use in malaria, 1057
Sulfamerazine, 1112. *See also* Sulfonamides
Sulfameter, 1112. *See also* Sulfonamides
Sulfamethazine, 1112. *See also* Sulfonamides
Sulfamethizole, 1111. *See also* Sulfonamides
Sulfamethoxazole, pharmacokinetics, 1730
　pharmacological properties and dosage, 1111. *See also* Sulfonamides
　structural formula, 1107
Sulfamethoxypyridazine, 1112. *See also* Sulfonamides
SULFAMYLON CREAM (mafenide acetate cream), 1112
Sulfanilamide, structural formula, 1107. *See also* Sulfonamides
Sulfapyridine, use in dermatitis herpetiformis, 1116. *See also* Sulfonamides
Sulfasalazine, pharmacological properties, dosage, and uses, 1112. *See also* Sulfonamides
Sulfates, particulate, toxicology, 1640
SULFATHALIDINE (phthalylsulfathiazole), 1112
Sulfathiazole, 1112
Sulfation factor, 1376
Sulfinpyrazone, 722–723, 932–933
　absorption, fate, and excretion, 933
　actions/effects on, platelet aggregation, 1361
　uric acid excretion, 932–933
　chemistry, 932
　history, 932
　preparations and dosage, 933
　untoward reactions and precautions, 933
　uses, gout, 722
　　hyperuricemia, 723
Sulfisoxazole, pharmacokinetics, 1731
　pharmacological properties and dosage, 1110. *See also* Sulfonamides
　preparations and routes of administration, 1111

structural formula, 1107
Sulfisoxazole acetyl, 1111
Sulfisoxazole diolamine, 1111
Sulfisoxazole and phenazopyridine, use in urinary tract infections, 1111, 1122
Sulfonamides, 1106–1119. *See also* Antimicrobial agents; Trimethoprim-sulfamethoxazole; individual agents
　absorption, 1109
　antibacterial spectrum, 1107–1108
　bacterial resistance, 1108–1109
　chemistry, 1107
　clinical classes, 1110
　distribution, 1109
　drug interactions, 1114
　excretion, 1110
　history, 1106
　mechanism of action, 1108
　metabolism, 1109–1110
　mixtures of sulfapyrimidines, 1111
　pharmacological properties of individual agents, 1110–1113
　protein binding, 1109
　synergists and antagonists, 1108
　toxic and untoward reactions, 1113–1114
　uses, 1114–1116
　　bacillary dysentery, 1115
　　burns, 1112
　　chancroid, 1116
　　inclusion conjunctivitis, 1115
　　leprosy, 1216
　　lymphogranuloma venereum, 1116
　　malaria, 1057
　　meningococcal infections, 1115
　　nocardiosis, 1115
　　ophthalmic infections, 1112, 1115
　　paracoccidioidomycosis, 1240
　　prophylactic, 1116, 1141
　　streptococcal infections, 1115
　　toxoplasmosis, 1116
　　trachoma, 1115
　　urinary tract infections, 1114–1115
Sulfondiethylmethane, legal regulations, 1671
Sulfones, 1214–1215
　absorption, distribution, and excretion, 1215
　antibacterial activity, 1214
　chemistry, 1214
　history, 1214
　preparations, routes of administration, and dosage, 1215
　untoward effects, 1214–1215
　uses, leprosy, 1216–1217
　　malaria, 1057
Sulfonmethane, legal regulations, 1671
Sulfonylureas, 1510–1514. *See also* individual agents
　chemistry, 1510
　duration of action, fate, and excretion, 1511–1512
　mechanism of action, 1511
　preparations and dosage, 1513
　reactions with alcohol, 387
　toxicity, 1512–1513
　use in maturity-onset diabetes, 1513–1514

Sulfoxone, structural formula, 1214. *See also* Sulfones

Sulfur, 956, 980–981

Sulfur dioxide, toxicology, 1639

Sulfurated lime, 980, 985

Sulfuric acid, toxicology, 1640

Sulindac, 707–708. *See also* Aspirin-like drugs
  absorption, fate, and excretion, 707
  chemistry, 707
  interactions with other drugs, 708
  pharmacological properties, 707
  preparations and dosage, 707
  toxic effects, 707
  uses, 708

Sulpiride, 397

Sunscreening agents, 959–960

Suramin, 1070–1071
  absorption, fate, and excretion, 1070
  chemistry and preparations, 1070
  filaricidal action, 1070
  routes of administration and dosage, 1070
  toxicity and precautions, 1071
  trypanocidal action, 1070
  uses, onchocerciasis, 1033, 1071
    trypanosomiasis, 1071

SURFACAINE (cyclomethycaine sulfate), 310

Surface-active agents, 951–963, 978–979. *See also* individual agents
  chemistry, 978
  germicidal properties, 978
  preparations, 978
  uses, 978–979

SURFAK (docusate calcium), 1009

SURITAL (thiamylal), 292

SUS-PHRINE (crystalline epinephrine suspension), 151

Sutilains, actions and uses, 962

SUX-CERT (succinylcholine chloride), 231

Sweet birch oil, 695

SYMMETREL (amantadine hydrochloride), 483, 1241

Sympathetic nervous system. *See* Autonomic nervous system

Sympathomimetic amines, centrally acting, abuse, 553–557

Sympathomimetic drugs, 138–175. *See also* Autonomic nervous system; individual agents
  absorption, distribution, and fate of noncatecholamines, 159
  actions/effects on, insulin secretion, 1500
  alpha and beta receptors, 139–140
  chemistry and structure-activity relationship, 141–143
  classification of actions, 138–141
  compensatory reflexes induced by, 140–141
  history, 138–139
  indirectly acting, 140–141, 157-158
  mechanism of direct action on effectors, 141
  mixed acting, 140, 157–158
  refractoriness to, 141
  release of stored norepinephrine, 140
  selective beta$_2$-receptor stimulants, 166–168
  sites and mechanism of action, 139–141
  uses, 168–172

  allergic disorders, 170–171
  bronchial asthma, 170–171
  cardiac arrhythmias and arrest, 170
  control of hemorrhage, 168
  decongestion of mucous membranes, 168–169
  enuresis, 172
  epilepsy, 172
  hyperkinetic syndrome, 172
  hypotension, 169
  local anesthesia, 169
  myocardial infarction, 169
  narcolepsy, 171
  obesity and weight reduction, 171–172
  ophthalmic, 171
  parkinsonism, 171
  psychogenic disorders, 172
  shock, 169–170

SYNALAR (fluocinolone acetonide), 1486

Synanon, 573

Synaptic transmission. *See* Autonomic nervous system

SYNCILLIN (phenethicillin potassium), 1137

SYNCURINE (decamethonium bromide), 231

SYNESTROL (dienestrol), 1428

SYNKAVITE (menadiol sodium diphosphate injection), 1594

SYNTHROID (levothyroxine sodium), 1406

SYNTOCINON (oxytocin injection), 938

Syphilis, choice of drugs in, 1092
  erythromycin in, 1225
  penicillin G in, 1139
  prophylaxis, penicillin G in, 1141
  tetracyclines in, 1190

Syrups, 1669

2,4,5-T, toxicology, 17, 1653

Tabun, history, 101
  structural formula, 105

TACE (chlorotrianisene), 1428

Tachyphylaxis, to sympathomimetic amines, 75

Taeniasis. *See* Cestodiasis

TAGAMET (cimetidine), 632

Talampicillin, 1145

Talbutal. *See also* Barbiturates
  chemistry, 351
  dosage, half-life, and preparations, 350

Talc, 953

TALWIN (pentazocine lactate injection), 526

Tamoxifen, 1304–1305, 1432. *See also* Antiestrogens
  use in neoplastic disease, 1254, 1304

TANDEARIL (oxyphenbutazone), 700

Tannic acid, status and toxicity, 955

TAPAZOLE (methimazole), 1411

Tapeworm infections. *See* Cestodiasis

TARACTAN (chlorprothixene), 410

Tardive dyskinesia, from antipsychotic drugs, 407, 412

Tars, 970

Tartar emetic. *See* Antimony potassium tartrate

Taurine, 246

TCDD, toxicology, 1653

Tea, 592, 603
TEEBACIN (aminosalicylate sodium), 1210
TEEBACIN ACID (aminosalicylic acid), 1210
TEEBACIN CALCIUM (aminosalicylate calcium), 1210
TEEBACIN KALIUM (aminosalicylate potassium), 1210
TEGOPEN (cloxacillin sodium), 1143
TEGRETOL (carbamazepine), 460
Temazepam. See also Benzodiazepines
    dosage and half-life, 350
TEMGESIC (buprenorphine), 528
Temporal arteritis, adrenocorticosteroids in, 1490
TEMPRA (acetaminophen), 704
TENSILON (edrophonium chloride), 112
TENUATE (diethylpropion hydrochloride), 172
TEPANIL (diethylpropion hydrochloride), 172
TEPP. See Tetraethyl pyrophosphate
Teprotide, 657
Terbutaline, 167-168. See also Sympathomimetic
        drugs
    dosage and preparations, 167
    pharmacological properties, 167
    receptor-type activity, 142
    structural formula, 142
    uses, 168, 170-171
Terpin hydrate and codeine elixir, 509
TERRAMYCIN (oxytetracycline hydrochloride), 1185
Tertiaryamylphenol, 969
Tertiarybutylphenol, 969
TESLAC (testolactone), 1458
TESSALON (benzonatate), 530
Testolactone, 1458
Testosterone, relative androgenic activity, 1448. See
        also Androgens
    structural formula and dosage, 1456
    synthesis and secretion, 1449-1451
Testosterone cypionate, 1456
Testosterone enanthate, 1456
Testosterone propionate, 1456
    use in neoplastic diseases, 1254, 1303-1304
Tetanus, barbiturates in, 360
    choice of drugs in, 1088
    curariform drugs in, 232
    diazepam in, 441
    erythromycin in, 1225
    paraldehyde in, 368
    penicillin G in, 1140
Tetrabenazine, 248, 249
Tetrabrom-o-methylphenol, 970
Tetracaine, structural formula, 301
Tetracaine hydrochloride, 309. See also Local anes-
    thetics
Tetrachlorodibenzo-p-dioxin. See TCDD
Tetrachloroethylene, 1026
    toxicology, 1646
Tetracycline. See also Tetracyclines
    absorption, distribution, and excretion, 1184
    dosage, 1185
    pharmacokinetics, 1731
    preparations and administration, 1185, 1186
    structural formula, 1181
Tetracyclines, 1181-1191. See also Antimicrobial
        agents; individual agents
    absorption, distribution, and excretion, 1183-1185
    antagonism to penicillin, 1183
    chemistry, stability, and assay, 1181
    dosage, 1185-1186
    effects on, intestinal flora, 1188-1189
        metabolism, 1188
        microbial agents, 1181-1183
        teeth and bone, 1187-1188
    Fanconi syndrome from, 1187
    history, 1181
    hypersensitivity reactions, 1188
    mechanism of antimicrobial action, 1183
    microbial resistance, 1183
    preparations and administration, 1185-1186
    source, 1181
    staphylococcal enteritis from, 1188-1189
    structural formulas, 1181
    suprainfection, 1188-1189
    toxicity, 1186-1189
    uses, 1189-1191
        acne, 1191
        actinomycosis, 1191
        amebiasis, 1062, 1068, 1191
        atypical mycobacterial infections, 1213
        blind-loop syndrome, 1191
        brucellosis, 1191
        chancroid, 1190
        cholera, 1190
        chronic obstructive pulmonary disease, 1191
        coccal infections, 1190
        Enterobacter aerogenes infections, 1190
        epididymitis, 1190
        Escherichia coli infections, 1190
        gonorrhea, 1190
        granuloma inguinale, 1190
        inclusion conjunctivitis, 1189
        leptospirosis, 1191
        lymphogranuloma venereum, 1190
        malabsorption disorders, 1190
        malaria, 1058
        mycobacterial infections, 1191
        Mycoplasma infections, 1190
        nocardiosis, 1191
        nonspecific urethritis, 1189
        psittacosis, 1189
        relapsing fever, 1191
        rickettsial infections, 1189
        Salmonella infections, 1190
        Shigella infections, 1190
        syphilis, 1190
        toxoplasmosis, 1191
        trachoma, 1189
        tropical sprue, 1191
        tularemia, 1190
        urinary tract infections, 1190
        Whipple's disease, 1191
        yaws, 1191
TETRACYN (tetracycline hydrochloride), 1185
Tetraethylammonium, 215
Tetraethylpyrophosphate, history, 100
    structural formula, 105
    use as insecticide, 104

Tetrahydrocannabinol, 560–563. *See also* Cannabis
  legal regulations, 1670
Tetrahydrocortisol, relative potency, duration of
  action, and equivalent dose, 1482
Tetrahydronaphthalene, 985
Tetrahydrouridine, 1281
Tetrahydrozoline, dosage and preparations, 168
  structural formula, 144
  use in nasal congestion, 168
Tetramethylammonium, 213–214
  structural formula, 213
Tetramisole, 1026
Tetrodotoxin, 65, 310–311
Thalidomide, 48, 1216
Thallium, toxicology, 1653
THAM (tromethamine), 869
THAM-E (tromethamine powder), 869
Thebaine, 496
Theobroma oil, 952
Theobromine, 592–593. *See also* Xanthines
Theophylline, 592–607. *See also* Xanthines
  pharmacokinetics, 1732
  preparations, 601
Theophylline ethylenediamine, 601
Theophylline olamine, 601
Theophylline sodium glycinate, 601
Therapeutics. *See also* Drug Interactions; Drugs;
    Patient Compliance; Toxicology
  individualization, 43–48
  principles, 40–55
THERIODIDE-131 (sodium iodide I 131), 1414
Thevetin, 730
Thiabendazole, 1027–1028
  absorption, fate, and excretion, 1027
  anthelmintic action, 1027
  chemistry, 1027
  preparations, route of administration, and dosage,
    1027
  toxicity and precautions, 1027–1028
  uses, 985, 1028
Thiacetazone, 1216
Thiambutosine, 1216
Thiamine, 1560–1566
  absorption, fate, and excretion, 1561–1562
  chemistry, 1560–1561
  history, 1560
  human requirement, 1561
  pharmacological actions, 1561
  physiological function, 1561
  preparations, 1562
  recommended dietary allowance, 1553
  symptoms of deficiency, 1561
  uses, alcoholic neuritis, 1563
    cardiovascular disease, 1563
    gastrointestinal disorders, 1563
    infantile beriberi, 1563
    Korsakoff's psychosis, 1563
    neuritis of pregnancy, 1563
    subacute necrotizing encephalomyelopathy,
      1563
    thiamine deficiency, 1563
    Wernicke's syndrome, 1563

Thiamylal. *See also* Barbiturates
  chemistry, 351
  use in intravenous anesthesia, 292
Thiazides. *See* Benzothiadiazides
2-(2-Thiazolyl)ethylamine, 610
Thienamycin, 1130
Thicthylperazine, use and dosage as antiemetic, 417
Thimerosal, 976
Thiobarbiturates, 351
Thioctic acid, 98
Thiocyanate, effect on thyroid, 1412
Thioguanine, 1287. *See also* Purine analogs
  use in neoplastic diseases, 1253, 1287
Thiopental. *See also* Barbiturates
  chemistry, 351
  use in intravenous anesthesia, 292–295
Thiopropazate, 406
Thioridazine. *See also* Antipsychotic agents
  chemistry, 409
Thioridazine hydrochloride, dosage forms, 409
  dose as antipsychotic, 409
  side effects, 409
Thiosulfate, uses, cyanide poisoning, 1651
  germicidal, 981
Thiotepa, 1260, 1268
  use in neoplastic disease, 1252, 1268
Thiothixene. *See also* Antipsychotic agents
  dosage forms, 410
  dose as antipsychotic, 410
  side effects, 410
  structural formula, 410
Thioxanthenes, 395, 396, 410. *See also* Antipsychotic
  agents
Thiphenamil, preparations and structural formula,
  132
THORAZINE (chlorpromazine), 408
Threadworm infections. *See* Strongyloidiasis
Thrombin, 955
Thrombocytopenia, adrenocorticosteroids in, 1301,
  1491
Thrombogenesis, 1347
Thrombokinase, 955
Thrombolytic agents, 1362
  uses, 1362, 1364
Thromboplastin, 955
Thrombosis, drug therapy, 1362–1364
Thromboxane A_2 (TXA$_2$), 669, 670. *See also* Prosta-
  glandins
Thromboxane B$_2$, 669, 670. *See also* Prostaglandins
Thromboxane synthetase, 669
Thymol, 969
THYPINONE (thyrotropin-releasing hormone), 1406
THYRAR (thyroid tablets), 1406
THYROCRINE (thyroid tablets), 1406
Thyroglobulin, 1398, 1406
Thyroid carcinoma, radioactive iodine in, 1416
  thyroid hormones in, 1408
Thyroid gland. *See also* Antithyroid drugs
  function tests, 1406
  hyperfunction, 1405
  hypofunction, 1405–1406
  ionic inhibitors, 1412

regulation of function, 1402
relation of iodine to function, 1403
Thyroid hormones, 1397–1408
  actions/effects on, cardiovascular system, 1404
    growth and development, 1403–1404
    lipid and carbohydrate metabolism, 1405
    metabolic rate, 1404
    plasma lipids, 844
  biosynthesis, 1398–1401
  chemistry, 1397–1398
  choice of preparation, 1406–1407
  comparative responses to thyroid preparations, 1407
  conversion of thyroxine to triiodothyronine, 1401
  degradation and excretion, 1402
  history, 1397
  measurement in plasma, 1406
  preparations, 1406
  regulation of synthesis, 1402
  secretion, 1400–1401
  storage, 1400
  structure-activity relationship, 1397–1398
  transport in blood, 1401
  uses, cretinism, 1407
    mild hypothyroidism, 1407
    myxedema, 1407
    myxedema coma, 1407
    nodular goiter, 1408
    simple goiter, 1408
    thyrotropin-dependent carcinoma, 1408
Thyroid tablets, 1406
THYROLAR (liotrix), 1406
Thyrotoxicosis, antithyroid drugs in, 1411
  iodide in, 1413
  propranolol in, 1412
Thyrotropin, 1387
  actions/effects on thyroid gland, 1402
  chemical properties, 1371
  hypothalamic regulation, 1390
Thyrotropin-releasing hormone, 1390
  preparation, 1406
  role as CNS transmitter, 253
Thyroxine, 1398, 1406. See also Thyroid hormones
THYTROPAR (thyrotropin), 1387, 1406
TIBIONE (amithiozone), 1216
Tic douloureux. See Trigeminal neuralgia
TICAR (ticarcillin disodium), 1147
Ticarcillin, 1146–1147. See also Penicillins
  pharmacokinetics, 1732
Ticrynafen, 910–911
  antihypertensive action, 805
Tienilic acid. See Ticrynafen
Timolol, 195–196
  structural formula, 189
  use in glaucoma, 113–114, 195
TIMOPTIC (timolol maleate), 195
TINACTIN (tolnaftate), 983
TINDAL (acetophenazine maleate), 409
Tinea infections, acrisorcin in, 984
  ammoniated mercury in, 976
  benzoic and salicylic acids ointment in, 984
  clotrimazole in, 983

griseofulvin in, 1238
haloprogin in, 983–984
miconazole in, 982–983
tolnaftate in, 983
undecylenic acid in, 982
Tinidazole, 1075
TITRALAC, 991, 993
TM10, 201
Tobacco, 212–213, 557–560. See also Nicotine
  chemical composition, 557–558
  chronic toxicity, 558–559
  history, 557
Tobramycin, 1175. See also Aminoglycoside antibiotics; Antimicrobial agents
  pharmacokinetics, 1733
  preparations, administration, and dosage, 1175
  structural formula, 1163
  untoward effects, 1175
  uses, 1175
TOFRANIL (imipramine hydrochloride), 424
TOFRANIL-PM (imipramine pamoate), 424
Tolamolol, 188, 196
Tolazamide, 1510–1514. See also Sulfonylureas
  duration of action, fate, and excretion, 1512
  preparations, 1513
Tolazoline, 183–184
  absorption, fate, and excretion, 184
  pharmacological properties, 183–184
  preparations, routes of administration, and dosage, 184
  structural formula, 183
  toxicity, side effects, and precautions, 184
  uses, 184
Tolbutamide, 1510–1514. See also Sulfonylureas
  duration of action, fate, and excretion, 1512
  pharmacokinetics, 1733
  preparations, 1513
TOLECTIN (tolmetin sodium), 709
Tolerance to drugs. See Drug abuse; individual agents
Tolfenamic acid, 708. See also Fenamates
TOLINASE (tolazamide), 1513
Tolmetin, 709–710. See also Aspirin-like drugs
  absorption, fate, and excretion, 709
  pharmacological properties, 709
  preparations and dosage, 709
  structural formula, 709
  toxic effects, 709
  uses, 710
Tolnaftate, 983
Toluene, toxicology, 1647
TOPICORT (desoximetasone), 1486
TOPSYN GEL (fluocinonide), 1486
TORECAN (thiethylperazine), 406
TORECAN MALEATE (thiethylperazine maleate), 417
Totaquine, 1057
Toxaphene, toxicology, 1650
TOXFILE (microfiche system for information on toxic substances), 1608
Toxicology, 1602–1659. See also Drugs, poisoning
  acute versus chronic, 1603
  allergic reactions, 1604

Toxicology (*Cont.*)
  animal tests of toxicity, 1606–1607
  definition, 2
  delayed toxicity, 1604–1605
  dose-effect relationship, 1602–1603
    probit analysis, 1603
  environmental toxicants, 1638–1659
  idiosyncratic reactions, 1604
  incidence of poisoning, 1607
  local versus systemic effects, 1605
  phototoxicity and photoallergy, 1605
  prevention and treatment of poisoning, 1608–1613
  principles, 1602–1614
  reversible and irreversible effects, 1605
  sources of information, 1608
  types of toxic effects, 1604–1606
Toxiferines, 220
TOXOGONIN (obidoxime chloride), 112
Toxoplasmosis, pyrimethamine in, 1050
  sulfonamides in, 1116
  tetracyclines in, 1191
Trachoma, choice of drugs in, 1093
  sulfonamides in, 1115, 1189
  tetracyclines in, 1189
Tragacanth, 951
TRAL (hexocyclium methylsulfate), 130
Tranquilizers. *See* Antianxiety drugs
Transcobalamins, 1334, 1335
Transferrin, 1315, 1316, 1318, 1321
Transfusion siderosis, deferoxamine in, 1634
TRANXENE (clorazepate), 440, 1671
TRANXENE-SD (clorazepate dipotassium), 440
Tranylcypromine, 428–430. *See also* Monoamine
    oxidase inhibitors
  mechanism of adrenergic action, 82
Tranylcypromine sulfate, preparations and dosage,
    424
TRASYLOL (aprotinin), 663
TRAVASE (sutilains ointment), 962
TRAVASOL (amino acid injection), 863
Traveler's diarrhea, tetracyclines in, 1190
TRECATOR-SC (ethionamide), 1209
Trench mouth, penicillin G in, 1140
Treponema pallidum infections, choice of drugs in,
    1092
Treponema pertenue infections, choice of drugs in,
    1092
TREST (methixene hydrochloride), 131
Tretinoin, 1591
  use in acne, 1591
Tretoquinol, 166
Triamcinolone. *See also* Adrenocorticosteroids
  preparations, 1485–1486
  relative potency, duration of action, and equiva-
    lent dose, 1482
Triamterene, 908–909. *See also* Diuretics
  absorption, distribution, and excretion, 908
  chemistry, 908
  clinical toxicity, 909
  mechanism of diuretic action, 908–909
  pharmacokinetics, 1734

  preparations, 909
  use as diuretic, 909
TRIAVIL (perphenazine–amitriptyline hydrochlo-
    ride), 424
Triazenes, use in neoplastic diseases, 1252, 1271
Triazolam. *See also* Benzodiazepines
  dosage and half-life, 350
  pharmacokinetics, 348
  structural formula, 340
TRIAZURE (azaribine), 1282
Tribromsalan, 981
Trichinosis, occurrence and treatment, 1032
Trichlormethiazide, structural formula, properties,
    and dosage, 900
Trichloroacetic acid, 956
Trichloroethane, toxicology, 1646
Trichloroethanol, 361
Trichloroethylene, 291–292
  toxicology, 1646
Trichlorophenoxyacetic acid. *See* 2,4,5-T
Trichomoniasis, metronidazole in, 1077
Trichophyton infections. *See* Tinea infections
Trichuriasis, occurrence and treatment, 1031
Triclocarban, 981
Triclofos sodium, chemistry, 361
  dosage, half-life, and preparations, 351
TRICLOS (triclofos sodium), 351
Triclosan, 969–970
Tricyclic antidepressants, 418–427. *See also* individ-
    ual agents
  absorption, distribution, fate, and excretion, 422–
    423
  actions/effects on, animal behavior, 420
    autonomic nervous system, 421–422
    brain amines, 420–421
    cardiovascular system, 422
    central nervous system, 419–421
    EEG, 420
    5-HT uptake, 638
    respiration, 422
    sleep, 420
  acute overdosage, 425–426
    treatment, 426
  anticholinergic activity, 127
  chemistry, 419
  history, 418–419
  interaction with other drugs, 426–427
  pharmacological properties, 419–427
  poisoning, physostigmine in, 116
  preparations and dosage, 424
  tolerance and physical dependence, 423
  toxic reactions and side effects, 423–426
  uses, alcoholism, 427
    depression, 434–435
    enuresis in childhood, 427
    obsessive-compulsive neurosis, 427
    phobic anxiety states, 427
TRIDESILON (desonide), 1486
Tridihexethyl, preparations and structural formula,
    131
TRIDIONE (trimethadione), 465

Triethylenemelamine, 1260, 1268. *See also* Alkylating agents
structural formula, 1260
use in neoplastic diseases, 1268
Triethylenephosphoramide, 1260
Triethylene*thio*phosphoramide, 1268. *See also* Alkylating agents
structural formula, 1260
use in neoplastic diseases, 1252, 1268
Triflualin, toxicology, 1654
Trifluoperazine. *See also* Antipsychotic agents
Trifluoperazine hydrochloride, dosage forms, 409
dose as antipsychotic, 409
side effects, 409
structural formula, 409
Trifluorothymidine, 1243
Triflupromazine. *See also* Antipsychotic agents
dosage forms, 408
side effects, 408
structural formula, 408
use and dose as, antiemetic, 417
antipsychotic, 408
Trigeminal neuralgia, carbamazepine in, 460
phenytoin in, 455
Trihexyphenidyl, chemistry, preparations, and dosage, 486
use in parkinsonism, 484-485
Triiodothyronine, 1398, 1406. *See also* Thyroid hormones
TRILAFON (perphenazine), 409
Trimedoxime, 112
Trimethadione, 464-465
absorption, distribution, biotransformation, and excretion, 463
anticonvulsant properties, 464
dosage, 465
effects on fetus, 471
history, 464
plasma concentration, 465
preparations and dosage, 465
structural formula, 464
toxicity, 465
use in epilepsy, 465, 469
Trimethaphan, 215-217. *See also* Ganglionic blocking agents
structural formula, 215
uses, hypertensive emergencies, 813
Trimethidinium, 215
Trimethobenzamide, use in preanesthetic medication, 270
Trimethoprim, 1048-1050
antimalarial actions and efficacy, 1048
chemistry, 1048
dihydrofolate reductase inhibition, 1049
history, 1048
pharmacokinetics, 1734
potentiation by sulfonamides, 1049
Trimethoprim-sulfamethoxazole, 1116-1119. *See also* Antimicrobial agents; Sulfonamides
absorption, distribution, and excretion, 1117
antibacterial spectrum, 1116

bacterial resistance, 1117
mechanism of action, 1116-1117
preparations, routes of administration, and dosage, 1118
toxic and untoward effects, 1118
uses, bacillary dysentery, 1119
bacterial endocarditis, 1119
brucellosis, 1119
gastrointestinal infections, 1119
genital infections, 1119
Pneumocystis carinii infections, 1119
prophylaxis, 1119
Pseudomonas infections, 1230
respiratory tract infections, 1118
Serratia infections, 1230
typhoid carriers, 1119
typhoid fever, 1119
urinary tract infections, 1118
Triorthocresyl phosphate, 111-112
Trioxsalen, chemistry, toxicity, and actions, 957
preparations and uses, 957
Tripelennamine, structural formula, 623. *See also* H₁-receptor blockers
Tripelennamine citrate, preparations and dosage, 628
Tripelennamine hydrochloride, preparations and dosage, 628
Triple dye, 980
Tripotassium dicitratobismuthate, 997
TRISOGEL, 991
TRISORALEN (trioxsalen), 957
Trisulfapyrimidines, 1111-1112. *See also* Sulfonamides
TROBICIN (sterile spectinomycin hydrochloride), 1228
TROCINATE (thiphenamil hydrochloride), 129
Tromethamine, 869
TRONOTHANE (pramoxine hydrochloride), 310
Tropic acid, 121
Tropicamide, ocular effects and uses, 134
preparations and structural formula, 132
Tropine, 121
Trypanosomiasis, furaltadone in, 1074
melarsoprol in, 1073
nifurtimox in, 1078
nitrofurazone in, 1074
pentamidine in, 1072
suramin in, 1071
tryparsamide in, 1074
Tryparsamide, 1074
use in trypanosomiasis, 1074
Trypsin, 961
Tryptamine, 564
Tryptophan, 351, 369, 636, 637
TUAMINE (tuaminoheptane sulfate), 168
Tuaminoheptane, dosage and preparations, 168
receptor-type activity, 142
structural formula, 142
use in nasal congestion, 168
TUBARINE (tubocurarine chloride), 230
Tuberculosis, amikacin in, 1212

Tuberculosis (*Cont.*)
  aminosalicylic acid in, 1209–1210
  capreomycin in, 1212
  chemoprophylaxis, 1213
  chemotherapy, 1212–1213
    atypical mycobacteria, 1213
    bacterial resistance, 1213
  choice of drugs in, 1091
  cycloserine in, 1210–1211
  ethambutol in, 1206–1207
  ethionamide in, 1208–1209
  isoniazid in, 1200–1203
  kanamycin in, 1211
  pyrazinamide in, 1208
  rifampin in, 1203–1206
  streptomycin in, 1207–1208
  viomycin in, 1211
Tubocurarine. *See also* Curare
  pharmacokinetics, 1735
  pharmacological actions, 223–228
  preparations and dosage, 230–231
  structural formula, 221
  use in diagnosis of myasthenia gravis, 115
Tularemia, choice of drugs in, 1090
  streptomycin in, 1173
  tetracyclines in, 1190
TXA$_2$. *See* Thromboxane A$_2$
TYLENOL (acetaminophen), 704
Typhoid carriers, ampicillin in, 1145
  trimethoprim-sulfamethoxazole in, 1119
Typhoid fever, ampicillin in, 1145
  chloramphenicol in, 1195
  choice of drugs in, 1089
  trimethoprim-sulfamethoxazole in, 1119
Typhus, choice of drugs in, 1092
  epidemic, chloramphenicol in, 1196
    tetracycline in, 1189
  murine, chloramphenicol in, 1196
    tetracyclines in, 1189
  scrub, chloramphenicol in, 1196
    tetracycline in, 1189
Tyramine, mechanism of adrenergic action, 82
  receptor-type activity, 142
  structural formula, 142
Tyrosine, precursor of norepinephrine, 72
Tyrosine hydroxylase, 72
TYZINE (tetrahydrozoline hydrochloride), 168

Ulcer. *See* Peptic ulcer
Ulcerative colitis, sulfasalazine in, 1112. *See also* Colitis
ULTRALENTE insulin (extended insulin zinc suspension), 1508, 1509
Undecylenic acid, 982
UNIPEN (nafcillin sodium), 1143
United States Adopted Name, 51, 1661
United States Pharmacopeia, 53–54
Upper motoneuron disorders, diazepam in, 441
Uracil mustard, 1267. *See also* Alkylating agents
  chemistry, 1258
  use in neoplastic diseases, 1252, 1267

Urea, 895–896
  preparations and dosage, 896
  toxicity, 896
  use as osmotic diuretic, 896
UREAPHIL (urea), 896
Ureaplasma urealyticum infections, choice of drugs in, 1092
URECHOLINE (bethanechol chloride), 95
Urethritis, choice of drugs in, 1092
  nonspecific, tetracyclines in, 1189
UREVERT (urea), 896
UREX (methenamine hippurate), 1120
Uricosuric agents, 929–934. *See also* individual agents
  pharmacological actions, 930–931
Uricosuric diuretics, 910–911. *See also* Diuretics; individual agents
Urinary retention, bethanechol in, 95–96
  neostigmine in, 113
Urinary tract antiseptics, 1119–1122
Urinary tract infections, ampicillin in, 1145
  carbenicillin indanyl in, 1146
  chloramphenicol in, 1196
  choice of drugs in, 1086
  gentamicin in, 1174
  methenamine in, 1120
  nalidixic acid in, 1121
  nitrofurantoin in, 1122
  oxolinic acid in, 1121
  phenazopyridine in, 1122
  polymyxin B in, 1230
  sulfonamides in, 1114–1115
  tetracyclines in, 1190
  trimethoprim-sulfamethoxazole in, 1118
Urine, alkalinization or acidification, 868
Urochloralic acid, 362
Urokinase, 1362
Ursodeoxycholic acid, 998, 999
Urticaria, adrenocorticosteroids in, 1490
  antihistamines in, 629
  sympathomimetic amines in, 171
USAN, 51, 1661
Uterine bleeding, dysfunctional, estrogens in, 1430
  progestins in, 1437
Uterine-stimulating agents, 935–950. *See also* individual agents
  experimental evaluation, 936
  physiological and anatomical considerations, 935–936
UTIBID (oxolinic acid), 1121
Uveitis, indomethacin in, 706

Vaccinia gangrenosa, methisazone in, 1242
Vaginitis, atrophic, estrogens in, 1430
Vagusstoff, 62–63
VALISONE (betamethasone valerate), 1484
VALIUM (diazepam), 296, 350, 440, 467, 1671
VALLESTRIL (methallenestril), 1428
VALMID (ethinamate), 350, 1671
VALPIN (anisotropine methylbromide), 130

Valproic acid, absorption, distribution, biotransformation, and excretion, 463
  chemistry, 462
  interactions with other drugs, 463
  pharmacokinetics, 1735–1736
  pharmacological effects, 462–463
  plasma concentrations, 463
  preparations and dosage, 463
  structural formula, 462
  toxicity, 463
  use in epilepsy, 464, 469–470
VANCERIL (beclomethasone dipropionate), 1484
VANCOCIN (sterile vancomycin hydrochloride), 1231
Vancomycin, 1230–1231. See also Antimicrobial agents
  absorption, distribution, and excretion, 1231
  antibacterial activity and mechanism, 1230
  chemistry, 1230
  dosage, 1231
  history and source, 1230
  mechanism of action, 1129
  pharmacokinetics, 1736
  preparations and administration, 1231
  toxicity, 1231
  uses, pseudomembranous colitis, 1227, 1231
    staphylococcal infections, 1231
    streptococcal endocarditis, 1231
VANIBASE, 952
Vanillylmandelic acid, 76 77
VANOBID (candicidin), 984
VANQUIN (pyrvinium pamoate), 1026
VANSIL (oxamniquine), 1022
VAPOROLE (amyl nitrite), 826
Vapors, toxicology, 1644–1647
Varicose ulcers, zinc oxide in, 977
Varicose veins, sclerosing agents in, 956
VARIDASE (streptokinase streptodornase), 961
Vascular disease, alpha-adrenergic blocking drugs in, 187
Vascular insufficiency, vasodilators in, 830–831
Vasoactive intestinal polypeptide, 663
  role as CNS transmitter, 253
VASOCON-A (antazoline phosphate), 628
VASODILAN (isoxsuprine hydrochloride), 831
Vasodilator drugs, 819–831. See also individual agents
Vasopressin. See Antidiuretic hormone
Vasopressin injection, 923
Vasopressin tannate, 924
Vasotocin, 916
VASOXYL (methoxamine hydrochloride), 166
V-CILLIN K (penicillin V potassium), 1137
VECTRIN (minocycline hydrochloride), 1185
Vegetable oils, 952
VEINAMINE (amino acid injection), 863
VELBAN (vinblastine sulfate), 1289
VELOSEF (cephradine), 1155
Venous thrombosis, anticoagulants in, 1363–1364
  dihydroergotamine in, 1363
  thrombolytic agents in, 1364
VENTAIRE (protokylol hydrochloride), 154
Ventricular tachycardia, bretylium in, 787

  disopyramide in, 778
  lidocaine in, 781
  phenytoin in, 783
  procainamide in, 776
  propranolol in, 785–786
  quinidine in, 772
  treatment, 769
VERACILLIN (dicloxacillin sodium), 1143
Verapamil, 828
Veratrum alkaloids, 808
VERMOX (mebendazole), 1018
VERSAPEN (hetacillin), 1145
VERSTRAN (prazepam), 350, 440, 1671
Vertigo, H_1-receptor blockers in, 629
Vesicants, 955
VESPRIN (triflupromazine hydrochloride), 408
VESTAL LPH, 969
VIBRAMYCIN (doxycycline hyclate), 1185
Vibrio cholerae infections, choice of drugs in, 1090
Vidarabine, 1242–1243, 1285
Vinblastine, 1287–1290. See also Vinca alkaloids
  clinical toxicity, 1289
  preparations, route of administration, and dosage, 1289
  use in neoplastic diseases, 1253, 1289
Vinca alkaloids, 1287–1290. See also Vinblastine; Vincristine
  absorption, fate, and excretion, 1288–1289
  actions/effects on kidney, 922
  chemistry, 1287
  cytotoxic actions, 1288
  history, 1287
  mechanism of action, 1288
  neurological actions, 1288
  structure-activity relationship, 1288
  use in neoplastic diseases, 1253, 1289–1290
Vincent's disease. See Trench mouth
Vincristine, 1287 1290. See also Vinca alkaloids
  clinical toxicity, 1289–1290
  preparations, route of administration, and dosage, 1289
  use in neoplastic diseases, 1253, 1289–1290
Vinyl ether, 291
VIOFORM (clioquinol), 1064
Viomycin, 1211
VIRA-A (sterile vidarabine), 1242
VIRA-A OPHTHALMIC (vidarabine ophthalmic ointment), 1242
Viral diseases, drugs for, 1240–1243
VISINE (tetrahydrozoline hydrochloride), 168
Vitamer, 1552
Vitamin A, 1583–1592
  absorption, distribution, fate, and excretion, 1588–1590
  bioassay and unitage, 1590
  chemistry and occurrence, 1583
  effects on tumor growth, 1584
  history, 1583
  human requirement, 1588
  hypervitaminosis, 1586–1588
  pharmacological actions, 1584
  physiological functions, 1584–1586

Vitamin A *(Cont.)*
  preparations, 1590–1591
  recommended dietary allowance, 1553
  retinol and epithelial structures, 1585, 1586
  role in visual cycle, 1585–1586
  signs and symptoms of deficiency, 1586
  uses, acne, 1591
    deficiency states, 1591
    prophylactic, 1591
Vitamin B complex, 1560–1576. *See also* individual
    vitamins
Vitamin B$_{12}$. *See* Cyanocobalamin
Vitamin B$_{12}$ with intrinsic factor concentrate, 1337
Vitamin C. *See* Ascorbic acid
Vitamin D, 1538–1545
  absorption, fate, and excretion, 1543
  actions/effects on, intestinal absorption of cal-
    cium, 1541
    kidney, 1525, 1541
    mobilization of bone salts, 1541
  chemistry and occurrence, 1539
  deficiency, 1542
  history, 1538
  human requirement, 1543–1544
  hypervitaminosis, 1542
  metabolic activation, 1540
    regulation, 1540
  preparations, 1544–1545
  provitamins, 1539
  recommended dietary allowance, 1553
  unitage, 1544
  uses, Fanconi syndrome, 1545
    hypoparathyroidism, 1545
    metabolic rickets and osteomalacia, 1545
    nutritional rickets, 1545
    renal osteodystrophy, 1545
Vitamin E, 1596–1598
  absorption, fate, and excretion, 1598
  assay and unitage, 1598
  chemistry, 1596
  history, 1596
  human requirement, 1598
  pharmacological actions, 1596
  physiological function, 1596
  preparations, 1598
  recommended dietary allowance, 1553
  symptoms of deficiency, 1597–1598
Vitamin K, 1592–1596
  absorption, fate, and excretion, 1593–1594
  assay and unitage, 1594
  history, 1592
  human requirement, 1593
  occurrence and chemistry, 1592
  pharmacological actions, 1592–1593
  physiological function, 1592–1593
  preparations, 1594
  provisional dietary allowance, 1555
  role in blood clotting, 1348, 1354–1355
  symptoms of deficiency, 1593
  toxicity, 1593
  uses, biliary obstruction or fistula, 1595

  drug-induced hypoprothrombinemia, 1595–
    1596
  hepatocellular disease, 1595
  hypoprothrombinemia of the newborn, 1594–
    1595
  inadequate intake or absorption, 1594–1595
  oral anticoagulant overdosage, 1358, 1359
Vitamins, 1551–1601. *See also* individual vitamins
  appropriate uses, 1552–1554
  federal regulations, 1554–1556
  general considerations, 1551–1558
  properties of water-soluble vitamins, 1564–1565
  provisional dietary allowances, 1555
  range of intakes, 1556–1558
  Recommended Daily Dietary Allowances, 1552–
    1554
  role in metabolism, 1562
  role in therapeutics, 1558
Vitiligo, methoxsalen in, 958
  monobenzone in, 959
  trioxsalen in, 958
VIVACTYL (protriptyline hydrochloride), 424
VOLEX (hetastarch injection), 862
Volume of distribution, definition, 21, 1676

Warfarin, 1353, 1357–1358. *See also* Anticoagulants,
    oral
  pharmacokinetics, 1737
  preparations and dosage, 1357–1358
  rodenticidal properties, 1652
Warts, cantharidin in, 956
Water, mechanism of diuresis, 893
  uses, 893
Water vapor, 335–336
Waxes, 953
Wegener's granulomatosis, adrenocorticosteroids in,
    1490
Weight reduction. *See* Obesity
Weil's disease, choice of drugs in, 1092
Wernicke's encephalopathy, 553
  thiamine in, 1563
WESTADONE (methadone hydrochloride), 519
Whipple's disease, tetracyclines in, 1191
Whipworm infections. *See* Trichuriasis
White lotion, 977, 981
White ointment, 952
White petrolatum, 952
White wax, 953
Whitfield's ointment, 984
Wills' factor, 1331
Wilms' tumor, dactinomycin in, 1291
  vincristine in, 1290
WILPO (phentermine hydrochloride), 172
Wilson's disease, penicillamine in, 1628
WIN GEL, 991
WINSTROL (stanozolol), 1458
Wintergreen oil, 695
Wolff-Parkinson-White syndrome, propranolol in,
    785
  quinidine in, 772

Wool fat, 952
Worm infections, treatment, 1031–1035
Wuchereria infections, occurrence and treatment, 1032–1033
WYAMINE (mephentermine sulfate), 164
WYCILLIN SUSPENSION (sterile penicillin G procaine suspension), 1137
WYDASE (hyaluronidase for injection), 960

Xanthine, structural formula, 592
Xanthine beverages, 603–604
Xanthines, 592–607. *See also* individual agents
  absorption, fate, and excretion, 600
  actions/effects on, blood vessels, 595
    cardiovascular system, 594–595
    central nervous system, 593–594
    cerebral circulation, 595
    coronary circulation, 595
    gastric secretion, 596–597
    heart, 594–595
    kidney, 596, 910
    metabolism, 597
    secretion, 596–597
    skeletal muscle, 596
    smooth muscle, 595–596
  cellular basis of action, 597–599
    relationship to adenosine, 598–599
    relationship to calcium ion, 598
    relationship to cyclic AMP, 598
  chemistry, 592–593
  history, 592
  mutagenic effects, 599–600
  preparations, 601
  relation to myocardial infarction, 600
  source, 592
  toxicology, 599–600
  uses, bronchial asthma, 602–603
    cardiac failure, 602
    chronic obstructive pulmonary disease, 603
    headache, 603
    hyperkinetic syndrome, 603
    respiratory stimulant, 603
XYLOCAINE (lidocaine hydrochloride), 309, 779
Xylometazoline, dosage and preparations, 168
  structural formula, 144
  use in nasal congestion, 168

Yaws, choice of drugs in, 1092
  tetracyclines in, 1191
Yeast infections. *See* Mycotic infections; individual agents
Yellow ointment, 952
Yellow wax, 953
Yersinia infections, chloramphenicol in, 1196
  choice of drugs in, 1090
YODOXIN (iodoquinol), 1064
Yohimbine, 186
YOMESAN (niclosamide), 1019

ZACTANE (ethoheptazine citrate), 517
ZACTIRIN (ethoheptazine citrate–aspirin), 518
ZARONTIN (ethosuximide), 461
ZAROXOLYN (metolazone), 900
ZEPHIRAN (benzalkonium chloride), 978
ZESTE (esterified estrogens), 1428
Zinc, recommended dietary allowance, 1553
Zinc acetate, 977
Zinc bacitracin, 1232
Zinc chloride, 977
Zinc gelatin, 953
Zinc oleate, 977
Zinc oxide, 953, 977
Zinc oxide and salicylic acid paste, 695, 977
Zinc oxide ointment, 977
Zinc oxide paste, 977
Zinc phenylsulfonate, 954
Zinc phosphide, toxicology, 1653
Zinc pyrithione, 957, 977
Zinc stearate, 953, 977
Zinc sulfate, 977
  use in acrodermatitis enteropathica, 1065
Zinc undecylenate, 982
ZINCON (zinc pyrithione), 957
Zineb, toxicology, 1655
Ziram, toxicology, 1655
Zirconyl hydroxychloride, 954
Zollinger-Ellison syndrome, cimetidine in, 632
ZOLYSE (chymotrypsin), 961
ZORANE 1/20, 1440
ZORANE 1.5/30, 1440
ZORANE 1/50, 1440
Zygomycetes infections, amphotericin B in, 1240
  flucytosine in, 1240
ZYLOPRIM (allopurinol), 721